Oxford Textbook of
Oncology

Project Administrator Sally Welham

Project Editor Dr Irene Butcher

Indexer Caroline Sheard

Production Controller Glen Fox

Development Editor Kate Martin

Design Manager Claire Walker

Typographer Jonathan Coleclough

Illustrations Technical Graphics Department, Oxford University Press

Publisher Alison Langton

Senior Editorial Advisers Professor Sir Michael Peckham
Professor Umberto Veronesi

volume **1**

Oxford Textbook of
Oncology
Second Edition

Edited by

Robert L. Souhami

*Principal, Royal Free and
University College London Medical School, London, UK*

Ian Tannock

*Professor of Medicine and Medical Biophysics,
Ontario Cancer Institute, Toronto, Canada*

Peter Hohenberger

*Professor of Surgery and Surgical Oncology,
Humboldt University, Berlin, Germany*

and

Jean-Claude Horiot

*Director, Centre de Lutte contre le Cancer George François Leclerc,
Dijon, France*

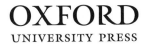

OXFORD
UNIVERSITY PRESS

OXFORD
UNIVERSITY PRESS

Great Clarendon Street, Oxford OX2 6DP

Oxford University Press is a department of the University of Oxford.
It furthers the University's objective of excellence in research, scholarship,
and education by publishing worldwide in

Oxford New York

Athens Auckland Bangkok Bogotá Buenos Aires Cape Town
Chennai Dar es Salaam Delhi Florence Hong Kong Istanbul Karachi
Kolkata Kuala Lumpur Madrid Melbourne Mexico City Mumbai Nairobi
Paris São Paulo Shanghai Singapore Taipei Tokyo Toronto Warsaw

with associated companies in Berlin Ibadan

Oxford is a registered trade mark of Oxford University Press
in the UK and in certain other countries

Published in the United States
by Oxford University Press Inc., New York

© Oxford University Press, 2002

British Library Cataloguing in Publication Data

Data available

Library of Congress Cataloguing in Publication Data

ISBN 0-19-262926 3
10 9 8 7 6 5 4 3 2 1

Typeset in Minion
by Latimer Trend & Company Ltd
Printed in Great Britain
on acid-free paper by
The Bath Press, Avon

Preface to the second edition

This second edition of the *Oxford Textbook of Oncology* follows the success of the first, published in 1995. Since that edition there have been remarkable developments in the basic and clinical science of cancer medicine. In this edition we have attempted to incorporate these advances, placing them in the context of the work of the practising clinician.

We have followed the example set by our predecessors in the previous edition by choosing authors from many different countries on the basis of their acknowledged expertise and excellence. We have developed, we hope, a style of explanation and illustration that is consistent throughout the text, so that the book looks and reads as a coherent work.

In the science chapters, which are in the early sections, we have attempted to explain and illustrate the biology on which cancer treatment increasingly depends for its conceptual framework. There have been major advances of understanding in molecular genetics, carcinogenesis, tumour growth and development, and the science of cancer treatment. We hope that these are described clearly enough for clinicians to see the relevance to clinical practice. Detailed examples of these general concepts are discussed in the tumour-specific chapters where the reader will also find discussion of the epidemiology and pathology of the individual tumours.

The sections which follow describe the principles of cancer treatment in its various forms. Here we have attempted to give the non-specialist oncologist a clear account of the practice of the different methods of cancer treatment. We have placed the chapters on symptomatic treatment at this point since we regard the control of symptoms as an extremely important aspect of cancer medicine which should be firmly understood by all those responsible for the care of patients.

The sections on specific tumours follow. Wherever possible we have tried to give a balanced account of what is an agreed approach to current diagnosis and therapy. Sometimes treatment choice is based on reliable evidence, but often it is not. We have asked our contributors to indicate, where possible, the strength of evidence that underlies the choice of treatment. The aim has been to present an account of modern practice indicating the prognosis and where further advances are needed. We hope that these chapters will be a synthesis of the modern approach to management of each tumour. Even in a large text such as this it is not possible to discuss all possible approaches in detail. There is a comprehensive reference list with each chapter that will provide the reader with suggestions for further reading.

A textbook such as this is a major undertaking. We could not have accomplished our work had we not had an excellent publishing team under Alison Langton at Oxford University Press. We give them our grateful thanks, especially to Irene Butcher and to the illustrators who have provided attractive and clear illustrations, often from rudimentary originals. Sally Welham has been as indispensable to the producion of this edition, as she was to the last. She has our heartfelt thanks.

October 2001

Robert L. Souhami
Ian Tannock
Peter Hohenberger
Jean-Claude Horiot

Preface to the first edition

The *Oxford Textbook of Oncology* is one of the highly successful series of textbooks produced by Oxford University Press of which the best known forerunner is the *Oxford Textbook of Medicine*. This textbook of oncology is the first new, major, and comprehensive textbook on cancer to appear for more than a decade and so is an important landmark for a wide readership. It comes at a crucially important time in the evolution of cancer treatment. During the past two to three decades some forms of cancer have become curable but many common cancers still pose an intractable problem. As in the health field generally, there is a high level of interest in primary and secondary prevention. However, the most important distinguishing feature in the 1990s is the explosive and far-reaching developments in the biological and physical sciences relevant to cancer.

In selecting the authorship of the chapters in the textbook, the editors have not drawn narrowly from one country but have been concerned to provide a wide range of expertise and a broad international perspective. The coverage is not only comprehensive but 'holistic', extending from advances in molecular genetics through to societal issues such as the support systems needed by cancer patients and their families.

Particular emphasis has been given to the integration of clinical oncology and science. In addition to the sections devoted to the scientific foundations of oncology, individual chapters included in the clinical sections make reference to aetiology and biology. The clinical sections are designed not only to instruct readers but to provide practical guidance to every day problems. In addition to common problems there is coverage of uncommon and rare tumours, less common presentations, and unusual complications of cancer and its treatment.

The expanding number of cancer journals, reviews, and books focusing on particular forms of diagnosis, on individual therapies, or on specific cancers, makes the place of the comprehensive reference source that maps the range of the oncology territory all the more important. The *Oxford Textbook of Oncology* will serve as a source of instruction and advice but also a pointer to some of the emergent areas such as the handling of genetic risk. The Textbook is designed to be relevant to a wide constituency within the general field of oncology including not only oncologists but clinicians whose day-to-day work includes the diagnosis and care of cancer patients. It will be relevant to oncologists in training as a reference source and for other clinicians in training. It will be of interest to scientists and to non-medical health professionals involved in the care of cancer patients. It will be of value to epidemiologists and behavioural scientists.

Many have helped in this important enterprise. John Wagstaff has been an unflagging source of support and his important contribution is gratefully acknowledged. The editors are also grateful for the help provided by Jonathan Waxman and Alberto Costa. We also wish to thank Pat Rice, Cyril Fisher, and Maureen Wagstaff for their editorial assistance. We owe a particular debt of gratitude to Sally Welham who has been closely involved with the Textbook since its inception and whose input, constructive advice, and hard work have greatly contributed to its succcess.

May 1995

Michael Peckham
Herbert Pinedo
Umberto Veronesi

Contents

Section 5 Complications of cancer

Contributors

Neil Aaronson Head, Division of Psychosocial Research and Epidemiology, The Netherlands Cancer Institute, Amsterdam
6.3 Quality of life

P. Abel Reader and Honorary Consultant Urologist, and Head of Section of Academic Urology, Imperial College of Science, Technology and Medicine, London, UK
13.1 Tumours of the prostate

Måns Åkerman Associate Professor and Senior Cytopathologist, Department of Pathology and Cytology, University Hospital, Lund, Sweden
3.2 Cytology and minimal sampling techniques

M. C. Aldridge Consultant in General and Gastrointestinal Surgery, Queen Elizabeth II Hospital, Welwyn Garden City, Hertfordshire, UK
10.8 Tumours of the biliary tract

David G. Allen Clinical Director of Surgical Services, Department of Gynaecological Oncology, Mercy Hospital for Women, Melbourne, Australia
12.1 Epithelial carcinoma of the ovary

P. L. Amlot Senior Lecturer/Honorary Consultant, Departments of Immunology and Clinical Oncology, Royal Free and University College Medical School, London, UK
5.4 Haematological complications of cancer

Barbara L. Andersen Professor, Departments of Psychology and Obstetrics and Gynecology, Ohio State University, Columbus, USA
12.9 Sexual dysfunction following cancer in women

I. Andrulis Senior Scientist, Samuel Lunenfeld Research Institute, Mount Sinai Hospital, Toronto, and Professor, University of Toronto, Ontario, Canada
1.1 Investigating the genetics of cancer

Maria Grazia Arena Department of Haematology and Oncology, Azienda Ospedali Riuniti, Reggio Calabria, Italy
3.7 Prognostic factors

S. Arnott Consultant Clinical Oncologist, London, UK
10.4 Colorectal cancer

Rodrigo Arriagada Consultant in Radiation Oncology, Instituto Radiomedicina, and Professor of Oncology, University of Santiago, Chile
14.3 Management of of non-small-cell lung cancer

D. Ash Consultant in Clinical Oncology, Cookridge Hospital, Leeds, UK
4.3.3 Interstitial and endoluminal radiation therapy

Philippe Autier Deputy Director, Division of Epidemiology and Biostatistics, European Institute of Oncology, Milan, Italy
8.1 Cutaneous malignant melanoma

Clifford C. Bailey Professor, Consultant Paediatric Oncologist, and Director of Research and Development, NHS Executive Northern and Yorkshire Research School of Medicine, Leeds, UK
18.1 Brain tumours in children

S. E. Baron-Hay Department of Medical Oncology, University of Sydney, New South Wales, Australia
20 Cancer of unknown primary site

Ann Barrett Professor of Radiation Oncology and Consultant Clinical Oncologist, University of Glasgow and Beatson Oncology Centre, UK
4.8 Total body irradiation

Richard Begent Ronald Raven Professor of Clinical Oncology, Royal Free and University College Medical School, London, UK
4.27 Targeted cancer therapy

A. C. Begg Head, Division of Experimental Therapy, The Netherlands Cancer Institute, Amsterdam
1.6 Growth and kinetics of human tumours

Robert S. Bell Vice President, Chief Operating Officer and Head of Surgical Services, Princess Margaret Hospital, Toronto, and Professor of Surgery, University of Toronto, Ontario, Canada
16.1 Sarcomas of the soft tissues

Tahar Benhidjeb Department of Surgery and Surgical Oncology, Universität Klinikum Charite, Robert-Roessle Klinik, Berlin, Germany
10.1 Oesophageal cancer

Christophe Bergeron Head, Oncologic Paediatric Department, Centre Leon Berard, Lyon, France
15.8 Hodgkin's disease in children

Thierry Berghmans Department of Internal Medicine and Medical Oncology, Institut Jules Bordet, Brussels, Belgium
4.10 Myelosuppression and infective complications

G. M. Besser Professor of Medicine, St Bartholomew's and The Royal London School of Medicine and Dentistry, Queen Mary College London; Head, Department of Endocrinology, St Bartholomew's and The Royal London NHS Trust, St Bartholomew's Hospital, London, UK
19.3 Pituitary tumours

Roy Bicknell Head of Molecular Angiogenesis Laboratory, Imperial Cancer Research Fund, Institute of Molecular Medicine, University of Oxford, UK
1.7 Angiogenesis and invasion

Peter Blake Consultant Clinical Oncologist and Head of Radiotherapy, Royal Marsden Hospital, London, UK
4.3.4 Intracavitary therapy
12.6 Carcinoma of the vagina

Carla Boccaccio Assistant Professor, Institute for Cancer Research (IRCC), University of Turin, Italy
1.4 Growth factors and cell signalling

J. D. Boice, Jr Oak Ridge National Laboratory, Biology Division, Oak Ridge, Tennessee, USA
2.3 Radiation carcinogenesis

J. J. Bonenkamp Department of Surgery, University Medical Centre Nijmegen, The Netherlands
10.2 Gastric cancer

Thierry Boon Director, Ludwig Institute for Cancer Research, Brussels Branch, and Professor, Catholic University of Louvain, Belgium
1.9 Tumour antigens

Chris Boshoff GlaxoWellcome Fellow, Wolfson Institute for Biomedical Research, University College London, UK
2.2 Viral carcinogenesis

Stephen G. Bown Professor of Laser Medicine and Surgery and Director of the National Medical Laser Centre, Royal Free and University College Medical School, London, UK
4.29 Photodynamic therapy and lasers in oncology

N. F. Boyd Head, Division of Epidemiology and Statistics, Ontario Cancer Institute, University Health Network and Professor of Medicine, University of Toronto, Ontario, Canada
11.1 The epidemiology of breast cancer

M. J. Boyer Head, Department of Medical Oncology, Royal Prince Alfred Hospital, Camperdown, Australia
13.5 Extragonadal germ-cell tumours

Michael Brada Reader and Consultant in Clinical Oncology, Royal Marsden Hospital, Sutton, Surrey, UK
5.5 Spinal metastatic disease
18.2 Tumours of the brain and spinal cord in adults

Vivien H. C. Bramwell Medical Director, Clinical Research Unit, London Regional Cancer Centre, Ontario, Canada
16.1 Sarcomas of the soft tissues

Eduardo Bruera Professor of Oncology, Alberta Cancer Foundation Chair in Palliative Medicine, University of Alberta, Edmonton, Canada
6.6 Care of patients who are dying, and their families

Robert Buckman Professor, Department of Medicine, University of Toronto and Medical Oncologist, Toronto-Sunnybrook Regional Cancer Centre, Ontario, Canada
6.5 Complementary medicine: challenges, lessons, and patients' expectations

Sue Burchill Scientific Director of Children's Cancer Research Laboratory, Leeds, UK
16.3 Ewing's sarcoma and the Ewing family of tumours

A. K. Burnett Professor of Haematology and Head of Department, University of Wales College of Medicine, Cardiff, UK
15.2 Acute leukaemias in adults

F. Calvo Hôpital Sud Lyon, Lyon, France
4.7.1 Intraoperative radiotherapy

Mario Campanacci* Scientific Director of the Istituti Ortopedici Rizzoli and Director of the First Orthopaedic Clinic of Bologna University, Italy
16.5 Malignant bone tumours other than osteosarcoma and Ewing's tumour

Stephen Cannon Middlesex Hospital, London, UK
16.4 Osteosarcoma

Antonino Carbone Professor; Scientific Director and Head, Division of Pathology, Centro di Riferimento Oncologico - IRCCS, National Cancer Institute, Aviano, Italy
15.14 Neoplastic complications of AIDS

Nicholas J. Cassisi Senior Associate Dean for Clinical Affairs, and Kenneth W. Grader Professor, Department of Otolaryngology, University of Florida College of Medicine, Gainsville, USA
9.1.4 Therapeutic principles in the management of head and neck tumours

Anna M. Cassoni Consultant Clinical Oncologist, Middlesex Hospital, London, UK
9.3 Tumours of the nasal cavity and paranasal sinuses

Jean-Charles Cerottini Professor and Director, Ludwig Institute for Cancer Research, Lausanne Branch, Epalinges, Switzerland
1.9 Tumour antigens

J. Chessells Leukaemia Research Fund Professor of Haematology and Oncology, Institute of Child Health, and Honorary Consultant Physician, Great Ormond Street Hospital for Children NHS Trust, London, UK
15.3 Acute leukaemia in childhood

D. Chevalier ENT and MN Surgery Service, University Hospital, Lille, France
9.7 Pharyngeal walls, hypopharynx, and larynx

Mary M. H. Cody Consultant Psychiatrist, The Mental Health Unit, Chase Farm Hospital, Enfield, Middlesex, UK
6.4 Support services for cancer patients

V. Peter Collins Professor of Histopathology and Morbid Anatomy, University of Cambridge, UK
18.2 Tumours of the brain and spinal cord in adults

Paolo M. Comoglio Director, Institute for Cancer Research (IRCC), University of Turin, Italy
1.4 Growth factors and cell signalling

K. C. Conlon Associate Chairman, Department of Surgery, Memorial Sloan Kettering Cancer Center, New York, USA
3.6 Laparoscopic staging for gastrointestinal malignancy

Alberto Costa Director, European School of Oncology, Milan, Italy
2.5 Cancer chemoprevention

M. Craanen Leiden University Medical Centre, The Netherlands
10.2 Gastric cancer

C. B. Croft Consultant ENT Head and Neck Surgeon, The Royal National Throat, Nose and Ear Hospital and The Royal Free Hospital, London, UK
9.8 Salivary glands

T. Crook Ludwig Institute for Cancer Research, Imperial College of Science and Medicine, St Mary's Hospital, London, UK
3.1 Molecular and cellular pathology of cancer

John Crown Consultant Medical Oncologist, St Vincent's University Hospital, Dublin, Ireland
4.21 Dose-intensive chemotherapy

D. C. Cunningham Consultant Medical Oncologist and Specialist in Gastrointestinal Cancer and Lymphoma, Royal Marsden Hospital, Sutton, Surrey, UK
10.6 Cancer of the pancreas

Giuseppe D'Aiuto Istituto per lo Studio e la Cura dei Tumori, Naples, Italy
2.5 Cancer chemoprevention

Maurizio D'Incalci Professor and Head, Department of Oncology, Istituto di Ricerche Farmacologiche 'Mario Negri', Milan, Italy
4.18 Vinca alkaloids, taxanes, and podophyllotoxins

Olav Dahl Professor and Senior Consultant, Department of Oncology, Institute of Medicine, Haukeland University Hospital, Bergen, Norway
4.6 Hyperthermia

Jack D. Davies* Professor, Southmead Hospital, Bristol, UK
11.2 The pathology of breast cancer

Richard H. de Boer Consultant Medical Oncologist, Cancer Services, Austin and Repatriation Medical Centre, Victoria, Australia
5.3 Paraneoplastic syndromes other than metabolic

S. de Jong Assistant Professor, Department of Medical Oncology, University Hospital Groningen, The Netherlands
4.20 Mechanisms of drug resistance

Pieter H. M. De Mulder Professor and Medical Oncologist, University Medical Centre, St Radboud, Nijmegen, The Netherlands
13.2 Bladder cancer

E.G.E. de Vries Professor of Medical Oncology, University Hospital Groningen, The Netherlands
4.20 Mechanisms of drug resistance

D. P. Dearnaley Reader in Prostate Cancer Studies, Institute of Cancer Research and Honorary Consultant in Clinical Oncology, Royal Marsden NHS Trust, Sutton, Surrey, UK
13.1 Tumours of the prostate

Andrea Decensi Director, Division of Chemoprevention, Istituto Europeo di Oncologia, Milan, Italy
2.5 Cancer chemoprevention

Gabriella Della Torre Senior Staff PhD, Istituto Nazionale Tumori, Milan, Italy
9.4 Tumours of the nasopharynx

Volker Diehl Professor and Director, Department of Internal Medicine I, University of Cologne, Germany
15.6 The cell biology of Hodgkin's disease

Luc Y. Dirix Department of Medical Oncology, University Hospital Gasthuisberg, Leuven, and Oncology Centre AZ St Augustinus, Antwerp, Belgium
5.2 Metabolic complications

---

* It is with much regret that we report the deaths of Mario Campanacci and Jack Davies during the preparation of this edition of the textbook.

Stanley Dische Visiting Professor in Oncology, University College London, UK
4.4.2 The programming of radiotherapy

Neil L. Dorward Consultant Neurosurgeon and Honorary Senior Lecturer, Royal Free Hospital, London, UK
18.2 Tumours of the brain and spinal cord in adults

M. Dowsett Professor of Biochemical Endocrinology at the Institute of Cancer Research and Head of the Department of Biochemistry, Royal Marsden Hospital, London, UK
4.25 Hormone therapy

Jean-Pierre Droz Professor of Medical Oncology, Lyon-RTH-Laennec School of Medicine and Head, Department of Medical Oncology, Centre Leon Berard, Lyon, France
13.3 Cancer of the kidney and ureter

Stephen Duffy Principal Scientist, Department of Mathematics, Statistics, and Epidemiology, Imperial Cancer Research Fund, London, UK
11.3 Mammographic screening: from the scientific evidence to practice

W. Duncan Professor of Radiation Oncology (retired), University of Edinburgh, UK
4.7.2 Particle radiotherapy

Rosalind A. Eeles Senior Lecture and Honorary Consultant in Cancer Genetics, Institute of Cancer Research and Royal Marsden NHS Trust, London, UK
1.3 Familial cancer

Alexander M. M. Eggermont Professor and Head of Department of Surgical Oncology, Daniel Den Hoed Cancer Centre, University Hospital Rotterdam, The Netherlands
8.1 Cutaneous malignant melanoma

Charis Eng Professor and Director, Clinical Cancer Genetics Program, Ohio State University Comprehensive Cancer Center, Columbus, USA
19.2 Medullary carcinoma of the thyroid

F. Eschwege Professor and Chief, Radiotherapy Department, Gustave Roussy Institute, Villejuif, France
9.7 Pharyngeal walls, hypopharynx and larynx

N.J. Espat Department of Surgery, Memorial Sloan Kettering Cancer Center, New York, USA
3.6 Laparoscopic staging for gastrointestinal malignancy

Lesley Fallowfield Professor in Psycho-Oncology, CRC Psychosocial Group, University of Sussex, Brighton, UK
6.2 Communication

Massimo Fanelli Division of Medical Oncology, Azienda Complesso Ospedaliero 'S. Filippo Neri', Rome, Italy
3.7 Prognostic factors

R. W. R. Farrell Consultant Otolaryngologist and Head and Neck Surgeon, North West London Hospitals Trust and West Hertfordshire Hospitals Trust; Honorary Consultant Head and Neck Surgeon, Royal Free Hospital, London, UK
9.8 Salivary glands

Peter Fayers Professor of Medical Statistics, University of Aberdeen, UK and Professor of Medical Statistics, Norwegian University of Science and Technology (NTNU)
6.3 Quality of life

Ian S. Fentiman Professor of Surgical Oncology, Guy's, King's and St Thomas's School of Medicine, Guy's Hospital, London, UK
5.1 Serous effusions

Aude Fléchon Clinical Instructor, Department of Medical Oncology, Centre Leon-Berard, Lyon-RTH Laennec School of Medicine, Lyon, France
13.3 Cancer of the kidney and ureter

Sophie D. Fosså Consultant in Medical Oncology and Radiotherapy, and Professor, National Radium Hospital, Oslo, Norway
13.7 Sexual dysfunction following pelvic malignancy in men

J. F. Fowler Emeritus Professor of Human Oncology and Medical Physics, University of Wisconsin at Madison, USA
4.7.2.0 Particle radiotherapy

Andreja Frilling Professor, Department for General Surgery and Transplantation, Essen, Germany
19.1 Carcinoma of the thyroid

R. J. M. Fry Consultant, Life Sciences Division, Oak Ridge National Laboratory, Tennessee, USA
2.3 Radiation carcinogenesis

Andrew Gallimore Department of Histopathology, University College and Royal Free School of Medicine, London, UK
9.1.2.0 Pathology of head and neck cancers

Giampietro Gasparini Professor and Director of Medical Oncology, Azienda Complesso Ospedaliero 'S. Filippo Neri', Rome, Italy
3.7 Prognostic factors

J. P. Gerard Professor, Hôpital Sud Lyon, Lyon, France
4.7.1 Intraoperative radiotherapy
10.5 Cancer of the anus

Alain Gerbaulet Head of Brachytherapy Service, Institut Gustave Roussy, Villejuif, France
9.5 Oral cavity
13.6 Tumours of the penis

Giuseppe Giaccone Professor, Department of Medical Oncology, Academic Hospital, Vrije Universiteit, Amsterdam, The Netherlands
14.5 Mesothelioma

Oliver Gimm Department of General, Visceral, and Vascular Surgery, Martin Luther University, Halle-Wittenberg, Germany
19.2 Medullary carcinoma of the thyroid

Christian Gisselbrecht Professor of Haematology and Head of Department of Haemato-Oncology, Hôpital St Louis, Paris, France
15.10 Non-Hodgkin's lymphoma in adults

Bengt Glimelius Professor, Section of Oncology, Department of Oncology, Radiology and Clinical Immunology, University Hospital, Uppsala, Sweden
10.9 Liver metastases

Aron Goldhirsch Director, Department of Medicine, European Institute of Oncology, Milan, Italy
11.7 Adjuvant therapy for breast cancer

John M. Goldman Professor and Chairman, Department of Haematology, Imperial College School of Medicine at Hammersmith Hospital, London, UK
15.4 Chronic myeloid leukaemia

Anthony H. Goldstone Professor and Director, North London Cancer Network, University College London Hospitals NHS Trust, UK
15.5 Chronic lymphatic leukaemia and other chronic lymphoid leukaemias

Peter Goldstraw Consultant Thoracic Surgeon, Royal Brompton Hospital, London, and Honorary Senior Clinical Lecturer, University of London, UK
14.3 Management of of non-small-cell lung cancer

Cesare Grandi Chief of Otolaryngology Unit, S. Chiara Hospital, Trento, Italy
9.4 Tumours of the nasopharynx
9.5 Oral cavity

Mel F. Greaves

Professor of Cell Biology and Director, Leukaemia Research Fund Centre, Institute of Cancer Research, London, UK
15.1 Biology of leukaemia

Anna Gregor Department of Clinical Oncology, Western General Hospital, Edinburgh, UK
14.4 Management of small-cell carcinoma of the lung

A. Grossman Professor of Neuroendocrinology, St Bartholomew's and The Royal London School of Medicine and Dentistry, St Bartholomew's Hospital, London, UK
19.4 Adrenal tumours

Richard Grundy Clinical Senior Lecturer in Paediatric Oncology, Institute of Child Health, University of Birmingham, UK
17.7 Rare tumours of childhood

B. A. Gusterson Professor and Head of Department of Pathology, Western Infirmary, Glasgow, UK
3.1 Molecular and cellular pathology of cancer

Jane Hall Director, Centre for Health Economics Research and Evaluation (CHERE), University of Sydney, Australia
7.4 Economic considerations for cancer clinicians

G. W. Hanks Professor of Palliative Medicine, University of Bristol, Bristol Haematology and Oncology Centre, UK
5.8 Cancer pain and its relief

Heine H. Hansen Professor, The Finsen Center, National University Hospital, Copenhagen, Denmark
14.4 Management of small-cell carcinoma of the lung

Ian R. Hart Professor and Head, Richard Dimbleby Department of Cancer Research/ICRF Laboratory, GKT School of Medicine, Rayne Institute, St Thomas's Hospital, London, UK
1.8 Metastasis

John A. Hartley Professor of Cancer Studies and Director, CRC Drug-DNA Interactions Research Group, Department of Oncology, Royal Free and University College Medical School, University College London, UK
4.14 Akylating agents

W. Hendry Previously Consultant Urologist, St Bartholomew's and Royal Marsden Hospitals, London, UK
13.4 Testicular tumours

J. M. Henk Consultant Clinical Oncologist, Royal Marsden Hospital, London, UK
9.10 Rare head and neck tumours
9.11 Tumours of the orbit

Robin Hesketh Senior Lecturer, Department of Biochemistry, University of Cambridge, UK
1.2 Oncogenes and tumour suppressor genes

Irene J. Higginson Professor of Palliative Care and Head, Department of Palliative Care and Policy, St Christopher's Hospice, London, UK
6.6 Care of patients who are dying and their families

Harald J. Hoekstra Professor of Surgical Oncology, Groningen University Hospital, The Netherlands
4.23 Regional chemotherapy

D. Hoelzer Professor of Internal Medicine and Director, Medical Clinic III, Goethe-University, Frankfurt, Germany
15.2 Acute leukaemias in adults

Heinz Höfler Director, Institute of Pathology, Munich, Germany
3.5 Staging

Peter Hohenberger Professor of Surgery and Surgical Oncology, Charite, Humboldt University, Berlin, Germany
4.1 Principles of surgical oncology
10.1 Oesophageal cancer

J. C. Horiot Professor of Radiation Oncology and Director, Centre de Lutte contre le Cancer, Centre Georges-François Leclerc, University of Dijon, France
9.6 Tumours of the oropharynx

A. Horwich Professor and Clinical Oncologist, Royal Marsden Hospital, Sutton, Surrey, UK
13.1 Tumours of the prostate
13.4 Testicular tumours

P. J. Hoskin Consultant Clinical Oncologist, Mount Vernon Hospital, Northwood, Middlesex and Reader in Oncology, University College London, UK
5.8 Cancer pain and its relief

David J. Howard Senior Lecturer and Honorary Consultant, Institute of Laryngology and Otology, University College London and The Royal National Throat, Nose, and Ear Hospital, London, UK
9.3 Tumours of the nasal cavity and paranasal sinuses

C. N. Hudson Emeritus Professor of Obstetrics and Gynaecology, St Bartholomew's and Royal London School of Medicine and Dentistry, London, UK
12.8 Sarcoma and melanoma of the female genital system

John Hungerford Consultant Ophthalmic Surgeon, Ocular Oncology Service, Moorfields Eye Hospital and St Bartholomew's Hospital, London, UK
8.2 Melanoma of the eye and orbit
17.3 Retinoblastoma

Robert D. Hunter Director of Clinical Oncology, Christie Hospital, Manchester, UK
12.3 Carcinoma of the cervix

Janet E. Husband Professor of Diagnostic Radiology, Royal Marsden Hospital, Sutton, Surrey, UK
3.3 Modern imaging in cancer managment

C. Irle Director, Haematology-Oncology, La Tour Hospital, Meyrin-Geneva, Switzerland
4.24 High dose chemotherapy and stem cell rescue

Peter G. Isaacson Professor of Histopathology, Royal Free and University College Medical School, University College London, UK
15.9 The pathology and biology of non-Hodgkin's lymphoma

R. James Professor and Director of Cancer Services for Kent, Maidstone and Tunbridge Wells NHS Trust, Maidstone, Kent, UK
10.5 Cancer of the anus

G. Jansen Biochemist, Department of Rheumatology, VU Medical Centre, Amsterdam, The Netherlands
4.16 Antimetabolites

J. R. Jass Professor and Head of Department of Pathology, University of Queensland School of Medicine, Brisbane, Australia
10.4 Colorectal cancer

Valerie Jenkins Senior Research Fellow in Psycho-Oncology, CRC Psychosocial Oncology Group, University of Sussex, Brighton, UK
6.2 Communication

Heikki Joensuu Professor of Oncology and Radiotherapy, Helsinki University Central Hospital, Finland
11.8 Treatment of locally advanced and metastatic breast cancer

N. W. Johnson Nuffield Research Professor of Dental Sciences, Royal College of Surgeons of England, and Professor of Oral Pathology and Director, WHO Collaborating Centre for Oral Cancer and Precancer, King's College London, UK
9.1.1 Epidemiology of premalignant and malignant lesions

Philip J. Johnson Chairman and Chief of Service, Department of Clinical Oncology, and Director of the Sir Y.-K. Pao Centre for Cancer, Chinese University of Hong Kong
10.7 Primary liver tumours

S. R. D. Johnston Senior Lecturer and Consultant Medical Oncologist, Royal Marsden Hospital and Institute of Cancer Research, London, UK
4.25 Hormone therapy

Adam Jones Specialist Registrar in Urology, Battle Hospital, Reading, UK
1.7 Angiogenesis and invasion

Andrew S. Jones Professor and Head of Department of Otolaryngology/Head and Neck Surgery, University of Liverpool, UK
9.9 Temporal bone malignancies

Colin H. Jones Senior Lecturer in Physics, Institute of Cancer Research, London, UK
4.3.4 Intracavitary therapy

Andrea Jox Department of Internal Medicine, University of Cologne, Germany
15.6 The cell biology of Hodgkin's disease

Ian Judson Honorary Consultant Medical Oncologist, Royal Marsden Hospital, London, UK
4.15 Cisplatin and analogues

Ulrich Keilholz Professor of Medicine, University Hospital Benjamin Franklin, Free University of Berlin, Germany
8.1 Cutaneous malignant melanoma

Lloyd R. Kelland Reader in Pharmacology, CRC Centre for Cancer Therapeutics, Institute of Cancer Research, Sutton, Surrey, UK
4.15 Cisplatin and analogues

Judith E. Kingston Senior Lecturer/Consultant in Paediatric Oncology, St Bartholomew's and The Royal London Hospitals, London, UK
17.3 Retinoblastoma

Andrew Kramar Biostatistician, Val d'Aurelle-Paul Lamarque Regional Cancer Centre, Biostatistics Unit, Montpellier, France
7.2 Endpoints

E. Kuipers Leiden University Medical Centre, The Netherlands
10.2 Gastric cancer

Janina Kulka Associate Professor, Second Department of Pathology, Semmelweis University of Medicine, Budapest, Hungary
11.2 The pathology of breast cancer

M. Laniado Specialist Registrar in Urology, Hammersmith Hospitals NHS Trust, London, UK
13.1 Tumours of the prostate

Thierry Le Chevalier Head, Department of Medicine, Institut Gustave Roussy, Villejuif, France
14.3 Management of of non-small-cell lung cancer

J. L. Lefebvre Chief, Head and Neck Department, Centre Oscar Lambret, Lille, France
9.6 Tumours of the oropharynx
9.7 Pharyngeal walls, hypopharynx, and larynx

Tristram H. J. Lesser Consultant ENT/Skull Base Surgeon, Department of Otorhinolaryngology, University Hospital Aintree, Liverpool, UK
9.9 Temporal bone malignancies

Ian Lewis Consultant Paediatric Oncologist, St James' University Hospital, Leeds, UK
16.3 Ewing's sarcoma and the Ewing family of tumours

Loren Lipson Chief, Division of Geriatric Medicine and Associate Professor of Medicine, Gerontology, Clinical Pharmacy, Medical Dentistry and Public Health, Occupational Science, and Occupational Therapy, University of Southern California, Los Angeles, USA
4.28 Cancer in the elderly: principles of treatment

Patrick Loehrer Professor of Medicine, Indiana University School of Medicine, Indianapolis, USA
14.6 Thymic tumours and their autoimmune associations

David Lowe Professor of Surgical Pathology, St Bartholomew's and The Royal London School of Medicine and Dentistry, London, UK
12.8 Sarcoma and melanoma of the female genital system

Laura Lozza Department of Radiotherapy, Istituto Nazionale per lo Studio e la Cura dei Tumori, Milan, Italy
9.4 Tumours of the nasopharynx

Elsebeth Lynge Professor of Epidemiology, Institute of Public Health, University of Copenhagen, Denmark
2.6 Cancer screening

Paolo Macchiarini Department of Thoracic and Vascular Surgery, Hôpital Marie Lannelonque, Paris Sud University, Paris, France
14.8 Uncommon intrathoracic tumours

Ian Magrath President, International Network for Cancer Treatment, Brussels, Belgium
15.11 The non-Hodgkin's lymphomas in children

Peter Maguire Professor of Psychiatric Oncology and Director of the CRC Psychological Medicine Group, Christie Hospital, Manchester, UK
6.1 Psychological sequelae of adult cancer and its treatment

M. Malone Consultant Histopathologist, Great Ormond Street Hospital for Children NHS Trust, London, UK
15.13 Histiocyte disorders

Jillian R. Mann Professor in Paediatric Oncology, The Children's Hospital, Birmingham, UK
17.5 Germ cell tumours of childhood

Robert Mansel Professor and Chairman of the Division of Hospital Based Specialities, University of Wales College of Medicine, Cardiff, UK
11.6 Local treatment and reconstruction

G. P. Margison Head, Cancer Research Campaign Carcinogenesis Group, Paterson Institute for Cancer Research, Christie Hospital Trust, Manchester and Senior Lecturer, University of Manchester, UK
2.1 Chemical carcinogenesis

M. Mason Professor of Clinical Oncology, University of Wales College of Medicine, Cardiff, UK
13.4 Testicular tumours

Philip Mayles Head of Physics, Clatterbridge Centre for Oncology, Bebington, Wirral, Merseyside, UK
4.3.2.0 External-beam radiation therapy

Jean-Jacques Mazeron Professor of Oncology, Paris University, France
9.5 Oral cavity

David R. McCready Leader, Breast Site, Department of Surgical Oncology, Princess Margaret Hospital, Toronto, Canada
11.4 Ductal carcinoma *in situ*

John R. McLaughlin Head, Division of Epidemiology and Biostatistics, Samuel Lunenfeld Research Institute, and Associate Professor, Department of Public Health Sciences, University of Toronto, Ontario, Canada
2.4 Principles of epidemiology

Howard L. McLeod Cancer Research Unit, The Medical School, University of Newcastle upon Tyne, UK
4.13 The pharmacology of anticancer drugs

William M. Mendenhall Professor, Department of Radiation Oncology, University of Florida, Gainesville, USA
9.1.4 Therapeutic principles in the management of head and neck tumours

Ben J. Mijnheer Head, Department of Clinical Physics, The Netherlands Cancer Institute, Amsterdam
4.3.1.0 Current practice of radiotherapy: physical basis

D.W. Miles Senior Lecturer and Honorary Consultant in Medical Oncology, Guy's and St Thomas's Hospital, London, UK
4.26 Biologically based therapies

Christopher Mitchell Consultant Paediatric Oncologist, John Radcliffe Hospital, Oxford, UK
17.4 Wilms' tumour

Indraneel Mittra Professor of Surgery and Consultant Surgeon and Scientist, Tata Memorial Hospital, Mumbai, India
11.5 Prognostic factors and staging

Roberto Molinari Head and Neck Surgical Oncology Division, Istituto Nazionale Tumori, Milan, Italy
9.4 Tumours of the nasopharynx

Silvio Monfardini Head, Division of Medical Oncology, Azienda Ospedale-Universita, Padua, Italy
15.14 Neoplastic complications of AIDS

Alessandro Morabito Azienda Ospedali Riuniti, Reggio Calabria, Italy
3.7 Prognostic factors

Gareth Morgan Professor of Haematology, Academic Unit of Haematology and Oncology, University of Leeds, UK
15.12 Myeloma

Tariq I. Mughal Consultant in Haematology and Medical Oncology and Senior Lecturer in Haematological Oncology, Royal Preston and Christie Hospitals, University of Manchester School of Medicine, UK
15.4 Chronic myeloid leukaemia

N. H. Mulder Professor, Department of Medical Oncology, University Hospital Groningen, The Netherlands
4.20 Mechanisms of drug resistance

Alastair J. Munro Professor of Radiation Oncology, Department of Surgery and Molecular Oncology, Ninewells Hospital and Medical School, Dundee, UK
9.2 Chemotherapy for head and neck cancer

Paul V. Murray Specialist Registrar in Chest Medicine, NE Thames Deanery, London, UK
14.2 Diagnosis and staging

Jan P. Neijt Department of Internal Medicine, Utrecht University Hospital, The Netherlands
12.1 Epithelial carcinoma of the ovary

David R. Newell Professor of Cancer Therapeutics, University of Newcastle upon Tyne, UK
4.13 The pharmacology of anticancer drugs

Edward S. Newlands Professor of Cancer Medicine, Imperial College School of Medicine, London, UK
12.2 Ovarian germ-cell and other rare ovarian tumours
12.5 Gestational trophoblastic tumours

Kees Nooter Senior Scientist, Department of Medical Oncology, Rotterdam Cancer Institute, The Netherlands
4.9 Principles of chemotherapy

Chris Norbury University Research Lecturer and Head, Cell Cycle Group, ICRF Molecular Oncology Laboratory, Weatherall Institute of Molecular Medicine, John Radcliffe Hospital, Oxford, UK
1.5 Control of the cell cycle and cell death

J. M. A. Northover Honorary Director, ICRF Colorectal Cancer Unit and Chairman, Department of Surgery, St Mark's Hospital for Intestinal and Colorectal Disorders, Harrow, Middlesex, UK
10.4 Colorectal cancer

Brian O'Sullivan Head, Sarcoma Section, Princess Margaret Hospital and Bartley-Smith Chair Associate Professor, Department of Radiation Oncology, University of Toronto, Canada
16.1 Sarcomas of the soft tissues

Odile Oberlin Paediatric Oncologist, Institut Gustave Roussy, Villejuif, France
15.8 Hodgkin's disease in children

P. Osin Department of Pathology, University College Hospital, London, UK
3.1 Molecular and cellular pathology of cancer

Jens Overgaard Professor and Head of Department, Danish Cancer Society Department of Experimental Clinical Oncology, Aarhus University Hospital, Denmark
4.6 Hyperthermia

H. Ozcelik Assistant Professor, Department of Laboratory Medicine and Pathobiology, University of Toronto, and Staff Scientist, Department of Pathology and Laboratory Medicine, Mount Sinai Hospital, Toronto, Ontario, Canada
1.1 Investigating the genetics of cancer

Eugenio Paci Chief, Unit of Clinical and Descriptive Epidemiology, Centre for the Study and Research on Cancer (CSPO), Florence, Italy
11.3 Mammographic screening: from the scientific evidence to practice

Anwar R. Padhani Consultant Radiologist, Paul Strickland Scanner Centre, Mount Vernon Hospital, Northwood, Middlesex, UK
3.3 Modern imaging in cancer managment

Fernando Paradinas Professor Emeritus, Imperial College School of Medicine, London, UK
12.2 Ovarian germ-cell and other rare ovarian tumours
12.5 Gestational trophoblastic tumours

U. Pastorino Director, Division of Thoracic Surgery, European Institute of Oncology, Milan, Italy
14.7 Surgical resection of pulmonary metastases

A. V. Patterson Senior Research Fellow, Auckland Cancer Society Research Centre, University of Auckland, New Zealand
4.4.1.0 Radiation sensitization: hypoxia related therapeutics

R. Pawson Senior Registrar, Department of Haematology, Royal Free Hospital, London, UK
5.4 Haematological complications of cancer

Giorgio Perilongo Associate Professor of Paediatrics, Division of Paediatric Haematology-Oncology, Department of Paediatrics, University Hospital of Padua, Italy
17.6 Hepatic tumours

A. R. Perry Academic Department of Haematology and Cytogenetics, Institute of Cancer Research, Sutton, Surrey, UK
3.1 Molecular and cellular pathology of cancer

G. J. Peters Associate Professor, Department of Medical Oncology, VU Medical Centre, Amsterdam, The Netherlands
4.16 Antimetabolites

T. Philip Director, Oncology Centre, Centre Leon Berard, Lyon, France
4.24 High dose chemotherapy and stem cell rescue

Piero Picci Director, Laboratory of Oncologic Research, Istituti Ortopedici Rizzoli, Bologna, Italy
16.5 Malignant bone tumours other than osteosarcoma and Ewing's tumour

Silvana Pilotti Head and Neck Surgical Oncology Division, Istituto Nazionale Tumori, Milan, Italy
9.4 Tumours of the nasopharynx

Jack Plaschkes Consultant in Paediatric Surgical Oncology, University Children's Hospital, Bern, Switzerland
17.6 Hepatic tumours

U. Plöckinger Department of Gastroenterology, Charite University Hospital, Humboldt University, Berlin, Germany
19.5 Neuroendocrine gastroenteropancreatic tumours

T. A. Plunkett Clinical Research Fellow, ICRF Breast Cancer Biology Group, Guy's Hospital, London, UK
4.26 Biologically based therapies

Pieter Postmus Professor, Pulmonary Department, VU Medical Centre, Amsterdam, The Netherlands
14.4 Management of small-cell carcinoma of the lung

A. C. Povey Senior Lecturer in Molecular Epidemiology, School of Epidemiology and Health Sciences, Medical School, University of Manchester, UK
2.1 Chemical carcinogenesis

Graziella Pratesi Assistant Professor, Laboratory of Preclinical Pharmacology, Istituto Nazionale dei Tumori, Milan, Italy
4.17 Antitumour antibiotics

Jon Pritchard Head of Paediatric Haematology and Oncology, King Faisal Specialist Hospital and Research Centre, Jeddah, Saudi Arabia
15.13 Histiocyte disorders

Kathy Pritchard-Jones Senior Lecturer in Paediatric Oncology, Royal Marsden Hospital and Institute of Cancer Research, Sutton, Surrey, UK
17.1 Molecular pathology of childhood cancer

Pamela Rabbitts St Bartholomew's Hospital, London, UK
14.1 Lung cancer: epidemiology, causation, genetics

D. Raghavan Professor of Medicine and Urology and Chief, Division of Medical Oncology, USC School of Medicine, Los Angeles, California, USA
4.28 Cancer in the elderly: principles of treatment
13.5 Extragonadal germ-cell tumours

Borghild Roald Professor of Pathology, Faculty of Medicine, University of Oslo, Norway
17.2 Neuroblastoma

A. G. Robertson Consultant in Clinical Oncology, Beatson Oncology Centre, Western Infirmary, Glasgow, UK
8.3 Skin cancer other than melanoma

Fausto Roila Medical Oncology Division, Policlinico Hospital, Perugia, Italy
4.11 Nausea, vomiting, and antiemetics

P. J. Ross Department of Medicine and the Gastrointestinal Unit, Royal Marsden Hospital, Sutton, Surrey, UK
10.6 Cancer of the pancreas

Marco Rosselli del Turco Epidemiological Unit, Centre for the Study and Prevention of Cancer, Florence, Italy
2.5 Cancer chemoprevention
11.3 Mammographic screening: from the scientific evidence to practice

Robin Rudd Consultant in Respiratory Medicine, St Bartholomew's Hospital, London, UK
14.1 Lung cancer: epidemiology, causation, genetics

R. C. G. Russell Consultant Surgeon, University College Hospitals, London, UK
10.6 Cancer of the pancreas

Gordon J. S. Rustin Professor and Director of Medical Oncology, Mount Vernon Hospital, Northwood, Middlesex, UK
3.4 Circulating tumour markers

M. P. Saunders Consultant Clinical Oncologist and Honorary Clinical Lecturer, Christie Hospital, Manchester, UK
4.4.1.0 Radiation sensitization: hypoxia related therapeutics

Michele Saunders Professor of Clinical Oncology, Mount Vernon Hospital, Northwood, London, UK
4.4.2.0 The programming of radiotherapy

Edward A. Sausville Associate Director, Screening Technologies Branch, Developmental Therapeutics Program, Division of Cancer Treatment and Diagnosis, National Cancer Institute, Frederick, Maryland, USA
4.22 New drug development

Pierre Scalliet Professor and Chief of Radiotherapy Department, Hôpital St Luc, University of Louvain, Belgium
13.2 Bladder cancer

Jan H. M. Schellens Professor and Medical Oncologist, The Netherlands Cancer Institute, Amsterdam
4.13 The pharmacology of anticancer drugs

Jean-Paul Sculier Professor and Chief of Medical Intensive Care, Institut Jules Bordet, Brussels, Belgium
4.10 Myelosuppression and infective complications

Michael J. Seckl Reader and Honorary Consultant in Medical Oncology, Charing Cross Hospital, London, UK
12.5 Gestational trophoblastic tumours

Peter Selby Professor of Cancer Medicine and Director, ICRF Clinical Centre at Leeds and Director, National Cancer Research Network, St James' Hospital, Leeds, UK
15.12 Myeloma

Hans-Jörg Senn Professor, Kantonsspital, St Gallen, Switzerland
11.7 Adjuvant therapy for breast cancer

Clare Shaw Chief Dietitian, Royal Marsden Hospital, London, UK
5.7 Therapeutic aspects of nutrition in cancer patients

Mary Sheppard Consultant Pathologist, Royal Brompton Hospital, London, UK
14.6 Thymic tumours and their autoimmune associations

Robert H. Shoemaker Chief, Screening Technologies Branch, Developmental Therapeutics Program, Division of Cancer Treatment and Diagnosis, National Cancer Institute, Frederick, Maryland, USA
4.22 New drug development

Tali Siegal Professor and Director of Neuro-Oncology Center, Hadassah Hebrew University Hospital, Jerusalem, Israel
5.5 Spinal metastatic disease

Tzony Siegal Director, Chosen Specialities Clinics and Chief of Spinal Surgery, Orthopaedic Department, Assuta Hospital, Tel Aviv, Israel

R. Sigal Professor of Radiology and Medical Imaging, Institut Gustave Roussy, Villejuif, France
9.1.3.0 Imaging of head and neck tumours
9.6 Tumours of the oropharynx

Anthony C. Silverstone Consultant Gynaecological Oncologist, University College London Hospitals, UK
12.4 Tumours of the endometrium and fallopian tube

Charles R. J. Singer Consultant Haematologist, Royal United Hospital, Bath, Avon, UK
15.5 Chronic lymphatic leukaemia and other chronic lymphoid leukaemias

Maurice L. Slevin Medical Oncologist, St Bartholomew's Hospital, London, UK
6.4 Support services for cancer patients

Ian E. Smith Professor of Cancer Medicine, Royal Marsden Hospital, Sutton, Surrey, UK
5.3 Paraneoplastic syndromes other than metabolic

Philippe Solal-Céligny Head of Department of Medical Oncology and Haematology, Centre J. Bernard, Le Mans, France
15.10 Non-Hodgkin's lymphoma in adults

Robert Souhami Principal, Royal Free and University College London Medical School, UK
16.3 Ewing's sarcoma and the Ewing family of tumours

David S. Soutar Consultant Plastic Surgeon, West of Scotland Plastic Oral and Maxillofacial Surgery Unit, Canniesburn Hospital, Glasgow, UK
8.3 Skin cancer other than melanoma

W. P. Soutter Reader in Gynaecological Oncology, Imperial College School of Medicine, Hammersmith Hospital, London, UK
12.7 Carcinoma of the vulva

Michele Spina Assistant to Professor, Division of Medical Oncology A, National Cancer Institute, Aviano, Italy
15.14 Neoplastic complications of AIDS

Stephen G. Spiro Professor and Head, Department of Respiratory Medicine, University College London Hospitals NHS Trust, UK
14.2 Diagnosis and staging

David Spooner Birmingham Children's Hospital, UK
18.1 Brain tumours in children

J. A. Squire J.C. Boileau Grant Chair in Oncologic Pathology and Associate Professor, Department of Laboratory Medicine and Pathobiology and Department of Medical Biophysics, University of Toronto, Ontario, Canada
1.1 Investigating the genetics of cancer

G. Gordon Steel Emeritus Professor of Radiobiology Applied to Radiotherapy, Institute of Cancer Research, Sutton, Surrey, UK
4.2 The biological basis of radiotherapy
4.3.4.0 Intracavitary therapy

M. C. G. Stevens CHC Professor of Paediatric Oncology, University of Birmingham, Birmingham Children's Hospital, UK
16.2 Malignant mesenchymal tumours of childhood

Charles Stiller Epidemiologist, Childhood Cancer Research Group, Department of Paediatrics, University of Oxford, UK
17.7 Rare tumours of childhood

Gerrit Stoter Chairman, Department of Medical Oncology, Rotterdam Cancer Institute (Daniel den Hoed Kliniek), Rotterdam, The Netherlands
4.9 Principles of chemotherapy

I. J. Stratford Professor of Pharmacy, Experimental Oncology group, Drug Action and Design, School of Pharmacy and Pharmaceutical Sciences, Manchester, UK
4.4.1 Radiation sensitization: hypoxia related therapeutics

Scott P. Stringer Professor and Vice-Chairman, Department of Otolaryngology, University of Florida College of Medicine, Gainesville, US
9.1.4 Therapeutic principles in the management of head and neck tumours

Simon B. Sutcliffe President and Chief Executive Officer, British Columbia Cancer Agency, Vancouver, Canada
4.12 Long-term follow-up

Hans Svensson Professor in Medical Radiation Physics at the University of Umea, Sweden
4.3.1 Current practice of radiotherapy: physical basis

J. W. Sweetenham Professor of Medicine, Division of Medical Oncology, University of Colorado Cancer Center, USA
15.7 Hodgkin's disease in adults

Diana Tait Consultant in Clinical Oncology, Royal Marsden Hospital and Senior Lecturer, Institute of Cancer Research, Sutton, Surrey, UK
4.3.2 External-beam radiation therapy

A. H. M. Taminiau Professor and Head, Oncological Orthopaedics, Leiden University, The Netherlands
5.6 Pathological fracture

Scott P. Tannehill University of Florida Shands Cancer Center, Gainsville, Florida, USA
9.1.4.0 Therapeutic principles in the management of head and neck tumours

M. H. N. Tattersall Professor of Cancer Medicine, University of Sydney
7.4 Economic considerations for cancer clinicians
20 Cancer of unknown primary site

David G. T. Thomas Professor of Neurosurgery, The National Hospital for Nervous Diseases, London, UK
18.2 Tumours of the brain and spinal cord in adults

Hilary Thomas Department of Gynaecological Oncology, Hammersmith Hospital, London, UK
12.7 Carcinoma of the vulva

Umberto Tirelli Professor and Director of Division of Medical Oncology A, National Cancer Institute, Aviano, Italy
15.14 Neoplastic complications of AIDS

Maurizio Tonato Professor and Director of the Medical Oncology Division, University Hospital, Perugia, Italy
4.11 Nausea, vomiting, and antiemetics

Valter Torri Head of Biometry Unit, Department of Oncology, Istituto di Ricerche Farmacologiche 'Mario Negri', Milan, Italy
7.1 Clinical trials and data management

C. Twelves Reader in Medical Oncology, CRC Department of Medical Oncology, Glasgow, UK
4.19 New anticancer drugs

Adrian P. M. van der Meijden Department of Urology, Groot Ziekengasthuis, Bosch Medicentrum, Den Bosch, The Netherlands
13.2 Bladder cancer

C. J. H. Van der Velde Head, Department of Gastrointestinal, Endocrine, and Oncological Surgery and Chairman, Dutch Gastric Cancer Group, Leiden University Medical Centre, The Netherlands
10.2 Gastric cancer

H. Van Krieken Professor, Department of Pathology, UMC St Radboud, Nijmegen, The Netherlands
10.2 Gastric cancer

Allan T. van Oosterom Professor and Director, Division of Oncology, University Hospitals, K.U. Leuven, Belgium
5.2 Metabolic complications

Hein van Poppel Professor and Head, Uro-Oncologic Clinic, UZ Sint Rafael, Leuven, The Netherlands
13.2 Bladder cancer

Jan B. Vermorken Professor of Oncology and Head of Department of Medical Oncology, University Hospital Antwerp, Belgium
12.1 Epithelial carcinoma of the ovary

Jaap Verweij Professor, Department of Medical Oncology, Rotterdam Cancer Institute (Daniel den Hoed Kliniek) and University Hospital, Rotterdam, The Netherlands
4.9 Principles of chemotherapy

Hans von der Maase Professor of Oncology, Aarhus University Hospital, Denmark
4.5 Combined radiotherapy and chemotherapy

David A. Walker Consultant Senior Lecturer, Paediatric Oncology, University Hospital, Nottingham, UK
17.7 Rare tumours of childhood

J. A. H. Wass Professor of Endocrinology, University of Oxford, UK
19.3 Pituitary tumours

J. Waxman Professor of Oncology, Imperial College London, UK
13.1 Tumours of the prostate

Jonathan Weiner Assistant Professor of Medicine, USC Norris Comprehensive Cancer Center, Los Angeles, USA
4.28 Cancer in the elderly: principles of treatment

Martin Werner Deputy Director, Department of Pathology, Technical University, Munich, Germany
3.5 Staging

Jeremy Whelan Consultant Medical Oncologist, Meyerstein Institute of Oncology, Middlesex Hospital, London, UK
16.4 Osteosarcoma

Leanne M. Wiedemann LRF Centre, Institute of Cancer Research, Chester Beatty Laboratories, London, UK
15.1 Biology of leukaemia

B. Wiedenmann Full Professor and Chief, Division of Hepatology and Gastroenterology, Department of Internal Medicine, Humboldt University, Berlin, Germany
19.5 Neuroendocrine gastroenteropancreatic tumours

T. Wiggers Professor and Surgeon, Department of Surgical Oncology, Groningen University Hospital, The Netherlands
10.3 Cancer of the small bowel

Nicholas Willcox Professor of Neuroscience, Weatherall Institute of Molecular Medicine, John Radcliffe Hospital, Oxford, UK
14.6 Thymic tumours and their autoimmune associations

Christopher J. Williams Co-ordinator, Cochrane Cancer Network, Institute of Health Sciences, Oxford, UK
7.3 The nature of evidence that can be used to make decisions in cancer care

N.S. Williams Professor of Surgery, St Bartholomew's and The London Queen Mary's School of Medicine and Dentistry, London, UK
10.4 Colorectal cancer

Jürgen Wolf Assistant Professor in Haematology/Oncology, University of Cologne, Germany
15.6 The cell biology of Hodgkin's disease

John R. Yarnold Reader and Honorary Consultant in Clinical Oncology, Academic Radiotherapy Unit, Royal Marsden Hospital, Sutton, Surrey, UK
4.3 Principles and practice of radiotherapy

Arthur Zimmermann Professor of Pathology and Head of Division of Clinical Histopathology, Institute of Pathology, University of Bern, Switzerland
17.6 Hepatic tumours

Franco Zunino Director, Laboratory of Preclinical Pharmacology, Istituto Nazionale dei Tumori, Milan, Italy
4.17 Antitumour antibiotics

1

Molecular and cell biology of cancer

1.1 Investigating the genetics of cancer

J. A. Squire, H. Ozcelik, and I. Andrulis

Introduction

Genetic technologies have made major advances in recent years, and both the power and sensitivity of methods in molecular biology have been greatly aided by the increasing number of genes discovered as part of the Human Genome Project.[1],[2] The fields of genetics and cancer overlap in many areas, and much of the success in our understanding of genetic defects in cancer cells has depended on the application of molecular methodologies. Some of the key methods used to identify and investigate genes associated with cancer are presented below. The reader is directed to more comprehensive texts for a full explanation of the methodologies and experimental details.[3],[4]

Positional cloning and gene discovery techniques

Basic methods of molecular genetic analysis

Restriction fragment length polymorphisms

Restriction enzymes recognize specific sequences in DNA. Thus any mutation within a recognition sequence will prevent that sequence from being recognized by that restriction enzyme. Mutations at sites recognized by restriction enzymes therefore lead to changes in the length of the fragments that are obtained after the digestion of DNA with such enzymes. Such mutations can occur as polymorphisms (i.e. changes in DNA that do not alter gene function) and when a polymorphism is present at a defined restriction enzyme site, it can be very useful for genetic analysis (Fig. 1(a)). Because such polymorphism leads to a difference in length of the fragments carrying the piece of DNA used for analysis, they are referred to as restriction fragment length polymorphisms. Such polymorphisms in DNA are inherited like any other genetic trait and can be used for linkage (see later) or loss of heterozygosity analysis of tumours (see later).

Blotting techniques

A widely used method for analysing the structure of DNA is the technique called 'Southern blotting',[3] which involves 'blotting' of DNA on to a supporting matrix. The Southern blot technique is outlined schematically in Fig. 1(b). The DNA to be analysed is cut into defined lengths using a restriction enzyme, and the fragments are separated by electrophoresis through an agarose gel. Under these conditions the DNA fragments are separated according to size, with the smallest fragments migrating farthest in the gel and the longest remaining near the origin. Pieces of DNA of known size are electrophoresed at the same time and act as a molecular weight scale. A piece of nylon membrane is then laid on top of the gel and a vacuum pump is used to draw fluid (containing the DNA) through the gel into the membrane. This suction causes the DNA to migrate from the gel to the nylon membrane, where it is immobilized and cannot diffuse further.

A common application of the Southern technique is to determine the size of the fragment in the DNA that carries a particular gene. For such an analysis, a cloned gene can be isolated and made radioactive. The nylon membrane containing all the fragments of DNA cut with a restriction enzyme is incubated in a solution containing the radioactively labelled gene. Under these conditions, the gene, usually called a probe, will anneal with homologous DNA sequences present on the membrane. Gentle washing will remove the single-stranded, unbound probe; hence the only DNA fragments remaining on the membrane containing radioactively labelled material will be those homologous sequences that hybridized with the labelled probe. To detect the region of the membrane containing the radioactive material, the nylon sheet is simply placed on top of a piece of X-ray film, enclosed in a dark container and placed at −70° C for several hours to expose the film. The film is then developed and the places where the radioactive material are located show up as dark bands.

An almost identical procedure can be used to characterize messenger RNA. In this case, RNA is separated by electrophoresis, transferred to nylon membranes; and probed with a labelled, cloned fragment of DNA. The technique is called 'Northern blotting' and is used to evaluate gross expression patterns of genes. An analogous procedure, called 'Western blotting' has also been devised to characterize proteins. Following separation by electrophoresis, the proteins are immobilized by transfer to a nylon sheet. To identify specific proteins, the sheet is incubated in a solution containing a specific antibody labelled with [125]I. The antibody will bind only to the region of the nylon containing the protein used to induce the antibody and the region of radioactivity can be located by the exposure of X-ray film.

More recently, non-radioactive labelling methods are becoming more popular for all types of blotting. In these systems, detection is achieved by labelling with reagents that undergo chemiluminescence when exposed to appropriate substrates. The emitted fluorescent light is then identified by short exposure to X-ray film, allowing the bands of interest to be identified.

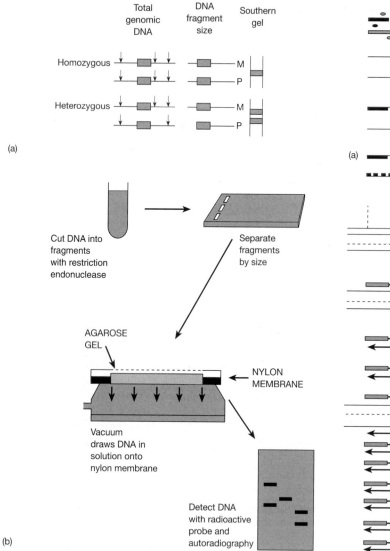

(a)

(b)

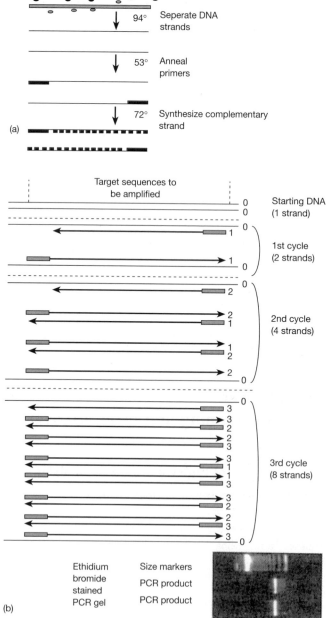

(a)

(b)

Fig. 1 (a) Restriction fragment length polymorphism analysis of DNA. In a normal cell, there are two copies of each piece of DNA, one derived from the maternal chromosome (M) and one from the paternal chromosome (P). The restriction sites for a specific restriction enzyme (designated by the arrows) are shown for each chromosome. Suppose that in an individual, the first restriction site to the right of a unique DNA sequence on the paternal chromosome has mutated and is missing. The result of this mutation is that the gene will be found on a smaller fragment of DNA from the maternal chromosome than from the paternal chromosome. Thus, a Southern blot of DNA from the cells will show two bands, one identifying the maternal chromosome and one identifying the paternal chromosome. (b) Analysis of DNA by Southern blotting. Schematic outline of the procedures involved in analysing DNA fragments by the Southern blotting technique. The method is described in more detail in the text.

Fig. 2 Schematic depiction of PCR. (a) Reaction sequence for one cycle of PCR. Each line represents one strand of DNA, the small rectangles are primers and the circles nucleotides. (b) The first three cycles of PCR shown schematically. (c) Ethidium bromide stained gel after 25 cycles of PCR. (See text for further explanation.)

Polymerase chain reaction (PCR)

PCR is an *in vitro* DNA amplification system that enables large amounts of DNA to be produced from very small amounts of starting material. The discovery of PCR technology eliminated the need for large number of cells to produce enough DNA and RNA for conventional molecular detection techniques. Additionally, it has improved and greatly simplified many of the early more cumbersome techniques of molecular biology required for isolating and analysing cloned genes.

PCR mimics the basic mechanism of DNA replication and involves a repeated cycling process made up of three defined stages, termed denaturation, annealing, and synthesis (see Fig. 2). In the first stage of denaturation the PCR reaction mixture is heated up (94° C), which denatures the double-stranded DNA molecules to form single strands.

In the annealing stage (50 to 60° C) the synthetic oligonucleotide primers recognize and bind to the complementary DNA regions of interest. During the synthesis stage, the thermostable Taq DNA polymerase enzyme extends the annealed primers, producing complementary copies of the initial single-strand DNA using deoxynucleotides (**dNTPs**) as building blocks. These three stages are usually repeated 25 to 35 cycles in 1 to 3 h producing DNA copies up to a million-fold. The products of PCR can then be subjected to any of the conventional methods of genetic analysis.

With a slight modification, RNA sequences can also be amplified using the PCR technique. It is first necessary to use the reverse transcriptase (**RT**) enzyme to make a complementary single-strand DNA copy (cDNA) of a mRNA prior to performing the PCR. Then, the cDNA is used as a template for a PCR reaction as described above; this technique is usually called RT–PCR. This technique is generally useful in the analysis of gene expression, specifically evaluating the levels of expression from different genes.[3] The RT–PCR technique also enables the detection of mRNA populations produced by alternative splicing or aberrant mechanisms including splicing mutations or chromosome rearrangements.

RT–PCR is ideal for the detection of tumours with reciprocal chromosome translocations as the fusion transcript generated by the rearrangement is only present in tumour cells and thus presents a unique substrate for RT–PCR detection. PCR technology is used increasingly to detect gene rearrangements and molecular markers for use in diagnosis and prognosis (reviewed in ref. 4).

Linkage analysis

Linkage analysis of human genes has utilized DNA from large well-documented families with a high incidence of a specific disease. If two genes are close together on a chromosome, they tend to be inherited together (i.e. they are 'linked'). Any two markers on a single chromosome can segregate (i.e. separate) through the phenomenon of meiotic recombination, but the closer the two genes are together on a chromosome, the less likely they are to be separated by a meiotic crossover. Thus, it is possible to map a new gene by looking for its linkage with other previously mapped genes. If several large families are available for analysis, one can also look for such recombination events and obtain an estimate of the distance of separation of two linked genes (Fig. 3). The distance between genes in a linkage map is given in recombination units or centiMorgans, and 1 cM equals a meiotic recombination frequency of 1 per cent in offspring, and is equivalent to about 1 million basepairs of human DNA. If there are several families or a very large family available for investigating linkage, this mapping technique can provide rapid and accurate information about gene localization. However, reliable results require the examination of many members of several families. Highly polymorphic DNA sequences have recently been recognized in which it is possible to recognize a large number of different alleles for a variety of genes that can be readily assayed by PCR.[3] These are the best markers to obtain initial information on linkage of a novel genetic trait such as the familial predisposition to cancer.

Loss of heterozygosity analysis

It is possible to compare DNA from a tumour to DNA isolated from normal white blood cells of the same individual, to determine whether there has been a specific deletion or loss of heterozygosity in the

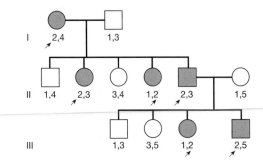

Fig. 3 Example of linkage to a disease trait using a highly polymorphic DNA sequence detectable by PCR. In this simple example the polymorphism is a DNA fragment length variation and five different alleles are possible. Polymorphisms can easily be identified by electrophoresis after performing PCR on DNA obtained from blood from each family member. It can be seen that allele 2 (arrowed) always segregates with the disease trait (solid symbols). In the example shown above allele 2 is tightly linked and no recombinants can be seen.

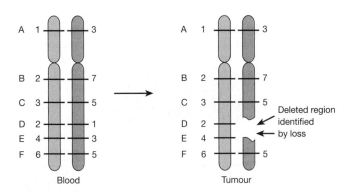

Fig. 4 Use of loss of heterozygosity analysis in mapping new tumour suppressor genes. Schematic depiction of loss of heterozygosity analysis using six highly polymorphic loci (A–F) evenly spaced along each homologue (shown as grey and white chromosomes). The numbers represent fragment sizes of each allele at polymorphic loci. Fragments lengths are measured by electrophoresis following PCR, and it can be seen that in this example all loci are constitutionally heterozygous, based on the analysis of the patient's blood. In contrast DNA from the tumour indicates that while loci A–C remain heterozygous, loci 'D' and 'E' have 'lost' allele '1' and '3', respectively, as a result of an interstitial deletion on the grey chromosome. By examining a large series of tumours in this way it would be possible to determine which locus maps closest to the region containing the unknown tumour suppressor gene.

tumour. Such changes are usually manifested as loss of one of the two heterozygous alleles when the tumour DNA is analysed by blotting techniques (see earlier). Sites of loss of heterozygosity can identify tumour suppressor genes: one copy of the normal gene is lost or mutated in the heterozygous state, and loss of the other copy may be associated with malignant transformation (see also Chapter 1.2) (Fig. 4). By screening a large series of paired blood and tumour samples with a panel of polymorphic markers (such as microsatellite markers—see section on the detection of point mutations) spaced across the genome, it has been possible to discover the chromosomal location of new tumour suppressor genes by loss of heterozygosity.

Once the smallest commonly lost region has been identified; it is then possible to use internet-based searches of human genome databases to evaluate each candidate gene that maps to this region. Comparative genomic hybdridization (see later) offers the potential for much easier screening and detection of deletions, but at present this technique lacks the resolution and the molecular precision required for identifying small deletions.

Fluorescence *in situ* hybridization (FISH) (see Plate 1)

FISH has become an essential tool for mapping genes and for the characterization of chromosome aberrations.[5] DNA probes, specific for a gene, chromosome segment, or whole chromosome 'paints', are labelled, usually by the incorporation of biotin and/or digoxigenin, and are then hybridized to metaphase chromosomes. Just prior to hybridization, metaphase chromosome spreads are heated briefly to approximately 75° C with 70 per cent formamide in buffered isotonic saline to denature the chromosomal DNA and the slides are incubated with the labelled DNA probe from the gene being studied. The DNA probe will re-anneal to the denatured piece of DNA at its precise location on the chromosome (see Fig. 5(a) and Plate 1). After washing off the unbound probe, the hybridized sequences are detected using avidin, which binds strongly to biotin, and/or antibodies to digoxigenin, coupled to fluorescein isothiocyanate, Texas Red, or another fluorochrome. The sites of hybridization are clearly visualized as fluorescent points of light where the probe is bound to chromatin. The advantage of FISH for gene mapping is that information is obtained directly about the positions of the probes in relation to chromosome bands or to other previously mapped reference probes.[4]

FISH can be performed on interphase nuclei from tumour biopsies or cultured tumour cells, which enables cytogenetic aberrations to be visualized without the need for obtaining good quality metaphase preparations. It is easy to detect massive changes in the copy number of oncogenes per cell. In Fig. 5(b) (Plate 1), the cytogenetic changes present when gene amplification has taken place are shown as magenta speckling in the dark blue nuclei. Numerical chromosome aberrations can also be detected using specific centromere probes which give two signals from normal nuclei but one signal when there is only one copy of the chromosome (monosomy). In Fig. 5(b) only one pale blue signal can be seen because the cell has only one copy of chromosome 1. Similarly, three signals would indicate that there was an extra copy (trisomy) of a particular chromosome. If the probes used for FISH are close to specific translocation breakpoints on different chromosomes, they will appear joined as a result of the translocation generating a 'colour fusion' signal (Fig. 5(c)). These procedures are particularly useful for rapid detection and enumeration of aberrations such as the various characteristic translocations present in leukaemias[6] thus providing immediate and directly quantitative diagnostic information.

Comparative genomic hybridization

For many types of malignancy, particularly solid tumours, it is not possible to select a suitable probe for FISH detection in metaphase or interphase nuclei. A new screening method called comparative genomic hybridization has been developed that allows investigators to produce a detailed map of the differences between chromosomes in different cells. This method detects increases (gene amplifications and chromosomal gains) or decreases (deletions or monosomies) of segments of DNA.[7] In typical comparative genomic hybridization experiments DNA from malignant cells and normal cells such as fibroblasts is labelled with two different fluorochromes and then hybridized simultaneously to normal chromosome metaphase spreads. Tumour DNA is labelled with biotin and detected with fluorescein (green fluorescence); the control DNA is labelled with digoxigenin and detected with rhodamine (red fluorescence). Regions of gain or loss of DNA sequences in the tumour, such as deletions, duplications, or amplifications, are seen as changes in the ratio of the intensities of the two fluorochromes along the target chromosomes (Fig. 5(d)). An amplified sequence will generate increased green fluorescence, whereas a deletion will shift the red/green ratio towards red. For low copy number amplifications and hemizygous deletions, this change in fluorescence ratio is difficult to distinguish by eye and requires specialized image analysis software. One disadvantage of comparative genomic hybridization is that it can only detect large blocks (>5 Mb) of over- or under-represented chromosomal DNA; balanced rearrangements such as inversions or translocations escape detection. Comparative genomic hybridization has gained wide acceptance as a new and promising approach for understanding the complex cytogenetic changes in solid tumours.[4]

Spectral karyotyping (SKY) and multi-fluor fluorescence *in situ* hybridization (M-FISH)

Recently, universal chromosome painting techniques have been developed in which it is possible to analyse all chromosomes simultaneously. Two essentially similar approaches have been developed: SKY[8] and M-FISH.[9] Both techniques are based on the principle of the differential display of coloured fluorescent chromosome-specific paints providing a complete analysis of the human chromosomal complement. Using combinations of 23 different coloured paints as a 'cocktail probe', subtle differences in fluorochrome labelling profiles after hybridization with this cocktail allows the computer to assign a unique colour to each chromosome pair. Thus, abnormal chromosomes in the karyotype of a tumour can be identified by the pattern of colour distribution along the axis of the chromosome so that rearrangements between different chromosomes will lead to a distinct transition from one colour to another at the position of the breakpoint (Fig. 5(e–g)). In contrast to comparative genomic hybridization, detection of such karyotype rearrangements using SKY and M-FISH is not dependent on change in copy number. This technology is particularly suited to solid tumours where the complexity of the karyotypes may often mask the presence of subtle chromosomal aberrations.

Gene enrichment techniques

In order to identify genes, whose expression is upregulated or downregulated in one cell type compared with another, several subtractive screening techniques have been developed. All methods rely on the principle that differential hybridization can be used to enrich for differentially expressed mRNA. The early subtractive hybridization methods were not efficient at identifying small differences in expression, and are both time-consuming and technically demanding. They have largely been superseded by faster and more convenient

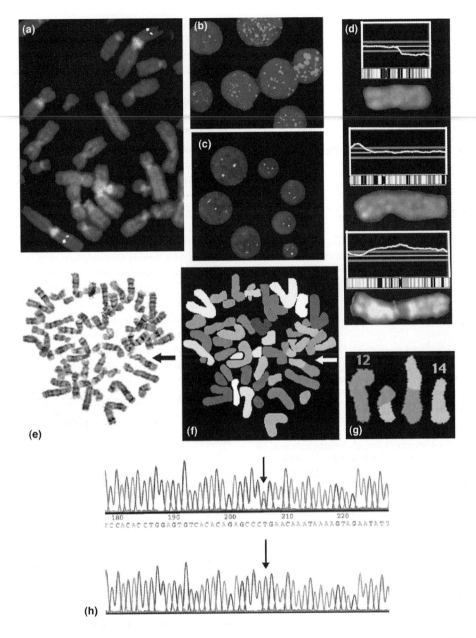

Fig. 5 (See Plate 1 for colour representation.) (a) Example of FISH mapping of a single copy genomic probe to chromosome 1. This is a DAPI (blue counterstain) banded normal metaphase preparation showing the location of positive signals (yellow signals) obtained with a cosmid probe containing an insert size of 40 kilobases of DNA from a gene on chromosome 1. A positive FISH signal is present on each chromatid of both pairs of chromosome 1 at band 1q25. (b) *MYCN* amplification in nuclei from neuroblastoma detected by FISH with a *MYCN* probe (magenta speckling) and a deletion of the short arm of chromosome 1. The signal (pale blue/green) from the remaining normal chromosome 1 is seen as a single spot in each nucleus. (c) Detection of a Philadelphia chromosome in interphase nuclei of leukaemia cells. All nuclei contain one green signal (BCR gene), one pink signal (ABL gene), and an intermediate fusion yellow signal because of the 9;22 chromosome translocation. (d) The comparative genomic hybridization analysis profile from a neuroblastoma cell line. Chromosome 1 shows an overall gain of DNA indicated by an increase in the level of green signal (bottom panel). In this cell line most of chromosome 1 was trisomic. Chromosome 2 has a strong green signal at band 2p24 due to amplification (50 copies/cell) of *MYCN* in the cell line (middle panel). The long arm of chromosome 6 shows a loss (deletion) of DNA and a shift towards the red signal (top panel). (e–g) SKY analysis of blood lymphocytes from a patient with a translocation. (e) One of the aberrant chromosomes can be seen by classical G-banding; (f) the same metaphase spread has been subjected to SKY; and (g) the 12;14 reciprocal translocation is identified. (h) Automated sequencing of BRCA2, the hereditary breast cancer predisposition gene. Each coloured peak represents a different nucleotide. The lower panel is a sequence of a wild-type DNA sample. The sequence of a mutation carrier in the upper panel contains a double peak (indicated by an arrow) in which the nucleotide 'T' in intron 17 located at 2 bp downstream of the 5' end of exon 18 is converted to a 'C'. This mutation results in aberrant splicing of exon 18 of the BRCA2 gene. The presence of a 'T' nucleotide in addition to the mutant 'C' implies that only one copy of the two BRCA2 genes is mutated in this sample.

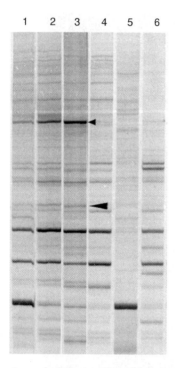

Fig. 6 Electrophoretic pattern following differential display PCR analysis of mRNA. Radioactive DNA fragments generated by RT–PCR are size fractionated by polyacrylamide gel electrophoresis and X-ray film is placed on top of the dried gel to display the 'bar code' profiles of the expressed genes in the mRNA pool. In this experiment the profiles of three different muscle tumours (lanes 1 to 3) are compared with the pattern generated by a related embryonal tumour of soft tissues (lane 4) and two unrelated tissues: spleen (lane 5) and liver (lane 6). Notice that some bands are common to all three muscle tumours and that the pattern is very similar to the embryonal tumour but quite distinct to the liver and spleen pattern. One band (short arrow) is very dark indicating it is highly expressed in all of the muscle tumours and another band (long arrow) is faintly expressed in the normal tissues and thus not differentially expressed.

PCR-based (see section on basic methods of molecular gentic analysis) approaches as described below.

Differential display

Differential display mRNA[10] is a form of RT–PCR in which the RT initiates cDNA synthesis from the very end of mRNA derived from a gene. Because all mammalian mRNAs have a tract of adenine residues at their 3′ end, it is possible to use an oligonucleotide containing several thymidine residues to hybridize to the majority of expressed genes in a population of mRNAs. If the oligonucleotide GATTTTTTTTTTTT is used as a primer, it will preferentially prime cDNA synthesis from the polyadenine tail of any mRNA whose 3′ end sequence ends in CT. The second primer is an arbitrary sequence of 10 bases that can bind to a random subset of sequences. The resulting amplification pattern produces a complex ladder of cDNA bands when separated using high resolution denaturing polyacrylamide gel electrophoresis (Fig. 6). Some applications of differential display analysis compare gene expression under different physiological conditions. Other approaches have studied expression at different developmental stages or have compared expression in

normal and malignant tissue.[10] These studies have identified a subset of genes whose expression patterns are different between the cell types.[11] By isolating specific bands from the gel, performing further cycles of PCR, and then checking the differential expression of the genes in the original cell populations, cDNA clones of differentially expressed genes can be obtained rapidly.

Representational difference analysis

Representational difference analysis is a PCR-coupled subtractive hybridization technique. Though similar in principle to conventional subtractive hybridization, its power to identify the differences between two populations of nucleic acids is far greater due to the PCR-based enrichment of the different sequences (Fig. 7). Representational difference analysis was originally used for the cloning of differences between two complex genomes.[12] With slight modifications and the addition of a reverse-transcription step, representational difference analysis can be used to isolate sequences that are differentially expressed.[13] Representational difference analysis has significant advantages over other molecular methods designed to enrich for expressed sequences. At the genomic level, representational difference analysis can be used to isolate polymorphic markers linked to a trait without prior knowledge of chromosomal location.[14] Representational difference analysis has been the most fruitful in cancer investigations, and has resulted in the identification of several cancer-related genes including transformation-related genes in oral cancer[15] and potential tumour-suppressor genes such as DMBT1 in malignant brain tumours[16] and PTEN in human brain, breast, and prostate cancer.[17]

Microarray analysis of genes

One of the important high-throughput technologies that has been developed to assess the expression of the increasing number of genes identified by the Human Genome Project is microarray analysis.[18] The approach involves the production of DNA arrays or 'chips' on solid supports for large-scale hybridization experiments. Two variants of the chip exist currently: in one format, DNA probe targets are immobilized to a solid inert surface such as glass and exposed to a set of fluorescently labelled sample DNAs; in the second format, an array of different oligonucleotide probes are synthesized *in situ* on the chip.[19] The array is exposed to labelled DNA samples; hybridized and complementary sequences are determined by digital imaging techniques. The resulting microarray, or 'DNA chip' technology allows large-scale gene discovery, expression, mapping, and sequencing studies as well as detection of mutations or polymorphisms. Microarrays of cDNAs have been used to study differential gene expression in bacteria, yeast, plant and human tissues, and cell lines.[20] This approach, in theory allows for the simultaneous analysis of the differential expression of thousands of genes at once and is having a major impact on understanding the dynamics of gene expression in cancer cells.[1]

A number of obstacles have to be overcome before microarray technology can be widely applied. First, several micrograms of good quality RNA derived from homogeneous tissue is required to generate sufficient cDNA to examine arrays. Secondly, simultaneous analysis of the level of expression of thousands of genes creates an enormous amount of complex interrelated bioinformatic data and consequent computational and statistical needs for interpretation.[21]

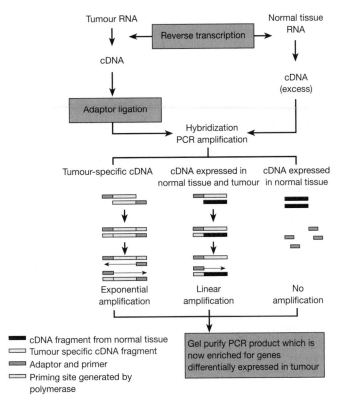

Fig. 7 Enrichment of tumour-specific cDNA by representational difference analysis. A simplified schematic depiction of the steps required to enrich for tumour-specific genes overexpressed in a tumour relative to control tissue using representational difference analysis. cDNA is made from RNA from tumour and from normal tissue by reverse transcriptase. To generate a suitable priming site for PCR in the cDNA derived from the tumour it is digested with a restriction enzyme that creates a small single-stranded DNA overhang adjacent to the enzyme cleavage site. Adaptor oligonucleotides are then added to the tumour cDNA and these will hybridize to this overhang region and provide a priming site for PCR amplification. An excess of cDNA derived from the normal tissue is then added to the mixture. Sequences derived only from the tumour RNA will be substrates for PCR and will exponentially increase in copy number relative to other genes present in the mixture. Other sequences will either linearly increase in copy number or will not have a priming site for PCR. In this way it is possible to isolate novel cDNA expressed in a tumour. Similarly, by reversing the procedure it is possible to isolate genes underexpressed in a tumour relative to a control tissue.

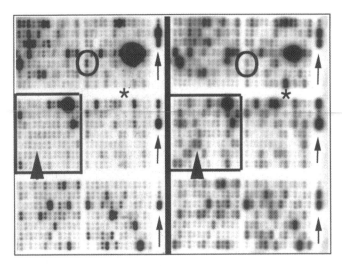

Fig. 8 Filter-based microarray analysis. Autoradiograms of Atlas™ (Clontech) cDNA expression array to demonstrate differential gene expression patterns by comparing dissected normal human squamous epithelial tissue (left panel) and a buccal cavity squamous cell carcinoma (right panel). Control household cDNA genes (arrowed) are used as reference target probes for normalization of the signal. As an example it can be seen that the boxed quadrant contains several genes (e.g. arrowhead) that are expressed at higher levels in tumour relative to normal squamous epithelial tissue. The cDNA signal above the asterisk is an example of a cell cycle gene overexpressed in tumour relative to normal in contrast to the encircled cDNA whose expression appears to be lower in tumour than in normal tissue (autoradiogram by courtesy of Dr Suzanne Kamel-Reid, Ontario Cancer Institute).

Thirdly, the biological relevance of subtle alterations in gene expression may not always have functional significance. Thus, until the inherent 'noise' in microarray systems is better understood it is likely to prove difficult to interpret more complex profiles of gene expression. Finally, most high-throughput systems are at present too costly to implement, except in large well-funded academic centres. However, simpler format microarray filter panels suited for radioactively labelled screening are being used in many research laboratories. In these commercial systems DNA from several hundred well-characterized genes with an established functional role in tumour biology have been bound to nylon filters (Fig. 8). While these microarray filter panels do not offer such a comprehensive screen as the systems described above, they provide a starting point for the simultaneous analysis of gene expression without the need for specialized imaging equipment.

Molecular characterization of genes

Detection of point mutations

Sequencing of DNA

The primary method for characterizing genes and the proteins that they encode is to determine the sequence of the DNA. The most frequently used method is dideoxy-chain termination.[22] For other methods of DNA sequencing see Ausubel *et al.*[3] The DNA template to be sequenced can be prepared in many ways; however, the most widely used approach is the sequencing of the PCR product.

DNA sequencing uses a method that is analogous to DNA replication *in vitro*. However, sequencing differs from DNA replication in that it uses dideoxynucleotide triphosphates (**ddNTPs**) in the reaction. DNA sequencing is carried out in four separate reactions each containing one of the four ddNTPs (i.e. ddATP, ddCTP, ddGTP, or ddTTP). In each reaction the sequencing primers bind and start the extension of the chain at the same place. The extended primers, however, terminate at different sites when dideoxynucleotides are incorporated (see Fig. 9). This will produce fragments of different size terminated at every nucleotide. Separation of the newly synthesized radioactive DNA on polyacrylamide gels allows visualization of each

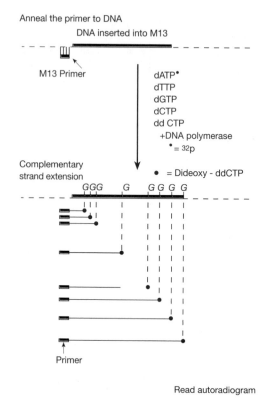

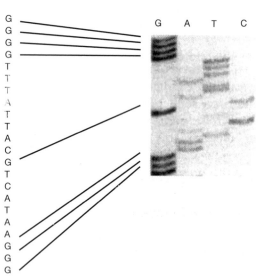

Fig. 9 Dideoxy-chain termination sequencing. The example shows an extension reaction to read the position of the nucleotide guanidine (see text for details).

fragment produced in the sequencing reaction. The use of polyacrylamide gels allows fragments differing by a single base to be separated. Usually a sequence of 200 to 500 bases can be read from a single gel.

Sequencing is usually performed by using automated sequencing systems utilizing fluorescent nucleotides and computerized sequence analysers. One of the most important advantages of this system is the automated detection of the sequencing results for data analysis.

The automated sequencing reaction is carried out in the same way as the manual sequencing except that the chain is labelled with fluorescent nucleotides and it is 'read' directly by the computer as each fragment migrates past an optical detector (Fig. 5(h)). The sequencing data are stored, analysed, and converted to DNA sequence by a computer.

Single-strand conformation polymorphism (SSCP)

SSCP is a commonly used technique for screening for mutations in cancer genes.[3] The technique is fast and easy to perform and detects regions with various types of DNA changes including single base substitutions. This technique relies on the property of single-stranded DNA having a tendency to adopt complex conformational structures stabilized by weak intramolecular hydrogen bonds. The electrophoresis conditions and temperature influence the conformation of sequences when DNA in a gel is subjected to an electric field, thus determining the migration patterns of different sequences. When a mutation is present in the DNA, this will affect the conformation of that sequence and will result in a different electrophoretic mobility relative to the wild-type sequences. In a typical SSCP experiment, PCR products are made in the presence of radiolabelled nucleotides using primers flanking the gene of interest. PCR products are heat denatured to form single strands and subjected to non-denaturing polyacrylamide electrophoresis. Control samples are run on the same gels so that differences from the wild-type electrophoretic pattern can be detected. The fragments with potential mutations or polymorphisms are detected as shifts from the wild-type control fragments (Fig. 10). As SSCP does not provide information about the nature of the change found, DNA sequencing must be performed on that region of the gene.

Protein truncation test

The protein truncation test is a very rapid and efficient method for detecting mutations that give rise to premature termination of protein synthesis from a gene.[23] These mutations consist of small deletions or insertions, splice errors, and changes to non-sense codons. The protein truncation test is a PCR-based technique where DNA or cDNA can be used as a template. PCR products in frame with the protein translation frame are amplified using primers specific to the gene of interest. One of the primers is designed to introduce sequences for RNA and consequent protein synthesis into the PCR product. Using an *in vitro* transcription/translation system, PCR products are copied into mRNA and consequently into the corresponding size of protein molecules. In the case of a truncation mutation within the PCR product, a shorter protein will be synthesized compared with control samples. The synthesized protein products are electrophoresed on polyacrylamide gel systems containing the detergent sodium dodecyl sulphate. The proteins resulting from truncation mutations migrate faster and are detected as bands on the polyacrylamide gel systems (Fig. 11).

Heteroduplex analysis

Heteroduplex analysis identifies mismatched bases formed when complementary strands of a mutant and its normal sequence are allowed to hybridize to form a double strand heteroduplex molecule. This PCR-based technique is sensitive enough to detect single base substitutions in a large tract of DNA; however, due to its efficiency

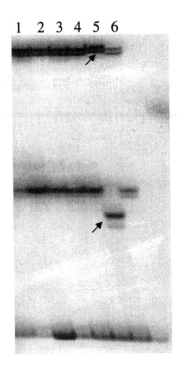

Fig. 10 SSCP analysis. Example using the p53-tumour suppressor gene. Exon 9 of the p53 gene has been PCR amplified in a series of tumour DNA samples obtained from breast cancer patients. The PCR products are subjected to non-denaturing polyacrylamide gels and electrophoresed at low temperatures (10 to 20° C). The band shifts in lane 5 indicate alterations in the gene sequence in exon 9 of the p53 gene. DNA sequencing for band shifts detected by SSCP is always carried out to identify the nature of the sequence alteration.

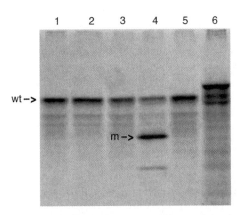

Fig. 11 The protein truncation test. Example using BRCA1 the hereditary breast and ovarian cancer gene. A region in exon 11 of BRCA1 gene has been analysed in a series of lymphocyte DNA samples from breast cancer patients. The wild-type protein products are indicated as 'wt'. The faster running product indicated as 'm' in lane 4 demonstrates the presence of a truncation mutation in this sample.

and simplicity, it has been more widely used in the detection of nucleotide insertions and/or deletions in heterozygous individuals. Heteroduplex formation is carried out by subjecting PCR products

to heat denaturation during which PCR molecules are separated into their single-stranded forms, followed by a cooling down step where single-stranded molecules re-anneal to form double-stranded molecules. Compared with homoduplex molecules where base pairing between the strands is complete, the mismatched heteroduplex molecules migrate much more slowly in polyacrylamide gels due to their shape, thus enabling the detection of the presence of mutations.

Microsatellite instability

Short repetitive DNA sequences or microsatellites, consisting of mono-, di-, tri-, and tetranucleotide repeats are widely distributed throughout the genome. These repeats are genetically unstable, undergoing alterations in length during DNA replication, either by expansion or contraction of the repeat sequences through many successive generations. Microsatellites form a great source of polymorphic genetic markers and have been used extensively in the construction of detailed linkage maps, and in the identification and characterization of genes related to specific diseases.

Microsatellite instability has been found to be associated with many sporadic and familial cancers, including hereditary non-polyposis colon cancer (see also Chapter 10.4).[24],[25] Hereditary non-polyposis colon cancer is caused by germline mutations in DNA mismatch repair genes. In the tumours of hereditary non-polyposis colon cancer patients, microsatellite instability is widespread, introducing many somatic mutations into the genome, thus probably affecting the function of genes important in colon carcinogenesis. Tumours exhibiting such instability are termed replication error positive. The replication error positive tumours can be identified by analysing a series of microsatellite repeat loci in the tumour and the normal tissue of the same individual. Oligonucleotide primers flanking the microsatellite loci are used for PCR amplification using radioactive isotopes or fluorescent dyes. Microsatellite instability, the change in the number of repeated units, can be observed by separating the alleles according to their size on the polyacrylamide gel electrophoresis system. The detection of an alteration in the size of a repeat in the tumour tissue in contrast to normal tissue indicates the presence of microsatellite instability in that tumour.

Yeast two-hybrid system

The yeast two-hybrid is a useful tool for studying interactions between proteins in an *in vivo* setting, as well as for identifying novel partners for proteins of interest.[26],[27] This powerful technique uses yeast as an expression system and takes advantage of the functional mechanisms of their transcription factors. Transcription factors contain a DNA-binding domain that recognizes and binds specific DNA sequences. Additionally, they have an activator domain that promotes transcription by interacting with and recruiting the necessary transcriptional machinery. The yeast two-hybrid system takes advantage of yeast transcription factors, such as the GAL4 protein, which consist of separable domains for DNA binding and transcriptional activation (see Fig. 12).

The yeast two-hybrid system can be used to study interactions between proteins in many ways. With this method, it is possible to determine the primary sequences needed for interaction between two protein partners. With this knowledge, one can predict the potential influence of specific amino acid alterations due to point mutations, on the interaction of a protein with its partner. Thus, it provides an

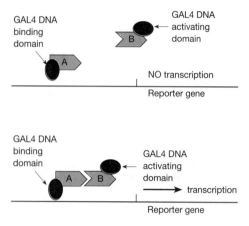

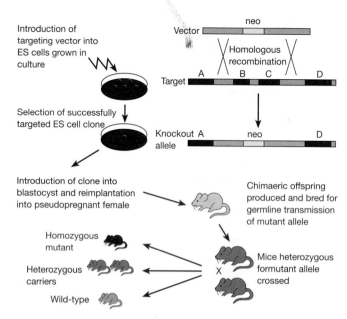

Fig. 12 Schematic depiction of yeast two-hybrid system. Reconstruction of the transcriptional activation ability of GAL4, a transcription factor in yeast with separable DNA-binding and DNA-activating domains. Hybrids containing either the DNA-binding or activating domain are not capable of initiating transcription (upper panel). A protein–protein interaction between two proteins A and B that can bind to the two domain of GAL4, brings the GAL4 domains together resulting in transcriptional activation of the downstream gene (lower panel).

Fig. 13 Gene targeting. The homologous region on the exogenous DNA is shown in grey, the selectable gene neomycin (neo) is hatched, and the target exons are black. The two recombination points are shown by 'X' and the exogenous DNA replaces some of the normal DNA of exons 'B' and 'C', thereby destroying its reading frame by inserting the small 'neo' gene. ES cells that have undergone a successful homologous recombination are selected as colonies in G418 because of the stable presence of the 'neo gene'. PCR primers for exons 'A' and 'D' are used to identify colonies in which an homologous recombination event has taken place. ES cells from such positive cells (dark colony) are injected into blastocysts, which are implanted into foster mothers (white). If germline transmission has been achieved, chimaeric mice are bred to generate homozygotes for the 'knocked out' gene.

ability to study whether a specific sequence variant in a cancer gene has a functional consequence and relevant clinical significance. Another application of a yeast two-hybrid system is that it can be used to screen cDNA expression libraries to identify proteins that interact with a given protein of interest. This approach is useful to identify important partners of proteins produced by cancer genes, which may help to identify molecular pathways in cancer.

Gene targeting and knockout mice

Gene targeting was developed as a method of site-directed *in vivo* mutagenesis in which a gene is intentionally targeted for a specific mutation. In this procedure, a cloned gene fragment is targeted to a particular site in the genome by a procedure called homologous recombination (reviewed in ref. 28). The technique relies on the ability of a cloned mammalian DNA fragments to undergo homologous recombination preferentially in a normal somatic cell at its naturally occurring germline position, thereby replacing the endogenous gene. The introduced mutation may result in the inactivation (or 'knocking-out') of gene expression or the alteration of gene expression to facilitate the study of gene function. The same approach can be used to correct a disease mutation in the mouse and restore normal function, thereby allowing therapeutic murine models to be developed.

An example of a typical targeting experiment is shown in Fig. 13. Initially the modified DNA is introduced into pluripotent stem cells derived from a mouse embryo (called ES cells). The frequency of homologous recombination is greatly influenced by a variety of factors such as the vector being used, the method of DNA introduction, the length of the regions of homology, and whether the targeted gene is expressed in ES cells. Homologous recombination with cloned sequences creates predictable novel DNA junctions in the genome, which can be conveniently detected by PCR. Oligonucleotide primers flanking the chosen site of recombination will only generate the correct sized PCR product if the expected DNA fragment at the site

of insertion is present. Once an ES cell line with the desired modification has been isolated and purified, ES cells are injected into a normal embryo where they often contribute to all the differentiated tissues of the chimeric adult mouse. If gametes are derived from the ES cells, then a breeding line containing the modification of interest can be established. Recent technological advances in gene targeting by homologous recombination in mammalian systems enable the production of mutants in any cloned gene.

Conclusions

Refinements in the techniques of molecular biology have allowed a rapid increase in the understanding of all aspects of tumour cell biology, and are being increasingly used in the analysis of clinical samples. Methods that allow the identification, isolation, and sequencing of genes have developed rapidly, providing a firm genetic basis for fundamental research related to the molecular changes that occur in malignancy. A number of novel technologies are providing detailed descriptions of the molecular rearrangements and functional abnormalities of genes in tumours. As the Human Genome Project approaches completion, more comprehensive molecular methods will be used to identify unique targets in human tumours for therapeutic intervention.

References

1. **Cole KA, Krizman DB, Emmert-Buck MR.** The genetics of cancer-a 3D model. *Nature Genetics*, 1999; **21**: 38–41.

2. **Strausberg RL, Dahl CA, Klausner RD.** New opportunities for uncovering the molecular basis of cancer. *Nature Genetics*, 1997; **16**: 415–416.

3. **Ausubel FM, *et al.*** *Current protocols in molecular biology.* New York: John Wiley, 2001.

4. **Dracopoli NC.** *Current protocols in human genetics.* New York: John Wiley and Sons, 2001.

5. **Verma RS, Babu A.** *Human chromosomes.* New York, McGraw-Hill, 1995.

6. **Rabbitts TH.** Chromosomal translocations in human cancer. *Nature*, 1994; **372**(6502): 143–9.

7. **Kallioniemi A, *et al.*** Comparative genomic hybridization for molecular cytogenetic analysis of solid tumors. *Science*, 1992; **258**(5083): 818–21.

8. **Ried T.** Images in neuroscience. Spectral karyotyping analysis in diagnostic cytogenetics. *American Journal of Psychiatry*, 1997; **154**(5): 594.

9. **Speicher MR, Gwyn Ballard S, Ward DC.** Karyotyping human chromosomes by combinatorial multi-fluor FISH. *Nature Genetics*, 1996; **12**(4): 368–75.

10. **Liang P, Pardee AB.** Differential display of eukaryotic messenger RNA by means of the polymerase chain reaction [see comments]. *Science*, 1992; **257**(5072): 967–71.

11. **Pienkowska M, *et al.*** Selection of probes for fluorescence in situ hybridization analysis by differential display polymerase chain reaction of mRNA from rhabdomyosarcoma. *Cancer Genetics and Cytogenetics*, 1996; **92**: 58–65.

12. **Lisitsyn N, Lisitsyn N, Wigler M.** Cloning the differences between two complex genomes. *Science*, 1993; **259**: 946–951.

13. **Hubank M, Schatz DG.** Identifying differences in mRNA expression by representational difference analysis of cDNA. *Nucleic Acids Research*, 1994; **22**(25): 5640–8.

14. **Lisitsyn NA, *et al.*** Direct isolation of polymorphic markers linked to a trait by genetically directed representational difference analysis. *Nature Genetics*, 1994; **6**: 57–63.

15. **Chang DD, Park NH, Denny CT, Nelson SF, Pe M.** Characterization of transformation related genes in oral cancer cells. *Oncogene*, 1998; **16**(15): 1921–30.

16. **Mollenhauer J, *et al.*** DMBT1, a new member of the SRCR superfamily, on chromosome 10q25.3–26.1 is deleted in malignant brain tumours. *Nature Genetics*, 1997; **17**: 32–9.

17. **Li J, *et al.*** PTEN, a putative protein tyrosine phosphatase gene mutated in human brain, breast, and prostate cancer [see comments]. *Science*, 1997; **275**(5308): 1943–7.

18. **Brown PO, Botstein D.** Exploring the new world of the genome with DNA microarrays. *Nature Genetics*, 1999; **21** (Supplement 1): 33–7.

19. **Bowtell DDL.** Options available-from start to finish-for obtaining expression data by microarray. *Nature Genetics*, 1999; **21** (Supplement 1): 25–32.

20. **Lander ES.** Array of hope. *Nature Genetics*, 1999; **21** (Supplement 1): 3–4.

21. **Bassett DE, Eisen MB, Boguski MS.** Gene expression informatics—it's all in your mine. *Nature Genetics*, 1999; **21**: 51–55.

22. **Sanger F.** Determination of nucleotide sequences in DNA. *Science*, 1981; **214**: 1205–10.

23. **Roest PA, Roberts RG, Sugino S, Van Ommen GJ, Den Dunnen JT.** Protein truncation test (PTT) for rapid detection of translation-terminating mutations. *Human Molecular Genetics*, 1993; **17**: 19–21.

24. **Aaltonen LA, *et al.*** Clues to the pathogenesis of familial colorectal cancer. *Science*, 1993; **260**: 812–16.

25. **Parsons R, *et al.*** Hypermutability and mismatch repair deficiency in RER+ tumour cells. *Cell*, 1993; **75**: 1227–36.

26. **Fields S, Song O.** A novel genetic system to detect protein-protein interactions. *Nature*, 1989; **340**: 245–46.

27. **Luban J, Goff SP.** The yeast two-hybrid system for studying protein-protein interactions. *Current Opinion in Biotechnology*, 1995; **6**: 59–64.

28. **Zimmer A.** Manipulating the genome by homologous recombination in embryonic stem cells. *Annual Review of Neuroscience*, 1992; **15**: 115–137.

1.2 Oncogenes and tumour suppressor genes

Robin Hesketh

It is now established that human cancers are principally genetic diseases, that is, they arise as a consequence of the accumulation of a set of mutational events that enable a specific clone of tumour cells to develop. For most cancers lethality is a consequence of subsequent metastasis of tumour cells from the site of the primary to colonize secondary locations in the body. The precise number of genetic changes required for these events remains unresolved for any cancer, but for adult cancers it is generally believed to range from five to 15. Genes that have been shown to have a functional association with specific cancers now number some 200 oncogenes and about 50 tumour suppressor genes.

This review begins with a definition of oncogenes and tumour suppressor genes followed by a brief summary of the major intracellular signalling pathways within which these genes are known to act. The function and clinical association of a select group of individual genes is then summarized to present the general principles discernible from our current knowledge of the molecular biology of human cancer without the complication of excessive detail. For more extensive discussion of individual genes the reader is referred to references cited in the text (short reviews where possible) and to books by Robin Hesketh.[1],[2]

Identification of oncogenes

Oncogenes were first identified in retroviruses capable of inducing tumours in animals and/or of transforming cells *in vitro* (e.g. avian leukosis virus and mouse mammary tumour virus). The oncogenes in retroviruses (e.g. v-*src*, v-*myc*) are homologous in sequence to normal cellular genes (proto-oncogenes, e.g. *Src*, *Myc*), which are highly conserved in evolution. It is now established that proto-oncogenes encode components of the signalling pathways which regulate cell proliferation and control the machinery of the cell cycle[3] (Fig. 1).

Despite their potent tumorigenic capacity in appropriate animal hosts, no retrovirus has yet been shown to be directly oncogenic in humans. However, it seems probable that the latent development of cancers that may follow infection by human T-lymphotropic viruses-1 and -2 or human immunodeficiency virus arises from subversion of normal cellular control mechanisms by the transcription factors encoded in their genomes (see also Chapter 2.2). Thus, for example, the human T-lymphotropic virus-1 *trans*-activating gene product TAX transforms cells *in vitro* and this correlates with the activation of JUN N-terminal kinases[4],[5] (JNKs; Fig. 2), which are components of

mitogen-activated protein kinase (**MAPK**) signalling pathways[6] (see also Chapter 1.5). A MAPK pathway is also activated by human immunodeficiency virus-1 envelope glycoproteins binding to the CD4 receptor.[7],[8]

Mechanisms of proto-oncogene activation

In the development of human cancers proto-oncogene activation may occur by mutation, DNA rearrangement (which includes loss or gain of entire chromosomes (aneuploidy), or chromosome translocation) or gene amplification[9] (Table 1). The mechanisms of amplification and chromosome translocation, respectively, can give rise to elevated cellular concentrations of the normal gene product or to the expression of new proteins created by the fusion of coding sequences from separate genes.

Point mutations, deletions, and insertions

Point mutations (or deletions or insertions of a few bases) may arise from the action of chemicals or radiation and give rise to dominantly acting oncogenes or cause loss of function of tumour suppressor genes. For example, the transfection experiments that originally revealed activated *RAS* genes in human tumours led to the finding that, for *RAS*, the transformation from normal proto-oncogene to oncogene arose from substitution of a single base, commonly resulting in the exchange of valine for glycine or glutamine for lysine at residues 12 or 61, respectively. In the tumour suppressor gene *P53* (*TP53*) over 5000 mutations have been identified: many of the point mutations affect p53 binding to DNA and hence the *trans*-activating capacity of the protein (i.e. its capacity to influence expression of other genes).

Gain/loss of chromosomes

Most major types of cancer show loss or gain of entire chromosomes and the changes involved may be extensive (e.g. up to 50 per cent) in terms of allelic loss. In addition to the examples given in Table 1 above, the genes of *RB1*, *P53*, and *APC* (*a*denomatous *p*olyposis *c*oli) (see below) are frequently lost in human cancers.

Translocation

The exchange of genetic material can occur between homologous or non-homologous chromosomes and can either be a balanced, reciprocal event or can involve loss of material from one or both junctions. Alternatively, inversion of segments within a chromosome

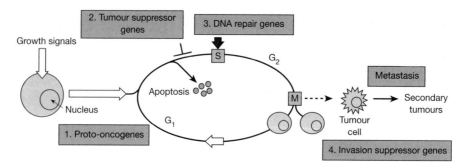

Fig. 1 Genetic signals in cancer development. Three broad functional categories may be distinguished within which mutations may arise: (1) and (2) pathways driving cell proliferation and controlling cell cycle progression and apoptosis (proto-oncogenes and tumour suppressor genes), (3) the occurrence of genetic instability through mutations in DNA repair genes, and (4) genes encoding proteins normally involved in the suppression of tissue invasion, the anomalous expression of which contributes to metastasis.

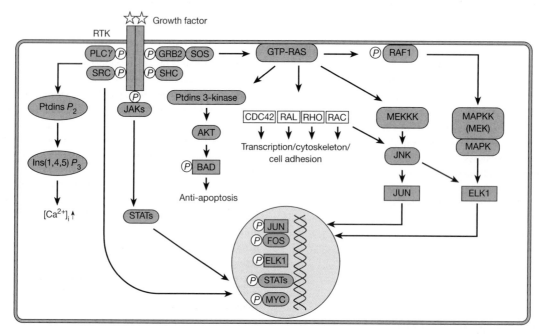

Fig. 2 Major intracellular signalling pathways controlling proliferation. Major signal transduction pathways that can emanate from activated receptor tyrosine kinases include the mitogen-activated protein serine/threonine kinase (**MAPK** or extracellular signal-regulated kinase (**ERK**)) pathway initiated via RAS and involving RAF1, MAPKK (also called MEK, (*MAP kinase* or *ERK kinase*)), and MAPKs (see text). Transcription factors that are targets for phosphorylation by MAPKs include ETS family proteins (ELK1), FOS, and JUN. A RAF1-independent pathway is also shown that leads to the activation of JUN N-terminal kinases (**JNKs** or stress-activated protein kinases, **SAPKs**). Receptor tyrosine kinases may also activate, directly or indirectly, phosphatidylinositol 3-kinase (**PtdIns 3-kinase**) and an antiapoptotic pathway (via the AKT serine kinase and BAD), phospholipase Cγ (**PLC**γ) leading to the hydrolysis of phosphatidylinositol 4, 5-bisphosphate (**PtdInsP₂**) and elevation of the free, intracellular concentration of calcium ([Ca^{2+}]$_i$), **SRC**, which is essential for the stimulation of DNA synthesis in response to platelet-derived growth factor (**PDGF**),[6] and members of the Janus family of protein kinases (Jak1, JAK2, JAK3, and TYK3) that phosphorylate on tyrosine residues various **STAT** (signal transducers and activators of transcription) transcription factor proteins.[5]

may occur without net loss, or interstitial deletions may give rise to shortened chromosomes.

In many solid tumours chromosome translocations appear to be random and manifest no pattern, even between histologically similar tumours. However, consistent rearrangements occur frequently in leukaemias and lymphomas and the genes involved in over 60 such translocations have now been defined. The majority of these encode transcription factors, the activities of which are altered as a consequence either of the formation of novel, chimeric proteins or of

the overexpression of the gene driven by anomalous regulatory sequences. Other classes of genes may be involved, however, and fusion proteins containing, for example, regions of cytokines, G proteins, stress response proteins, a clathrin assembly protein, mitochondrial proteins, cell death proteins, RNA binding proteins, and DNA binding proteins have been defined.

In chronic myeloid leukaemia the malignant cells in 95 per cent of cases express the chromosome translocation t(9;22)(q34;q11) involving *ABL* (that encodes a tyrosine kinase), which also occurs in

Table 1 Mechanisms of oncogene activation

Genetic event	Genetic change	Example
1. Base changes	Point mutations/deletions/insertions	*KRAS* mis-sense mutations in ~80% of pancreatic tumours.
2. Aneuploidy	Loss/gain of whole chromosome	Loss of chromosome 10 (*PTEN*) in glioblastomas. Trisomy (+*MET*) in papillary renal carcinoma.
3. Chromosome translocation	Fusion of non-contiguous segments	ABL C-terminus (*ABL* chromosome 9) to BCR N-terminus (*BCR* chromosome 22) in CML. *MYC* (8q24) to IgH (14q32) in Burkitt's lymphoma.
4. Chromosome amplification	Multiple (up to 1000 copies) amplification of regions 0.5–10 Mb	*NMYC* in 30% of advanced neuroblastomas.

25 per cent of adult acute lymphocytic leukaemias. Transgenic mouse studies indicate that this translocation is the initiating event in chronic myeloid leukaemia. The hybrid *BCR-ABL* gene encodes the BCR-ABL fusion protein, which has elevated tyrosine kinase activity and transforming capacity. BCR/ABL can bind to a number of intracellular proteins that are involved in transmitting mitogenic signals from the membrane to the nucleus of cells. These include p120*CBL*, the SH2/SH3 protein CRK, phosphatidylinositol-3' kinase, and GRB2/SOS1. One consequence of these interactions is the activation of pathways controlled by the RAS proto-oncogene, including the JNK pathway (see Fig. 2 and also Chapter 1.5). This suggests that the oncogenic activation of RAS could contribute to the development of chronic myeloid leukaemia and indeed abnormal expression of *RAS* and *MYC* as well as mutations in the tumour suppressor genes *RB1* and *P53* have been detected in the blast crisis of chronic myeloid leukaemia, *P53* mutations arising with high frequency. Furthermore, a variety of other chromosomal rearrangements may occur in chronic myeloid leukaemia each of which generates putative, aberrant transcription factor activity. Thus diverse molecular defects may contribute to the pathogenesis of chronic myeloid leukaemia and an equivalent progression has been defined in the development of acute lymphocytic leukaemia from myelodysplastic syndrome.

Gene amplification

An increase in gene copy number by amplification of specific DNA sequences occurs frequently in tumour cells, although it has not been shown to occur during normal mammalian cell development. Regions up to several megabases in length can be involved and these often include proto-oncogenes. The process expands the number of copies of a gene, which can lead to excess production of oncogene message and protein. Amplification appears to be mainly associated with the epidermal growth factor receptor (*EGFR*), *MYC* and *RAS* families, and the 11q13 locus. Amplification is thought to play a part in the later stages of cancer, generally appearing in cells that have metastasized. This is consistent with evidence that loss of the tumour suppressor gene *P53*, also generally a late event in tumour development, may be permissive for amplification. p53-dependent

growth arrest is exquisitely sensitive to the presence of only a few double strand breaks.[10] Inactivation of p53 permits immortalized non-tumorigenic cells and primary fibroblasts to replicate in the presence of chromosome breaks and to exhibit high rates of gene amplification.

The 11q13 locus, which includes the cyclin D1 gene, is amplified in about 20 per cent of human breast carcinomas and also in bladder tumours. Approximately 50 per cent of breast tumours examined immunohistochemically have revealed excessive levels of cyclin D1, and elevation of both cyclin D1 and cyclin D3 has been detected in the absence of increased levels of mRNAs.[11] Surprisingly, however, enhanced cyclin D1 expression appears to correlate with extended periods of remission and increased overall survival rates, whereas poor prognosis correlates with reduced levels of cyclin D1.[12] This suggests that cyclin D1 may be a useful prognostic indicator, but also that other factors, most probably *RB1* status, are more critical regulators of cell behaviour.

Oncogene activation and oxidative DNA damage

In the main, oncogene activation is the result of somatic events (i.e. what we do to ourselves) rather than hereditary genetic causes transmitted by mutation in the germline. It is, in other words, a consequence of evolution (mutation and selection) within the body of one animal. The epidemiological evidence supporting this conclusion is now overwhelming and it is widely known, for example, that in the Western world smoking and dietary factors each contribute to approximately 30 per cent of all cancer deaths (see also Chapter 2.1). Although the molecular mechanisms are far from understood, it seems probable that the major effects are manifested by the promotion of damage to DNA. Oxidative lesions in DNA are normally repaired with great efficiency by DNA repair enzymes but nevertheless accumulate with time and constitute the principal cause of cancers, essentially diseases of old age. Oxidative damage to DNA is also increased by the actions of the immune system in destroying infectious agents (viruses, parasites, and bacteria). Thus, for example, although the DNA tumour viruses that are oncogenic in humans (hepatitis B virus, Epstein–Barr virus, and some types of papillomavirus, see Chapter 2.2) appear to modulate proto-oncogene-controlled proliferation pathways;[13],[14] the chronic liver inflammation that follows hepatitis B virus infection is also associated with increased DNA damage arising from nitric oxide and superoxide generated by cells of the immune system. The catabolism of superoxide radicals into hydrogen peroxide and molecular oxygen is catalysed in human cells by three forms of superoxide dismutases. There is considerable evidence that manganese superoxide dismutase is important in suppressing the development of cancers: ectopic expression of manganese superoxide dismutase can reverse the malignant phenotype[15] and mutations in the manganese superoxide dismutase promoter may account for its reduced expression in some cancer cells.[16]

DNA mismatch repair genes

Mutations arising from errors during replication or as a result of the action of mutagenic agents are normally rectified by two major repair systems, mismatch repair and nucleotide-excision repair, respectively. Defects in mismatch repair were first shown to play a part in cancer development through the identification of alterations in the length of polyadenine 'microsatellite' sequences in colorectal cancers. Microsatellites are short, repetitive sequences of DNA (up to 6 bp with between 10 and 50 copies) that are stably inherited, vary from individual to individual, and have a relatively low inherent mutation rate. Failure of the strand-specific mismatch repair system to recognize and/or repair replication errors due to slippage by strand misalignment constitutes a 'mutator mechanism' for cancer development that is identifiable by the presence of ubiquitous, somatic microsatellite mutations. Defective nucleotide-excision repair genes were identified in patients with high susceptibility to skin cancers following exposure to ultraviolet radiation (see also Chapter 2.3).

MSH2, MSH3, and MSH6 are genes that encode members of the MutS DNA mismatch repair protein superfamily. MLH1, PMS1, and PMS2 are members of the MutL/HexB DNA mismatch repair family. Mutations in each of these human genes have now been identified in the germline of hereditary non-polyposis colon cancer families (see also Chapter 10.4). At least 40 per cent of hereditary non-polyposis colon cancer kindreds are associated with germline mutations in MSH2. Mutations in mismatch repair genes are associated with a mutator phenotype in which spontaneous mutagenesis is enhanced at many loci, predisposing to cancer development.[17] Microsatellite length heterogeneity is present in colon tumours, classified as replication error positive, showing that somatic genomic instability may be a very early event in the development of these tumours. A significant proportion of sporadic colorectal cancers with microsatellite instability have somatic mutations in MSH2 and microsatellite instability has also been detected in gynaecological sarcomas.

It is noteworthy that mutations in P53, APC, and KRAS are associated with malignant transformation but not with microsatellite instability.[18] This suggests that, although loss of function of mismatch repair genes clearly promotes genetic instability, the acquisition of mutations in major growth regulatory genes may equally well enhance malignant transformation. This is consistent with the conclusion that acquisition of the mutator phenotype is only one pathway to carcinogenesis and that selection without increase in the intrinsic mutation rate is also sufficient to account for the evolution of tumours through selective clonal expansion.[19]

Discovery of tumour suppressor genes

The existence of what are now variously known as tumour suppressor genes, recessive oncogenes, anti-oncogenes, or growth suppressor genes was originally inferred from the finding that when tumorigenic and non-tumorigenic cells were fused in culture the resulting hybrids were generally non-tumorigenic. When such hybrid cells do give rise to tumours in animals, this usually involves the loss of a specific chromosome derived from the non-tumorigenic cell. These observations suggest the existence of tumour suppressor genes, the normal function of which is to govern cell proliferation, and indicate that when non-tumorigenic hybrids are formed genetic complementation may be occurring such that the tumour suppressor function is supplied by the fusion partner. The two best understood tumour suppressor genes are the retinoblastoma (RB1) gene and P53. RB1 provides the classical model for a recessive tumour suppressor gene in that both paternal and maternal copies of the gene must be inactivated for the tumour to develop. For P53 and some other tumour suppressor genes, mutation at one allele may be sufficient to alter cell phenotype.

Growth factors, receptors, and proliferation signal transduction pathways

The properties of growth factors, their receptors, and of pathways that transmit signals from the cell membrane to the nucleus are described in detail in Chapter 1.5. The central features of these signalling pathways are that the interaction of polypeptide growth factors with their cognate receptors promotes receptor dimerization and activation of the intrinsic catalytic activity of the receptor (usually a tyrosine kinase).[20],[21] This results in receptor trans-phosphorylation, and interaction of specific adapter proteins or cytoplasmic enzymes with phosphotyrosyl residues initiates the activation of intracellular signalling pathways (Fig. 2). Of these, the most fully resolved is the MAPK pathway in which activation of receptors leads to activation of the RAS oncoprotein to its guanosine triphosphate (GTP) bound form. Activated RAS in turn recruits a serine/threonine kinase encoded by another oncogene, RAF1, to the plasma membrane, thereby activating a serine/threonine kinase cascade which leads to the phosphorylation of target transcription factors and activation of the gene expression programme associated with proliferation (see also Chapter 1.5).

The schematic pathway summary of Fig. 2 illustrates a number of complexities associated with growth regulation that have emerged in recent years: (a) multiple pathways may be activated in the same cell (e.g. by different growth factors); (b) pathways may include points of signal divergence (e.g. RAS); and (c) pathways may converge (e.g. the transcription factor ELK1 can be phosphorylated either by MAPK or JNK). These factors raise the question of how the integrated response to signals received by membrane receptors is generated in a cell-specific manner. This question is not fully resolved but it

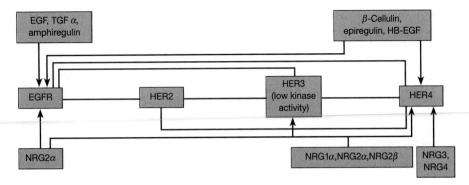

Fig. 3 Epidermal growth factor receptor (**EGFR**) family and ligands. Red lines connecting the receptors indicate that all possible heterodimeric complexes can exist, as well as homodimers. The receptor specificity of families of ligands is shown (black lines): EGF, transforming growth factor (**TGF**) -α, and amphiregulin interact specifically with the EGFR; β-cellulin, epiregulin, and heparin-binding EGF-like growth factor α (**HB-EGF**) with EGFR and HER4; neuregulin (**NRG**) -2α with EGFR, HER3, and HER4; NRG1α and NRG2β with HER3 and HER4. Two other neuregulins, NRG3 and NRG4 act through HER4.[26]

appears to derive from combinations of the following factors: (a) tissue specificity of at least one component in a given pathway; (b) the action of 'scaffold' proteins[22] that associate with pathway components to generate multi-enzyme complexes with enhanced transduction capacity for a specific signal; (c) regulation of transcription factor activity by multiple phosphorylation; (d) heterodimerization of transcription factors; (e) the existence of subfamilies of target transcription factors in turn having differential DNA binding specificity;[23] and (f) inter-pathway regulation (e.g. the negative regulation of the growth inhibitory transforming growth factor-β response by interferon-γ).[24]

Oncoprotein functions

The epidermal growth factor receptor family

The EGFR family (EGFR, HER2, HER3, and HER4) form a complex set of transmembrane signalling proteins that function by ligand-induced dimerization[25] (see also Chapter 1.5). All 10 possible homodimeric and heterodimeric combinations can occur, and over 18 ligands with differing specificity for EGFR, HER3, and HER4 are known. No ligand specific for HER2 has been identified but it appears to be a critical component in the signal relay system activated by ligand binding to the other family members (Fig. 3).

Activated EGFR family proteins associate via their phosphotyrosyl residues with a wide variety of cytosolic proteins such that receptor activation leads to the stimulation of RAS and the MAPK (ERK) and Jun kinase (JNK/SAPK) pathways (Figs 2 and 19; see Chapter 1.5 for more details).

Major deletions in the human EGFR that remove ligand binding capacity and confer constitutive phosphorylation on the protein have been detected in brain and lung tumours and in a high proportion of breast and ovarian tumours examined. This form of the receptor thus resembles retroviral v-ERBB (Fig. 4). It is constitutively associated with other proteins that can initiate intracellular signalling pathways, although it does not significantly activate the RAS-MAPK pathway that is associated with cellular transformation.

The *EGFR* gene is amplified by up to 50-fold in some primary tumours, including about 20 per cent of bladder and primary breast tumours. In the latter, *EGFR* amplification correlates strongly with early recurrence and death in lymph node-positive patients. Overexpression of EGFR occurs in pituitary adenomas and correlates with tumour aggressiveness. Increased expression of EGFR (and of HER2, HER3, and HER4) has also been detected in papillary thyroid carcinomas.

Mutations have not been detected in human *HER2* but it is overexpressed with high frequency in breast, stomach, ovarian, and bladder cancers and its overexpression or amplification has been detected in a variety of other cancers. In lymph node positive or node negative breast cancer patients there is a strong correlation between *HER2* amplification and poor prognosis, although the evidence that *HER2* promotes metastasis is controversial. Breast cancer cell lines that overexpress *HER2* have increased activity of the MAPK pathway.[27] There is an inverse correlation between *HER2* overexpression and oestrogen receptor expression in invasive cancer. The introduction of *HER2* cDNA into breast cancer cells expressing low levels of HER2 results in downregulation of oestrogen receptor and stimulates oestrogen-independent growth that is insensitive to tamoxifen.[28] Thus oestrogen resistance may arise from long-term suppression of the oestrogen receptor by HER2-mediated pathways.

HER3 is expressed in some carcinomas and, with low frequency, in sarcomas. Increased expression of HER3 and HER4 has been shown to be associated with the prognostically favourable oestrogen receptor positive phenotype of breast cancer.[29]

RET

RET tyrosine kinase is the receptor for glial-cell-line-derived neurotrophic factor and it is essential for some aspects of neuronal differentiation. In common with other receptor tyrosine kinases, receptor dimerization promotes activation of JNKs and MAPKs/ERKs via recruitment of coupling proteins. Activated RET may also recruit phospholipase Cγ, an interaction that is essential for manifestation of the full activity of at least some forms of oncogenic RET.[30]

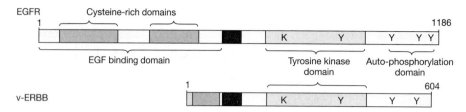

Fig. 4 Structures of epidermal growth factor receptor (**EGFR**) and v-ERBB. The transforming activity of avian erythroblastosis virus arises from v-*erbB*, which encodes a truncated form of the EGFR that has lost the ligand binding domain and remains constitutively active as a protein tyrosine kinase, independent of EGF. v-ERBB has also lost a C-terminal region that includes an autophosphorylation site, presumed important for normal function.

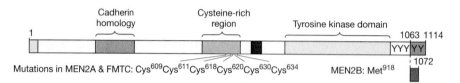

Fig. 5 Structure of RET receptor tyrosine kinase. An alternatively spliced C-terminus is represented. Y indicates C-terminal tyrosine phosphorylation sites. The major germline mutations in multiple endocrine neoplasia type 2A (**MEN2A**) and familial medullary thyroid carcinoma (FMTC) are shown, each resulting in the substitution of a cysteine residue, as is the point mutation associated with multiple endocrine neoplasia type 2B (**MEN2B**) and also with sporadic medullary thyroid carcinoma (**MTC**). Other rare mutations have been reported in sporadic medullary thyroid carcinoma and MEN2B.

RET is the first oncoprotein detected in which dominantly acting point mutations initiate human hereditary neoplasia. Germline mutations in *RET* cause multiple endocrine neoplasia type 2A (**MEN2A**) and type 2B (**MEN2B**) and familial medullary thyroid carcinoma (Fig. 5). Mis-sense, frameshift, and complex mutations also occur in *RET* in both familial and isolated cases of Hirschsprung's disease (congenital aganglionic megacolon).[31],[32]

The major mutations that have been detected result in constitutive kinase activation, either by direct modulation of catalytic activity or by induction of ligand-independent homodimerization. Directed expression of the MEN2B mutation (Met^{918}→Thr) in the developing sympathetic nervous system and in the adrenal medulla of mice causes benign neurological tumours histologically identical to human ganglioneuromas.[33] These neoplasms resemble benign neuroglial tumours that arise from the expression of activated *Ras* in the developing sympathetic nervous system. However, the levels of activated MAPK in tissues expressing high levels of RET^{MEN2B} are not significantly increased, suggesting that this form of activated tyrosine kinase receptor may stimulate an alternative signalling pathway.

A variety of oncogenic forms of RET also arise from chromosomal translocations (RET-PTC1 to RET-PTC5) and these are particularly associated with papillary thyroid carcinomas. Rearrangements of *RET* are highly prevalent in thyroid tumours of children exposed to fall-out from the Chernobyl reactor accident.[34]

SRC

SRC is a membrane-bound tyrosine kinase (Fig. 6), the activity of which increases markedly as cells pass through mitosis.[35] This appears to be an indirect effect of CDC2 (CDK1)/cyclin B1 (see Chapter 1.6), which phosphorylates the N-terminus of SRC causing a conformational change that renders the C-terminal regulatory tyrosine residue (Tyr^{527}) susceptible to phosphatase activity, thereby activating

SRC kinase. Transgenic mouse studies indicate some functional redundancy between the closely related members of the SRC family, SRC, FYN, and YES, and the activity of the latter two also rises during mitosis. Potentially important substrates of SRC are a protein involved in RNA processing, and RAF1, which is activated during mitosis and is stimulated by activated SRC (see Fig. 2). As RAF1 stimulates the MAPK pathway, MAPK activity, necessary for both meiotic maturation and growth factor signalling, may also be required for mitotic progression. More recently, it has been shown that active SRC is essential for the stimulation of DNA synthesis in response to PDGF. Blockade of the G$_1$–S phase transition by inhibition of SRC is reversible by overexpression of *Myc*, but not by the early response genes *Fos* and/or *Jun*, suggesting that SRC kinases may control *Myc* transcription.

These findings imply that src may play a crucial part in both progression through the G$_1$ phase and in mitosis. In addition, in a human prostate carcinoma cell line, transforming growth factor-β (which usually inhibits cell proliferation) downregulates the expression and activity of SRC and causes a concomitant increase in the level of unphosphorylated SHC protein, which may negatively regulate RAS activity. In transformed rat fibroblasts, transforming growth factor-β promotes degradation of activated SRC protein; this transforming growth factor-β-activated proteolysis of an essential mitogenic signalling component may have parallels with the activation of interleukin-1β-converting enzyme-like protease in the induction of apoptosis. In cells under hypoxic conditions, however, levels of *SRC* mRNA and kinase activity rise. This is associated with activated transcription of vascular endothelial growth factor (**VEGF**), a powerful stimulator of angiogenesis (see Chapter 1.8), and indicates that SRC may play a part in neovascularization during tumour development. These observations, together with the powerful tumorigenic capacity of oncogenic SRC in animals, suggest that *SRC* might be a frequent target for anomalous expression in human cancers. However, although increased SRC kinase activity has been reported in some colon cancers,

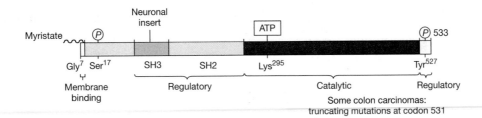

Fig. 6 Structure of SRC tyrosine kinase. All SRC family proteins are myristylated at Gly^2, which contributes to membrane anchoring; all share sequences throughout the src homology domains 1 (the tyrosine kinase catalytic region; SH1), 2 (SH2), and 3 (SH3), and all have the capacity to be regulated by phosphorylation of a common C-terminal tyrosine residue (Tyr^{527} in SRC). Ser^{12} and Ser^{17} are phosphorylated by protein kinase C and cyclic adenosine monophosphate-dependent protein kinase, respectively. Lys^{295} is essential for adenosine triphosphate (**ATP**) binding. In normal avian and rodent neurons and in some human neuroblastomas an alternative splicing mechanism inserts six amino acids in the SH3 domain.

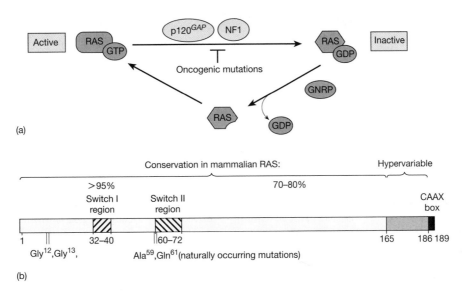

Fig. 7 (a) The RAS molecular switch. Conversion between the active (guanosine triphosphate (**GTP**) bound) and inactive (guanosine diphosphate (**GDP**) bound) forms of RAS is represented. GTP hydrolysis of normal RAS is promoted by GTPase activating proteins (**GAPs**) (p120GAP and NF1): GDP release is stimulated by guanine nucleotide releasing proteins (**GNRP**). (b) Structure of RAS protein. Cross-hatched regions indicate the switch regions. Switch I (or the 'effector domain') is the region in which substitutions reduce the biological effects of ras proteins in both mammalian and yeast cells, but do not affect GTP binding or hydrolysis. Switch I is essential for the stimulation of GTPase activity by GAP. Mutations in this region reduce the direct interaction that occurs between RAS and RAF1. The Switch II region, together with Switch I, forms the two domains that undergo large conformational changes upon exchange of bound GDP for GTP. Cys^{186} in the CAAX box is essential for transforming activity. Naturally occurring activating point mutations at codons 12, 13, 59, or 61 inhibit GTP hydrolysis; such oncogenic mutations, therefore, lock the GTP-RAS complex in an active form. Residues 184 to 186 include sites of fatty acid attachment.

skin tumours, and breast carcinomas, the only identified mutation is a truncation at codon 531 that activates SRC in 12 per cent of a sample of advanced human colon cancers.[36] This mutant form of SRC is tumorigenic and metastatic in nude mice.

RAS and RAF1

RAS proteins are molecular switches that are transiently activated in response to ligand-stimulated receptor tyrosine kinases by conversion from the guanosine diphosphate (GDP) bound form to the GTP bound form (Fig. 7(a) and 7(b); see also Chapter 1.5). The control of RAS activity is complex and may involve at least four classes of proteins: (a) GTPase-activating proteins (**GAPs**), which increase the rate of hydrolysis of GTP; (b) guanine nucleotide releasing proteins

(also called guanine nucleotide exchange factors[37]); (c) guanine nucleotide dissociation inhibitors; and (d) suppressors of RAS. RAF1 binds directly to RAS and the control of its activity is also complex. Several different wild-type and oncogenic RAS complexes have been crystallized to provide the first atomic descriptions of proto-oncogenes and oncogenes.[38],[39]

In addition to the receptors for EGF and PDGF, a large number of tyrosine kinase receptors activate RAS, including those for colony stimulating factor-1 (CSFR1/fms), neurotrophins (TRK), hepatocyte growth factor (MET), stem cell factor (KIT), and fibroblast growth factor[40] (see also Chapter 1.5). RAS-GTP activates RAF1 by the formation of a complex,[41] promoting the translocation of RAF1 to the plasma membrane and its hyperphosphorylation. RAF1 kinase is a component of the cascade that transmits signals from activated

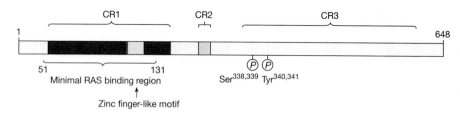

Fig. 8 Structure of RAF1. Conserved region (**CR**) 1 contains a zinc finger-like (transcription factor binding) motif; CR2 is conserved in virtually all forms of RAF and interacts directly with RAS proteins, binding RAS-GTP with a 1000-fold greater affinity than RAS-GDP[47] and inhibiting RAS-GAP activity. Phosphorylation of Ser[338/339] is essential for RAS signalling; amino acids 340 and 341 are major tyrosine phosphorylation sites.

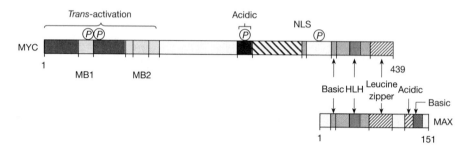

Fig. 9 Structure of MYC and MAX. The conserved sequences MYC box 1 (**MB1**) and 2 (**MB2**) lie within the *trans*-activation domain (i.e. that which binds to DNA to promote transcription of specific genes). The regions of MYC protein that are essential for apoptosis are identical to those required for co-transformation, autosuppression, and inhibition of differentiation, namely part of the N-terminus (amino acids 7 to 91 and 106 to 143), the helix–loop–helix (**HLH**) region (371 to 412) and the leucine zipper (414 to 433). The major site for casein kinase II phosphorylation, hyperphosphorylated during mitosis, is in the central acidic domain. NLS: nuclear localization signal. The RB1-related protein p107 forms a specific complex with the N-terminal *trans*-activation domain of MYC, which promotes MYC phosphorylation. Thr[58] and Ser[62] are phosphorylated by MAPKs and their phosphorylation modulates *trans*-activation by MYC. Thr[58] is frequently mutated in Burkitt's lymphoma: Glu[39], Ser[62], and Phe[138] are additional mutational hot spots in Burkitt and AIDS-related lymphoma. Residues 2, 11, 20, 140, 142, and 144 are potential casein kinase II phosphorylation sites in MAX.

growth factor receptor tyrosine kinases to MAPKs, as described in Chapter 1.5.

As Fig. 2 indicates, in addition to the linear pathway represented by RAS, RAF1, MEK, and MAPKs, alternative signalling mechanisms emanate from RAS or bypass it. Thus in some cell types at least full transformation by oncogenic RAS requires the activation by RAS of members of the RHO/RAC family of small guanosine triphosphatases (**GTPases**) that are involved in the organization of the cytoskeleton.[42],[43]

Mutations in the *RAS* family (*HRAS1*, *KRAS2*, and *NRAS*) are associated with a wide range of cancers. In all cancers the average incidence of *RAS* mutations is approximately 15 per cent, but in pancreatic carcinomas, for example, *KRAS2* mutations occur in 95 per cent of tumours and in colorectal carcinoma the reported range is from 20 per cent to 50 per cent. In general, mutations in *RAS* reduce its GTPase activity, the oncogenic protein thus remaining in an active, GTP-bound state. One consequence of this would be the sustained activation of the RAF-MAPK pathway (Fig. 2). Amplified genes may also have undergone mutation and, for *KRAS2* at least, there is evidence that amplification of the normal gene may occur in parallel with mutation of that gene.

The minisatellite region of *HRAS1* also appears to be mutated in some cancers. Minisatellites are tandem arrays of between 14 and 100 bp in length that are often polymorphic in the number of tandem repeats (hence referred to as variable number of

tandem repeats (**VNTRs**) or variable tandem repetitions (**VTRs**)). Minisatellites are dispersed throughout the genome and often occur just upstream or downstream of genes (or within introns). Many VNTR loci display dozens of alleles. The *HRAS1* minisatellite (VTR) comprises 30 to 100 copies of a 28 bp consensus repeat. There are four common and 25 rare alleles, the latter being more than twice as common in the genotypes of cancer patients than they are in normal individuals.[44] The VTR binds the constitutively expressed forms of the transcription factor NF-——B, suggesting that, by providing a tandem array of binding sites, this region may regulate transcription of both *HRAS1* and possibly other genes. Individuals with rare alleles of the *HRAS1* VTR who also carry an hereditary mutation in the *BRCA1* gene have an increased risk of ovarian cancer but not of breast cancer.

The MAPK pathway is constitutively activated in a wide range of primary human tumours as a consequence of the activation of upstream signalling proteins.[45] However, the human HT1080 fibrosarcoma and DLD-1 colon carcinoma cell lines, which express oncogenic *NRAS* and *KRAS* alleles respectively, differ in the activation of the MAPK pathway.[46] Thus HT1080s show activation of both the RAS/RAF/MEK/ERK pathway and of JNK (Fig. 2), whereas DLD-1 cells do not, suggesting that the latter utilize a distinct RAS-dependent signalling pathway(s).

RAF genes encode serine/threonine protein kinases and RAF1 is positively regulated by serine/tyrosine phosphorylation (Fig. 8). RAF1

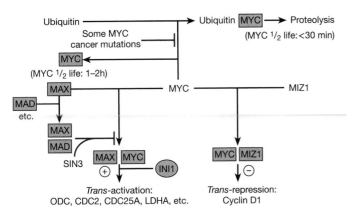

Fig. 10 Transcriptional control by MYC. MYC forms heterodimers with MAX that *trans*-activate a number of genes required for cell proliferation by binding to CAC(G/A)TG DNA sequences. These include ornithine decarboxylase (*ODC*), *CDC2*, *CDC25A* (encoding the phosphatase that activates CDC2), and lactate dehydrogenase (*LDHA*) (see also Fig. 19). Transcription is regulated in part by the function of MAX homodimers or heterodimers (with MAD, MXI1, MNT) that interact with SIN3 protein and repress transcription. MYC can also associate with some *trans*-activators (e.g. MIZ1) to repress transcription. Normal MYC undergoes ubiquitin-mediated proteolysis, which confers a short half-life. A number of mutations, arising for example in Burkitt's lymphoma, inhibit this degradative pathway and substantially increase the stability of MYC.

exists in a complex with the heat shock protein Hsp90 and this association is essential for RAF1 stability and cellular localization. Phosphorylated RAF1 also associates with the SH2 domains of FYN, SRC, and other proteins. *RAF1* is amplified in some non-small cell lung cancers and it is overexpressed in many small cell lung cancers. Deletions and translocations in the region of the *RAF1* locus (3p25) are associated with some human malignancies, including small cell lung carcinoma and renal carcinoma.

MYC

The MYC proteins (MYC, MYCN, and MYCL) each contain basic, helix–loop–helix, and leucine zipper domains that are each characteristic of a major class of transcription factors (Fig. 9). Each forms heterodimers with the protein MAX (which also contains all three motifs) that bind specifically to DNA as *trans*-activating complexes (i.e. complexes that activate the transcription of other genes). MAX expression is independent of MYC and MAX may thus regulate transcription of genes independently of Myc. However, other leucine zipper proteins (MAD/MXI1) form heterodimers with MAX that repress transcription (Fig. 10).

MYC is essential for normal cell proliferation and high levels of expression accelerate growth.[48],[49] Correspondingly, *Myc* expression is usually downregulated at the onset of differentiation and constitutive expression interferes with normal differentiation. However, in the absence of appropriate growth factors, MYC expression drives the induction of programmed cell death (apoptosis). Nevertheless, there are some exceptions to these general correlations (e.g. a variety of types of rapidly proliferating embryonic cells have little or no *Myc* expression and it is not expressed in dividing germ cells).

Although MYC is essential for cell proliferation and generally has been shown to regulate transcription of a wide variety of genes *in*

vitro, the biochemical connections between proto-oncogene signalling pathways and the machinery of cell cycle control have been difficult to resolve. MYC has long been known to activate ornithine decarboxylase, which is necessary for cell proliferation, but other critical targets have remained elusive. Recently, however, it has emerged that MYC can *trans*-activate both cyclin D1 and, indirectly, cyclin A, both of which are components of cyclin-dependent kinases that control passage through the cell cycle (see Chapter 1.6). Additionally, MYC/MAX directly *trans*-activates *CDC25A* that encodes a phosphatase mediating the activation of cyclin-dependent kinases. CDC25A itself has oncogenic capacity and its expression pattern during the cell cycle closely resembles that of MYC. Both CDC25A and CDC25B have been shown to be overexpressed in a high proportion of head and neck cancers. Consistent with these critical roles in driving DNA replication and cell division, *MYC* is repressed as a component of p53-mediated growth arrest. This observation appears consistent with the recent finding that MYC binds to BRCA1, the tumour suppressor gene product that is probably responsible for about one-third of families having multiple cases of breast cancer (see Chapter 1.4). BRCA1 appears to play a part in maintaining genomic integrity and one component of this mechanism may be the inhibition of MYC-driven proliferation.

An additional property of MYC is its capacity to activate directly the catalytic subunit of telomerase (**TERT**). Telomerase is a ribonucleoprotein DNA polymerase responsible for the synthesis of telomeres, which are short, tandem repeats of the hexanucleotide 5'-TTAGGG-3' at the ends of each chromosome. Telomerase is expressed in human germline cells and in certain stem cells but is not detectable in most somatic cells.[50] The growth arrest process associated with ageing (senescence) usually correlates with a decrease in telomere length and a consequence of the activation of oncogenes or the ablation of tumour suppressor genes is that senescence controls may be over-ridden. Thus, between 85 and 90 per cent of human primary tumours examined express telomerase (thus enabling them to avoid senescence), whereas only about 25 per cent of benign tumours do so.[51] In tumour cell lines telomerase activity reaches a maximum in S phase and a variety of inhibitors of cell cycle progression also inhibit telomerase activity.[52] The activation of TERT by MYC thus links the control of cell proliferation with the maintenance of chromosome integrity in normal and neoplastic cells,[53] although TERT cannot substitute for MYC in transforming primary rodent fibroblasts.[54]

Amplification and/or overexpression of *MYC* commonly occurs in a wide range of tumours. Mutations in the protein sequence are not necessary to render myc oncogenic, although when they do occur they may enhance pathogenicity. *MYCN*, which is primarily expressed in neuronal cells during embryogenesis, is amplified in neuroblastomas and also in retinoblastomas, astrocytomas, gliomas, and small cell lung carcinomas. *MYCN* expression correlates with the appearance of the more severe forms of cervical intraepithelial carcinoma (types II and III) and with increased metastasis in the advanced stages of neuroblastoma (see also Chapter 17.2). Amplification of the *MYC*-related gene, *MYCL1*, has also been detected in small cell lung carcinoma.

The most common genetic rearrangements in B-cell lymphomas (see Chapter 15.10) involve *MYC* (8q24) or *BCL2* (18q21.3). The translocations in Burkitt's lymphoma give rise to a *MYC* gene adjacent to one of three immunoglobulin loci, most commonly IgH (14q32).

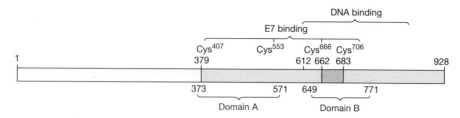

Fig. 11 Structure of the retinoblastoma protein (RB1). The binding regions for human adenovirus E1A protein, SV40 large T antigen, and the E7 oncoprotein of human papillomavirus 16 are shown. RB1 also binds cyclins D2, D3, B1, and C. These cyclins and the DNA oncoproteins show sequence homology only over the small putative RB1-binding region (the Leu-X-Cys-X-Glu sequence motif). RB1 also binds to Epstein–Barr nuclear antigens 2 and 5. The 'binding pocket' includes eight cysteine residues divided between domains A and B. The A and B pockets can interact directly to form the repressor motif that binds to E2F proteins to inhibit their *trans*-activating function. RB1 contains at least 12 distinct serine or threonine phosphorylation sites and its phosphorylation state is a critical determinant of progression through the cell cycle, with inhibition of RB1 phosphorylation causing cell cycle arrest (Fig. 12).

In the less common variants one of the immunoglobulin light chain loci (Ig— (2p12) or Igλ (22q11)) translocates to a position 3' of *MYC* on chromosome 8. In each type of translocation *MYC* expression is deregulated as a result of juxtaposition to immunoglobulin constant region gene segments, non-translocated *MYC* being transcriptionally silent. The translocated gene may also suffer damage that increases mRNA stability and/or acquire mutations that modulate function. Translocations involving *BCL2* and IgH generally activate *BCL2*, promoting cell survival and resistance to apoptosis. Three-way translocations involving *BCL2*, *MYC*, and IgH also occur in which the IgH allele not associated with the t(8;14) translocation drives the expression of *BCL2*. However, translocations in which *MYC* is activated and *BCL2* is inactivated also occur. Thus, although the deregulation of *BCL2* would be expected to prolong survival of the affected pre-B cells and hence increase the probability of activation of other oncogenes, including *MYC*, leukaemias can develop in the absence of functional BCL2. A translocation involving *MYC* and the T-cell receptor-α chain has also been detected in a B-cell lymphoma.

Tumour suppressor genes

The retinoblastoma gene (*RB1*) and E2F1

The retinoblastoma protein (RB1) functions as a signal transducer, connecting the cell cycle clock with transcriptional control mechanisms mediating progression through the first phase of the cell cycle (Figs 11 and 12; see Chapter 1.6). The broad transcriptional effects of RB1 are mediated by its inhibition of transcription factors that are required for the expression of genes involved in DNA replication and by repressing transcriptional activation by RNA polymerases I, II, and III. Thus RB1 regulates the overall biosynthetic capacity of the cell and its loss not merely releases a brake at the G_1/S phase transition but drives proliferation and hence chromosome duplication and the accumulation of mutations. *RBL1* (p107) and *RBL2* (p130) are related genes with distinct but overlapping functions.[56]

RB1 binds to many cellular proteins but the most critical appear to be the E2F family of transcription factors. The hypophosphorylated form of RB1 associates with E2F (Figs 11 and 12) and this complex is dissociated by phosphorylation of RB1 by cyclin D1-CDK4, cyclin E-CDK2, or cyclin A-CDK2 (or by E1A, SV40 T antigen or human papillomavirus E7 binding to RB1). The RB1-E2F complex is present

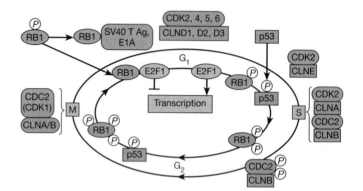

Fig. 12 Cell cycle control by the retinoblastoma protein (RB1), p53, and E2F1. Phosphorylation of RB1 in G_1 releases transcriptional repression by E2F1 to activate key cell cycle progression genes (*MYC*, *CDC2*, etc.). The major cyclin-dependent kinases (**CDKs**) and associated cyclins (**CLNs**) that control progression through the cell cycle are shown. These complexes are in turn regulated by the cyclin-dependent kinase inhibitors (**CDIs**) that comprise **WAF1** (wild-type p53-activated fragment 1), **KIP1**, **KIP2**, and the **INK4** (inhibitor of CDK4) family. CDIs act with differing specificities to inhibit the activity of CDKs, and WAF1/KIP1 proteins play an additional part as positive regulators of cyclin D-dependent kinases.[55] CDIs are therefore potential tumour suppressor proteins. Two common variants of WAF1 occur in both tumours and normal cells and mutations have been detected in prostate cancer, breast carcinoma, and transitional cell carcinoma. Homozygous deletion of *INK4A* is one of the most common genetic events in primary tumours and the *INK4A* locus is rearranged, deleted, or mutated in about 75 per cent of tumour cell lines (see Chapter 1.6).

in the G_1 phase of the cell cycle and functions as a transcriptional repressor. RB1 binding inhibits the *trans*-activation function of at least three (E2F1, E2F2, E2F3) of the six known members of the E2F family of transcription factors that are required for S phase.[57] E2F1 is an oncoprotein in that its coexpression with that of other oncogenes can cause transformation, and E2F1 alone can induce DNA synthesis in serum-starved cells, properties it shares with MYC. Major proliferation-associated genes regulated by E2F1 include *MYC*, *MYCN*, *MYB*, *CDC2*, dihydrofolate reductase, thymidine kinase, and *EGFR*. Remarkably, however, E2F1 also has the characteristics of a tumour suppressor gene. Mice in which E2F1 has been deleted show tissue-specific hyperplasia and develop a variety of tumours. The molecular basis for this complex behaviour is unclear, although it presumably reflects tissue-specific regulation of transcription by E2F1. E2F1 itself is not essential for normal development but its loss leads to subtle aberrations with ageing in some tissues, notably testicular atrophy. However, in the reproductive tract and lung, loss of E2F1 promotes aggressive tumour formation, with lymphomas also developing, apparently as a result of loss of apoptosis of thymocytes.

A further mechanism by which RB1 can repress transcription of genes containing E2F sites is through association with the enzyme histone deacetylase (HDAC).[58] HDAC1 binds to the RB1 pocket and, for some promoters, trans-repression is dependent on histone deacetylase activity. For other promoters, however, repression occurs by direct inhibition of transcription factor activity independent of HDACs.

The *RB1* gene is defective in all retinoblastomas. Major deletions occur in 15 to 40 per cent of cases: in addition, point mutations throughout the gene, deletions in the promoter, intronic mutations, and hypermethylation in the 5' region of the gene have each been shown to cause functional inactivation. Individuals with inherited retinoblastoma are also susceptible to malignant tumours in mesenchymal tissues, often osteosarcomas or soft tissue sarcomas. Inactive *RB1* alleles are very common in small cell lung carcinoma, and they occur in 20 to 30 per cent of non-small cell lung cancers, bladder and pancreatic carcinomas, and in human breast carcinomas.

P53, MDM2, and ARF

In normal cells p53 is expressed at extremely low levels (about 1000 molecules/cell), but it is strongly induced by cellular stress (e.g. DNA damage, hypoxia, or nucleotide deprivation), the concentration increasing by five- to 100-fold in most transformed and tumour cells. p53 functions principally as a transcription factor (Fig. 13), regulating genes that cause cell cycle arrest in G_1 when the genome is damaged. Elevated levels of p53 may also drive apoptosis.

The activity of p53 is negatively regulated by direct interaction with the **MDM2** (murine double minute 2) protein and also by phosphorylation.[60],[61] MDM2 binds within the activation domain of p53 (Fig. 14[62]) and formation of this complex inhibits trans-activation by p53. This interaction also targets p53 for degradation as a result of the ubiquitin ligase activity of MDM2, which is inhibited by association with ARF, the product of the *a*lternative *r*eading *f*rame situated within the *INK4A* locus.[63]–[65] Oncogenic changes (e.g. expression of oncogenic MYC, RAS, or E1A or loss of RB1) that activate E2F1 result in the upregulation of ARF and hence cause cell cycle arrest or apoptosis. Thus ARF functions as part of a p53-dependent fail-safe mechanism to protect cells from oncogenic changes that tend to cause abnormal proliferation. Mice in which *Arf*, but not *Ink4a*, is deleted spontaneously develop tumours at an early age and *Arf* itself is therefore a *bona fide* tumour suppressor gene. Phosphorylation of Ser^{15} occurs in response to DNA damage and this inhibits interaction with MDM2 and hence promotes trans-activation by p53. A functionally similar effect also arises as a result of phosphorylation or acetylation in the C-terminal domain following DNA damage, which relieves the trans-repression normally exerted by this highly basic region.

MDM2 also links functionally the activities of p53 and RB1 through its capacity to form trimeric complexes with the two tumour suppressor proteins. MDM2 preferentially binds to hypophosphorylated RB1 and the MDM2-RB1 interaction is essential for RB1 to inhibit both the antiapoptotic function of MDM2 and MDM2-dependent p53 degradation.[66] However, RB1/MDM2/p53 complexes remain active in that MDM2-induced block of p53-dependent transcription still occurs. This implies that trans-activation by wild-type p53 is not required for p53-dependent apoptosis. The association of RB1 with MDM2 also relieves the RB1 suppression of the E2F trans-activating function and MDM2 directly contacts E2F1 to stimulate its transcriptional activity. Thus MDM2 not only releases a proliferative block by silencing p53 but augments proliferation by stimulating an S-phase-inducing transcription factor.

Mutations in the single copy *P53* gene causing loss of protein function are the most frequent genetic changes yet shown to be associated with human cancers.[67] Point mutations, deletions, or insertions in *P53* occur in about 70 per cent of all tumours. The point mutations occur almost entirely in the central region of the protein that has been revealed by X-ray diffraction to bind to DNA. The most frequently mutated residues lie in the regions that directly contact DNA but other mutations modulate function by affecting the overall three-dimensional structure of the protein. The rare, autosomal dominant Li-Fraumeni syndrome arises from *P53* mutations inherited through the germline: 50 per cent of the carriers develop diverse cancers by 30 years of age, compared with 1 per cent in the normal population. In general, however, *P53* mutations are somatic and occur with high frequency in all types of lung cancer, in over 60 per cent of breast tumours and in about 40 per cent of brain tumours (astrocytomas), frequently in combination with the activation of oncogenes. The region deleted in chromosome 17p in most colorectal neoplasms includes *P53*.

APC

The *APC* (*a*denomatous *p*olyposis *c*oli) gene (Fig. 15) is mutated in the germline of patients with familial adenomatosis polyposis. In familial adenomatosis polyposis the development of hundreds of colonic polyps in early life leads, in untreated individuals, to colorectal cancer[68] (see also Chapters 1.4 and 10.4). APC binds as a homodimer to β-catenin that mediates signal transduction from E-cadherin cell surface adhesion proteins (Fig. 19). Targets of β-catenin include MYC[69] and cyclin D1.[70] The majority of mutations identified in *APC*[71] inactivate the gene product by truncation. Mutant forms of APC in colorectal tumours are unable to associate with β-catenin and hence cannot downregulate its trans-activation function. Hence loss of APC promotes the expression of MYC and cyclin D1, which are key regulators of cell proliferation. Conversely, ectopic expression of *APC* reduces CDK2 activity and causes concomitant G_1 arrest. APC is phosphorylated by glycogen synthase kinase 3β, which regulates the interaction of APC with β-catenin. Colorectal tumours expressing wild-type APC have activating mutations in the β-catenin gene.[72] Mutations in the β-catenin gene have also been detected in malignant ovarian carcinomas[73] and skin tumours.[74]

BRCA1 and BRCA2

Mutations in *BRCA1* and *BRCA2* predispose to breast cancer and together they are probably involved in about two-thirds of familial breast cancer, approximately 5 per cent of all cases. *BRCA1* is probably responsible for about one-third of families having multiple cases of breast cancer alone but for 80 per cent of families in which there is both breast cancer and epithelial ovarian cancer. Inheritance of a *BRCA1* mutation carries about a 60 per cent risk of breast cancer for

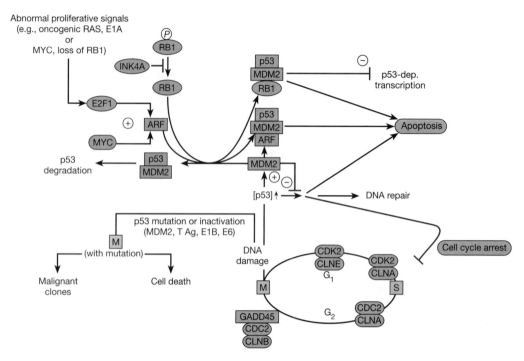

Fig. 13 Regulation of p53 activity. DNA damage elevates cellular p53 levels: *trans*-activation by wild-type, but not mutant, p53 can then cause cell cycle arrest, promote DNA excision repair, or drive apoptosis.[59] p53 also represses *MYC* and *BCL2* (antiapoptosis). *Trans*-activation by wild-type p53 is prevented by mutant p53 proteins or by adenovirus E1B, SV40 T antigen, or human papillomavirus-16 E6 protein, the latter targeting p53 for ubiquitin-mediated degradation. **MDM2** (murine double minute 2) is a critical negative regulator of p53 activity, promoting its ubiquitination and degradation. However, MDM2-induced p53 degradation is blocked by the action of **ARF** (alternative reading frame), which forms a trimeric p53/MDM2/ARF complex.

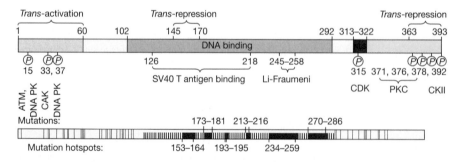

Fig. 14 Structure of p53. *Trans*-activation occurs via the N-terminal domain and there are two *trans*-repression domains, one of which is the basic C-terminal regulatory region. Major phosphorylation sites that regulate the activity of p53 include targets for the ataxia telangiectasia protein (**ATM**), DNA-activated protein kinase (**DNA PK**), cyclin-activated kinase complex (**CAK**), cyclin-dependent kinases (**CDK**; Ser315 in the nuclear localization signal), protein kinase C (**PKC**), and casein kinase II (**CKII**). The lower figure shows the distribution of identified p53 mutations.[62] Hot spots are shown as orange bars, including the region encoded by exon 7 in which germline mutations mainly occur in the autosomal dominant Li-Fraumeni syndrome.

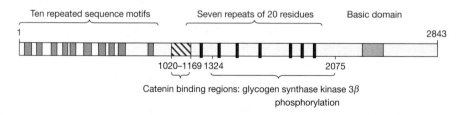

Fig. 15 Structure of **APC** (*adenomatous polyposis coli*). Amino acids 312 to 412 are deleted in an alternatively spliced form that utilizes exon 9a: a variety of other isoforms have been detected. APC contains multiple serine phosphorylation, glycosylation, and myristylation sites.

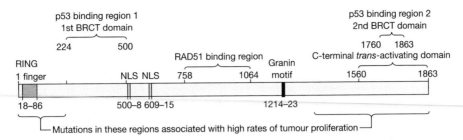

Fig. 16 Structure of BRCA1. The N-terminal region contains a C_3HC_4 zinc finger similar to those of many DNA-binding proteins. Two BRCT domains of BRCA1 interact with p53 and the second of these also recruits CBP/p300-associated histone acetyltransferase activity, which acetylates p53, thereby promoting *trans*-activation. Multiple alternative splicing patterns occur. NLS: nuclear localization signal.

that individual by age 50 and an 80 to 90 per cent lifetime risk (see Chapter 1.4).

BRCA1 (Fig. 16) and BRCA2 are putative transcription factors that undergo cell cycle-dependent phosphorylation that is maximal in S and M phases. BRCA1 *trans*-activates expression of the cyclin-dependent kinase inhibitor *WAF1* in a p53-independent manner and it inhibits cell cycle progression into S phase when transfected into human cancer cells. Both BRCA1 and BRCA2 bind to RAD51, which mediates DNA double strand break repair and meiotic recombination. BRCA1 and BRCA2, therefore, have potential roles in the regulation of transcription and DNA repair.[75]

Studies using transgenic mice show that both BRCA1 and BRCA2 are required for cell proliferation during embryogenesis. Despite this paradoxical behaviour, *BRCA1* and *BRCA2* are *bona fide* tumour suppressor genes, recent evidence indicating that not only are they functionally inactivated in a high proportion of hereditary breast cancers but that *BRCA1* expression is reduced in many sporadic breast cancers. The fact that mice in which the *Brca1* gene has been deleted are hypersensitive to γ-irradiation indicates that BRCA1 plays a part in maintaining genomic integrity, although massive chromosomal abnormalities arise only if p53 is also deleted or mutated. It is noteworthy that a form of *BRCA1* lacking exon 11 is produced in normal animals, which suggests that alternative splicing of this gene may be an important mechanism in development, as established for the Wilms' tumour suppressor gene, *WT1*.

Over 100 mutations in *BRCA1* have been detected and the majority are predicted to result in truncation to a functionally inactive form. Numerous truncating mutations have also been identified in *BRCA2*. There is a significant correlation between the location of BRCA1 mutations and the relative risk of breast or ovarian cancer within a family. Mutations in the N-terminal four-fifths of the protein carry a significant predisposition to ovarian cancer, whereas C-terminal mutations are strongly associated with breast cancer. This suggests that mutant BRCA1 may function in a tissue-specific manner as a tumour suppressor protein or alternatively that mutant BRCA1 is capable of exerting dominant negative effects by interacting directly with wild-type BRCA1 protein in a manner similar to that observed with p53 or APC.

NF1

The most frequent forms of neurofibromatosis are peripheral neurofibromatosis (**NF1**) and central neurofibromatosis (**NF2**). NF1 (von Recklinghausen neurofibromatosis) affects about 1 in 3500 individuals

and arises in cells derived from the embryonic neural crest, causing benign growths, including neurofibromas and café-au-lait spots on the skin, phaeochromocytomas, malignant Schwannomas, and neurofibrosarcomas. Between 30 per cent and 45 per cent of NF1 patients have learning disabilities. A variety of mis-sense and truncating mutations have been identified in the *NF1* gene.[76] These are generally inactivating and there are no evident hot spots.

The *NF1* gene product (neurofibromin) contains a GAP-related domain so that one consequence of *NF1* inactivation is to render cells exquisitely sensitive to agents that raise cellular levels of RAS-GTP. This occurs in tumour cells from patients with type 1 neurofibromatosis, even though the p120GAP protein is present and presumably causes constitutive activation of RAS signalling pathways. This may be a consequence of the much higher affinity (300-fold) for RAS of NF1 by comparison with p120GAP. However, it is evident from transgenic studies that p120GAP and neurofibromin co-operate during embryonic development. Thus the functional balance between NF1 and other GAP proteins is unclear and it is possible that NF1 may operate by alternative mechanisms, for example, by mediating differentiation in a RAS-regulated manner so that loss of NF1 promotes cell proliferation.

VHL

Von Hippel-Lindau (**VHL**) disease is a dominantly inherited familial cancer syndrome with variable expression and with age-dependent penetrance that predisposes individuals most frequently to haemangioblastomas of the central nervous system and retina, renal cell carcinoma, and pheochromocytoma.[77] The incidence at birth is at least 1/36 000. VHL is one of the major tumour suppressor genes in human renal cell carcinomas, particularly in the clear cell subtype of renal cell carcinoma (Fig. 17). Usually one allele is mutated (or methylated) and the other deleted. VHL protein binds specifically to the elongin B and C subunits of elongin (SIII), a heterotrimer (transcriptionally active subunit A and positive regulatory subunits B and C) that activates transcription by RNA polymerase II. VHL activity is probably normally regulated by casein kinase II phosphorylation and the major deletions or insertions in the gene that occur with high frequency in VHL are presumed to inactivate it, thereby minimizing interruptions in the activity of RNA polymerase and increasing the rate of transcription of genes involved in proliferation. Genes implicated in cancers that are regulated in part by control of transcriptional elongation include *MYC*, *MYCN*, *MYCL1*, and *FOS*.

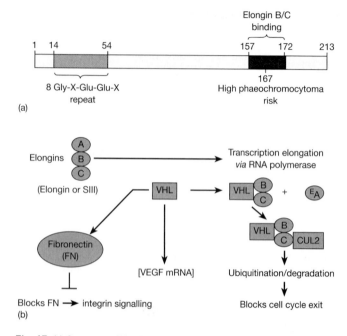

Fig. 17 (a) Structure of Von Hippel-Lindau (**VHL**) protein. VHL contains a tandemly repeated acidic domain (Gly-X-Glu-Glu-X). Met[54] is an alternative initiation codon and residues 54 to 213 also have tumour suppressor function, all known VHL mutations falling within this sequence. The region binding to elongin B and C is frequently altered by germline mutations in VHL kindreds. The most common mutation (codon 167) confers a high risk of phaeochromocytoma. (b) Functions of VHL. Specific VHL binding to elongins B and C inhibits transcription by RNA polymerase II. CUL-2, encoded by a member of the cullin multigene family, specifically associates with the trimeric VHL-elongin B–C complex *in vitro* and *in vivo* and targets VHL for degradation. Nearly 70 per cent of naturally occurring cancer-predisposing mutations of VHL disrupt this interaction. In VHL-associated and in sporadic haemangioblastomas, vascular endothelial growth factor (**VEGF**) is secreted (see Fig. 19). Wild-type VHL protein inhibits *VEGF* promoter activity and the loss of this activity may be responsible for the development of VHL.[78] VHL also interacts with fibronectin (**FN**), which inhibits both assembly of the extracellular fibronectin matrix and fibronectin signalling via integrin receptors.

Major deletions or insertions in the gene occur with high frequency (>12 per cent) in VHL patients. Over 40 different germline mutations encompassing mis-sense, non-sense, frameshift insertions/deletions, in-frame deletions, and a splice donor site mutation have been identified. In sporadic renal cell carcinomas VHL mutations are frequent (57 per cent) and varied. Mutations in VHL have also been detected in lung cancer, mesothelioma, gliomas, and in sporadic central nervous system haemangioblastomas. Hypermethylation of a normally unmethylated CpG island in the 5' region of *VHL*, detected in 19 per cent of one sample of renal cell carcinomas, silences the gene.[79]

WT1

Wilms' tumour is an embryonal renal neoplasm that occurs in sporadic and (very rarely) in familial forms and affects 1 in 10 000 children. It is the most common solid tumour of childhood, but combined chemotherapy and radiotherapy gives cure rates of more than 80 per cent. Approximately 2 per cent of Wilms' tumours occur

in association with aniridia (cf. 1/50 000 in the general population), genitourinary anomalies, and mental retardation (**WAGR** syndrome) in which deletions of 11p13 were first detected. WAGR, Beckwith–Wiedemann syndrome, and Denys–Drash syndrome confer hereditary susceptibility to Wilms' tumour[80] (see Chapter 17.4).

WT1 proteins are members of the zinc finger protein transcription factor family that may play a crucial part in normal genitourinary development (Fig. 18). They act through WT1 consensus binding sites to repress transcription of a variety of genes, including *BCL2*, *PDGFA*, *IGF2*, and *IGF1R*, the latter being a key mechanism by which WT1 suppresses cell growth.

Deletions or point mutations in *WT1* occur in Wilms' tumour and in Denys–Drash syndrome. These abolish DNA binding and hence repression of target genes. Insulin-like growth factor 2 is considered to be of particular importance in this context because it encodes an autocrine growth factor expressed at high levels in this paediatric tumour. *IGF2* is expressed from the paternal allele in normal human fetal tissue but relaxation of genomic imprinting appears to contribute to the development of Wilms' tumour. The various isoforms of WT1 can form dimers: germline mutations that give rise to Denys–Drash syndrome do so by antagonizing transcriptional repression by wild-type WT1. Like p53, therefore, WT1 can exhibit dominant negative behaviour.

Chromosomal translocation involving *WT1* has been detected in the desmoplastic small round cell tumour.[82] Loss of WT1 expression has been reported in 40 per cent of a sample of breast tumour cells,[83] suggesting that *WT1* may act as a tumour suppressor gene for breast carcinoma.

Invasion suppressor genes

The development of primary tumours is contingent upon the expression of an appropriate combination of genetic events involving oncogenes and tumour suppressor genes, as exemplified above. However, for tumours to evolve into malignant, metastatic forms additional changes in cellular gene expression are required that affect intercellular adhesion, the capacity to invade and migrate through surrounding tissues and angiogenesis at secondary sites (see Chapter 1.9). A large number of proteins have been implicated in the acquisition of metastatic potential, including cadherins, the immunoglobulin superfamily, integrins, matrix metalloproteinases, tissue inhibitors of metalloproteinases, the serine, cysteine and aspartic proteinases and heparanase, a variety of putative metastasis-suppressor genes (e.g. *NME1*, *NME2*, *KAI1*, and *ELM1*) and the ubiquitous cell surface glycoprotein CD44. It is notable that the vast majority of the data indicate that these cell surface and secreted proteins undergo modulation of expression levels as invasive capacity is acquired, rather than being directly altered by genetic alterations.

One of the factors most consistently implicated in invasion is E-cadherin, a member of a multigene family of transmembrane glycoproteins that mediate Ca^{2+}-dependent intercellular adhesion, cytoskeletal anchoring, and signalling that are thought to be essential for the control of morphogenetic processes, including myogenesis.[84] Cadherins preferentially interact with themselves in a homophilic manner in connecting cells. E-cadherin associates with three cytoplasmic proteins, α-, β-, and γ-catenin, and its cytoplasmic tail is

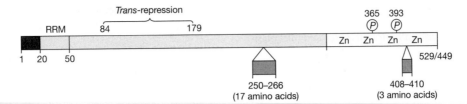

Fig. 18 Structure of WT1. WT1 is a member of the early growth response family. The N- and C-termini of the early growth response family are not highly conserved, but the zinc finger domains show strong homology. The family contain an N-terminal RNA recognition motif (**RRM**), present in all WT1 isoforms, that may be responsible for the interaction of WT1 with a number of spliceosomal proteins.[81] Four different WT1 zinc finger proteins arise as a consequence of alternative splicing of *WT1*, the most abundant form of the protein in both Wilms' tumour and normal kidney being that with both the 17 and 3 amino acid insertions. The −17 amino acid forms either repress or activate transcription. Ser[365] and Ser[393] are phosphorylated (by protein kinase A or protein kinase C), which inhibits DNA binding.

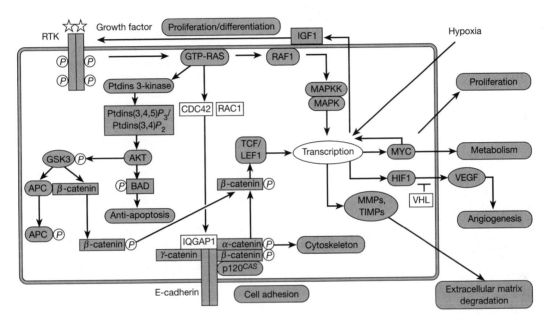

Fig. 19 Cellular responses during tumour development. Activation of the AKT serine/threonine kinase mediated by phosphatidylinositol 3-kinase (**PtdIns 3-kinase**) promotes phosphorylation both of the BCL family member BAD, which inhibits apoptosis, and also of glycogen synthase kinase 3β (**GSK3β**). GSK3β in turn phosphorylates both APC and β-catenin, releasing β-catenin to form an active complex with transcription factors of the lymphoid enhancer factor (**LEF1**)/T-cell factor (**TCF**) family. Genes known to be activated by β-catenin/TCF include *MYC*, *CLND1* (cyclin D1), and the metalloproteinase matrilysin.[85] Anomalous expression of other matrix metalloproteinases (**MMPs**) and of tissue inhibitors of metalloproteinases (**TIMPs**) is also associated with metastasis. MYC itself functions as a transcription factor to activate key cell cycle genes (*CDC2*, *CDC25A*) and glycolytic enzyme genes.[86] Hypoxic stress activates the transcription factor hypoxia-inducible transcription factor 1 (**HIF1**), a key target of which is the angiogenic agent vascular endothelial growth factor (**VEGF**). The small guanosine triphosphatases CDC42 and RAC1 act, possibly directly, on IQGAP1, which associates with both E-cadherin and β-catenin and in response to activated CDC42 or RAC1 promotes the dissociation of α-catenin from E-cadherin complexes with resultant decrease in cell–cell adhesion.[87] IQGAP1 binds to CDC42; however, in the presence of Ca²⁺ it dissociates to attach to calmodulin.[88]

linked via α- and β-catenin, with which the tumour suppressor gene product APC also interacts, to the actin cytoskeleton (Fig. 19).

The E-cadherin/catenin complex is a potent inhibitor of invasion, expression of which declines as most epithelial tumours (comprising 80 to 90 per cent of all human cancers) become metastatic. Loss or truncation of components is frequently associated with transition to invasive phenotype and poor prognosis for many human cancers. A high frequency (53 per cent) of impaired E-cadherin expression has been detected in primary breast cancers[89] where loss of one allele followed by mutation of the second allele is associated with invasive tumours, although this appears to be confined to infiltrative lobular carcinomas and is not detectable in infiltrative ductal or medullary carcinomas.[90] Mutations have also been detected in endometrial and ovarian carcinomas.[91] In a transgenic mouse model of pancreatic β-cell carcinogenesis loss of E-cadherin expression coincides with the transition from well differentiated adenoma to invasive carcinoma. Complete loss or markedly reduced expression of α- or β-catenin has been detected in some cancer cell lines.[92],[93] In a variety of human colon cancer cell lines αE-catenin (*CTNNA1*) is mutated and genetic instability due to loss of function of the *MSH6* mismatch repair gene results in invasive variants in which the second *CTNNA1* allele is mutated.[94]

Figure 19 schematizes the important part played by the E-cadherin/catenin complex in tumour development, together with other major biochemical events associated with tumorigenesis and metastasis. Activation of the phosphatidylinositol 3-kinase signalling pathway can release β-catenin from complexes with APC to promote transcription of genes required for both proliferation (*MYC*) and metastasis (*MMP7*). Changes in E-cadherin/catenin expression, discussed above, may modulate cell–cell interactions.

Solid tumours usually contain substantial hypoxic regions. A critical cellular response to hypoxia is the activation of the transcription factor hypoxia-inducible transcription factor 1. Hypoxia-inducible transcription factor 1 activates transcription of VEGF, a powerful angiogenic protein, by a mechanism that involves accumulation of *SRC* mRNA and activation of SRC kinase.[95] Hypoxia-inducible transcription factor 1 also upregulates glycolytic enzymes, thereby stimulating anaerobic glycolysis in solid tumours. VHL is a negative regulator of the hypoxia-inducible mRNAs, including those of *VEGF* and the glucose transporter *GLUT1*.[96] Figure 19 thus illustrates the extent to which the molecular mechanisms have been revealed that permit cells to mount an integrated biochemical response to the requirements of driving proliferation and overcoming apoptosis, undergoing migration, and promoting neovascularization, together with major adaptations of metabolism, thereby permitting tumour development and metastasis.

References

1. Hesketh R. *The Oncogene Handbook*. London and San Diego: Academic Press, 1994.

2. Hesketh R. *The Oncogene and Tumour Suppressor Gene FactsBook*, 2nd edn. San Diego and London: Academic Press, 1997.

3. Bishop JM. Cancer: the rise of the genetic paradigm. *Genes and Development*, 1995; 9: 1309–15.

4. Xu X, *et al.* Constitutively activated JNK is associated with HTLV-1 mediated tumorigenesis. *Oncogene*, 1996; 13: 135–42.

5. Ihle JN. Signaling by the cytokine receptor superfamily in normal and transformed hematopoietic cells. *Advances in Cancer Research*, 1996; 68: 23–65.

6. Barone MV, Courtneidge SA. Myc but not Fos rescue of PDGF signalling block caused by kinase-inactive Src. *Nature*, 1995; 378: 509–12.

7. Hodge DR, *et al.* Binding of c-Raf1 kinase to a conserved acidic sequence within the carboxyl-terminal region of the HIV-1 Nef protein. *Journal of Biological Chemistry*, 1998; 273: 15727–33.

8. Popik W, Hesselgesser JE, Pitha PM. Binding of human immunodeficiency virus type 1 to CD4 and CXCR4 receptors differentially regulates expression of inflammatory genes and activates the MEK/ERK signaling pathway. *Journal of Virology*, 1998; 72: 6406–13.

9. Lengauer C, Kinzler KW, Vogelstein B. Genetic instabilities in human cancers. *Nature*, 1998; 396: 643–9.

10. Huang L, Clarkin KC, Wahl GM. Sensitivity and selectivity of the DNA damage sensor responsible for activating p53-dependent G_1 arrest. *Proceedings of the National Academy of Sciences USA*, 1996; 93: 4827–32.

11. Russell A, Thompson MA, Hendley J, Trute L, Armes J, Germain D. Cyclin D1 and D3 associate with the SCF complex and are coordinately elevated in breast cancer. *Oncogene*, 1999; 18: 1983–91.

12. Gillett C, *et al.* Cyclin D1 and prognosis in human breast cancer. *International Journal of Cancer*, 1996; 69: 92–9.

13. Lee YI, *et al.* The human hepatitis B virus transactivator-gene product regulates Sp1 mediated transcription of an insulin-like growth factor II promoter 4. *Oncogene*, 1998; 16: 2367–80.

14. Lee Y-H, Yun Y. HBx Protein of Hepatitis B Virus Activates Jak1-STAT Signaling. *Journal of Biological Chemistry*, 1998; 273: 25510–15.

15. St Clair DK, Wan XS, Kuroda M, Vichitbandha S, Tsuchida E, Urano M. Suppression of tumor metastasis by manganese superoxide dismutase is associated with reduced tumorigenicity and elevated fibronectin. *Oncology Reports*, 1997; 4: 753–7.

16. Xu Y, *et al.* Mutations in the promoter reveal a cause for the reduced expression of the human manganese superoxide dismutase gene in cancer cells. *Oncogene*, 1999; 18: 93–102.

17. Kolodner R. Biochemistry and genetics of eukaryotic mismatch repair. *Genes and Development*, 1996; 10: 1433–42.

18. Heinen CD, Richardson D, White R, Groden J. Microsatellite instability in colorectal adenocarcinoma cell lines that have full-length adenomatous polyposis coli protein. *Cancer Research*, 1995; 55: 4797–9.

19. Tomlinson IPM, Novelli MR, Bodmer WF. The mutation rate and cancer. *Proceedings of the National Academy of Sciences USA*, 1996; 92: 14800–3.

20. Marshall CJ. Specificity of receptor tyrosine kinase signalling: transient versus sustained extracellular signal-regulated kinase activation. *Cell*, 1995; 80: 179–85.

21. Porter AC, Vaillancourt RR. Tyrosine kinase receptor-activated signal transduction pathways which lead to oncogenesis. *Oncogene*, 1998; 17: 1343–64.

22. Tapon N, Nagata K, Lamarche N, Hall A. A new Rac target POSH is an SH3-containing scaffold protein involved in the JNK and NF-——B signalling pathways. *EMBO Journal*, 1998; 17: 1395–404.

23. Wasylyk B, Hagman J, Gutierrez-Hartmann A. Ets transcription factors: nuclear effectors of the Ras-MAP-kinase signaling pathway. *Trends in Biochemical Sciences*, 1998; 23: 213–16.

24. Ulloa L, Doody J, Massagué J. Inhibition of transforming growth factor-β/SMAD signalling by the interferon-γ/STAT pathway. *Nature*, 1999; 397: 710–13.

25. Riese DJ, Stern DF. Specificity within the EGF family ErbB receptor family signaling network. *BioEssays*, 1998; 20: 41–8.

26. Harari D, *et al.* Neuregulin-4: a novel growth factor that acts through the ErbB-4 receptor tyrosine kinase. *Oncogene*, 1999; 18, 2681–9.

27. Janes PW, Daly RJ, deFazio A, Sutherland RL. Activation of the Ras signalling pathway in human breast cancer cells overexpressing *erb*B-2. *Oncogene*, 1994; 9: 3601–8.

28. Pietras RJ, *et al.* HER-2 tyrosine kinase pathway targets estrogen receptor and promotes hormone-independent growth in human breast cancer cells. *Oncogene*, 1995; 10: 2435–46.

29. Knowlden JM, *et al.* c-*erb*B3 and c-*erb*B4 expression is a feature of the endocrine responsive phenotype in clinical breast cancer. *Oncogene*, 1998; 17: 1949–57.

30. Borrello MG, *et al.* The full oncogenic activity of Ret/ptc2 depends on tyrosine 539, a docking site for phospholipase Cγ. *Molecular and Cellular Biology*, 1996; 16: 2151–63.

31. Edery P, *et al.* Mutations of the *RET* proto-oncogene in Hirschsprung's disease. *Nature*, 1994; 367: 378–80.

32. Romeo G, *et al.* Point mutations affecting the tyrosine kinase domain of the *RET* proto-oncogene in Hirschsprung's disease. *Nature*, 1994; 367: 377–8.

33. Sweetser DA, *et al.* Ganglioneuromas and renal anomalies are induced by activated RET[MEN2B] in transgenic mice. *Oncogene*, 1999; 18: 877–86.

34. Klugbauer S, Demidchik EP, Lengfelder E, Rabes HM. Molecular analysis of new subtypes of *ELE/RET* rearrangements, their reciprocal transcripts and breakpoints in papillary thyroid carcinomas of children after Chernobyl. *Oncogene*, 1998; 16: 671–5.

35. Taylor SJ, Shalloway D. Src and the control of cell division. *BioEssays*, 1996; 18: 9–11.

36. Irby RB, *et al.* Activating *SRC* mutation in a subset of advanced human colon cancers. *Nature Genetics*, 1999; 21: 187–90.

37. Sprang SR, Coleman DE. Invasion of the nucleotide snatchers: structural insights into the mechanism of G protein GEFs. *Cell*, 1998; 95: 155–8.

38. Wittinghofer F. Three-dimensional structure of p21^H-*ras* and its implications. *Seminars in Cancer Biology*, 1992; 3: 189–98.

39. Scheffzek K, *et al.* The Ras-RasGAP complex: structural basis for GTPase activation and its loss in oncogenic Ras mutants. *Science*, 1997; 277: 333–8.

40. Kerkhoff E, Rapp UR. Cell cycle targets of Ras/Raf signalling. *Oncogene*, 1998; 17: 1457–62.

41. Campbell SL, Khosravi-Far R, Rossman KL, Clark GJ, Der CJ. Increasing complexity of Ras signaling. *Oncogene*, 1998; 17: 1395–414.

42. Kauffmann-Zeh A, *et al.* Suppression of c-Myc-induced apoptosis by Ras signalling through PI(3)K and PKB. *Nature*, 1997; 385: 544–8.

43. Van Aelst L, D'Souza-Schorey C. Rho GTPases and signaling networks. *Genes and Development*, 1997; 11: 2295–322.

44. Trepicchio WL, Krontiris TG. Members of the rel/NF-—B family of transcriptional regulatory proteins bind the HRAS1 minisatellite DNA sequence. *Nucleic Acids Research*, 1992; 20: 2427–34.

45. Hoshino R, *et al.* Constitutive activation of the 41-/43-kDa mitogen-activated protein kinase signaling pathway in human tumors. *Oncogene*, 1999; 18: 813–22.

46. Plattner R, *et al.* Differential contribution of the ERK and JNK mitogen-activated protein kinase cascades to Ras transformation of HT1080 fibrosarcoma and DLD-1 colon carcinoma cells. *Oncogene*, 1999; 18: 1807–17.

47. de Rooij J, Bos JL. Minimal Ras-binding domain of Raf1 can be used as an activation-specific probe for Ras. *Oncogene*, 1997; 14: 623–5.

48. Bouchard C, Staller P, Eilers M. Control of cell proliferation by Myc. *Trends in Cell Biology*, 1998; 8: 202–6.

49. MYC review articles: *Oncogene*, 1999; 18: 2914–3016.

50. Mehle C, Piatyszek MA, Ljungberg B, Shay JW, Roos G. Telomerase activity in human renal cell carcinoma. *Oncogene*, 1996; 13;161–6.

51. Greider CW. Telomerase activity, cell proliferation, and cancer. *Proceedings of the National Academy of Sciences USA*, 1998; 95: 90–92.

52. Zhu X, *et al.* Cell cycle-dependent modulation of telomerase activity in tumor cells. *Proceedings of the National Academy of Sciences USA*, 1996; 93: 6091–5.

53. Wu KJ, *et al.* Direct activation of *TERT* transcription by c-MYC. *Nature Genetics*, 1999; 21: 220–4.

54. Greenberg RA, *et al.* Telomerase reverse transcriptase gene is a direct target of c-Myc but is not functionally equivalent in cellular transformation. *Oncogene*, 1999; 18: 1219–26.

55. Sherr CJ, Roberts JM. CDK inhibitors: positive and negative regulators of G1-phase progression. *Genes and Development*, 1999; 13: 1501–12.

56. Mulligan G, Jacks T. The retinoblastoma gene family: cousins with overlapping interests. *Trends in Genetics*, 1998; 14: 223–229.

57. Dyson N. The regulation of E2F by pRB-family proteins. *Genes and Development*, 1998; 12: 2245–62.

58. Luo RX, Postigo AA, Dean DC. Rb interacts with histone deacetylase to repress transcription. *Cell*, 1998; 92: 463–73.

59. Adams JM, Cory S. The Bcl-2 protein family: arbiters of cell survival. *Science*, 1998; 281: 1322–6.

60. Prives C. Signaling to p53: Breaking the MDM2-p53 circuit. *Cell*, 1999; 95: 5–8.

61. Freedman DA, Levine AJ. Regulation of the p53 protein by the MDM2 oncoprotein—thirty-eighth G.H.A. Clowes memorial award lecture. *Cancer Research*, 1999; 59: 1–7.

62. Walker DR, *et al.* Evolutionary conservation and somatic mutation hotspot maps of p53: correlation with p53 protein structural and functional features. *Oncogene*, 1999; 18: 211–18.

63. Haber DA. Splicing into senescence: the curious case of p16 and p19^{ARF}. *Cell*, 1997; 91: 555–8.

64. Fuchs SY, Adler V, Buschmann T, Wu X, Ronai Z. Mdm2 association with p53 targets its ubiquitination. *Oncogene*, 1998; 17: 2543–7.

65. Honda R, Yasuda H. Association of p19^{ARF} with Mdm2 inhibits ubiquitin ligase activity of Mdm2 for tumor suppressor p53. *EMBO Journal*, 1999; 18: 22–7.

66. Hsieh J-K, Chan FSG, O'Connor DJ, Mittnacht S, Zhong S, Lu X. RB regulates the stability and the apoptotic function of p53 via MDM2. *Molecular Cell*, 1999; 3: 181–93.

67. Soussi, T. *P53 data base at*: http: //perso.curie.fr/Thierry.Soussi/

68. Kinzler KW, Vogelstein B. Lessons from hereditary cancer. *Cell*, 1996; 87: 159–70.

69. He T-C, *et al.* Identification of c-*MYC* as a target of the APC pathway. *Science*, 1998; 281: 1509–12.

70. Tetsu O, McCormick F. β-catenin regulates expression of cyclin D1 in colon carcinoma cells. *Nature*, 1999; 398: 422–26.

71. Soussi T. *APC data base at*: http: //perso.curie.fr/Thierry.Soussi/

72. Sparks AB, Morin PJ, Vogelstein B, Kinzler KW. Mutational analysis of the APC/β-catenin/Tcf pathway in colorectal cancer. *Cancer Research*, 1998; 58: 1130–4.

73. Palacios J, Gamallo C. Mutations in the β-catenin gene (*CTNNB1*) in endometrioid ovarian carcinomas. *Cancer Research*, 1998; 58: 1344–7.

74. Chan EF, Gat U, McNiff JM, Fuchs E. A common human skin tumour is caused by activating mutations in β-catenin. *Nature Genetics*, 1999; 21: 410–13.

75. Zhang H, Tombline G, Weber BL. BRCA1, BRCA2, and DNA damage response: collision or collusion? *Cell*, 1998; 92: 433–6.

76. Leone PE, *et al.* NF2 gene mutations and allelic status of 1p, 14q and 22q in sporadic meningiomas. *Oncogene*, 1999; 18: 2231–9

77. Kaelin WG, Maher E. The VHL tumour-suppressor gene paradigm. *Trends in Genetics*, 1998; 14: 423–6.

78. Mukhopadhyay D, Knebelmann B, Cohen HT, Ananth S, Sukhatme VP. The von Hippel-Lindau tumor suppressor gene product interacts with Sp1 to repress vascular endothelial growth factor promoter activity. *Molecular and Cellular Biology*, 1997; 17: 5629–39.

79. Herman JG, *et al.* Silencing of the VHL tumor-suppressor gene by DNA methylation in renal carcinoma. *Proceedings of the National Academy of Sciences USA*, 1994; 91: 9700–4.

80. Rauscher FJ. The WT1 Wilms tumor gene product: a developmentally regulated transcription factor in the kidney that functions as a tumor suppressor. *FASEB Journal*, 1993; 7: 896–903.

81. Kennedy D, Ramsdale T, Mattick J, Little M. An RNA recognition motif in Wilms' tumour protein (WT1) revealed by structural modelling. *Nature Genetics*, 1996; 12: 329–32.

82. Kim J, Lee K, Pelletier J. The DNA binding domains of the WT1 tumor suppressor gene product and chimeric EWS/WT1 oncoprotein are functionally distinct. *Oncogene*, 1998; 16: 1021–30.

83. Silberstein GB, Van Horn K, Strickland P, Roberts CT, Daniel CW. Altered expression of the WT1 Wilms tumor suppressor gene in human breast cancer. *Proceedings of the National Academy of Sciences USA*, 1997; 94: 8132–7.

84. Christofori G, Semb H. The role of the cell-adhesion molecule E-cadherin as a tumour-suppressor gene. *Trends in Biochemical Sciences*, 1999; 24: 73–6.

85. Crawford HC, *et al.* The metalloproteinase matrilysin is a target of β-catenin transactivation in intestinal tumors. *Oncogene*, 1999; 18: 2883–91.

86. Dang CV, Semenza GL. Oncogenic alterations of metabolism. *Trends in Biochemical Sciences*, 1999; 24: 68–72.

87. Kuroda S, *et al.* Role of IQGAP1 a target of the small GTPases Cdc42 and Rac1 in regulation of E-cadherin-mediated cell-cell adhesion. *Science*, 1998; 281: 832–5.

88. Ho Y-D, John L Joyal, Zhigang Li, Sacks DB. IQGAP1 integrates Ca^{2+}/calmodulin and Cdc42 signaling. *Journal of Biological Chemistry*, 1999; **274**: 464–70.

89. Oka H, *et al.* Expression of E-cadherin cell adhesion molecules in human breast cancer tissues and its relationship to metastasis. *Cancer Research*, 1993; **53**: 1696–701.

90. Berx G, *et al.* E-cadherin is a tumour/invasion suppressor gene mutated in human lobular breast cancers. *EMBO Journal*, 1995; **14**: 6107–15.

91. Risinger JI, Berchuck A, Kohler MF, Boyd J. Mutations of the E-cadherin gene in human gynecologic cancers. *Nature Genetics*, 1994; **7**: 98–102.

92. Kawanishi J, Kato J, Sasaki K, Fujii S, Watanabe N, Niitsu Y. Loss of E-cadherin-dependent cell-cell adhesion due to mutation of the β-catenin gene in a human cancer cell line HSC-39. *Molecular and Cellular Biology*, 1995; **15**: 1175–81.

93. Pierceall WE, Woodard AS, Morrow JS, Rimm D, Fearon ER. Frequent alterations in E-cadherin and α- and β-catenin expression in human breast cancer cell lines. *Oncogene*, 1995; **11**: 1319–26.

94. Vermeulen SJ, *et al.* The αE-catenin gene (*CTNNA1*) acts as an invasion-suppressor gene in human colon cancer cells. *Oncogene*, 1999; **18**: 905–15.

95. Ellis LM, *et al.* Down-regulation of vascular endothelial growth factor in a human colon carcinoma cell line transfected with an antisense expression vector specific for c-src. *Journal of Biological Chemistry*, 1998; **273**: 1052–7.

96. Lonergan KM, *et al.* Regulation of hypoxia-inducible mRNAs by the von Hippel-Lindau tumor suppressor protein requires binding to complexes containing elongins B/C and Cul2. *Molecular and Cellular Biology*, 1998; **18**: 732–41.

1.3 Familial cancer

Rosalind A. Eeles

Introduction

For many centuries, cancer has been known to 'run in families'. It was described in Roman times and Broca, in 1866, described familial breast cancer in his wife's family.[1] In one sense, all cancer is genetic at the cellular level since genetic changes occur when a normal cell is transformed into a cancer cell; however, these changes are usually somatic (they only occur in the cancer cells and are not present in normal cells). A proportion of the common cancers (usually 5 to 10 per cent)[2] occur in individuals with a germline genetic alteration which confers an increased risk of cancer development. This is termed 'genetic predisposition to cancer' and the genetic alterations occur in every somatic cell in the body, as they are in the germline. Such alterations can also be passed on to offspring since, on average, half the gametes will contain the genetic alteration.

The clustering of more than one case of cancer within a family ('familial cancer') can occur for several reasons:

1. Clustering may occur due to chance; this is particularly seen with the common cancers. The higher the prevalence of a disease, the more likely it is that clustering will occur in families due to chance alone.
2. Individuals in the same family may share the same carcinogenic environmental exposures.
3. There may be a cancer-predisposition gene in the family accounting for familial clustering.

When is familial cancer more likely to be due to a cancer-predisposition gene in the family?

The markers of the presence of a cancer-predisposition gene in a familial cluster are:

- the clustering together of cancers at sites that are normally rare in the general population (for example, the association of medullary thyroid cancer with phaeochromocytoma in the multiple, endocrine-neoplasia type 2 syndrome);
- young age of onset relative to the general population;
- the occurrence of the same type of cancer on more than one occasion in the same individual (for instance, bilateral breast cancer; multiple colonic cancer);

- the presence of multiple cases of cancer in several individuals on the same side of a family.

How should familial cancer be assessed by the clinician?

Taking a full family history is central to the practice of the management of familial cancer. Family history-taking is part of normal medical history-taking; however in patients with cancer, family history should be ascertained as far as possible out to third-degree relatives (a first-degree relative is one generation away from the individual studied; for example, a parent, sibling, or child). The individuals with cancer should be noted in a family tree (see Fig. 1).

Standard notation is:

Male:	Square	□
Female:	Circle	○
Deceased:	Diagonal line through symbol	
Proband:	Arrow indicates individual who is giving the family history	↗

However, the standard notation for shading symbols does vary, so a legend indicating the notation used by the doctor who took the history should be attached to medical reports of the family tree.

Studies have shown that recall of family history is superior for first-degree relatives compared to that for more distant relatives, and recall of a family history for breast cancer is approximately 90 per cent accurate.[3],[4] However, accuracy falls for cancer at more indeterminate sites such as ovarian cancer, which is often reported as 'abdominal' or 'stomach' (this has an approximately 17 per cent miscall rate).[4] Verification of diagnosis would therefore be important in individuals such as the one with 'abdominal cancer' depicted in Fig. 1 since if this were shown to be ovarian cancer, the family shown in Fig. 1 would have breast/ovarian syndrome.

Not all cancer family clinics verify all breast cancer cases because of the high accuracy of recall and the fact that recall is more likely to be an over-recall, since mastectomy may have been performed for benign disease. This would result in an over-screening of 5 to 10 per cent of patients and it is often not cost-effective to verify all breast cancer cases. An exception would be if an individual wishes to undertake more extreme measures such as prophylactic surgery; cases of Munchausen's by proxy (individuals passing a fictitious family history of cancer on to other family members in order to provoke them to take preventive measures) have been reported, although these are rare (less than 1 per cent).[4] Douglas *et al.*[4] showed that

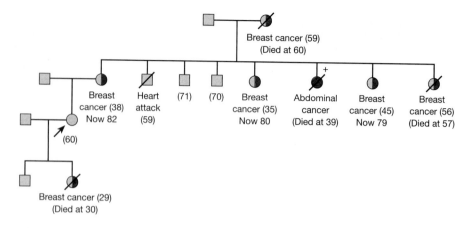

Fig. 1 A sample family tree (pedigree) demonstrating a family history of cancer. The chance that this family has a cancer-predisposition gene is > 95 per cent. Tracing the diagnosis of the abdominal cancer (+), via the Cancer Registry or medical record, verified that this was ovarian cancer, which indicates that this family has breast/ovarian cancer syndrome. This family is very likely to have a mutation in BRCA1 or BRCA2 (see text). Key: □, ○ unaffected; ■, ● affected with cancer (site specified); ◨, ◖ affected with breast cancer; → proband. Numbers are ages at death, or cancer diagnosis, or current age.

verification of all family histories in their cancer genetics clinic resulted in an 11 per cent change in recommendations for management, and that most of the changes were related to the verification of cancers at abdominal sites.

Penetrance

As can be seen in Fig. 1, the presence of a cancer-predisposition gene does not always result in cancer development. The proband (arrowed) has a very high chance of carrying the breast cancer-predisposition gene as she is the intervening individual between two cases: her mother and her daughter. (There are two prerequisites: one is that there is a predisposition gene present at all, which is very likely with the presence of six cases of breast cancer, and the second is that the proband's daughter is a gene carrier, which is very likely because of her very young age of disease onset.) The risk that a mutation in a cancer-predisposition gene in a gene carrier (the person who carries the mutation) gives rise to the development of the disease is called 'penetrance', and the fact that many cancer-predisposition genes do not universally result in cancer development is termed 'incomplete penetrance'.

Some cancer-predisposition syndromes have extremely high penetrance, for example familial polyposis coli has virtually 100 per cent penetrance for the development of colonic cancer by the age of 35.[5]

Genetic heterogeneity

Familial clustering of the same type of cancer may be due to more than one type of cancer-predisposition gene. This is termed 'genetic heterogeneity'. For example, familial breast cancer, in which there are clusters of four or more cases of breast cancer at 60 years of age or younger in the same lineage, may be due to either BRCA1 or BRCA2 (breast cancer genes 1 and 2). However, calculations from the Breast Cancer Linkage Consortium, which collates international data from breast cancer families,[6] have suggested that 63 per cent

of cancers in such families are due to either BRCA1 or BRCA2. There are, therefore, breast cancer families with numerous young cases (which are therefore likely to harbour a cancer-predisposition gene) which are due to a gene(s) that remains to be discovered: this gene has been named BRCA3.

Genotype–phenotype correlations

The genotype is the genetic make-up of an individual or cell (the DNA code) and the phenotype is the physical or biochemical effect of the genotype (for example, the occurrence of a certain type of cancer in an individual with a genetic alteration that predisposes to cancer). Different phenotypes may arise from different genetic alterations within the same gene. This is termed a genotype–phenotype correlation. An example is the multiple, endocrine-neoplasia type 2 syndrome (MEN2): MEN2A is the association of medullary thyroid cancer, phaeochromocytoma, and hyperparathyroidism; and MEN2B is the association of medullary thyroid cancer, a Marfanoid habitus, and mucosal neuromas. Both are caused by germline mutations (genetic alterations) in the RET proto-oncogene. MEN2A, in many cases, is caused by mutations in the extracellular, cysteine-rich region of the RET protein, whereas virtually all MEN2B families have an alteration at one specific part of the RET proto-oncogene which codes for the intracellular tyrosine kinase portion of the protein (see Chapters 1.2 and 1.4).

Not all cancer-predisposition genes display this genotype–phenotype phenomenon but, when it is present, it can be useful for genetic counselling to advise families about the phenotypic risk.

The importance of ascertaining the patient's genetic origin

Studies of the genetic changes present in the genotypes of populations from different geographical areas are starting to demonstrate that

Table 1 Some of the 'rare' genetic syndromes associated with an increased risk of malignancy and their mode of inheritance

Syndrome	Neoplasia or malignancy	Risk (%)[a]	Mode[b]	Chromosomal location[c]	Gene name
Neurofibromatosis type 1	Plexiform neurofibroma, optic glioma, neurofibrosarcoma	4–5	D	17q	NF1
Neurofibromatosis type 2	Acoustic neuroma (vestibular schwannoma)		D	22q	NF2
	– bilateral	86			
	– unilateral	6			
	Meningioma	45			
	Spinal tumours	26			
	Astrocytomas	4			
	Ependymomas	3			
Von Hippel–Lindau	Cerebellar haemangioblastoma	35–84	D	3p	VHL
	Retinal angioma	41–70			
	Renal-cell carcinoma	25–69			
	Phaeochromocytoma	15			
	Renal, liver, and pancreatic cysts	16–50			
Ataxia telangiectasia	Lymphoma	60	R	11q	ATM
	Leukaemia	27			
Bloom syndrome	Many sites Immunodeficiency	80	R	15q	BLM
Cowden syndrome	Breast cancer	30–50	D	10q	PTEN
	Thyroid cancer	15			
	Bowel cancer	?3			
	Multiple hamartomas of skin, tongue and bowel	100			
Basal-cell naevus/Gorlin's syndrome	Basal-cell carcinoma	80	D	9q	PTCH
	Ovarian fibroma	17			
	Medulloblastoma	4			
	Falx calcification, bifid ribs, macrocephaly	85			

[a] Lifetime risk of neoplasia or cancer.

[b] Mode of inheritance is classified as 'autosomal dominant' (D) or 'autosomal recessive' (R).

[c] Chromosomal arms: p, short arm; q, long arm.

NA, not available.

mutations in some cancer-predisposition genes are more common in certain populations, particularly those from less-outbred ethnic groups. Examples are the presence of a specific alteration in the breast cancer 2 gene, BRCA2, in the Icelandic population (there is a deletion of five bases in the central part of the gene);[7] and the presence of specific alterations in the Ashkenazi Jews, two in BRCA1 and one in BRCA2.[8],[9]

Recognizing 'patterns' of familial cancer

Certain genetic syndromes are associated with an increased risk of cancer in addition to other features of the syndrome. These are listed in Table 1. Other familial cancer syndromes consist predominantly of clustering of cancers at either one or at associated sites (Table 2). The ability to recognize the clustering of cancers at different sites as

being part of a syndrome is an important part in recognizing familial cancer; for example, the association of breast and ovarian cancer in a familial cluster is highly indicative of a breast/ovarian-predisposition gene.

Mechanisms of action of cancer-predisposition genes

Many cancer-predisposition genes are tumour-suppressor genes (see Chapter 1.2). Alterations have to occur in both copies of the gene for cancer to develop, since if the normal copy is present it acts to suppress the tumorigenic effect of the mutated copy or allele (the so-called tumour-suppressor gene model (Knudson's 'two-hit' hypothesis)).[11] In rare instances (MEN2 and familial papillary renal cancer) there is no loss of the normal allele in the copy at the same

Table 2 Syndromes associated with an increased risk of malignancy where the major feature associated with the syndrome is the development of cancer

Syndrome name	Malignancies	Risk (%)[a]	Mode	Chromosomal location	Gene name
Familial melanoma	Melanoma	53	D	9p	CDKN2 (P16)
Familial polyposis coli	Large bowel cancer Cancer of the upper GI tract Desmoid	~ 100 5 20	D	5q	APC
Breast/ovary cancer syndrome	Breast Ovary Colon Prostate	85 44–60 6 6	D	17q	BRCA1
Site-specific breast cancer	Breast Ovary Prostate Pancreas Other cancers, e.g. cutaneous and ocular melanoma, gall bladder, bile duct, Fallopian tube, stomach	85 27 14 4 ? <1	D	13q	BRCA2
Hereditary non-polyposis colorectal cancer (HNPCC)			D	2p 3p 2p 3p 2q 7q	hMSH2 HMLH1 hMLH6 TGFβ PMS1 PMS2
Lynch type 1	Site-specific colon only	70 (Some studies suggest a lower penetrance in women)			
Lynch type 2	Colon Endometrium Ovary Gastric biliary tract Transitional-cell carcinoma of the renal pelvis Melanoma Head and neck Brain Small bowel	70–80 43 9–19 < 10			
Muir–Torré syndrome	As HNPCC with skin lesions Keratoacanthoma/sebaceous cysts		D	2p	hMSH2
Turcot's syndrome	Brain tumour Very early-onset colon cancer (< 20 years) with café-au-lait patches	?	D/R	2p 3p 5q 7q	hMSH2 hMLH1 APC PMS2
Hereditary prostate cancer	Prostate	85	DR/X-linked	1q24 1q42 1p36 Xq 17p	HPC1 (not yet cloned) PCAP (not yet cloned) CAPB (not yet cloned) ? HPC2 (cloned)
Li–Fraumeni syndrome	Sarcoma Early-onset breast cancer Brain tumour Leukaemia Adrenocortical tumour Other cancers	24 in children 74 in men 95 in women	D	17p	TP53
Multiple endocrine neoplasia type 1	Parathyroid, endocrine pancreas, pituitary	70	D	11q	MEN-1
Multiple endocrine neoplasia type 2	Medullary carcinoma of thyroid Phaeochromocytoma (type 2A)	70 50	D	10q	RET
Retinoblastoma	Retinoblastoma Osteosarcoma Other cancers	90 6 8	D	13q	Rb1

[a] The risk is either the 'lifetime risk', as quoted in the reference articles (see ref. 10), or the 'risk to age 70 years' in those studies which have performed detailed age-specific calculations. Where possible, risks by set ages or per site are given; in the absence of such figures a 'syndrome' penetrance estimate is provided. These risks are approximate and may vary between different populations with different mutation profiles.

position as the cancer-predisposition gene on the second chromosome. Such syndromes are caused by a mutation in a dominant oncogene.[12],[13]

Genes that are responsible for the control of fundamental aspects of cell growth (e.g. parts of the cell cycle) are called 'gatekeepers',[14] for instance the *APC* gene mutations which cause familial polyposis coli. Others maintain the genetic stability of the cell. These are called 'caretakers': an example being *p53* mutations which may cause the Li–Fraumeni syndrome. Alterations in these genes result in genetic instability. Other genes are called 'landscapers'—an example is the *PTEN* gene, mutations of which cause Cowden syndrome. Such genes alter the tissue or landscape structure. This is why Cowden syndrome, for example, consists of multiple hamartomas.

Research approaches to discover cancer-predisposition genes

When a cancer-predisposition gene is thought to cause familial clustering, several approaches can be used to locate the gene. Once located and characterized (cloned), direct gene analysis can then be offered in the clinical setting.

Cytogenetic alterations

Gross chromosomal changes can be seen on cytogenetic analysis. Rarely, study of a constitutional chromosomal alteration, seen on cytogenetic analysis in an individual who has an unusually early onset of cancer and other unusual phenotypic features, can indicate the location of a cancer-predisposition gene. The chromosomal study of a man with mental retardation and polyposis led to the finding of a loss of part of chromosome 5, subsequently found to be the location of the polyposis gene, *APC*.[15]

Linkage analysis

The concept of genetic linkage was first recognized by Gregor Mendel, who noted that certain characteristics of his experimental plants tended to be co-inherited. The explanation for this became clear once it was recognized that chromosomes contain the genetic material and that two traits are linked only if the corresponding genes for them reside close together on the same chromosome (see Chapter 1.1).

The search for cancer-predisposition genes using linkage studies relies on collections of families containing numerous cases of the same cancer type, and the co-inheritance of genetic markers with the disease is said to show evidence of linkage if the co-inheritance is greater than would be expected by chance. An example is the co-inheritance of the gene for retinoblastoma with certain forms of the esterase D gene as it is nearby on the same chromosome. This is expressed as a so-called LOD score (*logarithm* to base 10 of the *od*ds). A LOD score is analogous to a *p* value in clinical trials, and a LOD of more than 3 is statistically significant and equivalent to odds of linkage of 1000 to 1 ($\log_{10} 1000 = 3$, LOD score > 3 is significant).

Phenotypic features

A physical characteristic associated with a cancer-predisposition syndrome may give a clue as to the location of the cancer-predisposition gene. For example, meningiomas are a feature of neurofibromatosis type 2 (*NF2*) and often show loss of one copy of chromosome 22, the site of the *NF2* gene.

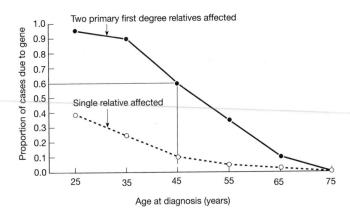

Fig. 2 Graph showing the probability that breast cancer is due to a predisposition gene by age at diagnosis (by courtesy of Professor D.T. Bishop, who used model from Ref. 17 to produce graph in Figure 2).

Association studies

A number of disease-susceptibility loci have been identified through the direct testing of candidate genes—looking for associations between particular alleles and disease—by comparing allele frequencies in affected individuals and matched controls; for example, variations in the *CYP17* gene which is involved in oestrogen metabolism. Feigelson *et al.*[16] have shown that there is an increased risk of breast cancer with certain variations in this enzyme.

Clinical implications

Cancer genetic counselling: aims

The aims of genetic counselling are to take an adequate family history, assess the risks of cancer using epidemiological models and other penetrance figures from mutation studies, and to outline the options for management of the increased risk. For example, when assessing the chance that an individual's family has a breast cancer predisposition, many clinics use the Claus model or CASH curves from the Cancer and Steroid Hormone study. This was a study of 4700 women who had breast cancer and whose family history was taken, Claus *et al.*[17] developed a model to estimate the chance that a cancer-predisposition gene was present in a particular cluster. It can be seen from Fig. 2 that if an individual has two close relatives (strictly first-degree relatives) with breast cancer at 45, there is a 60 per cent chance that there is a breast cancer-predisposition gene present (graph shown courtesy of Professor D. T. Bishop).[17]

Not all breast cancer clusters are due to mutations in *BRCA*1 or *BRCA*2. Tables published by the Breast Cancer Linkage Consortium and other studies provide data about the chance that a mutation will be found in *BRCA*1/2.[6],[18]–[21] This can be summarized using Tables 3(a) and (b).[21],[22] Figures 3(a) and (b) show the penetrance (risk of development of cancer) for breast or ovarian cancer if a *BRCA*1 or *BRCA*2 mutation is present respectively. The penetrance figures in

Table 3(a) Proportion of single cases due to *BRCA1* by age (estimated from the gene frequency)

Age	Breast (%)	Ovary (%)
20–29	7.5	5.9
30–39	5.1	5.6
40–49	2.2	4.6
50–59	1.4	2.6
60–69	0.8	1.8
20–69	1.7	2.8

From Ford *et al.*,[21] with permission.

Table 3(b) Threshold for probability of *BRCA1/2* mutation being present in cluster/single cancer cases

Chance that a mutation is present (%)*	Clinical description of cancer cluster/case
< 10	All single cases of breast or ovarian cancer
10	Single breast cancer cases < 35 years
> 10–≤ 30	≥ 2 breast cancer cases < 50 years 1 breast cancer < 40 years in an Ashkenazi
≤ 50	3 breast cancer cases < 50 years 4 breast cancer cases, no ovarian cancer 1 breast and ovarian cancer
> 50	> 1 breast and ovarian cancer ≥ 4 cases of female breast cancer < 60 years ≥ 4 cases female and ≥ 1 case male breast cancer

From Langston *et al.*;[18] Shattuck-Eidens *et al.*;[20] Ford *et al.*,[6] Mitchell and Eeles.[22]

*NB: The chance of detecting a mutation is lower because: at least 15% of mutations are regulatory, i.e. are not in the coding region of the gene which is the area tested; and the genetic screening methods are about 80% sensitive.

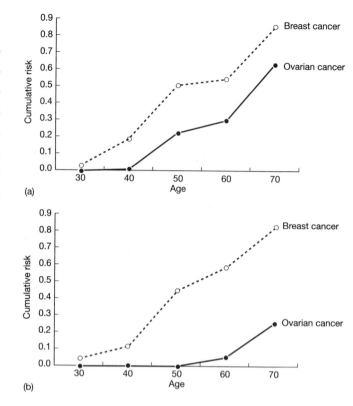

Fig. 3 (a) Penetrance curves showing the risk of breast and ovarian cancer by age in individuals who are carriers of cancer-causing mutations in the *BRCA1* gene. (b) Penetrance curves showing the risk of breast and ovarian cancer by age in individuals who are carriers of cancer-causing mutations in the *BRCA2* gene.

Figs 3(a) and (b) outline the overall penetrance, taking into account all families with mutations in *BRCA1/2* from a worldwide analysis.[6] When a cluster is identified that has a high chance of having an alteration in *BRCA1* or *BRCA2*, the specific alteration present in that particular cluster has to be identified. Over 100 alterations have been described in both these genes and submitted to a World Wide Web database (the Breast Cancer Information Core). Figures 4(a) and (b) show the positions at which alterations have been found in different families. There are some preliminary data suggesting that different alterations may confer different cancer risks. For example, those nearer the 5′ end of *BRCA1* may have a higher ovarian risk than those at the 3′ end.[23]

Traditionally, counselling has been non-directive; only management options and information about risk are presented to the patient, without a specific recommendation about which option to follow.[24] However, as more management options are having proven benefit in cancer genetics, counselling is becoming more directive.

How should cancer genetic counselling be structured?

As in many other areas of oncology, the multidisciplinary team approach is being increasingly used in cancer genetic counselling clinics. Most clinics are located within or in close association with a genetic screening service; however, cancer genetic counselling requires training in both genetics and oncology.

In many parts of Europe, counselling is traditionally led by medically qualified personnel. However, in the United Kingdom and the United States, genetic counsellors/clinical nurse specialists in cancer genetics counselling are starting to conduct much of the routine counselling, working with the medical personnel who provide the medical back-up and may provide the formal risk assessment by the cancer genetics team.

Risk perception

One of the primary reasons for identifying hereditary cancer is to enable family members to be targeted for advice on risk. This raises the important issue of the process of giving risk information. The adoption of preventive strategies may depend on the individual's perception of risk; for example, Croyle *et al.*[25] have shown that individuals at a perceived increased risk of heart disease were more

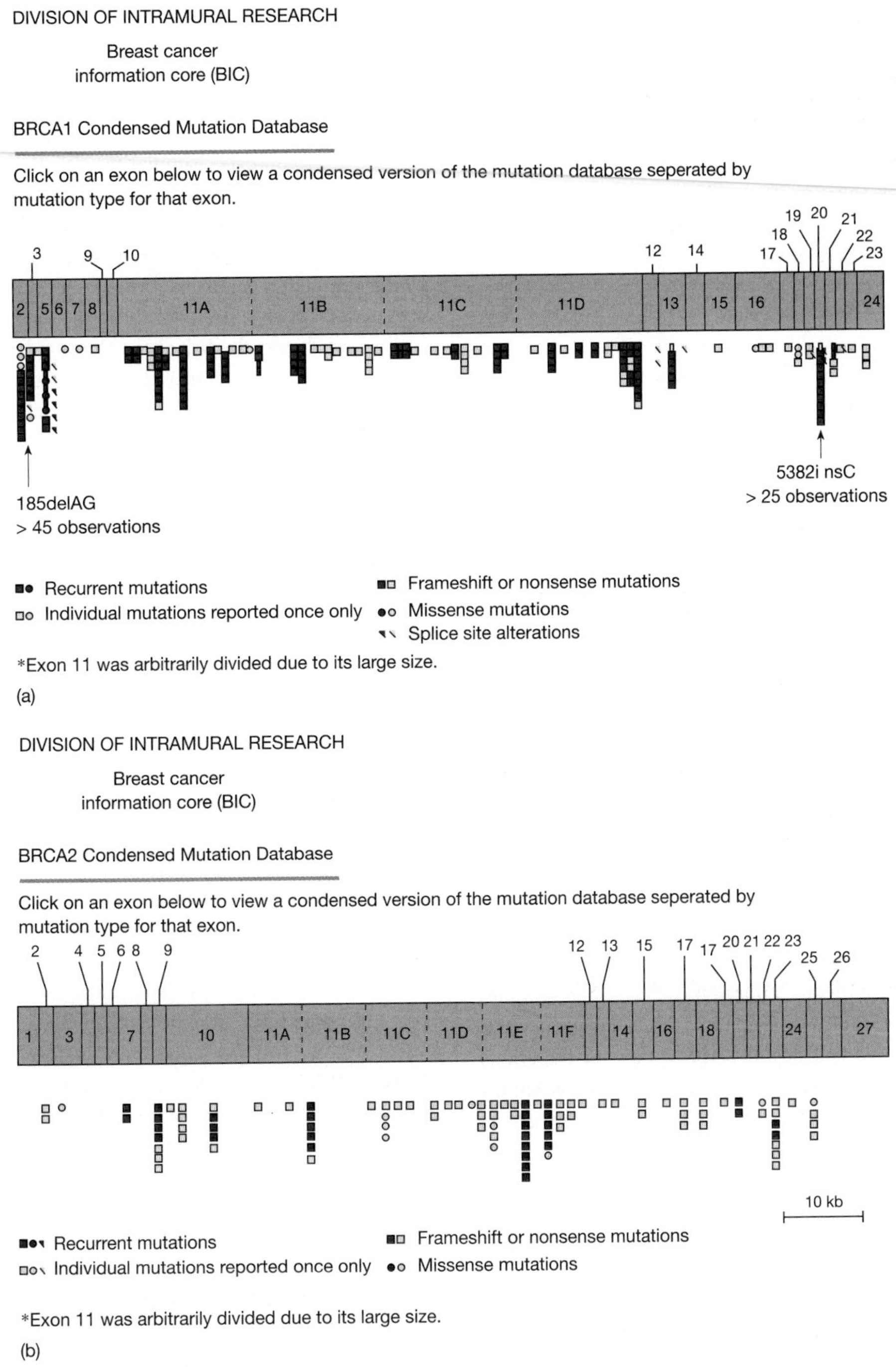

Fig. 4 (a) *BRCA*1 Information Core Mutation Database (BIC) showing the wide spectrum of positions and types of mutations within *BRCA*1 found in different families worldwide. Although some mutations are described more often than others ('hotspots'), e.g. the Ashkenazi Jewish alteration at the beginning and end of *BRCA*1, the mutation spectrum is wide and a specific alteration has to be identified within a familial cluster, prior to offering an unaffected member genetic testing. (b) *BRCA*2 Information Core Mutation Database (BIC) showing the wide spectrum of positions and types of mutations within *BRCA*2. Although some mutations are described more often than others ('hotspots') e.g. the Ashkenazi Jewish alteration at position 6174 of *BRCA*2 the mutation spectrum is wide and a specific alteration has to be identified within a familial cluster, prior to offering an unaffected member genetic testing.

likely to express their intentions to modify their lifestyle than those who perceived themselves to be at the same risk as the general population. The understanding and retention of this information may depend on the format in which it is presented and the individual's attitudes to risk. Even with the recent advances in the cloning of several cancer-predisposition genes, incomplete penetrance (i.e. not all gene carriers develop cancer, they are however at increased risk) means that known gene carriers still have to comprehend that they are at a certain level of risk, but that the development of cancer still has an element of uncertainty.

Risk information is often complex and can be expressed in various ways. It is current practice in genetic counselling clinics, and the more recent specialized cancer family clinics, to convey risk information numerically, either as a risk of developing disease per year, or risk by a certain age.[26] The risk value is often either given as a percentage risk or a '1 in x' value. However, information for the risk of developing cancer can be presented in several ways:

Numerical	Risk per year
	Risk by a certain age
	1 in x value or percentage format
	Relative risk corrected for age
General categorization	High/moderate/low risk
	The problem with this concept is that different individuals and doctors assign the same risk levels to different categories.
Situation analogy	A situation carrying an equivalent risk without any numerical information, e.g. the chances of picking an ace if one card is chosen blind from a card pack.
The risk figure measure	Risk of developing cancer
	Risk of not developing cancer
	Risk of death from cancer (this is very rarely given in clinics as it is perceived as too distressing).

The optimal format for conveying risk information is unknown. Studies have examined whether women correctly assess their level of risk,[27] but few have examined the best way to present genetic information to those who may be at increased risk of familial cancer, and it is unclear whether clients understand the rather complex explanations or how much of this information they remember. There are data suggesting that women do not wish to have or remember numerical information. For example, 98 per cent of women attending a cancer family clinic because of a family history of breast cancer could not remember their percentage annual risk, even when this was given both verbally in the clinic and by follow-up letter. They were somewhat better at providing feedback on their own lifetime risk, but 35 per cent gave an incorrect figure. More importantly though, they were able to report the category of their risk (low, medium, high) with reasonable accuracy, but this did not relate to their perception that they were more or less likely to develop cancer. This suggests that clients have a poor understanding of the risk information being given.[28]

Green and Brown[29] have suggested that the qualitative aspect of risk is more important than the quantitative aspect, and Sorensen et al.[30] suggested that many individuals do not remember or understand the genetic information given. Leonard et al.[31] claim that 'clients are bad at probabilistic reasoning and find quantitative risk estimates difficult to understand'. However, this finding contrasts with that of Josten et al.,[32] who reported from a cancer family clinic in Wisconsin that 'clients say that a number gives them boundaries rather than having an ambiguous sense of being high risk'. Interestingly, 5 to 10 per cent of individuals in this American study did not wish to be given numerical risk information.

The individual's background information, sociodemographic factors (e.g. educational level), and psychological profile could conceivably alter the optimal method of risk presentation since these can act as barriers to adequate information content.[33],[34]

Much of the research on the perception of risk has been undertaken in industrial contexts. Familiarity with the risk has been shown to lower the perception of the risk level. For example, the perception of radiation risk by people living near nuclear power plants is lower than in those not living near to such installations.[35] However, in cancer families, it is possible that a larger cancer burden (the number, age at diagnosis, and closeness of the relationship with the cancer cases) may distort the risk above the true level.[31],[36] Many people in cancer families erroneously think they have a 100 per cent risk of developing cancer, the only uncertainty being when the disease will occur. Lerman et al.[34] have reported that members of cancer families distort their risk, even when their family history consists of only one affected relative.

Vlek[37] claims there are five factors underlying perception of risk, namely:

(1) the potential degree of harm or lethality associated with the risk;
(2) the controllability through safety/rescue measures (i.e. prevention/early detection);
(3) the number of people exposed (this would equate to the cancer burden in the family);
(4) the familiarity with the effects of the risk; and
(5) the degree of voluntariness of exposure to the risk.

There are reports suggesting that those at highest risk adopt a lower rate of health preventive measures due to avoidance behaviours instigated by high levels of anxiety.[38]

From studies of lung cancer, there is some evidence that the perceived risk of **not** developing cancer is different from that expected from the perceived risk of **developing** the disease.[39] For example, a BRCA1 carrier has a lifetime risk (by 80 years of age) of developing breast cancer of 85 per cent, and therefore has a 15 per cent chance of *not* developing the disease. However, many women still believe that this risk level (i.e. the 15 per cent chance of not getting the disease) means they will inevitably develop breast cancer by the age of 80.

If cancer family clinics are to provide a useful service it is important to ensure that those counselled understand the risk information and advice they are given. Lack of understanding of their risk could impact on their ability to use this information when making decisions about the future management of their health, and may also affect their mental health if cancer-related worries are increased through misunderstanding information given in the clinic.

Medical history and examination

It must be established from the history and examination whether the patient is an affected or an at-risk member of the family, and the patient should be questioned on any symptoms indicative of cancer or congenital abnormalities. Initial clinical examination involves looking for any dysmorphic features and congenital anomalies. The skin should be carefully examined as many cancer syndromes are associated with dermatological features such as: pigmentary abnormalities, for example freckles on the lip in Peutz–Jeghers syndrome, café-au-lait

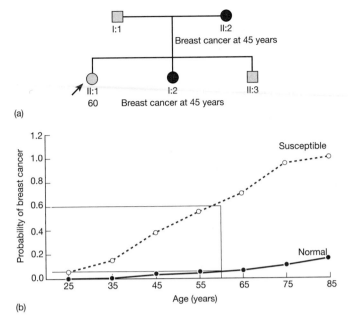

Fig. 5 (a) Example of a pedigree where an individual aged 60 has consulted regarding her breast cancer risk (for calculation see text). (b) The penetrance of any breast cancer risk gene using the Claus genetic model based on an epidemiological study from which modelling of gene risks was performed.

patches in neurofibromatosis I or Turcot's syndrome, and basal cell naevi in Gorlin's syndrome. Skin tumours, such as the epidermoid cysts seen in FAP (familial adenomatous polyposis), keratoacanthomas seen in the Muir–Torré syndrome, or tricholemmomas of Cowden's syndrome, can be indicators that the individual is very likely to be a gene carrier before confirmation by formal DNA genetic testing.

Discussion of cancer susceptibility and risks

This part of the interview involves communicating to the patient the results of the pedigree assessment, the risk assessment, and clinical examination. If a particular diagnosis is made, then information about that disease is given.

Those attending genetic clinics may have a very rudimentary knowledge of genetics, and it is important that they have a simple explanation of Mendelian genetics and how their risk has been assessed. A simple explanation of how cancer develops as a result of somatic genetic events is also sometimes helpful. In this way, patients may understand more of the information they are given. If they are being given empirical risks then one should offer to explain the method by which these figures are derived.

The first estimation is that of the chance of the familial cluster being due to a genetic predisposition. This is called the prior probability of a genetic predisposition gene being present, an illustration of the determination of which is shown in Figs 2 and 5. Figure 5(a) shows the breast cancer family history or pedigree being considered. The proband seeking risk advice is aged 60 and is unaffected, but has two first-degree relatives with breast cancer aged 45. From Fig. 2, which

shows curves drawn from the Claus model from the CASH study, it can be seen that the chance that two first-degree relatives have been affected with breast cancer at 45 is 60 per cent. The prior probability of a gene being present in this cluster is therefore 60 per cent. The chance that the proband has inherited the gene is therefore half of this, as half the genetic component is inherited from each parent; the prior probability that the proband is susceptible, in other words is a gene carrier, is therefore half of 60 per cent or 30 per cent (0.3; Table 4). Since the chance of not being a carrier (non-susceptible) is 1 minus the chance of being a carrier, then the chance of being non-susceptible (a non-gene carrier) is 1 minus 0.3 which equals 0.7.

The posterior probability in this instance is the chance that someone has inherited the breast cancer-predisposition gene present in the familial cluster, taking into account their position in the family tree and their current status, that is to say the fact that the proband is unaffected at 60 years of age. This is calculated using the penetrance curves. The penetrance curves from the Claus model are shown in Fig. 5(b) and if the proband is susceptible (a gene carrier) then the chance that they are unaffected at 60 years of age is 0.4 (the penetrance curve shows that the chance of developing the disease by the age of 60 is 60 per cent or 0.6, and therefore the chance of being unaffected is 1 – 0.6, or 0.4). If the proband is a non-carrier then the chance of being unaffected at 60 years of age is extremely high as the penetrance is only 4 per cent, hence the chance of being unaffected is 0.96. The posterior probability is the multiplied product of the susceptible column divided by the multiplied product of the non-susceptible column plus the product of the susceptible column. In this example, the posterior probability (best estimate based on available information) of being a gene carrier is 0.15.

This is a simple example of a Bayesian calculation. But such calculations can become very complicated if several generations are involved, or if there are intervening generations of unaffected individuals between affected individuals such as in the pedigree shown in Fig. 1. Laptop risk packages are now available to perform these calculations; however, as they are very model-dependent, knowledge of the problems associated with the models is very important to determine whether the risks are being under- or overestimated. An example is the recent Cyrillic laptop risk package which uses the Claus model, the problem here being that it underestimates the contribution of bilateral breast cancer or ovarian cancer to the overall cancer risk in breast cancer families. This is due to the fact that in this particular model, generated from an epidemiological study, bilateral breast cancer and ovarian cancer were not markers of higher genetic risk. This is now known not to be true from other studies.

If there are no data or the data have elements of uncertainty, then this must also be discussed. Sometimes familial clustering of cancers does not fit any particular syndrome, yet the cancer geneticist has a clinical impression that there may be something unusual occurring. If it is no more than a clinical judgement, then this must be made clear. Having a risk figure is useful for the clinician as this will dictate what management options are available, but it may only be useful to patients if they are put into context, that is to say in relation to the population risk of specific cancers (see above). In particular, the age range at which the greatest risk occurs must be discussed, to facilitate management choices such as the timing of prophylactic surgery or screening programmes.

Discussion of the possibilities for screening and prevention should follow. Suggested screening protocols are shown in Table 5. The

Table 4 Determination of residual risk for patients

	Susceptible	Non-susceptible
Prior probability (from Fig. 2)	0.30	0.70
Disease-free at 60 years	0.40	0.96
Posterior probability	$(0.30 \times 0.40)/(0.3 \times 0.4) + (0.7 \times 0.96) = 0.15$	0.85

i.e. The chance that the proband in Fig. 4(a) has a breast cancer predisposition gene is 15%.

scientific validity of any particular strategy should be explored since not all protocols have been proven to reduce mortality but others are proven. In some instances (e.g. MEN2 and thyroidectomy), prophylactic surgery needs to be discussed, but this must be approached with caution as some patients are frightened or even horrified at the suggestion. They may feel that this is confirmation from the doctor that their risk of cancer is unacceptably high, and may accentuate any fears they may have of the disease and its treatment.

Throughout the interview, it is important to be sensitive to any psychopathology that may be occurring. Frequently, there will have been bereavement due to the premature death of close relatives, particularly if this was a parent or a child. Unresolved bereavement may make it difficult for people to accept their own risks and make decisions about their own management. In addition, patients are sometimes unable to cope with their worries. Referral for formal psychological counselling may resolve these problems. Of particular concern are those individuals who have prophylactic surgery because of excess anxiety but who, while being temporarily relieved, often return at a later date with further cancer phobic symptoms. A psychological assessment and counselling should be strongly suggested before prophylactic mastectomy.

Predictive genetic testing

The number of cancer susceptibilities that have been mapped by genetic linkage is steadily increasing. In theory, direct mutation analysis is now possible for many different cancer-predisposition genes, but many are still performed in research laboratories and will need to be translated into diagnostic genetic laboratories in the next few years (Table 6). The mutation spectra (positions at which alterations have been found in different families) of *BRCA*1 and *BRCA*2 are shown in Fig. 4. This illustrates that the spectrum of alterations in both genes is very wide, unless the individual being tested is from a relatively closed genetic group (such as the Ashkenazi Jewish population). The mutation has to be first identified to ascertain which alteration is responsible for the familial clustering, and this is done by testing an affected individual. Only then can DNA testing be offered to unaffected individuals, as the alteration present in the family is then known. This allows DNA analysis to be carried out and individuals with a susceptibility gene can be identified before the development of the disease (presymptomatic genetic testing). In late-onset genetic disease susceptibilities, there is a consensus view that children (here classified as those aged under 18 years) should not be tested, unless there is to be a therapeutic intervention or change in management. However, some cancer susceptibilities do require

screening during childhood; for instance, screening for familial polyposis coli usually starts in early teenage years by sigmoidoscopy. DNA testing before this time will allow half the individuals to avoid having this invasive procedure. Testing would therefore seem entirely reasonable, particularly as preventive treatment by prophylactic surgery has been demonstrated to be a successful cancer prevention strategy in this disease. The value of testing for other cancer susceptibilities, where the role of screening and prevention is unknown, is more debatable. Many of the issues are relevant to testing for other adult-onset genetic diseases, such as Huntington's chorea where prevention is not possible. It has been demonstrated that using a set protocol for individuals having predictive testing for Huntington's chorea helps to minimize the problems experienced, and allows the individual to have time to decide if they really want the test and for what reason.[40]

There may be many reasons why individuals may wish to have a predictive test. They may want to know if they have the gene before having children, or to make plans for their own future. Some wish to make choices concerning prophylactic surgery or participation in screening or chemoprevention studies.

Facing a high risk of the development of cancer is particularly difficult for some people. Often there have been several deaths from the disease in the family, and since there is often a parent who died when the individual being counselled was in his/her teens, memories can be particularly painful. Since there may already be a great deal of anxiety about the disease, it may be very traumatic to find that the chance of having the gene for early onset of cancer is high. It is therefore recommended that a formal psychological protocol is followed when offering predictive testing for all cancer-predisposition genes.[41]

The genetic testing procedure involves several phases. Initially, the pros and cons and accuracy of the test are explained to the individual. These are the differences a positive and negative test result would make to the cancer risk if the gene being tested is indeed the cause of the cancers in the family, the ending of uncertainty, and the provision of more data on which to base decisions about clinical management and lifestyle. Potential disadvantages are psychological morbidity (although many clients are already very anxious) and the insurance implications. In the United Kingdom, all results of genetic tests currently have to be declared in the same way as any other medical test when seeking insurance. At present, the insurance companies do not actively request that these tests are performed. Following a statement in 1997 from the Association of British Insurers, genetic test results are not taken into account if they are detrimental to a person's insurance position if they are applying for an insurance policy for life coverage or for a mortgage of £100 000 or less.

Table 5 Screening protocols (for guidance only; different clinics may have individual minor alterations for this schema)

Disease	Screen	Age (years) at start of screen/range for screening
von Hippel–Lindau Affected	Annual: physical examination Urine testing Direct ophthalmoscopy Fluorescein angiography 24-h urinary VMA Renal ultrasound 3-yearly: MRI brain scan CT kidneys (more frequent if multiple cysts)	
von Hippel-Lindau At-risk relatives	Annual: physical examination Urine testing Direct ophthalmoscopy Fluorescein angiography 24-h urinary VMA Renal ultrasound 3-yearly: MRI brain scan CT kidneys (more frequent if multiple cysts) 5-yearly: MRI brain scan	5 upwards 5 upwards 10–60 20–65 15–24 20–65 40–60
Familial polyposis	Offer total colectomy with ileorectal anastomosis	Teenager (see below)
Affected	Annual: rectal stump screening (if conserved in surgery) 3-yearly: upper gastrointestinal endoscopy (annually if polyps found)	 20 upwards
Familial polyposis	Offer genetic analysis if possible	11 (polyps are rare before this age)
At-risk relatives	Annual: sigmoidoscopy Perform colonoscopy when polyps found on sigmoidoscopy and arrange colectomy	until 40
Gorlin's syndrome Affected (at-risk children usually have abnormal skull radiographs by 5 years)	Annual: dermatological examination 6-monthly: orthopantomogram for jaw cysts Examination of infants for signs of medulloblatoma (some advocate MRI **but not** CT due to radiosensitivity)	Infants upwards
MEN Type 2	Offer genetic screening if possible, if positive perform prophylactic thyroidectomy Annual: plasma calcium, phosphate, and parathormone Pentagastrin test Thyroid ultrasound Abdominal ultrasound and CT 24-h urinary VMA/blood catecholamines	5 8–70
MEN1	Annual: symptom enquiry (dyspepsia, diarrhoea, renal colic, fits, amenorrhoea, galactorrhoea) Examination Serum calcium Parathormone Renal function Pituitary hormones (PL, GH, ACTH, FSH, TSH) Pancreatic hormones (gastrin, VIP, glucagon, neurotensin, somatostatin, pancreatic polypeptide) Lateral skull radiograph for pituitary size or MRI for pituitary adenomas	5
Wilms' tumour At-risk individuals	3-monthly: renal ultrasound 6-monthly: renal ultrasound	Birth–8 years 8–12

Table 5 *continued*

Disease	Screen	Age (years) at start of screen/range for screening
Retinoblastoma (siblings and offspring of affected)	Offer genetic screening if possible 1-monthly: retinal examination without anaesthetic 3-monthly: retinal examination under anaesthetic 4-monthly: retinal examination under anaesthetic 6-monthly: retinal examination without anaesthetic Annual: retinal examination without anaesthetic Annual examination for sarcoma	 Birth–3 months 3 months–2 years 2–3 years 3–5 years 5–11 years Early teens for life
Li-Fraumeni	Annual: breast examination ?MRI (under investigation) Annual: examination	18–60 Lifelong
NF1 Affected NF2 At-risk relatives	Annual: examination Visual field assessment Offer genetic screening if possible Annual: examination Ophthalmoscopy for congenital cataracts Annual: audiometry Brainstem auditory-evoked potentials 3-yearly: MRI brain	Lifelong Childhood 10–40
Lynch I syndrome	2-yearly: colonoscopy	25 upwards
Lynch II syndrome	2-yearly: colonoscopy Annual: pelvic examination and ovarian and endometrial ultrasound and CA125 Some screen for other cancers in kindreds such as skin and urothelial malignancy Annual: mammography	25 upwards 30 upwards 35 upwards 35 upwards. Its use depends on amount of breast cancer in family
Muir–Torré syndrome	2-yearly: colonoscopy	25 upwards
Turcot's syndrome	2-yearly: colonoscopy	20 upwards
Colon cancer in a single relative aged < 45 years	5-yearly colonoscopy (3-yearly if polyps are found)	35 upwards
Familial melanoma	Annual: skin examination General sun-avoidance advice	Teenager upwards
Breast/ovarian syndrome	Annual: mammography Annual: pelvic examination Transvaginal ultrasound CA125	35 upwards or 5 years younger than youngest case (not less than 25–30) 35 upwards (30 if young ovarian cancer case in family)
Familial breast cancer	Annual: mammography	35 upwards or 5 years younger than youngest case (not less than 25)
Familial ovarian cancer	Annual: pelvic examination Transvaginal ultrasound CA125	30–35 upwards
Familial prostate cancer	Annual: serum prostate-specific antigen Digital rectal examination	50 upwards or 5 years young than youngest case (minimum age 40)
Familial testicular cancer	Regular testicular self examination	Late teens–50

From ref. 10 with permission.

Table 6 Location of and status of testing for cancer predisposition genes

Disease	Location	Mutation analysis available
Breast/ovarian	17q21	BRCA1
Familial breast cancer/male breast cancer	13q12	BRCA2
von Hippel–Lindau	3p25	VHL (research only)
Familial adenomatous polyposis	5q21	APC
Gorlin's syndrome	9q22	PTCH (research only)
Multiple endocrine neoplasia type 2	10q11	RET
Multiple endocrine neoplasia type 1	11q13	MEN1 (research only)
Wilms' tumour	11p13	WT1 (research only)
Retinoblastoma	13q14	RB1
Li–Fraumeni	17p13	TP53
Neurofibromatosis I	17q11	NF1 (research only)
Neurofibromatosis II	22q12	NF2
Lynch syndrome I	2p22	hMLH1
Lynch syndrome II	3p21	hMSH2

In certain circumstances, testing can be advantageous since some individuals in affected families are denied insurance to cover a cancer diagnosis. A negative test in such individuals may enable them to obtain insurance, although then of course, the urgency for the insurance may be removed.

There is a concurrent psychological assessment with the first counselling session. The client is then given a period of reflection (usually a minimum of 1 month) to decide whether or not to have the test; if they decide to proceed, they are seen again to discuss their reasons for wishing to do so. It is only then, and after obtaining written, informed consent, that a blood sample is collected for testing. The disclosure session is carefully planned so that the client knows how long they will have to wait for the result, at the same time they are advised to bring a supportive person to the consultation when the result is given. Following this, they are reviewed at intervals to ensure they are having no psychological problems.

Management of an increased risk of cancer due to a cancer-predisposition gene

In general, management strategies fall into four categories.

Screening

The aim of screening is to provide an earlier diagnosis. Screening strategies may need to be started earlier, be offered more frequently, or be offered for cancer sites where they would not normally be offered to the general population. An example is screening for ovarian cancer which is not usually offered to the general population, but would be offered from the age of 35 annually to a woman with a family history of two first-degree relatives with ovarian cancer at any age (see Table 5).

Chemoprevention

This is the administration of medication to healthy individuals to try to reduce the frequency of the development of cancer (see Chapter 2.5). There are currently several trials of chemoprevention for the common cancers, but no medication has so far been proven to be protective. For example, an American study showed that tamoxifen reduces the incidence of breast cancer in women at increased risk of the disease,[42] but this finding was not replicated in two European trials.[43],[44] The reason for the difference is unknown, although it is possible that the United Kingdom trial consisted of women at a higher genetic risk than the American trial. Whether tamoxifen is less effective in women with a genetic predisposition to breast cancer, rather than a hormonal predisposition, is unknown.

Prophylactic surgery

Prophylactic surgery is already offered routinely in certain syndromes, such as MEN2A where prophylactic thyroidectomy is offered from 5 years of age [45] in gene carriers. In this syndrome, testing is offered to children as it alters their management.

Prophylactic colectomy or colectomy with ileorectal anastomosis is offered to individuals with familial adenomatous polyposis.[46]

The role of prophylactic mastectomy in breast cancer families is more controversial, although early studies suggest a protective effect.[47] However, the proportion of carriers of the breast cancer-predisposition gene was unknown in the series that underwent prophylactic mastectomy.[47] Bilateral oophorectomy reduces breast cancer risk in BRCA1/2 carriers.[49]

Lifestyle changes

There is substantial interest in the interactions between genetic changes and environmental influences. Narod et al.[48] have shown that the oral contraceptive pill reduces the incidence of ovarian cancer in carriers of the breast cancer-predisposition genes BRCA1/2. Studies are in progress to investigate the influence of other changes in lifestyle in carriers of these genes.

Cancer prognosis

There are conflicting data as to whether cancer occurring in a carrier of a cancer-predisposition gene has a different prognosis from sporadic cancers occurring in the general population.

Watson et al.[50] have shown that colon cancers occurring in hereditary, non-polyposis, colorectal cancer patients have a better prognosis. It is postulated that, because the underlying genetic defect is a mismatch repair defect, the tumour cells cannot repair DNA damage induced by therapeutic agents as well as those tumour cells arising in individuals without a mismatch repair defect.

The data for breast cancer in BRCA1 carriers are conflicting. Some studies suggest a worse prognosis.[51] Others suggest no difference.[52]–[54]

Does genetic risk assessment/genetic testing alter cancer management?

The use of cancer risk assessment to alter cancer management is in its infancy, but individuals with a cancer-predisposition gene will be at risk of multiple cancers, either at other sites from the primary or at risk of a new primary. For example, someone with a germline mutation in the BRCA1 gene carries a 64 per cent lifetime risk of developing a second primary breast cancer and a 44 to 60 per cent risk of developing primary ovarian cancer.[6]

Individuals with breast cancer who have a BRCA1 mutation may therefore be considered for bilateral mastectomy and prophylactic oophorectomy. The latter can be part of their overall cancer management as adjuvant treatment[55] and also provides prophylaxis to reduce the risk of ovarian cancer.[56] Furthermore, the recognition of syndromes with an increased tumour incidence after radiation, e.g. Gorlin's syndrome, can provide indications for avoiding this modality.[57]

Cancer genetics is a rapidly expanding subspecialty within oncology. Within the Calman–Hine model of the delivery of cancer services in the United Kingdom, individuals with a family history of cancer can be triaged so that the highest risk individuals who can be offered predictive genetic testing should be seen by a cancer geneticist working closely with the regional genetics service. A knowledge of cancer genetics will be required of every oncologist so that they can apply this to the management of oncological patients whose prognosis, treatment, or risk of further cancers may be altered by the presence of a cancer-predisposition gene.

References

1. Broca PP. *Traites des tumeurs*. Paris: Asselin, 1866.

2. Easton D, Peto J. The contribution of inherited predisposition to cancer incidence. *Cancer Surveys*, 1990; **9**(3): 395–416.

3. Love RR, Evans AM, Josten DM. The accuracy of patient reports of a family history of cancer. *Journal of Chronic Diseases*, 1985; **38**(4): 289–93.

4. Douglas FS, O'Dair LC, Robinson M, Evans DG, Lynch SA. The accuracy of diagnoses as reported in families with cancer: a retrospective study. *Journal of Medical Genetics*, 1999; **36**(4): 309–12.

5. Bülow S. Familial adenomatous polyposis. *Annals of Medicine*, 1989; **21**(4): 299–307.

6. Ford D et al. Genetic heterogeneity and penetrance analysis of the BRCA1 and BRCA2 genes in breast cancer families. The Breast Cancer Linkage Consortium. *American Journal of Human Genetics*, 1998; **62**(3): 676–89.

7. Thorlacius S et al. Study of a single BRCA2 mutation with high carrier frequency in a small population. *American Journal of Human Genetics*, 1997; **60**(5): 1079–84.

8. Neuhausen S et al. Recurrent BRCA2 6174delT mutations in Ashkenazi Jewish women affected by breast cancer. *Nature Genetics*, 1996; **13**(1): 126–8.

9. Tonin P et al. Frequency of recurrent BRCA1 and BRCA2 mutations in Ashkenazi Jewish breast cancer families. *Nature Medicine*, 1996; **2**(11): 1179–83.

10. Eeles RA, Ponder BAJ, Easton DF and Horwich A (ed.). *Genetic predisposition to cancer*. London: Chapman and Hall, 1996.

11. Knudson AG, Jr. Hereditary cancer, oncogenes, and antioncogenes. *Cancer Research*, 1985; **45**(4): 1437–43.

12. Mulligan LM, Gardner E, Smith BA, Mathew CG, Ponder BA. Genetic events in tumour initiation and progression in multiple endocrine neoplasia type 2. *Genes Chromosomes and Cancer*, 1993; **6**(3): 166–77.

13. Zbar B, Lerman, M. Inherited carcinomas of the kidney. *Advances in Cancer Research*, 1998; **75**: 163–201.

14. Kinzler KW, Vogelstein B. Cancer-susceptibility genes. Gatekeepers and caretakers. *Nature*, 1997; **386**(6627): 761–3.

15. Bodmer WF et al. Localization of the gene for familial adenomatous polyposis on chromosome 5. *Nature*, 1987; **328**(6131): 614–16.

16. Feigelson HS et al. A polymorphism in the CYP17 gene increases the risk of breast cancer. *Cancer Research*, 1997; **57**: 1063–5.

17. Claus EB, Risch N, Thompson WD. Genetic analysis of breast cancer in the cancer and steroid hormone study. *American Journal of Human Genetics*, 1991; **48**(2): 232–42.

18. Langston AA, Malone KE, Thompson JD, Daling JR, Ostrander EA. BRCA1 mutations in a population-based sample of young women with breast cancer. *New England Journal of Medicine*, 1996; **334**(3): 137–42.

19. Shattuck-Eidens ED et al. A collaborative survey of 80 mutations in the BRCA1 breast and ovarian cancer susceptibility gene. Implications for presymptomatic testing and screening. *Journal of the American Medical Association*, 1995; **273**(7): 535–41.

20. Shattuck-Eidens ED et al. BRCA1 sequence analysis in women at high risk for susceptibility mutations. Risk factor analysis and implications for genetic testing. *Journal of the American Medical Association*, 1997; **278**(15): 1242–50.

21. Ford D, Easton, DF, Peto J. Estimates of the gene frequency of BRCA1 and its contribution to breast and ovarian cancer incidence. *American Journal of Human Genetics*, 1995; **57**(6): 1457–62.

22. Mitchell, G and Eeles RA. Cancer Topics, 1999; **11**: 1–7.

23. Gayther S et al. Variation of risks of breast and ovarian cancer associated with different germline mutations of the BRCA2 gene. *Nature Genetics*, 1997; **15**: 103–5.

24. Harper PS. *Practical genetic counselling*, 3rd edn. Wright, Butterworth, 1988.

25. Croyle RT, Sun YC, Louie DH. Psychological minimization of cholesterol test results: moderators of appraisal in college students and community residents. *Health Psychology*, 1993; **12**(6): 503–7.

26. Kelly PT. Informational needs of individuals and families with hereditary cancers. *Seminars in Oncology Nursing*, 1992; **8**(4): 288–92.

27. Evans DG, Burnell LD, Hopwood P, Howell A. Perception of risk in

women with a family history of breast cancer. *British Journal of Cancer.* 1993; **67**(3): 612–14.

28. **Lloyd S** *et al.* Familial breast cancer: a controlled study of risk perception, psychological morbidity and health beliefs in women attending for genetic counselling. *British Journal of Cancer,* 1996; **74**(3): 482–7.

29. **Green CH, Brown RA.** Counting lives. *Journal of Occupational Accidents.* 1978; **2**: 55.

30. **Sorensen JR, Swazey JP, Scotch NA.** Reproductive past, reproductive futures: genetic counselling and its effectiveness. *Birth defects: original article series.* New York: Alan Liss, 1981; 1–17.

31. **Leonard CO, Chase GA, Childs B.** Genetic counselling: a consumers' view. *New England Journal of Medicine.* 1972; **287**(9): 433–9.

32. **Josten DM, Evans AM, Love RR.** The cancer prevention clinic: a service program for cancer-prone families. *Journal of Psychosocial Oncology,* 1985; **3**: 5–20.

33. **Merz JF, Fisdhoff B.** Informed consent does not mean rational consent. *Journal of Legal Medicine,* 1990; **11**: 321–50.

34. **Lerman C, Daly M, Masny A, Balshem A.** Attitudes about genetic testing for breast-ovarian cancer susceptibility. *Journal of Clinical Oncology,* 1994; **12**(4): 843–50.

35. **Guedeney C, Mendel G.** *L'Angoisse Atomique et les Centres Nucleaires.* Paris: Payot, 1973.

36. **Ardern-Jones A.** Living with a cancer legacy the experience of hereditary cancer in the family. 1998; Institute of Cancer Research, London University, MSc thesis.

37. **Vlek C.** Risk assessment, risk perception and decision making about courses of action involving genetic risk: an overview of concepts and methods. *Birth Defects Original Article Series,* 1987; **23**(2): 171–207.

38. **Kash KM, Holland JC, Halper MS, Miller DG.** Psychological distress and surveillance behaviors of women with a family history of breast cancer. *Journal of the National Cancer Institute.* 1991; **84**(1): 24–30.

39. **McNeil BJ, Pauker SG, Sox-HC J, Tversky A.** On the elicitation of preferences for alternative therapies. *New England Journal of Medicine,* 1982; **306**(21): 1259–62.

40. **Tyler A, Ball D, Craufurd D.** Presymptomatic testing for Huntington's disease in the United Kingdom. The United Kingdom Huntington's Disease Prediction Consortium. *British Medical Journal,* 1992; **304**(6842): 1593–6.

41. **Watson M** *et al.* Psychosocial impact of testing (by linkage) for the *BRCA1* breast cancer gene: an investigation of two families in the research setting. *Psycho-Oncology,* 1996; **5**: 233–9.

42. **Fisher B** *et al.* Tamoxifen and chemotherapy for lymph node-negative, estrogen receptor-positive breast cancer. *Journal of the National Cancer Institute,* 1997; **89**(22): 1673–82.

43. **Veronesi U** *et al.* Prevention of breast cancer with tamoxifen: preliminary findings from the Italian randomised trial among hysterectomised women. Italian Tamoxifen Prevention Study. *Lancet,* 1998; **352**(9122): 93–7.

44. **Powles T** *et al.* Interim analysis of the incidence of breast cancer in the Royal Marsden Hospital tamoxifen randomised chemoprevention trial. *Lancet,* 1998; **352**(9122): 98–101.

45. **Lallier M** *et al.* Prophylactic thyroidectomy for medullary thyroid carcinoma in gene carriers of MEN2 syndrome. *Journal of Pediatric Surgery,* 1998; **33**(6): 846–8.

46. **Nyam DC** *et al.* Ileal pouch–anal canal anastomosis for familial adenomatous polyposis: early and late results. *Ann Surgery,* 1997; **226**(4): 514–19.

47. **Hartmann LC** *et al.* Efficacy of bilateral prophylactic mastectomy in women with a family history of breast cancer. *New England Journal of Medicine,* 1999; **340**(2): 77–84.

48. **Narod SA** *et al.* Oral contraceptives and the risk of hereditary ovarian cancer. Hereditary Ovarian Cancer Clinical Study Group. *New England Journal of Medicine,* 1998; **339**: 424–8.

49. **Rebbeck T** *et al.* Breast cancer risk after bilateral prophylactic oophorectomy in BRCA1 mutation carriers. *Journal of the National Cancer Institute* 1999; **91**: 1475–9.

50. **Watson P** *et al.* Colorectal carcinoma survival among hereditary nonpolyposis colorectal carcinoma family members. *Cancer,* 1998; **83**(2): 259–66.

51. **Johannsson OT, Ranstam J, Borg A, Olsson H.** Survival of BRCA1 breast and ovarian cancer patients: a population-based study from southern Sweden. *Journal of Clinical Oncology,* 1998; **16**(2): 397–404.

52. **Foulkes WD, Wong N, Rozen F, Brunet JS, Narod SA.** Survival of patients with breast cancer and BRCA1 mutations. *Lancet,* 1998; **351**(9112): 1359–60. [Letter]

53. **Verhoog LC** *et al.* Survival and tumour characteristics of breast-cancer patients with germline mutations of *BRCA1. Lancet,* 1998; **351**(9099): 316–21.

54. **Lee JS** *et al.* Survival after breast cancer in Ashkenazi Jewish BRCA1 and BRCA2 mutation carriers. *Journal of the National Cancer Institute,* 1999; **91**(3): 259–63.

55. **Early Breast Cancer Trialists' Collaborative Group** Systemic treatment of early breast cancer by hormonal, cytotoxic, or immune therapy. 133 randomised trials involving 31,000 recurrences and 24,000 deaths among 75,000 women. *Lancet,* 1992; **339**(8784): 1–15.

56. **Struewing JP** *et al.* Prophylactic oophorectomy in inherited breast/ ovarian cancer families. *Journal of the National Cancer Institute Monograms,* 1995; **17**: 33–5.

57. **O'Malley S, Weitman D, Olding M, Sekhar L.** Multiple neoplasms following craniospinal irradiation for medulloblastoma in a patient with nevoid basal cell carcinoma syndrome. *Journal of Neurosurgery,* 1997; **86**(2): 286–8.

1.4 Growth factors and cell signalling

Paolo M. Comoglio and Carla Boccaccio

Introduction

In a pluricellular organism, cells form tissues that maintain size, structure, and function appropriate to the organism as a whole. An extensive control-signalling network co-ordinates activities of every single cell, such as metabolism, movement, proliferation, differentiation, and death. These signals include proteins secreted by other cells—which diffuse freely in the extracellular environment—as well as membrane-bound macromolecules and components of the extracellular matrix. Due to their chemical nature, signals from proteins are transmitted across the plasma membrane by binding and activating transmembrane receptors.

Stimulation of cell growth and differentiation—functions that alter at the time of malignant transformation—mostly occurs via extracellular signals known as growth factors and cytokines. Growth factors are high affinity ligands for transmembrane receptors belonging to the family of receptor tyrosine kinases (RTK) and will be described in this chapter together with factors that inhibit proliferation and favour differentiation (the transforming growth factor-β family) via receptors endowed with serine–threonine kinase activity. Cytokine receptors that are involved in control of the haematopoietic system are described in Chapter 15.1.

The kinase activity of growth factor receptors is strictly regulated and is usually inhibited under basal conditions. Binding of a growth factor to the extracellular domain of the receptor removes this inhibition and triggers a biochemical signalling cascade inside the cytoplasm. The cell reacts with immediate (minutes) and late (hours/days) responses that affect both its structure and functions. These include transient modifications as well as dramatic and/or irreversible changes, sustained by expression of previously quiescent genes and *de novo* protein synthesis, necessary for cell differentiation and proliferation.

Growth factors affect the function of the 'cell cycle clock', a mechanism made up of nuclear regulators called cyclins, cyclin-dependent kinases, and cyclin inhibitors, that control the passage through the critical 'restriction point' towards DNA duplication and cell division (see Chapter 1.6). Growth factors stimulate cyclin expression to drive DNA synthesis. However, they can also block growth, by stimulating the expression of cyclin inhibitors, thus favouring the exit of the cell from the proliferation cycle and promoting differentiation. Cell cycle control is intimately connected with regulation of cell death. When DNA duplication is incorrect, or DNA is damaged, a replicating cell is programmed to 'commit suicide' to prevent transmission of genetic errors to its progeny. Growth factors can interfere with this process.

Signal transduction is the entire process that controls the flow of information from an extracellular signal across the plasma membrane and cytoplasm to the cell nucleus where gene transcription and DNA duplication are controlled. Many growth factors, their receptors, and the intracellular proteins mediating signal transduction are products of proto-oncogenes,[†] also known as cellular oncogenes. Their mutated, or aberrantly expressed counterparts—called 'activated' oncogenes—can induce neoplastic transformation *in vitro* and contribute to onset and progression of human tumours (see Chapter 1.2).

This chapter will focus on the physiological functions of growth regulating molecules to reveal how cancer may arise from the inappropriate activation of processes which—under physiological conditions—regulate life and death of normal cells.

Growth factors

Most growth factors in their mature form are soluble polypeptides. Some notable exceptions, such as ephrins, are transmembrane proteins (Table 1). They are usually small, having a molecular weight typically between 5 and 30 kDa and often derive from inactive precursors via a proteolytic cleavage. Precursors can be either larger transmembrane proteins or soluble polypeptides. In some cases, single genes (such as those for neuregulins type 1 and 2) encode for a number of different splice variants (i.e. polypeptides encoded by different segments of the same gene), producing molecules with slightly different specificities. The discovery of an increasing number of growth factors has allowed identification of families that bind, with a certain degree of promiscuity, to matching families of receptors.

Cells that produce growth factors do not form specific tissues or organs, such as the endocrine glands that secrete polypeptide hormones. Often they are interspersed in tissues in close contact with cells expressing the corresponding receptors. Thus, growth factors released into the extracellular space rapidly find their targets, and so acting in a 'paracrine' manner. However, like hormones, they are also found circulating in the blood and reach organs far from their source (Fig. 1).

Sometimes cells producing a growth factor also express its specific receptor. This condition, which allows for autocrine stimulation, although known to occur under physiological conditions (e.g. production of interleukins by lymphocytes) can be responsible for uncontrolled self-stimulation of cells to proliferate and for tumorigenesis. Autocrine loops associated with neoplastic transformation have been found involving platelet derived growth factor (PDGF) and fibroblast growth factor (FGF). A homologue of the PDGF-B chain is encoded

Table 1 Structure and biological activities of growth factors coupled to RTKs

Growth factor (GF)	Structure	Activity	Receptor (R)
EGF (epidermal GF)	Soluble 6 kDa protein results from cleavage of a 130 kDa transmembrane active precursor	Mitogenic for epithelial cells	EGFR (ErbB-1)
TGF-α (transforming GF-α)	Soluble 6 kDa protein results from proteolytic cleavage of a 25 kDa palmitoylated precursor	Mitogenic for epithelial cells	EGFR (ErbB-1)
Amphiregulin	14–22 kDa glycoproteins	Mitogenic	EGFR (ErbB-1)
HB-EGF (heparin binding-EGF)	14–20 kDa soluble proteins derived from proteolytic cleavage of a transmembrane precursor	Mitogenic, chemoattractant	EGFR/ErbB-4
Betacellulin	32 kDa soluble glycoprotein derived from proteolytic cleavage of a membrane-bound precursor	Mitogenic for pancreatic and breast cells	EGFR/ErbB-4
Nrg-1 (neuregulins 1), incl. NDF (neu differentiation factor), ARIA (acetylcholine receptor inducing activity), heregulin, and GGF (glail growth factor); Nrg-2	*NRG1* gene encodes at least 12 splice-variants isoforms; mature factors are 42–59 kDa glycoproteins derived from proteolytic cleavage of membrane-bound precursors	Mammary gland morphogenesis, heart, glia, and nervous system development	ErbB-3/ErbB-4
IGF-1 (insulin-like GF-1), insulin	7.5 kDa single chain secreted peptides	Cell proliferation, differentiation, and survival	Insulin R/IGF-1R
PDGF (platelet derived growth factor) -AA, -AB, -BB	30 kDa disulpide bonded homo/heterodimers; proteolytic processing of prepropeptides to give 16–18 kDa (PDGF-A) and 12 kDa (PDGF-B) mature forms	Chemotaxis, mitogenesis	PDGFR-α/PDGFR-β
SCF (stem cell growth factor)	31–36 kDa glycoproteins; transmembrane and proteolytically cleaved soluble forms	Proliferation, differentiation, migration, and survival of haemopoietic, melanogenic, and gametogenic cells	Kit
CSF-1 (colony stimulating factor-1)	70–90 kDa homodimeric glycoprotein; transmembrane and proteolytically cleaved soluble forms	Proliferation of macrophage/monocyte lineage; embryo implantation	Fms
Flt-3L	Transmembrane form and soluble 30 kDa disulphide-linked heterodimer	Proliferation/survival of haemopoietic progenitor cells	Flt-3
FGF (fibroblast GF) 1–9	17–30 kDa single chain secreted glycoproteins; soluble and proteoglycan associated	Mitogenic, neurotrophic, angiogenic	FGFR1–4
VEGF (vascular endothelial GF) -A, -B, -C	35–45 kDa homo/heterodimeric glycoproteins; heparin proteoglycan binding isoforms	Mitogenic and morphogenic for endothelial cells	VEGFR1–3
Angiopoietin	70 kDa glycoprotein	Assembly of non-endothelial wall components	Tie-2
HGF (hepatocyte GF)	Secreted inactive single chain precursor transformed by proteolytic cleavage in an active disulphide-linked heterodimers (30 + 60 kDa)	Mitogen, motogen, and morphogen for epithelia, endothelia, and mesenchymal cells	Met
MSP (macrophage stimulating protein)	Secreted inactive precursor cleaved in an active, two-chains dimer (25 + 45 kDa)	As above	Ron
GDNF (glial-derived neurotrophic factor)	20 kDa disulphide-linked homodimer	Survival factor for epithelial and neuronal cells	GDNFR/Ret complex
NGF (nerve GF), BDNF (brain-derived neurotrophic factor), NT (neurotrophin) -3, -4, -5	15–25 kDa active homodimers derived from inactive precursors	Mitogen, differentiative, and survival factors for neurones	Trk A-B-C
Ephrin A1–5	21–28 kDa soluble and GPI-linked forms	Axon guidance and repelling cues in the neuronal development	Eph A1–8
Ephrin B1–3	34 kDa transmembrane proteins	As above	Eph B1–6
Gas6	75 kDa secreted protein	Mitogenic and survival factor for haematopoietic and nervous cells	Axl/Sky

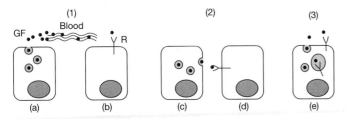

Fig. 1 How polypeptide growth factors (GF) reach their receptors (R). (1) represents endocrine secretion, typical of hormones, in which cell A releases a factor into the blood circulation, thus allowing it to reach distant cells (B); (2) represents paracrine stimulation, the most common among growth factors, in which a cell (C) secretes the polypeptide in the extracellular environment, where it binds an adjacent cell (D), usually of a different type; (3) represents autocrine stimulation, in which the same cell (E) expresses the growth factor and its receptor. Encounters between the two molecules can take place either outside or (very rarely) inside the cell, during protein synthesis (intracrine stimulation). Autocrine stimulation is mostly pathological and can contribute to cellular transformation.

by the viral oncogene v-*sis* of the simian sarcoma virus; the virus infects cells expressing the PDGF receptor, causing them to concomitantly produce its ligand. Here, interaction between a growth factor and its receptor can also take place inside the cell, provoking further generation of the growth signal.[1] Members of the FGF family (FGF3, known also as Int-2, FGF-4, known also as Hst, and FGF-8) can be aberrantly expressed as a consequence of proviral insertion of the mouse mammary tumour virus. Autocrine loops are thus generated, contributing to the development of breast tumours in affected mice.[2]

Transcription of genes encoding growth factors, their synthesis, and release may be constitutive or regulated by a number of specific signals (growth factors, cytokines, and hormones) that are still poorly understood. However, responsiveness to growth factors is mostly controlled at the target level, since the cells modulate the expression of the specific receptors. An additional level of control relies on the possibility of converting an inactive growth factor precursor into an active one by proteolytic cleavage at the surface of the target cell, as in the case of hepatocyte growth factor (HGF) (Fig. 2).[3]

Every cell type usually expresses a variety of growth factor receptors, and biological responses are the result of a combination of multiple, concomitant, and sequential stimuli. Induction of mitosis is (at least) a two-step process where quiescent cells (resting in the so-called G0 phase of the cell cycle) must first be recruited into the early G1 phase by 'competence' factors (such as PDGF). Later, the cells are induced to complete the preparatory phase and to start DNA synthesis (entering the S phase) by 'progression' factors such as epidermal growth factor (EGF) or insulin-like growth factor-1 (IGF-1). The relationship between growth factor signalling and progression during the cell cycle is described in detail in Chapter 1.5.

The attempt to assign a specific, restricted, and invariant biological response to every growth factor has failed. It has emerged that the same molecule can elicit profoundly different effects, such as proliferation and differentiation. The response depends on the target cell type and/or on the intensity and the duration of the stimulus.[4],[5] However, receptor binding to growth factor is both selective and high-affinity, indicating that the identity of the signal must be preserved when it crosses the plasma membrane.

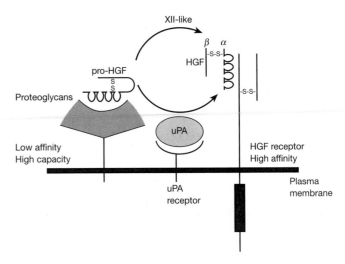

Fig. 2 Activation of HGF single-chain precursor at the cell surface. Biologically inactive pro-HGF is bound to heparan-sulphate proteoglycans that form a low affinity and high capacity reservoir. Urokinase-type plasminogen activator, bound to its specific transmembrane receptor, performs proteolytic cleavage transforming pro-HGF into the active α-β disulphide-linked heterodimer. This binds and activates its high-affinity tyrosine kinase receptor. Proteolytic conversion of pro-HGF into the active form is performed also by a factor homologous to coagulation factor XII (XII-like) circulating in the blood.

Receptor tyrosine kinases (RTKs) are built in functional modules

Growth factor receptors are protein tyrosine kinases that form a super-family sharing common basic structures (Fig. 3(a)): they encompass an N-terminal extracellular moiety, a single hydrophobic region spanning the plasma membrane, and a cytoplasmic domain endowed with regulatory and catalytic tyrosine kinase activity. A single polypeptide chain forms most of the known receptors. Exceptions are the sub-families of the insulin receptor (tetrameric) and of the HGF receptor (dimeric).

Schematically, RTKs are organized into five functional domains:

1. The **extracellular domain**, containing the high-affinity binding site for the growth factor. It encompasses some hundreds of amino acids, including glycosylation sites, cysteine residues (responsible for protein folding), and distinctive structural motifs.

2. The **transmembrane domain**, invariably containing about 25 hydrophobic residues embedded in the membrane lipid bilayer.

3. The **juxtamembrane domain** located in the cytoplasm, which starts with several basic amino acid residues, functioning as a stop-transfer signal during receptor protein synthesis and membrane localization. It includes about 50 amino acids and is endowed with important regulatory functions.

4. The **catalytic domain**, responsible for tyrosine kinase activity. It is composed of about 250 amino acids and, in some cases, is split into two subdomains by a non-catalytic regulatory region.

5. The **C-terminal tail**, including up to 200 amino acid residues; its length and function are variable in different receptors. This segment binds intracellular signal transducers after receptor activation.

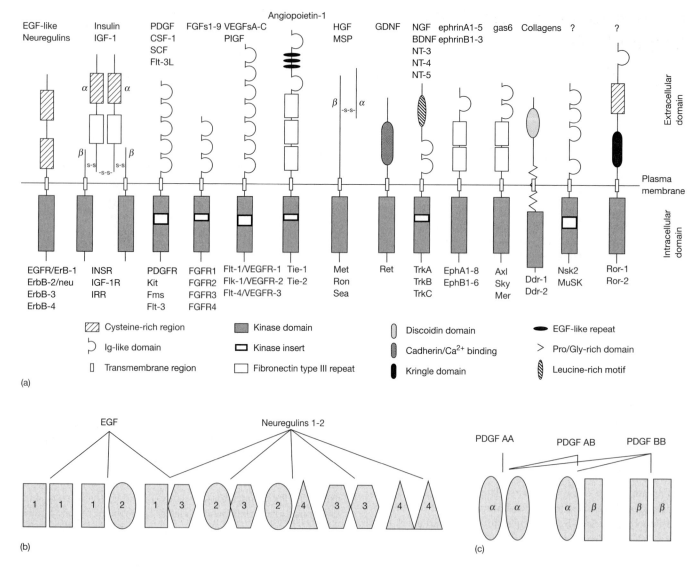

Fig. 3 (a) Receptor tyrosine kinases are classified into families according to the structural features of the extracellular domain that contains various combinations of protein motifs. Representative members for each subfamily are indicated, together with their corresponding ligands. For a detailed description see text. (b) Dimers formed by members of the epidermal growth factor receptor family (1: ErbB1; 2: ErbB2; 3: ErbB3; 4: ErbB4, following binding of ligands of the epidermal growth factor family (EGF and neuregulins). (c) Dimers formed by the two members, α and β, of the platelet-derived growth factor receptor family, following binding by different types of platelet-derived growth factors (PDGF AA, AB or BB).

Members of the tyrosine kinase receptor super-family share high homology in their transmembrane and catalytic domains. On the contrary, extracellular domains are very different and show various combinations of structural motifs. On the basis of these features, receptors can be grouped into families (Fig. 3(a)), in which members share similar patterns of extracellular structural motifs and a high degree of homology in the catalytic domain. These extracellular motifs have two basic functions. Some participate in the formation of complex tridimensional configurations to ensure binding site stability and specificity for growth factors. Other motifs mediate receptor dimerization, which is critical for kinase activation and signal transduction (see later). Moreover, in some instances, the extracellular domain mediates low-affinity interactions with other molecules present on the cell surface or in the extracellular matrix that can modulate receptor binding.[6]

Every receptor family has a corresponding growth factor family (Table 1 and Fig. 3(a)). As a rule, every receptor binds with high affinity to one single factor. There are, however, exceptions: some receptors bind more than one structurally related factor and some factors can bind different members of the same receptor family. Simultaneous ligand binding by two different receptor types is one of the possible mechanisms leading to formation of receptor heterodimers within the same family.[7]

The extracellular domain identifies receptor families

The epidermal growth factor receptor (EGF) family is characterized by two cysteine-rich regions in the extracellular domain (Fig. 3(a)). The cysteine residues form a number of disulphide bridges surrounding and stabilizing the tridimensional structure of the binding site. This family includes at least four members: the EGF receptor or ErbB-1 (mol. wt. 175 kDa), ErbB-2/neu, ErbB-3, and ErbB-4, which are expressed by cells of epithelial, mesenchymal, or glial origin. These receptors bind mitogenic factors belonging to the EGF and to the neuregulin families. The first includes EGF itself, a soluble peptide of 53 amino acids, TGF-α (transforming growth factor-α), amphiregulin, HB-EGF (heparin binding-EGF), and betacellulin. The second family includes the splice-variant proteins encoded by the NRG1 gene (heregulins, neu differentiation factor (NDF), acetylcholine receptor inducing activity (ARIA), glial growth factor (GGF), and others) and by the recently discovered NRG2 gene. The EGF-like factors bind directly to the EGFR/ErbB-1, but recruit the other receptor family members, promoting formation of EGFR homodimers or heterodimers with ErbB-2, or -3, or -4. Neuregulins bind directly ErbB-3 or -4 and recruit ErbB-1 and -2 as coreceptors, resulting again in homo- or heterodimers (Fig. 3(b)).[7],[8] These receptors, in particular EGFR and ErbB-2, have been found amplified and overexpressed in various tumours, including gliomas and breast and ovarian carcinomas.[9],[10] In experimental animal models, a point mutation in the transmembrane domain of ErbB-2 (also known as the product of the neu oncogene) leads to uncontrolled activation of the receptor kinase and is associated with tumours of the nervous tissues.[11]

The insulin receptor is the prototype of a family of tetrameric receptors, including the insulin-like growth factor-1 (IGF-1) receptor, the insulin-receptor related (IRR), and the product of the ROS gene. They are composed of two extracellular α chains bound to each other by disulphide links; every α chain (about 125 kDa) is covalently linked to a β chain (about 80 kDa) that crosses the plasma membrane and contains the tyrosine kinase domain (Fig. 3(a)). The α and the β chains are encoded by a single gene and are synthesized as a single precursor that undergoes proteolytic cleavage after formation of the interchain disulphide bonds. The extracellular domains of the whole family contain cysteine-rich regions, similar to those of the EGF receptors, and regions of homology with fibronectin III (an extracellular matrix protein) (Fig. 3(a)). The insulin receptor mediates mostly metabolic effects; the IGF-1 receptor, which binds insulin-like growth factor-1 with high affinity and insulin with lower affinity, transduces mitogenic stimuli.

The platelet-derived growth factor (PDGF) receptor is a member of a family characterized by extracellular domains encompassing five homology regions with the immunoglobulin loops (Ig) (Fig. 3(a)). There are two similar forms of PDGF receptor, named α and β (both 180 kDa). PDGF is a polypeptide formed by two chains, A (17 kDa) and B (16 kDa), covalently linked as homo- as well as heterodimers. Both chains bind the PDGF receptor. Since the A chain binds only the α receptor type, and the B chain binds both α and β, PDGF AA can induce only α receptor homodimers, while PDGF AB induces both α–β heterodimers and α homodimers. PDGF BB induces all three dimer combinations (Fig. 3(c)). PDGF is a powerful mitogen for a number of cell types, mainly of mesenchymal origin, and can

elicit effects on the cytoskeleton leading to cell movement through its β receptor isoform.[12] A fusion protein between the cytoplasmic domain of the PDGF receptor β and a dimerizing motif encoded by a gene named TEL is found as the product of the t(5;12) translocation in patients with chronic myelomonocytic leukaemia.[13]

The PDGFR family also includes the products of the proto-oncogenes KIT, FMS, and FLT-3. KIT encodes the receptor for SCF (stem cell growth factor), known also as Steel factor, that plays a key role in the development of haematopoietic cells, melanocytes, and germlines.[14] Cases of mastocytosis and myelodysplastic haematological disorders bear a point mutation in the catalytic domain of the Kit tyrosine kinase. Families with germline mutations of KIT develop stromal gastrointestinal tumours.[15],[16] FMS encodes the receptor for CSF-1 (colony stimulating factor-1); the product of FLT-3 is the receptor of a ligand (Flt-3L) that is involved in regulation of haematopoiesis. Mutations of FMS have been found in patients with myelodysplastic syndrome.[17]

The fibroblast growth factor (FGF) receptor family members are characterized by three extracellular regions (IgI–III), again homologous with the immunoglobulin loops (Fig. 3(a)). The IgI domain is separated from the IgII by a sequence rich in acidic residues. Four homologous receptors encoded by different genes are known: FGFR-1, -2, -3, and -4 (each about 100 kDa). Moreover, additional forms of FGFR-1 and -2 result from alternative splicing of the exons which encode the extracellular domain. These variants may contain different sequences in the IgIII loop (IIIa, -b, or -c) that are critical to determine binding specificity to the different members of the fibroblast growth factor family. The acidic FGF (aFGF or FGF-1) binds with high affinity both FGFR-1 and -2 either containing IIIb- or IIIc-type sequences. The basic FGF (bFGF or FGF-2) is a quite specific ligand for receptors containing IgIIIc-type sequences. KGF (keratinocyte growth factor) is a specific ligand for FGFR-2, containing IgIIIb-type sequences. FGF-3 (encoded by the INT-2 oncogene), FGF-4 (encoded by the HST oncogene), and FGF-5 to -9 are other members of this family. The matching receptors for these ligands are still unclear.[18],[19] Biological responses to FGF receptors, observed in a wide variety of cell types, include proliferation, motility, and angiogenesis.[20]

The members of the vascular-endothelial growth factor (VEGF) receptor family are characterized by the presence of seven Ig-like domains in the extracellular domain, similar to those found in PDGF and FGF receptors (Fig. 3(a)). Three members have been identified (about 200 kDa): VEGFR-1 (known also as Flt-1), VEGFR-2 (also called Flk-1 or KDR), and VEGFR-3 (or Flt-4). Angioblasts and endothelial cells specifically express these receptors that mediate mitogenic and morphogenic signals required for blood vessel formation. VEGFR-2 plays a key role during the early developmental stages of the primary vascular plexus (vasculogenesis), whereas VEGFR-1 and other receptors intervene later, during formation of new capillaries in a process called angiogenesis.[21] The ability to form new vessels is critical for a tumour mass to receive nourishment, survive, and expand, and is currently under intense investigation as a key target for cancer therapy[22] (see Chapter 1.8). At present, four ligands for the VEGF receptors have been isolated: vascular endothelial growth factor A (VEGF-A), -B, -C, and placental growth factor (PlGF). These are all dimeric glycoproteins that display high amino acid similarity with PDGF. VEGF-A binds to VEGFR-1 and -2, VEGF-C to VEGFR-2 and -3, PlGF is specific for VEGFR-1, while VEGF-B is likely to be the ligand for still unknown receptors.[23]

Another family of receptors specifically involved in blood vessel formation includes the tyrosine kinases encoded by TIE-1 and TIE-2/TEK. The extracellular domain of these molecules contains a combination of Ig-like regions, fibronectin III repeats, and EGF homology motifs (Fig. 3(a)). The ligand of Tie-2 is angiopoietin-1, a regulator of assembly of non-endothelial components of blood vessel walls.[24]

The hepatocyte growth factor (HGF) receptor is encoded by the MET proto-oncogene. It is the prototype of a family of heterodimeric proteins, formed by an extracellular α chain (50 kDa) and a transmembrane β chain (150 kDa), linked by disulphide bonds (Fig. 3(a)). The α–β chains derive from proteolytic cleavage of a single precursor (190 kDa), encoded by a single transcript. The ligand, HGF, compared to other growth factors, is a relatively large and complex molecule formed by two disulphide-linked chains (α and β). The α chain (30 kDa) shares high homology with the blood clotting cascade enzymes and contains the binding site for the receptor. The β chain (60 kDa) is homologous to the serine proteases, but lacks enzymatic activity. The mature form of HGF derives from a single-chain inactive precursor that is ubiquitously present in the extracellular matrix. Conversion to the active form takes place at the cell surface following proteolytic cleavage catalysed by the urokinase-type plasminogen activator. There is a second pro-HGF-converting enzyme in serum, homologous to coagulation factor XII (Fig. 2). HGF, known also as scatter factor, exerts pleiotropic responses: it stimulates 'invasive growth' (a process that combines proliferation and active migration across the extracellular matrix) of a number of cell types, among which are epithelia, endothelia, osteoblasts, myoblasts, and erythroid precursors.[25] This receptor family encompasses another two members, encoded by the RON and sea proto-oncogenes. The Ron ligand is macrophage stimulating protein (MSP), which is similar in structure and biological functions to HGF. The Sea ligand has yet to be identified. The MET oncogene is affected by point mutations in the intracellular catalytic domain in hereditary and sporadic papillary kidney cancers.[26] Moreover, it is overexpressed in a number of carcinomas of the thyroid, the ovary, and gastrointestinal tract, and it is amplified in their liver metastases.[27],[28]

The RET oncogene encodes a receptor characterized by the presence of a rather short extracellular domain containing a homology region with the intercellular adhesion molecule cadherin (Fig. 3(a)). Under physiological conditions, the Ret tyrosine kinase is activated by a peculiar mechanism: the glial-derived neurotrophic factor (GDNF) binds with high affinity to a receptor that is linked to the plasma membrane only with a lipid sequence (glycosylphosphatidyl-inositol (GPI)). The complex between GDNF and its GPI-linked receptor recruits the transmembrane Ret and activates intracellular signal transduction.[29] RET is responsible for hereditary autosomal dominant cancer syndromes, the multiple endocrine neoplasia (MEN 2A and 2B), and familial medullary thyroid carcinomas.[30] Germline mutations found in MEN affect cysteine residues in the extracellular domain as well as intracellular residues that cause receptor activation and signal transduction in the absence of the ligand. Inactivating mutations of Ret are responsible for the congenital Hirschprung disease, caused by incomplete development of gut innervation.[31] In sporadic papillary thyroid carcinomas, somatic rearrangements have been found in which the Ret intracellular domain is fused with

cytoplasmic proteins capable of inducing constitutive dimerization and kinase activation.[32]

The nerve growth factor (NGF) receptor family includes the tyrosine kinases encoded by the three related genes: TRK-A, -B, and -C (each about 145 kDa). They are characterized by an extracellular domain containing an N-terminal leucin-rich domain and two Ig-like loops (Fig. 3(a)). The NGF receptor family includes the high affinity receptors for the so-called neurotrophins (NGF, neurotrophin (NT)-3, -4, -5, and brain-derived neurotrophic factor (BDNF)), that play a key role in growth, differentiation, and survival of neurones and are mitogenic for some non-nervous cells.[33] Trk-A mediates the effects of NGF, Trk-B is a receptor for BDNF and NT-4 /-5, and Trk-C is a receptor for NT-3. Interestingly, in neural cancer cells, Trk-A and -C may have a tumour-suppressor effect, by induction of apoptosis. Increased expression of Trk-A or Trk-C correlates with a favourable prognosis in neuroblastoma and, respectively, medulloblastoma.[34],[35] In contrast, TrkB expression in neuroblastoma stimulates cell survival, invasiveness, and resistance to vinblastine chemotherapy.[36] Neurotrophins also bind a low-affinity transmembrane receptor, p75NTR, structurally unrelated to the Trk family and devoid of enzymatic activities. p75NTR seems to exert complex effects, either synergizing or antagonizing Trk-A. It acts as coreceptor for NGF, increasing intracellular signalling that leads to differentiation and/or survival. However, in the presence of low levels of TrkA activity, or in its absence, p75 stimulates apoptosis via a signalling pathway shared with the tumour necrosis factor receptor/Fas receptor.[37],[38]

The Eph family of receptor tyrosine kinases encompasses at least 14 members that fall into two subclasses (EphA1–8 and EphB1–6). The extracellular domain includes an N-terminal Ig-like motif, which contains the ligand binding site, followed by a cysteine-rich region and two fibronectin III repeats (Fig. 3(a)). Their ligands, ephrins, are membrane-bound molecules classified into two groups: ephrins A1–5, are anchored by a glycosylphosphatidyl-inositol (GPI) and bind Eph A; ephrins B1–3, contain a transmembrane and a short cytoplasmic domain and bind Eph B. Interaction of ligands and receptors occurs with a high degree of promiscuity and generates a repelling signal between adjacent cells that directs movement of neuronal axons towards their targets.[39],[40] The Eph family plays a role during formation of different embryonic boundaries in the neuronal compartments and in the transition area between arteries and veins.[41],[42]

The tyrosine kinase encoded by the AXL/UFO gene is the prototype of a family that includes Sky and Mer. The extracellular domain of these receptors contains two Ig-like motifs and two fibronectin III repeats (Fig. 3(a)). Their common ligand is gas6, a soluble protein related to the anticoagulation factor protein 6. The receptor family is involved in control of haematopoietic and nervous development.[43]

Receptors encoded by DDR-1 and -2 genes form a family characterized by a domain that is strongly homologous to discoidin 1 (a protein of the amoeba Dictyostelium discoideum). Recently, the search for their ligands gave a surprising result: both receptors are activated by extracellular matrix collagens. In particular, Ddr-1 is activated by types I, II, III, V, and XI collagen, while Ddr-2 is activated mainly by type I and III. Because the ligands are insoluble, activation of the tyrosine kinase is slower and more prolonged than that of receptors coupled to soluble ligands. Since their affinity for collagens is low, Ddr-1 and -2 probably form supermolecular complexes including integrins, the high affinity receptors for collagens.[44] Ddr-1 is over-expressed in epithelial tumours, where it may be responsible for expression of extracellular-matrix proteases that favour tumour invasion and metastasis.[45]

Finally, Nsk2/MuSK and Ror-1 and -2 are the prototypes of two other distinct families of tyrosine kinase receptors (Fig. 3(a)), whose ligands are still unknown.

The intracellular receptor domain

The region spanning the plasma membrane of the RTKs consists of about 25 hydrophobic amino acids connecting the extracellular with the intracellular domain. Although this transmembrane domain has a mainly structural role, a single point mutation can dramatically alter the tyrosine kinase activity of the receptor. For example the *ERBB-2/neu* oncogene, which encodes a member of the EGF receptor family, is constitutively activated due to a point mutation that causes substitution of a hydrophobic amino acid (valine) with a negatively-charged residue (glutamate).[11]

The juxtamembrane region of growth factor receptors corresponds to the sequence separating the catalytic from the transmembrane domain. It is conserved between receptors belonging to the same family. This region is involved in transmodulation of receptor activity by neighbouring signalling molecules, receptors, or transducers. Phosphorylation of serine residues in the juxtamembrane domain of EGF or HGF receptors results in down-modulation of the kinase activity. In the case of the EGF receptor, serine phosphorylation also inhibits binding between the extracellular domain and the growth factor, probably due to conformational changes of the entire molecule. Phosphorylation of the juxtamembrane domain is catalysed by the serine–threonine kinase protein kinase C (PKC). In turn, this is activated by diacylglycerol and Ca^{++} ions, both released into the cytoplasm after activation of the phosphoinositide cycle, which in turn is stimulated by activation of growth factor receptors. In this way, receptor stimulation causes a concomitant negative feedback. Moreover, tyrosine residues critical for signal transduction are located in the juxtamembrane domain of the PDGF receptor.[46]

The whole intracellular domain is highly conserved among RTKs, sharing up to 90 per cent homology within members of the same family.[47] Homology is concentrated in the **catalytic domain**, which includes about 250 amino acids and is flanked, or in some cases interrupted, by regulatory regions. Sequence alignment has revealed that there are 13 residues conserved in most RTKs, with some exceptions, such as ErbB3. Notably, the latter is not an active protein kinase. Crystal structure resolution of insulin and FGF receptor fragments has allowed delineation of models for the general structure of the catalytic domains. Figure 4 shows two lobes delimiting a cleft.[48],[49] In the central cleft, the protein substrate and the complex ATP-Mg^{++} ions are brought together, and the phosphotransfer reaction takes place. The N-terminal lobe contains a glycine-rich motif (Gly-X-Gly-X-X-Gly)‡ and the lysine residue (Lys 1110)§ critical for binding ATP. The lobular structure is stabilized by a conserved glutamate (Glu 1127) that forms a salt bridge¶ with the lysine in which mutations completely abolish the enzymatic function. Protruding into the central cleft is the 'catalytic loop', characterized by the sequence His-Arg-Asp-Leu-Ala-Ala-Arg-Asn (residues 1202–1209), in which the aspartate is the catalytic base, while the amino acids that follow

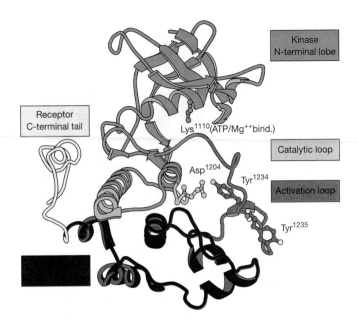

Fig. 4 Schematic representation of the conserved catalytic domain of tyrosine kinase receptors. The program Modeler was used to a draw a putative model based on the crystal structure of the insulin receptor kinase (by courtesy of Dr L. Pugliese). Conserved amino acids, critical for the phosphotransfer reaction, are indicated. Their numbers refer to the HGF receptor sequence. The N-terminal and the C-terminal lobes of the kinase domain delimit a cleft in which the two substrates, ATP (bound by Lys^{1110}) and tyrosine residues (recognized by the catalytic loop), come into contact. The activation loop contains tyrosines that, upon phosphorylation, increase the V_{max} of the kinase reaction. For a detailed description see text.

allow the tyrosine substrate to be recognized. Moving towards the C-terminal moiety, other conserved residues are found. The aspartate (1222), in the sequence Asp-Phe-Gly, functions as an Mg^{++} ion chelator. The glutamate (1253) and the arginine (1327) form ionic bridges that stabilize the two lobes. The aspartate (1265) stabilizes the catalytic loop.[6] The region of the C-terminal lobe between aspartate (1222) and glutamate (1253) contains a second loop, known as the 'kinase activation loop'. In the vast majority of receptors, this includes one to three conserved tyrosines (1234–1235) endowed with regulatory functions (see below). Point mutations found in *MET*, *RET*, or *KIT* oncogenes, which are responsible for sporadic and hereditary cancers, affect mostly amino acids located in the kinase activation loop. These mutations unleash the kinase activity in the absence of ligands.

Activation of receptor tyrosine kinases

Unbound receptor monomers are free to float in the lipid bilayer of the plasma membrane, where random reciprocal contacts occur in proportion to the number of receptor molecules present. For most receptors, ligand binding induces a conformational change in the receptor extracellular domain that stabilizes intermolecular interactions leading to formation of receptor dimers. Some ligands, such as PDGFs or VEGFs, are symmetrically bifunctional, that is capable of simultaneously binding two receptor molecules, thus fastening the receptor pair. In the case of the insulin receptor family,

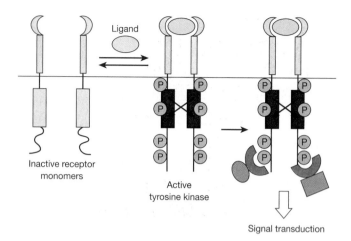

Ligand

Inactive receptor
monomers

Active
tyrosine kinase

Signal transduction

Fig. 5 Model of activation of tyrosine kinase receptors. Reversible ligand binding to the extracellular domain induces receptor dimerization and allosteric modifications that trigger the receptor enzymatic activity. A reciprocal tyrosine phosphorylation between the two partners occurs. Upon association to phosphotyrosines (pink circles), mediated by SH2 domains (pink C), transducer proteins are activated and propagate the signal inside the cell.

two identical receptor subunits, each formed by one α and one β polypeptide, are already covalently dimerized by disulphide links: the ligand probably induces a conformational change from the inactive to an active state.[50] In some cases, dimer formation requires complex interactions with other membrane-associated molecules. FGF-1 and -2 induce receptor dimerization only in the presence of heparan sulphate proteoglycans.[51]

Dimerization stabilizes the active state of the intracellular tyrosine kinase and brings its favourite substrate—the intracellular domain of another receptor—into its proximity. In this way, receptor *trans*-autophosphorylation takes place (Fig. 5). Tyrosine phosphorylation occurs both inside and outside the catalytic domain. Crystal structure analysis has demonstrated that, in the insulin receptor, the conserved tyrosine residue in the activation loop of the catalytic domain exerts a regulatory role. When the receptor is unbound, this tyrosine prevents exogenous protein substrates from accessing the catalytic site. However, steric hindrance inhibits *cis*-autophosphorylation of this residue. After ligand binding and receptor dimer formation, *trans*-phosphorylation of this tyrosine takes place and shifts the equilibrium towards a conformation that allows binding of exogenous substrates. This regulatory mechanism is probably shared by other receptor families, including those of the insulin receptor, HGFR, FGFR, and NGFR/Trk-A. In the case of HGFR, phosphorylation of the conserved two tyrosine residues in the activation loop (1234–1235) up-regulates the catalytic functions of the kinase.[49]

Trans-autophosphorylation of the receptor molecules outside the catalytic domain occurs at multiple sites including the kinase insert (when present), the juxtamembrane domain, and the C-terminal tail. Phosphorylation of these residues forms docking sites that are recognized with high affinity by cytoplasmic signal transducers that contain specific domains (see below).[52],[53] Creation of such docking sites through *trans*-autophosphorylation is probably an absolute requirement for receptor signal transduction inside the cell. Tyrosine kinase activation in the absence of receptor *trans*-autophosphorylation

is not enough to trigger a biological effect. This has been formally proven for the HGF receptor (encoded by the *MET* oncogene), which has a single transducer docking site made of two closely spaced tyrosines (1349–1356) in its C-terminal tail. In transgenic mice, mutation of these two tyrosines into phenylalanines results in a Met kinase which is perfectly active but devoid of any functional signalling, as seen in knock-out mice where the gene has been deleted.[54]

Tyrosine phosphorylation of the transducer docking site is also crucial for the oncogenic potential of RTKs. As mentioned, mutations in the kinase activation loop of the *MET* oncogene, associated with cases of kidney cancer, unleash the tyrosine kinase activity and result in loss of substrate specificity. However, when the two tyrosines of the transducer docking site are substituted with phenylalanines, the *in vitro* transforming ability and the biological activities mediated by the mutated Met kinase are completely abolished.[55]

Receptor tyrosine kinases recruit signal transducers that bind phosphotyrosine

Intracellular signalling proteins bind to phosphorylated receptors with high affinity by means of specific modules contained in their sequence. The most common is the so-called SH2 (Src homology region 2) domain that binds short peptide motifs invariably including a phosphotyrosine residue (pTyr). Specificity in intermolecular recognition is conferred by the three to five amino acid residues that follow pTyr. Specific association of different SH2-containing transducers dictates which signalling pathway will be activated.[56]

Crystallography and nuclear magnetic resonance have resolved structures of SH2 domains in detail and their functional properties have been elucidated. The SH2 domain is a compact structure encompassing about 100 residues. In its N-terminal moiety a pocket contains positively-charged amino acids, including a conserved arginine, that bind the negatively charged phosphate group of pTyr. Hydrophobic residues provide additional stability by interacting with the aromatic portion of the tyrosine side chain. Structural studies, complemented by screening of peptide libraries, have clarified that the C-terminal half of the SH2 domain recognizes the three amino acids that follow phosphotyrosine (Fig. 6). This allows high affinity association between distinct SH2-containing proteins and specific phosphotyrosines within the receptor sequence.[57] As a rule, the majority of RTKs contain a number of tyrosines that are phosphorylated following receptor activation, located in the C-terminal tail and in the juxtamembrane or in the kinase insert. Each of these phosphotyrosines is followed by a different consensus and binds preferentially only one SH2-containing transducer. For example in the PDGF receptor, the sequence pTyr-Val-Pro-Met binds specifically to the SH2 of the regulatory subunit p85 of phosphatidylinositol-3 kinase (PI-3K), while the sequence pTyr-Ile-Ile-Pro binds to the SH2 of phospholipase C-γ1.[58] As a notable exception among RTKs, the HGF receptor concentrates, in a unique two-phosphotyrosine 'multifunctional' consensus sequence, the capability of activating multiple transducers.[59]

Another peptide module besides the SH2 domain implied in recognizing phosphotyrosine-containing motifs is the PTB (phosphotyrosine binding) domain. Less common than SH2, PTB interacts

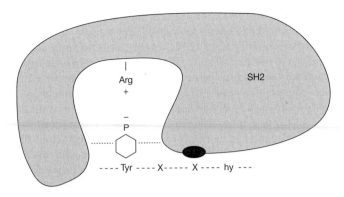

Fig. 6 Interaction between an SH2 domain and peptide sequences containing phosphotyrosine. In the N-terminal moiety of SH2 a pocket contains amino acids including a conserved arginine (Arg) whose positive charge (+) form ionic bridges with the negatively charged phosphate group (P–) bound to tyrosine (Tyr). Additional stability is provided by hydrophobic interactions (dotted lines) among the aromatic side-chain (hexagon) of tyrosine and hydrophobic residues in the SH2 pocket. The three amino acids that follow phosphotyrosine are recognized by the C-terminal moiety of SH2. The first and, in particular, the second residue (X indicates whatever amino acid) are critical to confer specific recognition (red oval) of a distinct SH2. The third residue is usually hydrophobic (hy).

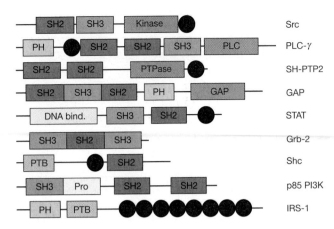

Fig. 7 Structure of signal transducer proteins that associate with activated tyrosine kinase receptors via phosphotyrosine binding domains (SH2 or PTB). Some are endowed with intrinsic enzymatic activities (dark grey box): Src (tyrosine kinase), PLC-γ (phospholipase), GAP (activation of GTPase), and SH-PTP2 (phosphatase), or are transcription factors that bind DNA (STAT). The others are adaptors that recruit to the receptor and to the plasma membrane other signalling proteins, described in detail in the text. The presence of tyrosine phosphorylation sites (red circles) and of conserved domains (SH3, Pro = proline rich motifs, PH), critical for intermolecular interactions and signal transduction, is indicated.

with high affinity with motifs in which pTyr is immediately preceded by the consensus sequence Asn-Pro-X. Hydrophobic amino acids located five to eight residues N-terminal to pTyr confer binding specificity. However, the PTB of some proteins can also recognize peptides where tyrosine is not phosphorylated. Therefore, PTB is considered essentially as a peptide recognition motif, serving a somewhat different purpose from SH2 domains. In fact PTB is mostly found in docking proteins ('adaptors', see below), such as Shc and IRS-1 (insulin receptor substrate-1), whose task is to recruit multiple signal transducers in the proximity of tyrosine kinase receptors before they are activated.[53]

Targeting signal transducers to the plasma membrane is crucial for joining the activated receptors. In some cases, this localization is achieved by a lipid molecule linked to the N- or to the C-terminus: examples are the transducers encoded by the *SRC* or the *RAS* oncogenes. We now know that PH (pleckstrin homology) domains can bind the negatively-charged groups of specific polyphosphoinositides found in the plasma membrane; this overcomes the requirement for lipid targeting and can couple the activity of inositol kinases and phosphatases to the regulation of intracellular signalling. PH domains are found in transducer molecules that either directly interact with RTKs or mediate further steps of downstream signalling. These include regulators of Ras and Rho small GTPase families (GTPase activating proteins; GTP/GDP exchangers such as SoS and Tiam1), phospholipases, kinases (PDK), and docking proteins (IRS-1).[53],[60]

Signal transducers that physically associate with activated receptors via SH2 domains are grouped into two main families (Fig. 7). One includes molecules endowed with intrinsic enzymatic activities, such as the Src family of cytoplasmic tyrosine kinases, phospholipase Cγ (PLC-Cγ), phosphotyrosine protein phosphatases (PTP), and GTPase activating proteins (GAP). This family can be extended to the recently discovered class of signal transducers that are, at the same time, activators of gene transcription (signal transducers and activators

of transcription, or STAT). The second family includes docking proteins playing a role of 'adaptors' devoid of intrinsic catalytic activity, whose function is to recruit signalling molecules to the activated receptor. Examples are Grb2 and Shc that couple the Ras pathway to the majority of RTKs, p85 that associates PI-3K to a number of receptors, and IRS-1, capable of recruiting multiple signal transducers to the insulin receptor family.[53]

Association with the activated RTKs stimulates the functions of the signal transducers in different ways. It can lower the Michaelis constant, K_m, for phosphorylation, making the transducer molecule a better substrate of receptor kinase activity. Tyrosine phosphorylation of the transducer usually causes its enzymatic activation, as in the case of PLCγ-1. However, phosphorylation of the SH-2 transducer does not always take place, as in the case of PI-3 kinase whose catalytic activity is stimulated by allosteric change. Finally, receptor binding relocalizes soluble cytosolic signalling proteins to the plasma membrane. Here they find substrates for enzymatic activity, as in the case of lipid kinases and hydrolases, or the GTP/GDP exchanger Sos. In all these cases phosphorylation of the receptor-associated transducer is dispensable.[6]

Signal transduction from receptor-associated molecules to the final effector targets, that is proteins that control gene expression (known as transcription factors), involves enzymatic cascades and second messenger production. Conserved recognition domains have been found that mediate supermolecular complex formation between signalling proteins. Among these, the best known and most common is the Src homology region 3 (SH3), a domain of about 60 amino acids that binds proline-rich sequences including characteristic Pro-X-X-Pro motifs. SH3 are present in almost all the above-mentioned SH-2 signal transducers (Fig. 7). Moreover, they are found in many cytoskeletal proteins, implicating a more general role in protein–protein interaction.[57]

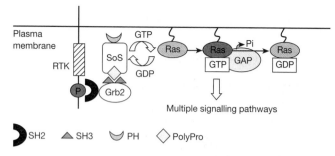

Fig. 8 Cycle of activation of Ras by RTKs. The adaptor Grb2 is constitutively associated with the guanine nucleotide releasing factor SoS through interaction between the SH3 domains of Grb2 and a polyproline motif (PolyPro) of SoS. Upon RTK activation, Grb2 binds receptor phosphotyrosine via SH2. SoS is thus recruited to the plasma membrane where Ras is located by means of a lipidic sequence. SoS exchanges GDP bound to inactive Ras with GTP. Ras coupled to GTP induces multiple signalling pathways (see Fig. 9). The cycle is completed when Ras hydrolyses GTP to GDP + inorganic phosphate (Pi) and reverts to its inactive GDP-bound state. This reaction is accelerated by GTPase activating proteins (GAP).

In signal transduction research there has been a substantial effort to couple a specific receptor, or at least a specific signalling pathway, to a given biological effect. Supposedly, pathways leading to proliferation, which correlate with the undifferentiated phenotype, are likely to be distinct from those that regulate differentiation. Until now, the attempt to find an unequivocal correlation between a specific signal transduction pathway and a unique biological event has failed. On the contrary, distinct receptors and pathways are found to cross-talk and reciprocally influence their responses. It is now thought that such effects are not a consequence of a single specific signal, but are mainly the result of a combination of events capable of overcoming a signalling threshold. In this context, it is easier to identify signals that are limiting factors for a biological response, rather than transducers which are capable—alone—of evoking specific events. Further consideration concludes that the same pathway may lead to different and even opposite results depending on whether activation is prolonged or transient, strong or weak.

The Ras pathway

Among signal transducers, the small GTP-ase Ras plays a central role in growth signalling and neoplastic transformation. First identified as the product of Harvey and Kirsten murine sarcoma retrovirus oncogenes, its cellular counterpart is found mutated and constitutively activated in a large number of human tumours. Ras is a small protein of 21 kDa (almost ubiquitously expressed) that associates to the plasma membrane via farnesyl, a lipidic sequence, which is added to its C-terminus. Ras functions as a molecular switch, cycling between an active GTP-bound state and an inactive GDP-bound state, the latter accumulating since Ras affinity for GDP is higher than for GTP.[61] After activation of the majority of RTKs, the level of GTP-bound Ras increases and triggers multiple signal transduction cascades (Fig. 8). Conversion from the inactive GDP-bound to the active GTP-bound form is stimulated by cytoplasmic proteins working as guanine nucleotide releasing factors (GNRFs) or GDP/GTP exchangers. The

best characterized GNRF, named SoS, contains polyproline motifs that are high-affinity ligands for the two SH3 domains contained in the adaptor molecule Grb2. Grb2 includes an SH2 domain, located between the two SH3 (Fig. 7), that preferentially binds the phosphorylated consensus sequence pTyr-X-Asn-Val. This is found in a large number of activated RTKs and in the Shc adaptor protein, which is also associated to phosphorylated RTKs (Fig. 7). Grb2 and SoS are likely to be preassociated in the cytoplasm. Following tyrosine phosphorylation, this complex is recruited to the receptor and thus to the plasma membrane, where SoS can interact with the Ras molecules.[62] After being activated by coupling to GTP, Ras hydrolyses it at a slow rate, reverting to its GDP-bound resting state. GTP-ase activating proteins (GAPs) that associate to phosphorylated receptors via SH2 domains increase Ras enzymatic activity, thus down-regulating Ras signalling. It is debatable whether GAPs also behave as Ras effectors, through binding and activation of Rho-GAP.[63] However, this latter is known to modulate the activity of the small GTP-ase Rho, which regulates organization of the actin cytoskeleton, inducing formation of stress fibres, which are bundles of filaments that traverse the cell and anchor to the plasma at adhesion sites named focal contacts.[64] Loss of the tumour suppressor gene *NF1*, which encodes a GAP protein called neurofibromin, is responsible for the familial tumour syndrome known as neurofibromatosis of Recklinghausen.[65]

Point mutations in the *RAS* oncogene are found frequently in a wide variety of cancers. These cause two major biochemical changes in the Ras proteins: impaired GTPase activity or facilitated GTP/GDP exchange. In both cases, the activated status of Ras is favoured and the following growth signalling is constitutively increased.[66]

Ras plays a key role in signal transduction by regulating a complex array of interconnected pathways leading to activation of transcription factors that promote expression of genes that control cell differentiation and proliferation. Moreover, Ras indirectly regulates protein synthesis, apoptosis, and cytoskeletal rearrangements (Fig. 9). Three main classes of Ras effectors are known to mediate such events *in vivo*. These include:

(1) the serine–threonine kinases involved in the mitogen-activated protein kinase (MAPK) and in the stress-activated protein kinase (SAPK) pathways (see below);

(2) phosphatidylinositol-3 kinase (PI-3K), which is also directly activated by RTKs via its regulatory subunit p85, and will be described below under 'Phospholipid signalling';

(3) the more recently found Ral guanine nucleotide exchange factors (RalGEFs).

Upon conformational change and recruitment to cell membranes, RalGEF acts as GTP/GDP exchanger for the small GTPase Ral. This in turn activates a kinase cascade as yet incompletely defined, which however is likely to stimulate the same transcription factors activated by the MAPK pathway. Ral is also involved in regulating vesicle transport and membrane traffic.[67]

Serine–threonine kinase cascades leading to the cell nucleus and influencing the cell cycle

The MAPK pathway is a cascade of serine–threonine kinase activation initiated by the Raf molecule (Fig. 9). This includes an N-terminal

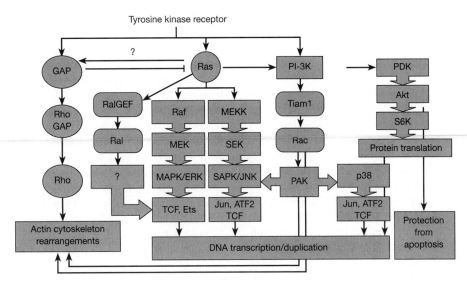

Fig. 9 Signalling pathways controlled by tyrosine kinase receptors through Ras. Block arrows indicate serine–threonine kinases. For detailed explanation see text.

binding region (CR1) that associates with the activated GTP-bound Ras, and a C-terminal (CR2) serine–threonine kinase domain. The mechanism of Raf activation is still poorly understood, but it is probable that it requires both recruitment to the cell membrane and serine–threonine phosphorylation. In the next step, Raf phosphorylates and activates kinases of the MEK (mitogen/extracellular-signal regulated kinase kinase) family, namely MEK-1 and -2. These are dual specificity threonine–tyrosine kinases (usually kinases are specific either for tyrosine or for serine–threonine). Prominent MEK substrates are the serine–threonine kinases known as MAPK (mitogen activated protein kinases), also referred to as ERK (extracellular signal regulated kinases). Two MAPK/ERKs are known, p44^{MAPK}/ERK1 and p42^{MAPK}/ERK2. Once activated, these translocate into the nucleus where they phosphorylate and modulate transcription factors, in particular those belonging to the ETs family.[68] This includes many homologous members, that can be grouped in two main subfamilies. One includes the Ets-1 and -2 proto-oncogene products, while the other encompasses Elk-1, Sap-1, and Net that form the so-called ternary complex factor (TCF).[69]

MAPKs phosphorylate a single threonine residue in the N-terminal region (known as 'pointed domain') of Ets-1 and Ets-2, and multiple serine and threonine residues in the transactivation domain of the three TCF components. Phosphorylated Ets co-operates with the transcription complex AP-1, a heterodimer including one member of the Fos proto-oncogene family coupled with one member of the Jun proto-oncogene family. The complex formed by Ets and AP-1 activates transcription through binding the gene promoter Ras responsive element (RRE). This mediates induction of transcription by Ras with high specificity and sensitivity.[69]

Following phosphorylation by MAPKs, TCF is activated to form a complex with SRF (serum response factor). This complex stimulates transcription through binding to the serum responsive element (SRE) present in the promoter of a number of 'immediately early genes' (genes induced by growth factors within tens of min after cell

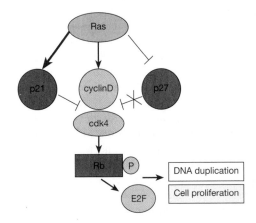

Fig. 10 The Ras pathway positively regulates cell cycle by induction of cyclin D transcription. This stimulates cdk 4 to phosphorylate Rb at multiple serine–threonine sites. Phosphorylated Rb releases transcription factors such as E2F. The final result is entry into the S phase of the cell cycle in which DNA duplication occurs. Moreover Ras down-regulates p27 that in turn inhibits the activity of cyclinD/cdk4 complex. On the contrary, intense and prolonged Ras activation (thick arrow) mainly induces p21 transcription, which is a cell cycle inhibitor, thus blocking progression toward DNA duplication. Positive regulators of the cell cycle are represented in dark pink, negative regulators in light pink.

stimulation). These include other transcription factors, such as members of the Fos family that form the AP-1 complex (see above) that further amplify the transcription response to Ras.[69]

A crucial link between transduction of the growth factor signal and control of the cell cycle is stimulation of cyclin D1 transcription through the Ras/MAPK/Ets pathway (Fig. 10). It is known that cyclin D1 expression is required for activation of cyclin-dependent kinase 4 (cdk4), whose main substrate is the protein encoded by the tumour suppressor gene Rb. Phosphorylation of Rb at many sites, induced by cdk4 and 6, is required for Rb inactivation and release of transcription factors such as E2F. Thus the cell moves beyond the so-called 'restriction point' of the cell cycle and starts to duplicate DNA (see also Chapter 1.6).[70]

Apart from stimulating positive regulators of the cell cycle, Ras also inhibits negative regulators of proliferation such as p27[Kip1](Fig. 10). This hampers the catalytic activity of the complexes formed by cdks and cyclins. MAPK phosphorylates p27, thereby inhibiting its activity and probably increasing its degradation. Paradoxically, the Ras pathway also up-regulates cell cycle inhibitors such as p21[Cip1], which is functionally and structurally related to p27 (Fig. 10). p21[Cip1] is probably induced at the transcription level, by complex mechanisms, following a sustained activation of the Ras/MAPK pathway.[70] This helps explain how Ras can regulate opposite events: its activation, when transient, stimulates proliferation probably by means of transcription of cyclin D. On the contrary, when intense and prolonged, Ras activation causes exit from the cell cycle, which allows differentiation programmes to take place, probably through induction of p21[Cip1].

A kinase cascade parallel to the Raf/MEK/ERK pathway is triggered by MEK kinase-1 (MEKK-1) (Fig. 9). *In vivo* this is not active on MEK, but on a homologous kinase named SEK (stress and extracellular signal regulated kinase). The ensuing step is phosphorylation and stimulation of the SAPK (stress-activated protein kinase) known also as JNK (Jun N-terminal kinase). This phosphorylates and activates a number of transcription factors, including the product of the Jun proto-oncogene, the member of TCF Elk-1, and ATF2. The SAPK pathway is strongly activated by inflammatory cytokines, interleukins, and a wide array of cellular stresses such as heat shock, and ultraviolet and ionizing radiations. On the contrary, it is poorly induced by growth factors. Triggering of the SAPK pathway involves both Ras and Rac, a small G-protein of the Rho family, which is activated mainly through PI3-kinase (see below). Rac stimulates a number of serine–threonine kinases including those of the PAK (p21RAS activated kinase) family. These phosphorylate and activate members of the SAPK pathway and a serine–threonine kinase known as p38RK (reactivating kinase), which in turn activates transcription factors including Elk-1 and Sap-1 (that join to from TCF), and ATF2.[64],[69] The outcome of induction of the SAPK pathway by growth factors is still controversial. On one hand, JNK seems to be essential for transformation by the tyrosine kinase receptor encoded by the *MET* oncogene.[71] On the other hand, it is likely that this pathway sustains induction of apoptosis by growth factors, as well as by cellular stressing events. In fact, Jun activation, which leads to formation and activation of the AP-1 complex, stimulates transcription of genes encoding for cytokines such as Fas ligand and tumour necrosis factor. These bind specific transmembrane receptors triggering a signal transduction cascade that controls apoptosis (see Chapter 1.6). Moreover, JNK can phosphorylate and inhibit Bcl-2, suppressing its activity of protection from apoptosis.[72]

Phospholipid signalling

The majority of activated receptor tyrosine kinases stimulate enzymes that generate lipid second messengers, namely phospholipase Cγ (PLCγ) and phosphatidylinositol-3 kinase (PI-3K).

PLCγ hydrolyses phosphatidylinositol-4,5-diphosphate (PI-4,5P$_2$) to diacylglycerol (DAG) and inositol 1,4,5 trisphosphate (IP$_3$) (Fig. 11). PLCγ contains two SH2 domains and an SH3 that allow association with cytoskeletal proteins (Fig. 7). Upon receptor binding, PLCγ undergoes tyrosine phosphorylation, which is required for its full enzymatic activation. Its product DAG is the physiological activator of enzymes belonging to the PKC (protein serine–threonine kinase C) family, which is involved in growth control and cellular transformation and is the target of tumour-promoting phorbol esters such as TPA. Some subtypes of PKC are also activated by PI-3K (see below). IP$_3$ binds to specific receptor channels in the internal membranes, mobilizing calcium from intracellular storage. How PLCγ is involved in signalling events leading to DNA duplication and cell division is still unclear.[6]

PI-3K has emerged as a key regulator of cell proliferation and survival and other activities supporting cell transformation and invasion of the extracellular matrix during tumour progression. A retrovirus-encoded PI-3K causes haemangiosarcomas in avians and can transform cell cultures.[73] PI-3 kinases form a superfamily of enzymes that phosphorylate phosphatidylinositols on the D3 position, forming D3 phosphoinositides. Three classes of PI-3K can be identified on the basis of substrate specificity.[74]

Class I PI-3K mainly phosphorylates PI(4,5)P$_2$ (the substrate of hydrolysis by PLCγ), thus forming the D3 phosphoinositide named phospatidylinositol (3,4,5) triphosphate, or PI(3,4,5)P$_3$. Class I PI-3K is associated with RTKs and with the complex formed by middle T antigen (the main transforming protein of polyomavirus) and pp60[Src] (the protein product of the *SRC* proto-oncogene). The best characterized class I member is a heterodimer consisting of a catalytic (p110) and a regulatory subunit (p85) containing both SH2 and SH3 domains (Fig. 7). Following p85 association with the phosphorylated receptor, p110 moves into proximity of the inner face of the plasma membrane where PI(4,5)P$_2$ is available for phosphorylation. Interestingly, RTKs can stimulate PI-3K either directly or indirectly. As mentioned previously, full activation of p110 seems to require additional allosteric modification through binding to the GTP-bound Ras protein.[74]

Recently, a number of D3 phosphoinositide targets have been identified, mostly involved in controlling cell survival, proliferation, and movement (Fig. 11). These targets contain the so-called pleckstrin (PH) domains that bind phosphorylated inositol lipids. A protein serine–threonine kinase, Akt/PKB, is directly activated by PI(3,4)P$_2$ and by phosphorylation performed by a kinase, PDK1, which is in turn activated by PI(3,4,5)P$_3$. Akt, the cellular counterpart of the retroviral oncogene v-*akt*, is responsible for PI 3-K-mediated protection against apoptosis. The Akt substrates, although still poorly understood, are known to include S6 Kinase (S6K) that, in turn, phosphorylates the S6 ribosomal subunit. S6K regulates protein translation upon mitogenic stimuli and plays a role in cell cycle progression from G1 to S phase.[75]

Other reported targets of PI-3K are the ε and λ family members of the protein serine–threonine kinase C (PKC). PI(3,4,5)P$_3$ can either directly affect PKC activity or recruit and localize its substrates at the plasma membrane, facilitating phosphorylation by PKCs. Again, the physiological relevance of activating PKC downstream of PI-3K is puzzling. Possibly, PKC modulates Raf activity, thus affecting the Ras pathway and the transduction of mitogenic stimuli (Fig. 11).[75]

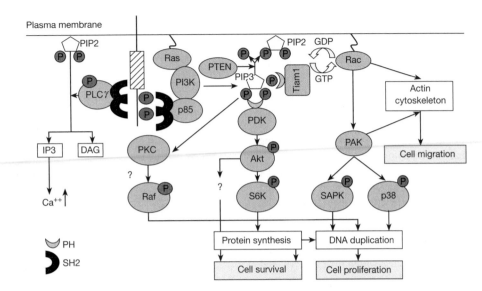

Fig. 11 Phospholipid signalling through activation of PLCγ and PI-3K. PIP2 is hydrolized by PLCγ to form IP3 and DAG. DAG activates PKC that possibly stimulates the Raf/MAPK cascade leading to DNA transcription and duplication. IP3 mobilizes Ca^{++} from intracellular stores increasing its cytoplasmic levels. PIP2 is phosphorylated at the D3 position by PI3-K to form PIP3. Phosphatidylinositides are dephosphorylated by PTEN phosphatase. PIP3 recruits and activates transducers containing PH domains. PDK activates a kinase cascade that controls protein synthesis and directly promotes cell survival. The GTP/GDP exchanger Tiam1 activates the small GTP-ase Rac that induces actin cytoskeleton rearrangements leading to cell migration, either directly or indirectly through PAK, a kinase that also regulates SAPK and p38, which in turn activate transcription factors responsible for control of cell proliferation. Red circles indicate that the molecule undergoes phosphorylation.

Finally, PI-3K is involved in controlling actin cytoskeletal re-arrangements and adhesion to the extracellular matrix, both of which are important for cell migration (Fig. 11). D3 phosphoinositides activate guanosine nucleotide exchange factors containing PH domains, including TIAM1.[75] This converts the small G-protein Rac into its active GTP-bound state. In several cell types Rac is required for formation of lamellipodia and membrane ruffles. These are thin protrusions of the plasma membrane supported by sheets of filamentous actin that lift off the substrate and fold backward during generation of cell movement.[64] Deregulation of Rac or TIAM1 activity is associated with the acquisition of an invasive and metastatic phenotype by tumour cells.[76] The effects of Rac on the actin cytoskeleton are likely to be mediated by downstream serine–threonine kinases, which are still poorly understood. Among these, a prominent role is played by PAK, mentioned above as a regulator of the SAPK pathway and of the p38/RK kinase.

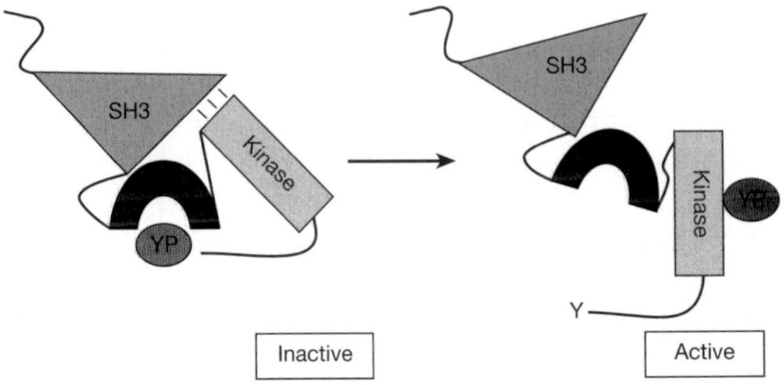

Non-receptor tyrosine kinases

The product of the *SRC* proto-oncogene, pp60[Src], is the prototype of a family of cytoplasmic protein tyrosine kinases encompassing at least 10 highly homologous members. On the basis of their pattern of expression, they are subdivided into three groups. Src, Fyn, and Yes are expressed in virtually every cell; Blk, Fgr, Hck, Lck, and Lyn are found mostly in haematopoietic cells. The Frk-related subgroup is expressed predominantly in epithelia. These enzymes are associated and activated by a number of transmembrane receptors, including the majority of RTKs, and regulate—by mechanisms largely unknown—cellular events including cell proliferation, survival, and invasiveness.

Fig. 12 Mechanism of Src activation. The inactive conformation of the kinase is stabilized by a C-terminal phosphotyrosine residue (red circle) that binds to the SH2 domain, while further interactions (short lines) between the kinase and the SH3 domain take place. Dephosphorylation of the C-terminal tyrosine releases the active conformation of the kinase that requires an additional tyrosine phosphorylation to be fully functional. For further details see text.

Src proteins (52–62 kDa) are composed of six distinct functional domains. From the N-terminus, there are a conserved domain (SH4), the unique region, an SH3, an SH2, a catalytic domain, and a short tail including a tyrosine residue. The SH4 domain is a brief sequence containing a myristilation signal (for coupling the protein to a fatty acid chain after translation) to allows targeting to cellular membranes. The unique region is the most variable among the Src family members. The SH3 and SH2 domains and the C-terminal tail participate in a complex intramolecular regulation of the Src catalytic activity (Fig. 12). In resting conditions, the C-terminal tyrosine, phosphorylated by the cytoplasmic kinase Csk, binds with high affinity the SH2

domain within the same molecule, favouring a closed, inactive conformation. This status is further stabilized by interactions among the
SH3, the kinase domain and a flanking region that contains a proline
rich motif. When the C-terminal tyrosine is dephosphorylated, by
means of a mechanism still poorly understood, the SH2 domain is
released and the kinase turns into the active form. To obtain full
enzymatic activity, tyrosine phosphorylation in the catalytic domain
is required.

Phosphotyrosines of ligand-activated RTKs compete for binding
to the Src SH2, displacing the inhibitory interaction with the C-
terminal tail. Association between Src and RTKs is followed by
phosphorylation of the tyrosine in the Src catalytic domain endowed
with up-regulation functions. Interestingly, the v-*src* transforming
oncogene, isolated from the Rous sarcoma virus, lacks the C-
terminal inhibitory moiety and displays constitutive kinase activation.

Redundancy of the Src family members within the same cell, and
the lack of specific inhibitors, makes difficult a definition of distinctive
biochemical and biological activities of these kinases. However, the
majority of the activated RTKs associate with—and activate—one or
more Src proteins. Use of dominant-negative mutants has demonstrated that soluble tyrosine kinases are required for full receptor
signalling. Although it is often difficult to discriminate between the
substrates phosphorylated directly by the RTKs and those subsequently
phosphorylated by Src, a large number of intracellular proteins are
putative Src targets. Among these the focal adhesion kinase is part
of a cytoplasmic signalling complex associated with the integrins that
controls cellular adhesion. Activated focal adhesion kinase, in turn,
recruits Grb2 and stimulates Ras and the ensuing pathways. During
generation of cell movement, Src induces formation of lamellipodia
and membrane ruffles. Again, this effect on the cytoskeleton is likely
to be mediated by induction of PI-3 K and Rac activity, both enhanced
in Src-transformed cells. Activation of Ras/MAPK and PI-3 kinase
pathways are required to obtain cell migration, proliferation, and
protection from apoptosis by Src.[77]

Phosphatases

Activated RTKs associate with SH-2-containing enzymes endowed
with phosphoprotein phosphatase activity that are candidates to
down-regulate tyrosine kinase signalling. Two main phosphotyrosine
phosphatases have been characterized, named SH-PTP1 and SH-
PTP2. The former is known also as PTP-1C or SHP or HCP, and is
expressed almost exclusively in haematopoietic cells and in some
epithelial tissues. In contrast, SH-PTP2 (also known as Syp or PTP-
2C) is present in most cell types. Both bind to phosphorylated RTKs
and are probably activated by phosphorylation. However, they seem to
play opposite roles in signal transduction: SH-PTP1 dephosphorylates
RTKs and seems to be involved in negative regulation. Unexpectedly,
SH-PTP2 appears to activate a positive signal transduction pathway,
which is still largely unknown. Possibly this involves dephosphorylation of the negative-regulatory phosphotyrosine of the
C-terminal tail of Src (see above).[6]

A recently-discovered member of the phosphatase family, named
PTEN, is the product of a tumour suppressor gene, whose mutations
are responsible for the inherited Cowden disease, a cancer syndrome
characterized by early onset of breast, thyroid, and brain tumours.

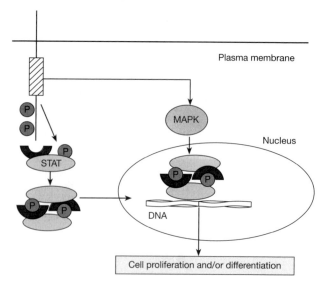

Fig. 13 Signal transduction and activation of transcription (STAT). STAT
molecules associate to activated receptors via their SH2 domain. They are
phosphorylated and form dimers stabilized by intermolecular SH2-
phosphotyrosine interactions. Dimers translocate into the nucleus where
they work as transcription factors, whose activity is further modulated by
MAPK. They regulate the expression of genes involved in the control of cell
proliferation and differentiation.

PTEN, although not endowed with SH2 domains, is likely to play
a prominent role in down-regulating tyrosine kinase receptor
signalling and acts on a wide array of downstream substrates. It
is capable of dephosphorylating phosphoserine, phosphotyrosine,
and the D3 phosphoinositides generated by PI-3K. The role of
mutated PTEN in tumorigenesis probably lies in its failure to
hydrolyse PIP3, which results in hyperactivation of the antiapoptotic
kinase Akt (Fig. 11).[78]

Signal transducers and activators of transcription (STAT)

RTKs activate a direct signalling pathway that stimulates gene transcription. This is mediated by molecules called signal transducers and
activators of transcription (STAT) a family of soluble proteins with
at least six members, named 1 to 6. First recognized as transducers
of cytokine receptors in the haematopoietic system, members 1, 3,
and 5 are widely expressed and implicated in RTK signal transduction
as well. They encompass an N-terminal DNA binding region, followed
by an SH3, an SH2, and a C-terminal tyrosine-containing sequence.
Upon phosphorylation, the C-terminal sequence binds, with high
affinity, the SH2 domain of another STAT molecule, forming homo-
or heterodimers (Fig. 13). Dimers translocate into the nucleus and
stimulate transcription of genes, largely unknown, involved both in
cell cycle control and differentiation. Among there are *FOS*, encoding
a transcription factor, and *WAF*-1, whose product negatively regulates
cell cycle progression. After cytokine receptor activation, STAT phosphorylation and the subsequent dimerization is performed by the

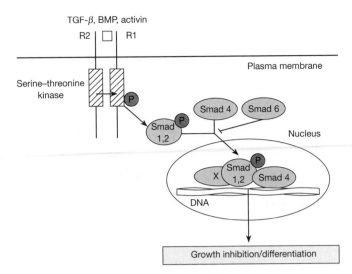

Fig. 14 Transforming growth factor-β (TGF-β) signalling. TGF-β family members (including activins and BMP) bind to a pair of serine–threonine kinase receptors (R1 and R2). R1 phosphorylates Smad1 or 2 and activates them to associate with Smad4. Smad6 is antagonistic and competes with Smad4 for this association. This complex translocates into the nucleus where it co-operates with other transcription factors (X) to induce expression of genes including cell cycle inhibitors. These mediate growth arrest and allow cell differentiation.

cytoplasmic kinases of a family named Jak. RTKs themselves can also directly phosphorylate and activate STAT. Moreover, fine-tuning of these molecules is achieved through serine phosphorylation performed by MAPK. In epithelial cells, STAT are transcription factors critical for differentiation.[79],[80]

The transforming growth factor-β (TGF-β) receptors and signal transduction pathways

As discussed above, polypeptides promoting cell proliferation and/or differentiation and related biological events, such as cell survival and movement, operate through receptor tyrosine kinases. Deregulation of the ensuing signal is likely to play a prominent role in cancer onset and progression. The TGF-β family is also implicated in cell cycle control, exerting mostly growth inhibitory effects following activation of receptor serine–threonine kinases (RSK). This family includes a large number of structurally-related polypeptides, comprising three main classes named TGF-βs, activins, and bone morphogenetic proteins (BMPs), which control organism development and homeostasis. Each factor binds specifically to a pair of transmembrane serine–threonine kinases called type I and type II receptor, respectively (Fig. 14). These are brought together by the ligand and probably form a heterotetrameric complex. Type II phosphorylates type I receptor, which, in turn, performs serine phosphorylation of exogenous substrates including the Smad proteins ('Smad' is the fusion of 'sma' and 'mad', the names of their homologues found in *Caenorhabditis elegans* and in *Drosophila*, respectively).[81]

Smads are, at the same time, signal transducers and transcription factors that fall into three structurally and functionally related classes. The first includes the so-called 'receptor-regulated Smads' that are direct substrates of SRKs. Smad1 and its relatives Smad5 and 8 are BMP type I receptor substrates, while Smad2 and 3 mediate TGF-β and activin type I receptor signalling. Smad4 is the prototype of the 'coSmad' class that is not a direct substrate of SRKs but forms a complex with receptor-phosphorylated Smads. These translocate into the nucleus and join to other transcription factors to control expression of specific genes. The third class includes the 'antagonistic' Smads 6 and 7 that compete with coSmads for association with receptor-activated Smads, thus blocking SRK signal transduction.

Smad proteins contain two conserved N-terminal and C-terminal domains known as 'Mad homology domain' 1 and 2 (MH1 and MH2) interspaced by a region of variable size and sequence. In resting conditions, MH1 and MH2 interact with each other causing the Smad molecule to fold, rendering it inactive. Upon SRK activation, the MH2 domain mediates physical association between Smad and SRK, it then undergoes phosphorylation on serine residues, and finally mediates formation of Smad multimeric complexes. When these are translocated into the nucleus, the MH1 domain of both receptor-regulated Smads and coSmads mediates DNA-binding activity, while MH2 activates gene transcription. Smad co-operates with transcription factors such as Fast-1, AP-1 (formed by factors encoded by the Fos or Jun oncogene families) and Sp-1. The Smad–Sp1 complex stimulates transcription of genes encoding cell cycle inhibitors such as $p15^{Ink4b}$ and $p21^{Cip1}$, thereby mediating TGF-β-induced growth arrest.[82] Cell cycle arrest allows terminal differentiation and is sometimes followed by apoptosis.

Alterations of TGF-β signalling pathways underlie many diseases. A gain of TGF-β activity is likely to play a central role in disorders characterized by accumulation of fibrotic matrix in lung, kidney, and liver parenchyma. On the other hand, the TGF-β family factors, their receptors, and Smads are considered tumour suppressor proteins, whose loss is observed in human cancer.[81] For example TGF-β type II receptor is inactivated by mutations in sporadic colon cancers with microsatellite instability.[83] This results from defects in DNA repair and leads to nucleotide deletions or additions in short repeated sequences (microsatellites) contained in many genes including the one for TGF-β type II receptor. Smad 4 was first identified as the product of a putative tumour suppressor gene (DPC4) frequently deleted or affected by inactivating mutations in pancreatic carcinoma.[84] Smad4 and 2 are also inactivated in a significant proportion of colorectal tumours and a small proportion of carcinomas of different types.[81]

Growth factor signalling results from integration of multiple pathways—a conclusion

Growth factors are a large family of soluble polypeptides that bind transmembrane receptors endowed with kinase activity. Receptor activation induces a number of biological effects including not merely proliferation, but also cell differentiation, migration, and protection from apoptosis. Paradoxically, under specific conditions growth factors can even cause growth arrest. Most growth factor-induced biological effects require expression of previously quiescent genes and *de novo* protein synthesis. Signals are conveyed from the extracellular environment where the factors bind to their receptors, into the nucleus where gene expression is controlled at the level of transcription by cascades of biochemical events known as signal transduction.

Although binding between ligand and receptor occurs with high affinity and is relatively specific, transduction inside the cell seems to break up the signal identity. In fact, cells express many different receptors and are concomitantly stimulated by combinations of extracellular signals. Each receptor can activate multiple transduction pathways simultaneously and vice versa, each signal transducer can be activated by distinct receptors. Pathways that were traditionally thought specific to given receptors are, on the contrary, shared by structurally and functionally unrelated superfamilies. Furthermore, cross-talk among distinct signalling cascades occurs to a wide extent and in multiple steps.

Thus, it is becoming clear that biological responses are not the effect of a single, specific transduction pathway but of co-operation among multiple signals, in which not only the quality but the intensity and duration of the signals are important to decide the final outcome. In some cases (e.g. Ras) activation may cause opposite effects depending on whether it is prolonged or transient, strong or weak. Co-operation goes together with redundancy: signalling pathways are partially overlapping and the lack of one is often compensated by others.

The signalling system that controls cell behaviour is sufficiently sophisticated to ensure fine integration of information from the environment and to compensate for dysfunction. Thus, to completely disrupt cell regulation, as occurs in cancer, it is evident that a number of hits (a minimum of four of five) are required in oncogenes and tumour suppressor genes that encode growth factors, their receptors, and signal transducers.

Notes

†   The following terms are widely accepted when describing genes or proteins: (1) human oncogenes are denoted in uppercase italics, e.g. *RAS*; (2) animal oncogenes in lowercase italics, e.g. *neu;* (3) proteins encoded by oncogenes in first letter uppercase then lowercase, e.g. Met.

‡   The following abbreviations indicate amino acid residues: Ala: alanine; Arg: arginine; Asn: asparagine; Asp: aspartate; Cys: cysteine; Gln: glutamine; Glu: glutamate; Gly: glycine; His: histidine; Ile: isoleucine; Leu: leucine; Lys: lysine; Met: methionine; Phe: phenilalanine; Pro: proline; Ser: serine; Thr: threonine; Trp: triptophan; Tyr: tyrosine; X: variable amino acid; Val: valine.

§   Numbers and position of residues refer to the sequence of the human HGF receptor.[55]

¶   Non-covalent ionic chemical bond between a negatively and a positively charged amino acid residue that stabilizes the tridimensional structure of the protein.

References

1.   **Waterfield MD, Scrace GT, Whittle N, *et al*.** Platelet-derived growth factor is structurally related to the putative transforming protein p28sis of simian sarcoma virus. *Nature*, 1983; **304**: 35–9.

2.   **Peters G, Brookes S, Smith R, Placzek M, Dickson C.** The mouse homolog of the hst/k-FGF gene is adjacent to int-2 and is activated by proviral insertion in some virally induced mammary tumors. *Proceedings of the National Academy of Science USA*, 1989; **86**: 5678–82.

3.   **Naldini L, Tamagnone L, Vigna E, *et al*.** Extracellular proteolytic cleavage by urokinase is required for activation of hepatocyte growth factor/scatter factor. *EMBO Journal*, 1992; **11**: 4825–33.

4.   **Cross M, Dexter TM.** Growth factors in development, transformation, and tumorigenesis. *Cell*, 1991; **64**: 271–80.

5.   **Sporn MB, Roberts AB.** Peptide growth factors are multifunctional. *Nature*, 1988; **332**: 217–19.

6.   **van der Geer P, Hunter T, Lindberg RA.** Receptor protein-tyrosine kinases and their signal transduction pathways. *Annual Review of Cell Biology*, 1994; **10**: 251–337.

7.   **Lemmon MA, Schlessinger J.** Regulation of signal transduction and signal diversity by receptor oligomerization. *Trends in Biochemical Sciences*, 1994; **19**: 459–63.

8.   **Burden S, Yarden Y.** Neuregulins and their receptors: a versatile signaling module in organogenesis and oncogenesis. *Neuron*, 1997; **18**: 847–55.

9.   **Fleming TP, Saxena A, Clark WC, *et al*.** Amplification and/or overexpression of platelet-derived growth factor receptors and epidermal growth factor receptor in human glial tumors. *Cancer Research*, 1992; **52**: 4550–3.

10.   **Horak E, Smith K, Bromley L, *et al*.** Mutant p53, EGF receptor and c-erbB-2 expression in human breast cancer. *Oncogene*, 1991; **6**: 2277–84.

11.   **Bargmann CI, Hung MC, Weinberg RA.** Multiple independent activations of the neu oncogene by a point mutation altering the transmembrane domain of p185. *Cell*, 1986; **45**: 649–57.

12.   **Heldin CH.** Structural and functional studies on platelet-derived growth factor. *EMBO Journal*, 1992; **11**: 4251–9.

13.   **Carroll M, Tomasson MH, Barker GF, Golub TR, Gilliland DG.** The TEL/platelet-derived growth factor beta receptor (PDGF beta R) fusion in chronic myelomonocytic leukemia is a transforming protein that self-associates and activates PDGF beta R kinase-dependent signaling pathways. *Proceedings of the National Academy of Science USA*, 1996; **93**: 14845–50.

14.   **Chabot B, Stephenson DA, Chapman VM, Besmer P, Bernstein A.** The proto-oncogene c-kit encoding a transmembrane tyrosine kinase receptor maps to the mouse W locus. *Nature*, 1988; **335**: 88–9.

15.   **Nagata H, Worobec AS, Oh CK, Chowdhury BA, Tannenbaum S, Suzuki Y, Metcalfe DD.** Identification of a point mutation in the catalytic domain of the protooncogene c-kit in peripheral blood mononuclear cells of patients who have mastocytosis with an associated hematologic disorder. *Proceedings of the National Academy of Science USA*, 1995; **92**: 10560–4.

16.   **Nishida T, Hirota S, Taniguchi M, *et al*.** Familial gastrointestinal stromal tumours with germline mutation of the KIT gene. *Nature Genetics*, 1998; **19**: 323–4.

17.   **Jacobs A.** Gene mutations in myelodysplasia. *Leukemia Research*, 1992; **16**: 47–50.

18.   **Fantl WJ, Johnson DE, Williams LT.** Signalling by receptor tyrosine kinases. *Annual Review of Biochemistry*, 1993; **62**: 453–81.

19.   **Burke D, Wilkes D, Blundell TL, Malcolm S.** Fibroblast growth factor receptors: lessons from the genes. *Trends in Biochemical Sciences*, 1998; **23**: 59–62.

20.   **Mason IJ.** The ins and outs of fibroblast growth factors. *Cell*, 1994; **78**: 547–52.

21.   **Risau W.** Mechanisms of angiogenesis. *Nature*, 1997; **386**: 671–4.

22.   **Hanahan D, Folkman J.** Patterns and emerging mechanisms of the angiogenic switch during tumorigenesis. *Cell*, 1996; **86**: 353–64.

23.   **Bussolino F, Mantovani A, Persico G.** Molecular mechanisms of blood vessel formation. *Trends in Biochemical Sciences*, 1997; **22**: 251–6.

24.   **Folkman J, D'Amore PA.** Blood vessel formation: what is its molecular basis? *Cell*, 1996; **87**: 1153–5.

25. Trusolino L, Pugliese L, Comoglio PM. Interactions between scatter factors and their receptors: hints for therapeutic applications. *Federation of American Societies for Experimental Biology Journal*, 1998; **12**: 1267–80.

26. Schmidt L, Duh FM, Chen F, Kishida T, Glenn G, Choyke P, *et al.* Germline and somatic mutations in the tyrosine kinase domain of the MET proto-oncogene in papillary renal carcinomas. *Nature Genetics*, 1997; **16**: 68–73.

27. Di Renzo MF, Olivero M, Ferro S, Prat M, Bongarzone, I, Pilotti S, *et al.* Overexpression of the c-MET/HGF receptor gene in human thyroid carcinomas. *Oncogene*, 1992; **7**: 2549–53.

28. Di Renzo MF, Olivero M, Giacomini A, Porte H, Chastre E, Mirossay L, *et al.* Overexpression and amplification of the met/HGF receptor gene during the progression of colorectal cancer. *Clinical Cancer Research*, 1995; **1**: 147–54.

29. Robertson K, Mason I. The GDNF-RET signalling partnership. *Trends in Genetics*, 1997; **13**: 1–3.

30. Hofstra RM, Landsvater RM, Ceccherini I, Stulp RP, Stelwagen T, Luo Y, *et al.* A mutation in the RET proto-oncogene associated with multiple endocrine neoplasia type 2B and sporadic medullary thyroid carcinoma [see comments]. *Nature*, 1994; **367**: 375–6.

31. Pasini B, Ceccherini I, Romeo G. RET mutations in human disease. *Trends in Genetics*, 1996; **12**: 138–44.

32. Grieco M, Santoro M, Berlingieri MT, *et al.* PTC is a novel rearranged form of the ret proto-oncogene and is frequently detected *in vivo* in human thyroid papillary carcinomas. *Cell*, 1990; **60**: 557–63.

33. Conover JC, Yancopoulos GD. Neurotrophin regulation of the developing nervous system: analyses of knockout mice. *Reviews in the Neurosciences*, 1997; **8**: 13–27.

34. Nakagawara A, Arima-Nakagawara M, Scavarda NJ, Azar CG, Cantor AB, Brodeur GM. Association between high levels of expression of the TRK gene and favorable outcome in human neuroblastoma. *New England Journal of Medicine*, 1993; **328**: 847–54.

35. Segal RA, Goumnerova LC, Kwon YK, Stiles CD, Pomeroy SL. Expression of the neurotrophin receptor TrkC is linked to a favorable outcome in medulloblastoma. *Proceedings of the National Academy of Science USA*, 1994; **91**: 12867–71.

36. Matsumoto K, Wada RK, Yamashiro JM, Kaplan DR, Thiele CJ. Expression of brain-derived neurotrophic factor and p145TrkB affects survival, differentiation, and invasiveness of human neuroblastoma cells. *Cancer Research*, 1995; **55**: 1798–806.

37. Kaplan DR, Miller FD. Signal transduction by the neurotrophin receptors. *Current Opinions in Cell Biology*, 1997; **9**: 213–21.

38. Segal RA, Greenberg ME. Intracellular signaling pathways activated by neurotrophic factors. *Annual Review of Neuroscience*, 1996; **19**: 463–89.

39. Drescher U. The Eph family in the patterning of neural development. *Current Biology*, 1997; **7**: R799–807.

40. Orioli D, Klein R. The Eph receptor family: axonal guidance by contact repulsion. *Trends in Genetics*, 1997; **13**: 354–9.

41. Flanagan JG, Vanderhaeghen P. The ephrins and Eph receptors in neural development. *Annual Review of Neuroscience*, 1998; **21**: 309–345.

42. Yancopoulos GD, Maisonpierre PC, Ip NY, *et al.* Neurotrophic factors, their receptors, and the signal transduction pathways they activate. *Cold Spring Harbor Symposium in Quantitative Biology*, 1990; **55**: 371–79.

43. Crosier KE, Crosier PS. New insights into the control of cell growth; the role of the Axl family. *Pathology*, 1997; **29**: 131–5.

44. Schlessinger J. Direct binding and activation of receptor tyrosine kinases by collagen. *Cell*, 1997; **91**: 869–72.

45. Vogel W, Gish GD, Alves F, Pawson T. The discoidin domain receptor tyrosine kinases are activated by collagen. *Molecular Cell*, 1997; **1**: 13–23.

46. Ullrich A, Schlessinger J. Signal transduction by receptors with tyrosine kinase activity. *Cell*, 1990; **61**: 203–12.

47. Hanks SK, Quinn AM, Hunter T. The protein kinase family: conserved features and deduced phylogeny of the catalytic domains. *Science*, 1988; **241**: 42–52.

48. Taylor SS, Knighton DR, Zheng J, Ten Eyck LF, Sowadski JM. Structural framework for the protein kinase family. *Annual Review of Cell Biology*, 1992; **8**: 429–62.

49. Hubbard SR, Mohammadi M, Schlessinger J. Autoregulatory mechanisms in protein-tyrosine kinases. *Journal of Biological Chemistry*, 1998; **273**: 11987–90.

50. Heldin CH. Dimerization of cell surface receptors in signal transduction. *Cell*, 1995; **80**: 213–23.

51. Schlessinger J, Lax I, Lemmon M. Regulation of growth factor activation by proteoglycans: what is the role of the low affinity receptors? *Cell*, 1995; **83**: 357–60.

52. Cohen GB, Ren R, Baltimore D. Modular binding domains in signal transduction proteins. *Cell*, 1995; **80**: 237–48.

53. Pawson T. Protein modules and signalling networks. *Nature*, 1995; **373**: 573–80.

54. Maina F, Casagranda F, Audero E, Simeone A, Comoglio PM, Klein R, Ponzetto C. Uncoupling of Grb2 from the Met receptor *in vivo* reveals complex roles in muscle development. *Cell*, 1996; **87**: 531–42.

55. Bardelli A, Longati P, Gramaglia D, *et al.* Uncoupling signal transducers from oncogenic MET mutants abrogates cell transformation and inhibits invasive growth. *Proceedings of the National Academy of Science USA*, 1998; **95**: 14379–83.

56. Songyang Z, Shoelson SE, Chaudhuri M, *et al.* SH2 domains recognize specific phosphopeptide sequences. *Cell*, 1993; **72**: 767–78.

57. Kuriyan J, Cowburn D. Modular peptide recognition domains in eukaryotic signaling. *Annual Review of Biophysics and Biomolecular Structure*, 1997; **26**: 259–88.

58. Songyang Z, Cantley LC. Recognition and specificity in protein tyrosine kianse-mediated signalling. *Trends in Biochemical Sciences*, 1995; **20**: 470–5.

59. Ponzetto C, Bardelli A, Zhen Z, *et al.* A multifunctional docking site mediates signaling and transformation by the hepatocyte growth factor/scatter factor receptor family. *Cell*, 1994; **77**: 261–71.

60. Lemmon MA, Ferguson KM, Schlessinger J. PH domains: diverse sequences with a common fold recruit signaling molecules to the cell surface. *Cell*, 1996; **85**: 621–4.

61. Lowy DR, Willumsen BM. Function and regulation of ras. *Annual Review of Biochemistry*, 1993; **62**: 851–91.

62. Pawson T, Schlessinger J. SH2 and SH3 domains. *Current Biology*, 1993; **3**: 434–42.

63. Marshall MS. Ras target proteins in eukaryotic cells. *Federation of American Societies for Experimental Biology Journal*, 1995; **9**: 1311–8.

64. Van Aelst L, D'Souza-Schorey C. Rho GTPases and signaling networks. *Genes and Development*, 1997; **11**: 2295–322.

65. Xu GF, O'Connell P, Viskochil D, *et al.* The neurofibromatosis type 1 gene encodes a protein related to GAP. *Cell*, 1990; **62**: 599–608.

66. Barbacid M. Ras genes. *Annual Review of Biochemistry*, 1987; **56**: 779–827.

67. Wolthuis RM, Bos JL. Ras caught in another affair: the exchange factors for Ral. *Current Opinions in Genetics and Development*, 1999; **9**: 112–17.

68. Campbell SL, Khosravi-Far R, Rossman KL, Clark GJ, Der CJ. Increasing complexity of Ras signaling. *Oncogene*, 1998; **17**: 1395–413.

69. Wasylyk B, Hagman J, Gutierrez-Hartmann A. Ets transcription factors: nuclear effectors of the Ras-MAP-kinase signaling pathway. *Trends in Biochemical Sciences*, 1998; **23**: 213–16.

70. Kerkhoff E, Rapp UR. Cell cycle targets of Ras/Raf signalling. *Oncogene*, **17**: 1998; 1457–62.

71. Rodrigues GA, Park M, Schlessinger J. Activation of the JNK pathway

is essential for transformation by the Met oncogene. *EMBO Journal*, 1997; **16**: 2634–45.

72. Basu S, Kolesnick R. Stress signals for apoptosis: ceramide and c-Jun kinase. *Oncogene*, 1998; **17**: 3277–85.

73. Chang HW, Aoki M, Fruman D, *et al*. Transformation of chicken cells by the gene encoding the catalytic subunit of PI 3-kinase. *Science*, 1997; **276**: 1848–50.

74. Vanhaesebroeck B, Leevers SJ, Panayotou G, Waterfield MD. Phosphoinositide 3-kinases: a conserved family of signal transducers. *Trends in Biochemical Sciences*, 1997; **22**: 267–72.

75. Toker A, Cantley LC. Signalling through the lipid products of phosphoinositide-3-OH kinase. *Nature*, 1997; **387**: 673–6.

76. Michiels F, Habets GG, Stam JC, van der Kammen RA, Collard JG. A role for Rac in Tiam1-induced membrane ruffling and invasion. *Nature*, 1995; **375**: 338–40.

77. Thomas SM, Brugge S. Cellular functions regulated by Src family kinases. *Annual Review of Cell and Developmental Biology*, 1997; **13**: 513–609.

78. Stambolic V, Suzuki A, de la Pompa JL, *et al*. Negative regulation of PKB/Akt-dependent cell survival by the tumor suppressor PTEN. *Cell*, 1998; **95**: 29–39.

79. Leonard WJ, O'Shea JJ. Jaks and STATs: biological implications. *Annual Review of Immunology*, 1998; **16**: 293–322.

80. Boccaccio C, Ando M, Tamagnone L, Bardelli A, Michieli P, Battistini C, Comoglio PM. Induction of epithelial tubules by growth factor HGF depends on the STAT pathway. *Nature*, 1998; **391**: 285–8.

81. Massague J. TGF-beta signal transduction. *Annual Review of Biochemistry*, 1998; **67**: 753–91.

82. Derynck R, Zhang Y, Feng XH. Smads: transcriptional activators of TGF-beta responses. *Cell*, 1998; **95**: 737–40.

83. Markowitz S, Wang J, Myeroff L, *et al*. Inactivation of the type II TGF-beta receptor in colon cancer cells with microsatellite instability. *Science*, 1995; **268**: 1336–8.

84. Hahn SA, Schutte M, Hoque AT, *et al*. DPC4, a candidate tumor suppressor gene at human chromosome 18q21.1. *Science*, 1996; **271**: 350–3.

1.5 Control of the cell cycle and cell death

Chris Norbury

Introduction

Tissue homeostasis is characterized by an exquisite balance between cell proliferation and cell death. Perturbation of this equilibrium, either through overproliferation or through failure of cell elimination, is the fundamental basis of all hyperplastic and neoplastic disease. This chapter surveys the molecular basis of cell cycle progression, which is absolutely required for cell proliferation, and apoptosis, which accounts for the vast majority of cell loss under normal physiological conditions. The high degree to which the molecular mechanisms involved have been conserved in evolution has allowed rapid exploration of these processes through the application of biochemistry and genetics to appropriate model organisms. Models for studies of cell cycle regulation include yeasts, fruit flies, and frog eggs, while the genetics of cell death were first defined in the nematode worm *Caenorhabditis elegans*. These models have been fundamental to our understanding of the analogous processes in human cells, as the latter are often not amenable to equivalently straightforward experimental techniques.

Cell cycle progression and links with cell growth controls

Cell cycle events

In most cell types, mitotic cell cycle progression consists of alternating rounds of chromosomal DNA replication (S-phase) and segregation of the chromosomes into two daughter cells in mitosis (M-phase).[1] The S- and M-phases are usually separated by gap phases (G_1 between M and S; G_2 between S and M; Fig. 1), although these are dispensable under circumstances where no increase in cell size is required; for example, in early embryogenesis. Exceptions to this general rule include differentiating megakaryocytes and trophoblasts, in which multiple discrete rounds of DNA replication are completed in the absence of mitosis. This programmed endoreduplication is probably necessary to support the dramatic cytoplasmic growth that is characteristic of these cell types. Unscheduled execution of this atypical cell cycle programme can be triggered in tumour cells by exposure to DNA damaging agents such as ionizing radiation or topoisomerase poisons, and may well contribute to tumour aneuploidy.[2]

Long-term withdrawal from the cell cycle can occur from either G_1 or G_2, depending on cell type, and can either be reversible (as in the cases of fibroblasts or resting T lymphocytes) or permanent (as it is for a wide variety of terminally differentiated cells). By contrast DNA replication and mitosis, the two major irreversible cell cycle events, are not subject to long-term interruptions under normal physiological conditions.

Linking cell size and the cell cycle

Increase in the size of human cells occurs in response to highly tissue- and cell-specific cues. If the appropriate signalling conditions are satisfied, bulk RNA and protein synthesis will be stimulated and cell size will increase accordingly. Growth controls operating at this level are quite distinct from the cell cycle controls governing accurate replication and segregation of the nuclear DNA. Cell growth control mechanisms are as diverse as the multitude of cell types themselves, while the events of DNA replication and mitosis are essentially identical in every cell. None the less, in many instances progression through the cell cycle has been found to be coupled to increase in cell size.[3] One view of this interrelationship would be that cell cycle progression is an inevitable, though indirect, consequence of increase in cell mass. Experimental evidence for oncogenic transformation as a result of overexpression of components of the protein synthetic machinery lends support to this idea.[4],[5] In these cases elevated levels of bulk protein synthesis (or some other aspect of increased cellular size) may be sensed by an intracellular mechanism that engages the cell cycle machinery to allow balanced growth of the transformed cell. Alternatively, cell cycle progression could depend upon the accumulation to a threshold level of one or more short-lived regulatory

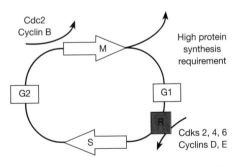

Fig. 1 Cell cycle events. Progression through the R point in late G_1 requires a high rate of protein synthesis and is controlled by G_1 Cdk/cyclin heterodimers. Once past the R point a cell is committed to completion of S-phase and, usually, mitosis (M). The G_2–M transition is controlled by the Cdc2/cyclin B protein kinase.

proteins. Such proteins would act as internal monitors of the translational activity of the cell, removing the requirement to invoke a direct sensor of total protein content or cell size. Cells which undergo hypertrophy in the absence of DNA replication or mitosis may simply fail to accumulate these regulatory proteins to the threshold level required for cell cycle progression. Conversely, early embryos may be programmed to synthesize high levels of the regulators, allowing rapid cell cycles in the absence of cell growth. Recent advances have identified cyclin proteins as cell cycle regulators that perform roles of this sort.

Cell cycle regulation

Commitment to S-phase entry

Irreversible commitment to enter the S-phase can occur several hours before the initiation of DNA replication itself. This commitment point is most widely known as the restriction (R) point,[6] defined as a step in G_1 beyond which a given cell remains committed to S-phase entry, regardless of subsequent growth factor deprivation or partial inhibition of protein synthesis. The R point can be considered as a point of integration or an interface between the diverse growth controls upstream and the universal biochemical events leading to DNA replication downstream.

Proteins of the cyclin family, notably cyclins D and E, appear to act as regulatory molecules governing R point commitment and the timing of DNA replication (Fig. 1).[7],[8] Accumulation of cyclin D1 in some cell types is absolutely dependent on the continued presence of growth factors, and experimentally enforced overexpression of cyclin D1 or E has the effect of advancing the onset of S-phase. Both cyclins are subject to ubiquitin-dependent proteolysis and have characteristically short half-lives, in line with predictions based on early experiments using protein synthesis inhibitors, which suggested that putative G_1/S regulators would have high turnover rates. Cyclin E is absolutely required for S-phase entry in at least one model organism, *Drosophila melanogaster*, in which ectopic cyclin E synthesis can induce complete additional rounds of DNA replication.[9]

Cyclin-dependent kinases and the G_1/S transition

The biochemical function of cyclins D and E is to form heterodimers with, and hence activate, members of the cyclin-dependent protein kinase (**Cdk**) family, specifically Cdk2, 4, and 6. Cdk activation during the G_1/S transition is presumed to result in phosphorylation of key protein substrates, leading in turn to modification of the biochemical properties of these substrates in such a way as to promote DNA replication.

The most intensively studied substrate of the cyclin D/E-dependent kinases is pRB, the tumour suppressor protein product of the retinoblastoma susceptibility gene[10] (see also Chapter 1.2). Investigation of this interaction has been hampered to some extent by the lack of any obvious equivalent of pRB in yeasts. One of the functions of hypophosphorylated pRB is to sequester transcription factors of the E2F family and therefore block E2F-dependent transcription in early G_1. Activation of cyclin D/E-dependent kinases in late G_1 results in pRB hyperphosphorylation and release of active E2F proteins. These heterodimerize with 'dimerization partner' (**DP**) proteins and drive

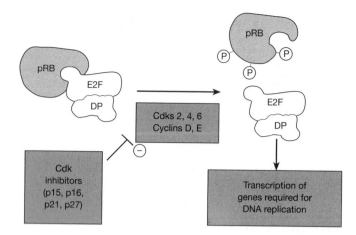

Fig. 2 Regulation of the G_1/S transition. In early G_1 the pRB protein is hypophosphorylated and sequesters transcription factors of the E2F/DP family. Phosphorylation of pRB by Cdk/cyclins results in the release of free E2F/DP heterodimers that drive S-phase-specific gene transcription. The Cdk/cyclin activities are inhibitable by a variety of Cdk inhibitor proteins that can block S-phase entry in response to diverse cues.

transcription of genes encoding enzymes necessary for 5'-deoxyribonucleotide synthesis and DNA replication itself (Fig. 2). Studies of murine embryonic fibroblasts support the idea that pRB is essential to R point control, as cells lacking pRB have a reduced requirement for serum growth factors and enter S-phase prematurely. Positive feedback control, ensuring the irreversibility of commitment to S-phase entry, is achieved through E2F-driven transcription of genes encoding G_1/S-phase-associated cyclins and Cdks. Inactivation of the G_1/S-phase Cdk/cyclin complexes is brought about, in part at least, by ubiquitin-dependent proteolysis of the cyclin subunits, which is promoted by cyclin phosphorylation at specific amino acid residues.

DNA replication

Human DNA replication involves temporally regulated initiation at 1000 to 10 000 bidirectional replication origin zones in each nucleus. The replication machinery is concentrated at 100 to 200 discrete foci within the nucleus, but there is no clear indication of which structural features of the DNA, if any, determine the positioning of origins in human cells. Much has been learned from precisely defined *in vitro* systems capable of recapitulating initiation from viral origins of replication, notably that of the simian virus SV-40.[11] Evidence from a number of other model systems strongly suggests that the Cdc6 protein and a complex consisting of multiple members of the 'minichromosome maintenance' (**Mcm**) protein family play key roles in the initiation process at human chromosomal replication origins (Fig. 3), although the biochemical functions of these proteins are not yet clear.[12],[13] The activity of cyclin A- and E-associated Cdk to phosphorylate key components of pre-replicative complexes including Cdc6 is also likely to be important at this stage.

All DNA sequences in the genome must be replicated once, but only once, in each cycle. The nuclear envelope plays an important part in this aspect of cell cycle regulation.[14],[15] Nuclear membrane disassembly in mitosis is required for preparation of the chromosomal replication origins for replicative activity in the subsequent cell cycle,

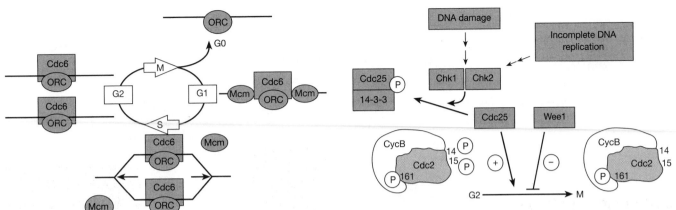

Fig. 3 Replication 'licensing'. Chromatin in G_1 cells is licensed for replication through recruitment of Mcm proteins to a pre-existing origin-recognition complex (ORC) associated with the Cdc6 protein. Initiation of replication is dependent on Cdk activities and results in the release of Mcm proteins from the chromatin. Re-recruitment of Mcm proteins at each of the replicated origins is only normally possible following breakdown of the nuclear envelope during mitosis. Entry into quiescence (G_0) is accompanied by loss of Cdc6 from the ORC.

Fig. 4 The G_2–M transition and mitotic checkpoints. Activation of the Cdc2/cyclin B heterodimer at the onset of mitosis is achieved by the Cdc25-catalysed removal of inhibitory phosphates (P) from Cdc2 residues T14 and Y15. Mitosis is inhibited by Wee1 and related protein kinases, which act to restore this inhibitory phosphorylation. Protein kinases of the Chk1/Chk2 family are activated in response to DNA damage or incomplete DNA replication, phosphorylate Cdc25 and may promote its sequestration by 14–3–3 proteins, inhibiting mitotic entry.

in a process that has been termed 'licensing'.[15] This process probably involves the association of Mcm proteins with a basal origin organizing complex on the chromatin. Once DNA synthesis has been initiated at a given origin, Mcm proteins are displaced from the chromatin in a manner that cannot be reversed until nuclear envelope breakdown in the subsequent M-phase. In this way initiation at any given origin of replication is limited to once per S-phase.

Mitosis

The cell cycle transition most clearly understood at the molecular level is the onset of mitosis (Fig. 4). To allow its accurate segregation into two daughter cells, the duplicated DNA in the G_2 nucleus has first to be condensed into discrete chromosomes. Other major mitotic events are disassembly of the nuclear membrane and underlying lamina, and reorganization of the microtubular cytoskeleton to form the spindle, the molecular machine which separates the replicated and condensed chromosomes. Further biochemical changes lead to disassembly of the nucleolus, vesicularization of the Golgi apparatus, and reorganization of the actin cytoskeleton. Remarkably, all of these events are brought about by the activation of a single protein kinase, the prototypic Cdk called Cdc2, which in its active form consists of heterodimers with A- or B-type cyclin proteins.[1],[3],[16]

Regulation of Cdc2 activity depends in part on the restriction of A and B cyclin synthesis to the S- and G_2/M-phases, but also on regulated cyclin proteolysis and phosphorylation of the kinase at three specific amino acid residues. Activating phosphorylation of Cdc2 at threonine residue 161 (T161) is performed by the Cdk-activating kinase (itself a Cdk) and is probably constitutive. Analogous phosphorylation events are required for the activation of G_1- and S-phase Cdks and are carried out by the same Cdk-activating kinase activity. Phosphorylation at T161 is coincident with, and probably serves to stabilize, Cdc2-cyclin A/B interaction. The heterodimeric protein kinase is then maintained in an inactive state by phosphorylation of

residues threonine 14 and tyrosine 15 (T14 and Y15) until the onset of mitosis, which is brought about by the abrupt dephosphorylation of T14 and Y15 and consequent activation of Cdc2. The inhibitory phosphorylation events are carried out by Wee1, a nuclear kinase largely specific for Y15, and Myt1, a membrane-associated enzyme with a substrate preference for T14. The Cdc25 family of protein phosphatases are responsible for the removal of phosphates from T14 and Y15. In an elegant positive feedback loop, Cdc2 is able to accelerate its own activation by phosphorylating and inhibiting Wee1 and simultaneously activating Cdc25. This mechanism forms the basis for the rapid increase in Cdc2 activity that ensures total cellular commitment to mitosis. Cyclin A/Cdc2 kinase activity appears slightly earlier than the cyclin B-associated kinase, and may play a 'priming' role, although the molecular basis for this is currently unknown. In addition to Wee1 and Cdc25, Cdc2 phosphorylates components of the nuclear lamina, constituents of the nucleolus and a number of other structural proteins. Further protein kinases may also be activated by Cdc2 in a phosphorylation cascade leading to mitotic chromatin condensation.

Inactivation of Cdc2-cyclin heterodimers is achieved by the ubiquitin/proteasome mediated proteolysis of the cyclin moiety. Conjugation of ubiquitin to cyclin B is performed by the anaphase-promoting complex, a multi-subunit ubiquitin ligase. This activity is also responsible for the targeting for proteolysis of other proteins, removal of which is required for the beginning of poleward chromosome movement in anaphase. Topoisomerase II is also essential at this stage, being required for the adenosine triphosphate-dependent decatenation of the replicated chromatids, without which the metaphase–anaphase transition would be impossible. Activation of the anaphase-promoting complex is, in part, dependent on Cdc2-mediated phosphorylation, such that this key mitotic kinase sows the seeds of its own destruction. Anaphase-promoting complex activity remains high from the onset of anaphase until the end of the G_1-phase in the subsequent cell cycle, a regulatory feature that ensures mitosis is followed by S-phase, rather than another mitosis.

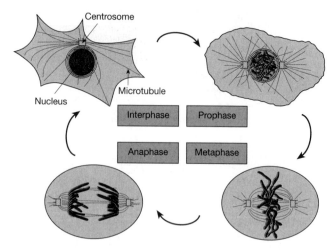

Fig. 5 The microtubular cycle. In early G₁ the interphase cell contains a single centrosome, from which a complex array of cytoplasmic microtubules is nucleated (top left). Centrosome duplication is completed by the time the cell enters mitotic prophase (top right). Chromosome condensation and nuclear envelope breakdown are accompanied by disassembly of the interphase microtubular array and the nucleation of spindle microtubules as the cell proceeds to metaphase (lower right). Loss of sister chromatid cohesion and shortening of the spindle microtubules drives chromosome segregation in anaphase (lower left).

Once anaphase is initiated and Cdc2/cyclin B kinase is inactivated, mitosis rapidly proceeds to completion through the poleward movement of the separated sister chromatids, reversal of mitosis-specific phosphorylation events and reformation of the nuclear envelope. Cytokinesis, the actin-dependent constriction of the neck between the nascent daughter cells, is apparently dependent on progression through mitosis, but is otherwise poorly understood in human cells. Rapid progress in studies of yeast cytokinesis is likely to illuminate the equivalent human processes in the near future.

The microtubular cycle

Distinct from, but closely co-ordinated with, the nuclear cell cycle, the ordered restructuring of the tubulin cytoskeleton plays a fundamental part in the accurate segregation of chromosomes (Fig. 5). Microtubular arrays are organized by the centrosomes, duplication of which begins at about the time of R point transition, but which is not complete until late G₂. Following Cdc2 activation in prophase, the interphase array of microtubules is disassembled prior to the formation of a bipolar spindle. By this stage the condensed, duplicated sister chromatid pairs are prepared for segregation by the assembly of a microtubule attachment site, the kinetochore, adjacent to each centromere. Microtubules nucleated at each of the duplicated centrosomes polymerize and depolymerize in a dynamic fashion until contact is established with a kinetochore, when the spindle microtubule in question becomes stabilized. The microtubule attachment site at each kinetochore contains adenosine triphosphate-dependent microtubule 'motor' proteins. As each pair of sister chromatids bears a pair of kinetochores, attachment of one of each pair to one of the two centrosomes allows the establishment of metaphase, with the pairs of sister chromatids aligned at the central plate, equidistant from the centrosomes. When all of the kinetochores are attached

to spindle microtubules the anaphase-promoting complex becomes activated in order to destroy sister chromatid cohesion and allow the onset of anaphase. This control mechanism involves Mad and Bub proteins in yeast, and related proteins probably act in similar ways to maintain chromosomal stability in human cells.[17],[18]

Cdk inhibitors

The activities of Cdks are limited in part by the abundance of specific inhibitor proteins. These fall into two groupings based on structural similarity either to the p21 product of the *CIP1/WAF1* gene or to the p16 protein. Synthesis of these proteins can be constitutive or inducible, for example by growth inhibitory factors such as transforming growth factor-β or in response to DNA damage.[19] The primary function of Cdk inhibitors would appear to be to set a threshold level for cyclin/Cdk complexes, above which they are free to phosphorylate their substrates. Members of the p21 family may also function in Cdk/cyclin heterodimer assembly and intracellular transport.

Regulated ubiquitin-dependent proteolysis of Cdk inhibitors has an important part in the control of cell cycle progression in human cells. As with the control of metaphase–anaphase progression, the key to the specific destruction of Cdk inhibitors in the G₁- and S-phase probably lies in a multi-subunit ubiquitin ligase, the SCF (Skp1/cullin/F-box) complex.

Checkpoint controls

Progression through the cell cycle is conditional upon 'checkpoint' regulatory mechanisms that serve to monitor a variety of intracellular events. These ensure, for example, that mitosis is not attempted until DNA replication has been completed and any remaining DNA damage has been repaired.[20] Additional checkpoints serve either to delay the onset of S-phase, to inhibit ongoing replication in response to DNA damage or to inhibit anaphase onset if spindle formation is inhibited. There is extensive overlap between the checkpoint pathways that are activated in response to S-phase inhibition and DNA damage. These signals are channelled through multiprotein complexes that include large protein kinases of the Atm/Atr family, resulting in activation of Chk1 and Chk2, functionally related downstream kinases.[21]–[23] These in turn phosphorylate Cdc25 and may promote its sequestration by phosphoprotein-binding proteins of the 14–3–3 family, resulting in inhibition of mitotic entry (Fig. 4).

Inhibition of S-phase entry following DNA damage is particularly well understood in human cells, and is absolutely dependent on the function of the tumour suppressor p53 (see also Chapter 1.2). Stabilization of p53 following detection of DNA lesions results in its transcriptional activation of the *WAF1/CIP1* gene encoding the Cdk inhibitor p21. Inhibition of G₁/S-phase Cdks following p21 induction is largely responsible for the DNA damage-induced block of progression into S-phase. The induction of p21 by p53 also reinforces the G₂ checkpoint, probably by direct p21-mediated inhibition of Cdc2/cyclin B. p53 regulation is complex, and its stability is determined in part by association with the Mdm2 protein, which targets p53 for nuclear export and ubiquitin-mediated proteolysis (see also Chapter 1.2). As the *MDM2* gene is itself transcriptionally activated by p53, a negative feedback loop is established that normally limits the abundance of p53. Disruption of the p53–Mdm2 interaction in response to cellular stress, either by p53 modification or by expression of p19ARF (an Mdm2-binding protein encoded by the *INK4A* gene, that also encodes the p16 Cdk inhibitor), blocks p53 degradation.

Cell cycle control in tumours

Loss of restriction point control

R point regulation is defective in many tumour cells.[24] Tumour cell lines are generally unable to arrest in a quiescent 'G$_0$' state when serum growth factors or amino acids are limiting, while primary fibroblasts and a number of other 'normal' cell types are able to arrest reversibly under these conditions. Loss of R point control in tumour cells can be achieved through the acquisition of any one of a variety of molecular lesions. These include loss of the pRB protein, overexpression of cyclin D1 or loss of Cdk inhibitors such as p16 that normally inhibit G$_1$/S-phase-specific Cdks.[10] Once R point control has been lost, it is likely that progression through the remainder of the cell cycle is usually constitutive.

The Cdk inhibitor p27 inhibits a variety of cyclin–Cdk complexes *in vitro* and is upregulated by cytokines such as transforming growth factor-β and by cell–cell contact, linking extracellular signals to the cell cycle.[19] Loss of contact inhibition and of response to transforming growth factor-β in transformed cells may imply frequent alteration of p27 function during tumorigenesis, although p27 mutations in human tumours are rare.[25] Unlike the related Cdk inhibitor p21, which is regulated primarily at the level of transcription, p27 is mainly regulated post-translationally by ubiquitin-dependent proteolysis.[26] Low p27 protein levels, apparently due to increased proteasome-dependent degradation, in common tumours such as colorectal and non-small cell lung carcinoma are associated with a poor prognosis,[27],[28] suggesting that p27 level may be a useful independent prognostic factor in a variety of tumour types. p27 degradation activity is not correlated with proteasome-mediated degradation of other substrates such as p21 and cyclin A, demonstrating that the substrate specificity of the ubiquitin/proteasome pathway is highly regulated.

Additional lesions, leading for example to reduction of the adhesion dependence of the cell or inhibition of the apoptotic death programme (see below), are required to complete the transformation process. In addition to cyclin D1, cyclins E, A, and B, Cdk2 and Cdc2 have also been reported to be overexpressed in a proportion of tumours.

Loss of checkpoint controls

Loss of p53 function is the commonest known lesion in cancer cells (see Chapter 1.3). As p53 is required for G$_1$ arrest in response to DNA damage, most tumour cells will be defective in this process.[29] This G$_1$ checkpoint defect is thought unlikely to contribute significantly to tumorigenesis *per se*, as the cells of mice lacking the p21 Cdk inhibitor are also largely defective in the G$_1$ checkpoint response; however, these animals are not cancer-prone, unlike those lacking p53. Tumours lacking p21 may behave differently from those in which p21 is still present following therapy, however, as long-term p21-mediated arrest in G$_1$ following DNA damage is associated with retention of cell viability, and hence with maintenance of tumour burden. Cells lacking p21, by contrast, appear more prone to DNA damage-induced death following therapy.[30],[31] Additional checkpoints controlled by p53 may contribute to its tumour suppressing

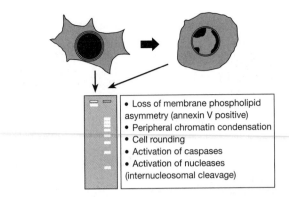

Fig. 6 Characteristic features of apoptosis. The onset of apoptotic death is accompanied by characteristic peripheral condensation of the chromatin, without nuclear envelope breakdown (top). Activation of nucleases in the dying cell (right) results in cleavage of the genomic DNA, preferentially in the internucleosomal spacer regions, leading to a characteristic 'ladder' on agarose gel electrophoresis (represented schematically, lower left). By contrast, genomic DNA from healthy cells (left) has a much lower mobility.

activity; these include regulation of centrosome replication[32] and a contribution towards the G$_2$ arrest induced by DNA damage.

Control of cell death

Apoptosis: cell death as a universal default pathway

Human development is accompanied not only by cell proliferation, but also by highly regulated cell death, for example in the developing brain or during digit formation in the early embryo.[33] Programmed cell death is accompanied by characteristic morphological and biochemical changes, including alteration in the phospholipid distribution in the plasma membrane, hyper-condensation of the chromatin at the nuclear periphery, and DNA fragmentation (Fig. 6). Ordered cell death of this sort, termed apoptosis, is a default pathway actively executed in response to withdrawal of cell-specific survival signals.[34] These signals can be mediated both by diffusible factors and by interactions between cell surface molecules and the extracellular matrix. The changes seen in apoptotic cells are distinguished from the more disorganized loss of cell structure seen in necrosis which, unlike apoptosis, also generally engages the inflammatory response.

Detection of apoptotic cells in mixed populations can be achieved by methods such as the TUNEL assay (terminal *T*dT-mediated d*UTP* nick end-labelling of the free 3' OH DNA ends generated by endonuclease activation), but this cannot distinguish apoptotic DNA fragmentation from other strand breaks, such as those that might occur in necrotic cells or cells exposed to DNA damaging agents. Alternative assays that are potentially more specific include cell surface binding of annexin V, a calcium-dependent phosphatidylserine-binding protein that can reveal loss of phospholipid asymmetry in the plasma membrane. Time-lapse videomicroscopy shows that apoptotic cell death can be very rapid, being completed in 20 min or less. This rapidity, combined with the engulfment of the resulting apoptotic bodies by phagocytosis, can lead to substantial underestimation of

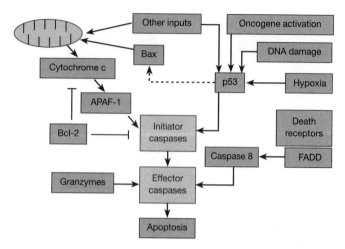

Fig. 7 Overview of apoptotic regulation. Initiator caspases can be activated by a variety of signals, some of which are transduced by pathways leading to p53 activation. Cytochrome c release from mitochondria (top left) can also contribute to caspase activation through APAF-1 binding. This process is promoted by Bax, which may be upregulated by p53, and is inhibited by Bcl-2 and related antiapoptotic proteins. Effector caspases can be activated independently by cytotoxic T-lymphocyte-derived granzyme proteases, or ligation of death receptors of the tumour necrosis factor receptor 1 family.

apoptotic rates following microscopic examination of fixed cell populations.[35]

Apoptosis and its regulation are highly relevant to tumour cell biology, as genetic lesions leading to diminished apoptosis may play a general role in tumorigenesis. In addition, many cancer therapies result in elevated levels of cancer cell apoptosis, although necrosis can also make a major contribution to tumour cell death, particularly in solid tumours.

A central role for caspases

Execution of apoptosis involves activation of members of a specialized family of *c*ysteine *asp*artyl prote*ases* (the caspases).[36],[37] The importance of these enzymes was first highlighted by genetic studies of *C. elegans*, which identified the *ced-3* gene product, a caspase, as being essential for developmentally regulated apoptotic cell deaths in this organism.[38] Regulation of apoptosis in human cells is substantially more complex than it is in *C. elegans*. Many different members of the human caspase family are involved in cell death, while others are involved in processes such as interleukin processing. Active caspases are heterodimeric, consisting of large and small subunits typically generated by caspase-mediated cleavage of a common precursor procaspase protein; there is therefore the potential for amplification of apoptotic signals through caspase proteolytic cascades. An apical regulatory role is played by certain caspases, notably caspases 8 and 9, with other members of the family performing effector roles downstream (Fig. 7). Target substrates of the caspases include a wide variety of intracellular proteins which contain cleavage sites containing aspartate residues in their amino acid sequences. On a random basis these sequences would be expected to be more frequent in large proteins than in smaller ones, so it is perhaps not surprising that the best characterized caspase substrates are large proteins such as poly-adenosine diphosphate ribose polymerase and DNA-dependent

protein kinase. The extent to which cleavage of specific proteins is responsible for the characteristic cellular changes seen in the apoptotic cell is not yet clear.

The Bcl-2 family

A second family of proteins playing key roles in the regulation of apoptosis includes Bcl-2, the product of a gene activated by t(14;18) chromosomal translocations in follicular lymphoma.[39] A Bcl-2 homologue in *C. elegans* is encoded by the *ced-9* gene and also functions as a suppressor of CED-3-mediated cell deaths. Additional Bcl-2-related proteins found in human cells have roles either in the promotion or inhibition of apoptosis. The mechanisms of action of these proteins remain somewhat controversial, but functional roles as membrane pores and regulators of caspase activation have been proposed. Members of the Bcl-2 family are capable of forming homo- and heterodimers, increasing the potential complexity of their regulation.

Mitochondria and cell death

Activation of caspase cascades can be triggered by a wide variety of physiological stimuli. While the activatory mechanisms involved are mostly poorly understood, in some cases release of cytochrome c from mitochondria appears to be an early step in caspase 9 activation.[40] Recapitulation of some aspects of the apoptotic programme *in vitro* is greatly stimulated by the addition of a mitochondrial fraction, and cytochrome c release from mitochondria is observed in apoptotic cells even if caspase activation is inhibited. Cytochrome c release stimulates the human APAF-1 protein (*a*poptotic *p*rotease *a*ctivating *f*actor 1), a structural relative of the pro-apoptotic CED-4 protein in *C. elegans*, to bind and activate procaspase 9. Surprisingly, mitochondrial release of cytochrome c does not seem to be a significant regulator of apoptosis in *C. elegans*.

Receptor-mediated death

Aside from withdrawal of survival signals, other physiologically important triggers of apoptosis include hypoxia, DNA damage, depletion of nucleotide pools, and engagement of 'death receptors' of the tumour necrosis factor receptor superfamily.[41] Death receptors are particularly important in the immune system, being required both for the removal of excess activated peripheral T cells and for the effective killing of target cells by cytotoxic T lymphocytes. The best-understood members of the death receptor family are CD95 (also known as Fas or Apo1) and the tumour necrosis factor receptor-1 itself. These are transmembrane proteins with cysteine-rich extracellular domains and intracellular regions that share a common structure termed the 'death domain'. The pro-apoptotic ligands for these receptors are homotrimeric peptides that are either soluble or expressed at the surface of an adjacent cell. Ligand-induced receptor clustering promotes the binding of a soluble cytosolic adaptor protein called FADD (*F*as-*a*ssociated *d*eath *d*omain), which itself contains a death domain as well as a caspase binding site, to the clustered death domains of the receptors. This in turn allows FADD-mediated oligomerization of procaspase 8 and self-activation of the caspase, followed by activation of effector caspases downstream (Fig. 7). The sensitivity of any given cell to receptor-mediated apoptosis depends on its inherent level of expression of the proteins involved in the pathway, probably modulated by the expression of 'decoy' receptors lacking intact intracellular death domains.

A further short-cut to caspase activation is taken during cytotoxic T-lymphocyte-mediated lysis of target cells. This type of cell death, which closely resembles apoptosis in its morphology, is accompanied by the release of perforin and lytic granules from the cytotoxic T lymphocytes. The granules contain 'granzyme' proteases that directly cleave and activate effector caspases. In many cases target cell lysis is therefore triggered by a combination of CD95 ligation and granzyme-mediated caspase activation.

p53-dependent apoptosis

In addition to its cell cycle regulatory functions discussed earlier, the p53 tumour suppressor protein is absolutely required for some forms of apoptosis, such as radiation-induced thymocyte death *in vivo*. Activation of p53 is thought to be central to the cellular decision of whether to arrest the cell cycle or to initiate cell death after exposure to DNA damage or other stresses (see also Chapter 1.2). Despite this, the mechanism of p53-induced apoptosis remains unclear. In some cases, p53-mediated transcriptional induction of the *BAX* gene, encoding a pro-apoptotic member of the Bcl-2 family, may be involved, but other targets and non-transcriptional apoptotic roles for p53 have also been proposed.[29]

Cells can die from any point of the cell cycle

Several experimental observations have led to the proposal that cell cycle progression is in some way linked to the initiation of apoptosis. Overexpression of proteins such as c-Myc that promote cell cycle entry has been found, for example, to drive cells into apoptosis if serum growth factors are simultaneously withdrawn.[42] A causal link between the onset of apoptosis and resumption of cell cycle progression in cells that have previously been arrested at the G_2 checkpoint in response to DNA damage has also been proposed. Nevertheless, apoptosis can be initiated from any point in the cell cycle, as well as from quiescent G_0 states. There is thus no 'hard-wired' connection between the cell cycle regulatory machinery and the molecules responsible for the onset of apoptotic death.

Oncogene co-operation *in vitro* may reflect selection during tumorigenesis for mutations leading both to the disruption of cell cycle regulation and to the inhibition of apoptosis. According to this 'dual key' hypothesis, a mutation at a single locus causing deregulation of cell cycle entry will also necessarily activate the default cell death pathway and lead to elimination of the mutant cell, rather than unrestrained proliferation. In this respect, oncogenes activated in isolation can also be regarded as tumour suppressor genes, as they serve to engage the apoptotic machinery and prevent proliferation. Support for this idea comes from $RB^{-/-}$ knockout mice, which die as early embryos, at least partly due to massive apoptosis in multiple tissues.

Cell death in tumours

Tumour cells can lose the requirement for survival signalling

Perhaps the clearest example of the contribution that failure of apoptosis can make to tumorigenesis is that of B-cell chronic lymphocytic leukaemia, which is characterized by a very low proliferation rate coupled with a dramatic reduction in the propensity for peripheral apoptosis relative to that of normal B cells. In adherent cell types, anchorage-dependence of cell growth generally reflects receptor-mediated inhibition of apoptosis. Loss of anchorage dependence is a common characteristic of solid tumours that is likely to be important in metastasis, as well as spatial disorganization during neoplasia. The histopathological observation of high rates of constitutive apoptosis in some solid tumours with high proliferative indices[43] underlines the genetic diversity of tumours (see also Chapter 1.6), and demonstrates that loss of dependence on survival factors is not an obligatory step in all instances of tumour progression.

Enhancing tumour cell specificity of cancer therapies

Improvements in the effectiveness of current therapies may be achieved by exploitation of the emerging knowledge of the genetic differences between tumour cells and their normal counterparts. All modes of conventional systemic cancer therapy that have been examined result in elevated levels of apoptosis, both in tumour cells and in tissues susceptible to therapy-related toxicity, such as bone marrow and intestinal epithelium. It is widely assumed that apoptosis is the primary cause of tumour cell death following therapy, though loss of long-term clonogenic potential is not necessarily associated with apoptosis in all cell types. The p53 status of tumour cells can determine the efficacy of cancer therapies *in vivo*, with maintenance of p53 function being associated with high rates of therapy-induced apoptosis and tumour regression.[44] Conversely, chemotherapy-induced apoptosis and loss of long-term viability can be inhibited in neuroblastoma and leukaemia cells by constitutive expression of Bcl-2,[45],[46] although this effect is dependent on cell type and apoptotic stimulus.

The most obvious general defect of cell cycle regulation in tumour cells is their lack of various checkpoint controls, particularly those dependent on functional activation of p53. It may be possible to exploit this generality, for example by using DNA damaging agents in combination with drugs that suppress still further the already weakened checkpoint responses of p53-compromised cells. On the other hand, cells lacking p53 function are likely to be relatively refractory to DNA damage-induced apoptosis.[44] Alternative strategies could involve direct stimulation of caspase cascades within cancer cells, as opposed to the indirect stimulation of these cascades induced by conventional therapies.

References

1. **Murray A, Hunt T.** *The cell cycle—an introduction.* Oxford: Oxford University Press, 1993.

2. **Waldman T, Lengauer C, Kinzler KW, Vogelstein B.** Uncoupling of S phase and mitosis induced by anticancer agents in cells lacking p21. *Nature,* 1996; **381**: 713–16.

3. **Norbury CJ, Nurse P.** Animal cell cycles and their control. *Annual Review of Biochemistry,* 1992; **61**: 441–70.

4. **Lazaris-Karatzas A, Montine KS, Sonenberg N.** Malignant transformation by a eukaryotic initiation factor subunit that binds to mRNA 5' cap. *Nature,* 1990; **345**: 544–7.

5. Sonenberg N. Translation factors as effectors of cell growth and tumorigenesis. *Current Opinion in Cell Biology*, 1993; 5: 955–60.

6. Pardee A. A restriction point for control of normal animal cell proliferation. *Proceedings of the National Academy of Sciences USA*, 1974; 71: 1286–90.

7. Ohtsubo M, Roberts JM. Cyclin-dependent regulation of G_1 in mammalian fibroblasts. *Science*, 1993; 259: 1908–12.

8. Resnitzky D, Gossen M, Bujard H, Reed SI. Acceleration of the G_1/S phase transition by expression of cyclins D1 and E with an inducible system. *Molecular and Cellular Biology*, 1994; 14: 1669–79.

9. Knoblich JA, Sauer K, Jones L, Richardson H, Saint R, Lehner CF. Cyclin E controls S phase progression and its down-regulation during *Drosophila* embryogenesis is required for the arrest of cell proliferation. *Cell*, 1994; 77: 107–20.

10. Sherr CJ. Cancer cell cycles. *Science*, 1996; 274: 1672–7.

11. Li JJ, Kelly TJ. Simian virus 40 DNA replication *in vitro*. *Proceedings of the National Academy of Sciences USA*, 1984; 81: 6973–7.

12. Coverley D, Laskey RA. Regulation of eukaryotic DNA replication. *Annual Review of Biochemistry*, 1994; 63: 745–76.

13. Madine MA, Khoo CY, Mills AD, Laskey RA. MCM3 complex required for cell cycle regulation of DNA replication in vertebrate cells. *Nature*, 1995; 375: 421–4.

14. Madine MA, Khoo CY, Mills AD, Mushal C, Laskey RA. The nuclear envelope prevents reinitiation of replication by regulating the binding of MCM3 to chromatin in *Xenopus* egg extracts. *Current Biology*, 1995; 5: 1270–9.

15. Blow JJ, Laskey RA. A role for the nuclear envelope in controlling DNA replication within the cell cycle. *Nature*, 1988; 332: 546–8.

16. Nurse P. Universal control mechanism regulating onset of M-phase. *Nature*, 1990; 344: 503–8.

17. Taylor SS, McKeon F. Kinetochore localization of murine Bub1 is required for normal mitotic timing and checkpoint response to spindle damage. *Cell*, 1997; 89: 727–35.

18. Cahill DP, *et al.* Mutations of mitotic checkpoint genes in human cancers. *Nature*, 1998; 392: 300–3.

19. Polyak K, *et al.* p27Kip1, a cyclin-Cdk inhibitor, links transforming growth factor-beta and contact inhibition to cell cycle arrest. *Genes and Development*, 1994; 8: 9–22.

20. Weinert T. DNA damage checkpoints update: getting molecular. *Current Opinion in Genetics and Development*, 1998; 8: 185–93.

21. Sanchez Y, *et al.* Conservation of the Chk1 checkpoint pathway in mammals: linkage of DNA damage to Cdk regulation through Cdc25. *Science*, 1997; 277: 1497–501.

22. Elledge SJ. Cell cycle checkpoints: preventing an identity crisis. *Science*, 1996; 274: 1664–72.

23. Matsuoka S, Huang M, Elledge SJ. Linkage of ATM to cell cycle regulation by the Chk2 protein kinase. *Science*, 1998; 282: 1893–7.

24. Pardee AB. G_1 events and regulation of cell proliferation. *Science*, 1989; 246: 603–8.

25. Ferrando AA, Balbin M, Pendas AM, Vizoso F, Velasco G, Lopez-Otin

C. Mutational analysis of the human cyclin-dependent kinase inhibitor p27kip1 in primary breast carcinomas. *Human Genetics*, 1996; 97: 91–4.

26. Pagano M, *et al.* Role of the ubiquitin-proteasome pathway in regulating abundance of the cyclin-dependent kinase inhibitor p27. *Science*, 1995; 269: 682–5.

27. Catzavelos C, Tsao MS, DeBoer G, Bhattacharya N, Shepherd FA, Slingerland JM. Reduced expression of the cell cycle inhibitor p27Kip1 in non-small cell lung carcinoma: a prognostic factor independent of Ras. *Cancer Research*, 1999; 59: 684–8.

28. Loda M, *et al.* Increased proteasome-dependent degradation of the cyclin-dependent kinase inhibitor p27 in aggressive colorectal carcinomas. *Nature Medicine*, 1997; 3: 231–4.

29. Levine AJ. p53, the cellular gatekeeper for growth and division. *Cell*, 1997; 88: 323–31.

30. Polyak K, Waldman T, He TC, Kinzler KW, Vogelstein B. Genetic determinants of p53-induced apoptosis and growth arrest. *Genes and Development*, 1996; 10: 1945–52.

31. Waldman T, *et al.* Cell-cycle arrest versus cell death in cancer therapy. *Nature Medicine*, 1997; 3: 1034–6.

32. Fukasawa K, Choi T, Kuriyama R, Rulong S, Vande Woude GF. Abnormal centrosome amplification in the absence of p53. *Science*, 1996; 271: 1744–7.

33. Jacobson MD, Weil M, Raff MC. Programmed cell death in animal development. *Cell*, 1997; 88: 347–54.

34. Raff MC. Social controls on cell survival and cell death. *Nature*, 1992; 356: 397–400.

35. Evan GI, *et al.* Induction of apoptosis in fibroblasts by c-myc protein. *Cell*, 1992; 69: 119–28.

36. Thornberry NA, Lazebnik Y. Caspases: enemies within. *Science*, 1998; 281: 1312–16.

37. Cryns V, Yuan J. Proteases to die for. *Genes and Development*, 1998; 12: 1551–70.

38. Hengartner MO. Programmed cell death in invertebrates. *Current Opinion in Genetics and Development*, 1996; 6: 34–8.

39. Adams JM, Cory S. The Bcl-2 protein family: arbiters of cell survival. *Science*, 1998; 281: 1322–6.

40. Green DR, Reed JC. Mitochondria and apoptosis. *Science*, 1998; 281: 1309–12.

41. Ashkenazi A, Dixit VM. Death receptors: signaling and modulation. *Science*, 1998; 281: 1305–8.

42. Evan G, Littlewood T. A matter of life and cell death. *Science*, 1998; 281: 1317–22.

43. Gaffney EF. The extent of apoptosis in different types of high grade prostatic carcinoma. *Histopathology*, 1994; 25: 269–73.

44. Lowe SW, *et al.* p53 status and the efficacy of cancer therapy *in vivo*. *Science*, 1994; 266: 807–10.

45. Miyashita T, Reed JC. Bcl-2 oncoprotein blocks chemotherapy-induced apoptosis in a human leukemia cell line. *Blood*, 1993; 81: 151–7.

46. Dole M, *et al.* Bcl-2 inhibits chemotherapy-induced apoptosis in neuroblastoma. *Cancer Res.*, 1994; 54: 3253–9.

Growth and kinetics of human tumours

A. C. Begg

Introduction

The rate of growth of a tumour can have important clinical consequences, as it will influence the natural history of the disease. It will determine the time from initiation to clinical symptoms, and from first symptoms to serious clinical problems. Furthermore, it will determine how long after treatment the tumour will take to recur if the treatment is unsuccessful. It may also determine the outcome of a treatment which takes several weeks or months to complete, such as in many radiotherapy or chemotherapy schedules. This is because continued cell production in fast proliferating tumours during treatment gaps may counteract cell killing from the treatment itself, reducing the chance of cure. Knowledge of a tumour's growth rate and growth potential can therefore be important for both prognosis and in treatment planning.

Basic principles

Growth patterns

Growth of a cell population resulting from each cell dividing into two daughters is fundamentally an exponential process. After each cell cycle time the cell population doubles. After X cell cycles, the number of cells will therefore be 2^X. After 30 cycles, for example, there will be 2^{30} (10^9) cells, so that one cell will have grown to mass of approximately 1 g. In a further 10 cycles there will be 2^{40} (10^{12}) cells, a mass of approximately 1 kg. Such growth is described by the simple equation:

$$N = N_0.2^X,$$

where N_0 is the initial number of cells and X is the number of cell cycles. If the cycle time, T_C, remains constant, this can also be expressed as:

$$N = N_0.2^{t/T_c}$$

$$\text{or } N = N_0.\exp(\ln2.\, t/T_C)$$

where t is the amount of time allowed for growth. An exactly analogous set of equations can be written for tumour volume, V, by substituting V and V_0 for N and N_0, assuming that the average cell volume and average density remain constant. Plotting either N or V

I would like to thank Dr Karin Haustermans for many useful discussions and critical comments on the manuscript.

on a log scale against time produces a linear curve (Fig. 1(b)), while a linear–linear plot gives the impression of a long silent interval and a sudden acceleration (Fig. 1(a)). Similar shapes are seen for plots of tumour diameter against time (Fig. 1(c),(d)), although the slope on a semi-log plot is one-third that for volume, since diameter is proportional to volume$^{0.33}$.

These equations will only apply if all cells remain cycling and no cells are lost from the population. In practice this almost never happens. Tumours tend to have an insufficient blood supply (see Chapter 1.7) resulting in nutrient and oxygen deficiencies, leading to some cells going out of cycle and also to cell death. In addition to nutrient deprivation, some tumours retain the differentiation pattern of the tissue of origin to a greater or lesser extent. This results in some cells differentiating into non-dividing cells which can continue to pre-programmed death. The effect of non-dividing cells will be considered first.

If there is a constant fraction of cells moving out of cycle at each division, growth will remain exponential but at a slower rate. For example, of the two daughter cells produced at each division, if on average only 1.5 remain in cycle and the other 0.5 become permanently non-dividing, then the population doubling time will not equal the cell cycle time but be $\ln2/\ln1.5 = 1.71$ times longer than T_C. In this situation, as well as there being a constant production of cycling cells, there will be a constant production of non-cycling cells. The cycling compartment is often termed the 'growth fraction' (**GF**) and will remain constant with time at 0.5 in this example. The effect of the GF is illustrated in Fig. 2 (upper panel), in which cell number has been plotted on a log scale versus number of cell cycles (proportional to time if the cell cycle time remains constant). Reducing the GF can have a large effect on tumour growth rate, as seen by the increase in doubling times indicated against each curve. Studies of tumours in experimental animals and in humans have shown that the GF is almost invariably less than 1.0 and varies markedly between tumours (Table 1, right column). High GF tumours will naturally grow faster for a given intrinsic cell cycling rate than those with low GFs. (See below for methods to measure T_C and GF.). The longer population doubling time resulting from a GF less than 100 per cent has been termed the 'potential' doubling time, or T_{POT}. It is thus a combination of T_C and GF, and would be equal to the actual volume doubling time if there were no cell loss (see below for equations and measurement methods).

Lack of nutrients or a terminal differentiation pathway can also lead to cell death. Necrosis and apoptosis (programmed cell death) are frequent in malignant tumours. If the dead cells remain in the

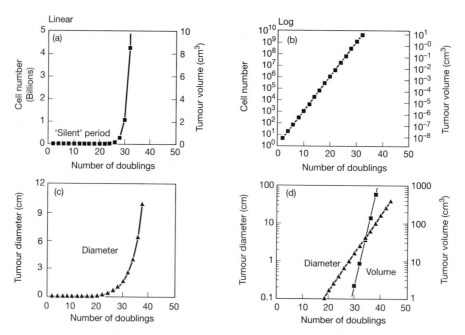

Fig. 1 Illustrations of exponential growth. On a linear scale (A), cell number and volume appear to remain undetectable for a large part of the tumour's growth history, followed by apparent rapid growth. On a semi-log plot (B), linear growth is observed, characterized by a constant doubling time. The tumour diameter (C) behaves similarly, although the slope on a log scale is one-third of that for volume (shown for comparison). The x-axis is number of doublings, which is proportional to time if the doubling time remains constant.

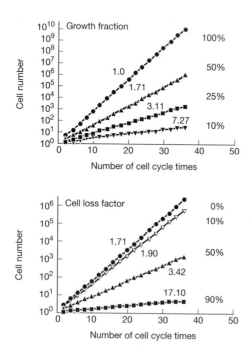

Fig. 2 Influence of the GF (upper) and cell loss (Ø; lower) on population growth rates. Lower GFs and higher cell loss factors result in slower growth and thus increased population doubling times. Numbers against each curve are the doubling times expressed in terms of number of cell cycles (equivalent to days if $T_C = 1$d). All curves in the lower panel have been calculated for a population with GF = 50 per cent.

tumour, they will contribute to tumour mass and could be regarded as part of the non-GF. However, cellular material which is lost from the tumour, either as intact cells or as lysed material, will slow the observed volume growth rate. Cell loss in kinetic terms usually means the loss of cell sized units of volume from the tumour mass. Cell loss can be described as a rate (K_L; fraction of cells lost per unit time) or as a fraction (Ø; cell loss rate as a fraction of the cell birth rate). Proliferating normal tissues are an obvious starting point for understanding the concept of cell loss. In the skin for example, cells in the basal layer proliferate, are pushed upwards through differentiating layers and are finally sloughed off at the surface. In adults, skin is a non growing organ, meaning that cell production is exactly balanced by cell loss. The cell loss factor is thus 1.0, or 100 per cent. This also applies to mucosa, for example in the oral cavity or intestinal tract. A reduction in cell loss with no change in production rate will result in overall growth, and thus the formation of a tumour. In most human solid tumours, cell loss factors have been found to be well over 50 per cent and often over 90 per cent (Table 2). These values are high, but because they are less than 100 per cent, progressive growth results. A tumour with no cell loss will have a volume doubling time 10 times shorter than a tumour with a cell loss factor of 90 per cent, such that only 10 per cent of cells produced effectively contribute to increasing the mass. The effect of increasing cell loss is illustrated graphically in Fig. 2 (lower panel). Loss of cells during growth can thus also be a major determinant of overall tumour growth rate. Cell loss is the cause of the difference between the 'potential' and 'volume' doubling times.

If the GF and cell loss factor remain constant, growth will remain exponential. In human tumours, exponential growth has been observed, but the period of observation without treatment is usually

Table 1 Cell kinetic parameters of human tumours obtained from *in vivo* labelling of patients with tritiated thymidine and performing labelled mitoses curve analyses (from data collated by Steel[1]). Phase times are median values. In two cases, the second wave was not pronounced enough to be able to calculate T_C.

Tumour type	Number of tumours	T_{G1} (h)	T_S (h)	T_{SG2} (h)	T_C (h)	GF (%)
Breast ca	2	19	20	6	51	61
Endometrial ca, ascites	1	50	48	7	113	25
Epithelioma	2	14	12	5	34	41
Malignant schwannoma	1	18	16	5	39	52
Maxillary antrum ca	1	8	11	4	23	64
Melanoma	2	37	21	5	70	25
Melanoma	3	19	14	7	47	70
Melanoma	1	20	19	8	56	59
Reticulum cell ca	1	32	14	5	53	14
Spindle cell epithelioma	1	38	10	7.5		82
Squamous cell ca	4	22	18	7	52	36
Stomach ca, ascites	1	17	19	3		58
Mean		*25*	*19*	*6*	*54*	*49*
Leukaemias:						
AML	2	37	19	3	64	24
AML/ALL	3	32	28	4	67	18
ALL	4	20	33	5	61	25
ALL	2	63	17	3	82	18
AMML	1	21	11	2	37	61
Plasma cell	1	37	16	2	57	47
Mean		*35*	*21*	*3*	*61*	*32*

AML = acute myeloblastic leukaemia.

ALL = acute lymphoblastic leukaemia.

AMML = acute myelomonocytic leukaemia.

ca = cancer.

quite short compared with the life history of the tumour. Often the volume doubling time becomes longer as the tumour increases in size. Examples of both patterns are shown in Fig. 3 for human lung tumours derived from serial measurements on chest radiography films. This can occur through a progressive decrease in the GF and/ or an increase in cell loss. This can be described mathematically by the Gompertz equation.[1]

Implications from growth patterns

Tumours exhibiting constant exponential growth will have long latency periods. A 1 g spherical tumour will have a diameter of about 1 cm and will probably be just detectable with current diagnostic procedures. Such a tumour will contain about 10^9 cells and will have undergone 30 doublings from the initial single cell. In only another 10 doublings, the tumour will be 1 kg (10^{12} cells) with a diameter of over 13 cm. In another three doublings, the tumour will be close to

10 kg with a diameter of just under 26 cm, a size which it is unlikely to reach without killing its host. Tumours can therefore often appear to be accelerating in the latter phase of growth, but this is simply their exponential nature. If anything, tumour growth will slow slightly during the clinical phase. Tumours therefore have a relatively long preclinical history during which they have the potential for metastatic spread. For example, an undetectable 1 mm diameter tumour with a potential doubling time of 5 days and a cell loss factor of 0.5 would shed more than 10 000 cells per day. Even if only a small fraction of these are live cells, the potential for seeding in this preclinical period is considerable.

A second implication from the above considerations, is that progressive growth can occur even if the intrinsic proliferation rate of the cells does not alter in the process of malignant transformation. If the cycle time remained the same as in the normal tissue of origin, but the tumour cells had a small increase in their capacity to survive by evading some of the normal differentiation or death controls, a

Table 2 Volume doubling times and cell loss factors of human tumours. Doubling times were mostly estimated from growth of lung metastases and represent median and ranges. Cell loss factors were estimated from T_{POT}, calculated from the thymidine labelling index on tumour biopsies and assuming $T_s = 15h$, and the volume doubling time (see text) (data from Steel).

Tumour type	Volume doubling time (days)	Cell loss factor (%)
Colorectal cancer	90 (60–170)	96
Squamous cell cancer head and neck	45 (33–150)	85
Bronchial cancer undifferentiated	90 (40–160)	97
Melanoma	52 (20–150)	73
Sarcoma	39 (16–78)	40
Lymphoma	22 (15–70)	29
Childhood tumours	20	82

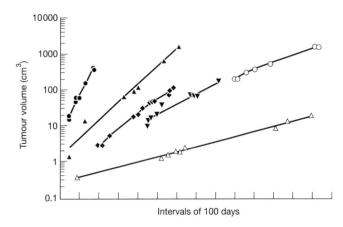

Fig. 3 Examples of growth rates of primary human lung carcinomas taken from serial chest radiographs (redrawn from Steel 1977[1]). Growth is near exponential in most cases, although also consistent with a small progressive growth reduction for some tumours.

progressively growing tumour mass could result. This would be manifested either by an increase in cell production rate caused by an increase in GF, or by the cell loss rate becoming less than the cell production rate. The latter might occur by overexpression of an anti-apoptotic gene such as *BCL-2*. Even minor evasions of the normal homeostatic controls would result in a tumour.

Measuring cell kinetics

Tumour volume

In order to measure the volume growth of a tumour, various techniques have been employed, the simplest being the use of callipers for accessible tumours such as metastatic skin nodules. Other methods for measuring tumour sizes include chest radiographs, computed tomography, nuclear magnetic resonance/magnetic resonance imaging, and other imaging techniques. With callipers, three orthogonal diameters are measured from which the volume can be estimated from the equation for an ellipse, namely:

$$V = \pi/6 . a.b.c, \text{ where } a, b, \text{ and } c \text{ are the three diameters,}$$

$$\text{or } V = \pi/6 . (\text{mean diameter})^3,$$

$$\text{or } V = \pi/6 . a.b^2, \text{ if the depth, } c, \text{ is difficult to measure.}$$

There are relatively few studies of the volume growth rates of human tumours as most new patients are treated within a matter of weeks after diagnosis. Even if at least two measurements are made before treatment, this time span is usually less than one doubling time (see below), rendering estimates of growth rate unreliable. The best data are from studies where the patients were for various reasons not treated and where several measurements were made over periods of months, either on primary tumours or lung metastases (see Fig. 3 for examples). Tumours of different sites grow on average at different rates, with primary colorectal tumours being some of the slowest growing tumours and lung metastases from lymphomas and teratomas being some of the fastest (Table 2). The shortest observed doubling times for solid tumours are about 3 weeks, while the longest are more than a year. The order of average growth rate from fast to slow are: embryonal tumours, lymphomas, sarcomas, squamous cell carcinomas, and adenocarcinomas. For each site and type, however, there is a wide range of growth rates (see ranges, Table 2).

To measure the underlying cell cycle kinetic parameters which determine the overall volume growth rate, several methods have been developed over the last four decades. The main ones involve counting mitoses, employing markers of DNA synthesis, and more recently, endogenous markers of proliferation.

Radiolabelled thymidine

The most obvious DNA synthesis marker is thymidine, the only one of the four DNA bases which doesn't occur in RNA. Thymidine itself can be radioactively labelled, usually with ^3H or ^{14}C. Detection is by autoradiography (photographic emulsion placed over cells or tissues on a microscope slide) or by liquid scintillation counting. The advantage of autoradiography over scintillation counting is that labelled and unlabelled cells can be distinguished, relationships with other structures, e.g. blood vessels, can be studied, and labelling in malignant and non-malignant tissues, distinguished by morphology, can be compared. Labelled cells are easier to detect than mitotic cells, and are more numerous because the duration of DNA synthesis (T_s) is longer than the duration of mitosis. The fraction of labelled cells (labelling index, **LI**) is a commonly studied cell kinetic parameter. In addition, cell cycle progression rates can be measured using the per cent labelled mitoses method.[1],[2] ^3H-TdR is injected into an animal or patient (which as a result of the rapid metabolism of thymidine gives almost instantaneous labelling of cells in the S phase), or for cells in tissue-culture by washing the tracer out after a few minutes. Samples are taken at a range of times and labelling of mitotic figures is measured. The fraction of mitoses which are labelled will rise and fall as the cohort of ^3H-TdR-labelled cells, initially in S, move into and out of mitosis. This pattern will be repeated one cell cycle later, although in practice the second wave is damped because of variability

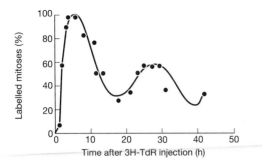

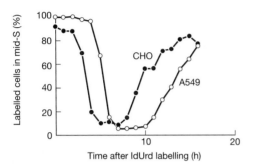

Fig. 4 Methods to measure cell cycle parameters. Upper panel: per cent labelled mitoses (PLM) curve for a subcutaneous mouse tumour using ³H-TdR and autoradiography. Lower panel: mid-S analysis for a hamster (Chinese hamster ovary) and a human tumour (A549) cell line using the thymidine analogue IdUrd and flow cytometric detection (non-radioactive). Thymidine or analogue were given as a pulse label and samples taken for analysis at the indicated times. In each case, the period between waves indicates T_C, curve damping indicates cycle phase variation, and both data sets can be analysed to yield estimates of all cycle phases (G₁, S, G₂/M). Compared with A549 cells, Chinese hamster ovary cells have a shorter S (shorter first wave) and a shorter cycle (earlier second wave). (Both data sets from the author.)

in cell cycle phase durations (Fig. 4, upper panel). From the frequency and width of the waves of labelled mitoses, the lengths of all phases of the cycle, together with their variations, can be determined.[1] This has been carried out a few times in the past on patients using multiple sampling after ³H-TdR injection. Tumour cell cycle times average just over 2 days in these studies (summarized in Table 1).

The disadvantages of these methods for studies on cancer patients are the need to administer radioactivity, the requirement for repeated biopsies, the long exposure times of the autoradiographs and the labour and skill required for the scoring. Alternative more rapid methods using thymidine analogues and flow cytometry are now used routinely (see below).

Flow cytometry

Flow cytometry consists of forcing cells in suspension to flow one by one past a light beam, usually from a laser.[3] Scattered light, either forwards or at 90°, can be quantified, giving information on cell size and granularity. More usefully, any fluorescent dyes the cells contain will be excited by the light beam, and the emitted fluorescence intensity quantified using photomultiplier tubes. Using optical filters, fluorochromes of several colours can be quantified simultaneously (Fig. 5). As antibodies can be conjugated with fluorochromes, antibody

staining can be readily detected, whether for surface, cytoplasmic, or nuclear antigens. Fluorescent dyes which bind particular cellular components can also be quantified; a good example being propidium iodide, a red fluorescent dye which binds DNA by intercalation. Total DNA content can then be measured by red fluorescence per cell. G₂ and M cells therefore have twice the red fluorescence of G₁ cells, with S phase cells having a range of intermediate values, giving a characteristic histogram from which the proportions of cells in these phases can be calculated (Fig. 6). Tumours are often aneuploid and show an extra peak (Fig. 6, right) corresponding to normal diploid cells in the tumour (e.g. fibroblasts and lymphocytes). Up to 10 000 cells per second can be analysed by flow cytometry, making this a rapid and quantitative method, avoiding the use of radioactivity. To obtain information about rates of progression through the cell cycle, other methods are necessary.

Thymidine analogues

Replacement of the methyl group of thymidine with a halogen atom of similar size such as iodine or bromine results in the analogues iododeoxyuridine (**IdUrd**) or bromodeoxyuridine (**BrdUrd**). Enzymes responsible for DNA synthesis cannot easily distinguish between thymidine and its analogues and so these are incorporated into DNA via the same pathway. Once in DNA, they can be detected with specific antibodies which recognize the small distortions caused by their incorporation.[4] The antibodies can in turn be labelled with an enzyme (usually a peroxidase) which allows immunohistochemical staining, or a fluorescent label (usually fluorescein isothiocyanate) for flow cytometry. In this way, all cells that have incorporated the analogue, i.e. those in the S phase, can be detected by a brown colour on immunoperoxidase-stained sections or by green fluorescence with flow cytometry. Thus the proportion of labelled cells represents those in S phase obtained by labelling with ³H-TdR.

For cell kinetic studies, BrUrd- or IdUrd-labelled cells are stained with a mouse antibody specific for the DNA-incorporated analogue, followed by an antimouse antibody conjugated with fluorescein iso-thiocyanate.[5] Cells are counterstained with propidium iodide giving total DNA content per cell. After flow cytometry, dot plots of IdUrd (or BrdUrd) green fluorescence against propidium iodide (DNA) red fluorescence show three subpopulations representing G₁ cells (low green and low red), G₂/M cells (low green and high red) and S phase cells (high green) (Fig. 7). This is a typical pattern for cells taken for analysis shortly (less than 1 h) after labelling. For samples taken at increasing times after pulse labelling, the patterns change, reflecting progression of labelled and unlabeled cells through the cycle.[6] Cells with different cell cycle times show different rates of change of these patterns. In the example shown in Fig. 7 for the rapidly growing cells (top panels), movement of the cells through the S phase is clearly visible by 3 h and by 6 h, all the unlabelled cells originally in G₁ have moved into the S phase, and all the labelled cells have moved out of S to G₂, or have divided and have returned to G₁. The slower growing cells have only reached in 6 h the position that the faster growing cells have reached in 3 h. All phases of the cell cycle can be obtained from these bivariate histograms, in a manner similar to the analysis of per cent labelled mitoses curves, except that the fraction of labelled cells in mid-S is measured instead of the fraction of labelled cells in mitosis (Fig. 4).[7],[8]

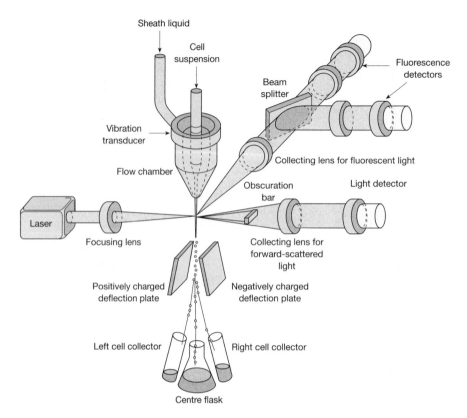

Fig. 5 Schematic illustration of a flow cytometer. Cells stained with fluorescent dyes pass in single file through a laser beam. The magnitude of scattered light and fluorescence of different colours is collected and recorded for each cell using optical filters and photomultiplier tubes. On some machines, cells with particular fluorescence and scatter characteristics can be physically sorted by charging the droplets containing the cells.

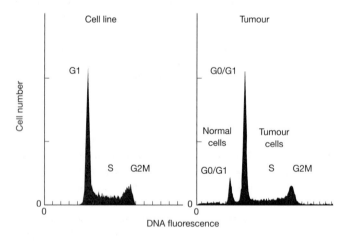

Fig. 6 DNA histograms of a cell line and an aneuploid human tumour measured by flow cytometry using red fluorescence of the DNA intercalating dye propidium iodide. The tumour also shows the presence of normal diploid cells. Histogram analysis can give the proportion of cells in G_1, S, and G_2M.

An alternative and related method makes use of fluorescence quenching of DNA binding dyes by BUrd or IdUrd incorporation.[9] This is also a powerful technique for cell cycle analysis of normal and perturbed populations, particularly in cell culture.

Relative movement

The relative movement (RM) method allows the duration of the DNA synthesis, T_S, LI, and T_{POT} to be estimated from one tissue sample.[10] This can be useful for clinical application where it is often difficult to take more than one biopsy. Several hours after intravenous injection of BrUrd or IdUrd a tumour biopsy is taken, fixed in ethanol, and a suspension of nuclei is subsequently made, stained and analysed by flow cytometry. The average position (red fluorescence) of the labelled cells which have not yet divided, relative to the positions of G_1 and G_2, is measured using computer-drawn windows around the appropriate subpopulations. The RM parameter is a DNA-content parameter defined to be zero for cells in G_1 and 1.0 for cells in G_2. As on average the labelled cells immediately after staining will be evenly distributed throughout the S phase, RM at that time will be approximately 0.5 (value assumed in the calculation). Subsequently, the cells progress towards G_2 and RM increases. RM can be measured in a sample taken a few hours (time t) after labelling, and a line is then plotted between RM = 0.5 at $t = 0$ and the measured RM at time t. This is extrapolated to the time required for RM to reach 1.0, which gives an estimate of the duration of DNA synthesis, T_S. The calculation assumes that the plot of RM versus time is linear, although theoretically it is curved. More rigorous mathematical ways to calculate T_S from RM have been described, taking into account this curvature.[11],[12] Other modifications have also been described for short sampling times[13] and to allow for a variable rate of DNA synthesis across the S phase.[14]

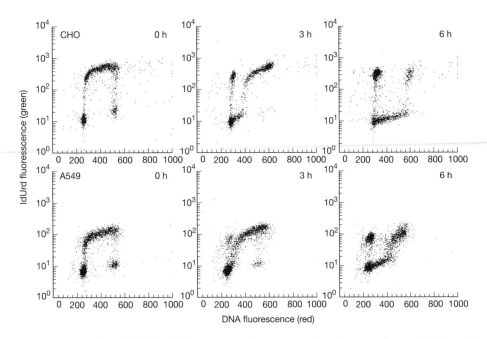

Fig. 7 Two parameter flow cytometry dot plots of IdUrd vs DNA content used to measure cell cycle progression rates in Chinese hamster ovary and A549 cell lines. Cells were pulse labelled with IdUrd and allowed to grow for the indicated times before analysis. Left-hand panels show the initial G_1, S, and G_2M populations which change with time in DNA content as they progress round the cycle. Progression rates can be estimated using the mid-S analysis method (see Fig. 4) or the RM method (see text).

Other methods

There are several other methods for measuring cell kinetics which, although useful, are not as widely used as those described above.

Double labelling techniques are those in which two thymidine analogues, e.g. IdUrd and BrdUrd, are administered separated by a few hours. Antibodies are available which can distinguish between the two analogues. The relative proportions of single- and double-labelled cells can be used to calculate T_S, which, coupled with the LI that can be concurrently measured, leads to estimates of T_{POT}.

IdUrd or BrdUrd can also be given continuously (constant exposure *in vitro*, continuous infusion *in vivo*), resulting in a progressive rise in the LI as G_1 cells enter S and become labelled and as S phase cells progress into M and divide (for principle, see ref.[1]). The rate of the LI increase can therefore be used to give quantitative information on rates of cell cycle progression, leading to estimates of T_S, LI, and hence T_{POT}.

Finally, the use of metaphase arrest agents can be used to study the rate of increase in the mitotic index (fraction of mitoses), the so-called stathmokinetic technique. The mitotic time and T_{POT} can be calculated from these data.

Proliferation markers

The use of thymidine analogues provides information on rates of cell cycle progression. A disadvantage for clinical studies is the need to administer a potentially toxic compound *in vivo*, although no acute or late toxicity has yet been observed for IdUrd or BrdUrd when used at low doses for cell kinetic studies. Alternative assays for proliferation have therefore been sought which do not require administration of an exogenous agent. There are several proteins which

are expressed in proliferating but not quiescent cells. Examples of these are DNA polymerase, histones H2 to H4, Ki67, proliferating cell nuclear antigen (**PCNA**), and some of the cyclins (see Chapter 1.5). Antibodies to these proteins can therefore be used to assess proliferation by immunohistochemistry or flow cytometry.

Ki67 is a nuclear protein associated with proliferating cells, which can be detected using the originally discovered antibody (Ki67), or by MIB1, an antibody against the same protein which allows better recognition on paraffin-embedded material.[15],[16] It is widely used to rank GFs of tumours and normal tissues under non-perturbed conditions,[17] although it is not reliable following cytotoxic treatment.

PCNA, an auxiliary protein for DNA polymerase delta, is involved in both DNA repair and DNA synthesis. When PCNA is tightly bound in the nucleus it is associated with DNA replication.[18] The fraction of PCNA-positive cells (tightly bound) is therefore a measure of the S phase fraction. PCNA is expressed in other phases of the cycle, however, where it is loosely bound in non-S phase cells.[19] The total (tight + loose) fraction of PCNA positive cells is then in principle a measure of the GF (all cycle phases). The tissue preparation technique will therefore influence the PCNA index, necessitating care in interpretation. As with Ki67, immunohistochemical methods or flow cytometry can be used for detection.

Several genes are only expressed in particular phases of the cycle, allowing their use as phase markers. Histones 3 and 4 are expressed in S phase,[20] as they are necessary for nucleosome assembly on newly synthesized DNA. Histone H3 expression has been used as a marker for the S phase and shown to correlate closely with thymidine or IdUrd/BrdUrd labelling index.[21]–[23] Gene expression is estimated from *in situ* hybridization with oligonucleotide or ribonucleotide probes specifically hybridizing to histone H3 mRNA. Use of a biotin- or digoxygenin-labelled probe allows detection with standard immunoperoxidase or immunofluorescence methods. This can be combined with IdUrd/BrdUrd labelling to give information on cycle phase times as well as phase fractions.

Cyclins, as their name suggests, are usually expressed in a cyclical fashion during the cell cycle. They control the transitions between cycle phases, e.g. G_1–S, G_2–M[24] (see Chapter 1.5). Cyclins activate specific kinases (enzymes which phosphorylate proteins) by forming complexes with them. Cyclins D and E are G_1 cyclins, cyclin A is mostly found in S, while cyclin B is found mostly in G_2. There are several subtypes of the B and D cyclins. The availability of antibodies to almost all known cyclins allows detection by immunohistochemical or flow methods. Cyclin B has been used as a marker of G_2 cells, and is also useful in distinguishing doublets of G_1 cells from true G_2 cells in flow cytometry. Cells containing cyclin A also tend to label with IdUrd/BrdUrd LI,[25] as would be expected for S phase cells.

Human tumour kinetics *in vivo* by thymidine analogue labelling

Kinetic information can be obtained by labelling human tumour biopsy material *in vitro* with ^{3}H-TdR or a thymidine analogue. Better information can be obtained by *in vivo* labelling, as this avoids potential artefacts of the *in vitro* procedure. Human tumours can be labelled by *in vivo* injection of IdUrd or BrdUrd with little or no toxicity at the low doses required for pulse-labelling kinetic studies.[26] Such studies on almost 2000 patients have shown a wide range in LI and T_{POT} between individual tumours, and between mean values for tumours in different sites, but with a narrower range for T_s (Table 3).

The presence of non-malignant cells in a tumour biopsy can disturb the accuracy of the estimates for the tumour cells. Attempts to overcome this have been made by using flow cytometry to measure T_S (described above) and combining it with the BrdUrd labelling index of tumour cells counted in tissue sections (immunoperoxidase), where tumour areas can be distinguished from stromal areas morphologically.[27] Alternatively, one can use a second antibody, if available, as a tumour marker, and measure the BrdUrd parameters only in those cells positive for the tumour marker. One such marker is cytokeratin for carcinomas.[7]

No method to directly measure T_C from one biopsy has been published, although if the GF is known it could be calculated from T_{POT}, as $T_C \simeq T_{POT}.GF$. A purported GF marker such as Ki67 (or MIB1) could be used for this purpose, although this may not give accurate estimates in all tumours.

Proliferation parameters

Relationship between parameters

The fraction of cells in a particular phase of the cell cycle will be determined by the length of that phase relative to the total cell cycle. For example, if T_S is 50 per cent of the cell cycle, then the LI (IdUrd/BrdUrd or ^{3}H-TdR) will be about 50 per cent for a population of dividing cells. If the mitotic time is 3 per cent of the cell cycle, then the mitotic index will be about 3 per cent, again assuming all cells are cycling. The IdUrd/BrdUrd LI will therefore always be higher

than the mitotic index, as T_S is considerably longer than T_M. PCNA and histone H3 label almost exclusively S phase cells and these indices should therefore be numerically close to the BrdUrd LI. Ki67 is expressed in all cell cycle phases, and should therefore give higher indices than BrdUrd, PCNA, or histone H3.

The three main factors contributing to tumour growth rate are the cell cycle time, the GF and the extent of cell loss. The potential doubling time, T_{POT} is defined as the cell number doubling time in the absence of cell loss, and is thus a combination of the cycle time and the GF. The three time parameters describing growth, from shortest to longest, are thus T_C, T_{POT} and T_D. Mathematically, the relationships between them are as follows.

$$T_{POT} \simeq T_C/GF.$$

It can also be shown[1] that:

$$T_{POT} = \lambda.T_s/LI$$

where (is a correction for the non-linear age distribution (proportionally more cells near the beginning than at the end of the cycle) and is usually between 0.8 and 1.0. This is a useful relationship, as T_S and LI can often be estimated from a single sample (see RM method above). For comparing or ranking human tumours, a constant value for φ is assumed. The relationship between T_{POT} and T_D is governed by cell loss.

The cell loss factor φ is the ratio of cell death rate to the cell birth rate.

$$\varphi = K_L/K_P$$

Expressed alternatively:

$$\varphi = 1 - T_{POT}/T_D,$$

$$\text{or } T_D = T_{POT}/(1 - \varphi)$$

It should be emphasized that the phase times and the cycle time are quite variable within a tumour due to microenvironmental variability (availability of oxygen and nutrients) and genetic heterogeneity.

Static versus dynamic parameters

Labelling indices for ^{3}H-TdR, IdUrd/BrdUrd, Ki67, PCNA, histone H3 and %S cells derived from DNA flow histograms are all static parameters as they say nothing about the rate of progression through the cell cycle. The IdUrd/BrdUrd LI is a function of the relative lengths of T_S and T_C, plus the GF. A LI of 20 per cent could arise from a T_S and T_C of 10 h and 50 h, respectively, but also from double these values. This assumes a linear age distribution and a 100 per cent GF. In practice neither will be true, but the principle remains. It is therefore not possible to derive phase times from a tumour LI. However, within the restrictions mentioned above, the LI provides a relatively robust proliferation parameter, and in some cases has been shown to correlate with outcome after therapy, demonstrating its prognostic significance.[26],[28]

Dynamic parameters involve times or rates. Thymidine or analogues can be used to define rates if another parameter is also measured. For BrdUrd or IdUrd and flow cytometry, the added parameter is DNA content. The rate of increase in DNA content of IdUrd-labelled cells allows the DNA synthesis time to be calculated (the RM method). Alternatively, measuring the flux of labelled cells across a mid-S window (cells with a DNA content halfway between

Table 3 Cell kinetic parameters of human tumours derived from *in vivo* labelling with BrUrd or IdUrd and flow cytometry (data derived from Rew and Wilson and Haustermans *et al.*) for the prostate data). The means or median values for parameters in each study were used to derive an overall mean and range for each site, if more than one study was done. The quoted rages thus represent variations between studies of medians or means. Ranges for individual tumours are larger. The total number of tumours studied is 1989.

Site		Number of patients	Number of studies	LI (%)	T_s (h)	T_{POT} (d)
Head and neck		712	9			
	Mean			9.6	11.9	4.5
	Range			(6.8–20.0)	(8.8–16.1)	(1.8–5.9)
CNS		193	3			
	Mean			2.6	10.1	34.3
	Range			(2.1–3.0)	(4.5–16.7)	(5.4–63.2)
Upper intestinal		183	6			
	Mean			10.5	13.5	5.8
	Range			(4.9–19.0)	(9.8–17.2)	(4.3–9.8)
Colorectal		345	5			
	Mean			13.1	15.3	4.0
	Range			(9.0–21.0)	(13.1–20.0)	(3.3.-4.5)
Breast		159	2			
	Mean			3.7	10.4	10.4
	Range			(3.2–4.2)	(8.7–12.0)	(8.2–12.5)
Ovarian		55	1			
	Mean			6.7	14.7	12.5
Cervix		159	2			
	Mean			9.8	12.8	4.8
	Range					(4.0–5.5)
Melanoma		24	1			
	Mean			4.2	10.7	7.2
Haematological:		106	3			
	Mean			13.3	14.6	9.6
	Range			(6.1–27.7)	(12.1–16.2)	(2.3–18.1)
Lung		27	1			
	Mean			9.9	10.5	8.2
Bladder		19	1			
	Mean			2.5	6.2	17.1
Renal cell ca		2	1			
	Mean			4.3	9.5	11.3
Prostate		5	1			
	Mean	1.4	11.7	28		

G_1 and G_2) allows determination of cell cycle phases and their variations (see Fig. 4).

Labelling patterns

Solid tumours invariably show heterogeneous labelling patters with kinetic markers such as ^{3}H-TdR or BrdUrd. One major cause of variation in proliferation within tumours is variation of nutrient supply. One obvious manifestation of this is a decrease in thymidine LI with increasing distance from a blood vessel.[29] The GF is highest closest to vessels and lowest for cells bordering necrosis which lack not only nutrients but also oxygen (Fig. 8).

In addition, a common observation in animal and human tumours labelled with BrdUrd or IdUrd is that some areas show relatively high labelling while others show no or low labelling, despite the presence of blood vessels. These regions may also be positive for an endogenous proliferation marker such as histone H3.[23] One likely cause is an interruption or reduction of flow in those blood vessels supplying the area, limiting access of thymidine or analogue. This is consistent with observations of cycling hypoxia and transient flow changes in many tumours, including in humans.[30]-[32] This may result in thymidine and analogue methods underestimating proliferative potential, although in most cases this is not likely to be a large problem as the fraction of temporarily closed or 'low flow' vessels is usually small.

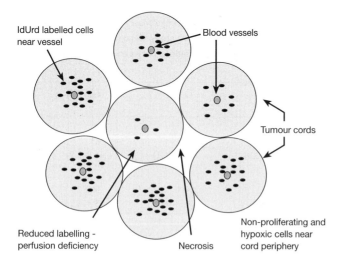

Fig. 8 Illustration of labelling patterns seen with thymidine or thymidine analogues. Two aspects of heterogeneity are seen; (a) most labelled cells are seen close to blood vessels, and (b) labelling around some blood vessels is lower than around others. The first is due to oxygen and nutrient diffusion limitations, combined with preferential uptake of thymidine by cells nearest vessels. The second is due to variations in blood flow, and thus oxygen/nutrient supply, in individual vessels.

Temporary cessation of nutrient/oxygen supply will probably temporarily halt or slow cycle progression,[33] and analogue labelling will reflect this.

Finally, in carcinomas, characteristic labelling patterns are often observed, including labelling in thin layers around the edge of tumour 'islands' or gland-like structures, akin to basal cell labelling in epithelia. Other tumours show random labelling, while some show intermediate patterns. These patterns, called marginal, intermediate, random, and mixed, can have prognostic significance for tumours treated with radiotherapy (other types of treatment have not been studied).[34] In this situation of heterogeneity due to differentiation, the non-labelled cells lead to lower values of LI and thus contribute, correctly, to estimates of the (non)-GF.

The problem of making measurements during treatment

After radiotherapy or chemotherapy, the cells which are killed often do not immediately disappear (e.g. by lysis or the late stages of apoptosis). These clonogenically dead cells can remain present for days, but are eventually doomed to die. There are no good ways of distinguishing a doomed cell from a survivor, either under the microscope or with flow cytometry. Doomed cells, however, are likely to exhibit different kinetics than survivors.[35] When counting an index microscopically (e.g. Ki67 or BrdUrd) or by flow cytometry after making a cell suspension, the doomed cells will contribute to the total, resulting in a potentially inaccurate measure of proliferation of surviving cells. This can be a large problem. A typical 2 Gy radiotherapy dose kills approximately half of the cells in a tumour of average radiosensitivity, so after 1 week (five doses) of a 6 to 7-week scheme, i.e. early in the schedule, the fraction of surviving cells

may be as low as 3 per cent (0.5^5). Up to 97 per cent of the cells may therefore be doomed, depending on the rate of their removal. Results of measurements made during or shortly after cytotoxic treatment should therefore be treated with caution if the purpose is to monitor kinetics of surviving cells.

Relevance for therapy

The overall treatment time for radiotherapy when given with curative intent is often 6 weeks or longer. Chemotherapy is given typically at intervals of 3 to 4 weeks and the total duration may be several months. These relatively long times provide opportunities for tumour cells which have survived the treatment up to that point to divide, depending on the length of the gaps occurring during the treatment schedule. This cell production (or 'repopulation') will offset cell kill and reduce the chance of cure.[36] This problem will be more acute for tumours with more rapid growth potential. Recent data from several trials of accelerated radiotherapy for head and neck cancer provide support for this notion,[37]–[39] showing that shorter schedules give consistently better tumour control. The most likely reason is reduced opportunities for repopulation in shorter treatments, although different reoxygenation patterns with more intense treatments cannot be ruled out. Accelerated repopulation can occur in some tumours as a result of treatment, so that, for example, if radiotherapy is administered some weeks after chemotherapy, the surviving tumour cells may be proliferating more rapidly after the regression caused by the chemotherapy than in untreated tumours.[36] It has been postulated that the effectiveness of the radiotherapy may be compromised by this increased repopulating ability, explaining some disappointing results of such dual modality therapies given sequentially in this way.[40]

Because of the suspected importance of repopulation rate, many studies have investigated whether proliferation-based assays can give useful prognostic information. DNA flow cytometry provides two readily obtained parameters, DNA ploidy and the fraction of cells in S phase (**SPF**). Aneuploid cells, i.e. those with abnormal DNA content, can be distinguished from cells with normal diploid DNA content (two copies of each chromosome) by an extra peak in the DNA histogram. Aneuploidy is a sign of genetic instability, involving chromosome duplications and often translocations. It is not a cell kinetic parameter but is usually measured together with SPF. A summary of the clinical utility of DNA content and SPF can be found in several special reports in *Cytometry* (1993; **14** (no. 5)). In general, aneuploidy is a weak negative prognostic indicator, although there are reports for both breast cancer and leukaemias (acute lymphoblastic leukaemia) that near diploidy (DNA index between 1 and 1.3) is a favourable indicator.[41],[42] DNA content changes indicate gross abnormalities only, and specific genetic changes affecting malignant behaviour and response to treatment cannot be monitored with this method, probably explaining its weakness as a predictor. SPF generally shows stronger associations with outcome, shown in several tumour sites, including breast, colon, prostate, and non-Hodgkin's lymphoma.[43],[44] Higher SPFs are usually associated with poorer outcome. SPF measurements are technically more difficult than for ploidy, and are probably equivalent to Ki67, PCNA, or cyclin A indices, where artefacts from cellular debris can be avoided more easily.

Immunohistochemical assays of endogenous proliferation markers such as Ki67 (or MIB1), PCNA, cyclins, and the cyclin-dependent kinase inhibitors have been investigated in numerous studies. In a review of the literature over the last 4 years, cyclin D1 appears to be one of the most consistent markers, with overexpression indicating a worse prognosis. Ki67, one of the most studied markers, showed significant correlations with outcome in only just over half of the studies. These included 18 different tumour sites and consequently a range of different treatment modalities. PCNA, p21 and p27 fared similarly. In breast cancer, there are several studies showing a relationship between outcome and either *in vitro* thymidine labelling index, mitotic index, or MIB1 index.[45]–[47] Some centres therefore incorporate a proliferation marker such as MIB1 or mitotic index into an overall prognostic indicator on which to make a treatment decision (high proliferation indicating a worse prognosis). (See Chapter 11.5 for critical review of prognostic factors in breast cancer.)

Exogenous proliferation markers such as the thymidine analogues BrdUrd and IdUrd have also been investigated as predictive markers for outcome after radiotherapy. The kinetic parameters are usually measured by flow cytometry on pretreatment biopsies. A recent pooled analysis of results for head and neck cancer from 11 centres showed that the potential doubling time, T_{POT}, showed no correlation with outcome. LI was significantly associated with local control in a univariate analysis ($p = 0.02$) but not in a multivariate analysis ($p = 0.16$).[26] Kinetic parameters measured in this way with present techniques therefore appear to provide only weak predictors.

A commonly held view is that faster proliferating cells or tissues are more sensitive to radiation. However, there is little evidence for a consistent relationship between cell proliferation rate and intrinsic sensitivity to radiation either from *in vitro* or animal studies. Faster growing tumours are likely to respond sooner after radiotherapy and are likely to recur sooner for a given level of cell kill than slow growing tumours (Fig. 9). This is simply a scaling of time and does not reflect differences in intrinsic sensitivity. The sensitivity to many drugs, however, is often related directly to proliferation rate in the sense that cycling cells are killed to a far greater extent than non-cycling cells[48],[49] (also see ref. 50). This is true for antimetabolites and also many alkylating and other agents. The ratio of doses for a given level of kill for slowly versus rapidly proliferating cells ranges between 1 and 2 for many alkylating agents, 2 to 5 for cyclophosphamide and bleomycin, while 5-fluorouracil and doxorubicin also show considerable specificity for rapidly growing cells. Tumour GF may therefore be an indicator of chemosensitivity for some drugs but not others. A higher proliferative activity can also be associated with a higher grade of malignancy, counteracting any positive correlation between GF and outcome. Competing factors for chemotherapy are thus sensitivity of cycling cells (positive), relationship between proliferation and malignancy grade (negative), and repopulation during long schedules (negative).

The cell cycle dependence of many drugs also provides a plausible explanation for the time course of myelosuppression and recovery after chemotherapy. Pluripotent stem cells are thought to proliferate slowly, committed stem cells proliferate relatively rapidly, while mature, differentiated cells of myelocytic, erythroid, and megakaryocyte lineages cease to proliferate. Cycle-dependent drugs like cyclophosphamide therefore have little immediate effect on peripheral blood counts, as committed stem cells will be unaffected and will remain for their respective life times. As they senesce and disappear,

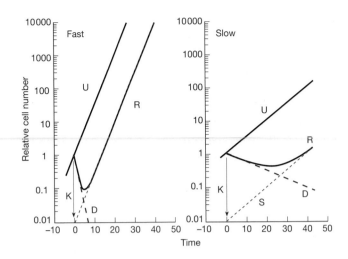

Fig. 9 Illustration of the differences between radiosensitivity and radioresponsiveness. Schematic treatment response of two tumours with different growth and regression rates (log cell number vs time in arbitrary units; irradiated at time 0). The left tumour grows rapidly and regresses rapidly after treatment, so this tumour would be regarded as rapidly responding. The right tumour grows and regresses slower, is therefore a slow responder and with less total volume reduction, but the cell kill (K) is the same, i.e. the radiosensitivity is identical. U = untreated, S = surviving cells, D = dead cells, R = recurrence (sum of dead and surviving cells).

they cannot be replaced from the immature precursor pool as these have been preferentially killed by the cycle-dependent drugs. They will in turn need to be replaced from the slowly proliferating, and therefore relatively protected, stem cells. Recovery times will therefore depend on the rates of maturation and expansion of stem cells through immature precursors to mature end-stage cells. Proliferation dependence of many chemotherapeutic agents is also evident by their action against other rapidly proliferating organs and cells such as the intestinal mucosa, gonads, and hair follicles. Radiotherapy is far less discriminating, as evidenced by the fact very slowly proliferating organs such as the kidney and spinal cord are highly sensitive to ionizing radiation. Rapidly proliferating tissues such as buccal and intestinal mucosa also suffer considerable damage after radiotherapy. Cell kinetics play a part here only in the time of expression, and not in absolute radiosensitivity, such that tissues with rapid turnover manifest their damage early after radiation (days to weeks) while slow turnover tissues manifest their damage late (months to years).

Some drugs and also ionizing radiation kill cells more effectively in some cell cycle phases than in others. This has led to the proposal that the synchronizing of cells in one phase of the cycle will allow scheduling of subsequent treatments to the time when the synchronized cohort enters a sensitive phase of the cycle. Efforts have largely failed due to the kinetic and physiological heterogeneity of tumours, to variable drug distribution within them and to the presence of non-cycling and hypoxic cells. Achieving high or adequate synchrony has therefore proved difficult or impossible.

Conclusions

Deregulated cell proliferation is a hallmark of cancer and its study is a prerequisite in understanding tumour growth patterns and response to therapy. Measurement techniques have become steadily more sophisticated and rapid, especially those using flow cytometry. The number of proliferation markers has also increased rapidly from the burgeoning knowledge of the molecular biology of the cell cycle. Application of cell kinetic methods has been crucial in understanding the time of response of tissues to radiotherapy, and both the time and the severity of response to chemotherapy. Cell proliferation, however, is but one factor determining outcome. The variability between studies on the prognostic value of almost all kinetic markers studied so far, emphasizes that one marker for one biological parameter is unlikely to provide strong prognostic information, although it will help to build up an overall picture of tumour grade and behaviour. Pretreatment measurements of proliferation using present techniques and presently available endogenous and exogenous markers so far provide relatively weak prognostic information when used as single parameters. However, repopulation rate is a factor of undoubted importance in determining outcome to both radiotherapy and chemotherapy in many tumours, as evidenced by clinical trials with varying overall treatment time. Development of better and more robust repopulation markers will help guide clinicians to choose optimum treatment schedules.

References

1. **Steel GG.** *Growth kinetics of tumours.* Oxford: Oxford University Press, 1977.

2. **Quastler H, Sherman FG.** Cell population kinetics in the intestinal epithelium of the mouse. *Experimental Cell Research,* 1957; **17**: 420–38.

3. **Shapiro HM.** *Practical flow cytometry.* New York: Wiley-Liss, 1995.

4. **Gratzner HG.** Monoclonal antibody to 5-bromo and 5-iododeoxyuridine: a new reagent for detection of DNA replication. *Science,* 1982; **218**: 474–5.

5. **Gray JW, Dolbeare F, Pallavicini MG, Beisker W, Waldman F.** Cell cycle analysis using flow cytometry. *International Journal of Radiation Biology and Related Studies in Physics, Chemistry and Medicine,* 1986; **49**: 237–55.

6. **Pallavicini MG, Summers LJ, Dolbeare FD, Gray JW.** Cytokinetic properties of asynchronous and cytosine arabinoside perturbed murine tumors measured by simultaneous bromodeoxyuridine/DNA analyses. *Cytometry,* 1985; **6**: 602–10.

7. **Begg AC, Hofland I.** Cell kinetic analysis of mixed populations using three-color fluorescence flow cytometry. *Cytometry,* 1991; **12**: 445–54.

8. **Gray JW, Bogart E, Gavel DT, George YS, Moore DH, 2d.** Rapid cell cycle analysis. II. Phase durations and dispersions from computer analysis of RC curves. *Cell Tissue Kinetics,* 1983; **16**: 457–71.

9. **Ormerod MG.** Analysis of cell proliferation using the bromodeoxyuridine/Hoechst-ethidium bromide method. *Methods in Molecular Biology,* 1997; **75**: 357–65.

10. **Begg AC, McNally NJ, Shrieve DC, Karcher H.** A method to measure the duration of DNA synthesis and the potential doubling time from a single sample. *Cytometry,* 1985; **6**: 620–6.

11. **White RA, Terry NH, Meistrich ML, Calkins DP.** Improved method for computing potential doubling time from flow cytometric data. *Cytometry,* 1990; **11**: 314–17.

12. **Terry NH, White RA, Meistrich ML, Calkins DP.** Evaluation of flow cytometric methods for determining population potential doubling times using cultured cells. *Cytometry,* 1991; **12**: 234–41.

13. **Ritter MA, Fowler JF, Kim Y, Lindstrom MJ, Kinsella TJ.** Single biopsy, tumor kinetic analyses: a comparison of methods and an extension to shorter sampling intervals. *International Journal Radiation Oncology, Biology, Physics,* 1992; **23**: 811–20.

14. **Baisch H, Otto U.** Intratumoral heterogeneity of S phase transition in solid tumours determined by bromodeoxyuridine labelling and flow cytometry. *Cell Proliferation,* 1993; **26**: 439–48.

15. **Torp SH.** Proliferative activity in human glioblastomas: evaluation of different Ki67 equivalent antibodies. *Molecular Pathology,* 1997; **50**: 198–200.

16. **Pinder SE, et al.** Assessment of the new proliferation marker MIB1 in breast carcinoma using image analysis: associations with other prognostic factors and survival. *British Journal of Cancer,* 1995; **71**: 146–9.

17. **Scott RJ, et al.** A comparison of immunohistochemical markers of cell proliferation with experimentally determined growth fraction. *Journal of Pathology,* 1991; **165**: 173–8.

18. **Morris GF, Mathews MB.** Regulation of proliferating cell nuclear antigen during the cell cycle. *Journal Biological Chemistry,* 1989; **264**: 13856–64.

19. **Wilson GD, Camplejohn RS, Martindale CA, Brock A, Lane DP, Barnes DM.** Flow cytometric characterisation of proliferating cell nuclear antigen using the monoclonal antibody PC10. *European Journal of Cancer,* 1992; **28A**: 2010–7.

20. **Stein GS, van Stein JL, Wijnen AJ, Lian JB.** Regulation of histone gene expression. *Current Opinion in Cell Biology,* 1992; **4**: 166–73.

21. **Dirks RW, Raap AK.** Cell-cycle-dependent gene expression studied by two-colour fluorescent detection of a mRNA and histone mRNA. *Histochemistry and Cell Biology,* 1995; **104**: 391–5.

22. **Konishi H, et al.** Histone H3 messenger RNA *in situ* hybridization correlates with *in vivo* bromodeoxyuridine labeling of S phase cells in rat colonic epithelium. *Cancer Research,* 1996; **56**: 434–7.

23. **Gown AM, et al.** Validation of the S phase specificity of histone (H3) *in situ* hybridization in normal and malignant cells. *Journal of Histochemistry and Cytochemistry,* 1996; **44**: 221–6.

24. **Pines J.** Cyclins, CDKs and cancer. *Seminars in Cancer Biology,* 1995; **6**: 63–72.

25. **Juan G, Li X, Darzynkiewicz Z.** Correlation between DNA replication and expression of cyclins A and B1 in individual MOLT-4 cells. *Cancer Research,* 1997; **57**: 803–7.

26. **Begg AC, et al.** The value of pretreatment cell kinetic parameters as predictors for radiotherapy outcome in head and neck cancer: a multicenter analysis. *Radiotherapy and Oncology,* 1999; **50**: 13–23.

27. **Bennett MH, et al.** Tumour proliferation assessed by combined histological and flow cytometric analysis: implications for therapy in squamous cell carcinoma in the head and neck. *British Journal of Cancer,* 1992; **65**: 870–8.

28. **Silvestrini R, Daidone MG.** Review of proliferative variables and their predictive value. *Recent Results in Cancer Research,* 1993; **127**: 71–6.

29. **Tannock IF.** The relation between cell proliferation and the vascular system in a transplanted mouse mammary tumour. *British Journal of Cancer,* 1968; **22**: 258–73.

30. **Pigott KH, Hill SA, Chaplin DJ, Saunders MI.** Microregional fluctuations in perfusion within human tumours detected using laser Doppler flowmetry. *Radiotherapy and Oncology,* 1996; **40**: 45–50.

31. **Chaplin DJ, Trotter MJ, Durand RE, Olive PL, Minchinton AI.** Evidence for intermittent radiobiological hypoxia in experimental tumour systems. *Biomedica Biochimica Acta,* 1989; **48**: S255–9.

32. **Brown JM.** Evidence for acutely hypoxic cells in mouse tumours, and a possible mechanism of reoxygenation. *British Journal of Radiology,* 1979; **52**: 650–6.

33. **Green SL, Giaccia AJ.** Tumor hypoxia and the cell cycle: implications for malignant progression and response to therapy. *Cancer Journal of Scientific American,* 1998; **4**: 218–23.

34. **Wilson GD, Dische S, Saunders MI.** Studies with bromodeoxyuridine

in head and neck cancer and accelerated radiotherapy. *Radiotherapy and Oncology*, 1995; **36**: 189–97.

35. Begg AC, Hofland I, Kummermehr J. Tumour cell repopulation during fractionated radiotherapy: correlation between flow cytometric and radiobiological data in three murine tumours. *European Journal of Cancer*, 1991; **27**: 537–43.

36. Withers HR, Taylor JM, Maciejewski B. The hazard of accelerated tumor clonogen repopulation during radiotherapy. *Acta Oncologica*, 1988; **27**: 131–46.

37. Saunders M, Dische S, Barrett A, Harvey A, Gibson D, Parmar M. Continuous hyperfractionated accelerated radiotherapy (CHART) versus conventional radiotherapy in non-small-cell lung cancer: a randomised multicentre trial. CHART Steering Committee. *The Lancet*, 1997; **350**: 161–5.

38. Horiot JC, *et al.* Accelerated fractionation (AF) compared with conventional fractionation (CF) improves loco-regional control in the radiotherapy of advanced head and neck cancers: results of the EORTC 22851 randomized trial. *Radiotherapy and Oncology*, 1997; **44**: 111–21.

39. Ang KK. Altered fractionation in the management of head and neck cancer. *International Journal of Radiation Biology*, 1998; **73**: 395–9.

40. Munro AJ. An overview of randomised controlled trials of adjuvant chemotherapy in head and neck cancer. *British Journal of Cancer*, 1995; **71**: 83–91.

41. Duque RE, Andreeff M, Braylan RC, Diamond LW, Peiper SC. Consensus review of the clinical utility of DNA flow cytometry in neoplastic hematopathology. *Cytometry*, 1993; **14**: 492–6.

42. Hedley DW. DNA Cytometry Consensus Conference. DNA flow cytometry and breast cancer. *Breast Cancer Research Treatment*, 1993; **28**: 51–3.

43. Hedley DW, Clark GM, Cornelisse CJ, Killander D, Kute T, Merkel D. Consensus review of the clinical utility of DNA cytometry in carcinoma of the breast. *Report of DNA Cytometry Consensus Conference on Cytometry*, 1993; **14**: 482–5.

44. Shankey TV, *et al.* Consensus review of the clinical utility of DNA content cytometry in prostate cancer. *Cytometry*, 1993; **14**: 497–500.

45. Tubiana M, *et al.* Kinetic parameters and the course of the disease in breast cancer. *Cancer*, 1981; **47**: 937–43.

46. Jansen RL, *et al.* MIB-1 labelling index is an independent prognostic marker in primary breast cancer. *British Journal of Cancer*, 1998; **78**: 460–5.

47. Thor AD, Liu S, Moore DH, 2, Edgerton SM. Comparison of mitotic index, *in vitro* bromodeoxyuridine labeling, and MIB-1 assays to quantitate proliferation in breast cancer. *Journal of Clin Oncology*, 1999; **17**: 470–7.

48. Twentyman PR, Bleehen NM. Changes in sensitivity to cytotoxic agents occurring during the life history of monolayer cultures of a mouse tumour cell line. *British Journal of Cancer*, 1975; **31**: 417–23.

49. Bruce WR, Meeker BE, Valeriote FA. Comparison of the sensitivity of normal hematopoietic and transplanted lymphoma colony-forming cells to chemotherapeutic agents administered *in vivo*. *Journal National Cancer Institute*, 1966; **37**: 233–45.

50. Tannock IF, Hill RP. *The basic science of oncology*. New York: McGraw-Hill, 1998.

51. Rew DA, Wilson GD. Cell production rates in human tissues and tumours and their clinical significance. *European Journal of Surgical Oncology*, 1999.

52. Haustermans KM, *et al.* Cell kinetic measurements in prostate cancer. *International Journal Radiation Oncology, Biology, Physics*, 1997; **37**: 1067–70.

Angiogenesis and invasion

Adam Jones and Roy Bicknell

Introduction

Angiogenesis is the growth of new blood vessels from existing vessels. Angiogenesis occurs in the physiological processes of wound healing, in the endometrium and ovary during the menstrual cycle,[1][2] and in pathologies such as psoriasis and diabetic retinopathy. There is now abundant evidence that the growth of solid tumours is also angiogenesis dependent.[3] Beyond a tumour size of 2–3 mm^2 diffusion of oxygen and nutrients is insufficient to support further growth, and generation of new blood vessels is required to supply nutrients to the tumour cells.

Stronger evidence for the role of angiogenesis in tumour biology includes:

(1) Cells transfected with angiogenic stimulators develop more vascular and larger tumours in mouse xenograft experiments than their parent cells.[4]

(2) Conversely, antiangiogenic strategies, e.g. neutralizing antibodies, mRNA anti-sense techniques, or transfection with inhibitors, lead to reduced tumour growth in animal models.

(3) The success of antiangiogenic treatments.

The degree of angiogenic activity in a tumour can be determined directly, by determining the degree of vascularization within that tumour, the intratumoral microvessel density, or indirectly by assaying known angiogenic stimulatory factors. Many models of angiogenesis have been developed, for example gene knockout mice deficient in specific angiogenic factors or receptors. The production of transgenic mice that spontaneously develop tumours has allowed the study of the role of angiogenesis in the progression from normal tissue to overt carcinoma. For example, mice with the SV40 large T oncogene expressed from the insulin promoter develop pancreatic tumours after undergoing an increase in angiogenesis.[5] Lastly, models such as the chick chorioallantoic membrane assay, the rabbit cornea, and the rodent sponge implant have allowed putative stimulatory and inhibitory molecules to be tested for their ability to induce or suppress vessel formation.

In addition to stimulators, many angiogenic inhibitors have been identified Angiogenesis is a dynamic balance of angiogenic stimulators and inhibitors mediating interactions between tumour cells, endothelial cells, and the surrounding extracellular matrix (Fig. 1). Understanding these interactions and the various controls of angiogenesis such as oncogenes and hypoxic regulation, points to antiangiogenesis becoming an extremely promising future therapy.

Intratumoral microvessel density

The vascular density of a tumour is demonstrated by immunostaining sections of that tumour with endothelial cell-specific antibodies such as those to von Willebrand factor or anti-CD31. While the overall vascular density is not a prognostic indicator, the intratumoral microvessel density is. The intratumoral microvessel density is considered to be the area of highest vascular density, which frequently occur in tumours as islands or 'hot spots'. Thus intratumoral microvessel density has been shown to be an independent prognostic factor in many tumours including breast, bladder, prostate, and lung.[6] However, only about three-quarters of such studies have confirmed such predictive value. This may be related to technical difficulties with antibody specificity and staining, or incorrect identification of 'hot spots' and vessels by the observer. Despite these reservations, intratumoral microvessel density appears to have a role in identifying high-risk patients and may aid individual tailoring of therapy. Recently quantification of intratumoral microvessel density was significantly correlated with the presence of occult bone marrow micrometastases in breast cancer patients.[7] Mechanistically, raised intratumoral microvessel density is detrimental to the patient in three main ways. Firstly, the increased number of vessels will supply increased oxygen and nutrients to support the tumour. Secondly, the increased availability of vessels will facilitate metastasis from that tumour, and lastly endothelial cells themselves are sources of angiogenic factors which

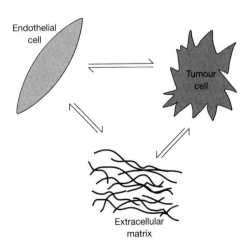

Fig. 1 Angiogenesis involves a complex interaction between endothelial cells, tumour cells, and the extracellular matrix.

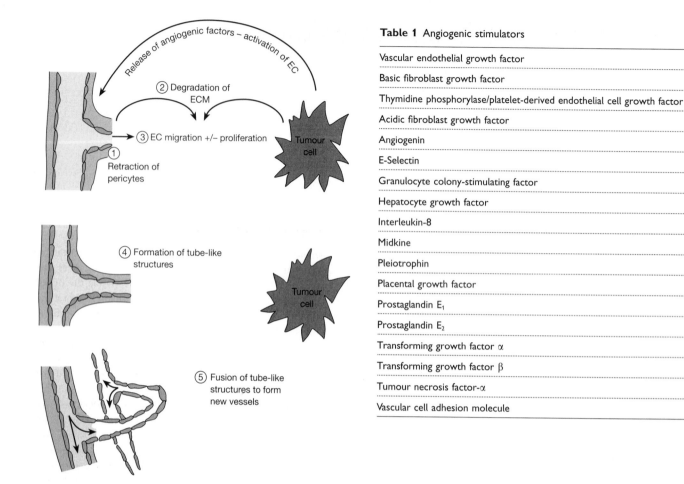

Fig. 2 Mechanisms of angiogenesis.

Table 1 Angiogenic stimulators

Vascular endothelial growth factor
Basic fibroblast growth factor
Thymidine phosphorylase/platelet-derived endothelial cell growth factor
Acidic fibroblast growth factor
Angiogenin
E-Selectin
Granulocyte colony-stimulating factor
Hepatocyte growth factor
Interleukin-8
Midkine
Pleiotrophin
Placental growth factor
Prostaglandin E$_1$
Prostaglandin E$_2$
Transforming growth factor α
Transforming growth factor β
Tumour necrosis factor-α
Vascular cell adhesion molecule

interact with tumour cells and the extracellular matrix to enhance angiogenesis. The greater the intravascular microvessel density the larger the number of endothelial cells available to secrete more factors.

The mechanism of angiogenesis

In response to an angiogenic stimulus a complex multistep process is initiated involving:

(1) Retraction of pericytes from the outer surface of endothelial cells.

(2) The release of proteases from stimulated endothelial cells which degrade extracellular matrix.

(3) Migration and usually proliferation of endothelial cells into the degraded extracellular matrix towards the angiogenic stimulus.

(4) Tubule formation.

(5) Fusion of tubules to form new vessels.

(6) Differentiation and stabilization of new vessels (Fig. 2).

Angiogenic stimulators

Many angiogenic factors have been identified and there have been several reviews of their properties (Table 1), see also Chapter 1.4.[8]

Elevated levels correlate with poor outcome in a number of tumours.

Basic fibroblast growth factor

The fibroblast growth factor (**FGF**) family consists of at least nine distinct but related members of which basic FGF (FGF-2) is the most extensively studied. Basic FGF is an 18 kDa molecule expressed in many organs and cultured cell types. It is a growth and migratory factor for endothelial cells, activities which are inhibited by specific antibodies to basic FGF. Endothelial cells themselves produce basic FGF and it may function in an autocrine fashion.

Basic FGF levels are higher in the urine of patients with bladder cancer and a number of other neoplasms. It is also highly expressed in Kaposi sarcoma lesions and its expression is upregulated in proportion to the degree of malignancy in human gliomas. However, despite abundant evidence for an association between basic FGF and tumour angiogenesis there are some reservations as to how important a part it plays. First, it is unclear how basic FGF is released from cells as it lacks a classic secretory signal. Secondly, basic FGF released by tumour cells can act in an autocrine manner to promote proliferation of carcinoma cells directly and thus some of the tumour growth-promoting effects of basic FGF may be independent of angiogenesis. Lastly, basic FGF often acts in synergy with other angiogenic factors whose actions may predominate.[9]

Vascular endothelial growth factor

Vascular endothelial growth factor (**VEGF**) is a multifunctional cytokine that promotes endothelial cell proliferation and migration *in vitro* and angiogenesis in various models. It also induces urokinase plasminogen activator (**uPA**), the urokinase plasminogen activator receptor (**uPAR**), and interstitial collagenase, all leading to degradation of the extracellular matrix which facilitates endothelial cell (as well as tumour cell) migration and invasion.

In addition, VEGF is a potent vascular permeability factor. Extravasation from leaky vessels of plasminogen which is converted by uPA (which VEGF also upregulates) leads to the production of plasmin adding further to the degradative local environment. Leaky vessels themselves also provide a ready portal for tumour dissemination.[10]

Differential splicing of the VEGF gene gives rise to four isoforms VEGF 206, 189, and the two major isoforms, VEGF 165, which is a 45-kDa homodimeric glycoprotein predominantly bound to the cell surface, and VEGF 121, which is more freely diffusible.

There are at least two VEGF receptor tyrosine kinases, Flt-1 (VEGFR1) and KDR (VEGFR2). Both are expressed primarily on vascular endothelial cells, although Flt-1 has been identified on monocytes. KDR can mediate the whole spectrum of VEGF activities whereas Flt-1 has more limited repertoire. Despite this, both are essential for angiogenesis as has been demonstrated by the vascular abnormalities and intrauterine death in knockout mice deficient for either Flt-1 or KDR.[11],[12] Further studies of knockout mice which lack the gene for VEGF confirm its critical importance in angiogenesis of embryogenesis with *in utero* death at E10.5. Also, a critical amount of VEGF is necessary for angiogenesis as evidenced by the vascular abnormalities and embryonic death seen when VEGF levels are reduced in knockout mice that retain a single copy of the gene for VEGF.[13],[14] These findings are remarkable as they suggest that while other factors play a part, VEGF is the essential vascular development factor, and in its absence no other gene will substitute.

In addition to elevated VEGF expression in many tumours, VEGF levels have been shown to have prognostic significance in breast, bladder, colon, and stomach cancer. Stronger evidence that VEGF plays a part in tumour behaviour rather than merely being a marker comes from a series of experiments where levels of VEGF are either enhanced or reduced and the effect of these manipulations tested in xenograft models. Transfection of the VEGF gene into MCF-7 breast cancer cells resulted in significantly increased expression compared with the wild-type cells. This had no effect on cell proliferation *in vitro* but when implanted subcutaneously in nude mice tumours derived from the transfected cells were faster growing and more vascular.[4] Opposite effects have been seen following transfection of an anti-sense construct to the VEGF′ gene into C6 glioma cells.[15] Neutralizing anti-VEGF antibodies have been used in colon, glioblastoma multiforme, and prostate cancer cell lines studied in xenograft models with significant inhibitory effects on tumour growth and angiogenesis.[10],[16] The use of a retrovirus to infect endothelial cells with a dominant negative mutant of the VEGF receptor (**VEGFR2**) interfered with signal transduction from the receptor and inhibited glioblastoma growth in a nude mouse model. Lastly, reversion from a malignant to a benign phenotype has been demonstrated by blocking VEGFR2, associated with disrupted angiogenesis and loss of invasion.[39] In addition to its obvious role in supplying tumours with oxygen and nutrients, angiogenesis now appears also to have a part in tumour invasion.

VEGF-C

Unlike VEGF which is angiogenic and acts directly on endothelial cells of blood vessels, VEGF-C is lymphangiogenic acting specifically on the endothelial cells of lymphatic vessels. Alitalo and colleagues achieved overexpression of VEGF-C in transgenic mice by linking the VEGF-C cDNA to a promoter which led to stimulation of gene expression in the basal cells of stratified squamous epithelium. This resulted in increased lymphatic endothelial cell proliferation and hyperplasia of the lymphatic vasculature.[17] VEGF-C may have a part in the lymphatic dissemination of tumours and VEGF-C mRNA has recently been reported in half of the malignancies studied.[18]

Angiopoietin-1 and Tie-2

Tie-1 and Tie-2/tek are both predominantly endothelial cell-specific receptor tyrosine kinases. Gene knockout mutations in mice have confirmed that they both have roles in blood vessel formation. Embryos lacking Tie-2 die by embryonic day 10.5 with abnormal vascular networks particularly in the myocardium. Tie-1 knockout mice die perinatally, with widespread oedema and haemorrhage. The oedema which begins in embryo is primarily due to loss of integrity of endothelial cells in blood vessels. Therefore Tie-1 appears to function in endothelial cell differentiation whereas Tie-2 is involved in angiogenesis.[19]

Gene knockout studies have confirmed that an important ligand for Tie-2 is angiopoietin-1 (Ang-1). There are differences between the role of VEGF/VEGFR1–VEGFR2 and Ang-1/Tie-2 in angiogenesis. Ang-1 fails to stimulate growth or migration of endothelial cells in culture. Expression of Tie-2 in embryogenesis follows that of VEGFR2 by about 24 h as does death of Tie-2 knockout mice as compared with VEGFR2 knockouts. At an ultrastructural level angiopoietin-1 knockout mice show disordered endothelial cell interactions with the surrounding extracellular matrix and surrounding pericytes.[20] It is therefore proposed that VEGF acts earlier in angiogenesis to promote new vessel growth and angiopoietin-1 acts later to stabilize these new vessels. Consistent with this hypothesis is the finding of dilated abnormal vessels in patients with venous malformations from two families with a gain of function mutation in the Tie-2 gene.[21]

Thymidine phosphorylase/platelet-derived endothelial cell growth factor

Thymidine phosphorylase is an enzyme in the nucleotide salvage pathway. It is also angiogenic and induces endothelial cell migration *in vitro* and blood vessel formation on the chick chorioallantoic membrane and in rabbit sponge models (for reviews see refs 22 and 23). Elevated levels of thymidine phosphorylase have been demonstrated in many tumours including bladder, breast, and ovarian cancers. In colorectal carcinoma thymidine phosphorylase correlates with Dukes stage and lymph node metastases and is prognostic for survival even after adjustment for Dukes stage and microvessel density.[24] Confirmatory evidence for the angiogenic activity comes from the reduction of blood vessel growth in the rodent sponge model using polyclonal antibodies to thymidine phosphorylase and the faster *in vivo* growth of MCF-7 breast cancer cells when transfected with the thymidine phosphorylase gene as compared with control cells.[25]

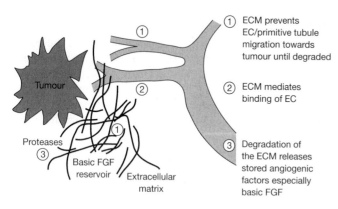

Fig. 3 Role of the extracellular matrix.

① ECM prevents EC/primitive tubule migration towards tumour until degraded

② ECM mediates binding of EC

③ Degradation of the ECM releases stored angiogenic factors especially basic FGF

Other angiogenic factors

A number of other angiogenic factors have been identified (Table 1), although less evidence exists as to their role in tumour biology.[26]

Extracellular matrix

The extracellular matrix is more than just a passive support for tumour and endothelial cells. It serves as (Fig. 3):

(1) A physical barrier.
(2) A source of angiogenic factors.
(3) A framework for cell adhesion.

The extracellular matrix—a physical barrier

Degradation of the extracellular matrix is essential for endothelial cell migration towards a tumour and for tumour invasion (see Chapter 1.9). uPA and matrix metalloproteinases are proteolytic enzymes critically involved in angiogenesis as well as tumour cell invasion. Urokinase plasminogen activator and its receptor uPAR expression are usually low in quiescent endothelium but upregulated by VEGF and basic FGF. Elevated levels of uPA and uPAR are prognostic in a number of tumours and correlations have been found between microvessel density and uPA. Antibodies against uPA and uPAR antagonists decrease matrix degradation. Prostate cancer cells transfected to overexpress the gene encoding the uPA inhibitor PAI-1 resulted in smaller, less vascular primary tumours and reduced liver and lung metastasis compared with parental wild-type cells in an athymic mouse model.[27] Furthermore, urokinase receptor antagonists reduce tubule formation in *in vitro* models and reduced tumour growth, microvessel density, and metastatic frequency in animal models.[28],[29]

Collagenase 6, a member of the matrix metalloproteinase family of extracellular matrix degradative enzymes, is produced by migrating endothelial cells. Expression of various members of the matrix metalloproteinase family is increased in many tumour tissues and surrounding stroma. Increased expression of natural tissue inhibitors of metalloproteinases has been associated with inhibition of angiogenesis *in vitro* and *in vivo* and inhibition of tumour cell invasion *in vitro* and lung metastasis *in vivo*.[30] These findings led to the development of

synthetic matrix metalloproteinase inhibitors which are reviewed below. Modification of extracellular matrix degradation is a promising therapeutic strategy.

Extracellular matrix and macrophages as sources of angiogenic factors

The extracellular matrix is a reservoir for angiogenic factors and cells associated with the extracellular matrix can release angiogenic factors. When basic FGF is bound to heparin it is inactive but protected from proteolytic degradation. Heparinase released by tumours and associated inflammatory cells will liberate and thus activate basic FGF.

Macrophages make up a considerable percentage of the total cellular mass within certain tumours, up to 50 per cent in some breast carcinomas. Macrophages influence angiogenesis and tumour invasion in three main ways: (a) release of angiogenic stimulators including VEGF, basic FGF and tumour necrosis factor-α; (b) modification of the extracellular matrix either by release of components of the extracellular matrix or degradative enzymes; (c) release of angiogenic inhibitors especially thrombospondin-1 (see below and ref. 31). Experimental inhibition of macrophage infiltration by interleukin-10 is correlated with reduced tumour growth and some of the antiangiogenic activity of the experimental drug linomide is thought to be due to the inhibition of both macrophage entry into tumours and their secretion of tumour necrosis factor-α.

In patients with invasive breast cancer, macrophage infiltration correlates with vascular grade and reduced relapse-free and overall survival and is an independent prognostic factor.[32] Owing to their multiple other functions, macrophages will probably be of limited use as a therapeutic target.

The extracellular matrix and cell adhesion

Cell adhesion molecules such as the integrins and cadherins are involved not only in cell adhesion but also in many aspects of angiogenesis including endothelial cell migration, tubule formation, and apoptosis.

Integrins

The integrins are a family of cell adhesion molecules that mediate cell to extracellular matrix interactions and participate in the regulation of adhesion, migration, invasion, and apoptosis of endothelial cells. This wide variety of responses is due to the large number of different integrins, each integrin heterodimer is made from one of 15α and 8β subunits. In addition, different integrins bind to different components of the extracellular matrix, and even to different regions within the same component molecule, to produce many cell cytoskeletal changes and transmembrane signalling. Thus, antagonism of the αvβ3 integrin inhibits angiogenesis induced by basic FGF but not VEGF while αvβ5 antagonists inhibit the angiogenic response to VEGF but not basic FGF.[33]

Integrin expression is upregulated by various angiogenic factors and also in proliferating rather than quiescent endothelial cells.[34] The monoclonal antibody LM609 targets the αvβ3 integrin and inhibits angiogenesis on the chick chorioallantoic membrane. In xenograft experiments with a human breast cancer cell line LM609 inhibited angiogenesis and reduced tumour invasion.[35] The αvβ3 integrin appears to be a key target. Not only does it mediate angiogenesis but it is also critical for endothelial cell survival by maintaining cell shape. When cells lose contact with the extracellular matrix they become rounded and this triggers apoptosis. At a molecular level, binding of αvβ3 blocks expression of the cell cycle inhibitor p21WAF1/CIP1 and increases the ratio of BCL-2 to BAX proteins. A high BCL-2/BAX ratio promotes cell survival.[36]

Tumour necrosis factor-α and interferon-γ reduce activation of the integrin αvβ3. In patients with metastatic melanoma these agents, in combination with melphalan, have been found to cause selective disruption of tumour vasculature, an effect that was associated with a 90 per cent complete response rate with isolated limb perfusion.[37] Decreased αvβ3-dependent endothelial cell adhesion resulting in apoptosis may explain these results.

Thus, due to their central role in the regulation of endothelial cell activity, integrins, especially the αvβ3 integrin, are promising therapeutic targets. The LM609 antibody has been humanized as 'vitaxin' and is now entering clinical trials.

The pex protein provides a link between the extracellular matrix functions of proteolysis and adhesion. Pex is a fragment of matrix metalloproteinase 2 which prevents its binding to the αvβ3 integrin and thereby inhibits its ability to breakdown collagen. Pex disrupts angiogenesis and tumour growth in the chorioallantoic assay. Pex is also found in tumours in conjunction with αvβ3 expression and may be an endogenous regulator of the invasive behaviour of new blood vessels.[38]

E-cadherin

E-cadherin is an important epithelial adhesion molecule frequently lost in cancers. Loss of E-cadherin expression has recently been shown to coincide with the transition from well differentiated adenoma to invasive carcinoma in a transgenic mouse model. The link between adhesion and gene expression has not been established, but stimulation of angiogenesis occurs in a similar model during transition from adenoma to carcinoma.

Natural inhibitors of angiogenesis

Known inhibitors of the process of angiogenesis are listed in Table 2.

Angiostatin

Occasionally patients will be seen in whom distant metastasis grow unexpectedly rapidly after surgical removal of the primary. Folkman and O'Reilly postulated that this phenomenon was due to a primary tumour releasing angiogenic stimulators that promoted its own growth, and angiogenic inhibitors, which by virtue of longer half lives, had a greater effect on the developing vasculature of distant secondaries thereby suppressing their growth. Using a Lewis lung carcinoma model, half the mice had primary tumours removed when they reached 1500 mm³ in size. These mice developed 10 times the number of visible surface lung metastasis and an increase in lung weight, indicative of total tumour burden, of 400 per cent compared with control mice whose primary tumour was left alone.[40] Control mice had avascular lung metastasis compared with the highly vascularized metastases in the other group. To confirm that this effect was due to a circulating angiogenesis inhibitor, serum and dialysed

Table 2 Angiogenic inhibitors

Natural

Angiopoietin-2

Angiostatin

Endostatin

Interferon-α.

Platelet factor 4

Retinoic acid

Thrombospondin-1

Tissue inhibitors of metalloproteinases

16 kDa prolactin fragment

Synthetic

Anti-epidermal growth factor antibodies

Anti-integrins

Anti-urokinase plasminogen activator receptor antibodies

Anti-VEGF antibodies

Batimastat/Marimastat

Bryostatin

Carboxyamido-triazole

CM 101

Dexrazoxane

Dominant negative receptors

Fragmin

Fumagillin analogues (ACM1470)

Linomide

Neovastat

Paclitaxel

Pentosan polysulphate

PEX

Soluble VEGF receptors

Squalamine

SU101

Suramin

Tecogalan

Thalidomide

Vitaxin

2-Methoxyoestradiol

concentrated urine was obtained from tumour-bearing animals. When given by intraperitoneal injection to animals that had the primary excised, there was again suppression of distant metastatic growth comparable with mice with intact primaries. By contrast normal mouse serum or urine given after removal of the primary did not prevent the rapid metastatic expansion previously seen.[40]

Pooled urine and serum from mice with primary tumours were separately purified to obtain a 38 kDa protein that inhibited endothelial cell proliferation. On microsequence analysis, this angiogenic inhibitor, named angiostatin, showed 98 per cent identity to an internal fragment of plasminogen. Elastase degradation of human plasminogen also released an internal fragment that also strongly inhibited endothelial cell proliferation in vitro. This human angiostatin inhibited vascularization and growth of metastases when given to mice whose primaries were removed with an efficiency equal to or greater than in mice where the primary tumour remained intact. Intact plasminogen, or saline control injections resulted in a significant increase in number of metastases and in lung weight. Furthermore, angiostatin specifically inhibited endothelial cell proliferation in vitro with no effect on the growth of Lewis lung carcinoma cells. Antibodies against this internal fragment of mouse angiostatin blocked anti-metastatic activity.[40]

Subsequently, angiostatin was shown to inhibit almost completely the growth of three human and three murine primary carcinoma cell lines implanted subcutaneously in athymic mice without obvious toxicity. Histological analysis of tumours revealed similar proliferative indices for control and angiostatin-treated tumours, but apoptotic indices increased five times in those receiving angiostatin. Thus angiostatin may act by inducing tumour dormancy, balancing tumour apoptosis, and proliferation.[41]

Gately and colleagues have demonstrated that PC3 human prostatic carcinoma cells convert plasminogen to angiostatin using uPA and free sulphydryl donors. This again highlights the interaction between tumour cells, endothelial cells, and the extracellular matrix. Furthermore, in a cell-free system the authors were able to generate angiostatin from plasminogen opening the door for potential large-scale production of angiostatin for therapeutic purposes.[42]

An alternative therapeutic strategy using angiostatin involves gene transfer by transfecting cDNA coding for angiostatin into cells. When this was performed in vitro into T241 fibrosarcoma cells, primary growth of xenografts derived from these cells was reduced by 77 per cent, and in about 70 per cent of mice lung metastases remained at the micrometastatic avascular stage.[43]

Endostatin

O'Reilly and Folkman have recently identified another angiogenesis inhibitor, endostatin, identical to the C-terminal fragment of collagen XVIII. Purified initially from a mouse haemangioendothelioma, endostatin specifically inhibits endothelial cell proliferation, and significantly reduced the growth of lung metastases in mice after removal of an implanted Lewis lung carcinoma primary. Furthermore, in a separate set of experiments, when endostatin was given to mice bearing isografts of either Lewis lung carcinoma, T241 fibrosarcoma, B16F10 melanoma or EOMA haemangioendothelioma, primary tumour growth was inhibited by greater than 99 per cent. Immunohistologically, these tumours demonstrate inhibition of angiogenesis and increased apoptotic indices with an unchanged proliferative index comparable with control tumours. This provides further support for the tumour dormancy theory. Tumours remained in the dormant state as long as endostatin was given but became vascularized, grew, and eventually killed the mice when endostatin treatment was stopped.[44]

The recurrence of tumours upon discontinuation of therapy would appear to be a barrier to potential clinical use, as treatment would have to be continuous. However, in a remarkable series of experiments endostatin was given in a pulsed manner to mice again bearing implanted Lewis lung carcinoma, T241 fibrosarcoma, or B16F10 melanoma tumours. Endostatin was stopped when tumours had regressed. Tumours were then allowed to regrow to their previous size and another course of endostatin was then given. This again resulted in tumour regression. The cycle was repeated for up to six courses whereupon there was no further regrowth of tumours. These experiments demonstrate that resistance did not develop to endostatin after repeated courses unlike treatment with cyclophosphamide or other conventional chemotherapeutic agents and that continuous therapy in humans may not be necessary[45] (Fig. 4). Time will reveal the true significance of these observations.

Thrombospondin-1

Thrombospondin-1 is another important endogenous inhibitor of angiogenesis. Secreted by a number of cell types, thrombospondin-1 has inhibitory effects in in vitro and in vivo assays of angiogenesis and reduces the growth of xenografted tumours when overexpressed following transfection into the tumour cells. Subcutaneous tumours derived from the human fibrosarcoma cell line HT1080 into which the gene for thrombospondin-1 had been transfected, inhibited the growth of experimental melanoma lung metastases, and also inhibited corneal angiogenesis induced by basic FGF pellets in these animals. Thrombospondin-1 was isolated from the plasma of these animals. Tumours derived from subclones of HT1080 that had been transfected with anti-sense constructs to thrombospondin-1 and which expressed very little thrombospondin-1 demonstrated only weak or no control over the growth of lung metastases.[46]

Angiostatin, endostatin, and thrombospondin-1 are powerful inhibitors of angiogenesis and show great promise as future therapeutic agents. Angiostatin and endostatin are fragments of larger molecules, plasminogen and collagen XVIII, which are themselves not anti-angiogenic, and the antiangiogenic activity of thrombospondin-1 resides with a fragment of the complete molecule. This suggests that proteolytic processing is a major mechanism for regulating angiogenesis. Finally a 16 kDa fragment of prolactin has also been identified which is antiangiogenic whereas the parent molecule is not.

Control of angiogenesis

Progression from normal tissue through pre-malignant to overtly malignant tumour has been studied in transgenic mice which develop spontaneous tumours. In these mice vascularization develops well before the emergence of invasive malignancy. For example in the K14-HPV16 transgenic mouse, all of the cells express the transforming gene of the human papilloma virus 16 and mice develop spontaneous epidermal squamous cell carcinomas. In these mice there is a progressive increase in expression of acidic fibroblast growth factor and VEGF with progression from normal through early phase hyperplasia to high-grade dysplastic pre-malignant epidermis. Similarly in the RIP-TAG mouse which develops spontaneous β islet cell tumours of

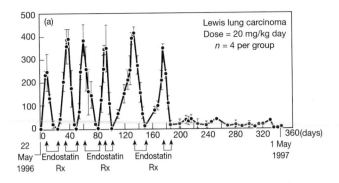

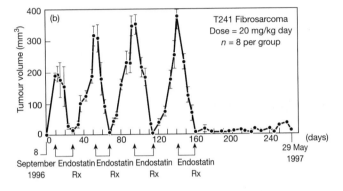

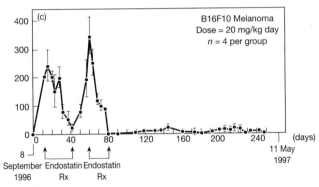

Fig. 4 Cycled endostatin therapy of tumours grown in the subcutaneous dorsa of mice. (a) Lewis lung carcinoma. When tumour volume reached 250–400 mm³, endostatin therapy was initiated. Tumours in four untreated animals grew to 10 005 ± 133 mm³ by day 27 (data not graphed). (b) T241 fibrosarcoma. Endostatin therapy was initiated when the mean tumour volume was 200 mm³ and in subsequent cycles when the tumour volume was greater than 300 mm³. Tumours in four untreated animals grew to 9127 ± 1183 mm³ by day 28. (c) B16F10 melanoma (a subclone of cells supplied by Isaiah Fidler, Houston). Endostatin therapy was initiated when the mean tumour volume was 230 mm³ for the initial cycle and at 350 mm³ for the second cycle. (Endostatin 20 mg/kg per day = 400 µg per 20 g mouse.) Tumours in four untreated animals grew to 7431 ± 1122 mm³ by day 41. (Reproduced from reference 45, with permission.)

the pancreas there is angiogenesis within a subset of islets at the hyperplastic stage prior to the progression to solid tumours.[47] A similar pattern is seen in patients with familial adenomatous polyposis coli during progression from early colonic adenomas to colonic carcinomas.[48]

Hypoxia

As blood vessels are required to provide increased oxygen and nutrients, it is not surprising that angiogenesis is stimulated by hypoxia and hypoglycaemia (Fig. 5). Clinically this is important, as enlarging tumours will inevitably develop ischaemic areas where metabolism of oxygen and glucose exceeds supply.

Several genes have been identified whose expression is stimulated by hypoxia and/or hypoglycaemia (Fig. 5). These include VEGF and specific enzymes on the glycolytic pathway such as lactate dehydrogenase A and glucose transporter 1. Expression of many of these genes is controlled by hypoxia inducible factor-1, which mediates transcriptional responses to hypoxia by binding to hypoxia response elements of the target gene. It is believed to play a major part in tumour vascularization, partly through upregulation of VEGF expression.[49] Furthermore, VEGF mRNA expression is not only upregulated but also stabilized by hypoxia. VEGF expression is also increased under conditions of hypoglycaemia.

Further evidence for the importance of the hypoxia signalling pathway in tumour growth *in vivo* has also been demonstrated using mouse hepatoma cell lines. Tumour cells with mutations in one of the two components of the hypoxia inducible factor-1 gene grow similarly to wild-type cells under aerobic conditions in monolayer culture. However, as xenografts they grew much more slowly than wild-type cells and show greatly reduced angiogenesis.[50] This is presumably due to failure of the cells to activate hypoxia inducible factor-1, and to produce VEGF in response to the hypoxia that occurs in these tumours.

Oncogenes

Evidence is now accumulating that sequential activation of oncogenes and inactivation of tumour suppresser genes not only plays an important part in freeing tumour cells from normal growth restraints that typify malignancy but also in the regulation of angiogenesis (Fig. 5). Oncogene activation affects angiogenesis by regulation of angiogenic factor and receptor expression, postreceptor signalling and extracellular matrix degradation.

VEGF is upregulated in association with activation of Ha-ras, fos, and V-src and downregulated with inactivation of the p53 tumour suppresser gene.[51] The kinase activity of the VEGF receptor, flk-1 is induced by mutations in the erbB2 oncogene and the homologous gene which encodes the epidermal growth factor receptor, as well as by increased levels of its ligands epidermal growth factor and transforming growth factor-α. These mutations and changes in expression are prognostic in a number of tumours including bladder and breast cancer.

The ras oncogene appears to be critical in angiogenesis. In signal transduction and endothelial cell activation, inactivation of the normal ras protein results in loss of directed cell migration. Furthermore, introduction of oncogenic ras into immortalized endothelial cells is associated with an increase in VEGF levels, bioactivity of matrix metalloproteinases, and a decrease in levels of tissue inhibitors of matrix metalloproteinases.[52]

A pro-angiogenic state is also achieved by reduction in angiogenesis inhibitors. Activation of the c-myc and c-jun oncogenes both lead to downregulation of thrombospondin-1. Reintroduction of various tumour suppresser genes including p53, the retinoblastoma gene and that associated with the von-Hippel Lindau syndrome has been

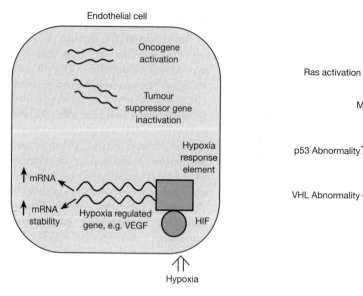

Fig. 5 Control of angiogenesis.

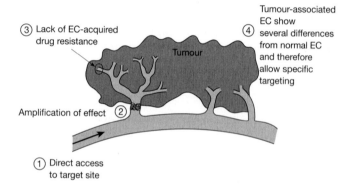

Fig. 6 Advantages of antiangiogenic therapy.

associated with either increased levels of angiogenic inhibitors or decreased levels of angiogenic stimulators.[53]

It may be possible to develop antiangiogenic therapy by targeting oncogenes. In this respect, blockade of the epidermal growth factor receptor has resulted in reduced angiogenesis and tumour growth *in vivo* as has inhibition by wortmannin[52] of phosphotidylinositol-3-kinase, a key molecule in a signalling pathway activated by ras. However, it is difficult to separate primary and secondary effects as any decrease in tumour growth will lead to a decrease in angiogenic stimulators. Thus cytotoxics are bound to have some antiangiogenic activity but the significance of this component in determining their antitumour activity is not clear.

Advantages of antiangiogenesis therapy

There are several potential advantages of antiangiogenic therapy over conventional treatments (Fig. 6). These include: (a) Enhanced drug delivery to the target site. An agent that acts primarily on the endothelium is given direct access to its target by intravenous administration. (b) Amplification of effect. Unlike targeting tumour cells where failure to destroy a proportion of the cells results in those cells proliferating and subsequent regrowth of the tumour, successful targeting of a few endothelial cells within a growing vessel may be sufficient to completely destroy that vessel. Likewise disruption of very few vessels may result in ischaemic necrosis of a substantial volume of tumour. Indeed it has been estimated that up to 10 carcinoma cells may depend on a single endothelial cell for effective perfusion. (c) Lack of endothelial cell drug resistance. Endothelial cells, unlike tumour cells, are genetically stable and are therefore less likely to have or to develop spontaneous mutations that result in drug resistance.[45] (d) Selective targeting of tumour endothelial cells is possible. Endothelial cells involved in the process of angiogenesis show several differences as compared with their normal counterparts. These differences, e.g. proliferatión rate and antigen expression, can be exploited so that antiangiogenic therapy attacks only the endothelial cells of tumours and not normal endothelium.

Tec-11 is a mouse monoclonal antibody against part of the transforming growth factor-α receptor. It binds strongly to endothelial cells in a number of tumours and only weakly if at all to endothelial cells in frozen sections from a panel of normal human tissues. It is postulated that these binding differences are related to the greater proliferation rate of tumour endothelial cells.[54] The proliferative rate of endothelial cells in tumours in mice is approximately 50 times that of endothelial cells in their normal tissues. The difference is less marked but still significant in human tumours.[55] Unfortunately Tec-11 and similar antibodies are not sufficiently selective yet to be exploited therapeutically and other potential endothelial specific antigens are being investigated including E-selectin and VEGF receptors.

Angiogenesis as a therapeutic target

Although the endothelial cell is ultimately the prime target, because of the complex interrelationships between endothelial cells, tumour

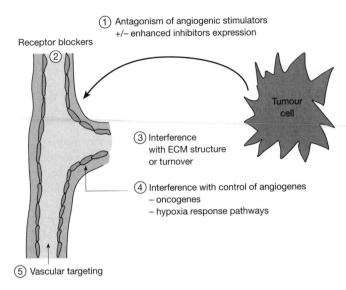

Fig. 7 Antiangiogenic strategies.

1. Antagonism of angiogenic stimulators +/– enhanced inhibitors expression

Receptor blockers
2.

Tumour cell

3. Interference with ECM structure or turnover

4. Interference with control of angiogenes – oncogenes – hypoxia response pathways

5. Vascular targeting

cells, and extracellular matrix, all of these can be attacked to disrupt some stage of angiogenesis. Therefore, an antiangiogenic effect can be achieved by targeting: (a) angiogenic stimulators; (b) angiogenic receptors; (c) extracellular matrix components; (d) extracellular matrix proteolysis; (e) control mechanisms of angiogenesis; or (f) the endothelial cell directly (Fig. 7).

Targeting angiogenic stimulators

Interferon-α

Interferon-α inhibits the production of basic FGF in a number of tumours. The natural history of haemangiomas of infancy is usually spontaneous regression over a number of years. If, however, these haemangiomas are very large they can be life threatening due to their complications. Interferon-α2A causes a significant regression in these cases.[56]

Thalidomide

Thalidomide is antiangiogenic, inhibiting basic FGF induced angiogenesis in the rabbit corneal assay. The well known teratogenicity may indeed be related to antiangiogenesis in the developing fetal limb bud.[57] Apart from this teratogenicity, however, thalidomide lacks significant systemic toxicity and is taken orally. Disease stabilization, albeit of short duration, has been demonstrated with hormone-resistant prostate cancer and a minimal radiographic response has been reported in two of 10 patients evaluable so far in a phase I glioma trial.[58]

Monoclonal antibodies to angiogenic stimulators

Anti-VEGF monoclonal antibodies have reduced tumour growth and angiogenesis in xenografts with glioblastoma and colon and prostate tumours.[59] Humanized anti-VEGF antibodies (Genentech) have recently finished phase I clinical trials where they have been found to be safe and are currently entering phase II trials (N. Ferrrara personal communication).

Suramin

Suramin, first synthesized over 80 years ago, has been used extensively for the treatment of trypanosomiasis. Among its multiple actions are inhibition of mitochondrial functioning, reduction in DNA polymerase activity and inhibition of the binding of VEGF and basic FGF to their receptors. Suramin has been used as a treatment for metastatic hormone-resistant prostate cancer, reducing prostate specific antigen by 50 per cent in about 30–40 per cent of patients and has resulted in some complete and partial responses, of short duration, in measurable disease. However, in these trials suramin has a narrow therapeutic window associated with significant toxicity including adrenal suppression and polyneuropathy at higher plasma concentrations.[60]

To avoid the problems of systemic toxicity alternative methods of administration are being investigated, where high local concentrations can be achieved, such as intravesically for recurrent superficial bladder cancer[61] and intraperitoneally for peritoneal tumours. Also derivatives of suramin have been developed which have equal or greater antiangiogenic activity but with reduced toxicity.[62]

One drawback of targeting specific angiogenic stimulatory factors is that angiogenesis may still be successfully achieved by the tumour using alternative factors. Targeting downstream effects of various angiogenic factors, such as postreceptor signalling pathways or endothelial cell/extracellular matrix interactions may prove more successful.

Targeting angiogenic receptors

1. Receptor blockers. SU-5416 (Sugen) is a synthetic VEGFR2 inhibitor. In animal models it is antiangiogenic and also reduces tumour growth. It is in phase I trials in patients with solid tumours.

2. Soluble receptor fragments. A variant of FLT-1 (VEGFR1) exists as a soluble truncated form, sFLT-1. This competes with the wild-type receptor for VEGF. The biological function of sFLT-1 is unclear, although it may be a physiological negative regulator of VEGF action.[63]

3. Dominant negative receptors. Using retroviral-mediated gene therapy techniques Millauer et al. induced expression of a dominant negative mutant form of VEGFR2. The formation of dimers with the endogenous receptor prevented signalling in response to VEGF binding. This resulted in reduced growth of glioblastoma multiforme cell lines in vivo.[64]

4. Carboxyamidotriazole. This interferes with calcium influx and cell signalling pathways. It inhibits angiogenesis in the chick chorioallantoic membrane and reduces both size and number of lung metastases after injection of HT-29 human colon cancer cell lines into the tail veins of nude mice.[65] Inhibition of postreceptor signalling pathways remains a further therapeutic target for angiogenesis therapy.

Targeting the extracellular matrix

1. Antibodies against integrins. As already seen the LM609 antibody to the integrin αVβ3 and other integrin antagonists can block angiogenesis and tumour invasion, induce endothelial cell apoptosis and cause tumour regression. Vitaxin is a humanized version of LM609 and is currently under evaluation in the

treatment of acquired immune deficiency syndrome (AIDS)-related Kaposi sarcoma. The LM609 antibody linked to a paramagnetic contrast agent has been used in combination with magnetic resonance imaging to detect angiogenesis *in vivo*.[66] This may prove a very useful non-invasive way of monitoring responses to various antiangiogenic therapies.

2. Doxorubicin and integrins. The coupling of doxorubicin to an αv integrin binding motif has been used to target drug delivery to areas of increased angiogenesis, thus allowing increased local concentration to be achieved with reduced systemic toxicity. This has resulted in enhanced efficiency and reduced toxicity as compared with free doxorubicin when given to athymic mice with breast cancer xenografts.[67]

3. Linomide. Linomide is a quinolone 3-carboxyamide. It inhibits angiogenesis in *in vitro* assays and *in vivo*, as measured by decreased microvessel density within tumours. It is undergoing evaluation in early clinical trials.[68]

Targeting proteolysis of the extracellular matrix.

1. Batimastat and Marimastat. Marimastat is a matrix metalloproteinase inhibitor, which reduces degradation of basement membranes and the extracellular matrix. Marimastat achieves high plasma levels after oral administration superseding its predecessor Batimastat which had poor water solubility. Marimastat treatment has resulted in reduced serum markers of malignancy in prostate, colon, pancreatic, and ovarian cancers.[69] Its major side-effects include musculoskeletal pain and frozen shoulder.

2. AGM 1470 (TMP 470). AGM 1470 is a semi-synthetic analogue of fumagillin that interferes with cell cycle progression and inhibits the metalloproteinase type II aminopeptidase (metAP-2). In AIDS-related Kaposi's sarcoma, partial responses have been reported in a proportion of patients at dose levels that are well tolerated and phase III trials are underway.[70]

Targeting control of angiogenesis

1. Oncogene inhibitors. As described earlier interference with oncogenes and their downstream signalling pathways may present therapeutic opportunities. Farnesyltransferase inhibitors block the activity of oncogenic-ras and antibodies against the epidermal growth factor receptor suppress angiogenesis and tumour proliferation in xenograft experiments.[71]

2. Targeting hypoxia response pathways. Hypoxically activated promoters have been used *in vitro* to increase the expression of the prodrug-activating bacterial enzyme, cytosine deaminase, which converts the prodrug 5-fluorocytosine to 5-fluorouracil resulting in increased cell death.[72] Such strategies may be of use *in vivo*. The ability to target tumour cells selectively with bioreductive drugs (i.e. those that require reduction for activation, such as timpazamine) on the basis of their hypoxic status has important implications. Not only are hypoxic cells a ready source of angiogenic factors, but they are also often resistant to radiotherapy and chemotherapy.

3. Induction of apoptosis. The precise mechanism of action of angiostatin and endostatin is unclear, although they do increase apoptotic indices within tumours. Phase I trials are about to start

with angiostatin and given the dramatic results in animal models where there was no appreciable toxicity, results are keenly awaited.

Targeting the endothelial cell directly

Vascular targeting is distinct from antiangiogenesis in that it is established tumour vessels rather than proliferating, migrating endothelial cells that are the target.

E-selectin and VEGFR2 are molecules that are overexpressed on tumour endothelium. As this expression is under the control of the respective promoters of these genes, the promoters can be used to direct expression of any gene specifically to the tumour endothelium, including chosen toxic genes.[73]

The inflammatory reaction responsible for some of the symptoms of respiratory distress syndrome in neonates is due to CM101, a group B haemolytic streptococcal exotoxin that binds to immature endothelium of the neonatal lung. However, CM101 also binds preferentially to tumour endothelium resulting in vessel disruption. Results from a phase I trial show some evidence of tumour regression using this agent.[74]

In a mouse model, a tumour endothelial specific marker has been induced experimentally. A bi-specific antibody, 'coaguligand', has been generated where one arm is directed against this endothelial marker and the other is linked to a truncated form of tissue factor. Intact tissue factor is involved in initiating the coagulation cascade. Upon binding of coaguligand to the tumour endothelial marker the truncated (inactive tissue factor) is brought into contact with cell surface phospholipids where it becomes activated and triggers the coagulation cascade. In mice with subcutaneous neuroblastomas intravenous coaguligand has resulted in specific thrombosis of tumour vessels and subsequent tumour necrosis with one-third of mice having complete tumour regressions.[75]

Criticisms of antiangiogenic therapy

Two major criticisms of antiangiogenic therapy are first, the potential interference with physiological angiogenesis and secondly, that the best results of most early clinical trials have shown disease stabilization rather than tumour response.

Angiogenesis is important in the physiological processes of wound healing, menstrual cycle, and embryogenesis. However, in the context of systemic treatment for malignancy these processes may not present major problems. Wound healing problems could be reduced by delaying antiangiogenesis therapy for a short while after surgery in much the same way as is done for chemotherapy or radiotherapy. Similarly menstrual cycle abnormalities and deliberate avoidance of pregnancy are common when conventional chemotherapy is used.

By depriving tumours of the blood supply necessary for growth, antiangiogenic therapy acts cytostatically rather than cytotoxically; consistent with this expectation are the results of many early clinical trials (described above) where success has often been disease stabilization rather than complete response. Such an effect might be satisfactory if lack of resistance and of toxicity make it possible to use prolonged antiangiogenic treatment. Quantifying such responses in clinical trials is difficult, and we may have to use additional endpoints such as reduced tumour blood flow or reduced levels of angiogenic factors in target tissues; otherwise, potentially useful agents may be discarded as providing no evidence of tumour response.

The way ahead

Combination therapy

Different antiangiogenic agents act on different components of the angiogenic process and therefore combinations of antiangiogenesis drugs might have synergistic effects. As our knowledge of different angiogenic stimulators and inhibitors, and understanding of the complex inter-relationships between endothelial cells, tumour cells, and extracellular matrix improves it may become possible to construct an angiogenic profile for individual patients and their tumours, and to tailor combination antiangiogenic therapy more specifically.

Combining antiangiogenic therapy with conventional chemotherapy, radiotherapy or hormonal therapy may have additional beneficial effects.[76] A more powerful antiangiogenic effect has recently been shown experimentally for combined angiostatin and ionizing radiation.[77] However, combinational therapy may present its own problems such as the reduction of access of chemotherapeutic drugs and decreased radioresponsiveness associated with increased hypoxia. In the clinical setting such effects need investigation in randomized clinical control trials.

Conclusions

In recent years angiogenesis has progressed from being a useful prognostic indicator to a realistic therapeutic target. Initial enthusiasm, slightly dampened when early trial results indicated predominantly cytostatic effects resulting in disease stabilization rather than complete response, has been reignited by the dramatic antitumour effects in the laboratory of the new wave of angiogenesis inhibitors. It will be of great interest to see whether these now translate to the clinic.

References

1. Ferrara N, *et al.* Vascular endothelial growth factor is essential for corpus luteum angiogenesis. *Nature Medicine*, 1998; 4: 336–40.

2. Rees MCP, Bicknell R. Angiogenesis in the endometrium. *Angiogenesis*, 1998; 2: 29–35.

3. Folkman J. What is the evidence that tumors are angiogenesis dependent? *Journal of the National Cancer Institute*, 1990; 82: 4–6.

4. Zhang H-T, *et al.* Enhancement of tumour growth and vascular density by transfection of vascular endothelial growth factor into MCF-7 breast carcinoma cells. *Journal of the National Cancer Institute*, 1995; 87: 213–18.

5. Hanahan D. Heritable formation of pancreatic β–cell tumors in transgenic mice expressing recombinant insulin/simian virus 40 oncogenes. *Nature*, 1985; 315: 115–21.

6. Weidner N, Sample JP, Welch WR. Tumor angiogenesis and metastasis—correlation in invasive breast carcinoma. *New England Journal of Medicine*, 1991; 324: 1–8.

7. Fox SB, *et al.* Association of tumour angiogenesis with bone marrow micrometastases in breast cancer patients. *Journal of the National Cancer Institute*, 1997; 89: 1044–9.

8. Bicknell R, Lewis CE, Ferrara N. *Tumour angiogenesis.* Oxford: Oxford University Press, 1997.

9. Pepper MS, Ferrara N, Orci L, Montestano R. Potent synergism between vascular endothelial growth factor and basic fibroblast growth factor in the induction of angiogenesis *in vitro*. *Biochemical and Biophysical Research Communications*, 1992; 189: 824–31.

10. Ferrara N, Davis-Smyth TD. The biology of vascular endothelial growth factor. *Endocrine Reviews*, 1997; 10: 4–25.

11. Fong GH, Rossant J, Gertsenstein M, Breitman ML. Role of the flt-1 receptor tyrosine kinase in regulating the assembly of vascular endothelium. *Nature*, 1995; 376: 66–70.

12. Shalaby F, *et al.* Failure of blood-island formation and vasculogenesis in Flk-1 deficient mice. *Nature*, 1995; 376: 62–6.

13. Ferrara N, *et al.* Heterozygous embryonic lethality induced by targeted inactivation of the VEGF gene. *Nature*, 1996; 380: 439–42.

14. Carmeliet P, *et al.* Abnormal blood vessel development and lethality in embryos lacking a single VEGF allele. *Nature*, 1996; 380: 435–9.

15. Saleh M, Stacker SA, Wilks AF. Inhibition of growth of C6 glioma cells *in vivo* by expression of antisense vascular endothelial growth factor sequence. *Cancer Research*, 1996; 56: 393–401.

16. Borgstrom P, Bourdon MA, Hillan KJ, Sriramarao P, Ferrara N. Neutralising anti vascular endothelial growth factor antibody completely inhibits angiogenesis and growth of human prostate carcinoma microtumours *in vivo*. *Prostate*, 1998; 35: 1–10.

17. Jeltsch M, *et al.* Hyperplasia of lymphatic vessels in VEGF-C transgenic mice. *Science*, 1997; 276: 1423–5.

18. Salven P, *et al.* Vascular endothelial growth factors vegf-b and vegf-c are expressed in human tumours. *American Journal of Pathology*, 1998; 153: 103–8.

19. Sato TN, *et al.* Distinct roles of the receptor tyrosine kinases Tie-1 and Tie-2 in blood vessel formation. *Nature*, 1995; 376: 70–4.

20. Suri C, *et al.* Requisite role of angiopoietin-1, a ligand for the Tie-2 receptor, during embryonic angiogenesis. *Cell*, 1996; 87: 1171–80.

21. Vikkula M, *et al.* Vascular dysmorphogenesis caused by an activating mutation in the receptor tyrosine kinase Tie-2. *Cell*, 1996; 87: 1181–90.

22. Brown N, Bicknell R. Thymidine phosphorylase, 2-deoxy-D-ribose and angiogenesis. *Biochemical Journal*, 1998; 334: 1–8.

23. Folkman J. What is the role of thymidine phosphorylase in tumour angiogenesis? *Journal of the National Cancer Institute*, 1996; 88: 1091–2.

24. Takebayashi Y, *et al.* Clinicopathological and prognostic significance of an angiogenic factor, thymidine phosphorylase in human colorectal carcinoma. *Journal of the National Cancer Institute*, 1996; 88: 1110–17.

25. Moghaddam A, *et al.* Thymidine phosphorylase is angiogenic and promotes tumour growth. *Proceedings of the National Academy of Sciences of the United States of America*, 1995; 92: 998–1002.

26. Nguyen M. Angiogenic factors as tumour markers. *Investigational New Drugs*, 1997; 15: 29–37.

27. Soff GA, *et al.* Expression of plasminogen activator inhibitor type 1 by human prostate carcinoma cells inhibits primary tumor growth, tumor-associated angiogenesis, and metastasis to lung and liver in an athymic mouse model. *Journal of Clinical Investigation*, 1995; 96: 2593–600.

28. Evans CP, Elfman F, Parangi S, Conn M, Cunha G, Schuman MA. Inhibition of prostate cancer neovascularisation and growth by urokinase-plasminogen activator receptor blockade. *Cancer Research*, 1997; 57: 3594–9.

29. Min HY, *et al.* Urokinase receptor antagonists inhibit angiogenesis and primary tumour growth in syngeneic mice. *Cancer Research*, 1996; 56: 2428–33.

30. Talbot DC, Brown PD. Experimental and clinical studies on the use of matrix metalloproteinase inhibitors for the treatment of cancer. *European Journal of Cancer*, 1996; 32A: 2528–33.

31. Polverini P. How the extracellular matrix and macrophages contribute to angiogenesis-dependent diseases. *European Journal of Cancer*, 1996; 32A: 2430–7.

32. Leek RD, Lewis CE, Whitehouse R, Greenall M, Clarke J, Harris AL.

Association of macrophage infiltration with angiogenesis and prognosis in invasive breast carcinoma. *Cancer Research*, 1996; **56**: 4625–9.

33. Friedlander M, Brooks PC, Shaffer RW, Kincaid CM, Varner JA, Cheresh DA. Definition of two angiogenic pathways by distinct αv integrins. *Science*, 1995; **270**: 1500–2.

34. Brooks PC. Role of integrins in angiogenesis. *European Journal of Cancer*, 1996; **32A**: 2423–9.

35. Brooks PC, Stromblad S, Klemke R, Visscher D, Sarkar FH, Cheresh DA. Anti-integrin, α,β₃ blocks human breast cancer growth. *Journal of Clinical Investigation*, 1995; **96**: 1815–22.

36. Stromblad S, Becker JC, Yebra M, Brooks PC, Cheresh DA. Suppression of p53 activity and p21^WAF1/CIP1 expression by vascular cell integrin α,β₃ during angiogenesis. *Journal of Clinical Investigation*, 1996; **98**: 426–33.

37. Ruegg C, Yilmaz A, Bieler G, Bamat J, Chaubert P, LeJeune FJ. Evidence for the involvement of endothelial cell integrin, α,β₃ in the disruption of the tumour vasculature induced by TNF and IFN-γ. *Nature Medicine*, 1998; **4**: 408–14.

38. Brooks PC, Silletti S, von Schalscha TL, Friedlander M, Cheresh DA. Disruption of angiogenesis by PEX, a noncatalytic metalloproteinase fragment with integrin binding activity. *Cell*, 1998; **92**: 391–400.

39. Skobe M, Rockwell P, Goldstein N, Vosseler S, Fusenig NE. Halting angiogenesis suppresses carcinoma cell invasion. *Nature Medicine*, 1997; **3**: 1222–7.

40. O'Reilly M, *et al*. Angiostatin: A novel angiogenesis inhibitor that mediates the suppression of metastases by a Lewis lung carcinoma. *Cell*, 1994; **79**: 315–28.

41. O'Reilly MS, Holmgren L, Chen CC, Folkman J. Angiostatin induces and sustains dormancy of human primary tumours in mice. *Nature Medicine*, 1996; **2**: 689–92.

42. Gately S, *et al*. The mechanism of cancer-mediated conversion of plasminogen to the angiogenesis inhibitor angiostatin. *Proceedings of the National Academy of Sciences of the United States of America*, 1997; **94**: 10868–72.

43. Cao Y, *et al*. Expression of angiostatin cDNA in a murine fibrosarcoma suppresses primary tumour growth and produces long term dormancy of metastases. *Journal of Clinical Investigation*, 1998; **101**: 1055–63.

44. O'Reilly M, *et al*. Endostatin: An endogenous inhibitor of angiogenesis and tumor growth. *Cell*, 1997; **88**: 277–85.

45. Boehm T, Folkman J, Browder T, O'Reilly MS. Antiangiogenic therapy of experimental cancer does not induce acquired drug resistance. *Nature*, 1997; **390**: 404–7.

46. Volpert OV, Lawler J, Bouck NP. A human fibrosarcoma inhibits systemic angiogenesis and the growth of experimental metastases via thrombospondin-1. *Proceedings of the National Academy of Sciences of the United States of America*, 1998; **95**: 6343–8.

47. Hanahan D, Christofori G, Naik P, Arbeit J. Transgenic mouse models of tumour angiogenesis: the angiogenic switch, its molecular controls, and prospects for preclinical therapeutic models. *European Journal of Cancer*, 1996; **32A**: 2386–93.

48. Rak J, Filmus J, Kerbel RS. Reciprocal paracrine interactions between tumour cells and endothelial cells: the 'angiogenesis progression' hypothesis. *European Journal of Cancer*, 1996; **32A**: 2438–50.

49. Carmeliet P, *et al*. Role of HIF-1 α in hypoxia-mediated apoptosis, cell proliferation and tumour angiogenesis. *Nature*, 1998; **394**: 485–90.

50. Maxwell PH, *et al*. Hypoxia-inducible factor-1 modulates gene expression in solid tumours and influences both angiogenesis and tumour growth. *Proceedings of the National Academy of Sciences of the United States of America*, 1997; **94**: 8104–9.

51. Rak J, *et al*. Mutant ras oncogenes upregulate VEGF/ VPF expression: implications for induction and inhibition of tumor angiogenesis. *Cancer Research*, 1995; **55**: 4575.

52. Arbiser JL, *et al*. Oncogenic H-ras stimulates tumour angiogenesis by

two distinct pathways. *Proceedings of the National Academy of Sciences of the United States of America*, 1997; **94**: 861–6.

53. Rastinejad F, Bouck NP. Oncogenes and tumour suppressor genes in the regulation of angiogenesis. In: Bicknell R, Lewis CE, Ferrara N (eds) *Tumour angiogenesis*. Oxford: Oxford University Press, 1997: 101–10.

54. Burrows FJ, Thorpe PE. Eradication of large solid tumours in mice with an immunotoxin directed against tumour vasculature. *Proceedings of the National Academy of Sciences of the United States of America*, 1993; **90**: 8996–9000.

55. Fox SB, *et al*. Relationship of endothelial cell proliferation to tumour vascularity in human breast cancer. *Cancer Research*, 1993; **53**: 4161–3.

56. Ezekowitz RAB, Mulliken JB, Folkman J. Interferon alpha-2a therapy for life threatening haemangiomas of infancy. *New England Journal of Medicine*, 1992; **326**: 1456–63.

57. D'Amato RJ, Loughnan MS, Flynn E, Folkman J. Thalidomide is an inhibitor of angiogenesis. *Proceedings of the National Academy of Sciences of the United States of America*.1994; **91**: 4082–5.

58. Fine HA, *et al*. A phase I trial of the antiangiogenic agent, thalidomide, in patients with recurrent high grade gliomas. *Proceedings of the American Society of Clinical Oncology*, 1997; **16**: 385a.

59. Warren R.S, Yuan H, Matli M.R, Gillett NA, Ferrara N. Regulation by vascular endothelial growth factor of human colon cancer tumorigenesis in a mouse model of experimental liver metastasis. *Journal of Clinical Investigations*, 1995; **95**: 1789–97.

60. Eisenberger M, *et al*. Suramin, an active drug for prostate cancer: interim observations in a phase I trial. *Journal of the National Cancer Institute*, 1993; **85**: 611–21.

61. Walther MM, Figg WD, Lineham WM. Intravesical suramin: a novel agent for the treatment of superficial transitional-cell carcinoma of the bladder. *World Journal of Urology*, 1996; **14**: S8–11.

62. Braddock PS, Hu D-E, Fan T-PD, Stratford IJ, Harris AL, Bicknell R. A structure-activity analysis of antagonism of the growth factor and angiogenic activity of basic fibroblast growth factor by suramin and related polyanions. *British Journal of Cancer*, 1994; **69**: 890–8.

63. Kendall RL, Thomas K.A. Inhibition of vascular endothelial growth factor by an endogenously encoded soluble receptor. *Proceedings of the National Academy of Sciences of the United States of America*, 1993; **90**: 10705–9.

64. Millauer B, Shawver LK, Plate KH, Risau W, Ullrich A. Glioblastoma growth is inhibited *in vivo* by a negative dominant Flk-1 mutant. *Nature*, 1994; **367**: 576–9.

65. Kohn EC, Sandeen MA, Liotta LA. In vivo efficacy of a novel inhibitor of selected signal transduction pathways including calcium, arachidonate and inositol phosphates. *Cancer Research*, 1992; **52**: 3208–12.

66. Sipkins DA, Cheresh DA, Kazemi MR, Nevin LM, Bednarski MD, Li KCP. Detection of tumour angiogenesis *in vivo* by α,β₃-targeted magnetic resonance imaging. *Nature Medicine*, 1998; **4**: 623–30.

67. Arap W, Pasqualini R, Ruoslahti E. Cancer treatment by targeted drug delivery to tumour vasculature in a mouse model. *Science*, 1998; **279**: 377–80.

68. Pawinsky A, *et al*. An EORTC phase II study of the efficacy and safety of linomide in the treatment of advanced renal cell carcinoma. *European Journal of Cancer*, 1997; **33**: 496–9.

69. Gore M, A'Hern R, Stankiewicz M, Slevin M. Tumour marker levels during marimastat therapy. *The Lancet*, 1996; **348**: 263.

70. Dezube BJ, *et al*. Fumagillin analogue in the treatment of Kaposi's sarcoma: a phase I AIDS clinical trial group study. AIDS clinical trial group no. 215 team. *Journal of Clinical Oncology*, 1998; **16**: 1444–9.

71. Ciardiello F, *et al*. Antitumour activity of combined blockade of epidermal growth factor receptor and protein kinase A. *Journal of the National Cancer Institute*, 1996; **88**: 1770–6.

72. **Dachs GU, et al.** Targeting gene expression to hypoxic tumour cells. *Nature Medicine*, 1997; **3**: 515–20.

73. **Jagger RT, Bicknell R.** Vascular targeting of anti-cancer gene therapy. In Bicknell R, Lewis CE, Ferrara N (eds) *Tumour angiogenesis*. Oxford: Oxford University Press, 1997: 357–76.

74. **Devore RF, et al.** Phase 1 study of the antineovascularization drug CM 101. *Clinical Cancer Research*, 1997; **3**: 365–72.

75. **Huang X, Molema G, King S, Watkins L, Edgington TS, Thorpe PE.** Tumour infarction in mice by antibody-directed targeting of tissue factor to tumour vasculature. *Science*, 1997; **275**: 547–50.

76. **Teicher B.** A systems approach to cancer therapy. *Cancer and Metastasis Reviews*, 1996; **15**: 247–72.

77. **Mauceri HJ, et al.** Combined effects of angiostatin and ionising-radiation in antitumour therapy. *Nature*, 1998; **394**: 287–91.

1.8 Metastasis

Ian R. Hart

Introduction

Metastasis, which is defined as the transfer of disease from one organ or part to another not directly connected with it, is the most clinically significant behavioural trait of malignant cancer. Surgical removal of the primary tumour, often combined with irradiation or chemotherapy, frequently offers successful treatment for neoplasia. However, dissemination of tumour cells commonly defeats such modes of treatment and cancer spread remains responsible for a large proportion of cancer deaths. Indeed, the fact that approximately 50 per cent of patients presenting with the common solid tumours already have metastatic disease at the time of presentation underlines the magnitude of the problem. Although spread may already have occurred by the time the physician sees the patient, so that opportunities for intervention have passed, it remains probable that a more complete understanding of the molecular and cellular mechanisms which contribute to tumour dissemination eventually will give rise to means of developing novel therapies. This chapter explores the proposed molecular and cellular mechanisms which underlie the phenomenon of tumour metastasis.

Mechanisms of metastasis

Cancer spread is a complex, multifactorial process where eventual outcome is dependent upon a series of sequential interactions between tumour and host. The major steps in the process are illustrated schematically in Fig. 1.

Following neovascularization (see Chapter 1.7) there is loss of tumour cell cohesion and disengagement of individual cells from the primary site. The disseminating cancer cell must then invade the surrounding stroma and enter the vasculature or lymphatic system. Entrance into these systems is followed by the release of individual cells or small emboli which must survive in the circulation before subsequently arresting in the capillary beds of distant organs. From here the disseminating cells must penetrate, and extravasate through, the arresting lymphatic or blood vessel walls. Finally, the newly established tumour focus must again induce a blood supply before growing to develop into a secondary cancer.

The reductionist approach to this multifactoral process has been to attempt to break it down into its composite parts and to analyse those molecules which play major roles in determining each of these steps. Because of apparent parallels between many of these interactions and those involved in the migratory behaviour of leucocytes during the process of inflammation, or indeed parallels with interactions

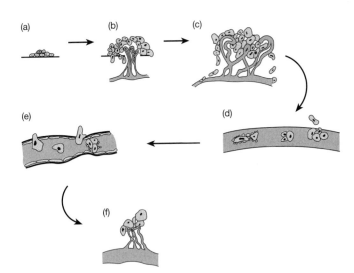

Fig. 1 Pathogenesis of metastasis (a) following the primary transformation of a normal epithelial cell, cohesion and normal cytoarchitecture is lost (b) in order for the tumour to grow beyond 2 mm^3 in size new blood vessels are induced from pre-existent host capillaries. These capillaries penetrate and cross the basement membrane. At the same time cells from the primary tumour mass disrupt the basement membrane and start to move through (c) losing cell–cell cohesion disseminating cancer cells move away from the constraints of the primary tumour, interacting with extracellular matrix proteins as they invade. Penetration into lymphatics or small blood capillaries occurs (d) following penetration tumours either grow at the site of intravasation or break away as small clumps or emboli which interact with each other or with cell components of the circulatory system (e) arresting either as a consequence of non-specific entrapment or as a consequence of specific cell–cell adhesion, tumour cells can either grow at the site of arrest or extravasate, again penetrating the basement membrane. (f) The requirement for secondary tumour growth necessitates the induction of a neovascular response from surrounding host tissue.

involved in the migration of endothelial cells during initiation of angiogenic responses, much of our knowledge regarding molecules putatively involved in regulating tumour spread has come from analyses of normal cells during these related processes.

Angiogenesis

The process of angiogenesis is described in Chapter 1.7. Here the point is made that, for tumours to grow to a size beyond approximately

2 mm³, there must be the induction of new vasculature. These blood vessels, derived from pre-existing capillaries or venules, are elicited from the surrounding host tissue in a process termed tumour angiogenesis. As the likelihood of metastasis occurring generally increases in direct proportion with the size of the tumour mass (with approximately 80 per cent of all cancers conforming to this rule) it is clear that angiogenesis must contribute not only to tumour growth *per se* but also to metastatic spread. Indeed the simple enumeration of microvessels in histological sections of tumours has proven to be a strong predictive marker of the probability of cancer dissemination.[1],[2] Coupled with the increase in microvessel density, which facilitates the access of greater numbers of disseminating cells to the microcirculation, there also is the fact that such vessels are leaky, and lack functional tight cell–cell adhesion, which therefore permits easier ingress of neoplastic cells.[3] The mechanisms of tumour-driven angiogenesis generally will not be covered in this chapter, but the concept of tumour latency as a consequence of angiogenic regulation will be discussed later as it has profound implications for the way in which metastatic disease may present.

Cell adhesion in the regulation of tumour spread

There are many parallels between normal leucocyte trafficking and tumour spread. Many of the cell–cell and cell–substrate interactions involved in both processes are regulated by changes in cellular adhesion. While the parallels are most evident in the later stages of tumour metastasis, i.e. the heterotypic clumping which can occur between peripheral leucocytes and neoplastic cells during embolization and the active adherence of arresting tumour cells to the endothelium of distant organs, the involvement of cell adhesion molecules in cancer spread extends across the spectrum of interactions. Thus the initial escape of a tumour cell from its primary location requires the loss of the cell–cell attachment which maintains tissue cohesion. In epithelial tumours this phenomenon is mediated largely by members of the cadherin family and in particular by E-cadherin. Equally, initial invasive behaviour may require the involvement of members of the integrin family of cell–surface molecules. A cartoon presenting the various family members of cell adhesion receptors is presented in Fig. 2.

Cadherins

Cadherins constitute a family of calcium-dependent, cell–cell adhesion molecules which predominately mediate homotypic cell–cell (i.e. between cells of the same type) interactions. They play a key part in determining tissue morphogenesis as well as in maintaining a differentiated phenotype. Cadherins are single-chain, transmembrane glycoproteins with a large extracellular region and a highly conserved cytoplasmic tail which interacts with the internal cytoskeleton via the linking intracellular proteins, α-, β-, and γ-catenin. Deletion of the cytoplasmic tail, or indeed loss, modification, or mutation of the catenins, abrogates cadherin activity thereby suggesting that the catenins have a major part in determining cadherin function.[4] Originally, it was shown that differentiated kidney epithelial cells adopted a fibroblastic morphology and became more invasive in collagen gels when E-cadherin activity was downregulated using

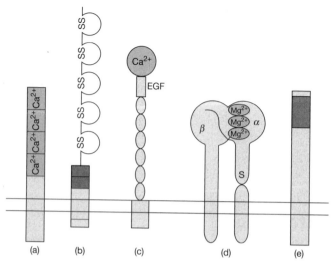

Fig. 2 Families of adhesion receptors. (a) Cadherin family. Single chain glycoproteins with an extracellular domain containing four repeats of approximately 110 amino acids with Ca²⁺ binding sites. The N-terminal 113 amino acids contain a conserved HAV sequence of importance in ligand binding and specificity. (b) Immunoglobulin superfamily. Characterized by varying numbers of immunoglobulin folds consisting of 70 to 100 amino acids stabilized by disulphide bonds. (c) Selectin family. Characterized by calcium-dependent (C-type) lectin domain at the N-terminus, followed by EGF-like repeats and varying numbers of repeats of a complement regulatory protein (CRP)-like domain. (d) Integrin family. Heterodimeric glycoproteins consisting of non-covalently associated α and β subunits. The α subunits consist of heavy and light fragments which are disulphide linked. The N-terminal region of the α subunit contains three (or four) cation binding sites. (e) CD44. Related to the cartilage proteoglycan core and link proteins at the N-terminal region, CD44 is the major cell surface receptor for hyaluronate.

monoclonal antibodies.[5] Moreover, the introduction of E-cadherin cDNAs into cell lines which lacked E-cadherin expression increased intracellular adhesion and decreased cell invasiveness.[5],[6] Concomitant with such experimental results there have been an increasing number of studies which have monitored both the immunohistochemical expression of E-cadherin and the integrity of the gene in various cancers. The majority of the immunocytochemical studies have found consistent loss of E-cadherin activity associated with poor prognosis, increased grade, and metastatic activity in several tumours, including prostate, stomach, bladder, colorectum, and pancreas (see references 7 to 9 for example).

Loss of E-cadherin protein, as detected by immunohistochemistry, may arise from a variety of mechanisms. The loss of heterozygosity at 16q22.1, where E-cadherin maps, is a frequent finding in breast cancer where it has been associated with the development of distant metastasis.[9] The majority of invasive lobular carcinomas of the breast fail to express any E-cadherin and this appears to relate to inactivation by truncation mutations throughout the extracellular domain, associated with loss of heterozygosity of the wild-type locus.[10] Similar mutations in E-cadherin in diffuse gastric carcinoma have been described implying that this means of losing E-cadherin function may be associated with a distinctive morphological pattern of invasive behaviour.

Equally, the finding that E-cadherin expression can be restored under experimental conditions or in metastases derived from E-cadherin negative primary tumours suggests that inactivation may occur through other mechanisms, such as promoter methylation.[11]

Simple loss of cadherin function is not the only means whereby cell–cell cohesion may be lost since there is a requirement for the catenins for optimal cadherin activity. It is not surprising therefore that reduction in α-catenin has been correlated with poor prognosis in some tumour types.

The recent finding that the adenomatous polyposis coli gene product associates with and binds to β-catenin[12] indicates that these intracellular linkage proteins may have a wider role in malignancy than simply serving as connectors between the cadherins and the internal actin cytoskeleton. Thus, in a recent series of reports, it has been shown that β-catenin binds to the DNA binding proteins of the T-cell factor-lymphoid enhancer family. In normal cells the adenomatous polyposis coli protein, in concert with glycogen synthase kinase, binds and regulates levels of free β-catenin by controlling the rate of degradation.[13],[14] However, in adenomatous polyposis coli-mutant cells the levels of β-catenin rise and, because this increase in β-catenin leads to a stable β-catenin–T-cell factor-lymphoid enhancer family complex, constitutively activate gene expression.[15] Some of the genes which are expressed as a consequence of these events are involved in inhibiting apoptosis or stimulating cellular proliferation; events likely to be of major significance in tumour development. Mutations in β-catenin can also activate this signalling pathway, so that the catenins may even act as oncogenes in terms of their capacity for determining unregulated cell growth. Such findings indicate that categorization of molecules into either the adhesive or the proliferative pathways is not always clear-cut, whereas the dysregulation of cell growth may be associated closely with alterations in normal adhesive/cohesive behaviour.

Integrins

The integrin family of cell surface receptors also plays a major part in a variety of different cellular functions. These activities include cell adhesion, migration during embryogenesis, thrombosis, and lymphocyte regulation.[16] Generally, this family of receptors mediates adhesion between cells and the extracellular matrix, although various members are involved in cell–cell interactions, mediated by binding to other cell adhesion molecules (**CAMs**) of the immunoglobulin superfamily.

The integrins are heterodimeric glycoproteins composed of α and β subunits which are non-covalently associated. Currently there are eight known β subunits and at least 14 α subunits which together are capable of generating an heterogeneous family of over 20 heterodimers. The precise combination of α and β subunits is responsible for ligand specificity. While, initially, it was thought that integrins functioned simply to link the cells to the various ligands it has become clear that these receptors serve as transducing molecules capable of influencing functions as diverse as migration, differentiation, and apoptosis through the generation of intracellular signals (see Chapter 1.4). Conversely, the integrin-expressing cell is able to activate or inactivate these molecules thus allowing rapid modulation and control of adhesive and de-adhesive activity.

Evidence for a major role for integrins in regulating the metastatic process comes from a range of experimental and clinical analyses,

but was inherent in Liotta's original description of the three steps necessary for the interaction of the invasive tumour cell with the basement membrane; i.e. attachment, matrix dissolution, and migration.[17] Immunohistochemistry of normal and malignant tissues has revealed differences in integrin expression levels associated with tumour development. While there is considerable heterogeneity in epithelial tumours with regard to the exact patterns of integrin expression it is clear that there are some consistent changes within different tumour types. Thus a reduction in the distribution of laminin and collagen receptors is a frequent observation in breast, pancreas, and lung cancers. Presumably the loss of attachment to the underlying basement membrane, which is composed largely of laminin and type IV collagen, associated with this downregulation may be important for facilitating tumour development. More intriguingly Natali *et al.*[18] have observed that normal levels of expression of the α6β4 laminin receptor may re-occur in breast cancer metastases in the lymph node even though the primary tumour expresses low levels. These observations, reminiscent of those already described for E-cadherin, suggest that processes such as clonal selection or host-dependent tissue-modulated changes in integrin expression may be occurring. Either there is an increased arrest or proliferation of a specific subset of integrin-expressing cells in the lymph nodes or, perhaps by mechanisms such as promoter methylation and de-methylation, there is local regulation of integrin expression.

The general downregulation of integrin levels with increasing malignancy which is observed in carcinomas is not a feature exhibited by all tumour types. Thus melanoma manifests a general upregulation of integrin expression as the tumours progress from the radial to the vertical growth phase and as metastatic disease develops.[19]

While integrins serve pre-eminently as cell–substrate adhesion molecules they may function also as cell–cell adhesion molecules and they then recognize members of the immunoglobulin superfamily. It is of interest then that α4β1, which serves to mediate leucocyte binding to V-CAM-1 (an inducible member of the immunoglobulin superfamily expressed on the surface of activated endothelium), has been found to be expressed at a higher level in more malignant, compared with more benign, melanomas. As α4β1/V-CAM-1 interactions are important in determining extravasation of leucocytes at sites of inflammation it is tempting to speculate that expression of α4β1 on melanoma cells is contributing to a similar type of behaviour during tumour spread (see Fig. 3).

Experimental studies examining the effect of overexpressing different integrin subunits in various recipient tumour cells have revealed a similar degree of complexity. Thus transfection of transformed Chinese hamster ovary cells with the fibronectin receptor, α5β1, reduced the migration and the proliferation rate of these cells to such an extent that they were rendered non-tumorigenic. Similarly the re-expression of α2β1 in a poorly differentiated mammary carcinoma caused the cells to revert to a more differentiated non-tumorigenic phenotype. These experimental data are consistent with the frequent downregulation of integrin expression observed in a variety of epithelial cancers. However, there are conflicting data which indicate that integrin–extracellular matrix interactions are a necessary component of metastasis formation and that increased malignancy may also be associated with increased integrin activity. Synthetic peptides corresponding to the integrin binding sites of extracellular matrix proteins blocked

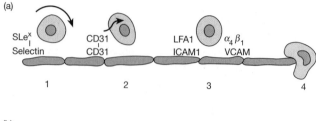

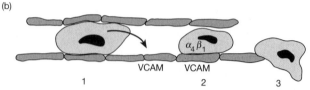

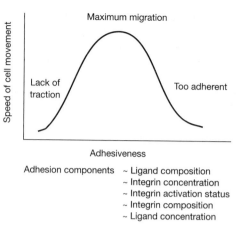

Fig. 3 Comparison of leucocyte arrest and extravasation with tumour cell (melanoma) arrest and extravasation. (a) Leucocyte: (1) inflammatory cytokines have induced endothelial cell adhesion molecules which interact with sialylated Lewis X antigens to initiate the rolling phenomenon; (2) CD31-mediated interactions trigger signals which activate integrins (conformational changes); (3) strong adhesion results from interaction between activated α4β1 integrin and cytokine-induced V-CAM; (4) transendothelial migration of leucocytes is induced. (b) Melanoma cell: (1) ectopic production of cytokines by tumour cell produces increased activation of endothelium with upregulation of V-CAM—this process is facilitated by the close interaction of a large neoplastic cell with a similar diameter capillary; (2) strong adhesion results from interaction between α4β1, which is in the constitutively active state when expressed by tumour cells, and V-CAM; (3) transendothelial migration of the melanoma cell is induced.

Fig. 4 Regulating events involved in controlling cellular migration. The rate of cell migration is a consequence of variation in adhesiveness; too 'sticky' and there is no movement, lack of 'stickiness' means lack of traction and there is no movement. Degree of adhesiveness which will relate to maximum migration is regulated by a number of cellular (integrin composition, concentration, and activation status) and host (ligand composition, ligand concentration) factors.

invasion *in vitro* of human melanoma lines. Moreover the decreased formation of lung tumour nodules in mice when such peptides (Arginine–Glycine–Aspartic acid or R-G-D) were co-injected with the tumour cells showed unequivocally that these receptors are involved in the localization of disseminating cancer cells.[20]

There is then an apparent paradox. In some human tumours the integrins appear to be downregulated in the later, more malignant stages whereas in other tumours, such as melanoma, there seems to be a requirement for the increased expression of these molecules in order for metastatic spread to occur. This paradox might be explained partially by our current understanding of the way that the third component of tumour cell invasion, i.e. migration, is regulated. This is dependent on interactions between a number of variables, including substrate and ligand density, the level of integrin expression and, perhaps most importantly, the ligand binding affinity or activation status of the integrin molecule (Fig. 4 and reference 21). These various parameters have a profound influence upon the behaviour of different tumour types while there also will be variation of their effects at different anatomical locations. For example, the nature of the substrate may vary from site to site while integrin expression level and activation state may be modulated by local cytokine concentrations. The complexity of these interactions indicates that immunohistochemical studies alone are unlikely to be totally informative about the functional activity and status of these molecules and may indicate why conflicting interpretations have been reported.

Immunoglobulin superfamily adhesion molecules

Members of the immunoglobulin superfamily of adhesion receptors contain one or more immunoglobulin-like domains. These molecules are involved both in homophilic and heterophilic interactions with a variety of ligands and play a major part in regulating embryonic neural development, wound healing, and inflammation. Particularly, these molecules play a major part in the process of leucocyte interaction with the endothelial wall thus determining the process of extravasation (Fig. 3). During an inflammatory reaction cytokines, such as tumour necrosis factor-α and interleukin-1, induce the expression of immunoglobulin superfamily members including I-CAM-1, I-CAM-2, V-CAM, and P-CAM on the endothelial wall. Here they interact with the integrins expressed on the leucocyte surface causing the cells to arrest following the selectin-induced rolling phenomenon (see Fig. 3). It has been argued that this physiological process provides a paradigm for the way in which haematogenous metastasis can occur. It is of interest therefore that tumour cells have been shown to produce and secrete cytokines capable of inducing CAMs on endothelial cells and, by doing so, stimulating tumour cell–endothelial cell adherence.[22] Equally, as I-CAM 1 has been characterized as a marker of progression in malignant melanomas and as it binds to the β2 integrins expressed on circulating leucocytes,[23] it is conceivable that an indirect interaction with leucocytes thus forming a large heterotypic cell clump may mediate adherence of the tumour cell to the endothelium (Fig. 1).

Selectins

Members of the selectin family initially were identified on platelets, leucocytes, and endothelium (P-, L-, and E-selectin respectively). The calcium-dependent lectin-like domain is situated at the distal end of the extracellular domain. This binds to the carbohydrate ligands sialylated Lewis^X and sialylated Lewis^A antigens, which are expressed on neutrophils and monocytes. During inflammation selectin expression is induced by cytokines and the low-affinity binding between these long molecules and the Lewis^X or Lewis^A antigens initiates leucocyte binding by 'tethering' and then stimulation of the rolling phenomenon; a process which is followed by arrest and extravasation mediated by integrin/immunoglobulin superfamily interactions. Again this process may serve as a paradigm for the mechanisms involved in tumour dissemination. Sialylated Lewis^X has been found to be expressed at the cell surface by carcinoma cells where it enables them to bind to activated endothelium. In colorectal cancer the increased expression of sialylated Lewis^X has been correlated with clinical stage and metastatic potential. These findings are consistent with the concept of circulating tumour cells behaving in an analogous fashion to circulating leucocytes. However, as illustrated in Fig. 3, there may be substantial differences between the behaviour of leucocytes undergoing laminar flow in vessels whose diameter is substantially greater than their own and the behaviour of large neoplastic cells, or emboli, forcing their way through vessels whose diameter is smaller than the dimensions of the deformable tumour cell. As cytokine release and stress or shear interactions with the endothelium may stimulate integrin–CAM interactions it is possible that there is no requirement for selectin-mediated arrest in tumour metastasis.

Other cell adhesion molecules

CD44, originally characterized as a lymphocyte homing receptor, is the major cell surface receptor for hyaluronate. That this molecule might play a part in determining metastatic spread was suggested by the work of Gunthert et al.[24] who showed that the metastatic proclivity of a rodent tumour was associated with expression of a specific CD44 isoform. A major way of generating different CD44 isoforms has been through regulated use of the complex gene which codes for this protein. The human gene has 20 exons, 10 of which are expressed by all cell types as the standard form (CD44s) and 10 of which are variably expressed to give rise to a number of variant forms (CD44v). The availability of antibodies to the products of the various exons of CD44 has led to a number of immunohistochemical studies of clinical material where, in general, this association between increased malignancy and variant exon usage, has been confirmed, although there still is debate over the general validity of these findings.

Mechanisms of tumour invasion

Two of the five general steps outlined in the Introduction as being involved in the pathogenesis of tumour spread depend upon the ability of the tumour cells to invade or infiltrate into areas of normal tissue. However, there is a third component of the invasive process apart from adherence and motility and that is tissue dissolution. There is evidence that tissue breakdown associated with tumour spread can result both from mechanical pressure and from the release of lytic enzymes.

Much tissue destruction may arise from the rapid proliferation of neoplastic cells leading to a build-up of pressure which results in sheets, or fingers, of tumour cells being forced along the lines of least mechanical resistance. Pressure from the growing mass also can occlude blood vessels leading to local tissue death as a consequence of anoxia. While in many instances the morphological appearance of malignant tumours conforms with this picture of root-like invasive

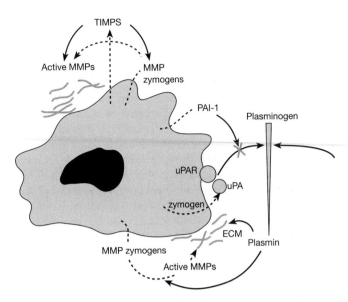

Fig. 5 Protease regulation in tumour cells. The production of inactive zymogens (pro-MMPs and pro-uPA) which require activation in the vicinity of the cell surface is counterbalanced by the production of inhibitors (e.g. TIMPs and PAI-1 and PAI-2).

growth there are also many observations that cannot be explained solely by this mechanism. There are numerous reports suggesting that the degradative activities of proteolytic enzymes, increase the invasiveness of cancers. There are three main families of proteases, categorized by the amino acid at their active site, thought to play a substantial part in tumour malignancy.

(1) The serine proteinases.

(2) The matrix metalloproteinases (**MMPs**).

(3) The aspartyl proteinases.

Regulation of enzyme activity is complex; a function not only of the level of expression of the enzyme itself but also of the concentration of activating and inhibiting factors in the local vicinity.

Urokinase plasminogen activator and its receptor

Urokinase plasminogen activator (**uPA**) probably is the most important member of the serine proteinase family and the uPA/urokinase plasminogen activator receptor (**uPAR**) system plays a key part in many physiological processes. Now, however, there are overwhelming indications that this system has a central role in the invasive behaviour of a range of tumour types. uPA is secreted as an inactive, single chain precursor or pro-uPA, which binds to a glycosyl phosphatidylinositol-linked membrane receptor (termed uPAR). Upon binding it is cleaved to an active two chain enzyme by membrane-bound plasmin and, in this form, it catalyses the conversion of plasminogen to plasmin. The broad-spectrum protease plasmin can, in turn, degrade circulating or tissue proteins directly as well as activate a range of enzymes, predominantly of the matrix metalloproteinase family (see Fig. 5). Eventual degradative activity against extracellular matrix components is the result of a cascade phenomenon with uPA controlling many of the downstream events.

The activity of uPA is regulated by at least four inhibitors the plasminogen activator inhibitors (PAI-1, PAI-2, and PAI-3) and protease nexin 1. PAI-1 is associated with the extracellular matrix protein vitronectin, which serves as a carrier molecule, and forms a complex with receptor-bound uPA. Upon formation of the complex it is internalized, partially degraded and the uPA is re-expressed on the cell surface. The conversion of receptor-bound pro-UPA to its active form proceeds at a substantially higher rate when uPA is bound to its receptor so that a cascade of proteolysis is initiated which is focused at the cell membrane. Immunohistochemical analyses of the uPA/uPAR system have found it to be located at the invasive edge of cancers as well as in the associated stromal cells. This observation of stromal cell involvement, which is a common feature for many proteolytic enzymes (see below), suggests that there are cell–cell-mediated or diffusion-based interactions between tumour and surrounding stroma. In many cancers levels of uPA, uPAR, and PAI-1 have emerged as strong prognostic indicators. In breast cancer, for example, higher tumour levels of uPA are associated with higher relapse rate and may even be a better indicator of disease-free survival than lymph node status, tumour size, or oestrogen receptor levels.[25] The apparently counter intuitive finding that PAI-1 is upregulated in cancers with a poorer prognosis[26] may be explained by the fact that, apart from inhibiting plasminogen activator activity, this molecule also plays a major part in stimulating the adhesive and migratory behaviour of tumour cells. Thus the contribution of this enzyme system to invasive and metastatic behaviour may not be attributable solely to a degradative capacity.

Matrix metalloproteinases

MMPs constitute a diverse family of zinc-dependent endopeptidases with a broad spectrum of activity. Originally, these enzymes were thought to be secreted only as inert molecules, maintained in the latent state by a distinctive PRCGVPD sequence in the pro-domain (letters represent individual amino acids), which upon activation, frequently by plasmin, are capable of degrading extracellular matrix and basement membrane components under physiologic conditions.[27] The family members also share a catalytic domain, containing the HEXGH motif, which is responsible for ligating the zinc required for catalytic function. Based upon their substrate specificity the secreted MMPs can be placed into different groupings. Thus, the collagenases are capable of degrading fibrillar collagen, the stromelysins exhibit a preference for proteoglycans and glycoproteins as substrates while the gelatinases, preferentially degrade non-fibrillar collagens and denatured collagens (gelatins).

More recently a group of transmembrane enzymes, the so-called membrane-type or MT-MMPs, have been described[28] and their major activity seems to relate to the cleavage, and hence activation, of Gelatinase A (MMP-2). Again, like the uPA/uPAR system, this spatial restriction of degradative activity appears to be important for localization of enzymatic function to the immediate vicinity of the invasive tumour cell.

While expression of the MMPs, in vitro, and presumably in vivo, can be modulated by a variety of growth factors and cytokines they also are regulated by activation (via plasmin for example) and such regulatory influences are likely to be anatomically dependent. Once

the MMPs are in their active form they are more susceptible to inhibition. This is not only by the general serum proteinase inhibitor, α_2-macroglobulin but also by a family of specific inhibitors termed tissue inhibitors of metalloproteinases (TIMPs).[29] Currently, four members (TIMP-1, -2, -3, and -4) of this family are known and these proteins, while all having in common the capacity to inhibit active MMPs, vary in terms of their tissue distribution and capacity to associate with latent MMPs.[27] During normal physiological processes MMP enzyme activity is regulated whereas during malignant disease regulation is disrupted such that there generally are increasing levels and numbers of MMPs associated with increasing tumour progression.[27]

Perhaps the most intensively investigated of these enzymes, with regard to involvement in metastasis, have been MMP-2 and MMP-9, or the gelatinases.[30] They are capable of degrading type IV collagen, a major structural component of the basement membrane, and this activity must be an essential component of the transition from carcinoma in situ to carcinoma where there is penetration of the basement membrane. The passage of disseminating cells into and out of small blood vessels must also involve penetration of the basement membrane and presumably relies on the involvement of these enzymes. Correlations between gelatinase expression and metastatic activity have been known for almost 20 years (see papers cited in reference 30). However, with the advent of in situ hybridization, it has become apparent that the source of these enzymes, and indeed of other protease groups, need not be the transformed cells themselves. Rather, adjacent normal stromal cells, presumably under the influence of the neoplastic cells, are the source of these enzymes, which may then be sequestered at the tumour cell surface or at the tumour focus–stromal cell interface.[31],[32]

The possibility of using synthetic inhibitors, which bind to the catalytic site of MMPs and thereby inhibit their activity, currently is under evaluation in clinical trials of agents such as Batimastat and Marimastat.[33] The invasive behaviour of endothelial cells, an essential component of angiogenesis, also is dependent on the activity of these enzymes[30] so that the therapeutic target for these drugs may also include tumour neovascularization (see Chapter 1.7).

Cathepsin D

Cathepsin D is a member of the aspartic proteinases which, has been shown to be an important prognostic factor in breast cancer.[34] This lysosomally located enzyme has little or no activity at or above pH 7.0 but breast cancer cell lines secrete high levels of the pro-form and in the acidic milieu of many tumours, such secretion might allow activity to contribute to the proteolytic cascade by facilitating activation of other proteinases. Even more intriguing is the possibility that, by modifying growth factors and their binding proteins, the major contribution of cathepsin D to tumour behaviour is by facilitating growth rather than invasive activity.[34]

Dissemination of tumour cells via lymphatics and blood vessels

Tumour cells may spread via lymphatics and blood vessels and there are numerous connections between the two systems such that disseminating tumour cells can move freely between them. It is well known, both from clinical observations and from experimental studies, that the mere presence of neoplastic cells in the circulation need not predict establishment of metastases. None the less with increasingly sophisticated techniques, such as reverse transcription–polymerase chain reaction and immunocytochemistry being utilized to quantitate the presence of residual disease[35] it is clear that the greater the number of disseminating cells in the circulation or bone marrow then the more likely it is that metastasis will occur eventually. The circulation is hostile to disseminating tumour cells and metastasis is an inefficient process (see below). However, some of the cellular interactions which do occur within the circulation may facilitate survival rather than induce cell death. For example, aggregation with other tumour cells, or with host cells such as lymphocytes and platelets, may result in the formation of larger cellular emboli which are more readily trapped in distant capillary beds. Presumably the cells in the interior of such emboli can better resist the turbulence and other traumatic effects of the circulation.

It is known that certain tumours frequently metastasize preferentially to specific organs.[36] Two contrasting hypotheses have been proposed to explain this selectivity. In the first the eventual site of metastatic development is considered to be a consequence of the anatomical location of the primary tumour. The number of viable tumour cells delivered to the first capillary bed encountered is the determining fact and this is a consequence of the draining lymphatic and vascular patterns of the primary tumour site. This mechanism undoubtedly is true for many tumours (hepatic metastases from colorectal cancer, for example) but does not explain all patterns of metastatic spread. For example, the kidney receives up to 25 per cent of cardiac output and yet this organ is involved infrequently in secondary tumour formation. Equally the tendency for breast carcinoma metastases to occur preferentially in the long bones can hardly be explained on the basis of draining vascular patterns. The work of Tarin *et al.*[37] who recorded autopsy findings on patients with inoperable carcinoma where peritoneovenous shunts were used to relieve abdominal pain from malignant ascites, has been important in a re-evaluation of this concept of anatomical location as the major cause of organ metastasis. While numerous viable, and presumably metastatically competent, cells were infused into the circulation via these shunts the post mortems revealed that the first organ capillary bed encountered was not necessarily the organ colonized by metastatic tumours.[37]

The original concept of Paget, that the fertile environment of the organ (the 'soil') allowed the compatible tumour cells (the 'seed') to grow, nowadays is supported by the known role that autocrine and paracrine factors play in the regulation of tumour cell proliferation. The observed differences in patterns of metastatic spread is, according to this hypothesis, a result of variations in growth stimulation or growth repression. Such variations might well reflect differences in local concentrations of these growth factors.

The third possible mechanism for determining patterns of organ-specific involvement rests upon the selective arrest and retention of metastatic cells as a consequence of specific ligand–receptor interactions. Such a selective process occurs in lymphocyte recirculation, a phenomenon which is analogous in many respects to tumour dissemination. Pasqualini and Rusolahti[38] have used the clever technique of *in vivo* delivery of Phage Display Libraries, to show that molecular variations occur which could regulate the specific trapping of tumour cells. Repeated *in vivo* selection of organ-homing phage was used to isolate recognition sequences for organ-specific address molecules on the luminal surfaces of endothelial cells.[38] The basis

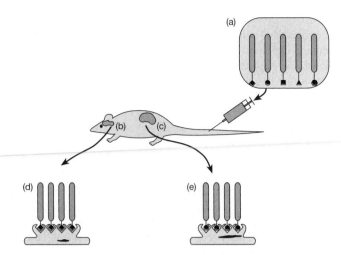

Fig. 6 *In vivo* organ targeting using phage display peptide libraries. Phage libraries where peptide sequences are displayed on the exterior surface of the phage virion (a) are injected intravenously into recipient mice. At times thereafter organs such as brain (b) or kidney (c) were removed, phage were recovered, amplified *in vitro* and re-injected to obtain enrichment. Sequencing of the inserts from organ-colonizing phage revealed dominant amino acid sequence motifs responsible for localizing to brain endothelium (d) or kidney epithelium (e). As the peptide sequences expressed by these phage are different the molecules which bind them must be different; the first indication of selective endothelial markers which could be important in organ-specific tumour metastasis.

of this approach is outlined in Fig. 6. The results showed unequivocally that there is molecular heterogeneity of the vascular endothelium and these molecular determinants are likely to play a part in organ-specific tumour spread. In subsequent experiments this approach has allowed the isolation of peptides which home specifically to tumour blood vessels and offers hope for the targeting of anticancer drugs specifically to the tumour vasculature.[39],[40]

The role of the immune system in metastasis

Any influence of the immune system on cancer growth is both subtle and complex (see Chapter 1.9). The existence of potentially immunogenic material, in the form of the primary tumour mass, might be expected to prime the host and to be effective in facilitating the elimination of small clumps of circulating cancer cells. Paradoxically however, the immune system appears not always to act so as to limit metastatic spread. Lymphocyte-tumour cell aggregation has been shown experimentally to increase the size of emboli and thus to increase the non-specific entrapment of neoplastic cells with a resultant increase in metastatic tumour burden. Moreover many of the white blood cells, such as leucocytes and monocytes, are the source of potent angiogenic factors necessary for the induction of tumour vascularization (see Chapter 1.7). Thus once arrest has occurred, or even when tumour cells are established in secondary organs, an immune response could have the undesirable effect of stimulating neovascularization and thereby stimulating cancer growth. These stimulatory effects may be deemed not to be the consequence of a specific immune response but simply represent the consequences of attributes of immune system cells. However, the role of specific immune responses on metastatic outcome remains uncertain even though the implicit assumption behind immunotherapy (Chapter 1.10) is that they must be for the patients' benefit.

The capacity of cytotoxic T lymphocytes to recognize foreign antigens only in the context of major histocompatibility class (**MHC**) I cell surface antigens means that the lack of MHC antigens or the lack of antigen processing in disseminating tumour cells may facilitate the evasion of a T-cell-based immune response. Thus, for example, downregulation of class 1 antigens as a consequence of the loss of the transporter associated with antigen processing (**TAP1** and **TAP2**) has been reported in a large percentage of high-grade breast carcinomas.[41] Equally, in malignant melanoma, it may be that mutations in the β_2-microgloblulin gene are responsible for the lack of class 1 gene expression at the tumour cell surface.[42]

It has been proposed that natural killer (**NK**) cells, in direct contrast to T lymphocytes, recognize the absence rather than the presence of class 1 antigens at the tumour cell surface.[43] Accordingly tumour cells which serve as the target for NK cell-mediated cytotoxicity are characterized by the absence or reduced expression of class 1 antigens.[44] An important subset of NK cells, so-called A-NK cells, are able to enter solid tissues and migrate to sites of metastasis where they are able to eradicate malignant cells.[45],[46] It would seem probable from these results therefore that, if the absence of class 1 molecules is a central feature in determining NK cytoxicity, increased HLA expression should occur during tumour progression.[47] Such a possibility seems at odds with studies showing that more malignant tumours have a reduction in class 1 antigen expression.[41],[42],[48] It may be that the failure to assay separately the products of individual loci within the MHC obscures these associations. Thus non-classical MHC encoded class 1 molecules HLA-E, HLA-F, and HLA-G (which are characterized by their low levels of expression and very limited polymorphism), may have different functional characteristics compared with the highly polymorphic classical class 1 molecules HLA-A, HLA-B, and HLA-C. The non-classical HLA-G product, for example, inhibits NK cell activity and is expressed aberrantly by malignant melanoma cells where it appears to serve as a means of escaping from immunosurveillance.[49] Equally it has been shown recently that HLA-E is the ligand for inhibitory CD94/NKG2A receptors on NK cells[50]; expression of this molecule at the cell surface will prevent NK lysis from occurring. Failure to monitor individually for these various products at the surface of tumour cells may provide an incomplete view of the likely relative sensitivity or resistance of such cells to the different effector cells of the immune system.

Equally the induction, suppression, or abrogation of MHC class I gene expression in progressed cancers is not the only means whereby metastasizing tumour cells can evade any putative immune surveillance mechanism. The requirement for co-stimulatory molecules to permit efficient cytotoxicity means that a variety of surface proteins must be expressed, both on the lymphocytes and on the target tumour cell, for T-cell killing to occur. The absence of such co-stimulatory molecules on the cell surface of metastasizing cancer cells represents a means whereby malignant neoplasms can evade the consequences of immune responses and much interest centres upon the possibility of reintroducing such target molecules into tumour cells in order to stimulate an effective immune response.

Complicating the issue considerably is the fact that the majority of direct investigations into the modulatory effect of the immune system on tumour spread have, of necessity, utilized rodent tumour lines. The relevance of these systems to the human situation has been questioned and it seems likely that any comparable effects in humans are likely to be far more subtle.

Tumour latency/dormancy

In many cancers, such as melanoma and breast carcinoma, a frequent clinical observation is that removal of the primary tumour is followed, often after an intervening period of several years or even decades, by the recurrence of overt neoplasia. It is presumed that malignant cells shed from the primary tumour mass must have remained dormant, although viable, throughout this period of time and that their gross appearance at this later date somehow represents the consequence of a shift in the balance between host and tumour.

It has been noted in certain animal models that the removal of the primary tumour, usually by surgery, may be accompanied by a sudden burst of metastatic development.[52] (See also Chapter 1.7.)

Although these two phenomena are not necessarily related they do share the fact that the ability of neoplastic cells to emerge from a dormant or latent state can have profound effects on metastatic behaviour. Working on this metastatic burst, induced by removal of the primary, Folkman's group[51]–[53] has suggested that the apparent suppressive effect of the primary tumour upon secondary tumour growth could be attributable to the production of an angiogenesis inhibitor.[52] This hypothesis was borne out by the purification of a circulating angiogenesis inhibitor, termed angiostatin, in the serum and urine of tumour-bearing mice.[52] Angiostatin, which is a 38-kDa fragment of plasminogen, appears to be one of a variety of natural cleavage products capable of exerting an anti-angiogenic effect (many of which are produced by enzymes involved in initiating the angiogenic response) and it may be that this is part of a general feedback mechanism to regulate neovascularization.[53] Clearly the sudden lack of any angiogenesis-suppressing agent, as a consequence of removal of the primary tumour for example, might cause a rapid burst in the growth of secondary tumours resulting from the rapid development of a new blood supply.

Gradual alterations in neovascularization might also account for the more clinically important phenomenon of true dormancy or latency. It has been observed, in experimental models, that it is the failure of solitary cells to initiate growth after extravasation and the failure of early micrometastatic deposits to continue growth into macroscopic foci which is the principal cause of metastatic inefficiency.[54] Disseminated foci therefore need to continue their growth beyond microscopic size and this could well implicate vascular development as the limiting factor. A recent report[55] has suggested that increased levels of specific hormones, such as occur physiologically with increasing age, might influence tumour development not through induced cellular proliferation but via the induction of a neovascular response. Thus Schiffenbauer and colleagues[55] reported that elevated levels of the gonadotrophins luteinizing hormone and follicle-stimulating hormone elevated the secretion of the angiogenic factor vascular endothelial growth factor. This elevated vascular endothelial growth factor secretion promoted the growth of ovarian carcinoma via induction of an angiogenic response, suggesting that hormonal therapy aimed at lowering circulating levels of gonadotrophins could

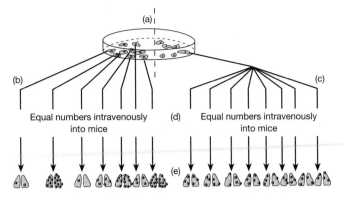

Fig. 7 Pre-existence of metastatic subpopulations within the parental cell population. Based on the experiment of Fidler and Kripke.[56] A culture of B16 murine melanoma cells (a) was split into two aliquots (b) and (c). One aliquot (b) was used to derive clonal lines from single cells while the other aliquot (c) was subdivided into further aliquots of multicellular origin. Either single-cell-derived clones or multi-cell-derived aliquots were adjusted to appropriate concentrations of cells and injected intravenously into the tail veins of recipient mice (10 animals per group). At a set time after injection animals were killed, lungs were removed and the number of lung tumour nodules was counted. While the various groups of mice injected with the multi-cell derived lines all had very similar levels of pulmonary tumour burden the various clones (established from single cells) showed marked and highly significant variability. Thus some clones gave rise to only a few lung nodules whereas other clones gave tremendous (100-fold) numbers of lung tumours for the input of similar cell numbers. Subcloning experiments showed that the clones initially bred true indicating that this was a genetically determined effect. The interpretation of this modified Luria-Delbruck fluctuation analysis was that subpopulations of tumour cells with high metastatic proclivity pre-existed within the parental population. This experiment has served as the major basis for attempting to identify genes whose expression may modulate metastatic spread.

Table 1 Metastasis-associated genes identified from comparison of metastatic and non-metastatic populations

Gene identified	Protein/function/homology
Decreased expression in metastatic population	
cystatin B	cysteine proteinase inhibitors
cystatin M	
KiSS-1	SH3 binding domain-signal transduction
Maspin	serine proteinase inhibitor
MRP1	motility related protein involved in cell migration
nm23	NDP kinase signal transduction
Increased expression in metastatic population	
Calcyclin	Calcium-binding protein
Caveolin-1	Membrane protein; involved in cholesterol influx/efflux
M-sema H	Semaphorin-chemorepellent
mts-1	Calcium-binding protein
Osteopontin	Bone sialoprotein. Adhesive glycoprotein
Stromelysin (transin)	Matrix metalloproteinase
Stromelysin-3	Matrix metalloproteinase

Source: modified from Chambers and Hill.

prolong remissions, in ovarian cancer at least, by extending tumour dormancy.[55]

Experimental models and approaches to metastasis

Perhaps the seminal experiment in metastasis research, and the one which has given rise to most studies aimed at identifying the genes involved in metastasis, was that of Fidler and Kripke.[56] These workers demonstrated that a subpopulation of metastatic cells pre-existed within the parental population (Fig. 7). Application of the correct selection pressure allowed the isolation of these pre-existent variant cells and facilitated the search for metastasis-associated genes by allowing the comparison of cells with different levels of metastatic activity but the same genetic background.

This experiment has not proven to be repeatable in all rodent tumour systems, perhaps as a consequence of instability in clonal behaviour, and this caused some controversy immediately after the initial publication. However, this study acted as a catalyst for efforts aimed at identifying and isolating genes controlling metastatic behaviour. Some of these genes are listed in Table 1 which is modified from an excellent review on mechanisms of metastasis.[57] Interestingly though, the results from these studies have confirmed the validity of the original conclusions drawn by Fidler and Kripke.[56] Thus nm23,

which has homology with the awd (abnormal wing disc) gene in *Drosophila* and which encodes for a nucleoside diphosphate kinase, originally was obtained by screening cDNA libraries from high metastatic and low metastatic subpopulations of a murine melanoma cell line.[58] However, quantitation of nm23 mRNA from human samples also revealed that there was a comparable downregulation of expression in the more advanced/progressed cancers.[59]

Equally caveolin-1 was isolated by differential display-polymerase chain reaction (DD) from genetically matched primary tumour- and metastasis-derived mouse prostate cancer cell lines.[60] Immunohistochemical analysis of protein expression revealed minimal caveolin expression in normal prostate epithelium, an increase in prostate cancer and a marked accumulation of positive staining in lymph node metastatic deposits.[60]

These results show that the utilization of rodent model systems, based on matched cell lines, can give rise to the identification of genes which are involved in human tumour progression and metastatic spread.

The major caveat about such an approach, based upon pure populations of cultured neoplastic cells, is that it ignores the contribution of normal host cells to the metastatic process. Stromelysin-3, a member of the MMP family (Table 1), was identified using subtractive hybridization of cDNA libraries prepared from invasive breast cancer or benign fibroadenoma.[31] Intriguingly, it was found that this gene was expressed not by the neoplastic cells themselves but by normal stromal fibroblasts in juxtaposition to the transformed cells.[31],[61] Utilization of cell lines, as distinct from whole tissue, would not have permitted identification of this important change in gene expression associated with metastatic activity.[31],[61] With the development of ever-more powerful techniques of gene expression analysis, such as DD or serial analysis of gene expression and the utilization of 'chip' technology,[62],[63] it is clear there will be a burgeoning of similar 'metastasis' genes in future years. What will be important to remember in both their isolation and their characterization is that such genes must influence tumour behaviour within the context of a responding host and that metastatic outcome is dependent upon a series of sequential interactions.

References

1. Weidner N, Semple JP, Welch WR, Folkman J. Tumor angiogenesis and metastasis-correlation in invasive breast carcinoma. *New England Journal of Medicine*, 1991; **324**: 1–8.

2. Ellis LM, Walker RA, Gasparini G. Is determination of angiogeneic activity in human tumours clinically useful? *European Journal of Cancer*, 1998; **34**: 609–18.

3. Brown JM, Giaccia AJ. The unique physiology of solid tumors. Opportunities (and problems) for cancer therapy. *Cancer Research*, 1998 **58**: 1408–16.

4. Shimazui T, *et al.* Prognostic value of cadherin-associated molecules (alpha-, beta-, and gamma-catenins and p120cas) in bladder tumors. *Cancer Research*, 1996; **56**: 4154–8.

5. Behrens J, Mareel M, Van Roy FM, Birchmeier W. Dissecting tumor cell invasion: epithelial cells acquire invasive properties after the loss of uvomorulin-mediated cell-cell adhesion. *Journal of Cell Biology*, 1989; **108**: 2435–47.

6. Chen H, Paradies NE, Fedor-Chaiken M, Brackenbury R. E-cadherin mediates adhesion and suppresses cell motility via distinct mechanisms. *Journal of Cell Science*, 1997; **110**: 345–56.

7. Dorudi S, Sheffield JP, Poulsom R, Northover JM, Hart IR. E-cadherin expression in colorectal cancer. An immunocytochemical and *in situ* hybridisation study. *American Journal of Pathology*, 1993; **142**: 981–6.

8. Dorudi S, Hanby AM, Poulsom R, Northover J, Hart IR. Level of expression of E-cadherin mRNA in colorectal cancer correlates with clinical outcome. *British Journal of Cancer*, 1995; **71**: 614–16.

9. Lindblom A, Rotstein S, Skoog L, Nordenskjold M, Larsson C. Deletions on chromosome 16 in primary familial breast carcinomas are associated with development of distant metastases. *Cancer Research*, 1993; **53**: 3707–11.

10. Berx G, *et al.* E-cadherin is inactivated by truncation mutations throughout its extracellular domain. *Oncogene*, 1996; **13**; 1919–25.

11. Hiraguri S, *et al.* Mechanisms of inactivation of E-cadherin in breast cancer cell lines. *Cancer Research*, 1998; **58**: 1972–7.

12. Behrens J, *et al.* Functional interaction of β-catenin with the transcription factor LEF-1. *Nature*, 1996; **382**: 638–42.

13. Su LK, Vogelstein B, Kinzler KW. Association of the APC tumor suppressor protein with catenins. *Science*, 1993; **262**: 1734–7.

14. Morin PJ, *et al.* Activation of β-catenin-Tcf signaling in colon cancer by mutations in β-catenin or APC. *Science*, 1997; **275**: 1787–90.

15. Korinek V, *et al.* Constitutive transcriptional activation by a β-catenin-Tcf complex in APC−/− colon carcinoma. *Science*, 1997; **275**: 1784–7.

16. Hynes RO. Integrins: versatility, modulation, and cell adhesion. *Cell*, 1992; **69**: 11–25.

17. Liotta LA, Rao CN, Barsky SH. Tumor invasion and the extracellular matrix. *Laboratory Investigation*, 1983; **49**: 636–49.

18. Natali PG, Nicotra MR, Botti C, Mottolese M, Bigotti A, Segattoo O. Changes in expression of alpha 6 beta 4 integrin heterodimer in primary and metastatic breast cancer. *British Journal of Cancer*, 1992; **66**: 318–22.

19. Marshall JF, Hart IR. The role of αv integrins in tumour progression and metastasis. *Seminars in Cancer Biology*, 1996; **7**: 129–38.

20. Humphries MJ, Olden K, Yamada KM. A synthetic peptide from fibronectin inhibits experimental metastasis of murine melanoma. *Science*, 1986; **233**: 467–70.

21. Palecek SP, Loftus JC, Ginsberg MH, Lauffenberger DA, Horwitz AF. Integrin-ligand binding properties govern cell migration speed through cell-substratum adhesiveness. *Nature*, 1997; **385**: 537–30.

22. Burrows FJ, *et al.* Influence of tumor-derived interleukin 1 on melanoma-endothelial cell interactions *in vitro*. *Cancer Research*, 1991; **51**: 4768–75.

23. Hart IR. Immune profile in metastasis. *Current Opinion in Immunology*, 1989; **1**: 900–3.

24. Gunthert U, *et al.* A new variant of glycoprotein CD44 confers metastatic potential to rat carcinoma cells. *Cell*, 1991; **65**: 13–24.

25. Duffy MJ, Reilly D, O'Sullivan C, O'Higgins N, Fennelly JJ, Andreasen P. Urokinase-plasminogen activator, a new and independent prognostic marker in breast cancer. *Cancer Research*, 1990; **50**: 6827–9.

26. Duggan C, Maguire T, McDermott E, O'Higgins N, Fennelly JJ, Duffy MJ. Urokinase plasminogen activator and urokinase plasminogen activator receptor in breast cancer. *International Journal of Cancer*, 1995; **61**: 597–600.

27. Chambers AF, Matrisian LM. Changing views of the role of matrix metalloproteinases in metastasis. *Journal of the National Cancer Institute*, 1997; **89**: 1260–70.

28. Sato H, Seiki M. Membrane-type matrix metalloproteinases (MT-MMPs) in tumor metastasis. *Journal of Biochemistry*, 1996; **119**: 209–15.

29. Declerck YA, Imren S. Protease inhibitors—role and potential therapeutic use in human cancer. *European Journal of Cancer*, 1994; **30**: 2170–80.

30. Liotta LA, Steeg PS, Stetler-Stevenson WG. Cancer metastasis and angiogenesis: An imbalance of positive and negative regulation. *Cell*, 1991; **64**: 327–36.

31. Basset P, *et al.* A novel metalloproteinase gene specifically expressed in stromal cells of breast carcinomas. *Nature*, 1990; **348**: 699–704.

32. Poulsom R, *et al.* Stromal expression of 72kda type IV collagenase (MMPa-2) and TIMP-2 mRNAs in colorectal neoplasia. *American Journal of Pathology*, 1992; **141**: 389–96.

33. Talbot DC, Brown PD. Experimental and clinical studies on the use of matrix metalloproteinase inhibitors for the treatment of cancer. *European Journal of Cancer*, 1996; **32**: 2538–3.

34. Rochefort H, Liaudet E, Garcia M. Alterations and role of human cathepsin D in cancer metastasis. *Enzyme and Protein*, 1996; **49**: 106–16.

35. Braun S, Muller M, Hepp F, Schlimok G, Riethmuller G, Pantel K. Micrometastatic breast cancer cells in bone marrow at primary surgery: Prognostic value in comparison with nodal status. *Journal of the National Cancer Institute*, 1998; **90**: 1099–100.

36. Paget S. The distribution of secondary growths in cancer of the breast. *The Lancet*, 1889; **i**: 571–3.

37. Tarin D, Price JE, Kettlewell MGW, Souter RG, Vass ACR, Crossley B. Mechanisms of human-tumor metastasis studies in patients with peritoneovenous shunts. *Cancer Research*, 1984; **44**: 3584–92.

38. Pasqualini R, Rusolahti E. Organ targeting *in vivo* using phage display peptide libraries. *Nature*, 1996; **380**: 364–6.

39. Arap W, Pasqualini R, Ruoslahti E. Cancer treatment by targeted drug delivery to tumor vasculature in a mouse model. *Science*, 1998; **279**: 377–80.

40. Rajotte D, Arap W, Hagedorn M, Koivunen E, Pasqualini R, Ruoslahti E. Molecular heterogeneity of the vascular endothelium

revealed by *in vivo* phage display. *Journal of Clinical Investigation*, 1998; **102**: 430–7.

41. Vitale M, *et al.* HLA class I antigen and transporter with antigen processing (TAP1 and TAP2) down-regulation in high-grade primary breast carcinoma lesions. *Cancer Research*, 1998; **58**: 737–42.

42. Hicklin DJ, Wang ZG, Arienti F, Rivolotini L, Parmiani G, Ferrone S. beta 2-microglobulin mutations, HLA class I antigen loss, and tumor progression in melanoma *Journal of Clinical Investigation*, 1998; **101**: 2720–9.

43. Karre K, Ljunggren HG, Piontek G, Kiessling R. Selective rejection of H-2-deficient lymphoma variants suggests alternative immune defense strategy. *Nature*, 1986; **319**: 675–8.

44. Karre K. Express yourself or die—peptides, MHC molecules, and NK cells. *Science*, 1995; **267**: 978–9.

45. Whiteside TL, Herberman RB. The role of natural-killer cells in immune surveillance of cancer. *Current Opinion in Immunology*, 1995; **7**: 704–10.

46. Okada K, *et al.* Elimination of established liver metastases by human interleukin 2-activated natural killer cells after locoregional or systemic adoptive. *Cancer Research*, 1996; **56**: 1599–608.

47. Karre K. How to recognize a foreign submarine. *Immunological Reviews*, 1997; **155**: 5–9.

48. Geertsen RC, Hofbauer GFL, Yue FY, Manolio S, Burg G, Dummer R. Higher frequency of selective losses of HLA-A and -B allospecificities in metastasis than in primary melanoma lesions. *Journal of Investigative Dermatology*, 1998; **111**: 497–502.

49. Paul P, *et al.* HLA-G expression in melanoma: A way for tumor cells to escape from immunosurveillance. *Proceedings of the National Academy of Sciences of the United States of America*, 1998; **95**: 4510–15.

50. Braud V, *et al.* HLA-E binds to natural killer cell receptors CD94/ NKG2A, B and C. *Nature*, 1998; **391**: 795–9.

51. Folkman J. Angiogenesis in cancer, vascular, rheumatoid and other disease. *Nature Medicine*, 1995 **1**: 27–31.

52. O'Reilly MS, *et al.* Angiostatin: a novel angiogenesis inhibitor that mediates the suppression of metastases by a Lewis lung carcinoma. *Cell*, 1994; **79**: 315–28.

53. O'Reilly MS, *et al.* Endostatin: an endogenous inhibitor of angiogenesis and tumour growth. *Cell*, 1997; **88**: 277–85.

54. Luzzi KJ, *et al.* Multistep nature of metastatic inefficiency—Dormancy of solitary cells after successful extravastion and limited survival of early micrometastases. *American Journal of Pathology*, 1998; **153**: 865–73.

55. Schiffenbauer YS, *et al.* Loss of ovarian function promotes angiogenesis in human ovarian carcinoma. *Proceedings of the National Academy of Sciences of the United States of America*, 1997; **94**: 13202–8.

56. Fidler IJ, Kripke ML. Metastasis results from pre-existing variant cells within a malignant tumor. *Science*, 1977; **197**: 893–5.

57. Chambers AF, Hill RP. Tumor progression and metastasis. In Tannock IF, Hill RP (eds), *The basic science of oncology*, 3rd edn. McGraw-Hill, Toronto, 1998.

58. Steeg PS, *et al.* Evidence for a novel gene associated with low tumor metastatic potential. *Journal of the National Cancer Institute*, 1988; **80**: 200–4.

59. Hartsough MT, Steeg PS. Nm23-H1: Genetic alterations and expression patterns in tumor metastasis. *American Journal of Human Genetics*, 1998; **63**: 6–10.

60. Yang G, *et al.* Elevated expression of caveolin is associated with prostate and breast cancer. *Clinical Cancer Research*, 1998; **4**: 1873–80.

61. Ahmad A, *et al.* Stromelysin-3: An idependent prognostic factor for relapse-free survival in node-positive breast cancer and demonstration of novel breast carcinoma expression. *American Journal of Pathology*, 1998; **152**: 721–8.

62. Liang P, Pardee AB. Differential display of eukaryotic messenger RNA by means of the polymerase chain reaction. *Science*, 1992; **257**: 967–71.

63. Zhang L, *et al.* Gene expression profiles in normal and cancer cells. *Science*, 1997; **276**: 1268–72.

1.9 Tumour antigens

Thierry Boon and Jean-Charles Cerottini

Introduction

Animal experimentation has demonstrated that T lymphocytes constitute an essential component of specific immune responses that produce tumour rejection. Recently, our understanding of the nature of the antigens recognized by T cells has made considerable progress and it appears now that there exists an effective T-cell-mediated immune surveillance capable of monitoring the genetic integrity of mammalian cells. Tumour-specific transplantation antigens that are recognized by T cells appear to be present on most if not all mouse tumours. To evaluate the prospects of specific immunotherapy of cancer, it is important to know whether human tumour cells also express antigens that are recognized by autologous T lymphocytes. We will review the mounting evidence in favour of the existence of cytolytic T cells with specific lytic activity for autologous tumour cells.

Tumour antigens recognized by T cells

Antigen recognition by T cells

T-cell antigen receptors

Although T cells, like B cells, originate in the bone marrow, only after migration to the thymus do they acquire receptors capable of recognizing antigen. This process requires a complex series of differentiation events, including rearrangement and expression of the genes encoding the T-cell antigen receptor (**TCR**) polypeptide chains. There are four distinct TCR chains (α, β, γ, and δ) which associate to form two different transmembrane heterodimers, α/β and γ/δ.

While α/β and γ/δ TCR are expressed on different T-cell subpopulations, both molecules are associated on the cell surface with the molecular complex referred to as CD3, which consists of five different polypeptide chains. In addition to the TCR–CD3 complex, thymic differentiation of T cells includes expression of two other cell-surface glycoproteins, CD4 and CD8, which play an important role in antigen recognition by α/β TCR-bearing (**αβ+**) cells. Expression of these glycoproteins on mature αβ+ T cells is mutually exclusive, thus allowing the identification of two distinct T-cell subsets, usually referred to as CD4+ and CD8+ subsets.

Like immunoglobulin heavy and light chains, each of the TCR chains has a variable and a constant region. While all the TCR molecules expressed by a given cell are identical, there is a high degree of diversity between the TCR variable regions found on different T cells, particularly in the αβ+ subpopulation.

The set of distinct TCR produced in an individual is usually referred to as the TCR repertoire. There is evidence that the TCR repertoire of peripheral αβ+ T cells is different from the initial repertoire expressed by αβ+ T cells in the thymus. This difference appears to result from selective mechanisms that take place in the thymus whereby T cells expressing TCR that recognize self components are eliminated, whereas T cells that bear TCR recognizing foreign antigens in association with self proteins encoded within the major histocompatibility complex (**MHC**) are positively selected. Although the mechanisms underlying this series of events are still poorly understood, there is evidence for the participation of thymic non-T cells, such as macrophages and/or dendritic cells, or epithelial cells in the negative or positive selection processes, respectively. Whether similar selective mechanisms are involved in the development of γδ+ T cells is unknown.

MHC restriction

It is well established that αβ+ T cells do not bind intact antigen in solution, but recognize on the surface of other cells antigenic peptides presented in association with proteins encoded by the MHC. This phenomenon is usually referred to as MHC-restricted recognition. The MHC products involved are the so-called class I molecules (HLA A, B, and C) and class II molecules (HLA DP, DQ, and DR). Both systems are extremely polymorphic, that is, there is a large number of allelic forms for each gene product. Each class I MHC molecule is made of a polymorphic transmembrane α-chain associated with an invariant chain, β_2-microglobulin. The extracellular portion of the α-chain has three domains, whereas β_2-microglobulin consists of a single, immunoglobulin-like domain. As revealed by X-ray crystallography, the three-dimensional structure of class I MHC molecules is characterized by a groove located on the membrane-distal portion of the molecule. The sides of the groove, which are provided by two α-helices, as well as the floor are derived from the first two extracellular domains of the α-chain. Comparison of class I amino acid sequences indicates that the polymorphism of these molecules is concentrated in residues at positions lining the floor and the sides of the groove. Thus there are local structural differences between grooves of class I MHC allelic products. Because the groove is a peptide-binding site, these structural differences may have profound effects on the set of peptides that can bind to individual class I molecules. Indeed, analysis of naturally occurring peptides eluted from MHC molecules reveals a strong bias for particular amino acids at positions that play a major role in the anchoring of peptides into the binding groove. This bias is relatively specific for a given MHC allelic product and thus defines a peptide motif for a given MHC molecule.

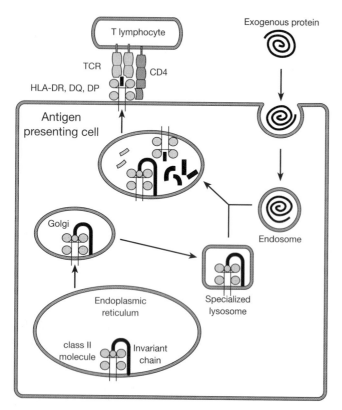

Fig. 1 T-cell recognition and antigen presentation by class II MHC molecules on antigen presenting cells.

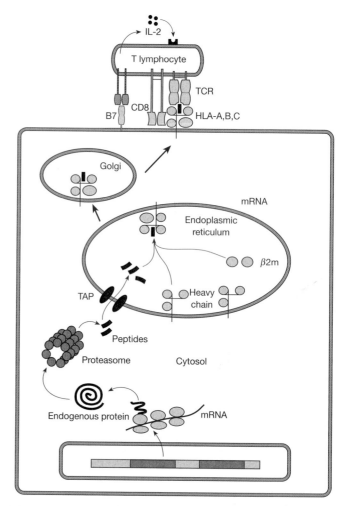

Fig. 2 T-cell recognition and antigen presentation by class I MHC molecules on target cells.

Class II MHC molecules consist of two distinct (α and β) polymorphic transmembrane chains which are non-covalently associated on the cell surface. This symmetrical arrangement contrasts with that of class I molecules. However, there is also a groove on the membrane distal portion of class II molecules to which both α- and β-chains contribute.

Although both MHC classes can present antigen to αβ+ T cells, there is a clear dichotomy in the MHC restriction exhibited by CD4+ and CD8+ subsets. CD4+ cells recognize antigen in association with class II molecules, whereas CD8+ cells recognize antigen in association with class I MHC molecules. For both CD4+ and CD8+ cells, antigen recognition by a given α/β TCR is restricted to a single peptide–MHC complex.

Antigen processing

The antigenic moieties recognized in association with class II MHC molecules are usually derived from soluble, exogenous proteins that have been captured by dendritic cells or other antigen-presenting cells. Receptor-mediated endocytosis, phagocytosis, and macropinocytosis all contribute to antigen uptake by class II MHC-expressing antigen-presenting cell. Presentation of class II-restricted antigen requires endosomal degradation of the captured protein into short peptides, followed by intracellular binding of the resulting antigenic peptides to class II molecules and transport of the peptide–MHC complexes to the cell surface (Fig. 1).[1] This series of events is usually referred to as antigen processing. Important features of the association between peptides and soluble class II MHC molecules

include selectivity (i.e. a given peptide binds to some class II molecules, but not to others) as well as diversity (i.e. a given class II MHC molecule binds a variety of peptides of diverse sequence). While selectivity results from structural differences in the peptide-binding site displayed by individual class II molecules, the observed diversity reflects the existence of a common binding motif in unrelated peptides that bind to the same class II molecule.

In contrast to class II-restricted T cells, class I-restricted T cells are usually directed against antigens that are synthesized within target cells, such as infectious virus-encoded proteins, minor histocompatibility antigens, and tumour-specific transplantation antigens. Presentation of class I-restricted antigen, like that of class II-restricted antigen, requires intracellular processing, binding of antigen-derived peptides to MHC molecules, and transport of the peptide–MHC complexes to the surface (Fig. 2).[2] Accordingly, any endogenously synthesized protein antigen, irrespective of its final destination (nucleus, cytosol, cell surface, or extracellular milieu), can potentially be presented in the form of a peptide bound to class I molecules. In addition, exogenously added synthetic peptides corresponding to linear segments of class I-restricted antigens can bind to 'empty' class I MHC molecules expressed at the cell surface and thus mimic endogenously produced antigenic determinants.

As nearly all class I-restricted T cells are cytolytic, an assay often used in studies of the antigenic peptides recognized by these cells is the lysis of appropriate target cells expressing the relevant class I molecules in the presence of exogenously added synthetic peptides. The use of synthetic peptides has revealed both diversity and selectivity in class I-restricted antigen presentation as it has for class II-restricted presentation. Antigenic peptides interact with some class I molecules, but not with others. Also, peptides from unrelated antigens have been shown to compete for binding to the same class I molecule.

The identification of common motifs which are responsible for peptide binding to a given class I molecule can be used to predict which peptides from a known protein sequence are likely to bind to a given class I MHC molecule and, hence, to be a potential source of antigenic peptides recognized by CD8 + T cells restricted to the same class I molecule.

It thus appears that the major function of both class I and class II MHC glycoproteins is to bind peptides derived from processed proteins and to display them on the cell surface. Given the extreme polymorphism of MHC molecules and the structural changes of the peptide-binding sites that are associated with this polymorphism, it is likely that the range of antigen-derived peptides that can be presented for recognition by $\alpha\beta$ + T cells will vary greatly from one individual to another. Moreover, for a given individual, recognition of particular peptide–MHC complexes will depend on the availability of $\alpha\beta$ + T cells expressing receptors capable of binding to these complexes.

Whether antigen recognition by $\gamma\delta$ + T cells is dependent on antigen processing and/or presentation by MHC products is unclear.

T-cell activation

Recognition of antigen by $\alpha\beta$ + T cells usually results in a complex process, usually referred to as activation, which eventually leads to cell division and acquisition of effector functions such as cytotoxicity and production of lymphokines. The TCR–CD3 molecular complex on the surface of T cells plays a central role in the initiation of this process, first by binding the relevant peptide–MHC complex displayed on the surface of antigen-presenting cell, and second by converting this event into a transmembrane signal which triggers intracellular activation events. In addition to the TCR–CD3 complex, other cell-surface glycoproteins contribute to the binding of T cells to antigen-presenting cells and/or to the transduction of activating signals. In particular, CD4 and CD8 molecules have been shown to bind to constant regions of class II and class I molecules, respectively. It has therefore been proposed that these two glycoproteins enhance the avidity with which CD4 + or CD8 + T cells interact with antigen-presenting cells. Other proteins involved in interactions of T cells with antigen-presenting cells include the so-called lymphocyte function associated antigen 1 (**LFA-1**) on T cells and its ligands, intercellular adhesion molecule 1 (**ICAM-1**) or ICAM-2 on antigen-presenting cells, as well as the CD2 protein and its ligand LFA-3. These interactions clearly play an important role in cell–cell adhesion, but it is conceivable that they also function in signal transduction. Indeed, there is evidence that at least two distinct signals are required for T-cell activation. The first signal originates from the interaction of the TCR–CD3 complex with its ligand, whereas the second signal may be provided by the interaction of costimulatory receptors and their ligands. One of the most important costimulatory receptors on T cells appears to be the CD28 molecule, the ligands for which consist of at least two members of the B7 family, B7–1 and B7–2, which are expressed on antigen-presenting cells, but usually not on tumour cells.

The dynamics of antigen-specific T-cell responses is characterized by rapid clonal expansion following T-cell activation. Clonal expansion of activated T cells is initiated at least *in vitro* by the interaction of interleukin 2 (**IL-2**) and its receptor. The elucidation of the cellular events involved in T-cell proliferation has greatly facilitated the development of methods allowing continuous culture of T cells *in vitro* as well as their cloning. The most commonly used approach is based on repeated exposure of T cells to antigen-bearing cells in the presence of IL-2. As discussed below, the availability of T-cell clones that can be maintained in culture indefinitely has played an essential role in studies concerning the specificity of T cells directed against tumour-associated antigens.

Clonal expansion of T cells is accompanied by the generation of effector cells and possibly memory cells and is followed *in vivo* by a contraction of the population of antigen-specific T cells, presumably by apoptosis of the effector cells. While little information exists on the dynamics of tumour-specific T cells elicited *in vivo*, two new methods have been developed recently that allow direct enumeration of such T cells in lymphoid tissues and peripheral blood from patients with cancer before and after specific immunization.[3] The first method, called enzyme-linked immunospot (**ELISPOT**) assay, takes advantage of the local release of cytokines, such as interferon-γ, by activated and/or memory T cells upon antigen recognition. While the ELISPOT assay allows the detection and enumeration of antigen-induced, cytokine-secreting T cells, the second method can be used to enumerate antigen-specific T cells irrespective of their functional state. This method is based on direct staining of antigen-specific T cells with fluorescent tetrameric complexes of MHC class I (or class II) molecules bearing the corresponding antigenic peptides. Application of these assays to the monitoring of T-cell responses to tumour antigens is in progress and is likely to provide further insight into the correlation, or lack thereof, between defined immune responses and clinical tumour responses.

Immune surveillance against tumours

Existence of tumour-specific transplantation antigens

Rodent tumours induced by viruses such as SV40, adenoviruses, or retroviruses express viral antigens that can elicit tumour rejection and that are recognized by MHC class I-restricted cytolytic T lymphocytes. These antigens are common to all tumours induced by the same virus in animals expressing the same major histocompatibility complex. Antigens that induce T-cell-mediated rejection responses are also generally present on tumours induced with chemical carcinogens or ultraviolet radiation.[4],[5] However, contrary to the viral antigens, these tumour-specific transplantation antigens show a very large diversity: each tumour expresses tumour-specific transplantation antigens that differ from those seen on other tumours, even when these tumours are induced in the same strain of mice and have the same histological type. In several systems, tumour-specific transplantation antigens have been found to elicit a cytolytic T-cell response.

The observation that tumours express tumour-specific transplantation antigens led to a revival of the theory of immune surveillance of cancer.[6] This hypothesis stated that the immune system evolved not only to eliminate foreign pathogens but also to recognize and destroy abnormal cells, such as cancer cells. It also proposed that most tumours were eliminated at a very early stage by immune rejection and that the development of cancer resulted from an occasional failure of the immune system. However, this hypothesis lost credibility when it became apparent that no general correlation could be made either in humans or in animals between immune depression and high tumour frequency.[7] Moreover, tumour transplantations carried out with spontaneous tumours, that is, tumours occurring without experimental interference, indicated that these tumours were incapable of eliciting any rejection response.[8] It was therefore claimed that tumour-specific transplantation antigens were an experimental artefact, unlikely to be found in human tumours.

It appears now that one should distinguish immunogenic tumour-specific transplantation antigens, which are capable on their own of eliciting an immune response, from non-immunogenic antigens, which can only serve as targets for an established response. That spontaneous tumours can express tumour-specific transplantation antigens of the second kind was demonstrated by using variant tumour cells expressing additional antigens. These variants were found to elicit a protective immune response against the original tumour cells. The protection showed specificity for the original spontaneous tumour and the immunized mice had cytolytic T-cell memory cells directed specifically against this tumour.[9] It appears, therefore, that the addition of new antigens on tumour cells enables the immune system to develop a response against a tumour-specific transplantation antigen which is too weak to elicit a response on its own. These additional antigens can be obtained by mutagen treatment, producing tum⁻ 'variants' that are rejected, or by transfection of genes coding for foreign antigens.[10],[11] From these findings, it appears likely that all rodent tumours, whatever their origin, express tumour rejection antigens against which a T-cell response can be elicited by immune manipulation. As discussed below, a similar situation appears to exist for human tumours.

Genetic mechanisms producing tumour-specific antigens

As discussed above, class I-restricted T cells recognize antigenic peptides derived from viral proteins that are synthesized within the target cell (Fig. 2). It is now clear in tumour cells that two major genetic mechanisms produce new antigens that are strictly tumour specific: gene mutation and gene activation (Fig. 3). Point mutations result in one amino acid change in a sequence coding for a potential antigenic peptide. This amino acid change enables the peptide to bind to an MHC class I molecule, whereas the normal peptide is unable to bind. Other amino acid changes produce a new epitope on a peptide that was already capable of binding to an MHC class I sequence. Whereas the T lymphocytes recognizing the normal peptide have been eliminated or paralysed by the natural tolerance processes, the new peptide can be recognized by a fresh set of cytolytic T cells. Several examples of potent new rejection antigens caused by point mutations were observed in tum⁻ variants, that is, tumour cell variants that are obtained by mutagenesis of mouse tumour cells and that have become incapable of producing progressive tumours because they are rejected by a potent T-cell-mediated response.[10] Several mouse tumour-specific antigens caused by mutations have now been identified.[12] The second mechanism is the activation of genes that are not expressed in normal cells but are expressed in some tumour

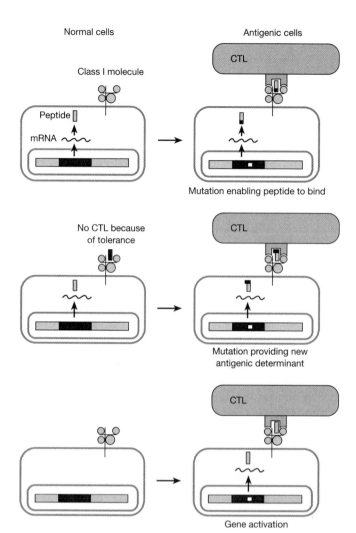

Fig. 3 Genetic mechanisms producing tumour-specific antigens.

cells. The first example was gene *P1A* which codes for a tumour-specific rejection antigen of mouse mastocytoma P815. This antigen is also present on the cells of several other mouse tumours.[13]

Human tumour antigens recognized by autologous cytolytic T lymphocytes

Antitumour cytolytic T cells

Antitumour cytolytic T lymphocytes have been derived from peripheral blood mononuclear cells of patients with cancer, and also from tumour-infiltrating lymphocytes, malignant effusions, and invaded lymph nodes.

Because they are readily available, peripheral blood leucocytes are a major source of lymphocytes for the study of autologous cytolytic T-cell responses. When T cells isolated from peripheral blood leucocytes are analysed immediately, they usually do not display significant cytolytic activity for autologous tumour cells. However, such cytolytic activity is often observed when peripheral blood leucocytes are cultured *in vitro* in the presence of irradiated autologous stimulator tumour cells. These mixed lymphocyte–tumour cultures (**MLTC**)

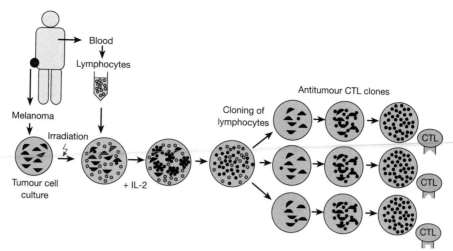

Fig. 4 Autologous mixed lymphocyte–tumour culture.

often show considerable proliferation of the lymphocytes (Fig. 4). Usually, IL-2 is added at a low concentration, which promotes lymphocyte growth without impairing the specificity of the cytolytic T-cell response. The responder lymphocytes of the MLTC are usually collected every week and restimulated with tumour cells. The cytolytic activity of the lymphocytes can be tested at this time. MLTC can often be continued for 30 to 40 days before the lymphocytes stop proliferating. The repeated stimulation of the lymphocytes requires the availability of a permanent culture of the autologous tumour.

Because melanomas give rise to permanent culture cell lines more often than other tumours, MLTC have been carried out for a large number of patients with melanoma. In many instances, the cultured lymphocytes show cytolytic activity after 2 or 3 weeks. This activity shows a degree of specificity for the autologous tumour cells: lysis of these cells is more efficient than lysis of autologous Epstein–Barr virus (**EBV**)-transformed B lymphocytes and lysis of K562 cells, which are targets for natural killer-like cytolytic activity. Usually, the antitumour specificity of the MLTC responder cells improves with time, presumably because the specific effectors multiply more actively than the non-specific effectors (Fig. 5). Similar results have been obtained with sarcomas and breast carcinomas. For some tumours which express low amounts of class I MHC molecules, it is necessary to treat the tumour cells with interferon to observe lysis by cytolytic T cells.

Human solid tumours are often infiltrated by T lymphocytes and the presence of these lymphocytes has been considered as an indication of host response against the tumour. T lymphocytes have been found in proportions varying from 15 to 70 per cent of the mononuclear cells recovered by enzymatic dissociation of the tumour tissue. The mixture of tumour-infiltrating lymphocytes and tumour cells has been incubated in medium supplemented with high concentrations of IL-2. At weekly intervals, the cells are harvested and resuspended in fresh medium, and the stimulator tumour cells progressively disappear from the culture. Some of these MLTC derived from melanoma tumours have produced cytolytic T cells showing specificity for autologous tumour cells.[14]

By diluting populations of antitumoral cytolytic T cells it is possible to obtain cytolytic T-cell clones, that is, stable populations of cytolytic

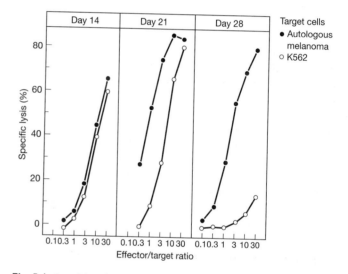

Fig. 5 Lytic activity of responder lymphocytes collected at days 14, 21, and 28 after the beginning of a culture with autologous melanoma cells. There is increasing specificity for the melanoma cells.

T cells derived *in vitro* from a single lymphocyte. These homogeneous cytolytic T-cell populations have proved to be essential tools for the assessment of cytolytic T-cell specificity and for the identification of their target antigen. As shown in Fig. 4, a number of antitumoral cytolytic T-cell clones of high lytic activity against the autologous melanoma cells were obtained. They were shown to have no activity against autologous fibroblasts, autologous EBV-transformed B cells, or cells like K562 that are very sensitive to lysis by natural killer cells (Fig. 6).

By incubating cytolytic T-cell clones with a large number of tumour cells it was possible to select, at a frequency of the order of 10^{-6}, tumour cells that had become resistant to the cytolytic T-cell clones. The resistant variants were interpreted to result from a loss of the antigen, a presumption that later proved to be true in many instances. Using a panel of cytolytic T-cell clones directed against the same

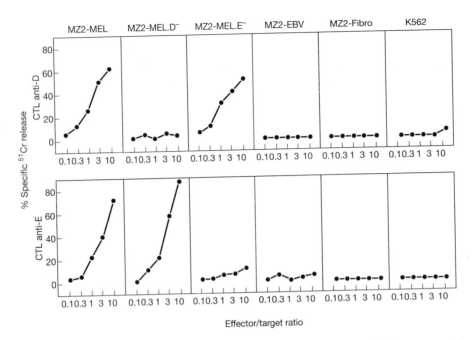

Fig. 6 Specificity of two antimelanoma autologous cytolytic T-cell clones. The lytic activity of the cytolytic T-cell clones was tested on an autologous melanoma line (MZ2-MEL), and on two antigen-loss variants (MZ2-MEL D⁻ and E⁻). Lysis was also measured on an autologous EBV-transformed B-cell line (MZ2-EBV) and fibroblast (MZ2-fibro), and also on an allogeneic melanoma (SK-MEL-29) and natural killer target K562. D⁻ and E⁻ lines were selected by *in vitro* immunoselection with the relevant cytolytic T cells.

tumour, it proved possible to show that most antigen-loss variants resistant to one cytolytic T-cell clone were still sensitive to lysis by most of the other clones directed against the same tumour (Fig. 6). This led to the important conclusion that human tumours carry not only one but several antigens recognized by autologous cytolytic T cells, probably more than five in most instances. This conclusion is of high relevance for the prospects of cancer immunotherapy.

Identification of human tumour antigens

Two methods have been used to identify the peptides presented to tumour-specific T cells. The first is a genetic approach based on the transfection of recombinant DNA libraries into cells expressing the MHC-presenting molecule, in order to isolate the gene encoding the antigen. The transfectants that express the antigen are identified by their ability to stimulate cytokine release by the relevant cytolytic T-cell clone (Fig. 7).[15] Once the gene has been isolated, the antigenic peptide is deduced from the sequence of the putative protein.

The second method is a biochemical purification of peptides eluted from the MHC class I molecules of the tumour cells. Tumour peptides are fractionated by high-pressure liquid chromatography, and the different fractions are then tested for their ability to sensitize target cells for lysis by relevant cytolytic T cells. The positive fraction is then further purified and sequenced. Peptide sequencing usually requires sophisticated mass spectrometry methods.[16] When post-translational modification of the protein occurs, the sequence of the peptide cannot be deduced from the sequence of the protein and the biochemical approach is then the only way to identify the natural epitope presented at the cell surface.[17] For instance, a tyrosinase antigenic peptide contains an aspartic acid which replaces a glycosylated asparagine residue because the deglycosylation also removes the amino group.

The list of antigens that is recognized by T cells in human tumour cells and that has been identified by the genetic approach is growing. Based on the pattern of expression of the parent protein, the antigens can be classified into four major groups: tumour-specific shared antigens, antigens produced by genes that are overexpressed in tumours, differentiation antigens, and antigens resulting from genetic mutations.

Tumour-specific shared antigens

Tumour-specific shared antigens are encoded by genes that are silent in most normal tissues but are activated in a number of tumours of various histological types. Prototype antigens of this group are those encoded by *MAGE* genes in humans. Additional human genes with a similar expression profile have been identified and are listed in Table 1. The only normal cells in which significant expression of genes of this category has been detected are placental trophoblasts and testicular germ cells.[18] Because these cells do not express MHC class I molecules, gene expression should not result in antigen expression and such antigens can be considered as strictly tumour-specific.[19]

The activation of the *MAGE* genes usually results from a demethylation of their promoter that correlates with genome-wide demethylation.[20],[21] Expression has been detected in substantial fractions of human tumours and the list of histological types of tumours expressing *MAGE* genes is increasing (Table 2).[22] Because they are shared by tumours expressing the genes and bearing the appropriate MHC type, these human antigens represent promising targets for cancer immunotherapy.

Some cytolytic T cells directed against breast, ovarian, and pancreatic carcinomas recognize an epitope of mucin, a surface protein

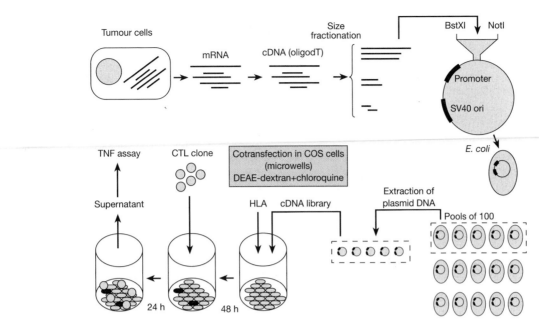

Fig. 7 The genetic approach used to identify human tumour antigens.

Table 1 Tumour-specific antigens shared by human tumours

Human gene	Normal expression	MHC	Peptide
MAGE-1	Testis	HLA A1	EADPTGHSY
		HLA Cw16	SAYGEPRKL
MAGE-3	Testis	HLA A1	EVDPIGHLY
		HLA A2	FLWGPRALV
		HLA B44	MEVDPIGHLY
MAGE-6	Testis	HLA Cw16	–
BAGE	Testis	HLA Cw16	AARAVFLAL
GAGE-1/2	Testis	HLA Cw6	YRPRPRRY
GAGE-3–6	Testis	HLA A29	–
RAGE-1	Testis	HLA B7	SPSSNRIRNT
GnTV[a]	None	HLA A2	VLPDVFIRC
mucin[b]	Lactating breast	Non-MHC-restricted	PDTRPAPGSTAPPAHGVTSA[c]

[a] Aberrant trancript of N-acetyl glucosaminyl transferase V (GnTV) that is found only in melanomas (Table 2).

[b] Overexpressed in 30 per cent of breast and ovarian carcinomas, and in a lower fraction of other carcinomas.

[c] MHC-unrestricted recognition of a repeated motif that is unmasked in tumours due to mucin underglycosylation.

composed of multiple tandem repeats of 20 amino acids. Whereas in normal cells mucin is heavily glycosylated, in these tumours the peptide repeats are unmasked by underglycosylation, resulting in cytolytic T-cell recognition. Remarkably, this recognition, which depends on the presence of multiple repeats, occurs in the absence of HLA restriction, presumably because the TCR binds directly to mucin protein. Mucin underglycosylation also occurs in breast duct epithelial cells during lactation, but only at the extracellular apical surface which normally is not accessible to T cells. These mucin antigens therefore appear to be very specific for tumour cells.[(23),(24)]

Antigens encoded by genes overexpressed in tumours

Lymphocytes infiltrating some ovarian carcinomas in patients who are HLA A2+ have been found to recognize a peptide derived from HER-2/neu, an oncogene expressed in normal tissues at low levels

Table 2 Expression in tumour samples of genes encoding T-cell antigens[a]

Histological type	Percentage of tumours expressing:					
	MAGE-1	MAGE-3	BAGE	GAGE-1,2	RAGE-1	GnTV
Melanomas						48
Primary lesions	16	36	8	13	2	
Metastases	48	76	26	28	5	
Non-small-cell lung carcinomas	49	47	4	19	0	0
Head and neck tumours	28	49	8	19	2	0
Bladder carcinomas	22	36	15	12	5	0
Sarcomas	14	24	6	25	14	0
Mammary carcinomas	18	11	10	9	1	0
Gastric carcinomas	29					
Oesophageal carcinomas[b]	53	47				
Prostatic carcinomas	15	15	0	10	0	0
Colorectal carcinomas	2	17	0	0	0	0
Renal cell carcinomas	0	0	0	0	2	0
Ovarian carcinomas[c]	28	17	15	31		
Neuroblastomas[d]	18	54				
Leukaemias and lymphomas	0	0	0	1	0	0

[a] Expression was measured by RT-PCR on total RNA using primers specific for each gene.

Data were compiled from refs 12, 14[b], 16[c], 17[d], and from data obtained at the Brussels branch of the Ludwig Institute.

and overexpressed in 30 per cent of breast and ovarian carcinomas.[22] Another gene named *PRAME* is overexpressed in almost all melanomas and in many other tumour types. It produces an antigen recognized by autologous cytolytic T cells.[22]

Differentiation antigens

A large number of cytolytic T cells directed against human melanoma were found to recognize not only a majority of melanomas but also normal melanocytes. The notion that such cytolytic T cells recognize melanocyte differentiation antigens was confirmed when the antigens were identified at the molecular level (Table 3). The first example was tyrosinase, a melanocyte protein that gives rise to different peptides that are presented either by class I or class II molecules to CD8 or CD4 T cells.[25]

The role of cytolytic T cells specific for such antigens in melanoma rejection is not clear, but is supported by the reported association of vitiligo with prolonged survival and spontaneous regression of melanoma.[26] Because melanocytes are also present in the choroid layer of retina, the potential ophthalmic toxicity of active immunotherapy targeted against these antigens needs to be evaluated very carefully.

B-cell lymphomas are monoclonal tumours derived from B cells. They express the idiotype corresponding to the antigen specificity of the parent B cell. T-cell responses against idiotypic epitopes have been reported.[27] Idiotypic immunoglobulins therefore represent a particular case of differentiation antigens that are unique to individual tumours.

Antigens resulting from mutations

Antigens of this third category correspond to peptides derived from regions of ubiquitous proteins that are mutated in tumour cells (Table 4). Two of these mutations affecting human genes *CDK4* and β-catenin may be involved in oncogenesis, since they were found in several human tumours and they have a demonstrated effect on the activity of the encoded proteins.[22] The CDK4 mutation prevents the protein from binding to its inhibitor, p16. This appears to alter the regulation of the cell cycle, favouring uncontrolled growth of the tumour cells. The β-catenin mutation results in stabilization of the protein which favours the constitutive formation of complexes with transcription factors, such as Lef-1. Constitutive β-catenin/Lef-1 complexes may result in persistent activation of as yet unidentified target genes, thereby stimulating cell proliferation or inhibiting apoptosis.[22] Another mutation which may antagonize apoptosis was identified recently with cytolytic T cells specific for a human squamous-cell carcinoma. The antigen is encoded by a mutated form of the *CASP-8* gene, which codes for protease caspase-8, also named FLICE or MACHα1. This protease is required for induction of apoptosis through the Fas and TNFR1 receptors, and the ability of the altered protein to trigger apoptosis appears to be reduced relative to the normal caspase-8.[22] Combined with the observations made with the CDK4 and β-catenin mutations, this suggests that a fraction of point mutations generating tumour antigens also play a role in tumoural transformation or progression.

Although the tumour antigens resulting from mutations are highly specific to the tumour, the fact that they are often unique prevents

Table 3 Differentiation antigens recognized by T cells on tumours

Tumour	Gene/protein	MHC	Peptide
Mouse melanoma	TRP-2	H-2 K^d	VYDFFVWL
Human melanoma	tyrosinase	HLA A2	MLLAVLYCL
		HLA A2	YMNGTMSQV
			YMDGTMSQV[a]
		HLA A24	AFLPWHRLF
		HLA B44	SEIWRDIDF
		HLA DR4	QNILLSNAPLGPQFP
			SYLQDSDPDSFQD
	Pmel17/gp100	HLA A2	KTWGQYWQV
		HLA A2	AMLGTHTMEV
		HLA A2	MLGTHTMEV
		HLA A2	ITDQVPFSV
		HLA A2	YLEPGPVTA[a]
		HLA A2	LLDGTATLRL
		HLA A2	VLYRYGSFSV
		HLA A2	SLADTNSLAV
		HLA A3	ALLAVGATK[a]
	Melan-A/MART-1	HLA A2	(E)AAGIGILTV[b]
		HLA A2	ILTVILGVL[a]
	gp75/TRP-1	HLA A31	MSLQRQFLR
	TRP-2	HLA A31	LLGPGRPYR
Other human tumours	CEA	HLA A2	YLSGANLNL
	PSA	HLA A2	FLTPKKLQCV
		HLA A2	VISNDVCAQV

[a] Natural peptide eluted from HLA molecules.

[b] Different cytolytic T cells preferentially recognize either the nonamer or the decamer.

Table 4 Tumour antigens resulting from mutations

Human gene/protein	Tumour	MHC	Peptide[a]
MUM-1	Melanoma	HLA B44	EEKL/VVLF
CDK4	Melanoma	HLA A2	ACDPHSGHFV
β-catenin	Melanoma	HLA A24	SYLDSGIHF
HLA-A2[b]	Renal cell carcinoma	–	–
bcr-abl (b3a2)	Chronic myeloid leukaemia	HLA DR4	ATGFKQSSKALQRPVAS[c]
CASP-8	Head and neck sqamous-cell carcinoma	HLA B35	–
KIAAO205	Bladder tumour	HLA B44	–

[a] The residue modified by the mutation is italicized.

[b] The mutation affects the HLA A2 gene itself.

[c] Peptide selected from the mutated sequence and used to stimulate cytolytic T cells in vitro.

their use as components of generic cancer vaccines. It is somewhat surprising that none of the frequently mutated oncogenes or tumour-suppressor genes, such as ras or p53, have been detected as targets of cytolytic T cells raised against tumour cells. However, synthetic ras and p53 mutant peptides have been used to generate cytolytic T cells

or rejection responses against tumours carrying the corresponding mutant genes.[22]

Myeloid leukaemias often express the chimeric protein bcr-abl, which results from a t(9;22) chromosomal translocation. CD4+ T cells, raised in vitro against a peptide centred on the fusion region of bcr-abl, were recently found to recognize HLA DR4 leukaemic blast cells expressing bcr-abl.[22] This indicates that another source of strictly tumour-specific antigens are the chimeric proteins encoded at the sites of chromosomal translocations. Because identical translocations occur frequently in certain types of leukaemias, these antigens might be shared by many leukaemias.

Viral antigens

Antigens derived from oncogenic viruses constitute another category of potentially useful tumour antigens. A number of viral antigens has been studied in detail in virally induced mouse tumours and shown to be relevant for tumour rejection. In humans, the best example is oncoprotein E7 of human papillomavirus 16 (HPV16), which is present in most cervical carcinomas. Tumour-specific cytolytic T cells have been elicited by *in vitro* sensitization with E7 peptides presented by HLA A2.[28]

Clinical perspectives

The identification of human tumour antigens recognized by cytolytic T cells opens new perspectives for cancer immunotherapy, based on therapeutic vaccination with defined antigens. Several strategies can be utilized for immunization, including peptides, proteins, DNA, recombinant viruses, or autologous dendritic cells exposed to peptides.

The first attempts to immunize patients against defined tumour antigens were undertaken in patients with B-cell lymphoma, who were immunized with the idiotypic epitope of the immunoglobulin expressed by their lymphoma cells. Tumour regressions were observed in several patients immunized with the idiotypic protein either conjugated to keyhole-limpet haemocyanin and mixed with adjuvant or pulsed on autologous dendritic cells.[29]–[31] Such treatment of B-cell lymphoma requires the preparation of a new vaccine for each patient.

The MAGE-like antigens can be used to develop common vaccines. Twenty-five patients with stage III and IV melanoma have received three subcutaneous injections of an antigenic peptide, encoded by *MAGE-3* and presented by HLA A1, in the absence of adjuvant. Tumour regressions have been observed in seven patients. No cytolytic T-cell response against the immunizing peptide could be detected in the blood of these patients.[32]

In another trial, a peptide of 105 amino acids, containing five repeated mucin epitopes, was injected with BCG into 67 patients with breast, colon, or pancreatic cancer. No clinical benefit was reported. However, an increase in the frequency of mucin-specific cytolytic T cells was seen in the blood of most patients.[24]

A number of patients have also been injected with peptides corresponding to melanoma differentiation antigens mixed with incomplete Freund's adjuvant or granulocyte–macrophage colony-stimulating factor (GM-CSF). In these studies, peptide-specific cytolytic T cells were obtained *in vitro* by restimulating blood lymphocytes from these patients with cells presenting the peptide.[33]–[35] Objective tumour regressions were documented in a few patients, and enhanced delayed-type hypersensitivity reactions were observed when GM-CSF was injected.

Eight patients with late-stage cervical cancer were vaccinated with a recombinant vaccinia virus expressing the E6 and E7 proteins of HPV16 and 18. No clinical side-effects were observed, nor was any clinical benefit reported. Each patient mounted an antivaccinia antibody response. An anti-HPV antibody response was observed in three patients and an HPV-specific cytolytic T-cell response in only one patient.[36]

Trials involving infusion of autologous dendritic cells pulsed with peptides encoded by *MAGE* or differentiation antigens have also produced clinical responses in a minority of patients.[37]

There can be little doubt that the coming years will witness a large number of clinical trials involving peptides, proteins, and recombinant defective viruses. These trials should establish whether improvements in the mode of immunizations will provide strong cytolytic T-cell responses and whether this will lead to regular clinical responses.

Tumour escape from T-cell response

On the basis of what we know about T-cell recognition, tumour cells could escape T-cell responses by decreasing their expression of either the tumour-specific antigenic peptides, the presenting HLA molecules, or also accessory binding molecules like ICAM-1.[38] Each of these possibilities can be expected to occur in some progressive tumour cell variants.

As described above, melanoma cell variants resistant to cytolytic T cells have been obtained *in vitro*. Some of these variants are most probably affected by mutations or deletions in the genes encoding for the antigenic peptides, whereas others appear to have lost the expression of class I molecules.

Many human tumours, such as small-cell lung carcinomas and neuroblastomas, express very low amounts of HLA molecules. In some instances, metastatic tumour cells seem to express less class I molecules than the primary tumours. This may be an important cause of escape from an immune response because the lack of the product of one allele should suffice to prevent presentation of the relevant antigenic peptide.

Burkitt's lymphoma provides an interesting example of tumour adaptation to immune constraints.[39] When normal B cells from patients were transformed *in vitro* with Epstein–Barr virus, these EBV-B cells could be used to stimulate *in vitro* a cytolytic T-cell response. Nevertheless, these cytolytic T cells failed to lyse effectively the virus-positive Burkitt's lymphoma cells. This appears to be due to lack of expression of all but one EBV antigen, and downregulation of the expression of HLA and accessory binding molecules.

It appears therefore that, like chemotherapy, immunotherapy of cancer will be confronted with the problem of resistant tumour cells. However, if human tumours express multiple tumour-specific transplantation antigens, this should make complete resistance difficult. Also, some non-specificity during an immune rejection response could help in the elimination of a few antigen-loss variants located in the mass of rejected tumour cells. After all, very large mouse tumours can be rejected completely even though antigen-loss variants arising from these mouse tumours have been observed.

Tumour antigens recognized by autologous antibodies

For many years, the search for human tumour antigens that are recognized by antibodies has been characterized by the use of antisera or, more recently, monoclonal antibodies obtained from animals immunized with human cancer cells (see Chapter 4.27). Despite extensive investigation, no bona fide tumour antigens have been identified by this approach. In addition to the use of heterologous antibodies, a considerable amount of work has been carried out to determine whether patients with cancer produce tumour-specific antibodies. To this end, a rigorous approach called autologous typing has been developed and applied to a large series of sera from patients with cancer.[40] While these studies provided evidence for the production of antibodies with specificity for autologous tumour cells in a few patients with cancer, no molecular characterization of the corresponding antigens could be obtained until recently. However, subsequent studies indicated that patients with cancer may often develop antibody responses against various oncoproteins expressed by tumour cells, such as Her-2/neu, p53, C-myc, C-myb, or ras[41] (see also Chapter 1.2). The greater incidence of antibodies with such specificity in patients with cancer compared with normal individuals suggests that release of intracellular oncoproteins by dying tumour cells may be responsible for their immunogenicity. Antibodies against tumour-associated cell surface proteins or carbohydrates have also been detected in sera from patients with cancer, thus indicating that human tumours may elicit multiple antibody responses in the autologous host.

In an attempt to substantiate these initial findings, a new approach has been developed recently which allows the unbiased search for tumour antigens recognized by antibodies present in autologous sera. This approach is called **SEREX**, for serological analysis of recombinant cDNA expression libraries of human tumours with autologous serum.[42] In a first step, a cDNA library is constructed from fresh tumour specimens, packaged into λ-phage vectors and expressed in *Escherichia coli*. In a second step, the recombinant proteins produced during lytic infection of the bacteria are transferred on to nitrocellulose membranes and identified as antigens by their reactivity with high-titre IgG antibodies present in autologous sera. In a third step, the nucleotide sequences of the cDNA inserts corresponding to the identified antigens are determined.

During the past 3 years SEREX has been applied to a wide range of human tumour types.[43] This survey has revealed a large array of tumour-associated antigens recognized by autologous antibodies, including known cytolytic T cell-defined tumour antigens, such as tyrosinase and MAGE-1. SEREX-identified antigens include other gene products that appear to elicit both humoral and cytolytic T-cell responses in patients with cancer. For example, the NY-ESO-1 antigen, which is selectively expressed in a proportion of different tumour types and in testis, has been found to be particularly immunogenic, with approximately 40 to 50 per cent of patients with tumours expressing this antigen developing an antibody response at some stage in the disease. Although it is not yet known what proportion of these patients also develop cytolytic T-cell responses against this antigen, there is evidence that such a dual response does exist.

Many SEREX-defined antigens are not strictly tumour-specific, but are only overexpressed in tumours. In some cases, there is evidence that tumour overexpression is caused by gene amplification. However, this does not apply to other antigens, which are expressed ubiquitously and at a similar level in cancer and normal tissues. Why such antigens elicit antibody responses only in patients with cancer has yet to be understood.

The clinical significance of antitumour antibodies in patients with cancer is unclear. From the limited amount of data available, it appears that antibodies against SEREX-defined antigens are usually detected in a small proportion of the patients bearing a tumour expressing the corresponding antigen and without any correlation to the tumour stage or tumour burden. As discussed above, the identification of cytolytic T cell-defined human tumour antigens has opened new perspectives for antigen-specific cancer immunotherapy. It is likely that future clinical trials along this line will include selected antibody-defined antigens in the formulation of cancer vaccines.

Summary

It is now clear that human tumour cells carry antigens that are not expressed on normal cells and that can be recognized by autologous T lymphocytes. This has opened the way for a systematic effort aimed at immunizing patients with cancer with defined tumour-specific antigens to induce immune rejection of their tumour. The observations made in clinical trials suggest that tumour rejection occurs occasionally as a result of therapeutic vaccination; but at this stage it is not yet possible to predict whether cancer immunotherapy will provide a major improvement in the treatment of cancer, because we have little understanding of what happens in immunized patients and in those who show tumour regression. Small-scale trials with all available forms of immunogens accompanied with a careful genetic analysis of tumour samples collected before and after treatment are, in our opinion, necessary for progress.

References

1. **Watts C.** Capture and processing of exogenous antigens for presentation on MHC molecules. *Annual Review of Immunology*, 1997; **15**: 821–50.

2. **Pamer E, Cresswell P.** Mechanisms of MHC class I-restricted antigen processing. *Annual Review of Immunology*, 1998; **16**: 323–58.

3. **Romero P, Cerottini JC, Waanders GA.** Novel methods to monitor antigen-specific cytotoxic T-cell responses in cancer immunotherapy. *Molecular Medicine Today*, 1998; **4**: 305–12.

4. **Klein G, Sjögren H, Klein E, Hellström KE.** Demonstration of resistance against methylcholanthrene-induced sarcomas in the primary autochthonous host. *Cancer Research*, 1960; **20**: 1561–72.

5. **Kripke ML.** Immunologic mechanisms in UV radiation carcinogenesis. *Advances in Cancer Research*, 1981; **34**: 69–106.

6. **Burnet FM.** A certain symmetry: histocompatibility antigens compared with immunocyte receptors. *Nature*, 1970; **226**: 123–6.

7. **Stutman O.** Immunodepression and malignancy. *Advances in Cancer Research*, 1975; **22**: 261–422.

8. **Hewitt H, Blake E, Walder A.** A critique of the evidence for active host defense against cancer based on personal studies of 27 murine tumours of spontaneous origin. *British Journal of Cancer*, 1976; **33**: 241–59.

9. **Van Pel A, Vessière F, Boon T.** Protection against two spontaneous mouse leukemias conferred by immunogenic variants obtained by mutagenesis. *Journal of Experimental Medicine*, 1983; **157**: 1992–2001.

10. **Boon T.** Antigenic tumor cell variants obtained with mutagen. *Advances in Cancer Research*, 1983; **39**: 131–51.

11. **Kobayashi H.** Modification of tumor antigenicity in therapeutics: increase in immunologic foreignness of tumor cells in experimental

model systems. In: Mihich E, ed. *Immunological Approaches to Cancer Therapeutics*, Vol. 13. John Wiley, New York, 1982, pp. 405–40.

12. Mumberg D, Wick M, Schreiber H. Unique tumor antigens redefined as mutant tumor-specific antigens. *Seminars in Immunology*, 1996; **8**: 289–93.

13. Lethé B, Van den Eynde B, Van Pel A, Corradin G, Boon T. Mouse tumor rejection antigens P815A and P815B: two epitopes carried by a single peptide. *European Journal of Immunology*, 1992; **22**: 2283–8.

14. Topalian SL, Solomon D, Rosenberg SA. Tumor-specific cytolysis by lymphocytes infiltrating human melanomas. *Journal of Immunology*, 1989; **142**: 3714–25.

15. De Plaen E, *et al.* Cloning of genes coding for antigens recognized by cytolytic T lymphocytes. In: Lefkovits I, ed. *The Immunology Methods Manual*. Academic Press, 1997: 692–718.

16. Cox AL, *et al.* Identification of a peptide recognized by five melanoma-specific human cytotoxic T cell lines. *Science*, 1994; **264**: 716–19.

17. Skipper JCA, *et al.* An HLA-A2-restricted tyrosinase antigen on melanoma cells results from posttranslational modification and suggests a novel pathway for processing of membrane proteins. *Journal of Experimental Medicine*, 1996; **183**: 527–34.

18. Takahashi K, Shichijo S, Noguchi M, Hirohata M, Itoh K. Identification of MAGE-1 and MAGE-4 proteins in spermatogonia and primary spermatocytes of testis. *Cancer Research*, 1995; **55**: 3478–82.

19. Haas GG Jr, D'Cruz OJ, De Bault LE. Distribution of human leukocyte antigen-ABC and -D/DR antigens in the unfixed human testis. *American Journal of Reproductive Immunology and Microbiology*, 1988; **18**: 47–51.

20. De Smet C, De Backer O, Faraoni I, Lurquin C, Brasseur F, Boon T. The activation of human gene MAGE-1 in tumor cells is correlated with genome-wide demethylation. *Proceedings of the National Academy of Sciences (USA)*, 1996; **93**: 7149–53.

21. Serrano A, Garcia A, Abril E, Garrido F, Ruiz-Cabello F. Methylated CpG points identified within MAGE-1 promoter are involved in gene repression. *International Journal of Cancer*, 1996; **68**: 464–70.

22. Van den Eynde B, van der Bruggen P. T cell-defined tumor antigens. *Current Opinion in Immunology*, 1997; **9**: 684–93.

23. Jerome KR, Domenech N, Finn OJ. Tumor-specific cytotoxic T cell clones from patients with breast and pancreatic adenocarcinoma recognize EBV-immortalized B cells transfected with polymorphic epithelial mucin cDNA. *Journal of Immunology*, 1993; **151**: 1654–62.

24. Barratt-Boyes SM. Making the most of mucin: a novel target for tumor immunotherapy. *Cancer Immunology and Immunotherapy*, 1996; **43**: 142–51.

25. Topalian SL, *et al.* Melanoma-specific CD4+ T cells recognize nonmutated HLA-DR-restricted tyrosinase epitopes. *Journal of Experimental Medicine*, 1996; **183**: 1965–71.

26. Rosenberg SA, White DE. Vitiligo in patients with melanoma: normal tissue antigens can be target for cancer immunotherapy. *Journal of Immunotherapy*, 1996; **19**: 81–4.

27. Wen Y-J, Lim SH. T cells recognize the VH complementarity-determining region 3 of the idiotypic protein of B cell non-Hodgkin's lymphoma. *European Journal of Immunology*, 1997; **27**: 1043–7.

28. Ressing ME, *et al.* Human CTL epitopes encoded by human papillomavirus type 16 E6 and E7 identified through *in vivo* and *in vitro* immunogenicity studies of HLA-A*0201-binding peptides. *Journal of Immunology*, 1995; **154**: 5934–43.

29. Hsu FJ, *et al.* Vaccination of patients with B-cell lymphoma using autologous antigen-pulsed dendritic cells. *Nature Medicine*, 1996; **2**: 52–8.

30. Hsu FJ, *et al.* Tumor-specific idiotype vaccines in the treatment of patients with B-cell lymphoma. Long-term results of a clinical trial. *Blood*, 1997; **89**: 3129–35.

31. Nelson EL, *et al.* Tumor-specific, cytotoxic T-lymphocyte response after idiotype vaccination for B-cell, non-Hogkin's lymphoma. *Blood*, 1996; **88**: 580–9.

32. Marchand M, *et al.* Tumor regressions observed in patients with metastatic melanoma treated with an antigenic peptide encoded by gene MAGE-3 and presented by HLA-A1. *International Journal of Cancer*, 1999; **80**: 219–30.

33. Salgaller ML, Marincola FM, Cormier JN, Rosenberg SA. Immunization against epitopes in the human melanoma antigen gp100 following patient immunization with synthetic peptides. *Cancer Research*, 1996; **56**: 4749–57.

34. Jäger E, *et al.* Granulocyte–macrophage-colony-stimulating factor enhances immune responses to melanoma-associated peptides *in vivo*. *International Journal of Cancer*, 1996; **67**: 54–62.

35. Cormier JN, *et al.* Enhancement of cellular immunity in melanoma patients immunized with a peptide from MART-1/Melan-A. *Cancer Journal from Scientific American*, 1997; **3**: 37–44.

36. Borysiewicz LK, *et al.* A recombinant vaccinia virus encoding human papillomavirus types 16 and 18, E6 and E7 proteins as immunotherapy for cervical cancer. *Lancet*, 1996; **347**: 1523–7.

37. Nestle FO, *et al.* Vaccination of melanoma patients with peptide- or tumor lysate-pulsed dendritic cells. *Nature Medicine*, 1998; **4**: 328–32.

38. Hämmerling GJ, Maschek U, Sturmhöfel K, Momburg F. Regulation and functional role of MHC expression on tumors. *Progress in Immunology*, 1989; **7**: 1071–8.

39. Klein G. Viral latency and transformation: the strategy of Epstein–Barr virus. *Cell*, 1989; **58**: 5–8.

40. Old LJ. Cancer immunology: the search for specificity. *Cancer Research*, 1981; **41**: 361–75.

41. Canevari S, Pupa SM, Menard S. 1975–1995 revised anti-cancer serological responses: biological significance and clinical implications. *Annals of Oncology*, 1996; **7**: 227–32.

42. Sahin U, Türeci O, Pfreundshuh M. Serological identification of human tumor antigens. *Current Opinion in Immunology*, 1997; **9**: 709–16.

43. Old LJ, Chen YT. New paths in human cancer serology. *Journal of Experimental Medicine*, 1998; **187**: 1163–7.

2

Aetiology, epidemiology, and prevention of cancer

2.1 Chemical carcinogenesis

G. P. Margison and A. C. Povey

Introduction

Our understanding of the mechanisms of human carcinogenesis is based on epidemiological studies, on investigations of inherited susceptibility syndromes and on animal, cell biological, and molecular experiments. A large number of organic and inorganic chemical agents, as well as viruses and ionizing and non-ionizing radiation have been shown to be capable of inducing cancers in a wide range of tissues in many species after administration by a variety of routes. Chemical carcinogens are generally also acutely toxic agents and can elicit a number of other biological responses including teratogenicity.

The majority of cancers probably result from non-lethal and irreversible genetic modifications in a single original cell that is thereby transformed, i.e. by mutations (broadly defined as any permanent change in the base sequence or coding properties of DNA). Molecular studies have shown that specific changes in specific genes, termed proto-oncogenes and tumour suppressor genes, are prerequisites for carcinogenesis. Consequently, the normal cellular functions and interactions of the products of these genes are a major focus of attention.

Following uptake by the host, many carcinogens undergo biotransformations of various kinds generally resulting in more reactive chemical species. This has led to the concept of inactive procarcinogens that undergo 'metabolic activation' to proximal or ultimate carcinogens. Most carcinogens act either directly or following metabolic activation, resulting in damage to DNA. These are collectively known as genotoxic agents and are commonly referred to as xenobiotic if they are exogenous in origin.

However, normal cells can contain DNA damage that is not attributable to exogenous agents and such endogenous ('background') DNA damage may contribute to carcinogenesis. Normally this damage is repaired effectively, or the cells are eliminated or suppressed by cellular or host control mechanisms. Therefore, agents may be carcinogenic, but not directly DNA damaging, by increasing the levels of the endogenous damage or by increasing the rate of proliferation or by attenuating the efficiency of these various cell and/or host-mediated cellular repair or elimination processes. Such agents are generally known as non-genotoxic carcinogens and/or co-carcinogens. A highly simplified generic scheme for some of these processes, many

of which are not single events but consist of stepwise changes, is presented in Fig. 1. In this scheme, it is evident that potential carcinogens, could act at several of the stages in carcinogenesis resulting in an increase in genotoxic damage and/or the suppression of cellular and/or host responses. Chemoprotective or chemopreventive agents can also act at one or more stages to suppress carcinogenesis (see Chapter 2.5).

This chapter will consider known human carcinogens, their identification, and the assessment of risk. It will expand on the scheme of Fig. 1 in terms of carcinogen processing and activation, the interactions of genotoxic agents with DNA, including human DNA, and their cellular consequences and the processes involved in multistage carcinogenesis.

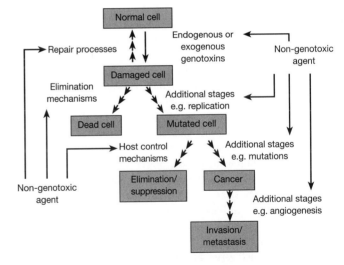

Fig. 1 General scheme for carcinogenesis. A normal cell may become damaged as a result of exposure to genotoxic agents (with or without metabolic activation) or endogenous processes. Cellular control mechanisms may reverse the modifications (repair) or eliminate the damaged cell via programmed cell death. If control at this level fails, the modified cell may survive and replicate to become mutated and further mutational or other changes may result in malignant transformation. Host control mechanisms may eliminate this cell or it might grow as a cancer and, if further control processes are ineffective, become invasive and metastatic and dependent on factors such as angiogenesis. As well as, or instead of acting directly as genotoxins, exogenous or endogenous agents may inhibit or enhance any of the control stages that are normally applied to modified cells. Carcinogenic agents may thus exert genotoxic or non-genotoxic effects or combinations of both.

The authors thank Dr Peter O'Connor and Dr Rhod Elder for reviewing the manuscript and Ian Tannock for his guidance and patience. GPM thanks the CRC for support. We apologize to the authors whose work has not been quoted.

Human carcinogens

Astute clinical observations together with epidemiological studies have shown that certain chemical agents or complex mixtures of agents, usually under conditions of prolonged or repetitive exposure, are carcinogenic in humans. These studies date back to the eighteenth century with the much quoted reports of Hill (snuff takers), Pott (soot exposure in chimney sweep's assistants), and von Soernmering (clay pipe smokers).[1] The evaluation of the carcinogenic risk to humans, initially of individual chemicals, and more recently of complex mixtures of chemicals and other agents such as viruses, parasites, and radiation has been undertaken by a number of organizations. The International Agency for Research on Cancer (IARC) have reviewed more than 800 agents and on the basis of both experimental animal studies and human data, 75 have been evaluated as being carcinogenic to humans.[2] These monographs also contain information on the production and use of the chemical agents and other biologically relevant data such as metabolism, distribution and mutagenicity in short-term tests.

Humans may be exposed to carcinogens through their occupation, environment, diet, lifestyle, or when they are treated for particular diseases. Occupational exposures that are known to cause human cancer include manufacturing processes, in which a specific or individual carcinogenic agent has not been identified (Table 1(a)) and those where cancer is thought to be due to specific chemical agents (Table 1(b)). Occupational cancers are induced in a relatively limited number of tissues, particularly lung, bladder, skin, and nasal cavity. In many cases the causative agents have been identified because of abnormally high levels of occupational exposure or because the agent causes a tumour that is rare. For example, asbestos causes mesothelioma and vinyl chloride, angiosarcoma of the liver. Many of these chemicals (e.g. asbestos, benzene, radon) can also be found in the normal environment but usually at much lower concentrations than in industrial or occupational settings. However, despite concerns aroused when clusters of, typically rare, cancers occur within a restricted geographical area over a limited period of time, there is at present only limited evidence that environmental (i.e. non-dietary, unavoidable non-lifestyle) exposures to chemical agents makes a significant contribution to human cancer. One possible exception to this may be passive smoking. Known 'natural' environmental carcinogens include solar radiation (skin cancer) and radon (lung cancer). Non-chemical human carcinogenic agents such as ionizing (e.g. X-rays) and non-ionizing (ultraviolet light) radiation and viruses are dealt with in Chapters 2.2 and 2.3.

Cancer incidence varies in different populations and, although genetic differences may account for some of this variation, environmental factors, particularly diet, are widely implicated in the modification of cancer incidence. Indeed, dietary components probably cause approximately one-third of all cancer deaths. The link between diet and human cancer has been determined largely by epidemiological studies of, for example, groups with special diets such as vegetarians, or migrant populations moving between regions of differing cancer incidence who attain the cancer incidence of the indigenous population by virtue of shifting to local diets.[3] Carcinogens may be present in the diet as a result of contamination (e.g. aflatoxins which cause liver cancer in humans), food processing (e.g. Chinese-style salted fish, the carcinogenic components of which

have yet to be identified, is a risk factor in nasopharyngeal cancer), or cooking (e.g. carcinogenic heterocyclic amines are formed during the cooking of red meat). However, dietary constituents can also inhibit carcinogenesis caused by chemical agents.[3]–[5] Thus, the relative balance of agents that can cause or inhibit cancer formation may be a key factor in diet-related carcinogenesis.

Tobacco smoke causes cancers not only in the lung, but also in a number of other tissues (bladder, pancreas and upper digestive tract) and smokeless tobacco products are similarly carcinogenic. Betel quid chewing, particularly with tobacco, causes cancers of the oral cavity. Tobacco smoke contains about 50 identified carcinogenic agents so that there is enormous potential for synergistic (and even antagonistic) effects. However, there is increasing evidence that lung cancer is associated primarily with a limited number of agents including polycyclic aromatic hydrocarbons, and bladder cancer with aromatic amines present in cigarette smoke. The relative risk of dying from lung cancer in smokers and the non-smoking spouses of smokers is proportional to the number of cigarettes smoked (Fig. 2)

Other lifestyle exposures, particularly the consumption of alcoholic beverages, have been shown to cause cancer of the oral cavity, pharynx, oesophagus, and liver. Furthermore, heavy alcohol drinking multiplies the risk of cancer from cigarette smoking, particularly the buccal cavity, pharynx, and oesophagus.[8]

A large number of pharmaceutical products, particularly but not exclusively cancer chemotherapeutic agents, cause human cancer in a variety of tissues (Table 2). Tumour type and induction time are related to particular drug or drug combinations used to treat the original tumour or disease[9],[10] and some have characteristic genetic changes (e.g. acute myeloid leukaemia after anthraclins or etoposide). Leukaemias and myelodysplastic syndrome are induced in more than 20 per cent of those Hodgkin's disease patients surviving after treatment, which includes lomustine (CCNU), and it has been estimated that up to 20 per cent of all acute myeloid leukaemia cases are iatrogenic (treatment-induced).[11] In a more recent example, autoimmune disease patients treated with azathioprine have been diagnosed with myelodysplasias and haematological neoplasms.[12] This iatrogenic carcinogenesis is of particular importance in clinical oncology where patients are treated with high doses of genotoxic drugs intended to kill cancer cells. However, it is also pertinent in the treatment of other conditions where specific drugs may be given over prolonged periods.

In the case of cancer, and perhaps also for autoimmune diseases, the patient is likely to have already succumbed to some unidentified aetiological factor that resulted in the induction of the primary tumour or the disease being treated. This may indicate a more general susceptibility that predisposes such patients to iatrogenic carcinogenesis. There are a number of genes with a variety of established and also unknown functions, specific mutations which clearly predispose humans to cancer induction.[13],[14] If such genes are related to susceptibility to iatrogenic cancers, then the treatment of affected patients who have good prospects of long-term survival must be considered carefully. In cancer treatment, there is an increasing use of high dose and adjuvant therapies and increasingly effective management of dose-limiting toxicities in normal tissues.[15] With the concomitant improvement in the long-term survival rates of treated patients, the danger is that the incidence of iatrogenic carcinogenesis and other delayed effects, such as lung fibrosis,[16],[17] are likely to increase.

Table 1 Occupational processes and chemicals found in an occupational setting that cause human cancer[2]

(a) Occupational processes

Process	Tumour site
Aluminium production	lung, bladder
Auramine manufacture	bladder
Boot and shoe manufacture and repair	nasal cavity, bladder
Coal gasification	skin (scrotum), lung, bladder
Coke production	skin (scrotum), lung, bladder
Furniture and cabinet making	nasal cavity
Haematite mining (underground with exposure to radon)	lung
Iron and steel founding	lung
Isopropanol manufacture (strong acid process)	nasal cavity, larynx
Paint (occupational exposure)	oesophagus, larynx, intrahepatic bile ducts
Magenta manufacture	bladder
The rubber industry	haemopoietic system, bladder
Strong inorganic mists containing sulphuric acid	larynx

(b) Chemicals found in an occupational setting

Agent	Tumour site
4-Aminobiphenyl	bladder
Arsenic compounds	skin, lung, liver, bladder, kidney, colon
Asbestos	lung, gastrointestinal tract
Benzene	haemopoietic system
Benzidine	bladder
Beryllium and beryllium compounds	lung
Bischloromethylether	lung
Coal-tars, coal-tar pitches	skin (scrotum), lung
Chromium (VI) compounds	lung
Mineral oils, untreated and mildly treated	skin (scrotum)
Mustard gas	lung, larynx
2-Napthylamine	bladder
Nickel compounds	nasal cavity, lung, larynx
Shale oils	skin (scrotum)
Silica crystalline (quartz, cristobalite)	lung
Soots, tars, and oils	lung, skin (scrotum)
Talc containing asbestiform fibres	lung
2,3,7,8-Tetrachlorodibenzo-p-dioxin	multi-site (lung)
Vinyl chloride	liver, brain, lung, haemopoietic system

Identification of human carcinogens

The incidence of most cancer types in the general population is usually very low and the identification of the aetiological factors involved have required epidemiological studies that have investigated the basis of higher than normal frequencies of certain cancers. These have been attributed to or associated with certain occupations or defined exposure groups (as in the case of pharmaceuticals, see above). In order to reduce the possible risk of cancer from agents of unknown human carcinogenicity, a number of different types of *in vitro* and *in*

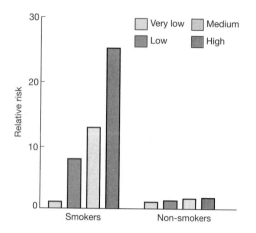

Fig. 2 Relative risk of dying from lung cancer in smokers and non-smokers exposed to spouses cigarette smoke. Data for smokers taken from a cohort of British physicians.[6] Consumption of cigarettes per day: very low = 0; low = 1 to 14; medium = 15 to 24; high = 25 +. Data for non-smokers taken from a cohort study of married non-smoking Japanese women.[7] Husbands' consumption of cigarettes per day: very low, non-smoking husbands; low = 1 to 14; medium = 15 to 19; high = >20.

During the 1960s and 1970s the long-term bioassay was developed to screen chemical agents for their carcinogenic potential. In essence, this involves the exposure of rats and mice (both male and female) to the maximum tolerated dose of the agent for 1 to 2 years. The incidence of tumours occurring in the exposed and control (non-exposed) animals is then determined. Known human carcinogens usually induce tumours under these conditions and the results of lifetime cancer tests in rodents are thus considered an indicator of potential human carcinogenicity. However, as well as using large numbers of animals, such tests are slow and expensive and despite extensive testing, there remain many chemicals that have not been examined in such bioassays. They also assume that the cellular responses occurring in the rodent are similar to those occurring in humans, and this is not always the case. Furthermore, certain cancers appear to be animal-specific. For example, oral administration of a number of different agents induces renal cancers in the male rat through the absorption of the test chemical via a male rat-specific α-2μ-globulin.[18] Whether there are equivalent human-specific mechanisms has not been established.[19]

An additional concern in the interpretation of such data on cancer induction in animals is that the high doses used may result in tissue toxicity. This can induce restorative hyperplasia, a promoting effect (see below) that may increase the frequency with which mutations lead to malignant transformation and cancer. At lower, non-toxic doses, such chemicals may not represent a carcinogenic hazard.[20] Human risk assessment requires an extrapolation of cancer incidence from these high-dose single agent animal studies to the typically

vivo assays that might predict such hazards have been explored: some indication of the potential genotoxicity of a compound may also be obtained from an examination of its chemical structure.

Table 2 Pharmaceutical products that cause human cancer

Agent	Tumour site
Analgesic mixtures containing phenacetin	urinary tract
Azathioprine	haemopoietic system, skin, liver
Busulphan (myleran)	haemopoietic system
Chlorambucil	haemopoietic system
Chlornaphazine	bladder
Cyclosporin	haemopoietic system
Cyclophosphamide	bladder, haemopoietic system
Diethylstilbestrol	uterus, vagina (in offspring)
Melphalan	haemopoietic system
8-Methoxypsoralen and ultraviolet	skin
Methyl CCNU	haemopoietic system
Oestrogen replacement therapy	endometrium
Oestrogens, steroidal	uterus, breast
Oral contraceptives (combined)	liver
Oral contraceptives (sequential)	endometrium
Tamoxifen	endometrium
Thiotepa	haemopoietic system
Treosulphan	haemopoietic system

CCNU = 1-(2-chloroethyl)-3-cyclohexyl-1-nitrosourea.

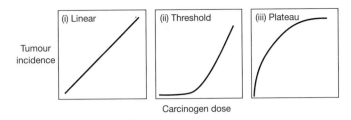

Fig. 3 Dose–response curves for the induction of cancers in experimental animals.[21] Examples of (i) linear and (ii) threshold relationships are observed for liver and bladder tumour induction, respectively, by administration of 2-acetylaminofluorine in the diet. A plateau relationship (iii) is observed for lung tumour induction by 4-(methylnitrosamino)-1-(3-pyridyl)-1-butanone.

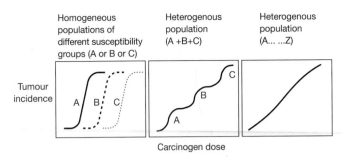

Fig. 4 Theoretical dose–response curves for carcinogenesis in different human populations.[23] Homogeneous populations may show 'classic' response curves while heterogeneous populations may demonstrate a stepwise increase in cancer incidence as a consequence of different susceptibility subgroups. As the number of these subgroups increases, the curve becomes smoother.

much lower dose, and mixed agent, human exposures. It is often assumed that there is a linear relationship between tumour response and exposure. Experimentally, three different types of dose curves have been observed: (i) a linear relationship with a carcinogen dose as seen in the induction of liver tumours by 2-acetylaminofluorene or aflatoxin B_1; (ii) a threshold dose effect as seen in the induction of bladder tumours by 2-acetylaminofluorene; and (iii) a plateau effect at high doses as seen in lung tumour induction by 4-(methyl-nitrosamino)-1-(3-pyridyl)-1-butanaone.[21] (Fig. 3).

Such non-linearities in the relationship between carcinogen dose and tumour incidence may result from the induction or saturation of enzyme activities (metabolic activation, DNA repair, etc.). For human risk assessment, it is generally considered that there is no safe (threshold) dose of a carcinogen. However, the presence of DNA repair mechanisms that have presumably evolved to deal with the potential detrimental effects of endogenous DNA damage (see later) does suggest that in practice there may be a threshold dose for chemical carcinogenesis. This would be the dose that produces damage in excess of that which can be eliminated by the repair system.

Because the human population has considerable interindividual variation in capacity for the metabolic activation of chemical carcinogens and in DNA repair rates,[22] thresholds, although present in individuals, might not be observed in a population. Therefore, collectively there may, in effect, be a linear relationship between tumour incidence and carcinogen dose[23] (Fig. 4).

Screening procedures for the *in vitro* identification of potential carcinogens and mutagens have been developed partly because of the problems associated with long-term bioassays.[24] Still the most widely known procedure is the Ames test which assesses the mutagenicity of chemicals, with or without exogenous metabolic activation systems (see below), usually a cell-free extract of rat liver, in a range of Salmonella bacterial strains engineered to detect specific types of mutations (Fig. 5).

Such assays are rapid and inexpensive but depend upon the property of a carcinogen to cause mutations. Not all mutagens are necessarily carcinogens, and neither are all carcinogens mutagenic in such systems. Mammalian cell mutation assays using the hypoxanthine phosphoribosyl transferase or thymidine kinase gene loci in heterozygous cells are essentially mammalian equivalents of the Ames test but rely more frequently on host cell, rather than exogenous, metabolic activation systems. *In vivo* and *in vitro* genotoxicity, measured as clastogenicity (i.e. damage to chromosomes) can be measured using

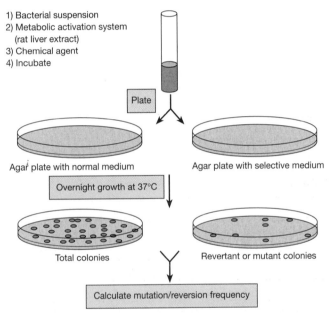

1) Bacterial suspension
2) Metabolic activation system (rat liver extract)
3) Chemical agent
4) Incubate

Plate

Agar plate with normal medium   Agar plate with selective medium

Overnight growth at 37°C

Total colonies   Revertant or mutant colonies

Calculate mutation/reversion frequency

Fig. 5 Schematic representation of the Ames test bacterial mutation assay. The relative mutagenic potencies of an agent is indicated by the number of colonies growing on a plate containing a toxic (selective) agent, relative to those on a non-selective plate. In a forward mutation assay, mutations of various types in one of several genes may give rise to resistant mutants. In a reverse mutation (reversion) assay, the bacteria harbour a gene that contains a defined mutation, often in a synthetic pathway, such that mutations that cause reversion back to the wild-type gene sequence enable the bacteria to grow on the selective medium.

chromosomal aberration and micronucleus assays. Potentially carcinogenic DNA damage that gives rise to 'unscheduled' DNA synthesis (i.e. non-semiconservative, or repair, synthesis) can be quantitated using radiolabelled DNA precursors, frequently using primary rat hepatocytes. More recently, the single-cell gel-electrophoresis technique (called the 'Comet' assay because of the appearance of the DNA) has been used to detect and quantitate DNA strand breaks arising from exposure to genotoxic agents. This assay is increasingly

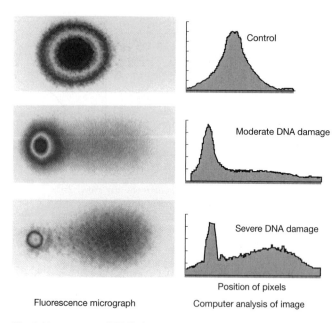

Fluorescence micrograph   Computer analysis of image

Fig. 6 Measurement of DNA damage by the single cell gel electrophoresis 'Comet' assay. Individual cells from chemical agent-treated cultures or animals are embedded in agarose gels, lysed, and subjected to electrophoresis under neutral or alkaline conditions. DNA strand breaks allow the DNA to migrate into the gel to an extent that is proportional to the number of strand breaks and this can be quantitated by computerized image analysis of individual cells in the gel (located by eye). The Y-axes indicate the integrated fluorescence intensity of the pixels on the corresponding micrographs. (See also Plate 1.)

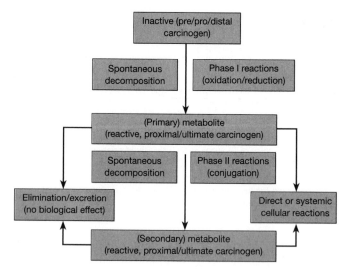

Fig. 7 Overall scheme for 'metabolic activation' of carcinogenic agents. Compounds that undergo spontaneous decomposition are referred to as 'direct-acting' because they do not require processing by cellular metabolic pathways.

used as a screen for genotoxic agents because it is very convenient, employs mammalian and often, human cells as targets and can be applied to *in vivo* exposures (Fig. 6 and see also Plate 1).

Transgenic mice and rats that have exogenous target genes inserted into their genome have been generated to identify and characterize potential human carcinogens *in vivo*. Following treatment of such animals, the DNA is isolated from tissues of interest and processed through bacteriophage. In this way, not only the relative potency (frequency of mutant phage plaques) but also the nature of the mutations induced (determined by DNA sequencing of plaque DNA) can be established. These models are particularly useful in examining tissue-specific genotoxic effects (e.g. ref. 25).

Carcinogen activation

The majority of known chemical carcinogens are unreactive *per se*, but are recognized by cellular enzymes as structural analogues of their physiological substrates and undergo enzymic processing. The normal function of such enzymes is considered to be the detoxification and elimination of potential cellular toxins. These reactions are mediated by so-called phase I enzymes, which generally oxidize or reduce the agent and convert it to a more water-soluble form. This can then be modified by phase II enzymes, which generally conjugate the primary metabolite and facilitate its elimination from the host (Fig. 7). When referring to exogenous chemical carcinogens, such processes are collectively known as 'metabolic activation' and agents

from different chemical classes may undergo both or either phase I and phase II processing. The inactive agents are referred to as pre-, pro-, distal, or indirect carcinogens and the metabolic processes generate intermediates that are called proximal or ultimate carcinogens to indicate that they are the biologically active species. Some agents undergo spontaneous chemical decomposition, usually hydrolysis, to generate active species, and these are referred to as 'direct-acting agents'. Other agents are carcinogenic *per se* without any biochemical intervention (e.g. DNA intercalating agents). The active species are generally short lived and can undergo reactions with many cellular molecules. Most of the reactions probably occur with water molecules in the cell. Reaction also occurs with proteins, lipids, and RNA but it is the reaction with DNA that is likely to have the greatest biological significance (see below).

A large number of enzymes participate in the phase I and phase II pathways of carcinogen metabolism.[26] (Table 3) Cytochrome p450 proteins (**CYP**) are the principal enzymes that catalyse the phase I oxidative metabolism of most endogenous (e.g. prostaglandins, hormones, steroids, aliphatic fatty acids) and exogenous chemicals (drugs, cigarette smoke components). More than 150 CYP enzymes have been identified and these have different substrate specificities with pronounced organ and interindividual differences in expression. The phase II enzymes include glutathione-S-transferases (**GST**), which detoxify metabolites by conjugating them with glutathione to produce hydrophilic products that are readily excreted. Other phase II processes are sulphation, glucuronidation, acetylation, methylation, and amino-acid conjugation. The balance between phase I and phase II enzymes plays a crucial part in determining the formation and fate of the ultimate carcinogen.

The principal site of metabolism is the liver, but many extrahepatic tissues also express the same or related enzymes capable of metabolizing carcinogens. In some cases, the agent can be activated in the liver, conjugated, and then transported to the extrahepatic tissue. Such 'transport' forms may then undergo further metabolism in the

Table 3 Enzymes that are known to be involved in carcinogen metabolism.

Enzyme*	Substrates
CYP1A1	polycyclic aromatic hydrocarbons
CYP1A2	arylamines, heterocyclic amines, aflatoxin B_1
CYP2A6	4-(methylnitrosamino)-1-(3-pyridyl)-1-butanone, *N*-nitrosodimethylamine, aflatoxin
CYP2E1	*N*-nitrosamines, butadiene, benzene, dihaloalkanes, styrene, vinyl chloride, urethane
CYP2D6	many therapeutic drugs, neurotoxins
GSTM1	polycyclic aromatic hydrocarbons, ethylene oxide, styrene
GSTT	dihaloalkanes
GSTP1	polycyclic aromatic hydrocarbons
NAT2	aromatic amines

*CYP, cytochrome P450; GST, glutathione-S-transferase; NAT, N-acetyl transferase.

form of deconjugation so that the target organ for tumour induction need not always be that in which the initial metabolic activation occurs.

Metabolic genotypes and phenotypes

A pivotal study was carried out in 1984, which suggested that individuals who were extensive metabolizes of the drug, debrisoquine, were more susceptible to lung cancer than poor metabolizers.[27] Since then, effort has been directed towards establishing the causes of variation in the levels of the activating enzyme (CYP2D6) and other metabolizing enzymes. A high degree of interindividual variability exists in the expression of these enzymes, partly due to polymorphisms within the encoding genes. Such polymorphisms can result in an absence of functional activity (e.g. GSTT1 and GSTM1), in the production of altered forms of the protein with either reduced or increased activity (e.g. CYP2D6), or in increased protein production (e.g. CYP1A1). Other polymorphisms have been described with unknown functional significance (e.g. CYP2E1) but which have been associated with altered cancer risk. Racial differences in the incidence of such genotypes may be one of the contributory factors underlying the different cancer incidence in different races.[28] Although genetic polymorphisms are associated with altered cancer risk, results from different epidemiological studies are often discordant, in part due to differences in study design.[29]

Cellular reactions of genotoxic agents

Carcinogens or their ultimate reactive species are usually unstable and indiscriminate in their reactions with cellular components: any molecule having a suitable electron configuration may become damaged. Damage to protein molecules is well documented and occurs with particular chemical groups on certain amino acids. Protein function can be affected[30] but in view of the many copies of the protein molecule that are present in cells, reaction with protein is unlikely to have a major biological impact. While a subtle change in a critical protein such as a DNA polymerase, or a protein controlling the expression of a particular gene could influence genome integrity,

relatively little work has been done in this area. Protein damage, particularly to haemoglobin, however, has been exploited as one of the monitors of exposure to carcinogens (e.g. ref. 31).

Direct reaction with lipid molecules is also known to occur. Lipid damage is of increasing interest because a variety of agents are known to induce oxidative stress responses that result in the lipid peroxidation pathway that gives rise to agents such as malondialdehyde that can induce DNA damage.[32]

Reaction with the cellular pool of DNA nucleotide precursors can occur and DNA replication and some pathways of DNA repair may provide opportunities for the incorporation of such damaged nucleotides into DNA (e.g. ref. 33). Enzymes have been identified recently that appear to have evolved specifically to avoid the incorporation of certain oxidized nucleotides into DNA by degrading the damaged DNA precursors.[34] These enzymes can be inhibited by carcinogenic metals which may provide a mechanism of carcinogenesis for such agents.[35] The extent to which nucleotide pool purging processes might also have evolved to prevent incorporation of other endogenously damaged nucleotides remains to be established.

DNA as the critical target for carcinogen action

The majority of chemical carcinogens can damage DNA and are referred to as genotoxic. DNA damage, probably occurring generally throughout the genome rather than in specific genes, can result in cell death and cells that survive exposure may have undergone various types of mutations, some of which may be manifested by inherited changes in specific genes. As there are only two copies of most genes per cell, in contrast to the many copies of most proteins, damage to DNA can be of critical biological importance.

DNA replication

While DNA damage sensors may function to effect cell cycle arrest to prevent replication of a damaged DNA template, they do not do so under all circumstances and replication of damaged DNA can take place. If a viable cell is produced, and the damage results in a change in the base sequence in a critical gene, the cell may acquire a malignant phenotype, usually following additional genetic changes that are a characteristic of genome instability. If this cell escapes any subsequent surveillance and elimination mechanisms, carcinogenesis may be the consequence (see Fig. 1).

Endogenous damage

Under normal physiological conditions, DNA is continuously undergoing damaging reactions.[36] Spontaneous depurination reactions can generate substantial levels of damage, for example between 10 000 and 200 000 base losses per genome per day has been proposed.[37],[38] DNA damage induced by reactive oxygen species, by lipid peroxidation-mediated endogenous aldehyde species, and by alkylating agents has now been demonstrated in DNA in control (non-treated) organisms and even in newborn animals. Indeed, human cells and tissues have been shown to contain sometimes substantial levels of DNA damage arising from such processes (see later) that may contribute to 'spontaneous' (perhaps more accurately, unidentified agent-induced) carcinogenesis. A current estimate suggests that in total approximately one million lesions are induced per genome per day by oxidation, depurination, and deamination.[39] The recent demonstration that certain DNA repair enzymes can act erroneously on normal DNA bases[40],[41] must also be considered as potentially contributing to the pool of endogenous damage.

Other types of endogenous damage can also be present in DNA. The so-called I-compounds,[36] which are adducts of unknown chemical structure, are detected in animal tissue DNA by sensitive procedures (see below) and while these can increase in abundance with animal age they do not increase following carcinogen exposure. This may be a consequence of any or a combination of the following: (i) they do not have the potential to cause adverse biological effects; (ii) cells can tolerate relatively high levels of this damage; (iii) no repair system has evolved to eliminate the damage; or (iv) the repair system is not expressed in the cell type in which the damage exists. Other DNA adducts are suspected to be innocuous because they do not interfere with normal base pairing, at least during DNA synthesis in vitro, are not substrates for any known DNA repair processes, or have not been found to be associated with any adverse cellular biological effects. An example of this would be the products of reaction with DNA phosphate residues (see below).

The DNA repair and damage sensing systems described below appear to have evolved to combat the potential adverse biological effects of DNA damage produced by physiological chemical processes (e.g. hydrolytic depurination) or by agents that are either endogenous (reactive oxygen species) or are present in the 'natural' environment. The latter includes ultraviolet light, ionizing radiation, and oxygen. The possibility that repair systems may also have evolved to deal with other DNA damage induced by naturally occurring chemical agents cannot be discounted.[37]

Exogenous agent-induced damage

The majority of carcinogens either directly, or after spontaneous decomposition or metabolic activation, induce damage in DNA. Initially, because of the relatively low level of adducts generated, DNA binding, and then the identity of DNA adducts were demonstrated by the use of synthetic radiolabelled agents of various kinds. Increasingly, damage-specific monoclonal or polyclonal antibodies and highly sensitive isotopic (e.g. ^{32}P-postlabelling) or non-isotopic methods (e.g. gas chromatography coupled to mass spectrometry, electrochemical, and fluorescence-based methods, membrane-based 'slot' or 'dot' blot methods) are being used directly or sometimes in combination with antibody-affinity enrichment steps (see ref. 42). These methods have the potential to detect specific DNA adducts at levels of approximately 1 adduct per 10^9 or10^{10} normal nucleotides (or even lower), that is one DNA adduct per cell. Damage-specific antibodies can also be used for the detection and quantitation of damage in fixed cells or tissues, that latter providing an assessment of the intracellular distribution of the damage. Some of these techniques are outlined in Fig. 8.

Methods that indicate only if damage is present in DNA, rather than identifying specific damage types, include the Comet and other assays used to screen for carcinogens (see above), pulse or graded electric field gel electrophoresis (both of these more frequently applied to damage detection following attack by reactive oxygen species), and polymerase chain reaction-based methods wherein damage prevents the amplification of DNA by forming non-coding lesions or preventing the passage of DNA polymerase.

The identified sites of reaction of several carcinogens or carcinogen groups with nucleotides in DNA are given in Table 4 and the structures of some of the most studied adducts are shown in Fig. 9 (see also ref. 43). Although certain of the adducts described below are likely to be important in human cancer risk, their quantitative impact is at present, far from being established.[44]

Perhaps the best characterized of the adducts are those resulting from the reaction of the straight chain unsubstituted alkylating agents of which methyl is the simplest and most widely studied. This is partly because representatives of the alkylating agents are direct-acting (i.e. they do not require metabolic activation) and their chemistry is well understood. Synthetic chemistry has therefore been used to prepare markers for identifying adducts produced in DNA in vitro and in vivo. Alkylating agents have thus been shown to react with the nitrogen and oxygen atoms in DNA resulting in 11 different base modifications (Fig. 10). In addition, reaction with the internucleotide phosphate residues results in two phosphotriester stereoisomers. Reaction at the 3'-hydroxyl termini can also occur.[45] Within the alkylating agents, there are differences in the mechanism of the reaction of the ultimate species with DNA that result in widely different relative amounts of the various products formed (considered in greater detail in refs 33 and 46).

While any nucleotide in DNA may be modified, the sequence context of a particular base can affect its reactivity with the attacking species by virtue of differences in electron density of particular sequences. This has been shown mainly with alkylating agents where central guanine residues in runs of guanine residues are found to be more frequently damaged than individual guanines (e.g. ref. 47), although other sequence-specific modifications can involve runs of pyrimidine bases.[48] This might account for mutational 'hot-spots' in genes involved in malignant transformation. Chromosome fragile sites may represent a special case of sequence-specific damage.

The initial damage to DNA may be followed by various spontaneous chemical reactions. These include: the hydrolytic loss of the modified base to generate apurinic or apyrimidinic sites, purine imidazole ring, and pyrimidine ring opening, DNA strand breaks and interstrand and/or intrastrand DNA cross-linking. Examples of agents generating the latter are the clinically used halo-substituted alkylating agents (e.g. CCNU and bischloroethylnitrosourea (BCNU)). These are probably cytotoxic principally via the formation of G:C DNA interstrand cross-links. However, while such cross-links are proposed as the lethal lesions, the molecular events leading to cell death have

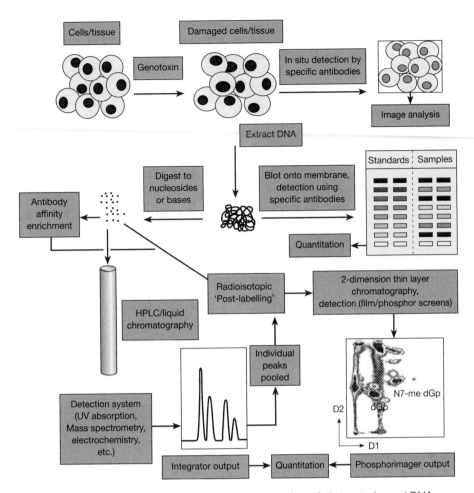

Fig. 8 Summary of some of the methodology applied for the detection and quantitation of specific lesions in damaged DNA.

yet to be defined. Furthermore, whether or not such cross-links can, in surviving cells, be responsible for malignant transformation or other late effects of treatment is also unclear.

The complexity of DNA damage produced by alkylating agents is probably exceeded only by agents that introduce oxidative damage into DNA. Ionizing radiation has usually been used to generate and characterize these lesions sometimes using pure nucleoside or nucleotide targets in aqueous solution. Here too the relative amounts of the various products can vary according to the damaging species. Chemical agents inducing similar damage include hydrogen peroxide, menadione, and other quinone-based agents, bleomycin, and lactams. As well as the direct DNA damage that such agents introduce into DNA, the lipid peroxidation cascade can produce additional DNA damage via degradation products such as malondialdehyde.

For most of the other classes of carcinogens, fewer reaction products in DNA have been identified (Table 4). However, for the alkylating agents, some of the minor but biologically significant products were originally not detected or identified because of their instability or the relatively small amounts generated. Therefore, unidentified minor products of the reaction of other agents with DNA may also emerge to be biologically important.

Certain oestrogens can cause genetic alterations through the formation of DNA damaging intermediates, modulating the formation of endogenous and/or dietary mutagenic agents or by binding to microtubules which disrupts tubulin assembly and induces aneuploidy.[49] However, hormones can affect carcinogenesis by epigenetic events such as the stimulation of cell proliferation and the heritable reprogramming of cellular differentiation. These events may be mediated by receptor-ligand binding.

In summary, there is usually a variety of DNA damage types arising as a consequence of exposure to single agents. Given that (i) endogenous damage is continuously generated, (ii) simultaneous exposure to multiple exogenous genotoxic agents damaging agents is essentially unavoidable, and (iii) any agent might also induce collateral damage via oxidation and/or lipid peroxidation pathways, the pattern of DNA damage in living cells is potentially enormously complex.

Human DNA damage

Adducts in DNA or other forms of DNA damage, have been detected in every human tissue examined (see Fig. 11).[50]

The levels of DNA damage observed as a result of non-iatrogenic exogenous exposures (e.g. in cigarette smokers) is of the order of 1 adduct per 10^7 to 10^9 normal DNA bases whereas that arising from endogenous exposures (e.g. reactive oxygen species) may be several orders of magnitude higher.[36],[50] There is considerable variation in

Table 4 Reaction sites of carcinogens with DNA

Carcinogen	Site of adduct formation[a]				
	G	**A**	**C**	**T**	**Phosphate**[b]
aflatoxin	**N7**				
4-aminobiphenyl	**C8**, N^2	C8			
benzene	1, N^2	1, N^6	3, N^4		
benzidine	**C8**, N^2				
2-napthylamine	**C8**, N^2	N^6			
vinyl chloride	**N7**, N^2, O^6	1, N^6	3, N^4		
ethylene oxide	**N7**, O^6	N3, N7, N1, N^6	N3	N3	
styrene oxide	**N7**, O^6, N^2	N1, N3, N^6	N3, N4, O^2	N3, $O4$	+
benzo[a]pyrene	N^2, N7	N^6	N^4		
acrolein	1,N^2				
IQ (2-amino-3-methylimidazo[4,5-f]quinoline)	**C8**, N^2				
PhIP (2-amino-1-methyl-6-phenylimidazo[4,5-b]pyridine)	**C8**, N^2				
Alkylating agents[c]	N3, **N7**, O^6	N1, N3, N7	O^2, N3	N3, O^2, O^4	+

[a] Normal font indicates reaction within a ring structure; italics and superscripts indicate reaction at an exocyclic group and the position of that group on the ring. Bold font indicates the most prevalent lesions.

[b] Indicates that reaction with phosphate residues has been demonstrated.

[c] Monofunctional agents of the general structure C_nH_{2n+1}. Bifunctional and polyfunctional agents are also known. Note: alkylating agents are often used as a clinical term to denote any compound that reacts with DNA.

the levels of adducts between different populations and indeed between different individuals. Mean levels of 8-hydroxydeoxyguanosine (formed predominantly by endogenous processes) in DNA from white blood cells have been reported to vary between about 0.1 and 40 adducts per 10^5 deoxyguanosine residues, that is a variation of approximately 400-fold. In contrast, the mean levels of bulky adducts in DNA from white blood cells of non-smokers varied from 0.2 to 7 adducts/10^8 normal nucleosides.[50] The levels of DNA adducts reflect not only the initial exposure but also a number of host factors, which are themselves subject to interindividual variation. These include the absorption of the carcinogen, its metabolic activation and deactivation (see above) and DNA repair activity (see below). Differences in sampling and analytical procedures may also account, in part, for such variation.[50]

Populations and individuals with high DNA adduct levels in a particular tissue may be at increased cancer risk and there is some epidemiological evidence to support this. Thus individuals living in Shanghai, China, who excreted AFB_1-N7-guanine adducts in their urine had almost a 10-fold higher risk of developing liver cancer than non-excretors.[51] The presence of DNA adducts in human tissues indicates that exposure to a particular agent has occurred and thus constitutes a risk factor in carcinogenesis. The quantitation of adducts may also be useful in identifying genetic and environmental factors that may influence adduct levels and, potentially, cancer risk. It would also allow an assessment of the effectiveness of intervention studies aimed at reducing the associated risk.

Consequences of DNA damage

One of the most challenging problems in understanding the mechanism of action of carcinogens has been to establish if particular biological responses can be attributed to a specific type of lesion in DNA. More recently, the question has become whether or not such a lesion is present in specific sequence(s) of a gene that is a critical target for carcinogenesis. The presence of mutations in oncogenes and tumour suppressor genes has been taken as evidence that DNA adducts were responsible for the mutations induced. However, it has been shown that such mutations can exist in target tissue DNA prior to carcinogen exposure and in this, and therefore possibly other, cases the carcinogen may act as a promoting agent (see below). Previously, the role of specific lesions was studied by isolation of DNA from treated cells or tissues and quantification of the individual lesion in relation to the endpoint being measured (e.g. induction of cancer[45]). Increasingly, specific antibodies are allowing lesions to be identified and quantified in tissue sections (see Fig. 8) and hence the events in individual cells are being examined in relation to their response to genotoxic agents.

The biochemical properties of individual lesions in DNA can also be examined *in vitro* using DNA that has been engineered or synthesized to contain a single modification, often in a specific nucleotide sequence. Such DNA is used to examine the coding properties of the lesion and its processing by purified proteins, crude cell extracts or following introduction into cultured mammalian cells. More recently,

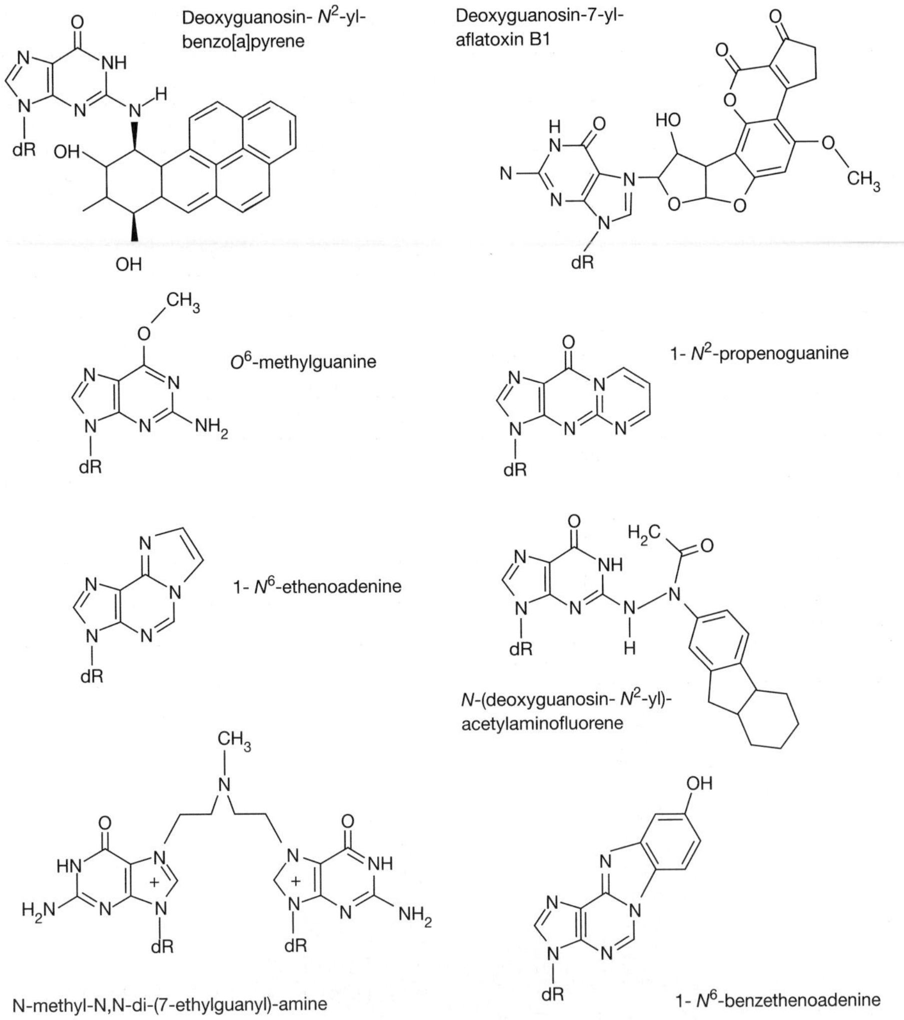

Fig. 9 Chemical structures of some of the commonly studied DNA lesions. Representative structures formed by the reaction of various carcinogens including the hydrocarbons (benzo[a]pyrene), aflatoxin-B1, the alkylating agents (methylating agents such as N-nitrosodimethylamine, chloroethylating agents such as vinyl chloride and malondialdehyde, a product of lipid peroxidation and the DNA cross-linking agent, nitrogen mustard), acetylaminofluorene, and the human carcinogen, benzene are shown. dR indicates the site of attachment to deoxyribose in DNA.

single gene deleted ('knockout') animals are being produced by targeted homologous recombination in embryonic stem cells in order to determine the contribution of specific gene products both to normal physiological development and to the biological effects of specific carcinogens. Increasingly such strains are also being cross-bred with other knockout strains to probe the effect of multiply deficient genotypes.[52],[53]

Cellular responses to DNA damage are presented in broad view in Fig. 12. DNA damage produced by endogenous or exogenous agents may be recognized by various cellular proteins. Recognition by damage sensor proteins may result in a series of events that ultimately increases the survival prospects of the cell or host by causing the recruitment and/or upregulation of DNA repair proteins, cell cycle arrest, and/or programmed cell death. Despite these protective systems, DNA replication can occur across a template that is damaged and, depending on the coding properties of the damage in

the template, this can result in duplex DNA that may contain a gapped or mutated daughter strand and persisting damage in the template strand. As mentioned, damaged nucleoside triphosphates might also be incorporated into DNA during replication and damage in the daughter strand may then be present. These DNA structures can invoke post-replicational cellular responses such as cell cycle arrest or cell death, but if another round of DNA replication occurs, a permanent change in the DNA base sequence may result. There are apparently no pathways for the repair of such heritable mutations presumably because they do not have any recognizable structural abnormalities.

Many of these processes, particularly damage sensing and cell cycle arrest, are under intense study and current understanding is likely to change as more factors and interactions are discovered. Nevertheless, some of the consequences of DNA damage are explored in greater detail below.

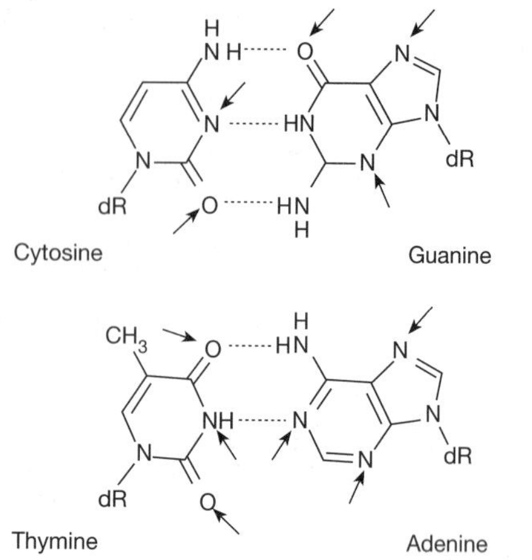

Alkylation product	N-Alkyl-N-nitrosourea	
	Methyl	Ethyl
3-Alkylguanine	<1	<1
O⁶-Alkylguanine	~6	~7
7-Alkylguanine	~65	~13
O²-Alkylcytosine	<1	<1
3-Alkylcytosine	<1	<1
O²-Alkylthymine	<1	~5
3-Alkylthymine	<1	<1
7-Alkylthymine	<1	~5
1-Alkyladenine	~2	~1
3-Alkyladenine	~7	~6
7-Alkyladenine	~2	~1
Phosphotriesters	~20	~70

Fig. 10 Sites of reaction of the potent carcinogenic alkylating agents, *N*-methyl-nitrosourea and *N*-ethyl-*N*-nitrosourea with DNA C:G and T:A base pairs. The inset indicates the relative amounts of the various products formed as a percentage of the total, figures in bold indicating the most abundant lesions.

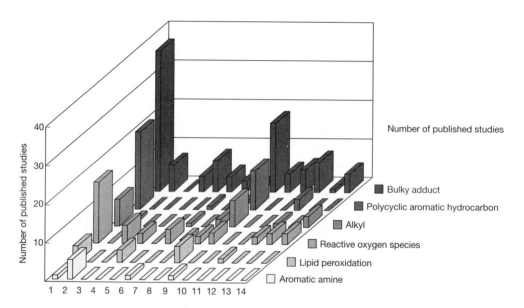

Fig. 11 Summary of the numbers of studies in which various types of DNA damage have been detected in DNA isolated from a wide range of human tissues.[50] 1, Blood; 2, bladder; 3, brain; 4, breast; 5, cervix; 6, colon; 7, kidney; 8, liver; 9, lung; 10, oral cavity; 11, pancreas; 12, placenta; 13, sperm; and 14, stomach.

Damage sensing and its consequences

An increasing number of genes are known to function as DNA damage sensors and subsequently to promote DNA repair and/or cell cycle arrest and/or cell death (see Figs 1 and 12). The precise mechanisms by which these pathways are invoked are still being elucidated, but they are determined by orchestrated intimate and highly specific protein–protein contacts and chemical modifications, principally phosphorylations. The archetypal sensor of DNA damage is the tumour suppressor gene p53, which has been termed the 'guardian of the genome' because of its ability to orchestrate other events. However, the picture is becoming less clear as the roles of other gene products are elucidated. Thus ATM, the gene mutated in

ataxia telangiectasia has been proposed as a sensor of oxidative damage[54] and it phosphorylates p53. However, it also interacts with many other protein factors and has thus been referred to as a hierarchical kinase.[55] DNA-dependent protein kinase binds to DNA double strand breaks in DNA and may phosphorylate p53. The products of the breast cancer susceptibility genes BRCA1 and BRCA2 have been implicated in cell cycle control and DNA repair and BRCA1 is required for transcription-coupled repair (see below) of oxidative damage in DNA.[56] Also, the carboxy-terminal regions of BRCA1 and BRCA2 interact with RAD51, suggesting a role in recombination repair (see below). The nuclear matrix, acting as a scaffold on which various components of the damage sensing and repair pathways may

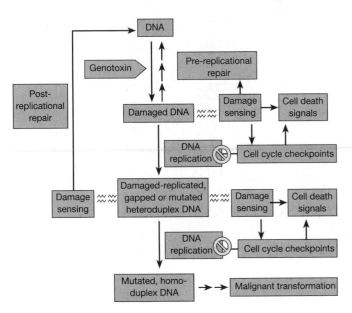

Fig. 12 Simplified view of the consequences of DNA damage. In this scheme the genotoxin can be either exogenous or endogenous and may also influence the other processes shown (see Fig. 1). A barred circle at the end of a line indicates inhibition of a process.

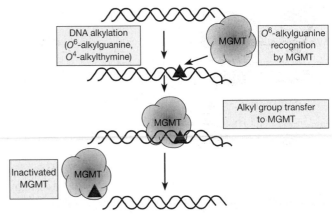

Fig. 13 Damage reversal by O^6-methylguanine-DNA-methyltransferase (MGMT). Repair is achieved by transfer of the alkyl group to a cysteine residue in the highly conserved pentapeptide PCHRV/I at the active site of the protein. O^6-alkylguanine-DNA-alkyltransferase-mediated repair is unique inasmuch as it does not involve breakage of the phosphodiester backbone in DNA.

reside or be recruited to has also been implicated to have a role in damage processing (e.g. ref. 57).

DNA repair

Many of the initial and secondary chemical changes introduced by chemical agents into DNA are recognized by cellular proteins that identify the size, shape, and charge of damage structures or the helix distortion they cause in DNA. It is these characteristics, as 'sensed' by a particular damage detection system or repair protein that determine if the damage is a suitable potential substrate for a particular repair enzyme or system, which then acts on the damage.[58] Where damaged is detected by sensors, these recruit appropriate repair proteins to the damage site. The repair processes, however, should be viewed as flexible and with overlapping substrate specificity rather than mutually exclusive, indeed the same substrate may be processed by two different repair pathways (e.g. ref. 59). As elaborated above, genotoxins generally produce a wide spectrum of DNA damage consisting of different lesions that can be repaired by different pathways. In some cases, binding of the repair protein to the damage can occur but subsequent steps can be slow if the chemical bonds that need to be modified are not in suitable positions. With the possible exception of the I-compounds (see above) the repair processes probably restore the vast majority of endogenously damaged DNA to its pre-damaged state. This is perhaps less likely to be the case with exogenously generated damage, given that the damage may sometimes be more abundant and less efficiently repaired because of substantial structural differences to endogenously produced damage.

There is very extensive information on the proteins currently known to be involved in the various DNA repair processes, their substrates, and inhibitors, their interactions with other cellular components, and the encoding genes and their expression. The components of some of the pathways have been identified by investigations

of patients with genetic predispositions to cancer that often involve increased sensitivity to ultraviolet or ionizing radiation as a consequence of defects in DNA damage processing (see Chapter 2.3 and Table 5). New information is continuously appearing and the current state of the art is presented in brief summary below.

Adduct removal/DNA damage reversal

A wide variety of alkyl group structures can be removed from the O^6-position of guanine or less efficiently from the O^4-position of thymine in DNA.[58] The protein molecule responsible operates by the stoichiometric transfer of the alkyl group to a cysteine residue in the active site of the protein itself, restoring the base to its predamaged state (Fig. 13). Because the protein is inactivated in the process, it is not a true enzyme and additional repair requires the *de novo* synthesis of new active protein.

The human version of the protein is called O^6-methylguanine-DNA-methyltransferase,[59] but because of its broad substrate specificity, is frequently referred to as O^6-alkylguanine-DNA-alkyltransferase. O^6-alkylguanine-DNA-alkyltransferase overexpressing mice are more resistant and null mutant ('knockout') mice are highly sensitive to carcinogenesis by appropriate alkylating agents.[60],[61] There is interest in clinical exploitation of this protein in cancer chemotherapy involving alkylating agents that kill cells via the formation of damage at the O^6-position of guanine in DNA. Possible approaches include tumour sensitization by inhibition of repair activity[62] or normal tissue protection, using gene therapy.[63]

Base excision repair

In the base excision repair pathway, the damaged base is recognized by one of a number of glycosylases (reviewed in Cunningham 1997[57] and Singer and Hang 1997[64]). These are true enzymes that generally act on low molecular weight DNA adducts (as opposed to higher molecular weight or 'bulky' lesions), purine or pyrimidine ring fission products and G:T and G:U mismatched bases produced by deamination of 5-methylcytosine and cytosine, respectively.

Table 5 Human syndrome genes involved in cancer predisposition and/or DNA repair

Syndrome (complementation group)	Gene
Xeroderma pigmentosum (A, B, C, D, E, F, G, and V)	XPA, XPB, XPC, XPD, XPE, XPF, XPG, and XPV
Cockayne's syndrome (A and B)	CSA and CSB
Trichothiodystrophy	TTD
Breast cancer susceptibility	BRCA1, BRCA2
Wilm's tumour	WT1
Ataxia telangiectasia	ATM
Autoimmune diseases	Ku70, Ku80
Familial adenomatous polyposis	APC
Fanconi's anaemia (8 complementation groups)	*FA-A, FA-C, FA-G
Gorlin's (basal cell naevus) syndrome	PTCH
Hereditary non-polyposis colorectal cancer	hMSH2, hMLH1, PMS1, PMS2
Li–Fraumeni	p53
Nijmegen breakage syndrome	NBS
Retinoblastoma	RB1
Severe combined immune deficiency	†DNAPKcs
Werner's syndrome	WRN
Bloom's syndrome	BLM

*Also known as FANCA, FANCC, and FANCG.

†cs = catalytic subunit.

The glycosylase hydrolyses the glycosylic bond between the damaged base and the deoxyribose residue, releasing the base and generating an apurinic or apyrimidinic site. The glycosylase can then be displaced by the apurinic apyrimidinic endonuclease, HAP1. This enzyme also recognizes apyrimidinic sites generated by spontaneous or damage-mediated base losses. HAP1 incises the DNA strand 5′ to the sugar ring. Repair can then proceed by alternative pathways of 'short patch' repair (Fig. 14), involving insertion of a single nucleotide, and 'long patch' involving the insertion of four to nine nucleotides. The enzyme, poly-adenosine-diphosphate-ribose polymerase, which binds to single and double strand nicks in DNA, may play a part in these processes.[65]

In short patch repair, the 5′-deoxyribose phosphate residue can be removed by the 5′-deoxyribose phosphodiesterase activity of DNA polymerase β. In other cases, glycosylases may have an AP-lyase activity that converts the deoxyribose ring to the aldehyde form, which is then acted upon by the 3′-phosphodiesterase activity of HAP1, or may also possess a function that removes the deoxyribose phosphate residue. These processes generate a suitable template for gap filling by insertion of a single nucleotide. DNA polymerase β then binds XRCC1 which recruits DNA ligase III to seal the remaining single-strand break. Reconstitution experiments have shown that the resulting gap is again filled by the DNA pol β pathway (Fig. 14).

Long patch repair is dependent upon proliferating cell nuclear antigen (**PCNA** (a homotrimeric protein likely forming a 'clamp' around the DNA)) and DNA polymerase δ. Reconstitution experiments show that the PCNA-dependent pathway also requires replication factor C (a heteropentameric protein), to load PCNA and DNA polymerase δ on to the DNA template, and flap endonuclease 1. This pathway results in the synthesis of a longer patch size of about six nucleotides causing the displacement of a short stretch of DNA, which is cleaved by flap endonuclease 1. Finally, the gap is sealed by DNA ligase I rather than XRCC1/DNA ligase III.

Nucleotide excision repair

Lesions that cause more substantial DNA helix distortion, classically thymine dimers (i.e. cross-linking of adjacent thymine bases caused by ultraviolet light) but also others such as the higher molecular weight 'bulky' adducts produced by polycyclic aromatic hydrocarbons[66] or inter and intrastrand DNA cross-links[67] are generally substrates for the nucleotide excision repair system. The factors involved in nucleotide excision repair differ in the initial stages according to whether or not it is acting generally upon DNA damage throughout the genome (global genome repair) or coupled to gene transcription (transcription-coupled repair). Several proteins, both singly and in combination, have been implicated in the initial step of damage recognition and confirmation, including XPA, RPA, XPE, and XPC-hHR23B.

Global genome repair

In one current model, global genome repair is initiated by the XPC–hHR23B protein complex. This recognizes the damage and this is 'confirmed' by the single strand binding protein XPA.[68] TFIIH is then recruited to the site. TFIIH is a complex of nine individual

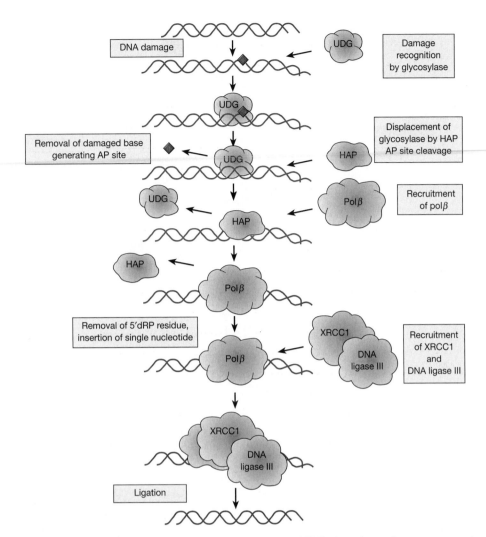

Fig. 14 Repair of DNA damage by the 'short patch' pathway of base excision repair. Uracil DNA glycosylase is shown as an example of the glycosylase enzyme initiating the process. Poly-adenosine-diphosphate-ribose polymerase, not shown in this scheme, may be involved prior to the DNA polymerase binding step in temporary gap sealing and repair factor recruitment.

proteins and two of its subunits, XPB and XPD are $3' \rightarrow 5'$ and $5' \rightarrow 3'$ DNA helicases, respectively. These unwind the DNA at the damaged site and facilitate access to other components of the pathway, while RPA (a heterotrimeric protein) binds to the undamaged strand, possibly to prevent nuclease action. This is followed by recruitment of the repair endonucleases, XPG and XPF–ERCC1, the endonuclease functions of which incise the phosphodiester backbone about six nucleotides 3' to the damage (XPG) followed by a second incision about 25 nucleotides 5' to the damage (ERCC1–XPF). This results in the removal of an approximately 30-nucleotide fragment (depending on the size and position of the lesion) containing the lesion. The resulting gap is filled by the concerted action of replication factor C, which then recruits PCNA. PCNA itself then recruits DNA polymerase δ or ε which fills the gap and then DNA ligase I, which rejoins the DNA strands. A consensus pathway is presented in Fig. 15. Recent reviews describe this process in more detail.[69],[70]

Transcription-coupled repair

Mutation induction by genotoxic agents is biased towards the non-transcribed strand of DNA and this is a consequence of more efficient repair of the transcribed strand via the coupling of NER to transcription. Transcription-coupled repair occurs when gene transcription by RNA polymerase II is stalled by a DNA lesion, usually considered to be one that causes helix distortion. The XPA protein may be involved in confirming that damage is present and repair is initiated by the transcription factor TFIIH. The Cockayne's syndrome group B (also known as ERCC6) and Cockayne's syndrome group A genes may be required for this process. The *hMSH2* and *BRCA*-1 gene products are required for the transcription-coupled repair of oxidative damage and the *hMLH1* or *hMSH2* gene products (see below) are needed for the repair of ultraviolet damage. The repair pathway then proceeds as described for global genome repair.

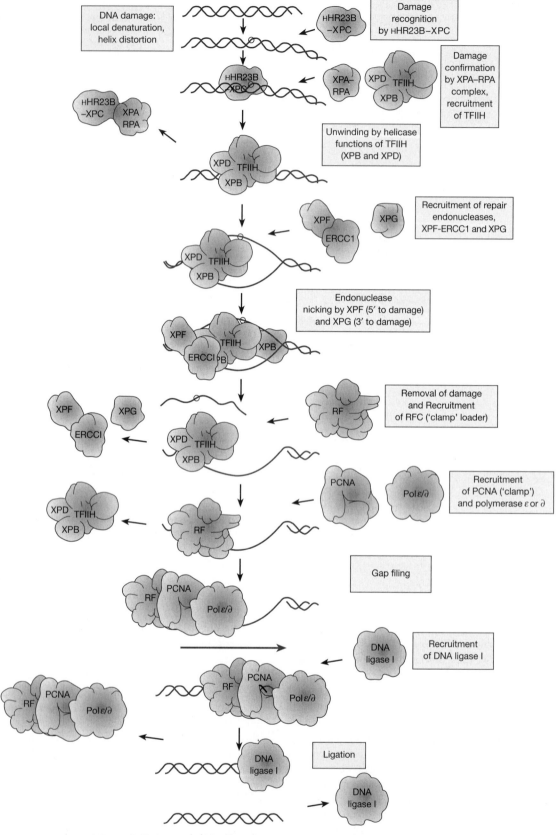

Fig. 15 Repair of DNA damage by the global genome repair pathway for nucleotide excision repair.

Postreplication mismatch repair

Following DNA replication of damaged DNA or of repetitive regions of undamaged DNA, structures can be produced that are substrates for the postreplication mismatch repair system (reviewed in Jiricny 1998[71] and Kolodner and Marsischky 1999[68]). This involves a number of gene products hMSH2, hMSH3, hMLH1, hPMS1, hPMS2, and hMSH6 (also known as the guanine-thymine mismatch binding protein) that operate to initiate strand-specific repair of DNA replication errors, including those produced by certain DNA adducts such as O^6AG (O^6-alkylguanine). Base–base mismatches or single base insertions are recognized by the hMSH2–hMSH6 heterodimer (**hMutSα**), while heteroduplexes containing two to four extra bases are substrates for the hMSH2–hMSH3 heterodimers (**hMutSβ**), although both hMSH6 and hMSH3 can operate independently in these processes. hMutSalpha also recognizes heteroduplexes containing cisplatin and O^6-methylguanine lesions. Mismatched bases and DNA up to 1 kb away from the mismatch are excised and while PCNA is implicated in this pathway, the precise nature of the excision, polymerization, and ligation steps have not yet been defined.

Recombination repair

Double strand breaks can be generated in DNA by oxidative damage, particularly ionizing radiation, and by attempts to replicate across single strand breaks in DNA. Repair of double strand breaks can be by homologous recombination repair or non-homologous (or 'illegitimate') end joining.[73],[74] The former is mediated by Rad51, Rad52, and Rad54 and may occur mainly in the late S/G$_2$ stage of the cell cycle. The gene mutated in AT (ATM) may be the initial damage sensor, phosphorylating c-Abl (and also p53). This in turn phosphorylates Rad51 enabling its interaction with Rad52 and thus the adenosine triphosphate-dependent pairing and strand exchange between homologous DNA molecules, which is stimulated by RPA. BRCA1 and BRCA2 are also needed for activation of homologous recombination. Non-homologous end joining can occur via two pathways: Ku70/Ku80/DNAPK$_{catalytic subunit}$, which appears to be the main pathway in invertebrates acting in the G$_1$/early S phase and the P95 (Nibrin, Nbs1) Mre11/Rad50 complex. Flap endonuclease 1 is also involved, as is Ligase IV, XRCC4, and probably Cockayne's syndrome group A and group B. In one model, Ku directs double strand breaks into the non-homologous end joining repair pathway, whereas Rad52 initiates repair by homologous recombination. However, the molecular interactions occurring during most of the repair processes described here are highly complex and much has yet to be resolved. Thus, the Fanconi's anaemia genes also appear to be involved in the fidelity of double strand break rejoining.[75]

Mutation

Despite the numerous repair systems present in cells to deal with DNA damage, heritable mutations can occur. Mutations are broadly defined as permanent changes in the base sequence of DNA and they can arise by the replacement, deletion, or insertion of DNA bases or the rearrangement, deletion, or amplification of DNA sequences.

Changes involving single base substitutions are point mutations. If they occur in protein coding regions, an abnormal amino acid may be encoded or a translation termination or novel initiation codon (non-sense mutations) might result. This may lead to the synthesis of an abnormal (mutated or truncated) protein molecule. Insertion or deletion of single or multiple bases can result in a change in the open reading frame of the encoded cDNA (frameshift mutations) that can also result in abnormal or truncated proteins. Small changes of this type occurring in the non-coding regions may result in incorrect splicing of pre-messenger RNA. Changes in the regulatory regions may influence the binding of regulatory or transcription molecules thus influencing the overall levels of protein expression. More extensive changes occur if long stretches of DNA are deleted or illegitimate sections of DNA are recombined and this can result in the complete loss of protein function or more subtle changes involving the loss of binding or functional domains. Gene amplification is a special case of mutation in which a large number of copies of a segment of DNA is produced.

In human tumours, the presence of a particular type of mutation, and its position within the mutated gene, may be a specific marker of exposure for a particular carcinogen and implicate specific base adducts as causative.[76] For example, dietary aflatoxin exposure has been correlated with a GC-TA transversion at codon 249 in p53 during liver carcinogenesis. Population differences in p53 mutational spectra may suggest different aetiological agents. In Qidong (China), the majority of hepatocellular tumours have a GC-TA transversion consistent with exposure to aflatoxin. However, in other areas of China, Japan, and Taiwan, tumours have a much lower prevalence of this specific mutation suggesting that other exposures are important.[77] GC-TA transversions, particularly at codons 157, 248, and 273, are common mutagenic events in lung tumours obtained from smokers. These mutations have a coding (non-transcribed) strand bias, which has been linked to the transcription-coupled repair of polycyclic aromatic hydrocarbon DNA-adducts formed in the transcribed strand.[76]

Much of the damage to total cellular DNA may be inconsequential as the majority of DNA is non-coding and has only a structural role. Of the coding and regulatory regions, there are two classes of genes, the proto-oncogenes or cellular oncogenes and the tumour suppressor genes, mutations in which appear to be prerequisites for carcinogenesis (see Chapter 1.3). Oncogenes have been identified over the past two decades as normal cellular homologues of the transforming oncogenic genes of viruses that are often involved in signal transduction pathways: mutation of a single copy of these genes usually results in a dominant phenotype. The normal function of the tumour suppressor genes seems to be to suppress the emergence of transformed cells and hence cancers; here homozygous mutation is usually required for transformation. Although changes in such genes are critical, it is increasingly accepted that mutations, or even phenotypic variations in expression of DNA repair genes, can attenuate cellular capacities for DNA repair and can result in increased mutation in oncogenes or tumour suppressor genes. In this context, repair genes are also a class of tumour suppressor genes.

Mutations of the type involving large deletions or recombination can result in visible changes in chromosome structures, including sister chromatid exchanges, rearrangements/translocations and deletions, and polyploidy and aneuploidy. These are very common in human cancers and may be mediated by recombination repair pathways.

Multistage carcinogenesis

In animal models of skin carcinogenesis, certain agents can cause critical changes in target cells that are insufficient to cause cancer;

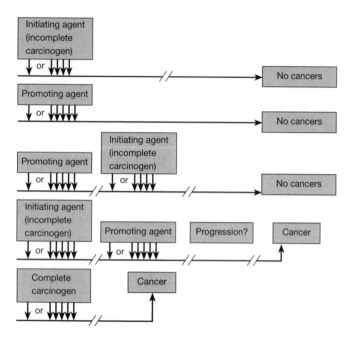

Fig. 16 Classical schemes of two-stage carcinogenesis. No tumours are generated if an initiator or promoter is administered alone or if the promoter is administered before the initiating agent. However, cancers are generated by administration of a promoter following an initiator or by a complete carcinogen. The scheme is further complicated by the reports of stage I and stage II promoters.

however, cancers can arise from such cells following repetitive administration of another agent that is not itself a carcinogen. This has given rise to the concept of initiators and promoters (or co-carcinogens) in carcinogenesis. A third stage, referred to as progression, has been ascribed to the transition from benign papilloma to malignant carcinoma. However, single applications of, usually, large and often toxic doses of single agents (chemicals or radiation) can be sufficient to induce cancers in animals. Here, the changes induced within the target cells that undergo transformation and possibly other host cells are more complex and extensive so that all of the prerequisites for carcinogenesis, including cell replication, are fulfilled after one exposure. In the two-stage hypothesis, such agents are considered 'complete' carcinogens, that is, they are able to act both as initiators and promoters (Fig. 16). This may be the situation in iatrogenic carcinogenesis in patients being treated for cancer and certain other diseases who have undergone single agent chemotherapy or radiotherapy, particularly with high-dose regimens, and in individuals who have been victims of industrial accidents or exposures. Paediatric and possibly adolescent cancers might also be a consequence of single or brief *in utero* exposure to genotoxic agents.

While initiators have been considered to be genotoxic agents and promoters non-genotoxic agents, the situation is clearly more complex as promoting agents have been shown to induce genotoxic damage or to increase the levels of endogenously produced damage. Promoters have also been considered to be general irritants and toxins that can kill cells and result in restorative hyperplasia. If a cell population contains 'spontaneously' (i.e. endogenously) mutated cells that have relative resistance to the toxic effects of the agent, this promoting effect can result in selective expansion of this population.

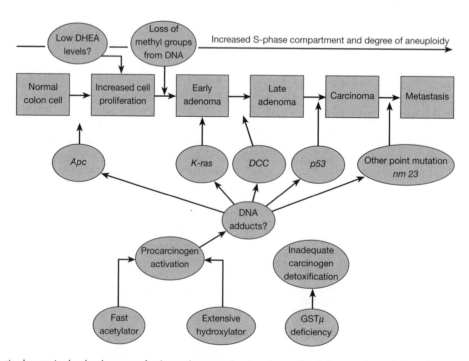

Fig. 17 Events and genetic changes in the development of colorectal cancer, showing the possible influence of metabolism phenotypes on DNA adduct formation and its contribution to the changes involved. Apc: adenomatous polyposis coli gene, DCC: deleted in colorectal carcinogenesis gene. (Adapted from Fearon and Vogelstein.[78])

In general, however, cancer in humans is most likely to be the consequence of multiple exposures to a combination of initiating/carcinogenic and promoting/co-carcinogenic agents, and their antagonists, over a protracted period of time. Mathematical analysis of the age-dependent increase in incidence of human tumours suggests that cancers arise as a multistep process requiring between 4 and 7 independent events. Thus tumorigenesis occurs in a series of stages that can be characterized by specific alterations in oncogenes and tumour suppressor genes involved in cell cycle control, cell signalling, DNA repair, and other processes. An example of this is presented in Fig. 17, which shows the progression of normal colonic cells through the various recognized stages to the appearance of metastatic colorectal cancer.

Conclusions

Chemical carcinogenesis in humans is a highly complex, multistep, multicomponent, and multifactorial process. The application of our increased understanding of chemical carcinogenesis and the development of new analytical procedures will help to identify those populations and individuals that are at increased cancer risk. Reducing the human cancer burden will require, for the majority of the population and at all stages of life, reduction of exposure to carcinogenic agents and the identification of populations/individuals at increased cancer risk, long before the tumour is clinically detectable. The possibility that specific diets or dietary components may be anticarcinogenic or protective by attenuation of the carcinogen activating systems and enhancement of the resistance mechanisms may be exploitable to reduce the impact of unavoidable exposures. However, tobacco is a good example of an avoidable risk and despite, or perhaps more accurately, because of, efforts by certain members of society, this carcinogen continues to make a major, but avoidable, contribution to the cancer burden in humankind.

References

1. Redmond DE Jr. Tobacco and cancer: the first clinical report, 1761. *New England Journal of Medicine*, 1970; **282**: 18–23.

2. *IARC Monographs on the Evaluation of the Carcinogenic Risk of Chemicals to Humans; 1970 to 1998.* Lyon, France: IARC.

3. World Cancer Research Fund/American Institute for Cancer Research. *Food nutrition and the prevention of cancer: a global perspective.* Washington: AICR, 1997.

4. Doll R. Nature and nurture: possibilities for cancer control. *Carcinogenesis*, 1996; **17**: 177–84.

5. Stewart BW, McGregor D, Kleihues P (eds). *Principles of chemoprevention.* IARC Scientific Publications No. 139. Lyon: IARC, 1996.

6. Doll R, Peto R. Mortality in relation to smoking: 20 years' observations on male British doctors. *British Medical Journal*, 1976; **2**: 1525–36.

7. Hirayama T. Non-smoking wives of heavy smokers have a higher risk of lung cancer: a study from Japan. *British Medical Journal*, 1981; **282**: 183–5.

8. *IARC monograph of the evaluation of the carcinogenic risk of chemicals to humans. Tobacco smoking.* IARC Scientific Publications No. 38. Lyon: IARC, 1986.

9. Gerson SL. Molecular epidemiology of therapy-related leukemias. *Current Opinion in Oncology*, 1993; **5**: 136–44.

10. Andersen MK, Johansson B, Larsen SO, Pedersen-Bjergaard J. Chromosomal abnormalities in secondary MDS and AML. Relationship to drugs and radiation with specific emphasis on the balanced rearrangements. *Haematologica*, 1998; **83**: 483–8.

11. Karp JE, Smith MA. The molecular pathogenesis of treatment-induced (secondary) leukemias: foundations for treatment and prevention. *Seminars in Oncology*, 1997; **24**: 103–13.

12. Kwong YL, Au WY, Liang RH. Acute myeloid leukemia after azathioprine treatment for autoimmune diseases: association with -7/7q-. *Cancer Genetics and Cytogenetics*, 1998; **104**: 94–7.

13. Knudson AG. Hereditary predisposition to cancer. *Annals of the New York Academy of Sciences*, 1997; **833**: 58–67.

14. Sarasin A, Stary A. Human cancer and DNA repair-deficient diseases. *Cancer Detection and Prevention*, 1997; **21**: 406–11.

15. Pettengell R. Expanding the role of blood progenitor cells. *Annals of Oncology*, 1995; **6**: 759–67.

16. O'Driscoll BR, Kalra S, Gattamaneni HR, Woodcock AA. Late carmustine lung fibrosis. Age at treatment may influence severity and survival. *Chest*, 1995; **107**: 1355–7.

17. Andrieu JM, *et al.* Ten-year results of a strategy combining three cycles of ABVD and high-dose extended irradiation for treating Hodgkin's disease at advanced stages. *Annals of Oncology*, 1998; **9**: 195–203.

18. Flamm WG, Lehman-McKeeman LD. The human relevance of the renal tumor-inducing potential of d-limonene in male rats: implications for risk assessment. *Regulatory Toxicology and Pharmacology*, 1991; **13**: 70–86.

19. Ashby J. The alpha2u-globulin discussion. *Environmental Health Perspectives*, 1998; **106**: A126.

20. Ames BN, Gold LS. Chemical carcinogenesis: too many rodent carcinogens. *Proceedings of the National Academy of Sciences USA*, 1990; **87**: 7772–6.

21. Poirier MC, Beland FA. DNA adduct measurements and tumor incidence during chronic carcinogen exposure in animal models: implications for DNA adduct-based human cancer risk assessment. *Chemical Research in Toxicology*, 1992; **5**: 749–55.

22. Perera FP. Molecular epidemiology: insights into cancer susceptibility, risk assessment, and prevention. *Journal of the National Cancer Institute*, 1996; **88**: 496–509.

23. Lutz WK. Dose-response relationship and low dose extrapolation in chemical carcinogenesis. *Carcinogenesis*, 1990; **11**: 1243–7.

24. Ashby J, Morrod RS. Detection of human carcinogens. *Nature*, 1991; **352**: 185–6.

25. Dean SW, Brooks TM, Burlinson B, Mirsalis J, Myhr B, Recio L, Thybaud V. Transgenic mouse mutation assay systems can play an important role in regulatory mutagenicity testing *in vivo* for the detection of site-of-contact mutagens. *Mutagenesis*, 1999; **14**: 141–51.

26. Idle JR, *et al.* The pharmacogenetics of chemical carcinogenesis. *Pharmacogenetics*, 1992; **2**: 246–58.

27. Ayesh R, Idle JR, Ritchie JC, Crothers MJ, Hetzel MR. Metabolic oxidation phenotypes as markers for susceptibility to lung cancer. *Nature*, 1984; **312**: 169–70.

28. Garte S. The role of ethnicity in cancer susceptibility gene polymorphisms: the example of CYP1A1. *Carcinogenesis*, 1998; **19**: 1329–32.

29. d'Errico A, Taioli E, Chen X, Vineis P. Genetic metabolic polymorphisms and the risk of cancer: a review of the literature. *Biomarkers*, 1996; **1**: 149–73.

30. Kroes RA, Abravaya K, Seidenfeld J, Morimoto RI. Selective activation of human heat shock gene transcription by nitrosourea antitumor drugs mediated by isocyanate-induced damage and activation of heat shock transcription factor. *Proceedings of the National Academy of Sciences USA*, 1991; **88**: 4825–9.

31. **Wild CP, Pisani P.** Carcinogen DNA and protein adducts as biomarkers of human exposure in environmental cancer epidemiology. *Cancer Detection and Prevention*, 1998; **22**: 273–83.

32. **Janero DR.** Malondialdehyde and thiobarbituric acid-reactivity as diagnostic indices of lipid peroxidation and peroxidative tissue injury. *Free Radical Biology and Medicine*, 1990; **9**: 515–40.

33. **Saffhill R, Margison GP, O'Connor PJ.** Mechanisms of carcinogenesis by alkylating agents. *Biochimica et Biophysica Acta*, 1985; **832** (Cancer Reviews) 111–45.

34. **Yakushiji H, et al.** Biochemical and physicochemical characterization of normal and variant forms of human MTH1; protein with antimutagenic activity. *Mutation Research*, 1997; **384**: 181–94.

35. **Porter DW, Yakushiji H, Nakabeppu Y, Sekiguchi M, Fivash MJ Jr, Kasprzak KS.** Sensitivity of *Escherichia coli* (MutT) and human (MTH1) 8-oxo-dGTPases to *in vitro* inhibition by the carcinogenic metals, nickel(II), copper(II), cobalt(II) and cadmium(II). *Carcinogenesis*, 1997; **18**: 1785–91.

36. **Marnett LJ, Burcham PC.** Endogenous DNA adducts: potential and paradox. *Chemical Research in Toxicology*, 1993; **6**: 771–85.

37. **Lindahl T.** Endogenous damage to DNA. *Philosophical Transactions of the Royal Society of London Series B Biological Sciences*, 1996; **351**: 1529–38.

38. **Nakamura J, Swenberg JA.** Endogenous apurinic/apyrimidinic sites in genomic DNA of mammalian tissues. *Cancer Research*, 1999; **59**: 2522–6.

39. **Holmquist GP.** Endogenous lesions, S-phase-independent spontaneous mutations, and evolutionary strategies for base excision repair. *Mutation Research*, 1998; **400**: 59–68.

40. **Berdal KG, Johansen RF, Seeberg E.** Release of normal bases from intact DNA by a native DNA repair enzyme. *EMBO Journal*, 1998; **17**: 363–7.

41. **Nicolas E, Beggs JM, Haltiwanger BM, Taraschi TF.** A new class of DNA glycosylase/apurinic/apyrimidinic lyases that act on specific adenines in single-stranded DNA. *Journal of Biological Chemistry*, 1998; **273**: 17216–20.

42. **Poirier MC.** DNA adducts as exposure biomarkers and indicators of cancer risk. *Environmental Health Perspective*, 1997; **105** (Suppl. 4): 907–12.

43. **Hemminki K, Dipple A, Shuker DEG, Kadlubar FF, Segerback D, Bartsch H.** *DNA adducts: identification and biological significance.* IARC Scientific Publications No. 125. Lyon: IARC, 1994.

44. **Nestmann ER, Bryant DW, Carr CJ.** Toxicological significance of DNA adducts: summary of discussions with an expert panel. *Regulatory Toxicology and Pharmacology*, 1996; **24**(1 Pt 1): 9–18.

45. **Margison GP, O'Connor PJ.** Biological consequences of reactions with DNA: Role of specific lesions. In Grover PL, Phillips DH (eds). *Chemical carcinogenesis and mutagenesis. Handbook of experimental pharmacology*, Vol. 94/1. Heidelberg: Springer, 1990; 547–71.

46. **Margison GP, O'Connor PJ.** Nucleic acid modification by N-nitroso compounds. In: Grover PL (ed.). *Chemical Carcinogenesis and DNA.* Vol. 1. Florida: CRC Press, 1979; 111–59.

47. **Hartley JA, Gibson NW, Kohn KW, Mattes WB.** DNA sequence selectivity of guanine-N7 alkylation by three antitumor chloroethylating agents *Cancer Research*, 1986; **46**: 1943–7.

48. **Broggini M, et al.** DNA sequence-specific adenine alkylation by the novel antitumor drug tallimustine (FCE 24517), a benzoyl nitrogen mustard derivative of distamycin. *Nucleic Acids Research*, 1995; **23**: 81–7.

49. **Huff J, Boyd J.** Barrett JC. *Cellular and molecular mechanisms of hormonal carcinogenesis: environmental influences.* New York: Wiley-Liss, 1996.

50. **Povey AC.** DNA adducts: endogenous and induced. *Toxicologic Pathology*, 2000; **29**: 405–14.

51. **Ross RK, et al.** Urinary aflatoxin biomarkers and risk of hepatocellular carcinoma. *Lancet*, 1992; **339**: 943–6.

52. **Friedberg EC, Meira LB, Cheo DL.** Database of mouse strains carrying targeted mutations in genes affecting cellular responses to DNA damage. *Mutation Research*, 1997; **383**: 183–8.

53. **Balmain A, Nagase H.** Cancer resistance genes in mice: models for the study of tumour modifiers. *Trends in Genetics*, 1998; **14**: 139–44.

54. **Rotman G, Shiloh Y.** The ATM gene and protein: possible roles in genome surveillance, checkpoint controls and cellular defence against oxidative stress. *Cancer Surveys*, 1997; **29**: 285–304.

55. **Lavin MF, Concannon P, Gatti RA.** Eighth international workshop on ataxia-telangiectasia. *Cancer Research*, 1999; **59**: 3845–9.

56. **Gowen LC, Avrutskaya AV, Latour AM, Koller BH, Leadon SA.** BRCA1 required for transcription-coupled repair of oxidative DNA damage. *Science*, 1998; **281**: 1009–12.

57. **Bouayadi K, van der Leer-van Hoffen A, Balajee AS, Natarajan AT, van Zeeland AA, Mullenders LH.** Enzymatic activities involved in the DNA resynthesis step of nucleotide excision repair are firmly attached to chromatin. *Nucleic Acids Research*, 1997; **25**: 1056–63.

58. **Singer B, Hang B.** What structural features determine repair enzyme specificity and mechanism in chemically modified DNA? *Chemcal Research and Toxicology*, 1997; **10**: 713–32.

59. **Tano K, Shiota S, Collier J, Foote RS, Mitra S.** Isolation and structural characterization of a cDNA clone encoding the human DNA repair protein for O^6-alkylguanine. *Proceedings of the National Academy of Sciences USA*, 1990; **87**: 686–90.

60. **Sakumi K, Shiraishi A, Shimizu S, Tsuzuki T, Ishikawa T, Sekiguchi M.** Methylnitrosourea-induced tumorigenesis in MGMT gene knockout mice. *Cancer Research*, 1997; **57**: 2415–18.

61. **Kawate H, et al.** Separation of killing and tumorigenic effects of an alkylating agent in mice defective in two of the DNA repair genes. *Proceedings of the National Academy of Sciences USA*, 1998; **95**: 5116–20.

62. **Dolan ME, Pegg AE.** O6-benzylguanine and its role in chemotherapy. *Clinical Cancer Research*, 1997; **3**: 837–47.

63. **Rafferty JA, et al.** Chemoprotection of normal tissues by transfer of drug resistance genes. *Cancer and Metastasis Reviews*, 1996; **15**: 365–83.

64. **Cunningham RP.** DNA glycosylases. *Mutation Research*, 1997; **383**: 189–96.

65. **Le Rhun Y, Kirkland JB, Shah GM.** Cellular responses to DNA damage in the absence of Poly(ADP-ribose) Polymerase. *Biochimemical and Biophysical Research Communications*, 1998; **245**: 1–10.

66. **Braithwaite E, Wu X, Wang Z.** Repair of DNA lesions induced by polycyclic aromatic hydrocarbons in human cell-free extracts: involvement of two excision repair mechanisms *in vitro*. *Carcinogenesis*, 1998, **19**: 1239–46.

67. **Chen ZP, et al.** Evidence for nucleotide excision repair as a modifying factor of O^6-methylguanine-DNA methyltransferase-mediated innate chloroethylnitrosourea resistance in human tumor cell lines. *Molecular Pharmacology*, 1997; **52**: 815–20.

68. **Sugasawa K, et al.** Xeroderma pigmentosum group C protein complex is the initiator of global genome nucleotide excision repair. *Molecular Cell*, 1998; **2**: 223–32.

69. **Wood RD, Shivji MK.** Which DNA polymerases are used for DNA-repair in eukaryotes? *Carcinogenesis*, 1997; **18**: 605–10.

70. **Lehmann AR.** Dual functions of DNA repair genes: molecular, cellular, and clinical implications. *Bioessays*, 1998; **20**: 146–55.

71. **Jiricny J.** Eukaryotic mismatch repair: an update. *Mutation Research*, 1998; **409**: 107–21.

72. **Kolodner RD, Marsischky GT.** Eukaryotic DNA mismatch repair. *Current Opinion in Genetic Development*, 1999; **9**: 89–96.

73. **Jeggo PA.** Identification of genes involved in repair of DNA double-strand breaks in mammalian cells. *Radiation Research*, 1998; **150** (Suppl. 5): S80–91.

74. **Kanaar R, Hoeijmakers JH, van Gent DC.** Molecular mechanisms of DNA double strand break repair. *Trends in Cell Biology,* 1998; **8:** 483–9.

75. **Escarceller M, *et al.*** Fanconi anemia C gene product plays a role in the fidelity of blunt DNA end-joining. *Journal of Molecular Biology,* 1998; **279:** 375–85.

76. **Greenblatt MS, Bennett WP, Hollstein M, Harris CC.** Mutations in the p53 tumor suppressor gene: clues to cancer etiology and molecular pathogenesis. *Cancer Research,* 1994; **54:** 4855–78.

77. **Lasky T, Magder L.** Hepatocellular carcinoma p53 G→T transversions at codon 249: the fingerprint of aflatoxin exposure? *Environmental Health Perspectives,* 1997; **105:** 392–7.

78. **Fearon ER, Vogelstein A.** Genetic model for colorectal tumorigenesis. *Cell,* 1990; **61:** 759–67.

2.2 Viral carcinogenesis

Chris Boshoff

Introduction

A substantial burden of human cancer worldwide is attributable to infection. Viral infections account for approximately 15 per cent of all human cancers. Cervical cancer, hepatocellular carcinoma, and Kaposi's sarcoma (**KS**), all caused by viruses, are some of the most important tumours in sub-Saharan Africa.

Leukaemia in chickens was first transmitted by 'an agent that passed through a filter' in 1908 and in 1911 Rous demonstrated the acellular transmission of a sarcoma.[1] In the 1930s Shope discovered oncogenic papillomaviruses in rabbits and in 1951 Gross discovered the first murine leukaemia virus. SV40 was discovered by Hilleman in 1960 as a contaminant of poliovirus vaccine grown in monkey kidney cultures. In 1964 Epstein, Achong, and Barr described a new human herpesvirus in Burkitt's lymphoma cell lines and this was the first link of a virus to a human cancer. At least four viral groups are now implicated in causing human cancer, i.e. hepatitis B virus (**HBV**), human T-cell leukaemia virus (**HTLV**-1), papillomaviruses, and gamma herpesviruses (Epstein–Barr virus (**EBV**) and KS-associated herpesvirus). Table 1 summarizes some of the major events of the twentieth century that contributed to our current understanding of the role of viruses in tumorigenesis.[1]–[13]

The insight that tumour viruses has provided into the regulatory control of cell division and intracellular signal transduction are even more important than the worldwide burden of viral-induced cancer: RNA splicing was discovered in DNA tumour viruses; oncogenes were first conceptualized and described in retroviruses; and the p53 tumour suppressor gene was first described as a protein that became bound to and sequestered by SV40 T antigen.

The interface between infection and malignancy is highlighted by the cancers prevalent in acquired immune deficiency syndrome (**AIDS**) (Table 2, see also Chapter 15.15). Human immunodeficiency virus (**HIV**)-infected individuals are specifically prone to cancer caused by viruses, e.g. EBV (lymphomas), papillomaviruses (squamous

Table 1 Chronological list of major discoveries of tumour viruses

Scientist/s (date/place)	Finding
Ellerman and Bang (1908/Copenhagen)	Transmitted by filtrates the erythromyeloblastic form of chicken leukaemia.
Rous (New York)	Transmitted first solid tumour, a chicken sarcoma, by a filtrate.
Shope (1933/New Jersey)	Transmitted rabbit papilloma by filtrates.
Bittner (1936/Maine)	Reported that the mouse mammary carcinoma agent is transmitted through the milk of nursing female mice.
Gross (1951/New York)	Discovered the mouse leukaemia virus.
Stewart and Eddy (1957/NIH)	Propagated the mouse parotid tumour virus, isolated by Gross in 1953, called it 'polyoma virus' and showed that it can induce tumours in mice, rats, and hamsters.
Friend (1956/New York)	A filterable agent could be passed serially in young weanling mice, inducing a leukaemia-like syndrome.
Sweet and Hilleman (1960)	Isolation of the 'vacuolating agent' from normal rhesus kidney cells.
Eddy (1962/NIH)	Virus present in normal rhesus monkey kidney cells (SV40), can induce sarcomas in new-born hamsters.
Trentin (1962/Houston)	Human adenovirus type 12 induces sarcomas in new-born hamsters.
Epstein, Achong, Barr (1964/London)	Virus particles shown in cultured lymphoblasts from Burkitt's lymphoma.
Churchill and Biggs (1967/London)	Discover the agent causing chicken neurolymphomatosis (Marek's disease).
Melèndez (1967/USA)	Isolation of *herpesvirus saimiri* from a squirrel monkey.
Gallo (1980/NIH)	Discovered viral production by a human T-cell leukaemia virus cell line (HTLV-1).
Chang and Moore (1994/New York)	Identify HHV-8 sequences by molecular technique in AIDS-KS biopsies.

Table 2 Tumours increased in patients with AIDS

Cancer type	Relative risk+	Viral link
Kaposi's sarcoma	310	HHV-8
Non-Hodgkin's lymphoma	113	EBV
Angiosarcoma	37	?
Anal cancer*	32	HPV
Leukaemias other than lymphoid and myeloid	11.0	?
Hodgkin's disease	8	?EBV
Leiomyosarcoma and other soft tissue sarcomas**	7	?EBV
Multiple myeloma	4.5	?
Primary brain cancer***	3.5	Papovaviruses
Testicular seminoma or malignant germinoma	2.9	?

+Adapted from ref. 90.

*Anal carcinoma is increased in gay men, even prior to HIV infection.

**EBV sequences described in smooth-muscle tumours from children with AIDS, including monoclonal EBV episomes in some cases.

***Predominantly malignant glioma or astrocytoma. The detection of papovavirus sequences in brain tumours remains unconfirmed.

EBV: Epstein–Barr virus.

HHV-8: Human herpesvirus-8.

HPV: Human papillomavirus.

carcinomas of skin and anogenital carcinoma), and KS-associated herpesvirus (lymphomas, multicentric Castleman's disease, and KS). The tumours with an increased incidence in HIV-infected individuals where a virus has not yet been described (Table 2) could still have a viral aetiology (unknown or known virus infection). Carcinogenesis is a multifactorial process and only a fraction of individuals infected with oncogenic viruses will develop a tumour, particularly in the absence of immunosuppression. Certain tumours with a known viral aetiology (e.g. nasopharyngeal and hepatocellular carcinoma) are not increased in AIDS, indicating that viral infection and immunosuppression, without co-factors, are not enough to precipitate the specific cancer. However, efficacious immunization against the primary infection would virtually eliminate the occurrence of the tumour with which the virus is associated. An effective vaccine against hepatitis B is available, whereas vaccines against EBV and human papilloma viruses are currently in clinical studies.

The oncogenic viruses are very diverse and include nearly all major families of DNA viruses that infect vertebrates (Table 3). DNA tumour viruses have been essential tools in dissecting out cellular transformation pathways. Of the RNA viruses, only retroviruses and the hepatitis C virus are implicated in tumorigenesis. Most tumorigenic retroviruses are members of the oncovirus subfamily and, of the genera in this subfamily, the most important is the type C virus genus: these include the mouse leukaemia and sarcoma viruses, feline leukaemia virus, avian leukosis viruses, bovine leukosis virus, and the human T-cell leukaemia/lymphoma viruses.[14]

Mechanisms of viral oncogenesis

The main feature of all tumour viruses is the ability to drive cellular proliferation that is not inhibited by the normal cellular or immune control mechanisms. This feature can be through direct or indirect mechanisms (Fig. 1).

When viruses enter cells, the cellular responses are comparable with that seen when oncogenes are transfected into cells: apoptosis, cell cycle arrest and/or increased host cell immunity; For example, the expression of oncogenic ras in primary human or rodent cells results in permanent G_1 arrest and is accompanied by accumulation of p53 and p16. Viruses employ countermeasures to these cellular responses to overcome cellular defence mechanisms[15] (see also Chapter 1.3).

A common strategy among oncogenic viruses is to provide their host cells with additional growth stimuli, thereby extending their proliferative capacity. Viral oncogenes can deregulate cell cycle control mechanisms by interfering with receptor-mediated signal transduction pathways and the function of nuclear cell cycle regulatory proteins (see Chapter 1.5). Several DNA viruses, for example, encode proteins which specifically target and inhibit both the retinoblastoma protein (**pRb**) and the p53 tumour suppressor pathways, involved in cell cycle regulation and apoptosis respectively[16] (Table 4 see also Chapter 1.6). By overriding growth-suppressive signals which control cell-cycle progression in untransformed cells, viruses promote the progression into the S-phase of the cell cycle (DNA synthesis), which is probably necessary for efficient replication of their viral genome.[16] A consequence of the deregulated progression through the cell cycle may be unlicensed cellular proliferation and ultimately transformation.

The induction of apoptosis is a common response of the host cell to viral infection. Deregulation of the host cell cycle machinery by viral-encoded proteins, leads to the upregulation of the tumour suppressor p53 which in turn activates genes encoding for proteins that mediate apoptosis such as Bax, Bik, and others of this family.[17] The p53 protein may also upregulate expression of death receptors such as CD95 (Fas, Apo-1) together with its ligand CD95L (FasL), which signal a cell to apoptose in response to signals from cytotoxic T lymphocytes or via an autocrine mechanism induced by soluble CD95L produced by the infected cell[18] (see also Chapter 1.6). It is therefore not surprising that some DNA tumour viruses encode proteins that can sequester and inactivate p53. In addition, some oncogenic human and primate herpesviruses encode homologues of cellular antiapoptotic proteins (i.e. bcl-2, interleukin (**IL**)-10, bcl-10, and FLICE inhibitory protein (**FLIP**)). Viral-encoded FLIP (**vFLIP**) is a new class of protein that interferes with apoptosis signalled through death receptors. vFLIPs are present in several herpesviruses and are also encoded by an oncogenic human pox virus.[18],[19] A cellular FLIP has also been identified.[20] Cellular and viral FLIPs act to inhibit an apoptosis pathway and cells expressing vFLIPs are protected against apoptosis induced by CD95 or by the tumour necrosis factor receptor.[21]

Our understanding of how viruses transform cells is advancing rapidly. It is well known that the tumour suppresser pRb (the retinoblastoma protein) is often a target of oncogenic viral proteins. The histone deacetylase HDAC1 forms a complex with pRb to repress the function of transcription factors and thereby inhibiting cell proliferation. Recently, it was shown that different viral oncoproteins

Table 3 Oncogenic DNA viruses

Virus family	Virus	Size	Host	Associated tumour	Associated risk factors
Hepadnavirus	Hepatitis B	3 kb	Primates, woodchucks	Liver cancer	In humans: alcohol, smoking, fungal toxins, hepatitis C virus
Papovavirus	SV40	5 kb	Monkey	Sarcomas (in rodents) ?Mesotheliomas (humans)*	Smoking, asbestos exposure
	Papilloma	7–8 kb	Human	Warts: anogenital, laryngeal, skin Anogenital carcinoma Skin, laryngeal, oesophageal carcinomas**	Immunosuppression Smoking, immunosuppression Sunlight, X-irradiation, immunosuppression
Adenovirus	Types 2,5,15	30–50 kb	Human	None in humans Hamsters: sarcomas	
Herpesvirus	EBV	130–250 kb	Human	Burkitt's lymphoma Post-transplant lymphoproliferation Nasopharyngeal carcinoma AIDS lymphoma ?Hodgkin's disease ?Smooth muscle tumours ?Gastric carcinoma	Malaria Immunosuppression Diet, HLA genotype HIV/immunosuppression Immunosuppression Immunosuppression
	HHV-8		Human	Kaposi's sarcoma Primary effusion lymphoma Plasmablastic variant of MCD	Immunosuppression, HIV (?Tat protein), ?HLA genotype

MCD, multicentric Castleman's disease.

*Controversial polymerase chain reaction (PCR) detection of SV40 sequences in this human tumour have been reported. It is suggested that the poliovirus vaccine, contaminated with SV40, introduced this agent into human populations.

**Although human papilloma virus (HPV) sequences have been detected in these squamous cell tumours, no causal link has yet been established.

such as papillomavirus E7, adenovirus E1A, and EBV nuclear antigen (EBNA)-5 can all disrupt the interaction between pRb and HDAC1,[22],[23] allowing transcription factors to initiate cell division.

Gamma herpesviruses

'*herpein*' Greek (to creep or crawl) refers to the characteristic skin lesions caused by herpes simplex and herpes zoster infections.

> O'er ladies lips, who straight on kisses dream,
> Which oft the angry Mab with blisters plagues,
> Because their breaths with sweetmeats tainted are.
> Shakespeare
> Romeo and Juliet c. 1595

Nearly 100 herpesviruses have been identified and almost all mammalian species have been shown to be infected by at least one member of the family. The known herpesviruses share a common virion architecture (Fig. 2) and four critical biological properties:

(1) all herpesviruses encode a large variety of enzymes involved in nucleic acid metabolism, DNA synthesis, and protein processing;

(2) the synthesis of viral DNA and assembly of the capsid occur mainly in the nucleus of infected cells;

(3) production of infectious virus progeny is generally accompanied by destruction of the infected cell (lytic infection);

(4) herpesviruses remain latent and persist for life in their hosts. Latent infection occurs in specific cell types which vary between viral types. The latent viral genomes take the form of circular episomes with only a fraction of viral genes expressed.

Members of the subfamily of gamma herpesviruses are characterised by their capacity to induce cell proliferation *in vivo*, resulting in transient or chronic lymphoproliferative disorders. They are large double-stranded DNA viruses and can infect and persist in lymphocytes. Gamma herpesviruses are widely disseminated in nature causing infection and disease in many species.

Epstein–Barr virus

EBV is the prototype of gamma herpesviruses. EBV is a highly transforming virus and EBV-infected B lymphocytes are highly immunogenic and elicit powerful cytotoxic T-cell lymphocyte responses[24] (Fig. 3). However, only a fraction of EBV-infected individuals will develop EBV-associated tumours and despite the interaction between autologous EBV-infected B cells and CD8+ T lymphocytes (i.e. cytotoxic T-cell lymphocyte), EBV persists in B lymphocytes. These two apparent paradoxes occur because of the downregulation of all growth transforming-associated viral proteins, which include those known to elicit cytotoxic T-cell lymphocyte responses, in persistently infected B lymphocytes.[25] Only EBV EBNA-1 is expressed in these cells. EBNA-1 is essential to maintain the stability and proliferation of the viral episome (unintegrated viral DNA)[26] and does not evoke an immune response. EBV-specific

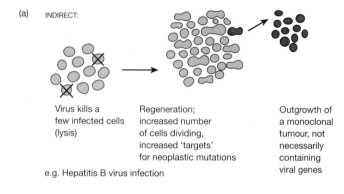

(a)   INDIRECT:

Virus kills a
few infected cells
(lysis)

Regeneration;
increased number
of cells dividing,
increased 'targets'
for neoplastic mutations

Outgrowth of
a monoclonal
tumour, not
necessarily
containing
viral genes

e.g. Hepatitis B virus infection

(b)   DIRECT:

Viral encoded protein initiates and maintains tumour growth

1. Viral oncogene is derived from normal cellular counterpart: (protooncogene)

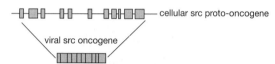

cellular src proto-oncogene

viral src oncogene

e.g. The viral oncogene of Rous sarcoma virus (v-src) is derived from many exons of the cellular src (c-src) proto-oncogene.

2. Viral oncogene has no related normal cellular counterpart:

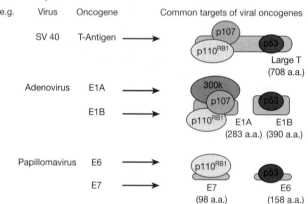

e.g.	Virus	Oncogene	Common targets of viral oncogenes
	SV 40	T-Antigen	p107, p110^{RB1}, p53, Large T (708 a.a.)
	Adenovirus	E1A	300k, p107, p110^{RB1}, E1A (283 a.a.)
		E1B	p53, E1B (390 a.a.)
	Papillomavirus	E6	p110^{RB1}, E7 (98 a.a.)
		E7	p53, E6 (158 a.a.)

3. Insertional mutagenesis:

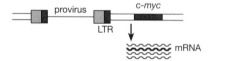

provirus   c-myc

LTR

mRNA

Provirus (e.g. avian leukaemia virus, ALV), is located upstream of the cellular *myc* gene. Viral long terminal repeat (LTR) is being used as a promoter for the transcription of high levels of *myc* gene messenger RNA.

Fig. 1 Mechanisms of viral oncogenesis.

cytotoxic T-cell lymphocytes are targeted against human leucocyte antigen (HLA) class 1-associated peptides derived from the EBNAs and the latent membrane proteins, with the notable exception of

EBNA-1. The choice of the viral target depends on the HLA phenotype of the responder.[27] A sufficient variety of immunogenic peptides can be presented by the HLA spectrum to provide immunosurveillance against uncontrolled growth of virally transformed immunoblasts.

In vitro, EBV infection of primary B lymphocytes efficiently induces continuous proliferation and transformation into permanent cell lines (called lymphoblastoid cell lines). These lymphoblastoid cell lines normally contain multiple episomal copies of the EBV genome.[28] Of the approximately 100 viral genes, only 13 genes are expressed in lymphoblastoid cell lines including the six nuclear proteins (EBNA-1 to -6), three membrane proteins (latent membrane proteins 1 to 3), and two non-translated RNAs (EBER 1 and 2) (reviewed in ref. 29). These transformation-associated viral proteins regulate the maintenance of episomal viral DNA and viral gene expression, drive cellular proliferation directly and through the transactivation of cellular oncogenes, and block apoptosis.

EBNA-1 is essential for the maintenance of the EBV genome in proliferating cells, whereas the other EBNAs and the latent membrane proteins are required for the transcriptional regulation, growth transformation and immortalization of infected B cells[29] (Fig. 3). EBNA-1 is required for the controlled replication of the EBV genome and is expressed in all known latently infected cells, irrespective of the cellular phenotype. EBNA-2 activates transcription of the viral latent membrane protein-1 and -2A genes as well as cellular genes, such as the proto-oncogene c-*fgr* and the gene encoding the B-cell activation antigen CD23, that are believed to play a part in EBV-induced B-cell growth transformation. EBNA-3, -4, and -6 (also called EBNA-3A, -3B, and -3C) are encoded by three genes that are tandemly placed in the EBV genome.[29] Because of their sequence similarity these proteins are likely to have similar functions in latent EBV infection and transformation. Latent membrane protein-1 stimulates the proliferation of B lymphocytes, can protect lymphoblastoid cell lines from apoptosis through the induction of bcl-2, and is defined as a viral oncogene, because it can transform cultured rodent fibroblasts and induces tumours in SCID mice.

Burkitt's lymphoma

The recognition of Burkitt's lymphoma and of its association with malaria and EBV infection is one of the great achievements of twentieth century medicine. After the Second World War, the Irish surgeon Denis Burkitt returned to Africa and studied a peculiar lymphoma common in African children (see also Chapter 15.12).[30] He noticed the specific geographical distribution (Fig. 4). His lecture tours on this topic brought him into contact with Anthony Epstein (at the Middlesex Hospital) who suspected an infective agent was the culprit. Epstein volunteered to look for viruses from Burkitt's lymphoma cell lines by electron microscopy and discovered the new herpesvirus.[7],[31]

Only EBNA-1 is expressed in Burkitt's lymphoma cells.[25] These cells thus represent the resting persistently infected B cells in the circulation. However, all Burkitt's lymphoma cells are in cell cycle and rapidly proliferating due to the universally present translocation of the c-*myc* gene[32],[33] (see also Chapter 1.3). This translocation brings c-*myc* under the control of an immunoglobulin gene locus preventing its downregulation and maintaining the proliferative state.

Table 4 Transforming genes of oncogenic viruses

Virus	HTLV-1	HPV-16	Adenovirus	SV40	EBV	HHV-8
Associated human malignancy	Adult T-cell leukaemia	Anogenital cancer	None	?None	Burkitt's lymphoma, NPC, HD	KS, PEL, MCD
Host cell type	T cells	Keratinocytes	Fibroblasts	Fibroblasts	B cells, epithelial cells	B cells, endothelial cells
Transforming genes	Tax	E6, E7	E1A, E1B	Large T, small t	EBNA-2, -3A, -3C, -LP, LMP-1	?cyclin, K1, ?K15, LNA-1

NPC: nasopharyngeal carcinoma.
HD: Hodgkin's disease.
KS: Kaposi's sarcoma.
PEL: primary effusion lymphoma.
MCD: multicentric Castleman's disease.

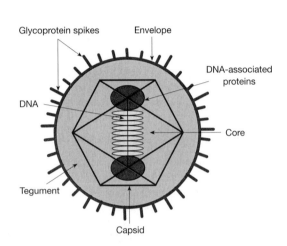

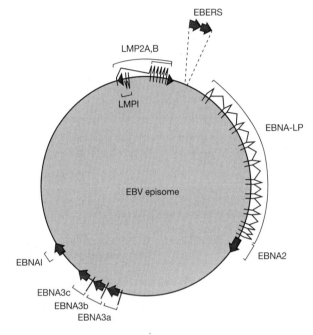

Fig. 3 The location and direction of transcription of the six EBNAs and the three latent membrane proteins are shown on the double-stranded viral DNA episome.

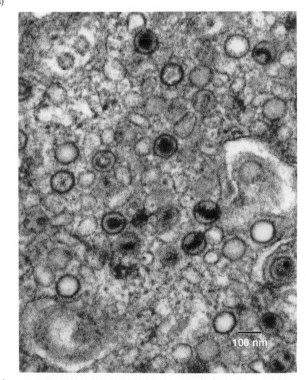

Fig. 2 (a) Schematic structure of a herpesvirus. (b) Electron micrograph of KS-associated herpesvirus particles in a primary effusion lymphoma cell (kindly provided by Dharam Ablashi, ABI Inc., USA).

This translocation 'accident' may therefore cause resting EBNA-1 expressing B cells to start proliferating.

The distribution of Burkitt's lymphoma in Africa coincides with the distribution of hyperendemic malaria. The association is further supported by the fact that the frequency of both diseases decrease with chloroquine prophylaxis. The immune dysregulation caused by malaria, including chronic stimulation of B cells and chronic antigen exposure, contributes to B-cell hyperplasia. Chronic B-lymphocyte hyperplasia increases the target cell population for aberrant recombinations. Malaria triggered B-cell hyperplasia with subsequent c-*myc*/immunoglobulin juxtaposition in conjunction with EBV driven cell proliferation are possibly enough to precipitate endemic Burkitt's lymphoma in Africa. The failure of EBNA-1 to induce an immune response and the downregulation of major histocompatibility complex class I proteins ensure immune evasion.[24]

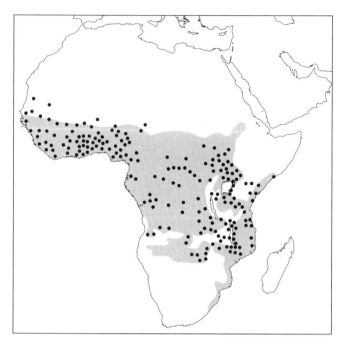

Fig. 4 The distribution of Burkitt's lymphoma as reported by Burkitt in 1962 (dots). The cases fall within the malaria belt (shaded area).

Table 5 Neoplasms associated with EBV infection and the EBV latent proteins expressed in these tumours

Tumour	EBV gene expression
Burkitt's lymphoma	EBNA-1
Nasopharyngeal carcinoma (NPC)	EBNA-1 LMP-1 LMP-2A[+]
Hodgkin's disease	EBNA-1 LMP-1, -2A, and -2B
PTLD*	EBNA-1–6 LMP-1, -2A, and -2B

*Post-transplant lymphoproliferative disease: EBV gene expression pattern is similar to that seen in *in vitro* EBV transformed B lymphoblastoid cell lines.

[+]Not always expressed in NPC.

Nasopharyngeal carcinoma (see also Chapter 9.4)

Cells in nasopharyngeal carcinomas express EBNA-1, but not the immunogenic EBNA-2 to -6 proteins (Table 5). Most cells also express latent membrane protein-1 and latent membrane protein-2. Latent membrane protein-1 is not always expressed, and this may reflect differences in viral expression dependent on the state of cellular differentiation. It seems that the virus enters epithelial cells from lytically infected lymphocytes trafficking through lymphoid-rich epithelium. Latent infection in normal epithelium has not been detected. The establishment of predominantly latent infection in epithelial cells could promote cellular proliferation and the progression from dysplasia to invasive carcinoma. Like Burkitt's lymphoma, co-factors are probably required to precipitate nasopharyngeal carcinoma. Animal data strongly support the epidemiological data that consumption of large quantities of salted fish (e.g. in southeast China) is one such important co-factor. Epidemiological data also support other factors such as the consumption of Chinese herbal teas, exposure to domestic wood fire, and possibly genetic predisposition.[34],[35]

Hodgkin's disease (see also Chapters 15.7–15.9)

The finding of clonal EBV in Reed Sternberg cells and the restricted pattern of latent viral gene expression in nearly 30 to 50 per cent of all cases throughout the world suggest that EBV is not only a passenger in this disease.[36] The presence of EBV in Reed Sternberg cells correlates with an increased expression of lymphocyte activation antigens, a decreased expression of the CD20 B-cell antigen and with expression of cytokines such as IL-10 and IL-6. Other evidence for a role of EBV is provided from both cohort and case–control studies in which a positive association between history of infectious mononucleosis and subsequent Hodgkin's disease is consistently reported. The role of EBV and of other co-factors remains to be elucidated.

Post-transplant lymphoproliferative disorder

Post-transplant lymphoproliferative disorders represent one of the most common complications of immunosuppression following an organ transplant. Post-transplant lymphoproliferative disorders also occur in some congenital immunodeficiencies, e.g. X-linked lymphoproliferative syndrome. These patients either develop a polyclonal mononucleosis-like syndrome or a clonal lymphoma. Phenotypically, post-transplant lymphoproliferative disorders resemble *in vitro* transformed lymphocytes, i.e. lymphoblastoid cell lines. These cells proliferate because of a lack of a cytotoxic T-cell lymphocyte response by an immunodeficient host and these tumours regress when immunosuppression is discontinued.[24]

Human herpesvirus-8

In 1872, the Hungarian dermatologist Moriz Kaposi published the case histories of five middle-aged and elderly male patients in Vienna with idiopathic multiple pigmented sarcomas of the skin.[37] For over 100 years, KS remained a rare curiosity to clinicians and cancer researchers, until its rapid increase in incidence in patients with AIDS.

Classic KS occurs predominantly in elderly male patients of southern European ancestry.[38] A high frequency is also seen in Israel and other Middle Eastern countries. This form of the disease is generally not as aggressive as the form originally described by Kaposi, for unknown, possibly immunological, reasons.

In some equatorial countries of Africa, KS (known as endemic KS) has existed for many decades, long preceding HIV[39] (Fig. 5). This form is found in younger patients as well as the elderly; the male/female ratio is >3 : 1. It is generally a more aggressive disease than classic KS, although less so than African AIDS-associated KS.[40] Endemic KS in African children is often associated with lymph node involvement only, and no skin lesions.

KS is also known to develop after an organ transplant (post-transplant or iatrogenic KS).[41] Patients of Mediterranean, Jewish, or

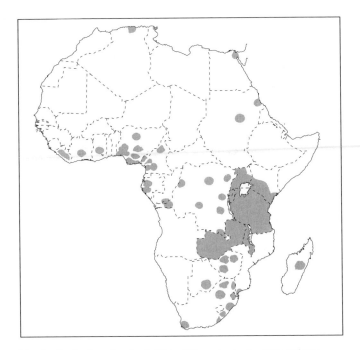

Fig. 5 Distribution of endemic KS in Africa prior to the HIV epidemic.

indicating that those at risk of KS have a higher viral load than those not at risk. To strengthen further the molecular epidemiologic association between HHV-8 and KS, it was demonstrated by polymerase chain reaction *in situ* hybridization, RNA *in situ* hybridization, and immunohistochemistry that HHV-8 is present in nearly all spindle cells (tumour cells) in KS lesions.[48] Furthermore, the vast majority of these cells are latently infected, suggesting that HHV-8, like other oncogenic viruses, is directly involved in driving or maintaining the proliferation of the tumour cells.

Primary effusion lymphoma

The emergence of primary effusion lymphoma (previously called body cavity-based lymphoma) as a new disease entity is linked to the identification of HHV-8: two groups recognized the unique aspects of some effusion-based lymphomas in patients with AIDS.[49],[50] The lymphoma cells in these patients were negative for most lineage-associated antigens, although immunoglobulin gene rearrangement studies indicated a B-cell origin. Karcher *et al.* (1992) further demonstrated the distinctiveness of the syndrome, reporting a high prevalence of EBV yet absence of c-*myc* rearrangements.[51] They also noted the tendency of the disease to remain confined to body cavities without further dissemination. Cesarman and colleagues (1995) found that HHV-8 was associated specifically with primary effusion lymphoma, but not with other high-grade AIDS-related lymphomas.[52]

Primary effusion lymphomas possess a unique constellation of features that distinguishes them from all other lymphoid malignancies: primary effusion lymphoma presents predominantly as malignant effusions in the pleural, pericardial, or peritoneal cavities usually without significant tumour mass or lymphadenopathy. These lymphomas occur predominantly in HIV-positive individuals with advanced stages of immunosuppression, but are occasionally seen in HIV-negative patients.

The majority, but not all, primary effusion lymphomas are co-infected with EBV, suggesting that the two viruses may co-operate in neoplastic transformation. Terminal repeat analysis indicates that EBV is monoclonal in most cases, implying that EBV was present in tumour cells prior to clonal expansion.

Multicentric Castleman's disease

Castleman's disease is a rare and usually polyclonal lympho-proliferative disorder of unknown aetiology.[53] The systemic variety is designated multicentric Castleman's disease (**MCD**) and is usually of the plasma-cell type. Interestingly, patients with MCD are at an increased risk to develop KS and certain B-cell lymphomas.

Soulier and colleagues (1995) were the first to report the presence of HHV-8 in MCD biopsies.[54] They found HHV-8 in all 14 lesions from HIV-positive French patients with MCD. Among HIV-negative cases seven of 17 lesions were positive for HHV-8.

HHV-8 is nearly universally present in HIV-positive individuals with MCD. Among MCD cases in immunocompetent hosts the presence of HHV-8 is restricted to about 40 per cent of cases. In MCD, HHV-8 is present in large immunoblastic-like cells (called plasmablasts) in the mantle zone. These plasmablasts express lambda light chain restriction and are not present in HHV-8 negative cases of MCD.[55] HHV-8 positive MCD is therefore specifically associated with a plasmablastic variant of Castleman's disease.

Arabian ancestry are over-represented among immunosuppressed patients who develop KS after a transplant.[38]

In 1981, the US Centers for Disease Control and Prevention became aware of an increased occurrence of two rare diseases in young gay men from New York City and California:[42] KS and *Pneumocystis carinii* pneumonia. This was the beginning of the AIDS epidemic and AIDS-KS is today the most common form of KS (see also Chapter 15.15).

Studies of AIDS case surveillance support the pre-AIDS data on the existence of a sexually transmissible KS cofactor: KS occurs predominantly in gay and bisexual men with AIDS, less commonly in those acquiring HIV through heterosexual contact, and rarely in AIDS patients with haemophilia or in intravenous drug users.[43],[44]

Chang and colleagues (1994) employed representational difference analysis to identify sequences of a new herpesvirus (human herpes-virus-8 (**HHV-8**), also called KS-associated herpesvirus) in AIDS-KS biopsies.[3] Representational difference analysis relies on cycles of subtractive hybridization and polymerase chain reaction amplification to enrich and isolate rare DNA fragments that are present in only one of two otherwise identical samples of DNA. This is a powerful technique which can detect small differences between complex genomes and has been used to identify DNA amplification in tumour tissues and the lack of tumour suppressor genes in cancers.[45],[46]

Kaposi's sarcoma

The first indication that HHV-8 is involved in the pathogenesis of KS was the detection of HHV-8 DNA by polymerase chain reaction in all forms of the disease. The virus is rarely detectable in non-KS tissues (except blood) from the same individual, indicating that viral load is highest in KS lesions. Furthermore, the detection of HHV-8 DNA by polymerase chain reaction in the peripheral blood of HIV-positive individuals predicts who will subsequently develop KS[47]

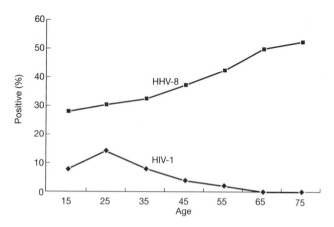

Fig. 6 The age-specific seroprevalence of HHV-8 (KS-associated herpesvirus) and HIV-1 among South African black cancer patients.

Seroprevalence

Northern Europe and North America

The seroprevalence of HHV-8 in the different HIV risk groups correlates with the incidence of KS: in the West, HHV-8 is found predominantly in HIV-positive gay men[56] and not in HIV-positive patients with haemophilia or HIV-positive intravenous drug users or heterosexuals.

In a cohort of men in San Francisco, it was shown that HHV-8 infection is associated with the number of homosexual partners and correlates with a previous history of a sexually transmitted disease (like gonorrhoea) and HIV infection,[57] suggesting that HHV-8 is sexually transmitted.

Mediterranean Europe

The incidence of classic KS is significantly higher in Italy than in the United Kingdom or the United States.[58] Similarly, the prevalence of antibodies to HHV-8 in blood donors in Italy is higher than rates reported in the United Kingdom and the United States.[59] Furthermore, the incidence of classic KS in Italy shows considerable regional variation and correlates with the prevalence of HHV-8.[59] The titre of anti-HHV-8 antibodies is highest in blood donors from the south, where the incidence of KS and the prevalence of HHV-8 is highest.[59] This is reminiscent of EBV infection, where a high anti-EBV antibody titre correlates with an increased risk of developing Burkitt's lymphoma or nasopharyngeal carcinoma.

Africa

In Africa, where KS rates are very high among HIV-positive individuals, the prevalence of antibodies to HHV-8 is higher than in the United Kingdom or the United States.[60] Early acquisition of HHV-8 in Africa is likely because KS occurs in African children. Serological evidence for mother-to-child transmission of HHV-8 in Africa has also been reported. In Africa, as in Mediterranean Europe, the prevalence of antibodies to HHV-8 increases steadily with age (Fig. 6).[60] Such an age distribution of infection is not typical for an agent that is predominantly sexually transmitted and suggests other routes of horizontal transmission in these endemic populations.

Captured genes

A substantial number of recognizable genes pirated from eukaryotic cellular DNA are encoded by HHV-8.[61] These include genes which encode dihydrofolate reductase, thymidilate synthetase, homologues of cyclin D and bcl-2, and proteins that may suppress the immune response. The structural proteins and viral enzymes which are common to most herpesviruses probably originated from an ancient progenitor of contemporary herpesviruses, whereas the recognizable cellular genes which occur sporadically in some herpesviruses, are probably more recent acquisitions from the host genome, and might support viral replication in a specific microenvironment (which for HHV-8 could be the microvasculature).[62] The captured genes have acquired unique properties which can give us insight into the biology of their cellular counterparts;[63] one reason why they have been the most studied proteins encoded by HHV-8.

HHV-8 cyclin

Cellular cyclins are critical components of regulation of the cell cycle (see Chapter 1.6): cyclins inactivate (by phosphorylation) various checkpoints throughout the cell cycle, allowing cells to enter DNA synthesis (S phase) or mitosis (M phase). Cyclins associate with their partners (the cyclin-dependent kinases, **CDKs**) to be fully active. The HHV-8 cyclin has highest sequence similarity to the cellular D-type cyclins. The HHV-8-cyclin forms active kinase complexes with CDK6[64] that phosphorylate pRb. Furthermore, unlike cellular D cyclin/CDK6 complexes, HHV-8-cyclin/CDK6 activity is resistant to inhibition by the CDK inhibitors (CKI) p16, p21, and p27.[65] Ectopic expression of v-cyclin prevents G_1 arrest imposed by each inhibitor and stimulates cell-cycle progression in quiescent fibroblasts.[65] HHV-8 cyclin/CDK6 also phosphorylates and inactivates p27,[66] the CKI known to be an effective inhibitor of cyclin E/CDK2 activity. This suggests that this viral cyclin can activate both of the pathways that are necessary for G_1/S-phase progression (i.e. cyclin D/CDK6 and cyclin E/CDK2, see Chapter 1.6).

The expression of the HHV-8-cyclin in latently infected spindle and primary effusion lymphoma cells, indicates a possible role in either the proliferation or the arrest of differentiation of these cells. Cyclin D1 expression, not cyclins E or A, inhibits the differentiation of immature myoblasts.[67] The E7 protein of HPV has also been shown to uncouple cellular differentiation and proliferation in human keratinocytes.[68] As KS spindle cells possibly represent undifferentiated endothelial cells, this role for the HHV-8 cyclin is an attractive hypothesis. Although EBV does not encode a cyclin homologue, the latent nuclear antigens induce cellular cyclin D2 expression.

Papillomaviruses

The papillomaviruses are small (~8 kbp) DNA viruses with circular, double-stranded genomes (Fig. 7). More than 80 distinct human papillomaviruses (**HPV**) have thus far been described. The majority of infections result in a benign proliferation of epithelial cells (warts). Cells are usually infected at the terminal stages of epithelial cell differentiation and lyse, so virus-induced proliferation is self-limiting

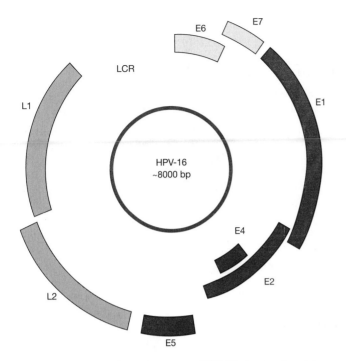

Fig. 7 The circular papillomavirus genome (HPV-16) showing the relative positions of six of the eight early viral genes (E1 to E7) and the two major late viral genes (L1 and L2). The E6 and E7 viral gene products are the tumour antigens expressed in human carcinomas (HPV oncogenes).

Table 6 Diseases associated with human papillomaviruses

Plantar warts (verruca vulgaris):	HPV-1, HPV-4
Hand warts (verruca vulgaris):	HPV-2, HPV-4, HPV-7
Papillomas of meat handlers:	HPV-7
Laryngeal papillomas and condylomas:	HPV-11
Genital warts (condyloma accuminata):	HPV-6, HPV-11, HPV-42
Bowenoid papulosis:	HPV-16
Epidermodysplasia verruciformis:	HPV-3, HPV-9, HPV-12, HPV-14, HPV-15
EV with malignant conversion:	HPV-5, HPV-8, HPV-10
Cervical cancer:	HPV-6, HPV-10, HPV-11, HPV-16, HPV-18, HPV-31, HPV-33, HPV-35, HPV-45,* HPV-52,** HPV-54**
Vulvar cancer:	HPV-10

HPV: human papillomavirus.

EV: Epidermodysplasia verruciformis.

HPV-16 and 18 are found in >90 per cent of *in situ* and invasive cervical cancer.

*HPV-45 in cervical cancer found predominantly in Africa.

**HPV-52 and 54 described mainly from Southeast Asia.

and does not progress to malignant transformation. However, a number of HPV types (so called oncogenic subtypes) are associated with human malignancies (Table 6).[69]

HPV was first proposed to be involved in the aetiology of genital warts in 1968.[70] Soon afterwards Zur Hausen suggested that cervical cancer might also be caused by HPV.[71],[72] Cervical cancer arises from the area of metaplasia between the squamous epithelium of the exocervix and the columnar epithelium of the endocervix (see Chapter 12.3). An infectious aetiology for cervical cancer was suggested by the observation that the most important risk factor for cervical cancer is the number of sexual partners. By polymerase chain reaction it has since been shown that more than 90 per cent of cervical cancers contain HPV sequences. HPV-16 is found in nearly 60 per cent and HPV-18 in 20 per cent of cervical cancers.[73] Other HPV types are also associated with cervical cancer, particularly in Africa and the Far East (Table 6).

As with EBV- and HHV-8-induced tumours, HPV sequences are present in the vast majority, if not all, tumour cells. A key step appears to be the random integration of viral DNA sequences into the genome of cells in the basal layer, i.e. the cells in which papilloma viruses normally persist.[74] As a result, as the cells move upwards from the basal epithelial layer to the surface, replication to new virus particles can no longer occur, and the normal progress of the virus infectious cycle has been interrupted. The integrated viral DNA may retain the capacity to express early genes (E6 and E7) and when these are switched on permanently, they continue to drive cellular proliferation. Secondary genetic changes occurring in these latently infected proliferating cells will ultimately give rise to clones of malignant cells.

HPV are detected frequently in pre-invasive cervical lesions (cervical intraepithelial neoplasia) and in general, the HPV detection rate increases with the severity of the lesion. The prevalence of HPV in cervical intraepithelial neoplasia grade III lesions is reported to be more than 70 per cent in 13 of 21 studies.[75]

As with other viral-induced cancers, co-factors are probably important in the pathogenesis: not all women with HPV-16 or -18 will progress to invasive cervical carcinoma.[75] Risk factors that could be involved include herpes simplex virus 2 infection, smoking, and possibly the contraceptive pill. Smoking-induced mutagenic DNA adducts have been found in cervical carcinoma cells.[75]

Some HPV types (e.g. 16, 18, 31, and 33) are termed high risk because they are found in lesions that often progress to malignant disease. Other types, such as 6 and 11, are termed low risk, only rarely giving rise to tumours. In most HPV-related cancers or cell lines, the E6 and E7 genes are actively transcribed. E6 and E7 can immortalize and transform human foreskin cells, indicating that they are viral oncogenes.[76] E6 and E7 DNA sequences from 'high-risk' subtypes are distinct from the sequences of 'low-risk' sub-types and are more 'oncogenic' *in vitro*. Like SV40 T antigen and the adenovirus-5 E1B 55 kDa protein, high-risk HPV E6 proteins can interact specifically with the p53 tumour suppressor protein. The interaction between p53 and high-risk HPV E6 protein results in rapid degradation of p53 through the ubiquitin-mediated proteolysis pathway. The aminoterminal domain of the HPV E7 protein is strikingly similar to regions of adenovirus E1A protein and the SV40 T antigen. The conserved regions of these oncogenic viral proteins bind to pocket proteins, a family of proteins that include pRb, p107, and p130. Complex formation between E7 and the pocket proteins results in

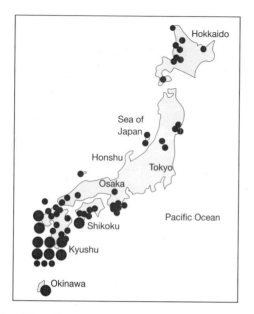

Fig. 8 Map of Japan showing the distribution of adult T-cell leukaemia. The larger dots represent areas with a higher incidence.

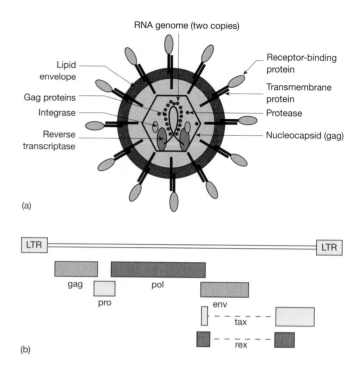

Fig. 9 (a) A retrovirus virion. Two RNA molecules—packaged with reverse transcriptase, integrase, gag proteins and protease—are surrounded by capsomeres (gag products) to form a nucleocapsid. This is enveloped in a lipid membrane. The lipid envelope is derived from the plasma membrane of the host cell. The env gene products make up the transmembrane subunit and the receptor-binding proteins that project out of the lipid envelope. (b) Schematic map of the HTLV-1 genome. The DNA provirus terminal repeated nucleotide sequences (long terminal repeats) bracketing the *gag*, *pro* (protease), *pol* (reverse transcriptase), and *env* genes. Tax and rex proteins regulate viral and cellular gene expression.

their functional inactivation. This may therefore contribute to the ability of E7 to induce DNA synthesis.

Some 40 years ago, cells from a particularly aggressive cervical cancer were the first human cancer cells to grow as an immortal cell line in culture. This cell line, called HeLa cells, became a popular source of human cells and indeed contaminated other cell cultures in many laboratories worldwide. At the time, no one associated cervical cancer with HPV. As the role of HPV in cervical cancer became established after nearly four decades of HeLa cells growing in laboratories, HPV-18 E6 and E7 were demonstrated in HeLa cells and shown to be expressed continuously. When the viral oncogenes E6 and E7 are turned off, the cells stop growing. After years in cell culture and in thousands of laboratories, this immortal and transformed cell line remains dependent upon HPV E6 and E7 proteins.

Human T-cell leukaemia virus-1

In 1977 Takatsuki and his colleagues reported that the pathology and clinical spectrum of certain T-cell leukaemias in Japanese adults can be described as one syndrome: adult T-cell leukaemia (see also Chapter 15.3). As with Burkitt's lymphoma, the geographical distribution of adult T-cell leukaemia in Japan (Fig. 8) suggested that genetic, environmental, and/or infectious agents are involved in the pathogenesis. Robert Gallo and colleagues at the NIH were the first (1980) to report the presence of a virus with reverse transcriptase activity from a T-cell lymphoma cell line. This was the first report of a human retrovirus and they called it HTLV-1. Hinuma (1982) and colleagues demonstrated retrovirus particles from an adult T-cell leukaemia cell line and it was soon shown that this agent is identical to HTLV-1.[77] Epidemiological studies in Japan showed that the distribution of adult T-cell leukaemia was similar to that of HTLV-1. Larger epidemiological studies also showed HTLV-1 in the coastal regions of central Africa

and, less frequently, in the Caribbean basin, Taiwan, and the aborigines of Papua New Guinea.[78] In all patients, HTLV-1 was associated with adult T-cell leukaemia and the viral isolates from these diverse geographical areas were almost identical. HTLV-1-infected tumour cells were grown from these patients in culture and shown to be immortal. Biologically, the link between adult T-cell leukaemia and HTLV-1 was confirmed when it was shown that when human T cells were incubated with HTLV-1, viral DNA could integrate into cellular DNA, express its viral proteins, and immortalize the cells for growth in culture.

HTLV-1 genome and gene products

HTLV-1 is a typical retrovirus: two copies of an RNA genome just over 9000 nucleotides long (Fig. 9) contain the *gag*, *pol*, and *env* genes surrounded by long terminal repeat sequences. *Gag* encodes three structural proteins that form the core of the virus, the *env* gene encodes proteins that make up the spikes that protrude from the lipid envelope surrounding the ribonucleoprotein core of the virus. *Pol* encodes the reverse transcriptase protein. One region of the HTLV-1 provirus encodes a set of two genes, which are not observed in avian or mouse retroviruses. These genes produce two viral proteins: tax and rex. Tax, acting upon the long terminal repeats adjacent to gag, promotes the transcription of gag-pol-env genes leading to the synthesis of more viral RNA chromosomes. Tax is therefore a transcriptional activator protein (reviewed in ref. 79). However, it was also shown that tax can stimulate the transcription of the cellular genes for IL-2 and the IL-2 receptor, both of which are required to initiate T-cell division. Furthermore, tax stimulates the transcription of other cellular genes including fos and the platelet-derived growth factor and of nuclear factor-κB, a key regulator of the cellular inflammatory and immune response. HTLV-1 immortalizes infected T cells *in vitro*, and when expressed in rat embryo fibroblasts also leads to cellular transformation. Tax therefore appears to be the principal HTLV-1 gene (oncogene) involved in tumorigenesis.

Characteristics of adult T-cell leukaemia

Adult T-cell leukaemia is found worldwide, but as described above clusters in certain ethnic groups and locations: the islands of Kyushu and Shikoku in southwestern Japan (Fig. 8), Caribbean basin, and black population in the southeastern United States. It is a malignant proliferation of CD4-positive T cells with a distinct T-cell morphology: vacuolated cells with lobulated nuclei and a high frequency of IL-2 receptor positive cells. Circulating antibodies to HTLV-1 are present in more than 90 per cent of patients and in their spouses. The onset of adult T-cell leukaemia is usually during adulthood. Clinically, there is frequent involvement of skin with lymphadenopathy and hepatosplenomegaly. Hypercalcaemia and lytic bone lesions are also frequent. The prognosis is very poor with few patients surviving more than 6 months.

Epidemiological studies have shown that HTLV-1 is transmitted from mother to child, either via passage of infected maternal T lymphocytes across the placenta, or via breast milk. HTLV-1 is also transmitted sexually via infected lymphocytes in semen or through blood products that contain lymphocytes. Only one in 1000 to 1 in 10 000 virus carriers over the age of 40 develops adult T-cell leukaemia. The incubation period to malignancy is therefore long and only a few infected will actually develop the disease.

All leukaemic cells contain at least one copy of the HTLV-1 provirus.[80] Non-transformed lymphocytes do not contain HTLV-1 sequences. The HTLV-1-positive malignant cells are clonal and each cell in the transformed lymphocyte clone contains virus integrated into the same site; however, this site varies from patient to patient. This indicates that HTLV-1 does not initiate malignancy by insertional mutagenesis or by activating a cellular oncogene at the site of integration. Transformation by HTLV-1 is mediated by transacting viral genes (especially tax) that activate the transcription of cellular growth genes.

Hepatitis B virus

Hepatitis B belongs to the hepadnavirus group, which also includes viruses of woodchucks, ducks, and squirrels. These agents contain a DNA genome that is partially double stranded and partially a single strand (Fig. 10). Under appropriate conditions, a DNA polymerase that is encoded by a viral gene can use the long DNA strand as a template and add nucleotides to the short DNA strand, making the entire genome a double-stranded helix. This occurs shortly after viral infection of a cell. The virus encodes four known genes and proteins: the hepatitis B surface antigen (**HBsAg**), the polymerase (P) gene,

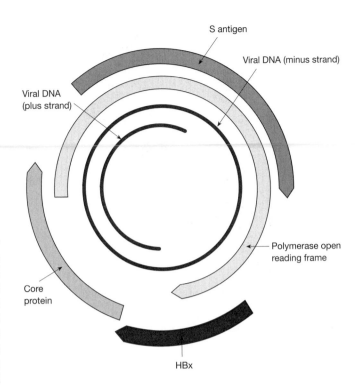

Fig. 10 Map of the HBV genome, showing the nucleotide sequences that encode the S antigen, the polymerase, the core protein, and the HBx protein.

the hepatitis B core antigen gene, and a fourth gene termed X that makes a protein not found in the virus particle. The viral genome is surrounded by a protein core, enclosed in turn by a lipid envelope from which protrudes lipoprotein spikes called the surface antigen (S antigen).

The HBV attaches to liver cells via the HBsAg. The virion core enzymes convert the partially single-stranded DNA to a complete, double-stranded DNA helix. The entire genome is then transcribed in the cell nucleus, producing an RNA that is a full-length copy of the viral DNA, as well as mRNAs of shorter length. The longest RNA transcript acts as a template for a reverse transcriptase that is also the DNA polymerase. This step is blocked by reverse transcriptase inhibitors that are being used to treat HBV infection. The reverse transcriptase copies the RNA template into a complementary DNA strand.

The most important routes of transmission in the West used to be via blood and blood products, but these are markedly reduced by the routine screening of donors and of blood. Today, the most important routes of transmission in the West are through needles shared among drug users and by heterosexual and homosexual venereal transmission. Close personal contact via body fluids such as saliva, and transmission from mother to new-born appear particularly important in developing countries where poor hygiene and socio-economic factors contribute to transmission.

The first clear example of serum hepatitis was reported in 1895 in Bremen, Germany. More than 10 per cent of shipyard workers receiving smallpox vaccine, administered by placing a drop of vaccine virus prepared from human lymph on the skin, which was then broken

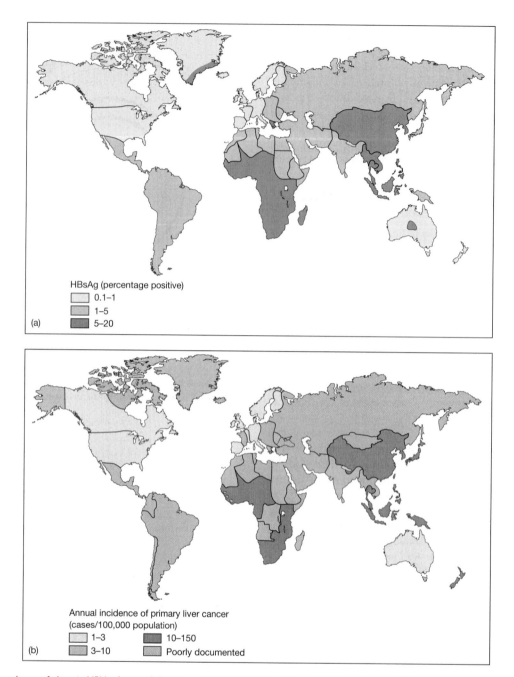

Fig. 11 (a) The prevalence of chronic HBV infection (HBsAg) worldwide. (b) The incidence of primary hepatocellular carcinoma correlates with the seroprevalence of HBsAg (a).

with a needle, developed jaundice and a hepatitis-like syndrome. The responses in individuals undergoing a primary infection with HBV vary significantly: mild and subclinical infections being the most common. The immune system appears to be responsible for liver damage. Both antibodies and CD8-positive T cells attack viral antigens on the surface of infected cells and kill large numbers of liver cells. About 2 to 10 per cent of adults with hepatitis B infections do not clear the virus, they continue to synthesize viral antigens, and this is termed chronic hepatitis. These patients continue to secrete large amounts of HBV in all body fluids.

HBV and hepatocellular carcinoma

The incidence of hepatocellular carcinoma (see also Chapter 10.7) correlates with the geographic prevalence of chronic carriers of HBV, who number 400 million worldwide (Fig. 11).[69] In the large prospective study by Beasley and colleagues, 22 707 Chinese men in Taiwan were followed over 6 years. Of this group, 3454 (15.2 per cent) were HBsAg positive. In the 6-year period, 116 died of hepatocellular carcinoma, and all but three of these patients were in the HBsAg-positive group. The risk of developing liver cancer was 105 to 217 times greater for HBsAg carriers than for non-carriers. On average, 1 in 322 HBsAg carriers died of liver cancer per year.

The mechanisms by which HBV induces liver cancer are not known precisely, but appear to be different from those in other viral-induced malignancies. One hypotheses is that chronic HBV infection leads to the continuous production of viral antigens, with elimination of infected cells by the immune system, subsequent liver cell re-generation, and again immune attack on newly infected cells. This constant stimulation of proliferation of liver cells lead to an increase in mutation rate, some of these mutations occurring in oncogenes, leading to cells being transformed (see Fig. 1). The cycle of cell death and regeneration, therefore, puts the host at risk for a higher incidence of cancer. The role of the virus is to promote this cycle.

An alternative hypothesis is that the X gene product (HBx protein), which promote transcription of viral and cellular genes, could be responsible for altering the expression of cellular genes involved in oncogenesis.[81] HBx is a 17-kDa protein that stimulates signal transduction pathways by acting in the cytoplasm. Studies have shown that HBx protein activates the Src family of tyrosine kinases, Ras and downstream Ras signalling pathways, including Raf, mitogen-activated protein (MAP) kinases and mitogen-activated ERK-activating kinase (MEK)[82] (see Chapter 1.5). HBx also binds to the C terminus of p53 and inhibit several p53 functions including transcriptional transactivation and apoptosis. However, in contrast to other viral oncogenes, the HBx gene does not transform cells *in vitro*. It is transcribed in only a fraction of hepatocellular carcinoma cells in-dicating that it cannot be directly involved in maintaining the pro-liferation of malignant cells.

Chronic infection of woodchucks with woodchuck hepatitis virus leads invariably, within 2 to 4 years, to the appearance of hepatocellular carcinoma. As in humans, this liver cancer is preceded by an extended period of chronic liver damage, probably resulting from the immune response to viral antigens. Woodchuck hepatitis virus infection is used as an animal model for studying the pathogenesis and treatment of human liver cancer.[83]

Aflatoxins

Epidemiological studies indicate that the consumption of food con-taminated with the mycotoxin aflatoxin B might act synergistically with HBV infection to induce primary liver cancer.[84],[85]

Hepatitis C virus

Hepatitis C virus (HCV) is an RNA virus associated with acute and chronic hepatitis and liver cirrhosis. Most patients with haemophilia that were treated with blood products prior to the use of virus-inactivation procedures were infected with HCV. As is true for HBV, the relative risk of hepatocellular carcinoma among persons with chronic HCV infection and cirrhosis is approximately 100 times the risk in uninfected persons. Persistent HCV infection is the cause of 70 per cent of the cases of hepatocellular carcinoma in Japan and approximately 30 to 50 per cent of the cases in the United States. In a cohort of 4865 haemophilic patients in the United Kingdom, the mortality from liver cancer was 5.6 times higher than that in the general population and this is probably due to hepatitis C infection.[86] HCV infection is also common among intravenous drug users.

Epidemiological studies from Taiwan have also indicated that HCV and HBV are interactive in inducing liver cancer.[87] In Korea, where mortality due to liver cancer is the highest in the world, HBV and HCV infection are independent risk factors. In low-endemic areas for HBV and HCV (e.g. Sweden), these viruses play a minor part in the pathogenesis of hepatocellular carcinoma, compared with alcohol-related cirrhosis. However, in patients with chronic HCV infection, alcohol abuse accelerates the onset of cirrhosis and hepatocellular carcinoma.

Treatment with interferon alpha and ribavirin does eradicate chronic HCV infection in some patients. It remains to be proven that this will lead to a reduction in the incidence of hepatocellular carcinoma in such patients.

Hepatitis G virus is also an RNA virus (flavivirus) and common in intravenous drug users.[88] It is associated with acute and chronic hepatitis, but has not yet been linked to the pathogenesis of hepato-cellular carcinoma. Hepatitis G virus infection does not appear to aggravate the course of chronic HBV or HCV infections.

There are more than 700 million individuals chronically infected with HBV and HCV in the world today. Safe and effective vaccines against HBV are available, although not yet used universally because of cost. An HCV vaccine is not yet available and may be difficult to develop because of the high variability of viral proteins. Global vaccination against these viruses will have a major impact on the incidence of primary liver cancer.[89]

Summary

Viruses cause some of the most common human cancers including cervical and hepatocellular carcinoma and KS. The world of the twenty-first century will be faced with new threats from emerging infectious agents and new disease manifestations of already known agents. A safe and effective vaccine against HIV should prevent a new wave of viral-driven malignancies. The increasing knowledge about the immune responses to virus-induced malignancy and the signalling pathways involved will also translate into new targets for drug therapies and immunotherapies for cancer.

References

1. Rous P. Transmission of malignant new growth by means of a cell free filtrate. *Journal of the American Medical Association*, 1911; **56**: 198.

2. Bittner JJ. Some possible effects of nursing on the mammary gland tumor incidence in mice. *Science*, 1936; **84**: 162.

3. Chang Y, *et al.* Identification of herpesvirus-like DNA sequences in AIDS-associated Kaposi's sarcoma. *Science*, 1994; **266**: 1865–9.

4. Churchill AE, Biggs PM. Agent of Marek's disease in tissue culture. *Nature*, 1967; **215**: 528–530.

5. Eddy BE, Borman GS, Grubbs GE, Young RD. Identification of the oncogenic substance in rhesus monkey kidney cell cultures as simian virus 40. *Virology*, 1962; **16**: 65–75.

6. Ellermann V, Bang O. Experimentelle leukamie bei huhnern. *Centralbl fur Bakt*, 1908; **46**: 595–609.

7. Epstein M, Achong B, Barr Y. Virus particles in cultured lymphoblasts from Burkitt's lymphoma. *The Lancet*, 1964; **i**: 702–3.

8. Friend C. Cell-free transmission in adult Swiss mice of a disease having the character of a leukemia. *Journal of Experimental Medicine*, 1957; **105**: 307–18.

9. Gross L. Spontaneous leukemia developing in C3H mice following inoculation, in infancy, with Ak-leukemic extracts, or Ak-embryos.

Proceedings for the Society of Experimental Biology and Medicine, 1951; **78**: 27–32.

10. Popovic M, *et al.* The virus of Japanese adult T-cell leukaemia is a member of the human T-cell leukaemia virus group. *Nature,* 1982; **300**: 63–6.

11. Shope RE. Infectious papillomatosis of rabbits. *Journal of Experimental Medicine,* 1933; **58**: 607–24.

12. Stewart SE, Eddy BE, Gochenour AM, Borgese NG, Grubbs GE. The induction of neoplasms with a substance released from mouse tumors by tissue culture. *Virology,* 1957; **3**: 380–400.

13. Trentin JJ, Yabbe Y, Taylor G. Tumor induction in hamsters by human adenovirus. *Proceedings of the American Association for Cancer Research,* 1962; **3**: 369.

14. Weiss RA, Teich N, Varmus H, Coffin J. *The molecular biology of tumor viruses: RNA tumor viruses.* New York: Cold Spring Harbor, 1984.

15. Weinberg RA. The cat and mouse games that genes, viruses, and cells play. *Cell,* 1997; **88**: 573–5.

16. Jansen-Durr P. How viral oncogenes make the cell cycle. *Trends in Genetics,* 1996; **12**(7): 270–5.

17. Sato T, *et al.* Interactions among members of the Bcl-2 protein family analyzed with a yeast two-hybrid system. *Proceedings of the National Academy of Sciences of the United States of America,* 1994; **91**(20): 9238–42.

18. Thome M, *et al.* Viral FLICE-inhibitory proteins (FLIPs) prevent apoptosis induced by death receptors. *Nature,* 1997; **386**(6624): 517–21.

19. Bertin J, *et al.* Death effector domain-containing herpesvirus and poxvirus proteins inhibit both Fas- and TNFR1-induced apoptosis. *Proceedings of the National Academy of Sciences of the United States of America,* 1997; **94**(4): 1172–6.

20. Irmler M, *et al.* Inhibition of death receptor signals by cellular FLIP. *Nature,* 1997; **388**: 190–5.

21. Nagata S. Apoptosis by death factor. *Cell,* 1997; **88**(3): 355–65.

22. Brehm A, Miska EA, McCance DJ, Reid JL, Bannister AJ, Kouzarides T. Retinoblastoma protein recruits histone deacetylase to repress transcription. *Nature,* 1998; **391**: 597–601.

23. Magnaghi-Jaulin L, *et al.* Retinoblastoma protein represses transcription by recruiting a histone deacetylase. *Nature,* 1998; **391**: 601–4.

24. Rickinson AB, Moss DJ. Human cytotoxic T lymphocyte responses to Epstein-Barr virus infection. *Annual Revue of Immunology,* 1997; **15**: 405–31.

25. Klein G. Epstein-Barr virus strategy in normal and neoplastic B cells. *Cell,* 1994; **77**(6): 791–3.

26. Yates JL, Warren N, Sugden B. Stable replication of plasmids derived from Epstein-Barr virus in various mammalian cells. *Nature,* 1985; **313**: 812–15.

27. de-Campos-Lima PO, Gavioli R, Zhang QJ, *et al.* HLA-A11 epitope loss isolates of Epstein-Barr virus from highly A11+ population. *Science,* 1993; **260**: 98–100.

28. Adams A, Lindahl T. Epstein-Barr virus genomes with properties of circular DNA molecules in carrier cells. *Proceedings of the National Academy of Sciences of the United States of America,* 1975; **72**: 1477–81.

29. Rickinson AB, Kieff E. Epstein-Barr virus. In: Fields BN, Knipe DM, Howley PM, eds. *Fields virology,* 3rd edn. Philadelphia: Lippincott, Raven Publishers, 1996: 2397–447.

30. Burkitt DP. A sarcoma involving the jaws in African children. *British Journal of Surgery,* 1958; **197**: 218–23.

31. Epstein MA, Henle G, Achong BG, Barr YM. Morphological and biological studies on a virus in cultured lymphoblasts from Burkitt's lymphoma. *Journal of Experimental Medicine,* 1965; **121**: 761–70.

32. Manolov G, Manolova Y. Marker band in one chromosome 14 from Burkitt lymphoma. *Nature,* 1972; **237**: 33–4.

33. Bernheim A, Berger R, Lenoir G. Cytogenetic studies on African Burkitt's lymphoma cell lines; t(8;14), t(2;8) and t(8;22) translocations. *Cancer Genet Cytogenet,* 1981; **3**: 307–15.

34. Yu MC. Nasopharyngeal carcinoma: epidemiology and dietary factors. *IARC Science-Publications* 1991; **105**: 39–47.

35. Zheng YM, *et al.* Environmental and dietary risk factors for nasopharyngeal carcinoma: a case-control study in Zangwu County, Guangxi, China. *British Journal of Cancer,* 1994; **69**: 508–14.

36. Armstrong AA, Weiss LM, Gallagher A. Criteria for the definition of EBV association in Hodgkin's disease. *Leukaemia,* 1992; **6**: 869–74.

37. Kaposi M. Idiopathisches multiples pigmentsarcom der haut. *Arch. Dermatol und Syphillis* 1872; **4**: 265–73.

38. Franceschi S, Geddes M. Epidemiology of classic Kaposi's sarcoma, with special reference to Mediterranean population. *Tumori,* 1995; **81**: 308–14.

39. Oettle AG. Geographic and racial differences in the frequency of Kaposi's sarcoma as evidence of environmental or genetic causes. In: Ackerman LV, Murray JF (eds) *Symposium on Kaposi's sarcoma.* Basel: Karger, 1962.

40. Bayley AC. Aggressive Kaposi's sarcoma in Zambia. *The Lancet,* 1984; **i**: 1318.

41. Penn I. Kaposi's sarcoma in immuno-suppressed patients. *Journal of Clinical and Laboratory Immunology,* 1983; **12**: 1–10.

42. Service PH. Kaposi's sarcoma and *Pneumocystis* pneumonia among homosexual men in New York City and California. *MMWR,* 1981; **30**: 305–8.

43. Beral V. Epidemiology of Kaposi's sarcoma. In: Beral V, Jaffe HW, Weiss RA (eds) *Cancer, HIV and AIDS.* New York: Cold Spring Harbor Laboratory Press, 1991: 5–22.

44. Beral V, Peterman TA, Berkelman RL, Jaffe HW. Kaposi's sarcoma among persons with AIDS: a sexually transmitted infection? *The Lancet,* 1990; **335**: 123–8.

45. Lisitsyn N, Lisitsyn N, Wigler M. Cloning the differences between two complex genomes. *Science,* 1993; **259**(5097): 946–51.

46. Lisitsyn NA, *et al.* Comparative genomic analysis of tumors: detection of DNA losses and amplification. *Proceedings of the National Academy of Sciences of the United States of America,* 1995; **92**: 151–5.

47. Whitby D, *et al.* Detection of Kaposi sarcoma associated herpesvirus in peripheral blood of HIV-infected individuals and progression to Kaposi's sarcoma. *The Lancet,* 1995; **346**(8978): 799–802.

48. Boshoff C, *et al.* Kaposi's sarcoma-associated herpesvirus infects endothelial and spindle cells. *Nature Medicine,* 1995; **1**(12): 1274–8.

49. Knowles DM, Inghirami G, Ubriaco A, Dalla-Favera R. Molecular genetic analysis of three AIDS-associated neoplasms of uncertain lineage demonstrates their B-cell derivation and the possible pathogenetic role of the Epstein-Barr virus. *Blood,* 1989; **73**: 792–9.

50. Walts A, E., Shintaku P, Said JW. Diagnosis of malignant lymphoma in effusions from patients with AIDS by gene rearrangement. *American Journal of Clinical Pathology,* 1990; **194**: 170–5.

51. Karcher DS, Dawkins F, Garrett CT. Body cavity-based non-Hodgkin's lymphoma (NHL) in HIV-infected patients: B-cell lymphoma with unusual clinical, immunophenotypic, and genotypic features. *Laboratory Investigation,* 1992; **92**: 80a.

52. Cesarman E, Chang Y, Moore PS, Said JW, Knowles DM. Kaposi's sarcoma-associated herpesvirus-like DNA sequences in AIDS-related body-cavity-based lymphomas. *New England Journal of Medicine,* 1995; **332**(18): 1186–91.

53. Castleman B, Iverson L, Menendez VP. Localized mediastinal lymph-node hyperplasia resembling thymoma. *Cancer,* 1956; **9**: 822–30.

54. Soulier J, *et al.* Kaposi's sarcoma-associated herpesvirus-like DNA

sequences in multicentric Castleman's disease. *Blood*, 1995; **86**(4): 1276–80.

55. Dupin N, *et al*. Distribution of HHV-8 positive cells in Kaposi's sarcoma, primary effusion lymphoma and multicentric Castleman's disease. *Proceedings of the National Academy of Sciences of the United States of America*, 1999; **96**: 4546–51.

56. Kedes DH, Operskalski E, Busch M, Kohn R, Flood J, Ganem D. The seroepidemiology of human herpesvirus 8 (Kaposi's sarcoma-associated herpesvirus): distribution of infection in KS risk groups and evidence for sexual transmission. *Nature Medicine*, 1996; **2**(8): 918–24.

57. Martin JN, Ganem DE, Osmond DH, Page-Shafer KA, Macrae D, Kedes DH. Sexual transmission and the natural history of human herpesvirus 8 infection. *New England Journal of Medicine*, 1998; **338**: 948–54.

58. Geddes M, Franceschi S, Balzi D, Arniani S, Gafa L, Zanetti R. Birthplace and classic Kaposi's sarcoma in Italy. *Journal of the National Cancer Institute*, 1995; **87**: 1015–17.

59. Whitby D, Luppi M, Barozzi P, Boshoff C, Weiss RA, Torelli G. KSHV seroprevalence in blood donors and lymphoma patients from different regions of Italy. *Journal of the National Cancer Institute*, 1998; **90**: 395–7.

60. Sitas F, *et al*. Antibodies against human herpesvirus 8 in black South African patients with cancer. *New England Journal of Medicine*, 1999; **340**: 1863–71.

61. Moore PS, Boshoff C, Weiss RA, Chang Y. Molecular mimicry of human cytokine and cytokine response pathway genes by KSHV. *Science*, 1996; **274**(5293): 1739–44.

62. Boshoff C. Coupling herpesvirus to angiogenesis. *Nature*, 1998; **391**: 24–5.

63. Boshoff C, Weiss RA. Kaposi's sarcoma-associated herpesvirus. In: Vande Woude G, Klein G (eds) *Advances in Cancer Research*. San Diego: Academic Press, 1998.

64. Godden-Kent D, *et al*. The cyclin encoded by Kaposi's sarcoma-associated herpesvirus (KSHV) stimulates cdk6 to phosphorylate the retinoblastoma protein and Histone H1. *Journal of Virology*, 1997; **71**: 4193–8.

65. Swanton C, Mann DJ, Fleckenstein B, Neipel F, Peters G, Jones N. Herpesviral cyclin/Cdk6 complexes evade inhibition by CDK inhibitor proteins. *Nature*, 1997; **390**: 184–7.

66. Ellis M, *et al*. Degradation of p27KIP cdk inhibitor triggered by Kaposi's sarcoma virus cyclin/cdk6 complex. *EMBO Journal*, 1999; **18**: 644–53.

67. Skapek SX, Rhee J, Spicer DB, Lassar AB. Inhibition of myogenic differentiation in proliferating myoblasts by cyclin D1-dependent kinase. *Science*, 1995; **267**: 1022–4.

68. Jones DL, Alani RM, Munger K. The human papillomavirus E7 oncoprotein can uncouple cellular differentiation and proliferation pathways in human keratinocytes by abrogating p21Cip1-mediated inhibition of cdk2. *Genes and Development*, 1997; **11**: 2101–11.

69. zur Hausen H. Viruses in human cancers. *Science*, 1991; **254**: 1167–73.

70. Dunn AEG, Ogilvie MM. Intranuclear virus particles in human genital wart tissue: observation on ultrastructure of the epidermal layer. *Journal of Ultrastructure Research*, 1968; **22**: 282–9.

71. Zur Hausen H, de Villiers EM, Gissmann L. Papillomavirus infection and genital cancer. *Oncology*, 1981; **12**: 124–8.

72. Zur Hausen H. Human genital cancer: synergism between two virus infections or synergism and initiating events? *The Lancet*, 1982; **ii**: 1370–2.

73. Lorinez AT, Temple GF, Kurman RJ, Jensen AB, Lancaster WD. Oncogenic association of specific human papillomavirus types with cervical neoplasia. *Journal of the National Cancer Inst*, 1987; **79**: 671–7.

74. Giri I, Danos O. Papillomavirus genomes: from sequence data to biological properties. *Trends in Genetics*, 1986; **2**: 227–32.

75. *The human papillomaviruses*. IARC Monographs on the evaluation of carcinogenic risks to humans. Lyon: IARC, 1995.

76. Yang Y, Okayama H, Howley PM. Bovine papillomavirus contains multiple transforming genes. *Proceedings of the National Academy of Sciences of the United States of America*, 1985; **82**: 1030–4.

77. Yoshida M, Miyoshi I, Hinuma Y. Isolation and characterisation of retrovirus from cells of human adult T-cell leukemia and its implication in the disease. *Proceedings of the National Academy of Sciences of the United States of America*, 1982; **79**: 2031–5.

78. Blattner WA, Kalyanaraman VS, Robert-Guroff M. The human type C retrovirus, HTLV, in blacks from the Caribbean region, relationship to adult T cell leukaemia/lymphoma. *The Lancet*, 1982; **ii**: 1277–8.

79. Yoshida M, Miyoshi I, Hinuma Y. Isolation and characterisation of retrovirus from cells of human adult T-cell leukemia and its implication in the disease. *Proceedings of the National Academy of Sciences of the United States of America*, 1982; **79**: 2031–5.

80. Yoshida M, Seiki K, Yamaguchi K, K. T. Monoclonal integration of human T cell leukaemia provirus in all primary tumours of adult T cell leukaemia suggests causative role of human T cell leukaemia virus in the disease. *Proceedings of the National Academy of Sciences of the United States of America*, 1984; **81**: 2534–7.

81. Kim CM, Koike K, Saito I, Miyamura T, Jay G. HBx gene of hepatitis B virus induces liver cancer in transgenic mice. *Nature*, 1991; **351**: 317–20.

82. Klein NP, Schneider RJ. Activation of Src family kinases by hepatitis virus HBx protein and coupled signaling to Ras. *Molecular Cell Biology*, 1997; **17**: 6427–36.

83. Ponzetto A, Forzani B. Animal models of hepatocellular carcinoma: hepadnavirus-induced liver cancer in woodchucks. *Italian Journal of Gastroenterology*, 1991; **23**: 491–493.

84. Bosch FX, Peers F. Aflatoxins: data on human carcinogenic risk. *IARC Science Publication*, 1991; **105**: 48–53.

85. Ozturk M. p53 mutation in hepatocellular carcinoma after aflatoxin exposure. *The Lancet*, 1991; **338**: 1356–9.

86. Darby SC, *et al*. Mortality from liver cancer and liver disease in haemophilic men and boys in the UK given blood products contaminated with hepatitis C. *The Lancet*, 1997; **350**: 1425–31.

87. Lu SN, *et al*. Different viral aetiology of hepatocellular carcinoma between two hepatitis B and C endemic townships in Taiwan. *Journal of Gastroenterology and Hepatology*, 1997; **12**: 547–50.

88. Diamantis I, Bassetti S, Erb P, Ladewig D, Gyr K, Battegay M. High prevalence and coinfection rate of hepatitis G and C infections in intravenous drug addicts. *Journal of Hepatology*, 1997; **26**: 794–7.

89. Prince AM. Prevention of liver cancer and cirrhosis by vaccines. *Clinics in Laboratory Medicine*, 1996; **16**: 493–505.

90. Goedert JJ, *et al*. Spectrum of AIDS-associated malignant disorders. *The Lancet*, 1998; **351**: 1833–9.

91. Rose TM, *et al*. Identification of two homologs of the Kaposi's sarcoma-associated herpesvirus (human herpesvirus 8) in retroperitoneal fibromatosis of different macaque species. *Journal of Virology*, 1997; **71**(5): 4138–44.

92. Desrosiers RC, *et al*. A herpesvirus of rhesus monkeys related to the human Kaposi's sarcoma-associated herpesvirus. *Journal of Virology*, 1997; **71**: 9764–9.

Radiation carcinogenesis

R. J. M. Fry and J. D. Boice, Jr

Introduction

Why has radiogenic cancer been studied so extensively? The reasons include: (1) The ubiquitous nature of radiation; all the earth's inhabitants have evolved and exist in a background of radiation. The combination of oxidative metabolism and naturally occurring radiation has ensured the conservation of genes required for repair of DNA that has been damaged by reactive oxygen species created by ionizing radiation and sunlight. The importance of the maintenance of the fidelity of DNA to life, and errors in repair to death, sometimes from cancer, have driven research with a very broad impact. (2) In addition to background radiation, especially that due to radon, large numbers of people are exposed to radiation for medical reasons or occupationally. Information about the risk posed by exposure became imperative with the birth of the nuclear age. The medical profession required knowledge about radiation protection for their patients and themselves and about how radiation could benefit therapy. (3) Exposed populations, especially the atomic bomb survivors, provided the possibility to study the risk of cancer. (4) The knowledge that has been obtained about (a) the interaction of radiation with DNA and other targets, which is probably the most extensive for any carcinogen, (b) the subsequent changes at a chemical and all levels of biological organization, and (c) the ability to measure and estimate dose. Radiation is a remarkable tool for investigating the mechanisms of carcinogenesis in general. However, knowledge of the events from the initial deposition of energy to the emergence of a cancer (Fig. 1) is incomplete.

This chapter is restricted to ionizing and ultraviolet radiation. Ionizing radiation may be electromagnetic, X or γ rays, or particulate electrons, protons, neutrons, alpha particles, and heavy ions.[1] The wavelengths of ultraviolet radiation range from 100 to 400 nm.

Interactions of ionizing radiation with tissue

The major source of ionizing radiation is natural background, which includes cosmic rays, terrestrial radiation, radon, and its decay products (Table 1). The contribution of exposures to radiation from medical uses varies considerably between developing and industrialized countries but is the major man-made source. In countries with a high level of health care, the annual effective dose from diagnostic examinations ranges from 0.3 to 2.2 mSv per person. The total estimated effective dose per person ranges from 0.02 mSv in the undeveloped countries to 0.7 mSv in those countries with the most developed health care. The average for the world is 0.3 mSv.[2]

Deposition of energy

The ability to remove electrons from atoms distinguishes ionizing radiation, such as X rays, from non-ionizing radiations, such as heat and ultraviolet radiation. The important difference between ionizing and non-ionizing radiations is in the deposition of the energy. Heat is absorbed uniformly whereas the deposition of energy from ionizing radiation is localized or clustered along the tracks of individual particles. Electromagnetic radiations are considered ionizing if the photon energy exceeds 124 eV (the minimum energy required to displace an electron), which corresponds to wavelengths less than 10^{-6} cm. The photon energy increases with decreasing wavelength. Electrons, protons, alpha particles, heavy charged ions (a component of cosmic rays), and uncharged neutrons are classified as particulate radiations.

The spatial distribution of ionizations produced by different radiations is the basis of the classification of radiation quality. For example, X and γ rays are said to be sparsely ionizing and alpha particles and neutrons are densely ionizing (Fig. 1). The energy transferred per unit length of the track, termed linear energy transfer (LET) in keV/μm is related to the relative biological effectiveness (RBE) of radiations.[3] The RBE increases with increasing LET, reaching a maximum at about 100 keV/μm. At this LET, the average separation of the ionizing events is about the diameter of the DNA helix and there is a high probability that a single track will cause a DNA double strand break. Energy absorbed in biological material can interact directly with targets in the cell, such as DNA, and initiate, by ionization or excitation, the events that result in a biological effect (Fig. 2). This is the so-called direct action of radiation and is the predominant process with high-LET radiations. Alternatively, the energy deposited in the cell may interact with water to produce free radicals that can diffuse a distance of about 4 nm and damage DNA by indirect action, characteristic of low-LET radiation (Fig. 2).

Ionizing radiation induces base damage, single and double-strand breaks in DNA, and other lesions (Fig. 1). Reactive oxygen species are produced by the normal cellular process of oxidative metabolism[4] at levels equivalent to those produced by high doses of radiation but with little or no consequences compared to radiation. What is different? The damage to DNA from endogenous free radicals is predominately to bases and is repaired with spectacular efficiency.[5] In contrast, the distribution of energy from ionizing radiation is primarily from secondary electrons and results in clusters of hydroxy

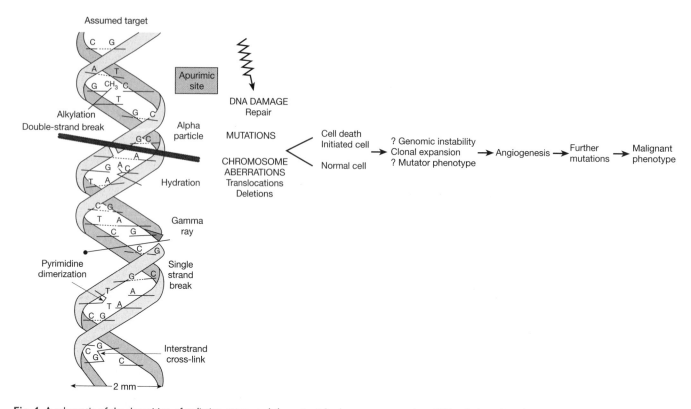

Fig. 1 A schematic of the deposition of radiation energy and the potential subsequent events. Low-LET radiations, X and γ rays are sparsely ionizing and the probability of inducing DNA double-strand breaks is low. In contrast, high-LET radiations, α particles, neutrons, and heavy ions produce a higher ratio of double-strand breaks to single-strand breaks than low-LET radiations.

Table 1 World average annual effective doses from natural sources (United Nations Scientific Committee on the Effects of Atomic Radiation[(2)])

Source	Worldwide average[a] annual effective dose[b] (mSv)
Cosmic rays	0.4
Terrestrial (external and internal)	0.7
Radon and decay products	1.3
Total	2.4[c]

[a] In some areas of the world the annual effective dose from cosmic rays may reach 2.0 mSv due to altitude and the effective dose from radon, and 10 mSv due to uranium deposits in the soil.

[b] Uniform whole-body exposures to radiation are rare. For example radiation from decay products of radon affects mainly the lung. Because of the significant differences in susceptibility of different organs to radiation-induced effects, absorbed doses are weighted by a factor that represents the relative contribution of the organ exposed to the total effect. The absorbed dose is also weighted for the radiobiological effectiveness of the radiation involved. The sum of the relevant weighted organ doses is known as the effective dose and is expressed in the SI unit sievert (Sv); 1 Sv = 100 rem. Radiation protection limits are expressed in terms of effective dose.

[c] The average annual effective dose in the United States is 3.6 mSv.

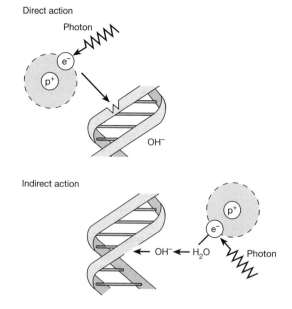

Fig. 2 A schematic of the indirect and direct action of radiation. Indirect action results from a hydroxyl radical (OH⁻) produced by a secondary electron and is characteristic of low linear energy transfer radiations. Damage to DNA can occur by direct action when energy from charged or uncharged particles is absorbed in the target, for example DNA. Atoms in the target may be excited or ionized, which starts the process leading to the DNA lesions. Direct action is characteristic of high-LET radiations.

radicals that in turn may cause localized multiple lesions in DNA.[6] These lesions are called multiply damaged sites and they consist of double and single DNA strand breaks and base damage. The latter two lesions are repaired rapidly and faithfully, but repair of double strand breaks is slower and, if part of complex lesions, the fidelity of the repair may be flawed. The probability of point mutations and chromosome aberrations increases with the complexity of the DNA lesion and the complexity increases with increasing LET, which explains why radiation with high LET is more efficient in causing biological effects (i.e. has a greater RBE).

Dose, dose response, dose fractionation, and dose rate

Dose

The fundamental unit quantity of radiation is absorbed dose, the energy absorbed per unit mass, which in the SI unit of joule per kilogram and has the special name gray (Gy); 1 gray = 100 rads. Dose may be specified at a point or, more commonly, averaged over an organ. Unfortunately, dose does not describe adequately the effect of very short range radiations such as alpha particles and Auger electrons. To investigate responses to these types of radiation at the cellular and subcellular level, it is necessary to determine the energy deposition at the micrometer or even nanometer scale.[7]

Dose response

The dose–response relationships of radiation-induced cancers vary among tissues. Therefore a number of different mathematical expressions could be fitted to the epidemiological and experimental data. There are two main approaches to dose–response models:

(1) to base the model on radiobiological considerations;
(2) to approximate empirically, for example, incidence as a function of dose, by simple mathematical functions.

A combination of the two approaches is used. The linear model, developed for point mutations, is the simplest and when modified for saturation of induction or cell inactivation is used to describe the response to high-LET radiation.

The linear–quadratic model was introduced to describe the induction of chromosome aberrations by low-LET aberrations as a function of dose (D) and is expressed as:

$$E = \alpha D + \beta D^2 \qquad (1)$$

where E is the probability of inducing a chromosome aberration, αD is the linear term, and βD^2 is the quadratic term. The linear term indicates the response to be predominantly due to single-track events, which are proportional to dose at low doses and low dose rates. With increasing dose and dose rates, two-track events become predominant and are proportional to the square of the dose, and the curve for the response bends upward (Fig. 3(a)). The dose response for high-LET radiation, such as neutrons, is linear, which implies the effect is caused by single track events (Fig. 3(a)). Linear, linear–quadratic, and quadratic dose responses have been considered applicable to data for the induction of different types of tumours. The dose response generally used in the estimation of the increase of radiation-induced cancer in epidemiological studies is a modified linear–quadratic response:

$$I(D) = (\alpha_0 + \alpha_1 D + \alpha_2 D^2)e^{-(\beta_1 D + \beta_2 D^2)} \qquad (2)$$

where $I(D)$ is the incidence corrected for intercurrent mortality, D is the dose, α_0 is the incidence in the unexposed population, α_1 and α_2 are coefficients for the linear and dose-squared terms for cancer induction and

$$e^{-(\beta_1 D + \beta_2 D^2)} \qquad (3)$$

is the probability of survival of neoplastically transformed cells where $\beta_1 D$ and $\beta_2 D^2$ are the linear and quadratic terms that describe the survival curve of the cells. High doses kill cells; however, the cell-killing term was based on a dose–response curve for the incidence of myeloid leukaemia not corrected for intercurrent mortality, which can overestimate the effect of cell killing[8] and was bell shaped. When the data were corrected for competing risks the curve was not bell shaped. The slope of the response decreased at high doses but did not become negative up to at least 4 Gy.

More importantly equation (2) is a simple description of a complex process such as radiation-induced carcinogenesis in which the effect of some of the factors, for example repair, must change with dose. Also, both the neoplastic transformation rate and cell killing are tissue dependent.

In experimental animals, the data from many types of tumours can be fitted to a linear–quadratic response. In contrast, with the exception of myeloid leukaemia, the dose–response curves for total cancers and individual types of tumours in the atomic bomb survivors[9] appear to be linear. It is not known why there is this difference.

Dose rate

A decrease of the dose rate of low-LET radiation reduces the carcinogenic effect. As the dose rate is reduced, the interval and spacing between individual depositions of energy or tracks increases. This results in a reduction of the probability of interaction of tracks and an increase in the probability of repair before an interaction, and thus reduces the effect (Fig. 3(a)).

As the dose rate is reduced a point is reached when lowering the dose rate further does not reduce the effect per unit dose. The effect is then dose-rate independent and total-dose dependent. The dose rate at which this occurs is dependent on the end point and the tissue. The United Nations Scientific Committee on the Effects of Atomic Radiation (UNSCEAR)[2] selected <0.05 mGy/min as the definition of a low dose rate.

There are no satisfactory data for the effect of dose rate on the induction of cancer in humans. Relevant experimental data are scanty but indicate that radiation exposure at low dose rates is perhaps five times less effective in causing cancer as the same total dose given at a high dose rate. An arbitrary low-dose-rate effectiveness factor (DREF) of two, which implies that there is a two-fold reduction in the probability of cancer induction at low dose rates compared to high dose rates, is used. For radiation protection purposes this reduction factor is the largest source of error in estimates of risk.[10]

A dose is considered protracted when it is both low dose rate and spread over a considerable time, perhaps weeks or months.

Dose fractionation

The epidemiological and experimental data indicate that the effects of fractionation of low-LET radiation in the reduction of the incidence

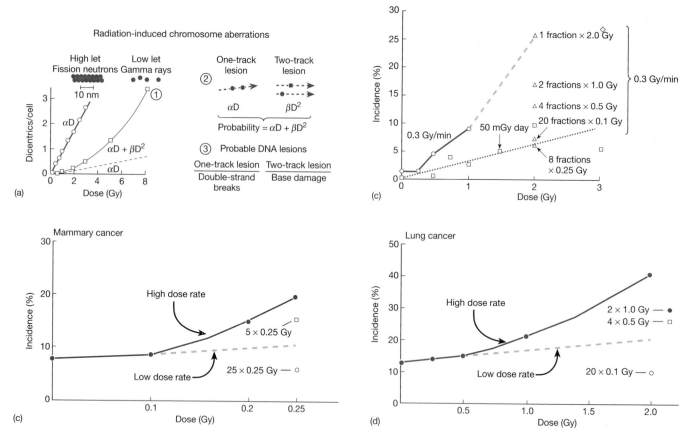

Fig. 3 (a) The probability of dicentric chromosome aberrations (which involves break in two separate chromosomes and result in a chromosome with two centromeres (dicentric)) as a function of dose of low and high-LET radiation, indicating the basis of the linear-quadratic dose–response model. (b) Dose response for induction of myeloid leukaemia in RFM mice by radiation.[11] (c) and (d) Dose responses for mammary cancer and lung cancer induced in BALB/c mice. (Adapted from ref 12). The radiation regimens are indicated.

of cancer as compared to the same total single dose are dependent on the dose per fraction and the tissue. If exposures to radiation are incurred in very small doses, about 0.01 to 0.5 Gy, depending on the tissue, or larger dose fractions are separated by adequate time for repair to occur, the carcinogenic effect is reduced. Fractionation reduces the induction of myeloid leukaemia and solid tumours in mice (Fig. 3).

An example of the tissue-dependent difference in the effect of fractionation is the exposure of patients with tuberculosis treated by pneumothorax. These patients underwent repeated examinations using fluoroscopy which involved multiple, small-dose fractions with high total doses, ranging up to about 18 Gy in the breast and about 24 Gy in the lung. Excess breast cancers but no excess lung cancers were observed.[13]

Fractionation appeared to reduce the incidence of lung cancer below that expected for a single dose but had little or no effect on the induction of breast cancer. The effect of dose fractionation in reducing the risk of radiation-induced cancer of the lung is supported by a comparison of the risk of lung cancer in the atomic bomb survivors exposed to a single high-dose-rate exposure and the fluoroscopy patients. For example the relative risk (observed/ expected) was 1.6 (1.3, 2.0) in the atomic bomb survivors compared to 1.00 (0.96, 1.07) for the fluoroscopy patients.[13]

Adaptive responses

Very low doses of low-LET radiation have been shown to reduce the induction of chromosome aberrations and other effects by subsequent exposure to higher doses, and this has been collectively referred to as an adaptive response.[14] The significance of these findings for these estimates of risk of cancer are not clear because the effect is transient. It has been suggested that adaptive responses are important in reducing the carcinogenic effect of ionizing radiation and that current estimates of risk are overestimates because the beneficial effect of adaptive responses are not taken into account.

Very low doses of radiation alter gene expression, including that of *TP53* which influences the processes of cell death by apoptosis and DNA repair (see Chapters 1.3 and 1.6). As yet, not enough information is available to factor adaptive responses into modelling of dose responses or the assessment of radiation risks.

Bystander effect

It has been assumed that the effect of radiation on cells is dependent on direct deposition of energy in the cell. Recently, it has been found that with alpha-particle radiation a much higher number of cells show sister chromatid exchanges[15] or altered expression of genes,

Table 2 Major epidemiological studies with quantitative estimates of radiation doses to specific organs and cancer risks[17],[18],[21],[22]

Type of exposure	Study
Radiotherapy for malignant disease	Cervical cancer[23],[24]
	Childhood cancer[26],[57]
	Breast cancer
	Endometrial cancer
	Hodgkin's disease[27]
	Bone marrow transplant[25]
Radiotherapy for benign disease	Ankylosing spondylitis[33]
	Benign gynaecological disorders
	Peptic ulcer[32]
	Breast disease
	Tinea capitis[30]
	Thymus[30]
	Tonsils[30]
	Haemangioma[31]
	Bone disease, radium-224
	Hyperthyroidism, iodine-131[43]
Diagnostic procedures	Tuberculosis, fluoroscopy[35],[36]
	Prenatal X-ray[37],[38]
	Thorotrast, thoron-232[39]
	Thyroid, iodine-131[42]
Occupation	Radium dial painters, radium-226[47]
	Underground miners[19]
	Radiologists[46]
	Nuclear workers[48],[52]
Atomic bomb	Japanese bomb survivors[9],[34]
	Marshall Islanders

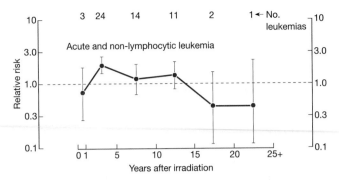

Fig. 4 Characteristic wave-like pattern of leukaemia risk over time since exposure among women treated with radiation for cervical cancer.[24]

including *TP53*, than are traversed by the particle.[16] This finding implies a bystander effect where damage in some cells leads indirectly to damage in neighbouring cells. Inhibition of gap junction communication between cells reduces the effect. These findings are important, in particular, for understanding the mechanism of induction of cancer by alpha particles.

Radiation epidemiology

There has been an evolution in the quality and sophistication of human studies of radiation effects, both in terms of quantifying cancer risk in relation to dose to specific organs and attempts to detect risk at relatively low levels of radiation exposure. The recent advances in radiation epidemiology have been compiled by the United Nations Scientific Committee on the Effects of Atomic Radiation,[17] in the Proceedings of the 1996 National Council on Radiation Protection and Measurements annual meeting,[18] and by the National Academy of Sciences Committee on the Biological Effects of Ionizing Radiation.[19] Based on such reports, national and international committees, such as the International Commission on Radiation Protection,[20] have set radiation protection guidelines for public and occupational exposures.

Important human studies with estimates of radiation dose to specific organs are listed in Table 2. While hundreds of studies have linked elevated cancer rates with medical radiation, only a few have been able to quantify risk by doses to specific organs. These human studies are discussed in more detail in the following sections.

Radiotherapy for cancer

Studies of medically-irradiated populations have provided substantial knowledge as to the carcinogenic effects of radiation, most notably an international study of cervical cancer patients.[23],[24] Other studies of second cancers providing important knowledge on radiation effects[22] include patients who developed breast cancer after radiotherapy for Hodgkin's disease, contralateral breast cancer after breast cancer, sarcomas after retinoblastoma and other childhood cancers, thyroid cancer after childhood cancer, and cancers after whole-body radiotherapy for bone marrow transplants.[22],[25],[26]

In large studies of cervical cancer patients treated with very high doses of ionizing radiation, it was predicted, based on studies of atomic bomb survivors, that several hundred extra cases of leukaemia would develop. Despite clinical blood evaluations and close observation of over 30 000 women in one series, however, no excess leukaemia was observed. When first reported in the 1960s, these large studies appeared to contradict current understanding of risk and suggested that radiation was not as effective in causing leukaemia as then believed, that cervical cancer patients might be immune to development of leukaemia, or that something peculiar in the way the radiation was delivered might be involved. Subsequently, larger studies using more sophisticated methods to estimate dose and risk provided a probable explanation, that is very high doses delivered to small volumes of tissue resulted in death of blood-forming stem cells such that neoplastic transformation could not occur.[23] Studies of several hundred thousand women with cervical cancer did eventually report a significant risk of leukaemia of about two-fold, which was attributed to the low dose scatter to bone marrow outside the irradiated pelvic area. A minimum latent period of about 2 years was seen and then risk was elevated for about 15 years before returning to normal levels; although the only significant elevation was seen 1 to 4 years after treatment (Fig. 4). The two-fold risk, at 7.5 Gy mean average dose to bone marrow, was substantially lower than the five-fold risk at 1 Gy observed among atomic bomb survivors, and the difference might be related to a combination of cell killing, the protraction of the irradiation (brachytherapy), the fractionation of the external beam

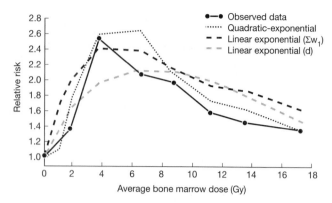

Fig. 5 Leukaemia dose–response relationship seen among women treated with radiation for cervical cancer.[21]

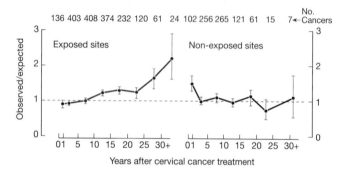

Fig. 6 Characteristic pattern of radiation-induced solid tumours over time since exposure, seen for heavily irradiated sites among cervical cancer patients treated with radiation.[24]

treatments, and the fraction of stem cells exposed during the partial-body exposures.

The leukaemia risk among cervical cancer patients was seen to increase with radiation dose averaged over the entire bone marrow up to about 4 Gy, and then decreased at higher levels, again suggesting that cell killing might predominate over transformation at such high doses (Fig. 5). A similar dose response was observed for radiation-induced chromosomal aberrations in circulating lymphocytes among cervical cancer patients. Lower risks of radiogenic leukaemia than expected, based on atomic bomb survivor data, have been confirmed in subsequent studies of patients treated with high-dose radiation for uterine cancer, breast cancer, and childhood cancer.[22] Such results offer a reasonable explanation as to why radiation-induced leukaemia appears to be a relatively rare occurrence after radiotherapy for cancer. In contrast, patients treated with high-dose alkylating agents are more frequently reported to develop excess numbers of leukaemia.

Another general characteristic of radiation-induced cancers is that the latent period, that is the time between exposure and the clinical detection of the malignancy, is relatively short for leukaemia (Fig. 6) and much longer for solid cancers.[17],[24] For irradiation in adulthood, the minimum latency for a solid tumour is about 5 to 9 years, and risk remains elevated for many years thereafter (Fig. 6).

Today, major advances in cancer therapy are allowing patients to live for many years and late effects of curative treatments are receiving greater attention. Thus, studies of long-term survivors of cancer will continue to provide quantitative information on radiation risks and perhaps lead to modifications in treatment approaches.

Radiotherapy and other factors

Only a few studies of interaction between factors that might increase cancer incidence have been conducted. Because of the increasing numbers of surviving cancer patients it is important to confirm whether radiotherapy and chemotherapy together enhance the risk of secondary leukaemia,[22] bone cancer,[26] and other tumours.

Studies of patients with Hodgkin's disease[27] and lung cancer[28] suggest that continued use of tobacco after radiotherapy potentiates the risk of secondary lung cancer. The extent to which radiotherapy and immunosuppression might interact to enhance the risk of cancer is not well-described,[17],[22] nor is the possible interaction between high-dose radiation and genetic predisposition.[29] It is also unclear whether low-dose indoor radon and cigarette smoking together enhance the risk of lung cancer, as seen in underground miners exposed to high levels of radon and radon decay products.[19]

Radiotherapy for benign disease

In years past, radiotherapy had been given to treat enlarged tonsils and thymus glands,[30] haemangiomas,[31] peptic ulcer,[32] ankylosing spondylitis,[33] and benign menstrual disorders.[17] These investigations have provided substantial knowledge on radiation-induced leukaemia and cancers of the thyroid, breast, and stomach. For example excess numbers of thyroid cancers appeared only among persons exposed under the age of about 15 years; irradiation of the newborn child resulted in excess breast cancer later in life; and leukaemia risks following protracted brachytherapy appeared somewhat lower than those following acute exposures.[17],[21] Significant excesses of stomach cancer that persisted to the end of life have been reported following radiation treatment for peptic ulcer in the 1940s.[32] Radiation combined with surgery appeared to enhance the development of stomach cancer, possibly mediated by hypoacidity and bile reflux. The relative risk estimates per Gy were similar to those reported from the studies of atomic bomb survivors, but the estimates of absolute excess risk were substantially different. The relative risk estimate for stomach cancer following irradiation for cervical cancer[23] is also more similar to the relative risk estimates among atomic bomb survivors[34] than the absolute risk estimates. These observations suggest that absolute estimates of radiation risk obtained from atomic bomb survivors for stomach cancer may not be applicable to Western populations, possibly related to the very high background rate of stomach cancer among Japanese. There is better agreement for relative risks (i.e. the ratio of risk in exposed compared to non-exposed populations).

Diagnostic uses of radiation

Other than background exposure due to radon, medical radiation from diagnostic procedures contributes the most to population exposure. Doses received by individual patients, however, are generally low and only a few studies have provided evidence of increased cancer rates. The first report that fractionated low-dose radiation (cumulating to large doses over several gray) could result in breast cancer later in life appeared in the 1960s and this was confirmed in the 1970s. The dose response was consistent with linearity, so that fractionating the cumulative dose over time did not appear to reduce risk much below that from more acute exposures.[35] The risk of breast cancer is seen to decrease with increasing age at exposure in practically all studies,[17] and risk appears minimal for postmenopausal women undergoing screenings with X-ray mammography. Large scale studies of tuberculosis patients have also failed to observe an increase in lung cancer despite substantial doses of the order of several gray, suggesting that the lung is relatively insensitive to the carcinogenic effects of radiation when the dose is delivered in many small fractions over a period of years.[36]

Since the reports in 1956 and 1958 that *in utero* radiation was associated with an increased risk of leukaemia and solid cancers during childhood, many epidemiological studies have been performed. Evidence for a causal association derives almost entirely from case-control studies (with their inherent biases, see Chapter 2. 4), whereas practically all cohort studies find no association, most notably the series of atomic bomb survivors exposed *in utero*.[37],[38] The evidence for an association of aetiological significance includes the consistency of findings in the case-control studies, the demonstration of a dose response, the reduction in risk seen over time apparently associated with a reduction of exposure dose, and the consistency with case-control studies of twins that minimize the possibility of selection bias.[37] The evidence against a causal relationship includes the absence of increased risk in any prospective study, the peculiar similarity in risk estimates (i.e. relative risks of about 1.5) for all solid cancers in childhood (e.g. Wilms' tumour, neuroblastoma, non-Hodgkin's lymphoma, brain cancer) despite the wide range of differences in occurrence and aetiology (suggesting an underlying bias in the case-control studies), and the minimal support from animal experiments.[38] There are few studies addressing the potential risk of adult cancer following intrauterine exposures, and the study of atomic bomb survivor is inconclusive. Despite these uncertainties, the medical profession has acted on the basis of a presumed risk for *in utero* exposures: ultrasound has largely replaced X-ray pelvimetry, and attempts to minimize fetal exposures are encouraged.

Radioactive thorium dioxide in colloidal solution (Thorotrast) has been used previously as a contrast agent for cerebral angiography and other radiographic examinations. Thorotrast is not excreted by the body and remains in the liver, bone marrow, and most body tissues. An alpha-particle emitter, Thorotrast was linked to very high risks of liver cancer and leukaemia, and to other cancers.[39] In some studies the cumulative risk of developing cancer after Thorotrast injection was over 80 per cent.

Medical and environmental radioactive iodines

There is an increasing understanding of radiation-induced thyroid cancer. Susceptibility, the type of tumour, and the mutations induced are age dependent. In a population of children (under 18 years of age) exposed to radioactive iodines from fallout from the Chernobyl accident, the rate of thyroid cancers, predominantly papillary carcinomas, was 13 per 10^4 (1986–1996) compared to a control level of 1 per 10^4.[40] About eight oncogenes or tumour suppressor genes have been associated with naturally-occurring thyroid cancers. In the papillary carcinomas in the children exposed to radiation, no mutations were found in *RAS* genes, in *TSH* receptor genes or in the exon of *TP53* that is commonly mutated. In contrast, about 60 per cent of the cancers showed rearrangement of the *RET* gene (see

Chapter 1.3 for information about these genes). *RET/PTC3* was the most frequent rearrangement of *RET* found.[41] Evidence suggests that a balanced intrachromosomal inversion, surmised to result from radiation-induced DNA double strand breaks, leads to a rearrangement involving the fusion of the *ELE* and *RET* genes.

It has been known since the 1950s that X-ray therapy in childhood resulted in high rates of thyroid cancer. Exposure of the thyroid gland in adult life, however, results in little if any cancer risk, whether from external photons[30],[40] or internal ^{131}I.[42] Large-scale studies of cancer incidence among patients administered diagnostic ^{131}I for scintillation scans have failed to reveal consistent evidence for an increased risk of thyroid cancer (mean dose 1 Gy). In addition to the strong modifying effect that age at exposure has on risk,[30],[34] the dose distribution in the thyroid gland and the relatively weak energy of the emitted beta particle during ^{131}I decay are other possible explanation for the absence of a radiation effect, that is the energy is deposited mainly in the colloid and does not reach the follicular cells. The low dose rate associated with the 8-day half-life of ^{131}I might also play a role if cellular damage has an opportunity to be repaired. Studies of large numbers of patients with hyperthyroidism treated with very high doses of ^{131}I have also failed to reveal any consistent excess of leukaemia or solid tumours.[43]

Mixed radionuclides of iodine, including those with shorter half-lives and more energetic beta emissions than those from ^{131}I, have been associated with increased risks of thyroid cancer, such as among the Marshallese Islanders exposed to fallout from a nuclear weapons test in 1954.[17],[21] Mixed radionuclides of iodine would uniformly irradiate the thyroid gland at a high rate, and probably contributed to the remarkable number of thyroid cancers seen among children after the reactor accident at Chernobyl.[44] Less than five deaths, however, have been attributed to thyroid cancer following the accident. The precise nature of the thyroid cancer risk among the residents near Chernobyl remains somewhat elusive and awaits dose–response evaluation; as well as clarification of the role of screening, the contribution of specific radionuclides, the modifying effect of endemic goiter, and the reasons for apparent urban–rural, country, and gender differences in risk. The reported sex ratio (male to female ratio) of incident thyroid cancer is near unity[44] and suggests that screening has made a substantial contribution to the reported excess of thyroid cancer. The sex ratio should be well below unity because females have both a higher background incidence of thyroid cancer than males and a higher risk of developing radiation-induced thyroid cancer. The high excess within 5 years of exposure is also much earlier than found in prior studies.[30] However, if the experience from X-irradiated populations holds, the excess of thyroid cancer would be predicted to continue far into the 21st century, and there should not be a levelling off or downturn in risk for many years. A downturn in the pattern of risk in the next 10 years would be consistent with a strong screening effect to explain the high number of excess cancers seen within the first 10 years of the accident.

A recent ecological survey attempting to link thyroid cancer mortality and incidence to estimated fallout doses of ^{131}I from weapons testing in the United States failed to find significant correlations overall or for exposures under the age of 5 when sensitivity is thought to be highest.[45] Interpretation is hindered by the substantial uncertainty in estimating thyroid dose some 40 years after exposure occurred, and the effect of population mobility. Children living in counties in the 1950s are unlikely to remain in the same counties for

40 years so that any correlation (or lack of) between estimated dose to thyroid and cancer occurrence is difficult to interpret. No increase in leukaemia has been attributed to Chernobyl radiation or to medical ^{131}I, in all likelihood because of the associated low bone marrow dose.

Occupation

The first cancer death attributable to radiation occurred in 1902 following occupational exposure to Thomas Edison's assistant, Mr Clarence Dally, who experienced substantial exposure during the development of the X-ray fluoroscope. Past studies of pioneering radiologists,[17],[46] underground miners,[19] and radium dial painters[47] contributed to our understanding of radiation effects and to the setting of radiation protection standards.[20] Occupational exposures today are generally low and any associated increases in cancer are difficult to detect.[48]

Workers at nuclear installations

Studies of workers within the nuclear industry may provide some validation of the risk estimates obtained from high dose and high dose rate investigations. Radiation doses are recorded for most workers and cumulative exposure for some might reach levels where adverse effects could be detected. Data from nearly 100 000 nuclear industry workers in three countries have been analysed and death due to leukaemia, but not other cancers, was significantly elevated.[48] Overall, only about nine of the nearly 4000 cancer deaths could be attributable to radiation. Despite the large numbers, even the combined series appear to have low statistical power to detect excess cancers related to the low doses received. Nonetheless, such studies can exclude the possibility that current risk estimates substantially underestimate risk at low doses.

Chernobyl

Few informative epidemiological studies have been published of the more than 600 000 workers sent to Chernobyl to clean up the contaminated environment and entomb the damaged reactor. No excess incidence of leukaemia or of other cancers was found among nearly 5000 workers from Estonia, and only death due to suicide was significantly elevated.[49] Thyroid screening of 2400 Estonian clean-up workers with ultrasound and subsequent needle biopsy of nodules revealed no radiation-related increase in thyroid disease.[18] A large group of Russian clean-up workers has been studied for leukaemia and thyroid cancer,[50] but interpretations are clouded because of apparent biases associated with special screening examinations and over-ascertainment (and misdiagnosis) among the workers and under-reporting of diagnoses in the general population used for comparison. Initial biological dosimetry studies of clean-up workers were generally consistent with estimates from physical dosimetry that the average dose received was about 10 cGy; however, more recent cytogenetic results based on fluorescent in situ hybridization (FISH) technology (see Chapter 1. 2) found little evidence for an increase in chromosomal aberrations among workers and suggested that mean doses might be lower than 10 cGy.[51] If the recent biodosimetry evaluations hold true, it will be difficult for even these larger studies to provide quantitative information on cancer risks.

Workers exposed to plutonium

Studies of large populations of workers exposed to low levels of plutonium find little correlation between plutonium exposure and cancer mortality.[17],[21] Recently, however, very-high-dose plutonium exposures have been reported to cause excess lung cancers among over 2300 workers at the Mayak radiochemical and plutonium production plants in Russia.[52] Mortality due to leukaemia was also elevated but was correlated with γ-ray doses and not plutonium exposure.

Radiologists and radiological technologists

Pioneering radiologists experienced increased rates of leukaemia and skin cancer in the years before the hazards of excessive radiation exposure were appreciated.[17],[21],[46] It was not uncommon, for example, for low white blood cell counts to be used as personal dosimeters to indicate that too much time was being spent with the X-ray apparatus.

Radiological technologists in more recent years are exposed to relatively low doses of radiation over long periods of time. The largest study to date of 145 000 technologists failed to identify a risk of leukaemia or breast cancer, although the data suggested a slight excess of breast cancer among women who worked during the 1940s when exposures might have been high.[53] Overall, the risk of cancer appears much lower than observed in studies of early radiologists who probably received substantially higher exposures.[46]

Radon

In 1556, Agricola described a mysterious lung disease afflicting miners of the Black Forest regions of Europe.[19] Inhaled radon and its decay products were subsequently indicted as the culprit. Studies of underground miners demonstrate convincingly that radon is a potent carcinogen, able to cause lung cancer and to interact with cigarette smoking in a way that enhances risk. Estimates from underground miners suggest that perhaps 10 to 14 per cent of all lung cancers in the general population may be related to breathing radon within homes. Radon in homes comes from the soil below. Uranium and the thorium in the soil eventually decay to radon, a radioactive gas, which percolates through the soil and collects in homes. Leukaemias and other cancers did not occur in excess among underground miners. Radon has not been linked to childhood leukaemia in studies involving radon measurements within homes.

It has been difficult to detect a risk of lung cancer due to radon levels in homes in case-control studies, in large part because the doses are low with an expected relative risk of only about 1.15 based on extrapolations from studies of miners. Further, other factors such as cigarette smoking are more important contributors to lung cancer risk with relative risks greater than 10-fold, and their effects are difficult to adjust for adequately. A recent meta-analysis was conducted of eight large case-control studies.[54] Although the reasons for heterogeneity in risk estimates among the studies could not be resolved, the combined estimate of risk at 150 Bq/m^3 (the level of radon that is close to the action level recommended in many countries for citizens to modify homes to reduce radon levels) was statistically significant at 1.14. Based on current evidence, the estimates of risk extrapolated from studies of underground miners appear to be valid at the lower radon levels experienced in homes.[19]

Atomic bomb survivors

The Japanese survivors of the atomic bombs dropped during World War II are at increased risk of developing cancer.[9],[17],[18],[21],[34] Risk was somewhat higher among children than adults, residents of Hiroshima than Nagasaki, and females than males. The elevated risk of cancer among survivors in Hiroshima may be related in part to a greater exposure to neutrons than in Nagasaki. The excess relative risk over time has remained constant for adults but is decreasing for survivors exposed as children. Many cancers have occurred in excess among atomic bomb survivors, including myelogenous leukaemia and cancers of the breast, thyroid, lung, stomach, colon, and others. Some cancers have not shown a significant increased rate of occurrence, including chronic lymphocytic leukaemia, T-cell leukaemia, non-Hodgkin's lymphoma, Hodgkin's disease, and cancers of the pancreas, rectum, cervix, testis, and prostate.

The dose response for leukaemia appears linear–quadratic whereas a straight line adequately fits the data for all solid cancers combined (c.f. Fig. 3). The linearity in the dose response for all solid cancers differs from animal studies and might be related to the effect of the small neutron component to dose, bias in reporting cause of death as cancer among low-dose survivors, errors in dosimetry, and/or the peculiar lumping of all cancers together despite various aetiologies and sensitivities to the induction of cancer by radiation. Approximately 500 cancers (7 per cent of all cancer deaths and 1 per cent of all deaths among the exposed populations) were attributed to radiation received from the atomic bombs. The risk of radiogenic leukaemia also appears to have run its course 40 years after exposure. Recent application of tumour registry data revealed excess cancers of the liver, thyroid, and skin.[34] Little additional information will be forthcoming on Japanese survivors older than about 40 years in 1945 since most have subsequently died. However, it will be well into the 21st century before lifetime risks among the young at exposure can be fully assessed.

Environmental exposure

Studies of populations exposed to high levels of natural background radiation have, in large part, been negative or non-informative.[17] In general, ecological studies are the weakest form of epidemiological research and have provided little insight into radiation risks. Some studies of populations living in areas of high natural background radiation in China and India have the advantage of estimating doses to individuals with some precision because there is little migration. However, the doses are generally low so that even large numbers of exposed persons have limited statistical power to detect effects.[17] A comprehensive study of women in China who lived their entire lives on radioactive sand due to high thorium content, for example, did not have problems of migration or uncertainty in dose estimates but failed to identify an increase in thyroid cancer or nodular disease.[17]

Studies of populations exposed to high levels of radioactive waste in the Southern Urals of Russia, however, are ongoing.[55] In 1957, a storage tank exploded (the Kyshtym accident) and released large amounts of radioactive waste, about one-quarter of that released from the Chernobyl accident. The population exposure, however, was not as great as that resulting from the dumping of high-level radioactive wastes from the Mayak nuclear facility into the Techa River prior to the accident. Excess leukaemia has been reported among the 28 000 residents along the river and doses as high as 400 cGy have been estimated. These studies have the potential for providing new information on the effects of ionizing radiation delivered chronically over time.

Radiation and genetic predisposition

The prevalence of known high penetrance mutations that predispose to cancer is less than 1 per cent in the general population and may account for 5 per cent of total cancers (see also Chapter 1.4). It is difficult to assess the increase in susceptibility for radiogenic cancers that may be associated with familial cancers. There are increased risks of radiation-induced cancer in persons with hereditary retinoblastomas[26],[56],[57] and nevoid basal cell cancer syndrome (NBCCS).[56] In breast cancer, in which the genetic contribution is relatively high, and in other familial cancers, the frequency of inherited mutations in known oncogenes or tumour suppressor genes is too low to have an impact on the assessment of radiation risk in the general population. Further, because of the high risk of spontaneous cancer in familial disorders, low doses of radiation are unlikely to influence cancer risk in the affected individual, whereas high doses from radiotherapy may be important.[56]

Ataxia telangiectasis (AT) is a rare, inherited syndrome caused by deficiency in DNA repair where cells are hypersensitive to cell killing by radiation. Children with this syndrome have a risk of cancer that is 100-fold that in the general population. Furthermore, the frequency of heterozygous mutations of the ATM gene (mutated in AT) in the general population is perhaps 1 per cent and the cells have a radiosensitivity to cell killing intermediate between that of homozygotes and controls. The impact of the heterozygous mutations on risk of cancer is disputed, from negligible to being involved in over 6 per cent of all breast cancers. There has not been a convincing demonstration that the heterozygotes have an increased sensitivity to induction of breast cancer by radiation in young women, an important question relative to the use of mammograms in the under 40 age group.[17],[56],[58]

Future research opportunities

Radiation epidemiology in the future should be able to clarify a number of important questions, notably the lifetime risk from exposures in childhood, the magnitude of the risk of second cancers following curative radiotherapy, the level of risk associated with radiation occupations in medicine and in the nuclear industry, as well as the effects of ^{131}I, plutonium, and radon. The study of the effects of chronic exposures is perhaps the most important research area for the future. Coupled with molecular analyses, there will also be new opportunities to study mechanisms of cancer induction, interactions with environmental carcinogens, or underlying genetic predispositions. It would be fascinating to learn whether radiations, either external or internal, could cause molecular signatures that implicates them uniquely as environmental causes of specific cancers. Emphasis should continue to be placed on studies of cancer survivors treated with radiotherapy since this group is rapidly becoming larger as a direct result of successful therapies. Studies of survivors of childhood cancer as well as the children exposed to the atomic bombs in Japan should make important contributions to our understanding of radiation carcinogenesis.

Mechanisms of radiation carcinogenesis

The induction of a permanent change in the control of the balance of cell proliferation, differentiation, and cell death is central to carcinogenesis. It is thought that the initial mutation is either in an oncogene(s) or tumour suppressor gene. Ionizing radiation induces a higher frequency of deletions than point mutations and deletions are more likely to inactivate tumour suppressor genes.

Recently, tumour suppressor genes have been classified into gate-keepers and caretakers.[59] Gatekeeper genes inhibit growth or increase the cell death rate. Examples of these genes are the adenomatous polyposis (APC) and retinoblastoma (RB1). Both copies of this type of suppressor gene must be inactivated to cause a tumour. It is proposed that inactivation of caretaker genes causes genomic instability and an increased mutation rate. Mismatch repair genes, MSH2 and MLH1, which are implicated in hereditary non-polyposis colorectal cancer (HNPCC) are considered caretaker genes (see Chapter 10.4). Loss of mismatch repair activity in a potential tumour cell may lead to genetic instability, leading to multiple mutations, which increase the probability of progression of the neoplastic process.

Initial events of tumourigenesis

The mutations associated with naturally-occurring cancers are also involved in radiogenic cancers. As yet, no specific radiation-induced lesion has been identified in solid cancers. In some leukaemias there are specific chromosome aberrations but they occur in both the radiation-induced and naturally-occurring leukaemias. Alterations in specific genes are associated with tumours in a number of specific tissues. For example, RET in thyroid, discussed above, and the patched gene (PTCH) in skin, discussed later, and BRCA1 and 2 in breast (see also Chapters 1.3 and 1.4).

The mutations and altered gene activity detected in radiation-induced tumours are not unique to radiation and the spectrum of induced changes is similar to that found in other tumours. An intensive search for specific mutations has been carried out, for example, in TP53 in lung cancers associated with exposure to alpha-particle radiation but no significant lesion has been identified. However, K-ras activation after exposure to either γ-rays or neutrons was shown to be characteristic of radiation-induced thymomas in AKR × RF/J/F$_1$ mice. N-ras genes were more frequently activated by chemical carcinogens.[60] In thymic lymphomas in RJ/F mice, the mutation spectra in the N-ras gene were different in tumours induced by γ-rays than in those included by neutrons.[61]

Overexpression but not amplification of c-myc was found in radiation-induced tumours in BCF$_1$ mice, especially in sarcomas,[62] and overexpression of several oncogenes was reported in osteo-sarcomas.[63] APC-deficient (min) mice are prone to the development of intestinal adenomas as a result of a germ line mutation of one of the two copies of the APC tumour suppressor gene. Ionizing radiation increased the number of tumours per mouse as compared to the unexposed mice. Thus, radiation may influence expression of spontaneous tumours and not initiation.[64]

A low incidence of myeloid leukaemia occurs spontaneously in a number of strains of mice and in all of the strains an incomplete translocation or an interstitial deletion in chromosome 2 is found. Radiation causes a dose-dependent increase and there is evidence that the changes in chromosome 2 initiate leukaemia.[65]

Because of the high frequency of mutations in TP53 in humans and Trp53 in mice in many types of tumours, the question arises whether it is an initial target for radiation carcinogenesis. Knockout mice deficient in Trp53 are more susceptible to both naturally-occurring and radiation-induced tumours.[66] This evidence alone does not indicate that the gene is an initial target. In many of the lymphomas induced in the knockout mice the wild type copy of the gene was lost. It was shown that in the cells of Trp53$^{+/-}$ mice there was a defect in G^2/M-phase checkpoint which leads to a radiation-induced loss or gain of chromosomes and it is suggested that chromosome 11 (the chromosome site of Trp53) may be the target.[67]

Genomic instability and mutator phenotype

Multiple chromosomal aberrations and mutations are found in cancers. The possibility that the multiplicity of lesions is a direct effect of a single exposure to radiation that causes a cancer is virtually nil. The very large number of mutations in cancer cells cannot be accounted for by known rates of radiation-induced mutation rates. Based on cell proliferation rates over a lifespan, a cell might acquire about three mutations but tumour cells may have hundreds. This discrepancy led to the suggestion by Loeb that acquisition of a mutator phenotype was a seminal change in cancer induction[68] and there is substantial evidence that radiation induces genomic instability.[69] At about the same time, Nowell suggested that the chromosomal aberrations and changes in number of chromosomes were caused by genomic instability and clonal selection that accelerated progression.[70]

A mutator phenotype is a term to describe the abnormal incidence of mutations that far exceeds the spontaneous mutation rate or that which could be induced by a single exposure to a carcinogenic agent such as ionizing radiation. The acquisition of a mutator phenotype may occur by different mechanisms. The recognition that ionizing radiation can induce genomic instability which might account for the multiplicity of mutations found in some cancer cells, and therefore the acquisition of what might be termed a mutator phenotype, is currently favoured as an explanation of some aspects of radiation carcinogenesis.

Ionizing radiation can cause mutations and chromosome instability in the progeny of normal cells many divisions after irradiation.[69] In mice there is an association between the probability of radiation-induced delayed chromosome aberrations and susceptibility for the induction of tumours.[71] The delayed development of mutations may provide an explanation of the latent period and of the large number of mutations in radiogenic cancers. High-LET radiations, such as alpha particles and heavy ions, are more effective than low-LET radiation in the induction of both genomic instability and carcinogenesis.

The frequency of genomic instability in bone marrow and other cells is not consistent with a specific mutation.[15] The probability of inactivating a specific gene, such as a mismatch repair gene, is less than 10^{-5}. Furthermore, four to six times as many cells show instability than are traversed by a single particle—the bystander effect discussed earlier.

The concept of genomic instability as an explanation for the multiplicity of mutations found in cancers is attractive especially since radiation can induce genomic instability, but the precise mechanisms that lead to radiation-induced cancer is not yet clear. Microsatellite instability is recognized as a feature of certain colon cancers. Mutations in repetitive sequences of genes associated with growth control may be important in a number of tissues and microsatellite instability may reflect the introduction of a mutator phenotype.

Multistage carcinogenesis

The consensus that cancer is a multistage process is based on:

(1) the observation that many cancers start as premalignant lesions, such as adenomas, and progress;

(2) there is more than one rate-limiting alteration;

(3) in some tumours a sequential appearance of mutations has been found in the progression of a cancer.

A single dose of radiation is a complete carcinogen and the latent period from exposure to the recognition of a cancer, while variable, can in humans be decades. For some types of cancer, such as breast, the majority of radiation-induced cancers appear at a time close to the age that the natural incidence of the specific cancer is rising and relatively independent of age at exposure. This suggests an influence of host factors.

Ionizing radiation induces a low frequency of complex damage that is repaired with difficulty and with errors. The result may be cell death or survival with chromosome aberrations, or other lesions resulting in mutations. Studies of radiation carcinogenesis have not provided any unique evidence for multistage carcinogenesis.

Ultraviolet radiation carcinogenesis

Introduction

There are three main types of skin cancer—basal cell carcinoma, squamous cell carcinoma (collectively referred to as non-melanoma carcinomas), and melanomas (see Chapters 8.1 and 8.3). Sunlight is implicated as a major cause in all three types of cancer. Basal cell carcinoma is the commonest neoplasm in Caucasians, accounting for about 80 per cent of the non-melanoma carcinomas, and squamous cell carcinoma about 20 per cent, and melanoma accounts for about 5 per cent of all skin cancers.[72]–[76]

Accurate annual incidence rates of non-melanoma skin cancer are difficult to obtain but the estimate for the United States in 1996 was about 800 000. The estimated new cases of melanoma for 1998 was 41 600. In Australia, the incidence of skin cancer was estimated in 1985 to be twice that of all other cancers. Incidence rates are increasing and most importantly melanoma is increasing at about 3 per cent per year in the United States.

Mortality rates from non-melanoma skin cancers are very low. Estimates of metastasis rates for basal cell carcinoma range from 0.003 per cent to 0.1 per cent, and for squamous cell carcinomas 1 per cent to 2 per cent.[75] It is estimated that 7300 of the 41 600 cases in the United States in 1998 will die from melanoma.[76]

Skin cancer and sun exposure

The evidence that exposures to the sun causes skin cancer in human includes:

(1) skin cancers occur more frequently in people who live in regions with high ambient solar irradiance and in those occupationally exposed;

(2) non-melanoma skin cancers occur most frequently on exposed sites, such as head, neck, and arms;

(3) pigmented skin is much less susceptible to non-melanoma skin cancers;

(4) lack of pigmentation, as in albinism, increases risk;

(5) high incidence at a young age in patients with xeroderma pigmentosum who are deficient in repair of ultraviolet radiation (UVR)-induced DNA damage induced by exposure to sunlight.

The incidence of skin cancer increases with increasing levels of ambient UVR. In the United States, the incidence of squamous cell carcinoma increases by 2 per cent to 4 per cent per 1 per cent increase in UVR, basal cell carcinomas by 1 per cent to 3 per cent, and melanomas by 0.5 per cent to 1 per cent.[76]

The closer to the equator, the greater the ultraviolet irradiance. In Australia, a nine-fold higher incidence of squamous cell carcinomas was observed in regions at latitudes less than 29°S compared to latitudes greater than 37°S. The increases in basal cell carcinomas and melanomas increased over three and two-fold respectively (Table 3).

The importance of exposure to the sun in the aetiology of melanoma has been questioned because melanomas frequently occur on less exposed areas of the body but this may be related to the importance of sunburn and intermittent recreational exposures, and not to the chronicity of exposures, which is important for non-melanoma carcinomas.

The risk of melanoma increases when children move to countries with high ambient solar irradiation but not when migration is at older ages. Both the high solar radiation and the greater susceptibility for melanoma at young ages appear to be involved.[77]

Concern about the effect of reduction of the ozone concentration in the stratosphere on diseases induced by UVR was raised as early as 1935. Recent estimates are that each 1 per cent decrease in ozone could increase the incidence of basal cell carcinomas by 2 per cent, squamous cell carcinomas by 3.5 per cent, and melanomas by 0.6 per cent.

The induction of photoproducts and dependence of DNA lesions on wavelength

In Fig. 7, the influence of wavelength on the molecular changes caused by UVR is shown. The wavelength influences the frequency of the lesions more than the type of lesion induced. The UVC radiation is not of importance as an environmental carcinogen because it is absorbed completely by the atmosphere. The amount of UVB radiation absorbed depends on the stratospheric ozone layer. UVA radiation is not absorbed by the atmosphere and penetrates deeper into the skin than UVB radiation.

UVC and UVB

The C5–C6 double bond of the pyrimidine bases in DNA (i.e. thymine and cytosine) is the most photochemically reactive and the commonest lesions are some form of dipyrimidine products (Fig. 7). The importance of (6–4) photoproducts (Fig. 7) has been demonstrated in a revertant xeroderma pigmentosum cell line capable of repairing these lesions but not cyclobutane pyrimidine dimers,[78] suggesting that cyclobutane pyrimidine dimers play an important, if not predominant, role in the biological effects of UVB radiation, including carcinogenesis. The predominant repair of the UVB radiation-induced lesions is by nucleotide excision repair. There are at least six distinct steps in nucleotide excision repair. The lesion is recognized, conformational changes in DNA occur, there is incision of the damaged strand on both sides of the lesion leaving the undamaged DNA strand

Table 3 Incidence of melanoma and non-melanoma in Australia in relation to latitude[77]

Latitude	Incidence per 100 000 person years		
	Melanoma	Basal cell carcinoma	Squamous cell carcinoma
<29°S	41	1182	421
29°–37°S	27	791	297
>37°S	19	323	47

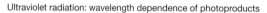

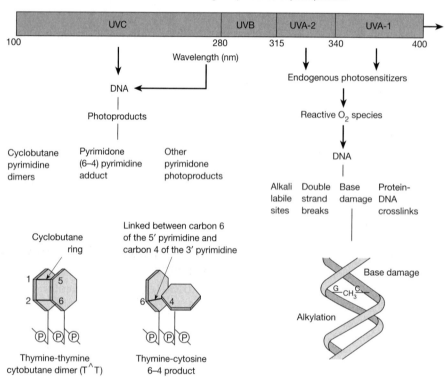

Fig. 7 A schematic of the dependence on wavelength of UV radiation for the induction of photoproducts.

intact, removal of the damage, DNA polymerase I activity and DNA synthesis replace the gap and finally the new DNA is sealed by a ligase to the pre-existing strand of DNA. In fish and marsupials, photoreactivation is a major mechanism of repair and this has been used to establish the central role of cyclobutane pyrimidine dimers in UVR-induced cancer in the opossum, *Monodelphis domestica* (Fig. 8). Photoreactivation reduces the number of cyclobutane pyrimidine dimers and the incidence of tumours.[79]

Repair of DNA damage induced by ionizing and UV radiation involves a large number of genes. Three main pathways have been identified and are identified by one of the prominent genes involved. For example, *RAD3* epistasis is responsible for nucleotide excision repair, *RAD52* group for double-stranded break repair and recombination, and the *RAD6* epistasis group for postreplication repair.

Xeroderma pigmentosum is a syndrome in which there is a deficiency in the repair of the DNA damage induced by sunlight. In xeroderma pigmentosum, the persistence of UVR-induced damage because of defective nucleotide excision repair is associated with a high incidence of skin cancer at a young age in areas exposed to sunlight (Fig. 9). The average age of a patient with non-melanoma skin cancer is about 60 years.[80] The difference in age distributions of the cancers indicates the debt we owe to evolution of repair of DNA damage by nucleotide excision repair. Excision repair eliminates many lesions including cyclobutane pyrimidine dimers and (6–4) photoproducts. In xeroderma pigmentosum, the postreplication process is also defective. In another rare syndrome with deficiency in DNA repair, trichothiodystrophy, the defect in nucleotide excision repair is associated with photosensitivity but not with excess skin

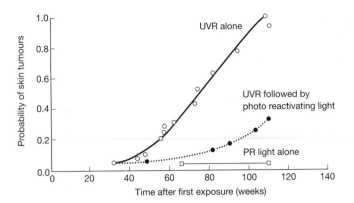

Fig. 8 Probability of skin tumours in *Monodelphis domestica* as a function of time after the first exposure to UVR (280–400 nm): ○- - -○; followed by exposure to 320–700 nm light: ○- - -○; and after exposure to 320–700 nm light: ..... .[79]

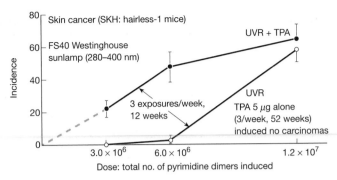

Fig. 10 Incidence of squamous cell carcinomas in SKH: hairless mice as a function of the cyclobutane pyrimidine dimers. UVR exposures, 3 per week for 12 weeks of 250, 500, and 1000 J/m²: ○- - -○. The same UVR regimen followed by treatments with 5 µg 12-0-tetradecanoylphorbol-13-acetate (TPA), 3 per week for 52 weeks: ○- - -○.[82] (Reproduced from Fry, 1984, with permission.)

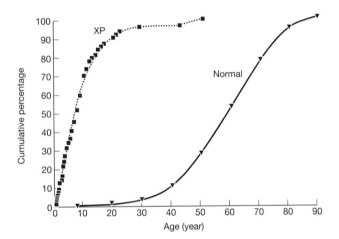

Fig. 9 Age at onset of cancer of the skin in xeroderma pigmentosum patients and in the general US population. (Reproduced from Kraemer 1997, with permission.[80])

shown in Fig. 7, the effects of the longer wavelengths are not caused by direct absorption of photons by DNA, as occurs with UVB, but by the production of reactive oxygen species. In contrast to UVB, base damage and DNA strand breaks predominate after exposure to UVA, but it is not known which of the DNA lesion(s) plays the major role in the mutations induced by UVA. In mouse skin, G:C to A:T transitions predominate but the frequency of induced *Trp53* mutations is less than with UVB.[81] UVA is able to induce skin cancer in mice, but it is not known how important UVA is in humans.

Non-melanoma skin cancers (see also Chapter 8.3)

Dose response

It was recognized in both epidemiological and experimental animal studies that multiple exposures to UVR were required to induce an excess of skin cancers and that the latent period was long. Experimental evidence indicates that the later exposures in a series influence the expression of the UVR-induced initiation; thus UVR acts not only as an initiator but also as a promoter.

The skin appears to have a remarkable ability to 'suppress' the progress from initiation to overt cancer. This interpretation is applicable to the data in Fig. 10. The curve for the relationship of the incidence of squamous cell carcinomas as a function of the total number of cyclobutane pyrimidine dimers, an appropriate biodosimeter, is curvilinear and suggests a threshold. The presence of initiated cells is revealed by their expression when promoted by repeated treatments with the promoter, 12-0 tetradecanoyl-phorbol-13-acetate (TPA) after the UV radiation regimen. The curve is shifted to the left.[82]

The interpretation of the findings in experimental animal studies has been supported by elegant molecular studies that are described below.

Squamous cell carcinoma

The two major photoproducts of UVB radiation are mutagenic. About 70 per cent of the mutations are cytosine to thymine (C → T)

cancer. The difference in susceptibility to cancer may be due to differences in the induction or repair of UVR-induced DNA photoproducts. Other explanations, such as differences in catalase levels and immune surveillance, have been proposed. Cockayne's syndrome is also a DNA repair deficient disease that shows no increased risk of skin cancer.

The role of the individual DNA photoproducts and their repair in UVR carcinogenesis remains unclear. It is like a complex lock where many of the tumblers have been turned by the investigator's key but not all of them.

UVA

UVA comprises the major fraction of the total spectral energy of solar UVR. Because of differences in their biological effects UVA has been divided into UVA2 (wavelength 315–340 nm), which has some similarity to UVB but is less effective in causing cancer, and UVA1 (340–400 nm), with quite different effects from those of UVB. As

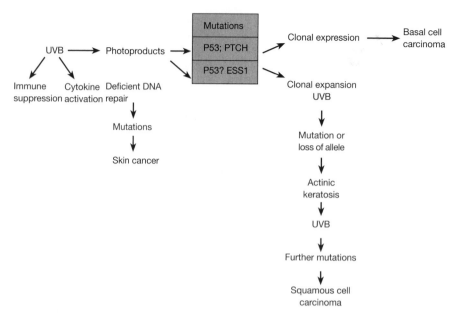

Fig. 11 Schematic of the mechanism of UVR-induced skin cancer. (Adapted from Brash, 1997.[84])

dipyrimidines (Fig. 7), 10 per cent are CC → TT, known as tandem-base changes.[83] Such specificity becomes important when the signature can be detected in genes such as *TP53* in skin tumours.[84]

The specific mutations which can be used to trace the history of the tumour has added an important temporal aspect. Over 50 per cent of human tumours show mutations in the tumour suppressor gene *TP53* and over 90 per cent of squamous cell carcinomas studied in the United States have a mutation somewhere in the *TP53* gene. Mutation hot spots occur, often at sites where photoproduct repair is slow. Mice with a mutation in *Trp53* are more susceptible to induction of tumours by UVR. In mice, *Trp53* mutations are found within 3 weeks of the onset of daily UVB irradiation and long before tumours are detected.[85] Mutation in the *TP53* gene is an early event in UVR-induced neoplastic transformation. However, patients with the Li–Fraumeni syndrome, with cells defective in *TP53*, there is a high incidence of cancer at several sites but not skin.

In the model of UVR carcinogenesis proposed by Brash and his colleagues (Fig. 11):

(1) *TP53* mutations are induced by UV photoproducts;

(2) with repeated exposures to UVR mutated cells undergo clonal expansion and further clones are induced;

(3) clonal expansion is enhanced by:

   (a) keratinocytes being killed by UVR (death by apoptosis, itself *TP53*-dependent, and detected by the presence of sunburn cells); and

   (b) the mutated cells having a greater resistance to the lethal effects of UVR;

(4) the enlarged, mutated cell population is a large target for further UVR-induced mutations and may obviate the need to involve the induction of a mutator phenotype;

(5) further mutations lead to progression to squamous cell carcinomas.[84]

Other effects of UVR, especially on the immune system must be taken into account in any complete model and hopefully, age dependency of susceptibility will be explained.

Immune surveillance is considered by some to be an important defence mechanism against malignancy. The finding that UVB radiation eliminated the capacity of the immune system to recognize and inhibit tumours induced by UVR in mouse skin[86],[87] led to a new field of research called photoimmunology. The reduction in the ability of the immune system to inhibit the development of tumours is considered an effect of UVB radiation that contributes to the cause of skin cancer by sunlight. The effects of UVB radiation are both local and systemic. Low doses of UVB radiation affect the ability of antigen presenting cells (Langerhans cells) to transfer antigenic signals to T cells in local lymph nodes effectively.

There may well be a number of pathways to the development of squamous cell carcinomas. The importance of the changes in genes and their sequence is not clear. Mutations of *TP53* have been reported in normal human skin exposed to sunlight;[88] the frequency of mutations in *TP53* varies from 10 to 60 per cent in squamous cell carcinomas; and premalignant lesions frequently have *TP53* mutations. Mutations in *RAS* are not a consistent finding, varying in frequency from 0 to 46 per cent.[89]

UVR and psoralens

Combined treatment with ultraviolet radiation (320–400 nm) and psoralen has been used in the treatment of psoriasis. In a therapeutic trial with a follow-up of 13 years, 25 per cent of the patients developed squamous cell carcinomas and only this type of skin cancer. Psoralen intercalates with DNA and with exposure to UVA psoralen–DNA crosslinks are formed. The diadducts cause cell killing, mutations, and are highly carcinogenic. A correlation between the number of psoralen–DNA crosslinks and the frequency of squamous cell carcinomas has been established experimentally.[90]

Basal cell carcinoma

The keratinocytes from which basal cell carcinomas arise are associated with the hair follicle and may be a distinct subpopulation. The tumour cells are diploid, there are no precursor lesions, and the circumscribed nature and absence of metastases are more those of an adenoma than a carcinoma.

Single gene disorders account for only 1 per cent of non-melanoma skin cancer but the naevoid basal-cell carcinoma syndrome (NBCCS), also known as Gorlin's syndrome, which is characterized by multiple basal cell carcinomas, has proven informative about the process of UVR-induced carcinogenesis. The keratinocytes in NBCCS are very susceptible to the induction of basal cell carcinoma by both UVR and ionizing radiation, but show no difference in survival from normal keratinocytes exposed to either type of radiation.[91] The gene PTCH is a human homologue of the Drosophilia patched (ptc) gene.[92] The role of this gene in the development of basal cell carcinoma is not known, but in Drosophilia ptc plays a role in the control of genes in cell–cell communication and the transforming growth factor-β signalling pathway. Experimental support for the role of PTCH was obtained from experiments with transgenic mice.

In about 50 per cent of sporadic basal cell carcinoma, mutations in PTCH with a C → T change, characteristic of UV mutagenesis, have been found. These findings indicate that PTCH is probably a target gene which plays an important role in UVR-induced basal cell carcinoma.

An interaction between X-rays and sunlight was found in patients treated in childhood for ringworm. A substantial excess of basal cell carcinoma was found in white but not black patients and preferentially in the areas of the skin exposed to both X-rays and UVR.[75] A similar interaction has been observed experimentally. It appears that exposure to sunlight promotes the cells initiated by X-rays.

Melanoma (see also Chapter 8.1)

A causal relationship between sunlight and melanoma has been established epidemiologically but the wavelengths of the UVR that induce melanoma are not known. Based on an action spectrum for induction of melanoma in a fish model and the assumption that its general form was the same as that for transforming human melanocytes, it was suggested that 90 to 95 per cent of melanomas in humans were induced by UVA.[93]

The first change in the development of melanoma is from a melanocyte to the naevus cell, which is similar in appearance but with chromosomal abnormalities. Development of a premalignant mole may lead to a primary melanoma, which subsequently invades locally and metastasizes.

Loss of heterozygosity occurs at loci on a number of chromosomes including 9p in the early stages of more than 50 per cent of melanomas.[94] Homozygous deletions of 9p21 occur later. About 10 per cent of malignant melanomas occur in individuals with a familial predisposition and a susceptibility locus has been assigned to chromosome 9p21. This site contains two genes: p16 and one that encodes the cdk inhibitor p15.[94] (see also Chapter 1.6). There is as yet no direct evidence that these molecular and chromosomal aberrations are induced by UVR. However, the excess incidence of melanomas in patients with xeroderma pigmentosum exposed to sunlight is considered evidence of the role of UVR.

In sporadic and familial melanoma, the specific mutations may be caused by double strand breaks and base damage induced by the reactive oxygen species produced by the UVA radiation. If these DNA lesions are involved, it is hard to explain the apparent resistance to the induction of melanomas by ionizing radiation.

Summary

Low-LET radiation is a relatively weak carcinogen. Estimates of risk have been obtained from data for the atomic bomb survivors who were exposed to whole-body single exposures at a high dose rate. About 7 per cent of all the cancer deaths in this population has so far been attributed to radiation. Radiation-induced cancers have a minimum latent period of 5 to 9 years and the excess risk may last 30 or more years. For leukaemias, the minimum latent period and the period of excess risk is shorter. Susceptibility for the induction of cancer varies with age, gender, and genetic background and among tissues. Lowering the dose rate and fractionating the dose reduce the carcinogenic effect.

There are less data for the carcinogenic effect of high-LET radiations, and they are limited to alpha particles from the progeny of radon, thorotrast, and plutonium. The differential deposition of radionuclides in specific tissues determines the type of cancers; lung cancer in the case of radon and plutonium, and liver cancer and leukaemia after injection of thorotrast.

Ionizing radiation induces tumours of the same types that occur naturally and no signature lesion has been identified. The mechanisms of carcinogenesis vary among tissues and, in particular, the factors that influence expression of the initiation of the events. The precise mutations and their sequence of appearance is not known for most tumours. It is clear that TP53 is commonly mutated in human tumours. The lack of TP53 increases the risk of tumours occurring and increases the susceptibility to induction by both ionizing and ultraviolet radiation. Chromosome aberrations are involved in leukaemagenesis and have been implicated in some solid cancers. Ionizing radiation causes deletions, which increases the probability of the loss of heterozygosity in genes involved in carcinogenesis, such as tumour suppressor genes. Genetic instability induced by radiation may contribute to the multiple mutations involved in cancer induction.

Non-melanoma skin cancer, the commonest cancer in Caucasians, is caused by sunlight. Specific lesions, cyclobutane pyrimidine dimers, which in xeroderma pigmentosum patients are not repaired, are associated causally with the induction of non-melanoma skin cancer. While UVB plays the predominant role in the induction of the initial mutations, UVA also plays a role in skin carcinogenesis.

The ability to eliminate or enhance the expression of various gene products in mice ensures that the mechanisms of carcinogenesis can be studied more easily and in greater detail that ever before.

References

1. **Johns HE, Cunningham JR.** *The physics of radiology.* 4th edn. Springfield: Charles C Thomas, 1983.

2. **United Nations Scientific Committee of the Effects of Atomic Radiation (UNSCEAR).** *Sources and effects of ionizing radiation.* Annex A. New York: United Nations, 1993.

3. **Barendsen GW.** Cellular and molecular mechanisms in radiation

carcinogenesis. In: Pecham MJ, Pinedo HM, Veronesi U, ed. *Oxford textbook of oncology.* New York: Oxford University Press, 1995: 151–9.

4. Beckman KB, Ames BN. Oxidative decay of DNA. *Journal of Biological Chemistry,* 1997; **272**: 19633–6.

5. Ward JF. Damage produced by ionizing radiation in mammalian cells: Identities, mechanism of formation and repairability. *Progress in Nucleic Acid Research and Molecular Biology,* 1988; **35**: 95–125.

6. Goodhead DT. Initial events in the cellular effects of ionizing radiations: Clustered damage in DNA. *International Journal of Radiation Biology,* 1994; **65**: 7–17.

7. Rossi H. Microdosimetry and its application in biology. In: Thomas RH, Perez-Mendez V, ed. *Advances in radiation protection and dosimetry in medicine.* New York: Plenum, 1980.

8. Upton AC. The dose-response relation in radiation-induced cancer. *Cancer Research,* 1961; **21**: 717–29.

9. Pierce DA, *et al.* Studies of the mortality of A-bomb survivors. Report 12, Part 1. Cancer 1950–1990. *Radiation Research,* 1996; **146**: 1–27.

10. National Council on Radiation Protection and Measurements. *Uncertainties in fatal cancer risk estimates used in radiation protection.* NCRP Report No. 126. Bethesda: National Council on Radiation Protection and Measurements, 1997.

11. Fry RJM. Effects of low doses of radiation. *Health Physics,* 1996; **70**: 823–7.

12. Ullrich RL, Jernigan MC, Satterfield LC, Bowles ND. Radiation carcinogenesis: time-dose relationships. *Radiation Research,* 1987; **111**: 179–84.

13. Howe GR. Overview of epidemiologic studies of radiation and cancer risk. In: Boice JD, Jr, ed. *Implications of new data on radiation cancer risk.* Proceedings No. 18. Bethesda: National Council on Radiation Protection and Measurements, 1997.

14. Wolff S. The adaptive response in radiobiology. *Environmental Health Perspectives,* 1998; **106**: 277–83.

15. Lorimore SA, *et al.* Chromosomal instability in the descendents of unirradiated surviving cells after alpha-particle irradiation. *Proceedings of the National Academy of Science, USA.* 1998; **95**: 5730–3.

16. Azzam I, de Toledo SM, Gooding T, Little JB. Intercellular communication is involved in the bystander regulation of gene expression in human cells exposed to very low fluences of alpha particles. *Radiation Research,* 1998; **150**: 497–504.

17. United Nations Scientific Committee on the Effects of Atomic Radiation. *Sources and effects of ionizing radiation. Annex I Epidemiology of radiation-induced cancer.* New York: United Nations, 2000.

18. Boice JD Jr, ed. *Implications of new data on radiation cancer risk.* Bethesda, MD: National Council on Radiation Protection and Measurements, 1997; 315 pp.

19. National Research Council Committee on the Biological Effects of Ionizing Radiation. *Health effects of exposure to radon (BEIR VI).* Washington, DC: National Academy Press, 1999.

20. International Commission on Radiological Protection. *1990 Recommendation of the International Commission on Radiological Protection.* Oxford: Pergamon Press, 1991.

21. Boice JD Jr, Land CE, Preston DL. Ionizing radiation. In: Schottenfeld D, Fraumeni JF Jr, ed. *Cancer epidemiology and prevention.* 2nd edn. New York: Oxford University Press, 1996: 319–54.

22. Curtis RE. Second cancers following radiotherapy for cancer. *NCRP Proceedings,* 1997; **18**: 79–94.

23. Boice JD Jr, *et al.* Radiation dose and second cancer risk in patients treated for cancer of the cervix. *Radiation Research,* 1988; **116**: 3–55.

24. Boice JD Jr, *et al.* Second cancer in relation to radiation treatment for cervical cancer: An international cancer registry collaboration. *Journal of the National Cancer Institute,* 1985; **74**: 955–75.

25. Curtis RE, *et al.* Solid cancers after bone marrow transplantation. *New England Journal of Medicine,* 1997; **336**: 897–904.

26. Tucker MA, *et al.* Bone sarcomas linked to radiotherapy and chemotherapy in children. *New England Journal of Medicine,* 1987; **317**: 588–93.

27. van Leeuwen FE, *et al.* Roles of radiotherapy and smoking in lung cancer following Hodgkin's disease. *Journal of the National Cancer Institute,* 1995; **87**: 1530–7.

28. Tucker MA, *et al.* Second primary cancers related to smoking and treatment of small-cell lung cancer. Lung Cancer Working Cadre. *Journal of the National Cancer Institute,* 1997; **89**: 1782–8.

29. Hisada M, Garber JE, Fung CY, Fraumeni JF Jr, Li FP. Multiple primary cancers in families with Li-Fraumeni syndrome. *Journal of the National Cancer Institute,* 1998; **90**: 606–11.

30. Ron E, *et al.* Thyroid cancer after exposure to external radiation: a pooled analysis of seven studies. *Radiation Research,* 1995; **141**: 259–77.

31. Lundell M, Hakulinen T, Holm LE. Thyroid cancer after radiotherapy for skin hemangioma in infancy. *Radiation Research,* 1994; **140**: 334–9.

32. Griem ML, *et al.* Cancer following radiotherapy for peptic ulcer. *Journal of the National Cancer Institute,* 1994; **86**: 842–9.

33. Weiss HA, Darby SC, Doll R. Cancer mortality following X-ray treatment for ankylosing spondylitis. *International Journal of Cancer,* 1994; **59**: 327–38.

34. Thompson DE, *et al.* Cancer incidence in atomic bomb survivors. Part II: Solid tumors, 1958–1987. *Radiation Research,* 1994; **137** (2 Suppl.): S17–67.

35. Boice JD Jr, *et al.* Frequent chest x-ray fluoroscopy and breast cancer incidence among tuberculosis patients in Massachusetts. *Radiation Research,* 1991; **125**: 214–22.

36. Howe GR. Lung cancer mortality between 1950 and 1987 after exposure to fractionated moderate-dose-rate ionizing radiation in the Canadian fluoroscopy cohort study and a comparison with lung cancer mortality in the atomic bomb survivor study. *Radiation Research,* 1995; **142**: 295–304.

37. Doll R, Wakeford R. Risk of childhood cancer from fetal irradiation. *British Journal of Radiology,* 1997; **70**: 130–9.

38. Boice JD Jr, Miller RW. Childhood and adult cancer following intrauterine exposure to ionizing radiation. *Teratology,* 1999; **59**: 227–33.

39. Andersson M, Carstensen B, Storm HH. Mortality and cancer incidence after cerebral arteriography with or without thorotrast. *Radiation Research,* 1995; **142**: 305–20.

40. Ron E. Thyroid cancer. In: Schottenfeld D, Fraumeni JF Jr, ed. *Cancer epidemiology and prevention.* 2nd edn. New York: Oxford University Press, 1996: 1000–21.

41. Rabes HM, Klugbauer S. Molecular genetics of childhood papillary thyroid carcinomas after irradiation: High prevalence of RET rearrangement. In: Schwab, Rabes S, Munk K, Hofschneider PH, ed. *Genes and environment in cancer.* Vol. 154. Berlin: Springer-Verlag, 1998: 248–64.

42. Hall P, Mattsson A, Boice JD Jr. Thyroid cancer following diagnostic administration of iodine-131. *Radiation Research,* 1996; **145**: 86–92.

43. Ron E, *et al.* Cancer mortality following treatment for adult hyperthyroidism. Cooperative Thyrotoxicosis Therapy Follow-up Study Group. *Journal of the American Medical Association,* 1998; **28**: 347–55.

44. Astakhova LN, *et al.* Chernobyl-related thyroid cancer in children of Belarus: a case-control study. *Radiation Research,* 1998; **150**: 349–56.

45. Gilbert ES, Tarone R, Bouville A, Ron E. Thyroid cancer rates and ^{131}I doses from Nevada atmospheric nuclear bomb tests. *Journal of the National Cancer Institute,* 1998; **90**: 1654–60.

46. Wang J-X, Inskip PD, Boice JD Jr, Li B-X, Zhang J-Y, Fraumeni JF Jr. Cancer incidence among medical diagnostic x-ray workers in China, 1950 to 1985. *International Journal of Cancer,* 1990; **45**: 889–95.

47. Fry SA. Studies of U.S. radium dial workers: an epidemiological classic. *Radiation Research,* 1998; **150** (5 Suppl.): S21–9.

48. Cardis E, *et al.* Effects of low doses and low dose rates of external ionizing radiation: cancer mortality among nuclear industry workers in three countries. *Radiation Research*, 1995; **142**: 117–32.

49. Rahu M, *et al.* The Estonian study of Chernobyl cleanup workers: II. Incidence of cancer and mortality. *Radiation Research*, 1997; **147**: 641–52.

50. Ivanov VK, *et al.* Case-control analysis of leukaemia among Chernobyl accident emergency workers residing in the Russian Federation 1986–1993. *Journal of Radiological Protection*, 1997; **17**: 137–57.

51. Littlefield LG, *et al.* Do recorded doses overestimate true doses received by Chernobyl cleanup workers? Results of cytogenetic analyses of Estonian workers by fluorescence *in situ* hybridization. *Radiation Research*, 1998; **150**: 237–49.

52. Koshurnikova NA, *et al.* The risk of cancer among nuclear workers at the 'Mayak' Production Association: preliminary results of an epidemiological study. *NCRP Proceedings*, 1997; **18**: 113–21.

53. Doody MM, Mandel JS, Lubin JH, Boice JD Jr. Mortality among U.S. radiologic technologists, 1926–1990. *Cancer Causes and Control*, 1998; **9**: 67–75.

54. Lubin, JH, Boice JD Jr. Lung cancer risk from residential radon: meta-analysis of eight epidemiologic studies. *Journal of the National Cancer Institute*, 1997; **89**: 49–57.

55. Kossenko MM, Degteva MO, Vyushkova OV, Preston DL, Mabuchi K, Kozheurov VP. Issues in the comparison of risk estimates for the population in the Techa River region and atomic bomb survivors. *Radiation Research*, 1997; **148**: 54–63.

56. International Commission on Radiological Protection. Genetic susceptibility to cancer. ICRP Publication 79. *Annals of the International Commission on Radiological Protection*, 1999; **28**: 1–157.

57. Wong FL, *et al.* Cancer incidence after retinoblastoma: radiation dose and sarcoma risk. *Journal of the American Medical Association*, 1997; **278**: 1262–7.

58. Lavin M. Role of the ataxia-telangiectasia gene (ATM) in breast cancer. A-T heterozygotes seem to have an increased risk but its size is unknown. *British Medical Journal*, 1998; **317**: 486–7.

59. Kinzler KW, Vogelstein B. Familial cancer syndromes: the role of caretakers and gatekeepers. In: Vogelstein B, Kinzler KW, ed. *The genetic basis of human cancer.* New York: McGraw-Hill, 1998: 241–2.

60. Guerrero I, Calzada P, Mayer A, Pellicer A. A molecular approach to leukemogenesis: mouse lymphomas contain an activated c-ras oncogene. *Proceedings of the National Academy of Science, USA*, 1984; **81**: 202–5.

61. Corominas M, *et al.* Ras activation in human tumors and in animal model systems. *Environmental Health Perspectives*, 1991; **93**: 19–25.

62. Niwa O, Enoki Y, Yokoro K. Overexpression and amplification of the c-myc gene in mouse tumors induced by chemicals and radiations. *Japanese Journal of Cancer Research*, 1989; **80**: 212–18.

63. Schön A, *et al.* Expression of protoncogenes in murine osteosarcomas. *International Journal of Cancer*, 1986; **38**: 67–74.

64. Haines JR, *et al.* Loss of heterozygosity in spontaneous and X-ray-induced intestinal tumors in F1 hybrid mice: evidence for sequential loss of apc(+) and dpc/4 in tumor development. *Genes Chromosomes Cancer*, 2000; **28**: 387–94.

65. Bouffler SD, Breckon G, Cox R. Chromosomal mechanisms in murine radiation acute myeloid leukaemugenesis. *Carcinogenesis.* 1996; **17**: 101–5.

66. Kemp CJ, Wheldon T, Belmain A. p53-deficient mice are extremely susceptible to radiation-induced tumorigenesis. *Nature Genetics*, 1994; **8**: 66–9.

67. Bouffler SD, Kemp CJ, Balmain A, Cox R. Spontaneous and ionizing radiation-induced chromosomal abnormalities in p53-deficient mice. *Cancer Research*, 1995; **55**: 3883–9.

68. Loeb LA. Cancer cells exhibit a mutator phenotype. In: Vande Woude GF, Klein G, ed. *Advances in cancer research.* Vol. 72. San Diego: Academic Press, 1998: 26–56.

69. Morgan WF, Kaplan MI, McGhee EM, Limoli CL. Genomic instability induced by ionizing radiation. *Radiation Research*, 1996; **146**: 247–58.

70. Nowell PC. The clonal evolution of tumor cell populations. *Science*, 1976; **194**: 23–8.

71. Ponnaiya B, Cornforth MN, Ullrich RL. Radiation-induced chromosomal instability in BALB/c and C57 Bl/6 mice: The difference is as clear as black and white. *Radiation Research*, 1997; **147**: 121–5.

72. Urbach F. Photocarcinogenesis: from the widow's coif to the p53 gene. *Photochemistry and Photobiology*, 1997; **655**: 1295–338.

73. Leigh IM, Bishop JAN, Kripke M L, eds, Skin Cancer. *Cancer Surveys*, 1996; **26**. [This issue consists of reviews on many aspects of skin cancer by various authors.]

74. Marks R. An overview of skin cancers: incidence and causation. *Cancer*, 1995; **75** (Suppl.): 607–12.

75. International Commission on Radiological Protection. *The biological basis for dose limitation in the skin.* ICRP report 59. *Annals of the International Commission on Radiological Protection*, 1991; **22**.

76. Landis SH, Murray T, Bolden S, Wingo PA. Cancer Statistics, 1998. *CA—A Cancer Journal for Clinicians*, 1998; **48**: 6–29.

77. Armstrong BK, Kricker A. Epidemiology of sun exposure and skin cancer. *Cancer Surveys*, 1996; **26**: 133–53.

78. Cleaver JE, Cortes F, Karentz D, *et al.* The relative biological importance of cyclobutane and (6–4) pyrimidine-pyrimidone dimer photoproducts in human cells: Evidence from a xeroderma pigmentosum revertant. *Photochemistry and Photobiology*, 1988; **48**: 41–9.

79. Ley RD, Applegate LA, Fry RJM, Sanchez AB. Photoreactivation of ultraviolet radiation-induced skin and eye tumors of *Monodelphis domestica. Cancer Research*, 1991; **51**: 6539–42.

80. Kraemer KM. Sunlight and skin cancer: Another link revealed. *Proceedings of the National Academy of Science, USA*, 1997; **94**: 11–14.

81. DeLatt JMT, DeGruijl FR. The role of UVA in the aetiology of non-melanoma skin cancer. *Cancer Surveys*, 1996; **26**: 173–91.

82. Fry RJM. Relevance of animal studies to the human experience. In: Boice JD Jr. and Fraumeni JF Jr. *Radiation carcinogenesis: epidemiology.* New York: Raven Press, 1984: 337–46.

83. Hutchinson F. Induction of tandem-based change mutations. *Mutation Research*, 1994; **309**: 11–15.

84. Brash D. Sunlight and onset of skin cancer. *Trends in Genetics*, 1997; **13**: 410–14.

85. Berg JW, *et al.* Early p53 alterations in mouse skin carcinogenesis by UVB radiation: Immunohistochemical detection of mutant p53 protein in clusters of preneoplastic epidermal cells. *Proceedings of the National Academy of Science, USA*, 1986; **93**: 274–8.

86. Daynes RA, Bernhard EJ, Barish MF, Lynch DH. Experimental photoimmunology: immunologic ramifications of UV-induced carcinogenesis. *Journal of Investigative Dermatology*, 1981; **77**: 77–85.

87. Kripke ML. Ultraviolet radiation and immunology: something new under the sun—presidential address. *Cancer Research*, 54: 6102–5.

88. Nakazkwa H, *et al.* UV skin cancer: Specific p53 gene mutation in normal skin as a biologically relevant exposure measurement. *Proceedings of the National Academy of Science, USA*, 1994; **91**: 360.

89. Rees JL. Skin cancer (Gorlin's syndrome) In: Vogelstein B, Kinzler KW, ed. *The genetic basis of human cancer.* New York: McGraw-Hill, 1998: 527–36.

90. Fry RJM, Ley RD, Grube D, Staffeldt F. Studies on the multistage nature of radiation carcinogenesis. In: Hecker E ed. *Carcinogenesis.* Vol 7. New York: Raven Press, 1982: 155–65.

91. Stacey M, Thacker S, Taylor AMR. Cultured skin keratinocytes from both normal individuals and basal cell naevus syndrome

patients are more resistant to γ-rays and UV light compared with cultured skin fibroblasts. *International Journal of Radiation Biology,* 1989; **56**: 45–58.

92. **Johnson RL,** *et al.* Human homolog of patched, a candidate gene for basal cell nevus syndrome. *Science,* 1994; **272**: 1668.

93. **Setlow RB, Grist E, Thompson K, Woodhead AD.** Wavelengths effective in induction of malignant melanoma. *Proceedings of the National Academy of Science, USA,* 1993; **90**: 6666–70.

94. **Kamb A, Erlyn M.** Malignant melanoma. In: Vogelstein B, Kinzler KW, ed. *The genetic basis of human cancer.* New York: McGraw-Hill, 1998: 507–18.

2.4 Principles of epidemiology

John R. McLaughlin

Introduction and fundamental concepts

People are the subject matter of 'epidemiology', as denoted by the term's Greek origin of '*epi*' (upon), '*demos*' (the people), and '*logos*' (study). In contrast, an individual patient is the immediate concern of a clinician, while cell systems or animal models are studied in the experiments of a basic scientist. All medical researchers share the goal of making advances that lead to improved health for people; however, it is the epidemiologist who targets groups of people for both observation and inference.

The purpose of this chapter is to introduce principles, concepts, and methods that are central to cancer epidemiology. Other chapters in this volume give detailed accounts of specific aetiological factors, particular types of cancer, and applications of epidemiological findings to cancer prevention and screening. This chapter describes fundamental epidemiological principles and their impact, including the scope of cancer epidemiology, the methods used in epidemiological research, challenges that are often faced in epidemiological studies, and finally, issues that must be considered in the interpretation and application of research findings.

Definition and scope of epidemiology

Epidemiology is defined as the study of the distribution and determinants of health-related states or events in human populations.[1] 'Cancer epidemiology' is the subdiscipline that focuses on one particular outcome of primary interest. Studies that focus on the 'distribution of disease' are referred to as 'descriptive epidemiology', whereas 'analytical epidemiology' refers to studies that examine the 'determinants of disease'. Descriptive epidemiology provides an indication of disease frequency, disease severity, and the burden of disease in society. In addition, descriptive studies that compare the distribution of disease between populations, such as international comparisons of cancer incidence rates, also provide clues about disease determinants that can be investigated in analytical epidemiological studies.

Epidemiological research can be further classified as 'classical' or 'clinical' epidemiology, where the former examines aetiology with cancer occurrence as the outcome, and the latter explores disease progression after diagnosis (Fig. 1). Other subdisciplines focus on particular 'determinants' or risk factors such as environmental, nutritional, occupational, or genetic epidemiology. Finally, studies may be classified according to the methods of measurement, such as in molecular epidemiology which incorporates molecular and cellular measurements.

The most important purpose of epidemiology is to identify 'determinants' of disease. When outcome is defined as disease occurrence, the determinants under investigation are aetiological factors (e.g. lung cancer occurs more frequently among smokers than non-smokers). Alternatively, in clinical epidemiological studies (Fig. 1), outcomes after diagnosis are examined, the determinants of which are indicators of prognosis or impact of treatment (e.g. lung cancer cases survive longer if they have early rather than late-stage disease).

The greatest contribution of epidemiology has been in identifying causes of serious diseases. The ultimate goal of improving health is achieved by applying this knowledge of disease causes in the planning, implementation, and evaluation of cancer control strategies. Epidemiology contributes particularly to the identification of high-risk populations, and ultimately, to the prevention of cancer. For example, the risk of lung cancer can be reduced after smoking cessation (i.e. primary prevention), or mortality due to cervical cancer can decrease after the introduction of screening programmes (i.e. secondary prevention).

A leading role for descriptive epidemiology is that by identifying the relative frequency and severity of health problems, priorities can be set for research and for planning medical and public health services. Epidemiology is also important in explaining local variations of disease, such as in the surveillance of a population for unusual patterns of disease (or associated exposures). Whereas surveillance programmes for many communicable diseases are effective in controlling outbreaks, for cancer and other diseases the goal of surveillance is primarily to provide a baseline for aetiological research or for the evaluation of interventions. Finally, in the process of enumerating disease occurrence, a subsidiary effect is that standardized methods of defining, measuring, and classifying disease have been developed, such as the International Classification for Diseases, which then benefits clinical practice, health care evaluation, and aetiological research.

Fundamental features of epidemiology

The epidemiological approach is distinctive in terms of several aspects of its objectives, methods, interpretation, and application.

Observational and experimental designs

Epidemiology employs predominantly observational rather than experimental research methods to study aetiology and disease progression. Although the experimental approach provides stronger

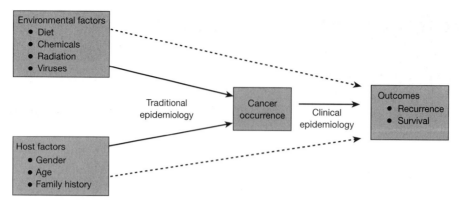

Fig. 1 The general approaches of classical and clinical epidemiology.

evidence, it is often not feasible or ethical, particularly when concerned with disease aetiology.[2] In contrast, randomized trials can be applied when an intervention has presumed benefits, such as in trials of cancer prevention, evaluations of screening programmes, and clinical epidemiology. However, it is in the development and application of non-experimental methods that epidemiology has had its greatest impact.

Specialized research methodology

The task of detecting causal relationships has necessitated the development of specialized research methods. Observational methods were needed to investigate rare diseases, to enable measurement of exposures and outcomes over a long period of time, and to examine the effects of multiple potential determinants simultaneously. Specialized methods were also needed to deal with potential biases, which rather than being seen as insurmountable flaws in all non-experimental research, are viewed as problems to be solved by the researcher through careful attention to research design, measurement, analysis, and interpretation.

Association and causation

There is seldom a simple one-to-one correspondence between cause and effect. For example, not all smokers get lung cancer, and not all who get lung cancer smoked (i.e. it is neither 'sufficient' nor 'necessary'). Nevertheless, tobacco use is now established as one of the component causes of lung cancer, where cause is defined as a factor that 'preceded the disease, and without which the disease either would not have occurred at all or would not have occurred until some later time.'[3] The identification of causes is an inferential process whereby associations that are detected between exposures and outcomes are interpreted with respect to guidelines that are suggestive of a causal role (see later).

Quantitative methods

To describe patterns of disease and risk factors among the individuals of a population, epidemiology relies heavily on probabilistic methods. A large amount of information can be summarized conveniently in descriptive statistics, such as in rates of incidence or mortality. Statistical methods are also used to test hypotheses about whether specific factors are associated with disease, and provide the basis for making inferences about a population from observations made on a sample. For example, to identify the causes of cancer, the risk (or probability) of cancer among individuals exposed to some factor that is suspected to cause (or protect against) cancer is compared with the risk of cancer in individuals not so exposed.

Uncertainty and confidence

Central to the epidemiological approach is the recognition that all observations are made with error: sources of error must be identified; the extent of uncertainty must be assessed; and as much as possible, error must be minimized. Other sources of uncertainty arise from the complexity of multifactorial disease processes, which makes them difficult to observe and measure. To account for these many types of uncertainty, epidemiological research relies on probabilistic scientific methods that demonstrate the contribution of chance (or random) variation by calculating standard deviations, confidence intervals, and test statistics. In additional, to guide the interpretation of research findings in the presence of uncertainty, a logical framework for causal reasoning is applied (see later).

Public interest and public health impact

The determinants of disease under investigation in epidemiological studies are often of concern to the general public, particularly with regard to the aetiological significance of environmental factors. Even if basic research involving *in vivo* or *in vitro* experiments demonstrates a causal mechanism with certainty, the value and impact of such a discovery will remain limited until it is also shown to affect people. Public health benefits can sometimes be achieved even if there is uncertainty about the causal role of an exposure, as exemplified by the work of John Snow, who achieved a marked reduction in the incidence of cholera by disabling a water pump in London in 1854, 25 years before the infectious agent was known. Similarly in cancer epidemiology, it was recognized in the 1960s that the risk of lung cancer could be reduced by discontinuing tobacco use, many years before an underlying biological mechanism was clearly established.

Methods of epidemiological research

Generation and testing of hypotheses

Epidemiology follows an iterative process whereby hypotheses are first developed to explain patterns of disease risk, and then tested in

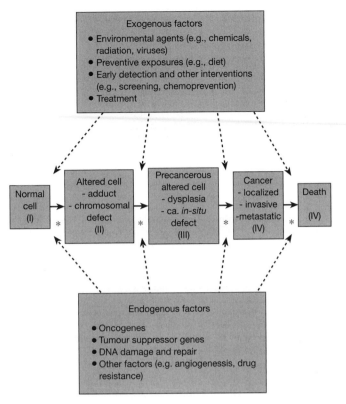

Fig. 2 A conceptual model of carcinogenesis where disease occurrence and progression is determined by exogenous and endogenous factors.

(i.e. a measure of internal dose in state II) would be classified as a form of 'exposure assessment'. Figure 2 shows that even if a single pathway is of primary interest, a wide range of other factors related to host susceptibility and exogenous factors may influence this pathway and may need to be controlled or otherwise accounted for.

Epidemiological measures for describing disease distribution

In summarizing the health experience of a population, the most basic measure of disease frequency or burden is a simple count of the total number of cases. In counting cancer cases, a distinction is made between incident and prevalent cases, where incidence refers to the number of new events, such as deaths or newly diagnosed cases, occurring in a defined population within a specified period of time. Prevalence is defined as the number of people with a given disease (or other condition), both newly and previously diagnosed, in a defined population at a designated time.

It is usually more meaningful to measure disease burden using a relative measure, whereby the disease frequency is considered in relation to the size of the population and the length of time in which events occurred. Risk is a widely used term that is defined as an individual's probability of suffering an adverse event in a specified time interval. If the period of observation is constant for all individuals, the risk of new disease can be summarized as a simple proportion:

Incidence proportion =

$$\frac{\text{(the cumulative number of new events during the interval)}}{\text{(the total number of people at the beginning of the interval)}};$$

which is sometimes referred to as the average risk, attack rate, or cumulative incidence. If the time interval is not fixed, the measure of disease burden must account for the variable duration of observation for each person, in addition to the total number of persons, and an incidence rate is used:

Incidence rate =

$$\frac{\text{(the number of new events over the period of observation)}}{\text{(the total amount of person-time observed)}};$$

where this denominator is the sum of the lengths of follow-up for all persons in the study. The patterns and trends of disease are usually summarized by annual rates, by fixing the length of observation at 1 year for each member of the population. Annual incidence rates provide an estimate of the proportion of the population that develops the disease (i.e. risk or cumulative incidence). Examples of worldwide incidence figures are provided later in the section on the descriptive epidemiology of cancer.

Prevalence is a function of both the incidence and duration of a disease or trait. In the situation of a relatively low prevalence (<10 per cent), this can be expressed by:

Prevalence rate = (incidence rate) × (mean duration).

For cancers with a high survival rate, prevalence is much higher than incidence, whereas prevalence is lower for cancers with poor prognosis (i.e. with short duration). Examples of prevalence rates are the number of individuals surviving with cancer at a point in time per 100 000 in the population, and the proportion of individuals in a population who smoke at a point in time. Disease prevalence is a useful measure of disease burden for planning health services. In

specific studies. The generation of hypotheses may arise from astute observations by a clinician who draws attention to a possible aetiological association, such as when a rare form of vaginal carcinoma was noted among the daughters of women exposed to diethylstilboestrol. Hypotheses may arise from descriptive epidemiological reports in which cancer rates are shown to vary by place or period, such as when rates of cutaneous malignant melanoma were observed to vary between geographic regions that differed in sunlight exposure. For disease processes where little is known about the determinants, hypotheses are sometimes generated by an exploratory epidemiological study that is conducted to check for associations among multiple factors for which there is no a priori reason for concern.

In the hypothesis testing phase, the risk of cancer among individuals exposed to some factor that is suspected to cause (or protect against) cancer is compared with the risk in individuals not so exposed. Alternatively, the risk of cancer recurrence or death can be compared between two groups defined according to the presence of a putative prognostic factor. Figure 2 depicts a multistage model of carcinogenesis and cancer progression. The wide range of hypotheses that can be tested in epidemiological studies can be derived from Fig. 2 by considering transitions between any combination of individual states. For example, a study of whether the exposure of a healthy individual (state I) to tobacco smoke (an exogenous factor) is associated with lung cancer risk (state IV) would be a traditional epidemiological study of an aetiological factor. An evaluation of whether smoking history was associated with serum cotinine level

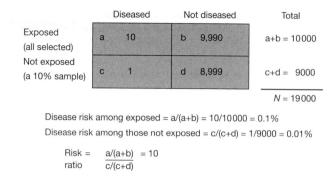

Disease risk among exposed = a/(a+b) = 10/10000 = 0.1%

Disease risk among those not exposed = c/(c+d) = 1/9000 = 0.01%

$$\text{Risk ratio} = \frac{a/(a+b)}{c/(c+d)} = 10$$

Fig. 3 A hypothetical cohort study in a community of 100 000 people, where all 10 000 exposed individuals are compared with a 10 per cent random sample of individuals who were not exposed. After following both groups for the occurrence of disease, risk and relative risk are estimated.

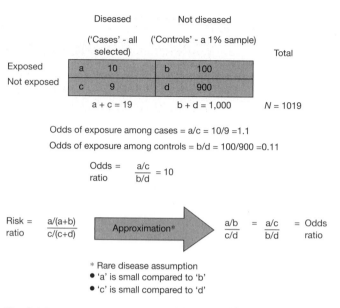

Odds of exposure among cases = a/c = 10/9 =1.1

Odds of exposure among controls = b/d = 100/900 =0.11

$$\text{Odds ratio} = \frac{a/c}{b/d} = 10$$

$$\text{Risk ratio} = \frac{a/(a+b)}{c/(c+d)} \quad \text{Approximation*} \quad \frac{a/b}{c/d} = \frac{a/c}{b/d} = \text{Odds ratio}$$

* Rare disease assumption
- 'a' is small compared to 'b'
- 'c' is small compared to 'd'

Fig. 4 A hypothetical case–control study in the same community as for the cohort study in Fig. 3, where all individuals with disease (19 'cases') are compared with a 1 per cent random sample of individuals who do not have the disease. After measuring exposure status in both groups, measures of risk (odds) and relative risk (odds ratio) are estimated.

contrast, aetiological studies refer to incidence because it is not affected by the many factors that influence survival after a diagnosis of cancer is made.

Epidemiological measures for detecting determinants of disease

Analytic studies search for disease determinants by comparing an observed course of events in a group with particular traits, to the level expected if the traits were not present. The ratio of the observed (O) to expected (E) frequency is a convenient summary measure of the strength of the association between risk and the traits that distinguish the groups. A ratio of 1.0 indicates that the observed frequency equals the expected frequency (i.e. that there is no association). This ratio directly measures 'relative risk' in the situation where both the numerator and denominator are risks, such as when two groups are compared in terms of the proportion who develop the outcome. The interpretation is similar when outcome is measured on different scales, thus ratios of rates (e.g. rate ratio) and counts (e.g. standardized mortality ratio) are also referred to as relative risk estimates.

Figure 3 shows how relative risk is calculated for a hypothetical cohort study (see later) conducted in a community with an overall population of 100 000. All of the 10 000 people who had the exposure of interest are compared with a 10 per cent random sample drawn from the remainder. The risk ratio indicates that the risk in the exposed group is 10 times greater than in the non-exposed group.

An alternate approach to studying whether there is an association between exposure and disease is to undertake a case–control study (see later). This design might include all 'cases' in this community, while taking a random sample of individuals who do not have the disease (i.e. the 'controls' shown in Fig. 4). As the probability of disease in each exposure group cannot be calculated, relative risk is estimated from an alternate measure of relative frequency: an odds, which is calculated as the ratio of the probabilities of an event's occurrence and non-occurrence. In the example the ratio of the odds for the diseased and non-diseased groups is 10, which equals the risk ratio obtained in the cohort study. Figure 4 also shows that in a cohort or a population, the odds ratio provides a valid estimate of relative risk when the disease is relatively rare (e.g. <20 per cent). Thus,

the odds ratio is an important indicator of strength of association, and is widely used in aetiological studies. Odds ratios are similar to 'likelihood ratios', which are used to interpret diagnostic tests in clinical research.[4]

Measurement error, random error, and bias

Accurate measurement is difficult to achieve in epidemiological studies. Exposure status is often determined by asking questions about events that took place many years earlier and, thus, some inaccuracies are inevitable. The determination of disease status, even when based on histological material, is also subject to error; thus, some incorrectly classified diseased and non-diseased individuals may be included in a study. Strategies used to minimize measurement error include the careful development, pretesting, and validation of data collection methods and instruments, and the use of independent assessments of exposure or disease status.

Even under ideal circumstances, some measurement error will remain, and the impact of this error on study results must be accounted for. Random error is a deviation between an observed value and a true value that is due only to chance. The concept of random error is central to the statistical analysis of data, such as in the assessment of whether an association arose by chance. This can be accomplished by statistical testing to assess whether the null hypothesis that there is no association can be rejected (i.e. relative risk equals 1.0). Confidence intervals (**CI**) provide further information as they indicate the range of relative risk estimates with which the data are consistent. A distinction should be made between the test of a specific a priori hypothesis as opposed to exploratory analyses of numerous potential risk factors because the latter could give rise to a statistical association by chance alone.

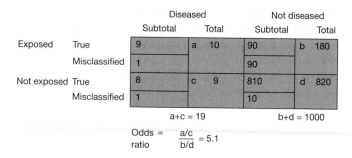

		Diseased			Not diseased	
		Subtotal	Total		Subtotal	Total
Exposed	True	9	a 10		90	b 180
	Misclassified	1			90	
Not exposed	True	8	c 9		810	d 820
	Misclassified	1			10	
		a+c = 19			b+d = 1000	

$$\text{Odds ratio} = \frac{a/c}{b/d} = 5.1$$

Fig. 5 Recalculation of the odds ratio in the hypothetical case–control study from Fig. 4 after incorporating 10 per cent random misclassification in the exposure measurement.

Measurement error may cause a study to be biased, in that the results or conclusions may systematically differ from the truth.[1] The usual effect of random measurement error on study results is to conceal or reduce the magnitude of true associations rather than to give rise to associations that are spurious. The effect of random error is demonstrated in Fig. 5, where it is assumed that exposure status was randomly misclassified in 10 per cent of subjects in the study shown in Fig. 4. This 'non-differential' misclassification affected both comparison groups equally, and resulted in underestimation of the relative risk, as the recalculated odds ratio (5.1) is lower than the original value (10). Although the attenuating effect of this type of misclassification is sometimes used to argue that true effects may be stronger than found in a particular study, the effect of measurement error is less predictable if it systematically differs between the main comparison groups, or if it affects other variables that are important predictors of the outcome (e.g. confounding variables). If measurement error is systematic or non-random, the resulting bias may give rise to results that either overestimate or underestimate true associations (also see later).

Research designs in epidemiology

Randomized trials

Randomized controlled trials, provide the strongest possible evidence that a causal relationship exists between an exposure and an outcome. The strength of this experimental approach arises because the randomization process used to allocate the exposure under investigation, should, on average, make the groups to be compared similar at the start of the study. Experimental studies are used less than observational designs because it is unethical to intentionally expose people to factors that may cause cancer or other adverse outcomes. Thus, randomized trials are limited to the investigation of exposures that may reduce the risk of cancer or other adverse outcomes, such as dietary modification, vitamin supplements, or cancer screening (see Chapters 2.5 and 2.6).

Cohort studies

Cohort studies differ from randomized trials in that the investigator cannot control the allocation of the primary exposure. In cohort studies, subsets of a given population are defined according to whether individuals are exposed to a factor suspected of increasing or decreasing risk. These subsets are followed forward in time and measurements are made to detect the newly occurring outcomes. At the end of follow-up, cancer risks in the exposed and non-exposed groups are compared and the relative risk due to exposure is calculated directly, as shown in Fig. 3.

The source population for a study of cancer aetiology may be the people living in a community or working in a particular occupation, with the main comparison groups then being defined according to exposures or traits such as lifestyle factors (e.g. smoking, diet), occupational factors, other environmental exposures, or genetic factors. In a clinical epidemiological study, the source population may be a series of cancer patients who serve as the cohort to be followed, in order to assess whether survival rates are related to features of their disease, history, or medical care.

In a prospective cohort study, cohort members are characterized with regard to risk factors at a baseline time, and are then followed over time using a surveillance mechanism that enables the detection of outcomes. This design has the advantage that exposure and outcome information can be updated repeatedly. A retrospective cohort study is possible if the exposure status can be determined historically, and if sufficient time has elapsed such that the outcome has occurred in a large number of subjects. If the outcome for a cohort study is a routinely and reliably reported event, such as death or the diagnosis of cancer, it may be possible to use record linkage to detect outcomes without contacting individuals. This has enabled very large cohort studies to be conducted, such as in the follow-up of workers in certain occupations and of patients who received specific medical interventions. For example, Fuchs et al.[5] reported recently on a cohort of approximately 90 000 nurses in the United States who completed a dietary assessment and were then followed for 16 years with cancer incidence being determined by contacting participants, while deaths were determined from death certificates.

Given that exposures cannot be assigned to individuals in cohort studies, the results may be open to more than one interpretation. Given that exposure is self-selected for many potential causes of cancer, such as occupation, cigarette smoking, and dietary practices, the finding of an association with cancer risk may mean either that these exposures are related causally or, alternatively, that the apparent effect is due to some form of selection bias, or to another attribute or exposure that introduced confounding (see later). Thus, care is required in designing, analysing, and interpreting cohort studies.

A major advantage of cohort studies is that they address directly the aetiological sequence of cause preceding effect. When carried out prospectively, it is feasible to measure exposure accurately, to characterize baseline cancer risk, and to follow the population for the development of multiple outcomes, including cancer. Cohort studies are efficient for studying rare exposures, because they can be designed to incorporate the most informative individuals (i.e. all who were exposed, but only a sample of the remainder). In clinical epidemiological studies of cancer patients, cohort designs can often be employed because the outcomes occur relatively frequently, the requisite periods of follow-up are shorter, and the patients are more likely to be followed over time. A limitation of the cohort design is that for rare outcomes (e.g. most cancers), these studies need very large numbers of subjects to have a good chance of detecting an association. Thus cohort studies of cancer aetiology tend to be large, time-consuming, and expensive, which has motivated the development of the more economical case–control design for the investigation of aetiological relationships.

Case–control studies

The design of a case–control study makes optimal use of the most informative individuals, the 'cases', while a representative sample is drawn from the remaining individuals (controls). A case–control study is nested within a cohort or population, and aims to provide information similar to that which would be observed if a cohort study could be conducted.

Although applied most frequently to study cancer incidence, the occurrence of any rare event can be studied in a case–control study. In a typical aetiological study, the source population is everyone living in a particular community, and a case series could include all new lung cancer cases that arise in that population over a specified period of time. Alternatively, if the source population is a series of cancer patients, then the 'case' definition could be the occurrence of adverse outcomes, such as non-response to therapy. Cases can be drawn from several sources, including hospital records, cancer registries, or clinics.

The control group for a case–control study consists of individuals who do not have the outcome of interest. This contrasts with the use of the term in randomized trials, where 'controls' do not have the exposure of interest. Controls must represent the population that gave rise to the cases, or more specifically, the distribution of exposures among controls must be the same as in the entire source population. Controls may be selected from hospitals, outpatient facilities, administrative records, or the general population using random-sampling techniques. Careful consideration must be given to the selection of cases and appropriate controls because there are many ways of introducing bias into the assessment of the relationship between exposure and disease (see later).

The retrospective measurement of exposure in case–control studies can be based on personal recall, available information from medical records or other databases, or biological specimens. In aetiological studies, questionnaires are used frequently to assess factors such as diet, occupational history, or personal habits, such as smoking history. Other factors, such as prior exposure to viruses or the influence of some aspect of the individual's phenotype or genotype on disease risk, may be assessed by direct examination or biomarkers.

Data analysis in case–control studies usually involves testing for differences in exposure frequency. Odds ratios provide valid estimates of relative risk when the outcome is uncommon (e.g. <15 to 20 per cent of population), which holds true for cancer incidence (Fig. 4). Furthermore, with appropriate sampling and analysis methods, case–control studies that compare rates rather than risks (or proportions) can also provide valid estimates regardless of the rarity of the outcome.

Case–control studies have particular advantages for investigating outcomes that are rare or that take many years to develop because recruitment focuses on the most informative individuals. This results in case–control studies having greater efficiency than cohort studies, as reflected in their smaller sample size, more rapid completion and lower costs. Certain limitations are shared by cohort and case–control studies, including the potential for selection biases that can challenge the comparability of groups in observational studies. The major additional challenge in case–control studies is the tendency for exposures to be misclassified, particularly when factors in the distant past must be recalled, and when there is no way to check the accuracy of this information.

Despite these disadvantages, case–control studies are frequently the only feasible means of assessing, in human populations, the validity of claims about the determinants of cancer risk. For example, Boffetta et al.[6] reported on a case–control study in which there was a slight, but not statistically significant, increase in the risk of lung cancer among those exposed to environmental tobacco smoke at work (odds ratio = 1.2, 95 per cent CI = 0.9 to 1.5). This study was carefully conducted, but it still had several limitations. Nevertheless, the rarity of lung cancer among non-smokers, the slow development of the outcome, and the small effect size make this a difficult relationship to study in humans by any other means. Thus, this case–control study will remain as the source of some of the best available evidence.

Other designs

Several designs for epidemiological research, such as ecological studies, cross-sectional studies, surveys, case series, and case reports, are used less frequently or make a smaller contribution due to their inherent limitations. An important hybrid design is where a case–control study is nested with a cohort study. If the cost of measuring exposures on all cohort members is prohibitively expensive (e.g. laboratory analysis of biomarkers in stored specimens), cost-effectiveness can be enhanced by measuring exposure for selected individuals, including the individuals who develop the cancer (cases) and a random sample of other cohort members who do not develop cancer (controls). A slight adaptation of this approach is the 'case-cohort' design, whereby cases are compared with a random sample of the whole cohort, which has the advantage of enabling the study of multiple outcomes. In addition, specialized applications of the standard designs are also used in genetic epidemiology, such as in cohort studies where instead of being selected from the general population, cohort members are selected from families. By comparing disease risk in families that differ in their genetic traits, while accounting for measured differences in environmental exposures, such genetic epidemiological studies can detect the relative contribution of both genetic and environmental risk factors.[7],[8]

Several epidemiology textbooks provide further detail regarding study design, conduct, and statistical analysis. Rothman and Greenland[3] provide a thorough review of theoretical and analytic matters, Kelsey et al.[9] focus on observational studies, while Brownson and Pettiti[10],[11] emphasize clinical outcomes research and health services evaluation.

Interpretation of results from epidemiological studies

The first steps in interpreting an epidemiological association are to assess whether it might have arisen from chance variation and to evaluate whether the internal validity of the study was diminished by bias or confounding. The role of chance variation can be addressed in an appropriately conducted statistical analysis. Questions about the impact of bias or confounding must be considered in the framework shown in Table 1, which serves as a guide in the evaluation of whether an observed association is causal.

Potential biases in epidemiological studies

A study is biased if deficiencies in measurement, study design, data collection, analysis, or interpretation lead to results or conclusions that systematically differ from the truth.[1] In contrast to random

Table 1 A framework for evaluating and interpreting a study of disease causation. (Adapted from Elwood 1998)

I. Are there alternative, non-causal explanations? (internal validity)
- Are the results affected by chance variation?
- Are the results affected by information bias?
- Are the results affected by selection bias?
- Are the results affected by confounding?

II. Do the results of a specific study meet the 'causal criteria?'
- Is there an appropriate temporal relationship?
- Is there a strong relationship?
- Is there a dose–response relationship?
- Are the results consistent within the study?
- Is the relationship specific within the study?

III. How do the results of one study relate to other evidence?
- Are the results consistent with other studies in this field?
- Is there a biologically plausible mechanism?
- Does the total evidence suggest specificity?
- Is the effect coherent with the known distribution of exposure and outcome?

IV. Are the results generalizable and relevant?
- Can the results be applied to the source population?
- Can the results be applied to other populations?
- Are the results relevant to the population?

error, which is likely to conceal true associations, bias distorts the truth by giving rise to results that either over- or underestimate associations. Thus, bias can create associations where none exist, or magnify or conceal associations that are genuine.

Biases can be classified according to whether they arise from the selection of subjects, or from the information that is collected. Within each of these general classes, many types of bias have been described.[1],[3],[12] A selection bias may occur if there are systematic differences in traits between those who are selected for study and those who are not. Table 2 lists subtypes of selection bias, including:

- *Detection bias* occurs if there are systematic differences in the way that subjects are identified or assessed. If an exposure gives rise to clinical symptoms or signs that resemble those of cancer it could cause clinicians to initiate a search for cancer. For example, drugs such as stilbestrol can cause endometrial bleeding and it was suggested that the association found between oestrogens and endometrial cancer arose in part because oestrogens caused endometrial bleeding which then caused occult cancers to be detected.

- *Lead-time bias* occurs if the follow-up of two groups does not begin at comparable times, such as when one group is selectively identified earlier in the natural history of the disease. For example, survival rates for patients with screen-detected disease may appear longer because they were detected earlier.

- *Response (or volunteer) bias* refers to the situation in which those who volunteer to participate in a study are systematically different from those who choose to not respond.

- *Berkson's (or admission rate) bias* may arise in a case–control study of hospitalized individuals if differential rates of admission apply to those with cancer who were exposed to a risk factor, as opposed to those with cancer who had no such exposure. For example, a case–control study of lung cancer could underestimate the adverse effect of smoking in the population if it compared lung cancer cases with hospitalized controls because smoking is associated with many reasons for hospitalization.

- *Length (also called prevalence-incidence or Neyman) bias* refers to a distortion of an aetiological association that arises if prevalent cases are used and exposure is related to survival after diagnosis. In this situation, an artefact may appear because long-term survivors are more likely to have the exposure. Recognition of the potential impact of this bias is the reason that incident cases are usually preferred for case–control studies of cancer aetiology. Length bias is an important consideration in observational clinical studies of patient outcomes after diagnosis. For example, Rubin *et al.*[13] reported that for women with ovarian cancer, survival rates were higher among BRCA1 mutation carriers compared with cases who did not have a family history of breast or ovarian cancer. Length bias is a potential problem here because the survival rate in the 'exposed' group may be overestimated as it is more likely for carrier status to be detected by genetic testing programmes when the index cancer case is alive. The ideal approach would be to conduct a

Table 2 Types of biases and their basic features

Type of bias	Features
Selection bias	
Detection bias	The likelihood of detecting the outcome systematically differs between subjects
Lead-time bias	Period of observation systematically differs because some are identified earlier
Response bias	Those who respond are systematically different from those who choose not to
Berkson's bias	Hospital admission rates systematically differ according to exposure and outcome
Length bias	If exposure is related to survival, its frequency systematically differs between prevalent and incident cases
Information bias	
Recall bias	Ability to remember past differs systematically between subjects
Measurement bias	Systematic error due to inaccurate measurement

prospective cohort study in which all incident cases in the population were tested for mutation status.

Information bias is defined as a distortion of study results due to differential accuracy of information relating to exposure or outcome between the comparison groups. Subtypes of information bias include:

- *Recall bias,* which is a potential problem in case–control studies, arises because diseased subjects are more likely to think about and recall previous exposure than non-diseased controls. For example, in aetiological studies, cancer cases may think more carefully about their past environmental exposures, and in genetic epidemiology, individuals who are themselves diseased are more likely to know about disease in other members of their family than are those who are not diseased.

- *Measurement bias* is a systematic error that occurs if measurements are made inaccurately. When misclassification is equivalent in each comparison group, results are biased towards finding no association, as shown in Fig. 5. It is also important to measure exposure and outcome events in the same way for each comparison group, in order to prevent the less predictable biasing effect of differential misclassification.

Each research design is susceptible to a particular set of biases. Selection bias is a potential problem for all observational studies, regardless of whether they employ a cohort or case–control design, because 'exposure' is self-selected rather than assigned. Information bias is of concern in all research designs, but is particularly important in observational studies due to the difficulties in the historical assessment of multifaceted environmental factors. Recall bias is the type of information bias to which case–control studies are particularly susceptible. A full discussion regarding biases and their effects is beyond the scope of this chapter and details should be sought in standard epidemiological texts.[3],[14]

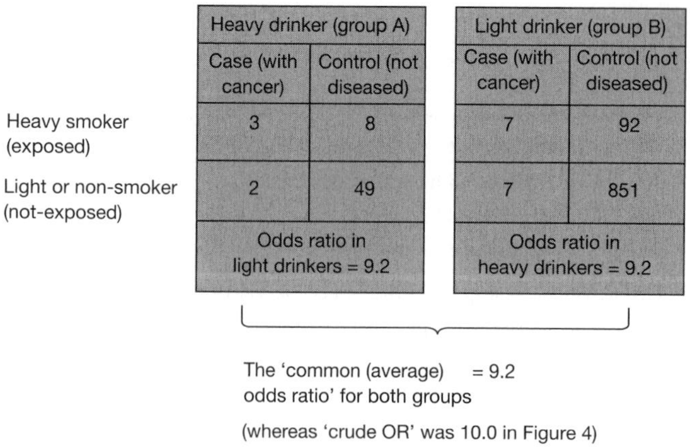

Confounding

Confounding is similar to bias in that it can produce spurious associations or mask associations that are real. A distinction is made because whereas bias is an issue related to study design or appropriate interpretation, confounding is an issue of alternative explanations for a study result. Confounding is defined as a distortion of the effect of an exposure on risk that arises because of an association with other factors that affect risk.[1] Thus, a confounding variable must satisfy two criteria: (a) it must be related to the risk of the outcome under study, and (b) it must be associated with the exposure of interest (but not be a consequence of exposure).

Alcohol ingestion is an example of a confounder when the risk of oesophageal cancer following exposure to cigarettes is under investigation. Both alcohol intake and smoking are risk factors for this disease, plus smokers are more likely to consume alcohol than are non-smokers. In studies of prognosis, confounding by differences in treatment may be important because the indications for particular treatments may be the same prognostic factors that are under investigation.

Confounding can be controlled during data analysis, whereas other sources of bias can be averted only in the design or conduct of a study. Confounding is detected and removed by examining whether the primary exposure-outcome relationship still exists when it is examined separately in each category of the confounder. For example,

Fig. 6 Confounding in a hypothetical case–control study of smoking and oesophageal cancer, where data from Fig. 4 are grouped according to a confounding variable (level of alcohol intake). Odds ratios for the effect of smoking are calculated for each group and then averaged to obtain the 'common odds ratio'. The difference between the 'common odds ratio' and the 'crude odds ratio' (from Fig. 4) indicated the presence of confounding.

the relationship between cigarette smoking and oesophageal cancer would be examined separately in subjects who are heavy drinkers and light drinkers of alcohol. This process is demonstrated in Fig. 6, as subjects in the hypothetical case–control study of Fig. 4 were grouped according to the potential confounder (e.g. alcohol intake, but this could be some other trait), the association was examined within these two groups, and then the average (or common) odds ratio across both groups was calculated. The common odds ratio of 9.2 is about 8 per cent smaller than the crude odds ratio of 10.0 (from Fig. 4). This indicates that after controlling for the confounding by the group variable (alcohol intake), the primary exposure (smoking) was still strongly associated with cancer risk, although the strength of its association was reduced slightly.

Confounding can be dealt with in the design of the study, as well as in data analysis. Selection of matched comparison groups that are alike with respect to the confounder ensures that any difference between them is not due to confounding by the matching variable. However, matching may cause an increase in both the cost and complexity of the study and it prevents an examination of the relationship between the confounder and the outcome. To identify confounding factors it is necessary to collect data on a wide range of factors in order to ensure that both established and potential risk factors can be accounted for.

Causal inference

Inference about whether an observed association is causal can be made following a logical framework in the form of a series of questions (Table 1). These questions focus initially on the design, analysis, and interpretation of a particular study, and then evaluates the results of the study in the context of other evidence. Important components of causal inference include the following.[3],[11],[15]

Temporality

The need for an exposure to precede disease is an indisputable requirement. The design of cohort studies involves detecting events that follow exposures, but the retrospective assessment of exposure in case–control studies makes the assessment of temporality more difficult. Temporal sequence is usually assured by enrolling incident rather than prevalent cases, and by recording information about exposures that occurred prior to the diagnosis. Owing to the long latency in the development of most cancers, the assessment may involve exposures that occurred many years before the diagnosis of cancer. Temporal patterns may also be examined in terms of how relationships change over time, such as in assessing whether risk varies by the period of exposure.

Strength of association

A stronger association between an exposure and cancer risk is more likely to be causal than a weaker association. Even if a strong association was affected by modest levels of bias or confounding, there is still likely to be an association after these factors are accounted for. Nevertheless, there are exceptions where weak associations are causal, and strong associations are due to other factors.

Dose–response relationship

Finding a relationship between an increasing level of exposure and increasing risk strengthens a causal interpretation. For example, with increasing amount smoked, there is an increase in carcinogen dose, and in biological damage, and consequently, a greater chance that cancer will develop. However, in some situations a simple linear relationship may not hold, such as with ionizing radiation, where a unidirectional relationship may only apply at lower doses (see Chapter 2.3).

Consistency

Within a study, consistency of a relationship can be demonstrated by analysing subgroups to see if the association is observed across a wide range of subjects. However, the strongest support for a causal relationship comes from consistency with other studies. Associations between an exposure and cancer that are demonstrated repeatedly by different investigators using different research methods, are more likely to be causal than are those where different methods generated different results. However, the same result obtained repeatedly from one research method does not necessarily strengthen it, because the same mistake may occur repeatedly. It is sometimes possible to assess consistency by conducting a meta-analysis that summarizes previous studies.

Biological plausibility

Associations between exposure and disease that agree with present knowledge about the reaction of cells and tissues to the exposure make it more plausible that the association is causal. However, the absence of supporting biological information may arise from the incomplete state of knowledge in the basic sciences.

Specificity

If an association is present between a single exposure and a single disease, this may support a causal interpretation; however, this seldom occurs in cancer studies. Cancer has many causal pathways, and most major causes of disease have a wide range of effects. Specificity only contributes to causal reasoning when it is present; absence of specificity is not important, as shown by the multitude of diseases that are associated with cigarette smoking.

Coherence

Causal inference may be indirectly supported by epidemiological observations on the distribution of the causes of disease, or by studies that examine a relationship from a different perspective. However, coherence offers weak support because it overlaps with plausibility and consistency, which contribute more directly to causal inference.

An overview of cancer epidemiology

Population-based statistics describe cancer patterns in terms of person, place, and time, which have implications regarding disease burden and underlying disease determinants. Examples of the most common types of cancer are reviewed to demonstrate the links between descriptive and analytical epidemiology.

Descriptive epidemiology of cancer

There are about 6.2 million deaths due to cancer worldwide in 1997, which accounted for 12 per cent of all deaths. This places cancer as the third most common cause of death after infectious and parasitic diseases, and circulatory diseases.[16] Estimates of worldwide cancer incidence can be derived from *Cancer incidence in five continents*,[17],[18] which contains data from cancer registries around the world. In 1990 there were approximately 8.1 million new cancer cases worldwide (excluding non-melanotic skin cancer), among which the five most frequent types were cancers of the breast, colon and rectum, cervix, stomach, and lung among females, and cancers of the lung, stomach, colon and rectum, prostate, and liver among males (Fig. 7). These types of cancer accounted for approximately 55 per cent of all cancers.

Cancer is a major concern in all nations, while the relative importance of particular types of cancer is highly variable (Fig. 8). The differences in distribution, which are particularly large for cancers of the prostate, liver, cervix, and colon–rectum, arise as a result of the combined effects of differences in population size, age structure, detection, reporting, and underlying aetiological factors. For example, prostate cancer is relatively more frequent in more developed countries because they have a larger proportion of older people and screening activities are common, whereas liver cancer is less frequent in part because one of the major aetiological factors (hepatitis B) is less prevalent.

A comparison of rates rather than counts (Fig. 9), provides a more valid comparison between countries because differences in population size are accounted for, and the process of age-standardization controls for the confounding influence of age. Figure 9 demonstrates the convention of referring to a large denominator of fixed size when expressing rates of rare diseases; for example, in the United States and Canada in 1990, the lung cancer incidence rates (age-standardized to the World Standard Population) were 70 per 100 000 males and 33 per 100 000 females.[18] The fact that lung cancer mortality rates are only slightly less than incidence rates indicates the severity of the disease, as most people who develop lung cancer will die from it relatively soon after the diagnosis. In contrast, the large

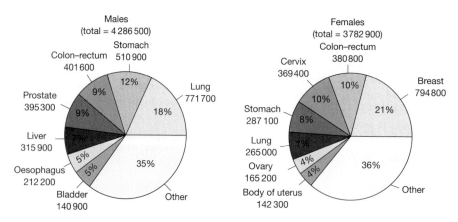

Fig. 7 Estimated number of new cancer cases and per cent distribution for leading types of cancer, by sex, worldwide in 1990. (Data source: Ferlay et al. 1998[18].)

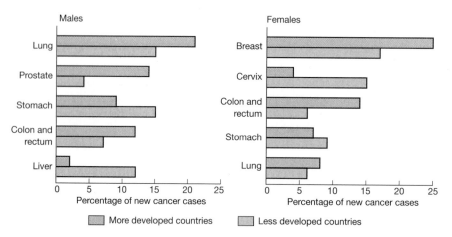

Fig. 8 The per cent distribution of new cases for the five most common types of cancer, by sex, for less developed and more developed countries in 1990. (Data source: Ferlay et al. 1998[18].)

difference between incidence and mortality rates for breast cancer among women, indicates that it has a more favourable prognosis.

Figure 9 shows a striking international variation in the frequency of the leading types of cancer, as lung cancer, breast cancer, and prostate cancer have incidence and mortality rates that are low in Asian and African countries, but high in northern Europe and America. There is a 10-fold variation in rates from lowest to highest for lung cancer and prostate cancer, and a fivefold variation for breast cancer.

While these large international differences in cancer incidence are due to a combination of genetic (inherited) and environmental factors, there are several lines of evidence that suggest that environment plays an important part, and consequently that cancer risks are modifiable. Strong evidence for the importance of environmental factors comes from the study of migrant populations, because for many types of cancer, groups of migrants who move from one country to another eventually acquire the cancer incidence of the country to which they moved. An example is seen for stomach cancer and prostate cancer among Chinese men, where men of Chinese ancestry living in Hawaii have a reported age-adjusted incidence of prostate cancer that is

about 30 times higher than that for men residing in Shanghai (Fig. 10). In contrast, the rate of stomach cancer is more than four times higher in Shanghai than Hawaii. For both types of cancer, the incidence rates are intermediate in Hong Kong, where certain features of lifestyle and health services are more 'Westernized'. The implication of such migrant studies is that the international variation in cancer rates, while being due partly to genetic differences between populations of each country, is also due to some feature of life in those countries.

Further evidence in support of the importance of environmental factors, and consequently, on the modifiability or preventability of cancer, is provided by observed variation in cancer rates within countries that exists between groups of people or over time. Time trends in incidence rates for the five most frequently diagnosed cancers (excluding non-melanoma skin cancer) are shown in Fig. 11 for Canada,[19] which is one of the few countries with total coverage of its population by a national cancer registry. Lung cancer incidence rates in men increased steadily until the mid-1980s, and then began to decline, whereas in women the rates are now about half as high as in men, but they continue to increase steadily. These patterns in lung cancer incidence follow, with a lag of about 20 years, the historical

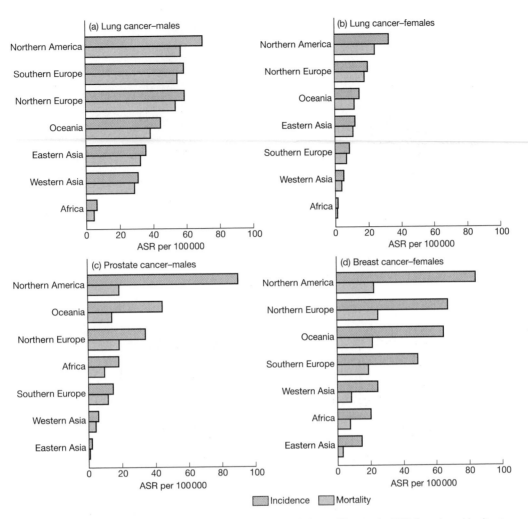

Fig. 9 International variation of in age-standardized incidence and mortality rates (ASR), by world region in 1990, for selected leading types of cancer (standardized to the World Population). (Data source: Ferlay *et al.* 1998[18].)

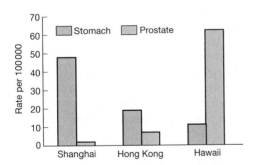

Fig. 10 Age-standardized incidence rates (standardized to the World Standard Population) for stomach cancer and prostate cancer among Chinese men in different countries, 1988 to 1992. (Data source: Parkin *et al.* 1997[17].)

patterns of tobacco use among both men and women. In the early 1990s there was a sharp increase in age-standardized incidence rates for prostate cancer, which can be attributed partly to the detection of occult cancer by screening for elevated serum levels of prostate-specific antigen; however, the recent down-turn in incidence suggests that the earlier detection achieved by the screening test has reached its maximal impact. Cancers of the bladder and uterus have lower incidence rates that have been stable, whereas there has been a small, but steady increase over time in the incidence of non-Hodgkin's lymphoma. The patterns depicted in Fig. 11 for Canada are similar to those seen in the United States.[20]

Even though incidence rates for all types of cancer combined have been relatively stable in many countries, caseloads continue to increase due to changes in the population. Figure 12 shows the trend in the number of new cancer cases among Canadian men over two decades, and depicts the relative contributions due to changes in the overall incidence rate, due to the increase in the number of men in the population, and due to the ageing of the population. Ageing of the population and increase in population size were the major determinants of the increase in incidence. Many countries have ageing populations similar to Canada's, and will face this pattern of continuously growing caseloads.

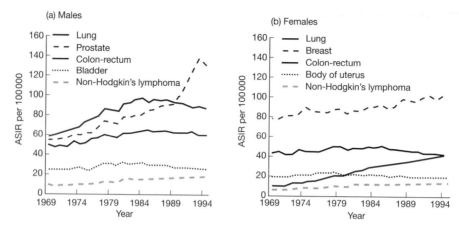

Fig. 11 Trends in age-standardized incidence rates (ASIR per 100 000) for the five most common cancers among men (A) and women (B), in Canada, 1964 to 1994. (Standardized to the World Standard Population; Adapted from National Cancer Institute of Canada, 1999[19].)

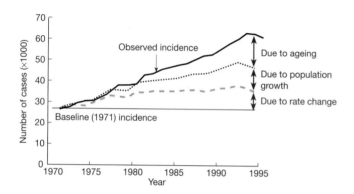

Fig. 12 The trend in the total number of newly diagnosed cancer cases among males in Canada, showing the relative contribution of changes in rates, population growth, and ageing of the population. (Adapted from National Cancer Institute of Canada, 1999[19].)

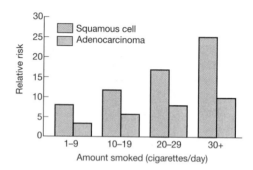

Fig. 13 The gradient of relative risk estimates for lung cancer among men, by number of cigarettes smoked per day and by histological type, with non-smokers as the baseline comparison group. (Adapted from Lubin and Blot 1984[25].)

Analytical epidemiology—demonstrated with lung cancer

The epidemiology of lung cancer is described to illustrate the application of analytical epidemiology, and the interpretation and implications of study results. Although tobacco smoke was suspected as a health hazard for almost 400 years, largely based on clinical observations, it was only in the 1930s when lung cancer mortality rates were seen to be increasing in England and the United States that scientific studies of the health effects of tobacco were initiated. By 1950, population-based data brought to light wide international variation in lung cancer mortality. At the same time, several retrospective epidemiological studies provided the first evidence, and these were followed by large prospective studies, such that by the mid-1950s there was strong evidence of a link between tobacco use and cancer.[21],[22] Ten years later there was epidemiological evidence that the risk of lung cancer declined after discontinuing smoking.

Throughout this period there was debate about whether tobacco smoke was a 'cause' of lung cancer, with major sources of uncertainty stemming from the absence of both experimental evidence and a definitive biological mechanism. In 1964, the landmark report on *Smoking and health* from the office of the United States Surgeon General, was the first demonstration of causation using the framework for causal inference outlined earlier.[23] Now there is overwhelming evidence that smoking causes cancer in humans,[24] based on: the strength and significance of associations, as lung cancer risk is 10 to 15-fold greater in smokers than non-smokers;[22] the consistency of findings in many epidemiological studies; the presence of strong dose–response relationships (Fig. 13);[25] and the more recently established biological mechanisms of carcinogens found in tobacco smoke.

Recent studies have examined the effects of lower levels of exposure to tobacco smoke. More than 35 case–control and five cohort studies have assessed the association between lung cancer and environmental tobacco smoke. Many studies did not detect statistically significant associations, partly because sample sizes were not sufficient to detect small differences in risk. However, when data from existing studies were combined in meta-analyses the relative risk of lung cancer was approximately 1.4 for the high category of measured exposures to second-hand smoke,[26] and 1.3 (95 per cent CI = 1.1 to 1.5) for non-smokers who lived with a smoker.[27]

Boffetta *et al.*[6] reported on a collaborative case–control study of the association between environmental tobacco smoke and lung cancer risk in non-smokers and light smokers, which involved 650 lung cancer cases and 1542 controls who were recruited at 12 cancer centres in seven countries. Key issues of this study are highlighted to demonstrate the application of the framework for critical appraisal shown in Table 1. Strengths of the study include that the investigators tried to maximize internal validity by developing and evaluating specialized questionnaires and by implementing systematic procedures. Nevertheless, the difficulties inherent in measuring environmental tobacco smoke exposure retrospectively and in maintaining standards across many collaborating centres make it possible that the study results suffered from slight information bias or selection bias. A strength of the study is that it accounted for the major potential confounding variables, which had a relatively small impact on the results. The role of chance was adequately explored in thorough statistical analyses, the details of which were clearly presented. For example, a weak, but not statistically significant, association was found between lung cancer risk and exposure to spousal and workplace environmental tobacco smoke, with an odds ratio of 1.14 (95 per cent CI = 0.88 to 1.47), and there was weak evidence of a dose–response relationship ($p = 0.01$ for trend test). Regarding the second set of criteria in Table 1, the results of Boffetta *et al.* are supportive of a causal relationship between environmental tobacco smoke and lung cancer in terms of dose–response and temporality, but not in terms of strength of association. Within the study, results were partially, but not completely, consistent as odds ratios were similar for workplace and spousal environmental tobacco smoke exposures, whereas an increased risk was not found for childhood exposures. With regard to the third set of criteria in Table 1, the most important features are that (a) the report is consistent with the meta-analyses and numerous individual studies that reported a slight increase in risk from spousal environmental tobacco smoke exposure, and (b) there is a plausible biological mechanism. Among the final criteria, the results of Boffetta *et al.* can be generalized most directly to the European populations that were studied, while inference beyond that would require additional supporting evidence. Finally, the relevance of the findings may be quite high, because even if the true increase in risk is modest, the high prevalence of environmental tobacco smoke exposure and the severity of the outcome would result in a serious burden of premature and preventable mortality in the population.

While the relationship between cigarette smoking and lung cancer is the most extensively documented aetiological relationship in cancer epidemiology, other risk factors for lung cancer have been identified, including ionizing radiation and certain occupational exposures, such as organic chemicals, heavy metals, and asbestos. Smoking is more prevalent and has a higher relative risk than other exposures. For example, smokers have a 10- to 15-fold greater risk of lung cancer than non-smokers,[22] whereas uranium miners who are exposed to radiation in the form of radon have a two- to fivefold increased risk.[28] Several dietary risk factors have been identified, such as low intake of vitamins A, C, and E, but results have been somewhat inconsistent and the protective effects of these vitamins have not been demonstrated in dietary intervention trials[29] (see also Chapter 2.5).

A possible role for genetic susceptibility as a determinant of lung cancer risk is suggested by the fact that not all who develop lung cancer are smokers, and lung cancer occurs more frequently in some families. Case–control studies found that lung cancer risk was two-to fourfold greater among individuals with a family history of lung cancer,[30],[31] a pattern which could be due to either genetic or shared environmental factors. Genetic–epidemiological analyses of pedigrees indicated subsequently that the familial pattern of lung cancer risk was consistent with Mendelian inheritance of an unknown susceptibility gene, the effect of which is expressed only in the presence of tobacco smoke.[32]

Molecular–epidemiological studies that searched for the presumed susceptibility genes focused initially on genes involved in the metabolism (e.g. cytochrome P-450 enzymes coded by CYP1A1, CYP2D6) and elimination (e.g. glutathione *S*-transferases, and *N*-acetyl-transferases) of carcinogens in tobacco smoke. In early studies of susceptibility, which relied on phenotypes such as the ability to metabolize debrisoquine, an increased risk of lung cancer was found among extensive metabolizers in some[33] but not all studies.[34] Subsequently, methods of genotyping were developed so that polymorphisms could be detected in the genes responsible for the metabolism of certain carcinogens contained in tobacco smoke. Using these methods, associations between certain metabolic genotypes and lung cancer risk were found to differ according to smoking status, which was more direct evidence of a 'gene–environment interaction'. As a further example of biologically supportive evidence, lung cancer cells grown in culture and exposed to benzo[*a*]pyrene, which is a toxin found in tobacco smoke, were shown to develop DNA adducts at mutational 'hotspots' in the p53 tumour suppressor gene.[35]

The final phase of an epidemiological review involves the development of strategies for reducing the burden of disease. Given the poor prognosis for most patients who develop lung cancer, and given that no method of early detection has been found that reduces mortality, primary prevention is the cancer control strategy with the greatest potential benefit. Prevention is more feasible for lung cancer than most cancers, because the cause of the majority of cases is known and is modifiable. While tobacco smoke is only one component of the web of environmental and genetic factors that lead to lung cancer, it is established as the predominant cause. Thus, tobacco control programmes are a major priority for decreasing the burden of lung cancer, and are required urgently due to the trends of increasing tobacco use in many countries.

Risk factors and the prospects for prevention

Analytic epidemiological studies have identified a wide range of environmental and genetic factors that are determinants of cancer risk in the population, examples of which are listed in Table 3.

Tobacco use

In addition to the causal role of tobacco smoke in lung cancer, it is associated with many other types of cancer, although not as strongly. Among the world's most common types of cancer, tobacco use is convincingly or probably associated with an increased risk of colorectal and cervical cancer (Table 3).[36] Most cancers of the lung, pleura, lip, oral cavity, pharynx, and larynx can be attributed to tobacco use, with estimated attributable risks of 80 to 90 per cent.[37],[38] For oesophageal cancer the attributable risk is approximately 75 per cent,

Table 3 Established risk factors (with probable or convincing evidence) for the leading types of cancer, worldwide. (Adapted from World Cancer Research Fund, 1997)

Type of cancer	Increases risk	Risk decreases
Lung	Smoking Asbestos exposure Occupational exposure (e.g. nickel, radon)	Vegetable and fruit intake Carotenoid intake
Breast	Family history (and germline BRCA1/2 mutations) Reproductive factors (e.g. nulliparity, late menopause) Rapid growth, greater height, and high body mass Alcohol Ionizing radiation	Vegetables and fruit intake
Stomach	Salt preserved food Infection with *Helicobacter pylori*	Vegetable and fruit intake Vitamin C
Colon–rectum	Smoking Family history or carrier of germline mutation Meat intake Alcohol use	Food refrigeration Physical activity Vegetable intake Aspirin
Liver	Alcohol intake Aflatoxin Hepatitis B and C viruses	
Cervix	Smoking Human papilloma virus	

while for bladder, kidney, and pancreas cancers it is in the range of 30 to 50 per cent. Doll and Peto concluded that across all sites combined, one-third of all cancer deaths in the United States could be prevented by removing the impact of smoking.[37]

Diet

Comprehensive surveys of epidemiological and experimental data have suggested a role of dietary constituents in many types of cancer. Dietary recommendations designed to lower cancer risk have included reducing fat intake to 30 per cent of total calories, including fruits, vegetables, and whole-grain cereals in the daily diet, minimizing consumption of salted and smoked foods, and drinking alcohol in moderation, if at all.[39] A recent re-evaluation of the evidence relating diet to cancer confirmed previously known relationships and elucidated some new ones (Table 4).[36] Diets high in vegetables and fruits, which are also high in fibre, antioxidants and other bioactive compounds, are associated with reduced risk of most, if not all, epithelial cancers (Table 4). Table 4 also shows that among the many types of cancer linked to diet, the direction of effects is uniform for each dietary component, which implies that even if interventions aim to reduce the risk for a specific cancer, benefits rather than hazards will also be expected for other types of cancer.

It may be difficult to distinguish between the effects of diet and other factors on cancer risk. In particular, while dietary recommendations may help to maintain body weight, this is also largely determined by regular physical activity, which itself is associated with a decreased risk of colon cancer (Table 3), and possibly of breast and lung cancer.[36] Similarly, alcohol is an established risk factor for many cancers, including cancers of the mouth, pharynx, larynx, oesophagus,

colon, rectum, and liver (Table 4). It probably also contributes to the risk of breast cancer (see Chapter 11.1).

The anticipated benefits have not been achieved in dietary intervention studies, such as the randomized trials of β-carotene supplements in which risk of lung cancer increased or remained unchanged.[29],[40] This finding could be explained if the aetiological effects of carotene were confounded by other factors, or if the benefits of carotene-containing foods were due to more than a single nutrient. Thus, recommendations regarding the prevention of cancer by dietary means have shifted away from interventions based on specific nutrients and supplements (e.g. carotenoids), focusing instead on whole foods (e.g. vegetables and fruit) in the context of an overall diet.[36]

Hormonal and reproductive factors

Reproductive and hormonal factors influence risk for cancers of the breast (Table 3), endometrium, and ovary. The risk of breast cancer and endometrial cancer is increased in women who have had fewer pregnancies, an earlier age of menarche, a later age of first pregnancy, and a later age of menopause, where this effect is thought to arise from prolonged exposures to the proliferative effects of endogenous oestrogens. Both oral contraceptives and postmenopausal oestrogens have been associated sometimes, but not consistently, with an increased risk of breast cancer (see Chapter 11.1).[41],[42],[43] An increased risk of endometrial cancer was seen among women who used oral contraceptives or oestrogen replacement therapies containing unopposed oestrogens, whereas the subsequent use of combinations that contained progestogen resulted in significantly reduced risks.[44] Ovarian cancer risk is also increased among women with low parity, but it is decreased in women who used oral contraceptives.[41] A

Table 4 A matrix of the impact of selected dietary components on cancer risk, by strength of evidence and direction of effect. (adapted from World Cancer Research Fund 1997)

Dietary factor	Cancer sites for which risk is:			
	Convincingly or probably decreased	Possibly decreased	Possibly increased	Convincingly or probably increased
Vegetable and fruit	Mouth, pharynx, larynx, oesophagus, lung, stomach, pancreas, colon, rectum, breast, bladder	Liver, ovary, endometrium, cervix, prostate, thyroid, kidney	–	–
Carotenoids and vitamin C (antioxidants)	Lung, stomach	Mouth, pharynx, oesophagus, pancreas, colon, rectum, breast, cervix	–	–
Fibre	–	Colon, rectum, breast, pancreas	–	–
Total and saturated animal fats	–	–	Colon, rectum, breast, endometrium, lung, prostate	–
Alcohol	–	–	Lung	Mouth, pharynx, larynx, oesophagus, liver, colon, rectum, breast

possible mechanism for this is that because pregnancy, breast-feeding, and oral contraceptive use decrease the number of ovulatory cycles, they reduce the likelihood of mitotic events that could arise during the epithelial repair and proliferation that follows every ovulation.

Radiation

Ionizing radiation is an established cause of cancer, with the epidemiological evidence being particularly convincing from large cohort studies of survivors of atomic bomb explosions in Japan, and individuals who received occupational or medical exposures to ionizing radiation (see Chapter 2.3). Many types of cancer are known to be caused by radiation, with the most firmly established dose–response relationships being for leukaemia and cancers of the thyroid, breast, lung, stomach, colon, bladder, oesophagus, and ovary.[45]

Other occupational exposures

Studies of occupationally exposed cohorts are useful in identifying environmental factors linked to cancer risk because effects are easier to detect among workers who have higher levels of exposure than in the general population. The identification of some rare forms of cancer among workers has prompted in-depth studies to search for aetiological factors. For example, the occurrence of angiosarcoma of the liver led to the identification of vinyl chloride as a risk factor,[41] and a rare form of lung cancer, mesothelioma, was linked to industrial exposures to asbestos (Table 3).

Viruses

The role of viruses in cancer aetiology has been established for only a few diseases (see Chapter 2.2). Associations are recognized between infection with hepatitis B virus and primary hepatocellular liver cancer, human papilloma virus, and cervical cancer (Table 3), and Epstein–Barr virus and Burkitt's lymphoma or nasopharyngeal cancer. There is substantial evidence from animal studies that other viruses cause cancer, but evidence in humans is lacking.

Familial aggregation and genetic factors

Epidemiological studies have demonstrated that many types of cancer exhibit a tendency to aggregate in families, such that close relatives of a cancer patient have a slightly increased risk for developing that form of cancer.[46] For certain types of cancer, inherited mutations in specific genes may increase the relative risk to more than a hundred-fold. Cancers for which potent cancer genes have been found include retinoblastoma (see Chapter 17.3), Wilms' tumour (see Chapter 17.4), breast cancer, ovarian cancer, colorectal cancer, and melanoma. While such inherited cancer genes are the most potent oncogenic influences in humans, they are rare and account for only a small proportion of the more common types of cancer.[47] For example, while inherited mutations in BRCA-1 convey a very high risk of breast or ovarian cancer for the small number of women affected, these account for approximately 5 per cent of all breast malignancies.[48]

Summary

Doll and Peto[37] evaluated the relative importance of risk factors and estimated the potential impact of possible interventions in terms of the proportion of deaths from specific cancers that could be prevented. This estimation was based on a review of the international variation in age-standardized death rates for major types of cancer and the relative risks associated with individual factors, including tobacco, diet, alcohol, reproductive and sexual behaviour, occupational and environmental exposures, infection, medical procedures, geophysical factors, and genetic factors. Doll and Peto estimated that the proportion of all cancer deaths in the United States that could be avoided through changes in specific environmental factors was 30 per cent for tobacco products, 35 per cent for dietary factors, 3 per cent for alcohol, and 4 per cent for occupational exposures. This methodology was used to conclude that a large proportion of common cancers in the Western world are potentially avoidable, and that the reduction of tobacco use has the single greatest potential for reducing the cancer burden.[37],[49],[50]

Features that enhance the potential impact of a cancer control strategy include: the exposure is common; the disease is serious; there is a strong association between exposure and disease; and the exposure status is modifiable in a way that is sustainable and acceptable to individuals. These principles underlie the differences in impact of population-based versus high-risk strategies: the latter may be highly relevant to individuals who manifest a risk factor, but the high-risk state is usually rare, which limits the potential impact on mortality in the population.[51] Complete knowledge of causal mechanisms is not required to achieve health benefits. For example, even though biological mechanisms of tobacco smoke carcinogenesis are not completely elucidated, reduction in tobacco use remains the most effective solution to achieve health benefits in the population.

Ethical isssues in epidemiological research

Ethical principles require that a researcher must aim to maximize benefits while minimizing risks to study participants, must respect privacy and autonomy, and must obtain consent that is appropriately informed. The observational designs that are predominant in epidemiology usually impart small or negligible hazards to individuals, while the benefits to participants may also be small. Thus, the ethical issues of primary concern in most epidemiological studies relate to privacy, freedom of choice, informed consent, and access to information.[52]

Data collection in many studies could be completed without directly contacting individuals, by referring to existing information in cancer registries, medical records, vital statistics, occupational records, or results of previous research or surveys. There has been an increase in the societal level of concern for privacy, due partly to the ease of electronic transfer of personal information. In addition, certain types of health information are highly sensitive, and there are well-founded concerns about security and confidentiality because if this information is used improperly, individuals may be adversely affected. For example, women who are found to carry a mutation in a breast cancer susceptibility gene, may be unable to obtain health or life insurance.

One response to concerns about privacy could be the requirement for individuals to give informed consent for each separate use of their archived health data. This may be appropriate for some research; however, in epidemiological studies of large populations over long periods, this is not feasible and could introduce serious selection bias. Another strategy is the removal of personal identifiers from health information that is made available to researchers; however, for many epidemiological studies information regarding individuals must be available so that personal exposures and outcomes can be compared. Thus, while these approaches protect privacy, they also impede analytical research that aims to benefit health. Accordingly, efforts must be taken to achieve a balance between the benefits to the public

that arise from health and medical research, and the important individual rights of privacy and autonomy.

Guidelines have been developed to assist institutions and individuals in weighing risks and benefits during the ethics review of a research plan (e.g. ref. 52). Regarding access to health records, the American College of Epidemiology has proposed that 'information collected during the course of health care and medical treatment may be disclosed to clinical investigators and health care researchers without a requirement for informed consent, if an Institutional Review Board rules that it is conducted in the public good, direct harm to individuals is unlikely, the individual will not be contacted, and individually identifiable data are not made public'.[53] Thus, it remains the investigator's responsibility to maintain strong safeguards against the inappropriate release or unintended use of research information.

Conclusions

In cancer epidemiology, disease patterns and determinants are studied in people using specialized research methods that rely largely on observational rather than experimental designs. These methods aim to overcome potential biases and confounding, to account for random error, and to deal with the multiplicity of factors that may contribute to risk. A fundamental component of the epidemiological approach is the framework for interpreting and applying research findings, whereby the quality of individual studies and the combined evidence is critiqued in order to assess whether an association is valid, causal, and important.

Historically, epidemiology made its greatest contribution in the identification of risk factors for disease occurrence, which formed the basis of programmes for primary prevention and early detection. Recently, the epidemiological approach has been applied increasingly and further developed in studies that have clinical, genetic, molecular, and other implications. There is optimism that the inclusion of measurements of biological processes in epidemiological studies will result in the discovery of new risk factors and gene–environment interactions, and in the elucidation of underlying causal mechanisms. However, health benefits can still be achieved even when biological mechanisms are not fully understood.

The principal task of epidemiology will continue to be the detection and measurement of disease determinants, so that groups of people can be identified who differ in their risk, which in turn gives direction for cancer control programmes. One of the challenges faced in modern epidemiology is in distinguishing between the relative merits of determinants that act at the level of the population, the individual, or the molecule. Similarly, it may be difficult to distinguish between the benefits of interventions that involve a population or that target individuals at high risk. However, there is a role for each strategy in balanced programmes and interventions that aim to reduce the cancer burden.

References

1. **Last JM** (ed.) *A dictionary of epidemiology.* New York: Oxford University Press, 1995.

2. **Hill AB.** Observation and experiment. *New England Journal of*

Medicine, 1953; **248**: 995–1001 (Reprinted in Greenland S, ed. *Evolution of epidemiologic ideas: annotated readings on concepts and methods*. Chestnut Hill, MA: Epidemiology Resources Inc., 1987).

3. Rothman KJ, Greenland S. *Modern epidemiology*. Philadelphia: Lippincott-Raven, 1998.

4. Sackett DL, Haynes RB, Guyatt GH, Tugwell P. *Clinical epidemiology: a basic science for clinical medicine*. Boston: Little, Brown and Co., 1991.

5. Fuchs CS, *et al*. Dietary fiber and the risk of colorectal cancer and adenoma in women. *New England Journal of Medicine*, 1999; **340**: 169–76.

6. Boffetta P, *et al*. Multicenter case-control study of exposure to environmental tobacco smoke and lung cancer in Europe. *Journal of the National Cancer Institute*, 1998; **90**: 1440–50.

7. Khoury MJ, Beaty TH, Cohen BH. *Fundamentals of genetic epidemiology*. New York: Oxford University Press, 1993.

8. Khoury MJ, Risch N, Kelsey JL (eds). Genetic epidemiology. *Epidemiologic Reviews*, 1997; **19**(1).

9. Kelsey J, Whittemore A, Evans A, Thompson D. *Methods in observational epidemiology*. New York: Oxford University Press, 1996.

10. Brownson R, Pettiti D. *Applied epidemiology: theory to practice*. New York: Oxford University Press, 1998.

11. Elwood M. *Critical appraisal of epidemiological studies and clinical trials*. London: Oxford University Press, 1998.

12. Sackett DL. Bias in analytic research. *Journal of Chronic Diseases*, 1979; **32**: 51–63.

13. Rubin S, *et al*. Clinical and pathological features of ovarian cancer in women with germ-line mutations of BRCA1. *New England Journal of Medicine*, 1996; **335**: 1413–16.

14. Breslow N and Day N. *Statistical methods in cancer research—Volume II—The design and analysis of cohort studies*. Lyon: International Agency for Research on Cancer, 1987.

15. Hill BA. *Principles of medical statistics*. New York: Oxford University Press, 1971

16. World Health Organization. *World health report 1998*. Geneva: World Health Organization, 1998.

17. Parkin DM, Whelan SL, Ferlay J, Raymond L, Young, J (eds). *Cancer incidence in five continents*, Vol. VII (IARC Scientific publications No. 143). Lyon: International Agency for Research on Cancer, 1997.

18. Ferlay J, Parkin DM, Pisani P. GLOBOCAN 1: Cancer Incidence and Mortality Worldwide in 1990 (www-dep.iarc.fr/dataava/globocan). Lyon, France: International Agency for Research on Cancer, 1998.

19. National Cancer Institute of Canada (NCIC). *Canadian cancer statistics—1999*. Toronto: NCIC 1999.

20. Ries LAG, *et al*. (eds). *SEER cancer statistics review, 1973–1991*. (http://www-seer.ims.nci.nih.gov). Bethesda: National Cancer Institute, 1998.

21. Hammond EC, Horn D. Smoking and death rates—report on forty-four months of followup of 187,783 men. *Journal of the American Medical Association*, 1958; **166**: 1294–308.

22. Doll R, *et al*. Mortality in relation to smoking: 40 years' observations on male British doctors. *British Medical Journal*, 1994; **309**: 901–11.

23. United States—Department of Health, Education and Welfare (US-DHEW). *Smoking and health: Report of the Advisory Committee to the Surgeon General of the Public Health Service*. Washington: Government Printing Office, 1964.

24. IARC (International Agency for Research on Cancer), *IARC Monographs on the evaluation of carcinogenic risks to humans*, Volume 38, *Tobacco smoke*. Lyon: IARC, 1986.

25. Lubin J, Blot WJ. Assessment of lung cancer risk factors by histologic category. *Journal of the National Cancer Institute*, 1984; **73**: 383–9.

26. Environmental Protection Agency (EPA). *Respiratory health effects of passive smoking: lung cancer and other disorders*. Washington DC: US-EPA, 1992.

27. Hackshaw AK, Law MR, Wald NJ. The accumulated evidence on lung cancer and environmental tobacco smoke. *British Medical Journal*, 1997; **13**: 980–8.

28. Lubin J, *et al*. Lung cancer in radon-exposed miners and estimation of risk from indoor exposure. *Journal of the National Cancer Institute*, 1995; **87**: 817–27.

29. Omenn G, *et al*. Effects of combination of beta carotene and vitamin A on lung cancer and cardiovascular disease. *New England Journal of Medicine*, 1996; **334**: 1150–5.

30. Tokuhata GK, Lilienfeld AM. Familial aggregations of lung cancer in humans. *Journal of the National Cancer Institute*, 1963; **30**: 289–312.

31. Shaw GL, *et al*. Lung cancer risk associated with cancer in relatives. *Journal of Clinical Epidemiology*, 1991; **44**: 429–37.

32. Sellers TA, *et al*. Effect of cohort differences in smoking prevalence on models of lung cancer susceptibility. *Genetic Epidemiology*, 1992; **9**: 261–71.

33. Caporaso NE, *et al*. Lung cancer and the debrisoquine metabolic phenotype. *Journal of the National Cancer Institute*, 1990; **85**: 1264–72.

34. Shaw GL, *et al*. Lung cancer risk associated with cancer in relatives. *Cancer Epidemiology Biomarkers and Prevention*, 1995; **4**: 41–9.

35. Denissenko MF, Pao A, Tang M, Pfeifer GP. Preferential formation of benzo[a]pyrene adducts at lung cancer mutational hotspots in P53. *Science*, 1996; **274**: 430–2.

36. World Cancer Research Fund. *Food, nutrition and the prevention: a global perspective*. Washington: American Institute for Cancer Research, 1997.

37. Doll R, Peto R. *The causes of cancer: quantitative estimates of avoidable risks of cancer in the United States*. Oxford: Oxford University Press, 1981.

38. United States—National Center for Health Statistics (US-NCHS). *Vital statistics of the United States, 1989. Volume II, Mortality*. Washington: United States Department of Public Health Service, 1991.

39. National Academy of Sciences. *Diet, nutrition and cancer*. Washington: National Academy Press, 1982.

40. Rowe PM. Beta-carotene takes a collective beating. *The Lancet*, 1996; **347**: 249.

41. IARC (International Agency for Research on Cancer), *IARC Monograph on the Evaluation of Carcinogenic Risks to Humans*—Supplement 7, *Overall Evaluations of Carcinogenicity: An Updating of IARC Monographs*, Volumes 1–42. Lyon: IARC, 1987.

42. Vessey MP: Exogenous hormones. In: Vessey MP, Gray M (eds). *Cancer risks and prevention*. Oxford: Oxford University Press, 1985: 166–94.

43. Collaborative Group on Hormonal Factors in Breast Cancer. Breast cancer and hormonal contraceptives: collaborative reanalysis of individual data on 53,297 women with breast cancer and 100,239 women without breast cancer from 54 epidemiological studies. *The Lancet*, 1996; **347**: 1713–27.

44. Grady D, *et al*. Hormone replacement therapy and endometrial cancer risk: a meta-analysis. *Obstetrics and Gynecology*, 1995; **85**: 304–13.

45. Committee on the Biological Effects of Ionizing Radiations, *Health effects of exposure to low levels of ionizing radiation (BEIR V)*, Washington, National Research Council, 1990.

46. Muller H, Weber W (eds). *Familial cancer*. Basel: Karger, 1985.

47. Li F. Familial aggregation. In Schottenfeld D, Fraumeni JF, Jr (eds). *Cancer epidemiology and prevention*. New York: Oxford University Press, 1996: 546–58.

48. Miki Y, *et al*. Isolation of BRCA1, the 17q-linked breast and ovarian cancer susceptibility gene. *Science*, 1994; **266**: 66–7.

49. Tomatis L, *et al*. (eds). *Cancer: causes, occurrence, and control*. Lyon: International Agency for Research on Cancer, 1990.

50. Shultz JM, Novotony TE, Rice DP. Quantifying the disease impact of cigarette smoking with SAMMECII software. *Public Health Reports*, 1991; 106: 326–33.

51. Rose G. Sick individuals and sick populations. *International Journal of Epidemiology*, 1985; 14: 32–8.

52. Council for International Organizations of Medical Sciences (CIOMS). *Ethics and Epidemiology: International Guidelines for Ethical Review of Epidemiological Studies.* Geneva: CIOMS, 1991.

53. Hiatt RA. American College of Epidemiology draft policy statement on privacy of medical records. *Epidemiology Monitor*, 1998; 19: 9–11.

2.5 Cancer chemoprevention

Andrea Decensi, Alberto Costa, Giuseppe D'Aiuto, and Marco Rosselli del Turco

Introduction

Chemoprevention is a recently introduced and rapidly growing area of oncology. The number of chemoprevention trials has increased substantially in just a few years, for there is no doubt that the prospect of being able to prevent cancer is universally attractive. The term chemoprevention was used in 1979 by Sporn and Newton who defined it as 'the prevention of cancer by the use of pharmacological agents that inhibit or reverse the process of carcinogenesis'.

Carcinogenesis is a complex and multistage process involving interactions between genes and environmental insults that ultimately affect cell proliferation and death. Chemoprevention focuses on intervening in the processes in the cascade of carcinogenic events to prevent the final progression to neoplastic disease, unlike chemotherapy, which concentrates on containing or eradicating cells that have already undergone malignant transformation. While chemotherapy is targeted at people with manifest disease, chemoprevention is directed at individuals who are apparently well, although those in high-risk groups could arguably have existing premalignant conditions. These important differences raise several considerations related to the design and execution of clinical trials of chemopreventive agents. Careful thought must be given to defining the sample population, to defining what is an acceptable intervention in a 'well' person, and what are valid endpoints for measuring outcome, for if the primary aim is to avoid malignancy, a successful intervention would need to be studied for many years.

The rationale behind many chemoprevention studies comes often, but not necessarily, from epidemiological and observational studies that look for an association between environmental factors and tumour occurrence. But environmental factors are hugely complex and dissecting out the primary causative factor within that association can be a long and frustrating task. It is notable that some important chemoprevention trials have contributed to our knowledge through totally negative findings.

This chapter discusses both the general considerations for chemoprevention trials and reviews intervention strategies that have been assessed for specific cancers.

Target populations

Epidemiological and genetic studies have allowed us to define high-risk groups for many malignancies. Risk may be conferred by inheritance of particular genes, such as the *APC* gene in colorectal cancer, or by exposure to known carcinogens, such as smoking and lung cancer.

However, there are many considerations in deciding whether high-risk groups are the most appropriate cohort for chemoprevention studies. If the sample population is a high-risk group there is an advantage in that the time to occurrence of a measurable endpoint may be more predictable and shorter. But there is also the question of how applicable results obtained from a high-risk group are to the general population. High-risk individuals could, by definition, already have premalignant changes. The preventive agent may then be treating this premalignancy and stopping its progression to overt cancer, rather than preventing premalignant changes from taking place. Although this distinction may be regarded as academic, since clinically the desired outcome is achieved, it makes the important mechanistic details of how chemopreventive agents are working difficult to elucidate.

Different target populations may be selected for studying different aspects of one cancer type. For example in breast cancer chemoprevention studies, a first level may involve primary prevention trials in a wide population of healthy women who have a higher, albeit moderate, risk for low-penetrance genetic factors (e.g. one first degree relative with breast cancer), or life-style (e.g. delayed pregnancies), or because of exposure to known promoting agents (e.g. hormone replacement therapy (HRT)). Due to limited statistical power, however, such studies are extremely costly. A second level could involve a limited population at very high risk because of highly penetrating genetic predisposition to cancer (e.g. *BRCA-1* and *BRCA-2* mutation carriers). Trials in this type of population may prove very efficient, but our limited understanding of the physiological function of these genes has so far prevented the rational choice of effective agents. A third level could involve secondary prevention trials in subjects with premalignant or early malignant lesions, for example breast atypical hyperplasia and lobular or ductal carcinoma *in situ* or microinvasive disease, or long-term survivors after adjuvant treatment.

Individuals with colorectal adenoma may also be viewed as an ideal cohort for chemoprevention. In fact, in many large bowel chemoprevention trials adenomas can have a double duty: they are used to identify subjects at risk for large bowel neoplasia, and also serve as endpoints. Many features of adenomas make them suitable for these tasks. Patients with adenomas are fairly numerous and easy to identify, furthermore, the 'adenoma–carcinoma' sequence suggests that adenomas are logical endpoints. The high risk of recurrence among adenoma patients means that a relatively modest number of subjects will suffice for an adequate statistical power. There are some limitations to the use of adenomas, however. Firstly, there is clearly heterogeneity of risk for subsequent cancer. Patients with only small adenomas may have rates of colorectal cancer that are not much greater than those of the normal population. Choosing the high-risk patients for preventive interventions makes sense from a risk–benefit point of view. However, from a population perspective, it may make more sense to answer the chemoprevention question in the numerous individuals who are each at small risk, but who collectively account for most of the cases of colorectal cancer.

Colon cancer can also provide an attractive setting for chemoprevention trails because of the frequency and variation of familial predisposition that is observed in this malignancy (see Chapter 10.4). Inherited colon cancer susceptibility varies from mild to severe. Conditions with extreme susceptibility include the autosomal dominantly inherited syndromes of familial adenomatous polyposis (FAP) and hereditary non-polyposis colorectal cancer (HNPCC). These are highly penetrant syndromes with extreme cancer risk. FAP arises from mutations of the *APC* gene and HNPCC from mutations of the mismatch repair genes. Specific and individual genetic diagnosis is now possible in both syndromes, thus allowing identification of genetically affected individuals for chemoprevention trials.

FAP accounts for less than 1 per cent of colon cancer, while HNPCC may be present in up to 5 per cent of cases. Familial clustering is common in the remainder of cases, which are often referred to as sporadic, but probably arise in part from inherited susceptibility. Epidemiological studies have shown that first-degree relatives have a two to four-fold increased risk of acquiring colon cancer compared to the general population. Ten per cent of individuals in the United States have a first-degree relative with colon cancer. This clinically identifiable, higher-risk group thus constitutes a large potential cohort for chemoprevention trials. However, recruiting specific high-risk populations may introduce unintentional biases if the individuals are alerted to their condition and have been educated about risk factors and lifestyle, such that they have already implemented risk-avoidance changes in lifestyle before the study has started.

The common familial cases of colon cancer can be further stratified by severity. A relative diagnosed under the age of 50 or two first-degree relatives affected with colon cancer confers an even greater risk for this malignancy, estimated to be four to six times that of the general population. Adenomatous polyps also precede the development of colon cancer in these categories, thereby providing a readily identifiable clinical endpoint to judge the effectiveness of chemoprevention.

Compliance in very long-term trials is an issue and will only be achieved if the medication is easy to take, the subject can appreciate the value of the study, and the follow-up studies are simple and convenient. But such large-scale undertakings can also yield huge amounts of data, and the effect of one or more chemopreventive agents on a variety of different cancers can be studied simultaneously. Indeed, observations on malignancies other than the primary target of the study have often brought unexpected bonuses, for example the Alpha-Tocopherol, Beta Carotene study (ATBC) examining the influence of vitamin E on lung cancer found positive effects on the incidence of prostate cancer.[1] Similarly, the study originally evaluating selenium for a chemoprotective role in skin cancer found positive effects on prostate, lung, and colon cancers,[2] and an investigation of fenretinide on breast cancer has shown encouraging results in ovarian cancer.[3] All these observations have formed the basis for further studies.

Table 1 Power to detect a 50 per cent decrease in breast cancer risk, all subjects followed up for 5 years, compliance 100 per cent

Rate per 1000	Number of women per group			
	1000	2000	3000	4000
2	0.24	0.43	0.59	0.72
4	0.43	0.72	0.87	0.95
6	0.59	0.87	0.96	0.99

The size and duration of a chemoprevention trial necessary to give a statistically meaningful result can be enormous. Table 1 shows how the power to detect a 50 per cent decrease in breast cancer risk is related to the number of cases and the sample size. So even in a high-risk population where the annual rate of breast cancer is approximately 6 per 1000 women, in order to obtain a reasonable statistical power of say 0.87, then 2000 women per arm would need to be studied over a 5-year period. These figures assume a 100 per cent compliance with the trial protocol, a figure that is far from realistic in a long-term study involving apparently well subjects. Calculations based on a 75 per cent compliance—a rate reported in several studies (see below)—show that the initial population would need to be increased from 2000 to 3600 subjects per arm. Such an undertaking may not be justified on the basis of currently available information and so preliminary information needs to be gathered from smaller studies of surrogate endpoints. If these are successful, they provide a stronger case for justifying a large trial.

Moreover, if an agent is to be given to huge numbers of people over extended periods then that agent must be of low toxicity, devoid of long-term effects, and effective at low doses. This makes long-established drugs, and naturally occurring vitamins and minerals attractive candidates for chemoprevention studies.

Surrogate endpoints in chemoprevention trials

Surrogate endpoints are biological markers or events that may be assessed or observed prior to the clinical appearance of the disease, and that bear some relationship to the development of that disease. They are intermediate in the sense that they occur sometime between a given intervention that affected the disease process and the time of the clinical diagnosis of the disease. The use of surrogate endpoint biomarkers in pivotal cancer chemoprevention trials may lead to a rational choice of agents which are likely to affect cancer incidence in subsequent phase III trials. For some malignancies there is a readily apparent natural surrogate marker. As mentioned, adenomatous polyps precede the development of colon cancer, thereby providing a readily identifiable clinical endpoint to judge the effectiveness of chemoprevention. However, there are complexities in considerations of the use of adenomas as endpoints of chemoprevention trials.

Adenomas that occur in prevention trials are generally small, and may not necessarily be associated with a greatly increased cancer risk. The issue for chemoprevention trials, however, is not only whether the endpoints are truly intermediate in the causal chain, but whether the intervention under study alters the adenoma recurrence risk to the same extent as it does for the colorectal cancer risk. This is a difficult matter to verify but the limited data available are encouraging. The epidemiology of colorectal adenomas (largely small adenomas) is similar in many regards to that for colorectal cancer itself. Thus to the extent that data are available, one can tentatively conclude that external influences affect adenomas and colorectal cancer similarly. But this must always remain a general consideration—whether chemopreventive agents act in the same way on the surrogate endpoint as they do on the progression of the neoplasm.

Histopathological markers

As cancer is a histopathological disease by definition (although driven by germline and somatic genetic alterations), histopathological markers closest to the incidence of invasive cancer both theoretically and demonstrably hold the greatest predictive value among the range of intermediate efficacy markers currently available for application in cancer prevention studies. Such markers may be reductions in the number, area, or grade of incident preinvasive neoplastic lesions (atypia of cytological specimens and dysplasia of histopathological specimens), and/or induced regression (decreases in number, area, or grade) of preinvasive neoplastic lesions. The utility and relevance of these markers are difficult to demonstrate definitively, because preinvasive neoplastic lesions are routinely excised as a part of the acceptable standard of care in the majority of instances, and because their risk for progression to invasive cancer is beyond the comfort level of most surgeons (e.g. ductal carcinoma-in-situ (DCIS), colorectal adenomas, cervical dysplasia, actinic keratoses, prostatic intraepithelial neoplasia (PIN)). In the case of colorectal cancer, the efficacy of these approaches is demonstrable; polypectomy certainly reduces the subsequent incidence of invasive disease, when assessed by the most rigorous methods consistent with ethical standards. The advancement of techniques such as computer-assisted image analysis that allow detection of early premalignant events and the ability to distinguish between metastases and de novo tumours will contribute greatly to chemoprevention studies.

In addition to histopathological surrogate endpoint biomarkers, markers which characterize fundamental pathophysiological alterations from relatively early points in neoplastic progression—therefore on subcellular, cellular, and early histological organizational levels—offer important mechanistic insights, including knowledge about key pharmacodynamic targets, and may represent tomorrow's validated efficacy biomarkers. Interruption in the balance of cellular population dynamics, such as cell proliferation, apoptosis, and sloughing, with progressive accumulation of cells, is a fundamental property of early neoplasia. Therefore, an important biomarker is 'incident' or clinically-observable masses of abnormal cells arising from normal-appearing, though actually abnormal, flat mucosa. Similarly, alterations in cellular morphology, which form the basis for the pathologist's designation of 'atypia' or 'dysplasia', are key early markers of the neoplastic process within cells and tissues (occurring both in observable masses of neoplastic cells and in the fields at risk), and are therefore appropriate characteristics to develop as markers of preventive efficacy. The nuclear polymorphism index, which characterizes tissue by several major features, including nuclear area, shape, texture, and nucleolar morphometry, are particularly important morphological features. The index is particularly useful when evaluated quantitatively by computer-assisted

Table 2 Rationale for the use of circulating IGF-1 as a surrogate biomarker for breast cancer

1. Mitogenic; antiapoptotic; tumorigenic in experimental systems
2. Stimulates normal mammary epithelial proliferation in primates
3. Mediates oestrogen effects in breast cancer cells
4. Activates oestrogen receptor pathway in the absence of E2
5. Has prognostic effect in breast cancer tissue
6. Modulated by tamoxifen and 4-HPR in vitro and in vivo
7. Reflects 4-HPR preventive activity
8. Predicts premenopausal breast cancer risk

image analysis; it is then the sum of the variances of the three measures. Ultimately, key genetic markers, or combinations of these, which predispose to neoplastic progression within fields of normally-appearing cells will be identified, and may be used as markers of preventive efficacy (e.g. homozygous APC alterations in the cellular population of the colorectum of an individual in the sporadic setting or in a genetically predisposed individual such as an FAP subject). Because these markers offer key mechanistic insights which can be applied to develop interventions, identify risk, or evaluate efficacy, investments in these markers are considered to be fundamental foundations to progress in preventing cancer.

Circulating plasma insulin-like growth factor-1 (IGF-l)

The IGF system plays a pivotal, permissive role in cell proliferation of both epithelial and mesenchymal tissues in at least three different ways: (1) it is highly mitogenic; (2) it protects normal and tumour cells from apoptosis; (3) it is required in several types of cells for the establishment and maintenance of the transformed phenotype and for tumorigenesis.[4] Large, well-conducted, long-term prospective studies have clearly shown that high circulating levels of IGF-1 and low levels of its major binding protein (IGFBP-3) are associated with a higher risk of developing subsequent premenopausal breast cancer,[5] prostate cancer,[6] lung cancer,[7] and colorectal cancer.[8],[9] This indicates that IGF-1 in the blood is a key regulator of cell and tumour growth for the vast majority of human epithelial cancers.[10] There is growing experimental, epidemiological, and clinical evidence that the IGF system is important in breast carcinogenesis. A summary of the rationale for the use of circulating IGF-l as a surrogate endpoint biomarker for breast cancer is provided in Table 2. In vitro, IGF-l is one of the most potent mitogens for breast cancer cell lines, where it mediates oestrogen action. Importantly, the interaction between IGF-l and oestrogen receptors is mutual, since IGF-l has been shown to function as a potent stimulatory factor of the oestrogen signalling pathway in the absence of oestrogen.[11]

Several studies have recently demonstrated that the anti-proliferative effect exerted by retinoids on breast cancer cell lines is mediated by the inhibition of IGF-stimulated growth. In humans, the synthetic retinoid fenretinide or 4-HPR was shown to modulate plasma IGF-l levels.[12] As IGF-1 can stimulate normal epithelial breast

Table 3 Relative risk of subsequent breast cancer by plasma IGF-1 levels

Case/control: 397 breast cancers/620 age-matched controls	
Time from blood collection to diagnosis	28 months (range 1–57)
All, top versus bottom quintile of IGF-1	RR = 0.99 (0.65–1.50)
Postmenopausal, top versus bottom quintile	RR = 0.85 (0.53–1.39)
Premenopausal, top versus bottom tertile	RR = 2.88* (1.21–6.85)
Premenopausal <50 years, top versus bottom tertile	RR = 7.28* (2.40–22.0)

From Hankinson *et al.*

*Adjusted for IGFBP-3

proliferation and promote breast cancer cell growth *in vitro* and *in vivo*, and because higher circulating IGF-1 levels have been found in women with breast cancer as compared to healthy controls, the change in IGF-1 levels may be considered as a potential surrogate endpoint of breast cancer inhibition.[13] As already noted, recent results from the Nurses' Health Prospective Study[5] indicate that premenopausal women with higher IGF-1 levels have an increased risk of developing breast cancer compared to women with lower levels (Table 3). Moreover, the observation that the modulation of IGF-1 by 4-HPR reflects its clinical effect on second primary breast cancers supports the role of this biomarker as a suitable surrogate endpoint in chemoprevention clinical trials of breast cancer.[13]

Both antioestrogens and retinoids can regulate IGF-1 synthesis in humans. Since they act through nuclear receptors belonging to the same steroid/thyroid/retinoid superfamily, it is likely that they interfere with IGF-1 through common pathways. For instance, oestrogens have been shown to regulate IGF-1 gene expression through the transcription factor AP-1, while retinoids can negatively regulate AP-1 responsive genes. Moreover, the hormonal regulation of IGF-1 synthesis appears to be complex, with oestrogens acting as dose-dependent stimulatory or inhibitory agents.[14] Specifically, physiological concentrations such as those achieved through transdermal HRT tend to increase IGF-1 levels, while pharmacological doses such as those achieved in the liver circulation after oral administration induce a decline of IGF-1 levels.

Mammographic density

There is a consistent line of evidence that a higher mammographic density is associated with an increased risk of breast cancer (>50 per cent RR = 4–5 compared to women with lucent mammograms; see also Chapter 11.1). There is a high degree of consistency among eight epidemiological studies that the higher category of breast density (>75 per cent) has an approximately five-fold increased risk of breast cancer compared to the lower category. This conclusion is mainly based on three prospective, nested, case-control studies (Table 4).[15]–[17] Thus, in contrast to the conflicting results provided by the qualitative classification of Wolfe, a quantitative assessment

(by visual inspection) of the percentage of breast density appears to be uniformly associated with an increased risk of breast cancer. Moreover, at variance with most other risk determinants, this factor may potentially be modified by some forms of intervention,[18],[19] providing the endpoint for new preventive interventions.

Dense breasts at mammography are associated with a higher incidence of early preneoplastic lesions (e.g. atypical hyperplasia and ductal carcinoma *in situ*) and are characterized by a predominant stromal component, supporting the contention that stromal–epithelial interactions play a significant role in breast carcinogenesis. The use of mammographic density above 50 per cent as an entry criterion for a chemoprevention trial can select a population with an incidence of breast cancer which is four to five times higher than the age-standardized incidence rate.[20] While visual (manual) quantification of density can readily be applied as an entry criterion for defining at-risk subjects, quantitative measurement of density by instrumental or computerized methods can more reliably be applied to assess variations during intervention.[15],[16]

Results from a randomized trial of low dietary fat intervention have shown that density can be modulated, particularly in the peri-menopausal group.[19] Tamoxifen has also been shown to be associated with a reduction of mammographic density in a recent pilot study.[18] By contrast, HRT can increase mammographic density by 17 per cent to 73 per cent according to different methods and studies. Thus, there is evidence for a hormonal regulation of mammographic density as well as for a modulation by active agents which can affect breast cancer risk, indicating that this factor may be another suitable surrogate endpoint for breast cancer in chemoprevention trials.

Chemoprevention strategies for specific cancers

Breast cancer

Tamoxifen studies

Tamoxifen is a non-steroidal triphenylethylene derivative which can be classified as a first generation selective oestrogen receptor modulator (SERM; see also Chapter 4.25). Tamoxifen is widely used for palliative endocrine treatment of advanced breast cancer and as adjuvant therapy to control micrometastatic relapse and new primaries in women treated surgically for early breast cancer. It has been investigated in three large, co-operative, phase III trials for prevention of breast cancer in at-risk women. The results of two of these studies, the Royal Marsden Tamoxifen Chemoprevention Trial and the Italian Tamoxifen Prevention Study, have recently been published in a preliminary form[21],[22] and the third, the National Surgical Adjuvant Breast and Bowel Project P-1 (NSABP P-1), has been reported in full.[23] These studies are summarized in Table 5. Besides breast cancer chemoprevention, these trials are investigating other possible benefits of tamoxifen suggested by previous clinical trials of adjuvant therapy, namely decreased cardiovascular morbidity and mortality, as well as prevention of osteoporosis in postmenopausal women.

The NSABP P-1 study, started in 1992, recruited 13 388 women who were at risk for breast cancer (i.e. were over 60 years old; were aged 35–59 with an increased risk for breast cancer (using the Gail algorithm) higher than 1.66 per cent in 5 years or had a history of lobular carcinoma *in situ*; Participants were randomized to tamoxifen

Table 4 Effect of per cent mammographic density on breast cancer risk in prospective studies

Author	n cases	n control	% density	Adjusted odds ratio	95% CI
Saflas 1991	67	58	45–65	3.8	2.1–3.6
	45	33	>65	4.3	2.1–8.8
Boyd	66	31	>75	6.1	2.8–13
Byrne	194	136	>75	4.4	3.1–6.1
	576	554	50–74	2.8	2.1–3.6
Kato	37	99 (pre)	>66	3.6	1.7–7.9
	48	81 (post)	>66	2.1	1.1–3.8

Table 5 Summary of breast cancer, endometrial cancer, and thromboembolic disease in randomized trials of tamoxifen and raloxifene

	Breast cancer prevention trial (BCPT)	Royal Marsden Hospital tamoxifen chemoprevention trial	Italian tamoxifen prevention trial
	n = 13 175	n = 2471	n = 5408
Subject characteristics	High breast cancer risk (age ≥ 60 or a combination of risk factors)	Family history of breast cancer; age 50 or in ≥ 2 relatives Median age 47 years	Women who have undergone hysterectomy (48% bilateral oophrectomy) Median age 51 years
Median follow-up	54.6 months	70 months	46 months
Breast cancer rate/1000 woman-years RR (95% confidence interval)	Invasive Placebo 6.8 Tamoxifen 3.4 RR = 0.51 (0.39 to 0.66)	All cases Placebo 5.0 Tamoxifen 4.7 RR = 1.1 (0.7 to 1.7)	All cases Placebo 2.3 Tamoxifen 2.1
Number and relative risk of ER + breast cancer	Placebo 130 Tamoxifen 41 RR = 0.31 (0.22 to 0.45)	Not available	Placebo 10 Tamoxifen 8
Number and relative risk of endometrial cancer	Placebo 15 Tamoxifen 36 RR = 2.53 (1.35 to 4.97)	Placebo 1 Tamoxifen 4	Not applicable
Number and rates of pulmonary emboli and venous thrombosis	Pulmonary emboli Placebo 6 Tamoxifen 18 RR = 3.0 (1.2 to 9.3) Venous thrombosis Placebo 22 Tamoxifen 35 RR = 1.60 (0.91 to 2.86)	DVT and PE Placebo 4 Tamoxifen 7	DVT and PE Placebo 4 Tamoxifen 7 Superficial phlebitis Placebo 9 Tamoxifen 33

or placebo. This trial gave such positive results that an interim analysis led to the early closure of the study.

It was shown that 20 mg/day of tamoxifen reduced the risk of invasive breast cancer by 49 per cent (two sided p<0.00001), with a cumulative incidence through 69 months of follow-up of 43.4/1000 in women in the placebo group and 22/1000 women in the treatment arm. The decreased risk occurred in women of all age groups: aged 49 years or younger (44 per cent); 50 to 59 years (51 per cent); and

60 years or older (55 per cent). Risk was also found to be reduced in women who had a history of lobular carcinoma *in situ* (56 per cent), or atypical hyperplasia (86 per cent), and those with any category of predicted 5-year risk. Tamoxifen reduced the risk of non-invasive breast cancer by 50 per cent (two sided p<0.002) and the occurrence of oestrogen-positive tumours by 69 per cent; it had no effect on oestrogen-negative tumours. Tamoxifen did not alter the rate of ischaemic heart disease, but did produce an overall 20 per cent

reduction in the incidence of osteoporitic bone fracture of the hip, radius (Colles'), and spine. Compared with the placebo group, however, women aged 50 or older receiving tamoxifen had a four-fold increased risk of early stage endometrial cancer, a three-fold increased risk of pulmonary embolism, and a significant excess of cataracts.[23] Notably, however, women aged 50 or younger had no increased incidence of adverse events. The decision to stop this trial was criticized by those who argued that the long-term effects of tamoxifen on the incidence of breast cancer and mortality will not be known. In other words, it will not be possible to distinguish delayed incidence (therapeutic effect on pre- or early malignant cells) from true disease eradication (prevention or reversal of initiation and promotion). This argument does not take into account: (1) the trial was not powered for mortality; (2) the informed consent included a statement on interim analyses and premature termination in case of striking differences; (3) the participants' safety is a greater priority than scientific advance.

Based on these findings, the Food and Drug Administration has approved the use of tamoxifen to reduce the risk of breast cancer in subjects at increased risk as assessed by the Gail model. This provides the first example of a medication approved and marketed as a cancer preventative agent, a concept which is likely to be expanded in clinical practice in the future.

The striking benefits of the NSABP P-1 trial do not seem to be confirmed by the European trials.[21],[22] The Italian study was a multicentre, double-blind, placebo-controlled chemoprevention trial, initiated in October 1992, to evaluate the effect of a daily dose of 20 mg oral tamoxifen for 5 years on the prevention of breast cancer in healthy women.[22] Eligible subjects were well women aged 35 to 70 years old who had prior hysterectomy for non-malignant conditions and the primary endpoint of this study is the incidence of breast cancer. Recruitment was stopped on December 31, 1997 with 5408 women randomized. Using the definition of drop out as the number of discontinuations other than major events, including women lost to follow-up, divided by the total number of women included in the analysis[24] the drop out rate for the Royal Marsden study was 35.5 per cent, for the NSABP P-1 study 28.8 per cent, and for the Italian study 20.7 per cent. In the Italian study, most women left for voluntary reasons other than side-effects (1.5 per 100 versus 0.5 per 100 who did leave because of side-effects). Moreover, several factors external to the study contributed to the high rate of withdrawal, including bad publicity in the media after the inclusion of tamoxifen in the list of class A carcinogens by the International Agency on Cancer Research (IARC) in 1996. Because this affected the rate of accrual, the Data Monitoring Committee advised that recruitment be stopped before the planned date. However, these data, rather than detracting from the findings, should underline the fact that maintaining compliance in the long-term is a formidable task even in an apparently highly motivated group and should be borne in mind when planning studies. Increasing public knowledge and appreciation of the value of chemoprevention trials can only help.

The preliminary results of the Italian study, after a median of 46 months, show no difference in the incidence of breast cancer between the two arms.[22] Of the 41 cases of breast cancer that have occurred so far, 22 cases were in the placebo group and 19 cases in the tamoxifen group. Among women on intervention from more than 1 year, there was a trend to a beneficial effect of tamoxifen (11 in the tamoxifen arm versus 19 in the placebo arm, p = 0.16). A border-line significant reduction of breast cancer was observed among women who were HRT users and received tamoxifen. Compared to the eight cases of breast cancer occurring among the 390 HRT users who were on placebo, there was one case of breast cancer among the 362 HRT users who were receiving tamoxifen (RR = 0.13, 95 per cent CI, 0.02–1.02). There was an increased risk of venous vascular events (38 women on tamoxifen versus 18 women on placebo, p = 0.0053), mainly consisting of superficial phlebitis, and 15 versus two cases of severe hypertriglyceridaemia in the tamoxifen and placebo arms, respectively (p = 0.0013).

As the combination of tamoxifen and transdermal HRT might reduce the risks and side-effects of either agent, their combined effect on several cardiovascular risk factors, including blood cholesterol levels, was tested within the trial.[25] Compared to small changes in the placebo group, tamoxifen was associated with changes in total, low density lipoprotein (LDL) and high density lipoprotein (HDL) cholesterol of –9 per cent, –14 per cent, and –0.8 per cent, respectively, which were similar in continuous HRT users and never HRT users. By contrast, the decrease induced by tamoxifen of total and LDL cholesterol was blunted by two-thirds in women who started HRT while on tamoxifen. Thus, the beneficial effects of tamoxifen on cardiovascular risk factors are unchanged in current HRT users, while they might be attenuated in women who start transdermal HRT while on tamoxifen. While tamoxifen can reduce the risk of breast cancer associated with HRT use, HRT could, on the other hand, reduce the tamoxifen's adverse events (i.e. vasomotor and urogenital symptoms and, possibly, endometrial cancer). These findings provide the background for future investigations of the combination of tamoxifen and HRT in order to reduce the risks while retaining the benefit of both agents.

An interim analysis of the United Kingdom pilot prevention trial has also been published.[21] In this study, 2494 healthy women, aged between 30 and 70, at increased risk of breast cancer because of family history were accrued between 1986 and 1996. They were randomized in a double-blind fashion to receive tamoxifen 20 mg/day of placebo for up to 8 years. The primary endpoint was the occurrence of breast cancer. After a median follow-up of 70 months, the results demonstrate the same overall frequency of breast cancer in both arms (tamoxifen 34, placebo 36, RR 1.06 (95 per cent CI 0.7–1.7), p = 0.8). Interestingly, women who were already on HRT (mostly by oral route) when they entered the trial showed an increased risk of breast cancer compared with non-users, while the subjects who started HRT while on trial had a significantly reduced risk.

Comparison of the preliminary results among the three studies[21]–[23] might seem to suggest that the efficacy of tamoxifen varies depending upon the type of population and the nature of the risk, for while the NSABP P-1 trial recruited women with a combination of genetic and reproductive risk factors for developing breast cancer, the United Kingdom study concentrated on those with a family history of breast cancer, and the Italian study enrolled women who had undergone a hysterectomy who would presumably be at a lower risk. Given the complexity of the issue, however, further results are clearly demanded.

In general, tamoxifen is well tolerated. Hot flushes and other vaginal symptoms are the most commonly reported side-effects; approximately 15 to 20 per cent more women receiving tamoxifen develop hot flushes attributable to the drug, compared with placebo. These symptoms appear more commonly among younger women despite the elevated levels of oestradiol and total oestrogens reported among premenopausal patients receiving tamoxifen.[26] The other, most frequently reported side-effects (15–20 per cent) are vaginal discharge and dryness, urinary disturbances secondary to urogenital atrophy, nausea, gastrointestinal disturbances, rapid pulse, and weight gain. Menstrual irregularities have also been observed. Antithrombin III activity is decreased in postmenopausal patients, and this may, in part, account for the increased risk of venous thromboembolic events that has been reported in two prevention trials.[22],[23] Thus, tamoxifen was reported to increase the incidence of deep vein thrombosis (DVT) and pulmonary emboli (PE) in all three trials (Table 5), but it must be remembered that these side-effects are common to all types of hormonal manipulations (including HRT, the pill, and other selective oestrogen receptor modulators (SERMs)). Ocular effects (retinal deposits, keratinopathy, cataract) have occurred at high doses; however, some recent reports suggest a lower incidence of such disorders at the chemopreventive trial dose of 20 mg/day.[27] As regards the increased risk of endometrial cancer associated with tamoxifen administration, the NSABP P-1 trial[23] has shown a four-fold increased risk of early-stage endometrial cancer in postmenopausal women in the tamoxifen group compared to the placebo group (36 versus 15, respectively). However, all cases except one in the placebo group were at an initial stage (FIGO stage I) and no death from endometrial cancer has been reported in the tamoxifen arm.

These considerations led to a study of the biological activity of tamoxifen with a view to establishing a dosing schedule with a better risk:benefit ratio.[28] The results indicated that a dose of 10 mg on alternate days, that is a 75 per cent reduction in the conventional dose of tamoxifen, does not affect the activity of the drug on a large number of biomarkers, including several surrogate markers of cardiovascular disease and circulating IGF-1, a likely surrogate marker for breast cancer. Future trials are thus warranted to assess the efficacy and the safety of tamoxifen at low doses. Finally, comparison of low-dose tamoxifen with novel selective oestrogen receptor modulators with potentially improved safety profiles could provide important clues for the choice of safe and effective preventive approaches for a wide range of oestrogen-related diseases.

Raloxifene

Raloxifene is another SERM that binds with high affinity and has agonist actions on oestrogen receptors in bone and those affecting lipid production, but has antagonists actions on receptors in breast and uterus. It has been demonstrated to maintain bone density and is used as an osteoporosis preventive agent and to lower LDL cholesterol in postmenopausal women without affecting the cholesterol.[29] It is potentially less hazardous than tamoxifen, since it has not been shown to induce endometrial cancer. However, it does produce blood clots, and its long-term efficacy and safety profile is unknown.

Raloxifene is currently undergoing investigation as a chemopreventive agent in breast cancer. A recent report of interim findings from the osteoporosis trials[30] showed that the incidence of newly diagnosed breast cancer was 1.7 per 1000 patient years for subjects receiving raloxifene, compared with 3.7 per 1000 patient years for those on placebo, giving a relative risk of 0.46 (CI = 0.28–0.75), corresponding to a 54 per cent reduction in incidence. Raloxifene had a marked effect on oestrogen-receptor-positive tumours, reducing their incidence by 70 per cent (RR 0.30; CI 0.24–0.64) with no effect on the incidence of oestrogen-receptors-negative tumours. The final

analysis of these data is awaited with interest. Raloxifine will be evaluated in comparison with tamoxifen in a large primary prevention trial in at-risk subjects in the United States. Other SERMs are also entering the field of clinical cancer prevention and a significant array of agents is likely to be tested in the next few years.

The synthetic retinoid fenretinide (N-(4-hydroxyphenyl) retinamide or 4-HPR)

Natural retinoids play a crucial role in cellular proliferation and differentiation, but their poor clinical tolerability has prevented the use of these compounds as cancer preventive agents. Toxic symptoms which may be acceptable in treating established cancer are not considered acceptable for reducing cancer risk. One of the less toxic vitamin A analogues studied for breast cancer chemoprevention is 4-HPR, a synthetic amide derivative of all-*trans* retinoic acid.[31] The inhibition of chemically-induced mammary carcinoma in rats by 4-HPR was first described in 1979.[32] On this basis, 4-HPR was proposed for chemoprevention trials in human breast cancer. This compound has been studied extensively and proved to be less toxic than many other retinoids.[31]

In contrast to retinoic acid, fenretinide selectively induces apoptosis rather than differentiation in several tumour cell systems and maintains a stable plasma concentration during prolonged administration. While its mechanism of action still remains unclear, recent studies indicate that fenretinide may be a selective retinoid receptor modulator which retains the inhibitory activity of retinoic acid on proliferative signals with an improved therapeutic index, an important limiting factor for other retinoids.[32] This selective binding to the nuclear receptors is likely to be the basis for its specific biological activities and its favourable pharmaceutical properties. Moreover, 4-HPR appears to be a potent inhibitor of the IGF system in breast cancer cell lines and this is an important mechanism of tumour cell growth inhibition by the retinoid.[33]

In recent years, 4-HPR has been shown to be active *in vitro* and *in vivo* against mammary, bladder, lung, ovary, cervix, neuroblastoma, leukaemia, and prostate preclinical models.[34] A characteristic feature of 4-HPR is the ability to inhibit cell growth through the induction of apoptosis rather than differentiation, an effect which is strikingly different from the parent compound all-*trans* retinoic acid and which may occur even in retinoic-acid-resistant cell lines. On the basis of the selective accumulation of 4-HPR in the human breast[32] and good tolerance in humans,[31] a phase III trial was started in 1987 aimed at reducing contralateral breast cancer. Briefly, 2972 women with a history of stage I breast cancer were randomized to 4-HPR 200 mg/day or no intervention for 5 years. The primary endpoint of the study was the occurrence of contralateral breast cancer as the first malignant event. The eligible women were diagnosed with stage I invasive breast cancer or DCIS within the previous 10 years and had undergone definitive surgery without adjuvant hormone or chemotherapy.

An interim analysis has shown that the number of cases of contralateral breast cancer was comparable in the two arms.[35] However, there was a beneficial trend in premenopausal women and a reversed trend in postmenopausal women. A test for interaction showed that the effect of 4-HPR is significantly modified by menopausal status. 4-HPR also reduced local recurrence in premenopausal women but not in postmenopausal women. The final results of this trial will be published shortly. Interestingly, modulation of plasma

IGF-1 levels by 4-HPR followed a similar pattern, that is IGF-1 levels were lowered in premenopausal women only.[12],[13]

The combination of tamoxifen and fenretinide

The concept of combining multiple agents with different activities to enhance activity and minimize toxicity has been pursued for quite some time in cancer chemoprevention research.[36] For instance, synergistic efficacy has been observed in animal studies of tamoxifen in combination with 4-HPR at lower, less toxic, doses.[37] A phase I trial of 20 mg/day tamoxifen in combination with increased doses of 4-HPR has recently been performed.[38] In a recent pilot study in at-risk women, the combination of tamoxifen 20 mg/day and 4-HPR 200 mg/day was also well tolerated.[39] Based on the encouraging results of previous clinical trials of tamoxifen and 4 HPR in premenopausal women,[23],[35] a trial of a combination of low-dose tamoxifen and fenretinide in premenopausal women at increased risk for breast cancer is currently underway.

Colorectal cancer

Activity of non-steroidal anti-inflammatory drugs in colon cancer prevention

Several recent studies have reported a 40 to 50 per cent decrease in the relative risk of colorectal cancer in persons who are continuous users of aspirin or other non-steroidal anti-inflammatory drugs (NSAIDs),[40] suggesting that these drugs may serve as effective cancer chemopreventive agents. However, prolonged use of NSAIDs results in untoward gastrointestinal side-effects that are probably due to inhibition of the production of gastric prostaglandins that play a crucial role in maintaining gastric mucosal integrity.

The azoxymethane-treated rat and Min/APC mice are used as complementary animal models of colorectal carcinogenesis. Several NSAIDs—piroxicam, sulindac, aspirin, ibuprofen, and others—have clear efficacy in these models resulting in 30 to 80 per cent reductions in the multiplicity and incidence of adenomas and cancer.[41] Though the protective effect appears class-related, there are reproducible differences in efficacy within the class. Whether these differences are relevant to humans is unknown. At a macroscopic level, NSAIDs prevent incident neoplasia (adenomas and carcinomas), cause adenomas to regress, and suppress the growth of carcinomas. Therefore, NSAIDs are effective when given 'early' (preceding adenoma formation), as well as 'late' (following the emergence of adenomas). On a cellular level, NSAIDs appear to increase the apoptotic index relative to proliferation of neoplastic cells, although molecular mechanisms responsible for this effect remain poorly defined.

More than 15 observational studies, using case-control, nested case-control, and prospective designs, have investigated the relationship between aspirin/NSAIDs and colorectal neoplasia. All but one suggest that NSAIDs are effective in lowering the incidence of human colorectal adenoma, reducing carcinoma incidence, and/or cancer-associated mortality, regardless of age, gender, country of residence, affected colorectal segment, or other underlying risk factors (e.g. diet, history of prior adenomas, socio-economic status). Potential confounding influences on aspirin's preventive efficacy have also been evaluated, such as a delay in cancer diagnosis by pain suppression and/or early detection by aspirin-induced gastrointestinal bleeding. These factors are considered extremely unlikely to account for the protective association. The preventive effects of aspirin may require extended periods of exposure; some investigations reported efficacy only with aspirin use of more than 10 years duration.

Since 1983, several non-randomized case-series and three small, randomized trials have reported the experiences of subjects with familial adenomatous polyposis (n = 150) treated with sulindac or indomethacin.[42] From these reports, it is clear that NSAIDs induce the regression of prevalent adenomas in this cohort, though complete regression of all adenomas is unlikely. The effect takes several months of exposure and requires continued administration. Three case reports of cancer occurring in familial adenomatous polyposis subjects taking sulindac suggest that a more effective chemopreventive agent, or combination of agents, may be necessary for optimal chemoprevention in this condition.

Despite this impressive body of evidence, NSAIDs are not prescribed for colorectal cancer prevention because of several key deficits in knowledge. We do not know which specific agent(s) is most effective and, more importantly, what dose or duration of treatment should be prescribed for this indication. In addition, traditional NSAIDs are associated with several well-known risks, including gastric irritation/ulceration, renal dysfunction, antiaggregatory effects in platelets, and liver dysfunction. Balancing the risks versus benefits of NSAIDs is a challenge in the preventive setting. Insights into the action of NSAIDs on their target enzyme, cyclo-oxygenase (COX) may hold clues to solving this dilemma.

Role of COX-2 and prostanoids in colon carcinogenesis

Cyclo-oxygenase catalyses the oxygenation of arachidonic acid to prostaglandin (PG) H_2 as the first step in the synthesis of prostaglandins, prostacyclins, and thromboxanes in mammalian cells. Two forms of the COX enzyme have been demonstrated. COX-1 is the major enzyme form found in healthy tissues; it is constitutively expressed and plays a role in thrombogenesis and in the homeostasis of the gastrointestinal tract and kidneys. COX-2 is a distinct isoform of COX-1 encoded by a different gene. It is inducible and up-regulated in states of pathology including inflammation and neoplasia, and has been associated with the elevated production of prostaglandins observed during inflammation, pain, and pyretic responses. The COX-2 gene belongs to a class of genes referred to as immediate early or early growth response genes which are expressed rapidly and transiently after stimulation of cultured cells by growth factors, cytokines, and tumour promoters; COX-2 expression is thus elevated in inflammatory cells and sites of inflammation. Most NSAIDs in current use inhibit both COX-1 and COX-2.

Previously, an increased COX-2 expression has been demonstrated in human colorectal adenocarcinomas when compared with normal, adjacent colonic mucosa;[43] these findings have been confirmed by the finding of elevated levels of COX-2 protein in colorectal tumours by western blotting and immunohistochemical staining. Markedly elevated levels of COX-2 mRNA and protein have also been observed in colonic tumours that develop in rodents after carcinogen treatment and in adenomas taken from Min mice. The observations of elevated COX-2 expression in three different models of colorectal carcinogenesis have led to the hypothesis that COX-2 expression may be related to colorectal tumorigenesis in a causal way. A recent report has demonstrated a 40 per cent reduction in aberrant crypt formation in carcinogen-treated rats given a selective COX-2 inhibitor.[44] Another study has provided genetic evidence which directly links

COX-2 expression to intestinal tumorigenesis. This recent report[45] demonstrated that *APC* mice develop hundreds of tumours per intestine. When these mice were bred with *COX-2* null mice there was an 80 to 90 per cent reduction in tumour multiplicity in the homozygous *COX-2* null offspring. Additionally, when the *APC* mice were treated with a highly selected COX-2 inhibitor, there was a marked reduction in tumour multiplicity. These results suggest that COX-2 may act as a tumour promoter in the intestine and that increased levels of COX-2 expression may result directly from disruption of the *APC* gene.

A further piece of compelling evidence for a role of COX-2 and prostanoids in colorectal cancer carcinogenesis, comes from a study of Yang *et al.*[46] This study compared the levels of five major stable metabolic products of the cyclo-oxygenase pathway in the normal-appearing mucosa and in adenomas of patients with familial adenomatosis polyposis to determine whether prostanoids are involved in the pathogenesis of colorectal adenomas. Of 12 patients tested, six had elevated levels of at least one prostanoid in the adenomas. More importantly, the relative levels of three prostanoids (prostaglandin (PG)D2, PGE2, and 6-keto-PGF1α) were elevated in adenomas compared to normal-appearing mucosa from the same patients, and the resulting ratios were correlated with the size of the adenoma. This elevation, however, was not observed until an adenoma reached an approximate size of 6 to 7 mm in diameter.

These observations support the hypothesis that increased *COX-2* expression, with the resultant elevation of prostanoid levels in adenomas, provides a potential mechanism for tumour promotion. If this is the case, selective inhibition of COX-2 could be chemopreventive. Several selective COX-2 inhibitors have recently been developed which are under evaluation both as alternatives to conventional NSAIDs in inflammatory conditions and as chemopreventive agents, these include celecoxib, nimesulide, and others.

Calcium as a chemopreventive agent in colorectal cancer

The fact that diet can influence the risk of colorectal cancer has been known for some time. There is a protective effect of fresh fruits and vegetables, while animal fats and red meat seem to increase risk.[47] It has been hypothesized that the carcinogenic activity of fat and meat derives from their stimulation of the production of bile acids, which are known carcinogens in animals. Calcium can bind bile acids and dietary calcium has been shown to be protective against bile-induced mucosal damage in experimental models. To assess these observations in humans a randomized, double-blind trial of the effect of dietary supplementation with calcium carbonate was undertaken in 930 subjects with a recent history of colorectal adenomas.[48] Follow-up endoscopies were conducted 1 and 4 years after the qualifying examination and the primary endpoint was the proportion of subjects in whom at least one adenoma was detected. The calcium carbonate group had a lower risk of recurrent adenoma. The adjusted risk ratio for any recurrence of adenoma with calcium as compared with placebo was 0.85 (95 per cent CI 0.74–0.98; $p = 0.03$). At least one adenoma was diagnosed in 127 (31 per cent) subjects in the calcium group and 159 (38 per cent) of subjects in the placebo group. The adjusted risk ratio was 0.81 (95 per cent CI 0.67–0.99). Thus these results show a significant, albeit modest, influence of calcium in reducing the risk of recurrent adenomas.

Lung cancer

Two major trials have been directed at the prevention of lung cancer by the chemopreventative agent β-carotene in well-nourished individuals: the Alpa-Tocopherol, Beta-Carotene (ATBC) Cancer Prevention Study[1] and the Beta-Carotene and Retinol Efficacy Trial (CARET).[49]

Previous epidemiological evidence had suggested that higher intake of vitamin E (alpha-tocopherol) and β-carotene (a precursor of vitamin A) was linked to a lower incidence of cancer, especially lung cancer, and cardiovascular disease. Basic research suggested plausible mechanisms by which this could occur, providing the impetus for randomized chemoprevention trials. The ATBC Study assigned 29 000 male Finnish smokers (aged 50–69 years) to receive β-carotene (20 mg/day), vitamin E (50 mg/day), a combination of both, or placebo, for an average of 6 years. The CARET study enrolled 18 000 men and women at high risk of lung cancer because of a history of cigarette smoking or occupational exposure to asbestos, and gave β-carotene (30 mg/day) in combination with retinol (25 000 IU/day) for an average of less than 4 years.

Both studies showed that β-carotene increased the risk of developing lung cancer in groups exposed to smoking or asbestos. Although the mechanism of this effect was not clear, it has been suggested that it is related to the reported pro-oxidant effect of β-carotene under high oxygen pressures and oxidative stress that occurs in the lungs of smokers.[50]

The detrimental effect of β-carotene appeared stronger (but not substantially different) in patients who smoked at least 20 cigarettes a day compared with a subset of moderate-intensity smokers (5–19 cigarettes per day) and was exacerbated by alcohol intake in the ATBC trial. No increase in the incidence of cancer due to β-carotene was seen in the subset of former smokers in the CARET study. There was also no evidence that β-carotene increases lung cancer risk in never or former smokers.

A further study has investigated the effects of β-carotene in a mixed population. The Physicians Health Study in the United States[51] randomized 22 071 male physicians to β-carotene (50 mg) or placebo on alternate days for an average of 12 years. Eleven per cent of the subjects were smokers and 39 per cent were former smokers, thus 50 per cent of the subjects had never smoked. In this broad population, supplementation with β-carotene produced neither benefit nor harm in terms of the incidence of cancer, cardiovascular disease, or death from all causes. Subset analyses of current or former smokers showed no significant differences in any of these endpoints. A reason for the differences between the findings of this trial and the two other major trials is not apparent, but this trial only included 2427 smokers half of whom would be randomized to placebo, so the lower subject numbers may have some bearing on the findings.

The above study also carried out concomitantly a secondary investigation of aspirin as a preventive agent on cardiovascular disease and cancer. The effects on heart disease were so striking that the aspirin intervention was terminated early. However, it was also noted that aspirin failed to affect the incidence of colorectal cancer—a result at variance with epidemiological studies showing a protective effect of aspirin on colorectal cancer.

These studies highlight the fact that intuitive extrapolation of epidemiological data into chemoprevention trials is not always successful. However, this may be because such observational studies are difficult to interpret, for although the association between β-carotene and a lower incidence of cancer may be present, how can it be shown whether the results were due to a high intake of β-carotene itself, other nutrients present in β-carotene-rich foods, other dietary habits, or other non-dietary aspects of lifestyle that accompany high intake of β-carotene? Moreover, the negative chemoprevention studies do not entirely contradict the epidemiological data. It was noted in both the ATBC and CARET trials that higher baseline plasma β-carotene levels were associated with lower rates of lung cancer. The consumption of foods rich in β-carotene (giving rise to these high plasma levels) could be regarded as markers of consumption of a protective diet rich in fruits and vegetables. The problem still remains of identifying these protective factors.

Skin cancer

Two well-designed chemoprevention trials have evaluated the preventative effects of selenium or retinol on skin cancer.[2],[52]

The study of selenium[2] gave definite negative results for the prevention of squamous cell carcinoma or basal cell carcinoma in 1312 patients with a history of non-melanoma skin cancer and living in regions of the United States where intake of selenium was naturally low. However, this study did show statistically significant effects of selenium in preventing prostate, lung, and colon cancers. The incidence of cancers were: prostate (selenium, n = 3; placebo, n = 13), lung cancer (selenium, n = 17; placebo, n = 31), colorectal cancer (selenium, n = 8; placebo, n = 19). Also the trial produced a statistically non-significant reduction in total mortality and a statistically significant reduction in total cancer mortality. These findings warrant further study of selenium as a chemopreventive agent.

A similar study assessed the value of oral retinol (25 000 IU) or placebo daily for 5 years in individuals who had a history of more than 10 actinic keratoses and at most two squamous cell or basal cell carcinomas.[52] A total of 2297 subjects were enrolled and followed for a median period of 3.8 years. The study showed that retinol was effective in preventing squamous cell carcinoma but not basal cell carcinoma.

All cancers

A study of nearly 30 000 subjects was carried out in Linxian, China.[53] Using a complex factorial design this study tested four main combined agent interventions of vitamins and minerals (retinol and zinc, riboflavin and niacin, vitamin C and molybdenum and β-carotene, vitamin E and selenium) over a 5-year period in this population who have a persistently low intake of several micronutrients. No statistically significant effect on cancer incidence was achieved by any intervention. Important secondary analyses, however, showed that the combination of selenium, β-carotene, and alpha-tocopherol was associated with a statistically significant lower total mortality rate (RR = 0.91; 95 per cent CI = 0.84–0.99), a 13 per cent reduction (borderline significant) in all cancer mortality rate (RR = 0.87; 95 per cent CI = 0.75–1.00) and a statistically significant lower mortality rate from stomach cancer (a major cancer in Linxian) (RR = 0.79; 95 per cent CI = 0.64–0.99). Although not definitive, these data do suggest that the combination of β-carotene, vitamin E, and selenium may affect the incidence of cancers, especially gastric cancer. It must be remembered though that this population had an initial poor intake of vitamins and minerals. It is possible that the lack of these nutrients confers a risk of developing

cancer that can be overcome by increasing the dietary intake. But that is not the same as saying that an additional intake of these vitamins and minerals by already well-nourished individuals will confer any active protection.

Retinoids

In addition to 4-HPR, several small studies have provided evidence that other retinoids have a protective function in several different types of cancer, especially in the prevention of second primary tumours. Since retinoids are effective in treating premalignant oral lesions, isotretinoin (13-cis-retinoic acid) (50–100 mg/m²) was investigated in comparison with placebo in 103 patients who were disease-free after treatment for squamous cell cancers of the pharynx, larynx or oral cavity.[54] While tumour recurrence was unaffected, the appearance of second primary tumours was significantly reduced in the isotrentinoin group (4 per cent versus 24 per cent; p = 0.005).

Another retinoid, polyprenoic acid, has been demonstrated to be effective in the prevention of second primary hepatomas.[55] In a study of 89 patients who were disease-free after resection of a primary hepatoma or percutaneous injection of ethanol, and who were randomly assigned to polyprenoic acid (600 mg/day) or placebo, the incidence of recurrent or new hepatomas was 27 per cent in the polyprenoic acid group compared with 49 per cent in the placebo group (p = 0.04) after a median follow-up of 38 months. A recent update of the trial has shown a significant advantage on mortality rate in the retinoid arm.

Retinol palmitate (30 000 IU/day for 12 months) was evaluated in comparison with no treatment in 307 patients with Stage I non-small cell lung cancer who had undergone curative surgery.[56] After a median follow-up of 46 months, recurrence of new primary tumours occurred in 37 per cent of the retinol palmitate group and 48 per cent of the controls. Second primary tumours occurred in 18 of the treated group and 29 patients in the control group developed 33 second primaries (p = 0.045).

Acitretin has been shown to reduce the incidence of squamous cell carcinoma in renal transplant patients.[57] Forty four patients with >10 keratotic skin lesions were randomized to placebo or acitretin (30 mg/day) for 6 months. In this period, 11 per cent of the active treatment group and 47 per cent of the placebos developed new squamous cell carcinomas (p = 0.01).

Topically applied all-trans-retinoic acid has also been shown to increase histological regression rate in women with moderate cervical intraepithelial hyperplasia (CIN II) from 27 per cent in the placebo group to 47 per cent in the retinoic acid group (p = 0.041).[58]

Collectively these studies provide evidence that retinoids may have a role in chemoprevention that warrants further investigation.

Negative studies

Twelve well-conducted trials have also provided useful definitive negative results (reviewed in Lippman et al.[59]). These have included: retinol and 13-cis-retinoic acid in squamous cell carcinoma and basal cell carcinoma of the skin; trials of riboflavin, retinol, and zinc in oesophageal dysplasia; trials of 13-cis-retinoic acid, etretinate, and β-carotene plus retinol in bronchial metaplasia; β-carotene in the prevention of large bowel adenoma; and the effect of β-carotene or folic acid in cervical dysplasia.

Future studies

It seems to be a common occurrence that chemoprevention trials that set out to investigate the specific interaction of a putative chemopreventive agent with a particular cancer provide equally useful data concerning other cancer types. Thus, the study evaluating the effect of selenium on the incidence of skin cancer[2] showed positive effects on prostate cancers. Similarly, the ATBC study of lung cancer[7],[60] showed a protective role for vitamin E on the incidence and mortality of prostate cancer; 99 cases of prostate cancer occurred in the group receiving 50 mg of vitamin E daily while 147 cases were seen in the control arm. The role of these two agents in protecting against prostate cancer is not clear but may be linked to their antioxidant role, their inhibition of cell proliferation, or promotion of apoptosis. A large phase III trial testing their combination is being planned.[61] These studies should provide the impetus to get to the 'final chapter in the story' of selenium, vitamin E, and prostate cancer.

Two ongoing, large-scale studies are investigating the prevention of second primary tumours of the head and neck and stage-I non-small cell lung cancer. Both studies are investigating the action of 13-cis-retinoic acid.[59]

Additionally, an international trial, Euroscan, is evaluating the effect of retinyl palmitate and n-acetyl cysteine in more than 2500 patients with early-stage cancer of the head and neck or early-stage non-small cell lung cancer.[62] The ongoing Prostate Cancer Prevention Trial is investigating the effect of finasteride, a testosterone analogue that competitively inhibits 5α-reductase, on the incidence of prostate cancer.[61]

The challenges of conducting well-designed and unequivocal trials in cancer chemoprevention are in some ways greater than the problems of assessing a new treatment for established disease. Disease prevention rather than palliation is an ambitions goal. However, this promising area of oncology is rapidly expanding and should provide some rewarding results in terms of reduction in cancer risk and mechanistic insights into the process of carcinogenesis.

References

1. **The α-Tocopherol, β-Carotene Cancer Prevention Study Group.** The effect of vitamin E and beta carotene on the incidence of lung cancer and other cancers in male smokers. *New England Journal of Medicine*, 1994; **330**: 1029–35.

2. **Clark LC, et al.** Effects of selenium supplementation for cancer prevention in patients with carcinoma of the skin. *Journal of the American Medical Association*, 1996; **276**:1957–63.

3. **De Palo G, et al.** Can ferentinide protect women against ovarian cancer? [letter]. *Journal of the National Cancer Institute*, 1995; **87**: 146–7.

4. **Baserga R.** The insulin-like growth factors I receptor: a key to tumor growth? *Cancer Research*, 1995; **55**: 249–52.

5. **Hankinson SE, et al.** Circulating concentrations of insulin-like growth factor-I and risk of breast cancer. *Lancet* 1998; **351**: 1393–6.

6. **Chan JM, et al.** Plasma insulin-like growth factor-I and prostate cancer risk: a prospective study. *Science*, 1998; **279**: 563–6.

7. **Yu H, Spitz MR, Mistry J, Gu J, Hong WK, Wu X.** Plasma levels of insulin-like growth factor I and lung cancer risk: a case-control analysis. *Journal of the National Cancer Institute*, 1999; **91**: 151–6.

8. **Ma J, et al.** Prospective study of colorectal cancer risk in men and

plasma levels of insulin-like growth factor (IGF)-I and IGF-binding protein-3. *Journal of the National Cancer Institute*, 1999; **91**: 620–5.

9. **Giovannucci E, et al.** Plasma insulin-like growth factor-I and binding protein-3 and risk of colorectal cancer and adenoma in women. *Proceedings of American Association for Cancer Research*, 1999; **40**: 211.

10. **Burroughs KD, Dunn SE, Barrett JC, Taylor JA.** Insulin-like growth factor-I: a key regulator of human cancer risk? *Journal of the National Cancer Institute*, 1999; **91**: 579–81.

11. **Kato S, et al.** Activation of the estrogen receptor through phosphorilation by mitogen protein kinase. *Science*, 1995; **270**: 1491–4.

12. **Torrisi R, et al.** The synthetic retinoid fenretinide lowers plasma 1GF-I levels in breast cancer patients. *Cancer Research*, 1993; **53**: 4769–71.

13. **Torrisi R, et al.** Effect of fenretinide on plasma IGF-1 and IGFBP-3 in early breast cancer patients. *International Journal of Cancer*, 1998; **76**: 787–90.

14. **Pollak M, et al.** Effect of tamoxifen on serum insulin-like growth factor I levels in stage I breast cancer patients. *Journal of the National Cancer Institute*, 1990; **82**: 1693–7.

15. **Saftlas AS, Hooover RN, Brimton LA, et al.** Mammographic densities and risk of breast cancer. *Cancer*, 1991; **67**: 2833–8.

16. **Boyd NF, et al.** Quantitative classification of mammographic densities and breast cancer risk: results from the Canadian National Breast Screening Study. *Journal of the National Cancer Institute*, 1995; **87**: 670–5.

17. **Byrne C, et al.** Mammographic features and breast cancer risk: effects with time, age, and menopause status. *Journal of the National Cancer Institute*, 1995; **87**: 1622–9.

18. **Kato I, Beinart C, Bleich A, Su S, Kim M, Toniolo PG.** A nested case-control study of mammographic patterns, breast volume, and breast cancer (New York City, NY, United States). *Cancer Causes and Control*, 1995; **6**: 431–8.

19. **Ursin G, Pike MC, Spicer DV, Porrath SA, Reitherman RW.** Can mammographic densities predict effects of tamoxifen on the breast? *Journal of the National Cancer Institute*, 1996; **88**: 128–9.

20. **Boyd NF, et al.** Effects at two years of a low-fat, high-carbohydrate diet on radiological features of the breast: results from a randomized trial. *Journal of the National Cancer Institute*, 1997; **89**: 488–96.

21. **Boyd NF, et al.** Mammographic densities as a criterion for entry to a clinical trial of breast cancer prevention. *British Journal of Cancer*, 1995; **72**: 476–9.

22. **Powles T, et al.** Interim analysis of the incidence of breast cancer in the Royal Marsden Hospital tamoxifen randomized chemoprevention trial. *Lancet*, 1998; **352**: 98–101.

23. **Veronesi U, et al.** Prevention of breast cancer with tamoxifen: preliminary findings from the Italian randomized trial among hysterectomized women. *Lancet*, 1998; **352**: 93–7.

24. **Fisher B, et al.** Tamoxifen for prevention of breast cancer: report of the National Surgical Ajuvant Breast and Bowel Project P-1 study. *Journal National Cancer Institute*, 1998; **90**: 1371–88.

25. **Veronesi U, Maisonneuve P, Costa A, Rotmensz N, Boyle P.** Drop-outs in tamoxifen prevention trials.[letter] *Lancet*, 1999; **353**: 244.

26. **Decensi A, et al.** Effect of tamoxifen and transdermal hormone replacement therapy on cardiovascular risk factors in a prevention trial. *British Journal of Cancer*, 1998; **78**: 572–8.

27. **Jordan VC, Fritz NF, Langan-Fahey S, Thompson M, Thomey DC.** Alteration of endocrine parameters in premenopausal women with breast cancer during long-term adjuvant therapy with tamoxifen as the single agent. *Journal of the National Cancer Institute*, 1991; **83**: 1488–91.

28. **Gorin MB, et al.** Long-term tamoxifen citrate use and potential ocular toxicity. *American Journal of Ophthalmology*, 1998; **125**: 493–501.

29. **Decensi A, et al.** Biological effects of tamoxifen at low doses in healthy women. *Journal of the National Cancer Institute*, 1998; **90**: 1461–7.

30. **Delmas PD**, *et al.* Effects of raloxifene on bone mineral density, serum cholesterol concentrations, and uterine endometrium in postmenopausal women. *New England Journal of Medicine*, 1997; **337**: 1641–7.

31. **Jordan VC**, *et al.* Raloxifene reduces incident primary breast cancers: integrated data from multicentre, double-blind, placebo-controlled, randomized trials in postmeopausal women. *Breast Cancer Research and Treatment*, 1998; **50**: 227.

32. **Costa A, Formelli F, Chiesa F, Decensi A, De Palo G, Veronesi U.** Prospects of chemoprevention of human cancers with the synthetic retinoid fenretinide. *Cancer Research* 1994; **54** (Suppl.): 2032–7.

33. **Fanjul A**, *et al.* A new class of retinoids with selective inhibition of AP-1 inhibits proliferation. *Nature*, 1994; **372**: 107–11.

34. **Moon RC, Thompson HJ, Becci PJ**, *et al.* N-(4-hydroxyphenyl)retinamide, a new retinoid for prevention of breast cancer in the rat. *Cancer Research*, 1979; **39**: 1339–46.

35. **Favoni RE**, *et al.*: Modulation of the insulin-like growth factor-I system by N-(4-hydroxyphenyl)retinamide in human breast cancer cell lines. *British Journal of Cancer*, 1998; **77**: 2138–47.

36. **Lotan R.** Retinoids and apoptosis: implications for cancer chemoprevention and therapy. *Journal of the National Cancer Institute*, 1995; **87**: 1655–7.

37. **De Palo G**, *et al.* A randomized trial of Fenretinide for the prevention of contralateral breast cancer. *Proceedings of the American Association for Cancer Research*, 1999; **40**: 304.

38. **Sporn MB.** Combination chemoprevention of cancer. *Nature*, 1980; **287**: 107–8.

39. **Ratko TA, Dentrisac CJ, Dinger NM, Thomas CF, Kelloff GJ, Moon RC.** Chemoprevention efficacy of combined retinoid and tamoxifen treatment following surgical excision of a primary mammary cancer in female rats. *Cancer Research*, 1989; **49**: 4472–6.

40. **Cobleigh MA**, *et al.* Phase I/II trial of tamoxifen with or without fenretinide, an analog of vitamin A, in women with metastatic breast cancer. *Journal of Clinical Oncology*, 1993; **11**: 474–7.

41. **Zujewski J**, *et al.* Pilot trial of tamoxifen (tam) and fenretinide (4-HPR) in women at high risk of developing invasive breast cancer. *Proceedings of the American Association for Cancer Research*, 1997; **38**: abs 1763.

42. **Smalley WE, DuBois RN.** Colorectal cancer and nonsteroidal anti-inflammatory drugs. *Advances in Pharmacology*, 1997; **39**: 1–20.

43. **Rao CV**, *et al.* Chemoprevention of colon carcinogenesis by sulindac, a non-steroidal anti-inflammtory agent. *Cancer Research*, 1995; **55**: 1464–72.

44. **Waddel WR, Gasner GF, Cerise EJ, Loughry RW.** Sulindac for polyposis of the colon. *American Journal of Surgery*, 1989; **157**: 175–8.

45. **Eberhart CE, Coffey RJ, Radhika A, Giardello FM, Ferrenbach S, DuBois RN.** Up-regulation of cyclooxygenase 2 gene expression in human colorectal adenomas and adenocarcinomas. *Gastroenterology*, 1994; **107**: 1183–8.

46. **Reddy BS, Rao CV, Seibert K.** Evaluation of cyclooxygenase-2 inhibitor for potential chemopreventive properties in colon carcinogenesis. *Cancer Research*, 1996; **56**: 4566–9.

47. **Oshima M**, *et al.* Suppression of intestinal polyposis in Apc delta716 Knockout mice by inhibition of cyclooxygenase 2. *Cell*, 1996; **87**: 803–9.

48. **Yang VW**, *et al.* Size-dependent increase in prostanoid levels in adenomas of patients with familial adenomatous polyposis. *Cancer Research*, 1998; **58**: 1750–3.

49. **Sandler RS.** Epidemiology and risk factors for colorectal cancer. *Gastroenterology Clinical of North America*, 1996; **25**: 717–35.

50. **Baron JA**, *et al.* Calcium supplements for the prevention of colorectal adenomas. *New England Journal of Medicine*, 1999; **34**: 101–7.

51. **Omenn GS**, *et al.* Effects of a combination of beta carotene and vitamin A on lung cancer and cardiovascular disease. *New England Journal of Medicine*, 1996; **334**: 1150–5.

52. **Omenn GS.** Chemoprevention of lung cancer: the rise and demise of beta-carotene. *Annual Review of Public Health*, 1998; **19**: 73–99.

53. **Hennekens CH**, *et al.* Lack of effect of long-term supplememattion with beta carotene on the incidence of malignant neoplasms and cardiovascular disease. *New England Journal of Medicine*, 1996; **334**: 1145–9.

54. **Moon TE**, *et al.* Effects of retinol in preventing squamous cell skin cancer in moderate-risk subjects: a randomized, double-blind, controlled trial. Southwest Skin Cancer Prevention Group. *Cancer Epidemiology Biomarkers and Prevention*, 1997; **6**: 949–56.

55. **Blot WJ**, *et al.* Nutrition intervention trials in Linxian, China: supplementation with specific vitamin/mineral combinations, cancer incidence, and disease-specific mortality in the general population. *Journal of the National Cancer Institute*, 1993; **85**: 1483–92.

56. **Hong WK**, *et al.* Prevention of second primary tumours with isotrentinoin in squamous-cell carcinoma of the head and neck *New England Journal of Medicine*, 1990; **323**: 795–801.

57. **Muto Y**, *et al.* Prevention of second primary tumours by an acyclic retinoid, polyprorenoic acid, in patients with hepatocellular carcinoma. Hepatoma Prevention Study Group. *New England Journal of Medicine*, 1996; **334**: 1561–7.

58. **Pastorino U**, *et al.* Adjuvant treatment of stage I lung cancer with hig-dose vitamin. *Journal of Clinical Oncology*, 1993; **11**: 1216–22.

59. **Bavinck JN**, *et al.* Prevention of skin cancer and reduction of keratotic skin lesions diuring acitretin therapy in renal transplant recipients: a double-blind, placebo-controlled study. *Journal of Clinical Oncology*, 1995; **13**:1933–8.

60. **Meyskens FL**, *et al.* Enhancement of regression of cervical intraepithelial neoplasia II (moderate dysplasia) with topically applied all-trans-retinoic acid: a randomized trial. *Journal of National Cancer Institute*, 1994; **86**: 539–43.

61. **Lippman SC, Lee J, Sabichi AL.** Cancer chemoprevention: progress and promise. *Journal of the National Cancer Institute*, 1998; **90**: 1514–28.

62. **Heinonen OP**, *et al.* Prostate cancer and supplementation with alpha-tocopherol and beta-carotene: incidence and mortality in a controlled trial. *Journal of the National Cancer Institute*, 1998; **90**: 440–446.

63. **Lippman SM.** Phase III cancer chemoprevention: focus on the prostate. In: Perry MC. *American Society of Clinical Oncology Education Book 36th Annual Meeting.* Lippincott Williams & Wilkins, Baltimore, 2000, pp. 32–41.

64. **Van Zandwijk N, Davesio O, Pastorino U**, *et al.* Euroscan, a randomized trial of vitamin A and N-acetylcysteine in patients with head and neck cancer or lung cancer. *Journal of the National Cancer Institute*, 2000; **92**: 977–86.

2.6 Cancer screening

Elsebeth Lynge

Purpose of cancer screening

Cancer develops in a stepwise way. At some point, symptoms such as blood in the stool or hoarseness, will bring the patient to the doctor. The earlier the cancer is diagnosed and treated, normally the better the prognosis of the patient. In cancer screening, this principle of early detection is extended to people without symptoms. Screening of people without symptoms allows detection of cancers at an early stage of invasiveness or even before they become invasive. Some early lesions can then be treated conservatively but very efficiently so that the patient can expect to live longer. Screening can then be beneficial for the patient. Figure 1 illustrates the expected time course for a cancer patient with the disease detected clinically as an invasive symptomatic disease, or detected by screening as an invasive non-symptomatic disease or as a preinvasive lesion.[1] The interval from the point in time when the lesion is detectable to the point in time when it would otherwise have been diagnosed as a clinical symptomatic disease is called the **sojourn time**, and the interval from detection by screening to clinical diagnosis is called the **lead time**. The length of the intervals may vary considerably for different types of cancer and for patients with a given disease. When a population is screened for a given cancer, a so-called **length bias** sampling of the incident cases is expected, as cases with a short sojourn time are less likely to be picked up in the screening.

Principles of screening

Screening gained emphasis in developed countries in the 1960s as evidenced, for example, 'by the controversies over cytological testing for cancer of the uterine cervix or regular medical check-ups for key executive personnel'. In 1968, the World Health Organization commissioned Wilson and Jungner to write their now famous principles of screening[2] (Table 1). These principles focused on screening for chronic diseases of adults and they were written primarily as a guide to public health agencies in developed countries.

The principles constituted a check list of preconditions to be fulfilled before a screening programme could be started. Most of the points addressed the importance and the natural history of the disease, the treatment possibilities, and the health care costs and organization. The remaining points addressed the screening test. The test should be suitable for screening, which means that it should have both a high **sensitivity** and a high **specificity**, concepts which will be defined later (see Fig. 4).

Table 1 Principles of screening

1.	The condition sought should be an important health problem.
2.	There should be an accepted treatment for patients with recognized disease.
3.	Facilities for diagnosis and treatment should be available.
4.	There should be a recognized latent or early symptomatic stage.
5.	There should be a suitable test for examination.
6.	The test should be acceptable for the population.
7.	The natural history of the condition, including development from latent to declared disease, should be adequately understood.
8.	There should be an agreed policy on whom to treat as patients.
9.	The cost of case-finding (including diagnosis and treatment of patients diagnosed) should be economically balanced in relation to possible expenditure on medical care as a whole.
10.	Case-finding should be a continuing process and not a 'once and for all' project.

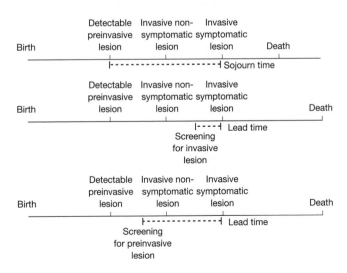

Fig. 1 Model of cancer disease detected without or with screening.

The principles of screening are still valid, but the experiences from the past 30 years show that it is not sufficient to check whether or not a screening activity fulfils certain preconditions. It is also necessary to evaluate whether or not a screening activity actually achieves its endpoint—reduction in disease-specific mortality or incidence.

Methods used in evaluation of cancer screening

If a population is screened with an effective method for early invasive disease and if the detected cases are treated appropriately, then the mortality from the disease in the population is expected to decrease. The key indicator for the effectiveness of screening is therefore decrease in disease-specific mortality. If the screening method also works for the detection of preinvasive lesions, then the incidence of the disease in the population is expected to decrease as well. A supplementary indicator for the effectiveness of screening is then a decrease in disease-specific incidence.

Over time, different methods have been used for evaluating the impact of screening activities on mortality and incidence. These methods will be presented below and illustrated with examples from the history of cancer screening.

Randomized controlled trials

Today, it is well established that the randomized, controlled trial is the proper way of testing a new medical procedure, including a new cancer screening test. Persons randomized to the screening group will be offered the screening test in combination with the normal treatment scheme for the particular disease. Persons randomized to the control group will be offered only the normal treatment scheme. To evaluate the outcome of the trial, both the screening group and the control group have to be followed from the time of randomization, and the key result is the estimated relative risk of the disease-specific mortality in the screening group compared with that of the control group.

Randomization may include only persons who have volunteered to take part in the study. If they all participate and if the screening test is not used in the control group, the trial will give a 'pure' estimate of the efficacy of the screening test. Randomization may also include all relevant persons living within an area. In this case a certain proportion of persons invited to screening may decline participation. If the screening test is, furthermore, already in use, for example as a diagnostic test, contamination is expected as some people in the control group may seek screening on their own initiative. The trial will then give an estimate of the effectiveness of the screening test when offered in a real population setting. The flow of events in a randomized, controlled trial including all relevant persons in an area is illustrated in Fig. 2.

The effect of faecal occult blood screening on mortality from colorectal cancer has been evaluated in four randomized controlled trials, in Minnesota, United States,[3],[4] in Göteborg, Sweden,[5],[6] in Nottingham, United Kingdom,[7] and in Fyn, Denmark,[8] see Table 2. The Minnesota trial included volunteers only and had a participation rate in the first round of about 80 per cent, whereas the other trials included all inhabitants and had participation rates in the first round from 53 to 67 per cent. The three trials including

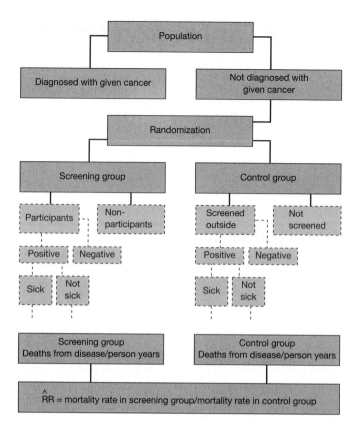

Fig. 2 Randomized, controlled trial of a screening test for a given cancer disease.

all inhabitants showed relative risks of colorectal cancer mortality in the screening group from 0.79 to 0.88 compared with the control group. The trial on volunteers showed surprisingly different results for those screened annually, relative risk 0.67, and for those screened biennially, relative risk 0.94. A meta-analysis of the four trials gave an overall relative risk of 0.84 (95 per cent confidence interval 0.77–0.93). The overall relative risk changed to 0.77 (95 per cent confidence interval 0.57–0.89) when it was adjusted for screening in the individual studies.[6]

Large, randomized, controlled trials can provide fairly accurate information about the number of lives expected to be saved following the implementation of a programme. Other benefits and negative side-effects of the screening can also be measured. The health care planners and the public are thus provided with adequate data for decision making. However, because they seek to detect relatively rare events, randomized trials require a large sample and long-term follow-up, and they are extremely expensive. The long time scale in the sequence of events in colorectal cancer screening illustrates problems that can be encountered in using randomized, controlled trials to make decisions about screening policies. Recruitment to the two last trials using faecal occult blood screening started in 1985 and the results were published in 1996. In the meantime, observational studies pointed to flexible sigmoidoscopy as probably a better screening tool for colorectal cancer.[9] Randomized, controlled trials using this test started in 1993[10],[11] but results will not be expected until about 2007.

Time trends in disease-specific mortality and incidence

Some new screening tests have been introduced prior to or without randomized, controlled trials. A broad range of epidemiological methods has then been used retrospectively to assess the effect of screening (see Chapter 2.4). For example the Pap smear for early detection of cervical cancer was widely used almost before the concept of the randomized, controlled trial was established. Time trends in cervical cancer mortality and incidence have since been used to assess the effectiveness of screening using the Pap smear.

In 1941, Papanicolaou and Traut[12] presented a 'simple, inexpensive method of diagnosis ... which could be applied to a large number of women in the cancer-bearing period of life'. The authors clearly stated that they were 'not yet in a position to offer a statistical proof of the reliability of this method of diagnosis, but we can say that in our experience it yields a high percentage of correct diagnoses when checked by tissue biopsies. There is evidence that a positive diagnosis may also be obtained in some cases of early disease'.

If the Pap smear worked for early detection of invasive disease, a decrease in cervical cancer mortality was to be expected in screened populations. If the Pap smear also worked for detection of preinvasive lesions, a decrease was to be expected in cervical cancer incidence. However, no one waited for the statistical proof, as the Pap smear was adopted widely throughout the world in the post war decades.

A mass screening programme started in Louisville, Kentucky, in 1956. Cervical cancer was the most frequent site of cancer among the low-income women in Louisville,[13] and about 10 years after the implementation of the programme it was possible to detect a decline in both the mortality and incidence of cervical cancer.[14] Another early programme started in British Columbia in 1949.[15] However, whether or not the programme here affected the cervical cancer mortality remained an unsettled issue for the next 25 years.[16] Some decline was seen, but this also occurred in other Canadian provinces. Evidence of an effect from the Canadian screening activity was seen when analysis of the regional trends in cervical cancer mortality from 1960–1962 to 1970–1972 indicated a possible association with the

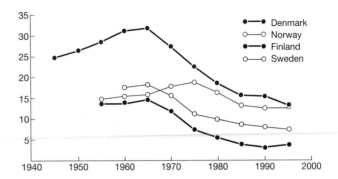

Fig. 3 Incidence of cervical cancer in the Nordic countries. Age standardized incidence rates per 100 000 (World Standard Population). Data source: Nordic Cancer Registries, personal communication, 1999.

regional screening activity in 1966.[17] In later years, this association was, however, not visible.[18]

The most convincing data for the effect of Pap smear screening came from the Nordic countries. In the late 1960s, organized screening programmes were established for all women in Finland, Iceland, and Sweden, for 40 per cent of women in Denmark, but for women in only one county in Norway. In the early 1970s, declining trends were seen in both the cervical cancer incidence[19] and mortality[20] in Finland, Iceland, Sweden, and Denmark, whereas the Norwegian trends increased. The Nordic data thus pointed to a clear association between the high screening coverage obtained in organized programmes and trends in incidence and mortality. An update of the Nordic incidence data shows a moderate, 10-year delayed decrease in cervical cancer incidence in Norway (Fig. 3). Opportunistic screening on a large scale started in Norway in the 1970s, while an organized, nationwide programme was introduced only in 1995.[21]

Cervical cancer has long been suspected of being, in part, a sexually transmitted disease. Frequent occurrence of certain types of human papillomavirus DNA (HPV-DNA) in tumour tissue was reported in

Table 2 Randomized, controlled trial on faecal occult blood screening for colorectal cancer

Location	Minnesota, US	Göteborg, Sweden	Nottingham, UK	Fyn, Denmark
Start of trial	1975	1982	1985	1985
Population	Volunteers	All inhabitants	Persons on GPs' lists	All inhabitants
Age	50–80	60–64	50–74	45–74
Screening interval	Annual + biennial	Two screens, 16–24 months	Biennial	Biennial
Number in each group	Ca. 15 500	Ca. 34 150	Ca. 75 000	Ca. 31 000
Participation in first round	Annual: 80% Biennial: 76%	63%	53%	67%
Years of follow-up	13	8.3	7.8	8.3
RR colorectal cancer (CRC) mortality	Annual: 0.67 (0.50–0.87) Biennial: 0.94 (0.68–1.31)	0.88 (0.69–1.12)	Verified as CRC: 0.85 (0.74–0.98) CRC on death certificate: 0.88 (0.76–1.01)	Verified as CRC: 0.79 (0.65–0.96) CRC + complications: 0.82 (0.68–0.99)

the late 1980s,[22] (see also Chapters 2.2 and 12.3). HPV-DNA has later been detected in virtually all samples of tumour tissue in a large collection from cervical cancer patients from around the world,[23] and both case–control[24] and cohort studies[25] have indicated HPV infection to be the key risk factor. An HPV-test has proved to be useful in the triage of women with minor abnormalities on the Pap smear,[26] and an HPV-test might therefore also be a tool in primary cervical cancer screening. Randomized trials with the HPV-test incorporated in primary screening are ongoing in Europe.

Survival of patients following diagnosis versus disease-specific mortality

The increase in mean survival for patients with screen-detected, as compared to clinically-detected, cancers should not be regarded as evidence of benefit for a screening programme. Both the gain in lead time, Fig. 1, and the tendency for screening to detect slower progressing cancers, length bias, cause such an effect.

For example the many chest radiographs taken for screening of tuberculosis after the Second World War showed that lung cancers could be detected in this way and early clinical data indicated a higher 5-year survival rate among patients having an asymptomatic lung cancer detected in this way than among patients with clinically-detected lung cancers. A non-randomized study showed, however, no effect on lung cancer mortality.[27] Detection and localization of occult lung cancers improved in the 1960s when a new method for processing of sputum and the flexible fiberoptic bronchoscope were developed. A large, randomized trial for lung cancer screening started in the United States in 1971 to determine 'whether detection of lung cancer can be improved by adding modern sputum cytological screening techniques to the examination at regular intervals by chest radiography',[28] but an unscreened control group was not included.

The dual screening group had a 5-year survival of nearly 55 per cent compared with 35 to 40 per cent in the chest radiograph only group, and even more remarkable was the difference between both groups and the 5-year survival of about 15 per cent among lung cancer patients in the general population. The authors were careful to emphasize caution in the interpretation of this finding.[29] Subsequent follow-up showed no statistically significant difference in lung cancer mortality between the dual screening group and the group screened with chest radiographs only.[30] There was no difference either in the lung cancer mortality in another part of the study where 4-monthly dual screening had been compared with the standard advice of annual dual screening.[31]

The United States study was unable to evaluate the potential benefit of annual chest radiographs alone and was 'designed under the belief than the annual chest radiograph did not produce a major impact on mortality from lung cancer',[32] and no effect was found of 4-monthly screening versus standard advice on annual screening. After completion of the study in 1986, some trialists, nevertheless, saw the longer survival among the patients in the trial as representing a real benefit and argued that 'elimination of routine chest radiographs would be equivalent to acceptance of total defeat in the treatment of lung cancer'.[33] The researchers were well aware of the pitfalls in using survival as an indicator of mortality, but it was difficult to accept this in practice. It is interesting that these comments were made 20 years after the possibilities for primary prevention of lung cancer through smoking cessation were well established.[34]

Lung cancer screening with annual chest radiographs is now part of the United States Prostate, Lung, Colon, and Ovarian Cancer Screening Trial,[11] where the outcome will be evaluated on the disease-specific mortality.

Case–control and cohort studies

The design of case–control and cohort studies, together with their inherent biases, is described in Chapter 2.4. Many screening tests have been evaluated in case–control studies, including Pap smears,[35] mammography,[36],[37] and chest radiographs.[38],[39]

The cases in a case–control study of, for example, mammography screening will be patients who die from breast cancer. The controls will typically be age-matched, but otherwise randomly selected women from the same area. The screening history of cases and controls can be assessed from medical records or questionnaires. The study will provide an estimate of the relative risk of dying from breast cancer among women ever screened compared with women never screened. A case–control study will thus, in principle, provide a test of the efficacy of the screening test. People included in case–control studies are, however, not randomized to the two exposure groups. A bias will be introduced in the study if non-screened women have a higher disease incidence than screened women, or if non-screened women have more lethal cancers than screened women.[40] In Sweden, women who do not participate in mammography screening programmes seem to be a selected group with a rather poor prognosis when they develop breast cancer.[41],[42] Data from case–control studies were useful in an initial assessment of the potential effect of mammography screening, but data from the randomized, controlled trials have now provided more reliable (less biased) evidence about the value of the screening procedure.

In the 1980s, data on time trends clearly indicated a beneficial effect of screening for cervical cancer. Few data were available, however, on the effect of different screening schedules, the key question being whether screening was needed annually or whether a similar protection could be obtained with less frequent screens.[43] To evaluate the optimal screening interval, data were collected from ten areas with well-established screening programmes.[44] The data collection was organized either as case–control or cohort studies. The cohort studies estimated the incidence of cervical cancer in women with negative smears by time since the last negative smear and by number of negative smears. Comparison was made with the incidence expected given that no screening had taken place. While the observed incidence could be calculated from screening and population data, the expected incidence given no screening had to be a 'guesstimate', for example the incidence in the area prior to implementation of the screening programme. However, given the lack of data from randomized, controlled trials on cervical cancer screening, these observational data provided a useful guide to screening policy, as they indicate that almost the same protective effect can be achieved with 3-yearly screening as with annual screening. Similar methods are now used to evaluate the incidence of interval cancers in breast cancer screening programmes.

Gray zone screening

The concept 'gray zone screening' is used to describe the situation where a diagnostic test starts to be used on a large scale on healthy people without prior evaluation of the potential benefits and risks.

Screening using serum levels of the prostate specific antigen (PSA) has never been evaluated in a randomized controlled trial. The dissemination of PSA testing in American men in the late1980s and 1990s is nevertheless the most rapid introduction of a cancer screening test ever seen on a population basis. Prostate cancer was in 1985 the second most common incident cancer in North American men.[45] Autopsy studies also showed that prostate cancer was often present as an occult disease.[46] During the period 1973 to 1986 the incidence of prostate cancer increased slightly in United States white men. Then, as a result of the widespread PSA testing, the incidence more than doubled from 1986 to 1992 but declined again from 1992.[47] Prostate cancer was the third most common incident cancer in western European men in 1985,[45] but Europe followed a much more conservative approach to PSA testing reflected in only slightly increasing incidence rates after 1985.

The possible treatment modalities (radical prostatectomy, radiation, hormone therapy, and watchful waiting) have not been evaluated in randomized, controlled trials. Observational studies indicate a high 10-year survival in patients with clinically localized prostate cancer treated conservatively with hormone therapy and/or watchful waiting.[48] The dissemination of PSA testing in the United States and the resulting increase in incidence of prostate cancer was accompanied by intensified treatment. The proportion of United States prostate cancer patients treated with radical prostatectomy increased from 9 per cent in 1974 to 29 per cent in 1993, and the proportion treated with radiation increased from 6 per cent to 39 per cent.[49] Side-effects of prostate cancer treatment are frequent with impotence occurring in most men treated by radical prostatectomy or radiation therapy, and incontinence also being a common problem (see Chapter 13.1).

The 'PSA adventure' in the United States happened 40 years after the introduction of the randomized, controlled trial as the proper test for new medical procedures, 20 years after publication of the Wilson and Jungner principles, and shortly after demonstration of the failure of lung cancer screening in the United States. When the PSA screening in United States men is evaluated according the Wilson and Jungner principles some observations can be made. First, prostate cancer is certainly an important health problem. Secondly, widespread prostate cancer screening was already ongoing using digital rectal examination. A survey in 1989 showed that 25 per cent of men over age 40 had annual digital rectal examination.[50] The question of whether or not to screen was not on the agenda, PSA was introduced in screening as 'a useful adjunct to rectal examination and ultrasonography'.[51] Thirdly, prostate cancers were perceived as slow growing tumours assumed to behave like breast cancers, where data on the effect of mammography screening on breast cancer mortality started to accumulate from randomized controlled trials in the mid 1980s.[52],[53] Fourthly, the PSA test was relatively cheap and the principles on 'available facilities' and 'balanced costs' are not of primary relevance in privately funded health care systems. In this setting, an entrepreneur spirit over-ruled scientific stringency, as illustrated by a statement from the Prostate Cancer Educational Council; 'We believed it was an ignored male disease. Thus [we] established the goal of encouraging men to be screened annually for prostate cancer. At that time, it was not known which age groups should be screened or whether use of the blood test for prostate specific antigen (PSA) had any value'.[50]

Table 3 Benefits and risks of mammography screening in women aged 50 to 69

Benefits	Risks
Decrease in breast cancer mortality	More years as cancer patient
Conservative treatment	False positive and false negative tests
	'Overtreatment' of carcinoma *in situ*
	Low dose radiation exposure
	Psychological side-effects

A trial of prostate cancer screening was undertaken in Quebec, Canada, in 1988 to 1996. However, only 23 per cent of the screening group participated, and 7 per cent of the control was screened. A 6 per cent decrease in prostate cancer mortality was reported in the screening group compared with the control group,[54] but this trial was so flawed in its design and analysis that no conclusion can be drawn from it. Large trials started in the United States in 1993[11] and in Europe in 1994,[55] where data on mortality are expected in about 2010. In the meantime, two data sources are available for evaluation. A series of nested case–control studies with stored serum samples and follow-up for cancer incidence indicates that PSA measurements can predict future occurrence of clinical prostate cancer.[56] The impact of the PSA screening can also be monitored by mortality time trends. A slight decrease is reported in the United States mortality rates for prostate cancer since 1991.[47] Regional data from the United States show, however, no clear correlation between previous increase in incidence and present mortality,[57] nor does a comparison between the incidence and the mortality trends in the United States and the United Kingdom.[58]

Benefits and risks

While a proven decrease in disease-specific mortality or incidence is a necessary condition for using a screening method, it is not a sufficient condition to justify use of the screen. A screening method might also have some negative side-effects. For the informed public of today, it is therefore necessary to present the potential benefits and potential risks of screening in a way which allows the individual citizen to decide on participation in screening programmes for her or himself.

Breast cancer screening with mammography for women aged 50 to 69 has been evaluated from this point of view in Denmark.[59] (see Table 3). The key benefit of mammography screening is a reduction in breast cancer mortality. Based on the Swedish randomized, controlled trials this is expected to be about 30 per cent among women aged 50 to 69 at their first invitation to mammography who have an initial participation rate of 85 per cent, are screened four to seven times, and have follow-up for 6 to 11 years.[60] Assuming a full effect from age of 50, this would, in Danish women, translate into a decrease in the risk of dying from breast cancer before age 85 from about 5 per cent to about 4 per cent. On the benefit side is also a potentially more conservative treatment since tumours are detected at a smaller size, although this is not well-elucidated based on data from the randomized trials.

Test Result	True disease status Sick (breast cancer confirmed)	Healthy	Total tested
Positive	True positive: 360	False negative: 1699	2059
Negative	False negative: 52	True positive: 28 251	28303
Total tested	412	29 950	30362

Number of 'true positive' includes women who tested positive and at surgery had invasive breast cancer or carcinoma *in situ* of the breast.

Number of 'false negative' estimated as the number of clinically diagnosed breast cancers in the interval between negative mammography and recall for screening after 2 years.

Sensitivity: 360/412 = 0.87
Specificity: 28251/29950 = 0.94

Fig. 4 True disease status and outcome of screening test, using data from first round of mammography screening in Copenhagen, Denmark.[65]

The negative effects of mammography screening include a longer period as a cancer patient due to the estimated lead time of 3 to 4 years.[61] Even conservative treatment has side-effects. Both lymph node dissection and radiation may cause damage to the nerves, oedema of the arm occurs in about one-third of patients, and radiation may affect the cosmetic quality of the breast-conserving surgery (see Chapter 11.6). Ten to twenty per cent of the tumours detected by screening are carcinoma *in situ* cases and not all of these would progress untreated to invasive cancers in the women's life time. Mammography involves low-dose radiation exposure, at the upper limit of about 2 mGy per screening film. Annual screening from age 50 with this dose has been estimated to induce 15 breast cancers in 100 000 women, where 1500 breast cancer deaths would be saved.[62] Current exposure levels are lower, but the data stress the need for thorough quality assurance of mammography equipment.

Mammography is not a perfect screening test. The proportion of women with false positive screening tests have varied from 0.7 per cent to 6.6 per cent in the first screening round and from 0.5 per cent to 5.2 per cent in the following rounds in various screening programmes.[59] The proportion of false negative tests can not be assessed directly, and the number of interval cancers is therefore used as an indicator. The number of interval cancers after 2 years as a percentage of breast cancer cases expected without screening has varied from 24 per cent in the Swedish WE-trial[61] to 42 per cent in two English programmes.[63],[64]

The sensitivity and specificity of mammography is calculated in Fig. 4, using data from the first round of the screening programme in Copenhagen, Denmark, where women aged 50 to 69 are offered biennial screening.[65] The importance of the specificity of a screening test is illustrated by the Copenhagen experience from the first three screening rounds, where about one-quarter of women following the entire programme is expected to get at least one false positive test. A much higher proportion of women with false positive tests has been reported from a programme in Maryland, United States.[66] False positive tests cause substantial anxiety that may persist for up to 18 months.[67],[68]

The need to provide individual citizens with information about both the benefits and risks of screening that allow them to make their own decision is now widely recognized. On cervical cancer, the joint director of the National Screening Committee for the United Kingdom says 'People need to be clear about the limitations and risks of screening, as well as the benefits. People are increasingly concerned about the adverse effects of health care and the balance between good and harm'.[69]

Monitoring screening programmes

The failure of the previous cervical cancer screening programme in England and Wales is a well known example of an unsuccessful public investment in cancer screening.[70] Screening of women aged 35 and over at 5-yearly intervals was recommended in 1966, and the number of smears increased from 700 000 in 1965 to 2 928 000 in 1980.[71] The programme might have contributed to the control of cervical cancer,[72] but the mortality rates in women under 35 years nevertheless started to increase in 1970 to 1974, by 1980 to 1983 the increase had spread to women under 45, and by 1985 to 1987 to women under 50.[73] Reasons for the failure of the screening programme were listed as: failure to reach the population at risk, lack of sensitivity of cervical screening, infrequently repeated screening, inadequate management of abnormalities detected, and ineffective treatment.[74] A major re-organization of cervical cancer screening started in England and Wales in 1988. A computerized call and recall programme was implemented together with management and quality assurance at all levels, and the payment of general practitioners was made dependent on their patients' compliance with the programme. National coverage is at present 85 per cent, and both the incidence and mortality from cervical cancer have decreased in the 1990s.[69]

Case–control studies have been suggested as a tool for monitoring the quality of screening programmes. Even when the benefits and negative side-effects of screening are well established in randomized, controlled trials, the customarization might be problematic. The results of the trial from a highly specialized centre might not be achieved in routine practice of less specialized centres. Cohort studies of the populations covered by the mammography screening programmes in Sweden and Finland show that they have achieved almost the same reduction in mortality[75],[76] as seen in the Swedish randomized, controlled trials,[60] indicating a successful technology transfer, although a reduction in mortality is still not visible in the national mortality statistics.[77]

Genetic screening

The identification of some of the genes underlying familial cancer syndromes has opened the possibility for genetic screening of family members. At an early age, members of cancer families can now be sorted into non-carriers and carriers of the cancer-causing mutations in these genes. Non-carriers can consider their cancer risk as being similar to that of the population at large. Carriers will know that they have a high probability of developing cancer at some point later in life.

Knowledge of disease penetrance is a crucial parameter for the carriers in order to decide on how to live with their carrier status. Several studies have been made of the disease penetrance of mutations in the *BRCA1* and *BRCA2* genes predisposing for familial breast cancer (see also Chapter 1.4). The initial studies were based on data from selected high risk families and indicated the cumulative breast cancer risk at age 70 to be 80 per cent or more in *BRCA1* and *BRCA2* mutation carriers.[78],[79] A study based on screening of volunteer Ashkenazi Jews indicated, however, the risk of cumulative breast cancer at age 70 to be 56 per cent in mutation carriers,[80] and a population-based study from Iceland indicated the cumulative breast cancer risk at age 70 to be 37 per cent in mutation carriers.[81] Disease progression and response to therapy are other parameters of importance for mutation carriers. It is, at present, uncertain whether or not hereditary breast cancers differ in these respects from sporadic breast cancers.

The healthy carriers of mutations in the *BRCA1* and *BRCA2* genes can, at present, choose between prophylactic mastectomy or frequent mammography or they can choose to live as the population at large. The available data offer poor guidance for mutation carriers to make an appropriate choice, and further data on disease penetrance, prognosis, and response to therapy are clearly warranted.

Expected effect of screening on cancer mortality

It is the purpose of cancer screening to save lives, and reduction in the disease-specific mortality is the key indicator for the success of screening. Such a reduction in disease-specific mortality has, so far, been documented only for Pap smear screening for cervical cancer,[20] mammography screening for breast cancer in women over 50,[60] and faecal occult blood screening for colorectal cancer.[4],[6]–[8]

Two attempts have been made to estimate the potential impact of population-based screening programmes on overall cancer mortality. In the estimate for the United States, the impact of screening on the number of cancer deaths in the year 2000 was calculated assuming introduction of nationwide screening programmes for cervical cancer and breast cancer in 1980. The simulation model indicated that these screening activities could result in a 3 per cent reduction in cancer deaths in 2000.[82] In the estimate for the Nordic countries, the impact of screening on the number of cancer deaths in 2013 to 2017 was calculated assuming an introduction in 1988 of nationwide screening programmes for cervical cancer, breast cancer, and colorectal cancer. This calculation, with a longer follow-up period and with colorectal cancer screening included, indicated that screening could result in a 6 per cent reduction in cancer deaths in 2013 to 2017.[83] Estimates such as these should be interpreted cautiously as they are based on a number of assumptions. It is noteworthy, however, that both of these estimates of the potential impact of screening are considerably lower than the estimates of the number of cancer deaths avoidable through primary prevention (see Chapter 2.5). In the United States calculation, this number was estimated to be in the range of 16 to 23 per cent of cancer deaths in 2000,[82] and for the Nordic countries to be 27 per cent of incident cancer cases in 2000.[84]

References

1. Walter SD, Day NE. Estimation of duration of a pre-clinical disease state using screening data. *American Journal of Epidemiology*, 1983; 118: 865–86.

2. Wilson JMG, Jungner G. *Principles and practice of screening for disease.* Public Health Papers 34. Geneva: World Health Organization, 1968.

3. Mandel J, *et al.* The University of Minnesota's Colon cancer control study: Design and progress to date. In: Chamberlain J, Miller AB, ed. *Screening for gastrointestinal cancer.* Toronto: Hans Huber Publishers, 1987: 17–24.

4. Mandel JS, *et al.* Reducing mortality from colorectal cancer by screening for fecal occult blood. *New England Journal of Medicine*, 1993; 328: 1365–71.

5. Kewenter J, Breving H, Engaras B, Haglind E, Ahren C. Results of screening, rescreening, and follow-up in a prospective randomised study for detection of colorectal cancer by fecal occult blood testing. Results for 68 308 subjects. *Scandinavian Journal of Gastroenterology*, 1994; 29: 468–73.

6. Towler B, Irwig L, Glasziou P, Kewenter J, Weller D, Silagy C. A systematic review of the effects of screening for colorectal cancer using the faecal occult blood test, Hemoccult. *British Medical Journal*, 1998; 317: 559–65.

7. Hardcastle JD, *et al.* Randomised controlled trial of faecal-occult-blood screening for colorectal cancer. *Lancet*, 1996; 348: 1472–7.

8. Kronborg O, Fenger C, Olsen J, Jørgensen OD, Søndergaard O. Randomised study of screening for colorectal cancer with faecal occult-blood test. *Lancet*, 1996; 348: 1467–71.

9. Atkin WS, Cuzick J, Northover JMA, Whynes DK. Prevention of colorectal cancer by once only sigmoidoscopy. *Lancet*, 1993; 341: 736–40.

10. Atkin WS, *et al.* Uptake, yield of neoplasia, and adverse effects of flexible sigmoidoscopy. *Gut*, 1998; 42: 560–5.

11. Gohagan JK, Prorok PC, Framer BS, Cornett JE. Prostate cancer screening in the prostate, lung, colorectal and ovarian cancer screening trial of the National Cancer Institute. *Journal of Urology*, 1994; 152: 1905–9.

12. Papanicolaou GN, Traut HF. The diagnostic value of varginal smears in carcinoma of the uterus. *American Journal of Obstetrics and Gynaecology*, 1941; 42: 193–206.

13. Christopherson WM. Cytologic detection and diagnosis of cancer. *Cancer*, 1983; 51: 1201–8.

14. Christopherson WM, Parker JE, Mendez WM, Lundin FE Jr. Cervix cancer death rates and cytologic screening. *Cancer*, 1970; 26: 808–11.

15. Fidler HK, Boyes DA, Worth AJ. Cervical cancer detection in British Columbia. *Journal of Obstetrics and Gynaecology of the British Commonwealth*, 1968; 75: 392–404.

16. Editorial. Cervical screening. *Lancet*, 1969; ii(7614): 255–6.

17. Miller AB, Lindsay J, Hill GB. Mortality from cancer of the uterus in Canada and its relationship to screening for cancer of the cervix. *International Journal of Cancer*, 1976; 17: 602–12.

18. Miller AB. Evaluation of the impact of screening for cancer of the cervix. In: Hakama M, Miller AB, Day NE, ed. *Screening for cancer of the uterine cervix.* Lyon: International Agency for Research on Cancer, 1986: 149–60.

19. Hakama M. Trends in the incidence of cervical cancer in the Nordic countries. In: Magnus K, ed. *Trends in cancer incidence.* Washington: Hemisphere publishing, 1982.

20. Läärä E, Day NE, Hakama M. Trends in mortality from cervical cancer in the Nordic countries: association with organised screening programmes. *Lancet*, 1987; i(8544): 1247–9.

21. Bjørge T, Skare GB, Slåttekjær PE, Melby W, Olsen M, Thoresen SØ. *Cervical cancer screening.* Olso: Kreftregisteret, 1994 [in Norwegian].

22. zur Hausen H. Papillomavirus in anogenital cancer as a model to understand the role of viruses in human cancers. *Cancer Research*, 1989; 49: 4677–81.

23. Bosch FX, *et al.* Prevalence of human papillomavirus in cervical cancer: a worldwide perspective. International biological study on

cervical cancer (IBSCC) study group. *Journal of the National Cancer Institute*, 1995; **87**: 796–802.

24. Muñoz N, *et al.* The causal link between human papillomavirus and invasive cervical cancer: a population based case-control study in Columbia and Spain. *International Journal of Cancer*, 1992; **52**: 743–9.

25. Kjær SK, *et al.* Human papillomavirus—the most significant risk determinant of cervical intraepithelial neoplasia. *International Journal of Cancer*, 1996; **65**: 601–6.

26. Cox JT, Lorincz AT, Schiffman MH, Sherman ME, Cullen A, Kurman RJ. Human papilloma virus testing by hybrid capture appears to be useful in triaging women with a cytologic diagnosis of atypical squamous cells of undetermined significance. *American Journal of Obstetrics and Gynecology*, 1995; **172**: 946–54.

27. Brett GZ. Earlier diagnosis and survival in lung cancer. *British Medical Journal*, 1969; **4**(678): 260–2.

28. Berlin NI, Buncher CR, Fontana RS, Frost JK, Melamed MR. The National Cancer Institute cooperative early lung cancer detection program. Results of the initial screen (prevalence). Early lung cancer detection: Introduction. *American Reviews of Respiratory Diseases*, 1984; **130**: 545–9.

29. Berlin NI, Buncher CR, Fontana RS, Frost JK, Melamed MR. The National Cancer Institute cooperative early lung cancer detection program. Results of the initial screen (prevalence). Early lung cancer detection: Summary and conclusions. *American Reviews of Respiratory Diseases*, 1984; **130**: 565–70.

30. Tockman MS, Frost JK, Stitik FP. Screening and detection of lung cancer. In: Aisner J, ed. *Lung cancer*. New York: Churchill Livingstone 1985: 25–40.

31. Fontana RS, Sanderson DR, Woolner LB, Taylor WF, Miller WE, Muhm JR. Lung cancer screening: The Mayo program. *Journal of Occupational Medicine*, 1986; **28**: 746–50.

32. Prorok PC, Miller AB, eds. *Screening for cancer.* Discussion on screening for lung cancer. Geneva: International Union Against Cancer, 1984: 136–42.

33. Flehinger BJ, *et al.* Screening for early detection of lung cancer in New York. In: Prorok PC, Miller AB, eds. *Screening for cancer.* Geneva: International Union Against Cancer, 1984: 123–35.

34. USDHEP. *Smoking and health: Report of the Advisory Committee to the Surgeon General of the Public Health Service.* PHS Publications no 1103. Washington DC: US Government Printing Office, 1964.

35. Clarke EA, Andersson TW. Does screening by Pap smears help prevent cervical cancer? A case-control study. *Lancet*, 1979; **ii**(8132): 1–4.

36. Verbeek ALM, Holland R, Stumans F, Hendriks JHCL, Mravunac M, Day NE. Reduction of breast cancer mortality through mass screening with modern mammography. First results of the Nijmegen project, 1975–1981. *Lancet*, 1984; **i**(8404): 1222–4.

37. Collette HJA, Rombach JJ, Day NE, Waard F de. Evaluation of screening for breast cancer in a non-randomised study (The DOM project) by means of a case-control study. *Lancet*, 1984; **i**(8388): 1224–6.

38. Ebeling K, Nischan P. Screening for lung cancer—results from a case-control study. *International Journal of Cancer*, 1987; **40**: 141–4.

39. Sobue T, Suzuki T, Naruke T. A case-control study for evaluating lung cancer screening in Japan. *International Journal of Cancer*, 1992; **50**: 230–7.

40. Cronin KA, Weed DL, Connor RJ, Prorok PC. Case-control studies of cancer screening: theory and practice. *Journal of the National Cancer Institute*, 1998; **90**: 498–504.

41. Gullberg B, Andersson I, Janzon L, Ranstam J. Screening mammography. *Lancet*, 1991; **337**: 244.

42. Lidbrink E, Frisell J, Brandberg Y, Rosendahl I, Rutqvist L-E. Non attendance in the Stockholm mammography screening trial: Relative mortality and reasons for non attendance. *Breast Cancer Research and Treatment*, 1995; **35**: 267–75.

43. Editorial. Intervals between Pap tests: a compromise. *World Health Forum*,1981; **2**: 533–40.

44. IARC Working group on evaluation of cervical cancer screening programmes. Screening for squamous cervical cancer: duration of low risk after negative results of cervical cytology and it's implication for screening policies. *British Medical Journal*, 1986; **293**: 659–64.

45. Parkin DM, Pisani P, Ferlay J. Estimates of the worldwide incidence of eighteen major cancers in 1985. *International Journal of Cancer*, 1993; **54**: 594–600.

46. Rietberger JBW, Schröder FH. Screening for prostate cancer—more questions than answers. *Acta Oncologica*, 1998; **37**: 515–32.

47. SEER Program of the National Cancer Institute. *SEER prostate cancer trends 1973–1995.* Washington DC: National Cancer Institute, 1999.

48. Chodak GW, *et al.* Results of conservative management of clinically localised prostate cancer. *New England Journal of Medicine*, 1994; **330**: 242–8.

49. Mettlin CJ, Murphy GP. Why is the prostate cancer death rate declining in the United States? *Cancer*, 1997; **82**: 249–51.

50. Crawford ED. Prostate cancer awareness work: September 22-to 28, 1997. *CA-A Cancer Journal for Clinicians*, 1997; **47**: 288–96.

51. Catalona WJ, *et al.* Measurement of prostate specific antigen in serum as a screening test for prostate cancer. *New England Journal of Medicine*, 1991; **324**: 1156–61.

52. Shapiro S, Strax P, Venet L. Periodic breast cancer screening in reducing mortality from breast cancer. *Journal of the American Medical Association*, 1971; **215**: 1777–85.

53. Tabár L, *et al.* Reduction in mortality from breast cancer after mass screening with mammography. *Lancet*, 1985; **i**(8433): 829–32.

54. Labrie F, *et al.* Screening decreases prostate cancer death: First analysis of the 1988 Quebec prospective randomised controlled trial. *Prostate*, 1999; **38**: 83–91.

55. Auvinen A, Rietberger JBW, Denis LJ, Schröder FH; Prorik PC. Prospective evaluation plan for randomised trials of prostate cancer screening. *Journal of Medical Screening*, 1996; **3**: 97–104.

56. Whittemore AS, Lele C, Friedman GD, Stamey T, Vogelman JH, Orrentreich N. Prostate specific antigen as predictor of prostate cancer in black and white men. *Journal of the National Cancer Institute*, 1995; **87**: 354–60.

57. Brawley OW. Prostate carcinoma incidence and patient mortality. The effects of screening and early detection. *Cancer*, 1997; **80**: 1857–63.

58. Sahibata A, Ma J, Whittemore AS. Prostate cancer incidence and mortality in the United States and the United Kingdom. *Journal of the National Cancer Institute*, 1998; **90**: 1230–1.

59. Sundhedsstyrelsen. *Early detection and treatment of breast cancer.* København: Sundhedsstyrelsen, 1997 [in Danish].

60. Nyström L, *et al.* Breast cancer screening with mammography: overview of Swedish randomised trials. *Lancet* 1993; **341**: 973–8.

61. Tabár L, Fagerberg G, Duffy SW, Day NE, Gad A, Gröntoft O. Update of the Swedish two-county program of mammograhis screening for breast cancer. *Radiology Clinics of North America*, 1992; **30**: 187–210.

62. European Commission. *European protocol on dosemetry in mammography.* Luxembourg: Office for Official Publications of the European Communities, 1996.

63. Woodman CHJ, Threlfall AG, Boggis CRM, Prior P. Is the three year breast screening interval too long? Occurrence of interval cancers in NHS breast screening programme's north western region. *British Medical Journal*, 1995; **310**: 224–6.

64. Day NE, *et al.* Monitoring interval cancers in breast screening programmes: the East Anglian experience. *Journal of Medical Screening*, 1995; **2**: 180–5.

65. Mammography Screening Evaluation Group, H:S Copenhagen Hospital Corporation. Mammography screening for breast cancer in

Copenhagen April 1991-March 1997. *APMIS*, 1998; **106** (suppl. 83): 1–44.

66. **Elmore JG, Barton MB, Moceri VM, Polk S, Arene PJ, Fletcher SW.** Ten year risk of false positive screening mammograms and clinical breast examination. *New England Journal of Medicine*, 1998; **338**: 1089–96.

67. **Ellman R, Angli N, Christians A, Moss S, Chamberlain J, Maguire P.** Psychiatric morbidity associated with screening for breast cancer. *British Journal of Cancer*, 1989; **60**: 781–4.

68. **Gram IT, Lund E, Slenker SE.** Quality of life following a false positive mammogram. *British Journal of Cancer*, 1990; **62**: 1018–22.

69. **NCS Cervical Screening Programme.** *Cervical screening programme, review 1998.* Sheffield: NHS Cervical Screening Programme, 1998.

70. **Editorial.** Cancer of the cervix: Death by incompetence. *Lancet*, 1985; ii(8451): 363–4.

71. **Roberts A.** Cervical cytology in England and Wales, 1965–1980. *Health Trends*, 1982; **14**: 41–3.

72. **Parkin DM, Nguyen-Dinh X, Day NE.** The impact of screening in the incidence of cervical cancer in England and Wales. *British Journal of Obstetrics and Gynaecology*, 1985; **92**: 150–7.

73. **Booth M, Beral V.** Cervical cancer deaths in young women. *Lancet*, 1989; i(8638): 616.

74. **Chamberlain J.** Reasons that some screening programmes fail to control cervical cancer. In: Hakama M, Miller AB, Day NE, ed. *Screening for cancer of the uterine cervix.* Lyon: International Agency for Research on Cancer, 1986: 161–8.

75. **Lenner P, Jonsson H.** Excess mortality from breast cancer in relation to mammography screening in northern Sweden. *Journal of Medical Screening*, 1997; **4**: 6–9.

76. **Hakama M, Pukkala E, Heikkilä M, Kallio M.** Effectiveness of the public health policy for breast cancer screening in Finland: population based cohort study. *British Medical Journal*, 1997; **314**: 864–7.

77. **Sjönell G, Ståhle L.** Health control with mammography does not reduce breast cancer mortality. *Läkartidningen*, 1999; **96**: 904–13 [in Swedish].

78. **Easton DF, Ford D, Bishop DT.** Breast cancer linkage consortium: breast and ovarian cancer incidence in BRCA1- mutation carriers. *American Journal of Human Genetics*, 1995; **56**: 265–71.

79. **Ford D, et al.** Genetic heterogeneity and penetrance analysis of the BRCA1 and BRCA2 genes in breast cancer families. *American Journal of Human Genetics*, 1998; **62**: 676–89.

80. **Struewing JP, et al.** The risk of cancer associated with specific mutations of BRCA1 and BRCA2 among Ashkenazi Jews. *New England Journal of Medicine*, 1997; **336**: 1401–8.

81. **Thorlacius S, et al.** Population-based study of risk of breast cancer in carriers of BRCA2 mutation. *Lancet*, 1998; **352**: 1337–9.

82. **Greenwald P, Sondik EJ, eds.** *Cancer control objectives for the nation 1985–2000.* National Cancer Institute Monographs 2. Bethesda, MD: NIH Publications, no 86–2880, 1986.

83. **Hristova L, Hakama M.** Effect of screening for cancer in the Nordic countries on deaths, costs and quality of life up to the year 2017. *Acta Oncologica*, 1996; **35** (suppl 9): 1–60.

84. **Olsen JH, et al.** Avoidable cancers in the Nordic countries. *APMIS*, 1997; **105** (suppl. 76): 1–146.

3

Diagnosis and investigative procedures

3.1   Molecular and cellular pathology of cancer

T. Crook, A. R. Perry, P. Osin, and B. A. Gusterson

Introduction

Although the role of the pathologist in the analysis of tumours is in a phase of rapid evolution, the same fundamental questions still exist. Can the tumour be allocated to a specific category according to defined classification systems? What is the degree of invasion and/or metastasis? Are there features which predict the prognosis and response to treatment? Are there clues to the aetiology of the tumour?

The traditional approach to such questions has been the histopathological examination of changes in tissue architecture. Immunocytochemistry has increased the ability of the cancer pathologist to identify markers of diagnostic and prognostic value, while the number of such markers is increasing as molecular biological techniques identify new alterations of protein expression in cancer. In addition, genetic analysis has linked many mutations to tumour type and tumour behaviour. There is now little doubt that molecular analysis of cancer genes and cancer proteins will have considerable clinical impact. Techniques for identifying protein and genetic changes in cancer are being refined; recent advances are allowing the automation of many procedures, and translation of these powerful techniques from the research laboratory into the diagnostic pathology laboratory is under way. It is our objective in this chapter to review the present and future impact of such advances in cellular and molecular biology on the pathological analysis of tumours.

Cancer genes and cancer proteins

At a molecular level, a tumour cell may be distinguished from its physiological neighbours by abnormalities in the structure or expression of certain genes. These genes may express features of the cell of origin, for example cytokeratins in squamous cell tumours or antigen receptors in B-cell malignancies. Alternatively, the abnormal genes may be fundamental to the cell's malignant behaviour and potential. Such tumour-associated genes fall into four distinct categories:

- oncogenes
- tumour suppressor genes
- DNA repair genes
- regulators of apoptosis.

In simple terms, oncogenes cause cells to proliferate, either by directly driving them through the cell cycle or by indirectly stimulating growth via receptor pathways. Oncogenes are normal cell proteins that become abnormally activated in malignant cells. Tumour suppressor genes are the converse, functioning in normal cells to oppose growth and proliferation they become abnormally inactivated in tumour cells when, in most cases, both alleles become non-functional. DNA repair genes may also become inactivated, causing accumulation of potentially damaging mutations. Finally, apoptosis regulators may promote cell survival when expressed abnormally in tumour cells, either by inactivation of proapoptotic genes or by activation of antiapoptotic genes. Current models of tumour development suggest that most, if not all, of these gene groups must be functionally altered during tumorigenesis.

Techniques

Preparation of tissue for analysis

Many techniques, including immunocytochemistry, DNA and RNA analysis, are optimized by appropriate harvesting of tissues. Some antigens are susceptible to proteolysis, and snap freezing in liquid nitrogen of all tissues should be encouraged, although formalin-fixed and paraffin-embedded tissues are still major sources of material for both diagnostic and research purposes. It is important that tumour material is collected in a way that prevents contamination by other cell types and without contact with RNA- and DNA-degrading enzymes. Microdissection of tissues can separate, for example, tumour from normal tissue, and may be used prior to DNA, RNA, or protein extraction. Laser microdissection and the use of optical tweezers enables the isolation of cells a few micrometres in diameter: such methods enable analysis of single cells from fresh, frozen, or paraffin-embedded tissue.[1]

Analysis of cancer proteins

Methods for the analysis of protein expression in tumours are generally immunological, requiring the production of antibody reagents specific for the protein of interest. The first step in the generation of such antibodies is to express the protein in an appropriate system such as bacteria or yeast; alternatively, synthesized peptides can be used.

T. Crook, P. Osin and B.A. Gusterson are supported by the registered charity Breakthrough Breast Cancer. Figure 1 was kindly provided by Dr Michael O'Hare, through a collaboration between Oxford Glycosciences and the Ludwig Institute for Cancer Research. Figure 2 was provided by Dr Jane Shipley. The image in Figure 3 is by courtesy of Affymetrix, Inc. (Santa Clara, CA).

Injection of the protein into experimental animals induces proliferation of B-lymphocyte clones which produce immunoglobulins directed against epitopes on the injected protein. Serum collected from the animal will contain a heterogeneous group of antibodies recognizing different epitopes of the protein, and such serum constitutes a polyclonal antibody. Alternatively, individual B-cell clones synthesizing antibody against a specific epitope can be isolated, immortalized by fusion with myeloma cells, and used as an unlimited source of that antibody: these antibodies are termed monoclonal.

Immunocytochemistry

Immunocytochemistry may be performed on frozen or paraffin-fixed sections, although not all antibodies can be used for both types of preparation. A dual-layer method is normally used, where the monoclonal or polyclonal antibody of choice is allowed to bind, with subsequent washing to remove background staining. A second layer of antibody, directed to the first antibody, is then applied: cross-species recognition is frequently used. The second layer is labelled for detection, for example with horseradish peroxidase. Polyclonal antibodies can demonstrate high sensitivity in immunocytochemical analysis because of the number of epitopes they recognize on the target protein; however, their specificity is often lower than that of monoclonal antibodies. Figure 1(a) shows an undifferentiated tumour, which the pathologist cannot diagnose. By staining the same tumour with an antibody that recognizes an epitope on the Ki-1 antigen (CD30) it is possible to diagnose a large cell lymphoma (Fig. 1(b)).

Western blotting

In this technique, a detergent extract of tissue is resolved on a denaturing sodium dodecyl sulphate/polyacrylamide gel. Under these conditions, the proteins in the tissue extract migrate as a function of their molecular weight, the effects of charge being minimized by the sodium dodecyl sulphate (detergent) present in the gel. Following electrophoresis, the proteins are transferred to a nitrocellulose filter where they become immobilized. Incubating this filter with antibodies to the protein of interest allows estimation of the steady-state level of that protein, provides information about the size of the protein, and may indicate the expression of abnormal forms of the protein. Such Western analysis is labour intensive, and requires the tissue of interest to be well preserved: it is usually inappropriate for studies of formalin-fixed, paraffin-embedded tissue sections. Moreover, Western blotting provides no information about the particular cell type in which expression is occurring, which may be important in the analysis of tumours which contain normal stromal tissue or lymphocyte infiltration. Such disadvantages limit the value of Western blotting in the routine analysis of tumours, and the enhanced sensitivity of immunocytochemistry, together with its applicability to both paraffin-embedded and frozen material, makes it the preferred technique.

Protein fingerprinting

Another approach is to investigate cell proteins by 'protein fingerprinting' using high-resolution, two-dimensional gel electrophoresis (Fig. 2). Proteins are electrotransferred on to an inert immobilizing matrix, fragmented by proteolysis or extracted by detergent, and the peptides generated separated by reverse-phase high-performance liquid chromatography. The method has previously been limited by

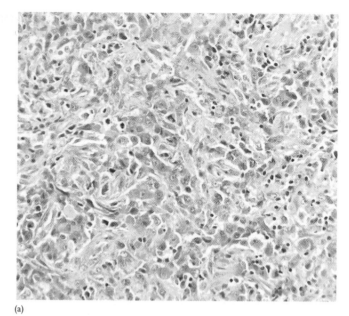
(a)

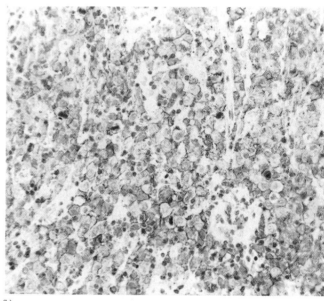
(b)

Fig. 1 (a) This shows a large celled undifferentiated tumour stained with haematoxylin and eosin. This can be diagnosed as a high grade cancer but there is a broad differential diagnosis, including an anaplastic carcinoma and lymphoma. (b) The same tumour, stained immunocytochemically with an antibody that recognizes an epitope on the Ki-1 antigen, shows the typical membrane staining seen in anaplastic large cell lymphomas.

difficulties in resolving protein spots and the absence of suitable databases. However, computer-assisted two-dimensional gel electrophoresis analysis, protein microsequencing technology, and mass spectrometry now enable rapid and reliable quantification, assessment of protein patterns, and direct sequencing of proteins. A further advantage is that differences in phosphorylation and glycosylation of proteins can be identified. A World Wide Web site containing comprehensive, updated, two-dimensional gel electrophoresis databases for different normal and tumour tissues should, in future, allow

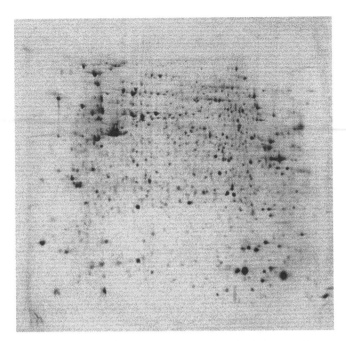

Fig. 2 This is an example of a two dimensional electrophoresis gel (2-D gel) of a protein extract of a human breast tumour. Each spot represents a different protein or a protein that has been modified by a process such as phosphorylation. The proteins are separated by size in the vertical dimension and by charge in the horizontal dimension. The sequence of the proteins can then be identified by mass spectrometry.

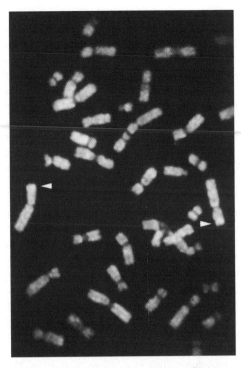

Fig. 3 Example of CGH analysis. The DNA from a neuroblastoma cell line and normal DNA were co-hybridized to normal metaphase chromosomes. The arrows indicate an amplicon on chromosome 2 corresponding to genomic amplification (multiple gene copies) of the NMYC gene. (See also Plate 1 for coloured representation.)

unification of methods and the construction of a general human protein index.[2] Such a database could be used for gene function analysis and for diagnostic and screening purposes, especially in the case of tumour-specific proteins.

Analysis of chromosomal abnormalities

Chromosomal abnormalities are frequently found in malignant cells. Many abnormalities are recurrent, and may be specific to tumour types, signifying underlying genetic abnormalities with direct involvement in tumorigenesis. Chromosome abnormalities are often multiple and complex in solid tumours: their analysis has historically been difficult using tissue sections, but the significance of particular changes is, with newer technology, becoming clearer. In haematological malignancies, individual cells are more easily analysed, abnormalities are found more straightforwardly, and many close associations between chromosome abnormalities, disease type, and prognosis have been identified.

Banding analysis

Detection of chromosome abnormalities has traditionally been performed through banding analysis of metaphase chromosomes. Cultured cells are treated with a microtubular toxin such as colchicene and the cells placed in hypotonic saline, where they swell, releasing their contents when dripped on to a microscope slide. The method has several disadvantages and subtle abnormalities may be missed. The t(12;21) translocation in childhood acute lymphoblastic leukaemia, for example, is not recognized by conventional cytogenetic techniques,

despite its being the commonest translocation in childhood leukaemia.[3] Metaphases may also be difficult to obtain in some malignant cells; indeed, in acute and chronic lymphoid malignancies, tumour cells are frequently resistant to mitogenic stimulation and metaphases are more likely to derive from normal cells, producing a falsely normal cytogenetic picture.

Fluorescent *in situ* hybridization-based techniques

In its simplest form, fluorescent *in situ* hybridization involves the hybridization of conjugated probes to metaphase chromosomes, and visualization of the probe by fluorescent microscopy. The analysis can be improved using charge coupled device cameras and computer imaging. Translocations can be detected using DNA probes for the chromosomal regions involved, labelled with different fluorescent colours that coalesce on juxtaposition, while chromosome aneuploidy can be determined using alpha satellite probes specific for centromeres. The main limitations of metaphase fluorescent *in situ* hybridization include the difficulty of obtaining metaphases from some tumour cells, the need to target specific abnormalities with specific probes, and the low resolution of hybridization, of the order of about 3 Mb.

Recent adaptations to the basic technique can help circumvent such problems.[4] Multicolour fluorescent *in-situ* hybridization, for example, utilizes 24 different colours or fluorochromes to 'paint' the individual chromosomes, enabling analysis of complex karyotypic abnormalities. Comparative genomic hybridization is a method particularly suited to the identification of numerical chromosome abnormalities, large deletions, and amplifications (Fig. 3).[5] The DNA produced and normal reference DNA are differentially labelled with fluorochromes and hybridized to normal metaphase chromosomes under competitor conditions with unlabelled DNA. A fluorescence ratio outside the normal range at a particular chromosome location is indicative of a change in copy number in that region. The major advantage of comparative genomic hybridization is the possibility of a whole genome screen in one experiment, and more than 1500 tumours have now been studied using comparative genomic hybridization. By combining the approach with the polymerase chain reaction (PCR) using degenerate oligonucleotide primers, analysis of archival material and small regions of specimens is now possible.[6],[7]

Interphase fluorescent *in situ* hybridization obviates the requirement for dividing tumour cells *in vitro*, and indeed can be used on frozen sections, although sectioning can cause loss of genomic material from the nucleus, and resolution is variable due to the complex folding of DNA. The combined use of fluorescent *in situ* hybridization and immunostaining (known as 'FICTION'), marries genetic abnormalities with cell phenotype, while other emerging techniques can correlate findings from morphology and fluorescent *in situ* hybridization at a cellular level. Finally, fibre-fluorescent *in situ* hybridization involves hybridization of probes to DNA fibres fixed on glass slides, allowing analysis with differently coloured contiguous probes, resulting in a 'colour barcode' of 250 kbytes or more. Breaks, deletions, and other rearrangements within such a barcode may thus be clearly defined.

Analysis of DNA abnormalilies

With the increased application of molecular biology, it has become clear that many mutations in cancer genes are not apparent at the cytogenetic level. As a result, it has become increasingly important to identify genes themselves, and relevant changes within their structure.

Southern blotting

Prior to the advent of PCR technology, molecular analysis of genetic change in human cancer was largely restricted to observation of gross alterations or deletions which could be detected by Southern blotting. In this technique, DNA is digested by restriction enzymes and the resulting fragments resolved by electrophoresis; the gel is then blotted on to filter paper, and the fragments probed with radiolabelled copies of the region of interest. In some cases, valuable information could be obtained from such studies. For example, the rearrangement caused by translocation of the c-*myc* oncogene to the Ig heavy chain locus in Burkitt's lymphoma could be detected by Southern blotting.[8] Similarly, amplification of *myc* in some tumours (for example N-*myc* in neuroblastoma) was easily identified.[9] At the single-nucleotide level, genes in which mutations occur at restricted locations could be studied by the use of a series of oligonucleotide probes, each complementary to a certain base substitution. Careful control of conditions permitted hybridization only of perfectly matched probes and thereby allowed identification of specific point mutations. This approach, although valuable when applied to the *ras* family of oncogenes, had limited applicability and was time-consuming and labour-intensive.[10]

The polymerase chain reaction (PCR) and related techniques

The PCR has revolutionized analysis of gene structure. The simplicity of the technique has allowed its widespread use in research laboratories

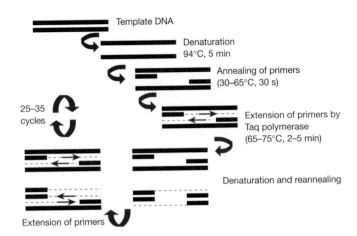

Fig. 4 The polymerase chain reaction. See text for explanation and applications.

and now in routine diagnostic pathology. The basis of the PCR is outlined in Fig. 4. In essence, the technique consists of a series of cycles in which DNA is subjected to sequential steps of denaturation by heating, annealing to oligonucleotide primers which flank the sequences to be amplified, and extension of the primers using a DNA polymerase. The discovery of thermostable DNA polymerases in bacteria living in hot springs obviated the requirement to add fresh enzyme after each denaturation step, and allowed the entire procedure to be performed in dedicated thermal cycling blocks with a single aliquot of enzyme. Since the initial description of the PCR, numerous modifications have been described and applied to problems in molecular pathology.

Screening for DNA sequence changes by PCR-based methods

The ability of the PCR to amplify large amounts of DNA from small samples has allowed the development of methods to analyse the sequence of individual genes in tumour series. In one of the first studies using the PCR, sequences encoding p53 were amplified from DNA, cloned into bacteriophage vectors, and mutations determined by sequencing mass cultures.[11] This revealed that *p53* mutation was a common event in many human tumours and prompted a great many studies of the sequence of potential cancer genes.

Detection of mutations has now been considerably simplified by screening techniques which detect the presence of mutations without necessitating sequencing of multiple clones for each tumour. This is particularly helpful in the analysis of DNA from tumours where the presence of contaminating normal tissue makes direct sequencing unreliable. One popular screening technique is single-strand conformation polymorphism analysis.[12] DNA is amplified by the conventional PCR, usually in the presence of a radioactive nucleotide to permit later detection of the amplified fragment. Following the PCR, the amplified DNA fragment is denatured by heating, then resolved on non-denaturing acrylamide gels. Fragments which contain sequence changes exhibit a pattern of altered mobility and can then be isolated and cloned for sequencing analysis. The sensitivity of single-strand conformation polymorphism analysis allows detection of mutant alleles at a frequency as low as 5 per cent. It has been extensively used in analysis of the structure of both tumour suppressor genes

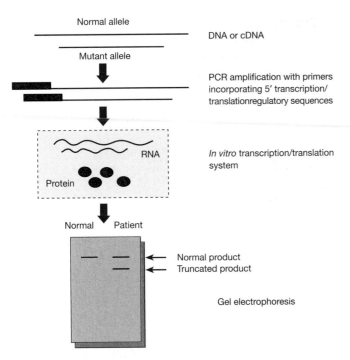

Normal allele

Mutant allele

DNA or cDNA

PCR amplification with primers incorporating 5′ transcription/translationregulatory sequences

RNA

Protein

In vitro transcription/translation system

Normal   Patient

Normal product
Truncated product

Gel electrophoresis

Fig. 5 The protein truncation test. The use of this test for detecting truncating mutations in DNA or RNA from human cancers is described in the text and in Powell *et al.*[13]

such as *p53* and *RB* (retinoblastoma gene), and oncogenes such as members of the *ras* family.

A second technique, particularly applicable to the analysis of genes with large coding sequences, is the protein truncation test (Fig. 5).[13] In this technique, the sequences of interest are amplified from genomic DNA or cDNA by PCR. The forward primer for the PCR incorporates sequences which bind bacteriophage RNA polymerase enzymes; thus, the addition of the amplified sequences to a transcription–translation reaction, in wheatgerm or reticulocyte lysate, results in the synthesis of protein encoded by the amplified sequences. The protein can then be resolved on a standard sodium dodecyl sulphate/polyacrylamide gel. The presence of truncating mutations in the amplified DNA is shown by the synthesis of proteins of lower molecular weight than those encoded by the wild-type sequence; the mutations can then be verified by sequencing. This approach is particularly useful for the analysis of genes in which truncating, rather than missense, mutations are the predominant form of genetic change.

Detection of loss of heterozygosity

The concept of a tumour suppressor gene was introduced by Knudson following studies of familial retinoblastoma.[14] Cells carrying one mutant and one wild-type allele of the *RB* gene were phenotypically normal, although there was an increased risk of cancer development. This led to a two-hit hypothesis of oncogenesis, where mutation in one allele of a tumour suppressor gene is followed by loss of the remaining wild-type allele, or 'loss of heterozygosity'. Since malignant change occurs only when both wild-type alleles of *RB* are lost, the term recessive oncogene, synonymous with tumour suppressor gene, is used by some investigators.

This scenario represents a paradigm for a large number of tumour suppressor genes and searches for sites of consistent loss of heterozygosity have proved helpful in localizing tumour suppressor genes. Before the PCR, such experiments relied on the use of restriction fragment length polymorphisms. Restriction fragment length polymorphisms occur as a result of point mutations, usually in noncoding regions of the genome, which vary between individuals. Restriction fragment length polymorphism analysis requires both tumour and normal tissue, and several micrograms of high-molecular-weight DNA for Southern blotting, which cannot be obtained from formalin-fixed tissue. Studies of solid tumour biopsies which contained a significant proportion of normal tissue were frequently unreliable, and although microdissection of normal and tumour tissues from the same tissue section overcame this problem, the low molecular weight and poor yield of the DNA often precluded the use of restriction fragment length polymorphisms analysis.

With the PCR came the identification of dinucleotide and trinucleotide repeats that have transformed studies of loss of heterozygosity in cancer. The repeats consist of variable numbers of reiterated di-, tri-, or tetranucleotides, called microsatellites. These simple repeats occur throughout the genome and are highly polymorphic. Moreover, the sizes of DNA fragments which contain these repeats are small enough to be easily amplified from formalin-fixed, paraffin-embedded, archival pathology specimens. Numerous markers are now available for each chromosomal arm and allelotyping of panels of tumours to find common sites of loss of heterozygosity can be easily performed.

Analysis of abnormalities of RNA

Meaningful DNA changes are usually confined to the coding and regulatory regions of genes. One approach to analysing cancer-related change is therefore to study abnormalities at the RNA level. RNA-based techniques suffer from two main problems: the easy degradation of RNA, and the difficulty in obtaining sufficient RNA, particularly in the analysis of low-abundance transcripts.

Northern blotting

Specific transcripts can be detected in RNA preparations by blotting and hybridization, using techniques similar to Southern blotting for DNA, but using denaturing conditions for electrophoresis. The method is time-consuming, easily subject to RNA degradation, and often relies on large amounts of tumour material without contaminating normal tissue. Small genetic changes cannot be detected, although some degree of quantification of RNA expression is possible. Generally, the advantages are outweighed by the disadvantages of this technique, and it has little place in the diagnostic pathology laboratory.

Reverse transcription PCR

In the reverse transcription PCR, RNA is isolated from the tissue of interest and converted into complementary DNA (cDNA) using a retroviral reverse transcriptase enzyme (Fig. 6). The cDNA then serves as a template for a PCR, the products of which can be visualized by resolution on agarose gels. The simplicity of the technique has made it an extremely popular method for the detection of gene expression but its use has been limited by difficulties in the quantification of products. Recent technology is overcoming this, using competitive methods or 'real-time PCR', where the rate of appearance of the product of the PCR is measured. This technique shows promise for

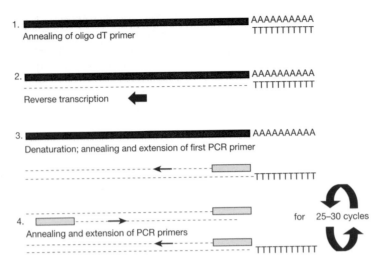

Fig. 6 Reverse transcription PCR. The use of this technique to detect gene expression, and its application to the analysis of human cancer is described in the text.

quantifying minimal residual disease and has allowed the development of automated, sensitive, high-throughput assays for detection of various degrees of gene expression at the RNA level.[15]

Representational difference analysis

Other modifications of the PCR have been applied to the identification of RNA differentially represented in two cell populations. Representational difference analysis, for example, has proved to be valuable in identifying infectious agents implicated in neoplasia. In this technique, genomic DNA is prepared from tumour and matched normal tissue and cut into small, blunt-ended fragments by restriction digestion. Short oligonucleotides, called adaptors, are then ligated on to the ends of the DNA from the tissue in which the novel sequences are being sought (almost always the tumour). The adapted DNA is then mixed with the normal DNA under conditions which favour hybridization of sequences common to the two populations. DNA sequences unique to the tumour fail to hybridize and can then be amplified by PCR using the sequences in the adaptors as priming sites. Such technology resulted in the identification of human herpesvirus type 8 as the likely causative agent of Kaposi's sarcoma.[16]

In situ hybridization

In situ hybridization is used to detect messenger RNA transcripts within fixed tissues or tissue sections. By this means, gene expression can be correlated with tissue architecture and areas of tumour infiltration. Probes are usually made with antisense RNA in which incorporation of labelled nucleotides enables localization of transcripts after hybridization. Labelling may be radioactive or non-radioactive. The method can give false-positive results due to non-specific background staining or hybridization to homologous transcripts; furthermore, low-level transcription cannot be detected. In addition, gene expression at the mRNA level does not necessarily correlate with expression at the protein level. For example, mRNA from the antiapoptosis gene *BCL2* is highly expressed in germinal centres and at lower levels in mantle zones, while the inverse is true for Bcl2 protein when analysed by immunocytochemistry.[17]

A more sensitive alternative to *in situ* hybridization is *in situ* PCR, where reverse transcription and/or PCR cycles are performed on spun cells or tissue sections. This method is unsuitable for assessing relative levels of expression because of the amplification effect of the PCR and because of cross-contamination from neighbouring tissues; however, it may be used to identify, for example, low-level viral DNA.

Applications

Immunostaining, PCR, and other techniques have become fundamental tools for addressing the key issues in cancer pathology: the nature of the tumour, the extent of the tumour, the behaviour of the tumour, and the cause of the tumour. The following are some of the most clinically relevant applications of such tools to the pathological analysis of tumours.

Immunohistochemistry in the diagnosis of undifferentiated tumours

Immunohistochemistry is of great value in the diagnosis of undifferentiated tumours when light microscopy is unable to discern diagnostic features. In adults, undifferentiated tumours are often composed of large pleomorphic cells that could originate from poorly differentiated carcinoma, anaplastic large cell lymphoma, amelanotic melanoma, or, less commonly, sarcoma. The problem of differentiating between those possibilities has been at least partially overcome by immunohistochemical detection of different cytoskeletal components, membrane conjugates, and leukocyte differentiation markers. Expression of cytokeratins strongly suggests an epithelial origin for the tumour, leukocyte common antigen is evidence of lymphoid origin, while expression of S100 protein and HMB45 is characteristic of malignant melanoma. Antibodies to tissue subtypes can further reduce the diagnostic possibilities. For example, a tumour negative for cytokeratin 7 and positive for cytokeratin 20 is very likely to be an adenocarcinoma of colonic origin, while cytokeratins 1 and 10 are expressed only in squamous epithelium. Detection of tumour-specific antigens by immunostaining is also possible for some tumours: monoclonal carcinoembryonic antigen suggests colorectal tumour, CA125 is associated with ovarian tumours, and human gonadotrophin with germ cell tumours. Differential diagnosis of small round blue cell tumours of childhood represents a similar challenge for the histopathologist, especially when the tumour presents as a metastasis in the viscera or bone marrow. Here, diagnostic possibilities may include haematological malignancies such as leukaemia or lymphoma, neuroblastoma, medulloblastoma, rhabdomyosarcoma, and nephroblastoma. Leukocyte common antigen would suggest lymphoid malignancy; nerve-cell-specific neurofilament is suggestive of a neuroectodermal tumour, and the markers of skeletal muscle differentiation, desmin and myoglobin, are indicative of rhabdomyosarcoma.

However, it is important to note that there is no antigen that is absolutely specific for any type of tumour, and neoplasms, especially when poorly differentiated, can show a wide range of aberrant protein expression: nephroblastoma, for example, can express markers of rhabdoid differentiation. Immunohistochemistry by no means replaces routine microscopic examination, but is a useful tool for verification of a suspected diagnosis.

Immunocytochemistry in the grading and staging of solid tumours

Most tumour grading systems include the analysis of cellular proliferation. In addition to the simple counting of mitotic figures in haematoxylin and eosin tissue sections, a number of immunocytochemically detectable markers of proliferation are now available to the pathologist. These include the nuclear antigen Ki67, expressed in all phases of the cell cycle except G_0, and proliferating cell nuclear antigen.

Staging of solid tumours may also be aided by immunocytochemical techniques, through assessment of dissemination of the tumour to distant sites such as lymph nodes and bone marrow. There is now good evidence that the presence of micrometastatic disease is strongly associated with the risk of relapse in tumours such as breast cancer.[18] In surgery for breast tumours, axillary lymph node dissection removes 10 to 30 nodes; generally, a single haematoxylin and eosin tissue section is examined from each for the presence of metastatic disease. This practice of sampling only a single section from each node results in a high false-negative rate and small micrometastases are likely to be undetectable. One approach to improving detection of micrometastatic disease is to seek expression of epithelial proteins such as keratins within potentially affected nodes. An early immunocytochemical study, using antibodies to cytokeratins and epithelial membrane antigen, detected micrometastases in 15 per cent of lymph nodes previously designated as tumour negative.[19] However, although this and other studies validated the principle of using specific protein markers in detection of micrometastases, the superior sensitivity of the reverse transcription PCR may prove more clinically useful.

Immunophenotyping in the classification of haematological disease

Many haematological malignancies are characterized by the expression of proteins that correspond to stages of differentiation in their normal physiological counterparts. Such cluster differentiation antigens are usually cell surface proteins. The pattern of cluster differentiation antigens is revealed by immunophenotyping, using monoclonal antibodies in combination with enzymatic staining or flow cytometry. Some antigens define broad groups such as myeloid or lymphoid, or B- or T-cell origin, while others serve to characterize disease type more specifically.

A widening repertoire of antigens and the increased use of flow cytometry have made the technique more powerful, and depending on the range of monoclonal antibodies selected for screening, phenotypic profiles can be established with important roles in determining diagnosis, risk group, and prognosis. Such profiles are increasingly being based upon variations in antigen density, quantitated by flow cytometry, rather than simply the presence or absence of antigen. Markers such as immunoglobulin light chains (— or λ) can also be used to establish the clonality of lymphoid cells.

A degree of caution is needed when interpreting the results of immunophenotyping. Individual antigens correlate poorly with disease type and prognosis. Although absent expression of certain adhesion molecules, such as cluster differentiation 44 (CD44) isoforms, has been associated with dissemination of lymphomatous disease, generally the overall pattern gives a much more reliable picture of tumour characteristics than any single cluster differentiation marker.[20] Furthermore, the choice of antigens used for screening is critical, and depends both on the clinical situation and on the results of morphological examination. Mantle cell lymphoma and chronic lymphocytic leukaemia, for example, have very similar immunophenotypes (and, indeed, morphologies) but can usually be distinguished by CD23 expression which is negative in mantle cell lymphoma—an important differential, considering the widely divergent prognoses for the two diseases.

Prognostic protein markers in solid tumours

As the number of potential genes of interest in cancer has grown, so has the number of antibodies available for investigation. Over the last 15 years, many antibodies to various cellular components have been claimed to be useful in diagnosis and prediction of tumour behaviour. Of these, only a limited number are routinely used—many other reagents have failed to live up to early expectations. Nevertheless, several extremely promising new markers with clear prognostic value have recently been described, and it is probable that at least a subset of these will soon be in routine use.

Perhaps one of the most exciting areas of progress in the histopathology of solid tumours has come from the immunocytochemistry of proteins involved in regulation of the cell cycle. A simplified model of the cycle is shown in Fig. 7. Proliferation follows an orderly progression controlled by the cyclin-dependent kinases and their regulatory subunits, the cyclins. The cyclins associate with, and activate, the cyclin-dependent kinases, which then phosphorylate substrates involved in progression of the cell cycle, amongst which the retinoblastoma protein (Rb) is pivotal. The activity of the cyclin/cyclin-dependent kinase complexes is inhibited by a group of proteins known as the cyclin-dependent kinase inhibitors which associate with the cyclin/cyclin-dependent kinase complexes. One group, the INK4 group, which includes p14^{ARF}, p15, p16^{INK4a}, and p18, specifically inhibits the CDK4 and CDK6 kinases which function in the G_1 phase of the cell cycle. The other group of cyclin-dependent

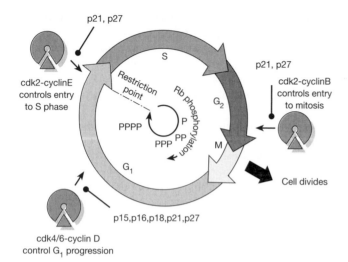

Fig. 7 A representation of the eukaryotic cell cycle. In this simplified model, progression through the cycle is regulated at key points by the state of phosphorylation of the retinoblastoma protein. This in turn is regulated by the relative activities of the cylin-dependent kinases (CDK) together with their associated regulatory subunits the cyclins, and the cyclin-dependent kinase inhibitors (CDKI) which include p15, p16, p18, p21, and p27. Many of these proteins have roles in human cancer.

kinase inhibitors includes p21^{Waf1}, p27^{Kip1}, and p57^{Kip2}. These cyclin-dependent kinase inhibitors are able to associate with all known cyclin/cyclin-dependent kinase pairs and thus affect progression through all phases of the cell cycle, acting as suppressors of proliferation.

It is now recognized that cell cycle proteins may have roles in neoplasia, and a number of recent studies have revealed that the expression of some of these proteins may be prognostically significant. For example, an increasing body of evidence has identified p27$Kip1$ as a powerful prognostic factor in a number of solid tumours. Initial reports revealed that breast cancer survival was significantly higher in patient groups which expressed p27^{Kip1} protein.[21] In a subsequent study, p27^{Kip1} expression in stage T1a and b small breast carcinomas was evaluated. P27^{Kip1} expression, with nodal status, was shown to be the only independent prognostic factor of many variables examined.[22] A similar study showed that p27^{Kip1} was an independent prognostic factor for colorectal cancer, lack of p27^{Kip1} expression being associated with poor prognosis.[23] These observations raised the possibility that analysis of p27^{Kip1} expression might be useful in selection of patients who would benefit from adjuvant therapy. Other studies revealed an association between the down-regulation of p27^{Kip1} and the development of colorectal metastases, and correlation of p27^{Kip1} with survival in non-small-cell lung cancer, Barrett's associated adenocarcinoma, and in prostate carcinoma.[24]–[27]

Whereas cyclin-dependent kinase inhibitors inhibit cell cycle progression, overexpression of cyclins promotes cell cycle progression. Expression of cyclin D1 has been correlated with favourable prognosis in breast cancer.[28] The simultaneous expression of cyclin D1 and the oestrogen receptor identifies tumours likely to respond to tamoxifen, whereas low-level expression of cyclin D1 increases the risk of relapse and death. To further explore the contribution of molecular predictive factors, clinically oriented randomized trials should not be conducted without translational research. However, at the moment clinical decisions relating to prognostic factors must still be based on those factors obtained from larger studies with longer follow-up than those available for cell cycle markers.[29] Other studies suggest that cyclin E may be a valuable prognostic factor in breast cancer.[30]

In addition to the clear importance of cell cycle promoters and inhibitors, other proteins may be of prognostic significance, for example cell receptors. Antibodies against both oestrogen receptors and progesterone receptors provide reliable evidence of expression in both frozen and formalin-fixed paraffin-embedded breast tissue sections, analysis giving a reasonable prediction of response to anti-endocrine therapy. Another type of marker is naturally produced serum autoantibody, directed to mutant proteins expressed in tumours. For example, the humoral antibody response to missense mutations in the *p53* gene can be immunocytochemically detected. Studies in lung cancer, in which *p53* mutation rates are as high as 70 per cent, have reported a prevalence of anti-p53 antibodies of 30 per cent, most being IgG.[31] The clinical utility of detecting these antibodies, and their role, if any, as indicators of early disease remains to be firmly established.

Prognostic protein markers in haematological malignancies

As for solid tumours, the expression of many cellular proteins has been studied for their prognostic value in haematological malignancies. Cell cycle regulators that have been associated with abnormal expression and poor outcome in leukaemias and lymphomas include p53, Rb, p27^{Kip1}, and cyclin D1.[32]–[35] Other proteins that may be prognostically important include the differentiation inhibitor factor nm23, increased expression of which may carry a worse prognosis in acute leukaemias.[36] Expression of the multidrug resistance protein p-glycoprotein in acute myeloid leukaemia confers resistance to cytotoxic therapies and a poor outcome, while in lymphomas, increased expression of Bcl2 appears to carry a poor prognosis.[37],[38] As a caveat, many studies of prognostic markers are in their early stages, and the relative importance of abnormalities in expression of these proteins remain, as in solid tumours, to be fully established.

Disease-associated cytogenetic changes

Analysis of large series of morphologically or histologically similar tumours can identify non-random genetic changes. One common abnormality in lymphoid malignancies, for example, is a translocation involving an immunoglobulin (Ig) locus or the T-cell receptor. The result of juxtaposing a distant gene to one of these loci is to place it under the influence of the Ig/T-cell receptor enhancer, resulting in a continuous transcriptional drive in B or T lymphoid cells. Genes translocated to these loci include:

- c-*myc* in Burkitt's lymphoma
- *CYCLIN D1* (*PRAD1*) in mantle cell lymphoma
- *BCL2* in follicular lymphoma
- *BCL6* in large cell lymphoma;
- *BCL10* in mucosa-associated lymphoid tissue (MALT) lymphoma
- *TAL1* and *TAL2* in T-cell acute lymphoblastic leukaemia (T-ALL).

Detection of such changes can define tumour subtypes and aid prognostic predictions. Screening may be performed by banding analysis of chromosomes, although fluorescent *in situ* hybridization can pinpoint the regions involved within chromosomes. Such techniques may also be applied to detection of quantitative changes in chromosome number, for example in acute lymphoblastic leukaemia where hyper- and hypodiploidy imply good and adverse prognoses respectively.[39]

Although solid tumours have historically been less amenable to karyotypic analysis, consistent genetic abnormalities can be identified. Genomic abnormalities in one of three chromosomal regions, gains in 1q,8q, loss of 13q, are detected by comparative genomic hybridization in 91 per cent of breast tumours.[40] In addition to their diagnostic contribution, these data have been used in the search for and identification of novel oncogenes (gains, amplifications) and tumour suppressor genes (losses of chromosomal material).[41],[42] Similarly, genomic profiles of familial tumour syndromes have been helpful in identifying hereditary cancer predisposition genes (see Chapters 11.2, 17.3, and 19.2).

Cytogenetic models of tumour progression

Comparison of patterns of changes in chromosomal copy number in tumours at different stages of progression (*in situ* versus invasive, primary tumour versus metastasis) provides information about the genetic relationship between these groups.[43] Differences in genomic changes characteristic of *in situ* and invasive carcinomas of the breast have been demonstrated, while the genetic profile of lobular carcinoma *in situ* and atypical lobular hyperplasia, using comparative genomic hybridization on microdissected glands, suggests that these lesions represent a single entity.[44]–[46] Such studies are contributing to an understanding of the relationship between intraepithelial lesions and their malignant potential.

The PCR in the analysis of solid tumours

Tumour involvement and occult metastases

An illustration of the diagnostic potential of the PCR is provided by the use of reverse transcription PCR in the preoperative diagnosis of papillary carcinomas of the thyroid.[47] In this study, RNA was isolated from material obtained during fine needle aspiration biopsy and subjected to reverse transcription to generate cDNA. The PCR was then used to amplify sequences encoding oncofetal fibronectin, which is known to be differentially expressed in thyroid cancer. In this study, the sensitivity of tumour diagnosis was 96.9 per cent and the specificity 100 per cent.

Another promising application of the PCR is in the detection of metastatic disease in the lymph nodes of patients with solid tumours. Such metastases represent the most important prognostic indicator in many common solid tumours, but histopathological analysis of lymph nodes is subject to a high false-negative rate. The reverse transcription PCR has shown particular promise in detection of axillary lymph node micrometastasis in breast cancer. Keratins occur in intermediate filaments in epithelial cells and RNA expression of one cytokeratin, K19, is reported to have value as a marker of breast cancer micrometastasis in axillary nodes.[48] Likewise, MUC-1 is a membrane-associated epithelial mucin overexpressed in breast cancer but absent from normal lymph nodes. A reverse transcription PCR for MUC-1 expression detects micrometastases in 15 per cent of histologically normal lymph nodes.[49] Further evidence of the superior sensitivity of reverse transcription PCR over routine histology was

afforded in a study which showed that detection of positive axillary lymph nodes increased from 26 per cent by histology to 66 per cent by reverse transcription PCR for carcinoembryonic antigen.[50] Recently, the use of the reverse transcription PCR for mammaglobin and carcinoembryonic antigen to detect metastatic disease in sentinel nodes of patients with breast cancer has shown exceptionally promising results.[51]

Other sites of occult tumour dissemination may allow analysis by PCR. Mutations in *p53*, which are likely to occur as late events in colorectal cancer, can be detected in the plasma of patients with Dukes stage C and D tumours and in the urine of patients with transitional cell carcinoma.[52],[53] Another clinically relevant illustration of the remarkable power of PCR-based technology was afforded by the identification of oncogenic *ras* mutations in the stools of patients with colorectal cancer.[54] In this study, DNA was purified from the faeces of patients with premetastatic colorectal tumors in proximal and distal colonic epithelium, which were known to contain mutations in K-*ras*. The same mutations were detectable in the stools of eight out of nine cases. Since mutation in K-*ras* is known to precede overt metastasis, this suggests one means by which a non-invasive molecular test can detect tumours at the stage at which they are surgically curable. For pancreatic tumours K-*ras* analysis of pancreatic juice may help to discriminate pancreatitis from cancer.

Microsatellite instability

The length of microsatellites is stably maintained in normal cells, but losses or gains commonly occur in human cancer.[55] Profound microsatellite instability was first observed in hereditary non-polyposis colon cancer and is associated with mutations in DNA repair genes. Microsatellite instability has also been demonstrated in many types of sporadic cancer, where it does not appear to commonly involve mutation in recognized repair genes.[56] Although microsatellite instability can inactivate tumour suppressor genes such as the type II TGF-β receptor gene and *BAX*, it most commonly occurs in non-coding regions of the genome and reflects a general susceptibility to mutation.

Because microsatellite instability is a phenomenon characteristic of cancer cells, analysis of microsatellites is being explored as a possible molecular marker for the presence of malignancy. Its great advantage is that the genetic alteration can be easily identified with one set of PCR primers. The sensitivity of microsatellite instability detection is about one neoplastic cell in 500 normal cells lacking the changes in microsatellite length: sufficient for the detection of tumour in many clinical situations.[57] Certain microsatellites are particularly susceptible to instability in human cancer, particularly tetranucleotide repeats; furthermore, whereas some markers are unstable in many tumour types, others show a tight specificity for particular types of disease, which may prove clinically useful. Initial studies have shown promise, microsatellite instability being detectable by PCR in urine, sputum, and surgical margins from patients with bladder, lung, and head and neck cancer.[58] One retrospective study, applying microsatellite instability analysis to urine samples of patients with bladder cancer, revealed a detection rate of over 90 per cent.[59] Another, prospective, study succesfully detected 10 out of 11 recurrent tumours, two of which showed microsatellite instability in advance of clinically detectable recurrence.[60]

Tumour viruses (see Chapter 2.2)

A number of viruses are linked to human tumours. Use of the PCR has had a profound effect on their study, by enhancing the sensitivity of detection in tumour tissue and in enabling the identification and cloning of new viruses from cancers. Both aspects are well illustrated by recent developments in the study of human papillomaviruses. These viruses, most notably types 16, 18, and 31, are strongly associated with anogenital neoplasia, which includes cervical, anal, and vulval squamous carcinomas. Cervical epithelium can be easily sampled and exfoliated cells examined for the characteristic morphological features of human papillomavirus infection. Such analysis forms the basis of the Papanicolaou smear which identifies women at risk of cervical dysplasia and carcinoma; however, cytology inevitably misses a significant proportion of abnormal smears. Recent studies have examined the potential for PCR-based analysis of human papillomavirus to supplement cytology and improve the sensitivity and specificity of traditional approaches.[61] PCR analysis for the presence of human papillomavirus sequences is already performed in addition to traditional cytology in some countries. The availabilty of degenerate PCR primers which allow the detection of multiple different human papillomavirus types in a single PCR is likely to increase its value in such routine diagnostic applications.[62]

PCR in the analysis of haematological malignancies

Mutations of diagnostic and prognostic significance

Genetic changes are best characterized at the molecular level, rather than relying on chromosomal analysis. In haematological malignancies, fusion oncogenes are common products of translocation in, for example, the Philadelphia chromosome, formed from the translocation of part of the long arm of chromosome 9 to chromosome 22. The translocation juxtaposes the *ABL* locus on chromosome 9 to the *BCR* locus on chromosome 22; the chimeric fusion gene, *BCR–ABL*, encodes an activated tyrosine kinase with both oncogenic and antiapoptotic functions. The *BCR–ABL* fusion is an almost invariable feature of chronic myeloid leukaemia and the same fusion, albeit with a different breakpoint and size of fusion protein, is also seen in a subset of acute lymphoblastic leukaemia, where it is associated with a particularly poor prognosis. Even when the Philadelphia chromosome is cytogenetically absent, PCR can reveal the *BCR–ABL* abnormality, and is now used routinely in diagnosis. Other chimeric fusion genes with prognostic significance may also be detected by reverse transcription PCR using primers designed from either side of the fusion gene, thereby avoiding amplification of non-adjacent genes. The disadvantage is that abnormalities must be specifically sought, although multiplex PCR enables several different abnormalities to be detected in one test.

There also appear to be some abnormalities that place patients in higher risk groups than their disease subtype might suggest. Those with high-grade non-Hodgkin's lymphoma, for example, may do worse if they carry rearrangements of c-*myc*, *BCL6*, or *BCL2*.[63] As in solid tumours, inactivation of tumour suppressor genes is becoming increasingly recognized in haematological malignancies: deletion of *p15* or *p16* may signify progression to higher-grade disease in non-Hodgkin's lymphoma and childhood acute lymphoblastic leukaemia.[64],[65] *p53* mutations are more frequent in relapsed leukaemia

than *de novo* leukaemia and appear to be linked to poor outcome in many haematological malignancies, while mutation of *WT1*, the Wilm's tumour gene, has been associated with a poor prognosis in acute myeloid leukaemia and possibly acute lymphoblastic leukaemia.[66],[67] Microsatellite instability has been identified in leukaemias and lymphomas, although not to the same degree as in solid tumours; its significance is not yet clear.[68]

Clonality analysis

Some haematological malignancies, particularly lymphomas at an early stage, are difficult to distinguish from reactive changes. Evidence of monoclonality provides supporting evidence for neoplastic disease when other findings are equivocal, and *IgH* and *TCR* gene rearrangements may be used to demonstrate the clonal origin of lymphoid cells. These can be rapidly detected by PCR amplification, which has generally replaced the more laborious method of Southern blotting. Clonality detection in myeloid malignancies may be achieved, in females only, by identifying heterozygosity of a polymorphism(s) in the X chromosomes, where each polymorphism is evenly represented in normal cell populations due to random X-chromosome methylation, but skewed towards one or other form in clonal populations. The polymorphism may be of a gene, microsatellite, or restriction fragment length. Problems with clonality analysis include false-positives due to normal oligoclonality, particularly associated with lymphocyte activation or age-related changes in myelopoiesis, and false-negative results due to presumed mutation of primer sites in malignant cells.[69]

A combination of microdissection and PCR has allowed the study of protein and genetic changes within single cells. This has particular application for Hodgkin's disease, where the malignant Reed–Sternberg cells represent fewer than 5 per cent of total cells, but single-cell PCR has been used to establish the clonality of these cells.[70]

Minimal residual disease

Haematological malignancies are particularly amenable to the monitoring of minimal residual disease. Sites of minimal residual disease such as blood and bone marrow are accessible to serial testing, and molecular abnormalities such as fusion genes, or clonal changes such as *Ig/TCR* rearrangements, can serve as useful disease markers. Sensitive techniques are required to detect minimal residual disease, and most are based on PCR methodology, although both fluorescent *in-situ* hybridization and quantitative flow cytometry have been used in this application. PCR has the advantage of being applicable to small amounts of material which can, if necessary, be drawn from archival specimens.

There are, however, problems with monitoring for minimal residual disease with PCR. Some molecular changes, previously associated with specific diseases, have now been detected in normal tissue, including the translocations t(4;11), usually associated with acute lymphoblastic leukaemia; t(14;18), the signature of follicular lymphomas, and t(9;22), the Philadelphia chromosome.[71]–[73] Nor does the presence of minimal residual disease necessarily predict relapse: for example, transcripts from the t(8;21) translocation in the M2 subtype of acute myeloid leukaemia persist long into remission.[74] Some of these problems may be circumvented by measuring serial changes and intervening only when there appears to be an increase in the amount of residual disease. Ideally this requires quantitative

GeneChip® P53 Probe Array Image

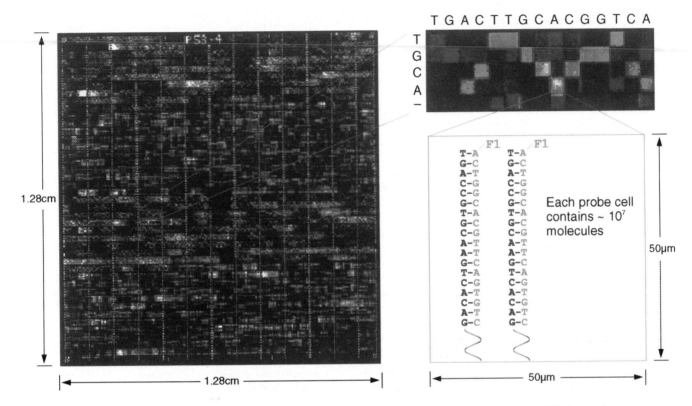

Fig. 8 This is an Affymetrix Gene Chip for the entire coding region of the human p53 tumour suppressor gene (exons 2–11). Probes on the array are arranged in sets of five. Each probe in the set is perfectly complementary to the reference sequence except for a mismatch position, called the 'substitution position'. At the substitution position, each of the four possible nucleotides (A,C,G,T) and a single base deletion are represented in the probe set.. Assay conditions optimize hybridization of the fluorescently labelled DNA target to the probe that best matches its sequence. This hybrid yields a higher fluorescence intensity relative to the four target:probe hybrid set. There are probe sets complementary to every base in the target gene, so each base along the gene is examined for the presence of mutant sequence (both missense and single base deletions). (See also Plate 2 for coloured representation.)

techniques, now possible with the advent of real-time PCR. One particular area in which monitoring of minimal residual disease has had direct therapeutic relevance has been in the care of patients after allogeneic bone marrow transplantation for chronic myeloid leukaemia.[75] In this situation, detection of *BCR–ABL* transcripts by reverse transcription PCR on bone marrow more than 6 months after transplantation is predictive of haematological relapse. If donor leukocytes are transfused at the point of molecular detection, patients may be restored to molecular remission without detectable *BCR–ABL* and with prolonged disease-free survival, whereas intervening at the time of frank haematological relapse carries a far worse prognosis.

The future: microarray technology

All human genes will be known and sequenced within the next few years. The next objective is to harness this information to improve methods of diagnosis, to identify new drug targets, and to identify inherited genetic differences that increase the risk of developing tumours.[76] Many companies have started to direct their attention to expression profiling at the protein level and, if the difficulties of sensitivity can be overcome, this may prove to be the best way forward for some applications.[77] Whilst these developments are taking place there are simpler ways that are already used to study large tumour series, including screening for loss of heterozygosity, mutation analysis, comparative genomic hybridization, and spectral karyotyping. The future is very exciting, but the explosion of data suggests that there will be a need to invest in as many people analysing the data as there are generating it.

One problem with tumour profiling is the huge number of potential cancer genes and cancer proteins that may have some clinical significance. Moreover, there is an intrinsic genetic instability in tumours, which leads to a strikingly high rate of genetic change: one estimate is that a new genetic anomaly occurs in a tumour in one out of every 10^5 tumour cells at each division.[78] Then there is the difficulty in correlating molecular abnormalities with clinical outcome, which requires good data management and, preferably, consensus in staging and treatment strategies. Creating adequate molecular and clinical databases is a rather formidable prospect, but large studies and pooling of information could establish the relative significance of molecular changes, allow a profile to be produced for any tumour, predict its response to treatment, and determine the best therapeutic strategy.

Technology to facilitate such an objective is now becoming available. A fundamental requirement is the ability to monitor the expression of numerous genes in parallel. One approach, pioneered by Vogelstein and co-workers, was termed serial analysis of gene expression.[79] An alternative approach which may eventually prove more applicable for routine use, involves the use of microarrays (Fig. 8). The first version of this technology utilized high-precision robots to print large numbers of cDNAs on to glass, with hybridization of radiolabelled cDNA prepared from total RNA. It demonstrated that such a system could allow measurement of differential expression of genes, including those of low abundance.

Microarray methods now under development depend on the ability to array full length cDNA or short oligonucleotides on glass slides, filters, or microchips at high density, by robotic imprinting or by *in situ* synthesis.[80],[81] The technology allows hundreds of thousands of individual spots to be put discretely in a 1 cm^2 array. In an open system, the objective is to identify new genes that are expressed, so a cDNA library is gridded out and then interrogated using RNA extracted from two different tissues, for example normal versus tumour. A closed system contains arrays of a single gene sequence, in order to identify point mutations in a DNA sample. All methods of analysis are based on the basic principles of hybridization and the probes used can be labelled with fluorochromes or radioactivity. Digital images are analysed by computer and different labelling intensities can give quantitative information. Obvious advantages of microarrays include their suitability for automation and their relatively low cost, which makes mass-production a feasibility.

The recently developed tissue microarrray technology will also prove a useful tool. The method is based on combining up to 1000 small tissue cylinders (0.6 mm in diameter), taken from a paraffin-embedded tissue block, into an array block. Serial sections taken from this array can then be used for detection of protein, DNA, or RNA targets by immunostaining, fluorescent *in-situ* hybridization analysis, or *in situ* hybridization. Large series of tumours can thus be studied in a short time.

The exploration of consistent changes in gene expression through microarrays will have implications for diagnosis and treatment. The expression patterns of genes with known function could be compared in different physiological and pathological conditions, while the profile of genes with unknown function could give a suggestion as to their possible biological role.[77] The first practical applications of microarrays are likely to be in the fields of diagnostic tests for mutations in genes such as *BRCA1* conferring tumour susceptibility, or in *p53* as an indicator of resistance to some forms of chemotherapy.[82]

References

1. Details on laser microdissection and its application can be found under the Human Genome Anatomy Project on the NCI Web Site (http://www.nci.nih.gov).

2. http://www.ludwig.edu.au/www/jpsl/jpslhome.htl (site under development).

3. Golub TR, *et al.* Fusion of the TEL gene on 12p13 to the AML1 gene on 21q22 in acute lymphoblastic leukaemia. *Proceedings of the National Academy of Sciences of the USA*, 1995; **92**: 4917–21.

4. Kluin PHM, Schuuring E. FISH and related techniques in the diagnosis of lymphoma. In: Wotherspoon AC (ed.) *Lymphoma cancer surveys*, vol. 30. New York: Cold Spring Harbor Laboratory Press, 1997: 3–20.

5. Kallionemi A, *et al.* Comparative genomic hybridisation for molecular cytogenetic analysis of solid tumours. *Science*, 1992; **258**: 818–21.

6. Telenius H, *et al.* Degenerate oligonucleotide-primed PCR: general amplification of target DNA by a single degenerate primer. *Genomics*, 1992; **13**: 718–25.

7. Speicher M, *et al.* Molecular cytogenetic analysis of formalin-fixed, paraffin-embedded solid tumours by comparative genomic hybridisation after DNA amplification. *Human Molecular Genetics*, 1993; **2**: 1907–14.

8. Erikson J, *et al.* Transcriptional activation of the translocated c-myc oncogene in Burkitt lymphoma. *Proceedings of the National Academy of Sciences of the USA*, 1983; **80**: 820–4.

9. Brodeur GM, *et al.* Amplification of N-myc in untreated human neuroblastomas correlates with advanced disease stage. *Science*, 1984; **2241**: 121–4.

10. Bos JL, *et al.* Prevalence of ras gene mutations in human colorectal cancers. *Nature*, 1987; **327**: 293–7.

11. Nigro JM, *et al.* Mutations in the p53 gene occur in diverse human tumour types. *Nature*, 1989; **342**: 705–8.

12. Orita M, *et al.* Detection of polymorphisms of human DNA by gel electrophoresis as single- strand conformation polymorphisms. *Proceedings of the National Academy of Sciences of the USA*, 1989; **86**: 2766–70.

13. Powell SM, *et al.* Molecular diagnosis of familial adenomatous polyposis. *New England Journal of Medicine*, 1993; **329**: 1982–7.

14. Knudson AG Jr. Mutation and cancer: statistical study of retinoblastoma. *Proceedings of the National Academy of Sciences of the USA*, 1971; **68**: 820–3.

15. Gerard CJ, *et al.* Improved quantitation of minimal residual disease in multiple myeloma using real-time polymerase chain reaction and plasmid-DNA complementarity determining region III standards. *Cancer Research*, 1998; **58**: 3957–64.

16. Chang Y, *et al.* Identification of herpesvirus-like DNA sequences in AIDS-associated Kaposi's sarcoma. *Science*, 1994; **266**: 1865–9.

17. Chleq-Deschamps CM, *et al.* Topographical dissociation of BCL2 messenger RNA and protein expression in human lymphoid tissues. *Blood*, 1993; **81**: 293–8.

18. Neville AM, *et al.* Occult axillary lymph-node micrometastases in breast cancer. *The Lancet*, 1990; **336**: 759.

19. Trojani M, *et al.* Micrometastases to axillary lymph nodes from invasive lobular carcinoma of the breast: detection by immunocytochemistry and prognostic significance. *British Journal of Cancer*, 1987; **56**: 838–9.

20. Jennings CD, Foon KA. Recent advances in flow cytometry: application to the diagnosis of haematological malignancy. *Blood*, 1997; **90**: 2863–92.

21. Porter PL, *et al.* Expression of cell-cycle regulators p27^{Kip1} and cyclin E, alone and in combination, correlate with survival in young breast cancer patients. *Nature Medicine*, 1997; **3**: 222–5.

22. Tan P, *et al.* The cell cycle inhibitor p27 is an independent prognostic marker in small (T1a,b) invasive breast carcinomas. *Cancer Research*, 1997; **57**: 1259–63.

23. Loda M, *et al.* Increased proteasome-dependent degradation of the cyclin-dependent kinase inhibitor p27 in aggressive colorectal carcinomas. *Nature Medicine*, 1997; **3**: 231–4.

24. Thomas GV, *et al.* Down-regulation of p27 is associated with development of colorectal adenocarcinoma metastases. *American Journal of Pathology*, 1998; **153**: 681–7.

25. Esposito V, *et al.* Prognsotic role of the cyclin-dependent kinase inhibitor p27 in non-small cell lung cancer. *Cancer Research*, 1997; **57**: 3381–5.

26. Singh SP, *et al.* Loss or altered subcellular localization of p27 in Barrett's associated adenocarcinoma. *Cancer Research*, 1998; **58**: 1730–5.

27. Yang RM, *et al.* Low p27 expression predicts poor disease-free survival in patients with prostate cancer. *Journal of Urology*, 1998; **159**: 941–5.

28. Gillett C, *et al.* Cyclin D1 and prognosis in human breast cancer. *International Journal of Cancer (Predictive Oncology)*, 1996; **69**: 92–9.

29. Nielsen NH, Emdin SO, Landberg G. Deregulation of G1 cyclins and pRb alterations in oestrogen receptor negative breast cancer with poor prognosis. *Proceedings of the American Association for Cancer Research*, 1996; **37**: 28.

30. Dou QP, Pardee AB, Keyomarsi K. Cyclin E- a better prognostic marker for breast cancer than cyclin D? *Nature Medicine*, 1996; **2**: 254.

31. Lubin R, *et al.* Serum p53 antibodies as early markers of lung cancer. *Nature Medicine*, 1995; **1**: 701–2.

32. Koduru PR, *et al.* Correlation between mutation in P53, p53 expression, cytogenetics, histologic type, and survival in patients with B cell non-Hodgkin's lymphoma. *Blood*, 1997; **90**: 4078–91.

33. Sauerbrey A, *et al.* Expression of the retinoblastoma tumor suppressor gene (RB-1) in acute leukemia. *Leukaemia and Lymphoma*, 1998; **28**: 275–83.

34. Vrhovac R, *et al.* Prognostic significance of the cell cycle inhibitor p27^{kip1} in chronic B-lymphocytic leukemia. *Blood*, 1998; **91**: 4694–700.

35. Hashimoto Y, *et al.* Intranuclear expression of cyclin D1 protein as a useful prognostic marker for mantle cell lymphoma. *Fukushima Journal of Medical Science*, 1997; **43**: 87–98.

36. Yokoyama A, *et al.* Evaluation by multivariate analysis of the differentiation inhibitory factor nm23 as a prognostic factor in acute myelogenous leukemia and application to other hematologic malignancies. *Blood*, 1998; **91**: 1845–51.

37. Leith CP, Willman CL. Prognostic markers in acute leukemia. *Current Opinion in Hematology*, 1996 **3**: 329–34.

38. Kramer MH, *et al.* Clinical significance of bcl2 and p53 protein expression in diffuse large B cell lymphoma: a population-based study. *Journal of Clinical Oncology*, 1996; **14**: 2131–8.

39. Chessels JM, *et al.* Cytogenetics and prognosis in childhood lymphoblastic leukaemia: results of MRC UKALL X. *British Journal of Haematology*, 1997; **99**: 93–100.

40. Tirkkonen M, *et al.* Molecular cytogenetics of breast cancer by CGH. *Genes, Chromosomes and Cancer*, 1998; **21**: 177–84.

41. Chen T, Sahin A, Aldaz CM. Deletion map of chromosome 16q in ductal carcinoma *in situ* of the breast: refining a putative tumour suppressor region. *Cancer Research*, 1996; **56**: 5605–9.

42. Courjal F, Theiller C. Comparative genomic hybridisation analysis of breast tumours with predetermined profiles of DNA amplification. *Cancer Research*, 1997; **57**: 4368–77.

43. James LA, Mitchell ELD, Menasce L, Varley JM. Comparative genomic hybridisation of ductal carcinoma *in situ* of the breast: identification of regions of DNA amplification and deletion in common with invasive breast cancer. *Oncogene*, 1997; **14**: 1059–65.

44. Kuukasjarvi T, *et al.* Genetic changes in intraductal breast cancer detected by comparative genomic hybridisation. *American Journal of Pathology*, 1997; **150**: 1465–71.

45. Nishizaki T, *et al.* Genetic alterations in lobular breast cancer by comparative genomic hybridisation. *International Journal of Cancer*, 1997; **74**: 513–17.

46. Lu YJ, *et al.* Comparative genomic hybridisation analysis of lobular carcinoma *in situ* and atypical lobular hyperplasia and potential roles for gains and losses of genetic material in breast neoplasia. *Cancer Research*, 1998; **58**: 4721–7.

47. Takano T, *et al.* Accurate and objective preoperative diagnosis of thyroid papillary carcinomas by reverse transcription-PCR detection of oncofetal fibronectin messenger RNA in fine-needle aspiration biopsies. *Cancer Research*, 1998; **58**: 4913–17.

48. Noguchi S, *et al.* Histologic characteristics of breast cancers with occult lymph node metastases detected by keratin 19 mRNA reverse transcription polymerase chain reaction. *Cancer*, 1996; **78**: 1235–40.

49. Noguchi S, *et al.* Detection of breast cancer micrometastases in axillary lymph nodes by means of reverse transcriptase-polymerase chain reaction: comparison between MUC-1 mRNA and keratin 19 mRNA amplification. *American Journal of Pathology*, 1996; **148**: 649–56.

50. Mori M, *et al.*Detection of cancer metastases in lymph nodes by reverse transcription polymerase chain reaction. *Cancer Research*, 1995; **55**: 3417–20.

51. Min CJ, Tafra L, Verbanac KM. Identification of superior markers for polymerase chain reaction detection of breast cancer metastases in sentinel lymph nodes. *Cancer Research*, 1998; **58**: 4581–4.

52. Mayall F, *et al.* Mutations of p53 gene can be detected in the plasma of patients with large bowel carcinoma. *Journal of Clinical Pathology*, 1998; **51**: 611–13.

53. Xu X, *et al.* Molecular screening of multifocal transitional cell carcinoma of the bladder using p53 mutations as biomarkers. *Clinical Cancer Research*, 1996; **2**: 1795–800.

54. Sidransky D, *et al.* Identification of ras oncogene mutations in the stool of patients with curable colorectal tumors. *Science*, 1992; **256**: 102–5.

55. Loeb LA. Microsatellite instability: marker of a mutator phenotype in cancer. *Cancer Research*, 1994; **54**: 5059–63.

56. Jackson AL, Loeb LA. The mutation rate and cancer. *Genetics*, 1998; **148**: 483–90.

57. Sidransky D. Nucleic acid-based methods for the detection of cancer. *Science*, 1997; **278**: 1054–8.

58. Mao L, *et al.* Microsatellite alterations as clonal markers for the detection of human cancer. *Proceedings of the National Academy of Sciences of the USA*, 1994; **91**: 9871–5.

59. Mao L, *et al.* Molecular detection of primary bladder cancer by microsatellite analysis. *Science*, 1996; **271**: 659–62.

60. Steiner G, *et al.* Detection of bladder cancer recurrence by microsatellite analysis of urine. *Nature Medicine*, 1997; **3**: 621–4.

61. Cuzick J, *et al.* Human papillomavirus testing in primary cervical screening. *The Lancet*, 1995; **345**: 1533–6.

62. Snijders PJ, Meijer CJ, Walboomers JM. Degenerate primers based on highly conserved regions of amino acid sequence in papillomaviruses can be used in a generalized polymerase chain reaction to detect productive human papillomavirus infection. *Journal of General Virology*, 1991; **72**: 2781–6.

63. Vitolo U, *et al.* Rearrangements of bcl-6, bcl-2, c-myc and 6q deletion in B diffuse large cell lymphoma: clinical relevance in 71 patients. *Annals of Oncology*, 1998; **9**: 55–61.

64. Drexler HG. Review of alterations of the cyclin-dependent kinase inhibitor INK4 family genes p15, p16, p18 and p19 in human leukemia-lymphoma cells. *Leukemia*, 1998; **12**: 845–59.

65. Heyman M, *et al.* Prognostic significance of p15INK4B and p16INK4 gene inactivation in childhood acute lymphocytic leukemia. *Journal of Clinical Oncology*, 1996; **14**: 1512–20.

66. Parry TE. The non-random distribution of point mutations in leukaemia and myelodysplasia—a possible pointer to their aetiology. *Leukaemia Research*, 1997; **21**: 559–74.

67. Bergmann L, *et al.* High level of Wilm's Tumor gene (wt1) mRNA in acute myeloid leukaemias are associated with a worse long-term outcome. *Blood*, 1997; **90**: 1217–25.

68. Gartenhaus RB. Microsatellite instability in hematologic malignancies. *Leukaemia and Lymphoma*, 1997; **25**: 455–61.

69. **Diss TC, Pan L.** Polymerase chain reaction in the assessment of lymphomas. In: Wotherspoon AC (ed.) *Cancer Surveys*, vol. 30. New York: Cold Spring Harbor Laboratory Press, 1997: 21–44.

70. **Kuppers R, Roers A, Kanzler H.** Molecular single cell studies of normal and transformed lymphocytes. In: Wotherspoon AC (ed.) *Cancer Surveys*, vol. 30. New York: Cold Spring Harbor Laboratory Press, 1997: 45–68.

71. **Uckun FM, *et al.*** Clinical significance of MLL-AF4 fusion transcript expression in the absence of a cytogenetically detectable t(4;11) (q21; q23) chromosomal translocation. *Blood*, 1998; **92**: 810–21.

72. **Limpens J, *et al.*** Lymphoma-associated translocation t(14;18) in blood B cells of normal individuals. *Blood*, 1995; **85**: 2528–36.

73. **Biernaux C, *et al.*** Detection of major bcr-abl gene expression at a very low level in blood cells of some healthy individuals. *Blood*, 1995; **86**: 3118.

74. **Miyamoto T, *et al.*** Persistence of multipotent progenitors expressing AML-ETO transcript in long-term remission patients with t(8;21) in acute myelogenous leukaemia. *Blood*, 1997; **87**: 4789–96.

75. **Hochhaus A, *et al.*** Molecular monitoring of residual disease in chronic myelogenous leukemia patients after therapy. *Recent Results in Cancer Research*, 1998; **144**: 36–45.

76. **Karp JE, Broder S.** Molecular foundations of cancer: new targets of intervention. *Nature Medicine*, 1995; **1**: 309–20.

77. **Strachan T, Abitol M, Davidson D, Beckmann JS.** A new dimension for the human genome project: towards comprehensive expression maps. *Nature Genetics*, 1997; **16**: 126–32.

78. **Tlsty TD, Margolin BH, Lum K.** Differences in the rates of gene amplification in nontumorigenic and tumorigenic cell lines as measured by Luria–Delbruck fluctuation analysis. *Proceedings of the National Academy of Sciences of the USA*, 1989; **86**: 9441–5.

79. **Velculescu VE, *et al.*** Serial analysis of gene expression. *Science*, 1995; **270**: 484–7.

80. **Marshall A, Hodgson J.** DNA chips: an array of possibilities. *Nature Biotechnology*, 1998; **16**: 27–31.

81. **Schafer AJ, Hawkins JR.** DNA variations and the future of human genetics. *Nature Biotechnology*, 1998; **16**: 33–9.

82. **Hacia JG, *et al.*** Detection of the heterozygous mutation in BRCA1 using high density oligonucleotide arrays and two-colour fluorescence analysis. *Nature Genetics*, 1996; **14**: 441–56.

3.2 Cytology and minimal sampling techniques

Måns Åkerman

A cytological, morphological diagnosis is based on the examination of individual cells, cell clusters, and minimal tissue fragments dislodged from their origin. For practical purposes, clinical cytology is divided into two types depending upon the means used to collect the cellular material:

1. Exfoliative cytology comprises all examinations performed on cells which are normally desquamated or exfoliated from epithelial, mesothelial, or synovial surfaces or forcibly detached by means of various devices.

2. Aspiration cytology (fine-needle aspiration cytology (FNAC), thin needle aspiration cytology, aspiration biopsy cytology) is the examination of cells collected by aspiration with the aid of thin needles and a syringe, often attached to a special device for one-handed manipulation.

Microscopic examination of cells in tumour diagnosis has been described since the beginning of the nineteenth century. However, the point at which exfoliative cytology was recognized as a simple and effective means for early diagnosis of malignancy came with the work of George Papanicolaou (1883–1962) who scientifically explored the method and introduced it into everyday clinical use.[1]

The use of FNAC can be traced back to 1850. The method was extensively used at the Memorial Hospital for Cancer and Allied Diseases in New York between 1920 and 1930 by Martin, Coley, and Ellis. Thanks to the experience and publications of pioneers Nils Söderström, Josef Zajicek, and Sixten Franzén, FNAC is widely recognized today as an inexpensive, rapid, simple, and highly accurate method for diagnosing malignant tumours in almost every body site. For a more comprehensive study of the history of clinical cytology the reader is referred to monographs.[2]

Exfoliative cytology

In an exfoliative cytological specimen the diagnosis is based on the examination of cells either desquamated or forcibly detached from their origin by means of mechanical devices such as spatulae, brushes, or jet washers. The collection of cells is often simple (Table 1, Fig. 1).

Preparation of the cellular material for microscopic examination

Fluids (effusions, urine, and cystic tumours) are either centrifuged in an ordinary centrifuge and the deposit smeared on slides or processed in a cytocentrifuge. When a fluid is processed in a cytocentrifuge, essentially equal number of cells are automatically distributed on one or several slides. Manual smearing is not necessary. This method is especially valuable when small amounts of fluid are to be investigated, for example cerebrospinal fluid. Brush and spatula specimens are gently smeared on slides.

Other methods of collecting the cells for microscopic examination are membrane filtration and processing of a cell block. Cell-block preparations are various methods by which the cells in the sample are collected in a small pellet, which then is fixed in formalin and processed as a small tissue sample—embedded in paraffin, blocked, and sectioned. The cellular material is thus transformed into a 'microbiopsy'. A cell block is a valuable preparation method when the cytological examination is supplemented with immunohistochemistry. Different cytology laboratories have different routines for the preparation of samples for examination and it is always advisable to ascertain how the laboratory requires the specimens to be prepared before sending them for analysis.

Routine fixation and staining methods are the same for exfoliative cytology and fine-needle aspiration cytology. Two methods are used:

1. The slides are dried in air and stained with May–Grünwald–Giemsa (MGG), Wright's stain, or Diff-Quik, using the same procedure as for haematology. Diff-Quik is a rapid stain (2–3 min).

2. The slides are wet fixed, immediately immersed in an alcoholic fixative (usually ethanol, 95 per cent). The alcoholic fixative may also be used as a coating fixative (spray-fix). After air-drying, the slides are stained with haematoxylin and eosin/erythrosin (HE) or according to Papanicolaou (Pap). Haematoxylin/eosin staining is carried out by a method similar to that used routinely for histopathological material. Haematoxylin and eosin/erythrosin staining may be performed rapidly; a slide can be examined within 7 to 8 min after smearing. The Pap method was originally devised by Papanicolaou to visualize the squamous epithelial cells in vaginal smears but is now widely used in all types of cytological material.[3]

Both fixation methods have their advantages and disadvantages. With air-drying, both cytoplasm and nucleus become flattened on the surface of the glass slide and the cell appears larger than a wet-fixed cell. In general, nuclear details including nucleoli are visualized excellently on wet-fixed smears and cytoplasmic details and matrix are very well demonstrated in air-dried smears. For a comprehensive comparison of the general properties of wet-fixed and air-dried smears see Orell *et al.*[3]

Table 1 Important targets for exfoliative cytology and the means by which the cells are collected

Body site	Collection method	Note
Body cavities and joints Effusions and exudates	Thoracocentesis Laparocentesis Joint aspiration	Spontaneously exfoliated cells; impossible to identify the site of the tumour
Central nervous system cerebrospinal fluid	Lumbar puncture	
Female genital tract vulva, vagina, cervix, endometrium	Spatula, brush, jet wash, various devices to scrape or aspirate the endometrial surface	A mixture of cells, spontaneously desquamated and forcibly removed; usually impossible to identify the site of the lesion
Respiratory tract	Sputum	Spontaneously desquamated cells; site of the lesion unknown
	Bronchial wash, bronchial lavage, bronchial brush	Cells removed from the lesion
Urinary tract	Voided urine	Spontaneously exfoliated cells
	Bladder wash	A mixture of cells, spontaneously desquamated and forcibly removed; site of the lesion unknown
Breast (nipple secretion)	Compression	Site of the lesion unknown
Ulcerations skin, vulva, nipple, lip, tongue, mouth	Spatula, brush	Forcibly removed cells from the lesion
Fresh tumour tissue	Touch preparation (imprint cytology)	

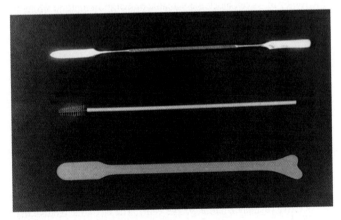

Fig. 1 Different types of devices used for cell collection in exfoliative cytology. From top to bottom: metal spatula, brush, wooden spatula.

Diagnosis in exfoliative cytology

With exfoliative cytology it is not possible to study the relationship between the tumour cells and stroma or the relationship of the tumour to the surrounding tissues. Important parameters in tumour diagnosis, such as extent and type of infiltration or intravascular growth, also cannot be determined by this method.

The cytopathologist is forced to base the diagnosis essentially on a thorough analysis of nuclear and cytoplasmic details. Nevertheless, it is possible, with a high grade of accuracy, not only to diagnose malignancy but also to identify different types of malignancies and to type-diagnose carcinomas in exfoliative specimens.[4]-[6] Clinically important examples are the diagnosis of squamous cell atypia (intra-epithelial cervical squamous neoplasia) as well as glandular cell

neoplasia in vaginal and endometrial samples and the subtyping of lung carcinoma in lung cytological specimens.[7],[8] Other examples are malignancy grading of bladder carcinoma and classification of carcinomas in exfoliative scrape cytology smears from small ulcerated superficial lesions suspected to be malignant in the skin, vulva, nipple, lips, tongue, and mouth. Tumours suitable for classical exfoliative cytological examinations are tumours originating from, or invading, epithelial and mesothelial surfaces and superficial ulcerated tumours.

Limitations of diagnosis

Spontaneously exfoliated cells may exhibit degenerative features which prevent the examination of important cytological parameters, such as variability in cell and nuclear size and shape, cell size relative to nuclear size, and chromatin structure. This phenomenon may be an important limitation in the subtyping of malignant cells in sputum cytology.

Other diagnostic pitfalls are the correct interpretation of reactive cellular and nuclear changes in epithelium secondary to inflammatory conditions, radiation, and chemotherapy[9],[10] as well as the correct interpretation of cells as malignant when they exhibit slight nuclear and cytoplasmic atypia.[11] A well-known example is the correct interpretation of reactive mesothelial versus neoplastic cells.[12]

Automation in exfoliative cytology

One of the most important examples of the valuable clinical use of exfoliative cytology is in mass screening programmes to detect cervical intraepithelial neoplasia. These programmes have played a major role in decreasing the occurrence of invasive cervix cancer in several countries.[13] However, a successful mass screening programme requires the examination of a large number of smears annually, with a high degree of accuracy. In order to increase the cost effectiveness of mass screening as well as to obtain an effective quality control by re-examination of smears to reduce the incidence of false negative cases, automated devices to screen cervical cytology slides have been an important research goal for over 30 years. Although a number of different systems have been invented only one, the PapNet system developed in 1989, has been widely tested.[14]–[16] At present, the PapNet system is one of the two systems approved by the Food and Drug Administration in the United States for rescreening negative slides. The PapNet system was developed as a supplementary test to overcome limitations of manual screening and rescreening of vaginal smears (Pap-smears). In this system, every cell on a slide is scanned and the 128 most abnormal cells are identified and displayed on the screen for ocular examination. The system is based on neural network processing. There is, however, still no system which is cost effective in the mass screening situation and, when it comes to diagnosis, superior to manual screening. For a comprehensive survey of computer-assisted cytology the reader is referred to a special issue of *Acta Cytologica*, 1998.[17]

Imprint (touch) preparations (imprint cytology)

A diagnostically valuable but overlooked subtype of exfoliative cytology is imprint cytology. Fresh samples from almost all types of tumour tissue are suitable for touch preparations. With a good touch imprint (the tissue sample not too forcibly pressed against the slide and not smeared), cellular and nuclear features are easy to study and the joint evaluation of imprint smears and tissue sections combines the classical parameters of histopathological diagnosis (relation of tumour to surrounding tissues, relation between tumour and stroma, extent and type of infiltration, intravascular growth, and tumour tissue pattern) with an excellent demonstration of tumour cell morphology.

The classic use of imprint cytology is in the diagnosis and classification of malignant lymphoma but according to the author's experience and others it is a valuable diagnostic adjunct in tumour diagnosis in general.[18]–[20] One particular use is in the differential diagnosis of the malignant, small, round cell tumours in childhood and adolescence (Fig. 2). Another use of imprint cytology is in the diagnosis of nipple discharge. The slide is gently pressed against the droplets of fluid which by palpation are forced onto the nipple. The majority of malignant tumours are suitable for imprint cytology. One exception is tumours with a collagenous or desmoplastic stroma where the yield often is poor. It is, however, always advisable to perform touch imprints on every unfixed tumour sample.

Fine-needle aspiration cytology (FNAC)

FNAC is a truly minimal sampling technique which, when applied optimally, offers a number of advantages compared to open surgical biopsy as well as coarse needle biopsy (core needle biopsy, thru-cut biopsy). Most aspirations can be performed on ambulatory patients. Incisions in the skin are never necessary. Local anaesthesia is not needed in most aspirations. One exception is aspirations of bone lesions when a partly destroyed cortex has to be breached. Another exception is FNAC in children when, depending on the clinical situation, local anaesthesia or a short general anaesthesia may be needed.

When aspirations are performed by cytopathologists or at hospitals with a department of pathology/cytology, rapid staining of the smear makes it possible to ascertain that sufficient material for diagnosis has been aspirated while the patient is waiting and a preliminary report is possible within 15 to 20 min. Fine-needle aspiration is the least tissue destructive of all biopsy methods, the risk for spread of tumour cells is negligible,[21] and severe complications rare. It is easy to collect cells from different parts of large tumours to diagnose tumour heterogeneity or to select another site when the sample at the first pass shows necrosis.

Coarse needle biopsy for histopathological examination of a thin tissue core (needle diameter usually 1.0–1.2 mm) is also an ambulatory, relatively simple method but a rapid diagnosis is less feasible, as is multiple sampling. A comparison of the advantages and disadvantages of fine-needle aspiration and coarse needle biopsy are given in Table 2. For optimal diagnostics both methods require technically good samples, which depends on the skill of the aspirator.

It is possible to aspirate and collect material from suspect lesions in every part of the body. Depending on the tumour, the aspirate consists of individual cells or a mixture of dispersed cells, cell clusters, and small tumour tissue fragments ('microbiopsies'). The technique, which is the same regardless of the site of the lesion, is based on three important points:

1. The lesion must be defined and it must be possible to put a thin needle into it.

2. At the same time as continuous aspiration the needle must be moved forwards and back in the lesion to tear off cells and small tissue fragments.

3. The aspirated cellular material must be smeared on glass slides in the best possible way for staining and microscopic examination.

In recent years, a modification of the technique has been proposed and tested. In lesions and tumours with an insignificant amount of stroma, it is possible to collect material for examination without aspiration by fine-needle capillary sampling. With this method it is sufficient to move the needle back and forth. Examples of common sites for sampling where this method is suitable are the thyroid gland, lymphnodes, testes, and stroma-poor breast lesions.[22],[23] The diagnostic accuracy is the same irrespective of sampling method.[24] Advantages of cell collection without aspiration are better perception of tumour consistency and control of the hand. According to our experience, there is less discomfort for the patient. This method is especially valuable when small, superficial tumours are needled.

Many cytopathologists often makes the first pass with the needle without aspiration, if the yield is none or poor the next passes are performed with aspiration. The needles are between 23 and 21 gauge; needles thicker than 21 gauge are not necessary. The basic technique of specimen collection is well described in various monographs.[3] Routine fixation and staining methods are the same as for exfoliative cytology.

Fine-needle aspiration was first used for a morphological diagnosis of palpable lumps; the main targets are breast tumours, followed by palpable lesions in the thyroid gland, enlarged lymph nodes, and tumours in general in the head and neck region. A relatively new target, still debated, is soft tissue tumour diagnosis.[25],[26]

With the aid of various imaging techniques, however, fine-needle aspiration can also be used to obtain material for microscopic examination from non-palpable, small and large lesions in every part

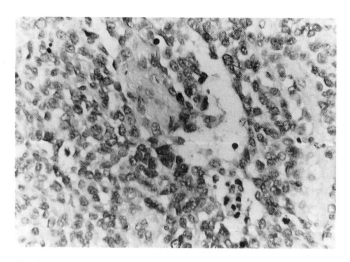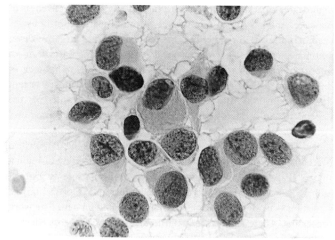

Fig. 2 Imprint cytology from a fresh tissue sample from alveolar rhabdomyosarcoma. In the imprint specimen (right) the morphology of the tumour cells is better evaluated than in the histological slide (left). The rhabdomyoblastic features (rounded and triangular cells, eccentric nuclei, dense cytoplasm) of the tumour cells are easier to recognize in the imprint section. (Left × 360; right × 900).

Table 2 Comparison between fine needle aspiration and coarse needle biopsy

	Fine needle aspiration	Coarse needle biopsy
Common parameters		
Ambulatory procedure		
General anaesthesia not necessary		
Minimal tissue trauma		
Technical skill necessary for optimal sampling		
Other parameters		
Multiple sampling (tumour heterogeneity)	+++	+
Rapid preliminary report (15–20 min)	+++	+ (frozen section 15–20 min)
Excellent cellular morphology	+++	+ – ++
Evaluation of tumour tissue pattern	–/+ +*	++ – +++
Useful for ancillary diagnostics	+ – +++**	+++

*A cellblock preparation may give information on tumour tissue pattern

**Depends on the yield

of the body. A typical example is stereotactic aspiration of small, non-palpable lesions discovered at mammography in mass screening for breast carcinoma.[27] Other common targets are mediastinal and lung tumours, tumours in the abdominal cavity, including in liver, pancreas, and kidney, and splenomegaly and non-palpable bone tumours.[28]–[32] Stereotactic fine-needle aspiration has also been used in the diagnosis of brain tumours.[33]

Fine-needle aspiration cytology diagnosis

Principally, there are the same prerequisites of diagnosis as in an exfoliative cytological smear. In general, a fine-needle aspirate consists of a mixture of dispersed cells, cell clusters, and, depending on the tumour type aspirated, small tumour tissue fragments ('micro-biopsies'). The overall pattern of the smear is a valuable diagnostic parameter in addition to the evaluation of nuclear and cytoplasmic details. Yet another important diagnostic criterion, especially in the

diagnosis of salivary gland, soft tissue, and bone tumours, is the evaluation of intercellular matrix substance.[26],[29],[34],[35]

Even when fine-needle aspiration cytology is used only as a screening instrument to determine benignity or malignancy, the final diagnosis should be based on the combined evaluation of clinical data, radiological investigations, if any, and the cytodiagnosis. This approach is the consensus for breast and thyroid lesions (clinical data, mammography and scintigraphy or ultrasound, respectively, and cytodiagnosis). Other examples of combined diagnostics are in the diagnosis of soft tissue and bone tumours.[26],[29]

Today, it is expected that a diagnosis based on an aspirate smear is not only reliable with regard to benignity and malignancy but also that it is possible, with a high degree of accuracy, to classify the tumour in question, including the type and malignancy grade. In hospitals with experienced cytopathologists, the combined evaluation of cytological examinations of routinely stained aspirate smears and clinical and radiological investigations, but omitting a biopsy, is, in the majority of cases, the basis for surgery for tumours in the breast, thyroid, lung, kidney, pancreas, and liver.

Traditionally, the search for reliable diagnostic criteria in the classification of tumours in fine-needle aspirates is achieved by comparative studies of smears and histological sections on the same tumour in a sufficient number of cases.[7],[34],[36],[37] Diagnostic features, permitting a confident type diagnosis, must be repetitive and reproducible. It is of paramount importance that such correlative cytological and histopathological studies are based on a correct histopathological diagnosis. The histopathologist has a crucial role in the accuracy of the cytological diagnosis.

Besides traditional tumour diagnosis, fine-needle aspiration smears may be used in malignancy grading and prognostication. Examples of these applications are in the evaluation of soft tissue sarcoma, non-Hodgkin's lymphoma, and breast carcinoma.[25],[38]–[40]

Accuracy of fine-needle aspiration diagnosis

The accuracy principally depends three important factors: the tumour site, the tumour type, and the experience of the cytopathologist. In general, the accuracy is 70 to almost 100 per cent for correctly distinguishing between a benign and a malignant cell population. This broad spectrum reflects variable diagnostic difficulties in various tumour entities. Examples of a high degree of accuracy in the classification of a tumour as benign or malignant are breast tumours, bone, and soft tissue tumours. Diagnostic difficulties in correctly classifying a tumour as benign or malignant are encountered in salivary gland carcinomas and neoplastic follicular thyroid lesions and some types of indolent non-Hodgkin's lymphomas. Tumour classification to type is, in experienced hands, high in the majority of non-Hodgkin's lymphoma, thyroid carcinoma (except differentiated follicular carcinoma), primary lung carcinoma, and the primary malignant bone tumours. Tumours that are difficult to subtype correctly are variants of salivary gland carcinoma and soft tissue tumours predominantly composed of spindle cells. In Table 3 examples of rates of insufficient aspirates and false diagnoses (in percentages) of tumours from various sites are listed.[29],[32],[41]–[49]

Limitations of diagnosis

There are two main limitations of a fine-needle aspiration cytodiagnosis; false diagnoses and difficulties in diagnosing preinvasive versus invasive carcinoma.

False diagnosis

There are three main causes of a false aspiration cytology diagnosis:

1. The sample was not collected from the tumour—a common reason for missing a palpable lump at aspiration is inexperience at palpation and needling. However, even experienced aspirators may miss small, movable tumours, especially those that are deep-seated. Ultrasound guided aspirations have proved to be helpful in the needling of thyroid lesions,[50] small deep-seated soft tissue tumours, and deep-seated lymph nodes in the neck. To avoid basing the diagnosis on material collected from the surrounding tissues it is imperative that the aspirator is experienced enough to evaluate whether the material might be consistent with the tumour in question (clinical data, palpatory findings). When rapid staining and examination of the smears from the first pass

with the needle is performed many such false diagnoses are avoided.

2. The cellular yield was poor or consisted of poorly preserved or necrotic cells, or the cells have been more or less destroyed due to bad smearing technique or inadequate or incorrect fixation. It unwise to base a definitive diagnosis on a poor yield unless the cells aspirated unequivocally meet the diagnostic criteria. When the cytopathologist performs the needling he or she is well aware of the importance of correct smearing and fixation techniques. Thus, for the clinician who performs fine-needle aspirations it is necessary not only to learn the aspiration technique but also how to correctly smear an aspirate and to follow the instructions from the laboratory on fixation methods.

3. The cells were misdiagnosed at the microscopic examination. The most common limitation of a correct diagnosis is misinterpretation of the cells at the microscopic evaluation. Like exfoliative cytology, reactive benign cellular changes may be misinterpreted as malignant. In addition to 'pseudomalignant' features in epithelium, reactive changes in mesenchymal tissues may fool the examiner. Typical examples are reactive changes in adipose tissue mimicking liposarcoma and in fibroblasts–myofibroblasts in the pseudomalignant benign soft tissue lesions (nodular fasciitis, proliferative fasciitis, and myositis) misdiagnosed as soft tissue sarcoma.[51] Postradiological cellular changes is another pitfall. A common example is in FNAC of breast when remaining palpatory findings after surgery and postoperative radiotherapy are needled.[52] On the other hand, there is risk of a false benign diagnosis in malignant tumours composed of uniform cells with bland nuclei or when the tumour cells appear essentially the same as normal cells from the organ in question. Nuclear Grade I breast carcinoma, differentiated follicular thyroid carcinoma, and synovial sarcoma are examples of malignancies which may be misinterpreted as benign lesions due to lack of malignant criteria in cells and nuclei (Fig. 3).

There are two important means to avoid a false diagnosis. In tumours with minimal or slight cellular atypia, parameters such as cellularity and cellular pattern are important to include in the microscopic assessment. Another is the shaping of the cytology report. When there is a doubt as to whether a tumour is benign or malignant it is often better return an inconclusive report ('not possible to determine')[26] rather than express various grades of uncertainty.

Diagnosis of preinvasive versus invasive carcinoma

This diagnostic problem is of especial clinical importance in the cytological evaluation of breast carcinoma. Cytological criteria predictive of invasiveness have, however, been proposed by Bondesson and Lindholm.[53] Diagnostic pitfalls in the cytological diagnosis which may lead to a false report are an obstacle to the use of cytology, especially when the definitive diagnosis is based on a cytological specimen. However, when the cytological examination is supplemented with complementary preparation methods and ancillary diagnostics a number of pitfalls may be avoided.

Complementary preparation methods

Aspirates suspended in a balanced salt solution and then processed in a cytocentrifuge are suitable for histochemical and immunohistochemical studies. When the yield is rich the processing of

Table 3 Accuracy of FNAC to diagnose correctly benign and malignant tumours in various sites; rates of false negative and false positive diagnoses and insufficient aspirates

Site	No. of cases	False negative (%)	False positive (%)	Insufficient aspirates (%)	Reference
Breast	3545	9.6	1.9	1.09	42
Breast	835	13	0.8	5.5	43
Breast	4110	3.9	0.3	6.4	44
Salivary gland	462	24	5	11	45
Salivary gland	438	45	24	2.3	46
Soft tissue	517	4.4	7	6	26
Bone	333*	1.5	1.6	6	29
Bone	300*	3	0.3	8	47
Thyroid	6346	2.4	0.3	20	48
Thyroid	308**	36	0	0.9	41
Lung	132***	0	0.8	not evaluated	32
Lymph node	266	11.3	0	12	49

*Primary bone tumours and metastases

**Solitary nodules

***Primary lung carcinoma

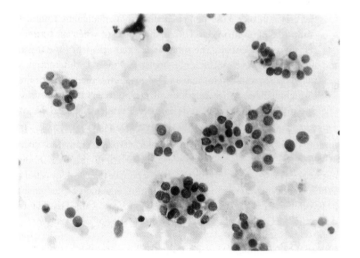 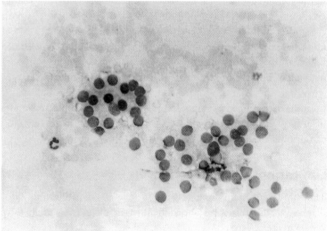

Fig. 3 Part of aspirate smears from thyroid follicular carcinoma (left) and thyroid follicular adenoma (right) showing similar nuclear characteristics and similar small follicular structures (left and right × 360).

a cell block for histopathological examination is a valuable complement to the cytological evaluation and the blocked material is well suited for immunohistochemical stainings[3],[54] (Fig. 4).

Adjunctive diagnostic methods in cytology

Today it is possible to make use of the same battery of adjunctive diagnostic methods as for a tissue sample. Table 4 summarizes current adjunctive methods.

Histochemistry

A number of histochemical stains may be used on cytological smears. The usefulness of histochemistry is exemplified by the following cases. Malignant melanoma may mimic almost every type of malignant tumour in an aspirate smear—a carcinoma-like epithelioid cell morphology, a sarcoma-like pleomorphic or fusiform cell pattern, or a lymphoma-like small cell population. A Masson–Fontana staining to vizualize melanin pigment may help in the differential diagnosis.

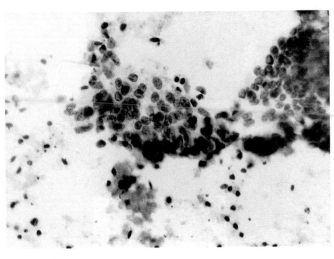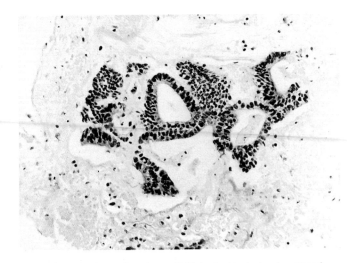

Fig. 4 Cell-block preparation from a fine-needle aspirate. FNAC from a bone metastasis from a colorectal carcinoma (left). In the blocked and sectioned part of the aspirate (right), the adenocarcinomatous origin of the lesion is easy to diagnose. (Left × 360, right × 90.) (Haematoxylin and eosin.)

Table 4 Adjunctive diagnostic methods to improve cytodiagnosis

Method	Diagnostic information
Histochemical stains: Masson-Fontana, Grimelius, Best's carmine, PAS, Alcian blue, hexamine-silver (Gomori), alkaline phosphatase	Melanin pigment, argentaffin pigment, glycogen, mucin, *Pneumocystis carinii*, fungi, osteoblastic origin
Immunohistochemical stains: immunofluoroscence (flow cytometry) peroxidase/anti-peroxidase alkaline phosphatase	Demonstration of various intracytoplasmic intermediary filaments, proteins, and cytoplasmic surface antigens, demonstration of clonal excess and hormonal receptors, proliferation activity
Electron microscopic examination	Demonstration of cytoplasmic organelles, filamentes or granulae; demonstration of cell junctions
DNA-ploidy analysis: flow cytometry image analysis	DNA-ploidy, proliferation activity
Morphometry	Demonstration of variation or uniformity in nuclear size and shape
Chromosomal analysis	Demonstration of diagnostic chromosomal aberrations
Molecular genetic analysis: FISH	Demonstration of diagnostic translocations
In situ amplification techniques	Demonstration of hybrid proteins in diagnostic chromosomal translocations; demonstration of virus infested cells

Stained smears may be destained and restained according to Masson–Fontana. Another example of the usefulness of histochemical staining is alkaline phosphatase staining of malignant bone tumours suspected to be osteosarcoma[29] (Fig. 5). A positive result excludes diagnostic pitfalls such as high-grade malignant chondrosarcoma, anaplastic large cell lymphoma, and metastases from carcinoma and melanoma in the differential diagnosis.

Immunohistochemistry

An extensive battery of antibodies is available for use on unstained smears or cytocentrifuge preparations. When cell blocks are prepared, a restricted range of antibodies is suitable, as for other formalin-fixed and paraffin-blocked tissue.[54]

The main diagnostic use of immunohistochemical stains is in the differential diagnosis of epithelial tumours, mesenchymal tumours, malignant melanoma, and malignant lymphoma. Immunohisto-chemistry is a valuable diagnostic adjunct in classification of the small round cell malignant tumours such as rhabdomyosarcoma, neuroblastoma, Ewing's sarcoma and precursor lymphoma in child-hood and adolescence, and in the type diagnosis of malignant lymphoma. Yet another valuable application is staining with anti-kappa and lambda antibodies to diagnose or refute light chain restriction in the differential diagnosis between benign lymphoid hyperplasia and indolent non-Hodgkin's lymphoma.[55] Another use of immunohistochemical staining is in the assessment of proliferative activity in malignant tumours, especially in the differential diagnosis of indolent and aggressive non-Hodgkin's lymphoma. In breast car-cinoma, fine-needle aspirates may be used for the demonstration of hormone receptor status and oncogene overexpression.[56],[57]

As aberrant expression of antigen may occur, for example keratin in leiomyosarcoma and anaplastic large cell lymphoma.[58],[59] Thus, the staining results must always be critically assessed and the final conclusion based on the combined evaluation of routine cytological examination and immunohistochemical staining. Flow cytometric analysis of fluorescence-labelled antibodies on tissue samples and bone marrow and blood samples is a well known and much used diagnostic adjunct in the diagnosis and type diagnosis of malignant lymphoma and leukaemia. A fine-needle aspirate or an effusion are excellent sources for a flow cytometric phenotyping in the diagnosis and subtyping of lymphoproliferative disorders. When the equipment

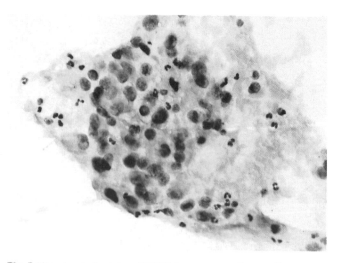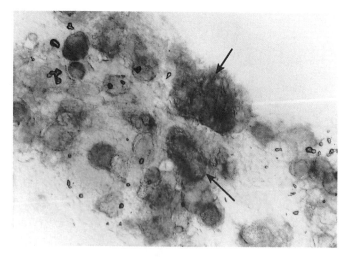

Fig. 5 Histochemical staining of FNAC from an osteosarcoma. The osteosarcoma cells are grouped in an epithelial-like cluster and show epithelioid features (left). In the alkaline phosphatase staining the cytoplasm of the osteosarcoma cells is strongly positive, obscuring the nucleus (arrow, right). (Left and right × 360.)

is accessible on the premises, a suspect non-Hodgkin's lymphoma may be rapidly classified within hours.

Immunohistochemistry is a much used adjunct method in FNAC. Its optimal use in diagnosis has, however, not yet been clarified.[60]

Electron microscopy

Although an electron microscopic examination is technically more complicated and more expensive than immunohistochemistry, an ultrastructural analysis is still a valuable diagnostic complement in selected diagnostic situations. Although immunohistochemistry has largely replaced electron microscopy in the differential diagnosis of low differentiated carcinoma, malignant melanoma, and large cell lymphoma, ultrastructural analysis is still an important diagnostic adjunct in soft tissue and bone tumour diagnosis.[61],[62] The type diagnosis of mesenchymal spindle cell tumours is a diagnostic dilemma in FNAC; the differential diagnosis between leiomyosarcoma, malignant peripheral nerve sheath tumour, monophasic synovial sarcoma, and fibrosarcoma is facilitated by electron microscopy as a supplement to immunohistochemistry as leiomyosarcoma does not always stain positively for desmin and malignant peripheral nerve sheath tumour does not always express S-100 protein. In FNAC, electron microscopic examination seems to be a better marker for monophasic synovial sarcoma than immunohistochemical analysis.[63]

The demonstration of osteoid is important in the diagnosis of osteosarcoma.[29],[64] The small round cell malignancies of childhood and adolescence (Ewing family of tumours, neuroblastoma, and alveolar rhabdomyosarcoma) all have different diagnostic ultrastructural features which may be easier to interpret than immunohistochemical stains[65] (Fig. 6).

DNA analysis

A DNA ploidy analysis is a valuable, yet limited, adjunct in the differential diagnosis between a benign or malignant tumour. An unequivocally non-diploid cell population favours a malignancy. However, a number of malignant tumours, even of high-grade malignancy, are composed of diploid cells.

DNA ploidy can be analysed either by flow or image cytometry.[66] As a flow cytometric analysis can be performed within 30 min of the aspiration it is very suitable when rapid results are necessary. However, cell-poor suspensions as well as aspirates from necrotic areas may cause a false diploid histogram.[67] Diploid flow histograms should be supplemented with an image cytometric ploidy analysis. Although image cytometry is a slower procedure (2–3 h), one advantage is that it is possible to examine routinely-stained smears, destain them, restain them with Feulgen staining and then perform the ploidy analysis.

Morphometry

Analyses of variations in nuclear size and nuclear configuration have been applied to various tumours and tumour-like conditions on exfoliative as well as aspirated specimens. The most important goal has been to evaluate whether a morphometric study might be of help in the differential diagnosis of benignity and malignancy.[68]

Chromosomal analysis

In recent years, a number of solid tumours, especially of mesenchymal origin and non-Hodgkin's lymphoma, have been found to have diagnostic chromosomal aberrations.[69],[70] It is possible to perform a karyotype analysis on fine-needle aspirates although the success rate is lower than in examination of tissue samples.[71],[72] The Ewing family of tumours, and synovial sarcoma, are tumours which harbour specific translocations of value in the differential diagnosis. Other tumour aspirates which may be of value to karyotype for definitive diagnosis are myxoid liposarcoma, alveolar rhabdomyosarcoma, anaplastic large cell lymphoma, and mantle cell lymphoma.

Molecular genetic analysis and *in situ* hybridization techniques

Dividing cells are not needed when these techniques are performed, and fewer cells are necessary than for a karyotype analysis. Thus,

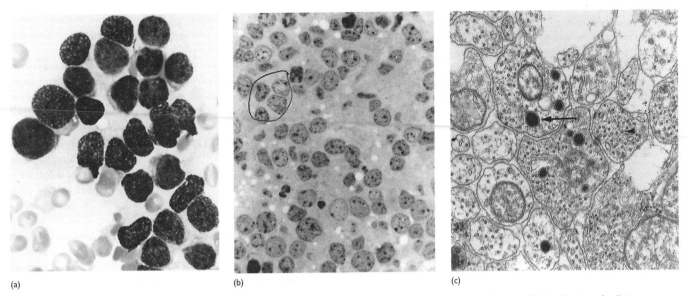

(a)   (b)   (c)

Fig. 6 The use of electron microscopic examination of fine-needle aspirate as an adjunct to light microscopic evaluation. (a) A collection of cells in an aspirate smear from an abdominal tumour in an infant. A number of differential diagnoses are possible, among them neuroblastoma (× 800). (b) Detail from the section of the embedded aspirate. The cells within the marked area are further processed for ultrastructural analysis. (c) Part of the cytoplasm from one of the cells at high magnification (× 31 500). Sectioned cytoplasmic processes containing neurosecretory granula (arrow) and sectioned neurotubuli (arrow head) strongly suggest a neuroblastoma.

these methods are well suited for fine-needle aspirates and other types of cytological specimens.[73] The genes involved in the translocations in a number of tumours with diagnostic aberrations (Ewing family of tumours, alveolar rhabdomyosarcoma, synovial sarcoma, myxoid liposarcoma, anaplastic large cell lymphoma, and mantel cell lymphoma) have been identified. By means of reverse transcriptase polymerase chain reaction (RT-PCR) applied on cellular samples it is possible to identify the specific translocation.[26],[74] Another application is the demonstration of virus-infected cells. Cytological preparations are well suited for the demonstration of chromosomal aberrations by means of fluorescence *in situ* hybridization (FISH).[75] Yet another clinically important example is the demonstration of Ki-ras point mutations in pancreatic juice in the diagnosis of pancreatic carcinoma.[76]

The use of adjunctive diagnostic methods is an important supplement to the routine cytological examination and many diagnostic pitfalls are avoided when they are part of the evaluation. When routine cytodiagnosis is supplemented with ancillary methods, the diagnostic accuracy may equal that of a biopsy specimen and definitive treatment can confidently be based on the fine-needle aspirate. Non-Hodgkin's lymphoma, and soft tissue and bone tumours are examples where a biopsy tissue diagnosis may be omitted before treatment.[26],[29],[38] By combining different specific methods it is also possible thoroughly to characterize a malignant tumour by FNAC.[74],[77]

However, omitting a pretreatment surgical biopsy for histopathological examination requires close co-operation between clinician and cytopathologist and experience in the various ancillary methods. An optimal use of FNAC as the definitive pretreatment diagnosis may require centralization of patients.[26]

Contraindications for the use of fine-needle aspiration

It is generally accepted that there are no absolute contraindications for fine-needle aspiration of superficial sites. A patient who is unwilling or can not co-operate is not suitable for fine-needle aspiration. When patients have bleeding disorders or are on anticoagulant therapy an appropriate medical consultation should be performed before aspiration of intra-abdominal targets, especially liver and spleen, and lung and mediastinum. It has been recommended that patients with suspected pheochromocytoma and echinoccus cysts should be aspirated with caution. It is debated whether fine-needle aspiration should be used in the diagnosis of suspected primary malignancies in the ovaries and testes and in candidates for curative hepatic surgery of liver tumours due to supposed tumour cell spread and the risk for implantation metastasis.

Critical analysis of the role of cytology in tumour diagnosis

Exfoliative as well as fine-needle aspiration cytology have been accepted for many years as valuable diagnostic methods. Debate continues about their usefulness, limitations, and efficacy. However, there are as yet few critical analyses of their role in the diagnosis, including the search for generally accepted procedures for sampling and reporting results. Diagnosis of intraepithelial cervical neoplasia is one of the oldest and most common targets for exfoliative cytology.

Table 5 Headings which are common to recommendations and guidelines in critical reviews of vaginal cytology, fine needle aspiration in general, and fine needle aspiration of breast tumours, thyroid lesions, and soft tissue tumours

Indication for examination
Patient consent
Technical aspects of sampling
Adequate yield
Reporting the result
Centralization or not of patients to tumour centre
Training programmes

However, it was not until 1988 that guidelines for sampling and reporting were proposed.[78]

With regard to fine-needle aspiration cytology the Papanicolaou Society of Cytopathology proposed guidelines for fine-needle aspiration procedures and reporting 1997.[79] A critical and thorough evaluation of FNAC of breast tumours was performed 1997 by a National Cancer Institute-sponsored international study group, resulting in recommended guide lines. So far, of all targets for fine-needle aspiration cytological diagnosis, only soft tissue tumours, breast lesions, and thyroid lesions have been the subject for critical reviews and recommended guidelines.[26],[80],[81] In Table 5 the most important points, common to all guide-lines, are listed.

Complications from the use of exfoliative cytology and fine-needle aspiration cytology

Exfoliative cytology produces virtually no complications except those that may be encountered when the sampling method is part of the routine procedure, such as centesis laparoscopy and thoracoscopy or lumbar puncture. The brushing or scraping of ulcerated epithelial surfaces or tumours causes very little discomfort.

In fine-needle aspiration cytology minor complications may occur but severe ones are infrequent[21] (Table 6). A slight haemorrhage, swelling, and tenderness may appear after aspirations of breast or the thyroid or salivary glands. Pneumothorax may occur in percutaneous aspirations of lungs, mediastinum, liver, and spleen. Pneumothorax may also occur as a rare complication when the target is small, firm, movable tumours in small breasts and in aspirations against movable lesions in supraclavicular and axillar regions. Pneumothorax requiring exsufflation is rare; in several series only 5 to 10 per cent of cases with pneumothoraces needed exsufflation.[82]–[84] The risk of intra-abdominal bleeding after transabdominal needling is small and only single cases have been reported. The stomach or intestinal wall may be penetrated in transabdominal aspirations but peritonitis, including bile peritonitis, are rare events. Edoute *et al.* reported two cases of peritonitis in 190 abdominal aspirations against palpable tumours and one case of fatal intraperitoneal haemorrhage in 492 liver aspirations in 406 patients.[30],[31]

The risk of disseminating malignant tumours by tumour cell spread in the needle track has been discussed extensively.[85] Risk factors for tumour implantation in the needle track have been proposed; large number of passes with the needle, needles coarser than 22 gauge, and fine-needle aspiration on intra-abdominal organs are the most common risk factors discussed. Case reports of implantation metastases after needling malignant tumours in the liver, pancreas, lung, and thyroid gland have been published. One target which has been much debated is fine-needle aspiration of malignant liver tumours in patients who are candidates for curative surgery.[86] The frequency of needle-tract seeding has, however, been reported to be between 0.003 and 0.009 per cent.[21] The general opinion is that this risk is negligible when aspirations are performed with a proper approach.

A rare problem is post-fine-needle aspiration tissue infarction, haemorrhage, and reactive cellular changes which may interfere with a subsequent histopathological examination.[87]

Table 6 Complications which are reported to be encountered with fine needle aspiration

Target	Complication	Note
Palpable tumours, various sites	Slight haemorrhage, swelling, tenderness	
Breast, lymph nodes in axillar fossae, thoracic wall	Pneumothorax	Especially when needling small, movable, firm tumours
Lung, mediastinum	Pneumothorax	A small, symptomless pneumothorax radiologically diagnosed after lung-aspiration is not uncommon; pneumothorax requiring exsufflation very rare
Spleen, liver	Pneumothorax, haemorrhage	Uncommon
Liver, pancreas	Implantation metastases	Uncommon
Abdominal tumours	Haemorrhage	Uncommon
Thyroid, lymph node	Post-FNA tissue infarction	Uncommon

Conclusions

Clinical cytology has proved to be a valuable diagnostic aid, not the least because the sampling methods are simple, inexpensive, causes minor discomfort to the patient, and enable a rapid, preliminary diagnosis possible before the patient has left the outpatient clinic. The challenge in the future is to improve the diagnosis with regard to tumour classification and prognosis by continuing correlative cytological–histological studies of tumours not yet cytologically classified. Other tasks are further research of the optimal diagnostic use of modern adjunctive methods on cytological specimens and critical examination of cytodiagnosis of various sites and tumours leading to universally-accepted guidelines for procedures, diagnosis, and reporting.

References

1. Papanicolaou GN, Traut HF. The diagnostic value of vaginal smears in carcinoma of the uterus. *American Journal of Obstetrics and Gynecology*, 1941; **42**: 193–205.

2. Naylor B. Cytopathology: the past, the present and a glimpse into the future. In: Gray W, ed. *Diagnostic cytopathology*. Edinburgh: Churchill Livingstone, 1995: 3–9.

3. Orell S. The techniques of FNA cytology. In: Orell S, Sterret FG, Walters M, Whitaker D, eds. *Fine needle aspiration cytology*. Edinburgh: Churchill Livingstone, 1992: 8–23.

4. Lan CS. Critical evaluation of the cytodiagnosis of fibrogastroendoscopic samples obtained under direct vision. *Acta Cytologica*, 1990; **34**: 217–220.

5. Lee KR, Manna EA, Jones MA. Comparative cytologic features of adenocarcinoma *in situ* of the cervix. *Acta Cytologica*, 1991; **35**: 117–26.

6. Wiener HG, Vooijs GP, van't Hof-Grootenboer B. Accuracy of urinary cytology in the diagnosis of primary and recurrent bladder cancer. *Acta Cytologica*, 1993; **37**: 163–9.

7. Erozan YS, Frost JK. Cytopathologic diagnosis of cancer in pulmonary material: a critical histopathologic correlation. *Acta Cytologica*, 1970; **14**: 560–5.

8. Liang XM. Accuracy of cytologic diagnosis and cytotyping of sputum in primary lung cancer: analysis of 161 cases. *Journal of Surgical Oncology*, 1989; **40**: 107–11.

9. Scoggins WG, Smith RH, Frable WJ, O'Donohue Jr WJ. False positive diagnosis of lungcarcinoma in patients with pulmonary infarcts. *Annals of Thoracic Surgery*, 1977; **24**: 480.

10. Shield PW, Daunter B, Wright RG. Post-irradiation cytology of cervical cancer patients. *Cytopathology*, 1992; **3**: 167–82.

11. Szyfelbein WM, Young RH, Scully RE. Adenoma malignum of cervix: cytologic findings. *Acta Cytologica*, 1984; **28**: 691–8.

12. Bedrossian C. Diagnostic problems in serous effusions. *Diagnostic Cytopathology*, 1998; **19**: 131–7.

13. Gustafsson L, Pontén J, Bergström R, Adami HO. International incidence rates of invasive cervical cancer before cytologic screening. *International Journal of Cancer*, 1997; **71**: 159–65.

14. Duggan MA, Brasker P. Paired comparison of manual and automated Pap test screening using the PapNet system. *Diagnostic Cytopathology*, 1997; **17**: 248–54.

15. Doorneward H, Woudt JMC, Strubbe P, van De Seip H, van Den Tweel. Evaluation of PapNet-assisted cervical re-screening. *Cytopathology*, 1997; **8**: 313–21.

16. Mitchell H, Medley G. Differences between false-negative and true-positive Papanicolaou smears on PapNet-assisted review. *Diagnostic Cytopathology*, 1998; **19**: 138–40.

17. Special issue, computer-assisted cytology. *Acta Cytologica*, 1998; **42**: 1–265.

18. Kjurkchiev G, Valkov I. Role of touch imprint and core biopsy for detection of tumor metastases in bone marrow. *Diagnostic Cytopathology*, 1998; **18**: 323–4.

19. Gaudin PB, Sherman ME, Brat DJ, Zahurak M, Erozan YS. Accuracy of grading gliomas on CT-guided stereotactic biopsies: a survival analysis. *Diagnostic Cytopathology*, 1997; **17**: 461–6.

20. Veneti S, Ionnaidou-Mouzaka L, Toufexi H, Xenitides J, Anastasiadis P. Imprint cytology. A rapid, reliable method of diagnosing breast malignancy. *Acta Cytologica*, 1996; **40**: 649–52.

21. Livraghi T, Damascelli B, Lombardi C, Spagnoli I. Risk in fine-needle abdominal biopsy. *Journal of Clinical Ultrasound*, 1983; **11**: 77–81.

22. Akhtar M, Ali M, Huq M, Faulkner C. Fine-needle biopsy: comparison of cellular yield with and without aspiration. *Diagnostic Cytopathology*, 1989; **5**: 162–5.

23. Madhuri KS, Maherbano MK, Sudhakar KB, Asha VK. Evaluation of fine needle capillary sampling in superficial and deep-seated lesions: an analysis of 670 cases. *Acta Cytologica*, 1998; **42**: 679–84.

24. Mair S, Dunbar F, Becker PJ, DuPlessis W. Fine needle cytology: is aspiration necessary? A study of 100 cases in various sites. *Acta Cytologica*, 1989; **33**: 809–13.

25. Willén H, Åkerman M, Carlén B. Fine needle aspiration (FNA) in the diagnosis of soft tissue tumours. A review of 22 years experience. *Cytopathology*, 1995; **6**: 236–47.

26. Åkerman M, Willén H. Critical review on the role of fine needle aspiration in soft tissue tumors. *Pathology Case Reviews*, 1998; **3**: 111–17.

27. Azavedo E, Svane G, Auer G. Stereotactic fine needle biopsy in 2594 mammographically detected non-palpable lesions. *Lancet*, 1989; **1**: 1033–6.

28. Al-Kaisi N, Siegler EE. Fine needle aspiration cytology of the pancreas. *Acta Cytologica*, 1989; **33**: 145–52.

29. Åkerman M, Domanski H. Fine needle aspiration (FNA) of bone tumours: with special emphasis on definitive treatment of primary malignant bone tumours based on FNA. *Current Diagnostic Pathology*, 1998; **5**: 82–92.

30. Edoute Y, Ben-Haim SA, Malberger E. Value of direct fine needle aspirative cytology in diagnosing palapble abdominal masses. *American Journal of Medicine*, 1991; **91**: 377–82.

31. Edoute Y, Tibon-Fischer O, Ben-Haim SA, Malberger E. Imaging-guided and non imaging-guided fine needle aspiration of liver lesions. Experience with 406 patients. *Journal of Surgical Oncology*, 1991; **48**: 246–51.

32. Mitchell ML, King DE, Bonfiglio TA, Patten Jr SF. Pulmonary fine needle aspiration cytopathology. A five year correlation study. *Acta Cytologica*, 1984; **28**: 72–6.

33. Willems JGMS, Alva-Willems JM. Accuracy of cytologic diagnosis of central nervous system neoplasms in stereotactic biopsies. *Acta Cytologica*, 1984; **28**: 243–9.

34. Klijanienko J, Viehl P. Fine needle sampling of salivary gland lesions 1. Cytology and histology correlation of 412 cases of pleomorphic adenoma. *Diagnostic Cytopathology*, 1996; **14**: 195–200.

35. Wakely PE, Geisinger KR, Cappelari JO, Silverman JF, Frable WJ. Fine-needle aspiration cytopathology of soft tissue: Chondromyxoid and myxoid lesions. *Diagnostic Cytopathology*, 1995; **12**: 101–5.

36. Dahl I, Åkerman M. Nodular fasciitis. A correlative cytologic and histologic study of 13 cases. *Acta Cytologica*, 1981; **25**: 215–23.

37. Walaas L, Kindblom L-G. Lipomatous tumors. A correlative cytologic and histologic study of 27 tumors examined by fine needle aspiration cytology. *Human Pathology*, 1985; **16**: 6–18.

38. Skoog L, Tani E. The role of fine-needle aspiration cytology in the diagnosis of non-Hodgkin's lymphoma. *Diagnostic Oncology*, 1991; **1**: 12–18.

39. Hunt CM, Ellis CW, Elston CW, Locker A, Pearson D, Blamley RW. Cytological grading of breast carcinoma—a feasible proposition. *Cytopathology*, 1990; **1**: 287–95.

40. Idvall I, Fernö M, Sigurdsson H, Åkerman M, Killander D. Fine needle aspiration cytology of breast carcinoma, pre-operative prognostic tool? *Breast*, 1995; **4**: 189–95.

41. Jayaram G. Fine needle aspiration cytologic study of the solitary thyroid nodule. Profile of 308 cases with histologic correlation. *Acta Cytologica*, 1985; **29**: 967–73.

42. Kline T, Joshi LP, Neal HS. Fine-needle aspiration of the breast: Diagnoses and pitfalls. A review of 3545 cases. *Cancer*, 1979; **44**: 1458–64.

43. Willis SL, Ramzay I. Analysis of false results in a series of 835 fine needle aspirates of breast lesions. *Acta Cytologica*, 1995; **39**: 858–64.

44. Arisio R, *et al*. Role of fine-needle aspiration biopsy in breast lesions. Analysis of a series of 4110 cases. *Diagnostic Cytopathology*, 1998; **18**: 462–7.

45. Lindberg L-G, Åkerman M. Aspiration cytology of salivary gland tumors: Diagnostic experience from six years of routine laboratory work. *Laryngoscope*, 1976; **86**: 584–94.

46. Atula T, Grenman R, Laippala P, Klemi P. Fine-needle aspiration biopsy in the diagnosis of parotid gland lesions. Evaluation of 438 biopsies. *Diagnostic Cytopathology*, 1996; **15**: 185–90.

47. Kreicbergs A, Bauer HF, Brosjö O, Lindholm J, Skoog L, Söderlund V. Cytologic diagnosis of bone tumors. *Journal of Bone and Joint Surgery* (British), 1996; **78-B**: 258–63.

48. Goellner JR, Chaib H, Grant CS, Johnson DA. Fine-needle aspiration cytology of the thyroid, 1980 to 1986. *Acta Cytologica*, 1987; **31**: 587–90.

49. Martelli G, *et al*. Fine needle aspiration cytology in superficial lymph nodes: an analysis of 266 cases. *European Journal of Surgical Oncology*, 1989; **15**: 13–16.

50. Lu C-P, Chang T-C, Wang C-Y. Serial changes in ultrasound-guided fine needle aspiration cytology in subacute thyroiditis. *Acta Cytologica*, 1997; **41**: 238–43.

51. Åkerman M. Reactive cellular changes in soft tissue. In: Goertller K, Feichter G E, Witte S, eds. *New frontiers in cytology. Modern aspects of research and practice*. Berlin: Springer-Verlag, 1988: 302–6.

52. Dornfield JM, Thompson SK, Shurbaji MS. Radiation induced changes in the breast: a potential diagnostic pitfall on fine needle aspiration. *Diagnostic Cytopathology*, 1992; **8**: 79–81.

53. Bondeson L, Lindholm K. Prediction of invasiveness by aspiration cytology applied to nonpalpable breast carcinoma and tested in 300 cases. *Diagnostic Cytopathology*, 1997; **17**: 315–20.

54. Nordgren H, Nilsson S, Runn AC, Pontén J, Bergh J. Histopathological and immunohistochemical analysis of lung tumors: description of a convenient technique for use with fine needle biopsy. *APMIS*, 1989; **97**: 136–42.

55. Sneige N, *et al*. Morphologic and immunocytochemical evaluation of 220 fine needle aspirates of malignant lymphoma and lymphoid hyperplasia. *Acta Cytologica*, 1990; **34**: 311–22.

56. Lönn U, Lönn S, Nylen U, Winblad G, Stenkvist B. Amplification of oncogenes in mammary carcinoma shown by fine-needle biopsy. *Cancer*, 1991; **67**: 1396–400.

57. Listrom MB, Fenoglio-Preiser CM. Immunohistochemistry in cytology. In: Koss L, ed. *Diagnostic cytology*. Philadelphia: J.B. Lippincott, 1992: 1532–60.

58. Miettinen M. Immunoreactivity for cytokeratin and epithelial membrane antigen in leiomyosarcoma. *Archives of Pathology and Laboratory Medicine*, 1988; **112**: 637–40.

59. Gustmann C, Altmannsberger M, Osborn M, Griesser H, Feller AC. Cytokeratin expression and vimentin content in large cell anaplastic lymphomas and other non-Hodgkin's lymphomas. *American Journal of Pathology*, 1991; **138**: 1413–22.

60. Saleh H, Masood S. Value of ancillary studies in fine-needle aspiration biopsy. *Diagnostic Cytopathology*, 1995; **13**: 310–15.

61. Fisher C. The value of electron microscopy and immunohistochemistry in the diagnosis of soft tissue sarcoma. A study of 200 cases. *Histopathology*, 1990; **16**: 441–54.

62. Kindblom L-G, Walaas L. Ultrastructural studies in the preoperative cytologic diagnosis of soft tissue tumors. *Seminars in Diagnostic Pathology*, 1986; **3**: 317–44.

63. Åkerman M, Willén H, Carlén B. Fine needle aspiration (FNA) of synovial sarcoma—a comparative histological-cytological study of 15 cases, including immunohistochemical, electron microscopic and cytogenetic examinations and DNA-ploidy analysis. *Cytopathology*, 1996; **59**: 589–92.

64. Waalas L, Kindblom L-G. Light and electron microscopic examination of fine-needle aspirates in the preoperative diagnosis of osteogenic tumors. A study of 21 osteosarcomas and two osteoblastomas. *Diagnostic Cytopathology*, 1990; **6**: 27–38.

65. Akhtar M, *et al*. Fine needle aspiration biopsy diagnosis of round cell malignant tumors of childhood. A combined light and electron microscopic approach. *Cancer*, 1985; **55**: 1805–17.

66. Bibbo M, Bartels P, Dytch H, Wied G. Cell image analysis. In: Bibbo M, ed. *Comprehensive cytopathology*. Philadelphia: WB Saunders, 1991: 965–83.

67. Fernö M, Baldetorp B, Åkerman M. Flow cytometric DNA ploidy analysis of soft tissue sarcomas. A comparative study of preoperative fine needle aspirates and postoperative fresh tissues and archival material. *Analytical and Quantitative Cytology and Histology*, 1990; **12**: 251–7.

68. van Diest P, Baak J. Morphometry. In: Bibbo M, ed. *Comprehensive cytopathology*. Philadelphia: WB Saunders, 1991: 946–64.

69. Choong PF, Rydholm A, Mertens F, Mandahl N. Musculoskeletal oncology. Advances in cytogenetics and molecular genetics and their clinical implications. *Acta Oncologia*, 1996; **36**: 245–54.

70. Kluin PHM, Vaandrager JW, van Krieken JM, Schuuring E. Chromosomal markers in lymphoma diagnosis. *Current Diagnostic Pathology*, 1996; **3**: 187–99.

71. Kristoffersson U, Olsson H, Åkerman M, Mitelman F. Cytogenetic studies in non-Hodgkin's lymphomas—results from fine-needle aspiration samples. *Hereditas*, 1985; **103**: 63–76.

72. Åkerman M, *et al*. Cytogenetic studies on fine needle aspiration samples from osteosarcoma and Ewing's sarcoma. *Diagnostic Cytopathology*, 1996; **15**: 17–22.

73. O—Leary JJ, Landers RJ, Chetty R. *In situ* amplification in cytological preparations. *Cytopathology*, 1997; **8**: 148–60.

74. Åkerman M, Åman P, Lindholm K, Carlén B. Primary Ewing's sarcoma of bone in a 73 year old man. Diagnosis by fine needle aspiration cytology, electron microscopy, immunocytochemistry and molecular genetic analysis. *Acta Cytologica*, 1995; **39**: 265–6.

75. Veltman J, Hopman A, Bot F, Ramaekers F, Manni J. Detection of chromosomal aberrations in cytologic brush specimens from head and neck squamous cell carcinoma. *Cancer (Cancer Cytopathology)*, 1997; **81**: 309–14.

76. Miki H, *et al*. Detection of c-Ki-ras point mutation from pancreatic juice. A useful diagnostic approach for pancreatic carcinoma. *International Journal of Pancreatology*, 1993; **14**: 145–8.

77. Hughes J, Caraway N, Katz R. Blastic variant of mantle-cell lymphoma: Cytomorphologic, immunocytochemical, and molecular genetic features of tissue obtained by fine-needle aspiration biopsy. *Diagnostic Cytopathology*, 1998; **19**: 59–62.

78. **The 1988 Bethesda System for Reporting Cervical/Vaginal Cytologic Diagnoses**. Developed and approved at the National Cancer Institute Workshop, Bethesda, Maryland, U.S.A. December 12–13, 1988. *Acta Cytologica*, 1989; **33**: 567–74.

79. **The Papanicolaou Society of Cytopathology task force on standards of**

practise. Guidelines of the Papanicolaou Society of Cytopathology for fine-needle aspiration procedure and reporting. *Diagnostic Cytopathology*, 1997; **17**: 239–47.

80. **National Cancer Institute Fine-needle Aspiration of Breast Workshop Subcommittees.** The uniform approach to breast fine-needle aspiration biopsy. *Diagnostic Cytopathology*, 1997; **16**: 295–312.

81. **The Papanicolaou Society of Cytopathology task force on standards of practise.** Guidelines of the Papanicolaou Society of Cytopathology for the examination of fine-needle aspiration specimens from thyroid nodules. *Diagnostic Cytopathology*, 1996; **15**: 84–9.

82. **Jamieson WRE,** *et al.* Reliability of percutaneous needle aspiration biopsy diagnosis of bronchogenic carcinoma. *Cancer Detection and Prevention*, 1981; **4**: 331–6.

83. **Lalli AF, McCormack LJ, Zelch M, Reich NE, Belovich D.** Aspireation of chest lesions. *Radiology*, 1978; **127**: 35–40.

84. **Westcott JL.** Direct percutaneous needle aspiration of localized pulmonary lesions. *Radiology*, 1980; **137**: 31–5.

85. **Roussel F, Dalion J, Benozio M.** The risk of tumoral seeding in needle biopsies. *Acta Cytologica*, 1989; **33**: 936–9.

86. **Jourdan JL, Stubbs RS.** Percutaneous biopsy of operable liver lesions: is it necessary or advisable? *New Zealand Medical Journal*, 1996; **109**: 469–70.

87. **Chan JKC, Tang SK, Tsang WYW, Lee KC, Batsakis JG.** Histologic changes induced by fine-needle aspiration. *Advances in Anatomic Pathology*, 1996; **3**: 71–90.

3.3 Modern imaging in cancer management

Anwar R. Padhani and Janet E. Husband

Introduction

Cancer imaging has become increasingly important in the management of patients with cancer, reflecting a growing need to evaluate disease status, not only at the time of diagnosis and staging, but also at regular intervals during follow-up. Close liaison between cancer clinicians and radiologists is essential if optimum utilization of imaging techniques is to be achieved. Technological advances in imaging techniques and cancer treatment options require constant reappraisal of imaging strategies. The choice of an imaging strategy or test is dependent on many factors, which include the information being sought, the availability and accuracy of imaging techniques, and the potential hazards to patients. Other factors determining imaging choice include the level of local expertise and enthusiasm. At a time of increasing demand for imaging resources and increasing healthcare costs, economic factors increasingly influence decisions regarding the most appropriate test in a given clinical situation.

This chapter reviews recent advances in imaging techniques and discusses methods used in assessing the clinical effectiveness of imaging technologies. We will then discuss imaging strategies in the management of patients with cancer according to diagnosis, staging, radiotherapy planning, monitoring response to treatment, and detection of relapse. Radiological imaging has a small but valuable place in screening for malignant disease, and this application will also be briefly considered.

Summary

- Diagnostic imaging is a rapidly evolving medical specialty based on technical innovations.
- Imaging continues to take on new clinical roles, thus requiring close co-operation between clinicians and radiologists for the optimal and appropriate use of imaging techniques.

We gratefully acknowledge the Cancer Research Campaign (CRC) for their ongoing, generous support of research within the Academic Department of Diagnostic Radiology at the Royal Marsden Hospital and Institute of Cancer Research, London. Mrs Janet MacDonald helped prepare the illustrations. We also acknowledge the many colleagues who have made helpful comments on the contents of the manuscript, including Professor MO Leach, Dr D MacVicar, Dr Adam Schwartz, Dr Vincent Khoo, and others.

Recent advances in imaging techniques

Imaging trends

Diagnostic imaging is perhaps the most rapidly evolving medical specialty and continues to take on new clinical roles. A number of general trends can be identified which together have made a substantial impact on clinical practice and research. One of the most impressive of these has been the ability to demonstrate anatomical and pathological information at ever-increasing spatial resolution. The technique of high-resolution computed tomography (**HRCT**) is able to resolve lung structures as small as 200 microns, thus allowing highly specific diagnoses such as lymphangitis carcinomatosis and invasive aspergillosis to be made. High-resolution magnetic resonance imaging (**MRI**) is able to depict individual nerves within the internal auditory canal and so enables the early detection of acoustic neuromas. Even so, it is important to recognize that, in most areas of the body, it is unusual to detect lesions less than 8 to 10 mm in diameter. Notable exceptions include lung lesions which can be identified on CT down to the size of 2 to 3 mm, and adrenal and some intracranial tumours (for example, acoustic neuromas) can be shown when only 5 mm in size. However, it should be borne in mind that there is a long 'silent interval' between conception of a tumour and its detection with imaging techniques.[1]

Imaging techniques have a variable ability to characterize lesions, particularly when small. The distinction of cysts from solid masses can be made with relative ease, but benign solid masses such as a haematomas or abscesses may have identical appearances to tumours. This variable ability to characterize lesion type is a major drawback of CT, but this also applies to other morphological imaging methods such as ultrasound and, to a lesser extent, MRI. Physiological imaging techniques have emerged to address the issue of limited tissue characterization. Anatomical techniques such as fluoroscopy, CT, and MRI are able to provide functional information to varying degrees. Nuclear medicine techniques, such as positron emission tomography (**PET**) and magnetic resonance spectroscopic (**MRS**) imaging, display predominantly physiological/metabolic but at lower spatial resolution.

With developments in computer hardware and software and digital image processing, it is now possible to fuse and display anatomical and functional images from the different modalities and so allow the spatial distribution of function to be assessed. Three-dimensional displays including virtual reality techniques (perspective rendering) are increasingly being used to diagnose and plan treatments, for example radiotherapy planning. Other imaging trends include faster

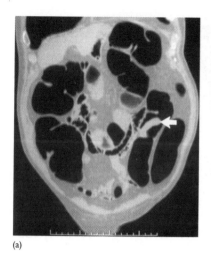

(a)

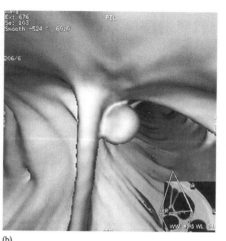

(b)

Fig. 1 (a)(b) Spiral CT reconstructed images. (a) Coronal multiplanar reconstruction of a multislice helical CT dataset, performed after air insufflation of the colon. A polyp (arrow) is visible in the descending colon. (b) Virtual reality endoscopic reconstruction showing the descending colon and polyp with its relation to a haustral fold.

data-acquisition times, such that it is now possible to freeze even the fastest physiological motions (for example, the heart beat) and it is currently even possible to observe neuronal brain activity by MRI techniques.

Advances in computed tomography

A number of advances have occurred in CT, the most significant of which are volumetric data acquisition, improvements in digital imaging processing, and, more recently, improvements in the ability to use CT for guided interventions in patients. Spiral CT (also called helical CT) is a relatively new technique that has now reached a level of maturity and availability. Volume data acquisition can be obtained as the patient is passed through a CT gantry at a constant rate (10 to 30 cm per second) while being irradiated. The ability to acquire motion-free images results from a number of technological advances, including improvements in X-ray tubes, multidetector technology, slip-ring engineering, and data-processing methods.[2]

Volume CT data acquisition has had a major impact on CT practice for a number of reasons. These include rapidity of data acquisition; the trunk can be examined in two breath-holds (30 s) on multislice systems. As data is acquired with suspended respiration, image misregistration and motion artefacts are eliminated allowing improved detection of focal lung and liver lesions. Respiratory misregistration refers to gaps in conventional CT data resulting from inconsistent repeated breath-holds which may result in missed lesions. The ability to slice directly through the middle of lesions thus eliminating neighbouring structures from the slice plane (minimizing partial volume effects) has improved the detection and characterization of focal lesions, particularly in the lung and liver.[3],[4] Spiral CT with intravenous contrast medium can be carried out reliably at optimal levels of vascular and parenchymal organ enhancement. The former has resulted in the development of a new CT application: CT angiography. This technique has already proved to be of value in demonstrating central pulmonary emboli with better specificity than radionuclide ventilation–perfusion (V/Q) scanning.[5] This technique has been found to be of value in the evaluation of patients with parenchymal lung disease suspected of having pulmonary emboli in whom V/Q scans are often indeterminate. With improved contrast

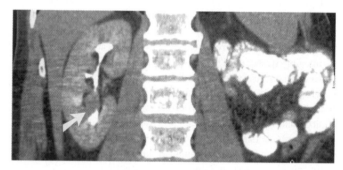

Fig. 2 Multislice CT evaluation of transitional carcinoma in the kidney. Coronal reconstruction from a multislice helical CT data acquisition shows a mass within the pelvi-calyceal system in the lower pole of the right kidney (arrow). There has been a previous left nephrectomy for a transitional carcinoma. These images were valuable for planning partial nephrectomy.

utilization, a decrease in contrast-dose usage is possible without sacrificing image quality. This is beneficial both economically and for patients with renal impairment, and results in fewer side-effects.

The ability of spiral CT to acquire overlapping slices without additional radiation exposure and the development of new interpolation algorithms that maintain section-sensitivity also represent major developments. These have resulted in the ability to obtain isotropic (cubic) voxels of data thus allowing improved multiplanar visualization and 3D image reconstructions. For example, virtual reality navigation can be applied to volume CT datasets to produce 'endoscopic-like' views of hollow organs, which may be useful in patients who are unsuitable for invasive endoscopic evaluation (Fig. 1).[6]–[8] Volume datasets are also helpful for treatment planning, for example in the surgical assessment of pancreatic cancer or in the selection of patients who are candidates for partial nephrectomy (Fig. 2). A disadvantage in volume data acquisition is the higher radiation dose. This is not intrinsic to the technique, but arises from the increased versatility of the technique which enables more complex examinations to be performed.

Summary

- Volumetric data acquisition using spiral or helical multislice technologies is the latest innovation in computed tomography.
- Potential patient benefits include rapid data acquisition, improved detection and characterization of lesions, optimal use of intravenous contrast-medium enhancement, and 3D imaging.
- Spiral CT is the preferred technique for detecting pulmonary and liver lesions prior to metastectomy and for surgical planning of pancreatic and renal cancer treatment.
- New roles for spiral CT include the detection of pulmonary emboli, CT angiography, and endoscopic viewing of hollow organs.

Advances in MR imaging

MRI has a number of imaging benefits, including superb soft tissue contrast, multiplanar and 3D image acquisition capability, freedom from bony artefacts, and high signal specificity. Other advantages include the absence of exposure to ionizing radiation (an important factor when imaging children, pregnant women, and the young with curable tumours) and the ability to acquire biological and physiological information. The latter includes macroscopic blood flow, tissue perfusion, capillary permeability, water diffusion, and even the ability to detect brain activation during motor, sensory, and other tasks. The disadvantages of MRI include the confines of the magnet, and the limited access to life-support and monitoring equipment. The presence of the magnetic field precludes examination of patients with heart valves and cardiac pacemakers, and examination times are still relatively long compared with CT.

There have been a number of advances in MR imaging which have occurred as a direct result of hardware and software developments together with improved and new contrast mechanisms.[9] The resolution of MRI has steadily improved hand in hand with a dramatic increase in the speed of image acquisition combined with motion-compensation techniques. The latter has resulted in the ability to examine restless patients and to image physiological events such as the heartbeat and tissue perfusion, and to observe neuronal brain activity. New contrast imaging characteristics can now be routinely imaged. These include magnetization transfer imaging which enables improved visualization of brain lesions after contrast-medium administration compared with conventional sequences. New sequences such as **FLAIR** (fluid-attenuated inversion recovery), which enable the distinction between bound and free water, have begun to replace conventional T_2-weighted sequences in specific circumstances such as in the diagnosis of multiple sclerosis. Brownian water motion imaging (diffusion imaging) has already found application in the early diagnosis of stroke[10] and may be of value in the assessment of brain tumours. There have also been important developments in coil technology, including the introduction of endocavitary coils. These endocavitary coils improve the signal-to-noise ratio allowing superb image quality for assessing the local extent of rectal, cervix, and prostate cancer.

A number of tissue-specific contrast agents have recently been introduced, or are in advanced clinical trials, which have potential application in patients with cancer. For example, liver-specific contrast media are now commercially available and clinical trials of contrast agents directed towards lymph nodes are at advanced stages of development.[11]–[13] These agents are already beginning to have an

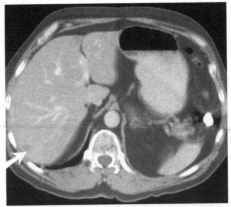

(a)

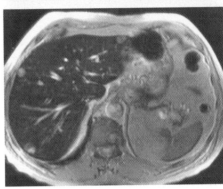

(b)

Fig. 3 MRI with a liver-specific contrast agent. (a) Axial CT image of the liver in a patient with metastatic colon cancer obtained in the portal phase of contrast enhancement. A metastasis is identified within segment VII (arrow). Other lesions are difficult to see. (b) Proton density-weighted, gradient-echo MR image of the liver at the same level performed after the administration of Ferumoxide contrast medium. Three deposits are seen. In total, three or four lesions were seen on CT, whereas seven lesions were visible on MRI.

impact on clinical practice. For example, liver-specific contrast agents that target hepatocytes or Kuppfer cells enable improved detection of focal lesions (Fig. 3).[14]–[16] The accuracy of contrast-enhanced MRI compared to CT arterioportography (**CTAP**) is currently under investigation. Moreover, because of results to date, it seems likely that these agents will have a significant impact on the surgical management of patients with colon cancer. Another recent development has been the incorporation of gadolinium or other lanthanide elements (with paramagnetic properties) into drugs with a view to imaging the biodistribution of the drug. A recent example of this is gadolinium texaphyrin, a tumour-selective radiosensitizer that has high selective uptake in brain tumours.[17]

Summary

- Recent advances include increased speed of data acquisition and the ability to visualize function superimposed on anatomical images.
- Functional measurements include tissue perfusion, permeability to micro- and macromolecules, observing Brownian motion of water molecules, and the detection of neuronal brain activity.
- New tissue-specific contrast agents include Kuppfer-cell and hepatocyte agents as well as lymph node-specific agents.

Table 1 Commonly used positron-emitting tracers

Radiotracer	Biological analogue	Measured response	Isotope half-life (min)
2-Deoxy-2(^{18}F)fluoro-D-glucose (FDG)	Glucose	Glucose metabolism Phosphorylation by hexokinase	110
5-(^{18}F)fluoro-DOPA	Dopamine	Amino acid metabolism	110
(^{18}F)Fluoromethyltyrosine	Tyrosine	Amino acid metabolism	110
(^{18}F)Fluoro-2′-deoxyuridine	Fluorodeoxyuridine	Nucleic acid metabolism	110
(^{18}F)fluoracyclovir	Acyclovir	Phosphorylation by thymidine kinase	110
(^{11}C)Acetate	Acetate	Fatty acid metabolism	20
(^{12}N)Ammonia	None	Tissue perfusion	10
(^{15}O)Water	Water	Tissue perfusion	2
(^{68}GA)EDTA	None	Capillary integrity; blood–brain barrier	60

• Ongoing developments will have a significant impact on cancer practice.

Advances in ultrasound

Ultrasound is an important diagnostic imaging modality for the evaluation of patients with cancer. For many applications, ultrasound is the ideal imaging modality as no patient preparation is required and contrast material is not usually administered. Most studies can be performed within 20 to 30 minutes and high-resolution portable units are also available. The lack of ionizing radiation makes ultrasound an attractive choice for assessing paediatric and gynaecological cancers. An additional advantage is the recent development of colour and power Doppler imaging, in which direct visualization of flow within blood vessels can be achieved without the need for contrast medium. However, ultrasound has a number of significant limitations. The diagnostic success of ultrasound is highly dependent on the skill and expertise of the operator. The lack of reproducibility using ultrasound (in part due to the use of non-orthogonal planes of imaging) is a significant limitation particularly for longitudinal studies. Abdominal ultrasound may be ineffective in patients who are obese, in those with fatty livers, and extensive bowel gas can preclude a full abdominal examination.

Ultrasound is an extremely efficient method for guiding percutaneous interventions such as biopsy, abscess drainage, and nephrostomy, because the needle insertion can be visualized directly in real-time. Ultrasound is also the initial imaging modality of choice when evaluating patients with biliary or renal disease, and for evaluation of the pelvis. Ultrasound is often used to clarify abnormalities seen by other imaging studies such as CT, MRI, and mammography.

Recent developments in transducer technology and colour Doppler imaging have significantly enhanced the role of ultrasound in cancer diagnosis. It is likely that continuing advances in ultrasound technology, such as 3D imaging, ultrasound contrast agents, and probe miniaturization,[18]–[22] will increase the effective use of ultrasound. Most current state-of-the-art systems are capable of performing high-resolution, grey-scale imaging as well as colour and spectral Doppler.

One of the major recent technological advances has been the development of advanced probe designs.[19] Specific examinations often require dedicated transducers that have both grey-scale resolution and colour Doppler sensitivity. The frequency of an ultrasound probe determines its clinical use. For example, high-frequency transducers (7 to 10 MHz) are used for near-field imaging of superficial structures; such probes have been incorporated into endoscopic devices for endoscopic ultrasound examination of the oesophagus, stomach, and rectum. These probes may be fitted with dedicated biopsy attachments. For routine abdominal imaging, however, a greater depth is required and lower frequency transducers (3 to 5 MHz) are used.

Colour Doppler sonography enables real-time visualization of blood flow with or without the use of ultrasound contrast agents.[20] Doppler information can be displayed graphically by the use of spectral Doppler analysis. The combination of real-time images and spectral Doppler analysis is sometimes referred to as Duplex scanning. Statistical analysis of the spectral Doppler waveform can be used to calculate indices of resistivity such as the pulsatility index. Waveform analysis has been used with mixed results to differentiate normal vessels from tumour neovascularity. Blood vessels within tumours lack a muscular coat and tone and result in prominent diastolic flow with a low pulsatility index. In contrast, hepatocellular carcinomas display high-velocity flow because of arteriovenous shunting. More recently, a number of limitations of Doppler imaging in the cancer setting have been noted and, in particular, it may not always be possible to differentiate malignant from benign lesions on the basis of tumour vascularity alone.

Summary

• Transducer technology and colour Doppler imaging has significantly advanced ultrasound diagnosis in cancer.

• Ultrasound contrast agents, probe miniaturization, and 3D imaging will increase the effective use of ultrasound.

Functional imaging techniques

Functional imaging techniques have a direct bearing on cancer practice. The current roles of positron-emission tomography (PET), dynamic contrast medium-enhanced MR imaging, and MR spectroscopy (MRS) will be discussed.

Positron-emission tomography (PET)

PET creates tomographic images that represent the metabolic activity of underlying tissue processes. Major developments that have enabled the successful implementation of this technique include radiopharmaceuticals that resemble endogenous biological compounds, quantification of tracer distribution, volume data acquisition, and whole-body tomographic imaging.

A number of radionuclides decay with the emission of a positron including carbon-11, nitrogen-13, oxygen-15, and fluorine-18. Each of these can be labelled to a variety of 'biologically interesting' pharmaceuticals whose kinetics can then be studied without disruption of metabolic pathways. A list of several commonly used positron-emitting radiotracers and their biochemical analogues is given in Table 1. The most commonly used PET radiotracer for tumour imaging is the glucose analogue 2-[F-18]fluoro-2-deoxy-D-glucose (**18-FDG**). This compound, which is a tracer for the glycolytic pathway, is important in cancer imaging for a number of reasons, including:

- the relatively long half-life of F-18 (110 min) allows feasible radiochemistry;
- the radionuclide may be produced in large quantities by small hospital-based cyclotrons;
- many common cancers, especially of the colon, lung, melanoma, lymphoma, and breast, are easily imaged using 18-FDG; and
- the biochemistry of cellular FDG uptake and metabolism is firmly understood.

FDG enters cells and is phosphorylated by hexokinase in a competitive process with glucose. Unlike glucose, little FDG-6-phosphate is then metabolized and does not diffuse out of the cells due to low membrane permeability. Thus, FDG-6-phosphate becomes trapped within the cells with high glucose metabolism. Tumour imaging with FDG relies on the premise that glucose metabolism is increased in malignant tumours.[23]

PET imaging is able to accurately measure the distribution of the radiotracer. The ability to semi-quantitatively analyse the uptake of the PET agent by the standardized uptake ratio (**SUR**) allows an objective method of reporting tracer uptake in a lesion. An SUR of more than 2.5 has been shown to be sensitive and specific in detecting malignant disease in the chest,[24] although visual analysis may be just as effective.[25] Another feature of PET is its ability to rapidly acquire a series of tomographic images through a volume of tissue. This is made possible through the design and arrangement of multiple rings of co-incident detectors in the PET camera. Rapid frame acquisition is also important for studying tracer kinetics and thus it is possible to measure tissue flow such as perfusion. PET cameras can also acquire tomographic whole-body images. By advancing the bed position relative to the scanner gantry at set time intervals, multiple sections can be acquired and large volumetric datasets can be displayed as orthogonal images.

18-FDG-PET has become an important tool in a number of clinical areas relevant to cancer practice and these will now be discussed.[26],[27]

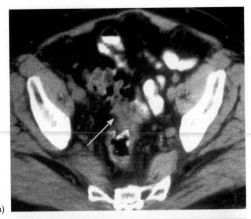

(a)

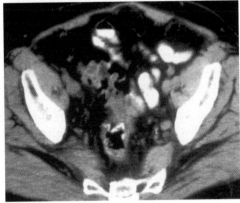

(b)

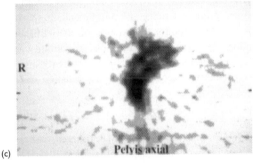

(c)

Fig. 4 Recurrent rectosigmoid carcinoma with unchanging CT appearance. (a) Axial CT image obtained 6 months after anterior resection for upper rectal cancer. Soft tissue thickening is identified adjacent to the surgical clips (arrow). Serum carcinoembryonic antigen (CEA) levels were normal. This image was interpreted as equivocal. (b) Ten months later, the patient was reinvestigated for a rising serum CEA level. Axial CT image through the pelvis at the same level shows no change in morphological appearances. (c) Axial FDG-PET image shows hypermetabolism at the site of the residual abnormality. At surgical resection, a proven recurrence was found.

Characterization of indeterminate lesions

Characterization of indeterminate lung lesions is a specific application for 18-FDG-PET. PET has shown high sensitivity for detecting malignant lung lesions (90 to 100 per cent), but specificity has been more variable (60 to 100 per cent) because benign inflammatory lesions may also take up 18-FDG.[24],[28]–[30] The ability to characterize lung lesions non-invasively has important clinical benefits including reductions in the costs and morbidity associated with biopsy and surgical sampling. Indeterminate adrenal masses are a common cause of clinical concern in patients with cancer. While experience in this area is currently limited, several studies have shown high sensitivity using 18-FGD-PET.[31],[32] One study has evaluated true indeterminate adrenal masses in patients with a variety of tumours and found 100 per cent sensitivity.[33]

Another important clinical area is the detection of local recurrence of colorectal carcinoma (Fig. 4). This has been extensively studied with 18-FDG-PET. In general, patients with recurrent colorectal malignancy have a high FDG uptake, whereas those patients with non-malignant masses, usually scars, do not. PET is superior to CT in detecting locally recurrent disease (95 per cent for PET and 65 per cent for pelvic CT).[23],[34] FDG-PET is also superior to conventional imaging in detecting unsuspected extrahepatic metastases including lymph node deposits and pulmonary metastases.[34],[35] Lai et al. reported that lesions detected using 18-FDG-PET alone resulted in a change in the clinical management in substantial numbers of patients.[35] No significant differences have been noted in the detection of hepatic metastatic lesions (98 per cent for PET and 93 per cent for CT and ultrasound) but experience in this area is currently limited.[34]

Many studies have evaluated the role of 18-FDG-PET in head and neck cancer and have found the technique highly accurate for the evaluation of the primary tumour and nodal metastases, but of limited overall usefulness. This paradox arises because competing imaging techniques such as CT and MRI already have very good accuracy. In special problem areas where 18-FDG-PET might be expected to offer unique advantages such as in screening for second lesions, searching for unknown primary lesions, or in differentiating benign from malignant salivary tumours, the results of FDG-PET have been disappointing.[36],[37] However, 18-FDG-PET is definitely superior to alternative methods of detecting tumour recurrence and in differentiating post-therapy sequelae such as radiation necrosis and fibrosis.[38]

Staging malignancies

Since PET allows the whole body to be imaged, it has the clear advantage of allowing global staging of tumours. Examples of such applications include mediastinal and adrenal staging, evaluation of lung cancer, and whole-body staging of patients with lymphoma. PET is able to demonstrate primary tumours in lung cancer, but its accuracy with regard to the local staging of disease compared with CT and MRI has not been fully determined. 18-FDG-PET is more accurate than CT in determining the presence or absence of intrathoracic, metastatic, lymph node disease.[39]–[42] This is because CT and MRI rely on nodal size alone to distinguish normal from abnormal nodes. PET is able to predict tumour absence in enlarged lymph nodes that are not FDG-avid (negative predictive value-100 per cent) and can show tumour in normal sized nodes (positive predictive value to 100 per cent).

Another disease that can be staged globally by 18-FDG-PET is lymphoma. PET appears to have an excellent accuracy for staging thoracoabdominal lymphomas regardless of tumour stage. It can detect disease in normal-sized lymph nodes and is also successful in being able to demonstrate the presence of extranodal disease (for example, bone marrow) that goes undetected by CT.[43],[44] 18-FDG-PET may also have a role in detecting residual active disease after the treatment of malignant lymphoma, but evidence of its power in

this regard is currently limited.[45],[46] Good sensitivities for the staging of other tumours, including breast cancer and melanoma, have also been documented.

Interestingly, the accuracy of 18-FDG-PET in staging prostate cancer is more limited. 18-FDG-PET has a high positive predictive value in detecting soft tissue lesions, but has a limited sensitivity (65 per cent) compared to routine bone scintigraphy in the identification of bony metastases.[47],[48] The latter occurs in metastatic bone disease possibly because the intrinsic high metabolic rate of normal marrow decreases the contrast with bony lesions.[49]

Monitoring response to treatment

One of the unique features of PET is the ability to directly measure changes in tissues or tumour metabolism that are induced by treatment. A Royal Marsden Hospital study[50] compared 18-FDG-PET and tumour size measurements on CT in 18 patients with liver metastases from colorectal cancer during the first month of chemotherapy. This study showed that PET was successfully able to discriminate responders from non-responders on a lesion-by-lesion basis and predicted overall patient treatment response. Similar studies have been performed in patients with hepatocellular carcinoma,[51] for head and neck tumours,[52] and in breast cancer.[53] Decreases in uptake by responding tumours can be observed as early as 45 min post-chemotherapy and changes in FDG metabolism occur far in advance of any shrinkage of tumour volume.[54] Usually, in non-responding patients, no significant decrease in FDG uptake is observed. However, a paradoxical increase in FDG uptake in the first few weeks of treatment occurs in some tumours[52],[55] that may be related to macrophage accumulation at sites of tumour-cell death.[56]

Summary

- PET represents the metabolic activity of underlying tissue processes such as glucose, oxygen, and amino acid metabolism or measures receptor-density status.

- Parameters assessable by PET may allow new clinical perspectives in the diagnosis and management of cancer as well as improving the understanding of tumour physiology and biochemistry.

- 18-FDG-PET is a tracer for the glycolytic pathway that already has widespread clinical application.

- Clinical applications for PET include the characterization of indeterminate lesions on conventional imaging, staging malignancy, and monitoring response to treatment.

- Research applications of PET include the evaluation of drug kinetics, and determination of the effect of treatment on tumour proliferation, physiology, and biochemistry.

Dynamic MR imaging

Many radiological studies are able to depict the increased vascularity of tumours. Recently, quantification of tumour vascularity using imaging methods, for example colour Doppler sonography and dynamic contrast medium-enhanced MRI (DCE-MRI) has been undertaken. Numerous studies have shown that malignant tumours frequently reveal faster and higher levels of enhancement when compared with normal surrounding tissues. This observation has been the basis for diagnostic contrast-medium MRI for many years. The introduction of fast imaging sequences and developments in tracer kinetic modelling for DCE-MRI studies now allow a fuller

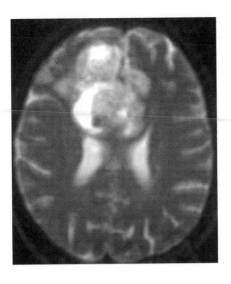
(a)

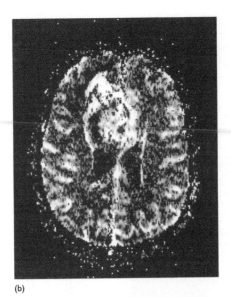
(b)

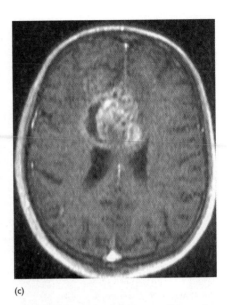
(c)

Fig. 5 Blood volume MRI imaging in oligodendroglioma. (a) Axial T_2-weighted MR image of a malignant cerebral oligodendroglioma. A large necrotic mass is seen in the right frontal lobe. The tumour extends across the midline. The high-signal regions seen within the tumour represent areas of necrosis. (b) Cerebral blood volume map at the same slice location. The tumour is noted to be markedly hypervascular with a blood volume equal or greater than the cortical grey matter. (c) Axial postcontrast-enhanced T_1-weighted image shows enhancement predominantly around the areas of necrosis, but there is little evidence of blood–brain barrier breakdown elsewhere within the tumour.

understanding of the physiological basis of contrast enhancement in human tumours. With optimal data collection, sequences can be designed to be sensitive to tissue perfusion and blood volume (so-called T_2^* methods) and/or permeability and extracellular leakage space (so-called T_1 methods). Such techniques permit the functional aspects of tumour neovascularity to be assessed *in vivo* non-invasively. Other advantages of MRI methods include good spatial resolution and the ability to incorporate physiological data acquisition into routine patient studies.

T_2^*-weighted imaging

Perfusion-weighted images can be obtained with 'bolus-tracking techniques' that analyse the passage of contrast material through a capillary bed.[57],[58] When a bolus of a paramagnetic contrast agent passes through a capillary bed, it produces magnetic field inhomogeneities that result in a decrease in the signal intensity of surrounding tissues. These signal alterations can be detected by T_2^*-weighted gradient-echo sequences (with long repetition and echo times employing low flip angles). The degree of signal loss is dependent on the vascular concentration of the contrast agent and microvessel density. Tracer kinetic principles can then be applied to provide estimates of tissue perfusion, for example relative blood volume (**rBV**), relative blood flow (**rBF**), and mean transit time (**MTT**).[59]

The signal loss observed with T_2^*-weighted sequences can be used qualitatively in clinical studies to characterize liver and breast lesions. In their studies, Ichikawa *et al.* were successfully able to discriminate between liver metastases, haemangiomata, and hepatocellular carcinoma on the basis of characteristic signal-intensity changes on ultrafast imaging sequences.[60] Kuhl *et al.* and Kvistad *et al.* have both used T_2^*-susceptibility contrast to improve the characterization of breast lesions. They showed strong, susceptibility mediated signal

loss in malignant breast disease compared to fibroadenomas which showed little or no T_2^* effects despite showing enhancement on T_1-weighted imaging.[61],[62] Quantitative imaging is currently restricted to normal brain and brain lesions with an intact blood–brain barrier (**BBB**), because the latter retains the contrast agent within the intravascular space. Relative cerebral blood volume (**rCBV**) mapping can be used to detect areas of increased vascularity in brain gliomas.[63] (Fig. 5). Areas of high tumour rCBV correlate with higher degrees of mitotic activity and vascularity. In non-gadolinium enhancing gliomas (namely those with an intact BBB), homogeneous low rCBV is found in the lowest grades whereas higher-grade tumours display both low and high rCBV components.[64] Relative CBV maps appear to have a high, negative predictive value in excluding the presence of high-grade tumour in untreated patients regardless of their enhancement characteristics on T_1-weighted MRI. Cerebral blood volume maps can therefore be used to direct stereotactic biopsy to areas of highest grade. Other potential uses of perfusion imaging in patients with brain tumours include determining prognosis and monitoring response to treatment.[65]

T_1-weighted imaging

Gadolinium chelates rapidly from the blood into the extracellular space of tissues at a rate determined by the permeability of the capillaries. The presence of contrast medium in the extracellular fluid space is visible on T_1-weighted images (short repetition and echo times employing large flip angles). The degree of enhancement seen on a series of T_1-weighted images acquired over a period of several minutes is dependent on a number of physiological and physical factors. These include microvessel density within a tumour, the permeability to micro- and macromolecules, and the volume of the extracellular leakage space. Vascular density in malignant tissues is

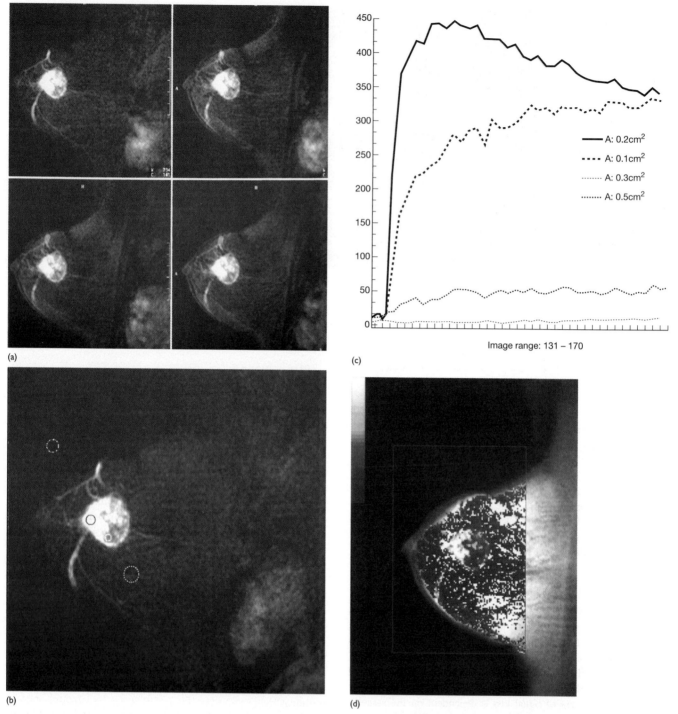

Image range: 131 – 170

Fig. 6 Dynamic contrast-enhanced MRI of breast carcinoma. (a) Sample frames from a sequential MRI study following intravenous administration of contrast medium in a patient with invasive ductal carcinoma. A large heterogeneously enhancing mass is visible. Numerous feeder vessels in the adjacent breast parenchyma are seen. (b) Regions of interest (**ROIs**) are placed in the tumour, within normal breast parenchyma and in background. (c) Time–signal-intensity curves from the ROIs demonstrated in (b). The solid line shows a sharp uptake, high peak, and rapid washout of contrast medium. The shape of the curve in the lower part of the tumour is different (slower rise, no washout). Heterogeneity of such time–signal-intensity curves is characteristic of malignant tumours. (d) Transfer constant map shows the permeability surface area product of the vasculature, displayed as a pixel map superimposed on the anatomical image (maximum transfer constant displayed is 2 min^{-1}) (see also Plate 1). Highly heterogeneous enhancement is also typical of cancer.

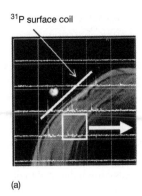

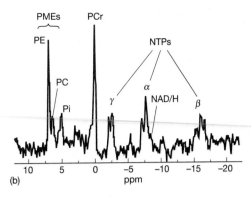

Fig. 7 Phosphorus MR spectroscopy of a soft tissue sarcoma. (a) A slice through a 3D spectral map from a proton-decoupled ^{31}P 3D spectroscopic imaging scan of a soft tissue sarcoma in the abdomen. The position of the ^{31}P surface coil is indicated and the reference standard in the coil housing is also visible. Spectra from voxels near the abdominal wall are characteristic of muscle, dominated by a strong phosphocreatine (PCr) signal at 0 p.p.m. (b) Deeper lying spectra, such as that in the highlighted voxel, are characteristic of tumour, with pronounced signal from phosphomonoesters (PMEs) at approximately 7 p.p.m. These MR-visible PMEs are precursors to cell-membrane formation and are elevated in many tumour types, possibly reflecting upregulated cell proliferation. In this study, the phosphoethanolamine (PE) and phosphocholine (PC) PME components have been resolved by the use of proton decoupling during the acquisition. Inorganic phosphate (Pi) and nucleoside triphosphate (NTP) signals are also visible. (By courtesy of Dr A.J. Schwarz, Institute of Cancer Research, London.)

higher than in normal parenchyma, but there is an overlap with benign lesions, including inflammatory and proliferative processes. In the brain, the capillary permeability is low due to the presence of an intact BBB, but is higher in normal extracranial tissues and in malignant lesions.

Analysis of enhancement seen on dynamic T_1-weighted images is a valuable diagnostic tool in a number of clinical situations. A well-established role is in lesion characterization, for example, in distinguishing benign from malignant breast and musculoskeletal lesions.[66]–[68] Simple observations from time–signal-intensity curves have shown that malignant tissues generally enhance early, with a rapid and large increase in signal intensity compared with benign tissues, which in general show a slower rise in signal intensity (Fig. 6). In the breast, sensitivities for discriminating benign from malignant lesions have been high but specificities have been more variable, with fibroadenomas sometimes demonstrating an enhancement pattern similar to that of invasive cancer.[69] Dynamic T_1-weighted MRI studies have also been found to be of value in staging bladder and prostate cancer.[70],[71] Dynamic MRI is also able to monitor the effects of treatment in patients with osteosarcomas and in breast, prostate, and cervix cancers.[72]–[75] Changes in contrast enhancement have been observed prior to changes in tumour volume. Currently, it is unclear whether such changes occur before changes in metabolism, which may be detectable by FDG-PET or MR spectroscopy. Contrast-enhanced, T_1-weighted studies also enable the early detection of tumour relapses within treated tissues.[76]–[78]

Summary

- Dynamic contrast-enhanced MRI is able to depict tissue perfusion and capillary permeability to micro- and macromolecules.

- Dynamic MRI can be used for lesion detection and characterization, to detect relapse in treated tissues, and to monitor the effects of treatment.

- Contrast-enhanced MRI is ideally suited for monitoring the effects of antiangiogenesis treatments.

Magnetic resonance spectroscopy

Magnetic resonance spectroscopy (**MRS**) is a powerful, non-invasive method for studying tumour biochemistry and physiology. Biochemical information obtained by MRS can be used to explore the metabolic characteristics of tumours and normal tissues. Spectral characteristics can also convey diagnostic information on the state of differentiation and grade of tumours. MRS can also be used to monitor the response of a tumour to therapy, and to follow the pharmacokinetics of some chemotherapeutic agents. Large-scale clinical trials are ongoing to define the clinical role of MRS. In this section we describe the basic principles of MR spectroscopy and review its possible clinical roles with respect to common nuclei that are observed in spectroscopic studies of cancer.[79],[80]

*Basic principles of nuclear magnetic resonance (**NMR**) spectroscopy*

Nuclear magnetic resonance is the physical phenomenon underlying both MR imaging and MRS. The essential difference between the two is that MRS measures signals from chemical compounds within tissues, whereas MR images tissue relaxation properties (T_1-spin lattice and T_2-spin–spin relaxation times). MRS is possible because resonance signals arise at slightly different frequencies, depending on the positions of the atomic nuclei that give rise to them in molecules. Nuclei in different local chemical (and hence magnetic) environments will resonate at unique frequencies that can be observed at different positions within a spectrum. The separation of the resonance frequencies is termed the 'chemical shift' and is quoted in the dimensionless units of parts per million (**p.p.m.**). Different chemical shifts allow the identification of individual components of the sample. Signals can be plotted as peaks on a normalized frequency scale, and the area under each peak is proportional to the concentration of atoms that gave rise to it. Thus, it is possible to obtain both qualitative and quantitative information on tissue biochemistry.

Most clinical MRS studies in cancer are concerned with signals from ^{31}P or ^{1}H atoms in endogenous metabolites, or ^{19}F signals from anticancer drugs. The greatest weakness of MRS is its low sensitivity, about 10^4 to 10^5 lower than MRI (depending on the nucleus in question). This is mainly because molecules of interest are present at much lower concentrations than tissue water (which gives rise to MRI signals), and also because nuclei other than ^{1}H give rise to inherently weaker signals. Consequently, only a small number of high-concentration metabolites can be detected. Fortunately, some of these metabolites (ATP, (phospho)choline, (phospho)creatine, lactate, N-acetylaspartate) are of great biological importance.

^{31}P magnetic resonance spectroscopy

The most commonly observed nucleus in MRS studies of extracranial tumours is ^{31}P. ^{31}P spectra are relatively simple and easy to interpret. Importantly, metabolically significant, phosphorus-containing compounds occur in living systems at high enough concentrations to be detectable by ^{31}P-MRS, thus providing an ideal method of monitoring tumour energetics. Observed metabolites typically include three resonances from the γ, α, and β phosphates of a nucleoside triphosphate (**NTP**) (predominantly ATP), inorganic phosphate (*Pi*), phosphocreatine (**PCr**) and pyridine dinucleotides (NAD$^+$ and NADH) (Fig. 7). Phospholipid metabolites observed include phosphomonoesters (**PME**) (consisting primarily of phosphocholine, PC and phosphoethanolamine, **PE**) and phosphodiesters (**PDE**) (glycerophosphocholine, **GPC**, and glycerophosphoethanolamine, **GPE**).

Tumour intracellular pH can be calculated from the chemical shift of the *Pi* signal, and using this technique it is now clear that tumour pH is slightly alkaline.[81] The acidic tumour pH measured by microelectrode techniques previously, appears to arise from lactic acid in the extracellular space.[82] Apparently, tumour cells maintain neutrality by pumping acidic ions into the extracellular compartment. Thus, the pH gradient across the tumour-cell membrane is reversed, in contrast to normal cells which are more acidic than their extracellular environment.

Human cancers are characterized by elevated PME, elevated PDE, and an alkaline pH (mean 7.2). Animal studies have shown that ^{31}P spectra acquired during the rapid tumour growth phase are quite different from spectra acquired during the nutritionally deprived phase, presumably as a result of decreased blood flow and the development of hypoxia.[83] Tumour acidification may also reflect poor vascularity, with poor clearance of H$^+$ ions produced by glycolysis. As PME and PDE resonances are related to cell-membrane turnover in tumours (PC and PE are membrane synthesis substrates and GPC and GPE are membrane breakdown products), alteration of these resonances can be used to probe membrane synthesis or membrane decomposition.[84] In addition, ^{31}P-MRS has been used to study changes in the energy and phospholipid metabolism of tumours during therapy.[85],[86] A review of treatment-induced changes in 61 tumour types showed that a decrease in PME occurred before measurable tumour shrinkage in 38 of 47 cases, that responded to chemotherapy or radiotherapy, but in only 1 of the 14 cases that did not respond.[85] Clinical trials are currently ongoing to assess the diagnostic and prognostic values of ^{31}P-MRS studies. Such studies will test the hypothesis that early changes in phospholipid metabolites may predict sensitivity or resistance to treatment.

^{1}H magnetic resonance spectroscopy

^{1}H-MRS allows the observation of several metabolites that are not detected by MRS of other nuclei. The major obstacle for ^{1}H-MRS is the high concentrations of tissue water and lipids, which must be suppressed to observe other metabolites. Most ^{1}H-MRS studies have therefore focused on the brain and intracranial pathologies, because little motion is present and many brain pathologies exhibit no lipid signals.[87] Typical resonances observed in brain at long echo times (for example, 135 to 270 ms) include N-acetylaspartate (**NAA**), total creatines (**tCr**), total cholines (**tCho**), alanine, and lactate. An echo time of 135 ms is commonly used to observe an inverted lactate peak, while resonances attributed to inositol, glucose, and mobile lipids may appear at short echo times (for example, 20 to 50 ms). Figure 8 shows ^{1}H spectra obtained from the white matter of a normal human brain and from a grade II astrocytoma.

A number of studies have shown that ^{1}H-MRS of human brain tumours differs significantly from those of normal brain tissue. NAA, is a specific neuronal marker that is not found in tumour tissue. In contrast, tCho is elevated in tumours; this signal is derived from free choline, PC, and GPC. PC is the substrate for membrane phospholipid synthesis, and when membranes are damaged, the visibility of lipid-bound choline groups is increased. Its elevation has also been attributed to increased cell-membrane synthesis within rapidly proliferating tissue. Creatine is used as a marker of normal brain-cell density and the creatine content of glioma tissue is considerably reduced. Alanine is sometimes observed in meningiomas,[88] suggesting that their metabolism involves transamination pathways and partial oxidation of glutamine rather than glycolysis.[89] Lactate, the end-product of anaerobic respiration, has been observed in cerebral metastases and glial brain tumours,[88] distinguishing them from meningiomas, neurinomas, and lymphomas. Lactate levels may correlate with the grade or type of tumour, though the absolute lactate level is dependent on the balance between production and clearance.[90]

Lipid resonances are frequently observed in brain tumour spectra[91] and arise from mobile lipid bilayers in intact membranes and other macromolecules. The amount of lipid has been correlated with the extent of necrosis[92] and grade of malignancy.[93] It has been suggested that ^{1}H-MRS can be used for the non-invasive assessment of tumour diagnosis and for grading brain gliomas.[94] Both these assessments are currently made by histological examination of biopsy material, the results of which may be erroneous due to sampling errors.

^{19}F magnetic resonance spectroscopy

There are no endogenous fluorine-containing compounds within the body, because of which there is no background signal. Numerous chemotherapeutic agents contain the ^{19}F nucleus as an essential component, allowing *in vivo* ^{19}F MRS to be used in both preclinical and clinical cancer studies for monitoring pharmacokinetics, or for assessing tumour biochemistry by using probe molecules. 5-fluorouracil (**5-FU**), a prodrug that is activated by anabolism to cytotoxic 5-fluoronucleotides and deactivated by catabolism predominantly in the liver, has been intensively studied by ^{19}F MRS.[95]–[97] 5-FU is used predominantly for the treatment of head and neck, breast, and gastrointestinal tumours. ^{19}F MRS can be used to monitor this therapy *in situ*. One study has shown a slower clearance of 5-FU from metastatic colon cancer ($t_{\frac{1}{2}}$ = 20 to 60 min) compared to blood (8

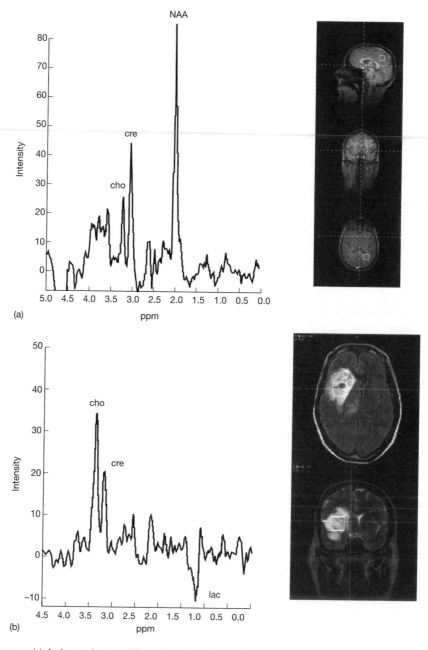

Fig. 8 Hydrogen MR spectroscopy. (a) A short echo time ($TE = 20$ ms) single voxel ^{1}H-MRS spectrum from the white matter of a normal subject. The location of the measured volume is shown in the T_2-weighted images. The major resonances are labelled. Cho, choline; cre, creatine; and NAA, N-acetylaspartate. (b) A long echo time ($TE = 135$ ms) single voxel ^{1}H-MRS spectrum obtained in a patient with a grade II glioma in the right parietal region. The location of the measured volume is shown in the T_2-weighted images. Cho, choline; cre, creatine; and lac, lactate. The pronounced lactate peak indicates poor prognosis. (By courtesy of Dr P Murphy, Institute of Cancer Research, London.)

to 20 min), a phenomenon known as 'tumour-trapping'.[98] Accumulation and retention of 5-FU within tumours has been correlated with tumour response.[98]–[100] 5-FU signals were observed in 78 to 100 per cent of responders but in only 8 to 23 per cent of nonresponders. ^{19}F MRS has been used for preclinical pharmacokinetic studies of other chemotherapeutic agents, such as antifolates or alkylating agents, and it can be used as an additional tool in drug development.[101],[102]

MR spectroscopy of cancer is able to give substantial insights into the metabolism of tumours *in vivo*. Despite this advantage, it has been slow to develop as a clinical tool. This has occurred for several reasons including the need for specialist hardware and software for data acquisition and analysis, measurement times are also relatively long compared to MRI examinations. There is yet no proven clinical application, and controversies continue on the procedures for performing, analysing, and interpreting MR spectra. However, the

Table 2 Fryback and Thornbury's hierarchical model of evaluating the efficacy of diagnostic images[105]

Level 1	Concerns the technical quality of images
Level 2	Addresses diagnostic accuracy, sensitivity, and specificity associated with the interpretation of images
Level 3	Focuses on whether the information produces change in the referring physician's diagnostic thinking
Level 4	Therapeutic efficacy, which concerns the effect on the patient management plan
Level 5	Efficacy studies measure (or compute) effect of the information on patient outcomes
Level 6	Analyses examine societal costs and benefits of a diagnostic imaging technology

enormous attraction to further probe cellular metabolic characteristics, particularly in the light of advances in drug development, will result in defining the appropriate role of MR spectroscopy.

Summary

- MRS is a powerful non-invasive method for studying tumour biochemistry and physiology.

- ^{31}P-MRS provides information on tissues energetics and pH; ^{1}H-MRS conveys information on cell-membrane synthesis and degradation, reflecting cellular proliferation and necrosis.

- MRS resonances can provide diagnostic information on tumour grade and are used to monitor tumour response to therapy.

- MRS has great potential to follow the pharmacokinetics of some chemotherapeutic agents.

Assessing imaging tests

Evaluating efficacy of imaging tests

New technology and spending on drugs have often been cited as major contributors to increased healthcare costs in many countries. Spending on new techniques is estimated to increase two- to three-fold, a rate that is in excess of the growth of other healthcare costs in the United States.[103] With the advent of evidence-based medicine and increasing cost constraints, the issue of the health benefits of high-technology imaging needs to be considered. The difficulties in evaluating a new imaging technology are well known[104] and a hierarchical systematic method of evaluation has been widely adopted.[105]–[107] (Table 2)

The technical performance of a new diagnostic test can usually be obtained from reports by innovators and product manufacturers. Many countries have independent agencies that evaluate such equipment, for example the Department of Health's Medical Device Agency in the United Kingdom. The relative accuracy of one imaging technique compared with another is also assessable. However, the results of comparative studies are not always clear-cut because the methods used for such evaluations differ from centre to centre. For example, many studies have compared the accuracy of clinical evaluation, ultrasound, and MRI in the staging of prostate cancer. The results of these studies show a wide range of sensitivity and specificity for the different techniques. For example, the Radiology Diagnostic Oncology Group (**RDOG**) compared body-coil MRI with transrectal ultrasound

(**TRUS**), and demonstrated a higher staging accuracy for MRI (69 per cent) than for TRUS (58 per cent).[108] A further RDOG study[109] utilizing the conventional body coil, fat-suppressed body coil, and endorectal coil (**ERC**) reported an overall accuracy for each technique of 61 per cent, 64 per cent, and 54 per cent, respectively. However, other groups have reported higher accuracy rates for the ERC, ranging up to 88 per cent.[110]–[112] The main reasons for these differing results are the age and level of equipment used and the expertise and enthusiasm of medical personnel in different evaluation centres. Furthermore, the selection of patients within a given study influences the results. For example, initial studies on the accuracy of MRI in staging prostate cancer revealed high levels of accuracy (more than 80 per cent)[113],[114] but had a relatively heavy burden of patients with advanced disease. With increasing recent awareness of prostate cancer, the incidence of screen-detected cancers (mostly early stage) is rising. Consequently, recent papers on the staging accuracy of early prostate cancer have been less encouraging.[108],[109]

An evaluation framework to assess the diagnostic and therapeutic impact of imaging technologies has been published.[115] However, few studies have appeared in this regard, with nearly all publications focusing on technical and diagnostic performance. Impact on health is most difficult to evaluate, particularly in cancer practice where diagnostic advances may occur in advance of the ability to treat the disease. In this situation, technological advances can further our understanding of cancer physiology and response to treatment and thus make an important contribution to patient management without demonstrating a direct impact on health.

Assessing the diagnostic accuracy of imaging tests

When a new radiological test is first assessed, its clinical role is not always appraised. The diagnostic performance of most imaging procedures is often based on the ability to correctly identify a disease of interest. In this section, the basic concepts of test performance and the strengths and weaknesses of their use in clinical decision-making will be illustrated. Interested readers are also invited to review Chapter 3.4 in this regard.

Diagnostic testing can be illustrated by a binary (2 × 2) table associating the test with the presence and absence of disease in patients (Table 3). The first column displays how the test performs on patients who have the disease in question, and the second column on those who do not have the disease. At the bottom of each column, the total number of patients who actually do and do not have the disease

Table 3 Decision matrix for analysing test results

Test outcome	Disease state Present	Absent	Total
Positive	True-positive (TP)	False-positive (FP)	TP + FP
Negative	False-negative (FN)	True-negative (TN)	FN + TN
Total	TP + FN	FP + TN	TP + TN + FP + FN

(according to the reference standard) is totalled. Displaying data in such a matrix assumes that the truth is capable of being known. The term 'gold standard' has been dropped, with increasing recognition that even the best reference standards, including histopathology, can be imperfect.[116]

A second assumption is that a diagnostic test must be positive or negative, a false assumption because many diagnostic tests yield continuous values. This is one of the first concepts that will be disregarded when discussing receiver-operator characteristic curves (see below). An important point to note is that these tests assess the diagnostic performance of the test in a specified clinical scenario (disease, condition) and may not be applicable more widely.

Intrinsic measures of test performance: sensitivity and specificity

Sensitivity: test performance on patients with the disease

The **sensitivity** of a test is its ability to correctly identify those patients with the disease under investigation; it is the probability that the test will be abnormal if the patient has the disease. The sensitivity of a test is also referred to as the true-positive predictive rate of the test. Thus 90 per cent sensitivity correctly identifies 90 per cent of those with the disease and misclassifies 10 per cent as normal.

$$\text{Sensitivity} = \frac{\text{true-positives}}{\text{true-positives} + \text{false-negatives}}$$

Specificity: test performance on non-diseased patients

The **specificity** of an investigation is the ability to correctly identify the absence of disease in those who do not have the disease, or is the proportion of patients without disease who have negative test results.

$$\text{Specificity} = \frac{\text{true-negatives}}{\text{false-positives} + \text{true-negatives}}$$

Thus, screening tests need to be of high sensitivity, whereas tests of high predictive value need to be highly specific. Both sensitivity and specificity are generally independent of disease prevalence and are called the intrinsic operating characteristics of the test. Sensitivity and specificity have several limitations, including little immediate clinical relevance and the fact that these two quantities cannot always be used to compare two tests. The latter occurs because sensitivity and specificity are intrinsically related to each other. As sensitivity increases, specificity decreases and vice versa. Furthermore, the sensitivity and specificity for a given diagnostic test may not be generalizable, varying from centre to centre depending on patient case-mix, experience of the observers, and the level of equipment.

The **accuracy** of a test is dependent on the sensitivity and specificity of a test and is defined as the number of correct results in all tests. This is also not valuable for comparison of tests because it is dependent on the proportion of diseased and non-diseased subjects in the study population.

$$\text{Accuracy} = \frac{\text{true-positives} + \text{true-negatives}}{\text{true-positives} + \text{true-negatives} + \text{false-positives} + \text{false-negatives}}$$

There are several pitfalls in the use of these diagnostic tests in clinical practice. The ability of a test to perform in any clinical situation is strongly influenced by the prevalence of the disease in the study population.[117] The predictive value of a test is an important index of actual test performance. The positive predictive value (**PPV**) of a test indicates the probability that the disease is actually present when the test is positive, and increases with increasing disease prevalence for a given sensitivity and specificity. It also increases with increasing specificity for a given prevalence.

$$\text{Posiive predictive value (PPV)} = \frac{\text{true-positives}}{\text{true-positives} + \text{false-positives}}$$

The negative predictive value (**NPV**) indicates the probability that the disease is absent when the test is negative.

$$\text{Negative predictive value (NPV)} = \frac{\text{true-negatives}}{\text{true-negatives} + \text{false-negatives}}$$

Thus NPV = 1-PPV

The negative predictive value increases with decreasing levels of disease prevalence for a given sensitivity and specificity, and increases with increasing sensitivity for a given prevalence.

It can be seen that reports quoting sensitivity and specificity values are more reliable than predictive values and accuracy estimates, both of which are influenced by regional variations in disease prevalence. Thus, it is possible for a test with high sensitivity and specificity to perform poorly in clinical practice when the disease prevalence is low.

Receiver-operating characteristics (ROC) analysis

Many diagnostic tests yield results that are continuous (for example, the normal short axis diameter of pelvic lymph nodes ranges between 7 and 10 mm)[118] or yield a number of interpretations (for example, test results graded as strongly positive, weakly positive, intermediate, weakly negative, and strongly negative). The latter variability occurs as a direct consequence of the inherent limitations of the test being used and the diagnostic criteria being applied. Furthermore, quoting

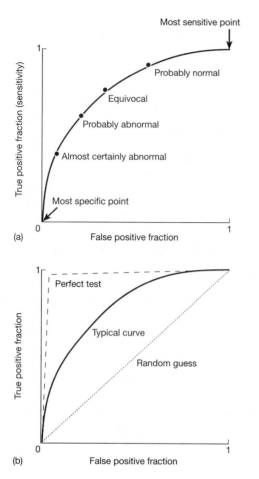

Fig. 9 ROC curves. (a) Stylized ROC curve; (b) ROC curves for random guessing and a perfect test compared.

True-positive fraction = sensitivity
True-negative fraction = specificity
False-positive fraction = 1-specificity
False-negative fraction = 1-sensitivity

To compare two or more imaging tests, a ROC curve is generated for each (Fig. 9(b)). Random guessing generates a straight diagonal line. A perfect test (one that completely separates those with and without disease) generates a curve with no false-positives and a 100 per cent sensitivity. In reality, a ROC curve is somewhere between the two. The more a ROC curve approximates to a perfect curve, the better its diagnostic performance.

A statistical test can be performed to determine whether two ROC curves are significantly different.[121] A commonly used procedure is to calculate the area under a ROC curve and make a comparison using a modified Wilcoxon rank-sum test. It can be shown that the area under the curve measures the probability that a pair of subjects, one with and the other without the disease, will be correctly identified by the test.

ROC analysis illustrates the fundamental principle that there is an inherent limit to the diagnostic discriminating power of a test. Once this limit has been reached, the interpreter can influence results. A ROC curve can be used to select the best cut-off criteria that allows an optimal predictive value at an acceptable cost (minimized false-negative and false-positive results). This is particularly relevant in the use of imaging tests used for staging patients with cancer where cut-off criteria for positive results are constantly being decided—for example, when one has to decide on the upper limit of normal size for normal lymph nodes on CT scans. The major limitation of ROC curves is that the information is of limited use in clinical decision-making.

Thus, we note that sensitivity and specificity are good intrinsic descriptors of test performance; however, they have limited clinical utility and cannot be used to compare two or more diagnostic procedures. ROC curves can be used to compare tests independent of reader variations and applied diagnostic criteria, but provide little clinically useful information. Predictive values provide the most important clinically useful information but are dependent on the prevalence of the disease in a population.

Summary

• Sensitivity measures how a diagnostic test performs in a defined population of patients who have a disease.
• Specificity measures how a diagnostic test performs in a defined population of patients who do not have the disease.
• Sensitivity and specificity are inherently related to each other.
• A sensitive test is more valuable in situations where false-negatives are undesirable. A specificity test is more valuable in situations where false-positives are undesirable.
• A sensitive test is more valuable in situations where we want to exclude a diagnosis. A specificity test is more valuable when there is a desire to identify the presence of disease.
• Positive predictive value indicates the meaning of a positive test.
• Negative predictive test indicates the meaning of a negative test.
• Predictive values are helpful in clinical decision-making.
• Predictive tests are only valuable for the population from which they are derived because of their dependence on the prevalence of the disease (pretest probability).

a single sensitivity and specificity to determine the overall usefulness of such tests can be inaccurate because it fails to take into account the variability of radiological interpretation; some readers apply more strict (under-readers) and others less strict (over-readers) criteria. In these situations the sensitivity and specificity of such tests is dependent on the cut-off value chosen for a positive and negative result. Receiver-operating characteristics (ROC) curves have been developed to efficiently display the relationship between sensitivity and specificity for tests with continuous outcomes.[119],[120] Such analyses can be helpful for comparing two or more imaging techniques for a range of observer interpretations.

A ROC curve is a curvilinear graph that plots the positive fraction (sensitivity) on the y-axis as a function of the false-positive fraction on the x-axis for a range of diagnostic criteria (Fig. 9(a)). A move towards the right on a ROC curve is equivalent to the use of less stringent criteria for determining the outcome of a test, thereby increasing sensitivity but decreasing specificity. A move towards the left results from using more strict criteria, thus increasing specificity and decreasing sensitivity. Note that the false-positive fraction equals 1-sensitivity and by reversing the scale of the x-axis, the x-axis becomes specificity. Thereby with new labels the ROC curve can now be called a 'sensitivity–specificity curve' as proposed by Brismar.[119]

- ROC curves provide a means of comparing diagnostic tests, independent of diagnostic criteria (strict or lax) that are used.

Imaging strategies

Radiologists need to be at the forefront of deciding which tests should be used for evaluating patients with malignant disease. Based on the above discussion, it can be seen that the proper use of imaging in patients with cancer is a complex issue and it is frequently impossible to give strict algorithms applicable to all centres. At best, only general guidelines can be initiated;[122]–[125] the specific role of general radiology, computed tomography, MRI, etc. being determined within a particular clinicoradiological environment. Widely adopted guidelines for individual cancer types in the United Kingdom are given in Table 4.

Imaging may be requested for the routine management of patients with cancer (service work) or for research studies. In the clinic, imaging may be requested as a routine investigation at the time of presentation for diagnostic and staging purposes.

For example, it is now well recognized that the survival of patients with lung cancer varies significantly in each of the TNM subcategories; a finding that is not surprising. However, Feinstein et al. found that when these patients were staged on clinical grounds alone (in other words without the benefit of ultrasound, CT, and nuclear medicine) the survival differences disappeared.[126] Imaging thus allows improved staging and treatment stratification. Imaging has also become a cornerstone for guiding diagnostic and therapeutic interventions, for example biopsy procedures, surgical planning, and for radiotherapy planning.

In those tumours where established treatments are available, imaging may be required to monitor therapeutic response. Imaging can also be used for the surveillance of patients who have no clinical evidence or imaging evidence of disease in order to identify relapse as early as possible. It is now clear that in a number of tumour types (for example, testicular teratoma and colorectal cancer) small-volume relapse can be managed successfully if an intensive programme of surveillance is performed. In addition, when there is a clinical suspicion of relapse, imaging can be used to confirm recurrence in a previously treated patient. The choice of an imaging test is dependent on the availability of imaging techniques, and also on their sensitivity in being able to detect and characterize recurrent disease in the presence of previously treated normal tissues which may have been damaged by therapy.

Another service role for imaging is aimed at the early detection of cancers, since most tumours are only detected late in their natural course. Such screening imaging tests may be directed either at the general population (for example, screening mammography for all women aged 50 to 65 years old) or at high-risk populations (for example, ultrasound screening of the pelvis in women with a strong family history of ovarian carcinoma).

Imaging also has a major role in supporting clinical trials of new therapeutic agents, and in this situation is used more frequently during the course of treatment as a tool for monitoring response and for management decisions. Imaging to support clinical trials is an increasingly important role for radiologists who have an interest in cancer. The high accuracy and reproducibility of cross-sectional imaging techniques (CT and MRI) makes them well suited to provide imaging endpoints as response parameters.

In the situations outlined above, not only is the imaging modality chosen dependent on the accuracy of the test but is also strongly influenced by local factors, which include the availability of equipment, expertise of medical and technical staff, and other demands made on imaging. It is not always possible to use the best imaging technique for every circumstance. However, it is important to adhere to good practice, and radiologists with their knowledge of diagnostic imaging techniques and interpretation of cancer can help to provide an optimal service within a given environment. When deciding protocols for given clinical situations, close collaboration between radiologists and clinicians is required. Such protocols should address the issues of the choice of imaging techniques for different tumour types, the timing in relation to treatment, and the timing of follow-up studies.

Screening techniques for cancer detection

The prevention and early detection of cancer are among the essential issues that must be addressed if significant improvements in patient survival rates are to be achieved. Several features make certain cancers suitable for screening. These include a substantial morbidity and mortality, high prevalence in a detectable preclinical stage, and the availability of effective treatments if cancer is detected. An ideal imaging test for screening large populations should possess a high level of sensitivity with an acceptable rate of specificity, employing technology that is widely available and relatively inexpensive. The technique should also be non-invasive or minimally invasive (including acceptable radiation burden) and be supported by competent technical and professional staff to obtain optimal images for interpretation.

Mammography is the only diagnostic imaging modality currently used to detect cancers in an asymptomatic population. This has occurred because of substantial advancements in technology, which have resulted in high-quality images at acceptable radiation dose and by increasing expertise for the interpretation of resultant images. No imaging test has been more studied than mammography (with or without clinical examination), and yet after more than 30 years of clinical trials, many questions remain unanswered. More than eight major trials have been conducted which have included half a million women.[127]–[132] This section is not the appropriate place for reviewing all these studies on breast cancer screening and interested readers are advised to refer to Chapter 11.3 for further information. Suffice to say that all trials have demonstrated consistent benefit for mammography in women in their 50s and 60s, but there is a lack of a statistically significant reduction in mortality for women in their 40s. Controversy continues on screening the latter group and screening for women in their 70s. Another area of controversy is the interval at which women should be screened. Recommendations on mammographic screening are not uniformly accepted and therefore the country guidelines, subject preferences, and clinical judgement should guide decisions on breast screening. Certainly, all women between the ages of 50 and 69 should be encouraged to undergo regular mammographic screening at regular intervals (1 to 3 years). Women at high risk in their 40s (and possibly 30s) should also be encouraged. Breast self-examination and clinical breast examination should be considered a supplement to mammography. It is likely that these recommendations will change in the future with new analyses of

Table 4 The Royal College of Radiologists, London, guidelines for imaging cancer patients (1998) ref. 123

Problem	Investigation	Recommendation (strength of evidence)	Comments
Parotid			
Diagnosis	US	Indicated [B]	To establish presence of a mass, particularly in superficial lesions
	MRI or CT	Indicated [B]	Useful in the deep portion of the gland and before complex surgery
Staging	MRI or CT	Indicated [B]	Especially when complex surgery contemplated; to clarify relations and involvement of deep lobe
Larynx			
Diagnosis	Imaging	Not indicated [B]	This is a clinical diagnosis
Staging	CT or MRI	Indicated [B]	MRI has the advantage of direct coronal imaging. MRI may eventually supersede
Thyroid			
Diagnosis	US or NM	Indicated [B]	Demonstrates morphology; allows guided aspiration for cytology or biopsy for histology. Some clinicians will proceed to aspiration with no imaging. NM may be appropriate if biopsy contraindicated. US-guided core biopsy is increasingly being used
Staging	CT or MRI	Indicated [B]	To assess local extent (e.g. retrosternal extension and nodes)
	NM	Indicated [B]	After thyroidectomy
Lung			
Diagnosis	CXR PA and Lat	Indicated [B]	But can be normal, particularly with central tumours
	CT	Specialized investigation [B]	Many centres proceed directly to bronchoscopy, which allows biopsy. CT is superior in identifying lesions responsible for haemoptysis
Staging	CT chest, upper abdomen	Indicated [B]	Despite limitations in specificity of nodal involvement, etc. Some centres perform NM for possible skeletal metastases
	MRI	Specialized investigation [B]	Assists in estimating local invasion of chest wall, particularly for apical and peripheral lesions and mediastinal invasion. Helps distinguish adrenal adenoma from metastasis.
	PET	Specialized investigation [B]	This single expensive investigation to identify small metastatic foci may save a lot of other investigations and inappropriate surgery
Oesophagus			
Diagnosis	Barium swallow	Indicated [B]	Before endoscopy in dysphagia
Staging	CT	Indicated [B]	Despite limitations in sensitivity and specificity of nodal involvement. Simpler than MRI for lung, liver, and intra-abdominal nodes
	Transoesophageal US	Indicated [A]	Increasing use of trans-oesophageal US for local staging where available
Primary liver lesion			
Diagnosis	US	Indicated [B]	The majority of lesions will be identified
	MRI or CT	Indicated [B]	If biochemical markers elevated and US is negative or liver very cirrhotic. Enhanced MRI and arterial-phase CT most accurate in delineating tumour extent
Staging	MRI or CT	Indicated [B]	MRI is probably the optimal investigation in assessing involved segments and lobes. CT arterial portography and intraoperative US useful where available
Secondary liver lesion			
Diagnosis	US	Indicated [B]	US will show the majority of metastases and guides biopsy
	CT or MRI	Indicated [B]	When US is negative and clinical suspicion high. MRI better for characterizing lesions. CT arterial portography is sensitive but not specific, however many now use triple-phase spiral CT techniques following intravenous enhancement. CT and MRI often part of other staging and follow-up protocols
Pancreas			
Diagnosis	US or CT or MRI	Indicated [B]	Much depends on body habitus. US usually successful in thin patients; CT better in the more obese. MRI for clarification of problems. Biopsy using US or CT. ERCP or MRCP may also be needed. Endoscopic US, where available, most sensitive

Table 4 *continued*

Problem	Investigation	Recommendation (strength of evidence)	Comments
Staging	CT or MRI abdomen	Indicated [B]	Especially if radical surgery contemplated. Wide local variation: some centres use angiography, others spiral CT; laparoscopy and laparoscopic US useful
Colon and rectum			
Diagnosis	Barium enema or colonoscopy	Indicated [B]	Much depends on local policy, expertise, and availability. Increased interest in CT of the colon
Staging	US	Indicated [B]	For liver metastases. Endoluminal US useful for local rectal spread
	CT or MRI abdomen, pelvis	Indicated [B]	Local preoperative staging to assess rectal lesions before pre-operative radiotherapy. Many centres now treat liver secondaries very aggressively, which may necessitate MRI and/or detailed CT. MRI and CT often complementary; both can assess other abdominal spread. Increasing interest in PET here
?Recurrence	US liver	Indicated [B]	For liver metastases. Some debate about the value of routine US follow-up in asymptomatic patients
	CT or MRI abdomen, pelvis	Indicated [B]	For liver metastases and local recurrence. Increasing interest in PET here
Kidney			
Diagnosis	US	Indicated [B]	US is good at distinguishing between cystic and solid masses
Staging	CT or MRI abdomen	Indicated [B]	For local extent, venous, nodal and ureteric involvement, opposite kidney, etc.
	CT chest	Not indicated routinely	The presence of lung metastases does not usually influence management. Increasing interest in PET
?Recurrence	CT abdomen	Indicated [B]	For symptoms suggesting relapse around nephrectomy bed. Routine follow-up not recommended
Bladder			
Diagnosis	Imaging	Not indicated [B]	Cytoscopy is the optimal (although not infallible, e.g. diverticulum) investigation
Staging	IVU	Indicated [B]	To assess kidneys and ureters for further urothelial tumours
	CT or MRI abdomen and pelvis	Indicated [B]	When radical therapy contemplated. MRI is probably more sensitive. CT widely used for radiotherapy planning
Prostate			
Diagnosis	Transrectal US	Indicated [B]	Some variation according to local availability and expertise. Transrectal US is widely used together with guided biopsies. Some interest in MRI and PET here
Staging	MRI/CT pelvis	Specialized [B] Investigation	Some variation in range of investigative and therapeutic policies. MRI with appropriate coils is sensitive for assessment before possible radical prostatectomy. Staging continued into the abdomen when pelvic disease found
	NM	Indicated [B]	To assess skeletal metastases, when PSA is significantly elevated
Testicle			
Diagnosis	US	Indicated [B]	Especially when clinical findings equivocal or normal
Staging	CT chest, abdomen, pelvis	Indicated [B]	Management now depends heavily on accurate radiological staging
Follow-up	CT abdomen	Indicated [B]	Some centres still routinely examine the chest as well, especially for patients without biochemical evidence of disease. Some debate as to whether whole pelvis imaging is needed at follow-up unless there are identified risk factors
Ovary			
Diagnosis	US	Indicated [B]	The majority of lesions are diagnosed by US (including transvaginal ultrasound with Doppler), laparoscopy, or laparotomy. Some are identified by CT/MRI investigations for abdominal symptoms. MRI useful for elucidating problems
Staging	CT/MRI	Specialized investigation [B]	Many specialists require CT or MRI in addition to staging by laparatomy. CT is still more widely available
Follow-up	CT abdomen, pelvis	Specialized [B]	Usually to assess response to adjuvant therapy. Also used, along with markers, to detect relapse

Table 4 *continued*

Problem	Investigation	Recommendation (strength of evidence)	Comments
Uterus: cervix			
Diagnosis	Imaging	Not indicated routinely [B]	Usually clinical diagnosis. MRI may assist in complex cases
Staging	MRI or CT abdomen and pelvis	Indicated [B]	MRI provides better demonstration of tumour and local extent. Also better for pelvic nodes. Para-aortic nodes and ureters must also be examined. Some centres now use transrectal US for local invasion
?Relapse	MRI or CT abdomen and pelvis	Specialized investigation [B]	MRI provides better information in the pelvis. Biopsy (e.g. of nodal mass) easier with CT
Uterus: Body			
Diagnosis	US or MRI	Indicated [B]	MRI can give valuable information about benign and malignant lesions
Staging	MRI or CT investigation	Specialized [B]	Both CT and MRI can show extrauterine disease. But MRI can also demonstrate intrauterine anatomy
Lymphoma			
Diagnosis	CT NM	Indicated [B]	CT good at evaluating nodal sites throughout the body. Also allows biopsy, although excision of whole node preferable where possible NM (gallium) can show foci of occult disease (e.g. mediastinum). PET used in some centres
Staging	CT chest, abdomen, pelvis	Indicated [B]	Depending on site of disease, head and neck may also need to be examined. Increasing interest in PET here
Follow-up	CT or MRI NM	Indicated [B] Specialized investigation [B]	Increasing role for MRI in long-term follow-up and residual masses Consider NM for gallium disease. Some centres use PET
Musculoskeletal tumours			
Diagnosis	X-ray + MRI	Indicated [B]	Imaging and histology complementary. Best before biopsy
Staging	MRI local disease + CT chest	Specialized investigation [C]	CT for lung metastases
Metastases from unknown primary tumour			
Diagnosis of primary lesion	Imaging	Not indicated routinely [C]	Rarely beneficial. Some exceptions for specialists, younger patients or favourable histology (see Section 20)

Table reproduced with kind permission from The Royal College of Radiologists, London; from RCR Working Party. Making the best use of a department of clinical radiology: guidelines for doctors (4th edn). London: The Royal College of Radiologists, 1998.[(123)]

Recommendations used are:

Indicated—the investigation(s) most likely to contribute to clinical diagnosis and management.

Not indicated routinely—this emphasizes that while no recommendation is absolute, the request requires cogent arguments for it.

Not indicated—supposed rationale for investigation is untenable.

Specialized investigation—complex or expensive investigations, requiring relevant clinical expertise. They need to be justified with discussion with a senior radiologist.

The strength of evidence is indicated by:

[A] randomized controlled trials (RCTs), meta-analyses, systematic reviews; or

[B] robust experimental or observational studies; or

[C] other evidence where the advice relies on expert opinion and has the endorsement of respected authorities.

Where there is conflicting data within a large body of excellent scientific reports, then the evidence is classified as [C].

international trials particularly for women in their 40s. Other imaging modalities are also undergoing clinical trials for screening women in selected patient groups (for example, dynamic contrast medium-enhanced MR imaging in women at high genetic risk of breast cancer).[(133),(134)]

The role of imaging techniques to screen for other tumours is increasingly being studied. Chest radiographs to screen for lung carcinoma or barium studies to screen for stomach and colon cancers are not employed in the general population, although there is a sporadic use in groups at high risk for these diseases. Similarly, there is interest in using ultrasound as a method for screening women with ovarian cancer and CT for the detection of hepatocellular carcinoma in patients with liver cirrhosis.[135],[136] A promising new technique for evaluation of the colon, which is currently undergoing feasibility studies, consists of reconstructing CT scans using a computer simulation technique (virtual colonoscopy). There is also renewed interest in screening for lung cancer, particularly in subjects at high risk of this disease. Previous studies performed in the 1970s showed a lack of survival benefit for lung cancer screening.[137]–[139] It has been suggested that the design, execution, and analysis of these studies were flawed. These factors together with the emergence of low-dose spiral CT as a technique for detecting lung lesions at a much smaller size has prompted investigators to reappraise lung cancer screening in high-risk groups.[140]

Summary

- Imaging techniques have the potential to screen for a number of primary tumours before they become clinically apparent.
- Mammography is the only diagnostic imaging modality currently used to detect cancers in an asymptomatic population.
- Promising new imaging techniques include low-dose spiral CT for detecting lung cancer and CT colonoscopy for colon polyp detection.

Diagnosis—suspected cancer

Imaging is essential for the diagnosis of all tumours that are not accessible to clinical evaluation or endoscopy. Although a precise histological diagnosis must be made before treatment is instigated, a diagnosis of 'malignancy' is frequently made based on imaging information alone. Those sites in which imaging plays a key role in diagnosis include the brain, breast, lungs and mediastinum, tumours arising from the abdominal organs, the retroperitoneum, and bones. Cancers of the head and neck and those arising from the pelvic organs, such as testicular cancer, bladder cancer, carcinoma of the cervix, and rectal cancer, are often detected by clinical examination.

The method of imaging chosen for investigation is largely determined by the physical capabilities of the imaging modality. Of all the imaging techniques, conventional radiography provides the highest spatial resolution. Radiography is therefore, best suited to studies of the gastrointestinal tract (barium studies), breast, and bone in which fine detail of the mucosal pattern or breast and bone architecture can be shown (Fig. 10). Conversely, CT has a higher density discrimination than conventional radiology and is, therefore, best suited for distinguishing small differences in density between soft tissue, fluid, fat, and other structures which cannot be demonstrated on conventional films (Fig. 11). Although ultrasound has the major advantage that ionizing radiation is not used, there are significant limitations (see also the section on 'Advances in ultrasound' above). Thus, ultrasound is often the initial diagnostic modality for evaluating the thyroid, parotid, testicle, and liver. The ultrasound beam cannot traverse bone or gas-containing viscera and is, therefore, an inappropriate technique for examination of the brain (except in the neonate) and the lungs. In the abdomen, gas-containing organs frequently make examinations difficult, but ultrasound remains the technique of first choice for evaluation of the pelvic organs.

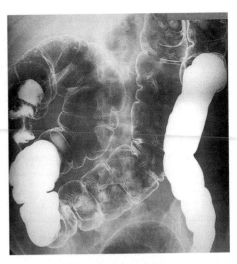

Fig. 10 Colon cancer. Apple core-like colonic carcinoma of the ascending colon in a patient with ulcerative colitis. Filiform polyposis is visible in the rest of the colon. The left colon is ahaustral due to previous colitis. Mucosal detail is excellent.

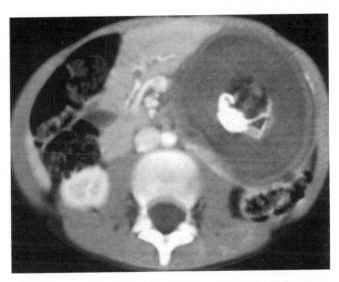

Fig. 11 Benign retroperitoneal teratoma. Axial CT image in a 7-year-old child showing a large mass in the left retroperitoneum. The mass is well defined, with high-density areas suggestive of bone together with low-density fatty areas. At surgical resection, this was shown to represent a benign retroperitoneal teratoma.

In many areas of the body, ultrasound and CT have overtaken radionuclide examinations because the specificity of radionuclide imaging is low. In some centres the technique is still used as a screening investigation for examination of the liver, thyroid, and brain. However, if an abnormality is found then further evaluation with CT (or ultrasound) is required before a definitive diagnosis can be made.

In the United Kingdom and in many other countries, where there is still limited access to magnetic resonance imaging (MRI), CT remains the first imaging procedure in the investigation of intracranial tumours in many centres. MRI is superior to CT for tumour detection, because of its inherent high sensitivity to altered brain tissue, and it can certainly better at demonstrating tumour extent. MRI is also superior to CT for evaluation of the posterior fossa due to the lack of beam-hardening artefacts. MRI has supplanted myelography for the detection and full assessment of spinal cord tumours, particularly following injection of intravenous contrast medium. However, MRI appears to be less reliable for the detection of small-volume, intradural spinal disease[141] and in patients with leukaemia and lymphoma. In patients with clinical suspected leptomeningeal disease with a negative MR examination, cerebrospinal fluid examination may yield positive cytology.[142]

Conventional fluoroscopy, ultrasound, and CT are useful techniques for **guiding** percutaneous biopsy. Diagnostic histological and cytological specimens can be obtained in over 90 per cent of tumours.[143] In general, fluoroscopy or ultrasound should be used if possible since biopsy under CT control is more expensive and time-consuming. CT guidance should be used in those situations when other methods are inappropriate, for example when biopsying retro-peritoneal nodes. Imaging guidance is also widely used to surgically guide the biopsy of suspected lesions. Examples include mammographic wire localization[144] and CT-guided wire localization of lung lesions prior to thoracoscopic resection.[145]

Staging

Accurate staging of patients with malignant disease is a fundamental part of their management and a major challenge for imaging. It is only by appreciating the local regional and systemic extent of the disease process that oncologists are able to make rational decisions regarding the most appropriate treatment strategy. The formulation of a management plan is dependent on the staging of the tumour as well as patient-specific factors such as performance status and patient preferences. Staging should achieve a definition of the local extent of the disease, including the precise anatomical site of the primary tumour, its relationship to vital organs, and the extent of local invasion into adjacent structures. Staging also allows an appreciation of the extent of regional spread via lymphatics or transcoelomically within body cavities, and the evaluation of the extent of haematogenous metastases at sites distant from the primary tumour.

Imaging is, justifiably, an integral part of staging patients with cancer and frequently results in the upstaging of clinical stage. Radiologists involved in cancer staging therefore need to have a thorough understanding of tumour behaviour and possible treatment options, as well as a detailed knowledge of the appropriate use, advantages, and limitations of the imaging techniques employed. In the United Kingdom, CT remains pivotal in the diagnosis and management of many patients with cancer. MR imaging installations still lag behind the number of CT scanners and, although MRI may be the technique of choice for a given tumour, imaging with this modality may frequently be impossible. In some cancers, the role of MRI has not been fully defined and no clear advantage of MRI over CT has been established (for example, renal cancer) whereas, in others, CT has clear advantages over MRI and remains the preferred technique (for example, lymphoma).

The TNM staging system is the internationally agreed, preferred method for staging most malignant tumours (see Chapter 3.5). It has

the advantages of being simple to apply, allows a concise and precise way of communicating information, is reproducible when applied to a large number of patients, and conveys prognostic information for treatment and decision-making. A few common tumours are not routinely staged using the TNM system: for example, Hodgkin's disease. Some tumours have no accepted staging in the TNM classification, for example brain tumours.

Local tumour spread (T category; see also organ-specific chapters)

The clinical staging of local tumour spread is frequently inaccurate, often resulting in an underestimation of disease extent. However, for some tumour types, clinical stage is more accurate than imaging in assessing local tumour extent. Indeed, for some tumours, clinical/surgical staging is the preferred method of evaluation, particularly for the early stages of disease—for example, head and neck tumours, melanoma, cervical carcinoma, and bladder cancer. Clinical staging with minimally invasive surgical techniques (for example, laparoscopy) is routinely undertaken for the operative assessment of stomach and pancreatic cancer, allowing better assessment of transcoelomic spread.[146] CT is ideally suited for assessing local tumour spread at a number of anatomical sites. In general, ultrasound is a less comprehensive modality because it frequently fails to delineate the complete tumour margin. Furthermore, ultrasound cannot assess certain anatomical sites such as the lung, mediastinum, and bone. Exceptions include endoscopic ultrasound, which is superior to both CT and MRI for assessing early, local tumour stage in hollow organs such as the oesophagus, stomach, and rectum.

The following tumours types have been selected for further discussion because they illustrate the major advantages and limitations of different imaging techniques used to stage cancers.

Head and neck cancers

The elegant display of facial anatomy in the axial and coronal plains has rendered CT a valuable technique for staging malignancies arising in this region. In **paranasal sinus tumours**, for example, extension of tumour into the ethmoid cells, the orbital apex, sphenoid sinus, pterygoid fossa, and the base of skull can be clearly delineated. This provides valuable information for surgeons and radiotherapists. CT frequently upstages the tumour extent compared to clinical evaluation. A major problem with CT is the presence of artefact arising from dental amalgam, which limits the usefulness of CT for evaluating tongue and oral cavity tumours. MR imaging now challenges the use of CT in the assessment of head and neck malignancy.[147],[148] This is because the superior contrast resolution and multiplanar imaging capability of MRI allows better detection and delineation of the intricate spread of tumours in this region. Furthermore, MRI can distinguish mucosal thickening and inflammation from tumour more reliably than CT.[149]

Modern imaging techniques have had a substantial impact on the management of tumours of the upper aerodigestive tract.[150] Imaging is an important adjunct to physical examination because it improves the adequacy of staging. Imaging also determines tumour resectability and the amount of surrounding tissue that must be resected to ensure adequate margins. As surgical resection of tumours in this region is often mutilating, an accurate assessment of soft tissue involvement is vital and clinical assessment of the depth of tumour invasion is

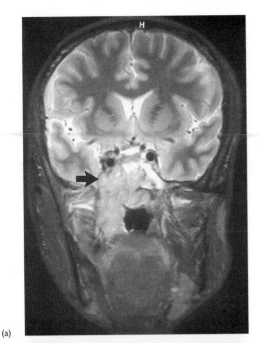

(a)

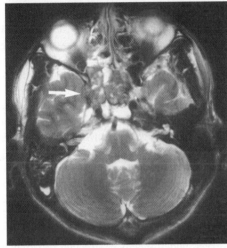

(b)

Fig. 12 Nasopharyngeal carcinoma. (a) Coronal STIR and (b) axial T_2-weighted MR images showing a large nasopharyngeal mass extending along the right wall of the pharynx. Extension of tumour into the posterior nasal space is visible on the axial images and there is tumour extension into the middle cranial fossa (arrows).

often inadequate (Fig. 12). In the assessment of carcinoma of the larynx, CT is often better than MRI at appraising cartilage involvement by tumour. MRI is more sensitive but less specific than CT in this regard.[151],[152] Spiral CT is also capable of higher resolution in delineating laryngeal anatomy.[153] In the majority of patients, cross-sectional imaging techniques allow a more comprehensive appreciation of the disease extent than laryngography,[154] and the accuracy of CT for staging laryngeal carcinoma can exceed 90 per cent in experienced hands.[155] Recently, MRI has challenged the use of CT in the assessment of laryngeal cancer. The main advantages of MRI over CT include its great sensitivity in detecting the extent of laryngeal invasion, and the coronal plane of imaging allows a better

assessment of transglottic spread. MRI is also superior in detecting vascular invasion, but cartilaginous invasion resulting in asymmetrical sclerosis assessed on CT remains the most sensitive indicator. One of the major drawbacks of MRI is motion artefact arising from swallowing movements and respiratory distress caused by obstructing tumours.

Renal tumours

Evaluation of renal masses deserves particular attention because CT has made a major contribution to preoperative assessment. Although intravenous urography (IVU) and ultrasound can solve most diagnostic problems, CT should be undertaken when ultrasound shows an atypical cyst requiring further evaluation since 5 to 7 per cent of all renal cancers may have a cystic component.[156] CT is better than ultrasound or IVU for identifying small renal neoplasms less than 3 cm in diameter. The overall staging accuracy of CT in staging renal carcinoma ranges between 72 and 90 per cent.[157] The accuracy of CT staging is enhanced by the use of the spiral or helical technique after rapid injection of intravenous contrast medium.[158] MRI is also a valuable method for staging renal carcinoma and is equally accurate to CT.[159],[160] Both CT and MR are able to evaluate perirenal extension, lymph node involvement, and macroscopic spread of tumour into the renal vein and inferior vena cava. The use of contrast medium and thin collimation allows CT assessment of renal vein invasion in over 95 per cent of cases.[161] The success of CT and MRI staging of renal carcinomas has resulted in the demise of arteriography, which is seldom used except for providing a vascular map to assist surgical resection, and for embolization to reduce tumour bulk. Ultrasound is less reliable for staging because overlying bowel gas often precludes adequate visualization of the renal vessels, inferior vena cava, and retroperitoneum.[162],[163]

Bladder cancer

This is well suited for staging with CT and MRI. Both techniques are more accurate in advanced than early disease. Clinical staging is more accurate in the evaluation of superficial bladder cancers. However, for invasive lesions, clinical staging has been shown to be inaccurate.[164] Bladder cancers invading the superficial and deep muscles usually produce bladder-wall thickening, but the distinction between superficial and deep-muscle invasion is impossible with CT.[165],[166] The most important role for CT is to distinguish tumours confined to the bladder wall from those that have spread into the perivesical fat. A smooth outer margin of the bladder wall suggests that the tumour is confined to the bladder, although the deep muscle may be invaded by tumour. An irregular, ill-defined, outer edge to the bladder wall with soft-tissue stranding into the perivesical fat raises the suspicion of perivesical disease (Fig. 13).[167],[168] Invasion of adjacent organs is frequently difficult to identify on CT when there is no clear fatty plane between such structures as the posterior bladder wall and rectum, prostate, uterine cervix, and vagina. Tumour may abut neighbouring organs without necessarily invading them. Other pitfalls include perivesical soft-tissue thickening resulting from oedema or infection (often as a result of cystoscopic resection). MRI is slightly superior to CT for staging bladder cancer; but in patients with obvious advanced disease, staging accuracies by both techniques are similar. MRI has the advantage of demonstrating perivesical extension and organ invasion in multiple planes and therefore determines the extent of disease better than CT. This information may be valuable for

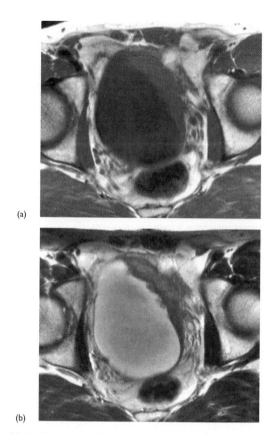

(a)

(b)

Fig. 13 Bladder cancer. (a) Axial T_1 and (b) T_2-weighted MR images of the bladder showing a large carcinoma with extravesical extension of disease (T3C disease).

radiotherapy planning but does not necessarily lead to a change in tumour stage.

Gynaecological cancer

The role of imaging in gynaecological cancer is well defined but relatively limited. Clinical staging of invasive carcinoma of the cervix by vaginal examination and examination under anaesthesia (EUA) has limitations, especially when there is parametrial spread. Clinical staging is highly accurate in patients with small-volume lesions confined to the cervix. Although not officially part of the FIGO system of staging (Federation of Obstetrics and Gynaecology), cross-sectional imaging techniques are increasingly being employed to assess parametrial spread. Both ultrasound and CT have application in the assessment of cervical cancer, but MRI has been shown to be the most consistently useful modality for all tumour stages and as accurate as contrast-enhanced CT for assessing nodal stage. It is also the most appropriate imaging method for staging carcinoma presenting during pregnancy. Endocavitary ultrasound is also successful in determining the maximal infiltration of tumour into the cervical tissues and in assessing tumour size. Local tumour staging by transrectal ultrasound compares favourably with the results of CT and MRI.[169] CT has a useful role in advanced carcinoma of the cervix and complements surgical staging. CT is more accurate with advanced-stage disease (over 90 per cent) than in early-stage disease (42 to 70 per cent) and is therefore not recommended for staging early tumours.[170],[171] A

particular limitation of CT is its overestimation of the size and extent of stage 1 disease because normal parametrial structures and inflammation can sometimes be misinterpreted as representing tumour. Understaging stage 2B and 3B tumours occurs because of the inability to visualize minimal and microscopic spread of tumour into parametrial structures. MRI demonstrates female genital tract anatomy in a way that was impossible to appreciate hitherto. The ability to image in oblique planes and the superior soft tissue contrast particularly on T_2-weighted images has given MRI an overall advantage over other techniques. A major advantage of MRI is the ability to delineate a high-signal tumour on T_2-weighted images on both sagittal and axial planes (Fig. 14).[172],[173] Positive contributions of MRI include the ability to detect the extent of tumour invasion into the endocervical canal and uterine body. However, MR staging accuracy of early-stage disease with minimal parametrial spread remains difficult. Its overall accuracy in detecting parametrial invasion is between 70 and 90 per cent and of assessing vaginal extension between 72 and 93 per cent.[172]–[175] Compared with CT, MRI offers significantly better evaluation of the tumour size, stromal invasion, and the local and regional extent of disease.

Prostate cancer

In prostate cancer, the primary aim is to determine whether the patient is a candidate for curative treatment based on locally confined disease. Digital rectal examination (**DRE**), transrectal ultrasound (**TRUS**), including TRUS-guided biopsy, CT and MRI are the important evaluation techniques. DRE plays a central role in staging and, although the findings of DRE are used widely, there is little data on the reliability of DRE for clinical staging. Data accumulated from prostatectomy specimens reveals that DRE underestimates the local extent of disease in 40 to 60 per cent of cases.[176]–[178] Transrectal ultrasound is an essential technique for the diagnosis of disease that also guides biopsies. The sensitivity for detecting capsular penetration lies between 20 and 85 per cent and specificity between 60 and 95 per cent.[108],[179],[180] There are a number of limitations of TRUS. About 10 to 30 per cent of tumours are isoechoic and therefore not all tumours are visible on ultrasound. Microscopic extension beyond the prostate capsule cannot be detected by TRUS.[181] TRUS is highly operator-dependent, with the diagnostic performance being determined by the experience of the ultrasonographer. There is also considerable inter- and intraobserver variability in the assessment of tumour stage. CT does not allow direct visualization of the prostate cancer and it is considered to be of little value in local staging.[182] The role of CT is limited to nodal staging, delineating advanced disease, and for radiotherapy treatment planning (see below). MRI provides the best depiction of anatomy of the prostate and seminal vesicles. The internal architecture of the prostate gland can clearly be delineated on T_2-weighted images and the prostate cancer is usually visible if greater than 5 mm in size. The accuracy of endorectal MRI to detect capsular penetration is highly variable, ranging from 33 to 80 per cent. The sensitivity of endorectal MRI for detecting seminal vesicle invasion ranges from 21 to 36 per cent.[183]–[187] There continues to be wide variation in opinion on the best treatment of limited prostate cancer and the role of imaging for staging still remains debatable. Most urologists use PSA, DRE, and TRUS with multiple biopsies for staging. There is insufficient data to indicate whether MRI improves outcome and is cost-effective.

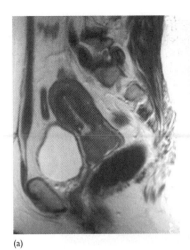

(a)

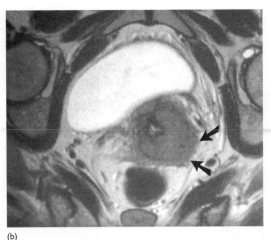

(b)

Fig. 14 Cervix carcinoma. (a) Sagittal and (b) true axial T_2-weighted images through the cervix in a patient with stage IIB cervix carcinoma. The normal architecture of the cervix is replaced by tumour and there is parametrial spread of disease visible on the axial images (b) (arrows).

Bone tumours

In the evaluation of primary bone tumours, the roles of radiologists and histopathologists are complementary. The morphological features of primary bone neoplasms are best demonstrated on plain radiographs. Bony destruction becomes visible on plain radiographs after 40 to 50 per cent loss of the medullary bone.[188],[189] The periosteum forms a barrier to the spread of tumour into surrounding soft tissues, and a periosteal response is often seen in the presence of the bony neoplasm or infection due to lifting and separation of the periosteum from the cortical bone. The staging role of imaging is to determine the intraosseous extent of the tumour and to detect the presence and extent of soft tissue involvement. CT has a well-defined role in the diagnosis of certain bone tumours, providing additional information over plain radiographs particularly in the spine and limb girdles. CT is the method of choice for surgical planning and detecting the preservation of an intact periosteum. The involvement of the soft tissues is characteristic but not diagnostic for malignant disease. The role of MRI in bone tumour diagnosis is limited, but contrast-enhanced MRI does allow the distinction of tumour from necrosis and oedema[190] and demonstrates tumour extension into soft tissues optimally.[191]

Lung cancer

Imaging plays an important role in the assessment of lung cancer. Local extent of the disease and histology of the tumour determine the prognosis of patients and appropriate therapeutic strategy. The TNM staging classification stresses a more aggressive surgical approach because the best chance of cure for patients with non-small-cell lung cancer (**NSCLC**) is surgical resection. It should be appreciated that even well-performed imaging disagrees with surgical findings in a significant proportion of patients. The surgical question is usually the identification of inoperable patients. A major role of staging using imaging techniques is therefore to differentiate unresectable disease (stage 3B and 4) from earlier stages. Stage 3B constitutes T4 tumours and those patients with N3 lymphadenopathy (involved lymph nodes in the contralateral mediastinum or supraclavicular fossa). T4 tumours are irresectable because of the degree of invasion of the vertebrae or of critical mediastinal structures (the heart, great vessels, trachea, and

oesophagus). In general, CT is the primary imaging modality used for tumour staging, with MRI having a secondary problem-solving role except for the evaluation of superior sulcus tumours. Both CT and MR are reasonably accurate in predicting limited (potentially resectable) mediastinal invasion. However, MRI is advantageous in specific regions, such as in determining the extent of bronchial involvement and for excluding some T4 features such as major vessel, oesophageal, and spinal involvement. The fundamental advantage of MRI relates to the ability to image in any plane and therefore to allow optimal assessment of the tracheal carina, aortopulmonary window, and aortic arch. However, both CT and MRI are less accurate in identifying patients with irresectable disease.[192] CT criteria for irresectability due to mediastinal invasion are hard to identify.[193],[194] The loss of fatty planes between tumour and mediastinal structures is often used as a criterion, but such an appearance may occur from image blurring caused by motion, fibrosis, or reactive inflammation. A large, prospective RDOG study comparing CT with MRI showed that MRI was more accurate in diagnosing mediastinal invasion in a small number of patients,[195] but other reports suggest that there is no overall advantage.[196],[197] Early studies also suggested that there was no significant difference in the ability of MRI or CT to detect chest wall invasion. Minimal chest wall invasion continues to be difficult to detect, although this may not be a significant limitation since *en bloc* resections are now feasible in selected patients. MRI is better than CT for evaluating the extent of chest wall involvement. CT is able to show bony destruction to advantage, but MRI is more helpful in evaluating early soft tissue disease invasion and bone marrow involvement. Thus the sensitivity for detecting chest wall invasion for CT ranges from 37 to 87 per cent and specificity ranges from 40 to 90 per cent.[198]–[203] The results of MRI studies are better in this regard.[195],[200],[203],[204] Recently, artificially induced pneumothorax and the movement of a tumour mass in relation to the mediastinum and chest wall during a series of deep breath-holds has also been investigated as a method of detecting minimal invasion.[205]–[209] However, problems in interpretation can occur due to the presence of benign pleural adhesions which result in intermediate specificities, limiting the accuracy of the technique. Promising reports have also appeared on ultrasound evaluation of chest wall invasion.[210],[211] These

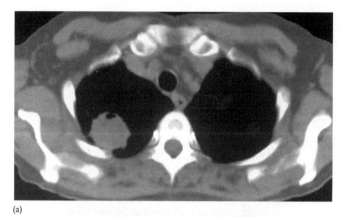

(a)

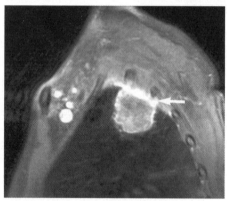

(b)

Fig. 15 Chest wall invasion by lung cancer. (a) Axial, non-enhanced CT image in a patient with non-small-cell lung cancer at the right lung apex. No chest wall invasion is seen (T category II). (b) Sagittal MR image following the administration of intravenous contrast medium. A fat-suppressed image has been obtained. Parietal and visceral pleural invasion is well demonstrated in this plane. Small fronds of tumour are seen beneath the third rib (arrow) (T category IIIA).

small studies suggest higher sensitivities and specificities with false-positive results occurring as a result of pleural adhesions. In the special case of superior sulcus tumours, MRI is superior to CT in detecting chest wall invasion, as well as in the evaluation of other neighbouring structures such as the brachial plexus, blood vessels, and the vertebral bodies (Fig. 15). MRI is the technique of choice for evaluating this tumour type because of multiplanar imaging capability and higher soft tissue contrast. Limitations of CT arise from the axial plane of imaging and from artefacts arising from neighbouring bony structures.

Oesophageal cancer

Any imaging technique that stages oesophageal cancer must be able to determine the depth of tumour penetration through the oesophageal wall, the presence of direct invasion into adjacent structures (especially the tracheobronchial tree and aorta), detect the presence of peri-oesophageal or regional lymphadenopathy, and identify metastases. The aim is to identify patients suitable for surgery as well as those in whom curative surgery is impossible due to mediastinal or abdominal disease. As individual layers of the oesophageal wall are not visualized on CT, oesophageal tumours are poorly staged and minimal mediastinal invasion is difficult to detect.[212] In patients with

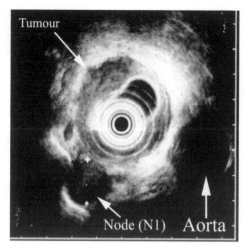

Fig. 16 Oesophageal ultrasound. Endoscopic axial ultrasound image of a T3 oesophageal cancer with an adjacent N1 lymph node. (By courtesy of Dr Z. Amin, Chelsea and Westminster Hospital, London.)

a lack of body fat, disease may be understaged because soft tissue density extending from the primary tumour cannot be identified. CT overstaging also occurs in about 30 per cent of cases thus depriving patients of potentially curative surgery.[213] Endoscopic ultrasound (EUS) has recently been evaluated for its ability to stage primary oesophageal cancers. Based on results to date, it appears that EUS is the single, most accurate method of assessing the local extent of oesophageal cancer (Fig. 16).[214]–[217] This is because it is able to visualize the layers of the individually and thus be able to predict tumour penetration into the submucosa and muscularis layers. The accuracy of EUS is dependent on the ability to traverse the primary tumour with the endoscope. This may be impossible in 20 to 40 per cent of patients.[218] Nevertheless, the accuracy of EUS ranges between 79 and 86 per cent.[214]–[217] Importantly, EUS can separate advanced tumours from early tumours (T4 versus T_1–3) with 97 per cent accuracy. Thus, it is suggested that conventional staging with CT be performed first to demonstrate advanced disease and to identify patients in whom a surgical approach should not be undertaken. In those with indeterminate findings and those with potentially limited disease, an EUS may be performed to assess local stage and invasion of adjacent nodes.

Gastric cancer

The ability of EUS to resolve individual layers of the gastric wall that closely parallel histological structure, makes it uniquely suited to evaluating the extent of penetration of gastric cancer. The overall accuracy of EUS is superior to CT in a number of studies, ranging from 89 to 92 per cent.[219]–[222] EUS therefore appears to be reliable in predicting resectability. However, EUS cannot visualize structures more than 6 cm from the probe, thus restricting the ability to assess perigastric lymph nodes. This limitation has reduced the accuracy for detecting lymph node involvement; nodal staging accuracy of 66 to 83 per cent.[217],[219],[220],[222] Therefore, in patients with gastric carcinoma in whom active management is considered (surgery or chemotherapy), CT is the best initial staging technique. Those patients considered resectable on CT should then undergo endoscopic ultrasound to define stage. Laparoscopic ultrasound, if available, may contribute to further staging information.

Colorectal cancer

In colorectal cancer, prognosis is strongly related to the depth of penetration of the carcinoma through the bowel wall, to the extent of lymphatic dissemination, and on the presence or absence of systemic metastases. Early studies suggested that the staging accuracy of CT was more than 90 per cent. More recently, the staging accuracy in patients with localized disease has been assessed. These studies show that CT is accurate in assessing advanced disease but that the staging accuracy for early disease (particularly differentiating T_2 from T3 lesions) is more limited.[223],[224] The major limiting factor is the inability of CT to distinguish between direct tumour infiltration into the pericolic fat and the desmoplastic reaction induced by a tumour. A large study by the RDOG reported on the performance of CT for local tumour staging in 314 patients (111 of whom had rectal cancers). This study showed that the accuracy of CT for predicting perirectal and pericolic tumour invasion was similar (74 per cent and 72 per cent, respectively).[225] The same study also reported on the performance of MRI in the same patients (using a standard body coil), where it found that the sensitivity for depicting perirectal or pericolic tumour invasion was between 49 and 37 per cent. Because MRI has a higher specificity in making this determination, the overall accuracy of the two techniques was similar. Recent advances in MRI include the availability of endorectal coils and the routine use of phased-array coils for pelvic imaging. Endorectal MRI is able to depict the layers of the rectal wall and can identify the muscularis propria. Studies evaluating this technique suggest an improved local tumour staging accuracy ranging from 79 to 92 per cent.[226]–[229] However, endorectal-coil MRI is unable to determine lymph node involvement and other imaging techniques are required to make this determination. Endorectal MRI is also uncomfortable and motion can degrade images thus limiting its usefulness. The staging accuracy of pelvic, phased-array coil MRI has recently been studied with encouraging results (Fig. 17).[230] Endorectal ultrasound is able to depict the layers of the rectal wall reliably, so allowing differentiation of the mucosa and the muscularis propria. The overall accuracy of this technique in assessing the depth of tumour penetration is higher than CT or body-coil MRI, ranging from 80 per cent to 85 per cent.[231]–[235] Application of EUS requires considerable expertise, with most studies indicating that overall staging accuracy increases substantially with experience. Endoscopic ultrasound is not feasible for some stenotic lesions or for bulky tumours and cannot be used for tumours proximal to the rectum.

Lymph node involvement—N category

The introduction of lymphography in the early 1960s was a major advance in radiology and a key investigative tool in the staging of many tumours, providing much information on the patterns of tumour spread and the behaviour of nodal deposits in response to treatment.[236] Lymphography is a technique that is able to visualize the internal architecture of lymph nodes directly. However, with the introduction of cross-sectional imaging techniques, this method of assessment has fallen out of favour for a number of reasons, including incomplete assessment (visualization) of lymph nodes that could be involved by tumour, and a low skill base of operators able to perform and interpret images. The accuracy of CT is similar to that of

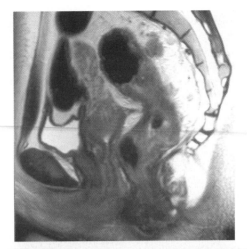

(a)

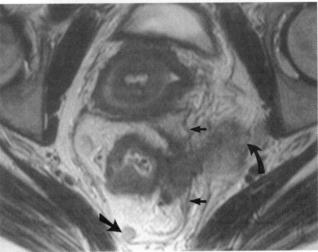

(b)

Fig. 17 Locally advanced rectal carcinoma. (a) Sagittal and (b) oblique axial MR images showing a large rectal carcinoma (T3) in the middle third of rectum. The axial images show tumour extension through the perirectal fat to the level of the mesorectal fascia (small arrows). Enlarged pararectal lymph nodes are seen in the presacral space (slanting arrow). A large necrotic lymph node is seen in the left internal iliac group (large arrow).

lymphography for detecting lymph node involvement from primary pelvic cancers. However, the demonstration of enlarged nodes directly and at sites not accessible to lymphography has resulted in lymphography being supplanted by CT and MR imaging.

Currently, the most widely available criterion for assessing lymph nodes is nodal size. Minor criteria include the site, number and tissue characteristics such as attenuation (on CT), signal intensity (on MRI), and echogenicity (on ultrasound). The currently accepted size criteria at common nodal sites is given in Table 5.[118],[237]–[241] The maximum short-axis diameter is usually chosen because it is less dependent on the position of lymph node in the scan plane than the long-axis. Size assessment methods are limited in their accuracy because sensitivity and specificity are determined by the size criterion chosen as the cutoff between normal and abnormal. Furthermore, it is not possible to detect microscopic disease in normal-sized nodes (false-negative result) or to distinguish enlarged hyperplastic (benign) from malignant

Table 5 Lymph node size at various anatomical sites: short-axis diameter, upper limits of normal

Site	Group	Short-axis size (mm)
Head and neck[237], [238]	Facial	Not visible
	Cervical	10 (<10 mm with central necrosis)
Axilla		10
Mediastinum[239]	Subcarinal	12
	Paracardiac	8
	Retrocural	6
	All other sites	10
Abdomen[240], [241]	Gastrohepatic ligament	8
	Porta hepatis	8
	Portacaval	10
	Coeliac axis to renal artery	10
	Renal artery to aortic bifurcation	12
Pelvis[118]	Common iliac	9
	External iliac	10
	Internal iliac	7
	Obturator	8

lymph nodes (false-positive results). For example, in patients with lung cancer, approximately 20 to 35 per cent of enlarged lymph nodes (more than 1 cm) are reactive and 7 per cent of normal-sized lymph nodes are involved by tumour.[242],[243] This limitation is important clinically. For example, in patients with lung cancer, operability is often determined by the lymph node status in the mediastinum. As imaging is limited in its accuracy to stage mediastinal lymph nodes, patients with tumours that are considered potentially resectable often undergo mediastinoscopy with lymph node sampling.

Experience with MRI to date has revealed no clear advantage of MRI over CT in the detection of enlarged nodes. With MRI, however, minimally enlarged nodes can be distinguished from blood vessels without the need for intravenous contrast medium. On occasion, this may facilitate the interpretation of difficult CT examinations. Clearly therefore, alternative, non-invasive means of assessing lymph node involvement by tumour are needed. Recently, lymph node-specific MR contrast agents based on iron oxide nanoparticles coated with low molecular weight dextran have been evaluated. This technique may emerge as an effective method of assessing lymph node involvement by tumour. The technique relies on the presence of normal lymphocytes within lymph nodes that aggregate small particles of iron oxide as part of their normal scavenging role. The presence of iron oxide particles within lymph nodes results in a decrease in the MR signal—a phenomenon seen in normal lymph nodes, but largely absent in lymph nodes involved by tumour. Initial studies with this agent were performed in patients with head and neck cancers and, recently, increasing experience has been obtained in patients with tumours of other body parts. The contrast agent has been found to be highly accurate (sensitivity 95 per cent, specificity 84 per cent) in patients with head and neck cancers[244] and although clinical experience in tumours at other sites is currently limited, encouraging results have been obtained.[11],[13]

Other means of lymph node assessment include surgical sampling, 18-FDG-PET, and lymphography. Surgical sampling has obvious disadvantages. These include the need for surgery (with its attendant costs and morbidity) and, in general, effective sampling cannot be performed without extensive surgery. 18-FDG-PET is a successful imaging technique capable of characterizing lymph nodes based on tissue metabolism (usually glucose) (see also above). 18-FDG-PET assessment of nodal disease is a successful technique with a high negative and positive predictive value (Fig. 18). Most studies have been performed for the evaluation of thoracic tumours[40],[41],[245] with few studies of the abdominal and pelvic organs.[246],[247]

Sentinel lymph node imaging is a novel approach that allows the identification of the lymph gland at highest risk of containing metastatic tumour (the sentinel gland). This is taken to represent the first lymph node to receive lymphatic drainage from a tumour; the assumption being that if the sentinel node is negative for tumour on microscopy, then an extensive lymph node dissection of regional lymph nodes is unnecessary. The identification of the sentinel lymph node can be performed via the use of blue dye injected around the primary tumour (e.g., in melanoma).[248] More recently, scintigraphic methods have been developed using technetium $^{99}Tc^m$ in serum albumin injected around a tumour, with the sentinel node being identified using a hand-held gamma detector. A recent study showed excellent correlation between the status of the sentinel lymph node and total nodal status in 97 per cent of women with breast cancer.[249] Interested readers are referred to disease-specific chapters on melanoma and breast cancer where further details can be found.

Summary

- Radiologists and oncologists need to understand the physiology of the lymphatic system and lymphatic drainage of each primary tumour.

- Size, site number, and tissue characteristics of nodes are important criteria for determining whether lymph nodes are normal or abnormal.

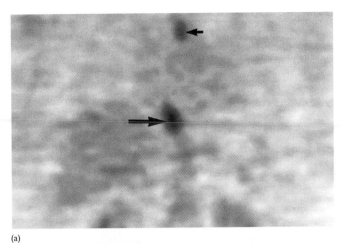

(a)

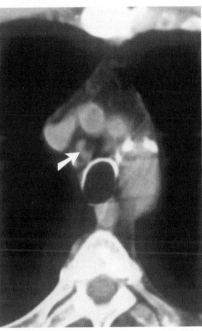

(b)

Fig. 18 Normal-sized mediastinal lymph node with biopsy-proven metastatic oesophageal carcinoma. (a) Coronal FDG-PET image showing hypermetabolism in a primary oesophageal tumour (large arrow). Focal upper mediastinal uptake of the FDG is also visible (small arrow). (b) Axial CT image taken just above the aortic arch shows a normal-sized, pretracheal lymph node with a central fatty hilus (arrow). A mediastinal biopsy of this lymph node was performed and showed microscopic metastatic disease. (By courtesy of Dr WL Wong, Mount Vernon Hospital, London.)

- Nodal size should be measured using the maximum short-access diameter (**MSAD**).
- Clusters of normal-sized asymmetrical nodes should be regarded with suspicion of harbouring metastases.
- Metastatic nodes may show central necrosis, cystic change, or calcification on CT. On MRI, there is considerable overlap between T_1 and T_2 relaxation times of benign and malignant nodes. High-frequency ultrasound may show nodal characteristics typical of a particular tumour (e.g. lymphoma).

- Intravenous contrast medium may result in nodal enhancement both on CT and on MRI.
- Contrast-enhanced imaging (using extracellular contrast agents and lymph node-specific agents) has the potential for differentiating enlarged benign from malignant lymph nodes.
- 18-FDG-PET is valuable for the detection of metastatic lymph nodes.
- Radiolabelled monoclonal antibodies are currently being investigated for the detection of tumour in normal-sized lymph nodes.
- Percutaneous biopsy of suspicious nodes is required in some patients, yielding diagnostic samples in 80 to 90 per cent of patients.

Distant metastases—M category

The most common sites for metastases are the lungs, skeletal systems, liver, and brain, and the preponderance of tumour spread to these sites influences the imaging approach.

Pulmonary metastatic spread

The most frequent pathway for pulmonary metastatic spread is by way of blood-borne tumour emboli. Metastases occurring via lymphatic spread, transbronchial aspiration, and bronchial arterial spread is less common. Lung metastases usually appear as well-defined nodules. Occasionally, the edges of metastatic deposits are ill-defined, particularly when the primary tumour is an adenocarcinoma, when haemorrhage occurs (for example, choriocarcinoma), or following treatment. Cavitation can occur in metastases from any malignancy but are particularly noted in those originating from tumours of squamous-cell type. Cavitation is not related to the size of metastases, but may be related to the liquefaction of keratin in squamous-cell carcinoma and mucoid degeneration in adenocarcinoma (Fig. 19). Thin-wall cysts (pulmonary lacunae) may occur at the site of treated metastases from non-seminomatous, germ-cell tumours. Calcification may be seen in metastases *de novo* or as a result of treatment; calcification in metastases from osteosarcoma and chondrosarcoma occur as part of the tumour matrix. Interlobular septal thickening, a highly specific sign of lymphangitis carcinomatosa, is attributed to irregular tumour growth within the septa with or without fibrosis (Fig. 20).

Although standard chest radiographs are the initial test for the detection of lung metastases, CT is currently the most sensitive technique for detecting pulmonary deposits. The sensitivity of CT is attributable to the lack of superimposition of intrathoracic structures and the high contrast between soft-tissue nodules and air-containing lung. The increased sensitivity of CT compared to plain radiographs is accompanied by a decreased specificity. The precise accuracy of CT is difficult to determine since surgical correlation has only been obtained in a limited number of studies. The specificity of CT is influenced by the type and stage of the underlying extrathoracic malignancy, but it also depends on the frequency of benign entities in the population. False-positive results occur from hamartomas, sarcoidosis, silicosis, histoplasmosis, intrapulmonary lymph nodes, small areas of fibrosis, tuberculosis, etc., all of which may be indistinguishable from metastatic disease. The smallest lesions are a real dilemma as they cannot be biopsied percutaneously and may not be palpable at surgery. Imaging features favouring metastases include:

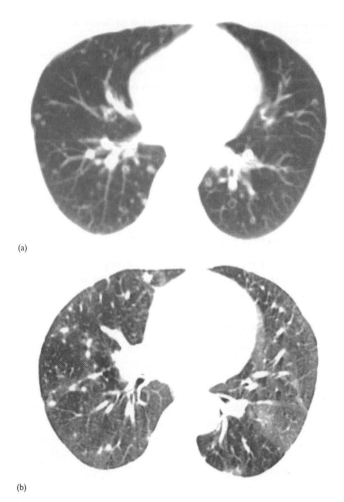

(a)

(b)

Fig. 19 Lung metastases. (a) Multiple cavitating metastases are seen in both lungs in this patient with metastatic rectal carcinoma. The presence of cavitation change does not correlate with the size of individual lesions. (b) High-resolution (1 mm cut) CT image through the lungs in a patient with metastatic breast cancer. Several irregular-edged, focal lesions are seen within both lungs which are characteristic of adenocarcinoma deposits.

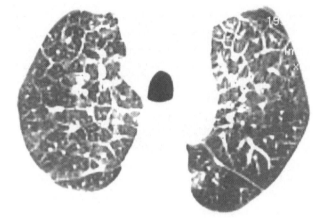

Fig. 20 Lymphangitis carcinomatosa. Axial high-resolution (1 mm cut) CT image through the lungs at the level of the aortic arch in a patient with metastatic prostate cancer. Bilateral, interlobular septal thickening and beading is seen. These appearances are characteristic for the interstitial spread of tumour within the lungs.

Summary

- Tumours with the highest incidence of lung metastases include choriocarcinoma, osteosarcoma, Ewing's' sarcoma, testicular teratomas, and thyroid cancer.
- Spread of tumour to the lungs is usually haematogenous, less commonly lymphatic.
- Over 80 per cent of lung metastases are in the periphery of the lung (> 60 per cent subpleural), and most commonly in the mid- and lower zones.
- Lymphangitis carcinomatosa arises most commonly from primary tumours of the lung, breast, and prostrate. Characteristic findings are demonstrated on high-resolution CT.
- Spiral CT is the most sensitive technique for the detection of lung metastases and is less specific than conventional CT.
- Indications for CT must take into consideration the findings on chest radiographs, the likely influence of results and management, and the propensity of the tumour to metastasize to the lungs.

Skeletal metastases

The purpose of imaging bone metastases is to identify the presence and extent of disease, evaluate complications such as spinal cord compression or fractures, and to monitor therapeutic response. Most bony metastases are asymptomatic, with over 90 per cent occurring within the distribution of the red bone marrow. Thus, in adults, the majority of metastases occur within the spine, shoulder, and pelvic girdles and the proximal limbs. The network of vertebral, epidural, and perivertebral veins plays a significant role in the transport of cancer cells to the vertebral column. Solitary metastases are uncommon, frequently occurring from renal or thyroid carcinomas. An accurate assessment of bony metastatic disease requires a combination of clinical evaluation, biochemical assessment, and appropriate imaging (Fig. 21).

^{99}Tc^{m}-diphosphonate (**MDP**) bone scanning has excellent sensitivity in the detection of bony metastases, with the advantage of being

the close relationship of nodules to an adjacent vessel; decreased density distal to a lesion; reticular changes surrounding a lesion; gross beading of the septal interstitium; spherical and ovoid shapes rather than linear or irregular shapes; and the absence of calcification.

The characterization of solitary pulmonary nodules in patients with known malignancy is a well-recognized diagnostic problem. In a large study of 800 patients who presented with an apparent solid nodule one or more years after detection and treatment of an extrathoracic malignancy, 63 per cent proved to be a new primary tumour with less than 25 per cent representing solitary metastases.[250] The likelihood of metastatic disease in such lesions depends on the histology of the primary tumour. In patients over 35 years of age, if the extrathoracic malignancy is a squamous carcinoma, the likelihood of a new lung primary tumour is about 65 per cent. If the extrathoracic malignancy is an adenocarcinoma, then the likelihood of a new tumour is about 50 per cent. For patients with sarcomas, a new solitary nodule is most likely to represent metastatic disease.

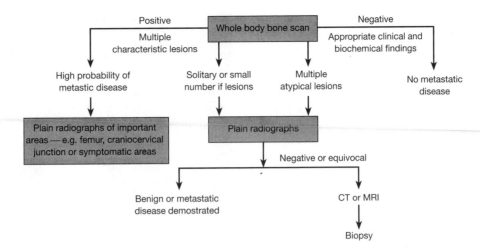

Fig. 21 Flow diagram for evaluating suspected metastatic bony disease.

able to visualize the whole skeleton. Bone scans can detect metastatic disease before they are evident on plain radiographs.[189],[251] As little as a 5 to 10 per cent change in the lesion to normal bone uptake ratio is required before an abnormal focus is seen on a bone scan. Bone scans have a low specificity and cannot distinguish benign from malignant causes of increased tracer uptake. They are reliable for detecting metastases from breast, prostate, lung, and kidney cancer but appear less reliable in patients with myeloma, lymphoma, and leukaemia where photopenic areas are observed. As a result, false-negative results are not uncommon.[251] False-positive examinations occur from trauma, infection, and metabolic disorders as well as from benign bone tumours. Conventional radiographs provide important information about cortical and trabecular bone but little information regarding the presence of lesions confined to the bone marrow. A 30 to 50 per cent reduction in bone density is required for lesions in cancellous bone to be visible on plain films. Osteolytic lesions are more difficult to identify than osteoblastic lesions. Fractures may occur when more than 50 per cent of the thickness of the long bone is involved radiographically.[252] Thus, although plain films are an insensitive method for detecting metastatic bony disease, they have the major advantage of being highly specific.

CT is not routinely used in the evaluation of metastatic bony disease; it is used instead for problem solving. Its roles include the characterization of bony lesions seen by other techniques particularly when MRI is unavailable (for example, for evaluation of solitary hot spots on a bone scan), planning decompression spinal surgery, and distinguishing benign from malignant vertebral collapse. CT is also valuable for guiding percutaneous bone biopsy. MRI is ideally suited for evaluating the bone marrow because it visualizes the bone marrow directly, has excellent soft tissue contrast, and multiplanar imaging capabilities. MRI has high sensitivity in the detection of bone marrow metastases even in the presence of normal radiographs and negative radionuclide bone scans.[253]–[255]

Vertebral collapse

In a patient with known malignancy, this poses diagnostic problems because the distinction of malignant and osteoporotic collapse cannot always be made on standard radiographs. A history of trauma and multiple areas of involvement in an elderly person suggest non-metastatic disease. The location of the collapsed vertebrae is also important because upper-thoracic vertebral collapse is more likely to be malignant than post-traumatic. On plain radiographs, uniform compression of the end plates is more likely to be due to osteopenia, whereas irregularity is more commonly seen with metastases. Both CT and MRI can be useful for distinguishing benign from malignant collapse. The presence of anterior or posterior cortical bony destruction, involvement of the pedicles, altered bone marrow attenuation or signal, and the presence of a paraspinal mass favours the diagnosis of malignant vertebral disease. Benign vertebral collapse is characterized by the presence of cortical fractures, retropulsion of bony fragments into the spinal canal, fractures within the cancellous bone, absence of bone destruction, and by a minimal, usually diffuse, paraspinal soft tissue mass (haematoma).

Summary

- Imaging plays a complementary role to clinical and biochemical evaluation of bony metastases.
- Radionuclide scans are the initial investigation of choice in the majority of patients.
- Screening with radionuclide studies for bone marrow metastases has a high yield in breast and prostate cancer.
- Plain radiographs should be used first to elucidate inconclusive radionuclide abnormalities.
- CT has a role in detecting lesions at sites difficult to assess on plain radiographs.
- CT is useful for guiding percutaneous biopsy.
- MRI is the most sensitive method currently available for detecting metastases and is moderately specific.
- CT and MRI are both useful for evaluating the cause of vertebral collapse.

Liver metastases

Liver metastases occur via the bloodstream. There is a latent period between the seeding of metastases and the time when they become manifest on clinical or imaging evaluation. For patients with clinical or biochemical evidence of metastatic liver disease, ultrasound should be used first. Liver metastases usually appear as low echogenic foci on ultrasound, and intravenous ultrasound contrast agents can improve the detection of focal liver lesions. Ultrasound provides a reliable assessment of the biliary tree and hepatic vasculature and will detect, localize, and characterize the majority of focal liver lesions. Intraoperative ultrasound remains the best imaging technique for detecting metastatic liver disease because it is able to identify very small lesions. In patients with unexpected or inconclusive sonographic findings, contrast-enhanced spiral CT is recommended. A single-phase acquisition (hepatic parenchymal phase) is adequate in the majority of patients, but a dual-phased CT study should be performed in patients suspected of harbouring hypervascular lesions. Hypervascular primary liver lesions include hepatoma and benign primary lesions such as fibronodular hyperplasia. Hypervascular metastases include those arising from islet-cell tumours of the pancreas, carcinoid tumours, melanoma, renal carcinoma, and phaeochromocytoma (Fig. 22). Most liver lesions are satisfactorily characterized by CT but in, case of doubt, MRI should be performed using both T_2-weighting and gadolinium enhanced T_1-weighted images. Patients who are candidates for surgical resections require super-paramagnetic iron oxide-enhanced MRI for maximal sensitivity (Fig. 3).[14]–[16] The more invasive procedure of CT arterioportography, though highly sensitive in detecting liver metastases, should be reserved for patients who are unable to undergo MRI and in those in whom MRI is inconclusive. CT arterioportography (CTAP) suffers from lower specificity because of flow effects which can have the appearance of metastases (pseudo-lesions) (Fig. 23).

Distinguishing benign focal liver lesions from metastases

When incidental liver lesions are discovered in patients with non-malignant disease, the likelihood of them being metastatic deposits is remote.[256] However, the appearance of small lesions appearing for the first time during surveillance after the initial treatment of malignant disease must be regarded with suspicion whatever their imaging appearances. Liver cysts are not uncommon and have characteristic features on ultrasound and MRI. Only a minority of metastases contain fluid and may thus be confused with cysts. Benign haemangiomas are found in up to 20 per cent of autopsies and are common in patients undergoing liver imaging for suspected metastatic disease. Most haemangiomas are irregular in shape but with clear-cut margins, and have characteristic ultrasound, CT, and MR appearances. Larger lesions may have atypical features due to the presence of central scarring. Small haemangiomas may have similar appearances to hypervascular metastases in the early phase of contrast enhancement, but the latter often show rapid washout of contrast medium. Areas of focal fatty change may also resemble metastatic disease, particularly when a nodular fatty infiltration is present.[257],[258] They can appear suspicious on ultrasound and on CT, but MRI is probably the most sensitive method of confirming focal fatty infiltration using the technique of in-phase and opposed-phase T_1 imaging (Fig. 24).

Summary

• The role of imaging includes the detection of lesions, distinguishing benign from metastatic disease, the selection of

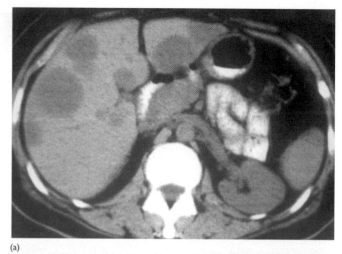

(a)

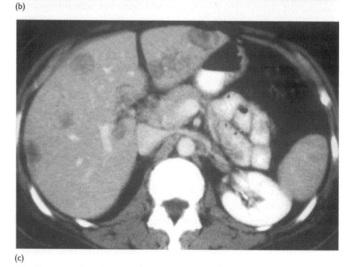

(b)

(c)

Fig. 22 Hypervascular metastases from a resected neuroendocrine pancreatic tumour. (a) Precontrast-enhanced CT image shows multifocal abnormalities within the liver compatible with metastatic disease. A pancreatic resection is seen. (b) Arterial phased image showing intense hypervascularity within individual lesions. (c) Image obtained in the portal phase of contrast enhancement. Note that the metastases have 'filled in' and appear smaller than on the precontrast-enhanced images. (By courtesy of Dr W. Teh, Northwick Park Hospital, London.)

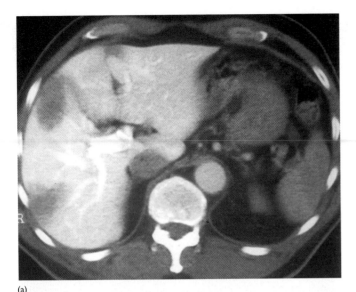

(a)

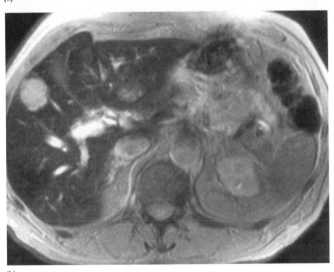

(b)

Fig. 23 Prominent flow effects on CT arterioportography (**CTAP**). (a) Axial CT image from arterioportogram showing three liver lesions. Note that the inferior vena cava, spleen, stomach, and bowel are not enhancing because injection of contrast medium is directly into the superior mesenteric artery. (b) Axial, proton density-weighted, gradient-echo MR image at the same level following ferumoxide contrast-medium administration. Only one lesion is seen. The other two lesions seen in Fig. (a) are flow effects, which are commonly seen during CTAP.

patients most eligible for surgical resection, and to assess response to treatment.

- Ultrasound and CT are the main diagnostic modalities for the evaluation of metastatic liver disease, and the roles for MR imaging include problem-solving and presurgical assessment.
- Multiphasic contrast-enhanced CT and MRI are useful techniques for liver lesion characterization and liver-specific, contrast-enhanced MRI is useful for presurgical liver assessment.

Brain metastases

Most occur late in the course of the natural history of the disease. Most brain metastases arise from lung cancer, breast, and melanoma, although other sources include renal and gastrointestinal tumours (Fig. 25). In a significant proportion of patients, the primary source may be unknown. MRI is the most sensitive imaging technique available for detecting brain metastases, but screening is undertaken in only select patient groups. Screening for metastases in non-small-cell lung cancer prior to thoracotomy can reveal asymptomatic brain metastases in 5 to 30 per cent of patients.[259],[260] The differential diagnosis of brain metastases includes primary brain tumours, infection, and haemorrhage. Meningeal deposits are usually seen in patients with leukaemia, non-Hodgkin's lymphoma, breast cancer, lung cancer, and malignant melanoma. Clinical features often non-specific and meningeal metastases are best demonstrated with contrast-enhanced MRI compared to CT (Fig. 26). Meningeal enhancement may also be seen in normal patients. Spinal cord compression is a common problem in patients with disseminated malignancy. Imaging of the whole spinal cord should be performed and MRI is the preferred imaging modality. A significant number of patients will have multiple levels of compression.[261],[262] (Fig. 27). Spinal meningeal disease is caused by invasion of the spinal nerve roots or by haematogenous spread to the leptomeninges. Patients frequently present with neurological features that do not point to a single specific site. Contrast-enhanced MRI is mandatory for the full evaluation of these patients.[263] Primary brain tumours may produce spinal seedlings and intramedullary metastases most commonly occur in breast and lung cancer and in malignant melanoma.

Adrenal metastases

Most adrenal metastases are asymptomatic and at autopsy may be seen in more than 25 per cent of patients. Demonstration of a secondary deposit renders the patient as having advanced disease. Benign adrenal tumours are also commonly found in the general population, and when an adrenal mass is seen even in a patient with a known carcinoma, the diagnosis is more likely to be an adenoma than a metastasis. Size alone is poor at distinguishing an adenoma from a metastatic deposit. Masses that are more than 3 cm are 90 to 95 per cent likely to be malignant, whereas those less than 3 cm are more likely to be benign.[264]–[265] Adrenal metastases have a variable appearance on CT and MRI. On CT, an attenuation value of 10 Hounsfield units (**HU**) without contrast-agent administration appears reliable in making this distinction. After contrast administration, early imaging is unreliable, but delayed CT (30 to 60 min) can be as effective as precontrast CT but using a cut-off value of 30 HU.[266] Chemical-shift MRI is equally specific in making this distinction, based on the well-known fact that adrenal adenomas contain lipid.[267]–[269] (Fig. 28). Both CT and MRI can reduce the need for biopsy of adrenal glands but when an adrenal mass cannot be characterized adequately, biopsy may still be required. (See also PET above).

Radiotherapy treatment planning

The ability of computer-assisted radiological techniques to produce two- (2D) and three-dimensional (3D) body images has transformed

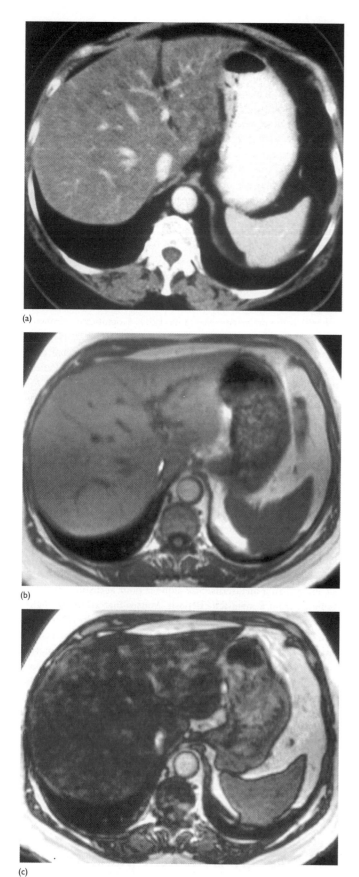

Fig. 24 Fatty infiltration mimicking metastatic disease. (a) Axial CT image in a patient with resected breast carcinoma and previous adjuvant chemotherapy. The patient was evaluated for abnormal liver function tests. There are diffuse areas of heterogeneity within liver parenchyma. No displacement of vessels is seen. The differential diagnoses lies between fatty infiltration and diffuse infiltrating metastatic disease. (b) Gradient-echo T_1-weighted image obtained in phase ($TE = 4.1$ ms) shows no abnormality. (c) Opposed phase image ($TE = 2.2$ ms) at the same slice location. Marked reduction in signal of the liver parenchyma is visible which is diagnostic of fatty infiltration. The areas of relative high signal on this image are areas of normal liver.

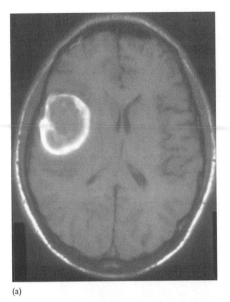 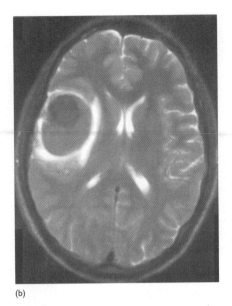 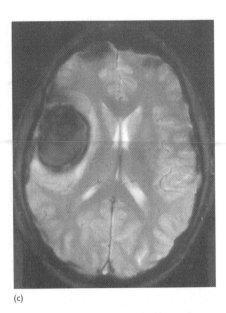

(a) (b) (c)

Fig. 25 Melanoma brain metastases. (a) Axial T_1-weighted image without intravenous contrast medium shows a large mass in the right cerebral hemisphere with a hyperintense rim suggestive of the presence of blood. (b) T_2-weighted image at the same slice position demonstrates the hyperintense high-signal area around the lesion (vasogenic oedema). (c) T_2^*-weighted, gradient-echo image shows a dark signal within the tumour mass and at its edge. This paramagnetic effect arises from the presence of melanin within the tumour and from the blood surrounding the mass.

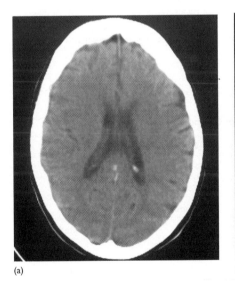 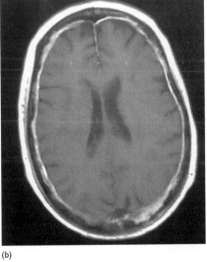

(a) (b)

Fig. 26 Metastatic breast carcinoma with meningeal tumour spread. (a) Axial CT imaging following contrast-medium administration fails to show meningeal enhancement. (b) Axial T_1-weighted MR image following contrast-medium administration shows marked, irregular enhancement of the meninges. Bony disease is also seen in the left parietal region.

the radiotherapy management of cancer. Imaging modalities such as CT and MRI provide complementary information for the localization and characterization of tumours and normal tissues (Table 6). Technological advances in these imaging modalities, in linear accelerator capabilities, computer workstations, and planning software have resulted in improved and sophisticated methods of treating patients with radiotherapy.

The evolution of conventional external-beam RT planning towards conformally designed treatments during the past decade has demanded improved methods to accurately assess the spatial relationship between

target volumes and surrounding tissues. The potential benefits of precise dose delivery while maximally sparing surrounding normal tissues are considerable. This is especially important in conformal RT, which often requires irregularly shaped treatment portals to produce an ideal 3D dose distribution from a range of planar and non-coplanar fields. It is well established that CT has made a dramatic impact on the accuracy of radiotherapy treatment planning in the past two decades.[270] This has resulted in improvements in the therapeutic ratio, either by minimizing normal tissue complications or, alternatively, allowing an increased dose and improved local

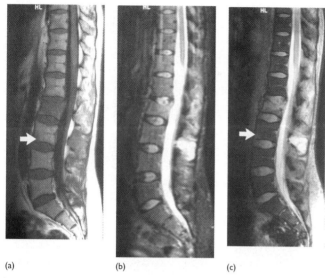

(a)   (b)   (c)

Fig. 27 Multiple metastases to the spine from breast cancer. (a) Sagittal T_1, (b) STIR, and (c) gradient-echo, T_2^*-weighted images show the presence of metastatic deposits within the vertebral bodies of L2, L3, and in the spinous process of L3. There is end-plate infraction of the vertebral body of L2, which is not of high signal on the STIR sequence but there is clear loss of trabecular bone visible on the gradient-echo T_2^* sequence. Loss of trabecular bone confirms metastatic disease. The large deposit within the spinous process of L3 is visible on all three sequences. An additional deposit is seen in the vertebral body of L3 anteriorly (arrow). No cord compression is identified.

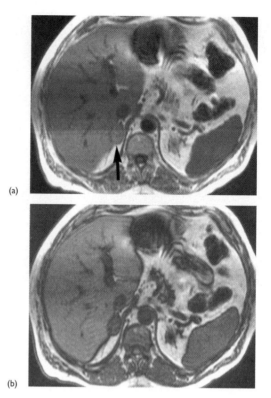

(a)

(b)

Fig. 28 Chemical-shift MR imaging of an indeterminate adrenal mass. (a) In phase ($TE = 4.1$ ms) and (b) opposed phase ($TE = 6.5$ ms) T_1-weighted MR images through the adrenal glands. Note that the right adrenal mass (arrow) decreases in signal on the opposed phase imaging. These appearances are characteristic for a lipid-containing adenoma.

control with currently acceptable levels of normal tissue toxicity. It has been postulated that if doses can be safely escalated by approximately 20 per cent, this may result in improvements in tumour control rates.[271] The development of MR imaging has introduced several added imaging benefits that may confer an additional advantage over the use of CT in RT planning and further improve the therapeutic ratio.[272]

Since radiotherapy plans are produced in the cross-sectional plane, CT has been extensively investigated as a method of providing accurate data for RT planning purposes. The advantages of CT include excellent image resolution, geometric image accuracy over large fields of view, electron-density information—important for dosimetry, excellent depiction of bony structures, and reasonable cost. Therefore, information regarding body contour, tumour localization, and normal anatomy are accurately depicted with CT, with multiple sections showing the tumour throughout its length. Coronal and sagittal reconstructions may be useful for defining tumour extent and has been most widely used for pelvic and intracranial tumours. CT also has the advantage that heterogeneity corrections can be made on a pixel-by-pixel basis.[273] This is important for the treatment of thoracic tumours because the radiation beam passes through aerated lung, and for the treatment of tumours of the pelvis when the beam traverses dense bone. Several studies have been conducted in which conventional methods of planning have been compared with CT.[274]–[277] Overall, these studies showed that treatment plans were altered in approximately 25 to 45 per cent of patients because of CT information. Consequently, CT is now the standard technique for planning tumours when precise information is required.

Table 6 Comparison of CT and MRI for radiotherapy planning[275]

Parameters	MRI	CT
Soft tissue contrast	Excellent	Moderate
Cortical bone contrast	Poor	Excellent
Image resolution	Good	Better
Functionality	Large	Limited
Scanning time	Long	Shorter
Electron density information	Nil	Present
Geometric image accuracy	Distortions present	Excellent
Multiplanar imaging	Available	Limited
Cost and availability	Higher/limited	Lower/wide

The technique of using CT for radiotherapy planning requires certain conditions. The scanner couch must be flat because the dish couch alters the body contour and the position of internal structures.[278] A large gantry aperture is required to permit complete visualization of the body contour, particularly in obese or large-sized

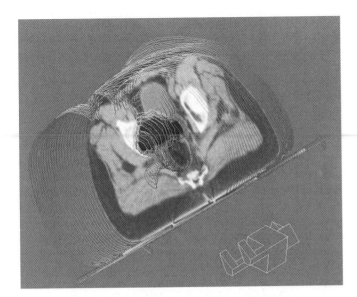

Fig. 29 3D CT radiotherapy planning. A 3D isodose distribution for prostate radiotherapy. (By courtesy of Dr V Khoo, Hammersmith Hospital, London.)

patients. Laser lights are used to align the patient in the treatment position during CT scanning and identical lights must be present on the treatment machine. The patient is then scanned through the region of the tumour. The centre of the tumour is related to a tattoo on the skin, which is marked with a therapy marker containing barium paste. This provides a skin reference point for the co-ordination of CT information with the eventual treatment set-up.

With CT, initial simulation and invasive techniques, such as cystography, are no longer required. The dimensions of the tumour recorded by CT are documented in three planes and a section through the centre of the tumour is chosen for planning. A hard-copy film of the chosen CT section may be enlarged to life size and the tumour, normal organs, and body contour traced from the image on to paper for planning. Alternatively, CT data can be transferred electronically to the radiotherapy planning computer. The radiotherapist then outlines the treatment volume using not only CT information but all available clinical and radiological evidence of disease. A physicist produces the radiotherapy plan from this information by superimposing the treatment beams directly on to the CT image (Fig. 29). The advantages of using a CT-integrated planning system are that the dose to individual structures is easily assessed, heterogeneity corrections can be obtained, magnification errors are minimized, and the process is less time-consuming.

MRI has not yet seriously challenged CT for RT planning in most anatomical sites.[279] The reasons for this include: the poor imaging of bone and the lack of electron-density information; the presence of intrinsic system-related and object-induced MR image distortions; and the paucity of widely available computer software to integrate and manipulate MR images accurately and reliably within existing RT planning systems. Despite these difficulties, MRI has complemented CT-based RT planning and in some regions of the body, especially the brain, where it is used with success. MRI can bring

major benefits in the RT planning process. These include superb soft tissue contrast which can be varied by changing the imaging sequence parameters. This can help evaluate the extent and margins of malignancies, especially those that infiltrate surrounding tissue such as muscle. The use of paramagnetic contrast agents has further increased its scope compared with CT especially in the evaluation of central nervous system lesions.

A feature of MRI is that cortical bone appears hypointense and does not give rise to an MR signal. This has both advantages and disadvantages for RT planning. Regions of the body that are surrounded by thick layers of bone will preferentially absorb X-rays from CT, so reducing soft tissue image quality and producing artefacts. This is particularly pronounced at the skull base. Compared with CT, MRI provides clear definition of the posterior fossa, brainstem, and lesions centred at bony prominences or those, such as the spinal cord, enclosed within bones. The disadvantages of not visualizing cortical bone relate to RT dosimetry and to poor co-registration of CT and MR image datasets. MRI can be acquired in any anatomical plane without loss of spatial resolution and allows 3D volumetric acquisition in a reasonable time. Furthermore, physiological and biological information can be obtained from other MR properties such as chemical shift, macroscopic blood flow, tumour blood volume, diffusion, permeability, and even brain activation. In the future, RT planning will have to take tissue function into account in order to minimize toxicity if dose-escalation treatments are to become the norm.

MRI has mostly been used for radiotherapy planning of tumours within the central nervous system as it is already the imaging modality of choice at this site. Intracranial movement is minimal and is largely governed by external motion of the skull vault which can be rigidly immobilized. Since the head can easily be placed within the central most homogeneous part of the MRI system, MRI distortions are small compared to the rest of the body. These factors, coupled with methods of image correction are effective for the head and have enabled MRI–CT-assisted RT planning. Numerous studies have shown that the addition of MRI can materially alter the radiation-volume, CT-based radiotherapy plans in 60 to 82 per cent of cases, as a direct result of improved definition of the tumour volume.[280] MRI is also currently being evaluated for radiotherapy planning of complex head and neck regions,[281]–[283] and for application in RT planning of lung and oesophageal cancer. Recently, MRI and CT have been used for radiotherapy planning of prostate cancer.[284] Improved organ definition, particularly of the prostatic apex, is an important advantage here. However, MR distortion may be more significant for larger anatomical regions and these issues need to be addressed prior to radiotherapy planning.

A number of other issues need to be resolved before MRI can be implemented into routine radiotherapy planning. These include the need for reliable distortion-correction algorithms to ensure accurate reproducible MRI data. Precise and dependable methods of fully automated image segmentation, correlation, and registration are also required. Quality assurance procedures are an inherent part of any RT planning system and these too need to be implemented. Although experience to date with MRI indicates a promising role in RT planning, much developmental work remains to be completed before its full potential is realized. Comparative and prospective clinical studies to determine the cost-effectiveness of MR radiotherapy planning and hence its ultimate clinical value will also be needed.

Summary

- CT planning improves the accuracy of defining tumour and target volumes and enables 3D-visualization of the target and normal structures.
- CT provides the basis for 3D dose calculations and conformal radiotherapy.
- Diagnostic radiology is critical to ensure that optimal imaging modalities are used and that interpretation of data is correct.
- Accurate construction of the target volume is the first step in attempting cure in patients with localized tumour treated with radiotherapy.
- Multimodality imaging and registration are powerful tools for yielding further improvements in the delivery of radiotherapy.
- Techniques are being developed to combine the improved tumour definition capabilities of MRI with the geometric accuracy and electron-density capabilities of CT in radiotherapy planning processes.

Assessing response to treatment

Monitoring the response of tumours to treatment is an integral and increasingly important function of radiologists working in oncological imaging. Imaging studies allow an objective method of quantifying tumour response to a variety of physical and pharmaceutical treatments. An important principle for the use of imaging in follow-up is that the same technique should be used for monitoring response as for staging the initial study. Decisions on the use of a particular imaging modality are influenced by progress in imaging evaluation and education, as well as developments in technology. Objective tumour shrinkage has been widely adopted as a standard endpoint to select new anticancer drugs for further study, as a prospective endpoint for definitive clinical trials designed to estimate the benefit of treatment in a specific group of patients, and is widely used in everyday clinical practice to guide clinical decision-making.

Standard size criteria for measuring therapeutic response were first proposed in 1981 and, although they have been adapted by various cancer organizations, they continue to be used largely unchanged.[285]–[287] It should be noted that the World Heath Organization (**WHO**), National Cancer Institute (**NCI**), and the European Organization for Research and Treatment of Cancer (**EORTC**) have recently adopted a new set of tumour response criteria (Response Evaluation Criteria in Solid Tumours—RECIST).[288] This followed a favourable report that compared the use of unidimensional to bidimensional measurements.[289] RECIST criteria are designed to replace existing WHO criteria and the two criteria are compared in Table 7. RECIST criteria provide guidance on the selection and measurement of lesions, allow assessment of response, and discuss imaging methods that can be used to measure lesions to reliably assess response.

There are many recognized limitations of size change as a tumour response variable. Where possible, a lesion should be measured bidimensionally by multiplying the largest diameter by its perpendicular size to give the product. Size changes for both response and progression are arbitrary and traditionally expressed as a percentage change from baseline. For example, a minimum of a 50 per cent reduction in lesion size (equivalent to a 75 per cent reduction in volume) is needed before a partial response to treatment can be documented. When multiple lesions are present, all the products are summed. In contrast, progressive disease is defined as an increase of 25 per cent in the size of one or more lesions or the appearance of new lesions(s). Measurements performed in this ways are laborious and there are numerous errors in obtaining tumour measurements. These arise from observer variations on the estimated position of the boundary of lesions. The edges of irregular or infiltrating lesions are often difficult to identify and, indeed, some tumours are impossible to measure, for example pulmonary lymphangitis carcinomatosa and ovarian carcinoma seeding into the peritoneal space. Furthermore, there is little consensus on whether necrosis and cystic change should be included or excluded when obtaining tumour measurements. The difficulty in distinguishing peritumoral fibrosis from tumour spread further confounds attempts at measurement. Measurement errors in estimating the size of small lesions can result in the misclassification of a significant number of patients. The current 25 per cent increase in the product has been shown by Lavin and Flowerdew to result in a one in four chance of declaring that progression has occurred when, in fact, the tumour is unchanged.[290]

So serious are these errors that 'independent review panels' are often employed by pharmaceutical companies to standardize the reporting of tumour response in clinical trials. Independent review panels can disagree with 'home radiologists' in 50 per cent of cases, with major disagreements occurring in up to 40 per cent of cases.[291] The causes for such disagreements include variations in the technique of examinations for obtaining images, lesion selection, and siting the edges of target lesions. Bidimensional size criteria do not take full account of tumour volume, particularly when one considers that state-of-the-art imaging machines can routinely acquire such information. However, 3D volume measurements are likely to encounter errors similar to bidimensional size measurements. A change in size may also be delayed chronologically, often requiring several treatments before a decision can be made on whether a treatment is effective. Reports from the functional imaging literature, particularly regarding PET, suggest that metabolic and physiological changes antecede size change.[292] For example, in patients with lymphoma responding to treatment, changes in energetics can be detected by 18-FDG-PET within hours,[293] whilst morphological changes are delayed in their appearance. Size changes may also fail to correspond to the patient's clinical condition. All of us have observed patients in whom there is obvious clinical progression (for example, deterioration of performance status, haematological indices, and tumour markers) but with no change in the size of marker lesions. Similarly, clinically inactive disease may be present with enlarging lesions, particularly in patients with non-seminomatous, germ-cell tumours.[294]

As a result, there is a pressing need to develop additional response parameters to overcome these limitations, and to address the growing need to monitor the response to treatment of a new generation of selective anticancer drugs. Cytotoxic chemotherapy is usually directed at molecular targets present in both normal and tumour tissues, and therefore toxicity to normal tissues limits this approach. Recent molecular understanding of the processes of tumour development

Table 7 Definitions of best response according to WHO* and RECIST**

Response category	WHO criteria[286] Change in the sum of products	RECIST[288] Change in sums of longest diameters
Complete response (CR)	Disappearance of all target lesions without any residual lesion; confirmed at 4 weeks	Disappearance of all target lesions; confirmed at 4 weeks
Partial response (PR)	50% or more decrease in target lesions, without a 25% increase in any one target lesion; confirmed at 4 weeks	At least 30% reduction in the sum of the longest diameter of target lesions taking as reference the baseline study; confirmed at 4 weeks
Stable disease (SD)	Neither PR nor PD criteria are met	Neither PR nor PD criteria are met, taking as reference the smallest sum of the longest diameter recorded since treatment started
Progressive disease (PD)	25% or more increase in the size of measurable lesion or appearance of new lesions	At least 20% increase in the sum of the longest diameter of target lesions, taking as reference the smallest sum longest diameter recorded since treatment started, or appearance of new lesions

* WHO: World Health Organization, Geneva, Switzerland[286]

**RECIST: Response Evaluation Criteria in Solid Tumours[288]

and metastasis have led to a number of new targets being identified for potential anticancer treatments. These targets are involved at one level or more in tumour biology, including tumour-cell proliferation and invasion, angiogenesis, and metastasis. Imaging studies may provide early evidence of drug activity, sometimes directed at the site of biological action. These may then be used as surrogate endpoints of drug efficacy to speed up the process of finding more effective drug combinations to enter into phase III trials.

So where should we look for new imaging response parameters? The clues are already here in what we can measure today and in new molecular imaging technologies.[295] Functional imaging parameters that reflect tumour vascularity, the microenvironment, and cell metabolism should be investigated as tumour response variables. These tumour features are inextricably linked in the majority of solid tumours because cancers cannot grow more than 1 mm^3 without acquiring additional nutrient support, usually via the recruitment of new vessels from the host.[295]–[297] Although the transition of dormant to active vascularization is not fully understood, it is clear that the metabolic microenvironment plays an essential role in tumour neoangiogenesis. Important metabolic factors include oxygenation, pH, metabolic and energetic status, and interstitial pressure and transport. These microenvironmental factors also have a direct effect on tumour cellular processes including gene expression and tumour proliferation, metastatic potential, and sensitivity to radiotherapy and anticancer drugs.[298],[299]

A variety of imaging techniques that assess cellular metabolic processes may act as potential tumour response variables. For example, ^{18}F-FDG-PET and [^{11}C]thymidine PET indicate glucose metabolism and the proliferative activity of tumours,[300] and ^{31}P-MRS and ^{1}H-MRS enable cellular energetics and the membrane turnover to be assessed.[80] Dynamic contrast medium-enhanced MRI provides insights into tumour perfusion, capillary permeability and leakage space is also being evaluated in such a role.[301] Other MR techniques are able to measure intracellular pH (^{31}P-MRS), water diffusion, and cell-membrane integrity (diffusion imaging). The development of novel

contrast agents will enable the distribution of extracellular pH to be mapped, and 18-fluoromidonidazole can be used as a PET imaging agent to measure tumour hypoxia non-invasively.[302] Furthermore, molecular imaging techniques currently being developed will enable us to image processes such as intracellular signalling, imaging of gene delivery and expression, and imaging of drug delivery. Some of these parameters have already been investigated for their potential as tumour response parameters but there have been few large correlative studies. Anatomical and multifunctional response assessment studies are difficult to perform because of costs, availability of equipment and expertise, lack of robust image registration procedures (particularly in extracranial applications), and time constraints that are acceptable to patients and institutional ethics committees. This is particularly the case where such evaluations have to be repeated to determine the optimal timing for the response of individual parameters. Thus, it is also evident that the parameters chosen for evaluation must be relevant to the biological action of the treatment being assessed. The importance of being able to perform such combined multifunctional and morphological examinations cannot, however, be over-emphasized; they will enable the co-registration of anatomical and functional data and so allow an appreciation of tumour heterogeneity, will enable correlation between different and diverse functional parameters (for example, correlation of MR lipid signals (necrosis) and tumour vascular permeability), and will allow longitudinal outcome studies to be performed. Such studies will also enable an improved understanding of aspects of tumour biology, treatment response, improve patient staging, treatment stratification, and determination of prognosis. These techniques will also have a central role in the evaluation of novel therapies, for example antiangiogenesis drugs and gene and antibody therapy.

Summary

• Imaging for cancer follow-up is of equal importance to imaging for the diagnosis and staging of malignancy.

- This same imaging technique should be used for follow-up throughout the course of the disease, and ideally this should be the same technique as used for staging.
- Imaging permits the evaluation of therapeutic response by measuring changes in volume and tumour composition.
- The plain radiographs remain central to the evaluation of tumour response in intrathoracic malignancy, primary breast cancer and bony tumours.
- CT is the mainstay of measuring changes in tumour volume with imaging.
- Regression rates are different for different pathological types of tumour. Measurement of tumour volume is difficult in irregular and diffuse tumours as well as those involving the hollow organs.
- Current criteria provide the standard for evaluating therapeutic response in terms of change of tumour size, but no consideration is given to the calculation of tumour volume or tumour composition.
- Contrast-enhanced MRI may provide information that reflects changes in tumour neovascularity.
- 18-FDG-PET imaging is likely to have a critical role in the clinical evaluation of therapeutic response when the technique becomes more widely available.

Evaluating residual disease

Evaluating residual disease after a primary course of treatment is important in two clinical circumstances. Persistent residual masses of considerable size may remain after apparent successful treatment, particularly in patients with seminoma, non-seminomatous germ-cell tumours (**NSGCT**), neuroblastoma, and lymphoma. Such masses may continue to regress for up to 2 years after completion of treatment,[303] and are a cause of concern because they are a potential site for relapse. For example, residual masses in the mediastinum may be seen in up to 80 per cent of patients with Hodgkin's disease and up to 40 per cent of patients with non-Hodgkin's lymphoma. Patients with residual disease are twice as likely to relapse when compared to those with no discernible disease (complete response). Additional treatments may be inappropriate for patients with 'sterilized disease'. Radiation for example, can result in long-term morbidity including a 15 per cent increase incidence of ischaemic heart disease, cardiomyopathy, and lung fibrosis.[304],[305] There is also a definite increased risk of secondary malignancies induced by radiotherapy. For example, in young women (under 20 years old) treated with mantle irradiation for Hodgkin's disease, there is a 40-fold increase in the incidence of breast cancer.[306] Another circumstance in which evaluation of residual disease becomes important is where residual disease is present and clinical relapse is suspected based on changing clinical symptoms or signs, or because of rising tumour markers. Examples of such a situation would include 'B symptoms' in patients with residual lymphoma masses or rising alphafetoprotein levels in patients with residual NSGCT masses. Early detection of the site of active disease may enable some of these patients to be salvaged with additional treatments.

There are several possible strategies for distinguishing 'active' from 'sterile' disease. This includes an analysis of morphological appearances. Features suggesting active disease include an invasive mass with ancillary features such as bony destruction. The presence

of additional lesions (local or distant) may also be valuable clues. A change in imaging appearances over a period can be a strong indicator of tumour recurrence. The signal intensity on MR imaging has been extensively investigated as a method for distinguishing 'active' from 'sterile' disease. The literature has focused on the evaluation of residual lymphoma masses and the evaluation of pelvic masses after rectal surgery. In residual lymphoma mass evaluation, a number of studies now suggest that the parameter of low-signal residual masses on T_2-weighted imaging is a reliable indicator of inactive disease.[307]–[311] For example, in the study of Spiers et al., 2 of 19 patients with low-signal masses relapsed on 1-year follow-up compared to 4 of 5 patients with high heterogeneous signal masses.[310] The presence of high signal is less reliable in determining the activity of the disease, particularly in the first 6 months after treatment. This is because a high signal on T_2-weighted MRI can also be caused by granulation tissue, necrosis, and cyst formation. In the evaluation of pelvic masses after surgery, the MR signal intensity of any residual masses is a less reliable indicator of active disease.[78],[312],[313] Recurrent rectal cancer may well be of dark signal on T_2-weighted imaging and ancillary findings (morphology and contrast enhancement) can provide additional information (Fig. 30).

Functional imaging techniques particularly DCE-MRI and FDG-PET appear to be useful in this clinical setting. Dynamic contrast-enhanced MRI has been found to be of value in determining the aetiology of residual disease in the pelvis and breast. The presence of early and rapid enhancement after the bolus administration of intravenous contrast medium is a good discriminator, complementing MR signal intensity and morphological features.[78],[312],[313] A major limitation is previous radiation treatment that can cause persistent enhancement of a scar long after treatments. 18-FDG-PET has been found to be superior to CT in detecting locally recurrent disease in the pelvis after colorectal cancer resection (95 per cent for PET and 65 per cent for pelvic CT).[23],[34] Ultimately, if non-invasive techniques are unable to distinguish 'active' from 'sterile' disease, then a biopsy will be required. Even biopsy in this clinical setting has inherent problems resulting from sampling and interpretation errors. Thus, while a positive biopsy may be useful, a negative biopsy may be less reliable.

Summary

- Residual masses of considerable size can be seen after treatment of lymphomas, germ-cell neoplasms, and neuroblastomas.
- Additional treatments of apparently sterilized disease can have important long-term complications.
- MRI has greater specificity than CT in distinguishing recurrent disease from fibrosis, but overlap of signal intensity on T_2-weighted images occurs.
- Dynamic contrast medium-enhanced MR imaging is a useful technique for evaluating residual disease, but delayed images may not be informative.
- Monoclonal antibody techniques and 18-FDG-PET may also be valuable for distinguishing active tumour from fibrosis.

Detection of relapse

The diagnosis of tumour relapse should be made as quickly and accurately as possible if further therapy is to be effective. Even if

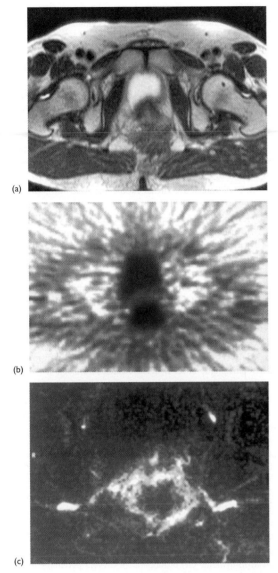

Fig. 30 Recurrent rectal cancer. (a) Proven rectal cancer recurrence in the pelvic floor (levator muscles) following anteroposterior resection. This T_2-weighted image demonstrates the presence of a mass behind the prostate with a dark signal intensity similar to that of muscle. (b) Axial FDG-PET image at the same level shows intense hypermetabolism at the site of the recurrent tumour. (c) Subtraction image from a dynamic contrast-enhanced MRI examination showing irregular ring-like enhancement in the tumour, a feature that is characteristic of tumour recurrence. Blood vessel enhancement is also seen. Note that the contrast medium has not yet been excreted into the urinary bladder.

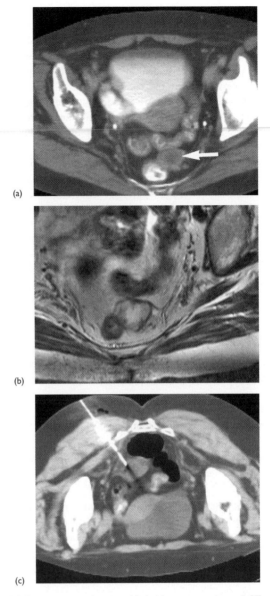

Fig. 31 Recurrent rectal cancer. (a) Axial contrast-enhanced CT scan with rectal contrast administration shows a left pararectal mass with a low-density centre (arrow). The uterus is visible behind the bladder. (b) Axial T_2-weighted MRI shows that this mass has a high-intensity centre. The differential diagnosis lies between recurrent disease and an infective or postsurgical complication. (c) Prone CT image showing a guided biopsy of the mass which confirmed tumour recurrence.

curative treatment is not an option, imaging can play an important role in defining the presence and extent of recurrence so that palliative treatment may be given appropriately. Disease relapse may be suspected because of:

(1) clinical symptoms and signs suggestive of recurrence;

(2) a rise in tumour marker estimations; and

(3) imaging features suggestive or diagnostic of relapse.

The imaging diagnosis of recurrent disease depends upon clinical presentation. In patients with clinical symptoms and signs suggestive of relapse, imaging is tailored to evaluate the local area where relapse is suspected as well as other anatomical sites which are known to be commonly involved. For example, in patients with prostate cancer who have been treated with pelvic radiotherapy, lymph node metastases usually recur in the retroperitoneum because the pelvic nodes have been 'sterilized'.[314] This emphasizes the importance of a full knowledge of the patient's previous treatment when searching for sites of relapse. Imaging itself may be the first technique to suggest relapse. This is commonly seen during routine imaging follow-up after treatment for lymphoma, testicular cancer, or colorectal cancer. An increase in nodal size or a soft tissue residuum may herald recurrent disease. In patients with a small increase in tumour size (less than 25 per cent), it is prudent to confirm this by a repeat study after a short interval of say 6 to 8 weeks.

One of the major problems in the detection of relapse is the distinction of post-treatment residual abnormalities from tumour. Baseline studies following treatment are helpful in distinguishing these entities since enlargement and change in shape of a residual mass suggests recurrence. A classic example is the distinction of postoperative fibrosis from tumour in patients with residual masses in the sacral hollow following surgery for colorectal cancer.[315]–[318] Follow-up CT examinations may show a change in the residual mass indicative of recurrence. In the absence of previous studies for comparison or other evidence of relapse such as raised serum markers, the diagnosis of relapse may be impossible.[318] Recurrent tumour may coexist with infection, abscess, or haematoma. In this situation further imaging with dynamic contrast MRI, immunoscintigraphy, and FDG-PET may help, but biopsy is often required (Fig. 31).[319]–[322]

Summary

- Disease relapse may be suspected on the basis of clinical symptoms and signs, rising tumour marker estimations, or imaging follow-up.
- A major problem of imaging is the distinction of post-treatment abnormalities from recurrent tumour. Infection and postsurgical change are further confounding factors.
- The distinction between recurrent tumour and fibrosis can be made on imaging if there is invasion of adjacent structures including bony involvement.
- Function imaging techniques such as dynamic contrast-enhanced MRI, immunoscintigraphy, and 18-FDG-PET may help to distinguish post-treatment residual abnormalities from tumour relapse.

Conclusions

In this review, an attempt has been made to give the reader a broad overview of the impact that modern imaging is making on the management of patients with cancer. There have been many exciting developments in imaging during the last two decades. Functional imaging techniques are likely to have a great clinical impact in the future, particularly in the efficacy assessment of selective anticancer drugs. Ongoing technological advances in imaging techniques and cancer treatment options will require constant reappraisal of imaging strategies in individual tumour types. Close liaison between cancer clinicians and radiologists will be essential if the optimum utilization of these imaging techniques is to be achieved.

References

1. Collins VP, Loeffler RK, Tivey H. Observations on the growth rates of human tumours. *American Journal of Roentgenology*, 1956; **76**: 988–1001.

2. Silverman PM, Cooper CJ, Weltman DI, Zeman RK. Helical CT: practical considerations and potential pitfalls. *Radiographics*, 1995; **15**: 25–36.

3. Buckley JA, *et al.* Pulmonary nodules: effect of increased data sampling on detection with spiral CT and confidence in diagnosis. *Radiology*, 1995; **196**: 395–400.

4. Urban BA, Fishman EK, Kuhlman JE, Kawashima A, Hennessey JG, Siegelman SS. Detection of focal hepatic lesions with spiral CT: comparison of 4- and 8-mm interscan spacing. *American Journal of Roentgenology*, 1993; **160**: 783–5.

5. Van Erkel AR, Van Rossum AB, Bloem JL, Kievit J, Pattynama EMJ. Spiral CT angiography for suspected pulmonary emboli: a cost effective analysis. *Radiology*, 1996; **201**: 29–36.

6. Jolesz FA, *et al.* Interactive virtual endoscopy. *American Journal of Roentgenology*, 1997; **169**: 1229–35.

7. Ogata I, Komohara Y, Yamashita Y, Mitsuzaki K, Takahashi M, Ogawa M. CT evaluation of gastric lesions with three-dimensional display and interactive virtual endoscopy: comparison with conventional barium study and endoscopy. *American Journal of Roentgenology*, 1999; **172**: 1263–70.

8. Vining DJ, Liu K, Choplin RH, Haponik EF. Virtual bronchoscopy. Relationships of virtual reality endobronchial simulations to actual bronchoscopic findings. *Chest*, 1996; **109**: 549–53.

9. Redpath TW. MRI developments in perspective. *British Journal of Radiology*, 1997; **70**: S70–80.

10. Fisher M, Albers GW. Applications of diffusion-perfusion magnetic resonance imaging in acute ischemic stroke. *Neurology*, 1999; **52**: 1750–6.

11. Harisinghani MG, *et al.* MR lymphangiography using ultrasmall superparamagnetic iron oxide in patients with primary abdominal and pelvic malignancies: radiographic–pathologic correlation. *American Journal of Roentgenology*, 1999; **172**: 1347–51.

12. Anzai Y, Brunberg JA, Lufkin RB. Imaging of nodal metastases in the head and neck. *Journal of Magnetic Resonance Imaging*, 1997; **7**: 774–83.

13. Bellin MF, *et al.* Lymph node metastases: safety and effectiveness of MR imaging with ultrasmall superparamagnetic iron oxide particles—initial clinical experience. *Radiology*, 1998; **207**: 799–808.

14. Hagspiel KD, *et al.* Detection of liver metastases: comparison of superparamagnetic iron oxide enhanced and unenhanced MR imaging at 1.5T with dynamic CT, intraoperative US and percutaneous US. *Radiology*, 1995; **196**: 471–8.

15. Seneterre E, *et al.* Detection of hepatic metastasis: ferumoxides-enhanced MR imaging versus unenhanced MR imaging and CT during arterial portography. *Radiology*, 1996; **200**: 785–92.

16. Reimer P, *et al.* Hepatic lesion detection and characterization: value of nonenhanced MR imaging, superparamagnetic iron oxide-enhanced MR imaging, and spiral CT-ROC analysis. *Radiology*, 2000; **217**: 152–8.

17. Viala J, Vanel D, Meingan P, Lartigau E, Carde P, Renschler M. Phases IB and II multidose trial of gadolinium texaphyrin, a radiation sensitizer detectable at MR imaging: preliminary results in brain metastases. *Radiology*, 1999; **212**: 755–9.

18. Whittingham TA. New and future developments in ultrasonic imaging. *British Journal of Radiology*, 1997; **70**: S119–32.

19. Rizzatto G. Ultrasound transducers. *European Journal of Radiology*, 1998; **27**: S188–95.

20. Cosgrove D. Echo enhancers and ultrasound imaging. *European Journal of Radiology*, 1997; **26**: 64–76.

21. Forsberg F, Merton DA, Liu JB, Needleman L, Goldberg BB. Clinical applications of ultrasound contrast agents. *Ultrasonics*, 1998; **36**: 695–701.

22. Hunerbein M, Totkas S, Ghadimi BM, Schlag PM. Preoperative evaluation of colorectal neoplasms by colonoscopic miniprobe ultrasonography. *Annals of Surgery*, 2000; **232**: 46–50.

23. Strauss LG, Conti PS. The applications of PET in clinical oncology. *Journal of Nuclear Medicine*, 1991; **32**: 623–48.

24. Patz EF Jr, *et al*. Focal pulmonary abnormalities: evaluation with F-18 fluorodeoxyglucose PET scanning. *Radiology*, 1993; **188**: 487–90.

25. Lowe VJ, Hoffman JM, DeLong DM, Patz EF, Coleman RE. Semiquantitative and visual analysis of FDG-PET images in pulmonary abnormalities. *Journal of Nuclear Medicine*, 1994; **35**: 1771–6.

26. Hoh CK, *et al*. PET in oncology: will it replace the other modalities? *Seminars Nuclear Medicine*, 1997; **27**: 94–106.

27. Schiepers C, Hoh CK. Positron emission tomography as a diagnostic tool in oncology. *European Radiology*, 1998; **8**: 1481–94.

28. Dewan NA, Reeb SD, Gupta NC, Gobar LS, Scott WJ. PET-FDG imaging and transthoracic needle lung aspiration biopsy in evaluation of pulmonary lesions. A comparative risk–benefit analysis. *Chest*, 1995; **108**: 441–6.

29. Gupta NC, Maloof J, Gunel E. Probability of malignancy in solitary pulmonary nodules using fluorine-18-FDG and PET. *Journal of Nuclear Medicine*, 1996; **37**: 943–8.

30. Knight SB, Delbeke D, Stewart JR, Sandler MP. Evaluation of pulmonary lesions with FDG-PET. Comparison of findings in patients with and without a history of prior malignancy. *Chest*, 1996; **109**: 982–8.

31. Erasmus JJ, *et al*. Evaluation of adrenal masses in patients with bronchogenic carcinoma using 18F-fluorodeoxyglucose positron emission tomography. *American Journal of Roentgenology*, 1997; **168**: 1357–60.

32. Lamki LM. Positron emission tomography, bronchogenic carcinoma, and the adrenals. *American Journal of Roentgenology*, 1997; **168**: 1361–2.

33. Boland GW, *et al*. Indeterminate adrenal mass in patients with cancer: evaluation at PET with 2-[F-18]-fluoro-2-deoxy-D-glucose. *Radiology*, 1995; **194**: 131–4.

34. Schiepers C, *et al*. Contribution of PET in the diagnosis of recurrent colorectal cancer: comparison with conventional imaging. *European Journal of Surgical Oncology*, 1995; **21**: 517–22.

35. Lai DT, *et al*. The role of whole-body positron emission tomography with [18F]fluorodeoxyglucose in identifying operable colorectal cancer metastases to the liver. *Archives of Surgery*, 1996; **131**: 703–7.

36. Greven KM, Keyes JW Jr, Williams DW 3rd, McGuirt WF, Joyce WT. Occult primary tumors of the head and neck: lack of benefit from positron emission tomography imaging with 2-[F-18]fluoro-2-deoxy-D-glucose. *Cancer*, 1999; **86**: 114–18.

37. McGuirt WF, *et al*. PET scanning in head and neck oncology: a review. *Head Neck*, 1998; **20**: 208–15.

38. Keyes JW Jr, Watson NE Jr, Williams DW 3rd, Greven KM, McGuirt WF. FDG PET in head and neck cancer. *American Journal of Roentgenology*, 1997; **169**: 1663–9.

39. Valk PE, *et al*. Staging non-small cell lung cancer by whole-body positron emission tomographic imaging. *Annals of Thoracic Surgery*, 1995; **60**: 1573–81.

40. Scott WJ, Schwabe JL, Gupta NC, Dewan NA, Reeb SD, Sugimoto JT. Positron emission tomography of lung tumors and mediastinal lymph nodes using [18F]fluorodeoxyglucose. The Members of the PET-Lung Tumor Study Group. *Annals of Thoracic Surgery*, 1994; **58**: 698–703.

41. Patz EF Jr, Lowe VJ, Goodman PC, Herndon J. Thoracic nodal staging with PET imaging with 18FDG in patients with bronchogenic carcinoma. *Chest*, 1995; **108**: 1617–21.

42. Sazon DA, *et al*. Fluorodeoxyglucose-positron emission tomography in the detection and staging of lung cancer. *American Journal of Respiratory and Critical Care Medicine*, 1996; **153**: 417–21.

43. Moog F, *et al*. Extranodal malignant lymphoma: detection with FDG PET versus CT. *Radiology*, 1998; **206**: 475–81.

44. Moog F, *et al*. Lymphoma: role of whole-body 2-deoxy-2-[F-18]fluoro-D-glucose (FDG) PET in nodal staging. *Radiology*, 1997; **203**: 795–800.

45. Cremerius U, Fabry U, Neuerburg J, Zimny M, Osieka R, Buell U. Positron emission tomography with 18F-FDG to detect residual disease after therapy for malignant lymphoma. *Nuclear Medicine Communication*, 1998; **19**: 1055–63.

46. de Wit M, Bumann D, Beyer W, Herbst K, Clausen M, Hossfeld DK. Whole-body positron emission tomography (PET) for diagnosis of residual mass in patients with lymphoma. *Annals of Oncology*, 1997; **8**: S57–60.

47. Shreve PD, Grossman HB, Gross MD, Wahl RL. Metastatic prostate cancer: initial findings of PET with 2-deoxy-2-[F-18]fluoro-D-glucose. *Radiology*, 1996; **199**: 751–6.

48. Yeh SD, *et al*. Detection of bony metastases of androgen-independent prostate cancer by PET-FDG. *Nuclear Medicine Biology*, 1996; **23**: 693–7.

49. Yao WJ, *et al*. Quantitative PET imaging of bone marrow glucose metabolic response to hematopoietic cytokines. *Journal of Nuclear Medicine*, 1995; **36**: 794–9.

50. Findlay M, *et al*. Noninvasive monitoring of tumor metabolism using fluorodeoxyglucose and positron emission tomography in colorectal cancer liver metastases: correlation with tumor response to fluorouracil. *Journal of Clinical Oncology*, 1996; **14**: 700–8.

51. Torizuka T, *et al*. Value of fluorine-18-FDG-PET to monitor hepatocellular carcinoma after interventional therapy. *Journal of Nuclear Medicine*, 1994; **35**: 1965–9.

52. Haberkorn U, *et al*. Fluorodeoxyglucose imaging of advanced head and neck cancer after chemotherapy. *Journal of Nuclear Medicine*, 1993; **34**: 12–17.

53. Wahl RL, Zasadny K, Helvie M, Hutchins GD, Weber B, Cody R. Metabolic monitoring of breast cancer chemohormonotherapy using positron emission tomography: initial evaluation. *Journal of Clinical Oncology*, 1993; **11**: 2101–11.

54. Hoekstra OS, van Lingen A, Ossenkoppele GJ, Golding R, Teule GJ. Early response monitoring in malignant lymphoma using fluorine-18 fluorodeoxyglucose single-photon emission tomography. *European Journal of Nuclear Medicine*, 1993; **20**: 1214–17.

55. Reisser C, Haberkorn U, Strauss LG. The relevance of positron emission tomography for the diagnosis and treatment of head and neck tumors. *Journal of Otolaryngology*, 1993; **22**: 231–8.

56. Reinhardt MJ, Kubota K, Yamada S, Iwata R, Yaegashi H. Assessment of cancer recurrence in residual tumors after fractionated radiotherapy: a comparison of fluorodeoxyglucose, l-methionine and thymidine. *Journal of Nuclear Medicine*, 1997; **38**: 280–7.

57. Rosen BR, *et al*. Susceptibility contrast imaging of cerebral blood volume: human experience. *Magnetic Resonance in Medicine*, 1991; **22**: 293–9.

58. Edelman RR, *et al*. Cerebral blood flow: assessment with dynamic contrast-enhanced T_2*-weighted MR imaging at 1.5 T. *Radiology*, 1990; **176**: 211–20.

59. Rempp KA, Brix G, Wenz F, Becker CR, Guckel F, Lorenz WJ. Quantification of regional cerebral blood flow and volume with dynamic susceptibility contrast-enhanced MR imaging. *Radiology*, 1994; **193**: 637–41.

60. Ichikawa T, Haradome H, Hachiya J, Nitatori T, Araki T. Characterisation of hepatic lesions by perfusion-weighted MR imaging with an echoplanar sequence. *American Journal of Roentgenology*, 1998; **170**: 1029–34.

61. Kuhl CK, *et al*. Breast neoplasms: T_2* susceptibility-contrast, first-pass perfusion MR imaging. *Radiology*, 1997; **202**: 87–95.

62. Kvistad KA, Lundgren S, Fjosne HE, Smenes E, Smethurst HB, Haraldseth O. Differentiating benign and malignant breast lesions with T_2*-weighted first pass perfusion imaging. *Acta Radiologicia*, 1999; **40**: 45–51.

63. Aronen HJ, *et al*. Cerebral blood volume maps of gliomas: comparison

with tumour grade and histologic findings. *Radiology*, 1994; **191**: 41–51.

64. Aronen HJ, *et al.* Echo-planar MR cerebral blood volume mapping of gliomas. Clinical utility. *Acta Radiologica*, 1995; **36**: 520–8.

65. Wenz F, *et al.* Effect of radiation on blood volume in low-grade astrocytomas and normal brain tissue: quantification with dynamic susceptibility contrast MR imaging. *American Journal of Roentgenology*, 1996; **166**: 187–93.

66. Appearance of various tissues and lesions. In *Contrast-enhanced MRI of the breast* (2nd edn) (ed. SH Heywang-Kobrunner, R Beck). Berlin: Springer-Verlag, 1996: 57–156.

67. Boetes C, *et al.* MR characterisation of suspicious breast lesions with a gadolinium-enhanced TurboFLASH subtraction technique. *Radiology*, 1994; **193**: 777–81.

68. Verstraete KL, De Deene Y, Roels H, Dierick A, Uyttendaele D, Kunnen M. Benign and malignant musculoskeletal lesions: dynamic contrast-enhanced MR imaging-parametric 'first-pass' images depict tissue vascularization and perfusion. *Radiology*, 1994; **192**: 835–43.

69. Brinck U, Fischer U, Korabiowska M, Jutrowski M, Schauer A, Grabbe E. The variability of fibroadenoma in contrast-enhanced dynamic MR mammography. *American Journal of Roentgenology, 1997*; **168**: 1331–4.

70. Barentsz JO, *et al.* Staging urinary bladder cancer after transurethral biopsy: value of fast dynamic contrast-enhanced MR imaging *Radiology*, 1996; **201**: 185–93.

71. Jager GJ, *et al.* Dynamic turboFLASH subtraction technique for contrast-enhanced MR imaging of the prostate: correlation with histopathologic results. *Radiology*, 1997; **203**: 645–52.

72. van der Woude HJ, *et al.* Osteosarcoma and Ewing's sarcoma after neoadjuvant chemotherapy: value of dynamic MR imaging in detecting viable tumor before surgery. *American Journal of Roentgenology, 1995*; **165**: 593–8.

73. Knopp MV, Brix G, Junkermann HJ, Sinn HP. MR mammography with pharmacokinetic mapping for monitoring of breast cancer treatment during neoadjuvant therapy. *Magnetic Resonance Imaging Clinics of North America*, 1994; **2**: 633–58.

74. Padhani AR, *et al.* Effects of androgen deprivation treatment on prostatic morphology and vascular permeability evaluated with MR imaging. *Radiology;* 2001; **218**: 365–74.

75. Mayr NA, *et al.* Tumor perfusion studies using fast magnetic resonance imaging technique in advanced cervical cancer: a new noninvasive predictive assay. *International Journal of Radiation Oncology, Biology and Physics, 1996*; **36**: 623–33.

76. Dao TH, Rahmouni A, Campana F, Laurent M, Asselain B, Fourquet A. Tumour recurrence versus fibrosis in the irradiated breast: differentiation with dynamic gadolinium-enhanced MR imaging. *Radiology*, 1993; **187**: 751–5.

77. Gilles R, *et al.* Assessment of breast cancer recurrence with contrast-enhanced subtraction MR imaging: preliminary results in 26 patients. *Radiology*, 1993; **188**: 473–8.

78. Kinkel K, *et al.* Dynamic contrast-enhanced subtraction versus T_2-weighted spin-echo MR imaging in the follow-up of colorectal neoplasm: a prospective study of 41 patients. *Radiology*, 1996; **200**: 453–8.

79. Leach MO. Introduction to *in vivo* MRS of cancer: new perspectives and open problems. *Anticancer Research*, 1996; **16**: 1503–14.

80. Robinson SP, Barton SJ, McSheehy PM, Griffiths JR. Nuclear magnetic resonance spectroscopy of cancer. *British Journal of Radiology, 1997*; **70**: S60–9.

81. Griffiths JR, Stevens AN, Iles RA, Gordon RE, Shaw D. 31P-NMR investigation of solid tumours in the living rat. *Bioscience Reports*, 1981; **1**: 319–25.

82. Griffiths JR. Are cancer cells acidic? *British Journal of Cancer*, 1991; **64**: 425–7.

83. Vaupel P, Kallinowski F, Okunieff P. Blood flow, oxygen and nutrient supply, and metabolic microenvironment of human tumors: a review. *Cancer Research*, 1989; **49**: 6449–65.

84. Tozer GM, Bhujwalla ZM, Griffiths JR, Maxwell RJ. Phosphorus-31 magnetic resonance spectroscopy and blood perfusion of the RIF-1 tumor following X-irradiation. *International Journal of Radiation Oncology, Biology and Physics, 1989*; **16**: 155–64

85. Negendank W. Studies of human tumors by MRS: a review. *NMR in Biomedicine*, 1992; **5**: 303–24.

86. Leach MO, *et al.* Measurements of human breast cancer using magnetic resonance spectroscopy: a review of clinical measurements and a report of localized 31P measurements of response to treatment. *NMR in Biomedicine, 1998*; **11**: 314–40.

87. Bruhn H, *et al.* On the interpretation of proton NMR spectra from brain tumours *in vivo* and *in vitro*. *NMR in Biomedicine*, 1992; **5**: 253–8.

88. Bruhn H, *et al.* Noninvasive differentiation of tumors with use of localized H-1 MR spectroscopy *in vivo*: initial experience in patients with cerebral tumors. *Radiology*, 1989; **172**: 541–8.

89. Manton DJ, Lowry M, Blackband SJ, Horsman A. Determination of proton metabolite concentrations and relaxation parameters in normal human brain and intracranial tumours. *NMR in Biomedicine, 1995*; **8**: 104–12.

90. Kugel H, Heindel W, Ernestus RI, Bunke J, du Mesnil R, Friedmann G. Human brain tumors: spectral patterns detected with localized H-1 MR spectroscopy. *Radiology*, 1992; **183**: 701–9.

91. Frahm J, Bruhn H, Hanicke W, Merboldt KD, Mursch K, Markakis E. Localized proton NMR spectroscopy of brain tumors using short-echo time STEAM sequences. *Journal of Computed Assisted Tomography, 1991*; **15**: 915–22.

92. Mountford CE, Tattersall MH. Proton magnetic resonance spectroscopy and tumour detection. *Cancer Surveys*, 1987; **6**: 285–314.

93. Kuesel AC, Sutherland GR, Halliday W, Smith IC. 1H MRS of high grade astrocytomas: mobile lipid accumulation in necrotic tissue. *NMR in Biomedicine, 1994*; **7**: 149–55.

94. Preul MC, *et al.* Accurate, noninvasive diagnosis of human brain tumors by using proton magnetic resonance spectroscopy. *Nature Medicine*, 1996; **2**: 323–5.

95. Koutcher JA, *et al. In vivo* monitoring of changes in 5-fluorouracil metabolism induced by methotrexate measured by 19F NMR spectroscopy. *Magnetic Resonance in Medicine*, 1991; **19**: 113–23.

96. Evelhoch JL. *In vivo* 19F nuclear magnetic resonance spectroscopy: a potential monitor of 5-fluorouracil pharmacokinetics and metabolism. *Investigational New Drugs*, 1989; **7**: 5–12.

97. Stevens AN, Morris PG, Iles RA, Sheldon PW, Griffiths JR. 5-fluorouracil metabolism monitored *in vivo* by 19F NMR. *British Journal of Cancer*, 1984; **50**: 113–17.

98. Findlay MP, *et al.* The non-invasive monitoring of low dose, infusional 5-fluorouracil and its modulation by interferon-alpha using *in vivo* 19F magnetic resonance spectroscopy in patients with colorectal cancer: a pilot study. *Annals in Oncology*, 1993; **4**: 597–602.

99. Presant CA, *et al.* Association of intratumoral pharmacokinetics of fluorouracil with clinical response. *Lancet*, 1994; **343**: 1184–7.

100. Schlemmer HP, *et al.* Drug monitoring of 5-fluorouracil: *in vivo* 19F NMR study during 5-FU chemotherapy in patients with metastases of colorectal adenocarcinoma. *Magnetic Resonance Imaging*, 1994; **12**: 497–511.

101. Newell DR, Maxwell RJ, Golding BT. *In vivo* and *ex vivo* magnetic resonance spectroscopy as applied to pharmacokinetic studies with anticancer agents: a review. *NMR in Biomedicine, 1992*; **5**: 273–8.

102. Workman P, Maxwell RJ, Griffiths JR. Non-invasive MRS in new anticancer drug development. *NMR in Biomedicine, 1992*; **5**: 270–2.

103. Holahan J, Dor A, Zuckerman S. Understanding the recent growth in

Medicare physician expenditures. *Journal of the American Medical Association*, 1990; **263**: 1658–61.

104. Fry IK. Who needs high technology? *British Journal of Radiology*, 1984; **57**: 765–72.

105. Fryback DG, Thornbury JR The efficacy of diagnostic imaging. *Medical Decision Making*, 1991; **11**: 88–94.

106. Thornbury JR, Fryback DG. Technology assessment–an American view. *European Journal of Radiology*, 1992; **14**: 147–56.

107. Thornbury JR Eugene W. Caldwell lecture. Clinical efficacy of diagnostic imaging: love it or leave it. *American Journal of Roentgenology*, 1994; **162**: 1–8.

108. Rifkin MD, *et al.* Comparison of magnetic resonance imaging and ultrasonography in staging early prostate cancer: results of a multi-institutional co-operative trial. *New England Journal of Medicine*, 1990; **323**: 621–6.

109. Tempany C, *et al.* Staging of prostate cancer with MRI: results of Radiology Oncology Diagnostic Group project—comparison of different techniques, including endorectal coil. *Radiology*, 1994; **192**: 47–54.

110. Schnall MD, Imai Y, Tomaszewski J, Pollack HM, Lenkinski RE, Kressel HY. Prostate cancer: local staging with endorectal surface coil MR imaging. *Radiology*, 1991; **178**: 797–802.

111. Huch Boni RA, *et al.* Optimization of prostate carcinoma staging comparison of imaging and clinical methods. *Clinical Radiology*, 1995; **50**: 593–600.

112. Hricak H, *et al.* Carcinoma of the prostate gland: MR imaging with pelvic phased-array coils versus integrated endorectal–pelvic phased-array coils. *Radiology*, 1994; **193**: 703–9.

113. Bezzi M, *et al.* Prostate carcinoma: staging with MRI at 1.5T. *Radiology*, 1988; **169**: 339–46.

114. Biondetti PR, *et al.* Clinical stage B prostatic carcinoma: staging with MR imaging. *Radiology*, 1987; **162**: 325–9.

115. Mackenzie R, Dixon AK. Measuring the effects of imaging: an evaluation framework. *Clinical Radiology*, 1995; **50**: 513–18.

116. Burton PR, Gurrin LC, Campbell MJ. Clinical significance not statistical significance: a simple Bayesian alternative to p values. *Journal of Epidemiology and Community Health*, 1998; **52**: 318–23.

117. Rosenquist CJ. Pitfalls in the use of diagnostic tests. *Clinical Radiology*, 1998; **40**: 448–50.

118. Vinnicombe SJ, Norman AR, Nicolson V, Husband JE. Normal pelvic lymph nodes: evaluation with CT after bipedal lymphangiography. *Radiology*, 1995; **194**: 349–55.

119. Brismar J. Understanding receiver-operating characteristic curves: a graphical approach. *American Journal of Roentgenology*, 1991; **157**: 1119–21.

120. Metz CE. ROC methodology in radiologic imaging. *Investigative Radiology*, 1986; **21**: 720–33.

121. Hanley JA, Neil BJ. A method of comparing the areas under receiver operator characteristic curves from the some cases. *Radiology*, 1983; **148**: 839–43.

122. Council, Royal College of Radiologists (1994). *The use of computed tomography in the initial investigation of common malignancies.* Royal College of Radiologists, London.

123. RCR Working Party. *Making the best use of a department of clinical radiology: guidelines for doctors* (4th edn). London: The Royal College of Radiologists, 1998.

124. American College of Radiology. *Appropriateness criteria for imaging and treatment decisions.* Reston, VA: American College of Radiology, 1995.

125. Board of the faculty of Clinical Radiology. The Royal College of Radiologists. *A guide to the practical use of MRI in oncology.* London: Royal College of Radiologists, 1999.

126. Feinstein AR, Hosin DM, Wells CK. The Will Roger's phenomenon. Stage, migration and new diagnostic techniques as a source of misleading statistics for survival in cancer. *New England Journal of Medicine*, 1985; **312**: 604–8.

127. Fletcher SW, Black W, Harris R, Rimer BK, Shapiro S. Report of the International Workshop on Screening for Breast Cancer. *Journal of National Cancer Institute*, 1993; **85**: 1644–56.

128. Tabar L, Duffy SW, Burhenne LW. New Swedish breast cancer detection results for women aged 40–49. *Cancer*, 1993; **72**: 1437–48.

129. Tabar L, Fagerberg G, Duffy SW, Day NE, Gad A, Grontoft O. Update of the Swedish two-county program of mammographic screening for breast cancer. *Radiological Clinics of North America*, 1992; **30**: 187–210.

130. Andersson I, *et al.* Mammographic screening and mortality from breast cancer: the Malmo mammographic screening trial. *British Medical Journal*, 1988; **297**: 943–8.

131. Alexander FE, *et al.* The Edinburgh randomised trial of breast cancer screening: results after 10 years of follow-up. *British Journal of Cancer*, 1994; **70**: 542–8.

132. Miller AB, Baines CJ, To T, Wall C. Canadian National Breast Screening Study: 2. Breast cancer detection and death rates among women aged 50 to 59 years. *Canadian Medical Association Journal*, 1992; **147**: 1477–88.

133. Kuhl CK, *et al.* Breast MR imaging screening in 192 women proved or suspected to be carriers of a breast cancer susceptibility gene: preliminary results. *Radiology* 2000; **215**: 267–79.

134. Brown J, *et al.* Magnetic resonance imaging screening in women at genetic risk of breast cancer: imaging and analysis protocol for the UK multicentre study. *Magnetic Resonance Imaging*. 2000; **18**: 765–76.

135. Andolf E, Jorgensen C, Astedt B. Ultrasound examination for detection of ovarian carcinoma in risk groups. *Obstetrics and Gynecology*, 1990; **75**: 106–9.

136. Henderson JM, Campbell JD, Olson R, Nelson RC. Role of computed tomography in screening for hepatocellular carcinoma in patients with cirrhosis. *Gastrointestinal Radiology*, 1988; **13**: 129–34.

137. Melamed MR, Flehinger BJ, Zaman MB, Heelan RT, Perchick WA, Martini N. Screening for early lung cancer. Results of the Memorial Sloan-Kettering study in New York. *Chest*, 1984; **86**: 44–53.

138. Kubik A, Parkin DM, Khlat M, Erban J, Polak J, Adamec M. Lack of benefit from semi-annual screening for cancer of the lung: follow-up report of a randomized controlled trial on a population of high-risk males in Czechoslovakia. *International Journal of Cancer*, 1990; **45**: 26–33.

139. Fontana RS, Sanderson DR, Woolner LB, Taylor WF, Miller WE, Muhm JR. Lung cancer screening: the Mayo program. *Journal of Occupational Medicine*, 1986; **28**: 746–50.

140. Henschke CI, *et al.* Early Lung Cancer Action Project: overall design and findings from baseline screening. *Lancet*, 1999; **354**: 99–105.

141. Barloon TJ, Yuh WT, Yang CJ, Schultz DH. Spinal subarachnoid tumor seeding from intracranial metastasis: MR findings. *Journal of Computed Assisted Tomography*, 1987; **11**: 242–4.

142. Yousem DM, Patrone PM, Grossman RI. Leptomeningeal metastases: MR evaluation. *Journal of Computed Assisted Tomography*, 1990; **14**: 255–61.

143. Welch TJ, Sheedy PF 2nd, Johnson CD, Johnson CM, Stephens DH. CT-guided biopsy: prospective analysis of 1,000 procedures. *Radiology*, 1989; **171**: 493–6.

144. Rissanen TJ, *et al.* Wire localized biopsy of breast lesions: a review of 425 cases found in screening or clinical mammography. *Clinical Radiology*, 1993; **47**(1): 14–22.

145. Thaete FL, Peterson MS, Plunkett MB, Ferson PF, Keenan RJ, Landreneau RJ. Computed tomography-guided wire localization of pulmonary lesions before thoracoscopic resection: results in 101 cases. *Journal of Thoracic Imaging*, 1999; **14**: 90–8.

146. Kriplani AK, Kapur BM. Laparoscopy for pre-operative staging and assessment of operability in gastric carcinoma. *Gastrointestinal Endoscopy*, 1991; **37**: 441–3.

147. Shapiro MD, Som PM. MRI of the paranasal sinuses and nasal cavity. *Radiological Clinics of North America, 1989*; **27**: 447–75.

148. Som PM, Shapiro MD, Biller HF, Sasaki C, Lawson W. Sinonasal tumors and inflammatory tissues: differentiation with MR imaging. *Radiology, 1988*; **167**: 803–8.

149. Lanzieri CF, Shah M, Krauss D, Lavertu P. Use of gadolinium-enhanced MR imaging for differentiating mucoceles from neoplasms in the paranasal sinuses. *Radiology, 1991*; **178**: 425–8.

150. Mukherji SK, Pillsbury HR, Castillo M. Imaging squamous cell carcinoma of the upper aerodigestive tract: what clinicians need to know. *Radiology, 1997*; **205**: 629–46.

151. Munoz A, *et al.* Laryngeal carcinoma: sclerotic appearance of the cricoid and arytenoid cartilage–CT-pathologic correlation. *Radiology, 1993*; **189**: 433–7.

152. Becker M, Zbaren P, Laeng H, Stoupis C, Porcellini B, Vock P. Neoplastic invasion of the laryngeal cartilage: comparison of MR imaging and CT with histopathologic correlation. *Radiology, 1995*; **194**: 661–9.

153. Mukherji SK, *et al.* Comparison of dynamic and spiral CT for imaging the glottic larynx. *Journal of Computed Assisted Tomography, 1995*; **19**(6): 899–904.

154. Archer CR, Sagel SS, Yeager VL, Martin S, Friedman WH. Staging of carcinoma of the larynx: comparative accuracy of CT and laryngography. *American Journal of Roentgenology, 1981*; **136**: 571–5.

155. Sagel SS, AufderHeide JF, Aronberg DJ, Stanley RJ, Archer CR. High resolution computed tomography in the staging of carcinoma of the larynx. *Laryngoscope, 1981*; **91**: 292–300.

156. Parienty RA, Pradel J, Parienty I. Cystic renal cancers: CT characteristics. *Radiology, 1985*; **157**: 741–4.

157. Zagoria RJ, Bechtold RE, Dyer RB. Staging of renal adenocarcinoma: role of various imaging procedures. *American Journal of Roentgenology, 1995*; **164**: 363–70.

158. McClennan BL. Oncologic imaging. Staging and follow-up of renal and adrenal carcinoma. *Cancer, 1991*; **67**: 1199–208.

159. Kabala JE, Gillatt DA, Persad RA, Penry JB, Gingell JC, Chadwick D. Magnetic resonance imaging in the staging of renal cell carcinoma. *British Journal of Radiology, 1991*; **64**: 683–9.

160. Hricak H, Thoeni RF, Carroll PR, Demas BE, Marotti M, Tanagho EA. Detection and staging of renal neoplasms: a reassessment of MR imaging. *Radiology, 1988*; **166**: 643–9.

161. Zeman RK, Cronan JJ, Rosenfield AT, Lynch JH, Jaffe MH, Clark LR. Renal cell carcinoma: dynamic thin-section CT assessment of vascular invasion and tumor vascularity. *Radiology, 1988*; **167**: 393–6.

162. Webb JA, Murray A, Bary PR, Hendry WF. The accuracy and limitations of ultrasound in the assessment of venous extension in renal carcinoma. *British Journal of Urology, 1987*; **60**: 14–17.

163. Levine E, Maklad NF, Rosenthal SJ, Lee KR, Weigel J. Comparison of computed tomography and ultrasound in abdominal staging of renal cancer. *Urology, 1980*; **16**: 317–22.

164. Whitmore WF Jr. Assessment and management of deeply invasive and metastatic lesions. *Cancer Research, 1977*; **37**: 2756–8.

165. Husband JE. Staging bladder cancer. *Clinical Radiology, 1992*; **46**: 153–9.

166. Bryan PJ, Butler HE, LiPuma JP, Resnick MI, Kursh ED. CT and MR imaging in staging bladder neoplasms. *Journal of Computed Assisted Tomography, 1987*; **11**: 96–101.

167. Morgan CL, Calkins RF, Cavalcanti EJ. Computed tomography in the evaluation, staging, and therapy of carcinoma of the bladder and prostate. *Radiology, 1981*; **140**: 751–61.

168. Koss JC, Arger PH, Coleman BG, Mulhern CB Jr, Pollack HM, Wein AJ. CT staging of bladder carcinoma. *American Journal of Roentgenology, 1981*; **137**: 359–62.

169. Yang WT, *et al.* Transrectal ultrasound in the evaluation of cervical carcinoma and comparison with spiral computed tomography and magnetic resonance imaging. *British Journal of Radiology, 1996*; **69**: 610–16.

170. Kilcheski TS, Arger PH, Mulhern CB Jr, Coleman BG, Kressel HY, Mikuta JI. Role of computed tomography in the presurgical evaluation of carcinoma of the cervix. *Journal of Computed Assisted Tomography, 1981*; **5**: 378–83.

171. Vick CW, Walsh JW, Wheelock JB, Brewer WH. CT of the normal and abnormal parametria in cervical cancer. *American Journal of Roentgenology, 1984*; **143**: 597–603.

172. Hricak H, Lacey CG, Sandles LG, Chang YC, Winkler ML, Stern JL. Invasive cervical carcinoma: comparison of MR imaging and surgical findings. *Radiology, 1988*; **166**: 623–31.

173. Togashi K, *et al.* Carcinoma of the cervix: staging with MR imaging. *Radiology, 1989*; **171**: 245–51.

174. Hawnaur JM, Johnson RJ, Buckley CH, Tindall V, Isherwood I. Staging, volume estimation and assessment of nodal status in carcinoma of the cervix: comparison of magnetic resonance imaging with surgical findings. *Clinical Radiology, 1994*; **49**: 443–52.

175. Cobby M, Browning J, Jones A, Whipp E, Goddard P. Magnetic resonance imaging, computed tomography and endosonography in the local staging of carcinoma of the cervix. *British Journal of Radiology, 1990*; **63**: 673–9.

176. Montie JE. Staging of prostate cancer. *Cancer, 1994*; **74**: 1–3.

177. Voges GE, McNeal JE, Redwine EA, Freiha FS, Stamey TA. Morphologic analysis of surgical margins with positive findings in prostatectomy for adenocarcinoma of the prostate. *Cancer, 1992*; **69**: 520–6.

178. Epstein JI, Pizov G, Walsh PC. Correlation of pathologic findings with progression after radical retropubic prostatectomy. *Cancer, 1993*; **71**: 3582–93.

179. Smith JA Jr. Transrectal ultrasonography for the detection and staging of carcinoma of the prostate. *Journal of Clinical Ultrasound, 1996*; **24**: 455–61.

180. Presti JC Jr, Hricak H, Narayan PA, Shinohara K, White S, Carroll PR. Local staging of prostatic carcinoma: comparison of transrectal sonography and endorectal MR imaging. *American Journal of Roentgenology, 1996*; **166**: 103–8.

181. Scardino PT, Shinohara K, Wheeler TM, Carter SS. Staging of prostate cancer. Value of ultrasonography. *Urological Clinics of North America, 1989*; **16**: 713–34.

182. Platt JF, Bree RL, Schwab RE. The accuracy of CT in the staging of carcinoma of the prostate. *American Journal of Roentgenology, 1987*; **149**: 315–18.

183. Tempany C, *et al.* Staging of prostate cancer: results of Radiology Diagnostic Oncology Group project comparison of three MR imaging techniques. *Radiology, 1994*; **192**: 47–54.

184. Chelsky MJ, Schnall MD, Seidmon EJ, Pollack HM. Use of endorectal surface coil magnetic resonance imaging for local staging of prostate cancer. *Journal of Urology, 1993*; **150**: 391–5.

185. Outwater EK, Petersen RO, Siegelman ES, Gomella LG, Chernesky CE, Mitchell DG. Prostate carcinoma: assessment of diagnostic criteria for capsular penetration on endorectal coil MR images. *Radiology, 1994*; **193**: 333–9.

186. Quinn SF, *et al.* MR imaging of prostate cancer with an endorectal surface coil technique: correlation with whole-mount specimens. *Radiology, 1994*; **190**: 323–7.

187. Jager GJ, *et al.* Local staging of prostate cancer with endorectal MR imaging: correlation with histopathology. *American Journal of Roentgenology, 1996*; **166**: 845–52.

188. Edelstyn GA, Gillespie PJ, Grebbell FS. The radiological demonstration of osseous metastases. Experimental observations. *Clinical Radiology, 1967*; **18**: 158–62.

189. Citrin DL, Bessent RG, Greig WR. A comparison of the sensitivity and

accuracy of the 99TCm-phosphate bone scan and skeletal radiograph in the diagnosis of bone metastases. *Clinical Radiology*, 1977; **28**: 107–17.

190. Bonnerot V, Charpentier A, Frouin F, Kalifa C, Vanel D, Di Paola R. Factor analysis of dynamic magnetic resonance imaging in predicting the response of osteosarcoma to chemotherapy. *Investigative Radiology*, 1992; **27**: 847–55.

191. Lang P, *et al.* Musculoskeletal neoplasm: perineoplastic edema versus tumor on dynamic postcontrast MR images with spatial mapping of instantaneous enhancement rates. *Radiology*, 1995; **197**: 831–9.

192. Martini N, *et al.* Comparative merits of conventional, computed tomographic, and magnetic resonance imaging in assessing mediastinal involvement in surgically confirmed lung carcinoma. *Journal of Thoracic and Cardiovascular Surgery*, 1985; **90**: 639–48.

193. Glazer HS, *et al.* Indeterminate mediastinal invasion in bronchogenic carcinoma: CT evaluation. *Radiology*, 1989; **173**: 37–42.

194. McLoud TC. CT of bronchogenic carcinoma: indeterminate mediastinal invasion. *Radiology*, 1989; **173**: 15–16.

195. Webb WR, *et al.* CT and MR imaging in staging non-small cell bronchogenic carcinoma: report of the Radiologic Diagnostic Oncology Group. *Radiology*, 1991; **178**: 705–13.

196. Laurent F, *et al.* Bronchogenic carcinoma staging: CT versus MR imaging. Assessment with surgery. *European Journal of Cardiothoracic Surgery*, 1988; **2**: 31–6.

197. Kameda K, Adachi S, Kono M. Detection of T-factor in lung cancer using magnetic resonance imaging and computed tomography. *Journal of Thoracic Imaging*, 1988; **3**: 73–80.

198. Pennes DR, *et al.* Chest wall invasion by lung cancer: limitations of CT evaluation. *American Journal of Roentgenology*, 1985; **144**: 507–11.

199. Pearlberg JL, *et al.* Limitation of CT in evaluation of neoplasm involving chest wall. *Journal of Computed Assisted Tomography*, 1987; **11**: 290–3.

200. Musset D, *et al.* Primary lung cancer staging: prospective comparative of MR imaging with CT. *Radiology*, 1986; **160**: 607–11.

201. Rendina EA, *et al.* Computed tomography for the evaluation of intrathoracic invasion by lung cancer. *Journal of Cardiovascular Surgery*, 1987; **94**: 57–63.

202. Ratto GB, *et al.* Chest wall involvement by lung cancer: computed tomographic detection and results of operation. *Annals of Thoracic Surgery*, 1991; **51**: 182–8.

203. Padovani B, *et al.* Chest wall invasion by bronchogenic carcinoma; evaluation with MR imaging. *Radiology*, 1993; **187**: 33–8.

204. Haggar AM, *et al.* Chest wall invasion by carcinoma of the lung. Detection by MR imaging. *American Journal of Roentgenology*, 1987; **148**: 1075–8.

205. Watanabe A, *et al.* Chest CT combined with artificial pneumothorax: value in detecting origin and extent of tumor. *American Journal of Roentgenology*, 1991; **156**: 707–10.

206. Yokoi K, *et al.* Tumor invasion of chest wall and mediastinum in lung cancer: evaluation with pneumothorax CT. *Radiology*, 1991; **181**: 147–52.

207. Murata T, *et al.* Chest wall and mediastinal invasion by lung cancer: evaluation with multisection expiratory dynamic CT. *Radiology*, 1994; **191**: 251–5.

208. Shirakawa T, Fukuda K, Miyamoto Y, Tanabe H, Tada S. Parietal pleural invasion of lung masses: evaluation with CT performed during deep inspiration and expiration. *Radiology*, 1994; **192**: 809–11.

209. Kuriyama K, *et al.* Pleural invasion by peripheral bronchogenic carcinoma; assessment with three-dimensional helical CT. *Radiology*, 1994; **191**: 365–9.

210. Suzuki N, Saitoh T, Kitamura S. Tumor invasion of the chest wall in lung cancer: diagnosis with US. *Radiology*, 1993; **187**: 39–42.

211. Sugama Y, Tamaki S, Kitamura S, Kira S. Ultrasonographic evaluation of pleural and chest wall invasion of lung cancer. *Chest*, 1988; **93**: 275–9.

212. Sondenaa K, Skaane P, Nygaard K, Skjennald A. Value of computed tomography in preoperative evaluation of resectability and staging in oesophageal carcinoma. *European Journal of Surgery*, 1992; **158**: 537–40.

213. van Overhagen H, *et al.* CT assessment of resectability prior to transhiatal esophagectomy for esophageal/gastroesophageal junction carcinoma. *Journal of Computed Assisted Tomography*, 1993; **17**: 367–73.

214. Hordijk ML, Zander H, van Blankenstein M, Tilanus HW. Influence of tumor stenosis on the accuracy of endosonography in preoperative T staging of esophageal cancer. *Endoscopy*, 1993; **25**: 171–5.

215. Rosch T, *et al.* Local staging and assessment of resectability in carcinoma of the esophagus, stomach, and duodenum by endoscopic ultrasonography. *Gastrointestinal Endoscopy*, 1992; **38**: 460–7.

216. Dittler HJ, Siewert JR. Role of endoscopic ultrasonography in esophageal carcinoma. *Endoscopy*, 1993; **25**: 156–61.

217. Grimm H, Binmoeller KF, Hamper K, Koch J, Henne-Bruns D, Soehendra N. Endosonography for preoperative locoregional staging of esophageal and gastric cancer. *Endoscopy*, 1993; **25**: 224–30.

218. Van Dam J, Rice TW, Catalano MF, Kirby T, Sivak MV Jr. High-grade malignant stricture is predictive of esophageal tumor stage. Risks of endosonographic evaluation. *Cancer*, 1993; **71**: 2910–17.

219. Botet JF, *et al.* Preoperative staging of gastric cancer: comparison of endoscopic US and dynamic CT. *Radiology*, 1991; **181**: 426–32.

220. Ziegler K, *et al.* Comparison of computed tomography, endosonography, and intraoperative assessment in TN staging of gastric carcinoma. *Gut*, 1993; **34**: 604–10.

221. Rosch T. Endoscopic ultrasonography. *Endoscopy*, 1994; **26**: 148–68.

222. Tio TL, Coene PP, Schouwink MH, Tytgat GN. Esophagogastric carcinoma: preoperative TNM classification with endosonography. *Radiology*, 1989; **173**: 411–17.

223. Freeny PC, Marks WM, Ryan JA, Bolen JW. Colorectal carcinoma evaluation with CT: preoperative staging and detection of postoperative recurrence. *Radiology*, 1986; **158**: 347–53.

224. Balthazar EJ, Megibow AJ, Hulnick D, Naidich DP. Carcinoma of the colon: detection and preoperative staging by CT. *American Journal of Roentgenology*, 1988; **150**: 301–6.

225. Zerhouni EA, *et al.* CT and MR imaging in the staging of colorectal carcinoma: report of the Radiology Diagnostic Oncology Group II. *Radiology*, 1996; **200**: 443–51.

226. Chan TW, *et al.* Rectal carcinoma: staging at MR imaging with endorectal surface coil. Work in progress. *Radiology*, 1991; **181**: 461–7.

227. Schnall MD, Furth EE, Rosato EF, Kressel HY. Rectal tumor stage: correlation of endorectal MR imaging and pathologic findings. *Radiology*, 1994; **190**: 709–14.

228. Pegios W, *et al.* MRI diagnosis and staging of rectal carcinoma. *Abdominal Imaging*, 1996; **21**: 211–18.

229. Joosten FB, Jansen JB, Joosten HJ, Rosenbusch G. Staging of rectal carcinoma using MR double surface coil, MR endorectal coil, and intrarectal ultrasound: correlation with histopathologic findings. *Journal of Computed Assisted Tomography*, 1995; **19**: 752–8.

230. Brown G, *et al.* Rectal carcinoma: thin-section MR imaging for staging in 28 patients. *Radiology*, 1999; **211**: 215–22.

231. Rifkin MD, Ehrlich SM, Marks G. Staging of rectal carcinoma: prospective comparison of endorectal US and CT. *Radiology*, 1989; **170**: 319–22.

232. Holdsworth PJ, *et al.* Endoluminal ultrasound and computed tomography in the staging of rectal cancer. *British Journal of Surgery*, 1988; **75**: 1019–22.

233. Beynon J, Mortensen NJ, Foy DM, Channer JL, Virjee J, Goddard P. Pre-operative assessment of local invasion in rectal cancer: digital examination, endoluminalsonography or computed tomography? *British Journal of Surgery*, 1986; **73**: 1015–17.

234. **Thaler W,** *et al.* Preoperative staging of rectal cancer by endoluminal ultrasound vs. magnetic resonance imaging. Preliminary results of a prospective, comparative study. *Diseases of the Colon and Rectum,* 1994; **37**: 1189–93.

235. **Harnsberger JR,** *et al.* The role of intrarectal ultrasound (IRUS) in staging of rectal cancer and detection of extrarectal pathology. *American Surgery,* 1994; **60**: 571–6.

236. **Macdonald JS.** The lymphographic diagnosis of malignancy. *Proceedings of the Royal Society of Medicine,* 1972; **65**: 719–80.

237. **Tart RP, Mukherji SK, Avino AJ, Stringer SP, Mancuso AA.** Facial lymph nodes: normal and abnormal CT appearance. *Radiology,* 1993; **188**: 695–700.

238. **van den Brekel MW,** *et al.* Cervical lymph node metastasis: assessment of radiologic criteria. *Radiology,* 1990; **177**: 379–84.

239. **Glazer GM, Gross BH, Quint LE, Francis IR, Bookstein FL, Orringer MB.** Normal mediastinal lymph nodes: number and size according to American Thoracic Society mapping. *American Journal of Roentgenology,* 1985; **144**: 261–5.

240. **Dorfman RE, Alpern MB, Gross BH, Sandler MA.** Upper abdominal lymph nodes: criteria for normal size determined with CT. *Radiology,* 1991; **180**: 319–22.

241. **Callen PW, Korobkin M, Isherwood I.** Computed tomographic evaluation of the retrocrural prevertebral space. *American Journal of Roentgenology,* 1977; **129**: 907–10.

242. **Aronchick JM.** CT of mediastinal lymph nodes in patients with non-small cell lung carcinoma. *Radiological Clinics of North America,* 1990; **28**: 573–81.

243. **Libshitz HI.** CT of mediastinal lymph nodes in lung cancer: Is there a 'state of the art'? *American Journal of Roentgenology,* 1983; **141**: 1081–5.

244. **Anzai Y,** *et al.* Initial clinical experience with dextran-coated superparamagnetic iron oxide for detection of lymph node metastases in patients with head and neck cancer. *Radiology,* 1994; **192**: 709–15.

245. **Avril N,** *et al.* Assessment of axillary lymph node involvement in breast cancer patients with positron emission tomography using radiolabeled 2-(fluorine-18)-fluoro-2-deoxy-D-glucose. *Journal of the National Cancer Institute,* 1996; **88**: 1204–9.

246. **Rose PG, Adler LP, Rodriguez M, Faulhaber PF, Abdul-Karim FW, Miraldi F.** Positron emission tomography for evaluating para-aortic nodal metastasis in locally advanced cervical cancer before surgical staging: a surgicopathologic study. *Journal of Clinical Oncology,* 1999; **17**: 41–5.

247. **Kosuda S, Kison PV, Greenough R, Grossman HB, Wahl RL.** Preliminary assessment of fluorine-18 fluorodeoxyglucose positron emission tomography in patients with bladder cancer. *European Journal of Nuclear Medicine,* 1997; **24**: 615–20.

248. **Morton DL,** *et al.* Technical details of intraoperative lymphatic mapping for early stage melanoma. *Archives Surgery,* 1992; **127**: 392–9

249. **Veronesi U,** *et al.* Sentinel-node biopsy to avoid axillary dissection in breast cancer with clinically negative lymph nodes. *Lancet,* 1997; **349**: 1864–7.

250. **Cahan WG, Shah JP, Castro EB.** Benign solitary lung lesions in patients with cancer. *Annals of Surgery,* 1978; **187**: 241–4.

251. **Tofe AJ, Francis MD, Harvey WJ.** Correlation of neoplasms with incidence and localization of skeletal metastases: An analysis of 1,355 diphosphonate bone scans. *Journal of Nuclear Medicine,* 1975; **16**: 986–9.

252. **Fidler M.** Incidence of fracture through metastases in long bones. *Acta Orthopaedica Scandinavica,* 1981; **52**: 623–7.

253. **Mehta RC, Wilson MA, Perlman SB.** False-negative bone scans in extensive metastatic disease: CT and MR findings. *Journal of Computed Assisted Tomography,* 1989; **13**: 717–19.

254. **Kattapuram SV, Khurana JS, Scott JA, el-Khoury GY.** Negative scintigraphy with positive magnetic resonance imaging in bone metastases. *Skeletal Radiology,* 1990; **19**: 113–16.

255. **Algra PR, Bloem JL, Tissing H, Falke TH, Arndt JW, Verboom LJ.** Detection of vertebral metastases: comparison between MR imaging and bone scintigraphy. *Radiographics,* 1991; **11**: 219–32.

256. **Jones EC, Chezmar JL, Nelson RC, Bernardino ME.** The frequency and significance of small (less than or equal to 15 mm) hepatic lesions detected by CT. *American Journal of Roentgenology, 1992*; **158**: 535–9.

257. **Yates CK, Streight RA.** Focal fatty infiltration of the liver simulating metastatic disease. *Radiology,* 1986; **159**: 83–4.

258. **Tang-Barton P, Vas W, Weissman J, Salimi Z, Patel R, Morris L.** Focal fatty liver lesions in alcoholic liver disease: a broadened spectrum of CT appearances. *Gastrointestinal Radiology,* 1985; **10**: 133–7.

259. **Yokoi K,** *et al.* Detection of brain metastasis in potentially operable non-small cell lung cancer: a comparison of CT and MRI. *Chest,* 1999; **115**: 714–19.

260. **Quint LE,** *et al.* Distribution of distant metastases from newly diagnosed non-small cell lung cancer. *Annals of Thoracic Surgery,* 1996; **62**: 246–50.

261. **Cook AM, Lau TN, Tomlinson MJ, Vaidya M, Wakeley CJ, Goddard P.** Magnetic resonance imaging of the whole spine in suspected malignant spinal cord compression: impact on management. *Clinical Oncology,* 1998; **10**: 39–43.

262. **Heldmann U, Myschetzky PS, Thomsen HS.** Frequency of unexpected multifocal metastasis in patients with acute spinal cord compression. Evaluation by low-field MR imaging in cancer patients. *Acta Radiologica,* 1997; **38**: 372–5.

263. **Loughrey GJ, Collins CD, Todd SM, Brown NM, Johnson RJ.** Magnetic resonance imaging in the management of suspected spinal canal disease in patients with known malignancy. *Clinical Radiology* 2000; **55**: 849–55.

264. **McGahan JP.** Adrenal gland: MR imaging. *Radiology,* 1988; **166**: 284–5.

265. **Candel AG, Gattuso P, Reyes CV, Prinz RA, Castelli MJ.** Fine-needle aspiration biopsy of adrenal masses in patients with extraadrenal malignancy. *Surgery,* 1993; **114**: 1132–6.

266. **Korobkin M, Brodeur FJ, Francis IR, Quint LE, Dunnick NR, Goodsitt M.** Delayed enhanced CT for differentiation of benign from malignant adrenal masses. *Radiology,* 1996; **200**: 737–42.

267. **Mitchell DG, Crovello M, Matteucci T, Petersen RO, Miettinen MM.** Benign adrenocortical masses: diagnosis with chemical shift MR imaging. *Radiology,* 1992; **185**: 345–51.

268. **Korobkin M,** *et al.* Adrenal adenomas: relationship between histologic lipid and CT and MR findings. *Radiology.,* 1996; **200**: 743–7.

269. **Outwater EK, Siegelman ES, Huang AB, Birnbaum BA.** Adrenal masses: correlation between CT attenuation value and chemical shift ratio at MR imaging with in-phase and opposed-phase sequences. *Radiology,* 1996; **200**: 749–52.

270. **Ling CC, Rogers CC, Morton RJ.** *Computed tomography in radiation therapy.* New York: Raven Press, 1983.

271. **Thames HD, Schultheiss TE, Hendry JH, Tucker SL, Dubray BM, Brock WA.** Can modest escalations of dose be detected as increased tumor control? *International Journal of Radiation Oncology, Biology and Physics,* 1992; **22**: 241–6.

272. **Consensus Conference.** Magnetic resonance imaging. *Journal of the American Medical Association,* 1988; **259**: 2132–8.

273. **Prasad SC, Pilepich MV, Perez CA.** Contribution of CT to quantitative radiation therapy planning. *American Journal of Roentgenology, 1981*; **136**: 123–8.

274. **Munzenrider JE, Pilepich M, Rene-Ferrero JB, Tchakarova I, Carter BL.** Use of body scanner in radiotherapy treatment planning. *Cancer,* 1977; **40**: 170–9.

275. **Ragan DP, Perez CA.** Efficacy of CT-assisted two dimensional treatment planning: analysis of 45 patients. *American Journal of Roentgenology, 1978*; **131**: 75–9,

276. **Goitein M,** *et al.* The value of CT scanning in radiation therapy

treatment planning: a prospective study. *International Journal of Radiation Oncology, Biology and Physics*, 1979; **5**: 1787–98.

277. **Dobbs HJ, Parker RP, Hodson NJ, Hobday P, Husband JE.** The use of CT in radiotherapy treatment planning. *Radiotherapy and Oncology*, 1983; **1**: 133–41.

278. **Hobday P, Hodson NJ, Husband J, Parker RP, Macdonald JS.** Computed tomography applied to radiotherapy treatment planning: techniques and results. *Radiology*, 1979; **133**: 477–82.

279. **Khoo VS, Dearnaley DP, Finnigan DJ, Padhani A, Tanner SF, Leach MO.** Magnetic resonance imaging (MRI): considerations and applications in radiotherapy treatment planning. *Radiotherapy and Oncology*, 1997; **42**: 1–15.

280. **Potter R, Heil B, Schneider L, Lenzen H, al-Dandashi C, Schnepper E.** Sagittal and coronal planes from MRI for treatment planning in tumors of brain, head and neck: MRI assisted simulation. *Radiotherapy and Oncology*, 1992; **23**: 127–30.

281. **Brown AP,** *et al.* Three-dimensional photon treatment planning for Hodgkin's disease. *International Journal of Radiation Oncology, Biology and Physics*, 1991; **21**: 205–15.

282. **Toonkel LM, Soila K, Gilbert D, Sheldon J.** MRI assisted treatment planning for radiation therapy of the head and neck. *Magnetic Resonance Imaging*, 1988; **6**: 315–19.

283. **Rudoltz MS, Ayyangar K, Mohiuddin M.** Application of magnetic resonance imaging and three-dimensional treatment planning in the treatment of orbital lymphoma. *Medical Dosimetry*, 1993; **18**: 129–33.

284. **Roach M 3rd, Faillace-Akazawa P, Malfatti C, Holland J, Hricak H.** Prostate volumes defined by magnetic resonance imaging and computerized tomographic scans for three-dimensional conformal radiotherapy. *International Journal of Radiation Oncology, Biology and Physics*, 1996; **35**: 1011–18.

285. **Miller A,** *et al.* Reporting results of cancer treatment. *Cancer*, 1981; **47**: 207–14.

286. *WHO handbook for reporting results of cancer treatment.* Geneva, Switzerland: World Health Organisation, 1979: offset publication No. 48.

287. **Hawthorn J.** *A practical guide to EORTC studies.* Brussels: European Organisation for the Research and Treatment of Cancer (EORTC), 1994.

288. **Therasse P,** *et al.* New guidelines to evaluate the response to treatment in solid tumors. European Organization for Research and Treatment of Cancer, National Cancer Institute of the United States, National Cancer Institute of Canada. *Journal of the National Cancer Institute*, 2000; **92**: 205–16.

289. **James K,** *et al.* Measuring response in solid tumors: unidimensional versus bidimensional measurement. *Journal of the National Cancer Institute*, 1999; **91**: 523–8.

290. **Lavin PT, Flowerdew G.** Studies in variation associated with the measurement of solid tumors. *Cancer*, 1980; **46**: 1286–90.

291. **Thiesse P,** *et al.* Response rate accuracy in oncology trials: reasons for interobserver variability. Groupe Francais d'Immunotherapie of the Federation Nationale des Centres de Lutte Contre le Cancer. *Jounal of Clinical Oncology*, 1997; **15**: 3507–14.

292. **Smith TA.** FDG uptake, tumour characteristics and response to therapy: a review. *Nuclear Medicine Communications*, 1998; **19**: 97–105.

293. **Hoekstra OS,** *et al.* Early treatment response in malignant lymphoma, as determined by planar fluorine-18-fluorodeoxyglucose scintigraphy. *Journal of Nuclear Medicine*, 1993; **34**: 1706–10.

294. **Husband JE, Hawkes DJ, Peckham MJ.** CT estimations of mean attenuation values and volume in testicular tumours: a comparison with surgical and histologic findings. *Radiology*, 1982; **144**: 553–8.

295. **Weissleder R.** Molecular imaging exploring the next frontier. *Radiology*, 1999; **212**: 609–14.

296. **Folkman J.** The role of angiogenesis in tumour growth. *Seminars in Cancer Biology*, 1992; **3**: 65–71.

297. **Folkman J.** Angiogenesis in cancer, vascular, rheumatoid and other disease. *Nature Medicine*, 1995; **1**: 27–31.

298. **Brown JM, Giaccia AJ.** The unique physiology of solid tumors: opportunities (and problems) for cancer therapy. *Cancer Research*, 1998; **58**: 1408–16.

299. **Tomida A, Tsuruo T.** Drug resistance mediated by cellular stress response to the microenvironment of solid tumors. *Anticancer Drug Design*, 1999; **14**: 169–77.

300. **Wells P, Harte RJA, Price P.** Positron emission tomography: a new investigational area for cancer research. *Clinical Oncology*, 1996; **8**: 7–14.

301. **Padhani AR.** Dynamic contrast-enhanced MRI studies in human tumours. *British Journal of Radiology*, 1999; **72**: 427–31.

302. **Koh WJ,** *et al.* Imaging of hypoxia in human tumors with [F-18]fluoromisonidazole. *International Journal of Radiation Oncology, Biology and Physics*, 1992; **22**: , 199–212.

303. **Williams MP,** *et al.* Computed tomography of the abdomen in advanced seminoma: response to treatment. *Clinical Radiology*, 1987; **38**: 629–33.

304. **Gustavsson A,** *et al.* Late cardiac effects of mantle radiotherapy in patients with Hodgkin's disease. *Annals of Oncology*, 1990; **1**: 355–63.

305. **Morgan G,** *et al.* Late cardiac, thyroid and pulmonary sequelae of mantle radiotherapy for Hodgkin's disease. *International Journal of Radiation Oncology, Biology and Physics*, 1985; **11**: 1925–31.

306. **Van Leeuwan F,** *et al.* Second cancer risk following Hodgkin's disease: a twenty year follow-up study. *Journal of Clinical Oncology*, 1994; **12**: 312–25.

307. **Rahmouni A,** *et al.* Lymphoma: monitoring tumor size and signal intensity with MR imaging. *Radiology*, 1993; **188**: 445–51.

308. **Hill M,** *et al.* Role of magnetic resonance imaging in predicting relapse in residual masses after treatment of lymphoma. *Journal of Clinical Oncology*, 1993; **11**: 2273–8.

309. **Nyman RS,** *et al.* Residual mediastinal masses in Hodgkin disease: prediction of size with MR imaging. *Radiology*, 1989; **170**: 435–40.

310. **Spiers AS, Husband JE, MacVicar AD.** Treated thymic lymphoma: comparison of MR imaging with CT. *Radiology*, 1997; **203**: 369–76.

311. **Maisey NR,** *et al.* Are 18fluorodeoxyglucose positron emission tomography and magnetic resonance imaging useful in the prediction of relapse in lymphoma residual masses? *European Journal Cancer*, 2000; **36**: 200–6.

312. **Muller-Schimpfle M,** *et al.* Recurrent rectal cancer: diagnosis with dynamic MR imaging. *Radiology*, 1993; **189**: 881–9.

313. **Blomqvist L, Fransson P, Hindmarsh T.** The pelvis after surgery and radio-chemotherapy for rectal cancer studied with Gd-DTPA-enhanced fast dynamic MR imaging. *European Radiology*, 1998; **8**: 781–7.

314. **Spencer JA, Golding SJ.** Patterns of lymphatic metastases at recurrence of prostate cancer: CT findings. *Clinical Radiology*, 1994; **49**: 404–7.

315. **Husband JE, Hodson NH, Parsons CA.** The role of computed tomography in recurrent rectal tumours. *Radiology*, 1980; **4**: 1–16.

316. **Reznek RH, White FE, Young JWR.** The appearances on computed tomography after abdomino-perineal resection for carcinoma of the rectum: a comparison between the normal appearances and those of recurrence. *British Journal of Radiology*, 1983; **56**: 237–40.

317. **Méndez RJ,** *et al.* CT in local recurrence of rectal carcinoma. *Journal of Computer Assisted Tomography*, 1993; **17**: 741–4.

318. **Sugarbaker PH,** *et al.* A simplified plan for follow-up of patients with colon and rectal cancer supported by prospective studies of laboratory and radiological test results. *Surgery*, 1987; **102**: 79–87.

319. **Haberkorn U,** *et al.* PET studies of fluorodeoxyglucose metabolism in patients with recurrent colorectal tumours receiving radiotherapy. *Journal of Nuclear Medicine*, 1991; **32**: 1485–90.

320. **Stomper PC, *et al.*** Detection of pelvic recurrence of colorectal carcinoma: prospective, blinded comparison of Tc-99m-IMMU-4 monoclonal antibody scanning and CT. *Radiology*, 1995; **197**: 688–92.

321. **Pema PJ, Bennett WF, Bova JG, Warman P.** CT vs MRI in diagnosis

of recurrent rectosigmoid carcinoma. *Journal of Computer Assisted Tomography*, 1994; **18**: 256–61.

322. **Beets G, *et al.*** Clinical value of whole-body positron emission tomography with [^{18}F]fluorodeoxyglucose in recurrent colorectal cancer. *British Journal of Surgery*, 1994; **81**: 1666–70.

3.4 Circulating tumour markers

Gordon J. S. Rustin

Introduction

Almost 80 years passed between the discovery of myeloma proteins by Bence Jones in 1848[1] and the discovery of human chorionic gonadotrophin and its association with trophoblastic tumours by Ascheim and Zondek in 1928.[2] In the interval many biochemical and endocrinological disturbances related to malignant disease were identified and some of these contribute to the initial diagnosis of some cancers.

A range of proteins and small peptides have since been identified as secreted products of solid tumours. Some have found clinical application as a means of monitoring the course of disease and as prognostic factors. Although large numbers of antigens have been identified in association with various cancers, only a few have so far been shown to have an impact on patient management (Table 1). New approaches to the identification of markers are likely to emerge from molecular genetic techniques, but there is no certainty that they will prove more specific and, therefore, potentially more sensitive than those identified so far. Although marker substances are considered in this chapter mainly in the context of serological monitoring, they have important applications in immunohistochemistry, immunoscintigraphy, and as targets for antibody-directed therapy. The optimal characteristics for a marker differ according to application, although some are valuable in multiple roles.

Ideally, secreted tumour markers would allow detection of the smallest mass of cells able to initiate the neoplastic process and this would require assays of high sensitivity to detect the tumour products diluted in body fluids.[3] In practice, the smallest mass of tumour that can be detected is determined less by the sensitivity of current assay methods than by the lack of uniqueness of the markers' association with cancer. Cross-reacting epitopes produced by normal tissues therefore determine the limit of sensitivity. The quantity of a marker produced per mean tumour cell must also affect sensitivity, although this is relative to the background level in blood or urine arising from non-tumour sources. The possibility that tumour-derived substances are antigenically distinct from the normal forms and, thus, identifiable as unique tumour-specific substances has long been entertained but not so far fulfilled.

Interpretation of tumour marker values is only secure when the antigen has been studied in detail with respect to its sources, its secretion and distribution in body fluids, degradation, and excretion. Clearly, the serum or urine concentration is a function of secretion and total clearance rates. Without such information the relationship between marker values and tumour burden is somewhat speculative, but the potential of biochemical products to reflect viable, marker-synthesizing cancer cells as opposed to tumour volume is part of their potential value.

A cancer cell population can range from four to greater than 10^{12} cells in man. In the case of human chorionic gonadotrophin and α-fetoprotein up to a 10^7-fold range of tumour activity may be measured. For other markers, only a 10^2- to 10^4-fold range of tumour burden can be monitored. The concentration of a marker in serum may vary widely between patients for a given tumour burden, but within the same patient serial marker values tend to reflect a less irregular relationship. Various factors can affect the relationship between tumour burden and marker concentration. Therapeutic substances including interferon, corticosteroids, cytotoxic agents, butyrate, and bromodeoxyuridine can modify the rate of synthesis or secretion by cells in cell culture but rarely lead to a change in serum levels in patients. Cytotoxic drugs may cause marker levels to rise temporarily through tumour cell lysis or through induction of differentiation of tumour cells.[4],[5]

It is evident that most existing markers are not sufficiently sensitive for screening purposes. The main exceptions at present are human chorionic gonadotrophin in screening the high-risk population of women who have hydatidiform mole and pentagastrin-stimulated levels of calcitonin to detect familial medullary carcinoma of the thyroid. α-Fetoprotein screening for hepatocellular carcinoma and catecholamine metabolite screening for neuroblastoma are less sensitive. Prostate-specific antigen is increasingly being used to screen for prostate cancer and CA 125 is used to screen women at high risk of ovarian cancer. When tumour markers are used for screening it

Table 1 Circulating markers of definite clinical value

Circulating marker	Tumours where most valuable
Human chorionic gonadotrophin (hCG)	Gestational trophoblastic, germ cell
α-Fetoprotein	Germ cell, hepatocellular
Carcinoembryonic antigen	Colorectal
CA 125	Ovarian
Prostate-specific antigen	Prostate
Lactate dehydrogenase	Germ cell
Squamous cell carcinoma antigen	Cervix

Table 2 Methods by which tumour markers are presented and defined

	Present	Absent
Assay positive	TP	FP
Assay negative	FN	TN
Sensitivity	$=\dfrac{TP}{TP+FN}\times 100$	
Specificity	$=\dfrac{TN}{FP+TN}\times 100$	
Positive predictive value	$=\dfrac{TP}{TP+FP}\times 100$	
Negative predictive value	$=\dfrac{TN}{FN+TN}\times 100$	

FP, false positive; FN, false negative; TP, true positive; TN, true negative.

should be remembered that the result of screening should be improved survival in the screened population. Diagnosing cancer earlier is a waste of resources unless there is also an improvement in quality and duration of life.

Tests for the presence of cancer

During the past 35 years there have been a series of claims put forward for general tests that predict the presence of cancer. There are problems related to such tests, in particular the false-positive test, which results in much anxiety and expenditure on radiological and other diagnostic examinations. The issues related to cancer tests have been reviewed elsewhere.[6] None of the tests which have been proposed have found an established place in clinical practice. On the basis that carcinogenesis probably involves multiple events in more than 200 different types of cell, the possibility of a single common phenotypic characteristic for cancer seems remote. However, it is now known that many patients with cancer have small numbers of circulating cancer cells or mutant DNA in their plasma.[7] It will only be a matter of time before commercial assays are available that can detect the most common cancer-related mutants in plasma DNA.

Definitions used in relation to tumour markers

In this chapter the sensitivity of a test is defined as the percentage of patients with a particular disease who have elevated marker levels and are therefore true positives (Table 2). Specificity is the percentage of patients without disease who have normal marker levels and are therefore true negatives. The positive predictive value is the percentage of positive results (i.e. elevated marker levels) which are true positives. Other terms frequently used are the false-positive rate, which is the percentage of patients without disease who have an elevated marker level, and the false-negative rate, which is the percentage of patients with disease who have a normal marker level. If one is observing a

trend in serial marker levels, the false-positive rate for marker response is the percentage of patients with no response clinically who have a fall in marker levels, and the false-negative rate is the percentage of patients with a clinical response who do not have a fall in marker levels.

Defining tumour response by change in tumour marker levels

Malignancies such as trophoblastic and germ cell tumours exhibit a good correlation between change in marker level and response or progression of the tumour. For these tumours a decline of marker level of a log or more is frequently used as a surrogate for response, which is usually measured according to change in tumour size as defined by groups such as the World Health Organization (WHO). Marker response is often defined as complete (fall to within normal range), greater than log fall, greater than 75 per cent fall, greater than 50 per cent fall, no change, or a rise. Precise definitions of response according to tumour markers are now being proposed for CA 125.[8] It is necessary to be aware of the proportion of marker changes that falsely predict a change in tumour status.

Human chorionic gonadotrophin and its subunits

Human chorionic gonadotrophin (hCG) comes closest to being the ideal tumour marker and will be discussed in more detail than other markers as the experience gained from its use is generally relevant to the marker field. The α- and β-subunits which constitute human chorionic gonadotrophin are the normal products of placental trophoblast and particularly of the syncytiotrophoblast. The α-subunit structure is shared with the α-subunit of luteinizing hormone, follicle-stimulating hormone, and thyroid-stimulating hormone. The β-subunit is unique but 80 per cent of its 145 amino acids are shared with the luteinizing hormone subunit. Immunoreactive hCG has also been identified in a variety of normal tissues in low concentration, including pituitary gland, liver, and colon.[9] Free α-subunit is detected mainly in late pregnancy and free β-subunit in early pregnancy.

Although desialylation of hCG does not affect its immunoreactivity, it reduces its biological activity in vitro and it accelerates clearance from blood in vivo. There have been many reports that hCG derived from the urine of patients with choriocarcinoma may differ from placental hCG through carbohydrate changes[10] and there may also be differences in hCG produced by other cells. Free β-subunit as well as intact hCG is produced by choriocarcinoma cells in vitro and by trophoblastic tumours in vivo.[11] The serum half-life of intact hCG is 16 to 24 h with the free subunit chains having much shorter half-lives.[12]

The assays used for hCG measurements are frequently described as β-hCG assays. These assays detect both intact hCG and β-hCG. Cross-reactivity with luteinizing hormone varies, but in most tests is now low. Measurements on serum tend to be less subject to interference than those on urine samples and time-corrected urine values tend to be approximately 50 per cent higher than those of serum. Normal non-pregnant serum values are generally less than 2 international units/litre (IU/l) but values up to 5 IU/l may occur.

Normal urine values are less than 30 IU/l.[13] β-Core fragment may be a major contributor to normal urine hCG but this has yet to be clearly defined and its importance may vary with the assay technique.

β-Core fragment

In addition to hCG, α-hCG, and β-hCG, pregnancy urine contains a fragment corresponding to residues 6 to 40 and 55 to 92 of β-hCG.[20] The fragment is present in WHO reference preparations of hCG and some widely used anti-β-hCG antibodies react with it.[21] β-Core fragment is found in urine but due to association with macromolecules is not detected in serum.[22] It can be detected by immunocytochemistry in syncytiotrophoblast tissue from placenta, hydatidiform mole, and choriocarcinoma, as well as over 90 per cent of non-trophoblast tissues. Elevated values of β-core fragment have been detected in urine from approximately 50 per cent of patients with gynaecological cancers.[23] It is too early to know whether this new marker will find a useful clinical role.

Ectopic production of hCG

The production of immunoreactive hCG by non-trophoblastic tumours has been recognized since the 1960s.[9] Carcinomas of the stomach, lung, pancreas (including islet cell tumours), colon, and bladder are frequent contributors. Although it can be argued that since normal tissues synthesize hCG, the term 'ectopic' is inappropriate, it is nevertheless a convenient distinction. In general though, with some exceptions, the serum values of hCG are only moderately raised in ectopic production and are rarely of great value for monitoring purposes. Exceptional cases with trophoblast-like differentiation may, however, be associated with high values and these are of interest because such tumours tend to be more aggressive but also more chemosensitive than non-hCG-producing tumours with similar sites of origin.[24] DNA fingerprinting has now shown that some patients with apparent choriocarcinoma that developed drug resistance contained no paternal chromosomal contribution and were in fact non-gestational tumours producing hCG ectopically.[25] Ectopic hormone production is not unique to malignancy and has been described in various forms of inflammatory bowel disease.

Gestational trophoblastic tumours

In patients with established trophoblastic tumours following any form of pregnancy, hCG is used to monitor the response to therapy and to detect the development of resistance or relapse after remission. As a rough guide, the limit of detection of hCG (less than 5 IU/l) corresponds with approximately 10^5 cells or less than 1 mm^3 of viable cells. Although this is more sensitive than any other detection system, it does not represent the endpoint for treatment, which is continued for about 6 weeks after hCG levels have reached the normal range. A plateau or rise in hCG levels indicates development of drug resistance.

There are two important diagnostic applications of hCG measurement. Serum:spinal fluid concentrations tend to be greater than 60:1 in the absence of brain metastases and ratios less than 60:1 indicate their presence unless sampled when serum values are falling rapidly.[14] Serum values in patients with choriocarcinoma which is clinically or radiologically apparent tend to be in the range 10^3 to 10^7 IU/l, but

in placental site trophoblastic tumours even bulky lesions are associated with levels that rarely rise above 10^2 to 10^3 IU/l.

Since hCG levels in patients with gestational choriocarcinoma reflect the body burden of viable tumour they constitute a significant prognostic factor, with high values contributing to high-risk status.[15]

Hydatidiform mole

Some patients with hydatidiform mole have higher concentrations of hCG in serum or urine than are found at the corresponding stage of normal pregnancy, but the diagnosis of hydatiform mole is now largely dependent on ultrasound scanning. Patients with hydatidiform mole (complete or partial) have an increased risk of choriocarcinoma. Although more than 90 per cent of hydatidiform moles die out spontaneously and although chemotherapy is generally effective in most patients with choriocarcinoma, it remains highly advantageous to identify patients with persisting molar tissue because treatment within 6 months of evacuation of the mole can involve relatively non-toxic chemotherapy. Patients with high levels of hCG (greater than 20 000 IU/l) more than 4 to 5 weeks after evacuation of a hydatidiform mole are a small subset requiring early intervention because they are at risk of uterine perforation. It has been shown that if hCG falls to the limit of detection within 56 days of evacuation then a 6-month follow-up period is generally adequate, but for those patients whose hCG becomes normal only after 56 days a 2-year follow-up remains advisable.[16] Patients who have had hydatidiform mole have a slightly increased risk of choriocarcinoma after any subsequent pregnancy and should have further hCG estimations at 4 and 12 weeks postpartum.

In monitoring the response of invasive mole or gestational choriocarcinoma to chemotherapy, it has long been noted that hCG levels may increase for several days before starting to fall. Tumour lysis or increased syncytial differentiation have been considered as possible mechanisms. The rate of fall of hCG values is a function of metabolic clearance and rate of synthesis and the lag before values fall is sometimes taken, mistakenly, to indicate drug resistance. The levelling out of values and rising serial values in the course of therapy do, however, indicate resistance. Following completion of therapy, hCG monitoring should be continued for at least 8 years.

Germ cell tumours

Germ cell tumours arising at any site may contain elements which produce hCG whether or not typical trophoblastic cells are identified morphologically. However, hCG is only a marker of part of the malignant cell population in germ cell tumours. In these tumours α-fetoprotein is equally important and lactate dehydrogenase may also be useful. However, some tumour elements may produce no detectable marker (Table 3).

As in the gestational tumours, the detection of drug resistance and the attainment of remission and early detection of relapses by marker measurements have become key components in management. Since Germa-Lluch et al.[18] first identified the prognostic significance of hCG, it has been shown that very high initial values or half-life of more than 3 days are among the strongest predictors of poor prognosis. An international germ cell collaborative group has produced a prognostic model based upon the management of 5862 patients with germ cell tumours.[19] This model uses three different ranges of hCG, α-fetoprotein, and lactate dehydrogenase as well as extent of disease on

Table 3 Tumour markers in metastatic non-seminomatous germ cell tumours

Marker	Proportion elevated	(%)	Range
hCG	421/760	55	40–68
α-Fetoprotein	439/716	61	59–74
α-Fetoprotein and/or hCG	414/515	80	70–92
Lactate dehydrogenase	639/1218	52	
Placental alkaline phosphatase	5/27	19	14–23

From ref.17.

scans to split patients into three prognostic groups and has superseded clinical staging for patient management (see Chapter 13.4). Approximately 10 per cent of seminomas are associated with elevated hCG levels produced by the syncytial giant cells seen in some of these tumours. Very high levels indicate a more aggressive tumour better treated as a non-seminomatous germ cell tumour.

α-Fetoprotein

The human gene for α-fetoprotein is located on chromosome 4 in a gene cluster with the albumin gene. α-Fetoprotein is synthesized by fetal yolk sac, liver, and intestine and in the fetus is the major serum protein acting as an albumin-like carrier protein.[26] In addition to its production in pregnancy, α-fetoprotein is present in small amounts (less than 10 µg/l) in normal serum and moderately elevated levels are seen in some patients with pancreatic, biliary, gastric, and bronchial cancers, as well as occasional patients with non-malignant hepatic disease where active hepatic regeneration is occurring. Increased amounts up to 10^7 µg/l are found in the serum of patients with hepatocellular carcinoma and with germ cell tumours of the testes, ovary, and midline structures, including mediastinum and pineal gland that contain yolk sac tissue (Table 3). α-Fetoprotein has a serum half-life of 4.5 days, so in patients with both yolk sac and choriocarcinomatous elements of germ cell tumour, hCG levels fall faster than α-fetoprotein levels.[5] High values of α-fetoprotein, like high values of hCG, reflect tumour burden and perhaps aggressiveness, and are of prognostic significance, so that values greater than 1000 µg/l indicate the need for more intensive therapy.[19] Yolk sac elements of germ cell tumours rarely metastasize to the brain so, in contrast to hCG, values of α-fetoprotein in the cerebrospinal fluid are not so useful.

One unfortunate aspect of α-fetoprotein as a tumour marker is that serum values occasionally increase as a result of chemotherapy.[27] Thus, after values have fallen in response to therapy they may start to increase again or, if initially normal, α-fetoprotein values may increase in the course of therapy to levels of 50 to 500 µg/l. Such levels may persist for many months after completion of therapy and do not necessarily indicate the presence of residual active tumour. This elevation is presumed to be the result of the action of methotrexate, platinum drugs, or etoposide on the liver.

Serum α-fetoprotein is elevated at presentation in 50 to 80 per cent of patients with hepatocellular carcinoma. In parts of the world such as China, where hepatocellular carcinoma is one of the most common malignant tumours, population screening by α-fetoprotein is justified as patients who have successful resection of a solitary, screen-detected tumour have a higher chance of long-term survival.[28] In low-risk areas such as the United Kingdom, serial α-fetoprotein estimation and ultrasound can be justified in high-risk groups including those with cirrhosis, chronic hepatitis B, or haemochromatosis. Although modest elevations of α-fetoprotein occur in about 20 per cent of patients with hepatitis, cirrhosis, biliary obstruction, and alcoholic liver disease, a massively elevated level in a patient with known cirrhosis is virtually diagnostic of hepatocellular carcinoma.

Placental alkaline phosphatase

An isoenzyme of alkaline phosphatase similar to that produced by the placenta was found in the serum of a patient with cancer by Fishman et al.[29] It is now known to be one of several phenotypic variants which are elevated in a variety of tumour tissues and in the serum of some patients with cancer. Assays using monoclonal antibodies are now available, but as several epitopes are recognized on the enzyme, different assays may recognize different variants. Testicular seminomas are the only tumours for which placental alkaline phosphatase assays have consistently shown a sensitivity of greater than 50 per cent,[17] but as levels are only raised in bulky tumours and fall to normal early in therapy, it is of marginal value as a serum marker.[30] The fact that it is membrane bound rather than secreted makes it more reliable as a histochemical marker of seminoma. If it is used to diagnose seminomas or dysgerminomas, it should be appreciated that elevated serum levels are found in people who smoke.

Carcinoembryonic antigen

This glycoprotein, with a molecular mass of approximately 200 000 Da, was first demonstrated using an antibody prepared by injection of an extract of human colon carcinoma into rabbits.[31] Once sensitive radioimmunoassays became available, it was found that serum carcinoembryonic antigen was elevated not only in carcinomas of the gastrointestinal tract and fetal digestive organs but also in a variety of other malignant and non-malignant conditions. The latter include severe benign liver disease, inflammatory lesions (particularly of the gastrointestinal tract), infections, trauma, infarction, collagen diseases, renal impairment, and smoking; low values are also found in the normal colon. However, higher concentrations are usually found in the serum of patients with gastrointestinal tumours than in the serum of patients with non-malignant conditions. Assays using both polyclonal and monoclonal antibodies are available, but assays using different antibodies may give different results and no method has so far been shown to be superior overall.

Diagnosis/screening

Serum carcinoembryonic antigen is elevated in fewer than 5 per cent of patients with Dukes grade A colorectal carcinoma, approximately a quarter of patients with Dukes grade B, 44 per cent of patients with Dukes grade C, and approximately 65 per cent of patients with distant metastases.[32] A high serum level may contribute to the diagnosis of cancer in patients presenting with gastrointestinal symptoms. The low incidence of raised values of serum carcinoembryonic antigen in early disease and the ability of benign conditions and smoking to cause raised concentrations indicates its lack of value in screening normal populations for colorectal cancer.[33] A study of carcinoembryonic antigen monitoring in patients with ulcerative colitis showed no benefit in earlier diagnosis of colorectal cancer.[34] It is also not reliable enough for monitoring patients with familial polyposis coli. Fifteen to fifty per cent of patients with colorectal polyps have been reported to have moderately raised carcinoembryonic antigen values with levels above five times the upper limit of the reference range suggesting the presence of carcinoma.[35],[36]

Prognosis/monitoring therapy

A raised preoperative serum carcinoembryonic antigen has been shown to be an important prognostic indicator in colorectal cancer, which is only in part due to its elevation being related to Dukes grade. However, no studies have yet shown benefit from adjuvant therapy based solely on an elevated preoperative value for carcinoembryonic antigen. The serum carcinoembryonic antigen value should fall to normal within 4 to 6 weeks of complete resection of a colorectal carcinoma. It should be remembered that 33 per cent of healthy persons with a smoking history have elevated carcinoembryonic antigen levels.[37] Levels usually rise with progressive disease and fall with response to chemotherapy or radiotherapy. If the carcinoembryonic antigen fails to decrease during radiotherapy, disease is likely to be found outside the radiation field, which may still be surgically resectable. Several studies have shown that survival is longer in patients who have a fall in serum carcinoembryonic antigen level during chemotherapy than in those in whom there is no change or an increase in levels.[38] The fall in levels presumably indicates tumour response. The predictive value of carcinoembryonic antigen detection of progressive disease in 17 patients was 100 per cent.[39] A confirmed rise of carcinoembryonic antigen on chemotherapy is sufficient evidence to stop or alter therapy.[33]

Patients with widespread metastases from many tumours, including carcinoma of the breast, stomach, bronchus, pancreas, oesophagus, cervix, ovary, and endometrium, may have elevated carcinoembryonic antigen levels, which can be used to monitor the response to therapy.

Early detection of recurrence

A rise in serum carcinoembryonic antigen can predict a recurrence of colorectal cancer 4 to 6 months before it is clinically detectable. One study of 311 patients showed that carcinoembryonic antigen was the first indicator of recurrent disease in 58 per cent of all patients and in 80 per cent of those with liver metastases.[40] The potential value of serial carcinoembryonic antigen monitoring after initial treatment is to detect solitary recurrences, which if resected results in improved survival. Many doctors believe that carcinoembryonic antigen testing should be performed every 2 to 3 months for 2 years or more in those patients for whom resection of liver metastases would be clinically indicated.[33] Non-randomized

studies suggest a higher resectable rate (45 to 55 per cent) in those on carcinoembryonic antigen monitoring than those on less intense monitoring (8 to 30 per cent).[41],[42] However, several randomized studies suggest no survival advantage from more intense follow-up.[43],[44] The preliminary results of the large prospective randomized CRC carcinoembryonic antigen second-look trial show no survival benefit from surgery after early detection of recurrence by rising carcinoembryonic antigen levels.[45] In that study 1447 patients were recruited and randomized between aggressive management including surgery or continued observation if an elevated carcinoembryonic antigen was detected. Further work is required to determine whether patients with just a rising carcinoembryonic antigen level would benefit from earlier chemotherapy.

CA 19.9

CA 19.9 is an antigen derived from a human colon adenocarcinoma cell line and defined by a monoclonal antibody designated 19.9. The epitope is structurally identical to the sialyated Lewis[a] antigen. Several commercial kits are available. Using an upper limit of normal of 37 IU/ml, only 0.6 per cent of blood donors but 15 to 36 per cent of patients with benign pancreatic, liver, and biliary tract diseases had elevated levels. Although elevated levels of CA 19.9 have been reported in as many as 75 per cent of patients with advanced colorectal carcinoma, most studies suggest that it is a less sensitive marker for colorectal carcinoma than carcinoembryonic antigen. However, it appears to be more sensitive than carcinoembryonic antigen for gastric and biliary tract carcinomas and is elevated in 70 to 89 per cent of patients with pancreatic carcinoma.[32],[46]

The main clinical value of CA 19.9 is in monitoring the response to therapy of patients with pancreatic and gastric carcinoma. Studies are required to show whether serial measurements can more accurately indicate disease response or progression than the currently used scans, which are often unreliable in upper gastrointestinal malignancies.

CA 50

CA 50 is another monoclonal antibody obtained by the immunization of mice with a colorectal carcinoma cell line. Part of the epitope that the CA 50 antibody recognizes is identical to the CA 19.9 epitope, but part can be present in patients who are Lewis[a] antigen negative, which is a potential advantage in those patients. It is therefore fairly similar to CA 19.9 but does appear to be elevated in the serum of more patients with malignancies outside the gastrointestinal tract, such as breast, lung, and prostate tumours.[47]

Breast carcinoma-associated mucins

Several groups have produced monoclonal antibodies to high molecular weight glycoproteins, described as mucins, derived from epithelial cells of the lactating breast. In some patients with cancer there is production of mucins with altered oligosaccharide attachments, but the protein core appears unchanged. Monoclonal antibodies have been produced to many different mucins with unique epitopes.

Unfortunately, measuring different mucins does not increase the percentage of patients with elevated levels. Antibodies that have been shown to be of value as serum tumour markers include 115D8 (which detects the MAM/6 antigen), DF3, human milk fat globulins 1 and 2, NCRC 11, B72.3, W1, M26, an antibody against mucin-like carcinoma-associated antigen, and an antibody against mammary surface antigen.[48] The most investigated mucin marker, referred to as CA 15.3, uses the 115D8 antibody for capture and the DF3 antibody as a tracer in a commercial kit. Elevated serum levels of CA 15.3 have been found in 12.5 per cent of women with benign breast disease, preoperatively in 11 per cent of women with operable breast cancer, and in 64 per cent of women with metastatic breast cancer.[49] The mucin-like carcinoma-associated antigen and the M26 markers have also been developed into commercial immunoassay kits and appear to have similar sensitivity to CA 15.3.

These mucin assays are of no value in screening because of their low sensitivity for the early stages of the disease. They are elevated in some patients with gynaecological cancers, which reduces their value when making a differential diagnosis. CA 15.3 elevation increases with increasing stage of disease and highest levels are seen in patients with liver or bone metastases.[50] Summation of results from 11 studies evaluating CA 15.3 in assessing response suggest that 66 per cent of patients show decreases in marker levels in the presence of responding disease, 73 per cent of patients show stable levels in the presence of stable disease, and 80 per cent show increasing levels in the presence of progressive disease.[33] Although mucin markers can be used to assess the response, particularly in patients with lesions such as bone metastases that are difficult to monitor, they are not accurate enough to be used alone to define response.

Several trials have shown that a rising CA 15.3 level during follow-up can detect relapse 2 to 9 months before clinical signs or symptoms develop.[33] A representative study of 205 patients demonstrated that rising CA 15.3 levels indicated recurrence in 73 per cent of those with a recurrence and in 6 per cent of those without a recurrence.[51] In view of the unproven value of early detection of recurrence, serum markers have no place at present in long-term follow-up assessments.

CA 125

The CA 125 antigen was originally defined by its reactivity with a murine monoclonal antibody raised by immunization with a human cell line derived from a serous cystadenocarcinoma of the ovary.[52] It is expressed on a glycoprotein of relatively high molecular mass (less than 200 000 Da). CA 125 is produced from derivatives of the coelomic epithelium, including the pleura, pericardium, peritoneum, fallopian tube, endometrium, and endocervix. It has been detected in many tissues and secretions, but not in the normal ovary. The antigen is present at the cell surface in more than 80 per cent of non-mucinous epithelial ovarian tumours and in a small percentage of many other tumours.[53] Shed antigen that reaches the blood has an apparent serum half-life of approximately 4.5 days.[52],[54]

There are several commercial assay kits available in the form of either an immunoradiometric assay or an enzyme-linked immuno-sorbent assay. In both assays the antibody to CA 125 is coated on a solid-phase immunoabsorbent and the multiple CA 125 epitopes on each antigen molecule enable the antigen to act as a bridge to the label.

Specificity

Using the immunoradiometric assay, the level of CA 125 was less than 35 IU/ml in 99 per cent and less than 65 IU/ml in 99.7 per cent of healthy blood-bank donors.[52] Levels above 35 IU/ml are frequently seen during the first trimester of pregnancy, with endometriosis, with cirrhosis (especially if ascites is present), and occasionally with a variety of other benign conditions.[55] Over 40 per cent of patients with advanced intra-abdominal neoplasms of diverse primary site and histology have elevated levels of CA 125. The newer CA 125 II assays utilize M11 as a capture antibody and the original OC 125 as a tracer, resulting in superior analytical performance including a lower upper limit of normal.

Sensitivity

Many studies have confirmed the initial report of over 80 per cent of patients with epithelial ovarian cancer having a CA 125 level greater than 35 IU/ml.[55],[56] The level is elevated preoperatively in over 90 per cent of women with stage III or stage IV disease but in only approximately 50 per cent with stage I disease. In women found to have residual tumour at a second-look operation, preoperative elevated levels are found in between 13 and 52 per cent of patients.

Clinical value

Diagnosis and screening

CA 125 has been investigated for its potential in screening well postmenopausal women,[57] but its low sensitivity for potentially curative stage I tumours suggests that alone it could only prevent a minority of ovarian cancer deaths and at great cost. A large randomized trial is currently investigating whether serial CA 125 screening with ultrasound in patients with elevated or rising levels can lead to improved survival. Apart from women at high risk of familial ovarian cancer, screening for ovarian cancer should not be offered to women outside a clinical trial. CA 125 has little diagnostic value for ovarian carcinoma, due to its poor specificity in women with abdominal symptoms or masses. However, a risk of malignancy index based on menopausal status, ultrasound findings, and CA 125 levels gave a sensitivity of 85 per cent and specificity of 98 per cent for diagnosing a malignant pelvic cancer among 143 women having a pelvic mass.[58]

Prognosis and response to treatment

Very high CA 125 levels prior to surgery are associated with a worse prognosis, but knowledge of this is unlikely to lead to any alteration in management. The exception is in women with stage 1 disease where a preoperative level greater than 65 IU/ml has been shown to be a powerful adverse prognostic indicator.[59] Such patients are candidates for chemotherapy rather than surveillance. Several groups have shown that the CA 125 level after one, two, or three courses of chemotherapy, a long half-life, or greater than sevenfold fall are the most important prognostic factors for survival. Prognostic information based on CA 125 should not be used to decide therapy, as in nearly 20 per cent of cases where CA 125 predicts a poor prognosis the patient has no cancer progression in the next 12 months.[60]

Serial CA 125 levels are currently the best way of monitoring response to therapy of carcinoma of the ovary (Fig. 1). CA 125 can also be useful during therapy of patients with ovarian germ cell and

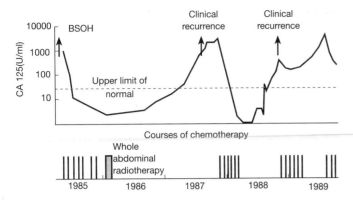

Fig. 1 CA 125 levels in a woman who had bilateral salpingo-oophorectomy and hysterectomy (BSOH) for advanced ovarian carcinoma. The CA 125 levels clearly demonstated responses to first- and second-line chemotherapy, an increase, indicating recurrent disease, occurring several months prior to clinical evidence of recurrence.

mixed mesodermal tumours. The occasional patient may have an early rise in levels due to tumour lysis despite responding[54] and levels can rise to above 100 IU/ml for several weeks after surgery. Recently, definitions for response based on serial CA 125 estimations have been proposed[8] and appear more accurate than scans for monitoring therapy. For use in clinical trials they have to be very precise and use mathematical logic in a computer program. Put simply, response according to CA 125 has occurred if either of the following criteria are applicable.

- Either a 50 per cent response has occurred if there is a 50 per cent decrease in serum CA 125 levels. There must be two initial elevated samples. The sample showing a 50 per cent fall must be confirmed by a fourth sample (requires four CA 125 levels).
- Or a 75 per cent response has occurred if there has been a serial decrease in serum CA 125 levels of more than 75 per cent over three samples (requires three CA 125 levels).

(In each, the final sample has to be at least 28 days after the previous sample). These definitions are particularly useful for clinical trials where they indicate which new treatments are active more easily and cheaper than by standard response criteria.

Detection of progression or relapse

A serial rise of CA 125 of more than 25 per cent appears the most accurate method of predicting progression of ovarian cancer during therapy and could lead to ineffective, toxic, and expensive therapy being withheld.[61] An elevated CA 125 prior to a second-look operation indicates a high chance of early progressive disease regardless of the second surgical procedure. A confirmed doubling from the upper limit of normal during follow-up predicts relapse with almost 100 per cent specificity.[62] There is controversy about the role of serial CA 125 measurements during follow-up with the anxiety from knowing CA 125 levels inducing 'CA 125 psychosis' in some patients. Although the use of CA 125 estimation to define progression may reduce the number of radiological investigations performed, there is no evidence at present that early reintroduction of chemotherapy or searching for a resectable site of relapse produces any survival benefit. A large Medical Research Council and EORTC trial is currently withholding

all serial CA 125 results from clinicians and patients during follow-up until the levels double. Patients are then randomized between immediate therapy or the clinician not being informed of the result so the patient continues on observation. Until the results of this trial are available, monitoring by CA 125 during follow-up should be discouraged.

Other markers for ovarian cancer

A number of other markers have been found to be elevated in a proportion of patients with ovarian carcinoma.[56] These include the breast carcinoma-associated mucins such as CASA, OVX1, and HMFG2, cytokeratin proliferation markers such as tissue polypeptide antigen, as well as placental alkaline phosphatase, TATI, CA 19.9, TAG 72.3, LASA, IAP, CSF, ferritin, NB/70K, and galactosyl transferase. None of these markers have yet been shown to be as useful clinically as CA 125. Attempts to combine these markers with CA 125 have, in some studies, increased the sensitivity but have not yet found widespread clinical approval.

Cytokeratin proliferation markers

The cytokeratin proliferation markers include tissue polypeptide antigen (TPA) which is a mixture of different cytokeratins, tissue polypeptide-specific antigen which is epitope M3 of TPA, and CYFRA 21–1 which is an assay for the detection of a soluble cytokeratin 19 fragment.[63] TPA is elevated in the serum in the majority of patients with advanced breast, ovarian, cervical, bladder, and colorectal carcinomas. As it can also be elevated in response to inflammation and in liver disease, but not in most patients with early cancer, it has little diagnostic value. Serial measurements appear to be useful for the evaluation of therapy and early detection of relapse. Because of its low specificity, it has been studied in combination with a variety of other markers. In colorectal cancer it fails to improve on the use of carcinoembryonic antigen alone. When used with CA 125 in patients with ovarian carcinoma there is a slight increase in sensitivity, enabling a slightly greater proportion of patients to be monitored by serial measurements. CYFRA 21–1 is elevated in the serum and urine of many patients with bladder cancer and may be used to provide prognostic information and for monitoring the clinical course.[64]

Lipid-associated sialic acid (LASA)

Interest in sialoglycolipids (gangliosides) as tumour markers was generated by the discovery that circulating levels of these compounds were elevated in tumour-bearing animals, suggesting that the lipid-bound sialic acid was of tumour origin. Elevated levels of a variety of gangliosides have been documented in tumours and serum from patients with several types of cancer. A more rapid assay method for measuring lipid-associated sialic acid rather than individual serum gangliosides has been developed by Dianon Systems Inc.[65] Elevated levels were found in the majority of patients with cancer, ranging from 77 per cent of 111 patients with breast cancer to 97 per cent of 36 patients with sarcoma, but the mean level in patients with cancer was less than twice that of controls. In patients with ovarian cancer, the sensitivity and specificity of lipid-associated sialic acid in combination with CA 125 is improved over either marker alone.

Tumour-associated trypsin inhibitor (TATI)

This compound, which is possibly identical to pancreatic secretory trypsin inhibitor, was originally identified and isolated from the urine of a patient with ovarian carcinoma. Although elevated serum levels have been found in patients with a variety of cancers, including pancreatic and ovarian cancer, a higher proportion of such patients have elevated urine levels. Six out of ten patients with mucinous ovarian tumours had elevated urine levels, suggesting that tumour-associated trypsin inhibitor could be of value in monitoring patients with normal CA 125 levels.

Squamous cell carcinoma-associated antigen

Kato and colleagues developed a radioimmunoassay based on a polyclonal antibody raised against an antigen called TA-4 that had been purified from a cervical cancer tissue homogenate. A kit for this assay using a monoclonal antibody is available. Using a cut-off such that 93 to 95 per cent of female controls are within the normal range, elevated serum levels are found in approximately 25 per cent of patients with FIGO stage I squamous cell carcinoma of the cervix, rising to over 80 per cent in those with stage III or IV disease.[66] This marker is not sensitive enough to detect microinvasive disease and is therefore of no value in screening. Elevated levels of squamous cell carcinoma-associated antigen have been found in 5 to 14 per cent of pregnant women and in over 50 per cent of patients with impaired renal function. A variety of other tumours, especially those of squamous histology, such as bronchial, oesophageal, head and neck, and anal, are associated with elevated serum levels of this antigen if the tumours are advanced.

Squamous cell carcinoma-associated antigen levels correlate well with the response to therapy in those who have initial elevated levels, but more data are required before one could reliably change therapy because of an inadequate fall. Patients who develop recurrent disease have a significantly higher pretreatment level than those without recurrence. In a large study of patients with stage 1B or IIA disease, Duk et al.[67] found by Cox regression analysis that the preoperative squamous cell carcinoma-associated antigen level was the only independent factor to affect survival. This suggests that squamous cell carcinoma-associated antigen and possibly other markers such as CA 125 could help to indicate which early stage patients have a poor prognosis and might benefit from combined modality therapy. The other useful role for squamous cell carcinoma-associated antigen is where rising levels are seen in patients with symptoms compatible with recurrent disease but in whom scans are clear. These patients must have recurrent disease.

Neurone-specific enolase

Neurone-specific enolase is a specific neuronal isomer of a widely distributed glycolytic enzyme. It is found not only in neural tissues but in all amine precursor uptake and decarboxylation cells. Radioimmunoassay kits are available. Although elevated tissue levels of neurone-specific enolase are found in many neuroendocrine tumours, elevated serum levels are rarely found except in patients with neuroblastoma and small cell lung cancer.[68] Elevated levels were found in 39 per cent of 38 patients with limited-stage small cell lung cancer and in 87 per cent of 56 patients with extensive-stage small cell lung cancer. High levels can be of diagnostic value, but false-positive values can be caused by lysed erythrocytes. As serial levels correlate closely with a response to therapy, neurone-specific enolase can be used to monitor treatment if serial chest radiographs are unsatisfactory.

Markers for prostatic cancer

Prostate-specific antigen

Prostate-specific antigen is the most useful tumour marker in patients with prostate cancer. It is a serine protease produced by prostate epithelium with the function of liquefying the gel which surrounds spermatazoa to enable them to become fully mobile. In serum, some prostate-specific antigen is found free but most is complexed to serine protease inhibitors, protein C inhibitor or α_1-antichymotrypsin. The prostate-specific antigen gene is on chromosome 19 and its expression is partly regulated by the presence of androgen. In the circulation prostate-specific antigen has a 2- to 4-day terminal half-life so serum levels rapidly reflect the rate of production. Prostate-specific antigen has superseded prostatic acid phosphatase as it is elevated in a higher proportion of men with prostate cancer.

Diagnosis, screening, and staging

Elevated serum levels of prostate-specific antigen (greater than 4 ng/ml) occur in about 53 per cent of men with intracapsular microscopic, and 77 per cent of men with intracapsular macroscopic prostatic cancer, but can also occur in 30 to 50 per cent of men with benign prostatic hypertrophy, a condition common in men of similar age group to those who develop prostate cancer.[69] The combination of prostate-specific antigen and digital rectal examination, followed by prostatic ultrasound in patients with abnormal findings, is commonly used for screening in the United States but is not recommended in the United Kingdom as there is so far no evidence of survival benefit from early detection of prostate cancer. There is a vocal debate raging, with those who advocate screening stating that an individual with early prostate cancer may be cured by radical surgery or radiotherapy. Those against screening point out that despite a 9 per cent chance of developing clinical prostate cancer during a man's life, there is only a 1 per cent chance of dying from it and we cannot predict which cancers will be aggressive, so most patients will suffer the side-effects of therapy without any benefit. Furthermore, about 40 per cent of those patients with prostate-specific antigen levels of 4.0 to 9.9 ng/ml at screening will already have tumour spread outside the prostate.[70]

Several methods are being used to improve diagnostic specificity. The best appears to be the measurement of the ratio of free to total prostate-specific antigen as more of this antigen is protein bound in patients with prostate cancer than those with benign prostatic hypertrophy. The ratio of free to total prostate-specific antigen is low (about 10 per cent) in prostate cancer compared with more than 16 per cent in benign prostatic hypertrophy and prostatitis. Using this ratio increases the specificity for diagnosing prostate cancer from 30 to 61 per cent.[71] The observation that with advancing age, prostate-specific antigen levels rise in parallel with the enlarging size of the prostate has led to age-specific reference ranges being produced for this antigen.[72] Thus if the upper limit of normal for men in their 40s was lowered to 2.5 ng/ml, more prostatic cancers would be detected, and if the upper limit of normal for men in their 70s was raised to 6.5 ng/ml, many men would be spared further diagnostic procedures. Prostate-specific antigen density and prostate-specific antigen density of the transition zone rely on ultrasound size estimations leading to lack of precision, but some centres have shown this measurement to improve specificity. Another method is based on the observation that prostate-specific antigen levels generally rise by more than 20 per cent per annum in cases of malignancy.[73] The prostate-specific antigen velocity calculated from serial levels can improve specificity but at the expense of delaying diagnosis.

Prostate-specific antigen levels cannot be used to predict whether there is capsular invasion. A recently studied research tool is to use the ultrasensitive reverse transcriptase polymerase chain reaction to detect prostate-specific antigen gene expression on circulating prostate cells.[74] This technique might improve staging by detecting pre-operatively those patients with extracapsular extension who do not benefit from radical surgery. Patients with prostate-specific antigen levels of less than 20 ng/ml can be assumed to have no bone metastases and do not necessarily need bone scans. However, not all patients with a prostate-specific antigen of greater than 20 ng/ml will have distant metastases. Lymph node metastases are usually associated with elevated prostate-specific antigen.

Prognosis, monitoring response, and detection of recurrence

As the prostate-specific antigen level correlates with prostatic volume and tumour differentiation, it is not surprising that a high pre-treatment level of antigen is associated with a poor prognosis. Prostate-specific antigen levels fall rapidly to normal after complete removal of tumour by radical prostatectomy. The rate of fall is slower after successful radiotherapy or endocrine therapy. Although part of the decline of prostate-specific antigen levels after androgen ablation can be attributed to decreased gene expression, those patients whose post-treatment prostate-specific antigen nadir is less than 4 ng/ml have a significantly longer remission duration than those whose post-treatment nadirs remain elevated.[75] Serial prostate-specific antigen levels are more sensitive and cheaper than bone scans for assessing response to hormonal therapy. Because so few patients with hormone-refractory prostatic cancer have objective responses to cytotoxic chemotherapy, it is difficult to determine whether prostate-specific antigen is an accurate surrogate marker of response in these patients. In a study of 103 patients treated with suramin, reduction of prostate-specific antigen levels had a weak prognostic significance with respect to survival.[76] A serial rise in prostate-specific antigen frequently precedes other evidence of disease progression in the patient with a past history of prostate cancer. The development of back pain in the presence of an elevated prostate-specific antigen level suggests the development of bone metastases.

Paraproteins

Monoclonal immunoglobulins detectable by serum electrophoresis (M proteins) occur in the serum and/or urine of 98 per cent of patients with myeloma. The malignant plasma cell mass correlates with serum M-protein levels, which can therefore be used to monitor the response to therapy. Evidence of radiological bone lesions and marrow infiltration is required to confirm the diagnosis of myeloma because M proteins are also found in patients with other B-cell neoplasms and in 0.9 per cent of asymptomatic adults over the age of 25. The prevalence of these proteins increases with age (Chapter 15.13).

Hormones

Several tumours of endocrine tissue can be diagnosed and their therapy monitored through the measurement of their eutopically produced hormones, which are increased following malignant transformation. Measurement of calcitonin and calcitonin gene-related peptide are used in the screening of families for medullary carcinoma of the thyroid. Screening for the catecholamine metabolites, vanillylmandelic acid and homovanillic acid, is used to detect neuroblastoma. Phaeochromocytomas and the 50 per cent of adrenal cortical carcinomas that are functional are other examples of endocrine tumours producing eutopic hormones. The many different gastrointestinal endocrine tumours which may be diagnosed by detection of increased levels of specific gut polypeptides are discussed elsewhere (Chapter 19.5).

Carcinoid tumours are also neuroendocrine tumours, which can be diagnosed and monitored by measurement of the serotonin metabolite 5-hydroxyindoleacetic acid in the urine. The measurement of ectopic hormones such as parathyroid hormone and parathyroid hormone-like protein is of clinical value in confirming the cause of hypercalcaemia rather than in monitoring tumours.

Tumour-associated markers

There are many circulating compounds which, despite being produced by normal rather than tumour cells, have been assessed for potential as tumour markers. The erythrocyte sedimentation rate can be used as a crude indicator of active disease in many patients with lymphoma and in myeloma. It may be an inaccurate guide for therapy as it can be influenced by too many factors. Acute-phase reactant proteins such as C-reactive protein, 1-acid glycoprotein, antichymotrypsin, and haptoglobin increase their plasma concentrations in response to a wide variety of stimuli. Although their levels have been reported to correlate with the progress of many tumours, especially lymphomas and leukaemias, it is debatable whether they add any useful clinical information.

Circulating immune complex concentrations are frequently elevated in malignant disease and have been shown to give prognostic indications. However, because of the many conditions in which they are elevated, the relationship between tumour burden and circulating immune complexes is not clear. Serum levels of β_2-microglobulins are elevated in a variety of malignancies and in renal impairment.

They have been shown to be a powerful prognostic indicator in patients with myeloma and lymphoma.

Polyamine levels in normal and tumour cells vary in response to cell growth, proliferation, and differentiation. Red cell and urinary spermadine and putricine levels have been shown to alter when tumours respond to chemotherapy, but their lack of specificity has prevented their general acceptance. Pteridines are produced by proliferating cells and activated T lymphocytes. The pteridine, neopterin, has been used both as a tumour marker and as an indicator of the effects of immune modulators. The tissue enzyme, lactate dehydrogenase, or its isoenzyme, hydroxybutyrate dehydrogenase, has been found to be useful for monitoring some patients with germ cell tumours not producing hCG or α-fetoprotein. Lactate dehydrogenase has also been found to be a useful prognostic indicator, especially in patients with germ cell tumours and lymphomas. Other tissue enzymes, such as γ-glutamyl transpeptidase and alkaline phosphatase, are sometimes useful for monitoring tumours.

New blood vessel development is required for tumour cell proliferation. It is not therefore surprising that elevated levels of angiogenic factors have been detected in the serum and urine of patients with various types of cancer. In one study 57 per cent of 132 patients with cancer had elevated levels of either basic fibroblast growth factor and/or vascular endothelial growth factor and levels tended to rise in those patients with tumour progression.[77] The introduction of antiangiogenesis and vascular targeting agents is likely to increase interest in these growth factors.

Conclusion

Hybridoma technology has led to a rapid increase in the number of circulating tumour markers that need to be evaluated clinically. The ever-increasing costs of health care make it mandatory that more studies are carried out to demonstrate how the use of new, as well as more established, tumour markers can make an impact on clinical decision-making. Most tumour markers are elevated in more than just one tumour type and are of limited diagnostic potential. However, a panel of markers can sometimes help in diagnosing the primary site of a metastatic tumour arising from a potentially treatable cancer, such as germ cell or prostatic cancer (see Section 20). Finding an elevated marker can help in monitoring therapy but should only be used in follow-up if its use has impact on survival. There is no doubt as to the value of human chorionic gonadotrophin and α-fetoprotein in the management of patients with trophoblastic or germ cell tumours, immunoglobulins in patients with myeloma, and CA 125 in patients with advanced ovarian cancer. The uncertainty as to the value of carcinoembryonic antigen in colorectal carcinoma, prostate-specific antigen in prostatic cancer, and mucins in breast carcinoma is partly due to the small amount of benefit derived from changing therapy as a result of tumour marker information. Improvements in therapy of the common solid tumours are likely to increase the need for tumour marker measurements. These measurements would, hopefully, lead to a reduction in the use of radiological and other tumour-imaging methods.

References

1. **Bence Jones H.** *Philosophical Transactions of the Royal Society of London*, 1848; **138**: 55–62.

2. **Ascheim S.** Early diagnosis of pregnancy, chorionepithelioma and hydatidiform mole by the Ascheim–Zondek test. *American Journal of Obstetrics and Gynecology*, 1930, **19**: 335.

3. **Bagshawe KD.** Comments on the measurement of HCG as a tumour specific substance. In: Holland JF, Hreschchyshyn MM, eds. *Choriocarcinoma*, UICC Monograph Series, Vol. 3. Berlin: Springer Verlag, 1967: 109–11.

4. **Bagshawe KD.** *Choriocarcinoma: the Clinical Biology of the Trophoblast and its Tumours.* London: Edward Arnold, 1969.

5. **Vogelzang NJ,** *et al.* Acute changes of α-feta protein and human chorionic gonadotrophin during induction chemotherapy of germ cell tumours. *Cancer Research*, 1982; **42**: 4855–61.

6. **Bagshawe KD.** Tumour markers: where do we go from here? *British Journal of Cancer*, 1983; **48**: 167–75.

7. **Mulcahy HE, Croke DT, Farthing MJG.** Cancer and mutant DNA in blood plasma. *Lancet*, 1996; **348**: 628.

8. **Rustin GJS,** *et al.* Defining response of ovarian carcinoma to initial chemotherapy according to serum CA 125. *Journal of Clinical Oncology*, 1995; **14**: 1545–51.

9. **Braunstein GD, Vaitukaitis JL, Carbone PP, Ross GT.** Ectopic production of human chorionic gonadotrophin by neoplasms. *Annals of Internal Medicine*, 1973; **78**: 39–45.

10. **Nishimura R,** *et al.* Characterisation of human chorionic gonadotropin in urine of patients with trophoblastic diseases by Western blotting using specific antibodies. *Japanese Journal of Cancer Research (Gann)*, 1987; **78**: 833–9.

11. **Gaspard U,** *et al.* Serum concentration of human chorionic gonadotropin and its α and β subunits. 2. Trophoblastic tumours. *Clinical Endocrinology*, 1980; **13**: 319–29.

12. **Wehmann RE, Nisula BC.** Metabolic and renal clearance rates of purified human chorionic gonadotropin. *Journal of Clinical Investigation*, 1981; **68**: 184–93.

13. **Borkowski A, Muquardt C.** Human chorionic gonadotropin in the plasma of normal, non-pregnant subjects. *New England Journal of Medicine*, 1979; **301**: 298–302.

14. **Bagshawe KD, Harland S.** Immunodiagnosis and monitoring of gonadotrophin producing metastases in the central nervous system. *Cancer*, 1976; **38**: 112–18.

15. **Bagshawe KD.** Risk and prognostic factors in trophoblastic neoplasia. *Cancer*, 1976; **38**: 1373–85.

16. **Bagshawe KD, Dent J, Webb J.** Hydatidiform mole in England and Wales 1973–1983. *Lancet*, 1986; **ii**: 673–7.

17. **Rustin GJS, Vogelzang NJ, Sleijfer DT, Nisselbaum SN.** Consensus statement on circulating tumour markers and staging of patients with germ cell tumours. In: *Prostate Cancer and Testicular Cancer*, EORTC Genito-urinary Group Monograph 7. New York: A.R. Liss, 1990: 277–88.

18. **Germa-Lluch JR, Begent RHJ, Bagshawe KD.** Tumour marker levels and prognosis in malignant teratoma of the testis. *British Journal of Cancer*, 1980; **42**: 850–5.

19. **The International Germ Cell Collaborative Group (IGCCG),** International Germ Cell Consensus Classification. A prognostic factor-based staging system for metastatic germ cell tumours. *Journal of Clinical Oncology*, 1997; **15**: 594–603.

20. **Birken S,** *et al.* The structure of human chorionic gonadotropin β core fragment from pregnancy urine. *Endocrinology*, 1988; **123**: 572–83.

21. **Wehmann RE, Blithe DL, Akar AH, Nisula BC.** β-Core fragments are contaminants of the World Health Organization Reference Preparations of human choriogonadotrophin and its α-subunit. *Journal of Endocrinology*, 1988; **117**: 147–52.

22. **Kardana A, Cole LA.** Serum hCG and β-core fragment is masked by associated macromolecules. *Journal of Clinical Endocrinology and Metabolism*, 1990; **71**: 1393–5.

23. Cole LA, Schwartz PE, Wang Y. Urinary gonadotropin fragments (UGF) in cancers of the female reproductive system. *Gynecologic Oncology*, 1988; **31**: 82–90.

24. Crawford SM, *et al.* Is ectopic production of human chorionic gonadotrophin (hCG) or α-fetoprotein (AFP) by tumour markers a marker of chemosensitivity? *European Journal of Cancer and Clinical Oncology*, 1986; **22**: 1483–7.

25. Fisher RA, *et al.* Gestational and nongestational trophoblastic tumours distinguished by DNA analysis. *Cancer*, 1992; **69**: 839–45.

26. Ruoslahtie E, Seppala M. α-Fetoprotein in cancer and fetal development. *Advances in Cancer Research*, 1979; **29**: 275–346.

27. Coppack S, *et al.* Problems of interpretation of serum concentrations of α-fetoprotein (AFP) in patients receiving cytotoxic chemotherapy for malignant germ cell tumours. *British Journal of Cancer*, 1983; **48**: 335–40.

28. Sato Y, *et al.* Early recognition of hepatocellular carcinoma based on altered profiles of α-fetoprotein. *New England Journal of Medicine*, 1993; **328**: 1802–10.

29. Fishman WH, Inglis NR, Stolbach LL, Krant MJ. A serum alkaline phosphatase isoenzyme of human neoplastic cell origin. *Cancer Research*, 1968; **28**: 150–4.

30. Nielson OS, *et al.* Is placental alkaline phosphatase (PLAP) a useful marker for seminoma? *European Journal of Cancer*, 1990; **26**: 1049–54.

31. Gold P, Freedman DS. Specific carcinoembryonic antigens of the human digestive system. *Journal of Experimental Medicine*, 1965; **122**: 468–81.

32. Begent RHJ, Rustin GJS. Tumour markers: from carcinoembryonic antigen to products of hybridoma technology. *Cancer Surveys*, 1989; **8**: 108–21.

33. American Society of Clinical Oncology. Clinical Practice Guidelines for the use of tumour markers in breast and colorectal cancer. *Journal of Clinical Oncology*, 1996; **14**: 2843–77.

34. Dilowari JB, Lennard-Jones JE, MacKay AM. Estimation of carcinoembryonic antigen in ulcerative colitis with special reference to malignant change. *Gut*, 1975; **16**: 255–60.

35. Doos WG, *et al.* CEA levels in patients with colorectal polyps. *Cancer*, 1975; **36**: 1996–2003.

36. Ziegenbein R, Jacobash KH, Pilgram G. Determination of CEA in plasma of patients with colorectal carcinoma and polyps. *Archiv für Geschwulstforschung*, 1980; **50**: 165–8.

37. Hansen J, *et al.* Carcinoembryonic antigen (CEA) assay: laboratory adjunct in the diagnosis and management of cancer. *Human Pathology*, 1974; **5**: 139–47.

38. Allen-Mersh TG, *et al.* Significance of a fall in serum CEA concentration in patients treated with cytotoxic chemotherapy for disseminated colorectal cancer. *Gut*, 1987; **28**: 1625–9.

39. Mayer RJ, *et al.* Carcinoembryonic antigen (CEA) as a monitor of chemotherapy in disseminated colorectal cancer. *Cancer*, 1978; **42**: 1428–33.

40. McCall JL, *et al.* The value of serum carcinoembryonic antigen in predicting recurrent disease following curative resection of colorectal cancer. *Diseases of the Colon and Rectum*, 1994; **37**: 875–81.

41. Bruinvels DJ, *et al.* Follow up of patients with colorectal cancer. *Annals of Surgery*, 1994; **219**: 174–82.

42. Minton JP, Hoehn JL, Gerber DM. Results of a 400 patient carcinoembryonic antigen second-look colorectal cancer study. *Cancer*, 1985; **55**: 1284–90.

43. Kjeldsen BJ, Kronborg O, Fenger C, Jorgensen OD. A prospective randomised study of follow-up after radical surgery for colorectal cancer. *British Journal of Surgery*, 1997; **84**: 666–9.

44. Shoemaker D, Black R, Giles L, Toouli J. Yearly colonoscopy, liver CT and chest radiography do not influence five year survival of colorectal cancer patients. *Gastroenterology*, 1998; **114**: 7–14.

45. Lennon T, Houghton J, Northover J on behalf of the CRC/NIH CEA Trial Working Party. *British Journal of Cancer*, 1994; **70**: 16.

46. Ritts RE Jr, *et al.* Initial clinical evaluation of an immunoradiometric assay for Ca 19-9 using the NCI serum bank. *International Journal of Cancer*, 1984; **33**: 339–45.

47. Holmgren J, *et al.* Detection by monoclonal antibody of carbohydrate antigen CA 50 in serum of patients with carcinoma. *British Medical Journal*, 1984; **228**: 1479–82.

48. Kenemans P, Bast RC, Yedema CA, Price MR, Hilgers J. CA 125 and polymorphic epithelial mucin as serum tumor markers. *Cancer Reviews*, 1988; **11–12**: 119–44.

49. Kufe D, *et al.* Differential reactivity of a novel monoclonal antibody (DF3) with human malignant versus benign breast tumours. *Hybridoma*, 1984; **3**: 223–32.

50. O'Brien DP, *et al.* CA1-53: a reliable indicator of metastatic bone disease in breast cancer patients. *Annals of the Royal College of Surgeons of England*, 1992; **74**: 9–12.

51. Safi F, *et al.* Comparison of CA1-53 in CEA in diagnosis and monitoring of breast cancer. *International Journal of Biological Markers*, 1989; **4**: 207–14.

52. Bast RC, *et al.* A radioimmunoassay using a monoclonal antibody to monitor the course of epithelial ovarian cancer. *New England Journal of Medicine*, 1983; **309**: 883–7.

53. Kabawat SE, Bast RC, Welch WR, Knapp RC, Colvin RB. Immunopathologic characterisation of a monoclonal antibody that recognises common surface antigens of human ovarian tumours of serous, endometroid and clear cell types. *American Journal of Clinical Pathology*, 1983; **79**: 1.

54. Canney PA, Moore M, Wilkinson PM, James RD. Ovarian cancer antigen CA 125: a prospective clinical assessment of its role as a tumour marker. *British Journal of Cancer*, 1984; **50**: 765–9.

55. Bast RC, Hunter V, Knapp RC. Pros and cons of gynecologic tumour markers. *Cancer*, 1987; **60**: 1984–92.

56. Tuxen MK, Soletormos G, Dombernowsky P. Tumor markers in the management of patients with ovarian cancer. *Cancer Treatment Reviews*, 1995; **21**: 215–45.

57. Jacobs I, *et al.* Prevalence screening for ovarian cancer in postmenopausal women by CA125 measurements and ultrasonography. *British Medical Journal*, 1993; **306**: 1030–4.

58. Jacobs I, Oram D, Fairbanks J, Turner J, Frost C, Grudzinskas J. Systematic evaluation of clinical criteria, ultrasonography and Ca 125 to achieve accurate preoperative diagnosis of ovarian cancer. *British Journal of Obstetrics and Gynaecology*, 1990; **97**: 922–9.

59. Nagele F, *et al.* Preoperative CA 125: an independent prognostic factor in patients with stage 1 epithelial ovarian cancer. *Obstetrics and Gynaecology*, 1995; **86**: 259–64.

60. Fayers PM, *et al.* The prognostic value of serum CA125 in patients with advanced ovarian carcinoma: an analysis of 573 patients by the Medical Research Council Working Party on Gynaecological Cancer. *International Journal of Gynecological Cancer*, 1993; **3**: 285–92.

61. Rustin GJS, Nelstrop A, Stilwell J, Lambert HE. Savings obtained by CA125 measurements during therapy for ovarian carcinoma. *European Journal of Cancer*, 1992; **28**: 79–82.

62. Rustin GJS, Nelstrop A, Tuxen MK, Lambert HJ. Defining progression of ovarian carcinoma during follow-up according to CA 125: a North Thames Ovary Group study. *Annals of Oncology*, 1996; **7**: 361–4.

63. Sundstrom BE, Stigbrand TI. Cytokeratins and tissue polypeptide antigen. *International Journal of Biological Markers*, 1994; **9**: 102–8.

64. Morita T, Kikuchi T, Hashimoto S, Kobayashi Y, Tokue A. Cytokeratin-19 fragment (CYFRA 21-1) in bladder cancer. *European Urology*, 1997; **32**: 237–44.

65. Katopodis N, Hirshaut Y, Geller NL, Stock CC. Lipid-associated sialic acid test for the detection of human cancer. *Cancer Research*, 1982; **42**: 5270–5.

66. **Kato H, Torigue T.** Radioimmunoassay for tumour antigen of human cervical squamous cell carcinoma. *Cancer,* 1977; **40**: 1621–8.

67. **Duk JM,** *et al.* Pretreatment serum squamous cell carcinoma antigen: a newly identified prognostic factor in early-stage cervical carcinoma. *Journal of Clinical Oncology,* 1996; **14**: 111–18.

68. **Carney DN,** *et al.* Serum neuron-specific enolase: a marker for disease extent and response to therapy of small-cell lung cancer. *Lancet,* 1982; ii: 583–5.

69. **Dorr VJ, Williamson SK, Stephens RL.** An evaluation of prostate-specific antigen as a screening test for prostate cancer. *Archives of Internal Medicine,* 1993; **153**: 2529–37.

70. **Catalona WJ,** *et al.* Measurement of prostate-specific antigen in serum as a screening test for prostate cancer. *New England Journal of Medicine,* 1991; **324**: 1156–61.

71. **Froschermaier SE, Pilarsky CP, Wirth MP.** Clinical significance of the determination of noncomplexed prostate-specific antigen as a marker for prostate carcinoma. *Urology,* 1996; **47**: 525–8.

72. **Oesterling JE, Lilja H.** Prostate-specific antigen: the value of molecular forms and age-specific reference ranges. In: Vogelzang NJ, Scardino PT, Shipley WU, Coffey DS, eds. *Comprehensive Textbook of Genitourinary Oncology.* Baltimore: Williams & Wilkins, 1996: 668–80.

73. **Pearson JD, Carter HB.** Natural history of changes in prostate specific antigen in early stage prostate cancer. *Journal of Urology,* 1994; **152**: 1743–8.

74. **Olsson CA,** *et al.* The use of RT-PCR for prostate-specific antigen assay to predict potential surgical failures before radical prostatectomy; molecular staging of prostate cancer. *British Journal of Urology,* 1996; **77**: 411–17.

75. **Miller JI,** *et al.* The clinical usefulness of serum prostate specific antigen after hormonal therapy of metastatic cancer. *Journal of Urology,* 1992; **147**: 956–61.

76. **Sridhara R, Eisenberger MA, Sinibaldi VJ, Reyno LM, Egorin MJ.** Evaluation of prostate-specific antigen as a surrogate marker for response of hormone refractory prostate cancer to suramin therapy. *Journal of Clinical Oncology,* 1995; **13**: 2944–53.

77. **Dirix LY,** *et al.* Elevated levels of the angiogenic cytokines basic fibroblast growth factor and vascular endothelial growth factor in sera of cancer patients. *British Journal of Cancer,* 1997; **76**: 238–43.

Staging

Martin Werner and Heinz Höfler

Staging

Cancer is characterized by the uncontrolled proliferation and, at least locally, aggressive growth of tumour cells. The expanding cancer cells are not usually detected before they have produced a clinically detectable mass with a volume of several mm³ or cm³. The neoplastic tissue may then still be confined to a particular organ or anatomical site. Often, however, there has already been invasion of surrounding organs or production of metastases. Appraising the extent of local invasion or distant metastasis of a tumour, i.e. staging, has become one of the most important elements in oncology. Tumour stage, besides the histogenetic classification and grading, determines the prognosis and guides decisions about therapy in an individual patient. Apart from the impact on treatment strategies or prognosis, staging also assists in evaluating the results of treatment, or in exchanging patient data between different hospitals or cancer centres. Moreover, correlation to the stage is necessary for the interpretation of results from investigations in oncological research.

Neoplasia may evolve in any organ or tissue of the human body. Each organ has a unique anatomical configuration and relationship to other organs, as well as its own particular supply from blood vessels and lymphatic channels. This implies site-specific differences in the patterns of both local spread and potential metastatic progress. The classification schemes for tumours by stage as proposed by national or international cancer committees and oncological associations, therefore, comprise specific recommendations for each organ or tissue.

Among the commonly applied schemes in oncology are the classifications proposed by the International Union Against Cancer (**UICC**), the American Joint Committee on Cancer (**AJCC**), and the Fédération Internationale de Gynécologie et d'Obstétrique (**FIGO**).[1]–[4] These classifications are the worldwide basis for the selection of an appropriate treatment by clinical staging, whereas pathological staging helps in assessing the prognostic factors. It is the aim of this chapter to explain the general rules of the most commonly used updated UICC TNM system.[1] Moreover, the problems of a variable interpretation hampering standardization, or of the differences that may emerge between the clinical and pathological staging, are discussed. Further detailed explanation of the TNM/pTNM classification, which is helpful when using the system on a daily basis, has been published by the UICC in the TNM supplement.[5] More information on the prognostic value of TNM staging is provided for cancer at most tumour sites in a UICC monograph.[6]

TNM classification—general rules

In 1997 the fifth edition of the TNM system was published, which corresponded exactly to the fifth edition of the *AJCC Cancer staging manual*.[1],[2] The updated TNM system is the result of a number of consultative editorial meetings by the members of the TNM Prognostic Factors Project Committee as well as national committees and international organizations. This close liason by all committees guarantees the overall acceptance of the classification system. It is a continuing objective of the UICC to revise the TNM system if major advances in diagnosis or treatment require reconsideration of the current classification.

In the TNM scheme, the term 'T' represents the primary tumour, 'N' the regional lymph nodes, and 'M' the distant metastases. In general, the dual TNM system defines for each site a pretreatment clinical classification and a postsurgical histopathological classification. The clinical classification (cTNM or TNM) is based on physical examination, imaging, endoscopy, and biopsy. Pathological classification is designated pTNM, and results from pathological (macroscopic and microscopic) evaluation of surgically resected specimens or biopsies. For most tumours, the standard surgical treatment includes the resection of both the primary tumour and the regional lymph nodes (Fig. 1) whereas distant deposits are only biopsied if there is clinical suspicion of metastasis. Therefore, pathological staging in the main describes the primary tumour and its regional lymph nodes.

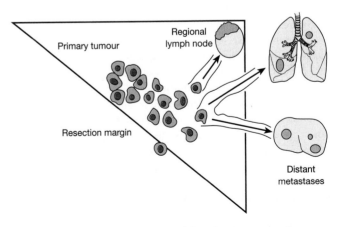

Fig. 1 In most tumour sites, resection of the primary tumour and dissection of regional lymph nodes is performed as standard therapy.

Primary tumour

The T/pT classification includes size and local invasion of the primary tumour. At some sites, penetration of the visceral serosa is an important criterion, i.e. penetration of the visceral pleura (lung) or peritoneum (e.g. stomach, colorectum). Cancer cells in effusions qualify for a higher pT category in ovarian carcinoma and lung. In liver and kidney, the microscopic evidence of tumour invasion to veins is a pT criterion. At some sites, multiple tumours may develop simultaneously, e.g. unilateral multicentric breast cancer or several colorectal carcinomas in patients with familial adenomatous polyposis. In these cases, the tumour with the highest category is classified and the multiplicity or number of tumours is indicated in parentheses, for instance pT3(m) or pT3(4).

The pT classification requires sufficient surgically resected tissue to determine the highest category, i.e. the entire tumour has to be removed and sent complete and without incisions to the pathologist for gross and microscopic examination. It is important that the incision of the tumour specimen is performed by the pathologist. If the pathologist receives a resection specimen which has already been cut, then exact determination of the pT classification and the tumour margins may be impossible. The situation is even worse if the incised specimen has been fixed, since retraction of the tissue occurs during fixation making the topographical assessment of the tumour and resection margins impossible. If the primary tumour cannot be assessed the category is TX.

Regional lymph nodes

The N/pN classification describes the absence or presence and extent of regional lymph node metastases. Complete resection of the regional lymph nodes by the surgeon and thorough sampling by the pathologist is necessary to ensure that the entire lymph node compartment containing all possible metastases has been removed. Therefore, for some sites the examination of a minimum number of lymph nodes is mandatory to define the postsurgical pN0 category, for instance 12 lymph nodes in colorectal, 10 in head and neck tumours with radical neck dissection, or six in thyroid, lung, vulva, or breast cancer. Otherwise, the classification is pNX. The numbers of lymph nodes required for the pN classification reflect the minimum numbers providing statistical significance at the different anatomical sites (Table 1). It is important that the pathologist's report mentions the ratio of regional lymph nodes with and without metastases. This ratio may also be added in parentheses to the pN classification, e.g. metastases in 2/14 regional lymph nodes: pN1(2/14).

Apart from the number of regional lymph nodes involved, the assessment of the greatest dimension of the metastasis (e.g. in head and neck tumours), and even of an extension beyond the lymph node capsule (in breast cancer) may be important. In breast cancer, small lymph node metastases (so-called micrometastases < 0.2 cm) are classified as pN1a. Micrometastases induce a stromal reaction within the lymph node (Fig. 2). In contrast, tumour cell emboli in the lymph node sinus, for example microinvolvement of the lymph node confined to endothelium-lined spaces, do not display reactions in the surrounding stroma. The latter situation is classified as pN0. The significance of a microinvolvement of regional lymph nodes has not yet been established, but there might

Table 1 Minimum number of lymph nodes required for the pN0 category[1]

Site	Number of lymph nodes
Lip and oral cavity	6
Pharynx	6
Larynx	6*/10†
Paranasal sinus	6*/10†
Salivary gland	6*/10†
Thyroid gland	6
Oesophagus	6
Stomach	15
Small intestine	6
Colon and rectum	12
Anal canal	12‡/6§
Liver	3
Gallbladder	3
Extrahepatic bile ducts	3
Pancreas	10
Lung	6
Skin	6
Breast	6
Vulva	6
Vagina	6§/10¶
Cervix	10
Corpus uteri	10
Ovary	10
Fallopian tube	10

*Selective neck dissection.

†Radical or modified radical neck dissection.

‡Perirectal–pelvic lymphadenectomy.

§Inguinal lymphadenectomy.

¶Pelvic lymphadenectomy.

be no difference from lymph nodes without tumour emboli within the sinus.[7,8]

Sentinel lymph nodes

A recent development is the application of sentinel lymph node biopsy to cN0 patients in order to investigate the regional lymph node(s) most likely to harbour metastases. With this approach, either a radioactive (^{99}Tc^m) or visual (isosulfan blue) tracer is injected into the area of the primary tumour. The tracer courses through the lymphatics to the regional lymph nodes, and the first (sentinel) lymph node labelled with the tracer can be detected intraoperatively. Currently, the first applications of sentinel lymphadenectomy are in melanoma and breast cancer.[9,10] Using radiolabelling, the sentinel

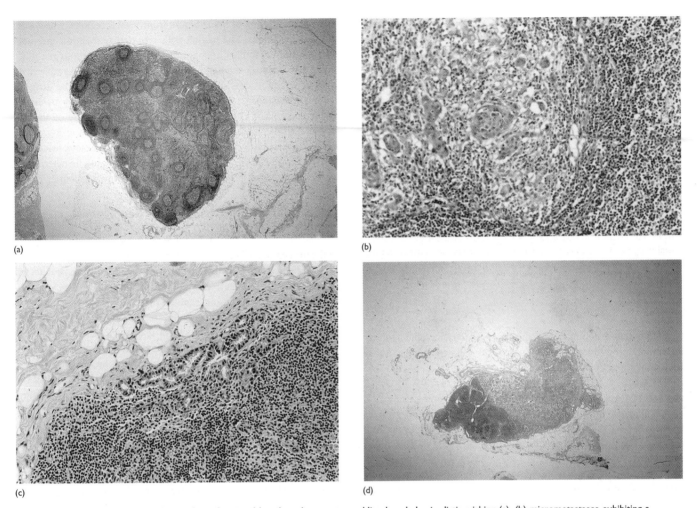

Fig. 2 The pN category reports the number of regional lymph node metastases. Histology helps in distinguishing (a), (b) micrometastases exhibiting a surrounding stromal reaction (= pN1) from (c) microinvolvement of tumour cells that are confined to the endothelial lined spaces (= pN0(it)). Lymph node metastasis (d) of a breast carcinoma less than 2 cm and with extension beyound the capsule (= pN1biii).

lymph node can be determined in more than 80 per cent of the breast cancer patients and has a highly predictive value for axillary lymph node status (< 90 per cent). However, extensive histo-pathological examination, for example in step sections, is necessary to exclude micrometastases.[11]

Apart from the examination of routinely stained serial sections, immunostaining for keratins may also be applied to paraffin sections of sentinel lymph nodes. This technique is helpful in quickly identifying small tumour cell groups. The discrimination between tumour microinvolvement (pN0) and micrometastasis (pN1, see above) is only possible by assessing a stromal reaction surrounding the tumour cells which is characteristic of true metastasis. So far, sentinel lymph nodes are not covered by the UICC classification since for most sites an examination of a certain number of lymph nodes is necessary for a valid pN category.

Distant metastases

Absence or presence of distant metastases is covered by the M/pM classification. This may also comprise cytology from the peritoneal cavity performed prior to surgery, except for ovarian cancer where it is classified in the T category. Apart from MX (distant metastasis cannot be assessed), there are only two categories, M0 for absence and M1 for presence of metastatic deposits. The exact localization of a metastasis can be specified by notating for instance PUL, OSS, or HEP for pulmonary, osseous, or hepatic metastasis respectively. Distant metastases should be confirmed by biopsy. If T4 tumours invade new areas of lymphatic dissemination, a lymph node metastasis in this new area should be designated as N1.

Stage grouping

Usually, after assessing the T, N, and M and/or pT, pN, and pM categories, these are grouped into stages. This final grouping comprises stages I to IV including substages. In general, the stage increases with the local and metastatic expansion of the tumour. In most organs, stage grouping is the predominant criterion for the choice of treatment. For instance, non-small-cell lung cancer tumours of stage I and II (or IIIa) are usually treated by surgical resection, whereas systemic chemo-therapy or radiation is applied to advanced stages III and IV. There is only one stage grouping for each anatomical site with the exception of thyroid gland tumours where—depending upon the histological

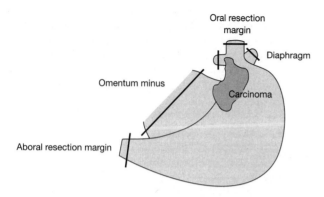

Fig. 3 The histopathological examination of the margins of a surgically removed tumour specimen includes a thorough sampling of all the resection margins. For instance, in gastrectomy specimens this includes the oral and aboral margins, i.e. the total circumference of the distal oesophagus and the proximal duodenum, and the margins close to the omentum minus and the diaphragm.

type—different groupings are defined for papillary or follicular, medullary, and undifferentiated carcinoma. No stage grouping exists so far for most ophthalmic tumours.

The term 'stage' applies to combinations of T, N, and M or pT, pN, and pM as well as to combinations of clinical and pathological TNM categories. Staging under certain circumstances may even be possible if the T or N categories cannot be determined.[5] In the fifth edition of the UICC TNM classification the stage grouping of tumours at most sites has been revised in order to give a better correlation with the clinical outcome for patients.[1] These revisions include tumours of the head and neck, salivary glands, lung, and soft tissues as well as some tumours of the digestive system and gynaecological and urological tumours. At some sites, only a few stage groups have been changed, for example in the stomach where the advanced stages III and IV have been newly defined. At other sites the stage grouping has been completely revised, for example the pancreas and fallopian tube.

R classification

The presence of residual (R) tumour after therapy is one of the best prognostic factors.[12] The R classification after surgical removal of the primary tumour includes the careful macroscopic and microscopic examination of the resection margins. Macroscopic evidence of residual cancer at the margin of a resection specimen not removed surgically is called R2. Optimally, macroscopic residual tumour is biopsied and assessed histologically. Tumour at the resection margin proved only histologically is defined as R1. A thorough sampling of all margins of a tumour specimen is necessary to obtain reliable results (Fig. 3). For a better identification of the definite resection margins in tissue sections, the margin may be marked by ink or 'Tippex' prior to sampling of the tissue blocks. The use of different dyes, for example black, blue, red, or green ink, is helpful in defining margins at varying anatomical locations. Depending on the tumour site, there may be some instances where histological examination of resection margins needs to be more extensive to exclude the presence of residual tumour. In lumpectomy specimens for breast cancer, for instance, the entire outer surface represents the resection margin.

Thorough sampling of tissue blocks from several regions is necessary in those specimens. The pathologist's report may mention the exact distance and anatomical topography of the closest tumour margin.

R2 also includes residual cancer at distant sites, for example liver, lung, or bone metastasis, that has not been removed by the surgeon. Distant metastasis may be confirmed in a small biopsy by histopathological examination. Residual tumour after non-surgical therapy is also classified as R2. The R classification cannot be assessed in a tumour resected in two or more parts which are not exactly orientated topographically (RX). The final R classification should be determined by the person who has access to all the data from a patient.

Additional classifications and descriptors

Serum tumour markers (see Chapter 3.4)

In the fifth edition of the TNM system, classification for some tumour sites has been revised to introduce serum markers that can be detected biochemically.[1] In germ cell tumours of the testis a new category designated S (serum tumour markers) has been added to the TNM scheme. The S classification uses the serum levels of LDH, human chorionic gonadotrophin, and alpha-fetoprotein in grouping the definite stage without influencing the anatomical categories. Similarly, the classification for gestational trophoblastic tumours incorporates serum levels of human chorionic gonadotrophin and duration of the disease as risk factors that have impact on the definite stage grouping.

L and V classification

Other optional classifications include the L and V classification for lymphatic and venous invasion respectively. Assessing the presence or absence of tumour cells (single or groups) within lymphatic or venous vessels requires an intensive microscopic examination of the primary tumour and the surrounding tissue, because the invasion of the vessel may be focal. Moreover, in thin-walled vessels the differentiation of lymphatic and venous channels can be difficult. After tissue fixation and processing, artificial spaces between tumour cell groups and the encircling tissue may be evident. These spaces are shrinkage artefacts and must not be mistaken for tumour invasion. Only tumour cells within channels unequivocally lined with endothelium can be classified as lymphatic or venous invasion. Immunohistochemistry with antibodies against endothelial cells (factor VIII, CD31) is helpful in proving true vessel invasion. However, the application of this method in routine pathological staging is not justified since for most tumours the prognostic significance of vessel invasion is still unclear.

r and y symbols

Important symbols that are used as prefix to the TNM or pTNM categories are r for recurrent tumours classified after a disease-free interval, and y for tumours staged during or following radiotherapy, chemotherapy, or multimodality therapy. The r symbol can be used for a chronological documentation of TNM/pTNM during the course of the disease.

C factor

The certainity (C) factor indicates the validity of the TNM classification which can be based upon different diagnostic methods. The use of the C factor comprising five degrees (C1 to C5) is optional.

The C factor increases with the validity of the diagnostic procedure applied. A TNM classification concluded from standard diagnostic means, for example inspection, palpation, or standard radiography, is designated as C1. Evidence from special diagnostic means such as more sophisticated radiographic, scintigraphic, or ultrasonographic imaging techniques as well as endoscopy combined with biopsy or cytology is defined as C2, and surgical exploration including biopsy or cytology as C3. Pathological examination is equivalent to C4 and evidence from autopsy is defined as C5. The appropriate degree of C may be added to the TNM scheme, for instance pT3C4, N2C1, M1C2.

Grading

Histopathological grading of the primary tumour is included in the UICC classification for most sites. Well-differentiated tumours which closely resemble the tissue of origin are designated as G1, and moderately differentiated tumours are headed G2. Poorly and un-differentiated tumours are denoted G3 and G4 respectively. Grades 3 and 4 can be combined as G3–G4. No grading exists for thyroid cancer, gestational trophoblastic tumours, or tumours arising in the testis. For epithelial tumours of the ovary, a grade GB has been added defining borderline malignancy. In small biopsies, a reliable grading may be difficult due to scanty tumour tissue. The same applies for biopsies with crush artefacts. In those cases, the grade should be designated as GX (grade of differentiation cannot be assessed).

In general, a variety of cytological and histological features, among them similarity to the tissue of origin, tissue architecture, nuclear pleomorphism, mitosis, or necrosis, are evaluated for assessing the tumour grade. Grading is subjective and requires substantial experience from the pathologist. For better standardization and to reduce interobserver variability, different semiquantitative methods of grading have been proposed for various tumours. For example, grading systems have been published for breast carcinoma, prostate carcinoma, and soft tissue tumours.[13]–[16] The pathologist's report should mention the grading system applied.

Staging after preoperative non-surgical therapy

For locally advanced tumours at several sites, for example oesophagus, stomach, colorectum, liver, breast, or soft tissue, down-categorizing ('down-staging') can be achieved by preoperative chemotherapy and/or radiation. In these cases, neoadjuvant treatment leads to a reduction or shrinkage of the tumour mass which may result in a reduced anatomical extent and lower pT category if compared with the T classification prior to therapy. Therefore, combined modality treatment may increase the percentage of complete (R0) tumour resection and survival time in patients with locally advanced cancer. In addition to its effect on the primary tumour or metastases, this treatment is also suggested to eliminate potential systemic micrometastases.

In order to estimate the response to preoperative therapy, the staging has to be assessed again after treatment. Inflammation and scarring in the tumour area may hamper the various imaging or endoscopic techniques.[17] Therefore, pathological staging is very important for accurately determining the effect of preoperative therapy. Careful macroscopic examination of the resection specimen and comprehensive or even complete histological analysis of the tumour area is necessary to assess the number of viable tumour cells left after therapy (ypT). Scarring and inflammation may also be evident in

regional lymph nodes, suggesting response to treatment in metastases. However, histopathology after preoperative therapy can only approximately estimate the initial pTNM category. The true stage prior to the initiation of therapy, which is almost invariably assessed by imaging procedures, cannot be reliably determined histopathologically. It is as yet unclear whether the prognosis of patients after down-categorizing of their tumour is according to the preoperative or post-therapeutic TNM stage.

Examples of staging

Correct application of the TNM/pTNM classification is obligatory for reliable staging. Table 2 gives an example of a chronological documentation of the clinical and pathological staging in a patient with colon cancer primarily treated by hemicolectomy. In the course of the disease he developed a liver metastasis that was resected. Another example for staging of a tumour after non-surgical treatment is demonstrated in Table 3. This patient with oesophageal cancer had received radiotherapy and chemotherapy prior to oesophagectomy.

It is obvious that the data for the TNM and the R classification are derived from different sources. In each patient the findings elaborated by physical examination, imaging, surgery, and histopathology contribute to the TNM coding. It is important that all experts involved in the investigation of a certain patient share their findings on the particular case. The ultimate TNM and R classification as well as the stage grouping should be performed by the person who has access to the most complete data. In cancer centres, tumour classification is often determined in clinicopathological conferences with experts from different fields reviewing each case.

Problems of clinical staging

Clinical staging is often hampered by the sensitivity of the methods applied, for example physical examination, imaging, and endoscopy. During the last two or three decades, a major impact on estimating the anatomical extent of cancer prior to treatment has come from a variety of newly established, more and more sensitive, imaging techniques. Sonography, computed tomography, nuclear magnetic resonance, positron emission tomography, and angiography enable the detection of tumours at various sites. Endoscopy and endoscopic sonography are well suited to the localization of tumours in several organs such as the gastrointestinal tract, bronchial tree, or larynx. However, histopathological examination remains the gold standard for the TNM classification as well as for several important features of cancer, including the differentiation and grade of a tumour, which influence the choice of treatment. For a better interpretation of the data, the C factor (see above) should be added to each TNM classification.

In a few circumstances the diagnosis of malignancy based upon clinical investigations may be difficult. Figure 4 gives an example of contradictory diagnoses by clinical and pathological staging. The resolution of imaging techniques, for example of endoscopic sonography or computed tomography in gastrointestinal tumours, may not be sufficient to enable exact determination of the depth of tumour invasion and local spread. Penetration of the visceral serosa, which is an important criterion of the T category in several tumours, is not evident using imaging techniques and can only be determined

Table 2 Chronological documentation of the TNM/pTNM classification in a patient with colon cancer

Date	TNM	Treatment	pTNM/R
June 1994	T2N0M0	Hemicolectomy	pT3pN1(2/24)pMX/R0
Sept. 1994	rT0N0M0		
Dec. 1994	rT0N0M0		
April 1995	rT0N0M0		
July 1995	rT0N0M1	Liver resection	rT0N0pM1(Liv)/R0
Oct. 1995	rT0N0M0		

Table 3 TNM/pTNM classification in a patient with oesophageal cancer

Date	TNM	Treatment	pTNM/R
Oct. 1997	T2N1M0	Radiotherapy and chemotherapy	
Dec. 1997	yT1N0M0	Oesophagectomy	ypT1pN0(0/11)pMX/R0
Feb. 1998	rT0N0M0		

histologically. Likewise, the presence of regional lymph node metastases has to be confirmed histologically, since small metastases or even the so-called micrometastases (< 0.2 cm) are only visible in tissue sections. Moreover, the resection margins after surgical removal to determine presence or absence of tumour (R classification) have to be examined histologically.

Another problem with clinical staging is that some hospitals or other diagnostic institutions may apply techniques that are less sensitive in defining the exact anatomical extent of tumours than those methods used in other centres. Moreover, the technical standard of the equipment used for a certain investigation may vary. These differences in the techniques and devices applied for assessing clinical stages have to be considered if stages from different hospitals are compared.

Problems of pathological staging

Assessing the precise anatomical extent of a primary tumour depends upon thorough macroscopic and histological examination of surgically resected specimens. At gross examination, several tissue blocks are chosen and further processed for microscopic analysis. The lack of uniform protocols for the sampling of tissue blocks from resected specimens accounts for the main discrepancies between institutions. Guidelines for tissue sampling in surgical specimens of different organs are increasingly being published.[18],[19] It is desirable for a better standardization of pathological staging that the tissue blocks should be picked from surgical resection specimens more methodically in different laboratories.

Sampling error may eventually result in an erroneous stage if the area defining the highest pT category has been missed. To ensure accurate staging, the tissue blocks taken from the primary tumour during macroscopic examination have to be chosen by an experienced pathologist. At several sites different histological tumour types with divergent prognostic values may be present, for example in the testis or the ovary. In those tumours, at least one tissue block per centimetre of tumour diameter has to be examined to exactly assess the tissue heterogeneity.

The pN classification requires histological examination of a certain number of lymph nodes for most organs (Table 1). Therefore, during gross examination a thorough search for small lymph nodes is necessary. The surgeon must also completely dissect the tissue containing the regional lymph nodes. This may be difficult at sites where a close anatomical relationship exists between the compartment of the regional lymph nodes and other important structures, for example in the adventitial tissue of the oesophagus or the axillary fat. However, it has to be emphasized that an extended lymphadenectomy contributes to the accuracy of staging. The better survival rates observed in studies with extended versus non-extended lymphadenectomy at some sites (e.g. stomach) can also be caused by migration to higher stages (the so-called Will Rogers phenomenon).[20],[21] The reason for the stage migration is that the extended lymphadenectomy leads to an increased number of lymph nodes examined histologically, which may result in a higher number of lymph node metastases if compared with non-extended lymphadenectomy.

For gross examination, lymph nodes may become more prominent after fixation of the tissue with picric acid. A rather cumbersome method is the extraction of lymph nodes by dissolving the fat. In general, lymph nodes with a diameter of more than 1 cm should be dissected into two or more parts and evaluated completely. The different areas of regional and distant lymph nodes in complex resection specimens must be marked by the surgeon, since the separation of the compartments may be difficult at gross examination.

No general agreement exists in the histological examination of the margins of resection specimens affecting the comparability of the R classification. Variations between different institutions are found in

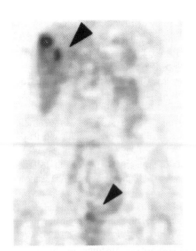

(a)

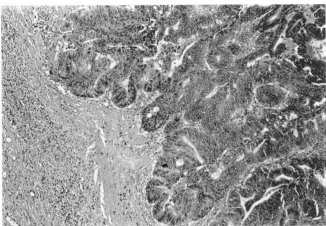

(b)

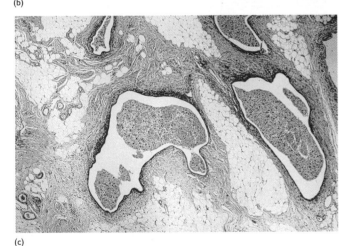

(c)

Fig. 4 (a) Positron emission tomograph for a patient with colorectal cancer treated by hemicolectomy 2 years previously. Metastatic tumour masses in the liver (above) and a mass in the proximity of the bladder (below) can be seen, suspected to be a local recurrence (see also Plate 1). Histology of the liver metastasis (b), and of the second lesion demonstating endometriosis (c). (By courtesy of Dr W. Weber.)

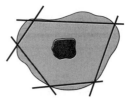
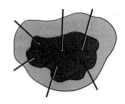

Fig. 5 Sampling of resection margins for histopathological examination. If the distance between the tumour and the margin of the specimen is more than 1 cm, tangential sections should be taken (left). Vertical sections are superior if the distance is less than 1 cm (right).

with and tangential sampling without direct relation to the tumour. The advantages are the possibility of measuring the exact distance between the tumour and resection margin in the vertical, and the ability to examine a larger area in the horizontal section. If at gross evaluation the distance between the tumour and the resection margin is more than 1 cm, tangential sectioning should be preferred (Fig. 5). It is necessary to ink the tumour margins in order to localize the true resection margins in histological sections.

Tumour and tissue banks

In addition to the pathological–anatomical features of a tumour covered by the TNM system, additional factors may become increasingly important for guiding decisions about therapy or estimating the prognosis. Among these, molecular genetic or biochemical tumour markers are mostly used in clinical trials and have not been determined routinely so far. However, some of these molecular markers can only be assessed in fresh and unfixed tissue and not after formaldehyde fixation and paraffin embedding, which is commonly used for storing pathological specimens. Therefore, the need for sampling of frozen tissue became evident, making high-quality DNA, RNA, and protein molecules available for diagnostic molecular analyses. To maintain a frozen tissue bank requires a pathologist who integrates it into the routine surgical pathology procedure.[22] Sampling of the tumour specimens should be performed by the pathologist who is responsible for the final pTNM classification. Because of the well known phenomenon of tumour heterogeneity, and of the striking variations in the tumour/stroma ratio in an individual tumour, a close relation between molecular analysis and histology is necessary. This can be achieved by either applying *in situ* techniques such as immunohistochemistry or *in situ* hybridization, or by microdissecting relevant tumour areas from histological sections which can be investigated by polymerase chain reaction techniques.[23]

References

1. Sobin LH, Wittekind Ch (ed.). *International Union against Cancer (UICC): TNM classification of malignant tumours* (5th edn). New York: Wiley-Liss, 1997.

2. Fleming ID, Cooper JS, Henson DE, Hutter RVP, Kennedy BJ, Murphy GP, O'Sullivan B, Yarbo JW (ed.). *American Joint Committee on Cancer: cancer staging manual*. Philadelphia: Lippincott, 1997.

3. Fédération Internationale de Gynécologie et d'Obstétrique (FIGO).

the number of tissue blocks sampled (e.g. in lumpectomy specimens) as well as the orientation of the selected sample in relation to the tumour. The two general possibilities of the latter are vertical sampling

Annual report on the results of treatment in gynecological cancer. *International Journal of Gynecology and Obstetrics*, 1989; **28**: 189–93.

4. Fédération Internationale de Gynécologie et d'Obstétrique (FIGO). Changes in gynecological cancer staging by the International Federation of Gynecology and Obstetrics. *American Journal of Obstetrics andGynecology*, 1990; **162**: 610–11.

5. Hermanek P, Henson DE, Hutter RVP, Sobin LH (ed.). *International Union against Cancer (UICC): TNM Supplement 1993*. Berlin: Springer, 1993.

6. Hermanek P, Gospodarowicz MK, Henson DE, Hutter RVP, Sobin LH (ed.). *International Union against Cancer: Prognostic factors in cancer*. Berlin: Springer, 1995.

7. Dowlatshahi K, Fan M, Snider HC, Habib FA. Lymph node micrometastases from breast cancer. *Cancer*, 1997; **80**: 1188–97.

8. Kerstelmeier R, Busch R, Fellbaum Ch, Böttcher K, Reich U, Siewert JR, Höfler H. Häufigkeit und prognostische Bedeutung von epitheloidzelligen Reaktionen und Mikrokarzinosen in den regionären Lymphknoten beim Magenkarzinom. *Pathologe*, 1997; **18**: 124–30.

9. Morton D, Wen DR, Wong JH, Economou JS, Cagle LA, Strorm FK, *et al*. Technical details of intraoperative lymphatic mapping for early stage melanoma. *Archives of Surgery*, 1992; **127**: 392–9.

10. Krag DN, Weaver D, Alex JC, Fairbank JT. Surgical resection and radiolocalization of sentinel lymph nodes in breast cancer using a gamma probe. *Surgical Oncology*, 1993; **2**: 335–9.

11. Jannink I, Fan M, Nagy S, Rayndu G, Dowlatshhi K. Serial sectioning of sentinel lymph nodes in patients with breast cancer: a pilot study. *Annals of Surgical Oncology*, 1998; **5**: 310–14.

12. Hermanek P, Wittekind C. Residual tumour R classification and prognosis. *Seminars in Surgical Oncology*, 1994; **10**: 12–20.

13. Bloom HJ, Richardson WW. Histological grading and prognosis in brest cancer. A study of 1049 cases of which 359 have been followed for 15 years. *British Journal of Cancer*, 1957; **11**: 359–77.

14. Gleason DF. Histologic grading of prostate cancer: a perspective. *Human Pathology*, 1992; **23**: 273–9.

15. Costa J, Wesley RA, Glatstein E, Rosenberg SA. The grading of soft tissue sarcomas: Results of a clinicopathologic correlation in a series of 163 cases. *Cancer*, 1982; **53**: 530–41.

16. Coindre JM, Trojani M, Contesso G, *et al*. Reproducibility of a histopathological grading system for adult soft tissue sarcoma. *Cancer*, 1986; **58**: 306–9.

17. Glaser F, Kuntz C, Schlag P, Herfarth C. Endorectal ultrasound for control of preoperative radiotherapy of rectal cancer. *American Surgeon*, 1993; **217**: 64–71.

18. Association of Directors of Anatomic and Surgical Pathology (ADASP). Recommendations for the reporting of resected neoplasms of the kidney. *Human Pathology*, 1996; **20**: 1005–7.

19. Association of Directors of Anatomic and Surgical Pathology (ADASP). Recommendations for the reporting of larynx specimens containing laryngeal neoplasms. *Virchows Archiv*, 1997; **431**: 155–7.

20. Feinstein AR, Sobin DM, Wells CK. The Will Rogers phenomenon. Stage migration and new diagnostic techniques as a source of misleading statistics for survival in cancer. *New England Journal of Medicine*, 1985; **312**: 1804.

21. Hermanek P. Will-Rogers-Phänomen—Fakt oder Fiktion? *Der Chirurg*, 1996; **67**: 769–70.

22. Naber SP, Smith LL, Wolfe HJ. Role of the frozen tissue bank in molecular pathology. *Diagnostic Molecular Pathology*, 1992; **1**: 73–9.

23. Becker I, Becker KF, Röhrl MH, Schütze K, Minkus G, Höfler H. Single-cell mutaion analysis from stained histological slides. *Laboratory Investigations*, 1996; **75**: 801–7.

Laparoscopic staging for gastrointestinal malignancy

N. J. Espat and K. C. Conlon

Introduction

Laparoscopy, and specifically laparoscopic staging, have become useful tools in the diagnosis, evaluation and staging of patients with gastrointestinal malignancies. This technology enables the determination of an appropriate course of therapy or surgical intervention that best benefits the individual patient based on the extent of their disease. It is the aim of this chapter to discuss the role for laparoscopic staging as an integral component of modern oncological patient care for tumours of the pancreas, oesophagus, stomach, liver, and intra-abdominal lymphoma.

A brief history

Physicians were able to perform limited body cavity examinations in the mid 1800s, with the aid of a device consisting of a hollow tube with refractive lenses.[1] Applications were initially limited to the bladder but through the investigative efforts of visionaries further use for this technique were developed. George Kelling, a German physician, is credited with making giant strides in the development of early organ examination. Kelling devoted most of his life to the development of techniques and instrumentation for the endoscopic evaluation of the upper gastrointestinal tract. In the later part of his extraordinary career, intra-abdominal whole organ visualization was achieved and was termed 'celioscopy'.[1],[2] Modern laparoscopy has been in development since that time. Although rudimentary by present standards, laparoscopes were developed for routine intra-abdominal evaluation, termed diagnostic laparoscopy. Popularized and used almost exclusively used for gynaecological abdominopelvic evaluation, beginning in the 1960s, laparoscopy has become a standard technique with a wide range of surgical interventions. Until the mid 1980s, the use of laparoscopy for procedures other than exploration was hampered by the limitations in available instrumentation.[1] The rapid progress in the development of laparoscopic instrumentation in the last decade has been the result of the introduction of the video computer chip in 1987. Driven by the success of Moertel in France, who is credited with performing the first laparoscopic cholecystectomy, laparoscopic technology has sprung forward at a breathtaking pace.[1],[3]

Laparoscopic staging: an overview

Laparoscopy provides visual access to body cavities through percutaneous trochars that are of a limited invasiveness, and as instrumentation has evolved so has the range of potential applications for this technology.

Laparoscopy for the examination and staging of patients with gastrointestinal malignancies has become a method to better select patients that will benefit from specific therapies.[3],[4] The principal goals for the laparoscopic evaluation of patients with an intra-abdominal malignancy are (1) to provide an accurate assessment by TNM staging (The American Joint Committee on Cancer (AJCC)); and (2) to guide appropriate therapy (see Table 1).[5]

Laparoscopic staging enables the accurate clinical staging of intra-abdominal malignancy through direct visualization, intraoperative ultrasound, and tissue acquisition for histological assessment. The need for accurate staging cannot be over emphasized, as this will determine what, if any, type of surgical intervention is required. Furthermore, it provides assessment for potential enrolment into an investigational trial. Accurate staging enables appropriate stratification of patients, which is necessary to validate the results of randomized clinical trials. In contrast, postoperative staging is based on the histopathology of the resected specimen, which yields useful information, including any need for adjuvant therapy, but does not enable the comparison or validation of different therapies.

An uncertain diagnosis, lacking tissue for histological examination, precludes patients with cancer from receiving treatment. Laparoscopy allows for the acquisition of tissue in these patients. The quality and quantity of tissue specimens that can be obtained by laparoscopic biopsy are superior to those from computed tomography (CT)-guided fine-needle aspiration.[6]

Optimal laparoscopic staging is achieved when it mimics the exploration that would be performed during exploratory laparotomy, with the benefit of avoiding the morbidity and recovery period.[6]

Table 1 Benefits of laparoscopic staging

Minimal invasion
Direct visualization for biopsy, access for intraoperative ultrasound
Access for diagnosis and accurate staging
Reduced morbidity as compared to open standard laparotomy
Reduced length of hospitalization following staging alone
Faster return to normal activity
Minimal delay for the administration of adjuvant therapy

Once the diagnosis is confirmed histologically and the patient is staged, the goal of surgical treatment should be to render the patient free of tumour (UICC stage R0). Towards this objective, laparoscopic staging facilitates the selection of patients that will benefit from an operation with curative intent rather than palliation. Furthermore, accurate disease staging and an R0 stage following resection have been shown by multivariate analyses to have the greatest impact on prognosis. Determination of clinical outcome is dependent on meticulous identification of prognostic factors in the preoperative setting.[7]

The staging accuracy by CT alone has been a matter of discussion in oncological staging. Dynamic, contrast-enhanced CT is the radiographic study of choice in the preoperative evaluation of patents with gastrointestinal tumours, particularly the pancreas. However, the resolution of this modality is limited to lesions that are larger than 2 to 3 mm, allowing for smaller lesions to be missed. CT has been demonstrated to have a high sensitivity in determining local regional extension of disease and vascular encasement, predicting unresectability in up to 100 per cent of patients. Despite this obvious benefit, CT is far less specific at determining resectability, and reports of accurate assessment of resectability in pancreatic tumour range from 57 per cent to 88 per cent.[8]–[10],[11] As such, many patients will still undergo a needless staging laparotomy.[12],[13]

A major advantage of staging laparoscopy for patients with gastrointestinal tumours is the prevention of unnecessary explorative laparotomies after CT scanning has demonstrated equivocal or potentially curative disease.[14] The identification of patients with advanced disease that do not require palliative surgical procedures is accurately performed through laparoscopic evaluation, obviating the need for open exploration in these patients.[15]

It would be difficult to overlook the rapid advancements in CT imaging but, despite progress, CT alone fails to stage disease accurately when compared to CT followed by laparoscopic staging.[16] Proponents of radiological evaluation as the sole preoperative staging modality heralded the new generation spiral CT scanners to have technical advantages over conventional CT scanners, however significant improvement was not achieved.[17] In comparison to CT evaluation alone, laparoscopic staging will identify subcentimetre hepatic, peritoneal, or omental tumour implants. CT alone is also of limited benefit for the assessment of lymph node metastases, organ invasion, or hepatic and peritoneal metastases.[17] Published series report that laparoscopic staging identifies disease in 22 to 48 per cent of patients who have no evidence of disseminated disease by CT.[4],[18]–[20] Additionally, peritoneal cytology from washings obtained at the time of laparoscopy will identify an additional 8 per cent of patients with micrometastases, not seen on CT.[21] Unfortunately, these patients with positive micrometastasis identified by cytology alone have an equally poor prognosis as those with visible metastases.[21]

Beyond the benefit of direct organ visualization and examination for radiographically inapparent disease, laparoscopy provides access for ultrasound evaluation. In this manner, deep parenchymal metastasis and vascular involvement can be identified.[22],[23]

In the sections that follow, laparoscopic staging for the assessment of pancreatic, oesophageal, gastric, and hepatic malignancy is presented. Discussion on the staging for pancreatic and gastric cancer is expanded, as the majority of the published literature reports on these subjects. Additionally, the role of laparoscopy in the management of intra-abdominal lymphoma is discussed.

Laparoscopic staging for pancreatic cancer

Pancreatic cancer is a malignancy with an unfavourable prognosis. Pancreatic adenocarcinoma will occur in 80 per cent of patients with pancreatic cancer and at the time of diagnosis only 10 per cent of patients have disease confined to the pancreas. Of the remaining patients, 40 per cent exhibit local spread and 50 per cent demonstrate distant disease.[12],[13] Surgical resection offers the only chance for long-term survival, but unfortunately less than 20 per cent of these patients are operative candidates. Accurate preoperative staging is important in determining which patients will be able to undergo curative resection.

Why laparoscopy?

Radiographically inapparent disease, such as occult peritoneal or hepatic metastasis, precludes curative resection. Without staging laparoscopy, the extent of the disease is unappreciated until after laparotomy has begun.[24]–[27] In patients with pancreatic cancer, who have a very limited expected median survival (less than 6 months), exploratory laparotomy may be associated with a significant perioperative morbidity, mortality, and diminished quality of life.[28],[29]

Warshaw et al. compared several different modalities in the preoperative assessment of pancreatic cancer.[16] Dynamic CT, magnetic resonance imaging (MRI), angiography, and laparoscopy were evaluated for accuracy in this study. Of 88 patients considered to have potentially curable disease, the accuracy of CT was 92 per cent in determining unresectability but only 56 per cent sensitive. Resectability was predicted in only 45 per cent of patients. CT scanning failed to identify liver metastasis in 23 patients. Angiography predicted 25 of 26 cases as being unresectable, with a sensitivity of only 66 per cent. The accuracy of predicting resectability was only 54 per cent. MRI results were similar to those of CT scan and offered no advantage. Laparoscopy identified liver and peritoneal metastasis in 22 of 23 cases and was correct in not identifying metastasis in 24 of 24 patients, with an overall 98 per cent accuracy of laparoscopy. Of the 19 cases in which no metastasis were seen, only eight proceeded to resection.

Simple laparoscopy

The modern experience with laparoscopy and pancreatic cancer began with the report of Ishida in 1983, where limited laparoscopic examination was done in 71 patients.[30] In this group of patients, hepatic metastasis were identified in 30 per cent and peritoneal disease noted in 41 per cent of patients. Cuschieri, in 1988, performed a study of immediately preoperative laparoscopy and then compared the results to open exploration.[15] Of the 51 patients, 42 were correctly staged as having unresectable disease by laparoscopy. However of the nine patients considered resectable by laparoscopy, only four underwent resection. Warshaw, in a separate series, performed laparoscopy in 40 patients.[31] Fourteen patients had positive findings at laparoscopy that resulted in a change in their operative management. Findings at laparoscopy included hepatic metastasis in six patients, peritoneal disease in seven, and a single omental implant. In the remaining 26 patients, three additional hepatic metastasis not identified by laparoscopy were identified at the time of operation. These studies, early in the modern era of laparoscopic staging, highlight the

Table 2 Frequency of hepatic metastases and resectability rate following laparoscopic staging for pancreatic cancer

Author		N	% liver metastases	% resected
Cuschieri	1988	73	70	44
Warshaw	1990	32	36	42
John	1995	40	45	46
Del-Castillo	1995	114	24	37
Conlon	1996	115	35	91

predictive value of simple laparoscopy and underscore the pitfalls of a negative examination.

CT scan combined with laparoscopy

Laparoscopic staging in conjunction with preoperative CT scanning has been shown to be an effective, accurate, and safe means of staging peripancreatic malignancy that has been previously validated by our group and others.[3],[21],[32],[33] While CT evaluation alone has been a useful and specific modality for the identification of unresectable disease in patients with pancreatic malignancy, as previously mentioned it has been more limited in the determination of resectability.[9],[10],[20],[34] CT staging is reported to yield erroneous preoperative assessment of the extent of disease in more than 50 per cent of patients, leading to an unnecessary laparotomy.[23],[35] CT evaluation as a predictor of resectability has been prospectively studied and demonstrated to be a poor predictor of resectability, and the use of laparoscopy following CT evaluation to detect sub-CT disease, and prevent needless laparotomy, has been advocated.[3],[20] Diagnostic laparoscopy without ultrasound or a multiport technique is reported to assess resectability in less than 40 per cent of patients. In sharp contradistinction, laparoscopic staging performed in manner that mimics open exploration exceeds 90 per cent accuracy at predicting resectability[3] (see Table 2).

At Memorial Sloan–Kettering Cancer Center, we have instituted multiport, extended laparoscopic technique for staging and assessment of resectability of peripancreatic tumours.[8] In our management algorithm (see Fig. 1), all patients undergo a contrast-enhanced dynamic CT scan of the abdomen, for determination of obvious unresectable disease, prior to proceeding to laparoscopy. Our laparoscopic staging technique, unlike previously published reports, mimics the surgical assessment of resectability performed at open exploration.

The technique of extended laparoscopic staging

An open technique is used to place a 10-mm periumbilical blunt port for the creation of a pneumoperitoneum in all cases. A 30° angled telescope is placed through this port. Trochars are placed in the right (10 mm) and left (5 mm) upper quadrants of the abdomen (Fig. 2). Positioning of the trochars is within the line of the planned incision if the patient is deemed resectable and laparotomy follows.

Initially, a four-quadrant examination of the peritoneal cavity is performed, searching for obvious peritoneal extension of disease.

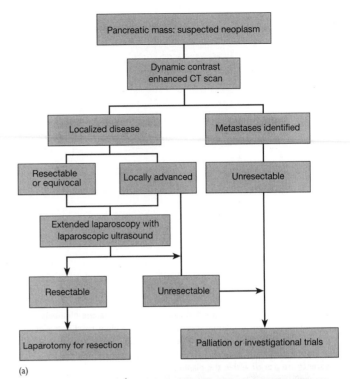

(a)

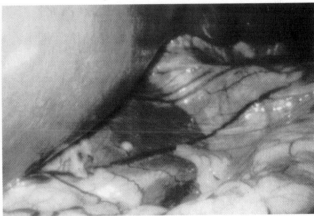

(b)

Fig. 1 (a) Algorithm for the staging and management of pancreatic malignancy. Dynamic thin-cut contrast enhanced CT scan of the abdomen is obtained for all patients. CT is an accurate modality to assess for unresectable disease. Only patients with equivocal findings or radiologically resectable disease progress to laparoscopic staging. Patients found to have unresectable disease do not undergo laparotomy, and should be considered for enrolment into investigational trials. (b) Pancreatic cancer—2 mm hepatic metastasis. This is the typical lesion missed by contrast radiographic imaging.

Peritoneal washings for cytological examination are collected after separately instilling 200 cc of saline into the right and left upper quadrants. The primary tumour is assessed, noting local extent, size, and fixation. The patient is then placed in a 20-degree reverse Trendelenburg position with 10 degrees of left lateral tilt. Next, the anterior and posterior surfaces of the right and left lobes of the liver are visually inspected. Palpation of the liver is achieved with the use of a 10-mm instrument. The liver is retracted anteriorly and the

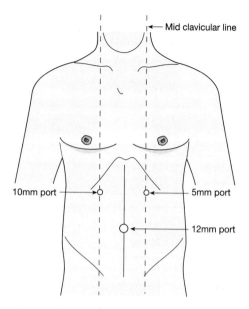

Fig. 2 Port placement for extended laparoscopic staging, the Memorial Sloan–Kettering Cancer Center approach. A 12 mm blunt trochar is placed via open technique into the periumbilical area. Bilateral subcostal incision is planned for pancreatic resection. Trochars in the right and left upper quadrants are placed within the planned incision line.

hepatoduodenal ligament is examined for gross adenopathy. The hilus of the liver is visualized; the foramen of Winslow is examined. At this point, periportal lymph node biopsy can be performed, if indicated. The patient is then repositioned into a 10-degree Trendelenburg position without tilt and the omentum is retracted into the left upper quadrant. The ligament of Treitz is visualized and the mesocolon is closely inspected. The gastrohepatic omentum is incised such that the caudate lobe of the liver, vena cava, and coeliac axis are exposed. Coeliac, portal, or perigastric nodes are sampled if necessary.

Laparoscopic ultrasound is then employed to evaluate the presence of non-surface hepatic lesions, peripancreatic tumour spread, and vascular invasion into the portal vein, superior mesenteric artery, or superior mesenteric vein.

Unresectability is determined if one or more of the following are confirmed histologically:

(1) hepatic, serosal, peritoneal, or omental metastasis;
(2) extrapancreatic extension of tumour;
(3) coeliac or high portal vein involvement by tumour;
(4) invasion or encasement of the coeliac axis, hepatic artery, or superior mesenteric artery.

Patients who are found to have portal or mesenteric vein involvement are considered potentially resectable and undergo exploration. In the absence of locally advanced or metastatic disease, a decision to proceed with pancreaticoduodenectomy is justified.

The Memorial Sloan–Kettering experience

Using this technique we have evaluated 442 consecutive patients with pancreatic and periampullary malignancies between December 1992 and December 1996, at Memorial Sloan-Kettering Cancer Center.[36]

Following radiological assessment including dynamic CT scan in all patients, 339 patients (77 per cent) were thought to be potentially resectable, 52 (12 per cent) were noted to be unresectable, and 51 (12 per cent) had equivocal findings. Of the 339 patients thought to have resectable disease, 303 patients underwent extended laparoscopic staging as described. Laparoscopic staging identified 48 patients with hepatic metastasis, 41 with extrapancreatic disease, 20 with nodal disease, and vascular invasion in another 37. Following laparoscopic assessment, 199 patients were deemed resectable, and of these 181 (91 per cent) were resected. Only 9 (19 per cent) were not resected after undergoing laparotomy. In this series, laparoscopic assessment provided a positive predictive index of 100 per cent, a negative predictive index of 91 per cent, and an accuracy of 94 per cent.

Laparoscopic ultrasound

Laparoscopic ultrasound is an integral part of the noteworthy improvement achieved in resectability following laparoscopic staging. Laparoscopy alone is limited by a two-dimensional assessment, such that intraparenchymal liver metastasis deep below the surface and retropancreatic vascular involvement may still be overlooked. Several authors have examined the use of laparoscopic ultrasound in conjunction with laparoscopic staging.[18],[19],[37],[38]

We have recently reported a prospective series of 90 patients with peripancreatic malignancy undergoing extended laparoscopic staging in combination with laparoscopic ultrasound.[18] Comparing conventional CT imaging, laparoscopic assessment alone, and laparoscopic assessment combined with laparoscopic ultrasound, this study demonstrated 98 per cent accuracy at predicting resectability for the combined approach. A single false positive was noted providing a positive predictive index of 100 per cent and a negative predictive index of 98 per cent.

Palliative bypass

Following the determination of unresectable disease, non-operative palliative interventions can subsequently be performed on an elective basis. In a series of 155 consecutive, prospectively followed patients undergoing laparoscopic staging at Memorial Sloan–Kettering Cancer Center, determined to have unresectable pancreatic adenocarcinoma, the role for prophylactic biliary or gastric bypass was examined. This group of patients included 40 with locally advanced and 115 with metastatic disease. Meticulous follow-up demonstrated that only 3 per cent of these patients subsequently required an open operation to treat a malignant obstruction. Although 10 per cent of the patients went on to require biliary decompression, in all cases but one this was accomplished using endoscopic stents. Only 3 patients had open gastric bypass performed. These findings suggest that there is no role for routine prophylactic bypass in the laparoscopically-staged, unresectable patient with pancreatic adenocarcinoma. We have recommended that open biliary bypass should be considered only for patients failing endoscopic decompression in the hands of an experienced operator, and that gastric bypass should be reserved for those patients with confirmed obstruction.[39]

Length of stay

Patients undergoing laparoscopic staging benefit from a decreased length of hospitalization since clearly long hospitalizations affect the quality of life in a patient population that has a life expectancy of approximately 6 months. Laparoscopic staging alone results in postoperative median hospitalization of 2 days.[3],[4] Further benefits of laparoscopic staging are the determination of the appropriate course of therapy and the avoidance of unnecessary surgical procedures.

Cost of laparoscopic staging

The perceived high cost of laparoscopic staging has been an issue for detractors the technique. In a prospective study conducted at Memorial Sloan–Kettering Cancer Center, the total costs for patients with pancreatic cancer undergoing open exploration were compared to patients undergoing laparoscopic staging prior to proceeding to laparotomy.[40] The results of this comparison were surprisingly significant in demonstrating the reduction in costs achieved by an initial laparoscopic staging. A 25 per cent reduction in total hospital charges was demonstrated in patients that first underwent laparoscopy. These savings were realized by avoiding the cost of unnecessary laparotomy and a reduced length of stay in the hospital.[40]

Laparoscopic staging for distal oesophageal and gastric–oesophageal junction cancer

Oesophageal cancer, specifically of the gastric–oesophageal junction, has been noted to have an increasing incidence of 10 per cent per year over the last decade. Over 70 per cent of patients with oesophageal cancer have lymph node metastasis at presentation, and the median survival for patients with metastatic disease is approximately 6 months.

At present, there is no accurate minimal procedure for the staging of mediastinal malignancy, with the exception of lung cancer via mediastinoscopy. For lower oesophageal carcinoma, staging studies on both sides of the diaphragm are necessary. Endoscopic oesophageal ultrasound is useful at determining tumour 'T' stage in combination with CT. However, laparoscopic staging provides a more accurate N and M stage for oesophageal cancer.[41]

The feasibility and efficacy of thoracoscopic and laparoscopic lymph node staging in oesophageal cancer was evaluated in a group of patients with biopsy-proven carcinoma of the oesophagus. Ultimately, 30 patients came to oesophagectomy, 17 of which had had combined thoracoscopic and laparoscopic evaluation. Evaluation of accuracy following resection was based on specimen pathology. Thoracoscopy was noted to understage nodal status, although it was 93 per cent accurate at detecting the presence of diseased nodes. The laparoscopic staging component was accurate in detecting lymph node metastases in 16 of 17 patients (94 per cent). Laparoscopic staging was accurate in detecting disease in unsuspected coeliac axis lymph nodes, missed by radiographic evaluation. This small experience with oesophageal staging suggests the need for further investigation for the role of combined thoracoscopy and laparoscopy.[42]

Adequate preoperative staging of patients with oesophageal and cardia carcinoma offers the potential for a rational choice of the therapy. The diagnostic value of laparoscopy compared to ultrasonography and CT in detecting intra-abdominal metastatic spread has been examined.[43],[44] Laparoscopic staging resulted in a change in the therapeutic approach for 10 per cent of patients with CT-missed peritoneal carcinomatosis. Laparoscopy showed a higher sensitivity than CT and ultrasonography in detecting peritoneal metastases (71 per cent versus 14 per cent versus 14 per cent, respectively), macroscopic nodal metastases (78 per cent versus 11 per cent versus 55 per cent), and liver metastases (86 per cent versus 71 per cent). These results suggest that laparoscopic staging is an effective diagnostic procedure in the preoperative staging of oesophageal and cardia carcinoma, avoiding unnecessary laparotomies and selecting the most appropriate treatment. No mortality or morbidity related to the laparoscopic procedure was experienced in this series.[45] Similar findings were reported by other groups, who assessed patients with gastric adenocarcinoma for intra-abdominal spread of malignancy using ultrasonography, CT, and laparoscopy. Laparoscopy was more sensitive in detecting hepatic, nodal, and peritoneal metastases. Ultrasonography and CT were particularly poor at detecting nodal and peritoneal metastases. There was no significant morbidity and no mortality associated with laparoscopy, which was more accurate in preoperative staging of gastric cancer than ultrasonography or CT.[43]

Evaluation for metastasis in a large series of 250 patients with cancer of the oesophagus and gastric cardia undergoing laparoscopic staging is also reported, with similar results. Metastases to the liver, peritoneum, omentum, stomach, and lymph nodes were discovered in 14 per cent of patients. Metastasis to the gastric wall or to the regional lymph nodes was noted in 10 per cent of patients. False negative findings from laparoscopic staging occurred in 4 per cent. Laparoscopic staging was found to be an effective procedure in pretherapy staging of oesophageal cancer.[44]

Further work, considering the role for CT alone or in conjunction with laparoscopy in the staging of upper gastrointestinal malignancies, was done in a group of patients with carcinoma of the oesophagus or gastric cardia. Determination of the sensitivity, specificity, and accuracy of laparoscopy, ultrasound, and CT for detecting intra-abdominal metastases was the aim of the study. Neither ultrasound nor CT detected any peritoneal metastases. Laparoscopy, in contrast, demonstrated a sensitivity of 89 per cent and an accuracy of 98 per cent. No morbidity or mortality associated with laparoscopy was encountered. The authors concluded that laparoscopic staging offers a safe, reliable method of evaluating intra-abdominal disease and may obviate the need for surgery in some patients.[46]

These series suggest that laparoscopic staging is superior for the detection of metastasis from oesophageal and gastric cardia lesions. Furthermore the procedure is safe, with minimal morbidity reported and avoids unnecessary operations.

Laparoscopic staging for gastric cancer

The majority of patients with gastric adenocarcinoma in the United States present with advanced disease. They are at high risk for intra-abdominal metastatic spread and optimal therapy depends on accurate preoperative evaluation.[4] Laparoscopic staging is useful for patient with gastric cancer that is not actively obstructed or actively haemorrhaging in order to provide appropriate care.[47] Laparoscopic staging in combination with ultrasound further enables accurate staging. The value of laparoscopic staging is further underscored as more than one-third of these patients have unsuspected metastatic disease at time of operation. Laparoscopy is highly accurate in detecting occult

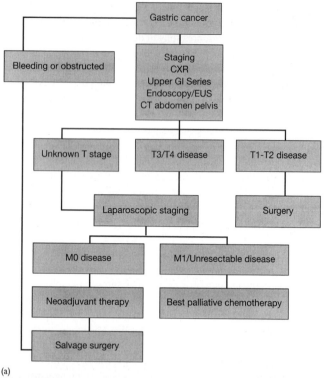

(a)

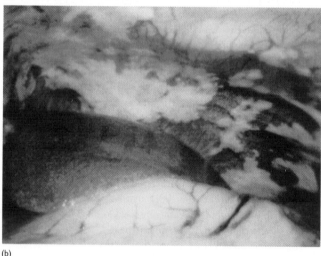

(b)

Fig. 3 (a) Gastric cancer management algorithm. Following the identification of gastric malignancy, evaluation for systemic disease is performed. Contraindications to laparoscopy include patients who are bleeding acutely or are obstructed. In the absence of radiographically-apparent metastasis, laparoscopic staging is performed. Patients having T1–T2 disease proceed to planned operation, while patients with advanced disease or metastasis are enrolled into investigational trials. Patients having M0 disease may be eligible to undergo salvage surgery following neoadjuvant therapy. (b) Gastric cancer—peritoneal metastasis. Commonly missed by conventional radiographic assessment, this thin, plaque-like peritoneal metastasis precludes resection.

metastases and identifies a unique population of stage IV patients who may benefit from newer, induction chemotherapeutic approaches while avoiding unnecessary laparotomy (Fig. 3). Combined CT and

laparoscopic staging is reported to yield a greater than 90 per cent resectability rate for patients operated on with curative intent.[47]

Technique for laparoscopic staging

Laparoscopic staging for gastric cancer is performed in a similar manner to that for pancreatic cancer. However, a significant difference is that in most cases laparoscopy is not performed immediately prior to operation. Only a minority of patients will present initially with early-stage disease, and laparoscopy identifies patients who may benefit from enrolment into neoadjuvant therapy trials. In general, laparoscopy is performed 1 week prior to planned resection, allowing for pathological examination of cytology and nodal biopsies.

An open technique is used to place a 10-mm periumbilical blunt port for the creation of a pneumoperitoneum; in all cases, three trochars are required. A 30-degree angled telescope is placed through the umbilical port, and the initial manoeuvre is the inspection of the peritoneal cavity, searching for obvious peritoneal extension of disease. Peritoneal washings for cytological examination are collected after separately instilling 200 cc of saline into the right and left upper quadrants. The primary tumour is then assessed, with examination of the liver and regional lymph nodes. Inspection of the ligament of Treitz, mesocolon, and small bowel follows. Laparoscopic ultrasound is then performed over the primary tumour to assess T stage and identify patients at high risk for early treatment failure. Patients with T1 or T2 lesions proceed to laparotomy, while patients with T3 and T4 lesions are considered for enrolment into investigational trials.[48]

The Memorial Sloan–Kettering experience

A prospective series of laparoscopic staging prior to laparotomy in 111 patients with gastric adenocarcinoma free of intra-abdominal metastatic disease based on preoperative CT scan was reported by Burke *et al.*[4] Laparoscopic staging enabled the identification of metastatic disease in 37 per cent of patients and accurately staged 94 per cent of the patients. Metastatic disease was identified with a sensitivity of 84 per cent and a specificity of 100 per cent. The most frequent site of metastasis was the peritoneum (72 per cent), followed by liver (9 per cent). Patients who underwent only laparoscopic staging were discharged in an average 1.4 days. This was significant when compared to the 6.5 days that patients having an exploratory laparotomy without resection were hospitalized. In this series, none of the patients undergoing only an initial laparoscopy returned for palliative surgery.[4]

Why laparoscopic staging?

TNM staging of gastro-oesophageal cancer is improved by the use of laparoscopy for the detection of occult metastases and endoscopic ultrasonography for T and possibly N staging. Laparoscopic ultrasonography may combine the strengths of both of these techniques. Comparison of TNM staging by means of laparoscopic ultrasonography, laparoscopy, and conventional CT has been reported. Validation of findings was by final pathological examination. Resectability for potential cure was determined by laparoscopic staging with intraoperative ultrasonography with a sensitivity of 100 per cent and a specificity of 91 per cent versus 100 per cent and 73 per cent for laparoscopy and 75 per cent and 60 per cent for CT, respectively. Overall TNM staging was 82 per cent accurate for laparoscopic staging with intraoperative ultrasonography versus 67 per cent for laparoscopy and 47 per cent for CT. T and N staging by laparoscopic staging and intraoperative ultrasonography were comparable to published results for endoscopic ultrasonography, and overall TNM staging was better.[49]

Prospective evaluation of immediately preoperative video laparoscopy compared to ultrasound/CT staging for gastric cancer is reported in a series that is currently in progress. TNM staging was used to compare the ultrasonography/CT findings and the laparoscopic findings with the pathological findings in resected specimens. The predictive value of laparoscopic staging was 86 per cent, with an overall staging accuracy of 69 per cent, compared to 33 per cent for ultrasonography/CT. On initial analysis of the data, laparoscopy appears the most specific method for detecting the resectability of the tumour, thus avoiding unnecessary laparotomies.[50]

Gastric cancer staging by laparoscopy in combination with ultrasound in the reviewed series is reported as being superior to either CT or endoscopic ultrasound alone. Laparoscopic staging has a high accuracy and specificity, and enables determination of resectability.

Hepatic malignancy

The careful examination of the liver is a component of the laparoscopic assessment of all gastrointestinal malignancies. Staging laparoscopy is an important advance that is also increasing resectability rates for hepatic tumours through laparoscopic detection of unresectable tumours.[51] Laparoscopic hepatobiliary surgery for benign conditions and biliary evaluation has advanced rapidly; however operations such as liver resections and biliary–enteric anastomosis are still under development.[52] As such, the staging and treatment of liver tumours through a laparoscopic approach continues to evolve with relatively little published information.

Assessment of hepatic lesions is based on whether the disease represents a primary hepatic tumour or if it is metastatic (Fig. 4). Consideration for resection of metastatic tumours will be dependent on the absence of systemic disease. For example in colorectal cancer metastasis to the liver, resectability is not assessed by laparoscopic examination. Rather, evaluation for recurrent disease by colonoscopy, extent of disease evaluation with chest radiograph, and review of the CT for obvious extrahepatic abdominal disease will guide the surgeon.

In contrast, a role for staging laparoscopy is emerging in the evaluation of primary hepatic tumours. Laparoscopic examination for cirrhosis precluding operative resection in the high-risk patient can be identified, as well as assessment or biopsy of regional lymph nodes heralding unresectability.[53] CT scanning alone only yields information about location and size of primary or satellite hepatic lesions. Laparoscopic assessment enables the examination of the abdominal cavity for extrahepatic disease gives a direct view for biopsy and diagnosis and, in combination with intraoperative ultrasonography, identifies radiographically-missed disease. Laparoscopic staging in combination with intraoperative ultrasonography is a far superior approach than CT alone or laparoscopy without intraoperative ultrasonography for hepatic lesions. With the use of laparoscopic intraoperative ultrasonography, primary or metastatic hepatic lesions can be accurately staged and operative intervention appropriately planned.[54],[55]

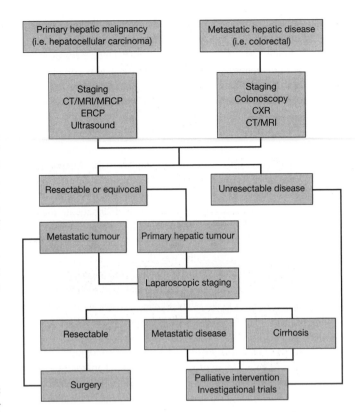

Fig. 4 Algorithm for the staging and management of hepatic malignancy. Resectability of primary and metastatic hepatic tumours is initially assessed radiographically. Metastatic lesions undergo disease-appropriate evaluation for systemic disease. For metastatic disease where laparoscopic assessment is appropriate and for primary hepatic cancers, laparoscopic staging is performed.

Extrahepatic lymph node examination identifies and enables the acquisition of nodal tissue for histology. This is important in selecting patients who will derive benefit from a major operation, since resection should proceed only when there is no evidence of lymph node metastasis. Information on tumour proximity to major hepatic veins and biliary structures will ultimately determine whether to proceed to laparotomy and the nature of the procedure to be performed.[56]

Laparoscopic staging performed immediately before a planned laparotomy can provide valuable information for management of liver and pancreas cancer. For evaluation of small liver and retroperitoneal malignancies, intraoperative ultrasonography performed by laparotomy is of proven value. It is technically possible to perform high quality ultrasonography through a laparoscopic cannula using high-resolution ultrasonographic transducers.[54]

The use of intraoperative ultrasonography evaluation in conjunction with open abdominal exploration of the liver provides relevant information for the staging and subsequent management of patients with liver tumours. The availability of the 5.0 to 7.5 MHz ultrasound transducer with multi-imaging capacity and spectral Doppler capabilities can provide similar information laparoscopically, thus avoiding unnecessary laparotomy. In a limited series of eight patients with hepatic lesions with no known extrahepatic disease or recurrence at the primary site, undergoing laparoscopy with intraoperative ultrasonography prior to major laparotomy, laparoscopy with intraoperative ultrasonography predicted unresectability in six of eight patients, all of whom were spared an unnecessary laparotomy.[55]

A resectability rate of 88 per cent for patients with hepatocellular carcinoma undergoing laparoscopic hepatic staging as compared to 68 per cent for patients undergoing open exploration has been reported. In this series, laparoscopic staging with intraoperative ultrasonography was used to determine resectability.[53]

Staging laparoscopy alone or combination with laparoscopic ultrasonography is being examined for its value in defining the extent of disease in patients with hepatobiliary malignancy. In this series, all patients were considered to have resectable tumours as determined by standard preoperative staging. Staging laparoscopy with ultrasonography predicted resectable tumours in 26 of 28 patients. Staging laparoscopy alone demonstrated previously-unrecognized, occult metastases in 11 patients (22 per cent). In 11 other patients (22 per cent) in whom laparoscopy alone was negative, laparoscopic ultrasonography (LUS) established unresectability from vascular invasion, lymph node metastases, or intra-parenchymal hepatic tumour. Unnecessary laparotomy can be safely avoided by laparoscopic staging combined with LUS in many patients with hepatobiliary malignancies.[57]

The impact of laparoscopic intraoperative ultrasonography guided biopsy was evaluated in a prospective fashion. Laparoscopy with intraoperative ultrasonography was performed on 18 consecutive patients with liver metastases considered to be surgically curable. New liver lesions with the potential to alter treatment were biopsied. Of 17 patients undergoing laparoscopic staging, biopsies were performed in 12 (71 per cent), extension of the surgical procedure was decided in four cases (24 per cent), and laparotomy was avoided in six cases (35 per cent). The accuracy for the preoperative staging was correct in 88 per cent. Liver lesions discovered by laparoscopic staging, which may result in a modification or cancellation of surgery, should be biopsied. Laparoscopic staging with intraoperative ultrasonography enables guidance for the biopsy of deep lesions.[58]

This combination of laparoscopy and ultrasonography was studied in 25 patients with known hepatic lesions, gallbladder carcinoma, or pancreatic cancer. Information obtained from this study resulted in a change in the surgical approach for 20 of these patients. Laparoscopic ultrasonography, although still in a preliminary phase of development, is a simple and reliable technique that will contribute to more accurate staging of intra-abdominal malignancy.[59]

Beyond staging, the laparoscope can be used for other, non-surgical therapies for the treatment of hepatic malignant disease. No longer is even a limited laparotomy necessary for cryoablative tumour treatment; with laparoscopy it can be performed under direct visualization.[60] Additionally, patients undergoing metastatic work-up for non-gastrointestinal malignancies derive benefit from laparoscopic hepatic assessment. A series of 125 patients with primary lung cancer undergoing 100 laparoscopic evaluations demonstrated the presence of metastatic liver lesions in 16 per cent of patients. Laparoscopic biopsy enabled histological confirmation of the diagnosis, thus guiding appropriate treatment. Most importantly, in 8 per cent of these patients laparoscopy yielded the diagnosis of metastasis not detected by other means. Laparoscopic staging found no false positives, was accomplished without complications, and well tolerated by the patients. In this patient population, the need for subsequent restaging can be met via laparoscopy.[61]

Lymphoma staging

Oncological surgical management of lymphoma has been changed by the introduction of minimally invasive laparoscopic staging techniques and instrumentation. The management of patients with Hodgkin's disease and non-Hodgkin's lymphoma is predicated on a definitive pathology diagnosis and accurate staging (Fig. 5). Historically, patients suspected to have Hodgkin's disease or non-Hodgkin's lymphoma underwent laparotomy-based staging and tissue collection. During the 1960s, laparotomy was used for staging to determine which patients were potentially curable.[62]

Collective reviews of laparotomy for the staging of lymphoma report a mortality rate that ranges from 0.3 per cent to 1 per cent. Major morbidity was reported to occur in 3 to 18 per cent of patients, while minor morbidity was reported as 6 to 9 per cent of patients. Morbidity-related delays in therapy occurred in 5 to 10 per cent of patients. In a separate series, the surgical morbidity was reported to be 26 per cent in a consecutive group of 133 patients.[63],[64] The significant morbidity associated with laparotomy led to the utilization of CT for the staging of patients with suspected lymphoma. However, CT demonstrates only the presence and size of lymph nodes. The combination of CT and CT-guided fine-needle aspiration for the diagnosis in these patients subsequently evolved.[65]

Prior to laparoscopic staging, tissue was obtained via laparotomy and/or CT-guided fine-needle aspiration biopsies.[66] While fine-needle aspiration is accurate at obtaining the diagnosis, with false-negative rates as low as 1 per cent,[6] the complex classification of lymphoproliferative disorders requires ample tissue for architectural analysis, immunophenotyping, and cytogenetic analysis that can not be obtained by fine-needle aspiration. Lack of adequate tissue prevents the determination of appropriate therapy regimens and prognostic risk stratification.[6]

Comparison of laparoscopy with open laparotomy staging demonstrated that patients undergoing laparoscopy recovered to oral intake faster, had shorter lengths of stay postoperatively, fewer complications, and had more total nodes harvested. Laparoscopic staging for patients with Hodgkin's disease is reported to be feasible, effective, and safe. Moreover, laparoscopic staging is oncologically equivalent and functionally superior to an open laparotomy approach.[67]

In the last 15 years, the use of laparoscopy for tissue collection and staging has been evolving.[8],[48],[65] Although initially laparoscopy was used for only for liver biopsies, newer instrumentation now enables the examination and collection of tissues from most parts of the abdominal cavity and the retroperitoneum.[68] Laparoscopic staging and biopsy has been demonstrated to be useful in the diagnosis, restaging, and reduction in the false negative rate of biopsies for the assessment of patients with lymphoma. However, the literature reports a more than 50 per cent false negative rate from biopsies. Subsequently, with the use of laparoscopic staging and biopsy, this rate has decreased to 8 per cent.[69] The capacity to perform multiple biopsies at different locations on the liver under direct visualization, as opposed to a single site biopsy as previously practised, is credited with this improvement.[69] The advantages of laparoscopy in the management of these patients are accurate diagnosis, no mortality, low morbidity, low false-negative rate, and shortened length of stay and rapid progression to therapy. Laparoscopy can be used to provide tissue safely for histological and molecular analysis without delaying therapy.[65]

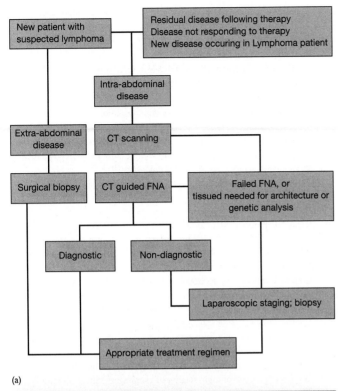

(a)

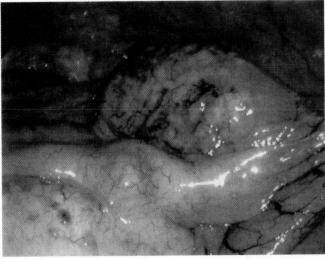

(b)

Fig. 5 (a) Algorithm for the management of the lymphoma patient. Patients having new or persistent intra-abdominal disease thought to be lymphoma should initially undergo radiological examination. Extra-abdominal disease can be assessed by surgical biopsy where appropriate. While CT-guided fine-needle aspiration is successful for biopsy, the quantity and quality of tissue is inferior for architectural and genetic studies. When fine-needle aspiration is not an option, or there is a requirement for tissue for special study, laparoscopy is useful. Furthermore, assessment of intra-abdominal viscera can be achieved. (b) Lymphoma—laparoscopic assessment of disease. Evident on CT scan, intra-abdominal lymphoma can be staged and appropriate tissue collected via laparoscopy.

Laparoscopic assessment and/or biopsy for patients with suspected or documented lymphoma should be considered when:[65]

(1) fine-needle aspiration cannot be performed;

(2) fine-needle aspiration is attempted but fails;

(3) tissue is needed for architecture, chromosomal, or other analysis;

(4) to differentiate between residual or recurrent disease following chemotherapy;

(5) when the disease does not respond to chemotherapy.

Summary

Laparoscopic staging techniques are becoming a standard approach in the assessment of patients with intra-abdominal malignancy. Laparoscopic staging is useful in patients with carcinoma of the lower third of the oesophagus for determining resectability or possible inclusion into neoadjuvant trials. Patients with gastric cancer at high risk for early failure, similarly benefit. The high frequency of advanced disease in patients with pancreatic cancer precludes resection in a majority of cases and laparoscopic staging can accurately assess resectability without laparotomy. Patients with new or residual intra-abdominal lymphoma benefit from a minimally invasive approach for accurate diagnosis and subsequent therapy, using a procedure that may repeated without major morbidity or mortality.

The potential patient benefit from laparoscopic staging prior to laparotomy include minimal surgical invasion with significant benefits for diagnosis and staging. In comparison to laparotomy, patients undergoing laparoscopy have reduced morbidity, decreased length of hospital stay, and faster return to normal activity. Most importantly, for patients who will go on to need additional non-operative therapy, laparoscopic staging results in only minimal postoperative delay prior to beginning adjuvant therapy.

References

1. Ahlgren M. [The 100th anniversary of laparoscopy. Earlier used in gynecologic diagnosis, now also in surgery]. *Lakartidningen*, 1997; **94**: 162–4.

2. Kelling G. Zur Colioskopie und Gastroskopie. *Archiv fur Klinische Chirurgie*, 1998; **126**: 226–8.

3. Conlon KC, Dougherty E, Klimstra DS, *et al.* The value of minimal access surgery in the staging of patients with potentially resectable peripancreatic malignancy. *Annals of Surgery*, 1996; **223**: 134–40.

4. Burke EC, Karpeh MS, Conlon KC, Brennan MF. Laparoscopy in the management of gastric adenocarcinoma. *Annals of Surgery*, 1997; **225**: 262–7.

5. Sendler A, Dittler HJ, Feussner H, *et al.* Preoperative staging of gastric cancer as precondition for multimodal treatment. *World Journal of Surgery*, 1995; **19**: 501–8.

6. Steel BL, Schwartz MR, Ramsy I. Fine needle aspiration biopsy in the diagnosis of lympadenopathy in 1103 patients. *Acta Cytology*, 1994; **38**: 76–81.

7. Siewert JR, Sendler A, Dittler HJ, Fink U, Hofler H. Staging gastrointestinal cancer as a precondition for multimodal treatment. *World Journal of Surgery*, 1995; **19**: 168–77.

8. Conlon KC, Dougherty E, Klimstra DS, *et al.* The value of minimal access surgery in the staging of patients with potentially resectable peripancreatic malignancy. *Annals of Surgery*, 1996; **223**: 134–40.

9. Fuhrman G, Charnsangavej C, Abbruzze SE, Martin R, Fenoglio C, Evans D. Thin-section contrast-enhanced computed tomography accurately predicts the resectability of malignant pancreatic neoplasms. *American Journal of Surgery*, 1994; **167**: 104–13.

10. Gulliver GM, Baker M, Cheng C. Malignant biliary obstruction: efficacy of thin section dynamic CT scan in determining resectability. *American Journal of Roentgenology, Radium Therapy and Nuclear Medicine*, 1992; **159**: 503–7.

11. Freeny PC, Traverso LW, Ryan JA. Diagnosis and staging of pancreatic adenocarcinoma with dynamic computed tomography. *American Journal of Surgery*, 1993; **165**: 600–6.

12. Brennan MF, Kinsella TJ, Casper ES. Cancer of the pancreas. In: DeVita VT, Hellman S, Rosenberg SA, ed. *Principles and practice of oncology*, 5th edn. Philadelphia: J.B. Lippincott, 1993: 849–82.

13. Carter D. Cancer of the pancreas. *Gut*, 1990; **31**: 494–6.

14. van Delden CO, van Dijkum EJ, Smits NJ, Gouma DJ, Reeders JW. Value of laparoscopic ultrasonography in staging of proximal bile duct tumours. *Journal of Ultrasound in Medicine*, 1997; **16**: 7–12.

15. Cuschieri A. Laparoscopy for pancreatic cancer: does it benefit the patient? *European Journal of Surgical Oncology*, 1988; **14**: 41–4.

16. Warshaw AL, Tepper JE, Shipley WU. Laparoscopy in the staging and planning of therapy for pancreatic cancer. *American Journal of Surgery*, 1986; **151**: 76–80.

17. Davies J, Chalmers AG, Sue-Ling HM, *et al.* Spiral computed tomography and operative staging of gastric carcinoma: a comparison with histopathological staging. *Gut*, 1997; **41**: 314–19.

18. Minnard EA, Conlon K, Hoos A, Dougherty E, Hann L, Brennan M. Laparoscopic ultrasound enhances the standard laparoscopy in the staging of pancreatic cancer. *Annals of Surgery*, 1998; **228**: 1–7.

19. John TG, Greig JD, Carter DC, Garden OJ. Carcinoma of the pancreatic head and periampullary region. Tumour staging with laparoscopy and laparoscopic ultrasonography. *Annals of Surgery*, 1995; **221**: 156–64.

20. Holzman M, Reitgen KL, Tyler D, Pappas T. The role of laparoscopy in the management of suspected pancreatic and periampulary malignancies. *Journal of Gastrointestinal Surgery*, 1997; **1**: 236–44.

21. Fernandez-del CC, Warshaw AL. Laparoscopy for staging in pancreatic carcinoma. *Surgical Oncology*, 1993; **2** (Suppl. 1):25–9.

22. Catheline JM, Champault G. [Ultrasonic laparoscopy in digestive diseases]. *Annales de Chirurgie*, 1996; **50**: 51–7.

23. Hann LE, Conlon KC, Dougherty EC, Hilton S, Bach AM, Brennan MF. Laparoscopic sonography of peripancreatic tumours: preliminary experience. *American Journal of Roentgenology*, 1997; **169**: 1257–62.

24. Geer R, Brennan M. Resection of pancreatic adenocarcinoma: prognostic indicators for survival. *American Journal of Surgery*, 1993; **223**: 279.

25. Harrison LE, Brennan MF. Portal vein involvement in pancreatic cancer: a sign of unresectability?. *Advances in Surgery*, 1997; **31**: 375–94.

26. Fernandez-del Castillo C, Rattner DW, Warshaw AL. Further experience with laparoscopy and peritoneal cytology in the staging of pancreatic cancer. *British Journal of Surgery*, 1995; **82**: 1127–9.

27. Cameron JL. Long-term survival following pancreaticoduodenectomy for adenocarcinoma of the head of the pancreas. *Surgical Clinics of North America*, 1995; **75**: 939–51.

28. de Rooj P, Rogatko A, Brennan M. Evaluation of palliative surgical procedures in unresectable pancreatic cancer. *British Journal of Surgery*, 1991; **78**: 1053–8.

29. Watanapa P, Williamson R. Surgical palliation for pancreatic cancer: developments during the past two decades. *British Journal of Surgery*, 1992; **79**: 8–20.

30. Ishida H. Peritoneoscopy and pancreas biopsy in the diagnosis of pancreatic diseases. *Gastrointestinal Endoscopy*, 1983; **29**: 211–18.

31. Warshaw AL, Gu ZY, Wittenberg J, Waltman AC. Preoperative staging and assessment of resectability of pancreatic cancer. *Archives of Surgery*, 1990; **125**: 230–3.

32. Conlon K, Minnard E. The value of laparoscopic staging in upper gastrointestinal malignancy. *Oncologist*, 1997; **2**: 10–17.

33. Fernandez-del Castillo C, Rattner DW, Warshaw AL. Standards for pancreatic resection in the 1990s. *Archives of Surgery*, 1995; **130**: 295–9.

34. Freeny PC. Cross-sectional imaging of the pancreas. *Baillieres Clinical Gastroenterology*, 1995; **9**: 135–51.

35. Harrison LE, Brennan MF. Portal vein resection for pancreatic adenocarcinoma. *Surgical Oncology Clinics of North America*, 1998; **7**: 165–81.

36. Merchant N, Conlon KC. Laparoscopic evaluation in pancreatic cancer. *Seminars in Surgical Oncology*, 1998; **15**: 155–65.

37. Murugiah M, Paterson-Brown S, Windsor JA, Miles WF, Garden OJ. Early experience of laparoscopic ultrasonography in the management of pancreatic carcinoma. *Surgical Endoscopy*, 1993; **7**: 177–81.

38. Bemelman WA, de WL, van DO, *et al.* Diagnostic laparoscopy combined with laparoscopic ultrasonography in staging of cancer of the pancreatic head region. *British Journal of Surgery*, 1995; **82**: 820–4.

39. Espat NJ, Brennan MF, Conlon KC. Laparoscopically staged patients with unresectable pancreatic adenocarcinoma do not require subsequent biliary or gastric bypass. *Journal of the American College of Surgeons*, 1999; **188**: 649–53.

40. Conlon K, Dougherty E, Brennan M. The economic effect of the introduction of laparoscopic staging for patients with adenocarcinoma of the pancreas: A prospective analysis of hospital charges. *Annals of Surgical Oncology*, 2000. (In review.)

41. Krasna MJ. Minimally invasive staging for esophageal cancer. *Chest*, 1997; **112**: 191S–4S.

42. Krasna MJ, Flowers JL, Attar S, McLaughlin J. Combined thoracoscopic/laparoscopic staging of esophageal cancer. *Journal of Thoracic and Cardiovascular Surgery*, 1996; **111**: 800–6.

43. Stell DA, Carter CR, Stewart I, Anderson JR. Prospective comparison of laparoscopy, ultrasonography and computed tomography in the staging of gastric cancer. *British Journal of Surgery*, 1996; **83**: 1260–2.

44. Dagnini G, Caldironi MW, Marin G, Buzzaccarini O, Tremolada C, Ruol. Laparoscopy in abdominal staging of esophageal carcinoma. Report of 369 cases. *Gastrointestinal Endoscopy*, 1986; **32**: 400–2.

45. Bonavina L, Incarbone R, Lattuada E, Segalin A, Cesana B, Peracchia. Preoperative laparoscopy in management of patients with carcinoma of the esophagus and of the esophagogastric junction. *Journal of Surgical Oncology*, 1997; **65**: 171–4.

46. Watt I, Stewart I, Anderson D, Bell G, Anderson JR. Laparoscopy, ultrasound and computed tomography in cancer of the oesophagus and gastric cardia: a prospective comparison for detecting intra-abdominal metastases. *British Journal of Surgery*, 1989; **76**: 1036–9.

47. Lowy AM, Mansfield PF, Leach SD, Ajani J. Laparoscopic staging for gastric cancer. *Surgery*, 1996; **119**: 611–4.

48. Conlon KC, Karpeh MS, Jr. Laparoscopy and laparoscopic ultrasound in the staging of gastric cancer. *Seminars in Oncology*, 1996; **23**: 347–51.

49. Finch MD, John TG, Garden OJ, Allan PL, Paterson-Brown S. Laparoscopic ultrasonography for staging gastroesophageal cancer. *Surgery*, 1997; **121**: 10–17.

50. D'Ugo DM, Coppola R, Persiani R, Ronconi P, Caracciolo F, Picciocchi. Immediately preoperative laparoscopic staging for gastric cancer. *Surgical Endoscopy*, 1996; **10**: 996–9.

51. Strasberg SM, Callery MP, Soper NJ. Laparoscopic surgery of the bile ducts. *Gastrointestinal Endoscopy Clinics of North America*, 1996; **6**: 81–105.

52. Strasberg SM, Callery MP, Soper NJ. Laparoscopic hepatobiliary surgery. *Progress in Liver Diseases*, 1995; **13**: 349–80.

53. Lo CM, Lai EC, Liu CL, Fan ST, Wong J. Laparoscopy and laparoscopic ultrasonography avoid exploratory laparotomy in patients with hepatocellular carcinoma. *Annals of Surgery*, 1998; **227**: 527–32.

54. Cuesta MA, Meijer S, Borgstein PJ, Sibinga ML, Sikkenk AC. Laparoscopic ultrasonography for hepatobiliary and pancreatic malignancy. *British Journal of Surgery*, 1993; **80**: 1571–4.

55. Barbot DJ, Marks JH, Feld RI, Liu JB, Rosato FE. Improved staging of liver tumours using laparoscopic intraoperative ultrasound. *Journal of Surgical Oncology*, 1997; **64**: 63–7.

56. Babineau TJ, Lewis WD, Jenkins RL, Bleday R, Steele GDJ, Forse RA. Role of staging laparoscopy in the treatment of hepatic malignancy. *American Journal of Surgery*, 1994; **167**: 151–4.

57. Callery MP, Strasberg SM, Doherty GM, Soper NJ, Norton JA. Staging laparoscopy with laparoscopic ultrasonography: optimizing resectability in hepatobiliary and pancreatic malignancy. *Journal of the American College of Surgeons*, 1997; **185**: 33–9.

58. Olivero G, Constans P, Solvignon F. Laparoscopy in the detection of hepatic metastasis of early bronchial cancer (100 laparoscopies). *Revue Francaise des Maladies Respiratoires*, 1980; **8**: 233–8.

59. Cuesta MA, Meijer S, Borstein J, Mulder L, Sikkenk AC. Laparoscopic ultrasonography for hepatobiliary and pancreatic malignancy. *British Journal of Surgery*, 1993; **80**: 1571–4.

60. Cuschieri A. Laparoscopic management of cancer patients. *Journal of the Royal College of Surgeons of Edinburgh*, 1995; **40**: 1–9.

61. Court-Payen M, Skjoldbye B, Struckmann J, Norgaard N, Pedersen IK, Bille-Brahe NE. [Hepatic metastases disclosed by laparoscopy and echographic laparoscopy. Impact of ultrasound-guided biopsy]. *Annales de Chirurgie*, 1997; **51**: 318–25.

62. Glatstein E, Guernesey JM, Rosenberg SA. The value of laparotomy and splenectomy in the staging of Hodgkin's disease. *Cancer*, 1969; **24**: 709–18.

63. Multani PS, Grossbard M. Staging laparotomy in the management of Hodgkin's disease: is it still necessary? *Oncologist*, 1996; **1**: 41–55.

64. Jockovich M, Mendenhall NP, Sombeck MD, Talbert Jl, Copeland EM, Bland KI. Long term complications of laparotomy in the management of Hodgkin's disease. *Annals of Surgery*, 1994; **219**: 615–24.

65. Mann B, Conlon KC, LaQuaglia M, Dougherty E, Moskowitz Ca, Zelenetz AD. Emerging role of laparoscopy in the diagnosis of lymphoma. *Journal of Clinical Oncology*, 1998; **16**: 1909–15.

66. Lefor AT, Flowers JL, Heyman MR. Laparoscopic staging of Hodgkin's disease. *Surgical Oncology*, 1993; **2**: 217–20.

67. Baccarani U, Brendan JC, Hiatt JR, *et al*. Comparison of laparoscopic and open staging in Hodgkin disease. *Archives of Surgery*, 1998; **133**: 517–22.

68. Salky BA, Bauer JJ, Gelernt I. The use of laparoscopy in retroperitoneal pathology. *Gastrointestinal Endoscopy*, 1988; **34**: 227–30.

69. Palmitano JB, Nicastro A, Castro RM, *et al*. [Hodgkin's disease and the liver. Study of 50 biopsies]. *Acta Gastroenterologica Latinoamericana*, 1984; **14**: 127–34.

70. Warshaw AL, Gu ZY, Wittenberg J, Waltman AC. Preoperative staging and assessment of resectability of pancreatic cancer. *Archives of Surgery*, 1990; **125**: 230–3.

71. John TG, Greig JD, Carter DC, Garden OJ. Carcinoma of the pancreatic head and periampullary region. Tumour staging with laparoscopy and laparoscopic ultrasonography. *Annals of Surgery*, 1995; **221**: 156–64.

3.7 Prognostic factors

Giampietro Gasparini, Maria Grazia Arena, Massimo Fanelli, and Alessandro Morabito

Introduction

The prognostic determinants for a patient with an invasive neoplastic disease are heterogeneous and often are tumour-type specific. The same variable may play a different prognostic role and may have diverse correlations with the other prognostic indicators in different tumour types. In general, the major prognostic indicators are related to the characteristics of the patient, the histopathology and biology of the tumour, and the efficacy of therapy.[1]

At the time of first diagnosis of neoplasia, some variables can be recorded such as: sex, age, general clinical conditions of the patient (i.e. performance status), and presence of concurrent or previous pathologies that may influence the possibility to treat the patient with the optimal antitumoral therapy. Certain neoplasia, such as Hodgkin's disease and lymphomas, may be accompanied by systemic symptoms such as weight loss, fever, and drenching night sweats (see Chapter 5.3). Indeed, paraneoplastic syndromes are frequent in lung, renal, and other cancers, and are characterized by inappropriate hormone production.

Subsequently, it is necessary to determine, by accurate physical examination and radiological investigation, the site of origin of the primary tumour and its extent of spread into the body in order to define the clinical stage of disease. For most solid tumours, the clinical stage of the tumour represents the single most important prognostic factor. The most frequently used method to classify the clinical (and pathological) stage of a solid tumour is based on a triad of elements: the dimension of the primary tumour (T); the locoregional lymphatic diffusion (N); and the presence of distant metastasis (M): the TNM system[2] (see Chapter 3.5).

For most solid neoplasia, the presence at diagnosis or the subsequent development of distant metastasis is the worst prognostic factor, which also interferes with the efficacy of therapy in terms of probability of response and outcome of the patient.

The definition of the pathological characteristics of the disease requires biopsy procedures to obtain material to assess:

(1) the exact histological type and grade of differentiation of the tumour;

(2) the pathological stage (of particular importance, for example, in the case of Hodgkin's disease, malignant lymphomas, ovarian and testicular cancers);

(3) after major surgical resection, to define the pathological T and N as well as the status of the margins of resection to establish whether the disease has been macroscopically eradicated by surgery (see Chapter 3.5).

The different histological subtypes of tumours require specific treatments so that most of the controlled clinical studies are restricted to clearly-defined eligibility criteria and sometimes must be conducted in variants of histological types of the same tumour (for example oesophageal cancer). Other more specific histopathological parameters have prognostic value only in some types of tumours, such as hormonal receptors and peritumoral vascular or lymphatic vessel invasion in breast cancer.[3],[4]

The histopathological material is the main source for the biological characterization of the tumour for the assessment of the so-called biological prognostic and predictive factors. In selected tumour types we also have the possibility to obtain prognostic information from circulating tumour markers. The prognostic value of abnormal levels of prostatic-specific antigen is well proven in patients with locally-advanced or metastatic prostate cancer, of carcinoembryonic antigen in patients with colorectal cancer, and of β-human chorionic gonadotropin and α-fetoprotein in testicular cancers. Also, lactate dehydrogenase is of prognostic importance, for example in malignant lymphomas and testicular cancers.[5]

For prognostic and predictive purposes new circulating biomarkers are currently under evaluation, such as extracellular domain of c-erbB-2. Also, some endothelial growth factors, such as basic fibroblast growth factor, hepatocyte growth factor, and the soluble isoforms of vascular endothelial growth factor, are promising in some tumour types such as breast and colorectal cancers[6] and warrant further investigation. These surrogate biomarkers, detectable by easy techniques, may be useful in assessing prognosis and in monitoring the activity of biologically-based treatments directed against each specific growth factor such as antibodies to c-erbB-2 or antiangiogenic agents.

Hayes *et al.*[7] proposed a tumour marker utility score called Tumour Marker Utility Grading System (TMUGS) that should assist clinician to determine the 'weight' of the prognostic factors. One component of TMUGS is the importance of the precise description of the tumour marker and of the assays used for its detection. Then, a semiquantitative scale (ranging from 0 to 3+) is proposed to quantify the clinical utility of the marker. A grade of '0' implies that the marker has no proven utility, while a grade '3 +' means that the marker needs to be used in routine clinical practice. Finally, the intermediate scores imply moderate evidence for the use of a certain marker.

Also the level of evidence (LOE) on which a decision is based is support for the evaluation of the significance of a prognostic indicator. LOE-I is provided by a single prospective, highly-powered study or from an overview or meta-analysis of studies each of which provides

Table 1 General prognostic factors

Factor	Examples of tumours in which the variable can be applied
Related to the characteristics of the patient	
Sex	Breast and lung cancers, soft tissue sarcomas, lymphomas are tumours with a tendency for better outcome in females
Age	Children and elderly patients have important differences in the compliance to therapy as compared with the adult (>18; <65 years old)
Performance status	All
Previous or concurrent pathologies	May require deviations from the optimal therapy
Socioeconomic level	All
Related to the characteristics of the tumour	
Site	All
Histological type	Testicular, breast and lung cancers, lymphomas
Grade of cell differentiation	Breast and lung cancers, sarcoma
Stage	All
Tumoral bulk	All
Biological characteristics	Breast, lung, head and neck cancers, leukaemias
Related to the therapy	
Complete surgical eradication	Most localized (early-stage) solid tumours
Adequate dose and schedule of radiation therapy, chemotherapy, or hormone therapy	All
Identification of the appropriate biological target	Patients treated with biologically-based treatments
Achievement of a complete remission	Lymphomas, leukaemias, testicular cancers
Compliance to therapy	All
Efficacy of salvage treatments in patients with recurrent disease	Testicular cancers, lymphomas, leukaemias

lower levels of evidence. LOE-II data derive from companion studies in which specimens are collected prospectively as part of prospective therapeutic trials. LOE-III includes the results obtained by retrospective studies.

Only those markers that are felt to be sufficiently strong to influence a therapeutic decision that results in improved clinical outcome for the patient are recommended. The authors[7] stated that TMUGS is not useful for deciding whether a marker is applicable to an individual patient but rather that it should be used to determine whether available data support the introduction of a novel tumour marker into routine clinical practice. By applying the TMUGS system,[7] the following circulating tumour markers are considered useful for monitoring the outcome of patients with metastatic disease: CA 15-3 and CA 27-29 for breast cancer, carcinoembryonic antigen for colorectal cancer, and prostatic-specific antigen for prostate cancer.

As far as predictive markers are concerned, it needs to be recognized that the compliance to therapy may differ among patients with the same tumour, stage, or other characteristics. It is common in clinical practice to see that the optimal anticancer treatment cannot be assigned in first instance to all the patients due to: advanced age, presence of associated diseases causing impaired functions of the organs metabolizing or eliminating specific drugs (that is hepatic and renal functions), allergy to drugs (for example taxanes), altered psychological status, pregnancy, reduced bone marrow reserve, etc.

The main general prognostic indicators, that is those which are more likely to be useful in different tumour types of solid neoplasia, are listed in Table 1. It should be noted when referring to results from large, prospective clinical trials that the characteristics of the patients in the trials may be different (in age, performance status,

concomitant severe diseases, etc.) from those of the general population in oncological units. The validity of prognostic factors is restricted to particular groups of patients when strict eligibility criteria have been used to select participants in a trial.

Prognostic factors and prognostic indexes

Prognostic factor

A variable determined at the time of diagnosis is of use in prognosis if it is capable of giving information on the natural history of a certain type of tumour. Therefore, a prognostic factor should be able to predict the clinical behaviour of the disease. The term prognostic factor should be applied when the patient is treated with radical, locoregional treatments alone (surgery or radiation therapy) but not if a systemic therapy is given. This distinction is important to avoid confusion with the category of 'predictive indicators' that are associated with the efficacy therapy.[8]

Recognizing a negative prognostic factor may contribute the potential cure of a disease by highlighting the limits of the current approach. An example is node-negative breast carcinoma. Approximately 70 to 75 per cent of the patients with node-negative, invasive breast carcinoma can be cured by surgery with or without radiation therapy alone and are disease-free at 10 years from surgery. However, about a quarter of the patients are at high risk and require systemic therapy to ameliorate the prognosis.[8] Some retrospective, and a few prospective, studies suggest that certain pathobiological variables are independent prognostic factors in node-negative breast cancer, including tumour size, expression of p53, and intratumoral vascularity (as a surrogate marker of angiogenesis).[1]

What is the appropriate clinical use of a prognostic factor? First, it can be used to give more detailed information in answer to the patient's questions about the future course of his or her disease. Second, it can be used to define the likelihood of recurrence and death of patients with the same tumour but with different pathobiological characteristics. Third, in relation to the level of risk, it can be used to assist a decision on the most appropriate procedures and intervals of follow-up after successful local therapy. Finally, it can be used to identify subgroups of patients with solid tumours characterized by different histological subtypes or grade of differentiation (such as ovarian, breast, lung cancers) with different outcomes within the same clinical or pathological stage who should be treated with different therapeutic approaches.

A new 'pure' prognostic factor should be tested in a homogeneous series of patients not treated with systemic therapy in order to verify whether it adds statistically-independent prognostic information when evaluated by a multivariate statistical model including the known, conventional prognostic variables. Such an approach should be performed initially in retrospective studies and then each new variable should be validated in clinical, controlled, prospective trials.[1],[8],[9]

Prognostic index

The development of a prognostic index is intended to identify an individualized, multiparametric variable obtained by a balanced combination of the prognostic factors considered in the model. A prognostic score can be obtained and used to define the category of risk to which an individual patient can be assigned. Examples of successful prognostic indices based on the TNM system[10] are in breast cancer by the Van Nuys classification,[11],[12] the Nottingham Breast Cancer Prognostic Index,[15] and the Aubele's Index[16] and in patients with liver metastases of colorectal carcinoma by the Nordlinger prognostic scoring system.[17]

All these prognostic indexes gave superior information compared to each of the individual prognostic indicator included in the score. For example the prognostic classification of breast ductal carcinoma *in situ* by the Van Nuys index includes three groups of patients, based on the presence or absence of high nuclear grade and comedo-type necrosis. The 8-year actuarial relapse–free survival for group 1 (non-high grade without comedo-type necrosis), group 2 (non-high grade with comedo-type necrosis), and group 3 (high grade with comedo-type necrosis) were 93 per cent, 84 per cent, and 61 per cent, respectively (p<0.05).[11],[12] The prognostic value of the index was superior to that of each of the two variables considered individually.

Similar results were reported by Elston et al. regarding the Nottingham index that includes the codetermination of tumour size, tumour grade, and lymph node status.[13] The prognostic value of the index was also evaluated prospectively and was found to be superior to that of each single variable tested.[14]

Another useful prognostic index is the Nordlinger score. A large cohort of 1568 patients with resected liver metastases from colorectal carcinoma was studied regarding the following variables: age, size of largest lesion, carcinoembryonic antigen level, stage of primary tumour, disease- free interval, number of liver metastases, and status of resection margins. Giving one point to each factor, three risk groups were identified: score equal to or less than 2; 3 to 4, and 5 to 7. The probability rates of 2-year overall survival were 79 per cent, 60 per cent, and 43 per cent respectively (p<0.005) and, overall, the prognostic power of the index was higher than that of each single variable.[17]

The main requirements for the correct development of a prognostic index are:

(1) availability of a large cohort of patients with similar characteristics enrolled in prospective, controlled, randomized studies with sufficiently long follow-up;

(2) complete information on the characteristics of each single prognostic factor (methodology of determination, standardization of the assay, type of distribution, and its association with the other variables);

(3) a statistical evaluation based on parametric multivariate analysis and a definition of the personalized prognostic score based on the likelihood of recurrence or death;

(4) validation of a new prognostic index by independent, prospective studies and the evaluation of the cost–benefit ratio for a wide application of the index prior to its routine use.[18]

Predictive indicators and predictive indexes

Predictive indicator

A variable, determined before therapy, is of predictive value if it gives information on the likelihood that a tumour is responsive (or resistant) to a specific treatment. Therefore, a predictive indicator should define the probability that a patient may benefit (or not) from the planned therapy.[8],[9] Appropriate clinical uses of a predictive indicator are:

(1) to optimize the individual therapeutic approach by identifying the best treatment on the basis of the characteristics of the patient and the tumour;

(2) to spare unnecessary toxicity and side-effects to patients with tumours that are likely to be resistant to a specific treatment.

As far as conventional, systemic anticancer therapy is concerned (that is hormone therapy, chemotherapy, immunotherapy), the settings to test new potential predictive indicators may be:

1. Neoadjuvant or palliative therapy in patients with advanced stages of disease. The analysis of the relationship between the predictive variables and the objective response to therapy or time to progression can be evaluated in a short time. Objective response is predictive of long-term clinical outcome in lymphomas, leukaemias, and also in solid tumours such as breast, lung, and colorectal cancers.[1]

2. Adjuvant therapy in patients with radical surgical resection of tumours. The analysis of the relationship between a predictive variable and the end-points of efficacy of adjuvant therapy (relapse-free survival, overall survival) requires long follow-up and controlled, prospective, clinical studies. Due to the partial efficacy of adjuvant treatments for solid tumours available at present and the toxicity related to chemotherapy, effective predictive indicators in this setting may significantly improve the future management and prognosis of these patients, and may

limit the problems related to the side-effects and toxicity of unnecessary or non-active treatments. The determination of the oestrogen receptor status for selection of patients with breast cancer to be treated with antioestrogens (that is tamoxifen) is the first example of a pathobiological predictive indicator in wide clinical use.[3] Other potentially useful predictive indicators currently under extensive clinical evaluation are parameters of cell proliferation (thymidine labelling index, S-phase fraction, growth fraction by Ki-67 or MIB-1), apoptosis (ratio bcl-2/bcl-x, bax; p53), angiogenesis (intratumoral vascularity, angiogenic factors), specific growth factors such as c-erbB-2 (HER-2/*neu*) or epidermal growth factor receptor, or markers of chemoresistance (MDR-1, P glycoprotein).[1]

The availability of a surrogate marker related to a molecular pathway of tumour progression, easily detectable with a standardized method, is the basis for the development of personalized treatments. Specific agents modulating biological pathways should only be administered after the characterization of the related predictive indicator (as a surrogate marker) in the tumour of individual patients.

Predictive index

At present, a validated predictive index capable of defining a score of prognostic indicators that can be used for individualized therapeutic decisions has been developed and validated only for chemotherapy in high-grade non-Hodgkin's lymphomas.[19] The current generation of prospective, randomized trials of adjuvant chemo–hormone therapy for high-risk breast cancer patients are evaluating, prospectively, in large, homogeneous series, multiple predictive indicators. An example is the TAX RP 56976-V-315 protocol from the Breast International Group of the National Surgical Adjuvant Breast and Bowel Project (NSABP). The aim is to validate the predictive value of certain markers already tested in retrospective studies and to define a personal predictive score for responsiveness or resistance to new schedules of adjuvant chemotherapy in patients with node-positive breast carcinoma.[1],[18] These trials are in progress and data is not yet available.

Recently, Bryant et al.[20] reported the results of the predictive value of S-phase fraction for outcome of patients with node-negative, oestrogen-receptor-positive breast cancer enrolled in the prospective NSABP protocol B-14, evaluating the therapeutic efficacy of adjuvant tamoxifen. The authors found that S-phase fraction was an independent predictor of relapse-free survival and overall survival in this cohort of cases.

The distinction between prognostic factor and predictive indicator is important, both from a theoretical point of view and also taking into account the substantial difference in the clinical application.[9] The following categories can be identified:

1. Prognostic but not predictive factors—examples are tumour size and the status of locoregional lymph nodes. In several solid tumours both these pathological parameters identify subgroups with different prognosis. However, the knowledge that a patient is at high risk because with a large primary tumour or lymph nodal metastasis is not of help for making specific and personalized therapeutic decisions.

2. Prognostic and predictive indicators—examples are oestrogen and progesterone receptors and expression of c-erbB-2 in breast cancer. All these markers have moderate prognostic value, but good predictive value for hormone therapy (oestrogen receptor),

chemotherapy (progesterone receptor, c-erbB-2), or for the anti-c-erbB-2 antibody (c-erbB-2 for Herceptin®).[3],[21],[22] Also certain parameters of tumour cell proliferation, such as thymidine labelling index or S-phase fraction by flow-cytometric assay, are both of prognostic and predictive value (mainly for chemotherapy) in some tumours such as breast, ovarian, and head and neck cancers.[23],[24]

3. Predictive but not prognostic indicators—this category of markers not represented at present. Some predictive markers under investigation are: degree of oxygenation of the tumour regarding radiosensitivity; thymidylate synthetase for sensitivity to 5-fluorouracil in patients with colorectal cancer; and MDR-1 for resistance to anthracyclines in various types of solid tumours.

Tables 2 and 3 summarizes the differences and discrimination between prognostic and predictive factor/index.

Methodological aspects

Laboratory assessment of prognostic and predictive markers

The majority of prognostic factors are measured by histopathology, immunohistochemistry, or biochemistry. Clinicians need to be informed as to the advantages and drawbacks of these methods and on the laboratory aspects that may influence the reliability, reproducibility, and evaluation of the results.[25]

Many pathological parameters are well established and their determination is highly standardized and reproducible among laboratories of different institutions. Examples include the classification of the dimension of the primary tumour, the method of analysis of lymph nodes, and the evaluation of the margins of surgical resection.

However, the classification of a tumour with regard to some special histological types may require an expert pathologist and sometimes the standard haematoxylin and eosin staining needs to be coupled with specific immunohistochemical or molecular biology assays, for example small cell lung carcinoma, lymphomas, and leukaemias. Other pathological parameters, such as peritumoral lymphatic or blood vessel invasion or histological grading, are potentially useful prognostic factors in some neoplasias (breast cancer, bladder cancer, sarcomas), but are not routinely used by all centres due to a lack of well-defined and standardized methods for their assessment and evaluation. Therefore, the results obtained in different laboratories regarding the above two markers are to be interpreted with caution because they may not be comparable.[4],[25]

Several prognostic and predictive biomarkers have been proposed in the last decade and the more common assays for their determination include: immunohistochemistry, immunoenzymatic, ELISA, or techniques of molecular biology such as *in situ* hybridization and the polymerase chain reaction (PCR). Much of our current knowledge on the clinical usefulness of novel biomarkers (that is p53, c-erbB-2, angiogenesis, markers of apoptosis) is from retrospective studies that often report inconclusive results due to methodological biases.[18] Potential factors that may negatively influence a prognostic or predictive assay are: inadequate specificity or sensitivity of the primary reagents (for example antibodies); technical problems related to the secondary reactions; lack of quality control for inter–intralaboratory variations; insufficient sample size; inadequate statistical analysis; large

Table 2 Prognostic indicator or index

Indicator	Index
It gives information on the natural behaviour of the disease in each patient	It includes more markers capable of defining a personalized prognostic score based on the individual probability of recurrence or death; the prognostic value of the index should be superior to that of each single marker tested
A 'pure' prognostic marker should be tested in a cohort of patients not treated with systemic therapy	The evaluation of the index requires a specific statistical approach base on parametric multivariate analysis applied to large series enrolled in prospective studies
To be clinically useful a new marker needs to add independent prognostic information when evaluated in models of multivariate analyses including the conventional prognostic factors	A new prognostic index needs to be validated by independent studies prior of its application in clinical practice

Table 3 Predictive indicator or index

Indicator	Index
It gives information on the probability that a patient may benefit from a specific therapy or, conversely, that a tumour is resistant to the treatment	It includes multiple factors to obtain a personalized score predictive of responsiveness or resistance to a specific treatment. The predictive value of the index should superior to that of each single marker tested
A proper evaluation of a predictive marker requires that the series of patients is prospectively treated with a homogeneous therapy	A proper evaluation needs the application of specific statistical parametric multivariate analysis in prospective, randomized clinical studies
Possible measures of efficacy of therapy for assessing a predictive indicator are: objective response, quality of life, time to progression, relapse-free survival, or a change in the molecular/cellular parameters for biological response modifier (BRM_s)	A new predictive index should be validated by independent studies prior of its application in clinical practice

heterogeneity in the characteristics of the tumours analysed; or, finally, lack of reproducibility and standardization of the entire method.[18]

In order to avoid methodological pitfalls in the determination of potentially useful prognostic and predictive markers, it is mandatory to perform prospective validations and comparative studies (for example ligand binding assay versus immunohistochemical methods for hormone receptors; immunoenzymatic assays versus immunohistochemistry for determination of specific molecules such as p53, c-erbB-2 protein, and vascular endothelial growth factor) by performing well-designed multicentre studies with centralized pathology review and quality control programmes as organized by the EORTC framework for sarcomas and other tumour types.

The potential clinical relevance of well-conducted research on new biological markers is of importance taking into account that:

1. The testing of new biological markers is made possible by advances in knowledge of the molecular mechanisms of tumour progression and metastasis. The development of a new biological prognostic factor is a multidisciplinary process involving geneticists, biologists, pathologists, and clinicians. A correct clinical assessment of a new marker can help not only to validate biological hypothesis or results of laboratory research but also to identify new potential targets for biologically-based anticancer treatments.

2. The identification of subgroups of patients with different risk by valid prognostic factors/indexes could permit more selective therapeutic approaches and more appropriate programmes of follow-up in patients with the same stage of disease. This may lead to an improvement in clinical results.

3. The identification of valid predictive factors of sensitivity (or resistance) to a certain treatment could spear unnecessary toxicity and side-effects in patients with resistant tumours or allow better therapeutic results in patients with sensitive tumours with a noticeable improvement of the benefit/costs ratio.

Importance of the clinical research

The features that may have an important impact on the results from studies of novel prognostic/predictive factors are: criteria of selection of the patients; criteria of assignment to therapy; sample of the cohort analysed; and the length of follow-up. Often, retrospective studies report results obtained in highly selected series (e.g. early-stage T1 No Mo breast cancer) or, on the contrary, on groups of cases that are too heterogeneous (e.g. mixed series of breast cancers inclusive of all histological types, T and N categories). Another type of bias is related to the heterogeneity of treatments given to the different subgroups of patients included in retrospective studies (e.g. patients with node-positive breast cancer treated with diverse adjuvant treatments).[1],[8],[18] The results of some studies on prognosis may be false-negative due to a too small cohort of cases analysed for the new marker with a consequently low power of the statistical tests or to a too brief period of observation with a consequently too low number of events.

The above considerations explain why the results of retrospective studies on novel biomarkers are at present poorly used for the routine management of cancer patients and why meta-analyses based on retrospective studies are feasible, but often inconclusive.[1],[8],[18] Only results from large, controlled, randomized, prospective studies have a chance of having important clinical impact, not only for novel therapeutic approaches but also for the development of new prognostic or predictive factors for clinical practice.

Statistical analysis

The following are the crucial points for a correct application of the statistical analyses in the evaluation of prognostic or predictive factors:

1. Distribution of the variable—it is important to distinguish between discontinuous (e.g. menopausal status, tumour size subgroups, histological grading categories) and continuous variables (e.g. hormone receptors, intratumoral vascularization, parameters of cell proliferation).[9],[18]

2. Definition of the cut-off value discriminating the positivity of a discontinuous variable—the cut-off point is to be assessed prospectively by appropriate and specific statistical procedures and not by using, for example, the mean or median value of the distribution of the variable. For continuous variables appropriate methods of evaluation are based on: regression splines, generalized additive or fractional polynomial models.[18]

3. Comparison of the outcome among different subsets of patients selected on the basis of the prognostic variable—the calculations of the survival curves are usually based on the Kaplan–Meier survival plots. However, a single Kaplan–Meier plot may be a summary of heterogeneous outcomes, so that the use of smoothing spline analysis are a more suitable method of analysis in certain situations.[20] Furthermore, some prognostic factors present a time-dependence of hazard ratios, so that the assumption of proportional hazard, which is the basis of the Cox analysis, is not tenable. Hilsenbeck et al.[26] have demonstrated, in a large cohort of patients with breast cancer, that the hazard ratios for oestrogen receptor, tumour size, and S-phase fraction change in time. In particular, the hazard ratios for tumour size and S-phase fraction were initially high but, subsequently, they rapidly decreased over time. As a consequence, both these markers have a strong prognostic value for early but not for long-term outcome. The data by Hilsenbeck et al.[26] and Bryant et al.[20] also suggest that the results of studies on prognostic factors with a too brief period of observation may lead to misinterpretations of the prognostic effect and that, in any case, they cannot yield to any definitive information on the prognostic value of marker.

4. A proper validation of a novel marker requires that a multivariate statistical analysis is performed in order to see if the new variable, when evaluated jointly with other covariates, retains an independent and significant statistical prognostic or predictive value.[1],[8],[18] The Cox proportional hazards regression model is the most commonly used multivariate statistical method. However, the Cox model is not applicable in all instances and other multivariate tests, such as regression trees, multiple testing, or neural networks, are more suitable in specific situations.[18]

Precise guidelines for the reporting of studies have recently been suggested by Altman and Lyman[18] in order to make the comparison between different studies more feasible and standardized.

Clinical guidelines

McGuire's research[27] has contributed greatly to our understanding of the importance of the methodological aspects in the clinical assessment of prognostic predictive factors. Regarding breast cancer, several authors[1],[8],[9],[27],[28] have suggested clinical guidelines for a proper clinical development of new markers with a clear distinction between retrospective and prospective testing and, more recently, between prognostic and predictive factors.[8],[9]

Besides the conventional parameters of outcome (relapse-free survival, overall survival) for prognostic factors or of therapeutic activity for predictive indicators (time to progression, objective response), the quality of life and the cost of care have also been recognized recently as valid endpoints to evaluate the validity and clinical usefulness of prognostic or predictive markers.[1],[9]

The TMUGS-plus system (described above) was recently proposed to determine whether available results support the routine clinical use of a certain marker classified as a weak, moderate, or strong prognostic factor on the basis of the clinical evidence available.[28] The recommendations suggested by Altman and Lyman,[18] coupled with the authoritative position taken by the American Society of Clinical Oncology (ASCO), should promote a more rigorous and fruitful approach to the clinical testing of new markers for prognostic or predictive purposes in the future. In fact, the unsatisfactory methodological approach to the clinical assessment of the biomarkers proposed in the last decade is a major cause of the scepticism of oncologists on the routine use of new biological markers for clinical practice. Therefore, potentially useful markers may be neglected because of the lack of a convincing methodology and of prospective validation.[25]

Below, we report examples of the clinical application of prognostic and predictive markers in two tumours types.

Breast cancer

The heterogeneity of the biological mechanisms that stimulate or suppress, via endocrine, autocrine, or paracrine pathways, the growth of breast cancer explain why TNM or any other single clinico-pathological feature do not have an absolute prognostic value in breast cancer.[29],[30] Axillary lymph nodes status remains the single strongest prognostic factor for recurrence, but its determination for prognostic purposes presents some limits:

1. The prognosis is related to the absolute number of involved nodes, so that only a total axillary clearance gives optimal information.

2. The increasing application of mammographic screening permits more frequent early diagnoses with a higher number of patients with small primary tumours. A significant association between the size of primary tumour and lymph nodal metastasis occurs. Therefore, there is an increasing number of patients with node-negative disease. This evidence, coupled with the expanding use of the procedure of the examination of the sentinel node, will probably reduce the need for axillary node dissection in the years to come.

3. At present, node status is also used in some centres as a discriminatory factor to evaluate the clinical usefulness of high-dose chemotherapy with bone marrow rescue for patients with more than 7/10 nodes involved. No controlled, large, prospective clinical trial has yet clearly demonstrated that the above approach

gives better results as compared to conventional adjuvant chemo-therapy. Indeed, node status is not a true predictive indicator because it is not able to predict response to specific drugs.

For all the above considerations, we need to identify additional prognostic and predictive markers.

The prognostic value of the clinical and conventional histo-pathological features is listed in Table 4.

Translation of basic research to the clinic setting has permitted the validation of the prognostic value of a large number of new biological markers during the last two decades. The prototype of biological markers is oestrogen receptor that, at present, remains the only one in widespread use. Two distinct types of oestrogen receptor (α and β), with diverse biological functions, have been identified recently. The traditional ligand binding assay measures both types, whilst new antibodies and immunohistochemical methods seem to be able to distinguish between the two.[3] Both oestrogen receptor and the related progesterone receptor are weak prognostic factors, but have strong predictive value for activity of the antioestrogen tamoxifen. The identification of oestrogen receptor-negative tumours spares the patients ineffective hormonal therapy. Conversely, the association of oestrogen receptor with efficacy of chemotherapy is inconsistent. Progesterone receptor has been found to have weak predictive value for adjuvant chemotherapy in some studies.[3]

Certain markers of cell proliferation have also been extensively evaluated. Most of the studies which included multivariate analysis in large series of patients found that high values of S-phase fraction[20] or thymidine labelling index are predictive of poor outcome in both node-negative and node-positive patients.[23] Widespread use of these markers of cell proliferation is, in part, limited by some methodological inconsistencies, lack of standardization and reproducibility (for S-phase fraction), or the need for a large quantity of fresh material (for thymidine labelling index).[1]

Novel biological markers of potential prognostic or predictive value include: p53, surrogate markers of angiogenesis (such as tumour vascularity or expression of angiogenic factors); cyclines; cell cycle inhibitor protein p27Kip1; type 1 tyrosine kinase growth factor receptor family (epidermal growth factor receptor, c-erbB-2, and others); markers of invasiveness (such as the urokinase plasminogen activator system, metalloproteinases, and tissue inhibitors of metallo-proteinases); laminin; integrins; and other markers listed in Table 4.[1]

The more promising results have been obtained with the de-termination of the following biological markers.

Intratumoral vascularization

Determination of microvessels using specific panendothelial markers (antibodies to CD31, CD34; fVIII-related antigen, etc.), immuno-histochemistry, identification of the vascular 'hot spot' (that is the area of highest vascular density within each single tumour), and the assessment of the absolute vascular count at light microscopy are surrogate markers of angiogenesis.[31] Approximately two-thirds of the published, retrospective studies that assessed the prognostic value of intratumoral vascularization documented a significant association of high vascularization with poor prognosis.[32]–[34]

p53

Most of the reported studies evaluated the expression of p53 by antibodies (pAb1801 and D07) directed to the p53 protein (mainly the mutated forms which are characterized by longer half-life) and

Table 4 Prognostic factors in operable breast cancer

Marker	Level of evidence
Clinical features	
age	weak
menopausal status	weak
timing of surgery	controversial
Histopathological indicators	
histological type	moderate
node status	high
tumour size	high
histological grade	moderate
peritumoral lymphatic and blood vessel invasion	controversial
Biological markers	
oestrogen receptor	moderate
progesterone receptor	weak
markers of cell proliferation	moderate
p53	inconclusive but promising
tumour vascularization and other markers of angiogenesis	inconclusive but promising
c-erbB-2	inconclusive but promising
EGFR	inconclusive but promising
plasminogen pathways	inconclusive but promising
nm23	controversial
cathepsin-D	controversial

immunohistochemistry. Even though different techniques, reagents, cut-off values for positivity, and criteria of evaluation have been used, two-thirds of the retrospective, published studies found that the patients with p53-immunoreactive tumours have poorer prognosis compared to those with p53-negative ones.[35] Alternative methods, but with high costs, have been tested with promising results.[36] The predictive value of p53 expression in patients treated with adjuvant chemotherapy or hormone therapy is controversial.[9],[35]

Markers of invasiveness

The determination, by immunohistochemical, immunoenzymatic, or ELISA methods, of the proteolytic pathways involved in degradation of extracellular matrix, tumour invasiveness, and angiogenesis is another promising approach. Both the urokinase plasminogen ac-tivator system and quantification of metalloproteinases have been tested in retrospective studies and most of the studies documented a prognostic usefulness.[37],[38] Because inhibitors of metalloproteinases are already in clinical evaluation, the assessment of the balance of levels of metalloproteinases and endogenous inhibitors of metallo-proteinases may also have predictive value for the therapeutic activity of such compounds.

Type I growth factor receptor family

The most studied markers in this category are epidermal growth factor receptor (EGRF) and c-erbB-2. Overall, about half of the retrospective studies found that the expression of each one of these two markers is associated with prognosis.[9],[21],[22],[39] The results of the predictive value of EGFR and c-erbB-2 positivity, which are both associated with hormone resistance in patients treated with tamoxifen, are more interesting.[40]–[42] The predictive value of c-erbB-2 for adjuvant chemotherapy remains suggestive but inconclusive, whilst a strong association between expression of c-erbB-2 and therapeutic activity of the anti-c-erbB-2 monoclonal antibody Herceptin® has been reported.[43],[44]

All the above markers still require more clinical evidence, based on prospective studies with standardization of the methodology and quality control programmes.

Bladder carcinoma

Tumour progression of this neoplasia is mainly affected by stage, histological grading, and depth of invasion. Lymph node involvement is the single most important prognostic indicator, and the median survival of patients with node-positive disease is 18 months. The following parameters are predictors of the likelihood of relapse in patients following radical cystectomy: hydronephrosis or elevated preoperative creatinine levels, anaemia, and age. Among the biological markers, retinoblastoma gene expression is altered in 30 to 40 per cent of patients with muscle-invasive bladder cancer and patients with absent or heterogeneous retinoblastoma expression have a significantly worse survival as compared to those with high expression levels. Alterations of the tumour suppressor gene p53 result in nuclear accumulation of inactive p53 protein and some studies demonstrated a poor outcome of patients with tumours with altered p53.[45] Cote et al.[45] found that adjuvant chemotherapy does not improve disease-free survival in patients with tumours lacking p53 expression. Similarly, p53-positivity in patients treated with neoadjuvant chemotherapy is associated with high risk of death.[46]

The level of expression of platelet derived endothelial cell growth factor, a potent angiogenic factor, was determined in 58 surgical specimens of bladder transitional cell carcinoma and compared with seven samples of normal urothelium by Mizutami et al.[47] The authors found that the median level of this angiogenic factor was 2.6 fold higher in tumours than in normal tissue and there was a significant correlation with stage progression and increased histology. Matrix metalloproteinases are important factors involved in degradation of the extracellular matrix and basement membrane, and are regulated by tissue inhibitors of metalloproteinases. Metalloproteinase-2 (MMP2) and tissue inhibitor of metalloproteinases-2 (TIMMP2) were evaluated in 41 bladder carcinomas by reverse transcriptase polymerase chain reaction analysis. Expressions of both MMP2 and TIMMP2 were more elevated in muscle-invasive pT2 bladder tumours than in pT1 tumours and were associated with decreased survival.[48]

Also, certain markers of angiogenesis have been provided to retain prognostic significance in invasive stages of bladder carcinoma. Two independent studies evaluated the prognostic value of intratumoral microvessel density. Dickinson et al.[49] used the panendothelial antibody anti-CD31 to immunostain the tumours of 45 patients. Multi-variate analysis showed that vascularization was an independent prognostic factor for overall survival. Bochner and colleagues[50] immunostained 164 tumours using the monoclonal antibody anti-CD34 and found that the patients with highly vascularized tumours had a significantly shorter relapse-free survival and overall survival than those with tumours characterized by low microvessel counts. The studies by O'Brien et al.[51] and Mizutani et al.[47] evaluated the prognostic value of expression of the angiogenesis factor thymidine phosphorylase (also known as platelet-derived endothelial cell growth factor) in primary bladder cancers.

O'Brien et al.[51] evaluated thymidine phosphorylase by immuno-histochemistry and western blot analysis in a series of 105 tumours, half of which had early-stage (pTa or p T1) tumours. The expression of thymidine phosphorylase was five-fold higher in tumours than in normal bladder mucosa. Tumour cell thymidine phosphorylase expression correlated with histological grade, but not with relapse-free survival or overall survival.

The study by Mizutani et al.[47] also demonstrated a higher level of expression of thymidine phosphorylase in bladder cancer as compared to normal bladder tissue and that the patients with Ta disease and low thymidine phosphorylase expression had a significant longer relapse-free survival than those with tumours with high thymidine phosphorylase expression. Finally, Grossfeld et al.[52] analysed thrombospondin-1 expression, a naturally occurring inhibitor of angiogenesis, in 163 patients with invasive transitional cell carcinoma of the bladder. Thrombospondin-1 was significantly associated with over-accumulation of p53 protein and microvessel density. The patients with thrombospondin-1 expression had a significantly longer overall survival than those without thrombospondin-1. Multivariated analysis showed that thrombospondin-1 retained prognostic significance after tumour stage, lymph node status, histological grade, and p53 status were included in the model.

Prospective research

Prognostic factors based on clinicopathologic characteristics are an integral part of the information needed for a proper management of cancer patients as the behaviour of neoplasia are often heterogeneous within the same stage of the same tumour type. However, the clinical testing of biological markers has been more controversial and disappointing as these have been conducted in retrospective studies not supported by a satisfactory methodology. As a consequence, at present, there is scepticism among oncologists on the use of novel biological markers for prognostic purposes.

The incorporation of novel prognostic markers into prognostic or predictive indexes is advocated instead of continuous research on new single indicators to enhance the ability to make decisions based on individualized scores of risk. The distinction between prognostic and predictive indicators is of increasing clinical importance, as predictive indicators are generally more useful than prognostic factors.[9] Often anticancer treatments are not effective in all patients, so that the knowledge that a therapy may or may not be effective is more important for the management of individual cancer patients than the mere information that the patient has good (or poor) prognosis.

The discovery of new surrogate markers that are potential targets for novel therapeutic approaches aimed at blocking tumour cell proliferation or induction of apoptosis, neutralizing growth factors, or inhibiting angiogenesis represents an integral part of the research for new treatments to improve the probability of cure of cancer patients. The availability of specific and sensitive surrogate markers predictive of efficacy of specific treatments will allow the possibility of improving the management of cancer patients by more individualized therapeutic approaches.[1] This opportunity may allow a more rationale use of conventional therapy as well as a proper testing of biologically-based anticancer treatments (such as: expression of c-erbB-2/HER-neu or epidermal growth factor receptor and therapy with specific neutralizing antibodies such as Herceptin®; tumoral vascularization or determination of endothelial growth factors/inhibitors and anti-angiogenic agents). Future translational research for identification of novel prognostic or predictive indicators will be more fruitful if supported by a more rigorous methodology for clinical testing, as suggested by the American Society of Clinical Oncology guidelines, Altman and Lyman's statistical recommendations, and the TMUGS-Plus system proposed by Hayes et al.[5],[18],[28]

It seems reasonable to hypothesize that the codetermination of surrogate predictive markers which are targets for sensitivity (or resistance) to conventional cytotoxic or hormonal agents coupled with the assessment of targets for biologically-based treatments is a valid strategy to improve the cure of cancer patients and to spare unnecessary toxicity and side-effects by applying more accurate criteria for the selection of patients for therapy.[1] The therapeutic options are increasing all the time and it may be presumed that a therapeutic synergism may occur between conventional and novel, biologically-based treatments.[53],[54] Therefore, a better co-ordination of research in the field of prognostic and predictive indicators, with standardization of the methods and quality controls is needed to contribute to a better management of cancer patients and to achieve the best therapeutic benefit of specific treatments.

References

1. Gasparini G. Prognostic variables in node-negative and node-positive breast cancer—editorial. *Breast Cancer Research and Treatment*, 1998; **52**: 321–31.

2. Sobin LH, Wittekind CH. *UICC:TNM classification of malignant tumours*. 5th edn. New York: John Wiley, 1997.

3. Osborne CK. Steroid hormone receptors in breast cancer management. *Breast Cancer Research and Treatment*, 1998; **51**: 227–38.

4. Page DL, Jensen RA, Simpson JF. Routinely available indicators of prognosis in breast cancer. *Breast Cancer Research and Treatment*, 1998; **51**: 195–208.

5. American Society of Clinical Oncology. Clinical practice guide-lines for the use of tumor markers in breast and colorectal cancer. *Journal of Clinical Oncology*, 1998; **14**: 2843–77.

6. Stearns V, Yamauchi H, Hayes DF. Circulating tumor markers in breast cancer: accepted utilities and novel prospects. *Breast Cancer Research and Treatment*, 1998; **52**: 239–59.

7. Hayes DF, Bast R, Desh CE, *et al.* A tumor marker utility grading system (TMUGS): a framework to evaluate clinical utility of tumor markers. *Journal of the National Cancer Institute*, 1996; **88**: 1456–66.

8. Gasparini G, Pozza F, Harris AL. Evaluating the potential usefulness of new prognostic and predictive indicators in node-negative breast cancer patients. *Journal of the National Cancer Institute*, 1993; **85**: 1206–19.

9. Henderson C, Patek AJ. The relationship between prognostic and predictive factors in the management of the breast cancer. *Breast Cancer Research and Treatment*, 1998; **52**: 261–88.

10. Fleming ID, Cooper JS, Henson DE, *et al. AJCC cancer staging manual*. 5th edn. Philadelphia: Lippincott-Raven, 1997.

11. Silverstein MJ, Poller DN, Waisman JR, *et al.* Prognostic classification of breast ductal carcinoma *in situ*. *Lancet*, 1995; **345**: 1154–7.

12. Silverstein MJ, Lagios MD, Craig PH, *et al.* A prognostic index for ductal carcinoma *in situ* of the breast. *Cancer*, 1996; **77**: 2267–74.

13. Elston CW, Gresham GA, Rao GS. The Cancer Research Compaign trial for early breast cancer: clinico–pathological aspects. *British Journal of Cancer*, 45, 655–62.

14. Todd JH, Dowle C, Williams MR, *et al.* Confirmation of a prognostic index in primary breast cancer. *Cancer*, 1987; **56**: 489–92.

15. Galea MH, Blamey RW, Elston CE, Ellis IO. The Nottingham Prognostic Index in primary breast cancer. *Breast Cancer Research and Treatment*, 1992; **22**: 207–19.

16. Aubele N, Auer G, Falkmer U, *et al.* Improved prognostication in small (pT1) breast cancers by image cytometry. *Breast Cancer Research and Treatment*, 1995; **36**: 83–91.

17. Nordlinger B, Guiguet M, Vaillant JC, *et al.* Surgical resection of colorectal carcinoma metastases to the liver. *Cancer*, 1996; **77**: 1254–62.

18. Altman DG, Lyman GH. Methodological challenges in the evaluation of prognostic factors in breast cancer. *Breast Cancer Research and Treatment*, 1998; **51**: 289–303.

19. Shipp MA. Prognostic factors in aggressive non-Hodgkin's lymphoma: who has 'high risk' disease? *Blood*, 1994; **83**: 1165–73.

20. Bryant J, Fisher B, Gündüz N, Costantino JP, Emir B. S-phase fraction combined with other patient and tumor characteristics for the prognosis of node-negative, estrogen-receptor-positive breast cancer. *Breast Cancer Research and Treatment*, 1998; **51**: 239–53.

21. De Placido S, Carlomagno C, De Laurentis M, Bianco AR. c-erbB2 expression tamoxifen efficacy in breast cancer patients. *Breast Cancer Research and Treatment*, 1998; **52**: 55–64.

22. Pegram MD, Pauletti G, Slamon DJ. HER-2/neu as a predictive marker of response to breast cancer therapy. *Breast Cancer Research and Treatment*, 1998; **52**: 65–77.

23. Amadori D, Silvestrini R. Prognostic and predictive value of thymidine labelling index in breast cancer. *Breast Cancer Research and Treatment*, 1998; **51**: 267–81.

24. Wenger CR, Clark GM. S-phase fraction and breast cancer: a decade of experience. *Breast Cancer Research and Treatment*, 1998; **51**: 255–65.

25. Gion M, Gasparini G. Biological and biochemical factors in the prognosis of breast cancer. In: Dixon JM, Sacchini V, eds. *Breast cancer: diagnosis and management*. European School of Oncology advanced education series. Elsevier, 2000 (in press).

26. Hilsenbeck SG, Ravdin PM, de Moor CA, Chamness GC, Osborne CK, Clark GM. Time-dependence of hazard ratios for prognostic factors in primary breast cancer. *Breast Cancer Research and Treatment*, 1998; **51**: 227–37.

27. McGuire WL, Clark GM. Prognostic factor and treatment decisions in axillary-node-negative breast cancer. *New England Journal of Medicine*, 1992; **326**: 1756–61.

28. Hayes DF, Trock B, Harris AL. Assessing the clinical impact of prognostic factors: when is 'statistically significant' clinically useful? *Breast Cancer Research and Treatment*, 1998; **51**: 305–19.

29. Dahiya R, Deng G. Molecular prognostic markers in breast cancer. *Breast Cancer Research and Treatment*, 1998; **52**: 185–200.

30. Hermanek P, Sobin LH, Fleming ID. What do we need beyond TNM? *Cancer*, 1996; **77**: 815–17.

31. Weidner N, Semple JP, Welch WR, Folkman J. Tumor angiogenesis and metastasis-correlation in invasive breast carcinoma. *New England Journal of Medicine*, 1991; **324**: 1–8.

32. Gasparini G, Harris AL. Clinical importance of the determination of tumor angiogenesis in breast carcinoma: Much more than a new prognostic tool. *Journal of Clinical Oncology*, 1995; **13**: 765–82.

33. Gasparini G. Clinical significance of the determination of angiogenesis in human breast cancer: Update of the biological background and overview of the Vicenza studies. *European Journal of Cancer*, 1996; **32A**: 2485–93.

34. Vermeulen PB, Gasparini G, Fox SB, *et al.* Quantification of angiogenesis in solid human tumours: an international consensus on the methodology and criteria of evaluation. *European Journal of Cancer*, 1996; **32A**: 2474–84.

35. Elledge RM, Allred DC. Prognostic and predictive value of p53 and

p21 in breast cancer. *Breast Cancer Research and Treatment*, 1998; **52**: 79–89.

36. **Bergh J, Norberg J, Sjögren S, Lindgren A, Holmberg L.** Complete sequencing of the p53 gene provides prognostic information in breast cancer patients, particularly in relation to adjuvant systemic therapy and radiotherapy. *Nature Medicine*, 1995; **1**: 1029–34.

37. **Grondal-Hansen J, Peters HA, van Putten WLJ, *et al.*** Prognostic significance of the receptor for urokinase plasminogen activator in breast cancer. *Clinical Cancer Research*, 1995; **1**: 1079–87.

38. **Toi M, Ishigaki S, Tominaga T.** Metalloproteinases and tissue inhibitors of metalloproteinases. *Breast Cancer Research and Treatment*, 1998; **52**: 113–24.

39. **Gullick WJ, Srinivasan R.** The type 1 growth factor receptor family: new ligands and receptors and their role in breast cancer. *Breast Cancer Research and Treatment*, 1998; **52**: 43–53.

40. **Nicholson S, Wright C, Sainsbury RC, *et al.*** Epidermal growth factor receptor as a marker for poor prognosis in node-negative breast cancer patients: neu and tamoxifen failure. *Journal of Steroid Biochemistry and Molecular Biology*, 1990; **37**: 811–14.

41. **Klijn JGM, Berns EMJJ, Bontebal M, Foekens J.** Cell biological factors associated with the response of breast cancer to systemic treatment. *Cancer Treatment Reviews*, 1993; **19**: 45–63.

42. **Wright C, Nicholson S, Angus B, *et al.*** Relationship between c-erbB2 protein product expression and response to endocrine therapy in advanced breast cancer. *British Journal of Cancer*, 1992; **65**: 118–21.

43. **Beselga J, Tripathy D, Mendelsohn J, *et al.*** Phase II study of intravenous recombinant human anti-p185 HER 2 monoclonal antibody in patients with HER2/neu-overexpressing metastatic breast cancer. *Journal of Clinical Oncology*, 1996; **14**: 737–44.

44. **Cobleigh MA, Vogel CL, Tripathy D, *et al.*** Efficacy and safety of herceptin (humanized anti-HER2 antibody) as a single agent in 22 women with HER2 overexpression who relapsed following chemotherapy for metastatic breast cancer. *Journal of Clinical Oncology*, 1998; **97a**: 376.

45. **Cote R, Esrig D, Groshen S, *et al.*** p53 and treatment of bladder cancer. *Nature*, 1997; **385**: 123–4.

46. **Sarkis A, Bajorin DF, Reuter VE, *et al.*** Prognostic value of p 53 Nuclear over expression in patients with invasive bladder cancer treated with neoadjuvant M-VAC. *Journal of Clinical Oncology*, 1995; **13**: 1384–90.

47. **Mizutami Y, Okada Y, Yoshida O.** Expression of platelet-derived endothelial cell growth factor in bladder carcinoma. *Cancer*, 1997; **79**: 1190–4.

48. **Kahayama H, Yokota K, Kurokawa Y, Murakami Y, Nishitami M, Kagawa S.** Prognostic value of matrix metalloproteinase-2 and tissue inhibitor of metalloproteinase-2 expression in bladder cancer. *Cancer*, 1998; **82**: 1359–66.

49. **Dickinson AJ, Fox SB, Persad RA, Hollyer J, Sibley GN, Harris AL.** Quantification of angiogenesis as an independent predictor of prognosis in invasive bladder carcinoma. *British Journal of Urology*, 1994; **74**: 762–6.

50. **Bochner BH, Cote RJ, Weidner N, *et al.*** Tumor angiogenesis is an independent prognostic indicator of invasive transitional cell carcinoma of the bladder. *Journal of the National Cancer Institute*, 1995; **87**: 1603–12.

51. **O'Brien T, Fox SB, Dickinson AJ, *et al.*** Expression of the angiogenic factor thymidine phosphorylase/platelet-derived endothelial cell growth factor in primary bladder cancers. *Cancer Research*, 1996; **56**: 4799–804.

52. **Grossfeld GD, Ginsberg DA, Stein JP, *et al.*** Thrombospondin-1 expression in bladder cancer: association with p53 alterations, tumor angiogenesis, and tumor progression. *Journal of the National Cancer Institute*, 1997; **89**: 219–27.

53. **Gasparini G, Harris AL.** Does an improved control of tumour growth require an anti-cancer therapy targeting both neoplastic and intratumoral endothelial cells? *European Journal of Cancer*, 1994; **30A**: 201–6.

54. **Gasparini G.** The rationale and future potential of angiogenesis inhibitors in neoplasia. *Drugs*, 1999; **58**: 17–38.

4

Scientific basis of cancer treatment

4.1 Principles of surgical oncology

Peter Hohenberger

Introduction

The majority of long-term cancer survivors have been cured largely because of the surgical removal of their solid tumour. Fewer patients are cured by radiotherapy, and fewer still by chemotherapy—Rosenberg calculated that about 43 per cent of such patients are cured by surgery, another 18 per cent by radiotherapy, and that another 6.5 per cent may profit from adjuvant and primary chemotherapy.[1] Even in the disseminated stages of disease, the surgical removal of isolated organ metastases may offer a realistic chance for cure, for example following resection of liver or lung metastases in patients with colorectal or other types of cancer. Therefore, one might assume that surgical oncology would attract major attention in the scientific community.

This is not the case, for it is the sessions on gene therapy or on new anticancer drugs that attract the largest attendance at national or international cancer conferences. However, gene therapy has yet to cure any patient who has cancer. Most trials in the field of oncology focus on new drugs, different drug schedules, combinations of drugs, or combinations of drugs with radiotherapy and/or surgery. These studies often address the question of whether chemotherapy or radiochemotherapy improves the results of surgery. Unfortunately, surgeons often do little more than contribute patients to such studies and perform the surgical procedure before or after the added treatment. Relatively few randomized trials have compared different surgical approaches in an attempt to determine the best available surgical treatment—for example, quadrantectomy plus radiotherapy versus mastectomy in breast cancer, gastrectomy with or without D2-lymphadenectomy for stomach cancer, or the comparison of open versus laparoscopic surgery for colorectal cancer. The performance of multicentre surgical trials is often hampered by difficulties in standardizing operative techniques between studies.

From a patient's point of view, the perception of surgical oncology is clearly different. Most patients confronted with an initial diagnosis of malignancy ask whether the lesion can be removed. Despite the need to undergo an operative procedure under general anaesthesia, this is widely regarded by patients as the preferred treatment option. They expect to fall asleep—undergo surgery—tolerate pain—be cured. The surgical removal of a tumour always implies the chance for cure. To undergo radiotherapy yields the question: 'It can't be operated upon?', indicating the fear that his/her case is 'beyond surgery'. The proposal to prescribe chemotherapy implies the possibility of disseminated disease.

The spectrum of cancer surgery ranges from very minor procedures (polypectomy, lumpectomy) to 'mega-operations' such as regional pancreatectomy, pelvic exenteration, or liver transplantation. The type of surgery performed depends on the biology and natural history of the tumour, the expected functional and cosmetic outcome, the skill of the individual surgeon, the efficacy and availability of other treatment modalities, the morbidity and mortality of the operation itself, and the patient's willingness to accept the associated risk(s).

Surgical oncology—definitions

As well as training and experience in the performance of major operations, an oncological surgeon must be familiar with the biology of cancer. A knowledge of the patterns and mechanisms of metastasis is essential for the selection of surgical and multimodality approaches to the treatment of patients with cancer.

How does the surgical oncologist differ from the general surgeon?

The surgical oncologist:

- has multidisciplinary training, combined with experience in performing sophisticated cancer operations;
- has expertise in screening and prophylaxis (prophylactic surgery of cancer), which necessitates familiarity with the epidemiology and natural history of different types of cancer;
- participates in specific training programmes, resulting in the establishment of standards of care in the surgical treatment of cancer;
- has a major involvement in prospective randomized trials, which is far more than just contributing surgical patients for adjuvant drug therapy; and
- follows the rules set out in Table 1 for best practice.

Specific definitions

Multivisceral resection

This implies the removal of neighbouring organs or structures to achieve complete resection of the primary tumour. Kausch–Whipple's procedure and pelvic exenteration are multivisceral resections.

Multimodality treatment

Multimodality treatment implies the combination of surgery with radiotherapy, chemotherapy, hyperthermia, immunotherapy, or any other therapeutic approach. Surgery may take place prior to, during,

Table 1 General rules in surgical oncology

1. Be aware when, in the course of the disease, the scheduled intervention will take place.

2. Try to accurately identify those patients who can be cured by local treatment alone.

3. In early cancer, limited methods must demonstrate their equality or superiority to more radical procedures prior to being translated from research into practice.

4. Try to select the local treatment that provides the best balance between local control and treatment-related morbidity.

5. Only radical resection with clear margins (R0-resection) is able to improve survival and the prognosis for the patient. This is the only approach allowing the patient to enter a period of disease-free survival.

6. Identify and recommend adjuvant treatment to the patient, which can improve local control and influence the development of metastatic disease.

7. Outcome analysis must not only focus on tumour-related issues but also on long-term problems related to the procedure.

8. When analysing treatment outcome, objective analysis as well as self-assessment by the patient is of value.

9. If surgical treatment seems to be required for patients in the late stage of their malignant disease, life expectation and quality of life prior to and after the surgical intervention needs to be addressed very carefully.

10. Patients scheduled for preoperative (neoadjuvant) multimodality treatment should be fit for an extended operation.

11. Timing of a surgical intervention may be required with respect to pretreatment measures, or if there is evidence of other confounding factors (e.g. menstrual cycle for breast cancer surgery)

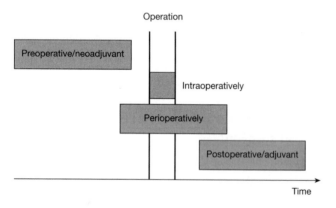

Fig. 1 Timing of multimodality treatment components related to a surgical procedure.

or after other treatment(s) (Fig. 1). This form of treatment requires specific knowledge of the other modalities, the effects of which will determine the optimal timing of surgery (Table 2). For example, the dose and schedule of radiotherapy (total radiation dose, conventional or hyperfractionated regimen) will influence the timing and nature of the operation. Immunocompromisation resulting from systemic chemotherapy may pose a particular risk, especially if hollow organs potentially contaminated by bacteria need to be resected. Skin damage following irradiation is not always a visible indicator of the extent of the radiation field. In patients scheduled to undergo surgery for tumour recurrence, this needs to be investigated to make sure there is undamaged tissue at the incision site to allow adequate wound healing (Fig. 2).

Guidelines

Practical guidelines for the primary treatment of cancers in different organs have been published by the Society of Surgical Oncology.[2]

These guidelines define the role of the surgeon in the initial management of major cancer sites. This educational release defines:

- guidelines for the early referral of patients to cancer specialists;
- the evaluation of symptomatic patients;
- required diagnostic procedures;
- surgical considerations about the method and extent of the operation; and
- other therapeutic considerations.

The surgeon has to provide essential information to the medical or radiation oncologist for postoperative adjunctive treatment, including the location of any residual tumour and the area at greatest risk for recurrence. Drawings of the newly created anatomy are useful for radiotherapy planning.

Questions to be asked by clinical research include: the criteria for patient selection for various procedures; the surgical technique and its associated morbidity, mortality, and functional outcome; quality control of studies; outcome analysis (trial endpoints); and economic considerations. Other questions also need to be addressed, for example regarding the use of isolated organ perfusion and fibroblast culture for improved closure following deep resections.

Historical landmarks

Most of these relate to the introduction of methods for performing more extensive operations without significant mortality and with acceptable morbidity. The contributions of Billroth (gastrectomy, 1860) Volkmann (rectal excision, 1878), Wertheim (hysterectomy, 1906), and Kausch and Whipple (duodenopancreatectomy 1935) cannot be overestimated. Robinson provides an excellent and detailed overview of the achievements of cancer surgery, tracing its history back to the resection of an osteosarcoma within a mandibular fragment found in East Africa and to Egyptian papyri reporting the removal of a limb tumour.[3] More recently, surgical approaches have focused

Table 2 Problems encountered with surgical procedures following preoperative radio- and/or chemotherapy

Positive effects of preoperative radio- and/or chemotherapy (neoadjuvant concept)
- tumour shrinkage (downstaging) improves resectability
- may sterilize the tumour boundaries
- may prevent tumour-cell spillage during operation
- may increase resection rate with clear margins (R0-resection)

Problems associated with immunocompromised patients (emergency and elective operations):
- anaemia and impaired bone marrow reserves
- neutropenia and lymphocytopenia
- impaired antibody production
- changes in microbial flora (fungal overgrowth in bacteria-contaminated organs due to antibiotics)
- translocation of bacteria facilitated (enterocolitis)
- collagen production by fibroblasts reduced

Potential for negative effects within surgical procedures:
- extent of tumour boundaries is sometimes more difficult to assess
- rate of anastomotic leakage in hollow organs may be increased (i.e. rectal or oesophageal cancer)
- delayed wound healing

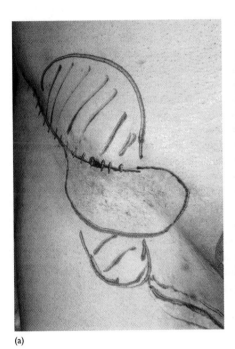

(a)

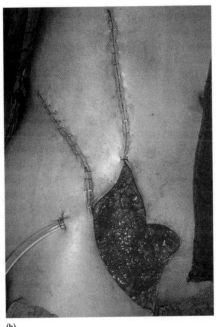

(b)

Fig. 2 Incision line for the removal of a sarcoma recurrence within an irradiated field of the right groin, to make sure that wound healing will take place from non-irradiated tissue. (a) Central area irradiation field (dashed area above and below shows the tumour extent); (b) wound closure from uninvolved skin and omentumplasty.

on minimizing the procedures or tailoring them to patients' individual risk factors.

A few landmarks in surgical oncology can be highlighted that do not focus on technical resectability alone:

- Halsted's radical mastectomy (1890) removed the breast and the lymph nodes *en bloc*, together with the minor and the major pectoralis muscles. This operation failed because it was based on the erroneous perception that breast cancer was a regional disease; of course, it is now recognized that breast cancer is a systemic

disease. Lesser surgery—see below—was later found to be as good as radical mastectomy.

- In 1967, Turnbull reported that the outcome for patients improved significantly after the adoption of the 'no-touch isolation technique' in colorectal surgery (Fig. 3). This result demonstrated that tumour cells can be spilt intraoperatively, and that the probability of locoregional recurrence can be decreased by paying attention to surgical technique.[61]

- Crile was the first to advocate the use of lesser surgery and to

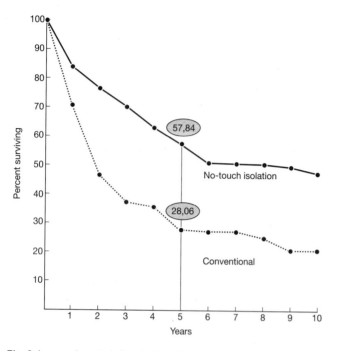

Fig. 3 Improved survival after the introduction of the 'no-touch isolation technique' by Turnbull. (Reproduced with permission from ref. 30.)

campaign against the use of radical mastectomy.[4],[5] Veronesi introduced quadrantectomy (later termed 'lumpectomy') and axillary lymph node dissection combined with irradiation of the remaining breast.[6] The Milan trials, and those inaugurated by Fisher and the **NSABP** (National Surgical Adjuvant Breast Project), demonstrated an equivalent outcome with less morbidity and improved cosmesis.[7]

- The most recent development of limiting axillary dissection to those patients with a positive sentinel lymph node or larger (T2) tumours, is a further step in the move away from using a radical procedure to a more tailored, individual approach (see Chapter 11.5).

- For almost a century, several surgeons and pathologists had suggested that the treatment of low rectal cancer required not merely resection of the primary tumour but also of its lymphatics.[8]–[10] The development of adequate resection margins and lymphatic clearance were described, and it was agreed that the treatment of rectal cancer could only be called 'radical' if a permanent colostomy was part of the procedure. During the 1970s and 1980s, the margin required for accepting an anterior resection as an adequate operation decreased.[11] Thorough investigations of lymphatic spread and consideration of anatomical and embryological features[12] have now made a low anterior resection including total mesorectal excision the treatment of choice.[13],[14] The most important event following Heald's publication on the mesorectum as the clue to pelvic recurrence, was not the description of the procedure but the education of a generation of surgeons to adopt his technique (see Chapter 10.4). This has led to improvement in the results of treatment and in the quality of life of patients.[15],[16] As a consequence, adjuvant trials of patients with rectal cancer need to be repeated to determine the contribution of radiotherapy

and/or chemotherapy when used with this newer type of operation.

- Knowledge of the vascular anatomy of the liver provided by Couinaud and Bismuth[17] greatly improved the outcome of liver surgery. Information on the segmentation of liver tissue according to the portal vein branches, resulted in segment-oriented resections and dramatically improved the control of bleeding, which had been the major problem connected with liver surgery (see Chapter 10.9). Improvements were seen in morbidity and mortality figures of both in the resection of metastases and of primary liver cancer.

- Enneking first defined the extent of the compartment that should be resected in the treatment of bone sarcomas.[18] This compartment includes the muscles originating proximal to the tumour and inserting distal to it; the whole compartment needs to be resected to completely excise locoregional spread. The definition of a compartment is also of value when planning surgery for the removal of an intracompartmental soft tissue sarcoma.

- Preservation of an organ, despite radical tumour surgery, has been one of the major achievements in recent years. Breast-conserving therapy is the most prominent example, but there is also evidence that amputation for sarcoma does not lead to a better survival than appropriate limb-sparing treatment (see Chapter 16.1).

- Combined radiochemotherapy has become the treatment of choice for primary anal cancer: this avoids abdominoperineal excision with a consequent colostomy as a first therapeutic approach.[19] For locally advanced laryngeal cancer, two randomized controlled trials have demonstrated that the combination of radiotherapy and chemotherapy, with surgical resection reserved for salvage, is as efficient as laryngectomy in terms of patient survival: this strategy allows preservation of the larynx and hence the patient's speech.[20],[21] Surgical removal or radiochemotherapy for squamous-cell cancer of the oesophagus seem to yield a similar outcome in terms of survival, but this has not been proven in a randomized trial (see Chapters 4.3. and 4.5).

- The safe application of recombinant, human, tumour-necrosis factor-alpha (**rhTNF-α**) in isolated limb perfusion is one of the first applications of biotherapy in humans.[22] This genetically engineered and potentially highly toxic molecule (which may cause septic shock when administered systemically) has proven effective in a well-defined disease, namely high-grade extremity sarcoma with extracompartmental extension (see Chapter 4.23).

Surgery for establishing tumour diagnosis

The development of computed tomography (CT) and magnetic resonance (MR) imaging combined with fine-needle aspiration or core biopsy has rendered surgery less necessary for establishing a diagnosis of malignant disease (see Chapter 3.2). Diagnostic laparoscopy (see Chapter 3.6) helps to avoid exploratory abdominal laparotomies. Only in a few situations where insufficient tissue can be obtained for adequate histological examination, is laparotomy still necessary; for example, this might be the case for retroperitoneal lesions or tumour recurrence within scar tissue, or if access to a malignancy is prevented by extensive adhesions.

Table 3 Technical rules for incisional biopsy or surgery for establishing tumour diagnosis

1. During surgical biopsy, scars should be placed carefully so that they can be removed as a part of the subsequent definitive surgical procedure: this is particularly important in surgery for soft tissue sarcoma and during staging laparoscopy where the ports for access to the abdominal cavity should be placed at standard incision lines (Figs 3 and 4).

2. During incisional biopsy no new tissue planes should be opened or contaminated by tumour cells, and haematoma must be avoided meticulously.

3. Obtaining representative tissue both for frozen-section and paraffin-embedded staining is essential (at least 2 × 2 cm × 1 cm in size).

4. Handling of the biopsy specimen (specific fixatives) needs to be planned carefully with the pathologist prior to the procedure.

Sometimes an incisional tumour biopsy is required (for example, soft tissue sarcomas and lymphomas) to obtain the necessary information for guiding treatment. Grading, and sometimes histological subtyping, can have a major influence in deciding which treatment should be chosen. Guidelines for performing an incisional biopsy are covered in Table 3 (see also Figs 4(a) and (b), and 5).

The spectrum of surgical oncology procedures with curative intent

Developments in molecular oncology have led to the detection of genetically determined malignancies. The multiple endocrine neoplasia (**MEN**) syndrome, familial adenomatosis polyposis (coli), or BRCA-1/2 associated breast cancer are examples where surgery may be required to remove high-risk organs. In addition to having a role in cancer prevention, the surgeon's skill may be used in the palliation of those patients with a heavy tumour load. The more common indication for surgical treatment is removal of the primary tumour with a curative intent. In addition to the issues directly linked to the goals and type of surgery, patients and their relatives need more than just surgical support (Table 4).

Consideration of the extent of tumour spread and total tumour burden is always a prerequisite for successful treatment. A rough estimate, gleaned from a variety of childhood tumours and animal experiments, suggests that a 5-cm tumour (volume of 120 to 150 ml) consists of approx. 3×10^{11} cells. Tumours at the detection threshold of 1 cm contain about 10^9 cells. For a locally advanced malignancy, surgical resection of 99.9 per cent of the tumour would decrease the tumour load from 10^{11} to 10^8 cells! (See Chapter 1.6.)

Surgery for preneoplastic conditions

Surgery for preneoplastic conditions, such as familial adenomatosis polyposis (coli) (**FAP**), cryptorchism, ulcerative colitis, or MEN-syndrome, deals with a tumour load of zero. The operative procedure must be radical, in the sense that no tissue bearing an increased risk of cancer is left behind. This is important in subcutaneous mastectomies or when performing a thyroidectomy for children with the MEN syndrome. The operation must be carried out without mortality and with an absolute minimum of morbidity. Functional consequences must be weighed against the risk of cancer development, for example during restorative proctocolectomy for FAP or for ulcerative colitis. Counselling patients and their relatives about the risk of cancer development and the morbidity associated with the procedure is an integral part of the surgeons' non-operative care. The

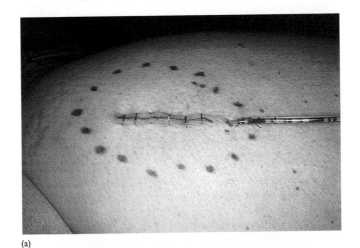
(a)

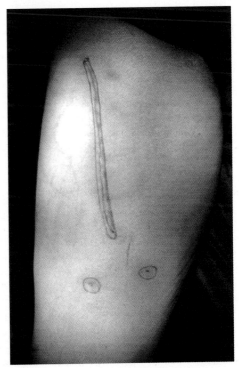
(b)

Fig. 4 (a) Proper incisional biopsy with drain exactly placed at the incision line. (b) Example of the improper localization of drains, this will require major skin excision during subsequent operation.

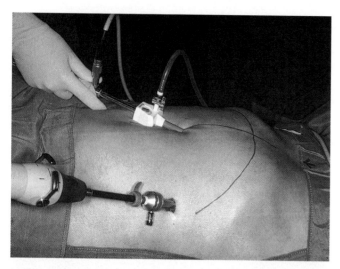

Fig. 5 Positioning of trocars at incision lines during diagnostic laparoscopy, required for subsequent laparotomies.

surgeon clearly needs to be familiar with the fundamentals of genetics and the analysis of genetic risk.

Surgery for early-stage cancer

This is dependent on knowing the extent of local tumour infiltration and the risk of lymphatic invasion or lymph node metastases. Endoluminal ultrasound in gastrointestinal tract cancer, intraoperative ultrasound and sophisticated MRI techniques in early hepatocellular cancer, or detailed measurements of the primary tumour in malignant melanoma (microinvasion) may enable the surgeon to decide whether limited surgery can be used instead of the standard procedure. However, a limited surgical approach is not feasible in other tumours such as cancer of the oesophagus or pancreas. Certain histological subtypes of tumours (for example, the signet-cell type of gastric cancer) are characterized by adverse biological properties, which put the patient at an increased risk of tumour recurrence after a limited surgical resection. In contrast, early bladder cancer that has not invaded the muscle wall may be treated successfully by transurethral resection, with or without the postoperative intravesical instillation of BCG (bacille Calmette–Guérin vaccine).

Standard oncological surgery

The overwhelming majority of tumours require the treatment of palpable, measurable, or visible masses. With such tumours the load is already substantial, but the tumour is limited to the organ in which it originates and no distant metastases can be detected. The patients hope for long-term survival or cure if they are fit enough undergo operation. Standard techniques such as partial or total mastectomy, hemicolectomy, anterior resection, nephrectomy, or lobectomy in the lung are representative examples.

The characteristic of this type of surgery is that the regional lymphatic drainage (axillary nodes for breast cancer, mesorectum for rectal cancer, hilar and paratracheal nodes in lung cancer, para-aortic nodes in kidney cancer) is resected together with the tumour-bearing organ. This is in contrast to the limited surgical approach to early-stage cancer, where limited lymphatic clearance and less-extensive

Table 4 The spectrum of surgical oncology procedures, tumour biological considerations, and specific issues of the surgeon–patient relationship

Tumour stage	Precancerous condition	Early cancer	Confined to original primary organ	Locoregionally advanced	Metastatic	Palliation intended
Typical examples	Cryptorchism MEN-syndrome Adenomatosis coli Ulcerative colitis	DCIS Polypous T1 colon T1-Barrett cancer	Gastric cancer Lung cancer Colorectal cancer	Sarcoma of the bone and soft tissues Rectal cancer Oesophageal cancer	Liver, lung metastases of colorectal cancer, ovarian cancer	Gastric outlet obstruction, Pain from distension or bone metastases Exulceration
Tumour load	Zero	Low (10^4–10^6 cells)	~10^8–10^{10}	10^{11}–10^{12}	>10^{12}	Few to >10^{12}
Type of surgery *– example*	Extremely low morbidity – thyroidectomy, – restorative proctocolectomy	Limited – endoscopic polypectomy – breast segmental excision	Standard (including regional lymphadenectomy) – gastrectomy, – anterior resection nephrectomy, – lung lobectomy	Specific combined-modality therapy – preoperative radiochemotherapy, – isolated limb perfusion followed by resection	Selective (cure sometimes possible) – liver resection – debulking and chemotherapy – intra-arterial chemotherapy	Individually tailored – intestinal bypass, – resection of exulcerated masses
Non-operative expectations of the surgeon by the patient	Counselling the patient and family	Prevention of second cancer Screening for genetic alterations	Coping Initiation of adjuvant treatment Follow-up	Interdisciplinary management Continued guidance of the patient	Discussing the hope for cure	Close cooperation with the palliation team

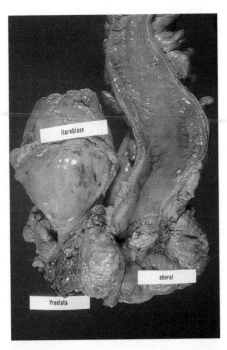

Fig. 6 Monobloc resection of rectal cancer invading to the prostate and bladder.

resection margins may sometimes be effective. Morbidity from these standard procedures should be low and mortality should be less than 5 per cent.

The surgical oncologist must also inform patients about adjunctive measures (postoperative adjuvant chemotherapy or radiotherapy) and assist them to cope with the results of surgery, particularly if organ function cannot be preserved or is lost due to perioperative complications (sexual function, voiding, swallowing, food intake, bowel movements). The aim of surgery at this stage of the disease is to provide a resection with clear margins (R0-resection according to the TNM classification, see Chapter 3.5).

Surgery for locally advanced disease

Patients presenting with locally advanced disease are characterized by invasion of the tumour into surrounding tissues beyond the organ in which it originates. These tumours are usually large and the tumour load is high. Tumours are often poorly differentiated and pose a considerable risk of distant metastases. When infiltrating beyond the borders of the organ, tumour cells often invade into nerve sheaths, perivascular tissue, or the lymphatics. Under these circumstances, surgery alone will rarely be able to achieve tumour control. The risk of local recurrence is high even if all visible, palpable, and detectable tumour is removed. This has been shown to be true for tumours of the breast, gastrointestinal tract (oesophagus, pancreas, or rectum), lung cancer, and sarcomas. Depending on the tumour location and histology, complete removal may be achieved using extended procedures (e.g. pelvic exenteration for rectal or bladder cancer, or pulmonary and thoracic wall resection for T4 lung cancer). Monobloc resection in this type of operation is a must! (Fig. 6). However, these procedures often result in major dysfunction for the patient and/or require allografts or tissue flaps for soft tissue reconstruction.

Whether a patient can be cured by extended surgery depends more on tumour biology than on the number of organs involved and their anatomical location. The results of treatment for locally advanced tumours can often be improved with a multimodality approach. In locally advanced breast, rectal, or oesophageal cancer, preoperative radio/chemotherapy is the treatment of choice. In squamous-cell cancer of the lung invading to the thoracic wall (Pancoast tumour), preoperative irradiation facilitates a radical resection with curative intent. Isolated limb perfusion may be employed followed by resection to improve tumour control in soft tissue sarcomas of the extremities. However, even if tumour resection is technically feasible, there are situations where this type of extended resection is contraindicated (for example, combined oesophageal and tracheal resection for T4-oesophageal cancer).

Combined modality therapy aims at:

- administering adjuvant treatment to those tissues with a good blood supply;
- sterilizing the tumour boundaries, thereby diminishing spillage of tumour cells intraoperatively;
- initiating tumour shrinkage ('downstaging'); and
- improving resectability and outcome.

The approaches described above have been labelled as 'mega-surgery'. However, it is not the 'mega' of the surgery that cures the patient but the thorough evaluation of the extent of the malignant spread and an interdisciplinary treatment plan. The successful management of these situations is an important step from 'oncological surgery' to 'surgical oncology'. It is essential that the surgeon knows and understands the interactions between the different treatment modalities and is experienced in the operation (Table 2). The increased risk of morbidity and mortality of surgical resection within a multidisciplinary treatment protocol needs to be evaluated and explained to the patient in advance, but this should be counterbalanced by an explanation of the potential gains of the approach. Furthermore, a surgeon's attitude towards multimodality treatment should be that, although his/her patient undergoes additional treatment (either prior to the operation and/or afterwards), the surgical treatment remains the key-procedure. Multimodality treatment is planned by a team of oncologists from different disciplines, but the surgeon remains a key member of the treatment team throughout.

Surgical treatment for metastatic disease

Over recent years, surgery for the treatment of metastatic disease has gained in popularity. The successful treatment of liver metastases from colorectal cancer or lung metastases from testicular or renal-cell cancer by metastectomy has raised the hope for cure. The status of disease progression should be judged by: the time interval from treatment of the primary tumour; the number, distribution, and size of metastases; and, for testicular tumours, the rate of increase in serum markers (see Chapter 13.4). Metastectomy may be used as an intent-to-cure-approach or as cytoreductive surgery. Both options require the appropriate selection of patients. Although the resection of liver or lung metastases has become standard treatment, morbidity and mortality remain important factors. The longer the interval between treatment of the primary tumour and the appearance of metastatic disease, the better the prognosis following metastectomy.[23],[24] Prospectively validated scoring systems may also be useful for selecting good-risk patients for curative metastectomy.[25]

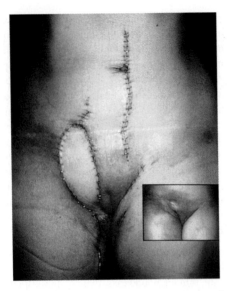

Fig. 7 Palliative removal of ulcerated lymph node metastases from vulvar cancer of the groin; and covering the soft tissue defect with a myocutaneous flap.

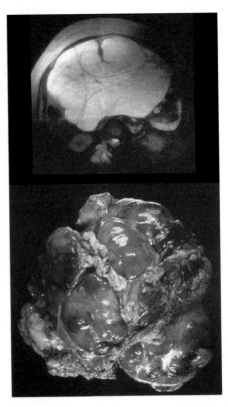

Fig. 8 Debulking surgery for metastatic liposarcoma initially originating in the thigh and with abdominal metastases. Above; CT appearances: below; operative specimen.

Cytoreductive surgery may be used in patients where chemotherapy (or another treatment modality) has proven efficacy. Limited morbidity from surgery is indispensable for such a combined approach. Tumour-cell repopulation may increase after debulking surgery, so that any delay in chemotherapy might outweigh the beneficial effects of surgery.

Surgery for palliation

In patients in whom a resection-for-cure intent is impossible, surgery may effectively relieve their symptoms (pain, distention, bleeding) and improve organ function (gastrointestinal transit), thereby improving the patient's quality of life and possibly prolonging life. Such surgical interventions are palliative. Unfortunately, no general recommendations can be given: the type, timing, and extent of surgery must be planned on an individual basis. Typical procedures include gastroenterostomy, biliodigestive anastomosis, enteric bypass, resection of ulcerated lymph node metastases (Fig. 7(a) and (b)), and debulking surgery (Fig. 8). The procedure carrying the lowest risk of morbidity and mortality for the patient is the best. Problems with wound healing or any other type of complication that prolong the patient's hospital stay or add morbidity must be avoided.

Surgical approaches to the treatment of obstructed hollow organs are in competition with endoscopical procedures. Generally, the less-invasive approach is preferable (for example, stent placement to restore oral food intake in patients with oesophageal cancer, see Chapter 10.1). Clinical decisions concerning palliative surgery are often more difficult to make than decisions regarding curative surgery; for instance, the life expectancy of the patient as well as the potential of other treatment options need to be discussed within a multi-disciplinary team.

Recently, the report of the National Confidential Enquiry on Perioperative Death in the United Kingdom suggested that 'surgeons are performing too many inappropriate and aggressive operations on patients who are frail or terminally ill'.[26] This report analysed data on patients who died within 30 days of a surgical procedure. The authors concluded that the decision to operate was sometimes not in the best interests of the patient. Other data from the literature confirm these findings; for example, perioperative mortality has been reported to exceed 10 per cent in patients who undergo exploratory laparotomy-only for gastric or pancreatic cancer.[27],[28] Patients with a minimal expectation of benefit from a procedure suffer most from its morbidity. A diagnostic laparoscopy prior to opening the whole abdomen is often advantageous (see Chapter 3.6).

Oncological emergencies

The easiest and most effective method for treating oncological emergencies (such as obstruction or perforation of the gastrointestinal tract, ureteral obstruction, pathological fracture, or spinal cord compression) should be chosen, irrespective of the tumour stage. For decision-making, the surgeon must possess sufficient oncological knowledge to be able to distinguish, for example, a vincristine-associated gastrointestinal-tract distention from an ileus due to a mechanical bowel obstruction. The decision to operate in such cases may be difficult, and often there is an ethical dilemma between improving the quality of life and prolonging the patient's suffering. If a terminally ill patient is dying of pneumonia, tracheostomy might be an adequate option. Whenever possible, a minimally invasive treatment for the control of symptoms should be considered (endoscopical or radiological interventions for a fistula, or treatment of a haemorrhage by embolization).

Surgery for reconstructive and rehabilitative procedures

There are a variety of complications of oncological treatments that require acute surgical intervention. Examples include radiation-induced side-effects such as osteoradionecrosis, proctitis, cystitis, or small bowel stricture. Chemotherapy may induce tissue necrosis due to the extravasation of cytotoxic drugs or abscess formation during neutropenia. Cutaneous or subcutaneous tissue necrosis often requires surgical intervention and resection of all damaged tissue, albeit after a time interval to await demarcation.

Major operations for cancer often sacrifice important organ function. Normally, reconstruction is already part of the operative strategy, with an interdisciplinary operative team working closely together. Immediate reconstruction helps patients accept the extent of a major surgical procedure and greatly assists with their psychological recovery. Breast reconstruction after mastectomy, continent ileostomy, or construction of a neobladder instead of a urinary diversion are common procedures. Generally, immediate reconstruction, compared to delayed tissue transfer, does not lead to increased morbidity or adversely affect treatment results, although it does prolong the procedure. The additional expenditure (blood transfusions, longer general anaesthesia, greater operative field for myocutaneous flaps; see Fig. 7(b)) is outweighed by the benefits of a one-step procedure, which is usually better tolerated by the patient than two procedures within a short time. Surgical multidisciplinary expertise, for tumour resection and tissue reconstruction, needs to be co-ordinated as close as possible.

A minority of patients undergo breast reconstruction after the primary operation. However, even if undertaken several months or years after mastectomy this is an important contribution to their quality of life (see Chapter 11.6). Restoration of sexual function with a penile prosthesis or construction of a neovagina are other examples. Transferring an abdominal colostomy to the perineum by constructing a neosphincter from the colorectal muscularis or using the gracilis muscle contributes to limiting the functional adverse effects of cancer surgery.[29] After surgical resection of a large sarcoma and loss of muscles resulting in joint arthrosis, transposing muscles from an agonistic to the antagonistic site may result in pain relief and salvage of the joint. Decisions regarding the use of these procedures need to be made with respect to the stage of disease and prognosis for each patient.

Surgical technique

Operative technique

In 1975 Turnbull described a 'no-touch isolation technique' to avoid tumour-cell dissemination during resection of the colon.[30] He referred to Cole's earlier investigations reporting the presence of cancer cells in the portal venous blood of a perfused, resected, cancerous segment of the human colon.[31] Cole's technique of colonic resection

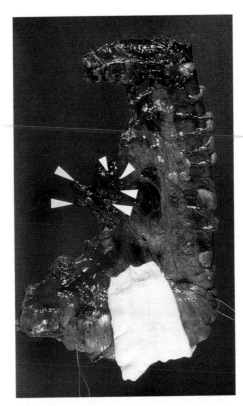

Fig. 9 No-touch isolation technique: resection specimen (left hemicolectomy) for cancer of the descending colon. Note the ligatures proximal and distant to the tumour, wrapping of the tumour due to its serosal invasion, and the centrally ligated vessels at the root of the inferior mesenteric artery for lymph node removal.

started with ligation of the vascular pedicle prior to operative manipulation. Turnbull pursued this approach, and compared his results with those of five surgeons at the Cleveland Clinic who continued to use the conventional technique of dividing the vessels after mobilizing the tumour. In the no-touch isolation technique the supplying artery is divided at its origin from the aorta centrally and the draining vein ligated to avoid the escape of tumour cells during intraoperative manipulation. The colonic lumen was occluded to eliminate intraluminal spillage and to prevent anastomotic recurrence. Wrapping the tumour with a cytocidal swab was intended to avoid scraping tumour cells off the serosal surface. Dissecting the central lymph nodes, and not just those of the mesocolon or paracolic nodes, avoided lymphatic spread (Fig. 9). Turnbull reported improved tumour control rates following colon resection (Fig. 3) and later for rectal and anal cancer.[32]

Most of the concepts mentioned above have been supported by subsequent investigations. Showers of tumour cells have been detected in the hepatic vein during the resection of liver tumours.[33] Rinsing the rectal stump prior to construction of the anastomosis has decreased the number of intraluminal recurrences.[34] In contrast, the results of small randomized trials have shown that extended locoregional lymphatic dissection has not improved patient survival, although local and regional recurrence rates have decreased.[35]–[38] The efficacy of wrapping a tumour penetrating to the serosal layer may be limited if tumour cells are already present in the peritoneal cavity. However,

Table 5 Technical principles of oncological surgery procedures

1. During surgery for the primary tumour, monobloc resection of the tumour and its lymphatic drainage area is the method of choice and should be carried out whenever possible. The opening of the lymphatics by separate incision lines carries the risk of inoculation or contamination with migrating tumour cells.

2. Tumour rupture during resection (e.g. fixed rectal cancer in the lower pelvis) must be considered as an incomplete resection, even if the pathologist describes clear margins.

3. According to WHO standards, the status concerning residual tumour is classified as R1.

4. Locally advanced tumours requiring multivisceral resection should also be resected monobloc. Generally, the tumour should be invisible during resection, i.e. the tumour surface should be covered by a plane of uninvolved tissue. When resecting tumours in difficult areas (retroperitoneum, pelvis) an incision line should be planned preoperatively using MRI or CT scanning to allow clear margins (Fig. 10).

5. The planned resection line should be used as a basis to decide whether reconstructive procedures are required.

6. If no such resection planes without tumour involvement can be defined, the resection will be incomplete and preoperative treatment by radiation and/or chemotherapy should be considered with the aim of downstaging the tumour or sterilizing its boundaries.

Table 6 Procedures in surgical oncology requiring specific training and expertise

Placement of in-dwelling catheters
- Central venous port
- Intra-arterial port (hepatic artery, splenic artery)
- Intraperitoneal catheter (Tenckhoff catheter)
- Intraperitoneal port systems

Extensive operative procedures
- Peritonectomy
- Hyperthermic peritoneal perfusion

Procedures requiring specific equipment and co-ordination of services
- Sentinel node biopsy
- Isolated limb perfusion

---

any unnecessary manipulation of the tumour during resection must be avoided. Adherence to Turnbull's philosophy requires only a minor effort, but it may have a major impact on the intraoperative dissemination of tumour cells (see also Table 5).

Specific technical approaches

There are special surgical techniques applied in cancer surgery exclusively (see Table 6).

Central venous port insertion

The insertion of a central venous port enables a stable vascular access for the delivery of systemic chemotherapy or parenteral nutrition. Appropriate management to avoid damage to the catheters, with the attendant risk for subsequent thrombosis, is mandatory. Furthermore, the oncology surgeon must be aware of the specific risks of hypercoagulability resulting in thrombosis, the risk of bleeding due to thrombocytopenia with periportal haematoma, and the increased risk of bacterial contamination in neutropenic patients. The site of the tumour is also important as mediastinal masses or lymph nodes may prevent correct placement of the catheter. The long-term function

and patency of the ports is improved if the insertion is carried out by an experienced surgeon.

Intra-arterial catheter placement

Proper positioning of an intra-arterial catheter for hepatic artery chemotherapy also requires experience and knowledge of the hepatic artery variations (see Chapter 4.23). Insertion of intraperitoneal catheters requires adequate positioning to allow infusional agents to disseminate throughout the abdominal cavity.

Isolated limb perfusion

Isolated limb perfusion for the treatment of malignant melanoma or soft tissue sarcoma confined to the limb is a demanding procedure, requiring an interdisciplinary work-up, technicians to operate a heart–lung machine, as well as the availability of an intensive care unit (for details see Chapters 4.23 and 16.1). Major problems with haemostasis can be encountered and preoperative work-up for cardiovascular disease is also required.

Peritonectomy for pseudomyxoma peritonei

This is an extremely demanding operation, where the decisive preoperative step must be a confirmed diagnosis. Performing a one-step peritonectomy or a multistep cytoreductive peritonectomy combined with intraperitoneal chemotherapy requires the services of an experienced surgical oncologist. This type of procedure should be performed in only a few centres per country to ensure that enough expertise can be gained and maintained.[39]

Sentinel node detection

The use of blue dye or radiolabelled colloids for detecting sentinel nodes is a technique used for intraoperatively mapping the lymphatic drainage of a tumour, and is predominantly used in cases of melanoma and breast cancer. For the procedure to be used safely and effectively, the surgeon must have undergone thorough training and performed at least 20 to 30 applications with a failure rate of less than 5 per cent. Prior to making clinical decisions (such as omitting lymphatic axillary dissection in breast cancer), 25 to 50 correct assessments should be required as the benchmark of competency.[40]

Interdisciplinary relationships and requirements

The decision to use different treatment modalities should be made by a team, preferably during an oncological case conference. In major comprehensive cancer centres, surgical oncologists, medical oncologists, radiation oncologists, pathologists, and diagnostic radiologists will all participate in a presentation of the patient's medical history, current findings, and discussion of treatment. The goals of treatment need to be agreed (palliation or cure), and the best available evidence should be used during the decision-making process. The wishes and physiological reserves of the patient, the experience of the surgeon and of other members of the therapeutic team, the available resources, and the urgency of intervention are all important determinants.

Within this multidisciplinary concept the term 'surgical oncology' is used to indicate that an experienced oncological surgeon will perform appropriate tumour resections. This may include general surgeons, orthopaedic surgeons, head and neck surgeons, gynaecological surgeons, thoracic surgeons, urological surgeons, neurosurgeons, and sometimes cardiovascular surgeons or transplantation surgeons.

A surgical oncologist is not necessarily the surgeon who is able to perform the most extensive procedure, but is the one who selects and administers the procedure likely to yield the best result. There is a responsibility for the surgical oncologist to be involved in adjuvant and neoadjuvant treatment protocols, and to be familiar with the general concepts of chemo-, radio-, and hormonal therapy. Surgical oncology as a specialty derives from the tradition that a surgeon should never become simply a technician. He/she needs to have a full understanding of the diagnosis, the indications for surgery, surgical procedures of choice, adjuvant programmes, the effects of different treatments upon patients, and a perception of the quality of life. To meet these demanding standards, surgeons must have knowledge of all aspects of malignant disease and its treatment, and must be able to meet medical oncologists, radiotherapists, pathologists, radiologists, cytologists, etc. as peers.

Quality control in surgical oncology

Several measures can be used to assess quality control (Table 7); for instance, the resectability rate, the proportion of patients resected with clear margins (R0-resection), and the rate of monobloc resections for T4 tumours. Other criteria include the proportion of patients receiving appropriate adjuvant treatment according to specific guidelines, and the proportion of patients being treated within clinical trials.

Examination of the resected specimen

Examination of the resected specimen or of tumour markers in the systemic circulation allows analysis of the completeness of any resection that claims to be radical (R0-resection).[41] Analysis of the resected specimen not only depends on the extent of clearance achieved by the surgeon, but also on the ability of the pathologist to assess lymph nodes and margins. Incomplete surgical removal will leave tumour behind. Inadequate examination by the pathologist will result in a false-negative assessment of the lymph node status. This can lead to poor survival in patients wrongly classified as node-negative, so that stage-adjusted survival rates with adequate surgery are compromised by inadequate pathology. Patients with false-negative nodes may not receive adjuvant treatment. In an analysis of the quality of rectal cancer surgery, these technical details and histopathological findings served as surrogate endpoints predicting late outcome.[42]

Postoperative morbidity and mortality

The incidence and type of postoperative morbidity and mortality represent further criteria for assessing the quality of surgery. The postoperative length of in-hospital stay, and/or stay on an intensive-care ward, is influenced by the age of the patients and emergency versus elective operations, as well as by tumour and patient-related factors and surgical skill. Significant differences between hospitals and surgeons regarding complication rates for colorectal cancer surgery have been reported; for instance, the rate of non-surgical complications ranged from 7 to 22 per cent and the rate of surgical complications from 3 per cent to 20 per cent. In a multicentre German analysis of both university and district hospitals, the relative risk for different institutions ranged from 0.54 to 2.29 (Fig. 11(a) and (b)).[43] A similar analysis in the United Kingdom showed a variation in R0-resection rates among surgeons of between 40 per cent and 76 per cent, a rate of anastomotic leakage between 0 per cent and 25 per cent, and postoperative mortality ranging from 8 per cent to 30 per cent. The corresponding differences in survival at 10 years in patients who underwent curative resection varied from 20 to 63 per cent.[44]

Local recurrence

Prominent in the above studies were differences in the local recurrence and disease-free survival rates. In most studies, local recurrence is a poor prognostic factor for subsequent survival. Local recurrence reflects the surgeon's ability to provide a complete resection, with the incidence of local recurrence almost always being related to the quality of the surgical procedure (Fig. 12(a)–(c)). In colorectal cancer, anastomotic recurrences located at the luminal site are clearly surgeon-related, which adherence to the principles of no-touch isolation would prevent. Inadequate lymphatic clearance will result in isolated lymphatic recurrences and patients may have to undergo clearance of the remaining lymphatic drainage area.[45] Disruption of the specimen, intraoperative tumour-cell spillage, and implantation of metastases are also surgeon-related.[46] The rate of tumour recurrence ranged from 5 per cent to 25 per cent and the 5-year survival (stage-corrected) from 48 per cent to 70 per cent in a study of seven German hospitals. The recurrence rate among individual surgeons, after taking the identified risk factors into account, varied from 0.56 to 2.03 for curative (R0) resections.[42]

Every effort should be made to minimize local recurrence. However, tumours may recur locally despite adequate margins and clearance of lymphatic drainage. This can be due to perineural or lymphatic tumour invasion and is associated with high-grade (G3) tumours. In almost all types of cancer the risk of locoregional recurrence in undifferentiated types of malignancy is significantly higher than in better differentiated lesions, even after R0-resection. If the surgical oncologist has kept to all the rules, local recurrence may be more a

Table 7 Approaches to quality control in surgical oncology

* Assess the resection specimen for completeness and margins
* Count nodes within the lymphatic drainage area to assess adequacy of clearance
* Control for serum parameters preoperatively versus postoperatively to assess completeness of the resection (e.g. calcitonin for medullary thyroid cancer, CEA for primary and metastatic colorectal cancer)
* Analyse the incidence of local recurrence
* Assess the type of local recurrence
* Calculate disease-free survival
* Analyse the incidence and type of postoperative morbidity (procedure-related, general complications)
* Assess postoperative mortality
* Calculate the length of in-hospital stay or stay on an intensive-care ward
* Compare local recurrence rate, disease-free survival, and overall survival rates between different centres
* Analyse functional outcome based on patient-completed questionnaires

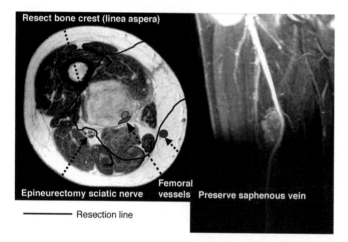

Fig. 10 Planning the resection procedure for locally advanced soft tissue sarcoma of the thigh after preoperative isolated limb perfusion. The femoral vessels need to be resected and reconstructed by autologous vein grafts; primary wound closure should be possible; the area at risk and closest to the tumour is the mediodorsal part of the femur (the linea aspera needs to be resected leaving the inserting fascial planes intact).

biological fact than a technical failure. Under these conditions survival is more dependent on distant metastases than on local recurrence.[47]

The surgeon as a prognostic factor

Since the early 1980s there have been reports of an intersurgeon variability in treatment results. In addition to the reported incidence for local recurrence described above, disease-specific and overall survival rates have also been reported[44],[48]–[50] (Table 8).

Comparisons made between surgical centres have revealed tremendous differences in survival and local recurrence rates for patients with colorectal and gastric cancer. A Canadian study of 680 patients involving 54 surgeons showed that surgeons performing less than 20 rectal cancer resections had a significantly higher risk for tumour-cell spillage, tumour rupture, and local recurrence than those performing

higher numbers of operations per year.[51] This was the second most significant factor for local recurrence, and translated into differences in disease-specific survival of the patients. Multivariate analysis with disease-specific mortality as an outcome variable showed that the extent of training followed by the stage of the disease, rectal perforation, and vascular or neural invasion of the tumour were the four most important factors. Very similar results were reported from the United Kingdom, with a broad variation of disease-specific survival and local recurrence between eight different surgeons.[44] There are also considerable differences between Dutch and Japanese hospitals in the outcome of patients following surgery for gastric cancer with curative intent.[52] A recent study of stage I epithelial ovarian cancer demonstrated that rupture of the cystic tumour during the operation adversely influenced five-year survival with a hazard ratio of 1.94 ($p = 0.002$).[53]

Prospective documentation of both tumour and patient-associated prognostic factors is necessary for correct evaluation of the surgeon's contribution to patient survival. Factors influenced by the surgeon relating to survival are an inadequate indication for surgery, inadequate surgical strategy, and deficits in surgical technique.

There has been much discussion on the influence of the volume of work on patient outcome.[54] Recommendations have been made that cancer services be organized with a minimal acceptable volume of work, since it has been demonstrated that the number of operations performed per year significantly influences the operative mortality for patients with oesophageal, pancreatic, and rectal cancer.[55]–[58] For pancreatic and colorectal cancer, a positive relationship was demonstrated between hospital volume of work and late survival in American university centres, New York hospitals, and those in the United Kingdom.[59]–[61]

It is sometimes difficult to separate the influence of hospital and surgeon workloads. There are cultural differences in providing medical services that tend to be surgeon/consultant-directed in the United Kingdom and the United States, whereas in Germany, France, and Sweden the hospital is at the frontline and not the individual surgeon.

Other analyses of surgery-related factors have evaluated workload, subspecialty training, and the experience of surgeons (trainees versus consultants). In some studies, neither consultant workload nor hospital throughput were identified as independently influencing patient

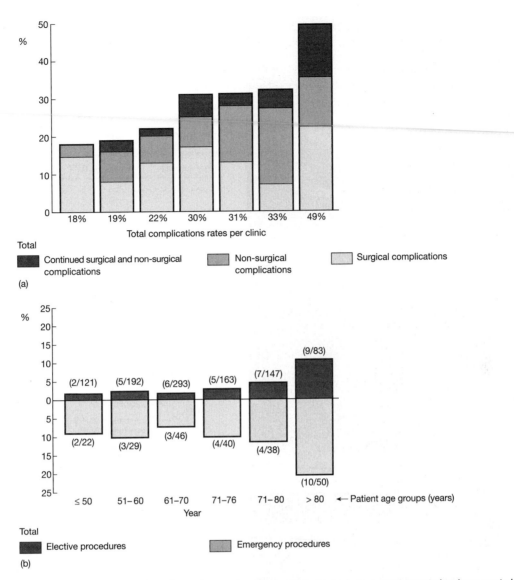

Fig. 11 Morbidity and mortality associated with surgery for colorectal cancer in seven hospitals. (a) Analysis separating surgical and non-surgical complications; (b) emergency versus elective procedures. (Taken from ref. 43 with permission.)

survival.[58] There is also evidence that properly supervised trainees can resect colorectal cancer without compromising long-term survival.[62] A Canadian analysis demonstrated that neither high workload nor subspecialty training alone resulted in best results, but the combination of training and experience yielded the best disease-free survival and lowest local recurrence rates (Fig. 13).[51]

The German analysis has shown that extensive personal experience in performing more than 50 colorectal resections per year may still be associated with a high local recurrence rate—some surgeons may learn from experience while others do not! Personal attitude, subspecialty training, and commitment, together with a thorough quality-control programme, are the most important factors in surgical oncology for optimizing the surgeon-related contribution to disease-specific outcome. This was demonstrated in a surgical training programme in Stockholm. Adopting the technique of total mesorectal

excision as a teaching initiative, the local tumour recurrence rates dropped from 15 per cent to 6 per cent and cancer-related deaths from 16 per cent to 9 per cent.[63] This finding resembles the results of Turnbull's initiative[4] for the surgical removal of colon cancer more than 40 years earlier (see above). A number of trials documenting the value of adjuvant chemo- or radiotherapy in colorectal cancer, and probably in other cancers, need to be challenged if surgical standards can be defined more accurately and are adopted by surgeons in high-volume cancer centres. Future studies examining the outcome for different types of cancer treated by primary surgery should consider the effect of surgeon-related factors. From a theoretical point of view, randomization stratified by surgeon-related factors should be part of the design of future clinical cancer trials. However, this approach is hardly feasible as one cannot ethically randomize patients to receive surgery that is expected to be inferior!

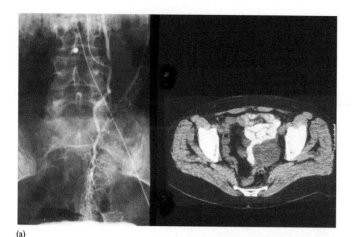

(a)

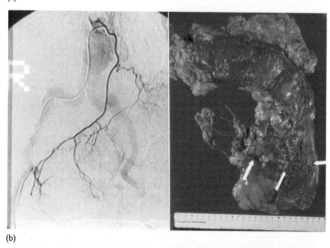

(b)

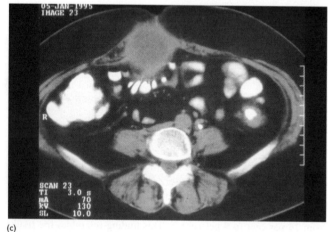

(c)

Fig. 12 Types of locoregional recurrences of colorectal cancer. (a) Anastomotic recurrence after anterior resection: tumour mass at the area of a stapled suture line. (b) Regional lymph node recurrence: angiogram reveals the arterial tree of the sigmoid colon preserved earlier; metastases occur in the mesentery distant to the anastomosis (arrows). (c) Implantation metastasis in the laparotomy scar.

Further aspects of outcome analysis

As well as disease-specific survival, the functional outcome of cancer operations and the morbidity relating to different treatments need to

Table 8 Comparison of outcome elements in patients undergoing resection for rectal cancer dependent on whether or not disruption of the tumour specimen took place intraoperatively

	Disruption/cell spillage	No signs	p value
Total group	n = 718	n = 53	
5-year survival	70 ± 5%	44 ± 17%	< 0.01
Subgroup pT2N0M0	n = 201	n = 15	
5-year survival	92 ± 0.7%	61 ± 30%	< 0.05

Adapted with permission from ref. 46.

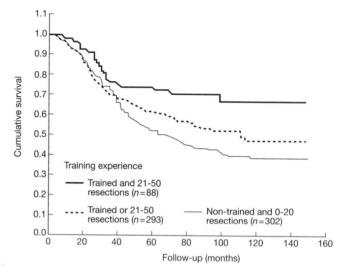

Fig. 13 Disease-specific survival in patients surgically treated for rectal cancer depending on the surgeons' caseload and training. (Taken from ref. 51 with permission.)

be evaluated. This is of particular interest in the treatment of lung cancer (pulmonary respiratory function), and in tumours of the pelvis (bladder, colorectum, genitourinary tract) where sexual function, voiding, and continence need to be addressed. If different treatment approaches result in similar disease-free survival rates but yield very different functional results (vocal cord preservation, swallowing, reflux), radical surgery may not be the best option.

The key issues in the treatment of soft tissue and bone sarcomas are limb function (including the need to use crutches or braces), walking ability, and limitations of movement. During follow-up visits the doctor usually, for example, asks the patient and analyses function by measuring the extent of flexion or extension of the joints. Anorectal manometry is used to assess sphincter function after surgery for low rectal cancer beyond exploring the patient's bowel movement habits. These examinations are thought to be 'objective', but may be biased by the doctor and/or by the patient—sometimes patients do not wish to induce disappointment in the physician who took so much care of them. There are often substantial discrepancies between the patient's self-assessment and the doctor's assessment (see Chapter 18.2). An example is given in Fig. 14 comparing the functional outcome in

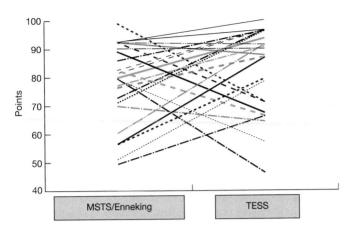

Fig. 14 Comparison of functional outcome in patients with extremity osteosarcoma analysed by the MSTS scale (a measure of impairment completed by the clinician) versus the Toronto Extremity Salvage Score (TESS, a patient self-report questionnaire regarding their physical disability). (Unpublished data.) See text for explanation.

patients with soft tissue sarcoma analysed by the doctor—according to the functional outcome scale of the Musculoskeletal Tumor Society (**MSTS**, see ref. 63)—with a patient self-assessment questionnaire. The latter, the Toronto Extremity Salvage Score (**TESS**, see ref. 64), asks the patients 30 questions regarding their daily activities and grades their limitations in performing those activities. There are similar estimations of the functional outcome between doctor and patient for some scales, but there are also very significant differences.

The surgical oncologist and evidence-based medicine

In the past, what we did clinically, we largely chose to do as individual practitioners. Now what we do is increasingly being directed by a growing variety of 'expert' groups, some of which are appointed by recognized and authoritative bodies, some of which are self-appointed'.[66] Evidence from randomized controlled trials (RCTs) cannot be translated from research into clinical routine crudely. Randomized trials may have restrictive entry criteria and poor generalizability, while comorbidity or social problems may severely influence the relative and absolute benefit claimed from such trials.

Surgical oncology is still a hierarchical, expert-knowledge-based discipline. In the past, operative techniques and radicality have only been investigated in rather small randomized trials, apart from the comparison of breast-conserving treatment versus mastectomy or the extent of lymphadenectomy in gastric cancer.[67] Operative strategies are almost always derived from the history of an institute or the 'school' of a prominent surgeon. A considerable number of myths still exist within surgical oncology, but only a few facts; hence, it will require serious efforts to increase the evidence from RCTs and to convert (or not) these myths into facts.

Evidence-based medicine (**EBM**) bases treatment decisions on the best available knowledge. However, this describes a rather idealistic scenario of clinical decision-making that does not mirror current routine. Not every decision can be made in the light of an exhaustive

EBM process. The vast majority of clinical decisions in surgical oncology are dictated by the presentation of a patient with a newly diagnosed tumour, or someone being referred for a symptomatic malignancy with the wish to have the tumour removed. Medical oncologists probably rely more on the outcomes of randomized controlled trials of different drug regimens than surgical oncologists rely on the results of RCTs of different operative techniques or stategies.

How can we change the communication between surgeons and patients to introduce some aspects of EBM? This seems to be easy when judging the value of adjuvant treatment. However, even interpretation of the first trial of adjuvant chemotherapy for colon cancer may be complex;[68] it was reported that the combination of 5-fluorouracil and levamisole reduced the mortality by 10 to 15 per cent, but this was in a group of patients with an unacceptably high, local recurrence rate of 22 per cent. It remains unclear whether adjuvant chemotherapy is effective if the local recurrence rate is less than 5 to 10 per cent. A rather scenario seems to develop in gastric cancer. The recently completed trial on adjuvant radiation and chemotherapy for resected adenocarcinoma of the stomach suggested significantly improved disease-free survival rates.[69] However, the local recurrence rate in the control group was unacceptable at 34 per cent. Interestingly, the same group had reported on 'inadequate documentation and resection for gastric cancer in the United States' 2 years earlier.[70] This surgical/human factor therefore needs to be taken into account.

There is also a problem in extrapolating EBM-derived results to individual patients. EBM may ignore the fact that clinical decisions involve the consideration of unique personal problems. This is clearly the case in surgical oncology where operative procedures are often performed knowing there is no EBM basis for the decision—but where, in the light of the surgeon's personal experience, the patient's clinical situation warrants the use of operative measures.

Surgery is a very experience-dependent domain, and attitude plays a major role. The less evidence there is that the type of planned operation is efficient, the more is a second opinion required. The wishes of the individual patient and his/her relatives may also influence the decision. The increasing emphasis on best evidence will inevitably mean that the dialogue between patient and surgeon will change, from a directive to a shared decision-making process. Although the key characteristics of shared decision-making may not be totally fulfilled, both parties should share information and agree on the proposed treatment (see also Chapter 3.6).

References

1. **Rosenberg SA.** Principles of cancer management: surgical oncology. *Cancer: principles and practice* (6th edn) (ed. SA Rosenberg, VT DeVita, S Hellman, SA Rosenberg). Philadelphia: Lippincott, Williams and Wilkins, 2001: 253–64.

2. **Society of Surgical Oncology.** *Practice guidelines for major cancer sites.* Arlington Heights, IL: SSO, 1997.

3. **Robinson JO.** History of surgical oncology. *Fundamentals of surgical oncology* (ed. JO Robinson, JR McKenna, GP Murphy). New York: Macmillan, 1986: 14–27.

4. **Crile G, Hoerr SO.** Results of treatment of carcinoma of the breast by local excision. *Surgery, Gynecology, Obstetrics,* 1971; **132**: 780–2.

5. Crile G. The case for local excision of breast cancer in selected cases. *Lancet*, 1972; **1**: 549–51.

6. Veronesi U, *et al.* Conservative treatment of breast cancer. A trial in progress at the Cancer Institute of Milan. *Cancer*, 1977; **39**(6 Suppl.): 2822–6.

7. Fisher B, *et al.* Findings from NSABP Protocol No. B-04—comparison of radical mastectomy with alternative treatments for primary breast cancer. I. Radiation compliance and its relation to treatment outcome. *Cancer*, 1980; **46**: 1–13.

8. Clogg HS. Cancer of the colon. A study of 72 cases. *Lancet*, 1908; **II**: 1007–11.

9. Dukes C. The spread of rectal cancer. *British Journal of Surgery*, 1930; **17**: 643.

10. Westhues H. *Die pathologisch-anatomischen Grundlagen der Chirurgie des Rektumkarzinoms.* Leipzig: Georg Thième, 1934.

11. Hohenberger P. Locoregional recurrence of rectal cancer: biological and technical aspects of surgical failure. *Recent Results in Cancer Research*, 1998; **146**: 127–40.

12. Heald RJ, Moran BJ. Embryology and anatomy of the rectum. *Seminars in Surgical Oncology*, 1998; **15**: 66–71.

13. Heald RJ, Husband EM, Ryall RD. The mesorectum in rectal cancer surgery—the clue to pelvic recurrence? *British Journal of Surgery*, 1982; **69**: 613–16.

14. Quirke P, Dixon MF. The prediction of local recurrence in rectal adenocarcinoma by histopathological examination. *International Journal of Colorectal Disease*, 1988; **3**: 127–31.

15. Enker WE, Thaler HT, Cranor ML, Polyak T. Total mesorectal excision in the operative treatment of carcinoma of the rectum. *Journal of the American College of Surgeons*, 1995; **181**: 335–46.

16. Arbman G, Nilsson E, Hallbook O, Sjodahl R. Local recurrence following total mesorectal excision for rectal cancer. *British Journal of Surgery*, 1996; **83**: 375–9.

17. Bismuth H. Surgical anatomy and anatomical surgery of the liver. *World Journal of Surgery*, 1982; **6**: 3–9.

18. Enneking WF, Spanier SS, Malawer MM. The effect of the anatomic setting on the results of surgical procedures for soft parts sarcoma of the thigh. *Cancer*, 1981; **47**: 1005–22.

19. Nigro ND, Vaitkevicius VK, Considine B. Combined therapy for cancer of the anal canal: a preliminary report. *Diseases of the Colon and Rectum*, 1974; **17**: 354–6.

20. Induction chemotherapy plus radiation compared with surgery plus radiation in patients with advanced laryngeal cancer. The Department of Veterans Affairs Laryngeal Cancer Study Group. *New England Journal of Medicine*, 1991; **324**: 1685–90.

21. Lefebvre JL, Chevalier D, Luboinski B, Kirkpatrick A, Collette L, Sahmoud T. Larynx preservation in pyriform sinus cancer: preliminary results of a European Organization for Research and Treatment of Cancer phase III trial. EORTC Head and Neck Cancer Cooperative Group. *Journal of the National Cancer Institute*, 1996; **88**: 890–9.

22. Lejeune F, *et al.* Rationale for using TNF alpha and chemotherapy in regional therapy of melanoma. *Journal of Cellular Biochemistry*, 1994; **56**: 52–61.

23. Long-term results of lung metastasectomy: prognostic analyses based on 5206 cases. The International Registry of Lung Metastases. *Journal of Thoracic and Cardiovascular Surgery*, 1997; **113**: 37–49.

24. Hohenberger P, Schlag P, Herfarth C. [Reoperation in colorectal carcinoma with curative intention.] *Schweizerische Medizinische Wochenschrift*, 1992; **122**: 1079–86.

25. Nordlinger B, *et al.* Surgical resection of colorectal carcinoma metastases to the liver. A prognostic scoring system to improve case selection, based on 1568 patients. Association Francaise de Chirurgie. *Cancer*, 1996; **77**: 1254–62.

26. United Kingdom national confidential enquiry into perioperative deaths. *British Medical Journal*, 1998; **317**: 1269.

27. Böttcher K, *et al.* [The epidemiology of stomach carcinoma from the surgical viewpoint. The results of the German Stomach Carcinoma Study 1992. The German Stomach Carcinoma Study Group]. *Deutsche Medizinische Wochenschrift*, 1993; **118**: 729–36.

28. Bakkevold KE, Kambestad B. Morbidity and mortality after radical and palliative pancreatic cancer surgery. Risk factors influencing the short-term results. *Annals of Surgery*, 1993; **217**: 356–68.

29. Schlag PM, Slisow W, Moesta KT. Seromuscular spiral cuff perineal colostomy: an alternative to abdominal wall colostomy after abdominoperineal excision for rectal cancer. *Recent Results in Cancer Research*, 1998; **146**: 95–103.

30. Turnbull-RBJ, Kyle K, Watson FR, Spratt J. Cancer of the colon: the influence of the no-touch isolation technic on survival rates. *Annals of Surgery*, 1967; **166**: 420–7.

31. Cole WH, Packard D, Southwick HW. Carcinoma of the colon with special reference to prevention of recurrence. *Journal of the American Medical Association*, 1954; 1549–53.

32. Turnbull-RB J. Current concepts in cancer. Cancer of the GI tract: colon, rectum, anus. The no-touch isolation technique of resection. *Journal of the American Medical Association*, 1975; **231**: 1181–2.

33. Koo J, *et al.* Recovery of malignant tumor cells from the right atrium during hepatic resection for hepatocellular carcinoma. *Cancer*, 1983; **52**: 1952–6.

34. Gertsch P, Baer HU, Kraft R, Maddern GJ, Altermatt HJ. Malignant cells are collected on circular staplers. *Diseases of the Colon and Rectum*, 1992; **35**: 238–41.

35. Pezim ME, Nicholls RJ. Survival after high or low ligation of the inferior mesenteric artery during curative surgery for rectal cancer. *Annals of Surgery*, 1984; **200**: 729–33.

36. Wiggers T, *et al.* No-touch isolation technique in colon cancer: a controlled prospective trial. *British Journal of Surgery*, 1988; **75**: 409–15.

37. Surtees P, Ritchie JK, Phillips RK. High versus low ligation of the inferior mesenteric artery in rectal cancer. *British Journal of Surgery*, 1990; **77**: 618–21.

38. Corder AP, Karanjia ND, Williams JD, Heald RJ. Flush aortic tie versus selective preservation of the ascending left colic artery in low anterior resection for rectal carcinoma. *British Journal of Surgery*, 1992; **79**: 680–2.

39. Sugarbaker PH. Surgical treatment of peritoneal carcinomatosis: 1988 Du Pont lecture. *Canadian Journal of Surgery*, 1989; **32**: 164–70.

40. Giuliano AE. See one, do twenty-five, teach one: the implementation of sentinel node dissection in breast cancer. *Annals of Surgical Oncology*, 1999; **6**: 520–1.

41. Hohenberger P, Schlag PM, Gerneth T, Herfarth C. Pre- and postoperative carcinoembryonic antigen determinations in hepatic resection for colorectal metastases. Predictive value and implications for adjuvant treatment based on multivariate analysis. *Annals of Surgery*, 1994; **219**: 135–43.

42. Hermanek P, Mansmann U, Altendorf HA, Riedl S, Staimmer D. [Comparative study of oncological outcome quality in colorectal carcinoma—ranking by surrogate endpoint?]. *Chirurg*, 1999; **70**: 407–14.

43. Riedl S, Wiebelt H, Bergmann U, Hermanek P. Postoperative complications and fatalities in surgical therapy of colon carcinoma. Results of the German multicenter study by the Colorectal Carcinoma Study Group. *Chirurg*, 1995; **66**: 597–606.

44. McArdle CS, Hole D. Impact of variability among surgeons on postoperative morbidity and mortality and ultimate survival. *British Medical Journal*, 1991; **302**: 1501–5.

45. Hohenberger P, Schlag P, Kretzschmar U, Herfarth C. Regional mesenteric recurrence of colorectal cancer after anterior resection or left hemicolectomy: inadequate primary resection demonstrated by angiography of the remaining arterial supply. *International Journal of Colorectal Disease*, 1991; **6**: 17–23.

46. Zirngibl H, Husemann B, Hermanek P. Intraoperative spillage of tumor cells in surgery for rectal cancer. *Diseases of the Colon and Rectum*, 1990; **33**: 610–14.

47. Trovik CS, *et al.* Surgical margins, local recurrence and metastasis in soft tissue sarcomas: 559 surgically-treated patients from the Scandinavian Sarcoma Group Register. *European Journal of Cancer*, 2000; **36**: 710–16.

48. Phillips RK, Hittinger R, Blesovsky L, Fry JS, Fielding LP. Local recurrence following 'curative' surgery for large bowel cancer: I. The overall picture. *British Journal of Surgery*, 1984; **71**: 12–16.

49. Köckerling F, Reymond MA, Altendorf HA, Dworak O, Hohenberger W. Influence of surgery on metachronous distant metastases and survival in rectal cancer. *Journal of Clinical Oncology*, 1998; **16**: 324–9.

50. Böttcher K, Siewert JR, Roder JD, Busch R, Hermanek P, Meyer HJ. [Risk of surgical therapy of stomach cancer in Germany. Results of the German 1992 Stomach Cancer Study. *Chirurg*, 1994; **65**: 298–306.

51. Porter GA, Soskolne CL, Yakimets WW, Newman SC. Surgeon-related factors and outcome in rectal cancer. *Annals of Surgery*, 1998; **227**: 157–67.

52. Yokota, *et al.* Disclosure of results of operations for gastric cancer in Japan. *Lancet*, 2000; **356**: 1689.

53. Vergote I, De Brabanter J, Fyles A, *et al.* Prognostic importance of degree of differentiation and cyst rupture in stage I invasive epithelial ovarian carcinoma. *Lancet*, 2001; **357**: 176–82.

54. Hillner BE, Smith TJ, Desch CE. Hospital and physician volume or specialization and outcomes in cancer treatment: importance in quality of cancer care. *Journal of Clinical Oncology*, 2000; **18**: 2327–40.

55. Begg CB, Cramer LD, Hoskins WJ, Brennan MF. Impact of hospital volume on operative mortality for major cancer surgery. *Journal of the American Medical Association*, 1998; **280**: 1747–51.

56. Lieberman MD, Kilburn H, Lindsey M, Brennan MF. Relation of perioperative deaths to hospital volume among patients undergoing pancreatic resection for malignancy. *Annals of Surgery*, 1995; **222**: 638–45.

57. Harmon JW, *et al.* Hospital volume can serve as a surrogate for surgeon volume for achieving excellent outcomes in colorectal resection. *Annals of Surgery*, 1999; **230**: 404–11.

58. Parry JM, Collins S, Mathers J, Scott NA, Woodman CB. Influence of volume of work on the outcome of treatment for patients with colorectal cancer. *British Journal of Surgery*, 1999; **86**: 475–81.

59. Birkmeyer JD, Warshaw AL, Finlayson SR, Grove MR, Tosteson AN. Relationship between hospital volume and late survival after pancreaticoduodenectomy. *Surgery*, 1999; **126**: 178–83.

60. Hannan EL, O'Donnell JF, Kilburn H, Bernard HR, Yazici A. Investigation of the relationship between volume and mortality for surgical procedures performed in New York State hospitals. *Journal of the American Medical Association*, 1989; **262**: 503–10.

61. Kee F, *et al.* Influence of hospital and clinician workload on survival from colorectal cancer: cohort study. *British Medical Journal*, 1999; **318**: 1381–5.

62. Singh KK, Aitken RJ. Outcome in patients with colorectal cancer managed by surgical trainees. *British Journal of Surgery*, 1999; **86**: 1332–6.

63. Martling AL, Holm T, Rutqvist LE, Moran BJ, Heald RJ, Cedermark B. Effect of a surgical training programme on outcome of rectal cancer in the County of Stockholm. Stockholm Colorectal Cancer Study Group, Basingstoke Bowel Cancer Research Project. *Lancet*, 2000; **356**: 93–6.

64. Enneking WF, Dunham W, Gebhardt MC, Malawer M, Pritchard DJ. A system for the functional evaluation of reconstructive procedures after surgical treatment of tumors of the musculoskeletal system. *Clinical Orthopedics*, 1993; **286**: 241–6.

65. Davis AM, Wright JG, Williams JI, Bombardier C, Griffin A, Bell RS. Development of a measure of physical function for patients with bone and soft tissue sarcoma. *Quality of Life Research*, 1996; **5**: 508–16.

66. Sniderman AD. Clinical trials, consensus conferences, and clinical practice. *Lancet*, 1999; **354**: 327–30.

67. Bonenkamp JJ, Hermans J, Sasako M, van de Velde CJ. Extended lymph-node dissection for gastric cancer. Dutch Gastric Cancer Group. *New England Journal of Medicine*, 1999; **340**: 908–14.

68. Moertel CG, *et al.* Levamisole and fluorouracil for adjuvant therapy of resected colon carcinoma. *New England Journal of Medicine*, 1990; **322**: 352–8.

69. Macdonald JS, *et al.* Postoperative combined radiation and chemotherapy improves disease-free survival (DFS) and overall survival (OS) in resected adenocarcinoma of the stomach and GE-junction. *Proceedings of the American Society of Clinical Oncology*, 2000; **19**(A1): 1a.

70. Estes NC, Macdonald JS, Touijer K, Benedetti J, Jacobson J. Inadequate documentation and resection for gastric cancer in the United States: a preliminary report. *American Surgeon*, 1998; **64**: 680–5.

4.2 The biological basis of radiotherapy

G. Gordon Steel

Introduction

One of the principal aims of radiation biology is to explain observed phenomena associated with the therapeutic uses of radiation. Much has been achieved and possible causes of failure have been well described. Modest results in exploiting this knowledge in the improvement of radiation therapy have been obtained and it may well be that further developments will follow.

Mechanisms of radiation cell killing

The absorption of radiation in biological tissues leads to the immediate production of ionized atoms and atoms raised into excited states. This leads, within 10^{-10} s, to the breakage of chemical bonds and the formation of free radicals, which proceed to react with cellular constituents. Some of these reactions are potentially damaging to the cell, others effectively inactivate the radicals. Free radicals have a very short lifespan and the amount of damage that remains (say, at 10^{-3} s after exposure) is the result of many competing, fast processes.

It is widely believed that the damage which is most significant for mutation and loss of cell viability is damage in DNA. This idea is supported by a number of differing sources of evidence. Local irradiation of parts of the cell show that the cell nucleus is much more sensitive than the cytoplasm. Short-range Auger-emitting isotopes such as ^{125}I, when specifically incorporated into DNA, are much more toxic than when incorporated into cytoplasmic membranes. Thymidine analogues such as bromodeoxyuridine, which become specifically incorporated into DNA, are efficient sensitizers of radiation cell killing. Not all parts of the genome are equally vulnerable to radiation damage. Some genes are more essential than others. The way DNA is packaged within the cell leads to some regions that, at any one time, are more accessible to repair enzymes than others. It is also now widely believed that certain types of interchromosomal interactions are more important than others in leading to cell death and mutation.

The spatial distribution of damage within the cell is not uniform. Energy deposition by sparsely ionizing radiations such as X- or γ-rays is in the form of electron tracks, at the end of which clusters of ionizations commonly occur (Fig. 1). There is some evidence that within repair-proficient cells the lesions that result from individual, well-separated ionizations may be repaired efficiently and that lethal events predominantly occur in ionization 'hot-spots'. The tracks produced by α-particles or the protons ejected by neutron irradiation are very dense; these are termed 'high-LET (linear energy transfer)

radiations'. Fewer cells are damaged by such radiation, per unit dose, but their damage tends to be serious and non-recoverable. The effects of high-LET radiation differ from those of low-LET radiation in other respects: there is less dependence on oxygen and less variation through the cell cycle. The radiobiological aspects of the therapeutic use of particle beams are covered elsewhere (Chapter 4.7.2).

When the DNA of cells is extracted and examined immediately after irradiation, a great deal of damage is apparent. On average, for every cell that is killed by low-LET radiation there may be over 1000 damaged bases, 1000 or more single-strand DNA breaks, and perhaps 40 double-strand breaks per cell. There may also be a smaller number of severe lesions comprising local, multiply-damaged sites. At body temperature, DNA damage disappears during the first hour or so after irradiation through the operation of repair processes. It seems likely, therefore, that cellular lethality is associated with the rare lesions that fail to repair. Whether a lesion causes cell death will depend on its severity and its location within the genome.

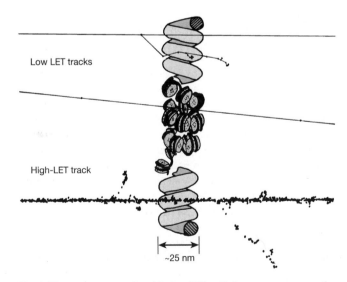

Low LET tracks

High-LET track

~25 nm

Fig. 1 The ionizations produced by low-LET radiations are, on average, far apart compared with the size of a DNA fibre but at the end of δ-ray tracks they are closer together and some occur in clusters. Highly ionizing heavy particles (such as protons produced by neutron irradiation) produce densely ionizing tracks, which deposit a large amount of energy on each passage through a DNA fibre. Reproduced from Goodhead, 1988, with permission.[1]

If cells are observed under the microscope during the few hours after irradiation it can be seen that they do not die immediately. They often proceed to mitosis, although the time at which they divide is delayed to an extent that depends on dose: this is called 'mitotic delay'. At division, chromosomal abnormalities become visible and some may be so severe that the cell will fail to complete mitosis. Cells that divide successfully (even through a number of cell cycles) may yet die at a subsequent mitosis. There is also evidence for an effect of radiation damage on the stability of the genome, leading to mutations and cell sterility appearing many cell generations later.[2]

Some cells, particularly those of the lymphoid system, undergo rapid cell death after irradiation. This has been called interphase cell death and more recently it has been recognized often to have the morphological and genetic characteristics of the process known as apoptosis. However, in most tissues the predominant mode of radiation-induced cell death is mitotic death.

Processing of radiation damage

Damage induced in DNA by exposure to radiation is subject to a series of enzymic processes that may either lead to successful repair or to the fixation of damage (that is 'misrepair'). The primary lesions involved in the mutagenic and lethal effects of far-ultraviolet (UV) radiation are thought to be pyrimidine dimers. Their repair involves the recognition of an altered base by glycosylase enzymes, which cut the deoxyribose backbone of the DNA strand leaving an apyrimidinic site that is then susceptible to attack by specific endonucleases. The repair of UV-induced damage involves the excision and resynthesis of a 'patch' of perhaps six to ten nucleotides. The repair of damage induced by ionizing radiation is less easy to characterize, reflecting the greater variety of lesions induced.

A variety of compounds have been found to interfere with the processing of DNA damage. Early studies used compounds known to inhibit normal DNA replication: antimetabolites such as cytosine arabinoside (Ara-C) and β-adenine arabinoside (β-Ara-A), hydroxyurea, which depletes nucleotide pools, and actinomycin and Adriamycin, which by intercalating DNA prevent unwinding and the access of repair enzymes. All these drugs have been shown to inhibit DNA repair in some cell systems. More specific inhibitors of enzymes have also been used, such as 3-aminobenzamide which inhibits poly(ADP-ribose) transferase, an enzyme that is critical for the ligation step in DNA repair.

The speed of DNA repair has been investigated by a variety of methods, including the rate of rejoining of strand breaks. This is found to be a multicomponent process in which the half-time of the fastest component may be a few minutes, with slower components ranging up to perhaps an hour.

DNA rejoining and DNA repair are not the same, for some rejoined breaks may have lost genetic information: the fidelity of rejoining may vary, yet this is essential for the restoration of gene function. This has been investigated by introducing into cells plasmids in which specific endonuclease cuts have been made in the DNA. By this means it has been found, for instance, that although fibroblasts of ataxia telangiectasia can successfully rejoin breaks in plasmid DNA, the process lacks fidelity and this may provide one explanation of the high radiosensitivity of these cells.

The processes involved in the repair of radiation-induced DNA damage are under the control of a large number of genes, sometimes collectively known as 'radiosensitivity genes'. The following list indicates the variety of genes that are involved:

(1) genes that control the activity of free-radical scavenging molecules (e.g. glutathione-s-transferases, superoxide dismutases, glutathione peroxidase);

(2) DNA repair genes controlling repair enzymes such as glycosylases, endonucleases, and kinases;

(3) genes involved in apoptosis, such as *TP53* and *bcl-2*;

(4) cell-cycle control genes.

There is considerable homology for many of these genes among the wide range of biological systems that includes bacteria, yeast, rodent cells, and human cells. Much of the laboratory research that aims to understand genetic processes in man is therefore carried out on the simpler, more primitive cell systems.

Cytogenetic mechanisms

During the past few years, attention has increasingly been directed at the relationship between chromosome aberrations and cell killing. Irradiated cells display a variety of chromosomal aberrations when they divide. These can take the form of breaks, exchanges between chromosomes, formation of ring structures, and many others. Some of these are 'stable', meaning that they do not lead to cell death and therefore persist through a number of cell generations. Those that do lead to cell death ('unstable' aberrations) usually involve the deletion and loss of a substantial chromosomal fragment. This can be the result of a 'terminal deletion' or of the formation of a 'dicentric' (that is the fusion product between two chromosomes, having two centromeres) which inevitably also leaves an 'acentric fragment'. Such an event involves the loss of many hundreds of genes and in diploid cells it will be lethal. It is widely perceived that interchromosomal interactions following radiation damage are therefore a major factor leading to cell death. Using the technique of fluorescent *in situ* hybridization (FISH) such interactions can now be followed in great detail and this may well throw light on how and when interchromosomal interactions occur. It is possible by 'interphase FISH' to visualize the domains occupied by individual chromosomes during interphase and to stain them in an identifiable colour. If the domains occupied by two particular chromosomes overlap, then the passage of a single charged particle through that region of the nucleus might lead to an interaction between the chromatin of the two chromosomes; if they do not overlap, then aberrations involving these two chromosomes would be unlikely.[3]

Concept of clonogenic tumour cells

A tumour is a complex biological structure consisting not only of cells that are frankly neoplastic or malignant but also of a variety of types of normal, non-neoplastic cells. A carcinoma has arisen from an epithelial tissue within which has developed a focus of cells that undergo uncontrolled growth. There is evidence that, in many tumours, neoplastic growth may begin from one transformed cell or that as a result of the early processes of cell selection the descendants of one cell tend to predominate; most tumours can therefore be described as 'unifocal'.

The parenchyma of a carcinoma consists of tumour cells that have resulted from neoplastic transformation in normal epithelial cells. In a well-differentiated tumour the normal maturation process of epithelial cells is to some extent maintained, with cells evolving from a proliferating phase, through a reversible resting phase, and eventually to a mature, non-proliferating, 'end-cell' status. This is why the tumour has a histological appearance that resembles its tissue of origin. Thus, even within the parenchyma, not all tumour cells are malignant (in the sense of cells retaining the ability to give rise to a new tumour).

The stroma is the supportive and vascular portion of the tumour. Various types of cells will be found and they are all normal (that is non-malignant) host cells. They are not neoplastic and they arise in the tumour as a result of three processes: by being overgrown by the invading tumour, by immigration from the rest of the body, or by proliferation within the tumour as a result of some stimulus emanating from the neoplastic cells. Many tumours contain substantial quantities of acellular material, in particular the products of necrosis and the products of cellular differentiation. Proliferating malignant cells often make up only a minor part of the total volume of a tumour, but these are the cells that provide the driving force for neoplastic growth and it is on these that therapeutic outcome depends.

We envisage that within the population of parenchymal tumour cells there is a subgroup of cells that have the capacity to produce a large family of descendants. These are the cells that can regrow the tumour if left intact at the end of treatment. We call these cells 'clonogenic', in other words 'colony-producing' cells. They are analogous to the stem cells of the bone-marrow: cells with infinite proliferative capacity, which give rise to progeny that differentiate into a variety of mature descendants. At the present time it is usually impossible to detect colony-forming cells *in situ* within a tumour; we can do this only in defined environments in tissue culture or (for transplantable rodent tumours) in transplantation sites.

The simplest example of a 'clonogenic assay' is *in vitro*—a suspension of tumour cells is prepared, taking care to avoid clumping, and portions are irradiated with a range of radiation doses, one being kept as a control. The irradiated and control suspensions are plated out in tissue culture under identical conditions and allowed to produce colonies. These are then counted, usually fixing the criterion for a countable colony at 50 cells; this choice implicitly defines the 'clonogenic cell' for the study in question. The fraction of plated cells that produces colonies is the 'plating efficiency' and the ratio of plating efficiencies in treated and control suspensions is the 'surviving fraction' of clonogenic cells (see Steel, 1997, for further details[4]).

What proportion of tumour cells are clonogenic? In some transplantable mouse tumours the proportion has been found to be high (over 10 per cent), but this is not known for any human tumour. Some authors have supposed that the clonogenic fraction could, in some radiocurable tumours, be below 0.1 per cent.

Survival of clonogenic cells

Although, as has been indicated in the previous section, radiation has many effects on a tumour cell population, the loss of colony-forming ability in clonogenic cells is thought to be the most important from the point of view of tumour eradication. As radiation dose is increased, the fraction of clonogenic cells that retain proliferative capacity decreases. The sensitivity of a cell population to radiation is well described by a 'cell survival curve'; that is, a plot of surviving fraction against dose. The shape of cell survival curves after irradiation

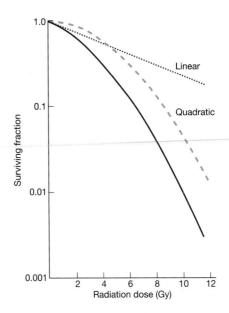

Fig. 2 Illustrating the two components that make up the linear-quadratic equation: the linear component is $(-\log S = \alpha d)$; the quadratic component is $(-\log S = \beta d^2)$.

has been the subject of extensive investigation, and a variety of models have been devised that are successful in fitting experimental data.[5],[6] The aim of seeking a universal theory of radiation cell killing is not yet realized.

Multitarget model

If a cell is assumed to have N targets, all of which have to be inactivated in order to kill the cell, then it follows that the survival curve will have a shoulder followed by an exponential tail: radiation dose has to be accumulated until it is likely that all N targets will be hit. For cells in which the value of N is large, a relatively large radiation dose has to be delivered before there is a significant likelihood that no target will remain intact. Backward extrapolation of the final slope to the survival axis (that is to zero dose) gives an intercept equal to N. The multitarget model produces survival curves that have zero initial slope; as this is in conflict with much experimental data the model is sometimes extended to include a component of single-hit killing, which steepens the initial slope.

Linear–quadratic model

This has the simple equation:

$$\text{Surviving fraction } (S) = \exp(-\alpha d - \beta d^2)$$
$$-(\log S) = \alpha d + \beta d^2$$

where *d* is the radiation dose. Surviving fraction is always less than unity, so $-(\log S)$ is a (positive) measure of radiation effect. The first term of the exponent thus describes a linear component of cell killing, the second a quadratic term. As shown in Fig. 2, the linear component defines the initial slope of the cell survival curve and the quadratic term defines its curvature. In contrast to the multitarget equation, the linear–quadratic model produces survival curves that bend continuously with increasing dose. What might be the mechanistic basis for such a model? A linear component of cell killing would result from the spatially random production of lesions, each of which is lethal. A quadratic component could result from the deposition of lesions that are non-lethal unless they undergo binary interaction; this notion has been widely discussed as a mechanism for shouldered cell survival curves.[7] One simple idea is that the linear component might result from the direct induction of a double-strand DNA break and the quadratic component from the production by separate ionizing particles of single-strand breaks, close enough together to interact and form a double-strand break.[8] However, at the radiation doses at which survival curves begin to bend (that is a few grays) the particle track density is not high enough to give a realistic probability of track coincidences within the scale of the DNA double helix (a few nanometers) and the elegant experiments of Goodhead, using low-energy X-rays, have confirmed that this explanation of the quadratic component is quantitatively unlikely.[9] Interaction between lesions on different chromosomes leading to the formation of an acentric fragment is a more plausible mechanism.

Repair saturation models

Here it is assumed that in the absence of repair, all radiation-induced lesions would be lethal and the survival curve would be steep and exponential. Cells are postulated to contain a substance or pool of substances ('Q-factor')[10] which are essential for the repair of radiation damage but are consumed in the process. At low radiation doses there is little damage and maximum availability of Q-factor: repair will therefore be almost complete. As dose increases, damage increases and the level of Q-factor falls: repair will therefore be progressively less effective. This approach thus provides a different explanation of the shoulder on cell survival curves, one that does not involve concepts of lesion interaction. The case for saturable repair models has been reviewed by Alper and Goodhead.[11],[12]

Lethal–potentially lethal damage model

Radiation is assumed to produce two different types of lesion: lethal lesions that cannot be repaired and potentially lethal lesions that lead to cell death only if they undergo binary interaction (otherwise they are fully repaired). This notion has been formulated mathematically.[13] In contrast to other models of radiation cell killing, this is a dynamic model: it incorporates rate constants for repair and fixation of potentially lethal lesions. It thus can predict not only the shape of the acute cell-survival curve but also the dose-rate effect, the effect of fractionation, and recovery from potentially lethal damage.

Tumour hypoxia and the oxygen effect

Three observations led to the widespread belief that hypoxia in tumours is a major cause of radioresistance. The first was that mammalian cells irradiated under hypoxic conditions are very resistant to radiation, requiring two to three times the radiation dose for a particular level of cell killing. The oxygen tension required for full resistance is very low, in the region of 0.1 per cent. The second observation was that focal necrosis is a common feature of tumours and the work of Thomlinson and Gray showed that this is observed at a rather standard distance (~150 μm) from patent blood vessels.[14] Subsequent calculations have confirmed their postulate that this

distance is determined by the diffusion distance of oxygen. The radiobiological implication is that at the boundary of necrosis there will be cells which are still alive but existing at a very low oxygen level. The third source of evidence was studies with oxygen electrodes.[15] When an oxygen-sensitive electrode is pushed through a tumour there usually is evidence for regions of reduced oxygen tension.

^{3}H-Misonidazole, which is preferentially bound to hypoxic cells, shows a patchy distribution within rodent and human tumours and provides a way of visualizing hypoxia in tissue sections. With this compound the results have shown clear evidence of hypoxia in most human carcinomas, but in surprisingly few sarcomas.[16]

Radiobiological studies on tumours in experimental animals have confirmed the picture of progressively developing hypoxia as tumours grow: tumours that are under approximately 1 mm in diameter have a radiosensitivity which is similar to that seen when the same cells are irradiated under oxic conditions in vitro.[17] Larger tumours have a similar sensitivity at low radiation doses, but show a resistant tail at high doses, the slope of which is consistent with the survival curve for tumours made totally hypoxic.

There is also considerable clinical evidence for an influence of hypoxia on the results of radiotherapy. Anaemic patients do less well than those with normal haemoglobin levels.[18],[19] Procedures that reduce the impact of hypoxia, such as hyperbaric oxygen or chemical radiosensitizers, have shown evidence of therapeutic gain (see below).

Reoxygenation

How is it possible that the objective evidence for hypoxia in tumours should be so strong, yet the benefits of efforts to beat hypoxic cells are so difficult to detect? The answer may lie in the phenomenon of 'reoxygenation'. During the early part of a course of fractionated radiotherapy the radiosensitive oxic cells will preferentially be killed and the hypoxic fraction of the viable survivors will increase. But as radiation-killed cells die and disappear it may well be that oxygen will diffuse further, increasing its availability to previously hypoxic cells. These will then increase in radiosensitivity. It must be emphasized that the concept of reoxygenation applies to surviving clonogenic cells. As treatment proceeds, such cells will form a diminishing proportion of the tumour volume, perhaps well below 1 cell in 1000. The tumour as a whole may or may not become better oxygenated.

Reoxygenation has been demonstrated in rodent tumours after large, single doses of radiation. If it occurs in human tumours it will tend to reduce the impact of hypoxia on the response to fractionated treatment given over a sufficiently long course. Shortening the treatment time, as is done in 'accelerated fractionation' or brachytherapy (see below) could, in some cases, lose the benefit of reoxygenation and hypoxia may thus become a more serious problem.

Efforts to overcome hypoxia

For many years hypoxia has been perceived as one of the most important reasons for failure in controlling tumours by radiation therapy. Approaches to overcome this cause of radioresistance have included the following:

1. Hyperbaric oxygen—patients were treated while lying in a high-pressure oxygen tank at a pressure of ~ 2 atmospheres. Although

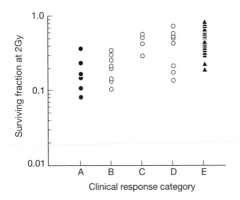

Fig. 3 The initial slope of *in vitro* cell survival curves for human tumour cells (indicated by the surviving fraction at 2 Gy) in relation to clinical response. The categories A to E are described in the text. Reproduced from Deacon *et al.*, 1984,[24] with permission.

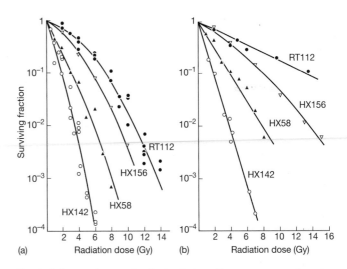

Fig. 4 Cell survival curves for the irradiation of human tumour cells under oxic conditions, illustrating the range of sensitivities that are observed (a) at high dose rate (~ 150 cGy/min), (b) at low dose rate (~ 2 cGy/min). HX142, neuroblastoma; HX58, pancreas carcinoma; HX156, cervix; RT112, bladder. Adapted from Steel *et al.*, 1987.[25]

now discontinued, this approach did show some therapeutic benefit.[20]

2. Improving oxygen delivery to tumours—the oxygen-carrying capacity of the blood can be increased by the injection of perfluorocarbons. Alternatively, the unloading of oxygen in tissues can be increased by the use of drugs that manipulate the oxygen dissociation curve.

3. Chemical radiosensitizers—a variety of drugs have been produced which mimic oxygen in its radiosensitizing effect on hypoxic cells. The best-known has been misonidazole. This underwent extensive clinical trials leading to the identification of some benefit, especially in head and neck cancers.[21],[22] Research continues into the development of improved radiosensitizing drugs.

4. High-LET radiations—one of the main rationales for developing new particle beams for radiotherapy was the fact that the effects of densely-ionizing beams are less influenced by the presence or absence of oxygen (see below). The gains from, for instance, neutron therapy have not been great and this approach is therefore not widely used.

A meta-analysis of 72 randomized clinical trials that sought to improve the results of radiotherapy by influencing tumour oxygenation using various approaches (9315 patients in all) has produced clear evidence for gain, particularly in head and neck cancers.[22]

Radiosensitivity of human tumour cells

For many years it was not appreciated that human tumour cells differ considerably in radiosensitivity. It was only during the 1970s that techniques for cloning human tumour cells in tissue culture became widely available. Fertil and Malaise were the first to draw attention to a possible correlation between the initial slope of the oxic cell survival curve and clinical radiocurability.[23] Figure 3 is taken from the review of published data by Deacon *et al.*[24] The five categories (A–E) represent categories of decreasing clinical radioresponsiveness (for instance A includes lymphoma, myeloma, and neuroblastoma; E includes glioma, melanoma, osteosarcoma). The ordinate is the surviving fraction for a dose of 2 Gy. Within each category the results

are scattered (as might be expected from different tumour types, different techniques, different laboratories) but there is a general tendency for a positive correlation in these data, consistent with Group A being more responsive than Group E. Group A cell lines have a mean survival of approximately 0.15; Group E has a mean of approximately 0.5. The clinical significance of this difference derives from the thought that if these survival values apply *in vivo* and if they are constant throughout a course of, for example, 30 fractions of radiotherapy, then the overall effect in Group A would be a highly curative surviving fraction of $(0.15)^{30} = 2 \times 10^{-25}$. In Group E the effect would be $(0.5)^{30} = 10^{-9}$. Although these are crude calculations, they do illustrate that the survival per 2-Gy dose might be an important determinant of the effects of fractionated radiotherapy.

The radiosensitivity of human tumour cells has therefore been a subject of considerable research interest. The range of sensitivities seen *in vitro* at high dose rate is illustrated in Fig. 4(a). Most of such data are well fitted by a linear–quadratic equation (Equation 1 above) and the full lines in the figure are of this form. It can be seen that among tumours of different types the radiation dose for a particular level of cell inactivation varies by perhaps a factor of roughly three. The effect of lowering the radiation dose rate is to amplify the differences between cell lines, as shown in Fig. 4(b) and as considered in the section on dose rate below. Low dose rate discriminates better than high dose rate between tissues of differing radiosensitivity.

The five Rs of radiobiology

The following five factors mainly determine the response of a tissue (normal or tumour) to fractionated radiotherapy. As originally described[26] there were four, but in view of the observations described in the previous section it seems important to add a fifth.

Repair (or recovery)

If a dose of radiation is split into two equal fractions separated in time, the effect is less than for the equivalent single dose. Elkind termed this 'recovery from sublethal damage'. Recovery is usually complete with a gap of 4 to 6 h but there is evidence for further slower recovery in some late-responding tissues such as the central nervous system.

Reassortment

Studies with synchronized cell populations have shown that radiosensitivity varies through the cell cycle, usually being maximal in G2 and mitosis, with a peak of resistance in the latter part of the S phase. As a result, a first dose of radiation will leave a surviving population that is non-uniformly distributed through the cell cycle. The effect of a second dose will depend on cell cycle progression (or 're-assortment'). For instance, a delay of a few hours may allow the cells that have survived within the S phase to move through into G2 where they will be more sensitive to a second treatment.

Repopulation

If the time between treatments is extended further, then a substantial proportion of the surviving cells may be able to go through mitosis, as a result of which their number will be greater at the time of a subsequent radiation dose. A greater dose will then be needed to counteract this repopulation. This may be particularly important over extended courses of fractionated radiotherapy to tumours that have a high proliferation rate.

Reoxygenation

As described above.

Radiosensitivity

This was described in the previous section and is, as it were, the baseline on which the other four Rs exert their effects. Two of them, when they occur, make the tumour or normal tissue more resistant to subsequent radiation doses (recovery, repopulation). The other two make it more sensitive (reassortment, reoxygenation).

Early and late normal tissue reactions

There are considerable differences in the extent and speed of response of normal tissues to radiation exposure. Tissues with a high rate of cell proliferation tend to be sensitive to radiation and to show the results of damage within a few days or weeks. These include the intestinal epithelium, mucosae of the mouth and oesophagus, bone marrow, and skin. The acute damage to these tissues may heal but eventually it may be followed by a later phase of tissue failure or necrosis. It is thought that this late phase of manifestation of damage may be due to radiation effects on the cells lining blood vessels or on other slowly proliferating cells of the stroma. In tissues that have a low rate of proliferation (for example lung, kidney, spinal cord), the early phase of damage is absent.

Four principal factors determine the radiation sensitivity of normal tissues:

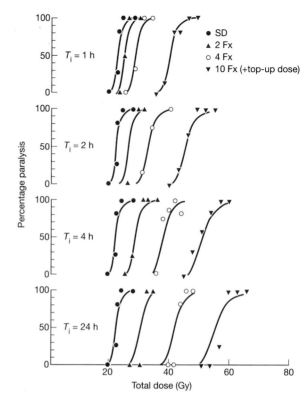

Fig. 5 Dose-response curves for damage to the rat spinal cord by single and fractionated doses of radiation. Two, four, or ten fractions (Fx) were given at intervals indicated by T_i. The 10 fraction treatments were followed by a top-up dose of 15 Gy. The results indicate the sparing effects of fractionation, as well as the fact that full recovery between fractions requires at least 4 h. (Reproduced from Ang et al., 1987,[30] with permission.)

1. The radiosensitivity of stem cells—clonogenic cell survival studies have demonstrated that among various epithelia in the mouse, radiosensitivity does not vary greatly. Some of the stem cells in bone marrow and testis are more radiosensitive and the target cells for damage to slowly renewing tissues are less sensitive.[27]

2. The extent of cellular depletion that can be tolerated before tissue function or integrity declines—in the intestinal epithelium, tissue failure is associated with approximately two decades of stem-cell depletion.

3. The volume of tissue irradiated—tolerance dose is greater for small rather than large irradiated volumes.[28] Volume is an important determinant of damage, partly because small damaged areas can more readily heal from the edges, but also because of its impact on the failure of an irradiated organ.

4. Fractionation—it is now recognized that the effect of changing the dose per fraction or the overall duration of radiotherapy differs between early- and late-reacting normal tissues, as described in the following section.

Dose–effect curves for damage to normal tissues are often very steep. This is illustrated in Fig. 5 for the irradiation of 2 cm lengths of the rat spinal cord. The effects of fractionation shown in these data will be referred to below. At the region of maximum steepness, the incidence of damage may increase from 20 to 80 per cent for a dose increase of only approximately 10 per cent. There is evidence that dose–effect curves are steeper for late-responding than early-responding normal tissues.[29]

New approaches to fractionation in radiotherapy

The experience of early radiotherapists, mainly in France and Austria, established the fact that when radiation treatment is protracted, either by fractionation or by lowering the dose rate, then a greater dose is required for the same level of effect. It was also found empirically that the therapeutic results were better for protracted irradiation than for a single dose (see Thames and Hendry, 1987; Bentzen and Overgaard, 1997, for historical reviews).[31],[32] Strandqvist, Cohen, and others formulated these relationships in so-called Strandqvist plots: the total radiation dose that gave a particular level of damage was plotted, on a logarithmic scale, against the duration of treatment, also on a log scale. 'Isoeffect curves' were plotted in this way both for effects on tumours and on normal tissues. The clinical data were of very limited precision and it appeared that they were consistent with a straight-line relationship on these double-logarithmic co-ordinates. This led these early investigators to postulate a power-law relationship between total dose and number of daily fractions for an isoeffect and this was formalized in the well-known 'NSD formula':[33]

$$\text{Total dose} = \text{NSD } T^{0.11} N^{0.24}$$

NSD is the nominal standard dose (which differs from one target tissue or isoeffect to another), T is the overall time in days, and N the number of fractions. This has widely been used to convert a prescribed dose for one schedule to that required with another. For damage to skin, using treatment courses that are neither very short nor very long, it is satisfactory. However, its predictions have not been found to be reliable for tissues other than skin, in particular for late-reacting normal tissues.[34] For a detailed critique of the NSD approach, see Bentzen and Overgaard.[32]

Ideas about fractionation based on the linear–quadratic equation

Starting in the early 1980s, there have been efforts to establish a more reliable system of time–dose calculations based on the linear–quadratic equation (Equation 1 above). The initial observation was that which is illustrated in Fig. 6: early-responding and late-responding normal tissues show a systematically different dependence on dose per fraction.[35] It was then recognized that the data obtained from fractionation studies on murine normal tissues conform to what would be expected if damage to the respective target cells followed a linear–quadratic equation. Specifically, the data fitted the relationship

$$\frac{1}{D} = \frac{\alpha}{E} + \frac{\beta}{E}d$$

where D is the total dose for a particular isoeffect (E), d is the dose per fraction, and α and β are the parameters of the linear–quadratic equation. Plots of $1/D$ against d are linear and allow the ratio α/β to be found from the ratio of intercept/slope. When these α/β ratios

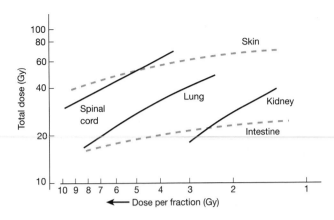

Fig. 6 Total dose for isoeffect as a function of dose per fraction, in a variety of normal tissues of the mouse. There is a systematic difference in the slope of these plots between late-responding tissues (full lines) and early-responding tissues (broken lines). After Thames *et al.*, 1982.[35]

Table 1 Some examples of α/β ratios for normal tissues and tumours

Tissue reaction	α/β ratio (Gy)
Early reactions	
Skin desquamation (mouse)	9–12
Skin desquamation (man)	~11
Intestine (mouse)	8–11
Mucosa (man)	8–15
Late reactions	
Spinal cord (rodents)	1.5–4.5
Spinal cord (man)	< 3.3
Brachial plexopathy (man)	~ 2–3
Telangiectasia (man)	2.5–3
Subcutaneous fibrosis (man)	~ 1.7
Pneumonitis (man)	3.3
Tumours, human	
Head and neck	7–16
Skin	~ 8.5
Melanoma, liposarcoma	~ 0.5

Extracted from Joiner and van der Kogel, 1997.[37]

were tabulated, it was found that the values for early-responding normal tissues were systematically higher than for the late-responding tissues (Table 1).

A high α/β ratio corresponds to a survival curve that is straighter than when the ratio is lower and it is this difference in curve shape that seems to lead to the different fractionation response of the various tissues.

This approach provides a more reliable way of calculating the effects of changing from one dose per fraction to another. First one

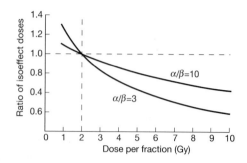

Fig. 7 Theoretical isoeffect curves relating total dose to dose per fraction for α/β ratios of 3 or 10 Gy (Equation 4). Total doses are normalized to that required in 2-Gy fractions. After Withers et al., 1983.[38]

must decide what is the reaction of normal tissues that limits treatment; then, from available data of the type shown in Table 1, the corresponding α/β ratio can be chosen.[36],[37] When an appropriate value for the α/β ratio has been selected, the following relationship then allows the calculation of a new total dose for a new dose per fraction:

$$\frac{D}{D_{ref}} = \frac{\alpha/\beta + d_{ref}}{\alpha/\beta + d}$$

where d_{ref} and D_{ref} are the dose per fraction and total dose for the reference treatment, and d and D are the corresponding values for the new treatment. The form of this relationship is shown in Fig. 7: the curves are flatter when the α/β ratio is high and they show greater curvature when it is low. As dose per fraction is increased, tissues with a low α/β ratio (the late-responding tissues) require a greater dose reduction than when the ratio is high. Similarly, as dose per fraction is reduced below the standard value of ~2 Gy, the late-responding tissues should be able to tolerate a higher total dose than the early-responding tissues.

Hyperfractionation

The ideas described in the previous paragraph have led to recent attempts to explore the therapeutic advantage of lowering the dose per fraction below ~ 2 Gy. It is reasoned that tumours, containing cells that on the whole proliferate fairly rapidly, might have α/β ratios, and thus a fractionation response, that resembles that of early-reacting normal tissues. There is experimental support for high α/β ratios from studies on mouse tumours,[39] and also from some studies on human cancer (Table 1). If this is the case, then lowering the dose per fraction below 2 Gy should allow the total dose for constant late reactions to be increased; this should increase tumour response, but of course at the price of a concomitant increase in early tissue damage.

To reduce the dose per fraction substantially without increasing the overall time usually requires more than one treatment per day. The term 'hyperfractionation' has come to be used for this style of treatment. It is essential that the fractions are kept far enough apart in time to allow full recovery, as indicated in the following subsection.

The magnitude of the potential gain can be judged from Fig. 7. If the tumour follows the curve for an α/β ratio of 3 Gy and the late reactions follow that for α/β = 10 Gy, then lowering the dose per fraction, for example, to 1.2 Gy increases the dose ratio for the tumour

by a factor of 1.07 and that for the normal tissue by a factor of 1.19. If the total dose were increased by 19 per cent using 1.2 Gy fractions, then the late radiation effects should be unchanged but the effective increase in dose to the tumour would be approximately 11 per cent. This estimate depends on the assumption that the α/β values are correct and that the linear–quadratic equation does work for doses per fraction as low as 1.2 Gy. Encouraging results from a randomized clinical trial of hyperfractionation in oropharyngeal cancer were published by Horiot et al.[40] Treatment with 70 fractions of 1.15 Gy (two fractions per day with a 4 to 6-h interval, total dose 80.5 Gy) produced a similar incidence of late tissue damage as a conventional schedule of 35 fractions of 2 Gy (70 Gy given in the same overall time of 7 weeks). However, the larger total dose in the hyperfractionated treatment produced a substantial increase of approximately 19 per cent in long-term local tumour control. The results of this study are in good agreement with the linear–quadratic model and support hyperfractionation as a way of increasing the therapeutic benefit in radiotherapy. See Chapter 4.4.2 for further details on the clinical results of hyperfractionation.

Accelerated radiotherapy

This is an alternative approach to the improvement of radiotherapy fractionation, though one that also involves the use of multiple fractions per day. The rationale is totally different. It is reasoned that the rate of repopulation by surviving clonogenic cells in some tumours may be so high as to negate significantly the effects of a course of radiotherapy of conventional duration. The cell proliferation rate in human tumours has been found to vary widely.[41] Furthermore, studies on experimental tumours have shown that clonogenic cells can repopulate faster than the pretreatment growth rate of the tumour.[42] For tumours where the repopulation rate is high, the appropriate response will be to treat over a shorter overall time. As with hyperfractionation, this will exacerbate acute reactions in normal tissues, for their tolerance of conventional therapy presumably depends in part on their ability to repopulate rapidly. Damage to late-responding normal tissues should not be increased by shortening the overall treatment time because their proliferation rate is lower and they are less sensitive to changes in treatment duration.

The simplest way to shorten the overall treatment time would be to increase the dose per fraction and give fewer fractions. This, however, would be a bad approach because (as is to be expected from Fig. 7) large doses per fraction have been found to produce a relative increase in late reactions in normal tissues.[36] The acceleration must therefore be achieved by keeping the dose per fraction within the normal range but by giving multiple fractions per day.

There have been a number of attempts to evaluate accelerated radiotherapy. The boldest is the continuous hyperfractionated accelerated radiotherapy (CHART) protocol of Saunders et al.[43] Fractions of 1.5 Gy were given three times per day (with a 6-h gap) for 12 consecutive days to patients with head and neck and bronchial tumours. The early results have been encouraging.[44]

The time interval between treatments must be carefully chosen when giving multiple fractions per day. Laboratory evidence suggests that the half-time for recovery of damage is in the region of 1.5 h and probably longer in the case of late-reacting normal tissues. This is well shown by the data on the rat spinal cord in Fig. 5. As the time interval between doses increases there is a progressive increase in the tolerance dose, for any chosen number of fractions. In this tissue there is an increase even when the interval went up from 4 to 24 h. For intervals of 4 h, recovery may therefore not be complete and damage will be greater than expected. While recognizing the logistical problems involved in performing multiple treatments per day in the clinic, it is important that the gap between treatments be kept as long as possible, preferably at least 6 h.

Bearing in mind the evidence that human tumours differ widely in proliferation rate, it seems likely that the benefits from accelerated radiotherapy will be in those that repopulate fastest. At the present time there is no way in which the speed of repopulation of surviving clonogenic cells can be determined in human tumours. What is being done, therefore, is to develop rapid methods for determining the pretreatment rate of cell proliferation in tumour biopsies and to assume that this may correlate with the repopulation rate. One widely explored approach is to give the patient an injection of a thymidine analogue (bromodeoxyuridine or iododeoxyuridine), which can be detected by flow cytometry and can give a measure of the S-phase fraction and the rate of passage of cells through the S phase.[45],[46]

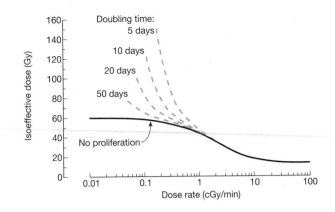

Fig. 8 Illustrating the dose-rate effect that results from repair and cell proliferation during radiation exposure. The lines show the calculated radiation doses that produce a fixed isoeffect. The full line shows the effect of repair without proliferation; the dashed lines show the additional sparing that results from proliferation with various doubling times.

The dose-rate effect: rationale for brachytherapy

A low dose rate can be viewed as the limiting case of hyper-fractionation: many small fractions given very frequently. Brachy-therapy therefore has distinct radiobiological advantages, as well as potential disadvantages.

Advantages:

(i) at a sufficiently low dose rate, this ultimate form of hyper-fractionation maximally spares late-responding normal tissues;

(ii) that is achieved within a short overall treatment time, thus giving minimal time for tumour-cell repopulation;

(iii) the geometric form of the radiation field exploits the volume effect in normal-tissue damage;

(iv) cell killing around an implanted source is very intense and provides a form of tumour debulking.

Disadvantages:

(i) the very non-uniform dose distribution risks the 'geometric miss' of some tumour cells;

(ii) the short overall treatment time may be inadequate to allow full reoxygenation of hypoxic tumour cells;

(iii) particularly with pulsed high dose-rate brachytherapy there is a temptation to treat too fast, thus losing the advantage listed as (i) above.

The effect of a single low dose-rate exposure will differ from that of the same dose given at high dose rate because the extended treatment time allows a number of biological processes to take place: these are the five Rs of radiobiology listed above. Over what range of dose rate will these biological processes act? This depends on their speed. A fast process can compete with rapid infliction of damage and will produce effects at high dose rate. As a rough guide we can compare the time the process takes (for example after a brief radiation exposure) with the exposure time at low dose rate. Repair is a fast

process, with a half-time in the region of 1 h in mammalian cells. At a dose rate of 1 Gy/min or more (typical of high dose-rate exposures in clinical and experimental radiotherapy) a dose of, for example, 2 Gy is delivered in 2 min and little recovery can occur during exposure. There will, therefore, be little effect of dose rate. Lowering the dose rate to 10 cGy/min increases the exposure time for 2 Gy to 20 min and some recovery will occur. Reduction by a further factor of 10 (to 1 cGy/min) gives an exposure time of over 3 h for 2 Gy and at this dose-rate recovery will be almost complete.

In contrast, proliferation is a much slower process. Cell cycle times for human cells are in the region of 2 to 4 days and only when the exposure time becomes a significant part of a day will this produce a significant effect. Figure 8 illustrates this in the form of calculated isoeffect curves for a cell population that has an α/β ratio of 3.7 Gy. The full line shows the sparing effect of repair (half-time 0.85 h) which occurs over the dose-rate range from around 20 cGy/min down to 0.2 cGy/min. The dashed lines show the effect of proliferation at various rates; this indicates the substantial sparing that may occur at very low dose rates in proliferating tissues.

The effect of reduced dose rate on cell survival was shown in Fig. 4. The shouldered survival curves at high dose rate become straight at a dose rate of around 1c Gy/min, reflecting the fact that the time-dependent processes which produce the shoulder can then proceed during exposure and even go to completion. An important observation, and one that has often been overlooked, is that there are wide differences among human tumour cells in the steepness of survival curves at low dose rate. In this example, taken from our own work,[25] the dose required for two decades of cell kill ranges by a factor of approximately seven. Note that cell lines from human tumours also differ in the magnitude of the dose-rate effect: resistant cell lines show considerable dose sparing but some radiosensitive lines (such as the HX142 neuroblastoma line) show little change of sensitivity with dose rate.

Studies on experimental animals have also found that the magnitude of the dose-rate effect differs from one normal tissue to another. Many tissues recover well from radiation damage and show a strong dose-rate effect. Bone marrow is perhaps the extreme example of a tissue whose stem cells show little dose-rate effect.

In evaluating the therapeutic implications of these observations it must be realized that the clinical use of low dose-rate irradiation (in interstitial or intracavitary therapy) is not primarily for radiobiological reasons but because these approaches lead to a better dose distribution within the tumour. Furthermore, the clinical choice is not between a single exposure at high dose rate or at low dose rate, but between fractionated high dose-rate treatment and a single (or a few) low dose-rate exposures. As indicated above, both of these ways of protracting radiation treatment exploit the same biological processes (principally recovery and repopulation) and in broad terms tissues that are well spared by one will also be spared by the other. Fowler has calculated, on the basis of the linear–quadratic model, equivalence relationships between fractionated and low dose-rate irradiation.[34] For a tumour with an α/β ratio of 10 Gy and a late-responding normal tissue with $\alpha/\beta = 3$ Gy, the relative effects of continuous exposure at approximately 0.5 Gy/h will be equivalent to 30 high dose-rate fractions of 2 Gy. The advantage of the continuous exposure is that it would be complete in 5 days. Low dose-rate radiotherapy is the most efficient way of maximizing recovery whilst keeping the treatment duration as short as possible. It is therefore theoretically attractive where tumour-cell repopulation is thought to be rapid.

Radiobiology of high linear energy transfer (LET) radiations

Most external-beam radiotherapy is done with X-rays, γ-rays, or high-energy electron beams. When absorbed in matter, these deposit energy by ionization and excitation of atoms diffusely throughout the irradiated volume. The ionizations are not random: as indicated at the start of this chapter the secondary electrons that are produced by these radiations form tortuous tracks that are at first sparsely ionizing but eventually produce small but dense clusters of ionizations. Nevertheless, such radiations are usually described as 'low linear energy transfer (LET)' radiations.

A variety of alternative radiation beams produced by modern particle accelerators are of potential interest to radiotherapy. Their attraction mostly lies in their physical properties, but they may also have radiobiological advantages.[47]

Physical properties of heavy-particle radiations

1. The Bragg peak. Heavy particles increase their ionizing density as they slow down and therefore the dose delivered by the primary beam tends to increase and reach a peak towards the end of the particle range. This should, in principle, be ideal for the treatment of deep-seated tumours. (Examples are protons, accelerated nuclei of helium, carbon neon, etc., π-mesons).

2. The paths of heavy particles are much straighter than for electrons. It is therefore easier to produce well-defined beams with good spatial resolution (protons probably provide the cheapest way of obtaining this advantage).

3. Slow neutrons (for instance, from a reactor) can generate the local release of highly ionizing α-particles on interaction with

boron in tissues. The exploitation of this depends on achieving sufficient selective uptake of boron into tumour cells.

Biological properties of heavy-particle radiations

1. High-LET radiations produce more cell killing per unit dose. This is expressed as a high relative biological effectiveness. There is less cellular recovery after high-LET radiation and cell survival curves are steep and relatively straight. In changing from low- to high-LET radiotherapy it is essential to have accurate information on the relative biological effectiveness, which also depends on the dose per fraction.

2. Low oxygen–enhancement ratio. The oxygen effect (see above) is much less marked with high-LET radiations. Oxygen enhancement ratio is defined as the ratio of radiation doses that produce the same level of effect under hypoxic/oxic conditions. This ratio tends to be approximately 2.5 to 3 for low LET radiations; it falls progressively with increasing LET to almost 1.0 for the most densely-ionizing beams. Hypoxic cells are therefore not resistant to high-LET radiation.

3. Less selective cell killing. Variation of radiosensitivity through the cell cycle is less marked with high- than with low-LET radiations. Differences between resistant and sensitive cell types are also less.

After many years of experimental and clinical investigation of high-LET radiotherapy, its therapeutic potential is still not entirely clear. The results of clinical trials were summarized by Withers[48]. A number of studies have shown benefit from neutrons in the treatment of salivary gland tumours, prostate tumours, and soft-tissue sarcomas. There is little evidence for benefit in other sites and in brain, pancreas, and bladder the results may have been worse than with photons.

Combination of radiotherapy and chemotherapy

The treatment of cancer patients with both radiotherapy and chemotherapy is widespread, although the biological effects and clinical benefit of combining these treatments are sometimes in doubt. Some advantages have clearly been demonstrated in a few diseases, and a wide variety of biological rationales have been adduced in favour of combined therapy.

Mechanisms that potentially could be exploited were classified by Steel and Peckham as follows:[49]

1. Spatial co-operation—an improvement in therapy that is achieved by one agent (drug or radiation) dealing with disease that is spatially missed by the other.

2. Simple addition of antitumour effects—to give two effective cytotoxic agents should kill more tumour cells than either alone, provided they do not antagonize one another. For benefit to be obtained in this way, it is critically important that the toxicities of drugs and radiation should not greatly overlap, that is that chemotherapy does not seriously reduce radiation tolerance or vice versa. Provided full single-agent doses can be maintained in the combination, it is not essential for the antitumour effects to

add perfectly: X plus any fraction of Y is, in principle, always greater than X alone.

3. Protection of normal tissues—especially the use of drugs that protect against radiation damage to normal tissues, in the absence of similar protection of tumour cells.

4. Enhancement of tumour response—the use of combinations that produce a greater antitumour response than would have been expected from the response achieved with the agents used separately. The detection of a greater-than-expected result is complicated by the theoretical problems of defining a synergistic response. These arise from the fact that dose–response curves for tumour response are almost always non-linear. The uncertainties associated with identifying synergism were described by Steel and Peckham in terms of isobolograms, within which an 'envelope of uncertainty' can be envisaged.[49]

Any one of these mechanisms by itself could give an improved therapeutic strategy compared with radiotherapy or chemotherapy used alone. A particular combination of drugs and radiation may simultaneously exploit more than one of the mechanisms.

A matter of particular interest is the extent to which the success of drug–radiation combinations depends on interactions between the effects of the two agents. By interaction we mean a situation in which treatment with one agent modifies the response of a tissue (normal or tumour) to the second agent. The first two mechanisms listed above specifically *exclude* interactive effects between the drugs and radiation. On the other hand, protection of normal tissues and enhancement of tumour response depend upon interactive effects.

In clinical practice, there is evidence in a few tumour types for the exploitability of spatial co-operation; it also seems likely that the simple addition of antitumour effects of drug and radiation chosen to give independent toxicity has given occasional benefit. The exploitability of interactive combinations is more in doubt. Interactions between cytotoxic drugs and radiation that lead to enhanced cell killing have been well demonstrated in some experimental systems, especially in tissue culture. The clearest demonstration is the cell survival shoulder-reducing property of the cytotoxic antibiotics when given soon before or soon after irradiation. This appears to be a universal property of these drugs, which have also been found to enhance radiation-induced damage in a variety of normal tissues. Enhanced tumour cell killing has also occasionally been seen with other drugs but not consistently in different experimental systems. Interactions seen *in vitro* have often not been reproduced *in vivo* and interactions seen in one tumour system have often not been confirmed in others.

In contrast, the increase in damage to normal tissues when some drugs are used with radiation has been well shown. The picture here is more predictable than for the antitumour effects and drugs that enhance the radiation effects on particular normal tissues have been clearly documented.

Time dependence of drug–radiation interactions

The timing of combined treatment is important and in general the greater the time interval between treatments, the less the combined toxicity. Extensive studies have been made on the time-dependence of effects on normal tissues in the mouse, employing the useful 'time-line' approach (reviewed by Steel).[50] Fixed doses of drug and radiation are chosen and given to animals, varying only the time interval

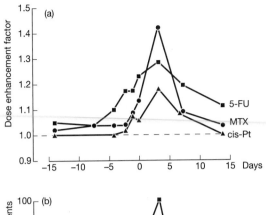

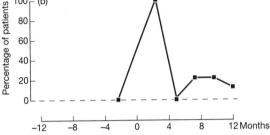

Fig. 9 Examples of time-line studies taken from the experimental and clinical literature. (a) Methotrexate (MTX), 5-fluorouracil (5FU), or cis-platinum combined with pelvic irradiation in mice (from Pearson and Steel, 1984).[51] (b) Proportion of patients with non-seminomatous testicular tumours treated with chemotherapy and irradiation who developed gastrointestinal or late skin damage. (Reproduced from Yarnold *et al.*, with permission.)[52]

between them. Measurement of damage to normal tissue (or tumour response) then gives a profile that shows times of maximum or minimum effect. Two examples of this are shown in Fig. 9. The upper diagram shows time-lines for pelvic irradiation in the mouse, combined with each of three different cytotoxic agents.[51] The ordinate indicates the dose-enhancement factor (that is, the ratio of radiation doses (without drug/with drug) that produce the same level of damage). Giving the drugs well before radiation produced little or no enhancement of damage; peak enhancement was seen for drug given during the first 7 days after irradiation; at longer intervals the effect declined.

Figure 9(b) shows one of the few examples of clinical time-line data.[52] This was assembled from historical experience in the treatment of testicular non-seminoma, mainly using the three-drug regimen of cis-platinum, vinblastine, and bleomycin. The proportion of patients showing subcutaneous or gastrointestinal damage was recorded and the results show an interesting parallel with the experimental data shown above, on a longer time scale.

When this same approach has been used on experimental tumours there has been little evidence of systematic peaks of response at or around the time of irradiation.[50] The therapeutic implication is that to give chemotherapy at or shortly after irradiation may be a poor therapeutic strategy; it may tend to enhance damage to normal tissues without a corresponding increase in tumour response. These experimental data therefore do not confirm the clinical experience in some diseases that concurrent radiotherapy/chemotherapy is preferable to a sequential protocol.

The clinically confirmed benefits of combined chemotherapy/radiotherapy have been few.[53],[54] They have been found in a small group of diseases that respond to chemotherapy alone. The moral seems to be that only when a drug or drug combination has the ability to eradicate occult disease or substantially to reduce the size of objectively measurable disease is there likely to be any demonstrable benefit from its use in conjunction with radiotherapy. The risk of increasing damage to normal tissues is considerable; combined therapy should therefore not be given without good reason. The immediate future probably lies in selecting drugs and patients in which a good chemotherapeutic response can be expected, whilst avoiding drugs that seriously enhance radiation damage to normal tissues. The scientific rationale is probably stronger for sequential than for concurrent radiotherapy/chemotherapy.

References

1. Goodhead DT. Spatial and temporal distribution of energy. *Health Physics*, 1988; **55**: 231–40.

2. Mothersill C. Genomic instability. *International Journal of Radiation Biology* (Special issue), 1998; **74**: 661–804.

3. Sachs RK, Chen AM, Brenner DJ. Review: proximity effects in the production of chromosome aberrations by ionizing radiation. *International Journal of Radiation Biology*, 1997; **71**: 1–20.

4. Steel GG. Clonogenic cells and the concept of cell survival. In: Steel GG, ed. *Basic clinical radiobiology*. 2nd edn. UK: Arnold, 1997.

5. Elkind MM, Whitmore GF. *The radiobiology of cultured mammalian cells*. London: Gordon and Breach, 1967.

6. Joiner MC. Models of radiation cell killing. In: Steel GG, ed. *Basic clinical radiobiology*. 2nd edn. UK: Arnold, 1997.

7. Kellerer AM, Rossi HH. The theory of dual radiation action. *Current Topics in Radiation Research Quarterly*, 1972; **8**: 85–158.

8. Chadwick KH, Leenhouts HP. A molecular theory of cell survival. *Physics in Medicine and Biology*, 1973; **18**: 78–87.

9. Goodhead DT. Inactivation and mutation of cultured mammalian cells by aluminium characteristic ultrasoft X-rays. *International Journal of Radiation Biology*, 1977; **32**: 43–70.

10. Alper T. *Cellular radiobiology*. Cambridge University Press, 1979.

11. Alper T. Keynote address: survival curve models. In: Meyn RE, Withers HR, ed. *Radiation biology in cancer research*. New York: Raven Press, 1980: 3–18.

12. Goodhead DT. Saturable repair models of radiation action in mammalian cells. *Radiation Research*, 1985; **104**: S58–67.

13. Curtis SB. Lethal and potentially lethal lesions induced by radiation—a unified repair model. *Radiation Research*, 1986; **106**: 252–70.

14. Thomlinson RH, Gray LH. The histological structure of some human lung cancers and the possible implications for radiotherapy. *British Journal of Cancer*, 1955; **9**: 539–49.

15. Cater DB, Silver IA. Quantitative measurements of oxygen tension in normal tissues and in tumors of patients before and after radiotherapy. *Acta Radiologica*, 1960; **53**: 233–56.

16. Urtasun RC. Tumour hypoxia, its clinical detection and relevance. In: Dewey WC, Edington M, Fry RJM, Hall EJ, Whitmore GF, ed. *Radiation research: a twentieth century perspective*. San Diego: Academic Press, 1992: 725–31.

17. Stanley JA, Shipley WU, Steel GG. Influence of tumour size on hypoxic fraction and therapeutic sensitivity of Lewis lung tumour. *British Journal of Cancer*, 1977; **36**: 105–13.

18. Dische S, Saunders MI, Warburton MF. Haemoglobin, radiation morbidity and survival. *International Journal of Radiation Oncology, Biology, Physics*, 1986; **12**: 1335–7.

19. Overgaard J, Hansen HS, Jorgensen K, Hansen MS. Primary radiotherapy of larynx and pharynx carcinoma—an analysis of some factors influencing local control and survival. *International Journal of Radiation Oncology, Biology, Physics*, 1986; **12**: 515–21.

20. Henk JM. Does hyperbaric oxygen have a future in radiation therapy? *International Journal of Radiation Oncology, Biology, Physics*, 1981; **7**: 1125–8.

21. Overgaard J. Sensitization of hypoxic tumour cells-clinical experience. *International Journal of Radiation Biology*, 1989; **56**: 801–11.

22. Overgaard J. Overcoming hypoxic cell resistance. In: Steel GG, ed. *Basic clinical radiobiology*. 2nd edn. UK: Arnold, 1997.

23. Fertil B, Malaise EP. Inherent cellular radiosensitivity as a basic concept for human tumor radiotherapy. *International Journal of Radiation Oncology, Biology, Physics*, 1981; **7**: 621–9.

24. Deacon J, Peckham MJ, Steel GG. The radioresponsiveness of human tumours and the initial slope of the cell survival curve. *Radiotherapy and Oncology*, 1984; **2**: 317–23.

25. Steel GG, Deacon JM, Duchesne GM, Horwich A, Kelland LR, Peacock JH. The dose-rate effect in human tumour cells. *Radiotherapy and Oncology*, 1987; **9**: 299–310.

26. Withers HR. The four R's of radiotherapy. *Advances in Radiation Biology*, 1975; **5**: 241–71.

27. Potten CS, Hendry JH. *Cytotoxic insult to tissue*. London: Churchill Livingstone, 1983.

28. Withers HR. Treatment volume and tissue tolerance. *International Journal of Radiation Oncology, Biology, Physics*, 1988; **14**: 751–9.

29. Thames HD, *et al.* Fractionation parameters for human tissues and tumours. *International Journal of Radiation Biology*, 1989; **56**: 701–10.

30. Ang KK, Thames H, van der Kogel AJ, van der Schueren. The rate of repair of radiation-induced damage in the rat spinal cord is dependent on the size of dose per fraction. *International Journal of Radiation Oncology, Biology, Physics*, 1987; **13**: 557–62.

31. Thames HD and Hendry JH. *Fractionation in radiotherapy*. UK: Taylor and Francis, 1987.

32. Bentzen SM, Overgaard J. Time-dose relationships in radiotherapy. In: Steel GG, ed. *Basic clinical radiobiology*. 2nd edn. UK: Arnold, 1997.

33. Ellis F. Dose, time and fractionation: a clinical hypothesis. *Clinical Radiology*, 1969; **20**: 1–7.

34. Fowler JF. Dose-rate effects in normal tissues. In: RF Mould, ed. *Brachytherapy 2*. Proceedings of the 5th International SELECTRON Users' Meeting 1988. Eersum, The Netherlands: Nucletron International, 1989: 26–40.

35. Thames HD, Withers HR, Peters LJ, Fletcher GH. Changes in early and late radiation responses with altered dose fractionation: implications for dose-survival relationships. *International Journal of Radiation Oncology, Biology, Physics*, 1982; **8**: 219–26.

36. Fowler JF. The linear-quadratic formula and progress in fractionated radiotherapy. *British Journal of Radiology*, 1989; **62**: 679–94.

37. Joiner MC, van der Kogel AJ. Linear-quadratic approach to fractionation and calculation of isoeffect relationships. In: Steel GG, ed. *Basic clinical radiobiology*. 2nd edn. UK: Arnold, 1997.

38. Withers HR, Thames HD, Peters LJ. A new isoeffect curve for change in dose per fraction. *Radiotherapy and Oncology*, 1983; **1**: 187–91.

39. Williams MV, Denekamp J, Fowler JF. A review of α/β ratios for experimental tumors: implications for clinical studies of altered fractionation. *International Journal of Radiation Oncology, Biology, Physics*, 1985; **11**: 87–96.

40. Horiot J-C, *et al.* Hyperfractionation versus conventional fractionation in oropharyngeal carcinoma: final analysis of a randomized trial of the EORTC cooperative group of radiotherapy. *Radiotherapy and Oncology*, 1992; **25**: 231–41.

41. Steel GG. *The growth kinetics of tumours*. Oxford University Press, 1977.

42. Stephens TC, Steel GG. Regeneration of tumors after cytotoxic treatment. In: Meyn RE, Withers HR, ed. *Radiation biology in cancer research.* New York: Raven Press, 1980.

43. Saunders MI, *et al.* Continuous hyperfractionated accelerated radiotherapy in locally advanced carcinoma of the head and neck region. *International Journal of Radiation Oncology, Biology, Physics,* 1989; 17: 1287–93.

44. Horiot J-C, Bontemps, P, van den Bogaert, W, *et al.* Accelerated fractionation compared to conventional fractionation improves loco-regional control in the radiotherapy of advanced head and neck cancers: results of the EORTC 22851 randomised trial. *Radiotherapy and Oncology,* 1997; 44: 111–121.

45. McNally NJ, Wilson GD. Cell kinetics of normal and perturbed populations measured by incorporation of bromodeoxyuridine and flow cytometry. *British Journal of Cancer,* 1986; 59: 1015–22.

46. Begg AC, *et al.* Predictive value of potential doubling time for radiotherapy of head and neck tumor patients: results from the EORTC cooperative trial 22851. *Seminars in Radiation Oncology,* 1992; 2: 22–5.

47. Joiner MC. Particle beams in radiotherapy. In: Steel GG, ed. *Basic clinical radiobiology.* 2nd edn. UK: Arnold, 1997.

48. Withers HR. Neutrons and other clinical trials: impossible dreams? *International Journal of Radiation Oncology, Biology, Physics,* 1987; 13: 1967–70.

49. Steel GG, Peckham MJ. Exploitable mechanisms in combined radiotherapy-chemotherapy: the concept of additivity. *International Journal of Radiation Oncology, Biology, Physics,* 1979; 5: 85–91.

50. Steel GG. The search for therapeutic gain in the combination of radiotherapy and chemotherapy. *Radiotherapy and Oncology,* 1988; 11: 31–53.

51. Pearson AE, Steel GG. Chemotherapy in combination with pelvic irradiation: a time-dependence study in mice. *Radiotherapy and Oncology,* 1984; 2: 49–55.

52. Yarnold JR, Horwich A, Duchesne G, Westbrook K, Gibbs JE, Peckham MJ. Chemotherapy and radiotherapy for advanced testicular non-seminoma. 1. The influence of sequence and timing of drugs and radiation on the appearance of normal tissue damage. *Radiotherapy and Oncology,* 1983; 1: 91–9.

53. Tannock IF. Combined modality treatment with radiotherapy and chemotherapy. *Radiotherapy and Oncology,* 1989; 16: 83–101.

54. Girling DJ, Parmar KB. Benefits and hazards of combined radiotherapy and chemotherapy in clinical oncology. In: Tobias JS, Thomas PRM, ed. *Current radiation oncology,* Vol. 3. UK: Arnold, 1997.

4.3 Principles and practice of radiotherapy

John R. Yarnold

Introduction

The success of radiotherapy depends on its ability to eradicate cancer without undermining the structure and function of surrounding normal tissues. Cancers differ in their response to ionizing radiation. Much of the difference seems to be accounted for by variation in tumour size and, by implication, the number of tumour clonogens. However, tumour size is not the whole story. For example, bulky (greater than 5 cm) germ cell tumours or lymphomas are eradicated locally with a higher likelihood than even small (less than 2 cm) malignant gliomas or melanomas. The common carcinomas and most sarcomas lie between these two extremes of radiocurability.[1],[2] The biological basis of these differences includes variations in tumour cell radiosensitivity and proliferation kinetics.

Using a standard schedule of treatment that delivers 2.0 Gy daily on 5 days of the week, the likelihood of eradicating the common carcinomas rises steeply above a minimum tumour dose. For example, as the total dose increases from 50 to 60 Gy in 2.0 Gy fractions, the chance of eradicating a 2 cm focus of squamous carcinoma rises from 50 to 90 per cent.[3],[4] There is a steep dose–response relationship for normal tissue effects as well. The ability to climb well up the tumour dose–response curve depends on staying low down on the corresponding curve for dose-limiting normal-tissue reactions (see Fig. 1). The definition of a dose-limiting adverse effect is based on everyday experience of what patients accept in exchange for prospects of cure. Many adverse effects are consistent with a good quality of life despite mild or moderate incapacity. Other complications are so devastating that a risk of 0.1 per cent may be considered unacceptable by the patient, for example, spinal cord injury. The dose intensity associated with the highest acceptable risk of serious complications in an organ or tissue is called the tolerance dose. Most dose-limiting complications associated with conventional radiotherapy (one fraction of 2.0 Gy daily, Monday to Friday) develop many months or years after radiotherapy, and are referred to as late effects. In special circumstances, mucosal reactions developing during or shortly after radiotherapy, so-called early effects, become dose-limiting. Either way, patients and doctors may vary in their opinions of what constitutes tolerance in a particular situation. The tolerance dose for late effects varies according to which organs are irradiated, the proportion of each organ lying within the high-dose zone, and the radiotherapy fraction size. The tolerance dose for early effects in self-renewal tissues such as skin and mucosa is profoundly influenced by overall treatment time. Where late effects are concerned, tissues in the eye, central nervous system, kidney, lung, and gastrointestinal tract tend to tolerate lower total doses than muscle, bone, subcutaneous tissue, and skin. Tolerance of early and late effects is also strongly influenced by radiotherapy technique and the timing of surgery and cytotoxic chemotherapy.

The need for higher radiation doses to larger tumours conflicts with the reduced ability of normal tissues to withstand them.[5] A schedule of 70 Gy in 2.0 Gy fractions may be safe for a T2 (2 to 5 cm) squamous carcinoma in the tonsillar fossa, but the same dose to a squamous carcinoma in a main bronchus risks fatal mediastinal complications. The reduced tolerance in the latter situation relates to differences in treatment volume and the types of normal tissues contained within it. There may be a planned reduction in the radiotherapy volume during the last week or so of curative treatment which confines radiotherapy to bulky disease at presentation (so-called shrinking field technique). The lower risk of complications associated with smaller radiotherapy volumes underpins much successful clinical practice, including brachytherapy techniques. At some tumour sites, the need for radiotherapy doses of greater than 70 Gy can be reduced by prior cytoreductive surgery, chemotherapy, or endocrine therapy. If reductions in radiotherapy volume are taken

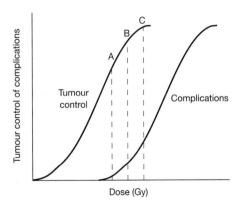

Fig. 1 Dose–response curves for tumour control of complications. The optimal dose (B) gives high tumour control with a low complication rate—further increases in dose (C) produce little improvement in control at the expense of a high complication rate. A suboptimal dose (A) significantly reduces tumour control. (Adapted, with permission, from Alan Horwich, ed. *Oncology, a Multidisciplinary Textbook*, 1st edn, Fig. 9.2, p. 120. London: Chapman & Hall, 1995.)

The author is grateful to Dr J.-P. Gerard for constructive comments on this manuscript.

too far, the price is an increased risk of tumour recurrence at the edges of the high-dose zone.

Pretreatment patient selection based on tumour stage and health status has a profound influence on radiotherapy outcome. This consideration makes it impossible to compare reliably the outcomes of different therapeutic approaches outside the context of prospective randomized trials. At several disease sites, radiotherapy and surgery offer comparable levels of tumour cure, and the choice of modality is dictated by the availability of resources, clinical expertise, patient preference, and medical traditions. Continued uncertainty relating to the contributions of different modalities can usually be traced to weak trial design, unreliable measures of morbidity, and low statistical power.[6]

Definition and actions of ionizing radiation

Ionizing radiation behaves either as photons (X-rays, γ-rays) or as subatomic particles (electrons, neutrons). All forms used in radiotherapy have the ability to penetrate tissue, where the physical energy is dissipated by multiple molecular interactions that convert a proportion into chemical change. Ionizing radiation is defined by the amount of energy absorbed per unit mass of tissue, and its unit is the gray (Gy); 1 Gy (100 cGy) corresponds to the absorption of 1 joule per kilogram of tissue.

The biological effects of ionizing radiation used in therapy can be traced to the random displacement of orbital electrons (ionization) from molecules in the path of a beam as it traverses tissue. The commonest interaction is between ionizing radiation and water, producing highly unstable and chemically reactive hydroxyl radicals. Hydroxyl radicals are involved in many kinds of chemical reactions in tissues, including damage to chromosomes.[7] Unrepaired DNA double-strand breaks are thought to be a potent cause of death in dividing cells. Other forms of cellular damage may be lethal in some cell types, including DNA or plasma membrane damage which triggers cell death by apoptosis.[8] Apoptosis is a genetically programmed response to cell damage that may underlie the unusual radiosensitivity of germ cells, lymphoid cells, and the neoplasms that arise from them.

Cell killing by radiotherapy is a fundamental determinant of clinical outcome, although the relationship between cell killing and tissue effect is powerfully modified by repopulation in many tumours and self-renewal normal tissues. For example, repopulation of tumour clonogens in squamous cell carcinoma of the bronchus compensates for a significant proportion of cell killing over a 6-week course of radiotherapy.[9],[10] Repopulation is also a feature of epidermis, gastrointestinal mucosa, and bone marrow, so-called early reacting normal tissues. The rapid proliferation kinetics in these tissues accounts for the early onset of side-effects and complete healing within weeks of finishing treatment.

Although there is a close relationship between radiation-induced cell killing and the responses of early reacting normal tissues, the responses of so-called late reacting normal tissues that make up the central nervous system, lung, liver, kidney, and musculoskeletal system are less straightforward. In these tissues, clinical symptoms and signs of radiotherapy damage appear over a period of years after radiotherapy. It is likely that unrepaired DNA double-strand breaks

in muscle cells or neurones do not lead directly to cell death because such cells are postmitotic and can function despite chromosome breaks. According to this model, the atrophy and fibrosis seen years after high-dose radiotherapy in many late reacting normal tissues are secondary to ischaemia as a result of radiation-induced death in capillary endothelium. Normal capillary endothelium has an extremely low mitotic index, so it may be many years before irradiated endothelial clonogenic cells attempt cell division and express the lethal radiation damage in their genomes.

Ionizing radiation is known to activate a genetically regulated stress response in cells and tissues within minutes of exposure, although this is not known to have clinical consequences in patients undergoing radiotherapy. This well-studied phenomenon illustrates a point that not all tissue responses to ionizing radiation are necessarily related to cell killing. In recent years, accelerated senescence and upregulation of collagen production in tissue fibroblasts exposed to X-rays has been postulated to underly the development of clinical fibrosis after radiotherapy.[11] Other postulated mechanisms of fibrosis involve the induction of fibrogenic cytokines, particularly transforming growth factor-β isoforms, by a chronic inflammatory response to necrosis in irradiated tissues.[12] Either way, tissue responses to radiotherapy involve the modulation of genetically regulated pathways that are rapidly becoming elucidated.

Sources of ionizing radiation used in radiotherapy

External radiotherapy

Most radiotherapy treatments use high-energy X-rays with good penetrative power generated by linear accelerators (see Fig. 2). A few are still given using cobalt-60 γ-rays (equivalent in penetration to 4 MV X-rays) or low-energy 300 kV X-rays. The X-ray source of a linear accelerator is mounted on a gantry that rotates in a 360° arc around a single point in space called the isocentre. During treatment, the couch and patient are manoeuvred with millimetre precision so that the centre of the patient's tumour is located at the machine isocentre. This ensures that treatment beams intersect the tumour from whichever angle the machine is operated.

The penetrative power of X-rays is described by the electrical potential in millions of volts needed across an X-ray tube in order to produce them. These voltages are much too high to be generated safely in a radiotherapy facility. The linear accelerator exploits other physical principles to produce a beam equivalent to an X-ray machine operating in the range of 4 to 20 million volts (**MV**), hence the descriptive term megavoltage radiation. The X-rays are emitted from a tungsten target a few millimetres in diameter in the head of the linear accelerator under bombardment by an intense stream of electrons. The beam emitted by the X-ray source diverges in air for about 100 cm before it achieves the cross-sectional dimensions needed for treatment (see Fig. 3). The 100 cm distance from the source of ionizing radiation to the patient is characteristic of what is referred to as external-beam radiotherapy, or teletherapy (tele = long distance). Because the tungsten target is not a perfect point source, the edges of the beam are not sharp, but have a penumbra several millimetres wide.

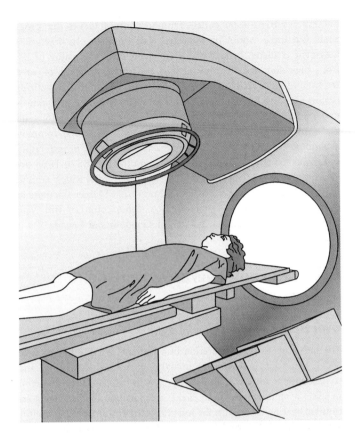

Fig. 2 Patient lying supine on treatment couch prior to treatment. The machine gantry rotates around the patient through 360° on a horizontal axis, enabling different angles of entry for different beams. The X-ray beam emerges from the head of the linear accelerator in the upper part of the figure. In the path of the exit beam in the lower right-hand corner of the figure is a detection device which records the intensity of the exit beam.

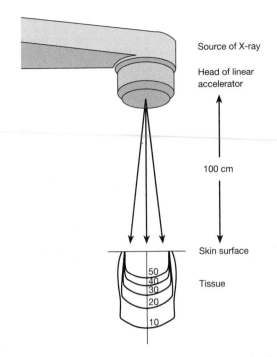

Fig. 3 Schema showing divergence of an X-ray beam as it emerges from the head of a linear accelerator with exponential attenuation beneath the skin surface. A 100 per cent isodose (maximum dose) is beneath the skin surface, at a depth depending on beam energy.

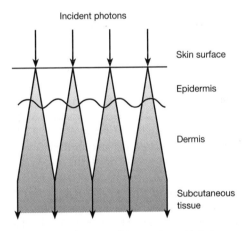

Fig. 4 Schema depicting photon tracks scattering orbital electrons predominantly in a forward direction beneath the skin surface. The electron density increases to a maximum at a depth depending on beam energy (approximately 1.5 cm for 6 MV X-rays).

X-ray beam divergence between source and tumour accounts for a reduction in beam intensity roughly in accordance with the inverse square law. Air molecules absorb (attenuate) very little of the beam, but as soon as the beam enters tissue, attenuation increases sharply (see Fig. 3). The absorption of X-rays in tissue is exponential, meaning that a fixed proportion of the energy is absorbed per unit length (centimetre depth) of tissue irradiated. This relationship is disturbed by air cavities in the lung and bowel which absorb less dose, and transmit correspondingly more. The contribution of divergence within the patient to reduced beam intensity is relatively modest compared with the absorption of energy by interaction with tissue water and other molecules.

Megavoltage X-rays deposit the maximum dose a centimetre or more beneath the skin surface depending on beam energy. This is because the orbital electrons displaced from tissue water and other molecules by X-rays as they penetrate skin are scattered forward in the path of the beam, depositing their energy in successive forward collisions with other orbital electrons beneath the skin surface (see Fig. 4). The forward accumulation of scattered electrons translates into a chain reaction of ionization events in cell nuclei beneath the skin surface. The relatively sparse ionizations in superficial layers account for the skin-sparing properties of megavoltage radiation, and explain why acute skin reactions are seldom dose-limiting. This useful

property stands in contrast to 'DXT', or kilovoltage X-rays (150 to 300 kV), now little used, which deposit the maximum energy in the skin.

Internal radiotherapy

Brachytherapy (brachy = short distance) exploits the inverse square law over distances of a few centimetres. Artificial radioactive sources are inserted directly into tumour tissues (interstitial therapy to the tongue or prostate, for example) or natural body cavities (intracavitary treatment to the uterine cavity or bronchus, for example). The adjacent tumours receive very high total doses of radiation, often in excess of 100 Gy, whilst the surrounding normal tissues receive a much lower dose. If the periphery of a tumour at 1 cm distance from central radioactive sources receives 100 Gy, the dose falls to roughly 25 per cent (25 Gy) 1 cm further away, in accordance with the inverse square law. Interstitial or intracavitary radiotherapy is very effective if access to the tumour can be gained and the tumour size is up to 5 cm diameter. Highly radioactive sources, usually iridium-192, deliver therapeutic doses to patients within minutes inside a specially protected treatment room. This form of treatment is called high dose-rate brachytherapy. An alternative mode of treatment involves a much lower dose rate, typically delivered continuously over a few days, which reproduces the kind of treatment historically delivered with radium.

Radiotherapy for clinical cure or symptom relief

Few tumour sites are beyond the reach of curative surgery, but there are important locations where radiotherapy is the treatment of choice, usually because organ or tissue function is better preserved. Early stage carcinomas of the head and neck, cervix uteri, bladder, and prostate are common examples. At other sites, radiotherapy contributes to patient cure in combination with surgery and/or cytotoxic therapies. Indications for curative radiotherapy are generally well defined by clinical trials. At some primary tumour sites, it is still unclear what contribution regional lymphatic control makes to cure. Recent data for early breast cancer seem to confirm the importance of local-regional control for long-term survival after several decades of uncertainty.[13],[14] The requirements for cure include the ability to encompass local-regional disease with radiotherapy beams without exceeding the ability of critical normal tissues to tolerate the prescribed dose. The absence of detectable haematogenous metastases at presentation is usually a crucial additional requirement. Ability to tolerate the early and late side-effects of radiotherapy is maintained into the ninth decade of life in the absence of intercurrent illness.[15],[16]

In borderline cases, it is a matter of judgment involving doctors and patient to decide that curative treatment is justified, or that risks and severity of early and late morbidity outweigh small prospects of cure. At chances of clinical cure below 5 per cent, the choice may be to treat with palliative intent. In ideal circumstances, the choice is discussed and agreed with the patient. In incurable patients expected to live a few years rather than a few months, it is common to prescribe high doses with the aim of eradicating local-regional disease responsible for symptoms, or of delaying tumour regrowth for the life of the patient. The practice is based on an impression that patients tend to have a more dignified death from intercurrent illness secondary to generalized metastases than from focal disabilities (obstruction, bleeding, pain) caused by uncontrolled local-regional disease. Exceptions include metastases in the central nervous system, for example, where focal disabilities are typically severe.

Palliative radiotherapy is usually confined to disease responsible for symptoms, so that the treatment volume is often smaller than in the curative setting, and associated with fewer acute side-effects. Ideally, the radiotherapy dose intensity would be adjusted to reflect the responsiveness of the patient's tumour, normal tissues, and prognosis, but these cannot be predicted with precision. In practice, a judgment is made, balancing the expected gains in quality of life from high-dose radiotherapy against treatment duration (4 to 6 weeks) and the severity of acute radiotherapy side-effects. In patients predicted to live for months rather than years, low-dose palliation is preferred on the basis that it often suffices for lifelong palliation, and that acute side-effects are kept to a minimum. In several common situations, such as the palliation of metastatic bone pain or respiratory symptoms from lung cancer, single doses in the range 8 to 10 Gy are of proven safety and effectiveness.[17],[18] Practices differ widely around the world, but the delivery of a small number of larger fractions in the palliative setting is characteristic of some countries with very heavy case-loads, including the United Kingdom and Canada.[19]

External radiotherapy treatment planning

Overview

The first stage in the preparation of a patient for radiotherapy is to decide what organs need to be included in the high-dose zone, and to locate them accurately in the patient (see Fig. 5). The next step is to select a radiotherapy beam (field) arrangement that encompasses tumour-bearing tissue with the least exposure of surrounding healthy tissues, such as the orbit or spinal cord. The selection is achieved with the help of powerful computer software, which uses anatomical information from X-ray computer tomography of the patient to calculate the optimal beam specifications. The energy, field dimensions, and angle of entry of each beam are adjusted to deliver an even distribution of radiation dose to the tumour. Steep downward dose gradients are required outside the edge of the high-dose zone. Artificial surface landmarks (for example, tattooed points) are established as reliable reference points for defining the point of entry of radiotherapy beams on a daily basis.

The accuracy of beam localization is usually verified using a simulator before a course of treatment starts. This diagnostic X-ray machine screens the patient, reproducing the beam sizes, shapes, and gantry angles of the treatment to be delivered on the linear accelerator (see Fig. 6). The simulator projects a transmission image of each beam ('beam's eye view') on a television monitor or diagnostic X-ray film. The beam's eye view of each radiotherapy field is verified by the prescribing clinician. Once radiotherapy is underway, the accuracy of beam localization continues to be checked regularly by an electronic detector array that measures the radiotherapy beam as it exits from the patient, and generates a transmission image of the treatment (see Fig. 2). This image can be visually compared with the corresponding image generated by the simulator before treatment, and with the image generated by the radiotherapy three-dimensional planning computer software. Imaging devices are being used increasingly to verify dosimetry *in vivo*, as well as to verify the accuracy of beam placement.

Defining the volume to be treated

The definitions and terms used to describe the treatment zone are agreed internationally.[20] All macroscopic disease to be included

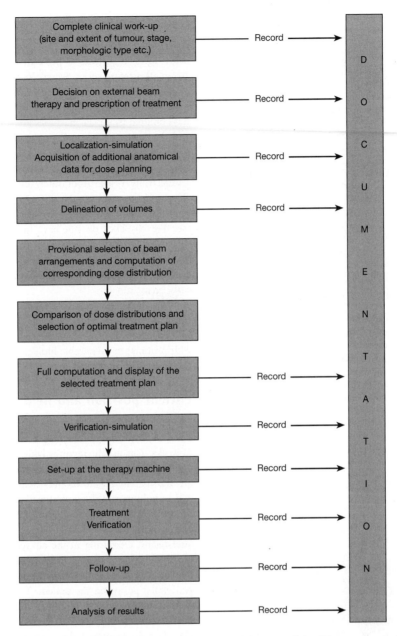

Fig. 5 Steps in the radiotherapy procedure. NB: There should be a continuous feedback between all the different steps. A difficulty at a given point may question all the decisions made at a previous step. (Reproduced, with permission, from the International Commission on Radiation Units and Measurements (ICRU) Report 50: *Prescribing, Recording, and Reporting Photon Beam Therapy*, Fig. 2.1. Issued 1 September 1993).

defines the gross tumour volume (see Fig. 7). A margin reflecting uncertainty about the extent of microscopic disease is added to create the clinical target volume. The gross tumour volume and clinical target volume are determined by clinical assessment, staging investigations, and by knowledge of the natural history of the disease. X-ray computed tomography and magnetic resonance imaging have revolutionized the accuracy of diagnosis and anatomical localization for radiotherapy in recent decades.[21] Limits of accuracy imposed by tissue movement, such as respiratory excursion, and technical factors are taken into account by adding a further margin to create the planning target volume. Finally, the high-dose envelope does not

conform exactly to the size and shape of the planning target volume, but tends to be larger. It is called the treatment volume.

The margins of treatment are often reduced in the last 2 weeks or so of curative radiotherapy, an approach referred to as a shrinking field technique. The rationale is that tumour control is usually limited by residual disease in the centre of the target volume, justifying a higher dose to this region. This involves one or several reductions in treatment volume in order to increase tolerance and minimize the risk of complications. After cytoreductive surgery or chemotherapy, the initial clinical target volume typically encompasses the original extent of disease at presentation, not the disease remaining after

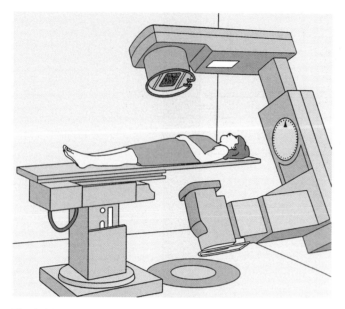

Fig. 6 Schema of radiotherapy simulator for comparison with Fig. 2. The source of X-rays in the upper part of the diagram emits diagnostic-quality X-rays which are imaged using the detector underneath the patient. Like the linear accelerator, the gantry is able to rotate on a horizontal axis through 360°. Regardless of gantry angle, the central axis of beams intersect at a fixed point in space called the isocentre. The patient is usually positioned so that the centre of the tumour corresponds to the machine isocentre.

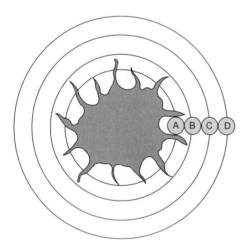

Fig. 7 Schema illustrating internationally agreed terms used to describe radiotherapy volumes. A, gross tumour volume, encompassing macroscopic cancer; B, clinical target volume, encompassing suspected microscopic disease; C, planning target volume, taking into account precision of treatment planning and delivery; D, treatment volume, the volume of tissue encompassed within a 90 per cent treatment radiation isodose.

cytoreduction. This reflects the observations that tumours do not necessarily shrink concentrically, and that microscopic foci often remain well beyond the margins of palpable disease.

Radiotherapy beam energy

A 6 MV X-ray beam delivers 100 per cent dose at about 1.5 cm depth below the skin surface, 90 per cent dose at 5 cm, and 70 per cent at 10 cm (the centre of an average patient) (see Fig. 8). Although the commonest X-ray energy is 6 MV, higher energies of 10 to 15 MV have higher penetrative powers and are helpful in large patients. γ-Rays emitted by cobalt machines are suitable for superficial tumours and the treatment of small or thin patients, although the relatively broad penumbra of the beam is a real disadvantage near critical structures such as the spinal cord and orbit.

Electrons are also produced by linear accelerators. Their penetrative characteristics resemble the behaviour of particles in that they reach a certain depth, typically several centimetres, and are fully absorbed (see Fig. 8). They do not have quite the same skin-sparing characteristics as megavoltage X-rays, so they are usually used to top up (boost) the total dose to superficial lesions, for example malignant cervical lymph nodes or the surgical bed after tumour excision for early breast cancer.

Other types of ionizing radiation, for example protons and neutrons, have specialized or research applications. Their potential advantages rest either on a favourable dose distribution (highly localized with protons) or favourable biological properties (no hypoxic radio-resistance with neutrons).

Patient position and field arrangements

The patient must be comfortable if the same treatment position is to be reproduced with millimetre precision on a daily basis over a period of weeks. This usually involves lying the patient supine with a variety of external supports ranging from simple pillows to body shells. Shells are transparent plastic moulds manufactured to fit the individual, and to hold part of the body (head and neck for instance) in a fixed position relative to the isocentre (point of intersection) of the X-ray beams. The position is reproduced on a daily basis using fixed laser beams crossfiring in the air space above the treatment couch. Electronic control of all couch movements enables the patient to be manoeuvred until fine pencil beams of laser light project across predefined points on the patient. These points are marked by small metal tags on supporting shells or by point tattoos on the skin introduced for the purpose. These surface reference points are displayed on X-ray computed tomographs or magnetic resonance images if marked appropriately. The accurately known relationships of two or three surface landmarks to a patient's tumour ensure that couch movement can bring the centre of the treatment volume to coincide exactly with the isocentre of the treatment machine.

The simplest arrangement is a single beam, suitable for superficial volumes such as skin cancers or rib metastases. The commonest palliative field arrangement uses two fields at 180° to each other, one directed to the front of the patient and the other to the back. This is called a parallel opposed field arrangement. Virtually all tissue between the two fields receives at least 90 per cent of the prescribed dose, including much non-target normal tissue. This is not a problem when palliative doses are prescribed, but large treatment volumes place limits on the total dose that can be given. Three or four intersecting beams are used for radical treatments because the high-dose volume is smaller than the corresponding volume encompassed by opposed fields. Apart from considerations of treatment volume, the optimal beam arrangement considers critical normal structures

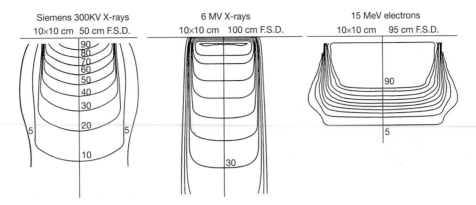

Fig. 8 Schema illustrating the differences in shape and penetration of low-energy (300 kV) orthovoltage X-rays, high-energy (6 MV) X-rays, and 15 MeV electrons; 10 × 10 refers to the field size and shape in centimetres; F.S.D., focus–skin distance, referring to the distance in centimetres between the X-ray source in the head of the machine and the skin surface.

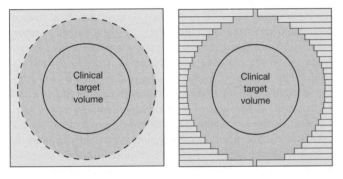

Fig. 9 Schema depicting how the treatment volume (cuboidal) can be made to conform more closely to the planning target volume (usually spheroidal) using a multileaf collimator. The horizontal bars represent thin tungsten leaves which move to designated positions in the X-ray beam under computer control. Irregular beam profiles can be generated to encompass irregular target volumes.

such as the eye, brainstem, and kidneys which may be excluded by particular combinations of beam number and direction.

Treatment volume and field shaping; conformal therapy

Most tumours are spheroidal, and the ideal treatment volume is therefore also spheroidal. In practice, the volumes generated by rectangular radiotherapy beams are cuboidal, with the consequence that more normal tissue is included in the corners of the cube than is necessary or desirable.[22] It has always been possible to manufacture and place thick lead-alloy shielding blocks in the path of the beam to shield small critical structures, but this technology is cumbersome and crude. Manually placed lead shielding blocks are rendered obsolete by multileaf collimators built into the head of modern linear accelerators. Multileaf collimators are arrays of tungsten 'fingers' that move into any position in the beam under microprocessor control, absorbing the beam in that location (see Fig. 9). The ability of modern linear accelerators to generate beams of spheroidal cross-section means that treatment volumes conform more closely to the ideal

target volume. This explains the term 'conformal radiotherapy', which aims to minimize the volume of normal tissue in the treatment zone by more accurate beam shaping. Virtually any cross-sectional beam shape can be generated and implemented under computer control within seconds on a daily basis, a very important technological advance (see Chapter 4.3.2).

Radiotherapy dose distribution (dosimetry)

Dosimetry is the study of radiation dose absorption in the patient. Dosimetry in its simplest form is demonstrated by a single beam directed at the patient perpendicular to the skin surface, as used to treat painful rib metastases or skin tumours, for example. Using 250 kV X-rays, the maximum (100 per cent) dose is deposited at the skin surface and falls off exponentially and rapidly beneath it, such that at 5 cm depth the absorbed dose is only 50 per cent of that at the skin surface (see Fig. 8). Using 6 MV X-rays, the absorbed dose is 70 per cent or so at the skin surface, accounting for the skin-sparing effect of high-energy X-ray beams. The absorbed dose increases to a maximum (100 per cent) at a depth of 1.5 cm below the skin surface, after which it falls off exponentially, to 90 per cent at 5 cm, and 50 per cent at 10 cm depth.

Two X-ray beams entering the patient from opposite sides of the body (parallel opposed fields) represent the commonest field arrangement used for palliative therapy, and for the first phase of some radical treatments as well. Provided the beam energy is high enough, the dose distribution is homogeneous, but all tissue between the two beams receives at least 90 per cent of the prescribed dose (see Fig. 10). For most high-dose treatments, more than two intersecting X-ray beams offer the most favourable dose distribution. The prescribed (100 per cent) dose is confined to the volume of overlap between all fields, with rapid fall in absorbed dose outside. The variation in absorbed dose inside the high-dose envelope (treatment volume) is kept within 10 per cent of that prescribed in accordance with international recommendations.[23] In the past, dose distribution was checked in a single cross-section through the centre of the treatment volume (called two-dimensional dosimetry). Nowadays, it is usual to check and modify the dose distribution at several levels above and below the central cross-section of the treatment volume (three-dimensional dosimetry) (see Fig. 11 and Plate 1). Three-dimensional

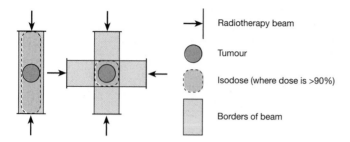

→	Radiotherapy beam
●	Tumour
(dashed)	Isodose (where dose is >90%)
(shaded)	Borders of beam

Fig. 10 Schema depicting size of the high-dose volume (dotted line) compared with the target volume (circle). The simple two-field arrangement shown on the left treats a large volume of tissue that lies outside the target volume, although simplicity and speed of treatment delivery offers advantages in palliative settings.

dosimetry is calculated using computerized algorithms based on anatomical information from X-ray computed tomography or other imaging modalities.[24] Multicolour displays present radiotherapy dose distributions in the patient in any cross-sectional plane selected, overlaid on X-ray CT or MRI images of normal structures and tumour tissue. This presents a detailed and vivid picture of radiation dose distribution in all tumour-bearing and healthy structures (see Fig. 12).

In order to achieve a uniform dose distribution across the treatment volume, the energy profile across each beam is often adjusted automatically to produce a beam that is less intense on one side of the beam axis than the other. The adjustment takes into account the angle of incidence of the beam to the skin surface, as well as the number, direction, and intensity of other beams. Computer technology has greatly increased the scope for individualizing beam profiles in recent years, further improving the evenness (homogeneity) of radiotherapy dose distributions.

Checking the treatment plan

Clinicians work closely with radiation physicists and radiographic technicians (radiographers) to prepare the optimal technical specification for each patient. This specification is a detailed account of every step in the treatment process, including all the machine settings. All calculations must be independently checked before final approval of a treatment plan by the clinician. Sophisticated electronic technology does not guarantee freedom from technical or human error, and secure checking procedures must be in place. Computer networking aids accurate electronic transfer of treatment data from the radiotherapy planning computer, via the simulator, to the linear accelerator.

Treatment verification and delivery

Ideally, the clinician, physicist, and radiographers are present to verify new treatments on the first day. In practice, responsibility falls chiefly to the radiographers to supervise treatment delivery on a day-to-day basis, although the physicists and clinicians must be available at any time to review any aspect of treatment. Field arrangements are checked by visual inspection and physical measurements of the crossfiring laser beams as they impinge on surface reference points, and of the white light beam that projects a visible image of the radiotherapy

beam on to the skin. Electronic monitoring of the exit radiotherapy beam is assuming greater importance as technology improves, since it can be used to generate anatomical pictures of the treatment as well as dose profiles as treatment is being delivered. Enough soft tissue and bony contrast can be seen on a television monitor or on hard-copy film to verify the correct positioning of each field in real time on a daily basis (see Fig. 13 and Plate 2). This technology, called megavoltage imaging, is now used routinely to monitor treatment accuracy, confirming precision to within 2 or 3 mm in most treatment settings.[25] Written protocols describing accuracy requirements and quality assurance are now implemented in all departments.[26]

Radiotherapy fractionation

Fraction size

Differences in the responses of tumours and normal tissues are exploited, not only by technical optimization of radiotherapy, but also by adjusting biological parameters, such as total dose, fraction size, and overall treatment time. Early in the twentieth century, pioneers of radiotherapy noted that the maximum exposure of a patient to X-rays could be safely increased if the total dose was divided into a series of smaller doses (fractions) given 24 h apart. The division of the total dose into smaller components is called fractionation. It was noticed that at many common cancer sites, fractionation spared the normal tissues at the expense of the tumour. In the treatment of squamous cell carcinoma of the skin, for example, a single exposure of 2000 roentgens (roughly 2000 cGy or 20 Gy absorbed dose in modern units) cured tumours only at the expense of severe acute skin reactions and marked scarring in later years. The same antitumour effect was achieved with milder acute skin reactions and much less late scarring by giving a series of smaller fractions, corresponding roughly to 60 Gy in 2.0 Gy fractions over 6 weeks.

The relationship between fraction size and tissue response is not linear.[27] In other words, a 10 per cent increase from 2.0 to 2.2 Gy per fraction does not cause a 10 per cent increase in tissue response. It often translates into a greater than 10 per cent increase in tissue response, measured as the probability of a specific complication or of tumour control, with variations in the quantitative relationships that are open to therapeutic exploitation. A schedule using fraction sizes larger than 2.0 Gy involves a lower total dose than a schedule using 2.0 Gy fractions, and vice versa. In treating squamous cell carcinomas in the head and neck, cervix uteri, or bronchus, for example, the rate of dose-limiting late complications appears to rise faster than the rate of increase in tumour control when fraction size increases above 2.0 Gy.[28] In these tumour sites, therapeutic ratio appears to be optimized if fraction sizes larger than 2.0 Gy are avoided. There may be further gains from fraction sizes of 1.5 to 1.8 Gy, in which case fractions have to be given more than once daily to prevent undue prolongation of overall treatment time.[29],[30] The use of fractions smaller than the conventional 2.0 Gy is called hyperfractionation.

Fraction sizes of 2.0 Gy remain the standard against which other fractionation schedules are compared. However, there is a tradition of using fewer, slightly larger, fractions (2.5 to 3.0 Gy) over a shorter overall treatment time for some curative treatments, particularly in the United Kingdom.[31]–[34] The use of fraction sizes larger than 2.0 Gy

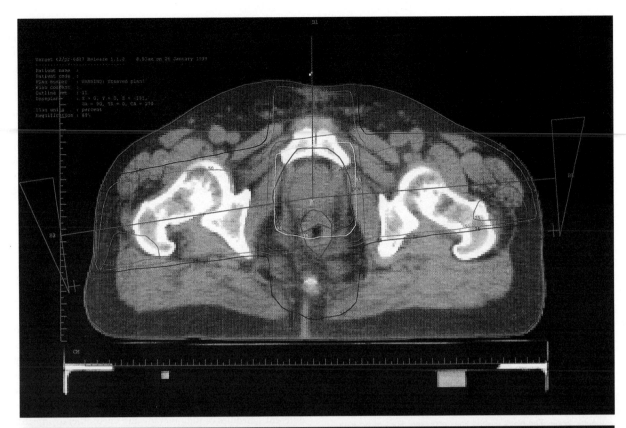

(a)

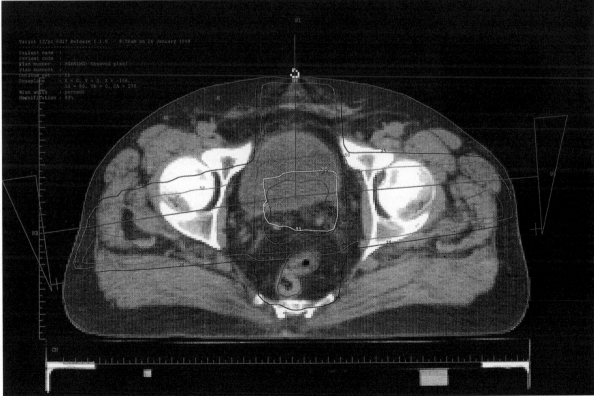

(b)

Fig. 11 Two transverse cross-sections of the pelvis generated by X-ray computer tomography in a patient with prostate cancer. The tomograms are used to define and outline the planning target volume. The non-target rectum is also outlined on contiguous anatomical sections, here shown through the centre (a) and upper (b) levels of the radiotherapy volume. X-ray absorption data derived from X-ray computer tomography have been used directly to calculate the radiotherapy isodose distributions. These are shown as dark lines in the figures, based on the intersection of one anterior and two wedged lateral radiotherapy fields. The white 95 per cent isodose encompasses the target volume at both levels (black outline inside 95 per cent isodose) (see also Plate 1).

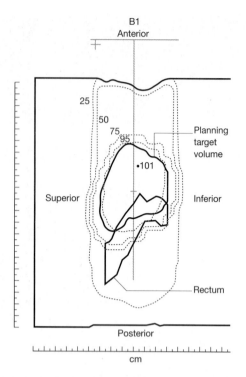

Fig. 12 Radiotherapy isodose curves through the planning target volume and rectum (solid red) reproduced in sagital section from Fig. 11. The straight grey line represents the central axis of the anterior field entering through the pubic bone. The black dashed lines represent lines of isodose. Note that the 95 per cent isodose curve almost entirely encircles the planning target volume, but avoids about 50 per cent of the rectum behind it, including the posterior rectal wall.

is called hypofractionation. Larger fractions (4 to 10 Gy) are a historical feature of many palliative schedules in the United Kingdom, where its convenience relates to fewer hospital visits and shorter overall treatment time.[17],[18] The other context where large fraction sizes are often used is in interstitial or intracavitary brachytherapy, where large single doses are highly practical and tolerance is maintained by the small volumes treated (a few hundred cubic centimetres compared with more than a thousand cubic centimetres in many external-beam treatments).

Treatment time

It is recognized that surviving clonogenic cells in some tumours not only continue to proliferate during radiotherapy, but also increase their rate of proliferation in response to cell death, in a similar way to self-renewing normal tissues.[9],[35] A certain proportion of each radiotherapy fraction, sometimes one-third, can be envisaged as compensating for tumour cell proliferation between exposures, including the weekends. Randomized clinical trials have tested the benefits of shortening the overall treatment time in tumour types, including squamous cell carcinoma of the head and neck, considered to have relatively fast proliferation rates.[36] This is achieved by giving two or three fractions per day, each fraction separated by 6 to 8 h, sometimes including weekends. This technique is called accelerated fractionation, reflecting the shorter overall treatment times. It is nearly always combined with hyperfractionation, in that individual fraction

sizes are usually 1.6 to 1.8 Gy. For example, in a recent trial of hyperfractionated, accelerated radiotherapy in squamous cell lung cancer which recorded superior local control and overall survival, the experimental arm delivered 36 fractions of 1.5 Gy over 12 days, compared with 30 fractions of 2.0 Gy over 6 weeks for the control arm.[37]

The total dose is slightly reduced when accelerated fractionation is used because normal epithelia (skin, buccal, oesophageal, and intestinal mucosa) have less time to repopulate during radiotherapy, and acute side-effects are more severe. It should be noted that mesenchymal cells, including vascular endothelium, do not repopulate significantly during several weeks of radiotherapy. Hence, variation in treatment time, in itself, has no significant effect on the severity of late normal-tissue atrophy and fibrosis.

Integrating radiotherapy with other modalities

Surgery and chemotherapy each enhance normal-tissue responses to radiotherapy. With chemotherapy, the enhancement depends on the drug and dose schedule.[38] The enhancement is influenced by scheduling, concurrent treatment being associated with the greatest enhancement of radiation adverse effects.[39] The difficulty of predicting the enhancement of early and late normal-tissue responses after different schedules of radiotherapy and chemotherapy means that, in the interests of safety, an interval of at least a few days is often left between exposure to each modality. Even so, an arbitrary reduction in total radiotherapy dose may be introduced to compensate for an elevated complication risk, particularly when anthracyclines are used.

The clinical benefits of combined chemoradiotherapy rely on enhanced tumour control, although this does not necessarily involve any interaction between drugs and radiotherapy at the tissue level.[40] For example, drugs may be given to eradicate microscopic metastases, as in early breast cancer, whilst the radiotherapy is given to eradicate local-regional disease.[14],[41] In other situations, such as locally advanced head and neck cancer, chemotherapy and radiotherapy are intended to interact locally in the control of bulky disease. In general, it has been very difficult to prove the benefits of combined chemotherapy and radiotherapy in the control of local-regional disease in common solid tumours.[42] A common feature of comparative trials is a higher rate of normal-tissue damage, as well as tumour control, in the combined modality arm, leaving it unclear whether a slightly higher dose in the radiotherapy alone arm would have achieved the same result.[43]

There are two situations where combined modality therapy has been unequivocally associated with therapeutic gain in terms of local tumour control without enhanced normal-tissue complications. The first is the combination of low-dose cisplatin and high-dose radiotherapy in squamous cell carcinoma of the bronchus, and the second is the combination of radiotherapy and fluorouracil in anal cancer.[44],[45] In the case of cisplatin, the drug acts as a radiosensitizer, not as a cytotoxic agent, and appears to sensitize tumour cells in preference to normal cells. In anal cancer, fluorouracil acts as a cytotoxic agent, which appears to interact with radiotherapy at the tissue, enhancing tumour response to a greater degree than normal-tissue responses.

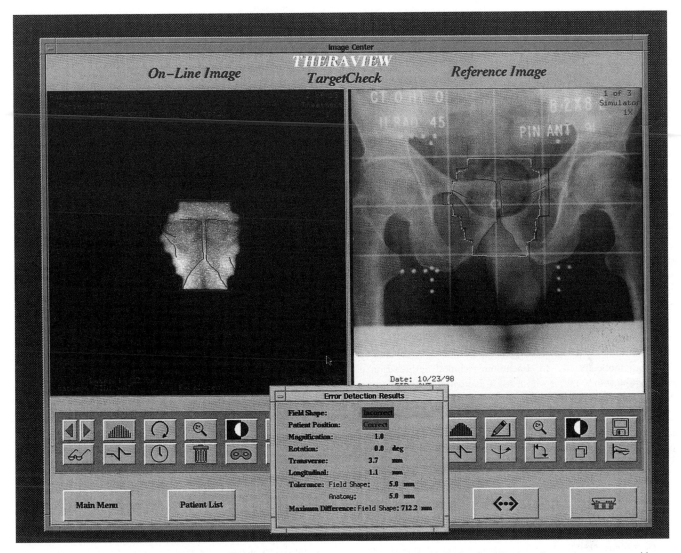

Fig. 13 TV monitor screen on a linear accelerator console of the patient represented in Figs 11 and 12. On the right, the reference image generated by a simulator show a 'beam's eye view' of the anterior field, shaped using a multileaf collimator. The bony outline of the pubis is used to verify the accuracy of field replacement during therapy by imaging the exit beam of the linear accelerator, shown in the on-line image on the left. These two views are compared and verified on a daily basis, with adjustments if defined tolerance limits are not met (see also Plate 2).

Management of adverse effects

Explanation and prevention achieve a great deal in the management of acute side-effects, defined as those that develop during, or shortly after, a course of radiotherapy. Acute side-effects can usually be related to cell depletion, although fatigue, nausea, and vomiting cannot be understood in these terms. For example, depletion of the basal layer of the epidermis accounts for desquamation of the skin that sometimes complicates curative therapy. Acute skin reactions can be unpleasant for a minority of patients, but are nearly always temporary. Maintained nutrition and fluid intake are particularly important when treating any part of the gastrointestinal tract, when specialist dietary advice and supervision are often needed. Dental and oral hygiene are particularly relevant for patients with head and neck cancer, in order to prevent infections that intensify mucositis. Other preventive measures against oral mucositis include the avoidance of alcoholic spirits and highly spiced food. Painful mucositis is palliated by a range of remedies, starting with aspirin mucilage. Skin desquamation is managed using gelatin-based applications that have transformed skin care in the last decade. Diarrhoea is managed in the usual way, with codeine phosphate or Motilium. Nausea and vomiting respond to the usual antiemetics, including 5-hydroxytryptamine antagonists. No specific measures are currently available to combat fatigue, other than rest. Late side-effects are much more difficult to manage, and can be made worse by inappropriate interventions. Surgery can be life saving in the removal of segments of necrotic bowel, for example. Otherwise, emphasis is placed on rehabilitation, including dietary advice, physiotherapy, pain control, and psychological support, depending on the clinical syndrome.

The future of radiotherapy

Advances in the technical basis of radiotherapy, including individualized three-dimensional treatment planning, conformal radiotherapy, beam intensity modulation, electronic megavoltage imaging, and patient positioning devices are all undergoing formal testing to establish therapeutic cost-effectiveness. Computer technology enables linear accelerators to be preprogrammed with complex treatment specifications capable of being implemented and verified to levels of accuracy previously undreamed of. These measures do not represent a plateau in expectations for future advances in radiotherapy, but they do represent a transformation in accuracy and sophistication.

Significant advances have been made with unconventional fractionation regimens based on sound biological principles and clinical data in lung cancer and head and neck cancer. Specific radiosensitization of tumour cells has been achieved by low-dose cisplatin in squamous cell carcinoma of the lung, and this combination may have other applications. However, prediction of normal-tissue responses based on biological assays is still in the future. Predictive tests of tumour proliferation, hypoxia, and cellular radiosensitivity also remain the subjects of intensive research. The contribution of cell and molecular biology over the last 40 years to the understanding of radiotherapy effects has been profound, but the clinical benefits have been modest so far. In conclusion, technical optimization of radiotherapy with X-rays is within reach. Biological optimization has exciting prospects, but still some way to go.

References

1. Deacon J, Peckham MJ, Steel GG. The radioresponsiveness of human tumours and the initial slope of the cell survival curve. *Radiotherapy and Oncology*, 1984; **2**: 317–23.

2. Steel G, Peacock JH. Why are some human tumours more radiosensitive than others? *Radiotherapy and Oncology*, 1989; **15**: 63–72.

3. Fletcher GH. Local results of irradiation in the primary management of localized breast cancer. *Cancer*, 1972; **29**: 545–51.

4. Fletcher GH. Clinical dose–response curves of human malignant epithelial tumours. *British Journal of Radiology*, 1973; **46**: 1–12.

5. Withers HR, Taylor JMG, Maciejewski B. Treatment volume and tissue tolerance. *International Journal of Radiation Oncology*, 1988; **14**: 751–9.

6. Bentzen S. Towards evidence based radiation oncology: improving the design, analysis, and reporting of clinical outcome studies in radiotherapy. *Radiotherapy and Oncology*, 1998; **46**: 5–18.

7. Iliakis G. The role of DNA double strand breaks in ionizing radiation-induced killing of eukaryotic cells. *BioEssays*, 1991; **13**: 641–8.

8. Illidge TM. Radiation-induced apoptosis. *Clinical Oncology*, 1998; **10**: 3–13.

9. Fowler J. How worthwhile are short schedules in radiotherapy? A series of exploratory calculations. *Radiotherapy and Oncology*, 1990; **18**: 165–81.

10. Fowler J, Lindstrom MJ. Loss of local control with prolongation in radiotherapy. *International Journal of Radiation Oncology, Biology, Physics*, 1992; **23**: 457–67.

11. Herskind C, Bentzen SM, Overgaard J, Overgaard M, Bamberg M, Rodemann HP. Differentiation state of skin fibroblast cultures versus risk of subcutaneous fibrosis after radiotherapy. *Radiotherapy and Oncology*, 1998; **47**: 263–9.

12. Tibbs MK. Wound healing following radiation therapy: a review. *Radiotherapy and Oncology*, 1997; **42**: 99–106.

13. Cuzick J, *et al.* Cause-specific mortality in long-term survivors of breast cancer who participated in trials of radiotherapy. *Journal of Clinical Oncology*, 1994; **12**: 447–53.

14. Overgaard M, *et al.* Postoperative radiotherapy in high-risk premenopausal women with breast cancer who receive adjuvant chemotherapy. *New England Journal of Medicine*, 1997; **337**: 949–55.

15. Pignon T, *et al.* Age is not a limiting factor for radical radiotherapy in pelvic malignancies. *Radiotherapy and Oncology*, 1997; **42**: 107–20.

16. Pignon T, Gregor A, Schaake-Konig C, Roussel A, van Glabbeke M, Scalliet P. Age has no impact on acute and late toxicity of curative thoracic radiotherapy. *Radiotherapy and Oncology*, 1998; **46**: 239–48.

17. Price P, Hoskin PJ, Easton D, Austin D, Palmer SG, Yarnold JR. Prospective randomised trial of single and multifraction radiotherapy schedules in the treatment of painful bony metastases. *Radiotherapy and Oncology*, 1986; **6**: 247–55.

18. Bleehen NM, Girling DJ, Fayers PM, Aber VR, Stephens RJ. Inoperable non-small-cell lung cancer (NSCLC): a Medical Research Council randomised trial of palliative radiotherapy with two fractions or ten fractions. *British Journal of Cancer*, 1991; **63**: 265–70.

19. Duncan G, Duncan W, Maher EJ. Patterns of palliative radiotherapy in Canada. *Clinical Oncology, The Royal College of Radiologists (London)*, 1993; **5**: 92–7.

20. International Commission on Radiation Units and Measurements (ICRU). *Definitions of terms and concepts. Prescribing, Recording, and Reporting Photon Beam Therapy*, Report no. 50. ICRU, 1993: 3–26. Bethesda, MD.

21. Goitein M, Abrams M. Multi-dimensional treatment planning: I. delineation of anatomy. *International Journal of Radiation Oncology, Biology, Physics*, 1983; **9**: 777–87.

22. Tait DM, Nahum A, Southall C, Chow M, Yarnold JR. Benefits expected from simple conformal radiotherapy in the treatment of pelvic tumours. *Radiotherapy and Oncology*, 1988; **13**: 23–30.

23. Goitein M. Causes and consequences of inhomogeneous dose distributions in radiation therapy. *International Journal of Radiation Oncology, Biology, Physics*, 1986; **12**: 701–4.

24. Hanks GE, *et al.* Dose escalation with 3D conformal treatment: five year outcomes, treatment optimization, and future directions. *International Journal of Radiation Oncology*, 1998; **41**: 501–10.

25. Mubata CD, Bidmead AM, Ellingham LM, Thompson V, Dearnaley DP. Portal imaging protocol for radical dose-escalated radiotherapy treatment of prostate cancer. *International Journal of Radiation Oncology, Biology, Physics*, 1998; **40**: 221–31.

26. Brahme A, *et al.* Accuracy requirements and quality assurance of external beam therapy with photons and electrons. *Acta Oncologica*, 1988; **Suppl. 1**: 7–15.

27. Joiner MC. Hyperfractionation and accelerated radiotherapy. In: *Basic Clinical Radiobiology*, 2nd edn. London: Arnold, 1997: 123–31.

28. Thames HD, *et al.* Fractionation parameters for human tissues and tumors. *International Journal of Radiation Biology*, 1989; **56**: 701–10.

29. Horiot JC, *et al.* Hyperfractionation versus conventional fractionation in oropharyngeal carcinoma: final analysis of a randomized trial of the EORTC cooperative group of radiotherapy. *Radiotherapy and Oncology*, 1992; **25**: 231–41.

30. Beck-Bornholdt HP, Dubben HH, Liertz-Petersen C, Willers H. Hyperfractionation: where do we stand? *Radiotherapy and Oncology*, 1997; **43**: 1–21.

31. Wiernik G, *et al.* Final report of the general clinical results of the British Institute of Radiology fractionation study of 3F/wk versus 5F/wk in radiotherapy of carcinoma of the laryngo-pharynx. *British Journal of Radiology*, 1990; **63**: 169–80.

32. Rezvani M, Alcock CJ, Fowler JF, Haybittle JL, Hopewell JW, Wiernik G. Normal tissue reactions in the British Institute of Radiology Study of 3 fractions per week versus 5 fractions per week in the treatment of

carcinoma of the laryngo-pharynx by radiotherapy. *British Journal of Radiology*, 1991; **64**: 1122–33.

33. Chappell R, Nondahl DM, Rezvani M, Fowler JF. Further analysis of radiobiological parameters from the first and second British Institute of Radiology randomized studies of larynx/pharynx radiotherapy. *International Journal of Radiation Oncology, Biology, Physics*, 1995; **33**: 509–18.

34. Yarnold JR, Price P, Steel GG. Non-surgical management of early breast cancer in the United Kingdom: radiotherapy fractionation practices. *Clinical Oncology*, 1995; **7**: 223–6.

35. Thames HD, Bentzen SM, Turresson I, Overgaard M, van den Bogaert W. Time–dose factors in radiotherapy: a review of the human data. *Radiotherapy and Oncology*, 1990; **19**: 219–35.

36. Horiot JC, *et al.* Accelerated fractionation (AF) compared to conventional fractionation (CF) improves loco-regional control in the radiotherapy of advanced head and neck cancers: results of the EORTC 22851 randomised trial. *Radiotherapy and Oncology*, 1997; **44**: 111–21.

37. Saunders M, Dische S, Barrett A, Harvey A, Gibson D, Parmar M. Continuous hyperfractionated accelerated radiotherapy (CHART) versus conventional radiotherapy in non-small-cell lung cancer: a randomised multicentre trial. *Lancet*, 1997; **350**: 161–5.

38. Markiewicz DA, *et al.* The effects of sequence and type of chemotherapy and radiation therapy on cosmesis and complications after breast conservation therapy. *International Journal of Radiation Oncology, Biology, Physics*, 1996; **35**: 661–8.

39. Yarnold JR, *et al.* Chemotherapy and radiotherapy for advanced testicular non-seminoma. *Radiotherapy and Oncology*, 1983; **1**: 91–9.

40. Steel G, Peckham MJ. Exploitable mechanisms in combined radiotherapy–chemotherapy: the concept of additivity. *International Journal of Radiation Oncology, Biology, Physics*, 1979; **5**: 85–91.

41. Ragaz J, *et al.* Adjuvant radiotherapy and chemotherapy in node-positive premenopausal women with breast cancer. *New England Journal of Medicine*, 1997; **337**: 956–62.

42. Tannock IF. Combined modality treatment with radiotherapy and chemotherapy. *Radiotherapy and Oncology*, 1989; **16**: 83–101.

43. Henk JM. Controlled trials of synchronous chemotherapy with radiotherapy in head and neck cancer: overview of radiation morbidity. *Clinical Oncology*, 1997; **9**: 308–12.

44. Schaake-Konig C, *et al.* Radiotherapy combined with low-dose *cis*-diammine dichloroplatinum (II) (CDDP) in inoperable nonmetastatic non-small cell lung cancer (NSCLC): a randomized three arm phase II study of the EORTC lung cancer and radiotherapy cooperative groups. *International Journal of Radiation Oncology, Biology, Physics*, 1990; **19**: 967–72.

45. Northover JMA, *et al.* Epidermoid anal cancer: results from the UKCCCR randomised trial of radiotherapy alone versus radiotherapy, 5-fluorouracil, and mitomycin. *Lancet*, 1996; **48**: 1049–54.

Aspects of radiotherapy

4.3.1 Current practice of radiotherapy: physical basis

Hans Svensson and Ben J. Mijnheer

Energy transfer by ionizing radiation to matter

The interaction of ionizing radiation with matter has been discussed in several textbooks.[1],[2] It is not the intention to repeat this information but instead to concentrate on facts of interest for the understanding of the biological effect and the dose distributions obtained by various radiation qualities.

Ionization and excitation

Soon after the discovery of X-rays by Conrad Röntgen in 1895, Henri Becquerel, in 1896, studied the properties of uranium minerals and found that the radiation emanated by the mineral discharged a charged electroscope. The ionizing properties of the rays were discovered.

The International Commission on Radiation Units and Measurements (ICRU) describes ionization as 'a process in which one or more electrons are liberated from a parent atom or molecule or other bound state'.[3] Therefore, ionizing radiation can be either charged particles, so-called direct ionizing radiation (e.g. electrons, protons), or uncharged particles, indirect ionizing radiation (e.g. photons, neutrons) capable of causing ionization. The cut-off energy below which radiation is non-ionizing depends on the properties of the material in which the interactions are taking place.

For ionizing radiation, the mean energy W expanded in a gas per ion pair formed is a very important factor in dosimetry. W is defined by the ICRU[4] as

$$W = E/N$$

where E is the initial kinetic energy of a charged particle that completely dissipated its energy in the gas and N is the mean number of ion pairs formed. This definition also applies for solids and liquids.

It is interesting to note that only about half of the energy transferred to matter goes into ionization. The other important energy transfer phenomenon is electronic excitation, in which an orbital electron in an atom or molecule is raised to a higher energy level, that is to an outer orbit. Also, excitations can have chemical and biological consequences.

A very small amount of energy is needed to produce an ion pair. W is about 34 eV for air. Thus an electron with an energy of 3.4 MeV would create about 100 000 ion pairs before all its energy is transferred to air. An irradiation giving 1 Gy to tissue would therefore produce as much as 2×10^{14} ion pairs per gram of air and roughly the same magnitude of ions in tissue. This is the reason why it is theoretically possible to 'hit' all cells in a tumour.

W-values are quite insensitive to the radiation quality; that is, charge, mass, and energy of the incident particle. Therefore, the relative contributions of energy transfer from ionization and from excitation are fairly constant for different types of radiation. This fact makes the absorbed dose (that is, energy absorption per unit mass) a suitable quantity for use in radiation biology, as it might be that ionization and excitation have different potential to create biological effect.

Two types of direct ionizing radiation are today used in radiotherapy—electrons and protons (heavier particles have been used on a very small scale in experimental radiotherapy). Protons are still used only at a few centres.

Electrons and protons

Electrons, in the energy range of interest in radiotherapy up to 50 MeV, lose most of their energy in collision with atomic electrons. Nuclear interactions are of importance at very high energies not used in therapy. Protons, instead, interact mainly with the nucleus. The interaction with atomic electrons results in excitation or ejection of electrons from the atomic shells. The ejected electron and the atom with the hole form an ion pair. If the ejected electron has enough energy, it can produce more ion pairs along its track. Such electrons are known as delta rays in Fig. 1.

The 'rate' of energy loss of a charge particle is described by the linear stopping power S defined by:

$$S = \frac{dE}{dl} \quad (MeV/cm)$$

where dE is the energy lost by the charged particle traversing a distance dl in a material (Fig. 1). The linear stopping power for electrons and protons are given in Table 1. S has a value close to 2 to 3 MeV/cm for electron energies in common use in therapy. The values are much higher for proton beams, especially at low energies.

The relative biological effects (RBE) for different types of radiations when delivering the same absorbed dose to a tissue depends on the 'rate' of energy loss of the particles. The linear energy transfer, LET, is the average energy locally imparted to the medium, dE, when

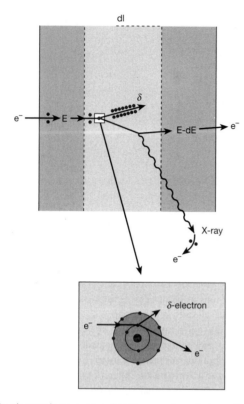

Fig. 1 An electron loses energy when it passes through tissue. Most of the energy will be expended through collision with atomic shell electrons, so called collision losses, see inserted figure. If the ejected electron has energy enough to collide and ionize another atom it is called δ-electron. Electron energy might also be absorbed through so-called radiation losses. X-rays are then produced. This is a fairly rare process in tissue. The lighter area in the figure symbolizes tissue. A thin slice, dl, in this tissue is enlarged. S = dE/dl is the stopping power.

traversing a distance, dl (Fig. 1). LET and S are thus close related physical quantities. The difference is that stopping-power values also include energy losses that are not locally absorbed, for example bremsstrahlung (X-ray) produced in the layer dl. In a strict definition of LET, one should therefore state what is meant by local imparted energy. In practice, this is of small importance as the RBE is only slowly varying with the LET. For electron radiation LET is usually approximated with the energy losses to electrons in the atomic shell (so called collision losses). S in Table 1 includes all losses. The small part that gives rise to energy transfer to bremsstrahlung is indicated in Table 1 in brackets. The collision energy loss for electrons varies between 1.9 and 2.1 MeV/cm in the energy range 0.5 to 50 MeV. For clinical protons the variation is instead between 6 and 400 MeV/cm.

In radiation biology, LET is given in units of keV/μm as the interest is to compare energy deposited in volumes corresponding to the size of sensitive structures in cells. (10 MeV/cm = 1 keV/μm).

Table 1 also includes ranges. The so called continuous–slowing down approximation has been used to calculate the range. This means that it gives the path length which an electron would travel in the course of slowing down, in an unbounded uniform water phantom if the rate of energy loss along the entire track was always equal to the mean rate of energy loss. As an example the range of a 10 MeV electron is 5 cm which is obvious as electrons of energies 0.5 to 10 MeV lose energy of at a mean rate of about 2 MeV/cm.

The LET of protons is thus very much depending on the particle energy. High energy protons of 125 MeV have a range of about 11 cm (Table 1). When this proton is travelling through the tissue it will successively lose energy, at small phantom depth with a rate of about 6 MeV/cm. When an energy of only 20 MeV is left it loses energy at a higher ratio, 26 MeV/cm. However, in the last 4 mm of its range the energy dissipation is very high, which will give rise to a so-called 'Bragg peak', that is a high dose in a narrow peak. In practice, this peak will be smoothen out as the path length and the depth of penetration vary between different particles. As most of the energy is delivered with moderate LET values the RBE of protons for practical therapy is only 10 to 20 per cent higher than that for electrons.

Table 1 Linear stopping powers and ranges for electrons and protons passing through water (≈ soft tissue); data from ICRU (for explanation see text)[5], [6]

Energy, E MeV	Electrons			Protons	
	Stopping power, S MeV × cm⁻¹		Range, cm	Stopping power, S MeV × cm⁻¹	Range, cm
0.5	2.0		0.2	413	0.9×10^{-3}
1.0	1.9		0.4	260	2.5×10^{-3}
2.0	1.9		1.0	157	7.6×10^{-3}
5.0	2.0	(0.1)	2.6	79	36×10^{-3}
10	2.1	(0.2)	5.0	46	0.1
20	2.5	(0.4)	9.3	26	0.4
30	2.7	(0.6)	13	18	0.9
50	3.3	(1.1)	19.8	12	2.2
125				6.1	11

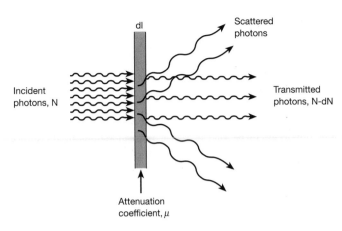

Fig. 2 The attenuation of photons in a material dl having the linear attenuation coefficient μ.

Photons and neutrons

Photons and neutrons (that is indirect ionizing radiation) traversing a distance in a medium undergo far fewer interactions than charged particles and the mean energy transfer is much larger per interaction. These are the only types of indirect ionization radiation used in radiotherapy.

In principle, photons can interact with the orbital electrons (photo-electric and Compton effects) or with the nucleus (pair production and photonuclear reactions). As a result, electrons or positrons will be produced, except in the rare cases when photonuclear reactions take place and neutrons, protons, or other particles can be emitted. However, photonuclear reactions are of minor importance for radiotherapy beams as the threshold for the process is several MeV for most materials. The cross-section (that is the probability for interaction) is also very small.

The number, dN, of N photons which experience interactions when traversing a distance dl in a material can be determined from the relationship

$$dN = \mu N dl$$

μ is called the linear attenuation coefficient (Fig. 2). The value of μ is a function of the photon energy and the atomic number of the material. It is of great importance to be able to compute the attenuation in different tissues (i.e. bone, muscle, lung) to determine the decrease in the number of photons (fluence) with the phantom depth and also the absorbed dose at different points in the patient. Values of μ can be found in textbooks in radiation physics.

Neutrons interact mainly with an atomic nucleus. The most important process in tissue is the interaction with hydrogen. The kinetic energy of the neutron will be divided between the hydrogen nucleus (i.e. the proton) and the neutron. As an example the average energy of the recoil proton from a 20-MeV neutron will be 10 MeV and this recoil proton will travel only about 1 mm in tissue (Table 1). Neutron radiation thus produces low energy protons with fairly high LET (Table 1). The RBE of clinical neutrons is therefore rather high, generally between 2 and 4. The value depends on several parameters such as the neutron energy, dose per fraction, and type of biological effect studied.

Dosimetry

Historical background

In the early days, the amount of radiation to the patient was described by the skin reaction. The radiotherapists investigated the irradiation time needed to produce skin erythema when using a certain X-ray unit in their department. The treatment was then generally divided into several fractions and each irradiation time corresponded to a partial skin erythema dose. One skin erythema dose corresponded roughly to an exposure of 800 röntgen (R) on the skin of the patient.[7]

Very early it was suggested that the 'amount' of radiation could be measured from the degree of interaction of radiation with matter. Holzknecht , in 1902, suggested the use of a chemical dosimeter; that is, a mixture of salts changing from yellow to green when exposed to X-rays.[8] A few years later Villard, in 1908, proposed the ionization chamber as a dosimeter.[9] However, these more objective ways of specifying the amount of radiation were taken into clinical use very slowly and very different real doses were applied by different departments. For instance in Sweden Sievert carried out ionization chamber measurements at the various radiotherapy departments in 1925.[10] He concluded 'It had been thought that the same dose was being given in all the röntgen therapy departments in the country but variations between 320 R and 1400 R were found.' An important step towards standardization was taken when the quantity exposure was adopted by the first International Radiology Congress in Stockholm in 1928. This quantity has survived although the unit has changed. Today ionization chambers are often calibrated by standardization laboratories with respect to exposure (or kerma), but the user is more interested in determining absorbed dose. Therefore, different conversion and correction factors are used by the medical physicists to determine the absorbed dose to water from measurements with an ionization chamber calibrated in exposure (or kerma).

Exposure, kerma, and absorbed dose

The definitions of radiation quantities are taken from the ICRU Report 33 in which much more detailed information can also be found.[3] A schematic description of the interaction processes underlying these definitions is given in Fig. 3.

The absolute measurements of the exposure for 'conventional' X-rays are performed using a free-air ionization chamber, in principle an open-ended, plane-parallel chamber with a collimator defining the cross-section of the air volume. At higher energies a graphite ionization chamber is used and the Bragg–Gray theory is applied. With present techniques it is difficult to measure exposure when the photon energies involved are greater than a few MeV or less than a few keV.

There is a trend to replace the use of the quantity exposure by kerma, an acronym for kinetic energy released to unit mass. This quantity is defined for any material (not only air as is the case for exposure). The kerma, K, is defined by dE_{tr}/dm where dE_{tr} is the sum of initial kinetic energies of all charged particles liberated by uncharged ionizing particles (X-rays, gamma radiation, and neutrons) in a material of mass dm:

$$K = dE_{tr}/dm$$

During the 1960s ^{60}Co units, linear accelerators, and betatrons came into common use in radiotherapy. It was then not possible to

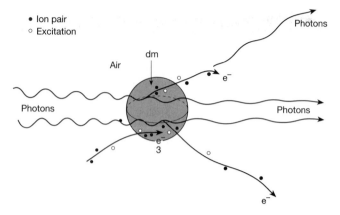

Fig. 3 Exposure X is the charge dQ of ions of one sign per mass dm of air, that is liberated from electrons 1 and 2 before they are stopped in air; that is, X = dQ/dm. The unit is C/kg (formerly röntgen; 1 R = 2.58 × 10⁻⁴ C/kg). Air kerma K_{air} is the energy dE_{tr} transferred to electrons 1 and 2 from photons per mass dm of air; that is $K_{air} = dE_{tr}/dm$. The unit is the gray (Gy). Kerma is defined for all materials (not only air) and for indirectly ionizing radiation (photons and neutrons). The absorbed dose D_m is the mean energy dε imparted by ionizing radiation to the matter of mass dm, that is, $D_m = d\varepsilon/dm$ and is that part of energy 'absorbed' inside the sphere of mass dm from electrons 1, 2, and 3. D_m is defined for all materials and types of ionizing radiation. The unit is the gray (Gy).

use the exposure for the physical specification of the treatment as absolute measurements were difficult to perform at energies above a few MeV. Thus, the absorbed dose to water was accepted as the quantity to which biological effects should be related.

The absorbed dose D is defined as dε/dm, where dε is the mean energy imparted by ionizing radiation to matter of mass dm:

$$D = d\varepsilon/dm$$

The unit of absorbed dose is the gray (Gy): 1 Gy = 1 J/kg. The energy imparted is subject to stochastic fluctuations which become significant if the number of charged particles incident on the mass dm is low. Therefore, in the definition of absorbed dose the mean value dε of the energy imparted to the matter of mass dm is used. The influence of stochastic variations is very pronounced if subcellular structures are considered, for example, DNA molecules. For example a structure in a cell with a diameter of 0.3 μm will, as a mean, only be 'hit' once when 1 Gy is delivered with photon or electron beams. In reality, this means that some structures will have several interactions and other none. With neutron radiation even fewer structures would, as a mean, be 'hit' with 1 Gy but those which are hit would instead get much larger energy transfer. These variations are of great importance in understanding the biological effects of different types of radiations and are dealt with in the field of microdosimetry.[11]

In reporting the absorbed dose it is always necessary to state the material. In the calibration of accelerator monitors, it is general practice to determine the absorbed dose to water even if the measurements are made in a plastic phantom. The absorbed dose to the plastic material might be somewhat different. Also, it is generally not considered that the absorbed dose to muscle and adipose tissue differs from that to water.

The international calibration system

For many reasons it is important to have an accurate and coherent world-wide metrology system in all radiotherapy centres. Thus, it is of great importance that the absorbed dose for different beam qualities can be measured in a consistent way in individual departments so that patients can be transferred from one treatment machine to another without changing the prescribed dose value. Of course it is also important to be able to repeat the calibrations in the future even if the centre replaces the dosimeter instrument. Furthermore, agreement in dose determination between different departments is essential as the success of radiotherapy depends very much on exchange of experience.

The policy in this field is generally set by the ICRU. Reports from the ICRU cover a very broad field which is often of direct use in radiotherapy, not only in the field of calibration but also for dose and target volume specification. Physical data recommended by the ICRU are generally applied in calibrations. For instance new evaluations of W and S by the ICRU resulted in changes in the exposure and air-kerma primary standards.

In a few countries, there are primary standard dosimetry laboratories that carry out 'absolute' determinations of exposure, air kerma, and absorbed dose. The primary standards dosimetry laboratories compare their standards at the Bureau International des Poids et Mesures in Paris and an international reference standard is set from these intercomparisons. Most countries do not have primary standards dosimetry laboratories. Instead, a secondary standard dosimetry laboratory calibrates instruments at the Bureau International des Poids et Mesures or at a primary standards dosimetry laboratory and supplies calibrations for hospitals. In many countries, there are regulations requiring that the dosimeters used for calibration of therapy beams should have a calibration that is 'traceable' to a primary standard.

Calibration of radiotherapy sources

One of the most important tasks of a medical physicist at a radiotherapy department is to calibrate the monitors of therapy sources (conventional X-ray units, ⁶⁰Co-units, accelerators) and source strengths of radionuclides used for brachytherapy. However, the radiation oncologist also has certain responsibilities; the degree differs owing to the organizational structure. It is not possible for the physicist to perform an adequate calibration if he or she is not well informed about the intended clinical use of equipment. Furthermore, the radiation oncologist has the direct responsibility for the patient, which means that he or she should to be well informed about the quality of the technical work that is directly related to patient treatments.

The ionization chamber is still considered to be the best dosimeter for careful calibrations in therapy beams. Large departments, at least, should have one ionization chamber system of high quality (so-called reference class instrument) that is calibrated at the national calibration laboratory (a secondary or primary standards dosimetry laboratory). A constancy check should be made regularly, preferably against a special check source. A log book should be kept that can be easily understood by an outside audit group. This system should then used to calibrate the field instruments at the centre.

Generally, the calibrations are made in terms of air kerma or exposure. Absorbed dose determinations at the reference point are then performed by applying a dosimetry protocol (for example the International Code of Practice).[12]

New accelerators should always be calibrated independently by at least two persons. Several accidents would have been avoided if this rule had been followed. However, some hospitals do not have two different teams for such measurements. In such cases a mailed dosimetry service (for example with a thermoluminescence dosimeter) could be used. The International Atomic Energy Agency (IAEA) has a mail dosimetry service intended mainly for developing countries. A similar service is provided in Europe by the European Society for Therapeutic Radiology and Oncology (ESTRO).

The calibration is generally carried out in several steps. The accelerator dose monitor is first calibrated to give the dose in a reference point, for example with photon radiation, source–skin distance (SSD) = 100 cm, field size 10 × 10 cm and phantom depth 10 cm in a water phantom. Measurements and calculations must then be performed so that accurate dose determinations can be made at a specified point in the centre of the target (tumour) volume or other points of interest, for instance in healthy organs at risk.

The accelerator monitor is situated in the head of the accelerator. Therefore this monitor responds to a different beam than that incident on the patient. Thus, at the patient level at the centre of the beam a large contribution of scattered radiation from the collimator, flattening filters, etc. situated in the head will contribute to the dose. This contribution is a function of the field size, addition of absorbing blocks to form the field, and also wedged filters. In open photon beams (i.e. without wedges) at a fixed source to skin distance, the field size dependence of the response of the monitor is often about 30 per cent for fields between 5 × 5 cm and 30 × 30 cm. It is obvious that it is very difficult to determine the dose even in a water phantom for the field size of interest with an accuracy of a few per cent which today is required in some radiotherapy. A procedure that could be followed has been recommended by an IAEA/ESTRO working group.[13] The dose to the reference point in the phantom is, in this report, measured in two steps. The scattered radiation from the accelerator head and that created in the phantom itself are determined separately. Similar procedures are also often used in computer dose planning systems for monitor unit computations. In all methods, a large number of measurements are, however, needed.

A dosimetry quality control programme should be set up for each new radiation unit. Regular checks must be performed of, for instance, the calibration of the accelerator dose monitor, the beam field uniformity, and the agreement between light and radiation fields. The contents of this programme must be adjusted to each type of radiotherapy machine and to the local conditions (see the section on quality control of teletherapy equipment).

Radiotherapy sources: external beam therapy

At present, most radiotherapy is carried out with linear accelerators.[14] However, in the future it will probably be useful to have also a ^{60}Co unit in some centres as this is a very reliable source giving an adequate beam for some treatments, such as head and neck and breast. Most radiotherapy centres are also equipped with conventional X-ray machines, often used for superficial therapy or palliative treatments.

The radiation energy of the photons used for treatment varies from approximately 0.01 MeV (10 keV) to 50 MeV. The specification of the beam energy for ^{60}Co units is very straightforward as photons (gamma rays) of two energies are delivered (1.17 and 1.33 MeV) and the mean energy is 1.25 MeV. The accelerating potential (in kV or MV) is often reported for conventional X-ray machines and accelerators to describe the beam quality as it is difficult to specify a spectrum of photons with different energies.

The IAEA defines low energy X-rays for potentials between 10 and 100 kV (0.03 mm Al < half-value layer ≤ 2 mm Al), medium energy X-rays between 100 and 300 kV (2 mm Al < half-value layer 3 mm Cu), and high energy X-rays for beams from accelerators.[12] Sometimes the term Grenz-ray therapy is used for potentials below approximately 20 kV, contact therapy for potentials between 40 and 50 kV, superficial therapy for potentials between 50 and 150 kV, orthovoltage therapy for potentials between 150 and 500 kV, and supervoltage for potentials over 500 kV. For beams from conventional X-ray machines it is also common to specify the radiation quality in terms of the half-value layer which is defined as the thickness of a specified material which, when introduced in the beam, reduces the exposure rate by a half. The half-value layer is used because it gives a better specification of the beam quality than the accelerating potential. Radiation beams with the same accelerating potential could have very different spectral distributions as these are influenced by the construction of the X-ray machine (for example type of rectifier and filtration).

Electrons in electron beams have a fairly narrow spectral distribution and the electron energy at the phantom surface is generally reported in MeV (see section on Beam quality, below).

^{60}Co units

The first ^{60}Co units were introduced in the early 1950s. The unit consists of a ^{60}Co source located near the centre of a lead-filled container. The source is either moved to an opening in the head or is fixed and a collimator is opened so that the radiation can emerge.[1] The ^{60}Co source delivers two gamma rays in a cascade of fairly high energies (1.17 and 1.33 MeV).

^{60}Co is produced by irradiating stable ^{59}Co with neutrons in a reactor. The ^{60}Co material is usually in the form of a solid cylinder, discs, or pellets and is contained inside a cylindrical stainless steel capsule sealed by welding. To prevent leakage, another similar capsule is used outside the first one. The diameter of the ^{60}Co source must be between 1 and 2 cm in order to give sufficient dose rate. This gives a fairly large geometric penumbra (i.e. a zone at the border of the treatment field that is only partly shadowed by the collimator) which is the major disadvantage of a ^{60}Co unit.

Multisource equipment is used for stereotactic 'radiosurgery' by a few centres (see the section stereotactic radiosurgery). ^{60}Co sources of diameter approximately 1 mm (therefore giving a very small penumbra) are positioned in a hemisphere so that all beams are directed towards a single point. For instance, the 'gamma knife' has 201 sources and covers targets from approximately 5 to 40 mm (that is, diameter of the sphere). A target point selected in the brain can be placed at the centre of the radiation focus. A dose of 60 Gy could be delivered to this point within 20 min.

Electron accelerators

The first 'megavolt' unit in clinical use in 1939 (at St Bartholomew's Hospital, London) was a special X-ray machine that could deliver 1000 kV (1 MV). A parallel development of different types of accelerators started at the end of the 1940s and the resonant transformer, van de Graaff generator, and betatron were brought into clinical use at the beginning of the 1950s. The betatron was the most successful of these constructions, and several hundred were used.

The clinical betatrons delivered electron beams with maximum energies of between 20 and 45 MeV. In principle, any electron energy from a few MeV up to the maximum energy could be obtained. The beam current was adequate for electrons to achieve a dose rate. However, the flattening was generally poor.[15] Furthermore, the dose rate for the X-ray beams was fairly low. This was because delivery of the same dose rate to the patient using X-ray beams required an intrinsic accelerator current approximately three orders of magnitude greater than that required with electron beams. However, a usable dose rate could be obtained very near the maximum energy, but still generally less than 1 Gy/min at a source–skin distance (SSD) of 1 m. These disadvantages, and the fact that the installation is very bulky, gave the linear accelerators a considerable edge in popularity over the betatrons.

It was possible to construct the linear electron accelerator because of the successful development of microwave generators (magnetrons or klystrons) during the Second World War. The first clinical accelerator began operating at Hammersmith Hospital, London, in 1953. Today more than 4000 linear accelerators are in use for radiotherapy throughout the world. The basic components of a linear accelerator are shown in Fig. 4, and their functions are briefly explained below.

Electrons are emitted from the electron gun (cathode) during short pulses and are initially accelerated in the injection part of the accelerator tube. In this part the electrons are correctly timed in synchronization with the maxima of the accelerating field set up by the microwaves. Bunches of electrons leave the injector spaced one wavelength apart at a speed close to that of light.

The accelerating energy is delivered by microwaves at approximately 3000 MHz (or 3.10^9 Hz: compare other types of electromagnetic radiations, for example television 3.10^6 Hz, infrared 3.10^{12} Hz, visible light 6.10^{14} Hz, ^{60}Co gamma rays 3.10^{20} Hz; 1 Hz = 1 cycle/s). The microwave source (magnetron of klystron) delivers microwaves during periods of 2 to 6 μs. Such periods (macropulses) are generally repeated with a pulse repetition frequency (prf) of 10 to 400 Hz. For instance if the macropulse is 5 μm and the prf is 100 Hz, the accelerator will then be energized for 0.5 ms during each second and the number of electron bunches during each macropulse will be 15 000 ($= 5 \times 10^{-6} \times 3 \times 10^9$).

Electron bunches travel at a speed close to that of light separated by a distance of 10 cm. Thus, the time structure of the radiation in a linear accelerator and a ^{60}Co unit is very different. This does not appear to influence the relative biological effectiveness of the radiation, although it is of concern in dose measurements as corrections for ion recombination may be needed in pulsed radiation.

Magnetrons or klystrons must be replaced at regular intervals and often represent the most expensive spare part of a linear accelerator. Magnetrons are generally used for smaller accelerators (below approximately 20 MeV). They generally have a lifetime of 1 to 3 years.

Klystrons are often more expensive but generally have a much longer lifetime and can deliver a higher power level.

The accelerator tube consists of a copper cylinder, the interior of which is divided by copper discs or diaphragms of varying aperture and spacing. This section is evacuated to a high vacuum. The microwaves are transported by a special waveguide from the source (klystron or magnetron) to the accelerator tube. In the travelling-wave type of accelerator the electron bunches are travelling forward in synchronization with the microwaves. This requires a load in the end of the accelerating structure to prevent reflection of the wave. The standing-wave type of accelerator makes use of the waves at both ends of the accelerating structure and produces stationary waves.

The travelling-wave design is simpler and produces an intrinsic electron beam with a somewhat narrower spectrum. However, the standing-wave system is more efficient and a shorter accelerating length can be used. The accelerating electrical field strength developed in a standing-wave structure may average as much as 0.15 MeV/cm whereas the travelling-wave often gives approximately half that value.

Small linear accelerators with accelerating potentials of 4 to 6 MeV are either mounted in the treatment head itself or in the gantry arm. The head mounting is compact as the accelerating tube is situated along the treatment beam axis, making bending magnets redundant. The accelerating structure needs to be of the standing-wave type in this case in order to attain an acceptable isocentre height (below approximately 130 cm).

Accelerators mounted in the treatment gantry must have a bending magnet. Treatment-gantry-mounted linear accelerators are made with energies up to approximately 25 MeV (that is, the electron energy). For still higher energies the accelerator tube needs to be fixed and a rotating-beam transport system must be used. Linear accelerators up to approximately 40 MeV have been used for therapy.

The microtron is a microwave-driven accelerator. The first clinical use was in the mid-1970s. Acceleration by the microwaves takes place in a simple cavity. A magnetic field forces the electrons to move in circular orbits and return to the cavity. The electrons receive an additional amount of energy, of approximately 0.5 MeV, for each passage of the cavity and the orbit radius increases on each passage. The principle is very simple but the large diameter of the magnet, approximately 2 m for 20 MeV, is a disadvantage. The magnet is stationary and the electrons are directed along tubes to the gantry and further to the treatment head. It is possible to use more than one treatment gantry with a single microtron as an electron beam with very small energy spread is produced which simplifies the beam transport. A further increase in energy is possible if the 'simple' accelerating cavity is replaced by a small linear accelerator. The magnet must now be constructed to give the electrons a race-track type of orbit with an increasing circumference with increasing number of passages of the linear accelerator. The first clinical accelerator of this type, the race-track microtron, was taken into clinical use in 1986. The accelerator is fairly compact and can give electron and X-ray beams with energies between 5 and 50 MeV in steps of 5 MeV.

In the electron mode, large uniform radiation fields are obtained either through scattering of the electrons in foils or through scanning using a magnet. A careful design of the flattening system is of great importance as the shape of the depth–dose curve, the uniformity and stability of the beam, and the dose rate are affected. Thus, scattering foils which are too thick may give uniform distributions near the phantom surface but deteriorate the dose distribution. Also, the

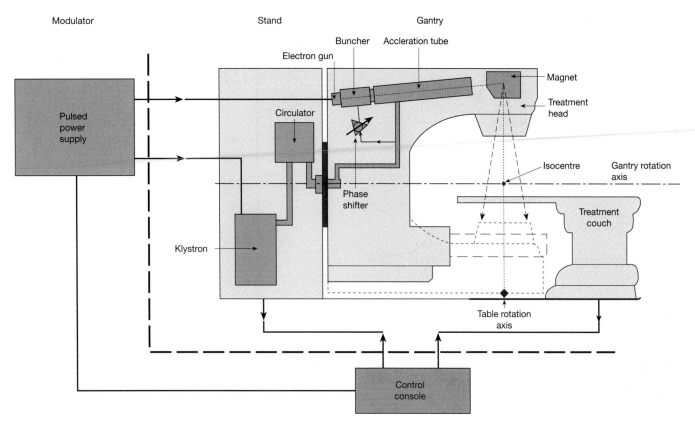

Fig. 4 Block diagram of a medical linear accelerator.

accelerator dose monitors and the collimators (often with special electron applicators or tubes) must be designed so that the scattering in these devices does not destroy the beams. Some manufacturers offer adjustable field size collimators for electron beams, which is to be preferred from the practical point of view.

In the X-ray mode, a target is introduced into the beam just after the bending magnet or just after the accelerating tube for gantry-mounted accelerator tubes. The target consists of a metal plate that is just thick enough to stop the electrons. Part of the energy loss in the target is due to bremsstrahlung production (X-rays). The scattering foils are replaced by a flattening filter. The function of this filter is different from the foil as it absorbs more radiation in the central beam than at distances from the centre. The filter is conical and generally absorbs between 60 and 90 per cent of the photons in the central part of the beam when uniform beams of dimensions 40 cm × 40 cm are required. Thus, the flattening filter thus reduces the 'output' from the accelerator. This is particularly inconvenient at very high photon energies as the unflattened field for such qualities is very peaked. Furthermore, high-energy electrons are produced in the filter from photon interactions which destroy part of the build-up. An interesting method of solving this problem is to use a scanning electron beam on the X-ray target to produce beams of a large size.[16]

Most modern therapy machines are isocentrically mounted with a target–isocentre distance of 100 cm. One critical parameter from the ergonomic point of view is the isocentre height over the floor. A height over approximately 130 cm is generally considered to be inconvenient.

Modern treatment machines often have often a special 'check and confirm' system which indicates whether the machine parameters (for example collimator and gantry angle, table height, dose monitor setting) are in agreement with the reference set-up. However, reproducible positioning of the patient on the treatment table is necessary to make the repetition of machine parameters meaningful. Laser indication on the patient is often used to make patient positioning reproducible. In addition, a good system for fixing the patient on the treatment table is very useful.

Beam quality

The choice of irradiation machines is a matter of both department practice and economic constraints. For instance some departments do not use electrons, but instead apply advanced treatment plans with multiple, high-energy photon beams. However, a broad choice of beam qualities certainly simplifies the optimization of a dose distribution.

The dose distribution from beams of the same nominal energy and field size may differ considerably owing to differences in the spectral distribution of the intrinsic accelerator beam and the design of scattering foils, flattening filters, and collimators. Therefore, the therapy centre should not purchase an accelerator based on such parameters as maximum available energies but instead request certain specifications regarding the dose distribution.

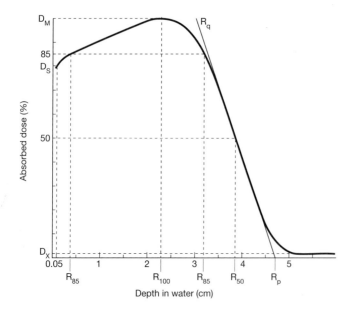

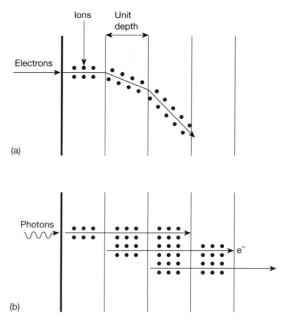

Fig. 5 Therapeutic depth–dose distribution with definitions of all parameters used in the text: D_M, level of maximum absorbed dose; D_s, surface dose measured at 0.5 mm depth; D_x, photon background; R_{100}, depth of dose maximum; R_{85}, therapeutic range; R_{50}, half-value depth; R_p, practical range.

Fig. 6 Schematic illustration of the build-up of absorbed dose at air–tissue interfaces. (a) Electron beam. The electrons traverse an increasing path length through each 'slice' with depth owing to scattering. The dose maximum is obtained when this is just balanced by loss of electrons due to absorption. The build-up of delta rays is not considered in the figure as this has a very small effect. (b) Photon beam. The number of electrons generated in each 'slice' at small photon depths is fairly constant. Therefore, the dose maximum is obtained at a depth corresponding to the range of the generated electrons. (In practice these electrons have different angles and energies and non-uniform energy deposition).

Figure 5 shows some parameters of special importance for electron beams. The skin (or surface) dose measured at 0.5 mm depth is generally approximately 80 per cent between 5 and 10 MeV (SSD = 1 m). It increases with energy and is approximately 90 per cent at energies over 20 MeV, but could be higher or lower depending on construction of the treatment head. The build-up is mainly due to the fact that electrons are travelling almost perpendicular to the phantom surface at small depths. At larger depths the mean deviation of the electrons from this direction will increase due to scattering in the phantom (patient), as indicated in Fig. 6. Therefore, the path length of the electrons through a traversing depth interval will increase with the depth, giving higher doses in each interval. A broad angular distribution at the skin surface, for instance owing to electron scattering in the collimator, will reduce this build-up.

The electron modality is frequently used in order to cover a depth interval from the near-skin region to a certain depth (the therapeutic range) with a uniform dose. A rapid fall-off of the depth dose is then desired. The therapeutic range is often taken as the depth of the 85 per cent isodose line. The therapeutic range R_{85} increases with the beam energy. However, very different values of R_{85} are obtained for accelerators with the same nominal energy. For instance with some accelerators having a very 'clean' electron beam (narrow energy and angular distribution) $R_{85} = 7$ cm is obtained with 22 MeV while 40 MeV is needed to obtain this R_{85} value with other accelerators.

The half-value depth R_{50} and the practical range R_p, as defined in Fig. 5, are related to the mean energy $\bar{E}_0$ and the most probable energy $E_{p,0}$ respectively of the electrons at the phantom surface. These energies are needed for dosimetry. In addition, it is general practice to specify the beam in a radiotherapy procedure by $E_{p,0}$. ($E_{p,0}$ is generally 1 MeV or a few MeV larger than $\bar{E}_0$). It is often sufficient

to estimate the energy in MeV at the phantom surface (or more correctly $E_{p,0}$) by multiplying the value of R_p in cmH_2O with a factor of 2.

The relative X-ray background D_x for electron beams is often a few per cent. The bremsstrahlung component is partly generated by electrons in the patient (or phantom) and partly due to contaminating X-rays from the accelerator (for example generated in scattering foils). The relative contribution of X-rays increases with electron energy but varies considerably for different accelerators. There will also be a bremsstrahlung component below heavy metal shields. A contamination of up to 7 to 9 per cent is obtained with some accelerators. This contamination is generally a minor problem in clinical practice, but could be of great significance in whole-body radiation of the skin where electron beams from several directions are used. The electrons will deposit their energy only in the superficial layer of malignant tissue but at greater depths a considerable dose will be given to healthy tissue because the X-rays are very penetrating.

Electrons have a very high probability of experiencing nuclear 'elastic' scattering. The electron scattering angles for a number of tissues and phantom materials have been tabulated as a function of the energy.[17] The scattering angle increases rapidly with the atomic number and with decreasing electron energy; that is, the values are higher for skeleton–cortical bone than for muscle and much higher for electrons of 5 MeV than for those of 20 MeV. The differences in the atomic numbers and densities of various tissues and cavities in a

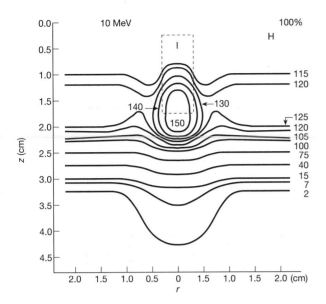

Fig. 7 Isodose diagram showing the effect of an air cavity I in a homogeneous tissue-equivalent material H. The irradiation was in the vertical direction with 10 MeV electrons. The normalization to 100 per cent was made at the phantom surface and not at dose maximum as is usually done. The hot spot behind the cavity and the cold spot at the side of the cavity should be noted. (Reproduced from Abou-Mandour and Harder (1978), with permission).[18]

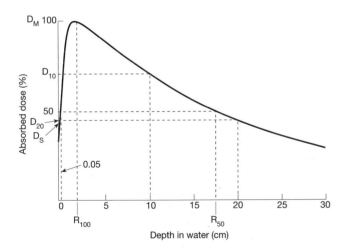

Fig. 8 Central axis depth–dose curve for a typical 10 MeV photon beam with definitions of all the parameters used in the text: D_M, maximum absorbed dose; D_s, surface dose measured at a depth of 0.5 mm; R_{100}, depth of dose maximum; R_{50}, half-value depth.

patient given an imbalance of in- and out-scattering which influences the dose distribution, particularly at low electron energies. In clinical practice, this could result in serious under- or overdosages close to a bone or air cavity (Fig. 7).

Figure 8 shows some parameters of special importance for photon beams. In this case, the build-up is due to the successive build-up of electrons in the phantom from photon interactions (see Fig. 6). The full build-up will be achieved at a depth approximately corresponding to the mean range of the electrons produced by the photons. Electrons generated in material outside the phantom, such as the air, collimator, and the beam-flattening filter, increase the surface dose. This contribution generally increases with the beam size. Therefore, the surface dose is dependent on the construction of the treatment head. In a typical accelerator air provides the greatest contribution up to approximately 10 MV, while the flattening filter is of greatest importance at higher energies. The shielding block holder (tray) and other material close to the patient may destroy the build-up. The depth of the dose maximum R_{100} is for a 10 cm × 10 cm field size and SSD = 100 cm is approximately 0.5 cm for ^{60}Co gamma rays, and increases from approximately 1.0 to 5.0 cm from 4 to 35 MV.[19] The R_{100} value is reduced if the incident beam is contaminated by electrons.

The depth of the 50 per cent depth dose R_{50} is sometimes used to describe the beam quality. R_{50} is approximately 12 cm for ^{60}Co gamma-ray beams (10 cm × 10 cm, SSD = 100 cm) and increases from approximately 13.5 cm to 26 cm between 4 and 45 MV.

Treatment planning

General remarks

Treatment planning is generally considered to be the series of procedures that begins after the diagnostic information has resulted in a decision to treat the patient with radiotherapy. The main steps in the treatment planning process are the acquisition of patient data, the definition of the target volume, the dose calculation for a particular beam arrangement, and the treatment simulation. For relatively simple treatment techniques, for example equally weighted anterior–posterior fields, manual planning is, and will be, used in a number of institutions. If the patient contour shows no large variation and if the target volume and critical organs have no strong curvatures, standard dose distributions can be used in combination with a hand calculation of the dose at the dose specification point as defined in ICRU Report 50.[20] Such a procedure yields adequate information in the central plane. For more complicated treatment techniques and/or if patient data have a more complex shape, computerized treatment planning is a prerequisite.

The computer is mainly used for two purposes: imaging and dose calculation. The imaging part is used for representation of patient data, including the delineation of the target volume and critical organs, and for representation of the results of the dose calculation. Treatment plans are generally presented in one plane but the rapid development of computer hard- and software makes it now possible to display three-dimensional relationships between isodose surfaces and anatomical structures. Special techniques have been developed for the viewing of a number of sections through the body of the patient simultaneously. Several computer graphics techniques, such as surface rendering of target volume and internal anatomy, shaded graphics, illumination from virtual light sources, highlighting of areas covered by the fields and colour-wash dose display, are implemented in commercial three-dimensional treatment planning systems. Beam's eye-view, BEV, is another type of display, showing anatomic and contour information from the point of view of the source (Fig. 9). BEV is extremely useful in selecting the most appropriate beam directions and position of shielding blocks, that is the maximum

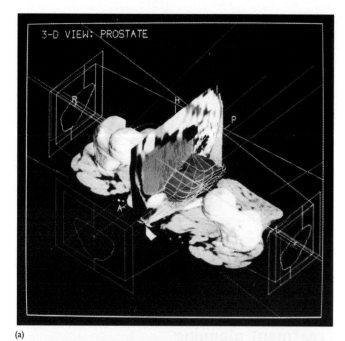

Fig. 9 (a)(b) Shape of beam defined by beam's eye view.

must find a solution for the two constraints: calculation accuracy and calculation time. Different solutions are possible. For instance a fast mode of an algorithm can be obtained by increasing the grid size. Once the beam directions, beam weights, and wedges have been chosen, the final dose calculation can be performed with a reduced grid size. Another aspect determining the time required for treatment planning is the co-operation between planning radiographer, physicist, and radiotherapist. The drawing of the target area and other regions of interest in different slices is a time consuming task and should be well integrated in the treatment planning process.

Evaluation and optimization of two-dimensional treatment plans is not a simple task. Both visual and mathematical procedures can be used while more recently the incorporation of radiobiological modelling for optimization purposes has been proposed.[21]–[23] Physical optimization considers only physical quantities, such as dose and volume, while biological optimization applies biological models, such as tumour control probability (TCP) and normal tissue complication probability (NTCP), to predict the treatment outcome. Current clinical experience is almost completely based on physical dose optimization. Only recently have several groups started to apply biological models to describe clinical results. A simple way to describe the final result is the use of P+, the probability of uncomplicated tumour control, as introduced by Brahme and colleagues. When the TCP and NTCP are statistically independent, P+ is equal to: TCP (1–NTCP). This approach has, however, to be considered carefully if other severe complications and/or inhomogeneous dose distributions are involved.

Dose–volume histograms provide a complete summary of the entire three-dimensional dose distribution. There are two types of dose–volume histograms—differential and integral—which both give the fractional volume as a function of either the dose or up to a specific dose value, respectively (Fig. 10). These dose–volume histograms can be used to compare rival treatment plans by ranking and improving them using physical and biological optimization methods. All evaluation or optimization models should be based on clinical data, particularly with respect to the dose–volume effect. The relationship between tumour control and normal tissue response on one hand and the inhomogeneous dose distribution on the other is, therefore, an important area for future research.

Accuracy of external photon beam dose calculations

As discussed in the section on dosimetric and geometric uncertainties, criteria for the accuracy of the dose calculation at relevant points in a patient relative to that at the reference point in a phantom can be formulated from the overall dose accuracy requirements. Uncertainties of 2 and 3 per cent, excluding the effect of heterogeneities, have been reported.[24],[25] In regions involving steep dose gradients, a requirement in the position of isodose lines is a better criterion. Values of 2 mm and 3 mm are recommended and even more severe constraints have been proposed by other authors.[24],[25]

Basically there are two different approaches to testing the accuracy of computer planning systems. Most commonly, the dose calculations of the treatment planning system are compared with measurements. Another approach is to compare the results of the treatment planning system with more sophisticated dose calculation procedures using first principles, for example Monte Carlo methods. The latter procedure is

separation between target volume and organs at risk. A BEV approach should, however, always be accompanied by a dose calculation for final judgement.

Dose calculation algorithms differ greatly with respect to their accuracy, speed, need for input data, and possibility to perform three-dimensional calculations. The continuous development of two-dimensional dose calculation algorithms resulted in a high degree of sophistication both with respect to accuracy and to interactivity, for dose calculations in the central plane in a large number of clinical situations. Nevertheless, there still exists a number of problem areas, even in two-dimensional dose calculations. Although approximate two-dimensional dose calculations in other planes are possible, these algorithms usually cannot be applied for accurate three-dimensional dose calculations. Three-dimensional treatment planning systems

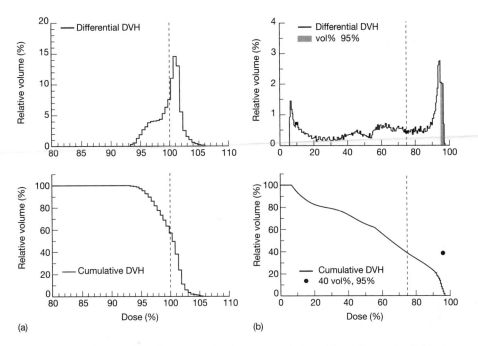

Fig. 10 Differential and integral (cumulative) dose–volume histograms of a planning target volume (a) and the rectal wall (b) of a treatment of a prostate cancer.

only applied if measurements are difficult to perform, for example in the region of lack of electronic equilibrium. Measurements can be compared with dose calculations from the treatment planning system using a standard set of measured beam data. Extensive tests of this kind have been performed by German and French physicists.[26],[27] This method avoids the necessity of making measurements by the user of the test program. It does require, however, the introduction of basic beam data in the system which is not directly of relevance for the clinic. For that reason tests based on a comparison of local beam data and local computer facilities have been performed by Dutch physicists.[28] These studies showed that the accuracy of dose calculation algorithms was quite acceptable for most treatment planning systems for a number of clinically-relevant situations. Outside the central part of the target volume and outside the central plane, there are, however, several situations where dose calculations are imperfect. Some of these problem areas will now be discussed in more detail.

Most algorithms have difficulties in predicting the dose at interfaces between materials having different density, that is where lack of electron equilibrium exists. The build-up region at air–tissue interfaces is such a region. Most dose calculations in treatment planning systems cannot be trusted in such a build-up region. This situation not only exists at the skin but also during the irradiation of small air cavities with small fields, for example for treatment of the larynx.[29],[30] Particularly if high photon energies are applied, a second dose build-up occurs in the tissue behind the air cavity due to lack of lateral electron equilibrium in the cavity (Fig. 11).

Most commercial treatment planning systems are unable to predict the effect on the dose distribution scattered back of electron from high atomic number materials irradiated by photon beams. These interfaces are created by metallic prostheses and dental materials in teeth inside the body as well as the skin and by the presence of

metallic surfaces at the beam exit side of the patient. The magnitude of this backscatter dose is a function of the photon beam energy, atomic number of the metal, and other factors such as distance to the tissue–metal interface. The increase in dose is 40 per cent or more (see Fig. 12) but the range of the backscattered electrons is small; about 2 mm of tissue (or polystyrene) is sufficient to absorb most of these electrons.

An important aspect of three-dimensional dose calculation algorithms is their ability to provide accurate dose estimates in non-central planes. A typical example where reliable dose calculations in off-axis planes are desirable is the treatment of breast cancer. In most two-dimensional systems deviations can be expected because the algorithms do not take the lack of scatter into account whereas more advanced, three-dimensional algorithms might yield better results. Accurate dose calculation is of utmost importance if the dose will be specified in an off-axis plane. Other areas where treatment planning in off-axis planes is particularly important is in the head and neck region, for mantle fields, and at the matchline of adjacent fields. Also during dose escalation studies using conformal therapy techniques, accurate knowledge of the 95 per cent isodose surface is required.

Tissue inhomogeneities will modify dose distributions obtained for homogeneous tissue (water) situations. The dose due to primary photons can usually be predicted in a relatively simple way but the dose due to scattered radiation is, however, modified in a less predictable way. Most commercial treatment planning systems apply relatively simple algorithms such as the effective attenuation method, the tissue–air ratio (TAR) method, or the power-law TAR method. These methods take only partly the scattered radiation component into account and therefore only give acceptable results under specific conditions. For instance if part of the lung is situated in the tangential field of breast irradiation, any of these simple algorithms gives satisfactory results and should be applied. On the other hand, it has

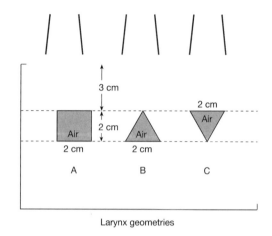

Larynx geometries

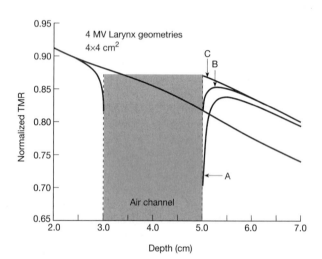

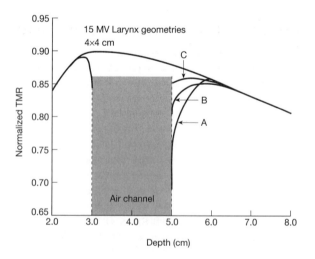

Fig. 11 Tissue–maximum ratio, TMR, measured in the presence and absence of air cavities of different dimensions representing larynx geometries for 4 MV and 15 MV X-rays (from Klein et al., 1993).[30]

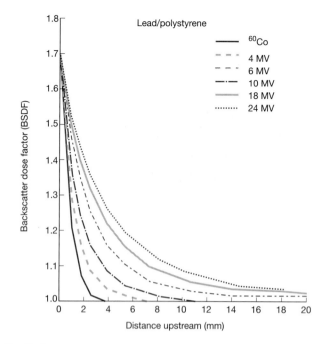

Fig. 12 Backscatter as a function of the distance upstream from a lead/polystyrene interface for different photon beam energies (from Das and Khan, 1989).[31]

been shown that these simple algorithms introduce large errors if applied for lung dose calculations during total body irradiation.[32] For moderate field sizes these lung dose correction factors are not very accurate but always give dose values more close to the actual dose than by not applying such a correction. For small field sizes the lack of lateral electron equilibrium causes a considerably lower dose than predicted by any of these algorithms, particularly at higher photon energies (Fig. 13). It is therefore advisable to omit lung dose corrections under these circumstances. Separation of primary and scattered radiation makes it possible, in principle, to take the scattered component into account in a more accurate way. Several of these more sophisticated inhomogeneity correction methods, as discussed in ICRU Report 42,[24] yield good results. A disadvantage of these algorithms is that they are quite slow in commercial treatment planning systems and need additional input data for the planning system (e.g. depth dose data for small field sizes). The question of electron equilibrium is also not addressed in these methods, thus giving the same discrepancies in build-up regions as the more simple algorithms.

Besides lung and air cavities, other inhomogeneities such as bone, fat, and metallic prostheses will influence the dose distribution. The errors made when no correction is applied for bone and fat is a function of the tissue thickness and photon beam energy: the higher the energy the smaller the error.[34] An error of several (2 to 5) per cent is made in the dose determination in the target volume if these tissues are assumed to be water like. The shadowing effect downstream of metallic hip prostheses can be quite substantial. An attenuation of as much as 50 per cent can be found under the prosthesis depending on the size and if it has either a hollow or solid femoral head. It is therefore recommended to avoid to irradiate the prosthesis; this is also because the interface dose would be high (Fig. 12).

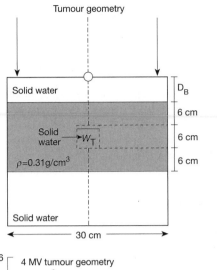

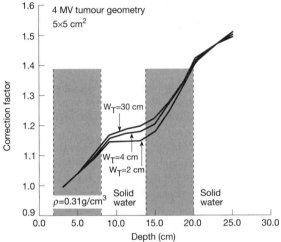

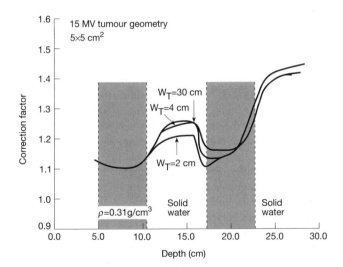

Fig. 13 Lung dose correction factor for 4 MV and 15 MV X-rays for a 5 × 5 cm² field as a function of depth below the surface of the phantom. The solid water area in the middle of the lung represents a tumour having different widths (from Rice *et al.*, 1988).[33]

If irradiation is unavoidable, information about the type and dimensions of the prosthesis, for instance obtained with a portal image to determine if it is hollow or solid, should be introduced in the treatment planning system for the determination of the inhomogeneity correction.

The determination of the absolute dose, that is the computation of the number of monitor units, is performed in some treatment planning systems by the system itself. In other systems this has to be done by the user, which requires another program with additional data including output factors, tray factors, wedge factors, and depth dose data for non-reference circumstances. This computation of the number of monitor units may introduce additional uncertainties if, for instance, the field size or depth dependence of wedge factors is not taken into account. Also, the calculation of monitor units for blocked fields is, in most planning systems, too simple. For accurate calculations it is necessary to separate the head scatter and phantom scatter components of the total dose. Using the same field size for both components may introduce considerable errors for some types of accelerators where the head scatter component is quite large. A similar, but usually smaller, problem exists for the presence of the tray on which the blocks are positioned. The dose reduction will be a function of the distance from the tray to the patient, whereas the skin dose will also strongly be influenced by the distance, field size, and beam energy. In a recent ESTRO booklet, a formalism has been presented for monitor unit calculations for simple geometries which takes a number of these effects into account.[35]

Finally, it has to be stressed that the dose specification procedure should be unambiguous and preferably follow the recommendations given in ICRU Report 50.[20] Any treatment protocol or publication of treatment results should not only report the dose at the dose specification point but also provide information on the treatment technique, the radiation quality, beam weighting, and corrections for heterogeneity.

Quality assurance of treatment planning systems

Although the need for quality assurance of planning systems is generally recognized, as elucidated more extensively in the section on Quality assurance below, and each institution performs a set of tests of its own planning system, it is only recently that extensive sets of recommendations have been formulated.[36],[37] In earlier decades, the scope of the decisions made with the treatment planning system mainly involved the dose calculation in one or a few planes. Now, however, with full three-dimensional planning available in many centres, there has been a huge increase in magnitude and complexity of treatment planning decisions, based on information from the treatment planning system. According to the American Association of Physicists in Medicine Task Group 53 Report[37] quality assurance of modern treatment planning systems should therefore include:

- quality assurance of the whole system including its software, procedures, and training;

- testing, documentation, and characterization of non-dosimetric aspects of planning;

- measurement, testing, and verification of the dosimetric aspects of the planning system;

- quality assurance of the clinical use of the system throughout the entire treatment planning process.

The main error sources of treatment planning systems are related to: (1) beam data acquisition and reconstruction; (2) patient data acquisition and representation; (3) algorithms for the dose computation and representation; and (4) hardware components. Quality control of these procedures will be discussed briefly.

1. First of all, accurate basic beam data (the beam data library) should be introduced in the system. Differences in the construction of the flattening filter and scattering foil, instability of the radiation beam, and energy variation over the field will result in different dose distributions for treatment machines having the same nominal energy. Regular comparison of measured dose distributions (depth dose data and dose profiles) with the basic beam data present in the treatment planning system is therefore necessary.[26],[38]

2. Special tests are required to check the accuracy in reproducing the geometric sizes of patient contours, as well as tissue density. Because CT data are usually transferred directly to the treatment planning system, it is necessary to check CT data first using a test phantom with well known values for contours and densities. In this way incorrect choice of window level and width and in the magnification factor can be discovered. Also, manual patient data input procedures (e.g. digitizing measured contours) need to be checked.

3. If dose calculation algorithms are tested, any deviation introduced by the basic beam data should first be established. A distinction should then be made between the accuracy of the dose calculation algorithm itself and the way the algorithm is implemented in the system. Any programming error should, in principle, be discovered by the manufacturer of the software but the testing of the program in a clinical environment might reveal unexpected errors. A number of tests is therefore required with different levels of complexity: single beams with varying dimensions, single beams with beam modifying devices, oblique incidence, body curvature, and inhomogeneities and multiple stationary and moving beams. The latter test procedure should be based on a set of treatment plans that are used frequently in the clinic. These checks should be carried out at regular intervals, after each new release of the software, or after modification of the hardware. Also, if a new set of data is added to the system the whole series of tests should be repeated because errors might be introduced at unexpected places.

4. Functional tests of all hardware components (central processing unit, printer, plotter, digitizer) should be performed. For this purpose test packages or special instructions in accompanying documentation should be provided by the companies. The accuracy of the input/output devices can be checked, for instance by entering a figure with particular dimensions or a body cross section and comparing the image displayed at the screen and the hard copy obtained from the plotter with the original drawing.

Finally, it should be noted that with the introduction of three-dimensional planning systems, quality control of hardware and software of these systems has become an increasingly important task. The development of checks to test both the geometric and dosimetric accuracy of three-dimensional systems is still at an early stage.

Special treatment techniques

Introduction

Conventional treatment with existing teletherapy equipment applies rectangular radiation fields with lengths varying between about 3 and 40 cm, source–skin distances varying between about 60 and 150 cm, and a limited number of beam shapes and directions. Currently available equipment and treatment planning systems have been designed for these purposes and can handle these situations often in a satisfying way although areas of concern still exist. There are, however, clinical situations that require more extreme values of field size and source–skin distance. For instance very small tumours can be treated with a number of small beams of diameter smaller than 3 cm (stereotactic radiosurgery). For total body irradiation (TBI), on the other hand, very large field sizes are needed. TBI often requires large source–skin distances, up to 5 m, whereas intraoperative radiotherapy (IORT) is generally applied at a distance to the target as short as possible.

Beam shaping is usually performed by positioning metal blocks in the beam. The heavy weight of these blocks and the labour intensive procedure makes the use of a multileaf collimator for this purpose very attractive (see section on Multileaf collimators, below). Improved dose distribution can sometimes also be obtained by applying beams with varying intensity over the field, and specific beam directions. The use of these unconventional field shaping techniques and beam directions require special dose calculation methods and quality assurance procedures. For these unconventional circumstances, special precautions have to be taken and the radiation physics aspects of these special treatment techniques will be discussed in this section.

Total body irradiation

The special problems in TBI can be summarized as follows: how can the patient be fitted in the treatment field, how can an adequate dose distribution be obtained over the whole body, and how can the dose to organs at risk be kept below tolerance levels? The solution to the first problem depends on the local circumstances (space and type of treatment facility available for TBI) and a large variety in methods of TBI exist (Fig. 14).[32] Dedicated units may consist of multiple sources, a sweeping beam, a moving couch, or a modified collimator. More often, however, existing teletherapy equipment is used for TBI which requires a solution for the local geometric constraints, that is the positioning of the patient in a treatment field of limited size and non-flat beam profiles. Usually anteroposterior treatments (AP-PA), lateral treatments, or a combination of both is employed to obtain a uniform dose distribution.

The factors that influence the dose distribution under TBI conditions are basically the same as those under conventional treatment conditions. Dose uniformity improves for higher photon energies (excluding the build-up region), smaller patient diameter, and larger treatment distance. If a maximum dose variation of 10 per cent is allowed, AP-PA treatments can be performed with most photon beams, even ^{60}Co gamma rays if large distances are applied. The use of lateral opposed fields for adults requires, however, at least 8 MV photon beams at large distances to get the same homogeneity. Due to variation in patient thickness, higher doses occur in thin body areas: the extremities and the neck. Tissue-equivalent bolus and simple one-dimensional compensators are, therefore, often used to

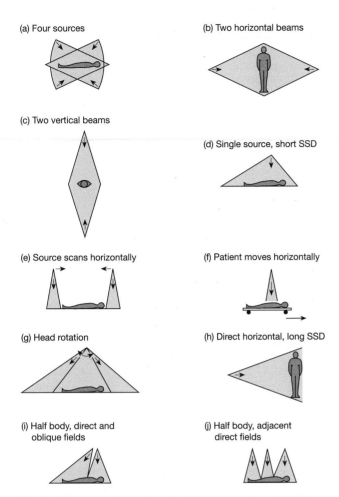

(a) Four sources

(b) Two horizontal beams

(c) Two vertical beams

(d) Single source, short SSD

(e) Source scans horizontally

(f) Patient moves horizontally

(g) Head rotation

(h) Direct horizontal, long SSD

(i) Half body, direct and oblique fields

(j) Half body, adjacent direct fields

Fig. 14 Different methods of total body irradiation. (From AAPM Report 17.)[32]

to select one of the algorithms for inhomogeneity correction (see section on Accuracy of external photon beam dose calculations, below). Due to its lower density, the lung dose will be higher than the prescribed TBI dose. Hence, if the lung dose is to be reduced by 15 to 20 per cent, shielding blocks or lung compensators have to be applied. This can be done by positioning standard shielding blocks for a fraction of the total treatment time, or by placing customized thin sheets of lead or other lung compensator material during the whole treatment session. Sometimes the arms are used as lung attenuators in lateral fields. Positioning of the arms is, however, not very reproducible and it might therefore be better to position the arm in another way and to use other lung shields.

The limitations of the presently available treatment planning systems, the accuracy of the positioning of lung shielding blocks and tissue compensators, for example in the neck/shoulder region, and movement of the patient can alter the dose distribution drastically. For these reasons *in vivo* dosimetry measurements are often applied to get the actual dose delivered to a patient (see section on *In vivo* dosimetry, below).

The dose specification during TBI is basically identical to the procedure recommended in the ICRU Report 50.[20] The TBI dose is often specified at the midline of the level of the umbilicus. The inhomogeneity in the dose distribution over the whole target volume, that is the whole body, should be specified, for example within +5 per cent and −10 per cent. Also, the dose to the lung should be specified, for instance as the dose to more than half the lung volume. In addition to a short description of the irradiation technique, the dose rate should also be specified because pulmonary complications might be dose rate dependent.

Stereotactic radiotherapy

The treatment of small brain tumours by using extremely small radiation fields was described over 40 years ago,[39] but has only been applied in a limited number of other institutions. By using a stereotactic frame, the target volume can be irradiated with small beams of photons with an accuracy of the order of 1 mm. This technique, which is called stereotactic radiosurgery if it is delivered in one fraction or stereotactic radiotherapy if given in a fractionated way, offers selected patients, mainly with brain tumours and arteriovenous malformations, an alternative to conventional surgery.

Two different approaches are possible to deliver the radiation to the target volume. The first procedure is a static method which consists of the delivery of a high radiation dose to a relatively small target volume by simultaneous treatment with a large number of ^{60}Co gamma-ray beams. Figure 15 shows this so called 'gamma knife', which consists of 201 hemispherically arrayed ^{60}Co sources. By blocking selected collimator openings, using different collimator helmets, and applying different exposure times, it is possible to optimize the dose distribution. The other, dynamic, procedure consists of the use of multiple arc therapy from a linear accelerator equipped with special collimators.[40] A stereotactic frame is used for localization of the target via CT or MRI. During treatment the patient's head is positioned and immobilized either on the radiotherapy couch or independently of the radiotherapy couch on a special stand. The entire system is then verified to check if the set up and alignment is correct to treat a specific target. This can be done by special devices or an

compensate for contour variation. The use of bolus has the advantage that the skin dose is high. It should be noted, however, that for these large TBI fields the surface dose is already much higher than for the conventional field sizes. Perspex sheets in front of the patient are sometimes applied to increase the skin dose even more.

The actual dose distribution in a patient treated in a large field is, in addition, determined by the variation in beam intensity and beam energy over the beam profile. Knowledge of these quantities is required to make reliable relative dose calculations in points outside the central plane. Most commercial two-dimensional treatment planning systems do not possess the capabilities to take these variations into account and are therefore not suitable for calculating dose distributions under TBI conditions. Another effect generally not fully considered in conventional treatment planning systems is the lack of lateral scatter in patients that are smaller than the dimensions of the beam. Experimental determination of the complex dose distribution characteristics of TBI techniques in human-shaped phantoms is therefore often applied.

Accurate knowledge of the dose to the lungs is very important during TBI because the dose–effect curves for lung damage are quite steep. Lung doses can be evaluated using measurements in heterogeneous phantom configurations. These data can then be used

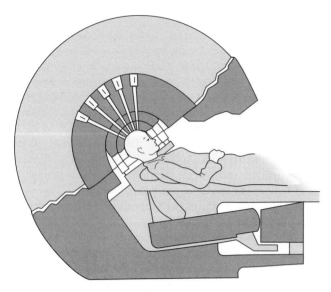

Fig. 15 The 'gamma knife'. The interchangeable collimator helmet is attached to the sliding bed. During treatment this helmet is linked with the stationary helmet in the shield for precise collimation of the gamma-ray beams to the target.

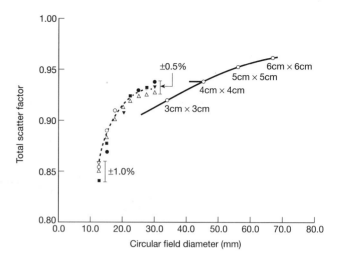

Fig. 16 Total scatter factor, that is the output at the depth of dose maximum relative to that of a 10 cm × 10 cm field, as a function of field size for small 6 MV X-ray beams defined by circular auxiliary collimators and square fields defined by the movable jaws. The different symbols indicate data obtained with ionization chambers of different sizes and LiF ribbons (from Rice *et al.*, 1987).[41]

anthropomorphic phantom in combination with film. Such a simulation is a prerequisite for this type of treatment because the mechanical tolerances of the gantry and the treatment couch may have a large influence on the actual dose distribution.

Dose distributions produced by these small beams are more difficult to measure than those delivered by conventional photon beams. First, large dose gradients are present thus requiring small detectors. Secondly, the lack of lateral electron equilibrium complicates the interpretation of the measured value because the detector has a finite size. Good agreement was obtained in off-axis ratios measured with thermoluminescence dosimetry, photographic film, and a small, 3.5 mm diameter ionization chamber.[41] By using a brass build-up cap, in-air measurements can be used to determine the collimator scatter as a function of field size. The measurements in the phantom yield the total phantom plus collimator scatter (Fig. 16).

These data show a strong dependence of the output on field size due to the lack of lateral equilibrium, which is of particular importance for very small field sizes and high photon energies. Another phenomenon resulting from this lack of electron equilibrium is the shift in the depth of dose maximum to the surface of the phantom for smaller field sizes.

The execution of small field radiotherapy requires a very careful delineation of the target volume, design of the treatment parameters, and quality control of the whole procedure. Stereotactic radiosurgery can therefore only be performed in a reliable way if close co-operation exists between neurosurgeons, radiotherapists, and radiation physicists.

Intraoperative radiotherapy

Intraoperative radiotherapy (IORT) is a specialized radiation technique for treating deeply situated cancers with large, single doses while avoiding irradiation of normal tissues. IORT is now employed alone or given as a boost to a course of fractionated external beam

therapy. IORT is not a new idea. It has been, and still is, applied with orthovoltage X-rays. However, interest in IORT has been renewed since electron beam radiation has been used, thus reducing the dose to healthy organs at the distal part of the target volume. After the pioneer work of Japanese investigators,[42] a number of institutions started to develop the technique. In some institutions, dedicated linear accelerators have been installed in an operating room for IORT use only. A review of the technical aspects and clinical results can be found elsewhere.[43]

One of the major problems with IORT is the exact positioning of the electron beam collimator with respect to the target volume. These cones not only define the treatment field but also serve to retract healthy organs outside the beam. Important practical aspects are the weight of these applicators and the visibility of the irradiated region when they are positioned. Although collimating systems are now commercially available, most institutions developed their own solution suitable for their specific situation. Generally, perspex cones are used, having a large variety of shapes, dimensions, and docking devices. The docking procedure is an important part of the IORT treatment because it should be easily performed in an operating room and have a good reproducibility. If, for instance, the gantry angle would deviate more than 2° from the intended angle, then unacceptable dose distributions might result. Before IORT is applied it is therefore necessary that there is a thorough understanding of the different factors influencing the dose distribution within the target volume and in the surrounding healthy tissues.

The primary electron beam characteristics, as valid for normal electron beam treatment, will be different for IORT due to possible modifications of the scattering-foil system, jaw settings of the X-ray collimators, and the presence of the cone. These changes will result in variations of the surface dose, field flatness, depth–dose curve, bremsstrahlung tail, and absolute output.[44] Due to the scatter of electrons against the collimator wall, high-dose regions may occur at

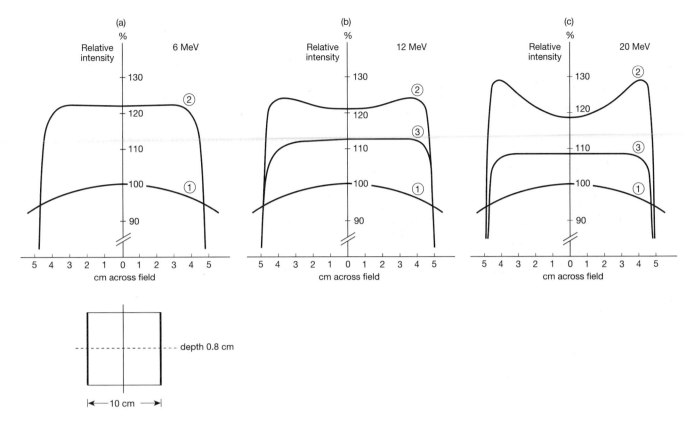

Fig. 17 Beam profiles at 0.8 cm depth of 6, 12, and 20 MeV electron beams, measured along the dashed line in the diagram. (1) Plain beam profile. (2) Profile with two applicator walls. (3) Profile with field defining frame. (From van der Laarse *et al.*, 1978).[45]

the edges of the field (Fig. 17). Customized shielding of part of the field by lead cut-outs or low melting point alloys is therefore applied. Special dose calculation programs, based on pencil beam algorithms, are available to determine the dose distribution as well as the output factor for these irregular field shapes. These programs can also be used to obtain the dose distribution for matching fields if more than one field is required to cover the entire target volume.

Dose distributions are generally known for specific beam directions and distances between the cone and the target volume. If variations in these parameters occur, for instance due to breathing, corrections in the dose calculation have to be applied. Air gap corrections as well as corrections for inhomogeneities such as lung and bone must be implemented in these dose calculation programs. These calculations should be verified with measurements for the situations encountered in clinical practice. It is, in addition, recommended to apply *in vivo* dosimetry during the actual IORT procedure to the patient.

Because a number of technical and physical, as well as biological and clinical, problems have to be solved, IORT is labour intensive. A wide range of specialized equipment and physics support, for example for dose calculations and measurements, is necessary. This technique therefore requires close collaboration of the surgeon, radiotherapist, and physicist.

Multileaf collimators

Beam shaping can be optimized by positioning standard lead blocks or customized low melting point alloys in the radiation field. In this

way conformation therapy can be performed using beam shapes either obtained from simple drawings on a simulator image or from CT images applying the beam's eye view projection (Fig. 9). A serious problem with these blocks is their heavy weight. The advent of high resolution multileaf collimators may largely eliminate the need for these blocks.

Several groups have studied the use of multileaf collimators as discussed, for instance, by Brahme.[46] The early devices consisted of a limited number of parallel-opposed adjustable rods where the leaf motion is linear, that is the beam divergency was not taken into account. More recent systems consist of double focused leaves thus giving a smaller penumbra, particularly for larger fields. The resolution of the field shape is limited by the number of leaves, resulting in a stair-case shape of the isodose lines (Fig. 18). The stair-case structure is, however, considerably smoothed at the 90 per cent and 10 per cent isodose level. Leakage of radiation between the individual leaves is another technical problem which has to be solved in order to obtain a high performance from the collimator system. From a theoretical study of the optimal settings of a multileaf collimator for static fields, Brahme concluded that the best possible orientation of the collimator is, in general, when the direction of motion of the leaves is parallel with the direction in which the target volume has its shortest cross section.[46]

Another application of multileaf collimators is to vary the intensity of stationary photon beams over the radiation field. By using the multileaf collimator in such a dynamic mode, fairly complex dose distributions can be generated. The lack of electron or photon scatter

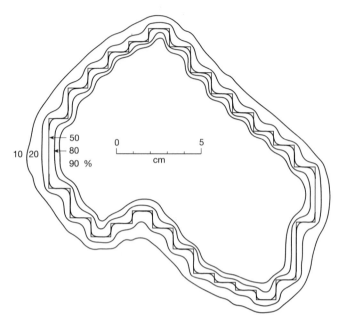

Fig. 18 Isodose distribution of a 20 MV X-ray beam at the depth of dose maximum. The field is defined by 26 leaves of a multileaf collimator (from Brahme, 1988).[46]

equilibrium near beam edges can, for instance, be compensated with this method by an increased incident fluence of primary photons. The exact movement of all the leaves can be calculated for a particular dose distribution from the elementary dose distribution of a single pair of leaves. This problem is related to the inverse treatment planning problem—which incident beams are required to produce the desired dose distribution in the target volume? The next, and even more complicated, problem is to combine dynamic multileaf collimators with moving beam therapy. It might take some time before the merits of such a method have been tested in clinical practice.

Quality assurance programmes

Introduction

Quality assurance is a concept generally applied in industry but was adapted and further developed for medical care. The aim of quality assurance is to guarantee the performance of a product or process within certain specifications. Quality control is the process of measurement and comparison with existing standards and the actions necessary to modify those parameters which are found lower than the accepted level of quality. Quality assurance has a more general meaning than quality control but both terms are sometimes also considered synonymous. Quality audit is a quality control or a review of the quality control system by an independent group of observers. These site reviews may identify a number of errors as has been observed, for instance, during dosimetry reviews.

The physical aspects of quality assurance programmes have been elucidated in a number of documents drafted by national and international organizations and at several symposia. The most important quality assurance programmes discussed in these reports are related to beam characteristics of treatment machines, to properties of simulators, CT scanners, and treatment planning systems, and to treatment verification procedures. Quality control programmes related to these subjects will be discussed in this section and in the section on Quality assurance of treatment planning systems, above.

Dosimetric and geometric uncertainties

Any quality control programme is related to the accuracy required for a particular application. It is obvious that not all types of radiotherapeutical treatment need the same level of accuracy. From a practical point of view it is, however, difficult to conceive several levels of accuracy in the same institution. Action levels should, therefore, be based on requirements for the treatments demanding the highest accuracy. However, the availability of resources (personnel for maintenance and quality control) and technical possibilities of the equipment (type and 'age') limit the accuracy that can be obtained with existing equipment.

There is an increasing amount of clinical evidence indicating that a high degree of accuracy in dose delivery is essential for the success of radiotherapy. This applies certainly for the dose level, but for the dose distribution (geometric accuracy) some clinical data are also available. As far as the dose level is concerned, a requirement for an accuracy of 3.5 per cent has been proposed (i.e. one standard deviation in the combined random and systematical uncertainty) in the dose value at the specification point or in the mean dose to the target volume.[25],[47] The latter authors discussed also extensively the effect of non-uniformity of the relative dose distribution on tumour control probability. From their considerations it can be concluded that for steep dose-effect curves, the actual dose distribution should be uniform within about ± 3 per cent. Combining this requirement for the relative dose distribution with the accuracy requirement for the dose delivery to the dose specification point, yields a dose accuracy requirement of about 5 per cent, one standard deviation, for other points in the target volume.

Information on the overall uncertainty in the actual dose delivery to the dose specification point has also been estimated by several groups.[25],[47] Although the details in these studies differ somewhat, an estimated overall uncertainty varying between about 4 per cent for photon beams and about 5 per cent for electron beams has been reported. The results of some dosimetry intercomparisons as presented as examples in Fig. 19 do suggest that the actual uncertainties are somewhat smaller. It should be noted, however, that the standard deviations observed in these studies, varying between 1.5 and 3 per cent, do not include the uncertainty in the absolute value of the physical parameters such as the stopping power. These dose intercomparisons were also performed with anthropomorphic phantoms. It can be expected that the uncertainty in the actual dose delivery to patients will be somewhat larger than those observed in these phantom studies.

These estimates of the overall uncertainty and the results of the dosimetry intercomparisons demonstrate that the 3.5 and 5 per cent accuracy requirements can only be realized for relatively simple treatment conditions. For more complicated treatment techniques higher uncertainties can be expected, particularly outside the central plane. Extensive quality control programmes of treatment machines,

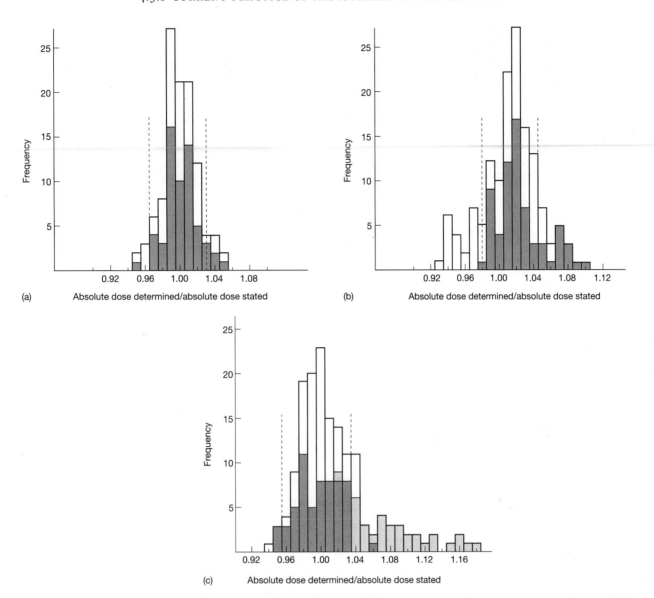

Fig. 19 Results of the EORTC dosimetry intercomparison (from Johansson *et al.*, 1986).[48] (a) The distribution of the ratio of determined to stated absorbed dose for ⁶⁰Co gamma-ray beams for different field sizes, beam modifiers, and depth for 20 machines. Lined bars represent square field sizes and the open bar beams with modifiers and rectangular field sizes. The vertical lines indicate the acceptable level of variation. (b) Distribution of the ratio of determined to stated absorbed dose for photon beams with qualities between 4 and 25 MV X-rays for different field sizes, beam modifiers, and depths for 24 accelerators. Lined bars represent accelerators with sealed monitor chambers and open bars unsealed monitor chambers. The vertical lines indicate the acceptable level of variation. (c) Distribution of the ratio of determined to stated absorbed dose for electron beams with qualities between 4 and 25 MeV at 15 accelerators. Open bars represent scattering foil machines. Lined bars represent scanning beam systems and dotted bars scanning beam systems without correction for recombination losses. The vertical lines indicate the acceptable level of variation.

dose calculation algorithms, and patient data are therefore required for these situations.

Only limited clinical information is available on the effect of random and systematic positioning errors on clinical outcome. These studies demonstrated a higher relapse rate in patients where shielding blocks had inadequate margins during their treatment, as revealed by portal film analysis. Theoretical considerations can also be used for estimating the effect of patient positioning errors on tumour control probability.[25] Formulating a requirement for the geometric accuracy from these clinical considerations is, however, a much more difficult problem than for the dose level. Estimates of the actual uncertainties

in beam set-up and patient set-up can also be considered. Figure 20 summarizes how these geometric uncertainties may interact.

Combining all the information, it seems reasonable to expect that the position of a field edge or shielding block with respect to the target volume should have an accuracy less than 5 mm, one standard deviation. Such a requirement is in line with the recommendations of the International Electrotechnical Commission (IEC) for the geometric tolerance of the radiation field, as discussed by Rassow.[50] It can be expected that the introduction of on-line portal imaging in the clinic will yield more quantitative information on the actual spatial uncertainty resulting from patient set-up, beam set-up, and

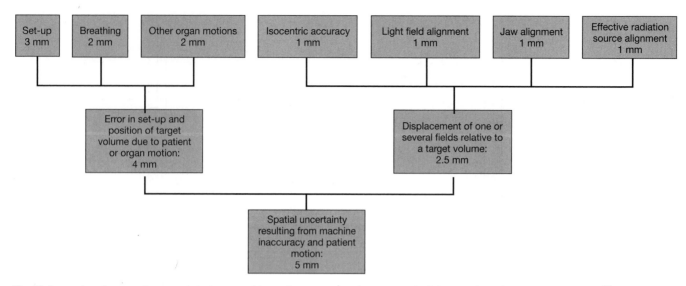

Fig. 20 Interaction of geometric uncertainties in external beam therapy expressed as one standard deviation (modified from AAPM, 1984).[49]

patient motion and may result in an improvement of the geometric accuracy.

Quality control of teletherapy equipment

After the installation of teletherapy equipment, a number of tests have to be performed to verify certain specifications of the machine's performance. These acceptance tests include mechanical tests, radiation beam tests, and radiation protection surveys. After the unit is accepted an extensive set of measurements have to be performed before the equipment can be placed in clinical service. These commissioning measurements are required for input to a treatment planning system and for tables used for different types of other calculations. Once the acceptance tests and commissioning measurements are completed and patient treatment has started, a quality control programme must be initiated. A quality control protocol should be available for each type of teletherapy equipment. It should specify the equipment and technique to be used, the frequency of these measurements, tolerance levels, and actions to be undertaken. Finally, it should state how all information is recorded. Table 2 gives, as an example, a summary of the type and frequency of tests that should be performed. These tests are required to check both the dosimetric and geometric properties of the beams.

The detailed specifications of such a quality control programme for teletherapy equipment will depend on the type of equipment, its clinical use, and the resources available. It is obvious that a large accelerator with many electron and photon energies used for co-operative clinical trials in an academic environment needs more quality control than a ⁶⁰Co unit used for simple treatments in a small hospital. A number of authors and organizations have formulated guidelines for quality control programmes.[25],[49],[51],[52] A comparison of these programmes shows that no single quality control programme can be proposed that is suitable for all radiotherapy centres in all countries. It is recommended that national organizations formulate minimal and ideal quality control programmes suitable for small and large radiotherapy centres, taking into account type of equipment, personnel, and funds available.

Table 2 Example of a quality control programme of teletherapy equipment

Daily
1. Output check at central axis
2. Beam alignment: light field size, position side lights (lasers) and position of isocentre
3. Check of mechanical and electrical safety systems, tests of machine parameter indicator lights and patient communication devices

Weekly
1. Dose calibration at central axis
2. Energy constancy
3. Field flatness/ symmetry
4. Light field—radiation field coincidence

Monthly
1. Monitor linearity and output at different gantry angles
2. Beam alignment at different gantry angles
3. Field flatness/ symmetry at different gantry angles
4. Wedge factors at different gantry angles
5. Energy at different gantry angles

Annually
1. Output for several field sizes
2. Depth dose characteristics for several field sizes
3. Treatment accessories

In order to perform quality control measurements, a large number of measurement techniques are available. These methods vary in sophistication, depending on the purpose of the measurement and the amount of time (and money) available. For instance for daily tests of beam alignment relatively simple devices can be used, such as a cubic box with a scale on it. Also the daily measurement of the radiation output of an accelerator can be performed with a straightforward technique. A block of plastic with a robust dosimeter, connected to a simple electrometer, is often employed. Such a relative

Table 3 Results of the dosimetry intercomparisons in the Nordic countries in 1971 and 1982; X is the percentage difference in the absorbed dose calibration by the local centre and the visiting team

Parameter[a]	^{60}Co γ rays		Low energy electrons		High energy electrons		High-energy X-rays	
	1971	1982	1971	1982	1971	1982	1971	1982
X	−0.4	−0.1	2.9	1.1	1.5	0.4	−0.6	−1.7
X_{max}	1.7	2.7	18	6	19	7	2.3	8
X_{min}	−1.5	−2.0	−6	−9	−7	−11	−13	−2
σ	1.0	1.4	8.1	2.7	8.7	3.4	5.9	2.3

[a] Mean, maximum positive and negative deviations, and standard deviations are given.[53]

output check should be related to an absolute dose determination using a calibrated ionization chamber under reference circumstances using a modern dosimetry protocol.

If the purpose of the measurement is not only to check the output but also other beam characteristics such as field flatness, beam symmetry, penumbral width, beam energy, and light field/ radiation field coincidence, then a number of devices are commercially available. Photographic film in combination with a scanning densitometer is frequently used for these tests. Such a scanning densitometer is often part of a sophisticated three-dimensional scanning system which is used for measuring and analysing beam data during the acceptance and commissioning tests and as part of the annual quality control programme. Also, photographic films can nowadays be digitized by means of a video camera after which computer analysis can be performed. Because it is very practical to have immediate information on these beam properties, other instruments have been developed that have an on-line response. Usually an array of a few, for instance five, ionization chambers or diodes is used for this purpose. More detailed profile measurements can be obtained with a linear array of a larger number of detectors (30 to 88 are nowadays commercially available). Regular calibration of all these devices is necessary to correct for changes in relative sensitivity of the detectors.

Quality control of the energy of the beam can be performed by checking the ratio of detector readings at two different depths in a phantom. Another approach, which can be used with an array of detectors, is the positioning of a wedge or a pair of wedges in the beam, which will change the beam profile as a function of beam energy. Such a system for quality control of the energy can be used both for X-ray and electron beams. Regular checks of the steering system of the accelerator also provides valuable information on the stability of the energy of the electrons accelerated in the machine.

It is important to note that these routine quality control measurements should be simple procedures which do not require much time. More extensive measurements using more sophisticated equipment are necessary after major repair of the equipment or at relatively long time periods.

Quality audit and dosimetry intercomparisons

In spite of a quality control programme it is possible that fairly large differences may occur between beam properties stated by the institution and those measured by a visiting team. An example is given in Table 3[53] showing that a large improvement occurred in

dosimetry in the Nordic countries in the period between the two intercomparisons. It should be noted, however, that considerable differences still existed in 1982, even between the stated dose values for different beam qualities within the same department.

Also in other countries, for example Belgium, France, Great Britain, the Netherlands, and Switzerland, dosimetry intercomparisons between radiotherapy institutions have been performed or are in progress. The distribution of the ratios of stated and measured dose values generally shows a Gaussian shape with an acceptable standard deviation (Fig. 19(a) and (b)). Such a small standard deviation was not only observed for photon beams under reference conditions (Fig. 19(b)) but also at the dose specification point for the irradiation of anthropomorphic phantoms.[38],[54],[55] This indicates that both the output determination of the accelerator and the dose calculation procedure using the treatment planning system did not introduce considerable errors, at least for relatively simple treatment techniques. In some situations, however, unacceptable discrepancies have been observed (Fig. 19 (c)). These large deviations occurred in centres having scanning electron beams without applying the appropriate correction procedure for the large recombination losses of ions produced in ionization chambers applied for the output determination. The dosimetry intercomparison performed by the Institute of Physical Sciences in Medicine (IPSM) in Great Britain revealed a considerable calibration error of a ^{60}Co.[55] Due to an arithmetic error, for 5 months patients had been receiving excess radiation doses of 25 per cent, which was discovered by the IPSM quality audit.

Quality audit is a prerequisite for institutions participating in interinstitutional clinical trials involving radiation therapy. In Europe, such activities have been performed by the EORTC Radiotherapy Group Quality Control Project. Some of the results obtained by Johansson et al.,[48] at the dosimetric part of the quality control carried out at 18 radiotherapy centres during the period 1982 to 1984, are presented in Fig. 19. The results show a larger spread for photon beams produced with accelerators compared to ^{60}Co gamma-ray beams and for electron beams compared to photon beams, particularly for accelerators having a scanning beam system. In the United States, the Radiological Physics Center (RPC) has performed this type of quality assurance since 1968, while the Radiation Therapy Oncology Group (RTOG) also reviews the validity of tumour dose statements for individual patients entering into multicentre clinical trials. It has been shown that the frequency of occurrence of protocol deviations for the accurate delivery of prescribed dose can be quite large.[56] Initial review of the plan of treatment resulted in a markedly improved level of data submitted in new protocol studies. The results of these quality audit programmes clearly demonstrate the importance of having a review of the quality control programme of teletherapy equipment by outside individuals.

In vivo dosimetry

There are many steps in the chain determining the dose delivery to a patient undergoing radiotherapy . Each of these steps may introduce an uncertainty. It is therefore worthwhile, and sometimes even necessary, to have an ultimate check of the actual treatment by using *in vivo* dosimetry. *In vivo* dose measurements can be divided into entrance dose measurements, exit dose measurements, and intracavity dose measurements.

Entrance dose measurements serve to check the output and performance of the treatment apparatus as well as the accuracy of patient set-up. Exit dose measurements serve, in addition, to check the dose calculation algorithm and to determine the influence of shape, size, and density variations of the body of the patient on the dose calculation procedure. Sometimes it is also possible to determine the intracavity dose in readily accessible body cavities such as the oral cavity, oesophagus, vagina, bladder, and rectum.

The two techniques that are most often used for *in vivo* dosimetry are thermoluminescence dosimetry and the use of silicon diodes. The advantages of thermoluminescence dosimeters are well known: their relatively small energy dependence (in the megavoltage energy range) and their small size without any cables to reading (or high voltage) equipment. Although there exists a vast amount of information on the theoretical aspects of thermoluminescence dosimetry, for example see Horowitz,[57] details about the practical aspects of the use of thermoluminescence dosimetry are scarce.[58]–[60] In order to obtain a high accuracy when using thermoluminescence dosimetry in the clinic, a number of tests are required as discussed in these reports. It is also important that each thermoluminescence dosimeter user should determine for her/his own thermoluminescence dosimetry material, read-out equipment, and anneal procedure the optimum procedure to obtain the highest accuracy and precision.

An important disadvantage of the use of thermoluminescence dosimetry is the delay between the irradiation and the result. For that reason silicon diodes are nowadays also applied in a number of institutions for *in vivo* dosimetry.[61] Due to the damage to the diode caused by irradiation, some properties will change with integrated dose. For this reason the calibration factor will, for instance, gradually change with time. Three basic physical properties of diodes are important for their clinical use: the energy dependence, the temperature dependence, and, for some diodes, the dose per pulse dependence of the sensitivity. In addition, the angular dependence and the distance between the diode and the patient's skin, particularly at the exit side, are important but give rise to negligible or small corrections if the diodes are positioned in the proper way. The energy and dose per pulse dependence do, however, require small correction factors for changes of the calibration factor with field size, SSD, patient thickness, and the presence of the wedge. Because not all diodes behave in a similar manner, even if they belong to the same badge, these correction factors have to be determined for each diode.

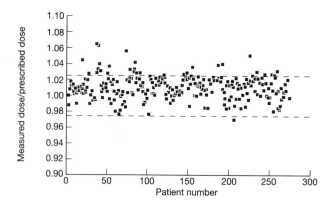

Fig. 21 Ratio of measured and prescribed dose at the dose specification point for treatment of prostate tumours. The action levels, $\pm$ 2.5 per cent, are indicated by dotted lines.

A very common use of *in vivo* dosimetry is the determination of the dose to a point in a patient outside the target volume. The dose to the eye, spinal cord, or rectum might be important if the target volume is situated close to these organs. Even if this distance is large, it is sometimes necessary to determine the dose delivered to the patient, for example the dose to the abdomen in case of treatment of a pregnant woman.

Most *in vivo* dosimetry measurements are, however, performed to check the dose to the target volume. The philosophy behind these measurements is, however, different. In order to check the overall accuracy, in a number of institutions, particularly in Scandinavian countries, entrance dose measurements using silicon diodes are performed at least once and sometimes more often, during each treatment series. Deviations larger than 3 per cent from the prescribed dose are considered to be meaningful for ^{60}Co gamma radiation whereas the corresponding figure for high-energy X-rays is 5 per cent. These action levels were chosen from an analysis of the observed discrepancies.

Another application of entrance dose measurements is the check of equipment performance. When an accelerator is, for particular reasons, not very stable, the difference between actual and intended dose values can be quite large. Entrance dose measurements will demonstrate these differences, which may occur under specific gantry angles while the routine output check, under zero degrees gantry angle, does not reveal any peculiarity.

The immediate availability of the dose value while the patient still is in treatment position, offers a possibility to trace directly the origin of a discrepancy between measured and intended dose. In this way inaccuracies of external contours and errors in patient set up, for example mistakes between isocentric and fixed SSD techniques, can be discovered and may result in modification of the treatment technique.[62]

By combining *in vivo* entrance and exit dose measurements with phantom measurements it is possible to separate the influence of machine performance, patient contour (and density), and inaccuracies of the dose calculation algorithms in the treatment planning system. In this way a number of small errors were discovered during an *in vivo* dosimetry programme of prostate cancer treatments using high dose–high precision techniques (Fig. 21).

An important application of *in vivo* dosimetry is during total body irradiation (TBI). In a similar way as under usual treatment conditions, the dose distribution varies as a function of a number of parameters such as beam energy, SSD, and patient diameter. However, most commercial treatment planning systems cannot calculate the dose under TBI conditions in a reliable manner. Consequently, it will be difficult to predict the actual dose delivered to the patient in the points of interest, for example to the lungs. Moreover, patient movement will influence the actual position of the patient under the sometimes special circumstances required for TBI (Fig. 14). It is therefore recommended to use *in vivo* dosimetry for determining the actual dose to the patient during TBI. In some institutions dosimeters are read out after part of the TBI treatment is given to the patient. The remaining dose is determined on the basis of the results of these *in vivo* dose measurements.

Portal imaging

Besides dosimetric errors, geometric errors are also of considerable importance in determining the outcome of a radiotherapeutic treatment. Once the target volume has been defined, patient positioning, beam arrangement, and field sizes have to be selected and confirmed. The geometric accuracy is limited by the uncertainties in a particular patient set-up, by uncertainties in the beam set-up, and can, in addition, be the result of movement of the patient, or more specifically, the target volume during the treatment. Patient set-up accuracy is mainly determined by the uncertainty in the position of external landmarks with respect to the target volume. A number of accessories are available to help the accurate and reproducible positioning of the patient, which should afterwards be checked at the simulator. If the patient is then transferred from the simulator to the treatment table, additional positioning errors of the patient with respect to the beam may occur. Regular inspection of patient alignment aids at both types of equipment is, therefore, important. Checks of beam alignment features such as isocentre indication, numerical field indication, and light field/ radiation field indication belong to the standard quality control programme of each institution (Table 2).

In order to verify the patient set-up with respect to the position of the radiation beam, portal imaging is often applied. By portal imaging the field placement during the actual treatment is checked relative to anatomical structures of the patient. Such a check is usually made at the beginning of the patient's treatment, repeated if the radiation fields are modified, and, in some centres, during the course of the treatment. Also, during the course of one treatment, it can be useful to have more than one check, for instance to observe the influence of swallowing and breathing on patient set-up.

At present, photographic films are commonly applied, but the quality of these images produced by high-energy photons is rather poor compared with conventional X-ray images. Several methods are available to optimize the quality of portal film images. In addition, portal film enhancement can be performed after digitizing the image, for example by means of a video camera, thus yielding a better visibility of relevant anatomical landmarks. Although portal film evaluation is usually performed on a light box, the techniques of digital portal image enhancement offer in principle the possibility to apply automated procedures to quantify differences between verification and simulation image.

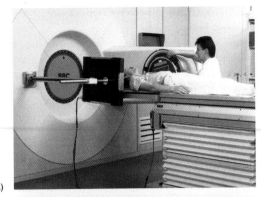

(a)

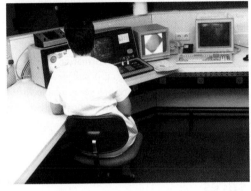

(b)

Fig. 22 (a) Portal imaging device mounted at the gantry of a linear accelerator for a lateral irradiation of the head. (b) Keyboard, control monitor, and image display monitor of the portal imaging device next to the operator's console at the accelerator.

Besides the poor quality of megavoltage X-ray films, another disadvantage of the film technique is its off-line character, which requires a certain amount of time before the result can be applied clinically. For this reason a number of groups have started the development of on-line portal imaging devices as recently reviewed by Boyer *et al.*[63] Three different approaches are now in the stage of clinical testing. In the first method, a metal plate/ phosphor screen combination is used to convert the photon beam intensity into a light image. The screen is viewed by a sensitive video camera using an angled mirror. A drawback of this approach is the bulkiness of the device as a result of the use of a mirror. Replacement of the mirror by a fibre-optic arrangement may result in a much flatter system having comparable properties. The second method is to scan the radiation beam by means of an array of radiation detectors (silicon diodes or scintillation detectors). Because the efficiency of these detectors is high, a good contrast resolution can be obtained with such a system. The mechanical motion of the system might be a disadvantage of this approach. In the third approach, a matrix of liquid-filled ionization chambers is used. A 256×256 light weight ionization chamber matrix was developed having outer dimensions similar to a film cassette (Fig. 22).

Recently, a new category of electronic portal imaging device has been developed consisting of a metal plate/ phosphor screen X-ray detector combined with an amorphous silicon flat panel array. The array acts like a large area light sensor and records the optical signals generated in the metal plate/ phosphor screen detector when irradiated by a megavoltage beam.[64]

An advantage of on-line imaging compared with the portal film technique is that the image is available a few seconds after the start of the irradiation. This allows, in principle, a quick decision about continuation of treatment if the comparison of portal image with simulator image does not show unacceptable discrepancies. This is of special importance if patients are entered into clinical trials, where a protocol violation can be detected at an early stage of the treatment. In addition, a series of images can be generated during a treatment session because images can be obtained with these devices in a few seconds. The availability of many portal images thus allows the analysis of dynamic aspects of patient irradiation such as patient or organ motion during treatment. An on-line image detector will be a very useful tool during the quality assurance of complicated treatment techniques, for example using computer controlled irradiations and during dose escalation studies using conformation therapy techniques.

The field of on-line portal imaging is still developing and many findings in research institutions are not yet available for large scale clinical use. Therefore, much work needs to be done before treatment set-up analysis by on-line portal imaging will be used on a routine base in the clinic.

References

1. Johns HE, Cunningham JR. *The physics of radiology.* 4th ed. Springfield, IL: Charles C Thomas Publisher, 1983.

2. Kahn FM. *The physics of radiation therapy.* Baltimore: Williams and Wilkins, 1984.

3. ICRU (International Commission on Radiation Units and Measurements). Report 33. *Radiation quantities and units.* Bethesda, MD: ICRU, 1980.

4. ICRU (International Commission on Radiation Units and Measurements). Report 31. *Average energy required to produce an ion pair.* Bethesda, MD: ICRU, 1979.

5. ICRU (International Commission on Radiation Units and Measurements). Report 37. *Stopping Powers for electrons and positrons.* Bethesda, MD: ICRU, 1984.

6. ICRU (International Commission on Radiation Units and Measurements). Report 49. *Stopping powers and ranges for protons and alpha particles.* Bethesda, MD: ICRU, 1993.

7. Wachsmann F, Dimotsis A. *Kurven und Tabellen für die Strahlentherapie.* Stuttgart: S Hirzel Verlag, 1957.

8. Holzknecht G. *Das Chromoradiometer.* Presentation at Congrès International d'Electrologie, 1902. Archives d'Electricité Mèdicale Tome X, 1902: 577.

9. Villard P. Instrument de mesure a lecture directe pour les rayons X. *Archives d'Electrologie Mèdicales*, 1908; **16**: 692–9.

10. Sievert RM. The institute of radiophysics. *Acta Radiologica*, 1965; **250** (Suppl.): 91–117.

11. ICRU (International Commission on Radiation Units and Measurements). Report 36. *Microdosimetry.* Bethesda, MD: ICRU, 1983.

12. IAEA (International Atomic Energy Agency). Technical Reports Series 277. *Absorbed dose determination in photon and electron beams. An international code of practice.* Vienna: IAEA, 1987.

13. ESTRO (European Society of Therapeutic Radiation Oncology). *Monitor unit calculation for high energy photon beams.* Leuven: Garant Publishers NV, 1997.

14. Diamond J, Hanks GE, Kramer S. The structure of radiation oncology

15. Svensson H, Hettinger G. Measurement of doses from high energy electron beams at small phantom depth. *Acta Radiologica*, 1967; **6**: 289–93.

16. Karlsson M, Svensson H, Nyström H, Stenberg J. The 50 MeV mace-track accelerator—a new approach to beam shaping and modulation. In: *Dosimetry in radiotherapy, proceedings of a symposium*, Vol. 2. Vienna: International Atomic Energy Agency, 1988: 307–20.

17. ICRU (International Commission on Radiation Units and Measurements). Report 35. *Radiation dosimetry: Electron beams with energies between 1 and 50 MeV.* Bethesda, MD: ICRU, 1984.

18. Abou-Mandour M, Harder D. Berechnung der Dosisverteilung schneller Elektronen in und hinter Gewebehomogenitäten beliebiger Breite II. *Strahlentherapie*, 1978; **154**: 546–54.

19. Brahme A, Svensson H. Radiation beam characteristics of a 22 MeV microtron. *Acta Radiologica*, 1979; **18**: 244–72.

20. ICRU (International Commission on Radiation Units and Measurements). Report 50. *Prescribing, recording and reporting photon beam therapy.* Bethesda, MD: ICRU, 1993.

21. Bortfeld T, Schlegel W, Dykstra C, Levengrun S, Preiser K. Physical versus biological objectives for treatment plan optimization. *Radiotherapy and Oncology*, 1996; **40**: 185.

22. Brahme A. Treatment optimization using physical and radiobiological objective functions. In: Smith AR, ed. *Radiation therapy physics.* Berlin: Springer-Verlag, 1995.

23. Webb S. *The physics of conformal radiotherapy: advances in technology.* Bristol: IOP Publishing, 1997.

24. ICRU (International Commission on Radiation Units and Measurements). Report 42. *Use of computers in external beam radiotherapy procedures with high-energy photons and electrons.* Bethesda, MD: ICRU, 1987.

25. Brahme A, Chavaudra J, Landberg T, Mccullough E, Nuesslin F, Rawlinson A, Svensson G, Svensson H. Accuracy requirements and quality assurance of external beam therapy with photons and electrons. *Acta Oncologica*, 1988; (Suppl. 1): 1–76.

26. Rosenow UF, Dannhausen H-W, Lubbert K, *et al.* Quality assurance in treatment planning. Report from the German task group. In: Bruinvis IAD, ed. *Proceedings of the 9th International Conference on the Use of Computers in Radiotherapy.* Amsterdam: North Holland, 1987: 45–8.

27. SFPH (Societé Française des Physiciens d'Hôpital). *Choix et évaluation des systèmes informatiques en radiothérapie.* Paris: Siège Institut Curie, 1989.

28. Wittkämper FW, Mijnheer BJ, van Kleffens HJ. Dose intercomparison at the radiotherapy centres in The Netherlands. 2. Accuracy of locally applied computer planning systems for external photon beams. *Radiotherapy and Oncology*, 1988; **11**: 405–14.

29. Epp ER, Boyer AL, Doppke KP. Underdosing of lesions resulting from lack of electronic equilibrium in upper respiratory air cavities irradiated by 10 MV X-ray beams. *International Journal for Radiation Oncology, Biology, Physics*, 1977; **2**: 613–19.

30. Klein EE, Rice RK, Chin LM, Mijnheer BJ. The influence of air cavities on dose distributions for photon beams. *International Journal of Radiation Oncology, Biology, Physics*, 1993; **27**: 419–27.

31. Das IJ, Khan FM. Backscatter dose perturbation at high atomic number interfaces in megavoltage photon beams. *Medical Physics*, 1989; **16**: 367–75.

32. AAPM (American Association of Physicists in Medicine). Report 17. *The physical aspects of total and half body photon irradiation.* New York: American Institute of Physics, 1986.

33. Rice RK, Mijnheer BJ, Chin LM. Benchmark measurements for lung dose corrections for X-ray beams. *International Journal for Radiation Oncology, Biology, Physics*, 1988; **15**: 399–409.

practices in the continental United States. *International Journal of Radiation Oncology, Biology and Physics*, 1988; **4**: 547–8.

34. Dutreix A. When and how can we improve precision in radiotherapy? *Radiotherapy and Oncology*, 1984; **2**: 275–92.

35. Dutreix A, Bjärngard BE, Bridier A, Mijnheer BJ, Shaw J, Svensson H. Monitor unit calculation for high energy photon beams. In: *ESTRO Booklet 3*. Leuven: Garant, 1997.

36. Van Dyk J, Barnett J, Cygler J, Shragge P. Commissioning and quality assurance of treatment planning computers. *International Journal of Radiation Oncology, Biology, Physics*, 1993; **26**: 261–73.

37. Fraass B, Doppke K, Hunt M, *et al.* American Association of Physicists in Medicine Task Group 53 Report: Quality assurance for clinical radiotherapy treatment. *Medical Physics*, 1998; **25**: 1773–829.

38. van Bree NAM, van Battum LJ, Huizenga H, Mijnheer BJ. Three-dimensional dose distribution of tangential breast treatment: a national dosimetry intercomparison. *Radiotherapy and Oncology*, 1991; **22**: 252–60.

39. Leksell L. The stereotaxic method and radiosurgery of the brain. *Acta Chirurgica Scandinavica*, 1951; **102**: 316–19.

40. Lutz W, Winston KR, Maleki N. A system for sterotactic radiosurgery with a linear accelerator. *International Journal of Radiation Oncology, Biology, Physics*, 1988; **14**: 373–81.

41. Rice RK, Hansen JL, Svensson GK, Siddon RL. Measurements of dose distributions in small beams of 6 MV X-rays. *Physics in Medicine and Biology*, 1987; **32**: 1087–99.

42. Abe M. Intraoperative radiotherapy—past, present and future. *International Journal for Radiation Oncology, Biology and Physics*, 1984; **10**: 1987–90.

43. Rich TA. Intraoperative radiotherapy. *Radiotherapy and Oncology*, 1986; **6**: 207–21.

44. Biggs PJ, Epp ER, Ling CC, Novack DH, Michaels HB. Dosimetry, field shaping and other considerations for intraoperative electron therapy. *International Journal of Radiation Oncology, Biology and Physics*, 1981; **7**: 875–84.

45. van der Laarse R, Bruinvis IAD, Nooman FD. Wall-scattering effects in electron beam collimation. *Acta Radiologica Oncologica*, 1978; **17**: 113–24.

46. Brahme A. Optimal setting of multileaf collimators in stationary beam radiation therapy. *Strahlentherapie und Onkologie*, 1988; **164**: 343–50.

47. Mijnheer BJ, Battermann JJ, Wambersie A. What degree of accuracy is required and can be achieved in photon and neutron therapy? *Radiotherapy and Oncology*, 1987; **8**: 237–52.

48. Johansson K-A, Horiot JC, van Dam J, Lepinoy D, Sentenac I, Sernbo G. Quality assurance control in the EORTC Cooperative Group of Radiotherapy. 2. Dosimetry intercomparison. *Radiotherapy and Oncology*, 1986; **7**: 269–79.

49. AAPM (American Association of Physicists in Medicine). Report 13. *Physical aspects of quality assurance in radiation therapy*. New York: American Institute of Physics, 1984.

50. Rassow J. Quality control of radiation therapy equipment. *Radiotherapy and Oncology*, 1988; **11**: 45–55.

51. HPA (Hospital Physicists Association). *Commissioning and quality assurance of linear accelerators*. Report No. 54. York, UK: IPSM Publications, 1988.

52. Kutcher G, *et al.* Comprehensive QA for radiation oncology: Report of AAPM Radiation Therapy Committee Task Group 40. *Medical Physics*, 1994; **21**: 581–618.

53. Svensson H. Quality assurance in radiation therapy: physical aspects. *International Journal of Radiation Oncology, Biology and Physics*, 1984; **10** (Suppl. 1):56–65.

54. Wittkämper FW, Mijnheer BJ, van Kleffens HJ. Dose intercomparison at the radiotherapy centres in The Netherlands. 1. Photon beams under reference conditions and for prostatic cancer treatment. *Radiotherapy and Oncology*, 1987; **9**: 33–44.

55. Thwaites DI, Williams JR, Aird EG, Klevenhagen SC, Williams PC. A dosimetry intercomparison of megavoltage photon beams in UK radiotherapy centres. *Physics in Medicine and Biology*, 1992; **37**: 445–61.

56. Wallner PE, Lustig RA, Pajak TF, *et al.* Impact of initial quality control review on study outcome in lung and head/neck cancer studies—review of the Radiation Therapy Oncology Group experience. *International Journal of Radiation Oncology, Biology and Physics*, 1989; **17**: 893–900.

57. Horowitz YS. TL dose response. In: *Thermoluminescence and thermoluminescent dosimetry*, Vol. 2. Boca Raton, Florida: CRC Press, 1984: 2–36.

58. Rudén B-I. Evaluation of the clinical use of TLD. *Acta Radiologica Therapy Physics, Biology*, 1976; **15**: 447–64.

59. HPA (Hospital Physicists Association). *Practical aspects of thermoluminescence dosimetry*, Report CRS 43. London: HPA Publications, 1984: 12–22.

60. NCS (Netherlands Commission on Radiation Dosimetry). *Proceedings symposium on thermoluminescence dosimetry*. Rijks Instituut voor Volksgezondheid en Milieuhygiene, Bilthoven, The Netherlands, 1988.

61. Rikner G, Grusell E. Patient dose measurements in photon fields by means of silicon semiconductor detectors. *Medical Physics*, 1987; **14**: 870–3.

62. Leunens G, van Dam J, Dutreix A, van der Schueren E. Quality assurance in radiotherapy by dosimetry. Entrance dose measurements, a reliable procedure. *Radiotherapy and Oncology*, 1990; **17**: 141–51.

63. Boyer AL, Antonuk L, Fenster A, *et al.* A review of electronic portal imaging devices (EPIDS). *Medical Physics*, 1992; **19**: 1–16.

64. Munro P, Bouius DC. X-ray quantum limited portal imaging using two-dimensional portal image registration. *Medical Physics*, 1998; **25**: 689–702.

4.3.2 External-beam radiation therapy

Philip Mayles and Diana Tait

Volume definition

External-beam radiotherapy is the most commonly employed means of delivering radiation to a tumour. For its successful application, a number of concepts have to be understood and a planning process carefully followed. The first objective for the radiotherapist is to decide what anatomical volume requires treatment. This is arrived at by taking into account the clinical and surgical findings, information pertaining to the extent of disease derived from imaging, and likely sites of microscopic involvement from knowledge of patterns of disease spread. This is referred to as the 'gross tumour volume',[1] although in many instances the tumour mass will have been removed surgically and the term therefore defines the volume of tissue at risk of malignant involvement (Fig. 1). However, because of the limitations of determining the margins of microscopic involvement, a biological margin is added around the tumour volume. The size of this margin is a clinical judgement that reflects the level of uncertainty about the precise extent of the disease. This is referred to as the 'clinical target volume'. A further internal margin may need to be applied for movement of the target associated with breathing or the cardiac cycle. The combination of these margins leads to the 'internal target

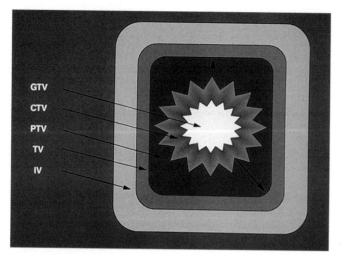

Fig. 1 ICRU Report 50.[1]

volume'.[2] Once this volume has been defined, taking account of the biological uncertainties, the question of technical uncertainties must be addressed. These arise because of the many stages involved in the planning and delivery of radiotherapy, and the errors that can be incurred at each stage. The potential errors are numerous, but include problems in tumour localization, simulator errors and inaccuracy, and lack of reproducibility in the treatment set-up. To allow for these a further margin, the technical margin, is allowed around the internal target volume and the tissue so enclosed is known as the 'planning target volume'. Data on patterns of relapse after local treatment provide useful information to assist in determining the extent of these margins which, combined, are usually in the region of 1 to 2 cm in all dimensions around the gross tumour volume.

The target volume defined by the radiotherapist may be irregular in outline, or have a concave border, but the limitations of collimation with conventional X-ray therapy confine the actual high-dose region to a more regular shape. This high-dose region is known as the 'treated volume'.[1]

These concepts underpin all radiotherapy planning but their precise application depends on the clinical setting and whether a treatment is palliative or radical in intent. Low-dose, palliative, treatments are generally well tolerated by normal tissues with little constitutional upset to the patients and so can usually be delivered using simple beam arrangements such as a direct field or parallel opposed fields. High-dose, radical or curative, treatments are very dependent on the dose to normal tissues and require much more complex beam arrangements in order to maximize the dose to the target volume whilst keeping the normal-tissue dose within the same limits. The capability to achieve this normal-tissue sparing has been revolutionized by technological developments in treatment planning and delivery and these provide the components for conformal therapy. This term, conformal therapy, is difficult to define precisely but, in general terms, it expresses the aim of conforming the shape of the high-dose volume to the shape of the target volume with maximal sparing of surrounding normal tissues. This conformation can be achieved by keeping planning margins, as defined in this section, as small as accuracy will permit, by increasing the number of treatment fields, by combining different energies and weightings, and by utilizing means of field blocking to provide shaped treatment volumes.

Radiotherapy planning

Treatment selection

Radiotherapy planning begins with the clinical assessment of the patient, at which point the treatment intent is defined; broadly classified as palliative, radical, or urgent. This selection decision should be based on protocol guidelines which take into account tumour type, tumour stage, patient symptoms, performance status, and normal-tissue function.

Patient position and immobilization

The selection of a treatment position is based on considerations of patient comfort as well as on technical issues. A comfortable position helps the patient to maintain the position throughout each fraction for the entire course of treatment and, thus, has a major impact on accuracy and reproducibility. Position also influences normal-tissue irradiation and simple manoeuvres can have a significant effect. For example, in irradiating the pelvis, having the patient lying prone encourages normal small bowel, the critical normal tissue that dictates the radiation dose that can be delivered to pelvic tumours, to fall away from the treatment volume.[3] This effect can be increased by treating the patient with a full bladder. In irradiating the neck area, neck extension can spare the floor of the mouth and submandibular glands, whilst in the chest, treating with the arms up above the head allows beams to come in through the side of the chest without first having to pass through the tissues of the arm. Technical considerations include the optimum beam arrangement and the capability of the treatment facility to achieve this.

When reproducibility is particularly critical, the patient may need some help to maintain the position and this has led to the development of a number of immobilization systems. In deciding the need for immobilization devices and the type of device to be used, the determining factor is the degree of accuracy required. This is dependent primarily on the proximity, and size, of critical organs. While a significant radiation dose to a small part of a large, sensitive organ may be acceptable, a dose to the same volume of a small organ such as the eye may have serious effects. In the thorax and abdomen, internal movement, and the limitations on the accuracy with which target structures can be defined, restrict the precision of immobilization required to about 5 mm. However, in treatments to the head and neck, proximity to the eyes and spinal cord requires an accuracy of about 2 mm and some form of immobilization device will be required. Immobilization may here be achieved with plastic beam direction shells, or more recently with a stereotactic frame.[4],[5] It must be emphasized that such devices only work satisfactorily if the patient is comfortable within them. When treating lesions close to the spinal cord in the trunk, immobilization may also become necessary. In this case a plaster cast, or bags of polystyrene that, when evacuated, form a rigid mould, may be used.[6] Such devices are increasingly being used for conformal therapy, where precise definition of target and normal tissue volumes demands a high degree of set-up accuracy and reproducibility.[7]–[9]

Reference landmarks

In order to relate the radiation beam to internal anatomical structures, skin landmarks are necessary. In radiotherapy of the trunk it is usual to make small, point tattoos on the patient's skin to provide a permanent record of the beam position. It is essential that these should be on a stable part of the body. Thus, when treating the pelvis it is better to use lateral tattoos rather than anterior ones, which may move during treatment because of respiration and between treatments because of changes in the patient's weight. To determine the beam position unambiguously relative to the target volume, it is necessary to define a three-dimensional coordinate system. For this the minimum requirement is three points to define the plane of treatment. However, because the human body is not rigid, it may be desirable to use additional points. For head and neck treatments the marks can be placed on the beam direction shell, but considerable care needs to be exercised when this is done because shrinkage of the tumour can change the relation of the shell to the target volume considerably.

Patient–machine alignment

This can be achieved with varying levels of sophistication.

Direct marking

This is usually done on the treatment set and can adequately define palliative fields to cover palpable disease or tender bone metastases, employing either single or parallel opposed fields. For skin cancers, using single fields with methods of superficial radiation, it is acceptable to apply fields using only the surface anatomy as a guide. However, in clinical situations where more penetrating radiation such as high-energy electrons are used, it is advisable to apply more sophisticated methods.

Simulator

In order to deliver a high radiation dose to a deep-seated tumour, the tumour must be irradiated from several directions; most high-energy treatment units are mounted so that the treatment machine and the patient support can rotate about a common centre (or isocentre).

The simulator is a diagnostic X-ray set with an image intensifier mounted on an isocentric gantry to simulate the movements possible with the treatment unit and enabling a beam's eye view of any field relative to the patient to be obtained. This allows alignment of beams based on the underlying bony anatomy. It also provides a means of assessing the feasibility of a complicated set-up. The screening facility allows real-time visualization of the movements of internal structures, which is especially important in the thorax. The contours of the patient are usually assessed manually, but more sophisticated, automatic methods are becoming more common,[10],[11] especially those based on videotape images of lines projected on to the patient's skin.[12],[13] Use of the simulator is also essential when CT data are not available. The simulator films provide a reference of the treatment for verification purposes.

Computed tomography

For accurate radiotherapy of deep-seated lesions, CT data are essential. These can show external and internal contours,[14]–[16] and also tissue density to allow more accurate dose calculations. Doses in the thorax

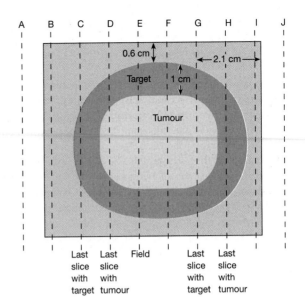

Fig. 2 The effect of CT slice spacing on the uncertainty in field localization. A tumour volume is shown as it intersects CT slices taken at 10-mm intervals. In defining a target volume with a margin of 10 mm round the tumour it has to be assumed that the tumour extends half way to the next slice. The field must clear the target by 6 mm to allow for the dose gradient at the beam edge. This margin will be too great at the right hand and too small at the left. The uncertainty may be reduced by reducing the slice interval.

may be in error by about 15 per cent when variations in tissue density are not taken into consideration.[17],[18] The practice of drawing lung contours freehand, based on drawings in anatomy books, may lead to similar inaccuracies because of individual variation in both the density of lung and its location. When defining a target volume based on CT data, several factors need to be considered:

1. It is essential that a system is devised to enable transfer of the coordinate system of the CT scanner to the radiotherapy treatment machine. Markers used for this purpose often cause artefacts on the CT images, which reduces their usefulness for diagnostic purposes. This is a particular problem where the scanning facility is provided entirely by the diagnostic radiology department, for whom the primary requirement is a clear image. When treating the head, these difficulties can be overcome by the use of a stereotactic reference frame. Originally these were screwed to the skull, but for a small sacrifice in precision, non-invasive versions have been developed.[19]

2. The accuracy achievable in identifying the sagittal extent of the target with CT is limited by the slice spacing. In Fig. 2, tumour has been identified on slices D to G, but it must be assumed that it extends at least half way to the next slice. It can be seen that there is an overall uncertainty of up to 2 cm in the length of the target volume. This uncertainty can only be reduced by closer spacing of the scans at the margins of the tumour.

3. It must be appreciated that it is not always possible to see the extent of the tumour on a CT image. In these circumstances it is necessary to make inferences. To assist in these, other imaging methods, such as magnetic resonance imaging (**MRI**), scintigraphy, and ultrasonography,[20] and more recently positron

emission tomography (**PET**), can be used. The geometric accuracy of the latter two of these methods of imaging is usually not sufficient for radiotherapy purposes, but they can be invaluable as an aid to interpreting the CT data.

4. It is common practice to confirm the CT localization with a simulator, but proper account must be taken of the divergence of the simulator beam when comparing CT images with radiographs. In particular the 'topogram' (sometimes called 'scanogram' or 'scout view') shows divergence in the transverse plane only, and an anterior structure that is aligned with a posterior structure on a topogram will not necessarily line up on a normal radiograph. This difficulty can be avoided if comparisons are limited to transverse planes through the centre of the X-ray beam. Provided that a good coordinate system can be devised, it is possible to omit the visit to the simulator altogether.

CT simulation

The transfer of the patient coordinate system to the treatment machine may be facilitated by the addition of a laser marking system to the CT scanner. Once the CT scans of the patient have been taken, the target volume can be outlined and its centre defined as the isocentre. The laser marking system can then be used to place tattoos on the patient's skin which can be used to set-up the patient for treatment.

Verification images can be produced by a computer projection through the CT density matrix with an appropriately divergent beam simulating the treatment field. This produces a 'digitally reconstructed radiograph'. This process is called CT, or virtual, simulation[21] and with a modern fast scanner can be very efficient. However, three problems must be borne in mind. The first is that movement of internal organs is not shown by the CT scanner (as compared with fluoroscopy on a simulator). Second, the CT scanning session may take place when the patient is feeling particularly nervous and tense so that the position does not accurately reflect the treatment position. Third, it is often not possible to replicate the treatment position (for example with patients needing breast treatment) with the restriction that the patient must be able to pass through the aperture of the CT scanner. This latter difficulty may be addressed by obtaining a CT scan in a conventional simulator, a facility referred to as simulator CT. Images so acquired are not of diagnostic quality and take about 1 min per slice to create, but can provide adequate localization of heart and lung for breast treatment planning, for example.

Volume shaping

The dose that can be delivered to a target volume by external-beam radiotherapy is limited by the radiation tolerance of adjacent normal tissues. The tolerance dose for specific organs is very variable and depends on other factors, such as the volume of the organ irradiated, the age of the patient, and the fractionation schedule employed. Reliable clinical information on dose–response for normal tissues is difficult to establish but, from the limited data available, it would seem that dose–response curves are steep within the dose range used for curative radiotherapy;[22],[23] it is therefore very likely that any increase in target dose will be accompanied by a significant increase in toxicity for normal tissues.

As a result of the delicate balance between the dose necessary to achieve local tumour control and that likely to produce unacceptable toxicity in normal tissues, the principle of radiotherapy planning is

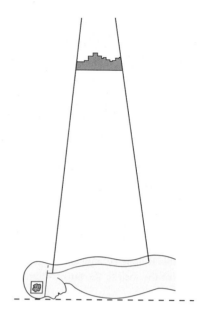

Fig. 3 Diagram showing the insertion of a tissue compensator to reduce the dose inhomogeneity caused by varying patient contour in treatment of the spinal cord.

to arrange for minimal dose to be delivered to the normal tissues, while maximizing the target volume dose.[24],[25] A number of traditional treatment techniques are designed to achieve this. For example, the use of multiple fields, compared with single or opposed fields, allows delivery of a higher dose at depth, with decreased dose to the normal tissue traversed by the beam. The use of shrinking fields and boosts are further techniques that allow the target dose to be increased. The introduction of standard-shaped lead blocks, within the beam, can be used to exclude, or at least reduce, the dose to adjacent normal tissues. Customized blocks, that is blocks constructed for an individual's treatment, have long been used, for example to protect the lungs in mantle irradiation. The accompanying requirements for accuracy of patient positioning and immobilization have been discussed above.

In addition to achieving a differential in dose between the target volume and normal tissues, the aim of planning is to produce as even a dose as possible within the target volume. However, curved body contours and tissue inhomogeneity, such as the presence of lung or bone, can lead to unacceptable variation of dose within, and around, the target volume. The placement of wedge filters and compensators within the path of the beam is a standard means of attempting to correct for this. For example, in irradiating the spinal cord by a fixed, posterior field, the dosimetry will vary according to the depth of the spinal cord within the body, and its distance from the radiation source. A maximum and minimum dose can be calculated for this, and should these differ by more than 10 per cent, a compensator will usually be constructed in an attempt to produce a more even dose distribution. Figure 3 shows an example of a compensator being used to improve the dose distribution where a radiation field is applied to a target at non-uniform depth.

The precise target volume may be irregular in outline, the shape depending on the tumour mass itself and the area of adjacent tissue considered to be at risk for microscopic spread. However, as standard

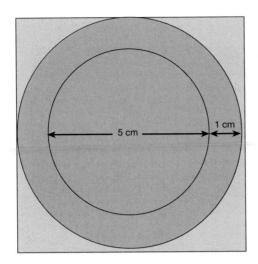

Fig. 4 Schematic representation of a rectangular field being used to cover a spherical target volume consisting of a 5-cm tumour volume with a 1-cm margin.

collimators define beams of rectangular cross-section, the high-dose volume, at depth within the patient, ends up being box shaped. This inevitably means that unnecessary normal tissue is included within the high-dose volume. Figure 4 is a schematic representation of the implication of this for the extent of normal tissue that is included. In this example, a 1-cm margin has been allowed around a 5-cm spherical tumour, and this target volume covered by a field 7 cm square. The volume of the treatment 'box' is 343 cm^3, which includes as much as 163 cm^3 of normal tissue outside the spherical target volume. In the condition shown it is relatively simple to place standard lead blocks in the corners of the beam, but in order to achieve maximum exclusion of normal tissues the blocks would have to have curved edges following the exact contour of the target volume. Under treatment conditions, where the target volume has an irregular outline in all dimensions, maximal exclusion of normal tissues requires very sophisticated planning.

The application of computers to radiotherapy has already had a marked impact on treatment approaches and promises great potential for improving geometric accuracy, dose uniformity, and reproducibility. This technological application enables the radiotherapist to refine traditional planning principles by allowing the size and shape of the high-dose zone to be tailored more closely to that of an ideal target volume, with maximal exclusion of surrounding normal tissue,[26] and this is what the term conformal therapy refers to.

This strategy enables a higher total dose to be delivered within the limits of tolerance of normal tissue, with the expectation of an improvement in local control and, for some tumour sites, in long-term survival.[27],[28] For example, failure of local control is an important cause of death at a number of primary cancer sites, including the head and neck region, uterine cervix, bladder, prostate, and rectum. Based on the data available from the results of salvage surgery at these sites, there is reason to be optimistic in supposing that more effective radiotherapy would indeed lead to improved survival.[29]

Target drawing

The principles of the International Commission on Radiological Units and Measurements (**ICRU**) Report number 50 form the basis for three-dimensional target definition in conformal therapy and for many treatment situations can be applied directly. However, in the setting of multimodality cancer treatment, which may employ any combination of surgery, radiotherapy, chemotherapy, endocrine therapy, and biological modifiers, there may need to be some further interpretation of these definitions.[30] The two most common situations are where surgery and/or chemotherapy have been used prior to radiotherapy.

Post-surgery

After surgery, the gross tumour volume has been removed, usually totally, but in doing so the areas of microscopic spread may have been modified and thus the clinical target volume will need to take account of this. For example, in a low carcinoma of the rectum, excised by anteroposterior resection, the perineum is a common area for tumour recurrence, presumably because of scar implantation at the time of surgery, and must be included in the target volume. In this and other postoperative situations, preoperative imaging can help in defining the target volume but has the major limitation of not being obtained with the patient in the treatment position. Furthermore, surgery will have influenced the relationship of the normal tissues. This is very apparent after lobectomy for lung cancer where the remaining lung expands to fill the space of that removed, and tissue, biologically unlikely to harbour tumour cells, may now lie in the 'tumour bed'. An additional complication after surgery is that venous and lymphatic drainage may be distorted and lead to aberrant pathways of spread. All these factors need to be carefully considered at the time of planning and as much information as possible regarding preoperative tumour status, surgical procedure, postoperative course, and postoperative imaging be obtained.

Post-chemotherapy

After chemotherapy, the problem is mainly one of the influence of change in gross tumour volume as a result of response to treatment. Unlike surgery, there should be no disruption or distortion of normal tissues and, consequently, no change in patterns of tumour spread. However, the question of the most appropriate volume to treat (i.e. the pre- or post-chemotherapy volume) is generally not known and is a difficult question to address. The greatest problem comes with highly chemosensitive tumours, such as lymphoma and small cell lung cancer, where initially bulky tumour may disappear completely on imaging. There is then an enormous difference in clinical target volume between the pre- and post-chemotherapy situations. For small cell lung cancer, although the question has not been addressed in a clinical trial, treatment of the smaller volume appears to be effective and incurs less toxicity than treating the original disease extent.[31]

Consistency of target drawing

Although the ICRU 50 definitions provide a basis for standardizing target drawing, there is still considerable scope for clinician variation in interpretation. This has been demonstrated in studies which provide the same clinical and imaging data to a number of radiotherapists and require them to define the target volume. Such studies have been performed for brain tumours[32] and for non-small cell lung cancer.[33]

There are a number of factors contributing to clinician variation and some, such as uncertainty of tumour extent on imaging, cannot be overcome until imaging techniques allow better differentiation between tumour and, for example, collapse (such as consolidation in the lung or postoperative change in the pelvis). However, margin consistency can be improved upon by utilizing software developments which allow a margin around the gross tumour volume to be drawn uniformly in all dimensions.[34],[35]

Three-dimensional planning

In conventional radiotherapy planning, the limits of the target volumes are defined in two dimensions on any one particular simulator X-ray film. The aim is then to plan the best arrangement of external beams to deliver the prescribed dose to this target volume, keeping the variation in dose in this region to within 10 per cent. However, assessment of dosimetry is often based on a single plane, conventionally the mid-plane, and fails to take into account the inhomogeneity throughout the entire target volume.[36] For example, after conservative surgery for breast cancer it is common to encompass the entire breast by tangential fields. The dosimetry is usually assessed in the mid-plane, with wedges selected to minimize the anterior hot spot produced by the reduced tissue in this area. However, this only attempts to correct for body contouring in one plane, while there is considerable variation in target thickness in the longitudinal axis. Depending on the patient's dimensions, this may produce marked inhomogeneities.[37] Multiple outlines can be taken to check dosimetry at different levels and this process is particularly important where critical normal-tissue structures dip in and out of the target volume, as is the case with the spinal cord in many head and neck treatments. However, this still only provides selected information and is very labour intensive.

Computer technology has revolutionized the way in which CT data can be assimilated for radiotherapy planning. The ability to reconstruct transaxial CT data and display the information in any chosen plane has made accessible the concept of three-dimensional planning.[38]–[40] Three-dimensional reconstructions of the target volume and normal tissues of interest can be viewed from any angle and, most importantly, the trajectory of any beam can be visualized through the body. This facility generates a beam's eye view, as obtained by simulator X-rays, but with unwanted tissue structures suppressed, and allows precise localization of the target volume and normal tissues within the beam's path (Fig. 5).

Customized blocks

Standard blocks, triangles and rectangles of lead, are a very crude means of excluding normal tissues. However, the construction of customized blocks from simulator X-ray films is not only time consuming, but also carries the potential danger of shielding tumour because only limited anatomical information is available. CT-based three-dimensional planning with beam's eye view display, enables customized blocks to be constructed using an enormous amount of information about normal tissues and their relationship to the target volume in many planes and at many levels. This obviously reduces the likelihood of a geographical 'miss', provided that the accuracy and reproducibility of the daily set-up on the treatment machine are assured.

Multileaf collimators

Another means of shaping radiotherapy fields is the multileaf collimator.[41]–[45] Standard collimators define the beam with straight edges so that the radiation field is either square or rectangular. However, collimators are now available that are made up of a number

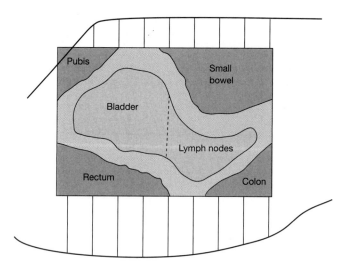

Fig. 5 Beam's eye view (BEV) showing target volume of bladder and nodes. The relationship of the adjacent blocked normal-tissue structures (pubis, rectum, small bowel, and colon) is shown as viewed by the path of this treatment beam.

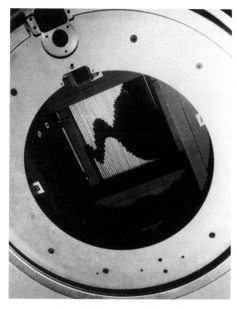

Fig. 6 An irregularly shaped field border as produced by a multileaf collimator (MLC).

of leaves, each capable of independent movement. Thus, depending on the number of leaves per collimator, the beam edge can be shaped as required (Fig. 6). Movement of individual leaves is under computer control and, thus, provides an automated alternative to placing customized blocks within the beam's path. Such a facility obviates the time and money involved in the processing of customized blocks, and reduces the setting-up time on the treatment machine.[46] It also permits better conformation to the target volume by use of an increased number of shaped fields.[47] However, this must be offset by the capital expenditure on the hardware and software, and by the

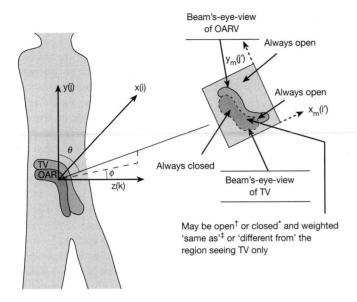

Fig. 7 The x, y, z coordinate system used to specify the dosimetry $D_{i,j,k}$, together with the relationship between this system and the position of the multileaf collimator. The multileaf collimator coordinates ^xM, ^yM, the leaves being parallel to the ^xM direction. The position of the multileaf collimator is such that a line from the origin of dose space to the centre of the face of the multileaf collimator makes an angle θ with the positive y axis and an angle φ with the positive z axis. The target volume (TV) is shown unshaded and the volume of organs at risk (OAR) is shown shaded in the patient. The figure also shows how the areas in the multileaf collimator space may be separately labelled depending on whether they 'connect' to only target volume, only organs at risk, target volume plus organs at risk, or other tissue. The dotted line represents the beam's eye view of the target volume (shown unshaded in the patient). Note the grey-scale values are merely convenient labels for display; they are not the beam weights which feature in the optimization. Key to footnote symbols: *, mode (a); $\neq$ mode (b); †, mode (c); ‡ modes (b) and (c).

increased maintenance and back-up required by such sophisticated machinery.

Intensity-modulated radiation therapy

Shaping the beam to conform to the shape of the target volume, as seen from the radiation source, will in general allow close conformation to target volumes, provided these volumes do not have concave surfaces. However, where there are concavities in the target surface, such as when a tumour is wrapped around the spinal cord or the brainstem, it is desirable to vary the intensity of the radiation across the beam. A simple approach is to divide each beam into two parts: one covering the whole target including sensitive normal tissues, if necessary, and the other excluding any sensitive normal tissues (Fig. 7).[47] The weight given to each part of the beam can be adjusted to minimize normal-tissue dose while maintaining acceptable uniformity within the target volume. In this way, normal-tissue sparing can be greatly improved. More sophisticated developments of this technique divide the field into a number of segments. This allows compensation for inhomogeneous tissue densities and even tighter conformation to the target volume.[48] For irradiation of small target volumes, a micro-multileaf collimator with 2-mm wide jaws (projected at the isocentre) has been developed.[49] By moving the collimator jaws while the radiation beam

is on, a very non-uniform beam intensity profile can be generated which can be used to produce a uniform dose distribution shaped to almost any target volume.

Planning for such treatments requires sophisticated computer techniques referred to as inverse planning. In traditional planning, beam directions and weights are selected by the planner, the dose distribution calculated, and the plan adjusted iteratively until it is considered satisfactory. In inverse planning, the required dose distribution is specified and then the beam configuration required to deliver that distribution is calculated by the computer.[50]

Delivery of dynamic therapy can be achieved using static fields with dynamic movement of the jaws of the micro-multileaf collimator to create an intensity-modulated beam, or the machine can be rotated around the patient while an appropriate irradiation field is generated. The latter is called tomotherapy.[51] The major areas of clinical interest for these techniques are the lung[27] and head and neck.[52],[53]

Limitations to accuracy

Introduction

With the increasing sophistication of radiotherapy treatment machines and the consequent moves towards more complicated set-ups, quality assurance is becoming of increasing importance. However, it is important to be aware of the inherent limitations to accuracy that no quality assurance programme can overcome.

1. The internal anatomy of patients may vary from day to day and from minute to minute. The relative position of organs in the pelvis varies with the state of the bladder.[54],[55] Similarly, kidney position varies with respiration and there are the obvious problems of cardiac and respiratory movement in the chest. These problems are not addressed by most studies of accuracy of set-up, which are generally based on relations to bony landmarks. The older published studies[56]–[58] were based on measurements from films exposed on the treatment machine, which are necessarily of poorer quality than diagnostic films. However, a number of commercial digital imaging systems that can be attached to a treatment machine are now in clinical use (Figs 8 and 9).[59]–[61] This not only allows an improvement in image quality, but also allows an image to be produced in almost real time. This offers, for the first time, the possibility of adjusting the patient's position before the treatment is given and of monitoring patient movement during a single fraction. Some progress has been made to producing CT images using the treatment machine (megavoltage CT).[62],[63] Although the images are of poorer quality than diagnostic CT, this facility enables the patient's position and the dosimetry to be compared directly with the original CT data and treatment plan, respectively.

2. Current imaging modalities are unable to identify the extent of microscopic tumour spread and it is often even difficult to define the macroscopic extent. This biological uncertainty means that a larger margin must be taken around visible tumours than would be necessary with precise microscopic tumour mapping. When localization is done without the aid of CT, or MRI, there is a substantial likelihood of missing the tumour.

3. Even when a treatment machine is mechanically adjusted to meet its specification, there must be some margin for error. Although

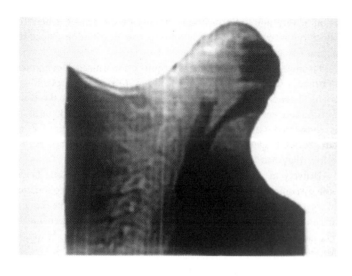

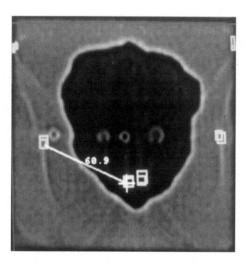

Figs 8 and 9 Use of commercial digital imaging systems attached to a treatment machine.

these errors are of a smaller order than those relating to localization, they may be about 2 mm for a modern accelerator and up to 4 mm for an older one.

Implications for target size

Studies of positioning[8],[9],[56]–[58],[64] indicate that an accuracy of 5 mm is a reasonable expectation, but that 10 mm errors are not uncommon. However, these studies are mainly based on variability in relation to the first treatment and do not take into account the uncertainties in the initial localization or movement of soft-tissue structures within the bony framework. The implication of this is that a margin of at least 10 mm around a tumour is essential unless very special precautions are taken to ensure accuracy.[65] In the head and neck region, this margin may have to be reduced because of proximity to sensitive normal tissues.

Dose measurements

It is difficult to do direct studies of the accuracy achieved in dosimetric terms. Factors such as scatter from areas of very high or very low tissue density are not well modelled by treatment planning systems,[36],[66] whose accuracy is largely assessed by measurements in water phantoms. However, as computer speeds increase, the potential calculation accuracy is constantly improving. Studies in anthropomorphic phantoms suggest that the accuracy achieved may be substantially worse in some situations than the 5 per cent called for by the ICRU.[67] In addition, it must be borne in mind that it is standard practice to allow a 10 per cent variation in dose over the target volume.

In addition to the inherent inaccuracies in treatments, there is also the possibility that machine failures or human errors may introduce substantial errors. These errors can be in both the location of the radiation beam in relation to the target and in the actual dose delivered. Megavoltage beam's eye view devices can help to eliminate geometric errors. The use of *in vivo* measurements, with diodes, is now being advocated as a way of picking up errors throughout the dosimetric chain.[68],[69] Unfortunately, this method of dosimetry is not entirely reliable. Diodes show energy, orientation, and temperature dependence, and more frequent recalibration is necessary than that required for most other methods of dosimetry.

Dose limitations

There have been no satisfactory studies of the extent to which these factors relating to accuracy compromise the success with which radiotherapy can be given. Attempts are beginning to be made to rectify this.[24],[65],[70],[71] These studies use data on normal tissue and tumour cells to compute 'normal-tissue complication probabilities' and 'tumour control probabilities'. The former determines the maximum acceptable dose and the latter the minimum. With the help of these concepts it may be possible to make a more realistic assessment of the expected benefit of recent advances.

Common treatment techniques

This section describes the application of common treatment techniques in clinical practice. The aim is to show the breadth of application of a few standard techniques to a multiplicity of treatment sites, the details of which can be found in the chapters on the relevant sites.

Single field

A single field arrangement, with the beam directed at the area for treatment, is used in several common clinical situations, both palliative and curative. Palliation of skin and subcutaneous deposits, and many bony metastatic sites, is achieved in this way. The same technique, but employing very different dose and fractionation schedules, is used to cure skin tumours and to boost areas of residual disease or high risk of microscopic disease. A common boost site is the tumour bed following wide local excision of an invasive breast cancer and a single electron field, of appropriate energy, will provide good coverage of the target volume whilst relatively sparing underlying lung. Similarly, high-dose radiotherapy to locoregional disease in the head and neck

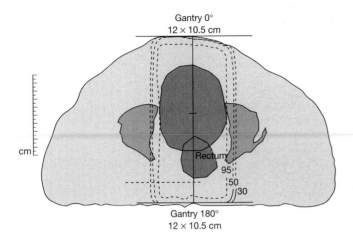

Gantry 0°
12 × 10.5 cm

cm

Rectum
95
50
30

Gantry 180°
12 × 10.5 cm

Fig. 10 Anteroposterior parallel opposed fields are often used for phase I or palliative treatments to the thorax. Here, they encompass a pelvic tumour where the volume taken in by the 95 per cent isodose should be compared with Fig. 4.

is often delivered by means of a single electron field, following larger field irradiation to a phase 2 volume. This technique provides a means of supplementing the dose to gross tumour, whilst sparing underlying structures such as the oesophagus and spinal cord.

Opposed fields

Single fields are not suitable for deep-seated sites in the thorax and abdomen for two reasons. First, an unacceptably high dose would need to be given at the skin surface in order to achieve a tumoricidal dose at a depth of 10 cm. Second, the dose would not be distributed evenly across the tumour, with a region of low dose at the point furthest from the site of beam entry. Two-field techniques enable the dose to be evenly distributed through the target volume.

The most common two-field arrangement consists of an anterior and a posterior field arranged exactly opposite each other. These anteroposterior parallel opposed fields are one of the most frequently used field arrangements in both palliative and curative settings (Fig. 10). With rectangular fields the high-dose volume is box shaped because it encompasses all the tissues between the rectangular portals. The high-dose volume is always much larger than the tumour, and this usually limits the total dose to the equivalent of 45 Gy in 4.5 weeks, delivered in daily fractions of 2 Gy. Although large volumes are suitable as a first phase of curative treatment, higher doses require a field arrangement that reduces the high-dose volume and avoids critical structures.

Thorax

Opposed fields are commonly used in the palliative treatment of symptomatic lung and oesophageal cancers. The basic rectangular field can be modified with simple lead blocks to shield one or more corners.

Palliative treatments encompass the radiologically visible disease in the chest with a margin of 1 to 2 cm. The dose is prescribed midway between the anterior and posterior skin surfaces on the central axis of the opposed beams. This field arrangement is simple to plan, technically easy to set up, and comfortable since the patient lies in the supine position.

A minority of patients with thoracic tumours merit high-dose treatment with curative intent and these require an altered field arrangement to reduce the high-dose volume and avoid critical structures such as the spinal cord (see below). Individually shaped lead blocks can be made to shield healthy lung in these circumstances.

Head and neck region

Opposed lateral fields are often used in head and neck cancer to irradiate midline structures where a single field would overdose the superficial tissues at the point of entry. However, the head and neck region in composed of a multiplicity of subsites each needing specific treatment planning. Although this relatively simple technique is appropriate for part of the treatment at a number of these sites, overall, irradiation of the head and neck is a complex procedure which is described in detail in the site-specific chapters elsewhere in the book.

Opposed fields in the head and neck region are suitable for doses up to an equivalent of 50 Gy in 5 weeks, delivered in daily fractions of 2 Gy. Higher doses are delivered by electron boosts to sites of residual disease or by interstitial implants.

Breast

Radiotherapy in early-stage breast cancer has assumed new importance in the era of breast conservation; local excision of the breast lump with narrow margins of healthy tissue is the treatment of choice rather than mastectomy. With the woman lying in a comfortable, supine position and her arms resting on or near the top of her head, opposed fields can be arranged to glance across the breast with minimal exposure of underlying lung or cardiac tissues. X-rays of 4 to 6 MV are ideal for their skin-sparing properties and good penetration. These are described as tangential fields to the breast and typically deliver the equivalent of 50 Gy in 5 weeks, in daily fractions of 2 Gy, before a boost to the tumour site using a single electron field.

Because there is less tissue in the region of the nipple than at the base of the breast, unmodified or 'open' fields deliver an uneven dose with a maximum dose in the nipple region. This can be overcome by inserting wedge-shaped tissue compensation into the beams (Fig. 11). This produces an even dose distribution in the coronal plane but does not modify inhomogeneity in the parasagittal plane, that is, above and below the central plane. Attempts to compensate for variation in the parasagittal plane are being evaluated and may become routine in the future if such a modification can be shown to improve cosmetic outcome.[72]

Brain

Cerebral secondaries are common and usually multiple. The whole brain is encompassed by opposed lateral fields with the patient lying supine. The fields are large rectangles, with the inferior border running from the superior orbital margin to the tip of the tragus. These surface landmarks define the base of the skull. Treatments delivered with curative intent to children with medulloblastoma requiring craniospinal irradiation, and those to selected individuals with gliomas, require highly reproducible positioning from day to day and a customized immobilization device is essential. The orbits are shielded by inserting lead blocks. Direct measurements of orbital dose are

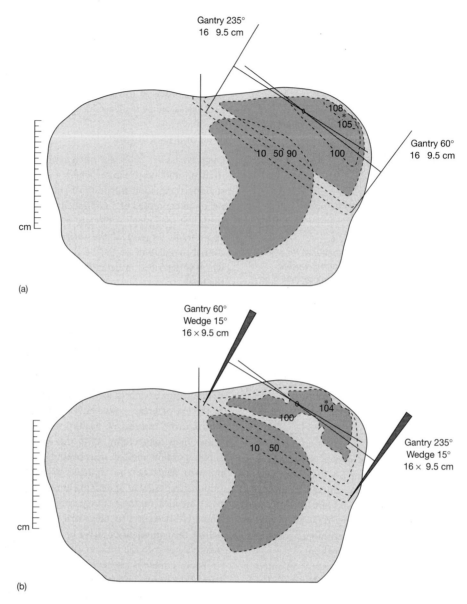

Fig. 11 Tangential fields to the breast following local excision of a T₁ breast cancer. In (a) unwedged fields are responsible for a steep dose gradient across the volume with the maximum dose anteriorly. Wedged fields in (b) compensate for breast curvature and restore a more homogeneous dose distribution.

made during treatment using lithium fluoride dose meters placed on the overlying skin.

Mantle and inverted Y

In the present era of effective systemic therapy, radiotherapy is much less commonly used as a sole, curative method in Hodgkin's disease and testicular cancer, but the 'mantle field' is still the preferred, curative treatment for patients with stage I or IIA Hodgkin's disease. The mantle is composed of two, very large, anteroposterior opposed fields with individually tailored lead blocks to shield the healthy tissues, especially the lungs. This large treatment volume limits the total dose to the equivalent of 40 Gy in 4 weeks, delivered in daily fractions of 2 Gy, which is curative for these highly radiosensitive tumours.

The same principle of large opposed fields is used to treat the para-aortic, iliac, and inguinal lymph nodes in some patients with Hodgkin's disease and germ cell tumours. Here, careful shielding is necessary to protect the kidneys as well as the intestines.

Wedge-pair and three-field techniques

The main disadvantage of opposed-field techniques for high-dose, curative treatments is that the high-dose volume is usually larger than it need be, corresponding to the full thickness of the patient between the portals of entry. At superficial sites, two fields can be angled at 90° to each other to reduce the high-dose zone and to avoid critical structures such as the spinal cord, orbit, or parotid glands. When radiotherapy is confined to a central target such as the oesophagus, bladder, or prostate, a better approach is to angle three or more fields so that they overlap only across the target volume. This confines the high-dose zone to the target volume.

Buccal cavity

A pair of anterior and lateral fields at an angle of approximately 90° to each other can be used for cancers in the head and neck region that are off midline, notably the parotid. At this site it is possible to deliver a high dose with curative intent from one side of the patient. This has the advantage of sparing the opposite parotid gland and avoids the unpleasant complications associated with absent salivation.

With an unwedged beam the dose is very uneven, with a maximum dose just beneath the skin and the dose falling off towards the anatomical midline. A pair of 45° wedges ensures a homogeneous dose distribution (Fig. 12).

Pelvis

Cancers of the bladder or prostate in the centre of the pelvis are best encompassed by three fields, an anterior and two lateral fields or an anterior and two posterior oblique fields (Fig. 13), or by four fields. The high-dose zone corresponds to the area of overlap of the fields in the centre of the pelvis. If opposed lateral fields are used, 45° wedges are inserted in the lateral beams with the thick edges anterior to ensure a homogeneous dose distribution. If fields are evenly spread, either at 60°, 90°, or 120°, wedges may not be needed. The patient lies supine during treatment and the placement of the lateral or posterior oblique fields should enable sparing of the posterior wall of the rectum. This reduces the severity of acute proctitis and the probability of late complications such as bleeding or stenosis.

Thorax

Similar three-field arrangements are commonly used for high-dose treatments to the oesophagus and bronchus. In these sites, the posterior oblique fields commonly traverse several centimetres of healthy lung tissue and there is less absorption of the radiation beam because of the air contained within it. Absorption in aerated lung is approximately 30 per cent of that in other soft tissues but is age dependent, being higher in young people and lower in elderly people. Corrections for the increased transmission of radiation through aerated lung tissue must be made to avoid overdosing structures in the centre of the chest. The density of lung measured in Hounsfield units on CT scan allows an accurate estimate of the appropriate correction for an individual patient.

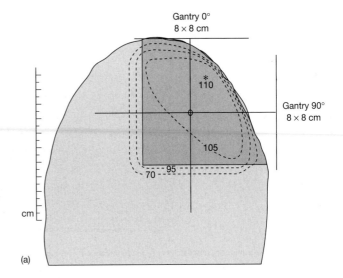

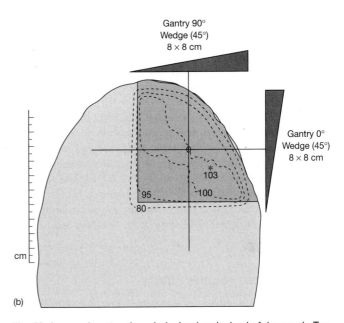

Fig. 12 A coronal section through the head at the level of the mouth. Two unwedged fields encompass a cancer on the anterolateral border of the tongue in (a), but the dose is uneven. In (b), wedged fields restore a homogeneous dose distribution to the target volume.

Clinical evaluation of computer technology in radiotherapy

The incorporation of computer technology into radiotherapy has been accompanied by increasingly sophisticated treatment planning. Attractive as this may be on theoretical grounds, such 'advances' need to be carefully evaluated clinically. As radiotherapy plans become more complicated, then the demands on accuracy at the various stages in the planning process increase, and daily reproducibility of set-up becomes critical. A further concern is the reliance placed on imaging to define these intricate treatment plans and it is important to bear in mind the limits of resolution for any particular imaging technique. Carefully designed studies are therefore required to define the role of the new technology and to ensure that there are real benefits to be had. There is at present a dearth of randomized controlled trials, partly because of the difficulty of justifying treating a larger volume of normal tissue when facilities are available to confine the radiation dose to the target tissue. However, there is growing evidence that conformal therapy is beneficial.

Patterns of relapse

An important part of the analysis of these techniques is the careful documentation of failure patterns, especially with regard to recurrence

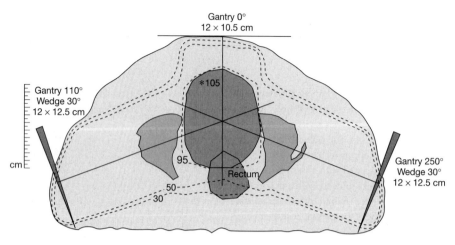

Gantry 0°
12 × 10.5 cm

Gantry 110°
Wedge 30°
12 × 12.5 cm

cm

*105

95

Rectum

50

30

Gantry 250°
Wedge 30°
12 × 12.5 cm

Fig. 13 A three-field plan encompassing a T$_3$ bladder cancer. The high-dose zone conforms well to the target volume, in contrast to the situation illustrated in Fig. 1.

at the edge of the treatment volume. There are two possible contributing factors in marginal recurrence: inaccuracy in tumour localization and failure of precision in treatment delivery. The latter can, and should, be carefully monitored in conformal therapy, using beam's eye view devices such as digital imaging and megavoltage CT. Provided that this is satisfactory, then a marginal recurrence can be presumed to be a reflection of inadequate tumour localization, a variable that is otherwise difficult to assess. Careful analysis of data such as these may lead to important modifications in the process of target volume localization. However, for some tumours such as low-grade gliomas[73] and non-small cell lung cancer,[74] tumour recurrence has been shown to occur within the treated volume and the use of conformal techniques to achieve higher doses may prove beneficial is such situations.[75]

Normal-tissue volume effects

The presence, and extent, of a volume effect for normal-tissue tolerance is an important concept that underpins the philosophy behind conformal therapy. For most tissues there are few data describing this in detail, but clinical experience shows that tolerance to higher doses is improved by reducing the volume of normal tissue within the high-dose zone. Computer analysis of normal-tissue dosimetry and its correlation with clinical effect will define the level of clinical significance of taking known volumes of a particular organ to a particular dose. This information can then be used to identify areas in which efforts to exclude normal tissues are most likely to result in clinical benefit. There are, however, certain clinical situations where the important normal tissue is invaded by tumour, or at least lies at the centre of the treatment volume, and its exclusion is therefore not possible without compromising the chance of local tumour control. In such circumstances it seems unlikely that conformal therapy will ever permit any useful increase in dose, but knowledge of such situations may provide important information on which to base clinical decisions such as the choice of treatment technique. For example, with bladder cancer, although normal bowel may be excluded from the treatment volume, it is still necessary to treat the bladder

itself, which then becomes the normal tissue critically limiting radiation dose. Any increase in dose will be accompanied by an incidence of bladder toxicity and raises the question of whether or not that level of toxicity in normal tissue is preferable to the surgical option of cystectomy.

Yarbro and Ferrans[76] compared quality of life of patients with prostate cancer treated surgically or with conventional radiotherapy. They found that urinary function was superior in patients treated with radiotherapy ($P = 0.0002$), whereas bowel function was superior in the surgical group ($P = 0.05$). Both groups reported poor sexual function, but in the surgical group this was worse ($P = 0.009$). The emphasis in radiotherapy should therefore be to reduce rectal doses and conformal radiotherapy might be expected to reduce bowel toxicity.

Undoubtedly, conformal techniques can reduce the volume of normal tissue taken to a high dose.[26],[77] In addition to planning exercises of this sort, clinical studies have utilized these techniques and have proceeded to dose escalation. Studies like this have been used to demonstrate a lower acute toxicity rate in patients who are conformally treated in conjunction with dose escalation compared with historic controls given conventional doses by conventional techniques.[78],[79] The possibility of giving a higher dose to the prostate using conformal therapy without the expected side-effects has been demonstrated in a number of studies[80]–[82] and similar results have been shown for lung.[83]

However, clinically and scientifically there are problems with directly comparing groups of patients of this sort and the only way to address the benefits derived from such techniques in a definitive way is to compare them, with conventional treatments, in the setting of a randomized trial. Such a trial was designed and implemented at the Royal Marsden Hospital in which patients undergoing pelvic radiotherapy were randomized to either conventional treatment or a conformal technique, utilizing customized blocks designed by beam's eye view, which allowed significant sparing of normal tissues.[84]–[86] The trial was originally designed to use acute toxicity as a means of demonstrating whether or not a reduction in the normal tissue irradiated would translate into a reduction in the normal-tissue effect

Table 1 Percentage of patients (within study group) with toxic effects of RTOG grade 0 to 4

	Conformal radiotherapy (n = 114)					Conformal radiotherapy (n = 111)					P for difference between groups	P for trend	Relative risk (95% CI)
	0	1	2	3	4	0	1	2	3	4			
Toxic effects on rectum (% of patients)													
Proctitis: rectal bleeding	66	31	3	0	0	49	39	11	0	1	0.009	0.002	1.37 (1.08–1.73)
Proctitis: pain	93	5	2	0	0	88	8	4	0	0	0.16	0.18	1.06 (0.98–1.16)
Total proctitis	63	32	5	0	0	44	41	14	0	1	0.004	0.0009	1.45 (1.12–1.87)
Diarrhoea	91	9	0	0	0	87	13	0	0	0	0.36	..	1.07 (1.11–1.94)
Worst rectal toxic effects	59	36	5	0	0	40	45	14	0	1	0.006	0.001	1.47 (1.11–1.94)
Toxic effects on bladder (% of patients)													
Haematuria	92	2	6	0	0	92	4	3	1	0	0.76	0.93	1.03 (0.95–1.12)
Cystitis	51	35	14	0	0	48	35	17	0	0	0.58	0.51	1.08 (0.82–1.41)
Incontinence	90	5	0	0	0	88	9	0	3	0	0.60	0.87	1.05 (0.95–1.16)
Worst bladder toxic effects	47	33	15	0	0	41	36	19	4	0	0.34	0.48	1.16 (0.86–1.57)

Table shows worst side-effects recorded during 2 years' follow-up. χ^2 compares grade 0 with grade 1 or greater toxic effects between the groups; relative risk compares grade 0 with grade 1 or greater toxic effects.

experienced by the patients. However, late toxicity data were also collected on patients in this trial. Results of the acute toxicity analysis failed to show any statistically significant differences between the two arms in terms of level of symptoms, or medication prescribed to counteract these symptoms. Despite this, analysis of late toxicity data has shown a significant reduction in the development of radiation-induced proctitis and bleeding in the patients treated with the conformal technique (Table 1). Encouragingly, there was no associated difference in terms of tumour control or survival between the two arms of the trial.[87] A European study[88] found significant benefits in reduction of acute anal toxicity. Another randomized study comparing 70 Gy given with conventional therapy and 78 Gy given conformally has been reported by Nguyen et al.,[89] where112 patients were sent questionnaires and of these 101 were evaluable. In spite of the dose difference, the conventional radiotherapy group had more moderate or major changes in bowel function (34 per cent compared with 10 per cent), more frequent bowel movements (47 compared with 27 per cent), and more urgent frequent bowel movements (37 compared with 18 per cent). Thus it has now been clearly demonstrated, in randomized trials, that implementation of conformal radiotherapy reduces radiation-related morbidity. The Royal Marsden study also emphasizes the inadequacy of acute side-effects as a proxy for the development of late radiation sequelae, which are the important effects in terms of long-term outcome of treatment and quality of life.

Tumour control

Most studies of increased dose are at the stage of carrying out dose-escalation phase II studies. For the prostate these have generally shown that increased doses are not necessary for patients with low prostate-specific antigen scores prior to treatment, but that improved local control can be achieved by increasing the dose if the prostate-specific antigen is more than10 ng/ml.[90],[91] Many studies of conformal therapy have now demonstrated that it is safe to increase the dose delivered to the prostate to between 74 and 80 Gy.[89] Delivery of such doses with conventional radiotherapy would lead to significantly increased complications. A recent report by Zelefsky et al.[92] of a large dose-escalation study in which 743 patients have been treated has produced good evidence of a dose response as shown in Fig. 14. The results presented here may be overoptimistic as they are likely to be associated also with improved treatment technique. However,

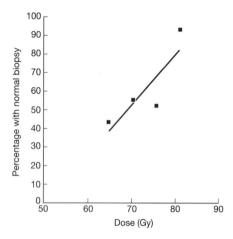

Fig. 14 Negative biopsy rate against dose[92]

Table 2 Outcome compared with dose for prostate cancer[95]

Dose range	Dose (Gy)	Freedom from failure (%)
Low	< 67	61
Intermediate	67–77	74
High	> 77	96

this result clearly shows the potential for improvement in therapy. Pollack and Zagars[93] also found that the actuarial freedom from failure was dose dependent when looking at retrospective data (Table 2). Hanks *et al.*[90] found that after 5 years the hazard of biochemical failure decreased by 8 per cent for each additional 1 Gy delivered.

It is, however, not clear whether improved local control of prostate cancer will translate into improved survival. The use of neutrons for treatment may be regarded as a form of dose escalation. A randomized study of neutron therapy for prostate cancer showed a significant increase in local control of prostate cancer at the expense of 11 per cent serious complications.[94] In this study most of the neutron treatments were given with rectangular fields. However, at the University of Washington a multileaf collimator was used and their complication rate was almost negligible.[95] This demonstrates, at least for neutrons, that a reduction in the volume of unnecessary normal tissue irradiated is beneficial. At present the improvement in survival has not reached significance in spite of lower prostate-specific antigen levels in the neutron arm,[96] although the high complication rates in this study may have influenced this. However, there is a significant improvement in survival[96] in the randomized study of mixed photon and neutron irradiation.[97] Prostate cancer is a slowly growing disease and a long follow-up is necessary to establish definitive results. Studies of dose escalation in lung cancer are at an earlier stage,[27] but evidence from the CHART study[98] shows that improvement in local control by a biological increase in dose produced significant improvement in survival. Armstrong *et al.*[27] have also demonstrated the possibility

of improved survival by applying conformal therapy to non-small cell lung cancer.

Resource implications

Important as the biological and clinical implications of conformal therapy are, an analysis of change in workload, compared with the use of standard techniques, is essential in the full evaluation. As conformal therapy is based on detailed knowledge of normal-tissue anatomy, adequate time must be spent on acquiring detailed images through the region of interest, and this may involve the use of multiple types of imaging, including CT, MRI, and PET. The information then has to be scrutinized by the radiotherapist, who defines the target volume and normal tissues of interest on every image, an exercise which is generally much more time consuming than traditional planning. Three-dimensional planning facilities provide the therapist with many more options in the approach to treatment, but again this means that the process is more lengthy than when applying a standard field arrangement to any particular tumour site. Once a treatment plan has been produced, the implementation of conformal therapy involves greater use of immobilization devices and of means for confirming the daily reproducibility of set-up. Although there are certainly many steps that involve an increase in workload, computer-controlled radiotherapy does save time and effort in certain areas. For example, it may avoid the manual construction of blocks and the time involved in lining up lead blocks on the treatment machine. In addition, wedges can be introduced and removed from the field in an automated fashion, so that it is not necessary for the radiographer to do this manually, or for there to be any interruption in the treatment for such adjustments to take place. Furthermore it can be shown that the reduction in normal tissue damage can reduce the overall cost of treatment.[28]

References

1. ICRU. *Prescribing, Recording and Reporting Photon Beam Therapy.* International Commission on Radiological Units and Measurements, Report No. 50. Bethesda, Maryland: ICRU, 1993.

2. Landberg T. Prescribing and reporting conformal radiotherapy. *ESTRO pre-meeting workshop on challenges in conformal radiotherapy, Nice.* Brussels: ESTRO, 1997.

3. Gallagher MJ, *et al.* A prospective study of treatment techniques to minimise the volume of pelvic small bowel with reduction of acute and late effects associated with pelvic irradiation. *International Journal of Radiation Oncology, Biology, Physics,* 1986; **12**: 1565–73.

4. Podgorsak EB, Oliver A, Pla M, Lefebvre PY, Hazel J. Dynamic stereotactic radiosurgery. *International Journal of Radiation Oncology, Biology, Physics,* 1988; **14**: 115–26.

5. Saunders WM, *et al.* Radiosurgery for arteriovenous malformations of the brain using a standard linear accelerator: rationale and technique. *International Journal of Radiation Oncology, Biology, Physics,* 1988; **15**: 441–7.

6. Jakobsen A, Iversen P, Gadeberg C, Hansen JT, Hjelm Hansen M. A new system for patient fixation in radiotherapy. *Radiotherapy and Oncology,* 1987; **8**: 145–51.

7. Blomgren H, Lax I, Naslund I, Svanstrom R. Stereotactic high dose fraction radiation therapy of extracranial tumours using an accelerator. Clinical experience of the first 31 patients. *Acta Oncologica,* 1995; **34**: 861–70.

8. Hanley J, *et al.* Measurement of patient positioning errors in three-dimensional conformal radiotherapy of the prostate. *International Journal of Radiation Oncology, Biology, Physics*, 1997; **37**: 435–44.

9. Mubata CD, Bidmead AM, Ellingham LM, Thompson V, Dearnaley DP. Portal imaging protocol for radical dose-escalated radiotherapy treatment of prostate cancer. *International Journal of Radiation Oncology, Biology, Physics*, 1998; **40**: 221–31.

10. Velkley DE, Oliver GD Jr. Stereo-photogrammetry for the determination of patient surface geometry. *Medical Physics*, 1979; **6**: 100–4.

11. Spicka J, Fleury K, Powers W. Polyethylene-lead tissue compensators for megavoltage radiotherapy. *Medical Dosimetry*, 1988; **13**: 25–7.

12. Amols HI. Input of treatment planning data via a video frame grabber. *Medical Physics*, 1989; **16**: 140–1.

13. Andrew JW, Aldrich JE, Hale ME, Berry JA. A video-based patient contour acquisition system for the design of radiotherapy compensators. *Medical Physics*, 1989; **16**: 425–30.

14. Battista JJ, Rider WD, Van Dyk J. Computed tomography for radiotherapy planning. *International Journal of Radiation Oncology, Biology, Physics*, 1980; **6**: 99–107.

15. Fuwa N, Norita K, Okumura E, Horikawa Y, Uchiyama Y, Suyama NI. The use of CT in the treatment of lung cancer with radiation therapy. *Gan No Rinsho*, 1987; **33**: 369–73.

16. Tsujii H, Kamada T, Matsuoka Y, Takamura A, Akazawa TI, Iric G. The value of treatment planning using CT and an immobilizing shell in radiotherapy for paranasal sinus carcinomas. *International Journal of Radiation Oncology, Biology, Physics*, 1989; **16**: 243–9.

17. Dobbs HJ, Parker R-P, Hodson NJ, Hobday P, Husband JE. The use of CT in radiotherapy treatment planning. *Radiotherapy and Oncology*, 1983; **1**: 133–41.

18. Muller-Runkel R, Kalokhe U. Impact of CT information on the treatment planning for lung tumours. *Medical Dosimetry*, 1989; **14**: 9–15.

19. Gill SS, Thomas DGT, Warrington AP, Brada M. Relocatable frame for stereotactic external beam radiotherapy. *International Journal of Radiation Oncology, Biology, Physics*, 1991; **20**: 599–603.

20. Chen OT, Pelizzari CA. Image correlation techniques in radiation therapy treatment planning. *Computerized Medical Imaging and Graphics*, 1989; **13**: 235–40.

21. Sherouse GW, Bourland JD, Reynolds K, McMurry HL, Mitchell TP, Chaney-EL. Virtual simulation in the clinical setting: some practical considerations. *International Journal of Radiation Oncology, Biology, Physics*, 1990; **19**: 1059–65.

22. Morrison R. The results of treatment of cancer of the bladder—a clinical contribution to radiobiology. *Clinical Radiology*, 1975; **26**: 67–75.

23. Duncan W, *et al.* An analysis of the radiation related morbidity observed in a randomised trial of neutron therapy for bladder cancer. *International Journal of Radiation Oncology, Biology, Physics*, 1986; **12**: 2085–92.

24. Lyman JT. Complication probability as assessed from dose–volume histograms. *Radiation Research*, 1985; **8**(Suppl.): S13–19.

25. Goitein M. Causes and consequences of inhomogeneous dose distributions in radiation therapy. *International Journal of Radiation Oncology, Biology, Physics*, 1986; **12**: 701–4.

26. Tait D, Nahum A, Southall C, Chow M, Yarnold JR. Benefits expected from simple conformal radiotherapy in the treatment of pelvic tumours. *International Journal of Radiation Oncology, Biology, Physics*, 1988; **13**: 23–30.

27. Armstrong J, *et al.* Promising survival with three-dimensional conformal radiation therapy for non-small cell lung cancer. *Radiotherapy and Oncology*, 1997; **44**: 17–22.

28. Perez CA, *et al.* Cost benefit of emerging technology in localised carcinoma of the prostate. *International Journal of Radiation Oncology, Biology, Physics*, 1997; **39**: 875–83.

29. Suit HD, *et al.* Potential for improvement in radiation therapy. *International Journal of Radiation Oncology, Biology, Physics*, 1988; **14**: 777–86.

30. Van Kampen M, Levegrun S, Wannenmacher. Target volume definition in radiation therapy. *British Journal of Radiology*, 1997.

31. Kupelian PA, Komaki R, Allen P. Prognostic factors in the treatment of node-negative nonsmall cell lung carcinoma with radiotherapy alone. *International Journal of Radiation Oncology, Biology, Physics*, 1996; **36**: 607–13.

32. Leunens G, Menten J, Weltens C, Verstraete J, van der Schueren E. Quality assessment of medical decision making in radiation oncology: variability in target volume delineation for brain tumours. *Radiotherapy and Oncology*, 1993; **29**: 169–75.

33. Valley J, Mirimanoff R. Comparison of treatment techniques for lung cancer. *Radiotherapy and Oncology*, 1993; **28**: 1698–73.

34. Stroom JC, Storchi PRM. Automatic calculation of three-dimensional margins around treatment volumes in radiotherapy planning. *Physics in Medicine and Biology*, 1997; **42**: 745–55.

35. Belshi R, Pontvert D, Rosenwald J-C, Gaboriaud G. Automatic three-dimensional expansion of structures applied to determination of the clinical target volume in conformal radiotherapy. *International Journal of Radiation Oncology, Biology, Physics*, 1997; **37**: 689–96.

36. Goitein M. Limitations of two-dimensional treatment planning programs. *Medical Physics*, 1982; **9**: 580–6.

37. Webb S, *et al.* Clinical dosimetry for radiotherapy to the breast based on imaging with the prototype Royal Marsden Hospital CT simulator. *Physics in Medicine and Biology*, 1987; **32**: 835–45.

38. Dwyer III SJ, Lee KR, Mansfield CR, Fritz SL, Anderson WH, Cook PN. Display strategies using CT scan data for radiation therapy planning. *Proceedings in Medical Information*, 1980; **80**: 9–13.

39. Smith AR, Purdy JA, eds. Three-dimensional photon treatment planning. Report of the collaborative working group on the evaluation of treatment planning for external photon beam radiotherapy. *International Journal of Radiation Oncology, Biology, Physics*, 1991; **21**(1).

40. Kessler ML, McShan DL, Fraass BA. Displays for three-dimensional treatment planning. *Seminars in Radiation Oncology*, 1992; **2**: 226–34.

41. Matsuda T. Clinical significance of computer-controlled conformation radiotherapy—from seven years experience. In: *Proceedings of the 8th International Conference on the Use of Computers in Radiation Therapy*. Silver Spring, USA: IEEE Computer Society Press, 1984: 474.

42. Perry H, Mantel J, Vieque DM, Higdon DL, Lefkofsky MM. Dynamic treatment: automation of a multi-leaf collimator. In: *Proceedings of the 8th International Conference on the Use of Computers in Radiation Therapy*. Silver Spring, USA: IEEE Computer Society Press, 1984: 479.

43. Ishigaki T, Sakuma S, Watanabe M. Computer-assisted rotation and multiple stationary irradiation technique. Newly designed overrunning multileaf collimators for conformation radiotherapy. *European Journal of Radiology*, 1988; **8**: 76–81.

44. Kallman P, Lind B, Eklof A, Brahrne A. Shaping of arbitrary dose distribution by dynamic multileaf collimation. *Physics in Medicine and Biology*, 1988; **33**: 1291–300.

45. Galvin JM, Smith AR, Lally B. Characterisation of a multileaf collimator system. *International Journal of Radiation Oncology, Biology, Physics*, 1993; **25**: 181–92.

46. Fernandez EM, Shentall GS, Mayles WPM, Dearnaley DP. The acceptability of a multileaf collimator as a replacement for conventional blocks. *Radiotherapy and Oncology*, 1995.

47. Webb S. Optimisation by simulated annealing of three-dimensional, conformed treatment planning for radiation fields defined by a multileaf collimator: II. Inclusion of two-dimensional modulation of

the X-ray intensity. *Physics in Medicine and Biology*, 1992; **37**: 1689–704.

48. Derycke S, Van Duyse B, De Gersem W, De Wagter C, De Neve W. Non-coplanar beam intensity modulation allows large dose escalation in stage III lung cancer. *Radiotherapy and Oncology*, 1997; **45**: 253–61.

49. Shiu AS, *et al.* Comparison of miniature multileaf collimation (MMLC) with circular collimation for stereotactic treatment. *International Journal of Radiation Oncology, Biology, Physics*, 1997; **37**: 679–88.

50. Reinstein LE, *et al.* A feasibility study of automated inverse treatment planning for cancer of the prostate. *International Journal of Radiation Oncology, Biology, Physics*, 1998; **40**: 207–14.

51. Mackie TR, *et al.* Tomotherapy: a new concept for the delivery of dynamic conformal radiotherapy. *Medical Physics*, 1993; **20**: 1709–19.

52. Eisbruch A, *et al.* Comprehensive irradiation of head and neck cancer using conformal multisegmental fields: assessment of target coverage and non-involved tissue sparing. *International Journal of Radiation Oncology, Biology, Physics*, 1998; **41**: 559–68.

53. Meeks SL, Buatti JM, Bova FJ, Friedman WA, Mendenhall WM, Ziotecki RA. Potential clinical efficacy of intensity-modulated conformal therapy. *International Journal of Radiation Oncology, Biology, Physics*, 1998; **40**: 483–95.

54. Althof, Hoekstra CJM, te Loo H-J. Variation in prostate position relative to adjacent bony anatomy. *International Journal of Radiation Oncology, Biology, Physics*, 1996; **34**: 709–15.

55. Melian E, *et al.* Variation in prostate position quantitation and implications for three-dimensional conformal treatment planning. *International Journal of Radiation Oncology, Biology, Physics*, 1997; **38**: 73–81.

56. Rabinowitz I, Broomberg, Goitein M, McCarthy K, Leong. Accuracy of radiation field alignment in clinical practice. *International Journal of Radiation Oncology, Biology, Physics*, 1985; **11**: 1857–67.

57. Griffiths SE, Pearcey RO, Thorogood J. Quality control in radiotherapy: the reduction of field placement errors. *International Journal of Radiation Oncology, Biology, Physics*, 1987; **13**: 1583–8.

58. Huizenga IA, Levendag PC, De-Poore PM, Visser AC. Accuracy in radiation field alignment in head and neck cancer: a prospective study. *Radiotherapy and Oncology*, 1988; **11**: 181–7.

59. Lam WC, Partowmah M, Lee DJ, Waram WD, Lam KS. On-line measurement of field placement errors in external beam radiotherapy. *British Journal of Radiology*, 1987; **60**: 361–5.

60. Van Herk M, Meertens H. A matrix ionisation chamber imaging device for on-line patient set-up verification during radiotherapy. *Radiotherapy and Oncology*, 1988; **11**: 369–78.

61. Shalev S, *et al.* Video techniques for on-line portal imaging. *Computerized Medical Imaging and Graphics*, 1989; **13**: 217–26.

62. Swindell W, Simpson RG, Oleson JR, Chen CT, Grubbs EA. Computed tomography with a linear accelerator with radiotherapy applications. *Medical Physics*, 1983; **10**: 416–20.

63. Brahme A, Lind B, Nafstadius P. Radiotherapeutic computed tomography with scanned photon beams. *International Journal of Radiation Oncology, Biology, Physics*, 1987; **13**: 95–101.

64. Huddart R, *et al.* Accuracy of pelvic radiotherapy: prospective analysis of 90 patients in a randomised trial of blocked versus standard radiotherapy. *Radiotherapy and Oncology*, 1996; **39**: 19–29.

65. Killoran JH, Kooy HM, Gladstone DJ, Welte FJ, Beard CJ. A numerical simulation of organ motion and daily setup uncertainties: implications for radiation therapy. *International Journal of Radiation Oncology, Biology, Physics*, 1997; **37**: 213–21.

66. el Khatib E, Battista JJ. Accuracy of lung dose calculations for large-field irradiation with 6-MV X-rays. *Medical Physics*, 1986; **13**: 111–16.

67. ICRU. *Determination of Absorbed Dose in a Patient Irradiated by Beams of X or Gamma Rays in Radiotherapy Procedures.* International Commission on Radiological Units and Measurements, Report No. 24. Bethesda, Maryland: ICRU, 1976.

68. WHO. *Quality Assurance in Radiotherapy.* Geneva: World Health Organization, 1988.

69. Burman C, *et al.* Planning, delivery, and quality assurance of intensity-modulated radiotherapy using dynamic multileaf collimator: a strategy for large-scale implementation for the treatment of carcinoma of the prostate. *International Journal of Radiation Oncology, Biology, Physics*, 1997; **39**: 863–73.

70. Brahme A. Dosimetric precision requirements in radiation therapy. *Acta Radiologica et Oncologica*, 1984; **23**: 379–91.

71. Brahme A, Agren AK. Optimal dose distribution for eradication of heterogeneous tumours. *Acta Oncologica*, 1987; **26**: 377–85.

72. Hansen VN, Evans PM, Shentall GS, Heeler SJ, Yarnold JR, Swindell W. Dosimetric evaluation of compensation in radiotherapy of the breast: MLC intensity modulation and physical compensators. *Radiotherapy and Oncology*, 1997; **42**: 249–356.

73. Rudoller S, *et al.* Patterns of tumour progression after radiotherapy for low grade gliomas: analysis from the computed tomography/magnetic resonance imaging era. *American Journal of Clinical Oncology*, 1998; **21**: 23–7.

74. Sibley GS, Jamieson TA, Marks LB, Anscher MS, Prosnitz LR. Radiotherapy alone for medically inoperable stage I non-small-cell lung cancer: the Duke experience. *International Journal of Radiation Oncology, Biology, Physics*, 1998; **40**: 149–54.

75. Sibley GS. Radiotherapy for patients with medically inoperable stage I nonsmall cell lung carcinoma: smaller volumes and higher doses—a review. *Cancer*, 1998; **82**: 433–8.

76. Yarbro CH, Ferrans CE. Quality of life of patients with prostate cancer treated with surgery or radiation therapy. *Oncology Nursing Forum*, 1998; **25**: 685–93.

77. Keus R, Noach P, deBoer R, Lebesque J. The effect of customised beam shaping on normal tissue complications in radiation therapy of parotid gland tumours. *Radiation Oncology*, 1991; **21**: 211–17.

78. Hanks GE, Schultheiss TE, Hunt MA, Epstein B. Factors influencing incidence of acute grade 2 morbidity in conformal and standard radiation treatment of prostate cancer. *International Journal of Radiation Oncology, Biology, Physics*, 1995; **31**: 25–9.

79. Vijayakumar S, *et al.* Acute toxicity during external beam radiotherapy for localised prostate cancer: comparison of different techniques. *International Journal of Radiation Oncology, Biology, Physics*, 1993; **25**: 359–71.

80. Sandler HM, Perez CA, Tamayo C, Ten-Haken RK, Lichter AS. Dose escalation for stage C (T3) prostate cancer: minimal rectal toxicity observed using conformal therapy. *Radiotherapy and Oncology*, 1992; **23**: 53–4.

81. Forman JD, Duclos M, Shamsa F, Porter AT, Orton C. Hyperfractionated conformal radiotherapy in locally advanced prostate cancer: results of a dose escalation study. *International Journal of Radiation Oncology, Biology, Physics*, 1996; **34**: 655–62.

82. Leibel SA, *et al.* Three-dimensional conformal radiation therapy in locally advanced carcinoma of the prostate: preliminary results of a phase I dose-escalation study. *International Journal of Radiation Oncology, Biology, Physics*, 1994; **28**: 55–65.

83. Robertson JM, *et al.* Dose escalation for non-small cell lung cancer using conformal radiation therapy. *International Journal of Radiation Oncology, Biology, Physics*, 1997; **37**: 1079–85.

84. Tait D, *et al.* Conformal radiotherapy of the pelvis: assessment of acute toxicity. *Radiotherapy and Oncology*, 1993; **29**: 117–26.

85. Mayles WPM, *et al.* The Royal Marsden Hospital pelvic radiotherapy trial: technical aspects and quality assurance. *Radiotherapy and Oncology*, 1993; **29**: 184–91.

86. Tait D, *et al.* Acute toxicity in pelvic radiotherapy; a randomised trial

of conformal versus conventional treatment. *Radiotherapy and Oncology*, 1997; **42**: 121–36.

87. Dearnaley D, Khoo V, Tait D, Yarnold J, Horwich A. Modification of radiation side-effects by conformal radiotherapy techniques in prostate cancer: a randomised trial. *Lancet*, 1999; **353**: 267–73.

88. Koper PC, *et al*. Acute morbidity reduction using 3dcrt for prostate carcinoma: a randomized study. *International Journal of Radiation Oncology, Biology, Physics*, 1999; **43**: 727–34.

89. Nguyen LN, Pollack A, Zagars GK. Late effects after radiotherapy for prostate cancer in a randomized dose–response study: results of a self-assessment questionnaire. *Urology*, 1998; **51**: 991–7.

90. Hanks GE, *et al*. Dose escalation with 3D conformal treatment: five year outcomes, treatment optimisation, and future directions. *International Journal of Radiation Oncology, Biology, Physics*, 1998; **41**: 501–10.

91. Stock RG, Stone NN, Tabert A, Iannuzzi C, DeWyngaert JK. A dose–response study for I-125 prostate implants. *International Journal of Radiation Oncology, Biology, Physics*, 1998; **41**: 101–8.

92. Zelefsky MJ, *et al*. Dose escalation with three-dimensional conformal radiation therapy affects the outcome in prostate cancer. *International Journal of Radiation Oncology, Biology, Physics*, 1998; **41**: 491–500.

93. Pollack A, Zagars GK. External beam radiotherapy dose response of prostate cancer. *International Journal of Radiation Oncology, Biology, Physics*, 1997; **39**: 1011–18.

94. Russell KJ, *et al*. Photon versus fast neutron external beam radiotherapy in the treatment of locally advanced prostate cancer: results of a randomized prospective trial. *International Journal of Radiation Oncology, Biology, Physics*, 1994; **28**: 47–54.

95. Austin-Seymour M, *et al*. Impact of a multi-leaf collimator on treatment morbidity in localized carcinoma of the prostate. *International Journal of Radiation Oncology, Biology, Physics*, 1994; **30**: 1065–71.

96. Rossi Jr CJ, *et al*. Particle beam radiation therapy in prostate cancer: is there an advantage? *Seminars in Radiation Oncology*, 1998; **8**: 115–23.

97. Forman JD, *et al*. Conformal mixed neutron and photon irradiation in localized and locally advanced prostate cancer: preliminary estimates of the therapeutic ratio. *International Journal of Radiation Oncology, Biology, Physics*, 1996; **35**: 259–66.

98. Saunders M, Dische S, Barrett A, Harvey A, Gibson D, Parmar M. Continuous hyperfractionated accelerated radiotherapy (CHART) versus conventional radiotherapy in non-small-cell lung cancer: a randomised multicentre trial. CHART Steering Committee [see comments]. *Lancet*, 1997; **350**: 161–5.

4.3.3 Interstitial and endoluminal radiation therapy

D. Ash

Introduction

The discovery of radium in 1898 opened up the possibility of treating cancer by inserting radioactive material into tumours rather than shining beams of radiation in from the outside. This has the big advantage of concentrating the radiation where it is needed and minimizing the dose elsewhere.

After preliminary work to standardize radium sources, techniques of implantation were developed in the 1930s and 1940s with simple rules to guide the placement of sources and a system for calculating the dose, which made it possible for implants to be performed safely for a wide variety of indications.[1],[2]

Unfortunately, radium is difficult and hazardous to handle and this, together with the development of new linear accelerators with electron capability, led to a fall in the use of brachytherapy. The discovery of artificial radioactive isotopes which are easier to handle and less of a problem for radiation protection and the development of afterloading techniques resulted in a resurgence in brachytherapy in the 1960s and 1970s.[3],[4] New remote afterloading technology, image-guided source placement, and computer dosimetry have now made brachytherapy even safer and more accurate and have also extended its use to sites like the oesophagus and bronchus which were previously inaccessible.

Advantages and disadvantages

The advantages of interstitial therapy include:

(1) close conformity between the target volume and the treated volume;

(2) rapid fall-off of dose to spare surrounding normal tissue;

(3) short overall treatment time which minimizes the opportunity for tumour repopulation; and

(4) low dose-rate radiation which is relatively sparing to normal tissue (this may not apply to fractionated high dose-rate implants).

The potential disadvantages of brachytherapy include:

(1) radiation exposure to personnel—manual afterloading techniques have significantly reduced the risk of radiation exposure and this is practically eliminated when remote afterloading is used;

(2) possible risk of infection and bleeding;

(3) general or local anaesthesia is usually needed to insert the sources or source carriers;

(4) patients usually need to be admitted to hospital; and

(5) implantation skills need to be acquired to achieve satisfactory implants.

Indications

Interstitial implants may be indicated under the following circumstances:

(1) as the sole radical treatment;

(2) as a boost after external-beam radiation;

(3) performed intraoperatively in association with surgery;

(4) as salvage treatment after previous failure of external-beam radiation; and

(5) for palliation.

Most interstitial implants are performed as part of a radical treatment approach but endoluminal brachytherapy for cancers of the oesophagus and bronchus can be used to provide simple and convenient palliative treatment.

Table 1 Radionuclides for interstitial therapy

Radionuclide	Half-life	Energy range (MeV)	Tenth-value layer (cm-Pb)
^{226}Ra	1620 years	0.19–2.43	5.0
^{137}Cs	30 years	0.66	2.2
^{192}Ir	74 days	0.30–0.61	1.5
^{222}Rn	3.8 days	0.05–2.45	5.0
^{198}Au	2.9 days	0.41–1.09	1.1
^{125}I	60 days	0.027–0.035	0.01
^{117}Pd	17 days	0.023–0.027	0.01

Contraindications

There are nearly always alternatives to brachytherapy and these should be considered in the following circumstances:

(1) tumour infiltrating or attached to bone;

(2) presence of active infection within the potential implant volume;

(3) target volume not definable; and

(4) tumour not properly accessible to achieve satisfactory implant geometry.

Types of implantation

Implants may be either removable or permanent and there are various means of brachytherapy delivery.

Removable implants

The vast majority of removable implants are performed with iridium-192, though caesium-137 needles are still used occasionally. This approach requires that the sources or source carriers remain in the patient for the duration of the implant and are removed once the prescribed dose has been delivered.

Most of these implants can now be performed with remote afterloading machines.

Permanent implants

The commonest isotopes used for permanent implants are iodine-125, palladium-117, and gold-198 seeds. These are left in the tissue implanted and gradually give off radioactivity until they become inert. As shown in Table 1, the activity of permanent seed implants is low so that radiation protection can be achieved with relatively simple measures. Permanent implants are not amenable to remote afterloading but the risk of radiation exposure to personnel is extremely low.

Delivery of brachytherapy

Interstitial

The radioactive material is implanted into the tumour and surrounding tissue, for example in the tongue or breast.

Endoluminal

The radiation source is placed within a normal anatomical lumen which may be the site of malignancy, for example the bronchus, oesophagus, or bile duct.

Endocavity

The radiation is inserted into a normal body cavity, most commonly the uterus and cervix.

Surface mould

The radiation is placed a few millimetres above the surface to be treated, for example the skin.

Dosimetry

Dosimetry systems for interstitial brachytherapy are in three parts. The first is a set of rules governing the distribution of radiation sources in order to achieve the optimum dose homogeneity within the target volume. The best known examples are those described in the Manchester and Paris systems of brachytherapy.[2],[5] The second part is a description of how to calculate and specify the dose for brachytherapy and the third a system for dose prescription.

The original systems were developed before computers were available. Since computerized dosimetry of brachytherapy has become widely used there have been several ways in which dose and volume for brachytherapy have been specified. For this reason the International Commission on Radiation Units has recently made recommendations on dose and volume specification for reporting interstitial therapy,[6] which should bring some consistency and comparability to centres practicing brachytherapy.

It is recommended that the following items should be reported when describing brachytherapy applications.

1. Description of volume

    (a) the gross tumour volume;

    (b) the clinical target volume; and

    (c) the treated volume.

2. Description of the sources

    (a) the radionuclide used;

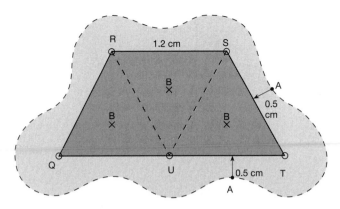

Fig. 1 The central plane of a five-line implant (QRSTU) in equilateral triangles.

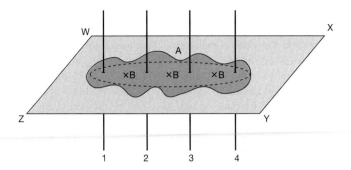

Fig. 2 A four-line implant (wires 1 to 4) has a central plane WXYZ. The mean of the dose rates at point B gives the mean central dose. The minimum target dose is shown at A and the target volume by the dotted line enclosed by the reference isodose.

(b) the type of source;

(c) the length of each source line used;

(d) the reference air kerma rate for each source; and

(e) the distribution of the strength within the source.

3. Description of the technique and source pattern

(a) the number of sources or source lines;

(b) separation between source lines and between planes;

(c) the geometrical pattern formed by the sources within the central plane of the implant, e.g. triangles or squares (Fig. 1);

(d) the surfaces in which the implant lies, i.e. planar or curved;

(e) whether the crossing sources are placed at one or more ends of a group of linear sources;

(f) the material of the inactive vector used to carry the radioactive sources; and

(g) the type of remote afterloading if used.

4. Description of the time pattern

Information on whether the radiation was continuous or non-continuous. If fractionated, there should be information on the radiation time of each fraction or pulse and the interval between fractions plus the overall treatment time.

5. Total reference air kerma (**TRAK**)

The TRAK is the sum of the reference air kerma rate for each source and the irradiation time for each source. This is analogous to the old concept of milligram hours.

6. Description of dose distribution, including

(a) the prescribed dose;

(b) the mean central dose, which is the arithmetic mean of the local minimum doses between sources in the central plane of the implant (Fig. 2); and

(c) the minimum target dose, which is defined as the minimum dose at the periphery of the clinical target volume.

When it is available, the following additional information should also be recorded.

1. The dimensions of the high-dose volumes, which are those encompassed by the isodose corresponding to 150 per cent of the mean central dose.

2. The dimension of any low-dose volume. This is often due to a geographical miss.

3. Dose uniformity data such as the spread in the individual minimum doses used to calculate the mean central dose in the central plane or a dose homogeneity index defined as the ratio of the minimum target dose to the mean central dose.

Dose rate and fractionation in brachytherapy

Until remote afterloading became available all brachytherapy was delivered continuously at low dose rate. Now, however, removable implants can be delivered with a wide variety of different dose rate and fractionation schedules. These include:

(1) continuous low dose rate with or without interruptions;

(2) single fraction, high dose rate;

(3) fractionated high dose rate; and

(4) pulsed.

When continuous low dose-rate implants were performed with radium needles it was recognized that higher dose rates were likely to be more biologically effective than low dose rates and a dose correction was therefore advised if the total dose was to be delivered in a shorter than expected overall treatment time.[7] Early experience with iridium-wire afterloading techniques suggested that a dose rate correction may not be necessary between 30 and 80 cGy/h.[8] Subsequent analysis of large numbers of patients has shown that there is indeed a dose rate effect. For head and neck cancer there is a significant increase in normal tissue complications in patients treated at dose rates of greater than 50 cGy/h compared with lower dose rates, and provided that more than 62.5 Gy total dose is given there is no significant increase in local control rates.[9] For breast cancer there is also a correlation between the probability of achieving local control with brachytherapy and the dose rate used, with higher local control at higher dose rates. It is more difficult, however, to draw correlations between dose-rate effects and normal-tissue morbidity in breast irradiation.[10]

The vast majority of high dose-rate brachytherapy is given either as a single fraction for palliation or as a boost after prior fractionated external-beam radiation. While it is recognized that high dose-rate brachytherapy is relatively more damaging to normal tissue than low dose rate in a way that is analogous to fraction size for external-beam radiation, this is not an issue for palliative treatments, which are well below tissue tolerance. For radical treatments, 66 to 75 per cent of the treatment is given with well-fractionated external-beam treatment so that the few fractions of high dose-rate brachytherapy are well tolerated. There is insufficient information at present to indicate the minimum number of fractions of high dose-rate brachytherapy that might be equivalent to continuous low-dose radiation given as the sole radical treatment.

Pulsed brachytherapy uses a single high-activity source (500 to 1000 mCi). It aims to simulate continuous low dose-rate treatment by stepping along the source carrier at 2.5- to 5-mm intervals in order to reproduce the distribution achieved from a continuous length of iridium. The single source steps through the whole of the implant in approximately 10 min to deliver a pulse of radiation. The pulses can be repeated hourly or at longer intervals. The aim is to deliver the same overall dose in the same overall treatment time but instead of giving the radiation continuously at low dose rate to give it in pulses.

The advantages of the pulsed dose-rate system are the following.

1. Only a single source needs to be prepared.
2. There is complete radiation protection.
3. The patient can be nursed and receive visitors safely between pulses.
4. It is possible to modify the dwell time at each step within the implant in order to optimize the dose distribution.
5. The dose rate per pulse or hour can be kept constant while source activity changes.

The radiobiology of pulsed brachytherapy is complex and the therapeutic ratio depends on knowledge of the relative half-times of repair of human tumours and normal tissues and the time between pulses. Hourly pulses of 50 cGy are likely to be very similar to continuous low dose-rate radiation. When pulse sizes increase and the duration between pulses increases to 3 h or more it is possible that there will be an increase in normal-tissue effect but it will require a lot of carefully collected clinical data to confirm this.[11],[12]

Clinical indications, techniques, and results

Interstitial therapy is of most value in relatively small tumours where radical curative treatment is the aim. It may also be used, however, to deliver a high-dose boost after previous external-beam radiation, and can often be of value as palliative treatment for relatively advanced, radioresistant primary tumours or for recurrences after previous external-beam radiation.

Oral cavity

T1 and small T2 carcinomas of the tongue and floor of mouth are ideal indications for brachytherapy because a very high local dose can be delivered while sparing surrounding normal tissue and achieving high local control rates.

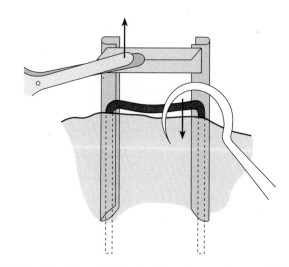

Fig. 3 After the radioactive hairpin has been inserted down the double guide, the guide itself is withdrawn while the crosspiece of the hairpin is held down on to the tissue surface with a Reverdin needle.

The two most commonly used techniques are the hairpin technique and the plastic tube loop technique.

Hairpin technique

The first phase of the implant is performed with inactive, stainless steel, slotted hairpin guides which are positioned in the tongue or floor of mouth and checked for parallelism by fluoroscopy. A stitch is passed under the hairpin guide and the radioactive hairpin is then inserted into the hairpin guide and held down while the guide is removed (Fig. 3). The stitch is then tied over the bridge of the hairpin to secure it in place. The separation between the limbs of the hairpin is fixed at 12 mm so the distance between each hairpin should be 12 to 14 mm to obtain the best homogeneous dose distribution (Fig. 4).

Plastic tube loop technique

For thicker lesions that cannot be encompassed within the 12-mm separation of hairpins, plastic tube loops can be used and also have the advantage of afterloading.

The loop is formed by passing a pair of hollow stainless steel needles through the skin into the oral cavity. A nylon cord is passed up one needle and down the other to form a loop. The stainless steel needles are removed and plastic tubing threaded over the nylon cord, which is then drawn round into the oral cavity to form the loop for afterloading. Two or three pairs of loops are constructed to cover the target volume using a separation of approximately 15 mm (Fig. 5).

The hairpin and plastic tube loop techniques are not suitable for remote afterloading. Straight line sources can be used for afterloading provided that the uppermost part of the plastic tube exits 4 or 5 mm above the mucosal surface and an optimization program is used to increase the dwell time in the top three source positions in order to ensure that the treatment isodose does not dip between the sources and fail to cover the tumour.[13]

The optimum results in terms of local control and avoidance of morbidity are achieved if the following guidelines are met.

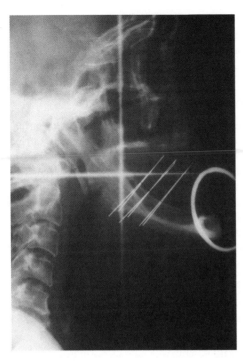

Fig. 4 Three double hairpins implanted into the lateral border of the tongue.

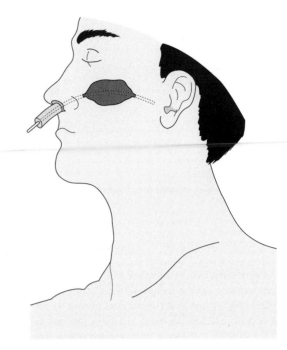

Fig. 6 Balloon catheter positioned in the nasopharynx for high dose-rate afterloading.

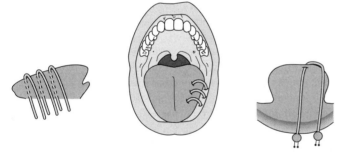

Fig. 5 Plastic tube loops in the tongue.

1. The reference dose rate should be less than 50 cGy/h.
2. Separation between sources should be 12 to 14 mm.
3. The minimum target dose should be 65 Gy.

For T1 and small T2 tumours of the oral cavity treated by brachytherapy alone the local control rate is 80 to 90 per cent. Approximately 20 per cent of patients may develop necrosis within the implant volume but the vast majority heal spontaneously.[14]

For T2 tumours, brachytherapy alone produces 80 to 90 per cent local control, but this falls to 40 to 50 per cent if brachytherapy is given as a boost after prior external-beam radiation. A full dose with brachytherapy is therefore preferable but, because there is approximately 30 per cent risk of occult node involvement, patients should be considered for selective neck dissection after their implant.[15],[16]

For those patients with larger tumours for whom surgery is not appropriate, brachytherapy should be used as a boost after 45 to 50 Gy to the primary site and lymph node areas.

Oropharynx

Tumours in the palate, tonsillar fossa, uvula, and base of tongue have a very high probability of spread to adjacent lymph nodes and it is therefore usual to treat with external-beam radiation in the first instance to deliver 45 to 50 Gy to the primary and regional nodes and to use the implant as a boost to deliver a further 20 to 25 Gy. This can be done either with a hairpin or loop technique. A local control rate of 88 per cent has been reported using these techniques for T1 and T2 tumours.[17]

Nasopharynx

Brachytherapy may have a role as a boost to the site of the primary during initial radical therapy or as salvage treatment for local recurrence.

A simple technique which can be performed under local anaesthesia to outpatients is one using nasal catheters within a balloon that can be positioned and inflated in the nasopharynx under fluoroscopic control. The catheters are connected to an afterloading machine and radiation is given at high dose rate in a fractionated course of treatment (Fig. 6).[18]–[20]

The treatment is most effective for those cases where the tumour is no more than 1 cm from the balloon surface in the nasopharynx. For radical treatment, two fractions of 5 Gy may be given at 1 cm from the balloon surface. For salvage treatment where brachytherapy is the only modality the treatment has to be given in several fractions, but the optimum number is not yet clear.

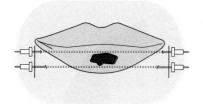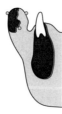

Fig. 7 Needle implant with template for cancer of the lip.

Lip

The lip is extremely well vascularized and tolerates radiation very well. Most tumours can be treated with an afterloading template-type implant (Fig. 7) and local control rates of over 95 per cent can be achieved with excellent cosmetic results in the vast majority of cases.[21] The incidence of lymph node involvement is low even for quite large tumours, but is higher in those cases where the tumour involves the commissure or the buccal mucosa. It is nevertheless not usual to give prophylactic treatment to the regional node areas.

Because of the excellent tolerance of the lip to radiation, it is sometimes possible to use an iridium wire implant to give a second radical treatment dose to salvage recurrences after previous external-beam radiation.

Neck nodes

Brachytherapy can be useful as a salvage treatment for patients who develop fixed malignant nodes in a previously irradiated area.

It is best to adopt an approach using surgical resection to remove as much tumour as possible combined with an iridium wire implant whereby plastic tubes are placed in the tumour bed over the likely site of residual disease. The surgical defect is covered with a vascularized flap which brings new blood supply to the previously irradiated tissue and the plastic tubes are afterloaded with iridium wire a few days after surgery.

Even though the patient has had previous irradiation, a dose of 60 Gy is necessary to achieve local control of disease and is usually well tolerated.

Skin cancer

The majority of skin cancers can be very adequately treated either by surgery or by superficial X-ray therapy or electron-beam radiation. There are some sites, however, where implant therapy allows a complex target volume to be covered more accurately and simply with interstitial rather than external-beam techniques and brings with it the advantages of a high rate of local control with excellent cosmesis. Brachytherapy can also be used for salvage of local recurrences within previously irradiated areas.

Cancers of the skin of the nose and nasal vestibule are a good indication for interstitial therapy and results in over 1600 cases have shown an overall local control rate of 93 per cent.[22] Cancers of the pinna can also be treated by brachytherapy and a 98 per cent

local control rate has been reported with good cosmesis and low complication rates.[23]

For some superficial skin cancers brachytherapy can be delivered in the form of a surface mould rather than as interstitial treatment.

Carcinoma of the prostate

As a result of testing for prostate-specific antigen, an increasing number of patients now present with localized carcinoma of the prostate which is suitable for radical local treatment. The disease is also being found increasingly in men under the age of 70.

Prostate cancer is not very sensitive to radiation and high doses need to be given to achieve local control. Brachytherapy provides the opportunity to give very high doses to the prostate with low doses to surrounding normal tissue and can often be done as a day case procedure. The indications for brachytherapy are similar to those for radical prostatectomy:

(1) life expectancy greater than 10 years;

(2) biopsy-proven adenocarcinoma;

(3) disease confined within the prostate capsule, i.e. T1 and T2;

(4) bone scan negative;

(5) CT or MRI negative with no evidence of pelvic node involvement; and

(6) prostate-specific antigen less than 30.

Initial experience with prostate implants was with radioactive iodine seeds inserted under direct vision into a prostate surgically exposed by retropubic incision.[24] It was difficult with this technique, however, to ensure even seed distribution within the prostate and the resulting hot spots and cold spots were responsible for late complications and failures.[25]

Over the last few years new techniques using ultrasound and template-guided needle placement which is performed percutaneously have shown that it is possible to achieve homogeneous dose delivery with a minimum of 160 Gy to the prostate capsule.[26],[27] Results to date show survival free from relapses of prostate-specific antigen which is equivalent to that for similarly staged patients treated by radical prostatectomy, but with a treatment that is much more convenient and with significantly less morbidity.[28]–[32]

Anal canal

The conventional surgical technique is abdominoperineal excision, which inevitably results in a permanent colostomy for all patients. It is now clear, however, that squamous carcinoma of the anal canal can be cured by radiation and the majority of patients are suitable for an attempt at conservative treatment. It is usual to treat by external-beam radiation in the first instance to cover the primary tumour and the drainage areas of the perirectal lymph nodes. The need to include areas drained by inguinal lymph nodes remains controversial.

The anal canal and, in particular, the perianal margin tolerate radiation poorly and it is important to use an implantation technique that avoids convergence and divergence of the radioactive sources. This can be achieved with a template, which ensures accurate positioning of the source through the period of implantation (Fig. 8).

It is not necessary for patients to have a colostomy before implantation but suitable bowel preparation is required. Six to eight

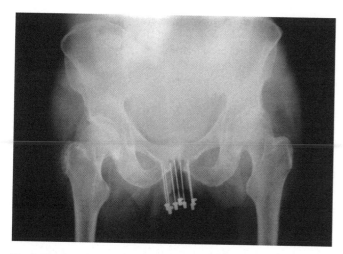

Fig. 8 Template implant for carcinoma of the anal canal.

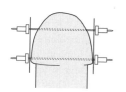 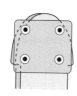 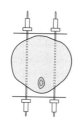

Fig. 9 Template implant for carcinoma of the penis.

weeks after external-beam radiation (to a dose of 30 to 40 Gy) the implant is made, using the template technique, to deliver a further 20 to 30 Gy. Papillon[33] has reported a 5-year survival of 68 per cent with these techniques. This is comparable with results that can be achieved by radical surgery, but the vast majority of patients have retained normal anal function.

It is now possible to achieve still higher rates of local control in anal carcinoma using a combination of external-beam radiation and cytotoxic chemotherapy. The complications associated with radical external-beam radiation in the perineum, however, are considerable. It may still be better, therefore, to use chemoradiation first and to complete treatment of the primary with an interstitial implant.

Penis

Radical or partial amputation is the conventional surgical treatment for these cases and provides good local control. The majority of patients, however, would prefer to avoid surgery and it is quite possible to cure cancer of the penis by radiation.

Tumours up to 3 cm in diameter are suitable for interstitial implantation using a template. Prior circumcision is essential and an indwelling urinary catheter is used during the period of implantation (Fig. 9).

The testicles and groins are protected from radiation by supporting the penis in a foam block. The usual dose is 65 Gy. After this there are 3 to 4 weeks of urethritis and skin reaction. When this has settled, urinary and sexual function return to normal in the vast majority of

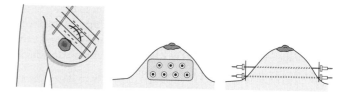

Fig. 10 Template implant to deliver a boost to the tumour bed after local excision of breast cancer.

patients. Meatal stenosis may occur in a few, but is usually amenable to simple dilatation.

Treatment by implantation shows a local control rate of 95 per cent.[34] The majority of sexually active patients retain their potency. These results suggest that for the patient with early carcinoma of the penis, neither their survival nor their chance of local control will be compromised by conservative treatment, and surgery should be reserved for salvage.

Carcinoma of the breast

Interstitial implants can be used in the management of breast cancer in a number of different ways, as described in the next three subsections.

As a boost to the tumour bed for conservative treatment of operable breast cancer

Some 80 to 90 per cent of recurrences after local excision of breast cancer are in the tumour bed. The volume of tissue around the excision site is therefore at higher risk of recurrence than other parts of the breast, and it is likely that the risk of recurrence can be reduced by giving a greater radiation dose. If high doses of radiation are given by transcutaneous external-beam techniques, skin tolerance will be exceeded and the cosmetic result will be impaired. Implantation techniques are therefore indicated in order to deliver a high dose to the deeper tissues at risk without damaging the skin and subcutaneous tissues. Implantation is usually best done with a template to achieve a two- or three-plane volume implant (Fig. 10), but at the periphery of the breast a single-plane implant using plastic tubing may be preferable. Some 10 to 14 days after external-beam radiation (to 45 to 50 Gy) the tumour bed is boosted with an implant that delivers an additional 20 to 25 Gy. Using such techniques the local control rate for T1 tumours is 93 per cent at 7 years and 89 per cent for T2 tumours.[35] Breast boosts may also be given effectively with high dose-rate remote afterloading.[36]

It is almost certainly not necessary to use an implant boost for all patients and it may be preferable to reserve implantation for patients who are at higher than usual risk of recurrence.[37] Conservative treatment is usually restricted to patients with tumours of less than 3 to 4 cm in diameter. For patients with larger tumours it is still possible to consider breast conservation and in these cases preoperative radiation is given with the tumour in place. The tumour residue is then excised and an implant carried out to the tumour bed at the time of the operation.

As a boost to residual tumour after radiotherapy for inoperable disease

Patients who present with large inoperable tumours require a very high dose of radiation in order to achieve local control. In these cases, treatment is therefore given by external-beam radiation in the first instance, and the dose to the residual tumour then boosted with an implant. In this way it is possible to increase the total dose to the centre of the tumour to 85 to 90 Gy, which has been shown to achieve a considerably higher rate of local control.[38]

As salvage for local recurrence

Chest wall recurrences after mastectomy and postoperative radiation are often the first sign of more widely disseminated disease and frequently occur in the form of diffuse dermal infiltration. For the less common patients who develop localized, apparently solitary recurrences in an irradiated field where simple surgery is not appropriate, implantation provides another opportunity for local control. A single-plane implant with the plastic tube technique is usually best and it is necessary to deliver at least 50 to 60 Gy in order to regain local control, which may be quite long lasting provided the patient is not affected by spread of disease elsewhere.

Intracranial tumours

Primary brain tumours are relatively resistant to radiation and it is not often possible to achieve local control by conventional doses of radiation given with external-beam techniques, even with multiple fields. Interstitial implantation is one way in which local radiation dose can be increased without intolerable damage to surrounding tissues but, until recently, this has been difficult to do because of problems of accurate tumour localization and of the placement of radioctive sources.

New techniques of stereotactic localization with computed tomography can, however, now allow safe and accurate implantation to be applied to a variety of malignant tumours in the brain. Interstitial implantation has a role in sites where surgery would be hazardous and has also been used for recurrences after previous surgery and external-beam radiation. The majority of treated patients have had gliomas, but some secondary tumours have also been treated. Tumours less than 5 cm in diameter have been selected for implantation, which has delivered doses of 60 to 100 Gy, often in conjunction with external-beam radiation.

Because the patients have been highly selected, it remains unclear what the place of implantation will come to be in relation to other treatment techniques for brain tumours; no randomized comparisons have been made. For selected gliomas, however, a median survival of 12 to 15 months has been claimed, with approximately 40 per cent of patients alive at 1 year.[39]-[42]

Cancer of the female reproductive tract

The main role for brachytherapy in these cancers is in intracavitary treatment for carcinomas of the cervix and uterus, which is described elsewhere. Interstitital treatment does, however, have a role under certain cirumstances, three of which are described in the next subsections.

Carcinoma of the vagina

It is usual to treat carcinomas of the vagina by external-beam radiation in the first instance. This will often cause sufficient regression of the primary tumour to allow it to be boosted by brachytherapy from an intravaginal, central source. Where the residual tumour is 1 cm or more in thickness, interstitial therapy may be indicated in order to extend the treated volume of the radiation deeper into the tissues. This can be achieved by interstitial implantation of iridium-wire hairpins or by using a template technique similar to that for carcinoma of the anal canal.

For some lesions a combination of a central vaginal source plus interstitial implantation is required. The higher dose that can be achieved by an interstitial implant boost is often of value in improving local control.

Urethra

The urethra and suburethral vulval mucosa are rarely the site of a primary tumour but more commonly involved by secondary deposits, particularly from endometrial carcinoma. After catheterization of the urethra a circumferential palisade of needles can be implanted, often with a template technique. Good palliation of these troublesome lesions can be achieved by this method.

Parametrium

Stages 2B and 3 carcinoma of the cervix are often associated with bulky disease that cannot be controlled by conventional doses of eternal-beam radiation. Techniques have been developed to boost the dose to the parametrium by an iridium-wire implant in selected cases in order to try and improve local control. Parametrial implants require rigid templates and often involve implantation of large volumes of tissue, when both sides are implanted simultaneously. There is a 10 to 20 per cent risk of serious complications, particularly in relation to the bladder base, small bowel, and ureter, but local recurrence rates have been reduced from approaching 50 per cent to around 25 per cent.[43]-[45]

Carcinoma of the bladder

Before the era of megavoltage radiation, implantation was frequently used in bladder cancers in order to achieve a high dose within a deep seated tumour. As megavoltage therapy improved and transurethral resection advanced, implantation gradually fell out of use. The exception to this general trend was in Rotterdam, where interstitial implantation with radium or caesium needles continued for a long time. A very large series of cases treated with radium-needle implants has shown unequalled local control in selected patients.[46] As local control remains a problem in a significant proportion of infiltrating bladder cancers, new afterloading techniques using iridium wire have been developed to try to achieve similar results but with less radiation exposure. These techniques have achieved a 5-year local control rate of 88.5 per cent in T1 and T2 tumours.[47],[48]

Soft tissue sarcoma

Local excision of soft tissue sarcomas is associated with a high rate of local recurrence, but it has been shown that conservative surgery plus radical postoperative radiotherapy can achieve results as good as those of mutilating radical surgery. One of the ways of achieving a high dose of localized radiation to the tumour bed after surgery for sarcoma is to make a perioperative implant where plastic tubes can be laid in the tumour bed for afterloading when the wound has been closed.[49],[50] There are problems in obtaining satisfactory geometry in many patients, but an implant used in this way can deliver a boost to the tumour bed if associated with wider field, external-beam radiation. Improvements in local control have been claimed for these techniques.[51],[52]

Carcinoma of the bronchus

The vast majority of bronchial carcinomas are not suitable for radical treatment and for those that can be completely resected surgically there is little evidence that adjuvant local therapy improves results. There may, however, be a small group of patients in whom minimal residual disease at surgery can be implanted at the time of operation and when this may contribute to cure. A subgroup in which this approach may be appropriate is that of superior sulcus tumours; these are often slowly growing and late to metastasize. A selected series of patients treated with perioperative iodine-125 implantation has shown a local control rate of 68 per cent for those implanted compared with 57 per cent for those treated conventionally.[53] Differences in survival were not statistically significant. In a larger group of patients who received perioperative iodine-125 implants for incomplete resection or positive mediastinal nodes, a 5-year survival of 6 per cent was achieved.[53]

The majority of patients with inoperable lung cancer are suitable for simple palliation only, particularly for symptoms of endobronchial obstruction and bleeding. High dose-rate afterloading machines have now been developed with fine catheters that can be positioned by fibreoptic endoscopy within endobronchial tumours. These are afterloaded with high-activity iridium-192 by remote control, which delivers a large dose of radiation directly to the tumour and 7.5 to 15 Gy at 0.5 cm from the source. It is often possible to treat patients in a single session without the need for general anaesthesia and very useful palliation has been reported with minimal morbidity.[54]–[57] It is also possible to use brachytherapy curatively for small tumours either with or without external-beam therapy.[58]

Carcinoma of the oesophagus

Similar high dose-rate afterloading techniques to those described for bronchial carcinoma can be used for inoperable tumours of the oesophagus. Good palliation can be achieved in one or two treatments with minimal morbidity and the majority of patients are suitable for this form of treatment.[59] As local recurrence remains a considerable problem in those patients in whom radical radiotherapy is attempted, there is reason to hope that local control can be improved for these patients by combining endocavity irradiation with external-beam techniques.[60]

Salvage therapy after previous radical radiotherapy

If there are recurrences after external-beam radiation it is rarely possible to reirradiate with external-beam techniques without a substantial risk of necrosis. Perhaps because of the radiobiological advantage of continuous low dose rate, it is possible to reirradiate with implant therapy in some clinical situations, when local control can be regained without exceeding the tolerance of normal tissue. In a series of 70 patients with new or recurrent oropharyngeal cancers arising in previously irradiated tissue an actuarial, local control rate of 60 per cent was achieved at 5 years. Twenty seven of these patients developed mucosal ulceration or necrosis, of which half were successfully managed conservatively.[61] When considering salvage therapy it is often tempting, because of the previous radiation, to give less than a radical dose, but where long-term control is the aim, this is rarely achieved with low doses and at least 60 Gy is required. Meticulous technique is necessary to avoid hot spots in such salvage implants and somewhat lower than usual dose rates may possibly make necrosis less likely.

Brachytherapy for benign disease

There are a number of indications where brachytherapy is of value in benign disease. The common link is in its role as a localized means of preventing or reducing stromal proliferation either from fibroblasts, smooth muscle cells, or new blood vessels.

Keloids

Keloid scars are not only unsightly but often itchy and painful. Simple surgical excision is followed by recurrence in over 80 per cent of cases.

Excision can be combined with brachytherapy by positioning a plastic tube in the suture line after excision of the keloid. Afterloading with iridium wire to deliver a dose of 15 Gy at 0.5 cm will reduce the recurrence rate down to approximately 20 per cent.[62]

Pterygium

Pterygium is a condition where a pad of connective tissue with blood vessels grows over the cornea. Simple excision is followed by recurrence in a high proportion of patients and can be significantly reduced by following excision with brachytherapy using a strontium plaque applied to the cornea.[63]

Peripheral vascular disease

Following balloon angioplasty of stenosed peripheral arteries, up to 50 per cent of patients may experience restenosis within a year of dilatation. This is thought to be due to neointimal proliferation initiated by the disrupted smooth muscle cells in the arterial wall.

Endovascular brachytherapy using an iridium-wire source that can be afterloaded into an arterial balloon catheter reduces the risk of restenosis down to approximately 20 per cent.[64]

Coronary artery disease

As for peripheral arteries, coronary artery angioplasty is commonly followed by restenosis. For small coronary arteries a β-radiation source is necessary and can be made small enough to pass into the predilated coronary artery. Like peripheral vessels the risk of restenosis is reduced by approximately 50 per cent.[65] Clinical trials are currently in progress to confirm the efficacy of endovascular brachytherapy.

References

1. **Quimby EH.** Dosage calculations in radium therapy. *American Journal of Roentgenology,* 1947; **57**: 622–7.

2. **Meredith WJ,** ed. *Radium Dosage: the Manchester System.* Edinburgh: Livingstone, 1949.

3. **Henschke UK, Hilaris BS, Mahan GD.** Afterloading in interstitial and

intracavitary radiation therapy. *American Journal of Roentgenology*, 1963; **90**: 386–95.

4. Pierquin B. *Precis de Curietherapie*. Paris: Masson, 1964.

5. Pierquin B, Dutreix A, Paine C, Chassagne D, Marinello G, Ash D. The Paris System in interstitital radiation therapy. *Acta Radiologica et Oncologica*, 1978; **17**: 33–47.

6. International Commission on Radiological Units and Measurements (ICRU). *Dose and Volume Specification for Reporting Interstitial Therapy*. Report No. 58. Washington, DC: ICRU Publications, 1997.

7. Patterson R. Studies in optimum dosage. *British Journal of Radiology*, 1952; **25**: 505–16.

8. Pierquin B, Chassagne D, Baillet F, Paine CH. Clinical observations on the time factor in interstitial radiotherapy using iridium 192. *Clinical Radiology*, 1973; **24**: 506–9.

9. Mazeron JJ, *et al.* Effect of dose rate on local control and complications in definitive irradiation of T1 to 2 squamous cell carcinomas of mobile tongue and floor of mouth with interstitital iridium 192. *Radiotherapy and Oncology*, 1991; **21**: 39–47.

10. Mazeron JJ, *et al.* Influence of dose rate on local control of breast carcinoma treated by external beam irradiation plus iridium 192 implant. *International Journal of Radiation Oncology, Biology, Physics*, 1991; **21**: 1173–7.

11. Brenner OJ, Hall EJ. Conditions for the equivalence of continuous to pulsed low dose rate brachytherapy. *International Journal of Radiation Oncology, Biology, Physics*, 1991; **20**: 181–90.

12. Fowler JF, Mount M. Pulsed brachytherapy: the conditions for no significant loss of therapeutic ratio compared with traditional low dose rate brachytherapy. *International Journal of Radiation Oncology, Biology, Physics*, 1992; **23**: 661–9.

13. Sethi T, Ash D, Flynn A, Workman G. Replacement of hairpin and loop implants by optimised straight line sources. *Radiotherapy and Oncology*, 1996; **39**: 117–21.

14. Mazeron JJ, Crook JM, Marinello G, Walop W, Pierquin B. Prognostic factors of local outcome for T1, T2 carcinomas of oral tongue treated by iridium 192 implantation. *International Journal of Radiation Oncology, Biology, Physics*, 1990; **19**: 281–5.

15. Pernot M, Malissard L, Aletti P, Hoffstetter S, ForVard JJ, Bey P. Iridium 192 brachytherapy in the management of 147 T2 N0 oral tongue carcinomas treated with radiation alone: comparison of two treatment techniques. *International Journal of Radiation Oncology, Biology, Physics*, 1992; **23**: 223–8.

16. Bachaud JM, *et al.* Radiotherapy for stage one and two carcinomas of the mobile tongue and/or floor of mouth. *Radiotherapy and Oncology*, **31**: 199–206.

17. Mazeron JJ, *et al.* Definitive radiation treatment for early stage carcinoma of the soft palate and uvula: the indications for iridium 192 implantation. *International Journal of Radiation Oncology, Biology, Physics*, 1987; **13**: 1829–37.

18. Wang CC, Busse J, Gitterman M. A simple afterloading applicator for intracavitary irradiation of carcinoma of the nasopharynx. *Radiology*, 1975; **115**: 737–8.

19. Teo PM, Kwan WH, Yu P, Lee WY, Leung SF, Choi P. A retrospective study of the role of intracavitary brachytherapy and prognostic factors determining local tumour control after primary radical radiotherapy in 903 non-disseminated nasopharyngeal carcinoma patients. *Clinical Oncology*, 1996; **8**: 160–6.

20. Slevin NJ, Wilkinson JM, Filby HM, Gupta NK. Intracavitary radiotherapy boosting for nasopharynx cancer. *British Journal of Radiology*, 1997; **70**: 412–14.

21. Pigneux J, Richard P, Lagarde C. The place of interstitial therapy using iridium 192 in the management of carcinoma of the lip. *Cancer*, 1979; **43**: 1073–7.

22. Mazeron JJ, *et al.* Radiation therapy of carcinomas of the skin of nose and nasal vestibule: a report of 1676 cases from the Group Europeen de Curietherapie. *Radiotherapy and Oncology*, 1989; **13**: 165–73.

23. Mazeron JJ, *et al.* Radiation therapy for carcinoma of the pinna using iridium 192 wires: a series of 70 patients. *International Journal of Radiation Oncology, Biology, Physics*, 1986; **12**: 1757–63.

24. Whitmore WF, Hilaris BS, Grabstald H, Batata MA. Implantation of iodine 125 in prostatic cancer. *Surgical Clinics of North America*, 1974; **54**: 887–95.

25. Fowler JE Jr, Barzell W, Hilaris BS, Whitmore WF Jr. Complications of iodine 125 implantation and pelvic lymphadenectomy in the treatment of prostatic cancer. *Journal of Urology*, 1979; **121**: 447–51.

26. Holm HH, Juul N, Pederson JF, Hansen H, Stroyer I. Transperineal I^{125} seed implantation in prostatic cancer guided by transrectal ultrasonography. *Journal of Urology*, 1983; **130**: 293–6.

27. Blasko JC, Ragde H, Schumacher D. Transperineal percutaneous iodine 125 implantation for prostate carcinoma using transrectal ultrasound and template guidance. *Endocurietherapy, Hyperthermia, Oncology*, 1987; **3**: 131.

28. Blasko JC, Grimm PD, Ragde H. Brachytherapy and organ preservation in the management of carcinoma of the prostate. *Seminars in Radiation Oncology*, 1993; **3**: 240–9.

29. Kaye KW, Olson DJ, Payne JT. Detailed preliminary analysis of iodine-125 implantation for localised prostate cancer using percutaneous approach. *Journal of Urology*, 1995; **153**: 1020–5.

30. Stock RG, *et al.* Prostate specific antigen findings and biopsy results following interactive ultrasound guided transperineal brachytherapy for early stage prostate carcinoma. *Cancer*, 1996; **77**: 2386–92.

31. Beyer DC, Priestley JB. Biochemical disease free survival following iodine-125 prostate implantation. *International Journal of Radiation Oncology, Biology, Physics*, 1997; **37**: 559–63.

32. Ragde H, *et al.* Brachytherapy for clinically localised prostate cancer: results at 7 and 8 year follow up. *Seminars in Surgical Oncology*, 1997; **13**: 438–43.

33. Papillon J. *Rectal and Anal Cancers*. Berlin: Springer Verlag, 1982.

34. Daly NJ, Douchez J, Combes PM. Treatment of carcinoma of the penis by iridium 192 wire implant. *International Journal of Radiation Oncology, Biology, Physics*, 1982; **8**: 1239–43.

35. Pierquin B, Mazeron JJ, Glaubiger D. Conservative treatment of breast cancer in Europe: Report of the Groupe Europeen de Curietherapie. *Radiotherapy and Oncology*, 1986; **6**: 187–98.

36. Hammer J, Seewald DH, Track C, Zoidl JP, Labeck W. Breast cancer: primary treatment with external beam radiation therapy and high dose rate iridium implantation. *Radiology*, 1994; **193**: 573–7.

37. Rathmell A, Ash D. Radiotherapy after conservative surgery for breast cancer: selective use of iridium 192 wire boost to tumour bed in high risk patients. *Clinical Oncology*, 1991; **3**: 204–8.

38. Arriagada R, Mouriesse H, Sarrazin D, Clark RM, DeBoer G. Radiotherapy alone in breast cancer. Analysis of tumour parameters, tumour dose and local control: the experience of the Gustave Roussy Institute and the Princess Margaret Hospital. *International Journal of Radiation Oncology, Biology, Physics*, 1985; **11**: 1751–7.

39. Halligan JB, Stelzer KJ, Rostomily RC, Spence AM, Griffin TW, Berger MS. Operation and permanent low activity iodine 125 brachytherapy for recurrent high grade astrocytomas. *International Journal of Radiation Oncology, Biology, Physics*, 1996; **35**: 541–7.

40. Mundinger F, *et al.* Long term outcome of 89 low grade brain stem gliomas after interstitital radiation therapy. *Journal of Neurosurgery*, 1991; **75**: 740–6.

41. Burnstein M, Laperierre N. Indications for brachytherapy for brain tumours. *Acta Neurochirurgica, Supplementum*, 1995; **63**: 25–8.

42. McDermott MW, Sneed PK, Gutin PH. Interstitial brachytherapy for malignant brain tumours. *Seminars in Surgical Oncology*, 1998; **14**: 79–87.

43. **Martinez A, Edmondson GK, Cox RS, Gunderson LL, Howes AE.** Combination of external beam irradiation and multiple site perineal applicator (MUPIT) for treatment of locally advanced or recurrent prostatic, anorectal and gynaecologic malignancies. *International Journal of Radiation Oncology, Biology, Physics*, 1985; **11**: 391–8.

44. **Aristizabel SA, Woolfitt B, Valencia X, Ocampo G, Surwit EA, Sim D.** Interstitial parametrial implants in carcinoma of the cervix stage IIB. *International Journal of Radiation Oncology, Biology, Physics*, 1987; **13**: 445–50.

45. **Erickson B, Gillin MT.** Interstitial implantation of gynaecological malignancies. *Journal of Surgical Oncology*, 1997; **66**: 285–95.

46. **Van der Werf-Messing BHP.** Cancer of urinary bladder treated by interstitial radium implant. *International Journal of Radiation Oncology, Biology, Physics*, 1979; **4**: 373–8.

47. **Mazeron JJ, et al.** Conservative treatment of bladder carcinoma by partial cystectomy and interstitial iridium 192. *International Journal of Radiation Oncology, Biology, Physics*, 1988; **15**: 1323–30.

48. **Wijnmaalen A, et al.** (1997). Muscle invasive bladder cancer treated by transurethral resection, followed by external beam radiation and interstitial iridium 192. *International Journal of Radiation Oncology, Biology, Physics*, 1997; **39**: 1043–52.

49. **Collins JE, Paine CH, Ellis F.** The treatment of connective tissue sarcomas by local excision followed by radioactive implant. *Clinical Radiology*, 1976; **27**: 39–41.

50. **Mills EED, Hering ER.** Management of soft tissue tumours by limited surgery combined with tumour bed irradiation using brachytherapy and supplemental teletherapy. *British Journal of Radiology*, 1981; **54**: 312–17.

51. **Devlin PM, Harrison LB.** Brachytherapy for soft tissue sarcomas. *Cancer Treatment and Research*, 1997; **91**: 107–28.

52. **Burmeister BH, Dickinson I, Bryant G, Doody J.** Intra-operative implant brachytherapy in the management of soft tissue sarcomas. *Australian and New Zealand Journal of Surgery*, 1997; **67**: 5–8.

53. **Hilaris BS, Martini N, Wong GY, Nori D.** Treatment of superior sulcus tumour (Pancoast tumour). *Surgical Clinics of North America*, 1987; **5**: 965–77.

54. **Hilaris BS, Martini N.** Interstitial brachytherapy in cancer of the lung: 20 years experience. *International Journal of Radiation Oncology, Biology, Physics*, 1979; **5**: 1951–6.

55. **Seagren FL.** Endobronchial irradiation: a review. *Endocurietherapy, Hyperthermia, Oncology*, 1986; **2**: 87–91.

56. **Gollins SW, Burt PA, Barber PV, Stout R.** Long term survival and symptom palliation in small primary bronchial carcinomas following treatment with intraluminal radiotherapy alone. *Clinical Oncology*, 1996; **8**: 239–46.

57. **Barber P, Stout R.** High dose rate endobronchial brachytherapy for the treatment of lung cancer: current status and indications. *Thorax*, 1996; **51**: 345–7.

58. **Gaspar LE.** Brachytherapy in lung cancer. *Journal of Surgical Oncology*, 1998; **67**: 60–70.

59. **Rowland CG, Pagliero KM.** Intracavitary irradiation in palliation of carcinoma of the oesophagus and cardia. *Lancet*, 1985; **ii**: 981–3.

60. **Schraube P, Fritz P, Wannenmacher MF.** Combined endoluminal and external irradiation of inoperable oesophageal carcinoma. *Radiotherapy and Oncology*, 1997; **44**: 45–51.

61. **Mazeron JJ, et al.** Salvage irradiation of oropharyngeal cancers using iridium 192 wire implant: 5 year results of 17 cases. *International Journal of Radiation Oncology, Biology, Physics*, 1987; **13**: 957–62.

62. **Peiffert D, et al.** Surgery and curietherapy of keloids. *Revue de Stomatologie et de Chirurgie Maxillo-Faciale*, 1995; **92**: 108–12.

63. **Pajonk F, Flick H, Mittelviefhaus H, Slanina J.** Post operative pterygium prevention by radiotherapy with strontium-90 β-rays. *Frontiers of Radiation Therapy and Oncology*, 1997; **30**: 259–64.

64. **Schopohl B, et al.** Ir192 endovascular brachytherapy for avoidance of intimal hyperplasia after percutaneous transluminal angioplasty and stent implantation in peripheral vessels; 6 years of experience. *International Journal of Radiation Oncology, Biology, Physics*, 1996; **36**: 835–40.

65. **Teirstein PS, et al.** Catheter based radiotherapy to inhibit restenosis after coronary stenting. *New England Journal of Medicine*, 1997; **336**: 1697–703.

4.3.4 Intracavitary therapy

Peter Blake, Colin H. Jones, and G. Gordon Steel

Introduction

Intracavitary therapy is 'brachytherapy', short-distance irradiation achieved by the insertion of sealed radioactive sources into body cavities. It has been confined largely to the treatment of gynaecological malignancies, particularly those of the cervix, vagina, and uterus, although there has been a small role for the use of conventional intracavitary sources in the treatment of some cancers of the nasopharynx.

With the development of high dose-rate systems using microsources, the range of body sites now amenable to intracavitary, intraluminal, and interstitial therapy is widening. In particular, experience is growing in the area of the intraluminal therapy of bronchial and oesophageal cancers, either for primary therapy alone, in combination with external radiotherapy, or as treatment for recurrence in a previously irradiated volume. Intraluminal therapy is discussed further in Chapter 4.3.3 and specific applications in the chapters on head and neck, gastrointestinal, and lung cancers.

Gynaecological intracavitary treatment

This type of treatment began very soon after the discovery of radium at the end of the nineteenth century as, before the development of megavoltage radiotherapy, external-beam treatment of central pelvic tumours was made difficult by poor penetration of orthovoltage X-rays. Some tumours in the body of the uterus, the cervix, and the vagina could be treated by internal irradiation from radioactive sources placed in the uterine cavity and vagina. This 'intracavitary' treatment was found to be sufficient to eradicate early disease and to be a convenient method of reducing tumour bulk prior to surgery for larger tumours. Inoperable tumours were treated by a combination of both intracavitary and external-beam treatment.

Naturally occurring radium was the first isotope used and several systems of placing intracavitary radium in the uterus, cervix, and vagina were developed. The most important of these were the 'Stockholm' and 'Paris' systems in which radium was carried in an intrauterine tube and specially shaped vaginal boxes and cylinders. These systems have been further developed over the years and, for safety reasons, radium has been replaced by caesium.

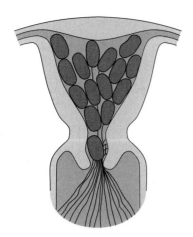

Fig. 1 Diagram of the arrangement of Heyman's capsules within the uterine cavity.

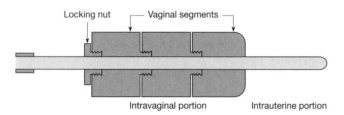

Locking nut — Vaginal segments —

Intravaginal portion   Intrauterine portion

Fig. 2 An intracavitary applicator for the irradiation of the vagina and body of uterus in continuity.

The dose distribution within the uterine cavity from an intrauterine tube and vaginal applicators was not suitable for the radical treatment of endometrial cancer. To irradiate the uterine wall, systems of packing the uterus with multiple radioactive sources were developed. Most widely used were 'Heyman's capsules'. These were metal capsules each containing a radium source, attached to long strings and were packed into the uterine cavity in a known order so that, at the completion of treatment, they could be withdrawn in reverse order. Great skill was needed to position the capsules to remain stable throughout the treatment period, to give a homogeneous dose to the uterine wall, and to avoid them becoming tangled (Fig. 1).

Tumours of the vagina or those of the cervix or endometrium extending into the lower two-thirds of the vagina could be irradiated using a vaginal obturator, often known as a 'Dobbie', of a variable length and diameter. This obturator was loaded centrally with a radioactive line source which, in some systems, could extend beyond the obturator to pass through the cervix into the uterine cavity as necessary (Fig. 2).

Active applicators may contain permanent sources or may be loaded with sources of a chosen activity for the individual patient (preloaded). However, a major development in intracavitary therapy has been the replacement of active applicators with hollow applicator tubes which, after being inserted and positioned correctly, are manually or remotely afterloaded with the radioisotope (usually caesium-137) only when the patient has returned to the ward.

Remote afterloading systems eliminate completely the irradiation of staff, allowing higher activity sources to be used so that intracavitary therapy can be administered over a shorter period of time. Shorter treatment times have the advantages of less discomfort for the patient, less morbidity from prolonged bed rest, the possibility of a greater patient throughput and, therefore, greater cost-effectiveness. However, the safe doses, determined empirically in the days of radium therapy, can no longer be used without modification if the dose rate is increased. Modern low dose-rate remote afterloading systems commonly use radioactive sources up to 3.5 times the activity of standard radium sources. Although the relationship between dose rate, tumour cell kill, and normal tissue tolerance is still not entirely clear, to produce a given amount of normal tissue damage the total dose delivered must be reduced as the dose rate increases. This is discussed in greater detail later in this chapter.

If very high-activity cobalt or iridium sources are used, then treatment times can be reduced to a few minutes, enabling patients to be treated as outpatients rather than inpatients and ensuring stability of the applicators during treatment. However, it is necessary not only to reduce the dose but also to divide the treatment into several fractions, which may pose problems in exactly reproducing the positioning of the applicators for each fraction.

Physical aspects of intracavitary therapy

Specification of radiation dose

In the earliest days of brachytherapy, radiation 'dose' was expressed simply in terms of milligrams-hour (mg-h; the quantity of radium in milligrams multiplied by the duration of treatment in hours). The roentgen unit (R) was introduced in 1928 for measuring the exposure due to X-rays and, subsequently, in 1937, to γ-photons. Traditionally, the activity of radium was described in terms of milligrams, but the formal unit of activity was the curie (Ci). More recently, with the introduction of SI units, the becquerel (Bq) has been adopted as the unit of activity: 1 Bq being the equivalent of 1 disintegration per second. Total reference air kerma has now replaced milligrams-hour.

The dose received by a patient describes the actual energy deposited in the tissue by the ionizing radiation. The unit of absorbed dose was defined by the International Commission on Radiological Units and Measurements (**ICRU**) as the gray (Gy), where 1 Gy = 1 J/kg. More recently, it has been recommended that absorbed dose measurement should be based on the concept of kerma (an acronym for kinetic energy released in the medium). In practice, for sources used in brachytherapy, kerma and absorbed dose are used interchangeably.

Table 1 summarizes details of the old and new dosimetric units. The advent of radionuclides other than radium and the development of computers for three-dimensional dosimetric studies have allowed optimization of the dose distribution to conform with the disease pattern in a way that was not possible when intracavitary brachytherapy was first used.

Intracavitary sources

Naturally occurring radium is one of the most dangerous radionuclides in medical use not only because of the very high energy of radiation emitted, requiring heavy shielding for staff protection, but also because the decay product of radium is radon gas, which is intensely radioactive and could contaminate a large area if not contained. Artificially produced radionuclides of cobalt, iridium, and caesium have solid

Table 1 Units of activity and dose

Quantity	Symbol	SI unit	Old unit	Relation
Activity	A	Bq	Ci	$1\ \mathrm{Ci} \equiv 37\ \mathrm{GBq}$
Dose	D	$\mathrm{Gy} \equiv \mathrm{J/kg}$	rad	$1\ \mathrm{rad} \equiv 10^{-2}\ \mathrm{Gy}$
Kerma	K	$\mathrm{Gy} \equiv \mathrm{J/kg}$	–	–
Kerma rate constant	Γ_δ	$\mu\mathrm{Gy/h}$ per $\mathrm{MBq.m^2}$	–	–
Exposure	X	C/kg	R	$1\ \mathrm{R} \equiv 2.58 \times 10^{-4}\ \mathrm{C/kg}$
Exposure rate constant	Γ^*_δ	$\mathrm{pA/kg}$ per $\mathrm{MBq.m^2}$	$\mathrm{R/h}$ per $\mathrm{Ci.m^2}$	$1\ \mathrm{R/h}$ per $\mathrm{Ci.m^2} = 1.937\ \mathrm{pA/kg}$ per $\mathrm{MBq.m^2}$

non-radioactive decay products and have three other important additional advantages over radium:

1. Cobalt-60, iridium-192, and to a lesser extent, caesium-137 can be produced at a much higher specific activity (i.e. with more radioactivity per gram) than radium. This allows for the production of smaller, high-activity sources.

2. The γ-ray emissions from caesium-137 and iridium-192 are of lower energies than those from radium, which makes for more convenient shielding of sources.

3. Iridium-192 also has the advantage that it can be produced in wire form; this has allowed the development of surface mould and interstitial therapy.[1]

Source strength

The strength of a radioactive source is specified in terms of the reference air kerma rate, which is defined as: the air kerma rate in air at a reference distance of 1 m corrected for attenuation and scatter in air, and is measured in micrograys/hour (μGy/h).

Low dose-rate sources have an activity within the range 0.5 to 2.5 GBq. It is good practice to measure these sources in a well-type ionization chamber against a source that has been calibrated by a National Standards Laboratory. Multiple sources of the same nominal strength will cover a range of strengths and these should be determined so that sources can be selected optimally for treatment. Higher-activity sources are also available for afterloading techniques. Table 2 summarizes the range of activities that are available.

Source dosimetry

Brachytherapy with radium led to the formulation of dose tables which enabled users to calculate the dose rate at specific distances from individual sources.[2]–[4]

Although experimental studies have shown that dose distributions local to implanted sources of less toxic radionuclides are not significantly different from those for radium sources of equivalent strength, this similarity does not necessarily prevail along the longitudinal axes of linear sources nor at distances greater than a few centimetres from the source (Table 3). If dose tables are to be used, it is necessary that appropriate checks are undertaken to ensure that dose calculations are valid for the technique that is being employed.

With the aid of computer planning it is now possible to compute complete dose distributions in several planes so it becomes possible to study not only the dose distribution throughout the target volume but also the dose to organs at risk and to lymph nodes.

Input data for an individual patient are normally obtained from orthogonal X-rays or some other radiographic method of obtaining three-dimensional information. The reconstruction technique should be tested to ensure that the method gives reliable results before being used for clinical dosimetry. Various source reconstruction techniques have been tested by Slessinger and Grigsby[6] and they showed that the accuracy of source reconstruction was usually within 3 mm.

As is the case in other radiotherapy techniques, the overall uncertainty in dose specification in brachytherapy can be subdivided into the uncertainty associated with localization and irradiation of the target volume and the uncertainty in dose determination. In external-beam therapy it is necessary to work within an uncertainty of dose specification of less than 5 per cent: whenever possible similar accuracy should be sought in brachytherapy. At this level of uncertainty the high-dose gradients in intracavitary therapy correspond to only small spatial differences (typically 1 to 2 mm). However, these differences might be significant, especially when clinical effects are dependent upon relatively small dosage differences. To meet the 5 per cent dose specification requirement it is necessary not only to know the strengths of the radioactive sources but also to be able to calculate the dose distribution around the sources inserted into the patient with a high degree of precision.

Manual gynaecological treatment systems

Although manual systems are now seldom used, it is on these that modern remote afterloading systems have been modelled.

In the 1920s and 1930s work at the Radiumhemmet in Stockholm and at the Curie Foundation in Paris resulted in the evolution of the Stockholm system[7] and the Paris system[8] for the treatment of uterine cancer. Although in both methods radium was inserted into the uterine canal and in the lateral fornices of the vagina, there were important differences in terms of the activity and distribution of the radium employed and also the duration of treatment.

Stockholm system

This method was introduced first by Gosta Forsell in 1914 and developed by Heyman.[7],[9] The technique has been described comprehensively by Kottmeier[10] and was based on the use of large amounts of heavily filtered radium (100 to 120 mg) for relatively short periods of time. The treatment was fractionated into two or three equal parts of between 20 and 24 h, with an interval of 1 week between the first and second application and a 2- to 3-week interval between the second and third application. The source configuration

Table 2 Source data for high dose-rate remote afterloading brachytherapy

Radionuclide	Activity	No. of sources	Type of source	Source diameter (mm)	Dose rate	Transfer mechanism
^{60}Co	4–20 GBq	20 variable	Pellet	2.5	High	Pneumatic, cable
^{137}Cs	0.5–1.5 GBq	48	Pellet	2.5	Low/medium	Pneumatic
^{137}Cs	0.75 GBq	Variable	Capsules	1.7	Low	Cable
^{137}Cs	30–250 MBq/cm	15	Ribbon	< 2.3	Low/medium	Pneumatic, cable
^{192}Ir	400 GBq	1	Cylinder	1.1 ($\times$ 5)	High	Cable
^{192}Ir	20–40 GBq	1	Cylinder	1.1 ($\times$ 5)	Pulsed	Cable
^{192}Ir	10 MBq/cm	15–20	Wire, ribbon	0.5/2.3	Low/medium	Pneumatic, cable

Table 3 Ratio of exposure in water to exposure in air calculated using the Meisberger polynomial[5]

Radionuclide	Distances from source (cm)				
	2	4	6	8	10
^{60}Co	0.974	0.940	0.897	0.853	0.813
^{137}Cs	0.977	0.966	0.937	0.900	0.856
^{192}Ir	1.018	1.013	0.996	0.967	0.925
^{226}Ra	0.985	0.960	0.929	0.894	0.860

resulted in high localized dose rates and high dose gradients near to the surface of the vaginal sources (Fig. 3). Treatments were highly individualized according to patient anatomy and extent of disease, but the accumulated dose to the bladder did not exceed 60 Gy and that in the rectum 50 Gy, with a maximum dose per insertion of 25 Gy. Many modifications to the classic Stockholm technique have been made.

Paris system

In this system irradiation was continuous over a period of about 6 to 8 days. A treatment consisted typically of two or three individual sources (one in each lateral fornix and sometimes one central source in front of the cervical os) and one intrauterine tube. The strength of each source was 10 to 15 mg of radium, so the total activity was 50 to 90 mg. The vaginal sources were in cylindrical 'corks' of approximately 20 mm in diameter, held in place in the lateral fornices by a 10-cm long metal spring connecting each cork (Fig. 4). The larger source–tissue distance of this method, compared with that of the Stockholm system, produced a great depth dose in surrounding tissue and tended to increase the dose delivered to pelvic nodes. The geometrical source configuration used in the Paris method has become the basis of numerous other systems in the evolution of intracavitary gynaecological brachytherapy, including the Manchester and Fletcher–Houston systems and most afterloading techniques.

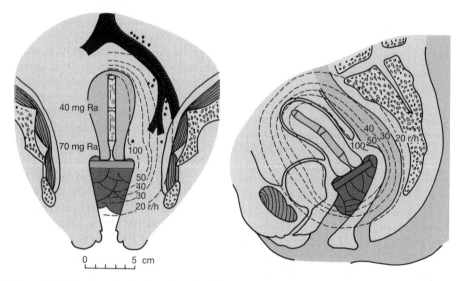

Fig. 3 Typical anteroposterior and lateral isodose distributions for a Stockholm intracavitary treatment.

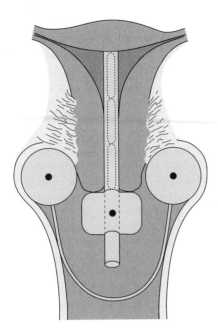

Fig. 4 Paris-type intracavitary applicators.

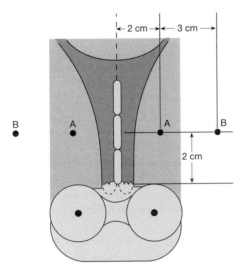

Fig. 5 The Manchester system points A and B.

Manchester system

The work of Tod[11] and Tod and Meredith[12] led to the conclusion that, in patients being treated with a fractionated Paris technique, the limiting dose was not the dose to the rectum or bladder, but the dose in the area where the uterine vessels cross the ureter, the 'paracervical triangle'. For the assessment of dosage, a point 2 cm lateral to the centre of the uterine canal and 2 cm from the mucous membrane of the lateral fornix in the plane of the uterus was selected and designated to be point 'A' (Fig. 5). A study of over 500 cases showed a clear relationship between the tolerance of normal tissues and the dose received in this area.

A further reference point, B, was also defined to be 5 cm from the midline and 2 cm up from the mucous membrane of the lateral fornix; this point not only gives the dose in the vicinity of the pelvic wall near the obturator node but also gives a good indication of the lateral spread of the effective dose.

The applicators used in the vagina were ovoids corresponding approximately to isodose surfaces for a radium tube 20 mm long, and were made of hard rubber. They were used in pairs and locked in position either by a spacer or by a washer; the former fixed the distance between the ovoids at 1 cm while the latter allowed them to lie almost in contact; the ovoids were 2, 2.5, and 3.0 cm in diameter. The uterine tubes were made from rubber in three different lengths capable of taking in line either one, two, or three radium tubes, each 2 cm long. Each tube was closed at one end and had a flange at the other to ensure that when it and the vaginal ovoids were packed into position, the intrauterine tube did not slip out during treatment.

The activity and arrangement of the sources were such as to ensure that the dose rate at point A was 53 R/h and the total dose for two equal insertions was 8000 R delivered in 144 h. The dose at point B was 25 to 30 per cent of the dose at point A. To achieve these requirements and to ensure that the dose to the vaginal mucosa remained acceptable, the Manchester system defined the number of 'units' of radium to be used in each ovoid and the tube size. The dose rates of point A were tabulated for uterine applicators and ovoids. The loadings for long, medium, and short intrauterine tubes were $10+10+15$ mg, $10+15$ mg, and 20 mg, respectively, with the higher-activity source in the fundus; typically, in SI units the dose rate at point A from the intrauterine source was 27 to 34 cGy/h. Large, medium, and small ovoids were loaded with 22.5, 20, and 17.5 mg of radium to give a dose rate of about 19 cGy/h. The dose rate to point A was obtained by adding the contributions from the tube and the ovoids. If an insertion was 'standard', the dose rate at point A for the ideal insertion determined the treatment time, even though the classic reference geometry might not be achieved. However, if an insertion was non-standard, for instance if a short (2 cm) intrauterine tube was used or if the vaginal applicators lay one above the other in the vagina, then the dose to point A should be reduced so as not to exceed the normal tissue tolerance.[13]

Fletcher–Houston system

This system is a development of the Manchester system using, in place of ovoids, colpostats which have separate handles that can be locked together by a scissor joint. This allows the vagina to be distended laterally, with a resultant increase in dose to the paracervical and parametrial tissues. Developed in the early 1950s by Fletcher, the treatment is determined by the volume of disease rather than the stage of disease.[14] Like other techniques, the amounts of both external irradiation and intracavitary irradiation are interdependent and careful attention is paid to the cumulative dose to the diseased tissue. The applicators have the same diameters as the Manchester ovoids but are slightly longer; they are cylindrical in shape rather than oval and the surfaces do not conform to isodose surfaces. Plastic jackets fit over the smallest metal applicator to achieve the necessary variation in size. Tungsten shielding is included in the base and top of the applicator to provide some protection to the anterior wall of the rectum and the base of the bladder. The vaginal applicator and uterine tube loadings are similar to those of the Manchester technique, but local microdosimetry is different due to the in-built shielding. The technique requires that careful consideration is given to anatomical features such as vault size, extent and volume of the tumour, length of uterine canal, and the anatomical position of the pelvic nodes.

Afterloading

Afterloading is the name given to techniques in which applicators or catheters are placed in a patient and subsequently loaded with radioactive sources. The method permits optimal positioning of the applicators without any associated radiation hazard. There are two essential requirements for a good afterloading system and rigorous quality assurance procedures must be adopted to ensure compliance with these requirements.

1. The design of the applicator must allow for the correct positioning of the source with respect to the tissue volume to be irradiated

2. It must be possible to position the sources reproducibly.

Manual afterloading techniques

Manual afterloading is now rarely used other than in developing countries where radioactive sources are loaded by hand into the applicators. Usually this occurs after the patient has had localizing radiographs and has returned to the ward, where protective lead shields are used to minimize radiation exposure of the staff. The method has been shown to be an effective means of radiation protection, except for staff who are exposed to radiation in the course of nursing the patient.

Afterloading techniques became popular principally after technical innovations by Henschke et al.[15] and the introduction of miniature caesium sources[16] which permitted the construction of flexible source trains. In 1966 Chassagne and Pierquin,[17] at the Institut Gustav Roussy, described a technique using a moulded plastic vaginal applicator afterloaded with caesium sources. This involved fabricating an acrylic mould for individual patients. The flexible source trains were inserted into the mould via guides. The mould is such a good fit that patients may be allowed to get out of bed for exercise during treatment; also, local hygiene is assured by daily vaginal irrigation via a special tube. In this method, the dose fractionation is based essentially on the Paris low dose-rate system.

A disposable manual afterloaded system developed commercially by Amersham International plc consists of uterine and ovoid tubes made of flexible polyvinyl tubing and ovoids, spacers, and washers made of high-impact polystyrene. The applicators, which are impregnated with barium, separate into sections which can be held together by a polystyrene disc through which the sections pass. Although the device is based on the Manchester system, in practice the principal axis of the ovoid sources lies at a different angle to that of the Manchester ovoids and allowance must be made for this difference when dose calculations are made.

Remote-controlled afterloading (low and medium dose rates)

Remote afterloading systems give staff complete protection from irradiation and several are available commercially. The sources can be in the form of a flexible spring, containing one or more capsules, attached to a cable, or can be multiple spherical radioactive beads, transferred pneumatically into the patient. Table 2 compares the principal characteristics of some of the equipment that is available.

There are three important methods of achieving low dose-rate afterloading, two of which are in common use. Each uses a different method of source transfer and has different applicators.

1. The CIS Curietron system is representative of a cable-driven static source system and makes use of preloaded flexible source trains which are transferred from the Curietron safe into the applicator using drive cables. The source train consists of caesium-137 sources and inactive spacers loaded into a stainless steel spring, closed at one end. The other end of the source train is sealed with a hook which serves to identify the source train and provides a means of connection to one of the drive cables. Nine source trains may be loaded into the Curietron at any one time, each of which is connected to an independently controlled drive cable. Users have to determine, at the time of manufacture, what source configuration will be required, and it is usual to have a selection of source trains (typically of length 5 to 80 mm, and of activity 0.5 to 10 GBq) kept in a separate, larger safe.

2. In the Nucletron Selectron machine, now the most common afterloading machine worldwide, the sources are in the form of 2.5-mm diameter spherical pellets. Source trains can be made up of a combination of 48 sources and inactive spacers. The number of sources and their positions in each train is independently programmable. Nucletron manufacture a three-channel and a six-channel low dose-rate/medium dose-rate caesium-137 machine. In both machines, sources are sorted magnetically and transferred pneumatically into stainless steel applicators in the patient via flexible pneumatic tubing. The machines are controlled remotely and all sources are withdrawn when the treatment time has expired or whenever someone enters the treatment room.

3. Less commonly used, the Buchler system is also mechanically driven by cable but makes use of a single radioactive source which oscillates in a predetermined manner to produce the required radiation dose distribution. During treatment the position of the source is controlled by a specially shaped programme disc which moves the source with constant frequency within the applicator over a path length of up to 200 mm. A three-channel system can be used to simulate two fixed ovoid sources and a uterine tube.

Remote-controlled afterloading (high dose rates)

High dose-rate afterloading can only be achieved using radioisotopes of very high specific activity. At present only cobalt (^{60}Co) and iridium (^{192}Ir) satisfy the requirements that an afterloading source emits radiation of a suitable energy, be solid, have solid decay products, be capable of being worked, be non-soluble, and yet be produced with a very high specific activity. Whereas cobalt sources, with a half-life of over 5 years, only need replacement on the basis of radioactive decay every 3 to 6 years, iridium sources have an inconveniently short half-life of only 74 days and require replacement every 3 to 4 months.

Much of the pioneer work in high dose-rate brachytherapy techniques was carried out with TEM Cathetron high dose-rate machines. These machines made use of preloaded flexible source trains, similar to the Curietron but using high-activity cobalt-60 sources, which were loaded from a source safe and transferred into applicators via drive cables. Nowadays, in Europe and the United States, the

Gammamed 12 and microSelectron HDR (Nucletron) machines are the most commonly used of the several that are available. Both use a small, high-activity iridium-192 cable-driven source which is programmed to move in a stepwise fashion with a variable dwell time at each position. The machine has also been adapted for use with a lower activity source to deliver pulsed brachytherapy.

The radiobiology of altered dose rates

The ICRU defines low, medium, and high dose-rate brachytherapy as follows:

Dose rate to the reference point:

0.4–2 Gy/h	low dose rate
2–12 Gy/h	medium dose rate
above 12 Gy/h	high dose rate

The dose rate to point 'A' from the classic Manchester system is 53 cGy/h and is, clearly, low dose-rate therapy.

However, modern remote afterloading machines have enabled higher-activity caesium sources to be used and dose rates are commonly between 150 and 180 cGy/h. Although this would still be low dose-rate therapy according to the ICRU definition, clinical experience has shown that a dose reduction is needed to maintain an isoeffect with standard dose-rate therapy. It has been suggested that the definitions be changed, so that dose rates which require a reduction in dose from those given by standard activity systems be classified as medium or high dose rates. However, with the current ICRU definitions, afterloading systems delivering a dose rate of less than 200 cGy/h should, correctly, continue to be referred to as low dose-rate systems. There is a much clearer dividing line between low and medium dose-rate systems using caesium and high dose-rate systems using cobalt or iridium.

Time–dose relationships in brachytherapy

The principal reasons for choosing interstitial or intracavitary radiotherapy in preference to external-beam treatment relate to dose delivery and dose distribution rather than to radiobiology. However, the question of whether low dose-rate irradiation itself carries a therapeutic advantage is an interesting one; there is a considerable volume of literature on the dose-rate effect both in tumours and in normal tissues, on the basis of which it would be difficult to claim an overall benefit or disadvantage.

Mammalian cells are usually less sensitive to irradiation at a low dose rate because protraction of exposure allows recovery and repopulation to take place. Recovery is a fast process with a half-time that is often in the range 0.5 to 1.5 h; repopulation is much slower, with doubling times that are unlikely to be less than 48 h. As a result of the large difference in the speed of these processes, recovery and repopulation will influence tissue damage (normal or malignant) over very different ranges of dose rate.[18] Broadly speaking, recovery will have an effect when the duration of exposure is a significant fraction of an hour, whereas repopulation will not be important unless the exposure time becomes a day or more. Thus, for dose rates from the few grays per minute used in external-beam treatment down to around 1 cGy/min, recovery will be the dominant modifying factor.

Below 1 cGy/min, repopulation will become important in any tissue where cell proliferation is taking place.

There are considerable differences in the extent of sparing in normal tissues as dose rate is reduced (reviewed by Steel et al.).[18] Haematopoietic tissues show little sparing; in other tissues the iso-effective dose increases by a factor of up to 1.5 at dose rates as low as 10 cGy/min and up to 2.0 or more at rates down to 1 cGy/min.

Among human tumour cells there is also clear evidence that the extent of low dose-rate sparing varies widely.[19] In some of the most radiosensitive cells there is little or no dose sparing down to 1 cGy/min; in more resistant cells the sparing factors at 1 cGy/min can, as with the normal tissues, range up to 2.0 or more. Tumour types that are treated by brachytherapy will probably have factors at the upper end of this range.

The effect of a dose-rate reduction on therapeutic index (i.e. ratio of tumour effect to normal-tissue damage) cannot be judged without specific information on the tissues in question. In broad terms, we may expect that for the types of tumours which are treated by brachytherapy the position will be similar to that with fractionated external-beam treatment: late-reacting normal tissues (low α/β ratio) will show large dose sparing; tumours that have higher α/β ratios will show less sparing and dose protraction should give an advantage.

Whether a low dose-rate exposure is better than a single high dose-rate treatment is not, of course, the clinically important question. Rather, we need to ask how a single low dose-rate exposure compares with fractionated treatment. In terms of 'recovery', for any dose per fraction in fractionated treatment there is a continuously administered dose rate at which the biological effects should be similar, independent of the α/β ratio.[20] However, if the tumour cells have a rapid rate of 'repopulation' then there could be an advantage in the continuous low dose-rate exposure. Treatment at low dose rate is the most efficient way of maximizing recovery while keeping the treatment duration as short as possible.

Variation in cell killing around an implanted radioactive source

The non-uniformity of the radiation field around an implanted source has important radiobiological consequences. Close to the source the dose rate is high and the cellular radiosensitivity will be given by the acute radiation survival curve. As we move away from the source, two changes take place: cells will be less sensitive at the lower dose rates, and within a given period of implantation the accumulated dose will also be less. These two factors lead to a very rapid change of cell killing with distance from the source. Within tissues close to the source the level of cell killing will be so high that cells of any radiosensitivity will be killed. Further out the effects will be so low that even the most radiosensitive cells will survive. Between these extremes there is a critical zone in which differential cell killing will occur. As shown by Steel et al.,[21] for cells of any given level of radiosensitivity there will be a cliff-like change from total cell kill to 100 per cent survival, taking place over a radial distance of a few millimetres. The distance of the cliff from the source is determined by the radiosensitivity of the cells at low dose rate, nearer for radioresistant cells and further away for radiosensitive cells.[22] This is illustrated in Fig. 6, which also indicates the difference between external-beam and implant radiotherapy. Only in a narrow zone around the source (where the surviving fraction changes from say

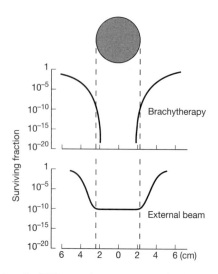

Fig. 6 Variation of cell kill around a point source of radiation. The source gives 0.87 Gy/min at 2 cm (i.e. 75 Gy in 6 days); there are 10^9 cells/cm^3, for which $\alpha = 0.35$ Gy^{-1}, $\beta = 0.035$ Gy^{-2} and the half-time for recovery = 1 h. The shaded area indicates the volume within which the surviving fraction is below 10^{-10}.

10^{-20} to 10^{-6}) will radiobiological considerations be of interest or importance.

Models of the dose-rate effect

It is frequently necessary to consider the therapeutic implications of a change in dose rate, either for continuous or fractionated exposure. The linear-quadratic approach[23] allows calculations to be made of the isoeffective total dose that results from a change in dose per fraction, assuming a particular value for the α/β ratio and also that complete recovery occurs between fractions.

The theoretical description of the response of cells and tissues to continuous irradiation at various dose rates began with the work of Oliver[24] and Szechter and Schwartz.[25] They calculated the dose-equivalent of sublethal damage from an initial dose increment and then assumed that this decayed exponentially. Although this was a purely empirical approach and no assumptions were made about the underlying cell survival curve, these models were successful in describing experimental data. Thames et al.,[26] Dale,[27] and Thames[28] followed the same approach but assumed that cell killing at high dose rate was described by a linear-quadratic equation. The resulting model could be applied both to fractionated treatment with short interfraction intervals and also to continuous irradiation at any dose rate. The basic equation was of the form:

$$E = \alpha.D + \beta.D^2.f(t)$$

where E is the level of effect, α and β are parameters of the linear-quadratic equation, D is the total dose, and f(t) is a function of time (either time between fractions or duration of continuous exposure). Note that the time-dependent recovery term modifies only the quadratic term in the linear-quadratic equation, a feature that is supported by experimental data.[19],[22]

This equation allows isoeffect relationships to be calculated, but unfortunately, the recovery half-time is seldom known in clinical situations, which limits the precision of calculations of this sort. Nevertheless, the development of mathematical models to extrapolate experience at low dose rate to higher dose rates and to pulsed brachytherapy provides a safer method of introducing these new technologies than existed before.[29]

Pulsed brachytherapy

The availability of computer-controlled high dose-rate afterloading systems provides the opportunity to deliver interstitial or intracavitary radiotherapy in a series of pulses. The gaps between pulses allow greater freedom for the patient and increased safety for nursing staff. In principle, any move away from continuous exposure towards closely spaced dose fractions carries a radiobiological disadvantage. This is equivalent to fractionation with a larger dose per fraction and the theoretical and experimental evidence that this will lead to a relative increase in late normal-tissue reactions is strong. The magnitude of this effect has been considered by Brenner and Hall,[30],[31] who conclude that for gaps of up to 60 min between pulses the radiobiological deficit may be acceptable and clinical trials have begun.[32]–[34]

Overall treatment time

A further warning about the use of high dose-rate afterloading systems relates to overall time. Reoxygenation of hypoxic tumour cells may occur to such an extent over a conventional 4- to 6-week course of radiotherapy that hypoxic cells may not be a serious problem. High dose-rate afterloading systems create the temptation to shorten the overall time and, if this is done, the greater will be the radioresistance due to hypoxia.

Clinical experience of altered dose rates

Increasing low dose rates

As referred to before, a major change in dose rate in intracavitary therapy occurred with the development of high-activity caesium microsources. The low dose-rate Selectron, a microprocessor-controlled, pneumatically operated system, was able to utilize these high-activity sources and became widely available in the late 1970s. When using the Manchester system of an intrauterine tube and two vaginal ovoids, these sources enable a dose rate of 180 cGy/h to point A to be achieved. One of the first centres to investigate the use of this increased dose rate was the Christie Hospital, Manchester. Over several years this centre has conducted one of the largest studies of the effects of increased dose rate in gynaecological intracavitary therapy.

In this study, patients with early stage carcinoma of the cervix have been treated with intracavitary therapy alone, using either the classic radium and caesium applicators or Selectron applicators. In the standard treatment 75 Gy was delivered to point A in two fractions over 10 days at 53 cGy/h, while the Selectron applicators delivered to point A at approximately 180 cGy/h. Four doses to point A were studied with the Selectron applicators—75, 70, 65, and 60 Gy—given as two fractions over 10 days. It would appear that to avoid a high incidence of normal-tissue damage a reduction in dose is needed, and this reduction lies between 10 and 15 per cent of the dose given at the standard dose rate. Within this dose range similar local control rates are seen.[35]

Using a high dose rate

Very high-activity cobalt sources were developed for high dose-rate intracavitary brachytherapy in the late 1960s. The machine most commonly used for this treatment was the Cathetron, which contained three source trains to allow Manchester-type treatment applicators to be used.

It was recognized that treatment would have to be fractionated to allow normal tissue repair, which takes place during low dose-rate intracavitary irradiation, to occur between fractions. In addition, unless a large number of fractions were used, a considerable dose reduction would be needed when using high dose rates.[36] Clinical work was then based on radiobiological models, but was soon tempered by clinical experience.[37]

Early trials of Cathetron therapy showed that, when used for preoperative irradiation in patients with cancer of the cervix, the eradication of disease, as assessed on the hysterectomy specimen, was the same for patients treated with either a reduced dose on the Cathetron or a conventional dose from radium sources.[38] However, the severe complication rate was significantly higher in the radium-treated patients than in those treated by the Cathetron. This was attributed to the superior stability of the Cathetron applicators over the short treatment time. This serves to illustrate the difficulty in comparing intracavitary treatments at different dose rates. Although a dose-rate effect may be present, this could be obscured by tissue reactions that are more dependent on the precise dose distribution due to the geometry of the sources.

Throughout the 1970s and early 1980s high dose-rate therapy continued in a small number of centres equipped with machines using high-activity cobalt sources. However, in the latter half of the 1980s new technology enabled very small sources of intense activity to be used for intracavitary therapy. These sources, made of iridium-192, could be manufactured with a diameter of less than 1 mm, allowing applicators to be of much smaller width (less than 4 mm) than was the case for either low dose-rate caesium sources or high dose-rate cobalt sources, where the diameter of the intrauterine tube needed to be at least 6 mm. This slenderness of applicator, apart from being attractive for gynaecological use because of the increased ease of insertion, has stimulated interest in intracavitary and intraluminal therapy at other sites.

Comparisons between low and high dose-rate treatment have mostly been either historical within one institution or concurrent between two separate treatment centres. In an excellent review of these comparative studies Karen Fu and Theodore Phillips[39] state:

'in reviewing the results in the literature, several problems became apparent to us: (a) dose specification between different centres was not standardised, (b) dosimetry systems and methods were variable, (c) there were technical variations including the type of applicators, use of protective shields, treatment positions etc., (d) dose-volume information was unavailable in most reports, (e) external beam dose or treatment time as well as the time sequence of external beam irradiation and intracavitary therapy were variable, (f) different methods of rectal and bladder dose measurements were used, (g) toxicity grading systems were not standardized, and (h) length of patient follow-up was variable. Thus, results between centres may not be comparable.'

Table 4 Regimens for combined external-beam and intracavitary therapy[41]

External-beam therapy:
45 Gy/20 f/4 weeks
Intracavitary therapy:
LDR 35 Gy pt A/1 f
or
HDR 17 Gy pt A/2 f
HDR 18 Gy pt A/2 f
HDR 19 Gy pt A/2 f

f, fractions; HDR, high dose rate; LDR, low dose rate; pt A, point A.

Table 5 Results of treatment: follow-up of 2 to 5 years[41]

	Low dose rate	High dose rate
Patients	220	203
Residual disease	22	23
Local control	189 (86%)	170 (84%)
Cervical recurrence	9	10
Parametrial recurrence	12	11
Pelvic control	177 (80%)	159 (78%)
Distant metastases	18	13
Overall control	159 (72%)	146 (72%)

However, these authors felt able to conclude that 'most of the non-randomised studies suggest similar survival, local-control and complication rates using fractionated remote afterloading HDR intracavitary brachytherapy combined with external beam irradiation for carcinoma of the cervix compared to historical or concurrent LDR controls'. This is the conclusion that Khoury et al.[40] came to in analysing the results of patients treated by the Cathetron between 1967 and 1974 and followed-up for as long as 16 years. They felt that the long-term results of high dose-rate treatment were similar to those obtained at other centres using low dose rates at that time.

Few centres have used the same time/dose/fractionation schemes, and the ideal for high dose-rate intracavitary therapy and its integration with external-beam irradiation has yet to be determined. However, one of the very few randomized studies comparing low with high dose-rate intracavitary therapy illustrates a successful regimen and gives some indication of how much the standard low dose-rate dose should be reduced when using high dose-rate therapy.

Sharma et al.[41] reported the results of treatment of 423 patients with carcinoma of the cervix. There were 220 assessable patients randomized into the low dose-rate arm of the study, while 203 assessable patients received high dose-rate treatment. The regimens are shown in Table 4. Patients received external-beam irradiation before intracavitary therapy to the doses shown. Follow-up was for between 2 and 5 years. There were some very minor differences in local control and the incidence of distant metastases, but the overall control rate of disease was 72 per cent in both groups (Table 5).

Table 6 Local failure related to intracavitary dose[41]

	Dose reduction factor	No.	Residual disease	Local recurrence	Total local failures	
					No.	%
LDR 35 Gy	–	220	22	9	31	14
HDR 17 Gy/2 f	49%	27	6	3	9	33
HDR 18 Gy/2 f	51%	35	3	1	4	11
HDR 19 Gy/2 f	54%	141	14	6	20	14

f, fractions; HDR, high dose rate; LDR, low dose rate.

There was a 17 per cent incidence of acute hyperaemia of the vagina seen with high dose-rate therapy, a problem not encountered after low dose-rate treatment, and 5.5 per cent incidence of late effects seen in the vagina after high dose-rate therapy while these problems occurred in only 2.5 per cent of the low dose-rate group. Urinary morbidity was approximately the same, while rectal problems, grades 2 and 3, were seen in 3 per cent of the low dose-rate group but in none of the high dose-rate group. Apart from the incidence of acute vaginal hyperaemia, there cannot be said to be any significant difference in the incidence of normal tissue effects in the two groups. It would appear, therefore, that the treatment regimens used in the low and high dose-rate groups were biologically very similar.

Within the high dose-rate group, three different intracavitary doses were used. The results of these three regimens are shown in Table 6 and, although the numbers are small, it would appear that, when given at a high dose rate, to reduce the low dose-rate dose to 49 per cent results in a high local failure rate.

In general, it has been found that to avoid an unacceptable normal-tissue complication rate or local recurrence rate, the dose given at the high dose rate should be in the region of 55 to 70 per cent of the dose given at the low dose rate, the fraction size should not exceed 8 to 10 Gy, and treatments should be between once and three times per week.

Intracavitary therapy dose prescription and dose recording

Intracavitary doses are specified according to the system of applicators used. If Manchester-type applicators are used, with an intrauterine tube and two vaginal ovoids, then the dose is prescribed to point A. This prescription point is 2 cm lateral to the cervical canal and 2 cm above the lateral fornix (Fig. 5). It is theoretically where the ureter crosses the uterine artery. In practice, point A is measured from the radiographs as 2 cm lateral to the centre of the intrauterine radioactive source and 2 cm above its lowest limit.

Other applicators require that the dose is prescribed in different ways, some to prescription points and others to tumour volumes. The prescription method for a particular type of intracavitary system cannot be extended from one system to another. With all intracavitary treatment, whether continuous low dose rate or fractionated high dose rate, the prescription should specify the total radiation dose to the prescription point or volume, the length of each treatment, the number of times the treatment is to be repeated, and the total time over which treatment is given.

In many cases the intracavitary treatment will be part of a combined approach, using external-beam therapy also. The external-beam dose must be expressed separately. An example of a radiotherapy prescription for the treatment of cervical carcinoma would be 50.4 Gy in 28 fractions delivered over 5.5 weeks (50.4 Gy/28 f/5.5 w) by external-beam therapy (8 MV X-rays) to the pelvis, using an anterior and two lateral fields, plus 22.5 Gy delivered over 22 h to point A from an intrauterine tube and two vaginal ovoids remotely afterloaded with caesium. A more specific prescription detailing field sizes, the use of wedge compensators and shielding blocks, and the length of the intrauterine tube and size of the vaginal ovoids, together with details of the distribution of radioisotope within these applicators and the dose rate at the prescription point is needed for the physics staff to calculate the exact dosimetry of a complete course of treatment.

The ICRU have issued specific recommendations for reporting intracavitary and interstitial therapy in gynaecology.[42],[43] Fundamental to these requirements is the need for dosimetry in orthogonal planes (Fig. 7). Most computer treatment planning systems facilitate this by means of data acquired from a pair of radiographs taken at different angles.

Dose and volume specification for reporting intracavitary brachytherapy in gynaecology

The dose gradient near to the sources is so high that the specification of the target dose to specific points of interest is less meaningful than for external-beam therapy. In Report number 38, the ICRU recommend the adoption of a dose volume specification which should be used in conjunction with the total reference air kerma for a patient's treatment. A record of absorbed dose at reference points related to organs at risk or to bony structures is also recommended, as well as details of the time–dose pattern. However, the recorded information will only be meaningful if the treatment technique employed has been fully documented, including information about the sources and the applicators.

Description of reference volume

The tissue volume encompassed by a reference isodose surface should be specified in reporting absorbed doses. There are three complementary aspects related to this requirement: the dose level, the

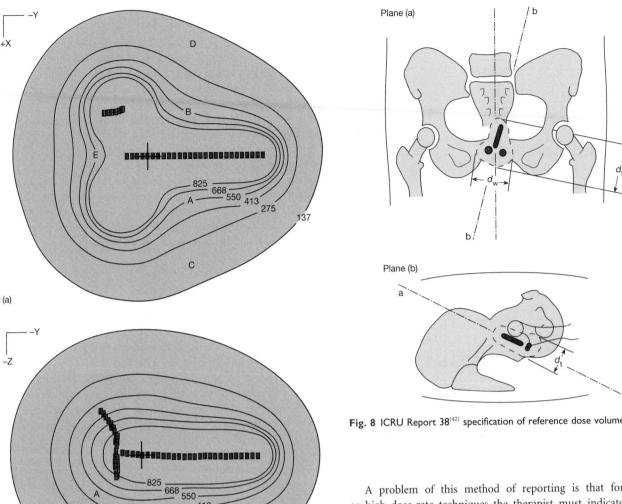

Fig. 7 Anteroposterior (a) and lateral (b) dose distribution of a Manchester insertion using a high dose-rate stepping iridium source.

Fig. 8 ICRU Report 38[42] specification of reference dose volume.

description of the reference volume, and the recording of dose to various reference points.

Dose level

For classic low dose-rate therapy an absorbed dose level of 60 Gy is widely accepted as the appropriate reference level. It is important to realize that this level is only chosen to facilitate reporting and is not advocated as a minimum tumour dose or other prescription level.

When more than one intracavitary insertion is made, the absorbed dose to consider is that resulting from all insertions. The time–dose pattern should be clearly stated. When intracavitary therapy is combined with external-beam therapy, the isodose level to be considered is the difference between 60 Gy and the dose delivered at the same location by external-beam therapy.

A problem of this method of reporting is that for medium or high dose-rate techniques the therapist must indicate the dose level he believes to be equivalent to 60 Gy delivered at low dose rate.

Reference volume

The combination of uterine sources and vaginal sources results in a pear-shaped distribution with its longest axis coincident with the intrauterine source. The reference volume is determined from radiographs of the intracavitary insertion (Fig. 8).

Absorbed dose at reference points

Recommended reference points include those relatively close to the sources but related to organs at risk, and those related to bony structures. Reference points close to the sources, often in regions of steep dose gradients, are not recommended.

The determination and specification of the absorbed dose close to organs at risk, such as the bladder and rectum, should either be measured or calculated. Chassagne and Horiot[44] described methods of determining points of reference for both organs, which have been extended from standard to novel systems.[45]

The bladder reference point is obtained using a Foley catheter with 7 cm³ of radio-opaque fluid in the balloon. The catheter is pulled downwards to bring the balloon against the urethra. On the lateral radiograph, the reference point is obtained on the posterior surface of the balloon on an anteroposterior line drawn through the centre of the balloon. On the frontal radiograph, the reference point is taken

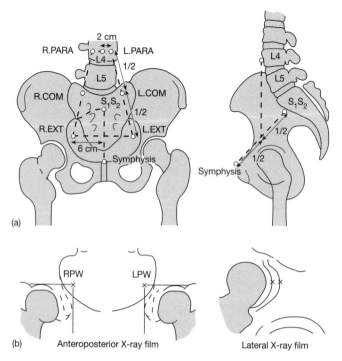

Fig. 9 ICRU Report 38[42] specification of reference points related to bony structures.

at the centre of the balloon. Barrilot *et al.*[46] have shown that ultrasound measurements can be used as an alternative.

For the rectal dose reference point: on the lateral radiograph, an anteroposterior line is drawn from the lower end of the intrauterine source (or from the middle of the intravaginal sources). On this the point is located 5 mm behind the posterior vaginal wall. The posterior vaginal wall is visualized, depending upon the technique, by means of an intravaginal mould or by opacification of the vaginal cavity with a radio-opaque gauze used for packing. On the anteroposterior radiograph this reference point is at the lower end of the intrauterine source or at the middle of the intravaginal sources.

Reference points related to bony structures include the lymphatic trapezoid[14] and the pelvic wall reference point.[47] Fig. 9(a) illustrates the basis of the location of the lymphatic trapezoid from anteroposterior and lateral radiographs. The six points of reference are the mid-external iliac lymph nodes (R EXT and L EXT), the low para-aortic area (R PARA and L PARA), and the low common iliac lymph nodes (R COM and L COM). The pelvic wall reference point can be visualized on an anteroposterior and a lateral radiograph (Fig. 9(b)) and related to fixed bony wall structures. This point is intended to be representative of the absorbed dose at the distal part of the parametrium and at the obturator lymph nodes. Evaluation of the absorbed dose at reference points related to well-defined bony structures and lymph node areas is particularly useful when intracavitary therapy is combined with external-beam therapy.

Differences in positioning of the applicators in relation to organs and reference points in patients undergoing multiple brachytherapy treatments require that these calculations are performed for each application and then summated.[48]

Clinical indications

The localized nature of the high-dose region around intracavitary sources makes their application most suitable for small tumours against which they can be closely positioned. Early stage Ib carcinoma of the cervix is such a tumour, where the sources can actually pass through and be abutted directly against the neoplasm (Fig. 5). Where malignant cells lie at a distance from intracavitary sources and are outside the high-dose region, a combination of external-beam treatment and intracavitary therapy is needed.

In gynaecological oncology, intracavitary irradiation is used particularly in the treatment of carcinoma of the cervix, as adjuvant therapy post-hysterectomy for patients with carcinoma of the endometrium, and for some patients with tumours of the vagina. While treatment details are included in specific chapters, the general principles of treatment using intracavitary therapy at these sites are as follows.

Carcinoma of the cervix

The treatment of carcinoma of the cervix most commonly involves intracavitary therapy in combination with external-beam irradiation, with applicators based on one of the classic systems. These all involve the insertion of an intrauterine tube and one or more vaginal applicators which are placed against the cervix. The dose rate is then highest in the region of the cervix and uterine cavity, and falls off most rapidly anteriorly and posteriorly. Laterally, the Paris, Manchester, and Fletcher–Houston systems create a pear-shaped dose distribution that delivers a higher dose rate to the parametria than to the rectum and bladder (Fig. 7).

Preoperative intracavitary treatment is rarely practised now, but was previously used to make surgery easier by reducing the size and vascularity of tumours. Nowadays, stage Ib tumours are usually operated upon without any radiotherapy. Both intracavitary and external-beam therapy are required for inoperable tumours or if pelvic nodal disease is suspected. External-beam therapy is the main modality of treatment and intracavitary therapy is used only to give a boost to the central disease. The techniques used to combine these two modalities vary widely.

One method is to deliver the external-beam treatment before the intracavitary therapy. The most individualized external-beam treatment may use three or four fields to treat a volume determined by anatomical landmarks, MRI, or CT scan to cover the groups of nodes at risk of involvement. Alternatively, a standard volume, for instance a 14 x 14-cm parallel opposed pair to the pelvis is used in some centres, especially in developing countries. When external-beam therapy is used prior to intracavitary therapy there is usually no central shielding. The dose that can subsequently be delivered by intracavitary therapy is limited by that already received by the dose-limiting normal tissues in the central pelvis, especially the rectum and bladder.

If intracavitary therapy is used before external-beam treatment, it has been customary to deliver a dose that is at least half of a radical intracavitary dose. This means that subsequent external-beam treatment is limited to a low dose, insufficient to treat the pelvic side walls, unless a central shield is used to spare those tissues that have already been heavily irradiated. The positioning of this central shield is extremely important. If the shield is slightly to one side of the intracavitary volume then, when summing the dose contributions from external-beam and intracavitary treatments, there is the risk of a relative overdosage on one side of the volume while there would be underdosage on the other side. This could lead to an increased risk of both normal-tissue damage and local recurrence. At its most sophisticated, the shield can be custom-built for the individual patient and can be positioned according to the dose distribution of the intracavitary therapy for that patient.

The advantages of using external-beam treatment before intracavitary therapy are, first, that there is no problem in locating a central shield, and second, that the tumour, in responding to external-beam treatment, shrinks towards the centre of the pelvis and is then better encompassed in the high-dose region around the sources. On the other hand, the advantage of using intracavitary therapy first is that a higher proportion of the central pelvic dose is from the intracavitary therapy and a much higher total dose is received by the tumour immediately around the sources.

There is increasing concern in the measurement and reporting of radiotherapy side-effects in all sites. However, this is particularly so in the treatment of gynaecological cancers with brachytherapy as the morbidity of a fistula or stricture in relation to a high dose region around the sources is considerable. In addition, it is vital that new technologies are introduced with rigorous monitoring of both early and late radiotherapy side-effects and brachytherapy is an area of rapid technological change. No one system of recording side-effects has universal acceptance and, in the past, systems tended to concentrate on early or late reactions or on those related to a particular modality of treatment. The production of the Franco-Italian glossary was an attempt to produce a tool for measuring all complications from all treatment modalities. Although the glossary can appear unwieldly, it can be used successfully.[49],[50] However, systems such as this need constant critical review to remain useful and, in general, are only effective for the prospective collection of toxicity data.[51]

Carcinoma of the endometrium

In most centres the standard treatment for endometrial carcinoma, after diagnosis at dilatation and curettage, is total hysterectomy, bilateral salpingo-oophorectomy, and adjuvant radiotherapy, based on histological risk factors. It is unusual for treatment by radiotherapy alone to be needed. However, for patients either physically or mentally unfit to undergo surgery, radical radiotherapy may be used.

The healthy uterine cavity is a triangular space when viewed in the anteroposterior plane and a slit in the lateral plane. However, when diseased, this cavity may be very distorted by tumour, uterine fibroids, or extrinsic compression. In addition to distortion of the cavity, the uterine wall may be of very variable thickness. To achieve a uniform dose distribution to the uterine wall can, therefore, be very difficult when using intracavitary sources and most regimens will rely on external-beam radiotherapy making the major contribution.

Heyman's capsules, mentioned in the introduction to this chapter, were an attempt to produce an even dose distribution to the uterine wall by utilizing many small point sources (Fig. 1). It is extremely difficult to achieve a satisfactory dose distribution by this method and the technique of insertion and withdrawal can be hazardous if active sources are used. Therefore, afterloading methods have been developed both for Heyman's capsules and for other intrauterine devices.

These other devices have mainly taken the form of two curved tubes curling into the uterine cornua, although multiple tubes, springing apart within the uterine cavity like the ribs of an umbrella, have also been used. Several of these devices have been developed to allow unequal radioisotope loading of the tubes so that, by using a CT scan of the uterus, the dose distribution can be designed to match the uterine wall. These afterloading systems are usually remotely operated and may deliver treatment at either low or high dose rates. Nevertheless, there is evidence that irradiation by a single line source within the uterine cavity can produce as good results as these more complex systems.[52]

Carcinoma of the vagina

Stage I carcinoma of the vagina and early stage II tumours, where there is minimal submucosal invasion, may be treated by interstitial implant using iridium wire. More deeply invasive tumours are usually most effectively treated by a combination of external-beam and interstitial irradiation. However, where lesions are circumferential around the vagina or where interstitial implant is technically difficult, as behind the pubic arch, intracavitary irradiation may be used either alone, in combination with external-beam treatment, or as part of a template-guided interstitial implant that incorporates a vaginal obturator.

The commonest tumours in the vagina are extensions from cervical and endometrial malignancies and are treated with external-beam radiotherapy and an intracavitary device that can irradiate the body of the uterus, cervix, and vagina with a line source (Fig. 2).

Future developments

The development of very high-activity microsources that can be remotely afterloaded into applicators has widened the scope of brachytherapy and has enabled tumours at previously inaccessible sites to be treated. In addition to the development of high dose-rate gynaecological treatments, intraluminal therapy has been a particular area of study.

Fine catheters can be passed through tumours in the upper nasal passages, nasopharynx, oesophagus, bronchus, urethra and ureter, and man-made passages, such as nephrostomy tracks. The slenderness of the catheters and the short time required to deliver the treatment make obstruction during the period of treatment much less of a problem than was the case with low dose-rate intraluminal therapy. Low dose-rate catheters were commonly as much as 1 cm in diameter and required to be in situ for several hours. High dose-rate catheters may be little more than 2 or 3 mm in diameter and need only be in place for a few minutes. Applicator design is a constant area of interest, both to improve local dosimetry and to widen the range of tumours that can be treated.

In gynaecological treatments, microprocessor-controlled source positioning and sophisticated planning computers enable optimization of dose distributions. This, particularly, requires very careful clinical assessment as the rules for both source positioning and dose prescription, derived empirically over many years, begin no longer to apply when tailor-made volumes are treated. However, the potential gains in local tumour control with a reduction in normal tissue damage could be considerable.

With the development of models of biological effectiveness, planning brachytherapy on the basis of radiation isodose volumes may be replaced by planning using biological isoeffect volumes.

In addition to investigating new sites for therapy and new methods of treatment planning, different methods of patient preparation are also being studied to allow treatment to be given without the need for a general anaesthetic or overnight stay in hospital.

Organizations such as the International Commission on Radiological Units and Measurements continue to develop better reporting systems for describing the radiotherapy, while others are developing reporting methods for the results of treatment and complications. This should improve communication between centres and allow improved sharing of and benefiting from clinical experience.

References

1. Pierquin B. *Precis de Curietherapie, Endocurietherapie et Plesiocurietherapie.* Paris: Masson, 1964.

2. Paterson R, Parker HM. A dosage system for γ-ray therapy. *British Journal of Radiology,* 1934; 7: 592–632.

3. Quimby EH. Dosage tables for linear radium sources. *Radiology,* 1944; 43: 572–7.

4. Meredith WJ, ed. *Radium Dosage, the Manchester System,* 2nd edn. Edinburgh: E.& S. Livingstone, 1967.

5. Meisberger LL, Keller RJ, Shalek RJ. The effective attenuation in water of the γ-rays of gold 198, iridium 192, caesium 137, radium 226 and cobalt 60. *Radiology,* 1968; 90: 953–7.

6. Slessinger ED, Grigsby PW. Verification studies of 3D brachytherapy source reconstruction techniques. In: Mould RF, ed. *Brachytherapy.* The Netherlands: Nucletron International BV, 1989: 130–5.

7. Heyman J. Technique in the treatment of cancer uteri at Radiumhemmet. *Acta Radiologica,* 1929; 10: 49–64.

8. Regaud C. Radiotherapy of carcinoma of the cervix uteri. Paris method. *American Journal of Roentgenology and Radium Therapy,* 1929; 21: 1.

9. Heyman J. The so-called Stockholm method and the results of treatment of uterine cancer at Radiumhemmet. *Acta Radiologica,* 1935; 16: 129.

10. Kottmeier HL. Surgical and radiation treatment of carcinoma of the uterine cervix. Experience by the current individualised Stockholm technique. *Acta Radiologica,* 1964; 43(Suppl. 2): 1.

11. Tod TF. Rectal ulceration following the radiation treatment of carcinoma of the cervix uteri. Pseudo carcinoma of the rectum. *Surgery, Gynaecology and Obstetrics,* 1938; 67: 617–31.

12. Tod MC, Meredith WJ. A dosage system for use in the treatment of cancer of the uterine cervix. *British Journal of Radiology,* 1938; 11: 809–24.

13. Meredith WJ, Massey JB. *Fundamental Physics of Radiology,* 3rd edn. Bristol: John Wright, 1977.

14. Fletcher GH. *Textbook of Radiotherapy,* 3rd edn. Philadelphia: Lea & Febiger, 1980.

15. Henschke UK, Hilaris BS, Mabian GD. Afterloading in interstitial and intracavitary radiation therapy. *American Journal of Roentgenology, Radium Therapy and Nuclear Medicine,* 1963; 90: 386–95.

16. Horwitz H, Kereiakes JG, Baker GK, Cluxton SE, Barett CM. An afterloading system utilizing caesium 137 for the treatment of carcinoma of the cervix. *American Journal of Roentgenology, Radium Therapy and Nuclear Medicine,* 1964; 91: 176–91.

17. Chassagne D, Pierquin B. La plesiocurietherapie du cancer du vagin par moulage plastique avec iridium 192—preparation non radio-active. *Journal de Radiologic et d'Electrologic,* 1966; 46: 89–93.

18. Steel GG, Down JD, Peacock JH, Stephens TC. Dose-rate effects and the repair of radiation damage. *Radiotherapy and Oncology,* 1986; 5: 321–31.

19. Steel GG, Deacon JM, Duchesne GM, Horwich A, Kelland LR, Peacock JH. The dose-rate effect in human tumour cells. *Radiotherapy and Oncology,* 1987; 9: 299–310.

20. Fowler JF. Dose-rate effects in normal tissues. In: Mould RF, ed. *Brachytherapy 2. Proceedings of the 5th International SELECTRON Users' Meeting 1988.* The Netherlands: Nucletron International BV, 1989: 26–40.

21. Steel GG, Kelland LR, Peacock JH. The radiobiological basis for low dose-rate radiotherapy. In: Mould RF, ed. *Brachytherapy 2. Proceedings of the 5th International SELECTRON Users' Meeting 1988.* The Netherlands: Nucletron International BV, 1989: 15–25.

22. Steel GG. Cellular sensitivity to low dose-rate irradiation focuses the problem of tumour radioresistance. (The ESTRO Breur Lecture.) *Radiotherapy and Oncology,* 1991; 20: 71–83.

23. Thames HD, Hendry JH. *Fractionation in Radiotherapy.* London: Taylor & Francis, 1987.

24. Oliver R. A comparison of the effects of acute and protracted γ-radiation on the growth of seedlings of *Vicia faba.* Part II. Theoretical calculations. *International Journal of Radiation Biology,* 1964; 8: 475–88.

25. Szechter A, Schwartz G. Dose-rate effects, fractionation, and cell survival at lowered temperatures. *Radiation Research,* 1977; 71: 593–613.

26. Thames HD, Withers HR, Peters LJ. Tissue repair capacity and repair kinetics deduced from multifractionated or continuous irradiation regimens with incomplete repair. *British Journal of Cancer,* 1984; 49(Suppl. VI): 263–9.

27. Dale RG. The application of the linear-quadratic dose–effect equation to fractionated and protracted radiotherapy. *British Journal of Radiology,* 1985; 58: 515–28.

28. Thames HD. An 'incomplete-repair' model for survival after fractionated and continuous irradiation. *International Journal of Radiation Biology,* 1985; 47: 319–39.

29. Dale RG, Jones B. The clinical radiobiology of brachytherapy. *British Journal of Radiology,* 1998; 71: 465–83.

30. Brenner DJ, Hall EJ. Fractionated high dose rate versus low dose rate regimens for intracavitary brachytherapy of the cervix. *British Journal of Radiology,* 1991; 64: 133–41.

31. Brenner DJ, Hall EJ. Conditions for the equivalence of continuous to pulsed low dose rate brachytherapy. *International Journal of Radiation Oncology, Biology and Physics,* 1991; 20: 181–90.

32. Vissier AG, van den Aardweg GJMJ, Levendag PC. Pulsed dose rate and fractionated high dose rate brachytherapy: Choice of brachytherapy schedules to replace low dose rate treatments. *International Journal of Radiation Oncology, Biology and Physics,* 1996; 34: 497–505.

33. Brenner DJ, Schiff PB, Huang Y, Hall EJ. Pulsed dose rate brachytherapy: design of convenient (daytime-only) schedules. *International Journal of Radiation Oncology, Biology and Physics,* 1997; 39: 809–15.

34. Rogers CL, Freel JH, Speiser BL. Pulsed low dose rate brachytherapy for uterine cervix carcinoma. *International Journal of Radiation Oncology, Biology and Physics,* 1999; 43: 95–100.

35. Hunter R. The Manchester experience with LDR variation in brachytherapy of cervix carcinoma. In: *International Brachytherapy, Report of the 8th International Brachytherapy Conference, Nice.* The Netherlands: Nucletron-Oldeft, 1995: 52–5.

36. Liversage WE. The application of cell survival theory to high dose-rate intracavitary therapy. *British Journal of Radiology,* 1966; 39: 338–49.

37. Joslin C, Smith C, Mallick A. The treatment of cervix cancer using high activity sources. *British Journal of Radiology,* 1972; 45: 257–70.

38. O'Connell D, Howard N, Hull MGR. Pre-operative irradiation of

uterine cancer using the Cathetron. In: Bates TD, Berry RJ, eds. *High Dose-rate Afterloading in the Treatment of Cancer of the Uterus.* London: *British Journal of Radiology,* Special Report No. 17, 1980: 1–10.

39. Fu KK, Phillips TL. High dose-rate versus low dose-rate intracavitary brachytherapy for carcinoma of the cervix. *International Journal of Radiation Oncology, Biology and Physics,* 1990; **19**: 791–6.

40. Khoury GC, Bulman AS, Joslin CAF. Long term results of Cathetron high dose rate intracavitary radiotherapy in the treatment of carcinoma of the cervix. *British Journal of Radiology,* 1991; **64**: 1036–43.

41. Sharma SC, Patel FD, Gupta BD, Negi PS, Aygagari S. Clinical trial of LDR versus HDR brachytherapy in carcinoma of the cervix. Report of the 6th International Selectron Users Meeting. *Selectron Brachytherapy Journal,* 1991; **5**: 75–9.

42. International Commission on Radiological Units and Measurements (ICRU). *Dose and Volume Specification for Reporting Intracavitary Therapy in Gynaecology.* Report No. 38. Washington, DC: ICRU Publications, 1985.

43. International Commission on Radiological Units and Measurements (ICRU). *Dose and Volume Specification for Reporting Interstitial Therapy.* Report No. 58. Washington, DC: ICRU Publications, 1997.

44. Chassagne D, Horiot JC. Propositions pour une définition commune des points de reference. *Journal de Radiologic et d'Electrologic,* 1977; **58**: 371–3.

45. Tan LT, Warren J, Freestone G, Jones B. Bladder dose estimation during intracavitary brachytherapy for carcinoma of the cervix using a single line source system. *British Journal of Radiology,* 1996; **69**: 953–62.

46. Barrilot I, Horiot JC, Maingon P, Bone-Lepinoy MC, Vaillant D, Feutray S. Maximum and mean bladder dose defined from ultrasonography. Comparison with the ICRU reference in gynaecological brachytherapy. *Radiotherapy and Oncology,* 1994; **30**: 231–8.

47. Chassagne D, Gerbaulet A, Dutreix A, Cosset JM. Utilisation pratique de la dosimetric par ordinateur en curietherapy gynecologique. *Journal de Radiologic et d'Electrologic,* 1977; **58**: 387–93.

48. Grigsby PW, Georgiou A, Williamson JF, Perez CA. Anatomic variation of gynaecologic brachytherapy prescription points. *International Journal of Radiation Oncology, Biology and Physics,* 1993; **27**: 725–9.

49. Pedersen D, Bentzen SM, Overgaard J. Reporting radiotherapeutic complications in patients with uterine cervical cancer. The importance of latency and classification system. *Radiotherapy and Oncology,* 1993; **28**: 134–41.

50. Sinistero G, Sismondi P, Rumore A, Zola P. Analysis of complications of cervix cancer treatment by radiotherapy using the Franco-Italian Glossary. *Radiotherapy and Oncology,* 1993; **26**: 203–11.

51. Shakespeare TP, Ferrier AJ, Holecek MJ, Jagavkar RS, Stevens MJ. Difficulties using the Franco-Italian Glossary in assessing toxicity of cervical cancer treatment. *International Journal of Gynaecological Cancer,* 1998; **8**: 51–5.

52. Potter K, Knocke TH, Kucera H, Weidinger B, Holler W. Primary treatment of endometrial carcinoma by HDR brachytherapy alone. In: *International Brachytherapy, Report of the 8th International Brachytherapy Conference, Nice.* The Netherlands: Nucletron-Oldeft, 1995: 195–6.

4.4 Programming of radiotherapy and sensitization

4.4.1 Radiation sensitization: hypoxia-selective therapeutics

M. P. Saunders, A.V. Patterson, and I. J. Stratford

Chronic and acute hypoxia

In 1955 Tomlinson and Gray published the results of a histological study of necrosis in fresh specimens of bronchial carcinoma. They observed that all tumour cords with a radius of greater than 200 μm had a necrotic centre, and that no tumour cord with a radius less than 160 μm showed any evidence of necrosis. These observations, combined with oxygen diffusion calculations, led to the hypothesis that the tissue oxygen tension would be essentially zero at a distance of 150 to 200 μm from a capillary. It was anticipated that along this limited diffusion distance would exist gradients of oxygen concentration, where cells could remain viable. This supposition was confirmed by Powers and Tolmach in 1963 who generated a biphasic cell-survival curve after irradiation of solid subcutaneous lymphosarcomas in mice to demonstrate that these tumours consisted of viable aerobic and hypoxic cells (as defined by a gas-phase oxygen concentration $(Po_2) \leq 1$ per cent $\equiv 7.6$ mmHg).

Later studies modelling the oxygen supply and tissue oxygenation in tumours,[1] as well as evaluation of oxygen diffusion distances in human xenograft models,[2] provided further evidence in support of the existence of chronic **diffusion-limited** hypoxia. Groebe and Vaupel[2] showed that radiosensitivity might be less than 10 per cent of maximum at intercapillary distances above 100 μm, and if intercapillary distances exceeded 140 μm, areas of radiobiological hypoxia extended right up to the arterial end of the microvessel. Direct intercapillary distance measurements in cervix uterus carcinomas have also been shown to predict for the presence of tissue hypoxia.[3]

In contrast with the blood supply to normal tissues, tumour vascular organization is often 'chaotic', consequently tumour blood flow through microvessels can be both intermittent and fluctuating. Transient **perfusion-limited** hypoxia is thought to arise not only from this abnormal vascular morphology, but also from geometric and viscous resistance to blood flow. Geometric and viscous resistances are primarily governed by the vessel diameter and the rheological properties of the blood, respectively.[4]

As a result of the altered vascular architecture, serious functional disturbances of the microflow are manifest, including arteriovenous-shunt perfusion, regurgitation and intermittent blood flow, and unstable speed and direction of flux. Geometric resistance to blood flow[5] may occur as a result of mechanical obstruction by micro- and macrothrombosis, erythrocyte sludging, transient plugging of microvessels by white blood cells, platelet aggregation, or the invasion and/or compression of the vessel lumen by surrounding neoplastic tissues.[4] Viscous resistance is influenced by many factors, including: haemoconcentration, aggregation of red blood cells, cell deformability, plasma viscosity, and plasma protein concentration.[6]

Using the Hoechst dye technique Chaplin et al.[7] showed that this phenomenon of non-perfusion was followed by reperfusion-induced transient hypoxia in transplanted murine tumours. The subsequent application of multichannel, laser Doppler microscopy conclusively demonstrated these dramatic fluctuations in blood flow in both xenografts[8] and the clinical setting.[8],[9] Using 300-μm diameter probes, fluctuations in erythrocyte flux have been recorded in tumour microregions with an estimated volume of 0.01 mm.[3] Initial studies in an undifferentiated murine sarcoma SaF xenograft model[10] recorded twofold changes or greater in 48 per cent of microregions examined over a 60-min period. Similar results (37 per cent) were seen in the human colon adenocarcinoma HT-29 xenograft model,[8] and in both systems over 50 per cent of the changes in blood flow occurred within 20 min.

Clinical analysis of both primary and recurrent breast carcinomas, as well as metastases to regional lymph nodes and skin from a variety of tumours of different histologies, revealed similar results.[8],[9] Of 66 human tumour microregions sampled, 26 per cent showed a change in erythrocyte flux by at least a factor of 2, while 58 per cent of the samples demonstrated a more than 1.5-fold change. The frequency of slower, more persistent fluctuations was greater than that seen in the earlier experimental systems. However, a high proportion of the changes measured still occurred within 20 min, and in at least 30 per cent of cases the change was reversed within the 60-min observation period. A factor of 2 reduction in perfusion could correspond to a 50 per cent reduction in blood flow in all the vessels contained in the probes' sampling volume, or at the other extreme, the complete closure of 50 per cent of the vessels contained within the microregion. Likewise, a 1.5-fold decrease would result if flow ceased in 30 per cent of the sampled vessels.

The development of laser Doppler microprobes has been crucial in the demonstration of the temporal nature of microregional fluctuations in tumour perfusion. While no system presently exists to measure temporal changes in tissue oxygenation directly, the observation that radiobiologically hypoxic cells can result from dynamic perfusion changes supports the inference that acute hypoxia, arising from changes in vascular flux,[7] can occur spatially and temporally on both a micro- and macroscopic scale. These disturbances in tumour blood flow are considered to be a major contributing factor to the presence of low Po_2 in human solid tumours.

Evidence for tumour hypoxia

In a review of published literature, Moulder and Rockwell[11] showed that 37 out of 42 experimental tumour models were found to contain hypoxic cells, with hypoxic fractions ranging from less than 1 per cent to 50 per cent. Although the proportion of hypoxic cells varied widely between tumour types, the average hypoxic fraction was in the region of 15 per cent. This figure does not indicate whether cells are permanently hypoxic, or whether they exist in a dynamic state of fluctuating oxygenation. Cater and Silver (1960) were the first to use the polarographic oxygen electrode to directly evaluate tumour oxygenation. Since then a series of studies in both experimental models and clinical trials have shown low or even zero oxygen partial pressures (Po_2) in malignant tissues.[12] Compared with the normal tissues, many human tumours are oxygen-deprived, with median Po_2 in tumours ranging from 1.3 to 3.9 per cent.[13] In contrast, median Po_2 in normal tissues are significantly higher, at 3.1 to 8.7 per cent. Of note, extreme values below 0.3 per cent Po_2 were found to be common in tumours but rare in normal tissues.[13] These observations are not universally consistent, and in a recent abstract Collingridge et al.[14] showed that oxygenation in normal brain tissue was similar to that found in gliomas. Using an Eppendorf Po_2 histograph, they documented the oxygenation in low- and high-grade tumours and the adjacent normal tissues in 18 anaesthetized patients. The average median Po_2 value was lower in high-grade tumours (4.0 mmHg (0.5 per cent Po_2) versus 12.9 mmHg (1.7 per cent Po_2)), but the oxygenation in the surrounding tissues was statistically similar. They concluded that the oedema created by the tumour may compromise the oxygenation in the adjacent normal tissues. Interestingly, the intratumoural values obtained in two conscious patients were much higher at 30.2 (4.0 per cent Po_2) and 40.1 mmHg (5.3 per cent Po_2). This may be due to the respiratory and cardiac depressant effects of the anaesthetics. As an extension to this work, Collingridge et al. are now accruing more patients to assess the influence of anaesthetics on tissue oxygenation. In an earlier study Sundfor et al.[15] evaluated the effect of propofol anaesthesia on the oxygenation of tumours as measured by the polarographic oxygen electrode. They plotted the frequency distributions of Po_2 in five patients with cervical carcinoma. From the pooled data, no difference in oxygenation was found, suggesting that anaesthesia did not effect the results obtained using this method.

Hypoxic cells and radiotherapy resistance

In experimental systems, hypoxic cells have been shown to be resistant to radiotherapy.[16],[17] Low, linear energy-transfer (**LET**) radiations,

such as X-rays, are sparsely ionizing and have an indirect action, generating free radicals such as OH•, e^-_{aq}, (hydrated electron), and H atoms that can react with DNA. Anoxic cells (defined as less than 10 p.p.m. of O_2) are approximately 2.5- to 3-fold more radioresistant than normoxic cells; that is to say, a 2.5- to 3-times larger radiation dose is required to achieve the same reduction in clonogenicity or effective tumour control. In general, a radical radiotherapy treatment is given in 2-Gy fractions (for example, 60 Gy in 30 fractions). At this fractionation, the oxygen enhancement ratio (**OER**) is lower at about 2.0, indicating that there is less oxygen dependency if tumours are treated in this manner.[18] However, even with this fractionation, tumours can still be relatively radioresistant.

Experimentally, half-maximal sensitivity (*K* value) is seen at about 0.3 per cent O_2 (3000 p.p.m. O_2, $\equiv$ 2.1 mmHg).[18] This phenomenon, known as the oxygen enhancement ratio, is thought to result from oxygen's ability to react with and chemically modify the initial radiation-induced DNA radical.[19] If oxygen is present it reacts with the ionized target molecules generating organic peroxide lesions, which are thought to be significantly less repairable forms of damage. For the 'oxygen fixation' effect to be observed, oxygen must be present during, or within a millisecond after, the radiation exposure.

The recent development of methodologies incorporating the technique of gas chromatography–mass spectrometry (**GC-MS**) has facilitated the detailed analysis of free radical-induced DNA damage.[20] This technique permits the measurement of a large number of products in the same sample of DNA or chromatin in a single analysis, and allows the chemical characterization and quantification of base-derived and sugar-derived products as well as of DNA–protein crosslinks. GC-MS analysis of chromatonized DNA following exposure to ionizing irradiation has demonstrated the formation of various pyrimidine-derived and purine-derived modified bases, the yields and characteristics of which have been shown to be dependent upon factors such as the type of irradiation, DNA conformation, and the direct radical environment. The modification of DNA bases through addition or abstraction by ionizing radiation-generated free radicals (for example, OH•, e^-_{aq}, H atom) is strongly influenced by the presence of an oxic versus an anoxic environment. The presence of oxygen increases the yields of most products with the exception of formamidopyrimidines. Some products (for example, 8-hydroxyguanine) are produced almost exclusively in the presence of oxygen, while others are produced under both conditions. When oxygen is present, peroxyl radicals are formed by the addition of molecular oxygen to sugar or base radicals of DNA. Further short-chain reactions of DNA radicals may occur but these will depend upon the types of radicals, their reaction partners, and the reaction environment. This results in the formation of a wide variety of final products through a spectrum of different mechanisms.

Clinical evidence for radioresistance

Tumour hypoxia is associated with poor radiotherapy results. In 1968, Kolstad measured the oxygen tension at the surface of cervical tumours with a polarographic electrode and demonstrated that tumours with oxygen concentrations between 0 and 9 mmHg had more local recurrences following radiotherapy than those above 9 mmHg.[21] Some 20 years later, Gatenby et al.[22] determined the oxygen concentration in head and neck nodal metastases with the polarographic electrode. They found that radiotherapy responders had significantly greater mean tumour oxygen concentrations than non-responders.

In 1993, Hockel et al.[23] published a paper showing that hypoxia was an indicator of poor prognosis in cervical carcinoma treated with radiotherapy. An updated analysis was published 3 years later confirming these findings.[24] A total of 44 patients with advanced cervical carcinoma received radiotherapy ($n = 29$), some with induction ($n = 11$) or concomitant ($n = 4$) chemotherapy. Tumour oxygenation status was determined using the Eppendorf histograph system. Two tracks were made in each tumour and between 25 and 35 oxygen measurements were taken from each track. The 23 patients with hypoxic tumours (< 10 mmHg) had a significantly worse disease-free survival (DFS) probability compared to patients with better oxygenated tumours ($p = 0.0484$).[23] In the follow-up study, Hockel et al.[24] evaluated the overall survival probability of patients with hypoxic cervical tumours, which were treated with either radiation or surgery. In total, 103 patients were included, all of whom had advanced cervical tumours (FIGO stage bulky Ib to IVb). The Kaplan–Meier method was used to show that the disease-free and overall survival of patients with hypoxic tumours was significantly worse, whether they were treated with primary surgery or radiotherapy. This suggested that tumour oxygenation was a strong prognostic indicator irrespective of the treatment modality.

A study carried out by Brizel et al.[25] evaluated the relationship between tumour hypoxia and the development of distant metastases in soft-tissue sarcomas treated with irradiation/hyperthermia. They showed that tumours which were hypoxic prior to treatment were significantly more likely to metastasize than those tumours that were well oxygenated. These observations support those of Hockel et al.,[24] emphasizing the importance of tumour hypoxia as an independent prognostic indicator.

Brizel et al.[26] subsequently evaluated the effect of tumour hypoxia on outcome, in patients with stage IV head and neck tumours treated with radiotherapy. Using a polarographic electrode, 28 patients underwent P_{O_2} measurements, prior to radiotherapy. A highly significant increase in DFS was found in patients with a median tumour P_{O_2} of more than 10 mmHg compared with those patients with more hypoxic tumours (78 versus 22 per cent; $p = 0.009$).

Indirect evidence to support the influence of oxygenation on radiation response comes from observations that show a correlation between a patient's haemoglobin concentration and tumour control. In a review of 33 trials in cervical, bladder, prostate, lung, and head and neck tumours, Overgaard and Horsman[27] deduced that a haemoglobin concentration in the upper regions of the normal range was associated with an increased probability of local control in the irradiated field. There was, however, no reduction in the incidence of distant metastases. As well as blood transfusions, another method aimed at reducing tumour hypoxia includes the use of perfluorochemical emulsions (that is, Fluosol). Evans et al.[28] demonstrated a long-term benefit when patients with high-grade gliomas received a combination of radiotherapy and Fluosol/oxygen breathing. This indirectly suggests that tumour hypoxia is a therapeutic hindrance and that alleviating it can lead to a beneficial radiotherapeutic effect.

Both direct and indirect experimental evidence has demonstrated that hypoxic tumours are radioresistant, and accumulating clinical evidence of the actual relationship between tumour oxygen status and outcome of treatment overwhelmingly points to tumour oxygenation as an **extremely important modifier** of the slope of the dose–response curve in some tumour types.

Hypoxic cells and chemotherapy resistance

The evidence for hypoxia leading to chemoresistance is less abundant than for radioresistance and comes mainly from preclinical work with oxygen enhancing systems. However, there are compelling reasons and considerable experimental suggestion[16],[23],[29]–[31] to anticipate that hypoxic cells are resistant to some types of cytotoxic drugs, not least because a high proportion of hypoxic cells are non-cycling and many chemotherapeutic agents are mitotic poisons. A 16-h exposure to hypoxia can reduce DNA synthesis by 80 to 90 per cent in vitro irrespective of the cell-cycle point,[32],[33] and probably provides marked protection from many commonly employed antimetabolites. This is evidenced by reports showing that exponentially growing cells in vitro, when rendered chronically hypoxic during drug exposure, are more resistant to many chemotherapeutic agents, particularly antimetabolites and DNA-interchelators. These include actinomycin D, doxorubicin, etoposide, mitoxantrone, vincristine, m-AMSA, taxol, 5-fluorouracil, arabinoside, procarbazine, streptonigrin, and bleomycin.[30] With redox-active agents such as bleomycin, streptonigrin, and etoposide, oxygen itself is directly involved in the mechanism of toxicity. Teicher[30] used colony-survival assays to show that FSaIIC fibrosarcoma cells were more resistant to treatment with bleomycin if they were exposed under hypoxic conditions. They also showed that the cytotoxicity of this drug could be increased if the exposure was carried out in an atmosphere of 95 per cent O_2 and 5 per cent CO_2 (carbogen). This later result was also confirmed in vivo, by demonstrating a growth delay if the bleomycin was administered whilst the animal was breathing carbogen or hyperbaric oxygen. A similar result with the topoisomerase II inhibitor, etoposide, was found by the same group using a perfluorochemical emulsion to reduce tumour hypoxia.[30] This combined treatment delayed tumour regrowth by 2.2 to 3.3 times that seen with etoposide alone in three in vivo models. This suggested that a reduction in tumour hypoxia, induced by the perfluorochemical emulsion, resulted in an increased sensitivity to etoposide. In another in vivo study,[30] the addition of a perfluorochemical emulsion followed by carbogen breathing increased the antitumour effect of the alkylating agent cyclophosphamide, as measured by growth delay.

However, for the majority of chemotherapeutic drugs, resistance is not strictly related to the direct absence of molecular oxygen per se, and is probably related to the induction of multiple early stress-response proteins, complex modulations of cell-cycle progression, and changes in recognition and/or response to DNA damage. This capacity for rapid adaptation also extends to the acquisition of temporary drug resistance as a posthypoxic characteristic. This transient phenomenon has been reported for doxorubicin, methotrexate, 5-fluorouracil, actinomycin-D, etoposide, BCNU, and cisplatin, in various murine and human cell-line models.[29],[30]

Hypoxia and genetic instability

Hypoxia not only provides an environment that directly facilitates drug resistance through the temporary induction of drug resistance-associated genes, but it can also encourage the evolution of stable phenotypic changes characteristic of permanent chemotherapeutic drug resistance. Hypoxia is an early event in tumour growth and provides a major selection mechanism for mutations that confer a survival advantage under hypoxia. Selection for mutant p53 has been demonstrated to occur following repeated cycles of hypoxia and reoxygenation *in vitro* and has been related to enhanced hypoxic cell survival *in vivo*.[34] Loss of functional p53 status appears to enhance certain types of genetic instability and has been linked to enhanced aneuploidy, gene amplification, and recombination events, all of which may then contribute to further tumour progression.[35] This phenomenon may be amplified by the fact that anoxia has been shown to enhance DNA strand breaks, perhaps providing a mechanism for further genomic instability. In addition, the mutation of p53 during tumour progression results in the elimination of certain signals that are proapoptotic. Consequently, some tumours can become inherently resistant to chemotherapy or radiation therapy-induced apoptosis. Thus hypoxia is a potent physiological stress that is thought to promote tumour progression, both driving and selecting for genetic diversity, to give rise ultimately to an aggressive neoplastic phenotype.[24],[33],[34],[36]

Experimental evidence supports the belief that increases in genetic instability and gene amplification can promote the generation of mutations that render individual cells less susceptible to treatment. A marked enhancement in the frequency of methotrexate resistance and dihydrofolate reductase (**DHFR**) gene amplification has been observed *in vitro*, with acquisition of resistance being related to the duration of both hypoxia and re-oxygenation. Furthermore, hypoxia was shown to enhance the frequencies of simultaneous resistance to methotrexate and doxorubicin, which was related to both DHFR and P-glycoprotein gene amplification.[37] This later example of gene overexpression may have therapeutic implications in the treatment of tumours with other drugs, such as vincristine, etoposide, and taxol, which are extruded from cells by the P-glycoprotein efflux pump.

Modifying factors to reduce tumour hypoxia

Cumulative evidence strongly indicates that tumour hypoxia promotes both radioresistance and chemoresistance, which can contribute to the inability to achieve tumour control. Consequently, many approaches have been developed to overcome this therapeutic hindrance. These include the use of hypoxic-cell radiosensitizers[38],[39] and, more recently, the combination of carbogen and nicotinamide (**ARCON:** accelerated radiotherapy with carbogen and nicotinamide).[40] In a meta-analysis of 83 randomized clinical trials involving 10 779 patients treated with hyperbaric oxygen, radiosensitizers, oxygen or carbogen breathing, and blood transfusions, the local control probability was improved by 4.7 per cent ($p < 0.00004$). The overall survival probability also showed a significant enhancement ($p < 0.05$), particularly in squamous-cell head and neck tumours.[27],[41] This result emphasized

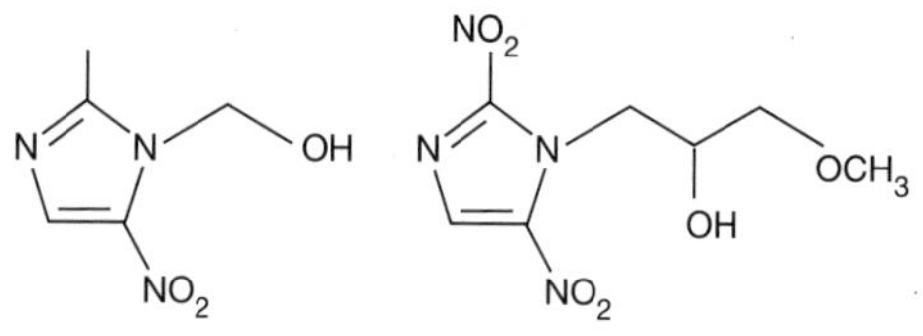

Fig. 1 Metronidazole and misonidazole.

the power of a meta-analysis, since most of the trials evaluated were not significant, although, when viewed together, there was an overall tendency towards a better outcome in the hypoxic modification arms. As with many studies, the main reason why most were unable to achieve significance was the small sample size. The median number of patients entered into the studies was only 84, when probably near to 1000 patients would be needed to show a significant result, particularly as only a proportion of the treated tumours would have been significantly hypoxic. This overview emphasized that hypoxia is a problem and that there may be a therapeutic gain by manipulating factors to reduce it.

Radiosensitizers are oxygen-mimetic agents that can substitute for oxygen in 'fixing' radiation-induced DNA damage. The antibiotic metronidazole was the first nitroheterocyclic drug investigated clinically as a hypoxic-cell radiosensitizer. The more active compound, misonidazole, was subsequently investigated, but overall the results were rather disappointing. This was possibly due to the neurological toxicity limiting the dose that could be administered (Fig. 1).

Less lipophilic analogues of misonidazole analogues were developed, including etanidazole and pimonidazole. However, a trial involving the latter drug had to be stopped since an interim analysis showed that patients in the treatment arm were faring less well than those in the control group. Nimorazole, a 5-nitroimidazole, was then developed and successfully used by the Danish head and neck cancer group (**DAHANCA**), in combination with radiotherapy, to provide an improvement in local control (49 per cent versus 33 per cent, $p = 0.002$).[42]

To date, none of the methods used to reduce tumour hypoxia have gained a place in the routine treatment of patients in the United Kingdom or the United States. In Denmark, however, the radiosensitizer nimorazole was used in the randomized study DAHANCA 5. Nimorazole was randomly allocated to patients with supraglottic and pharyngeal carcinomas treated with irradiation. A highly significant benefit in terms of local control and disease-free survival was shown.[43] In a follow-up paper[42] there was still a significant and important improvement in local control (49 versus 33 per cent; $p = 0.002$), but no difference in overall survival was found. The fact that it has not gained a place in other areas of the world may reflect both the scepticism of other clinicians and an unwillingness to change.

Targeting hypoxia

Rather than aiming to eliminate tumour hypoxia, an attractive alternative is to **exploit** this unique physiological difference for

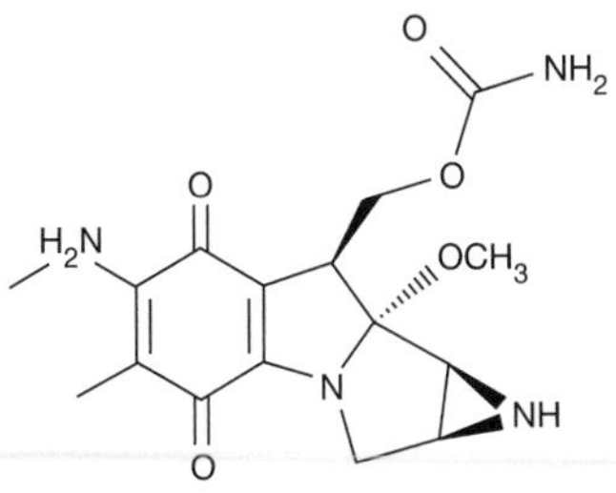

Fig. 2 Mitomycin C.

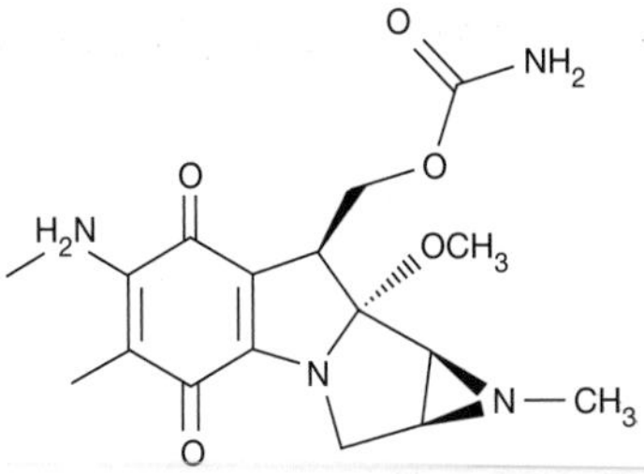

Fig. 3 Porfiromycin.

therapeutic gain. Treatments that focus on hypoxic tissues can selectively target solid neoplasias, whilst sparing normal well-oxygenated tissues. Bioreductive agents are a broad class of compounds that provide this selective cytotoxicity towards hypoxic cells, at concentrations well below that required for their radiosensitizer effects.

Bioreductive drugs

Bioreductive drugs can be separated into three main classes: nitroimidazoles; N-oxides; and quinones. All require activation by endogenous reductases such as DT-diaphorase (DTD), xanthine oxidase (XO), aldehyde dehydrogenase (ALDH), cytochrome b_5 reductase (b5R), cytochrome P-450 (CYP450), and cytochrome P-450 reductase (P450R). Reductive metabolism is initiated by the transfer of a single electron to the hypoxic cytotoxin. Enzymes that can preferentially donate one electron include CYP450, P450R, b5R, and XO. Consequently, bioreductive prodrugs are metabolized to highly cytotoxic products that can strand-break, crosslink, or intercalate DNA. The process of metabolic reduction is reversed by oxygen, such that the cytotoxic metabolites are rapidly back-oxidized to their parent compound. Superoxide radicals are derived from the action of this one-electron 'futile cycle' and are considered to be less toxic than the activated drug, due to the abundance of cellular reactive-oxygen detoxifying mechanisms, most notably the superoxide dismutase(s) and catalase combinations.

The rate at which a hypoxic cytotoxin is metabolized will be determined by both the presence of the relevant reductase(s) and the ability of the drug to act as a substrate for this reducing enzyme(s). It follows that cells with a high expression of a particular enzyme will be more sensitive to treatment with a bioreductive drug that is activated by the reductase. Thus hypoxic cytotoxins can selectively target tumours that have regions of low oxygen tension which predispose to radiotherapeutic resistance.[44]

Quinones (mitomycin C, porfiromycin, and EO9 for example)

Mitomycin C (MMC, Fig. 2)

MMC, the prototype bioreductive drug, was isolated from *Streptomyces caespitosus*. It has been used in the treatment of cancer for nearly 20 years and has gained a place in the therapy of a number of solid tumours, including lung and breast cancer. It has three cytotoxic groups (aziridine ring, carbamate, and quinonics) and requires either a one- or two-electron reduction for its activation.

DTD is thought to be the major two-electron reductase involved in the bioactivation of MMC. This pathway is oxygen-independent,

which may contribute to the low selectivity MMC exhibits towards hypoxic cells.[45] MMC can also be efficiently activated by the one-electron reducing enzyme P450R, and this enzyme is an important contributor to the hypoxic activation of this quinone.[46] Recent studies have also identified an NADPH-dependent, mitochondrial, one-electron reductase that contributes significantly to the metabolism of MMC and appears to be more efficient than DTD at metabolizing MMC.[47] Importantly, mitochondria have been identified as a critical target for MMC toxicity, suggesting that the activity of these reductases may be of considerable therapeutic relevance.[48]

However, it is unclear whether the one-electron or two-electron reduced forms of MMC, or both, are responsible for cytotoxicity, and mechanisms have been proposed for either the semiquinone or hydroquinone as the toxic species. The mechanism is further complicated by the potential involvement of both species with O_2-driven auto-oxidation, and by the possibility of both disproportionation and comproportionation reactions between the quinone and its reduced forms.[49],[50]

A randomized study in squamous-cell carcinoma of the head and neck looking at the role of postoperative radiation therapy, with or without mitomycin C, was published by Weissberg *et al.*[51] The drug was administered soon after the start of 5 weeks of radiotherapy, and some patients received a second dose 6 weeks later. From a cohort of 117 patients, an increase in the actuarial disease-free survival (DFS) was found in those given the combined treatment, compared with patients receiving radiotherapy alone (75 per cent versus 49 per cent; $p < 0.07$; median follow-up > 5 years). It was concluded that a treatment benefit was obtained without a significant increase in toxicity related to the mitomycin C. The dose-limiting toxicity includes prolonged myelosuppression, pulmonary fibrosis, cardiotoxicity, and nephrotoxicity. Because of these side-effects, other bioreductive drugs with a better therapeutic index have been sought.

Porfiromycin (methyl-MMC, Fig. 3)

Porfiromycin is an analogue of MMC and has a greater aerobic/hypoxic differential cytotoxicity than MMC.[52] Compared to MMC, which has an approximately twofold selective toxicity towards hypoxic cells, porfiromycin exhibits a broader tenfold oxic/hypoxic differential cytotoxicity. This superior hypoxia-selectivity is predominantly due to a lowering of the aerobic toxicity, and has been shown to be related to the lower incidence of DNA crosslinks generated by porfiromycin under aerobic conditions. Porfiromycin is activated by both one- and two-electron reductases[46] and, like MMC, it is the single-electron reduction pathway that confers the hypoxia-selective properties of

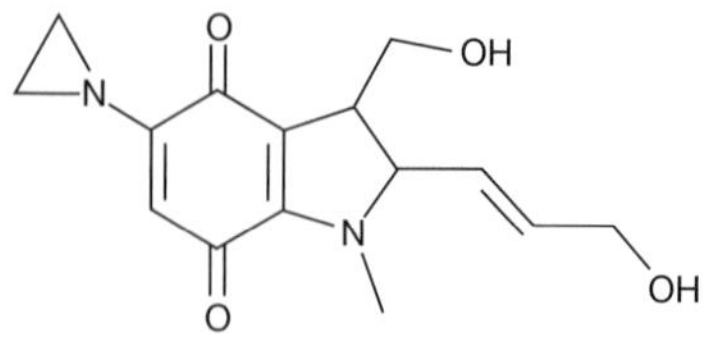

Fig. 4 The indoloquinone EO9.

this agent. Several one-electron reductases have been evaluated as important contributors to this oxygen-sensitive metabolism.[46],[49] The semiquinone radical generated by one-electron reduction is thought to be the dominant cytotoxic species.[49],[50]

In a phase I toxicity study, porfiromycin was given concomitantly with radiotherapy to patients with head and neck tumours. This study was later extended into a phase III comparison of radiotherapy plus porfiromycin to radiotherapy plus MMC, again in patients with head and neck tumours. The early results suggested that the toxicity profile was acceptable and the trial is presently ongoing.[53]

EO9 (Fig. 4)

EO9 is a synthetic indolequinone which was originally synthesized by Oostveen and Speckman in 1987. Even though it is an analogue of MMC, it has been shown to differ both *in vitro* and *in vivo* in its antitumour profile and is less myelosuppressive than MMC.[54] It is a much better substrate for both rat and human DTD and is considerably more active under hypoxic conditions.[55],[56] A hypoxic/aerobic differential of approximately 30-fold has been demonstrated by Adams *et al.*[57]

EO9, like MMC, is subject to both one- and two- electron reductive metabolism to the semi- and hydroquinone, respectively. However, details of the relative contributions of cellular reductases, and their respective contributions to aerobic versus hypoxic cytotoxicity, have only recently begun to emerge (Fig. 5).

Early studies identified DTD as an important enzyme for the metabolism of EO9, and bioactivation of EO9 by purified DTD resulted in DNA single-strand breaks.[55] The suggestion of a role for DTD in EO9 cytotoxicity was confirmed by Robertson *et al.*[56] when a good correlation was demonstrated between the sensitivity of a panel of human cell lines to aerobic EO9 exposure and intracellular DTD activity *in vitro*. Reduction of EO9 by purified DTD has been shown to result in either DNA single-strand breaks,[55],[58] or DNA alkylation and crosslinking[59],[60] and as such there is disagreement in the literature as to the nature of the cytotoxic lesions generated under aerobic conditions.[61],[62] Butler *et al.*[61] demonstrated that the hydroquinone was rapidly back-oxidized to EO9 under aerobic conditions with the concomitant production of H_2O_2, suggesting reactive oxygen species (**ROS**) formation (particularly OH•) would be the dominant cause of DNA damage. This must question the ability of the hydroquinone, formed directly by DTD-dependent metabolism, to generate significant crosslinking in intact cells. Perhaps in studies where correlations were observed between the cytotoxicity of EO9 in air and DTD expression, the effect was mediated via ROS. Yet, Walton *et al.*[55] observed that superoxide dismutase did not prevent the

formation of single-strand breaks, implying that alkylation was initiating the DNA-damaging effect. Whatever the mechanism, direct evidence that human DTD is relevant to EO9 toxicity in whole cells has recently been provided by transfection of human NQO1 cDNA into Chinese hamster ovary (**CHO**) cells. Clones expressing high levels of DTD were sensitized to aerobic EO9 exposure.[63]

Robertson *et al.*[56] also demonstrated that in cells with high DTD levels, treatment with EO9 under hypoxic conditions did not provide significant additional cytotoxicity, whereas cells with low DTD levels were markedly sensitized to EO9 in hypoxia. This is consistent with a dominant oxygen-insensitive role for DTD in the metabolism of EO9,[55],[59] but in the absence of DTD, alternative oxygen-sensitive, one-electron processes will contribute to cytotoxicity, but only under low oxygen tensions. In agreement, it has been demonstrated that an inverse correlation exists between the hypoxic cytotoxicity of EO9 and DTD activity in two independent panels of human cell lines.[55],[56]

The importance of one-electron reductases in the bioactivation of EO9 was exemplified using the HT-29 and BE cell-line pair.[64] Under hypoxia, the DTD-rich HT-29 cells demonstrated only a 2.9-fold increase in cytotoxicity, while the DTD-deficient BE cell line became 1000- to 3000-fold more sensitive to EO9 exposure. The relationship between aerobic potency of EO9 has subsequently been correlated to DNA damage in these cell lines.[59] BE cells showed a dramatic 30-fold increase in the extent of crosslinks formed under hypoxic conditions, supporting the relevance of one-electron reduction in EO9 cytotoxicity under low oxygen tension.

More importantly *in vivo* studies have also demonstrated that EO9 functions as a hypoxia-selective cytotoxin.[57] While EO9 was inactive against the KHT sarcoma in mice as a single agent, it could strongly potentiate the action of 10-Gy X-irradiation. This effect was much larger for EO9 than MMC, and appeared to be related to the superior hypoxic cytotoxicity ratio of EO9 against KHT cells *in vitro*. It was concluded that since 10 Gy was sufficient to eradicate the aerobic fraction of the xenograft, this implied that EO9 was functioning as a hypoxic cytotoxin. In support, a greater than additive effect was seen in four types of rat tumours when EO9 was administered postirradiation.[65] *In vivo* studies have attempted to correlate tumour response to EO9 with reductive enzyme profile, but no relationship has been found for either DTD, P450R, or b_5R activities.[62] However, tumour sensitivity *in vivo* was shown to be related to the overall ability of tumour homogenates to catabolize EO9 under hypoxic conditions ($r^2 = 0.86$; $p = 0.07$), but not so clearly under aerobic conditions ($r^2 = 0.82$; $p = 0.17$). The severity and extent of hypoxia within these xenograft models was not determined, so interpretation of the data is difficult.

EO9 has completed phase I and phase II clinical evaluations in non-small-cell lung cancer (NSCLC).[66],[67] Unfortunately, these trials failed to demonstrate any significant antitumour activity, although enzyme levels were not measured. The reason for this, may be partly due to the design of these studies. Patients in both trials were treated with EO9 alone. It is perhaps inappropriate to evaluate any hypoxic cytotoxin as a single agent, since only the hypoxic subpopulation of a tumour will be treated. Better results might have been achieved by combining the treatment with radiotherapy, in a similar approach to the studies with porfiromycin and tirapazamine.

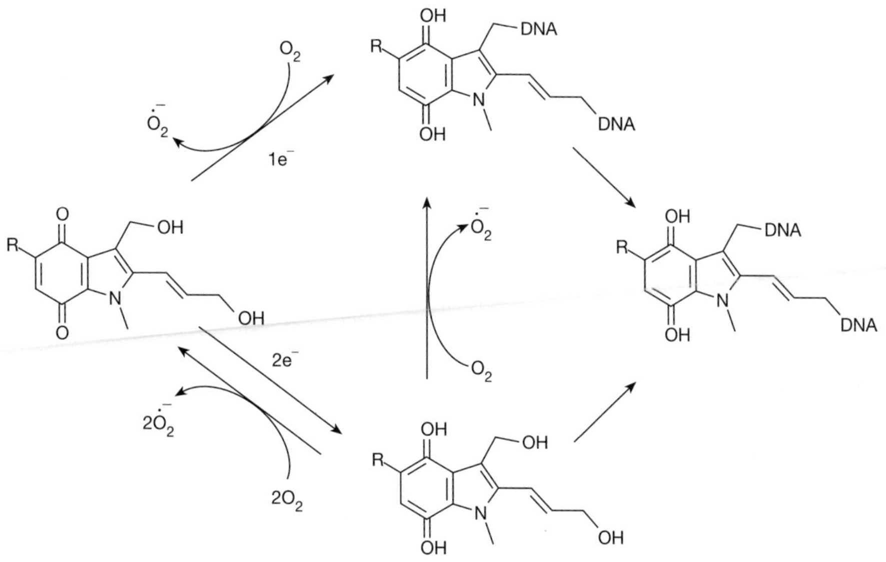

Fig. 5 Proposed differential oxygen-sensitivity of indolequinone metabolism by one- or two-electron reduction pathways.

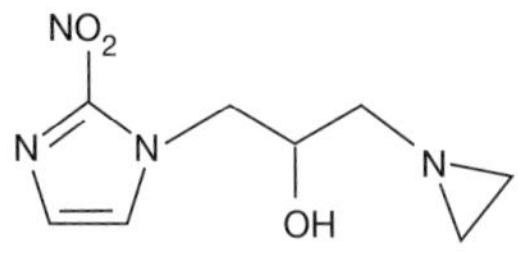

Fig. 6 RSU1069.

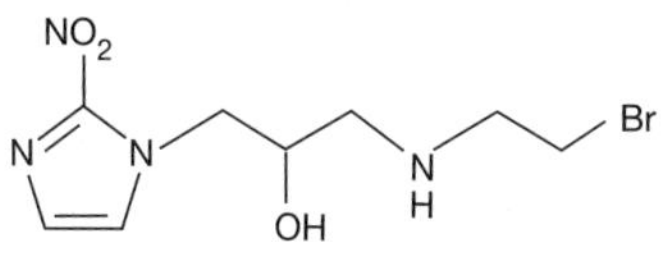

Fig. 7 RB6145.

Nitroimidazoles (for example, RSU1069 and its prodrug RB6145)

RSU1069 (Fig. 6)

RSU1069 is a dual-function 2-nitroimidazole which was developed as an aziridinyl derivative of misonidazole.[44] It is both a radio-sensitizer, like the structurally related misonidazole, and an alkylating agent due to the presence of an aziridine ring. It is activated by one-electron reductases, to give rise to a nitroso radical. This process is reversed by back-oxidation. In aerobic conditions it is a typical monofunctional alkylating agent, probably due to the reactivity of the aziridine ring. In hypoxic regions, one-electron reduction of the nitro group creates another cytotoxic side-chain making RSU1069 a bifunctional alkylating agent. This bifunctionality is believed to be responsible for both the high hypoxic to aerobic cytotoxic differential and the substantial radiosensitizing activity. It is up to 100 times more toxic to hypoxic cells than to aerobic ones.[68] RSU1069 went into clinical trials in 1986, but because of considerable gastrointestinal toxicity it was not evaluated any further in patients[69] (prior to the advent of newer antiemetics such as 5-HT$_3$ antagonists).

RB6145 (Fig. 7)

RB6145 is a chemical prodrug of RSU1069. It retains both the radiosensitization and bioreductive properties of RSU1069, but was considerably less toxic in animal studies.[70] RB6145 is metabolized *in vivo* with 30 per cent conversion to RSU1069.[71],[72] In experimental models, when RB6145 was given at three times the dosage of RSU1069

Fig. 8 Tirapazamine.

it was just as effective but less toxic.[70] CI-1010, the *R*-enantiomer of RB6145, caused marked retinal toxicity in mice, rats, dogs, and monkeys. Because of this serious side-effect, RB6145 will not be entering clinical trials in humans. Retinopathy may arise as a consequence of the retina becoming hypoxic during visual inactivity and could be related to drug-induced lethargy in animal models.

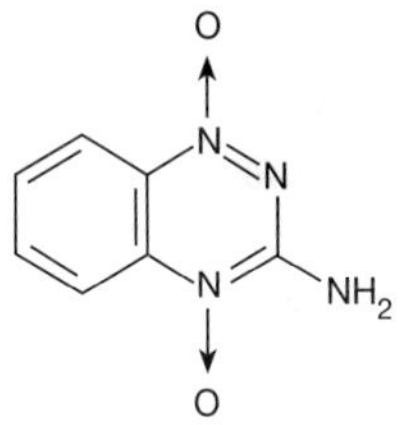

Benzotriazine-di-N-oxides

Tirapazamine (SR4233/WIN59075) (Fig. 8), the lead compound in this class of cytotoxins, was developed by Zeman *et al.*[73] It is activated by one-electron reduction to a nitroxide radical intermediate, before detoxification by a further chemical reduction to SR4317.[74] A further two-electron reduction leads to the formation of another non-toxic

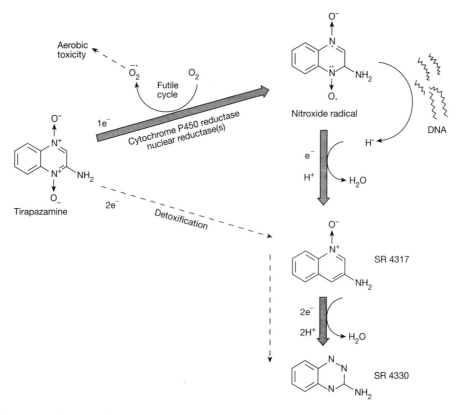

Fig. 9 Proposed mechanism of tirapazamine metabolism by one- and two-electron reduction.

metabolite, SR4330 (Fig. 9). Under hypoxic conditions, the radical is thought to abstract a hydrogen atom from DNA to produce single- and double-strand breaks, leading to chromosomal defects. These aberrations are significantly more difficult to repair than those produced by X-rays.[75],[76]

Tirapazamine exhibits considerable selective cytotoxicity, with oxic/hypoxic differentials in the order of 30- to 300-fold in most murine and human cell lines.[73],[77] None the less, tirapazamine is also toxic to aerobic cells. The mechanism of oxic toxicity is likely to be related to the instability of the cytotoxic radical, which is back-oxidized to the parent compound in the presence of oxygen. This example of redox cycling results in the concurrent generation of superoxide radicals, which are less cytotoxic than the drug-radical species.[74]

Multiple enzymes are capable of reducing tirapazamine to its two-electron reduction product, SR4317.[74],[78]–[80] However, the relative contributions of these enzymes with respect to cytotoxic drug-radical formation is unclear, and furthermore, between 30 and 60 per cent of the tirapazamine consumed remains unaccounted for.[81] The majority of the studies on tirapazamine metabolism have concentrated on microsomal activation, since this is the site of greatest enzyme activity. Walton and Workman[78] showed that anaerobic reduction of tirapazamine by mouse liver microsomes was 40 times greater than that which could be achieved by cytosolic-dependent reduction. The microsomal one-electron reductase, cytochrome P-450 reductase, has been identified as an important determinant of the rate of hypoxic metabolism and cytotoxicity of tirapazamine.[82]

However, it has been suggested that microsomal metabolism of tirapazamine is of little or no consequence to the outcome of cellular toxicity, due to the labile nature of the radical species. It is proposed that only nuclear activation of tirapazamine is relevant, with respect to the generation of tirapazamine radicals that ultimately give rise to the lethal DNA damage.[83] However, since multiple micro-environmental factors could influence the relative contributions of the nuclear and microsomal reductases, this supposition remains unproven.[81]

Preclinical studies have concentrated on combining tirapazamine with either irradiation[84] or other chemotherapeutic drugs such as cisplatin and cyclophosphamide.[85] Clinical studies followed this productive approach,[86],[87] and tirapazamine is currently in phase II and III clinical trials as an adjunct to cisplatin-based chemotherapy or radiotherapy. Recent results have shown a dramatic survival advantage if patients with non-small-cell lung cancer were treated with tirapazamine and cisplatin, compared to cisplatin mono-therapy.[88]

Predicting the clinical response to tirapazamine (TPZ)

Since the enzymology of TPZ is unresolved, the alkaline 'comet' single-cell gel electrophoresis technique, which measures the level of DNA single-strand breaks in individual cells following TPZ treatment, is probably the current method of choice for predicting the clinical response of individuals.[89] Using the functional endpoint of DNA damage as a predictive marker, a measure of both the oxygen tension and the activity of single-electron reductases within individual cells

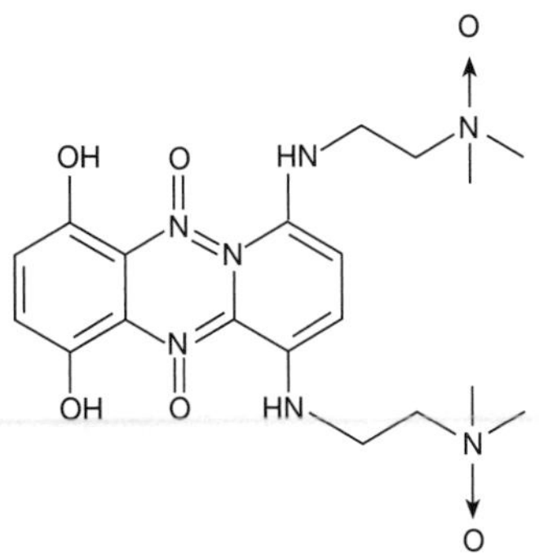

Fig. 10 AQ4N.

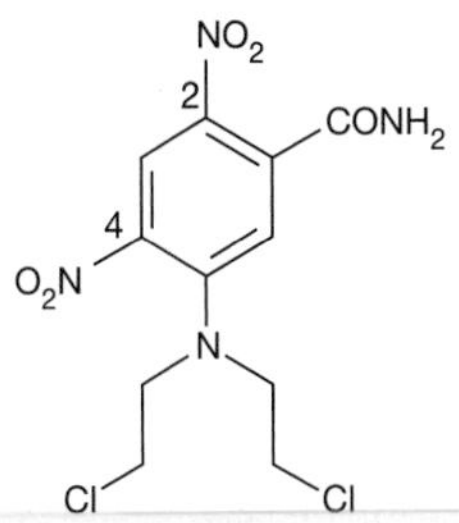

Fig. 11 SN23862.

can be determined. This overcomes the difficulty in knowing how to interrelate independent measurements of enzyme activity with oxygen tension. Moreover, a knowledge of the possible influences of sub-cellular localization of key reductases at different oxygen tensions becomes unimportant.

The utility of this approach has been demonstrated *in vitro* and *in vivo*[89]–[91] and has confirmed that DNA single-strand breaks correlate with cytotoxicity in both human and murine cell lines and xenograft models. Olive and colleagues[89] found the comet assay to be an adequate predictor of the surviving fraction in xenograft models if samples were collected within 1 h of TPZ administration. A similar relationship between DNA single-strand breaks at 60 min and cell survival was reported by Simm and colleagues[90] in a murine cell line *in vitro*. These relationships were measurable at clinically relevant doses of TPZ, with the high levels of DNA single-strand break formation allowing accurate detection, yet with the background DNA damage being comparatively minimal. However, variations in the cell's ability to repair DNA damage could complicate interpretation[75] and the apparent inability of the technique to predict interactive toxicity with radiation may prove to be a limitation.[91]

Ultimately, a knowledge of the key reductive enzymes responsible for tirapazamine metabolism in humans could allow targeting of this drug to patients who have tumours with favourable enzyme profiles and Po_2 dependence.[81] This together with non-invasive tumour imaging techniques using non-toxic hypoxic markers (that is, ^{19}F MRI) would facilitate rational patient selection prior to tirapazamine treatment. Such an approach could have considerable advantages over the intrinsically invasive nature of tissue sampling necessary for comet-assay measurements.

Other bioreductive cytotoxins in development

AQ4N (Fig. 10)

AQ4N is an aliphatic di-*N*-oxide analogue of mitoxantrone, which is metabolized by a concerted two-electron reduction to AQ4M and then to AQ4. Despite the absence of a detectable one-electron intermediate, metabolic reduction is readily inhibited by oxygen. The mechanism of inhibition may involve competition between oxygen and AQ4N for reducing species.[92] This active metabolite, AQ4, is a DNA-affinic topoisomerase II inhibitor. Raleigh *et al.*[93] used a panel of human liver microsomes to establish the role of the different CYP450 isoenzymes in the metabolism of this prodrug. They showed that the anaerobic metabolism of AQ4N was mediated by the 3A group of enzymes,

which are overexpressed in a wide range of human tumours.[81] They therefore suggested that this would allow tumour-specific activation of this bioreductive prodrug. AQ4N is currently being evaluated in a phase 1 study.

SN23862 (Fig. 11)

This is a 2,4-dinitrobenzamide mustard that has two nitro groups on the aromatic ring to raise the reduction potential sufficiently to allow enzymatic nitroreduction. Reduction of a nitro group at either the 2 or 4 positions causes a redistribution of electron density leading to a major increase in cytotoxicity. This has been described as an 'electronic switch', whereby reduction of the nitro group leads to a rearrangement of the electron density in the molecule to activate a latent moiety.[94] So far, 20 nitrogen mustard analogues derived from SN23862 have been developed, four of which are potentially superior to CB1954 for activation by *Escherichia coli* nitroreductase.[95] These novel prodrugs are activated by reduction to generate diffusible cytotoxins, and are currently being evaluated for application in combination with gene therapy.

A recent publication by Wilson *et al.*[96] examined the possibility of bioreductive drugs that can be activated by ionizing radiation. It was proposed that these so-called radiation-activated cytotoxins (**RAC**) would not have the same limitations found with conventional bioreductive drugs. For example, metabolism would not be dependent on a tumour's enzyme profile and activation should be completely suppressed by molecular oxygen, so preventing normal tissue toxicity. Radiolysis of water by ionizing radiation generates three primary radical species, including an aquated electron (e^-_{aq}). It was postulated that this product would reduce prodrugs that had reduction potentials too low for enzymatic reduction. Nitroarylmethyl quaternary (**NMQ**) ammonium salts have a number of features that make them a model for RAC development. Early results suggested that, although the NMQ salts were still enzymatically reduced, activation and cytotoxicity was increased further by ionizing radiation.

Increasing tumour hypoxia to enhance bioreductive drug activity

Hypoxic cytotoxins can be particularly effective when used in combination with ionizing radiation to target both the aerobic and hypoxic cell populations. Yet methods aimed at selectively **increasing** tumour hypoxia have also been evaluated as an alternative strategy, with the intention of expanding the therapeutic target for bioreductive drugs. In principle, this has been achieved in experimental systems by clamping the base of the tumour to reduce tumour blood flow, or by the use of vasoactive agents, such as hydralazine. This latter drug is believed to work by decreasing tumour blood flow relative to normal tissues.

Left-shift agents such as **BW12C** and **BW589C** stabilize oxy-haemoglobin and thus reduce oxygen delivery to tissues. Because of the asymmetry of the displacement of the oxygen dissociation curve, the relative change in oxygenation is greater in tumours than in normal tissues. An increase in a tumour radiobiological hypoxic fraction was found after BW12C was administered to mice with RIF-1 or KHT tumours. In a phase 1 study, BW12C was administered to patients with gastrointestinal tumours prior to treatment with MMC, in an attempt at increasing the cytotoxicity of this bioreductive drug.[97] A later paper also evaluated the oxygenation in tumours and normal tissues using the polarographic electrode system.[98] The BW12C infusion resulted in a significant reduction in oxygenation in both accessible tumours and subcutaneous tissues. While no associated increase in toxicity was found, efficacy was also unaltered. This may be related to the poor selectivity of MMC for hypoxic cells.

In a study by Butler et al.,[99] **RB6145** was given together with nitro-L-arginine. This latter drug inhibits the production of the vasodilator nitric oxide and therefore can be considered to be a vasoconstrictor. Nitro-L-arginine was administered within 1 h of an intraperitoneal injection of RB6145 into mice bearing KHT tumours. The tumours were removed 24 h later and a series of clonogenic assays was set up. Survival of tumours treated with both RB6145 and nitro-L-arginine was significantly reduced, compared to those treated with either drug alone. This data suggested that the nitro-L-arginine caused tumour hypoxia, thereby enhancing the toxicity of RB6145. This study emphasized the possibility that manipulation of the tumour environment to create greater tumour hypoxia can provide therapeutic benefit.

Agents such as flavone acetic acid (**FAA**) and its analogue 5,6-dimethylxanthenone-4-acetic acid (**DMXAA**) can selectively damage tumour vasculature by induction of tumour-necrosis factor alpha (**TNFα**). This in turn leads to selective tumour hypoxia. FAA has been administered together with MMC to treat B16 melanoma xenografts in C57BL/6NCrj mice.[100] Tumour blood flow was significantly reduced compared to muscle blood flow, which remained unchanged. The greatest antitumour effect was found when FAA was given 1 h after MMC, although the maximum enhancement was seen when this treatment was also combined with hyperthermia. FAA has been used as a single agent in clinical trials but lacked significant antitumour activity.

DMXAA is a more potent cytokine inducer than FAA, suggesting that it may cause greater tumour hypoxia and antitumour effect. At high doses used to treat murine xenografts, it caused extensive haemorrhagic necrosis, but the tumours tended to recur.[101] It has entered clinical trials as a single agent but may be more effective when combined with other modalities of treatment. Wilson et al.[102] treated RIF-1 and MDAH-MCa-4 xenografts with a combination of DMXAA and ionizing radiation. They found that the sequencing of administration was critical, the greatest antitumour effect occurring when the drug was given immediately after a single fraction of radiotherapy. It was suggested that the hypoxia induced after administration of DMXAA was short-lived and that surviving cells were able to reoxygenate sufficiently to become radiosensitive. Treatment with fractionated radiotherapy appeared less effective than with single fractions. It was suggested that this was due to the therapeutic effect of fractionated radiotherapy being less influenced by tumour hypoxia.

Combretastatins are a group of compounds isolated from the African bush willow, *Combretum caffrum*. They are structurally similar to colchicine and interfere with microtubule activity so inhibiting cell growth and proliferation. The prodrug combretastatin A-4 disodium phosphate is more water-soluble than the natural combretastatins and has been used recently in a number of preclinical studies. The active metabolite has been shown to selectively damage proliferating endothelial cells found in tumours, leading to vascular shutdown and hypoxia.[103] Li et al.[104] administered combretastatin A-4 disodium phosphate within 1 h after a 15-Gy dose of ionizing radiation. Tumour necrosis was seen histologically and even with the prodrug alone, an increase in tumour cell kill was evident. They showed that the combined therapy significantly reduced tumour survival compared to treatment with radiation alone. Also, from the shape of the survival curve, they suggested that combretastatin A-4 disodium phosphate had a major effect on the radioresistant hypoxic-cell population.

Bioreductive drugs as prodrugs for GDEPT

Gene-directed, enzyme-prodrug therapy (**GDEPT**) requires the transfer of therapeutic DNA into target cells in order to facilitate the expression of metabolic 'suicide' enzymes. The utility of this tumour-targeted 'molecular chemotherapy' is usually dependent upon the specificity of suicide-gene delivery and/or appropriate neoplasia-specific gene expression. Such controlled therapeutic gene targeting is designed to confer conditional sensitivity in the presence of an appropriate prodrug. A prodrug is defined as a chemical that is inert in the free state, but which, once activated, is converted to a cytotoxic species.

Most GDEPT paradigms utilize non-mammalian enzymes in combination with selective prodrug substrates to restrict metabolism to genetically modified cells. In contrast, bioreductive prodrugs are activated by enzymes that can be present in both tumour and normal tissues, but cytotoxicity is restricted by the presence of oxygen. Evidence suggests that tumour-specific expression of these reductive enzymes is very heterogeneous, even in tumours of the same subtype.[81] It has been proposed that the overexpression of oxygen-sensitive reductive enzymes in tumours would lead to enhanced activation of bioreductive drugs, thereby targeting hypoxic malignant tissues.[82]

A well-recognized, oxygen-inhibitable reductase is the flavoprotein NADPH:cytochrome P-450 reductase (**P450R**). Normally P450R shuttles electrons from NADPH via its FAD and FMN prosthetic groups to cytochrome P-450, cytochrome b_5, or heme oxygenase. Of the various mammalian single-electron reductases, P450R has the most appropriate one-electron equivalent redox couples to facilitate the transfer of single electrons to artificial electron acceptors with a range of redox potentials.[105] Under aerobic conditions P450R exists exclusively as a stable semi-quinone radical (FAD-FMNH•), which enables it to donate single electrons to any prodrug with an appropriate one-electron reduction potential.[105],[106] The rate of reduction is strongly determined by the value of the one-electron reduction potential of the substrate.[49],[107] This dependence implies that thermodynamic factors predominate, such that the interaction between

P450R and its substrate involves a simple outersphere electron-transfer mechanism, with no appreciable binding of the compound to the enzyme. Consequently, P450R is very promiscuous and can catalyse the oxygen-inhibited activation of the majority of bioreductive prodrugs, including the nitroaromatic, aromatic N-oxide, and quinone 'triggered' agents.[29],[49],[82] Such broad prodrug flexibility, coupled with the intrinsic hypoxia-selectivity of bioactivation may be of significant clinical value when utilizing this form of redox-sensitive enzyme/prodrug paradigm. Further, if the therapeutic application of an oxygen-inhibited reductase is **combined** with selective tissue expression using hypoxia-responsive transcriptional elements, it would provide an attractive and novel strategy for targeting oxygen-deprived tumour cells using gene therapy.

The 'bystander' effect

As an extension of the original concept of bioreductive drugs as prodrugs activated under low tissue Po_2 to kill hypoxic cells, it has been proposed that these agents might ideally provide a bystander effect.[108],[109] The 'bystander' effect can be defined as an amplification of the effects of a prodrug beyond the cell in which it was activated.[110] Since systemic or local delivery of therapeutic genes is unlikely to target all tumour cells *in vivo*, it is considered advantageous that a prodrug should kill not only cells expressing the enzyme but also surrounding non-transfected cells. Thus incomplete infection of tumour cells can still achieve total cell kill.

By releasing a diffusible cytotoxin upon reductive activation, bioreductive prodrugs can selectively utilize the population of hypoxic cells present in most solid tumours. Providing the activated prodrug is sufficiently stable to diffuse away from its site of generation, the requirement for an appropriate reductive environment for prodrug metabolism will contribute significantly towards the therapeutic specificity of a GDEPT strategy. Of the four main redox-sensitive 'trigger' systems, only the nitroaromatic prodrugs have been extensively developed as hypoxia-activated diffusible prodrugs capable of killing oxygenated bystander cells.[29],[94],[108],[109] More recently, hypoxia-activated diffusible prodrugs based upon the indolequinone 'trigger' of EO9 have also been proposed and are currently in development.[111]

Hypoxia-response elements

A range of promoter/enhancer sequences have been characterized for application in gene therapy, potentially allowing the tightly regulated expression of therapeutic genes within neoplastic tissues. Targeted gene expression can be achieved using tissue- or disease-specific promoters, or alternatively through exploiting transcriptional elements that are responsive to physiological conditions unique to solid-tumour microenvironments, including glucose-deprivation and hypoxia.[112] The recent observations that hypoxia-responsive elements (HREs), found within a number of genes,[113] can specifically regulate transcription in response to biological hypoxia, has suggested that HRE-dependent expression of therapeutic enzymes might be one approach to exploiting a unique characteristic of tumour physiology. Such an HRE-driven GDEPT strategy could be applied to a broad range of solid tumours of variable tissue origin and histology, and might fulfil an important therapeutic goal.

The molecular basis of HRE-dependent transcriptional regulation

Hypoxia-enhancer regions have been found in a number of genes including erythropoietin (EPO),[114] vascular endothelial growth factor,[115] and a number of proteins involved in glucose metabolism, including: phosphoglycerate kinase-1, aldolase A, enolase 1, lactate dehydrogenase A, pyruvate kinase M, phosphofructokinase L, and glucose transporter-1.[113],[116]–[119] Among the genes encoding glycolytic enzymes, regulation by hypoxia is isozyme-specific in a way that correlates with their increased expression in malignant cells.[116],[117]

The erythropoietin (**EPO**) gene HRE was the first enhancer to be characterized in detail. A minimal 24 base-pair (bp) sequence 3′ of the coding region has been defined as sufficient for hypoxia response (less than 1 per cent O_2). The EPO-derived hypoxia-response element was subsequently reported to confer O_2-dependent transcription, independent of orientation, distance, and homologous or heterologous promoter context, and was universally functional in mammalian cells.[120] The nuclear transcription factor, hypoxia-inducible factor 1 (**HIF-1**), was shown to specifically interact with the HRE of EPO.[121] Mutations of the EPO enhancer that prevented HIF-1 binding also eliminated the hypoxic induction of EPO reporter genes. Further studies demonstrated that hypoxia-mediated induction of transcription could be improved by reducing the distance between the enhancer and promoter, and increased further by inserting multiple copies of the 24-bp sequence.[122] The finding that hypoxically inducible activity of the EPO HRE was widespread in mammalian cells implied that an oxygen-sensing mechanism was present in non-EPO producing cells, and suggested that HIF-1 was a universal transcription factor that served to regulate other oxygen-dependent genes.

Hypoxia inducible factor-1 (HIF-1)

Hypoxia-inducible factor-1 is a heterodimer (HIF-$1\alpha/\beta$) that has been shown to transcriptionally regulate oxygen-responsive genes that contain hypoxia-response elements (HREs).[123]–[125] Oxygen-dependent control of HIF-1 is predominantly achieved by changes in the proteolytic stability and *trans*-activation capacity of the HIF-1α subunit, while HIF-1β is constitutively expressed.[125] As implied, the HIF-1α subunit is regulated at the post-mRNA level, being continuously synthesized and degraded under normoxic conditions.[126] Degradation is mediated, at least in part, by the ubiquitin–proteasome system that is regulated through a defined regulatory domain.[127] Stabilization is dependent upon redox-induced changes, which is complimented and amplified by post-translational changes in transactivation capacity probably involving other redox and protein phosphorylation events.[126],[127] Ultimately, transcriptional activation will depend upon an interrelated series of events, including nuclear accumulation, dimerization, DNA binding, cofactor recruitment, and transactivation.

Oxidative metabolism and the cellular response to hypoxia

Oxygen tension influences whether ATP will be produced primarily by aerobic respiration-linked phosphorylation, or by catabolic reactions that generate ATP at the substrate level. Oxidative phosphorylation is far more efficient than substrate-level phosphorylation

Table 1 Sequences of various hypoxia-response elements

EPO	mouse	GGGCCCT	*ACGTGC*	TGCCTCG	**CATG**	GC
EPO	human	GGGCCCT	*ACGTGC*	TGTCTCA	**CACA**	GC
PGK-1	mouse	ATTTGTC	*ACGTCC*	TGCACGA	**CGCG**	AG
LDH-A	mouse	CCAGCGG	*ACGTGC*	GGGAACC	**CACG**	TG
GLUT-1	mouse	TCCACAG	*GCGTGC*	CGTCTGA	**CACG**	CA

EPO, erythropoietin; PGK-1, phosphoglycerate kinase-1; LDH-A, lactate dehydrogenase-A; GLUT-1, glucose-transporter-1.

in capturing the redox energy of reduced substrates, with the oxygen-dependent tricarboxylic (Krebs) cycle generating an 18-fold greater equivalent yield of ATP than the anaerobic glycolytic (Embden–Meyerhof) pathway. Utilization of the primary cellular nutrients, glucose and fatty acids, to provide pyruvate for subsequent processing by oxidative phosphorylation, is far more energetically favourable than the generation of lactate by anaerobic glycolysis. Thus oxygen deprivation in solid-tumour tissues impacts upon the pathways of glucose utilization and so will elicit an adaptive physiological response at the cellular level.

A rapid increase in glucose utilization occurs upon inhibition of mitochondrial function (Pasteur effect). Consequently, long-term cellular adaption occurs, with increases in the biosynthetic rate of the genes encoding both high-capacity facilitated glucose transport (primarily Glut-1 and -3),[128] and glycolytic metabolism, including: phosphofructokinase-L and -M, pyruvate kinase-M, aldolase-A and -C, phosphoglycerate kinase-1 (**PGK-1**), enolase-1, and lactate dehydrogenase A.[113],[116]–[119] The induction of glycolytic enzymes in response to oxygen deprivation is isozyme-specific, reflecting the specific catalytic functions of various isoforms.[117] Webster[129] showed that in cells grown under 2 per cent oxygen for 72 h, there is a two- to fivefold increase in steady-state mRNA and transcription for lactate dehydrogenase, pyruvate kinase, triose phosphate isomerase, and aldolase.

Firth *et al.*[113] demonstrated that the murine PGK-1 gene was regulated by hypoxia, with similar characteristics to that of the EPO gene. They defined an 18-bp sequence of DNA in the promoter region of the PGK-1 gene that had close homology to the EPO HRE. The sequences of various HREs are now well defined, with an HRE core and a second conserved sequence being required for functionality (Table 1).

Applications of hypoxia-driven gene therapy

Dachs and colleagues[130] utilized a trimer of the PGK-1 HRE, linked to the thymidine kinase, 9–27, or PGK-1 promoters, to regulate the expression of the surface 'reporter' protein CD2. A control plasmid contained the 9–27 interferon-responsive promoter linked to CD2, but without the enhancer elements. These constructs were stably transfected into the HT1080 cell line and the response to different degrees of hypoxia evaluated. Each of the clonal cell lines that contained the PGK-1 HRE-driven expression vectors showed marker gene induction (CD2) in response to 2 per cent Po_2 or less. At 1 per cent Po_2 gene induction was approximately 2-fold, whereas under catalyst-induced anoxia this induction reached a maximum of 6.4-fold with the 9–27 promoter and 4-fold with the thymidine kinase

promoter. The gene for *E. coli* cytosine deaminase was also driven by the 9–27 promoter under the control of the PGK-1 enhancer. This enzyme converts the prodrug 5-fluorocytosine (5-FC) to the cytotoxic antimetabolite, 5-fluorouracil (5-FU). Under hypoxic conditions, the HT1080 transfectants showed increased cytosine deaminase activity and were five times more sensitive to 5-FC than the parental cell line. This suggested that 5-FC had been converted to 5-FU by cytosine deaminase under these conditions.

These results showed that it was possible to modulate the transcription of a gene by inserting regulatory sequences responsive to hypoxia within a heterologous promoter context. In a similar strategy, HREs from the PGK-1 gene were ligated upstream from a minimal thymidine kinase (sTK) promoter driving the cDNA for P450R.[131] This vector was transfected into the HT1080 human fibrosarcoma cell line and a stable clone generated. After a 24-h incubation under anoxic conditions a threefold rise in P450R activity was found compared to the same clone under aerobic conditions ($p < 0.001$). This clone was significantly sensitized to tirapazamine, but only following the hypoxic preinduction of P450R ($p = 0.03$). Similar experiments employing a more robust SV40 early-gene promoter in place of the sTK promoter markedly improved the amplitude of P450R expression, increasing the differential sensitivity (oxic:anoxic cytotoxicity ratio) of the 2-nitroimidazole, RSU1069, from 34- to 250-fold. This HRE-driven activating system might equally be applied in combination with any of the nitro- or indolequinone-triggered prodrugs.[95],[111] These data suggest that a highly specific strategy could be developed to target hypoxic regions in tumours.

Combining the intrinsic hypoxia-selective nature of bioreductive prodrugs in concert with an HRE-regulated GDEPT strategy that utilizes an oxygen-inhibited activation step should ensure that cytotoxicity is rigorously restricted to hypoxic tissues. By exploiting a physiological property of solid tumours (rather than a genetic property), this therapeutic strategy has the potential to be applied to many cancers of diverse genetic and tissue origins.[112] Furthermore, where tumour hypoxia is heterogeneous, fluctuating, or even absent, agents are now becoming available that will selectively generate acute reductions in tumour oxygenation. Thus coupling bioreductive prodrugs with hypoxia-dependent gene therapy could allow a highly focused attack to be made on hypoxic cells in solid tumours.

References

1. **Degner FL, Sutherland RM.** Mathematical modeling of oxygen supply and oxygenation in tumour tissues: prognostic, therapeutic and

experimental implications. *International Journal of Radiation Oncology, Biology, Physics*, 1988; **15**: 391–7.

2. Groebe K, Vaupel P. Evaluation of oxygen diffusion distances in human breast cancer xenografts using tumour-specific *in vivo* data: role of various mechanisms in the development of tumour hypoxia. *International Journal of Radiation Oncology, Biology, Physics*, 1988; **15**: 691–7.

3. Awwad HK, Naggar M, Mocktar N. Intercapillary distance measurement as an indicator of hypoxia in carcinoma of the cervix uteri. *International Journal of Radiation Oncology, Biology, Physics*, 1986; **12**: 1329–1333.

4. Jain RK. Determinants of tumour blood flow. *Cancer Research*, 1988; **48**: 2641–58.

5. Boucher Y, Jain RK. Microvascular pressure is the principal driving force for interstitial hypertension in solid tumors: implications for vascular collapse. *Cancer Research*, 1992; **52**: 5110–14.

6. Sevick EM, Jain RK. Viscous resistance to blood flow in solid tumors: effect of hematocrit on intratumor blood viscosity. *Cancer Research*, 1989; **49**: 3513–19.

7. Chaplin DJ, Olive PL, Durrand RE. Intermittant blood flow in a murine tumour: radiobiological effects. *Cancer Research*, 1987; **47**: 597–601.

8. Hill SA, *et al.* Microregional blood flow in murine and human tumours assessed using laser Doppler microprobes. *British Journal of Cancer*, 1996; **74**(Suppl. 27): 260–3.

9. Powell MEB, Hill SA, Saunders MI, Hoskin PJ, Chaplin DJ. Human tumor blood flow is enhanced by nicotinamide and carbogen breathing. *Cancer Research*, 1997; **57**: 5261–4.

10. Chaplin DJ, Hill SA. Temporal heterogeneity in microregional erythrocyte flux in experimental solid tumours. *British Journal of Cancer*, 1995; **71**: 1210–13.

11. Moulder JE, Rockwell S. Hypoxic fractions of solid tumors: experimental techniques, methods of analysis, and a survey of existing data. *International Journal of Radiation Oncology, Biology, Physics*, 1984; **10**: 695–712.

12. Sutherland RM, Ausserer WA, Murphy BJ, Laderoute KR. Tumor hypoxia and heterogeneity: challenges and opportunities for the future. *Seminars in Radiation Oncology*, 1996; **6**(1): 59–70.

13. Vaupel P. Oxygenation of solid tumours. In *Drug resistance in oncology* (ed. BA Teicher) New York: M Dekker, 1993: 59–85.

14. Collingridge DR, Piepmeier JM, Knisely JPS, Rockwell S. Polarographic measurement of oxygen tension in human brain gliomas. *International Journal of Radiation Oncology, Biology, Physics*, 1998; **42**(Suppl. 1): 267. (Abstract)

15. Sundfor K, Lyng H, Kongsgard U, Trope C, Rofstad EK. Polarographic measurement of pO-2 in cervix carcinoma. *Gynecological Oncology*, 1997; **64**: 230–6.

16. Rockwell S, Moulder JE. Hypoxic fractions of human tumors xenografted into mice: a review. *International Journal of Radiation Oncology, Biology, Physics*, 1990; **19**: 197–202.

17. Moulder JE, Rockwell S. Tumor hypoxia: its impact on cancer therapy. *Cancer Metastasis Reviews*, 1987; **5**: 313–41.

18. Hall EJ. *Radiobiology for the radiologist* (4th edn). Philadelphia: JB Lippincroft, 1994.

19. Zhang H, Koch CJ, Wallen CA, Wheeler KT. Radiation-induced DNA damage in tumours and normal tissues. III. Oxygen dependence of the formation of strand breaks and DNA–protein crosslinks. *Radiation Research*, 1995; **142**: 163–8.

20. Dizdaroglu M. Chemical determination of free radical-induced damage to DNA. *Free Radicals and Biological Medicine*, 1991; **10**: 225–42.

21. Kolstad P. Intercapillary distance, oxygen tension and local recurrence in cervix cancer. *Scandinavian Journal of Clinical and Laboratory Investigation*, 1968; **Suppl. 106**: 145–57.

22. Gatenby RA, *et al.* Oxygen distribution in squamous cell carcinoma metastases and its relationship to outcome of radiation therapy. *International Journal of Radiation Oncology, Biology, Physics*, 1988; **14**: 831–8.

23. Hockel M, *et al.* Intratumoral Po_2 predicts survival in advanced cancer of the uterine cervix. *Radiotherapy Oncology*, 1993; **26**: 45–50.

24. Hockel M, Schlenger K, Aral B, Mitze M, Schaffer U, Vaupel P. Association between tumor hypoxia and malignant progression in advanced cancer of the uterine cervix. *Cancer Research*, 1996; **56**: 4509–15.

25. Brizel DM, *et al.* Tumor oxygenation predicts for the likelihood of distant metastases in human soft tissue sarcoma. *Cancer Research*, 1996; **56**: 941–3.

26. Brizel DM, Sibley GS, Prosnitz LR, Scher RL, Dewhirst MW. Tumour hypoxia adversely affects the prognosis of carcinoma of the head and neck. *International Journal of Radiation Oncology, Biology, Physics*, 1997; **38**: 285–9.

27. Overgaard J, Horsman MR. Modification of hypoxia-induced radioresistance in tumours by the use of oxygen and sensitizers. *Seminars in Radiation Oncology*, 1996; **6**: 10–21.

28. Evans RG, Kimler BF, Morantz RA. Lack of complications in long-term survivors after treatment with fluosol and oxygen as an adjuvant to radiation therapy for high grade brain tumours. *International Journal of Radiation Oncology, Biology, Physics*, 1993; **26**: 649–52.

29. Wilson WR. Tumour hypoxia: challenges for cancer chemotherapy. In *Cancer biology and medicine* (ed. MJ Waring, AJ Ponder). Lancaster: Kluwer Academic, 1992: Vol. 3; 87–131.

30. Teicher BA. Hypoxia and drug resistance. *Cancer Metastasis Reviews*, 1994; **13**: 139–68.

31. Grau C, Overgaard J. Effect of cancer chemotherapy on the hypoxic fraction of a solid tumour measured using a local tumour control assay. *Radiotherapy and Oncology*, 1988; **13**: 301–9.

32. Krtolica A, Ludlow JW. Hypoxia arrests ovarian carcinoma cell cycle progression, but invasion is unaffected. *Cancer Research*, 1996; **56**: 1168–73.

33. Graeber TG, Peterson JF, Tsai M, Monica K, Fornace AJ, Giaccia AJ. Hypoxia induces accumulation of p53 protein, but activation of a G1-phase checkpoint by low oxygen conditions is independent of p53 status. *Molecular and Cellular Biology*, 1994; **14**: 6264–77.

34. Graeber TG, *et al.* Hypoxia-mediated selection of cells with diminished apoptotic potential in solid tumours. *Nature*, 1996; **379**: 88–91.

35. Hartwell LH, Kastan MB. Cell cycle control and cancer. *Science*, 1994; **266**: 1821–8.

36. Hill RP. Tumour progression: potential role of unstable genomic changes. *Cancer Metastasis Reviews*, 1990; **9**: 137–45.

37. Rice GC, Ling V, Schimke RT. Frequencies of independent and simultaneous selection of Chinese hamster cells for methotrexate and doxorubicin (adriamycin) resistance. *Proceedings of the National Academy of Sciences USA*, 1987; **84**: 9261–4.

38. Adams GE. Hypoxic cell sensitizers for radiotherapy. In *Cancer, a comprehensive treatise* (ed. FF Becker). New York: Plenum Press, 1976: 181–223.

39. Stratford IJ. Concepts and development in radiosensitization of mammalian cells. *International Journal of Radiation Oncology, Biology, Physics*, 1992; **22**: 529–32.

40. Chaplin DJ, Horsman MR, Aoki DS. Nicotinamide, fluosol DA and carbogen: a strategy to reoxygenate acutely and chronically hypoxic cells *in vivo*. *British Journal of Cancer*, 1991; **63**: 109–13.

41. Overgaard J. Importance of tumour hypoxia in radiotherapy: a meta-analysis of controlled clinical trials. *Radiotherapy and Oncology*, 1992; **24**: Abstract S64.

42. Overgaard J, *et al.* A randomised double-blind phase III study of nimorazole as a hypoxic radiosensitiser of primary radiotherapy in supraglottic larynx and pharynx carcinoma. Results of the Danish head

and neck cancer study (DAHANCA) protocol 5–85. *Radiotherapy and Oncology*, 1998; **46**: 135–46.

43. Overgaard J, *et al.* Nimorazole as a hypoxic radiosensitiser in the treatment of supraglottic larynx and pharynx carcinoma. First report from the Danish Head and Neck Cancer Study (DAHANCA) protocol 5–85. *Radiotherapy and Oncology*, 1991; **20**: 143–9.

44. Adams GE, Stratford IJ, Edwards HS, Bremner JCM, Cole S. Bioreductive drugs as post-irradiation sensitizers: comparison of dual function agents with SR 4233 and the mitomycin C analogue EO9. *International Journal of Radiation Oncology, Biology, Physics*, 1992; **22**: 717–20.

45. Workman P, Stratford IJ. The experimental development of bioreductive drugs and their role in cancer therapy. *Cancer Metastasis Reviews*, 1993; **12**: 73–82.

46. Belcourt MF, Hodnick WF, Rockwell S, Sartorelli AC. Differential toxicity of mitomycin C and porfiromycin to aerobic and hypoxic Chinese hamster ovary cells overexpressing human NADPH: cytochrome c (P-450) reductase. *Proceedings of the National Academy of Sciences USA*, 1996; **93**: 456–60.

47. Spanswick VJ, Cummings J, Smyth JF. Enzymology of mitomycin-C metabolic-activation in tumor-tissue—characterisation of a novel mitochondrial reductase. *Biochemical Pharmacology*, 1996; **51**: 1623–30.

48. Pritsos CA, Biggs LA, Gustafson DL. A new cellular target for mitomycin C: a case for mitochondrial DNA. *Oncology Research*, 1997; **9**: 333–7.

49. Powis G. Metabolism and reactions of quinoid anticancer agents. *Pharmacology and Therapeutics*, 1987; **35**: 57–162.

50. Keyes SR, *et al.* Role of NADPH: cytochrome c reductase and DT-diaphorase in the biotransformation of mitomycin C. *Cancer Research*, 1984; **44**: 5633–43.

51. Weissberg M, *et al.* Randomised clinical trial of mitomycin C as an adjunct to radiotherapy in head and neck cancer. *International Journal of Radiation, Oncology, Biology, Physics*, 1989; **17**: 3–9.

52. Rockwell S, Keyes SR, Sartorelli AC. Preclinical studies of porfiromycin as an adjunct to radiotherapy. *Radiation Research*, 1988; **116**: 100–13.

53. Haffty BG, *et al.* Bioreductive alkylating agent porfiromycin combination with radiation therapy for the management of squamous cell carcinoma of the head and neck. *Radiation Oncology Investigations*, 1997; **5**: 235–45.

54. Hendriks HR, *et al.* EO9: a novel bioreductive alkylating indoloquinone with preferential solid tumour activity and lack of bone marrow toxicity in preclinical models. *European Journal of Cancer*, 1993; **29A**: 897–906.

55. Walton MI, Smith PJ, Workman P. The role of NAD(P)H: quinone reductase (EC 1.6.99.2, DT-diaphorase) in the reductive bioactivation of the novel indoloquinone antitumor agent EO9. *Cancer Communications*, 1991; **3**: 199–206.

56. Robertson N, Haigh A, Adams GE, Stratford IJ. Factors affecting sensitivity to EO9 in rodent and human tumour cells *in vitro*: DT-diaphorase activity and hypoxia. *European Journal of Cancer*, 1994; **30A**: 1013–19.

57. Adams GE, Stratford IJ. Bioreductive drugs for cancer therapy: the search for tumor specificity. *International Journal of Radiation Oncology, Biology, Physics*, 1994; **29**: 231–8.

58. Phillips RM. Bioreductive activation of a series of analogues of 5-aziridinyl-3-hydroxymethyl-1-methyl-2-[1H-indole-4,7-dione] prop-beta-en-alpha-ol (EO9) by human DT-diaphorase. *Biochemical Pharmacology*, 1996; **52**: 1711–18.

59. Bailey SM, *et al.* Involvement of DT-diaphorase (EC 1.6.99.2) in the DNA cross-linking and sequence selectivity of the bioreductive anti-tumour agent EO9. *British Journal of Cancer*, 1997; **76**: 1596–603.

60. Maliepaard M, Wolfs A, Groot SE, De Mol NJ, Janssen LHM. Indoloquinone EO9: DNA interstrand cross-linking upon reduction by

DT-diaphorase or xanthine oxidase. *British Journal of Cancer*, 1995; **71**: 836–42.

61. Butler J, Spanswick VJ, Cummings J. The autooxidation of the reduced forms of EO9. *Free Radical Research*, 1996; **25**: 141–8.

62. Cummings J, Spanswick VJ, Gardiner J, Ritchie A, Smyth JF. Pharmacological and biochemical determinants of the antitumour activity of the indoloquinone EO9. *Biochemical Pharmacology*, 1998; **55**: 253–60.

63. Gustafson DL, Beall HD, Bolton EM, Ross D, Waldren CA. Expression of human NAD(P)H: quinone oxidoreductase (DT-diaphorase) in chinese hamster ovary cells: effect on the toxicity of antitumor quinones. *Molecular Pharmacology*, 1996; **50**: 728–35.

64. Plumb JA, Workman P. Unusually marked hypoxic sensitization to indolequinone EO9 and mitomycin C in a human colon-tumour cell line that lacks DT-diaphorase activity. *International Journal of Cancer*, 1994; **56**: 134–9.

65. Smitskamp-Wilms E, Hendriks HR, Peters GJ. Development, pharmacology, role of DT-diaphorase and prospects of the indolequinone EO9. *General Pharmacology*, 1996; **27**: 421–9.

66. Schellens JH, *et al.* Phase I and pharmacologic study of the novel indoloquinone bioreductive alkylating cytotoxic drug E09. *Journal of the National Cancer Institute*, 1994; **86**: 906–12.

67. Pavlidis N, *et al.* A randomized phase II study with two schedules of the novel indoloquinone EO9 in non-small-cell lung cancer: A study of the EORTC early clinical studies group (ECSG). *Annals of Oncology*, 1996; **7**: 529–31.

68. Stratford IJ, O'Neill P, Sheldon PW, Silver ARJ, Walling JM, Adams GE. RSU 1069: a nitroimidazole containing an aziridine group—bioreduction greatly increases cytotoxicity under hypoxic conditions. *Biochemical Pharmacology*, 1986; **35**: 105–9.

69. Horwich A, Holliday SB, Deacon JM, Peckham MJ. A toxicity and pharmacokinetic study in man of the hypoxic radiosensitiser RSU-1069. *British Journal of Radiology*, 1986; **59**: 1238–40.

70. Bremner JC. Assessing the bioreductive effectiveness of the nitroimidazole RSU1069 and its prodrug RB6145: with particular reference to *in vivo* methods of evaluation. *Cancer Metastasis Reviews*, 1993; **12**: 177–93.

71. Jenkins TC, *et al.* Synthesis and evaluation of alpha-[[(2-haloethyl)amino]methyl]-2- nitro-1H-imidazole-1-ethanols as prodrugs of alpha-[(1-aziridinyl)methyl]-2- nitro-1H-imidazole-1-ethanol (RSU-1069) and its analogues which are radiosensitizers and bioreductively activated cytotoxins. *Journal of Medicinal Chemistry*, 1990; **33**: 2603–10.

72. Binger M, Workman P. Pharmacokinetic contribution to the improved therapeutic selectivity of a novel bromoethylamino prodrug (RB 6145) of the mixed-function hypoxic cell sensitizer/cytotoxin alpha-(1-aziridinomethyl)-2-nitro-1H-imidazole-1-ethanol (RSU 1069). *Cancer Chemotherapy and Pharmacology*, 1991; **29**: 37–47.

73. Zeman EM, Brown JM, Lemmon MJ, Hirst VK, Lee WW. SR-4233: a new bioreactive agent with high selective toxicity for hypoxic mammalian cells. *International Journal of Radiation, Oncology, Biology, Physics*, 1966; **12**: 1239–42.

74. Lloyd RV, Duling DR, Rumyantseva GV, Mason RP, Bridson PK. Microsomal reduction of 3-amino-1,2,4-benzotriazine 1,4-dioxide to a free radical. *Molecular Pharmacology*, 1991; **40**: 440–5.

75. Biedermann KA, Wang J, Graham RP, Brown JM. SR4233 cytotoxicity and metabolism in DNA repair-competent and repair-deficient cell cultures. *British Journal of Cancer*, 1991; **63**: 358–62.

76. Wang J, Biedermann KA, Brown JM. Repair of DNA and chromosome breaks in cells exposed to SR4233 under hypoxia and to ionising radiation. *Cancer Research*, 1992; **52**: 4473–7.

77. Stratford IJ, Stephens MA. The differential hypoxic cytotoxicity of bioreductive agents determined *in vitro* by the MTT assay. *International Journal of Radiation Oncology, Biology, Physics*, 1989; **16**: 973–6.

78. Walton MI, Workman P. Enzymology of the reductive bioactivation of

SR 4233: a novel benzotriazene di-N-oxide hypoxic cytotoxin. *Biochemical Pharmacology*, 1990; **39**: 1735–42.

79. Walton MI, Wolf CR, Workman P. The role of cytochrome P450 and cytochrome P450 reductase in the reductive bioactivation of the novel benzotriazine di-N-oxide hypoxic cytotoxin 3-amino-1,2,4-benzotriazine-1,4-dioxide (SR 4233, WIN 59075) by mouse liver. *Biochemical Pharmacology*, 1992; **44**: 251–9.

80. Cahill A, White INH. Reductive metabolism of 3-amino-1,2,4-benzotriazene-1,4-dioxide (SR 4233) and the induction of unscheduled DNA synthesis in rat and human derived cell lines. *Carcinogenesis*, 1990; **11**: 1407–11.

81. Patterson AV, Saunders MP, Chinje EC, Patterson LH, Stratford IJ. Enzymology of tirapazamine metabolism: a review. *Anti-Cancer Drug Design*, 1998; **13**: 541–73.

82. Patterson AV, Saunders MP, Chinje EC, Talbot DC, Harris AL, Stratford IJ. Overexpression of human NADPH: cytochrome c (P450) reductase confers enhanced sensitivity to both tirapazamine (SR4233) and RSU1069. *British Journal of Cancer*, 1997; **76**: 1338–47.

83. Evans JW, Yudoh K, Delahoussaye YM, Brown JM. Tirapazamine is metabolised to its DNA-damaging radical by intranuclear enzymes. *Cancer Research*, 1998; **58**: 2098–101.

84. Brown JM, Lemmon MJ. Potentiation by the hypoxic cytotoxin SR4233 of cell killing produced by fractionated irradiation of mouse tumours. *Cancer Research*, 1990; **50**: 7745–9.

85. Dorie MJ, Brown JM. Tumour-specific schedule dependent interaction between tirapazamine (SR 4233) and cisplatin. *Cancer Research*, 1993; **53**: 4633–6.

86. Rodriguez GI, *et al*. A phase I/II trial of the combination of tirapazamine and cisplatin in patients with nonsmall cell lung cancer (NSCLC). *Proceedings of the Annual Meeting of the American Society of Clinical Oncology*, 1996; **15**: 382.

87. Lee D, *et al*. Concurrent tirapazamine and radiotherapy for advanced head and neck carcinomas: a phase II study. *International Journal of Radiation Oncology, Biology, Physics*, 1998; **42**: 811–15.

88. Gatzemeier U, Rodriguez G, Treat J, von Roemeling R, Viallet J, Rey A. Tirapazamine–cisplatin: the synergy. *British Journal of Cancer*, 1998; **44**(Suppl. 4): 15–17.

89. Olive PL, Vikse CM, Banath JP. Use of the comet assay to identify cells sensitive to tirapazamine in multicell spheroids and tumors in mice. *Cancer Research*, 1996; **56**: 4460–7.

90. Simm BG, Van Zijl PL, Brown JM. Tirapazamine-induced DNA damage measured using the comet assay correlates with cytotoxicity towards hypoxic tumour cells *in vitro*. *British Journal of Cancer*, 1996; **73**: 952–60.

91. Simm BG, Menke DR, Dorie MJ, Brown JM. Tirapazamine-induced cytotoxicity and DNA damage in transplanted tumors: relationship to hypoxia. *Cancer Research*, 1997; **57**: 2922–8.

92. Patterson LH. Rationale for the use of aliphatic N-oxides of cytotoxic anthraquinones as prodrug DNA binding: a new class of bioreductive agent. *Cancer Metastasis Reviews*, 1993; **12**: 119–34.

93. Raleigh SM, Wanogho E, Burke MD, McKeown SR, Patterson LH. Involvement of human cytochromes P450 (CYP) in the reductive metabolism of AQ4N, a hypoxia activated anthraquinone di-N-oxide prodrug. *International Journal of Radiation Oncology, Biology, Physics*, 1998; **42**: 763–7.

94. Simm BG, Denny WA, Wilson WR. Nitro reduction as an electronic switch for bioreductive drug activation. *Oncology Research*, 1997; **9**: 357–69.

95. Friedlos F, Denny WA, Palmer BD, Springer CJ. Mustard prodrugs for activation by *Escherichia coli* nitroreductase in gene-directed enzyme prodrug therapy. *Journal of Medicinal Chemistry*, 1997; **40**: 1270–5.

96. Wilson WR, Tercel M, Anderson RF, Denny WA. Radiation-activated prodrugs as hypoxia-selective cytotoxins: model studies with nitroarylmethyl quaternary salts. *Anti-Cancer Drug Design*, 1998; **13**: 663–85.

97. Dennis IF, Ramsay JR, Workman P, Bleehen NM. Pharmacokinetics of BW12C and mitomycin C, given in combination in a phase I study in patients with advanced gastrointestinal cancer. *Cancer Chemotherapy and Pharmacology*, 1993; **32**: 67–72.

98. Falk SJ, Ramsay JR, Ward R, Miles K, Dixon AK, Bleehen NM. BW12C perturbs normal and tumour tissue oxygenation and blood flow in man. *Radiotherapy and Oncology*, 1994; **32**: 210–17.

99. Butler SA, Wood PJ, Cole S, Adams GE, Stratford IJ. Enhancement of bioreductive drug toxicity in murine tumours by inhibition of the activity of nitric oxide synthase. *British Journal of Cancer*, 1997; **76**: 438–44.

100. Takeuchi H, Baba H, Maehara Y, Sugimachi K, Newman R. Flavone acetic acid increases the cytotoxicity of mitomycin C when combined with hyperthermia. *Cancer Chemotherapy and Pharmacology*, 1996; **38**: 1–8.

101. Lash CJ, *et al*. Enhancement of the antitumour effects of the antivascular agent 5,6-dimethylxanethenone-4-acetic acid (DMXAA) by combination with 5-hydroxytryptamine and bioreductive drugs. *British Journal of Cancer*, 1998; **78**: 439–45.

102. Wilson WR, Li AE, Cowan DSM, Siim BG. Enhancement of tumour radiation response by the anti-vascular agent 5,6-dimethylxanthenone-4-acetic acid. *International Journal of Radiation Oncology, Biology, Physics*, 1998; **42**: 905–8.

103. Dark GG, Hil SA, Prise VE, Tozer GM, Pettit GR, Chaplin DJ. Combretastatin A-4, an agent that displays potent and selective toxicity towards tumour vasculature. *Cancer Research*, 1997; **57**: 1829–34.

104. Li L, Rojiani A, Siemann DW. Targeting tumour vasculature with combretastatin A-4 disodium phosphate: effects on radiation therapy. *International Journal of Radiation Oncology, Biology, Physics*, 1998; **42**: 899–903.

105. Vermilion JL, Coon MJ. Purified liver microsomal NADPH-cytochrome P-450 reductase. *Journal of Biological Chemistry*, 1978; **253**: 2694–704.

106. Yasukochi Y, Peterson JA, Masters BSS. NADPH-cytochrome c (P450) reductase. *Journal of Biological Chemistry*, 1979; **254**: 7097–104.

107. Butler J, Hoey BM. The one-electron reduction potential of several substrates can be related to their reduction rates by cytochrome P-450 reductase. *Biochimica Biophysica Acta*, 1993; **1161**: 73–8.

108. Denny WA, Wilson WR. Bioreducible mustards—a paradigm for hypoxia-selective prodrugs of diffusible cytotoxins (HPDCs). *Cancer Metastasis Reviews*, 1993; **12**: 135–51.

109. Denny WA, Wilson WR, Hay MP. Recent developments in the design of bioreductive drugs. *British Journal of Cancer*, 1996; **74**(Suppl. 27): 32–8.

110. Pitts JD. Cancer gene therapy—a bystander effect using the gap junction pathway. *Molecular Carcinogenesis*, 1994; **11**: 127–30.

111. Jaffar M, Everett SA, Naylor MA, Robertson N, Stratford IJ. Targeting hypoxia with a new generation of indolequinones. *Anti-Cancer Drug Design*, 1998; **13**: 593–609.

112. Dachs GU, Dougherty GJ, Stratford IJ, Chaplin DJ. Gene therapy—the hypoxic cell as a target. *Oncology Research*, 1998; **9**: 313–25.

113. Firth JD, Ebert BL, Pugh CW, Ratcliffe PJ. Oxygen-regulated control elements in the phosphoglycerate kinase 1 and lactate dehydrogenase A genes: similarities with the erythropoietin 3' enhancer. *Proceedings of the National Academy of Sciences USA*, 1994; **91**: 6496–500.

114. Goldberg MA, Gaut CC, Bunn HF. Erythropoietin mRNA levels are governed by both the rate of gene transcription and posttranscriptional events. *Blood*, 1987; **77**: 271–7.

115. Goldberg MA, Schneider TJ. Similarities between the oxygen sensing mechanism regulating the expression of vascular endothelial growth

factor and erythropoietin. *Journal of Biological Chemistry*, 1994; **269**: 4355–9.

116. Ebert BL, Firth JD, Ratcliffe PJ. Hypoxia and mitochondrial inhibitors regulate expression of glucose transporter-1 via distinct *cis*-acting sequences. *Journal of Biological Chemistry*, 1995; **270**: 29083–9.

117. Ebert BL, Gleadle JM, O'Rourke JF, Bartlett SM, Poulton J, Ratcliffe PJ. Isozyme specific regulation of genes involved in energy metabolism by hypoxia, cobalt, and desferrioxamine: similarities with the regulation of erythropoietin. *Journal of Biochemistry*, 1995; **313**: 809–14.

118. Semenza GL, Roth PH, Fang HM, Wang GL. Transcriptional regulation of genes encoding glycolytic enzymes by hypoxia-inducible factor 1. *Journal of Biological Chemistry*, 1994; **269**: 23757–63.

119. Semenza GL, *et al.* Hypoxia response elements in the aldolase A, enolase 1, and lactate dehydrogenase A gene promoters contain essential binding sites for hypoxia-inducible factor 1. *Journal of Biological Chemistry*, 1996; **271**: 32529–37.

120. Maxwell PH, Pugh CW, Ratcliffe PJ. Inducible operation of the erythropoietin 3' enhancer in multiple cell lines: evidence for a widespread oxygen-sensing mechanism. *Proceedings of the National Academy of Sciences USA*, 1993; **90**: 2423–7.

121. Wang GL, Semenza GL. General involvement of hypoxia-inducible factor 1 in transcriptional response to hypoxia. *Proceedings of the National Academy of Sciences USA*, 1993; **90**: 4304–8.

122. Pugh CW, Ebert BL, Ebrahim O, Maxwell PH, Ratcliffe PJ. Analysis of *cis*-acting sequences required for operation of the erythropoietin 3' enhancer in different cell lines. *Annals of the New York Academy of Sciences*, 1994; **718**: 31–9.

123. Dachs GU, Stratford IJ. The molecular response of mammalian cells to hypoxia and the potential for exploitation in cancer therapy. *British Journal of Cancer*, 1996; **74**(Suppl. 27): 126–32.

124. Bunn HF, Poyton RO. Oxygen sensing and molecular adaption to hypoxia. *Physiology Reviews*, 1996; **76**: 839–55.

125. O'Rourke JF, *et al.* Hypoxia response elements. *Oncology Research*, 1997; **6–7**: 327–32.

126. Salceda S, Caro J. Hypoxia-inducible factor 1alpha (HIF-1α) protein is rapidly degraded by the ubiquitin-proteasome system under normoxic conditions. *Journal of Biological Chemistry*, 1997; **272**: 22642–7.

127. Pugh CW, O'Rourke JF, Nagao M, Gleadle JM, Ratcliffe PJ. Activation of hypoxia-inducible factor-1; definition of regulatory domains within the alpha subunit. *Journal of Biological Chemistry*, 1997; **272**: 11205–14.

128. Pessin JE, Bell GI. Mammalian facilitative glucose transporter family: structure and molecular regulation. *Annual Reviews in Physiology*, 1992; **54**: 911–30.

129. Webster KA. Regulation of glycolytic enzyme RNA transcriptional rates by oxygen availability in skeletal muscle cells. *Molecular and Cellular Biochemistry*, 1987; **77**: 19–28.

130. Dachs GU, Patterson AV, Firth JD, Ratcliffe PJ, Stratford IJ, Harris AL. Targeting gene expression to hypoxic tumor cells. *Nature Medicine*, 1997; **3**: 515–20.

131. Saunders MP, Patterson AV, Ratcliffe PJ, Harris AL, Stratford IJ. Using gene therapy to selectively activate bioreductive drugs in tumours. *Proceedings of the Annual Meeting of the American Association for Cancer Research*, 1998; **39**: Abstract 3490.

4.4.2 The programming of radiotherapy

Michele I. Saunders and Stanley Dische

Introduction

When radiotherapy is given with the object of cure, treatment is most commonly given daily from Monday to Friday, using an individual dose increment of between 1.8 Gy and 2 Gy, and over a period of 6 to 8 weeks total doses between 60 Gy and 72 Gy are achieved. The higher the dose, the greater is the probability of eradication of all tumour cells so it is the tolerance of the normal tissues which limits the total dose which can be reached. Early reactions, which usually begin within 3 to 4 weeks of commencement of treatment, normally settle within 3 to 4 weeks of its conclusion; they are often troublesome but almost invariably settle completely. It is the late changes, appearing more than 6 months later which limit the total dose of radiation that can be given.

When radiotherapy is given for palliation, the situation is very different. It is possible to obtain regression sufficient to relieve symptoms with much lower total doses. When the volume to irradiate is small, an adequate dose may be given in a single treatment but with larger volumes a short fractionated course of 1 to 2 weeks may be employed. With the relatively low total doses used, the incidence of late changes in normal tissues is minimal in the inevitably short survival of these patients.

New knowledge concerning tumour cell proliferation, the influence of the overall duration of treatment, and the probability of tumour eradication and the relationship between fraction size and the incidence of late morbidity have led clinical oncologists to look again at conventional radiotherapy to determine if a manipulation of the dose per fraction, the number of fractions, and overall time could improve the results of radiotherapy.

Tumour cell proliferation during a course of radiotherapy

Tumour cell kinetics

When untreated human tumours are observed over a period of time, their size increase relatively slowly. Volume doubling times commonly range from 25 to 100 days.[1] In the past, clinical oncologists have not been concerned that cellular proliferation during a course of radiotherapy was a serious problem. Knowledge of the cell kinetics of human tumours now suggests there may be a considerable discrepancy between events occurring at the cellular level and the observation of a good response as indicated by reduction in tumour bulk.

It was in radiobiology that the technique employing tritiated thymidine was developed to study cell kinetics but it was, however, a demanding one, taking a number of weeks to complete.[2] The burden of radioactivity using carbogen labelling limited studies to elderly patients with advanced disease. In 1985, Begg *et al.* reported a new approach. They gave a small dose of bromodeoxyuridine (BUdR), initially to animals and then to humans, and performed a biopsy of the tumour 4 to 6 h later. With the use of a cell sorter, the

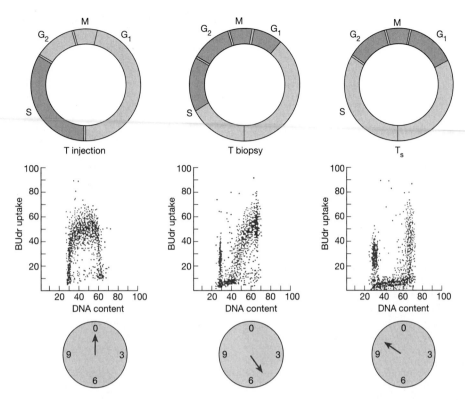

Fig. 1 Immediately after injection, only cells in S phase show BUdR incorporation in this diploid population. At the time of biopsy, in this case at 5 h, there has been progression of the labelled cohort and some have passed through mitosis and have entered G_1. The relative movement of the cells still in S phase can be used, with the method developed by Begg et al.,[3] to calculate the length of S phase (T_s). At 10 h, the duration of T_s in this case, all labelled cells have left S phase and are now in G_2 and M or, having divided, are in G_1.[4],[10] (By courtesy of Drs G.D. Wilson and M.H. Bennett.)

labelling index and the duration of the DNA synthetic period (T_s), could be calculated from the redistribution of the BUdR labelled cells round the cell cycle in the time between injection and biopsy. Furthermore, they obtained a result within 24 h (Fig. 1). From these values could be calculated the potential cell doubling time (T_{pot})—a measure of the proliferative activity of tumour cells, taking into account the presence of dividing and non-dividing cells but assuming an absence of cell loss.[3] Extensive study in human tumours has shown that the T_{pot} ranges widely from 2 to 12 or more days (Fig. 2).[4],[5] In squamous cell carcinomas in the uterine cervix or in the head and neck region, the majority of tumours appear to have the potential to double their cell number in 5 or fewer days. An extension of the technique to the counting of labelled cells in a histological preparation has shown that there are areas within the tumour where potential proliferation rates are even higher: many squamous cell cancers in the head and neck region have areas where the T_{pot} may be less than 2 days (Fig. 3).[6]

Normally, spontaneous cell loss due to differentiation, apoptosis, and degeneration due to nutritional deprivation accounts for the 10 to 20-fold differences observed between cellular and volume doubling times.[7]

When tumour cells are destroyed by radiotherapy or cytotoxic chemotherapy, this situation is likely to be greatly altered.[8] When a squamous cell carcinoma is given a 2-Gy radiation dose, half the tumour cells may be destroyed. At the end of the first week of

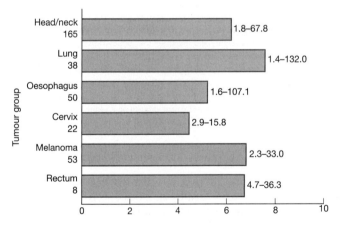

Fig. 2 Median potential cell doubling time (T_{pot}) (days) of human tumours. The number of cases studies and the range of T_{pot} found are also shown (Wilson et al. 1988; Dische et al. 1989).[4],[10]

conventional treatment therefore, the number of surviving tumour cells may be less than 5 per cent of the original number. With cell destruction occurring at such a rate it seems most probable that the high spontaneous cell loss occurring in the unperturbed tumour will be greatly reduced and the tumour cells may realize their full

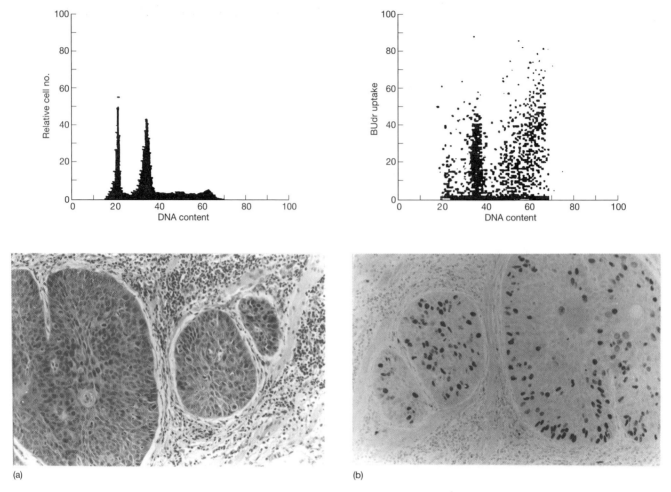

Fig. 3 A man aged 62 presented with a 3-cm tumour of the right side of the anterior two-thirds of the tongue that was 7 cm in maximum diameter. It penetrated deep into the musculature of the tongue and also extended on to the floor of the mouth. There was, however, no evidence for glandular invasion or distant metastasis. The patient was given BUdR and a biopsy taken. The DNA profile (top left) revealed a subpopulation of cells with an abnormal DNA content, showing a peak of 35 units, the normal diploid cells are seen at 20 units. The distribution of BUdR labelling in relation to the DNA content of the tumour is shown (top right) and indicates that proliferation was mainly associated with the aneuploid cells. The labelling index was 16.8 per cent and the duration of S phase was calculated to be 13.4 h. From these values it was calculated that the potential cell doubling time (T_{pot}) was 2.7 days, suggesting that the tumour was one that had a capacity for rapid cellular proliferation. The histological appearance (bottom left) was that of a grade 3 squamous cell carcinoma. Using immunohistochemistry (bottom right) the cells that had taken up the BUdR can be clearly seen. The mean labelling index, as shown histologically, was calculated to be 20.1 per cent. The patient was treated by continuous, hyperfractionated, accelerated radiotherapy (CHART) with complete regression and died due to intercurrent disease at 7 years without return of tumour (Bennett et al. 1992).[6] (By courtesy of Drs G.D. Wilson and M.H. Bennett.)

reproductive potential.[9],[10] The resulting cellular repopulation may, in fact, be further accelerated by an increase in growth fraction of the surviving tumour cells and a reduction in cycle time. In these circumstances, repopulation may occur at a faster rate than that suggested by the cell kinetics determined prior to treatment.

Overall treatment time and tumour control

Maciejewski and his colleagues in 1983 were first to show the importance of overall treatment time in determining the outcome.[11] In a series of 500 patients with head and neck tumours, there was a highly significant inverse relationship between the duration of treatment and the possibility of local tumour control. In an analysis of 310 patients with T3 or T4 squamous cell carcinoma of the larynx, they found that in the patients given comparable doses, as calculated using the nominal standard dose (NSD) equation, local control rates decreased from around 80 per cent at overall treatment times of 32 to 35 days, to only 16 per cent at 56 to 63 days. A similar association has since been shown in many analyses of the influence of overall time on the results of radiotherapy in head and neck cancer.[12]–[16] Similar findings have now been reported in tumours of the skin,[17] bladder,[18] non-small cell lung cancer,[19] cervix,[20] and breast.[21]

All these analyses give strong support to the view that overall time is important to radiation response and therefore to the view that cellular repopulation during treatment is a major determinant of tumour control. The size of the effect and the consistency with which it has been demonstrated is impressive but some reservations must be expressed concerning these analyses of data gathered retrospectively. Prolongation of the duration of treatment is not necessarily a random process: patients with more aggressive and more advanced disease may be more distressed by reactions and so treatment may be more protracted. This has been overcome by an analysis of the influence of overall time upon tumour control in the patients treated conventionally in the randomized trial of continuous, hyperfractionated, accelerated radiotherapy (CHART) in head and neck cancer which showed a margin of advantage but this did not reach conventional levels of statistical significance.[22] The use of a rest period during a course of radiotherapy has long been employed as a means of allowing the patient to recover from severe, early reactions. It has, however, been shown by Overgaard that this prolongation of overall time leads to impaired tumour control without sparing late morbidity in normal tissues, giving strong confirmation to the views concerning tumour cell repopulation.[23]

Onset of repopulation

Great importance to the design of schedules to overcome the hazard of cellular repopulation is knowledge as to when this process commences. In a number of animal systems, the acceleration of tumour growth after irradiation has been determined using single treatments and fractionated courses; the time to repopulation has shown considerable variation but commonly begins between 7 and 21 days after initiation of treatment.[24],[25]

In the normal bone marrow, repopulation may commence in as short a time as 8 to 10 h after exposure to radiation, but only after 14 days in the skin.[7],[26] It is possible that there is a relationship between the latent interval seen in a normal tissue before cellular depletion by radiation results in a proliferation of normal cells and the response time of tumours derived from the same normal tissue. The simple concept that tumour cells are different from normal ones in that their growth is free from control mechanisms, has long been discarded. Research in oncogenes and growth factors, using techniques now available in molecular biology, reveal a complexity of control mechanisms. So far, however, there is little to guide the clinician as to time of initiation of repopulation from these molecular studies.

Withers *et al.* researched the literature reporting the results of radiotherapy in head and neck cancer and found 59 sets of data where they were able to estimate the dose to achieve 50 per cent local control. In calculating this, they expressed the dose given as if it had been applied in 2-Gy fractions.[9] They found evidence that repopulation in squamous cell carcinoma in the head and neck region commences after a lag-period of 3 to 4 weeks from initiation of radiotherapy. This work has had much influence upon those working in the field but remains controversial. Further analyses of the same material by Bentzen and Thames, failed to show a lag before repopulation commenced.[27]

In many of the analyses of overall time upon tumour control in head and neck cancer, repopulation has been assumed to begin 4 weeks after commencement of radiotherapy and it has been shown that a dose increment of the order of 0.6 Gy per day is required in order to negate the cellular proliferation. This is consistent with a 4-day clonogen doubling time.[9],[12]

Fractionation and normal tissue change

In the 1920s and 30s the benefit of radiotherapy was increased by moving from a single or a few large treatments to daily treatments given over a period of many weeks. Tumour control was increased and morbidity reduced but the total radiation dose given in many small fractions needed to be raised—for example a dose of 20 Gy in a single treatment must be elevated to a total of 60 to 65 Gy when treatment is given in 30 fractions over 6 weeks.[28] Strandqvist[29] proposed a mathematical formula to relate total dose and overall time to skin tolerance. Subsequently, it was found that the effect of fraction number as well as overall time and total dose must be included in the equation and this was incorporated in the NSD model introduced by Ellis in 1969.[30] The formula became a valuable tool but it later became evident that when less than 10 fractions were given, late effects in normal tissues were greater than predicted.[31]

A number of other approaches have been proposed but during the last decade the linear quadratic formula has become favoured:[32],[33]

$$E = nd \left(1 + \frac{d}{\alpha\beta} \right)$$

Where E = effect, n = number of fractions, d = dose give per fraction; α and β are the linear and quadratic coefficients.

It has been shown that, at clinically relevant doses, tumours and early-reacting tissues respond to ionizing radiation dominantly with a linear relationship between dose and effect—the linear or α component. In the late-reacting tissues, in the clinically relevant dose range, an important part of the effect is related to the square of the individual dose given—the β or quadratic element. The important implication of this linear quadratic model is that by giving radiotherapy in many small doses there should be a further sparing of the changes in late reacting tissues but little alteration in the response in the early-reacting, normal tissues and of the response of tumour.

The reduced incidence of late normal tissue injury with the use of a small dose per fraction, or its corollary increase in late tissue injury after the use of a large dose per fraction, has been demonstrated in many analyses of clinical data related to sites such as the spinal cord,[34],[35] the uterine cervix,[36] the skin,[37] bone,[38] and the pericardium and the mediastinum.[39]

Increased tolerance to radiation dose with the use of many small fractions in the management of tumours in the head and neck has been confirmed by work at the University of Florida, Gainesville,[40] by the European Organization for Research and Treatment of Cancer Fractionation Trial (EORTC),[41] and also by the results of the Radiation Therapy Oncology Group (RTOG) Protocol 8313.[42] In all three trials, considerably higher total doses of radiation were tolerated when small doses of 1.15 to 1.2 Gy were given twice daily and in two this appeared to lead to improved tumour control.[40],[43] Similar findings have been reported by Edsmyr *et al.*[44] in the radiotherapy of carcinoma of the bladder (Fig. 4).

There have, however, been some reports where it would appear that tumour control rates in head and neck cancer have been maintained using a reduced number of fractions at high dose, with a reduction in total dose, without any increase in the incidence of late damage.[45],[46] Overall treatment times for the hypofractionated arms,

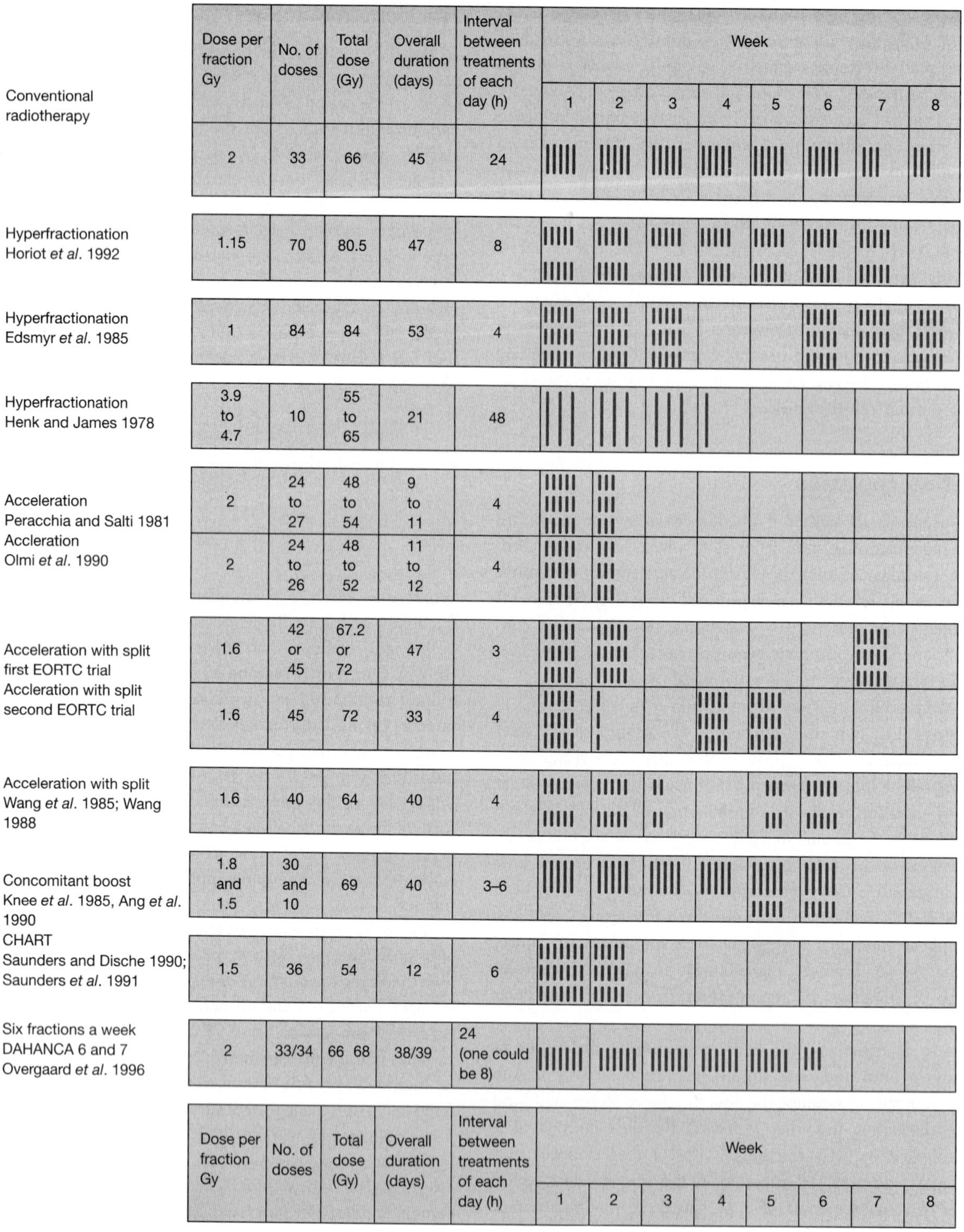

	Dose per fraction Gy	No. of doses	Total dose (Gy)	Overall duration (days)	Interval between treatments of each day (h)	Week 1–8
Conventional radiotherapy	2	33	66	45	24	(schedule chart)
Hyperfractionation Horiot et al. 1992	1.15	70	80.5	47	8	(schedule chart)
Hyperfractionation Edsmyr et al. 1985	1	84	84	53	4	(schedule chart)
Hyperfractionation Henk and James 1978	3.9 to 4.7	10	55 to 65	21	48	(schedule chart)
Acceleration Peracchia and Salti 1981	2	24 to 27	48 to 54	9 to 11	4	(schedule chart)
Accleration Olmi et al. 1990	2	24 to 26	48 to 52	11 to 12	4	(schedule chart)
Acceleration with split first EORTC trial	1.6	42 or 45	67.2 or 72	47	3	(schedule chart)
Accleration with split second EORTC trial	1.6	45	72	33	4	(schedule chart)
Acceleration with split Wang et al. 1985; Wang 1988	1.6	40	64	40	4	(schedule chart)
Concomitant boost Knee et al. 1985, Ang et al. 1990	1.8 and 1.5	30 and 10	69	40	3–6	(schedule chart)
CHART Saunders and Dische 1990; Saunders et al. 1991	1.5	36	54	12	6	(schedule chart)
Six fractions a week DAHANCA 6 and 7 Overgaard et al. 1996	2	33/34	66 68	38/39	24 (one could be 8)	(schedule chart)
	Dose per fraction Gy	No. of doses	Total dose (Gy)	Overall duration (days)	Interval between treatments of each day (h)	Week 1–8

Fig. 4 Altered fractionation schedules.

however, were much reduced to range between 16 and 21 days and the results may therefore be, in part, explained by a reduction of the chance for repopulation and partly also by the overall poor survival of the patients in these studies, leading to poor sensitivity for late effects. The British Institute of Radiology trial of three fractions versus five fractions, which included 734 patients with squamous cell cancer in the larynx and hypopharynx, similarly failed to show significant differences in survival, local tumour control, need for laryngectomy, or in morbidity.[47] This pioneering study allowed each centre to choose its own dose level. There was wide variation in the treatments regimens employed leading inevitably to a low sensitivity. There was, in fact, a 14 per cent benefit to the five fractions per week over three in terms of freedom from tumour recurrence and in the need for laryngectomy. If these levels had been statistically significant, both the patient and clinician would have favoured five rather than three fractions per week.

The interfraction interval

In order to give an increased number of treatments (hyperfractionation), or to reduce overall duration of treatment (acceleration), more than one fraction must be given on each treatment day. After radiation treatment some of the damage induced is irreversible but some can be repaired. Sufficient time must be given for the repair to be complete in the normal tissues otherwise there will be an accumulation of incomplete repair and an increase in biological effect. As it is change in the late-responding tissues which is the most important factor limiting the total dose that may be given in a course of radiotherapy, the choice of an appropriate interfraction interval is extremely important.

The time course for repair of sublethal injury varies from tissue to tissue and for each more than one process with differing time courses may be involved.[48],[49] In the animal models, the time taken for 50 per cent of sublethal injury to be repaired has largely ranged from 30 to 90 min. In a compromise in gaining the maximum amount of repair and the practical problems associated with the organization of treatment more than once per day, interfraction intervals have usually ranged from 4 to 8 h. Nguyen et al.,[50] however, gave seven treatments per day at 2-h intervals to patients with head and neck cancer. The 2-h interfraction interval is the shortest recorded in a clinical study and may be the explanation for a very high and unacceptable incidence of postradiation morbidity, which exceeded 50 per cent in some groups. In a RTOG study of twice daily treatment, those cases where the interfraction interval was less than 4.5 h showed a significantly higher incidence of late morbidity when compared with those treated with an interval greater than 4.5 h.[42] Although some of the earlier studies did employ an interfraction interval of 4 h when more than one treatment was given per day, in more recent work, interfraction intervals of at least 6 h and sometimes 8 h have been employed.

In 1989, an unexpected incidence of radiation myelitis was encountered using the CHART regimen with accelerated radiotherapy over 12 days and an interfraction interval of 6 h (see below).[51] With the small dose per fraction and low total dose employed, the linear quadratic equation suggested that there was a reduced rather than elevated risk of myelopathy. No further cases have been reported after a reduction in the total dose permitted to the spinal cord. Radiation myelopathy was also reported from Toronto in patients who had also received accelerated radiotherapy.[52] These clinical experiences led to further laboratory experiments which suggested that there was a component of repair of sublethal injury in spinal cord in dogs which exceeded 4 h.[53],[54] This, in part, suggested the reason for the clinical incidence of radiation myelopathy.

A review of the CHART data together with all the clinical data now available, including in particular that from trials using other schemes of accelerated radiotherapy by Saunders, Bentzen, and Dische (in preparation), suggests that, in general, half-times of repair of sublethal injury in the human may be longer than in the animal models and range from 4 to 5 h. As in the animal models, half-times of repair in spinal cord are longer than those for other tissues: an even longer half-time of repair, perhaps exceeding 8 h, may exist in the human spinal cord and so may fully account for the radiation myelopathy observed in the CHART pilot study.

Studies of altered fractionation

Hyperfractionation

The evidence suggesting a reduction in the incidence of late tissue change with the use of small doses per fraction encouraged clinical trials of hyperfractionation in which the overall duration of treatment was maintained but two or more treatments, each with a dose considerably smaller than the conventional 1.8 to 2 Gy, were given on each treatment day. An early trial was that performed at the Radiumhemmet by Littbrand and colleagues, in 1971 to 1978, in carcinoma of the bladder.[44] Essentially, three treatments were given each day of 1.0 Gy and compared with the daily treatment of 2 Gy; total doses of 84 Gy and 64 Gy resulted. Hyperfractionation gave a significantly greater survival and a margin of greater local tumour control without an increase in morbidity.

A randomized, controlled clinical trial in oropharyngeal carcinoma was performed by the EORTC.[41] Twice daily treatment using an individual dose of 1.15 Gy was compared with a daily dose of 2 Gy. Both were given over the same overall period of 7 weeks, achieving total dose of 80.5 Gy in 70 fractions compared with 70 Gy in 35 fractions. Acute reactions were slightly more troublesome in the hyperfractionated group but late reactions were similar, supporting the hypothesis that a low dose per fraction is associated with a lower incidence of late injury so enabling higher tumour doses to be achieved without raising the overall risk of morbidity. Primary tumour control was significantly improved in the hyperfractionated group where 5-year local tumour control was 59 per cent compared with 40 per cent in the standard conventional arm ($p = 0.02$). There was a smaller margin of improved survival ($p = 0.05$).[55] This is an important achievement as the surgical salvage and high intercurrent mortality seen in trials involving head and neck cancer reduce the survival benefit which can be obtained. At Gainesville the results of treatment using a very similar regimen showed advantage when compared retrospectively with those seen in previous patients with tumours at all sites within the head and neck region.[56] In a phase I/II trial conducted by the Radiation Therapy Oncology Group, fractions of 1.2 Gy were given twice per day for 5 days per week and patients were assigned to achieve total doses of 67.2 Gy, 72.0 Gy, 76.8 Gy, and later 81.6 Gy. The highest dose of 81.6 Gy, which was given over a period of just under 7 weeks, was found to give an incidence of late effects no greater than with the other arms and similar to that expected using conventional daily treatments.[42] This regimen has been chosen as one of the four arms of a RTOG trial in head and neck cancer which has just been completed with a total accrual of 1200 patients, however the results are not yet available.

In the management of brain tumours, a statistically significant improvement in survival was achieved in the management of grade 3 and 4 gliomas using a hyperfractionated regimen in a randomized trial against conventional treatment without apparent increase in morbidity.[56]

Pure hyperfractionation therefore has been shown to be of advantage in the management of certain tumours. Only a limited adoption of hyperfractionation in the routine management of patients with head and neck cancer has, however, followed. The economic and social burden of doubling the number of treatments and requiring patients to wait long periods within a treatment centre or to travel twice in one day, has been a deterrent.

Further studies of hyperfractionation include a new EORTC trial in which tumours at all sites in the head and neck are included and treatment is given in combination with cytotoxic chemotherapy. The recently concluded, but not yet reported, RTOG study included a hyperfractionated arm.

Pure acceleration

A simple acceleration of a conventional course of treatment by giving 2-Gy fractions on two or more occasions on each day has been attempted by a number of workers. In a pilot study in bladder cancer, a standard 30 fraction course of radiotherapy using 2-Gy increments was given in twice daily treatments over a period of 3 weeks. An increase in acute and, in particular, in late morbidity led to a reduction in the total dose in order to achieve tolerance.[57] In patients with head and neck cancer, 2-Gy increments were given three times a day and the whole course completed within 2 working weeks. Despite a reduction in total dose to the range 54 to 56 Gy, acute reactions were very troublesome and a number of cases failed to heal. The incidence of late morbidity was high with rates of severe complication exceeding 25 per cent in the survivors.[58],[59] Tumour control rates did not appear, in these pilot studies, to be improved. Lamb et al.[60] reduced the dose per fraction to 1.8 Gy and treated three times per day to achieve a total dose of 58 Gy in 3.5 working weeks. Acute morbidity was troublesome and required supportive measures for nutrition, however, there were promising tumour control rates and a randomized, controlled clinical trial was initiated.

In the management of locally advanced non-small cell lung cancer, 60 Gy in 2-Gy fractions were similarly given in a period of 3 weeks in a four arm study where there was a subrandomization to the addition of chemotherapy.[61] There was some increase in acute and late reactions in the patients in the accelerated arm. Follow-up has not shown an advantage in terms of survival or local tumour control to acceleration.[62]

It seems, therefore, that pure acceleration where standard individual doses of 2 Gy are given twice or thrice daily leads to some increase in morbidity. Commonly, total doses have to be reduced and this approach has not shown proven advantage.

Acceleration using a split course

Difficulties in achieving a satisfactory total dose when using normal dose increments between 1.8 and 2 Gy led to the use of smaller dose increments combined with a rest period during treatment (split course). Van der Schueren and his group observed the reactions in patients with head and neck cancer given accelerated radiotherapy and established a regimen in which 1.6 Gy was given three times daily for 2 working weeks.[63],[64] Marked reactions commenced over the following weekend and a gap of 4 weeks was then allowed for this to settle before giving further treatment over 4 to 5 days using three times daily treatment and the same individual dose fraction. A total dose of 67 to 72 Gy was achieved in an overall duration of 7 weeks. A randomized, controlled trial performed by the EORTC compared this scheme, with and without misonidazole, against daily fractionated radiotherapy over 7 weeks to a total dose of 72 Gy.[65] The study, which included 523 patients, revealed similar tumour control in all three arms without significant difference in the incidence of late morbidity.[66] It is noteworthy that the overall duration of treatment was similar for all groups and repopulation during the 4-week gap may well have resulted in such a tumour burden that the final dose was inadequate to eradicate all tumour.

A further EORTC study incorporated a shorter gap, earlier in the course, so that the overall duration of treatment was reduced from 7 to 5 weeks. The same total dose of 72 Gy was achieved. A total of 512 patients with T2, T3, and T4 cancer in the head and neck region, with the exception of hypopharynx, was included. There was a 13 per cent gain in local tumour control at 5 years ($p = 0.02$) and there was trend ($p = 0.06$) for improved survival. Severe, late damage occurred in 14 per cent of the patients in the accelerated arm compared with 4 per cent in the conventionally treated cases. Although significantly improved tumour control was achieved, the incidence of late toxicity has not led to adoption of this regimen.[55],[67]

The combination of a acceleration with a rest period was employed by Wang et al. who, in twice daily treatments, gave increments of 1.6 Gy and began a rest period in the middle of the third week so that the final boost completed therapy in 6 weeks. In phase II studies including tumours at a number of sites within the head and neck region, improved tumour control was observed when comparison was made with previously treated cases.[68],[69] This regimen was tested in the four-arm study of the RTOG which is now complete and awaiting analysis.

Concomitant boost

Commonly in the management of head and neck tumours by radiotherapy, treatment is first given to a large volume which includes areas at risk of microscopic involvement but in the final phase a small volume containing only the area of known involvement with a modest margin is given a boost dose. In this way the smallest volume is given the highest dose so as to minimize late radiation morbidity.

At the MD Anderson Hospital, Houston the overall duration of treatment has been reduced from 7.5 to 6 weeks by giving the boost as a second treatment in the day during a main course of treatment.[70] Following pilot studies when the boost was given during various phases in the main treatment, it was found that the best results were achieved by giving it during the last 2 weeks. The results of a pilot study in oropharyngeal carcinoma have yielded promising results and this technique formed an arm of the RTOG trial awaiting analysis.[71]

Hyperfractionation of accelerated radiotherapy

A 20-fraction regimen of radiotherapy given over 4 weeks has been standard in the management of head and neck cancer at the Princess Margaret Hospital in Toronto. In a prospective, randomized trial, 336 patients received either the established 51 Gy in 20 fractions over 4 weeks or 58 Gy in 40 fractions over 4 weeks, 1.45 Gy being given twice daily.[72] A total of 336 patients with advanced laryngeal or pharyngeal carcinoma were included in the trial, which was completed in 1995. A margin of improved locoregional control has been demonstrated for the hyperfractionation arm but this is not statistically significant. Recognizing the modest increase in total dose achieved in the hyperfractionation arm, the margin of benefit would seem to be appropriate and the result therefore in keeping with those reported of accelerated radiotherapy using different regimens in patients with head and neck cancer.

Continuous, hyperfractionated, accelerated radiotherapy (CHART)

At the Cancer Treatment Centre at Mount Vernon, in a collaboration with colleagues at the Gray Laboratory, a novel scheme of continuous, hyperfractionated, accelerated radiotherapy (CHART) was devised with the objective of improving tumour control and reducing the incidence of late effects in normal tissue.[73] Once commenced, treatment was to be continued every day until its conclusion. In the head and neck region all regimens of accelerated radiotherapy result in the appearance of marked mucosal reactions to the 13th or 14th days after initiation of radiotherapy and therefore it seemed best to complete treatment in 12 days. In this way, there would no problem of attempting to continue through reactions which would be allowed to heal without the inhibition given by further irradiation. During such a short overall period of treatment little, if any, repopulation of tumour cells would be permitted to occur.[74]

In the CHART regimen therefore, radiotherapy is given three times each day, with an interval of 6 h between fractions, on 12 consecutive days including the weekend. The pilot study was commenced in January 1985, using a dose increment of 1.4 Gy, but with good tolerance this was soon elevated to 1.5 Gy, so that in 36 treatments a total dose of 54 Gy was achieved. A total of 263 patients, mainly with head and neck and non-small cell lung cancer, were entered into the pilot study which was concluded in March 1990 when randomized trials were commenced.[51],[74]

The radiation reactions which appeared in mucosae soon after treatment was completed were marked, but on the whole well tolerated. In some cases, final healing of small areas of mucosa, usually in the tongue, was delayed for several months but all finally resolved. Acute reactions in skin were unexpectedly reduced. Radiation myelitis was, however, an unexpected late complication in five patients. The permitted radiation dose to the spinal cord using this regimen was reduced and no further cases of radiation myelitis have presented.[71]

In other normal tissues the anticipated reduction in the incidence of late changes has been demonstrated. Skin given full radiation doses with conventional radiotherapy does not normally recover to regrow hair but this has been observed in some patients given CHART where the skin received the full dose.[75] Observation of the patients suggested that 1 to 2 years after completion of treatment, there was a greater degree of recovery of parotid function in the CHART cases than previous experience with conventional radiotherapy had given. A study of parotid and whole salivary flow gave confirmation to the view that there was reduced late change in the parotid after CHART.[76]

When comparison was made with the results of previous patients treated conventionally for advanced head and neck cancer, there was evidence for improved primary tumour control and in 76 patients with locally advanced non-small cell lung cancer, there was significant improvement in primary tumour control and in survival when comparison was made again with previously treated cases.[75],[77]

After considering these findings, in a joint Medical Research Council, Cancer Research Campaign, and Department of Health initiative, multicentre trials in non-small cell lung cancer and head and neck tumours were established to compare CHART with conventional radiotherapy. A total of 1481 patients were entered into these studies between April 1990 and April 1995.[78]

In the head and neck study there was, overall, a small margin of advantage in primary tumour control but this did not reach statistical significance.[79] In the control of nodal disease, there was a very small margin in favour of conventional treatment. In T3, T4 laryngeal carcinoma however, there was a large margin in favour of CHART. As in the pilot study the immediate reactions were more troublesome in the CHART arm but were quite well tolerated and settled sooner than those in the conventionally treated patients. Nine different parameters of late radiation change were analysed and in five there was a significant reduction in the CHART arm compared with conventional radiotherapy.

When considering all 563 cases including in the trial in non-small cell lung cancer, the survival at 2 years in the CHART cases was 30 per cent compared with 21 per cent for conventional, giving a 22 per cent reduction in the risk of death ($p = 0.008$). Local tumour control was also improved ($p = 0.033$).[80] Squamous cell carcinoma accounted for 81 per cent of the cases, here at 2 years, 33 per cent of the CHART patients were alive compared with 20 per cent of the conventionally treated cases, giving a reduction in the risk of death of 30 per cent ($p = 0.0007$); this was associated with improved local tumour control ($p = 0.012$). As in the head and neck study, morbidity was closely observed and here it appeared equal in both arms of the trial. While both head and neck and non-small cell lung cancer patients received the same total dose with CHART of 54 Gy, in the conventional arms different total doses for conventional radiotherapy were adopted, recognizing the normal tissue tolerance of the tissues and the volumes irradiated in the management of the two areas: the total dose was 66 Gy for the head and neck cases and 60 Gy for the non-small cell lung cancer cases, given in both in 2 Gy fractions. Differences in morbidity may be due to this, and perhaps also the differences in tumour control.

An elevation in total dose given with the CHART regimen has been attained by extending into a third week when also it was possible to omit the week ends (CHARTWEL = CHART week end less). This has easily been possible in treating the chest for dysphagia due to treatment; this reaction first appears late in the third week—5 or 6 days later than the reaction in the mucosae of the head and neck. A total dose of 60 Gy in 40 fractions has been tolerated and the work continues.[81] Other tumour sites have been treated including the rectum. The combinations with cytotoxic chemotherapy and with brachytherapy are discussed below.

Acceleration by treating six or seven times per week

In the Danish Head and Neck Cancer Group (DAHANCA) trials 6 and 7, in carcinoma of larynx and pharynx, six treatments were given per week , either with an extra attendance on Saturday or by giving a second treatment on another day of the week.[82] Total doses ranging from 66 to 68 Gy were identical in the two arms and so the essential difference between the two arms was 7 days in the overall duration. Those patients with laryngopharyngeal and oropharyngeal carcinoma all received, in addition, the hypoxic cell sensitizer nimorazole as indicated by the previous DAHANCA study. Nimorazole was not administered to the patients with laryngeal cancer.

A preliminary report gives an improvement in local regional tumour control of 10 per cent in the accelerated arm and similar morbidity levels in both arms of the trial. Clear therapeutic benefit is therefore emerging from this study.[82]

In a pilot study of treatment in 2 Gy fractions on 7 compared with 5 days of the week performed by Skladowski et al.,[83] which reduced the overall time from 7 to 5 weeks, an unacceptable incidence of late radiation change prompted a reduction of individual doses to 1.8 Gy. Similar changes were made in the control arm and in both some prolongation of overall time was made in order for this to be achieved. Morbidity is now acceptable and tumour control in the accelerated arm appears to be considerably improved.

Further directions of research

Brachytherapy and accelerated treatment

Brachytherapy has a long established place in the management of patients with accessible tumours of limited volume. When a single exposure is employed the overall treatment times are less than 7 days, so brachytherapy is a form of accelerated treatment. A protracted, low dose rate will spare late effects in the normal tissues in a similar way to hyperfractionation using external beam therapy.[84]

The combination of external beam with intracavity or interstitial implantation is often employed in the management of oral and uterine cervix tumours. A T2 N0 carcinoma of the tongue may be treated by external beam therapy and a dose of 44 Gy given in 2-Gy fractions over a period of 4.5 weeks, followed by an implantation of radioactive sources so as to give a further 40 Gy in a period of 4 days. Because of the treatment reaction which will be evident at the conclusion of the external beam therapy, a rest period must usually be allowed for this to settle before the implantation can be performed, but a 2 or 3-week interval must allow tumour cell repopulation. With the CHART regimen, it has been possible to perform the implant immediately after external beam therapy given three times per day for 9 days, introducing radioactive sources on the 10th day for a period of 2 to 3 days.[85] In this way all treatment is given continuously and completed to a total dose of 60 Gy before mucosal reactions develop on the 13th or 14th day from the beginning of all treatment.

Cytotoxic chemotherapy and accelerated radiotherapy

The combination of cytotoxic chemotherapy with radiotherapy to improve primary tumour control and/or eliminate subclinical metastatic disease, has been employed in the management of tumours at many sites. In a limited number of tumour situations clear margins of benefit been achieved but, where there has been an interval between the giving of the two modalities, as in neoadjuvant treatment, results have tended to be disappointing (see Chapter 4.5). The most promising

results have been reported when chemotherapy and radiotherapy are given concurrently; however, margins of increased tumour control must be measured against any increase in the incidence or severity of early and late reactions due to radiotherapy. It is in keeping with our knowledge of the cell kinetics of human tumours that incorporating an interval between radiotherapy and chemotherapy will allow tumour cell proliferation which may negate the benefit of combined treatment. Accelerated radiotherapy does give the potential for shorter interruptions but an increase in morbidity may limit this approach.

Hypoxia and accelerated radiotherapy

The radioresistance of the hypoxic tumour cell has been recognized since the 1930s but despite many clinical trials of methods to overcome hypoxia, such as hyperbaric oxygen and the chemical sensitizing agents, only limited progress has been made. An overview of all the trials has, however, shown that such methods do give significant advantage in tumour control though the margin is a modest one.[86]

A process of reoxygenation is believed to occur during fractionated radiotherapy when surviving hypoxic cells move to take over the blood supply of the well-oxygenated tumour cells which, being radiosensitive, are destroyed.[87] In this way the success of conventional radiotherapy in tumours known to contain hypoxic cells can be explained. The time scale of reoxygenation in human tumours is poorly understood but it does seem probable that reoxygenation will be less efficient when the overall duration of treatment is much reduced.

A hypoxic tumour is often described as one that has outstripped its blood supply due to its rapid growth. It seems, therefore, probable that tumour which has a capacity to proliferate rapidly is also one which shows radioresistance due to hypoxia. The combination of accelerated radiotherapy with breathing of carbogen to overcome chronic hypoxia and nicotinamide to reduce acute hypoxia (ARCON) has been introduced into clinical trial after promising laboratory study.[41] Pilot studies have been performed in a number of sites using a range of regimens.[88],[89] The management of gliomas has been disappointing but here an increased sensitization of the normal tissues can be expected and may account for some of the findings. In head and neck cancer, the most striking result has been achieved by the Nijmegen group in the management of advanced laryngeal cancer with 100 per cent complete regression rate and an 87 per cent control rate at 3 years in a series of 62 patients with advanced disease.[90] The use of ARCON in carcinoma of the bladder has also given evidence for improved tumour control.[91] Multicentre trials of ARCON in larynx and bladder are now being planned.

Surgery and postoperative radiotherapy

Any residual tumour cells within a field of surgery may be expected to proliferate rapidly in the vascular conditions which exist in the operative field during the weeks following surgery. It follows, therefore, that the interval between surgery and radiotherapy should be as short as possible and that an accelerated treatment should give a better result than a conventional one. Evidence to support both these hypotheses have emerged from a randomized trial completed at Houston.[92],[93]

The prediction of the tumours likely to benefit from accelerated treatment

In a study of tumour cell kinetics of patients receiving CHART in the pilot study, it was noted that benefit appeared to occur in those squamous carcinomas in the head and neck region showing a differentiated appearance rather than those where it was undifferentiated.[94] In a comparison of the results of split-course therapy with uninterrupted treatment across two randomized studies, it appeared that protraction of treatment by the use of a split impaired the response of differentiated tumours that made no difference to those that were undifferentiated.[95] To this evidence can be added a subanalysis of the CHART trial in head and neck cancer where it was shown that the differentiated tumours showed significant benefit to CHART whereas the undifferentiated tumours showed a similar margin in favour of conventional radiotherapy, though this was not significant because of the fewer number of undifferentiated tumours included.[79]

This evidence suggested that those tumours which most closely resemble the original squamous epithelium, a normal tissue which has an ability to proliferate rapidly, may retain this characteristic so that cellular repopulation during treatment may be a major problem when conventional radiotherapy is employed. The undifferentiated tumours may have lost this ability and here protracted radiotherapy, going to the highest radiation dose possible, may be the preferred policy. The bringing together of a database which will include a number of the randomized trials of accelerated radiotherapy may give further evidence on this important point. There is, therefore, a real possibility that selection of patients for specific regimens will allow greater overall benefit to be achieved.

In addition to histologically differentiation, other prognostic factors are undergoing study, including molecular markers in order to determine subgroups of tumours which may do better or do worse with the different programmes of treatment. There was initially promise that tumour cell kinetic studies in the individual patient performed prior to radiotherapy might give such prognostic information, however, in extensive study, the potential cell doubling time (T_{pot}) has not proved to be a prognostic marker of value.[96] A significant correlation between the labelling index and response to accelerated treatment has been demonstrated. However, a significant margin in a large study may not indicate sufficient specificity to allow a prognostic factor to be of value in an individual case.[97]

Accelerated radiotherapy and morbidity

The higher incidence of neural damage using accelerated radiotherapy must be recognized when accelerated treatment is being considered. In other tissues, reduced late damage may be attained but, as has been discussed, the margin is less than might be expected from a simple application of the linear quadratic model. Longer half-lives of repair of sublethal injury in human as compared with animal models may be the cause.

An unexpected advantage of accelerated radiotherapy was shown in the CHART pilot study, and confirmed in the randomized study, with regard to early and late reaction in the skin. This has meant the use of full bolus in patients is difficult to plan because of gross irregularity of contour due to previous surgery.[98] Reactions only occasionally progress to moist desquamation, heal rapidly, and lead to minimal late radiation change. Such a technique does allow for effective and accurate radiotherapy, particularly in the postoperative condition, and is an unexpected benefit of this accelerated radiotherapy. It is of interest that when the period of treatment was extended beyond 14 days using CHARTWEL, skin reactions became more severe. It seems probable, therefore, that to gain this benefit accelerated radiotherapy must be completed in no more than 12 days (unpublished observations).

Accelerated fractionation, tumour site, cure or palliation

The bulk of our knowledge as to the value of altered fractionation has been obtained in the management of squamous cell cancer in the head and neck region. There is some evidence to support the importance of repopulation in squamous cell cancer in other sites, in particular the lung where CHART showed significant advantage in a randomized trial and also in those sites where concurrent chemotherapy seems advantageous and where overall time can be related to the chance of successful radiotherapy.

There is little evidence to guide us as to the importance of repopulation in breast cancer. Some evidence suggests that where a boost treatment using brachytherapy is employed after external beam treatment, a better result is achieved when the interval between the two treatments is short, so supporting the concept of repopulation as an important factor in the postoperative breast situation.[21]

In carcinoma of cervix, there is similar evidence suggesting that a gap between external beam therapy and the boost brachytherapy may lead to impairment of results and certainly with a squamous cell carcinoma, this can be expected.[20] Accelerated radiotherapy to the pelvis, however, has been associated with increased normal tissue reaction. The CHART regimen has been employed for advanced and recurrent rectal cancer with promise, in a pilot study, and this work continues.[99]

Tumours such as prostatic cancer, where low proliferation rates have been demonstrated in tumour cell kinetic studies, are unlikely to benefit from accelerated treatment and studies reported to date give confirmation of this.[100]

Although in one randomized trial of accelerated hyperfractionation performed in supratentorial malignant gliomas, benefit was achieved compared with conventional treatment, the margin was small.[56] In other trials of accelerated radiotherapy in brain tumours, no clear result has so far been achieved and the area remains one for study.

Attention has naturally been concentrated upon the curative situation. In palliation, however, the reduction of the burden of attendance for the patient and of the cost to the cancer centre make hypofractionation attractive. In tumours known to show rapid tumour cell proliferation, the combination of hypofractionation with acceleration seems best, if practical.

Low dose hyper-radiosensitivity—ultrafractionation

Until recently, there was only limited laboratory data on tumour cell survival using individual dose fractions below 1 Gy as accurate measurement of cell survival at such low doses of radiation was not possible. Now, the fluorescent activator cell sorter (FACS) and the dynamic microscopic imaging processing scanner (DMIPS) have become available. Application of these techniques has shown a new and surprising excess cell kill at doses below 1 Gy relative to that predicted by the linear quadratic model. This phenomenon has been called 'low-dose hyper-radiosensitivity'.[101]

The data now available suggests that hyper-radiosensitivity is more commonly observed and is quantitatively greater in radioresistant tumour cell lines, including resistant human tumour cell lines, than in normal tissues. Theoretically, a therapeutic gain factor as high as 2.0 may be attained in the management of certain radioresistant tumours.[102]

There is now evidence that hyper-radiosensitivity does occur in human skin[103] and a clinical investigation to exploit hyper-radiosensitivity is underway. Radiation doses of the order of 0.5 Gy will need to be given three times per day and through the weekend in order to simulate in the clinic the conditions which have been shown in the laboratory to give benefit. Lower total doses may be appropriate so courses may not need to be extended beyond 5 weeks.[104] It will be some years before it can be shown if the promise of ultrafractionation will be possible in the clinic.

Conclusions

- There is now good evidence to show that cellular repopulation during a course of radiotherapy is an important factor determining the result in the management of squamous cell cancer in the head and neck and also in the lung.

- Acceleration and a dose elevation using hyperfractionation have been shown clear improvements in local tumour control in the radiotherapy of head and neck cancer. The CHART regimen has been shown to be best management in non-small cell lung cancer.

- The accumulation of data from fractionation studies, including the as yet unreported four-arm RTOG study, will, within the next few years, help to establish the best radiotherapy for head and neck cancer. Analyses of combined databases should yield valuable information. In other tumour sites, more trials are needed to explore the potential for improving the results of radiotherapy with new programs of treatment.

- The prediction of those tumours where repopulation is a major factor in determining success or failure will help gain the greatest benefit for the individual patient.

- The half-time for recovery of sublethal injury in the human may be longer than those in the animal—even 24 h may not be sufficient for full recovery to occur. Some of the disappointments in the results of trials are likely to be related to this.

- As with all approaches to improve the results of treatment in oncology, increased tumour control must be balanced against any increase in early and late morbidity.

- There are other causes for radiation failure and methods to overcome them must be integrated with the work in fractionation. An example now giving promise of benefit is the combination of acceleration, carbogen, and nicotinamide (ARCON).

- The translation of the results of laboratory studies and careful analyses of clinical data has led to the modification of the scheduling of radiotherapy and this is advancing patient care. Progress is never as rapid or as steady as the enthusiasts in the field would wish; there are disappointments as well as achievements. The value of

collaborative clinical trials performed at a very high standard has clearly been demonstrated and future advance will only follow intensified international collaboration.

References

1. **Charbit A, Malaise EP, Tubiana M.** Relation between the pathological nature and the growth rate of human tumors. *European Journal of Cancer*, 1971; 7: 707–15.

2. **Howard A, Pelc SR.** Synthesis of deoxyribonucleic acid in normal and irradiated cells and its relation to chromosome breakage. *Heredity*, 1953; 6: 261–73.

3. **Begg AC, McNally NJ, Shrieve DC, Kärcher HA.** A method to measure the duration of DNA synthesis and the potential doubling time from a single sample. *Cytometry*, 1985; 6: 620–6.

4. **Wilson GD, McNally NJ, Dische S, Saunders MI, Des Rochers C, Lewis AA, Bennett MH.** Measurement of cell kinetics in human tumours *in vivo* using bromodeoxyuridine incorporation and flow cytometry. *British Journal of Cancer*, 1988; 58: 423–31.

5. **Wilson GD.** Limitations of the bromodeoxyuridine technique for measurement of tumour proliferation. In: Beck-Bornholdt HP, ed. *Current topics in clinical radiobiology of tumors.* Berlin: Springer-Verlag, 1993; 27–43.

6. **Bennett MH, Wilson GD, Dische S, Saunders MI, Martindale CA, O'Halloran A.** Tumour proliferation assessed by combined histological and flow cytometric analysis: implications for therapy in squamous cell carcinoma in the head and neck. *British Journal of Cancer*, 1992; 65: 870–8.

7. **Denekamp J.** *Cell kinetics and cancer therapy.* Springfield: Thomas, 1982.

8. **Tubiana M.** Repopulation in human tumours—a biological background for fractionation in radiotherapy. *Acta Oncologica*, 1988; 27: 83–8.

9. **Withers HR, Taylor JMG, Maciejewski B.** The hazard of accelerated tumour clonogen repopulation during radiotherapy. *Acta Oncologica*, 1988; 27: 131–46.

10. **Dische S, Saunders MI, Bennett MH, Wilson GD, McNally NJ.** Cell proliferation and differentiation in squamous carcinoma. *Radiotherapy and Oncology*, 1989; 15: 19–23.

11. **Maciejewski B, Preuss-Bayer G, Trott K-R.** The influence of the number of fractions and of overall treatment time on local control and late complication rate in squamous cell carcinoma of the larynx. *International Journal of Radiation Oncology Biology Physics*, 1983; 9: 321–8.

12. **Taylor JMG, Withers HR, Mendenhall WM.** Dose-time considerations of head and neck squamous cell carcinomas treated with irradiation. *Radiotherapy and Oncology*, 1990; 17: 95–102.

13. **Barton MB, Keane TJ, Gadalla T, Maki E.** The effect of treatment time and treatment interruption on tumour control following radical radiotherapy of laryngeal cancer. *Radiotherapy and Oncology*,1992; 23: 137–43.

14. **Van den Bogaert W, Van Der Leest A, Rijnders A, Delaere P, Thames H, Van der Schueren.** Does tumor control decrease by prolonging overall treatment time or interrupting treatment in laryngeal cancer? *Radiotherapy and Oncology*, 1995; 36: 177–82.

15. **Fein DA, Lee WR, Hanlon AL, Ridge JA, Curran WJ, Coia LR.** Do overall treatment time, field size, and treatment energy influence local control of T1-T2 squamous cell carcinomas of the glottic larynx? *International Journal of Radiation Oncology Biology Physics*, 1996; 34: 823–31.

16. **Robertson C, Robertson G, Hendry JH, *et al.*** Similar decreases in local tumor control are calculated for treatment protraction and for

interruption in the radiotherapy of carcinoma of the larynx in four centers. *International Journal of Radiation Oncology Biology Physics*, 1998; **40**: 319–29.

17. Hliniak A, Maciejewski B, Trott K-R. The influence of the number of fractions, overall treatment time and field size on the local control of cancer of the skin. *British Journal of Radiology*, 1983; **56**: 596–8.

18. Maciejewski B, Majewski S. Dose fractionation and tumour repopulatoin in radiotherapy for bladder cancer. *Radiotherapy and Oncology*,1991; **21**: 163–70.

19. Koukourakis M, Hlouverakis G, Kosma L, *et al.* The impact of overall treatment time on the results of radiotherapy for nonsmall cell lung carcinoma. *International Journal of Radiation Oncology Biology Physics*, 1996; **34**: 315–22.

20. Perez CA, Grigsby PW, Castro-Vita H, Lockett MA. Carcinoma of the uterine cervix I. Impact of prolongation of overall treatment time and timing of brachytherapy on outcome of radiation therapy. *International Journal of Radiation Oncology Biology Physics*, 1995; **32**: 1275–83.

21. Dubray B, Mazeron JJ, Simon JM, *et al.* Time factors in breast carcinoma: influence of delay between external irradiation and brachytherapy. *Radiotherapy and Oncology*, 1992; **25**: 267–72.

22. Robertson G, Parmar M, Foy C, Saunders M, Dische S. Overall treatment time and the conventional arm of the CHART trial in the radiotherapy of head and neck cancer. *Radiotherapy and Oncology*, 1999; **50**: 25–8.

23. Overgaard J, Hjelm-Hansen M, Vendelbo Johansen L, Anderson AP. Comparison of conventional and split-course radiotherapy as primary treatment in carcinoma of the larynx. *Acta Oncologica*, 1988; **27**: 147–52.

24. Trott K-R, Kummermehr K. What is known about tumour proliferation rates to choose between accelerated fractionation or hyperfractionation? *Radiotherapy and Oncology*, 1985; **3**: 1–10.

25. Pavy JJ, Rojas A, Hodgkiss RJ, Wilson GD, Collier JM, Kelleher EJ. Proliferation in CaNT tumours during and after fractionated radiotherapy assessed by local control, clonogenic survival and cell kinetics. *Proceedings of the British Institute of Radiology*, 1990; **63**: 587.

26. Vassort F, Winterholer M, Frindel E, Tubiana M. Kinetic parameters of bone marrow stem cells using *in vivo* suicide by tritiated thymidine or by hydroxyurea. *Blood*, 1973; **41**: 789–96.

27. Bentzen SM, Thames HD. Clinical evidence for tumor clonogen regeneration: interpretations of the data. *Radiotherapy and Oncology*, 1991; **22**: 161–6.

28. Del Regato JA. Fractionation: a panoramic view. *International Journal of Radiation Oncology Biology Physics*, 1990; **19**: 1329–31.

29. Strandqvist M. Studieren über die cumulative Wirkung der Roentgenstrahlen bei Franktionierung. *Acta Radiologica* (Stockholm), 1944; Suppl. **55**.

30. Ellis F. Dose, time and fractionation: a clinical hypothesis. *Clinical Radiology*, 1969; **20**: 1–7.

31. Thames HD, Hendry JH. *Fractionation in radiotherapy*. London: Taylor and Francis, 1987.

32. Barendsen GW. Radiobiology of neutrons. *International Journal of Radiation Oncology Biology Physics*, 1982; **8**: 2103–8.

33. Fowler JF. The linear-quadratic formula and progress in fractionated radiotherapy. *British Journal of Radiology*, 1989; **62**: 679–94.

34. Wara WM, Phillips TL, Sheline GE, Schwade TG. Radiation tolerance of the spinal cord. *Cancer*, 1975; **35**: 1558–62.

35. Dische S, Martin WMC, Anderson P. Radiation myelopathy in patients treated for carcinoma of the bronchus using a six fraction regime of radiotherapy. *British Journal of Radiology*, 1981; **54**: 29–35.

36. Sealy R. *Advances in medical oncology*, Vol 6. Oxford/New York: Pergamon, 1979: 223.

37. Turresson I, Notter G. The influence of the overall treatment time in radiotherapy on the acute reactions: comparison of the effects of daily and twice-a-week fractionation on human skin. *International Journal of Radiation Oncology Biology Physics*, 1984; **10**: 608–18.

38. Overgaard M. Spontaneous radiation-induced rib fractures in breast cancer patients treated with postmastectomy irradiation—a clinical radiobiological analysis of the influence of fraction size and dose-response relationships on late bone damage. *Acta Oncologica*, 1988; **27**: 117–22.

39. Cossett JM, Henry-Amar M, Girinski T, Malaise E, Dupouy N, Dutreix J. Late toxicity in Hodgkin's disease—the role of fraction size. *Acta Oncologica*, 1988; **27**: 123–30.

40. Parsons JT, Cassisi NJ, Million RR. Results of twice-a-day irradiation of squamous cell carcinoma of the head and neck. *International Journal of Radiation Oncology Biology Physics*, 1984; **10**: 2041–51.

41. Horiot J, Le Fur R, N'Guyen T, *et al.* Hyperfractionation versus conventional fractionation in oropharyngeal carcinoma: final analysis of a randomized trail of the EORTC cooperative group of radiotherapy. *Radiotherapy and Oncology*, 1992; **25**: 231–41.

42. Cox JD, Pajak TF, Marcial VA, *et al.* ASTRO plenary: interfraction interval is a major determinant of late effects, with hyperfractionated radiation of carcinomas of upper respiratory and digestive tracts: results from Radiation Therapy Oncology Group Protocol 8313. *International Journal of Radiation Oncology Biology Physics*, 1991; **20**: 1191–5.

43. Horiot JC, Van den Bogaert W, Ang KK, *et al.* European Organization for Research and Treatment of Cancer trials using radiotherapy with multiple fractions per day. In: Vaeth JM, Meyer J, eds. *Time, dose and fractionation in the radiation therapy for cancer*. Basel: Karger, 1988: 99–104.

44. Edsmyr F, Andersson L, Esposti PL, Littbrand B. Nilsson B. Irradiation therapy with multiple small fractions per day in urinary bladder cancer. *Radiotherapy and Oncology*, 1985; **4**: 197–203.

45. Henk JM, James KW. Comparative trial of large and small fractions in the radiotherapy of head and neck cancers. *Clinical Radiology*, 1978; **29**: 611–16.

46. Weissberg JB, Son YH, Percarpio B, Fischer JJ. Randomized trial of conventional versus high fractional dose radiation therapy in the treatment of advanced head and neck cancer. *International Journal of Radiation Oncology Biology Physics*, 1982; **8**: 179–85.

47. Rezvani M, Alcock TJ, Fowler JF, Haybittle JL, Hopewell LW, Wiernik G. A comparison of the normal tissue reactions in patients treated with either 3F/wk or 5F/wk in the BIR (British Institute of Radiology) trial of radiotherapy for carcinoma of the laryngopharynx. *International Journal of Radiation Biology*, 1989; **56**: 717–20.

48. Fowler JF. What next in fractionated radiotherapy? *British Journal of Cancer*, 1984; **49** (Suppl. 6):285–300.

49. Thames HD. An 'incomplete repair' model for survival after fractionated and continuous irradiations. *International Journal of Radiation Biology*, 1985; **47**: 319–39.

50. Nguyen TD, Demange L, Froissart D, Panis X, Loirette M. Rapid hyperfractionated radiotherapy. Clinical results in 178 advanced squamous cell carcinomas of the head and neck. *Cancer*, 1985; **56**: 16–19.

51. Dische S, Saunders MI. Continuous, hyperfractionated, accelerated radiotherapy (CHART). An interim report upon late morbidity. *International Journal of Radiation Oncology Biology Physics*, 1989; **16**: 67–74.

52. Wong CS, Van Dyk J, Simpson WJ. Myelopathy following hyperfractionated accelerated radiotherapy for anaplastic thyroid carcinoma. *Radiotherapy and Oncology*, 1991; **20**: 3–9.

53. Landuyt W, Fowler J, Ruifrok A, Stuben G, van der Kogel A, van der Schueren E. Kinetics of repair in the spinal cord of the rat. *Radiotherapy and Oncology*, 1997; **45**: 55–62.

54. Ang KK, Jiang GL, Guttenberger R, Thames HD, Stephens LC, Smith CD, Feng Y. Impact of spinal cord repair kinetics on the practice of

altered fractionation schedules. *Radiotherapy and Oncology*, 1992; **25**: 287–94.

55. **Horiot JC, Bontemps P, Begg AC, et al.** New radiotherapy fractionation schemes in head and neck cancers. The EORTC trials: a benchmark. In: Kogelnik HD, Sedlmayer F, eds. *HoHHHHHHProgress in radio-oncology VI.* Bologna: Monduzzi Editore, 1998: 735–41.

56. **Shin KH, Urtasun RC, Fulton D, et al.** Multiple daily fractionated radiation therapy and misonidazole in the management of malignant astrocytoma. *Cancer*, 1985; **56**: 758–60.

57. **Cole DJ, Durrant KR, Roberts JT, Dawes PJ, Yosef H, Hopewell JW.** A pilot study of accelerated fractionation in the radiotherapy of invasive carcinoma of the bladder. *British Journal of Radiology*, 1992; **65**: 792–8.

58. **Peracchia G, Salti C.** Radiotherapy with thrice-a-day fractionation in a short overall time; clinical experiences. *International Journal of Radiation Oncology Biology Physics*, 1981; **7**: 99–104.

59. **Olmi P, Cellai E, Chiavacci A, Fallai C.** Accelerated fractionation in advanced head and neck cancer: results and analysis of late sequelae. *Radiotherapy and Oncology*, 1990; **17**: 199–207.

60. **Lamb DS, Spry NA, Gray AJ, Johnson AD, Alexander SR, Dally MJ.** Accelerated fractionation radiotherapy for advanced head and neck cancer. *Radiotherapy and Oncology*, 1990; **18**: 107–16.

61. **Ball D, Bishop J, Smit J, et al.** A phase III study of accelerated radiotherapy with and without carboplatin in nonsmall cell lung cancer: an interim toxicity analysis of the first 100 patients. *International Journal of Radiation Oncology Biology Physics*, 1995; **31**: 267–72.

62. **Ball D, Bishop J, Smith J, et al.** A phase III study of conventional and accelerated radiotherapy (RT) with and without carboplatin in unresectable non small cell lung cancer (NSCLC). *Radiotherapy and Oncology*, 1996; **40** (Suppl. 1):S61.

63. **Van den Bogaert W, Van der Schueren E, Horiot J-C, Chaplain G, Arcangeli G, Gonzale D, Svoboda V.** The feasibility of high-dose multiple daily fractionation and its combination with anoxic cell sensitizers in the treatment of head and neck cancer. *International Journal of Radiation Oncology Biology Physics*, 1982; **8**: 1649–55.

64. **Vanuytsel L, Ang KK, Vandenbussche L, Vereecken R, Van der Schueren E.** Radiotherapy in multiple fractions per day for prostatic carcinoma: the complications. *International Journal of Radiation Oncology Biology Physics*, 1986; **12**: 1589–95.

65. **Van den Bogaert W, Van der Schueren E, Horiot J-C, et al.** Early results of the EORTC randomized clinical trial on multiple fractions per day (MFD) and misonidazole in advanced head and neck cancer. *International Journal of Radiation Oncology Biology Physics*, 1986; **12**: 587–91.

66. **Van den Bogaert W, van der Schueren E, Horiot JC, et al.** The EORTC randomized trial on three fractions per day and misonidazole (trial no: 22811) in advanced head and neck cancer: long-term results and side effects. *Radiotherapy and Oncology*, 1995; **35**: 91–9.

67. **Horiot J-C, Bontemps P, van den Bogaert W, et al.** Accelerated fractionation (AF) compared to conventional fractionation (CF) improves loco-regional control in the radiotherapy of advanced head and neck cancers: results of the EORTC 22851 randomized trial. *Radiotherapy and Oncology*, 1997; **44**: 111–21.

68. **Wang CC.** Local control of oropharyngeal carcinoma after two accelerated hyperfractionation radiation therapy schemes. *International Journal of Radiation Oncology Biology Physics*, 1988; **14**: 1143–6.

69. **Wang CC, Blitzer PH, Suit H.** Twice-a-day radiation therapy for cancer of the head and neck. *Cancer*, 1985; **55**: 2100–4.

70. **Knee R, Fields RS, Peters LJ.** Concomitant boost radiotherapy for advanced squamous cell carcinoma of the head and neck. *Radiotherapy and Oncology*, 1985; **4**: 1–7.

71. **Ang K, Peters L.** Concomitant boost radiotherapy in the treatment of head and neck cancers. *Seminars in Radiation Oncology*, 1992; **2**: 31–3.

72. **Cummings BJ, Keane TJ, Pintillie M, et al.** A prospective randomized trial of hyperfractionated versus conventional once daily radiation for advanced squamous cell carcinomas of the larynx and pharynx. *Radiotherapy and Oncology*, 1996; **40** (Suppl. 1):S30.

73. **Saunders MI, Dische S.** Radiotherapy employing three fractions in each day over a continuous period of 12 days. *British Journal of Radiology*, 1996; **59**: 523–5.

74. **Dische S, Saunders MI.** The rationale for continuous, hyperfractionated, accelerated radiotherapy (CHART). *International Journal of Radiation Oncology Biology Physics*, 1990; **19**: 1317–20.

75. **Saunders MI, Dische S, Grosch EJ, Fermont DC, Ashford RFU, Maher EJ, Makepeace AR.** Experience with CHART. *International Journal of Radiation Oncology Biology Physics*, 1991; **21**: 871–8.

76. **Leslie MD, Dische S.** Parotid gland function following accelerated and conventionally fractionated radiotherapy. *Radiotherapy and Oncology*, 1991; **22**: 133–9.

77. **Saunders MI, Dische S.** Continuous, hyperfractionated, accelerated radiotherapy (CHART) in non-small cell carcinoma of the bronchus. *International Journal of Radiation Oncology Biology Physics*, 1990; **19**: 1211–15.

78. **Saunders MI, Dische S, Barrett A, Parmar MKB, Harvey A, Gibson D, on behalf of CHART Steering Committee.** Randomised multicentre trials of CHART vs conventional radiotherapy in head and neck and non-small-cell lung cancer: an interim report. *British Journal of Cancer*, 1996; **73**: 1455–62.

79. **Dische S, Saunders M, Barrett A, Harvey A, Gibson D, Parmar M, on behalf of the CHART Steering Committee.** A randomised multicentre trial of CHART versus conventional radiotherapy in head and neck cancer. *Radiotherapy and Oncology*, 1997; **44**: 123–36.

80. **Saunders M, Dische S, Barrett A, Harvey A, Gibson D, Parmar M, on behalf of the CHART Steering Committee.** Continuous hyperfractionated accelerated radiotherapy (CHART) versus conventional radiotherapy in non-small-cell lung cancer: a randomised multicentre trial. *Lancet*, 1997; **350**: 161–6.

81. **Saunders MI.** The role of novel radiotherapy schedules in the curative treatment of non-small cell lung cancer. *Lung Cancer Therapy*, 1997; **15**: 507–9.

82. **Overgaard J, Sand Hansen H, Sapru W, et al.** Conventional radiotherapy as the primary treatment of squamous cell carcinoma (SCC) of the head and neck: A randomized multicenter study of 5 versus 6 fractions per week—preliminary report from the DAHANCA 6 and 7 trial. *Radiotherapy and Oncology*, 1996; **40** (Suppl. 1):S31(110).

83. **Skladowski K, Maciejewski B, Golen M, Pilecki B, Przeorek W, Tarnawski R.** Randomized clinical trial of 7-day-continuous accelerated irradiation (CAIR) of head and neck cancer. Preliminary report on three-year tumour control and normal tissue toxicity. *Radiotherapy and Oncology*, 2000; **55**: 101–10.

84. **Steel GG, Down JD, Peacock JH, Stephens TC.** Dose-rate effects and the repair of radiation damage. *Radiotherapy and Oncology*, 1986; **5**: 321–31.

85. **Goodchild K, Hoskin PJ, Dische S, Pigott K, Powell MEB, Saunders MI.** Continuous, hyperfractionated, accelerated radiotherapy (CHART) treatment and brachytherapy in patients with early oral or oropharyngeal carcinomas: a prospective review of outcome and morbidity. *Radiotherapy and Oncology*, 1999; **50**: 29–31.

86. **Overgaard J, Horsman MR.** Overcoming hypoxic cell radioresistance. In: Steel GG, ed. *Basic clinical radiobiology.* New York: Arnold 1997: 141–51.

87. **Thomlinson RG.** Reoxygenation as a function of tumor size and histopathological type. In: Bond VP, Suit HD, Marcial V, eds. *Time and dose relationships in radiation biology as applied to radiotherapy.* New York: Brookhaven National Laboratory Report 50203, 1970:242–54.

88. **Kaanders JHAM, Stratford MRL, Liefers J, Dennis MF, van der Kogel**

AJ, van Daal WAJ, Rojas A. Administration of nicotinamide during a five-to seven-week course of radiotherapy: pharmacokinetics, tolerance, and compliance. *Radiotherapy and Oncology*, 1997; **43**: 67–73.

89. Saunders MI, Hoskin PJ, Pigott K, Powell MEB, Rojas AM, Stratford M. A Phase I/II study of ARCON (accelerated radiotherapy with carbogen and nicotinamide) in locally advanced head and neck disease. *British Journal of Cancer*, 1996; **74** (Suppl. 28):044.

90. Kaanders JHAM, Pop LAM, Marres HAM, Liefers J, van den Hoogen FJA, van Daal WAJ, van der Kogel AJ. Accelerated radiotherapy with carbogen and nicotinamide (ARCON) for laryngeal cancer. *Radiotherapy and Oncology*, 1998; **48**: 115–22.

91. Hoskin PJ, Saunders MI, Phillips H, *et al.* Carbogen and nicotinamide in the treatment of bladder cancer with radical radiotherapy. *British Journal of Cancer*, 1997; **75**: 260–3.

92. Ang KK, Trotti A, Garden AS, Foote RL, Morrison WH, Geara FB, Peters LJ. Overall time factor in postoperative radiation: results of a prospective randomized trial. *Radiotherapy and Oncology*, 1996; **40** (Suppl. 1):S30 (108).

93. Awwad HK, Shouman T, Loyayef M, Begg A, Wilson G, Eissa S. Accelerated hyperfractionation (AHF) compared to conventional fractionation in the postoperative radiotherapy of locally advanced head and neck cancer: influence of proliferation. *Radiotherapy and Oncology*, 1998; **48** (Suppl. 1):S17 (65).

94. Wilson GD, Dische S, Saunders MI. Studies with bromodeoxyuridine in head and neck cancer and accelerated radiotherapy. *Radiotherapy and Oncology*, 1995; **36**: 189–97.

95. Hansen O, Overgaard J, Hansen HS, *et al.* Importance of overall treatment time for the outcome of radiotherapy of advanced head and neck carcinomas: dependency on tumor differentiation. *Radiotherapy and Oncology*, 1997; **43**: 47–51.

96. Begg AC, Hofland I, Van Glabekke M, Bartelink H, Horiot JC. Predictive value of potential doubling time for radiotherapy of head and neck tumour patients: Results from the EORTC Cooperative Trial 22851. *Seminars in Radiation Oncology*, 1992; **2**: 22–5.

97. Begg AC, Haustermans K, Hart AA, *et al.* The value of pretreatment cell kinetic parameters as predictors for radiotherapy outcome in head and neck cancer: A multicenter analysis. *Radiotherapy and Oncology*, 1998; **50**: 13–23.

98. Saunders MI, Dische S, Barrett A, Harvey A, Griffiths G, Parmar M. Continuous, hyperfractionated, accelerated radiotherapy (CHART) versus conventional radiotherapy in non-small cell lung cancer: mature data from the randomised multicentre trial. *Radiotherapy and Oncology*, 1999; **52**: 137–48.

99. Glynne-Jones R, Saunders MI, Hoskin P, Phillips H. A pilot study of continuous, hyperfractionated, accelerated radiotherapy in rectal adenocarcinoma. *Clinical Oncology*, 1999; **11**: 334–9.

100. Fowler JF, Ritter MA. A rationale for fractionation for slowly proliferating tumors such as prostatic adenocarcinoma. *International Journal of Radiation Oncology Biology Physics*, 1995; **32**: 521–9.

101. Joiner MC, Marples B, Johns H. The limitation of the linear-quadratic model at low doses per fraction. In: Beck-Bornholdt HP, eds. *Medical radiology. Current topics in clinical radiobiology of tumours.* Berlin: Springer-Verlag, 1993:51–66.

102. Joiner MC, Short SC, Lambin P, Marples B. Effect of low doses per fraction: cellular studies. *Radiotherapy and Oncology*, 1998; **48** (Suppl. 1):S4 (12).

103. Turesson I, Johansson K-A, Nyman J, Florgegard M, Wahlgren T. A clinical study of the effect of low dose per fraction. *Radiotherapy and Oncology*, 1998; **48** (Suppl. 1):S4 (15).

104. Saunder MI. Clinical superfractionation. *Radiotherapy and Oncology*, 1998; **48** (Suppl. 1):S8 (28).

4.5 Combined radiotherapy and chemotherapy

Hans von der Maase

Introduction

Numerous combinations of cancer chemotherapeutic drugs and radiation treatment have been used in the last three decades in the management of patients with a variety of solid tumours. The aim of using combined modality treatments is to improve local and/or systemic control; however, this must be considered within the concept of the therapeutic index taking into consideration the effects on critical normal tissues. Thus, a therapeutic gain by combining radiation treatment and cancer chemotherapeutic drugs can only be obtained by an improved tumour response with less enhancement of toxicity or by reduced toxicity with less reduction of the tumour response. Such a therapeutic gain may be achieved by one of four potentially exploitable modes of action.[1]

1. Enhancement of tumour response in excess of enhancement of critical normal tissue damage.
2. Normal tissue protection if the tumour cells are not similarly protected.
3. Independent cell kill without overlapping critical toxicity profiles.
4. Spatial cooperation, which indicates that the two treatment modalities affect different tumour sites, i.e. eradication of the local tumour by radiation and eradication of systemic tumour cells by the chemotherapeutic regimen.

Modes 1 and 2 represent true drug–radiation interactions where one modality modifies the effect of the other, i.e. sensitization or protection. Specific antitumour activity of the drug by itself is not necessarily required. A therapeutic gain by these two modes of action has been demonstrated in experimental studies;[2] however, until now this has had no major clinical implications. Modes 3 and 4 are non-interactive. It is essential that both the chemotherapeutic drug regimen and the radiation treatment are effective and that the combined treatment can be administered with acceptable toxicity. A pure additive effect by independent cell kill is illustrated in Fig. 1. The major limitation for the success of these approaches is the generally poor to modest efficacy of chemotherapeutic drugs in many solid tumours in adults. Furthermore, most drug–radiation combinations are associated with enhanced normal tissue reactions. However, spatial cooperation and independent cell kill are the mechanisms that are most likely to lead to a therapeutic gain in clinical practice.

Experimental studies

Tumours in animals, including xenografts in nude mice, have different growth rates and other important properties as compared with human tumours. So, although experimental studies in tumours may provide important information about possible drug–radiation interactions, the results of combined modality treatment for experimental tumours are not likely to be predictive for effects in clinical practice. In contrast, combined schedules with risk of increased toxicity in humans may be predicted from reactions in normal tissues of experimental animals.[3]

Mechanisms of drug–radiation interactions

The combined use of cancer chemotherapeutic drugs and radiation has been demonstrated to enhance the antitumour effect in a variety of experimental *in vitro* and *in vivo* studies. The mechanisms by which these interactions occur are seldom known in detail. Possible mechanisms that can explain the interactive processes are summarized briefly as follows (for reviews see Hill and Bellamy,[4] Fu and Phillips,[5] and Steel[2],[6]).

A true radiosensitizing effect reflected by a drug-induced increase of the slope of the radiation dose–response curve (Fig. 1) has been observed rarely. It has been demonstrated for a few drugs such as actinomycin D and cisplatin, but is not a consistent finding. Inhibition

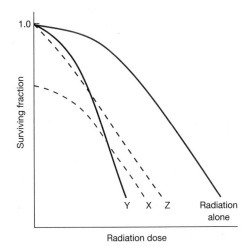

Fig. 1 Cell survival curves for radiation alone and for radiation combined with drug *x* indicating a pure additive effect (non-interactive); combined with drug *y* indicating a true radiosensitizing effect reflected by a drug-induced increase of the slope; and combined with drug *z* indicating inhibition of repair of radiation damage reflected by a reduced shoulder with an unchanged slope of the dose–response curve.

of repair of radiation damage will also modify the radiation dose–response curve by changing the shoulder (Fig. 1), and is also a form of 'radiosensitization'. Several drugs, including actinomycin D, doxorubicin, and cisplatin, have been found to inhibit repair of sublethal damage or potentially lethal radiation damage. This mechanism is of particular interest in clinical practice where drug-induced inhibition of repair between successive dose fractions will result in increased cell killing. Unfortunately, there is no evidence that such an effect acts selectively in tumours as compared with normal tissues. So, there is no net therapeutic gain.

The effects of both chemotherapy and radiotherapy may be cell cycle dependent and cycle phase dependent. As both treatment modalities may induce cell cycle synchronization, in theory, drugs and irradiation might be sequenced in order to treat the tumour cells in the most sensitive phase of the cell cycle. However, variability in cell cycle phase duration, differences of duration of drug action, and other factors have prevented this from being implemented in clinical practice.

Repopulation of surviving cells between radiation dose fractions may limit damage to normal tissues, but may also prevent eradication of tumours. Many anticancer drugs inhibit proliferation and may reduce repopulation. Thus, concurrent chemotherapy and radiotherapy may lead to an enhanced tumour effect even with minimal cell killing by the drug itself (Fig. 2(a)). However, therapeutic gain is only achieved if this effect is tumour specific. As an example, inhibition of tumour-specific growth factor receptors might lead to therapeutic gain. In contrast, if chemotherapy is given before radiotherapy, this might enhance repopulation before and during radiation treatment and thereby induce a decreased tumour effect (Fig. 2(b)).

Bioreductive agents such as mitomycin C and the experimental drug tirapazamine are activated under hypoxic conditions and are selectively cytotoxic to hypoxic cells.[7] As these cells are generally resistant to radiotherapy, the combination of such drugs and radiation treatment might lead to an enhanced tumour response.

Shrinkage of a tumour following one treatment modality may improve blood and oxygen supply, induce recruitment of non-cycling cells and increase the frequency of proliferating cells, which may enhance the effect of the second treatment modality. A reduction of tumour size by one treatment also means that there are fewer cells to be killed by the other. Debulking of a tumour by chemotherapy might also allow the size of a subsequent radiation field to be reduced, and thus, limit normal tissue damage. However, in most clinical situations, chemotherapy is not able to eradicate all tumour cells in the involved area, and the radiation field should encompass the initial gross tumour volume.

Normal tissues reactions

Normal tissue reactions following combinations of radiotherapy and chemotherapy depend on several factors such as the specific drug and drug dose, the radiation dose, dose rate and fractionation regimen, the time intervals and sequence of the two treatment modalities and the specific tissue in question. The possible interactions are numerous and difficult to evaluate in clinical studies. Therefore, most detailed knowledge about the combined effects of radiotherapy and chemotherapy is derived from experimental studies. Reviews of experimental normal tissue data include the articles by Phillips and Fu,[8] Steel[2] and von der Maase.[3],[9]

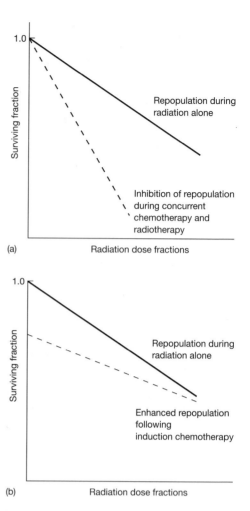

Fig. 2 (a) Concurrent radiotherapy may inhibit repopulation of surviving cells between radiation dose fractions and lead to an enhanced tumour effect (or enhanced normal tissue effect) even with no, or minimal, cell killing by the drug itself. (b) Induction chemotherapy may lead to tumour response, but subsequently also to enhanced repopulation before and during radiation treatment and thereby induce an overall decreased tumour effect compared with that following radiation alone.

Most studies of normal tissue reactions following combined radiotherapy and chemotherapy are focused on early responding tissues, and more data on late toxicity are needed. It seems, however, that the radiation-modifying effects of drugs are most pronounced for early normal tissue reactions as compared with late toxicity.

In the following, experimental studies of the combined effects of radiotherapy and chemotherapy in selected normal tissues of rats and mice are summarized. The radiation-modifying effect of drugs was, whenever possible, quantified by use of the so-called dose-modifying factor (**DMF**) defined as the radiation dose required to produce a specific effect when given alone relative to the radiation dose required to produce the same effect when combined with a drug (Fig. 3). A DMF value of 1 indicates no effect on radiation response (0) and a DMF value below 1 a protective effect (−). Generally, minor enhancement of radiation response (+) indicates DMF values below 1.2, moderate enhancement (++) indicates DMF values between

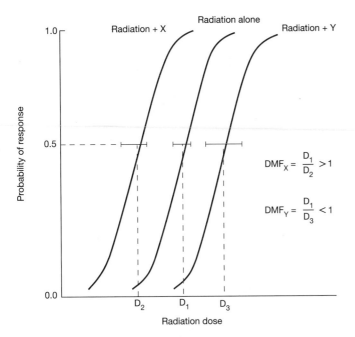

Fig. 3 Dose–response curves illustrating the doses required to achieve a specific endpoint for radiation alone and for radiation combined with drug *x* and drug *y*. Bars represent 95 per cent confidence limits for the specified doses. The DMF value for drug *x* is above 1 indicating enhancement of the radiation response whereas the DMF value for drug *y* is below 1 indicating a protective effect.

1.2 and 1.4, and pronounced enhancement ($+++$) indicates DMF values above 1.4 (Table 1).

For comparison with the experimental results, available clinical data on the radiation-modifying effects of drugs are indicated for each normal tissue.

Skin

Many drugs have been shown to enhance radiation-induced skin reactions.[3] The most pronounced effect has been observed for bleomycin. Other drugs that enhance acute skin reactions include actinomycin D, doxorubicin, cisplatin, methotrexate, and mitomycin C. The radiation-modifying effect has generally been most pronounced for drug administration at the same time as or a few hours before irradiation. Actinomycin D and doxorubicin have also enhanced the radiation response when given 3 days after a fractionated course of irradiation.[10]

In clinical practice, actinomycin D and doxorubicin are known to enhance skin reactions including induction of the so-called recall phenomenon.[8],[11],[12] Bleomycin is also known to enhance skin reactions and mucositis.[13],[14] In a randomized study, cisplatin administered concurrently with radiotherapy for patients with head and neck cancer enhanced the frequency of severe mucositis compared with that of radiation alone.[15] Methotrexate may also enhance skin reactions in clinical practice,[16] whereas cyclophosphamide and 5-fluorouracil seem to have no effect on radiation-induced skin reactions.[16]–[19] Thus, skin reactions in clinical practice seem to be qualitatively in accordance with experimental results (Table 1).

Oesophagus

Actinomycin D, doxorubicin, and cisplatin have shown a pronounced enhancement of the radiation response in oesophagus when administered 2 h before radiation. Carmustine (BCNU) and bleomycin have also been shown to enhance oesophageal toxicity.[20],[21]

In accordance with the experimental results, actinomycin D, doxorubicin, cisplatin, and bleomycin have been shown to enhance the radiation response in the oesophagus of humans.[8],[14],[22],[23] The combination of cisplatin and 5-fluorouracil administered concurrently with irradiation has also been shown to enhance oesophagitis in a randomized study.[24]

Intestine

Most drugs enhance the acute radiation response in the intestinal tract.[3] The effect has generally been most pronounced following simultaneous treatment. Actinomycin D and doxorubicin have also enhanced the effect when administered after radiotherapy.[20] Cytosine arabinoside is the only drug known to have a protective effect against intestinal toxicity when given 12 h before irradiation.[25] Cyclophosphamide and vincristine appear to have minimal effects on radiation-induced toxicity in the intestinal tract.[3]

Pearson and Steel[26] have investigated a series of drugs in combination with pelvic irradiation. They found a totally different time dependency. Doxorubicin, lomustine (CCNU), cisplatin, cyclophosphamide, cytosine arabinoside, etoposide, 5-fluorouracil, and methotrexate all enhanced the radiation response with the most pronounced effect when drugs were given 3 days after pelvic irradiation. The evaluation was based on lethality and may thus involve more than just intestinal toxicity.

Only a few studies have investigated the effect of combined chemotherapy and radiotherapy on late toxicity in the intestinal tract. Studies have concentrated on cisplatin, which causes no enhancement of late radiation damage.[27],[28]

Clinically, actinomycin D, doxorubicin, bleomycin, and 5-fluorouracil have been found to enhance gastrointestinal toxicity, especially when given concurrently with radiation treatment.[8],[14],[18],[19],[22] Yarnold et al.[29] observed a time dependency similar to the experimental data reported by Pearson and Steel.[26] Thus, the risk of subcutaneous fibrosis, gastrointestinal damage, and haematological toxicity in patients with testicular cancer was most pronounced for chemotherapy administered after radiotherapy, as compared with that following the reverse sequence of the combined treatment modalities.[29]

Lung

In the lungs, actinomycin D, doxorubicin, bleomycin, and cyclophosphamide have resulted in a pronounced enhancement of radiation-induced damage, whereas cytosine arabinoside, 5-fluorouracil, hydroxurea, and methotrexate had no effect.[3] Enhancement of the radiation response was generally most pronounced for drug administration simultaneous with or after irradiation. No effect on radiation-induced lung reactions was observed for cisplatin in two studies using single doses,[30],[31] whereas cisplatin enhanced the radiation response when given 3 days before fractionated irradiation.[32] Lockhart et al.[33] have studied a series of drugs in combination with hemithoracic irradiation, and found that cyclophosphamide enhanced the radiation response whereas in this study doxorubicin, carboplatin, and vinblastine had no significant effect on the radiation-induced lung reactions.

Table 1 Dose-modifying effects* of drugs in selected normal tissues of experimental animals

Drugs	Normal tissue						
	Skin	Oesophagus	Intestine	Lung	Kidney	Bladder	Haemopoietic tissue
Actinomycin D	+	+ + +	+ +	+ +			
Doxorubicin	+	+ + +	+ +	+ + +			+ +
BCNU	+	+ +	+ +	−	+ +		
Bleomycin	+ +	+	+ + +	+ + +			0
Cisplatin	+	+ + +	+ +	0/+	+ +	+ +	+ + +
Cyclophosphamide	−/0	−/0	0	+ + +	0	+ + +	+ +
Cytosine arabinoside		−		0	0		+ +
5-Fluorouracil	0		+ +	0			+ + +
Hydroxurea	+		+	0			+ +
Methotrexate	+		+ +	0			0
Mitomycin C	+		+	+	0		+ + +
Vincristine		0	0/+	+	0		

*The dose-modifying effects of the drugs are indicated for drug administration resulting in the most pronounced effect on the radiation response, i.e. for drug administration at the same time as irradiation for all tissues except haemopoietic tissue where the effect of drug administration after irradiation has been indicated.

0, no effect on radiation response; +, enhancement, i.e. combined effect more pronounced than that of radiation alone; +, minor, + +, moderate, + + +, pronounced; −, protection, i.e. combined effect less pronounced than that of radiation alone.

In accordance with the experimental results, actinomycin D, doxorubicin, bleomycin and cyclophosphamide have been shown to increase pulmonary toxicity when combined with thoracic irradiation.[14],[16],[34]–[36] Especially actinomycin D and bleomycin have caused a high incidence of fatal complications following simultaneous drug–radiation administration. Cisplatin did not influence lung toxicity in combination with irradiation when evaluated in a randomized study.[23]

Kidney

BCNU and cisplatin have been shown to enhance renal damage when administered before, at the same time as and after renal irradiation as compared with the effect of radiation alone.[37],[38] Renal tolerance to cisplatin was reduced after previous renal irradiation and the effect became more severe with increasing radiation–drug intervals.[39] Clinically, one should be cautious with cisplatin administered together with renal irradiation and in cases with prior radiotherapy of parts of the kidneys.

Bladder

Cyclophosphamide enhanced the early as well as late radiation response in the bladder, whereas cisplatin primarily enhanced the late response.[40] The effect of cyclophosphamide was pronounced even when administered 9 months before or after irradiation.[41]

In a retrospective analysis of patients with bladder cancer, cisplatin administered concomitantly with radiotherapy had apparently no significant impact on bladder toxicity as compared with that following radiotherapy alone.[42]

Haemopoietic tissue

All investigated drugs with the exception of bleomycin and vincristine enhanced the radiation response in haemopoietic tissue.[3] The radiation-modifying effect is extremely time dependent. Enhancement of the radiation response was most pronounced for drug administration simultaneous with or after irradiation, whereas drug administration before radiation may even have a protective effect. For example, methotrexate had a protective effect when administered 1 to 3 days before irradiation, no effect as a simultaneous treatment, and a pronounced enhancement of the radiation response when administered 1 to 3 days after irradiation.[43] A radioprotective effect of drug administration 1 to 3 days before irradiation has also been shown for cyclophosphamide and cytosine arabinoside.[44] The radioprotective effect is probably mediated by drug-induced enhancement of the recovery of haemopoietic stem cells after whole body irradiation. Yan et al. have shown a similar time dependency for cyclophosphamide to protect against total body irradiation.[45]

Clinically, it is a well known experience that doses of drugs which induce major haematological toxicity often have to be reduced in patients with prior radiotherapy to areas with bone marrow involvement.

Chemotherapy combined with low dose rate radiotherapy

Sherman et al.[46] observed that the radiation-modifying effect of doxorubicin on oesophageal and lung toxicity was more pronounced in combination with low dose rate as compared with high dose rate irradiation. Lochhart et al.[47] reported that the effect of low dose rate irradiation to cause less damage to normal tissues as compared with high dose rate irradiation was abolished when cyclophosphamide was administered before irradiation. Similarly, cyclophosphamide has been shown to enhance radiation-induced lung damage when administered 1 day before low dose rate irradiation followed by bone marrow transplantation, whereas the drug had no effect in combination with high dose rate irradiation.[48] However, no enhancement of the radiation response was apparently found in two other studies using low dose rate irradiation.[49],[50]

More studies are warranted to evaluate the combined effect of drugs and low dose rate irradiation, because the risk that drugs may reduce the sparing effect of low dose rate irradiation has important clinical implications.

A summary of radiation-modifying effects of drugs in different normal tissues is indicated in Table 1. The most pronounced effects have been found when drugs were administered simultaneously with irradiation in accordance with clinical observations.[3] One exception from this pattern of time dependency is haemopoietic tissue with the most pronounced enhancement of radiation response for drug administration after irradiation. In contrast, combined effects in experimental tumours are, generally, less time dependent than in normal tissues.[2],[3],[9]

Clinical studies

Treatment strategies

The combination of cancer chemotherapeutic drugs and radiation in clinical practice is based on three different strategies.

1. Concurrent treatment.
2. Alternating regimens.
3. Sequential treatment divided into:
   a. induction chemotherapy (pre-radiation or neoadjuvant chemotherapy), or
   b. postradiation chemotherapy (adjuvant chemotherapy).

Concurrent treatment

The main rationale for administering radiotherapy and chemotherapy concurrently is to obtain a therapeutic gain either by enhancement of the tumour response as a true drug–radiation interaction or by independent cell kill. The main problem is the risk of a substantial increase of acute toxicity, which may require a reduction of the total radiation dose and also of the drug doses. If so, it is important to question whether an apparent therapeutic gain was due to the combined modality approach or whether the same result could have been achieved by one of the two treatment modalities—usually radiation—if administered in an optimal way.

In general, it is important to compare combined radiotherapy and chemotherapy with radiotherapy alone at equal levels of toxicity; however, it is often difficult to predict doses that will give equivalent toxicity, especially as this will depend on both the radiation regimen, the chemotherapeutic regimen, and the irradiated critical normal tissues. Furthermore, it is likely that there will be differences for acute and late reactions. Although more data on late responding tissues are warranted, increases in late toxicity following combined radiotherapy and chemotherapy seem to be less pronounced as compared with acute normal tissue reactions.

Alternating regimens

The rationale for this approach is to achieve therapeutic gain by independent cell kill. The advantage is that both modalities can be administered early without the same degree of enhanced toxicity as seen with concurrent treatment. Thus, temporal separation of the treatment modalities allows normal tissue recovery and both modalities can often be delivered in full doses. However, each treatment is administered as a split course with the risk of decreased efficacy.

Sequential treatment

Temporal separation of radiotherapy and chemotherapy often makes it possible to avoid enhanced normal tissue reactions. A therapeutic gain is most likely to occur by spatial cooperation. Advantages and disadvantages depend on the sequence between the two treatment modalities.

Induction chemotherapy

Chemotherapy is administered initially in order to reduce tumour bulk and to eradicate occult metastatic tumour cells. Tumour shrinkage may result in a reduced hypoxic cell fraction and, thus, increase the effect of subsequent radiation treatment. The disadvantages include a delay in delivering an effective local treatment and the possibility of chemotherapy-induced accelerated regeneration of tumour cells (Fig. 2(b)). These possible disadvantages are likely to be most important with modest to poor efficacy of the chemotherapeutic regimen.

Postradiation chemotherapy

This approach is used primarily to eradicate tumour cells outside the radiation field, although chemotherapy may also have an effect on residual tumour cells within the irradiated area. The main problem is that delayed application of systemic treatment may result in the development of drug resistant cell clones. Furthermore, the radiation-induced normal tissue damage may decrease tolerability of subsequent chemotherapy.

Results of combined radiotherapy and chemotherapy

The following is a review of combined modality treatment in tumours of adults. Conclusions will be based on high levels of evidence, i.e. on results from larger randomized studies and meta-analyses. However, literature-based overviews as compared with patient-based meta-analyses may overestimate the effect of new treatment options compared with that of conventional treatment strategies.[51],[52]

Brain tumours (see also Chapter 18.2)

The most common malignant tumour types are the poorly differentiated anaplastic astrocytomas and glioblastomas. Surgery ranging from biopsy to radical resection followed by postoperative radiation treatment is generally considered the standard treatment, but the prognosis for these patients is still dismal. The main problem is failure to achieve local control as primary brain tumours do not metastasize outside the central nervous system. The rationale for combining chemotherapy with radiation treatment is, thus, to enhance the local tumour response. Most trials have investigated the effect of concurrent administration of radiotherapy and chemotherapy, and most investigated drugs have been within the nitrosourea group.

Table 2 Brain tumours: randomized phase III studies of postoperative radiotherapy and chemotherapy in malignant gliomas

Reference (first author)	Number of evaluable patients	Treatment groups	Survival outcome
Walker (1978)[53]	222	Surgery alone RT BCNU RT + BCNU	RT better then surgery alone
Walker (1980)[54]	358	MeCCNU RT RT + MeCCNU RT + BCNU	RT + CT better, than CT alone
EORTC (1981)[55]	116	RT RT + CCNU/VM-26	No difference
Green (1983)[56]	527	RT + Methylprednisolone RT + BCNU RT + PCZ RT + BCNU/Methylprednisolone	No difference
Hatlevoll (1985)[57]	244	RT ± MISO RT ± MISO + CCNU	No difference
Nelson (1988)[58]	554	RT (60 Gy) RT (70 Gy) RT + BCNU RT +MeCCNU/DTIC	No difference
Trojanowsky (1988)[59]	198	RT RT + CCNU	No difference
EORTC (1991)[60]	246	RT RT + CIS	No difference
Halperin (1993)[61]	249	RT + AZQ RT + BCNU	No difference
Hildebrand (1994)[62]	255	RT RT + DBD/BCNU	RT + chemotherapy better than RT alone
Halperin (1996)[63]	327	RT RT + MMC→BCNU ± 6MP	No difference
Roberts (1998)[64]	674	RT RT + PCZ/CCNU/VCR	No difference

5FU, 5-fluorouracil; 6MP, 6-mercaptopurine; AZQ, diaziquone; BCNU, carmustine; BLM, bleomycin; CA, cytosine arabinoside; CARBO, carboplatin; CCNU, lomustine; CIS, cisplatin; CMV, cisplatin, methotrexate, and vinblastine; CTX, cyclophosphamide; DBD, dibromodulcitol, DOX, doxorubicin; EPO, etoposide; IFOS, ifosfamide; LV, leucovorin; MeCCNU, methyl lomustine; MISO, misonidazole; MMC, mitomycin C; MTX, methotrexate; PCZ, procarbazine; RT, radiotherapy; VBL, vinblastine; VCR, vincristine; VDS, vindesine; VM-26, teniposide.

The results of the 12 largest randomized phase III studies are summarized in Table 2.

Many of these trials have not used an intention-to-treat analysis of survival and have also other methodological problems. The majority of trials have failed to show a statistically significant improvement of survival by the addition of chemotherapy. Improved survival was reported only in the study by Hildebrand *et al.*[62] comparing radiation combined with dibromodulcitol and BCNU with radiation alone. In contrast to the general lack of survival benefit, most of the combined treatment regimens resulted in increased toxicity.

Improved survival has been observed in two other randomized studies,[65],[66] which included only a small number of patients. In another small randomized phase III trial, postradiation chemotherapy with CCNU, procarbazine, and vincristine was superior to postradiation BCNU in patients with anaplastic gliomas.[67] There

is also a published literature-based overview of 16 randomized clinical studies involving more than 3000 patients.[68] The analysis showed an absolute improvement in survival by the use of additional chemotherapy of 10.1 per cent at 1 year and 8.6 per cent at 2 years with no long-term benefit. Although this may point on a modest effect on survival by use of chemotherapy together with postoperative radiotherapy for malignant gliomas, this effect should be regarded as unproven because of the methodological problems of constituent trials. Furthermore, the recent large randomized study from the Medical Research Council (**MRC**) in the United Kingdom showed no difference in survival for combined treatment as compared with radiation alone. A total of 647 patients with high-grade gliomas were randomized to receive either radiotherapy alone or radiotherapy plus a combination of procarbazine, CCNU, and vincristine following surgery. Median

Table 3 Head and neck cancer. Randomized phase III studies of concurrent radiotherapy and chemotherapy in locally advanced squamous cell carcinoma of the head and neck

Reference (first author)	Number of evaluable patients	Treatment groups	Survival outcome
Lo (1976)[72]	136	RT RT + 5FU	RT + 5FU better than RT alone
Stefani (1980)[73]	150	RT RT + hydroxurea	No difference
Shanta (1980)[74]	157	RT RT + BLM	RT + Bleomycin better than RT alone
Vermund (1985)[75]	222	RT RT + BLM	No difference
Fu (1987)[76]	104	RT RT + BLM→BLM/MTX	RT + chemotherapy better than RT alone
Gupta (1987)[77]	313	RT RT + MTX	No difference
Eschwege (1988)[78]	199	RT RT + BLM	No difference
Sanchiz (1990)[79]	577	RT RT + 5FU	RT + 5FU better than RT alone
Keane (1993)[80]	209	RT RT + MMC/5FU	No difference
Browman (1994)[81]	175	RT RT + 5FU	RT and 5FU better than RT alone
Haffty (1997)[82]	195	RT RT + MMC	RT + MMC better than RT alone
Jeremic (1997)[83]	159	RT RT + CIS RT + CARBO	RT + CIS or carboplatin better than RT alone
Wendt (1998)[84]	270	RT RT + CIS/5FU/LV	RT + chemotherapy better than RT alone
Al-Sarraf (1998)[85]	185	RT RT + CIS→CIS/5FU	Only nasopharyngeal cancer RT + chemotherapy better than RT alone
Brizel (1998)[86]	116	RT RT + CIS/5FU→CIS/5FU	Trend for combined treatment better than RT alone
Calais (1999)[87]	226	RT RT + CARBO/5FU	Only oropharyngeal cancer, RT + chemotherapy better than RT alone

For abbreviations please see footnote to Table 2.

survival was 9.5 months for radiation alone and 10 months for the combined modality treatment.[64]

More effective drugs are needed to obtain a major improvement for patients with malignant gliomas. Presently, surgery and postoperative radiotherapy should be considered standard treatment for these patients.

Head and neck cancer (see also Chapters 9.2–9.7)

Squamous cell carcinomas of the head and neck grow locally and metastasize to regional lymph nodes whereas haematogenous metastases are generally rare and usually a late event. The exception is nasopharyngeal cancer where distant metastases are more common. Thus, the main rationale for combining radiotherapy and chemotherapy in most patients with squamous cell cancers of the head and neck is to obtain therapeutic gain by independent cell kill and not by spatial cooperation.

The addition of chemotherapy to radiation with or without surgery has been investigated in several randomized studies.

Induction chemotherapy has been investigated with the aim of avoiding mutilating surgery without influencing survival and in order to improve survival. Two studies[69],[70] have addressed the question as to whether induction chemotherapy with cisplatin and 5-fluorouracil could be useful for larynx preservation. Both trials demonstrated that it was possible to avoid laryngectomy in the majority of patients with advanced laryngeal cancer without jeopardizing survival. However, larynx preservation can also be achieved by using radiotherapy alone and reserving surgery for patients with residual or recurrent tumours. Thus, it is not known whether induction chemotherapy increases the probability of larynx preservation.

The effect of induction chemotherapy on survival has been investigated in several randomized trials, most of which have not shown any survival benefit.[52],[71] Sixteen randomized phase III trials comparing concurrent radiotherapy and chemotherapy with radiotherapy alone with more than 50 patients per randomization group have been published (Table 3). More than half of these studies have demonstrated a statistically significant improvement of survival in favour of the combined modality treatment. The potential survival benefit from additional concurrent chemotherapy was also found in three literature-based meta-analyses,[88]–[90] whereas the same overviews found either a minimal[89] or no significant effect for induction chemotherapy.[88],[90] The effect of sequence has also been investigated in four randomized studies.[91]–[94] Overall, these studies have demonstrated an advantage for concomitant radiotherapy and chemotherapy as compared with sequential treatment.

In a recent patient-based meta-analysis of 10 741 patients randomized in 63 studies, there were no survival benefits for induction chemotherapy and postradiation chemotherapy. There was, however, a statistically significant absolute survival benefit at 5 years of 8 per cent from use of concomitant chemotherapy,[95] although this is obtained at the expense of enhanced toxicity.[90] It is possible that the survival benefit of adding chemotherapy could instead be achieved by increasing the radiation dose, or by use of hyperfractionated irradiation.[96]

In conclusion, radiotherapy and/or surgery is still the standard treatment for squamous cell carcinoma of the head and neck. Concurrent radiotherapy and chemotherapy with cisplatin or carboplatin with or without 5-fluorouracil may be the treatment of choice in selected patients and for patients with nasopharyngeal cancer this approach may be considered standard treatment.

Small cell lung cancer (see also Chapter 14.4)

The main treatment for patients with small cell lung cancer is combination chemotherapy. The question has been whether radiotherapy should be added to chemotherapy in patients with limited stage small cell lung cancer. Several randomized trials have shown that chest irradiation can improve local control whereas improved survival in single studies has not been obtained. However, two meta-analyses based on 11 and 13 studies, respectively, have demonstrated a statistically significant absolute survival benefit of 5.4 per cent at 2 to 3 years.[97],[98] Thus, the addition of chest irradiation in patients with limited disease seems justified, but when should radiation then be given? Five randomized phase III studies have addressed the question of early versus delayed chest radiation (Table 4). There are many differences between these studies with respect to both the chemotherapeutic regimen, the radiation dose levels, whether radiotherapy and chemotherapy was given concurrently or sequentially and whether prophylactic cranial irradiation was also given. These differences may hamper a valid conclusion. In general, the data

support a treatment strategy of using chemotherapy combined with early thoracic irradiation. Whether this should be applied concurrently, sequentially, or as an alternating regimen should be further clarified.

Several randomized studies have demonstrated a statistically significant reduction in the rate of brain metastases following prophylactic cranial irradiation (PCI).[104]–[106] However, no single study has obtained a statistically significant survival benefit following PCI. This has been attributed to the limited number of patients in these trials, but even in the two largest phase III studies with 294[107] and 314 patients,[108] the possible survival benefit was not statistically significant. The majority of patients die because of progression of the systemic disease, and one should probably look for a survival benefit of PCI in the group of patients with the best prognosis. Such a strategy is supported by the results from a recent meta-analysis on 987 patients in complete remission, where the use of PCI resulted in a statistically significant improved 3-year survival rate from 15.3 per cent to 20.7 per cent.[109] Further studies should address the selection of patients for PCI and the optimal dose and schedule.

Non-small cell lung cancer (see also Chapter 14.3)

The effect of chemotherapy either given concurrently with radiation treatment or as induction chemotherapy followed by radiotherapy in unresectable stage III non-small cell lung cancer has been investigated in several randomized phase III studies (Table 5). Most trials have used cisplatin- or carboplatin-based chemotherapy.

Studies of concomitantly administered radiotherapy and chemotherapy have shown either no difference in survival or improved survival for the combined treatment strategy as compared with that of radiation alone (Table 5). In a study by Jeremic et al.[115] patients were randomized to hyperfractionated radiation treatment alone or with concurrently administered carboplatin and etoposide. There was a significantly improved survival in patients receiving combined radiotherapy and chemotherapy with a 4-year survival rate of 23 per cent versus 9 per cent for patients receiving radiation alone.[115]

The majority of studies of induction chemotherapy have demonstrated a significantly improved survival for the combined treatment strategy (Table 5). In the Cancer and Leukemia Group B trial updated by Dilllmann et al. in 1996,[121] patients were randomized to radiation alone versus two cycles of induction chemotherapy with cisplatin and vinblastine followed by radiotherapy. The 5-year survival rate for the combined modality was 17 per cent versus 6 per cent for patients receiving radiation alone.[121]

There have been three published patient—or literature-based meta-analyses, which taken together indicate that the addition of chemotherapy reduces the risk of death by about 10 per cent and results in an absolute improvement in the 2-year survival of about 4 per cent.[122]–[124]

The addition of chemotherapy to radiotherapy has resulted in a small but definite survival benefit. The optimal combined modality treatment has not been defined. Toxicity is greater from concurrent chemotherapy and radiotherapy as compared with that of induction chemotherapy followed by radiotherapy, which supports the use of induction chemotherapy. The incorporation of promising new agents such as paclitaxel, vinorelbine, and gemcitabine may further improve survival for patients with locally advanced non-small cell lung cancer and randomized trials addressing these questions are in progress.[125],[126]

Table 4 Small cell lung cancer (SCLC): randomized phase III studies of chemotherapy combined with either early (ECI) or delayed (LCI) chest irradiation in SCLC

Reference (first author)	Number of evaluable patients	Treatment groups	Survival outcome
Perry (1987)[99]	270	ECI from day 1 LCI delayed 9 weeks	Borderline advantage for LCI
Murray (1993)[100]	308	ECI delayed 3 weeks LCI delayed 15 weeks	ECI better than LCI
Takada (1996)[101]	228	ECI from day 1 LCI delayed 12 weeks	ECI seems to be better than LCI
Work (1997)[102]	199	ECI from day 1 LCI delayed 18 weeks	No difference
Jeremic (1997)[103]	107	ECI from day 1 LCI delayed 6 weeks	ECI better than LCI

Table 5 Non-small cell lung cancer (NSCLC): randomized phase III studies of either concurrent chemotherapy and radiotherapy (C) or induction chemotherapy (I) followed by radiotherapy in NSCLC

Reference (first author)	Number of evaluable patients	Treatment groups	Combined schedule	Survival outcome
Soresi (1988)[110]	95	RT RT + CIS	C	No difference
Schaake-Koning (1992)[111]	331	RT RT + CIS daily	C	Combined treatment better than RT alone
Trovó (1992)[112]	146	RT RT + CIS	C	No difference
Blanke (1995)[113]	215	RT RT + CIS	C	No difference
Jeremic (1995)[114]	169	RT RT + CARBO/EPO (two schedules)	C	Combined treatment better than RT alone
Jeremic (1996)[115]	131	RT RT + CARBO/EPO	C	Combined treatment better than RT alone
Mattson (1988)[116]	238	RT CIS/DOX/CTX→RT	1	No difference
Morton (1991)[117]	114	RT MTX/DOX/CTX/MeCCNU→RT	1	No difference
Le Chavalier (1992)[118]	353	RT VDS/CTX/CIS/CCNU→RT	1	Combined treatment better than RT alone
Wolf (1994)[119]	78	RT + CIS IFOS/VDS/→RT + CIS	1	Combined treatment better than RT ± CIS
Sause (1995)[120]	452	RT (two schedules) CIS/VBL→RT	1	Combined treatment better than RT alone
Dillman (1996)[121]	155	RT CIS/VBL→RT	1	Combined treatment better than RT alone

For abbreviations please see footnote to Table 2.

Breast cancer (see also Chapter 11.7)

Several randomized studies have shown that adjuvant chemotherapy and endocrine treatment after surgery improve survival of patients with breast cancer[127],[128] (see Section 11). The role of adjuvant radiotherapy after mastectomy has also been evaluated in several randomized studies. Until recently, these studies have demonstrated that postoperative radiotherapy reduces the frequency of loco-regional recurrences with no statistically significant improvement in overall survival.[129],[130] However, a large nation-wide Danish study has now demonstrated that radiotherapy after mastectomy in high-risk pre-menopausal patients receiving adjuvant chemotherapy significantly improves overall survival.[131] A total of 1708 patients were randomized to receive either eight cycles of chemotherapy with cyclophosphamide, methotrexate, and 5-fluorouracil (**CMF**) plus radiotherapy or nine cycles of CMF alone. The frequency of loco-regional recurrences with or without distant metastases was 9 per cent following the combined modality treatment and 32 per cent following CMF alone. The 10-year overall survival rates were 34 per cent and 48 per cent in two groups of patients, respectively ($p < 0.0001$). These results are supported by the Vancouver study[132] of 318 randomized patients, although the overall survival benefit did not reach statistical significance ($p = 0.07$). Improvement of overall survival has also been reported for the addition of radiotherapy to adjuvant tamoxifen in postmenopausal patients.[133] These studies point to the importance of achieving control of both loco-regional and systemic disease and are examples of a therapeutic gain obtained by combined radiotherapy with chemotherapy or endocrine treatment by spatial cooperation. The need for a combined modality approach is further emphazised because more and more patients are treated by lumpectomy (instead of mastectomy) where adjuvant radiotherapy is standard.

In the Danish and Vancouver studies of premenopausal patients, the radiotherapy was administered either between the first and second course of CMF[131] or between the fourth and fifth course of CMF.[132] However, the optimal combined modality regimen has yet to be found. One randomized study has shown an increased risk of loco-regional failure and a decreased risk of distant metastases but no significant overall survival benefit following chemotherapy given before radiotherapy compared with the opposite sequence of the two treatment modalities.[134]

Oesophageal cancer (see also Chapter 10.1)

The prognosis for patients with oesophageal cancer is dismal. The treatment options have been surgery and/or radiotherapy with no proven superiority of either of these treatment modalities. Seven randomized studies have addressed whether combined radiotherapy and chemotherapy can improve the outcome for patients with loc-alized oesophageal cancer (Table 6). Four of these studies compared combined radiotherapy and chemotherapy with radiation alone whereas preoperative radiotherapy and chemotherapy was compared with surgery alone in the three other studies. The number of patients was rather small in the majority of trials, and the radiation dose was suboptimal in some of them. This is especially critical in the study by Roussel et al.[138] where radiotherapy was the definitive local treatment. In two of the studies, chemotherapy was only administered as a single course.[135],[136] In the study by Herskovic et al.[137] patients were randomized to radiation alone with a total dose of 64 Gy versus radiation at a lower dose of 50 Gy plus four courses of cisplatin and 5-fluorouracil administered concomitantly with the radiation treatment. In the updated report,[24] the median survival was 14.1 months for radiotherapy plus chemotherapy and 9.3 months for radiation alone, and the corresponding 5-year survival rates were 27 per cent and 0 per cent, respectively. They subsequently treated 69 patients with the same combined modality regimen and maintained the superior results. Toxicity, especially oesophagitis, was enhanced in the combined modality group.[24]

Three randomized trials have investigated the effect of preoperative combined radiotherapy and chemotherapy (Table 6). Survival was improved following the combined treatment strategy in one of these studies.[140] Chemotherapy consisted of two courses of cisplatin and 5-fluorouracil administered concomitantly with radiation at a total dose at 40 Gy. The 3-year survival rate was 32 per cent for the combined modality group and 6 per cent for surgery alone.[140]

In conclusion, encouraging results of concomitantly administered radiotherapy and chemotherapy in patients with localized oesophageal cancer have been achieved. Such a strategy may be the treatment of choice in selected patients, although the optimal dose and schedule of the combined modality treatment has yet to be clarified.

Gastric cancer

Surgery is the treatment of choice in resectable gastric cancer (see Chapter 10.2). Radiotherapy and/or chemotherapy has no significant impact on survival.[142] These treatment modalities should only be used within clinical trials.

Pancreatic cancer (see also Chapter 10.6)

The studies of radiation alone versus combined radiotherapy and chemotherapy in resectable and unresectable pancreatic cancer have generally included only a small number of patients. As indicated in the review by Tannock,[52] some studies have suggested a survival benefit whereas other studies did not. The survival outcome is uniformly poor. More effective drugs are necessary to improve the treatment results in patients with pancreatic cancer. Studies of new combined treatments such as the combination of radiotherapy and gemcitabine are ongoing.[143]

Rectal cancer (see also Chapter 10.4)

Surgery is the main treatment of patients with cancer of the rectum. Adjuvant radiotherapy administered either before or after surgery has generally resulted in increased local control whereas survival has been improved in some and not in other studies.[144] Four randomized trials have evaluated the addition of chemotherapy to radiotherapy as adjunctive treatment to surgery (Table 7). One randomized trial has investigated preoperative radiotherapy with or without 5-fluoro-uracil and found survival following the combined treatment to be inferior to preoperative radiotherapy alone.[145] Two trials have in-vestigated the effect of postoperative radiotherapy with or without 5-fluorouracil + methyl CCNU.[146],[147] In the trial by the Gastro-intestinal Tumour Study Group,[146] patients were also randomized to surgery alone and postoperative chemotherapy alone. The combined treatment improved disease-free survival compared with that fol-lowing surgery alone, but there was no significant improvement of overall survival.[146] In the study by Krook et al.[147] the 5-year overall survival following combined treatment was 57 per cent versus 48 per

Table 6 Oesophageal cancer: randomized phase III studies of radiotherapy and chemotherapy in localized cancer of the oesophagus

Reference (first author)	Number of evaluable patients	Treatment groups	Survival outcome
Andersen (1984)[135]	82	RT (63 Gy) RT (55 Gy) + BLM	No difference
Araújo (1991)[136]	59	RT (50 Gy) RT (50 Gy) + 5FU/MMC/BLM	No difference
Herskovic (1992)[137] Al-Sarraf (1997)[24]	123	RT (64 Gy) RT (50 Gy) + CIS/5FU	RT + chemotherapy better than RT alone
Roussel (1994)[138]	221	RT (40 Gy) RT (40 Gy) + CIS	No difference
Le Prise (1994)[139]	86	Surgery RT (20 Gy)→CIS/5FU→surgery	No difference
Walsh (1996)[140]	113	Surgery RT (40 Gy) + CIS/5FU→surgery	Improved survival following combined treatment
Bosset (1997)[141]	282	Surgery RT (37 Gy) + CIS→surgery	No difference

For abbreviations please see footnote to Table 2.

Table 7 Rectal cancer: randomized phase III studies of radiotherapy and chemotherapy in rectal cancer

Reference (first author)	Number of evaluable patients	Treatment groups	Survival outcome
Boulis-Wassif (1984)[145]	247	Preoperative RT Preoperative RT/5FU	RT alone better than RT + 5FU
Gastrointestinal Tumor Study Group (1985)[146]	202	Surgery alone Postoperative 5FU/MeCCNU Postoperative RT Postoperative RT + 5FU/MeCCNU	Combined treatment improved disease-free, but not overall, survival
Krook (1991)[147]	204	Postoperative RT Postoperative RT + 5FU/MeCCNU	Combined treatment better than RT alone
Wolmark (2000)[148]	694	Postoperative 5FU/MeCCNU/VCR Postoperative RT + 5FU/MeCCNU/VCR Postoperative 5FU/Leucovorin Postoperative RT + 5FU/Leucovorin	Combined treatment not better than CT alone

For abbreviations please see footnote to Table 2.

cent following postoperative radiotherapy alone. The effect of postoperative radiotherapy and chemotherapy has also been compared with the effect of postoperative chemotherapy alone with no significant difference in disease-free or overall survival.[148] Overall, there has been no consistent improvement of survival by use of combined radiotherapy and chemotherapy. Therefore, it is not clear why the National Cancer Institute Consensus Conference has concluded that patients with rectal cancer should be offered combined radiotherapy and 5-fluorouracil-based chemotherapy as standard postoperative treatment.[149] Hopefully, the problem will be solved by the many randomized trials of combined modality treatment in rectal cancer that are in progress.[150]

Cancer of the anal canal (see also Chapter 10.5)

Concomitantly administered radiotherapy and chemotherapy has been widely used in the treatment of epidermoid cancers of the anal canal. The most frequent investigated chemotherapeutic regimens have included 5-fluorouracil and mitomycin C. Non-randomized studies have suggested that combined treatment improves loco-regional control and increases the frequency of patients with retained

Table 8 Cancer of the anal canal: randomized phase III studies of concomitant radiotherapy and chemotherapy in epidermoid anal cancer

Reference (first author)	Number of evaluable patients	Treatment groups	Survival outcome
UKCCCR (1996)[152]	562	RT RT + 5FU/MMC	Combined treatment improved colostomy-free and cancer-specific survival No difference in overall survival
Bartelink (1997)[153]	103	RT RT + 5FU/MMC	Combined treatment improved colostomy-free survival. No difference in overall survival
Flam (1996)[154]	291	RT + 5FU RT + 5FU/MMC	Inclusion of MMC improved colostomy-free survival. No difference in overall survival.

For abbreviations see footnote to Table 2.

anorectal function.[151] Furthermore, it appears that concomitantly administered radiotherapy and chemotherapy is more effective than sequential treatment.[151]

The results of three randomized studies of combined radiotherapy and chemotherapy in epidermoid anal cancer have been published (Table 8). Two studies have investigated the effect of 5-fluorouracil and mitomycin C administered concomitantly with radiotherapy versus radiotherapy alone.[152],[153] One study has investigated mitomycin C in addition to concomitantly administered radiotherapy and 5-fluorouracil.[154] In the UKCCCR Anal Cancer Trial Working Party study, the local failure rate following radiotherapy alone was 59 per cent versus 36 per cent following the combined treatment, but there was no survival advantage. Early morbidity was more frequent in the combined treatment group, whereas there was no difference in late morbidity.[152] In the European Organization for Research and Treatment of Cancer (**EORTC**) study,[153] the addition of chemotherapy also improved the loco-regional control and colostomy-free survival, whereas there was no overall survival benefit. The 5-year survival rate for the entire patient population was 56 per cent. Late side-effects were similar in the two treatment groups.[153] In the Radiation Therapy Oncology Group (**RTOG**)/Eastern Cooperative Oncology Group trial, the addition of mitomycin C to radiotherapy and 5-fluorouracil resulted in a higher colostomy-free survival (71 per cent versus 59 per cent) with no significant difference in overall survival. Toxicity was greater in the group of patients receiving mitomycin C.[154]

Thus, the combination of concurrent radiotherapy and chemotherapy with 5-fluorouracil and mitomycin-C has improved colostomy-free survival but not overall survival. However, as preservation of anorectal function is very important, this combined modality approach may be considered the treatment of choice in patients with locally advanced epidermoid cancer of the anal canal.

Renal cell carcinoma

Standard treatment for patients with renal cell carcinoma remains surgery (see Chapter 13.3). The addition of radiotherapy and/or chemotherapeutic drugs or other antineoplastic agents has not been shown to be of any benefit.

Bladder cancer (see also Chapter 13.2)

A number of studies have evaluated the effect of combined modality treatment with radiation and drugs (Table 9). Most studies have investigated the effect of induction chemotherapy. Only one of these studies has suggested improved survival for the combined modality treatment and this was only obtained in a subgroup analysis for patients with T3 and T4 tumours.[157] In the large MRC/EORTC study[158] patients were randomized to receive local treatment only versus combined chemotherapy with cisplatin, methotrexate, and vinblastine (**CMV**) followed by the same local treatment. Among the 975 randomized patients, local treatment was radiation alone in 414 patients, cystectomy alone in 484 patients, and preoperative radiotherapy followed by cystectomy in 77 patients. The addition of CMV did not improve survival compared with that following any of the local treatments alone.[158]

One small randomized study has investigated the effect of concurrent cisplatin and radiotherapy versus radiotherapy alone.[160] The loco–regional control was improved in the combined modality group without a statistically significant effect on overall survival.[160]

There is a meta-analysis of single agent cisplatin as induction chemotherapy or administered concurrently with local definitive treatment versus local definitive treatment alone, in most cases radiotherapy.[162] The analysis was based on individual data from 479 patients from four randomized studies, and showed no significant impact on survival.[162]

Concurrently administered chemotherapy and radiotherapy with or without induction chemotherapy has also been used with the purpose of selecting patients for bladder preservation. In most cases, induction chemotherapy has consisted of two cycles of CMV followed by single agent cisplatin administered concomitantly with radiation treatment up to a total dose of 40 to 45 Gy. Responders have then continued to 60 to 70 Gy, whereas non-responders have been recommended cystectomy. This strategy has resulted in bladder preservation in about 40 to 50 per cent of patients,[163]–[165] but randomized studies are needed to evaluate the effect of this bladder preservation strategy as compared with radiation alone.

The standard treatment of patients with locally advanced muscle-invasive bladder cancer remains cystectomy or radiation treatment.

Table 9 Bladder cancer: randomized phase III studies of radiotherapy and chemotherapy in muscle invasive bladder cancer

Reference (first author)	Number of evaluable patients	Treatment groups	Combined schedule	Survival outcome
Shearer (1988)[155]	376	RT MTX→RT→MTX	I + P	No difference
Wallace (1991)[156]	255	RT CIS→RT	I	No difference
Malmström (1996)[157]	311	RT + cystectomy CIS/DOX→RT + cystectomy	I	Combined treatment better than RT + cystectomy in T3/T4 tumours
MRC/EORTC (1999)[158]	975	Local treatment* CMV→local treatment*	I	No difference
Shipley (1997)[159]	126	RT + CIS CMV→RT + CIS	I + C	No difference
Coppin (1996)[160]	99	RT RT + CIS	C	No difference
Richards (1983)[161]	110	RT RT→DOX/5FU	P	No difference

For abbreviations see footnote to Table 2.

*Local treatment: cystectomy or radiotherapy or radiotherapy plus cystectomy.

Prostatic cancer (see also Chapter 13.1)

In locally advanced prostatic cancer, the use of induction endocrine treatment before radiotherapy may reduce the rate of local recurrence.[166] In one of two large randomized studies from the RTOG,[167] 456 evaluable patients with T2–T4 tumours were randomized to receive a luteinizing hormone-releasing hormone agonist (goserelin) plus antiandrogen treatment with flutamide for 2 months before and during radiotherapy versus radiotherapy alone. In the other RTOG trial,[168] 977 patients with T3 tumours, N1 disease or positive margins after prostatectomy were randomized to receive either continuous goserelin treatment together with radiotherapy or radiotherapy alone. Both trials demonstrated significantly improved local control for the combined modality treatment with no improvement in overall survival.[167],[168] However, follow-up is still relatively short for observation of possible differences in mortality.

In an EORTC/NCIC study,[169] 401 evaluable patients with locally advanced prostatic cancer were randomized to radiotherapy alone versus radiotherapy plus goserelin for 3 years. In this study, both local control and overall survival were improved in the group of patients receiving combined treatment compared with that following radiotherapy alone.[169]

These results are encouraging, but it is possible that endocrine treatment alone might give similar results. Several studies are addressing this question.

Testicular germ cell cancer (see also Chapter 13.4)

Following orchidectomy, patients with stage I disease may be managed by close surveillance. Otherwise, patients with seminoma stage I and stage IIA and B are offered radiation treatment, whereas patients with more advanced seminomas and non-seminomatous tumours are offered chemotherapy. There are no routine indications for applying combined radiotherapy and chemotherapy, either concurrently or sequentially.

Ovarian cancer

Following initial surgery, chemotherapy is the treatment of choice for patients with ovarian cancer FIGO stages II to IV (see Chapter 12.1). Although additional radiotherapy in combination with chemotherapy or radiotherapy alone has been used in patients with stage II and III disease, this is not regarded as part of the standard treatment.

Cancer of the corpus uteri

Postoperative radiotherapy after hysterectomy in patients with deeply invasive endometrial cancer is used routinely in some centres and has been abandoned in others (see Chapter 12.4). There are no data to support the use of additional chemotherapy or endocrine treatment.

Cancer of the cervix uteri (see also Chapter 12.3)

Radiotherapy has until recently been the standard treatment for locally advanced cervical cancer. The addition of chemotherapy with the aim of improving survival by increasing local tumour control and/or by eradicating tumour cells outside the pelvic area has been studied extensively.[170],[171]

The largest randomized studies are summarized in Table 10. Hreshchyshyn et al. found that hydroxurea administered concomitantly with radiotherapy resulted in a statistically significant improvement of response, progression-free survival, and overall survival,[172] but the study has been criticized for a series of methodological problems.[170] A subsequent large randomized study comparing radiotherapy with misonidazole and the same regimen with concomitantly administered hydroxurea found no difference.[175] Similarly, survival improvement was not demonstrated in three other phase III studies of concurrent radiotherapy and chemotherapy.[173],[174],[176] Recently, however, five large randomized phase III studies have demonstrated a statistically significant survival benefit by using concomitant cisplatin-based

Table 10 Cancer of the cervix uteri: randomized phase III studies of either concurrent chemotherapy and radiotherapy (C) or induction chemotherapy (I) followed by radiotherapy in cervical cancer

Reference (first author)	Number of evaluable patients	Treatment groups	Combined schedule	Survival outcome
Hreshchyshyn (1979)[172]	104	RT RT + hydroxurea	C	Combined treatment better than RT alone
Runowicz (1989)[173]	151	RT RT + CIS/MTX/CA/VCR	C	No difference
Mickiewicz (1991)[174]	100	RT RT + MMC/5FU/CIS	C	No difference
Stehman (1993)[175]	296	RT + MISO RT + MISO + hydroxurea	C	No difference
Thomas (1998)[176]	221	RT (two schedules) RT (two schedules) + 5FU	C	No difference
Keys (1999)[177]	369	RT RT + CIS	C	Improved survival following combined treatment
Peters (2000)[178]	243	RT RT + CIS/5FU	C	Improved survival following combined treatment
Morris (1999)[179]	386	RT RT + CIS/5FU	C	Improved survival following combined treatment
Rose (1999)[180]	526	RT + hydroxurea RT + CIS RT + hydroxurea/CIS/5FU	C	Improved survival following CIS-containing combined treatment
Whitney (1999)[181]	368	RT + hydroxurea RT + CIS/5FU	C	Improved survival following RT + CIS/5FU
Wong (1999)[182]	220	RT RT + epirubicin	C	Improved survival following combined treatment
Chauvergne (1993)[183]	151	RT MTX/CA/VCR/CIS→RT	I	No difference
Souhami (1991)[184]	107	RT BLM/VCR/MMC/CIS→RT	I	RT alone better than combined treatment
Tattersall (1992)[185]	71	RT CIS/VBL/BLM→RT	I	No difference
Kumar (1994)[186]	184	RT BLM/IFOS/CIS→RT	I	No difference
Tattersall (1995)[187]	260	RT CIS/epirubicin→RT	I	RT alone better than combined treatment
Sundfør (1996)[188]	94	RT CIS/5FU→RT	I	Trend for combined treatment better than RT alone

For abbreviations see footnote to Table 2.

chemotherapy.[177]–[181] In the study of Keys et al.,[177] patients with bulky stage IB cervical cancer were randomized to radiation alone or radiation with weekly cisplatin. Treatment was in all cases followed by hysterectomy. The 4-year survival rate was 83 per cent in the group receiving combined treatment versus 74 per cent in the radiation alone group.[177] Peters et al.[178] randomized patients with stage IA2 to IIA, who were initially treated with radical hysterectomy and pelvic lymphadenectomy, to receive either radiation alone or radiation plus

four courses of cisplatin and 5-fluorouracil with the two first courses administered concomitantly with radiation therapy. Overall survival was significantly improved by the addition of chemotherapy.[178] Similarly, Morris et al.[179] have shown that concurrent administration of cisplatin and 5-fluorouracil significantly improved survival in patients with stage IIB to IVA compared with that following radiation alone with a 5-year survival rate of 73 per cent and 58 per cent, respectively.[179] Two other large randomized studies did not include a group of patients receiving radiation alone, but instead the standard treatment group received radiation and hydroxurea.[180],[181] In the study by Rose et al.[180] this group of patients was compared with either radiation plus weekly cisplatin or a three-drug combination of hydroxurea, 5-fluorouracil, and cisplatin administered concurrently with radiotherapy in patients with stage IIB to IVA cervical cancer. Survival was equivalently improved for both these schedules with a relative risk of death of about 0.60 compared with that following radiation combined with hydroxurea alone.[180] Similarly, Whitney et al.[181] have shown that radiation treatment with concurrently administered cisplatin and 5-fluorouracil significantly improved survival compared with that of radiation plus hydroxurea in the same patient categories (stage IIB to IVA).[181] Furthermore, Wong et al.[182] have reported that patients with bulky stage I, II, and III cervical cancer receiving epirubicin with and after radiotherapy had a better survival than patients receiving radiation alone.[182] The addition of concurrently administered chemotherapy in these studies was generally associated with increased toxicity which, however, was manageable and the combined treatment was in all cases well tolerated.[177]–[182]

For induction chemotherapy, only one study has shown a trend to survival benefit (Table 10). Sundfør et al.[188] compared radiation alone with induction chemotherapy with cisplatin and 5-fluorouracil followed by radiotherapy and obtained 5-year survival rates of 57 per cent and 70 per cent, respectively ($p = 0.07$). Two other randomized studies of induction chemotherapy showed a significantly reduced survival in the group of patients who received the combined treatment schedule compared with that following radiation alone.[184],[187] In the remaining phase III studies, no significant differences were obtained (Table 10).

There have also been two randomized studies of the effect of postoperative adjuvant radiotherapy and chemotherapy. In the study by Tattersall et al.[189] postoperative radiotherapy was compared with postoperative radiotherapy combined with cisplatin, vinblastine, and bleomycin. Curtin et al.[190] compared postoperative chemotherapy with cisplatin and bleomycin versus postoperative radiotherapy and the same chemotherapeutic regimen. No significant survival differences were obtained in either of these two studies.[189],[190]

In conclusion, cisplatin-based chemotherapy—either cisplatin alone or cisplatin combined with 5-fluorouracil administered concurrently with radiotherapy should be considered standard treatment in patients with locally advanced cancer of the cervix uteri. The use of adjuvant chemotherapy administered after operation or radiation treatment should not be applied outside clinical trials.

Malignant melanoma (see also Chapter 8.1)

Radiation treatment in patients with malignant melanoma may be used in specific situations, primarily as a palliative treatment modality. The addition of chemotherapy, especially cisplatin administered concurrently with radiotherapy, has been investigated, but there are no randomized studies. Thus, there is no indication for combined radiotherapy and chemotherapy in malignant melanoma outside of clinical trials.

Sarcomas (see also Chapter 16.1)

Although the combination of radiotherapy and chemotherapy is used in selected patients, there is no evidence of superiority of the combined treatment strategy in patients with sarcomas. As Ewing's sarcoma is both sensitive to radiotherapy and chemotherapy, most treatment protocols include both modalities. In this specific tumour type, there is some evidence that, at least in larger tumours, there may be a local control advantage after combined chemotherapy and radiotherapy compared with that following combined chemotherapy and surgery.[191] In soft tissue sarcomas, limb sparing is obtained in many patients by the use of adjuvant radiotherapy, but the role of adjuvant chemotherapy remains controversial.[192] A recent, large patient-based meta-analysis of the effect of adjuvant chemotherapy compared with local treatment alone showed improved relapse-free survival with no significant effect on overall survival.[193]

Hodgkin's lymphoma (see also Chapter 15.8)

Hodgkin's lymphomas are highly sensitive to both radiotherapy and chemotherapy, and these treatment options administered as single modalities or in combination will cure the majority of patients with early-stage Hodgkin's disease. Two patient-based meta-analyses have assessed the value of an initial combined treatment strategy.[194],[195] In the overview by Specht et al.[195] the value of combined treatment versus radiotherapy alone was analysed whereas Loeffler et al.[194] have analysed the effect of combined treatment versus chemotherapy alone.

Specht et al.[195] analysed data for 1688 patients with early-stage Hodgkin's disease in 13 trials. They found that the addition of chemotherapy to radiotherapy halved the 10-year failure risk (16 per cent versus 33 per cent), but did not have a significant overall survival benefit. The reason is that salvage chemotherapy at relapse is more effective following radiotherapy alone than following initial combined treatment.[195] Specht et al. also found that use of less extensive radiotherapy increased the risk of failure compared with that of more extensive radiotherapy (43 per cent versus 31 per cent), but without decreasing overall survival.[195]

In the meta-analysis by Loeffler et al.[194] patients with Hodgkin's disease of all stages were included. The role of radiotherapy combined with chemotherapy compared with the same chemotherapeutic regimen was analysed based on 918 patients from seven trials. The addition of radiotherapy improved the 10-year overall relapse-free rate by 11 per cent (62 per cent versus 51 per cent) with no significant effect on overall survival. They also analysed trials evaluating whether the combination of chemotherapy and radiotherapy can be substituted by chemotherapy alone using either more cycles of the same chemotherapeutic regimen or alternative regimens containing additional drugs. This analysis was based on 837 patients from seven trials. There was no difference with respect to tumour control, but 10-year overall survival was significantly decreased in the group of patients receiving radiotherapy. This difference was probably due to an increased frequency of toxic events in the group of patients receiving combined chemotherapy and radiotherapy.[194]

In conclusion, patients with early-stage Hodgkin's disease may be offered either radiotherapy alone and salvage chemotherapy at relapse or initial combined radiotherapy and chemotherapy. The radiation treatment may be less extensive with the use of reduced radiation fields. Patients with advanced-stage Hodgkin's disease should be offered primarily chemotherapy alone with additional radiotherapy reserved for specific indications.

Non-Hodgkin's lymphomas (see also Chapter 15.10)

Miller et al.[196] have published the results from the South-West Oncology Group (SWOG) comparing chemotherapy with combined chemotherapy and radiotherapy in patients with localized, intermediate- or high-grade non-Hodgkin's lymphomas. They randomized 401 eligible patients to receive either eight cycles of cyclophosphamide, doxorubicin, vincristine, and prednisone (**CHOP**) or three cycles of CHOP followed by radiation treatment of involved-fields. Three cycles of CHOP plus radiotherapy significantly improved progression-free survival (77 per cent versus 64 per cent) and overall survival (82 per cent versus 72 per cent) compared with that following eight cycles of CHOP. Furthermore, life-threatening toxicities were reduced from 40 per cent following CHOP × 8 to 30 per cent following CHOP × 3 plus radiotherapy.[196] Thus, a strategy of combining less extensive chemotherapy with involved-field radiotherapy seems to be an effective treatment option in patients with localized non-Hodgkin's lymphomas.

Conclusions and future aspects

The combined effects of radiotherapy and chemotherapy are extremely complex. Experimental studies are important to achieve a better understanding of basic mechanisms of drug–radiation interactions and normal tissue reactions in experimental animals may be predictive for clinical outcome. The most serious toxic reactions should be expected when drugs are administered concurrently with or shortly after irradiation, and from the use of drugs that are toxic by themselves to the normal tissue in question. It is advisable to test new drug–radiation combinations experimentally before implementation in clinical practice.

Clinically, the use of a combined modality approach with radiotherapy and chemotherapy has for many years been an attractive challenge, but, with rather disappointing results for tumours of adults. It is encouraging that recent years have provided high-level evidence about the effects of combined radiotherapy and chemotherapy for a series of tumour types. Therapeutic gain by spatial cooperation has been demonstrated for small cell lung cancer, breast cancer, and lymphomas and by independent cell kill for non-small cell lung cancer, oesophageal cancer, cancer of the anal canal, cancer of the cervix uteri, and selected patients with head and neck cancer. The results obtained demonstrate the importance of large, well designed randomized trials and patient-based meta-analyses. These studies have also (and as importantly) demonstrated areas where combined radiotherapy and chemotherapy is ineffective, e.g. brain tumours. In these and many other tumour types, new effective drugs are needed to improve clinical outcome. Drugs such as paclitaxel[197],[198] and gemcitabine[199],[200] may have the potential to improve the therapeutic index when combined with radiotherapy. Another approach is to develop experimental agents with specific properties that can complement radiotherapy, such as tirapazamine, which is selectively toxic to hypoxic cells.[7] A therapeutic gain might also be achieved by selective normal tissue protection. Ongoing studies with drugs like amifostine[201],[201] may clarify whether a therapeutic gain can be obtained by this mode of action.

Close cooperation between experimental and clinical research within this complex area is of utmost importance. Experimental and clinical data should be considered cautiously when planning drug–radiation combinations, and regimens which have not been established as standard treatments should only be applied within the context of a clinical study.

References

1. **Steel GG, Peckham MJ.** Exploitable mechanisms in combined radiotherapy-chemotherapy: The concept of additivity. *International Journal of Radiation Oncology, Biology, Physics*, 1979; **5**: 85–91.

2. **Steel GG.** The search for therapeutic gain in the combination of radiotherapy and chemotherapy. *Radiotherapy and Oncology*, 1988; **11**: 31–53.

3. **von der Maase H.** Complications of combined radiotherapy and chemotherapy. *Seminars in Radiation and Oncology*, 1994; **2**: 81–94.

4. **Hill BT.** Overview of experimental laboratory investigations of antitumor drug–radiation interactions. In: Hill BT, Bellamy AS (eds). *Antitumor drug–radiation interactions*. Boca Raton, FL, CRC, 1990: 225–46.

5. **Fu KK, Philips TL.** Biologic rationale of combined radiotherapy and chemotherapy. *Hematology/Oncology Clinics of North America*, 1991; **5**: 737–52.

6. **Steel GG.** Combination of radiotherapy and chemotherapy: principles. In: Steel GG (ed.). *Basic clinical radiobiology*. London: Edward Arnold, 1997: 184–94.

7. **Boyer MJ.** Bioreductive agents: a clinical update. *Oncology Research*, 1997; **9**: 391–5.

8. **Philips TL, Fu KK.** Quantification of combined radiation therapy and chemotherapy effects on critical normal tissues. *Cancer*, 1976; **37**: 1186–200.

9. **von der Maase H.** Experimental studies on interactions of radiation and cancer chemotherapeutic drugs in normal tissues and a solid tumour. *Radiotherapy and Oncology*, 1986; **7**: 47–68.

10. **Lelieveld P, et al.** The effect of treatment in fractionated schedules with the combination of x-irradiation and six cytotoxic drugs on the RIF-1 tumor and normal mouse skin. *International Journal of Radiation Oncology, Biology, Physics*, 1985; **11**: 111–21.

11. **Cassady JR, et al.** Radiation–Adriamycin interactions: Preliminary clinical observations. *Cancer*, 1975; **36**: 946–9.

12. **Aristizabal SA, et al.** Adriamycin-irradiation cutaneous complications. *International Journal of Radiation Oncology, Biology, Physics*, 1977; **2**: 325–31.

13. **Forastiere AA, et al.** Radiotherapy and bleomycin-containing chemotherapy in the treatment of advanced head and neck cancer: Report of six patients and review of the literature. *International Journal of Radiation Oncology, Biology, Physics*, 1981; **7**: 1441–50.

14. **Overgaard J, Grau C.** Interactions between bleomycin and x-irradiation In: Hill BT, Bellamy AS (eds). *Antitumor drug–radiation interactions*. Boca Raton, FL, CRC, 1990: 53–67.

15. **Bachaud JM, et al.** Combined postoperative radiotherapy and weekly cisplatin infusion for locally advance squamous cell carcinoma of the head and neck: Preliminary report of a randomized trial. *International Journal of Radiation Oncology, Biology, Physics*, 1991; **20**: 243–6.

16. **Fowle B.** Interactions of chemotherapy and radiation in the treatment of nonmetastatic breast cancer. In: Meyer JL, Vaeth JM (eds). *Radiotherapy/chemotherapy interactions in cancer therapy. Frontiers of Radiation Therapy and Oncology*. Basel: Karger, 1992; **26**: 95–114.

17. **Bentzen SM, et al.** Early and late normal-tissue injury after postmastectomy radiotherapy alone or combined with chemotherapy. *International Journal of Radiation Biology*, 1989; **56**: 711–15.

18. **Thomas PRM, et al.** Toxicity associated with adjuvant postoperative therapy for adenocarcinoma of the rectum *Cancer*, 1986; **57**: 1130–4.

19. **Overgaard M, et al.** A randomized feasibility study evaluating the effect of radiotherapy alone or combined with 5-fluorouracil in the treatment of locally recurrent of inoperable colorectal carcinoma. *Acta Oncologica*, 1993; **32**: 547–53.

20. **Philips TL, Wharam MD, Margolis LW.** Modification of radiation injury to normal tissues by chemotherapeutic agents. *Cancer*, 1975; **35**: 1678–84.

21. Philips TL. Small animal model systems for testing combined modality treatment effects on normal tissue. *Frontiers of Radiation Therapy and Oncology*, 1979; **13**: 6–8.

22. Philips TL, Fu KK. Acute and late effects of multimodal theapy on normal tissues. *Cancer*, 1977; **40**: 489–94.

23. Schaake-Koning C, *et al.* Radiotherapy combined with low-dose cis-diammine dichloroplatinum (II) (CDDO) in inoperable nonmetastatic non-small cell lung cancer (NSCLC): a randomized three arm phase II study of the EORTC lung cancer and radiotherapy cooperative groups. *International Journal of Radiation Oncology, Biology, Physics*, 1990; **19**: 967–72.

24. Al-Sarraf M, *et al.* Progress report of combined chemoradiotherapy versus radiotherapy alone in patients with esophageal cancer: an intergroup study. *Journal of Clinical Oncology*, 1997; **15**: 277–84.

25. Phelps TA. Cytarabin (Ara-C) induced radioresistance of mouse jejunal stem cells following single or fractionated doses of radiation. *International Journal of Radiation Oncology, Biology, Physics*, 1980; **6**: 1671–7.

26. Pearson AE, Steel GG. Chemotherapy in combination with pelvic irradiation: a time dependence study in mice. *Radiotherapy and Oncology*, 1984; **2**: 49–55.

27. Dewit L, Oussoren Y, Bartelink H. Early and late damage in the mouse rectum after irradiation and cis-diamminedichloroplatinum (II). *Radiotherapy and Oncology*, 1987; **8**: 57–69.

28. Julia AM, *et al.* Concomitant evaluation of efficiency, acute and delayed toxicities of combined treatment of radiation and CDDP on an in vivo model. *International Journal of Radiation Oncology, Biology, Physics*, 1991; **20**: 347–50.

29. Yarnold JR, *et al.* Chemotherapy and radiotherapy for advanced testicular non-seminoma. *Radiotherapy and Oncology*, 1983; **1**: 91–9.

30. Peckham MJ, Collis CH. Clinical objectives and normal tissue responses in combined chemotherapy and radiotherapy. *Bulletin du Cancer (Paris)*, 1981; **68**: 132–41.

31. von der Maase H, Overgaard J, Vaeth M. Effect of cancer chemotherapeutic drugs on radiation-induced lung damage in mice. *Radiotherapy and Oncology*, 1986; **5**: 245–57.

32. Tanabe M, Godat D, Kallman RF. Effects of fractionated schedules of irradiation combined with cis-diamminedichloroplatinum II on the SCCVII/ST tumor and normal tissues of the C3H/KM mouse. *International Journal of Radiation Oncology, Biology, Physics*, 1987; **13**: 1523–32.

33. Lockhart SP, Down JD, Steel GG. Mouse hemothoracic irradiation and its interaction with cytotoxic drugs. *Radiotherapy and Oncology*, 1992; **24**: 177–85.

34. Cohen IJ, *et al.* Dactinomycin potentiation of radiation pneumonitis: a forgotten interaction. *Pediatric Hematology and Oncology*, 1991; **8**: 187–92.

35. Catane R, *et al.* Pulmonary toxicity after radiation and bleomycin: a review. *International Journal of Radiation Oncology, Biology, Physics*, 1979; **5**: 1513–8.

36. Trask CWL, *et al.* Radiation-induced lung fibrosis after treatment of small cell carcinoma of the lung with very high-dose cyclophosphamide. *Cancer*, 1985; **55**: 57–60.

37. Moulder JE, Fish BL. Influence of nephrotoxic drugs on the late renal toxicity associated with bone marrow transplant conditioning regimens. *International Journal of Radiation Oncology, Biology, Physics*, 1991; **20**: 333–7.

38. Stewart FA, Oussoren Y, Bartelink H. The influence of cisplatin on the response of mouse kidney to multifraction irradiation. *Radiotherapy and Oncology*, 1989; **15**: 93–102.

39. Stewart FA, Luts A, Begg AC. Tolerance of previously irradiated mouse kidneys to cis-diamminedichloroplatinum (II). *Cancer Research*, 1987; **47**: 1016–21.

40. Lundbeck F, Oussoren Y, Stewart FA. Early and late damage in the mouse bladder after radiation combined with cyclophosphamide or cisplatinum, evaluated by two different functional assays. *Acta Oncologica*, 1993; **32**: 679–87.

41. Edrees G, Luts A, Stewart F. Bladder damage in mice after combined treatment with cyclophosphamide and x-rays. The influence timing sequence. *Radiotherapy and Oncology*, 1988; **11**: 349–60.

42. Sauer R, *et al.* Efficacy of radiochemotherapy with platin derivatives compared to radiotherapy alone in organ-sparing treatment of bladder cancer. *International Journal of Radiation Oncology, Biology, Physics*, 1998; **40**: 121–7.

43. von der Maase H. Interactions of drugs and radiation in haemopoietic tissue assessed by lethality of mice after whole-body irradiation. *International Journal of Radiation Biology*, 1985; **48**: 371–80.

44. Millar JL, Blackett NM, Hudspith BN. Enhanced postirradiation recovery of the haemopoietic system in animals pretreated with a variety of cytotoxic agents. *Cell and Tissue Kinetics*, 1978; **11**: 543–53.

45. Yan R, Peters LJ, Travis EL. Cyclophosphamide 24 h before or after total body irradiation: Effects on lung and bone marrow. *Radiotherapy and Oncology*, 1991; **21**: 149–56.

46. Sherman DM, *et al.* The effect of dose-rate and adriamycin on the tolerance of thoracic radiation in mice. *International Journal of Radiation Oncology, Biology, Physics*, 1982; **8**: 45–51.

47. Lochart SP, Down JD, Steel GG. The effect of low dose-rate and cyclophosphamide on the radiation tolerance of the mouse lung. *International Journal of Radiation Oncology, Biology, Physics*, 1986; **12**: 1437–40.

48. Varekamp AE, de Vries AJ, Zurcher C. lung damage following bone marrow transplantation. II Contribution cyclophosphamide. *International Journal of Radiation Oncology, Biology, Physics*, 1987; **13**: 1515–21.

49. Fu KK, Rayner PA, Lam KN. Modification of the effects of continuous low dose-rate irradiation by concurrent chemotherapy infusion. *International Journal of Radiation Oncology, Biology, Physics*, 1984; **10**: 1473–8.

50. Fu KK, Lam KN. Early and late effects of cisplatin and radiation at acute and low dose-rates on the mouse skin and soft tissues of the leg. *International Journal of Radiation Oncology, Biology, Physics*, 1991; **20**: 327–32.

51. Stewart LA, Parmar MKB. Meta-analysis of the literature or of individual patient data: Is there a difference? *Lancet*, 1993; **341**: 418–22.

52. Tannock F. Treatment of cancer with radiation and drugs. *Journal of Clinical Oncology*, 1996; **12**: 3156–74.

53. Walker MD, *et al.* Evaluation of BCNU and/or radiotherapy in the treatment of anaplastic gliomas. *Journal of Neurosurgery*, 1978; **49**: 333–43.

54. Walker MD, *et al.* Randomized comparisons of radiotherapy and nitrosoureas for the treatment of malignant glioma after surgery. *New England Journal of Medicine*, 1980; **303**: 1323–9.

55. EORTC. Evaluation of CCNU, VM-26 plus CCNU, and procarbazine in supratentorial brain gliomas. *Journal of Neurosurgery*, 1981; **31**: 55–27.

56. Green SB, *et al.* Comparisons of carmustine, procarbazine and high-dose methylprednisone as additions to surgery and radiotherapy for the treatment of malignant glioma. *Cancer Treatment Reports*, 1983; **67**: 121–32.

57. Hatlevoll R, *et al.* Combined modality treatment of operated astrocytomas <grade 3 and 4. A prospective and randomized study of misonidazole and radiotherapy with two different radiation schedules and subsequent CCNU chemotherapy. Stage II of a prospective multicenter trial of the Scandinavian Glioblastoma Study Group. *Cancer*, 1985; **56**: 41–7.

58. Nelson F, *et al.* Combined modality approach to treatment of malignant gliomas—Re-evaluation of RTOG 7401/ECOG 1374 with long-term follow-up. *NCI Monographs*, 1988; **6**: 279–84.

59. Trojanowsky T, *et al.* Postoperative radiotherapy and radiotherapy combined with CCNU chemotherapy for treatment of brain gliomas. *Journal of Neurooncology*, 1988; **6**: 285–91.

60. EORTC Brain Tumor Group. Cisplatin does not enhance the effect of radiation therapy in malignant gliomas. *European Journal of Cancer*, 1991; **27**: 568–71.

61. Halperin EC, Gaspar L, Imperato J, Salter M, Herndon J, Dowling S. An analysis of radiotherapy data from the CNS cancer consortium's randomized prospective trial comparing AZQ to BCNU in the treatment of patients with primary malignant brain tumors. *American Journal of Clinical Oncology*, 1993; **16**: 277–83.

62. Hildebrand J, *et al.* Adjuvant therapy with dibromodulcitol and BCNU increases survival of adults with malignant gliomas. *Neurology*, 1994; **44**: 1479–83.

63. Halperin EC, *et al.* A phase III randomized prospective trial of external beam radiotherapy, mitomycin C, Carmustine, and 6-mercaptopurine for the treatment of adults with anaplastic glioma of the brain. *International Journal of Radiation Oncology, Biology, Physics*, 1996; **34**: 793–802.

64. Roberts JT, Thomas DGT, Bleehen NM, Abram P, *et al.* MRC randomised trial of adjuvant chemotherapy in high grade glioma (HGG) —BR05. *Radiotherapy and Oncology*, 1998; **48** (Suppl. 1): 77 (Abstract 304).

65. Solero CL, *et al.* Controlled study with BCNU vs. CCNU as adjuvant chemotherapy following surgery plus radiotherapy for glioblastoma multiforme. *Cancer Clinical Trials*, 1979; **2**: 43–8.

66. Afra D, Kocsis B, Dobay J, Eckhardt S. Combined radiotherapy and chemotherapy with dibromodulcitol and CCNU in the postoperative treatment of malignant gliomas. *Journal of Neurosurgery*, 1983; **59**: 106–10.

67. Levin V, *et al.* Superiority of post-radiotherapy adjuvant chemotherapy with CCNU, procarbazine, and vincristine (PVC) over BCNU for anaplastic gliomas: NCOG 6G61 final report. *International Journal of Radiation Oncology, Biology, Physics*, 1990; **18**: 321–4.

68. Fine HA, Dear KBG, Loeffler JS, Black PM, Canellos GP. Meta-analysis of radiation therapy with and without adjuvant chemotherapy for malignant gliomas in adults. *Cancer*, 1993; **71**: 2585–97.

69. The Department of Veterans Affairs Laryngeal Cancer Study Group. Induction chemotherapy plus radiation compared with surgery plus radiation in patients with advanced laryngeal cancer. *New England Journal of Medicine*, 1991; **24**: 1685–90.

70. Lefebvre JL, *et al.* (for the EORTC Head and Neck Cancer Cooperative Group). Larynx preservation in pyriform sinus cancer: Preliminary results of a European organization for research and treatment of cancer phase III trial. *Journal of the National Cancer Institute*, 1996; **88**: 890–9.

71. Bourhis J, Eschwege F. Radiotherapy-chemotherapy combinations in head and neck squamous cell carcinoma: Overview of randomized trials. *Anticancer Research*, 1996; **16**: 2397–402.

72. Lo TCM, *et al.* Combined radiation therapy and 5-fluorouracil for advanced squamous cell carcinoma of the oral cavity and oropharynx: a randomized study. *American Journal of Roentgenology, Radium Therapy and Nuclear Medicine*, 1976; **126**: 229–35.

73. Stefani S, Chung TS. Hydroxyurea and radiotherapy in head and neck cancer—Long term results of a double-blind prospective study. *International Journal of Radiation Oncology, Biology, Physics*, 1980; **6**: 1398.

74. Shanta V, Krishnamurthi S. Combined bleomycin and radiotherapy in oral cancer. *Clinical Radiology*, 1980; **31**: 617–20.

75. Vermund H, *et al.* Bleomycin and radiation therapy in squamous cell carcinoma of the upper aero-digestive tract: a phase III clinical trial. *International Journal of Radiation Oncology, Biology, Physics*, 1985; **11**: 1877–86.

76. Fu KK, *et al.* Combined radiotherapy and chemotherapy with bleomycin and methotrexate for advanced inoperable head and neck cancer: Update of Northern California Oncology Group randomized trial. *Journal of Clinical Oncology*, 1987; **5**: 1410–18.

77. Gupta NK, Pointon RCS, Wilkinson PM. A randomized clinical trial to contrast radiotherapy with radiotherapy and methotrexate given synchronously in head and neck cancer. *Clinical Radiology*, 1987; **38**: 575–81.

78. Eschwege F, *et al.* Ten year results of randomized trial comparing radiotherapy and concomitant bleomycin to radiotherapy alone in epidermoid carcinomas of the oropharynx: Experience of the European Organization for the Research and Treatment of Cancer. *National Cancer Institute Monographs*, 1988; **6**: 275–8.

79. Sanchiz F, *et al.* Single fraction per day versus two fractions per day versus radiochemotherapy in the treatment of head and neck cancer. *International Journal of Radiation Oncology, Biology, Physics*, 1990; **19**: 1347–50.

80. Keane TJ, *et al.* A randomized trial of radiation therapy compared to split course radiation therapy combined with mitomycin C and 5 fluorouracil as initial treatment for advanced laryngeal and hypopharyngeal squamous carcinoma. *International Journal of Radiation Oncology, Biology, Physics*, 1993; **25**: 613–8.

81. Browman GP, *et al.* Placebo-controlled randomized trial of intravenous infusional 5-fluorouracil during standard radiotherapy in locally advanced head and neck cancer. *Journal of Clinical Oncology*, 1994; **12**: 2648–53.

82. Haffty BG, *et al.* Chemotherapy as an adjunct to radiation in the treatment of squamous cell carcinoma of the head and neck: Results of the Yale Mitomycin Randomized Trials. *Journal of Clinical Oncology*, 1997; **15**: 268–76.

83. Jeremic B, *et al.* Radiation therapy alone or with concurrent low-dose daily either cisplatin or carboplatin in locally advanced unresectable squamous cell carcinoma of the head and neck. a prospective randomized trial. *Radiotherapy and Oncology*, 1997; **43**: 29–37.

84. Wendt TG, *et al.* Simultaneous radiochemotherapy versus radiotherapy alone in advanced head and neck cancer: a randomized multicenter study. *Journal of Clinical Oncology*, 1998; **16**: 1318–24.

85. Al-Sarraf M, *et al.* Chemoradiotherapy versus radiotherapy in patients with advanced nasopharyngeal cancer: Phase III randomized intergroup study 0099. *Journal of Clinical Oncology*, 1998; **16**: 1310–17.

86. Brizel DM, *et al.* Hyperfractionated irradiation with or without concurrent chemotherapy for locally advanced head and neck cancer. *New England Journal of Medicine*, 1998; **338**: 1798–804.

87. Calais G, *et al.* Randomized trial of radiation therapy versus concomitant chemotherapy and radiation therapy for advanced-stage oropharynx carcinoma [see comments]. *Journal of the National Cancer Institute*, 1999; **91**: 2081–6.

88. Stell PM. Adjuvant chemotherapy in head and neck cancer. *Seminars in Radiation and Oncology*, 1992; **2**: 195–205.

89. Munro AJ. An overview of randomised controlled trials of adjuvant chemotherapy in head and neck cancer. *British Journal of Cancer*, 1995; **71**: 83–91.

90. El-Sayed S, Nelson N. Adjuvant and adjunctive chemotherapy in the management of squamous cell carcinoma of the head and neck region: a meta-analysis of prospective and randomized trials. *Journal of Clinical Oncology*, 1996; **14**: 838–47.

91. SEGOG. A randomized trial of combined multidrug chemotherapy and radiotherapy in advanced squamous cell carcinoma of the head and neck. *European Journal of Surgical Oncology*, 1986; **12**: 289–95.

92. Adelstein D, *et al.* Simultaneous versus sequential combined technique therapy for squamous cell head and neck cancer. *Cancer*, 1990; **65**: 1685–91.

93. Merlano M, *et al.* Randomized comparison of two chemotherapy, radiotherapy scheme for stage III and IV unresectable squamous cell carcinoma of the head and neck. *Laryngoscope*, 1990; **100**: 531–42.

94. Taylor S, *et al.* Randomized comparison of neoadjuvant cisplatinum and fluorouracil infusion followed by radiation versus concomitant treatment in advanced head and neck cancer. *Journal of Clinical Oncology*, 1994; **12**: 385–95.

95. Pignon JP, Bourhis J, Domenge C, Designe L. Chemotherapy added to locoregional treatment for head and neck squamous-cell carcinoma: three meta-analyses of updated individual data. MACH-NC Collaborative group. Meta-Analysis of Chemotherapy on Head and Neck Cancer. *Lancet*, 2000; **355**: 949–55.

96. Horiot JC, *et al.* Hyperfractionation versus conventional fractionation in oropharyngeal carcinoma: final analysis of a randomized trial of the EORTC cooperative group of radiotherapy. *Radiotherapy and Oncology*, 1992; **25**: 231–41.

97. Warde P, Payne D. Does thoracic irradiation improve survival and local control in limited-stage small-cell carcinoma of the lung. A meta-analysis. *Journal of Clinical Oncology*, 1992; **10**: 890–5.

98. Pignon JP, *et al.* A randomized combined modality trial in small cell carcinoma of the lung. Comparison of combination chemotherapy-radiation therapy versus cyclophosphamide-radiation therapy effects of maintenance chemotherapy and prophylactic whole brain irradiation. *New England Journal of Medicine*, 1992; **327**: 1618–24.

99. Perry MC, Eaton WL, Propert KJ, *et al.* Chemotherapy with or without radiation therapy in limited small-cell carcinoma of the lung. *New England Journal of Medicine*, 1987; **316**: 912–18.

100. Murray N, *et al.* Importance of timing for thoracic irradiation in the combined modality treatment of limited-stage small-cell lung cancer. *Journal of Clinical Oncology*, 1993; **11**: 336–44.

101. Takada M, Fukuoka M, Furuse K, *et al.* Phase III study of concurrent versus sequential thoracic radiotherapy in combination with cisplatin and etoposide for limited stage small cell lung cancer: a randomized study. *Proceedings of the American Society for Clinical Oncology*, 1997; **15**: 372 (Abstract).

102. Work E, *et al.* Randomized study of initial versus late chest irradiation combined with chemotherapy in limited-stage small-cell lung cancer. *Journal of Clinical Oncology*, 1997; **15**: 3030–7.

103. Jeremic B, *et al.* Initial versus delayed accelerated hyperfractionated radiation therapy and concurrent chemotherapy in limited small-cell lung cancer: a randomized study. *Journal of Clinical Oncology*, 1997; **15**: 893–900.

104. Kristjansen PEG, Hansen HH. Prophylactic cranial irradiation in small cell lung cancer—an update. *Lung Cancer Supplement*, 1995; **3**: 23–40.

105. Ball DL, Matthews JP. Prophylactic cranial irradiation: More questions than answers. *Semininars in Oncology*, 1995; **5**: 61–8.

106. Gregor A. Prophylactic cranial irradiation in small-cell lung cancer: Is it ever indicated? *Oncology*, 1998; **12** (Suppl. 2): 19–24.

107. Arriagada R, *et al.* Prophylactic cranial irradiation for patients with small-cell lung cancer in complete remission. *Journal of the National Cancer Institute*, 1995; **87**: 183–90.

108. Gregor A, *et al.* Prophylactic cranial irradiation is indicated following complete response to induction therapy in small-cell lung cancer: Results of a multicentre randomised trial. *European Journal of Cancer*, 1997; **33**: 1752–8.

109. Auperin A, *et al.* Prophylactic cranial irradiation for patients with small-cell lung cancer in complete remission. Profylactic Cranial Irradiation Overview Collaborative Group. *New England Journal of Medicine*, 1999; **341**: 476–84.

110. Soresi E, *et al.* A randomized clinical trial comparing radiation therapy versus radiation therapy plus cis-dichlorodiammine platinum (II) in the treatment of locally advanced non-small cell lung cancer. *Seminars in Oncology*, 1988; **15** (Suppl. 7): 20–5.

111. Schaake-Koning C, *et al.* Effects of concomitant cisplatin and radiotherapy on inoperable non-small-cell lung cancer. *New England Journal of Medicine*, 1992; **326**: 524–30.

112. Trovó MG, *et al.* Radiotherapy versus radiotherapy enhanced by cisplatin in stage III non-small-cell lung cancer. *International Journal of Radiation Oncology, Biology, Physics*, 1992; **24**: 11–5.

113. Blanke C, *et al.* Phase III trial of thoracic irradiation with or without cisplatin for locally advanced unresectable non-small cell lung cancer: a Hoosier Oncology Group protocol. *Journal of Clinical Oncology*, 1995; **13**: 1425–9.

114. Jeremic B, *et al.* Randomized trial of hyperfractionated radiation therapy with or without concurrent chemotherapy for stage III non-small-cell lung cancer. *Journal of Clinical Oncology*, 1995; **13**: 452–8.

115. Jeremic B, *et al.* Hyperfractionated radiation therapy with or without concurrent low-dose daily carboplatin/etoposide for stage III non-small-cell lung cancer: a randomized study. *Journal of Clinical Oncology*, 1996; **14**: 1065–70.

116. Mattson K, *et al.* inoperable non-small cell lung cancer: radiation with or without chemotherapy. *European Journal of Cancer and Clinical Oncology*, 1988; **24**: 477–82.

117. Morton RF, *et al.* Thoracic radiation therapy alone compared with combined chemoradiotherapy for locally unresectable non-small cell lung cancer. *Annals of Internal Medicine*, 1991; **115**: 681–6.

118. Le Chevalier T, *et al.* Radiotherapy alone versus combined chemotherapy and radiotherapy in nonresectable non-small-cell lung cancer: First analysis of a randomized trial in 353 patients. *Journal of the National Cancer Institute*, 1991; **83**: 417–23.

119. Wolf M, *et al.* Radiotherapy alone versus chemotherapy with ifosfamide/vindesine followed by radiotherapy in unresectable locally advanced non-small cell lung cancer. *Seminars in Oncology*, 1994; **21** (Suppl. 4): 42–7.

120. Sause W, *et al.* Radiation Therapy Oncology Group (RTOG) 88–08 and Eastern Cooperative Oncology Group (ECOG) 4588: Preliminary results of a phase III trial in regionally advanced, unresectable non-small-cell lung cancer. *Journal of the National Cancer Institute*, 1995; **87** (3): 198–205.

121. Dillman RO, *et al.* Improved survival in stage III non-small-cell lung cancer: seven-year follow-up of Cancer and Leukemia Group B (CALGB) 8433 trial. *Journal of the National Cancer Institute*, 1996; **88**: 1210–5.

122. Marino P, Preatoni A, Cantoni A. Randomized trials of radiotherapy alone vs. combined chemotherapy and radiotherapy in stages III a and III b non-small-cell lung cancer: a meta-analysis. *Cancer*, 1995; **76**: 593–601.

123. Non-small Cell Lung Cancer Collaborative Group. Chemotherapy in non-small cell lung cancer: a meta-analysis using updated data on individual patients from 52 randomised clinical trials. *British Medical Journal*, 1995; **311**: 899–909.

124. Pritchard RS, Anthony SP. Chemotherapy plus radiotherapy compared with radiotherapy alone in the treatment of locally advanced, unresectable, non-small-cell lung cancer: a meta-analysis. *Annals of Internal Medicine*, 1996; **125**: 723–9.

125. Bunn PA, Vokes EE, Langer CJ, Schiller JH. An update on North American randomized studies in non-small cell lung cancer. *Seminars in Oncology*, 1998; **4** (Suppl. 9): 2–10.

126. Giaccone G, Manegold C, Rosell R, Gatzemeier U, Quoix E. An update on European randomized studies in non-small cell lung cancer. *Seminars in Oncology*, 1998; **4** (Suppl. 9): 11–7.

127. Early Breast Cancer Trialists' Collaborative Group. Systemic treatment of early breast cancer by hormonal, cytotoxic, or immune therapy: 133 randomised trials involving 31,000 recurrences and 24,000 deaths among 75,000 women. *Lancet*, 1992; **339**: 71–85.

128. Bonadonna G, Valagussa P, Moliterni A, Zambetti M, Brambilla C. Adjuvant cyclophosphamide, methotrexate, and fluorouracil in node-positive breast cancer: the results of 20 years of follow-up. *New England Journal of Medicine*, 1995; **332**: 01–906.

129. Cuzick J, *et al.* Cause-specific mortality in long-term survivors of

breast cancer who participated in trials of radiotherapy. *Journal of Clinical Oncology*, 1994; **12**: 447–53.

130. **Early Breast Cancer Trialists' Collaborative Group.** Effects of radiotherapy and surgery in early breast cancer: an overview of the randomized trials. *New England Journal of Medicine*, 1994; **333**: 1444–55 [Erratum, *New England Journal of Medicine*, 1996; **334**: 1003].

131. **Overgaard M, et al.** (for the Danish Breast Cancer Cooperative Group 82b Trial): Postoperative radiotherapy in high-risk premenopausal women with breast cancer who receive adjuvant chemotherapy. *New England Journal of Medicine*, 1997; **336**: 949–55.

132. **Ragaz J, et al.** Adjuvant radiotherapy and chemotherapy in node-positive premenopausal women with breast cancer. *New England Journal of Medicine*, 1997; **337**: 956–62.

133. **Overgaard M, et al.** Postoperative radiotherapy in high-risk postmenopausal breast-cancer patients given adjuvant tamoxifen. Danish Breast Cancer Cooperative Group, DBCG 82c randomised trial. *Lancet*, 1999; **353**: 1641–8.

134. **Recht A, et al.** The sequencing of chemotherapy and radiation therapy after conservative surgery for early-stage breast cancer. *New England Journal of Medicine*, 1996; **334**: 1356–61.

135. **Andersen AP, et al.** Irradiation, chemotherapy and surgery in oesophageal cancer: a randomized clinical study. *Radiotherapy and Oncology*, 1984; **2**: 179–88.

136. **Araújo CMM, et al.** A randomized trial comparing radiation therapy versus concomitant radiation therapy and chemotherapy in carcinoma of the thoracic oesophagus. *Cancer*, 1991; **67**: 2258–61.

137. **Herskovic A, et al.** Combined chemotherapy and radiotherapy compared with radiotherapy alone in patients with cancer of the esophagus. *New England Journal of Medicine*, 1992; **326**: 1593–8.

138. **Roussel A, et al.** Results of the EORTC-GTCCG phase III trial of irradiation vs. irradiation and CDDP in inoperable oesophageal cancer. *Proceedings of the American Society for Clinical Oncology*, 1994; **13**: 199 (Abstract).

139. **Le Prise E, et al.** A randomized study of chemotherapy, radiation therapy, and surgery versus surgery for localized squamous cell carcinoma of the oesophagus. *Cancer*, 1994; **73**: 1779–84.

140. **Walsh TN, et al.** A comparison of multimodal therapy and surgery for esophageal adenocarcinoma. *New England Journal of Medicine*, 1996; **335**: 462–7.

141. **Bosset JF, et al.** Chemoradiotherapy followed by surgery compared with surgery alone in squamous-cell cancer of the esophagus. *New England Journal of Medicine*, 1997; **337**: 161–7.

142. **Bonenkamp HJ, et al.** Adjuvant therapy after curative resection for gastric cancer: Meta-analysis of randomized trials. *Journal of Clinical Oncology*, 1993; **11**: 1441–7.

143. **Regine WF, Abrams RA.** Adjuvant therapy for pancreatic cancer: Back to the future. *International Journal of Radiation Oncology, Biology, Physics*, 1998; **42**: 59–63.

144. **Freedman GM, Coia LR.** Adjuvant and neoadjuvant treatment of rectal cancer. *Seminars in Oncology*, 1995; **22**: 611–24.

145. **Boulis-Wassif S, et al.** Final results of a randomized trial on the treatment of rectal cancer with preoperative radiotherapy alone or in combination with 5-fluorouracil, followed by radical surgery. Trial of the European Organization on Research and Treatment of Cancer Gastrointestinal Tract Cancer Cooperative Group. *Cancer*, 1984; **53**: 1811–18.

146. **Gastrointestinal Tumor Study Group.** Prolongation of the disease-free interval in surgically treated rectal carcinoma. *New England Journal of Medicine*, 1985; **312**: 1465–72.

147. **Krook JE, et al.** Effective surgical adjuvant therapy for high-risk rectal carcinoma. *New England Journal of Medicine*, 1991; **324**: 709–15.

148. **Wolmark N, et al.** Randomized trial of postoperative adjuvant chemotherapy with or without radiotherapy for carcinoma of the rectum: National Surgical Adjuvant Breast and Bowel Project Protocol R-02. *Journal of National Cancer Institute*, 2000; **92**: 361–2.

149. **NIH Consensus Conference.** Adjuvant therapy for patients with colon and rectal cancer. *Journal of the American Medical Association*, 1990; **264**: 1444–50.

150. **Minsky BD.** Current and future directions in adjuvant combined-modality therapy of rectal cancer. *Oncology*, 1997; **11** (Suppl. 10): 61–8.

151. **Cummings BJ.** Concomitant radiotherapy and chemotherapy for anal cancer. *Seminars in Oncology*, 1992; **19** (Suppl. 11): 102–8.

152. **UKCCCR Anal Cancer Trial Working Party.** Epidermoid anal cancer: results from the UKCCCR randomised trial of radiotherapy alone versus radiotherapy, 5-fluorouracil, and mitomycin. *Lancet*, 1996; **348**: 1049–54.

153. **Bartelink H, et al.** Concomitant radiotherapy and chemotherapy is superior to radiotherapy alone in the treatment of locally advanced anal cancer: results of a phase III randomized trial of the European Organization for Research and Treatment of Cancer Radiotherapy and Gastrointestinal Cooperative Groups. *Journal of Clinical Oncology*, 1997; **15**: 2040–9.

154. **Flam M, et al.** Role of mitomycin in combination with Fluorouracil and radiotherapy, and of salvage chemoradiation in the definitive nonsurgical treatment of epidermoid carcinoma of the anal canal: Results of a phase III randomized intergroup study. *Journal of Clinical Oncology*, 1996; **14**: 2527–39.

155. **Shearer RJ, et al.** Adjuvant chemotherapy in T3 carcinoma of the bladder. A prospective trial: Preliminary report. *British Journal of Urology*, 1988; **62**: 558–64.

156. **Wallace DM, et al.** Neo-adjuvant (pre-emptive) cisplatin therapy in invasive transitional cell carcinoma of the bladder. *British Journal of Urology*, 1991; **67**: 608–15.

157. **Malmström PU, et al.** Five-year followup of a prospective trial of radical cystectomy and neoadjuvant chemotherapy: Nordic Cystectomy Trial I. The Nordic Cooperative Bladder Cancer Study Group. *Journal of Urology*, 1996; **155**: 1903–6.

158. *International collaboration of trialists.* Neo-adjuvant cisplatin, methotrexate, and vinblastine chemotherapy for muscle-invasive bladder cancer: a randomised controlled trial. *Lancet*, 1999; **354**: 533–40.

159. **Shipley WU, et al.** Phase III trial of neoadjuvant chemotherapy in patients with invasive bladder cancer treated with selective bladder preservation by combined radiation therapy and chemotherapy: inital results of Radiation Therapy Oncology Group 89-03. *Journal of Clinical Oncology*, 1998; **16**: 3576–83.

160. **Coppin CM, et al.** Improved local control of invasive bladder cancer by concurrent cisplatin and preoperative or definitive radiation. The National Cancer Institute of Canada Clinical Trials Group. *Journal of Clinical Oncology*, 1996; **14**: 2901–7.

161. **Richards B, et al.** Adjuvant chemotherapy with doxorubicin (Adriamycin) and 5-fluorouracil in T3, NX, M0 bladder cancer treated with radiotherapy. *British Journal of Urology*, 1983; **55**: 386–91.

162. **Ghersi D, et al.** Does neoadjuvant cisplatin-based chemotherapy improve the survival of patients with locally advanced bladder cancer: a meta-analysis of individual patient data from randomized clinical trials. *British Journal of Urology*, 1995; **75**: 206–13.

163. **Tester W, et al.** Neoadjuvant combined modality program with selective organ preservation for invasive bladder cancer: Results of Radiation Therapy Oncology Group phase II trial 8802. *Journal of Clinical Oncology*, 1996; **14**: 119–26.

164. **Shipley WU, Zietman AL, Kaufman DS, Althausen AF, Heney NM.** Invasive bladder cancer: treatment strategies using transurethral surgery, chemotherapy and radiation therapy with selection for bladder conservation. *International Journal of Radiation Oncology, Biology, Physics*, 1997; **39**: 937–43.

165. **Fellin G, et al.** Combined chemotherapy and radiation with selective organ preservation for muscle-invasive bladder carcinoma. A single-institution phase II study. *British Journal of Urology*, 1997; **90**: 44–9.

166. Pollack A, Zagars GK. Androgen ablation in addition to radiation therapy for prostate cancer: is there true benefit. *Seminars in Radiation and Oncology*, 1998; **2**: 95–106.

167. Pilepich MV, *et al.* Androgen deprivation with radiation therapy compared with radiation therapy alone for locally advanced prostatic carcinoma: a randomized comparative trial of the radiation therapy oncology group. *Urology*, 1995; **45**: 616–23.

168. Pilepich MV, *et al.* Phase III trial of androgen suppression using goserelin in unfavorable-prognosis carcinoma of the prostate treated with definitive radiotherapy: Report of the Radiation Therapy Oncology Group protocol 85–31. *Journal of Clinical Oncology*, 1997; **15**: 1013–21.

169. Bolla M, *et al.* Improved survival in patients with locally advanced prostate cancer treated with radiotherapy and goserelin. *New England Journal of Medicine*, 1997; **337**: 295–300.

170. Perez CA, Grigsby PW, Chao CKS. Chemotherapy and irradiation in locally advanced squamous cell carcinoma of the uterine cervix: a review. *Seminars in Radiation and Oncology*, 1997; 7 (Suppl. 2): 45–65.

171. Shueng PW, Hsu WL, Jen YM, Wu CJ, Liu HS. Neoadjuvant chemotherapy followed by radiotherapy should not be a standard approach for locally advanced cervical cancer. *International Journal of Radiation Oncology, Biology, Physics*, 1998; **40**: 889–96.

172. Hreshchyshyn MM, *et al.* Hydroxyurea or placebo combined with radiation to treat stages IIIB and IB cervical cancer confined to the pelvis. *International Journal of Radiation Oncology, Biology, Physics*, 1979; **5**: 317–22.

173. Runowicz CD, *et al.* Concomitant cisplatin and radiotherapy in locally advanced cervical carcinoma. *Gynecologic Oncology*, 1989; **34**: 395–401.

174. Mickiewicz E, *et al.* Chemotherapy (CT) + radiotherapy (RT) vs. radiotherapy alone in cervical cancer stage IIab to Iba, a randomized study. *Proceedings of the American Society for Clinical Oncology*, 1991; **10**: 192 (Abstract).

175. Stehman FB, *et al.* Hydroxyurea versus misonidazole with radiation in cervical carcinoma: Long-term follow-up of a Gynecologic Oncology Group trial. *Journal of Clinical Oncology*, 1993; **11**: 1523–8.

176. Thomas G, *et al.* A randomized trial of standard versus partially hyperfractionated radiation with or without concurrent 5-fluorouracil in locally advanced cervical cancer. *Gynecologic Oncology*, 1998; **69**: 137–45.

177. Keys HM, *et al.* Cisplatin, radiation and adjuvant hysterectomy compared with radiation and adjuvant hysterectomy for bulky stage IB cervical carcinoma. *New England Journal of Medicine*, 1999; **340**: 1154–61.

178. Peters WA, *et al.* Concurrent chemotherapy and pelvic radiation therapy compared with pelvic radiation therapy alone as adjuvant therapy after radical surgery in high-risk early-stage cancer of the cervix. *Journal of Clinical Oncology*, 2000; **18**: 1606–13.

179. Morris M, *et al.* Pelvic radiation with concurrent chemotherapy compared with pelvic and para-aortic radiation for high-risk cervical cancer. *New England Journal of Medicine*, 1999; **340**: 1137–43.

180. Rose PG, *et al.* Concurrent cisplatin-based radiotherapy and chemotherapy for locally advanced cervical cancer. *New England Journal of Medicine*, 1999; **340**: 1144–53.

181. Whitney CW, *et al.* Randomized comparison of fluorouracil plus cisplatin versus hydroxurea as an adjunct to radiation therapy in stage IIB–IVA carcinoma of the cervix with negative par-aortic lymph nodes: a gynecologic oncology group and southwest oncology group study. *Journal of Clinical Oncology*, 1999; **17**: 1339–48.

182. Wong LC, *et al.* Chemoradiation and adjuvant chemotherapy in cervical cancer. *Journal of Clinical Oncology*, 1999; **17**: 1339–48.

183. Chauvergne J, *et al.* Neoadjuvant chemotherapy of stage IIb or III cancers of the uterine cervix. Long-term results of a multicenter randomized trial of 151 patients. *Bulletin of Cancer*, 1993; **80**: 1069–79.

184. Souhami L, *et al.* A randomized trial of chemotherapy followed by pelvic irradiation therapy in stage IIIB carcinoma of the cervix. *Journal of Clinical Oncology*, 1991; **9**: 970–7.

185. Tattersall MHN, Ramirez C, Coppleson M. A randomized trial comparing platinum-based chemotherapy followed by radiotherapy alone in patients with locally advanced cervical cancer. *International Journal of Gynecology and Cancer*, 1992; **2**: 244–51.

186. Kumar L, *et al.* Chemotherapy followed by radiotherapy versus radiotherapy alone in locally advanced cervical cancer: a randomized study. *Gynecologic Oncology*, 1994; **54**: 307–15.

187. Tattersall MH, *et al.* Randomized trial of epirubicin and cisplatin chemotherapy followed by pelvic radiation in locally advanced cervical cancer. Cervical Cancer Study Group of the Asian Oceanian Clinical Oncology Association. *Journal of Clinical Oncology*, 1995; **13**: 444–51.

188. Sundførd K, *et al.* Radiotherpay and neoadjuvant chemotherapy for cervical carcinoma: a randomized multicenter study of sequential cisplatin and 5-fluorouracil and radiotherapy in advanced cervical carcinoma stage 3B and 4A. *Cancer*, 1996; **77**: 2371–8.

189. Tattersall MHN, Ramirez C, Coppleson M. A randomized trial of adjuvant chemotherapy after radical hysterectomy in stage Ib-IIa cervical cancer patients with pelvic lymph node metastases. *Gynecologic Oncology*, 1992; **46**: 175–81.

190. Curtin JP, *et al.* Adjuvant chemotherapy versus chemotherapy plus pelvic irradiation for high-risk cervical cancer patients after radical hysterectomy and pelvic lymphadenectomy (RH-PLND): a randomized phase III trial. *Gynecologic Oncology*, 1996; **61**: 3–10.

191. Sailer SL. The role of radiation therapy in localized Ewing's sarcoma. *Seminars in Radiation and Oncology*, 1997; **7**: 225–35.

192. Verweij J, Pinedo HM, Suit HD (eds). *Soft tissue sarcomas: present achievements and future prospects.* Boston: Kluwer, Academic Publishers, 1997.

193. Sarcoma Meta-analysis Collaboration. Adjuvant chemotherapy for localised resectable soft-tissue sarcoma of adults: meta-analysis of individual data. *Lancet*, 1997; **350**: 1647–54.

194. Loeffler M, *et al.* Meta-analysis of chemotherapy versus combined modality treatment trials in Hodgkin's disease. *Journal of Clinical Oncology*, 1998; **16**: 818–29.

195. Specht L, Gray RG, Clarke MJ, Peto R. Influence of more extensive radiotherapy and adjuvant chemotherapy on long-term outcome of early-stage Hodgkin's disease: a meta-analysis of 23 randomized trials involving 3,888 patients. *Journal of Clinical Oncology*, 1998; **16**: 830–43.

196. Miller TP, *et al.* Chemotherapy alone compared with chemotherapy plus radiotherapy for localized intermediate- and high-grade non-Hodgkin's lymphoma. *New England Journal of Medicine*, 1998; **339**: 21–6.

197. Gerard CR, Jones JM, Schiff PB. Taxol and radiation. *Journal of the National Cancer Institute*, 1993; **85**: 89–94.

198. Minarik L, Hall E. Taxol in combination with acute and low dose rate irradiation. *Radiotherapy and Oncology*, 1994; **32**: 124–8.

199. Shewach DS, Lawrence TS. Radiosensitization of human solid tumor cell lines with gemcitabine. *Seminars in Oncology*, 1996; **23** (Suppl. 10): 65–71.

200. Lawrence TS, Eisbruch A, Shewach DS. Gemcitabine-mediated radiosensitization. *Seminars in Oncology*, 1997; **2** (Suppl. 7): 24–8.

201. Capizzi RL. Amifostine: The preclinical basis for broad-spectrum selective cytoprotection of normal tissues from cytotoxic therapies. *Seminars in Oncology*, 1996; **4** (Suppl. 8): 2–17.

202. Tannehill SP, Mehta MP. Amifostine and radiation therapy. Past, present, future. *Seminars in Oncology*, 1996; **4** (Suppl. 8): 69–77.

Hyperthermia

Olav Dahl and Jens Overgaard

Introduction

Knowledge about heat treatment of tumours is as old as written medical texts. In the Edwin Smith surgical papyrus, which was probably the first medical text and which dates back more than 5000 years, a description is given of a patient with a tumour in the breast which was treated with hyperthermia (cautery).[1] Similar procedures have since been used throughout recorded history. The current interest in hyperthermia can probably be ascribed to the German physician W. Busch who, in 1886, described a patient with a facial sarcoma which disappeared after severe infection with erysipelas which caused prolonged high fever. This and similar observations led the New York surgeon William B. Coley to develop his 'mixed bacterial toxin', thereby becoming the father of both the modern use of hyperthermia and of non-specific immunotherapy for the treatment of cancer. Concurrently others applied local hyperthermia directly. Thus the Swedish physician F. Westermark reported in 1898 that moderately elevated temperatures (< 45 °C) could induce significant regression and even disappearance of cervical carcinomas.[2] The positive interaction of hyperthermia with radiation was known about at the beginning of the twentieth century, but as radiotherapy techniques developed there was less need for additional therapies until the role of radiotherapy reached a plateau. George Hahn and others have provided experimental evidence for the positive interaction of hyperthermia and drugs.[3],[4]

The biological rationale for the interaction of hyperthermia with radiation and drugs in experimental studies is sound, both *in vitro* and in animals. The major obstacles towards clinical use have been the problems of applying heat to tumours more than 3 cm below the skin in local applications and focusing the heat towards tumours within the body for regional heating. Heating technology is still far from ideal, but during the last decades substantial improvement has occurred, both in heating devices and in the ability to predict the individual heating pattern by accurate simulation of energy deposition in models of the patient. Several phase III clinical studies have now been published.

This chapter is intended to give an overview of the biological rationale for and the current clinical experience of local and regional hyperthermia, especially in combination with radiation as currently applied in oncology.

Biological effects

Cellular effects of hyperthermia

Heat alone

Moderate heat treatment (approximately 41 to 45 °C) is able to destroy malignant and normal cells *in vitro* when applied for some time. The mechanisms of this destruction are complex and involve damage to nuclei, membranes, and cytoplasmic components.[3],[5]–[7]

Sensitivity to hyperthermia varies greatly between different cell lines, but as a whole there is no specifically enhanced sensitivity in malignant cells. Most experimental studies have been made with rodent cell lines, which in general seem to be somewhat more sensitive to hyperthermia than human cells, but otherwise do not differ from them qualitatively.[8],[9]

Thermal damage to cells depends on the temperature and the heating time and appears to follow a well-established Arrhenius plot indicating a specific inactivation energy, which is in accord with the

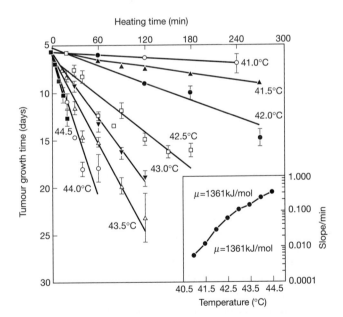

Fig. 1 Tumour growth time as a function of heating time for a solid mouse mammary carcinoma heated in the range 41.0 to 44.5 °C *in vivo*. Tumour growth time was the time taken for tumours to regrow to five times their pretreatment size. Each datum point represents the mean ± standard error of the mean. Inset: time–temperature plot showing the slope of the dose–response curves as a function of heating temperature. Based on the slope values, the activation energy (μ) was calculated by Arrhenius analysis. (Redrawn from Lindegaard and Overgaard.[5])

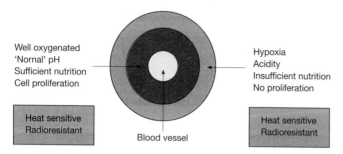

Fig. 2 Schematic illustration of the microenvironment in tumours as a function of insufficient vascularization and its influence on the sensitivity to hyperthermia and irradiation.

effect being due to protein and membrane damage rather than to primary DNA damage (Fig. 1). Other factors such as variation within the cell cycle may also affect heat-induced cell death.[10]

Heat-induced damage is also strongly influenced by the extra-cellular environment. Thus, a milieu characterized by deprived nutritional conditions, including chronic hypoxia, increased acidity, and starvation leading to reduced ATP content, promotes hyperthermic damage (Fig. 2).[6],[11],[12] This is not, as with radiation damage, an oxygen effect. In fact, acute hypoxia or hypoxic conditions persisting for a reasonable time in an otherwise normal environment do not seem to influence the degree of hyperthermic damage. The main factor responsible for the enhanced cell death is probably the increased acidity, and as a whole, cells situated in a deprived environment seem to be considerably more sensitive to hyperthermia than cells under physiological conditions. Since such a deprived environment normally only exists in solid tumours, this enhanced sensitivity is a major factor behind the rationale for applying hyperthermia to the treatment of solid tumours.

Thermal tolerance is the phenomenon by which one heat treatment induces a temporary resistance to subsequent heating.[3],[13] If two heat treatments are separated by a short interval and thermal tolerance has been induced by the first, the second treatment may be of very little value. The magnitude and kinetics of thermal tolerance depend on the heat trauma and differ between various tumours and tissues. It is therefore impossible to predict the exact magnitude of thermal tolerance for a given treatment. Thermal tolerance has been observed in all tissues in which it has been investigated, and must be considered to be a general phenomenon when heat is applied in a fractionated scheme.

Interaction with radiation *in vitro*

Hyperthermia enhances the effect of radiation on cells in culture (hyperthermic radiosensitization). This effect occurs primarily when the radiation is given during hyperthermia (simultaneous treatment); any interval between the two reduces the effect but without qualitative change. The effect is complex, involving both an increase in direct radiosensitivity, depending on temperature and heating time, and a reduced accumulation of sublethal damage resulting in a smaller shoulder to the survival curve.[14] After irradiation there is a reduced variation in sensitivity to hyperthermia as a function of the phase of the cell cycle, as the effect of combined treatment tends to be most pronounced in phases that are most resistant to radiation. The repair of potentially lethal damage can also be reduced by additional heat

treatment. Interestingly, the oxygen effect does not seem to be affected; thus the response to radiation in oxygenated and acutely hypoxic cells seems to be equally sensitized by hyperthermia. There may also be a direct hyperthermic effect independent of the radiation.

Interaction with chemotherapy *in vitro*

The effect of most chemotherapeutic agents is enhanced at elevated temperature.[3],[4] There is no single mechanism that can explain the interaction with drugs. Thus, the effect may include altered drug uptake through the cell membranes, altered chemical reactions within the cells, changes in enzymes activating or inactivating the drugs, or greater susceptibility of the cells towards drugs during hyperthermic stress. In several cell systems more cells die by apoptosis after hyperthermia than without hyperthermia. Furthermore, the effect of the drug may be strongly modified by the cellular environment, especially pH.[3] Examples of drugs which are not enhanced by hyperthermia are antimetabolites (5-fluorouracil, methotrexate), etoposide, taxanes, and vinca alkaloids.

Effect of hyperthermia *in vivo*

Effect of heat on tumours and tissues *in vivo*

In addition to the direct cellular effect of hyperthermia, the response *in vivo* is influenced by various physiological adaptations which cause the response in normal tissues and tumours to differ.[6],[15],[16] This specific hyperthermic cytotoxicity is seen as the direct killing of cells by heat in a deprived microenvironment characterized by insufficient blood supply, with subsequent poor nutrition, and increased acidity due to anaerobic metabolism and the accumulation of lactic acid and other waste products. Cells situated in such areas are highly sensitive to hyperthermia and can be destroyed by heat treatment that does not cause significant damage to cells in a 'normal' environment. Such environmental deprivation does not normally occur in normal tissue, thus favouring a selective effect in tumours.

It is characteristic that hyperthermic cell destruction, both in normal tissues and in tumours, occurs within hours of treatment. Thus the damage is dominated by interphase cell death due to necrosis and apoptosis rather than reproductive cell death seen after radiation. This rapid tissue destruction occurs even faster in tumours within a deprived environment.

Late-occurring heat damage additional to this acute cell destruction has not been described. Thus, the direct heat effect occurs promptly and any subsequent damage appears to be a direct consequence of the acute trauma. This may be the basis for the immediate pain relief often observed after local hyperthermia. After systemic heating, a substantial increase in endorphins may also reduce pain.

In rodents, hyperthermia induces an increase in blood flow, which at higher temperatures is followed by a temperature-dependent decrease in blood flow, especially in tumours.[17],[18] Thus it is possible to achieve relatively higher temperatures in tumours than in normal tissues. Mild hyperthermia may increase blood flow and thus enhance the oxygen content of tissues.[19] However, there is also evidence that tissue oxygen rapidly returns to normal values after the treatment.[20]

Interaction with radiation *in vivo*

Heat interacts with radiation *in vivo* through two different mechanisms: hyperthermic radiosensitization and direct hyperthermic cytotoxicity.[21],[22]

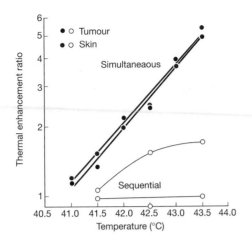

Fig. 3 Thermal enhancement ratio (TER) as a function of temperature in a solid mouse mammary carcinoma and its surrounding skin. Hyperthermia was given for 1 h either simultaneously (full symbols) or 4 h after irradiation (open symbols). The thermal enhancement ratio was calculated as the dose of radiation alone relative to the dose of radiation combined with heat to obtain the given endpoint. (Partially redrawn from Overgaard.[21])

Hyperthermic radiosensitization, expressed as the thermal enhancement ratio (Fig. 3), is most prominent with the simultaneous application of heat and radiation but is of the same magnitude in both tumour and normal tissue. Such treatment will not increase the therapeutic ratio unless the tumour is heated to a higher temperature than the normal tissue. As mentioned above, hyperthermia also has a direct cytotoxic effect, which is especially pronounced in some solid tumours. Moderate heat treatment alone can, almost selectively, destroy tumour cells in a nutritionally deprived, chronically hypoxic and acidic environment. Because cells in a hypoxic environment are the most radioresistant ones, a smaller radiation dose is probably needed to control these cells when combined with hyperthermia. Whereas the cytotoxic effect of heat is independent and has no relation to the timing of the radiation treatment, heat-induced radiosensitization is strongly dependent upon the sequence and interval between the application of the two methods.[21] Maximal sensitization is achieved by true simultaneous treatment (radiation in midheating) and any interval between the two treatments decreases the sensitization, which normally disappears with intervals longer than a few hours (Fig. 3). Thus, if critical normal tissues are heated, the cytotoxicity is best utilized if the heat is given at least 3 to 4 h after irradiation. The magnitude of both the sensitizing and the cytotoxic effect depends on the temperature and heating time. The effect is far more pronounced for radiosensitization. The cytotoxic effect is smaller, but with moderate heat treatment the effect can be directed selectively towards tumour cells in a deprived environment, whereas cells in a normal milieu seem not to suffer any heat damage.

The dual biological effect leaves us with two strategies for applying hyperthermia as an adjuvant to radiotherapy. One is as a radiosensitizing agent enhancing the effect of ionizing radiation in heated tissues. This strategy is probably only valid if hyperthermia and radiation are applied simultaneously. The other strategy utilizes the specific cytotoxic effect on radioresistant cells and is achieved by sequential treatment. From a practical point of view, true simultaneous

treatment is very difficult to achieve with external heating, and the major effect of the combined treatment will have to rely on hyperthermic cytotoxicity. Due to the relatively low blood flow in tumours, the direct cytotoxic effect may be more pronounced in tumours than in normal tissues. In practice simultaneous hyperthermia and radiation are usually achieved only by interstitial therapy.

The biological rationale has been documented in a few clinical studies comparing the effects of simultaneous and sequential treatments in various superficial tumours and normal tissues. The correlation between the biological rationale and the clinical data is impressive.[22] The only divergence between the biological rationale and the clinical data is that the quantitative difference between simultaneous and sequential treatment is less in clinical studies than would be expected from animal studies. In particular it should be noted that when hyperthermia is given in close association with radiotherapy there is a risk of enhancing the radiation damage to normal tissue. In most studies hyperthermia is in practice applied for logistical reasons about 30 min after the radiation. There may be somewhat more pronounced local side-effects with additional side-effects specific to hyperthermia, like erythema, isolated blisters, and burns. There is no documented increase of late radiation effects when radiation is combined with hyperthermia.

Interaction with chemotherapy *in vivo*

The principle behind combining hyperthemia and chemotherapy has been investigated in several experimental tumour systems and these studies have generally confirmed the theoretical rationale.[3],[23] Enhancement of the effect of the drug induced by hyperthermia is characteristically observed if the treatments are given simultaneously, i.e. the drug is administered immediately before the heating, whereas the drug does not seem to enhance the hyperthermic damage. If any interval is allowed between the two modalities, the effect is normally at most additive. There may be different target populations for the two methods, and hyperthermia (at low temperatures) may enhance the effect of the drug by increasing uptake and pharmacokinetics variables or may modify the action through the various mechanisms described above for *in vitro* conditions. For a combination of local or regional hyperthermia with drugs there seems to be an enhanced effect without an undue increase in local side-effects. One should, however, be careful in applying hyperthermia together with a drug in organs where drug-specific side-effects occur. Whole-body hyperthermia has previously been associated with a range of major side-effects. These have now been reduced by better heating methods. It appears that the combination of drugs with whole-body hyperthermia increases the efficacy of the drugs, at the expense of somewhat more side-effects. Whether this approach is better than increasing the drug dose alone remains to be shown in controlled trials.

Technical aspects of hyperthermia

The ideal requirement is that the tumour volume should be uniformly heated (to temperatures above 42 to 43 °C) without creating thermal damage in the surrounding normal tissue. Furthermore, a reasonably accurate measurement of the temperature of the tumour in time and space is needed for proper assessment of the treatment. These requirement are rather difficult to satisfy for the following reasons:

(1) The complex geometry of many tumours makes it difficult to heat the whole tumour in one session.

(2) The blood flow is a major factor in establishing the final temperature distribution and it is largely unknown, difficult to predict, and hard to measure.

(3) Present electromagnetic heating devices for superficial tumours give their best performance in the first few centimetres from the surface, making heating of tumours deeper than 3 cm a technological challenge. Ultrasound reaches deeper, but ultrasound is reflected by air or causes overheating of bone.

(4) Invasive thermometry is limited to relatively few points for practical and ethical reasons.

Nevertheless, technical advances have been made over recent years. In the following sections the main technical aspects will be dealt with briefly. More detailed information can be obtained from recent reviews.[24],[25]

Heat delivery techniques

In most cases either electromagnetic or acoustic methods are used. Tissue has electrical and acoustic resistivity, which means that when a local current density or pressure is applied, absorption will take place. This absorption will give rise to a local increase in temperature proportional to the absorption density, and equilibrium will usually be achieved after 5 to 10 min. The equilibrium or steady state temperature will depend on the cooling (usually applied at the surface through a water bolus), the applied total power, the geometry, the local blood flow, and the thermal properties of the tissue. In some instances the treatment is limited by patient tolerance, often due to local hotspots.

Non-invasive methods for superficial heating

Capacitive heating

The simplest technique for the heating of superficial tumours is to apply low-frequency currents from an electrode on the surface or through a surface bolus, so-called capacitive heating. The other pickup electrode may be large and remote from the region of interest. The technique is quite effective for genuine surface heating because the heating also penetrates depthwise, but if there are fat layers in between the electrodes a large part of the power is delivered to the fat, owing to its greater resistivity. Another drawback is that there may be high electric fields near the edges, so care must be taken to avoid surface burns. Capacitive heating therefore really requires skin cooling (10 °C) and a subcutaneous fat layer less than 1 cm.[26] This method is also widely used in Japan for deep heating, but 21 per cent of the patients have side-effects like pain during heating, later burns, or fat induration.[27]

Radiating applicators

Well-designed radiating applicators avoid the above-mentioned problems. The design usually causes the radiated electric field to run parallel to the fat–muscle interface, thus avoiding the problem of heating the fat and making it easy to match the applicator to the generator so the available power is used. A variety of electromagnetic applicators have been designed over the years for a range of frequencies from 27 to 2450 MHz, encompassing open circular or rectangular waveguides and horns, microstrip antennas, spirals, arrays of smaller applicators, and other arrangements. Based on knowledge of plane-wave propagation in tissue it may be shown that the penetration is largest at the lower frequencies and of the order of 1 cm at the highest frequencies. However, the effective penetration for a given aperture size is to a large extent independent of frequency, due to near-field effects, so for a single applicator the choice of frequency is not so important. Some increase in penetration may be achieved by having a converging phase front in the aperture instead of a diverging one, which, for example, is characteristic of horn antennas.

Ultrasound

Ultrasound is as effective as other methods in heating surface tumours, but the ultrasound waves are scattered from bones and air-filled cavities making it impractical for some regions. The pain threshold may also be lower for ultrasound when there is absorption in bone tissue.

It is often difficult to match the shape of the tumour area with the geometry of the applicator, so attempts have recently been made to cover the surface with a mosaic of relatively small applicators with overlapping heating patterns, thus accommodating irregular shapes. A very important advantage of this arrangement is that the power in the individual elements may be controlled independently, so that an inhomogeneous distribution of blood flow may be counteracted. These mosaic arrays have been used for both electromagnetic and acoustic radiators. A newly developed alternative is to use one scanning applicator over the surface, where the speed of scanning and dwell-time over various areas may be controlled automatically by a computer. Several focused applicators allow heating at considerable depths (8 to 10 cm).

Invasive methods

Invasive techniques have the great advantage that the heating volume may be closely fitted to the tumour volume.

Radiofrequency needle electrodes

The most common invasive technique allows a low-frequency radiofrequency current to flow between needles, commonly called radiofrequency needle electrodes. The frequency is typically a few megahertz, but in principle it could be done at even lower frequencies, although it is customary to avoid frequencies below 50 kHz in order not to interfere with normal body signals. The current flow is transverse to the needle axis with the density highest near the needle, where the temperature will peak. Direct cooling of the needles may push the maximum temperature away from the needle surface. It is important to keep the needles parallel in order to have some axial uniformity. Advantages of the technique are its simplicity, that the length of the needles may be chosen according to the size of the treatment volume, and the possibility of combining the treatment with brachytherapy.

Microwave antennas

A more sophisticated technique is to use the needles as microwave antennas, that is, the inner conductor of a thin coaxial cable is used as a transmitting antenna. One antenna may work alone, in contrast to the radiofrequency needles, but the power density (and temperature) is still largest near the surface of the antenna, resulting in a rather local heating effect. Furthermore, there is some variation along the antenna, making it difficult to utilize the length efficiently, in contrast to the

Table 1 Physical parameters for electromagnetic and ultrasound heating of tissue (data from Hand and ter Haar[28])

Type of wave		Frequency (MHz)	Wavelength (cm)			Penetration depth (cm)		
			In muscle	In fat	In bone	In muscle	In fat	In bone
EM:	RF	0.5–30	610–61	~2000–218	~2000–219	130–14	~1000–160	~1000–160
	µwave	300–1000	11.9–4.1	41–12.6	41–12.6	3.9–2.4	32.1–14.3	32.1–14.3
		2450	1.8	5.2	5.2	1.7	11.2	11.2
US		0.5–5	0.3–0.03	0.3–0.03	0.6–0.06	12–1.2	20–2.0	3–0.09

Abbreviations: EM = electromagnetic; US = ultrasound; RF = radiofrequency; µwave = microwave.

radiofrequency needles. The main advantage is that several antennas may work synchronously in an array. The fields add coherently in phase and, as the fields add with N, the number of elements in the array, the power adds as N squared. Thus, it is possible to have maximum power away from the surface of the antenna for the treatment of a larger volume. This has been used successfully in the treatment of brain tumours, with four elements forming an array.

Other invasive techniques

There are other invasive techniques under development, including the use of small ferromagnetic implants which are heated through an external time-varying magnetic field or a technique that uses hot water through thin pipes. These methods rely on thermal conduction into the tissue, as there is no heat production in the tissue. The piped water method is especially interesting because it allows heating with simultaneous treatment by external beam irradiation.

Non-invasive methods for deep (regional) heating

Electromagnetic heating

Deep electromagnetic heating is restricted to frequencies below approximately 100 MHz, as the penetration of higher frequencies is too small. Such low frequencies indicate a large wavelength, making focusing difficult, hence the name regional heating. As for interstitial techniques, the penetration may be improved by using an array, in this case around the body with the electric field parallel to the body axis. In early versions of this technique all the elements, typically four, were excited with equal power and equal phase, giving relatively uniform heating over the cross section. A disadvantage is that large volumes of water are required as the bolus and coupling medium. New versions with the antennas in an elliptical arrangement have permitted smaller bolus pressures. In the first generation of applicators there were no degrees of freedom except by placing the patient in an off-centre position. In newer systems the number of rows of antennas has increased to eight, and the length is divided into three. Thus 24 separate antennas can be individually regulated allowing the individual radiators to have arbitrary amplitude and phase, making it possible to manipulate the power distribution and to some extent the temperature distribution. The total power needed for a given treatment may also be reduced. Another variant is use of a ring applicator around the body with a radiant annular gap between two antennae.

It is important to know that the penetration of electromagnetic waves is dependent on the frequency applied (Table 1), but it also varies strongly according to the type of tissue through which the waves pass. By definition the penetration depth is the depth in centimetres which reduces the amplitude of the wave to e^{-1} (37 per cent) of its value at the surface.[28] At this depth the energy deposition has decreased to e^{-2} (14 per cent) of its value at the surface. In practice the penetration depth of a clinical surface applicator is given as the depth at which it reaches 25 per cent of its maximum specific absorption rate (SAR). One of the problematic physical restrictions for heat deposition is that the longer the wavelength of an electromagnetic wave, the better its tissue penetration, but then the possibility of focusing the energy is reduced.

Ultrasound

The acoustic properties of tissue are different from its electromagnetic properties in the sense that the attenuation per wavelength is much smaller. This means that it is possible using ultrasound to have rather small focal regions of the order of millimetres at depths of more than tens of centimetres. In general such a small hotspot is not an advantage in itself, but by mechanical scanning and focusing very good results may be achieved at depth, even close to bone, because the power decays quickly behind a focus.

Thermometry

Hyperthermia is defined as the deposition of heat energy to achieve temperatures above 41 °C in tumours. The clinical effect of hyperthermia is therefore closely related to the thermal parameters (the minimum or maximum temperature) obtained in the malignant tumour.[29],[30] However, descriptions of thermal dose including both the temperature and time are superior to simple temperature recordings.[31] The heat dose is generally expressed as the cumulative equivalent minutes (CEM) at 43 °C for at least 90 per cent of the measured points (CEM 43 °C T_{90}, the tenth percentile) or as CEM 43 °C T_{min} (the lowest temperatures measured in the tumour), according to a well-established formula.[32]–[34] The CEM 43 °C exhibits the strongest correlation with immediate tumour response and durable local control in recurrent or metastatic breast cancer and for malignant melanomas (Fig. 4).[35] Invasive thermometry is mandatory to obtain the necessary temperature information for these calculations.

Use of invasive thermometry caused 64 per cent of the treatment-related complications when pelvic catheters were inserted by a transgluteal computed tomography (CT) guided technique and left *in situ* for the whole treatment period.[36] The catheters frequently had to be removed. By a similar technique for most patients, 19 per cent

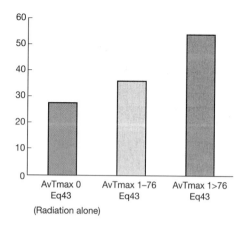

Fig. 4 Local control of malignant melanoma at 5 years posttreatment as a function of heat dose expressed as average maximal temperature (AvTmax) from each heating session expressed according to the CEM 43 °C formula. Tumours treated by radiation alone serve as controls. (Based on data presented by Overgaard et al.[30])

of catheters had to be removed due to side-effects.[37] However, the local problems were strongly correlated with the dwell time of the catheters and never occurred for dwell times of less than 5 days. In 300 patients with 1491 deep-heating sessions, the incidence of complications was 11 per cent, of which 4 per cent were scored as serious.[34] In this study only 2 per cent of catheter complications occurred in pelvic/abdominal sites when the catheters were removed after each session, in contrast to 11 per cent of catheter complications for various carcinomas where the catheters were left in place. This study underlined that the thermometry data were useful for steering the power deposition for regional heating, and that thermometry data from the first heating session could be used to determine if the patients were suitable for further heating. In Bergen we remove all catheters after each session. We place two or three catheters into the tumours through rectal and vaginal mucous membranes or directly percutaneously into the tumours before each heating session. After having treated 50 patients with pelvic tumours for more than 250 sessions, we have had no serious complications—only three small instances of bleeding after removal of the catheters—and no local infections. We therefore strongly advocate the use of invasive thermometry by transient insertion of catheters to ensure control of the temperature during hyperthermia.

For clinical studies of hyperthermia we recommend careful quality assurance procedures.[38] The guidelines of the European Society for Hyperthermic Oncology and the Radiation Therapy Oncology Group, which all emphasize thermometry, should be followed.[39]–[43] The recording of temperature is still a must for scientific use of hyperthermia. Only exceptionally (in superficial bladder tumours and small tumours close to major vessels) may tumour-related endoluminal thermometry replace intratumoral thermometry. It is also important that the actual thermometry system selected is properly calibrated to give reliable recordings to within 0.1 °C. A possible future approach may be non-invasive thermometry using the proton shift of magnetic resonance (MR) obtained during heating. In a pilot study of four patients, a close

correlation between fibreoptic temperature measurements and corrected MR thermometry measurements was observed.[44] In Europe such MR-based non-invasive thermometry during regional heating with the BSD 2000 heating device is currently under investigation in Munich and Berlin. The spatial resolution is about 1 cm^3 and the thermal resolution 0.5 °C.[45] Another approach is the use of microwave radiometry.[46]

Clinical results

Hyperthermia alone

Hyperthermia alone has been used for many tumour types, using different methods and schedules. In summary, the overall rate of response to heat alone was 42 per cent, with a complete response rate of 12 per cent, among 515 patients treated in 22 different studies published in the 1970s and 1980s.[47] The response to hyperthermia alone may occur very rapidly, typically within 1 to 2 weeks, but unfortunately the duration of response is transitory. The main problem is that local tumours can only be eradicated at high temperatures, which simultaneously cause significant damage to surrounding normal tissues. Due to the cost of equipment and manpower, hyperthermia alone is rarely indicated for palliative reasons only. However, both in curative and palliative therapy hyperthermia may substantially increase the effect of other modalities like radiation and chemotherapy and should therefore be considered as part of a combined modality strategy for treatment of cancer. In this review we focus on recently published phase III studies with locally advanced tumours at different tumour sites.

Hyperthermia and radiation

The use of heat as an adjuvant to radiation treatment of local and regional disease is promising. The indications for hyperthermia in clinical radiotherapy are twofold. First, hyperthermia may be included in the primary treatment of locally advanced tumours, where improved local control is expected to result in subsequent improved cure rates and better survival.[22],[48] Secondly, hyperthermia has an evident role in palliative treatment when combined with radiation, especially for recurrent tumours in previously irradiated areas. There are still technical limitations on heat delivery, and homogeneous heating of a defined tumour volume is a goal rather than an achievable fact. However, some tumour types at specific sites have repeatedly shown an improved response to combined treatment with heat and radiation in such a way that we expect this treatment to become an established first-line treatment for certain indications. It should be remembered that current clinical practice is based upon a substantial number of phase I/II studies and also some phase III studies.[22] When the dose–effect curves for radiation alone are compared with isodose curves for radiation and heat, a consistent shift to the left can be observed with a therapeutic enhancement rate of about 1.5 to 1.6 (Fig. 5).

Superficial tumours

Primary treatment offered to patients with a relatively long life expectancy must be optimal. Hyperthermia should consequently only be added to those radiation treatment schedules already known to

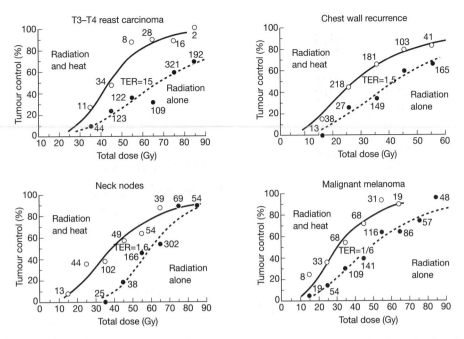

Fig. 5 Dose–response relation for advanced breast carcinoma (top left), recurrent breast carcinoma (top right), advanced neck nodes (bottom left), and malignant melanoma (bottom right) treated with radiation or combined radiation and hyperthermia. The total doses for breast and head and neck carcinomas were normalized assuming daily fractions of 2 Gy and an alpha/beta ratio of 25 Gy; for malignant melanoma the alpha/beta ratio was considered to be 2.5 Gy. (See Overgaard for further details.[22])

be as effective as possible. The combined therapy is therefore based on radiotherapy administered by a standard daily fractionation schedule, adding heat once or twice a week. Particular attention should be paid to possible hyperthermic increase of the radiation effect in normal tissues. If excess heating of normal tissues can be avoided, the heat treatment should preferably be given simultaneously or immediately after radiation, because some radiosensitization by heat may add to the destruction of tumours by heat alone. Otherwise, an interval of approximately 3 to 4 h is recommended between radiation and hyperthermia to avoid any sensitization of the radiation response in normal tissue.[22]

Superficial tumours of varying histology

Generally hyperthermia increases the complete response rate when combined with radiation compared with that obtained with radiation alone or in historical controls.[22] An important multi-institutional study including 307 patients treated with different heating techniques failed to support an earlier promising phase II study.[49] Radiation was administered as 32 Gy divided into eight fractions, and hyperthermia was aimed at achieving a temperature of 42 °C for 45 to 60 min. The results were similar in both groups, with an overall complete response in 30 per cent of patients treated with radiotherapy alone and in 32 per cent in the combined group. In a subgroup analysis for tumours of less than 3 cm in diameter, however, there was an improved complete response rate for combined therapy— 62 per cent for breast and 67 per cent for other tumours localized on the trunk and extremities compared with 40 per cent after radiotherapy alone. The explanation proposed by the authors is that they often failed to treat deeper lesions properly due to limitations in their heating devices. In contrast, lesions greater than 3 cm in

diameter showed no difference in response between the two treatment groups. One may also question the actual radiation schedule used. This negative study has had a great influence on the interest in hyperthermia as a clinical modality in the United States. The study has clearly demonstrated the need for careful quality assurance procedures in hyperthermia.

Malignant melanoma

Hyperthermia aimed at achieving a temperature of 43 °C for 60 min was added to hypofractionated radiotherapy in the treatment of superficial metastasic and recurrent malignant melanoma; radiotherapy consisted of a radiation dose of 8 or 9 Gy in three fractions with an interval of 4 days.[50] The study was organized by the European Society for Hyperthermic Oncology and recruited 70 patients with 139 lesions. The complete response rate in the combined group was 62 per cent, almost twice as high as after radiotherapy alone (35 per cent; $p < 0.05$). The 2-year local control rate was also significantly improved: 46 versus 28 per cent (Fig. 6). When paired lesions were analysed within the same patients, there was significantly better response in the combined treated group ($p < 0.014$).[30] In a multivariate analysis the CEM 43 °C and radiation dose corresponded with the response rate.

Breast cancer

Recurrent breast cancer frequently causes local discomfort and can easily be recognized by patients, thus increasing their psychological distress. In a small randomized study including 18 patients with multiple skin metastases from breast carcinomas, hyperthermia at 41 to 45 °C for 45 min was administered 0.5 to 4 h after irradiation, fractionated as 3 Gy × 10.[51] The objective response rate was significantly enhanced in the combined group (57 per cent complete

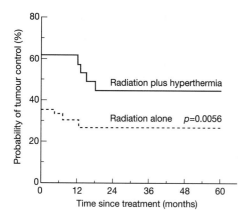

Fig. 6 Probability of tumour control after treatment with radiation alone or radiation plus hyperthermia for recurrent or metastatic malignant melanoma. (Reproduced from Overgaard *et al.* with permission from *The Lancet.*[50])

response and 32 per cent partial response) compared with radiotherapy alone (25 per cent complete response and 25 per cent partial response) ($p = 0.004$).

The results of five randomized controlled studies including 306 breast cancer patients with both locally advanced and recurrent tumours have been jointly published.[52] The 171 patients treated with combined therapy exhibited a complete response rate of 59 per cent in contrast to 41 per cent in 135 patients given radiotherapy alone ($p < 0.001$). Thus the enhancement effect of combined therapy favoured such treatment by an odds ratio of 2.3. There was a substantially better and longer duration of response in recurrent tumours compared with locally advanced primary tumours, probably reflecting better heating of the more superficial tumours located on the chest wall rather than larger primary tumours within the breast tissue. Tumours at a depth of less than 3 cm had a complete response rate of 60 per cent in contrast to 38 per cent for deeper tumours. Primary tumours and tumours outside previously irradiated areas had a 61 per cent complete response rate after radiation doses above 40 Gy, in contrast to a complete response rate of 46 per cent for tumours localized in previously irradiated areas where only 28 Gy were administered in eight fractions. The difference is therefore probably related to higher radiation doses. The tumour size also influenced the response: of tumours less than 16 cm², 70 per cent exhibited a complete response compared with only 45 per cent of tumours occupying larger areas. These authors also noted that the tumours regressed more rapidly in the combined treatment group than after radiation alone. For extensive recurrences it is possible to obtain 95 per cent complete response with radiation and overlapping hyperthermia fields if the fields are separated by at least 3 days to avoid thermal tolerance.[53] In some centres in The Netherlands combined treatment is now offered as standard to patients with breast cancer recurring in previously irradiated areas.[54]

Head and neck lymph nodes

Radiotherapy is the treatment of choice for inoperable lymph node metastases from squamous cell carcinomas of the head and neck.

Several phase II studies have clearly indicated a benefit for hyperthermia added to radiotherapy.[22],[55],[56] In a phase III trial, 44 patients with cervical N3 lymph nodes were randomized into two groups.[57] One group had radiation alone—67.5 Gy, given as 2 to 2.5 Gy daily—or the same radiation dose combined with hyperthermia aimed at a minimum temperature of 42 to 42.5 °C for 30 min. An interim analysis of the first 36 tumours revealed better tumour control in the combined group, and the study was therefore prematurely closed for ethical reasons. A long-term follow-up analysis confirmed that adjuvant hyperthermia improved the local control at 5 years to 69 per cent compared with 24 per cent in the radiation alone group ($p = 0.015$).[57] The 5-year survival rate was also significantly improved: 53 per cent in the combined group versus 0 in the radiation alone group ($p = 0.02$). The addition of cisplatin (20 mg/m²/week) did not further enhance the response or survival.[58]

A similar study from India, including 65 patients with lymph node metastases from different primary head and neck cancers, showed improved tumour control in the combined group, particularly for patients with advanced disease.[59] In stage III disease 58 per cent had a complete response and 25 per cent a partial response after combined therapy versus 20 per cent and 40 per cent respectively after radiation alone ($p < 0.05$). For stage IV disease a complete response of 70 per cent and partial response of 29 per cent were observed after combined therapy versus 37 per cent and 25 per cent respectively after radiotherapy alone ($p < 0.05$). Long-term results have not yet been published.

A third phase III randomized study on treatment of neck nodes was organized by the European Society for Hyperthermic Oncology. This study had to be closed because of slow recruitment. There was no difference in initial response (53 versus 50 per cent complete response) or local control (33 versus 31 per cent) in the radiation arm and radiation combined with hyperthermia respectively.[60]

The role of hyperthermia in head and neck nodes should be further studied. The varying results may reflect problems of heat delivery, especially for deep-seated tumours, difficulties in proper heating of tumours with curved surfaces, and the particular anatomy of the head and neck with its bony structures and air cavities.

Salivary gland tumours

In a study of 10 advanced and 10 recurrent parotid carcinomas (15 primaries and five nodal recurrences), radiation doses of 66 and 30 Gy respectively were combined with twice-weekly hyperthermia by local heating to 42.0 °C for 30 min.[61] An initial favourable response, 80 per cent complete response and 20 per cent partial response, transformed to a 5-year local recurrence-free survival of 62 ± 13 per cent. A small pilot study including four patients (six tumour sites) with adenoid cystic carcinoma of the salivary glands supported these findings.[62] All gave a complete response after radiation combined with heat. Two of the patients remained in long-term local control after 42 and 63 months.

Interstitial thermoradiotherapy

By combining brachytherapy and hyperthermia the same catheters can be used for both radiation and heating of localized tumours. The different heating techniques, radiofrequency heating, microwaves, ferromagnetic seeds, or hot water sources, have recently been extensively reviewed.[63] A complete response was obtained in 55 to

65 per cent of cases and a partial response in another 25 to 30 per cent. The late toxicity was on average 8 per cent (range 4 to 17 per cent). In some series of primary tumours the complete response rate was above 80 per cent. Head and neck cancer, breast tumours, pelvic malignancies such as uterine cervix and rectum, and skin cancer have been treated in these phase I/II studies.

There were no differences in any endpoint (complete response 53 and 55 per cent, 2-year survival 34 and 35 per cent) in a randomized phase III study including recurrent or persistent tumours, mostly head and neck and pelvic tumours given radiation alone or radiation with heat.[64]

In a recently published randomized trial on patients with glioblastoma multiforme, interstitial hyperthermia (30 min at 42.5 to 50 °C) was administered to one group before and after a brachytherapy boost of 60 Gy at 0.4 to 0.6 Gy/h added to external radiotherapy of 59.4 Gy in 1.8 Gy fractions.[34] Despite the small numbers (39 patients had radiation alone and 40 radiation plus hyperthermia), the time to progression (from 33 to 44 weeks respectively; $p = 0.045$) and survival (from 76 to 85 weeks respectively; $p = 0.02$) was significantly improved in those patients receiving the radiation plus hyperthermia. The 2-year survival probability was enhanced from 15 to 31 per cent. There was somewhat more toxicity in the heated group, especially grade 1 and 2 neurological changes, but overall the toxicity was mild to moderate.

Generally, the technique of interstitial hyperthermia seems to be more effective than most other methods of heat application, but this may reflect the selection of smaller tumours for implantation as smaller volume and the minimum temperature are independent variables for a complete response.[65] Further confirmatory randomized studies are therefore warranted.

Oesophageal cancer

Despite the oesophagus being localized centrally in the body, tumours start in the superficial squamous cell layer. They are therefore easily accessible by intracavitary heating devices. Oesophageal carcinoma is one of the commonest cancers in Asia. In Japan the group of Sugimachi has performed several randomized studies on preoperative or definitive treatment using hyperthermia combined with radiation alone, or radiation plus either bleomycin or cisplatin.[66]–[70] These phase III studies have shown that hyperthermia both increases local tumour control and improves survival in both advanced cases and early stages combined with surgical resection. Chinese studies have reported excellent results after combinations of radiation, chemotherapy, and hyperthermia.[71],[72] It is difficult to really assess the contribution of hyperthermia in a complex setting where different radiation and chemotherapy regimens are used, together with variable selection of patients for surgery. A problem for conduction of phase III trials in Western countries is that this disease is so rare that no single institution with ready access to hyperthermia equipment will be able to recruit sufficient patients to confirm the interesting Japanese data.

Malignant lymphoma

Combination chemotherapy is the cornerstone of curative treatment for malignant lymphoma. However, some patients with cutaneous locations and early lymph node manifestation of non-Hodgkin's lymphoma are treated by radiotherapy. Among patients with paired lesions (five cutaneous lymphomas, 14 mycosis fungoides, and seven Kaposi's sarcomas), a complete response was obtained in respectively four of five, 11 of 14, and four of seven lesions treated by hyperthermia and radiation, in contrast to one of five, two of 12, and three of seven after radiation alone.[73] Local lymphomas, many failing to respond to radiotherapy or recurring after previous radiotherapy or chemotherapy, have also been included in four small pilot studies.[74]–[76] Despite a relatively low radiation dose combined with local hyperthermia, local tumour control was obtained in 37 out of 42 patients, giving an overall response rate of 88 per cent (99 per cent confidence interval of 66 to 97 per cent). Most of the patients did not have local recurrence for the rest of their lives. These pilot studies deserve further clinical testing in localized lymphomas where a local curative or palliative response cannot be granted by current radiation or chemotherapy treatments alone.

Hyperthermia in deep-seated tumours

Modern imaging techniques like CT, MR, and ultrasound provide better localization of tumours for radiotherapy planning. Modern radiotherapy equipment including linear accelerators and treatment planning systems allows better deposition of the radiation energy. Therefore an increased response may be expected from radiotherapy alone. As an example the 5-year survival rate for stage III cervical cancer increased from 25 per cent in 1973 to 47 per cent in 1983.[77] However, particularly bulky cervical cancers with diameters above 6 cm remain a challenge.[78],[79] Despite giving a high radiation dose of 85 Gy for stage IIB and III cervical tumours, pelvic failure occurred in 35 to 50 per cent of cases.[80] In a small randomized study in stage II and III cervical cancer, the same radiation regimen (brachytherapy combined with external radiation) alone or combined with hyperthermia did not increase the side-effects.[81] Local tumour control was observed in 14 out of 20 evaluable cases in the combined group, in contrast to 11 of 22 in the control group.

These findings were substantiated by a subgroup analysis of about 100 patients included in a Dutch prospectively randomized study.[82] The local control rate increased from 57 per cent after radiation alone to 83 per cent when radiation was combined with hyperthermia in advanced cervical carcinoma. This response transferred into an improved survival rate, which increased from 27 per cent to 52 per cent after 3 years' follow-up (Fig. 7). It is of particular interest that most of the patients were negatively selected with many bulky tumours having diameters above 6 cm. Cisplatin should possibly be added to the combination (see below).

In total the Dutch study included 360 pelvic tumours (bladder cancer, cervical cancer, and mostly recurrent rectal cancer).[82] The patients received full-dose external radiotherapy to a total dose of 65 Gy for rectal cancer, 56 Gy for bladder cancer, and 66 Gy for cervical cancer, including brachytherapy. The original heating was delivered by the BSD 2000 system in Rotterdam, the Amsterdam four-waveguide applicator system in Amsterdam, and the Utrecht coaxial TEM applicator in Utrecht. Hyperthermia was given once per week during the period of external radiotherapy for a total of five treatments. After a heating-up period of a maximum of 30 min, the hyperthermia treatment continued for 60 min. Despite the fact that 9 per cent of the patients randomized to hyperthermia did not, for various reasons, actually receive the allocated treatment, a significant improvement in durable local control was observed with an initial complete response rate of 39 per cent after radiotherapy alone and

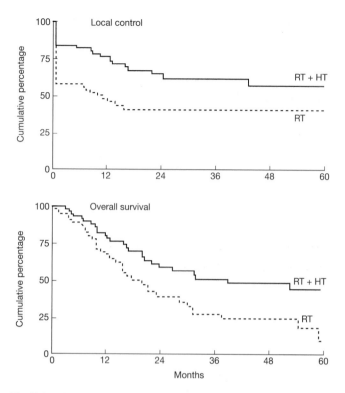

Fig. 7 Local tumour control and overall survival among 100 patients with cervical carcinomas included in the Dutch Deep Hyperthermia Trial (data from January 1998). (With permission from J van Der Zee.)

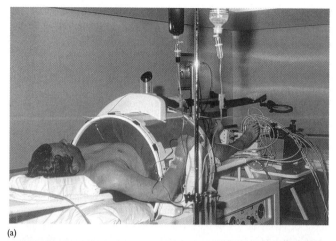

(a)

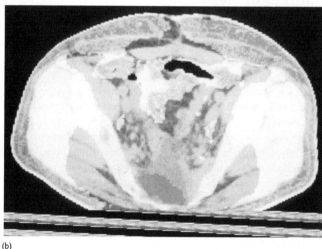

(b)

Fig. 8 (a) A patient undergoing deep microwave hyperthermia for locally advanced rectal cancer using a phase array system.[85] (b) Heat distribution shown following invasive thermometry. (Illustration provided by Professor P. Wust, Department of Diagnostic Radiology and Radiation Oncology, Chatité, Humboldt University of Berlin, Germany.) (See also Plate 1.)

56 per cent in the combined arm ($p = 0.005$). The overall 3-year survival was also significantly improved, from 24 per cent following radiotherapy to 31 per cent following combined treatment ($p = 0.014$).

A new surgical technique, total mesorectal excision, has reduced the local recurrence rate for operable rectal cancer to the order of 5 per cent. Until more data are provided, hyperthermia should be limited to combinations with radiation for locally advanced or recurrent rectal cancers where positive results have been published in small series.[83],[84] A German phase II trial in patients with locally advanced (T3/4) rectal cancer has recently been published.[85] Thirty-seven patients received hyperthermia using the BSD 2000 system combined with 45 Gy of radiotherapy and chemotherapy (350 mg/m² 5-fluorouracil plus 5 mg leucovorin) (Fig. 8 and see also Plate 1). The resection specimens from five patients showed no viable tumour (pathologically confirmed complete response rate of 14 per cent) and none of the patients developed a local recurrence after resection with clear margins at a follow-up of 38 months. However, to assess the contribution of hyperthermia to long-term tumour control we must await the results of the ongoing randomized trial (preoperative radiochemotherapy with and without hyperthermia). On the other hand, an Australian group have failed to demonstrate any difference in a small randomized study with 73 eligible patients with locally recurrent or unresectable primary adenocarcinomas of the rectum.[86]

Hyperthermia and chemotherapy

Cytotoxic drugs can be administered as systemic intravenous therapy targeting all cancer cells within the body, as a local perfusion to the extremities and liver, or as intracavitary administration (intraperitoneally and into the bladder). It is practical to distinguish between systemic chemotherapy combined with local or regional hyperthermia, isolated hyperthermic perfusion, and whole-body hyperthermia combined with systemic drugs. The background for the combination of hyperthermia and cytotoxic drugs is based on solid experimental data.[3],[4],[87]

Systemic chemotherapy combined with local or regional hyperthermia

The rationale for this combination is to exploit the effect of hyperthermia to increase the effect of a systemic drug at a site where there is a tumour bulk or where previous experience has shown that tumour tends to recur after chemotherapy alone.

Soft tissue sarcomas

High-grade soft tissue sarcomas tend to recur locally and exhibit a high frequency of distant metastases. Multimodal treatment with pre- and postoperative combination chemotherapy and local radiotherapy and surgery has improved local control, especially for limb tumours, while high-grade sarcomas located in other areas still have a poor prognosis. The Munich group has combined systemic chemotherapy with regional hyperthermia.[88],[89] In their first studies ifosfamide was infused during regional hyperthermia while the drug etoposide was administered 1 day before hyperthermia, based on animal studies showing that this drug may have a reduced effect when combined with hyperthermia.[90] Some patients previously demonstrating resistance to ifosfamide achieved local tumour control when the same drug was combined with hyperthermia. There was a correlation between the intratumour temperature and the response rate. The feasibility of the procedure and the initial complete response rate was acceptable. The second 1991 protocol combined regional hyperthermia with etoposide, doxorubicin, and ifosfamide for 4 days every third week, with hyperthermia administered on days 1 and 4.[89] A clinical objective response was obtained in 42 per cent of 59 patients. Six tumours exhibited a histopathological complete response at the time of surgery. It is noteworthy that 63 per cent (37 out of 59) of the patients with a poor prognosis included in the trial showed no evidence of disease after an observation time of 34 months. We have also tested this regimen in Bergen and seen some striking clinical effects. The Munich group has proposed an interesting explanation for this improved disease-free survival. In the laboratory they have demonstrated that after hyperthermia heat shock proteins are transferred to the cell membrane where they may serve as receptors for natural killer T cells.[91] These studies have supported an ongoing multicentre study by the European Organization for Research on Treatment of Cancer (protocol 62961) and the European Society for Hyperthermic Oncology. In this phase III study chemotherapy with etoposide, ifosfamide, and doxorubicin is given with and without regional hyperthermia to patients with high-grade primary or recurrent tissue sarcoma with defined poor prognostic factors before and after locoregional therapy with surgery or radiation.

Bladder cancer

Superficial *in situ* bladder cancer is often treated by instillation of a solution of a cytotoxic drug or bacille Calmette–Guérin. In a small randomized study 40 mg mitomycin-C in 50 ml water was administered into the bladder, the solution was changed after 30 min, and the combined group received simultaneous hyperthermia for 1 h with 915 MHz administered by a microwave applicator in the bladder.[92] The temperature measured at the superficial layer of the bladder wall was 42.5 to 45.5 °C. Despite most of the patients having failed prior therapy, a pathological complete response was documented in 66 per cent of the 29 patients in the combination group in contrast to only 22 per cent of 23 patients in the chemotherapy alone group ($p < 0.01$). After a follow-up period of 37 months, superficial transitional cell carcinoma of the bladder had recurred in 27 per cent of the hyperthermia group against 39 per cent after chemotherapy alone.

Cervical cancer

The use of induction chemotherapy and a combination of radiotherapy and chemotherapy have until now not produced improved result in cervical cancer. However, recent publications indicate that radiation combined with concurrent weekly cisplatin or cisplatin combined with 5-fluorouracil every third week improves local control and survival.[93]–[96] Hyperthermia enhances the effect of cisplatin generally, and a 52 per cent response rate is reported after hyperthermia combined with cisplatin in pelvic recurrences of cervical carcinomas failing previous radiotherapy.[4],[97] In a Japanese randomized study, local hyperthermia increased the response rate of a combination of bleomycin and mitomycin-C from 40 per cent to 84 per cent in primary tumours, and from 17 per cent to 45 per cent in recurrent vulvar and vaginal carcinomas.[98] Hyperthermia may therefore be considered in addition to a combination of radiation and cisplatin, as a trimodal approach, to further improve the control of locally advanced cervical carcinomas.

Hyperthermic perfusion with cytotoxic drugs

Malignant melanoma (see also Section 8)

Treatment by normothermic perfusion with melphalan has a long tradition for malignant melanoma of the extremities. In a non-randomized comparison, 47 per cent of 203 patients obtained a complete response after drug alone, while the heated perfusion of melphalan yielded 82 per cent complete response in 22 patients.[99] In a phase II study a complete response rate of 65 per cent and a partial response rate of 26 per cent were obtained in 24 tumours.[100] A corresponding very high response rate was obtained when mild hyperthermia (temperature 40 to 40.5 °C for 90 min) was combined with high-dose tumour necrosis factor-α, interferon-γ, and melphalan. This regimen yielded a complete response of 90 per cent and a partial response of 10 per cent in 29 patients.[101] It is noteworthy that 18 of these patients had failed previous isolated perfusion with melphalan or cisplatin. A later report confirmed a complete response rate of 91 per cent of 53 patients after tumour necrosis factor-α and interferon-γ plus melphalan, in contrast to a complete response rate of 52 per cent after melphalan alone under mild hyperthermic conditions.[102] The main problem with therapy with tumour necrosis factor-α is that the duration of the antitumour effect is relatively short, with relapses after 3 to 4 months in many patients.[103]

Two randomized controlled studies have compared mild (39 to 40 °C) hyperthermic perfusion with melphalan (0.9 to 1.5 mg/kg body weight for the lower and 0.45 to 1.0 mg/kg body weight for the upper extremities) for 60 min as an adjuvant therapy after surgery with surgery alone.[104],[105] The German study was prematurely closed due to improved disease-free survival in the perfusion group. There was a recurrence rate of 11 per cent of 53 patients in the perfusion group in contrast to 49 per cent after surgery alone ($p < 0.01$).[105] The difference in all subgroups based on tumour thickness was significant. The survival was also significantly ($p < 0.01$) improved after perfusion, but survival rates in the control group were very much worse than usually observed. In the Swedish study, 17 per cent of patients remained free of recurrence after surgery alone, in contrast to 30 per cent in the group given perfusion prior to surgery.[106] Despite the significantly improved disease-free survival ($p = 0.04$), there was no difference in survival among the 69 patients included in this trial. A problem with these two studies is that one group had both hyperthermia and drug while the control group had surgery alone. A design where one group had normothermic perfusion and one group hyperthermic perfusion is necessary to assess the true role of hyperthermia in this setting.

A review of published phase II studies concluded that the data from studies of hyperthermic perfusion with melphalan indicated a 10 per cent improved survival at 5 years.[99] A large randomized multicentre study accumulating 832 assessable patients with primary cutaneous melanoma more than 1.5 mm thick failed to show any difference in time to distant metastases or overall survival.[106] The occurrence of transit metastases was reduced from 7 to 3 per cent, and the occurrence of regional lymph node metastases in patients without elective lymph node dissection was reduced from 13 to 7 per cent. Based on this large study, adjuvant mild hyperthermic perfusion with melphalan alone can hardly be recommended as a routine therapy in the clinic.

Soft tissue sarcoma

Hypethermic isolated perfusion has also been used as a preoperative procedure for advanced or recurrent limb sarcomas. For sarcomas a 5-year survival rate of 70 per cent and a local recurrence rate of 14 per cent were obtained in phase II studies.[107] Using a combination of melphalan and tumour necrosis factor-α combined with isolated hyperthermic (40 to 40.5 °C) limb perfusion for soft tissue sarcomas, high clinical and even higher pathological responses, 29 per cent and 53 per cent respectively, were observed in 186 patients with recurrent sarcomas treated at eight European centres.[108]

Whole-body hyperthermia and systemic drugs

A major obstacle to successful cancer therapy is the development of systemic metastases in the majority of cancer sites. Experimental studies have indicated that hyperthermia is able to increase the effect of many cytotoxic drugs. It has been established that most patients can tolerate a systemic temperature of about 41.8 °C for several hours, and a substantial number of phase I/II studies have explored the role of whole-body hyperthermia at 41.8 °C combined with various systemic drugs.[109]–[111] Newer techniques using hot water chambers for heating are better tolerated than earlier techniques, and conscious patients can now be treated without significant patient distress. Whole-body hyperthermia has until now chiefly been applied to patients with tumours at very advanced stages. It is expected that whole-body hyperthermia will become a treatment modality for increasing the response in chemosensitive tumours. The fact that hyperthermia is able to purge bone marrow used for transplantation makes this option especially interesting. Long-duration mild hyperthermia may also cause tumour destruction by stimulation of apoptosis or other immunological mechanisms, but the clinical results of this strategy is still limited.[112]

Side-effects of hyperthermia

For superficial heating, blisters and burns were previously a problem. With proper use of a bolus—circulation of cooling water within a plastic bag—for cooling of the superficial skin layers and correct coupling between the applicator and the body, thermal burns are now more rarely seen.

In earlier versions of regional heating devices, patients were frequently caused general distress by irradiation to large volumes by stray electromagnetic radiation, and heating sessions had frequently to be terminated due to local pain caused by hot-spots at tissue boundaries.[113]–[115] Development of reliable treatment planning systems has provided the means to steer the energy deposition and

excessive heating of fat tissue in the perineum can be avoided with proper use of additional bags containing saline.[116],[117] Deep heating is therefore currently feasible with acceptable patient discomfort. Only a limited increase in side-effects has occurred for combinations of hyperthermia with radiation. When combining hyperthermia with drugs one should be aware of possible aggravation of drug-specific organ effects in the heated organ system.

Conclusion

Hyperthermia is currently an accepted clinical modality which has evolved from being a treatment of last hope for advanced cases into a treatment which enhances the effect of radiation and drugs in patients where current therapy is often failing. It can also be combined with surgery in many instances as patients may harbour residual tumour tissue at small sites. It is particularly important not to judge the final results of a therapy on the basis of initial clinical response alone since one frequently finds that patients with no objective response, or only a partial response, after therapy show complete disappearance of the tumour cells upon histological examination. Hyperthermia has been shown to be of proven benefit in several clinical phase III studies. It should, however, still be regarded as an experimental therapy the merits of which should be further explored.

References

1. **Overgaard J.** History and heritage—an introduction. In: Overgaard J (ed.) *Hyperthermic oncology*, vol 2. London: Taylor and Francis, 1985: 3–8.

2. **Dahl O, Overgaard J.** A century with hyperthermic oncology in Scandinavia. *Acta Oncologica*, 1995; **34**: 1075–83.

3. **Hahn GM.** *Hyperthermia and cancer.* New York: Plenum, 1982.

4. **Dahl O.** Interaction of heat and drugs *in vitro* and *in vivo*. In: Seegenschmiedt MH, Fessenden P, Vernon CC (ed.) *Medical radiology—diagnostic imaging and radiation oncology*, vol 1. Berlin: Springer, 1995: 103–21.

5. **Lindegaard JC, Overgaard J.** Factors of importance for the development of the step-down heating effect in a C3H mammary carcinoma *in vivo. International Journal of Hyperthermia*, 1987; **3**: 79–91.

6. **Urano M, Douple E.** Thermal effects on cells and tissues. In: Urano M, Douple E, eds. *Hyperthermia and oncology*, vol 1. Utrecht: VSP, 1988.

7. **Dewey WC.** The search for critical targets by heat. *Radiation Research*, 1989; **120**: 191–204.

8. **Hahn GM, Nina SC, Elizaga M, Kapp DS, Anderson RL.** A comparison of thermal responses of human and rodent cells. *International Journal of Radiation Biology*, 1989; **56**: 817–25.

9. **Woo SY, et al.** Heterogeneity of heat response in murine, canine and human tumors: Influence of predictive assays. *International Journal of Radiation Oncology, Biology, Physics*, 1991; **20**: 479–88.

10. **Dewey WC, et al.** Cell biology of hyperthermia and radiation. In: Meyn RE, Withers HR (ed.) *Radiation biology in cancer research.* New York: Raven, 1980: 589–621.

11. **Gerweck LE, Nygaard TG, Burlett M.** Response of cells to hyperthermia under acute and chronic hypoxic conditions. *Cancer Research*, 1979; **39**: 966–72.

12. **Overgaard J, Nielsen OS.** The role of tissue environmental factors on

the kinetics and morphology of tumor cells exposed to hyperthermia. *Annals of the New York Academy of Sciences*, 1980; **335**: 254–80.

13. Overgaard J, Nielsen OS. The importance of thermotolerance for the clinical treatment with hyperthermia. *Radiotherapy and Oncology*, 1983; **1**: 167–78.

14. Overgaard J. Fractionated radiation and hyperthermia: Experimental and clinical studies. *Cancer*, 1981; **48**: 1116–23.

15. Overgaard J, Poulsen HS. Effect of hyperthermia and environmental acidity on the proteolytic activity in murine ascites tumor cells. *Journal of the National Cancer Institute*, 1977; **58**: 1159–61.

16. Horsman MR, Overgaard J. Thermal radiosensitization in animal tumours: The potential for therapeutic gain. In: Urano M, Douple E (ed.) *Hyperthermia and oncology*, vol 2. Utrecht: VSP, 1989; 113–45.

17. Song CW. Effect of local hyperthermia on blood flow and microenvironment: A review. *Cancer Research*, 1984; **44**: 4721s–4730s.

18. Reinhold HS, Endrich B. Tumour microcirculation as a target for hyperthermia. *International Journal of Hyperthermia*, 1986; **2**: 111–37.

19. Song CW, Griffin RJ, Shakil A, Iwata K, Okajima K. Tumor pO_2 is increased by mild temperature hyperthermia. *Hyperthermic Oncology*, 1996; **II**: 783–5.

20. Horsman MR, Overgaard J. Can mild hyperthermia improve tumour oxygenation? *International Journal of Hyperthermia*, 1997; **13**: 141–7.

21. Overgaard J. Simultaneous and sequential hyperthermia and radiation treatment of an experimental tumor and its surrounding normal tissue *in vivo*. *International Journal of Radiation Oncology, Biology, Physics*, 1980; **6**: 1507–17.

22. Overgaard J. The current and potential role of hyperthermia in radiotherapy. *International Journal of Radiation Oncology, Biology, Physics*, 1989; **16**: 535–49.

23. Dahl O. Hyperthermia and drugs. In: Watmough DJ, Ross WM (ed.) *Hyperthermia. Clinical and scientific aspects*. Glasgow: Blackie, 1986: 121–53.

24. Field SB, Hand JW. *An introduction to the practical aspects of clinical hyperthermia*. London: Taylor and Francis, 1990.

25. Seegenschmiedt M, Fessenden P, Vernon C, eds. *Thermoradiotherapy and thermochemotherapy. Vol 2, Clinical applications*. Berlin: Springer, 1995: 1–420.

26. Rhee JG, Lee CKK, Osborn J, Levitt SH, Song CW. Precooling prevents overheating of subcutaneous fat in the use of RF capacitive heating. *International Journal of Radiation Oncology, Biology, Physics*, 1991; **20**: 1009–15.

27. Kakehi M, Ueda K, Mukojima T, *et al*. Multi-institutional clinical studies on hyperthermia combined with radiotherapy or chemotherapy in advanced cancer of deep-seated organs. *International Journal of Hyperthermia*, 1990; **6**: 719–40.

28. Hand JW, ter Haar G. Heating techniques in hyperthermia. I. Introduction and assessment of techniques. *British Journal of Radiology*, 1981; **54**: 443–66.

29. Oleson JR, Dewhirst MW, Harrelson JM, Leopold KA, Samulski TV, Tso CY. Tumor temperature distributions predict hyperthermia effect. *International of Radiation Oncology, Biology, Physics*, 1989; **16**: 559–70.

30. Overgaard J, Gonzalez Gonzalez D, Hulshof MCCH, *et al*. Hyperthermia as an adjuvant to radiation therapy of recurrent or metastatic malignant melanoma. A multicenter randomized trial by the European Society for Hyperthermic Oncology. *International Journal of Hyperthermia*, 1996; **121**: 3–20.

31. Leopold KA, Dewhirst M, Samulski T, *et al*. Relationships among tumor temperature, treatment time, and histopathological outcome using preoperative hyperthermia with radiation in soft tissue sarcomas. *International Journal of Radiation Oncology, Biology, Physics*, 1992; **22**: 989–98.

32. Field SB, Morris CC. The relationship between heating time and temperature: Its relevance to clinical hyperthermia. *Radiotherapy and Oncology*, 1983; **1**: 179–86.

33. Sapareto SA, Dewey WC. Thermal dose determination in cancer therapy. *International Journal of Radiation Oncology, Biology, Physics*, 1984; **10**: 787–800.

34. Sneed PK, Dewhirst MW, Samulski T, Blivin J, Prosnitz LR. Should interstitial thermometry be used for deep hyperthermia? *International Journal of Radiation Oncology, Biology, Physics*, 1998; **40**: 1015–17.

35. Kapp DS, Cox RS. Thermal treatment parameters are most predictive of outcome in patients with single tumor nodules per treatment field in recurrent adenocarcinoma of the breast. *International Journal of Radiation Oncology, Biology, Physics*, 1995; **33**: 887–99.

36. van der Zee J, Peer-Valstar JN, Rietveld PJM, de Graaf-Strukowska L, van Rhoon GC. Practical limitations of interstitial thermometry during deep hyperthermia. *International Journal of Radiation Oncology, Biology, Physics*, 1998; **40**: 1205–12.

37. Wust P, Gellermann J, Harder C, *et al*. Rationale for using invasive thermometry for regional hyperthermia of pelvic tumors. *International Journal of Radiation Oncology, Biology, Physics*, 1998; **41**: 1129–37.

38. Hornsleth SN, Frydendal L, Mella O, Dahl O, Raskmark P. Quality assurance for radio frequency regional hyperthermia. *International Journal of Hyperthermia*, 1997; **13**: 169–85.

39. Hand JW, Lagendijk JJW, Bach Andersen J, Bolomey JC. Quality assurance guidelines for ESHO protocols. *International Journal of Hyperthermia*, 1989; **5**: 421–8.

40. Dewhirst MV, Phillips TL, Samulski TV, *et al*. RTOG quality assurance guidelines for clinical trials using hyperthermia. *International Journal of Radiation Oncology, Biology, Physics*, 1990; **18**: 1249–59.

41. Waterman FM, Dewhirst MW, Fessenden P, *et al*. RTOG quality assurance guidelines for clinical trials using hyperthermia administered by ultrasound. *International Journal of Radiation Oncology, Biology, Physics*, 1991; **20**: 1099–107.

42. Emami B, Stauffer P, Dewhirst MW, *et al*. RTOG quality assurance guidelines for interstitial hyperthermia. *International Journal of Radiation Oncology, Biology, Physics*, 1991; **20**: 1117–24.

43. Lagendijk JJW, van Rhoon GC, Hornsleth SN, *et al*. ESHO quality assurance guidelines for regional hyperthermia. *International Journal of Hyperthermia*, 1998; **14**: 125–33.

44. Carter DL, MacFall JR, Clegg ST, *et al*. Magnetic resonance thermometry during hyperthermia for human high-grade sarcoma. *International Journal of Radiation Oncology, Biology, Physics*, 1998; **40**: 815–22.

45. Dewhirst MW, Prosnitz L, Thrall D, *et al*. Hyperthermic treatment of malignant diseases: Current status and a view toward the future. *Seminars in Oncology*, 1997; **24**: 616–25.

46. Chive M. Use of microwave radiometry for hyperthermia monitoring and as a basis for thermal dosimetry. In: Gautherie M (ed.) *Methods of hyperthermia control*. Berlin: Springer, 1990: 112–28.

47. Overgaard J, Bach Andersen J. Hyperthermia. In: Peckham M, Pinedo H, Veronesi U (ed.) *Oxford textbook of oncology*, 1st edn, vol. 1. Oxford: Oxford University Press, 1995: 823–35.

48. Kapp DS. Site and disease selection for hyperthermia clinical trials. *International Journal of Hyperthermia*, 1986; **2**: 139–56.

49. Perez CA, Pajak T, Emami B, Hornback NB, Tupchong L, Rubin P. Randomized phase III study comparing irradiation and hyperthermia with irradiation alone in superficial measurable tumors. *American Journal of Clinical Oncology*, 1991; **14**: 133–41.

50. Overgaard J, Gonzalez Gonzalez D, *et al*. Randomised trial of hyperthermia as adjuvant to radiotherapy for recurrent or metastatic malignant melanoma. *The Lancet*, 1995; **345**: 540–3.

51. Lindholm C-E, Kjellen E, Nilsson P, Hertzman S. Microwave-induced hyperthermia and radiotherapy in human superficial tumours: Clinical results with a comparative study of combined treatment versus radiotherapy alone. *International Journal of Hyperthermia*, 1987; **3**: 393–411.

52. Vemon CC, Hand JW, Field SB, *et al*. Radiotherapy with or without

hyperthermia in the treatment of superficial localized breast cancer: Results from five randomized controlled trials. *International Journal of Radiation Oncology, Biology, Physics*, 1996; **35**: 731–44.

53. Engin K, Tupchong L, Waterman FM, *et al.* Multiple field hyperthermia combined with radiotherapy in advanced carcinoma of the breast. *International Journal of Hyperthermia*, 1995; **10**: 587–603.

54. van der Zee J, van der Holt B, Rietveld P, *et al.* Reirradiation combined with hyperthermia in recurrent breast cancer results in a worthwhile local palliation. *British Journal of Cancer*, 1999; **79**: 483–90.

55. Arcangeli G, Barni E, Cividalli A, *et al.* Effectiveness of microwave hyperthermia combined with ionizing radiation: Clinical results on neck node metastases. *International Journal of Radiation Oncology, Biology, Physics*, 1980; **6**: 143–8.

56. Valdagni R, Kapp DS, Valdagni C. N3 (TNM–UICC) metastatic neck nodes managed by combined radiation therapy and hyperthermia: Clinical results and analysis of treatment parameters. *International Journal of Hyperthermia*, 1986; **2**: 189–200.

57. Valdagni R, Amichetti NI. Report of long-term follow-up in a randomized trial comparing radiation therapy and radiation therapy plus hyperthermia to metastatic lymphnodes in stage IV head and neck patients. *International Journal of Radiation Oncology, Biology, Physics*, 1994; **28**: 163–9.

58. Amichetti M, Graiff C, Fellin G, *et al.* Cisplatin, hyperthermia. and radiation (trimodal therapy) in patients with locally advanced head and neck tumors: A phase I-II study. *International Journal of Radiation Oncology, Biology, Physics*, 1993; **26**: 801-7.

59. Datta NR, Bose AK, Kapoor HK, Gupta S. Head and neck cancers: Results of thermoradiotherapy versus radiotherapy. *International Journal of Hyperthermia*, 1990; **6**: 479–86.

60. Overgaard J, van der Zee J, Vernon C, Gonzalez DG, Arcangeli G. Thermoradiotherapy of malignant tumors. European randomized multicenter trials evaluating the effect of adjuvant hyperthermia in radiotherapy. In: Kogelnik HD (ed.) *Progress in radio-oncology V.* Bologna: Monduzzi, 1995: 507–13.

61. Gabriele P, Amichetti M, Orecchia R, Valdagni R. Hyperthermia and radiation therapy for inoperable or recurrent parotid carcinoma. A phase I/II study. *Cancer*, 1995; **75**: 908–13.

62. Bamett TA, Kapp DS, Goffinet DR. Adenoid cystic carcinoma of the salivary glands. *Cancer*, 1990; **65**: 2648–56.

63. Seegenschmiedt MH, Klautke G, Seidel R, Stauffer P. Clinical practice of interstitial thermoradiotherapy. In: Seegenschmiedt M, Fessenden P, Vernon C, eds. *Thermoradiotherapy and thermochemotherapy. Vol 2, Clinical applications.*. Berlin: Springer, 1995: 207–62.

64. Emami B, Scott C, Perez CA, *et al.* Phase III study of interstitial thermoradiotherapy compared with interstitial radiotherapy alone in the treatment of recurrent or persistent human tumors: A prospectively controlled randomized study by the Radiation Therapy Oncology Group. *International Journal of Radiation Oncology, Biology, Physics*, 1996; **34**: 1097–104.

65. Seegenschmiedt MH, Martus P, Fietkau R, Iro H, Brady LW, Sauer R. Multivariate analysis of prognostic parameters using interstitial thermoradiotherapy (IHT-IRT): Tumor and treatment variables predict outcome. *International Journal of Radiation Oncology, Biology, Physics*, 1994; **29**: 1049–63.

66. Ueo H, Sugimachi K. Preoperative hyperthermochemoradiotherapy for patients with esophageal carcinoma or rectal carcinoma. *Seminars in Surgical Oncology*, 1990; **6**: 8–13.

67. Sugimachi K, Kitamura K, Baba K, *et al.* Hyperthermia combined with chemotherapy and irradiation for patients with carcinoma of the oesophagus—A prospective randomized trial. *International Journal of Hyperthermia*, 1992; **8**: 289–95.

68. Sugimachi K, Kuwano H, Ide H, Toge T, Saku M, Oshiumi Y. Chemotherapy combined with or without hyperthermia for patients

with oesophageal carcinoma: A prospective randomized trial. *International Journal of Hyperthermia*, 1994; **10**: 485–93.

69. Kitamura K, Kuwano H, Watanabe M, *et al.* Prospective randomized study of hyperthermia combined with chemoradiotherapy for esophageal carcinoma. *Journal of Surgical Oncology*, 1995; **60**: 55–8.

70. Maehara Y, Kuwano H, Kitamura K. Matsuda H, Sugimachi K. Hyperthermochemoradiotherapy for esophageal cancer. *Anticancer Research*, 1992; **12**: 805–10.

71. Li DJ, Wang CQ, Qiu SL, Shao LF. Intraluminal microwave hyperthermia in the combined treatment of esophageal cancer: A preliminary report of 103 patients. *National Cancer Institute Monograph*, 1982; **61**: 419–21.

72. Hou B-S, Xiong Q-B, Li D-J. Thermo-chemo-radiotherapy of esophageal cancer. A preliminary report of 34 cases. *Cancer*, 1989; **64**: 1777–82.

73. Kim JH, Hahn EW. Clinical and biological studies of localized hyperthermia. *Cancer Research*, 1979; **39**: 2258–61.

74. Kim JH, Hahn EW, Antich PP. Radiofrequency hyperthermia for clinical cancer therapy. *National Cancer Institute Monographs*, 1982; **61**: 339–42.

75. Petersen IA, Kapp DS. Local hyperthermia and radiation therapy in the retreatment of superficially located recurrences in Hodgkin's disease. *International Journal of Radiation Oncology, Biology, Physics*, 1990; **18**: 603–11.

76. Donato V, Zurlo A, Nappa M, *et al.* Multicentre experience with combined hyperthermia and radiation therapy in the treatment of superficially located non-Hodgkin's lymphomas. *Journal of Experimental Clinical Research*, 1997; **16**: 87–90.

77. Komaki R, Brickner TJ, Hanlon AL, Owen JB, Hanks GE. Long-term results of treatment of cervical carcinoma in the United States in 1973, 1978 and 1983: Patterns of care study (PCS). *International Journal of Radiation Oncology, Biology, Physics*, 1995; **31**: 973–82.

78. Takeshi K, Katsuyuki K, Yoshiaki T, *et al.* Definitive radiotherapy combined with high-dose-rate brachytherapy for stage III carcinoma of the uterine cervix: Retrospective analysis of prognostic factors concerning patient characteristics and treatment parameters. International *Journal of Radiation Oncology, Biology, Physics*, 1998; **41**: 319–27.

79. Kapp KS, Stuecklschweiger GF, Kapp DS, *et al.* Prognostic factors in patients with carcinoma of the uterine cervix treated with external beam irradiation and Ir-192 high-dose-rate brachytherapy. *International Journal of Radiation Oncology, Biology, Physics*, 1998; **42**: 531–40.

80. Perez CA, Grigsby PW, Chao KSC, Mutch DG, Lockett MA. Tumor size, irradiation dose, and long-term outcome of carcinoma of uterine cervix. *International Journal of Radiation Oncology, Biology, Physics*, 1998; **41**: 307–17.

81. Sharma S, Sandhu APS, Patel FD, Ghoshal S, Gupta BD, Yadav NS. Side-effects of local hyperthermia: Results of a prospectively randomized clinical study. *International Journal of Hyperthermia*, 1990; **6**: 279–85.

82. van der Zee J, González González D, van Rhoon GC van Dijk JDP, van Putten WLJ, Hart AAM. Comparison of radiotherapy alone with radiotherapy plus hyperthermia in locally advanced pelvic tumours: a prospective, randomised, multicentre trial. *The Lancet*, 2000; **355**: 1119–25.

83. Berdov BA, Menteshashvili GZ. Thermoradiotherapy of patients with locally advanced carcinoma of the rectum. *International Journal of Hyperthermia*, 1990; **6**: 881–90.

84. You Q-S, Wang R-Z, Suen G-Q, *et al.* Combination preoperative radiation and endocavitary hyperthermia for rectal cancer: Long-term results of 44 patients. *International Journal of Hyperthermia*, 1990; **9**: 19–24.

85. Rau B, Wust P, Hohenberger P, Löffel J, Hünerbein M, Gellermann J, Below C, Riess H, Felix R, Schlag PM. Preoperative hyperthermia

combined with radiochemotherapy in locally advanced rectal cancer. A phase II clinical trial. *Annals of Surgery*, 1998; **227**: 380–9.

86. Trotter JM, Edis AJ, Blackwell JB, *et al.* Adjuvant VHF therapy in locally recurrent and primary unresectable rectal cancer. *Australasian Radiology*, 1996; **40**: 298–305.

87. Dahl O. Mechanisms of thermal enhancement of chemotherapeutic cytotoxicity. In: Urano M, Double E (ed.) *Hyperthermia and oncology*, vol. 4. Utrecht: VSP, 1994: 9–28.

88. Issels RD, Prenninger SW, Nagele A, *et al.* Ifosfamide plus etoposide combined with regional hyperthermia in patients with locally advanced sarcomas: A phase II study. *Journal of Clinical Oncology*, 1990; **8**: 1818–29.

89. Issels RD, Mittermüller J, Gerl A, *et al.* Improvement of local control by regional hyperthermia combined with systemic chemotherapy (ifosfamide plus etoposide) in advanced sarcomas: Updated report on 65 patients. *Journal of Cancer Research and Clinical Oncology*, 1991; **117** (suppl. IV): S141–SI47.

90. Voth B, Sauer H, Wilmanns W. Thermostability of cytostatic drugs *in vitro* and thermosensitivity of cultured human lymphoblasts against cytostatic drugs. *Recent Results in Cancer Research*, 1988; **107**: 170–6.

91. Multhoff G, Botzler C, Wiesnet M, *et al.* A stress-inducible 72-kDa heat-shock protein (HSP72) is expressed on the surface of human tumor cells, but not on normal cells. *International Journal of Cancer*, 1995; **61**: 272–9.

92. Colombo R, Lev A, Da Pozzo LF, Freschi M, Gallus G, Ricatti P. A new approach using local combined microwave hyperthermia and chemotherapy in superficial transitional bladder carcinoma treatment. *Journal of Urology*, 1995; **153**: 959–63.

93. Thomas GM. Improved treatment for cervical cancer—concurrent chemotherapy and radiotherapy. *New England Journal of Medicine*, 1999; **340**: 1198–200.

94. Rose PG, Bundy BN, Watkins EB, *et al.* Concurrent cisplatin-based radiotherapy and chemotherapy for locally advanced cervical cancer. *New England Journal of Medicine*, 1999; **340**: 1145–53.

95. Morris M, Eifel PJ, Lu J, *et al.* Pelvic radiation with concurrent chemotherapy compared with pelvic and para-aortic radiation for high-risk cervical cancer. *New England Journal of Medicine*, 1999; **340**: 1198–200.

96. Keys HM, Bundy BN, Stehman FB, *et al.* Cisplatin, radiation, and adjuvant hysterectomy compared with radiation and adjuvant hysterectomy for bulky stage IB cervical carcinoma. *New England Journal of Medicine*, 1999; **340**: 1154–61.

97. Rietbroek R, Schilthuis M, Bakker P, *et al.* Phase II trial of weekly locoregional hyperthermia and cisplatin in patients with previously irradiated recurrent carcinoma of the uterine cervix. *Cancer*, 1997; **79**: 935–43.

98. Fijiwara K, Kohno I, Sekiba K. Therapeutic effect of hyperthermia combined with chemotherapy on vulvar and vaginal carcinoma. *Acta Medica Okayama*, 1987; **42**: 55–62.

99. Cumberlin R, DeMoss E, Lassus M, Friedman M. Isolation perfusion for malignant melanoma of the extremity: A review. *Journal of Clinical Oncology*, 1985; **3**: 1022–31.

100. Lejeune FJ, Deloof T, Ewalenko P, *et al.* Objective regression of unexcised melanoma in-transit metastases after hyperthermic isolation perfusion of the limbs with melphalan. *Recent Results in Cancer Research*, 1983; **86**: 268–76.

101. Liénard D, Lejeune FJ, Ewalenko P. In transit metastases of malignant melanoma treated by high dose rTNFalpha in combination with interferon-γ and melphalan in isolation perfusion. *World Journal of Surgery*, 1992; **16**: 234–40.

102. Lejeune F, Liénard D, Eggermont A, *et al.* Clinical experience with high-dose tumor necrosis factor alpha in regional therapy of advanced melanoma. *Circulatory Shock*, 1994; **43**: 191–7.

103. Vaglini M, Belli F, Ammatuna M, *et al.* Treatment of primary or relapsing limb cancer by isolation perfusion with high-dose alpha-tumor necrosis factor, gamma-interferon, and melphalan. *Cancer*, 1994; **73**: 483–92.

104. Ghussen F, Krüger I, Groth W, Stützer H. The role of regional hyperthermic cytostatic perfusion in the treatment of extremity melanoma. *Cancer*, 1988; **61**: 654–9.

105. Hafström L, Rudenstam C-M, Blomquist E, *et al.* Regional hyperthermic perfusion with melphalan after surgery for recurrent malignant melanoma of the extremities. *Journal of Clinical Oncology*, 1991; **9**: 2091–4.

106. Koops HS, Vaglini M, Suciu S, *et al.* Prophylactic isolated limb perfusion for localized high-risk limb melanoma: Results of a multicenter randomized phase III trial. *Journal of Clinical Oncology*, 1998; **16**: 2906–12.

107. Cavallere R, Di Filippo F, Cavallere F, *et al.* Clinical practice of hyperthermic extremity perfusion in combination with radiotherapy and chemotherapy. In: Seegenschmiedt MH, Fessenden P, Vernon CC (ed.) *Thermoradiotherapy and thermochemotherapy*, vol. 2. Berlin: Springer, 1995: 323–45.

108. Eggermont AMM, Schraffordt Koops H, *et al.* Isolated limb perfusion with tumor necrosis factor and melphalan for limb salvage in 186 patients with locally advanced soft tissue extremity sarcomas. *Annals of Surgery*, 1996; **224**: 756–65.

109. Bull JM, Lees D, Schuette W, *et al.* Whole body hyperthermia: A phase-I trial of a potential adjuvant to chemotherapy. *Annals of Internal Medicine*, 1979; **90**: 317–23.

110. Wiedemann GJ, Robins HI, Gutsche S, *et al.* Ifosfamide, carboplatin and etoposide (ICE) combined with 41.8°C whole body hyperthennia in patients with refractory sarcoma. *European Journal of Cancer*, 1996; **32A**: 888–92.

111. Robins H, Rushing D, Kutz M, *et al.* Phase I clinical trial of melphalan and 41.8 degrees C whole-body hyperthermia in cancer patients. *Journal of Clinical Oncology*, 1997; **15**: 158–64.

112. Sakaguchi Y, Makino M, Kaneko T, *et al.* Therapeutic efficacy of long-duration low-temperature whole body hyperthermia when combined with tumor necrosis factor and carboplatin in rats. *Cancer Research*, 1994; **54**: 2223–7.

113. Sapozink MD, Gibbs FA Jr, Egger MJ, Stewart JR. Regional hyperthermia for clinically advanced deep-seated pelvic malignancy. *American Journal of Clinical Oncology*, 1986; **9**: 162–9.

114. Pilepich MV, Myerson RJ, Emami BN, Perez CA, Leybovich L, von Gerichten D. Regional hyperthermia: A feasibility analysis. *International Journal of Hyperthermia*, 1987; **3**: 347–51.

115. Emami B, Myerson RJ, Scott C, Gibbs F, Lee C, Perez CA. Phase I/II study, combination of radiotherapy and hyperthermia in patients with deep-seated malignant tumors: Report of a pilot study by the Radiation Therapy Oncology Group. *International Journal of Radiation Oncology, Biology, Physics*, 1991; **20**: 73–79.

116. Paulsen KD, Jia X, Sullivan JM Jr. Finite element computations of specific absorption rates in anatomically conforming, full-body models for hyperthemia treatment analysis. *IEEE Transactions on Biomedical Engineering*, 1993; **40**: 933–45.

117. Hornsleth SN. Radiofrequency regional hyperthermia. *European Doctorate (Ph.D.)*. Aalborg University, 1996.

4.7 **Specialized techniques**

4.7.1 **Intraoperative radiotherapy**

J. P. Gerard and F. Calvo

Introduction—definition

Intraoperative radiation therapy (IORT) refers to the delivery of irradiation during a surgical operation. This technique aims at delivering a higher effective dose to the tumour (or tumour bed) while preventing radiation complication by surgically displacing radiosensitive, normal organs and tissues. One of the most common forms of IORT at the present time is the use of electron beams (intraoperative electron radiation therapy, IOERT). Data generated with IOERT will be the major interest of this chapter. It is also possible to perform IORT with brachytherapy, either with low or high-dose-rate radioactive sources. The use of a low energy photon beam (50–100 KV) is unusual nowadays.

History

One of the first report of IORT was published in 1905. It described the case of a non-resectable stomach cancer which was directly exposed, during surgery, to irradiation with orthovoltage X-rays.[1] A recent report has described a European IORT-like procedure combining tumour resection and fractionated IORT in 1905.[2] During the period from 1925 to 1935, IORT was used in many centres due to the poor depth dose curve of the X-rays available at this time. With the advent of the telecobalt machine, IORT was discontinued after 1950. Abe *et al.*, in Kyoto, pioneered a new approach with an electron beam used for IORT.[3],–[5] In Japan, IOERT was used between 1970 and 1980 with a single high-dose irradiation (30–40 Gy) to treat, predominantly, gastric and pancreatic carcinoma.[4],[6] In the early 1980s several clinical programmes of IOERT were developed in the United States.[7],[8] Experimental studies were performed on animals, usually dog, to assess the tolerance of the normal tissues to escalating doses of IOERT with or without external irradiation.[9]–[13] Randomized trials were initiated at the National Cancer Institute.[7],[12],[14] Unfortunately, none of these phase III trials were able to accrue enough patients to give a strong level of evidence on clinical results. In Europe, Calvo *et al.* developed an active programme in Spain, initially in Pamplona and later in Madrid. Between 1980 and 1990, many IOERT facilities were opened in Germany, France, Italy, Austria, Norway, Sweden, and others. Up to now, more than 10 000 patients have been treated with IOERT throughout the world and reported in the literature.

Rationale for IORT

In industrialized countries, it is assumed than one-third of the population will be affected by cancer in the coming century. If one takes the example of France, it is estimated that every year 60 per cent of the patients with cancer will die from their disease (140 000 deaths). In one-third of these cancer-related deaths there is a component of local tumour recurrence responsible for this treatment failure.[15] Local control of the primary tumour is a mandatory condition for cure, although it is not always the only condition.[16] The impact of local control on the overall survival depends on the site of the primary tumour. It is crucial for brain tumours and less significant for melanoma of the skin or breast cancer. Local control appears more and more as an essential factor for long-term survival in abdominopelvic tumours.[17] Surgery remains the most efficient treatment for local disease control. Radiation therapy, with doses of 45 to 50 Gy in 5 weeks, as an adjuvant treatment, is efficient for control of subclinical, residual, malignant disease after complete, gross tumour resection (R1–R0 surgery). Such a radiation dose range is often close to the tolerance limit of normal organs and tissues contained in the abdominopelvic region. Sterilization of gross residual or unresected malignant lesion (carcinoma or sarcoma), requires radiation doses of 65 to 75 Gy to achieve long-term, local control. Such a high dose range is hazardous when delivered with external beam radiation therapy (EBRT) alone.

The aim of IORT is to overcome the tolerance of the normal tissues and to increase the precision of the radiation dose deposited in the target volume. Taking advantage of the surgical approach, it is possible to selectively irradiate the lesion or risk area and to deliver a high single dose with complete protection of the mobile, uninvolved organs and tissues surrounding the tumour. On the other hand, IORT delivers a single dose which yields no differential effect between normal tissues and cancer cells. It is the reason why IORT is very seldom performed as a single procedure. In most centres, IORT is considered to be boost technique and is associated with an EBRT. It has been demonstrated that a boost dose of 10 to 15 Gy after EBRT of 45 to 55 Gy is able to improve significantly the local control.[16] It is the aim of IOERT to deliver safely this extra dose.

IOERT facilities and techniques

IORT with electrons is performed with a linear accelerator. The energy of the electrons usually varies between 6 and 20 MeV. The percentage depth dose of electrons collimated with an IORT applicator is generally lower than electrons with a standard collimation system. To irradiate non-resectable, gross tumours of 2 or 3 cm thickness, electrons of 15 to 18 MeV must be used. The linear accelerator must be equipped with a dedicated adaptor for insertion of applicators. According to the volume to be irradiated, different localizers or applicators are used. Plexiglass or steel are acceptable materials. The lower end is either straight or in several bevelled angulations. Different accessories (equalizing filters, shields, bolus materials, etc.) are used to conform the dose deposited to the target volume. Each applicator and accessory needs an individualized dosimetric calibration before being accepted for clinical use, which is a time consuming procedure for the physics department.[18]–[21]

In most centres, IOERT is performed in a surgical operating room where the cone is positioned, or its position simulated, to irradiate precisely the target volume and protect the normal tissue (Fig. 1). The cone is fixed in the appropriate position with a rigid, articulated arm connected to the operating table. Dressings may help prevent organs at risk (e.g. small bowel) being close to the cone. Sterile plastic sheets cover the cone and wound to keep the whole procedure aseptic. Optical systems are helpful to control the accurate positioning of the cone. The patient is transported under general anaesthesia from the operating room to the linear accelerator room (Fig. 2). The distance and the transportation system can vary depending on the institution. Connection between the cone and the adaptor can be done mechanically (hard docking) or by an optical alignment procedure (soft docking). A misalignment of 5° between the central axis of the electron beam and the central axis of the cone can cause a 20 per cent reduction and or inhomogeneity of dose distribution in the treated volume. Thermoluminescent detectors can be used to control the delivery of the correct dose (*in vivo* dosimetry).[18],[19],[21] Irradiation time lasts between 5 and 15 min depending on the dose, the applicator size, and the electron energy. Close surveillance of the patient is performed during the irradiation by the anaesthesiology team outside the accelerator room using a close-circuit TV monitoring system (Fig. 3). After irradiation, the patient is moved back to the operating room, were the applicator is removed and the surgical procedure is completed. In some institutions, a dedicated linear accelerator has been installed in the operating room itself. Small, mobile linear accelerators, delivering only electrons, are being developed by some industrial companies (Fig. 4). These mobile linear accelerators will deliver electrons with energies ranging from 6 to 12 MeV. The radioprotection requirements of such a machine will be minor as it only delivers electron beams. A mobile linear accelerator for IOERT could be moved between hospitals or between operating rooms, as required. This would be a useful innovation for the development of this technique.[22],[23]

Experimental and biological background

Many different experimental studies, predominantly in the dog, have been performed in the United States.[11]–[13] One of the aims of these

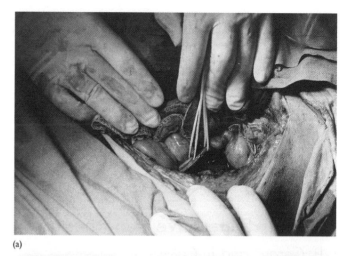

(a)

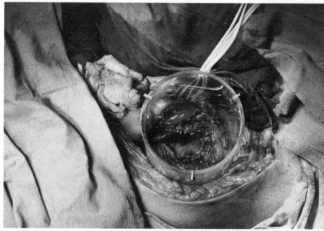

(b)

Fig. 1 (a) Definition of the tumour bed area in an extraoseous Ewing's sarcoma in partial response after induction chemotherapy. Mobile structures (ureter, small bowel, and colon) are ready to be displaced from the electron beam. (b) IOERT applicator positioned in the target volume with protection of normal, uninvolved tissues and organs (8 cm in diameter; 30° bevelled).

studies was to evaluate the tolerance of various normal tissues and organs to a single, high dose of electrons, with or without fractionated external beam radiotherapy in the range 45 to 50 Gy. Clinical data published in the past 20 years have confirmed the good tolerance of the large vessels to high single doses.[10] On the other hand, some organs appear dose-limiting to high single dose. Predominant IOERT-sensitive structures in clinical trials are peripheral nerves,[24] ureters,[25] bile ducts, oesophagus, and duodenum. Bone necrosis, with vertebral collapse or sacral necrosis, have been described by different authors.[26],[27] Sensory or motor neuropathy is a limiting side-effect of IOERT in the abdomen, pelvis, and extremities. Grade 3 pain or weakness can be seen after a delay of 2 to 4 months. It is related to the dose delivered and the length of nerve irradiated.[24] Radiation-induced neuropathy is not always easy to distinguish from neurological tumour compression (Table 1).

The biological effectiveness of a single dose of IOERT is not yet well understood. It is considered equivalent to twice or three times

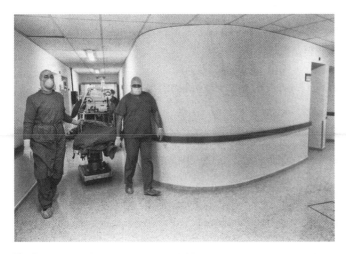

Fig. 2 Transportation procedure for IOERT: the patient is moved on the surgical table and a supplemental device holds the transportable respirator and anaesthesia monitors.

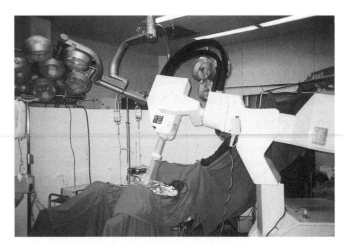

Fig. 4 Small, transportable linear accelerator, NOVAC 7, in clinical use (July, 1998).

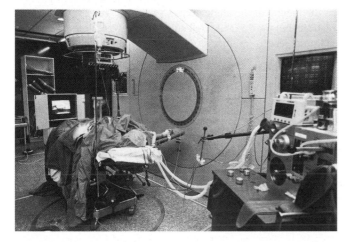

Fig. 3 IOERT procedure prepared: the patient is under general anaesthesia and is monitored; the electron applicator is positioned in the anatomical target volume; close circuit TV is connected for visual control in the linear accelerator room.

Table 1 Normal tissue tolerance of IOERT—experimental and clinical data

Tissue	Maximum tolerance dose (Gy)	Tissue lesions
Good tolerance		
Aorta–vena cava	40	Wall fibrosis
Portal vein anastomosis	35	Wall stenosis
Bronchial stump	35	Fistula
Bladder	30	Ureterovesical stenosis
Trachea	30	Fibrosis
Muscle	25	Fibrosis–atrophy
Non-dissected ureter in dogs	20	Stenosis
Average tolerance		
Normal ureter in man	20	Stenosis
Bile duct	20	Stenosis
Heart	20	Fibrosis
Lung	20	Fibrosis
Small bowel	20	Stenosis
Bone	20	Necrosis
Poor tolerance		
Oesophagus	15	Stenosis
Peripheral nerve	15	Neuropathy
Large bowel	15	Perforation–stenosis
Kidney	15	Atrophy
Dissected ureter	15	Stenosis–fistula

the numeric value of the dose given with a standard fractionated schedule. A single dose of 10 Gy is close to 20 or 30 Gy in 2 or 3 weeks. A single dose of 20 Gy is close to 40 to 60 Gy in 4 to 6 weeks. When a single dose of 15 Gy of IOERT is added to a dose of 45 Gy of fractionated EBRT, the 'total equivalent biological dose' is estimated to be in the range of 75 to 90 Gy in 8 to 9 weeks. During the past decade, after analysing the data on local control and toxicity from the most relevant clinical experiences, there has been a trend toward reducing the dose of IOERT. In the context of association with doses of 45 to 50 Gy from EBRT, the following doses of IOERT can be recommended: after a R0 resection 10 to 12 Gy; after a R1 resection (microscopic residual disease) 13 to 15 Gy; after a R2 resection doses of 16 to 20 Gy can be given to a gross tumour mass. The sequencing of EBRT and IORT is also the subject of investigation. It is often discussed at the time of a multidisciplinary consultation. Whenever

it is thought possible, preoperative EBRT should be preferred. This has the advantage of an improved tolerance, preventing seeding, and better treatment programme compliance. In cases of small tumour size, it is sometimes preferred to start with surgery to have a proper localization of the disease. In the past, reirradiation of a previously irradiated area was usually considered impossible but this is no longer a standard recommendation. In the pelvis for recurrent disease in an irradiated area, it appears possible to give a second irradiation with a moderate total dose of 30 to 35 Gy, EBRT with an IOERT boost of 10 to 20 Gy.[28] Different approaches are being developed to enhance the effect of IOERT using chemotherapy, hyperthermia, or oxygen.[29]

Patient selection and evaluation endpoints

IORT may be proposed whenever the standard treatment programme, including the best combination of surgery, irradiation, and chemotherapy, gives a local failure rate of 15 to 20 per cent or higher. The approach is used essentially when the treatment is given with a curative intent. It is contraindicated in presence of disseminated disease. The patient should be in good general condition and operable. Full inform consent must be obtained, due to the intense nature treatment with an IORT component. In practice, IORT is proposed most often in the treatment of abdominopelvic cancers, in tumour stages in which local failure is frequent, with a relatively low rate of distant metastases. These anatomical cavities limit the doses of irradiation to 50 to 55 Gy due to the tolerance of the small bowel, kidney, spinal cord, and rectum.

When IORT is proposed in association with a R0 or R1 resection to control subclinical residual disease, it is impossible without a randomized trial to have a high level of evidence of the effectiveness of this treatment. Randomized trial is the appropriate methodology to assess the relevance of a treatment aimed at subclinical disease control. In the field of IORT, such randomized trials have, so far, been very difficult to run. However, when IORT is proposed to treat gross tumour deemed to be unresectable by experienced surgeons, the assessment of results is simple. In such a situation, it is well known that EBRT with doses of 45 to 55 Gy is unable to give long-term control. The tumours with no resection or gross residual disease are the best model to evaluate the relevance of IORT after palliative surgery. Even when combined chemoradiotherapy and extensive resection are proposed, the R2 surgery provides good evidence of the merit of this technique. Local control should be considered the endpoint utilized to evaluate IORT efficacy. It is well know that local control is not an easy endpoint to measure accurately. Statistically, local control is not independent from metastases and the estimate of local control values with time is difficult. Overall survival in R2 surgery remains the best evaluable endpoint to assess the value of IORT contribution to cure.

Results of IORT

The results of IOERT will be discussed first for recurrent tumours. As stated above, local recurrence is a good model to evaluate this procedure because complete gross tumour resection is often impossible in such a situation and long-term survival is unusual. On the other hand, it is difficult in recurrent tumours series to eliminate selection bias.

The place of IOERT in the initial, radical treatment of a primary cancer will then be analysed. Often recurrent and primary lesions are analysed together. This is confusing as these two disease situations have a completely different natural history. Primary tumours usually give better results in terms of local control and survival but they are often treated with a R0 resection. There are few centres with more than 1000 patients treated with IOERT. The Mayo Clinic in Rochester has the largest experience with this technique and its results are quoted below.

IOERT and local relapse

Uterine cancer

Between 1983 and 1995, a series of 54 patients (origin tumour site: cervix uteri, 36; endometrium, 14; vagina, 3; ovary, 1) were treated at the Mayo Clinic. At the time of surgery, after maximum debulking 16 had gross residual tumours. The median IOERT dose was 17.5 Gy. At 3 years, the actuarial local control rate was 54 per cent; the 5-year actuarial overall survival was 27 per cent. In cases of R0–R1 surgery, the 5-year overall survival was 37 per cent and in cases of R2 it was 10 per cent. In 15 patients, IOERT and EBRT was delivered for a recurrence in a previously irradiated pelvis (dose 50 Gy). No severe radiation toxicity was observed and the survival rates were similar to those seen in patients without prior EBRT.[30] In Lyon between 1987 and 1993, a series of 54 patients were treated with the same combination of EBRT and IOERT. The 5-year overall survival was 28 per cent for endometrial carcinomas (11 cases) and 18 per cent for carcinomas of the uterine cervix (43 cases). For 33 patients with R2 resection, the 5-year overall survival was 17 per cent. There was one postoperative death and 6 grade 3 complications (two sensory neuropathies, one ureteral stenosis, one rectovaginal fistula, one rectal necroses, and one lumbar vertebral collapse).[31] The University Clinic of Navarra reported 17 per cent 5-year survival and 10 out of 18 patients locally controlled.[32],[33] Similar results have been published by other centres.[34],[35] Review of the literature shows that after pelvic relapse the overall 5-year survival rate for R2 lesions does not exceed 5 per cent. This clinical situation appears as a good model to demonstrate the effectiveness of IOERT. Although selection bias cannot be eliminated, it is highly probable that IOERT increases two or three-fold the chance of long-term survival in these non-resectable pelvic relapses with an acceptable rate of toxicity.

Colorectal cancer

Locoregional relapses fixed to the pelvic cavity or abdominal wall after radical surgery have poor prognosis. IOERT after incomplete gross resection appears to be able to give some local control and long-term survival. Between 1981 and 1995, 123 patients were treated at the Mayo Clinic for local recurrence with no prior irradiation. All patients were treated with EBRT (45 to 55 Gy) with or without 5-fluorouracil-containing chemotherapy and IOERT (10 to 20 Gy) without adjuvant chemotherapy. The 5-year overall survival for R1 and R2 surgery was 24 and 18 per cent, respectively. Without IOERT, the historical series at the Mayo for similar patients showed a 5-year overall survival of 5 per cent.[28],[36]–[38] The last published up-data of the experience in Pamplona identified 27 patients treated with recurrent disease (including previous pelvic radiotherapy) with a projected 5-year survival of 18 per cent.[39] Equivalent results,[13],[40],[41] sometimes not as good,[42],[43] have been published by groups in Boston, Norway, and Italy. In France, a series of 73 patients from five institutions was pooled. The local control rate was 61 per cent when EBRT and IOERT were combined. Severe grade 3 neuropathy was the main toxicity noticed for such pelvic IOERT.[42] In conclusion, in patients with recurrent cancer in the pelvis or paraortic lymph node, IOERT with EBRT may be beneficial when compared to EBRT alone and may offer a modest but real chance of cure.

Retroperitoneal soft tissues sarcomas

With surgery alone the local relapse rate for recurrent retroperitoneal soft tissue sarcoma is 75 per cent or more[44] even if combined with EBRT, which is difficult to deliver safely in doses exceeding 45 to 50 Gy. This is a typical situation where IOERT can improve local control and survival. At the Mayo Clinic between 1981 and 1995, 44 patients with recurrent retroperitoneal soft tissue sarcoma were treated with wide resection and IOERT (median dose 15 Gy) and EBRT (median dose 46 Gy).[45],[46] The majority (66 per cent) of the tumours were high grade sarcoma. Local control was observed in 27 patients (61 per cent). The 5-year overall survival was 42 per cent. In nine cases, only R2 surgery was possible. Grade 3 peripheral neuropathy developed in five patients (11 per cent). Calvo, in Spain, treated 12 cases of recurrent retroperitoneal soft tissue sarcoma. Local control was achieved in seven patients and the 5-year survival rate was 20 per cent. A clear benefit is observed when using IOERT in comparison with EBRT alone.[47]

Miscellaneous relapses

In many different sites, IOERT has been used for local relapse. This include local relapse of cancer of the kidney,[36] cancer of the head and neck,[48],[49] lymph node relapse in the mediastinum or lumbar region,[50] brain tumours,[51] bone sarcomas,[52] paediatric tumours.[53] All these series are inhomogeneous but they have in common a high local control rate with acceptable toxicity in R2 resection.

IOERT for relapse in a previously irradiated area

This represents a challenging clinical and therapeutic situation which is seen increasingly. Irradiation is often used in the initial treatment of carcinoma of the rectum and of the uterine cervix. Pelvic recurrences of these two cancers present the oncologist with a problem. Until recently, it was a rule not to reirradiate the pelvis. The dose of EBRT is kept below 40 Gy and the dose of IOERT can be increased to 15 Gy for R0–R1 resection and 20 to 23 Gy for R2 resection. Such a reirradiation can be proposed for patients with strict selection—young age, good general condition, small well-localized malignant disease relapse, and no distant metastases after a careful work up. The volume treated with EBRT should be kept as small as clinically possible.

IOERT and primary tumour

Abdominopelvic tumour

Gastric cancer

When assessed at autopsy or second-look surgery, the sites of tumour recurrence in gastric carcinoma after radical surgery a high rate of local and regional relapse in the celiac regions was found. In patients dying from gastric cancer, a component of locally progressive tumour was found in 50 per cent.[54],[55] This is a strong argument for trying to improve local disease control with IOERT in gastric cancer. Four randomized trials (Table 2) have been performed using IOERT alone following surgery in gastric cancer. The trials of Abe and Chen have shown a significant benefit in overall survival for patient with stage III–IV treated with IOERT.[3],[6],[56] A more recent trial in Germany, using the same technique, has not reproduced such results in a recent

interim analysis.[57] There has been increased postoperative mortality and morbidity with IOERT but improved local control (91 per cent versus 83 per cent) and specific survival in stage III patients. In the United States, a phase III trial was stopped before sufficient accrual of patients was reached. A small benefit in terms of local control without survival impact was noticed.[14] None of these four trials have really convinced the medical community of the possible benefit of IOERT. Many methodological flows and bias were present in these trials which weakened the level of evidence. One of the main criticism made of the non-American trials was the use of IOERT alone with single doses in the range of 30 to 40 Gy without EBRT. In Pamplona, a pilot study was conducted in 48 patients combining EBRT (46 Gy in 1.8 to 2 Gy fractions) and IOERT (15 Gy) with or without chemotherapy. In stages III–IV disease, local control appears to be increased and two patients with R2 resection were long-term survivors.[58] This group have up-dated long-term results in patients with serosal and/or nodal involvement; at 10 years locoregional control and survival rates were 89 and 38 per cent, respectively.[55] In Lyon between 1986 and 1994, 82 patients were treated with the same association of IOERT and postoperative EBRT. A four-field box technique was used to irradiate the celiac region to a dose of 46 to 50 Gy. There was no attempt to irradiate the splenic hilum. The 5-year overall survival was 82 per cent for 26 pN0 patients and 52 per cent for 31 pN1–2 patients; two patients died, at 3 and 6 months, from intestinal haemorrhage with a questionable relation to IOERT.[59],[60] The recent experience of Ogata favours the use of a large field of IOERT with a cone of 9 cm diameter.[61]

There is still a lack of strong evidence to say that IOERT should be a standard component of treatment in gastric cancer. Other approaches, such as extended lymphatic dissection or adjuvant chemotherapy, are under investigation at the present time. There is a strong need for well-designed, randomized trials to test its contribution. The role of adjuvant EBRT plus chemotherapy with or without IOERT is a promising field to be explored.

Cancer of the pancreas

Resectable tumour In resectable primary cancer of the pancreas a phase III randomized trial has been performed at the National Cancer Institute, Bethesda. Only 24 patients were included. Randomization was performed at the time of a Whipple operation and compared IOERT alone (20 Gy) with EBRT alone (50 Gy/5 weeks). At 3 years, two patients were alive in the group with IOERT and none in the EBRT group. This trial was, of course, not conclusive.[12] In Lyon between 1987 and 1994, 19 patients underwent duodenopancreatectomy with IOERT (median dose 15 Gy) followed by EBRT (46 Gy/4.5 weeks). Postoperative death was nil. Two patients were alive with no evidence of disease at 5 years. Median survival time was still modest (11 months) with a 4-year overall survival of 20 per cent.[62],[63] Despite IOERT and combined treatment, 5-year survivors are unusual.

Non-resectable tumour Non-resectable tumour is a frequent situation in cancer of the head of pancreas. The median survival time ranges from 3 to 6 months and IOERT is usually performed with a palliative intent. As in other tumour sites, the results are improved if IOERT is associated with EBRT.[63] An universal antalgic effect has been clearly demonstrated.[64] In some series, possibly due to selection bias, median survival time between 10 and 12 months have been reported with occasional survivors after 3 years.[65] Despite combined aggressive

Table 2 IOERT randomized trials in gastric cancer

	Surgery alone	IOERT	p value
Abe, Japan 1964–1986: 211 patients			
Stage I–II	54 patients	44 patients	NS
Stage III–IV	56 patients	57 patients	<0.05
Stage I–II 5-year overall survival	85%	75%	
Stage III–IV 5-year overall survival	21%	43%	
Chen, China 1972–1988: 200 patients			
Stage III–IV	100 patients	100 patients	<0.05
5-year overall survival	30%	65%	
Kramling, Germany 1988–1996: 108 patients			
Stage I–II	43 patients	40 patients	
Stage III–IV	22 patients	23 patients	NS
Operative mortality	1.5%	7.5%	NS
Local recurrence	4 patients	1 patient	NS
Mean survival time	33 months	28 months	
Sindelar, United States 1978–1984: 41 patients (16 surgery alone; 25 IOERT)			
Toxicity G3–5	10 patients	10 patients	
Local recurrence	9 patients	2 patients	<0.01
5-year overall survival	3 patients	2 patients	

treatment with chemotherapy or elective liver irradiation, survival remains very poor and it remains questionable to propose such a heavy treatment for only few months of life. It is possible that bypass, with IOERT and a short course of EBRT, in patients with M0 lesions represent one of the best palliative treatment.

Preoperative irradiation with or without IOERT One of the reasons of the poor prognosis of cancer of the pancreas is the high incidence of liver metastasis and peritoneal failure, rapidly occurring in the course of the disease. In an attempt to increase survival rates and improved patients selection some institutions are initiating the treatment with combined EBRT and chemotherapy. If metastases developed during the first few months the treatment is oriented toward symptomatic palliation, but if after restaging the patient is operable, surgery is proposed with, if possible, duodenopancreatectomy. In Houston, in a series of 51 patients, 38 were operated. In 30 cases, a Whipple operation was possible with IOERT. There was no sterilized specimen and the median survival time was 18 months. At the Mayo Clinic, in 27 patients with unresectable patients after such a preoperative EBRT and restaging, patients receiving IOERT had a median survival time of 14.6 months with one patient alive at 5 years.[64]

Fixed rectal cancer (T4)

Despite combined EBRT, chemotherapy, and extensive surgery, such large tumours fixed to the pelvic lateral wall or sacrum (or prostate) are difficult to control locally. As surgery is often a R2 resection, IOERT appears as an attractive treatments indication. Several pilot studies, including between 10 and 100 patients, have been reported with encouraging results.[66]–[69] The EBRT component is given preoperatively (with or without 5-fluorouracil- containing chemotherapy) to doses ranging from 45 to 55 Gy to the posterior pelvis, usually with the patient in a prone position and a three or four-fields technique. The dose of IOERT depends on the amount of residual disease after maximal resection (between 10 and 22 Gy). At Massachusetts General Hospital Boston, in a series of 42 patients, the 5-year overall survival was 43 per cent. This result was superior to historical control experiences.[70] At the Mayo Clinic in a series of 56 patients, the 5-year overall survival was 46 per cent with an actuarial 3-year local failure rate of 16 per cent. At 3 years distant metastases were present in half of the patients.[29] A randomized trial is ongoing in France including T3–4 rectal adenocarcinoma treated with preoperative EBRT (40 Gy/4 weeks) with or without IOERT. A identical phase III trial is being proposed in the Netherlands. These results tend to show that T4 rectal cancers are a very good indication for IOERT. Here also, toxicity was described as peripheral neuropathy and sacral bone necrosis.[70] The Spanish group studying IORT updated the multi-institutional experience with preoperative chemoradiation (45 to 50 Gy plus 5-fluorouracil first and last 5 days of irradiation), radical surgery, and presacral electron boost (10 to 15 Gy) in T3–T4–Nx primary rectal cancer. The indication of IOERT was considered an adjuvant radiation boost. One local recurrence (outside the IORT-boosted region) was observed in 76 consecutive patients analysed and treated in a period of 12 years. Actuarial survival was projected 72 per cent at 7 years follow-up.[71]

Colon cancer

At the Mayo Clinic between 1974 and 1994, out of 103 patients with advanced colon cancer, 11 were treated with IOERT and EBRT. The rate of local failure in this group was 11 per cent compared with 82 per cent when IOERT was not delivered. The 5-year overall survival of the 11 patients was 76 per cent. Although selection bias is possible, these results are promising and further studies should be carried out.[72]

Cancer of gall bladder, extrahepatic bile ducts, and liver

Todoroki reported a series of 37 patients with stage IV adenocarcinoma of the gall bladder treated with surgical resection plus IOERT (mean dose 20.9 Gy), followed by EBRT (mean dose 40 Gy). The 5-year overall survival was 9 per cent. In a historical control group, when no IOERT was given, the 5-year overall survival was 0 per cent. It was mainly patients with R1 resection whom benefited from IOERT.[73],[74] In Germany[75] and the United States,[76] pilot studies have explored the feasibility of IORT in the management of cancer of bile duct and liver.

Retroperitoneal soft tissue sarcoma

With surgery alone, the local recurrence rate is reported as high as 60 to 80 per cent. Postoperative EBRT cannot deliver safely doses over 45 Gy in large abdominal fields, which would be required for treatment of such a poorly radiosensitive tumour.

A randomized trial was conducted at the National Cancer Institute and included 35 patients with retroperitoneal soft tissue sarcoma.[7],[77] The control group was treated with surgery and postoperative EBRT (60 Gy split course). The experimental group was treated with surgery and IOERT (20 Gy) followed by EBRT (40 Gy). There was no difference in the 5-year overall survival (49 per cent). In the IOERT group, there was a significant improvement in local control, in field freedom for recurrence (60 versus 20 per cent), and reduction in radiation chronic enteritis (15 versus 50 per cent). Between 1981 and 1995 at the Mayo Clinic, 43 patients with retroperitoneal soft tissue sarcoma were treated with wide excision and IOERT (median dose 12.5 Gy) with pre- or postoperative EBRT (median dose 47 Gy).[46] The 5-year overall survival was 53 per cent with a local control in two-thirds of the patients. Grade 3 peripheral neuropathy developed in four patients (9 per cent). The histological cellular grade of the sarcoma did not affect the local control or survival rate. In Europe[47],[78] and in Boston,[44] similar, encouraging results have been published. One open question is to know what to do after an initial R0 (or R1) resection for a retroperitoneal soft tissue sarcoma. Is it necessary to perform second-look surgery with IOERT plus EBRT or only EBRT? Careful follow-up of the patient with sonography and CT scan and reservation of surgery and IOERT only for a local recurrence is an alternative strategy that should be prospectively evaluated.

Bladder cancer

The technique of IOERT for urinary bladder cancer was described by Shipley et al.[79] IOERT is performed at the time of cystotomy. The cone is easily positioned on the trigone or on the fixed part of the bladder. This IOERT procedure can be associated with a preoperative combined chemoradiotherapy. In Lyon between 1988 and 1994, a series of 24 patients (20 T2, four T3) were treated. A first line EBRT was given (48 Gy/5 weeks), combined in 14 patients with concomitant chemotherapy (methotrexate, vinblastine, cisplatinum, MVC). The median dose of IOERT was 15 Gy with an applicator size of 7 cm in diameter. The 4-year overall survival was 64 per cent. A local relapse in the bladder was seen in three cases and one was salvaged by a subsequent total cystectomy. In three patients a grade 2 bladder necrosis or ureteral stenosis was observed. The technique appears well adapted for tumour of the fixed part of the bladder.[80] The group in Pamplona published high tumour sterilization rates in muscle-invasive bladder cancers using preoperative radiotherapy, IOERT (15 Gy), and programmed cystectomy.[81] These downstaging results were similar to the concomitant use of induction chemotherapy: 71 per cent pT0.

Uterine cervix cancer T3b

Involvement of the tumour into the whole parametrium and fixation to the pelvic wall is a characteristic of T3b cervix cancer. The standard treatment is exclusive radiotherapy. Despite high irradiation doses (EBRT plus brachytherapy) the rate of local disease progression is close to 40 per cent. Surgery is not recommended because, as in T4 rectal cancer, it is very often impossible not to leave gross tumour in the pelvis at the time of resection. In Lyon from 1988 to 1995, 28 patients with advanced carcinomas of the cervix stage T2b (12 patients) or T3b (16 patients) were treated with a combined approach including surgery. In 14 patients, pelvic lymph node involvement was present initially. The treatment protocol in this pilot study was EBRT (with or without concomitant 5-fluorouracil-cisplatinum in 13 patients) with a median dose of 46 Gy followed by a cervicovaginal Iridium-192 brachytherapy (15 Gy). After a rest period of 3 to 4 weeks, radical surgery was performed (Wertheim III with or without lymphadenectomy) with IOERT boost directed to the pelvic side wall resection limit of the parametrium. The dose of IOERT ranged from 12 to 18 Gy according to the amount of residual disease present after resection. The 5-year overall survival was 52 per cent. The rate of local relapse in the pelvis was 22 per cent. Severe grade 3 toxicity was observed in 13 per cent of cases, either related to surgery (urinary bladder) or radiotherapy (neuropathy, ureteral fistula). These preliminary results could lead to a reappraisal of the role of surgery in T3b uterine cervix carcinoma.[31],[82] At the University Clinic of Navarra in Pamplona, 26 locally advanced patients treated from 1985 to 1997 with preoperative chemoradiation (45–50 Gy, cisplatin plus 5-fluorouracil intravenous infusion days 1 to 4 and 21 to 25 of irradiation), radical surgery plus IOERT to the parametrial resection margin spaces (10–15 Gy), and no brachytherapy, achieved a pelvic control rate of 93 per cent and 5-year disease free survival rate of 76 per cent. IORT-related complications included neuropathy[3] and chronic pelvic pain.[3] Ureteral changes were also seen, but its origin appears to be multifactorial.[32],[83]

Extra-abdominopelvic tumour

Pilot studies with IOERT have been conducted in nearly all the anatomical sites. The aim was always to improve local control in situations where the rate of local relapse remains high with standard treatment.

Malignant brain tumour

Many different pilots studies have been published in the United States, Japan, and Europe.[51],[84] Histological subtypes included were: glioblastoma, low grade glioma, and metastases. The treatment was an association of local resection with EBRT (10 to 20 Gy) followed by EBRT (40 to 60 Gy). Tolerance was described acceptable in most of reports. Some conclusions were encouraging but the level of evidence is still weak.

Head and neck tumours

For tumours of the glossotonsillar sulcus or floor of the mouth extensive surgery and IOERT have been performed in the United States,[85] France,[86] and Germany.[87] Increased local control were reported with low toxicity. In cases of local relapse in a previously irradiated area, IORT appears feasible. In a series of 47 patients with primary or nodal recurrence, Rate et al.[88] reported a 2-year overall survival rate of 55 per cent and a local control rate of 61 per cent without significant toxicity. The data from Pamplona has been reported from a group of 31 patients treated in an 11-years period, including 23 cases with recurrent disease (half of them in previously irradiated area). Extensive debulking surgery plus IOERT with or without EBRT and reconstruction of the tissue defect with muscle–cutaneous flap, locally controlled disease in 16 patients and projected a 5-year survival rate of 19 per cent.[48]

Breast cancer

The technique of IOERT for boosting of the tumour bed at the time of lumpectomy was initially described in Toledo.[89] A dose of 10 to 15 Gy is given to the tumour bed with the advantage of a shorter course of postoperative breast irradiation. In a series of 50 patients Dubois et al. were able to reproduce this treatment in T1 and small T2 tumours with good local control and excellent tolerance.[90]

Intrathoracic tumours

In non-small cell lung cancer, IOERT has been performed in three different situations: on the hilum, bronchial stump, and mediastinum for tumours of the main bronchus with lymph nodes involvement or R2 resections;[50] on the primary tumour when resection was deemed unfeasible due to respiratory insufficiency;[91] and on the thoracic wall for T3 lesions with adhesions to ribs or pleura.[92] The experience of adding an IOERT boost component to the multimodal management of pancoast tumours proved to be feasible at the University Clinic of Navarra, with local control rates of 91 per cent and 5 year survival around 50 per cent.[93] The last up-dated publication of multimodal therapy in stage III non-squamous-cell lung cancer including an IOERT component achieved a thoracic control rate of 76 per cent in 55 patients treated with neoadjuvant containing chemotherapy.[94] Although local control appeared to be improved, long-term overall survival remained modest. The dose of IOERT to the oesophagus or trachea must not exceed 12 Gy if a large portion of these organs are included in the treated volume. A pilot study to treat malignant mesothelioma has been undertaken at the University of California at San Francisco. A group of five patients were treated in 1995 to 96 with pleurectomy and complete decortication to remove all visible, macroscopic disease. The IOERT conducted at the completion of resection typically encompassed three fields (average 10 Gy/field) with 6 to 9 MeV electrons to include major fissures, the diaphragm, and the pericardium. Postoperative conformal therapy was given postoperatively (doses from 40 to 65 Gy). No severe toxicity was observed. Effusion and dyspnoea were controlled in all patients. More patients and longer follow-up are needed to evaluate this strategy.

Extremities sarcomas

Several pilot studies in the United States and Europe have been conducted, including large number of patients with soft tissue sarcomas of the extremities.[95],[96] When large tumours with R1 resection are present, IOERT brings encouraging results. Calvo in Spain and the Mayo Clinic used a similar protocol with a preoperative or postoperative EBRT (50 Gy) and wide excision with IOERT boost to the tumour bed area (10 to 15 Gy). Local control rate with a good function of the preserved limbs was reported in 90 per cent of the cases.[97] Bone tumours in the pelvis are not amenable for complete, gross resection and IOERT might be of benefit for local tumour control promotion.[52]

Paediatric tumours

A large series from Haase et al. at the Denver Children's Hospital has been published.[53] A local control rate of 75 per cent was achieved in 48 patients with malignancy and 91 per cent in 11 patients with benign but locally aggressive, recurrent tumours. Histologies were variable (neuroblastoma, desmoid, soft tissue sarcoma, Wilm's tumour). One of the striking results of this series was the low radiation toxicity of this treatment which is of prime importance in children.[98] Bone sarcoma in paediatric patients treated with an IOERT component obtained local control rates of 80 per cent in 16 Ewing's sarcoma patients and 94 per cent in 22 with osteosarcoma.[98],[99] Leavey et al. treated 24 neuroblastoma patients and reported 67 per cent local control.[100]

Level of evidence

The data presented in Chapter 4.7 demonstrate that IOERT in combination with surgery, EBRT, and chemotherapy is feasible with an acceptable level of acute and late morbidity. The dose escalation possible with IOERT has lead to new radiation side-effects such as radiation neuropathy and bone necrosis which appeared as limiting factors for this technique. The clinical benefit of IOERT has not yet been demonstrated with a strong level of evidence. Promotion of local control seems to be obtained in most of pilot studies and/or phase I–II oriented trials. In fact, local control is not a reliable endpoint because it is often difficult to measure with accuracy and it is not a good surrogate for overall survival. This is especially true in pilot, non-randomized studies. The benefit in terms of overall survival remains questionable. Phase I–II studies cannot provide good evidence of an improvement in overall survival. Although comparisons with historical series tend to show that IOERT provides a better overall survival in rectal or uterine cancer,[29]–[31],[70] the level of evidence remains very weak.

Randomized trials are difficult to perform with IOERT but some have been reported, mainly in gastric cancer (Table 2). These trials claimed significant improvement in local control or overall survival. Unfortunately, small number of patients, methodology, deviation or lack of good peer review publication dot not provide total confidence in the presented data and clinical practice has not been deeply influenced by these results. From a methodological point of view, patients treated with R2 resection may provide the best level of evidence for a clinical benefit of IOERT. There is at the present time a large number of papers reporting more than 100 patients with such incomplete gross resection and with survival exceeding 5 years and with acceptable radiation toxicity.[4],[13],[39],[45],[73],[95] As it is commonly recognized that disease in such patients cannot be locally controlled with standard radiation therapy (with or without chemotherapy), these results should be analysed as a good evidence of the effectiveness of IOERT.

Present recommendations and future prospects

As the level of evidence for the benefit of IOERT is not yet very strong, this procedure must still be considered to be in the field of clinical research. It is clear that large, randomized trials are still difficult to conduct due to the small number of centres with an active IOERT programme in the world. These centres should be strongly encouraged to design and conduct phase III trials. Results of the ongoing French trial in rectal cancer may, in a few years, bring interesting data. Recurrent pelvic cancer, which is a frequent situation, could be an interesting field for a randomized trial.

Outside of clinical trials, it should be recommended to used IOERT only as a local boost in association with an EBRT. The dose for subclinical disease after R0 or R1 resection should be close to 12 Gy to avoid, as much as possible, radiation neuropathy. As IOERT is an invasive and aggressive treatment, strict selection is needed to use this procedure, mostly in a curative intent situation. One of the most relevant clinical situation is when there is a high likelihood of incomplete gross surgery (R2 resection) in a patients with only locoregional tumour with no distant metastases.

One of the main limitation for the development of IOERT is the reluctance of many surgeons (due to logistic difficulties) to operate far from their own operating room. The recent design in the United States and Italy of mobile linear accelerators, which should be able to be transported from one hospital to another, should solve this problem and encourage new enthusiasm in institutions engaged in cancer research.[22],[23]

Such mobile units should be truly mobile so as to be easily transported from one operating room to another. Careful radio-protection control should be in place when using a linear accelerator delivering only electron beams between 6 and 12 MeV to avoid exceeding the legal authorized dose to the environment. Such a mobile unit should be used only under the supervision and responsibility of a radiotherapy department with the assistance of an experienced radiophysics unit and the presence at the time of surgery of a radiation oncologist.

Intraoperative irradiation can also be performed with low-dose rate or high-dose rate brachytherapy techniques. The relative merits of IOERT and brachytherapy are beyond the scope of this chapter. Both techniques aim at the same goal—increasing the dose to the tumour bed to improve local control without severe radiation toxicity. Experience gained in a variety of clinical situations, technical developments, radioprotection requirements, and financial costs, will in the coming years help to define the pros and cons between these different approaches of IORT.

Since the discovery of X-rays a century ago, it has been demonstrated that whenever a higher radiation dose could be delivered to the tumour without increasing the rate of severe side-effects this resulted in a therapeutic gain through better local malignant disease control.[15] Technological radiotherapy research is aiming at increasing the selectively of the dose deposited, such as three-dimensional conformal therapy, radiosurgery, and brachytherapy. IOERT is a development in line with this technological progress. A technical solution must be found for all surgeons to have access to IOERT whenever a clinical situation required it. Research should also be oriented toward biological improvement of IOERT dose-escalation possibilities (oxygen effect, hyperthermia, sensitizer gene therapy, etc.). A combined approach with chemotherapy and systemic therapy will be necessary to overcome the problem of distant metastases, which will continue to be one of the major issues in contemporary oncology.

References

1. Beck C. External roentgen treatment of internal structures. Eventration treatment. *New York State Medical Journal*, 1909; **89**: 621–2.

2. Casas FA, Ferrer F, Calvo FA. European historical role of intraoperative radiation therapy (IORT): a case report from 1905. *Radiotherapy and Oncology*, 1997; **43**: 323–5.

3. Abe M, Shibamoto YT, Akahashi M. Intraoperative radiotherapy in carcinoma of the stomach and pancreas. *World Journal of Surgery*, 1987; **11**: 549–464.

4. Abe M, Takahashi M. Intraoperative radiotherapy: the japanese experience. *International Journal of Radiation Oncology Biology Physics*, 1981; **7**: 863–8.

5. Abe M, Takahashi M, Shibamoto Y, Ono K, Onoyama Y, Torizuka K. Application of intraoperative radiation therapy to refractory cancers. *Annals of Radiology*, 1989; **6**: 493–4.

6. Takahashi M, Abe M. Intraoperative radiotherapy for carcinoma of the stomach. *European Journal of Surgical Oncology*, 1986; **12**: 247–50.

7. Kinsella TJ, Sindelar WF, Lack E, Glatstein E, Rosenberg SA. Preliminary results of a randomized study of adjuvant radiation therapy in resectable adult retroperitoneal soft tissue sarcoma. *Clincal Oncology*, 1988; **6**: 18–25.

8. Noyes RD, Weiss SM, Krall JM, Sause WT, Owens JR, Wolkov HB, *et al.* Surgical complications of intraoperative radiatrion therapy: the radiation therapy oncology group experience. *Journal of Surgical Oncology*, 1992; **50**: 209–15.

9. Arimoto T, Takamura A, Tomita M, Kanero Y. IORT for esophageal carcinoma. Significance of IORT dose for the incidence of fatal tracheal complication. *International Journal of Radiation Oncology Biology Physics*, 1993; **27**: 1063–7.

10. Hoopes PJ, Gilette EL, Withrow WJ. Intraoperative irradiation of the canine abdominal aorta and vena cava. *International Journal of Radiation Oncology Biology Physics*, 1987; **13**: 715–22.

11. Kinsella TJ, Sindelar WF, De Luca AM. Treshold dose for peripheral nerve injury following intraoperative radiotherapy (IORT) in a large animal model. *International Journal of Radiation Oncology Biology Physics*, 1988; **15**: 205.

12. Sindelar WF, Kinsella TJ. Randomized trial of intraoperative radiotherapy in resected carcinoma of the pancreas. *International Journal of Radiation Oncology Biology Physics*, 1986; **12**: 148.

13. Willett CG, Shellito PC, Tepper JE, Eliseo R, Convery K, Wood WC. Intraoperative electron beam radiation therapy for recurrent locally advanced rectal or rectosigmoid carcinoma. *Cancer*, 1991; **67**: 1504–8.

14. Sindelar WF, Kinsella TJ, Tepper JE, *et al.* Randomized trial of intraoperative radiotherapy in carcinoma of the stomach. *American Journal of Surgery*, 1993; **165**: 178–87.

15. Tubiana M. The role of local treatment in the cure of cancer. *European Journal of Cancer*, 1992; **28A**: 2061–9.

16. Suit HD. Local control and patient survival. *International Journal of Radiation Oncology Biology Physics*, 1992; **23**: 653–60.

17. Gerard JP, Romestaing P, Sentenac I. La radiothérapie per opératoire. *Revue du Praticien*, 1989; **69**: 45–8.

18. Beteille D, Setzkorn R, Prevost H, Dusseau L, Missous O, Dubois JB. Laser heating of thermoluminescents plates: application to IORT. *Medical Physics*, 1996; **23**: 1–4.

19. Dubois J.B. La radiothérapie per-opératoire dans le traitement des cancers. *Annales de Chirurgie*, 1989; **43**: 785–9.

20. Gerard JP, Sentenac I, Gilly F, *et al.* Le point sur la radiothérapie per opératoire. *La Lettre du Cancérologue*, 1993; **2**: 3–8.

21. Palta J, Biggs P, Hazle J, Huq M, Dahl R, Ochran T, *et al.* IORT electron beam. Technique, dosimetry and dose specification: report of task force 48 of the radiation therapy committee, American Association of Physicists in Medicine. *International Journal of Radiation Oncology Biology Physics*, 1995; **33**: 725–46.

22. Meurk ML, Goer D, Spalek G. The mobetron. A new concept for IORT. *Frontiers of Radiation Therapy and Oncology*, 1997; **31**: 65–70.

23. Zonca C, Fossati V, Basso Ricci S, Soriani A, Begnozzi L. Preliminary studies for clinical application of Novac 7. A mobile IOERT unit. *Frontiers of Radiation Therapy and Oncology*, 1997; **31**: 60–4.

24. Shaw EG, Gunderson LL, Martin JK, Beart RW, Nagorney DM, Podratz KC. Peripheral nerve and ureteral tolerance to intraoperative radiation therapy: clinical and dose-response analysis. *Radiotherapy and Oncology*, 1990; **18**: 247–55.

25. McChesney Gilette SL, Gilette EL, Powers BE, Park RD, Withrow SJ. Ureteral injury following experimental intraoperative radiation. *International Journal of Radiation Oncology Biology Physics*, 1989; **17**: 791–8.

26. De Ranieri J, Crouet H, Levy C, *et al.* Radiothérapie abdomino pelvienne per opératoire par électrons à dose unique. *Presse Medicale*, 1984; **15**: 839–41.

27. Powers BE, Gilette EL, Mc Chesney SL, Withrow SJ, le Couteur RA. Bone necrosis and tumor induction following experimental intraoperative irradiation. *International Journal of Radiation Oncology Biology Physics*, 1989; **17**: 559–67.

28. Haddock MG, Gunderson LL, Nelson H, Cha RM, Devine R, Dozois R. IORT for locally recurrent colorectal cancer in previously irradiated area. *Frontiers of Radiation Therapy and Oncology*, 1997, **31**: 243–4.

29. Gunderson LL, Nelson H, Martenson JA, *et al.* Locally advanced primary colorectal cancer. IORT and external beam irradiation + 5 FU. *International Journal of Radiation Oncology Biology Physics*, 1997; **37**: 601–14.

30. Garton GR, Gunderson LL, Webb MJ, *et al.* Intraoperative irradiation in gynecologic cancer: Uptate of the Mayo clinic experience. *International Journal of Radiation Oncology Biology Physics*, 1997; **37**: 839–43.

31. Gerard JP, Dargent D, Raudrant D, Braillon G. Place de la radiothérapie per opératoire dans le traitement des cancers de l'utérus. *Bulletin du Cancer Radiotherapie*, 1994; **81**: 186–95.

32. Calikins, Lester S, Stehman F, Clinez H, Calvo F. Intraoperative radiotherapy in advanced or recurrent gynecologic cancer. *Annals of Radiology*, 1989; **32**: 501–3.

33. Martinez Monge R, Jurado M, Azinovic I, *et al.* Intraoperative radiotherapy in recurrent gynecological cancer. *Radiotherapy and Oncology*, 1993; **28**: 127–33.

34. Mahe MA, Cuilliere JC, Guillard Y, Cussac A, Brunet TG, Lisbona A. Radiothérapie intra operatoire dans les récidives et les formes avancées du cancer du col utérin. *Bulletin du Cancer*, 1993; **80**: 500–1.

35. Mahe MA, Gerard JP, Dubois JB, *et al.* IORT in recurrent carcinoma of the uterine cervix: report of the french IORT group on 70 patients. *International Journal of Radiation Oncology Biology Physics*, 1996; **34**: 21–6.

36. Frydenberg M, Gunderson LL, Hahn G, Fieck J, Zincke H. Preoperative external beam radiotherapy followed by cytoreductive and intraoperative radiotherapy for locally advanced primary or recurrent renal malignancies. *Journal of Urology*, 1994; **152**: 15–21.

37. Gunderson LL, Martin J K, Beart RW, *et al.* Intraoperative and external beam irradiation for locally advanced colorectal cancer. *Annals of Surgery*, 1988; **207**: 52–60.

38. Suzuki K, Gunderson LL, Devone RM, Weaver A, Dozois RR, Illstrup DM, *et al.* Intraoperative irradiation after palliative resection for locally recurrent rectal cancer. *Cancer*, 1995; **75**: 939–52.

39. Abuchaibe O, Calvo FA, Azinovic I, Aristu J, Pardo F, Alvarez-Cienfugos J. Intraoperative radiotherapy in locally advanced recurrent colorectal cancer. *International Journal of Radiation Oncology Biology Physics*, 1993; **26**: 859–67.

40. Calvo FA, Algarra SM, Azinovic I, *et al.* Intraoperative radiotherapy for recurrent and/or residual colorectal cancer. *Radiotherapy and Oncology*, 1989; **15**: 133–40.

41. Eble MJ, Kallinowski F, Wulf J, Lehnert T, Wannenmacher M. Moderate dose IORT and EBRT in locally advanced or recurrent rectal cancer. *Hepato-Gastroenterology*, 1994; **41**: 21 [Abst].

42. Bussieres E, Gilly FN, Rouanet P, *et al.* Recurrences of rectal cancers: results of a multimodal approach with IORT. *International Journal of Radiation Oncology Biology Physics*, 1996; **34**: 49–56.

43. Holm T, Blomqvist L, Cedermark B, Lundell G, Wilking N. Multimodality approach including IORT in the treatment of primary unresectable and locally recurrent rectal carcinoma. *Hepato-Gastroenterology*, 1994; **41**: 21 [Abst].

44. Willett CG, Suit HD, Tepper JE, *et al.* Intraoperative electron beam radiation therapy for retroperitoneal soft tissue sarcoma. *Cancer*, 1991; **68**: 278–83.

45. Gunderson LL, Nagorney DM, Mc Llrath DC, *et al.* External beam and intraoperative electron irradiation for locally advanced soft tissue sarcomas. *International Journal of Radiation Oncology Biology Physics*, 1993; **25**: 647–56.

46. Petersen I, Haddock M, Donohue J, Nagomey O, Gunderson L, Grill J. Use of IORT in the management of retroperitoneal and pelvic soft tissue sarcomas. *International Journal of Radiation Oncology Biology Physics*, 1996, **36**: 185 [Abst].

47. Calvo F, Azinovic I, Martinez-Monge R, Aristu J, Amillo S, Berian J. Intraoperative radiotherapy for the treatment of soft tissue sarcomas of central anatomical sites. *Radiation Oncology Investigations*, 1995; **3**: 3096.

48. Martinez Monge R, Azinovic I, Alcade J, *et al.* IORT in the management of locally advanced or recurrent head and neck cancer. *Frontiers of Radiation Therapy and Oncology*, 1997; **31**: 122–5.

49. Ratto C, Sofo L, Valentini V, Nulera P, Crucitti F. Treatment of primary and recurrent rectal cancer with multimodal approach including IORT. *Hepato-Gastroenterology*, 1994; **41**: 21–2 [Abst].

50. Calvo F, Ortiz De Urbina D, Abuchaibe O, Azinovic I, Aristu J, Santos M, Llorens R. IORT during lung cancer surgery: early clinical results. *International Journal of Radiation Oncology Biology Physics*, 1990; **19**: 103–9.

51. Willich N, Prott F, Schuller P, Wagner W, Paltovic S, Morgenroth C, *et al.* Pilot study of IORT for malignant brain tumors. *Hepato-Gastroenterology*, 1994; **41**: 16 [Abst].

52. Hoekstra HS, Sindelar W, Szabo B, Kinsella T. Hemipelvectomy and IORT for bone sarcomas of the pelvic girdle. *Hepato-Gastroenterology*, 1994; **41**: 5 [Abst].

53. Haase GM, Meagher DP Jr, McNeely LK, Daniel WE, Poole MA, Blake M, *et al.* Electron beam intraoperative radiation therapy in pediatric neoplasms. *Cancer*, 1994; **74**: 738–45.

54. Guillemin F, Malissard L, Aletti P, Bey P. IORT for carcinoma of the stomach. A five year pilot study. In: Abe M, ed. *Intra operative radiation therapy. Proceedings of the Third International Symposium on IORT.* Pergamon Press, 1991: 199–200.

55. Martinez Monge R, Calvo FA, Azinovic I, *et al.* Patterns of failure and long term results in high risk resected gastric cancer treated with postoperative radiotherapy with or without intraoperative electron boost. *Journal of Surgical Oncology,* 1997; **66**: 24–9.

56. Chen GX, Song SB. Evaluation of IORT for gastric carcinoma. Analyse of 247 patients. In: Abe M. *Intraoperative radiation therapy. Proceedings of the Third International Symposium on IORT.* Pergamon Press, 1991: 190–1.

57. Kramling HJ, Willich N, Cramer C, Wilkowski R, Schildberg FW. IORT for gastric cancer. Intermediate results after 4 years. *Revista de Medicina de la Universidad de Navarra,* 1998; **42**: 47.

58. Calvo FA, Aristu JJ, Azinovic I, *et al.* Intraoperative and external radiotherapy in resected gastric cancer: updated report of a phase II trial. *International Journal of Radiation Oncology Biology Physics,* 1992; **24**: 729–36.

59. Coquard R, Gilly FN, Romestaing P, *et al.* IORT combined with limited lymph node resection in gastric cancer. An alternative to extended dissection ? *International Journal of Radiation Oncology Biology Physics,* 1997; **39**: 1093–8.

60. Gilly FN, Gerard JP, Braillon G, *et al.* Radiothérapie per opératoire dans les adénocarcinomes gastriques. A propos de quarante cinq cas. *Annales de Chirurgie,* 1993; **43**: 234–9.

61. Ogata T, Araki K, Matsuura K, Yoshida S. A 10 years experience of IORT for gastric cancer and a new surgical method of creating a wider irradiation field. *International Journal of Radiation Oncology Biology Physics,* 1995; **32**: 341–7.

62. Coquard R, Gilly FN, Romestaing P, *et al.* IORT in resected pancreatic cancer: feasibility and results. *Radiotherapy and Oncology,* 1997; **44**: 271–5.

63. Gilly F, Beaujard N, Carry F, Braillon G, Gerard JP. IORT in pancreatic cancer. *Frontiers of Radiation Therapy and Oncology,* 1997; **31**: 41–3.

64. Garton GR, Gunderson LL, Nagorney DM, *et al.* High dose preoperative external beam and intraoperative irradiation for locally advanced pancreatic cancer. *International Journal of Radiation Oncology Biology Physics,* 1993; **27**: 1153–7.

65. Mohiuddin M, Stevens JH, Rosato F, Schritcht A, Cantor R, Bierman W. IORT in the combined modality management of pancreatic cancer. *Hepato-Gastroenterology,* 1994; **41**: 20 [Abst].

66. Baulieux J, Gerard JP. Cancer du rectum localement avancé. Intérêt de la rpo. *Journal of Medicine,* Lyon, 1995; **75**: 9–14.

67. Sischy B. Intraoperative electron beam radiation therapy with particular reference to the treatment of rectal carcinomas. Primary and recurrent. *Diseases of the Colon and Rectum,* 1986; **29**: 714–18.

68. Valentini V, Cellini N, Sofo L, Ratto C, Crucitti F. Chemoradiation therapy and IORT in locally advanced rectal cancer: preliminary results in 36 patients. *Frontiers of Radiation Therapy and Oncology,* 1997; **31**: 213–16.

69. Wiig J, Tveit K, Gierchsky K, Olsen D. IORT for primary inoperable and locally recurrent rectal cancer. *Hepato-Gastroenterology,* 1994; **41**: 22 [Abst].

70. Willett cg, Shellito PC, Tepper JE, Eliseo R, Convery K, Wood WC. Intraoperative electron beam radiation therapy for primary locally advanced rectal and rectosigmoid carcinoma. *Journal of Clinical Oncology,* 1991; **9**: 843–9.

71. Azinovic I, Calvo FA, Santos M, *et al.* Intense local therapy in primary rectal cancer: multi-institutional results with preoperative chemoradiation therapy plus IORT. *Frontiers of Radiation Therapy and Oncology,* 1997; **31**: 196–9.

72. Schild SE, Gunderson L, Haddock MG, Wong W, Nelson H. The treatment of locally advanced colon cancer. *International Journal of Radiation Oncology Biology Physics,* 1997; **37**: 51–8.

73. Todoroki T, Iwasaki Y, Kawamoto T, Nakamura K. Resection combined with IORT for stage IV gallbladder carcinoma. *World Journal of Surgery,* 1991; **15**: 357–66.

74. Todoroki T, Iwasaki Y, Okamura T, *et al.* IORT for advanced carcinoma of the biliary system. *Cancer,* 1980; **46**: 2179–84.

75. Willborn K, Sauerwein W, Erhard J, Eigler F, Sack H. IORT for carcinoma of the extrahepatic bile ducts. *Frontiers of Radiation Therapy and Oncology,* 1997; **31**: 173–6.

76. Monson JRT, Donohue JH, Gunderson LL, Nagormey DM, Bender CE, Wieand HS. Intraoperative radiotherapy for unresectable cholangiocarcinoma: the Mayo clinic experience. *Surgical Oncology,* 1992; **1**: 283–90.

77. Sindelar WF, Kinsella TJ, Chen PW, *et al.* Intraoperative radiotherapy in sarcomas of the retroperitoneum: final results of a prospectively randomized clinical trial. *Archives of Surgery,* 1993; **128**: 402–10.

78. Bussieres E. , Stockle E, Richaud P, Avril A, Kind M, Kantor G, Coindre JM, Bui B. Retroperitoneal soft tissue sarcomas: a pilot study of IORT. *Journal of Surgical Oncology,* 1996; **62**: 49–56.

79. Shipley WV, Kaufman D, Prout G. IORT in patients with bladder cancer. *Cancer,* 1987, **60**: 1485–8.

80. Hulewicz G, Roy P, Coquard R, *et al.* La radiothérapie per opératoire dans le traitement conservateur des cancers infiltrants de vessie. *Progrès en Urologie,* 1997, 7: 229–34.

81. Calvo FA, Aristu JJ, Abuchaibe O, *et al.* Intraoperative and external preoperative radiotherapy in invasive bladder cancer: effect of neoadjuvant chemotherapy in tumor downstaging. *American Journal of Clinical Oncology,* 1993; **16**: 61–6.

82. Dargent D, Gerard J.P, Adeleine P. Place de la radiothérapie intra opératoire dans le traitement du cancer utérin. *Journal of Obstetrics and Gynecology,* 1993, 1: 120–7.

83. Jurado M. Intraoperative radiotherapy (IORT) in locally advanced and recurrent cervical cancer. *Revista de Medicina de la Universidad de Navarra,* 1998; 17 (Supp. 1):54.

84. Dobellbower R, Carter D, Lokshina A, McCutchan P. IORT for intracranial neoplasms. *Hepato-Gastroenterology,* 1994; **41**: 16 [Abst].

85. Garret P, Rate W, Hamaker R, Ducan T, Pugh N, Ross D, *et al.* IORT in head and neck cancer with tongue invasion. *Hepato-Gastroenterology,* 1994; **41**: 7–8 [Abst].

86. Schmitt T, Prades JM, Pinto N, Puel G, Talabard JN, Martin C. IORT on a part of radiosurgical treatment for locally advanced oropharyngeal carcinomas. *Hepato-Gastroenterology,* 1994; **41**: 8 [Abst].

87. Nilles-Schendera A, Stoll P, Fromhold H, Schilli W. IORT in floor of the mouth cancer. *Frontiers of Radiation Therapy and Oncology,* 1997; **31**: 102–4.

88. Rate W, Garret P, Hamaker R, Pugh N, Charles G. IORT for recurrent head and neck cancer. *Cancer,* 1991; **67**: 2738–40.

89. Holliis W, Merrick M, Dobelbower J. IORT for early breat cancer: a novel technique. *Hepato-Gastroenterology,* 1994; **41**: 5 [Abst].

90. Dubois JB, Hay MH, Gely S, Saint Aubert B, Rouanet P, Pujol H. IORT in breast carcinomas. *Frontiers of Radiation Therapy and Oncology,* 1997; **31**: 31.

91. Juettner FM, Arian-Schad K, Porsch G, *et al.* Intraoperative megavolt radiation therapy combined with external radiation in nonresectable non-small cell lung cancer: preliminary report. *International Journal of Radiation Oncology Biology Physics,* 1990; **18**: 1143–50.

92. Guibert B, Mulsant P, Romestaing P, Chambon M, Rochette C, Gerard JP. IORT in thorasic surgery. *Hepato-Gastroenterology,* 1994; **41**: 15 [Abst].

93. Martinez Monge R, Herreros J, Aristu JJ, *et al.* Combined treatment in superior sulcus tumors. *American Journal of Clinical Oncology,* 1994; **17**: 317–22.

94. Aristu JJ, Rebollo J, Martinez Monge R, *et al.* Cisplatin, mitomycin and vindesine followed by intraoperative and postoperative radiotherapy for stage III non small cell lung cancer: final results of a

phase II study. *American Journal of Clinical Oncology*, 1997; **20**: 276–81.

95. **Dubois JB, Debrigode C, Hay M,** *et al.* IORT in soft tissue sarcoma. *Radiotherapy and Oncology*, 1995; **34**: 160–3.

96. **Eble MJ, Lehnert TH, Schwarzbach M,** *et al.* IORT for extremity sarcomas. *Frontiers of Radiation Therapy and Oncology*, 1997; **31**: 146–50.

97. **Petersen I, Gareton G, Pritchard P, Sim F, Rock M, Gunderson L.** IORT in the treatment of extremity soft tissue sarcoma. *Hepato-Gastroenterology*, 1994; **41**: 3 [Abst].

98. **Halberg FE, Harrison M, Salvatierra O, Longaker M, Wara W, Phillips T.** IORT for Wilm's tumor *in situ* or *ex vivo. Cancer,* 1991; **67**: 2839–43.

99. **Calvo FA, Ortiz de Urbina D, Sierrasesumaga L,** *et al.* Intraoperative radiotherapy in the multidisciplinary treatment of bone sarcomas in children and adolescents. *Medical Pediatric Oncology*, 1991; **19**: 478–85.

100. **Leavey PJ, Odom LF, Poole M,** *et al.* Intraoperative radiation therapy in pediatric neuroblastoma. *Medical Pediatric Oncology*, 1997; **28**: 424–8.

4.7.2 Particle radiotherapy

W. Duncan and J. F. Fowler

Introduction

The particle beams of main interest in radiotherapy are electrons, protons, and neutrons. Beams of 'heavy particles' (heavier than protons, in the nuclear mass range from helium-4 to neon-20) are of less practical interest and are only available in two or three centres in the world. These latter, and negative pi mesons, have become less interesting for oncology treatment than protons in the last decade. So for more details about them the reader is referred to the corresponding chapter, by the same authors, in the first edition of this Oxford Textbook of Oncology or the detailed books by Bewley, Fowler, or Raju.[1]–[3]

All charged particles have the physical, dose-planning, advantage that the beams are limited in maximum depth of penetration, depending on their energy and mass. Tissues deeper than the tumour need not be irradiated. This is in contrast with standard X-ray (photon) beams which are gradually attenuated and always deliver some radiation beyond the tumour. Electron beams, for this reason, are often used to treat superficial tumour sites, such as chest wall, or to boost the dose distribution of intricate sites within the oral cavity. Proton beams can provide almost ideally sharp-edged dose distributions, and their use is slowly increasing, but is limited by the capital cost of the equipment. All particle beams require high-energy accelerators. Those which accelerate electrons can produce either a beam of high energy X-rays (photons) or electrons. Such linear accelerators (linacs) are standard in most radiotherapy departments today. Larger machines such as cyclotrons, circular or stadium-shaped synchrotrons, or extended linear accelerators are necessary to accelerate protons or the heavier particles to the energy of 200 to 250 million electron volts (MeV) per nucleon which is necessary for adequate tissue penetration.

Electron beams

Electron beams are commonly used in cancer treatment, being available as an alternative output to the photon beam from many standard linear accelerators, switchable within minutes. The range of an electron beam in centimetres is roughly half the energy in million volts of the electron beam in the machine. Electrons are therefore used in routine treatments to improve, often greatly, the dose distribution for certain individual tumours.

Proton beams

Some half-dozen countries now have at least one proton beam treatment facility and another dozen proton centres are being planned with proposed start-up times before the end of the year 2002. They are of increasing interest in radiotherapy because their dose distributions in tissue have the sharpest edges of all the particle beams, and because machines to accelerate them are smaller and cheaper than for the heavier nuclear particles (see below). Proton beams have given good results in the treatment of ocular melanoma (only 70 MeV is needed), of tumours close to brainstem or spinal cord, and of small lesions in the brain, including arteriovenous malformations, as described in the clinical sections below. For deep seated lesions, a proton beam of 200 to 250 MeV is needed. The number of patients treated with proton beams exceeds 8500 in Boston (United States), 3000 in Moscow (Russia), and 5000 in Loma Linda, California (United States).

The associated physics necessary for accurate beam direction and localization of the treatment volume has pioneered improved localization procedures for all photon radiotherapy, such as 'beam's eye viewing' in general treatment planning.

The advantage of proton beams lies entirely in their good physical dose distribution (Fig. 1). The dose falls laterally from 90 per cent to 20 per cent within a few millimetres. Radiobiological properties are not different from those of conventional photon beams. No extra damage is caused to hypoxic cells, and no less repair occurs of the repairable component of radiation damage. At the end of the proton track, when the particle has slowed down, a dose peak occurs (the well-known Bragg peak). Since this is only a few millimetres long it

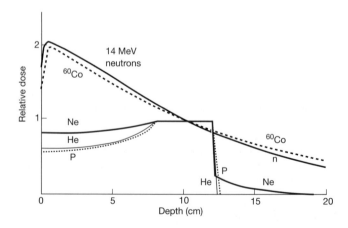

Fig. 1 Depth–dose distributions of various types of beam in tissue (Tobias *et al.* 1971).[4]

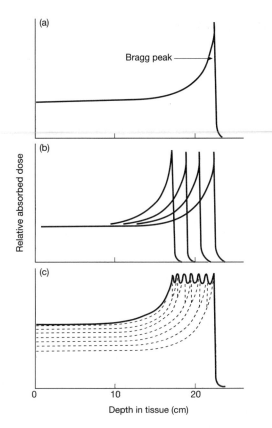

Fig. 2 Depth–dose distribution of a charged particle (ion) beam, showing the Bragg peak: (a) single energy, (b) four energies, showing altered ranges, (c) multiple energies, arranged to cover a target or tumour volume at depth (Fowler 1981).[2]

has to be 'spread out' to cover a tumour of several centimetres depth, losing much of its height relative to the dose earlier in the track (Fig. 2). This is done by varying the energy of the proton beam, from just reaching the proximal edge to covering the distal edge of the tumour, during each treatment. The resulting dose distribution is, however, very much better than that obtainable from any other type of beam.[5]

An advantage of protons over heavier particles is that there is less dose beyond the maximum range of the protons. A small component of dose is projected beyond the maximum range of heavier particles by spallation: the forward projection of disintegration products of nuclear collisions along the particle track. This effect, and the even smaller sideways projection of similar nuclear fragments, is less for proton beams than for the heavier particles. The lower cost of the smaller accelerator for protons than for the heavier particles has already been mentioned. Compared with the standard linear accelerators or cobalt-60 machines in radiation oncology departments everywhere, of course a proton beam installation would be several times more expensive. It is not impossible that a large future demand for proton accelerators would result in economies of construction costs—this has happened before in other fields.

Neutron beams

There are two contrasting kinds of neutron beam, slow and fast. Fast neutrons are generated by modest-sized cyclotrons, usually of 40 to

70 MeV energy in order to give at least as good tissue penetration as cobalt-60 or 4 to 6 MV photon beams. Protons are accelerated on to a beryllium target, and the resulting forward-transmitted neutron beam is attenuated exponentially in tissue as in the case of X-ray beams, because neutrons, like photons, are uncharged. There are no advantages in the physical dose distributions, which are comparable or marginally inferior to photon beams, in part because fast neutron targets are larger than those for X-rays. The potential advantages are purely radiobiological, and the practical magnitude of them is still under debate:

1. Tumour cells which are radioresistant because they are hypoxic are less resistant to neutrons than to photons, in comparison with a given level of damage to normally-oxygenated tissues, that is to non-tumour tissues.

2. Cells which are radioresistant due to very slow proliferation (long G1 phase of the cell cycle) are less radioresistant to neutrons than to photons, relative to the average radiosensitivity of other cells. The treatment of prostate tumours is an obvious application of this potential advantage.

Both of these potential advantages stem from the same basic reason. Neutron beams consist partly of 'high-LET' radiation (high linear energy transfer, high ionizing density along the tracks of the secondary particles). High-LET radiation causes a higher proportion of irrepairable damage in the DNA of cells and tissues, and a correspondingly smaller proportion of repairable 'sublethal' damage. Therefore there is little difference between biological damage with and without the radiosensitizer oxygen present, and between the different phases of the cell cycle, in contrast to low-LET radiation where much larger differences occur. This difference between the greater effectiveness of high than low-LET radiation because less repair can occur is represented by the term relative biological effectiveness, RBE. The higher the ionizing density of the particle tracks the higher will be the RBE. A high RBE, such as 2, means that a given dose of high-LET radiation is twice as damaging as the same physical dose of photons.

However, much confusion has been caused in the past because RBE also depends on the dose per fraction, being highest for lowest fraction sizes. RBE is also tissue dependent, being especially high for the slowly-proliferating, late-responding, normal organs in which life-threatening, late complications can occur. This major point, the greater radiobiological effect on slowly rather than on rapidly proliferating tissues, is vital. It leads to an obvious potential disadvantage of fast neutron beams.

This disadvantage is due to exactly the same reason as the second potential advantage listed above—the greater damage to slow-growing tumours. Late-responding normal tissues, which are the tissues that proliferate slowly, are relatively more vulnerable to high-LET radiation injury. Low-LET radiation (photons or electrons) are remarkably good at sparing late-responding normal tissues from damage when the usual small daily doses of radiation are employed. However, this good sparing is reduced when high-LET radiation is used. This gives neutrons a tendency to cause a relatively high proportion of late complications for a given tumour effect. That is their main disadvantage, and the trend can be seen clearly in the summary, below, of clinical results of neutron therapy. It can be overcome by a careful restriction of the total dose, but the therapeutic window is in principle narrow, and for some types of tumour probably non-existent. The disadvantage could, in principle, also be partially counteracted by giving neutron treatments in shorter overall times—such as in 4 weeks instead of 6 or 7 weeks—but attempts to confirm this by clinical evidence have not succeeded. Neutron therapy is now used rarely, some half-dozen centres in the world being in action. The physical and radiobiological properties of fast neutron beams are described in detail in Bewley's excellent book.[1]

Slow neutrons from nuclear reactors: boron neutron capture therapy

Several groups are investigating or developing clinical facilities to use the interaction of a tumour-seeking drug containing boron or gallium with slow neutrons emerging from a high-flux nuclear reactor. This general approach is called boron neutron capture therapy (BNCT) because B was the first element to be so used, due to its high capture cross section for slow neutrons. The slow neutrons themselves cause relatively little biological effect, but on capture by a B or Ga nucleus they cause disintegration, projecting a short-range, high-LET alpha particle out of the nucleus. The damage is highly local, within a few cell diameters.

The value of this strategy obviously depends on a high uptake of the drug containing B or Ga in the tumour relative to the uptake in surrounding normal tissues. Slow neutron beams diffuse widely in tissue, so the benefit of sharp beam edges is not present, in contrast with protons or even photons. Neutron beams with epithermal energies have better tissue penetration than the lower-energy thermal neutron beams, but few nuclear reactors can produce epithermal beams of sufficient intensity. Favoured sites for BNCT are brain and, with thermal neutron beams, malignant melanoma. For the latter tumours uptake of a specific boron-containing drug can be high. BNCT is practised or planned in half a dozen countries.[6]

Heavy ion beams

Heavy ions—heavier than protons—include helium, carbon, silicon, neon, and argon beams. They all have Bragg peaks which can be projected controllably to many centimetres depth in tissue, and these peaks contain a proportion of high-LET radiation. However, the peaks become progressively less sharp as the mass of the particle increases, so that the advantageous ratio of high dose in the spread-out peak to lower dose along the entrance track is not as good as for protons. Further, the heavier particles have more tendency to break up en route, thus projecting lighter particles beyond the desired range. They nevertheless have better physical depth doses than photons or neutrons, together with the radiobiological differences from photons due to high LET that were described above for fast neutrons. These radiobiological advantages (and disadvantages) are minimal for helium-4 beams, and approach in magnitude to those of fast neutrons only for neon-20 or the even heavier argon-40 ions.

Beams of accelerated helium nuclei were extensively used at Berkeley, California from 1957 to 1992, mainly for lesions in the brain including pituitary irradiations and arteriovenous malformations. Over 2000 patients were treated, with good results. In addition, heavier particles from the Bevalac accelerator at Berkeley were also investigated from 1975 to 1992, leading to the use of beams of carbon-12 and neon-20 ions for radiotherapy of 433 patients with malignant tumours in several body sites. Follow-up reports of these clinical results are being published by Dr J. Castro and his colleagues, as reviewed below. These 'heavy particles' have slightly less physical advantages progressively with increasing nuclear mass, in terms of dose in the spread-out peak relative to dose in the overlying track of the entering particles.

The heavy ion beam in Berkeley was closed in 1992, although results are still being published. Heavy ions are currently (1998) being used for radiotherapy actively at the National Institute for Radiological Sciences in Chiba, Japan[7] and were just beginning to be used clinically at the GSI, Darmstadt, Germany in the summer of 1998. Proton beams have more widespread support in the international oncology community. For those who are interested, further information about proton and other heavy particle beams is regularly updated on the Internet at the Particles Newsletter Web Site:

http://neurosurgery.mgh.harvard.edu/hcl/ptles.htm

Negative Pi mesons

There was a time, in the 1960s, when negative pi mesons appeared to be promising for radiotherapy. They have a mass equal to 230 electrons, that is about 1/8 of that of a proton. They traverse tissue depositing ionization at low LET but at the end of their range they are captured into an (oppositely charged) nucleus in tissue, which then disintegrates, ejecting several alpha particles, neutrons, or protons and a beryllium nucleus, in the form of a 'star' of partly high-LET radiation locally in the tumour. They are produced at low yield by very high energy proton beams, 600 to 800 MeV, and are therefore expensive to produce. Few accelerators large enough to produce them exist anywhere. Three pion facilities were developed in the 1970s, in Los Alamos, United States, in Vancouver, Canada, and in Villigen, Switzerland but none is now producing negative pi mesons for therapy. Two of them are, however, using proton beams for radiotherapy. Apart from the expense and difficulty of pion production, a fundamental disadvantage was that the high-LET component of the 'star' region amounted to only about 20 per cent of the total dose. Negative pi mesons thus gave dose distributions which were no better than carbon ions, not as good as protons, and with only a small radiobiological difference from protons or photons. Further details can be found in the books by Fowler and Raju.[2],[3]

Summary of the physics and radiobiology of particle beams

An overview of the relative physical and radiobiological differences of the particle beams is given in Fig. 3. This was published originally by Dr A. Koehler of the Harvard cyclotron team and reproduced by Raju in his admirably detailed book.[3] The biological differences of high LET from photons are plotted upwards on the Y axis, and the physical depth dose advantages are plotted horizontally along the X axis. Fast neutron beams have the highest RBE but only ordinary depth dose characteristics. Protons have the best depth dose characteristics, but only ordinary radiobiological factors, just like photons. The lighter 'heavy particle beams', such as carbon or silicon ions,

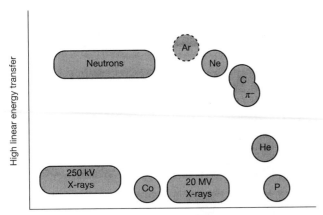

Fig. 3 Biological advantages of high-LET radiation (plotted upward) versus physical depth–dose advantages of the various types of beam discussed (Raju 1980).[3]

have a combination of these potential advantages, as shown in Fig. 3.

Clinical evaluation of particle therapy

Fast neutrons

Fast neutron therapy was first tested clinically in 1938. The neutron beam (d(16) + Be) was produced by a novel particle accelerator known as a 'cyclotron' which had just been developed at Berkeley, California by E.O. Lawrence and W. Livingstone. Dr Robert Stone, the senior clinical investigator, was assisted in his research by Dr John Larkin. A group of 250 patients, mostly with locally advanced cancers, was selected for treatment between 1938 and 1941, when the programme came to an end. The results of this carefully planned and well documented clinical study are described in Stone's Janeway Memorial Lecture of 1948.[8] His clinical appraisal was remarkably perceptive. He reported that many advanced cancers had been successfully treated, particularly cancers of the salivary glands, prostate, and some arising in secondary neck nodes. However, late, normal tissue complications were severe and commonly observed. There was little difference between the radiation dose needed to control these cancers and the dose which produced serious, late morbidity. Eighteen patients had lasting cancer control but all had distressing, severe, late neutron-related complications. Stone concluded that neutrons were no more efficacious than X-ray (photon) therapy and were regularly associated with unacceptably severe, late effects.

A re-evaluation of fast neutron therapy was stimulated by the description of the ' oxygen effect' by L H Gray *et al.* in 1953.[9] Many cancers were known to contain hypoxic cells that, being relatively radioresistant, were thought to be a possible cause of failure after photon therapy. They had demonstrated that the cytocidal effects of neutrons were reduced much less by tumour hypoxia than were the effects of photons. Neutron therapy studies were begun in 1965 at the Hammersmith Hospital, London where the first Medical Research Council (MRC) Cyclotron Unit was built. The radiobiological and clinical reports from the MRC Cyclotron Unit were all highly optimistic about the advantages of fast neutron therapy. In particular, they blamed late complications on the use of too few fractions each of too high a neutron dose instead of multiple small fractions. Their advocacy of high-LET radiotherapy led to a huge investment in related research and development throughout the world. In the United States alone this amounted to over $70 million.

In the following 30 years, over 15 000 patients have been treated with fast neutrons. Only about 1000 of these have been recruited to randomized clinical trials. Many of the trials have failed to recruit adequate numbers of patients to have the statistical power to answer the questions posed. The assessment of neutron therapy also has been made difficult because of the physical and technical limitations of the neutron generators used in the early clinical trials. These limitations have included the unreliable performance or irregular availability of the machines, the poor penetrating power of the neutron beams, low dose rates, fixed treatment heads, and inadequate range of available field sizes. The later hospital-based neutron therapy machines provide adjustable isocentric beams and depth–dose profiles similar to standard Mega-voltage equipment.

Another difficulty in the evaluation of neutron therapy has been the different fractionation regimes used in the randomized treatment groups. When two radiation modalities of different quality are to be compared in a randomized clinical trial the design of the study should require, ideally, that the overall treatment times should be similar in each treatment group. Accelerated fractionation may improve local tumour control rates of 'head and neck' cancers and cancers at other sites. Fast neutrons have commonly been scheduled over 4 weeks, following the original regime used at the Hammersmith Hospital. In contrast, the photon therapy with which neutrons are to be compared has been given, commonly, in an overall time of 5 to 7 weeks. This difference makes it impossible to establish if an observed difference in outcome is truly a qualitative effect of the radiation rather than an avoidance of tumour cell proliferation in the shorter treatment time.

An essential requirement in the design of these trials is to ensure, by careful pilot studies, that the incidence and severity of late radiation-related morbidity, is similar in the experimental and control groups of patients. Only if this condition is achieved may a valid comparison be made of the efficacy of the two treatments on tumour control. This has seldom been satisfied in randomized trials of neutron therapy.

Head and neck cancers

The study of neutron therapy has concentrated mostly on the treatment of squamous cell cancers of the upper foregut region. There have been eight randomized (phase III) trials of head and neck cancers. Five trials have compared neutrons alone with standard photon irradiation, while three have compared a combined photon and neutron regime with photons alone. The results are summarized in Fig. 4.

The first trial was reported from the MRC Cyclotron Unit in London.[10] A group of 134 patients with various head and neck cancers were recruited to the study. The results demonstrated a four-fold, highly significant, increase in local tumour control rates after neutron treatment (76 per cent) compared with photons (19 per cent). However, the late radiation morbidity reported subsequently[11] gave an estimate of the incidence of serious complications to be significantly higher after neutrons (21 per cent) than observed after

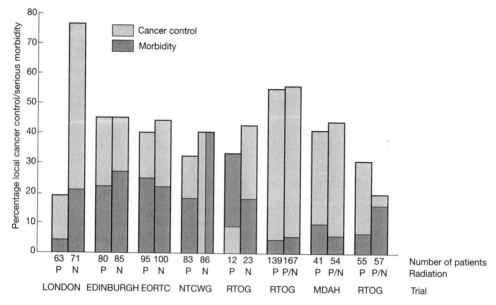

Fig. 4 Head and neck cancer trials (P = photon, N = neutron).

photons (4 per cent). The morbidity after neutrons was so severe that 28 per cent of patients who had lasting local tumour control died directly as a result of late radiation complications. No late radiation-related deaths were observed in the group of patients treated with photons, as one would expect. The mortality rates were similar in both treatment groups. There was no good evidence that neutron therapy was better than higher dose photons. The higher local tumour control rates observed after neutrons were offset by the increase in serious, late, radiation-related morbidity.[12]

The Radiation Therapy Oncology Group (RTOG) in the United States reported the results of a randomized trial[13] which compared a combined schedule of photons (three fractions per week) plus neutrons (two fractions per week) with standard Mega-voltage photon therapy. The treatment times (7 weeks) were similar in both arms of this study. The analysis of the results of 306 of the 322 patients randomized, demonstrated similar tumour control rates (55 per cent versus 56 per cent) and similar normal tissue morbidity (5 per cent and 6 per cent) in both treatment groups. Also there was no significant difference in survival rates.

The MD Anderson Hospital completed a similar trial which compared a combined regime of two fractions neutrons/week plus three fractions photons/week with standard photon therapy. Ninety-five patients were randomized; 54 to have the mixed-schedule neutrons and 41 to have photons alone. None was excluded from the analysis.[14] The local tumour control rates were similar in both groups, 44 per cent in the neutron group and 41 per cent in the photon group. Survival rates were also similar. Serious, late morbidity was observed in 7 per cent of neutron-treated patients and 10 per cent after photons alone.

The RTOG undertook a randomized trial of fast neutrons alone versus photons for patients with unresectable head and neck cancer. The study was designed to recruit patients similar to those entered into the 'mixed beam' RTOG trial but was closed prematurely because of poor accrual. Only 40 patients were randomized and the results of a group of 35 patients considered to be 'eligible' were published.[15]

However, the analysis is uninformative because of the small number of patients. There were only 12 in the photon group and 23 in the neutron group; very few patients survived 2 years. The mortality was similar in both groups. The local control rates at 1 year (43 per cent with neutrons, 9 per cent with photons) were significantly different, statistically. However, the local cancer control rates were similar (52 per cent versus 42 per cent) after salvage surgery. The morbidity rates were not significantly different. The photon results are unacceptably poor in that the tumour control was only 9 per cent (at 1 year) and was associated with an incidence of serious morbidity of 33 per cent.

An Edinburgh trial[16],[17] compared neutrons of similar energy to that of the MRC Cyclotron Unit, London, with Mega-voltage photon therapy. Both treatments were given in 20 daily fractions over 4 weeks. The treatment protocols were designed to produce similar levels of late radiation-related complications. One hundred and twenty patients with squamous cell cancer of the 'head and neck' region were randomized to receive either neutrons alone or photons. The results showed that lasting tumour control was achieved in 45 per cent of patients in both arms of the trial. In the final analysis the late radiation-related morbidity was slightly lower in the photon-treated group (20 per cent) compared with the neutron treated group (27 per cent) but the difference was not statistically significant. Survival rates were also similar in the two treatment groups.

A European Organization for the Research and Treatment of Cancer (EORTC) collaborative trial combined the experience of radiation oncology centres at Amsterdam, Edinburgh, and Essen.[18] The protocol was similar to that described above for the Edinburgh trial. One hundred and ninety-five patients were randomized and all were subjected to analysis. Local control in head and neck cancer was observed to be 40 per cent after photons and 44 per cent after neutron therapy. Late radiation morbidity was also similar in the two treatment groups, 24 per cent after photons and 21 per cent after neutrons. No significant difference was observed in survival rates.

A RTOG trial (78–08) compared a boost of either photons or neutrons after a standard course of wide-field photon irradiation.[19] A total of 118 patients with untreated squamous cell cancer of the head and neck region was entered into the study. The analysis included 57 patients treated with the neutron boost and 58 with photons. The local cancer control was similar, 20 per cent in the neutron group and 31 per cent in the photon group. Serious, late morbidity was not significantly different, 16 per cent after neutrons and 7 per cent after the photon boost. Survival was also similar in the two randomized groups.

The final randomized trial of head and neck cancer was conducted by the Neutron Therapy Collaborative Working Group (NTCWG). This multicentre international study compared high energy neutrons from hospital-based facilities with Mega-voltage photon therapy. Neutron therapy was given in 12 fractions over 4 weeks, that is similar to the Hammersmith regime. The neutron dose was adjusted for the higher beam energy of these modern facilities and a target absorbed dose of 20.4 Gy was specified. The photon schedule was 70.0 Gy in 35 daily fractions over 7 weeks. A total of 178 patients were randomized of which 169 were the subject of analysis.[20] The local tumour control was similar in both treatment groups, 32 per cent after photons and 37 per cent after neutrons. The actuarial survival rates were also similar in both groups. There was a statistically significant difference in the radiation-related serious morbidity which was only 18 per cent in the photon group compared with 40 per cent in the neutron group. It was concluded that fast neutrons, employing high energy beams, good techniques, and accelerated fractionation, are no better than standard Mega-voltage photon therapy.

In none of the eight randomized trials has neutrons been demonstrated to be superior to photons when the balance of local tumour control rates and the incidence of serious, late complications are taken into account. Mega-voltage photon therapy is more efficacious than neutrons in the management of epidermoid cancers of the head and neck region.

Salivary gland tumours

It is considered by some radiation oncologists that inoperable malignant tumours arising in the major or minor salivary glands are better treated by neutrons than by photons. This claim depends largely on the anecdotal evidence of uncontrolled clinical studies and historical reviews reported from the United States and Europe.[21],[22] These reports suggest that neutron therapy is much better on average (60 per cent local control rates) than the results of historical photon therapy series (30 per cent control rates). Such comparisons are, of course, unsafe. There is no certainty that the clinical or treatment variates were similar in the neutron and photon groups that are compared. Many of these advanced, inoperable tumours were treated in the past with palliative rather than radical intent. This is difficult to determine retrospectively because radiation morbidity is often poorly reported or not recorded at all.

One randomized trial was initiated by the RTOG neutron therapy group (RTOG 76–08). Regrettably the study was closed prematurely because patient accrual was so poor. The results of the trial were published[23],[24] but the analysis contributes little to our scientific evaluation of the efficacy of neutron therapy. Only 32 patients were randomized of whom seven (22 per cent) were excluded from the analysis. In the neutron-treated group of 13 patients, 56 per cent had

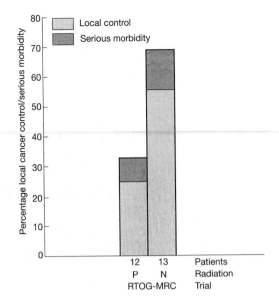

Fig. 5 Inoperable salivary gland tumours (P = photon, N = neutron).

lasting local tumour control compared with 25 per cent in the photon-treated group of 12 patients. The absolute difference in failures rates (four with neutrons, nine with photons) is not statistically significant. A logrank analysis of the time to failure does show a significant difference between the two groups. However, the serious, late radiation morbidity was also much higher in the neutron group (69 per cent) compared with that observed in the photon-treated group (33 per cent), a highly significant difference (Fig. 5). Survival was so poor that only 40 per cent of patients survived 2 years; the difference in survival between the two groups is not significant.

There is therefore no sound evidence from this trial that there is any qualitative advantage of neutron therapy compared with photons in treating malignant salivary gland tumours.

Non-small cell lung cancer

The results of the first randomized trial of neutrons for non-small cell lung cancer were reported from Berlin-Buch in 1982.[25] This is a unique study in that the local tumour control rates were based on the histological assessment of the treatment volume at autopsy. A total of 201 patients were entered into the study. The local tumour control was significantly higher in the group of patients treated with a combined schedule of neutrons and photons (39 per cent) than with photons alone (20 per cent). No data were reported on the radiation morbidity rates. However, mortality was significantly higher in the neutron-treated group than in the photon-treated group. No patient in the neutron group survived 2 years whereas 7 per cent of patients given photon therapy were alive at 5 years. The investigators considered that excessive, late, radiation-related morbidity may have been the cause of the observed increased mortality in the neutron-treated group.[26]

A Heidelberg trial recruited 115 patients with squamous cell cancer of the lung. This began as a randomized trial but the unreliable performance of the D-T neutron generator determined that the process of randomization had to be abandoned. The report does

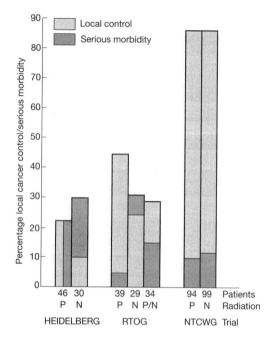

Fig. 6 Lung cancer trials (P = photon, N = neutron).

record the observations made on two groups of eligible patients, well-balanced for prognostic variates, that were treated and followed-up according to strict protocol.[27] Thirty were treated with neutrons and 46 with photons. It was demonstrated that the group of patients treated with photons had a better local tumour control rate (22 per cent versus 10 per cent) and better survival than the group treated with neutrons (Fig. 6).

An RTOG randomized trial of inoperable non-small cell lung cancer compared neutron therapy alone, combined neutrons and photons, and standard photon irradiation in three groups.[28] A total of 113 patients were randomized but only 102 were included in the definitive analysis. The local tumour control rates were higher in the group of 39 patients treated with photons alone (44 per cent) than in the groups treated with neutrons (27 per cent). (Fig. 6) The serious radiation-related morbidity was significantly higher in the groups treated wholly or in part with neutrons (24 per cent) than in the photon-treated group (5 per cent). Four patients treated with neutrons developed radiation myelitis; none in patients treated with photons. No fatal complications were recorded in the group of patients treated with photons; five patients (8 per cent) of the neutron-treated patients died of radiation-related morbidity. The survival rates were similar in the three treatment groups.

The final trial to be reported of neutrons for patients with non-small cell lung cancer was conducted by the Neutron Therapy Collaborative Working Group (NTCWG).[29] High energy neutron therapy was given in a dose of 20.4 Gy in 12 daily fractions in 4 weeks. This accelerated regime was compared with Mega-voltage photon therapy delivered as 66.0 Gy in 33 daily fractions. Two hundred patients with inoperable non small-cell lung cancer were recruited to the study. The analysis of results was based on the observations of 193 patients, 94 treated with photons and 99 with neutrons. Clinical and radiological assessment of local tumour failure was similar (about 13 per cent) in the two randomly allocated treatment groups (Fig. 6).

Overall survival was also similar in the two groups. The serious, late, radiation-related morbidity was similar in site, incidence, and severity in the two groups (about 11 per cent). A subgroup analysis of survival data suggested that patients with squamous cell cancer of the lung may have been more effectively treated with neutrons. However, this hypothesis has never been put to the test of validation in a prospective clinical trial. The evidence from all these trials indicates that neutrons offer no advantage compared with photons in treating inoperable lung cancer.

Cervix cancer

Two randomized trials have been conducted on the use of neutrons in the treatment of patients with locally advanced cancer of the uterine cervix. The first results reported were those of an RTOG study.[30] One hundred and fifty six patients were randomized to be treated either by photons (50.0 Gy in 25 fractions) or by a combined schedule of neutrons and photons in the same overall time. Both groups received similar supplementary treatment either with in-tracavitary radio-cobalt applications or external photon beam therapy. The published analysis included 146 patients. The local tumour rates at 2 years were not significantly different in both treatment groups (52 per cent after photons, 45 per cent after neutrons) (Fig. 4). The difference observed in late morbidity (11 per cent after photons, 19 per cent after neutrons) was also similar. The neutron generators used in this trial had either low energy beams or a technical performance inferior to that of Mega-voltage photon machines; most neutron machines had a fixed horizontal beam. When high energy neutron generators, with movable beams, were commissioned in the United States another randomized trial was opened to compare standard photon therapy and neutrons alone. The trial did not receive the support of oncologists and was abandoned after 2 years when it had accrued very few patients.

A team from the National Institute of Radiological Sciences in Japan has also reported the results of a randomized trial of cervical cancer.[31] Treatment options compared photons alone with a combined neutron/photon regime. The local control rates and mortality were similar in the two treatment groups. The report did not include data on late, radiation-related complications and so the two treatments cannot be compared objectively.

Rectal cancer

The role of neutrons in the management of locally advanced or recurrent adenocarcinoma of the rectum has been examined in two small, randomized trials. In these studies the effects of low energy neutron beams alone were compared with photons. In a trial conducted in Edinburgh[32] the local tumour control rates were similar in both randomized groups but the radiation morbidity was significantly higher in the neutron-treated group (17 per cent) compared with the photon group (6 per cent). In Amsterdam, the trial included patients with inoperable rectal cancer and advanced bladder cancer.[33] This study is difficult to evaluate because of its design and the vagaries of the randomization process. Two different neutron doses were employed (17.0 Gy versus 19.0 Gy in 20 fractions); and there were almost five times as many patients with rectal cancer who were allocated to receive photon therapy, presumably by chance. However, there was no significant difference in the pelvic tumour control rates between the photon group and the group which received the lower of the two neutron dose levels. Morbidity was also similar in the two groups.

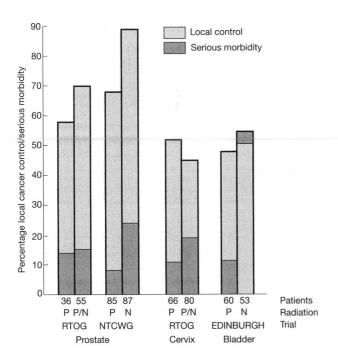

Fig. 7 Pelvic cancer trials (P = photon, N = neutron).

In the group of patients that were given the higher neutron dose the tumour control rate increased to 37 per cent (from 7 per cent) but the serious, late, radiation morbidity also had increased, unacceptably, from 7 per cent to 23 per cent. The survival rates of patients treated with photons were significantly higher than those observed in the neutron-treated patients.

Bladder cancer

Transitional cell carcinoma of the bladder has been the subject of three randomized trials of low-energy neutron therapy. None has demonstrated an advantage of neutrons compared with photons. In all of these trials an unacceptably high incidence of severe, late, radiation-related complications was observed. In Edinburgh, local tumour control rates were similar (about 50 per cent) in both treatment groups[34] (Fig. 7). In Manchester, the local tumour control rates have not been reported.[35] The serious, late, radiation morbidity following neutron therapy was significantly higher than after photons in both the Edinburgh trial (55 per cent versus 12 per cent) and the Manchester trial (44 per cent versus 8 per cent) (Fig. 7). The results of the Amsterdam trial, referred to above, led to similar conclusions. Patients who were treated with photons for transitional cell cancer of the bladder were observed to have a significantly higher survival than those given neutron therapy.

In this context reference has to be made to the randomized trials of pelvic cancers conducted at the MRC Cyclotron Unit at Clatterbridge Oncology Centre, England. The cyclotron there generates high energy neutrons and is equipped with an isocentric treatment head and movable jaws. The trials of patients with pelvic cancers were closed at Clatterbridge prematurely in February 1990. This decision was taken on the advice of the Data Monitoring Committee that had received an interim analysis showing a statistically significant increase in mortality in the group of patients with cancer

of the cervix, bladder, or rectum treated with neutrons.[36] The local cancer control and late radiation-related morbidity rates were similar in the two randomized treatment groups. No reason could be given to explain the large difference observed in the morality rates between the photon and neutron-treated groups and this has never been explained.

Prostate cancer

two randomized trials of neutron therapy for inoperable prostate cancer have been completed in the United States. The first trial compared a combined schedule of neutrons (two fractions per week) and photons (three fractions per week) with Mega-voltage photons alone. Both regimes were given in 35 fractions over 7 weeks. A total of 95 patients were randomized, of whom four were later excluded from the trial.[37] In the analysis 55 patients were allocated to the neutron group and 36 to receive photons alone. The locoregional tumour control rates were determined actuarially at 10 years to be 70 per cent in the neutron group compared with 58 per cent in the group treated with photons alone (Fig. 7). The difference in the 'time to locoregional failure' curves between the two groups was statistically significant by logrank analysis. This difference was reflected in the overall survival (46 per cent versus 29 per cent) and cause-specific survival rates (55 per cent versus 43 per cent) being significantly higher in the neutron-treated group. The serious, late radiation morbidity was similar in both groups (about 13 per cent). This was a small study in that the 'control' group consisted of only 36 patients. It did demonstrate a real advantage in terms of both improved local tumour control and survival to the group of patients treated with the combined neutron/photon regime.

This successful trial was followed in the United States by another randomized trial designed to compare high energy neutrons alone with standard Mega-voltage photon therapy. Neutron therapy was delivered in 12 fractions over 4 weeks (20.4 Gy) and the photons in 35 fractions in 7 weeks (70.0 Gy). Patients eligible had high grade T2 and T3/4; N0/1 prostate cancer. None had evidence of metastatic disease. At the close of recruitment 178 patients had been randomized.[38] Six patients were excluded from subsequent analysis. The actuarial locoregional control rates were 89 per cent in the neutron group and 68 per cent in the photon-treated group ($p = 0.01$). The serious, late radiation morbidity was significantly higher in the neutron-treated patients (24 per cent) compared with 8 per cent in the photon group ($p < 0.01$) (Fig. 7). The authors claim that neutron irradiation was 'significantly superior' therapeutically to photons. However, the increase in locoregional tumour control may be seen to be offset by the increase in serious, late radiation morbidity. An increase in therapeutic ratio has therefore not been demonstrated for this neutron regime. The overall and cause-specific mortality rates were similar in the two randomized groups. The analysis has shown a highly significant difference in the proportion of patients with elevated prostate specific antigen (PSA) levels at 5 years in the two groups. By this criterion, 45 per cent in the photon group failed compared with 17 per cent in the neutron group. At the time of reporting, the distant failure rates were similar in both treatment groups. Longer follow-up surveillance is required to explain this interesting observation.

The authors draw attention to their finding that the late radiation-related complications were significantly lower in patients randomized to receive neutrons who were treated on machines with movable jaws and with plans delivering precisely controlled treatment volumes. A reduction of the high-dose volume may decrease the incidence of radiation complications but it also carries the increased risk of higher locoregional failure. The superiority of fast neutrons alone in treating inoperable prostate cancer remains to be proved.

Brain tumours

Brain gliomas have been the subject of four randomized trials. Ninety-seven patients with supratentorial gliomas were included in trials of neutrons alone versus Mega-voltage photon therapy.[39],[40] In 221 patients the randomization was between standard photon therapy and a combined regime of neutrons and photons.[41],[42] In the analysis of the results of these trials, the observed median survival rates were similar in the randomly allocated groups. In all the trials, the investigators observed severe demyelinization in the brain within the treatment volume irradiated with neutrons. In the small number of patients examined by autopsy, there were regular reports of white matter destruction in normal brain, although tumour necrosis was observed in some patients. No evidence was provided that there was a safe therapeutic window for the treatment of supratentorial gliomas with fast neutrons. The neutron dose required to kill glioma cells is similar to that which produces irreversible white matter destruction in normal brain.

Bone and soft tissue sarcomas; malignant melanoma

It has been suggested that neutrons may be better that photons in treating bone and soft tissue sarcomas and malignant melanoma. These claims are based on single-centre, uncontrolled series; no controlled trials have been conducted to evaluate the role of neutrons in treating these tumours. There is no good evidence to conclude that neutrons have any qualitative advantage over photons in treating these tumours and they do carry the risk of serious, late complications.

Conclusions on fast neutron therapy

It is clear from the evidence of controlled clinical trials that, in general, cancers are more effectively and more safely treated by photons than by neutron irradiation. Neutron therapy regimes, delivering small dose fractions, do not deal any more effectively with hypoxic tumour cells or take better advantage of their reoxygenation during a course of radiotherapy than photons. It was also suggested subsequently that slowly growing tumours, such as the adenoid cystic carcinoma and prostatic adenocarcinoma, rather than hypoxic tumours, may be a more appropriate indication for neutron therapy. The evidence on which to base such a recommendation is not convincing.

There is no conclusive evidence to support the routine use of fast neutrons in clinical radiotherapeutics. They should be advised to be used only in phase III, randomized clinical trials. However, other improvements in oncology and radiotherapeutics have reduced the imperative there once was for starting new trials of sites such as salivary gland and prostate cancers. There are now less than six fast neutron therapy facilities in operation around the world and it is evident that this treatment modality is of less interest to radiation oncology than it was. Its risks are generally seen to outweigh its theoretical advantages.

Boron neutron capture therapy

Boron capture neutron therapy (BNCT) was first proposed in 1936 but it continues to remain part of experimental radiotherapeutics and has failed, as yet, to realize its theoretical potential.[43] BNCT depends for its efficacy on being able to achieve a selective, uniform uptake in tumours of a neutron capture compound, such as boron compounds, which have a high affinity for thermal neutrons. Absorption of these low energy neutrons is much more likely in boron nuclei than in nuclei of other elements in tissues. The nuclear reactions that follow, result in the disintegration of the stable 10-boron nucleus with the production of a helium nucleus (alpha particle) and a lithium nucleus. Both are very densely ionizing radiations with a range of only a few cell diameters (9 µm). The lethal effects of the radiation should then be confined to the tumour cells with little, if any, damage to surrounding normal tissues. It is estimated that the radiotherapeutic gain could be as much as three-fold.

The ideal boronated compound has not yet been found. A more promising compound currently being evaluated in boron-ophenylalanine-fructose, which does show selective uptake in glioma cells. The pharmacokinetics of these compounds are complex but details of the microcirculation, within tumours, and of the macro-circulation in respect of relative boron levels in tumour and normal tissues have to be determined by reliable measurement techniques. This is essential for the consistent and safe delivery of prescribed doses and to obtain the best possible radiotherapeutic gain.

Thermal neutrons have a very poor penetration in tissues which is a great limitation to their clinical usefulness. Epithermal neutrons have better penetrating qualities in tissues (50 mm) where they are slowed or 'thermalized'. Thermal and epithermal neutrons are usually produced from a nuclear reactor and clinical facilities have had to be built around them. Compact proton accelerators, designed to produce epithermal neutrons, which are suitable for installation in hospital-based BNCT facilities, may soon be available.

The principal clinical interest has so far focused on the treatment of brain gliomas and cutaneous melanoma, tumours relatively resistant to photons. Only phase I/II trials, which include very small numbers of patients, have been carried out in Japan and the United States.[43] Currently a phase I EORTC study of BCNT for postoperative gliomoblastoma is being undertaken at the European high flux reactor at Petten. No randomized trial of BCNT has been conducted.

At present, there is insufficient clinical evidence to make any scientific judgement about how valuable this approach may prove to be. Its potential usefulness depends entirely on the efficiency of the pharmacological agents used to concentrate the boron in the tumour rather than in normal tissues. The subject remains full of interest and expectation.[43] However, it is proving very difficult to demonstrate a convincing role for this complex and expensive approach to cancer therapy.[44]

Negative pi-mesons

Densely ionizing radiations may be delivered to tumours by beams of accelerated charged particles such as pions or heavy ions (neon, argon, and silicon). These charged particles have the physical advantage of delivering much improved dose distributions compared with photons or neutrons, as well as the biological characteristics of high-LET radiation.[2],[3]

Pion therapy requires extremely large, complex and expensive beam generation and delivery systems. Only three facilities have established formal clinical programmes. These were located in the United States at the Los Alamos Medical Pion Facility, in Villigen, Switzerland at the Paul Scherrer Institute, and in Vancouver, Canada at the Tri-Universities Meson Facility. About 1200 patients were recruited to clinical studies of pion therapy between 1974 and 1996, of whom only about 160 have been included in randomized trials. Only at the Tri-Universities Meson Facility, in association with the Vancouver Clinic of the British Columbia Cancer Control Agency, have randomized, clinical trials been completed successfully.

Most of the patients treated at the Los Alamos Medical Pion Facility were involved in dose-ranging studies.[45] Ninety-six patients were able to be given what were considered to be radical doses of irradiation before the programme was closed in 1981. These patients had very advanced stages of disease; most had cancers of head and neck, brain, prostate, or pancreas. Some patients with head and neck cancers and others with prostate cancer were thought to have responded well, but after critical appraisal no better than would have been expected with photons.[46]

The clinical studies at the Paul Scherrer Institute in Switzerland, which began in 1982, followed closely those conducted at Los Alamos. Their further experience provided no evidence that pions had a therapeutic advantage compared with photons. Indeed, the clinical investigators reported that an unacceptably high incidence of serious, late morbidity was observed in patients treated for bladder cancer.[47] The clinical programme closed in 1993.

At the Tri-Universities Meson Facility clinical studies, beginning in 1982, focused on patients with gliomas and cancers of the bladder and prostate. The first randomized trial at Vancouver evaluated pions in the treatment of supratentorial astrocytomas (grades 3 and 4). Eighty-four patients were randomized, of whom three were ineligible for analysis.[48] At that time the median follow-up was 4 years (range 1 to 7 years). The median survival was similar in both groups, 41 weeks for pions and 43 weeks for photons. The radiation-related morbidity was also similar in the two treatment groups.

Their second randomized trial concerned the role of conformal pion therapy for inoperable prostate cancer (T3/4, N0, M0). This trial recruited 219 patients, two of whom were excluded from the analysis of results. The pion therapy was given in 15 fractions over 3 weeks (36.0–37.5 Gy); photons in 32/33 fractions over 6.5 weeks (64.0–66.0 Gy). The local tumour control rates were similar in both treatment groups; 56 per cent after pions and 64 per cent after photons at 5 years. The overall and cause-specific survival were similar in both groups. The serious, late radiation-related morbidity was also similar in both groups. It was noted that late 'grade 2' complications were observed to be significantly higher in the photon group of patients. It is of interest that acute bladder reactions were significantly worse in the pion group, presumably because of the accelerated treatment schedule. No enhanced therapeutic efficacy was demonstrated with pions.[49]

Claims have been made by the investigators at the Paul Scherrer Institute that soft-tissue and bone sarcomas may be advantageously treated with pions using conformal therapy techniques.[50] However, it is impossible to make any scientific judgement of the clinical validity of these observations. Pion therapy, from the evidence of limited clinical experience, does not offer any therapeutic advantage compared with good photon therapy, and it is very much more expensive.

Argon, neon, silicon, and carbon ion beams

Heavy charged-particle therapy has been evaluated at the University of California, Lawrence Berkeley Laboratory since 1979.[51] The clinical team there has examined the therapeutic applications of these accelerated heavy ions, but only neon, argon, and silicon ions, within the Bragg peak, have low oxygen enhancement ratio (OER) values similar to those of fast neutron beams. The use of argon ions is compromised by particle fragmentation and relatively high RBE values in the entrance region compared with those in the Bragg peak region. Silicon ions would seem to offer the best combination of achieving both improved dose distribution and low OER values compared with photons but have not been tested clinically.

Neon irradiation was subjected to phase I/II trials at the Lawrence Berkeley Laboratory in which 239 patients with many different types of tumours were assessed.[52] Evaluation is made more difficult in that, because of technical problems, the neon radiation was usually combined with photons and/or helium ions. It was reported that some clinical results were encouraging,[53] just as with the early experience of neutrons. However, randomized trials were never begun and the clinical programme was closed in 1992.

Carbon ions are also classed as high-LET radiation but their specific ionization is not sufficiently dense to yield OER values as low as neutrons or pions, and in biological terms are more comparable to helium ions or protons. They do offer a good physical advantage of improved dose distributions. It remains to be demonstrated whether carbon ions will prove to be of any special advantage compared with helium ion and proton beam therapy.

Helium ions and protons

These charged particles have the biological characteristics similar to orthovoltage photons. However, being charged particles most of their energy is deposited within the terminal, Bragg peak, region of their tracks through tissues. Consequently the target-absorbed dose can be concentrated at a precise depth while sparing the overlying tissues.[54] The precision of the enhanced distribution of dose, using 'wide' radiation beams (that is, produced by scattering through a foil rather than by using a pencil beam) may allow critical normal tissues and vital organs to be effectively shielded from high radiation doses that would threaten to exceed normal tissue tolerance. The improved treatment planning makes it possible to deliver safely much higher doses of radiation to the well-defined target volume than would be tolerable with photon radiation. These applications of proton and helium ion beams are now routinely employed for the treatment of cancers located at the base of skull and cervical spine.[55] The results of their further evaluation in the management of paravertebral tumours and pituitary tumours must be awaited. Multiple, wide-beam techniques using only the plateau region, rather than the spread Bragg peak, to cover the tumour volume, also have been employed to increase further the accuracy of the target-absorbed dose, because the depth of the Bragg peak is difficult to achieve accurately.

Proton treatments may be designed to be given as an additional 'boost' dose to the tumour volume in combination with photon therapy. It is considered that higher tumour control rates may be achieved in this way without any increase in late, normal tissue morbidity. Studies of patients with inoperable tumours of the prostate and rectum and other locally advanced tumours are being conducted to determine whether these techniques do offer real advantage in their management.

The enhanced precision of dose distribution that is possible allows techniques known as 'radiosurgery' to be employed. These techniques use pencil beams of radiation which are focused on a small lesion so that a very high, localized dose of radiation may be safely delivered; doses much larger than would otherwise be tolerable by critical normal tissues. Radiosurgery with proton beams or helium ions has been established as a safe and highly effective treatment of choroidal melanomas.[56],[57] Choroidal haemangiomas and intracranial arterio-venous malformations may also be successfully treated in this way using protons. Their clinical superiority over photons using similar techniques has however, yet to be established.

Proton therapy requires large, expensive particle accelerators, generating 150 to 250 MeV protons and other complex beam direction and treatment planning equipment for their safe and reliable clinical application. It is estimated that proton therapy may cost two or three times that of comparable photon therapy. The exploitation of these sophisticated radiotherapeutic techniques has been pioneered with protons at the Harvard Cyclotron Laboratory, in association with Massachusetts General Hospital, since 1959 and with heavy charged particles at the University of California, Lawrence Berkeley Laboratory, since 1957. In Europe, much of the early development of proton therapy was carried out at the University of Uppsala in Sweden. Work with heavy ions continues in Japan and it began in Germany in 1998. It is estimated that about 15 000 patients have been treated by high energy proton irradiation over the last 30 years. About 25 proton therapy facilities are now in operation in the United States and Canada, Europe, Japan, and South Africa. A specially designed North-east Proton Therapy Centre, based on a 235-MeV isochronous cyclotron, is being built at the Massachusetts General Hospital, Harvard Medical School.

Choroidal melanoma

The treatment of this tumour by proton beam therapy (or helium ions) is now routinely used around the world, and is considered to be the treatment of choice for many patients. Patients are treated by focusing a pencil beam of radiation on to the precisely localized tumour by means of stereotactic beam direction techniques. Treatment is usually given in a small number of fractions (about five) over 8 to 10 days. Results are excellent in achieving a high probability of lasting tumour control (about 95 per cent), often with retention of good visual acuity.[57],[58] The risk of subsequent enucleation depends on the size of the tumour and the retention of visual acuity also depends on the distance of the lesion from the fovea. Reasonable vision may be preserved, in general, in about 70 per cent of patients with small tumours and in 40 per cent of those with tumours larger than 3.0 mm diameter. Late complications, such neovascular glaucoma, may require enucleation in about 15 per cent of patients within 5 years, and 20 per cent in a 10-year period. The lens receives a substantial dose of radiation and about 40 per cent of patients may develop posterior subcapsular opacities within 3 years of treatment. Tumour recurrence is observed in only about 5 per cent of patients.

Chordomas and chondrosarcomas

Greatly improved results, compared with photons, have been demonstrated in treating chordomas and chondrosarcomas arising at the base of the skull and in the upper cervical vertebrae with wide-field proton or helium ion beams.[59] Computer-based three-dimensional treatment planning and rigorous beam direction techniques are employed to achieve precise localization of the irradiated volume and avoid sensitive neural and endocrine tissues. These techniques allow much higher doses to be delivered to these sites than would be possible with photon radiation. Remarkably high local control rates (70 per cent) have been observed. These excellent results have been obtained in treating carefully selected tumours which have allowed complete sparing of the critical normal tissues. They therefore should not be compared directly with historical series of photon therapy which often will have included large lesions for which the dose prescribed may have been greatly compromised by the radiation tolerance of the central nervous system. However, the remarkable results that are regularly achieved by these special techniques have established proton and helium-ion therapy as the elective treatment for these life-threatening, inoperable tumours.

Prostate cancer

It is suggested, with some confidence, that the local control of prostate cancer may be greatly increased, without increasing normal tissue morbidity, by delivering higher doses of charged particles such as protons or helium ions to a well-circumscribed tumour volume. Shipley et al.[60] have reported the results of one randomized trial of high-dose radiotherapy using a proton therapy boost compared with conventional dose irradiation with Mega-voltage photons. Over many years, 202 patients with locally advanced (stage T3–4) prostate cancer were recruited to this study. Patients first received 50.4 Gy photon therapy to the pelvis. They were then were randomized to have either additional standard photon treatment of 16.8 Gy or conformal proton therapy to a dose of 25.2 Gy (an increase of 12.5 per cent). The local tumour control rates at 5 years were similar (about 86 per cent) in the two treatment groups. However, the serious, late radiation-related complications were significantly higher in the group of patients which was given the high-dose conformal proton therapy. No significant difference was observed in overall or cause-specific survival rates. This high-dose proton therapy regime clearly was not beneficial in that the late morbidity was increased unacceptably while locoregional cancer control was not improved. Other randomized trials are planned but it will be many years before their results can be evaluated. Meanwhile, conformal radiotherapy using Mega-voltage photon beams is being developed rapidly in several centres.

Conclusions on heavy charged particle therapy

Amongst the range of charged particles, helium, heavy ions, and protons that have been evaluated only protons appear to show continuing promise for a substantiated role in clinical radio-therapeutics. Their physical advantages are clear, even though progress in conformal photon therapy, with inverse dose planning, is beginning to make clinicians wonder if photons may prove one day to be as good as protons.

Protons have been shown to be have important advantages in treating a number of selected, rather uncommon, tumours. There is good evidence, although not conclusive, that protons are more effective than photons in treating chordomas and other tumours arising at the base of the skull and in upper cervical spine. Protons have an established role in treating choroidal melanomas and are considered to be the treatment of choice for many of these lesions.

High energy proton facilities would best be provided in a small number of large, comprehensive cancer centres where knowledge and expertise in treating selected tumours and other lesions would be concentrated. The clinical indications for proton therapy and the highly sophisticated techniques employed must continue to be developed and evaluated. There is a need for much more evidence from phase III randomized clinical trials about the possible advantages of protons compared with the best conformal photon radiotherapy.

References

1. Bewley DK. *The physics and radiobiology of fast neutron beams.* Bristol: Institute of Physics Publishing, Medical Science Series, 1989.

2. Fowler JF. *Nuclear particles in cancer treatment.* Medical physics handbooks No. 8. Bristol: (Institute of Physics) Adam Hilger, 1981.

3. Raju MR. *Heavy particle radiotherapy.* New York: Academic Press, 1980.

4. Tobias CA, Lyman JT, Lawrence JH. Heavy particle beams in radiotherapy. *Progress in Atomic Medicine. Recent Advances in Nuclear Medicine,* vol. 3 (Lawrence JH, ed). New York: Grune and Stratton, 1971: 167–218.

5. Lin R, Hug EB, Schaefer RA, Miller DW, Slater JM, Slater JD. Conformal proton radiation therapy of the posterior fossa. *International Journal of Radiation Oncology, Biology and Physics,* 2000; **48**: 1219–26.

6. Soloway AH, Barth RF, Carpenter DE, eds. *Advances in neutron capture therapy.* New York: Plenum, 1993.

7. Sasaki Y. *National Institute of Radiological Sciences annual report.* Science and Technology Agency, Chiba-shi 263–8555 Japan, March 1998.

8. Stone RS. Neutron therapy and specific ionisation: Janeway Memorial Lecture. *American Journal of Roentgenology,* 1948; **59**: 771–85.

9. Gray LH, Conger AD, Ebert M, Hornsey S, Scott OCA. The concentration of oxygen dissolved in tissue at the time of irradiation as a factor in radiotherapy. *British Journal of Radiology,* 1953; **26**: 638–48.

10. Catterall M, Sutherland I, Bewley DK. First results of a randomised clinical trial of fast neutrons compared with X or gamma rays in treatment of advanced tumours of the head and neck. *British Medical Journal,* 1975; **280**: 653–6.

11. Catterall M, Bewley DK, Sutherland I. Second report on results of a randomised clinical trial of fast neutrons compared with X or gamma rays in treatment of advanced cancers of the head and neck. *British Medical Journal,* 1977; **1**: 1642.

12. MRC Neutron Therapy Working Group. A comparative review of the Hammersmith (1971–75) and Edinburgh (1977–82) neutron therapy trials of certain cancers of the oral cavity, oropharynx, larynx and hypopharynx. *British Journal of Radiology,* 1986; **59**: 429–40.

13. Griffin TW, David R, Laramore GE, Hussey DH, Hendrickson FR, Rodriguez-Antunez A. Mixed beam radiation therapy for unresectable squamous cell carcinoma of the head and neck: the results of a randomised RTOG study. *International Journal of Radiation Oncology, Biology and Physics,* 1984; **19**: 2211–15.

14. Maor MH, Hussey DH, Barkley HT, Peters LJ. Neutron therapy for head and neck cancer: II. Further follow-up on the M D Anderson TAMVEC randomised trial. *International Journal of Radiation Oncology, Biology and Physics,* 1983; **9**: 1261–5.

15. Griffin TW, David R, Hendrickson FR, Maor MH, Laramore GE. Fast neutron radiation therapy for unresectable squamous cell carcinomas of the head and neck: the results of a randomised RTOG study. *International Journal of Radiation Oncology, Biology and Physics,* 1984; **19**: 2217–23.

16. Duncan W, Orr JA, Arnott SJ, Jack WJL, Kerr GR, Williams JR. Fast neutron therapy for squamous cell carcinoma in the head and neck region: results of a randomised trial. *International Journal of Radiation Oncology, Biology and Physics,* 1987; **13**: 171–8.

17. MacDougall RH, Orr JA, Kerr GR, Duncan W. Fast neutron therapy for squamous cell carcinoma of the head and neck: final report of the Edinburgh randomised trial. *British Medical Journal,* 1990; **301**: 1241–2.

18. Duncan W, Arnott SJ, Battermann JJ, Orr JA, Schmitt G, Kerr GR. Fast neutrons in the treatment of head and neck cancers; results of a multi-centre randomised clinical trial. *Radiotherapy and Oncology,* 1984; **2**: 293–300.

19. Maor MH, *et al.* Evaluation of a neutron boost in head and neck cancer. Results of a randomised RTOG trial 78–08. *American Journal of Clinical Oncology,* 1986; **9**: 61–6.

20. Maor MH, *et al.* Fast neutron therapy in advanced head and neck cancer: a collaborative international randomised trial. *International Journal of Radiation Oncology, Biology and Physics,* 1995; **32**: 599–604.

21. Buchholtz TA, Laramore GE , Griffin BR, Kohn WJ, Griffin TW. The role of fast neutron radiation therapy in the management of advanced salivary gland malignant neoplasms. *Cancer,* 1992; **69**: 2779–88.

22. Krull A, *et al.* European results in neutron therapy of malignant salivary gland tumors. *Buletin du Cancer, Radiotherapie,* 1996; **83** (Suppl.): 125–9s.

23. Laramore GE, *et al.* Neutron versus photon irradiation for unresectable salivary gland tumors: Final report of an RTOG-MRC randomised clinical trial. *International Journal of Radiation Oncology, Biology and Physics,* 1993; **27**: 235–40.

24. Stelzer KJ, *et al.* Fast neutron radiotherapy. The University of Washington experience. *Acta Oncologica,* 1994; **33**: 275–80.

25. Eichhorn HJ. Results of a pilot study on neutron therapy with 600 patients. *International Journal of Radiation Oncology, Biology and Physics,* 1982; **8**: 1561–5.

26. Eichhorn HJ, Lessel A, Dalluge KH, Huttner J, Welker K, Grunan H. Pilot study on neutron therapy: Part I. The applicability of neutron therapy. *Radiobiologia Radiotherapia,* 1981; **22**: 262–92.

27. Schnabel K, Vogt-Moykopf J, Berberich W, Abel U. Vergleich einer Neutronen -mit einer Photonenbestrahlung des Bronchialkarzinoms. *Strahlentherapie Onkologie,* 1983; **159**: 458–64.

28. Laramore GE, *et al.* Fast neutron and mixed beam radiotherapy for inoperable non-small cell carcinoma of the lung. Results of a RTOG randomised study. *American Journal of Clinical Oncology,* 1986; **9**: 233–43.

29. Koh WJ, *et al.* Neutron vs photon radiation therapy for inoperable non-small cell lung cancer: results of a multi-center randomised trial. *International Journal of Radiation Oncology, Biology and Physics,* 1993; **27**: 499–505.

30. Maor MH, *et al.* Neutron therapy in cervical cancer: results of a Phase III RTOG study. *International Journal of Radiation Oncology, Biology and Physics,* 1988; **14**: 885–91.

31. Tsunemoto H, Morita S, Sarons S, Dino Y, Yoo Y. Present status of fast neutron therapy in Asian countries. *Stralentherapie Onkologica,* 1989; **165**: 330–6.

32. Duncan W, Arnott SJ, Jack WJL, Orr JA, Kerr GR. Results of two randomised clinical trials of neutron therapy in rectal adenocarcinoma. *Radiotherapy and Oncology,* 1987; **8**: 191–8.

33. Battermann JJ. Results of fast neutron therapy for advanced tumours of the bladder and rectum. *International Journal of Radiation Oncology, Biology and Physics,* 1988; **8**: 2159–64.

34. Duncan W, *et al.* A report of a randomised trial of d(15)+Be neutrons compared with mega-voltage Xray therapy of bladder cancer. *International Journal of Radiation Oncology, Biology and Physics,* 1985; **11**: 2043–9.

35. Pointon RS, Read G, Greene DA. A randomised comparison of photons and 15 MeV neutrons for the treatment of carcinoma of the bladder. *British Journal of Radiology,* 1985; **58**: 219–24.

36. **Errington RD, et al.** High energy neutron therapy for pelvic cancers: study stopped because of increased mortality. *British Medical Journal,* 1991; **301**: 1045–50.

37. **Laramore GE, Krall JM, Thomas FJ, Griffin TW, Maor MH, Hendrickson FR.** Fast neutron radiotherapy for locally advanced prostate cancer: results of an RTOG randomised study. *International Journal of Radiation Oncology, Biology and Physics,* 1985; **11**: 1621–6.

38. **Russell KJ, et al.** Photon versus fast neutron external beam radiotherapy in the treatment of locally advanced prostate cancer: results of a randomised prospective trial. *International Journal of Radiation Oncology, Biology and Physics,* 1994; **28**: 47–54.

39. **Catterall M, et al.** Fast neutrons compared with mega-voltage X-rays in the treatment of patients with supra-tentorial glioblastomas: a controlled pilot study. *International Journal of Radiation Oncology, Biology and Physics,* 1980; **6**: 261–6.

40. **Duncan W, et al.** Report of a randomised pilot study of the treatment of patients with supra-tentorial gliomas using neutron irradiation. *British Journal of Radiology,* 1886; **59**: 373–7.

41. **Griffin TW, et al.** Fast neutron radiation therapy for glioblastoma multiforme: Results of a RTOG randomised trial. *American Journal of Clinical Oncology,* 1983; **1**: 661–7.

42. **Duncan W, et al.** The results of a randomised trial of mixed-schedule (neutron/photon) irradiation in treatment of supra-tentorial grade III and IV astrocytoma. *British Journal of Radiology,* 1986; **59**: 379–83.

43. **Various authors.** Edition dedicated to boron capture neutron therapy. *International Journal of Radiation Oncology, Biology and Physics,* 1994; **28**: 1059–217.

44. **Laramore GE, Spence M.** Boron neutron capture therapy for high grade glioma of the brain: a cautionary note. *International Journal of Radiation Oncology, Biology and Physics,* 1996; **36**: 241–6.

45. **Kligerman MM, von Essen CF, Khan MK, Smith AR, Sternhagen CJ, Sala JM.** Experience with pion radiotherapy. *Cancer,* 1979; **43**: 1043–51.

46. **von Essen CF, Bagshawe MA, Bush SE, Smith AR, Kligerman MM.** Long-term results of pion therapy at Los Alamos. *International Journal Radiation Oncology, Biology and Physics,* 1987; **13**: 1389–98.

47. **Studer UE, Gerber E, Zimmermann A, Kraft R, von Esssen CF.** Late results in patients treated with pi-mesons for bladder cancer. *Cancer,* 1993; **71**:439–47.

48. **Pickles T, et al.** Pion radiation for high grade astrocytoma: results of a randomized study. *International Journal of Radiation Oncology, Biology and Physics,* 1997; **37**: 491–7.

49. **Pickles T, et al.** Pion conformal radiation of prostate cancer: results of a randomised study. *International Journal Radiation Oncology, Biology and Physics,* 1999; **43**: 47–55.

50. **Greiner R, et al.** Pion irradiation at Paul Scherrer Institute. Results of dynamic treatment of unresectable soft tissue sarcoma. *Strahlentherapie Onkologie,* 1990; **166**: 30–3.

51. **Castro JR.** Results of heavy ion radiotherapy. *Radiation Environmental Biophysics,* 1995; **34**: 45–8.

52. **Linstadt DE, Castro JR, Phillips TL.** Neon ion irradiation. Results of the Phase I and II clinical trials. *International Journal of Radiation Oncology, Biology and Physics,* 1991; **20**: 761–9.

53. **Castro JR, et al.** Neon heavy charged particle radiotherapy of glioblastoma of the brain. *International Journal of Radiation Oncology, Biology and Physics,* 1997; **38**: 257–61.

54. **Suit HD, Griffin TW, Castro JR, Verhey LJ.** Particle radiation therapy research plan. *American Journal of Clinical Oncology,* 1988; **11**: 330–41.

55. **Slater JM, Slater JD, Archambeau JO.** Proton therapy for cranial base tumors. *Journal of Craniofacial Surgery,* 1995; **6**: 24–6.

56. **Munzenrider JE, et al.** Conservative treatment of uveal melanoma: Probability of eye retention after proton therapy. *International Journal of Radiation Oncology, Biology and Physics,* 1988; **15**: 553–8.

57. **Castro JR, et al.** Fifteen years experience of helium ion therapy for uveal melanoma. *International Journal of Radiation Oncology, Biology and Physics,* 1997; **39**: 989–96.

58. **Desjardins L, et al.** Resultats preliminaires de la protontherapie du melanome de la choroide au Centre de Protontherapie d'Orsay (CPO): les 464 premiers cas. *Cancer Radiotherapie,* 1997; **1**: 222–6.

59. **Hug EB, Fitzek MM, Liebsch NJ, Munzenrider JE.** Locally challenging osteo- and chondrogenic tumors of the axial skeleton: results of combined proton and photon radiation therapy using three-dimensional treatment planning. *International Journal of Radiation Oncology, Biology and Physics,* 1995; **31**: 467–76.

60. **Shipley WU, et al.** Advanced prostate cancer: the results of a randomised comparative trial of high dose irradiation boosting with conformal protons compared with conventional irradiation using photons alone. *International Journal of Radiation Oncology, Biology and Physics,* 1995; **32**: 3–12.

4.8   Total body irradiation

Ann Barrett

Introduction

The first machine for whole body radiotherapy treatment was designed by a German physicist, Dessauer, in 1905, only 8 years after the discovery of X-rays. There are reports of responses to whole body irradiation in patients with leukaemia and lymphomas from as early as 1907.[1] A special total body irradiation (TBI) machine was installed at the Memorial Hospital, New York in 1931, and results using a whole body dose of 25 per cent of an erythema dose were reported from 1932 to 1942.[2],[3]

Doses were limited to approximately 3 Gy, until Thomas *et al.*[4] reported the effectiveness of intravenous infusion of bone marrow in overcoming haemopoietic toxicity. The recognition of leucocyte histocompatibility antigens led to safer bone marrow transplantation,[5] and improved management of graft-versus-host disease made it possible to consider treatment for the majority of patients who do not have a fully compatible sibling.[6]

Initially patients with the most radiosensitive tumours, such as leukaemias and lymphomas, were treated.[7] The indications for systemic irradiation have now extended to many other types of cancer.

A scientific basis for total body irradiation has been difficult to establish because many interacting factors affect the outcome of treatment. Unless bone marrow support is given after TBI, patients will die from bone marrow failure before they develop toxicity in other systems. Such haematopoietic support, however, produces problems such as graft-versus-host disease which may, in turn, influence complications such as interstitial pneumonitis in which radiation plays an important part. It is also difficult to determine how much radiotherapy contributes to control of disease in a multimodality treatment. Comparison of results between centres where many aspects of patient management may differ is also difficult. In the last 10 years, studies undertaken in the large number of patients recorded by the International and European Bone Marrow Transplant Registries, and the continuing experimental work of the Seattle Group, have improved our understanding of the best way to give whole body irradiation.[8],[9]

Aims of total body irradiation

At doses of 6 to 15 Gy, total body irradiation will produce bone marrow ablation. For benign disease, TBI may be used to produce enough immunosuppression to allow infused marrow or stem cells to engraft so that the underlying defect can be corrected. For patients with diffuse malignancies, the aim is to eradicate malignant cells by high-dose, systemic radiotherapy (with chemotherapy) and to rescue the patient from the inevitable bone marrow toxicity by bone marrow transplantation or stem cell infusion.

Thus, in the first situation, the therapeutic agent is the transplant and in the second, the high-dose therapy (including TBI). Obviously, the optimal scheduling of TBI for the two situations may be different. Chemotherapy alone is often adequate to permit marrow engraftment in patients with benign disease, although the increased immune suppression which can be obtained by adding TBI is sometimes necessary after rejection of a first graft or when HLA matching is less close. For malignant disease, relapse remains a major problem and ways of intensifying treatment safely are still being sought.

For each disease treated, choosing the best treatment means taking into account:

(1) the target cell population (i.e. the normal immune system or a malignant cell population);
(2) the biological behaviour and radiation response characteristics of the target cell population;
(3) the dose needed to achieve the planned effect;
(4) the most appropriate schedule of TBI;
(5) the interaction of radiation with other agents used in patient management;
(6) the probable complications.

Types of 'rescue' after high-dose therapy

In the early days of high-dose therapy, bone marrow was used for 'rescue' and could be obtained from a number of sources. Identical twin grafts (syngeneic bone marrow) are well tolerated by the recipient, but may be associated with a higher rate of relapse because of loss of a 'graft-versus-leukaemia' effect. This may offset the advantage of a lower incidence of transplant-related complications. Allogeneic grafts from a fully compatible family member are preferable, although these may cause graft-versus-host disease. The scope of high-dose therapy has been widened by using partly compatible family members or fully compatible unrelated donors, although graft-versus-host disease and rejection are problems. T cell depletion of allogeneic 'mismatched' or unrelated grafts reduces graft-versus-host disease, but leads to a high incidence of graft rejection and leukaemic relapse.

Reinfusion of autologous marrow (harvested during remission) has been widely used. Persisting malignant cells may, however, be returned to the body and lead to relapse. 'Purging' the marrow *in vitro* to remove tumour cells may improve outcome.[10] However, it is difficult to eliminate all tumour cells from the patient and this probably remains the major cause of relapse.

More recently, peripheral blood progenitor cells harvested after stimulation by appropriate colony stimulating factors have been used to ensure engraftment. Allogeneic peripheral blood stem cells from a sibling donor may also be used satisfactorily.[11] Autologous peripheral blood progenitor cells may be purged to remove tumour cells, or particular progenitor cell populations can be expanded *in vitro* before infusion.[12] Such manipulation may lead to an increased risk of graft failure. Cord blood has also been used to provide stem cells for engraftment.

Indications for high-dose therapy with TBI

Leukaemia

Most intensive treatments with haemopoietic support are undertaken for leukaemia.

Acute lymphocytic leukaemia

Children with acute lymphocytic leukaemia at high risk of relapse should be considered for treatment in first complete remission. Allogeneic matched, related donors are used when available, but allogeneic unrelated, matched or related, partially mismatched grafts may be considered for those at higher risk. Other children in the standard risk group are considered for transplantation if they relapse after second complete remission. In this group long-term survivals of 50 to 70 per cent may be expected.[13] Relapse remains a major problem and attempts to intensify preparative regimens have usually been more toxic without improving survival.

In adults, results are less satisfactory because of high relapse and complication rates (4-year actuarial survival rates of 30–40 per cent) and bone marrow transplantation is reserved for those with Ph + disease or those in second remission.[14]

Acute non-lymphocytic leukaemia

Patients with acute myeloid leukaemia may be transplanted in first remission if they have a matched sibling donor. Relapsing patients should be considered for autologous bone marrow or peripheral blood progenitor cells, or unrelated matched donor bone marrow support after high-dose therapy in second remission. Disease free survivals of 50 to 80 per cent at 5 years can be expected in a group of selected, young patients.[15]

Chronic myeloid leukaemia

Allogeneic bone marrow transplantation after high-dose therapy is the only curative option for patients with chronic myeloid leukaemia, although it is only feasible in younger patients. If patients are transplanted in chronic phase within 1 year of diagnosis using cyclophosphamide/busulfan or cyclophosphamide/TBI, 5-year survival rates between 40 and 70 per cent are obtained. Outcome of transplantation later in chronic phase, or in accelerated phase disease, is much poorer and the procedure is ineffective in patients treated in blast crisis. Benign primitive progenitor cells from marrow obtained early in the disease may be used for marrow reconstitution after remission induction.[16]

Non-Hodgkin's lymphoma

High grade

A large number of patients with lymphoma have been treated with autologous bone marrow transplantation at different stages of their disease. Patients with intermediate or high grade disease with poor prognostic features (bone marrow or central nervous system involvement and high LDH levels) may be transplanted in first completed remission. Patients in second remission whose disease remains sensitive to chemotherapy may also be transplanted with good results to give improvement in long-term survival rates from 20 to 50 per cent.[17] Relapse rates are higher when autologous marrow is used and although the transplant related morbidity is higher with allogeneic transplants, they may offer the advantage of a graft-versus-lymphoma effect since progression rates are lower in patients who develop chronic graft-versus-host disease. Because of the toxicity of this treatment, it is more suitable for young patients (less than 55 years).[18]

Low grade

Patients with short first or second remission from chemotherapy or those in whom only partial remission can be obtained may have improved survival after high-dose therapy and autografting.[19] However, this should not be the first approach because of the risk of myelodysplasia after transplantation, and the long natural history of the disease. There is no clear evidence of benefit from graft purging. Allogeneic transplantation may improve control rates.[20]

Hodgkin's disease

Patients with high risk or relapsed Hodgkin's disease may also be appropriately treated by high-dose chemotherapy with or without TBI.[21] Early transplantation is recommended to avoid drug resistant disease developing and to minimize cumulative toxicity.

Multiple myeloma

Young patients (less than 55 years) with good initial response to chemotherapy should be considered for high-dose therapy with peripheral blood progenitor cells or autologous bone marrow, or allogeneic transplant following high-dose therapy with melphalan alone or with TBI. A plateau in survival at approximately 40 per cent has been reported. Regimens containing TBI appear to give better results than those using chemotherapy alone. Patients relapsing after high-dose therapy with TBI may still have prolonged survival.[22]

Other tumours

Patients with stage 4 neuroblastomas with poor prognostic factors (aged more than 1 year or with n-*myc* amplification) may be treated with high-dose therapy after conventional chemotherapy.[23]

Patients with disseminated Ewing's sarcoma, primitive neuroectodermal tumour (PNET), or rhabdomyosarcoma, where conventional treatment has a low chance of producing cure, are now being transplanted in well-defined research protocols.

Selected young patients with breast cancer may benefit from high-dose therapy and some studies are treating patients with high-grade brain tumours in this way, usually with chemotherapy alone. In patients with solid tumours such as these, radiotherapy is used for local control rather than as part of the conditioning for high-dose therapy. Use of TBI in these situations remains experimental.

Techniques for total body irradiation

To obtain a large enough field to encompass the whole body using a conventional treatment unit, the machine must be used with an extended source–patient distance, as the largest field size available at normal working distances is usually of the order of only 40 cm². Under these working conditions, data obtained for standard treatments cannot be used and simple extrapolation is inaccurate. Depth–dose data must be obtained by direct measurement in a finite phantom at the extended distance used. The flatness of the beam at extended source–patient distance must be determined. Scatter contributed from walls, floor, and treatment couch must also be directly measured and will be different for each treatment room. Dose distributions can be calculated from tissue–air ratios or computed tomographic density measurements. Special TBI planning systems have been developed which incorporate anatomical information from CT scanning with parameters of dose calculation, such as depth, backscatter, tissue thickness, thickness of inhomogeneity, off axis distance, and source to skin distance, to give accurate predictions of dose distribution.[24],[25]

In vivo dosimetry can be performed with thermoluminescent lithium fluoride monitors, diodes, or other *in vivo* dosimeters and only these direct readings will fully take into account variations in body dimensions at different levels, differences between individual patients, the effect of positioning of the body with regard to the beam and the loss of internal scatter because the field is larger than the patient.

The maximum field sizes that can be obtained depend on the size and geometry of the treatment room and are often unsatisfactorily small, even when the patient is treated lying along the diagonal of the beam to increase the effective field size. Many centres will have no choice of machine for total body irradiation and will have to use either cobalt or linear accelerator equipment chosen primarily by the characteristics of the room in which it is situated. The patient may need to be confined within the available field size by a device such as a specially designed treatment chair or a perspex box of the same dimensions as the field size.[26]–[28]

With the patient in the supine position and treating with lateral fields, a more homogenous dose distribution may be obtained using higher energies of photons, such as 18 MV. If lung shielding is used and the patient treated with anteroposterior/ posteroanterior fields, 6 MV irradiation may give a more satisfactory distribution.[29] There is no clinical evidence of a difference in outcome of treatment whether a cobalt machine or linear accelerator at various energies is used.[30]

Homogeneity

By analogy with conventional radiation treatment, it has been assumed that the aim of total body irradiation should be to obtain as homogenous a dose as possible to the whole body. If open and unmodified beams are used, inhomogeneities of up to 15 per cent may be found. In thinner regions of the body, such as the neck and ankles, doses may be larger than midabdominal doses by up to 15 per cent. Doses in the lung are variable, but may be up to 10 per cent higher because

of increased transmission in air. Doses to the head may be low because they may be within the penumbral region if the field size is small or because of loss of internal scatter. The patient's position also affects dose distribution. For example, flexion of the neck to bring the chin on to the chest will reduce doses to the neck, and lung doses may be modified by varying the position of the arms.

Many centres use compensators to decrease doses to the lung or lower limbs or bolus around neck or ankles to act as compensators. Lung shields are used either as compensators to limit the lung dose to that received elsewhere in the body or to reduce the dose even lower to minimize pulmonary complications of total body irradiation. Some centres have considered applying shielding to the kidneys or liver to limit late toxicity.[31]

Boosts

The assumption that homogeneity is desirable may be questioned. The most effective treatment may be one which delivers the highest dose feasible to the areas most likely to contain disease. In practice, this approach has been used when boosts are given to various parts of the body known to harbour residual disease or to areas at high risk because of poor chemotherapy access. Anecdotal reports suggest reduced probability of relapse in testes, brain, and spleen when doses to these sites are boosted with 4 to 6-Gy fractionated over 2 to 4 days, but there is no firm data from clinical trials to support this approach.[32]

Boost to nodal areas

With the increasing use of high-dose therapy in the treatment of lymphomas, additional treatment to initial or residual areas of nodal disease may be considered advisable since, after bone marrow transplantation, most lymphoma relapses occur in sites of previous disease. Local radiotherapy may be given before or after high-dose chemotherapy or TBI. Full therapeutic doses (35 Gy) have been reasonably well tolerated after bone marrow transplantation, although leucopenia and mucositis may be troublesome.[33] It may be more convenient to plan to deliver boosts to local nodal areas before TBI using doses of 20 Gy to involved sites. Particular care should be taken with mediastinal irradiation which may result in pneumonitis.[34]

Shielding

Lung shielding

Lung shielding is used by approximately 80 per cent of European centres[27] undertaking total body irradiation. Lead blocks are usually made individually for each patient, from suitable planning films or from CT measurements, to cover the lung from the clavicle to the dome of the diaphragm following the inner contour of the chest wall. Some techniques shield the lung for the main part of the TBI treatment and then add a boost to the bone-marrow-containing ribs using electrons.[35] This is a complex arrangement and additional lung dose from the electron boost is inevitable. Scattered irradiation within the lung may also be significant, but it is difficult to quantify.

Shields are placed either close to the machine head, which may make alignment with the patient difficult, or in direct contact or very close to the patient. Positioning may then be more accurate, but may cause some discomfort to the patient. It is difficult to ensure the accuracy of shielding especially if treatments are prolonged or if patients are restless or unco-operative; the proximity of the mediastinum, liver, and spleen, to which full doses must be given, makes accuracy very important.

Shielding is only effective for, at most, 60 per cent of the lung volume; 30 per cent lies within the mediastinal fields and 5 per cent in the apex where shielding is difficult, although lung doses may be the highest.[36] For this reason and because of concerns about accuracy in placing shields, some centres prefer to use no lung shielding, but to restrict lung doses to those known to be within tolerance.

A reduction in the incidence of interstitial pneumonitis when shielding was introduced has been claimed by many groups, but often this change coincided with a reduction in effective whole body doses by fractionation or more careful measurement of lung doses. It is not clear whether the development of interstitial pneumonitis can be provoked by high doses to part of the lung only or whether partial protection is effective. The benefit of lung shielding, except to provide compensation if homogeneity of treatment is being sought, therefore is unproven. Similar rates of interstitial pneumonitis are reported by groups using techniques with and without lung shielding.[30]

Specific techniques

Most groups giving total body irradiation treatments use a standard cobalt unit or linear accelerator (4–18 MV) operating at a source–skin distance of approximately 4 m, which will usually give field sizes from 128 to 160 cm. Within this field size, patients may lie supine, on their side, or be seated with knees bent up on a special chair.

Perspex of up to 2 cm in thickness is placed next to the patient, both on the beam side (entry) to prevent skin sparing, which would occur with high energy radiation and is undesirable because leukaemic cells may infiltrate the skin, and on the exit side to absorb backscatter from walls, which increases skin dose without adding usefully to midplane doses.[24]

Special total body irradiation units have been installed in a number of centres. In Toronto, a single source, wide-angled collimator unit permits large field irradiation at a short treatment distance. Dual source treatment facilities have been available for many years in Seattle, where two opposing cobalt sources are mounted on floor rails to allow adjustment of treatment distances as sources decay.[7] The patient is placed between the two horizontal beams. At the Royal Marsden Hospital in London, dual cobalt sources were mounted vertically to provide field sizes of 2×0.65 m at 2 m source–skin distance; in Boston, Massachusetts, two 4 MV linear accelerators similarly mounted give field sizes of 80×220 cm. These special facilities provide the possibility for varying the parameters of treatment which are fixed with most single source units because of field size constraints.[28],[37]

Where there is no room large enough for total body irradiation, some centres have used a scanning cobalt beam to cover the whole body. This has the theoretical disadvantage that not all the malignant cell population is being irradiated at the same time and that the incident dose rate is higher than when whole body treatments are given at extended distances. In practice, there is no evidence to suggest that this technique is less effective, although a higher incidence of interstitial pneumonitis has been reported with a sweeping beam technique than with a static beam.[38]

Most patients are treated with posteroanterior and anteroposterior fields because the increased thickness of the body when lateral fields are used leads to less satisfactory dose distributions. This effect is less obvious in children. High energy linear accelerators (~18 MV) may give a better dose distribution if lateral fields are used to treat the supine patient. If vertical treatment units are used with the patient supine, it is possible to place lung shielding more accurately. With the patient lying on his side, careful positioning of the arms may contribute to compensation for increased lung transmission.

Some centres in the United States and Europe have adopted the technique first developed at the Memorial Hospital in New York where patients are treated standing, supported by a modified bicycle seat and arm supports, with lung shields suspended from their shoulders. Additional boost treatments are then given with electrons to the chest wall to increase the dose to bone-marrow-bearing ribs.[35]

From analysis of treatment results notified to the International and European Bone Marrow Transplant Registries, there is no evidence for superiority of one treatment technique over another and factors such as the dose given and the scheduling of total body irradiation are likely to be much more important.[30]

Total lymphoid irradiation

Total lymphoid irradiation may be used in organ engraftment to produce immune suppression without the lung toxicity of total body irradiation.[39] Initially, beneficial symptomatic response in autoimmune diseases, such as systemic lupus erthymatosis and rheumatoid arthritis, was reported,[40] but these responses may be short lived and a relatively high incidence of secondary B-cell malignancy suggests that this approach should be used with caution. Total lymphoid irradiation has been used for conditioning patients with aplastic anaemia after graft rejection, but it is a complicated technique and offers little advantage over low-dose total body or thoracoabdominal irradiation. With total lymphoid irradiation, doses of 20 to 34 Gy with conventional daily fractionation have been used. It has also been used in some centres before or after total body irradiation to produce additional immune suppression for patients receiving T-cell depleted marrow grafts.

Shaped fields such as a mantle and inverted Y (used more commonly in the treatment of Hodgkin's disease) or thoracoabdominal fields with lung shielding may be used to deliver doses of 5 to 6 Gy.

Scheduling of total body irradiation

It is difficult to decide from published data whether there is a best regimen for total body irradiation. Schedules must be compared using effects on all the endpoints shown in Table 1. Only a few clinical trials have addressed questions of radiation scheduling. Often the effect on only one endpoint is described. Obviously, if a patient dies early of failure of engraftment, the effect of that TBI schedule on later endpoints cannot be determined. It is theoretically possible to calculate an optimum schedule using data from large series of patients treated with TBI and alpha and beta ratios for each of the normal tissues and tumour population. In practice, because of variabilities shown in Table 2, it has been difficult to claim superiority of one treatment over another and most of the schedules in current use have been shown empirically to be reasonably well tolerated (Table 3).

Bone marrow stem cells have a limited capacity to repair sublethal damage and the typical cell survival curve means that little effect is

Table 1 Endpoints for comparison of TBI schedules

Target	Endpoint	Time to endpoint
Immune system	engraftment	2–3 weeks
Malignant cells	disease control	variable
Normal tissues		
lung	pneumonitis	up to 100 days
eye	cataract	3 years
kidney	nephritis	variable, up to many years
other organs		variable, up to many years

Table 2 Factors affecting outcome of TBI

Variation of radiosensitivity

1. Of individual normal tissues and organs
(a) in same patient
(b) between patients

2. Of tumour cells
(a) between patients
(b) in different diseases

expected from changes in radiation schedule.[41] There are some data suggesting increased sensitivity to fractionated treatments;[42] nevertheless, overall the effect of variation in dose rate and fractionation are insignificant for the killing of normal bone marrow cells which represent a very radiosensitive population. Bone marrow ablation before donor engraftment can be achieved with doses of 6 Gy—doses below the level at which lung damage will occur. Scheduling is therefore not critical if normal stem cell death is the only consideration.

Graft-versus-host disease is minimized by *in vitro* manipulation of harvested bone marrow to reduce T cell numbers. The use of T-cell-depleted bone marrow, however, results in an increased rate of graft rejection and leukaemic relapse, and conditioning has to be intensified to overcome this problem. The cell responsible for graft rejection has not yet been identified. Various lymphocyte subsets are known to have different *in vitro* radiosensitivities,[43] but further studies are needed to determine how to manipulate these factors most effectively.

Leukaemic cells are highly radiosensitive with a low capacity for accumulation and repair of sublethal damage.[44] Changes in dose rate or fractionation would therefore be expected to cause little effect, but fractionation over a period of 5 days could lead to a reduction in log cell kill if doubling times are short (of the order of 2.5 days). There is some evidence of increased survival of leukaemic cells *in vitro* when radiation is given as a split course compared with continuous radiation to the same dose.

Various groups have shown that increasing the dose of radiation produces increased tumour cell kill. In a study of escalating single fraction low dose rate total body irradiation in 238 patients at the Royal Marsden Hospital, London, a lower relapse rate was noted after 10.5 than 9.5 Gy, although at a higher dose of 11.5 Gy any benefit in preventing leukaemic relapse was off-set by a high early death rate from lung damage. Similarly the Seattle Group showed a lower rate of leukaemic relapse after 15.7 Gy compared with 12 Gy, although at the expense of a higher transplant-related mortality.[9],[45] However, for other tumour types whose radiobiological characteristics are different, dose should not be considered in isolation.[46] Other biological factors, such as total body burden of tumour, may outweigh any possible advantage of increasing dose within the range permitted by normal tissue toxicity.

Normal tissues

A direct effect of increasing total radiation dose on the incidence of damage in various normal tissues can also be demonstrated.[47],[48] Considerable sparing of damage to lung may be achieved in single fraction treatments by lowering the dose rate, but regimens using small dose per fraction are likely to be best since, for equivalent toxicity, single fraction dose rates would have to be very low leading to unreasonably long treatment times. Fractionated TBI is therefore now widely used, although there is still variation in the dose given per fraction. If fractionated radiotherapy is used, it is likely that most benefit will be obtained by using small doses per fraction (less than 2 Gy), although even lower fraction sizes (1.2 Gy) may be beneficial in terms of lung sparing and are clinically feasible and effective.[35] Within the range of dose used per fraction, little additional benefit is gained using a low dose rate rather than the standard output of most machines, although additional sparing with very low dose rates has been reported experimentally. Similar dose–response curves and beneficial effect of fractionation in reducing late damage have been shown for liver, kidney, and lens.

In summary, toxicity to normal tissue, efficacy against tumour population and feasibility in terms of delivery, must all be considered

Table 3 Current well-tolerated TBI schedules

Study group	Regimen (Gy)	Fraction size (Gy)	Time (days)	Dose specification point
Seattle[45]	13.20 children 14.40 adults	1.2	3	abdomen
UK MRC	14.40	1.8	4	max. lung
Memorial[35]	13.20 (with lung shielding and electron boost)	1.2	4	abdomen

Table 4 Acute complications of TBI

Complication	Threshold dose (Gy)	Time of onset	Duration	Permanent sequelae
Vomiting	2–3	1.5–8 hours	4 days	none
Diarrhoea	2–3	4–5 days	10–20 days	malabsorption (rare)
Hypotension	5–6	during treatment	transient	none
Pyrexia	?	during treatment	transient	none
Parotitis	3–4	first 24 h	6–12 months	dry mouth
Raised amylase	?	first 24 h	6 days	none
Fall in lymphocyte count	1	60% by 13 hours 30 h half-life	1 year	susceptibility to infection
Fall in thyroid-stimulating hormone levels	10	6–12 months	permanent	none ? susceptibility to thyroid cancer
Alopecia	10	10 days	regrowth 6–12 months	

as well as overall treatment time and time between fractions. Regimens shown in Table 3 all offer the advantages of high dose, low dose per fraction, and reasonable overall treatment time and therefore appear to be the most satisfactory at present. Further experience in treating patients with other tumours may lead to a change in these recommendations, but the parameters of normal tissue toxicity will not change so that any modifications are likely to be small.

Drug–radiation interactions

TBI is only one element of the conditioning regimen and drug radiation interactions may alter the effectiveness or toxicity of a particular schedule. Cyclophosphamide 120 mg/kg given on days 4 and 3 before TBI, as recommended initially by the Seattle group,[7],[9] has been widely used. Since disease relapse remains a major problem, attempts have been made to intensify conditioning by modifying radiation dose and fractionation or by adding different chemotherapeutic agents. Conditioning with chemotherapy alone may be used, as with the Santos schedule of cyclophosphamide/busulphan.[49] Both TBI and busulfan are potent stem cell killers and similar results are obtained with either regimen, although the spectrum of morbidity is different.[50] The optimum schedule must be determined taking all these factors into consideration.[51]–[53]

For a radiation oncologist, one of the persisting challenges is to assist in developing more effective, less toxic preparatory regimens. In many cases, the effects of individual drugs given with radiation are well known and potentially toxic drugs such as cytosine arabinoside, methotrexate, and cisplatin can be avoided. As new drugs are developed and added to conditioning regimens, constant vigilance and careful observation are needed to detect any unforeseen interactions.

Table 5 Biochemical measurements not affected acutely by TBI

Serum urea
Electrolytes
Liver function tests
Calcium, phosphate
Alkaline phosphatase
T_3, T_4

Complications of total body irradiation
Acute effects

Acute effects are shown in Table 4. Vomiting is less marked after fractionated than single fraction treatments. Children under 10 experience less vomiting than adults. Vomiting may be precipitated by movement and general discomfort and reduced by fasting, antiemetics, and steroid administration.[54],[55] Parotitis is followed by xerostomia which may persist for up to a year after treatment, although salivation may be stimulated by pilocarpine.[56] Careful attention to dental hygiene is necessary to prevent further complications. Graft-versus-host disease exacerbates the oral sequelae of treatment.[57] Table 5 shows biochemical parameters which are unaffected by TBI.

Late effects

Late effects on lung, liver, kidney and heart are detailed in Table 6. Interstitial pneumonitis and graft-versus-host disease are the two most important factors contributing to early death. Fever, dyspnoea, cough, and hypoxia are associated with characteristic X-ray changes

Table 6 Late effects after TBI

Organ	Permanent sequelae
Lung	Interstitial pneumonitis, fever, dyspnoea, cough, reduced DLCO
Liver	Veno-occlusive disease, weight gain, jaundice, abdominal pain, hepatomegaly
Kidney	Radiation nephritis, hypertension, haematuria, impaired renal function
Heart	Rarely occurs Myocardial fibrosis, constrictive pericarditis, possibly premature coronary artery disease

Table 7 Factors increasing the risk of pneumonitis after transplantation

Increasing TBI dose
High dose rate, single fraction TBI
Intensity of immune suppression
Degree of HLA incompatibility
Graft-versus-host disease
Infection
Older age
Poor performance status
Long interval from diagnosis to transplant

of diffuse interstitial infiltrates, and lung function testing shows a reduction in diffusing capacity. The clinical syndrome is due to an accumulation of activated T cells in the lungs with an associated population of macrophages and neutrophils.[58] There is an increase in cells expressing messenger RNA for inflammatory proteins such as tumour necrosis factor-α, interleukin-1-β, and transforming growth factor-β. The host MLC class II expressing cells are increased in lung tissue after TBI and this process is potentiated in patients undergoing allogeneic transplant or those with a lesser degree of matching whereas it is rare with syngeneic transplants or autologous grafts. These acute changes lead on to type 2 pneumocyte proliferation and collagen deposition with fibrosis.

Many factors will interact with radiation damage to increase the risk of interstitial pneumonitis. Up to 40 per cent of cases are associated with infection, which may be diagnosed by bronchial alveolar lavage or by lung biopsy. Characteristic viral inclusion bodies of CMV or other infective agents may be isolated. In approximately 60 per cent of patients with interstitial pneumonitis, no infectious agent can be isolated and a diagnosis of idiopathic pneumonitis is made. Factors increasing the risk of interstitial pneumonitis are shown in Table 7.[59]

In the International Bone Marrow Transplant Registry series, patients with none of these factors had an 8 per cent probability of developing interstitial pneumonitis compared with 94 per cent in patients with all these factors. There was no evidence from this study of an advantage for fractionated radiation in reducing pneumonitis and no dose–response relationship was detected for radiation doses to lung between 5.6 and 12.8 Gy.[30]

Methotrexate appears to have more direct toxicity for lung than cyclosporin. This may be because of a potentiating effect of radiation damage. The cyclosporin syndrome of adult respiratory distress may be seen after renal toxicity has developed from high-dose treatment. Increasing age may increase risk of pneumonitis because there is a greater likelihood of prior infection with cytomegalovirus. Graft-versus-host disease also increases the risk of pneumonitis by immunological and infective processes.

The lack of correlation in the study above of pneumonitis with total dose contrasts strongly with data presented by Keane et al.[47] who showed a clear dose response relation over the range of 7 to 10 Gy. This may have been obscured in the data from the International Bone Marrow Transplant Registry by different ways of reporting doses or by the fact that some of the schedules were delivering doses below the threshold for lung damage.

Liver

Liver damage in recipients of bone marrow transplants may be related to the conditioning regimen, to graft-versus-host disease, or to infection either previously or newly acquired. The clinical picture of radiation or chemotherapy associated liver damage develops within a few weeks of treatment with weight gain, jaundice, abdominal pain, hepatomegaly, ascites, and, in severe cases, encephalopathy. This condition is associated with a high mortality rate and is more often seen after preparation of patients with busulfan than with TBI.[60]

Histopathological changes are of veno-occlusive disease. The terminal hepatic venules and sublobular veins are narrowed by sub-endothelial fibrosis and thickening with trapping of cells, including hepatocytes, within the lumen resulting in obstruction to sinusoidal blood flow. Although factors other than radiation are usually more important in its causation, the incidence is reported to be lower after fractionated than high-dose-rate single fraction TBI. Low-dose heparin and tissue plasminogen activators such as alteplase have been used to try to reduce the severity of this problem. Spontaneous resolution within 3 to 4 weeks may occur.[60]

Kidney

There are many factors which may contribute to renal damage during the preparation for and recovery from bone marrow transplantation including the use of chemotherapeutic agents such as ifosfamide, antibiotics, and cyclosporin.

Tests of glomerular function after bone marrow transplant/TBI usually show only minor impairment. Tubular defects and haemolytic uraemic syndrome are more likely to occur, but are related more to drugs than to radiation exposure.[61] Endothelial injury is characteristic of acute radiation nephropathy which is related to dose of radiation. The doses used for TBI should be below the threshold for overt damage. Although renal failure is a common problem of multifactorial aetiology after bone marrow transplantation, it is difficult to quantitate precisely the contribution of TBI. Miralbell however has shown a dose-dependent effect in his patients.[31]

Radiation nephritis is a well-recognized entity after local field irradiation to doses in excess of 20 Gy and may occur many years after exposure. The first report of radiation nephritis after total body irradiation was by Bergstein et al.[62] Two children developed hypertension, haematuria, and impaired renal function 6 months after treatment. Histologically, the kidney showed expanded mesangial zones, thickening of capillary and arteriolar walls, focal areas of tubular atrophy, and interstitial oedema and fibrosis. One of the patients had received cyclosporin and acyclovir, drugs with known renal toxicity. Tarbell et al.[63] found evidence of renal dysfunction in 11 out of 29 survivors of transplantation for acute lymphoblastic leukaemia or neuroblastoma between 1980 and 1986. Conditioning regimens had included drugs with renal toxicity such as cisplatin, teniposide, and ifosfamide. Patients presented with anaemia, haematuria, and a rising creatinine: biopsy in two patients showed changes consistent with radiation nephritis or the haemolytic uremic syndrome.

It thus appears that the tolerance of the kidney to radiation may be diminished when multiagent chemotherapy is used concomitantly and that children may be especially susceptible. Because of the late onset of radiation nephritis, this problem may increase in severity with longer follow-up of survivors of bone marrow transplantation.

Eye

Marked changes are observed in transplanted patients who develop chronic graft-versus-host disease with keratoconjunctivitis and changes in lacrimal gland secretions. Retinitis may result from conditioning with cytosine arabinoside and TBI. In uncomplicated survival after total body irradiation, the only change to be observed is the development of cataract. In the Seattle series reported in 1984,[64] the risk of developing cataract was 18 per cent and 19 per cent in patients treated with chemotherapy or fractionated total body irradiation and 80 per cent in those receiving single fraction total body irradiation. All cases were bilateral and the risk increased for 3 years after transplantation before stabilizing. Surgical excision was necessary in half the patients. Chronic graft-versus-host disease and steroid therapy were also associated with a higher risk of developing cataracts. With low-dose-rate, single-fraction, total body irradiation, the incidence is lower than after high-dose-rate, single-fraction treatments, but higher than with fractionated irradiation, being of the order of 58 per cent at 10 years.[65]

Teeth

Disturbances in tooth development and size are seen after bone marrow transplant with TBI with a severity inversely proportional to age at the time of treatment.[66]

Central nervous system damage

A syndrome of somnolence with lassitude, anorexia, nausea, and sometimes vomiting, may be expected at about 6 weeks after TBI. A similar picture is seen after cranial irradiation for acute lymphocytic leukaemia and is believed to be due to transient demyelination. No treatment is needed as the condition improves spontaneously (within 7 to 10 days). It does not correlate with any persisting or late damage.

Leukoencephalopathy may occur within days or months of transplantation and may be related to drug administration (especially high-dose methotrexate), radiation, or viral infection. It is uncommon after total body irradiation unless previous cranial irradiation has been given and the incidence is inversely correlated with age. The characteristic appearance on computed tomographic scanning is of dilated ventricles, cerebral atrophy, hypodense areas, and calcification.

Damage to the spinal cord has been reported anecdotally but is rare.

By extrapolation from results of prophylactic cranial irradiation for leukaemia, impairment of cognitive function and learning ability would be expected, although there are few detailed long-term studies yet.[67]

Quality of life

Quality of life after bone marrow transplantation may be impaired. In a study from Toronto, many patients reported low grade symptoms such as fatigue, pain, joint stiffness, and sleep disturbance. Patients studied at less than 3 years from the time of transplant experienced considerable impairment, while longer-term survivors were indistinguishable from the normal population in most areas studied. However, 81 per cent of patients overall were satisfied with the health related quality of life after treatment and 94 per cent were prepared to recommend a transplant for somebody in similar circumstances.[68]

Hormonal changes

Gonadal function

Gonadal function and fertility are known to be affected by high-dose chemotherapy and total body irradiation. The degree of impaired function depends on age, sex, and dose and type of therapeutic agent used.

In adult women, the usual pattern seen after TBI is ovarian failure with amenorrhoea, low plasma oestradiol levels with raised gonadotrophins, and infertility. Low androgen levels may be found, probably also resulting from ovarian damage. A direct effect on the adrenal gland may occur although no abnormalities of plasma cortisol levels have been reported. Since androgen is needed to sustain increased muscle activity during exercise, low levels may help to explain the easy fatiguability reported by patients after TBI.[69]

In very young but postpubertal females, ovarian recovery may be seen in 10 to 25 per cent at 2 to 7 years after bone marrow transplant. Recovery is not affected by hormone replacement therapy and this may be temporarily discontinued to assess whether recovery has occurred. It is possible that this group of patients may undergo early menopause (as has been reported after chemotherapy).

In men, the most common pattern is of infertility (due to a direct effect on the testes) but with normal testosterone and gonadotrophin levels. If additional radiation is given by a testicular boost so that total doses are greater than 20 Gy, testosterone levels may be low with raised gonadotrophins and replacement therapy may then be necessary.

Studies in prepubertal children suggest that many boys and some girls receiving TBI may progress normally through puberty. Young age at the time of treatment may be relatively protective. Most boys will probably be azoospermic, but patients who progress through puberty with normal gonadotrophin and sex hormone levels may be fertile.[70],[71]

Although the probability of fertility cannot yet be accurately predicted, pregnancies have been reported after TBI given to males and females. No abnormalities in offspring of these patients have been reported, although the rate of spontaneous abortion may be increased.[72]

Thyroid function

The most common abnormality seen after bone marrow transplant with TBI conditioning is compensated or overt hypothyroidism with elevated thyroid-stimulating hormone levels with or without low free serum thyroxine or tri-iodo thyronine levels. Thyroid abnormalities, which are commonly first detected between 12 and 60 months after treatment, have been reported in 2 to 56 per cent of patients treated with TBI, but hypothyroidism may also occur in up to 10 per cent of patients conditioned without TBI.[73] Replacement therapy is given early to try to reduce the risk of induction of thyroid malignancy.

Growth

Growth may be affected by TBI in two ways:

(1) by damage to the hypothalamus and pituitary gland leading to impaired growth hormone production;

(2) by a direct effect on the epiphyseal plate leading to early epiphyseal fusion.

Studies comparing effects of TBI with thoracoabdominal irradiation have shown that the central effect is the most significant. Cranial irradiation given before TBI increases the risk of failure of growth hormone production.[74]

Normal levels of growth hormone may be maintained after TBI, especially if this is fractionated, or a pattern of normal plasma levels with low growth hormone peaks after stimulation may be seen. Growth hormone should be administered if growth hormone levels are measured to be low, if there is a low growth hormone peak after two stimulation tests, and a loss of height SDS of one SD or more (shown by measurement of sitting rather than standing height). Low growth hormone peaks have been reported in 20 to 70 per cent of patients and graft-versus-host disease and poor nutritional status increase the risk of growth hormone failure. Administration of growth hormone at an early stage as soon as growth velocity starts to fall off prevents further decrease in height, although 'catch-up' growth does not occur.

Appropriate sex hormone administration is also essential to obtain the full growth potential of the pubertal growth spurt.

Heart

Cardiac toxicity is not a major problem after total body irradiation, although it has been observed after high-dose cyclophosphamide therapy. Myocardial fibrosis and constrictive pericarditis are late effects occurring many years after conventional radiotherapy, and careful follow-up of patients receiving total body irradiation is necessary to determine whether these same complications will develop. In one study of 28 patients with leukaemia, serial echocardiography and radionuclide ventriculography showed abnormalities in only four, in whom the resting ejection fraction was reduced after treatment. Animal studies have shown acute changes in the pattern of isoenzymes in mice after total body irradiation and these enzyme changes may lead to functional alterations. On the basis of experience from conventional radiotherapy it seems possible that coronary artery disease or myocardial infarction may occur at an earlier age than normal in this patient population.[75]

Second tumour induction

In the first year or two after bone marrow transplantation, the commonest malignancies seen are recurrence of the original disease or lymphoproliferative disorders which seem to be related to immune suppression and Epstein Barr virus infection.[76]

A large study from the Seattle Group and the International Bone Marrow Transplant Registry has followed nearly 20 000 patients treated with bone marrow transplantation to determine the risk of developing a new solid cancer; 9501 patients survived longer than 1 year and 73 per cent of the patients had had TBI as part of the initial conditioning for bone marrow transplant; 3200 patients have survived for 5 years or more and in this group 80 second tumours were diagnosed. These included 17 carcinomas of the buccal cavity or pharynx, 11 brain tumours, 11 melanomas, eight thyroid carcinomas, nine bone and connective tissue tumours, and three liver tumours. The overall risk of developing a second tumour was inversely related to the age at the time of bone marrow transplant and directly related to time since treatment, original tumour type, and dose of radiation.[77]

Risk in children treated before the age of 10 was increased 36.6 times and at age 20 to 29, 4.6 times, whereas over the age of 39 the risk was nearly the same as in a normal population. Cumulative incidence was 0.7 per cent at 5 years, 2.2 per cent at 10 years, and 6.7 per cent at 15 years. Patients with acute lymphocytic leukaemia were most likely to develop brain tumours whereas melanoma occurred more often in those treated for acute myeloid leukaemia. Patients treated with thoracoabdominal or total body irradiation had a higher risk than those conditioned without radiation. No difference was seen whether TBI was given as a single fraction or in several fractions. The risk of brain tumours was highest in those who had received cranial as well as total body irradiation (nine of the 13 patients with brain tumours).

Other factors which are possibly associated with increased risk may be determined by immunological abnormalities: T cell depletion possibly related to melanoma induction, immune abnormalities with oral mucositis and chronic graft-versus-host disease for buccal cavity tumours, cyclosporin administration (for skin tumours), papilloma virus infection in squamous cell carcinomas of skin and buccal mucosa. Buccal cavity tumours are commonest in men. The three parotid tumours observed were mucoepidermoid carcinomas—the type also observed in survivors of the atomic bomb.

It is interesting to compare this pattern of second tumour incidence with that seen after treatment of leukaemia without bone marrow transplant when the cumulative incidence of second tumours at 20 years is 2.9 to 4 per cent. A similar pattern of brain, thyroid, skin, and connective tissue tumours occurs, but the greatest risk (27 times expected) is of brain tumours in those treated with cranial irradiation.[78]

These data underline the risks of radiation and the need for prolonged follow-up. Patients should be encouraged to avoid exposure to known carcinogens (such as tobacco) which may potentiate the effects of radiation.

Further research is still needed to determine when TBI will improve outcome of intensive therapy for poor prognosis diseases, how it should best be given, and what the long-term sequelae will be. Individualization of TBI treatments on the basis of normal tissue and tumour radiosensitivities may eventually be possible to optimize outcome.

References

1. Chaoul H, Lange K. Ueber Lymphogranulomatose und ihre Behandlung mit Röntgenstrahlen. *Munchener Medizinische Wochenschrift*, 1923; **23**: 725–7.

2. Heublein AC. A preliminary report on continuous irradiation of the entire body. *Radiology*, 1932; **18**: 1051–62.

3. Medinger FG, Craver LF. Total body irradiation with review of cases. *American Journal of Röntgenology and Radiotherapy*, 1942; **48**: 651–71.

4. Thomas ED, Lochte HL, Luw C, Ferrebee JW. Intravenous infusion of bone marrow in patients receiving radiation and chemotherapy. *New England Journal of Medicine*, 1957; **257**: 495–6.

5. Dausset J, Nenna A. Présence d'une leuco-agglutinine dans le serum d'un cas d'agranulocytose chronique. *Comptes Rendues de la Société Biologique*, 1952; **146**: 1539–41.

6. Kernan NA, *et al.* Analysis of 462 transplantations from unrelated donors facilitated by the National Marrow Donor Programme. *New England Journal of Medicine*, 1993; **328**: 593–602.

7. Thomas ED, *et al.* Marrow transplantation for acute nonlymphoblastic leukemia in first remission. *New England Journal of Medicine*, 1979; **301**: 597–9.

8. Bortin MM, Horowitz MM, Rimm AA. Progress report from the International Bone Marrow Transplant Registry. *Bone Marrow Transplant*, 1992; **10**: 113–22.

9. Petersen FB, *et al.* Marrow transplantation following escalating doses of fractionated total body irradiation and cyclophosphamide. *International Journal of Radiation Oncology, Biology, and Physics*, 1992; **23**: 1027–103.

10. Brenner MK, *et al.* Gene marking after bone marrow transplantation. *European Journal of Cancer*, 1994; **30A**: 1171–6.

11. Korbling M, Huh YO, Durett A, *et al.* Allogeneic stem cell transplantation: peripheralization and yield of donor-derived primitive hemopoietic progenitor cells(CD34+ Thy-1dim) and lymphoid subsets,and possible predictors of engraftment and graft-versus-host disease. *Blood*, 1995; **86**: 2842–8.

12. Moolten DN. Peripheral blood stem cell transplant: future directions. *Seminars in Oncology*, 1995; **22**: 271–90.

13. Barrett AJ, *et al.* Bone marrow transplantation from HLA- identical siblings as compared with chemotherapy for children with acute lymphoblastic leukemia in a second remission. *New England Journal of Medecine*, 1994; **331**: 1253–8.

14. Zhang MJ, Hoelzer D, *et al.* Long term follow up of adults with acute lymphoblastic leukaemia in first remission treated with chemotherapy or bone marrow transplantation. *Annals of Internal Medicine*, 1995; **123**: 428–31.

15. Zittoun RA, Mandelli IF, Willemze R, *et al.* Autologous and allogeneic bone marrow transplantation compared with intensive chemotherapy in acute myelogenous leukaemia. *New England Journal of Medicine*, 1995; **332**: 217.

16. Applebaum FR, Clift R, Radich J, Anasetti C, Buckner CD. Bone marrow transplantation for chronic myelogenous leukaemia. *Seminars in Oncology*, 1995; **22**: 405–11.

17. Philip T, *et al.* Autologous bone marrow transplantation as compared with salvage chemotherapy in relapses of chemotherapy-sensitive non-Hodgkin's lymphoma. *New England Journal of Medecine*, 1995; **333**: 1540–5.

18. Sweetenham JW, *et al.* High dose therapy and bone marrow transplantation for intermediate and high grade non-Hodgkin's lymphoma in patients aged 55 years and over: results from the European Group for Bone Marrow Transplantation. *Bone Marrow Transplantation*, 1994; **14**: 981–7.

19. Rohatiner A, *et al.* Myeloablative therapy with autologous bone marrow transplantation as consolidation therapy for recurrent follicular lymphoma. *Journal of Clinical Oncology*, 1994; **12**: 1177–84.

20. van Besien KW, Khouri IF, Giralt SA, *et al.* Allogeneic bone marrow transplantation for refractory and recurrent low grade lymphoma: the case for aggressive management. *Journal of Clinical Oncology*, 1995; **13**: 1096–102.

21. Nademanee A, *et al.* High dose chemotherapy with or without total body irradiation followed by autologous bone marrow and/or peripheral blood stem cell transplantation for patients with relapsed and refractory Hodgkin's disease. Results in 85 patients with analysis of prognostic factors. *Blood*, 1995; **85**: 1381.

22. Varterasian M, *et al.* Transplantation in patients with multiple myeloma. *American Journal of Clinical Oncology*, 1997; **20**: 462–6.

23. Stram DO, *et al.* Consolidation chemoradiotherapy and autologous bone marrow transplantation versus continued chemotherapy for metastatic neuroblastoma: A report of two concurrent Children's Cancer Group studies. *Journal of Clinical Oncology*, 1996; **14**: 2417–26.

24. Van Dam J, Rijnders A, Vanuytsel L, Zhang HZ. Practical implications of backscatter from outside the patient on the dose distribution during total body irradiation. *Radiotherapy and Oncology*, 1988; **13**: 193–201.

25. Sánchez-Nieto B, Sánchez-Doblado F, Terrón JA.. A CT-aided PC-based physical treatment planning of TBI: a method for dose calculation. *Radiotherapy and Oncology*, 1997; **42**: 77–85.

26. Barrett A. Total body irradiation (TBI) before bone marrow transplantation in leukaemia. *British Journal of Radiology*, 1982; **55**: 562–5.

27. Quast U. Total body irradiation—a review of treatment techniques in Europe. *Radiotherapy and Oncology*, 1987; **9**: 91–106.

28. Lutz WR, Dougan PW, Bjarngard BE. Design and characteristics of a facility for total body and large field irradiation. *International Journal of Radiation Oncology Biology Physics*, 1988; **15**: 1035–40.

29. Ekstrand K, Greven K, Wu Q. The influence of x-ray energy on lung dose uniformity in total body irradiation. *International Journal of Radiation Oncology Biology Physics*, 1997; **38**: 1131–6.

30. Bortin MM, Kay HE, Rimm AA, Gale RP. Factors associated with interstitial pneumonitis after bone marrow transplantation for acute leukaemia. *Lancet*, 1982; ii: 437–9.

31. Miralbell R, *et al.* Renal toxicity after allogeneic bone marrow transplantation. *Journal of Clinical Oncology*, 1996; **14**: 579–85.

32. Lapidot T, Singer TS, Salomon O, Terzi A, Schwartz E, Reisner Y. Booster irradiation to the spleen following total body irradiation. *Journal of Immunology*, 1988; **141**: 2619–24.

33. Abrams RA, Liu PJC, Ambinder RF, *et al.* Hodgkin and non-Hodgkin lymphoma: local-regional radiation therapy after bone marrow transplantation. *Radiology*, 1997; **203**: 865–70.

34. Rosalia M, *et al.* High dose cyclophosphamide, fractionated total body irradiation with involved field irradiation and autologous bone marrow transplantation in malignant lymphoma. *Leukemia and Lymphoma*, 1996; **20**: 249–57.

35. Shank B, Chu FCH, Dinsmore R, *et al.* Hyperfractionated total body irradiation for bone marrow transplantation. Results in seventy leukemia patients with allogeneic transplants. *International Journal of Radiation Oncology Biology Physics*, 1983; **9**: 1607–11.

36. Dutreix J, *et al.* Biologic and anatomic problems of lung shielding in whole-body irradiation. *Journal of the National Cancer Institute*, 1986; **76**: 1333–5.

37. Lewis MA, Rosenbloom ME. A double-headed cobalt-60 unit for large field irradiation. *British Journal of Radiology*, 1988; **61**: 1192–5.

38. Kim TH, Rybka WB, Lehnert S, Podgorsak EB, Freeman CR.

Interstitial pneumonitis following total body irradiation for bone marrow transplantation using two different dose rates. *International Journal of Radiation Oncology Biology Physics*, 1985; **11**: 1285–91.

39. Slavin S, Narrastek E, Weshler Z, Brautbar C, Rachmilewitz EA, Fuks Z. Bone marrow transplantation for severe aplastic anaemia in HLA identical siblings using total lymphoid irradiation and cyclophosphamide. *Transplantation Proceedings*, 1983; **15**: 668–70.

40. Strober S, *et al.* Efficacy of total lymphoid irradiation in intractable rheumatoid arthritis. *Annals of Internal Medicine*, 1985; **102**: 441–9.

41. Senn JS, McCulloch EA. Radiation sensitivity of human bone marrow cells measured by a cell culture method. *Blood*, 1970; **35**: 56–60.

42. Tarbell NJ, Amato DA, Down JD, Mauch P, Hellman S. Fractionation and dose rate effects in mice—a model for bone marrow transplantation in man. *International Journal of Radiation Oncology Biology Physics*, 1989; **13**: 1065–9.

43. Uckun FM, Chang WS, Nesbit M, Kersey JH, Ramsay NKC. Immunophenotype predicts radiation resistance in T-lineage acute lymphoblastic leukemia and T-lineage non-Hodgkin's lymphoma. *International Journal of Radiation Oncology Biology Physics*, 1992; **24**: 705–12.

44. O'Donoghue JA. Fractionated versus low dose rate total body irradiation. Radiobiological considerations in the selection of regimes. *Radiotherapy and Oncology*, 1986; **7**: 242–7.

45. Demirer T, *et al.* Allogeneic marrow transplantation following cyclophosphamide and escalating doses of hyperfractionated total body irradiation in patients with advanced lymphoid malignancies. *International Journal of Radiation Oncology Biology Physics*, 1995; **32**: 1103–9.

46. Peters IJ, Withers HR, Cundiff JH, Dicke KA. Radiobiological considerations in the use of total body irradiation for bone marrow transplantation. *Radiology*, 1979; **131**: 243–7.

47. Keane TJ, Van Dyke J, Rider WD. Idiopathic interstitial pneumonia following bone marrow transplantation: the relationship with total body irradiation. *International Journal of Radiation Oncology Biology Physics*, 1981; **7**: 1365–70.

48. Ringden O, *et al.* Increased mortality by septicaemia, interstitial pneumonitis and pulmonary fibrosis among bone marrow transplant recipients receiving an increased mean dose rate of total irradiation. *Acta Radiologica et Oncologica*, 1983; **22**: 421–8.

49. Santos GW, Tutscha PJ, Brookmayer R. Marrow transplantation for acute non-lymphocytic leukemia after treatment with busulphan and cyclophosphamide. *New England Journal of Medecine*, 1983; **309**: 1347.

50. Ringden O, Ruutu T, Remberger M. A randomized trial comparing busulphan and total body irradiation in allogeneic marrow transplant recipients with hematological malignancies. *Transplantation Proceedings*, 1994; **26**: 1831–2.

51. Gordon BG, Warkentin PI, Strandjord SE, *et al.* Allogeneic bone marrow transplantation for children with acute leukemia: long-term follow-up of patients prepared with high-dose cytosine arabinoside and fractionated total body irradiation. *Bone Marrow Transplantation*, 1997; **20**: 5–10.

52. Hjiyiannakis P, Mehta J, Milan S, Powles R, Hinson J, Tait D. Melphalan, single fraction total body irradiation and allogeneic bone marrow transplantation for acute leukemia: Review of transplant related mortality. *Leukemia and Lymphoma*. 1997; **25**: 565–72.

53. Kumar M, Saleh A, Rao PV, *et al.* Toxicity associated with high dose cytosine arabinoside and total body irradiation as conditioning for allogeneic bone marrow transplantation. *Bone Marrow Transplantation*, 1997; **19**: 1061–4.

54. Westbrook C, Glaholm J, Barrett A. Vomiting associated with whole body irradiation. *Clinical Radiology*, 1987; **38**: 263–6.

55. Spitzer TR, Bryson JC, Cirenza E, *et al.* Randomized double blind placebo controlled evaluation of oral ondansetron in the prevention of nausea and vomiting associated with fractionated total body irradiation. *Journal of Clinical Oncology*, 1994; **12**: 2432–8.

56. Barrett A, Jacobs A, Kohn J, Rayman J, Powles RL. Changes in serum amylase and its isoenzymes after whole body irradiation. *British Medical Journal*, 1982; **285**: 170–1.

57. Dahllöf G, Bågesund M, Ringdén O. Impact of conditioning regimens on salivary function, caries-associated microorganisms and dental caries in children after bone marrow transplantation. A 4-year longitudinal study. *Bone Marrow Transplantation*, 1997; **20**: 479–83.

58. Nakayama Y, Makino S, Fukuda Y, Min K, Shimizu A, Ohsawa N. Activation of lavage lymphocytes in lung injuries caused by radiotherapy for lung cancer. *International Journal of Radiation Oncology Biology Physics*, 1996; **34**: 459–67.

59. Pino Y, Torres JL, Bross DS, *et al.* Risk factors in interstitial pneumonitis following allogeneic bone marrow transplantation. *International Journal of Radiation Oncology Biology Physics*, 1982; **8**: 1301–7.

60. Baglin TP. Veno-occlusive disease of the liver complicating bone marrow transplantation. *Bone Marrow Transplantation*, 1994; **13**: 1–4.

61. Patzer L, *et al.* Renal function after conditioning therapy for bone marrow transplantation in childhood. *Medical and Pediatric Oncology*, 1997; **28**: 274–83.

62. Bergstein J, Andreoli SP, Provisor AJ, Yum M. Radiation nephritis following total body irradiation and cyclophosphamide in preparation for bone marrow transplantation. *Transplantation*, 1986; **41**: 63–6.

63. Tarbell NJ, Guinan EC, Niemeyer C, Mauch P, Sallan SE, Weinstein JH. Late onset of renal dysfunction in survivors of bone marrow transplantation. *International Journal of Radiation Oncology Biology Physics*, 1988; **15**: 99–104.

64. Deeg HJ, *et al.* Cataract after total body irradiation and marrow transplantation: a sparing effect of dose fractionation. *International Journal of Radiation Oncology Biology Physics*, 1984; **10**: 957–64.

65. Fife K, Milan S, Westbrook K, Powles R, Tait D. Risk factors for requiring cataract surgery following total body irradiation. *Radiotherapy and Oncology*, 1994; **33**: 93–8.

66. Nasman M, Forsberg C-M, Dahllof G. Long term dental development after treatment for malignant disease. *European Journal of Orthodontics*, 1997; **19**: 151–9.

67. Peper M, Schraube P, Kimmig B, Wagensommer C, Wannenmacher M, Haas R. Long term cerebral effects of total body irradiation and quality of life. *Recent Results in Cancer Research*, 1993; **130**: 219–30.

68. Sutherland HJ, *et al.* Quality of life following bone marrow transplantation: a comparison of patient reports with population norms. *Bone Marrow Transplantation*, 1997; **19**: 1129–36.

69. Hovi L, Tapanainen P, Saarinen-Pihkala UM, Siimes MA. Impaired androgen production in female adolescents and young adults after total body irradiation prior to BMT in childhood. *Bone Marrow Transplantation*, 1997; **20**: 561–5.

70. Sarafoglou K, Boulad F, Gillio A, Sklar C. Gonadal function after bone marrow transplantation for acute leukemia during childhood. *Journal of Pediatrics*, 1997; **130**: 210–16.

71. Sanders JE. Pubertal development of children with marrow transplantation before puberty. *Journal of Pediatrics*, 1997; **130**: 174–5.

72. Sanders JE, *et al.* Pregnancies following high-dose cyclophosphamide with or without high-dose busulfan or total body irradiation and bone marrow transplantation. *Blood*, 1996; **87**: 3045–52.

73. Toubert M, *et al.* Short- and long-term follow-up of thyroid dysfunction after allogeneic bone marrow transplantation without the use of preparative total body irradiation. *British Journal of Haematology*, 1997; **98**: 453–7.

74. Huma Z, Boulad F, Black P, Heller G, Sklar C. Growth in children after bone marrow transplantation for acute leukemia. *Blood*, 1995; **86**: 819–24.

75. Kupari M, Volin L, Suokas A, Timonen T, Hekali P, Ruutu T. Cardiac involvement in bone marrow transplantation. *Bone Marrow Transplantation*, 1990; 5: 91–8.

76. Darrington DL, *et al.* Incidence and characterization of secondary myelodysplastic syndrome and acute myelogenous leukemia following high-dose chemo-radiotherapy and autologous stem-cell transplantation for lymphoid malignancies. *Clinical Oncology*, 1994; 12: 2527–34.

77. Curtis RE, *et al.* Solid cancers after bone marrow transplantation. *New England Journal of Medicine*, 1997; 336: 897–904.

78. Nygaard R, *et al.* Second maligant neoplasms in patients treated for childhood leukaemia. *Acta Paediatrica Scandinavica*, 1991; 80: 1220–8.

4.9 Principles of chemotherapy

Jaap Verweij, Kees Nooter, and Gerrit Stoter

Introduction

The treatment of cancer is one of the best examples of a multidisciplinary approach to treatment in medicine. Surgery and radiotherapy are frequently still the primary choice of treatment for patients with malignant tumours. However, since 60 to 70 per cent of patients with cancer will develop metastatic disease during their lifetime despite local control of their cancer, for most patients cancer has to be considered as a systemic disease, requiring systemic treatment. The development of systemic therapy over the last few decades has therefore created an important role for medical oncologists in the care of patients with cancer. The types of systemic treatment available to the medical oncologist are continually expanding with newly emerging pharmacological and biological therapies that have clinical activity. We can predict that the role of medical oncology will become increasingly important in the near future.

Every medical oncologist must be aware of the rationale for choosing specific drugs, combinations of drugs, or combinations of different types of treatment. This chapter summarizes the scientific basis of chemotherapy, and addresses important issues in the development of new approaches using molecular targets in a more sophisticated way to try to obtain tumour cell kill or dormancy.

Principles of chemotherapy

As indicated above, in the majority of patients with cancer, chemotherapy will be considered for use at some time during the course of their illness, either aiming at cure, prolongation of life, and/or palliation (Fig. 1).

The design of chemotherapy regimens is based on specific knowledge about cell cycle kinetics, pharmacokinetics, biochemical–pharmacological factors, and empirical knowledge of the responsiveness of specific tumours to specific drugs.

Cellular principles of chemotherapy

For cytotoxic treatment the following characteristics of tumour growth are important in determining outcome:

- cell cycle time
- tumour doubling time
- growth fraction
- tumour size or the number of cells in the population.

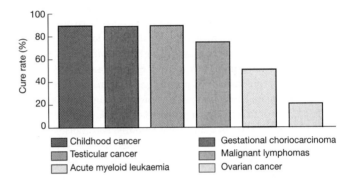

Fig. 1 Cure rates with chemotherapy in some human tumours.

- Childhood cancer
- Testicular cancer
- Acute myeloid leukaemia
- Gestational choriocarcinoma
- Malignant lymphomas
- Ovarian cancer

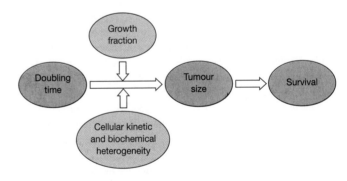

Fig. 2 Cancer dynamics.

Decades ago Skipper *et al.*[1] found that the doubling time of proliferating murine cancer cells is constant, forming a straight line on a semilog plot. Death of the animals resulted when the malignant cells reached a critical fraction of body weight. Since other experiments[2] had shown that a single surviving cell leads to treatment failure, and there is still no evidence that normal levels of host defence are capable of eliminating a few remaining tumour cells, for a given amount of chemotherapy survival was related to tumour size at the time of diagnosis (Fig. 2).

These studies were performed in model systems showing logarithmic (exponential) growth. All of the cells were in cycle and dividing, with no cells in a resting phase, and the cell number doubling at a tumour-specific rate. While knowledge based on these model characteristics is important, the rules only apply to the cells in the proliferation compartment. Unfortunately, only a few human cancers have a large proportion of such responsive proliferating cells. In most tumours there is a large non-proliferating compartment. The growth fraction is the fraction of cells within the total tumour that are actively dividing.[3]

Most human tumours are diagnosed when they are relatively large and kinetically heterogeneous. Due to a variety of factors such as poor vascularity, hypoxia,[4] and competition for nutrients, they exhibit decelerating growth at this stage. Larger tumours contain a high fraction of slowly- or non-dividing cells (termed G_0 cells) and as a consequence the growth fraction is low. Therefore, in treating human tumours, the fractional cell kill hypothesis probably does not apply as well as in animal tumour models. Non-proliferating cells are less sensitive to antineoplastic agents, particularly because they have time to repair the damaged DNA. As many antineoplastic agents are most effective against rapidly dividing cells, the cell-kinetic situation at tumour diagnosis is unfavourable for treatment with most drugs.

Unlike the tumour models used by Skipper, and related to the fact that the proliferating cell population is distinct from the non-proliferating population, human tumours are thought to follow a different growth pattern. Attempts have been undertaken to describe human tumour growth by mathematical models. Two available models are the so-called gompertzian growth model and the exponential growth model. The primary distinction between the two models is that in the gompertzian growth kinetics the growth fraction of the tumour is not constant but decreases exponentially with time. Exponential growth implies that the time taken for a tumour to double its volume is constant. A significant problem is that most tumours only become clinically manifest by approximately 10^9 tumour cells, representing the last part of the tumour's growth curve. Thus, estimating growth curves of human primary tumours based on multiple time points of tumour volume appeared to be difficult, if not impossible. Overall, the available data suggest that the gompertzian growth model is the most probable model. The gompertzian growth curve is sigmoid in shape on a log scale.

The dynamics of this curve are as follows. As indicated, small tumours have the largest growth fraction; but since total cell number is small, even a large growth fraction yields only a small increase in tumour cell number.[5] In the middle portion of the curve, growth reaches a maximum because, although neither the total cell number nor the fraction of proliferating cells is at a maximum, their product does reach a maximum (at about one-third of maximum tumour volume). At the end of the curve, the total cell number is very large but the growth fraction is at a minimum, probably because the number of anoxic and necrotic cells has reached a maximum and the curve reaches a plateau as the tumour approaches the lethal volume.

Since the fractional cell kill effect applies only to the proliferating fraction, it is evident that the best opportunity to achieve total cell kill is in the early part of the curve when the growth fraction is at a maximum. We will observe the maximum measurable tumour response at the midportion of the curve where growth rate is greatest. This is the most appropriate stage to study activity of drugs against a particular tumour. A comparable kill of proliferating cells at the upper part of the curve will be unlikely to show a measurable response because the overall growth rate is so small, and this accounts in part for the therapeutic refractoriness of large human tumours.

Reduction of tumour mass by surgery, radiotherapy, or cell cycle non-specific drugs might stimulate slowly dividing cells to become more rapidly dividing, thereby increasing susceptibility to therapy. Thus, an initially slowly responding tumour may become more responsive to therapy with continued treatment.

Apart from cell-kinetic heterogeneity, biochemical cellular heterogeneity of human tumours may also negatively influence the potential of cure. Although most human tumours evolve from a single clone of malignant cells,[6] more recent studies have shown that this homogeneity does not persist during further stages of tumour growth, presumably as a result of somatic mutation of the original tumour line. More advanced human tumours are composed of cell types with differing morphological and biochemical characteristics.[7] As modelled in studies on gene amplification,[8],[9] such spontaneous mutations occur at a predictable frequency of 1 per 10^5 to 10^6 cell divisions. When non-homogeneous tumour cells are exposed to drugs, sensitive tumour cells will be destroyed while resistant cells will survive and proliferate.[10] As a result, tumour cell kill tends to decrease with subsequent courses of treatment, as resistant cells are selected. Paradoxically, normal tissues never change their level of sensitivity to chemotherapy, emphasizing an important qualitative characteristic of the cancer cell.

Pharmacological principles of chemotherapy

The scheduling of drug treatments is based on both practical and theoretical considerations. Intermittent cycles of treatment are used

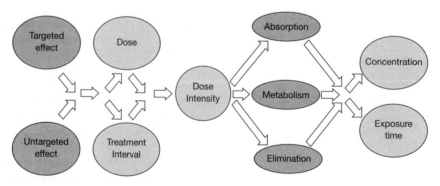

Fig. 3 Pharmacodynamics in cancer chemotherapy.

to allow periods of recovery of normal tissues. This strategy aims at retreatment with full therapeutic doses as frequently as possible in keeping with the fractional cell kill hypothesis, but also allowing the normal tissues to recover from the unintended effects of cytotoxic treatment (Fig. 3). The outcome of chemotherapy will obviously largely depend on the overall intrinsic sensitivity of the treated tumour.

Fractional cell kill means that a given drug concentration applied for a defined time period will kill a constant fraction of the total cell population, independent of the absolute number of cells. In other words, each treatment cycle kills a specific fraction (percentage) of the remaining cells. Since this fraction is never 100 per cent, a single drug administration will never be sufficient to eradicate a tumour completely. Therefore treatment results will also be a direct function of:

- the drug concentration and exposure time and
- the frequency of repeating treatment.

Drug concentration and exposure time will be dependent on pharmacological factors such as drug absorption, metabolism, and elimination. These will have to be considered in general in determining the dose, schedule, and route of drug administration. In addition, interpatient variations in pharmacokinetic parameters are usually large and this may be one reason for the inconsistency in responses of 'sensitive' tumours.

An important source of the interindividual variability in pharmacokinetics is the variable oral absorption of some drugs. Other important factors such as renal or hepatic dysfunction can cause delayed elimination of drug resulting in increased toxicity. To avoid such an increase in toxicity, doses of drugs will have to be modified, depending on their route of elimination. Because the interindividual variation in pharmacokinetics is not always predictable on the basis of renal or hepatic function, direct measurement of plasma drug concentrations may provide a better guide for dosage adjustment to ensure adequate and safe drug exposure. Reliable assays, mainly using high-pressure liquid chromatography, are available for most antineoplastic agents.

How frequently one is able to repeat dosing is, as stated, largely dependent on the unintended side-effects. Various normal tissues have a relatively high growth fraction and are therefore also susceptible to the effects of cytotoxic treatment. The time required for these normal tissues to recover from the effect of cytotoxic therapy will determine how rapidly a cycle of treatment can be repeated. The type of side-effect and patient tolerance will be important factors.

Dose intensity

Most cancer chemotherapeutic agents *in vitro* and *in vivo* exhibit a steep dose–response curve. Consequently, it is considered desirable to administer them in humans at the highest possible dose-intensity, since in theory even small reductions in dose would lead to substantial reductions of tumour cell kill. The importance of dose intensity in tumour responsiveness in humans was first suggested in heavily criticized retrospective analyses performed by Levin and Hryniuk[11] and others.[12] These investigators suggested dose–response correlations for 5-fluorouracil in colon cancer, cisplatin in ovarian cancer, adriamycin in breast cancer, and vincristine in Hodgkin's disease. Subsequently, for some of these, prospective randomized trials of relatively small sample size have supported or refuted the concept.

It is generally accepted that the most important measure of drug exposure would be the area under the curve in a plot of local tumour drug concentration against time. Obviously there is a hierarchy ranging from simple plasma levels of unbound and activated drug (where appropriate), to activated drug concentrations within the target tumour cell. Unfortunately, there are scarcely any data from humans to suggest that plasma drug levels do correlate with tumour levels. Further, there may be confounding factors such as drug interactions by activation of the cytochrome P450 system,[13] which is frequently involved in drug metabolism. This might lead to one drug altering the metabolism of others. Patterns of excretion, drug metabolism, protein binding, and third-space sequestration in general will also affect drug levels in tumour tissue. Still, even with an agent such as methotrexate where we have extensive experience with human dose levels that correlate with toxicity, there is no good correlation between dose level and antitumour efficacy. The question of the therapeutic importance of dose intensity is more likely to be resolved through careful clinical trials than by meticulous pharmacological studies.

Dose intensity of treatment is usually expressed as average dose per week (mg/m² per week) over each course of treatment. Dose intensity can also be calculated for the total length of treatment and it can be calculated for each drug in a combination or for the total of drugs used. Dose intensity, as said, is considered as a correlate of tumour exposure to drug. An increase in dose intensity can be achieved in the following ways.

Local drug application

Dose intensity can be increased by local drug application in various ways.

1. Direct intrathecal administration of drugs such as methotrexate or cytarabine enables a higher local dose in a sanctuary site.
2. Hepatic artery or portal vein infusion in theory allows an increased drug concentration to liver primary or secondary tumours.[14]
3. Intra-arterial perfusion can be used for limb melanomas and soft tissue sarcomas.
4. Intraperitoneal chemotherapy is effective for ovarian cancer.[15],[16]

Dose intensification using local administration in uncontrolled studies has suggested improved response rates. However, with the exception of intrathecal therapy in acute lymphocytic leukaemia and intraperitoneal therapy for ovarian cancer, none of the regional methods has been reported in randomized trials to produce a longer survival than conventional systemic methods of drug administration.

An increase of the dose per administration

The dose per administration can be increased without changing the intervals between administrations.

One such method to increase tumour cell kill is to use doses of chemotherapy that cause prolonged bone marrow suppression and to rescue the host either with autologous bone marrow harvested before treatment or with allogenous marrow from a histocompatible donor. The latter approach has the advantage of infusing marrow that is free of malignant cells, but the disadvantage that marrow donated by a second person contains lymphocytes that may cause so-called graft-versus-host disease, a potentially lethal complication. Recently it has become clear that blood stem cells also circulate in peripheral blood. These circulating stem cells can be harvested before chemotherapy and then autoinfused after high-dose chemotherapy (so-called peripheral stem cell transplantation). This technique is certainly simpler and has largely supplanted collection of autologous bone marrow.

With the use of high-dose chemotherapy, new dose-limiting toxicities to organs other than bone marrow emerge, such as nitrosourea toxicity to lung, kidneys, or liver.[17],[18] For this reason its use is still limited to certain classes of drugs. Moreover, these severe toxicities to other organs still render marrow-ablative high-dose chemotherapy difficult to use in repeated cycles, whatever the salvage technique. This is important because of the earlier indicated fact that a single cycle of chemotherapy usually fails to eradicate the complete solid tumour. Finally, as also previously indicated, it is not at all clear that a linear relationship exists between the dose of drug and tumour cell kill for all drugs and all tumours. In tumour models, with a high growth fraction, increased cell kill results from higher drug doses, but in human tumours, cell kill may well be limited to the relatively low fraction of cells in active proliferation. To date, marrow-ablative chemotherapy in humans has only been shown effective in leukaemias and lymphomas, tumour types with high growth fractions and intrinsic sensitivity to chemotherapy.

Shortening treatment intervals

This method has been used, especially in solid tumours, as another way of increasing dose intensity.

The introduction of drugs such as the 5-hydroxytryptamine-3 antagonist antiemetics and the haematopoietic growth factors has greatly facilitated this approach. Although weekly[19] or biweekly administration of relatively high doses of drugs previously given at 3- to 4-week intervals seems feasible and yields interesting results in uncontrolled trials, it is far too early to conclude if the resulting increases in dose intensity produce an increase in cure rate.

Principles of combination chemotherapy

As a consequence of somatic mutations, tumour cell kill tends to decrease with subsequent courses of treatment, as genetically resistant cell types are selected out. For this reason single-agent treatment is rarely curative. Therefore, and for a variety of other reasons discussed here, cancer chemotherapy is most frequently given as a combination of different drugs. Favourable and unfavourable interactions between drugs must be considered in developing such combination regimens. These interactions may be pharmacokinetic, cytokinetic, or biochemical, and influence the effectiveness of the components of the combination. The theoretical and sometimes proven superiority of combination chemotherapy over single-agent treatment is derived from the principles listed in Table 1.

Activity as a single agent

Drugs with at least activity as a single agent should be selected. Because of primary resistance (see later), which is frequent for any single agent even in the most responsive tumours, complete response rates of single agents rarely exceed 20 per cent.

Different mechanisms of action

Drugs with different mechanisms of action should be combined. The various anticancer agent classes have different targets in the cell

Table 1 Principles of combination chemotherapy

Use drugs active as a single agent
Use drugs with different mechanisms of action
Use drugs with different mechanisms of resistance
Use drugs with different side effects
Be aware of drug–drug interactions

(Table 2; see also Chapter 4.13). Thus, even if a certain target cannot be exploited in a given tumour cell, another target might. Even if tumours are initially sensitive, they usually rapidly acquire resistance after drug exposure. This is probably due to selection of pre-existing resistant tumour cells in the biochemically heterogeneous tumour cell population. In other words, the chemotherapy destroys the sensitive cell population, but is less effective against the non-sensitive population of cells that subsequently is able to continue expanding. In addition, cytotoxic drugs themselves appear to increase the rate of mutation to resistance, at least in tumour models.[20] The use of multiple agents with different mechanisms of action enables independent cell killing by each agent. Cells that are resistant to one agent might still be sensitive to the other drug(s) in the regimen, and might thus still be killed. Known patterns of cross-resistance must be taken into consideration in the design of drug combinations.

Different mechanisms of resistance

Drugs with different mechanisms of resistance should be combined. Resistance to many agents may be the result of mutational changes unique to those agents. However, in other circumstances a single mutational change may lead to resistance to a variety of different drugs. The number of potential mechanisms of resistance is continually increasing and is partly drug dependent.

The most investigated form of multidrug resistance is the one mediated by increased expression of the P170 membrane glycoprotein (**PGP**). Primary (intrinsic) overexpression of this protein has been identified in tumours derived from healthy tissues in which the protein also occurs.[21] Secondary (acquired) overexpression has also been found following chemotherapy in various diseases. PGP mediates the efflux of drugs such as anthracyclines, vinca alkaloids, epipodophyllotoxins, and various others, all derived from natural resources. PGP-mediated active efflux results in decreased intracellular drug levels resulting in decreased cell kill. Agents that compete for the protein such as calcium-channel blockers, cyclosporin, and various synthetically produced drugs can, at least in models, reverse the effect of PGP (Fig. 4). The clinical relevance of this type of resistance and its reversal is still unclear.

A second potentially important type of resistance relates to altered drug binding to topoisomerase II. This is an enzyme known to induce breaks in double-stranded DNA in the presence of drugs such as epipodophyllotoxins and anthracyclines.[22],[23] However, again little is known about the clinical relevance of topoisomerase II resistance.

Third, for several of the classic alkylating agents (cisplatin, cyclophosphamide, melphalan) resistance appears to be related to enhanced repair of drug-induced DNA damage.

Table 2 Chemotherapeutic agents by mechanism of action

Class	Target	Drug(s)
Antimetabolites	Thymidylate synthase	5-Fluorouracil, 5-fluorodeoxyuridine (5-FUDR)
	Dihydrofolate reductase	Methotrexate
	DNA polymerase	Cytarabine
	Ribonucleotide reductase	Hydroxyurea
	Phosphoribosylpyrophosphate aminotransferase	6-Mercaptopurine, 6-thioguanine
	Adenosine deaminase	Pentostatin
	Deoxycytidine triphosphate	Gemcitabine
Alkylating agents		
Nitrogen mustards		Mechlorethamine, cyclophosphamide, melphalan, ifosfamide, chlorambucil
Nitrosoureas		Carmustine (BCNU), lomustine (CCNU), semustine (methyl-CCNU), streptozocin, chlorozotocin
Platins		Cisplatin, carboplatin
Others		Thiotepa, hexamethylmelamine, busulphan, dacarbazine, procarbazine
Topoisomerase II inhibition		Etoposide, teniposide
Topoisomerase I inhibiton		Irinotecan, topotecan
Antitumour antibiotics		
	Alkylation + topisomerase II inhibition	Doxorubicin, daunorubicin, mitoxantrone, darubicin, epirubicin, amsacrine
	Alkylation after bioreduction	mitomycin C
Intercalating agents	RNA synthesis	Dactinomycin, mithramycin
	Uncertain mechanisms	Bleomycin
Spindle poisons		
Vinca alkaloids		Vincristine, vinblastine, vindesine, navelbine
Taxanes		Taxol, taxotere

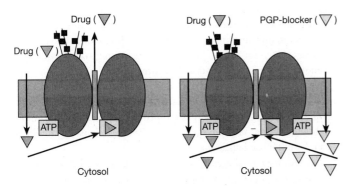

Fig. 4 P-glycoprotein: action and inhibition. The blocking agent binds to the cytoplasmic binding site of the drug, inhibiting its efflux.

There are many other mechanisms of resistance, including alterations in target proteins (e.g. dihydrofolate reductase with altered affinity for methotrexate) and carrier-mediated drug uptake (e.g. reduced folate). In the heterogeneous human tumours, there are frequently various mechanisms of resistance that play a role. Reversing only one of these is unlikely to yield a major impact. Resistance reversal is therefore pursued in only limited numbers of tumours.

Because of the presence of drug-resistant mutants at the time of clinical diagnosis, the earliest possible use of drugs that are not cross-resistant is recommended to avoid the selection of double mutants by sequential chemotherapy. Adequate cytotoxic doses of drugs have to be administered as frequently as possible to achieve maximal kill of both sensitive and moderately resistant cells. Less desirable alternatives are the use of different regimens in alternating cycles of therapy or the use of multiple cycles of one regimen given to the point of maximal response, followed by a second regimen.

Table 3 Drug interactions in combination chemotherapy

Antagonism of antitumour effect
  L-Asparaginase prior to methotrexate
  5-Fluorouracil prior to methotrexate

Enhancement of antitumour effect
  Nitroimidazoles enhance alkylating agent activity
  Leucovorin increases 5-fluorouracil inhibition of thymidylate synthase
  Methotrexate increases both 5-fluorouracil and cytarabine activation
  Inhibitors of pyrimidine synthesis enhance 5-fluorouracil incorporation
  into RNA

Reversal of drug resistance
  Calcium-channel blocker inhibit efflux by P-glycoprotein

Prevention or reversal of toxicity
  Allopurinol blocks 5-fluorouracil activation by normal tissues
  Leucovorin prevents methotrexate toxicity
  Deoxycytidine prevents toxicity of cytarabine

Different dose-limiting toxicities

If possible, drugs with different dose-limiting toxicities should be combined. In the case of non-overlapping toxicity it is more likely that each of the drugs can be used at full dose and thus the effectiveness of each agent will be maintained in the combination. Unfortunately, for many cytotoxic agents the side-effects frequently involve myelosuppression. If there is overlapping myelotoxicity, arbitrary scales of dose adjustment according to bone marrow toxicity can be used, or haematopoietic growth factors can be added to reduce the risk related to myelosuppression. Clearly, drugs that lack bone marrow toxicity, such as vincristine, cisplatin, and bleomycin, are favoured to combine with myelosuppressive agents. Drugs with renal or hepatic side-effects in theory can alter the elimination of other agents through these routes and therefore must be used with caution in combinations. For example, cisplatin causes renal toxicity and is known to alter the pharmacokinetics of other agents (such as methotrexate or bleomycin) that depend on renal elimination as their primary mechanism of excretion. If cisplatin is given before methotrexate, as in the treatment of bladder or head and neck cancer, careful monitoring of renal function, adequate hydration before and after administration of methotrexate, and dose adjustment for methotrexate are essential to ensure that delayed methotrexate excretion does not lead to severe drug toxicity.

Cell cycle-related and biochemical interactions

Cell cycle-related and biochemical interactions between drugs can also be used to design combinations. Examples of drug interactions are listed in Table 3.

Provided that the drugs used are active in a particular disease, knowledge of cell kinetics can be used to consider initiation of therapy with agents that are not specific for cell cycle (the alkylating agents and nitrosoureas), first to reduce tumour bulk and second to recruit slowly dividing cells into active DNA synthesis. Once the latter is achieved, therapy can be continued within the same cycle of treatment with agents specific for cell cycle phase (such as methotrexate or the fluoropyrimidines) that mainly affect cells during periods of DNA synthesis. Further, repeated courses with S-phase-specific drugs, such

as cytosine arabinoside and methotrexate, that block cells during the period of DNA synthesis, are most effective if they are administered during the rebound rapid recovery of DNA synthesis that follows the period of suppression of DNA synthesis.[24] For cytosine arabinoside, for instance, this occurs approximately 10 days after the first treatment with this agent.

An example of biochemical interaction suggesting a rational sequencing of drugs is shown by the experimental demonstration that the sequence of 5-fluorouracil and methotrexate seems crucial to the cytotoxicity of this combination. *In vitro*, if methotrexate precedes 5-fluorouracil by at least 1 h,[25] synergistic results are obtained. This may be due to an increased activation of 5-fluorouracil to its nucleotide form. The opposite sequence of drug administration leads to antagonism due to block of the thymidylate synthase pathway induced by 5-fluorouracil. Through this block the intracellular folates are preserved in their active tetrahydrofolate form, which diminishes the effect of the methotrexate block of dihydrofolate reductase.

Agents that lack intrinsic antitumour activity but, for instance, enhance the intracellular activation or target binding of the cytotoxic agent or inhibit the repair of lesions produced by the cytotoxic drug may also modulate the activity of cytotoxic agents. For example, leucovorin (5-formyltetrahydrofolate) enhances 5-fluorouracil binding to thymidylate synthase.[26]

It is important to realize that none of the suggested interactions, with the possible exception of 5-fluorouracil and leucovorin, has yielded clinical activity that is superior to simultaneous use of the same drugs. This could be a result of other confounding interactions or simply of the fact that the appropriate clinical trials have not been performed. Importantly, there is a tremendous paucity of pharmacokinetic interaction studies of commonly applied combination regimens. Recently it has been shown that cisplatin affects the pharmacokinetics of drugs such as taxol and topotecan, and consequently it is, for instance, universally recommended to administer taxol before cisplatin, which happens to be the sequence with the highest tumour cell kill *in vitro*.

Based upon the given considerations, combinations have been developed that are curative in diseases such as the malignant lymphomas, acute lymphocytic leukaemia, testicular cancer, and various cancers of childhood.

For patients with metastatic disease, combination chemotherapy is used with the overall strategy of giving repeated cycles of the regimen over a finite time period. The tumour response is then assessed. If the tumour has progressed, treatment is discontinued. If there has been tumour regression or stabilization, continuation of treatment is considered. If there has been complete clinical disappearance of the tumour, discontinuation of treatment is considered.

In an attempt to improve the long-term disease-free survival rate and cure rate, for some indications the basic strategy of cyclic chemotherapy has been modified in three ways.

First, combinations of drugs that are not cross-resistant have been used to maintain complete remission induced with the initial combination. This strategy has not improved survival in solid tumour treatment, but has been successful in preventing relapse in childhood acute lymphocytic leukaemia.

Second, hormonal agents, such as oestradiol, have been used with the aim of stimulating hormone-responsive cells into active DNA synthesis and thus rendering these cells susceptible to the effect of cell cycle-specific drugs. Such an approach is effective in experimental

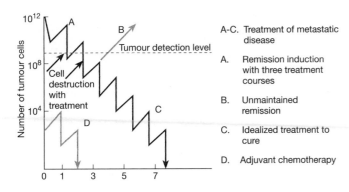

Fig. 5 The principle of adjuvant chemotherapy as opposed to treatment of measurable disease.

models but has not yet shown any benefit in human solid tumours.

Finally, the still relatively limited success rate of chemotherapy in metastatic solid tumours has meant that the search for new, and hopefully more effective, drugs continues. Examples will be discussed later in this chapter.

Adjuvant and neoadjuvant systemic therapy

Drug therapy is also used to benefit patients who exhibit no evidence of residual disease after initial therapy, but are at high risk of relapse (adjuvant therapy), or those with bulky primary disease to reduce this bulk preceding local therapy (neoadjuvant therapy).

Adjuvant therapy

There are two major reasons why adjuvant chemotherapy might be considered: (i) the high rate of recurrence after surgery for some, apparently localized tumours and (ii) the failure of systemic therapy or combined modality treatment to cure patients with clinically apparent metastatic disease. These issues may in turn be related to the following three points.

First, once the tumour bulk is reduced to clinically undetectable levels with local therapy, the number of cells yet to be destroyed by subsequent chemotherapy is relatively small, in contrast to the large numbers of cells in the case of clinical metastatic disease. According to the principles of log cell kill in the first situation, the likelihood of completely eradicating the remaining tumour cells is much higher than in the latter (Fig. 5).

Second, as mentioned earlier, there is evidence from tumour models that supports the hypothesis that tumours are most sensitive to chemotherapy at their earliest stages of growth. This is thought to be related to their high growth fraction (most cells are in active progression through the cell cycle), shorter cell cycle times, and therefore greater fractional cell kill for a given dose of drug.[27] Once tumours progress to clinical detectability, their growth fraction falls, the cell cycle time lengthens, and they become much less sensitive to treatment.

Third, there is a relationship between tumour bulk and tumour cell resistance. The probability of the occurrence of resistant cells in

a tumour population is a function of the total number of cells present. Therefore, subclinical (occult) tumours rather than clinically detectable tumours are more likely to be cured by a specific schedule or type of chemotherapy.

On the other hand, there are obviously potential disadvantages of adjuvant chemotherapy that have to be taken into account. They relate to immediate, short-, and long-term side-effects of such treatment. Since a fraction of patients receiving adjuvant treatment is already cured by the primary surgical procedure they would therefore experience needless toxicity and risks if treated with adjuvant therapy. Clearly, it would be preferable to avoid adjuvant therapy in these patients, but unfortunately, there is no proven method at present to identify the patients 'cured' by primary local therapy. The immediate side-effects obviously relate to potentially lethal infectious complications from neutropenia, bleeding, and less hazardous but very inconvenient side-effects such as alopecia and nausea and vomiting. The latter side-effects are still the worst in the patients' perception.[28] Late complications such as carcinogenicity and irrecoverable sterility assume greater importance, but neither risk has been adequately quantified for all drugs and combinations. The risks of other late effects such as bone marrow hypoplasia from alkylating agents and nitrosoureas, the cardiotoxicity of doxorubicin, neurotoxocity of platins and taxanes, and pulmonary toxicity of bleomycin and the nitrosoureas should obviously not outweigh the potential benefits. In balancing these risks with the outcome as far as tumour eradication is concerned, adjuvant chemotherapy has become a standard of care in many cancers of childhood, the breast, the colon, and the ovary.

Neoadjuvant therapy

If chemotherapy is used as initial treatment, preceding a form of local therapy, it is called 'neoadjuvant therapy' or 'induction therapy'. Such neoadjuvant chemotherapy has attracted increasing attention in the treatment of some adult solid tumours. Factors related to the response to neoadjuvant chemotherapy are similar to those that may affect adjuvant chemotherapy, namely growth rate, presence of drug resistance, and tumour mass.

The potential benefits of neoadjuvant chemotherapy involve the control of the primary tumour as well as of potential micrometastases. There are several potential advantages for control of the primary tumour.[8],[29]

First, local reduction of the tumour may facilitate the use of more conservative surgery and/or radiotherapy. This can be especially important in situations where loss of functional use and cosmetic appearance can be devastating to the patient, which is for instance the case in head and neck tumours and sarcomas.

Second, administering chemotherapy prior to the local therapy avoids the potential of poor distribution and penetration of drug at the tumour site due to the compromised vascularity that may result from surgery and/or radiation therapy.

Third, cytotoxic drugs can be combined concurrently with radiation therapy to increase the local control rate. This approach has been especially effective in head and neck cancer (see Section 9). The effect is not due solely to radiosensitization.

Fourth, post-chemotherapy surgery offers a unique opportunity to assess the correlation between clinical tumour response measurements and actual pathological changes.

Fifth, the response of the primary tumour to chemotherapy may reflect the response of micrometastases and therefore influence further patient management.

Concerning the control of micrometastases, it is possible that these are only generated after the primary tumour attains a threshold size. At this point metastatic variants develop at a fast rate.[30] This process is similar to the one discussed previously for the occurrence of spontaneous mutants. Both possibilities favour the use of chemotherapy as early as possible. On the other hand, some data suggest that clinically undetectable metastases may initially be indolent with low growth fraction, which would make them less susceptible to chemotherapy.[29]

The disadvantages of neoadjuvant chemotherapy are similar to those mentioned for adjuvant chemotherapy. Additional disadvantages may be:

(1) selection of drug-resistant clones;

(2) an increase in toxicity from subsequent therapies;

(3) a failure of cytotoxic agents to reduce the primary tumour significantly, thereby possibly allowing further subclinical progression of disease; and

(4) a loss of the advantage of attacking micrometastases after surgery when they may exhibit more favourable cell kinetics.

Nevertheless, the use of neoadjuvant chemotherapy certainly holds promise for the treatment of several solid tumours in man.

Apart from the already mentioned relation between the response to neoadjuvant chemotherapy and subsequent radiotherapy, the response to neoadjuvant chemotherapy may also select a group of patients who will achieve prolonged disease-free survival. It is conceivable that well-designed clinical trials on neoadjuvant chemotherapy could show further correlations between initial response and ultimate outcome (i.e. survival) which, in combination with other prognostic factors, could alter the management of certain diseases.[29] As a result of studies involving neoadjuvant chemotherapy, in combination with either surgery or radiation therapy, such treatment has become the standard of care in some groups of patients with diffuse large-cell lymphomas, osteosarcomas and other paediatric cancers, limited small-cell lung cancers, and head and neck cancers.

New molecular targets for systemic anticancer therapy

Recently, molecular biology studies have significantly expanded our knowledge concerning the cellular mechanisms that turn normal cells into tumour cells. The role of oncogenes and tumour suppressor genes in these processes is becoming increasingly clear. Inactivation of tumour suppressor genes by mutation, deletion, or whole chromosome loss, and/or activation of oncogenes by chromosomal translocation or amplification of point mutation[31],[32] have both been linked with disease progression[33],[34] and/or a poor prognosis. These findings have triggered the development of new drugs, such as those that interfere with specific molecules participating in signal transduction pathways involved in tumorigenesis. In addition, this knowledge of the genes involved in tumour development can be used for targeted gene therapy, which is discussed in Chapter 4.27. Furthermore, important information concerning the role of stromal factors and angiogenesis in tumour growth has become available and

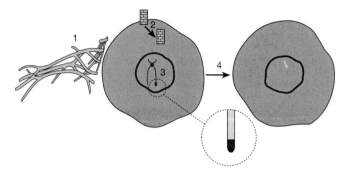

Fig. 6 Targets for new drugs: (1) inhibition of angiogenesis, (2) inhibition of intracellular signal transduction, (3) inhibition of telomerase, and (4) inhibition of stromal factors.

subsequently these have also become targets for development of drug therapy (Fig. 6).

Signal transduction

A large number of dominant cellular oncogenes and tumour suppressor genes continue to be identified. These oncogenes and tumour suppressor genes encode proteins that are involved in the various pathways through which cells sense their environment and subsequently respond to it (cell signalling), particularly with respect to controlling cell proliferation, differentiation, and death.[35]–[39] These proteins participate in each of the crucial steps in the transfer of information, from growth factors which bind to receptors at the cellular membrane, to the read out of specific genes. They can be classified into:

· growth factors themselves

· membrane receptors

· intracellular transducers, and

· nuclear transcription factors.

Ideally, removal of proliferation-promoting signals from cancer cells would force the tumour cell into a non-cycling G_0-like state, leading to an overall inhibition of the growth of the tumour. Frequently, in tumour growth these proteins are overexpressed or hyperactive. Hence, direct inhibition of these overstimulated transduction pathways might result in a relatively greater inhibition of tumour growth than growth of normal tissues,[40]–[43] where there is no overstimulation. In view of this mechanism of inhibition, we may expect that cell signal transduction inhibitors will have a cytostatic rather than a cytotoxic effect. They are designed to block proliferation but will not necessarily kill tumour cells as is the case with classic cytotoxic drugs or radiation. Because of this cytostatic effect, and in view of the possibility that growth-arrested cells could escape from the pharmacological blockade, we have to anticipate that signal transduction inhibitors will have to be administered chronically and, depending on their half-life, probably daily.

The biochemical specificity that can be achieved will be greater the closer to the membrane receptor the drug acts. However, the likelihood of a bypass of the blockade as a result of input from alternative signalling pathways is also greater in these circumstances. In contrast, the further down the transduction pathway the drug acts, the greater the likelihood of toxicity will be as a result of simultaneous

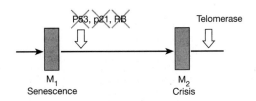

Fig. 7 Absence/mutation of tumour suppressor genes enables cells to keep dividing beyond mortality stage 1 (M1). Telomerase enables cells to keep dividing beyond mortality stage 2 (M2).

inhibition of many signal transduction pathways. However, blockade of individual genes would in theory not suffer from these weaknesses. Considerable effort is now focused on the development of inhibitors of receptor thyrosine kinase and ras, which are on the 'direct' path from receptors to transcription factors, and on protein kinase C, which is a major factor in signalling 'cross-talk'. In addition, many other potential targets in these pathways are being explored.

One of the methods is the use of antisense drugs. Antisense oligodeoxynucleotides are complementary to a targeted mRNA. These have been shown, *in vitro* and *in vivo*, to be able to shut off expression of activated oncogenes.[44] Antisense molecules are chemically synthesized oligomers that specifically block the translational process by hybridization, preferably to the translation initiation site of the specific mRNA. Oligonucleotides designed to hybridize to specific mRNA sequences have been used to inhibit the expression of a variety of viral- and cellular-encoded proteins and clinical trials have recently started.[45]

Notwithstanding the abovementioned likelihood of achieving cytostasis (or cell dormancy), there are also data to suggest that in cells with deregulated oncogenes, removal of the proliferation signals can induce a programmed cell death or apoptosis.[46] Thus, signal transduction inhibitors in theory could also have some indirect cytotoxic effects.

Telomerase inhibitors

Telomeres are end regions of eukaryotic chromosomes. They protect free DNA ends from end-to-end fusions and exonucleocytic degradation.[47] Telomeres may be important for homologue pairing and recombination,[48] for inhibiting expression of several non-essential genes,[49] and for premeiotic chromosomal movement in eukaryotes.[50] During each cell division the two DNA strands separate and daughter strands are synthesized in a slightly different manner on the leading and the lagging strand, with replication respectively in a continuous and a discontinuous fashion. The result is an 'end replication imbalance',[51],[52] leading to a loss of 50 to 200 base pairs with every cell division.[53] This eventually shortens telomeres to a length that activates an antiproliferative mechanism termed mortality stage 1 (M1). At this stage, senescence of cells occurs due to a DNA-damage signal that induces p53, p21, and retinoblastoma gene product (pRB) activity.[54] As a consequence, telomere shortening serves as a 'mitotic clock'[55] and restricts the number of possible cell divisions to between 50 and 70,[56] thereby contributing to cellular ageing. In some cells, mortality stage 1 is bypassed and these cells continue to divide until telomeres become critically shortened in mortality stage 2, or M2 (Fig. 7). At this latter stage, a specialized DNA polymerase called

telomerase appears in many immortalized cells, and neutralizes its internal RNA template to synthesize the telomeric sequence, thereby compensating for the loss of original telomeric DNA due to the incomplete replication. Further shortening of telomeres is prevented and stabilization of their length is achieved, which contributes to immortalization. Telomerase activity is repressed in most normal human tissues but is abundantly present in various tumours,[57] thereby presenting a potentially unique target of anticancer therapy.

There appears to be a gradual increase in telomerase activity from early- to late-stage tumours.[57] Agents that inhibit telomerase are now in development. Because they are most likely to shorten telomeres critically only after a lag period, this may lead to senescence in a small proportion of cells and a slight theoretical increase in doubling time of non-senescent cells. Thus, given as a short-term single-agent treatment their effect will be negligible. However, when given long-term following effective cytotoxic therapy they might be useful, because high proliferation rates in small tumours might lead to larger numbers of senescent cells due to critically shortened telomeres and eventually to tumour eradication.

Angiogenesis

The growth of new blood capillaries from pre-existing vessels is called angiogenesis. This process is fundamental to a variety of physiological and pathophysiological processes, including cancer. Under normal circumstances, angiogenesis is tightly controlled through an appropriate balance between an increased production of stimulatory factors and a concomitant decreased production of inhibitors. Normally, for instance in wound repair, angiogenesis is a process that occurs over a restricted time following which the proliferating endothelial cells rapidly return to their usual state of quiescence.[58] However, the development and maintenance of many diseases are dependent on the persistence of this process and the loss of normal regulatory mechanisms, and the growth of solid tumours is one of them. Angiogenesis and neovascularization have been shown to be a crucial step in the dissemination and further progression of malignant disease.[59],[60] By inhibiting the factors involved in angiogenesis, the growth of solid tumours and their metastases can be potently suppressed in tumour models. In tumour-bearing mice the use of angiogenesis inhibitors, apart from inducing a state of cell dormancy, has even induced a regression of established tumours and cures. However, the value of this concept has not yet been proved in humans.

Protease inhibitors

Proteolytic degradation of the extracellular matrix by extracellular proteases is necessary for tumour cells to be able to penetrate the basement membrane, the tissues, gain access to blood vessels, exit them again, and colonize at distant sites (metastases). In addition, angiogenesis (see above) also involves active proteolytic degradation of the extracellular matrix by invasive endothelial cells.[61]

The fact that proteases are localized preferentially in adjuvant stromal cells, rather than in invasive tumour cells, suggests that the production of proteases by the surrounding stromal cells can be triggered by tumour cells.[62] Thus, tumour cells are able to increase proteolytic activity without increasing their own production and secretion of proteases, and they can concentrate and activate proteases in the pericellular space. The four classes of endopeptidases that play a role in these processes are:

- serine
- cysteine
- aspartyl and
- metalloproteinases.[61]

Metalloproteinases in turn can be classified into:

- collagenases
- gelatinases
- stromelysins and
- membrane-type metalloproteinases.[61]

Tumour cells can achieve optimal matrix degradation by stimulating production of a variety of proteases. This enables them to escape attempts to restore the production and secretion of proteases in tumours. Direct or indirect inhibition of proteases may represent important ways to inhibit tumour cell proteolysis.[63] In drug development, it may be important to target more than one family of proteases.

In tumours there appears to be a temporal local imbalance between the levels of activated enzymes and their naturally occurring inhibitors. For instance, the proportion of active metalloproteinases overwhelms the local inhibitory activity surrounding the tumour, which results in a breakdown of the extracellular matrix. This in turn facilitates the direct expansion and local invasion of the primary tumour, the movement of tumour cells across the vascular basement membrane, and the invasion and local growth of metastases. Metalloproteinase activity also contributes to the invasive in-growth of new blood vessels, a requisite for malignant tumour growth.

Metalloproteinase inhibitors were the first protease inhibitors to enter clinical trials.[61] They were initially developed as potential antimetastatic agents.[61] However, studies in tumour models have shown they also directly suppress growth and development of lymphatic metastases. The antiangiogenic features of these drugs may relate to the inhibition of haematogenous metastases.[64]

Importantly, preclinical studies suggest that metalloproteinase inhibitors and cytotoxic agents may act synergistically.[65]

General issues

The preclinical data on the inhibitors of these new targets indicate that they act as cytostatic drugs. Thus, while a regression of tumour induced by follow-up mechanisms cannot be ruled out, the aim of their use would be primarily to generate a state of tumour dormancy by halting proliferation, and thus creating progression arrest. Therefore, the anticipated necessity of long-term treatment administration requires minimal side-effects and an easy administration schedule in order to maximize drug compliance. In contrast to cytotoxic agents, the recommended dose for these new inhibitors will therefore not be the maximally tolerated dose, but a dose with an optimal biological effect.

References

1. Skipper HE. Historic milestones in cancer biology: a few that are important to cancer treatment (revisited). *Seminars in Oncology*, 1979; 6: 506–14.

2. Furth J, Kahn MC. The transmission of leukemia of mice with a single cell. *American Journal of Cancer*, 1937; 31: 276–82.

3. Mendelsohn ML. The growth fraction: a new concept applied to tumors. *Science*, 1960; 132: 1496.

4. Tannock IF. The relationship between proliferation and the vascular system in a transplanted mouse mammary tumor. *British Journal of Cancer*, 1968; 22: 258–73.

5. Norton L, Simon R. The Norton–Simon hypothesis revisited. *Cancer Treatment Reports*, 1986; 70: 163–9.

6. Fialkow PJ. Clonal origin of human tumors. *Biochimica et Biophysica Acta*, 1976; 458: 283–321.

7. Shapiro JR, Shapiro WR. Clonal tumor cell heterogeneity. *Progress in Experimental Tumor Research*, 1984; 27: 49–66.

8. Goldie JH, Coldman AJ. A mathematic model for relating the drug sensitivity of tumors to their spontaneous mutation rate. *Cancer Treatment Reports*, 1979; 63: 1727–33.

9. Schimke RT. Gene amplification in cultured mammalian cells. *Cell*, 1984; 37: 705–13.

10. Curt GA, Chabner BA. Gene amplification in drug resistance: of mice and men. *Journal of Clinical Oncology*, 1984; 2: 62–4.

11. Levin L, Hryniuk WM. Dose intensity analysis of chemotherapy regimens in ovarian carcinoma. *Journal of Clinical Oncology*, 1987; 5: 756–67.

12. Longo DL, *et al.* Twenty years of MOPP therapy for Hodgkin's disease. *Journal of Clinical Oncology*, 1986; 4: 1295–306.

13. Alberts DS, Peng YM, Chen HS, Struck RF. Effect of phenobarbital on plasma levels of cyclophosphamide and its metabolites in the mouse. *British Journal of Cancer*, 1978; 38: 316–24.

14. Kemeny N, Schneider A. Regional treatment of hepatic metastases and hepatocellular carcinoma. *Current Problems in Cancer*, 1989; 13: 197–284.

15. Howell SB. Intraperitoneal chemotherapy for ovarian carcinoma. *Journal of Clinical Oncology*, 1988; 6: 1673–5.

16. Alberts DS, *et al.* Phase III study of intraperitoneal cisplatin (CDDP)/ intravenous cyclophosphamide (CPA) vs i.v. CDDP/i.v. CPA in patients with optimal disease stage III ovarian cancer: a SWOG-GOG-ECOG Intergroup study. *Proceedings of the American Society of Clinical Oncology*, 1995; 14: 273.

17. Tchekmedyian NS, *et al.* High-dose chemotherapy without autologous bone marrow transplantation in melanoma. *Journal of Clinical Oncology*, 1986; 4: 1811–18.

18. Philips GL, *et al.* Intensive 1.3-bis(2-chloroethyl)-1 nitrosourea (BCNU) (NSC-4366650) and cryopreserved autologous marrow transplantation for refractory cancer. A phase I–II study. *Cancer*, 1983; 52: 1792–802.

19. Planting ASTh, Van der Burg MEL, De Boer-Dennert M, Stoter G, Verweij J. Phase I/II study of a short course of weekly cisplatin in patients with advanced solid tumors. *British Journal of Cancer*, 1993; 68: 789–92.

20. Rice GC, Hoy C, Schimke RT. Transient hypoxia enhances the frequency of DHFR gene amplification in Chinese hamster ovary cells. *Proceedings of the National Academy of Sciences (USA)*, 1986; 83: 5978–82.

21. Fojo AT, *et al.* Expression of a multidrug-resistance gene in human tumors and tissues. *Proceedings of the National Academy of Sciences (USA)*, 1987; 84: 265–9.

22. Pommier Y, *et al.* Altered DNA topoisomerase II activity in Chinese hamster cells resistant to topoisomerase II inhibitors. *Cancer Research*, 1986; 46: 3075–81.

23. Deffie AM, Batra JK, Goldenberg GJ. Direct correlation between topoisomerase II activity and cytotoxicity in adriamycin-sensitive and -resistant P388 leukemia cell lines. *Cancer Research*, 1989; 49: 58–62.

24. Vaughan WP, Karp JE, Burke PJ. Two-cycle-times sequential chemotherapy for adult acute nonlymphocytic leukemia. *Blood*, 1984; 64: 975–80.

25. Cadman E, Heimer R, Davis L. Enhanced 5-fluorouracil nucleotide formation after methotrexate administration: explanation for drug synergism. *Science*, 1979; **205**: 1135–7.

26. Grem JL, *et al.* An overview of the current status and future directions of clinical trials with fluorouracil and folinic acid. *Cancer Treatment Reports*, 1987; **71**: 1249–64.

27. Salmon SE. Kinetics of minimal residual disease. *Recent Results in Cancer Research*, 1979; **67**: 5–15.

28. De Boer-Dennert M, *et al.* Patient perception of the side-effects of chemotherapy: the influence of 5HT3 antagonists. *British Journal of Cancer*, 1997; **76**: 1055–61.

29. Frei E, Miller D, Clark JR., Fallon BG, Ervin TJ. Clinical and scientific consideration in preoperative (neoadjuvant) chemotherapy. *Recent Results in Cancer Research*, 1986; **103**: 1–5.

30. Hill RP, Chambers AF, Ling V. Dynamic heterogeneity: rapid generation of metastatic variants in mouse B16 melanoma cells. *Science*, 1984; **224**: 998–1000.

31. Huang H-JS, *et al.* Suppression of the neoplastic phenotype by replacement of the RB gene in human cancer cells. *Science*, 1988, **242**: 1563–6.

32. Baker SJ, Markowitz S, Fearon ER, Wilson JKV, Vogelstein B. Suppression of human colorectal carcinoma cell line growth by wild type p53. *Science*, 1990; **249**: 912–15.

33. Bishop JM. The molecular genetics of cancer. *Science*, 1987, **235**: 305–11.

34. Alitalo K, Schwab M. Oncogenes amplification in tumor cells. *Advances in Cancer Research*, 1986; **47**: 235–81.

35. Weinberg RA. Tumor suppressor genes. *Science*, 1991; **254**: 1138–45.

36. Cantley LC, *et al.* Oncogenes and signal transduction. *Cell*, 1991; **64**: 281–302.

37. Lewin B. Oncogene conversion by regulatory changes in transcription factors. *Cell*, 1991, **64**: 303–12.

38. Aaronson S. Growth factors and cancer. *Science*, 1991; **254**: 1146–53.

39. Lane DP. A death in the life of p53. *Nature*, 1993; **362**: 786–7.

40. Gesher A. Toward selective pharmacological manipulation of protein kinase C—opportunities for the development of novel anti neoblastic agents. *British Journal of Cancer*, 1992; **66**: 10–19.

41. Grunicke HH, Uberall F. Protein kinase C modulation. *Seminars in Cancer Biology*, 1992; **3**: 351–60.

42. Kikkawa U, Kishimoto A, Nishizuka Y. The protein kinase C family: heterogeneity and its implications. *Annual Review of Biochemistry*, 1989; **58**: 31–44.

43. Weinstein IB, *et al.* Roles of specific isoforms of protein kinase C in growth control and cell transformation. *Proceedings of the American Association of Cancer Research*, 1993; **34**: 611–12.

44. Kitada S, Takayama S, DeRiel K, Tanaka S, Reed JC. Reversal of chemoresistance of lymphoma cells by antisense-mediated reduction of bcl-2 gene expression. *Antisense Research and Development*, 1994; **4**: 71–9.

45. Webb A, *et al.* Bcl-2 antisense therapy in patients with non-Hodgkin lymphoma. *Lancet*, 1997; **349**: 1137–41.

46. Dive C, Evans CA, Whetton AD. Induction of apoptoses—new targets for cancer chemotherapy. *Seminars in Cancer Biology*, 1992; **3**: 417–27.

47. McClintock B. The fusion of broken ends of chromosomes following nuclear fusion. *Proceedings of the National Academy of Sciences (USA)*, 1942; **28**: 458–63.

48. Zakian VA. Telomeres: beginning to understand to end. *Science*, 1995; **270**: 1601–7.

49. Lustig AJ. Involvement of the silencer and UAS binding protein RAP1 in regulation of telomere length. *Science*, 1990; **250**: 549–53.

50. Chikashige Y, *et al.* Telomere-led premeiotic chromosome movement in fission yeast. *Science*, 1994; **264**: 270–3.

51. Watson JD. Origin of concatameric T4 DNA. *Nature*, 1972; **239**: 197–201.

52. Olvonikov AM. A theory of marginotomy. *Journal of Theoretical Biology*, 1971; **41**: 181–90.

53. West MD. The cellular and molecular biology of skin aging. *Archives of Dermatology*, 1994; **130**: 87–95.

54. Wright WE, Shay JW. Time, telomeres and tumors: Is cellular senescence more than an anticancer mechanism? *Trends in Cell Biology*, 1995; **5**: 293–7.

55. Harley CB, Vaziri H, Counter CM, Allsopp RC. The telomere hypothesis of cellular aging. *Experimental Gerontology*, 1992; **27**: 375–82.

56. Hayflick L. The limited *in vitro* lifetime of human diploid cell strains. *Experimental Cell Research*, 1965; **37**: 614–36.

57. Sharma S, *et al.* Preclinical and clinical strategies for development of telomerase and telemere inhibitors. *Annals of Oncology*, 1997; **8**: 1063–74.

58. Denekamp J. Vasculature as a target for tumor therapy. In: Hammersen F, Hudkicka O, eds. *Progress in Applied Microcirculation.* Basel: Karger Publishers, 1984: 8–38.

59. Folkman J. Tumor angiogenesis. In: Mendelsohn J, Israel MA, Liotta LA, eds. *The Molecular Basis of Cancer.* Philadelphia: WB Saunders, 1995: 206–32.

60. Holmgren L, O'Reilly MS, Folkman J. Dormancy of micrometastases: balanced proliferation and apoptosis in the presence of angiogenesis suppression. *Nature Medicine*, 1995; **1**: 149–53.

61. Denis LJ, Verweij J. Matrix metalloprotease inhibitors: present achievements and future prospects. *Investigational New Drugs*, 1997; **15**: 175–85.

62. Basset P, *et al.* A novel metalloproteinase gene specifically expressed in stromal cells of breast carcinomas. *Nature*, 1990; **348**: 699–704.

63. Vassalli JD, Pepper MS. Tumour biology. Membrane proteases in focus. *Nature*, 1994; **370**: 14–15.

64. Brown PD, Giavazzi R. Matrix metalloproteinase inhibition: a review of anti-tumour activity. *Annals of Oncology*, 1995; **6**: 967–74.

65. Anderson IC, Shipp MA, Docherty AJP, Teicher BA. Combination therapy including a gelatinase inhibitor and cytotoxic agents reduces local invasion and metastasis of murine Lewis lung carcinoma. *Cancer Research*, 1993; **53**: 2087–91.

4.10 Myelosuppression and infective complications

Thierry Berghmans and Jean-Paul Sculier

Introduction

Myelosuppression is one of the commonest complications of cancer and its treatment. Its occurrence is favoured by neoplastic infiltration of the bone marrow. It is usually induced by anticancer treatment consisting mainly of chemotherapy, but also by radiotherapy (conventional or isotopic). The leading causes of death in patients with cancer are infection and haemorrhage. In early retrospective studies,[1]–[5] 10 to 41 per cent of deaths were due to infection. In a trial in which 230 granulocytopenic patients were randomized between two broad-spectrum antibiotic combinations, overall mortality directly attributable to infection was 8 per cent (19 of 230).[6] In the same retrospective series,[1]–[5] haemorrhage, associated or not with thrombocytopenia, was the cause of death in up to 41 per cent of patients. The intensity of anticancer treatment is increasing with the use of autologous or allogeneic bone marrow transplantation, intensive chemotherapy, concomitant administration of chemotherapy and radiotherapy, and the introduction of new agents that cause profound immunosuppression, such as nucleoside analogues. The frequency and degree of myelosuppression are therefore expected to become more important.

It is difficult to evaluate the economic consequences of febrile neutropenia and haemorrhage in cancer patients. Frequently, these patients are hospitalized for other reasons when such complications occur. However it is probable that, compared with a patient who did not develop febrile neutropenia or haemorrhage, the treatment costs will be high because of increased hospitalization, laboratory analyses, radiological tests, treatment such as intravenous infusion, broad-spectrum antibiotics, transfusions, total parenteral nutrition, and intensive care, and nursing or other professional services.[7] In a retrospective analysis, Leese *et al.* determined the cost of one febrile neutropenia episode to be £2068, with hospital costs accounting for 57.8 per cent, drug treatment 25.8 per cent, and diagnostic tests 16.4 per cent.[8]

In this chapter, we will review the preventive and therapeutic aspects of the complications of myelosuppression as well as the risk factors and the mechanisms of susceptibility of this pathological condition. For this purpose, data have been interpreted according to an evidence-based-medicine methodology.

Evidence-based methodology

The evidence-based-medicine methodology has been adapted from the methods reported in the Pulmonary Artery Catheter Consensus Conference[75] and is summarized in Tables 1 and 2. Five levels of evidence have been defined, ranging from large, well-conducted, randomized trials to case reports and expert opinion. Meta-analyses, particularly useful in case of no clear response to multiple non-large randomised trials, are considered as level II evidence. Advice has been graded from A to E according to the level of evidence available in the literature. Some of the best published trials will be cited as references for further reading.

Neutropenia

Potential complications and risk factors

The neutrophil has a key role in host defence. In uninfected patients, the production and elimination of neutrophils are balanced. When infection occurs, chemotactic agents are generated. Neutrophils are released from the bone marrow and migrate into the infected site. The cellular neutrophil defence mechanisms are activated. Infectious agents are destroyed by a complex process including phagocytosis, followed by release of granules into the phagocytic vesicle, resulting in killing of the organism.

The relationship between neutropenia and the risk of severe infections has been established by Bodey *et al.*[9] The risk of developing infectious complications depends on the duration and level of neutropenia. These two variables also predict the severity of the infection. With a neutrophil count above 1000/mm^3, the risk of developing an infection is very low and similar to normal patients. As the number of neutrophils falls below this value, the incidence of infection rapidly increases and becomes a major risk when the neutrophil count is below 100/mm^3. This is of particular importance because infections have been shown to be the main direct cause of death in patients developing febrile neutropenia treated by empirical antibiotherapy.[6]

All patients with neutropenia do not have the same risk of developing complications despite a similar neutrophil count. In a prospective series of cancer patients with febrile neutropenia,[10] serious medical complications such as hypotension, respiratory failure, altered mental status, congestive heart failure, and cardiac arrhythmia occurred in 27 per cent and death in 8 per cent. In this series the factors predicting serious complications were shown to be those reported in a prior, retrospective study.[11] Four prognostic groups could be defined in multivariate analysis: (1) inpatient status; (2) outpatient status with serious concurrent, independent comorbidity; (3) patients with uncontrolled cancer; (4) all other patients. Multiple complications (17 per cent) and death (10 per cent) were common among patients in groups 1 to 3 but did not occur in group 4 patients.

Table 1 Guidelines for the management of the management of the patients with chemotherapy-induced bone marrow failure

	Solid tumours	Haematological malignancies	Bone marrow transplantation
Prevention			
Neutropenia related infection			
Short duration	none	none	none
Long duration			
Bacterial infection	Quinolone or cotrimoxazole + penicillin or macrolide	Quinolone or cotrimoxazole + penicillin or macrolide	Quinolone or cotrimoxazole + penicillin or macrolide
Fungal infection	none	+ fluconazole	+ fluconazole
Viral infection	none	none	+ acyclovir, + ganciclovir if risk of CMV infection
Pneumocystis	none	none	+ cotrimoxazole
G or GM-CSF	To reduce the duration and severity of neutropenia if this is predicted to be of long duration		
Environment	Protective isolation for long-duration neutropenia		
Thrombocytopenia	Platelet transfusions if platelet count <10 000/mm³		
Anaemia	Erythropoietin if platinum-derivative-containing chemotherapy and if economically possible		
Treatment			
Febrile neutropenia	Empirical antibacterial antibiotics		
Initial approach	New β-lactams (+ aminoglycoside if signs of severity)		
Secondary approach	Assess clinical response and infection documentation		
Microbiological documentation	Antimicrobial therapy adaptation		
Fever persistence without documentation	Add: aminoglycoside if severe signs of sepsis vancomycin on day 4 to cover Gram-positive cocci infection amphotericin B on day 7 to cover fungal disease		
Duration of therapy	Assess neutrophils count and fever response: afebrile and >500/mm³: stop afebrile and <500/mm³: stop on day 7 if low risk patient, others continue persistent fever and <500/mm³: continue for 2 weeks and reassess		
Complementary measures	Management in ICU if severe sepsis, septic shock, or other organ failures		
Bleeding due to thrombocytopenia	Platelet transfusion		
Severe anaemia	Red cell transfusion		

In a large series of febrile neutropenic patients with bacteraemic episodes,[12] factors predicting bacteraemia in a logistic regression analysis were found to be: antifungal prophylaxis, duration of granulocytopenia before fever, platelet count, highest fever, shock, and presence and location of initial signs of infection. Shock was associated with Gram-negative bacteraemia and signs of infection at a catheter site were predictive of Gram-positive bacteraemia. In another prospective study[13] 'superinfection', defined as any infection either occurring during antibiotic therapy or developing within 1 week after antibiotic discontinuation, was associated with a crude mortality of 48 per cent. In a multivariate analysis, risk factors for 'superinfection' were: longer duration of profound neutropenia, lack of use of quinolones as prophylaxis, presence of a central venous catheter, and persistence of fever after 3 days of antibiotic therapy.

Neutropenia is frequently associated with other conditions predisposing to infections. Host's defence defects can be associated with the neoplasm or its treatment. Both cellular (T lymphocyte) and humoral (B lymphocyte) immune deficiencies as observed with leukaemia or bone marrow transplantation. Host's defences may be breached by neoplastic obstruction of viscera (respiratory, gastrointestinal, and urinary), by disruption of cutaneous and mucosal barriers, and by invasive procedures and blood product transfusion.[14] The principal pathogens occurring in immunocompromised patients are listed in Table 3.

Clinical features of neutropenia

There are several manifestations of infections that can occur in neutropenic patients—fever, bacteraemia, sepsis, septic shock, multiple organ failure, and adult respiratory distress syndrome, with or without a clinically and/or microbiologically apparent source. Bacteraemia in critically ill patients is associated with a poorer

Table 2 Levels of evidence and grading of advice

Levels of evidence

I	Large, randomized trials with clear-cut results; low risk of false-positive (α) error or false-negative (β) error
II	Small, randomized trials with uncertain results; moderate to high risk of false-positive (α) and/or false-negative (β) error; meta-analyses
III	Non-randomized, contemporaneous controls
IV	Non-randomized, historical controls
V	Case series, uncontrolled studies, and expert opinion

Grading of advice

A	Supported by at least two level I investigations without contradictory data from other studies of level I evidence
B	Supported by only one level I investigation
C	Supported by level II investigations only
D	Supported by at least one level III investigation
E	Supported by level IV or level V evidence

Table 3 Host defence defects and associated pathogens (reprinted from Ref. 14 with permission)

Defect	Bacteria	Fungi	Viruses	Parasites
Neutropenia	Gram-negative bacilli *Ps. aeruginosa* *E. coli* *Klebsiella pneumoniae* *Enterobacter* spp. Gram-positive cocci *Staph. aureus* *Staph. epidermidis* *Streptococcus* spp. *Corynebacterium* spp.	*Candida* spp. *Torulopsis glabrata* *Aspergillus* spp. Mucoraceae		
Cellular immune deficiency	*Listeria monocytogenes* *Mycobacterium* spp. *Nocardia asteroides* *Legionella pneumophila*	*Candida* spp. *Cryptococcus neoformans*	Herpes simplex Varicella zoster Cytomegalovirus Epstein–Barr virus	*Pneumocystis carinii* *Toxoplasma gondii* *Cryptosporidium* *Strongyloides stercoralis*
Humoral immune deficiency	*Streptococcus pneumoniae* *Haemophilus influenzae* Staphylococci Streptococci			
Visceral neoplastic obstruction	Colonizing bacteria	*Candida* spp. *Aspergillus* spp.		
Disruption of barriers	Staphylococci Streptococci *Ps. aeruginosa* Gram-negative enteric bacilli	*Candida* spp.	Herpes simplex	
Invasive procedures	Staphylococci *Corynebacterium* spp. Gram-negative bacilli	*Candida* spp.		
Blood product transfusion			Hepatitis B, C, and other Cytomegalovirus AIDS	

prognosis when occurring in patients with comorbidities such as active malignancy.[15] Sepsis is a poor prognostic factor in patients presenting with haematological malignancies.[14] Despite the important place of neutrophil in the pathogenesis of adult respiratory distress syndrome and multiple organ failure, these complications may occur in profoundly granulocytopenic patients, suggesting that other cells such as macrophages, platelets, clotting factors, kinins, or cytokines (interleukin-1 or tumour necrosis factor-α) could play a role.[14] None of these manifestations is specifically associated with a particular pathogen. Sepsis or septic shock can occur in the presence of bacteria (Gram positive and negative), as well as of fungal pathogens and, although rare, *Pneumocystis carinii* infections.

During the last three decades, the epidemiology of bacterial infections has changed. Initially, more than 80 per cent of documented bacteraemias were due to Gram-negative organisms, with enterobacteria and *Pseudomonas aeruginosa* representing the commonest pathogens incriminated in bacteraemia or major infections.[16] Nowadays, Gram-positive bacteria are increasing in frequency and are documented in around 50 per cent of the microbiologically-documented febrile neutropenic episodes (Table 3). *Streptococcus viridans*, *Staphylococcus aureus*, and coagulase-negative staphylococci are the most frequent pathogens. This may be due to an increased use of invasive procedures and permanent, tunnelled, subcutaneous catheters, to the administration of chemotherapeutic regimens which frequently disrupt mucosal barriers favouring bacterial invasion, and to the prescription of quinolones for prophylactic purposes.[14] It is possible, as suggested in an empirical antibiotherapy trial,[17] that the course of staphylococcal infections, without clinically obvious manifestations, can be more indolent than Gram-negative bacterial ones.

Many micro-organisms can be the source of respiratory failure in granulocytopenic patients. Pneumonia can be due to bacteria, Gram-negative as well as positive, fungal pathogens such as *Aspergillus*, virus, and *Pneumocystis carinii*.

Pneumonia due to *Pneumocystis carinii* is generally associated with a cellular immunodeficiency as observed with bone marrow transplant or steroid therapy. It is rarely documented in solid tumour patients not undergoing transplantation. Patients present with fever, dry cough, and progressive respiratory failure with hypoxia and hypocapnia, although more aggressive courses have been described. Diffuse interstitial perihilar infiltrates are the principal, although not specific, radiological characteristics of this infection (Figs 1 and 2). In some cases, chest radiographs can be normal. Nodules, cavitations, and pneumothorax have been described. Untreated, the mortality is greater than 50 per cent. Treatment consists of the administration of high doses of cotrimoxazole. Aerosolized or intravenous pentamidine is one of the therapeutic alternatives.

Viral infections occur frequently during some periods of the year, such as winter for influenza or spring and autumn for respiratory syncytial virus (RSV). Prodromal symptoms are generally non-specific with fever, cough, or rhinorrhea for the most commonest pathogens such as influenza, parainfluenza 1, 2, and 3, some herpesvirus such as HHV-6, adenovirus, and RSV. Thereafter, infection can disseminate to the lungs and induce diffuse bilateral pneumonitis with a poor prognosis despite intensive treatment. Epidemics due to RSV have been reported in transplantation centres. Antiviral treatments are now available such as acyclovir, ganciclovir, and foscavir for *herpes*

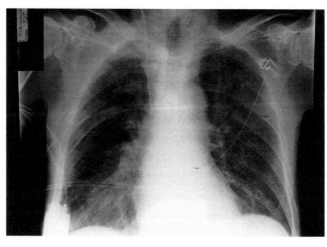

Fig. 1 Chest radiograph of a patient with pulmonary *Pneumocystis carinii* infection showing bilateral, diffuse lung interstitial infiltrates.

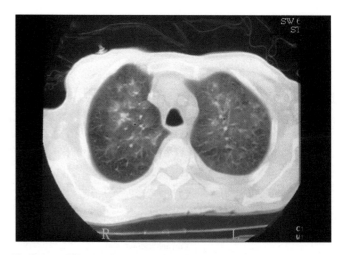

Fig. 2 Lung CT scan of a patient with pulmonary *Pneumocystis carinii* infection showing diffuse interstitial and alveolar infiltrates.

viridae, vidarabine, zanamivir, and amantadine for influenza, and ribavirine for RSV.

Cytomegalovirus (CMV) is a serious cause of pulmonary infections following allogeneic bone marrow transplants. Infection is diagnosed by the isolation of CMV from a clinical site, principally blood, urine, and throat. CMV disease is defined by the concomitant documentation of an infection and clinical manifestations. Unlike HIV patients, CMV disease in allogeneic transplanted patients occurs almost exclusively in the lungs. When CMV pneumonia is established the prognosis is poor and the risk of death is as high as 90 per cent. Treatment involves the use of ganciclovir or foscavir and the administration of immune globulins.

Herpes infections (HSV-1 and 2) are generally characterized by reactivation of mucositis (oral or genital). In immunocompromised patients, varicella can be manifested by a generalized infection associated with a particular poor prognosis.

Fungal infections are predominantly due to *Candida* spp. and *Aspergillus* spp., although new pathogens have been described recently such as *Fusarium* spp., *Penicillium* spp., *Mucormycoses*, and others. Manifestations are extremely various: fungaemia, pneumonia, cutaneous infection, cystitis and pyelonephritis, and catheter infections. Fungal pneumonia is frequently due to *Aspergillus* spp. The diagnosis of this infection is difficult and is the reason why amphotericin B is frequently added to empirical antibiotherapy in neutropenic patients with fever. Clinical signs of aspergillus pneumonia can be scanty—fever, cough, progressive respiratory failure, and chest pain are the most prominent. Haemoptysis, which can be life-threatening, is a major complication. Although treatment is available the prognosis of this infection is poor and with death in up to 80 per cent of cases. Other localizations of aspergillus infection have been described such as sinuses and brain. Treatment is with amphotericin B. In order to reduce the side-effects observed with this drug, new liposomal formulations have been developed but their exact role remains to be defined. New agents, such as intravenous itraconazole and voriconazole, are currently being investigated. Surgery can be performed in some subgroups of patients presenting with a very high risk of haemorrhage.[18]

Candida infections are principally associated with fungaemia and pneumonia. Others sources of infection, such as catheter devices or urinary tract, are also observed. The particularity of candida infections is the emergence of non-albicans strains, such as *Candida krusei*, *C. glabrata*, and *C. parapsilosis*, with different susceptibilities to fluconazole, itraconazole, and amphotericin B.

Granulocytopenic patients can develop acute abdominal pain. The most frequent cause, which is often a diagnosis of exclusion, is neutropenic enterocolitis. This condition includes a wide spectrum of complications from transient bowel oedema to frank infarction of tissue. The syndrome variously consists of fever, watery diarrhoea, and diffuse or localized abdominal pain. In most cases, medical treatment will be initiated with bowel rest, gastrointestinal decompression, broad-spectrum antibiotics, and nutritional support. Close observation is mandatory. Surgery will be indicated in case of perforation, abscess, pneumatosis intestinalis, massive bleeding, obstruction, or persisting sepsis. Prognosis is influenced by the duration of neutropenia and overall mortality can range between 8 and 60 per cent.[14]

The diagnosis of an infection in a granulocytopenic patient can be difficult. Around one-third of neutropenic fevers will be microbiologically documented, another third will be clinically diagnosed. The remaining third, including non-infectious causes of fever (transfusion, tumoural lysis syndrome), will not be firmly diagnosed. Sample collection and culture are the same in immunocompetent and compromised patients, but in granulocytopenic patients with fever there is a need to multiply the number and the sites of samplings. In neutropenic fever, blood cultures (at least two samples from different sites), urine, throat, and rectal samples must be cultured. Other sampling must be adapted to the clinical situation, such as skin biopsies or bronchoalveolar lavage.

Management of neutropenic fever will imply prevention and rapid treatment. In the presence of grave signs such as renal failure or low blood pressure, admission to an intensive care unit is needed. In the literature there are only case reports and series and retrospective studies on the role of critical care for the cancer patient with bone marrow failure complications including sepsis.[19] The published data

show a benefice in favour of the use of life support techniques in these situations. The use of inotropic and ventilation supports and early treatment of hypotension and oliguric renal failure is similar to immunocompetent patients, taking into account the isolation procedures and the coagulation disorders and thrombocytopenia frequently observed in myelosuppressed patients.

Prevention

Prophylactic antibiotherapy (Table 4)

Antibacterial therapy

Many randomized trials have assessed the prevention of bacterial infections by oral antibiotic administration in neutropenic patients. The majority of these trials were double-blind, placebo-controlled but few included a large number of patients. Antibacterial prevention consisted of non-absorbable antibiotics (such as gentamicin and vancomycin), trimethoprim–sulfamethoxazole (cotrimoxazole), or quinolones. These were found effective, mainly in term of reduction of occurrence of infection and bacteraemia, but not for the prevention of fever or for overall mortality. Table 4 summarizes the levels of evidence. Large, randomized trials are available only for the evaluation of trimethoprim–sulfamethoxazole.[20],[21] Meta-analyses have been performed on the trials testing oral quinolones.[22],[23] In a meta-analysis of 18 trials including 1408 patients, quinolones have been shown to significantly reduce the relative risks of Gram-negative bacterial infections to 0.21, of microbiologically documented infections to 0.65, and of total infections to 0.54.[23]

The different oral antibacterial antibiotic policies have been compared in multiple randomized trials, often of a small size. Cotrimoxazole and quinolones appeared to have similar effects in term of overall occurrence of febrile neutropenia, infections, or bacteraemia or of mortality.[24] However, cotrimoxazole tended to offer a better protection against Gram-positive infections while quinolones provided a better prevention of Gram-negative complications. Many small randomized studies have shown that both policies have a better preventive effect than oral non-absorbable antibiotics.

The addition of an oral, systemic antibiotic against Gram-positive cocci has been shown to offer a selective protection against streptococcal and other Gram-positive infections, without reducing the overall infectious complication rate and without decreasing overall mortality. Two large randomized trials have established this effect for the macrolide roxithromycin[25] and for oral penicillin V.[26]

The problem created by antibiotic prophylaxis is the development of resistance and the occurrence of Gram-negative bacteria resistant to quinolones or cotrimoxazole. Moreover, with the used fluoroquinolones, more streptococcal infections have been documented. The potential benefit of antibiotic prophylaxis can thus be counterbalanced by the emergence of resistant pathogens. New trials, comparing placebo to prophylaxis, using new antibiotics with improved Gram-positive and negative spectra, need to be performed in order to determine the exact role of this approach.

Antifungal therapy

Various antifungal agents have been investigated by multiple controlled studies in the neutropenic patient, particularly in situations with prolonged leucopenia, as in acute leukaemia or after bone marrow transplantation. The two agents for which the most consistent data are available are amphotericin B and fluconazole (Table 4).

Table 4 Level of evidence of effectiveness of prophylactic antibiotherapy

Prophylactic policy	Grade (see Table 2)	Recommendation
Oral antibacterial antibiotics versus none		
non-absorbable antibiotics	C	beneficial
trimethoprim–sulfamethoxazole (cotrimoxazole)	A	beneficial
quinolones	C	beneficial
Comparison of oral antibacterial antibiotics		
cotrimoxazole versus quinolones	B	equivalent
cotrimoxazole versus non-absorbable antibiotics	C	first better
quinolones versus non-absorbable antibiotics	C	first better
Oral antibiotics against Gram-positive coccal infections		
penicillin V versus none	B	beneficial
macrolide versus none	B	beneficial
Antifungal antibiotics versus none		
(a) superficial fungal infections		
intravenous amphotericin B	C	no benefit
fluconazole	A	beneficial
(b) systemic fungal infections		
intravenous amphotericin B	C	probably beneficial
fluconazole	C	probably beneficial
Antiviral drugs		
(a) against herpes simplex		
acyclovir	C	beneficial
ganciclovir	C	possibly beneficial
(b) against herpes zoster		
acyclovir	C	possibly beneficial
ganciclovir	C	no benefit
(c) against cytomegalovirus		
acyclovir	C	no benefit
ganciclovir	C	beneficial
Cotrimoxazole prevention of *Pneumocystis carinii* infection	B	beneficial

Amphotericin B, when systemically administered, is probably effective in preventing systemic fungal infection.[27] Fluconazole, an orally absorbable triazole agent, has been definitively demonstrated to prevent superficial mycotic infections in large randomized trials[28]–[30] but its impact on the prevention of systemic infection is much less evident. None of these approaches had a significant impact on mortality. The number of trials comparing the various antifungal agents is too small to allow unequivocal conclusions. Taking the data from randomized trials, antifungal prophylaxis could be recommended to patients with a high risk of fungal infection, such as those with haematological malignancies or treated by bone marrow transplantation who will have a long period of myelosuppression. For solid tumours, no firm guideline can be recommended and, except for clinical trials, fungal prophylaxis should not be routinely administered. The type of prophylaxis must be adapted to the ecology of the hospital, to the type of fungi found in the surveillance culture, and to the capacity of the patients to take the medications by the oral route.

Antiviral therapy

Acyclovir and ganciclovir have been assessed in bone marrow transplantation patients for the prevention of viral infections due to herpes simplex, herpes zoster, and cytomegalovirus. As summarized in Table 4, acyclovir is mainly effective against herpes simplex virus while ganciclovir is able to prevent cytomegalovirus infections but with non-negligible renal and haematological toxicity. Their impact on mortality is doubtful, possibly due to the relatively small size of the controlled trials. Only preventive administration of acyclovir can be recommended in patients treated with allogeneic bone marrow transplantation to prevent CMV reactivation. Oral ganciclovir is poorly absorbed and its efficacy has not been proven. In these patients, regular samples (one or two times per week) of blood, throat, and urine must be taken and cultured for CMV. If a culture becomes positive, even in the absence of clinical manifestations of infection, treatment with intravenous ganciclovir (5 mg/kg twice per day for 14–21 days) or, in case of resistance or intolerance, with foscavir (60 mg/kg three times per day for 14–21 days) must be administered. This approach has led to a reduction in the incidence of established CMV disease. No prophylaxis is recommended for solid tumours and haematological malignancies not treated by allogeneic bone marrow transplantation.

Anti-Pneumocystis carinii therapy

Prophylactic administration of oral cotrimoxazole has been shown to prevent *Pneumocystis carinii* pneumonitis, mainly in patients with acute lymphoblastic leukaemia.[31] It can be administered at a dose

Table 5 Prevention of infection by haematological growth factors in the neutropenic patient

Question	GM-CSF		G-CSF	
	Grade of advice	Recommendation	Grade of advice	Recommendation
Solid tumours				
duration of neutropenia	B	reduction	A	reduction
level of neutropenia	B	reduction	A	reduction
febrile neutropenia rate	B	no reduction	B	reduction
infection incidence	B	no reduction	B	no reduction
treatment mortality	B	no reduction	B	no reduction
overall toxicity	B	unchanged	B	unchanged
overall survival	B	unchanged	B	unchanged
Lymphoma				
duration of neutropenia	B	reduction	B	reduction
nadir of neutropenia	B	reduction	A	reduction
febrile neutropenia rate	B	no reduction	A	no reduction
infection incidence	C	possibly yes	B	possible reduction
overall toxicity	B	increased	A	increased
overall survival	B	unchanged	A	unchanged
Leukaemia				
leukaemia regrowth stimulation	A	no	A	no
duration and severity of neutropenia	A	reduction	A	reduction
febrile neutropenia rate	C	no reduction	B	no reduction
infection incidence	B	no reduction	B	no reduction
overall toxicity	B	increased	B	increased
overall survival	B	unchanged	B	unchanged
Bone marrow transplantation				
duration of neutropenia	A	reduction	B	reduction
febrile neutropenia rate	C	no reduction	B	no reduction
infection incidence	C	no reduction	C	no reduction
immediate mortality	C	unchanged	C	unchanged
overall survival	C	unchanged	C	unchanged
overall toxicity	C	worse	C	unchanged

of 160 mg trimethoprim/ 800 mg sulfamethoxazole, once per day, three times a week. In case of contraindications, it can potentially be replaced by aerosolized pentamidine or dapsone in bone marrow transplantation patients.

Haematological growth factors (Table 5)

Granulocyte-macrophage (GM-CSF) and granulocyte (G-CSF) colony-stimulating factors are haematological growth factors implicated in the physiological production of granulocytes. Both have been produced by genetic engineering and assessed in clinical trials for their ability to protect against myelosuppression induced by chemotherapy. The interpretation of the results of the published trials is difficult because their designs are somewhat different. The trial objectives have been to prevent febrile neutropenia, to shorten the duration of the neutropenic episode, to allow greater dose intensity of chemotherapy, or to decrease mortality.

G-CSF

Recombinant human G-CSF has been derived from the bacterium *Escherichia coli* (r metHu G-CSF or filgrastim) and from Chinese hamster ovary cells (rHuG-CSF or lenograstim). Dose-finding studies have established that the optimal dosage is 2 or 5 µg/kg subcutaneously,

a higher dosage does not improve the degree or duration of neutropenia and its consequences.

Solid tumours In the first randomized study performed in patients with small-cell lung cancer treated by chemotherapy and published in 1991 by Crawford et al.,[32] a significant reduction of neutropenia, duration of neutropenia, need for antibiotics, days of hospitalization, and incidence of infections was observed in the group treated with G-CSF. These results were only partially confirmed in subsequent studies. A criticism is the particularly high incidence of febrile neutropenia in the placebo group due to the myelosuppressive chemotherapy compared to the incidence observed in general practice. This may have lead to an overestimate of the efficacy of G-CSF in the treatment of solid tumours. According to the published literature, including a meta-analysis of randomized trials in small-cell lung carcinoma, G-CSF has been shown to reduce the duration and the level of the neutropenia, as well as the risk of developing febrile neutropenia,[33] in patients receiving chemotherapy. G-CSF can probably enhance the relative dose intensity of chemotherapy. However, it does not change the incidence of infection, the mortality, or the overall survival. It is well tolerated. Slight bone pain, easily manageable, occurs frequently.

Lymphoma The effect of G-CSF in patients with lymphoma treated by chemotherapy is similar to that observed for solid tumours, except that some trials have shown a reduction in the number and severity of documented infections.[34] Toxicity is increased by the occurrence of bone pain but this side-effect is mild. It should be noted that in all trials G-CSF has been shown to improve the dose intensity of the chemotherapy.

Acute leukaemia G-CSF has been investigated in various types of leukaemia (mainly acute myeloid and lymphoblastic) and has been shown to be safe by multiple, controlled, randomized trials in patients with remission of the disease.[35] No blastic stimulation was observed in these randomized studies. As in solid tumours, it reduces the duration and the severity of neutropenia, without clear impact on the overall occurrence of infections and survival. The absence of effect on the incidence of infection may be due to the long duration of neutropenia. It may be partly counterbalanced by a possible reduction in the duration of febrile neutropenic episodes. This is subject to caution, because these significant reductions were not found in all the trials and, when significant, they were not the primary objective and had only an exploratory value. The augmentation of dose intensity is not reflected in the response rate nor survival, disease-free survival, or mortality in the majority of the publications.

Bone marrow transplantation Multiple, usually relatively small, randomized trials have been published on the effect of G-CSF in patients undergoing bone marrow transplantation (mainly autologous). The drug has been shown to reduce the duration of neutropenia and the duration of hospitalization.[36] It is well tolerated but has no significant effect on infection incidence or survival.

GM-CSF

Recombinant human GM-CSF has been derived from the yeast *Saccharomyces cerevisiae* (sargramostim) or from the bacterium *Escherichia coli* (molgramostim). GM-CSF has been shown to enhance the proliferation of granulocyte and macrophage precursors, resulting in an increase in functionally mature granulocytes and macrophages. Many controlled trials have tried to determine its effectiveness in the prevention of chemotherapy-induced neutropenia and its infectious complications. Dosages varied between 5 and 10 µg/kg per day or 250 µg/m² subcutaneously. The principal side-effects consisted of flu-like symptoms (fever, myalgias, and chills), rash, bone pain, hypersensitivity reaction, and fluid retention. An acute respiratory failure can occur at the first dose. In some trials, GM-CSF has been associated with increased thrombocytopenia. A possible causal relationship has been suggested between GM-CSF and the development of pleuritis, pericarditis, cardiac arrhythmia, hypotension, confusion, anorexia, fatigue, and gastrointestinal discomfort.

Solid tumours GM-CSF has been shown, in almost all trials, to reduce the nadir and the duration of the neutropenia. However, it had no significant effect on the occurrence of febrile neutropenia and infections. Mortality related to chemotherapy was not reduced and overall tolerance to chemotherapy not improved.[37] Moreover, toxicity in the GM-CSF arms was frequently statistically significantly enhanced. This was due to local reactions at the injection site rather than haematological complications such as thrombocytopenia or non-haematological side-effects such as anorexia, degradation of the general status, oedema, thromboembolism, fever, pain, skin rash, and gastrointestinal disturbances.[38] Toxic deaths, attributable or not to the administration of the cytokine, were also more frequently observed.[38] The number of adequate trials is still limited, and more studies with good methodology and a large number of patients are needed to give definitive recommendations. At this time, preventive administration of GM-CSF in solid tumours is not recommended except in clinical trials.

Lymphoma One large trial has shown a reduction in the duration and severity of chemotherapy-induced neutropenia in non-Hodgkin lymphoma, with a marginal effect in favour of a reduction in infection occurrence but without overall survival improvement, despite an improvement in complete response rate in the high-risk subgroup.[39] The chemotherapy was COP-BLAM (cyclophosphamide, doxorubicin, bleomycin, vincristine, procarbazine, prednisolone) and the number of assessable patients was 172. Other randomized trials, including a lower number of patients presenting either with Hodgkin and/or non-Hodgkin lymphomas were performed using a CHOP (cyclophosphamide, Adriamycin, vincristine, prednisolone) chemotherapy programme or autologous bone marrow transplantation. Similar effects on duration and severity of induced neutropenia were found. No firm conclusion can be drawn from these very small trials on survival, occurrence of fever, or infection. Toxicity was generally significantly higher in the GM-CSF arms. GM-CSF cannot be recommended for routine prophylaxis in lymphomas.

Acute myelogenous leukaemia GM-CSF does not stimulate the regrowth of leukaemia.[40] When administered after chemotherapy it reduces the duration and severity of neutropenia. There is no clear effect on the occurrence of fever and infection and no improvement in overall survival. Overall toxicity is increased by the side-effects of GM-CSF (rash, thrombocytopenia, fluid retention).

Bone marrow transplantation Many controlled trials have assessed the role of GM-CSF in patients with a haematological malignancy and undergoing cytoreductive conditioning regimens followed by allogeneic or autologous bone marrow transplantation or transplantation of peripheral blood stem cells. The drug has been shown to be clearly effective[23] in reducing the duration of neutropenia and thus the length of hospitalization. No consistent effect on infectious complications or mortality has been observed. Among 14 randomized trials in which information on infectious complications is available, only two have demonstrated a reduction in infections in the GM-CSF arm.[41],[42] In three trials[41]–[43] a reduction in bacterial infection was noted in subgroup analyses. There were some explanations for the absence of an impact of GM-CSF on survival and mortality. It could have been due to the duration and severity of neutropenia which, despite their reduction by GM-CSF, remained long and severe, persistently predisposing patients to infections. Secondly, engrafted patients might die from their malignant disease or other complications such as haemorrhage despite intensive supportive therapy. Further, the number of patients included in these trials was low and may be too low to detect a significant survival difference between the treatment arms. In some studies, there was an increased toxicity due to GM-CSF with a capillary leak syndrome, rash, and perhaps organ dysfunction.

CSF comparisons

Data comparing GM-CSF and G-CSF are limited. A randomized trial failed to show clinically significant difference between sargramostim and filgrastim in a series of cancer patients undergoing chemotherapy.[44]

Table 6 Effect of protective isolation

Endpoint	Answer	Grade (see Table 2)
Febrile neutropenia occurrence	Decreased	C
Documented infection occurrence	Decreased	C
Immediate mortality	Decreased	C
Tumour response to chemotherapy	Unchanged	C
Overall survival	Unchanged	C

In conclusion, the routine use of G-CSF and GM-CSF, out of clinical trials, is not recommended for solid tumours for which the expected duration of neutropenia is short. The use of these factors can be considered when neutropenia will have a long duration or when it will be necessary to maintain or enhance dose intensity of the chemotherapy. In these cases, the benefit of the growth factors must be compared to the potential risk of reactivation of the disease (acute leukaemia), the side-effects, and the costs of the treatment.

Isolation (Table 6)

Protective isolation can be carried out by placing patient in a single room or a laminar-airflow room. In the 1970s many small, controlled trials assessed this procedure for patients with haematological malignancies. They showed a reduction in the occurrence of febrile neutropenia and documented infections and probably in the immediate mortality. Although most did not show long-term benefits, the largest study[45] suggested a benefit for the isolation procedure, with increased leukaemia response and improved overall survival.

Hospitalized patients with profound ($<100/mm^3$) and prolonged neutropenia should be settled in isolation rooms. No firm guideline, based on the literature review, can be given on the type of isolation. Mask, gowns, and gloves are recommended although their use has not been extensively studied. Regular hand washing, before and after each visit, is mandatory. For patients with less profound neutropenia or those who are ambulatory, no precise guideline can be drawn from the literature.

Infectious complications

Empirical antibiotherapy for febrile neutropenia

Empirical antibiotherapy was introduced in the 1960s for the management of febrile neutropenia. This therapeutic policy was shown to be effective in comparison with the administration of antibiotics only when there was documented infection and isolation of the pathogen. The bacteria targeted by the treatment are the aerobic Gram-negative bacilli, particularly *Escherichia coli*, *Klebsiella pneumoniae*, and *Pseudomonas aeruginosa*. The last is the most difficult to control and is the main cause of death due to Gram-negative bacilli. The choice of the drugs has thus been influenced according to activity against *Pseudomonas*, with the introduction of combinations comprising an anti-*Pseudomonas* β-lactam (such as carbenicillin or ticarcillin) and an aminoglycoside (such as gentamicin or more recently amikacin).[46]

Multiple controlled and uncontrolled trials of variable quality, over the last three decades, have investigated the best antibiotic regimen for febrile neutropenia. The main questions that have been, or are still are being addressed with reference to drugs in current use are: Should an aminoglycoside be added to the β-lactam? Should a glycopeptide be added to the basic β-lactam regimen? Is a monotherapy with a single antibacterial antibiotic sufficient? What is the best β-lactam to administer? Can quinolones be used? Is empirical antifungal therapy justified? Which antifungal agent should be chosen for that indication? Table 7 summarizes the main answers to these questions, the topic having been the subject of recent evidence-based medicine guidelines.[47]

Antibacterial antibiotics

The role of the aminoglycoside in the antibacterial combination has been investigated in multiple trials but, due to the study design or to methodological problems, the question cannot be answered with a high grade of certainty. Their theoretical advantages are a better protection against infection by Gram-negative bacteria (particularly *Pseudomonas aeruginosa*), a synergistic effect against these pathogens, and a reduction in the development of resistance. The addition of aminoglycosides adds to toxicity. An aminoglycoside-based therapy has not been shown to improve the results, in terms of infection control or mortality, when the drug is added or compared to, regimens containing a third or fourth generation cephalosporin or a so-called anti-*Pseudomonas* penicillin such as piperacillin-tazobactam, imipenem, or meropenem.[48],[49] When used, aminoglycosides can be safely prescribed with a once-per-day schedule[50] and a short course (3 days) is as effective as a long course, except in cases of Gram-negative bacteraemia.[51] They have to be avoided if other potentially nephrotoxic drugs, such as cisplatin or cyclosporin, are administered. If they are not part of the initial treatment, it is recommended to add them on an empirical basis if there is a clinical deterioration with signs of sepsis.

The incidence of Gram-positive cocci infections, including *Staphylococcus sp.* and *Streptococcus sp.*, has increased in neutropenic patients. This observation has lead to the addition of antibiotics to which these pathogens are usually sensitive. The glycopeptides, vancomycin and teicoplanin, fulfil this criterion. A series of randomized trials have investigated this therapeutic strategy without demonstrating a positive impact on overall mortality or mortality due to infection. There is, however, an improvement in the response rate of fever, and perhaps clinically documented infections, but toxicity is significantly increased.[17] These infections appear to be adequately treated if antibiotherapy is subsequently adapted according to the results of microbiological tests or if the glycopeptides are added after a few days of non-responding fever. There seemed to be no major difference between the two available drugs, vancomycin and teicoplanin, according to a large randomized study.[52]

A monotherapy empirical regimen with a new β-lactam has been compared to combined regimens containing a β-lactam and/or an aminoglycoside and/or a glycopeptide. Results have been equivalent if the new β-lactam is a third or fourth generation cephalosporin[48] such as ceftazidime, ceftriaxone, or cefepime, or a penicillin or penem such as imipenem/cilastatin, meropenem, or piperacillin/tazobactam.[49],[53] Toxicity may be decreased by monotherapy, depending on the drugs used in combination therapy.

The best monotherapy regimen has been investigated in controlled trials comparing penems and last generation cephalosporins.[54],[55] Drugs mainly examined were imipenem, meropenem, and ceftazidime.

Table 7 Effect of empirical antibiotherapy in the treatment of febrile neutropenia: recommendations supported by grade A to C advice

Assessed treatment	Control treatment	Control of infection			Effect on mortality		Toxicity
		Fever	Clinically documented	Microbiologically documented	Overall mortality	Mortality directly due to infection	
Antibacterial antibiotics							
aminoglycosides + new β-lactam(s)	new β-lactams	= (C)	= (C)	= (C)	= (C)	= (C)	increased (B)
glycopeptides + new β-lactams	new β-lactams	improved (B)	= (C)	= (C)	= (A)	= (A)	increased (A)
monotherapy (new β-lactams)	combinations	= (C)	= (C)	= (C)	= (C)	= (C)	decreased (B)
new penems or penicillins	3rd/ 4th generation cephalosporins	= (B)	= (B)	= (B)	= (B)	= (B)	increased (C)
quinolones	β-lactams + aminoglycoside	worse (C)	= (C)	worse (C)	= (C)	= (C)	= (C)
Antifungal antibiotics							
amphotericin B	no amphotericin	= (C)		improved (C)	= (C)	decreased (C)	increased (C)
fluconazole	amphotericin B	= (C)		= (C)	= (C)	= (C)	decreased (C)

= is equivalent; grade of advice in parentheses.

There was no major difference, imipenem was sometimes reported as more active but also more toxic, without significant effect on mortality.

The β-lactams have also been compared within a given combination. Randomized trials have been conducted assessing different cephalosporins (ceftriaxone or cefepime versus ceftazidime) or a penicillin (such as ticarcillin or piperacillin) versus a cephalosporin (ceftazidime or cefoperazone). Results showed no significant difference between any of these drugs.[50],[56]

The quinolones, such as norfloxacin, ofloxacin, and ciprofloxacin, have also been assessed in monotherapy and in combination therapy. These antibiotics appeared to be less effective than the more classical ones, with significantly lower response rates.[57]

The duration of the antimicrobial therapy has been studied in prospective but uncontrolled trials, suggesting that intravenous antibiotics can be stopped if the infection is controlled and the fever has disappeared, even if the neutrophils have not recovered. In case of fever of unknown origin, prospective randomized trials have shown that for subgroups of patients, antibiotics can be stopped after 3 or 7 days if the fever has resolved (level of evidence: C). This has still to be definitively assessed by appropriate randomized trials. The 1997 guidelines of the Infectious Diseases Society of America[47] proposed that if the patient is afebrile within 3 days of treatment, the treatment should be stopped on day 7, except in high-risk patients whose absolute neutrophil count remains below 500/mm³ on day 7.

Finally, a few trials have evaluated the management of the febrile neutropenic patient on an ambulatory basis. This approach seems to be feasible but will require further large, well-conducted randomized trials before it is considered to be a safe practice.

Antifungal agents

The role of empirical antifungal therapy has been the subject of much less investigation than empirical antibacterial therapy in febrile neutropenic patients. Various drugs have been assessed in this situation: amphotericin B (Fungizone®), various lipid soluble formulations of amphotericin B (including Ambisome®), fluconazole, and ketoconazole. The topic has been the subject of a meta-analysis.[58] There seemed to be no survival benefit for antifungal agents given empirically to patients with cancer complicated by febrile neutropenia. However, when administered empirically to neutropenic patients with a fever not responding to antibacterial antibiotics, amphotericin B has been shown able to reduce significantly mortality due to fungal infection.[59] The published studies, however, are small and require confirmation by adequate randomized trials. It should be noted that the toxicity is increased, particularly when Fungizone® is used.

Empirical antifungal treatments have been compared. Fluconazole seemed to give similar results to amphotericin B, with a decreased toxicity.[60] It should, however, be pointed out that fluconazole offers no protection against *Aspergillus* sp. and should thus be avoided in centres where this pathogen is a frequent cause of infection and in patients who have a past history of aspergillosis. Ambisome® seemed to offer advantages in term of efficacy and toxicity in comparison to Fungizone® in a randomized study requiring further confirmation.[61]

Other therapies (Table 8) for febrile neutropenia

Haematological growth factors

G-CSF[62] and GM-CSF[63] have been assessed in randomized trials in patients with established febrile neutropenia when given in addition

Table 8 Role of therapies other than antibiotics in the management of the patient with febrile neutropenia receiving empirical antimicrobial treatment

Treatment modality	Neutropenia duration	Fever control	Infection control	Effect on mortality	Toxicity
G-CSF administration	decreased (A)	increased (C)	= (C)	= (A)	= (A)
GM-CSF administration	decreased (B)	= (B)	= (C)	= (B)	= (C)
Leucocytes transfusion			increased (C)	decreased (C)	
Intravenous immune globulin	= (C)	increased (C)	= (C)	= (C)	
Management of severe complications in ICU				decreased (E)	

= is equivalent; ICU: intensive care unit: grade of advice in parentheses.

to empirical antibiotherapy. This policy has resulted in a significant reduction of neutropenia duration and, for G-CSF, in a better control of fever. However, control of infection and mortality were not improved. Toxicity was not increased by the administration of the growth factors. Guidelines of the Infectious Diseases Society of America[47] and of the American Society of Clinical Oncology[64] do not recommend the routine use of CSFs in the febrile neutropenic patient.

Leucocytes transfusions

Leucocytes transfusions were the subject of multiple randomized trials in the 1970s. A recent meta-analysis has reviewed these results for the prevention of infection in the neutropenic patient.[65] There was a significant reduction in the risk of infection, mortality, and death due to infection in transfused patients. Granulocyte transfusions were also shown to be effective in cases of Gram-negative bacteraemia in the neutropenic patient,[66] with a significantly improved survival. This policy merits new investigation, particularly with the recent development in haematological technology and with the availability of haematological growth factors. Obviously, there is a correlation between neutrophil recovery and cure of infection. In some instances, there is a need to have a large number of leucocytes appear rapidly at the infection site. This cannot be achieved by growth factors which will take, at least, some days to enhance the neutrophil count. Because of the risks of granulocyte transfusions (graft-versus-host disease, anaphylactic or immunological reactions, infection), their place in the treatment of febrile neutropenia remains to be defined.

Immune globulin administration

Immune globulin administration has been extensively investigated in the bone marrow transplantation patient for the prevention of cytomegalovirus (CMV) infection and interstitial pneumonitis and was shown to be effective in both CMV-negative and CMV-positive transplant recipients.[67] The number of trials in febrile neutropenia is very limited. A small randomized study[68] assessed their role in children in addition to antibiotics in febrile neutropenia and showed no benefit. It can be recommended that, in allogeneic bone marrow transplant patients, immune globulin is administered in addition to antiviral prophylaxis. For patients without globulin deficiency, new trials are needed to define the place of such an approach.

Thrombocytopenia

Potential complications and risk

Severe, potentially lethal, bleeding is a frequent problem in oncology, especially in patients with leukaemia or treated by chemotherapy. In a retrospective analysis of 438 patients with acute leukaemia,[69] bleeding occurred on admission in 38 per cent of the patients and during the first month in 11 per cent. Twenty-six fatal haemorrhages were documented, mainly intracranial, followed in frequency by the gastrointestinal tract. Thrombocytopenia is, in these patients, the main cause predisposing to bleeding. The risk is considered as clinically significant if the platelet count is below 50 000/mm³ but can occur at higher levels in cases of associated thrombocytopathy or coagulopathy, such as disseminated intravascular coagulation or toxic effect of drugs on platelets.

Bleeding prevention (Table 9)

Platelet transfusions

In case of severe thrombocytopenia, two policies are possible: 'wait and see' and prophylactic platelet transfusions. In the first, platelets are only transfused if bleeding occurs. In the second, the objective is to maintain the platelet count above a threshold associated with a low risk of spontaneous haemorrhages. Randomized trials conducted in the 1970s have shown the superiority of the prophylactic transfusion policy.[70] The time to first bleeding episode is significantly longer and the number of bleeding episodes significantly reduced. The threshold below which platelets have to be transfused has also been the subject of randomized trials[71] and a level of 10 000 platelets/mm³ has been shown as safe as 20 000/mm³, with the advantage of requiring significantly fewer platelet transfusions in the absence of fever or infection, in the absence of bleeding, and when invasive procedures were not planned.

Multiple platelet transfusions can result in alloimmunization with the risk that the patient becomes refractory to transfusions. This risk can be minimized by application of the threshold of 10 000 platelets per mm³ for transfusion, the use of single donors, and removal of leucocytes prior to transfusion. It is particularly high in cases of bone marrow transplantation. In the bone marrow transplantation patient,

Table 9 The role of transfusions and growth factors in the management of thrombocytopenia and anaemia

	Response	Grade of advice
Thrombocytopenia		
Bleeding prevention:		
platelet transfusion if platelet count <10 000/mm³	bleeding reduction	A
thrombopoietin administration	unknown	E
Bleeding treatment:		
platelet transfusion	bleeding control	A
Anaemia		
Prevention: erythropoietin administration	reduced need for transfusion	C
Treatment: red cell transfusions	correction	A

platelets will have to be irradiated (to avoid possible graft-versus-host disease transmitted by leucocytes present in the transfusion) and deleucocytized in CMV-negative bone marrow transplantation recipients (to avoid cytomegalovirus transmission).

Thrombopoietin

Thrombopoietin is the growth factor of megakaryocytes. It has been produced for clinical administration by recombinant technology. The first feasibility trials have shown that its administration to patients is safe and stimulates platelet production.[72] Further adequate, randomized trials are necessary to determine its effectiveness in the management of chemotherapy-induced thrombocytopenia.

Bleeding treatment (Table 9)

The treatment of bleeding due to chemotherapy-induced thrombocytopenia is the transfusion of platelets accompanied by the transfusion of red cells, and the correction of associated causes such as infection and risk factors such as duodenal ulcer. Platelets should be given as rapidly as possible, according to the same rule as for preventive administration. The volume of transfusion will depend on the severity of the bleeding and on the platelet count that will be obtained. In practice, one standardized platelet concentrate (= 1 unit) will contain around 0.5×10^{11} platelets and one pack obtained by apheresis 2 to 8×10^{11} platelets. Advantages of apheresis are the reduction in the risk of alloimmunization and infection and the possible resolution of unsuccessful transfusion in alloimmunized patients. Leucocytes should be removed and, according to the particular situation of the patient, the sample tested for CMV, irradiated (reducing the risk of post-transfusional graft-versus-host disease), and tested for HLA compatibility or plasma removed in case of plasma allergy or IgA deficiency. The prescription is 1 unit/10 kg (or 5 kg in cases of major bleeding) with respect of the ABO rules. Transfusion is considered as unsuccessful if less than 30 per cent of the platelets are found in the circulation after 1 h or 20 per cent the day following the transfusion. The potential complications of platelets transfusion are anti-HLA and antierythrocyte immunization, graft-versus-host disease, red cell haemolytic reactions, and infectious transmissions.

Anaemia

Potential complications and risks

Severe anaemia may result in complications such as cardiac failure, acute pulmonary haemodynamic oedema, angina pectoris, myocardial infarction, mental confusion, cerebrovascular accidents, cardiovascular collapse, and peripheral circulatory insufficiency. The risk is higher when the anaemia is more acute. It is thus very important that the haemoglobin level does not fall below a threshold, usually fixed at 8 g/dl. Two policies are possible: prophylactic administration of erythropoietin to avoid reaching this threshold or transfusion of red cells when the threshold is reached or if the patient presents with related symptoms.

Prevention: erythropoietin (Table 9)

Erythropoietin is the growth factor for the red cell precursors and has been produced for clinical purposes by recombinant technology. Randomized trials have shown its effectiveness in reducing the need for red cell transfusion in patients treated by platinum derivatives[73] but there is an economic problem because the drug is much more expensive than transfusions.[74] Potential advantages of erythropoietin are ambulatory management and absence of complication. Disadvantages are necessity of repeated drug injections, slow action, and failure in some patients.

Treatment: red cell transfusions (Table 9)

Transfusion is the only available and effective treatment for anaemia. It is less expensive than erythropoietin administration but it has the inconveniences of requiring hospital admission and is associated with the potential complications of transfusion reactions or transmission infection such as viruses (HIV, hepatitis B, C, G, for example). In order to decrease the risk of infection, especially in patients requiring multiple transfusions, removal of leucocytes must be part of the routine of red blood cell administration. Transfusions reactions must be prevented by close compatibility between donors and receivers. A search for particular alloimmunization must be made in cases of unsuccessful transfusion.

References

1. Houten L, Reilley AA. An investigation of the cause of death from cancer. *Journal of Surgical Oncology*, 1980; **13**: 111–6.

2. Klastersky J, Daneau D, Verhest A. Causes of death in patients with cancer. *European Journal of Cancer*, 1972; **8**: 149–54.

3. Ostrow S, Diggs CH, Sutherland J, Wiernik PH. Causes of death in patients with non-Hodgkin's lymphoma. *Cancer*, 1981; **48**: 779–82.

4. Kefford RF, Cooney NJ, Woods RL, Fox RM, Tattersall MHN. Causes of death in an oncology unit. *European Journal of Cancer and Clinical Oncology*, 1981; **17**: 1117–24.

5. Klastersky J, Weerts D, Gompel C. Causes of death in acute non-lymphocytic leukemia. *European Journal of Cancer*, 1975; **11** (Suppl.): 21–7.

6. Sculier JP, Weerts D, Klastersky J. Cause of death in febrile granulocytopenic cancer patients receiving empiric antibiotic therapy. *European Journal of Cancer and Clinical Oncology*, 1984; **20**: 55–60.

7. Goa KL, Bryson HM. Recombinant granulocyte-macrophage colony-stimulating factor (rGM-CSF). An appraisal of its pharmacoeconomic status in neutropenia associated with chemotherapy and autologous bone marrow transplant. *Pharmacoeconomics*, 1994; **5**: 56–77.

8. Leese B, Collin R, Clark DJ. The costs of treating febrile neutropenia in patients with malignant blood disorders. *Pharmacoeconomics*, 1994; **6**: 233–9.

9. Bodey GP, Buckley MB, Freireich EJ. Quantitative relationships between circulating leukocytes and infection in patients with acute leukemia. *Annals of Internal Medicine*, 1966; **64**: 328–40.

10. Talcott JA, Siegel RD, Finberg R, Goldman L. Risk assessment in cancer patients with fever and neutropenia: a prospective, two-center validation of a prediction rule. *Journal of Clinical Oncology*, 1992; **10**: 316–22.

11. Talcott JA, Finberg R, Mayer RJ, Goldman L. The medical course of cancer patients with fever and neutropenia. *Archives of Internal Medicine*, 1988; **148**: 2561–8.

12. Viscoli C, *et al.* Factors associated with bacteraemia in febrile, granulocytopenic cancer patients. *European Journal of Cancer*, 1994; **30A**: 430–7.

13. Nucci M, *et al.* Risk factors and attributable mortality associated with superinfections in neutropenic patients with cancer. *Clinical Infectious Diseases*, 1997; **24**: 575–9.

14. Sculier JP. Indications for intensive care in the management of infections in cancer patients. In: Klastersky J, ed. *Infectious complications of cancer*. Norwell, MA: Kluwer Academic Publishers, 1995: 233–44.

15. Pitter D, Thiévent B, Wenzel RP, *et al.* Importance of pre-existing comorbidities for prognosis of septicemia in critically ill patients. *Intensive Care Medicine*, 1993; **19**: 265–72.

16. Klastersky J. Treatment of neutropenic infection: trends towards monotherapy. *Support Care Cancer*, 1997; **5**: 365–70.

17. European Organization for Research and Treatment of Cancer (EORTC) International Antimicrobial Therapy Cooperative Group and the National Cancer Institute of Canada-Clinical Trials Group. Vancomycin added to empirical combination antibiotic therapy for fever in granulocytopenic cancer patients. *Journal of Infectious Diseases*, 1991; **163**: 951–8.

18. Bernard A, Caillot D, Casasnovas O, *et al.* Intérêt de la chirurgie dans le traitement de l'aspergillose pulmonaire invasive chez les patients neutropéniques. *Revue des Maladies Respiratoires*, 1998; **15**: 49–55.

19. Brunet F, *et al.* Is intensive care justified for patients with haematological malignancies? *Intensive Care Medicine*, 1990; **16**: 291–7.

20. EORTC International Antimicrobial Therapy Project Group. Trimethoprim-sulfamethoxazole in the prevention of infection in neutropenic patients. *Journal of Infectious Diseases*, 1984; **150**: 372–9.

21. Pizzo PA, Robichaud KJ, Edwards BK, Schumaker C, Kramer BS, Johnson A. Oral antibiotic prophylaxis in patients with cancer: a double-blind randomized placebo-controlled trial. *Journal of Pediatrics*, 1983; **102**: 125–33.

22. Cruciani M, *et al.* Prophylaxis with fluoroquinolones for bacterial infections in neutropenic patients: a meta-analysis. *Clinical Infectious Diseases*, 1996; **23**: 795–805.

23. Engels EA, Lau J, Barza M. Efficacy of quinolone prophylaxis in neutropenic cancer patients: a meta-analysis. *Journal of Clinical Oncology*, 1998; **16**: 1179–87.

24. Donnelly JP, Maschmeyer G, Daenen S, on behalf of the EORTC-Gnotobiotic Project Group. Selective oral antimicrobial prophylaxis for the prevention of infection in acute leukaemia—ciprofloxacin versus co-trimoxazole plus colistin. *European Journal of Cancer*, 1992; **28A**: 873–8.

25. Kern WV, Hay B, Kern P, Marre R, Arnold R. A randomized trial of roxithromycin with acute leukemia and bone marrow transplant recipients receiving fluoroquinolone prophylaxis. *Antimicrobial Agents and Chemotherapy*, 1994; **38**: 465–72.

26. International Antimicrobial Therapy Cooperative Group of the European Organization for Research and Treatment of Cancer. Reduction of fever and streptococcal bacteremia in granulocytopenic patients with cancer. *Journal of the American Medical Association*, 1994; **272**: 1183–9.

27. Perfect JR, *et al.* Prophylactic intravenous amphotericin B in neutropenic autologous bone marrow transplant recipient. *Journal of Infectious Diseases*, 1992; **165**: 891–7.

28. Goodman JL, *et al.* A controlled trial of fluconazole to prevent fungal infections in patients undergoing bone marrow transplantation. *New England Journal of Medicine*, 1992; **326**: 845–51.

29. Winston DJ, *et al.* Fluconazole prophylaxis of fungal infections in patients with acute leukemia. *Annals of Internal Medicine*, 1993; **118**: 495–503.

30. Slavin MA, *et al.* Efficacy and safety of fluconazole prophylaxis for fungal infections after marrow transplantation—a prospective, randomized, double-blind study. *Journal of Infectious Diseases*, 1995; **171**:1545–52.

31. Hughes WT, *et al.* Successful chemoprophylaxis for Pneumocystis carinii pneumonitis. *New England Journal of Medicine*, 1977; **297**: 1419–26.

32. Crawford J, Ozer H, Stoller R, *et al.* Reduction by granulocyte colony-stimulating factor of fever and neutropenia induced by chemotherapy in patients with small-cell lung cancer. *New England Journal of Medicine*, 1991; **325**: 164–70.

33. Messori A, Trippoli S, Tendi E. G-CSF for the prophylaxis of neutropenic fever in patients with small cell lung cancer receiving myelosuppressive antineoplastic chemotherapy: meta-analysis and pharmacoeconomic evaluation. *Journal of Clinical Pharmacy and Therapeutics*, 1996; **21**: 57–63.

34. Gisselbrecht C, *et al.* Placebo-controlled phase III study of lenograstim (glycosylated recombinant human granulocyte colony-stimulating factor) in aggressive non-Hodgkin's lymphoma: factors influencing chemotherapy administration. *Leukemia and Lymphoma*, 1987; **25**: 289–300.

35. Heil G, *et al.* A randomized, double-blind, placebo-controlled, phase III study of filgrastim in remission induction and consolidation therapy for adults with de novo acute myeloid leukemia. *Blood*, 1997; **90**: 4710–18.

36. Gisselbrecht C, *et al.* Placebo-controlled phase III trial of lenograstim in bone-marrow transplantation. *Lancet*, 1994; **343**: 696–700.

37. Steward WP, *et al.* Effects of granulocyte-macrophage colony-stimulating factor and dose intensification of V-ICE chemotherapy in small-cell lung cancer: a prospective randomized study of 300 patients. *Journal of Clinical Oncology*, 1998; **16**: 642–50.

38. Bunn PA, Crowley J, Kelly K, *et al.* Chemoradiotherapy with or without granulocyte-macrophage colony stimulating factor in the treatment of limited-stage small-cell lung cancer: a prospective phase III randomized study of the Southwest Oncology Group. *Journal of Clinical Oncology*, 1995; **13**: 1632–41.

39. Gerhartz HH, *et al.* Randomized, double-blind placebo-controlled, phase III study of recombinant human granulocyte-macrophage colony-stimulating factor as adjunct to induction treatment of high-grade malignant non-Hodgkin's lymphomas. *Blood*, 1993; **82**: 2329–39.

40. Stone RM, *et al.* Granulocyte-macrophage colony-stimulating factor after initial chemotherapy for elderly patients with primary acute myelogenous leukemia. *New England Journal of Medicine*, 1995; **332**: 1671–7.

41. Nemunaitis J, *et al.* Phase III randomized, double-blind placebo-controlled trial of rhGM-CSF following allogeneic bone marrow transplantation. *Bone Marrow Transplantation*, 1995; **15**: 949–54.

42. Nemunaitis J, Rabinowe SN, Singer JW, *et al.* Recombinant granulocyte-macrophage colony-stimulating factor after autologous bone marrow transplantation for lymphoid cancer. *New England Journal of Medicine*, 1991; **324**: 1773–8.

43. Advani R, Chao NJ, Horning SJ, *et al.* Granulocyte-macrophage colony-stimulating factor (GM-CSF) as an adjunct to autologous hemopoietic stem cell transplantation for lymphoma. *Annals of Internal Medicine*, 1992; **116**: 183–91.

44. Beveridge RA, *et al.* Randomized trial comparing the tolerability of sargramostin (yeast-derived RhuGM-CSF) and filgrastim (bacteria-derived RhuG-CSF) in cancer patients receiving myelosuppressive chemotherapy. *Support Care Cancer*, 1997; **5**: 289–98.

45. Rodriguez V, *et al.* Randomized trial of protected environment—prophylactic antibiotics in 145 adults with acute leukemia. *Medicine*, 1978; **57**: 253–66.

46. Schimpff S, Satterlee W, Youg VM, Serpick A. Empiric therapy with carbenicillin and gentamicin for febrile patients with cancer and granulocytopenia. *New England Journal of Medicine*, 1971; **284**: 1061–5.

47. Hughes WT, *et al.* 1997 guidelines for the use of antimicrobial agents in neutropenic patients with unexplained fever. *Clinical Infectious Diseases*, 1997; **25**: 551–73.

48. De Pauw BE, Deresinski SC, Feld R, Lane-Allman EF, Donnelly JP for the Intercontinental Antimicrobial Study Group. Ceftazidime compared with piperacillin and tobramycin for the empiric treatment of fever in neutropenic patients with cancer. A multicenter randomized trial. *Annals of Internal Medicine*, 1994; **120**: 834–44.

49. Cometta A, *et al.* Monotherapy with meropenem versus combination therapy with ceftazidime plus amikacin as empiric therapy for fever in granulocytopenic patients with cancer. *Antimicrobial Agents and Chemotherapy*, 1996; **40**: 1108–15.

50. The International Antimicrobial Therapy Cooperative Group of the European Organization for Research and Treatment of Cancer. Efficacy and toxicity of single daily doses of amikacin and ceftriaxone versus multiple daily doses of amikacin and ceftazidime for infection in patients with cancer and granulocytopenia. *Annals of Internal Medicine*, 1993; **119**: 584–93.

51. The EORTC International Antimicrobial Therapy Cooperative Group. Ceftazidime combined with a short or a long course of amikacin for empirical therapy of gram-negative bacteremia in cancer patients with granulocytopenia. *New England Journal of Medicine*, 1987; **317**: 1692–8.

52. Menichetti F, *et al.* Effects of teicoplanin and those of vancomycin in initial empirical antibiotic regimen for febrile, neutropenic patients with hematologic malignancies. *Antimicrobial Agents and Chemotherapy*, 1994; **38**: 2041–6.

53. Deany NB, Tate H. A meta-analysis of clinical studies of imipenem-cilastatin for empirically treating febrile neutropenic patients. *Journal of Antimicrobial Chemotherapy*, 1996; **37**: 975–86.

54. The Meropenem Study Group of Leuven, London and Nijmegen. Equivalent efficacies of meropenem and ceftazidime as empirical monotherapy of febrile neutropenic patients. *Journal of Antimicrobial Chemotherapy*, 1995; **36**: 185–200.

55. Freifeld AG, *et al.* Monotherapy for fever and neutropenia in cancer patients: a randomized comparison of ceftazidime versus imipenem. *Journal of Clinical Oncology*, 1995; **13**: 165–76.

56. Cometta A, *et al.* Piperacillin-tazobactam plus amikacin versus ceftazidime plus amikacin as empiric therapy for fever in granulocytopenic patients with cancer. *Antimicrobial Agents and Chemotherapy*, 1995; **39**: 445–52.

57. Meunier F, *et al.* Prospective randomized evaluation of ciprofloxacin versus piperacillin plus amikacin for empiric antibiotic therapy of febrile granulocytopenic cancer patients with lymphomas and solid tumors. *Antimicrobial Agents and Chemotherapy*, 1991; **35**: 873–8.

58. Gotzsche PC, Johansen HK. Meta-analysis of prophylactic or empirical antifungal treatment versus placebo or no treatment in patients with cancer complicated by neutropenia. *British Medical Journal*, 1997; **314**: 1238–44.

59. EORTC International Antimicrobial Therapy Cooperative Group. Empiric antifungal therapy in febrile granulocytopenic patients. *American Journal of Medicine*, 1989; **86**: 668–72.

60. Viscoli C, *et al.* Fluconazole versus amphotericin B as empirical antifungal therapy of unexplained fever in granulocytopenic cancer patients: a pragmatic, multicentre, prospective and randomised clinical trial. *European Journal of Cancer*, 1996; **32A**: 814–20.

61. Prentice HG, *et al.* A randomized comparison of liposomal versus conventional amphotericin B for the treatment of pyrexia of unknown origin in neutropenic patients. *British Journal of Haematology*, 1997; **98**: 711–8.

62. Maher DW, *et al.* Filgrastim in patients with chemotherapy-induced febrile neutropenia. A double-blind, placebo-controlled trial. *Annals of Internal Medicine*, 1994; **121**: 492–501.

63. Vellengo E, *et al.* Randomized placebo-controlled trial of granulocyte-macrophage colony-stimulating factor in patients with chemotherapy-related febrile neutropenia. *Journal of Clinical Oncology*, 1996; **14**: 619–27.

64. American Society of Clinical Oncology. Recommendations for the use of hematopoietic colony-stimulating factors: evidence-based, clinical practice guidelines. *Journal of Clinical Oncology*, 1994; **12**: 2471–508.

65. Vamvakas EC, Pineda AA. Determinants of the efficacy of prophylactic granulocyte transfusions: a meta-analysis. *Journal of Clinical Apheresis*, 1997; **12**: 74–81.

66. Herzig RH, Herzig GP, Graw RJ Jr, Bull MI, Ray KK. Successful granulocyte transfusion therapy for gram-negative septicemia. A prospective randomized controlled study. *New England Journal of Medicine*, 1977; **296**: 701–5.

67. Bass EB. Efficacy of immune globulin in preventing complications of bone marrow transplantation: a meta-analysis. *Bone Marrow Transplantation*, 1993; **12**: 273–82.

68. Sumer T, Abumelha A, Al-Mulhim I, Al-Fadil M. Treatment of fever and neutropenia with antibiotics versus antibiotics plus intravenous gammaglobulin in childhood leukemia. *European Journal of Pediatrics*, 1989; **148**: 401–2.

69. Törnebohm E, Lockner D, Paul C. A retrospective analysis of bleeding complications in 438 patients with acute leukaemia during the years 1972–1991. *European Journal of Haematology*, 1993; **50**: 160–7.

70. Murphy S, *et al.* Indications for platelet transfusion in children with acute leukemia. *American Journal of Hematology*, 1982; **12**: 347–56.

71. Rebulla P, *et al.* The threshold for prophylactic platelet transfusions in adults with acute myeloid leukemia. *New England Journal of Medicine*, 1997; **337**: 1870–5.

72. Basser RL. Thrombopoietic effects of pegylated recombinant human megakaryocyte growth and development factor (PEG-rHuMGDF) in patients with advanced cancer. *Lancet*, 1996; **348**: 1279–81.

73. **Spaëth D, Marchal C, Blanc-Vincent MP.** Standards, options et recommandations pour l'utilisation de l'érythropoïétine en cancérologie. *Bulletin du Cancer,* 1998; **85**: 337–46.

74. **Sheffield R, Sullivan SD, Saltiel E, Nishimura L.** Cost comparison of recombinant human erythropoietin and blood transfusion in cancer chemotherapy-induced anemia. *Annals of Pharmacotherapy,* 1997; **31**: 15–22.

75. **Pulmonary Artery Catheter Consensus Conference Participants.** Pulmonary artery catheter consensus conference: consensus statement. *Critical Care Medicine,* 1997; **25**: 910–25.

Nausea, vomiting, and antiemetics

Maurizio Tonato and Fausto Roila

Introduction

Nausea and vomiting are generally considered the most distressing side-effects of cancer chemotherapy. Good control of these symptoms is therefore a very important endpoint in cancer medicine and contributes to a substantial improvement in the quality of life of patients with cancer. Emesis is a complex phenomenon characterized by three components: vomiting, nausea, and retching, which are often, but not always, interrelated. Three types of chemotherapy-induced emesis can be identified: (i) acute emesis, which occurs soon after chemotherapy administration; (ii) delayed emesis, which has arbitrarily been defined as emesis beginning 24 h after chemotherapy administration that can persist for 6 to 7 days; and (iii) anticipatory emesis, which can occur before a subsequent course of chemotherapy. Although these are arbitrary distinctions, the three types of emesis are probably distinct phenomena and give rise to different therapeutic problems.

The incidence and severity of nausea and vomiting in patients receiving chemotherapy vary depending on the type of chemotherapy and patient's characteristics such as sex, age, previous experience of chemotherapy, alcohol intake, experience of emesis during pregnancy, and motion sickness. The emetogenic potential of various chemotherapeutic agents differs and a classification of different risk categories is useful, though difficult to define because it is based on criteria that are not always objective.

Despite these limitations, a four-level classification has recently been agreed (Table 1).[1] In the last few years, much progress has been made in antiemetic therapy, mainly due to a better understanding of the mechanisms of nausea and vomiting induced by chemotherapy and to the introduction of new, more active drugs. In this chapter the results of this progress in terms of standardization of optimal therapy in different clinical settings are outlined. For each clinical problem the level of consensus recently expressed by the subcommittee for antiemetics of the Multinational Association of Supportive Care in Cancer (**MASCC**) during the Perugia Conference (April 28–29, 1997) is also reported.[1]

Pathophysiology and neuropharmacology of chemotherapy-induced emesis

Emetic pathways (Fig. 1)

Chemotherapy-induced emesis is a multifactorial and complex phenomenon. Different pathways and a variety of receptors are involved in the mechanisms by which chemotherapeutic agents cause nausea and vomiting, so no single antiemetic agent is effective in every kind of emesis.

Our current knowledge of the emetic phenomena has evolved from studies on animal models showing that two distinct centres in the brain are involved in the control of emesis. The first, known as the chemoreceptor trigger zone, is in the area postrema situated in a circumventricular structure at the caudal end of the fourth ventricle and accessible to humoral stimuli from blood or cerebrospinal fluid. The other, known as the vomiting centre, is in the nucleus tractus solitarius, which is the main integrative nucleus for visceral and some somatic functions receiving inputs from abdominal vagal afferents. It is subjacent to the area postrema and responsible for the control and co-ordination of the mechanisms involved in emesis. Interaction between the chemoreceptor trigger zone and chemotherapy involves the release of various neurotransmitters that activate the vomiting centre. The chemoreceptor trigger zone cannot initiate emesis independently but only through stimulation of the vomiting centre. In addition to the chemoreceptor trigger zone, three other sources of afferent input to the vomiting centre have been identified: the vestibular system, the pharynx, and cortical structures. The vestibular apparatus of the middle ear appears to play a part primarily in motion sickness and does not seem to be important for chemotherapy-induced nausea and vomiting. The afferent input from the pharynx and gastrointestinal tract travels to the vomiting centre and to the chemoreceptor trigger zone along the vagus nerve or via sympathetic pathways stimulated by products of small intestine cell damage. Electrical stimulation of the cerebral cortex, hypothalamus, and thalamus can also evoke emesis and these areas appear to have important roles in anticipatory emesis.[2]

Neuropharmacology of emesis

Various neuroreceptors have been identified in or around the area postrema and in the gastrointestinal tract, including dopamine, serotonin, histamine, noradrenaline, apomorphine, neurotensin, substance P, angiotensin II, vasoactive intestinal polypeptide, gastrin, vasopressin, thyrotrophin-releasing hormone, and leucine-encephalin. By blocking dopamine D_2 receptors which are abundant in the area postrema the emetic response can be abolished, but there is little evidence of a role for peripheral D_2 receptors in the process of emesis. The precise role of histamine H_1 and muscarinic cholinergic receptors identified in the nucleus tractus solitarii in chemotherapy-induced emesis is unclear although antagonists of histamine and acetylcholine can abolish emesis associated with motion sickness.

Table 1 Approximate emetogenic potential of single chemotherapy agents*

Degree of emetogenicity	Agent
High	Cisplatin ≥ 50 mg/m^2
	Mechlorethamine
	Streptozocin
	Cyclophosphamide >1500 mg/m^2
	Carmustine >250 mg/m^2
	Dacarbazine
Moderate to high	Cisplatin <50 mg/m^2
	Cytarabine >1 g/m^2
	Carboplatin
	Ifosfamide
	Carmustine ≤ 250 mg/m^2
	Hexamethylmelamine (oral)
	Cyclophosphamide ≤ 1500 mg/m^2
	Anthracyclines
	Topotecan
	Irinotecan
	Procarbazine (oral)
	Methotrexate >250 mg/m^2
	Cyclophosphamide (oral)
	Mitoxantrone
Low to moderate	Taxoids
	Etoposide
	Methotrexate >50 mg/m^2 <250 mg/m^2
	Mitomycin
	Gemcitabine
	Fluorouracil <1000 mg/m^2
Low	Bleomycin
	Busulfan
	Chlorambucil (oral)
	2-Chlorodeoxyadenosine
	Fludarabine
	Hydroxyurea
	Methotrexate ≤ 50 mg/m^2
	L-phenylalanine mustard (oral)
	6-Thioguanine (oral)
	Vinblastine
	Vincristine
	Vinorelbine

*With kind permission from Kluwer Academic Publishers.[1]

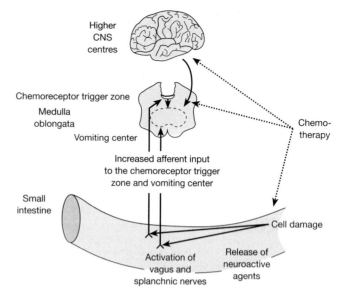

Fig. 1 Proposed pathways of chemotherapy-induced emesis. Chemotherapeutic drugs may induce emesis through cell damage in the gastrointestinal tract, direct action on medullary centres (the vomiting centre and the chemoreceptor trigger zone), or learned (cortical) responses. CNS, central nervous system. (Adapted from Grunberg and Hesketh. Control of chemotherapy-induced emesis. *New England Journal of Medicine*, 1993; **329**: 1790–6.)

Chemotherapy may cause release of serotonin from the enterochromaffin cells in the upper gastrointestinal mucosa. The released serotonin stimulates emesis via both the vagal 5-HT$_3$ receptors and the greater splanchnic nerve which then signal to the vomiting centre, as well as by directly activating 5-HT receptors stimulating centrally the area postrema.[3]

In experimental studies in animals some antiemetic drugs such as sulpiride or domperidone, which are potent antagonists of dopamine (D$_2$) receptors, have been shown to be ineffective in the prevention of cisplatin-induced nausea and vomiting, while selective 5-HT$_3$ receptor antagonist induced a high rate of complete protection from vomiting. The 5-HT$_3$ receptor antagonist is considered to exert its action by interrupting the vomiting reflex in two ways: by blocking the stimulus reaching the vomiting centre via the vagal nerve and by reducing the detection and integration of incoming information in the vomiting centre. The poor efficacy of 5-HT$_3$ receptor antagonists in man in the delayed phase does not exclude a role for 5-HT, acting on some other receptor, in this phase of the response. This form of emesis may also be due to direct bowel inflammation. Finally, it is also possible that the antineoplastic agents act on different sites and stimulate different receptors so that a combination of antiemetic agents may produce better results than single drugs.

Prevention of emesis due to highly emetogenic drugs

This category is mainly represented by cisplatin (Table 1) which, when used at doses greater than 50 mg/m^2, induces nausea and

It seems that no one neurotransmitter is responsible for every kind of chemotherapy-induced nausea and vomiting, but 5-hydroxy-tryptamine (5-HT) receptors are particularly important in the pathophysiology of acute vomiting whereas others may be important in the pathophysiology of nausea and delayed emesis. 5-HT receptors have been classified into three main types with evidence of subtypes in some of them. One of these, the type 3 (5-HT3) receptor, appears to have a determinant role in the process of emesis. Eighty per cent of the body content of serotonin is contained on vagal afferent neurones and in other neurones in the gastrointestinal tract and it has also been identified in the area postrema, in the nucleus tractus solitarii, and presynaptically on vagal afferent terminals in the medulla.

vomiting in almost 100 per cent of patients. Vomiting usually begins 2 to 3 h after its administration, reaches its maximal intensity after 5 to 6 h, and thereafter appears only sporadically. However, delayed emesis, beginning 24 h after chemotherapy, is an additional problem in 20 to 85 per cent of patients treated with this drug.

The schedule of cisplatin administration is also important. Lengthening the duration of its infusion from 1 to 8 h results in a significant decrease in vomiting episodes and when the drug is administered in divided doses during consecutive days a tolerance to the emetic effect is observed. In fact, nausea and vomiting may peak during the first 2 days of chemotherapy but then gradually decrease until they disappear on days 4 or 5.

Acute emesis

Before the introduction of the 5-HT₃ receptor antagonists, an intravenous combination of high-dose metoclopramide plus dexamethasone and diphenhydramine or lorazepam was the most efficacious anti-emetic prophylaxis for cisplatin-induced acute emesis, with complete protection from vomiting being obtained by about 60 per cent of patients.[3]

With the use of intravenously administered 5-HT₃ receptor antagonists (ondansetron, granisetron, tropisetron, and dolasetron), complete protection from cisplatin-induced acute emesis can be achieved in 40 to 60 per cent of patients.[4]

Several large randomized clinical trials have shown that the combination of a 5-HT₃ receptor antagonist with dexamethasone significantly increases the antiemetic activity, with complete protection from acute vomiting being reported by 70 to 90 per cent of patients.[5]

To identify the best antiemetic regimen for the prevention of cisplatin-induced acute emesis, two large, double-blind, randomized studies have compared a 5-HT₃ receptor antagonist plus dexamethasone with a combination of high-dose metoclopramide plus dexamethasone and diphenhydramine or lorazepam.[6],[7] The rate of complete protection from vomiting and nausea was significantly greater with ondansetron plus dexamethasone with respect to the metoclopramide combination in both studies. The tolerability was better with ondansetron plus dexamethasone. Furthermore, with the metoclopramide combination, complete protection from vomiting significantly decreased from the first to the third cycle of chemotherapy, while there was no such decrease in protection with ondansetron plus dexamethasone, although protection from nausea also decreased significantly with this regimen.[8]

The combination of a 5-HT₃ receptor antagonist plus dexamethasone should therefore be considered the antiemetic of choice for the prevention of cisplatin-induced acute emesis.

Preliminary data also suggest that the addition of a dopamine antagonist (metopimazine) to a 5-HT₃ receptor antagonist increases the antiemetic efficacy with respect to the 5-HT₃ antagonist used alone.[9] These findings should therefore be further explored in randomized clinical trials evaluating the possible increase of antiemetic efficacy where metopimazine is added to standard therapy.

Despite the existence of some pharmacological differences among 5-HT₃ antagonists,[10] their efficacy and tolerability has been found similar in several double-blind comparative trials.[11] The choice is therefore influenced largely by the acquisition cost, although this parameter can be difficult to calculate. Despite the fact that the optimal dose, schedule, and route of administration of the 5-HT₃

Table 2 Dosage and schedule of 5-HT₃ antagonists in cisplatin-induced emesis*

Agent	Daily dose	Schedule	Route
Ondansetron	8 mg	Single dose	Intravenous
	24 mg	Single dose	Oral
Granisetron	10 µg/kg	Single dose	Intravenous
	2 mg	Single dose	Oral
Tropisetron	5 mg	Single dose	Intravenous
Dolasetron	1.8 mg/kg	Single dose	Intravenous
	200 mg	Single dose	Intravenous

*With kind permission from Kluwer Academic Publishers.[1]

antagonists have been evaluated in several trials,[12] contradictory data have been obtained and there is an even wider variability in the 'approved' single intravenous dose.

For example, in the United States the approved dose of ondansetron is 32 mg or approximately 0.45 mg/kg, that is, four times higher than the dose of the same antiemetic generally used in Europe (8 mg). For granisetron, the generally used dose in the United States is 1 mg or 10 µg/kg while in Europe the dose currently used is 3 mg or 40 µg/kg. The Perugia Conference reached a consensus on the doses of 5-HT₃ receptor antagonists and the results of such agreement are reported in Table 2.

Preliminary data also suggest that the oral route is equivalent to intravenous administration. In two large double-blind studies, oral granisetron (2 mg) achieved results similar to intravenous ondansetron (32 mg)[13] and oral ondansetron (24 mg) to intravenous ondansetron (8 mg).[14] Furthermore, good results were shown in a pilot study using an oral combination of dolasetron and dexamethasone.[15] The optimal dose of dexamethasone was not identified, but it has recently been demonstrated, in a double-blind randomized trial, that 20 mg intravenously was superior to 4, 8, or 12 mg given intravenously.[16]

Delayed emesis

Nausea and vomiting occurring in patients more than 24 h after cisplatin administration has been defined as delayed emesis. The incidence varies from 20 to 93 per cent of patients in different studies, and the intensity is maximal on days 2 and 3 after chemotherapy.[4]

A double-blind trial[17] has shown that the combination of orally administered metoclopramide plus dexamethasone has better antiemetic activity with respect to dexamethasone alone or placebo and these results have subsequently been confirmed by another study.[18] However, despite treatment with the above-mentioned combination of drugs, 45 to 50 per cent of cisplatin-treated patients still suffer from delayed emesis.[19] The optimal dose and schedule of dexamethasone and metoclopramide has not been identified. In both studies a dose of 0.5 mg/kg of metoclopramide administered four times a day was used. However, a study evaluating the optimal dosage of metoclopramide for prevention of cisplatin-induced delayed emesis showed that 20 mg of metoclopramide given four times a day for 7 days is the maximum tolerated dose without the concomitant use of diphenhydramine.[20]

Table 3 Antiemetic treatments of choice in different clinical situations*

Problems	Treatment of choice
Single high dose of cisplatin (≥ 50 mg/m^2)	
Acute emesis	5-HT$_3$ antagonist + dexamethasone
Delayed emesis	Dexamethasone + metoclopramide, or a 5-HT$_3$ antagonist
Single dose of carboplatin, doxorubicin, epirubicin, or cyclophosphamide	
Acute emesis	5-HT$_3$ antagonist + dexamethasone
Delayed emesis	Dexamethasone or 5-HT antagonist, or 5-HT$_3$ antagonist + dexamethasone

*With kind permission from Kluwer Academic Publishers.[1]

The role of 5-HT$_3$ receptor antagonists in the prevention of cisplatin-induced delayed emesis has been evaluated in a number of trials, but only two of them were methodologically sound and provided reliable, albeit controversial, results. Ondansetron was shown in one study to give approximately 35 per cent complete protection from delayed vomiting, which was not much different from the 25 per cent achieved by placebo,[21] whereas, in the other study, the combination of granisetron plus dexamethasone was shown to be of similar efficacy to dexamethasone alone.[22] Recently, a study comparing the activity of ondansetron against metoclopramide, both combined with dexamethasone in the prevention of cisplatin-induced delayed emesis, has shown that the two treatments offer similar protection from delayed emesis, although ondansetron plus dexamethasone may be preferred in patients who suffer from acute vomiting. This study also showed that optimal control of acute emesis is essential to achieve good protection from delayed nausea and vomiting, irrespective of the antiemetic treatment received.[23]

To date, the most effective regimen to prevent cisplatin-induced delayed emesis has been shown to be the combination of dexamethasone with either metoclopramide or a 5-HT$_3$ receptor antagonist, beginning their administration 24 h after chemotherapy and for a minimum of 72 h (Table 3). The level of consensus expressed by the experts of the Perugia Conference on this topic and concerning the above-mentioned combination therapy was considered high.[1]

Prevention of emesis induced by moderately highly emetogenic chemotherapy

This category of drugs is mainly represented by intravenous cyclophosphamide, doxorubicin, epirubicin, and carboplatin used alone or in some combination (Table 1).

The pattern of emesis after their administration is characteristic. Cyclophosphamide induces a late onset of emesis (about 10 to 12 h after its administration). When cyclophosphamide is combined with doxorubicin, the time to onset of vomiting is shorter (6 to 8 h). Carboplatin induces a pattern of emesis similar to that of cyclophosphamide (emesis begins about 6 to 7 h after its administration).

Acute emesis

Corticosteroids such as dexamethasone (8 mg intravenously before chemotherapy, plus 4 mg orally repeated every 6 h for four doses) or methylprednisolone (40 to 125 mg intravenously or intramuscularly starting before chemotherapy and continuing every 6 h for three doses) give complete protection from vomiting in about 60 to 80 per cent of patients. Contrasting results have been shown in studies which have compared the efficacy of corticosteroids with that of metoclopramide, but corticosteroids were always found to be better tolerated.[4]

The development of 5-HT$_3$ antagonists stimulated a number of comparative trials. When used alone, these compounds have been shown to have superior antiemetic activity with respect to older drugs, such as metoclopramide, alizapride, or phenothiazines, and similar efficacy when compared with dexamethasone (dexamethasone 8 mg intravenously plus 4 mg orally every 6 h starting at the same time as chemotherapy).[24],[25]

Interestingly, one of these studies demonstrated that the combination of a 5-HT$_3$ antagonist with dexamethasone is significantly more efficacious than dexamethasone or granisetron alone (complete protection from acute vomiting being achieved in 93, 71, and 72 per cent of patients, respectively) and its antiemetic activity persists during three consecutive cycles of chemotherapy.[25],[26] In two other trials ondansetron combined with dexamethasone was shown to be superior to the combination of metoclopramide plus dexamethasone.[27],[28]

Therefore, the combination of a 5-HT$_3$ antagonist plus dexamethasone can provide optimal prevention of acute emesis and this conclusion was also confirmed by a high level of consensus at the Perugia Conference.[1]

Delayed emesis

Only a few studies have been specifically planned to evaluate the prevention of delayed emesis induced by cyclophosphamide, carboplatin, epirubicin, or doxorubicin. Oral ondansetron (8 mg twice a day) as well as oral dexamethasone (4 mg twice a day) and oral dolasetron (200 mg once daily) with or without corticosteroids on days 2 to 5 after chemotherapy have been found to be efficacious, with delayed emesis being prevented in approximately 40 to 60 per cent of patients.[29]–[31]

In these patients the degree of protection from acute emesis has a great influence on the occurrence of delayed emesis. In fact, in one study the overall incidence of delayed vomiting and moderate–severe nausea was reported to be less than 20 per cent if patients did not have acute vomiting and moderate–severe nausea and about 55 to 75 per cent if they did.[32] Therefore, prophylactic treatment should be received by those patients having a significant chance of suffering from delayed emesis. In this case, oral dexamethasone alone, or a 5-HT$_3$ antagonist or their combination, beginning 24 h after chemotherapy and continuing for a minimum of 72 h, should be administered.

Prevention of emesis induced by low emetogenic chemotherapy

Very few controlled studies have been carried out in patients treated with low–moderate and low emetogenic chemotherapy (Table 1). It is therefore impossible to identify the optimal antiemetic treatment.[1]

In clinical practice a prophylactic antiemetic treatment, especially with a 5-HT$_3$ receptor antagonist, is not recommended unless the existence of well-established prognostic factors or previous experience with chemotherapy-induced emesis make it necessary. In this case, antiemetic treatment should be prescribed on an individual patient basis.

Refractory emesis and rescue antiemetic therapy

There are no clear definitions of the terms refractory emesis and rescue antiemetic therapy.[1] Rescue antiemetic treatment is often referred to as antiemetics given on demand to a patient with emesis. No randomized double-blind trials have investigated antiemetics in this setting.

A few trials have investigated patients with refractory emesis defined as emesis in the previous cycle of chemotherapy, but without emesis before the subsequent cycle of chemotherapy (no anticipatory emesis). In two randomized trials, metopimazine improved the efficacy of ondansetron[33] and of ondansetron plus methylprednisolone[34] in patients with refractory emesis, but more data are needed before definite conclusions can be drawn.

Anticipatory emesis

As anticipatory emesis develops when frequent and/or severe post-treatment nausea and vomiting have occurred, the best preventative treatment is optimal control of post-chemotherapy emesis. In one study, evaluating 1385 patients prior to the fourth chemotherapy cycle, the prevalence of anticipatory nausea was around 20 per cent with approximately one-third of all patients experiencing symptoms at least once by the fourth treatment. Approximately 8 per cent of patients had at least one occurrence of anticipatory vomiting during this period.[35]

Contrasting data have so far been published on the incidence and severity of anticipatory nausea and vomiting before and after the introduction of the 5-HT$_3$ antagonists in clinical practice.[36],[37]

The pharmacological agents currently used cannot provide complete protection from anticipatory nausea and vomiting. One clinical study showed that low-dose oral alprazolam may be a potentially useful treatment (0.5 to 2 mg)[38] although, unfortunately, the efficacy of this drug tended to decrease as chemotherapy treatment continued. Several studies have also demonstrated the efficacy of systematic desensitization and hypnosis against anticipatory nausea and vomiting.[39],[40]

The most efficacious strategy against anticipatory emesis is therefore represented by a multidisciplinary approach, including the best possible pharmacological control of acute and delayed nausea and vomiting, drugs as needed to decrease anxiety, and supportive behavioural treatment (systematic desensitization, hypnosis).

Emesis induced by high-dose chemotherapy

High-dose chemotherapy followed by haematopoietic stem cell transplantation provides a unique challenge in the prevention and management of emesis. Few published data exist to define the magnitude of this problem as well as the best preventive intervention.

The natural history of emesis following different regimens of high-dose chemotherapy is even less well established. A very high rate of early and delayed nausea and vomiting, however, has been documented in most published trials evaluating the toxicities of high-dose chemotherapy regimens for bone marrow transplantation.

Three small randomized trials involving the 5-HT$_3$ antagonists have been published. In one, ondansetron was shown to be superior to metoclopramide and droperidol.[41] In another, continuous infusion of chlorpromazine was comparable with continuous infusion of ondansetron, but ondansetron was significantly less toxic.[42] The third study showed no statistically significant difference in the control of emesis between granisetron and 'standard' antiemetic therapy.[43]

Although the 5-HT$_3$ antagonists have some efficacy in the prevention of acute emesis, further studies are necessary to determine their optimal dosage and timing as well as their combination with dexamethasone or other drugs. At present, no therapy has convincingly been shown to control delayed emesis induced by high-dose chemotherapy.

Radiotherapy-induced emesis

The incidence and severity of radiotherapy-induced emesis is related to the site, the field size, and the dose of radiotherapy. Total body irradiation and irradiation of the upper part of the abdomen or of the whole abdomen are considered the most emetogenic regimens in radiotherapy. The emetogenic potential is moderate in radiotherapy of the thorax, pelvis, and lower half of the body, and low in radiotherapy of the head and neck, extremities, brain, and skin.

Before the advent of the 5-HT$_3$ antagonists, the few trials carried out demonstrated only a moderate control of emesis with older antiemetic drugs (complete protection from vomiting in approximately 50 per cent of patients submitted to moderately emetogenic radiotherapy but only poor control for highly emetogenic radiotherapy).

Convincing data exist from comparative studies that the 5-HT$_3$ antagonists have superior antiemetic efficacy with respect to placebo, metoclopramide, prochlorperazine, and a combination of metoclopramide, dexamethasone, and lorazepam in the prevention of emesis induced by moderately and highly emetogenic radiotherapy.[44]

Despite a possible increase in antiemetic efficacy when 5-HT$_3$ antagonists are combined with corticosteroids (complete control of emesis in 86 per cent of cases), the data are too preliminary to reach a definitive conclusion regarding this drug combination.[44]

Further studies are required to evaluate optimal dosing and timing of the 5-HT$_3$ antagonists as well as their combination with other antiemetic drugs.

Future perspectives

In Table 3 recommendations for antiemetic therapy in relation to the different chemotherapeutic agents and to the type of emesis (acute or delayed) are reported. Improvements in the prevention of chemotherapy-induced nausea and vomiting can come from new drugs or a new combination of drugs obtained through the achievements of clinical research based on sound methodology. It is also desirable that the knowledge acquired during the last few years find the widest possible clinical application in order to provide the best available antiemetic treatment for every patient undergoing chemotherapy. Unfortunately, however, it is not always easy to transfer these results into clinical practice.[45] At the same time, it is necessary to pursue new avenues of research to solve definitively the problems of emesis induced by cancer treatments.

Recently, basic research has introduced the possibility that substance P may be partly responsible for emesis induced by chemotherapy. Substance P, a regulatory peptide, induces vomiting and binds to the NK1 (neurokinin) neuroreceptor. Compounds that block the NK1 receptor lessen emesis after cisplatin, ipecac, copper sulphate, apomorphine, and radiation therapy. The NK1 receptor antagonist, PD 154075, has shown complete protection from cisplatin-induced acute and delayed emesis in 100 per cent of ferrets.[46] The first pilot study with the NK1 receptor antagonist CP-122,721 used in cancer patients was published in 1997[47] showing definite activity against acute and delayed emesis after cisplatin. These NK1 receptor antagonists may also provide additive benefit in acute emesis and nausea control when combined with a 5-HT₃ receptor antagonist and dexamethasone.

The addition of such compounds to well-established standard antiemetic therapy could be useful, but this hypothesis needs to be demonstrated in well-designed clinical trials.

References

1. Antiemetic Subcommittee of MASCC. Prevention of chemotherapy and radiotherapy-induced emesis: results of the Perugia Consensus Conference. *Annals of Oncology*, 1998; **9**: 811–19.

2. Andrews PLR. The mechanism of emesis induced by chemotherapy and radiotherapy. In: Tonato M, ed. *Anti-emetics in the Supportive Care of Patients* (ESO monograph). Berlin: Springer 1996: 3–24.

3. Andrews PLR, Naylor J, Joss A. Neuropharmacology of emesis and its relevance to anti-emetic therapy. Consensus and controversies. *Supportive Care in Cancer*, **6**: 197–203.

4. Del Favero A, Roila F, Tonato M. Reducing chemotherapy-induced nausea and vomiting. Current perspectives and future possibilities. *Drug Safety*, 1993; **9**: 410–28.

5. Roila F, Tonato M, Ballatori E, Del Favero A. Comparative studies of various antiemetic regimens. *Supportive Care in Cancer*, 1996; **4**: 270–80.

6. Italian Group for Antiemetic Research. Ondansetron + dexamethasone versus metoclopramide + dexamethasone + diphenhydramine in prevention of cisplatin-induced emesis. *Lancet*, 1992; **340**: 96–9.

7. Cunningham D, *et al.* Optimum anti-emetic therapy for cisplatin-induced emesis over repeat courses: ondansetron plus dexamethasone compared with metoclopramide, dexamethasone plus lorazepam. *Annals of Oncology*, 1996; **7**: 277–82.

8. Italian Group for Antiemetic Research. Difference in persistence of efficacy of two antiemetic regimens on acute emesis during cisplatin chemotherapy. *Journal of Clinical Oncology*, 1993; **11**: 2396–404.

9. Herrstedt J, Sigsgaard T, Handberg J, Schousboe BMB, Hansen M, Dombernowsky P. Randomized, double-blind comparison of ondansetron versus ondansetron plus metopimazine as antiemetic prophylaxis during platinum-based chemotherapy in cancer patients. *Journal of Clinical Oncology*, 1997; **15**: 1690–6.

10. Andrews PL, Bhandari P, Davey PT, Bingham S, Marr HE, Blower PR. Are all 5-HT₃ receptor antagonists the same? *European Journal of Cancer*, 1992; **28A**(Suppl. 1): 2–6.

11. Roila F, Ballatori E, Tonato M, Del Favero A. 5-HT₃ receptor antagonists: differences and similarities. *European Journal of Cancer*, 1997; **33**: 1364–70.

12. Gandara DR, Roila F, Warr D, Edelman MJ, Perez EA, Gralla RJ. Consensus proposal for 5-HT₃ antagonists in the prevention of acute emesis related to highly emetogenic chemotherapy. Dose, schedule, and route of administration. *Supportive Care in Cancer*, 1998; **6**: 237–43.

13. Gralla RJ, Popovic W, Strupp J, Culleton V, Preston A, Friedman C. Can an oral antiemetic regimen be as effective as intravenous treatment against cisplatin: results of a 1054-patient randomized study of oral granisetron versus intravenous ondansetron. *Proceedings of the American Society of Clinical Oncology*, 1997; **16**: 52a.

14. Krzakowski M, Graham E, Geodhals L, Pawlieki M, Yelle L, Joly F. Control of acute cisplatin-induced nausea and emesis using a once daily oral treatment regimen of ondansetron plus dexamethasone. *European Journal of Cancer*, 1997; **33**(Suppl. 8): 19.

15. Kris MG, *et al.* Prevention of acute emesis in cancer patients following high-dose cisplatin with the combination of oral dolasetron and dexamethasone. *Journal of Clinical Oncology*, 1997; **15**: 2135–8.

16. Italian Group for Antiemetic Research. Double-blind, dose-finding study of four intravenous doses of dexamethasone in the prevention of cisplatin-induced acute emesis. *Journal of Clinical Oncology*, 1998; **16**: 2937–42.

17. Kris MG, Gralla RJ, Tyson LB, Clark RA, Cirrincione C, Groshen S. Controlling delayed vomiting: double-blind, randomized trial comparing placebo, dexamethasone alone, and metoclopramide plus dexamethasone in patients receiving cisplatin. *Journal of Clinical Oncology*, 1989; **7**: 108–12.

18. Moreno I, *et al.* Comparison of three protracted antiemetic regimens for the control of delayed emesis in cisplatin-treated patients. *European Journal of Cancer*, 1992; **28A**: 1344–7.

19. The Italian Group for Antiemetic Research. Cisplatin-induced delayed emesis: pattern and prognostic factors during three subsequent cycles. *Annals of Oncology*, 1994; **5**: 585–9.

20. Grunberg SM, Ehler E, McDermed JE, Akerley WL. Oral metoclopramide with or without diphenhydramine: potential for the prevention of late nausea and vomiting induced by cisplatin. *Journal of the National Cancer Institute*, 1988; **80**: 864–8.

21. Navari RM, *et al.* Oral ondansetron for the control of cisplatin-induced delayed emesis: a large, multicenter, double-blind, randomized comparative trial of ondansetron versus placebo. *Journal of Clinical Oncology*, 1995; **13**: 2408–16.

22. Latreille J, *et al.* Use of dexamethasone and granisetron in the control of delayed emesis for patients who receive highly emetogenic chemotherapy. *Journal of Clinical Oncology*, 1998; **16**: 1174–8.

23. The Italian Group for Antiemetic Research. Ondansetron versus metoclopramide, both combined with dexamethasone, in the prevention of cisplatin-induced delayed emesis. *Journal of Clinical Oncology*, 1997: **15**: 124–30.

24. Jones AL, *et al.* Comparison of dexamethasone in the prophylaxis of emesis induced by moderately emetogenic chemotherapy. *Lancet*, 1991; **338**: 483–7.

25. The Italian Group for Antiemetic Research. Dexamethasone, granisetron or both for the prevention of nausea and vomiting during

chemotherapy for cancer. *New England Journal of Medicine*, 1995; **332**: 1–5.

26. **The Italian Group for Antiemetic Research.** Persistence of efficacy of three antiemetic regimens and prognostic factors in patients undergoing moderately emetogenic chemotherapy. *Journal of Clinical Oncology*, 1995; **13**: 2417–26.

27. **Soukop M, et al.** Ondansetron compared with metoclopramide in the control of emesis and quality of life during repeated chemotherapy for breast cancer. *Oncology*, 1992; **49**: 295–304.

28. **Du Bois A, et al.** A randomized, double-blind, parallel-group study to compare the efficacy and safety of ondansetron (GR38032F) plus dexamethasone with metoclopramide plus dexamethasone in the prophylaxis of nausea and emesis induced by carboplatin chemotherapy. *Oncology*, 1997; **54**: 7–14.

29. **Kaizer L, et al.** Effect of schedule and maintenance on the antiemetic efficacy of ondansetron combined with dexamethasone in acute and delayed nausea and emesis in patients receiving moderately emetogenic chemotherapy: a phase III trial by the National Cancer Institute of Canada Clinical Trial Group. *Journal of Clinical Oncology*, 1994; **12**: 1050–7.

30. **Koo WH, Ang PT.** Role of maintenance oral dexamethasone in prophylaxis of delayed emesis caused by moderately emetogenic chemotherapy. *Annals of Oncology*, 1996; **7**: 71–4.

31. **Pater JL, et al.** The role of the 5-HT$_3$ antagonists ondansetron and dolasetron in the control of delayed onset of nausea and vomiting in patients receiving moderately emetogenic chemotherapy. *Annals of Oncology*, 1997; **8**: 181–5.

32. **The Italian Group for Antiemetic Reseach.** Delayed emesis induced by moderately emetogenic chemotherapy: do we need to treat all patients? *Annals of Oncology*, 1997; **8**: 561–7.

33. **Herrstedt J, Sigsgaard T, Boesgaard M, Jensen TP, Dombernowsky P.** Ondansetron plus metopimazine compared with ondansetron alone in patients receiving moderately emetogenic chemotherapy. *New England Journal of Medicine*, 1993; **328**: 1076–80.

34. **Lebeau B, et al.** The efficacy of a combination of ondansetron, methylprednisolone and metopimazine in patients previously uncontrolled with a dual antiemetic treatment in cisplatin-based chemotherapy. *Annals of Oncology*, 1997; **8**: 887–92.

35. **Morrow GR, Roscoe JA.** Anticipatory nausea and vomiting: models, mechanisms and management. In: Dicato M, eds. *Medical Management of Cancer Treatment Induced Emesis*. London: Martin Dunitz, 1997: 149–66.

36. **Aapro MS, Kirchner V, Terrey JP.** The incidence of anticipatory nausea and vomiting after repeat cycle chemotherapy: the effect of granisetron. *British Journal of Cancer*, 1994; **69**: 957–60.

37. **Morrow GR, Roscoe JA, Hynes HE, Flynn PJ, Pierce HI, Burish T.** Progress in reducing anticipatory nausea and vomiting: a study in community practice. *Supportive Care in Cancer*, 1998; **6**: 46–50.

38. **Razavi D, et al.** Prevention of adjustment disorders and anticipatory nausea secondary to adjuvant chemotherapy: a double-blind, placebo-controlled study assessing the usefulness of alprazolam. *Journal of Clinical Oncology*, 1993; **11**: 1384–90.

39. **Morrow GR, Arsenau JC, Asbury RF, Bennett JM, Boros L.** Behavioral treatment for the anticipatory nausea and vomiting induced by cancer chemotherapy. *New England Journal of Medicine*, 1982; **306**: 431–2.

40. **Zeltzer LK, Dolgin M, Le Baron S, LeBaron C.** A randomized, controlled study of behavioral intervention for chemotherapy distress in children with cancer. *Pediatrics*, 1991; **88**: 34–42.

41. **Agura ED, et al.** Anti-emetic efficacy and pharmacokinetics of intravenous ondansetron infusion during chemotherapy conditioning for bone marrow transplant. *Bone Marrow Transplantation*, 1995; **16**: 213–22.

42. **Bosi A, et al.** Ondansetron versus chlorpromazine for preventing emesis in bone marrow transplant recipients: a double-blind randomized study. *Journal of Chemotherapy*, 1993; **5**: 191–6.

43. **Okamoto S, et al.** Granisetron in the prevention of vomiting induced by conditioning for stem cell transplantation: a prospective randomized study. *Bone Marrow Transplantation*, 1996; **17**: 679–83.

44. **Feyer PC, Stewart AL, Titlbach OJ.** Aetiology and prevention of emesis induced by radiotherapy. *Supportive Care in Cancer*, 1998; **6**: 253–60.

45. **The Italian Group for Antiemetic Research.** Transferability to clinical practice of the results of controlled clinical trials: the case of antiemetic prophylactic treatment for cancer chemotherapy-induced nausea and vomiting. *Annals of Oncology*, 1998; **9**: 759–65.

46. **Singh K, Field MJ, Hughes J, et al.** The tachykinin NK1 receptor antagonist PD 154075 blocks cisplatin-induced delayed emesis in the ferret. *European Journal of Pharmacology*, 1997; **321**: 209–16.

47. **Kris MG, Radford JE, Pizzo BA, Inabinet R, Hesketh A, Hesketh PJ.** Use of an NK1 receptor antagonist to prevent delayed emesis after cisplatin. *Journal of the National Cancer Institute*, 1997; **89**: 817–18.

4.12 Long-term follow-up

Simon B. Sutcliffe

The teratogenic effects of cancer treatment

Teratogenesis is the production of physical (and functional) defects due to postconception exposure to any agent(s) that increases the incidence of a congenital anomaly in the developing fetus or embryo. Teratogens may act directly (genotoxic) through interaction with DNA or with macromolecules that then react with DNA, for example radiation therapy, cytotoxic chemotherapeutic agents, or through epigenetic mechanisms wherein the teratogen does not itself damage DNA but causes alterations that, in turn, predispose to the induction of a congenital anomaly, for example disruption of hormonal, growth, or immunological regulation. Several factors are essential to the understanding of the teratogenic impact of a therapeutic intervention: the stage of gestation (gestational age) at exposure, the dose of the teratogen (as a function of one-time, cumulative, or 'area-under-the-curve'), and the mode of biological action of the teratogen. In many circumstances this information is incomplete, particularly with respect to the mode of action of the teratogen. Furthermore, whilst consistent interpretation can be applied to controlled observations regarding teratogen exposure in lower mammalian species, the interpretation of human teratogenesis due to therapy for cancer is confounded by the rarity of the event, the termination of many pregnancies exposed in the first trimester without medical report, the consistency of reporting either normal or abnormal outcomes of exposed pregnancies, the anecdotal and uncontrolled nature of reports of human exposure during pregnancy, the individual interplay of maternal age, gestational age, therapy modality(ies), and genetic background, and the natural high frequency of embryonic loss in early pregnancy.

The stages of fetal development

The stages of fetal development are listed below and are shown in Fig. 1.

- The preimplantation period—weeks 1 and 2 postconception: At this stage, the zygote progresses through cell division to become a multicellular organism prior to implantation at the blastocyst stage. It is insensitive to the teratogenic and growth-retarding effects of radiation, but shows the greatest degree of sensitivity to the lethal effects of irradiation (intrauterine cell death).
- Embryogenesis—weeks 3 to 8 postconception: During this period of early organogenesis, the embryo is very sensitive to the lethal, teratogenic, and growth-retarding effects of irradiation, but may recover to varying degrees from the growth-retarding effects in the fetal and postpartum period. The major impact of teratogens during this phase is expressed as major morphological abnormalities that may result in intrauterine death or congenital abnormalities in the fetus.
- The fetal period—weeks 9 to 38 (term) postconception: The fetal period is characterized by growth and development on a background of formed organ systems. Exposure to teratogens during the fetal phase results in growth retardation, impaired functional development, and mental retardation without major morphological abnormalities. Whilst organogenesis is substantially complete, development of the central nervous system continues well into the second trimester. In addition, migration and maturation of germ cells within the fetal gonad continues throughout the fetal period.

The effects of a teratogen may be evident following exposure, for example preimplantation cell death, embryonic death, or the production of morphological abnormality. Other effects may only become evident postpartum or in childhood, adolescence, or adult life, for example neuronal depletion, infertility, tissue hypoplasia, neoplasia, or shortening of reproductive lifespan or total lifespan. In addition, the mechanisms of teratogenesis may include the induction of cytogenetic abnormalities and somatic mutations, as well as indirect impacts upon both embryo/fetus and placenta encompassing angiogenesis, endocrine dysfunction, growth, and differentiation.[2],[3]

Teratogenic impact of diagnostic and therapeutic interventions for cancer in pregnancy

Surgery

Surgery can usually be performed safely during the second and third trimesters of pregnancy and is without direct teratogenic effect. Important considerations, however, relate to the teratogenic potential of drugs and anaesthetics used in the operative and perioperative period, the adverse impact of hypoxia or hypotension from supine positioning and vascular compression by the gravid uterus, and the increased risk of thromboembolic events associated with decreased venous flow in the lower extremities consequent on immobility and/or pelvic venous congestion. An increased risk of premature labour is recognized in association with intra-abdominal surgery in pregnancy.

Radiation

X-rays (diagnostic), and gamma-rays (radio-isotope imaging and therapeutic) are of short wavelength, are highly penetrating,

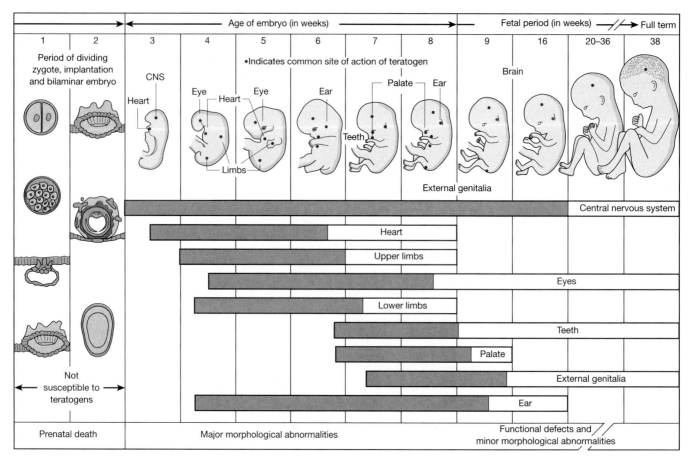

Fig. 1 Schematic illustration of the critical periods in human development. Coloured areas denote highly sensitive periods. The white indicates stages that are less sensitive to teratogens. (Reprinted from Moore[1] with permission.)

and produce ionization in tissues with subsequent electrochemical reactions that have the capability to damage DNA. Diagnostic ultrasound utilizes non-ionizing 'radiation' at an energy spectrum below the level that may cause tissue disruption. Similarly, magnetic resonance imaging creates anatomical images through electromagnetic fields that have no ionizing potential.

The frequency and magnitude of the effects of ionizing radiation on the fetus are related to the absorbed fetal dose, the type of radiation, and the gestational age at exposure. The principal risks include embryonic lethality, structural malformations, growth impairment, mental retardation, carcinogenesis, and hereditary defects.[4] The relationship of these risks to gestational age at exposure and a summary of risk as a function of radiation dose are shown in Tables 1 and 2 respectively.[5]–[10] Although a substantial part of the data source refers to observations arising from radiation exposure from radioactive fall-out at Hiroshima and Nagasaki, direct observation from 26 children receiving therapeutic irradiation at various stages of gestation substantiate the principal findings in rodents and human atomic bomb survivors (Fig. 2).[7] In this series, the radiation doses were fairly large (air exposure of more than 250 R with no upper limit stated), and the observed abnormalities consistent, i.e. structural malformations in weeks 4 to 11, growth retardation, microcephaly, and mental retardation predominantly in weeks 11 to 16, but also in

weeks 16 to 20. The apparent absence of any effect of radiation exposure in weeks 1 to 3 and weeks 20 to term must be considered with caution given the limited number of observations, the principal effect in weeks 1 to 3 being embryonic lethality, and the limited follow-up information on the survivors examined at 3 months to 16 years of age.

Exposure of the embryo/fetus to radiation in current oncological practice may occur during diagnostic evaluation, therapeutic external beam radiation, or therapeutic administration of radionuclides. Estimated fetal doses from diagnostic radiological procedures are: chest radiograph 0.01 to 0.05 mGy; abdominal flat plate 2.5 to 3 mGy; intravenous pyelogram 4 to 6 mGy; lower gastrointestinal series 8 to 10 mGy; lymphogram 10 to 15 mGy; computed tomogram of abdomen and pelvis 10 to 50 mGy. Such doses are well below the generally applied standard of 100 mGy exposure during the first trimester of pregnancy for consideration of a therapeutic abortion.[11] Whilst they are also well below the 'thresholds' for increased probability of a significant effect at various stages of gestation (Table 2), multiple or cumulative exposure could approach these levels, and the 'thresholds' must be considered estimates rather than absolute data points. A responsible position with respect to exposure to diagnostic X-rays during pregnancy would accept those procedures that are necessary to establish a management decision to the benefit of the

Table 1 Risk associated with irradiation during fetal development[5]

	Preimplantation	Organogenesis	Early fetal	Mid-fetal	Late fetal
Postconception time (days)	0–8	9–50	51–105	106–175	> 175
Postconception time (weeks)	1	2–7	8–15	16–25	> 25
Effects:					
Lethality	+ + +	+	+	−	−
Gross malformations	−	+ + +	+	+	−
Growth retardation	−	+ + +	+ +	+	+
Mental retardation	−	−	+ + +	+	−
Sterility	−	+	+ +	+	+
Cataracts	−	+	+	+	+
Other neuropathology	−	+ + +	+	+	+
Malignant disease	−	+	+	+	+

− No observed effect. + Demonstrated effect. + + Readily apparent effect. + + + High incidence.

Table 2 Risk in relation to radiation dose during fetal development. (After Brent[5] and Stovall et al.[4])

	Preimplantation	Organogenesis	Early fetal	Mid-fetal	Late fetal
Postconception time (days)	0–8	9–50	51–105	106–175	> 175
Postconception time (weeks)	1	2–7	8–15	16–25	> 25
Principal effects	Lethality	Growth retardation	SMR	SMR.	Growth retardation
		SHS without mental retardation	SHS	Growth retardation	Carcinogenesis
		Major malformations	Growth retardation Sterility	Carcinogenesis Sterility	Sterility
Index effect	Lethality	SHS	SMR	SMR	Carcinogenesis
Radiation dose for index effect*	Threshold: 0.1 Gy LD50: 1 Gy	Threshold: > 0.1 Gy 40% risk at 0.5 Gy	Threshold: 0.12 Gy 40% risk per Gy ≈ 50% at 1 Gy.	Threshold: 0.65 Gy 20% at 1 Gy	? 14% per Gy
Data source	Rat[3]	Human[6],[7]	Human[7],[8]	Human[6],[7]	Human[9]

SMR = severe mental retardation. SHS = small head size.

*Radiation doses for principal effects are commonly acute single exposures. Fractionation of the dose would probably reduce the risk.[10]

mother and/or child, but any exposure that does not directly contribute to an informed decision is neither warranted nor considered 'safe'.

The radiation dose that would be experienced by the embryo/fetus during maternal therapeutic irradiation can be established prior to the initiation of therapy through detailed reconstructive dosimetry. The principal parameters influencing absorbed dose include beam energy, field size, and distance from the edge of the beam to the reference point for dose measurement. Representative plots of absorbed dose in relation to distance from the field edge are shown as a function of beam energy for a standard field size (Fig. 3(a)) and as a function of field size for a single beam energy (Fig. 3(b)). The distance from the field edge requires correlation with an appropriate reference point relating to the fetus—commonly the uterine fundus—

although it is recognized that there will be an inconstant relationship between fetal anatomy and beam edge due to fetal movement and growth during planned fractionated radiation therapy. Figure 4 depicts fundal height (gestational age) in relation to the lower border of a supradiaphragmatic parallel-opposed (panel a) and an upper abdominal parallel-opposed pair of radiation fields (panel b), with superimposition of absorbed dose estimates for ^{60}Co and 6 MV photons as a percentage of the dose at the midplane in the centre of the radiation field. In this example, a mantle field to treat supradiaphragmatic Hodgkin's disease to a tumour dose of 35 Gy would result in a dose of approximately 0.1 to 0.11 Gy (6 mV photons) or 0.24 to 0.25 Gy (^{60}Co) for a fundal height of 12 weeks' gestation. Second-trimester exposure could result in doses up to 1 to 2 per cent of the tumour dose, i.e. 0.35 to 0.70 Gy (6 MV, ^{60}Co respectively).

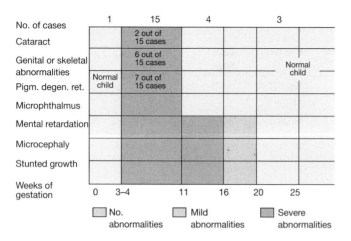

Fig. 2 Tentative timetable of abnormalities in man induced by irradiation of the fetus during various stages of gestation. (Reprinted with permission from Dekaban.[7])

Clearly, these doses are well within the range for a significant risk of damage during the first trimester (0.1 to 0.5 Gy), and for damage during any trimester (> 0.5 Gy).

In circumstances where maternal external beam radiation therapy is considered an appropriate intervention, every consideration should be given to minimization of the fetal dose. Reduction of external radiation scatter from photon leakage through the treatment head of the machine and from scatter from collimators and beam modifiers may be addressed through the design of appropriate external shielding, recognizing the practical aspects of extensive external lead shielding of sufficient thickness to absorb high-energy photons.[4] Published reports of radiation therapy for women with supradiaphragmatic Hodgkin's disease complicated by pregnancy confirm the previously described dose estimates, namely:

- First trimester of pregnancy—fetal dose estimate 14.4 cGy ± 0.7 cGy.[12]

- Second trimester of pregnancy—fetal dose estimates without shielding 11 to 58 cGy, with 9 mm thick external abdominal lead shielding 7 to 47 cGy, and with 5 cm external beam shielding 10 cGy to the fundus and 3 cGy to the pubis for a target dose of 35 Gy.[13],[14]

Fetal dose estimates based upon phantom dosimetry have also been established for the use of tangential photon beams as would commonly be applied in the management of breast cancer.[15] For ^{60}Co beams, the maximum dose to the fetus for a target dose of 5000 cGy would be 14, 45, and 201 cGy for 8, 20, and 36 weeks gestational age (minimum distance from fetus to field centre 40, 24, and 9 cm). Maximum fetal dose estimates for 6 to 25 MV photon beams are 3, 12, and 143 cGy for equivalent gestational age (maximum distance between fetus and field centre).

Radio-iodine (^{131}I) is an established component of the treatment of differentiated epithelial thyroid carcinoma, a condition well represented in women during child-bearing years. Orally administered radio-iodine results in low whole-body radiation dose as well as a high thyroid dose due to beta emission concentrated within the thyroid gland or functioning metastases. In the absence of functioning pelvic metastases, the anticipated whole-body fetal radiation dose from therapeutic ^{131}I administration to the mother would be small (0.25 cGy to the fetus for an administered dose of 3700 MBq).[16] However, the potential for underestimation of fetal dose using medical internal radiation dose tables has been identified consequent upon the demonstration of prolonged retention of isotope within the gestating uterus, with an estimated dose range of 5.3 to 15.8 cGy for an administration of 3700 MBq radio-iodine ^{131}I.[17] The fetal thyroid dose for the same administered dose was estimated to be 90 to 900 Gy. Pathological examination of the fetus following termination of pregnancy at the 24th to 25th week of pregnancy (in this case following inadvertent administration of ^{131}I without knowledge of pregnancy) demonstrated substantial necrobiotic destruction of the thyroid follicular epithelium with extensive fibrosis. Lesser changes were noted in the testes and adrenal glands.[16] The establishment of a non-pregnant state is clearly a mandatory precaution prior to

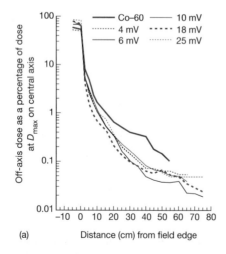

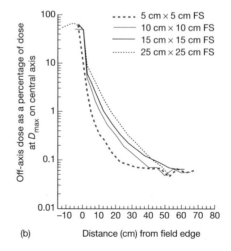

Fig. 3 Representative plots of total absorbed dose in a phantom normalized to 100 per cent on the central axis at depth of maximum dose: (a) for a 10 × 10 cm² field using ^{60}Co X-rays and 4, 6, 10, 18, and 25 MV photons at 10 cm depth; (b) for 4 MV photons for field sizes of 5 × 5, 10 × 10, 15 × 15, and 25 × 25 cm² at 10 cm depth. (Reprinted with permission from Stovall et al.[4])

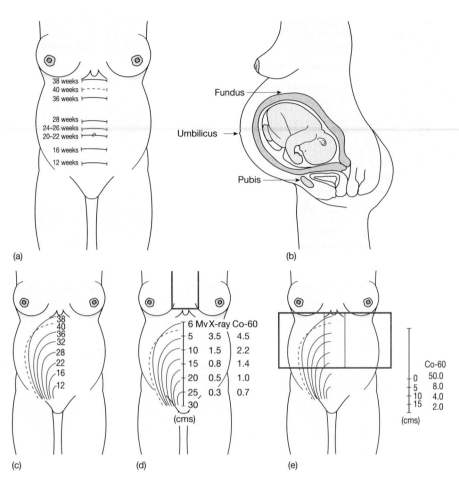

Fig. 4 (a) Anterior schematic diagram indicating fundal height at various times during pregnancy. (b) Lateral schematic diagram of a full-term fetus. (c) Fundal height by gestational age. (d) Radiation dose expressed as a percentage of the midplane dose in the centre of the radiation field for both 6 MV X-rays and ^{60}Co photon irradiation. The radiation field is a 'mantle' parallel-opposed pair of fields with the lower border at the xiphisternum. (e) Radiation dose expressed as a percentage of the midplane dose in the centre of the radiation field for ^{60}Co photons. The radiation field is a large upper abdominal parallel-opposed pair of fields with the lower border at the umbilicus.

administration of radio-iodine to women within their child-bearing years.

Chemotherapy

Systemic chemotherapy for the treatment of cancer is intended to achieve cell death through interference with replication or through induction of programmed cell death. It would, therefore, be predicted that these agents would have teratogenic potential. This has been the experience with their use during controlled testing in other mammalian species and in uncontrolled anecdotal experience in humans. A comprehensive analysis of the pharmacology of anticancer drugs is presented in Chapters 4.13 to 4.19, and experience of their use in pregnancy can be found in Wiebe and Sipila.[18] The principles underlying the impact of anticancer drugs administered during pregnancy may be developed according to two key issues:

* The total therapeutic exposure of the embryo/fetus, i.e. the drugs administered (dose, schedule, single agent, and/or combinations) and their mechanism of action.
* The gestational age of the embryo/fetus.

The drug exposure of the embryo/fetus is principally determined by passive transplacental diffusion of agents from the maternal circulation to the fetus. Accordingly, factors to be considered include (Table 3):

* The maternal exposure—the drug concentration × time (area under the curve) recognizing the influence of the pharmacokinetics of the pregnant state upon the area under the curve for all agents administered.

* The physiochemical properties of the agents administered, namely:

  (i) Molecular weight—small molecular weight (less than 1000 Da and especially less than 600 Da) favours penetration.

  (ii) Degree of protein binding—the active agent is non-protein bound. Lower protein binding increases the availability of active agents for transfer.

  (iii) Lipophilicity—the more lipophilic (fat soluble) the agent, the greater the degree of transplacental penetration.

  (iv) Degree of ionization—non-ionized agents transfer more readily.

Table 3 Clinical pharmacokinetics of chemotherapeutic agents in pregnancy. (Adapted from Wiebe and Sipila.[18])

Pharmacokinetic parameter	Maternal factors	Fetal factors
Volume of distribution	Up to 50% increase in plasma volume	
Peak drug concentration	Influenced by route of administration Decreased due to dilutional effect	
Half-life	Influenced by protein binding, absorption, elimination, third space	
ACU*	Variable	
Drug absorption	Reduced gastric emptying Constipation Variable oral absorption	
Enterohepatic circulation	May be increased, enhancing bioavailability	
Protein binding	Increase in plasma proteins Increased protein binding of drug	
Renal clearance	Increased GFR† and renal plasma flow in pregnancy	
Hepatic clearance	Increase mixed function oxidase system in pregnancy	Decreased mixed function oxidase and glucuronide conjugation systems in fetal liver
Third space	Amniotic fluid sequestration of water-soluble agents, e.g. methotrexate, cis-platinum	
pH effects		Lower pH favours retention of basic drugs
P-glycoprotein	Expression in gravid uterus may selectively exclude agents from the placentofetal blood pool	

* Area under the curve.

† Glomerular filtration rate.

Given these properties, the majority of cytotoxic agents have high membrane penetration and would be expected to achieve equilibrium levels between mother and fetus (studies suggest a 90 per cent equilibrium after 15 min of fetal exposure to constant maternal drug levels). Lesser membrane penetration would be expected for heavily protein-bound agents, for example vinca alkaloids, and high molecular weight agents, for example L-asparginase, interferons.

• Fetal factors influencing the area under the curve for agents administered (see Table 3).

Clinical experience with anticancer drugs administered during the course of human pregnancy documents the use of agents representative of all major classes of agents reviewed in Chapters 4.14 to 4.18. This experience includes single agents and combination regimens in current use for Hodgkin's disease (MOPP (mechlorethamine, vincristine, procarbazine, prednisone) and derivatives, ABVD (doxorubicin, bleomycin, vinblastine, dacarbazine)), non-Hodgkin's lymphoma (CHOP (cyclophosphamide, doxorubicin, vincristine, prednisone); CHOP-bleo (CHOP + bleomycin)), acute leukaemias (daunorubicin, doxorubicin, epirubicin-mitoxantrone, m-AMSA (amsacrine), cytosine arabinoside, thioguanine, etoposide), endodermal sinus tumours (vincristine, actinomycin-D, cyclophosphamide, doxorubicin), and adult neuroblastoma (cis-platinum and etoposide).[19]–[24] More recent additions include all-*trans* retinoic acid in the treatment of acute promyelocytic leukaemia, and α-interferon for management of chronic-phase chronic myeloid leukaemia.[25]–[27] The interpretation of their use in pregnancy relates to the second key issue, namely gestational age at the time of exposure. As with the assessment of risk of radiation exposure there are several factors which make precise determination of the risk of chemotherapy difficult. These include a spontaneous abortion rate of 25 per cent in the general population, a background population risk of congenital malformations in pregnancy of 3 per cent for all births, and many other events with the potential to influence pregnancy outcome which may be unrecorded, for example other drug exposure (both prescription and illicit), smoking, and alcohol abuse. The cumulative experience identifies a risk of 17 to 23 per cent of fetal malformations arising as a result of first trimester exposure to single-agent and/or combination chemotherapy.[19] Experience during second- and third-trimester pregnancies is not associated with structural malformations, based upon a large number of observations encompassing multiple agents and regimens for a variety of maternal conditions. Whilst this observation would imply that cancer chemotherapy carries a significant risk of fetal structural malformation when administered in the first trimester, but is 'safe' in the second and third trimester, this latter implication requires considerable caution. 'Safety' cannot be equated with outcomes other than absence of structural malformation based upon the observational literature available. Other effects are important, such as the acute complications of fetal distress, haematological compromise, and hormonal insufficiency. There are other potential longer-term effects requiring prolonged follow-up, including physical and mental development, fertility, cancer risk, and total lifespan.

Other considerations in relation to antineoplastics in pregnancy include the use of support medications (limited use of 5-HT$_3$-antagonist antiemetics and leucocyte growth factors has been reported without adverse incident), and the predictable and observable teratogenic risks associated with recently introduced biological therapies for cancer. Limited experience is available with interferons, no data are available for targeted immunological therapies, and it would be predicted that antiangiogenesis agents might have adverse teratogenic impacts during all phases of gestation.

Considerations in the management of the pregnant patient with cancer

The management of the pregnant patient with cancer poses a unique dilemma in as much as decisions have an impact on both mother and fetus—an interdependent unit wherein the mother is the beneficiary of decisions maximizing the probability of cancer control during the pregnancy, whilst the fetus passively accrues therapy-related morbidity and mortality risks with no benefit other than the survival of the mother to a gestational age appropriate for delivery. In this circumstance, decision-making requires the participation, understanding, and support of the patient and family, as well as an experienced and well-informed clinical team to advise and supervise all aspects of care during the antenatal, delivery, and postnatal period. Reviews of these aspects of management of the pregnant patient with cancer are available.[20],[28]–[30] In deciding on a management strategy the important issues for consideration include:

- The natural history of the malignancy, the projected benefits of cancer therapy for the mother, and the anticipated impacts of deferring a treatment decision until parturition.
- The influence of pregnancy upon the natural history of the cancer.
- The influence of the cancer upon maternal and fetal health during the course of the pregnancy. In this consideration, fetal health is contingent upon maternal survival until a gestational age appropriate for fetal delivery—a fetal age of greater than 30 weeks to ensure a high probability of fetal survival. The risk of fetal metastasis from maternal malignancy appears to be of little practical clinical importance.[31] Factors mitigating against fetal metastases include the 'barrier' effect of the placenta—whilst sequestration of malignant cells may be seen in the maternal circulation of the placental villi, invasion of the villous circulation and involvement of the fetal circulation is very rarely recorded. In addition, the maternal malignancy is a 'foreign graft' within a fetus whose immune system begins development within the second trimester.
- The impact of disease evaluation, investigation, and staging upon appropriate therapeutic decision-making for the mother, and upon fetal health. This issue largely relates to radiological and/or radionuclide evaluation for correct attribution of disease stage as a basis for maternal therapy, and the risks of fetal teratogenesis or future cancer risk for the exposed fetus consequent upon radiation exposure.
- The influence of cancer treatment upon the fetus—the potential consequences of surgery, radiation, and systemic therapy upon the fetus in terms of teratogenesis, growth and development, and carcinogenesis must be addressed.
- Difficulties in antenatal care:

(i) Maternal—nutrition, dentition, oral and/or vaginal candidiasis, emesis, constipation, psychosocial support.

(ii) Fetal—intrauterine growth monitoring, prompt recognition of fetal distress and access to fetal blood sampling as appropriate.[26],[32],[33]

- Problems relating to childbirth. In addition to the obstetric considerations relating to the timing and mode of delivery, the impact of maternal therapy upon blood count nadirs requires co-ordination between oncologist and obstetrician. Fetal blood counts may parallel those of the mother, or may demonstrate suppression of haemopoesis unrevealed by maternal counts.[34] Following delivery, detailed evaluation of the neonate is mandatory to establish physical health and potential complications of therapy, e.g growth retardation, issues related to a 'small-for-dates' baby, issues related to premature delivery, analysis of blood counts, hormone profiles if necessary (e.g. adrenal suppression related to maternal steroid exposure, hypothyroidism, etc.), and chromosome analysis to reveal any cytogenetic impacts of exposure to therapeutic agents during pregnancy.

- Difficulties relating to postnatal care:

(i) In the mother these include completion of disease investigation and management; suppression of lactation and avoidance of breast feeding if maternal chemotherapy is to continue, because chemotherapeutic agents are transferred into breast milk. Advice on contraception will be needed, particularly if maternal therapy is to continue. This may be because of the uncertainty of maternal prognosis soon after completion of therapy or because of concerns regarding potential therapy-induced damage to ova which is manifested as higher fetal loss in the 12-month period following cancer treatment.[35]

(ii) In the infant/child/adolescent—attention to growth, mental and physical development, endocrine function, and gonadal function.

Long-term outcomes related to cancer treatment and pregnancy

Although many of the concerns surrounding cancer treatment during pregnancy are related to maternal and fetal health during the course of the pregnancy, following childbirth there may be problems related to the long-term health of both mother and child.

Maternal health

Management decisions made during pregnancy may have an effect on long-term maternal outcome. Following delivery, any previous compromise of management of the tumour, such as limited evaluation of the spread of the disease and modifications of therapy, require re-evaluation to establish that optimal management is achieved now that there are no continuing concerns about *in utero* fetal health.

The impact of therapy on future reproductive potential, for example the effect of cancer therapy on ovarian function (see below), will need to be considered.

Health of the child

Longer-term follow-up of children exposed to cancer therapy *in utero* has not identified any additional physical or mental developmental issues other than those due to early gestational exposure.

There are no data regarding the fertility potential of adults exposed to cancer therapy agents *in utero*. Sterility in other mammalian species has, however, been noted with exposure to radiation (100 cGy) during early organogenesis to late fetal periods.[5] The data derived from patients treated for cancer in childhood and adolescence, and in adults of reproductive age (see below), suggest that it is likely that there will be retention of gonadal function in a fetus exposed to radiation or chemotherapy that has been optimized in accordance with current practices in pregnancy.

Risk of teratogenesis in pregnancies in adults who have been exposed during fetal life

There are no direct data which measure the risk of fetal malformation in those who have been exposed to cancer treatment during fetal life. Women who conceive within 1 year of completing chemotherapy for gestational trophoblastic neoplasms have a higher rate of fetal loss, implying that there is potentially a late effect of chemotherapy in adults on subsequent fetal development.[35] However, there does not appear to be an appreciable risk of teratogenesis in pregnancies following chemotherapy in childhood.[36]

Late cancer risk

Data on carcinogenesis as a result of radiation exposure *in utero* have been derived from case–control epidemiological studies comparing the frequency of prenatal X-ray exposure in children dying from cancer with that of matched controls.[37] Other case–control studies have assessed the frequency of prenatal X-ray exposure on cancer incidence in twin versus singleton pregnancies (where radiological exposure *in utero* was greater for twins than for singleton pregnancies).[38] Japanese cohort studies have examined observed cancer incidence in survivors exposed *in utero* to atomic radiation compared with the general population matched for age, sex, and year. These studies establish an excess cancer risk following prenatal radiation exposure. The observed cancer incidence is 640 cases/10 000/Gy of fetal dose for ages 0 to 14 years, 55 cases/10 000/Gy fetal dose for ages 4 to 15, and 223 cases/10 000/Gy fetal dose for ages 4 to 39 years.[39] The observation of premature death wholly attributable to cancer risk, maximally expressed in those aged less than 10 years at the time of A-bomb exposure, directly supports the concern regarding cancer induction as a consequence of total body irradiation *in utero*.[40] To date, information relating to cancer risk following exposure to chemotherapy *in utero* is limited by sample size and follow-up; however, such limited observations would suggest that cancer induction is not a measurable concern so far.

Children of parents who have been treated in childhood

Within the limitations of the sample size and duration of follow-up of reported studies, there is no clinically detectable increase in mutational injury, expressed as congenital anomalies and/or childhood cancer, in the offspring of survivors of exposure to cancer therapy in childhood and in adulthood who maintain fertility after cancer therapy.[41]–[44]

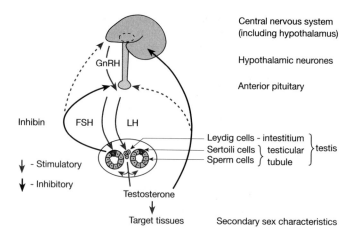

Fig. 5 Schematic illustration of male reproductive physiology. Gonadotrophin-releasing hormone (**GnRH**) is produced by the hypothalamus and transported to the anterior pituitary gonadotrophic cells via the pituitary portal system. Under the influence of GnRH, FSH (follicle stimulating hormone), and LH (luteinizing hormone) are synthesized and released by the anterior pituitary. FSH acts on Sertoli cells within the testicular tubule to produce androgen binding protein. Testosterone is produced by Leydig cells within the intertubular tissue of the testis, extrinsic to the tubule, under the influence of LH. Testosterone enhances spermatogenesis and drives male secondary sex characteristics. Testosterone acts via a feedback loop on the hypothalamus, and possibly on the anterior pituitary, to regulate LH production. Sertoli cells secrete inhibitors to regulate FSH production by the anterior pituitary, and possibly by regulation of hypothalamic GnRH secretion.

Effects of cancer treatment on fertility

Reproductive physiology

Sperm production in the male takes place throughout postpubertal life from a constantly renewing germinal epithelium with a maturation cycle time of approximately 3 months. Within the seminiferous tubule, all stages of germ cell maturation arise from an identifiable stem cell. The germinal epithelium is maintained by production of follicle-stimulating hormone (**FSH**) in the pituitary and is regulated by a negative-feedback mechanism through inhibin production in the seminiferous tubule (Fig. 5). Androgen production by the testes takes place through an anatomically distant mechanism—the Leydig cells—whose function is regulated by production of luteinizing hormone (**LH**) in the pituitary and negative-feedback control through production of testosterone in the Leydig cells. Injury to the testes may result in depletion of the germinal epithelium, the extent and duration of which will reflect loss of the stem cell compartment, and in failure of biosynthesis of androgenic steroid hormone. The two processes are not, however, totally interdependent. Treatment-induced azoospermia does not necessarily imply diminished or absent hormone production and is not synonymous with functional castration. Male fertility is most effectively measured by semen analysis: volume of ejaculate, sperm concentration ('normal value' $> 20 \times 10^6$/ml), sperm mobility ('normal value' > 50 per cent motile sperm), and percentage of abnormal forms ('normal value' > 30 per cent sperm of normal morphology).[45] Levels of FSH are a less accurate surrogate measure

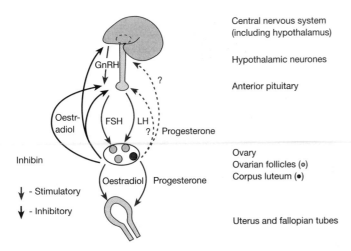

Fig. 6 Schematic illustration of female reproductive physiology. The hypothalamus produces gonadotrophin-releasing hormone (**GnRH**) which is transported to the gonadotrophic cells of the anterior pituitary through the pituitary portal system. GnRH stimulates the production and pulsatile release of FSH (follicle stimulating hormone) and LH (luteinizing hormone). Granulosa cells of the ovarian follicle produce oestradiol under the influence of FSH. Oestradiol provides feedback inhibition of FSH and GnRH production by the pituitary and hypothalamus respectively, along with inhibins produced by the ovary. Oestradiol has stimulatory effects upon the breast, uterus, vagina, and distal urethra. Progesterone is produced by the corpus luteum following ovulation. A negative-feedback loop for progesterone control of gonadotrophins and GnRH at the anterior pituitary and hypothalamic level has been postulated.

of male fertility, elevated levels correlating with deficient, defective, or absent spermatogenesis.

The ovarian germ cells are a non-renewing population, of maximal number *in utero* and decaying to approximately 400 at menopause. Depletion takes place through anovulatory maturation and attrition prior to the menarche, and by maturation, degeneration, and ovulation during reproductive life. In normally menstruating women, ovarian function depends upon production of FSH in the pituitary to stimulate the ovarian follicular granulosa cells to produce oestradiol (Fig. 6). Negative-feedback regulation of FSH takes place through oestradiol. The production of oestrogen and progesterone by the ovarian follicle is entirely dependent upon the cyclic maturation of the oocyte. Therapy that induces damage to the oocyte depletes a fixed and ever-declining cell population. Furthermore, loss of the germinal epithelium of the ovary results in failure of production of ovarian steroid hormone, thus producing functional castration.

Fertility assessment in women consists of a menstrual history, including menopausal symptoms, and measurement of levels of FSH. Persistent amenorrhoea in the presence of sustained elevation of FSH implies ovarian failure (menopause).

As the gonad affects endocrine and reproductive function in both sexes, treatment-induced damage may result in a number of clinical problems. These include endocrine dysfunction, with physiological and psychosexual implications, changes in gonadal size, architecture, and cellular content impacting upon fertility and reproductive lifespan,

and, theoretically, the induction of germ-line mutations predisposing to hereditary illness.

The impact of cancer on fertility and gonadal function

While considerable attention has been directed to the effects of cancer therapy, the presence of cancer, independent of therapy, may have an adverse impact upon gonadal function.

Semen analysis in untreated males with Hodgkin's disease has revealed reductions in sperm count to levels of less than 20×10^6/ ml in up to 50 per cent of those surveyed, poor motility levels and an elevated proportion of abnormal forms, endocrine evidence of impaired spermatogenesis and compensated biochemical hypogonadism, and confirmation by biopsy of oligospermia and abnormal epithelial maturation.[46]–[48] These changes correlate with fever, advanced stage, and possibly with immunological dysfunction.[48],[49] Similar findings of greater magnitude have been noted in males with untreated testicular cancer, and have been attributed variously to cryptorchidism, a primary germ cell disorder, raised βhCG (β-human chorionic gonadotrophin), carcinoma *in situ*, raised scrotal temperature, and immunological mechanisms.[46],[50]–[52] Biochemical hypogonadism has also been noted frequently in males with advanced non-gonadal cancer.[53]

Cryopreservation of sperm and artificial insemination is widely available to counteract the effect of cancer therapy upon spermatogenesis.[54] However, the high proportion of males with Hodgkin's disease or testicular cancer with poor semen quality, or inadequate post-thaw motility, means that cryopreservation is problematic for many patients unless special techniques are used for sperm purification and concentration, or to increase the chances of oocyte fertilization from poor-quality semen, for example intracytoplasmic sperm injection for *in vitro* fertilization.[48],[55]

Cyclical ovarian activity is influenced by many factors such as critical body mass, stress, and emotional state. Advanced non-gynaecological cancers (e.g. leukaemias) may also involve the ovary and uterus directly, resulting in secondary amenorrhoea. In most circumstances there is, however, little information regarding ovarian dysfunction as a consequence of untreated malignancy, although assessment of the luteal phase of the menstrual cycle in women with untreated breast cancer, or in premenopausal women at higher risk of developing breast cancer, have suggested a higher rate of anovulatory cycling.[56]–[59]

The effect of the untreated disease state as a cause of gonadal dysfunction may be demonstrated by the return of menstrual activity or recovery of spermatogenesis following institution of therapy.

Although the ovary is more resistant to the effects of cancer therapy than the testis, certain therapeutic interventions predict a high probability of ovarian failure. The available techniques for preservation of human oocytes require the harvest of oocytes under ultrasound guidance following artificial stimulation of the ovary to produce several oocytes. This remains experimental, with limited general availability. Of potential future interest is the technique of cryopreservation of ovarian cortical strips which can subsequently be reimplanted on the ovarian pedicle. Embryo storage, whilst possible, is again of limited practicality due to the time required to acquire sufficient oocytes, the availability of a parental partner, and the general availability of the technology.

Cancer treatment and gonadal function

Radiation therapy and testicular function

The unique sensitivity of the male germinal epithelium to radiation has been clearly demonstrated in carefully constructed single-dose exposure experiments in human 'volunteers'.[60] Morphological evidence of spermatogonial injury was evident with single doses as low as 10 cGy. Such studies also indicated the maturational cycle of spermatogenesis to be approximately 70 days.[61] Given the low threshold for accumulation of dose without expression of injury, these studies infer that fractionated radiation exposure is probably more damaging than acute exposure of equivalent-total dose.

Several retrospective studies have defined the probability of damage to the germinal epithelium and subsequent recovery following therapeutic irradiation for non-gonadal tumours.[62] Although the interpretation of these studies is made difficult by a number of variables, for example the state of the epithelium prior to therapy and the duration of follow-up since therapy, it can be deduced that if the testis receives fractionated total doses of less than 150 cGy this will result in temporary oligospermia or azoospermia, with probable recovery over a 2- to 3-year period. Prolonged azoospermia with a low likelihood of recovery may be expected with received doses in excess of 300 to 350 cGy. Testicular doses of 150 to 300 cGy will result in severe oligospermia or azoospermia, which may be prolonged without certainty of recovery, particularly at the higher end of the dose range.[63],[64]

For radiation fields not encompassing the testes, the radiation dose to the testes from a therapeutic treatment can be established by direct measurement, for example by thermoluminescence dosimetry, or by estimation under simulated clinical conditions in a 'mock' human phantom. The testicular dose derives predominantly from internal radiation scatter within the body and is determined by field size, beam energy, and depth of the tissue of interest within the radiation volume. The principal determinant, however, is the distance of the testis from the beam edge. Based upon these parameters, tabular or graphic representation of gonadal dose as a percentage of tumour dose can be derived (Fig. 7).[65]

In clinical practice, large supradiaphragmatic radiation fields may contribute 1 to 2 per cent of the tumour dose to the testis, resulting in minor temporary abnormalities without permanent sequelae. With abdominal radiation fields, the distance from the beam edge to the testis is critical. Fields above the pelvic brim may contribute 1.5 to 4 per cent of the tumour dose; those involving the pelvis, particularly if inguinal or femoral regions are included, may result in a scatter dose in excess of 10 per cent of the tumour dose, with resultant prolonged oligospermia or azoospermia if no attempts are made to minimize the scatter dose to the testes.

The principal component of gonadal dose derives from the anterior beam, given that the testes are predominantly an anterior structure in a supine patient. With an appropriately constructed lead shielding device, the testicular dose can be reduced by at least 75 per cent, resulting in a gonadal dose of approximately 1 to 2.5 per cent of the

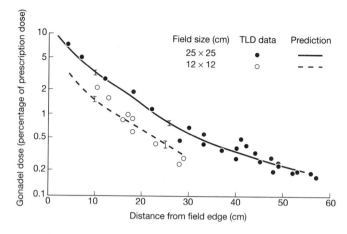

Fig. 7 Comparison of scatter dose to the unshielded testis obtained with thermoluminescent dosimeters on patients (open and full circles), and prediction from mock human phantoms (solid and dashed lines). Data apply to opposed field treatment with 6 MeV photons at a depth of 0.25 cm below the skin surface. (Reprinted with permission from Shapiro et al.[65]).

tumour dose applied to a large abdominopelvic radiation field.[66],[67] Such dose reduction is compatible with early recovery of normal spermatogenesis.[66],[67]

Whilst scattered radiation dose to the testes is of considerable importance in terms of spermatogenesis, synthesis of androgen by the Leydig cells is not adversely influenced by doses of this magnitude. Biochemical hypogonadism may, however, follow therapeutic testicular irradiation where doses in excess of 20 Gy are employed.[68],[69]

The testicular dose due to therapeutic ^{131}I administration for thyroid carcinoma is approximately 0.16 to 3.2 × 10^{-8} cGy/Bq ^{131}I administered. Such doses would not be of clinical relevance other than with repeated ^{131}I exposure and/or functioning pelvic metastases.[70],[71] Testicular exposure of less than 1 per cent of the tumour dose would result from source leakage following intracranial radiation using gamma-knife radiosurgery.[72]

Radiation and ovarian function

Many of the data defining the sensitivity of the ovary to irradiation are indirect, being a compilation of experience of radiation inducing premature menopause and retrospective studies of the effects of scattered radiation used in the treatment of non-gonadal malignancy.[62] The data indicate that the ovary is relatively more resistant to the damaging effects of radiation than the testis. This increased capacity to absorb radiation without expression of injury suggests that fractionated radiation is probably less injurious than a single exposures of equivalent dose. It is also apparent that a dose–response relationship with age exists, with younger women generally requiring higher doses to produce permanent amenorrhoea. Thus, women in their late reproductive years have a high probability of radiation castration with ovarian doses in excess of 4 Gy (400 cGy). A dose of 4 Gy would probably not influence ovarian function in a child or adolescent, and would result in permanent amenorrhoea in fewer than 50 per cent of women treated in early reproductive life.[73] Doses in excess of 10 Gy (1000 cGy) will cause ovarian failure in the majority of adult women, although even this dose does not necessarily guarantee castration in an individual exposed during childhood.[73] The dose range of 4 to 8 Gy (400 to 800 cGy) carries the most uncertainty for prediction of ovarian failure, with indication that permanent amenorrhoea will occur in more than 50 per cent of women exposed in their reproductive years.[74]–[76] Critical factors influencing retention of ovarian function, therefore, are age at exposure, ovarian dose (> 5 Gy), and use of gonadotoxic chemotherapy.[76]

In the clinical context, irradiation fields above the diaphragm (e.g. a mantle field for supradiaphragmatic Hodgkin's disease) contribute less than 1 per cent of the tumour dose to the ovaries for both ^{60}Co and higher-energy beams. For a standard para-aortic field (lower beam edge 10 cm from the ovary), measured doses of approximately 2 to 2.5 per cent of the tumour dose (high-energy and ^{60}Co respectively) are recorded.[77] The lack of any clinical impact of such exposure in women receiving mantle and para-aortic fields (calculated scatter to the pelvis at the ovaries 3.2 Gy) has been reported following 38 normal pregnancies in 18 women of a cohort of 36, aged 10 to 40 years at the time of diagnosis.[78]

Radiation fields encompassing the pelvis inevitably result in ovarian exposure to the full tumour dose unless surgical transposition of the ovaries has been performed. The site of ovarian relocation in relation to the proposed irradiation field is relevant. Transposition to the iliac crests results in a three- to four-fold reduction in ovarian dose compared with central pelvic location behind the uterus.[79] The potential benefits of oophoropexy must be weighed against the potential disadvantages. Unsatisfactory or unstable ovarian relocation may preclude adequate external shielding, and potential compromise to the ovarian blood supply may follow mobilization of the ovarian artery. Oophoropexy must therefore be an integral part of the overall management plan with the specific objective of preservation of ovarian function.[80]

The use of radio-iodine for the treatment of thyroid cancer does not result in a clinically significant ovarian dose (in the absence of functioning pelvic metastases) in the context of a discernible impact upon long-term risk of infertility or birth defects.[81] The measured ovarian dose from ^{131}I ranges from 0.16 to 3.2×10^{-8} cGy/Bq ^{131}I.[82]

Ovarian dose (and fetal dose) from radiation scatter during ^{60}Co or high-energy X-ray radiation therapy using a tangential breast treatment technique appropriate for unilateral breast cancer varies according to breast size (radiation field size) and distance between the inferior beam edge and the ovary (point of reference). Maximum estimates range from approximately 0.078, 0.037, and 0.013 per cent of the tumour dose for a ^{60}Co beam at distances of 30, 40, and 50 cm between beam edge and ovary—doses which are substantially below the threshold for any foreseeable impact on ovarian function.[83] Similarly, the source leakage dose from gamma-knife radiosurgery is not of clinical relevance to ovarian function.[72]

Chemotherapy and testicular function

Single-agent chemotherapy

There is a substantial literature documenting the effects of single-agent chemotherapy upon gonadal function in a range of neoplastic and non-neoplastic conditions.[84] As a broad generalization, the effects of chemotherapy are predominantly expressed on the germinal epithelium. They depend on the cell cycle activity of the agent(s), their principal action being on actively dividing cell populations rather than resting (G_0) or slowly proliferating cells, and are related to cumulative dose. Alkylating agents (cyclophosphamide, chlorambucil (> 400 mg), busulfan, melphalan, nitrogen mustard), have been most actively studied and appear to be particularly damaging to spermatogenesis with prolonged or permanent azoospermia following cumulative exposure to cyclophosphamide (> 11 g) and chlorambucil (> 400 mg). Late recovery of spermatogenesis is possible, however, and cumulative dose estimates and biopsy evidence of an absent germinal epithelium are not absolute evidence of permanent sterility.

There is less information for other classes of cytotoxic drugs employed as single agents. Methotrexate, in conventional or high doses, and 5-fluorouracil appear to have temporary effects upon spermatogenesis that are fully recoverable, as might be predicted for cycle-specific agents influencing rapidly dividing cell populations. Similarly, the vinca alkaloids appear to have little, if any, adverse, long-term impact upon spermatogenesis. Other agents, for example doxorubicin, cis-platinum, and etoposide as components of multiagent combinations, are associated with transient, but fully recoverable, effects. Corticosteroids may have adverse effects upon sperm density and motility, with evidence of arrested spermatogenesis that is recoverable after therapy.

Multiagent chemotherapy

Regimens for lymphoma

The effects of the MOPP, MOMP (mechlorethamine, vincristine, methotrexate, prednisone), and CVP (cyclophosphamide, vincristine, prednisone) regimens for adult males with lymphoma were initially reported in 1973, with evidence of azoospermia in the majority and some degree of recovery in fewer than 50 per cent of patients studied.[85] The MOPP experience was confirmed with the **MVPP** (mechlorethamine hydrochloride, vinblastine sulphate, procarbazine, and prednisolone) regimen, which revealed complete germinal aplasia during the 12-month period following completion of chemotherapy as evidenced by raised gonadotrophins, azoospermia, and absence of spermatogenesis on testicular biopsy (Fig. 8). A variable degree of compensated biochemical hypogonadism was also present.[86] Azoospermia and elevated FSH were evident by the third cycle of therapy, indicating damage to the epithelium from the start of therapy, the expression of azoospermia being consistent with the 70-day maturation cycle of spermatogenesis (Fig. 9).[87] Subsequent studies indicate a low (< 20 per cent) probability of recovery of spermatogenesis, with follow-up periods ranging from 2 to 12.5 years.[88] Similar findings are reported for the COPP (cyclophosphamide, vincristine, procarbazine, prednisone) regimen (six to ten cycles) for advanced Hodgkin's disease.[89] Factors associated with the less gonadotoxic impact of MOPP (or its analogues) appear to be reduction or omission of procarbazine, a reduction in the number of cycles of MOPP therapy through combination with radiation, or alternation with a less gonadotoxic regimen.[90]–[92]

More recently, other regimens have been introduced for the treatment of advanced Hodgkin's disease. The ABVD regimen has shown superior efficacy to MOPP in controlled trials, and is much less gonadotoxic with a greater than 75 per cent probability of recovery of spermatogenesis.[93],[94] Other regimens of established efficacy in phase II or single arm/institution settings include **VEEP** (vincristine, epirubicin, etoposide, and prednisolone), **Stanford V** (a three-cycle regimen comprising doxorubicin, vinblastine, mechlorethamine, vincristine, bleomycin, etoposide, and prednisolone), and **NOVP** (nitoxantrone, vincristine, vinblastine, and prednisolone).[95]–[97] All

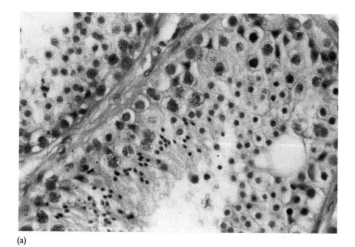

(a)

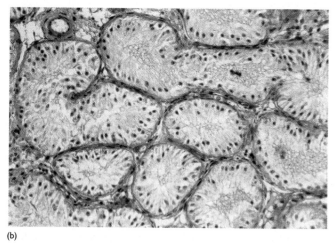

(b)

Fig. 8 (a)(b) Histological appearance of the testis: (a) before treatment and (b) after treatment for Hodgkin's disease, showing germ cell aplasia.

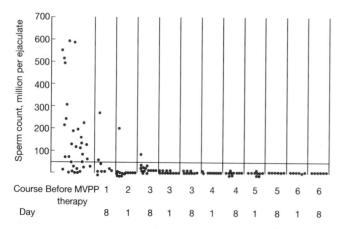

Fig. 9 Semen analysis indicating sperm counts before and during MVPP (mechlorethamine hydrochloride, vinblastine sulphate, procarbazine, and prednisolone) therapy. (Reprinted with permission from Chapman et al.[87])

regimens are associated with high rates of recovery of spermatogenesis.

Less information is available regarding the impact of chemotherapy for non-Hodgkin's lymphoma upon gonadal function. The commonly used **CHOP** (cyclophosphamide, doxorubicin, vincristine, prednisolone) regimen with bleomycin and other agents, including interferon and radiation, was reported to cause azoospermia in all patients, with subsequent recovery of spermatogenesis in 35 of 51 patients over 5 years. Pelvic radiation and cumulative cyclophosphamide dosages greater than $9.5\,g/m^2$ were associated with a higher risk of permanent sterility.[98] The **VAPEC-B** (vincristine, doxorubicin, prednisolone, etoposide, cyclophosphamide, and bleomycin) regimen was associated with the presence of spermatozoa in 13 of 14 patients examined at a median of 13.5 months (range 5 to 30 months) since completion of therapy. All seven patients with non-Hodgkin's lymphoma treated with 11 weeks of VAPEC-B had sperm counts in excess of $10 \times 10^6/ml$ at a median of 20 months (10 to 30 months) after therapy, suggesting that this regimen causes little permanent damage to the germinal epithelium.[99]

The initial belief that the prepubertal state conveys possible protection against the gonadotoxic effects of alkylating agents or MOPP chemotherapy appears to be without justification.[100],[101] The disparity may be in the interpretation of FSH levels in the pre- and postpubertal states, wherein the germinal epithelium feedback loop in prepubertal boys is through androgen, as opposed to inhibin in the adult.[102]

Regimens for testicular germ cell tumours

Interpretation of the effects of chemotherapy on spermatogenesis is confounded by the fact that approximately 50 per cent of patients have evidence of impaired spermatogenesis before treatment, that all factors having an impact upon pretreatment testicular function may or may not be reversible with therapy, and that a number of variations within the standard cis-platinum based therapy regimens have been reported. Clinical observation indicates that regimens incorporating platinum, etoposide, and bleomycin principally affect the germinal epithelium with a high probability of functional recovery of spermatogenesis.[103]–[107] A recent analysis of risk factors that predict the recovery of sperm count identified the prechemotherapy sperm count to be the strongest determinant. Also of importance was the lesser gonadotoxicity of carboplatin compared with cis-platinum. Vinca alkaloids, no longer commonly used in first-line regimens, were independently associated with recovery of spermatogenesis.[107] The number of cycles of therapy (all incorporating platinum compounds), and the cumulative dose of cis-platinum also correlate with the probability and time course of recovery of spermatogenesis.[104],[105],[107] A predictive model with 25 per cent, 45 per cent, and 82 per cent probabilities of recovering spermatogenesis by 2 years postchemotherapy, based upon prechemotherapy sperm count and number of cycles of therapy, has been proposed (Table 4).[107]

Regimens for acute leukaemia

The gonadal toxicity of regimens for acute leukaemia depends on the duration of therapy, cumulative exposure to alkylating agents, testicular infiltration by leukaemia, and radiation (either as scatter from craniospinal fields or from total body irradiation in the context of bone marrow transplant). The prepubertal state is not protective of gonadotoxic effects. In boys with acute lymphoblastic leukaemia receiving regimens incorporating vincristine, prednisolone, 6-mercaptopurine, and methotrexate along with L-asparaginase, doxorubicin, cytosine, arabinoside, and cyclophosphamide, Lendon et al.

Table 4 Probability of recovery of spermatogenesis (in per cent) by 2 years after orchidectomy and cis-platinum or carboplatinum based combination chemotherapy according to pretreatment sperm count in men treated for testicular germ cell cancers (adapted from Lampe et al.[107])

Pretreatment sperm count	Less than four cycles of treatment		More than four cycles of treatment	
	Carbo	Cis	Carbo	Cis
Normospermia: > 10 × 10⁶/ml	82%	45%	45%	25%
Oligospermia: (1–9) × 10⁶/ml	82%	45%	45%	25%
Azoospermia: < 1 × 10⁶/ml	45%	25%	25%	25%

reported a reduced tubular fertility index, interstitial fibrosis, and thickening of the tubular basement membrane compared with the testicular histology of those dying before or within 3 weeks of commencing chemotherapy.[108] Age, pubertal status, and total dose of cytotoxics, other than cyclophosphamide and cytosine arabinoside (> 1 g/m²), were not related to the tubular fertility index. Basal and stimulated gonadotrophin and testosterone levels were similar to age-matched controls, as noted by others.[102],[108] An autopsy study of predominantly postpubertal males with acute and chronic leukaemias receiving a variety of chemotherapeutic agents reported significantly decreased spermatogenic activity and tubular fertility index and increased interstitial fibrosis in the majority of cases compared with matched controls. No clear correlation was noted between the severity of changes and the sexual maturity of the patient, type of leukaemia, dose or type of chemotherapy, or time since the last dose of chemotherapy. Notwithstanding these observations, histological evidence of residual reproductive potential was evident in 65 per cent of patients.[109]

The use of maintenance chemotherapy using cyclophosphamide, 6-mercaptopurine, and methotrexate for up to 3 years after induction of remission in patients with acute lymphoblastic leukaemia was associated with considerably more gonadotoxicity than the use of a standard induction regimen without prolonged maintenance therapy for acute non-lymphoblastic leukaemia, the latter group demonstrating recovery of normal spermatogenesis.[110]

Bone marrow transplantation with preparative regimens incorporating total body irradiation, whether single dose or fractionated, at levels currently employed (commonly 10 to 12 Gy in five to six fractions, twice daily) will result in universal azoospermia with almost no expectation of recovery, although very rare circumstances of oligospermia and paternity have been recorded.[111],[112]

Chemotherapy and ovarian function

Single-agent chemotherapy

The effects of single-agent chemotherapy on ovarian function during the treatment of renal, rheumatological, and neoplastic disease have shown alkylating agents to be the most frequent cause of ovarian dysfunction, and that older age at the time of exposure and cumulative dose (particularly protracted, continuous alkylator therapy) correlated with the probability of ovarian failure.[84] Ovarian dysfunction has been

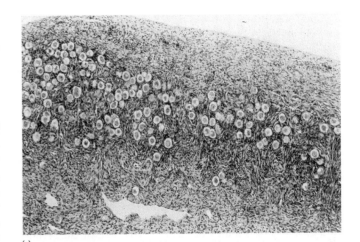

(a)

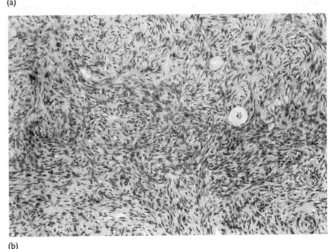

(b)

Fig. 10 Histological appearance of the ovary, (a) before treatment and (b) after chemotherapy for Hodgkin's disease, showing gross follicular destruction.

variously described in terms of amenorrhoea, elevated gonadotrophins with low serum or urinary oestrogens, and arrested follicular maturation or absence of ova on ovarian biopsies (Fig. 10). Recovery of regular menses was noted, even after prolonged amenorrhoea, but

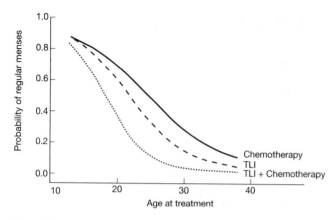

Fig. 11 Probability of regular menses after chemotherapy, total lymphoid irradiation (TLI), and total lymphoid irradiation and chemotherapy, according to age at time of treatment. (Reprinted with permission from Horning et al.[114])

was generally restricted to women in their early reproductive lifespan at the time of exposure.

Multiagent chemotherapy

Regimens for lymphoma

The MOPP, MVPP, and COPP regimens are associated with an incidence of ovarian failure highly correlated with age at the time of exposure.[113]–[117] Whilst return of regular menses may occur following therapy-induced amenorrhoea, this is more characteristic of those treated at a young reproductive age (Fig. 11).[114] Permanent amenorrhoea affects the majority of women treated in their late twenties or older, and progressive ovarian dysfunction and failure continue even after completion of therapy.[113] Given that the oocyte population has no renewable stem cell components and that damage due to chemotherapy adds to the inevitability of follicular atresia throughout the reproductive years, the principal endpoint of the effect of therapy is 'functional remaining ovarian lifespan', rather than the presence of regular menstrual activity or fertility at any given point in time.

As in the male, the MOPP regimen and its derivatives appear to be particularly gonadotoxic, probably related to the nitrogen mustard and the chronic oral procarbazine exposure. The ABVD regimen was reported to have no associated loss of ovarian function in a small number of women compared with an incidence of 50 per cent in a population of similar age exposed to MOPP chemotherapy.[93] Experience with the Stanford V (doxorubicin, vinblastine, mechlorethamine, vincristine, bleomycin, etoposide, prednisone) regimen in 19 premenopausal women revealed amenorrhoea in the majority during therapy, with resumption of regular menses in all patients 1 to 3 months after therapy. Permanent amenorrhoea occurred in a 43-year-old patient 1 year after therapy.[96] The occurrence of pregnancy with normal fetal outcomes in those with regular menses after therapy is regularly recorded, but the endpoint of relevance in relation to therapy is reproductive capacity, i.e. functional remaining ovarian lifespan, rather than ability to conceive after therapy.[113]

The importance of loss of menstrual activity due to therapy pertains not only to fertility and reproductive capacity, but also to the impact of the resultant premature, artificial menopause on psychological, psychosexual, and physical health.[118]

Regimens for germ cell tumours

Pregnancy and mutational events in the offspring have been recorded as a measure of outcome of therapy for women with gestational trophoblastic disease treated over the period 1958 to date.[119]–[126] All classes of cytotoxic drugs have been used, both cycle-specific and cycle-independent, alone and in combination, and for both metastatic germ cell tumours and those apparently confined to the uterus and pelvis. The mean age of patients was in the mid-twenties, with a relatively small proportion over the age of 30 years. The literature is very consistent in showing that chemotherapy regimens for gestational trophoblastic neoplasms (including combination therapy with cisplatinum and etoposide) do not appear to be associated with induction of a premature menopause or ovarian failure, are compatible with preservation of fertility in the majority of women, and are not associated with any detectable increase in the incidence of congenital abnormalities or demonstrable cytogenetic abnormalities in subsequent offspring.[126]

Regimens for breast cancer

Chemotherapeutic agents reported in the adjuvant setting for women with breast cancer include single alkylating agents (cyclophosphamide, melphan) and the combination of cyclophosphamide, methotrexate, and 5-fluorouracil (CMF) and its variants with doxorubicin (CAF or AC). The risk of development of treatment-induced ovarian failure is related to the age of the patient and the total cumulative dose of drug(s), with younger patients having a greater likelihood of retaining menstruation after therapy.[127]–[129] The incidence of CMF-induced amenorrhoea was 54 per cent in women aged less than 40 years compared with 96 per cent in those over 40 years, with return of menses in 23 per cent and 4 per cent respectively.[129] Similarly, the probability of early menopause 3, 5, and 10 years following adjuvant therapy was 18 per cent, 27 per cent, and 58 per cent respectively.[130]

Separate considerations in relation to breast cancer include the role that therapy-induced castration might play in relation to beneficial disease-related outcomes, the potential impact of pregnancy upon the natural history of occult or previously treated breast cancer, and the role of hormonal replacement therapy following premature, symptomatic menopause (see Section 11).

Regimens for acute leukaemia

There is little information regarding ovarian function and modern therapy for acute leukaemia. In principle, it would be anticipated that the clinical variables of age at exposure, cumulative exposure, and chronic alkylator use would be risk factors for ovarian failure. Autopsy studies have revealed no significant difference between the number of primary follicles in ovaries of patients compared with age-matched controls. The number of secondary follicles was markedly decreased in both pre- and postpubertal patients, indicative of the arrest of maturation without loss of germ cells.[109] Normal progression through puberty was noted in the majority of girls undergoing therapy for acute leukaemia, with pubertal status at the time of therapy being the principal determinant of ovarian dysfunction.[131] Age greater than 25 years and the use of continuous low-dose alkylator therapy characterized the greater than 50 per cent probability of ovarian failure in patients treated with various regimens for haematological and related malignancies.[132]

There may be retention of menstrual activity after high-dose chemotherapy. This is age related, with 100 per cent recovery in those aged less than 26 years and approximately 30 per cent recovery in those aged more than 26 years.[133] The addition of total body irradiation adds, predictably, to the ovarian failure rate (return of menses in 9 of 76 younger patients and in 0 of 68 older women).[133] Within the dose ranges employed for total body irradiation, those at the higher range (10 to 13.2 Gy) almost invariably result in ovarian failure with no discernible impact upon hypothalamic–pituitary function.[112] At lower dose levels (5 to 8 Gy), pregnancies have been reported in patients undergoing transplantation for acute leukaemia, particularly during childhood or early reproductive years.[134]

Management of the gonadal consequences of chemotherapy and radiotherapy[135]

There is now sufficient information available to enable us to predict gonadal injury following radio- or chemotherapy. In the use of these treatments it is essential to consider the potential effects upon ovarian or testicular function.

Counselling

The impact of malignant disease and its treatment upon fertility and hormonal function should be openly discussed. Neither patients nor their partners or those within the social environment of the patient may understand that changes in sexual function, interpersonal relationships, and self-esteem may be due to altered gonadal physiology resulting from treatment.[118] Psychosocial and psychosexual consequences are common, may be profound, and yet neither may be acknowledged by patient, partner, or physician, or attributed to the diagnosis and treatment of cancer (see Chapter 6.1). If fertility is retained, questions regarding the appropriateness of pregnancy in the context of the natural history of disease and the potential consequences for the fetus are paramount (see above).[136] Anticipated loss of fertility for either sex carries implications regarding the appropriateness of contraceptive practice, the remaining functional ovarian lifespan in women in relation to age at treatment and drugs/regimens employed, and, for males, the issue of recovery time from treatment-induced acute azoospermia.

Planned avoidance or minimization of therapeutic gonadal injury

In deciding upon the most effective treatment strategy (e.g. adjuvant chemotherapy or radiation), the anticipated benefits of treatment must be weighed against the adverse impact upon the gonads. The least gonadotoxic drugs/regimen should be selected without compromising efficacy or, if there has been such compromise, this should be acknowledged by physician and patient. All necessary steps should be taken to shield the gonads from unnecessary exposure to radiation.

Germ cell cryopreservation

Sperm banking is an appropriate consideration for all male patients undergoing gonadotoxic therapy who express continued interest in fertility. Even when the semen is of poor quality, sperm banking should be considered given the improved prospect of fertility with the advent of advanced *in vitro* fertilization techniques. Unfortunately, human oocyte/zygote cryopreservation techniques remain experimental and of limited practicality and availability.

Techniques available to subfertile/infertile couples after cancer treatment

Where cryopreserved sperm are available, artificial insemination is a readily available technique. Where there is neither stored sperm nor likely recovery of spermatogenesis, anonymous donor sperm matched for racial and physical characteristics is accessible for intracervical or intrauterine injection at the time of ovulation.

In vitro fertilization may be employed as a means of enhancing prospects for fertilization. Ova, retrieved under ultrasound guidance following artificial stimulation of multiple follicles, may be harvested from a female patient with functioning ovaries, or in the circumstance of ovarian failure, donor oocytes may be obtained. Cryopreserved or fresh sperm, from partner or donor, may be employed in admixture culture, or through micromanipulative techniques, for example intracytoplasmic sperm injection. Such embryo implantation techniques require the administration of exogenous hormonal supports to maintain the early pregnancy in the mother with ovarian failure.

Adoption remains an alternative means of acquiring a family for infertile couples for whom *in vitro* fertilization techniques are unsuccessful or not preferred.

Hormonal replacement therapy

For women experiencing a premature, artificial menopause due to cancer therapy (established by lack of menses and sustained hormonal correlation), hormone replacement therapy is appropriate to address psychosexual/sexual wellbeing unless other medical contraindications prevail, for example coagulopathy, thromboembolic disorders etc. Hormone replacement therapy also addresses issues related to bone mineralization and concerns about premature development of coronary artery disease. Replacement with oestrogen and progesterone preparations is usual, using oral, patch, or implant preparations. Where preparations without cyclic breakthrough are employed for medical or personal preference, regular gynaecological supervision is appropriate. Hormone replacement therapy in women with breast cancer requires separate specialist consideration (see also Section 11).

Therapy-induced hypogonadism in the male is uncommon, and may be established through demonstration of subnormal testosterone levels in the presence of elevated luteinizing hormone. Where biochemical hypogonadism exists, hormone replacement therapy is appropriate. Issues relating to reduced potency in the presence of normal sex hormone levels are more common and necessitate psychological and urological evaluation.

Approaches to prevention of loss of gonadal function using germ cell maturation arrest

Attempts to prevent loss of germinal epithelium during cancer therapy have been employed based upon the premise that rapidly dividing cells are more sensitive to cytotoxic therapy and that arrest of maturation of germinal epithelium during therapy may protect against therapeutic injury. In both males and females there have been attempts to arrest epithelial maturation of the primary follicle or spermatogenesis, commonly using non-pulsatile, chronic treatment with supraphysiological doses of LHRH analogues to suppress the pituitary–gonadal axis. The results of several clinical studies have failed to substantiate the hypothesis, and no evidence for protection against the severity and duration of therapy-related injury to the germinal epithelium has been established.[137]

Second malignancies

The past decade has witnessed a decline in overall cancer mortality in the United States. For most common cancers, improvements in survival have been modest and consistent and amount to approximately 1 to 2 per cent per year. For other less common tumour types, including Hodgkin's disease, germ cell tumours, and childhood cancer, improvements have been substantial. Currently, the gains in reduction in mortality rate exceed those of incidence. Fewer people are dying of their cancer and life expectancy for the majority of patients with cancer is increasing. Accordingly the prevalence of cancer within the population is increasing. The price of this success is the increasing burden of late effects of disease and/or therapy—the consequences of enhanced survival. Such late effects include reproductive, endocrine, cardiac, and psychosocial consequences, and also the increased risk of developing additional cancers.

The development of a cancer subsequent to initial diagnosis and therapy of a first cancer has traditionally been assumed to be a late consequence of treatment, i.e. secondary, and hence due to therapy. The development of more than one primary cancer is now increasingly recognized to have both constitutional and acquired predisposing factors. These factors are multiple, probably highly interrelated, and include the following.

Genetic predisposition[138],[139]

Cancer is a genetic disease. The major classes of clinically relevant cancer-causing genes are oncogenes: genes normally expressed in cell growth and proliferation that cause cancer when over-expressed, amplified, or mutated; tumour suppressor genes that normally regulate cell growth and proliferation and contribute to malignancy when their negative regulatory controls are lost through deletion or mutation; and DNA repair genes which identify and repair DNA mismatches following DNA replication and prior to mitosis. Aberrant function of these genes, most commonly through mutations, characterizes both common sporadic cancer and hereditary/familial cancer. When such mutations are in the germline DNA such traits are transmitted to future progeny. The resulting cancer predisposition may follow

mendelian inheritance patterns—hereditary cancer—or reflect clustering of cases within a family without a definitive inheritance pattern—multigene or multifactorial cancer. Sporadic, or acquired, cancer reflects the acquisition of mutations in cancer-causing genes within somatic cells, i.e. it is not transmissible to future progeny through the germline.

Hereditary predisposition to cancer, as determined by marked familial clustering or mendelian inheritance patterns, is thought to contribute to 5 to 10 per cent of cancer incidence. Although this is a relatively small component of overall cancer incidence, it assumes particular importance in two contexts: firstly, the identification of predisposed individuals through genetic screening, counselling, and early preventative or therapeutic strategies, and secondly, the prevalence within the population of genetic predisposition in survivors of a first cancer diagnosis who remain at increased risk of developing second or subsequent cancers within target tissues characteristic of the predisposition syndrome.

Familial clustering may also be characteristic of cancer thought to be predominantly environmental in origin. This clearly may be indicative of common exposure to known carcinogens or agents damaging DNA within families. It may, however, also have an underlying genetic basis due to inherited polymorphisms resulting in varying levels of function of xenobiotic metabolizing enzymes (oxidation and conjugation hepatic enzymes conducting phase I and II metabolism functions), and/or DNA repair gene functions. It may also reflect the interaction of a number of genes with lower penetrance.

Common aetiology

Data from several sources including mutational assays, animal models, and epidemiological surveys have established associations between environmental and lifestyle exposures that confer an increased risk for specific cancers. Such exposures include dietary risk factors, for example animal fat, alcohol, lifestyle, and occupational risk factors, for example tobacco smoking, sun exposure, ionizing radiation, various chemicals and minerals.

The risk of a second smoking-related cancer in survivors of an initial cancer arising in the upper aerodigestive tract is well established. The reduction in risk of subsequent cancer consequent upon cessation of smoking is also established. The role of environmental or occupational risk factors for a second malignancy is particularly relevant for patients with a smoking-related upper aerodigestive malignancy, bowel cancer, cutaneous melanoma, or clearly defined work-place exposure to known carcinogens.

Ionizing radiation[140]–[142]

Humans have evolved in an environment of constant background exposure to ionizing radiation from cosmic and terrestrial sources. This background radiation constitutes approximately 80 per cent of total population exposure, the remaining 20 per cent being predominantly from diagnostic and therapeutic exposures. The contribution of background radiation to excess cancer risk is unknown and is largely unmodifiable other than by residence in areas of known high or low background levels.

Exposure to ionizing radiation by accidental or therapeutic exposure has been clearly shown to increase cancer risk. Such evidence has been obtained from Japanese atom bomb survivors, fluoroscopic procedures in patients treated with artificial pneumothorax for pulmonary tuberculosis, and therapeutic exposure during the treatment of benign and malignant conditions. The following general points are important with regard to the cancer-inducing potential of ionizing radiation:

- Qualitative and quantitative aspects of the radiation, for example linear energy transfer of radiation, total dose, dose per fraction, and dose rate.

- The volume of exposure and the differing sensitivity of the organs/tissues within the radiated volume.

- Person-related attributes: age at time of exposure, with excess risk being greater for exposure at earlier ages, genetic predisposition to enhanced radiation sensitivity as in retinoblastoma gene mutations, ataxia telangiectasia (*AT* gene mutations), or aberrant DNA repair syndrome.

- The latent period for induction of cancer is long. Whether the excess risk in persons exposed at a young age is constant over their lifetime is unknown.

Radiation is known to induce chromosomal aberrations, cause single- and double-strand DNA breaks, give rise to mutations in somatic cells, and to influence gene expression. Whether radiation induces specific mutations distinguishable from other carcinogens is unknown.

Therapeutic radiation as currently practised would appear not to be a powerful carcinogen, and the benefits of radiotherapy for a malignancy outweigh concerns regarding the risk of radiation-induced secondary cancer. This risk is, however, particularly germane in the following circumstances:

- radiation for benign conditions, where the benefits of therapeutic radiation are unclear

- in younger age groups

- in combined modality therapies, using very large radiation fields (e.g. total body irradiation)

- with unconventional dose fractionation schedules

- in individuals genetically predisposed to enhanced radiation sensitivity.

Genetically determined radiation sensitivity in circumstances other than hereditary syndromes is currently being defined.

Cancer chemotherapy[143]–[145]

Chemotherapeutic agents for cancer share the common properties of known carcinogens in causing cell damage through their effects on DNA. This fundamental property is intrinsic to their cytotoxic effect on tumour cells. Their carcinogenic effects have been established over the past three decades consequent upon the ability to achieve remission of disease and prolongation of life for patients with an increasing number of tumour types.

It is well established that treatment with alkylating agents and nitrosoureas is associated with an increased risk of myelodysplasia and acute myeloid leukaemia, particularly in the 10 years following exposure. Podophyllotoxins (etoposide; tenoposide), often in combination with alkylating agents or anthracycline, may also be associated with secondary acute myeloid leukaemia. Alkylating agents have the general property of forming covalent linkages with chemical groups on biological molecules that have an excess of electrons (alkylation).

Excess second cancer risk has been recorded with the use of melphalan as an adjuvant therapy for node-positive breast cancer, methyl-CCNU as an adjuvant for gastrointestinal cancer, and MOPP therapy or derivatives (nitrogen mustard, vincristine, procarbazine, prednisolone) for advanced Hodgkin's disease. The most frequently observed second malignancy following alkylator chemotherapy is acute myeloid leukaemia. In the Stanford series of second malignancies reported after treatment for Hodgkin's disease, the relative risk for all cancers was 6.4 (relative risk for acute myeloid leukaemia 144; non-Hodgkin's lymphoma 35; all solid tumours 4.3). Attribution of the cause of a second cancer following treatment for Hodgkin's disease is complex in as much as radiation therapy, chemotherapy, and underlying cellular immune deficits may all be implicated. Restricting the observation to patients treated for Hodgkin's disease with radiation alone, the relative risk of acute myeloid leukaemia was increased at 17.5, but substantially less than the relative risk of 360 for chemotherapy alone. Second solid tumours have also been observed in the Hodgkin's cohort after initial therapy. Increased relative risks were seen for lung and pleural malignancies, breast cancer, melanoma, soft tissue sarcomas, salivary gland, and thyroid cancers. Again the independent roles of radiation, chemotherapy, and immunodeficiency are difficult to distinguish. Several of the solid tumours occur within, or at the margins of, radiation fields, implicating radiation as a major contributor to the second cancer. The long latency is also consistent with a radiogenic aetiology. However, in the case of breast cancer as a second cancer, the relative risk following chemotherapy and radiation (relative risk 6.3; 95 per cent confidence interval 3.1 to 11.6) was substantially higher than for those treated with radiation alone (relative risk 0.8; 95 per cent confidence interval 0.1 to 2.5). Younger age at the time of treatment was the principal factor affecting risk of subsequent breast cancer.

Immunodeficiency

The development of cancers on a background of cellular immunodeficiency is well established for the genetically determined (congenital) immunodeficiency states, in those who are subject to therapeutic immunosuppression for organ transplantation, and with the acquired immunodeficiency syndrome (**AIDS**). Tumours commonly seen in such patients include lymphomas, epithelial skin cancers, and Kaposi's sarcoma in the AIDS group. An underlying contribution of Epstein–Barr virus and human herpesvirus 8 to these malignancies is also established.

Cellular immunodeficiency is a component of the natural history of untreated Hodgkin's disease. Following therapy, long-standing deficits in cell-mediated immune function are recognized clinically and in *in vitro* assay systems. An excess risk of epithelial skin cancers was recorded in Hodgkin's disease cohorts prior to the use of chemotherapeutic agents, and occasional reports of non-endemic Kaposi's sarcoma were also noted. Acute myeloid leukaemia was not seen in the era prior to chemotherapy, although the median survival for patients with Hodgkin's disease for this period was approximately 3 years.

The role of cellular immunodeficiency in the development of second cancers in patients with Hodgkin's disease may be of particular relevance in the excess risk of non-Hodgkin's lymphoma. The lack of significant histological evidence of host immune response in secondary cutaneous melanomas after therapy for Hodgkin's disease has been linked speculatively to the underlying cellular immunodeficiency state.

Co-incidence

Second cancers may also happen by chance in the absence of any of the factors defined above. Although statistical techniques to determine relative and absolute risks for second cancers are based upon comparison of observed and expected events in test and control populations, the possibility of random events is not precluded.

To put the situation into perspective: risk of a second cancer is a late effect, i.e. it is a consequence of survival. To be eligible to develop a second cancer, one has to survive the first cancer. Much of the risk of a second cancer is related directly to treatment, and the modalities of therapy are unlikely to change profoundly within the next one to two decades. However, the prevalence of treated cancer in the population is increasing, and there is an increasing awareness of the factors that may modify predisposition to cancer, either primary or secondary, for example genetic, lifestyle, behaviour, etc. Accordingly, attention must be focused on strategies to minimize second cancer risk. These are discussed in the following subsections.

Genetic testing

Our knowledge of cancer predisposition genes is incomplete at present. Relevant mutations in known genes are being defined. Precise information regarding the penetrance of specific mutations and the efficacy of interventions is limited. The impacts of mutations within families and in the normal population are currently the subject of epidemiological research. Accordingly, genetic testing for cancer predisposition in an individual having a primary cancer is currently appropriate only in the circumstance of known hereditary syndromes or strong familial clustering. The American Society of Clinical Oncology has published guidelines for appropriate use of genetic testing.[146] The categories for testing include:

- Families with hereditary syndromes in which the results of genetic testing, either positive or negative, would change medical care. This category comprises the cancer predisposition syndromes associated with mendelian inheritance patterns, primarily autosomal dominant syndromes, for which some of the relevant genes have been identified. Genetic testing as a basis for clinical management should be considered a current standard of care for such individuals.

- Families with heritable syndromes with a high probability of linkage to known genes for cancer susceptibility in which identification of the carrier status is presumed to be important. Examples of such syndromes include hereditary non-polyposis colon cancer, hereditary breast–ovarian cancer, and Li–Fraumeni syndrome.

- Individuals without a family history of cancer, or families with heritable syndromes in which only a small percentage of members have germline mutations, or individuals for whom the identification of a mutation carries no known established medical benefit. In these circumstances, genetic testing is without established clinical application.

Thus, for those who do not have a precedent for familial predisposition to cancer, there would appear to be no clinical rationale for the use of genetic testing to identify individuals more highly predisposed to developing a second cancer. There would, however, appear to be a strong role for research into the association between therapy, mutations, and subsequent cancer development within the various classes of cancer predisposition genes (oncogenes, tumour suppressor, and mismatch repair genes) and the polymorphisms associated with genes subserving activation, inactivation, and metabolism of potential carcinogens.

Lifestyle and behaviour

The overwhelming environmental risk factor for development of cancer is tobacco smoke, being causally implicated in cancer of the lung, upper aerodigestive tract, pancreas, kidney, and bladder. Weaker associations exist for dietary animal fat and red meat with colon and prostate cancer, and for breast and colon cancer with moderate/high alcohol intake. Cervical cancer is causally associated with early age of sexual activity, number of partners, and infection with human papilloma virus. Counselling on cessation of smoking should be mandatory for individuals surviving one smoking-related cancer and dietary and lifestyle advice, as appropriate, to risk-related behaviours.

Screening and early detection

The premise for population screening for disease incorporates the availability of a test of appropriate sensitivity and specificity, the ability to detect occult, asymptomatic disease, and the availability of procedures that can favourably influence the outcome if applied earlier in the natural history of disease. These criteria are met by mammographic screening for breast cancer in women over 50 years of age, by cervical cytology testing for cervical neoplasia, and by faecal occult blood testing for bowel cancer. Inasmuch as individuals exposed to therapy for a primary cancer constitute a higher-risk group for developing second cancer, particularly those exposed in childhood and young adult life, increased attention to screening for breast, cervix, and bowel cancer following control of the primary tumour is appropriate.

Chemoprevention[147]

Survival after a first primary tumour carries an increased risk of a second primary tumour, as a consequence of genetic, therapy-related, or common environmental carcinogen exposure. Predisposition to a second cancer is presumed to reflect genomic instability and therapy-related mutations—molecular events enhancing the initiation of a tumour or facilitating progression of a 'damaged' cell to the malignant phenotype. In theory, knowledge of the molecular basis of these events could enable development of therapeutic preventive strategies (chemoprevention), employing pharmacological or natural agents that could block the damage to DNA leading to initiation of carcinogenesis, or to reverse or inhibit the progression of premalignant cells to the invasive phenotype.

The inhibition of tumour development by the selective action of synthetic agents upon specific molecular targets has been demonstrated in a number of clinical research settings:

- Regulation of retinoid receptors using retinoids. Retinoids are required for the proper differentiation of the upper aerodigestive and tracheobronchial epithelium. Loss of retinoid receptors is characteristic of malignant tumours of the upper aerodigestive and respiratory tracts, and may be restored using retinoids with reversal of the development of premalignant epithelial lesions.

- Inhibition of colon carcinogenesis with cyclo-oxygenase-2 inhibitors. Cyclo-oxygenase-2 overexpression is a characteristic early event in colon carcinogenesis, giving rise to increased formation of prostaglandins from arachidonic acid. Suppression of apoptosis appears to be one consequence of cyclo-oxygenase-2 over-expression. Clinical studies with cyclo-oxygenase-2 inhibitors demonstrating prevention of adenoma formation in genetically predisposed individuals suggest that non-toxic, selective molecular inhibitors will have broad applicability in the prevention of bowel cancer.

- Regulation of hormone receptors in breast cancer. Tamoxifen, an anti-oestrogen, has been shown to reduce the incidence of development of primary breast cancer in high-risk women, and to reduce the incidence of contralateral breast cancer in women treated with tamoxifen for a primary breast cancer. The target for tamoxifen is the oestrogen receptor, a membrane receptor whose activation by oestrogen gives rise to transcriptional events resulting in modulation of genes regulating growth, differentiation, and apoptosis. Further clinical studies in the chemoprevention of breast cancer are employing selective modulators of oestrogen receptors expressing anti-oestrogen effects in breast and uterine tissue whilst retaining the oestrogenic properties in bone mineralization and lipid metabolism. Similar conceptual approaches are being employed in prostate cancer using finasteride to inhibit androgen receptors.

The study of chemopreventative agents will require the characterization of molecular pathways of carcinogenesis, and the derivation of intermediate markers of DNA damage and their functional consequences, for example DNA aneuploidy, loss of heterozygosity, p53 mutations, and growth factor expression. Biomarkers of increased carcinogenic risk will help to define those more likely to develop cancer and measure the effectiveness of therapeutic interventions within a relatively short time frame.

The increased risk of development of a second cancer within the same organ system, or at other sites, in patients surviving a first cancer defines a population in whom research studies of chemoprevention are appropriate.

Surveillance

For the majority of patients completing therapy, the most immediate threat posed by cancer is that of recurrent disease. The probability of recurrence of a tumour is usually greatest in the first few years following therapy, with a declining probability thereafter. The utility of regular surveillance with scheduled investigations has been questioned for most cancers, given that reporting by patients of symptoms or signs of recurrence has a much higher probability of defining recurrence than periodic imaging or laboratory medicine examinations.[148]

As a second malignancy, acute myeloid leukaemia is most commonly seen in the decade following therapy. The incidence declines rapidly thereafter. Second solid cancers have a longer latency, with an accumulating incidence with time and no period beyond which there is no risk. It might reasonably be inferred that routine surveillance and investigation to detect a second solid tumour would also have a low probability of timely detection relative to a patient's report of symptoms or signs of illness. This position should, however, not detract from:

- The appropriate use of screening procedures to detect occult disease in those at higher risk of developing cancer as outlined above.
- The role of patient education, information, and counselling about healthy lifestyles, risk behaviours, and awareness of symptomatology to be brought to early medical attention.
- The continued search for biomarkers of predisposition that might be a more effective surveillance tool than routine general imaging or blood tests.

Characterization of treatment-related risk

Although a number of predisposing factors for second malignancy have been defined, those related to treatment are the most significant. The carcinogenic impact of radiation therapy has been relatively poorly characterized for current clinical applications. Knowledge of the carcinogenic risks of chemotherapy for cancer relate principally to alkylating agents and to regimens of more historic interest. Current treatment philosophies employing combined modality or adjuvant therapy and the use of biological substances of various modes of action affecting tumour biology and host constitution are likely to increase substantially. Accordingly, continued vigilance is required to characterize the late effects of current and future therapies.

References

1. **Moore KL** (ed.). *The developing human.* Philadelphia: Saunders, 1988.
2. **Russell LB.** X-ray induced developmental abnormalities in the mouse and their use in the analysis of embryologic patterns. *Journal of Experimental Zoology,* 1950; **114**: 545–601.
3. **Roux C, Horvath C, Dupuis R.** Effects of pre-implementation low dose radiation on rat embryos. *Health Physics,* 1983; **45**: 993–9.
4. **Stovall M, et al.** Fetal dose from radiotherapy with photo beams: Report of AAPM Radiation Therapy Committee Task Force No. 36. *Medical Physics,* 1995; **22**: 63–82.
5. **Brent RL.** The effects of embryonic and fetal exposure to x-ray microwaves, and ultrasound. *Clinical Journal of Obstetrics and Gynecology,* 1983; **26**: 484–510.
6. **Otake M, Schull WJ.** Radiation-related small head sizes among prenatally exposed survivors. *International Journal of Radiation Biology,* 1992; **63**: 255–70.
7. **Dekaban AS.** Abnormalities in children exposed to X-radiation during various stages of gestation: tentative timetable of radiation injury to the human fetus, Part 1. *Journal of Nuclear Medicine,* 1968; **9**: 471–7.
8. **Schull WJ.** Report of Risk Task Group of Committee 1. Ionizing radiation and the developing human brain. *Annals of the IRCP.* Pergamon: New York, 1991.
9. **National Research Council, Committee on the Biological Effects of Ionizing Radiations.** Health effects of exposure to low levels of ionizing radiation. *Beir V Report.* Washington, DC: National Academy, 1990: 359–60.
10. **National Council on Radiation Protection.** Influence of dose and its distribution in time on dose-response relationships for low-LET radiations. *NCRP Report 64.* Bethesda, MD: National Council on Radiation Protection, 1980.
11. **Hammer-Jacobsen E.** Therapeutic abortion on account of X-ray examination during pregnancy. *Danish Medical Bulletin,* 1959; **6**: 113–22.
12. **Friedman E, Jones GW.** Fetal outcome after maternal radiation treatment of supradiaphragmatic Hodgkin's disease. *Canadian Medical Association Journal,* 1993; **149**: 1281–3.
13. **Cygler J, Ding GX, Kendal W, Cross P.** Fetal dose for a patient undergoing mantle field irradiation for Hodgkin's disease. *Medical Dosimetry,* 1997; **22**: 135–7.
14. **Leung JT, Kuan R, Patel V.** Radiotherapy for Hodgkin's disease in

pregnancy. *Australasian Radiology*, 1996; **40**: 146–8. (See also: *Australasian Radiology*, 1996; **40**: 101–3 and *Australasian Radiology*, 1997; **41**: 407–9.)

15. **Van Der Giessen PH.** Measurement of the peripheral dose for the tangential breast treatment technique with Cobalt[60] gamma radiation and high energy X-rays. *Radiotherapy and Oncology*, 1997; **42**: 257–64.

16. **Whitehead E, Shalet SM, Blackledge G, Todd I, Crowther D, Beardwell CG.** Uterine radiation dose from open sources: the potential for underestimation. *European Journal of Nuclear Medicine*, 1990; **17**: 94–5.

17. **Arndt D, et al.** Radio-iodine therapy during an unknown remained pregnancy and radiation exposure of the fetus. *Strahlenther Onkology*, 1994; **170**: 408–14.

18. **Wiebe VJ, Sipila PEH.** Pharmacology of antineoplastic agents in pregnancy. *Critical Reviews in Oncology/Hematology*, 1994; **16**: 75–112.

19. **Doll DC, Ringenberg S, Yarbro JW.** Management of cancer during pregnancy. *Archives of Internal Medicine*, 1988; **148**: 2058–64.

20. **Barnicle MM.** Chemotherapy and pregnancy. *Seminars in Oncology Nursing*, 1992; **8**: 124–32.

21. **Aviles A, Diaz-Magueo JC, Talavera A, Guzmán R, Garcia EL.** Growth and development of children of mothers treated with chemotherapy during pregnancy: current status of 43 children. *American Journal of Hematology*, 1991; **36**: 243–8.

22. **Kim DS, Park MI.** Maternal and fetal survival following surgery and chemotherapy of endodermal sinus tumour of the ovary during pregnancy: a case report. *Obstetrics and Gynecology*, 1989; **73**: 503–7.

23. **Metz SA, Day TG, Pursell SH.** Adjuvant chemotherapy in a pregnant patient with endodermal sinus tumour of the ovary. *Gynecologic Oncology*, 1989; **32**: 371–4.

24. **Arango HA, Katter CS, Decesare SL, Fiorica JV, Lyman GH, Spellacy WN.** Management of chemotherapy in a pregnancy complicated by a large neuroblastoma. *Obstetrics and Gynecology*, 1994; **84**: 665–8.

25. **Sham RL.** All *trans*-retinoic acid-induced labour in a pregnancy patient with acute promyelocytic leukemia. (letter). *American Journal of Hematology*, 1996; **53**: 145.

26. **Terada Y, Shindo T, Endoh A, Watanabe M, Fukaya T, Yajima A.** Fetal arrhythmia during treatment of pregnancy-associated acute promyelocytic leukemia with all *trans*- retinoic acid and favourable outcome (letter). *Leukemia*, 1997; **11**: 454–5.

27. **Baer MR.** Letter to the Editor: Normal full term pregnancy in a patient with chronic myelogenous leukemia treated with a-interferon. *American Journal of Hematology*, 1991; **37**: 66.

28. **Sutcliffe SB.** Treatment of neoplastic disease during pregnancy: Maternal and fetal effects. *Clinical Investigative Medicine*, 1985; **8**: 333–8.

29. **Allen HH, Nisker J.** *Cancer in pregnancy.* Cambridge: Cambridge University Press, 1996.

30. **Koren G, Lishner M, Farine D (ed.).** *Cancer in pregnancy.* Cambridge: Cambridge University Press, 1996..

31. **Rothman LA, Cohen CJ, Astarloa J.** Placental and fetal involvement by maternal malignancy. A report of rectal carcinoma and review of the literature. *American Journal of Obstetric Gynecology*, 1973; **166**: 1023–34.

32. **Hsu K-F, Chang C-H, Chou C-Y.** Sinusoidal fetal heart rate pattern during chemotherapy in a pregnant woman with acute myelogenous leukemia. *Journal of the Formosan Medical Association*, 1995; **94**: 562–5.

33. **Morishita S, Imai A, Kawabata I, Tamaya T.** Acute myelogenous leukemia in pregnancy: fetal blood sampling and early effects of chemotherapy. *International Journal of Gynecology and Obstetrics*, 1994; **44**: 273–7.

34. **Murray NA, Acolet D, Deane M, Price J, Roberts IAG.** Fetal marrow suppression after maternal chemotherapy for leukemia. *Archives of Disabled Children*, 1994; **71**: F209–F210.

35. **Rustin GJS, Booth M, Dent J, Salt S, Rustin F, Bagshawe KD.** Pregnancy after cytotoxic chemotherapy for gestational trophoblastic tumours. *British Medical Journal*, 1984; **288**: 103–6.

36. **Green DM, Zevon MA, Lowrie G, Seigelstein N, Hall B.** Congenital anomalies in children of patients who received chemotherapy for cancer in childhood and adolescence. *New England Journal of Medicine*, 1991; **325**: 141–6.

37. **Muirhead CR, Kneale GW.** Prenatal irradiation and childhood cancer. *Journal of Radiological Protection*, 1989; **9**: 209–12.

38. **Rodvall Y, Pershagen G, Hrubec Z, Ahlbom A, Petersen NL, Boice JD Jr.** Prenatal X-ray exposure and childhood cancer in Swedish twins. *International Journal of Cancer*, 1990; **46**: 362–5.

39. **Yoshimoto Y, Kato H, Schull WJ.** Risk of cancer among children exposed *in utero* to A-bomb radiations 1950–1984. *The Lancet*, 1988; **2**: 665–9.

40. **Schull WJ, Kato H.** Malignancies and exposure of the young to ionizing radiation. *Cancer Bulletin*, 1982; **34**: 84–9.

41. **Li FP, Fine W, Jaffe N, Holmes GE, Holmes, FF.** Offspring of patients treated for cancer in childhood. *Journal of the National Cancer Institute*, 1979; **62**: 1193–7.

42. **Mulsihill JJ, et al.** Cancer in the offspring of long term survivors of childhood and adolescent cancer. *The Lancet*, 1987; **2**: 813–17.

43. **Green DM, Fiorello A, Zevon MA, Hall B, Sargelstein N.** Birth defects and childhood cancer in offspring of survivors of childhood cancer. *Archives of Pediatric Adolescent Medicine*, 1997; **151**: 379–83.

44. **Senturia YD.** The teratogenic effect of cancer treatment.In: Peckham M, Pinedo H, Keronesi U (ed.) *Oxford textbook of oncology.* Oxford: Oxford University Press, 1995: 2343–8.

45. **World Health Organization.** *Laboratory manual for the examination of human semen and sperm/cervical mucus interactions.* Cambridge: Cambridge University Press, 1992: 107.

46. **Hendry WF.** Semen analysis in testicular cancer and Hodgkin's disease: pre and post treatment findings and implications for cryoprevention. *British Journal of Urology*, 1983; **55**: 769–73.

47. **Chapman RM, Sutcliffe SB, Malpas JS.** Male gonadal dysfunction in Hodgkin's disease. A prospective study, *Journal of the American Medical Association*, 1981; **245**: 1328–8.

48. **Redman JR.** Semen cryopreservation and artificial insemination for Hodgkin's disease. *Journal of Clinical Oncology*, 1987; **5**: 233–8.

49. **Marmor D, Elefant E, Dauchez C, Rouk C.** Semen analysis in Hodgkin's disease before the onset of treatment. *Cancer*, 1986; **57**: 1986–7.

50. **Hansen PV, Trykker H, Andersen J, Helkjaer PE.** Germ cell function and hormonal status in patients with testicular cancer. *Cancer*, 1989; **64**: 956–61.

51. **Carroll PR.** Fertility status of patients with clinical stage 1 testes tumour on a surveillance protocol. *Journal of Urology*, 1987, **138**: 70–2.

52. **Van der Maase H.** Carcinoma *in situ* of contralateral testes in patients with testicular germ cell cancer: A study of 27 cases in 500 patients. *British Medical Journal*, 1986; **293**: 1398–401.

53. **Chlebowski RJ, Heber D.** Hypogonadism in male patients with metastatic cancer prior to chemotherapy. *Cancer Research*, 1982; **42**: 2495–8.

54. **Scammell GE.** Cryopreservation of semen in men with testicular tumour or Hodgkin's disease: results of artificial insemination of their partners. *The Lancet*, 1985; **ii**: 31–2.

55. **Sanger WG, Armitage JO, Schmidt MA.** Feasibility of semen cryopreservation in patients with malignant disease. *Journal of the American Medical Association*, 1980; **244**: 789–90.

56. **Chapman RM, Sutcliffe SB, Malpas JS.** Cytotoxic induced ovarian failure in women with Hodgkin's disease 1. Hormone function. *Journal of the American Medical Association*, 1979; **242**: 1877–81.

57. **Whitehead E.** The effect of combination chemotherapy on ovarian

function in women treated for Hodgkin's disease. *Cancer*, 1983; 52: 988–93.

58. **Grattarola R.** The premenstrual endometrial pattern of women with breast cancer: a study of progestational activity. *Cancer*, 1964; 17: 1119–22.

59. **Bulbrook RD.** Plasma oestradiol and progesterone levels in women with varying degrees of risk of breast cancer. *European Journal of Cancer*, 1978; 14: 1369–75.

60. **Rowley MJ, Leach DR, Warner GA, Heller CG.** Effect of graded doses of ionizing radiation on the human testes. *Radiation*, 1974; 59: 665–78.

61. **Heller CG, Clermon Y.** Spermatogenesis in man: an estimate of its duration. *Science*, 1963; 140: 184–5.

62. **Ash P.** The influence of radiation on fertility in man. *British Journal of Radiology*, 1980; 53: 271–8.

63. **Pedrick TJ, Hoffe RT.** Recovery of spermatogenesis following pelvic irradiation for Hodgkin's disease. *International Journal of Radiation Oncology and Biological Physics*, 1986; 12: 117–21.

64. **Cantola GM, Keller JW, Henzler M, Rubin P.** Effect of low dose testicular irradiation on sperm count and fertility in patients with testicular seminoma. *Journal of Audiology*, 1994; 15: 608–13.

65. **Shapiro E, et al.** Effects of fractionated irradiation on endocrine aspects of testicular function. *Journal of Clinical Oncology*, 1985; 3: 1232–9.

66. **Fraas BA, Kinsella TJ, Harrington FS, Glatstein E.** Peripheral dose to the testes: the design and clinical use of a practical and effective gonadal shield. *International Journal of Radiation Oncology and Biological Physics*, 1985; 11: 609–15.

67. **Sutcliffe SB.** Infertility and gonadal function in Hodgkin's disease. In: Selby P, McElwain TJ (ed.) *Hodgkin's disease*. Oxford: Blackwell Scientific, 1987; 343–4.

68. **Brauner R, Caltabiano P, Rappaport R, Lexerger G, Schaison G.** Leydig cell insufficiency after testicular irradiation for acute lymphoblastic leukemia. *Hormone Research*, 1988; 30: 14–114.

69. **Castillo LA, Craft AW, Kernaham J, Evans RGB, Aynsley-Green A.** Gonadal function after 12.Gy testicular irradiation in childhood acute lymphoblastic leukemia. *Medical and Pediatric Oncology*. 1990; 18: 185–9.

70. **Handelsman, DJ, Turtle JR.** Testicular damage after radioactive iodine (^{131}I) therapy for thyroid cancer. *Clinical Endocrinology*, 1983; 18: 465–72.

71. **Ahmed SR, Shalet SM.** Gonadal damage due to radioactive iodine (^{131}I) for thyroid carcinoma. *Postgraduate Medical Journal*, 1985; 61: 361–2.

72. **Berk HW, Larner JM, Spaulding C, Agarwal SK, Scott MR, Steiner L.** Extracranial absorbed doses with gamma knife radiosurgery. *Stereotactic Functional Neurosurgery*, 1993; 61 (Supplement 1): 164–72.

73. **Stillman RJ, et al.** Ovarian failure in long term survivors of childhood malignancy. *American Journal of Obstetrics and Gynecology*, 1981; 139: 62–6.

74. **Thomas PRM, et al.** Reproductive and endocrine function in patients with Hodgkin's disease: effects of oophoropexy and irradiation. *British Journal of Cancer*, 1976; 33: 226–31.

75. **Ray GR, Trueblood HW, Enright LP, Kaplan HS, Nelson TS.** Oophoropexy: a means of preserving ovarian function following pelvic megavoltage radiotherapy for Hodgkin's disease. *Radiology*, 1970; 96: 175–80.

76. **Haie-Meder C, et al.** Radiotherapy after ovarian transposition: ovarian function and fertility preservation. *International Journal of Radiation Oncology, Biology, and Physics*, 1993; 25: 419–24.

77. **Niroomand-Rad A, Cumberlin R.** Measured dose to ovaries and testes from Hodgkin's fields and determination of genetically significant dose. *International Journal of Radiation Oncology, Biology, and Physics*, 1993; 25: 745–51.

78. **Madsen BL, Guidice L, Donaldson SS.** Radiation-induced premature menopause: a misconception. *International Journal of Radiation Oncology, Biology, and Physics*, 1995; 32: 1461–4.

79. **Sharma SC, Williamson JF, Khan FM, Lee CKK.** Measurement and calculation of ovary and fetus dose in extended field radiotherapy for 10 MV X-rays. *International Journal of Radiation Oncology, Biology, and Physics*, 1981; 7: 843–6.

80. **Gabriel DA, Bernard SA, Lambert J, Groom RD III.** Oophoropexy and the management of Hodgkin's disease: A resolution of the risks and benefits. *American Medical Association—Archives of Surgery*, 1986; 121: 1083–5.

81. **Smith MB, Xue H, Takahashi H, Cangir A, Andrassy RJ.** Iodine 131 thyroid ablation in female children and adolescents: long-term risk of infertility and birth defects. *Annals of Surgical Oncology*, 1994; 1: 128–31.

82. **Briere J, Philippon B.** Absorbed dose to ovaries or uterus during ^{131}I therapy of cancer or hyperthyroidism. *International Journal of Applied Radio Isotopes*, 1979; 30: 643–71.

83. **Van der Giessen, PH.** Measurement of the peripheral dose for the tangential breast treatment technique with Cobalt 60 gamma radiation and high energy X-rays. *Radiotherapy and Oncology*, 1997; 42: 257–64.

84. **Sieber SM, Adamson RH.** Toxicity of antineoplastic agents in man : chromosomal observations, anti-fertility effects, congenital malformations and carcinogenic potential. *Cancer Research*, 1975; 22: 57–155.

85. **Sherins RJ, DeVita VT.** Effect of drug treatment for lymphoma on male reproductive capacity. *Annals of Internal Medicine*, 1973; 79: 216–20.

86. **Chapman RM, Sutcliffe SB, Rees LH, Edwards CRW, Malpas JS.** Cyclical combination chemotherapy and gonadal function. Retrospective study in males. *The Lancet*, 1979; i: 285–9.

87. **Chapman RM, Sutcliffe SB, Malpas JS.** Male gonadal dysfunction in Hodgkin's disease. A prospective study. *Journal of the American Medical Association*, 1981; 245: 1323–8.

88. **Waxman JM, et al.** Gonadal function in Hodgkin's disease: Long term follow-up of chemotherapy. *British Medical Journal*, 1982; 285: 1612–13.

89. **Charak BS, et al.** Testicular dysfunction after cyclophosphamide–vincristine–procarbazine–prednisolone chemotherapy for advanced Hodgkin's disease. *Cancer*, 1990; 65: 1903–6.

90. **Roeser HP, Stocks AE, Smith AJ.** Testicular damage due to cytotoxic drugs and recovery after cessation of therapy. *Australian and New Zealand Journal of Medicine*, 1978; 8: 250–4.

91. **Da Cunha MF, Merstrich ML, Fuller LM.** Recovery of spermatogenesis after treatment for Hodgkin's disease: limiting dose of MOPP chemotherapy. *Journal of Clinical Oncology*, 1984; 2: 571–7.

92. **Viviani S, et al.** Testicular dysfunction in Hodgkin's disease before and after treatment. *European Journal of Cancer*, 1991; 27: 1389–92.

93. **Viviani S, et al.** Gonadal toxicity after combination chemotherapy for Hodgkin's disease. Comparative results of MOPP vs ABVD. *European Journal of Cancer Clinical Oncology*, 1985; 21: 601–5.

94. **Kulkarni SS, Sastry PSRK, Sarkia TK, Parikh PM, Gopal R, Advani SH.** Gonadal function following ABVD therapy for Hodgkin's disease. *American Journal of Clinical Oncology*, 1997; 20: 354–57.

95. **Hill M, et al.** Evaluation of the efficiency of the VEEP regimen in adult Hodgkin's disease with assessment of gonadal and cardiac toxicity. *Journal of Clinical Oncology*, 1995; 13: 387–95.

96. **Bartlett NL, Rosenberg SA, Hoppe RT, Hancock SL, Horning SJ.** Brief chemotherapy, Stanford V and adjuvant radiotherapy for bulky or advanced stage Hodgkin's disease: A preliminary report. *Journal of Clinical Oncology*, 1995; 13: 1080–8.

97. **Meistrich ML, Wilson G, Mathur K, et al.** Rapid recovery of spermatogenesis after mitoxantrone vincristine, vinblastine, and

prednisone chemotherapy for Hodgkin's disease. *Journal of Clinical Oncology*, 1997; **15**: 3488–95.

98. Pryzant RM, Meistrich ML, Wilson G, Brown B, McLaughlin P. Long-term reduction in sperm count after chemotherapy with and without reduction therapy for non-Hodgkins' lymphoma. *Journal of Clinical Oncology*, 1993;**11**: 239–47.

99. Radford JA, Clark S, Crowther D, Shalet, SM. Male fertility after VAPEC-B chemotherapy for Hodgkin's disease and non-Hodgkin's lymphoma. *British Journal of Cancer*, 1994; **69**: 379–81.

100. Sherins RJ, Olweny CLM, Ziegler JL. Gynaecomestia and gonadal dysfunction in adolescent boys treated with combination chemotherapy for Hodgkin's disease. *New England Journal of Medcine*, 1978; **299**: 12–16.

101. Heikens J, Behrendt H, Adriannse R, Berghout A. Irreversible gonadal damage in male survivors of pediatric Hodgkin's disease. *Cancer*, 1996; **78**: 2020–4.

102. Shalet S. Testicular function after combination chemotherapy in childhood for acute lymphoblastic leukemia. *Archives of Disease in Childhood*, 1981; **56**: 275–8.

103. Drasga R. Fertility after chemotherapy for testicular cancer. *Journal of Clinical Oncology*, 1983; **1**: 179–83.

104. Peterson PM, Hanson SW, Giwercman A, Rorth M, Skakkabaek NE. Dose-dependent impairment of testicular function in patients treated with cisplatin-based chemotherapy for germ cell cancer. *Annals of Oncology*, 1994; **5**: 355–8.

105. Stephenson WT, Poirier SM, Rubin L, Einhorn LH. Evaluation of reproductive capacity in germ cell tumour patients following treatment with cisplatin, etoposide and bleomycin. *Journal of Clinical Oncology*, 1995; **13**: 2278–80.

106. Pont J, Albrecht W. Fertility after chemotherapy for testicular germ cell cancer. *Fertility and Sterility*, 1997: **68**: 1–5.

107. Lampe H, Horwich A, Norman A, Nicholls J, Dearnaley DP. Fertility after chemotherapy for testicular germ cell cancers. *Journal of Clinical Oncology*, 1997; **15**: 239–45.

108. Lendon M, *et al.* Testicular histology after combination chemotherapy in childhood for acute lymphoblastic leukemia. *The Lancet*, 1978; **ii**: 439–41.

109. Kuhajda FP, Haupt HM, Moore GW, Hutchins GM. Gonadal morphology in patients receiving chemotherapy for leukemia. Evidence for reproductive potential and against a testicular tumour sanctuary. *American Journal of Medicine*, 1982; **72**: 759–67.

110. Waxman J, Terry YA, Reish LH, Lister TA. Gonadal function in men treated for acute leukaemia. *British Medical Journal*, 1983; **287**: 1093–4.

111. Sanders JE, *et al.* Late effects on gonadal function of cyclophosphamide, total body irradiation, and marrow transplantation. *Transplantation*, 1983; **36**: 252–5.

112. Littley MD, Shalet SM, Morgenstern GR, Deakin DP. Endocrine and reproductive dysfunction following fractionated total body irradiation in adults. *Quarterly Journal of Medicine*, 1991; **278**: 265–74.

113. Chapman RM, Sutcliffe SB, Malpas JS. Cytotoxic-induced ovarian failure in women with Hodgkin's disease: i hormone function. *Journal of the American Medical Association*, 1979; **242**: 1877–81.

114. Horning SJ, Hoppe RT, Kaplan HS, Rosenberg SA. Female reproductive potential after treatment for Hodgkin's disease. *New England Journal of Medicine*, 1981; **304**: 1377–82.

115. Schilsky RL, *et al.* Long term follow-up of ovarian function in women treated with MOPP chemotherapy for Hodgkin's disease. *American Journal of Medicine*, 1981; **71**: 552–6.

116. Whitehead E, *et al.* The effect of combination chemotherapy on ovarian function in women treated for Hodgkin's disease. *Cancer*, 1983; **52**: 988–93.

117. Kreuser ED, Xiros N, Hetzel WD, Heimpel H. Reproductive and endocrine capacity in patients treated with COPP chemotherapy for Hodgkin's disease. *Journal of Cancer Research and Clinical Oncology*, 1987; **113**: 260–6.

118. Chapman RM, Sutcliffe SB, Malpas JS. Cytotoxic-induced ovarian failure in women with Hodgkin's disease: ii Effects on sexual function. *Journal of the American Medical Association*, 1979; **242**: 1882–4.

119. Van Thiel D, Ross GT, Lipsett MB. Pregnancies after chemotherapy of trophoblastic neoplasms. *Science*, 1970; **169**: 1326–7.

120. Ross, GT. Congential anomalies among children born of mothers receiving chemotherapy for gestational trophoblastic neoplasms. *Cancer*, 1976; **37**: 1043–7.

121. Rustin GJS, Booth M, Dent J, Salt S, Rustin F, Bagshawe KL. Pregnancy after cytotoxic chemotherapy for gestational trophoblastic tumours. *British Medical Journal*, 1984; **288**: 103–6.

122. Adewole IF, Rustin GJS, Newlands ES, Dent J, Bagshawe KL. Fertility in patients with gestational trophoblastic tumours treated with etoposide. *European Journal of Cancer Clinical Oncology*, 1986; **22**: 1479–82.

123. Ayhau A, Ergeneli MH, Yuce K, Yapar EG, Kisnisçi AH. Pregnancy after chemotherapy for gestational trophoblastic disease. *Journal of Reproductive Medicine*, 1990; **35**: 522–4.

124. Song HZ, Pao-chen Wu, Yuan-e W, Xiu-yu Yang, Shu-ying Dong. Pregnancy outcomes after successful chemotherapy for choriocarcinoma and invasive mole : long term follow-up. *American Journal of Obstetrics and Gynecology*, 1988; **158**: 538–45.

125. Kfer JJ, Iversen T. Malignant trophoblastic tumours in Norway. Fertility rate after chemotherapy. *British Journal of Obstetrics and Gynecology*, 1990; **97**: 623–5.

126. Cohen MM, Gerbie AB, Nadler HL. Chromosomal investigation in pregnancies following chemotherapy for choriocarcinoma. *The Lancet*, 1971; **ii**: 219.

127. Reichman BS, Green KB. Breast cancer in young women: Effect of chemotherapy on ovarian function, fertility and birth defects. *National Cancer Institute Monographs*, 1994; **16**: 125–9.

128. Sutton R, Buzdar AU, Hortobagyl GN. Pregnancy and offspring after adjuvant chemotherapy in breast cancer patients. *Cancer*, 1990; **65**: 847–50.

129. Bonadonna G, Valagussa P. Adjuvant systemic therapy for resectable breast cancer. *Journal of Clinical Oncology*, 1985; **3**: 259–75.

130. Valagussa P, De Candis D, Antonelli G, Bonadonna G. Reproductive potential after adjuvant chemotherapy for breast cancer. *Recent Results in Cancer Research*, 1996; **140**: 277–83.

131. Siris ES, Leventhal BG, Viatukartis JL. Effects of childhood leukaemia and chemotherapy on puberty and reproductive function in girls. *New England Journal of Medicine*, 1976; **294**: 1143–6.

132. Beard MEJ, Clark VA. Ovarian failure following cytotoxic therapy. *New Zealand Medical Journal*, 1984; **97**: 759–62.

133. Sanders JE, *et al.* Ovarian function following marrow transplantation for aplastic anemia or leukaemia. *Journal of Clinical Oncology*, 1988; **6**: 813–18.

134. Samuelsson A, Fuchs T, Simonsson B, Bjorkholm M. Successful pregnancy in a 28 year old patient autografted for acute lymphoblastic leukemia following myeloablative treatment including total body irradiation. *Bone Marrow Transplantation*, 1993; **12**: 659–60.

135. Royal College of Physicians/Royal College of Radiologists. Management of gonadal toxicity resulting from the treatment of adult cancer. *Report of a Working Party of the Joint Council for Clinical OncologyUnited Kingdom*, 1998.

136. Bandyk EA, Gilmore MA. Perceived concerns of pregnant women with breast cancer treated with chemotherapy. *Oncology Nursing Forum*, 1995; **22**: 975–7.

137. Kreuser ED, Klingmuller D, Thiel E. The role of LHRH analogues in protecting gonadal functions during chemotherapy and irradiation. *European Journal of Urology*, 1993; **23**: 157–64.

138. **Offit K.** *Clinical cancer genetics, risk counseling and management.* New York: Wiley-Liss, 1998: 21–211.

139. **Claus EK.** The genetic epidemology of cancer. In: Ponder BAJ, Cavenee WK, Soloman E (ed.) *Genetics and cancer: a second look.* New York: Cold Spring Harbor Laboratory Press, 1995: 13–26.

140. **Rauth AMR.** Radiation carcinogenesis. In: Tannock IF, Hill RP (ed.) *The basic science of oncology* (2nd edn). New York: McGraw Hill, 1992: 119–35.

141. **Fry RJM.** Radiation carcinogenesis: current issues and future prospects. In: Tobias JS, Thomas PR (ed.) *Current radiation oncology,* vol. 2. London: Arnold, 1996: 68–87.

142. **Hall EJ.** Radiation carcinogenesis. In: *Radiobiology for the radiologist* (4th edn). Philadelphia: Lippincott, 1994: 323–50.

143. **Tannock IF.** Biological Properties of anti cancer drugs. In: Tannock IF, Hill RP (ed.) *The basic science of oncology* (2nd edn). New York: McGraw Hill, 1992: 302–16.

144. **Tucker MA.** Solid second cancer following Hodgkin's disease. *Hematology and Oncology Clinics of North America,* 1993; 7: 389–400.

145. **Henry-Amar M, Dietrich PY.** Acute leukemia after the treatment of Hodgkin's disease. *Hematology and Oncology Clinics of North America,* 1993; 7: 369–88.

146. **Statement of the American Society of Clinical Oncology: Genetic testing for cancer susceptibility.** *Journal of Clinical Oncology,* 1996; **14**: 1730–6.

147. **Hong WK, Sporn MB.** Recent advances in chemoprevention of cancer. *Science,* 1997; **278**: 1073–7.

148. **Brigden ML.** Evidence-based follow-up testing of treated cancer patients—what does the literature support? *Annals of the Royal College of Physicians and Surgeons of Canada,* 1999: 32: 281–90.

The pharmacology of anticancer drugs

David R. Newell, Howard L. McLeod, and
Jan H. M. Schellens

Introduction and definition of terms

There are two features of cancer chemotherapy that combine to make the use of anticancer drugs a particularly challenging area of therapeutics. Firstly, anticancer drugs have very small therapeutic indices, so that the window between a dose that is active and one that produces life-threatening toxicity is usually narrow. Indeed, anticancer therapy is often deemed to have been inadequate if toxicity is not produced. In more chemoresistant tumour types (e.g. lung and colorectal) responses are seen in less than 50 per cent of patients, despite the occurrence of toxicity in the majority of individuals, and in such cases the therapeutic index of the drug or drugs used, the ratio of a toxic to an active dose, is less than unity for the overall patient population. The second factor that complicates use of the anticancer drugs is the time delay between drug administration and drug effect, both for activity and most toxicities. The majority of drug regimens involve multiple cycles of therapy and responses are often not observed until after the second or third course of treatment. Similarly, dose limiting toxicities are usually not apparent until 1 to 2 weeks after drug administration. Thus the clinical effects of drug treatment cannot be used to guide dosing at the time of drug administration, and in this respect cancer chemotherapy is distinct from many other therapeutic areas. For example in antihypertensive therapy and anaesthesia blood pressure and consciousness, respectively, can be used to determine the dose that is effective yet safe in each individual patient.

Given the dual challenge of the small therapeutic indices of anticancer drugs and the time delay between administration and effect, as well as the common and life-threatening nature of the disease being treated, an understanding of the pharmacology of anticancer drugs is particularly important. With such an understanding it is in principle possible to treat each patient with the drugs that are most likely to be of benefit, and at doses and with schedules which are unlikely to produce unacceptable toxicity. Furthermore, during the evaluation of novel therapeutics, pharmacological studies are essential to ensure that potentially active drug levels are being achieved in patients, in comparison to preclinical data, and that the drug is interacting with its intended target. Thus pharmacological studies play a key role in both optimizing the efficacy of established therapies and evaluating new treatments; the two general approaches being pursued to develop improved cancer chemotherapies.

As with all areas of therapeutics, there are two general aspects to the pharmacology of anticancer drugs: pharmacokinetics and

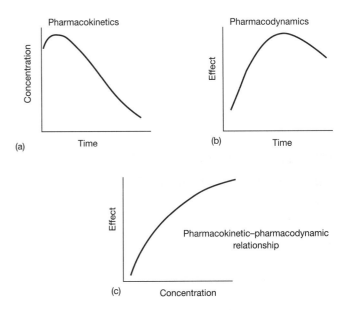

Fig. 1 Schematic representation of (a) pharmacokinetics, (b) pharmacodynamics, and (c) pharmacokinetic–pharmacodynamic relationships.

pharmacodynamics. Pharmacokinetics describes the time course and the fate of a drug in the body in relation to its absorption, distribution, metabolism, and excretion. In practical terms, pharmacokinetics describes 'what the body does to the drug'. Conversely, pharmacodynamics describes the time course of drug action, or 'what the drug does to the body', which in the case of anticancer drugs is antitumour activity and toxicity. As shown in Fig. 1, pharmacokinetic (Fig. 1(a)) and pharmacodynamic (Fig. 1(b)) analyses both have time as the independent variable, and one aim of pharmacological studies is to integrate pharmacokinetic and pharmacodynamic data to establish pharmacokinetic–pharmacodynamic relationships. In pharmacokinetic–pharmacodynamic relationships (Fig. 1(c)), the pharmacokinetic parameter (e.g. plasma drug concentration) is the independent variable and, provided the relationship between dose and the pharmacokinetic parameter is understood, dosing can be adjusted in order to achieve (activity) or avoid (toxicity) a given pharmacodynamic effect.

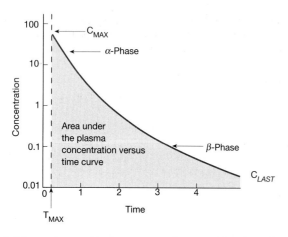

Fig. 2 Primary pharmacokinetic parameters determined from logarithmic plasma concentration versus time plots.

Pharmacokinetic principles, parameters, and calculations

Primary pharmacokinetic parameters

Primary pharmacokinetic parameters are those which are derived directly from the measured concentration versus time data. In graphical representations of concentration versus time data (e.g. Fig. 1(a)), it is usual to plot the concentration data using a logarithmic scale (Fig. 2). The change in drug concentration with time often follows first-order kinetics, that is the rate of change is dependent on the drug concentration with the rate being greatest at higher concentrations (see below, equation 13). By using a logarithmic axis for the concentration data, first-order processes appear as straight lines, and the number of straight line components in the logarithmic plasma concentration versus time profile reflects the number of distinct phases in the disposition of the drug. The primary pharmacokinetic parameters that can be derived directly from the concentration versus time plot are illustrated in Fig. 2 and include the following:

C_{max} the maximum concentration observed—units of concentration (e.g. mg/ml, μg/ml, μM);

T_{max} the time of the maximum concentration—units of time (e.g. min, h);

Half-lives   the time taken for the plasma concentration to decrease by half during each of the log-linear concentration decay phases—units of time (e.g. min, h);

AUC   the area under the concentration versus time curve—units of concentration × time (e.g. mg/ml × min, μM × h).

The half-life $(t_{1/2})$ for each phase in the plasma concentration versus time curve is indicated by a Greek letter, starting with α as the first phase after C_{max} followed by β, etc.; the last phase being described as the terminal phase with an associated terminal half-life. Where the slope of the concentration versus time curve is calculated by non-linear regression analysis, that is using the raw and not the logarithmically-transformed concentration data, $t_{1/2}$ is calculated by

dividing the natural logarithm of 2 (0.693) by the first-order rate constant (k) derived by non-linear regression analysis:

$$t_{1/2} = 0.693/k \tag{1}$$

The AUC is a particularly important pharmacokinetic parameter as it provides, in a single value, a measure of drug exposure. For many anticancer drugs activity is dependent on the total exposure, that is the product of drug concentration and duration of incubation *in vitro*, and AUC *in vivo*. AUC is also used in calculating a number of secondary pharmacokinetic parameters (see below), and in dose escalation trials where it is important to determine whether or not there is a linear relationship between dose and AUC (see below). AUC can be calculated by a number of methods, of which the trapezoidal (equation 2) and log-trapezoidal (equation 3) are both the simplest and the least influenced by assumptions related to pharmacokinetic models:

$$AUC = \Sigma \ (1/2(C_{n-1} + C_n)(t_n - t_{n-1})) + C_{last}/k \tag{2}$$

$$AUC = \Sigma \ ((C_{n-1} + C_n)(t_n - t_{n-1}) \ / \ (\ln C_{n-1} + \ln C_n)) + C_{last}/k \tag{3}$$

Where C_n is the concentration at each time point t_n and C_{n-1} is the concentration at the previous time point t_{n-1}, C_{last} is the concentration at the last time point at which the drug is detectable, and k is the terminal phase first-order rate constant.

Primary pharmacokinetic parameters are often the most important and can have a direct impact on patient care—there are now a large number of examples where the toxicities of anticancer drugs have been related to the plasma C_{max}, plasma AUC, or time above a given plasma drug concentration. Similarly, the activity of certain cancer chemotherapeutics has been related to AUC. With respect to drug scheduling, primary pharmacokinetic parameters are again of direct practical value; for example T_{max} and $t_{1/2}$ can dictate the interval between doses. As a general guide, drugs should be administered at intervals which are no less than 4 × the terminal phase half-life, if drug accumulation (i.e. rising levels with successive doses) is to be avoided. Drug concentrations in the plasma should be at most 6.25 per cent of the C_{max} after four half-lives: that is they will be 50 per cent after $1 \times t_{1/2}$, 25 per cent after $2 \times t_{1/2}$, 12.5 per cent after $3 \times t_{1/2}$, and 6.25 per cent after $4 \times t_{1/2}$.

Although the vast majority of primary pharmacokinetic parameters are derived from plasma concentration versus time analyses, this is largely due to the technological and ethical difficulties inherent in obtaining tumour or normal tissue data. Recent methodological advances have provided new approaches to obtaining tumour and normal tissue data (see below), and pharmacokinetic modelling can also generate values for tissue concentrations. In theory, tumour and sensitive normal tissue drug concentrations should relate more closely to activity and toxicity, respectively, than plasma data. However, this theory has rarely been put to the test.

Secondary pharmacokinetic parameters

Secondary pharmacokinetic parameters are calculated from the primary parameters described above. Depending on the pharmacokinetics of the drug, and the type of calculation and/or pharmacokinetic model employed, a very large number of secondary pharmacokinetic parameters can be derived. However, in many cases, these parameters have little if any clinical relevance or physiological meaning. Furthermore, the accuracy of secondary parameters can be hard to determine and difficult to verify by direct experimentation. Two secondary parameters are, however, of direct clinical relevance: clearance and bioavailability.

Clearance

The clearance of a drug is a measure of the rate of drug removal from the body, the higher the clearance the more rapid the elimination of the drug. The units of clearance are volume per unit time (e.g. ml/min or l/h), and clearance can be thought of as the volume of the space into which the drugs distributes that is cleared of all drug molecules per unit time. Glomerular filtration rate, the volume of plasma water removed by the kidneys per unit time, is the physiological process most directly analogous to drug clearance. The clearance of anticancer drugs can be due to renal, metabolic, or biliary processes (see below) which combine to determine the total clearance of a drug from the plasma. For a drug that has been administered intravenously as a bolus dose or short infusion, total drug clearance can be readily determined by the equation:

$$\text{Clearance} = \text{Dose/AUC} \qquad (4)$$

Depending on whether dose is absolute (e.g. mg or g) or normalized for body size (e.g. mg/m^2 or mg/kg), the clearance will either be absolute (e.g. ml/min or l/h) or normalized (e.g. ml/min/m^2 or ml/min/kg). Clearance values for different drugs vary over a wide range; however, the value for cardiac output is generally an upper limit (2–3 l/min/m^2 in adults). Where the value for the clearance of a drug is close to that of the cardiac output, there is almost complete extraction of the drug from the blood stream during the first pass through the body following systemic administration. Although plasma drug AUC values can be calculated following non-systemic or extravascular administration, for example oral or intramuscular dosing, it is not valid to calculate the clearance from these AUCs. Following non-systemic administration, the absorption of the drug may not be 100 per cent and hence the dose entering the circulation may not be the dose given to the patient.

For drugs being given as a constant rate intravenous infusion, and where a steady state plasma concentration is reached, clearance can be calculated as:

$$\text{Clearance} = \text{Dose Rate/Steady State Concentration} \qquad (5)$$

The clearance of a drug is probably the single most important pharmacokinetic parameter. For drugs with equal activity against their targets, clearance will determine the dose of a drug that will be required; drugs subject to rapid clearance needing larger doses to achieve and maintain active levels. Interindividual differences in drug clearance explain much of the variation between patients in drug tolerance, and the above clearance equations (equations 4 and 5) form the basis of approaches to pharmacologically-guided dosing (PGD). As discussed below, PGD seeks to compensate for interindividual pharmacokinetic and pharmacodynamic variation and can involve the use of the two clearance equations to determine the dose required to achieve a target AUC or steady state level (see equation 21).

Provided that drug elimination mechanisms are not being saturated, drug clearance should be independent of the dose given. However, if the value for drug clearance is dependent on the dose given, the pharmacokinetics of the drug are said to be 'non-linear' or saturable (see equations 18 and 19). Information on the linearity of pharmacokinetics is critical in Phase I dose escalation trials.

Bioavailability

The bioavailability of a drug is the fraction of the dose administered which reaches the systemic circulation when the agent has not been given by the intravenous route (e.g. by oral or intramuscular administration). If the bioavailability of a drug is either poor or variable then the non-intravenous route should not be used. This is particularly important in cancer chemotherapy where relatively small changes in drug bioavailability may result in a given dose being either ineffective or lethal.

The bioavailability of a drug is the ratio of the AUC following dosing by the non-intravenous extravascular route to the AUC following intravenous dosing:

$$\text{Bioavailability (\%)} = \text{AUC}_{\text{non-intravenous}}/\text{AUC}_{\text{intravenous}} \times 100 \qquad (6)$$

If the same doses (e.g. mg or mg/m^2) are not used for both intravenous and non-intravenous dosing the pharmacokinetics of the drug must be known to be linear over the relevant concentration range, and the AUC values dose-normalized appropriately, for the bioavailability calculation to be valid.

Pharmacokinetic models

Pharmacokinetic models have been developed to enable calculation of a variety of pharmacokinetic parameters,[1] and four types are frequently applied, based on different underlying concepts: non-compartmental, compartmental, physiological, and population models. Each of these models is associated with specific advantages and limitations.

Non-compartmental models

The non-compartmental method is the most simple and robust model for calculating pharmacokinetic parameters. As described above, the non-compartmental model is appropriate for calculation of the AUC (equations 2 and 3)[2]. As indicated in equations 2 and 3, to obtain the final part of the AUC after the last measured concentration–time point the curve should be extrapolated to infinity using the equation:

$$\text{Extrapolated area} = C_{\text{last}}/k \qquad (7)$$

Where C_{last} is the plasma concentration at the latest measured time-point and k is the slope of the concentration–time curve (Fig. 2).

Compartmental models

In contrast to non-compartmental models, compartmental models involve assumptions about the distribution of the drug in the body, that is the body is assumed to be composed of one or more theoretical compartments. The drug is directly introduced into the blood or central compartment by intravenous administration, or it reaches the central compartment after extravascular administration, for example following oral, rectal, dermal, intrathecal, or intranasal application. Subsequently, the drug will be distributed homogeneously over a given volume, called the apparent volume of distribution.

In a one-compartment model it is assumed that the body is composed of one compartment and that after administration the drug is instantaneously distributed within this compartment. The volume of the distribution (V, units of volume i.e. l, l/m^2, or l/kg) is the apparent volume needed to account for all the drug in the body (A) given the concentration at time zero (C_0):

$$V = A/C_0 \qquad (8)$$

The decline of the plasma concentration in the elimination phase can be described by the linear equation:

$$\ln C = \ln C_0 - kt \qquad (9)$$

Where $\ln C$ is the natural logarithm of the plasma concentration at time t, C_0 is the plasma concentration at time 0, and k is the elimination rate constant (time^{-1}).

Equation 9 can be rewritten as:

$$C = C_0 \times e^{-kt} \qquad (10)$$

and by multiplying by V as:

$$A = Dose \times e^{-kt} \qquad (11)$$

Differentiating equation 10 results in:

$$dA/dt = -k Dose \times e^{-kt} \qquad (12)$$

and, by combining equations 11 and 12, in the important relationship:

$$dA/dt = -kA \qquad (13)$$

Equation 13 reveals that the rate of change of the amount of drug in the body is proportional to the amount present, which is termed a first-order process.

Equation 9 can be used to obtain the important terminal or elimination half-life ($t_{1/2}$), the time taken for the concentration in plasma to decrease by 50 per cent, that is for C_0 to drop to $0.5 \times C_0$.

$$t_{1/2} = (\ln C_0 - \ln [0.5 C_0])/k = \ln 2/k = 0.693/k \qquad (14)$$

For many drugs the shape of the plasma concentration–time curve shows a rapid initial decline followed by one or more slower phases. The initial decline represents distribution from the blood compartment to other tissues, and the terminal phase represents the elimination of the drug from the central compartment after redistribution of the drug back into the plasma. For most drugs, distribution to other tissues and diffusion back into the plasma are linear and passive processes determined by concentration gradients, tissue binding, the perfusion of deep tissues, and the permeability of tissue membranes. The plasma concentration at time 't' for a two-compartmental model after an intravenous bolus administration (Fig. 3) can be written by:

$$C_{(t)} = Ae^{-\alpha t} + Be^{-\beta t} \qquad (15)$$

and for a three-compartmental model by:

$$C_{(t)} = Ae^{-\alpha t} + Be^{-\beta t} + Ce^{-\gamma t} \qquad (16)$$

For a three-compartment model the AUC can be calculated by:

$$AUC = A/\alpha + B/\beta + C/\gamma \qquad (17)$$

The advantage of using compartmental pharmacokinetics is that modelling the concentration–time curve according to equations 15 or 16 enables assessment of a range of pharmacokinetic parameters as outlined, for example, in Fig. 3 for a two-compartmental model. The disadvantage is that if the pharmacokinetics of the drug are

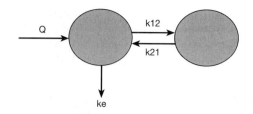

Fig. 3 Theoretical two-compartmental model with volume of distribution V_c of the central compartment and V_p of the peripheral or deep compartment and elimination rate constant k, and inter-compartmental rate constants k_{12} and k_{21}.

not optimally described by the chosen model, the AUC and other parameters defined in the model may be inaccurate.

An important prerequisite for an unbiased estimate of pharmacokinetic parameters is that clearance is due to non-saturable processes. However, elimination by metabolism, biliary, or renal tubular secretion may be saturable, and under these conditions the rate of change of the plasma concentration can be described by the Michaelis–Menten equation:

$$dC/dt = -Vmax \times C/(Km + C) \qquad (18)$$

Where Vmax is the maximum velocity of clearance and Km the Michaelis–Menten constant, a measure of the affinity of the metabolizing enzyme or transport protein for the drug.

If $C \gg Km$, equation 18 can be written as:

$$dC/dt = Vmax \qquad (19)$$

The rate of change of the plasma concentration when $C \gg Km$ is a constant equal to Vmax and independent of concentration C (a zero-order process and non-linear pharmacokinetics). Estimates of pharmacokinetic parameters tend to be biased under the circumstances of non-linear pharmacokinetics.

Physiological models

Compartmental pharmacokinetic models are based on the assumption that drug absorption and disposition can be described by one or more theoretical compartments. The true complexity of all associated pharmacokinetic processes is, however, far greater than can be described by these simple models. In physiological models, attempts are made to take normal or abnormal anatomic characteristics and physiological processes into consideration. Distribution characteristics for the organs of the body may be different from each other. In addition, the clearance of the drug from each organ may differ. Furthermore, blood flows and clearance from each organ are used instead of rate transfer constants. These characteristics are modelled in the physiological approach to pharmacokinetics and the resulting models are often very complex. Furthermore, physiological pharmacokinetic models require detailed experimental data to enable estimation of all parameters. One example of a physiological model is that described by Dedrick and colleagues for cisplatin.[3]

Population models

The population approach is a powerful alternative to classical or standard compartmental and non-compartmental pharmacokinetic

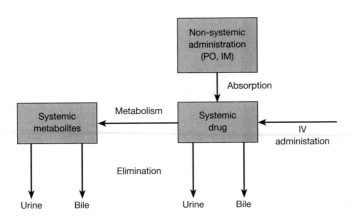

Fig. 4 Major mechanisms for the clearance of anticancer drugs.

models, and is based on statistical theory.[4] All drugs exhibit pharmacokinetic variability, and population pharmacokinetics describes this variability in terms of factors which are termed fixed and random effects.[4],[5] The fixed effects are the population average values of pharmacokinetic parameters and may be a function of demographic and biochemical characteristics, such as weight, height, age, gender, renal and liver function, as well as of environmental factors such as concomitant drug therapy. Random effects are those due to inter- and intrapatient variability, and quantify the amount of pharmacokinetic variability not explained by the fixed effects. Population analyses can be performed by applying the Non-linear Mixed Effects Model programme NONMEM (Beal and Sheiner 1980), which treats the population as a unit of analysis rather than the individual. In general, the population method requires less data per individual, but more individuals are needed for a useful analysis than in a classical pharmacokinetic study. Estimation of fixed and random effects allows the design of dosing regimens in subpopulations of patients at risk, for example those with renal or hepatic dysfunction, and adaptive dosing by using Bayesian feedback techniques.[5]

Drug clearance mechanisms

Anticancer drugs are cleared from the body by metabolism, renal elimination, and/or biliary clearance (Fig. 4).

Metabolism

Many drugs are lipid soluble and undergo biotransformation to more water soluble products prior to excretion in the urine and/or bile. The main site of drug metabolism is the liver, although other organs (e.g. the gut, lung, and kidney) can metabolize xenobiotics. In addition, many of the enzymes responsible for drug metabolism are also found in tumour tissue, although the significance of intratumoural drug metabolism is not well established. Drug metabolism can involve two different phases—phase I (oxidation) and phase II (conjugation). Some anticancer drugs are prodrugs, that is they have no inherent biological activity, and therefore require metabolic activation (e.g. cyclophosphamide, ifosfamide, dacarbazine, procarbazine, 5-fluorouracil, capecitabine, 6-mercaptopurines, cytosine arabinoside, gemcitabine).

The enzymes (mono-oxygenases or mixed function oxidases) responsible for oxidation and other analogous phase I reactions are sited in the hepatic endoplasmic reticulum and are collectively termed cytochrome P450, due to the presence of the iron-containing cytochrome (CYP) which absorbs light at 450 nm when complexed with carbon monoxide. Although phase I oxidative metabolites may be inert, many have biological activity. The classic example of drug metabolism in cancer chemotherapy is cyclophosphamide, which undergoes a complex series of metabolic steps forming at least six metabolites of varying cytotoxic (e.g. phosphoramide mustard) and toxic (e.g. acrolein) potential.[6] Products of phase I reactions (oxidized metabolites) may be excreted directly or further metabolized by conjugation (phase II metabolism). The activities of phase I enzymes can be increased by enzyme inducers (e.g. phenobarbitone, phenytoin, carbamazepine), or reduced by inhibitors (e.g. ketoconazole), and this forms the basis of some important drug interactions. For example the clearance of etoposide and busulfan can be more rapid in patients on anticonvulsants, leading to potentially subtherapeutic drug concentrations.[7]

Phase II conjugation reactions involve the addition of an endogenous group, such as glucuronic acid or sulphate, to the parent drug or its oxidized metabolite. Nearly all conjugates are inert; notable exceptions in cancer medicine are morphine 6-glucuronide and irinotecan glucuronide. Larger acidic conjugates, for example glucuronides, are excreted in the bile, whereas those with a molecular weight below 500 are usually excreted in the urine. Following biliary excretion, metabolites can be deconjugated by bacterial flora in the gut lumen and the parent drug or metabolite may then be reabsorbed.

Individual patients have their own complement of enzymes with overlapping substrate specificities. The levels of these enzymes are genetically controlled, but they are also effected by environmental factors, such as age, nutritional status, disease, smoking (tobacco and marijuana), alcohol consumption, and concomitant drugs. For example infants and young adults often eliminate drugs more rapidly than adults. Hepatic mono-oxygenase activity gradually diminishes in old age, but the activity of phase II enzymes appears to be maintained in the elderly. Oxidation reactions can be less efficient in the presence of severe metastatic liver disease and in malnourished patients. Conjugation mechanisms, however, are often preserved even in hepatic cirrhosis. Dosage adjustment in patients with liver disease is crude as abnormalities of hepatic function tests relates poorly to changes in metabolic capacity (see below).

Renal elimination

Drugs are handled by the kidneys in three major ways. For all drugs the free fraction in plasma is filtered at the glomerulus. In addition, some drugs are actively extracted from the plasma and secreted into the lumen of the proximal tubule, whereas others are passively reabsorbed in the distal tubule. Individual compounds may be subjected to one or more of these processes and active secretion increases the rate of renal clearance of drugs and passive reabsorption reduces it. Overall renal clearance is therefore equal to the sum of the rates of elimination by filtration and secretion minus the rate of reabsorption. Only the free drug fraction in the plasma can be filtered, and the renal clearance of a drug by filtration is therefore equal to the unbound fraction in plasma multiplied by the glomerular filtration rate. For active secretion there are separate transport systems for acids (e.g. methotrexate) and bases, and competition can occur between drugs utilizing these systems. For example probenecid will potentiate methotrexate toxicity, by competing for and reducing tubular secretion and hence renal clearance. Similarly, cimetidine can also block the tubular secretion of anticancer drugs. For carboplatin, whose renal clearance is solely due to glomerular filtration, renal function is used to individualize patient dosage (see below).

Biliary clearance

Drugs can be excreted by hepatocytes into the bile, usually as conjugates, and acidic drugs or metabolites with molecular weights exceeding 500 are likely to follow this route (e.g. irinotecan glucuronide). Biliary excretion provides a backup pathway when renal function is impaired. Reabsorption of drugs excreted in the bile may lead to an enterohepatic cycle which can maintain plasma levels and prolong their action.

Influence of protein binding

Once a drug reaches the systemic circulation it may be bound to circulating proteins, of which albumin is the most important although α_1-acid glycoprotein can be important for basic drugs (see below). Most drugs must be unbound (free) to have a pharmacological effect. However, protein binding is clinically relevant for only a few drugs of which the most important is etoposide.[8],[9] For protein binding to be of clinical relevance, three criteria must be met:

1. Plasma protein binding must be extensive and high affinity; if the drug is weakly or <90 per cent bound to plasma proteins, protein binding will have little impact on the amount of unbound drug in circulation (i.e. the amount of drug that is available for distribution to the site of action).

2. Tissue distribution must be limited; if the distribution of a drug into tissues is extensive drug displaced from plasma protein binding sites will be mopped-up by tissue binding.

3. Variation in binding must occur in patients; only when something changes the level of protein binding of a drug can its action change.

Factors which can alter protein binding include hypoalbuminaemia (albumin <25 g/l), renal failure (in which the affinity of proteins for drugs can be altered), and displacement by other drugs. Only following displacement by other drugs is the change in protein binding likely to be sudden. In the other cases, the changes are gradual and alone are unlikely to alter the effects of a drug, because clearance from the body will prevent the build up of a high free-drug concentration in the plasma. However, the above factors can alter the relationship between the total plasma concentration of a drug and its unbound concentration, which may not be detected in pharmacokinetic studies as most drug assays measure total, not free, drug concentrations.

Pharmacodynamic principles and parameters

Conventional drugs and conventional parameters

Toxicity parameters

Conventional anticancer drugs are cytotoxic agents, that is they exert their biological action by inducing tumour cell kill. Unfortunately, the cytotoxic effect is not specific to tumour cells and normal cells

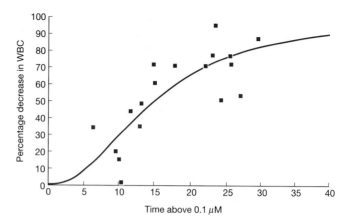

Fig. 5 Relationship between the pharmacokinetics (time-period above 0.1 μM in plasma) of paclitaxel and dose-limiting leucocytopenia (WBC).[10]

are also affected. Typically, rapidly dividing tissues, such as the bone marrow, the epithelial layer of the gastrointestinal tract, and hair follicles, are most sensitive to the effects of conventional anticancer agents. The classical toxicity profile therefore includes: myelosuppression (leucopenia, thrombocytopenia, and/or anaemia), nausea, vomiting, diarrhoea, and hair loss. Myelosuppression may be associated with clinical signs and symptoms, including infection and fever, nose bleeding, spontaneous haematomas, and fatigue, and results in a reduction of cell counts in the peripheral blood. The lowest level (nadir) of the leucocyte (granulocyte) and/or thrombocyte count is generally achieved at day 10 to 14, after which the counts recover to normal or baseline values. Hair loss can develop 14 to 21 days after the administration of the first cycle of chemotherapy, although not all conventional cytotoxic agents induce alopecia.

For many conventional anticancer drugs significant logarithmic or sigmoidal relations exist between the AUC and the per cent decrease in leucocyte and granulocyte counts. The latter is generally expressed as the per cent decrease in absolute neutrophil count (ANC):

$$\%NC = \frac{ANC\ at\ start - ANC\ at\ Nadir}{ANC\ at\ start} \times 100 \qquad (20)$$

Figure 5 shows an example of a pharmacokinetic–pharmacodynamic relationship for paclitaxel-induced leucopenia.[10]

Conventional anticancer drugs may also cause non-antiproliferative toxicities. For example cisplatin, vinca alkaloids, and taxanes induce sensory neuropathy. Neurotoxicity is typically related to the cumulative dose of the anticancer agent and can be disabling for a patient, extending to motor neurotoxicity if high cumulative doses are given. For cisplatin most patients experience sensory loss and paraesthesias after doses of more than 300 to 350 mg/m². Neurotoxicity may even increase after discontinuation of cisplatin therapy and reach a maximum at 3 to 6 months. Subsequently, the clinical signs tend to recover, at least partly. Ototoxicity is frequent following cisplatin, and results in tinnitus and progressive hearing loss, which is nonreversible. The development of neurotoxicity can show scheduledependency; paclitaxel infusions of long duration (24 h) are significantly less neurotoxic than the short infusions (1–3 h).

Other toxicities which may be induced by cytotoxic drugs include renal tubular damage and dysfunction (cisplatin), congestive heart failure (anthracyclines), diarrhoea (irinotecan), haemorrhagic cystitis (cyclophosphamide and ifosfamide), hepatic toxicity (gemcitabine, methotrexate), nail toxicity (taxanes), and hand-foot syndrome (5-fluorouracil). These drug-specific toxicities are often related to the cumulative dose and/or absolute dose per course and may not be related to the cytotoxic mechanism of action of the drug. Furthermore, subpopulations of patients may be at risk for certain toxicities due to a genetically determined inability to eliminate the drug, for example 5-fluorouracil treatment in patients with dihydropyrimidine dehydrogenase deficiency will induce severe diarrhoea and myelosuppression (see below).

Efficacy parameters

Tumour cell kill resulting in a reduction of tumour volume is the primary effect of conventional anticancer drugs. Therefore, direct tumour measurements are carried out at the start of treatment and during follow-up in order to monitor the clinical effect of therapy. Tumour response is defined as complete (100 per cent disappearance of all tumour) or partial (at least 50 per cent reduction of tumour volume), no change (i.e. stable disease), or progressive disease (at least 25 per cent increase in tumour volume compared to baseline). However, tumour shrinkage may not be an appropriate pharmacodynamic marker, particularly for drugs with non-cytotoxic mechanisms of action (see below).

As an alternative to tumour shrinkage, tumour markers can sometimes be used to monitor activity. Tumour markers are endogenous compounds, usually small glycoproteins, which are also present at low levels in certain normal tissues, where their cellular function is often unknown. Some markers reach high levels in fetal tissues (e.g. α-fetoprotein) or in placental tissue or during pregnancy (e.g. β-human chorionic gonadotrophin). Established and useful tumour markers for monitoring treatment include: α-fetoprotein and β-human chorionic gonadotrophin in germ cell tumours, CA125 in ovarian cancer, prostate specific antigen in prostate cancer, CA15.3 in breast cancer, carcinoembryonic antigen in colorectal cancer (and some other epithelial tumours), thyroglobulin in thyroid cancer, and α-fetoprotein in primary liver cell cancer. From a pharmacodynamic perspective, tumour markers can be extremely valuable as they may provide a quantitative measure of otherwise subclinical antitumour effects.

Drugs with novel non-cytotoxic mechanisms

Recent insights into the molecular and cellular pathology of cancer have provided a plethora of new targets against which to direct drug therapy. Drugs with novel targets are similar to conventional agents with respect to pharmacokinetics, that is they are subject to the same absorption, distribution, metabolism, and elimination pathways, but dissimilar in terms of pharmacodynamics. It is widely anticipated that drugs which exploit the molecular and cellular pathology of cancer should be markedly less toxic to normal tissues than cytotoxic agents, as well as having greater activity. As a consequence, the occurrence or absence of normal tissue toxicity due to antiproliferative action (e.g. haematological or gastrointestinal) cannot be used to determine whether or not, respectively, active drug levels are being achieved. Instead of normal tissue toxicity, drug-specific pharmacodynamic markers are needed to ensure that potentially active drug levels are being achieved and maintained. Summaries of recently developed therapeutics which attempt to exploit the molecular and cellular pathology of cancer have been published.[11]–[13]

Drugs directed at the molecular pathology of cancer

At the molecular genetic level, a contemporary view of cancer is that it is a disease in which there is loss of tumour suppresser gene function (by mutation or deletion, e.g. p53 and Rb), gain of oncogene expression (by mutation, amplification, or over-expression, e.g. ras and c-erbB-2), and activation of immortality genes (e.g. telomerase). Loss of p53 function is often cited as the most common genetic defect in cancer,[14] and one mechanism by which p53 causes cell cycle arrest is via the expression of peptide cyclin dependent kinase inhibitors, such as p21. Two small molecule inhibitors of cyclin dependent kinases that are in early clinical trials are flavopiridol and UCN-01, and the former had dose limiting toxicities of secretory diarrhoea and hypotension,[15] that is side-effects distinct from those of conventional cytotoxic drugs. Haematological toxicity was mild and sporadic. With the staurosporine derivative UCN-01, unpredicted high-affinity binding to human α₁-acid glycoprotein was encountered in the Phase I trial which resulted in very slow plasma clearance and a very small volume of distribution.[16] In contrast, UCN-01 was extensively distributed and rapidly cleared from the plasma in mice, rats, and dogs. This latter result illustrates how a conventional pharmacokinetic parameter, protein binding, can have a major impact on the properties of a novel cancer therapeutic. More generally, surrogate pharmacodynamic markers for cyclin dependent kinase inhibition would be valuable, and non-invasive detection of the inhibition of ^{11}C-thymidine incorporation by positron emission tomography (PET, see below) may be one approach.

A large number of inhibitors of mitogenic oncogene products have been developed and certain of these are in early clinical trials. For example, SU101 is an inhibitor of platelet-derived growth factor receptor tyrosine kinase, a growth factor receptor which is stimulated via an autocrine loop in glioblastoma.[17] In a Phase I clinical trial, SU101 was found to be rapidly converted to a metabolite (SU0020) which is a previously-described inhibitor of dihydro-orotate dehydrogenase, and hence an antiproliferative antimetabolite. This result illustrates the potential impact of pharmacokinetics, metabolism in this case, on the pharmacodynamics of compounds with novel mechanisms of action. A more generic approach to the inhibition of mitogenic oncogene signalling is the use of antisense oligonucleotides, and the anti-c-raf-1 antisense ISIS 5132 has recently undergone clinical evaluation.[18] The Phase I trial of ISIS 5132 did not define a maximally tolerated dose; however, it was nevertheless shown that there was a persistent reduction in c-raf-1 expression in peripheral blood mononuclear cells in two patients who experienced prolonged stable disease. In the case of antisense therapies, measurement of target gene transcript levels represents an exquisitely specific pharmacodynamic marker, although data on tumours are preferable to those from blood cells. More generally, the study with ISIS 5132 shows that with signal transduction modifiers it is not necessary to define or use maximally tolerated doses in order to achieve biological effects, which again contrasts with conventional clinical practice for cytotoxic drugs.

Drugs directed at the cellular pathology of cancer

To enable a primary tumour to reach a clinically-detectable size and establish secondary deposits angiogenesis and metastasis must take place, and a number of agents designed to prevent these events are in early clinical trials. The fumigillin analogue TNP-470 is an antiangiogenic drug where, in a Phase II trial in renal-cell cancer, only one partial response was observed in 33 patients.[19] This latter result illustrates the difficulty of evaluating the activity of compounds which, at best, prevent tumour growth and do not cause regressions. Ultimately, the use of such agents is likely to be in adjuvant treatment following primary therapy. However, it is unlikely that there will be a commitment to large Phase III trials in order to establish efficacy in the absence of convincing data from surrogate pharmacodynamic markers. In the case of the antiangiogenic and antimetastatic matrix metalloproteinase inhibitor Marimastat, attempts were made to use decreases in the rate of tumour marker rise in order to choose the appropriate dose for Phase III trials.[20] However, a subsequent Phase III trial in pancreatic cancer was negative, and the use of histological or imaging methods such as magnetic resonance (MR) or PET may provide more appropriate pharmacodynamic data for antiangiogenic drugs (see discussion by Boral et al.[12]).

In summary, it is already clear that pharmacological studies will also play a key role in the development of drugs targeted at the molecular and cellular pathology of cancer. In particular, robust and validated surrogate pharmacodynamic markers will be needed if these new agents are to be appropriately evaluated, and biopsy- or imaging-based early clinical trials may become mandatory.

Practical implications and applications of pharmacokinetics and pharmacodynamics in cancer chemotherapy

Conventional drugs in routine use

Variable absorption following extravascular drug administration

Inter- and intrapatient variation in pharmacokinetics after intravenous administration by bolus injection or infusion is caused by variability in drug disposition, that is distribution, metabolism, and elimination. However, after administration by an extravascular route variation in absorption kinetics can also contribute to the pharmacokinetic variability. Consequently, variability between and within patients is almost without exception more pronounced after administration of an extravascular dose than after intravenous administration of the same drug. The variability can be caused by a number of different mechanisms. For the oral route, instability at the pH values encountered in the gastrointestinal tract (e.g. melphalan), saturation of uptake (e.g. methotrexate), and poor dissolution characteristics (e.g. etoposide) can result in variable systemic exposure. Interaction with food components or other drugs may also significantly increase variability. Furthermore, partial or complete gastrectomy, or motility disorders may result in reduced or slower absorption of oral drugs.

A recently identified source of low and variable oral bioavailability is the affinity of certain drugs (e.g. etoposide and paclitaxel) for the membrane-bound drug transporter P-glycoprotein. Similarly, high affinity for the cytochrome P450 drug metabolizing enzyme system, and in particular for the CYP3A family, may also contribute to interpatient variability in systemic exposure after oral administration. Combined with P-glycoprotein (and possibly other but as yet unidentified drug transporters), cytochrome P450 constitutes a highly efficient system which protects the body from exposure to xenobiotics. During the first-pass through the liver high and variable extraction of a drug can result in variable and low systemic exposure. However, first pass metabolism can also result in the formation of toxic metabolites. For example oral ifosfamide appears to result in the formation of a neurotoxic first-pass metabolite, possibly chloroacetaldehyde, and hence the drug should not be given via this route.

Although oral administration is convenient, the use of this route is limited to a relatively small number of cytotoxic drugs that display consistent and adequate bioavailabilty (i.e. chlorambucil, temozolomide, low-dose methotrexate, and mecaptopurine). Non-cytotoxic anticancer drugs requiring protracted dosing would definitely benefit from being given orally (e.g. antiangiogenic and antimetastatic agents) and novel approaches may extend the list of cytotoxic agents that can be given by this route (see below).

Drug interactions

Although anticancer agents are one of the most toxic classes of medications prescribed, there is relatively little information available about clinically-relevant drug interactions.[21] Pharmacokinetic drug interactions have been described, including alterations in absorption, catabolism, and excretion. For example the bioavailability of 6-mercaptopurine is increased by coadministration of allopurinol or methotrexate. Induction of etoposide, teniposide, and busulfan clearance by anticonvulsants results in a lower systemic exposure that could reduce efficacy. As indicated above, alterations in methotrexate renal elimination have been observed with concurrent probenecid administration. Pharmacodynamic interactions at the cellular levels have also been described with a number of anticancer drug combinations, for example 5-fluorouracil and methotrexate; however, only rarely have clinical correlates been established, for example the greater potency, and possibly activity, of 5-fluorouracil when administered with folinic acid. Although drug interactions among commonly used anticancer agents have been identified, this remains an under-investigated area of anticancer pharmacology.

Pharmacogenetics

Variable drug metabolism due to a genetic basis is often called polymorphic drug metabolism because of the identification of multiple clinical groups with a unique pattern of elimination. For example, early studies with isoniazid identified slow and fast acetylators who were susceptible to different pharmacological and toxic effects. However, there are relatively few examples of relevance to oncology (Table 1).[22] Approximately 10 per cent of Caucasian populations are heterozygous for low thiopurine methyltransferase activity, while 1/300 are completely deficient.[23] Such completely deficient individuals cannot metabolize 6-mercaptopurine or azathioprine efficiently, leading to severe or fatal haematological toxicity. A less frequent, but equally important, polymorphism involves 5-fluorouracil inactivation by dihydropyrimidine dehydrogenase.[24] The molecular basis for many of these poor metabolizer phenotypes has been detailed and DNA-based tests using the polymerase chain reaction (PCR) are

Table 1 Clinically important drug metabolism polymorphisms

Enzymes	Number of drug substrates	Poor metabolizers (Caucasians)	Human gene cloned?	Clinical substrates /probes
Debrisoquin hydroxylase (CYP2D6)	>30	5–10%	yes	dextromethorphan
N-acetyltransferase	>15	50%	yes	caffeine
Mephenytoin hydroxylase (CYP2C19)	3–5	5%	yes	omeprazole
Thiopurine methyltransferase	>3	0.33%	yes	6-mercaptopurine
Dihydropyrimidine dehydrogenase	2 +	1–3%?	yes	5-fluorouracil

available at research centres. The frequency of poor metabolizers for many of these polymorphic enzymes differs significantly between ethnic groups. For example, 2 per cent of Southwest Asians subjects (Indian, Pakistani, Sri Lankan) are heterozygous for low thiopurine methyltransferase activity alleles compared to 10 per cent of British Caucasians.

Influence of renal and hepatic insufficiency

A large number of factors can lead to variation in the pharmacokinetics of anticancer agents, including patient age, hepatic metastases, prior therapy, and nutritional status. In patients with renal impairment, dosages of drugs which usually undergo extensive renal elimination (>50 per cent) should be reduced. Such drugs include methotrexate, cisplatin, and carboplatin (see below). In addition, previous therapy with cisplatin, and to a lesser extent methotrexate, can predispose a patient to poor renal function and altered pharmacokinetics. Measurement of hepatic dysfunction is less accurate than measurement of renal function. Liver function test values 3 to 5 times that of normal can be associated with greater systemic exposure (reduced clearance) for drugs with a high degree of hepatic metabolism, but liver function tests cannot be readily used to individualize patient therapy.[25] Elevated bilirubin concentrations are also used as general criteria for dosage modifications, but have not been developed into accurate guidelines. More quantitative approaches, such as the MEGX (monoethylglycinexylidide) test, have shown correlation with systemic clearance and may be useful strategies for optimizing drugs whose pharmacological activity is heavily influenced by liver function.

Dose selection and pharmacologically-guided dosing

Pharmacologically-guided dosing (PGD) seeks to use pharmacological data to select the most appropriate drug(s), dose(s), and schedule(s) for the treatment of each patient, with the aim of maximizing the chances of activity whilst at the same time minimizing the risk of unacceptable toxicity. In practice, the selection of drugs is primarily based on prior clinical experience of the treatment of similar patients, both with respect to the tumour (type, stage, and grade) and the characteristics of the individual (e.g. age, prior therapy, intercurrent

disease, etc.). In selecting agents for combination therapy, demonstrated single agent activity and non-overlapping toxicities, mechanisms of action, and resistance profiles are the primary factors taken into account.

Chemosensitivity testing is an alternative approach to prior experience in the selection of drugs, in which tumour cells from each patient are screened *ex vivo* for sensitivity to a broad range of agents and the most active drugs subsequently used to treat the patient.[26] However, the majority of patients entered onto prospective chemosensitivity testing trials have failed, for a variety of reasons, to receive the drug treatment identified *in vitro* as being potentially the most active. Furthermore, in those patients who did receive the drug(s) which were predicted to be the most active, the impact on overall survival was often not adequately addressed. Given the additional complication of how best to perform the *in vitro* equivalent of combination therapy, and the difficulty of interpreting data from combination experiments, it is unlikely that chemosensitivity testing in cancer chemotherapy will ever assume the role it has in antimicrobial therapy.

Once a drug or drug combination has been chosen, the schedule and dose must be selected. For the majority of cytotoxic drugs, the need to administer doses that are toxic to normal dividing tissues dictates the use of intermittent cycles of therapy, such as the very common 3 or 4-week dosing interval to allow for bone marrow recovery (see above). Within each cycle, bolus, daily, or infusional therapy can be used and the choice is dictated by the class of drug, as well as patient convenience and resource issues. For most alkylating agents and platinum complexes, the choice of administration schedule does not influence the maximally tolerated dose greatly, whereas for antimetabolites infusional administration often decreases the maximally tolerated dose and may alter the dose limiting toxicity, for example in the case of 5-fluorouracil. With antibiotics and plant alkaloids (topoisomerase inhibitors and tubulin binding agents) the impact of the schedule of administration on the maximally tolerated dose and the nature of the dose limiting toxicity is compound specific.[27]

Having identified the drug and the schedule of administration, the next step is to prescribe the dose to be given, and there are three general options:

(1) empirical dosing;

(2) adaptive dosing;

(3) empirical or adaptive dosing with feedback control.

In empirical dosing, all patients receive the same absolute dose of a drug (e.g. in mg or g), and this is the standard method of treating adults with most diseases other than cancer. With adaptive dosing, the characteristics of each patient are considered prior to therapy and the information used to select what is predicted to be the most appropriate dose for each individual. Examples of factors that can be used in adaptive dosing are age, renal and hepatic function, and concomitant drug therapy; surrogates for body size, drug elimination, and drug interactions, respectively.

Cancer chemotherapy is unusual in that body surface area is widely used as a parameter for adaptive dosing. The rationale for using surface area stems from the observation that, for cytotoxic drugs, maximally tolerated doses in different species are similar if doses are normalized to surface area (e.g. mg/m^2), but highly discrepant if body-weight-normalized (e.g. mg/kg) or absolute (e.g. mg) doses are compared. The pharmacological basis for the comparability of surface-area-normalized maximally tolerated doses is two-fold; factors which affect drug clearance such as tissue blood flow, renal function, hepatic function, and metabolic rate scale according to surface area, as does the extracellular fluid volume and hence volume of distribution. It should be noted that not all cytotoxic drugs have comparable mg/m^2 maximally tolerated doses across species, antimetabolites being a notable exception due to the requirement for intracellular activation, and their modulation by endogenous DNA precursors (nucleosides and bases).

Although adaptive dosing using surface area is still standard practice in cancer chemotherapy, its use is based largely on habit rather than evidence of clinical benefit,[28] with the important exception of paediatric oncology where doses obviously need to be scaled to body size. Thus, in adults, it would almost certainly be as safe, and certainly more simple and cost effective, if initial drug doses were absolute (i.e. fixed total mg doses). Subsequent dosing of each patient should be based on experience gained during the first cycle of therapy, and this is the third approach to dosing; empirical or adaptive dosing with feedback control.

Empirical or adaptive dosing with feedback control uses pharmacodynamic and/or pharmacokinetic data from the first cycle of therapy to adjust doses on subsequent courses. The most commonly used pharmacodynamic parameter is toxicity, and doses are often reduced in the face of unacceptable side-effects. However the converse, dose escalation in the face of insufficient toxicity, rarely happens and as a result many tumours may be under-treated due to under-dosing. Guidelines for the systematic use of toxicity to guide feedback dosing in cancer chemotherapy have been proposed; that is prime dose, modified dose, and toxicity-adjusted dose (PMT dosing),[29] although these have yet to be widely adopted. Due to the delay between dosing and antitumour effects as measured by conventional clinical endpoints (e.g. tumour shrinkage), it is not possible to use activity to guide dosing. However, imaging techniques such as PET and MR may in the future allow real-time efficacy monitoring and dose adjustment (see below).

Feedback control using pharmacokinetic data (also termed therapeutic drug monitoring) is based on the observation that there are large interindividual differences in drug clearance for most drugs, typically three-fold for the majority of patients and 10-fold at the extremes. The implication of such pharmacokinetic variability is that,

given equivalent tumour and normal tissue sensitivity, optimal doses may vary by a factor of 10 between individuals. Indeed, it has been argued that rather than defining maximally tolerated doses in Phase I clinical trials with cytotoxic drugs, maximum tolerated systemic exposures should be identified.[30] Maximum tolerated systemic exposures can have units of AUC, steady state, or time above a given plasma concentration. The only cancer drug that is routinely dosed on the basis of systemic exposure is the platinum complex carboplatin,[31] where adaptive dosing on the basis of pretreatment renal function is used to identify the absolute dose needed for each patient (see below). Only in exceptional cases (e.g. anephric patients and those with variable renal function) is it necessary with carboplatin to use feedback control as well.

Pharmacologically-guided dosing in Phase I–II trials

Phase I–II trials are the first time a new drug or drug combination is subjected to clinical evaluation. Endpoints in early clinical trials with cytotoxic drugs have historically been the identification of the maximally tolerated dose and dose limiting toxicity (Phase I) and the level of activity in defined tumour types (Phase II). However, these endpoints are no longer appropriate, particularly for non-cytotoxic drugs, and more contemporary endpoints for Phase I–II trials, which could be more appropriately described as pharmacological studies, are:

(1) definition of the relationship between drug dose and pharmacokinetics, both in patients and in relation to preclinical data;

(2) demonstration that systemic drug levels can be achieved that are associated with activity in preclinical models;

(3) confirmation of drug–target interaction, preferably in tumour tissue;

(4) description of pharmacokinetic–pharmacodynamic relationships.

On the basis of such information, it should be possible to conclude whether or not the new treatment is likely to effect its intended target at tolerated doses, and hence whether or not further clinical evaluation is warranted.[32],[33] Pharmacokinetic information is also of practical value in guiding dose escalation in early clinical trials, where it is important to minimize the number of patients treated with doses that are too low to be potentially active or alternatively too high to be safe.[34] During the latter stages of early clinical trials, it may be possible to use population analyses to identify pharmacokinetic–pharmacodynamic relationships, and recent studies with docetaxel are an excellent example.[35]

Pharmacologically-guided dosing (PGD) in Phase II–III trials and routine practice

Realization that interindividual differences in drug clearance result in some patients receiving inadequate doses and others toxic doses, when treatment is based solely on surface area, has led to PGD Phase II-III trials. In these trials PGD in the form of adaptive dosing (on the basis of surface area) with feedback control (on the basis of plasma drug clearance data) has been compared to conventional surface area-based dosing. As a prelude to PGD trials it is necessary to establish that there is:

(1) significant interpatient variation in drug clearance, and that interpatient variation exceeds intrapatient variability;

(2) a relationship between pharmacokinetic and pharmacodynamic (response or toxicity) variability;

(3) a clinically-feasible method of drug level monitoring and dose adjustment (i.e. PGD);

(4) less variation in systemic drug exposure (AUC, steady state levels, Cmax, or trough) when PGD is implemented.

If these four criteria are not met then PGD is unlikely to be superior in terms of outcome (efficacy and/or toxicity) than surface area-based dosing. Landmark studies by Evans and colleagues in the treatment of childhood acute lymphoblastic leukaemia (ALL) are an excellent example of the application of PGD where, in a randomized Phase III trial, it was shown that PGD with methotrexate, teniposide, and cytarabine improved outcome in children with B-lineage disease.[36] In other studies, for example cisplatin and 5-fluorouracil for the treatment of head and neck cancer,[37] PGD has resulted in more consistent and manageable toxicity without compromising antitumour activity.

As indicated previously, carboplatin is the only drug in routine clinical use where dosing is based on a target systemic exposure (AUC), rather than surface area-based or absolute doses. During early clinical trials it was recognized that there was substantial inter-individual variation in the clearance of carboplatin, and that the variation was due to differences in renal function. It was shown that renal elimination was the major route of carboplatin clearance (>80 per cent of the dose in individuals with normal renal function), and that the mechanism of renal elimination was glomerular filtration. These pharmacokinetic data allowed a simple dosing formula to be defined which gives the absolute carboplatin dose (mg) required to achieve a target AUC (mg/ml $\times$ min)[31]:

$$\text{Dose (mg)} = \text{Target AUC (mg/ml} \times \text{min)} \times [\text{GFR (ml/min)} + 25] \qquad (21)$$

Where GFR is the glomerular filtration rate and 25 is a constant (in adults) to account for non-renal clearance. Particular attention needs to be paid to the method used to determine the GFR, and estimates calculated on the basis of plasma creatinine alone can give inaccurate and biased results. A number of studies have shown that GFR-based dosing results in more predictable carboplatin AUC values and toxicity, and GFR-based dosing is now the recommended way to administer the drug.[38]

Molecular determinants of anticancer drug pharmacodynamics

As depicted in Fig. 6, the relationship between the dose of a drug and the ultimate clinical outcome of treatment is influenced by factors that are both 'upstream' and 'downstream' of the drug target. Upstream factors include systemic pharmacokinetics, cellular transport, and intracellular activation and inactivation. Downstream factors are those that determine the response of a cell to a given level and duration of drug–target interaction, and amongst these factors apoptotic propensity as dictated by tumour suppresser gene status may be particularly important. In the case of downstream factors, molecular lesions responsible for tumour development, that is tumour suppresser gene loss and/or oncogene activation, may also influence

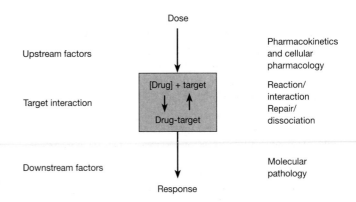

Fig. 6 Schematic representation of the factors which influence the relationship between drug dose and tumour response.

response to therapy. In addition to upstream and downstream factors, the level and structure of the drug target, and the reversibility of drug–target interactions (e.g. DNA repair), can also determine activity.

A large number of studies have attempted to define the prognostic significance of upstream factors, drug target levels, and downstream parameters for specific drug treatments. Whilst to date these studies have been largely correlative in nature, it is widely predicted that in the future such information will be used to select the drugs, schedules, and doses needed to treat each patient's tumour most effectively. In the following sections specific examples are given where information on drug target levels and downstream determinants of response is being, or could be, used to guide therapy. Cellular upstream factors are usually described as drug resistance mechanisms, and examples of clinically-relevant parameters are described in Chapter 4.20.

Drug target levels

The antimetabolite 5-fluorouracil is one of the most extensively used and studied cancer drugs. 5-Fluorouracil displays activity in breast and gastrointestinal malignancies and has at least three potential loci of action: inhibition of thymidylate synthase following conversion to fluorodeoxyuridine monophosphate (FdUMP), incorporation into RNA as fluorouridine triphosphate (FUTP), and uptake into DNA as fluorodeoxyuridine triphosphate (FdUTP). The observation that response rates in colorectal cancer are generally increased by the coadministration of folinic acid (leucovorin), biochemical modulation that increases thymidylate synthase inhibition, suggests that thymidylate synthase is an important target for 5-fluorouracil in patients. Thus the relationship between response to 5-fluorouracil-based therapy and thymidylate synthase levels has been investigated in a number of studies and a consensus is emerging that low thymidylate synthase levels are related to a better outcome in established disease.[39]–[41]

A more contemporary example of the importance of the drug target levels is c-erbB-2 expression in breast cancer. The expression of c-erbB-2 is associated with poor prognosis in breast cancer. However, the anti-c-erbB-2 monoclonal antibody trastuzumab has been shown to have activity as a single agent and in combination with cytotoxic drugs that is superior to cytotoxic drug treatment alone.[42],[43] FDA-approved methods of measuring c-erbB-2 expression have been defined[44] and, in general, advances in molecular diagnostics will need to keep pace with therapeutics if new agents are to be rationally used in routine practice.

Oncogene expression

In addition to being novel targets for therapeutic intervention, oncogene expression can also influence the outcome of treatment with conventional cytotoxic drugs. For example retrospective analyses of two large series of breast cancer patients suggest that c-erbB-2 expression confers sensitivity to doxorubicin containing therapy, in a dose-dependent manner.[45],[46] However, the reasons for the association between c-erbB-2 expression and chemosensitivity have not been defined, and for other oncogenes no such relationships have been observed, for example K-ras mutations in lung cancer and response to ifosfamide, carboplatin, and etoposide.[47]

Tumour suppresser gene status and apoptotic propensity

Although p53 is well established as the tumour suppressor gene whose function is most frequently disrupted in human cancers, its role as a prognostic indicator and determinant of response to cytotoxic therapy remains controversial.[14] In human tumour cell lines, in vitro sensitivity to the majority of DNA-interactive cytotoxic drugs is enhanced by the presence of a functional p53 pathway.[48] However, retrospective analyses of the relationship between p53 status and outcome in clinical trials have produced conflicting results.[49] Two factors that could obscure potential relationships are the nature of the p53 assay used (e.g. immunohistochemistry, partial or complete gene sequencing) and the type and numbers of cytotoxic drugs in the chemotherapy. In two studies using single agent therapy and gene sequencing, that is doxorubicin for breast cancer[50] and carboplatin for ovarian cancer,[51] higher response rates were observed in patients with wild-type p53. The addition of taxanes (paclitaxel or docetaxel) to combinations used in breast and ovarian cancer may limit the value of prospective trials to evaluate p53-based therapy stratification, as the activity of the taxanes does not appear to be influenced by p53 status.[48] An additional complication with p53-based treatment stratification is that activation of wild-type p53 can either cause apoptosis or cell cycle arrest, in a cell-type-specific manner, and it is not clear which of these events relate to clinical response. Although p53 pathway function is undoubtedly an important potential pharmacodynamic determinant of drug action, it is not clear at present how best to use a knowledge of p53 status in the management of individual patients.

Whilst p53 has been the major focus of studies on relationships between the molecular pathology of tumours and chemosensitivity, other important apoptotic pathways and factors have also been identified. For example, pro-(e.g. bax) and anti-(e.g. bcl-2) apoptotic factors which regulate cytochrome C-mediated caspase activation have been shown in some cases to be related to response or resistance, respectively.[52] The concept of a tumour cell being inherently resistant to apoptosis, and hence to chemotherapy, would be consistent with clinical experience; however, it is not clear how current cytotoxic treatment options would be guided by such information.

Novel approaches to optimizing and studying pharmacokinetics and pharmacodynamics in cancer chemotherapy

Optimizing oral administration

Absorption enhancement

Recently, a number of mechanisms underlying the poor oral bioavailability of anticancer drugs have been unravelled (see above). This understanding has initiated research to optimize oral administration through the development of pro-drugs and/or the coadministration of selective absorption enhancers. One of the successful approaches has been the development of the 5-fluorouracil prodrug capecitabine, which undergoes enzymatic conversion in the gut and liver to 5'dFCR, and in tumour and liver into the 5-fluorouracil prodrug 5'dFUR by cytidine deaminase. Subsequently, metabolism by pyrimidine nucleoside phosphorylase, which is expressed at high levels in tumour tissue, results in formation of 5-fluorouracil.[53] Other approaches designed to improve the oral bioavailability of 5-fluorouracil are coadministration with inhibitors of the pyrimidine catabolizing enzyme, dihydropyrimidine dehydrogenase (e.g. ethynyluracil), or the use of a 5-fluorouracil prodrug (e.g. UFT).

Combinations of oral anticancer drugs which have high affinities for P-glycoprotein (e.g. paclitaxel and docetaxel) and a P-glycoprotein blocker, such as cyclosporin A, can also significantly increase systemic exposure.[54] Similarly, for drugs with a high affinity for CYP3A, coadministration of an effective CYP3A inhibitor can substantially increase systemic exposure, and may reduce interpatient AUC variability. For example the HIV protease inhibitor ritonavir is an effective CYP3A inhibitor which has been used to increase the systemic exposure of the coadministered protease inhibitor saquinavir.

Patient compliance

For oral drugs, non-compliance represents a major source of variability in pharmacokinetics. Non-compliance can be multifactorial: permanent or temporary discontinuation of drug intake, or inadequate scheduling of intake. Non-compliance can be substantially reduced by careful instruction of the patient, use of diary cards, home psychological support, and exercise in pill taking.[53] Electronic devises are available for checking compliance, and assessment of urinary drug and/or metabolite levels can also be helpful.

Novel approaches to studying plasma pharmacokinetics

Population methodology and limited sampling models

Population pharmacokinetic–pharmacodynamic analyses allow assessment of the clinical relevance of pharmacokinetic variability and the identification of subpopulations at risk of over- or underexposure. The population approach is based on the analysis of a large data set of patients with, generally, sparse sampling (1–4 blood samples) of each patient. As an example, application of population analyses during the development of docetaxel in 640 patients revealed important pharmacokinetic–pharmacodynamic relationships.[35] First course AUC was a significant predictor of febrile neutropenia and of time to progression in patients with non-small cell lung cancer. In addition, clearance of docetaxel was reduced in patients with moderate hepatic dysfunction. Consequently, these patients are at increased risk of developing neutropenia and dose adjustments should be made at start of treatment (i.e. adaptive dosing based on hepatic function). The population approach is increasingly regarded as an essential tool in the drug development process.

Analytical methodology

The provision of reliable pharmacokinetic data requires analytical methodology that is:

1. Specific—the compound being detected should be the intended analyte.

2. Precise, accurate, and unbiased—the concentration determined should be the true value.

3. Sensitive—pharmacologically active concentrations should be detectable.

4. Reproducible—the concentration of drug detected in a given sample should be the same regardless of the analytical run in which it is determined.

Appropriate guidelines for these criteria have been published.[55]

Most analytical methods combine a chromatographic separation (e.g. liquid–solid or gas–liquid chromatography) with spectral detection (e.g. UV or mass spectroscopy). Although instrumentation of increasing sophistication and sensitivity is being developed, an additional feature of an analytical method is that it should be robust. High performance liquid chromatography (HPLC) with UV detection is a well tried and tested method, and satisfies the above criteria for most anticancer drugs. HPLC is ideally suited to the analysis of drugs in biological fluids such as plasma and urine, and for compounds that lack a UV chromophore, or where additional sensitivity is required, on-line mass spectrometry is increasingly the method of detection of choice.

Novel approaches for studying tumour pharmacokinetics and pharmacodynamics

Pharmacological studies have conventionally been restricted to those that can be performed with readily accessible body fluids such as blood and urine. While such studies can give information on systemic pharmacology (e.g. total body pharmacokinetics and normal tissue pharmacodynamics), they do not generally provide data on tumour drug concentrations or the interaction of a drug with its intended target in cancer cells. Without such tumour data it is not possible to interpret fully the results of clinical trials. For example, a drug could be inactive clinically because of an inadequate level and/or duration of drug target interaction, and in such a case the drug target could still valid for intervention. Conversely, the observation of clinical activity does not validate a drug target, as the compound may be acting via an alternative mechanism. As indicated previously, for novel compounds that act by non-cytotoxic mechanisms where tumour shrinkage cannot be expected, tumour pharmacodynamic studies are essential during the early stages of clinical development and there are two approaches to obtaining such data: tumour biopsy studies and non-invasive imaging.

Tumour biopsy studies

Histopathological studies on tumour material taken at diagnosis remain the mainstay of cancer diagnosis. The use of light microscopy provides information on tissue structure and morphology, and the advent of immunohistochemistry has allowed the expression of specific cancer-related proteins to be determined. Where these proteins are drug targets (e.g. erbB-2, see above), the information can be used to select patients for specific therapies. An advantage of immuno-histochemistry is that it provides information on the distribution of protein levels across a tumour sample; however, a limitation is that only a small number of proteins can be studied. One approach to broadening the number of targets measured is to study mRNAs and use genomic technologies (e.g. DNA chips) to detect levels of thousands of gene transcripts.[56] Coupled to evolving proteomic techniques and laser microdissection to study specific areas within tumours, molecular tumour profiling can provide information on each patient's tumour which could then be used to stratify therapies.[57] Ultimately, it is anticipated that the therapies offered to a patient will be ones targeted to the specific molecular lesions detected by tumour profiling.

In order to obtain post-treatment pharmacological data, it is necessary in most settings to undertake a second biopsy procedure, which has associated with it risks and ethical issues. The notable exception is leukaemia and there are many excellent examples of pharmacological studies on leukaemic cells with antimetabolites that have led to clinical studies of PGD, for example those with methotrexate[58] and cytarabine,[59] and also preliminary data with alkylating agents.[60]

Non-invasive methodology

The alternative to post-treatment biopsies for pharmacological studies of tumour tissue is the use of non-invasive imaging techniques. The two methodologies that are currently available are magnetic resonance imaging and spectroscopy (MRI/MRS), and positron emission tomography (PET). The two techniques are complimentary, and both have their strengths and weaknesses. MRI can provide information on structure and, following the administration of paramagnetic tracers such as Gd-DTPA to measure blood flow, function. MRS can provide information on the distribution of drugs within the body and their chemical form; however, the technique has inherently poor sensitivity (mM drug concentrations are generally required) and the drug must contain a paramagnetic nucleus at a high abundance. The most abundant isotope of fluorine (^{19}F) is paramagnetic and as a consequence fluorine-containing drugs, notably 5-fluorouracil, have been popular choices for MRS studies. A major advantage of MR is that it does not require the administration of radioactive isotopes and hence avoids the associated health and regulatory issues. An example where MRS has been shown to provide useful tumour pharmacokinetic data in patients is the detection of 5-flurouracil retention in the tumours of patients responding to drug treatment, as opposed to those who did not.[61]

In contrast to MRS, PET is extremely sensitive, requiring only tracer doses to give detectable signals. Furthermore, the simultaneous emission of two γ-rays at 180 degrees on positron annihilation allows excellent spatial resolution and localization of the isotope within the patient. However, PET does require the administration of radioactivity and the half-lives of the more widely used isotopes are very short, for example ^{18}F 110 min and ^{11}C 20 min. Such rapid radiochemical decomposition places severe constraints on the synthetic chemistry that can be used for PET labelling, and the duration of studies once the isotope has been administered to the patient. A generic antiproliferative pharmacodynamic PET marker is ^{11}C-thymidine, which is currently being evaluated in patients, and ^{18}F-5-fluorouracil has already been used to study the biochemical modulation of the drug in tumours in patients by N-(phosphonoacetyl)-L-aspartic acid (PALA), folinic acid, and α-interferon.[62] Given the potential of both ^{19}F-MR and ^{18}F-PET, there is a strong case for the inclusion of a fluorine atom at a pharmacologically innocuous and synthetically accessible site in all drug molecules.

Conclusion

For the foreseeable future chemotherapy will continue to be the only realistic means of treating the majority of patients with disseminated cancer. An understanding and the application of pharmacological principles, as outlined and illustrated in this chapter, will be central to both the optimization of the use of existing drugs and the introduction of new agents designed to exploit the molecular and cellular pathology of cancer.

References

1. **Rowland M, Tozer THN.** *Clinical pharmacokinetics: concepts and applications.* 3rd edn. Baltimore: Williams and Wilkins, 1995.

2. **Gibaldi M, Perrier D.** *Pharmacokinetics.* 2nd edn. New York: Marcel Dekker, 1982.

3. **Farris FF, Dedrick RL, King FG.** Cisplatin pharmacokinetics: Applications of a physiological model. *Toxicology Letters,* 1888; **43**: 117–37.

4. **Beal SL, Sheiner LB.** The NONMEM system. *American Statistician,* 1980; **34**: 118–9.

5. **Whiting B, Kelman AW, Grevel J.** Population pharmacokinetics. Theory and clinical practice. *Clinical Pharmacokinetics,* 1986; **11**: 387–401.

6. **Ren S, Kalhorn TF, McDonald GB, Anasetti C, Appelboum FR, Slattery JT.** Pharmacokinetics of cyclophosphamide and its metabolites in bone marrow transplantation patients. *Clinical Pharmacology and Therapeutics,* 1998; **64**: 289–301.

7. **Rodman JH, Murry DJ, Madden T, Santana VM.** Altered etoposide pharmacokinetics and time to engraftment in pediatric patients undergoing autologous bone marrow transplantation. *Journal of Clinical Oncology,* 1994; **12**: 2390–7.

8. **Joel SP, Shah R, Clark PI, Slevin ML.** Predicting etoposide toxicity: relationship to organ function and protein binding. *Journal of Clinical Oncology,* 1996; **14**: 257–67.

9. **Stewart CF, Arbuck SG, Fleming RA, Evans WE.** Changes in the clearance of total and unbound etoposide in patients with liver dysfunction. *Journal of Clinical Oncology,* 1990; **8**: 1874–9.

10. **Huizing MT, et al.** Pharmacokinetics of paclitaxel and metabolites in a randomised comparative study in platinum-pretreated ovarian cancer patients. *Journal of Clinical Oncology,* 1993; **11**: 2127–35.

11. **Baringa M.** From bench top to bedside. *Science,* 1997; **278**: 1036–9.

12. **Boral AL, Dessain S, Chabner BA.** Clinical evaluation of biologically targeted drugs: obstacles and opportunities. *Cancer Chemotherapy and Pharmacology,* 1998; **42** (Suppl. 2):S3–21.

13. **Fahraeus R, Fischer P, Krausz, Lane DP.** New approaches to cancer therapies. *Journal of Pathology,* 1999; **187**: 138–46.

14. **Kirsch DG, Kastan MB.** Tumor-suppressor p53: implications for tumor development and prognosis. *Journal of Clinical Oncology,* 1998; **16**: 3158–68.

15. **Senderowicz AM, et al.** Phase I trial of continuous infusion flavopiridol, a novel cyclin-dependent kinase inhibitor, in patients with refractory neoplasms. *Journal of Clinical Oncology,* 1998; **16**: 2986–99.

16. **Fuse E, et al.** Unpredicted clinical pharmacology of UCN-01 caused by specific binding to human α_1-acid glycoprotein. *Cancer Research,* 1998; **58**: 3248–53.

17. **Eckhardt SG, et al.** Phase I and pharmacologic study of the tyrosine kinase inhibitor SU101 in patients with advanced solid tumours. *Journal of Clinical Oncology,* 1999; **17**: 1095–104.

18. **Stevenson JP, et al.** Phase I clinical/pharmacokinetic and pharmacodynamic trial of the c-*raf*-1 antisense oligonucleotide ISIS 5132 (CGP 69846A). *Journal of Clinical Oncology,* 1999; **17**: 2227–36.

19. **Stadler WM, Kuzel T, Shapiro C, Sosman J, Vlark J, Vogelzang NJ.** Multi-institutional study of the angiogenesis inhibitor TNP-470 in metastatic renal carcinoma. *Journal of Clinical Oncology,* 1999; **17**: 2541–5.

20. **Nemunaitis J, et al.** Combined analysis of studies of the effects of the matrix metalloproteinase inhibitor Marimastat on serum tumor markers in advanced cancer: Selection of a biologically active and tolerable dose for longer-term studies. *Clinical Cancer Research,* 1998; **4**: 1101–9.

21. **McLeod HL.** Clinically relevant drug-drug interactions in oncology. *British Journal of Clinical Pharmacology,* 1998; **45**: 539–44.

22. **Iyer L, Ratain MJ.** Pharmacogenetics and cancer chemotherapy. *European Journal of Cancer,* 1998; **34**: 1493–9.

23. **Lennard L.** Therapeutic drug monitoring of antimetabolic cytotoxic drugs. *British Journal of Clinical Pharmacology,* 1999; **47**: 131–43.

24. **Milano G, McLeod HL.** Can dihydropyrimidine dehydrogenase impact 5FU-based treatment? *European Journal of Cancer,* 2000; **36**: 37–42.

25. **Donelli MG, Zucchetti M, Munzone E, D'Incalci M, Crosignani A.** Pharmacokinetics of anticancer agents in patients with impaired liver function. *European Journal of Cancer,* 1998; **43**: 33–46.

26. **Cortazar P, Johnson BE.** Review of the efficacy of individualized chemotherapy selected by *in vitro* drug sensitivity testing for patients with cancer. *Journal of Clinical Oncology,* 1999; **17**: 1625–31.

27. **Lokich J, Anderson N.** Dose intensity for bolus versus infusion chemotherapy administration: Review of the literature for 27 anti-neoplastic agents. *Annals of Oncology,* 1997; **8**: 15–25.

28. **Ratain MJ.** Body-surface area as a basis for dosing of anticancer agents: science, myth or habit? *Journal of Clinical Oncology,* 1998; **16**: 2297–8.

29. **Gurney H.** Dose calculation of anticancer drugs: A review of the current practice and introduction of an alternative. *Journal of Clinical Oncology,* 1996; **14**: 2590–611.

30. **Evans WE, et al.** Concept of maximum tolerated systemic exposure and its application to Phase I-II studies of anticancer drugs. *Medical and Pediatric Oncology,* 1991; **19**: 153–9.

31. **Calvert AH, et al.** Carboplatin dosage: prospective validation of a simple formula based on renal function. *Journal of Clinical Oncology,* 1989; **7**: 1748–56.

32. **Eisenhauer EA.** Phase I and II trials with novel anticancer agents: endpoints, efficacy and existentialism. *Annals of Oncology,* 1998; **9**: 1047–52.

33. **Gelman KA, Eisenhauer EA, Harris AL, Ratain MJ, Workman P.** Anticancer agents targeting signalling molecules and the cancer cell environment: challenges for drug development? *Journal of the National Cancer Institute,* 1999; **91**: 1281–7.

34. **Collins JM, Grieshaber CK, Chabner BA.** Pharmacologically guided phase I clinical trials based upon preclinical drug development. *Journal of the National Cancer Institute,* 1990; **82**: 1321–6.

35. **Bruno R, *et al.*** Population pharmacokinetics/pharmacodynamics of docetaxel in Phase II studies in patients with cancer. *Journal of Clinical Oncology*, 1998; **16**: 187–96.

36. **Evans WE, Relling MV, Rodman JH, Crom WR, Boyett JM, Pui C-H.** Conventional compared with individualized chemotherapy for childhood acute lymphoblastic leukemia. *New England Journal of Medicine*, 1998; **338**: 499–505.

37. **Fety R, *et al.*** Clinical impact of pharmacokinetically-guided dose adaptation of 5-fluorouracil: Results from a multicentric randomised trial in patients with locally advanced head and neck carcinomas. *Clinical Cancer Research*, 1998; **4**: 2039–45.

38. **Alberts DS, Dorr RT.** New perspectives on an old friend: optimizing carboplatin for the treatment of solid tumours. *Oncologist*, 1998; **3**: 15–34.

39. **Johnson TS, *et al.*** Thymidylate synthase expression and response to neoadjuvant chemotherapy in patients with advanced head and neck cancer. *Journal of the National Cancer Institute*, 1997; **89**: 308–13.

40. **Lenz H-J, *et al.*** P53 point mutations and thymidylate synthase messenger RNA levels in disseminated colorectal cancer: an analysis of response and survival. *Clinical Cancer Research*, 1998; **4**: 1243–50.

41. **Aschele C, *et al.*** Immunohistochemical quantification of thymidylate synthase expression in colorectal cancer metastasis predicts for clinical outcome in fluorouracil-based chemotherapy. *Journal of Clinical Oncology*, 1999; **17**: 1760–70.

42. **Ross JS, Fletcher JA.** The HER-2/*neu* oncogene in breast cancer: prognostic factor, predictive factor, and target for therapy. *Oncologist*, 1998; **3**: 237–52.

43. **Goldenberg MM.** Trastuzumab, a recombinant DNA-derived humanized monoclonal antibody, a novel agent for the treatment of metastatic breast cancer. *Clinical Therapeutics*, 1999; **21**: 309–18.

44. **Jacobs TW, Gown AM, Yaziji H, Barnes MJ, Schnitt SJ.** Specificity of Hercep test in determining HER-2/*neu* status of breast cancer using the United States Food and Drug Administration-approved scoring system. *Journal of Clinical Oncology*, 1999; **17**: 1983–7.

45. **Thor AD, *et al.*** ErbB-2, p53, and efficacy of adjuvant therapy in lymph node-positive breast cancer. *Journal of the National Cancer Institute*, 1998; **90**: 1346–60.

46. **Paik S, *et al.*** ErbB-2 and response to doxorubicin in patients with axillary lymph node-positive, hormone receptor-negative breast cancer. *Journal of the National Cancer Institute*, 1998; **90**: 1361–70.

47. **Rodenhuis S, *et al.*** Mutational activation of the K-*ras* oncogene and the effect of chemotherapy in advanced adenocarcinoma of the lung: a prospective study. *Journal of Clinical Oncology*, 1997; **15**: 285–91.

48. **O'Connor PM, *et al.*** Characterization of the p53 tumour suppressor pathway in cell lines of the National Cancer Institute anticancer drug screen and correlations with the growth-inhibitory potency of 123 anticancer agents. *Cancer Research*, 1997; **57**: 4285–300.

49. **Ruley HE.** P53 and response to chemotherapy and radiotherapy. In: DeVita VT, Hellman S, Rosenberg SA, eds. *Important advances in oncology 1996*. Philadelphia: Lippincott-Raven Publishers, 1996: 37–55.

50. **Aas T, *et al.*** Specific P53 mutations are associated with *de novo* resistance to doxorubicin in breast cancer patients. *Nature Medicine*, 1996; **2**: 811–4.

51. **Calvert AH, *et al.*** Carboplatin and paclitaxel, alone and in combination: Dose escalation, measurement of renal function, and role of the p53 tumor suppressor gene. *Seminars in Oncology*, 1999; **26** (Suppl. 2):90–4.

52. **Schmitt CA, Lowe SW.** Apoptosis and therapy. *Journal of Pathology*, 1999; **187**: 127–37.

53. **DeMario MD, Ratain MJ.** Oral chemotherapy: rationale and future directions. *Journal of Clinical Oncology*, 1998; **16**: 2557–67.

54. **Meerum Terwogt, *et al.*** Co-administration of cyclosporin enables oral therapy with paclitaxel. *Lancet*, 1998; **352**: 285.

55. **Shah VP.** Analytical methods validation: Bioavailability, bioequivalence and pharmacokinetic studies. *Journal of Pharmaceutical Sciences*, 1992; **81**: 309–12.

56. **Gerhold D, Rushmore T, Caskey CT.** DNA chips: Promising toys have become powerful tools. *Trends in Biochemical Sciences*, 1999; **24**: 168–73.

57. **Kononen J, *et al.*** Tissue microarrays for high-throughput molecular profiling of tumor specimens. *Nature Medicine*, 1998; **4**: 844–7.

58. **Synold TW, *et al.*** Blast cell methotrexate-polyglutamate accumulation *in vivo* differs by lineage, ploidy, and methotrexate dose in acute lymphoblastic leukemia. *Journal of Clinical Investigation*, 1994; **94**: 1996–2001.

59. **Plunkett W, Iacoboni S, Estey E, Danhauser L, Liliemark JO, Keating MJ.** Pharmacologically directed Ara-C therapy for refractory leukemia. *Seminars in Oncology*, 1985; **12** (Suppl. 3):20–30.

60. **Frank AJ, Proctor SJ, Tilby MJ.** Detection and quantification of melphalan-DNA adducts at the single cell level in hematopoietic tumor cells. *Blood*, 1996; **88**: 977–84.

61. **Presant CA, *et al.*** Association of intratumoural pharmacokinetics of fluorouracil with clinical reponse. *Lancet*, 1994; **343**: 1184–7.

62. **Harte RJA, *et al.*** Tumor, normal tissue, and plasma pharmacokinetic studies of fluorouracil biomodulation with N-phosphonacetyl-L-aspartate, folinic acid, and interferon alpha. *Journal of Clinical Oncology*, 1999; **17**: 1580–9.

4.14 Alkylating agents

John A. Hartley

Introduction

The antitumour alkylating agents, the oldest class of anticancer drugs, were introduced into the clinic over 50 years ago. They remain among the most widely administered and effective anticancer agents, being important components of many combination chemotherapy regimens, and of high-dose chemotherapy with stem cell support.

Historically, the successful, early clinical trials with the nitrogen mustard mechlorethamine were stimulated by early observations with the First World War chemical warfare agent sulphur mustard gas. In 1919, Krumbhaar and Krumbhaar documented a delayed myelo-suppression and lymphoid aplasia in addition to the vesicant action of sulphur mustard to the skin, conjuctiva, and respiratory tract.[1] Subsequently Gilman, Goodman, Philips, and Dougherty showed mechlorethamine to be less toxic than sulphur mustard in animal studies and to produce dramatic regressions in murine lympho-sarcomas.[1],[2] The first cancer patients were treated in 1942 and in 1946, when studies on nitrogen mustards were declassified, several reports were published indicating clinical activity in Hodgkin's disease, lymphoma, and chronic lymphocytic and myelocytic leukaemia.[3],[4] Thus the development of alkylating agents represents an excellent example of the rational application of a serendipitous observation and the first example where a knowledge of the properties of cancer cells was applied to drug design.

The range of structures of the clinically used alkylating agents is extensive. In fact, since the early success with mechlorethamine, many thousands of analogues have been synthesized with the aim of achieving enhanced therapeutic activity or a different range of tumour response.

Although chemically reactive, alkylating agents should not be seen as totally indiscriminate chemical toxins. The formation of covalent adducts on cellular DNA is the mechanism common to all the antitumour alkylating agents and, given their chemical reactivity, it is perhaps surprising that a valuable therapeutic index can be achieved in many situations. These drugs, however, can have widely differing tumour specificities, potencies, and toxicity profiles. Indeed, within the same class of agents, for example the nitrogen mustards, even small differences in the non-alkylating portions of the drugs can lead to marked differences in properties such as chemical reactivity, cellular uptake, pharmacokinetic behaviour, metabolic bioactivation and de-toxification, and cross-resistance patterns. Because of these differences and the nature of the target of these drugs, it is possible to use alkylating agents in combination and achieve additive and, with careful scheduling, synergistic tumour cell killing.

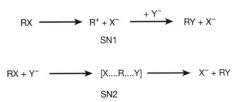

Fig. 1 The chemistry of alkylation showing the two extremes of S_N1 and S_N2 reactions (see text).

Molecular pharmacology of alkylating agents

Chemistry of alkylating agents

In purely chemical terms, an alkylating agent is defined as a compound capable of replacing a proton in another molecule by an alkyl cation. An alkylation reaction can occur by two extreme mechanisms—S_N1 and S_N2 (Fig. 1). In S_N1 reactions the rate limiting step is the initial formation of a reactive, positively charged intermediate which can then react rapidly with an electron-rich nucleophile. Such reactions follow first-order kinetics with a rate that depends on the concentration of the alkylating agent. In contrast, S_N2 reactions which follow second-order kinetics and depend on both the concentration of the alkylating agent and the nucleophile, involve a transition state involving both reactants. The clinically useful agents include drugs that alkylate through an S_N1 mechanism (e.g. nitrogen mustards), agents that alkylate through an S_N2 mechanism (e.g. busulfan), and some compounds that alkylate through reactions with characteristics of both an S_N1 and an S_N2 mechanism. Although it would be expected that differences in the alkylation reaction mechanism might influence the nature of the biological nucleophiles affected by a given drug, the practical consequences are not obvious, possibly because of the complicated interactions which can take place in the cellular milieu. However, the overall chemical reactivity does have a bearing on pharmacological outcome.

The chemistry of the alkylation reaction by the nitrogen mustard mechlorethamine is illustrated in Fig. 2. The initial step is an internal S_N1 cyclization to form a highly reactive, positively charged aziridinium ion with the loss of a chloride ion. The positively charged aziridinium ion is then able to react with electron-rich centres (nucleophiles). This process can be repeated with the other chloroethyl arm of the

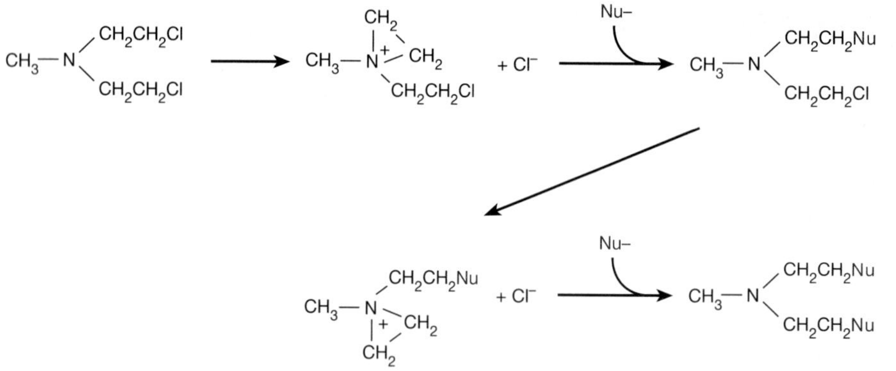

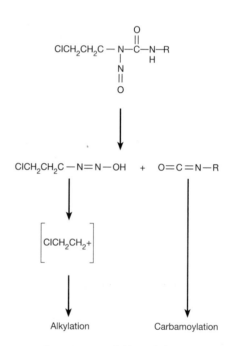

Fig. 2 Mechanism of alkylation by the nitrogen mustard mechlorethamine. Initial loss of a chloride ion produces a reactive aziridinium ion which can react with a nucleophile (Nu⁻) to form a covalent adduct. Loss of a second chlorine can produce a reaction with a second nucleophile. If both nucleophiles are DNA bases, a DNA crosslink results.

drug and a second nucleophile. As a result of their ability to produce two alkylation events, agents of this type are termed bifunctional alkylating agents. It should be emphasized that the transfer of the alkyl (or substituted alkyl) group to the target molecule (usually replacing a hydrogen atom) is a chemical reaction involving the formation of a covalent bond with biological nucleophilic sites and therefore is distinct from the type of non-covalent interaction seen with other DNA interacting antitumour agents such as the intercalating agents.

Several alkylating agents used clinically are close derivatives of mechlorethamine. Where the substituent group in place of the simple methyl group in mechlorethamine attracts electrons the loss of chlorines is discouraged, the azidirinium ion forms less readily, and the alkylating agent is chemically less reactive. The aromatic nitrogen mustards melphalan and chlorambucil, for example, are more stable than mechlorethamine which has a half-life of only a few minutes in aqueous solution. This makes these aromatic nitrogen mustards easier to handle and less vesicant than the aliphatic mechlorethamine. Oral administration is also possible. Two other clinically important nitrogen mustards, cyclophosphamide and ifosfamide, are chemically inert (much more so than melphalan and chlorambucil) and require oxidative metabolic activation in the liver to a circulating metabolite, followed by conversion to the ultimate reactive species as part of a complex series of biochemical transformations.

Agents such as thio-TEPA contain aziridine rings analogous to the aziridinium ion of the nitrogen mustards although they are less reactive because they are uncharged. In this case, the ring system is very sensitive to acid in which a protonated and more reactive structure is formed. Quinone-containing agents such as diaziquone and mitomycin C have the added advantage that alkylation is facilitated by the change in electron distribution when the non-aromatic quinone is reduced either chemically or enzymatically to an aromatic semi-quinone or hydroquinone. These agents are often referred to as bioreductive alkylating agents. An attractive feature of such drugs is that they can be activated more efficiently in the hypoxic cells which commonly occur in poorly vascularized tumour tissues.[5] Drugs containing *N*-methyl groups, including the melamine hexamethylmelamine and the dimethyltriazene dacarbazine (DTIC), require hepatic oxidative hydroxylation of the *N*-methyl moieties to

Fig. 3 Spontaneous decomposition of chloroethylnitrosoureas to produce both alkylating and carbomoylating species. Alkylation results from the chloroethyldiazohydroxide which can chlorethylate nucleophilic sites on DNA.

generate DNA reactive species. Recent derivatives of these drugs (for example, trimelamol and temozolamide) can liberate the active product spontaneously. The chloroethylnitrosoureas which include bischloroethylnitrosourea (BCNU, carmustine), cyclohexylchloroethylnitrosourea (CCNU, lomustine), and methyl-CCNU (semustine) can decompose to form a variety of reactive intermediates, including the chloroethyldiazohydroxide which can chloroethylate nucleophilic sites on DNA (Fig. 3). In addition, many chloroethylnitrosoureas also decompose to form isocyanates which can engage in carbamoylation reactions with proteins (Fig. 3). Detailed descriptions of the chemistry of the alkylating agents can be found in several reviews.[6],[7]

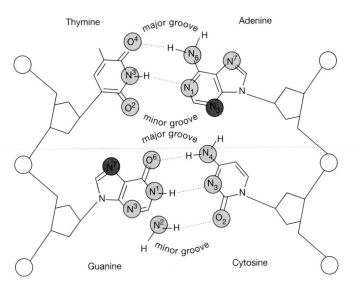

Fig. 4 Sites of reaction on the bases of DNA by simple alkylating agents. Numerous potential reaction sites have been identified (colour) in all four DNA bases, although not all have equal reactivity. In general, the ring nitrogens of the bases are more nucleophilic than the oxygens with the N7-position of guanine (in the major groove of DNA) and the N3-position of adenine (in the minor groove of DNA) being the most reactive (full colour).

These highly reactive, small molecules can bind covalently to electron-rich nucleophilic sites on large or small biological molecules. The favourite atoms as alkylation sites are sulphur, nitrogen, oxygen, and phosphorus, in particular those contained within sulphydryl, hydroxyl, carboxyl, acetyl, phosphoryl, amino, and imidazole groups. These agents, therefore, have the potential to enter into a large variety of chemical reactions with many important biological molecules, including DNA, RNA, and proteins.

Molecular mechanism of action

Alkylating agents can react with a variety of electron-rich nucleophiles present in the body. Reaction with water and thiols, such as glutathione, will protect the cell from damage. Drug molecules which escape this fate can damage biological macromolecules such as proteins and nucleic acids. The alkylation of cellular DNA is, however, linked to the cytotoxic, carcinogenic, and mutagenic affects of this class of agent. Numerous potential reaction sites for alkylation have been identified in all four DNA bases, although not all of them have equal reactivity.[8] Nucleophilic centres in DNA bases that are the most reactive to alkylating agents are shown in Fig. 4. In general, the ring nitrogens of the bases are more nucleophilic than the oxygens with the N7 position of guanine (in the major groove of DNA) and the N3 position of adenine (in the minor groove of DNA) being the most reactive. In addition, alkylation of oxygen in phosphodiester linkages can occur resulting in the formation of phosphotriesters.

It seems natural to suppose that highly electrophilic compounds will target the most nucleophilic sites on the DNA and that, in the absence of perturbing steric effects, the reaction would be largely governed by the molecular electrostatic potential of the attacked site. Calculations of the molecular electrostatic potential clearly demonstrate that the most negative potentials on the bases are situated

in the vicinity of N7 for guanine and N3 for adenine.[9] Indeed, the most negative site anywhere within the bases of DNA is at the guanine N7 position which is considerably more negative than the corresponding site on adenine. However, although the most frequent site of alkylation of DNA by most alkylating agents is the N7 position of guanine, not all guanines may be alkylated to the same extent. The negative electrostatic potential of the N7 position of a particular guanine is influenced by its flanking bases.[9] For example a guanine flanked by other guanine residues has the most negative electrostatic potential and will preferentially undergo electrophilic attack. A guanine flanked by cytosines is the least susceptible to alkylation. As a result, alkylation by simple agents such as mechlorethamine is preferentially targeted towards guanine-rich regions of DNA.[10]

Although many agents give a similar pattern of alkylation to mechlorethamine, the chemical structure of the non-reactive portion of an alkylating agent can influence the sequence specificity of the alkylation reaction. For example two nitrogen mustard analogues, uracil mustard and quinacrine mustard, have been shown to alkylate preferentially at 5'-PyGC (Py = pyrimidine) and 5'-GG/TPu (Pu = purine) sequences respectively.[11] Although these patterns of DNA base sequence specificity were originally derived from applications of DNA sequencing technology to the analysis of alkylation reactions on naked DNA, the same patterns of sequence specificity have been shown to be preserved in intact cells.[12]

Although a small number of clinically used alkylating agents have only one reactive group and are therefore monofunctional, the majority are bifunctional. Since the demonstration by Ross, Haddow, and coworkers over 40 years ago that bifunctionality was an essential prerequisite for potent cytotoxicity and antitumour activity in many instances (e.g. the nitrogen mustards), it was proposed that the formation of covalent crosslinks was a critical event. The possible modes of interaction of bifunctional agents with DNA are shown in Fig. 5. The formation of crosslinks requires an initial reaction to form a monoadduct. The second alkylation event to form the crosslink is often slow and not all monoadducts go on to form crosslinks. For many agents the ratio of monoadducts to crosslinks is at least 20:1 and often higher.[13] Such monoadducts may be mutagenic and carcinogenic. Crosslinking involving DNA can be on the same strand of DNA (intrastrand), between the two strands of DNA (interstrand), or between a base on DNA and a reactive group on a protein (DNA–protein).

DNA interstrand crosslinks and DNA–protein crosslinks can be detected in mammalian cells at pharmacologically relevant doses of bifunctional alkylating agents by the technique of alkaline elution developed by Kohn,[14] and DNA intrastrand crosslinks have been measured indirectly.[15] Although the relative contribution of the latter has been hard to assess, considerable evidence points to the interstrand crosslink as being the critical cytotoxic lesion. For example the extent of interstrand crosslinking generally correlates well with the cytotoxic activity of members of the nitrogen mustard class.[16] Indeed, for the three nitrogen mustards melphalan, chlorambucil, and benzoic acid mustard, which have very different chemical reactivities, the order of reactivity based on hydrolysis rate (i.e. reaction with water) or reaction with simple chemicals, is chlorambucil > melphalan > benzoic acid mustard. In tumour cells in culture, however, the order of cytotoxicity was found to be melphalan > chlorambucil > benzoic acid mustard, which is the same order as the efficiency of the three compounds to

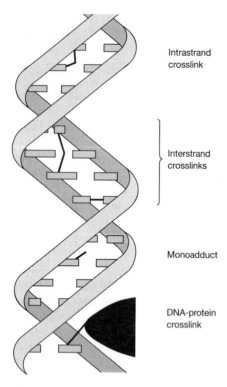

Intrastrand
crosslink

Interstrand
crosslinks

Monoadduct

DNA-protein
crosslink

Fig. 5 Types of reaction possible by bifunctional alkylating agents on DNA. The critical cytotoxic lesion is generally considered to be the interstrand crosslink which can span two or more base pairs (as in the case of nitrogen mustards) or form within a base pair (as in the case of the chloroethylnitrosoureas). Crosslinks are, however, formed much less frequently than monoadducts.

produce DNA interstrand crosslinks in the cells, or indeed in isolated DNA.[17]

In a series of dimethanesulphonates with increasing length of methylene bridge, a correlation has been found between ability to form interstrand crosslinks (but not DNA–protein crosslinks) and cytotoxicity. The hexamethylene bridged compound rather than the clinically used tetramethylene member, busulfan, is optimum for both interstrand crosslinking and cytotoxicity.[18] Cells possessing high levels of the enzyme guanine O6-alkyltransferase remove the critical DNA monoadduct produced by chloroethylnitrosoureas and prevent the formation of interstrand crosslinks by these drugs. These cells are much more resistant to killing by the drugs than cells lacking this enzyme, even though drug uptake and formation of DNA–protein crosslinks is equivalent in both cell types.[19],[20]

DNA can accommodate interstrand crosslinks of different lengths. For most nitrogen mustards the crosslink contains five atoms (seven in the case of ifosfamide) and would require a separation of approximately 8 Å between two guanine N7 positions. Physical molecular modelling predicts that in a 5′-GC sequence the guanine N7 positions would be closest to this distance, with the distance being further in the reverse 5′-CG sequence. Surprisingly, experimental evidence using oligonucleotides of defined sequence indicate that, although mechlorethamine can form interstrand crosslinks in a 5′-GC site, the preferred sequence was 5′-GNC with the crosslink therefore spanning three base pairs.[21] In order to accommodate such a crosslink the DNA must therefore be highly distorted.

The guanine N7 position is in the major groove of DNA. Crosslinks can also be formed in the minor groove of DNA. For example the bioreductive alkylating agent mitomycin C, following reduction, produces a metabolite which alkylates and crosslinks between guanine-N2 positions in the minor groove at the sequence 5′-CG.[22]

The interstrand crosslink formed by the chloroethylnitrosoureas is much shorter than that produced by the nitrogen mustards and contains only two atoms. Two crosslink products have been isolated from DNA treated with chloroethylnitrosoureas.[23] The guanine N7 to guanine N7 crosslinked product formed is generally assumed to be the result of an intrastrand crosslink. The other product is a crosslink between guanine and cytosine through the N1 and N3 positions, respectively, and is the result of an interstrand crosslink. The steps to the formation of this product are shown in Fig. 6. Following the initial, rapid alkylation at the guanine O6 position the crosslink can take several hours to form. This gives time for this adduct to be repaired by the enzyme guanine O6-alkyltransferase, thus preventing crosslink formation. The level of this enzyme is therefore a major determinant of sensitivity to chloroethylnitrosoureas, but not to bifunctional alkylating agents which form interstrand crosslinks through other positions on the DNA.[24] A more detailed account of the interactions of alkylating agents with DNA can be found elsewhere.[25]

Cellular consequences of DNA damage by alkylating agents

The uptake of alkylating agents into cells is generally by simple passive diffusion, although the transport of mechlorethamine and melphalan is by active, carrier-mediated processes involving the choline and specific amino acid transport systems, respectively. Once inside the cell, covalent adduct formation on cellular DNA is the mechanism of cytotoxicity common to all antitumour alkylating agents. Formation of DNA monoadducts may cause a variety of structural alteration to the DNA such as base ring openings. DNA single strand breaks can occur via depurination. Numerous DNA repair enzymes are present to correct the DNA damage[26] but can, in some cases, produce further damage such as base deletions or the formation of DNA strand breaks as a result of endonuclease attack. If not further processed correctly, DNA strand breaks can persist and subsequent chromosomal rearrangements can occur. The formation of DNA single strand breaks is involved in the cytotoxic action of monofunctional alkylating agents which cannot form DNA crosslinks.

It is assumed that bulky DNA monoadducts, and in particular unrepaired DNA crosslinks, will interfere with DNA replication and transcription by blocking DNA and RNA polymerases, as has been demonstrated *in vitro*. The repair of alkylation damage is complex and different adducts produced by the same drug may be repaired by different mechanisms. For example, the monoadducts produced by mechlorethamine may be repaired primarily by the base excision repair mechanism involving specific DNA glycosylases. The DNA interstrand crosslinks formed by this agent, however, may be repaired by a process involving initially the more complex mechanism of nucleotide excision repair, but also it appears to involve the mechanism of recombination.[26] The removal of DNA alkylation damage is further complicated by the finding that DNA repair is heterogeneous within the genome.[27] With mechlorethamine preferential repair of adducts is observed in a transcriptionally active gene compared to a silent

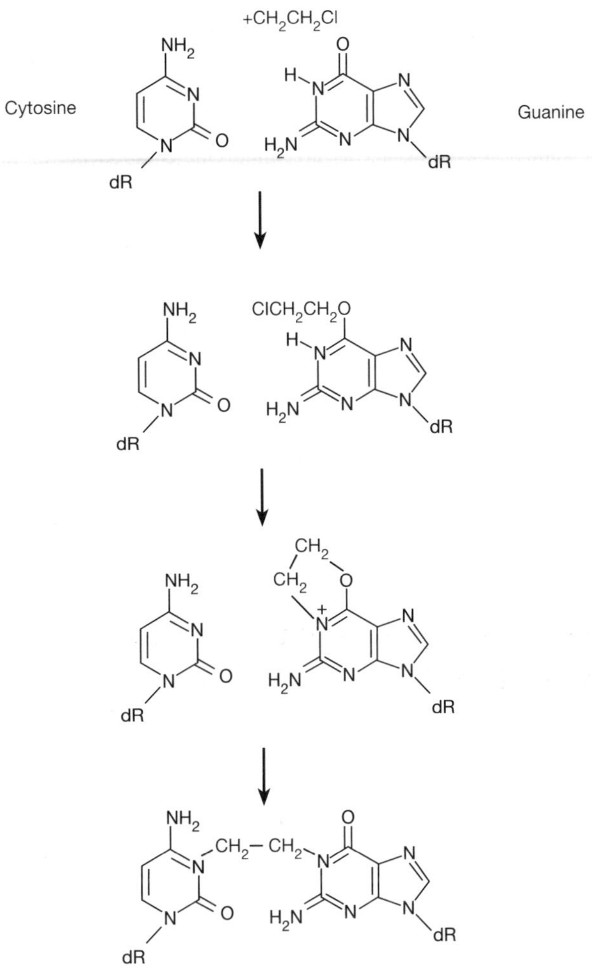

Table 1 Mechanisms of cellular resistance to alkylating agents

Decreased drug uptake	
Alteration in DNA repair capacity:	increase in guanine O6-alkyltransferase increased removal of DNA interstrand crosslinks loss of DNA mismatch repair
Increase in detoxification pathways:	elevation in cellular thiols, e.g. glutathione elevation in specific glutathione S-transferases
Alteration in apoptotic pathways	

Fig. 6 Steps to the formation of a G–C crosslink by the chloroethylnitrosoureas. An initial alkylation at the O6 position of guanine is followed by an internal cyclization reaction to form the unstable intermediate 1,06-ethanoguanine. Reaction then occurs with the cytosine on the opposite strand of the DNA to form the crosslink. Although adducts at the N7 position of guanine (7-chloroethylguanine and 7-hydroxyethylguanine) are the most abundant adducts formed by the chloroethylnitrosoureas it is the initial reaction at the O6 position of guanine that is most critical for antitumour activity.

many (but not all) chemotherapeutic alkylating agents compared with the plateau phase.

Clearly several types of DNA damage produced by alkylating agents, and in particular the DNA interstrand crosslink, are cytotoxic to cells. In many cell types the efficiency of a drug to induce such crosslinks is directly related to its cytotoxicity. However, although the production and repair of DNA interstrand crosslinks and other forms of DNA damage are very important, this is not the whole story and the DNA damage response process linking the drug-target interaction to cell death is only starting to be understood in detail. In a series of Burkitt lymphoma cell lines, sensitivity to mechlorethamine varies by up to five-fold with no correlation with DNA crosslinking or its repair. Cell death, by apoptosis, was linked to differences in processes subsequent to DNA damage or removal of crosslinks, in particular cell cycle effects and associated signalling pathways.[30] In several experimental systems the expression of p53 has been shown to critically influence response to DNA damage by alkylating agents. Cells with mutant p53 can demonstrate resistance to these drugs. Expression of the antiapoptotic gene *bcl-2* may also result in decreased sensitivity to chemotherapeutic alkylating agents.

Chemotherapeutic alkylating agents such as the nitrogen mustards are both mutagenic and carcinogenic in a variety of test systems, including the classic McCann and Ames tests. They induce sister chromatid exchanges and other chromosomal alterations. Transformation of cells in culture can occur and tumours can be induced in laboratory animals following nitrogen mustard administration. Clinically the use of alkylating agent drugs is associated with a higher risk of developing second neoplasms, particularly leukaemia.[31]

Cellular resistance to alkylating agents

Cellular resistance to alkylating agents can occur by several mechanisms summarized in Table 1. Some of these mechanisms are general in nature, while others are specific to particular alkylating agents. As a result cross-resistance between different alkylating agents is not always seen supporting the clinical use of combinations of alkylating agents in some cases, for example in a high dose setting. In some situations, however, multiple mechanisms of resistance can develop simultaneously.

Clearly, alterations in the apoptotic pathways found in tumours can be responsible for intrinsic and acquired resistance to alkylating

gene, and coding regions also undergo more efficient repair than non-coding sequences.[28]

The production of various forms of DNA damage, particularly unrepaired DNA interstrand crosslinks and strand breaks, leads to cell cycle arrest. This allows time for the cell to attempt to repair the damaged template. Although there are variations through the cell cycle, cell killing is observed throughout.[29] Indeed, alkylating agents are generally regarded as being cell cycle phase non-specific. Both fast and slow growing cells can be killed by alkylating agents, although generally rapidly growing cells are more sensitive. There is a greater sensitivity *in vitro* of cells during the exponential phase of growth to

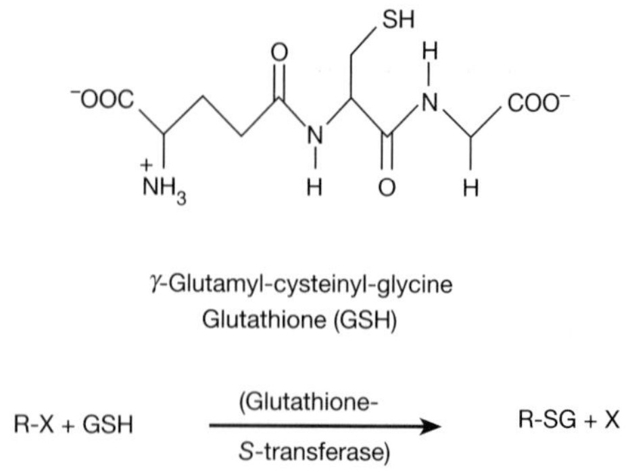

γ-Glutamyl-cysteinyl-glycine
Glutathione (GSH)

R-X + GSH →(Glutathione-S-transferase)→ R-SG + X

Fig. 7 Glutathione and its reaction with alkylating agents.

agents. The increased ability of tumour cells to repair certain types of DNA damage may also be important in determining chemosensitivity. For example guanine O6-alkyltransferase is a major determinant of sensitivity to the chloroethylnitrosoureas and increased expression confers resistance to this class of agent, but not to bifunctional alkylating agents which form interstrand crosslinks through other positions on the DNA. Furthermore, chronic lymphocytic leukaemia cells from patients who have acquired resistance to nitrogen mustards show elevated repair of melphalan-induced DNA interstrand crosslinks in vitro compared to those from sensitive or untreated patients.[32] Conversely, cells that are deficient in mismatch repair are more resistant than normal cells to killing by some alkylating agents.[33] Mutations in mismatch repair genes, which have been found in hereditary non-polyposis colon cancer and certain sporadic tumours, could lead not only to increased genetic instability (a mutator phenotype), but also to an increased resistance to certain types of DNA damage.

Mechanisms which prevent the alkylating agent from reaching DNA can also contribute to resistance. Most clinically used alkylating agents are not substrates for the P-glycoprotein efflux pump and, as a result, cross-resistance is not seen in multidrug resistant cells. Drug uptake can, however, be reduced by other mechanisms; for example cells resistant in vitro to either mechlorethamine or melphalan have been shown to have altered or mutated active transport carriers.[34],[35] A more general resistance mechanism to alkylating agents results from elevation of cellular thiols, in particular glutathione. Glutathione-mediated detoxification pathways play a central role in the inactivation and elimination of xenobiotics, including many clinically used alkylating agents. γ-Glutamylcysteine synthetase catalyses the rate-limiting step in de novo synthesis of glutathione and increased glutathione levels can be related to increased activity of this enzyme. Reaction of alkylating agents with glutathione can be facilitated by certain glutathione-S-transferases (Fig. 7). These represent a multigene family of enzymes and can be elevated in resistant cells.[36] The α, μ, and π classes appear to be the major glutathione-S-transferase isozymes involved in anticancer drug resistance. The α isozyme appears particularly important for nitrogen mustards such as chlorambucil and melphalan, whereas the μ isozyme may be more relevant for chloroethylnitrosoureas.[36] However, transfection experiments have not fully confirmed the significance of the GSTs in drug resistance.

Clinical pharmacology of alkylating agents

General properties

Survival curves of cell lines exposed to alkylating agents in vitro usually show an exponentially increased cell killing with increasing dose in what is often referred to as 'first order' or 'pseudo first order' cell killing. Alkylating agents are important components of many high-dose regimens, with melphalan, cyclophosphamide, and ifosfamide being used most commonly. Overall, alkylating agents are generally classified as proliferation-dependent but, as discussed previously, proliferation rate alone does not account for differences in cell survival between tumour cell lines. Clinically these agents are, however, most toxic towards rapidly dividing cells, with general side-effects occurring in bone marrow, gastrointestinal mucosa, and hair follicles. The ability of alkylating agents also to kill more slowly proliferating (and even quiescent) cells at high doses is often seen as a considerable advantage over other classes of cytotoxic agent which are cell cycle dependent.

Different classes of alkylating agent, and different members within a particular class resulting from changes in the non-alkylating portion of the molecule, can have very different patterns of pharmacokinetic biodistribution and normal tissue toxicity. Drugs which show little or no differential cell killing effect between rapidly and more slowly growing cells tend to produce more prolonged myelosuppression. Thus, whereas with cyclophosphamide complete haematological recovery has occurred 3–4 weeks following treatment, this can take 6 weeks with busulfan due to the more slowly proliferating stem cell compartment receiving relatively more damage. With both drugs intermittent therapy is therefore generally used rather than prolonged, continuous dosing. Because of the widely differing potencies, toxicities, and disease selectivities of different alkylating agents, it is possible to use them in combination to achieve additive, and with careful scheduling, synergistic cell killing.

Nitrogen mustards (Table 2)

Mechlorethamine (Fig. 8)

The prototype bifunctional alkylating agent mechlorethamine is now rarely used clinically. It is still incorporated as part of treatment regimens for Hodgkin's disease, for example MOPP (mechlorethamine, vincristine, procarbazine, and prednisone), although even in this indication it has been replaced by other alkylating agents such as chlorambucil. Mechlorethamine has also been shown to be effective when applied topically to treat mycosis fungoides. It is transported into cells by the choline transporter, and is highly reactive chemically. It decays rapidly in aqueous solution and body fluids with a half-life of only a few minutes. Its pharmacokinetics have not been investigated. The principal dose-limiting toxicity of mechlorethamine is myelosuppression. The drug is highly vesicant causing skin ulceration if extravasation occurs. It must be given through a well-sited cannula through a fast-running infusion.

Melphalan (Fig. 9)

Melphalan is the amino acid phenylalanine derivative of mechlorethamine and was originally synthesized with the rationale that some

Table 2 Nitrogen mustards

Name	Major approved indications	Route	Typical dosage and administration	Major toxicities
Mechlorethamine	Hodgkin's disease, mycosis fungoides	IV	0.4 mg/kg (10–12 mg/m^2) every 4–6 weeks; 6 mg/m^2 on days 1 and 8 every 4 weeks (MOPP)	Neutropenia, thrombocytopenia, nausea and vomiting, phlebitis
Melphalan	Multiple myeloma, ovarian carcinoma	PO	1 mg/kg total dose over 5 days, every 4–5 weeks	Neutropenia, thrombocytopenia
		IV	8 mg/m^2 every 4–5 weeks	
		IV high dose	40–200 mg/m^2	Neutropenia, mucositis, nausea and vomiting
Chlorambucil	Chronic lymphocytic leukaemia, low grade lymphomas, Hodgkin's disease, multiple myeloma	PO	0.1–0.2 mg/kg (4–10 mg total) daily for 3–6 weeks	Neutropenia
Cyclophosphamide	Leukaemias, Hodgkin's disease, Burkitt's lymphoma, breast and ovarian carcinomas, sarcomas	PO	50–100 mg/m^2 daily	Leukopenia, nausea and vomiting
		IV	1000–1500 mg/m^2 every 3 weeks	Alopecia, haemorrhagic cystitis
		IV high dose	2000–7000 mg/m^2 over 1–4 days	Thrombocytopenia, cardiotoxicity
Ifosfamide	Soft tissue sarcomas, Ewing's sarcoma, non-small cell lung cancer	IV	1200–2400 mg/m^2/day for 3 days every 3 weeks; 500 mg/m^2/day as single dose	Haemorrhagic cystitis (prevented with mesna), myelosuppression, nausea and vomiting, alopecia, CNS toxicity
		IV high dose	3000–4000 mg/m^2 on days 1–4	As above but of increased incidence and degree

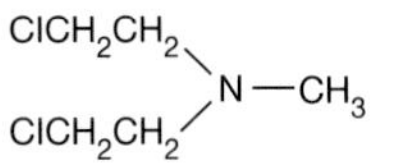

Fig. 8 Mechlorethamine.

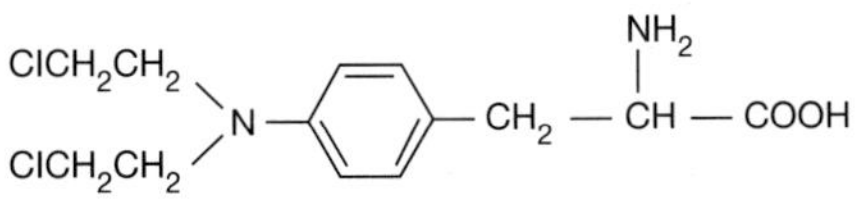

Fig. 9 Melphalan.

selectivity to tumour cells might be achieved since they are actively proliferating and therefore more actively undergoing protein synthesis than non-proliferating cells. Uptake into cells is through an active, amino acid carrier-mediated process. It is non-vesicant, and is inactivated by chemical hydrolysis to monohydroxy and dihydroxy melphalan. Approximately 15 per cent of the drug is extracted intact in the urine. The drug can be given both intravenously and orally and the pharmacokinetics of both routes of administration have been studied in humans. Oral bioavailability is low (20–50 per cent) and highly variable. The plasma half-life is around 90 min for oral dosing and biphasic for intravenous dosing with an initial half-life of 6 to 8 min and a terminal half-life of 40 to 75 min.

Melphalan has significant activity in multiple myeloma either as a single agent or in combination with prednisone or vincristine and other alkylating agents such as cyclophosphamide. In addition, melphalan given intravenously has activity, either alone or in combination with other drugs, in high dose bone marrow or stem cell transplant regimens for breast, ovarian, and testicular cancers and multiple myeloma.

Haematological suppression, including both leucopenia and thrombocytopenia, is the dose limiting toxicity of melphalan. The nadir counts are at 10 to 24 days following administration. In the high dose/ stem cell transplant setting, toxic effects include mucositis, nausea and vomiting, diarrhoea, and alopecia. Skin rashes, allergic reactions, haemolytic anaemia, vasculitis, and pulmonary fibrosis have been reported as toxicities in small numbers of patients. As with many alkylating agents, melphalan is oncogenic. In ovarian cancer patients the increase in risk of developing acute non-lymphocytic leukaemia is two to three-fold higher for melphalan compared to cyclophosphamide.[37]

Chlorambucil (Fig. 10)

Chlorambucil is the phenylbutyric acid derivative of mechlorethamine and, like melphalan, was synthesized over 30 years ago during attempts to produce more effective and specific analogues. It is relatively stable in aqueous solution and, in contrast to mechlorethamine and melphalan, enters cells by simple diffusion. Chlorambucil is well absorbed on oral administration and is given by this route. The usual

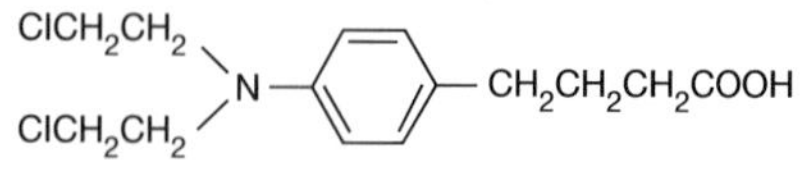

Fig. 10 Chlorambucil.

dosage is 4 to 10 mg daily in chronic lymphocytic leukaemia and it is generally administered as a single agent or with prednisone. The range of bioavailability of chlorambucil given orally is 56 to 100 per cent. The half-life for chlorambucil in the circulation is around 90 min. The drug is rapidly converted to its major metabolite aminophenylacetic acid. In addition, the butyric acid side-chain of chlorambucil can be metabolized by a mitochondrial β-oxidation pathway forming phenylacetic acid mustard. This process and the extensive plasma protein binding (>90 per cent) of chlorambucil affect the therapeutic index.

Chlorambucil has shown activity against a range of human malignancies but is used primarily for the long-term treatment of chronic lymphocytic leukaemia, low-grade lymphomas, Hodgkin's disease, and multiple myeloma. The major dose-limiting toxicity is myelosuppression but the drug has few acute toxicities and as a result finds particular clinical utility in the elderly. Several studies have described a high incidence of secondary leukaemias in patients treated with chlorambucil for several years.[38],[39]

Cyclophosphamide (Fig. 11)

Cyclophosphamide is the most widely used antitumour alkylating agent. It was originally designed as an inert prodrug which would be converted to a reactive nitrogen mustard in tumours by the action of phosphoamidase enzymes. These enzymes had been shown to be over-expressed in a variety of solid tumours. The drug was found to have significant antitumour activity against animal tumours and rapidly found its way into clinical practice, demonstrating activity against a wide variety of human tumours. As a prodrug, cyclophosphamide is non-toxic towards most tumour cells in culture and would, therefore, not have been selected through current *in vitro*-based screens. It is now clear that the route of activation is not through the mechanism originally proposed and the drug undergoes the complex series of metabolic and spontaneous steps illustrated in Fig. 11.

The initial metabolism of cyclophosphamide is in the liver by cytochrome P450 to produce 4-hydroxycyclophosphamide which enters the circulation and tissues. A variety of activation/ deactivation reactions can then occur. 4-hydroxycyclophosphamide exists in equilibrium with aldophosphamide which can either be deactivated by the enzyme aldehyde dehydrogenase to form carboxyphosphamide, or be broken down spontaneously to form phosphoramide mustard and acrolein. Phosphoramide mustard is the bifunctional alkylating species believed to be the active antitumour agent produced by cyclophosphamide. Acrolein, which is excreted intact in the urine, is responsible for the bladder toxicity of the drug. Inactivation of acrolein in the urine can be achieved by administration of sodium-2-mercaptoethane (mesna) which prevents urotoxicity. A second site of deactivation is the conversion of 4-hydroxycyclophosphamide to 4-ketocyclophosphamide by the enzyme aldehyde oxidase. Clearly a selective antitumour effect would be favoured if a greater level of

deactivation occurred in host tissue including the bone marrow. Differences in the level of aldehyde dehydrogenase are believed to be particularly critical in this respect.

Cyclophosphamide is used in combination chemotherapy regimens for the treatment of many haematological and solid tumours including Hodgkin's disease, non-Hodgkin's lymphoma, Burkitt's lymphoma, cancers of the breast, bladder, lung, cervix, and ovary, and sarcomas. It can be administered intravenously or orally. The drug has a good oral bioavailability of around 90 per cent. The pharmacokinetics of the parent molecule cyclophosphamide have been studied and the plasma half-life found to be 4 to 6.5 h.

The usual dose-limiting toxicity of cyclophosphamide is dose-dependent myelosuppression, mainly leucopenia. The leucocyte nadir and time of recovery is more rapid than with many other alkylating agents. Nausea and vomiting are common and alopecia is severe in over half of all patients treated by either the oral or intravenous route. Haemorrhagic cystitis can arise due to the accumulation of acrolein in the urinary tract and can be prevented or treated with hydration and administration of mesna.

Cyclophosphamide is an important drug in high-dose chemotherapy, either alone or in combination with bone marrow or stem cell transplantation for treatment of lymphomas and solid tumours. The pharmacokinetics of high-dose cyclophosphamide do not differ significantly from those of standard dose treatments. Cardiotoxicity can occur at these high doses by an unknown mechanism. Cyclophosphamide is also used as an imunosuppressant.

Ifosfamide (Fig. 12)

Ifosfamide belongs to the same oxazaphosphorine class of nitrogen mustards as cyclophosphamide. In the case of ifosfamide, one of the 2-chloroethyl groups is located on the nitrogen atom of the oxazaphosphorine ring. Like cyclophosphamide it is a prodrug and is activated by hydroxylation in the liver. This process is less efficient than with cyclophosphamide. This changes the pharmacokinetics of the drug so that ifosfamide activation is significantly slower and more inactive metabolites are produced. In particular, chloracetaldehyde is a major metabolic product with ifosfamide which may contribute to the neurotoxicity sometimes seen with this agent.

Ifosfamide has a broad antitumour activity. It is particularly useful in the treatment of soft tissue sarcomas and has produced responses in non-small cell lung cancer. It is administered intravenously and is less myelosuppressive than cyclophosphamide. Ifosfamide has a plasma half-life of 7 to 15 h. In the absence of mesna it produces dose-limiting haemorrhagic cystitis and can be associated with a severe, but usually reversible, neurotoxicity.

Nitrosoureas (Table 3)

BCNU (Fig. 13)

Several clinically useful nitrosoureas resulted from extensive synthesis programmes based on the finding in the late 1950s and early 1960s that 1-methyl-3-nitrosoguanidine and 1-methyl-1-nitrosourea had antileukaemic activity. Most of these drugs incorporate a 2-chloroethyl moiety which is essential for DNA crosslinking ability. A distinguishing feature is the extreme lipophilicity of these agents which facilitates uptake into the central nervous system. Although they share many of the features of the nitrogen mustards, their mechanism of DNA

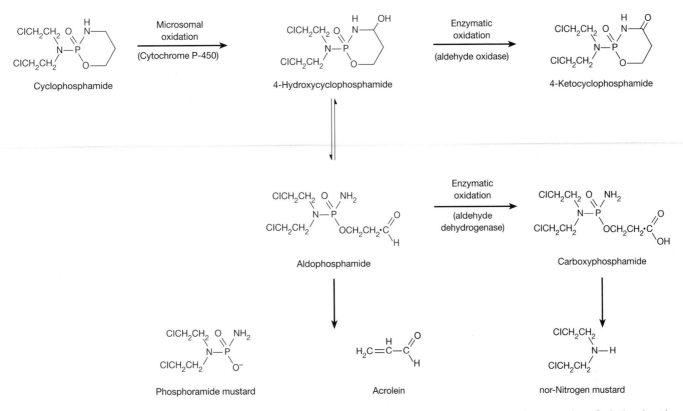

Fig. 11 Cyclophosphamide and its metabolism. The route to the ultimate alkylating species, phosphoramide mustard, is shown in colour. Cyclophosphamide is a prodrug and initial metabolism occurs in the liver to produce 4-hydroxycyclophosphamide. This exists in equilibrium with aldophosphamide which can break down spontaneously to form phosphoramide mustard and acrolein. Deactivation can occur by oxidation of either 4-hydroxycyclophosphamide or aldophosphamide.

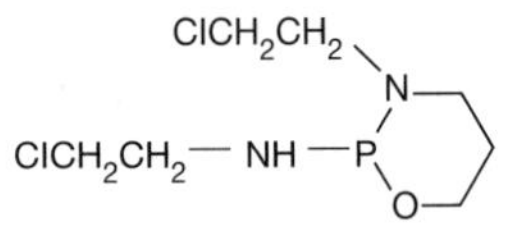

Fig. 12 Ifosfamide.

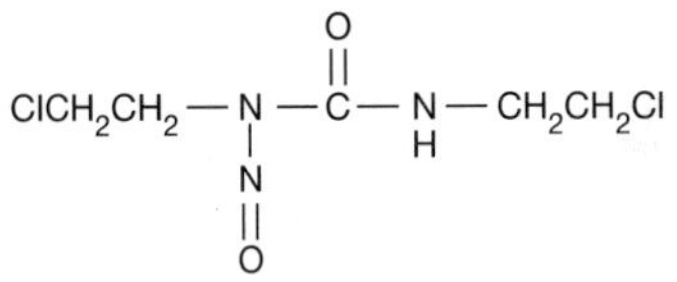

Fig. 13 BCNU.

Table 3 Nitrosoureas

Name	Major approved indications	Route	Typical dosage and administration	Major toxicities
BCNU	Brain tumours, multiple myeloma, lymphomas	IV	200 mg/m² every 6 weeks	Myelosuppression, nausea and vomiting, hepatotoxicity, pulmonary fibrosis
		IV high dose	300–600 mg/m²	Pulmonary (interstital pneumonitis and fibrosis), hepatotoxicity
CCNU	Brain tumours, Hodgkin's disease	PO	100–130 mg/m² every 6–8 weeks	Myelosuppression, nausea and vomiting, nephrotoxicity
MeCCNU	as CCNU	PO	125–200 mg/m² every 6 weeks	as CCNU
Streptozotocin	Pancreatic islet cell carcinoma, malignant carcinoid	IV	500 mg/m² for 5 days every 6 weeks	Nephrotoxicity, nausea and vomiting, acute hypoglycaemia, pain at injection site

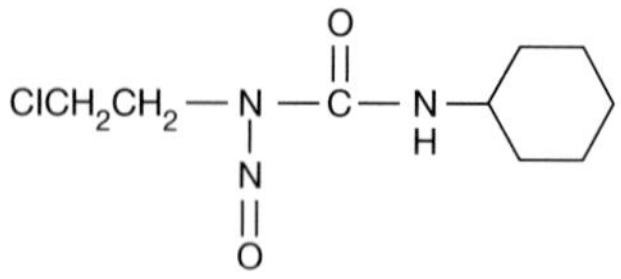

Fig. 14 CCNU.

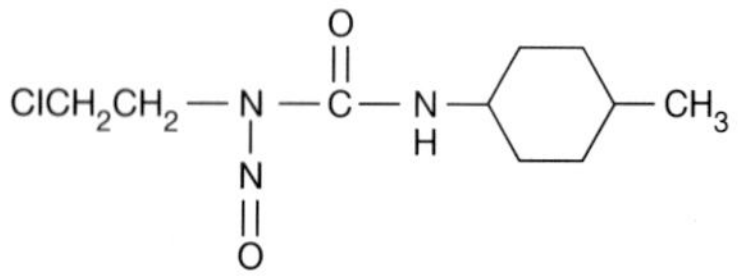

Fig. 15 MeCCNU.

Fig. 16 Streptozotozin.

alkylation is distinct and they only exhibit partial cross-resistance in experimental systems (see above).

BCNU (carmustine) rapidly decomposes in aqueous solution and when given intravenously has a plasma half-life of around 20 min. It is rapidly metabolized by the liver. Because of its rapid appearance in the cerebrospinal fluid it is used in the treatment of brain tumours. It is also used in the treatment of lymphomas, multiple myeloma, malignant melanoma, and in some high-dose/ bone marrow and stem cell transplant regimens. The dose limiting toxicity is haematopoietic and is relatively delayed and prolonged. Prolonged BCNU treatment can also result in pulmonary fibrosis. In the high-dose setting hepatotoxicity and pulmonary toxicity are dose limiting and veno-occlusive disease occurs.

CCNU (Fig. 14)

CCNU (lomustine) differs from BCNU in having a cyclohexyl ring in place of one of the chloroethyl groups. This modification makes CCNU much more lipophilic than BCNU and it is more effective in some settings. It is given orally and it is used to treat primary brain tumours usually in combination with other drugs. Extensive first pass metabolism occurs to produce metabolites which are 4-hydroxylated on the cyclohexyl ring. These metabolites have similar properties to the parent drug and they are together responsible for the antitumour activity. The half-life of the metabolites is approximately 2 h.

The dose-limiting toxicity of CCNU is a delayed myelosuppression, which may be prolonged. A dose-dependent nephrotoxicity occurs with prolonged administration.

MeCCNU (Fig. 15)

MeCCNU (semustine) differs in structure from CCNU only in that it has a methyl group at the 4 position on the cyclohexyl ring. This modification prevents the metabolic 4-hydroxylation that occurs in the liver with CCNU. Although more active in several preclinical models, MeCCNU is generally equipotent or less potent than other chloroethylnitrosoureas in the clinic. It is metabolized by hepatic mixed function oxidases to hydroxylated metabolites that retain alkylating ability. It is more lipophilic than CCNU and readily crosses the blood–brain barrier. Delayed and prolonged myelosuppression is the dose-limiting toxicity.

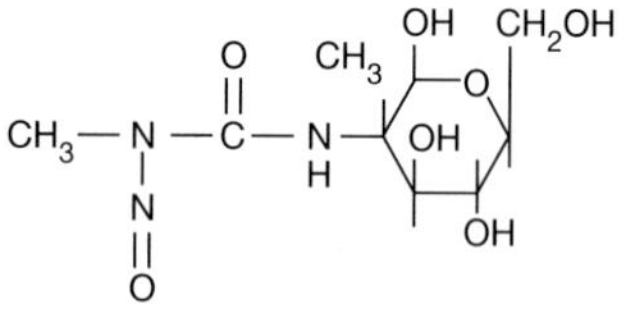

Streptozotocin (Fig. 16)

Streptozotocin is a naturally occurring nitrosourea isolated from *Streptomyces achromogenes*. It is more hydrophilic than the other clinically used nitrosoureas and differs also in being a monofunctional alkylating agent. Methylation at the O6 position of guanine is essential for its action. This compound was shown to be diabetogenic in animals. As a result of its sugar moiety an important aspect of the drugs distribution is its uptake and retention in pancreatic β cells. Clinically, streptozotocin is used mainly to treat islet cell tumours of the pancreas and malignant carcinoid. When administered as a single agent, myelosuppression is not a dose-limiting toxicity. There is cumulative nephrotoxicity, severe cumulative nausea and vomiting, and pain is experienced at the injection site.

Alkylalkanesulphonates (Table 4)

Busulfan (Fig. 17)

The dimethanesulphonate busulfan is more stable than chlorambucil and melphalan and produces DNA crosslinks directly. In contrast to nitrogen mustards and chloroethylnitrosoureas, it has a more marked effect on myeloid stem cells than lymphoid cells. As a result, it is used at standard doses in the treatment of chronic myelogenous leukaemia. In addition, it is used at high dose with cyclophosphamide in allogenic and autologous transplantation in the treatment of refractory leukaemias, lymphomas, and some paediatric solid tumours.

Busulfan is well absorbed from the gastrointestinal tract and is orally administered. In adults, the oral absorption proceeds by zero-order kinetics with a mean lag time of around 40 min and a duration of around 2 h. The half-life of the drug, at both normal and high dose, is around 2.5 h. It readily penetrates into the central nervous system.

The nadir of myelosuppression with busulfan can be very long compared to other bifunctional alkylating agents. The nadir granulocyte count is at 11 to 30 days and recovery usually requires 34 to 54 days. Interstitial pulmonary fibrosis or 'busulfan lung' is a rare late toxicity which can occur up to 10 years after treatment. Hyperpigmentation can also be seen as a complication of therapy.

Treosulfan (Fig. 18)

Although treosulfan is structurally related to busulfan, the activation pathway of both drugs is quite different. Unlike busulfan, which alkylates as a primary methanesulfonate, treosulfan is a prodrug for epoxy compounds and converts non-enzymatically to L-diepoxybutane via the corresponding monoepoxide under physiological conditions (Fig. 18). DNA alkylation and interstrand crosslinking are

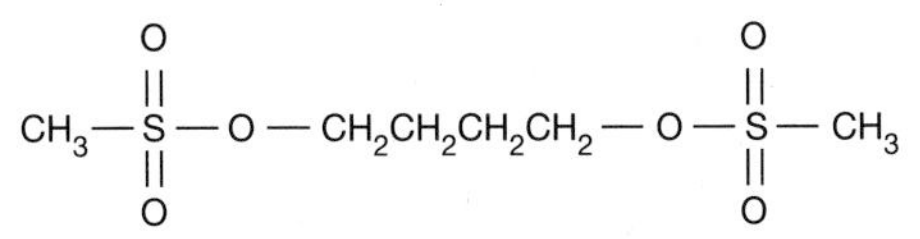

$$CH_3-\overset{\overset{O}{\|}}{\underset{\underset{O}{\|}}{S}}-O-CH_2CH_2CH_2CH_2-O-\overset{\overset{O}{\|}}{\underset{\underset{O}{\|}}{S}}-CH_3$$

Fig. 17 Busulphan.

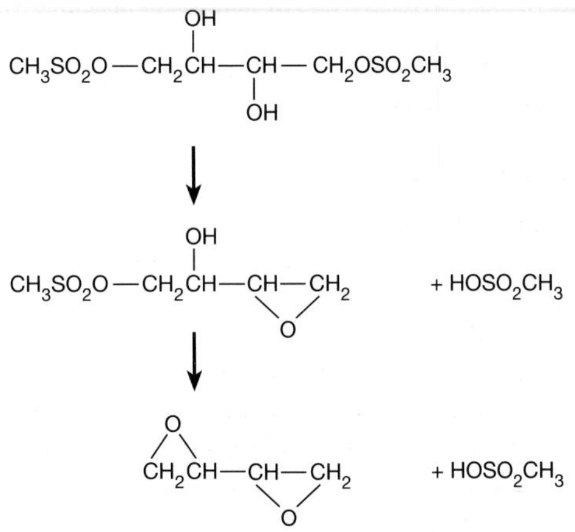

$$CH_3SO_2O-CH_2\overset{\overset{OH}{|}}{CH}-\overset{\underset{|}{OH}}{CH}-CH_2OSO_2CH_3$$

↓

$$CH_3SO_2O-CH_2\overset{\overset{OH}{|}}{CH}-CH-CH_2 \quad + HOSO_2CH_3$$

↓

$$CH_2CH-CH-CH_2 \quad + HOSO_2CH_3$$

Fig. 18 Treosulfan and its spontaneous pH-dependent activation into the diepoxide, L-diepoxybutane via a monoepoxide.

produced from the resulting epoxide compounds. Synthesized more than 30 years ago, treosulfan possesses a broad spectrum of antitumour activity *in vivo* but has been limited clinically to the treatment of ovarian carcinoma. Toxicological evaluation and clinical experience, however, has shown no significant non-haematological toxicity and the drug is therefore being re-evaluated as a candidate for high-dose chemotherapy with autologous stem cell reinfusion.

Aziridines (Table 5)

Thio-TEPA (Fig. 19)

Thio-TEPA (N,N'-,N''-triethylenethiophosphoramide) was recognized as an antitumour agent in the 1950s. Its metabolism and decomposition are complex but the major metabolite *in vivo* is TEPA (triethylenephosphoramide) (Fig. 19) which is much less stable. Indeed thio-TEPA may act as a prodrug for the TEPA formed in the liver. The plasma half-life of thio-TEPA is between 1 and 2 h but the

metabolite is more persistent such that the overall area under the curve for TEPA is 5 to 10-fold greater than for thio-TEPA.

Thio-TEPA has activity in a variety of malignancies including leukaemia, Hodgkin's disease, and ovarian, breast, and bladder cancers, but has not been widely incorporated into combination chemotherapy. The drug can be administered by any parenteral route and is used in the intravesical treatment of bladder tumours. Dose-limiting toxicity is myelosuppression but the drug is characterized by its relative lack of non-haematological toxicity. As a result it has been incorporated into high-dose regimens with bone marrow transplantation. At high dose, toxicities include mucositis, hepatotoxicity, and neuropathy.

Mitomycin C (Fig. 20)

Mitomycin C is the prototype bioreductive alkylating agent. It is a natural product isolated from *Streptomyces caespitosus*. It is activated by reduction of the quinone moiety and alkylation and crosslinking occurs in the minor groove of DNA. It is used in a number of combination chemotherapy protocols, particularly in the treatment of gastric cancer. In addition, it can be used intraperitoneally or, more commonly, by direct intravesical administration in the treatment of superficial bladder cancer. It is absorbed poorly through the bladder and therefore provides an effective local therapy. Bone marrow suppression, which can be prolonged, is the dose-limiting toxicity. The degree and duration of myelosuppression depends on the total cumulative dose. Mitomycin C is administered intravenously and is a potent vesicant. Precautions should be taken to avoid extravasation during administration. Among the other toxicities unique to mitomycin C is vasculitis with manifestations ranging from haemolytic–uraemic syndrome to veno-occlusive disease. When given in combination with an anthracycline, mitomycin C can enhance the cardiotoxic effect of the anthracycline. An interstitial pneumonitis can also occur. Nausea and vomiting are frequent toxicities.

Diaziquone (Fig. 21)

The search for compounds that could be activated by reduction preferentially in hypoxic tumour cells led to the evaluation of a range of aziridinyl-containing compounds including diaziquone (AZQ). This compound can undergo reduction of the quinone moiety which enhances the reactivity of the two aziridine rings. The drug is lipophilic and readily crosses the blood–brain barrier. In clinical trials diaziquone was active either alone or in combination with BCNU in brain tumours.[40] On intravenous administration, the drug is rapidly distributed and eliminated. Brain tumour levels reach between 48 and

Table 4 Alkyalkanesulphonates

Name	Major approved indications	Route	Typical dosage and administration	Major toxicities
Busulfan	Chronic myelogenous leukaemia	PO	4–8 mg daily	Neutorpenia, interstitial pulmonary fibrosis, hyperpigmentation of skin
		high dose	4 mg/kg/day for 4 days	Hepatotoxicity, nausea and vomiting
Treosulfan	Ovarian cancer	PO	1g/day for 4 weeks	Myelosuppression
		IV	5–15 g every 1–3 weeks	Myelosuppression

Fig. 19 Thio-TEPA (left) and its major metabolite TEPA (triethylenephosphoramide) (right).

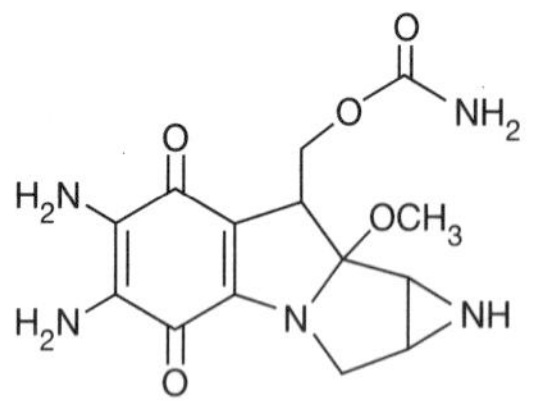

Fig. 20 Mitomycin C.

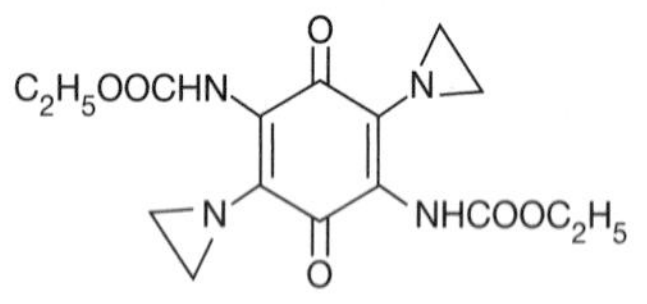

Fig. 21 Diaziquone.

85 per cent of plasma levels. The dose-limiting toxicity of diaziquone is myelosuppression and with thrombocytopenia a frequent occurrence.

N-methyl type compounds (Table 6)

Hexamethylmelamine (Fig. 22)

Hexamethylmelamine was first synthesized in the 1950s and undergoes metabolism by hepatic microsomal enzymes to produce hydroxylated and demethylated intermediates. The half-life of hexamethylmelamine is 3 to 10 h. The major metabolite is N-hydroxymethylpenta-methylmelamine (Fig. 22). The relatively stable melamines produced are assumed to be the active metabolites of hexamethylmelamine because of their ability to alkylate DNA, and their polyfunctionality could allow DNA crosslink formation. Formaldehyde is produced during enzymatic N-demethylation. The formation of active metabolites by hepatic enzymes is much less efficient in humans than in mice.

Hexamethylmelamine has a poor aqueous solubility and is only available for oral administration. Oral absorption is variable with peak levels after 0.5 to 3 h. It has demonstrated activity as a single agent and in combination against bronchial, cervical, and breast cancers and lymphomas, but is most commonly used in the management of ovarian cancer. Troublesome nausea and vomiting limit its usefulness and other toxicities include peripheral neuropathies and central nervous system effects.

Trimelamol (Fig. 23)

In an attempt to overcome some of the limitations of hexa-methylmelamine, several analogues have undergone clinical trials. Pentamethylmelamine is much more water soluble but trials were disappointing and it was found to be as emetic as hexa-methylmelamine. The hydroxymethyl analogue trimelamol was developed as a fully activated analogue of hexamethylmelamine which would bypass the relatively inefficient metabolic activation seen in humans. Significant activity was demonstrated against refractory ovarian cancer and the drug was less emetic and neurotoxic than pentamethylmelamine. The mode of action of trimelamol has not

Table 5 Aziridines

Name	Major approved indications	Route	Typical dosage and administration	Major toxicities
Thio-TEPA	Intravesical treatment of bladder, tumours, ovarian cancer, breast cancer	IV	0.3–0.4 mg/kg every 1–4 weeks	Myelosuppression
		intravesical	30–60 mg/week × 4	Lower abdominal discomfort, bladder irritability
		IV high dose	500–1125 mg/m^2	Mucositis, hepatotoxicity, neuropathy
Mitomycin C	Gastric cancer, bladder cancer	IV	10–20 mg/m^2 every 6–8 weeks	Myelosuppression, nausea and vomiting, tissue necrosis after extravasation, nephrotoxicity, haemolytic–uraemic syndrome, interstitial pneumonitis, cardiotoxicity, veno-occlusive disease
Diaziquone	Brain tumour	IV	18–20 mg/m^2 days 1 and 8 of 28 day cycle; 8 mg/m^2/day for 5 days	Myelosuppression, thrombocytopenia

Table 6 *N*-methyl type compounds

Name	Major approved indications	Route	Typical dosage and administration	Major toxicities
Hexamethylmelamine	Ovarian cancer	PO	Single agent 260 mg/m² days 1–14 Combination 150–200 mg/m² days 1–14 every 4 weeks (4 divided daily doses)	Nausea and vomiting, central and peripheral neurotoxicity
Procarbazine	Hodgkin's disease	PO	100 mg/m² days 1–14 every 4 weeks	Myelosuppression, nausea and vomiting
Dacarbazine	Malignant melanoma, Hodgkin's disease	IV	250 mg/m² days 1–5 every 3–4 weeks	Nausea and vomiting, myelosuppression
Temozolomide	High grade glioma	PO	150–250 mg/m² days 1–5 every 4 weeks	Myelosuppession, nausea and vomiting

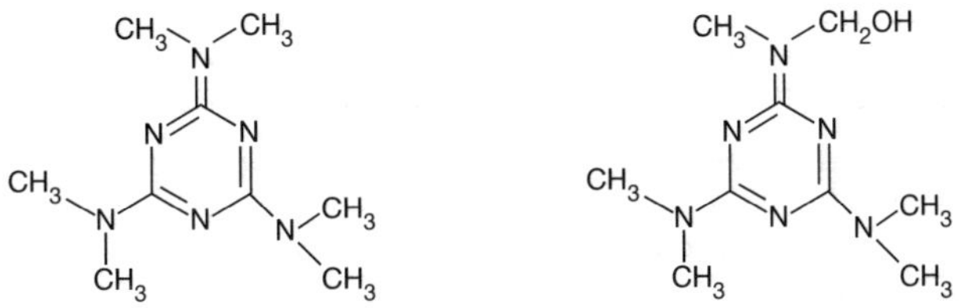

Fig. 22 Hexamethylmelamine (left) and its major metabolite *N*-hydroxymethylpentamethylmelamine (right).

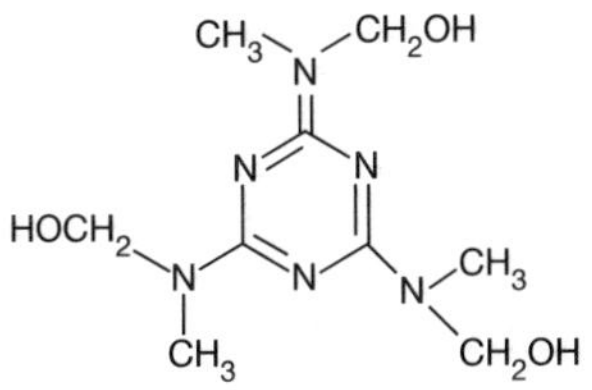

Fig. 23 Trimelamol.

been fully established and various mechanisms have been suggested. The formation of DNA interstrand crosslinking has however been clearly demonstrated, but extensive DNA–protein crosslinking is also observed due to the action of released formaldehyde.

Procarbazine (Fig. 24)

Procarbazine was originally synthesized as an inhibitor of monoamine oxidase but was found in animals to have antitumour activity. It is an *N*-methyl-substituted hydrazine and, following oxidation of the hydrazine in the liver, it undergoes a complex series of enzymatic and chemical breakdown steps to produce DNA alkylating species. It has a half-life of 10 min. The cytotoxicity of procarbazine is generally assumed to be mediated by methylation of DNA, probably via the O6 position of guanine.

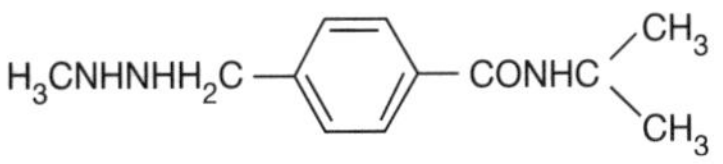

Fig. 24 Procarbazine.

Clinically, procarbazine is used most commonly in the treatment of Hodgkin's disease but is also used in combination with other drugs for lymphomas and brain tumours. It is given orally. Dose-limiting toxicity is delayed myelosuppresion, mainly thrombocytopenia. Because of its potential to inhibit monoamine oxidase it has potentially negative drug and food interactions. For example effects of CNS depressants, sympathomimetic drugs, and tricyclic antidepressants are increased. Interaction with tyramine-rich foods can cause hypertensive crisis, tremor, and palpitations. With concomitant alcohol, antabuse-like activity with severe gastrointestinal toxicity and headache can result.

Dacarbazine (DTIC) (Fig. 25)

Dacarbazine requires metabolic activation to produce alkylating species. The active metabolite produced during *N*-demethylation by hepatic cytochrome P450 is 5-(3-methyltriazen-1-yl) imidazole-4-carboxamide (MTIC). This can then eliminate the reactive methyldiazonium ion as a methylating intermediate (Fig. 25). Dacarbazine therefore acts as a monofunctional alkylating agent and methylation at the O6 position of guanine is assumed to be the primary cytotoxic event. Cells or xenografts with low levels of guanine O6-alkyltransferase are more sensitive to dacarbazine than those with high levels and, when given clinically, dacarbazine depletes levels of this enzyme in peripheral blood cells. The drug is light sensitive and can be broken down to form toxic species.

Dacarbazine has single agent activity against malignant melanoma with reported partial remission rates of up to 30 per cent. It is also active as a single agent in Hodgkin's disease and is used in combination regimens for Hodgkin's disease and soft tissue sarcomas. The drug is administered intravenously and the dose-limiting toxicity is myelosuppression with nausea and vomiting occurring in 90 per cent of patients.

Temozolomide (Fig. 26)

Temozolomide was synthesized to generate the active metabolite of dacarbazine, MTIC, spontaneously and therefore overcome the

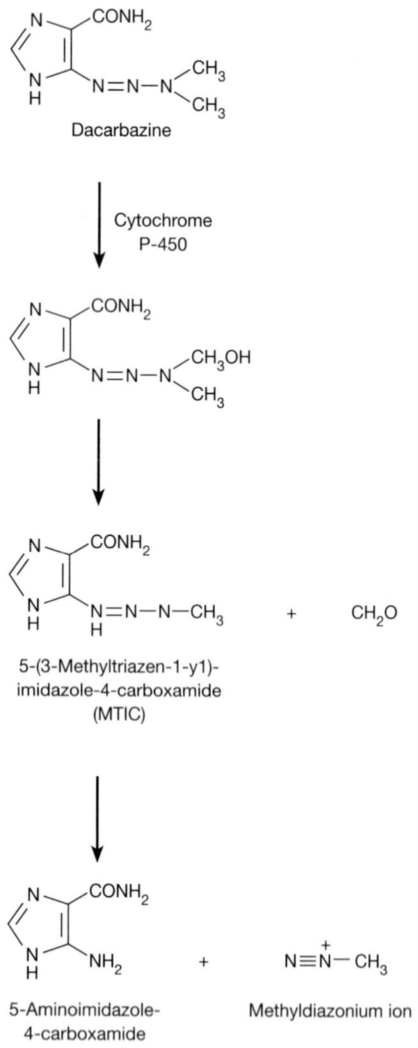

Fig. 25 Dacarbazine (DTIC) and its metabolism to produce 5-(3-methyltriazen-1-yl) imidazole-4-carboxamide (MTIC). MTIC can then eliminate the reactive methyldiazonium ion.

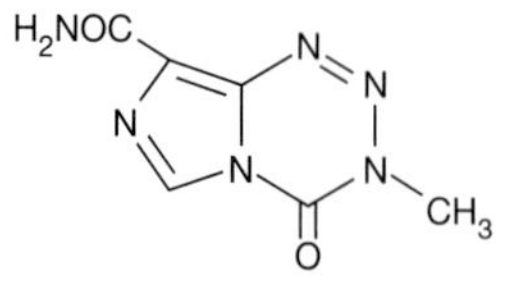

Fig. 26 Temozolomide.

relatively inefficient *N*-demethylation step in humans. Temozolomide similarly acts as a monofunctional alkylating agent with methylation at the O6 position of guanine being essential for its action. The drug can be given orally and activity in melanoma and high grade glioma was demonstrated in a phase I trial involving oral administration daily for 5 days. Subsequent phase II trials in recurrent or progressive

high-grade glioma produced objective responses and tolerable side-effects.[41] The dose limiting toxicity is myelosuppression.

New approaches and future prospects

Despite the important place antitumour alkylating agents have in cancer chemotherapy they are far from ideal drugs. Improvements in their clinical use may come from a number of approaches, including the more optimal and rational use of existing drugs either alone or in combination, the use of novel alkylators which may be more selective in their action, or by using strategies to deliver the drugs more effectively to the tumour site. Clearly, a detailed understanding of the molecular, cellular, and clinical pharmacology of alkylating agents is required in order to achieve these aims.

The more effective use of existing alkylating agents may come from the rational application of new drug combinations which are not cross-resistant, or whose combined mechanisms produce additive or synergistic effects. The optimization of pharmacokinetic exposure with individual patients using therapeutic drug monitoring approaches may also be feasible.[42] In addition, methods are becoming available which allow the detection and quantitation of the critical adducts produced by alkylating agents, and their repair, in the clinical setting. For example a modification of the single cell gel electrophoresis (comet) assay allows the formation and repair of the DNA interstrand crosslinks produced by bifunctional alkylating agents to be monitored in peripheral blood and in tumour material.[43] High-dose strategies employing bone marrow transplantation supported by haemopoietic growth factors continue to be evaluated.

Understanding the mechanisms which make some tumours inherently sensitive (or resistant) to DNA damaging agents is an important goal with the ultimate aim of producing strategies to overcome inherent or acquired resistance. Potential approaches to overcoming resistance pharmacologically are being pursued. Examples are the use of agents which deplete cellular protectors such as glutathione (e.g. L-buthionine (SR)-sulfoximine (BSO)) and agents which modulate DNA repair (e.g. inhibition of guanine O6-alkyl-transferase by O6-benzylguanine). Advances in the understanding of the signalling pathways that control the responses to DNA damage, such as cell cycle arrest and apoptosis, may also provide important opportunities for pharmacological intervention to enhance the effectiveness of alkylating agents. Antiangiogenic agents have also been shown to potentiate the effects of cytotoxic agents in animal models,[44] and the development of bioreductive alkylating agents which would undergo preferential activation in the hypoxic regions of solid tumours remains of interest.[5] Considerable medicinal chemistry effort has gone into the design and synthesis of thousands of analogues of currently used alkylating agents. Although some advantages can be gained, it is unlikely that simple analogues of existing agents would confer more than minimally incremental value, particularly against the refractory, major solid tumours.

Conventional, clinically used alkylating agents lack selectivity on several levels. In addition to generally lacking selectivity to tumour over normal tissue, they are not selective for binding to their biological target, DNA, and when binding to DNA does occur the number of critical lesions, such as DNA interstrand crosslinks, may be small compared to other DNA lesions which do not contribute to antitumour activity but which may add to early and late toxicity. There is, therefore, much scope in designing novel agents or strategies which can overcome these limitations and enhance the selectivity of alkylating agent–DNA interactions.

In an attempt to target alkylation more efficiently to DNA, several types of DNA-affinity or DNA-directed alkylating agents have been synthesized. For example DNA intercalating ligands or polyamines have been used to carry attached alkylating groups to the DNA.[45],[46] Although many of these agents have shown enhanced cytotoxic potency *in vitro* over the corresponding non-targeted alkylating agent and activity *in vivo*, none of these agents have been evaluated clinically. Other alkylating agents with a high affinity for DNA have been derived from the extremely cytotoxic antibiotic CC-1065 originally isolated from *Streptomyces zelensis* in the mid-1970s. Although CC-1065 was too toxic in animal systems, three analogues with an improved therapeutic index, adozelesin, bizelesin, and carzelesin, are in clinical trial. These potent agents, like CC-1065, bind with high affinity to the minor groove of DNA and alkylate at the N3 position of adenine.[47] Unlike most clinically used alkylating agents that alkylate preferentially in G/C-rich sequences, these agents preferentially bind to A/T-rich regions of DNA.

Highly efficient DNA interstrand crosslinking agents have also been rationally designed and synthesized. For example the linking of two pyrrolo[2,1-c][1,4]benzodiazepine natural product antitumour antibiotic units together with an appropriate flexible linker produced the highly efficient interstrand crosslinking agent DSB-120. The irreversible crosslinks produced by this agent occur between two guanine bases within the minor groove via their exocyclic N2 atoms. In contrast to the interstrand crosslinks produced by most conventional bifunctional alkylating agents, those produced by DSB-120 cause minimal distortion to the DNA and appear difficult to be recognized and repaired in cells.[48] Several analogues of DSB-120 are currently undergoing preclinical evaluation.

In addition to having a greater selectivity for DNA, and for producing critical cytotoxic DNA lesions, many of the agents described above are also highly selective for certain sequences of DNA. For example DSB-120 spans six base pairs and actively recognizes and crosslinks a central 5′-GATC sequence. The novel agent tallimustine, which has recently undergone clinical trials, contains a conventional nitrogen mustard attached to the highly A/T sequence-selective, natural product distamycin A. Tallimustine binds non-covalently in the minor groove with high affinity to A/T-rich sequences but alkylates selectively within the sequences 5′-TTTTG̲G and 5′-TTTTG̲A (where alkylation occurs in the minor groove at the N3-position of the underlined base).[49] Agents which can deliver alkylating groups selectively to longer DNA sequences are being developed by both conventional medicinal chemistry and novel combinatorial chemistry-based approaches. What is clear is that enhanced sequence-specific alkylation can produce enhanced cytotoxic potency and that alkylation within different sequence contexts can lead to differences in biological response. In addition, the mechanisms of recognition and repair, and the resulting downstream responses to the DNA alkylation produced by these novel agents, appear to differ from those of conventional chemotherapeutic alkylating agents. A key question is whether enhancing sequence-specific alkylation will ultimately translate into an improved therapeutic index clinically.

Several strategies attempt to target alkylating agents more selectively to tumours. In addition to the locoregional administration of drugs, techniques of drug delivery that exploit the abnormal

tumour vasculature in solid tumours, including enhanced permeability and retention, are being evaluated. These include delivery systems based on polymers, liposomes, and microparticulates. Alternative approaches utilize antibodies targeted to tumour-associated antigens. Particularly promising with respect to alkylating agents is the approach of antibody-directed enzyme prodrug therapy (ADEPT) which is currently undergoing clinical evaluation.[50] In this two-phase system, an enzyme conjugated to a tumour-selective antibody is allowed to localize to the tumour prior to the administration systemically of a prodrug which is converted by the enzyme to an active agent at the tumour site. Ultimately, if proven to have real clinical utility, this approach will further benefit from the design of prodrugs of the novel types of lesion- and sequence-selective agents discussed above.

As opportunities to utilize the potential of gene-based therapies advance, there will be possibilities to exploit this technology to enhance the clinical effectiveness of chemotherapeutic alkylating agents. One possibility being actively pursued would involve expressing prodrug-activating-genes selectively in tumour cells. Alternatively, drug resistance genes (e.g. guanine O6-alkyltransferase) could be delivered to dose-limiting normal tissues such as the bone marrow. Although high-dose therapy would still be limited by second organ toxicity, the advantage over conventional bone marrow transplantation would be the opportunity to give multiple, high-dose treatments over a relatively short period.

References

1. **Karnofsky DA.** Summary of results obtained with nitrogen mustard in the treatment of neoplastic disease. *Annals of the New York Academy of Sciences*, 1958; **68**: 899–914.

2. **Calabresi P, Parks RE Jr.** Alkylating agents, antimetabolites, hormones and other antiproliferative agents. In: Goodman LS, Gilman A, eds. *The pharmacological bases of therapeutics*. New York: MacMillan, 1975: 1254–68.

3. **Goodman LS, Wintrobe MM, Dameshek W, Goodman MJ, Gilman A, McLennan MT.** Nitrogen mustard therapy; use of methyl-bis(beta-chloroethyl)amine hydrochloride and tris(betachloroethyl) amine hydrochloride for Hodgkin's disease, lymphosarcoma, leukemia and certain allied and miscellaneous disorders. *Journal of the American Medical Association*, 1946; **132**: 126–32.

4. **Gilman A, Philips FS.** The biological actions and therapeutic applications of the chloroethyl amines and sulphides. *Science*, 1946; **103**: 409–15.

5. **Workman P, Stratford IJ.** The experimental development of bioreductive drugs and their role in cancer therapy. *Cancer and Metastasis Reviews*, 1993; **12**: 73–82.

6. **Wilman DEV (ed).** *Chemistry of antitumour agents.* Glasgow: Blackie, 1990.

7. **Farmer PB.** Metabolism and reactions of alkylating agents. In: Powis G. ed. *International encyclopedia of pharmacology and therapeutics.* Section 141. Oxford: Pergamon, 1994:1–77.

8. **Singer B.** Sites in nucleic acids reacting with alkylating agents of differing carcinogenicity or mutagenicity. *Journal of Toxicology and Environmental Health*, 1977; **2**: 1279–95.

9. **Pullman A, Pullman B.** Molecular electrostatic potential of the nucleic acids. *Quarterly Reviews in Biophysics*, 1981; **14**: 289–380.

10. **Mattes WB, Hartley JA, Kohn, KW, Matheson DW.** GC-rich regions in genomes as targets for DNA alkylation. *Carcinogenesis*, 1988; **9**: 2065–72.

11. **Mattes WB, Hartley JA, Kohn KW.** DNA sequence selectivity of

guanine-N7 alkylation by nitrogen mustards. *Nucleic Acids Research*, 1986; **14**: 2971–87.

12. Hartley JA, Bingham JP, Souhami RL. DNA sequence selectivity of guanine-N7 alkylation by nitrogen mustards is preserved in intact cells. *Nucleic Acids Research*, 1992; **20**: 3175–8.

13. Brendel M, Ruhland A. Relationship between functionality and genetic toxicology of selected DNA-damaging agents. *Mutation Research*, 1984; **133**: 51–85.

14. Kohn KW, Ewig RAG, Erickson LC, Zwelling LA. Measurement of strand breaks and crosslinks in DNA by alkaline elution. In: Friedberg EC, Hanawalt PC, eds. *DNA repair: a laboratory manual of research techniques*. New York: Marcel Dekker, 1981: 379–404.

15. Chun EHL, Gonzales L, Lewis FS, Jones J, Rutman RJ. Differences in the *in vivo* alkylation and crosslinking of nitrogen mustard sensitive and resistance lines of Lettre-Ehrlich ascites tumors. *Cancer Research*, 1969; **29**: 1184–94.

16. O'Connor PM, Kohn KW. Comparative pharmacokinetics of DNA lesion formation and removal following treatment of L1210 cells with nitrogen mustards. *Cancer Communications*, 1990; **2**: 387–94.

17. Sunters A, Springer CJ, Bagshawe K, Souhami RL, Hartley JA. The cytotoxicity DNA crosslinking ability and DNA sequence selectivity of the aniline mustards melphalan, chlorambucil, and 4-[bis(2-chloroethyl)amino]benzoic acid. *Biochemical Pharmacology*, 1993; **32**: 2297–301.

18. Bedford P, Fox BW. DNA-DNA interstrand crosslinking by dimethanesulphonic acid esters. *Biochemical Pharmacology*, 1983; **32**: 2297–301.

19. Erickson LC, Bradley MO, Ducore JM, Ewig RAG, Kohn KW. DNA crosslinking and cytotoxicity in normal and SV40 transformed human cells treated with antitumor nitrosoureas. *Proceedings of the National Academy of Sciences USA*, 1980; **77**: 467–71.

20. Erickson LC, Laurent G, Sharkey NA, Kohn KW. DNA crosslinking and monoadduct repair in nitrosourea-treated human tumour cells. *Nature*, 1980; **288**: 727–9.

21. Millard JT, Raucher S, Hopkins PB. Mechlorethamine crosslinks deoxyguanosine residues at 5'-GNC sequences in duplex DNA fragments. *Journal of the American Chemical Society*, 1990; **112**: 2459–60.

22. Tomasz M, Lipman R, Chowdary C, Pawlak J, Verdine GL, Nakanishi K. Isolation and structure of a covalent crosslink adduct between mitomycin C and DNA. *Science*, 1987; **235**: 1204–8.

23. Ludlum DB. DNA alkylation by the haloethylnitrosoureas: nature of modifications produced and their enzymatic repair or removal. *Mutation Research*, 1990; **233**: 117–26.

24. D'Incalci M, Citti L, Taverna P, Catapano CV. Importance of the DNA repair enzyme O6-alkyl guanine alkyltransferase (AT) in cancer chemotherapy. *Cancer Treatment Reports*, 1988; **15**: 279–92.

25. Hartley JA. Selectivity in alkylating agent-DNA interactions. In: Neidle S, Waring MJ, eds. *Molecular aspects of anticancer drug-DNA interactions*. Macmillan, Basingstoke, UK. 1993: 1–31.

26. Friedberg EC, Walker GC, Siede W. *DNA repair and mutagenesis*. Washington DC. ASM Press, 1995.

27. Hanawalt PC. Heterogeneity of DNA repair at the gene level. *Mutation Research*, 1991; **247**: 203–11.

28. Wassermann K, Kohn KW, Bohr VA. Heterogeneity of nitrogen mustard-induced DNA damage and repair at the level of the gene in Chinese hamster ovary cells. *Journal of Biological Chemistry*, 1990; **265**: 13906–13.

29. Tannock IF. Experimental chemotherapy and concepts related to the cell cycle. *International Journal of Radiation Biology*, 1986; **49**: 335–55.

30. O'Connor PM, *et al.* Relationship between DNA crosslinks, cell cycle, and apoptosis in Burkitt's lymphoma cell lines differing in sensitivity to nitrogen mustard. *Cancer Research*, 1991; **51**: 6550–7.

31. Schmahl D, Habs M, Lorenz M, Wagner L. Occurrence of second tumours in man after anticancer drug treatment. *Cancer Treatment Reviews*, 1982; **9**: 167–94.

32. Torres-Garcia SJ, Cousineau L, Caplan S, Panasci L. Correlation of resistance to nitrogen mustards in chronic lymphocytic leukemia with enhanced removal of melphalan-induced DNA crosslinks. *Biochemical Pharmacology*, 1989; **38**: 3122–3.

33. Fink D, Aebi S, Howell SB. The role of DNA mismatch repair in drug resistance. *Clinical Cancer Research*, 1998; **4**: 1–6.

34. Goldenberg GJ, Vanstone CL, Israels LG, Ilse D, Bihler I. Evidence for a transport carrier of nitrogen mustard in nitrogen mustard-sensitive and -resistant L5178Y lymphoblasts. *Cancer Research*, 1979; **30**: 2285–91.

35. Moscow JA, Swanson CA, Cowan KH. Decreased melphalan accumulation in a human breast cancer cell line selected for resistance to melphalan. *British Journal of Cancer*, 1993; **68**: 732–7.

36. Tew KD. Glutathione-associated enzymes in anticancer drug resistance. *Cancer Research*, 1994; **54**: 4313–20.

37. Green MH, *et al.* Melphalan may be a more potent leukaemogen than cyclophosphamide. *Annals of International Medicine*, 1986; **105**: 360–7.

38. Lerner HJ. Acute myelogenous leukemia in patients receiving chlorambucil as long-term adjuvant chemotherapy for stage II breast cancer. *Cancer Treatment Reports*, 1978; **62**: 1135–9.

39. Berk PD, Goldberg JD, Silverstein MN. Increased incidence of acute leukemia in polycythemia vera associated with chlorambucil. *New England Journal of Medicine*, 1981; **304**: 441–3.

40. Schold SC, Mahaley MS, Vick NA. Phase II diaziquone-based chemotherapy trials in patients with anaplastic supratentorial astrocytic neoplasms. *Journal of Clinical Oncology*, 1987; **5**: 464–9.

41. Newlands ES, Stevens MF, Wedge SR, Wheelhouse RT, Brock C. Temozolamide: a review of its discovery, chemical properties, pre-clinical development and clinical trials. *Cancer Treatment Review*, 1997; **23**: 35–61.

42. Workman P, Graham MA (eds). *Cancer surveys. Vol 17, Pharmacokinetics and cancer chemotherapy*. New York: Cold Spring Harbor Press, 1993.

43. Hartley JM, Spanswick VJ, Gander M, Giacomini G, Whelan J, Souhami RL, Hartley JA. Measurement of DNA crosslinking in patients on ifosfamide therapy using the single cell gel electrophoresis (comet) assay. *Clinical Cancer Research*, 1999; **5**: 507–12.

44. Teicher BA, Sotomayer EA, Huang ZD. Antiangiogenic agents potentiate cytotoxic cancer therapies against primary and metastatic disease. *Cancer Research*, 1992; **52**: 6702–4.

45. Denny WA. DNA-interacting ligands as anti-cancer drugs: prospects for future design. *Anti-cancer Drug Design*, 1989; **4**: 241–63.

46. Holley JL, Mather A, Collis PM, Hartley JA, Bingham JP, Cohen GM. Selective targeting of tumour cells and DNA by a chlorambucil-spermidine conjugate. *Cancer Research*, 1992; **52**: 4190–5.

47. Reynolds VL, Molineux JJ, Kaplan DJ, Swenson DH, Hurley LH. Reaction of the antitumor antibiotic CC-1065 with DNA. Location of the site of thermally induced strand breakage and analysis of DNA sequence specificity. *Biochemistry*, 1985; **24**: 6228–37.

48. Smellie M, Kelland L, Thurston DE, Souhami RL, Hartley JA. Cellular pharmacology of novel linked anthramycin-based sequence selective DNA minor groove crosslinking agents. *British Journal of Cancer*, 1994; **70**: 48–53.

49. Broginni M, Coley H, Mongelli N, *et al.* DNA sequence specific adenine alkylation by the antitumour drug tallimustine (FCE24517), a benzoyl nitrogen mustard derivative of distamycin. *Nucleic Acids Research*, 1995; **23**: 183–9.

50. Bagshawe KD. Towards generating cytotoxic agents at cancer sites. *British Journal of Cancer*, 1989; **60**: 275–81.

4.15 Cisplatin and analogues

Ian Judson and Lloyd R. Kelland

History and discovery of cisplatin

The parent compound, and for many years the only clinically available anticancer drug cis-dichlorodiammine platinum (II), or cisplatin, remains one of the most commonly prescribed agents with a very broad spectrum of activity. It was discovered serendipitously by Rosenberg[1] while investigating the effects of electric currents on bacteria that caused a filamentous growth pattern and growth inhibition. These effects were found to be due to complexes formed by an interaction between the platinum electrodes and growth medium. Neutral complexes were found to have relatively selective effects on cell division and proved to have broad antitumour activity in mouse model tumour systems. Of these, cisplatin was found to be the most active and was taken forward into clinical trials.

Phase I studies were carried out in the early 1970s by Wiltshaw and colleagues in London[2] and Higby and colleagues in New York.[3] Although antitumour activity was reported in tumours such as refractory testicular teratoma and ovarian cancer, the incidence of severe side-effects such as nausea and vomiting and kidney damage was initially unacceptable. Cvitkovic and colleagues[4] demonstrated that hyperhydration with isotonic saline ameliorated the nephrotoxicity and allowed the drug to be administered repeatedly, albeit with a gradual deterioration in renal function. Other side-effects including vomiting, peripheral neuropathy, tinnitus, and high-tone hearing loss have proved much more difficult to manage, although the advent of 5-hydroxytryptamine type 3 (5-HT$_3$) antagonists has made nausea and vomiting less of a problem.[5]

Chemistry

Cisplatin is a neutral square planar coordination complex with two chloride and two ammonia ligands in the cis-configuration (Fig. 1). Early structure–activity studies in tumour-bearing mice showed that the trans-isomer of cisplatin is devoid of antitumour activity.[6] Platinum exists in two main oxidation states, Pt^{2+} usually designated Pt(II) as in cisplatin and carboplatin or Pt^{4+} designated as Pt(IV) as in JM216 (see below). In platinum (IV) complexes there are six bonds and ligands, four in a square planar configuration and two located axially directly above and below the platinum, thus producing an octahedral configuration.

The chemical properties of the platinum complexes are largely dependent upon the relative displacement reactions of the various ligands. Whereas some bonds (such as those to the nitrogens in cisplatin, or sulphur) are essentially irreversible under physiological conditions, the stability of bonds to halogens and to aquo (H$_2$O) is much lower. The loss of the chlorine atoms is critical to the antitumour properties of cisplatin. The presence of relatively high chloride concentrations in extracellular fluid (approximately 100 mmol) suppresses the formation of mono- and diaquo species while intracellular chloride concentrations are lower (approximately 4 mmol) thereby allowing their formation. Since the mono- and diaquo species are far more reactive and better leaving groups than chlorines, this allows reactions with critical cellular nucleophiles, especially DNA (see below).

Mechanisms of action and resistance

Following the introduction of cisplatin into the clinic, it was soon apparent that many tumours exhibited intrinsic resistance to this drug (e.g. colorectal, non-small cell lung cancers) while others acquired resistance during courses of chemotherapy (e.g. some ovarian and small cell lung cancers). This prompted laboratory-based investigations aimed at determining the mechanisms by which cisplatin exerts its antitumour effects and how tumour resistance occurs.

DNA as the target for the antitumour effects of cisplatin

It is generally believed that cisplatin exerts its antitumour properties through binding to DNA, where specific adducts have been

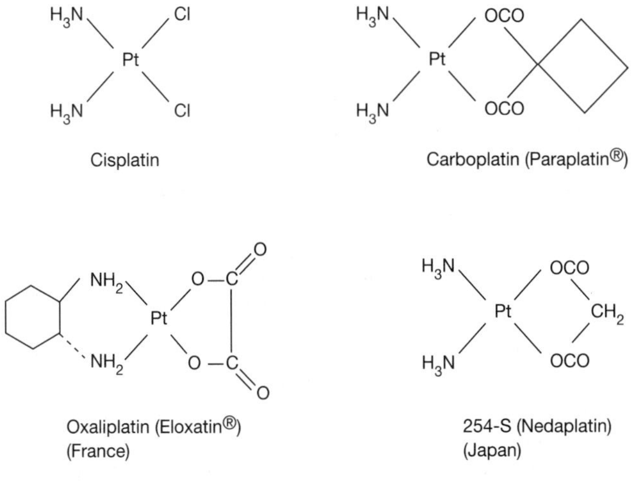

Fig. 1 Platinum drugs currently registered for use.

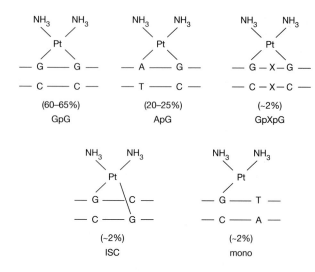

Fig. 2 Binding of cisplatin to DNA.

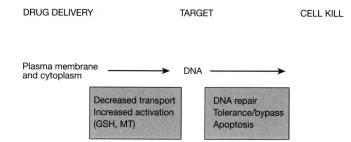

Fig. 3 Mechanisms of resistance to cisplatin.

identified.[7],[8] Cisplatin reacts with the N7 position of the imidazole ring of guanines (**G**) or adenines (**A**) on DNA to form a variety of monofunctional or, importantly, bifunctional adducts which then block replication and/or prevent transcription (Fig. 2). The most common adduct of cisplatin (60 to 65 per cent) involves binding to adjacent deoxyguanosines along the same strand of DNA (the GpG 1,2-intrastrand adduct). Other identified adducts include the ApG 1, 2-intrastrand (20 to 25 per cent), and low numbers of GpXpG and ApXpG 1,3-intrastrand, monofunctional, DNA–protein cross-links and G–G interstrand cross-links. Both the GpG and ApG 1,2-intrastrand adducts unwind DNA by 13° whereas the GpXpG 1,3-intrastrand adduct unwinds DNA by 23°; bending of the DNA double helix is similar (32 to 35°) for all three types of adduct. Further evidence for DNA as the target of cisplatin's antitumour effects is provided by observations that: (i) cells from patients with diseases where DNA repair processes have been biochemically characterized as deficient (e.g. xeroderma pigmentosum) are hypersensitive to cisplatin; (ii) correlations have been shown between levels of platinum–DNA adducts in peripheral blood lymphocytes and disease (or toxicity) response in patients receiving cisplatin (or carboplatin); and (iii) the high-resolution crystal structure of double-stranded DNA containing the GpG 1,2-intrastrand adduct[9] and the nuclear magnetic resonance (NMR) solution structure of a G–G interstrand cross-link[10] have been elucidated (and see ref. 8 for a review).

There still remains debate, however, as to which of the above described adducts on DNA are of most importance in mediating tumour cell killing. Support for a role for the predominant 1,2-intrastrand adducts arises from findings that the inactive *trans*-isomer of cisplatin (transplatin) is sterically unable to form these adducts and that these adducts are relatively poorly removed from DNA compared with 1,3-intrastrand and monofunctional adducts. On the other hand, although interstrand cross-links represent only a small proportion of the overall adducts, studies have shown a relationship of cell killing or resistance to numbers or repair of interstrand cross-links (see reference 8 for a review). The adducts formed by carboplatin on DNA are essentially the same as those formed by cisplatin although, to obtain equivalent levels, 20- to 40-fold higher concentrations are required in cell lines, reflecting the much slower rate of aquation for carboplatin.[11]

Resistance to platinum drugs

Mechanism of resistance studies have generally used human tumour cell lines repeatedly exposed *in vitro* to cisplatin. In such cell lines, two broad causes of resistance have been observed: (i) those preventing adequate drug from reaching the target DNA and (ii) a failure in cell death to occur post-binding of platinum to DNA (Fig. 3; see ref. 12 for a recent review). Decreased drug transport and increased intracellular detoxification through increased levels of thiols, especially glutathione or metallothioneins, represent the major causes of inadequate drug reaching DNA. Post-DNA binding mechanisms of resistance include increased DNA repair of adducts and an ability to tolerate greater levels of DNA damage with a concomitant failure to engage programmed cell death (apoptotic) pathways. While much has been elucidated using *in vitro* models, the relative importance of these multifactorial mechanisms in the clinic is less clear.

Inadequate platinum binding to DNA

Most *in vitro* models of acquired cisplatin resistance exhibit a decrease in platinum accumulation, typically two- to fourfold. It is generally believed that this is due to reduced drug uptake rather than increased drug efflux (the commonly described P-glycoprotein multidrug resistance efflux pump is not overexpressed in cisplatin-resistant tumours). However, the mechanism by which cisplatin enters cells is not fully understood and appears to involve both passive diffusion and facilitated transport, possibly through a gated channel (see reference 13 for a review). The uptake of cisplatin is not saturable or inhibited by structural analogues. However, at least a proportion of uptake is energy dependent and can be modulated by pharmacological agents, such as the Na^+,K^+-ATPase inhibitor ouabain and the membrane interactive antifungal agent amphotericin. While there have been occasional reports of alterations in levels of proteins in transport-deficient cells with acquired cisplatin resistance, there are no universally accepted platinum transport proteins identified to date. Recently, interest has focused on the protein **cMOAT** (canalicular multispecific organic anion transporter) or **MRP2**, a member of the ATP-binding cassette family of transport proteins, which has been shown to be overexpressed in some cisplatin-resistant cells exhibiting a platinum transport defect.[14]

Intracellular inactivation of platinum drugs may occur through binding to thiol-containing species, namely the cytoplasmic tripeptide glutathione or metallothioneins, a class of cysteine-rich isoproteins of low molecular weight. Many platinum-resistant cell lines exhibit relatively high levels of intracellular glutathione compared with their sensitive counterparts and a direct interaction between 1 mol of platinum complexed with 2 mol of glutathione has been shown in tumour cells.[15] Glutathione levels showed a significant correlation with cisplatin sensitivity in our own panel of eight human ovarian carcinoma cell lines exhibiting a 100-fold range in intrinsic sensitivity and cells could be sensitized to platinum drugs by depleting glutathione levels with buthionine sulphoximine.[16] Increased levels of metallothioneins have been described in at least some cell lines with acquired cisplatin resistance and, moreover, transfection of human metallothionein-II$_A$ cDNA into cells conferred over fourfold resistance to cisplatin.[17]

Post-platinum–DNA binding

A variety of proteins have been described that recognize and bind to platinum DNA damage. These damage recognition proteins include the XPA–RPA complex, non-histone chromatin HMG1 and HMG2, human upstream binding factor hUBF, histone H1, the TATA box-binding protein TBP, and hMSH2 and may either assist in the removal and repair of such damage or, conversely, shield damage from repair proteins.[8],[18] Removal of platinum–DNA lesions is widely believed to occur mainly by nucleotide excision repair, where an ATP-dependent multiprotein complex removes the damage in the form of an oligonucleotide of 27 to 29 nucleotides (see reference 18 for a review).

There is evidence of increased nucleotide excision repair of platinum–DNA adducts contributing to resistance to platinum drugs and, conversely, defective nucleotide excision repair contributing to the hypersensitivity of some cell lines. Increased removal of platinum from the overall genome of resistant cell lines relative to parent sensitive lines has been observed in several models. Furthermore, nucleotide excision repair can occur preferentially in actively transcribed genes relative to the overall genome (transcription coupled repair). Increased gene-specific repair of cisplatin interstrand crosslinks has been reported in cisplatin-resistant human ovarian cancer cell lines.[19] Increased levels of RNA encoding another protein involved in nucleotide excision repair, ERCC1, have been associated with clinical resistance to platinum drugs in patients with ovarian cancer.[20] A defect in another protein involved in nucleotide excision repair, XPG, in mouse leukaemia cells, caused hypersensitivity to cisplatin and recently, the hypersensitivity of testicular germ cell tumours to cisplatin-induced DNA damage has been attributed to reduced XPA protein leading to poor removal by nucleotide excision repair.[21] The possibility of enhancing the therapeutic effect of cisplatin by combining with drugs which effect nucleotide excision repair of platinum DNA damage is being explored with aphidicolin (an inhibitor of DNA polymerases) and gemcitabine.

The HMG-box proteins, including HMG1 and HMG2, bind selectively to DNA modified by cisplatin but not to that modified by the inactive isomer transplatin. In contrast to the nucleotide excision repair proteins, HMG1 has been shown to inhibit the repair of the GpG 1,2-intrastrand major DNA adduct of cisplatin by human excision nuclease *in vitro*.[22] A model for the role of the HMG proteins involving shielding of adducts from repair proteins has been proposed.

Increased tolerance to platinum DNA damage is a phenomenon reported in some resistant tumours. Enhanced replicative bypass, the ability of the replication complex to synthesize DNA past a cisplatin-induced adduct, has been shown to occur in some cisplatin-resistant cells.[18],[23] Although not much is known of the underlying cellular pathways leading to increased tolerance, one component involves dysfunction of a second DNA repair process, mismatch repair.[18],[23] This is a recently described, although incompletely elucidated, ATP-dependent repair process involving at least five proteins (MLH1, MSH2, MSH3, MSH6, and PMS2) and responsible for correcting misincorporated nucleotides. Loss of mismatch repair has been associated with low-level (approximately twofold) resistance to cisplatin and carboplatin, but interestingly, not to oxaliplatin or JM216.[24] Moreover, the hMSH2 protein recognizes cisplatin-induced GpG 1, 2-intrastrand adducts on DNA. Furthermore, some tumour cell lines with acquired cisplatin resistance have been shown to have lost mismatch repair activity, primarily due to defects in the hMLH1 subunit.[18],[23],[24] Mismatch repair defects in hMutSα (heterodimer of hMSH2 and hMSH6) or hMutLα (heterodimer of hMLH1 and PMS2) have been shown to contribute to an increase in replicative bypass of cisplatin adducts.[23] Drug resistance in tumours deficient in mismatch repair is then thought to occur by preventing futile cycles of translesion synthesis and mismatch correction.

Following the binding of platinum to DNA, various other genes and proteins have been implicated in determining cellular sensitivity and resistance. These include those involved in mediating programmed cell death or apoptosis (the *p53* tumour suppressor gene, the *bcl2* family, c-*myc*, and *ras* genes).[25] Cells exposed to cisplatin (and other platinum drugs) show the morphological and biochemical characteristics of apoptosis, namely chromatin condensation, membrane blebbing, and DNA fragmentation.[26] The possible importance of the *p53* gene (one of the most commonly altered in human cancers) in determining the sensitivity of tumour cells to cisplatin (and other DNA-damaging drugs) is highlighted in studies with the National Cancer Institute 60 cell line drug-screening panel. Cells with mutant *p53* sequence were more resistant to cisplatin than those possessing wild-type p53 function.[27] The *bcl2* family of genes encodes a group of pro- (e.g. BAX) and anti-apoptotic (e.g. BCL2, BCL-X$_L$) proteins which form homo- and heterodimers with one another. Relative levels of pro- and anti- apoptotic proteins may function as a cell survival/ cell death rheostat to influence cell sensitivity and resistance to apoptosis-inducing drugs such as cisplatin.

Clinical pharmacology of cisplatin

The pharmacokinetics of platinum complexes are usually studied by measuring total platinum, which includes that bound to proteins, and ultrafiltrable platinum, which represents active drug. Initial clearance of cisplatin is rapid, with a distribution half-life ($T_{\frac{1}{2}}\alpha$) of 13 min and elimination half-life ($T_{\frac{1}{2}}\beta$) of 43 min; however, due to the reaction of the drug with plasma proteins, the terminal elimination half-life ($T_{\frac{1}{2}}\gamma$) is prolonged at 5.4 days.[28] Cisplatin is secreted by the renal tubule, which may in part account for its nephrotoxicity.

A number of agents, principally thiols, have been developed in the hopes of preventing toxicities such as neuropathy and nephrotoxicity by detoxifying active species in the tissues. If this occurred preferentially in the kidneys, for example, an improvement in therapeutic index might occur, but the concern has always remained that this approach might reduce the antitumour efficacy of cisplatin. Amifostine was developed initially as a radioprotective agent. It may also protect against the side-effects of chemotherapy and is said to be less activated in tumour tissue than at other sites such as bone marrow or kidney giving rise to improved selectivity. A randomized trial in which patients with ovarian cancer were treated with cisplatin plus cyclophosphamide with or without amifostine has shown equivalent antitumour activity with reduced cumulative toxicity in the amifostine group.[29] Hypertonic saline may also reduce the level of aquated platinum species allowing larger doses to be given without renal failure. Unfortunately, dose escalation to 200 mg/m^2 leads to other, serious toxicities, including severe motor neuropathy, loss of colour vision, and blindness.[30]

Clinical antitumour spectrum of cisplatin

When first introduced into clinical practice, cisplatin had the greatest impact on cancers of the testis and ovary and remains a key component of treatment for these diseases. Since that time a multitude of combination chemotherapy studies has been performed with virtually all other anticancer agents. Other tumour types for which cisplatin represents a major part of therapy include squamous cancers of the head and neck and cervix, small cell and non-small cell lung cancer, urothelial cancer, and to a somewhat lesser extent cancers of the upper gastrointestinal tract.

One particular drug combination deserves special mention. Paclitaxel was identified by the National Cancer Institute of the United States as a promising anticancer drug in their screens. Early trials demonstrated activity against platinum-refractory ovarian cancer.[31] A phase III trial was conducted by the Gynecologic Oncology Group, study GOG 111, which demonstrated superior progression-free and overall survival for patients with stage III ovarian cancer treated with cisplatin plus paclitaxel compared with cisplatin plus cyclophosphamide.[32] These results have been confirmed by a European–Canadian study[33] and there is a broad consensus that cisplatin plus paclitaxel represents a significant advance in the treatment of advanced ovarian cancer.[34]

Registered platinum analogues

The chemical structures of the platinum complexes currently registered, carboplatin, oxaliplatin (registered in France), and 254-S (registered in Japan), are shown in Fig. 1. The development of cisplatin analogues was prompted by the combination of unique antitumour activity and severe cumulative, irreversible toxicities associated with cisplatin. In general the reactivity, or rate of hydrolysis of platinum complexes is proportional to their overall toxicity, especially to the kidney and nervous system.[11],[35] In addition to the need for less toxic alternatives to cisplatin the problem of drug resistance was a major impetus to analogue development.

Carboplatin

Carboplatin was developed during a systematic search for compounds which retained the antitumour spectrum and level of activity of cisplatin with a reduced level of toxicity. Two of the compounds developed by Cleare and colleagues[36] were tested clinically, iproplatin

and carboplatin, but carboplatin appeared superior in a human tumour xenograft test, while lacking kidney toxicity.[35]

Early clinical trials with carboplatin performed by Calvert et al.[37] confirmed the improved toxicity profile of the compound. At conventional doses it does not cause renal impairment, is not ototoxic, and has been only rarely reported to cause neuropathy. It is significantly less emetic than cisplatin. Since there is no requirement for saline hydration to protect against renal damage, carboplatin treatment is much more convenient for the patient. The dose-limiting toxicity proved to be myelosuppression, principally thrombocytopenia, and antitumour activity was demonstrated in a variety of tumour types including cancers of the ovary and lung.

Clinical pharmacology of carboplatin

Carboplatin (cis-diammine-1,1-cyclobutane dicarboxylate platinum (II)) is a much more stable molecule in which platinum forms part of a six-membered ring. It has a much slower rate of aquation and subsequent cross-link formation than cisplatin.[11] The plasma elimination is similar to that of cisplatin; $T_{1/2}\alpha$: 22 min, $T_{1/2}\beta$: 116 min, and $T_{1/2}\gamma$ 5.8 days.[38] However, it is not renally secreted. It probably enters cells as the intact drug and is also largely eliminated in the urine due to glomerular filtration as the intact molecule. As a result, carboplatin clearance is largely defined by the glomerular filtration rate. This observation led to the development of dosing formulas based on renal function of which that of Calvert et al.[39] is the most widely employed. This is based on glomerular filtration rate being measured by the elimination of ^{14}C-labelled EDTA, a more accurate measurement of glomerular filtration rate than creatinine clearance and superior to the 'calculated creatinine clearance' methods, such as that of Cockroft and Gault. The Calvert formula has been validated prospectively and allows the drug exposure in terms of the area under the concentration times time curve (**AUC**) to be defined by the glomerular filtration rate plus a constant equal to the non-renal clearance:

Dose (mg) = AUC (mg/ml.min)
[glomerular filtration rate (ml/min) + 25]

This does not predict for toxicity since it does not allow for other factors such as prior exposure to marrow toxic treatment. Studies have shown that carboplatin AUC correlates with bone marrow toxicity and retrospective studies, in which AUC was calculated based on a knowledge of glomerular filtration rate and actual dose administered, have suggested a threshold for antitumour efficacy.[40] Prospective studies have so far failed to prove a benefit for dose intensities in excess of AUC 7 every 4 weeks.

Antitumour activity of carboplatin

Randomized trials have demonstrated equivalent activity between cisplatin and carboplatin both as a single agent and in drug combinations in the treatment of ovarian cancer.[41] These studies did not calculate carboplatin dosage according to renal function and might be regarded as suboptimal. In the majority of cases patients had suboptimally debulked disease. For example, in the study reported by Swenerton et al.[42], cisplatin at 75 mg/m^2 or carboplatin at 300 mg/m^2 was given in combination with cyclophosphamide at 600 mg/m^2 every 4 weeks for six cycles. The results were similar to the first such study reported by Taylor et al.[43] using the single agents at 100 mg/

m² and 400 mg/m², respectively. A meta-analysis has subsequently combined data from 10 studies and confirmed equivalence in the treatment of suboptimally debulked disease.[44]

In contrast, four studies were performed in which carboplatin replaced cisplatin in combination with etoposide with or without bleomycin for the treatment of good-risk germ cell tumours and demonstrated cisplatin to be superior. Although initial response rates tended to be similar, relapse-free survival favoured cisplatin in each case.[41]

In the case of other tumour types the situation is less clear, but carboplatin appears to be equally effective in the treatment of small cell lung cancer where the disease is extensive, with some reservations about the subset of patients with limited disease in whom there are some data supporting the use of cisplatin. In non-small cell lung cancer both cisplatin and carboplatin are widely used in a variety of drug combinations. Carboplatin may be favoured owing to its lower toxicity in this palliative setting. Recently, platinum complexes in combination with gemcitabine and paclitaxel have been shown to be active and comparative trials with cisplatin or carboplatin in combination with paclitaxel are underway.

Comparative trials of cisplatin or carboplatin with 5-fluorouracil in the treatment of head and neck cancer tend to support the use of cisplatin, including one neoadjuvant trial in which the cisplatin arm showed both a superior response rate and 5-year survival.[45] The lack of comparative data precludes definitive statements regarding cancers of the bladder, cervix, endometrium, and upper gastrointestinal tract and further studies are required in these diseases.

The combination of carboplatin with paclitaxel is worthy of special note. The dose-limiting toxicity of carboplatin is principally thrombocytopenia, while for paclitaxel given by short infusion it is neutropenia. When given in combination, thrombocytopenia is less than with carboplatin alone, the dose interval for carboplatin can be reduced to 3 weeks, and both drugs can be administered at their respective standard doses, or greater.[46]–[48] In this context carboplatin also appears highly active against urothelial cancer[49] and other tumour types, such as endometrial cancer.[50]

Oxaliplatin (Eloxatin®)

One of the most important goals in the development of analogues to cisplatin was the ability to overcome drug resistance. The observations by Burchenal et al.[51] that agents in which the ammine ligands were replaced by a diaminocyclohexane group were active against cisplatin-resistant cell lines, such as the P388 murine leukaemia, led to the development of a range of such agents, a number of which underwent clinical testing. These included a platinum (IV) complex with four chlorine atoms, initially called tetraplatin, subsequently ormaplatin. This proved highly neurotoxic and also nephrotoxic and failed to demonstrate clinical activity against cisplatin-resistant tumours. Oxaliplatin, however, while it has not been tested in this setting, does appear to have a somewhat different spectrum of antitumour activity.[52] This agent has shown activity in advanced colorectal cancer both as a single agent[53] and in combination with 5-fluorouracil. Claims have been made in favour of chronomodulation using programmable pumps to deliver 5-fluorouracil and folinic acid maximally at 4.00 a.m. and oxaliplatin at 4.00 p.m. Using this regimen the activity was higher, with an objective response rate of 53 per cent, and toxicity was less compared with

standard daily infusion protocols.[54] Responses may be obtained in patients whose disease is refractory to standard 5-fluorouracil plus leucovorin regimens.[55] Oxaliplatin produces a curious pattern of neurotoxicity, including facial dysaesthesia which may be provoked by exposure to cold. Peripheral sensory neuropathy may also occur, but is rarely dose limiting. The drug does not cause significant nephrotoxicity. Oxaliplatin clearly represents a significant advance in the treatment of advanced colorectal cancer and its potential has yet to be determined.

254-S (Nedaplatin®)

This compound has only been studied in Japan. Thrombocytopenia is the dose-limiting toxicity although occasional severe nephrotoxicity has been reported. Phase II studies have shown activity in a similar range of tumour types responsive to cisplatin.[56]

Analogues in development

During the 1990s, the main focus of new platinum drug development has been on designing agents for oral administration and/or capable of circumventing one or more of the above-described mechanisms of tumour resistance to cisplatin (e.g. overcoming transport defects, decreasing drug inactivation by thiols, varying DNA-binding properties). Emphasis has been placed upon the establishment and use of human tumour cell lines and xenografts representative of both intrinsic and acquired cisplatin resistance and characterized in terms of their major mechanism(s) of resistance.[57] Cell lines with acquired resistance that is of defined mechanisms have been established and incorporated within new platinum drug discovery cascades.[58] A variety of novel agents have been discovered, some of which are now in clinical trial.

JM216 (BMS 182751)

JM216 (bis acetato amminedichloro(cyclohexylamine) platinum (IV)) was developed as a cisplatin analogue for oral administration. As both cisplatin and carboplatin require administration by injection, such a drug should improve patient convenience and, if combined with other oral agents, allows the possibility of fractionated combination chemotherapy treatment on an outpatient basis. Synthetic efforts concentrated on a novel class of platinum complex, the ammine/amine (or 'mixed amine') platinum (IV) dicarboxylates possessing lipophilic axial ligands and asymmetric carrier ligands. Studies using an in vitro panel of human ovarian carcinoma cell lines showed that this class of complex exhibited selective cytotoxicity to intrinsically cisplatin-resistant cell lines.[58]

JM216 was selected for phase I clinical trial on the basis of the following encouraging preclinical properties: oral antitumour activity comparable with that of intravenously administered cisplatin or carboplatin against a panel of human ovarian carcinoma xenografts;[59] lack of specific organ toxicity, with myelosuppression being dose limiting in mice; and the ability to overcome acquired cisplatin resistance in three out of six human tumour cell lines (whereas ormaplatin exhibited partial or full cross-resistance in all six).[59] Mechanistic studies have shown that JM216 is capable of circumventing cisplatin resistance due to one of the three main mechanisms of resistance, namely reduced drug accumulation.

In phase I clinical trials JM216 demonstrated saturable oral bio-availability, dose-limiting myelosuppression, and a lack of nephro-, oto-, or neurotoxicity. A five times daily regimen proved to be most suitable for phase II evaluation.[60] JM216 is currently undergoing phase III evaluation.

JM473/AMD473/ZD0473

Phase I clinical trials with ZD0473 (cis-amminedichloro(2-methyl-pyridine) platinum (II)) began at the Royal Marsden NHS Trust Hospital in November 1997. The chemical rationale for the synthesis of ZD0473 was based on developing a platinum compound with reduced susceptibility to inactivation by elevated intracellular thiol concentrations, a commonly observed feature of cisplatin-resistant tumours (see above). This was achieved by increasing steric bulk at the platinum centre using the 2-methylpyridine carrier ligand.

ZD0473 has been shown to possess a number of promising preclinical properties.[61],[62] These include circumvention of acquired cisplatin resistance in vitro in human ovarian tumour lines where resistance is due to one or more of reduced drug accumulation, increased glutathione, and enhanced DNA repair. ZD0473 has been shown to possess distinct DNA-binding properties from those of cisplatin. Moreover, significant in vivo antitumour activity was observed against some ovarian tumour xenografts with acquired cisplatin resistance by both the intraperitoneal and oral routes of administration. Finally, the toxicity profile of ZD0473 in mice is reminiscent of carboplatin with myelosuppression being dose limiting and no detectable nephro- or neurotoxicities.

BBR3464

Farrell and coworkers have recently described a novel charged trinuclear platinum complex, BBR3464, which entered clinical trial during 1998.[63] The molecule contains two trans-PtCl(NH3)2 units linked by a NH2(CH2)6(NH2-trans-Pt(NH3)2-NH2(CH2)6NH2 diamine chain. BBR3464 forms long-range interstrand cross-links on DNA, is up to 100-fold more potent than cisplatin in vitro, and showed in vivo antitumour activity, independent of p53 status, in a range of human tumour xenografts.

Liposomal cisplatin

A 'stealth' liposomal platinum complex, SPI-077, has recently entered clinical trial in an attempt to improve upon the drug delivery and distribution properties of free cisplatin. To date, no acute myelo- or nephrotoxicities have been reported; the drug's pharmacokinetics are clearly different from those of free cisplatin.[64]

trans-Platinum complexes

A major paradigm for structure–activity relationships of platinum complexes is that trans-platinum complexes are inactive as antitumour agents.[6] However, during the 1990s at least three independent groups have described trans-platinum compounds, some endowed with promising in vitro antitumour properties. These include comparable cell-killing properties to those of cisplatin, retention of potency against some cells with acquired cisplatin resistance, and distinct DNA-binding properties. One trans-platinum complex, JM335 (trans-ammine (cyclohexylaminedichlorodihydroxo) platinum (IV)) showed

marked in vivo antitumour efficacy against both murine and human subcutaneous tumour models.[65] To date, however, no trans-platinum complex has reached clinical trial.

Summary

Since its introduction into clinical practice almost 30 years ago, the metal coordination complex cisplatin has made a significant impact in the chemotherapeutic treatment of many solid adult malignancies, especially testicular and ovarian cancers. Carboplatin is a second-generation, less toxic analogue, with a broadly similar spectrum of antitumour activity. Another analogue, oxaliplatin, has shown some antitumour efficacy against colorectal cancer. The first orally available platinum complex, JM216, is currently in clinical trial. Cisplatin exerts its antitumour effects through binding to DNA. Some tumours fail to respond to cisplatin through mechanisms either involving insufficient drug reaching the target DNA (decreased drug transport, increased cytoplasmic detoxification) and/or increased DNA repair or increased tolerance to platinum-induced DNA damage. Platinum drugs designed to overcome some or all of these resistance mechanisms are now entering early clinical trial.

References

1. **Rosenberg B.** Fundamental studies with cisplatin. *Cancer*, 1985; **55**: 2303–16.

2. **Wiltshaw E, Carr B.** *Cis*-platinum(II)diammine-dichloride. In: Connors TA, Roberts JJ, eds. *Platinum Coordination Complexes in Cancer Chemotherapy*. Heidelberg: Springer-Verlag, 1974: 178–82.

3. **Higby DJ, Wallace HJ Jr, Holland JF.** *Cis*-dichlorodiammineplatinum (NSC-119875): a phase I study. *Cancer Chemotherapy Reports*, 1973; **57**: 459–63.

4. **Cvitkovic E, Spaulding J, Bethune V, Martin J, Whitmore WF.** Improvement of *cis*-dichlorodiammineplatinum (NSC 119875): therapeutic index in an animal model. *Cancer*, 1977; **39**: 1357–61.

5. **Kidgell AE, Butcher ME, Brown GW.** Antiemetic control: 5-HT3 antagonists: review of clinical results, with particular emphasis on ondansetron. *Cancer Treatment Reviews*, 1990; **17**: 311–17.

6. **Connors TA, Cleare MJ, Harrap KR.** Structure–activity relationships of the antitumor platinum coordination complexes. *Cancer Treatment Reports*, 1979; **63**: 1499–502.

7. **Fichtinger-Schepman AM, van der Veer JL, den Hartog JH, Lohman PH, Reedijk J.** Adducts of the antitumour drug *cis*-diamminedichloro platinum(II) with DNA: formation, identification and quantitation. *Biochemistry*, 1985; **24**: 707–13.

8. **Comess KM, Lippard SJ.** Molecular aspects of platinum–DNA interactions. In: Neidle S, Waring M, eds. *Molecular Aspects of Anticancer Drug–DNA Interactions*, Vol 1. London: Macmillan Press, 1993: 134–68.

9. **Takahara PM, Rosenzweig AC, Frederick CA, Lippard SJ.** Crystal structure of double-stranded DNA containing the major adduct of the anticancer drug cisplatin. *Nature*, 1995; **377**: 649–52.

10. **Huang H, Zhu L, Reid BR, Drobny GP, Hopkins PB.** Solution structure of a cisplatin-induced DNA interstrand cross-link. *Science*, 1995; **270**: 1842–5.

11. **Knox RJ, Friedlos F, Lydall DA, Roberts JJ.** Mechanism of cytotoxicity of anticancer platinum drugs: evidence that *cis*-diamminedichloroplatinum(II) and *cis*-diammine-(1,1-cyclobutanedicarboxylato)platinum(II) differ only in the kinetics of their interaction with DNA. *Cancer Research*, 1986; **46**: 1972–9.

12. **Johnson SW, Ferry KV, Hamilton TC.** Recent insights into platinum drug resistance in cancer. *Drug Resistance Updates*, 1998; **1**: 243–54.

13. **Gately DP, Howell SB.** Cellular accumulation of the anticancer agent cisplatin: a review. *British Journal of Cancer*, 1993; **67**: 1171–5.

14. **Kool M, et al.** Analysis of expression of cMOAT (MRP2), MRP3, MRP4 and MRP5, homologues of the multidrug resistance associated protein gene (MRP1), in human cancer cell lines. *Cancer Research*, 1997; **57**: 3537–47.

15. **Ishikawa T, Ali-Osman F.** Glutathione-associated *cis*-diamminedichloro platinum(II) metabolism and ATP-dependent efflux from leukemia cells. *Journal of Biological Chemistry*, 1993; **268**: 20116–25.

16. **Mistry P, Kelland LR, Abel G, Sidhur S, Harrap KR.** The relationships between glutathione, glutathione-*S*-transferase and cytotoxicity of platinum drugs and melphalan in eight human ovarian carcinoma cell lines. *British Journal of Cancer*, 1991; **64**: 215–20.

17. **Kelley SL, Basu A, Teicher BA, Hacker MP, Hamer DH, Lazo JS.** Overexpression of metallothionein confers resistance to anticancer drugs. *Science*, 1988; **241**: 1813–15.

18. **Chaney SG, Sancar A.** DNA repair: enzymatic mechanisms and relevance to drug response. *Journal of the National Cancer Institute*, 1996; **88**: 1346–60.

19. **Zhen W, et al.** Increased gene-specific repair of cisplatin interstrand cross-links in cisplatin-resistant human ovarian cancer cell lines. *Molecular and Cellular Biology*, 1992; **12**: 3689–98.

20. **Dabholkar M, Bostick-Bruton F, Weber C, Bohr VA, Egwuagu C, Reed E.** ERCC1 and ERCC2 expression in malignant tissues from ovarian cancer patients. *Journal of the National Cancer Institute*, 1992; **84**: 1512–17.

21. **Koberle B, Masters JRW, Hartley JA, Wood RD.** Defective repair of cisplatin-induced DNA damage caused by reduced XPA protein in testicular germ cell tumours. *Current Biology*, 1999; **9**: 273–6.

22. **Huang JC, Zamble DB, Reardon JT, Lippard SJ, Sancar A.** HMG-domain proteins specifically inhibit the repair of the major DNA adduct of the anticancer drug cisplatin by human excision nuclease. *Proceedings of the National Academy of Sciences (USA)*, 1994; **91**: 10394–8.

23. **Vaisman A, et al.** The role of hMLH1, hMSH3 and hMSH6 defects in cisplatin and oxaliplatin resistance: correlation with replicative bypass of platinum–DNA adducts. *Cancer Research*, 1998; **58**: 3579–85.

24. **Fink D, et al.** The role of DNA mismatch repair in platinum drug resistance. *Cancer Research*, 1996; **56**: 4881–6.

25. **Lowe SW, Ruley HE, Jacks T, Housman DE.** P53-dependent apoptosis modulates the cytotoxicity of anticancer agents. *Cell*, 1993; **74**: 957–67.

26. **Eastman A.** Activation of programmed cell death by anticancer agents: cisplatin as a model system. *Cancer Cells*, 1990; **2**: 275–80.

27. **O'Connor PM, et al.** Characterization of the p53 tumor suppressor pathway in cell lines of the National Cancer Institute anticancer drug screen and correlations with the growth inhibitory potency of 123 anticancer agents. *Cancer Research*, 1997; **57**: 4285–300.

28. **Vermorken JB, et al.** Pharmacokinetics of free and total platinum species after short term infusion of cisplatin. *Cancer Treatment Reports*, 1984; **68**: 505–13.

29. **Kemp G, et al.** Amifostine pretreatment for protection against cyclophosphamide-induced and cisplatin-induced toxicities: results of a randomized control trial in patients with advanced ovarian cancer. *Journal of Clinical Oncology*, 1996; **14**: 2101–12.

30. **Ozols RF, et al.** High-dose cisplatin in hypertonic saline. *Annals of Internal Medicine*, 1984; **100**: 19–24.

31. **Rowinsky EK, Donehower RC.** The clinical pharmacology of paclitaxel (TAXOL) *Seminars in Oncology*, 1992; **20**(Suppl. 3): 16–25.

32. **McGuire WP, et al.** Cyclophosphamide and cisplatin compared with paclitaxel and cisplatin in patients with stage III and stage IV ovarian cancer. *New England Journal of Medicine*, 1996; **334**: 1–6.

33. **Stuart G, et al.** Updated analysis shows a highly significant improved overall survival (OS) for cisplatin–paclitaxel as first line treatment of advanced ovarian cancer: mature results of the EORTC-GCCG, NO-COVA, NCIC CTG and Scottish Intergroup trial. *Proceedings of the American Society of Clinical Oncology*, 1998; **17**: abstract 1394.

34. **Adams M, et al.** Chemotherapy for ovarian cancer—a consensus statement on standard practice. *British Journal of Cancer*, 1998; **78**: 1404–6.

35. **Harrap KR.** Preclinical studies identifying carboplatin as a viable cisplatin alternative. *Cancer Treatment Reviews*, 1985; **12**: 21–33.

36. **Cleare MJ, Hydes PC, Hepburn DR, Malerbi BW.** Antitumour platinum complexes: structure activity relationships. In: Prestyko AW, Crooke ST, Carter SJK, eds. *Cisplatin: Current Status and New Developments*. New York: Academic Press, 1980: 149–70.

37. **Calvert AH, Harland SJ, Newell DR, Siddik ZH, Harrap KR.** Phase I studies with carboplatin at the Royal Marsden Hospital. *Cancer Treatment Reviews*, 1985; **12**: 51–7.

38. **Elferink F, et al.** Pharmacokinetics of diammine (1,1-cyclobutane dicarboxylato) platinum(II) (carboplatin) after intravenous administration. *Cancer Treatment Reports*, 1987; **71**: 1231–7.

39. **Calvert AH, et al.** Carboplatin dosage: prospective evaluation of a simple formula based on renal function. *Journal of Clinical Oncology*, 1989; **7**: 1748–56.

40. **Jodrell DI, et al.** Relationship between carboplatin exposure and tumour response and toxicity in patients with ovarian cancer. *Journal of Clinical Oncology*, 1992; **10**: 520–8.

41. **Go RS, Adjei AA.** Review of the comparative pharmacology and clinical activity of cisplatin and carboplatin. *Journal of Clinical Oncology*, 1999; **17**: 409–22.

42. **Swenerton K, et al.** Cisplatin–cyclophosphamide versus carboplatin–cyclophosphamide in advanced ovarian cancer: A randomized phase III study of the National Cancer Institute of Canada Clinical Trials Group. *Journal of Clinical Oncology*, 1992; **10**: 718–26.

43. **Taylor AE, et al.** Long-term follow-up of the first randomized study of cisplatin versus carboplatin for advanced epithelial ovarian cancer. *Journal of Clinical Oncology*, 1994; **12**: 2066–70.

44. **Aabo K, et al.** Chemotherapy in advanced ovarian cancer: an overview of randomized clinical trials. *British Medical Journal*, 1991; **303**: 884–93.

45. **de Andres L, et al.** Randomized trial of neoadjuvant cisplatin and fluorouracil versus carboplatin and fluorouracil in patients with stage IV-M0 head and neck cancer. *Journal of Clinical Oncology*, 1995; **13**: 1493–500.

46. **du Bois A, et al.** Cisplatin/paclitaxel versus carboplatin/paclitaxel as first-line chemotherapy in ovarian cancer: interim analysis of an AGO Study Group trial. *Proceedings of the American Society of Clinical Oncology*, 1997; **16**: abstract 1272.

47. **Neijt JP, et al.** Randomized phase III study in previously untreated epithelial ovarian cancer FIGO stage IIB, IIC, III, IV, comparing paclitaxel–cisplatin and paclitaxel–carboplatin. *Proceedings of the American Society of Clinical Oncology*, 1997; **16**: abstract 1259.

48. **McGuire WP, Ozols RF.** Chemotherapy of advanced ovarian cancer. *Seminars in Oncology*, 1998; **25**: 340–8.

49. **Vaughn DJ, et al.** Paclitaxel plus carboplatin in advanced carcinoma of the urothelium: an active and tolerable outpatient regimen. *Journal of Clinical Oncology*, 1998; **16**: 255–60.

50. **Vasuratna A, et al.** Prolonged remission of endometrial cancer wth paclitaxel and carboplatin. *Anticancer Drugs*, 1998; **9**: 283–5.

51. **Burchenal JH, Iranai G, Kern K, Lokys L, Turkevich J.** 1,2-Diaminocyclohexane platinum derivatives of potential clinical value. *Recent Results in Cancer Research*, 1980; **74**: 146–55.

52. **Rixe O, et al.** Oxaliplatin, tetraplatin, cisplatin and carboplatin: spectrum of activity in drug-resistant cell lines and in cell lines of the

National Cancer Institute's Anticancer Drug Screen Panel. *Biochemical Pharmacology*, 1996; **52**: 1855–65.

53. **Becouarn Y, *et al.*** Phase II trial of oxaliplatin as first-line chemotherapy in metastatic colorectal cancer patients. Digestive Group of French Federation of Cancer Centers. *Journal of Clinical Oncology*, 1998; **16**: 2739–44.

54. **Levi FA, *et al.*** Chronomodulated versus fixed-infusion-rate delivery of ambulatory chemotherapy with oxaliplatin, fluroruracil, and folinic acid (leucovorin) in patients with colorectal cancer metastases: a randomized multi-institutional trial. *Journal of the National Cancer Institute*, 1994; **86**: 1608–17.

55. **Machover D, *et al.*** Two consecutive phase II trials of oxaliplatin (L-OHP) for treatment of patients with advanced colorectal carcinoma who were resistant to previous treatment with fluoropyrimidines. *Annals of Oncology*, 1996; **7**: 95–8.

56. **Akaza H, *et al.*** Phase II study of *cis*-diammine(glycolato)platinum, 254-S, in patients with advanced germ-cell testicular cancer, prostatic cancer, and transitional-cell carcinoma of the urinary tract. *Cancer Chemotherapy and Pharmacology*, 1992; **31**: 187–92.

57. **Kelland LR, Jones M, Abel G, Valenti M, Gwynne JJ, Harrap KR.** Human ovarian carcinoma cell lines and companion xenografts: a disease oriented approach to new platinum anticancer drug development. *Cancer Chemotherapy and Pharmacology*, 1992; **30**: 43–50.

58. **Kelland LR, Murrer BA, Abel G, Giandomenico CM, Mistry P, Harrap KR.** Ammine/amine platinum (IV) dicarboxylates: a novel class of platinum complex exhibiting selective cytotoxicity to intrinsically cisplatin-resistant human ovarian carcinoma cell lines. *Cancer Research*, 1992; **52**: 822–8.

59. **Kelland LR, *et al.*** Preclinical antitumor evaluation of bis-acetato-ammine-dichloro cyclohexylamine platinum (IV): an orally active platinum drug.. *Cancer Research*, 1993; **53**: 2581–6.

60. **McKeage MJ, *et al.*** Phase I and pharmacokinetic study of an oral platinum complex given daily for 5 days in patients with cancer. *Journal of Clinical Oncology*, 1997; **15**: 2691–700.

61. **Holford J, Sharp SY, Murrer BA, Abrams M, Kelland LR.** *In vitro* circumvention of cisplatin resistance by the novel sterically hindered platinum complex AMD473. *British Journal of Cancer*, 1998; **77**: 366–73.

62. **Raynaud FI, *et al.*** Cis-Amminedichloro(2-methylpyridine) platinum (II) (AMD473), a novel sterically hindered platinum complex: *in vivo* activity, toxicology, and pharmacokinetics in mice. *Clinical Cancer Research*, 1997; **3**: 2063–74.

63. **Pratesi G, *et al.*** Complete lack of cross-resistance of cisplatin-resistant tumors to a novel charged trinuclear platinum complex: p53-independent antitumor efficacy. *Proceedings of the American Association of Cancer Research*, 1997; **38**: A2078.

64. **DeMario MD, *et al.*** A phase I study of liposome-formulated cisplatin (SPI-77) given every 3 weeks with patients with advanced cancer. *Annals of Oncology*, 1998; **9**(Suppl. 2): A466.

65. **Kelland LR, *et al.*** A novel *trans*-platinum coordination complex possessing *in vitro* and *in vivo* antitumor activity. *Cancer Research*, 1994; **54**: 5618–22.

4.16 Antimetabolites

G. J. Peters and G. Jansen

Introduction

Antimetabolites are agents that interfere with normal metabolism due to their structural similarity to normal intermediates in the synthesis of RNA and DNA precursors. They can serve as substrates for enzymes, inhibit enzymes, or do both. Due to differences in metabolism between normal cells and cancer cells, many antimetabolites have the potential to act with a certain degree of specificity on cancer cells. In the last decades, the focus of research has been directed to enhancing the selectivity of antimetabolites by the design of rational combinations including the use of biochemical modulation. The latter implies the pharmacological manipulation of intracellular pathways of a drug, with the aim of improving the therapeutic index. The design of rational combinations has only been possible due to our increasing knowledge of normal nucleotide metabolism, the mechanism of action of antimetabolites, and that of other anticancer agents. Information about the metabolism of antimetabolites and their effects on normal metabolism is, however, incomplete. Although this type of knowledge is even scarcer for solid tumours, the use of advanced detection techniques, invasive and non-invasive, has greatly contributed to a better insight into the drug metabolism of solid tumours.

In this chapter the mechanism of action of commonly used antimetabolites is discussed, as well as those factors which influence their activity such as route and schedule of administration, drug disposition, and biochemical modulation by other drugs or natural compounds.

Targets of antimetabolites

Antimetabolites act upon or interfere with several steps in normal metabolism. Figure 1 shows the pathways of pyrimidine (deoxy)-nucleotide synthesis and the site of action of several antimetabolites. The concept of a key enzyme has proven to be useful in the design of antimetabolites.[1] A key enzyme catalyses an essential step in a metabolic pathway (Table 1), but this also implies that inhibition of such an essential step may not only affect the function of cancer cells but also that of normal rapidly dividing cells. Clinically, this is manifested by the serious haematological and gastrointestinal toxicities caused by antimetabolites. Table 2 gives a list of some antimetabolites

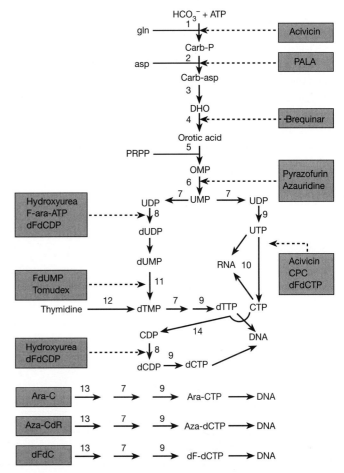

Fig. 1 Schematic representation of pyrimidine nucleotide synthesis showing the targets of several antimetabolites. The enzymes catalysing these reactions are: 1, carbamyl-phosphate synthetase; 2, aspartate transcarbamylase; 3, dihydro-orotase; 4, DHO dehydrogenase; 5, orotate phosphoribosyltransferase (OPRT); 6, orotidine 5′-monophosphate (OMP) decarboxylase; 7, mononucleotide kinases; 8, ribonucleotide reductase; 9, nucleoside diphosphate kinase; 10, CTP synthetase; 11, thymidylate synthase; 12, thymidine kinase I; 13, deoxycytidine kinase; 14, 5′-nucleotidase. Note: Asp = aspartate; carb-P = carbamyl-phosphate; DHO = dihydro-orotic acid; PRPP = 5-phosphoribosyl-1-pyrophosphate; PALA = N-phosphonacetyl-L-aspartate; CPC = cyclopentenyl cytosine; CTP = cytidine 5′-triphosphate.

We thank A. M. B. Paalman for excellent secretarial assistance and K. Smid for preparation of the figures.

Table 1 Properties of a key enzyme (a key enzyme may exhibit either one or more of these properties)

A key enzyme has a unique biological role
It determines the rate of a pathway
It determines the direction of a pathway
It is the first or last enzyme in a pathway
It is the final enzyme of two common pathways
A key enzyme is a pathway
It catalyses a one way reaction

A key enzyme has a complicated regulation
It is a target of feedback regulation
A key enzyme has usually a multiple regulation
A key enzyme has allosteric properties

and the respective enzymes or pathways with which they interfere. It should be noted, however, that most successful (i.e. registered and clinically used) antimetabolites interfere with a key enzyme. Examples are 5-fluorouracil, methotrexate, 6-mercaptopurine, 1-β-D-arabino-furanosylcytosine (**ara-C**), 2',2'-difluoro-2'-deoxycytidine (gemcitabine); the unsuccessful antimetabolite N-phosphonacetyl-L-aspartate (**PALA**) inhibits aspartate transcarbamylase, which is not a key enzyme. The activity of this enzyme in most cell lines and tissues is 10 to 1000 times higher than the preceding and next enzymes in the pyrimidine *de novo* pathway.[1],[2] Most antimetabolites interfere with RNA and/or DNA synthesis. Due to their potential interference with DNA synthesis, either by inhibition or incorporation, most antimetabolites induce DNA damage leading to apoptotic cell death. However, antimetabolites may also interfere with other processes such as glycosylation, synthesis of phospholipids, and metabolic processes in cellular organelles such as mitochondria, nucleus, or lysosymes, either directly, by the subcellular localization of enzymes or through the role of cytochrome c in induction of apoptosis.[3]–[8]

Antifolates

Approximately 50 years ago, the first antimetabolite to be used in the clinic was the antifolate aminopterin, which was subsequently

Table 2 Targets of several antimetabolites

Antimetabolite	Target	Effect
5-Fluorouracil	Thymidylate synthase* RNA synthesis*	Depletion dTTP Processing impaired
Methotrexate	Dihydrofolate reductase*	Depletion reduced folates
Tomudex/ZD1694	Thymidylate synthase*	Depletion dTTP
Ara-C	DNA polymerase*	Inhibition DNA synthesis Incorporation DNA
Azadeoxycytidine	DNA polymerase*	Differentiation induction
Gemcitabine	Incorporation into DNA Incorporation into RNA dCMP deaminase CTP synthetase* Ribonucleotide reductase*	Inhibition DNA synthesis Depletion dATP, dGTP, dCTP Disturbance normal nucleotides (Self)-potentiation
Hydroxyurea	Ribonucleotide reductase*	Depletion deoxynucleotides
Deoxycoformycin	Adenosine deaminase*	Accumulation dATP
Fludarabine	Ribonucleotide reductase*	Accumulation F-ara-ATP Depletion dCTP, dATP
Cladribine	Ribonucleotide reductase*	Accumulation Cl-dATP;
6-Mercaptopurine	Purine de novo*, depletion GTP Incorporation DNA	Depletion dATP, dCTP Inhibition DNA
6-Thioguanine	Incorporation DNA	Inhibition DNA
Tiazofurin	IMP dehydrogenase*	Depletion GTP
Acivicin	IMP dehydrogenase* Carbamyl phosphate synthetase* CTP synthetase*	Depletion GTP Depletion pyrimidine nucleotides Depletion CTP
PALA	Aspartate transcarbamylase	Depletion pyrimidine nucleotides

*Indicates key enzyme or pathway.

PALA: phosphonoacetyl-L-aspartate.

Natural folates

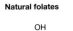

Folic acid   5-CH₃THF   5-CHOTHF (LV)

DHFR

MTX   EDX   TMQ

TS

ZD1694   ZD9331   AG337

GARTFase

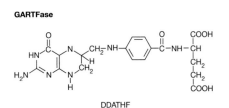

DDATHF   AG2034   LY231514 (MTA)*

Fig. 2 Chemical structures of folic acid, reduced folate cofactors, and antifolate inhibitors of dihydrofolate reductase, thymidylate synthase, and glycinamide ribonucleotide transformylase (GARTFase). * LY231514 is referred to as a multitargeted antifolate (MTA) since it can inhibit dihydrofolate reductase and GARTFase beyond its primary target thymidylate synthase (TS).

substituted by methotrexate.[9]–[11] Antifolates are structural analogues of the essential vitamin folic acid (Fig. 2). In eukaryotic cells, natural reduced folate cofactors, e.g. 5-methyltetrahydrofolate and 5-formyltetrahydrofolate, are essential as one-carbon donors in a variety of biosynthetic reactions, including the biosynthesis of amino acids (methionine, serine), purine biosynthesis *de novo*, and synthesis of thymidylate for DNA/RNA synthesis. Furthermore, folates serve as one-carbon donors in methylation reactions by which they can control gene expression, and therefore the functional activity of proteins, lipids, and hormones.[11],[12] Since the introduction of methotrexate to the clinic in the 1950s, a number of antifolates have been developed, but none of them has proven to be superior to methotrexate. Recently, however, knowledge of the factors that contribute to the clinical activity of methotrexate, for example membrane transport, intracellular retention, and target enzyme inhibition, has provided a basis for the rational design and synthesis of a second and third generation of antifolates.[11],[13]–[16] Several of these promising folate analogues have entered clinical pratice or are now under clinical investigation.[14],[17]–[23] It is not clear whether these compounds will substitute for methotrexate in the near future, but they may have an additional role in the treatment of specific types of cancer, for the circumvention of acquired resistance to methotrexate, or in other diseases such as rheumatoid arthritis.[24] Analogues may also have fewer side-effects than methotrexate. A series of excellent reviews on the various aspects of methotrexate have been published.[11],[13],[19],[25]–[32] Several steps in the metabolism and mechanism of action of methotrexate have to be considered (Table 3) and will be dealt with in separate sections.

Transport of methotrexate

Transport of methotrexate is a critical factor in its chemotherapeutic efficacy. Methotrexate has to be transported across the cellular membrane into the cell and the drug has to be retained in the cell. The intracellular concentration of methotrexate is the result of a dynamic equilibrium between influx and efflux. Methotrexate can enter the cell

Table 3 Mechanism of cellular resistance to methotrexate and secondary effects mediated by methotrexate

Resistance to methotrexate
Defective methotrexate influx/increased methotrexate efflux
Degradation to 7-OH-methotrexate
Impaired polyglutamylation
Less efficient binding of methotrexate to dihydrofolate reductase
Extent and retention of inhibition of dihydrofolate reductase
Alteration in folate homeostasis (expanded folate pools)
Purine and/or pyrimidine nucleoside salvage

Secondary effects of methotrexate
Dihydrofolate polyglutamates inhibit purine *de novo* and thymidylate synthase
Inhibition of thymidylate synthase and AICAR transformylase by methotrexate polyglutamates
Polyglutamates of 7-OH-methotrexate can bind to dihydrofolate reductase
Polyglutamylation of 7-OH-methotrexate can inhibit thymidylate synthase and AICAR transformylase
Polyglutamates of 10-formyl-dihydrofolate can inhibit thymidylate synthase and GAR transformylase
Alterations in cytosolic and mitochondrial folate pools

AICAR, aminoimidazole carboxamide; GAR, glycinamide ribonucleotide.

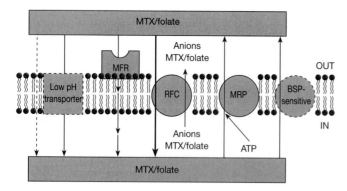

Fig. 3 Internalization and efflux routes for natural folates and folate analogues; the reduced folate carrier is the predominant route for uptake of (anti)folates in malignant cells. Membrane folate receptor (MFR) can play a role in specific tumour types. The clinical relevance of a third route, a low-pH transporter is as yet unclear. Passive diffusion of methotrexate/folates may proceed at very high extracellular concentrations.[32] One efflux route for natural folates and folate analogues is the influx carrier, reduced folate carrier, which can function bidirectionally. A second route is via members of the multidrug resistance protein (MRP) family. This route is inhibitable by probenecid. Finally, a third route is inhibitable by bromosulfophthalein (BSP). The molecular identity of this route is as yet unknown.

via several processes that may operate exclusively or simultaneously in mammalian cells (Fig. 3(a)).[15],[33],[34]

The reduced folate carrier

The reduced folate carrier mediates inward transport of folates and antifolates in most neoplastic cells.[32],[35],[36] The human reduced folate carrier is a glycosylated integral membrane protein with a molecular mass of 80 to 120 kDa.[37]–[39] The reduced folate carrier protein is encoded by the *RFC1* gene, localized on chromosome 21 (21q22.2–q22.3).[40],[41] The transport kinetic properties of the reduced folate carrier display a characteristic profile of high-affinity transport for reduced folate cofactors ($K_m = 1$–3 μM) and methotrexate ($K_m = 2$–26 μM) but a poor affinity for transport of folic acid ($K_m = 200$–400 μM).[32],[35],[36] Constitutive functional reduced folate carrier activity has been demonstrated in a variety of tumour cell lines of different origin.[32],[36],[42]–[44] In general, reduced folate carrier activity is relatively high in undifferentiated neoplastic and fetal tissues, whereas its activity declines upon cellular maturation/differentiation. In addition, functional reduced folate carrier activity can be subject to metabolic regulation as changes in the cellular folate and purine status can downregulate transport activity.[39],[45]

The membrane folate receptor/membrane-associated folate binding protein

Membrane folate receptors are structurally different from the reduced folate carrier since they reside in the outer layer of the plasma membrane by means of a linkage via a glycosylphosphatidyl inositol anchor attached to the C terminus of the protein.[46] Membrane folate receptors are glycosylated membrane proteins (molecular weight 38–44 kDa) with a high affinity for folic acid ($K_d = 0.1$–1 nM); the affinity of the receptor for reduced folate cofactors and methotrexate is approximately threefold and 100-fold lower, respectively, compared with folic acid.[15],[34],[46]–[48] Currently, at least three membrane folate receptor isoforms have been identified which are encoded by membrane folate receptor genes localized on chromosome 11 (q13.3–q13.5).[49],[50] These isoforms differ in their binding affinity for folates and antifolates.[32],[48] The exact mechanism of membrane folate receptor-mediated uptake of (anti)folate compounds is still an unresolved and controversial issue. At least two different pathways for membrane folate receptor-mediated transport have been described. The first pathway is the classical receptor-mediated endocytosis route via clathrin-coated pits, a second route is via potocytosis.[51]–[53]

Membrane folate receptors are expressed in many tissues of both normal and malignant origin, in primary cell cultures, and in a variety of established tumour cell lines.[54]–[58] The expression of membrane folate receptor isoforms is tissue specific and can often be upregulated in neoplastic tissues.[54],[55],[59] Membrane folate receptor appears to be constitutively overexpressed in ovarian carcinoma.[54],[56],[57],[60] Over-expression of membrane folate receptor in neoplastic tissues is currently being exploited for therapeutic targeting with:

- monoclonal antibodies directed to membrane folate receptor[61]–[64]
- folate-conjugated macromolecules (cytotoxins, anticancer drugs, antisense oligodeoxyribonucleotides, radionuclides)[65]–[68]
- high-affinity binding antifolates.[15]

Other transport routes

An (anti)folate transporter that displays optimal activity at a pH below 7.4 has been described in a limited number of neoplastic cells.[69],[70] This low-pH transporter has relatively similar affinities for methotrexate, reduced folates, and folic acid. Transport of methotrexate via this route is tenfold higher at pH 6.2 than at pH 7.4. The clinical relevance of this transport protein remains to be established.

Passive diffusion

Passive diffusion may contribute to the uptake of methotrexate in high-dose regimens (> 1 g methotrexate/m^2) as it increases linearly with the extracellular methotrexate concentration.[27],[71]

Antifolate efflux

Over the past decade, multiple efflux routes for methotrexate have been identified in leukaemia cells and characterized based on differences in the potency of a series of selected inhibitors. In murine L1210 and human CCRF-CEM leukaemia cells at least three separate efflux routes are discernible (Fig. 3(b)).[72]–[76] One efflux route (system I) can be the reduced folate carrier itself which can function bi-directionally.[77] The other two routes display direct dependence on ATP for efflux and can be differentially inhibited by bromosulfophtalein (system II) and probenecid (system III). The relative contribution of each of these systems is dependent on the cell line and on energy.[73],[78] Recently, insight in the molecular identity of these (anti)folate efflux pumps was obtained from observations by Saxena and Henderson, Hooijberg et al., and Kool et al. who demonstrated that some multidrug resistance proteins could mediate antifolate drug extrusion.[79]–[83] In particular, transfection of cells with multidrug resistance protein 1, 2, or 3 conferred resistance to methotrexate when exposed for short time periods, during which this drug was not converted to long-chain polyglutamate forms.[80],[81] Inhibition of multidrug resistance protein-mediated efflux by probenecid could reverse the resistance phenotype.[80] A number of recent studies have underlined that the (in)activity of efflux routes can contribute significantly to the biological activity of antifolates. Schlemmer and Sirotnak demonstrated a large differential in efflux efficiency for folic acid and antifolates like methotrexate in L1210 leukaemia cells;[84] folic acid displayed relatively slow efflux rates compared with methotrexate. In Chinese hamster ovary cells, defective folate efflux of folic acid resulted in increased intracellular levels of folates which abolished the biological activity of a number of polyglutamatable and lipophilic antifolates.[5],[85]

Since multidrug resistance proteins are constitutively expressed in a variety of neoplastic cells and tissues, it is conceivable that drug extrusion via a multidrug resistance protein contributes to methotrexate resistance in clinical specimens.[83],[86]–[88]

Transport-related antifolate resistance

Transport-related resistance is considered to be a common mechanism of resistance to methotrexate. The majority of cases of transport defects refer to decreased methotrexate uptake as a result of decreased expression of reduced folate carrier or altered transport kinetic properties (increased K_m or decreased V_{max}) of the reduced folate carrier.[11],[19],[28],[29],[32],[36],[43],[44],[89]–[92] Several mutations in the rodent reduced folate carrier gene have been described which result in single amino acid substitutions at different sites of the predicted transmembrane domain of the reduced folate carrier protein.[93]–[96] These mutations result in a marked impairment in methotrexate uptake. Single/double mutations have also been reported in the human RFC1 gene which result in premature termination of translation which disrupts expression of reduced folate carrier protein.[97] Recently it has been shown that some mutations in the murine and human reduced folate carrier gene selectively enhance transport (decreased K_m) of natural folates (leucovorin and folic acid) over folate analogues such as methotrexate.[92],[95],[98],[99] Cells harbouring these reduced folate carrier mutations preserved their accumulation of reduced folate cofactors but had impaired antifolate uptake.

Transport-related mechanisms of resistance to methotrexate observed in vitro can also be common mechanisms of clinical resistance to methotrexate.[11],[29],[32],[37],[44],[100] Whitehead et al. demonstrated that decreased methotrexate accumulation and conversion to long-chain polyglutamate forms was a factor linked to poor prognosis in acute lymphoblastic leukaemia.[101],[102] Methotrexate accumulation appeared to be correlated with ploidy, especially hyperdiploid blasts with three or four copies of chromosome 21, but could not explain differences in methotrexate–polyglutamate accumulation between B-lineage and T-lineage acute lymphoblastic leukaemia.[41],[103] In newly diagnosed acute lymphoblastic leukaemia approximately 5 to 15 per cent of patients showed evidence of impaired (more than 1.8-fold reduction) methotrexate transport; in relapsed acute lymphoblastic leukaemia this number increased to 20 to 60 per cent of samples.[37],[91],[104] Although a wide variability (up to 100-fold) in reduced folate carrier mRNA expression has been noted in leukaemic cells, impaired methotrexate transport was found to be correlated with a decreased expression of reduced folate carrier mRNA.[91],[103],[105]

Transport-related resistance to methotrexate can also be due to increased expression of membrane folate receptor.[15],[47],[54],[55],[59] Due to the high affinity of folate binding protein for the natural folates (both reduced and oxidized) and a poor affinity for methotrexate, tumour cells in vitro and in vivo can grow at physiological folate levels and are resistant to therapeutic concentrations of methotrexate.

A better understanding of the molecular, biochemical, and functional properties of the various influx and efflux mechanisms will hopefully contribute to a further improvement in the clinical efficacy of antifolates.

Folate homeostasis

A growing body of evidence suggests that a cancer patient's cellular folate status is an important parameter determining the toxicity and antitumour activity of folate-based chemotherapeutic drugs.[106],[107] Expanded intracellular folate pools, which may abrogate antifolate sensitivity, may arise either from specific mutations in the reduced folate carrier gene, resulting in the synthesis of a structurally altered reduced folate carrier protein with increased folate uptake, or from

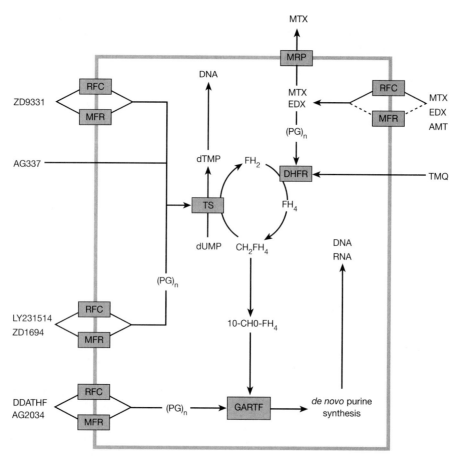

Fig. 4 Schematic presentation of reduced folate carrier- and membrane folate receptor-mediated inward transport of methotrexate and novel antifolates, multidrug resistance protein-mediated drug extrusion, metabolism of natural folates and antifolates, and intracellular targeting of dihydrofolate reductase, thymidylate synthase, and GARTFase. The efficiency of reduced folate carrier and membrane folate receptor transport of antifolates is depicted by a full line (representing a major transport route) or a broken line (representing a minor transport route). Regarding intracellular targeting of antifolates, only the primary targets of the antifolates are depicted. It should be taken into account that polyglutamate forms of antifolates can inhibit additional enzymes in folate metabolism. These interactions are not illustrated for the sake of clarity. (Taken in part from Jansen and Pieters.[31])

impaired folate efflux.[85],[92],[94],[95],[98] Conversely, decreased intracellular folate pools, which can confer toxic effects, may arise due to increased folate efflux mediated by multidrug resistance protein.[80] Indeed, several studies have pointed out that dietary folates or folate supplementation have a marked impact on the therapeutic activity of antifolates.[108]–[110]

Intracellular metabolism

Inhibition of dihydrofolate reductase

Once inside the cell, methotrexate binds rapidly to the target enzyme dihydrofolate reductase located in the cytoplasm (Fig. 4); this enzyme catalyses the reduction of dihydrofolate to tetrahydrofolate. Inhibition will lead to a depletion of the reduced folates, 5,10-methylene-tetrahydrofolate, a precursor for the *de novo* synthesis of dTMP, 5,10-methenyl-tetra-hydrofolate, and 10-formyl-tetrahydrofolate, a substrate for both glycinamide ribonucleotide transformylase and 5-amino-4-imidazole carboxamide ribonucleotide transformylase, enzymes involved in the *de novo* synthesis of purine nucleotides.[11],[111],[112] Methotrexate is a competitive inhibitor

of dihydrofolate reductase with respect to dihydrofolate and forms a ternary complex consisting of dihydrofolate reductase–NADPH–methotrexate.[113] The binding affinity of methotrexate to the enzyme is considerably influenced by the oxidation–reduction state and the availability of NADPH to stabilize the complex. Since the cellular level of dihydrofolate reductase is in excess of the requirements of the cell for reduced folates, tetrahydrofolate synthesis continues until more than 95 per cent of the enzyme is inhibited. Since dihydrofolate competes with methotrexate for the binding sites, methotrexate has to be present in excess. So, binding of methotrexate to the complex essentially determines the extent of inhibition of dihydrofolate reductase; changes in the conformation of dihydrofolate reductase, for example by substitution of phenylalanine at position 31, decreased the tight binding of methotrexate to dihydrofolate reductase.[114]

Polyglutamylation

Naturally occurring folates and antifolates such as methotrexate can be extensively metabolized to polyglutamate derivatives in an ATP-dependent reaction catalysed by the enzyme folylpoly-γ-glutamate synthetase.[115],[116] Folylpoly-γ-glutamate synthetase is localized in the cytosol and mitochondria where it catalyses the addition of multiple (up to seven to 10) negatively charged glutamate residues to the γ-carboxyl group of (anti)folate compounds.[117],[118] Polyglutamylation of (anti)folates prolongs intracellular retention because rapid efflux is prevented. Consequently, defective polyglutamylation due to low folylpoly-γ-glutamate synthetase activity has been associated with methotrexate resistance.[119]–[122] Polyglutamate formation has been characterized in a variety of cell lines from normal and neoplastic murine and human tissues.[123] Polyglutamate synthesis is dependent on the concentration of the drug and the duration of the exposure. Both Pizzorno et al. and Braakhuis et al. demonstrated that the difference in sensitivity of several squamous cell carcinonoma cell lines to methotrexate is dependent on the times for which the cells were exposed to methotrexate.[124],[125] A short exposure to high-dose methotrexate (comparable to a bolus injection) was moderately effective in the synthesis of polyglutamates. At a continuous exposure to a lower concentration of methotrexate more polyglutamates were formed which were retained for longer.

Clinical studies for childhood leukaemia have shown that the efficacy of accumulating high levels of methotrexate polyglutamates is an important factor for the outcome of treatment with methotrexate.[101],[102],[126]–[130] Children with high levels of methotrexate polyglutamates in their leukaemic blasts had an improved 5-year survival compared with children who had a lower accumulation.[101] The efficacy of methotrexate polyglutamylation appeared to be better in acute lymphoblastic leukaemia cells from the B lineage than from the T lineage.[127],[131],[132] This was associated with a constitutively higher folylpoly-γ-glutamate synthetase activity in B cells than in T cells. In addition, B cells exhibited a significant post-treatment upregulation in folylpoly-γ-glutamate synthetase activity that was observed to only a minor extent for T-lineage acute lymphoblastic leukaemia cells. The responsiveness of acute lymphoblastic leukaemia cells to methotrexate has been associated with extensive polyglutamylation, whereas defective methotrexate polyglutamylation is a major cause of inherent methotrexate resistance in acute myeloid leukaemia.[11],[29],[126],[132],[133] In acute myeloid leukaemia cells, Longo et al. observed a twofold higher K_m value (decreased affinity) for folylpoly-γ-glutamate synthetase with a methotrexate substrate than for folylpoly-γ-glutamate synthetase enzyme.[134] In a comparative study for acute lymphoblastic leukaemia, Synold et al. and Masson et al. demonstrated that high-dose methotrexate treatment regimens improved the accumulation and polyglutamylation of methotrexate as compared with a low-dose methotrexate protocol.[128],[129] Whitehead et al. also observed that hyperdiploid lymphoblasts accumulated significantly higher levels of methotrexate polyglutamates than did aneuploid or diploid lymphoblasts.[102] Patients with hyperdiploid lymphoblasts have an improved prognosis, possibly because of their enhanced sensitivity to methotrexate-based chemotherapy. It is interesting that the rate of synthesis of methotrexate polyglutamates is relatively low in bone marrow and gut epithelium, which are tissues known to be dose-limiting for toxicity.[135]–[137]

The formation of methotrexate polyglutamates allows the accumulation of intracellular drug levels far above levels that would exist under normal equilibrium. Methotrexate polyglutamates are at least as potent as the normal methotrexate monoglutamate in their capacity to inhibit dihydrofolate reductase. In addition, methotrexate polyglutamates appear to dissociate less rapidly from the enzyme than

the monoglutamate. For example, for methotrexate pentaglutamate the dissociation half-life of the dihydrofolate reductase ternary complex was ten times longer than for methotrexate monoglutamate.[138]

Besides the formation of polyglutamate forms, cells contain a catabolic pathway that mediates the breakdown of polyglutamate forms of (anti)folates. The enzyme responsible for this process is γ-folylpolyglutamate hydrolase and is localized in the lysosome.[139]–[141] Rhee et al. demonstrated that a sevenfold increase in the activity of γ-folylpolyglutamate hydrolase enzyme was partly responsible for the resistance to methotrexate in a subline of the rat hepatoma H35 cell line.[142] In leukemic blast cells, it appeared that the ratio of folylpoly-γ-glutamate synthetase to γ-folylpolyglutamate hydrolase activity was the best predictive index for the formation of methotrexate polyglutamates.[132],[143] The ability of cancer cells to form polyglutamates and to retain them intracellularly is one of the major determinants of sensitivity or resistance to antifolate treatment.

Indirect effects

In addition to the inhibitory effect on dihydrofolate reductase, methotrexate polyglutamates, but not the monoglutamate, are potent inhibitors of other enzymes which require folate, including thymidylate synthase and aminoimidazolecarboximide (AICAR) transformylase (Table 3). Furthermore, the methotrexate-induced inhibition of dihydrofolate reductase leads to an accumulation of dihydrofolate which can also be polyglutamated. Dihydrofolate polyglutamates can also directly inhibit de novo purine synthesis.[144] Inhibition of the de novo purine synthesis can lead to an increase in the concentration of 5-phosphoribosyl-1-pyrophosphate. Sant et al. provided evidence that not only are the above-mentioned enzymes being inhibited but that amidophosphoribosyltransferase, the first enzyme from the de novo purine synthesis, may be the principal site of inhibition.[145] The pentaglutamate from dihydrofolate appeared to be a potent non-competitive inhibitor of the enzyme isolated from L1210 leukaemia cells with an inhibition constant of 3.4 μM. These results indicate that non-dihydrofolate reductase targets are attractive for the development of new antifolates in antineoplastic therapy. Biochemical and clinical evaluation of this second generation of antifolates will be discussed in a following section.

Degradation to 7-OH-methotrexate

Another pathway in the metabolism of methotrexate is that of hydroxylation to 7-OH-methotrexate catalysed by aldehyde oxidase. This enzyme has been demonstrated in the livers of many mammalian species and in a number of malignant cells and cell lines. 7-OH-methotrexate has been demonstrated at high levels in plasma and urine after injection of moderate to high doses of methotrexate. 7-OH-methotrexate can interfere with the cytotoxicity of methotrexate at several levels. 7-OH-methotrexate is not cytotoxic to methotrexate-sensitive cells, but does affect the influx and efflux of methotrexate itself, thus reducing the sensitivity to methotrexate.[146],[147] This may be a factor in the resistance to methotrexate. 7-OH-methotrexate does not bind to dihydrofolate reductase, but is a substrate for polyglutamylation. The pentaglutamate of 7-OH-methotrexate is capable of binding to dihydrofolate reductase. It has also been demonstrated that the higher polyglutamates of 7-OH-methotrexate can inhibit thymidylate synthase and AICAR transformylase.[148] These interesting properties of 7-OH-methotrexate may either contribute to cytotoxicity in for example the liver or kidney, or may add to the antitumour effect.

Cell kill by methotrexate and salvage

The ultimate effect of methotrexate is a depletion of reduced folates followed by either depletion of thymidine nucleotides and/or purine nucleotides, resulting in a so-called thymineless or purineless state, respectively.[149] This will lead to 'unbalanced growth', a state in which RNA and protein synthesis can continue, but DNA synthesis and consequently cell division are inhibited. This corresponds to a state of S-phase arrest, which has to persist for several hours to result in cell death.[150] The contribution of each of these pathways to cell kill probably varies with cell type. Thus, both exogenous purines and thymidine can prevent the cytotoxicity of methotrexate, and it has been suggested that this may be selective.[151] Preformed purines and thymidine are part of the diet and are released from dying cells.[152] They can contribute to purine and pyrimidine nucleotide synthesis via the salvage pathways and may represent an inherent form of resistance to methotrexate.[153],[154]

The depletion of dTTP can lead to an additional effect in the mechanism of action of methotrexate and folate depletion, i.e. the misincorporation of dUTP into DNA, causing DNA lesions.[155]–[158] Misincorporated dUTP will be recognized by uracil glycosylase and excised, leading to strand breaks. It has been postulated that the latter effect may be the ultimate cause of cell death after exposure to methotrexate, since this event may induce activation of poly(ADP-ribose) polymerase, subsequently leading to depletion of NAD, and that of ATP.[159] The ultimate result will be an inability to phosphorylate, to synthesize RNA, DNA, and protein, and to maintain membrane integrity, leading to cell death.

It has become evident that following depletion of intracellular folates and/or purines/pyrimidines, methotrexate can induce the process of programmed cell death (apoptosis) which is controlled by various cell cycle-related genes, e.g. p53, the retinoblastoma (Rb) gene, c-*myc*, p21, and bcl-2.[8],[160]–[163] Malignant cells lacking functional p53 display resistance to many anticancer drugs due to a common impairment to go into apoptosis.[8],[164]–[166] Transfection of wild-type p53 in p53-null HL-60 cells conferred sensitivity to multiple drugs, including the antifolate ZD1694.[163] Mutation or hyperphosphorylation of Rb causes it to lose its ability to bind to and inactivate E2F. E2F is a transcription factor for dihydrofolate reductase and thymidylate synthase. Consequently, the activity of these enzymes is increased. This mechanism of resistance to methotrexate in human sarcoma cells was reversed by transfection of the Rb gene.[162]

Clinical pharmacology of methotrexate

Methotrexate is one of the few antineoplastic agents for which a relationship between plasma drug levels and cytotoxicity has been established.[153],[167]–[172] It is common, therefore, to monitor plasma levels of methotrexate in order to identify patients at high risk for toxicity and to adapt therapy. Toxicity is a function of dose and exposure. Exposure to levels higher than 0.02 μM (the concentration threshold) for longer than 42 h (the time threshold) is associated with high toxicity. Posttreatment with leucovorin will 'rescue' normal tissues without significantly affecting the antitumour effect. Methotrexate is toxic to rapidly proliferating tissues such as bone marrow and gastrointestinal mucosa, especially at high doses. Nausea, vomiting,

mucositis, transient encephalopathy, and anorexia may accompany high-dose methotrexate therapy. Nephrotoxicity is frequently observed with high doses of methotrexate. Intrathecal therapy with methotrexate has been associated with central nervous system toxicity.

Analysis and elimination

The various methods for measurement of methotrexate include an enzyme inhibition assay using dihydrofolate reductase, a competitive protein binding assay (using dihydrofolate reductase as the binding protein), a radioimmunoassay, and an enzyme-linked immunoassay.[173] These assays may lack selectivity since the immunoassays also detect methotrexate metabolites; however, they are sensitive and convenient for routine clinical use. High-performance liquid chromatography is very selective and discriminates between methotrexate and 7-OH-methotrexate.

Methotrexate is administered to patients via several routes and a number of different schedules are used.[174],[175] The plasma pharmacokinetics of intravenous methotrexate over a conventional (up to 100 mg/m^2) and moderate (100–1000 mg/m^2) dose range generally follows a three-phase disappearance pattern. An elimination phase with a half-life of 2 to 3 h and a terminal phase of elimination with a half-life of 8 to 10 h follow the short distribution phase. The drug is eliminated almost exclusively by renal excretion.[176] Methotrexate is filtered through the glomerulus, reabsorbed in the proximal tubule (which can be blocked by probenecid), and secreted by the distal tubule. Most methotrexate is excreted unchanged within 6 h. The clearance of methotrexate equals or exceeds that of creatinine but is not entirely predictable. In plasma, 50 to 60 per cent of methotrexate is protein bound. In a comparative study in a dose range of 0.5 to 33.6 mg/m^2, Borsi and Moe observed a disproportionate increase of the steady state concentration, both in serum and cerebrospinal fluid.[177] In children from 1 to 4 years steady state plasma concentrations of methotrexate were lower while the volume of distribution was higher (27 litres/m^2 compared with 16 litres/m^2) compared with older subjects. Clearance at 0.5 g/m^2 was higher (146 ml/min/m^2) than at doses from 3 to 33.6 g/m^2 (about 50 ml/min/m^2).

Since methotrexate is a weak organic acid that is negatively charged at neutral pH, and since it has limited lipid solubility, it will diffuse slowly across physiological membranes. In the cerebrospinal fluid, or third-space compartments, such as pleural effusions and ascites fluid, penetration will therefore be low. Due to a low rate of reabsorption methotrexate will, however, accumulate in third-space fluids. In cerebrospinal fluid methotrexate levels are only 3 per cent of those in plasma, but these levels will also be maintained for longer.

A number of agents alter protein binding (salicylates, tetracycline, probenecid, etc.), but many of these agents also compete with methotrexate for renal tubular secretion.[178] The concomitant use of methotrexate with, for example, salicylates may therefore reduce the clearance and increase the toxicity.

High-dose methotrexate

The administration of methotrexate at high doses (1–33 g/m^2) with leucovorin rescue has been used as a therapeutic strategy for several tumour types since its initial use for osteogenic sarcoma.[179] Theoretically, the rationale for high-dose methotrexate has several attractive features:[11],[129],[169],[175]

(1) At high drug levels a transport deficiency can be overcome.

(2) High free intracellular methotrexate may overcome decreased inhibition of dihydrofolate reductase.

(3) High methotrexate levels may increase polyglutamate formation.

(4) High-dose methotrexate will prolong the exposure time of cells to a toxic drug concentration.

(5) Normal cells may be rescued from the effects of methotrexate and tumour cells not.

(6) High-dose methotrexate will lead to cytocidal drug levels in cerebrospinal fluid.

Despite these appealing features, the role of high-dose methotrexate in the treatment of human cancer remains undefined and controversial.[27],[180] The optimum dose of methotrexate, schedule of leucovorin rescue, and the clinical indications have not been well established. For treatment of recurrent childhood acute lymphoblastic leukaemia, high-dose methotrexate appeared not to be superior to low-dose/intermediate-dose methotrexate.[181] Winick *et al.* showed that fractionated doses of oral methotrexate were equally active in achieving a similar event-free survival for childhood leukaemias as other high-dose, schedules.[182] However, other studies by Niemeyer *et al.*, Reiter *et al.*, and Mahoney *et al.* demonstrated a better clinical outcome with the high-dose methotrexate versus the low-dose methotrexate regimens.[171],[172],[183],[184] Given the marked individual differences in systemic clearance of methotrexate, Evans *et al.* showed that an individualized rather than a generalized dosing scheme for methotrexate should be considered to further improve clinical outcome.[169] There are only two settings in which high-dose methotrexate can have a potential benefit, as adjuvant chemotherapy for osteogenic sarcoma and for diseases where penetration of the drug into sanctuary sites (e.g. the central nervous system) is essential. For instance in childhood acute lymphoblastic leukaemia high-dose methotrexate has been useful in preventing central nervous system relapses.

High-dose methotrexate schedules produce very high initial plasma levels of methotrexate (10 μM to 1 mM), which are sustained at levels higher than 1 μM for 12 to 30 h.[129] A steady state gradient of 30:1 exists between plasma and cerebrospinal fluid over a large dose range, so with high-dose methotrexate cytocidal levels will be reached.[175],[177],[185] All schedules require leucovorin to prevent life-threatening toxicity. Hydration and administration of sodium bicarbonate are required to prevent nephrotoxicity. This might result from precipitation of methotrexate or 7-OH-methotrexate in the renal tubules, since these compounds are relatively insoluble at acid pH. Leucovorin has to be given when methotrexate is higher than a certain threshold level at a certain time point (Table 4). Different schedules of high-dose methotrexate will require an adapted leucovorin rescue. The original Jaffe regimen began leucovorin rescue 2 h after methotrexate administration. However, evidence is accumulating that rescue can be delayed for up to 24 h after methotrexate administration. Delaying the start of leucovorin may also make rescue of tumour cells less likely whilst minimizing toxicity to normal cells. Borsi *et al.* presented evidence that reduction of the dose of leucovorin below 15 mg/m² may increase the efficacy of high-dose methotrexate, while remaining safe in preventing treatment-related toxicity.[186]

Other schedules

Methotrexate is also given at moderate doses (100–1000 mg/m²), and such schedules are generally well tolerated when administered frequently, with no metabolic adaptation being observed.[171],[172],[177],[187]

Plateau methotrexate levels were about 7 μM. This schedule may be an alternative to high-dose methotrexate.

Methotrexate is frequently administered orally in the maintenance therapy of acute lymphoblastic leukaemia in children and currently also for treatment of rheumatoid arthritis but at lower doses.[24],[26],[129],[168],[178],[182] Absorption is variable, but at doses of less than 25 mg/m² the drug shows a good bioavailability, at doses above 50 mg/m² the bioavailability is only 20 to 50 per cent. Peak levels of 1 μM are observed between 1 and 5 h after drug administration at optimal absorption. Levels remain above 0.1 μM for about 6 h. Patients with a good absorption appeared to have fewer relapses than in those where it was poor. Balis *et al.* investigated subcutaneous administration as an alternative to oral therapy and observed that this route is convenient and produces essentially 100 per cent bioavailability.[188] At 40 mg/m² oral dosing resulted in only one-third of the exposure which occurred with the subcutaneous route. Thus for maintenance therapy the subcutaneous route is to be preferred, since bioavailability is more reproducible.

The use of hyperosmotic agents, such as mannitol, offers the possibility of opening the blood–brain barrier and allowing a greater penetration of chemotherapeutic agents to intrathecal and intracerebral neoplasms. The use of mannitol may also lead to increased accumulation of drug in the cerebral cortex and thus to enhanced neurotoxicity.[189] Another approach to the prophylaxis and treatment of meningeal leukaemia is the use of intrathecal methotrexate at a fixed dose of 12 mg. The half-life of intrathecal methotrexate is about 6 to 12 h, but appeared to be longer in patients who experienced neurotoxicity, especially when it was given in combination with irradiation. Irradiation induces an increase in the permeability of the blood–brain barrier leading to an increased concentration of methotrexate in brain tissue.[190]

Novel antifolates

The recognition that impaired transport, impaired polyglutamylation, and/or increased dihydrofolate reductase activity are common mechanisms of intrinsic and acquired clinical resistance to methotrexate has initiated the design and synthesis of a new generation of antifolates that could overcome one or more of these mechanisms of methotrexate resistance.[11],[13],[14],[19],[20],[31],[191]–[194] Moreover, these novel antifolates may circumvent the toxic effects of methotrexate (see the section on the clinical pharmacology of methotrexate). Characteristic features of these novel antifolates are:

(1) Their improved transport efficiency via the reduced folate carrier and/or the membrane folate receptor.

(2) No dependency on carrier- or receptor-mediated transport pathways for cell entry.

(3) Prolonged intracellular retention (due to improved polyglutamylation via folylpoly-γ-glutamate synthetase).

(4) Targeting of enzymes in folate metabolism other than dihydrofolate reductase, e.g. thymidylate synthase and GARTFase.

Table 5 and Figs 2 and 4 present an overview of the chemical structures, efficiency of transport and polyglutamylation, and current status of clinical evaluation of a number of novel antifolates.

The novel antifolates can be divided into three groups:

(1) Those depending on reduced folate carrier/membrane folate receptor transport and polyglutamylation by folylpoly-γ-glutamate synthetase (EDX (edatrexate), AMT, GW1843, ZD1694,

Table 4 Example of high-dose methotrexate therapy; prevention/reversal of toxicity[26],[27],[174],[175]

1. Prehydration and urinary alkalinization: 12 h before methotrexate administration with sodium bicarbonate to prevent nephrotoxicity. Check pH ($\geq$7 at time of administration)

2. Jaffe regimen; 1.5–7.5 g/m$^{(2)}$ over a 6-h infusion. Continue hydration

3. Start leucovorin rescue after 2–24 h after end of infusion (15 mg/m$^{(2)}$, every 6 h for seven doses)

4. Monitor plasma methotrexate levels every 48 h and adjust leucovorin therapy; levels > 0.5 μM require leucovorin rescue (see table below)

Drug level	Dose of leucovorin (every 6 h × eight doses)
0.5 μM	15 mg/m$^{(2)}$
1 μM	100 mg/m$^{(2)}$
2 μM	200 mg/m$^{(2)}$

Table 5 Transport and polyglutamylation properties, and clinical status of methotrexate versus novel antifolates in cancer chemotherapy

Antifolate	Target enzyme	Affinity RFC†	Affinity MFR†	Affinity FPGS†	Clinical phase	Reference
Methotrexate	DHFR	+ +	+	+ +		Bertino[11]
Trimetrexate	DHFR	–	–	–	II–III	Lin et al.,[662] Bertino,[11] Gorlick and Bertino[175]
Edatrexate	DHFR	+ + + +	+	+ + +	III	Grant et al.,[195] Schornagel et al.[17]
Aminopterin (AMT)	DHFR	+ + + +	+	+ + +	I–II	Smith et al.,[130] Ratliff et al.[199]
ZD1694	TS	+ + + +	+ + +	+ + + +	II–III	Cocconi et al.,[23] Hughes et al.[206]
LY231514	TS(+)‡	+ + + +	+ + +	+ + +	I–II–III	Rinaldi,[214] Shih et al.,[203],[204] Calvert and Walling[21]
ZD9331	TS	+ + + +	+ + +	–	I–II–III	Jackman et al.,[208] Boyle et al.[210]
AG337	TS	–	–	–	I–II–III	Rafi et al.,[18] Hughes and Calvert[205]
DDATHF	GARFTase	+ + + +	+ + + +	+ + +	I	Mendelsohn et al.[201]
AG2034	GARFTase	+ + + +	+ + +	+ + +	I–II	Boritzki et al.[202]

Further details can be found in various chapters of the book Jackman AL (ed.) 1999 *Antifolate drugs in cancer therapy* (Totowa, NJ: Humana Press). See also Jackman and Judson,[30] Peters and Ackland,[19] Gorlick et al.,[29] and Rustum et al.[20]

†Data from Westerhof et al.[15]

‡LY231514 is also referred to as multitargeted antifolate (MTA, ACIMTA) to illustrate that this compound inhibits, beyond TS, also DHFR and GARFTase.

Abbreviations: FPGS = folylpoly-γ-glutamate synthetase; RFC = reduced folate carrier; DHFR = dihydrofolate reductase; TS = thymidylate synthase; MFR = membrane folate receptor; GARTF = glycinamide ribonucleotide transformylase.

LY231514/ multitargeted antifolate, DDATHF, and AG2034). These antifolates may overcome methotrexate resistance due to more efficient transport and polyglutamylation.[130],[195]–[206]

(2) Antifolates that depend on reduced folate carrier transport for cell entry but do not require polyglutamylation (PT523, ZD9331).[207]–[210] These antifolates may overcome methotrexate resistance because of impaired polyglutamylation due to a low folylpoly-γ-glutamate synthetase or increased γ-folylpolyglutamate hydrolase activity.

(3) The groups of lipophilic antifolates (TMQ, AG337) that do not require reduced folate carrier-/membrane folate receptor-mediated transport and polyglutamylation. These antifolates can enter cells by passive/facilitated diffusion and therefore have the potential to circumvent transport-related and polyglutamylation-related methotrexate resistance.[126],[175],[205],[211] All antifolate inhibitors of thymidylate synthase and GARFTase can overcome methotrexate resistance associated with elevated dihydrofolate reductase activity.[11],[14],[15],[192],[212],[213]

The new generation of antifolates (edatrexate (EDX), Raltitrexed/ZD1694, LY231514/multitargeted antifolate) has shown promising activity in phase II to III clinical trials for the treatment of head and neck squamous cell carcinoma, colorectal carcinomas, and non-small cell lung cancer.[17],[21],[23],[214] Dose limiting toxicities for these novel antifolates include: for datrexate, stomatitis, skin toxicity, and hair loss;[17] for multitargeted antifolate, neutropenia, thrombocytopenia, and fatigue;[214],[215] and for ZD1694/Raltitrexed; diarrhoea, nausea, vomiting, neutropenia, and hepatic toxicity.[216],[217] Other rationally designed novel antifolates (GW1843, AG337, ZD9331, and AG2034) are currently being evaluated in phase I to II clinical trials.[18]–[20],[210],[218] At present it is unknown whether these novel antifolates will be superior to methotrexate as a single agent or whether they may display efficacy in drug combination regimens. In this respect, it is has been recognized that enhanced antitumour activity of novel antifolates may be achieved through decreasing host toxicity by administering oral folic acid or leucovorin.[109],[110]

Fluoropyrimidines

For several decades 5-fluorouracil and other fluoropyrimidines have been used in the treatment of advanced colorectal cancer, other tumours of the gastrointestinal tract, breast cancer, and head and neck cancer.[20],[219],[220] Clinical application of 5-fluorouracil is changing. Currently, 5-fluorouracil is not usually used as a single agent (as such the objective response rate for colorectal cancer was usually less than 20 per cent). *In vitro* studies have now clearly demonstrated that the cytotoxicity of 5-fluorouracil can be enhanced by biochemical modulation—the combination of 5-fluorouracil with an agent which can interfere with its mechanism of action.[220]–[224] *In vivo* such a combination should increase its antitumour properties in a selective manner. Biochemical modulation studies with 5-fluorouracil have exploited the complex mechanism of action of 5-fluorouracil with the aim of achieving a selective enhancement of its activity. These studies have led to the development of combinations of 5-fluorouracil with leucovorin, with the ultimate aim of circumventing either intrinsic or acquired resistance to 5-fluorouracil. More recently several new compounds, such as the antifolate thymidylate synthase inhibitor Tomudex, the topoisomerase inhibitor irinotecan (CPT-11), gemcitabine, and the platinum analogue oxaliplatin, have been combined successfully with 5-fluorouracil in the treatment of various diseases.

Mechanisms of action and resistance

Activation and inactivation

5-Fluorouracil is an analogue of uracil (Fig. 5) but due to its additional resemblance to orotic acid and thymine, the drug uses the same pathways as these natural substrates. 5-Fluorouracil is transported into the cell either by a high-affinity nucleobase carrier or by passive diffusion.[225] Nucleoside transporters are unlikely to contribute to nucleobase transport. In order to be active 5-fluorouracil has to be converted to one of its nucleotides (Fig. 6). These are:

- 5-Fluorouridine-5′-triphosphate (FUTP), which can be incorporated into RNA
- 5-Fluoro-2′-uridine-5′-triphosphate (FdUTP), which can be incorporated into DNA

- 5-Fluorouridine-5′-diphosphate (FUDP) sugars, which may interfere with glycosylation of proteins and lipids
- 5-Fluoro-2′-deoxyuridine-5′-monophosphate (FdUMP), which is an inhibitor of thymidylate synthase, a key enzyme in the *de novo* synthesis of the pyrimidine deoxynucleotide 2′-deoxythymidine-5′-triphosphate (dTTP), a direct precursor for the synthesis of DNA.

Disturbances in one of these conversions can lead to resistance to 5-fluorouracil.[154],[220] Thus the activity of the anabolism pathways (either directly via orotate phosphoribosyltransferase or indirectly via the pyrimidine nucleoside phosphorylase and kinase) has been associated with the cytotoxic effects of 5-fluorouracil. Cellular transport of 5-fluorouracil itself has not been shown to limit its cytotoxicity but it has been demonstrated that transport deficiency of its nucleoside analogue floxuridine, can lead to resistance.

Initial studies on 5-fluorouracil resistance concentrated on its activation pathways (Table 6). Indeed, it was recognized in several model systems that a low activity of uridine kinase and uridine phosphorylase (and the channelled uridine phosphorylase–uridine kinase) and orotate phosphoribosyltransferase were related to resistance to 5-fluorouracil.[226]–[230] In *in vivo* models both high uridine phosphorylase activity and high orotate phosphoribosyltransferase activity were related to 5-fluorouracil sensitivity.[231],[232] However, Ardalan *et al.* observed low 5-phosphoribosyl-1-pyrophosphate levels in 5-fluorouracil-resistant tumours and a higher activity of 5-phosphoribosyl-1-pyrophosphate synthetase sensitive tumours, indicating an important role for orotate phosphoribosyltransferase since 5-phosphoribosyl-1-pyrophosphate is the cosubstrate for this enzyme in activation of 5-fluorouracil.[233] Activation of 5-fluorouracil via uridine phosphorylase also requires the action of uridine kinase, which is usually limiting.[222],[234],[235] More evidence for the importance of the orotate phosphoribosyltransferase pathway was obtained by Holland *et al.* who showed that injection of the uridine phosphorylase inhibitor benzylacyclouridine together with 5-fluorouracil resulted in the accumulation of FUR in the tumour, whereas no FUR was observed when 5-fluorouracil was injected as a single agent.[236] This means that FUR should be formed as a degradation product of FUMP, and indicates the existence of a futile cycle 5-fluorouracil → FUMP → FUR → 5-fluorouracil. This can be considered as some 'hidden' depot of 5-fluorouracil in the tumour responsible for the long retention of 5-fluorouracil in tissues.[237] High activity of the orotate phosphoribosyltransferase pathway is essential for 5-fluorouracil activation.[222] Thus, 5-fluorouracil resistance is determined by a combination of several factors such as decreased activation of 5-fluorouracil, increased breakdown of 5-fluorouracil, its nucleosides, and its nucleotides, and aberrations in thymidylate synthase activity (see later).[154],[224] These factors may be different for each cell or tumour type.

5-Fluorouracil can be inactivated by degradation to 5-fluoro-dihydrouracil in a reaction catalysed by dihydropyrimidine dehydrogenase with NADPH as the cosubstrate. 5-Fluorodihydrouracil is degraded further to fluoroureidopropionate and subsequently to fluoro-β-alanine, NH_3, and CO_2. Conversion of fluoro-β-alanine to fluoroacetate has been related to neurotoxicity.[238] However, fluoro-β-alanine itself was shown to cause neurotoxicity, manifested by a direct action on myelin-inducing vacuole formation and a necrosis/softening-like change of the brainstem.[239] Fluoro-β-alanine itself can

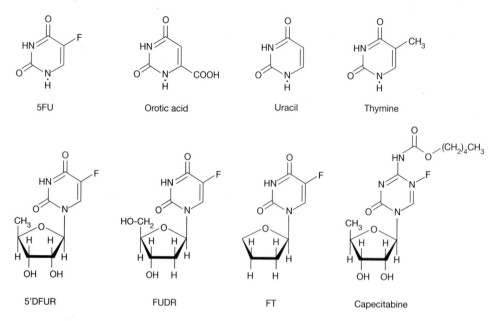

Fig. 5 Structural formula of 5-fluorouracil compared with its normal counterparts, orotic acid, uracil, and thymine; and of the 5-fluorouracil analogues 5'DFUR (Doxifluridine), FUDR (Floxuridine), Ft (Ftorafur, tegafur), and Capecitabine (Xeloda).

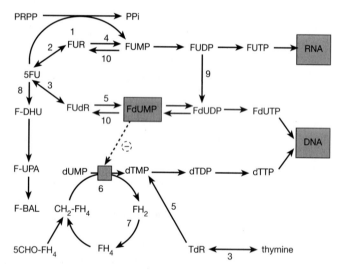

Fig. 6 Schematic representation of 5-fluorouracil metabolism with possible sites responsible for resistance. Resistance can be due to an increase of the target enzyme (thymidylate synthase), a decrease in activation, or an increased inactivation (of 5-fluorouracil itself to F-DHU or of the 5-fluorouracil nucleotides 5-fluorouridine-5'-monophosphate (FUMP) or FdUMP to the nucleosides 5-fluorouridine (FUR) and floxuridine). Inhibition of thymidylate synthase by FdUMP is represented by a Θ and a bar. The boxes indicate that a low accumulation (FdUMP) or decreased incorporation (RNA, DNA) can limit the action of 5-fluorouracil. Enzymes catalysing these reactions are: 1, orotate phosphoribosyltransferase; 2, uridine phosphorylase; 3, thymidine phosphorylase; 4, uridine kinase; 5, thymidine kinase; 6, thymidylate synthase; 7, dihydrofolate reductase; 8, dihydropyrimidine dehydrogenase; 9, ribonucleotide reductase; 10, 5'-nucleotidases and phosphatases. F-DHU = 5-fluorodihydrouracil; FUPA = fluoroureidopropionate; F-BAL = α-fluoro-β-alanine; PRPP = 5-phosphoribosyl-1-pyrophosphate; TdR = thymidine.

Table 6 Mechanisms of resistance to 5-fluorouracil (modified from Peters and Jansen[154] and Peters and Köhne[224])

Decreased accumulation of activated metabolites
Decreased activation
Increased inactivation
Increased inactivation of 5-fluorouracil nucleotides

Target-associated resistance
Decreased RNA effect
Altered effect on thymidylate synthase
  Aberrant enzyme kinetics
  Increased dUMP levels
  Decreased FdUMP accumulation
  Decreased stability of ternary complex
  Depletion of intracellular folates
  Decreased polyglutamylation of folates
  Recovery and enhanced enzyme synthesis
  Gene amplification
  Enzyme induction

Pharmacokinetic resistance
The drug does not reach the tumour
Disease state affects drug distribution
Increased elimination

also form conjugates with bile acids such as cholate and chenodeoxycholate.[240]–[242] These conjugates may have a role in the hepatic and biliary toxicity that develops in patients receiving hepatic arterial infusions of fluoropyrimidines. 5-Fluorouracil degradation occurs in all tissues, including tumours, but is most abundant in the liver and to a lesser extent in the kidney.[243],[244] Thus, the liver plays an important role in degradation and elimination of 5-fluorouracil. In patients, large amounts of the breakdown products have been demonstrated in plasma and urine. Breakdown products have also been demonstrated in the liver with ^{19}F nuclear magnetic resonance.[245]

Inhibition of 5-fluorouracil degradation can enhance the availability of 5-fluorouracil to other tissues, including the tumour. Initial studies used the ability of natural substrates of dihydropyrimidine dehydrogenase to modulate 5-fluorouracil. However, thymidine, a precursor of thymine, did not improve the therapeutic index of 5-fluorouracil, while in rats toxicity was increased.[246],[247] Thymidine also interferes at other sites of 5-fluorouracil metabolism. Uracil, the other natural substrate of dihydropyrimidine dehydrogenase, has been developed more successfully as a modulator of 5-fluorouracil catabolism. When administered orally with Ftorafur in a molar ratio of 4:1 (**UFT**, uracil with Ftorafur), it has a similar activity against advanced colorectal cancer as standard intravenous push 5-fluorouracil regimens in combination with leucovorin.[224]

Impaired 5-fluorouracil degradation due to a deficiency of dihydropyrimidine dehydrogenase results in a dramatic increase in 5-fluorouracil toxicity, leading to death.[248]–[250] Therefore clinical trials with synthetic inhibitors of 5-fluorouracil degradation have been performed carefully, taking into account that toxicity might increase. Several new types of inhibitors of dihydropyrimidine dehydrogenase, such as ethynyluracil (eniluracil) and 5-chloro-2,4-dihydropyridine have been developed.[251]–[254] Ethynyluracil is a so-called suicide inhibitor which acts by inactivation of the enzyme. The other compounds are competitive inhibitors of dihydropyrimidine dehydrogenase. Several preclinical and clinical studies now show that these compounds have a comparable activity when given orally in combination with either 5-fluorouracil or Ftorafur, compared with standard 5-fluorouracil regimens.

Inhibition of thymidylate synthase

Inhibition of thymidylate synthase by FdUMP is considered to be the main mechanism for the action of 5-fluorouracil (Fig. 6). Several mechanisms of resistance to 5-fluorouracil have been attributed to alterations in thymidylate synthase.[154] Characteristics of the thymidylate synthase enzyme have been described in detail by others.[255],[256] Thymidylate synthase catalyses the conversion of dUMP to dTMP, for which 5,10-methylenetetrahydrofolate serves as a methyl donor. FdUMP acts as a potent competitive inhibitor of thymidylate synthase with dUMP. The inhibition by FdUMP is mediated by the formation of a covalent ternary complex between FdUMP, thymidylate synthase, and 5,10-methylenetetrahydrofolate, while the retention of inhibition is also dependent on the ratio between free dUMP and FdUMP levels.[257],[258] A low sensitivity to 5-fluorouracil has been related to a rapid disappearance of FdUMP. A high dUMP concentration or limited binding of FdUMP to thymidylate synthase may reduce retention of the inhibition of thymidylate synthase.

The stability of the ternary complex is highly dependent on the availability of 5,10-methylenetetrahydrofolate or one of its polyglutamates.[258] Leucovorin can increase the availability of methylenetetrahydrofolate (Fig. 6). After transfer across the membrane, mediated by the reduced folate carrier, leucovorin will be metabolized to methylenetetrahydrofolate, which will undergo polyglutamylation and thus enhance inhibition of thymidylate synthase.[32],[259],[260] A decreased activity of folylpoly-γ-glutamate synthetase and altered binding of FdUMP to thymidylate synthase have been associated with 5-fluorouracil resistance.[48],[257],[261]–[263] In the absence of methylenetetrahydrofolate or one of its polyglutamates, FdUMP forms an unstable binary complex, which results in poor inhibition.[257],[263]–[265] In addition disturbed folate pools lead to intrinsic resistance as well as a high level of enzyme before treatment.[257],[262],[265],[266] Gene amplification of thymidylate synthase and mutations in the gene lead to acquired resistance.[263],[267]–[269] Thus, changes in the thymidylate synthase gene at the DNA level (e.g. mutations or gene amplification) are clearly associated with acquired resistance to fluoropyrimidines.

Expression of thymidylate synthase under physiological conditions is related to the cell cycle, with a high activity during the S phase.[270] The translation of thymidylate synthase mRNA appears to be controlled by its end product, the thymidylate synthase protein, in an autoregulatory manner. However, when thymidylate synthase is bound to a ternary complex, the protein can no longer regulate its synthesis, leading to the observed increase. Thus, inhibition of thymidylate synthase in vitro, either by the formation of the ternary complex between FdUMP, the enzyme, and 5,10-methylenetetrahydrofolate or by specific thymidylate synthase inhibitors such as ZD1694, disrupts the regulation of enzyme synthesis, which is manifested as an increase in thymidylate synthase protein expression.[271]–[273] This increase is not accompanied by an increase in thymidylate synthase mRNA or by a change in the stability of the enzyme. p53 mRNA translation can also be regulated by thymidylate synthase protein, while wild-type p53 protein can also inhibit thymidylate synthase promotor activity.[274],[275] Thus regulation of induction of thymidylate synthase is a very complicated process, which may be even more disrupted (more induction) in cells with mutated p53 than with wild-type p53 (low induction). The 5-fluorouracil-induced increase could be prevented by interferon-γ.[271] A similar increase in thymidylate synthase has also been observed in vivo in murine tumours.[276],[277] This increase could be prevented by leucovorin or by the use of a high dose of 5-fluorouracil.[224] These mechanisms probably play a role in the observed enhancement of sensitivity to 5-fluorouracil and may reverse resistance to 5-fluorouracil.

Inhibition of thymidylate synthase in primary human colon tumours and in liver metastases is retained for at least 48 to 72 h after a bolus injection of 500 mg/m^2 of 5-fluorouracil;[266],[278] in 19 patients responding to hepatic artery infusion of 5-fluorouracil inhibition of thymidylate synthase was two- to threefold higher and enzyme levels were two- to threefold lower than in 21 patients not responding. In breast cancer patients binding of FdUMP and the effect of methylenetetrahydrofolate decreased during development of resistance.[279] These results demonstrate that the analysis of biochemical parameters in tumour biopsies obtained at both short and longer time periods after 5-fluorouracil administration gives valuable information about the in vivo mechanism of action of the drug in patients' tumours.

5-Fluorouracil incorporation into RNA

In most cells and tissues 5-fluorouracil will be incorporated into all classes of RNA, including ribosomal, transfer, and messenger RNA; however, in tumour cells incorporation takes place particularly into nuclear RNA.[280] In several model systems in vitro the amount of 5-fluorouracil in RNA was correlated with sensitivity to 5-fluorouracil;[281] in vivo the antitumour effect of 5-fluorouracil, together with the gastrointestinal cytotoxicity, was also related to the amount of 5-fluorouracil in RNA.[282],[283] Cytotoxicity due to incorporation of 5-fluorouracil into RNA is mainly determined by the incorporation of 5-fluorouracil into nuclear RNA.[284] At drug concentrations which do not impair transcription, methylation of 4S nuclear RNA appeared to be impaired;[284] this was possibly associated with an impaired processing of nuclear RNA to cytoplasmic RNA.[281],[285],[286] A major point of discussion is whether incorporation of 5-fluorouracil into RNA or inhibition of thymidylate synthase (see below) is the major factor responsible for antitumour activity. Since in vitro and in vivo incorporation of 5-fluorouracil into RNA is concentration and dose dependent respectively, it was postulated that incorporation of 5-fluorouracil into RNA is related to the antitumour effect since the antineoplastic activity is also dose dependent.[287] However, the extent and duration of in vivo thymidylate synthase inhibition is also dose dependent.[277] A higher dose of 5-fluorouracil (enabled by uridine protection) enhanced antitumour activity, and was associated with a longer duration of inhibition of thymidylate synthase than the lower dose, but without an increase in the incorporation of 5-fluorouracil into RNA.[224] Similar to these in vivo studies, in vitro studies also indicate that uridine does not influence incorporation of 5-fluorouracil into RNA, while withdrawal of 5-fluorouracil does not diminish incorporation of 5-fluorouracil into RNA.[288] Thus thymidylate synthase inhibition, and its downstream effects, seems to be the most important factor determining antineoplastic activity.

Similar findings have been obtained in samples from patients. In patients who received either 5-fluorouracil alone or 5-fluorouracil with leucovorin, the incorporation into RNA was similar but the inhibition of thymidylate synthase was significantly increased in the leucovorin group. Furthermore the incorporation of 5-fluorouracil in the RNA of patients with a partial or complete response was not significantly different from that in non-responders, but the extent of thymidylate synthase inhibition was.[278] There is, on the other hand, substantial evidence that the side-effects of 5-fluorouracil are related to its incorporation into RNA, since a decrease in the incorporation of 5-fluorouracil into RNA due to the presence of uridine was associated with a decrease in the extent of side-effects of 5-fluorouracil.[289],[290] In summary, information is accumulating that the antitumour activity of 5-fluorouracil is predominantly related to the inhibition of thymidylate synthase, rather than to its incorporation into RNA.

DNA directed effects of 5-fluorouracil

5-Fluorouracil can exert an effect on DNA either by its incorporation or by inducing a deoxynucleotide imbalance (decrease of dTTP and increase of dUTP, Fig. 6). Incorporation of 5-fluorouracil into DNA has long been considered to be a very unlikely event, and thus not to contribute to 5-fluorouracil cytotoxicity. FdUTP can be formed intracellularly but its concentration remains very low, since it is hydrolysed by dUTPase, while FdUTP incorporated into DNA may be removed by uracil-DNA glycosylase in a similar manner to the removal of uracil from DNA. Due to the inhibition of thymidylate synthase, the dTTP concentration is usually depleted while that of dUTP increases.[234],[288],[291] These conditions cause an imbalance in deoxyribonucleotides and may favour incorporation of both dUTP and FdUTP into DNA. The importance of dUTPase in the cytotoxicity of 5-fluorouracil has been demonstrated by comparison of cell lines with high and low levels of dUTPase and by transfection of the gene in cells with a low level of dUTPase. It was evident from these studies that a high level of expression of dUTPase can prevent cytotoxicity of 5-fluorouracil.[292],[293] Despite the action of dUTPase, 5-fluorouracil

can be incorporated into DNA and a relationship between incorporation of 5-fluorouracil and cytotoxicity has indeed been postulated.[294] It seems that both misincorporation of 5-fluorouracil into DNA and the excision of these residues can be responsible for cell death. 5-Fluorouracil can induce DNA strand breaks through its misincorporation, but also because of inefficient DNA repair (due to the lack of dTTP) of normally occurring defects in purine and pyrimidine residues.[295] More insight in the role of DNA damage caused by treatment with 5-fluorouracil was obtained by analysis of the effect of interferon-α on the formation of both single- and double-strand breaks.[296],[297] Interferon-α increased both types of strand breaks, a mechanism which was possibly responsible for the enhanced cytotoxic effect of that combination compared with 5-fluorouracil alone.

A major factor in the induction of DNA damage is the occurrence of an imbalance in the pool of deoxyribonucleotides; this seems to be a normal phenomenon and is probably related to cell death. This process has been investigated in more detail in cell systems deficient in thymidylate synthase. Thymidine depletion due to a deficiency of thymidylate synthase leads to a depletion of dTTP but an increase in dATP, resulting in G_1 S arrest.[298]–[300] Cells with a p53 wild-type phenotype died by apoptosis, while mutant p53 cells with relatively high Bax and Fas (Apo-1, CD95) expression went in cytostasis.[301] Since apoptosis could be induced by an anti-Fas antibody, colon cancer cells seem to have a functional Fas-mediated apoptosis pathway, which may be regulated by wild-type p53.[302] This indicates a regulating role for thymidylate synthase expression due to its (auto)-regulation by itself and p53. Altered regulation of essential cell-cycle checkpoints by, for example, the phosphorylation status of the retinoblastoma protein and its complex with E2F, may also play a role in this process.[162]

Predictive parameters for response to 5-fluorouracil treatment

Results of both in vitro and in vivo models and in patients indicate that the pretreatment level of several target enzymes involved in the metabolism of 5-fluorouracil might predict the response to 5-fluorouracil.[303],[304] The large variation in both the activity levels of thymidylate synthase enzyme and the expression of thymidylate synthase mRNA in human colorectal cancer observed in pre- and posttreatment samples supported this hypothesis.[266],[278],[305]–[307] In patients, treatment with 5-fluorouracil or its derivatives may induce thymidylate synthase levels due to enhanced thymidylate synthase translation, with no change in levels of thymidylate synthase mRNA.[266],[279],[308] Patients with colon cancer and a low expression of thymidylate synthase mRNA were more likely to respond to protracted 5-fluorouracil infusions or hepatic artery infusions with 5-fluorouracil or floxuridine, in a similar way to patients with stomach cancer.[306],[309]–[311] Intensive immunohistochemical staining for thymidylate synthase was associated with a shorter survival in patients with rectal cancer, head and neck cancer, and breast cancer treated with (neo)adjuvant chemotherapy.[312]–[314] For patients with metastatic colon cancer, no relation between response and intensity of thymidylate synthase staining was observed, possibly because the patients were being treated for advanced disease but thymidylate synthase expression was measured in primary tumours.[315] These studies indicate that pretreatment measurement of thymidylate synthase levels may predict whether patients are more likely to respond to fluoropyrimidine-containing treatment regimens.

In addition to thymidylate synthase levels there is accumulating evidence that tumoural dihydropyrimidine dehydrogenase levels can also predict response to 5-fluorouracil. A high level of dihydropyrimidine dehydrogenase (both enzyme and mRNA) in human tumour xenografts was found to be significantly correlated with a low sensitivity to 5-fluorouracil treatment.[316] A relationship has been shown between dihydropyrimidine dehydrogenase activity and 5-fluorouracil sensitivity in a panel of 19 cell lines of various tumours and in tumour samples from patients with head and neck cancer.[317],[318] The combination of both dihydropyrimidine dehydrogenase and thymidylate synthase expression was shown by Danenberg et al. to be a strong predictive parameter for response to 5-fluorouracil treatment, but Etienne et al. found no relationship between this combination and outcome of treatment (5-fluorouracil with cisplatin) in patients with head and neck cancer.[319],[320] The combination of mutant p53 and high thymidylate synthase levels was shown to be a poor prognostic parameter in colon cancer and a low expression of both the excision repair crosscomplementing and thymidylate synthase gene was associated with poor response to a cisplatin–5-fluorouracil combination regimen in gastric cancer.[321]–[323]

Clinical pharmacology of 5-fluorouracil

Analysis and elimination

For the last decades the most widely used method of measuring plasma 5-fluorouracil has been high-performance liquid chromatography with UV absorption as the detection method.[173] Currently concentrations of 5-fluorouracil down to 0.1 μM can be measured.[173],[324]–[326] A lower detection limit for 5-fluorouracil (3 nM) can be achieved with derivatization followed by gas chromatography mass spectrometry.[237],[327],[328] Most pharmacokinetic studies have been terminated within 3 h, when the plasma concentration falls below the detection limit of high-performance liquid chromatography. With gas chromatography mass spectrometry plasma concentrations can be followed for at least 24 h after injection.

The pharmacokinetics of single-dose 5-fluorouracil administered as an intravenous bolus injection in doses varying between 300 and 600 mg/m^2 has been studied most extensively and are summarized in Table 5.[153],[220],[329],[330] Peak levels of 5-fluorouracil can reach the millimolar range, with a subsequent rapid decline. 5-Fluorouracil is rapidly distributed over all tissues. The total clearance is rather high (Table 7), comparable with the flow through the liver, but hepatic extraction has been estimated at 50 per cent.[331] The kidneys contribute to elimination both by degradation and active renal secretion, with about 20 per cent of 5-fluorouracil being excreted as the parent drug.[324] In addition the lungs may also contribute significantly to clearance of 5-fluorouracil.[324],[329] Collins et al. have shown that a saturable two-compartment model can be used to describe the disappearance kinetics of 5-fluorouracil for the first hour.[332] However, in a third compartment plasma levels fluctuated from 3 nM to 0.1 μM between 4 and at least 24 h.[327] It is most likely that this 5-fluorouracil represents efflux from the tissues; 5-fluorouracil tumour levels vary from 2 to 10 μM between 2 and 48 h after administration of a 500 mg/m$^{(2)}$ bolus injection of 5-fluorouracil, while 5-fluorouracil is retained for a long period in RNA which may form a depot for 5-fluorouracil.[237],[277],[278] Wolf et al. demonstrated with ^{19}F nuclear magnetic

Table 7 Pharmacokinetic parameters of 5-fluorouracil

Bolus injection at 400–900 mg/m^2	
Half-life β	9–20 min
Half-life γ	2–7 h
Volume of distribution	14–54 litres
Clearance from plasma	50–140 litres/h
Peak levels	1 mM
Continuous infusion	
Steady state levels	1–71 μM
Clearance from plasma	54–420 litres/h
Oral adminnistration	
Steady state levels	0.5–10 μM
Half-life β (dependent on DPD inhibitor)	2–4 h

DPD = dihydropyrimidine dehydrogenase.

resonance that the half-life in tumours (0.5–2.1 h) was considerably longer than that in plasma (9–20 min).[245] The background for this difference has not yet been identified, although it has been demonstrated that a decrease in the intratumoural pH can increase the elimination half-life of 5-fluorouracil in the tissue.[333] Mainly for practical reasons, 5-fluorouracil is increasingly being given as a short-term infusion over 10 to 30 min instead of a bolus over 2 to 4 min. This may result in lower peak levels of 5-fluorouracil and may even decrease the response rates to the treatment.[334],[335] 5-Fluorouracil push injection appears to be a more efficient administration technique.

Non-linearity of 5-fluorouracil kinetics is related to the saturation of 5-fluorouracil catabolism.[324],[327],[329],[331],[336] Peak plasma levels of the first catabolite, 5-fluorodihydrouracil, were found to be between 20 and 40 μM with a terminal half-life of 40 to 60 min.[336],[337] Using ^{19}F nuclear magnetic resonance the other catabolites have been demonstrated in human plasma.[338] Cumulative urinary excretion of the catabolites showed that fluoro-β-alanine was the major catabolite followed by fluoroureidopropionate, while 5-fluorodihydrouracil excretion was minimal. Sweeny et al. and Malet-Martino et al. observed that one of the major breakdown products of 5-fluorouracil was a bile acid conjugate of fluoro-β-alanine.[240],[338] This conjugate may contribute to liver toxicity after intrahepatic treatment of liver metastasis with fluoropyrimidines.[242]

Comparison of schedules

Continuous intravenous administration of 5-fluorouracil has been investigated in various schedules; the length and frequency of which give rise to large differences in the maximum tolerable dose and toxicity. Generally mucositis is dose limiting for infusions, with bolus injections mainly causing myelosuppression;[329] the hand–foot syndrome occurs rather frequently with continuous infusion.[339]–[341] For continuous 5-fluorouracil infusion a much larger clearance value (2–6 litres/min) than for intravenous bolus administration has been observed.[332] The high pulmonary extraction may account for this elimination, but the liver and kidney also contribute to clearance.[324],[329],[332] For colorectal cancer Lokich et al. demonstrated a higher response rate for continuous infusion (30 per cent) versus weekly bolus injection (7 per cent);[342] however, overall survival was comparable. In a meta-analysis with data from 1219 patients from six randomized studies the response rate for continuous infusions

Table 8 Results of meta-analyses and randomized studies in colorectal cancer using several 5-fluorouracil schedules (modified from Peters and Köhne[224])

Schedule	No of trials	No of patients	Response (CR/PR)	p-value	Median survival (months)	p-value	Reference
5-FU alone versus 5-FU/LV	9	1381	11% versus 23%	<0.001	11.0 versus 11.5	0.57	Meta-analysis 1992[594]
Systemic 5-FU or FUDR versus HAI FUDR	5	391	14% versus 41%	<0.001	12.2 versus 16.0	0.14	Meta-analysis 1996[663]
5-FU bolus versus 5-FU CI	6	1219	14% versus 22%	<0.001	11.3 versus 12.1%	0.04	Meta-analysis 1998[340],[341]
5-FU$_{24h}$ + LV†		91	44%		16.2		Köhne et al.[606]†
5-FU$_{24h}$ + IFN‡		90	18%	<0.05	12.7	<0.04	Köhne et al.[606]
5-FU$_{24h}$ + IFN + LV§		49	27%		19.6		

†5-FU$_{24h}$: 2600 mg/m^2 + LV 500 mg/m^2 2 h, weekly × 6.

‡5-FU$_{24h}$: 2600 mg/m^2 + IFN 3 MU s.c. three times per week, weekly × 6.

§5FU$_{24h}$: 2600 mg/m^2 + LV + IFN, weekly × 6.

5-FU = 5-fluorouracil; LV = leucovorin; FUDR = Floxuridine; CI = continuous infusion; IFN = interferon-α; HAI = hepatic arterial infusion; CR = complete response; PR = partial response; s.c. = subcutaneously; MU = million units.

was 22 per cent compared with 14 per cent for various 5-fluorouracil bolus schedules without leucovorin ($p = 0.0002$) with a slightly increased survival (Table 8).[340],[341]

An interesting circadian pattern in the plasma concentration of 5-fluorouracil has been observed during protracted continuous 5-fluorouracil infusion, with the peak in the 5-fluorouracil concentration at 11 a.m. and the trough at 11 p.m.[343],[344] The value of the peak/trough ratio was about 5. A circadian pattern was also observed in mice.[345] The concentrations of 5-fluorouracil were the inverse of the circadian pattern of the catabolic enzyme dihydrouracil dehydrogenase. Circadian rhythms of metabolism have been described in mice.[346],[347] However, recent data indicate that under less controlled conditions (i.e. in the majority of cancer patients) the circadian pattern of dihydropyrimidine dehydrogenase is less consistent, although a circadian pattern of 5-fluorouracil plasma concentration is still present.[348],[349] These data suggest that continuous infusion of 5-fluorouracil should not be given at a constant rate, but according to a circadian pattern, using programmable pumps in order to minimize host toxicity.[350] Programmed 5-fluorouracil and leucovorin administration with the peak at 4 a.m., combined with oxaliplatin (peak in the afternoon) showed a clear advantage compared with flat administration, with responses rates of 51 per cent compared with 29 per cent.[351] Currently more randomized studies are ongoing in order to demonstrate whether this difference is due to the circadian administration.

A large variability in bioavailability for orally administered 5-fluorouracil, between 28 and 100 per cent, has been observed; this may be related to a saturable hepatic catabolism but also to an additional first-pass effect.[324],[329],[332] Because of these variabilities, 5-fluorouracil alone should not be given via the oral route. However, in the last decade the development of orally administered drugs, including 5-fluorouracil (pro)drugs has progressed rapidly. Currently various forms of oral formulation are being evaluated in the clinic;

these formulations are either based on a combination of 5-fluorouracil (or prodrug) with a dihydropyrimidine dehydrogenase inhibitor, or on a prodrug selectively activated in the tumour. Plasma concentrations of these formulations are generally comparable with that for continuous infusions and vary depending on the drug combination and the frequency with which the drug is given.[352]–[355] The formulations with a dihydropyrimidine dehydrogenase inhibitor include uracil with Ftorafur, S-1 (Ftorafur with 5-chloro-2,4-dihydropyridine and oxonic acid), and 5-fluorouracil with ethynyluracil.[19],[352],[355] Capecitabine is a prodrug of Doxifluridine which is activated by thymidine phosphorylase which has a higher activity in tumour tissues.[222],[356]–[358] In contrast to the former group, capecitabine causes the hand–foot syndrome, typical for continuous infusions. Since plasma levels are in the same range, this indicates that degradation products of 5-fluorouracil (absent in the combinations with dihydropyrimidine dehydrogenase inhibitors) may be responsible for this specific type of toxicity.

5-Fluorouracil is also being given intrahepatically by portal or arterial infusions for the treatment of liver metastases. Hepatic extraction and the rate of infusion determine the systemic availability. Rapid intrahepatic arterial infusions at a high dose (1000 mg/m^2/day) result in relatively low hepatic extractions of 20 to 60 per cent and a high systemic availability.[331] At a slow infusion rate and/or lower doses (780 mg/m^2/day) hepatic extraction was greater than 90 per cent with a low systemic toxicity.[324] Kemeny performed several studies on floxuridine in combination with several agents, all consistently showing an improved response rate and survival for the hepatic artery infusion arm.[359] Although floxuridine has a pharmacokinetic advantage (better extraction) over 5-fluorouracil, response rates for administration of 5-fluorouracil or floxuridine as single agents are comparable (around 40 per cent).[360] A meta-analysis of seven randomized studies comparing hepatic artery infusion with floxuridine with intravenous therapy with floxuridine or 5-fluorouracil demonstrated a better response rate (41 per cent compared with 14 per cent respectively) and a survival advantage.[340],[341] Hepatic artery infusion is advised for patients with liver metastases.

Intraperitoneal infusions offer the possibility of achieving higher drug concentrations and of maximizing exposure of tumours within the abdominal cavity, leading to effective treatment of not only the liver metastases (via the portal vein) but also of peritoneal metastases. Intraperitoneal 5-fluorouracil can be administered via peritoneal dialysis or by using implantable devices. Hepatic extraction was calculated to be 67 per cent, while a 2- to 3-log difference was observed between peritoneal and plasma 5-fluorouracil concentrations.[361] With a constant infusion the mean steady state level of 5-fluorouracil in the intraperitoneal cavity was 622 μM.[362] Total body clearance ranged from 0.9 to 16.5 litres/min, similar to continuous intravenous systemic infusions of 5-fluorouracil. Clearance decreased with increasing 5-fluorouracil concentration which is consistent with saturable or non-linear 5-fluorouracil pharmacokinetics. At present intraperitoneal infusions are not often used for administration of 5-fluorouracil.

Evidence is accumulating that there is a relationship between 5-fluorouracil pharmacokinetics and toxicity and/or response. In an intrapatient dose-escalation study Van Groeningen et al. determined the pharmacokinetics of 5-fluorouracil and related this to clinical toxicity using a logistic regression model.[327] At an area under the plasma versus time curve of more than 18 mg/h/litre the risk of toxicity was about 50 per cent. In a retrospective study Santini et al. concluded that the area under the curve from days 0 to 3 of a 5-day continuous infusion was predictive for toxicity.[363] In a subsequent prospective study this information was used to adapt dosage in the second half of the cycle. A relationship between the area under the curve and the response rate was postulated. The latter may, however, also be a relationship between dose intensity and response. Such a correlation has been demonstrated previously.[287] Trump et al. established a relationship between the 5-fluorouracil dose, the steady state plasma concentration, and the percentage of reduction in white blood cells, as well as the frequency of stomatitis.[364] In this study 5-fluorouracil was given to 47 patients as a 3-day continuous infusion in a dose range from 185 to 3600 mg/m^2/day in combination with dipyridamole at 7.7 mg/kg/day. Also, for oral formulations, a relation was found between 5-fluorouracil plasma levels and gastric intestinal toxicity.[352]

Two major approaches have been taken to individualize 5-fluorouracil-based therapy in patients. In the first the dose of 5-fluorouracil is adapted following measurement of 5-fluorouracil at the first administration in order to reach a target concentration. In a prospective study patients with head and neck cancer were randomized to receive a standard 96 h infusion (4 g/m^2) with cisplatin, or a 5-fluorouracil dose adjusted according to the 5-fluorouracil concentration under the curve.[365] In the latter arm the 5-fluorouracil dose was significantly reduced in subsequent cycles. Both haematological (neutropenia and thrombopenia) and non-haematological (mucositis) side-effects were significantly more frequent in the standard dose arm; response rates were comparable. This study shows the value of individual adaptation of the 5-fluorouracil dose based on pharmacokinetics. A second approach includes the measurement of dihydropyrimidine dehydrogenase activity in white blood cells before treatment in order to identify those patients (1 to 3 per cent) at risk of developing more or less serious toxicity.[250] Katona et al. observed that patients with high dihydropyrimidine dehydrogenase activity were at a lower risk of developing toxicity than those with low dihydropyrimidine dehydrogenase activity;[366] in this latter group a reduction in the 5-fluorouracil dose was necessary. The first approach may actually also identify patients with potentially low dihydropyrimidine dehydrogenase activity, since plasma levels are likely to be increased substantially in this group of patients.

Other fluoropyrimidines

A number of analogues have been developed since the initial synthesis of 5-fluorouracil; some of them replaced 5-fluorouracil in general clinical practice, especially when given orally in a combination. Floxuridine was one of the first analogues; however, the drug was too toxic for systemic administration but was very suitable for intra-arterial administration for the treatment of liver metastasis.[367] More than 90 per cent of floxuridine is removed in its first pass through the liver, thus preventing systemic toxicity.[331] The drug can, however, also be administered as a bolus injection. In an animal model system it was shown that bolus injection was more effective than continuous infusion.[277],[368] In this schedule floxuridine partly acts as a prodrug for 5-fluorouracil; resulting in a more prolonged inhibition of thymidylate synthase than 5-fluorouracil alone.

Another analogue is 5'-deoxy-5-fluorouridine (doxifluridine), which cannot be phosphorylated directly, but has to be phosphorylysed to 5-fluorouracil.[369] It has been demonstrated that pyrimidine nucleoside phosphorylases (thymidine and/or uridine phosphorylase) have to be present in the tumour and it was considered that the drug would be more selective for tumours with a high thymidine phosphorylase activity. It has, however, been demonstrated that other factors in the activation of the compound may also determine its antitumour effect.[370] The drug has a comparable or nearly comparable antitumour effect to 5-fluorouracil itself in advanced colorectal cancer, but its clinical use has been hampered by its neuro- and cardiotoxicity.[371] Several trials with oral doxifluridine have been initiated and indicate that the drug may have clinical use when given orally.

In the last decade several prodrugs of doxifluridine have been developed and one of these, capecitabine (Fig. 5) has been evaluated extensively in the clinic.[356] Capecitabine can also be administered orally, but requires several sequential activation steps: removal of the carbamate group by carboxyl esterase, followed by deamination by cytidine deaminase to doxifluridine and subsequent phosphorylysis to 5-fluorouracil. In several human cancer xenograft models Capecitabine was more active than 5-fluorouracil or uracil with Ftorafur, and was also more active in several 5-fluorouracil-resistant models. In clinical trials capecitabine has shown a response rate of 21 to 24 per cent in metastatic colorectal cancer and 20 per cent in heavily pretreated paclitaxel-resistant breast cancer patients.[372],[373] Pharmacokinetic studies showed that capecitabine is rapidly and extensively absorbed (81 per cent) with a T_{max} of less than 1 h after fasting and 1 to 2 h after food intake.[353],[374] It is rapidly metabolized via 5'-deoxyfluorocytidine and doxifluridine to 5-fluorouracil. In tumour samples taken from patients treated with capecitabine, tumour tissue concentrations were 2.5-fold higher than in normal tissues. Considering the interesting profile of combinations (additive to synergistic with 10 to 12 other anticancer agents) and the increased thymidine phosphorylase (TP) activity in tumours the drug is certainly of interest for various types of malignancies.

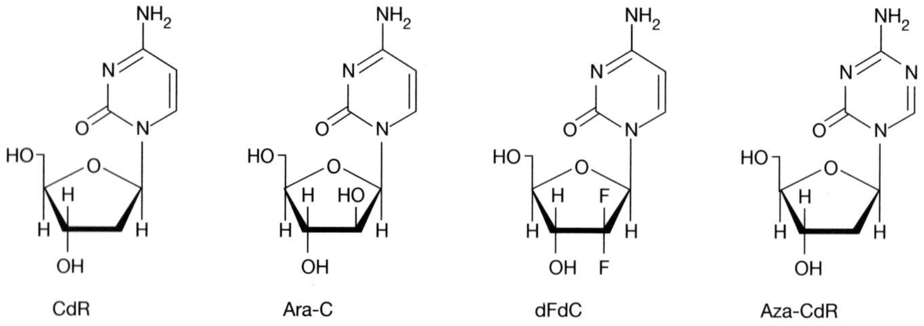

CdR   Ara-C   dFdC   Aza-CdR

Fig. 7 Structural formulae of ara-C, dFdC and 2′-deoxy-azacytidine (aza-CdR) compared with deoxycytidine (CdR).

Ftorafur (1,2-tetrahydrofuranyl-5-fluorouracil) acts as a depot form for 5-fluorouracil and produces little myelosuppression, but significant gastrointestinal toxicity and neurotoxicity. The drug is well absorbed orally in contrast to 5-fluorouracil itself. Conversion to 5-fluorouracil may occur predominantly in tumour cells and the liver and is predominantly catalysed by cytochrome P450 2A6, although a role for thymidine phosphorylase has also been postulated.[324] Ftorafur is not given as a single agent but only in biochemical modulation regimens, which enable oral formulation forms, such as uracil with Ftorafur and S-1 (Ftorafur with 5-chloro-2,4-dihydropyridine and oxonic acid).

Cytidine analogues

Several cytidine and deoxycytidine analogues have been synthesized in the past and tested for their potential clinical use. The most successful agent is ara-C which is used as first-line treatment in acute myeloblastic leukaemia and (non)-Hodgkin's lymphoma.[375]–[379] Ara-C differs from deoxycytidine by a modification in the 2′ position of the sugar moiety (Fig. 7). Other cytidine analogues differ by substitutions in either the base-part of the molecule or the sugar moiety. Since leukaemic cells can be obtained relatively easily, several *in vivo* pharmacological studies have been conducted with these cells in relation to the antileukaemic effect, but studies with solid tumours are limited.[376]–[378]

Mechanism of action and resistance

As an analogue of deoxycytidine, ara-C shares the same metabolic pathways with this nucleoside. In order to be activated, ara-C has to be transported into the cell. Membrane transport of ara-C is mediated by facilitated diffusion via a family of transport carrier systems for nucleosides.[380]–[382] The human equilibrative nucleoside transporter (hENT1; previously termed *es*) is responsible for 80 per cent of ara-C influx in human leukaemic blast cells. Since the rate of membrane transport of most nucleosides is usually high compared with subsequent phosphorylation, this step is considered not to be limiting for the activity of ara-C. However, in the situation where plasma levels of ara-C are low (at a 'standard dose' of ara-C about 0.5 μM) the drug has to compete with other nucleosides for the transport carrier, and influx of ara-C may then be low. A correlation has been observed between the rate of ara-C influx and the clinical response

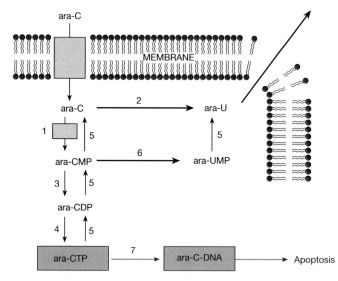

Fig. 8 Schematic presentation of metabolic pathways of ara-C, including possible resistance factors. The enzymes catalysing these reactions are: 1, deoxycytidine kinase; 2, deoxycytidine deaminase; 3, nucleoside monophosphate kinase; 4, nucleoside diphosphate kinase; 5, 5′-nucleotidases and phosphatases; 6, dCMP deaminase; 7, DNA polymerase. The hatched bars represent an impaired transport across the cellular membrane and a deficiency of deoxycytidine kinase. The fat arrows denote an increased deamination. The boxes (ara-CTP and ara-C-DNA) indicate that a low accumulation and incorporation into DNA can limit the action of ara-C.

to ara-C/daunomycin therapy.[383] Impaired transport may be overcome by the use of high-dose ara-C where high plasma levels (10–200 μM) can be achieved. At these concentrations passive diffusion is more important.[375],[384],[385] In addition, efflux of ara-C may limit its cytotoxic effect, and a useful approach to increasing the retention of ara-C within the cell, thus enhancing its cytotoxic effects, may be to combine it with a nucleoside transport inhibitor.[386]

For biochemical activation ara-C is dependent on phosphorylation catalysed by deoxycytidine kinase and subsequently by nucleotide kinases (Fig. 8). It has been demonstrated that ara-C is not active in deoxycytidine kinase-deficient cell lines (Table 9).[387]–[389] The triphosphate **ara-CTP** is the active metabolite of ara-C. The K_m of ara-CTP and dCTP for DNA polymerase are in the same range and so ara-CTP can act as a weak competitive inhibitor of DNA

Table 9 Factors related to resistance to ara-C

Transport, either influx or efflux
Decreased activation due to a deficiency of deoxycytidine kinase
Increased inactivation:
    enhanced deamination of ara-C to ara-U
    enhanced deamination of ara-CMP to ara-UMP
    enhanced degradation of ara-CTP
Increased dCTP pools which:
    compete with the ara-CTP for incorporation into DNA
    inhibit deoxycytidine kinase catalysed phosphorylation of ara-C
Increase in CTP synthetase yielding more CTP and subsequently dCTP
Altered DNA polymerase
Increase of DNA repair
In leukaemia protection by increased bcl-2 levels

polymerase.[377],[390] Ara-C is also incorporated into DNA, in which the drug behaves as a relative chain terminator.[391] Both replication and DNA repair are inhibited. The major effect of cytarabine is probably inhibition of the elongation of DNA.[392]

There is increasing evidence that cytarabine can induce apoptosis. Inhibition of colony formation by cytarabine could be enhanced by a combination with both granulocyte/monocyte colony stimulating factor and interleukin 3, which was associated with an increase in the degree of apoptosis, and correlated with the enhanced expression of the *c-jun* transcriptional activator.[393],[394] This effect is mediated by the interaction of an activated *c-jun* protein with its own promotor.[395] In the National Cancer Institute's *in vitro* screening panel an increased sensitivity to ara-C was observed in cells with an activated *ras* oncogene compared with cells with wild-type *ras* alleles; induction of apoptotic cell death was efficient in cells with activated *ras* oncogenes.[396] There is accumulating evidence that an increased expression of *bcl-2* protein in myeloid leukaemia is associated with a decrease in therapy-induced apoptosis, reduced patient survival, and *in vitro* autonomous growth of leukaemic cells.[397],[398] In *bcl-2* transfected cells a decreased sensitivity to ara-C and a lower percentage of apoptosis was observed. Ara-C treatment did not change *bcl-2* levels, and the accumulation of ara-CTP and its incorporation into DNA were not changed.[398] This indicates that high intracellular levels of *bcl-2* operate distally to inhibit the final apoptotic pathway. Various kinases may be involved in this process; Chelliah *et al.* observed an increase in ara-C-induced apoptosis by the protein kinase C activator bryostatin in human leukaemia HL-60 cells.[399] In contrast, dysregulation of the cyclin-dependent kinase inhibitor p21 increased susceptibility of U937 cells to ara-C-induced apoptosis associated with mitochondrial perturbations implicated in the activation of the apoptotic protease cascade, such as caspase-3 activation.[400] It is therefore clear that not only factors involved in drug activation and degradation, but also several factors in the apoptotic pathway determine sensitivity to cytarabine.

Accumulation and retention of ara-CTP and its incorporation into DNA have been shown by several authors to be the main factors determining the cytotoxic effect.[376],[377],[388],[390],[401]–[404] *In vitro* studies have clearly shown that an initially high accumulation of ara-CTP, a long retention, and a high incorporation into DNA determine the sensitivity of cells in culture. In addition Rustum *et al.* have shown a relationship between an initially high accumulation of ara-CTP and

long retention in leukaemic lymphoblasts and the response rate and duration of response.[403],[405] Plasma ara-C levels and ara-CTP formation are not related, which implies that there is great variability in the levels of activating enzymes.[406],[407] In addition it has been observed that in several patients ara-CTP formation continued after the end of the infusion and declined thereafter with a half-life of 3 to 4 h.[406],[407] The retention of ara-CTP appears to be a critical factor in the response of patients to ara-C treatment. Preisler *et al.* showed a correlation between ara-CTP retention and the duration of complete remission in acute myelogenous leukaemia.[408] One of the reasons for giving high-dose ara-C treatment is to enhance ara-CTP formation; however, Plunkett *et al.* showed that ara-CTP formation in leukaemic blasts during ara-C treatment is saturated at plasma levels reached at a dose of 0.5 to 1 g/m², which is considerably lower than a standard high dose of 3 g/m² ara-C (see the section on clinical pharmacology).[409]

Cells are maximally sensitive during the S phase, in which DNA synthesis is active. Ara-C is, however, also active in other phases of the cell cycle. Thus generally ara-C can be considered as an S-phase-specific drug and in model systems 60 per cent of cells can accumulate in the S phase.[410],[411] The number of cells eliminated by ara-C will therefore depend upon cell kinetic properties. A blockade has been noted in the progression of S-phase cells into the G_2 phase, but a progression delay at the G_1–S boundary has also been noted. The difference may depend on the concentration of ara-C and the exposure time. In patients treated with ara-C, evidence has also been obtained that cells are arrested in the S phase.[412]

Role of drug degradation

In addition to its metabolic activation ara-C can also be inactivated by deamination. Ara-C itself can be deaminated by (deoxy)cytidine deaminase, while the monophosphate ara-CMP is a substrate for dCMP deaminase. Ara-CTP can be degraded by direct dephosphorylation. It is clear that degradation can determine the cytotoxic action of ara-C. For ara-C, and other cytidine analogues, it has been demonstrated that degradation of the drug by deamination may decrease its antitumour activity.[401],[413],[414] Forced expression of deoxycytidine deaminase by transfection of the gene will result in resistance to cytarabine and other deoxycytidine analogues.[415]–[417] The deaminated product is not cytotoxic. It was postulated that in leukaemic cells the ratio between the deaminase and the kinase determines the response to ara-C.[413],[414] It was shown that in responding patients the deaminase/kinase ratio was low, while in non-responders it was high. Jahnsstreubel *et al.* demonstrated that responding patients had a lower median deaminase activity than non-responding patients.[418] There was, however, a large variation in enzyme activities. In addition, not only deamination of the drug itself but also that of ara-CMP by dCMP deaminase may limit the activity of ara-C.[401]

For ara-C it has been demonstrated that ara-U (1-β-D-arabino-furanosyl-uracil) can have pronounced effects on the metabolism and cytotoxicity of ara-C.[419] Preincubation of cells with the deaminated product ara-U enhanced the cytotoxicity of ara-C by increased phosphorylation to ara-CTP and incorporation into DNA. Furthermore the synthesis of CDP-choline was enhanced. Sasvari-Szekely *et al.* postulated that formation of CDP-choline and subsequent synthesis of phospholipids may be affected by ara-C treatment.[4]

Clinical pharmacology of Ara-C

Measurement of ara-C is done by either a simple, rapid, and specific immunoassay or by high-performance liquid chromatography which has the advantage of determining both ara-C and its deaminated product ara-U.[420],[421]

Ara-C is not administered orally because of the presence of cytidine deaminase in the liver and the high first-pass elimination in the liver. Ara-C has been given intravenously over a wide range of doses.[153],[375],[376] The standard or conventional dose varies from 100 to 200 mg/m^2 daily and is given by intermittent injection or by continuous infusion over 5 to 10 days. The steady state plasma concentration is generally in the range of 0.1 to 0.5 μM and the clearance is about 134 litres/m^2.[422] Males have a significantly faster clearance than females. Clearance was correlated with the pretreatment white blood cell blast count.[422]

In the high-dose protocols the drug is administered at 2 to 3 g/m^2 every 12 h times 12, resulting in peak concentrations in the range of 100 μM ara-C, which fall rapidly with a half-life α of 7 to 20 min and a half-life β of 0.5 to 2 h. Ara-U is rapidly formed from ara-C, and peak levels are found within 15 min of ara-C administration and are about 100 μM. The half-life of ara-U is much longer than that of ara-C, being of the order of 0.5 to 6 h. The parent drug is rapidly distributed into total body water, while levels in the cerebrospinal fluid reach about 50 per cent of that in plasma. About 70 per cent of the ara-C is excreted in the urine in the form of ara-U. In children the rate of conversion of ara-C to ara-U increases with age.[423] High-dose ara-C, compared with standard doses, appears to give comparable or greater efficacy in induction of remission in acute myelogenous leukaemia, but some individuals are resistant to conventional dosing and may obtain a remission with higher doses.[375],[385] In other leukaemic diseases favourable results have been found with high-dose ara-C. Since high-dose ara-C treatment leads to high drug levels in the cerebrospinal fluid, this regimen may provide an adequate prophylaxis for treatment of central nervous system leukaemia.

In summary, high-dose ara-C can overcome impaired transport and may enhance intracellular ara-CTP pools, although this may be disputable and cells at the boundary of G$_1$–S may be more sensitive to high-dose ara-C.

The toxicity of standard dose ara-C is expressed as nausea, vomiting, hair loss, and pancytopenia. In several patients, the so-called 'ara-C syndrome' is observed, consisting of fever, myalgia, joint and bone pain, chest pain, a maculopapular rash, and kerato-conjunctivitis.[385] Occasionally, standard-dose ara-C causes 'ara-C lung', acute pancreatitis, and peritonitis. With high-dose ara-C the incidence of these toxicities increases, as has for instance clearly been shown for the severity of skin signs, gastrointestinal toxicity, and ocular signs.[424] Eye toxicity may be related to inhibition of DNA synthesis. The use of deoxycytidine drops might be a rational way to prevent this side-effect.[385] Dose-limiting toxicity of high-dose ara-C consists of central nervous system dysfunction (especially cerebellar). Pericarditis and peripheral neuropathies have also been reported with high-dose ara-C. The pathogenesis of the pulmonary side-effects is not clear, although some evidence has been presented that the incidence and severity are more pronounced with high-dose ara-C. An 'ara-C lung' is characterized by (sub)acute respiratory failure accompanied by diffuse changes on chest radiographs and the diagnosis is usually made when other explanations (such as infection) can be excluded.

There is some interest in very low-dose ara-C (20 mg/m^2/day).[425],[426] Very low steady state plasma levels were observed, below the level (100 nM ara-C) assumed to be required for cytotoxicity. It has been postulated that ara-C may act as a differentiation-inducing agent at these low doses.[427]

Cytarabine analogues

Several analogues or depot forms of ara-C have been synthesized, in order to prevent catabolism of ara-C. Ara-C has been enclosed in liposomes and several conjugates (N^4-acyl-analogues, ara-C esters, cyclocytidine) have been synthesized.[428] All these compounds have the same mechanism of action as ara-C since they have to be converted to ara-CTP. Promising preclinical results have been obtained, with a better therapeutic index then ara-C. The application of an ara-C prodrug may enable the administration of these drugs as an oral formulation, while the nature of several of these compounds will result in a longer retention of ara-C in body fluids. An example is ara-CMP stearate.[429] Other prodrugs of ara-C contain lipophilic sidechains in either the base or in the sugar.[430]–[432] Such molecules can enter cells by a transporter-independent mechanism and possibly act as a depot form intracellularly, as evidenced by a twofold increase in the half-life of ara-CTP.[430],[433] Such properties might make these analogues suitable for the treatment of solid tumours, but the compounds still require further clinical investigation.

5-Aza-2′-deoxycytidine

5-Aza-2′-deoxycytidine (aza-CdR) is a cytidine analogue (Fig. 7) with a different mechanism of action which has undergone extensive clinical evaluation. Both 5-azacytidine (aza-CR) and aza-CdR have significant activity in leukaemia, but aza-CdR has shown more toxicity.[434],[435] Aza-CdR is active in experimental leukaemia and human acute myelogenous leukaemia.[436],[437] Aza-CR is activated by uridine-cytidine kinase to the monophosphate aza-CMP and subsequently to the triphosphate aza-CTP, which can be incorporated into RNA and can cause defective protein synthesis and polyribosomal degradation. Aza-CTP can also be incorporated into DNA, thus causing inhibition of DNA methylation which may explain its ability to induce differentiation of both normal and malignant cells. Resistance in murine leukaemic cells develops through deficiency of uridine-cytidine kinase. Aza-CdR is activated by deoxycytidine kinase to aza-dCMP, which is converted to aza-dCTP and incorporated into DNA. Similar to aza-CR it can inhibit DNA methylation and induce differentiation.[438] Aza-CdR causes dramatic effects on chromosomes, such as decondensation of chromatin structure, chromosome instability, and advance in replication timing.[439]

Both aza-CR and aza-CdR are removed rapidly from the plasma by metabolic clearance (deamination to the uridine derivative) and chemical decomposition by ring cleavage. The latter effect may contribute to the lethal effects of both compounds after incorporation into macromolecules. The most interesting clinical activity of the drug has been observed in chronic lymphatic leukaemia.

2′2′-Difluoro-2′-deoxycytidine (gemcitabine)

Mechanism of action

Gemcitabine (Fig. 7) is a deoxycytidine analogue with pronounced activity against several solid tumours, including non-small cell lung cancer, pancreatic cancer, ovarian cancer, and bladder cancer. This is

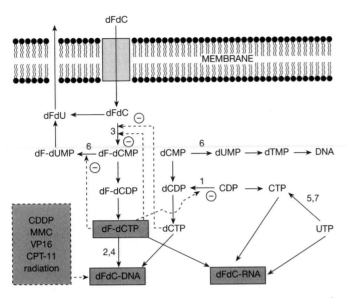

Fig. 9 Metabolism of gemcitabine (dFdC) and targets for combinations with other drugs and radiation: 1, ribonucleotide reductase; 2, repair of DNA damage; 3, decreased feedback inhbition of dCK by dCTP which will selfpotentiate metabolism of dFdC; 4, dFdCTP incorporation into DNA; 5, inhibition of CTP synthetase; 6, inhibition of dCMP deaminase by dFdCTP, which will selfpotentiate, but also decrease dUMP levels, enhancing inhibition of thymidylate syntase by FdUMP; 7, normal nucleotides will be in imbalance, similar to deoxynucleotides. Abbreviations: CDDP = cisplatin; MMC = mitomycin-C; VP16 = etoposide; CPT-11 = irinotecan.

modes of action of gemcitabine. Ribonucleotide reductase can be inhibited by the diphosphate, gemcitabine-DP, which not only prevents reduction of CDP to dCDP but also that of ADP to dADP, resulting in a depletion of dCTP and dATP.[458]-[460] Since dCTP is a feedback regulator of deoxycytidine kinase, its depletion will enhance gemcitabine activation, while the depletion of dATP will inhibit DNA repair. Another effect of gemcitabine is the gemcitabine-TP-mediated inhibition of dCMP deaminase, which is even enhanced because of the decreased concentration of dCTP, an allosteric activator of this enzyme.[444],[461] Finally, gemcitabine-TP is an inhibitor of CTP synthetase, which will lead to an increase in the concentration of the substrate UTP and a depletion of CTP, potentiating the incorporation of gemcitabine-TP into RNA and DNA.[462],[463] In addition to these effects gemcitabine treatment of cells increases the concentration of ATP.[449],[463] Collectively, the various effects of gemcitabine result in a unique pattern of selfpotentiation.

Gemcitabine shows a heterogenous effect on the cell cycle which seems to be dependent on the cell type. In leukaemic cells gemcitabine causes an accumulation in early S phase, but in human HL-60 leukaemic cells gemcitabine decreased the S-phase fraction from 38 to 24 per cent with an accumulation of cells in the G_1/G_0 phase from 31 to 74 per cent.[440],[453] In several solid tumour cell lines the effects were variable, with a transient accumulation in early S phase in colon and pancreatic cancer cells.[459],[460] In prostate and non-small cell lung cancer cells a decrease in S-phase cells was observed.[456],[457] Under all conditions gemcitabine induced apoptosis not only in leukaemic cells but also in cells from various histological subtypes, such as myeloma cells, SW1573 lung cancer cells, HT-29 colon cancer cells, and non-small cell lung cancer cells.[455],[457],[459],[464] In the National Cancer Institute's *in vitro* screening panel gemcitabine sensitivity was increased in cells with an activated *ras* oncogene compared with cells with wild-type *ras* alleles, which was the most predominant form for non-small cell lung cancer cells; induction of apoptotic cell death was efficient in cells with activated *ras* oncogenes.[396] Apparently the mechanism of cell death differs between the various cell types. This also indicates varying roles for the DNA repair mechanism.

Clinical pharmacology of gemcitabine

Several phase I clinical trials with gemcitabine have been performed which showed a strong schedule dependence. With the daily times five schedule severe hypotension was observed at the maximally tolerated dose of 12 mg/m², with the twice weekly schedule the maximally tolerated dose was 65 mg/m², while with the weekly schedule this dose was 960 mg/m² and in the two-weekly schedule 5700 mg/m².[465]-[468] The weekly schedule has been evaluated extensively in phase II trials and is now widely used in clinical practice for treatment of pancreatic cancer and non-small cell lung cancer, usually in combination with cisplatin.[469],[470] A 24-hour infusion (at the maximally tolerated dose of 180 mg/m²) given weekly resulted in a similar response rate as the 30-minute weekly infusion (about 20 per cent in non-small cell lung cancer).[471] This schedule dependency was also observed in preclinical *in vitro* and *in vivo* studies (see above).

Pharmacokinetics of gemcitabine was generally comparable with that of ara-C, with a rapid initial half-life of about 12 min.[467],[472] Peak plasma concentrations of gemcitabine at the maximum tolerated dose in this schedule were about 100 μM; in the two-weekly schedule these concentrations were 400 to 500 μM.[153] Urinary excretion could be attributed mainly to 2′,2′-difluorodeoxyuridine, which accounted

in clear contrast to the other deoxycytidine analogues ara-C and aza-CdR. Gemcitabine was selected out of a panel of 2′,2′-difluoronucleosides because of its excellent preclinical activity against a number of experimental tumours and human xenografts, which was very schedule dependent.[440]-[443] Daily and weekly administration were not effective; the most active schedules were every third day times four and weekly 24 h infusions.

The metabolism of gemcitabine is well understood and in several aspects is similar to that of other deoxynucleoside analogues (Fig. 9).[154],[444] Membrane transport is mediated by facilitated diffusion catalysed by human equilibrative nucleoside transporter 1.[382],[445] Subsequent activation of gemcitabine to its mononucleotide is catalysed by deoxycytidine kinase; however, gemcitabine is also a substrate for the mitochondrial thymidine kinase 2.[389],[446] The accumulation of the active metabolite, the triphosphate gemcitabine-TP, is higher than that of ara-CTP.[389],[445] The elimination of gemcitabine-TP is biphasic with a very long terminal half-life (depending on the cellular system it may be even more than 24 h).[447] The activity of gemcitabine is strongly correlated with the extent of gemcitabine-TP formation, its incorporation into DNA, and its inhibition of DNA synthesis.[447]-[449] Gemcitabine is predominantly found in internucleotide linkage in DNA. After incorporation into DNA, DNA polymerase is slowed down, but at least one more nucleotide is incorporated before final termination of chain elongation. This 'masked chain termination' prevents exonucleases from recognizing and excising gemcitabine. The extent of incorporation into DNA and its subsequent inhibition is dependent on the tumour.[449],[450]

Gemcitabine is also incorporated into RNA and induces apoptosis.[449],[451]-[457] This latter effect may be related to the multiple for about 77 per cent of the administered dose.[(467),(473)] The dose-limiting toxicity of the weekly schedule appeared to be mainly myeloid. This schedule is currently used for treatment of non-small cell lung cancer and pancreatic cancer. The myelosuppression, predominantly neutropenia and leukopenia, is usually mild and short-lived. Transaminase increases are common, but are rarely dose limiting; renal toxicity is mild. Gastrointestinal toxicities occur but are generally mild. There is a higher incidence of flu-like syndromes and oedema, but they are generally mild.[(474)] Formation of gemcitabine-TP in mononuclear cells appeared to be saturable, with a biphasic elimination similar to that observed in cell lines.[(475)] Since phosphorylation of gemcitabine by deoxycytidine kinase is a saturable process and because of the schedule dependence in various preclinical studies, infusion times of the drug have been increased in patients with a fixed rate of 10 mg/m²/min;[(476)] infusion time could be increased to 8 h with a proportional increase in gemcitabine-TP accumulation. Because of its relatively mild toxicity profile, its broad activity profile, and synergistic/additive activity with many drugs, gemcitabine is currently being evaluated in many combinations (both chemo- and radiotherapy) in various malignancies.[(450),(477)–(479)] Toxicities of the combinations are dependent on the drug with which gemcitabine is combined; for example in combination with cisplatin, thrombocytopenia and myelosuppression increase.

Other pyrimidine antimetabolites

A number of pyrimidine antimetabolites have been synthesized in the past (see Fig. 1), most of which were directed at an enzyme of the pyrimidine *de novo* pathway. None of them, however, has shown clinical activity compared with established chemotherapy, but several of these agents have added considerably to our understanding of normal nucleotide synthesis and metabolism in both normal and malignant cells. Most of the agents were inactive at the maximum tolerated dose, but several of these compounds may have a clinical application at a low biochemically active dose. For PALA several clinical trials have been performed in combination with 5-fluorouracil.[(221)] Although initial trials were negative because the dose of the active agent, 5-fluorouracil, was lowered, a potentially better therapeutic index for PALA–5-fluorouracil may be obtained at lower PALA doses compared with 5-fluorouracil alone.[(480)]

The same might hold for Brequinar, a potent inhibitor of the pyrimidine *de novo* enzyme dihydro-orotic acid dehydrogenase, resulting in a clear uridine depletion after administration to animals and patients.[(481)] Although clinically inactive as a single agent, the compound can potentiate the activity of 5-fluorouracil in animal models, and this potentiation appeared to be schedule dependent.[(482),(483)] Clinical studies with the combination showed that Brequinar decreased uridine levels at a non-toxic dose, which makes the latter combination feasible and worth further evaluation.[(484)]

Acivicin, a glutamine analogue which inhibits both glutamine-utilizing enzymes from the pyrimidine *de novo* pathway (Table 1), may also have clinical utility as part of a biochemical modulation schedule.[(1)] The same is true for 3-deazauridine, an inhibitor of CTP synthesis.[(485)] Another inhibitor of CTP synthetase is the triphosphate of cyclopentenyl cytosine, which affects selectively replicating cells.[(486)] In a phase I trial severe hypotension was observed, which seems to occur more often with pyrimidine antimetabolites and which may

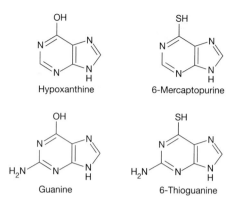

Fig. 10 Structural formulas of the thiopurines 6-mercaptopurine and 6-thioguanine compared with their normal counterparts hypoxanthine and guanine.

be controlled by a different schedule or administration procedure.[(487),(488)] Currently pyrimidine antimetabolites are widely used for many malignancies, usually in combination. It should be kept in mind that their activity and toxicity is usually very schedule dependent, a property which should also be taken in consideration in their early preclinical and evaluation.

In recent years several cytidine analogues have been developed with a different target from those mentioned above. An example is (E)-2′-deoxy-2′-(fluoromethylene) cytidine which is a potent irreversible inhibitor of ribonucleotide reductase.[(489)] This compound has excellent *in vivo* antitumour activity with the ability to induce *in vivo* apoptosis.[(490)] In addition this compound has strong radiosensitization activity.[(491)] 2′-Deoxy-2′-methylidenecytidine (**DMDC**) is a deoxycytidine analogue which is highly resistant to cytidine deaminase but which has similar mechanisms of action to gemcitabine.[(358),(492)] The antitumour activity of DMDC, which can be given orally, was better in tumours with a higher cytidine deaminase activity than that of gemcitabine. Deoxycytidine concentrations were also low in tumours with a high cytidine deaminase activity, precluding rescue of DMDC by deoxycytidine.

In the last years interest in L-nucleosides has increased considerably; These compounds are recognized by the normally occurring enzymes. One such a compound β-L-dioxolane-cytidine, has excellent *in vitro* and *in vivo* activity and may be a lead compound for the development of more L-nucleosides.[(493)]

Thiopurines

The thiopurines 6-mercaptopurine and 6-thioguanine are analogues of the normal purine metabolites hypoxanthine and guanine (Fig. 10) and are different from the parent compounds in having an SH group attached at the sixth position of the molecule. Since their synthesis and initial characterization, they have been used and are still used for remission induction therapy and maintenance therapy of acute lymphocytic leukaemias of childhood and in acute myelogenous leukaemia.[(494)] No activity of thiopurines against solid tumours has

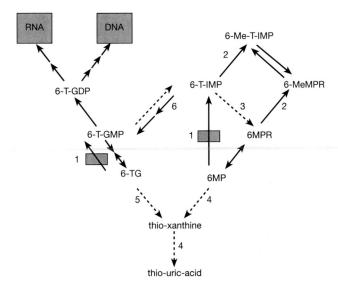

Fig. 11 Schematic presentation of metabolism of the thiopurines including potential resistance mechanisms. Bars represent resistance due to a decreased activity of this pathway (hypoxanthine-guanine phophoribosyltransferase); boxes include targets related to resistance due to a decreased stability (RNA and DNA) and dashed lines due to increased degradation. Enzymes catalysing these reactions are: 1, hypoxanthine-guanine phophoribosyltransferase; 2, thiopurine methyltransferase; 3, nucleotidases and phosphatases; 4, xanthine oxidase; 5, guanine deaminase; 6, IMP dehydrogenase. Abbreviations: 6MPR = 6-mercaptopurine riboside; 6-MeMPR = methyl-mercaptopurineriboside; 6-Me-T-IMP = methyl-thio-IMP; 6-T-IMP = thio-IMP; 6-T-GMP = thio-GMP; 6-T-GDP = thio-GDP.

been shown. Thiopurines are usually administered in combination with methotrexate.

Mechanism of action and resistance

Uptake and activation

The similarity of these compounds to the normal purine bases hypoxanthine and guanine means that thiopurines share common metabolic pathways with their physiological counterparts.[494]–[498] They penetrate cells easily and are excellent substrates for a number of enzymes in purine metabolism, both in the anabolic and catabolic pathways (Fig. 11). Hypoxanthine-guanine phosphoribosyl transferase, a key enzyme in the purine salvage pathway, also catalyses the essential activation of both 6-mercaptopurine and 6-thioguanine to their nucleotide derivatives, 6-thio-**IMP** (inosine 5′-phosphate) and 6-thio-**GMP** (guanosine 5′-phosphate) respectively.[1],[2] The activity of hypoxanthine-guanine phosphoribosyl transferase and the availability of its cofactor 5-phosphoribosyl-1-pyrophosphate are therefore critical factors in the cytotoxic activity of both 6-mercaptopurine and 6-thioguanine (Table 10). Since 6-thio-IMP can be converted to 6-thio-GMP, 6-mercaptopurine can actually be considered as a prodrug for 6-thioguanine. 6-Thio-GMP will be phosphorylated to 6-thio-**GDP** (guanosine 5′-diphosphate), and subsequently to 6-thio-**GTP** (guanosine 5′-triphosphate), which can be incorporated into RNA.

In addition, it has been reported that 6-mercaptopurine is an inhibitor of cellular RNA synthesis and that 6-thio-ITP can inhibit both RNA polymerase I and II.[499] 6-Thio-GDP is also a substrate

for ribonucleotide reductase, catalysing the reduction to 6-thio-dGTP, which can be incorporated into DNA, leading to a delayed cytotoxic action.[500] Incorporation into DNA can also lead to strand breaks which have been related to cytotoxicity.[501] The incorporation of the nucleophilic 6-thioguanine also makes DNA more sensitive to alkylation.[502] 6-Thioguanine can cause gross unilateral chromatid damage, probably due to malfunction of 6-thioguanine-containing DNA as a replication template.[503]

Role of thiopurine methyltransferase and 6-thioguanine nucleotide accumulation

Both the thiopurines 6-mercaptopurine and 6-thioguanine can be methylated to 6-methyl- mercaptopurine and 6-methyl- thioguanine by transfer of the methylgroup of S-adenosyl-methionine catalysed by thiopurine methyltransferase followed by phosphorylation. The accumulation of 6-methyl-thio-IMP is more pronounced and rapid at 10 µM than at 2 µM 6-mercaptopurine, resulting in a decrease in S-adenosyl-methionine, affecting other methylation reactions, such as hypomethylation of newly formed DNA.[504] Purine *de novo* nucleotide synthesis is inhibited by methylated mononucleotides preventing the cells from progressing into G_2–M phases.[505]

The activity of thiopurine methyltransferase varies considerably between patients, and its contribution to cytotoxicity has been a matter of discussion.[498],[506] The activity of red blood cell thiopurine methyltransferase was found to be inversely related to the thiopurine nucleotide content in the erythrocytes of leukaemia patients.[498],[506] Neutropenia was correlated with a high concentration of red blood cell thioguanine nucleotides.[507] In addition, 17 of 19 patients who had relapsed had a thioguanine nucleotide content below the group median. Children who fail to form adequate concentrations of thioguanine nucleotides are at higher risk of treatment failure.[498],[508] The extent of thioguanine nucleotide formation is dose dependent, while wide variations in thioguanine nucleotides may be indicative of non-compliance to therapy.[509],[510]

The role of thiopurine methyltransferase in the therapeutic efficacy of thiopurine has been studied in great detail. Thiopurine methyltransferase activity is controlled by a single genetic locus with two alleles, one for low and one for high activity.[498],[511],[512] There are pharmacogenetic differences between various ethnic populations associated with gene sequence polymorphisms.[512] Several mutant genes have now been identified which are associated with thiopurine methyltransferase deficiency.[512],[513] The wild type does not differ between ethnic populations, but thiopurine methyltransferase variant allele frequencies vary. Thiopurine methyltransferase deficiency is inherited as an autosomal recessive trait in 1 out of 300 individuals. In general 89 per cent of the population has a high activity and 11 per cent an intermediate activity, which is associated with large interindividual variations in thiopurine toxicity and efficacy. Thiopurine methyltransferase levels are usually measured in red blood cells but levels are correlated with that in normal lymphocytes, platelets, kidneys, liver, and also with that in leukaemic blasts before treatment.[511] Thiopurine methyltransferase levels usually increase during treatment.[498],[511] Although a negative association has been found between thioguanine nucleotide accumulation in red blood cells and thiopurine methyltransferase activity, in leukaemic blast cells a high thiopurine methyltransferase activity may lead to accumulation of toxic metabolites, which may inhibit purine *de novo* synthesis. The latter pathway does not exist in red blood cells. Additional studies in blast

Table 10 Factors related to resistance to thiopurines

Decreased activation:
decreased activity of (HGPRT)
decreased accumulation and retention of thionucleotides
Increased inactivation:
inactivation to thioxanthine and thiouric acid
increased breakdown of activated nucleotides, catalysed by phosphatases and/or 5'-nucleotidases
Methylation of thiopurines:
in cell lines high concentrations of 6-methyl-IMP potentiate cytotoxicity
in patients increased thiopurine methyl transferase has been associated with more relapses
Increased DNA repair

HGPRT = hypoxanthine-guanine phosphoribosyltransferase.

cells from patients are needed to determine the extent to which thiopurine methyltransferase may mediate toxicity in blast cells.

Regulatory effects

The close similarity of 6-mercaptopurine and 6-thioguanine to the normal purine bases means that they not only use the same metabolic pathways but also exert a number of similar regulatory functions. Firstly, 6-mercaptopurine is a competitive inhibitor of hypoxanthine-guanine phosphoribosyl transferase for guanine and hypoxanthine. Secondly, 6-mercaptopurine also inhibits the cleavage of inosine and guanosine to hypoxanthine and guanine respectively, a reaction which is catalysed by purine nucleoside phosphorylase. 6-Mercaptopurine, therefore, regulates its own phosphoribosylation. Thirdly, both 6-thio-IMP and 6-methyl-thio-IMP are strong inhibitors of the first enzyme (5-phosphoribosyl-1-pyrophosphate amido phosphoribosyl transferase) in the purine *de novo* synthesis of nucleotides (Fig. 11). This is similar to the feedback inhibition of IMP, but 6-methyl-thio-IMP is a better inhibitor than both 6-thio-IMP and IMP. 6-Thio-GMP does not inhibit the purine *de novo* pathway.[495] As a result of the inhibition of 5-phosphoribosyl-1-pyrophosphate amido phosphoribosyltransferase, 5-phosphoribosyl-1-pyrophosphate will not be used in the *de novo* purine pathway and its concentration will increase. The accumulated 5-phosphoribosyl-1-pyrophosphate can be used for increased synthesis of 6-thio-IMP; so-called 'self-enhancement'. In addition to the increased 5-phosphoribosyl-1-pyrophosphate availability the concentration of the purine nucleotides will decrease, causing a delay of cells in the S phase.

6-Thio-IMP is a non-competitive inhibitor of adenylosuccinate synthetase and a competitive inhibitor of adenylosuccinate lyase; these enzymes catalyse the subsequent steps in the conversion of IMP to AMP. Inhibition is only observed at high concentrations of 6-thio-IMP. In addition, 6-thio-IMP is also an inhibitor of IMP dehydrogenase, the first step in the conversion of IMP to GMP. This inhibition is mediated by the formation of a disulphide bond between its mercaptogroup and that of the enzyme. Another effect of 6-mercaptopurine was reported by Mojena *et al.*.[514] It was demonstrated that 6-mer-captopurine could inhibit purified 6-phosphofructo-2-kinase from either rat liver or bovine heart, possibly by formation of a disulphide bond between 6-mercaptopurine and a reactive thiol group(s) on the enzyme, responsible for the catalytic activity. Reducing agents such as mercaptoethanol or dithiothreitol reversed the effect. These data provide additional evidence that the effects of 6-mercaptopurine are

multifactorial. It can be concluded that 6-mercaptopurine is able to interfere with a number of reactions in purine nucleotide synthesis, most of them actually leading to a enhanced activation of the drug itself.

Inhibition of *de novo* synthesis of purine nucleotides is usually not sufficient to cause cytotoxicity, since it has been demonstrated that these events are reversible. The site of the cytotoxic effect of both 6-mercaptopurine and 6-thioguanine is therefore most likely to be their incorporation into DNA, and to a lesser extent into RNA. Since DNA itself, and precursors of DNA, is mainly assembled in the S phase of the cell cycle, it follows that 6-mercaptopurine and 6-thioguanine are drugs specific to the phase of the cell cycle. Accumulation of cells in S phase has been repeatedly demonstrated.[505],[515] This S-phase arrest may result in apoptosis. 6-Mercaptopurine is able to evoke rapid apoptotic cell death, which is associated with a decrease in the ratio between bcl-2/bax.[516] Since at short exposures to the drugs cells may continue to cycle it follows that prolonged exposure may be necessary in order to achieve optimum cell killing by 6-mercaptopurine and 6-thioguanine.

Role of drug degradation

6-Mercaptopurine and 6-thioguanine are excellent substrates for purine salvage enzymes as well as for catabolic enzymes. This also holds for the nucleotide derivatives. Substantial quantities of 6-mercaptopurine are converted to 6-thioxanthine and subsequently to 6-thiouric acid. Both these reactions are catalysed by xanthine oxidase, and are subject to inhibition by allopurinol. 6-Thioguanine can also be converted to 6-thioxanthine in a reaction catalysed by guanine deaminase. In addition, methylated thiopurines may be oxidized to sulphonic products, with liberation of inorganic sulphate. It is clear that extensive degradation of 6-mercaptopurine and 6-thioguanine may limit the bioavailability of the drugs; thus interindividual differences in catabolism might appear as resistance to the drug. The activity of the catabolic enzymes is abundant in most normal tissues, but the enzyme is absent from normal lymphocytes and leukaemic lymphoblasts. In addition xanthine oxidase is downregulated in tumours.[1] Inhibition of xanthine oxidase by allopurinol will enhance the bioavailability of 6-mercaptopurine. Since thiopurine methyltransferase converts 6-thioguanine to the inactive methyl-6-thioguanine, it may in this regard be considered as a breakdown enzyme. Degradation of thiopurines can therefore be an important process in limiting the bioavailability of these drugs. The absence, for example, of xanthine oxidase in leukaemic cells, however, adds to the selectivity of thiopurine therapy.

Another important feature in the degradation of thiopurines is the breakdown of the active nucleotides, catalysed by either phosphatases and/or 5'-nucleotidases. Resistance to thiopurines has been observed in cell lines with increased concentrations of a membrane-bound phosphatase.[517] In patients, the relation between phosphatase activity and response is less clear. Zimm et al. observed a marked increase in phosphatase activity in only two out of 10 patients with acute lymphoblastic leukaemia at the time of relapse.[518] Patients with common acute lymphoblastic leukaemia and a 5'-nucleotidase-positive phenotype had a lower probability of continuous complete remission than those with a 5'-nucleotidase-negative phenotype.[519] In a larger group of patients with common acute lymphoblastic leukaemia and pre-B-cell acute lymphoblastic leukaemia, those with a high ecto-5'-nucleotidase activity had a low probability of continuous complete remission.[520] It has been hypothesized that high ecto-5'-nucleotidase activity will cause dephosphorylation of exogenous nucleotides (derived from dying cells for example) to nucleosides, which will subsequently enter the cells and bypass the inhibition of the purine de novo pathway and decrease the cytotoxicity of the thiopurine nucleotides.[2],[521] In addition it is clear that a high activity of cytosolic 5'-nucleotidase will cause an extensive degradation of thiopurine nucleotides.

Clinical pharmacology of thiopurines

Investigation of pharmacokinetics using high-performance liquid chromatography has been hampered by a lack of either sensitivity or selectivity, due to the presence of interfering compounds in plasma or oxidation of the drug. The latter can be prevented by addition of a reducing agent. Technical advances have further improved sensitivity.[522]–[524] 6-Mercaptopurine is generally admininistered orally to patients and its absorption is about 50 per cent. Peak concentrations after oral 6-mercaptopurine are less than 1 µM and are highly variable.[525] The coadminstration of allopurinol, an inhibitor of xanthine oxidase, increased peak plasma levels and the area under the curve about fivefold for orally administered 6-mercaptopurine, but not for intravenous 6-mercaptopurine. This differential effect is probably attributable to the inhibition by allopurinol of the first-pass effect in the liver. At identical doses of 100 mg/m² 6-mercaptopurine reached fourfold higher plasma concentrations than 6-thioguanine, but the concentration of red blood cell thioguanine nucleotides was sevenfold higher for the 6-thioguanine group.[526] However, in the 6-mercaptopurine group more methylated nucleotides were formed than in the 6-thioguanine group, indicating that 6-mercaptopurine might exert its cytotoxic effects not only via thioguanine nucleotides.[526] Thrombocytopenia was dose-limiting for the 6-thioguanine group, but not for the 6-mercaptopurine group.[527] Absorption of 6-thioguanine is more erratic, and this drug is usually administered intravenously.[496]

Due to the variable absorption resulting in considerable interpatient variation in the pharmacokinetics of oral 6-mercaptopurine, intravenous administration of the drug is currently being investigated more intensively.[497] The main use of intravenous 6-mercaptopurine is probably not in its administration as a single agent, but in combination with methotrexate. In addition intravenous administration of 6-mercaptopurine might also affect its distribution. Jacqzaigrain

et al. found a concentration of about 3.8 µM of 6-mercaptopurine in the cerebrospinal fluid after intravenous administration but a concentration of less than 0.18 µM after oral administration.[528] In addition accumulation of thioguanine nucleotide increased rapidly. The mechanism of action might shift, since a higher dose might increase the extent of formation of methyl-thio-IMP thus enhancing the inhibition of the purine de novo synthesis.

Large interindividual variations in the pharmacokinetics of oral 6-mercaptopurine have been reported in maintenance therapy.[529] Evidence has been obtained suggesting that plasma levels of 6-mercaptopurine, determined during therapy, may be related to the risk of relapses and myelotoxicity, with a low area under the curve being predictive for a greater chance of relapse.[530],[531] Other drugs and food intake may interfere with drug uptake.[532],[533] Drug degradation as discussed above is responsible for the majority of drug elimination. 6-Thioxanthine and 6-thiouric acid are not only found in the plasma, but also the nucleosides of the thiopurines.[525],[534] These metabolites may be of clinical importance. The plasma secondary half-life β for 6-mercaptopurine varies from 20 to 60 min and that of 6-thioguanine from 80 to 90 min.

6-Mercaptopurine is well tolerated at doses up to 100 mg/m² per day. Doses for maintenance therapy of 50 to 75 mg/m²/day are common in clinical practice. Since 6-mercaptopurine and 6-thioguanine are both incorporated into DNA, rapidly dividing cells of the bone marrow and the gut epithelium are more susceptible to their cytotoxic effects. Myelosuppression is dose dependent but complete recovery is usually observed. Reversible hepatotoxicity is observed, while mucositis and gastrointestinal toxicities are mild and acceptable. Cholestatic jaundice occurs dose dependently (more frequent at doses of more than 2.5 mg/kg) and can be a serious problem when given together with methotrexate. 6-Mercaptopurine therapy should be withdrawn until hepatotoxicity is resolved and subsequent dose reduction should be considered.

Other purine analogues

In addition to the thiopurines there are number of other purine analogues (Table 1 and Fig. 11) which act upon purine nucleotide synthesis and/or use purine enzymes for activation. One group of compounds consists of the inhibitors of the de novo synthesis of purine nucleotides such as the antifolates methotrexate and dideazatetrahydrofolate; and the amino acid analogues, such as azaserine and acivicin. A second group of purine antimetabolites consists of adenosine analogues, such as 9-β-D-arabinofuranosyl-adenine (ara-A) and deoxycoformycin. A third group of antipurines consists of the inhibitors of IMP dehydrogenase, such as tiazofurin. As yet the purine de novo inhibitors have not shown a significant antitumour and/or antileukaemic activity which is any better than that of the 'standard' agents. For the adenosine analogues and tiazofurin more promising data have been reported and are discussed below.

Adenosine analogues

Ara-A and fludarabine

Ara-A (Fig. 12) itself is not active and has to be phosphorylated to its triphosphate, this reaction being catalysed by adenosine kinase and deoxycytidine kinase and subsequently by nucleotide kinases (Fig.

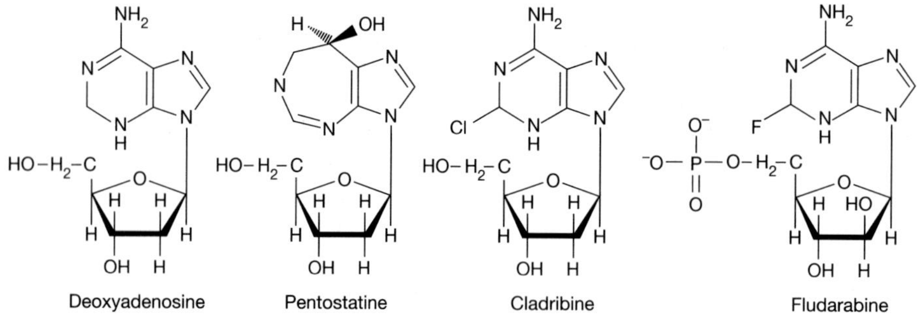

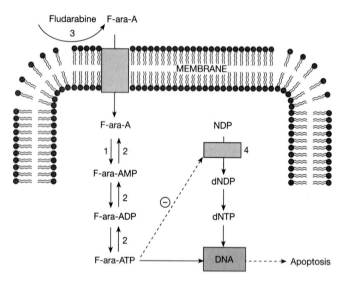

Fig. 12 Structural formulae of deoxyadenosine and its analogues fludarabine, cladribine, and pentostatine.

Fig. 13 Schematic presentation of metabolism of fludarabine including resistance mechanisms. Fludarabine has to be dephosphorylated outside the cell to F-ara-A in order to be taken up by the cell; inside the cell F-ara-A will be rephosphorylated. F-ara-ATP is a potent inhibitor of ribonucleotide reductase, represented by a bar. Both incorporation of F-ara-ATP and an imbalance in deoxyribonucleotide pools will affect DNA synthesis (box), ultimately leading to apoptotic cell death. NDP = nucleoside diphosphate; dNDP = deoxynucleoside diphosphate; dNTP = deoxynucleoside triphosphate. Enzymes catalysing these reactions are: 1, deoxynucleoside kinases (including deoxycytidine kinase); 2, nucleotidases and phosphatases; 3, extracellular nucleotidases and phosphatases; 4, ribonucleotide reductase.

13).[(496),(535),(536)] The triphosphate ara-ATP is an inhibitor of DNA polymerase. Ara-A possesses potent antitumour activity against animal tumours, but its clinical applicability is hampered by its low solubility and its rapid deamination catalysed by adenosine deaminase. The analogue 2-fluoro-ara-AMP (fludarabine) is more soluble, but to enter the cell it has to be dephosphorylated by an ecto-5′-nucleotidase, which is present on most cells. The product, 2-fluoro-ara-A, is not deaminated, and its phosphorylation is catalysed by deoxycytidine kinase.[(535)] The triphosphate derivative is a potent inhibitor of DNA polymerase and ribonucleotide reductase and can be incorporated into both RNA and DNA.[(537)] The triphosphate derivative is a potent inhibitor of DNA primase, resulting in inhibition of primer RNA synthesis, while inhibition of DNA ligase I results in inhibition of DNA synthesis[(538),(539)]

In lymphocytes isolated from patients with chronic lymphocytic leukaemia 2-fluoro-ara-A has been shown to be a potent inducer of apoptosis.[(540)] This seems to correlate with the disease status of the patient. Both ara-A and 2-fluoro-ara-AMP are cell phase-specific drugs and progression of the cells through the S phase is inhibited.[(541),(542)]

Fludarabine is highly toxic against both normal and malignant lymphoid and myeloid cells. Exposure to fludarabine also resulted in a decrease in bcl-2 expression and an increase in apoptosis.[(542)] Downregulation of bcl-2 may be correlated with response to treatment.[(543)] In initial clinical trials with high doses of fludarabine (50–150 mg/m²/day for 5–7 days), neutropenia and a high degree of central nervous system toxicity were observed[(496),(544)] At lower doses (25–50 mg/m²/day for 2–5 days) the compound is highly active against chronic lymphocytic leukaemia. Response rates of more than 70 per cent have been reported with only mild and reversible toxicity, which have been confirmed in a randomized study comparing fludarabine with cyclophosphamide–doxorubicin–prednisone. Remission rates were 60 and 44 per cent respectively.[(545),(546)]

After administration fludarabine is rapidly dephosphorylated and is only detectable for 2 to 4 min. Peak plasma concentrations of the metabolite F-ara-A are reached at the end of the infusion and have a short initial half-life of 5 min, followed by an intermediate phase with a half-life of 1 to 2 h, while the terminal elimination phase has a half-life of 10 to 30 h. At longer infusions only two elimination phases are observed.[(536)] Pharmacokinetics are linear and elimination is largely by renal excretion.

Deoxycoformycin

The discovery of a causal association between severe immune disorders and deficiencies in two enzymes of purine metabolism, adenosine deaminase and purine nucleoside phosphorylase, stimulated research into purine metabolism in lymphoid cells and tissues (Fig. 14).[(2),(496),(547)] A deficiency of adenosine deaminase is selectively toxic for T lymphocytes and it was reasoned that inhibition of adenosine deaminase would also be toxic for T-cell leukaemia. Adenosine deaminase catalyses the deamination of adenosine and deoxyadenosine to inosine and deoxyinosine (Fig. 11). Several inhibitors of adenosine deaminase have been isolated from natural sources or synthesized. Deoxycoformycin (pentostatin) is a very potent, tight

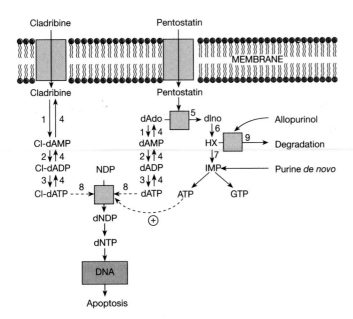

Fig. 14 Schematic presentation of the metabolism of cladribine and the effect of pentostatin on purine metabolism. Cladribine and pentostatin are taken up by facilitated diffusion. Enzymes catalysing the reaction are: 1, deoxycytidine kinase; 2, nucleoside monophosphate kinase; 3, nucleoside diphosphate kinase; 4, 5'nucleotidases and phosphatases; 5, adenosine deaminase; 6, purine nucleoside phosphorylase; 7, hypoxanthine–guanine phosphoribosyl transferase; 8, ribonucleotide reductase; 9, xanthine oxidase.

binding, irreversible inhibitor of adenosine deaminase (Fig. 12).[548] Inhibition of adenosine deaminase will lead to accumulation of deoxyadenosine which will be phosphorylated to dATP, a potent inhibitor of ribonucleotide reductase. This will lead to inhibition of DNA synthesis. In addition DNA repair is inhibited, resulting in accumulation of DNA strand breaks. Adenosine deaminase is widely distributed in human tissues, but non-lymphoid tissues lack the necessary kinase enzyme and do not accumulate dATP.[547] dATP is therefore selectively accumulated in lymphoid cells. Deoxycoformycin is even more specific for T cells, possibly due to the high ratio of deoxyadenosine kinase activity compared with 5'-nucleotidase. Thus, human trials with deoxycoformycin were initiated against leukaemia, mostly T-cell acute lymphoblastic leukaemia, but were disappointing because of high toxicity at the applied doses (>10 mg/m²/week, administered either as a daily schedule or a weekly dose).[496],[547] Toxicity consisted of haemolytic anaemia, acute tubular necrosis, and liver abnormalities.[549] However, some short-term remissions were observed in T-cell acute lymphoblastic leukaemia, which is resistant to conventional cytotoxic chemotherapy. At lower doses (4 mg/m² biweekly) toxicity is low, but the drug is active against hairy cell leukaemia at these doses. Overall response rates are 96 to 100 per cent, while complete remission may be achieved in 59 to 96 per cent of cases. It has been observed that patients refractory to interferon-α can respond to deoxycoformycin.[550]

Deoxycoformycin has a biphasic elimination with an initial half-life between 30 and 85 min and a terminal half-life varying from 3 to 9 h.[550] Peak plasma concentrations varied from 12 to 120 nM, and between 30 and 50 per cent of the drug is excreted unchanged in the urine. The obvious pharmacodynamic action is inhibition of adenosine

deaminase, associated with an increase in deoxyadenosine concentrations, which in turn results in an increase in dATP in erythrocytes and leukaemia cells.[536]

2-Chloro-2'-deoxyadenosine

2-Chloro-2'-deoxyadenosine (**CdA**) is an adenosine analogue (Fig. 12) resistant to deamination by adenosine deaminase; the drug requires phosphorylation catalysed by deoxycytidine kinase, and deoxycytidine could prevent CdA-induced growth inhibition.[552] Exposure of leukaemic cells to CdA results in a stimulation of deoxycytidine kinase, which results in selfpotentiation.[553] In order to exert its cytotoxic action the drug requires intracellular accumulation of CdA nucleotides (Fig. 14), which can be incorporated into DNA and interfere with DNA polymerases and ribonucleotide reductase.[554],[555] This results in a depletion of deoxyribonucleotides and an inhibition of DNA synthesis. The latter effect is possibly related to its efficient use by DNA polymerases, resulting in an inhibition of further chain extension. Its mechanism of action also involves the induction of apoptosis, as was observed in lymphocytes from patients with either hairy cell leukaemia or chronic lymphocytic leukaemia.[540],[556] The drug is active against a number of leukaemic cell lines in nanomolar concentrations, but no activity has been demonstred against lines from non-lymphoid solid tumours.[557]

CdA has shown clinical activity against lymphoproliferative diseases and is very active against hairy cell leukaemia (85 per cent complete remission), including in patients refractory to interferon-α.[558]–[560] In 40 patients with low-grade lymphocytic lymphomas, an overall response rate of 43 per cent was achieved, with eight patients a complete response and nine a partial responses.[561] In 36 previously treated patients with low-grade non-Hodgkin's lymphoma an overall response rate of 42 per cent (partial response 16 per cent) was observed.[562] Activity (47 per cent response) was also observed in children with acute myeloid leukaemia, as well as in patients with B-cell chronic lymphocytic leukaemia resistant to fludarabine.[563],[564] In 20 untreated patients an overall response of 85 per cent was observed with a 7-day schedule.[565] For pretreated patients the overall response was lower.[560],[566] Although the triphosphate of CdA is considered to be the active metabolite, no relationship has been found between its intracellular concentration and response to treatment.[567] Accumulation of CdA triphosphate has been found to be related to maximum plasma CdA concentration. The dose-limiting toxicity (at 0.7 mg/kg/course) is mainly myelosuppression and nephrotoxicity.

CdA is given as a 2 h infusion, over five consecutive days (0.14 mg/kg/2 h) or as a 7-day continuous infusion (total dose 0.7 mg/kg). During the 2-h infusion the CdA concentration was about 200 nM, and plasma elimination half-lives were about 35 min and 6.7 h for the α and β phases respectively.[568] During the 24-h infusion steady state plasma concentrations were about 22 nM; the areas under the time versus concentration curves were comparable for the two schedules. Steady state levels at a 5-day infusion of 8.9 mg/m²/day were 34.6 nM.[563] The concentration in cerebrospinal fluid was about 15 per cent of that in plasma. Renal clearance accounts for about half of the total clearance. Oral administration of 0.14 or 0.28 mg CdA/kg as a phosphate-buffered salt solution resulted in a bioavailability of 48 and 55 per cent respectively.[569] Subcutaneous administration had a 102 per cent bioavailability. Peak plasma concentrations after intravenous, oral, and subcutaneous administration of 0.14 mg drug/kg were about 169, 53 and 318 nM. The interpatient variability after

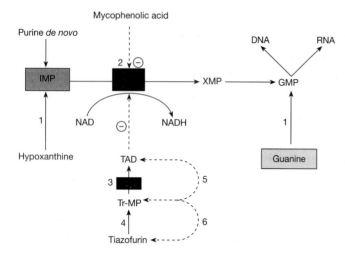

Fig. 15 Schematic representation of the metabolism of tiazofurin and mycophenolic acid and possible resistance mechanisms. Bars represent resistance mechanisms either by an increase of the target enzyme (IMP dehydrogenase) or a decrease in activation (NAD pyrophosphorylase). Dashed lines represent resistance due to an increased inactivation. Other possible factors involved in resistance are in boxes (IMP, NAD, guanine). Enzymes catalysing these reactions are: 1, hypoxanthine-guanine phosphoribosyl transferase (HGPRT); 2, IMP dehydrogenase; 3, NAD pyrophosphorylase; 4, adenosine kinase and/or a phosphotransferase; 5, TADase, a phosphodiesterase; 6, nucleotidases and phosphatases. TR-MP = tiazofurin monophosphate; TAD = tiazofurin adenine dinucleotide.

administration of the oral solution was no greater than that after intravenous administration.

Inhibitors of IMP dehydrogenase

A number of inhibitors of IMP dehydrogenase has been studied for their potency as antitumour agents.[570] The IMP dehydrogenase inhibitor mycophenolic acid was not active. Another inhibitor is tiazofurin (2-β-D-ribofuranosylthiazole-4-carboxamide), a thiazole C nucleoside, which has shown considerable activity in a number of tumour models. The drug shows activity in leukaemia.[571] Tiazofurin is metabolized to its monophosphate and subsequently to its diphosphate, tiazofurin adenine dinucleotide (TAD), an analogue of NAD$^+$ (Fig. 15).[572] TAD is a strong competitive inhibitor of IMP dehydrogenase leading to a depression of GTP and dGTP concentrations and to inhibition of cell proliferation.[573] Inhibition of IMP dehydrogenase with tiazofurin has been associated with induction of differentiation, probably by the downregulation of the c-ras gene consequent upon depletion of GTP.[574] Tiazofurin has shown a synergistic interaction with a number of different drugs including taxol and gemcitabine.[575] In a tiazofurin-resistant cell line NAD levels were decreased, which was accompanied by an increased sensitivity to temozolomide alone; since NAD is a substrate for poly(ADP-ribose) polymerase, this may affect DNA repair.[576]

Phase I studies with tiazofurin have shown that neurotoxicity is a dose-limiting side-effect.[577] Drug response has been shown to depend on the extent of inhibition of IMP dehydrogenase and the depletion of GTP. Patients with leukaemia who showed a response were those with considerable GTP depletion and inhibition of IMP

dehydrogenase in the lymphoblasts.[571] The most consistent responses were seen in patients with myeloid blast crisis of chronic myeloid leukaemia.[578],[579]

Combinations of antimetabolites and biochemical modulation

Our extensive knowledge about the mechanism of action of antimetabolites and the metabolism of normal purine and pyrimidine precursors, together with the relatively mild toxicity profile of antimetabolites, makes this group of cytostatic agents very attractive for combination with each other or with other anticancer agents.[580] A specific purpose behind combining drugs is biochemical modulation, which involves the pharmacological manipulation of the intracellular pathways of a drug. Unlike classical combination chemotherapy, which requires the combination of two or more active drugs, biochemical modulation may involve the combination of two active drugs, but also that of one inactive modulating drug and an active drug, or the combination of an active drug with a modulating normal metabolite. The aim of all these combinations is to selectively increase the cytotoxicity to tumour cells and/or a selective protection of normal cells. Many extensive reviews on different subjects of biochemical modulation have been published.[154],[220],[221],[224],[377]–[379],[580]–[588]

Numerous combinations have been tested (see the above-mentioned reviews), but not all have been clinically successful. Table 11 gives an overview of combinations which are either in common use, have been tested in clinical trials with positive results, or have good prospects. A number of clinical trials have suffered from bad scheduling. It has already been pointed out by Martin and Leyland-Jones and O'Dwyer that a good 'translation' of preclinical data to the clinic is essential for there to be a positive outcome.[221],[580],[587] Initial screening of potential combinations is usually performed in cell culture, with cells which have a doubling time varying between 12 and 48 h. The next step should be testing on animal tumours which have a doubling time varying from 2 to 15 days. Unfortunately this step is often omitted. The last step is introduction of the combination into the clinic, where tumours have a doubling time varying from several days to several months. Scheduling may need some adaptation, and apparently negative trials have sometimes been the result of using the wrong schedule. The time interval and sequence of administration are very important, since the wrong sequence can result in antagonism instead of the required synergism. For that purpose it is recommended that clinical studies are accompanied, whenever possible, by mechanistic studies in the target tissue, the tumour, or in surrogate tissues to analyse the molecular targets. White blood cells are often suitable for these purposes. Sequences mentioned in Table 6 are the effective schedules. Several of the combinations mentioned in this table have already been discussed in previous sections.

Biochemical modulation of 5-fluorouracil

Scheduling of leucovorin and 5-fluorouracil may be important in order to achieve adequate potentiation of the effect of 5-fluorouracil. In vitro studies have not shown a clear schedule dependency for the combination with 5-fluorouracil, but the combination of floxuridine followed by leucovorin was not effective.[589] In vivo studies in mice

Table 11 Relevant biochemical modulation combinations (modified from Peters et al.[587])

Modulators	Mechanism of modulation
PALA → 5-FU	Enhanced 5-FU anabolism in tumours
5-FU → uridine	Protection of myeloid tissues by interference with 5-FU-RNA
LV +/→ 5-FU	Increased stabilization of the ternary complex
Interferon +/→ 5-FU	Increased FdUMP leading to enhanced inhibition of thymidylate synthase; increased DNA damage
Methotrexate →5-FU	Increase of PRPP leading to increased anabolism of 5-FU
TMQ → 5-FU/LV	Increase of PRPP leading to increased anabolism of 5-FU; bypass reduced folate carrier
HD methotrexate → LV	Bypass of folate depletion
Methotrexate →6-MP	Increase of PRRP leading to enhanced 6-MP anabolism
Allopurinol + 6-MP	Decrease of 6-MP catabolism
Eniluracil + 5-FU	Better absorption of oral 5-FU; inhibition DPD
Uracil or CDHP + Ft	Better absorption Ft; inhibition DPD
Oxaliplatin + 5-FU	DNA directed?; thymidylate synthase
SN-38 or CPT-11 → 5-FU	More DNA damage; thymidylate synthase inhibition?
Dipyridamole ←/+ 5-FU	Inhibition of efflux of (5-FU) nucleosides
Dipyridamole ← ara-C	Permit entry of ara-C; delayed dipyridamole will prevent efflux of ara-C
Dipyridamole + methotrexate	Prevention influx nucleosides to protect rescue by e.g. thymidine
Deoxycytidine + ara-C	Selective inhibition of ara-C phosphorylation in normal bone marrow
Fludarabine → ara-C	Increased ara-C anabolism and formation of ara-CTP
Gemcitabine → cisplatin	Increased adduct formation and retention incorporation into DNA

The arrows indicate the sequence; + indicates simultaneous administration.

Abbreviations: PALA = phosphonoacetyl-L-aspartate; 5-FU = 5-fluorouracil; LV = leucovorin; PRPP = 5-phosphoribosyl-1-pyrophosphate; 6-MP = 6-mercaptopurine; HD = high dose; CDHP = 5-chloro-2,4-dihydropyridine; DPD = dihydropyrimidine dehydrogenase; Ft = ftorafur

bearing colon tumours have indicated that administration of leucovorin after 5-fluorouracil is less effective than pretreatment or simultaneous administration.[590]

The combination of 5-fluorouracil with leucovorin is based on the stabilization of the ternary complex between FdUMP, thymidylate synthase, and CH_2-tetrahydrofolate (Fig. 6). The bioavailability of the latter is increased by leucovorin administration. After transfer across the membrane mediated by the reduced folate carrier, leucovorin will be metabolized to CH_2-tetrahydrofolate.[32] Although intermediates of the metabolic pathway of leucovorin to CH_2-tetrahydrofolate can also support the formation of the ternary complex, CH_2-tetrahydrofolate is the most active substrate.[259] Polyglutamates of CH_2-tetrahydrofolate, which are formed by the action of folylpoly-γ-glutamate synthetase, will enhance inhibition of thymidylate synthase.[591] In general prolonged exposure of cells also led to a 1.5 to twofold increased enhancement of the cytotoxicity of 5-fluorouracil and 5-fluoro-2′-deoxyuridine by 1 to 10 μM leucovorin.[224] Lower concentrations of leucovorin are generally not sufficient to potentiate the effects of 5-fluorouracil or FUDR, while higher concentrations generally do not enhance the effect.[303] There are fewer *in vivo* studies on modulation of 5-fluorouracil by leucovorin, usually limited to the description of the antitumour effect but not including mechanistic studies.[589] 5-Fluorouracil alone shows a clear tumour-dependent

thymidylate synthase inhibition, followed by a two- to threefold induction after 2 to 3 weeks.[276],[277],[283],[592] The potentiation of the antitumour activity of 5-fluorouracil by leucovorin given before 5-fluorouracil in several murine tumours was associated with a prevention of the induction of thymidylate synthase and with a more pronounced inhibition of thymidylate synthase by leucovorin plus 5-fluorouracil compared with 5-fluorouracil alone.[276] Thus, *in vivo* modulation of 5-fluorouracil with leucovorin seems to be related to prolonged inhibition of thymidylate synthase and prevention of thymidylate synthase induction.

A number of different schedules have been used successfully in phase III trials—biweekly, weekly, and daily administrations, as well as 24-h, 48-h, and continuous infusions (Table 12).[593]–[595] The schedules in which leucovorin is injected as a bolus, thus preventing accumulation of leucovorin and subsequently of polyglutamates, appear to be less effective, in line with the preclinical observations. Leucovorin has to be administered at a certain threshold dose allowing sufficient accumulation of the drug. The lower response rate in the study of Petrelli *et al.* may be related to the long interval between administration of leucovorin and 5-fluorouracil, while in the study of O'Connell, 5-fluorouracil was injected immediately after leucovorin.[596],[597] It is most likely that, in the first study, leucovorin would have been eliminated at the time of 5-fluorouracil injection, while

Table 12 Efficacy of various 5-fluorouracil combination regimens in untreated patients with colorectal cancer (see text for references)

Schedule	Phase	No of patients	Response (CR/PR)	Median survival (months)
LV + oxaliplatin + 5-FU:				
chronomodulated	II, III	284	55%†	19
(a) flat infusion	III	140	30%†	16
(b) without oxaliplatin		100	16%	19
CPT-11 + 5-FU$_{24h}$	I, II	26	62%	
TMQ + 5-FU + LV	II	61	48%	
UFT + LV	II, II	66, 177	36%, 36%	
Capecitabine	II	68	24%	
5-FU + eniluracil	II	23	30%	

†Difference significant $p < 0.05$, in three different phase III studies, compared with either flat infusion (two studies) or without oxaliplatin (one study).

Phase I, II: CPT-11 80–120 mg/m²; LV 500 mg/m² + 5-FU$_{24h}$ 1800–2600 mg/m², weekly × 6.

Phase II: TMQ 110 mg/m² plus LV 200 mg/m², d1; plus 5-FU 500 mg/m² and 50 mg LV p.o. q6 h ×7 d2.

Abbreviations: 5-FU = 5-fluorouracil; LV = leucovorin; CR = complete response; PR = partial response; UFT = uracil with ftorafur; d1 = day1; p.o = orally; q6h × 7 d2 = every 6 h for 7 times starting at day 2.

Schedules are those advised by the manufacturer.

this would not be the case with the simultaneous injection of leucovorin and 5-fluorouracil. Although low-dose leucovorin seems to be better than high-dose leucovorin, it has to be noted that the 5-fluorouracil dose was lower in the high-dose leucovorin regimen.[598] It may be concluded that the best way to administer leucovorin is as an infusion, thus allowing accumulation of folates and folylpolyglutamates in the tissues: 5-fluorouracil has to be administered either immediately after leucovorin or during the infusion of leucovorin. Administration of 5-fluorouracil weekly or five times daily every 4 or 5 weeks generally gave the same results. Several meta-analyses consistently demonstrated a benefit for a combination of leucovorin and 5-fluorouracil compared with 5-fluorouracil alone in terms of response rate, but a benefit in terms of increased survival was not always evident, and when observed was only moderate.[340],[341],[594],[595] Toxicity of the combination of leucovorin and 5-fluorouracil is more severe than that of 5-fluorouracil alone. In particular, diarrhoea and stomatitis are increased. Oral administration of leucovorin has also been demonstrated to result in a potentiation of 5-fluorouracil.[599] Some phase II clinical trials of 5-fluorouracil in combination with the pure active isomer L-leucovorin demonstrated a similar activity, and both forms can be used interchangeably.[600]

Initial evidence was obtained that interferon-α can be used as a biochemical modulator, possibly acting by enhancement of the downstream effects of inhibition of thymidylate synthase.[601] Interferon-α increased the extent of DNA strand break formation induced by 5-fluorouracil, which was even more pronounced for the triple combination of 5-fluorouracil, leucovorin, and interferon-α;[296],[297] interferon did not enhance the inhibition of thymidylate synthase. Although it was initially postulated that interferon-α could increase the concentration of FdUMP this was not confirmed in a large panel of colon cancer cell lines.[297] The effects of interferon-α are completely different from those exerted by interferon-γ, which seems to be related to regulation of the expression of thymidylate synthase.[271],[272]

Initial clinical studies demonstrated a beneficial effect of interferon-α on the antitumour activity of 5-fluorouracil.[601],[602] However, subsequent randomized studies did not demonstrate any benefit for the addition of interferon-α to 5-fluorouracil alone.[603] Interestingly, interferon-α altered the pharmacokinetics of 5-fluorouracil, leading to an increase in the area under the 5-fluorouracil concentration–time curve and a decrease in 5-fluorouracil clearance compared with that of 5-fluorouracil–leucovorin. Also in a triple combination of 5-fluorouracil, leucovorin, and interferon-α a high response rate of 54 per cent was initially observed in two independent trials with 44 and 28 patients respectively.[604],[605] Since 5-fluorouracil with leucovorin and interferon-α did not show an advantage over leucovorin and 5-fluorouracil in a randomized study, it was argued that only leucovorin had a modulating effect.[606] Studies in colon cancer cell lines indicate that modulation of 5-fluorouracil by interferon-α is not a general phenomenon, but only occurs in specific cell lines, and sometimes only under specific growth conditions.[297] The combination of 5-fluorouracil with interferon-α is no longer being evaluated in clinical studies.

Combinations of 5-fluorouracil with methotrexate gave controversial results in the clinic, possibly due to a neutralization of the effects of methotrexate by leucovorin, resulting in a net modulation by leucovorin, or competitive inhibition by leucovorin of methotrexate uptake.[224],[607] Trimetrexate is a lipophilic inhibitor of dihydrofolate reductase, which does not use the reduced folate transport system, cannot be polyglutamated, and does not compete with leucovorin for cellular uptake and metabolism.[32],[608] Romanini *et al.* showed that leucovorin can enhance the cytotoxicity of trimetrexate and the metabolism of 5-fluorouracil intracellularly (increased 5-fluorouracil activation), as well as enhancing the inhibition of thymidylate synthase.[609] These results formed the basis for clinical studies on a combination of trimetrexate with 5-fluorouracil and leucovorin. This combination had activity in previously treated patients, with a response rate of approximately 20 per cent, and a rsponse rate of about 50 per cent in untreated patients.[610] These studies are an elegant example how a rational combination can be based on preclinical studies, combining increased 5-fluorouracil activation with enhanced inhibition of thymidylate synthase.

The combination of phosphoroacetyl-L-aspartate (**PALA**) and 5-fluorouracil is an example of the combination of an inactive drug with an active drug. Only a low dose of PALA is required to obtain the biochemical effect necessary for increased anabolism of 5-fluorouracil. By inhibition of pyrimidine *de novo* synthesis (Fig. 1) PALA can enhance the availability of 5-phosphoribosyl-1-pyrophosphate, thus increasing the anabolism of 5-fluorouracil and its incorporation into RNA.[580] In several phase II clinical trials the response rate for this combination varied from 33 to 43 per cent, but in larger randomized studies these effects were not confirmed.[306],[480],[611],[612]

For the combination 5-fluorouracil and uridine it is essential that the natural non-toxic nucleoside is given after 5-fluorouracil in order to selectively rescue normal bone marrow.[585],[613] Too short an interval may influence the antitumour effect of 5-fluorouracil. In clinical studies both orally and intravenously administered uridine could reverse 5-fluorouracil-induced leukopenia, allowing the administration of higher doses of 5-fluorouracil, confirming the preclinical studies.[580],[613]–[616] These studies also demonstrated that uridine prevented the incorporation of 5-fluorouracil into RNA.[289],[580] Delayed uridine administration has also been shown to protect against gastrointestinal toxicity in murine models due to selective protection of 5-fluorouracil-induced apoptosis in the gut.[617],[618] In clinical studies a selective protective effect on the normal tissues and an enhanced antitumour effect was observed, not only with uridine but also with PN401, a uridine prodrug that can be given orally.[615],[619]

The use of inhibitors of dihydropyrimidine dehydrogenase allows administration of 5-fluorouracil (or one of its prodrugs) as an oral formulation, since degradation is almost completely prevented. This results in 5-fluorouracil concentrations in the micromolar range. The most widely used formulation at this moment is UFT, in which uracil is combined with Ftorafur in a 4:1 molar ratio.[224],[620] This formulation has been refined, resulting in S-1, which is a combination of Ftorafur, 5-chloro-2,4-dihydropyridine, and oxonic acid in a molar ratio of 1:0.4:1.[224],[352],[621] 5-Chloro-2,4-dihydropyridine is a potent reversible inhibitor of dihydropyrimidine dehydrogenase and oxonic acid has the same effect on orotate phosphoribosyltransferase;[622] since oxonic acid accumulates specifically in normal gut, this will reduce gastrointestinal toxicity.[621] In another formulation 5-fluorouracil is combined with ethynyluracil, a suicide inhibitor of dihydropyrimidine dehydrogenase.[354],[623] All these formulations have shown clinical activity (Table 12) in various tumour types, which is usually comparable with that found with modulated 5-fluorouracil bolus schedules and probably also continuous infusions. The main advantage is the convenient oral administration of these formulations.

Other combinations with 5-fluorouracil

Since FdUMP and the new antifolates bind at different sites of the enzyme, studies combining 5-fluorouracil with new antifolate thymidylate synthase inhibitors have been started. At the molecular level it was observed that AG337, polyglutamates of ZD1694, and multitargeted antifolate enhanced the binding of FdUMP to thymidylate synthase;[624] this was associated with an additive cytotoxicity, DNA damage, and thymidylate synthase inhibition in several colon cancer cell lines, similar to sequential studies of ZD1694 followed by 5-fluorouracil.[625] Such studies have formed the basis for ongoing clinical studies, which indicate a response rate higher than that for either agent alone.

Previous preclinical and clinical studies with 5-fluorouracil and cisplatin indicated a potential beneficial effect of the combination, although the results were contradictory, possibly depending on the mechanism of interaction and the tumour type.[626] Continuous infusion of 5-fluorouracil with cisplatin is effective in head and neck cancer, but not in colon cancer.[627] However, a new platinum analogue, oxaliplatin, was active as a single agent in colon cancer and did not show renal toxicity.[628] Oxaliplatin in combinations was superior to various other treatment regimens. Oxaliplatin was synergistic with 5-fluorouracil in preclinical studies, and the combination entered clinical development.[629],[630] The most impressive results were obtained by Levi *et al.* who included oxaliplatin in a chronotherapy trial with leucovorin and 5-fluorouracil (peak at night), resulting in a response rate of 55 per cent compared with 29 per cent for flat infusion.[351] Oxaliplatin is also being evaluated in other schedules with 5-fluorouracil, which all indicate a positive of effect of the combination, compared with several leucovorin–5-fluorouracil schedules.

Another compound which shows a favorable effect in combination with 5-fluorouracil is irinotecan, a topoisomerase I inhibitor, which as a single agent has a similar response rate in colorectal cancer to 5-fluorouracil. Irinotecan is converted to its active metabolite SN-38. Generally irinotecan followed by 5-fluorouracil was highly synergistic in the *in vitro* studies, while simultaneous addition was additive; the reverse sequence gave contradictory results.[631]–[635] *In vivo* studies with colon cancer xenografts showed no effect or additivity at simultaneous administration, but sequential administration resulted in a better antitumour effect than each compound alone. Guichard *et al.* demonstrated that pretreatment with irinotecan prolonged thymidylate synthase inhibition.[633] Irinotecan induced a blockage of cells in the S phase, which increased the incorporation of 5-fluorouracil into DNA. DNA damage was increased in the schedule in which irinotecan was administered before 5-fluorouracil.[635] 5-Fluorouracil given before irinotecan, however, increased the uptake of irinotecan into HT29 cells.[633] Substantial evidence therefore exists that irinotecan and 5-fluorouracil can be synergistic and that the effect may be related to thymidylate synthase.

In clinical studies the combined use of irinotecan and 5-fluorouracil regimens resulted in a response rate higher than that for either agent alone.[224],[304] The administration of irinotecan before 5-fluorouracil seemed to be preferable to that of 5-fluorouracil before irinotecan, which is in line with the preclinical results. Topoisomerase inhibitors can also be combined with Raltitrexed; preclinical studies indicated that sequential exposure to SN-38 followed by Ralitrexed produced synergistic toxicity.[636] Interestingly this sequence (the topoisomerase inhibitor last) was also optimal for most of the combinations.

Cytarabine combinations

An interesting combination is that of fludarabine and cytarabine; both compounds require activation catalysed by deoxycytidine kinase. Fludarabine can increase the activity of this enzyme thus leading to an increase in ara-CTP accumulation, whereas the triphosphate of the purine analogue is a potent inhibitor of ribonucleotide reductase. In leukaemic lymphocytes from patients with chronic lymphocytic leukaemia the fludarabine-induced increase in ara-CTP was 1.5-fold and 1.8-fold in leukaemic acute lymphoblastic leukaemia cells, with no effect on plasma cytarabine concentration, deamination, or elimination of cellular ara-CTP.[637],[638] In addition to the potentiating effects of fludarabine it has also been demonstrated that growth factors can enhance the cytotoxic effect of ara-C;[411],[639],[640] granulocyte/monocyte colony stimulating factor is particularly effective in this respect, resulting in increased accumulation of ara-CTP and increased incorporation into DNA.[411],[640] The combination of granulocyte/monocyte colony stimulating factor, fludarabine, and ara-C (the FLAG regimen) is one of the most active regimens in acute myeloid leukaemia, with response rates of up to 70 per cent.

It has been shown that deoxycytidine may selectively inhibit phosphorylation of ara-C in normal bone marrow cells and to a lesser extent in leukaemic cells.[641]–[643] Concentrations of deoxycytidine which increase to up to 10 µM in plasma during chemotherapy may be high enough to inhibit phosphorylation of ara-C.[643] In vitro this difference enabled protection from cytarabine by deoxycytidine of normal myeloid progenitor cells, but not of leukaemic progenitor cells. Administration to patients of levels of deoxycytidine as high as 22 g/m^2/day for 5 days was essentially non-toxic.[644] In combination with deoxycytidine the dose of cytarabine could be increased to 14 g/m^2/day, at which only mild toxicities were observed.[645] These clinical trials in which the metabolism of cytarabine is modulated either in the tumour cell or in normal tissues all need further evaluation.

Gemcitabine combinations

Mechanistic studies on gemcitabine demonstrated that the drug affects DNA repair mechanisms. These properties make gemcitabine an ideal candidate for combination with anticancer agents which either cause direct damage to DNA or form DNA adducts. Preclinical studies clearly demonstrated synergism between gemcitabine and cisplatin in ovarian, non-small cell lung cancer, head and neck cancer, and colon cancer cell lines.[450],[646]–[650] Gemcitabine increased the formation of DNA–platinum adducts but, in the combination, the accumulation of gemcitabine triphosphate was decreased. However, cisplatin induced an increase in incorporation of gemcitabine into DNA, which was related to the extent of DNA–platinum adduct formation.[450] In cisplatin-resistant cell lines a decreased repair of DNA–platinum adducts was observed in gemcitabine-treated cells. Pretreatment with gemcitabine generally gave the best results. In vivo studies with head and neck xenografts, murine colon, and non-small cell lung cancer also demonstrated an at least additive, and in some lines a more than additive, effect of gemcitabine and cisplatin.[647],[651],[652]

Following the studies with cisplatin, many other drugs have been evaluated for their potential synergistic interaction with gemcitabine. Additive to slightly synergistic effects have been observed for etoposide, vindesine, topotecan, mitomycin-C, 5-fluorouracil, multitargeted antifolate, and taxol, but usually the effects were less pronounced.[457],[587],[648],[649],[653],[654] For etoposide the effects may be related

to repair of DNA damage.[653] Gemcitabine induced a decrease in dUMP concentration, which may explain a synergistic effect with 5-fluorouracil and multitargeted antifolate.[587] Gemcitabine is a potent radiosensitizer; an effect which is postulated to be related to the decrease in dATP.[478],[654] Although the extent of radiosensitization correlated with the decrease in dATP it is possibly one major factor but not an ultimate determinant.[459]

In addition to the above-mentioned mechanistic interaction, gemcitabine and cisplatin have non-overlapping toxicity patterns and are both active in non-small cell lung cancer. Several phase I and II studies have been performed, which consistently showed a better effect for the combination (a response rate of up 58 per cent) compared with each drug alone (response rates of about 20 per cent).[470],[479],[655],[656] This is in excellent agreement with the preclinical studies.[587] Gemcitabine–cisplatin is now considered to be one of the better treatment options for non-small cell lung cancer, but the combination has also shown good results in the treatment of bladder cancer, ovarian cancer, and pancreatic cancer. Gemcitabine and cisplatin have a schedule-dependent pharmacokinetic interaction. In white blood cells cisplatin increased the accumulation of gemcitabine triphosphate when given 24 h before gemcitabine, whereas retention of DNA–platinum adducts tended to be increased when gemcitabine was given before cisplatin.[477]

Other clinical combinations include paclitaxel, doxorubicin, etoposide, and 5-fluorouracil.[587],[657] Interestingly, paclitaxel increased and shifted the peak of white blood cell gemcitabine triphosphate in a dose-dependent fashion. Clinical studies with gemcitabine as a radiosensitizer are ongoing in various diseases.[658] This application is very much dependent on the dose of gemcitabine and the interval of drug administration and radiation. A short interval and/or high dose of gemcitabine before radiation can result in lethal toxicity. The best efficacy is observed with lower doses of gemcitabine. These studies clearly demonstrate that development of new combinations with gemcitabine will benefit from thorough knowledge of the metabolism, mechanism(s) of action, resistance profile, and the mode of interaction of gemcitabine with other compounds.

Other combinations

The combination of methotrexate and 6-mercaptopurine is common in the treatment of childhood leukaemia, but it has been postulated that the optimal schedule is usually not given.[497],[659] Methotrexate stimulates 6-mercaptopurine metabolism.[659],[660] In a sequential methotrexate–6-mercaptopurine schedule all 59 patients entered remission; three relapsed after 2 to 3 years.[661] Schmiegelow et al. demonstrated that the pharmacokinetics of methotrexate and 6-mercaptopurine may have a significant influence on the risk of relapse;[508] a low accumulation of both thioguanine nucleotides and methotrexate-polyglutamates were related to a shorter event-free survival.

Dipyridamole-based combinations suffer from the complication that dipyridamole itself will be bound in the plasma and might be inactive.[153] The use of other nucleoside transport inhibitors might circumvent this problem. Nucleoside transport inhibitors do not inhibit the uptake of the base 5-fluorouracil, but inhibit the efflux of active nucleosides. Grem and Fischer demonstrated that the enhancing effect of dipyridamole on the activity of 5-fluorouracil was based on the inhibition of the efflux of the 2′-deoxy-5-fluorouridine, thus increasing the intracellular concentration of its monophosphate, FdUMP.[583] In combination with ara-C the nucleoside transport inhibitor should be administered after ara-C in order to permit entry of ara-C and subsequently prevent efflux. In combination with methotrexate and, for example, PALA or acivicin, influx of external nucleosides will be prevented, which can inactivate the drug by supplying alternative precursors for nucleotide synthesis.

References

1. Weber G. Biochemical strategy of cancer cells and the design of chemotherapy: GHA Gloves Memorial Lecture. *Cancer Research*, 1983; **43**: 3466–92.

2. Peters GJ, Veerkamp JH. Purine and pyrimidine metabolism in peripheral blood lymphocytes. *International Journal of Biochemistry*, 1983; **15**: 115–23.

3. Peters GJ, Pinedo HM, Ferwerda W, De Graaf TW, Van Dijk W. Do antimetabolites interfere with the glycosylation of cellular glycoconjugates? *European Journal of Cancer*, 1990; **26**: 516–23.

4. Sasvári-Széleky M, Spasokoukotskaja T, Staub M. Deoxyribocytidine is salvaged not only into DNA but also into phospholipid precursors. IV. Exogenous deoxyribocytidine can be used with the same efficacy as (ribo)cytidine for lipid activation. *Biochemical and Biophysical Research Communications*, 1993; **194**: 966–72.

5. Jansen G, Barr HM, Kathmann I, et al. Multiple mechanisms of resistance to polyglutamatable and lipophilic antifolates in mammalian cells: role of increased folylpolyglutamylation, expanded folate pools, and intralysosomal drug sequestration. *Molecular Pharmacology*, 1999; **52**: 761–9.

6. Wang L, Hellman U, Eriksson S. Cloning and expression of human mitochondrial deoxyguanosine kinase cDNA. *FEBS Letters*, 1996; **390**: 39–43.

7. Hatzis P, Al-Madhoon AS, Jülligs M, Petrakis TG, Eriksson S, Talianidis I. The intracellular localization of deoxycytidine kinase. *Journal of Biological Chemistry*, 1998; **273**: 30239–43

8. Brown JM, Wouters BG. Apoptosis, p53 and tumor cell sensitivity to anticancer agents. *Cancer Research*, 1999; **59**: 1391–9.

9. Farber S, Diamond LK, Mercer RD, Sylvester RF, Wolf JA. Temporary remissions in acute leukemia in children produced by folic acid antagonist, 4-aminopteroyl glutamic acid (aminopterin). *New England Journal of Medicine*, 1948; **238**: 787–93.

10. Jukes TJ. Searching for magic bullets: early approaches to chemotherapy-antifolates, methotrexate. *Cancer Research*, 1987; **47**: 5528–36.

11. Bertino JR. Ode to methotrexate. *Journal of Clinical Oncology*, 1993; **11**: 5–14.

12. Kisliuk RL. Folate biochemistry in relation to antifolate selectivity. In: Jackman AL (ed.) *Antifolate drugs in cancer therapy*. Totowa, NJ: Humana, 1999: 13–36.

13. Bertino JR, Sobrero A, Mini E, Moroson BA, Cashmore A. Design and rationale for novel antifolates. *National Cancer Institute Monographs*, 1987; **5**: 87–91.

14. Jackman AL, Calvert AH. Folate-based thymidylate synthase inhibitors as anticancer drugs. *Annals of Oncology*, 1995; **6**: 871–81.

15. Westerhof GR, Schornagel JH, Kathmann I, et al. Carrier- and receptor-mediated transport of folate antagonists targeting folate-dependent enzymes: correlates of moleculare structure and biological activity. *Molecular Pharmacology*, 1995; **48**: 659–71.

16. Takemura Y, Jackman AL. Folate-based thymidylate synthase inhibitors in cancer chemotherapy. *Anti-cancer Drugs*, 1997; **8**: 3–16.

17. Schornagel JH, Verweij J, De Mulder PHM, et al. Randomized phase III trial of edatrexate versus methotrexate in patients with metastatic and/or recurrent squamous cell carcinoma of the head and neck: a European organization for research and treatment of cancer head and neck cooperative group study. *Journal of Clinical Oncology*, 1995; **13**: 1649–55.

18. Rafi I, Taylor GA, Calvete JA, et al. Clinical pharmacokinetic and pharmacodynamic studies with the non-classical antifolate thymidylate synthase inhibitor 3,4-dihydro-2-amino-6-methyl-4-oxo-5-(4-pyridylthio)-quinazoline dihydrochloride (AG337) given by 24-hour continuous intravenous infusion. *Clinical Cancer Research*, 1995; **1**: 1275–84.

19. Peters GJ, Ackland SP. New antimetabolites in preclinical and clinical development. *Expert Opinion Investigational Drugs*, 1996; **5**: 637–79.

20. Rustum YM, Harstrick A, Cao S, et al. Thymidylate synthase inhibitors in cancer therapy: direct and indirect inhibitors. *Journal of Clinical Oncology*, 1997; **15**: 389–400.

21. Calvert AH, Walling JM. Clinical studies with MTA. *British Journal of Cancer*, 1998; **78**: 35–40.

22. Kaye SB. New antimetabolites in cancer chemotherapy and their clinical impact. *British Journal of Cancer*, 1998; **78**: 1–7.

23. Cocconi G, Cunningham D, van Cutsem E, et al. Open, randomized, multicenter trial of raltitrexed versus fluorouracil plus high dose leucovorin in patients with advanced colorectal cancer. *Journal of Clinical Oncology*, 1998; **16**: 2943–52.

24. Cronstein BN. Molecular therapeutics. Methotrexate and its mechanism of action. *Arthritis and Rheumatism*, 1996; **39**: 1951–60.

25. Schornagel JH, McVie JG. The clinical pharmacology of methotrexate. *Cancer Treatment Reviews*, 1983; **10**: 53–75.

26. Jolivet J, Cowan KH, Curt GA, Clendeninn NJ, Chabner BA. The pharmacology and clinical use of methotrexate. *New England Journal of Medicine*, 1983; **309**: 1094–104.

27. Ackland SP, Schilsky RL. High-dose methotrexate: A critical reappraisal. *Journal of Clinical Oncology*, 1987; **5**: 2017–31.

28. Sirotnak FM. Determinants of resistance to antifolates: biochemical phenotypes, their frequency of occurrence and circumvention. *National Cancer Institute Monographs*, 1987; **5**: 27–35.

29. Gorlick R, Goker E, Trippett T, Waltham M, Banerjee D, Bertino JR. Intrinsic and acquired resistance to methotrexate in acute leukemia. *New England Journal of Medicine*, 1996; **335**: 1041–8.

30. Jackman AL, Judson IR. The new generation of thymidylate synthase inhibitors in clinical study. *Expert Opinion Investigational Drugs*, 1996; **5**: 719–36.

31. Jansen G, Pieters R. The role of impaired transport in (pre)clinical resistance to methotrexate: insights on new antifolates. *Drug Resistance Updates*, 1998; **1**: 211–18.

32. Jansen, G. Receptor- and carrier-mediated transport systems for folates and antifolates. In: Jackman AL (ed.) *Antifolate drugs in cancer therapy*. Totowa, NJ: Humana, 1999: 293–321.

33. Westerhof GR, Jansen G, Van Emmerik N, et al. Membrane transport of natural folate and antifolate compounds in murine L1210 leukemia cells: Role of carrier- and receptor-mediated transport systems. *Cancer Research*, 1991; **51**: 5507–13.

34. Westerhof GR, Rijnboutt S, Schornagel JH, Pinedo HM, Peters GJ, Jansen G. Functional activity of the reduced folate carrier in KB, MA104 and IGROV-I cells expressing folate binding protein. *Cancer Research*, 1995; **55**: 3795–802.

35. Goldman ID, Matherly LH. The cellular pharmacology of methotrexate. *Pharmacological Therapeutics*, 1985; **28**: 77–102.

36. Sirotnak FM. Obligate genetic expression in tumor cells of a fetal membrane property mediating 'folate' transport: biological significance and implications for improved therapy of human cancer. *Cancer Research*, 1985; **45**: 3992–4000.

37. Matherly LH, Taub JW, Ravindranath Y, et al. A. Elevated dihydrofolate reductase and impaired methotrexate transport as

elements in methotrexate resistance in childhood acute lymphoblastic leukemia. *Blood*, 1995; **85**: 500–9.

38. Freisheim JH, Ratnam M, McAlinden TP, *et al*. Molecular events in the membrane transport of methotrexate in human CCRF-CEM leukemia cells. *Advances in Enzyme Regulation*, 1992; **32**: 17–31.

39. Jansen G, Mauritz R, Assaraf YG, *et al*. Regulation of carrier-mediated transport of folates and antifolates in methotrexate-sensitive and resistant leukemia cells. *Advances in Enzyme Regulation*, 1997; **35**: 59–76.

40. Moscow JA, Gong M, He R, *et al*. Isolation of a gene encoding a human reduced folate carrier (RFC1) and analysis of its expression in transport-deficient, methotrexate-resistant human breast cancer cells. *Cancer Research*, 1995; **55**: 3790–4.

41. Belkov VM, Krynetski EY, Schuetz JD, *et al*. Reduced folate carrier expression in acute lymphoblastic leukemia: Mechanism for ploidy but not lineage differences in methotrexate accumulation. *Blood*, 1999; **93**: 1643–50.

42. Ratnam M, Freisheim JH. Proteins involved in the transport of folates and antifolates by normal and neoplastic cells. In: Picciano MF, Stokstad ELR, Gregory JF (ed.) *Folic acid metabolism in health and disease*. New York: Wiley-Liss, 1990: 91–120.

43. Matherly LH. Mechanisms of receptor-mediated folate and antifolate membrane transport in cancer chemotherapy. In: Georgopapadakou NH (ed.) *Drug transport in antimicrobial and anticancer chemotherapy*. New York: Marcel Dekker, 1995: 453–524.

44. Moscow JA. Methotrexate transport and resistance. *Leukemia and Lymphoma*, 1998; **30**: 215–24.

45. Jansen G, Westerhof GR, Jarmuszewski MJA, Kathmann I, Rijksen G, Schornagel JH. Methotrexate transport in variant human CCRF-CEM cells with elevated levels of the reduced folate carrier: selective effect on carrier-mediated transport of physiological concentrations of reduced folates. *Journal of Biological Chemistry*, 1990; **265**: 18272–7.

46. Antony AC. The biological chemistry of folate receptors. *Blood*, 1992; **79**: 2807–20.

47. Jansen G, Schornagel JH, Westerhof GR, Rijksen G, Newell DR, Jackman AL. Multiple transport systems for the uptake of folate-based thymidylate synthase inhibitors. *Cancer Research*, 1990; **50**: 7544–8.

48. Wang X, Shen F, Freisheim JH, Gentry LE, Ratnam M. Differential stereospecificities and affinities of folate receptor isoforms for folate compounds and antifolates. *Biochemical Pharmacology*, 1992; **44**: 1898–902.

49. Ragoussis J, Senger G, Trowsdale J, Campbell IG. Genomic organization of the human folate receptor genes on chromosome 11q13. *Genomics*, 1992; **14**: 423–30.

50. Shen F, Ross JF, Wang X, Ratnam M. Identification of a novel folate receptor, a truncated receptor, and receptor type β in hematopoietic cells: cDNA cloning, expression, immunoreactivity, and tissue specificity. *Biochemistry*, 1994; **33**: 1209–15.

51. Rijnboutt S, Jansen G, Posthuma G, Hynes JB, Schornagel JH, Strous GJAM. Endocytosis of GPI-linked membrane folate receptor-α. *Journal of Cell Biology*, 1996; **132**: 35–47.

52. Anderson RGW, Kamen BA, Rothberg KG, Lacey SW. Potocytosis; sequestration and transport of small molecules by caveolae. *Science*, 1992; **255**: 410–11.

53. Anderson RGW. Caveolae: where incoming and outgoing messages meet. *Proceedings of the National Academy of Sciences of the United States of America*, 1993; **90**: 10909–13.

54. Ross JF, Chaudhuri PK, Ratnam M. Differential regulation of folate receptor isoforms in normal and malignant tissues *in vivo* and in established cell lines. *Cancer*, 1994; **73**: 2432–43.

55. Ross JF, Wang H, Behm FG, Mathew P, Wu M, Booth R, Ratnam M. Folate receptor type b is a neutrophilic lineage marker and is differentially expressed in myeloid leukemia. *Cancer*, 1999; **85**: 348–57.

56. Weitman SD, Lark RH, Coney LR, Fort DW, Frasca V, Zurawski VR, Kamen BA. Distribution of the folate receptor GP38 in normal and malignant cell lines and tissues. *Cancer Research*, 1992; **52**: 3396–401.

57. Weitman SD, Weinberg AG, Coney LR, Zurawski VR, Jennings DS, Kamen BA. Cellular localization of the folate receptor—potential role in drug toxicity and folate homeostasis. *Cancer Research*, 1992; **52**: 6708–11.

58. Garin-Chesa P, Campbell I, Saigo PE, Lewis JL, Old LJ, Rettig WJ. Trophoblast and ovarian cancer antigen LK26. Sensitivity and specificity in immunopathology and molecular identification as as a folate-binding protein. *American Journal of Pathology*, 1993; **142**: 557–67.

59. Reddy JA, Haneline LS, Srour EF, Antony AC, Clapp DW, Low PS. Expression and functional characterization of the β-isoform of the folate receptor on CD34 + cells. *Blood*, 1999; **93**: 3940–8.

60. Campbell IG, Jones TA, Foulkes WD, Trowsdale J. Folate-binding protein is a marker for ovarian cancer. *Cancer Research*, 1991; **51**: 5329–38.

61. Crippa F, Bolis G, Seregni E, Gavoni N, *et al*. Single dose intraperitoneal radioimmunotherapy with the murine monoclonal antibody I-131 MOv18: Clinical results in patients with minimal residual disease of ovarian cancer. *European Journal of Cancer*, 1995; **31A**: 686–90.

62. Canevari S, Stoter G, Arienti F, *et al*. Regression of advanced ovarian carcinoma by intraperitoneal treatment with autologous T lymphocytes retargeted by a specific monoclonal antibody. *Journal of the National Cancer Institute*, 1995; **87**: 1463–9.

63. Kranz DM, Patrick TA, Brigle KE, Spinella MJ, Roy EJ. Conjugates of folate and anti-T-cell receptor antibodies specifically target folate-receptor positive tumor cells for lysis. *Proceedings of the National Academy of Science of the United States of America*, 1995; **92**: 9057–61.

64. Molthoff CFM, Klein-Gebbinck J, Verheijen R, Kenemans P, Jansen G. Membrane folate-receptor mediated binding and internalization of (anti)folate-Mov18-immunoconjugates. *Tumor Targeting*, 1996; **2**: 140–1.

65. Leamon CP, Low PS. Delivery of macromolecules into living cells: a method that exploit folate receptor endocytosis. *Proceedings of the National Academy of Science of the United States of America*, 1991; **88**: 5572–6.

66. Wang S, Lee RJ, Cauchon G, Gorenstein DG, Low PS. Delivery of antisense oligodeoxyribonucleotides against the human epidermal growth factor receptor into KB cells with liposomes conjugated to folate via polyethylene glycol. *Proceedings of the National Academy of Science of the United States of America*, 1995; **92**: 3318–22.

67. Mathias CJ, Wang S, Lee RJ, Waters DJ, Low PS, Green MA. Tumor-selective radiopharmaceutical targeting via receptor-mediated endocytosis of gallium-67-deferoxamine-folate. *Journal of Nuclear Medicine*, 1996; **37**: 1003–8.

68. Reddy JA, Low PS. Folate-mediated targeting of therapeutic and imaging agents to cancers. *Critical Reviews in Therapeutic Drug Carrier Systems*, 1998; **15**: 587–627.

69. Henderson GB, Strauss BP. Characteristics of a novel transport system for folate compounds in wild type and methotrexate-resistant L1210 cells. *Cancer Research*, 1990; **50**: 1709–14.

70. Assaraf YG, Babani S, Goldman ID. Increased activity of a novel low pH folate transporter associated with lipophilic antifolate resistance in Chinese hamster ovary cells. *Journal of Biological Chemistry*, 1997; **273**: 8106–11.

71. Bender RA. The membrane transport of methotrexate. In: Periti P (ed.) *High dose methotrexate, pharmacology, toxicity and chemotherapy*. Firenze: Editrice Giuntina, 1979: 23–35.

72. Henderson GB, Tsjui JM. Transport routes utilized by L1210 cells for the influx and efflux of methotrexate. *Journal of Biological Chemistry*, 1984; **259**: 1526–31.

73. Henderson GB, Tsjui JM, Kumar HP. Characterization of the

individual transport routes that mediate the influx and efflux of methotrexate in CCRF-CEM human lymphoblastic cells. *Cancer Research*, 1986; **46**: 1633–8.

74. Henderson GB, Tsjui JM. Identification of the bromosulphothalein-sensitive efflux route for methotrexate as the site of action of vincristine in the vincristine-dependent enhancement of methotrexate uptake in L1210 cells. *Cancer Research*, 1988; **48**: 5995–6001.

75. Sirotnak FM, O'Leary DF. The issues of transport multiplicity and energetics pertaining to methotrexate efflux in L1210 cells addressed by an analysis of cis and trans effects of inhibitors. *Cancer Research*, 1991;. **51**: 1412–17.

76. Schlemmer SR, Sirotnak FM. Energy-dependent efflux of methotrexate in L1210 leukemia cells—evidence for the role of an ATPase obtained with inside-out plasma membrane vesicles. *Journal of Biological Chemistry*, 1992; **267**: 14746–52.

77. Zhao R, Seither R, Brigle KE, Sharina IG, Wang PJ, Goldman ID. Impact of overexpression of the reduced folate carrier (RFC1), an anion exchanger, on concentrative transport in murine L1210 leukemia cells. *Journal of Biological Chemistry*, 1997; **272**: 21207–12.

78. Dembo M, Sirotnak FM, Moccio DM. Effects of metabolic deprivation on methotrexate transport in L1210 leukemia cells: further evidence for separate influx and efflux systems with different energetic requirements. *Journal of Membrane Biology*, 1984; **78**: 9–17.

79. Saxena M, Henderson GB. Identification of efflux systems for large anions and anionic conjugates as the mediators of methotrexate efflux in L1210 cells. *Biochemical Pharmacology*, 1996; **51**: 975–82.

80. Hooijberg JH, Broxterman HJ, Kool M, et al. Antifolate resistance mediated by the multidrug resistance proteins MRP1 and MRP2. *Cancer Research*, 1999; **59**: 2532–5.

81. Kool M, Van der Linden M, De Haas M, et al. MRP3, an organic anion transporter able to transport anti-cancer drugs. *Proceedings of the National Academy of Science of the United States of America*, 1999; **96**: 6914–19.

82. Cole SP, Bhardwaj G, Gerlach JH, et al. Overexpression of a transporter gene in a multidrug-resistant human lung cancer cell line. *Science*, 1992; **258**: 1650–4.

83. Kool M, de Haas M, Scheffer GL, Scheper RJ, et al. Analysis of expression of cMOAT (MRP2), MRP3, MRP4, and MRP5, homologues of the multidrug resistance-associated protein gene (MRP1), in human cancer cell lines. *Cancer Research*, 1997; **57**: 3537–47.

84. Schlemmer SR, Sirotnak FM. Structural preferences among folate compounds and their analogues for ATPase-mediated efflux by inside-out plasma membrane vesicles derived from L1210 cells. *Biochemical Pharmacology*, 1995; **49**: 1427–33.

85. Assaraf YG, Goldman ID. Loss of folic acid exporter function with markedly augmented folate accumulation in lipophilic antifolate-resistant mammalian cells. *Journal of Biological Chemistry*, 1997; **272**: 17460–6.

86. Nooter K, Westerman MA, Flens MJ, et al. Expression of the multidrug-resistance associated protein (MRP) gene in human cancers. *Clinical Cancer Research*, 1995; **1**: 1301–10.

87. Van Triest B, Pinedo HM, Telleman F, Van der Wilt CL, Jansen G, Peters GJ. Cross-resistance to antifolates in multidrug resistant cell lines with P-glycoprotein or multidrug resistance protein expression. *Biochemical Pharmacology*, 1997; **53**: 1855–66.

88. Den Boer ML, Pieters R, Kazemier KM, et al. Relationship between major vault resistance protein, MRP, P-gp expression and drug resistance in childhood leukemia. *Blood*, 1998; **91**: 2092–8.

89. Wong S, Proefke SA, Bhushan A, Matherly LH. Isolation of human cDNAs that restore methotrexate sensitivity and reduced folate carrier activity in methotrexate-transport defective Chinese hamster ovary cells. *Journal of Biological Chemistry*, 1995; **270**: 17468–75.

90. Williams FMR, Flintoff WF. Isolation of a human cDNA that complements a mutant hamster cell defective in methotrexate uptake. *Journal of Biological Chemistry*, 1995; **270**: 2987–92.

91. Gorlick R, Goker E, Trippett T, et al. Defective transport is a common mechanism of acquired resistance in acute lymphocytic leukemia and is associated with decreased reduced folate carrier expression. *Blood*, 1997; **89**: 1013–18.

92. Jansen G, Mauritz R, Drori S, Sprecher H, et al. A structurally altered human reduced folate carrier with increased folic acid transport mediates a novel mechanism of antifolate resistance. *Journal of Biological Chemistry*, 1998; **273**: 30189–98.

93. Brigle KE, Spinella MJ, Sierra EE, Goldman ID. Characterization of a mutation in the reduced folate carrier in a transport defective L1210 murine leukemia cell line. *Journal of Biological Chemistry*, 1995; **270**: 22974–9.

94. Zhao R, Assaraf YG, Goldman ID. A mutated murine reduced folate carrier (RFC1) with increased affinity for folic acid, decreased affinity for methotrexate, and an obligatory anion requirement for transport function. *Journal of Biological Chemistry*, 1998; **273**: 19065–71.

95. Zhao R, Assaraf YG, Goldman ID. A reduced folate carrier mutation produces substrate-dependent alterations in carrier mobility in murine leukemia cells and methotrexate resistance with conservation of growth in 5-formyltetrahydrofolate. *Journal of Biological Chemistry*, 1998; **273**: 7873–9.

96. Roy K, Tolner B, Chiao JH, Sirotnak FM. A single amino acid difference within the folate transporter encoded by the murine RFC-1 gene selectively alters its interaction with folate analogues—implications for intrinsic antifolate resistance and directional orientation of the transporter within the plasma membrane of tumor cells. *Journal of Biological Chemistry*, 1998; **273**: 2526–31.

97. Gong M, Yess J, Connolly T, et al. Molecular mechanism of antifolate transport-deficiency in a methotrexate-resistant MOLT-3 human leukemia cell line. *Blood*, 1997; **89**: 2494–9.

98. Tse A, Brigle K, Taylor SM, Moran RG. Mutations in the reduced folate carrier gene which confer dominant resistance to 5,10-dideazatetrahydrofolate. *Journal of Biological Chemistry*, 1998; **273**: 25953–60.

99. Tse A, Moran RG. Cellular folates prevent polyglutamylation of 5,10-dideazatetrahydrofolate. *Journal of Biological Chemistry*, 1998; **273**: 25944–52.

100. Matherly LH, Taub JW. Methotrexate pharmacology and resistance in childhood acute lymphoblastic leukemia. *Leukemia and Lymphoma*, 1996; **21**: 359–68.

101. Whitehead VM, Rosenblatt DS,Vuchich MJ, Shuster JJ, Witte A, Beaulieu D. Accumulation of methotrexate and methotrexate polyglutamates in lymphoblasts at diagnosis of childhood acute lymphoblastic leukemia: a pilot prognostic factor analysis. *Blood*, 1990; **76**: 44–9.

102. Whitehead VM, Vuchich MJ, Lauer SJ, et al. Accumulation of high levels of methotrexate polyglutamates in lymphoblasts from children with hyperdipoid (> 50 chromosomes) B-lineage acute lymphoblastic leukemia: A Pediatric Oncology Group study. *Blood*, 1992; **80**: 1316–23.

103. Zhang L, Taub JW, Williamson M, et al. Reduced folate carrier gene expression in childhood acute lymphoblastic leukemia: Relationship to immunophenotype and ploidy. *Clinical Cancer Research*, 1998; **4**: 2169–77.

104. Trippett T, Schlemmer S, Elisseyeff Y, et al. Defective transport as a mechanism of acquired resistance to methotrexate in patients with acute lymphocytic leukemia. *Blood*, 1992; **80**; 1158–62.

105. Rots MG, Willey JC, Jansen G, et al. mRNA expression levels of methotrexate resistance related proteins in childhood leukemia as determined by a standardized competitive template based RT-PCR method. *Leukemia*, 2000; **14**; 2166–75.

106. John W, Picus J, Blanke CD, et al. Activity of multitargeted antifolate

(pemetrexed disodium, LY231514) in patients with advanced colorectal carcinoma: results from a phase II study. *Cancer,* 2000; **88**: 1807–13.

107. Niykiza C, Walling J, Thornton D, Seitz D, Allen R. LY231514 (MTA): relationship of vitamin metabolite profile to toxicity. *Proceedings of the American Society for Clinical Oncology*, 1998; abstract 2139.

108. Schmitz JC, Grindey GB, Schultz RM, Priest DG. Impact of dietary folic acid on reduced folates in mouse plasma and tissues. Relationships to dideazatetrahydrofolate sensitivity. *Biochemical Pharmacology*, 1994; **48**: 319–25.

109. Smith GK, Amyx H, Boytos CM, Duch DS, Ferone R, Wilson HR. Enhanced antitumor activity for the thymidylate synthase inhibitor 1843U89 through decreased host toxicity with oral folic acid. *Cancer Research*, 1995; **55**: 6117–25.

110. Alati T, Worzalla JF, Shih C, *et al.* Augmentation of the therapeutic activity of lometrexol [(6R-)5,10-dideazatetrahydrofolate] by oral folic acid. *Cancer Research*, 1996; **56**: 2331–5.

111. Benkovic SJ. The transformylase enzymes in *de novo* purine biosynthesis. *Trends in Biological Science*, 1984, **9**: 320–2.

112. Matherly LH, Barlowe CK, Philips VM, Goldman ID. The effects of 4-aminoantifolates on 5-formyltetrahydrofolate metabolism in L1210 cells. *Journal of Biological Chemistry*, 1987; **262**: 710–17.

113. Waltham MC, Holland JW, Robinson SC, Winzor DJ, Nixon PF. Direct experimental evidence for competitive inhibition of dihydrofolate reductase by methotrexate. *Biochemical Pharmacology*, 1988; **37**: 535–9.

114. Taira K, Benkovich SJ. Evaluation of the importance of hydrophobic interactions in drug binding to dihydrofolate reductase. *Journal of Medicinal Chemistry*, 1988; **31**: 129–37.

115. McGuire JJ, Hsieh P, Coward JK, Bertino JR. Enzymatic synthesis of folylpolyglutamates. *Journal of Biological Chemistry*, 1980; **255**: 5776–88.

116. Garrow T, Admon A, Shane B. Expression cloning of a human cDNA encoding folylpoly(γ-glutamate) synthetase and determination of its primary structure. *Proceedings of the National Academy of Sciences of the United States of America*, 1992; **89**: 9151–5.

117. Lin BF, Huang RFS, Shane B. Regulation of folate and one-carbon metabolism in mammalian cells. 3. Role of mitochondrial folylpoly-γ-glutamate synthetase. *Journal of Biological Chemistry*, 1993; **268**: 21674–8.

118. Chen L, Qi H, Korenberg J, Garrow TA, Choi YJ, Shane B. Purification and properties of human cytosolic folylpoly-γ-glutamate synthetase and organization, localization, and differential splicing of its gene. *Journal of Biological Chemistry*, 1996; **271**: 13077–87.

119. Pizzorno G, Mini E, Coronnello M, *et al.* Impaired polyglutamylation of methotrexate as a cause of resistance in CCRF-CEM cells after short term, high-dose treatment with this drug. *Cancer Research*, 1988; **48**: 2149–55.

120. McCloskey DE, McGuire JJ, Russell CA, *et al.* Decreased folylpolyglutamate synthetase activity as a mechanism of methotrexate resistance in CCRF-CEM human leukemia sublines. *Journal of Biological Chemistry*, 1991; **266**: 6181–7.

121. Drake JC, Allegra CJ, Moran RG, Johnston PG. Resistance to Tomudex (ZD1694): Multifactorial in human breast and colon carcinoma cell lines. *Biochemical Pharmacology*, 1996; **51**: 1349–55.

122. McGuire JJ, Russell CA. Folylpolyglutamate synthetase expression in antifolate-sensitive and -resistant human cell lines. *Oncology Research*, 1998; **10**: 193–200.

123. Gates S, Worzalla JF, Shih C, Grindey GB, Mendelsohn LG. Dietary folate and folylpolyglutamate synthetase activity in normal and neoplastic murine tissues and human tumor xenografts. *Biochemical Pharmacology*, 1996; **52**: 1477–9.

124. Pizzorno G, Chang Y-M, McGuire JJ, Bertino JR. Inherent resistance of human squamous carcinoma cell lines to methotrexate as a result of decreased polyglutamylation of this drug. *Cancer Research*, 1989; **49**: 5275–80.

125. Braakhuis BJM, Jansen G, Noordhuis P, Kegel A, Peters GJ. Importance of pharmacodynamics in the antiproliferative effect of the antifolates methotrexate and 10-ethyl-10-deazaaminopterin in squamous cell carcinoma of the head and neck. *Biochemical Pharmacology*, 1993; **46**: 2155–61.

126. Lin JT, Tong WP, Trippett TM, *et al.* Basis for natural resistance to methotrexate in human acute non-lymphocytic leukemia. *Leukemia Research*, 1991; **15**: 1191–6.

127. Barredo J, Synold TW, Laver J, *et al.* Differences in constitutive and post-methotrexate folylpolyglutamate synthetase activity in B-lineage and T-lineage leukemia. *Blood*, 1994; **84**: 564–9.

128. Synold TW, Relling MV, Boyett JM, *et al.* Blast cell methotrexate-polyglutamate accumulation *in vivo* differs by lineage, ploidy, and methotrexate dose in acute lymphoblastic leukemia. *Journal of Clinical Investigation*, 1994; **94**: 1996–2001.

129. Masson E, Relling MV, Synold TW, *et al.* Accumulation of methotrexate polyglutamates in lymphoblasts is a determinant of antileukemic effects *in vivo*. *Journal of Clinical Investigation*, 1996; **97**: 73–80.

130. Smith A, Hum M, Winick NJ, Kamen BA. A case for the use of aminopterin in treatment of patients with leukemia based on metabolic studies of blasts *in vitro*. *Clinical Cancer Research*, 1996; **2**: 69–73.

131. Galpin AJ, Schuetz JC, Masson E, *et al.* Differences in folylpolyglutamate synthetase and dihydrofolate reductase expression in human B-lineage versus T-lineage leukemic lymphoblasts: mechanisms for lineage differences in methotrexate polyglutamylation and cytotoxicity. *Molecular Pharmacology*, 1997; **52**: 155–63.

132. Rots MG, Pieters R, Peters GJ, *et al.* Role of folylpolyglutamate synthetase and folylpolyglutamate hydrolase in methotrexate accumulation and polyglutamylation in childhood leukemia. *Blood*, 1999; **93**: 1677–83.

133. Rots MG, Pieters R, Kaspers GJ, *et al.* Differential methotrexate resistance in childhood T- versus common/preB-acute lymphoblastic leukemia can be measured with by an *in situ* thymidylate synthase inhibition assay, but not by the MTT assay. *Blood*, 1999; **93**: 1067–74.

134. Longo GSA, Gorlick R, Tong WT, Ercikan E, Bertino JR. Disparate affinities of antifolates for folylpolyglutamate synthetase from human leukemia cells. *Blood*, 1997; **90**: 1241–5.

135. Fry DW, Anderson LA, Borst M, Goldman ID. Analysis of the role of membrane transport and polyglutamation of methotrexate in gut and Erlich tumor *in vivo* as factors in drug sensitivity and selectivity. *Cancer Research*, 1983; **43**: 1087–92.

136. Fabre I, Fabre G, Goldman ID. Polyglutamylation, an important element in methotrexate cytotoxicity and selectivity in tumor versus murine granulocytic progenitor cell *in vitro*. *Cancer Research*, 1984; **44**: 3190–5.

137. Barredo J, Moran RG. Determinants of antifolate cytotoxicity: folylpolyglutamate synthetase activity during cellular proliferation and development. *Molecular Pharmacology*, 1992; **42**: 687–94.

138. Jolivet J, Chabner BA. Intracellular pharmacokinetics of methotrexate polyglutamates in human breast cancer cells: selective retention and less dissociable binding of 4-NH$_2$-10-CH$_3$-pteroylglutamate4 and 4-NH$_2$-10-CH$_3$-pteroylglutamate 5 to dihydrofolate reductase. *Journal of Clinical Investigations*, 1983; **72**: 773–8.

139. O'Connor BM, Rotundo RF, Nimec Z, McGuire JJ, Galivan J. Secretion of γ-glutamyl hydrolase *in vitro*. *Cancer Research*, 1991; **51**: 3874–81.

140. Yao R, Schneider E, Ryan TJ, Galivan J. Human γ-glutamyl hydrolase: cloning and characterization of the enzyme expressed *in vitro*. *Proceedings of the National Academy of Sciences of the United States of America*, 1996; **93**: 10134–8.

141. Barrueco JR, O'Leary DF, Sirotnak FM. Metabolic turnover of

methotrexate polyglutamates in lysosomes derived from S180 cells. *Journal of Biological Chemistry*, 1992; **267**: 15356–61.

142. **Rhee MS, Wang Y, Nair MG, Galivan J.** Acquisition of resistance to antifolates caused by enhanced γ-glutamyl hydrolase activity. *Cancer Research*, 1993; **53**: 2227–30.

143. **Longo GSA, Gorlick R, Tong WP, Lin S, Steinherz P, Bertino JR.** γ-Glutamyl hydrolase and folylpolyglutamate synthetase activities predict polyglutamylation of methotrexate in acute leukemias. *Oncology Research*, 1997; **9**: 259–63.

144. **Allegra CJ, Hoang K, Yeh GC, Drake JC, Baram J.** Evidence for direct inhibition of *de novo* purine synthesis in human MCF-7 breast cells as a principal mode of metabolic inhibition by methotrexate. *Journal of Biological Chemistry*, 1987; **262**: 13520–6.

145. **Sant ME, Lyons SD, Phillips L, Christopherson RI.** Antifolates induce inhibition of amido phosphoribosyltransferase in leukemia cells. *Journal of Biological Chemistry*, 1992; **267**: 11038–45.

146. **Fabre G, Fabre I, Matherly LH, Cano J, Goldman ID.** Synthesis and properties of 7-hydroxymethotrexate polyglutamyl derivatives in Ehrlich ascites tumor cells *in vitro*. *Journal of Biological Chemistry*, 1984; **259**: 5066–72.

147. **Fabre G, Matherly LH, Fabre I, Cano J, Goldman ID.** Interactions between 7-hydroxymethotrexate and methotrexate at the cellular level in the Ehrlich ascites tumor *in vitro*. *Cancer Research*, 1984; **44**: 970–5.

148. **Sholar PW, Baram J, Seither R, Allegra CJ.** Inhibition of folate-dependent enzymes by 7-OH-methotrexate. *Biochemical Pharmacology*, 1988; **37**: 3531–4.

149. **Houghton PJ.** Thymineless death. In: Jackman AL (ed.) *Antifolate drugs in cancer therapy*. Totowa, NJ: Humana Press, 1999: 423–35.

150. **Jackson RC.** Unresolved issues in the biochemical pharmacology of antifolates. *National Cancer Institute Monographs*, 1987; **5**: 9–15.

151. **Schornagel JH, Leyva A, Pinedo HM.** Is there a role for thymidine in cancer chemotherapy? *Cancer Treatment Reviews*, 1982; **9**: 331–52.

152. **Traut TW.** Physiological concentrations of purines and pyrimidines. *Molecular and Cellular Biochemistry*, 1994; **140**: 1–22.

153. **Peters GJ, Schornagel J, Milano GA.** Clinical pharmacokinetics of antimetabolites. *Cancer Surveys*, 1993; **17**: 123–156.

154. **Peters GJ, Jansen G.** Resistance to antimetabolites. In: Schilsky RL, Milano GA, Ratain MJ (ed.) *Principles of antineoplastic drug development and pharmacology*. New York: Marcel Dekker, 1996: 543–85.

155. **Kunz BA, Kohalmi SE, Kunkel TA, Matthews CK, McIntish EM, Reidy DA.** Deoxyribonucleoside triphosphate levels: a critical factor in the maintenance of genetic stability. *Mutation Research*, 1994; **318**: 1–64.

156. **Blount BC, Mack MM, Wehr CM, et al.** Folate deficiency causes uracil misincorporation into DNA and chromosome breakage: Implications for cancer and neuronal damage. *Proceedings of the National Academy of Sciences of the United States of America*, 1997; **94**: 3290–5.

157. **James SJ, Miller BJ, Basnakian AG, Pogribny IP, Pogribny M, Muskhelishivili L.** Apoptosis and proliferation under conditions of deoxynucleotide pool imbalance in liver of folate/methyl deficient rats. *Carcinogenesis*, 1997; **18**: 287–93.

158. **Aherne GW, Brown S.** The role of uracil misincorporation in thymineless death. In: Jackman AL (ed.) *Antifolate drugs in cancer therapy*. Totowa, NJ: Humana Press, 1999: 409–21.

159. **Berger NA.** Cancer chemotherapy: new strategies for success. *Journal of Clinical Investigation*, 1986; **78**: 1131–5.

160. **Denis N, Kitzis A, Kruh J, Dautry F, Corcos D.** Stimulaton of methotrexate resistance and dihydrofolate reductase gene amplification by c-myc. *Oncogene*, 1991; **6**: 1453–7.

161. **Kwok JBJ, Tattersall MHN.** DNA fragmentation, dATP pool elevation and potentiation of antifolate cytotoxicity in L1210 cells by hypoxanthine. *British Journal of Cancer*, 1992; **65**: 503–8.

162. **Li WW, Fan J, Hochhauser D, et al.** Lack of functional retinoblastoma protein mediates increased resistance to antimetabolites in synthesis in human soft tissue sarcoma cell lines. *Proceedings of the National Academy of Sciences of the United States of America*, 1995; **92**: 10436–40.

163. **Ju JF, Banerjee D, Lenz HJ, et al.** Restoration of wild-type p53 activity in p53-null HL-60 cells confers multidrug sensitivity. *Clinical Cancer Research*, 1998; **4**: 1315–22.

164. **Lowe SW, Ruley HE, Jacks T, Housman DE.** p53-dependent apoptosis modulates the cytotoxicity of anticancer agents. *Cell*, 1993; **74**: 957–67.

165. **Lowe SW, Bodis S, McClatchey A, et al.** p53 status and the efficacy of anticancer therapy *in vivo*. *Science*, 1994; **266**: 807–10.

166. **Pritchard DM, Hickman JA.** Genetic determinants of cell death and toxicity. In: Jackman AL (ed.) *Antifolate drugs in cancer therapy*. Totowa, NJ: Humana Press, 1999: 437–51.

167. **Stoller RG, Hande KR, Jacobs SA, Rosenberg SA, Chabner BA.** Use of plasma pharmacokinetics to predict and prevent methotrexate toxicity. *New England Journal of Medicine*, 1977; **297**: 630–4.

168. **Relling MV, Fairclough D, Ayers D, et al.** Patient characteristics associated with high-risk methotrexate concentrations and toxicity. *Journal of Clinical Oncology*, 1994; **12**: 1667–72.

169. **Evans WE, Relling M, Rodman JH, Crom WR, Boyett JM, Pui CH.** Conventional compared with individualized chemotherapy for childhood acute lymphoblastic leukemia. *New England Journal of Medicine*, 1998; **338**: 499–505.

170. **Rubnitz JE, Relling MV, Harrison PL, et al.** Transient encephalopathy following high-dose methotrexate treatment in childhood acute lymphoblastic leukemia. *Leukemia*, 1998; **12**: 1176–81.

171. **Mahoney DH, Shuster JJ, Nitschke R, et al.** Intermediate-dose intravenous methotrexate with intravenous mercaptopurine is superior to repetitive low-dose oral methotrexate with intravenous mercaptopurine for children with lower-risk B-lineage acute lymphoblastic leukemia: A Pediatric Oncology Group phase III trial. *Journal of Clinical Oncology*, 1998; **16**: 246–54.

172. **Mahoney DH, Shuster JJ, Nitschke R, et al.** Acute neurotoxicity in children with B-precursor acute lymphoid leukemia: An association with intermediate-intravenous methotrexate and intrathecal triple therapy—a Pediatric Oncology Group study. *Journal of Clinical Oncology*, 1998; **16**: 1712–22.

173. **Tjaden UR, De Bruijn EA.** Chromatographic analysis of anticancer drugs. *Journal of Chromatography—Biomedical Applications*, 1990; **531**: 235–94.

174. **Chu E, Allegra CJ.** Antifolates. In: Chabner BA, Longo DL (ed.) *Cancer chemotherapy and biotherapy*. Philadelphia, PA: Lippincott Raven, 1996: 109–48.

175. **Gorlick R, Bertino JR.** Clinical pharmacology and resistance to dihydrofolate reductase inhibitors. In: Jackman AL (ed.) *Antifolate drugs in cancer therapy*. Totowa, NJ: Humana Press, 1999: pp 37–57.

176. **Bleyer WA.** The clinical pharmacology of methotrexate. *Cancer*, 1978; **41**: 36–51.

177. **Borsi JD, Moe PJ.** A comparative study on the pharmacokinetics of methotrexate in a dose range of 0.5 g to 33.6 g/m² in children with acute lymphoblastic leukemia. *Cancer*, 1987; **60**: 5–13.

178. **Balis FM.** Pharmacokinetic drug interactions of commonly used anticancer drugs. *Clinical Pharmacokinetics*, 1986; **11**: 223–35.

179. **Jaffe N.** Recent advances in the chemotherapy of metastatic osteogenic sarcoma. *Cancer*, 1972; **30**: 1627–31.

180. **Kamen BA, Winick NJ.** High dose methotrexate therapy: insecure rationale. *Biochemical Pharmacology*, 1988; **37**: 2713–15.

181. **Henze G, Fengler R, Hartmann R, et al.** Six-year experience with a comprehensive approach to the treatment of recurrent childhood acute lymphoblastic leukemia (ALL-REZ BFM 85). A relapse study of the BFM group. *Blood*, 1991; **78**: 1166–72.

182. **Winick N, Shuster JJ, Bowman WP, et al.** Intensive oral methotrexate

protects against lymphoid marrow relapse in childhood B-precursor acute lymphoblastic leukemia. *Journal of Clinical Oncology*, 1996; **14**: 2803–11.

183. Niemeyer CM, Gelber RD, Tarbell NJ, *et al*. Low-dose high dose methotrexate drug remission induction in childhood acute lymphoblastic leukemia (Protocol 81–01 update). *Blood*, 1991; **78**: 2514–19.

184. Reiter A, Schrappe M, Ludwig WD, *et al*. Chemotherapy in 998 unselected childhood acute lymphoblastic leukemia patients. Results and conclusions of the multicenter trial ALL-BFM 86. *Blood*, 1994; **84**: 3122–33.

185. Chu E, Johnston PG, Grem JL, *et al*. Antimetabolites. *Cancer Chemotherapy and Biological Response Modifiers*, 1994; **15**: 1–31.

186. Borsi JD, Wesenberg F, Stokland T, Moe PJ. How much is too much? Folinic acid rescue dose in children with acute lymphoblastic leukaemia. *European Journal of Cancer*, 1991; **27**: 1006–9.

187. Parker RI, Forman EN, Krumm KF, Abeel MJ, Martin HF. Pharmacokinetics and toxicity of frequent intermediate dose methotrexate infusions. *Therapeutic Drug Monitoring*, 1986; **8**: 393–9.

188. Balis FM, Mirro J Jr, Reaman GH, *et al*. Pharmacokinetics of subcutaneous methotrexate. *Journal of Clinical Oncology*, 1988; **6**: 1882–6.

189. Shapiro WR, Voorhies RM, Hiesiger EM, Sher PB, Basler GA, Lipschutz LE. Pharmacokinetics of tumor cell exposure to [^{14}C] methotrexate after intracarotid administration without and with hyperosmotic opening of the blood–brain barriers in rat brain tumors: A quantitative autoradiographic study. *Cancer Research*, 1988; **48**: 694–701.

190. Storm AJ, Van der Kogel AJ, Nooter K. Effect of X-irradiation on the pharmacokinetics of methotrexate in rats: alteration of blood–brain barrier. *European Journal of Cancer and Clinical Oncology*, 1985; **21**: 759–64.

191. Fry DW, Jackson RC. Biological and biochemical properties of new anticancer folate antagonists. *Cancer and Metastasis Reviews*, 1987; **5**: 251–70.

192. Hum MC, Kamen BA. Folate, antifolates, and folate analogs in pediatric oncology. *Investigational New Drugs*, 1996; **14**: 101–11.

193. Van Triest B, Pinedo HM, Van Hensbergen Y, *et al*. Thymidylate synthase as predictive parameter for sensitivity to 5FU and folate-based TS inhibitors in 13 non-selected colon cancer cell lines. *Clinical Cancer Research*, 1999; **5**: 645–55.

194. Rots MG, Pieters R, Peters GJ, *et al*. Circumvention of methotrexate resistance in childhood leukemia subtypes by rationally designed antifolates. *Blood*, 1999; **94**: 3121–8.

195. Grant SC, Kris MG, Young CW, Sirotnak FM. Edatrexate, an antifolate with antitumor activity: A review. *Cancer Investigation*, 1993; **11**: 36–45.

196. Duch DS, Banks S, Dev IK, *et al*. Biochemical and cellular pharmacology of 1843U89, a novel benzoquinazoline inhibitor of thymidylate synthase. *Cancer Research*, 1993; **53**: 810–18.

197. Jackman AL, Taylor GA, Gibson W, *et al*. ICI D1694, a quinazoline antifolate thymidylate synthase inhibitor that is a potent inhibitor of L1210 tumor cell growth *in vitro* and *in vivo*: A new agent for clinical study. *Cancer Research*, 1991; **51**: 5579–86.

198. Jackman AL, Kelland LR, Kimbell R, *et al*. Mechanisms of acquired resistance to the quinazoline thymidylate synthase inhibitor ZD1694 (Tomudex) in one mouse and three human cell lines. *British Journal of Cancer*, 1995; **71**: 914–24.

199. Ratliff AF, Wilson J, Hum M, *et al*. Phase I pharmacokinetic trial of aminopterin in patients with refractory malignancies. *Journal of Clinical Oncology*, 1998; **16**: 1458–64.

200. Mendelsohn LG, Shih C, Schultz RM, Worzalla JF. Biochemistry and pharmacology of glycinamide ribonucleotide transformylase inhibitors: LY309887 and lometrexol. *Investigational New Drugs*, 1996; **14**: 287–94.

201. Mendelsohn LG, Worzalla JF, Walling JM. Preclinical and clinical

202. Boritzki TJ, Bartlett CA, Zhang C, *et al*. AG2034: A novel inhibitor of glycinamide ribonucleotide transformylase. *Investigational New Drugs*, 1996; **14**: 295–303.

203. Shih C, Chen VJ, Gosset LS, *et al*. LY231514, a pyrolo[2,3-d]-pyrimidine-based antifolate that inhibits multiple folate-requiring enzymes. *Cancer Research*, 1997; **57**: 1116–23.

204. Shih C, Thornton DE. Preclinical pharmacology studies and the clinical development of a multitargeted antifolate, MTA (LY231514). In: Jackman AL (ed.) *Antifolate drugs in cancer therapy*. Totowa, NJ: Humana Press, 1999: 183–201.

205. Hughes A, Calvert AH. Preclinical and clinical studies with the novel thymidylate synthase inhibitor nolatrexed dihydrochloride (Thymitaq®, AG337). In: Jackman AL (ed.) *Antifolate drugs in cancer therapy*. Totowa, NJ: Humana Press, 1999: 229–41.

206. Hughes LR, Stephens TC, Boyle FT, Jackman AL. Ratitrexed (Tomudex®), a highly polyglutamatable antifolate thymidylate synthase inhibitor: design and preclinical activity. In: Jackman AL (ed.) *Antifolate drugs in cancer therapy*. Totowa, NJ: Humana Press, 1999: 147–65.

207. Rhee MS, Galivan J, Wright JE, Rosowsky A. Biochemical studies on PT523, a potent nonpolyglutamatable antifolate, in cultured cells. *Molecular Pharmacology*, 1994; **45**: 783–91.

208. Jackman AL, Kimbell R, Aherne GW, *et al*. The cellular pharmacology of an *in vivo* activity of a new anticancer agent, ZD9331: A water-soluble, non-polyglutamatable quinazoline-based inhibitors of thymidylate synthase. *Clinical Cancer Research*, 1997; **3**: 911–22.

209. Rosowsky A. Development of nonpolyglutamatable DHFR inhibitors. In: Jackman AL (ed.) *Antifolate drugs in cancer therapy*. Totowa, NJ: Humana Press, 1999: 59–100.

210. Boyle FT, Stephens TC, Averbuch SD, Jackman AL. ZD9331: preclinical and clinical studies. In: Jackman AL (ed.) *Antifolate drugs in cancer therapy*. Totowa, NJ: Humana Press, 1999: 243–60.

211. Varney MD, Marzoni GP, Palmer CL, *et al*. Crystal-structure-based design and synthesis of benz<cd>indole-containing inhibitors of thymidylate dynthase. *Journal of Medicinal Chemistry*, 1992; **35**: 663–76.

212. Li WW, Tong WP, Bertino JR. Antitumor activity of antifolate inhibitors of thymidylate and purine synthesis in human soft tissue sarcoma cell lines with intrinsic resistance to methotrexate. *Clinical Cancer Research*, 1995; **1**: 631–6.

213. Mauritz R, Bekkenk MW, Rots MG, *et al*. *Ex vivo* activity of methotrexate versus novel antifolate inhibitors of dihydrofolate reductase and thymidylate synthase against childhood leukemia cells. *Clinical Cancer Research*, 1998; **4**: 2399–410.

214. Rinaldi DA. Overview of phase I trials of multitargeted antifolate (MTA, LY231514). *Seminars in Oncology*, 1998; **26**: 82–8.

215. O'Dwyer PJ, Nelson K, Thornton DE. Overview of phase II trials of MTA in solid tumours. *Seminars in Oncology*, 1999; **26** (suppl.) 6: 99–104.

216. Guansekara NS, Faulds D. Raltitrexed. A review of its pharmacological properties and clinical efficacy in the management of advanced colorectal cancer. *Drugs*, 1998; **55**: 423–35.

217. Smith GK, Bigley JW, Dev IK, Duch DS, Ferone R, Pendergast W. GW1843, a potent, noncompetitive thymidylate synthase inhibitor: preclinical and preliminary clinical studies. In: Jackman AL (ed.) *Antifolate drugs in cancer therapy*. Totowa, NJ: Humana Press, 1999: 203–27.

218. Moertel CG. Chemotherapy of colorectal cancer. *New England Journal of Medicine*, 1994; **330**: 1136–42.

219. Pinedo HM, Peters GJ. 5-Fluorouracil: Biochemistry and pharmacology. *Journal of Clinical Oncology*, 1988; **6**: 1653–64.

220. Leyland-Jones B, O'Dwyer P. Biochemical modulation: Application of

laboratory models to the clinic. *Cancer Treatment Reports*, 1986; **70**: 219–29.

221. Peters GJ, Van Groeningen CJ, Laurensse EJ, Pinedo HM. A comparison of 5-fluorouracil metabolism in human colorectal cancer and colon mucosa. *Cancer*, 1991; **68**: 1903–9.

222. Weckbecker G. Biochemical pharmacology and analysis of fluoropyrimidines alone and in combination with modulators. *Pharmacology and Therapeutics*, 1991; **50**: 367–424.

223. Peters GJ, Köhne CH. Fluoropyrimidines as antifolate drugs. In: Jackman AL (ed.) *Antifolate drugs in cancer therapy*. Totowa, NJ: Humana Press, 1999: 101–45.

224. Griffith DA, Jarvis SM. Nucleoside and nucleobase transport systems of mammalian cells. *Biochimica et Biophysica Acta*, 1996; **1286**: 153–81.

225. Sköld O. Studies on resistance against 5-fluorouracil. IV Evidence for an altered uridine kinase in resistant cells. *Biochimica et Biophysica Acta*, 1963; **73**: 160–2.

226. Reichard P, Sköld O, Klein G, Revesz L, Magnussen P-H. Studies on resistance against 5-fluorouracil. I Enzymes of the uracil pathway during development of resistance. *Cancer Research*, 1962; **22**: 235–43.

227. Tezuka M, Sugiyama H, Tamemasa O, Inara M. Biochemical characteristics of a 5-fluorouracil-resistant subline of P388 leukemia. *Japanese Journal of Cancer Research (GANN)*, 1982; **73**: 70–6.

228. Reyes P, Hall TC. Synthesis of 5-fluorouridine 5′-phosphate by a pyrimidine phosphoribosyltransferase of mammalian origin. II. Correlation between the tumor levels of the enzyme and the 5-fluorouracil-promoted increase in survival in tumor-bearing mice. *Biochemical Pharmacology*, 1969; **18**: 2587–90.

229. Kessel D, Hall TC. Wodinsky I. Nucleotide formation as a determinant in 5-fluorouracil response in mouse leukemias. *Science*, 1966; **145**: 911–13.

230. Schwartz PM. Moir RD, Hyde CM, Turek PJ, Handschumacher RE. Role of uridine phosphorylase in the anabolism of 5-fluorouracil. *Biochemical Pharmacology*, 1985; **34**: 3585–9.

231. Houghton JA, Houghton PJ. Elucidation of pathways of 5-fluorouracil metabolism in xenografts of human colorectal adenocarcinoma. *European Journal of Cancer and Clinical Oncology*, 1983; **19**: 807–15.

232. Ardalan B, Villacorte D, Heck D, Corbett T. Phosphoribosyl pyrophosphate, pool size and tissue levels as a determinant of 5-fluorouracil response in murine colonic adenocarcinomas. *Biochemical Pharmacology*, 1982; **31**: 1989–92.

233. Peters GJ, Laurensse E, Leyva A, Lankelma J, Pinedo HM. Sensitivity of human, murine and rat cells to 5-fluouracil and 5′-deoxy-5-fluouridine in relation to drug-metabolizing enzymes. *Cancer Research*, 1986; **46**: 20–8.

234. Peters GJ, Laurensse E, Leyva A, Pinedo HM. Purine nucleosides as cell-specific modulators of 5-fluorouracil metabolism and cytotoxicity. *European Journal of Cancer and Clinical Oncology*, 1987; **23**: 1869–81.

235. Holland SK, Bergman AM, Zhao Y, Adams ER, Pizzorno G. ¹⁹F NMR monitoring of in vitro tumor metabolism after biochemical modulation of 5-fluorouracil by the uridine phosphorylase inhibitor 5-benzylacyclouridine. *Magnetic Resonance in Medicine*, 1997; **38**: 907–16.

236. Peters GJ, Lankelma J, Kok RM, et al. Prolonged retention of high concentrations of 5-fluorouracil in human and murine tumors as compared with plasma. *Cancer Chemotherapy and Pharmacology*, 1993; **31**: 269–76.

237. Koenig H, Patel A. Biochemical basis for fluorouracil neurotoxicity. *Archives of Neurology*, 1970; **23**: 155–60.

238. Okeda R, Shibutani M, Matsuo T, Kuroiwa T, Shimokawa R, Tajima T. Experimental neurotoxicity of 5-fluorouracil and its derivatives is due to poisoning by the monofluorinated organic metabolites, monofluoroacetic acid and α-fluoro-β-alanine. *Acta Neuropathologica*, 1990; **81**: 66–73.

239. Sweeny DJ, Barnes S, Heggie G, Diasio RB. Metabolism of 5-fluorouracil to an *N*-cholyl-2-fluoro-β-alanine conjugate: previously unrecognized role for bile acids in drug conjugation. *Proceedings of the National Academy of Sciences of the United States of America*, 1987; **84**: 5439–43.

240. Malet-Martino M-C, Bernadou J, Martino R, Armand JP. ¹⁹F NMR spectrometry evidence for bile acid conjugates of α-fluoro-β-alanine as the main biliary metabolites of antineoplastic fluoropyrimidines in humans. *Drug Metabolism and Disposition*, 1987; **16**: 78–84.

241. Zhang R, Barnes S, Diasio R. Disposition and metabolism of 2-fluoro-beta-alanine conjugates of bile acids following secretion into bile. *Biochimica et Biophysica Acta*, 1991; **1096**: 179–86.

242. Naguib FNM, El Kouni MH, Cha S. Enzymes of uracil catabolism in normal and neoplastic human tissues. *Cancer Research*, 1985; **45**: 5405–12.

243. Ho DH, Townsend L, Luna ML, Bodey GP. Distribution and inhibition of dihydrouracil dehydrogenase activities in human tissues using 5-fluorouracil as a substrate. *Anticancer Research*, 1986; **6**: 781–4.

244. Wolf W, Presant CA, Servis KL, et al. Tumor trapping of 5-fluorouracil: In vivo ¹⁹F-NMR spectroscopic pharmacokinetics in tumor-bearing humans and rabbits. *Proceedings of the National Academy of Sciences of the United States of America*, 1990; **87**: 492–6.

245. Woodcock TM, Martin, DS, Damin LAM, Kemeny NE, Young CW. Combination clinical trials with thymidine and fluorouracil: A phase I and clinical pharmacological evaluation. *Cancer*, 1980; **45**: 1135–43.

246. Engelbrecht C, Lungquist I, Lewan L, Ynger T. Modulation of 5-fluorouracil metabolism by thymidine: In vivo and in vitro studies on RNA-directed effects in rat liver and rat hepatoma. *Biochemical Pharmacology*, 1984; **33**: 745–50.

247. Tuchman M, Stoeckeler JS, Kiang DT, O'Dea RF, Ramnaraine ML, Mirkin BL. Familial pyrimidinemia and pyrimidimuria associated with fluorouracil toxicity. *New England Journal of Medicine*, 1985; **313**: 245–9.

248. Harris B, Carpenter J, Diasio R. Severe 5-fluorouracil toxicity secondary to dihydropyrimidine dehydrogenase deficiency—a potentially more common pharmacogenetic syndrome. *Cancer*, 1991; **68**: 499–501.

249. Milano G, Etienne M-C. Individualizing therapy with 5-fluorouracil related to dihydropyrimidine dehydrogenase: Theory and limits. *Therapeutic Drug Monitoring*, 1996; **18**: 335–40.

250. Daher GC, Naguib FNM, El Kouni MH, Zhang R, Soong SJ, Diasio RB. Inhibition of fluoropyrimidine catabolism by benzyloxybenzyluracil: Possible relevance to regional chemotherapy. *Biochemical Pharmacology*, 1991; **41**: 1887–93.

251. Porter DJT, Chestnut WG, Merrill BM, Spector T. Mechanism-based inactivation of dihydropyrimidine dehydrogenase by 5-ethynyluracil. *Journal of Biological Chemistry*, 1992; **267**: 5236–42.

252. Porter DJT, Spector T. Dihydropyrimidine dehydrogenase—kinetic mechanism for reduction of uracil by NADPH. *Journal of Biological Chemistry*, 1993; **268**: 19321–7.

253. Shirasaka T, Nakano K, Takechi T, et al. Antitumor activity of 1 M Tegafur–0.4 M 5-chloro-2,4-dihydroxypyridine–1 M potassium oxonate (S-1) against human colon carcinoma orthotopically implanted into nude rats. *Cancer Research*, 1996; **56**: 2602–6.

254. Danenberg PV. Thymidylate synthetase—a target enzyme in cancer chemotherapy. *Biochimica et Biophysica Acta*, 1977; **473**: 73–92.

255. Carreras CW, Santi DV. The catalytic mechanism and structure of thymidylate synthase. *Annual Reviews of Biochemistry*, 1995; **64**: 721–62.

256. Berger SH, Hakala MT. Relationship of dUMP and FdUMP pools to inhibition of thymidylate synthase by 5-fluorouracil. *Molecular Pharmacology*, 1984; **25**: 303–9.

257. Houghton JA, Torrance PM, Radparvar S, Williams LG, Houghton PJ. Binding of 5-fluorodeoxyuridylate to thymidylate synthase in human colon adenocarcinoma xenografts. *European Journal of Cancer and Clinical Oncology*, 1986; **22**: 505–10.

258. Van der Wilt CL, Pinedo HM, De Jong M, Peters GJ. Effect of folate diastereoisomers on the binding of 5-fluoro-2'-deoxyuridine-5'-monophosphate to thymidylate synthase. *Biochemical Pharmacology*, 1993; **45**: 1177–9.

259. Radparvar S, Houghton PJ, Houghton JA. Effect of polyglutamylation of 5,10-methylenetetrahydrofolate on the binding of 5-fluoro-2'-deoxyuridylate to thymidylate synthase purified from a human colon adenocarcinoma xenograft. *Biochemical Pharmacology*, 1989; **38**: 335–42.

260. Bapat AR, Zarov C, Danenberg PV. Human leukemic cells resistant to 5-fluoro-2'deoxyuridine contain a thymidylate synthase with lower affinity for nucleotides. *Journal of Biological Chemistry*, 1983; **258**: 4130–6.

261. Priest DG, Ledford SE, Doig MT. Increased thymidylate synthetase in 5-fluorodeoxyuridine resistant cultured hepatoma cells. *Biochemical Pharmacology*, 1980; **29**: 1549–53.

262. Berger SH, Barbour KW, Berger FG. A naturally occurring variation in thymidylate synthase structure is associated with a reduced response to 5-fluoro-2'-deoxyuridine in a human colon tumor cell line. *Molecular Pharmacology*, 1988; **34**: 480–4.

263. Spears CP, Gustavsson BG, Berne M, Frosing R, Bernstein L, Hayes AA. Mechanisms of innate resistance to thymidylate synthase inhibition after 5-fluorouracil. *Cancer Research*, 1988; **48**: 5894–900.

264. Yin MB, Zakrzewski SF, Hakala MT. Relationship of cellular folate cofactor pools to the activity of 5-fluorouracil. *Molecular Pharmacology*, 1983; **23**: 190–7.

265. Peters GJ, Van der Wilt CL, Van Groeningen CJ, Meijer S, Smid K, Pinedo HM. Thymidylate synthase inhibition after administration of 5-fluorouracil with or without leucovorin; implications for treatment with 5-fluorouracil. *Journal of Clinical Oncology*, 1994; **12**: 2035–42.

266. Jenh CH, Geyer PK, Baskin F, Johnson LF. Thymidylate synthase gene amplification in fluorodeoxyuridine-resistant mouse cell lines. *Molecular Pharmacology*, 1985; **28**: 80–4.

267. Berger SH, Jenh CH, Johnson LF, Berger FG. Thymidylate synthase overproduction and gene amplification in fluorodeoxyuridine-resistant human cells. *Molecular Pharmacology*, 1985; **28**: 461–7.

268. Clark JL, Berger SH, Mittelman A, Berger FG. Thymidylate synthase overproduction gene amplification in a colon tumor resistant to fluoropyrimidine chemotherapy. *Cancer Treatment Reports*, 1987; **71**: 261–5.

269. Navelgund LG, Rossana C, Muench AJ, Johnson LF. Cell cycle regulation of thymidylate synthetase gene expression in cultured mouse fibroblasts. *Journal of Biological Chemistry*, 1980; **255**: 7386–90.

270. Chu E, Koeller D, Casey J, *et al.* Autoregulation of human thymidylate synthase messenger RNA translation by thymidylate synthase. *Proceedings of the National Academy of Sciences of the United States of America*, 1991; **88**: 8977–81.

271. Chu E, Koeller D M, Johnston PG, Zinn S, Allegra CJ. Regulation of thymidylate synthase in human colon cancer cells treated with 5-fluorouracil and interferon-gamma. *Molecular Pharmacology*, 1993; **43**: 527–33.

272. Keyomarsi K, Samet J, Molnar G, Pardee AB. The thymidylate synthase inhibitor, ICI-D1694, overcomes translational detainment of the enzyme. *Journal of Biological Chemistry*, 1993; **268**: 15142–9.

273. Chu E, Allegra CJ. The role of thymidylate synthase as an RNA binding protein. *Bioassays*, 1996; **18**: 191–8.

274. Lee Y, Johnson LF, Chang LS, Chen Y. Inhibition of mouse thymidylate synthase promoter activity wild-type p53 tumor suppressor protein. *Experimental Cell Research*, 1997; **234**: 270–6.

275. Van der Wilt CL, Pinedo HM, Smid K, Peters GJ. Elevation of thymidylate synthase following 5-fluorouracil treatment is prevented by the addition of leucovorin in murine colon tumors. *Cancer Research*, 1992; **52**: 4922–8.

276. Van Laar JAM, Van der Wilt CL, Smid K, *et al.* Therapeutic efficacy of fluoropyrimidines depends on the duration of thymidylate synthase inhibition in the murine colon 26-b carcinoma tumor model. *Clinical Cancer Research*, 1996; **2**: 1327–33.

277. Peters GJ, Van der Wilt CL, Van Groeningen CJ, *et al.* Effect of different leucovorin formulations on 5-fluorouracil induced thymidylate synthase inhibition in colon tumors and normal tissues from patients in relation to response to 5-fluorouracil. In: Pfleiderer W, Rokos H (ed.) *Chemistry and biology of pteridines and folates (Proceedings of the 11th International Symposium)*. Berlin: Blackwell Science, 1997: 145–50.

278. Swain SM, Lippman ME, Egan EF, Drake JC, Steinberg SM, Allegra CJ. Fluorouracil and high-dose leucovorin in previously treated patients with metastatic breast cancer. *Journal of Clinical Oncology*, 1989; **7**: 890–9.

279. Mandel HG. The target cell determinants of the antitumor actions of 5-FU: does FU incorporation into RNA play a role. *Cancer Treatment Reports*, 1981; **65**: 63–71.

280. Cory JG, Breland JC, Carter GL. Effect of 5-fluorouracil on RNA metabolism in Novikoff hepatoma cells. *Cancer Research*, 1979; **39**: 4905–13.

281. Spiegelman S, Sawyer R, Nayak R, Ritzi E, Stolfi R, Martin DS. Improving the antitumor activity of 5-fluorouracil by increasing its incorporation into RNA via metabolic modulation. *Proceedings of the National Acadamy of Sciences of the United States of America*, 1980; **77**: 4966–70.

282. Houghton JA, Houghton PJ, Wooten RS. Mechanism of induction of the gastrointestinal toxicity in the mouse by 5-fluorouracil, 5-fluorouridine and 5-fluoro-2'-deoxyuridine. *Cancer Research*, 1979; **39**: 2406–13.

283. Glazer RI, Hartman KDA. The effect of 5-fluorouracil on the synthesis and methylation of low molecular weight RNA in L1210 cells. *Molecular Pharmacology*, 1980; **17**: 245–9.

284. Will CL, Dolnick BJ. 5-fluorouracil augmentation of dihydrofolate reductase gene transcripts containing intervening sequences in methotrexate-resistant KB cells. *Molecular Pharmacology*, 1986; **29**: 643–8.

285. Ghosal K, Jacob ST. An alternative molecular mechanism of action of 5-fluorouracil, a potent anticancer drug. *Biochemical Pharmacology*, 1997; **53**: 1569–75.

286. Hryniuk WM, Figueredo A, Goodyear M. Applications of dose intensity to problems in chemotherapy of breast and colorectal cancer. *Seminars in Oncology*, 1987; **14** (suppl. 14): 3–11.

287. Ren Q, Van Groeningen CJ, Hardcastle A, *et al.* Determinants of cytotoxicity with prolonged exposure to fluorouracil in human colon cancer cells. *Oncology Research*, 1997; **9**: 77–88.

288. Peters GJ, Van Dijk J, Laurensse E, *et al. In vitro* biochemical and *in vivo* biological studies of uridine 'rescue' of 5-fluorouracil. *British Journal of Cancer*, 1988; **57**: 259–65.

289. Sawyer RC, Stolfi RL, Spiegelman S, Martin DS. Effect of uridine on the metabolism of 5-fluorouracil in the CD8F1 murine mammary carcinoma system. *Pharmaceutical Research*, 1984; **2**: 69–75.

290. Curtin NJ, Harris AL, Aherne GW. Mechanism of cell death following thymidylate synthase inhibition: 2'-deoxyuridine-5'-triphosphate accumulation, DNA damage, and growth inhibition following exposure to CB3717 and dipyridamole. *Cancer Research*, 1991; **51**: 2346–52.

291. Canman CE, Lawrence TS, Shewach DS, Tang HY, Maybaum J (1993). Resistance to fluorodeoxyuridine-induced DNA damage and cytotoxicity correlates with an elevation of deoxyuridine triphosphatase activity and failure to accumulate deoxyuridine triphosphate. *Cancer Research*, 1993; **53**: 5219–24.

292. Canman CE, Radany EH, Parsels LA, Davis, MA, Lawrence TS, Maybaum J. Induction of resistance to fluorodeoxyuridine cytotoxicity and DNA damage in human tumor cells by expression of *Escherichia coli*. *Cancer Research*, 1994; **54**: 2296–8.

293. Sawyer RC, Stolfi RL, Martin DS, Spiegelman S. Incorporation of 5-fluorouracil into murine bone marrow DNA *in vivo*. *Cancer Research*, 1984; **44**: 1847–51.

294. Shuetz JD, Diasio RB. The effect of 5-fluourouracil on DNA chain elongation in intact bone marrow cells. *Biochemical and Biophysical Research Communications*, 1985; **133**: 361–7.

295. Houghton JA, Morton CL, Adkins DA, Rahman A. Locus of the interaction among 5-fluorouracil, leucovorin, and interferon-alpha-2A in colon carcinoma cells. *Cancer Research*, 1993; **53**: 4243–50.

296. Van der Wilt CL, Smid K, Noordhuis P, Aherne GW, Peters GJ. Biochemical mechanisms of interferon modulation of 5-fluorouracil activity in colon cancer cells. *European Journal of Cancer*, 1997; **33**: 471–8.

297. Ayasawa D, Shimizu K, Koyama H, Takeishi K, Seno T. Accumulation of DNA strand breaks during thymineless death in thymidylate synthase-negative mutants of mouse FM3A cells. *Journal of Biological Chemistry*, 1988; **258**: 12448–54.

298. Houghton JA, Tillman DM, Harwood FG. Ratio of 2′-deoxyadenosine-5′-triphosphate/thymidine-5′-triphosphate influences the commitment of human colon carcinoma cells to thymineless death. *Clinical Cancer Research*, 1995; **1**: 723–30.

299. Houghton JA, Harwood FG, Tillman DM. Thymineless death in colon carcinoma cels is mediated via Fas signalling. *Proceedings of the National Academy of Sciences of the United States of America*, 1997; **94**: 8144–9.

300. Houghton JA, Harwood FG, Bibson AA, Tillman DM. The Fas signaling pathway is functional in colon carcinoma cells and induces apoptosis. *Clinical Cancer Research*, 1997; **3**: 2205–9.

301. Tamura T, Aoyama N, Saya H, *et al*. Induction of Fas-mediated apoptosis in p53-transfected human colon carcinoma cells. *Oncogene*, 1995; **11**: 1939–46.

302. Peters GJ, Van der Wilt CL, Van Groeningen CJ. Predictive value of thymidylate synthase and dihydropyrimidine dehydrogenase. *European Journal of Cancer*, 1994; **30A**: 1408–11.

303. Van Triest B, Peters GJ. Thymidylate synthase: A target for combinations and determinant of chemotherapeutic response in colorectal cancer. *Oncology*, 1999; **57**: 179–94.

304. Leichman L, Lenz H-J, Leichman CG, *et al*. Quantitation of intratumoral thymidylate synthase expression predicts for resistance to protracted infusion of 5-fluorouracil and weekly leucovorin in disseminated colorectal cancers: Preliminary report from an ongoing trial. *European Journal of Cancer*, 1995; **31A**: 1306–10.

305. Leichman CG, Fleming TR, Muggia FM, *et al*. Phase II study of fluorouracil and its modulation in advanced colorectal cancer: A Southwest Oncology Group study. *Journal of Clinical Oncology*, 1995; **13**: 1303–11.

306. Horikoshi T, Danenberg KD, Stadlbauer TH, *et al*. Quantitation of thymidylate synthase, dihydrofolate reductase, and DT-diaphorase gene expression in human tumors using the polymerase chain reaction. *Cancer Research*, 1992; **51**: 108–16.

307. Omura K, Kawakami K, Kanehira E, *et al*. The number of 5-fluoro-2′-deoxyuridine-5′-monophosphate binding sites and the reduced folate pool in human colorectal carcinoma tissues—changes after tegafur and uracil treatment. *Cancer Research*, 1995; **55**: 3897–901.

308. Kornmann M, Link KH, Lenz HJ, *et al*. Thymidylate synthase is a predictor for response and resistance in hepatic artery infusion chemotherapy. *Cancer Letters*, 1997; **118**: 29–35.

309. Davies MM, Johnston PG, Kaur S, Allen-Mersh TG. Colorectal liver metastasis thymidylate synthase staining correlates with response to hepatic arterial floxuridine. *Clinical Cancer Research*, 1999; **5**: 325–8.

310. Lenz H-J, Leichman CG, Danenberg KD, *et al*. Thymidylate synthase mRNA level in adenocarcinoma of the stomach: A predictor for primary tumor response and overall survival. *Journal of Clinical Oncology*, 1996; **14**: 176–82.

311. Johnston PG, Fisher ER, Rockette HE, *et al*. The role of thymidylate synthase expression in prognosis and outcome of adjuvant chemotherapy in patients with rectal cancer. *Journal of Clinical Oncology*, 1994; **12**: 2640–7.

312. Johnston PG, Mick R, Recand W, *et al*. Thymidylate synthase expression and response to neoadjuvant chemotherapy in patients with advanced head and neck cancer. *Journal of the National Cancer Institute*, 1997; **89**: 308–13.

313. Pestalozzi BC, Peterson HF, Gelbert RD, *et al*. Prognostic importance of thymidylate synthase expression in early breast cancer. *Journal of Clinical Oncology*, 1997; **15**: 1923–31.

314. Findlay MPN, Cunningham C, Morgan G, Clinton S, Hardcastle A, Aherne GW. Lack of correlation between thymidylate synthase levels in primary colorectal tumours and subsequent response to chemotherapy. *British Journal of Cancer*, 1997; **75**: 903–9.

315. Ishikawa Y, Kubota T, Otani Y, *et al*. Dihydropyrimidine dehydrogenase activity and messenger RNA level may be related to the antitumor effect of 5-fluorouracil on human tumor xenografts in nude mice. *Clinical Cancer Research*, 1999; **5**: 883–9.

316. Beck A, Etienne MC, Chéradame S *et al*. A role for dihydropyrimidine dehydrogenase and thymidylate synthase in tumor sensitivity to fluorouracil. *European Journal of Cancer*, 1994; **30A**: 1517–22.

317. Etienne MC, Cheradame S, Fischel JL, *et al*. Response to fluorouracil therapy in cancer patients: The role of tumoral dihydropyrimidine dehydrogenase therapy. *Journal of Clinical Oncology*, 1995; **13**: 1663–70.

318. Salonga D, Danenberg KD, Johnson M, *et al*. Colorectal tumors responding to 5-fluorouracil have low gene expression levels of dihydropyrimidine dehydrogenase, thymidylate synthase and thymidine phosphorylase. *Clinical Cancer Research*, 2000; **6**: 1322–7.

319. Etienne MC, Pivot X, Formento JL, *et al*. A multifactorial approach including tumoural epidermal growth factor receptor, p53, thymidylate synthase and dihydropyrimidine dehydrogenase to predict treatment outcome in head and neck cancer patients receiving 5-fluorouracil. *British Journal of Cancer*, 1999; **79**: 1864–9.

320. Lenz HJ, Danenberg KD, Leichman CG, *et al*. p53 and thymidylate synthase (TS) expression in untreated stage II colon cancer: Association with recurrence, survival and tumor site. *Clinical Cancer Research*, 1998; **4**: 1227–34.

321. Lenz HJ, Hayashi K, Salonga D, *et al*. p53 point mutations and thymidylate synthase messenger RNA levels in disseminated colorectal cancer: An analysis of response and survival. *Clinical Cancer Research*, 1998; **4**: 1243–50.

322. Metzger R, Leichman CG, Danenberg KD, *et al*. ERCC1 mRNA levels complement thymidylate synthase mRNA levels in predicting response and survival for gastric cancer patients receiving combination cisplatin and fluorouracil chemotherapy. *Journal of Clinical Oncology*, 1998; **16**: 309–16.

323. El Sayed YM, Sadée W. The fluoropyrimidines. In: Ames MM, Powis G, Kovach JS (ed.) *Pharmacokinetics of anticancer agents in humans*. Amsterdam: Elsevier, 1983: 209–27.

324. Gamelin E, Boisdron-Celle M, Turcant A, Larra F, Allain P, Robert J. Rapid and sensitive high-performance liquid chromatographic analysis of halogenopyrimidines in plasma. *Journal of Chromatography B*, 1997; **695**: 409–16.

325. Ackland SP, Garg MB, Dunstan RH. Simultaneous determination of dihydrofluorouracil and 5-fluorouracil in plasma by high-performance liquid chromatography. *Analytical Biochemistry*, 1997; **246**: 79–85.

326. Van Groeningen CJ, Pinedo HM, Heddes J, *et al*. Pharmacokinetics of 5-fluorouracil assessed with a sensitive mass spectrometric method in patients during a dose escalation schedule. *Cancer Research*, 1988; **48**: 6956–61.

327. Matsushima E, Yoshida K, Kitamura R, Yoshida K-I. Determination of S-1 (combined drug of tegafur, 5-chloro-2, 4-dihydroxypyridine and potassium oxonate) and 5-fluorouracil in human plasma and urine

using high-performance liquid chromatography and gas chromatography-negative ion chemical ionization mass spectrometry. *Journal of Chromatography B*, 1997; **691**: 95–104.

328. Myers CE. The pharmacology of fluoropyrimidines. *Pharmacology Reviews*, 1981; **33**: 1–15.

329. Diasio RB, Harris BE. Clinical pharmacology of 5-fluorouracil. *Clinical Pharmacy*, 1989; **6**: 215–37.

330. Ensminger WD, Rosowsky A, Raso V, *et al.* A clinical pharmacologic evaluation of hepatic arterial infusion of 5-fluoro-2'-deoxyuridine and 5-fluorouracil. *Cancer Research*, 1978; **38**: 3784–92.

331. Collins JM, Dedrick RL, King FG, Speyer JL, Myers CE. Non-linear pharmacokinetic models for 5-fluorouracil in man. *Clinical Pharmacology and Therapeutics*, 1980; **28**: 235–46.

332. Guerquin-Kern J-L, Leteurtre F, Croisy A, Lhoste J-M. pH dependence of 5-fluorouracil uptake observed by in vivo ^{31}P and ^{19}F nuclear magnetic resonance spectroscopy. *Cancer Research*, 1991; **51**: 5770–3.

333. Larsson, P-A, Carlsson G, Gustavsson B, Graf W, Glimelius B. Different intravenous administration techniques for 5-fluorouracil. *Acta Oncologica*, 1996; **35**: 207–12.

334. Glimelius B, Jakobsen A, Graf W, *et al.* Bolus injection (2–4 min) versus short-term (10–20 min) infusion of 5-fluorouracil in patients with advanced colorectal cancer: A prospective randomised trial. Nordic Gastrointestinal Tumour Adjuvant Therapy Group. *European Journal of Cancer*, 1998; **34**: 674–8.

335. De Bruijn EA, Van Oosterom AT, Tjaden UR, Reeuwijk HJEM, Pinedo HM. Pharmacology of 5'-deoxy-5-fluorouridine in patients with resistant ovarian cancer. *Cancer Research*, 1985; **45**: 5931–5.

336. Heggie GD, Sommadossi JP, Cross DS, Huster WJ, Diasio RD. Clinical pharmacokinetics of 5-fluorouracil and its metabolites in plasma, urine and bile. *Cancer Research*, 1987; **46**: 2203–6.

337. Malet-Martino MC, Martino R, Lopez A, *et al.* New approach to metabolism of 5'deoxy-5-fluorouridine in humans with fluorine-19 NMR. *Cancer Chemotherapy and Pharmacology*, 1984; **13**: 31–5.

338. Poorter RL, Peters GJ, Bakker PJM, *et al.* Intermittent continuous infusion of 5-fluorouracil and low dose oral leucovorin in patients with gastrointestinal cancer—relationship between plasma concentrations and clinical parameters. *European Journal of Cancer*, 1995; **31A**: 1465–70.

339. Meta-Analysis Group in Cancer. Efficacy of intravenous continuous infusion of fluorouracil compared with bolus administration in advanced colorectal cancer. *Journal of Clinical Oncology*, 1998; **16**: 301–8.

340. Meta-Analysis Group in Cancer. Toxicity of fluorouracil in patients with advanced colorectal cancer: effect of administration schedule and prognostic factors. *Journal of Clinical Oncology*, 1998; **16**: 3537–41.

341. Lokich JJ, Ahlgren JD, Gullo JJ, Philips JA, Fryer JG. A prospective randomized comparison of continuous infusion fluorouracil with a conventional bolus schedule in metastatic colorectal carcinoma: a Mid-Atlantic Oncology Program study. *Journal of Clinical Oncology*, 1989; **7**: 425–32.

342. Harris BE, Song R, Soong S-J, Diasio RB. Relationship between dihydropyrimidine dehydrogenase activity and plasma 5-fluorouracil levels with evidence for circadian variation of enzyme activity and plasma drug levels in cancer patients receiving 5-fluorouracil by protracted continuous infusion. *Cancer Research*, 1990; **50**: 197–201.

343. Fleming RA, Milano G, Thyss A, *et al.* Correlation between dihydropyrimidine dehydrogenase activity in peripheral mononuclear cells and systemic clearance of fluorouracil in cancer patients. *Cancer Research*, 1992; **52**: 2899–902.

344. Codacci-Pisanelli G, Van der Wilt CL, Pinedo HM, *et al.* Antitumor activity, toxicity and inhibition of thymidylate synthase of prolonged administration of 5-fluorouracil in mice. *European Journal of Cancer*, 1995; **31A**: 1517–25.

345. El Kouni MH, Naguib FNM, Park KS, Cha S, Darnowski JW, Soong

S-J. Circadian rhythm of hepatic uridine phosphorylase activity and plasma concentration of uridine in mice. *Biochemical Pharmacology*, 1990; **40**: 2479–85.

346. Naguib FNM, Soong S-J, El Kouni MH. Circadian rhythm of orotate phosphoribosyltransferase, pyrimidine nucleoside phosphorylases and dihydrouracil dehydrogenase in mouse liver: possible relevance to chemotherapy with 5-fluoropyrimidines. *Biochemical Pharmacology*, 1993; **45**: 667–73.

347. Grem JL, Yee LK, Venzon DJ, Takimoto CH, Allegra CJ. Inter- and intrainvidual variation in dihydropyrimidine dehydrogenase activity in peripheral blood mononuclear cells. *Cancer Chemotherapy and Pharmacology*, 1997; **40**: 117–25.

348. Van Kuilenburg ABP, Poorter RL, Peters GJ, *et al.* No circadian variation of dihydropyrimidine dehydrogenase, uridine phosphorylase, β-alanine and 5-fluorouracil during continuous infusion of 5-fluoruoracil. *Advances in Experimental Medicine and Biology*, 1998; **431**: 815–16.

349. Roemeling RV, Hrushesky WJM (1987). Circadian pattern of continuous FUDR infusion reduces toxicities. *Advances in Chronobiology Part B*, 1987; **227**: 357–73.

350. Lévi F, Zidani R, Misset J-L, for the International Organization for Cancer Chronotherapy. Randomised multicentre trial of chronotherapy with oxaliplatin, fluorouracil, and folinic acid in metastatic colorectal cancer. *The Lancet*, 1997; **350**: 681–6.

351. Van Groeningen CJ, Peters GJ, Schornagel JH, *et al.* Phase I clinical and pharmacokinetic study of oral S-1 in patients with advanced solid tumors. *Journal of Clinical Oncology*, 2000; **18**: 2772–9.

352. Reigner B, Verweij J, Dirix L, *et al.* Effect of food on the pharmacokinetics of capecitabine and its metabolites following oral administration in cancer patients. *Clinical Cancer Research*, 1998; **4**: 941–8.

353. Schilsky RL, Hohneker J, Ratain MJ, *et al.* Phase I clinical and pharmacologic study of eniluracil plus fluorouracil in patients with advanced cancer. *Journal of Clinical Oncology*, 1998; **16**: 1450–7.

354. Hirata K, Horikoshi N, Okazaki M, *et al.* Pharmacokinetic study of S-1, a novel oral fluorouracil anti-tumor drug. *Clinical Cancer Research*, 1999; **5**: 2000–5.

355. Miwa M, Ura M, Nishida M, *et al.* Design of a novel oral fluoropyrimidine carbamate, capecitabine, which generates 5-fluorouracil selectively in tumours by enzymes concentrated in human liver and cancer tissue. *European Journal of Cancer*, 1998; **34**: 1274–81.

356. Ackland SP, Peters GJ. Thymidine phsophorylase: Its role in sensitivity and resistance to anticancer drugs. *Drug Resistance Updates*, 1999; **2**: 205–14.

357. Miwa M, Eda H, Ouchi KF, Keith DD, Foley LH, Ishitsuka H. High susceptibility of human cancer xenografts with higher levels of cytidine deaminase to a 2'-deoxycytidine antimetabolite, 2'-deoxy-2'-methylidenecytidine. *Clinical Cancer Research*, 1998; **4**: 493–7.

358. Kemeny N. Chemotherapy for colorectal carcinoma—one small step forward, one step backward. *Journal of Clinical Oncology*, 1995; **13**: 1287–90.

359. Van Laar JAM, Van Groeningen CJ, Ackland SP, Rustum YM, Peters GJ. Comparison of 5-fluoro-2'-deoxyuridine to 5-fluorouracil; and their role in the treatment of advanced colorectal cancer. *European Journal of Cancer*, 1998; **34**: 296–306.

360. Speyer JL, Collins JM, Dedrick RL, *et al.* Phase I and pharmacological studies of 5-fluorouracil administered intraperitoneally. *Cancer Research*, 1980; **40**: 567–72.

361. Gyves J. Pharmacology of intraperitoneal infusion 5-fluorouracil and mitomycin C. *Seminars in Oncology*, 1985; **12** (suppl. 4): 29–32.

362. Santini J, Milano G, Thyss A, *et al.* 5-FU therapeutic monitoring with dose adjustments leads to an improved therapeutic index in head and neck cancer. *British Journal of Cancer*, 1989; **59**: 287–90.

363. Trump DL, Egorin MJ, Forrest A, Willson, JKV, Remick S, Tutsch

KDA. Pharmacokinetic and pharmacodynamic analysis of fluorouracil during 72-hour continuous infusion with and without dipyridamole. *Journal of Clinical Oncology*, 1991; **9**: 2027–35.

364. Fety R, Rolland F, Barberi-Heyob M, *et al.* Clinical impact of pharmacokinetically-guided dose adaptation of 5-fluorouracil: results from a multicentric randomized trial in patients with locally advanced head and neck carcinomas. *Clinical Cancer Research*, 1998; **4**: 2039–45.

365. Katona C, Kralovanszky J, Rosta A, *et al.* Putative role of dihydropyrimidine dehydrogenase in the toxic side effect of 5-fluorouracil in colorectal cancer patients. *Oncology*, 1998; **55**: 468–74.

366. Kemeny N. Review of regional therapy of liver metastases in colorectal cancer. *Seminars in Oncology*, 1992; **19** (suppl. 3): 155–62.

367. Van Laar JAM, Durrani FA, Rustum YM. Antitumor activity of the weekly intravenous push schedule of 5- fluoro-2′-deoxyuridine +/– N-phosphonacetyl-L-aspartate in mice bearing advanced colon carcinoma 26. *Cancer Research*, 1993; **53**: 1560–4.

368. De Bruijn EA, Van Oosterom AT, Tjaden UR. Site-specific delivery of 5-fluorouracil with 5-deoxy-5-fluorouridine. *Regimens of Cancer Treatment*, 1989; **2**: 61–76.

369. Peters GJ, Braakhuis BJM, de Bruijn EA, Laurensse EJ, van Walsum M, Pinedo HM. Enhanced therapeutic efficacy of 5′deoxy-5-fluorouridine in 5-fluorouracil resistant head and neck tumours in relation to 5-fluorouracil metabolizing enzymes. *British Journal of Cancer*, 1989; **59**: 327–34.

370. Alberto P, Mermillod B, Germano G, *et al.* A randomized comparison of doxifluridine and fluorouracil in colorectal carcinoma. *European Journal of Cancer and Clinical Oncology*, 1988; **24**: 559–63.

371. Frings S, Hoffman-La Roche AG. Capecitabine—a novel oral tumoractivated fluoroupyrimidine. *Onkologie*, 1998; **21**: 451–8.

372. Ishikawa T, Fukase Y, Yamamoto T, Sekiguchi F, Ishitsuka H. Antitumour activities of a novel fluoropyrimidine, N-4-pentyloxycarbonyl-5′-deoxy-5-fluorocytidine (capecitabine). *Biological and Pharmaceutical Bulletin*, 1998; **21**: 713–17.

373. Budman DR, Meropol NJ, Reigner B, *et al.* Preliminary studies of a novel oral fluoropyrimidine carbamate—capecitabine. *Journal of Clinical Oncology*, 1998; **16**: 1795–802.

374. Bolwell BJ, Cassileth PA, Gale RP. High dose cytarabine: a review. *Leukemia*, 1988; **2**: 253–60.

375. Plunkett W, Gandhi V. Pharmacokinetics of arabinosylcytosine. *Journal of Infusional Chemotherapy*, 1992; **2**: 169–76.

376. Plunkett W, Gandhi V. Cellular pharmacodynamics of anticancer drugs. *Seminars in Oncology*, 1993; **20**: 50–63.

377. Rustum YM, Raymakers RAP. 1-Beta-arabinofuranosylcytosine in therapy of leukemia—preclinical and clinical overview. *Pharmacology and Therapeutics*, 1992; **56**: 307–21.

378. Grant S. Ara-C: Cellular and molecular pharmacology. *Advances in Cancer Research*, 1998; **72**: 197–233.

379. Paterson ARP, Kolassa N, Cass CE. Transport of nucleoside drugs in animal cells. *Pharmacology and Therapeutics*, 1981; **12**: 515–36.

380. Sirotnak FM, Barrueco JR. Membrane transport and the antineoplastic action of nucleoside analogues. *Cancer and Metastasis Reviews*, 1987; **6**: 459–80.

381. Mackey JR, Baldwin SA, Young JD, Cass CE. Nucleoside transport and its significance for anticancer drug resistance. *Drug Resistance Updates*, 1998; **1**: 310–24.

382. Wiley JS, Jones SP, Sawyer WH, Paterson ARP. Cytosine arabinoside influx and nucleoside transport sites in acute leukemia. *Journal of Clinical Investigation*, 1982; **69**: 479–89.

383. Capizzi RL, Yang JL, Rathmell JP, *et al.* Dose-related pharmacologic effects of high-dose ara-C and its self-potentiation. *Seminars in Oncology*, 1985; **12** (suppl. 3): 65–75.

384. Peters WG, Colly LP, Willemze R. High-dose cytosine arabinoside: pharmacological and clinical aspects. *Blut*, 1988; **56**: 1–11.

385. Chan TCK. Augmentation of 1-β-D-arabinofuranosylcytosine cytotoxicity in human tumor cells by inhibiting drug efflux. *Cancer Research*, 1989; **49**: 2656–60.

386. Bhalla K, Nayak R, Grant S. Isolation and characterization of a deoxycytidine kinase-deficient human promyelocytic leukemic cell line highly resistant to 1-β-D-arabinofuranosylcytosine. *Cancer Research*, 1984; **44**: 5029–37.

387. Kufe D, Spriggs D, Egan M, Munroe D. Relationships among ara-CTP pools, formation of (ara-C)DNA and cytotoxicity of human leukemic cells. *Blood*, 1984; **64**: 54–58.

388. Bergman AM, Pinedo HM, Jongsma APM, *et al.* Decreased resistance to gemcitabine (2′,2′-difluorodeoxycytidine) of cytosine-arabinoside resistant myeloblastic murine and rat leukemia cell lines: Role of altered activity and substrate specificity of deoxycytidine kinase. *Biochemical Pharmacology*, 1999; **57**: 397–406.

389. Momparler RL, Onetto-Pothier N. Drug resistance to cytosine arabinoside. In: Kessel D (ed.) *Resistance to antineoplastic drugs*. Boca Raton, FL: CRC Press, 1989: 354–67.

390. Townsend A, Cheng YC. Sequence specific effects of ara-5-aza CTP and ara-CTP on DNA synthesis by purified human DNA polymerases *in vitro*: visualisation of chain elongation on a defined template. *Molecular Pharmacology*, 1987; **32**: 330–9.

391. Ross DD, Cuddy DP, Cohen N, Hensley DR. Mechanistic implications of alterations in HL-60 cell nascent DNA after exposure to 1-beta-D-arabinofuranosylcytosine. *Cancer Chemotherapy and Pharmacology*, 1992; **31**: 61–70.

392. Bhalla K, Tang C, Ibrado AM, *et al.* Granulocyte-macrophage colony-stimulating factor/interleukin-3 fusion protein (pIXY-321) enhances high-dose ara-C-induced programmed cell death or apoptosis in human myeloid leukemia cells. *Blood*, 1992; **80**: 2883–90.

393. Brach MA, Herrmann F, Kufe DW. Activation of the AP-l transcription factor by arabinofuranosylcytosine in myeloid leukemia cells. *Blood*, 1992; **79**: 728–34.

394. Brach MA, Kharbanda SM, Herrmann F, Kufe DW. Activation of the transcription factor kB in human KG-1 myeloid leukemia cells treated with 1-β-D-arabinofuranosylcytosine. *Molecular Pharmacology*, 1992; **41**: 60–3.

395. Koo H-M, Monks A, Mikheev A, *et al.* Enhanced sensitivity to 1-β-D-arabinofuranosylcytosine and topoisomerase II inhibitors in tumor cell lines harboring activated ras oncogenes. *Cancer Research*, 1996; **65**: 5211–16.

396. Guedez L, Suresh A, Tung F, Zucali J. Quantitation of resistance to cytosine arabinoside by myeloid leukemic cells expressing bcl-2. *European Journal of Haematology*, 1996; **57**: 149–56.

397. Bullock G, Ray S, Reed JC, *et al.* Intracellular metabolism of ara-C and resulting DNA fragmentation and apoptosis of human AML HL-60 cells possessing disparate levels of bcl-2 protein. *Leukemia*, 1996; **10**: 1731–40.

398. Cheliah J, Freemerman AJ, Wu-Pong S, Jarvis WD, Grant S. Potentiation of ara-C-induced apoptosis by the protein kinase C activator bryostatin 1 in human leukemia cells (HL-60) involves a process dependent upon c-myc. *Biochemical Pharmacology*, 1997; **54**: 563–73.

399. Wang Z, Van Tuyle G, Conrad D, Fisher PB, Dent P, Grant S. Dysregulation of the cyclin-dependent kinase inhibitor p21WAF/CIP1/MDA6 increases the susceptibility of human leukemia cells (U937) to 1-β-D-arabinofuranosylcytosine-mediated mitochondrial dysfunction and apoptosis. *Cancer Research*, 1999; **59**: 1259–67.

400. Fridland A, Verhoef V. Mechanism for ara-CTP catabolism in human leukemic cells and effect of deaminase inhibitors on this process. *Seminars in Oncology*, 1987; **14** (suppl. 1): 262–8.

401. Plunkett W, Hug V, Keating MJ, Chubb S. Quantitation of 1-β-D-arabinofuranosylcytosine 5′-triphosphate in the leukemic cells from

bone marrow and peripheral blood of patients receiving 1-β-D-arabinofuranosylcytosine therapy. *Cancer Research*, 1980; **40**: 588–91.

402. Rustum YM, Preizler HD. Correlation between leukemic cell retention of 1-β-D-ara-binofuranosylcytosine 5′-triphosphate and response to therapy. *Cancer Research*, 1979; **39**: 42–9.

403. Colly LP, Richel DJ, Arentsen-Honders MW, Starrenburg CWJ, Edelbroek PM, Willemze R. A simplified assay for measurement of cytosine arabinoside incorporation into DNA in ara-C-sensitive and -resistant leukemic cells. *Cancer Chemotherapy and Pharmacology*, 1990; **27**: 151–6.

404. Rustum YM, Danhauser L, Luccioni C, Au JLS. Determinants of response to antimetabolites and their modulation by purine and pyrimidine metabolites. *Cancer Treatment Reports*, 1981; **65**: 73–82.

405. Liliemark JO, Plunkett W, Dixon DO. Relationship of 1-β-D-arabinofuranosylcytosine in plasma to 1-β-D-arabinofuranosylcytosine 5′-triphosphate levels in leukemic cells during treatment with high-dose 1-β-D-arabinofuranosylcytosine. *Cancer Research*, 1985; **45**: 5952–7.

406. Hiddemann W, Schleyer E, Unterhalt M, Kern W, Büchner T. Optimizing therapy for acute myeloid leukemia based on differences in intracellular metabolism of cytosine arabinoside between leukemic blasts and normal mononuclear blood cells. *Therapeutic Drug Monitoring*, 1996; **18**: 341–9.

407. Preisler HD, Rustum Y, Priore RL. Relationship between leukemic cell retention of cytosine arabinoside triphosphate and the duration of remission in patients with acute non-lymphocytic leukemia. *European Journal of Cancer and Clinical Oncology*, 1985; **21**: 23–30.

408. Plunkett W, Liliemark JO, Adams TM, *et al.* Saturation of 1-beta-D-arabinofuranosylcytosine 5′-triphosphate accumulation in leukemia cells during high-dose 1-beta-D-arabinofuranosylcytosine therapy. *Cancer Research*, 1987; **47**: 3005–11.

409. Karon M, Chirakawa S. The locus of action of 1-β-D-arabinofuranosylcytosine in the cell cycle. *Cancer Research*, 1970; **29**: 687–96.

410. Powell BL, Wang L-M, Gregory BW, Case LD, Kucera GL. GM-CSF and asparaginase potentiate ara-C cytotoxicity in HL-60 cells. *Leukemia*, 1995; **9**: 405–9.

411. Drenthe-Schonk A, Holdrinet R, Van Egmond J, Wessels H, Haanen C. Cytokinetic changes after cytosine arabinoside in acute myeloid leukemia. *Leukemia Research*, 1981; **5**: 89–96.

412. Colly LP, Peters WG, Richel D, Arentsen-Honders MW, Starrenburg CWJ, Willemze R. Deoxycytidine kinase and deoxycytidine deaminase values correspond closely to clinical response to cytosine arabinoside remission induction therapy in patients with acute myelogenous leukemia. *Seminars in Oncology*, 1987; **14** (suppl. 1): 257–61.

413. Mejer J, Nygaard P. Cytosine arabinoside phosphorylation and deamination in acute myeloblastic leukemia cells. *Leukemia Research*, 1978; **2**: 127–31.

414. Schröder JK, Kirch, C, Flasshove M, *et al.* Constitutive overexpression of the cytidine deaminase gene confers resistance cytosine arabinoside *in vitro*. *Leukemia*, 1996; **10**: 1919–24.

415. Neff T, Blau A. Forced expression of cytidine deaminase confers resistance to cytosine arabinoside and gemcitabine. *Experimental Hematology*, 1996; **24**: 1340–6.

416. Eliopoulos N, Cournoyer D, Momparler RL. Drug resistance to 5-aza-2′-deoxycytidine, 2′,2′-difluorodeoxycytidine, and cytosine arabinoside conferred by retroviral-mediated transfer of human cytidine deaminase cDNA into murine cells. *Cancer Chemotherapy and Pharmacology*, 1998; **42**: 373–8.

417. Jahnsstreubel G, Reuter C, Landwehr UAD, *et al.* Activity of thymidine kinase and of polymerase alpha as well as activity and gene expression of deoxycytidine deaminase in leukemic blasts are correlated with clinical response in the setting of granulocyte-macrophage colony-stimulating factor-based priming before and during TAD-9 induction therapy in acute myeloid leukemia. *Blood*, 1997; **90**: 1968–76.

418. Yang J-L, Cheng EH, Capizzi RL, Cheng Y-C, Kute T. Effect of uracil arabinoside on metabolism and cytotoxicity of cytosine arabinoside in L5178Y murine leukemia. *Journal of Clinical Investigation*, 1985; **75**: 141–6.

419. Piall EM, Aherne W, Marks VM. A radioimmunoassay for cytosine arabinoside. *British Journal of Cancer*, 1979; **40**: 548–56

420. Linssen P, Drenthe-Schonk A, Wessels H, Haanen C. Determination of cytosine arabinoside and uracil arabinoside in human plasma by high performance liquid chromatography. *Journal of Chromatography*, 1981; **332**: 371–8.

421. Fleming RA, Capizzi RL, Rosner GL, *et al.* Clinical pharmacology of cytarabine in patients with acute myeloid leukemia: A Cancer and Leukemia Group B study. *Cancer Chemotherapy and Pharmacology*, 1995; **36**: 425–30.

422. Periclou AP, Avramis VI. NONMEM population pharmacokinetic studies of cytosine arabinoside after high-dose and after loading bolus followed by continuous infusion of the drug in pediatric patients with leukemias. *Cancer Chemotherapy and Pharmacology*, 1996; **39**: 42–50.

423. Herzig RH, Wolff SN, Lazarus HM, Philips GL, Karanis C, Herzig GP. High-dose cytosine arabinoside therapy for refractory leukemia. *Blood*, 1983; **62**: 361–9.

424. Kreis W, Chaudri F, Chan K, *et al.* Pharmacokinetics of low-dose 1-β-D-arabinofuranosylcytosine given by continuous intravenous infusion over twenty-one days. *Cancer Research*, 1985; **45**: 6498–501.

425. Spriggs D, Griffin J, Wisch J, Kufe D. Clinical pharmacological of low dose cytosine arabinoside. *Blood*, 1985; **65**: 1087–9.

426. Papayannopoulou T, Torrealbu de Ron A, Veith R, Knitter G, Stamatoyannopoulous S. Arabinosylcytosine induces fetal hemoglobin in baboons by perturbing erythroid cell differentiation kinetics. *Science*, 1984; **224**: 617–19.

427. Hong CI, Bernacki RJ, Hui S-W, Rustum Y, West CR (1990). Formulation, stability, and antitumor activity of 1-β-D-arabinofuranosylcytosine conjugate of thioether phospholipid. *Cancer Research*, 1990; **50**: 4401–6.

428. Schleyer E, Braess J, Ramsauer B, Unterhalt M, *et al.* Pharmacokinetics of ara-CMP-stearate (YNK01): phase I study of the oral ara-C derivative. *Leukemia*, 1995; **9**: 1085–90.

429. Horber DH, Schott H, Schwendener RA (1995). Cellular pharmacology of N4-hexadecyl-1-β-D-arabinofuranosylcytosine in the human leukemic cell lines K-562 and U-937. *Cancer Chemotherapy and Pharmacology*, 1995; **36**: 483–92.

430. Breistol K, Balzarini J, Sandvold ML, *et al.* Antitumor activity of P-4055 (elaidic acid-cytarabine) compared to cytarabine in metastatic and s.c. human tumor xenograft models. *Cancer Research*, 1999; **59**: 2944–9.

431. Peters GJ, Voorn DA, Kuiper CM, *et al.* Cell specific cytotoxicity and structure-activity relationship of lipophilic 1-β-D-arabinofuranosylcytosine (ara-C) derivatives. *Nucleosides and Nucleotides*, 1999; **18**: 877–8.

432. Balzarini J, Degreve B, Andrei G, *et al.* Superior cytostatic activity of the ganciclovir elaidic acid ester due to the prolonged intracellular retention of ganciclovir anabolites in herpes simplex virus type 1 thymidine kinase gene-transfected tumor cells. *Gene Therapy*, 1998; **5**: 419–26.

433. Glover AB, Leyland-Jones BR. Biochemistry of azacytidine: a review. *Cancer Treatment Reports*, 1987; **71**: 959–64.

434. Glover AB, Leyland-Jones BR, Chun HG, Davies B, Hoth DF. Azacytidine: 10 years later. *Cancer Treatment Reports*, 1987; **71**: 737–46.

435. Richel DJ, Colly LP, Lurvink E, Willemze R. Comparison of the antileukemic activity of 5-aza-2′-deoxycytidine and arabinofuranosylcytosine in rats with myelocytic leukaemia. *British Journal of Cancer*, 1988; **58**: 730–3.

436. Richel DJ, Colly LP, Lurvink E, Willemze R. Activity of 5 aza-2′-deoxycytidine in ara-c-resistant and sensitive leukemia. *Contributions to Oncology*, 1989; **37**: 20–9.

437. Momparler RL, Côté S, Eliopoulos N. Pharmacological approach for optimization of the dose schedule of 5-aza-2′-deoxycytidine (decitabine) for the therapy of leukemia. *Leukemia*, 1997; **11** (suppl. 1): 1–6.

438. Haaf T. The effcts of 5-azacytidine and 5-azadeoxycitidine on chromosome structure and function: implications for methylation-associated cellular processes. *Pharmacology and Therapeutics*, 1995; **65**: 19–46.

439. Hertel LW, Boder GB, Kroin JS, *et al.* Evaluation of the antitumor activity of gemcitabine (2′,2′-defluoro-2′-deoxycytidine). *Cancer Research*, 1990; **50**: 4417–22.

440. Braakhuis BJ, Van Dongen GAMS, Vermorken JB, Snow GB. Preclinical in vivo activity of 2′,2′-difluorodeoxycytidine (gemcitabine) against head and neck cancer. *Cancer Research*, 1991; **51**: 211–14.

441. Boven E, Schipper H, Erkelens CAM, Hatty SA, Pinedo HM. The influence of schedule and the dose of gemcitabine on the anti-tumour efficacy in experimental human cancer. *British Journal of Cancer*, 1993; **68**: 52–6.

442. Veerman G, Ruiz van Haperen VWT, Vermorken JB, *et al.* Antitumor activity of prolonged as compared with bolus administration of 2′,2′-difluorodeoxycytidine *in vivo* against murine colon tumors. *Cancer Chemotherapy and Pharmacology*, 1996; **38**: 335–42.

443. Plunkett W, Huang P, Xu YX, Heinemann V, Grunewald R, Gandi V. Gemcitabine: metabolism, mechanisms of action, and self-potentiation. *Seminars in Oncology*, 1995; **22** (suppl. 11): 3–11.

444. Heinemann V, Hertel LW, Grindey GB, Plunkett W. Comparison of the cellular pharmacokinetics and toxicity of 2′,2′-difluorodeoxycytidine and 1-β-D-arabinofuranosylcytosine. *Cancer Research*, 1988; **48**: 4024–31.

445. Wang L, Munch-Petersen B, Herrstrom Sjoberg A, *et al.* Human Thymidine kinase 2: molecular cloning and characterisation of the enzyme activity with antiviral and cytostatic nucleoside substrates. *FEBS Letters*, 1999; **443**: 170–4

446. Ruiz van Haperen VWT, Veerman G, Eriksson S, *et al.* Development and characterization of a 2′,2′-difluorodeoxycytidine-resistant variant of the human ovarian cancer cell line A2780. *Cancer Research*, 1994; **54**: 4138–43.

447. Huang P, Chubb S, Hertel LW, Grindey GB, Plunkett W. Action of 2′2′-difluorodeoxycytidine on DNA synthesis. *Cancer Research*, 1991; **51**: 6110–17.

448. Ruiz van Haperen VWT, Veerman G, Vermorken JB, Peters GJ. 2′,2′-Difluoro-deoxycytidine (gemcitabine) incorporation into RNA and DNA from tumour cell lines. *Biochemical Pharmacology*, 1993; **46**: 762–6.

449. Van Moorsel CJA, Pinedo HM, Veerman G, *et al.* Mechanisms of synergism between cisplatin and gemcitabine in ovarian and non-small cell lung cancer cell lines. *British Journal of Cancer*, 1999; **35**: 808–14.

450. Huang P, Plunkett W. A quantitative assay for fragmented DNA in apoptotic cells. *Analytical Biochemistry*, 1992; **207**: 163–7.

451. Huang P, Plunkett W. Fludarabine- and gemcitabine-induced apoptosis, incorporation of analogs into DNA is a critical event. *Cancer Chemotherapy and Pharmacology*, 1995; **36**: 181–8.

452. Santini V, Dippolito G, Bernabei PA, Zoccolante A, Ermini A, RossiFerrini P. Effects of fludarabine and gemcitabine on human acute myeloid leukemia cell line HL 60: Direct comparison of cytotoxicity and cellular ara-C uptake enhancement. *Leukemia Research*, 1996; **20**: 37–45.

453. Bouffard DY, Momparler RL. Comparison of the induction of apoptosis in human leukemic cell lines by 2′2′-difluorodeoxycytidine (gemcitabine) and cytosine arabinoside. *Leukemia Research*, 1995; **19**: 849–56.

454. Gruber J, Geisen F, Sgonc R, *et al.* 2′,2′-difluorodeoxycytidine (gemcitabine) induces apoptosis in myeloma cell lines resistant to steroids and 2-chlorodeoxyadenosine (2-CdA). *Stem Cells*, 1996; **14**: 351–62.

455. Cronauer MV, Klocker H, Talasz H, *et al.* Inhibitory effects of the nucleoside analogue gemcitabine on prostatic carcinoma cells. *Prostate*, 1996; **28**: 172–81.

456. Tolis C, Peters GJ, Ferreira CG, Pinedo HM, Giaccone G. Cell cycle disturbances and apoptosis induced by topotecan and gemcitabine on human lung cancer cell lines. *European Journal of Cancer*, 1999; **35**: 796–807.

457. Heinemann V, Xu Y-Z, Chubb S, *et al.* Inhibition of ribonucleotide reduction in CCRF-CEM cells by 2′,2′-difluorodeoxycytidine. *Molecular Pharmacology*, 1990; **38**: 567–72.

458. Shewach DS, Hahn TM, Chang E, Hertel LW, Lawrence TS. Metabolism of 2′2′-difluoro-2′-deoxycytidine and radiation sensitization of human colon carcinoma cells. *Cancer Research*, 1994; **54**: 3218–23.

459. Lawrence TS, Chang EY, Hahn TM, Hertel LW, Shewach DS. Radiosensitization of pancreatic cancer cells by 2′,2′-difluoro-2′-deoxycytidine. *International Journal of Radiation Oncology Biology Physics*, 1996; **34**: 867–72.

460. Heinemann V, Xu Y-Z, Chubb S, *et al.* Cellular elimination of 2′2′-difluorodeoxycytidine 5′-triphosphate, a mechanism of self-potentiation. *Cancer Research*, 1992; **52**: 533–9.

461. Heinemann V. Gemcitabine—a modulator of intracellular nucleotide and deoxynucleotide metabolism. *Seminars in Oncology*, 1995; **22** (suppl. 11): 11–18.

462. Smitskamp-Wilms E, Pinedo HM, Veerman G, Ruiz van Haperen VWT, Peters GJ. Postconfluent multilayered cell line cultures for selective screening of gemcitabine. *European Journal of Cancer*, 1998; **34**: 921–6.

463. Haveman J, Rietbroek RC, Geerdink A, Vanrijn J, Bakker PJM. Effectof hyperthermia on the cytotoxicity of 2′,2′-difluorodeoxycytidine (gemcitabine) in cultured SW1573 cells. *International Journal of Cancer*, 1995; **62**: 627–30.

464. O'Rourke TJ, Brown TD, Havlin K, *et al.* Phase I clinical trial of gemcitabine given as an intravenous bolus on 5 consecutive days. *European Journal of Cancer*, 1994; **30A**: 417–18.

465. Martin C, Lund B, Anderson H, Thatcher N. Gemcitabine: once-weekly schedule active and better tolerated than twice-weekly schedule. *Anticancer Drugs*, 1996; **7**: 351–7.

466. Abbruzzese JL, Grunewald R, Weeks EA, *et al.* A Phase I clinical, plasma, and cellular pharmacology study of gemcitabine. *Journal of Clinical Oncology*, 1991; **9**: 491–8.

467. Vermorken JB, Guastalla JP, Hatty SR, *et al.* Phase I study of gemcitabine using a once overy 2 weeks schedule. *British Journal of Cancer*, 1997; **11**: 1489–93.

468. Lund B, Kristjanssen PEG, Hansen HH. Clinical and preclinical activity of 2′,2′-difluorodeoxycytidine (gemcitabine). *Cancer Treatment Reviews*, 1993; **19**: 45–55.

469. Van Moorsel CJA, Peters GJ, Pinedo HM. Gemcitabine: Future prospects of single-agent and combination studies. *The Oncologist*, 1997; **2**: 127–34.

470. Anderson H, Thatcher N, Walling J, Hansen H. A phase I study of a 24 h infusion of gemcitabine in previously untreated patients with inoperable non-small-cell lung cancer. *British Journal of Cancer*, 1996; **74**: 460–2.

471. Storniolo AM, Allrheiligen SR, Pearce HL. Preclinical pharmacologic and phase I studies of gemcitabine. *Seminars in Oncology*, 1997; **24** (suppl. 7): 2–7.

472. Edzes HT, Peters GJ, Noordhuis P, Vermorken JB. Determination of the antimetabolite gemcitabine (2′,2′-difluoro-2′-deoxycytidine) and of

2′,2′-difluoro-2′-deoxyuridine by ^{19}F nuclear magnetic resonance spectroscopy. *Analytical Biochemistry*, 1993; **214**: 25–30.

473. **Green MR**. Gemciabine safety overview. *Seminars in Oncology*, 1996; **23** (suppl. 10): 32–5.

474. **Grunewald R, Abbruzzese JL, Tarassoff P, Plunkett W**. Saturation of 2′,2′-difluorodeoxycytidine 5′-triphosphate accumulation by mononuclear cells during a phase I trial of gemcitabine. *Cancer Chemotherapy and Pharmacology*, 1991; **27**: 258–62.

475. **Grunewald R, Kantarjian H, Du M, Faucher K, Tarassoff P, Plunkett W**. Gemcitabine in leukemia, a phase I clinical plasma and cellular pharmacology study. *Journal of Clinical Oncology*, 1992; **10**: 406–13.

476. **Van Moorsel CJA, Kroep JR, Pinedo HM, *et al.*** Pharmacokinetic schedule finding study of the combination of gemcitabine and cisplatin in patients with solid tumors. *Annals of Oncology*, 1999; **10**: 441–8.

477. **McGinn CJ, Shewach DS, Lawrence TS**. Radiosensitizing nucleosides. *Journal of the National Cancer Institute*, 1996; **88**: 1193–203.

478. **Abratt RP, Sandler A, Crinò L, *et al.*** Combined cisplatin and gemcitabine for non-small cell lung cancer: Influence of scheduling on toxicity and drug delivery. *Seminars in Oncology*, 1998; **25** (suppl 9): 35–43.

479. **O'Dwyer PJ, Paul AR, Walczak J, Weiner LM, Litwin S, Comis RL**. Phase II study of biochemical modulation of fluorouracil by low dose PALA in patients with colorectal cancer. *Journal of Clinical Oncology*, 1990; **8**: 1497–503.

480. **Peters GJ, Schwartsmann G, Nadal JC, *et al.*** *In vivo* inhibition of the pyrimidine *de novo* enzyme dihydroorotic acid dehydrogenase by Brequinar sodium (DUP-785; NSC 368390) in mice and patients. *Cancer Research*, 1990; **50**: 4644–9.

481. **Pizzorno G, Wiegand RA, Lentz SK, Handschumacher RE**. Brequinar potentiates 5-fluorouracil antitumor activity in a murine model colon 38 tumor by tissue-specific modulation of uridine nucleotide pools. *Cancer Research*, 1992; **52**: 1660–5.

482. **Peters GJ, Kraal I, Pinedo HM (1992)**. *In vitro* and *in vivo* studies on the combination of Brequinar sodium (DUP-895; NSC 368390) with 5-fluorouracil; effects of uridine. *British Journal of Cancer*, 1992; **65**: 229–33.

483. **Buzaid AC, Pizzorno G, Marsh JC, *et al.*** Biochemical modulation of 5-fluorouracil with Brequinar: results of a phase I study. *Cancer Chemotherapy and Pharmacology*, 1995; **36**: 373–8.

484. **Moriconi WJ, Slavik M, Taylor S**. 3-Deazauridine (NSC 126849): An interesting modulator of biochemical response. *Investigational New Drugs*, 1986; **4**: 67–84.

485. **Kang G, Cooney DA, Moyer JD, *et al.*** Cyclopentenyluridine and cyclopentenylcytidine analogues as inhibitors of uridine-cytidine kinase. *Journal of Biological Chemistry*, 1989; **264**: 713–18.

486. **Politi PM, Xie F, Dahut W, *et al.*** Phase I clinical trial of continuous infusion cyclopentenyl cytosine. *Cancer Chemotherapy and Pharmacology*, 1995; **36**: 513–23.

487. **Viola JJ, Agbaria R, Walbridge S, *et al.*** *In situ* cyclopentenyl cytosine infusion of the treatment of experimental brain tumors. *Cancer Research*, 1995; **55**: 1306–9.

488. **Baker CH, Banzon J, Bollinger JM, *et al.*** 2′-Deoxy-2′-methylenecytidine and -2′-deoxy-2′2′-difluorocytidine 5′diphosphates: potent mechanism-based inhibitors of ribonucleotide reductase. *Journal of Medicinal Chemistry*, 1991; **34**: 1879–84.

489. **Bitonti AJ, Bush TL, Lewis MT, Sunkara PS**. Response of human colon and prostate tumor xenografts to (E)-2′-deoxy-2′-(fluormethylene) cytidine, an inhibitor of ribonucleotide reductase. *Anticancer Research*, 1995; **15**: 1179–82.

490. **Sun L-Q, Li Y-X, Guillou L, Mirimanoff R-O, Coucke PA**. Antitumor and radiosensitizing effects of (E) -2′-deoxy-2′-(fluoromethylene) cytidine, a novel inhibitor of ribonucleoside diphosphate reductase, on human colon carcinoma xenografts in nude mice. *Cancer Research*, 1997; **57**: 4023–8.

491. **Eda H, Ura M, Ouchi KF, Tanaka Y, Miwa M, Ishitsuka H**. The antiproliferative activity of DMDC is modulated by inhibition of cyticin deaminase. *Cancer Research*, 1998; **58**: 1165–9.

492. **Grove KL, Guo X, Liu S-L, Gao Z, Chu CK, Cheng Y-C**. Anticancer activity of β-L-dioxolane-cytidine, a novel nucleoside analogue with the unnatural L configuration. *Cancer Research*, 1995; **55**: 3008–11.

493. **Elion GB**. The purine path to chemotherapy. *Science*, 1989; **244**: 41–7.

494. **Paterson ARP, Tidd DM**. 6-Thiopurines. In: Sartorelli AC, Johns DJ (ed.) *Handbook of experimental pharmacology*, vol. 38(2). Berlin: Springer, 1975: 384–403.

495. **Riscoe MK, Brouns MC, Fitchen JH**. Purine metabolism as a target for leukemia chemotherapy. *Blood Reviews*, 1989; **3**: 162–73.

496. **Pinkel D**. Intravenous mercaptopurine: life begins at 40. *Journal of Clinical Oncology*, 1993; **11**: 1826–31.

497. **Lennard L, Lilleyman JS**. Individualizing therapy with 6-mercaptopurine and 6-thioguanine related to the thiopurine methyltransferase genetic polymorphism. *Therapeutic Drug Monitoring*, 1996; **18**: 328–34.

498. **Kawahata RT, Chuang LF, Holmberg CA, Osburn BI, Chuang RY**. Inhibition of human lymphoma DNA-dependent RNA polymerase activity by 6-mercaptopurine ribonucleoside triphosphate. *Cancer Research*, 1983; **43**: 3655–9.

499. **Tidd DM, Paterson ARP**. A biochemical mechanism for the delayed cytotoxic reaction of 6-mercaptopurine. *Cancer Research*, 1974; **34**: 738–46.

500. **Christie NT, Drake S, Meyn RE, Nelson JA**. 6-Thioguanine-induced DNA damage as a determinant of cytotoxicity in cultured Chinese hamsters ovary cells. *Cancer Research*, 1984; **44**: 3665–72.

501. **Bodell WJ, Morgan WF, Rasmussen J, Williams ME, Deen DF**. Potentiation of 1,3-bis(2-chloroethyl-1-nitrosuorea) (BCNU)-induced cytotoxicity in 9L cells by pretreatment with 6-thioguanine. *Biochemical Pharmacology*, 1985; **34**: 515–20.

502. **Maybaum J, Mandel HG**. Unilateral chromatid damage: a new basis for 6-thioguanine cytotoxicity. *Cancer Research*, 1983; **43**: 3852–6.

503. **Lambooy LHJ, Leegwater PAJ, Vandenheuvel LP, Bokkerink JP, Deabreu RA**. Inhibition of DNA methylation in malignant molt F4 lymphoblasts by 6-mercaptopurine. *Clinical Chemistry*, 1998; **44**: 556–9.

504. **Bökkerink JPM, Stet EH, De Abreu RA, *et al.*** 6-Mercaptopurine: Cytotoxicity and biochemical pharmacology in human malignant T-lymphoblasts. *Biochemical Pharmacology*, 1993; **45**: 1455–63.

505. **Lennard L, Lilleyman JS**. Are children with lymphoblastic leukemia given enough 6-mercaptopurine? *The Lancet*, 1987; **ii**: 785–7.

506. **Lennard L, Lilleyman JS**. Variable mercaptopurine metabolism and treatment outcome in childhood lymphoblastic leukemia. *Journal of Clinical Oncology*, 1989; **7**: 1816–23.

507. **Schmiegelow K, Schroder H, Gustafsson G, *et al.*** for the Nordic Society for Pediatric Hematology and Oncology. Risk of relapse in childhood acute lymphoblastic leukemia is related to RBC methotrexate and mercaptopurine metabolites during maintenance chemotherapy. *Journal of Clinical Oncology*, 1995; **13**: 345–51.

508. **Lennard L, Welch J, Lilleyman JS**. Mercaptopurine in childhood leukaemia: the effects of dose escalation on thioguanine nucleotide metabolites. *British Journal of Clinical Pharmacology*, 1996; **42**: 525–7.

509. **Lennard L, Welch J, Lilleyman JS**. Intracellular metabolites of mercaptopurine in children with lymphoblastic leukaemia: a possible indicator of non-compliance? *British Journal of Cancer*, 1995; **72**: 1004–6.

510. **McLeod HL, Relling MV, Liu Q, Pui C-H, Evans WE**. Polymorphic thiopurine methyltransferase in erythrocytes is indicative of activity in leukemic blasts from children with acute lymphoblastic leukemia. *Blood*, 1995; **85**: 1897–902.

511. **Otterness D, Szumlanski C, Lennard L, *et al.*** Human thiopurine methyltransferase pharmacogenetics: Gene sequence polymorphisms. *Clinical Pharmacology and Therapeutics*, 1997; **62**: 60–73.

512. Loennechen T, Yates CR, Fessing MY, Relling MV, Krynetski EY, Evans WE. Isolation of a human thiopurine s-methyltransferase (TPMT) complementary DNA with a single nucleotide transition A719G (TPMT-*-3C) and its association with loss of TPMT protein and catalytic activity in humans. *Clinical Pharmacology and Therapeutics*, 1998; **64**: 46–51.

513. Mojena M, Bosca L, Rider MH, Rousseau GG, Hue L. Inhibition of 6-phosphofructo-2-kinase activity by mercaptopurines. *Biochemical Pharmacology*, 1992; **43**: 671–8.

514. Wotring LL, Roti JL. Thioguanine-induced S and G2 blocks and their significance to the mechanism of cytotoxicity. *Cancer Research*, 1980; **40**: 1458–62.

515. Hortelano S, Bosca L. 6-mercaptopurine decreases the bcl-2/bax ratio and induces apoptosis in activated splenic B lymphocytes. *Molecular Pharmacology*, 1997; **51**: 414–21.

516. Lee MH, Huang Y-M, Sartorelli AC. Alkaline phosphatase activites of 6-thiopurine-sensitive and -resistant sublines of sarcoma 180. *Cancer Research*, 1978; **38**: 2413–18.

517. Zimm S, Reaman G, Murphy RF, Poplack DG. Biochemical parameters of mercaptopurine activity in patients with acute lymphoblastic leukemia. *Cancer Research*, 1986; **46**: 1495–8.

518. Veerman AJP, Hogeman PHG, Van Zantwijk CH, Bezemer PD. Prognostic value of 5′-nucleotidase in acute lymphoblastic leukemia with the common ALL phenotype. *Leukemia Research*, 1985; **9**: 1227–9.

519. Pieters R, Huismans DR, Loonen AH, Peters GJ, Hählen K, Veerman AJP. Relation of nucleotidase and phosphatase activities with drug resistance and clinical prognosis in childhood leukemia. *Leukemia Research*, 1992; **16**: 873–80.

520. Pieters R, Veerman AJP. The role of 5′-nucleotidase in therapy-resistance of childhood leukemia. *Medical Hypotheses*, 1988; **27**: 77–80.

521. Tidd DM, Dedhar S. Specific and sensitive combined high performance liquid chromatographic-flow fluorometric assay for intracellular-6-thioguanine metabolites of 6-mercaptopurine and 6-thioguanine. *Journal of Chromatography*, 1978; **145**: 237–46.

522. Ding TL, Benet LZ. Determination of 6-mercaptopurine and azathioprine in plasma by high-performance liquid chromatography. *Journal of Chromatography*, 1979; **163**: 281–8.

523. De Abreu RA, Van Baal JM, Schouten TJ, Schretlen EDAM. High-performance liquid chromatographic determination of plasma 6-mercaptopurine in clinically relevant concentrations. *Journal of Chromatography*, 1982; **227**: 526–33.

524. Zimm S, Grygiel JJ, Strong JM, Monks TJ, Poplack DG. Identification of 6-mercaptopurine riboside in patients receiving 6-mercaptopurine as a prolonged intravenous infusion. *Biochemical Pharmacology*, 1984; **33**: 4089–92.

525. Erbs N, Harms DO, Jankaschaub G. Pharmacokinetics and metabolism of thiopurines in children with acute lymphoblastic leukemia receiving 6-thioguanine versus 6-mercaptopurine. *Cancer Chemotherapy and Pharmacology*, 1998; **42**: 266–72.

526. Lancaster DL, Lennard L, Rowland K, Vora AJ, Lilleyman JS. Thioguanine versus mercaptopurine for therapy of childhood lympyoblastic leukaemia—a comparison of haematological toxicity and drug metabolite concentrations. *British Journal of Haematology*, 1998; **102**: 439–43.

527. Jacqzaigrain E, Nafa S, Medard Y, Bessa E, Lescoeur B, Vilmer E. Pharmacokinetics and distribution of 6-mercaptopurine administered intravenously in children with lymphoblastic leukaemia. *European Journal of Clinical Pharmacology*, 1997; **53**: 71–4.

528. Lafolie P, Hayder S, Björk O, Ahstrom L, Liliemark J, Peterson C. Large interindividual variations in the pharmacokinetics of oral 6-mercaptopurine in maintenance therapy of children with acute leukaemia and non-Hodgkin's lymphoma. *Acta Paediatrica Scandinavica*, 1986; **75**: 797–803.

529. Hayder S, Lafolie P, Björk O, Peterson C. 6-Mercaptopurine plasma levels in children, with acute lymphoblastic leukemia: relation to relapse risk and myelotoxicity. *Therapeutic Drug Monitoring*, 1989; **11**: 617–22.

530. Koren G, Ferrazini G, Sulh H, *et al*. Systemic exposure to mercaptopurine as a prognostic factor in acute lymphocytic leukemia in children. *New England Journal of Medicine*, 1990; **323**: 17–21.

531. Douglas I, Lister TA. The effect of food on the oral administration of 6-mercaptopurine. *Cancer Chemotherapy and Pharmacology*, 1986; **18**: 90–1.

532. Burton NK, Barnett MJ, Aherne GW, Evans J, Douglas I, Lister TA. The effect of food on the oral administration of 6-mercaptopurine. *Cancer Chemotherapy and Pharmacology*, 1986; **18**: 90–1.

533. Schouten TJ, De Abreu RA, Schretlen EDAM, Van Baal JM, Van Leeuwen MB, De Vaan GAM. 6-Mercaptopurine: high-dose 24-h infusions in goats. *Journal of Cancer Research and Clinical Oncology*, 1986; **112**: 61–6.

534. Verhoef V, Sarup J, Fridland A. Identification of the mechanism of activation of 9-β-D-arabinofuranosyladenine in human lymphoid cells using mutants deficient in nucleoside kinases. *Cancer Research*, 1981; **41**: 4478–83.

535. Plunkett W, Gandhi V. Pharmacology of purine nucleoside analogues. *Hematology Cell Therapy*, 1996; **38**: S67–S74.

536. Parker WB, Bapat AR, Shen JX, Townsend AJ, Cheng YC. Interaction of 2-halogenated dATP analogs (F, Cl, and Br) with human DNA polymerase, DNA primase, and ribonucleotide reductase. *Molecular Pharmacology*, 1988; **34**: 485–92.

537. Catapano CV, Chandler KB, Fernandes DJ. Inhibition of primer RNA formation in CCRF-CEM leukemia cells by fludarabine triphosphate. *Cancer Research*, 1991; **51**: 1829–35.

538. Yang S-W, Huang P, Plunkett W, Becker FF, Chan JYH. Dual mode of inhibition of purified DNA ligase I from human cells by 9-β-D-arabinofuranosyl-2-fluoroadenine triphosphate. *Journal of Biological Chemistry*, 1992; **267**: 2345–9.

539. Robertson LE, Chubb S, Meyn RE, *et al*. Induction of apoptotic cell death in chronic lymphocytic leukemia by 2-chloro-2′-deoxyadenosine and 9-beta-D-arabinosyl-2-fluoroadenine. *Blood*, 1993; **81**: 143–50.

540. Dow LW, Bell DE, Poulakos L, Fridland A. Differences in metabolism and cytotoxicity between 9-β-arabinofuranosyl-2-fluoroadenine in human leukemic lymphoblasts. *Cancer Research*, 1980; **40**: 405–10.

541. Petersen AJ, Brown RD, Gibson J, *et al*. Nucleoside transporters, bcl-2 and apoptosis in CLL cells exposed to nucleoside analogues *in vitro*. *European Journal of Haematology*, 1996; **56**: 213–20.

542. Gottardi D, De Leo AM, Alferano A, *et al*. Fludarabine ability to down-regulate Bcl-2 gene product in CD5+ leukaemic B cells, *in vitro/in vivo* correlations. *British Journal of Haematology*, 1997; **99**: 147–57.

543. Chun HG, Leyland-Jones B, Cheson BD. Fludarabine phosphate: A synthetic purine antimetabolite with significant activity against lymphoid malignancies. *Journal of Clinical Oncology*, 1991; **9**: 175–88.

544. Keating MJ, Kantarjian H, O'Brien S, *et al*. Fludarabine: a new agent with marked cytoreductive activity in untreated chronic lympocytic leukemia. *Journal of Clinical Oncology*, 1991; **9**: 44–9.

545. Johnson S, Smith AG, Loffler H, *et al*. Multicentre prospective randomised trial of fludarabine versus cyclophosphamide doxorubicin and prednisone (CAP) for treatment of advanced-stage chronic lymphocytic leukaemia. The French Cooperative Group on CLL. *The Lancet*, 1996; **347**: 1432–8.

546. Kefford RF, Fox RM. Purinogenic lymphocytotoxicity: Clues to a wider chemotherapeutic potential for the adenosine deaminase inhibitors. *Cancer Chemotherapy and Pharmacology*, 1983; **10**: 73–8.

547. Klohs WD, Kraker AJ. Pentostatin—future directions. *Pharmacological Reviews*, 1992; **44**: 459–77.

548. Cheson BD. Infectious and immunosuppressive complications of purine analog therapy. *Journal of Clinical Oncology*, 1995; **13**: 2431–48.

549. Ho AD, Thaler J, Madelli F, *et al.* Response to pentostatin in hairy-cell leukemia refractory to interferon-alpha. *Journal of Clinical Oncology,* 1989; 7: 1533–8.

550. Smyth JF, Paine RM, Jackman AL, *et al.* The clinical pharmacology of the adenosine deaminase inhibitor 2'deoxycoformycin. *Cancer Chemotherapy and Pharmacology,* 1980; 5: 93–101.

551. Carson DA, Wasson DB, Kaye J, *et al.* Deoxycytidine kinase-mediated toxicity of deoxyadenosine analogs toward malignant human lymphoblasts *in vitro* and toward murine L1210 leukemia *in vivo. Proceedings of the National Academy of Sciences of the United States of America,* 1980; 77: 6865–9.

552. Sasvári-Széleky, Spasokoukotskaja T, Szóke, Csapó Z, *et al.* Activation of deoxycytidine kinase during inhibition of DNA synthesis by 2-chloro-2'-deoxyadenosine (cladribine) in human lymphocytes. *Biochemical Pharmacology,* 1998; 56: 1175–9.

553. Plunkett W, Saunders PP. Metabolism and action of purine nucleoside analogs. *Pharmacology and Therapeutics,* 1991; 49: 239–68.

554. Chunduru SK, Appleman JR, Blakley RL. Activity of human DNA-polymerases α and β with 2-chloro-2'-deoxydenosine 5'-triphosphate as a substrate and quantitative effects of incorporation on chain extension. *Archives of Biochemistry and Biophysics,* 1993; 302: 19–30.

555. Carson DA, Wasson DB, Esparza LM, Carrera CJ, Kipps TJ, Cottam HB. Oral antilymphocyte activity and induction of apoptosis by 2-chloro-2'-arabino- fluoro-2'-deoxyadenosine. *Proceedings of the National Academy of Sciences of the United States of America,* 1992; 89: 2970–4.

556. Carson DA, Wasson DB, Taetle R, Yu A. Specific toxicity of 2-chlorodeoxyadenosine toward resting and proliferating human lymphocytes. *Blood,* 1983; 62: 737.

557. Piro LD, Carrera CJ, Beutler E, Carson DA. 2-Chlorodeoxyadenosine: an effective new agent for the treatment of chronic lymphocytic leukemia. *Blood,* 1988; 72: 1069–73.

558. Piro LD, Carrera CJ, Carson DA, Beutler E. Lasting remissions in hairy-cell leukemia induced by a single infusion of 2-chlorodeoxyadenosine. *New England Journal of Medicine,* 1990; 322: 1117–21.

559. Saven A, Piro LD. 2-Chlorodeoxyadenosine: A potent antimetabolite with major activity in the treatment of indolent lymphoproliferative disorders. *Hematology Cell Therapy,* 1996; 38: S93–S101.

560. Kay AC, Saven A, Carrera CJ, *et al.* 2-Chlorodeoxyadenosine treatment of low-grade lymphomas. *Journal of Clinical Oncology,* 1992; 10: 371–7.

561. Liliemark J, Porwit A, Juliusson G. Intermittent infusion of cladribine (CdA) in previously treated patients with low-grade non-Hodgkin's lymphoma. *Leukemia Lymphoma,* 1997; 25: 313–18.

562. Santana VM, Mirro J, Kearns C, Schell MJ, Crom W, Blakley RL. 2-Chlorodeoxyadenosine produces a high rate of complete hematologic remission in relapsed acute myeloid leukemia. *Journal of Clinical Oncology,* 1992; 10: 364–70.

563. Juliusson G, Elmhornrosenborg A, Liliemark J. Response to 2-chlorodeoxyadenosine in patients with B-cell chronic lymphocytic leukemia resistant to fludarabine. *New England Journal of Medicine,* 1992; 327: 1056–61.

564. Saven A, Lemon RH, Kosty M, Beutler E, Piro LD. 2-Chlorodeoxyadenosine activity in patients with untreated chronic lymphocytic leukemia. *Journal of Clinical Oncology,* 1995; 13: 570–4.

565. Tallman MS, Hakimian D, Zanzig C, *et al.* Cladribine in the treatment of relapsed or refractory chronic lymphocytic leukemia. *Journal of Clinical Oncology,* 1995; 13: 983–8.

566. Albertioni F, Lindemalm S, Reichelova V, *et al.* Pharmacokinetics of cladribine in plasma and its 5'-monophosphate and 5'-triphosphate in leukemic cells of patients with chronic lymphocytic leukemia. *Clinical Cancer Research,* 1998; 4: 653–8.

567. Liliemark J, Juliusson G. On the Pharmacokinetics of 2-chloro-2'-deoxyadenosine in humans. *Cancer Research,* 1991; 51: 5570–2.

568. Liliemark J, Albertioni F, Hassan M, Juliusson G. On the bioavailability of oral and subcutaneous 2-chloro- 2'-deoxyadenosine in humans—alternative routes of administration. *Journal of Clinical Oncology,* 1992; 10: 1514–18.

569. Geijssen GJ, Pieters R, Veerman AJP, Pinedo HM, Peters GJ. Do inhibitors of IMP dehydrogenase have a future in cancer chemotherapy? *International Journal of Purine Pyrimidine Research,* 1991; 2: 17–26.

570. Weber G, Jayaram HN, Lapis E, *et al.* Enzyme-pattern-targeted chemotherapy with tiazofurin and allopurinol in human leukemia. *Advances in Enzyme Regulation,* 1988; 27: 405–33.

571. Cooney DA, Jayaram HN, Gebeyehu G, *et al.* The conversion of 2-β-ribofuranosylthiazole-4-carboxamide to an analogue of NAD with potent IMP dehydrogenase-inhibitory properties. *Biochemical Pharmacology,* 1982; 31: 2133–6.

572. Jayaram HN, Cooney DA, Glazer RI, Dion RL, Johns DG. Mechanism of resistance to the oncolytic C-nucleoside 2-β-ribofuranosylthiazole-4-carboxamide (NSC 286193). *Biochemical Pharmacology,* 1982; 31: 2557–60.

573. Olah E, Natsumeda Y, Ikegami T, *et al.* Induction of erythroid differentiation and modulation of gene expression by tiazofurin in K-562 leukemia cells. *Proceedings of the National Acadamy of Science of the United States of America,* 1988; 85: 6533–7.

574. Weber G, Prajda N, Abonyi M, Look KY, Tricot G. Tiazofurin—molecular and clinical action. *Anticancer Research,* 1996; 16: 3313–22.

575. Boulton S, Kyle S, Durkacz BW. Low nicotinamide mononucleotide adenylyltransferase activity in a tiazofurin-resistant cell line—effects on NAD metabolism and DNA repair. *British Journal of Cancer,* 1997; 76: 845–51.

576. Balis FM, Lange BJ, Packer RJ, *et al.* Pedriatic phase I trial and pharmacokinetic study of tiazofurin (NSC 286193). *Cancer Research,* 1985; 45: 5169–72.

577. Tricot G, Jayaram HN, Weber G, Hoffman R. Tiazofurin: Biological effects and clinical uses. *International Journal of Cell Cloning,* 1990; 8: 161–70.

578. Tricot G, Weber G. Biochemically targeted therapy of refractory leukemia and myeloid blast crisis of chronic granulocytic leukemia with tiazofurin, a selective blocker of inosine 5'-phosphate dehydrogenase activity. *Anticancer Research,* 1996; 16: 3341–7.

579. Martin DS. Biochemical modulation: perspectives and objectives. In: Harrap KR, Connors TA. (eds.) *Proceedings of the eighth Bristol-Myers Symposium on Cancer Research. New Avenues in Developmental Cancer Chemotherapy.* London: Academic Press, 1987; 113–62.

580. Grem JL, Hoth OF, Hamilton JM, King SA, Leyland-Jones B. Overview of current status and future direction of clinical trials with 5-fluorouracil in combination with folinic acid. *Cancer Treatment Reports,* 1987; 71: 1249–64.

581. Grem JL, King SA, O'Dwyer PJ, Leyland-Jones B. Biochemistry and clinical activity of N-(phosphonacetyl)-L-aspartate: a review. *Cancer Research,* 1988; 48: 4441–54.

582. Grem JL, Fischer PH. Enhancement of 5-fluorouracil anticancer activity by dipyrimadole. *Pharmacotherapy,* 1989; 40: 349–71.

583. Darnowski JW, Handschumacher RE. Enhancement of fluorouracil therapy by the manipulation of tissue uridine pools. *Pharmacology and Therapeutics,* 1989; 41: 381–92.

584. Klubes P, Leyland-Jones B. Enhancement of the antitumor activity of 5-fluorouracil by uridine rescue. *Pharmacological Therapeutics,* 1989; 41: 289–302.

585. Peters GJ, Van Groeningen CJ. Clinical relevance of biochemical modulation of 5-fluorouracil. *Annals of Oncology,* 1991; 2: 469–80.

586. Peters GJ, Van der Wilt CL, Van Moorsel CJA, Kroep JR, Bergman

AM, Ackland SP. Basis for effective combination cancer chemotherapy with antimetabolites. *Pharmacological Therapy*, 2000; **87**; 227–53.

587. Mini E, Trave F, Rustum YM, Bertino JR. Enhancement of the antitumor effects of 5-fluorouracil by folinic acid. *Pharmacology and Therapeutics*, 1990; **47**: 1–19.

588. Van der Wilt CL, Peters GJ. New targets for pyrimidine antimetabolites for the treatment of solid tumors. Part 1, thymidylate synthase. *Pharmacy World and Science*, 1994; **16**: 84–103.

589. Nadal JC, Van Groeningen CJ, Pinedo HM, Peters GJ. Schedule-dependency of *in vivo* modulation of 5-fluorouracil by leucovorin and uridine in murine colon carcinoma. *Investigational New Drugs*, 1989; **7**: 163–72.

590. Radparvar S, Houghton PJ, Houghton JA. Characteristics of thymidylate synthase purified form a human colon adenocarcinoma. *Archives of Biochemistry and Biophysics*, 1988; **260**: 342–50.

591. Spears CP, Shahinian AH, Moran RG, Heidelberg C, Corbett TH. *In vivo* kinetics of thymidylate synthetase inhibition in 5-fluorouracil-sensitive and -resistant murine colon adenocarcinomas. *Cancer Research*, 1982; **42**: 450–6.

592. Arbuck SG. Overview of clinical trials using 5-fluorouracil and leucovorin for the treatment of colorectal cancer. *Cancer*, 1989; **63**: 1036–44.

593. Piedbois P, Buyse M, Rustum Y, *et al*. Modulation of fluorouracil by leucovorin in patients with advanced colorectal cancer: Evidence in terms of response rate. *Journal of Clinical Oncology*, 1992; **10**: 896–903.

594. Köhne-Wömpner CH, Schmoll HJ, Harstrick A, Rustum YM. (1992). Chemotherapeutic strategies in metastatic colorectal cancer—an overview of current clinical trials. *Seminars in Oncology*, 1992; **19**: 105–25.

595. Petrelli N, Douglas HO Jr, Herrera L, *et al*. The modulation of fluorouracil with leucovorin in metastatic colorectal carcinoma: A prospective randomized phase III trial. *Journal of Clinical Oncology*, 1989; **7**: 1419–26.

596. O'Connell MJ. A phase III trial of 5 fluorouracil and leucovorin in the treatment of advanced colorectal cancer: A Mayo Clinic/North Central Cancer Treatment Group study. *Cancer*, 1989; **63**: 1026–30.

597. Poon MA, O'Connell MJ, Wieand HS, *et al*. Biochemical modulation of fluorouracil with leucovorin: Confirmatory evidence of improved therapeutic efficacy in advanced colorectal cancer. *Journal of Clinical Oncology*, 1991; **9**: 1967–72.

598. Hines JD, Adelstein DJ, Spiess JL, Giroski P, Carter SG. Efficacy of high-dose oral Leucovorin and 5-Fluorouracil in advanced colorectal carcinoma: Plasma and tissue pharmacokinetics. *Cancer*, 1989; **63**: 1022–5.

599. Machover D, Grison X, Goldschmidt E, *et al*. Fluorouracil combined with the pure (6S)-stereoisomer of folinic acid in high doses for treatment of patients with advanced colorectal carcinoma—a phase-I-II study. *Journal of the National Cancer Institute*, 1992; **84**: 321–7.

600. Wadler S, Lembersky B, Atkins M, Kirkwood J, Petrelli N. Phase II trial of fluorouracil and recombinant interferon alfa-2a in patients with advanced colorectal carcinoma: An Eastern Cooperative Oncology Group study. *Journal of Clinical Oncology*, 1991; **9**: 1806–10.

601. Pazdur R. Fluuorouracil and recombinant interferon alfa-2a in advanced gastrointestinal neoplasms. *British Journal of Haematology*, 1991; **79** (suppl. 1): 56–9.

602. Kosmidis PA, Tsavaris N, Skarlos D *et al*. Fluorouracil and leucovorin with or without interferon alfa-2b in advaced colorectal cancer: analysis of a prospective randomized phase III trial. Hellenic Cooperative Oncology Group. *Journal of Clinical Oncology*, 1996; **14**: 2682–7.

603. Grem JL, Jordan E, Robson ME, *et al*. Phase-II Study of fluorouracil, leucovorin, and interferon alfa-2a in metastatic colorectal carcinoma. *Journal of Clinical Oncology*, 1993; **11**: 1737–45.

604. Sinnige HAM, Buter J, Devries EGE, *et al*. Phase I-II study of the

addition of alpha-2A interferon to 5-fluorouracil leucovorin—pharmacokinetic interaction of alpha-2A interferon and leucovorin. *European Journal of Cancer*, 1993; **29A**: 1715–20.

605. Köhne CH, Schöffski P, Wilke H, *et al*. Effective biomodulation by leucovorin of high dose infusional fluorouracil given as a weekly 24-hour infusion: Results of a randomized trial in patients with advanced colorectal cancer. *Journal of Clinical Oncology*, 1998; **16**: 410–26.

606. Van der Wilt CL, Braakhuis BJM, Pinedo HM, De Jong M, Smid K, Peters GJ. Addition of leucovorin in modulation of 5-fluorouracil with methotrexate: potentiating or reversing effect? *International Journal of Cancer*, 1995; **61**: 672–8.

607. Jackson RC, Fry DW, Boritzki TJ, *et al*. Biochemical pharmacology of the lipophilic antifolate, trimetrexate. *Advances in Enzyme Regulation*, 1984; **22**: 187–206.

608. Romanini A, Li WW, Colofiore JR, Bertino JR. Leucovorin enhances cytotoxicity of trimetrexate/fluorouracil, but not methotrexate/fluorouracil, in CCRF-CEM cells. *Journal of the National Cancer Institute*, 1992; **84**: 1033–8.

609. Conti JA, Kemeny N, Seiter K, *et al*. Trial of sequential trimetrexate, fluorouracil, and high-dose leucovorin in previously treated patients with gastrointestinal carcinoma. *Journal of Clinical Oncology*, 1994; **12**: 695–700.

610. Ardalan B, Singh G, Silberman H. A randomized phase I and II study of short-term infusion of high-dose fluorouracil with or without *N*-(phosphonacetyl)-L-aspartic acid in patients with advanced pancreatic colorectal cancers. *Journal of Clinical Oncology*, 1988; **6**: 1053–8.

611. Kemeny N, Conti JA, Seiter K, *et al*. Biochemical modulation of bolus fluorouracil by PALA in patients with advanced colorectal cancer. *Journal of Clinical Oncology*, 1992; **10**: 747–52.

612. Van Groeningen CJ, Peters GJ, Leyva A, Laurensse EJ, Pinedo HM. Reversal of 5-fluorouracil-induced myelosuppression by prolonged administration of high-dose uridine. *Journal of the National Cancer Institute*, 1989; **81**: 157–62.

613. Van Groeningen CJ, Peters GJ, Pinedo HM. Reversal of 5-fluorouracil-induced toxicity by oral administration of uridine. *Annals of Oncology*, 1993; **4**: 317–20.

614. Seiter K, Kemeny N, Martin D, *et al*. Uridine allows dose escalation of 5-fluorouracil when given with *N*-phosphonacetyl-L-aspartate, methotrexate, and leucovorin. *Cancer*, 1993; **71**: 1875–81.

615. Peters GJ, Van Groeningen CJ, Laurensse EJ, Pinedo HM. Thymidylate synthase from untreated human colorectal cancer and colonic mucosa: Enzyme activity and inhibition by 5-fluoro-2′-deoxyuridine-5′-monophosphate. *European Journal of Cancer*, 1991; **27**: 263–7.

616. Bagrij T, Kralovanszky J, Gyergyay F, Kiss E, Peters GJ. Influence of uridine treatment in mice on the protection of gastrointestinal toxicity caused by 5-fluorouracil. *Anticancer Research*, 1993; **13**: 789–94.

617. Pritchard DM, Watson AJM, Potten CS, Jackman AL, Hickman JA. Inhibition of uridine but not thymidine of p53-dependent intestinal apoptosis initiated by 5-fluorouracil: Evidence of the involvement of RNA perturbation. *Proceedings of the National Academy of Sciences of the United States of America*, 1997; **94**: 1795–9.

618. Kelsen DP, Martin D, O'Neil J, *et al*. Phase I trial of PN401, an oral prodrug of uridine, to prevent toxicity from fluorouracil in patients with advanced cancer. *Journal of Clinical Oncology*, 1997; **15**: 1511–17.

619. Unemi N, Takeda S, Tajima K *et al*. Studies on combination therapy with 1-(tetrahydro-2 furanyl)-5-fluorouracul plus uracil. I. Effect of coadministration of uracil on the antitumor activity of 1-(tetrahydro-2-furanyl)-5-fluorouracil and the level of 5-fluorouracil in AH 130 bearing rats. *Chemotherapy*, 1981; **29**: 164–75.

620. Takechi T, Nakano K, Uchida J, *et al*. Antitumor activity and low intestinal toxicity of S-1, a new formulation of oral tegafor, in experimental tumor models in rats. *Cancer Chemotherapy and Pharmacology*, 1997; **39**: 205–11.

621. Tatsumi K, Fukushima M, Shirasaka T, Fujii S. Inhibitory effects of pyrimidine, barbituric acid and pyridine derivatives on 5-fluorouracil degradation in rat liver extracts. *Japanese Journal of Cancer Research (GANN)*, 1987; **78**: 748–55.

622. Cao S, Rustum YM, Spector T. 5-Ethynyluracil (77C85): modulation of 5-fluorouracil efficacy and therapeutic index in rats bearing advanced colorectal carcinoma. *Cancer Research*, 1994; **54**: 1507–10.

623. Van der Wilt CL, Kuiper CM, Peters GJ. Combination studies of antifolates with 5-fluorouracil in colon cancer cell lines. *Oncology Research*, 1999; **11**; 383–91.

624. Longo GSA, Izzo J, Chang YM, *et al.* Pretreatment of colon carcinoma cells with tomudex enhances 5-fluorouracil cytotoxicity. *Clinical Cancer Research*, 1998; **4**: 469–73.

625. Van der Wilt CL, Van Laar JAM, Gyergyay F, Smid K, Peters GJ. Biochemical modification of the toxicity and the anti-tumour effect of 5-fluorouracil and cis-platinum by WR-2721 in mice. *European Journal of Cancer*, 1992; **28A**: 2017–24.

626. Tobias JS. Current role of chemotherapy in head and neck cancer. *Drugs*, 1992; **43**: 333–45.

627. Mathe G, Kidani Y, Segeguchi M, *et al.* Oxalato-platinum or L-OHP, a third-generation platinum complex: an experimental and clinical appraisal and preliminary comparison with cis-platinum and carboplatinum. *Biomedicine and Pharmacotherapy*, 1989; **43**: 237–50.

628. Raymond E, Buquetfagot C, Djelloul S, *et al.* Antitumor activity of oxaliplatin in combination with 5-fluorouracil and the thymidylate synthase inhibitor AG337 in human colon, breast and ovarian cancers. *Anti-Cancer Drugs*, 1997; **8**: 876–85.

629. Fischel JL, Etienne MC, Formento P, Milano G. Search for the optimal schedule for the oxaliplatin/5fluorouracil association modulated or not by folinic acid—preclinical data. *Clinical Cancer Research*, 1998; **4**: 2529–35.

630. Houghton JA, Cheshire PJ, Hallman JDN, *et al.* Evaluation of irinotecan in combination with 5-fluorouracil or etoposide in xenograft models of colon carcinoma cell lines. *Clinical Cancer Research*, 1996; **2**: 107–18.

631. Guichard S, Cassac D, Hennebelle I, Bugat R, Canal P. Sequence dependent activity of the irinotecan-5FU combination in human colon cancer nodel HT-29 *in vitro* and *in vivo*. *International Journal of Cancer*, 1997; **73**: 729–34.

632. Guichard S, Hennebelle I, Bugat R, Canal P. Cellular interactions of 5-fluorouracil and the campthothecin analogue CPT-11 (irinotecan) in a human colorectal carcinoma cell line. *Biochemical Pharmacology*, 1998: **55**: 667–76.

633. Mullany S, Svingen PH, Kaufmann SH, Erlichman C. Effect of adding the topoisomerase I poison 7-ethyl-10-hydroxycamptothecin (SN-38) to 5-fluorouracil and folinic acid in HCT-8 cells—elevated dTTP pools and enhanced cytotoxicity. *Cancer Chemotherapy and Pharmacology*, 1998; **42**: 391–9.

634. Mans DRA, Grivicich I, Peters GJ, Schwartsmann G. Sequence-dependent growth inhibition and DNA damage formation in differentially drug-sensitive human colon carcinoma cell lines by irinotecan and 5-fluorouracil at combinations of low, fixed doses with higher, varying doses. *European Journal of Cancer*, 1999; **35**: 1851–61.

635. Aschele C, Baldo C, Sobrero AF, Debernardis D, Bornmann WG, Bertino JR. Schedule-dependent synergism between raltitrexed and irinotecan in human colon cancer cells *in vitro*. *Clinical Cancer Research*, 1998; **4**: 1323–30.

636. Gandhi V, Kemena A, Keating MJ, Plunkett W. Fludarabine infusion potentiates arabinosylcytosine metabolism in lymphocytes of patients with chronic lymphocytic leukemia. *Cancer Research*, 1992; **52**: 897–903.

637. Gandhi V, Estey E, Keating MJ, Plunkett W. Fludarabine potentiates metabolism of cytarabine in patients with acute myelogenous leukemia during therapy. *Journal of Clinical Oncology*, 1993; **11**: 116–24.

638. Smith MA, Singer CRJ, Pallister CJ, Smith JG. The effect of haemopoietic growth factors on the cell cycle of AML progenitors and their sensitivity to cytosine arabinoside *in vitro*. *British Journal of Haematology*, 1995; **90**: 767–73.

639. Reuter C, Auf der Landwehr U, Schleyer E, *et al.* Modulation of intracellular metabolism of cytosine arabinoside in acute myeloid leukemia by granulocyte-macrophage colony-stimulating factor. *Leukemia*, 1994; **8**: 217–25.

640. Bhalla K, Cole J, MacLaughlin W, *et al.* Effect of deoxycytidine on the metabolism and cytotoxicity of 5-aza-2′-deoxycytidine and arabinosyl 5-azacytosine in normal and leukemic human myeloid progenitor cells. *Leukemia*, 1987; **1**: 814–19.

641. Grant S, Bhalla K, Gleyzer M. Interaction of deoxycytidine and deoxycytidine analogs in normal and leukemic human myeloid progenitor cells. *Leukemia Research*, 1986; **10**: 1139–40.

642. Cohen JD, Strock DJ, Teik JE, Katz TB, Marcel PD. Deoxycytidine in human plasma: Potential for protecting leukemic cells during chemotherapy. *Cancer Letters*, 1997; **116**: 167–75.

643. Bhalla K, Birkhofer M, Grant S, *et al.* Phase I clinical and pharmacologic study of deoxycytidine. *Leukemia*, 1988; **2**: 709–10.

644. Grant S, Baker M, Bhalla K. Phase I study of a continuous infusion of high-dose ara-C in conjunction with a fixed dose of 2′-deoxycytidine (IND 28108) in patients with refractory leukemia: An interim report. *Leukemia*, 1993; **7**: 1933–8.

645. Bergman AM, Ruiz van Haperen VWT, Veerman G, Kuiper CM, Peters GJ. Symergistic interaction between gemcitabine and cisplatin *in vitro*. *Clinical Cancer Research*, 1996; **2**: 521–30.

646. Peters GJ, Bergman AM, Ruiz van Haperen VWT, Veerman G, Kuiper CM, Braakhuis BJM. Interaction between cisplatin and gemcitabine *in vitro* and *in vivo*. *Seminars in Oncology*, 1995; **22** (suppl. 11): 72–9.

647. Van Moorsel CJA, Veerman G, Bergman AM, Guechev A, Vermorken JB, Postmus PE, Peters GJ. Combination chemotherapy studies with gemcitabine. *Seminars in Oncology*, 1997; **24**: (suppl. 7): 17–23.

648. Kanzawa F, Saijo N. *In vitro* interaction between gemcitabine and other anticancer drugs using a novel three-dimensional model. *Seminars in Oncology*, 1997; **24** (suppl. 7): 8–16.

649. Tsai CM, Chang KT, Chen JY, Chen YM, Chen MH, Perng RP. Cytotoxic effects of gemcitabine-containing regimens against human non-small cell lung cancer cell lines which express different levels of p185neu1. *Cancer Research*, 1995; **56**: 794–801.

650. Braakhuis BJM, Ruiz van Haperen VWT, Boven E, Veerman G, Peters GJ. Schedule dependent antitumor effect of gemcitabine in *in vivo* model systems. *Seminars in Oncology*, 1995; **22** (suppl. 11): 42–6.

651. Van Moorsel CJA, Pinedo HM, Veerman G, Vermorken JB, Postmus PE, Peters GJ. Scheduling of gemcitabine and cisplatin in Lewis lung tumour bearing mice. *European Journal of Cancer*, 1999; **35**: 808–14.

652. Van Moorsel CJA, Pinedo HM, Veerman G, *et al.* Combination chemotherapy studies with gemcitabine and etoposide in non-small cell lung and ovarian cancer cell lines. *Biochemical Pharmacology*, 1999; **57**: 407–15.

653. Van Putten JWG, Groen HJM, Smid K, Peters GJ, Kampinga HM. Endjoining deficiency and radiosensitation induced by gemcitabine. *Cancer Research*, 2001; **61**; 1585–91.

654. Crinò L, Scagliotti G, Marangolo M, *et al.* Cisplatin–gemcitabine combination in advanced non-small cell lung cancer. A Phase II study. *Journal of Clinical Oncology*, 1997; **15**: 297–303.

655. Abratt RP, Bezwoda WR, Goedhals L, Hacking DJ. Weekly gemcitabine (days 1, 8, 15) with monthly cisplatin (day 15): active combination chemotherapy for advanced non-small cell lung cancer. *Journal of Clinical Oncology*, 1997; **15**: 744–9.

656. Kroep JR, Giaccone G, Voorn DA, *et al.* Gemcitabine and paclitaxel; pharmacokinetic and pharmacodynamic interactions in patients with non-small cell lung cancer. *Journal of Clinical Oncology*, 1999; **17**; 2190–7.

657. **Vokes EE, Gregor A, Turrisi AT.** Gemcitabine and radiation therapy for non-small cell lung cancer. *Seminars in Oncology,* 1998; **25** (suppl. 9): 66–9.

658. **Bökkerink JPM.** Sequence-, time and dose-dependent synergism of methotrexate and 6-mercaptopurine in malignant human T-lymphoblasts. *Biochemical Pharmacology,* 1986; **35**: 3549–55.

659. **Giverhaug T, Loennechen T, Aarbakke J.** Increased concentrations of methylated 6-mercaptopurine metabolites and 6-thioguanine nucleotides in human leukemic cells *in vitro* by methotrexate. *Biochemical Pharmacology,* 1998; **55**: 1641–6.

660. **Camitta B, Leventhal B, Lauer S,** *et al.* Intermediate-dose intravenous methotrexateand mercaptopurine therapy for non-T, non-B acute lymphocytic leukemia of childhood: a Pediatric Oncology Group study. *Journal of Clinical Oncology,* 1989; **7**: 1539–44.

661. **Lin JT, Bertino JR.** Update on trimetrexate, a folate antagonist with antineoplastic and antiprotozoal properties. *Cancer Investigation,* 1991; **9**: 159–72.

662. **Meta-Analysis Group in Cancer.** Reappraisal of hepatic arterial infusion in the treatment of nonresectable liver metastasis from colorectal cancer. *Journal of the National Cancer Institute,* 1996; **88**: 252–8.

4.17 Antitumour antibiotics

Franco Zunino and Graziella Pratesi

Introduction

Antitumour antibiotics include a variety of natural compounds belonging to different chemical classes and characterized by different mechanisms of action. Although a large number of antitumour antibiotics have been identified (anthracyclines, actinomycins, bleomycins, mithramycins, enediyne antibiotics, and ansamycins), only a few are established antitumour agents available for treatment of human tumours. Since the most effective agents are anthracyclines (which are DNA intercalating agents), several structurally related synthetic agents have been developed. Anthracenediones and anthrapyrazoles are the best known series of synthetic intercalating agents with a relevant activity against some tumour types. Like anthracyclines, synthetic intercalators are known to be topoisomerase II poisons. Because of their similarity in structure and mechanism of action, such agents are considered in this chapter.

Anthracyclines

Anthracyclines represent a major class of antitumour antibiotics. The most effective member, doxorubicin, is one of the most widely used antitumour agents because of its broad spectrum of antitumour activity. The clinical success of daunorubicin and doxorubicin, the first generation of anthracyclines, has stimulated an intensive effort in the synthesis of analogues or structurally related compounds.[1] In spite of the preclinical development of a large number of agents of this class, only a small number of anthracyclines or intercalating agents are available for clinical use (Fig. 1). A rational drug design and analogue development was originally limited by a lack of precise information on the molecular and cellular basis of drug efficacy. Structure–activity relationship studies indicated that the presence of a planar ring system, allowing DNA intercalation (Fig. 2), is a necessary condition but not sufficient for optimal drug activity. Several lines of evidence indicate that the external binding moieties of the drug molecules (i.e. sugar residue and the cyclohexane ring A) may be critical for interaction with the cellular target.[2] More recently, novel, third-generation analogues emerged from a rationally based approach and a preclinical evaluation oriented to tumour type.[3],[4]

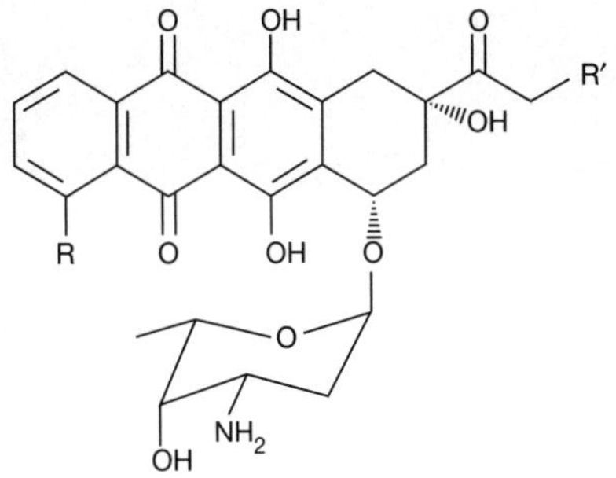

Daunorubicin and doxorubicin

Daunorubicin and doxorubicin, developed in the 1960s, were the first anthracyclines to be found clinically effective. The two prototype

Daunorubicin,	R = OCH$_3$,	R′ = H
Doxorubicin,	R = OCH$_3$,	R′ = OH
Idarubicin,	R = H,	R′ = H

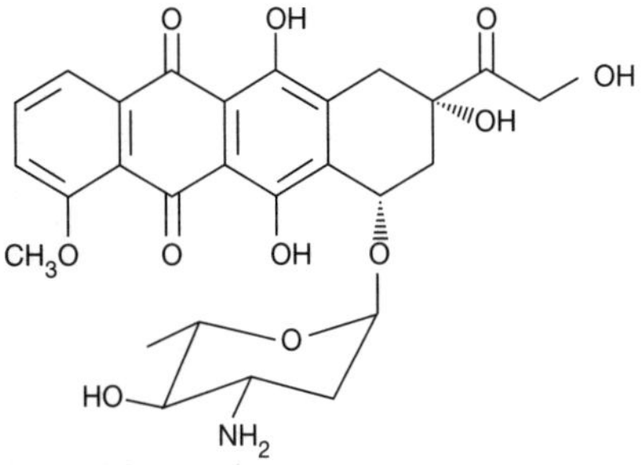

Epirubicin

Fig. 1 The chemical structures of clinically available anthracyclines.

anthracyclines are natural compounds originally isolated from *Streptomyces* species. Doxorubicin is produced by a variant of *Streptomyces peucetius* (var. *caesius*) exposed to the mutagen N-nitroso-N-methylurethane. The basic structure of anthracyclines consists of a tetracyclic aglycone linked to an amino sugar. In an attempt to improve the therapeutic and pharmacological properties of the natural compounds, a number of modifications of the basic structure were taken into consideration, including changes or substitutions of the C-9 side chain, the amino sugar, or the aglycone moiety.[1] Indeed, each of these moieties has been implicated in critical interactions with the cellular target (Fig. 3). No analogue to date has shown an activity clearly superior to doxorubicin, which remains the best anthracycline.[5]

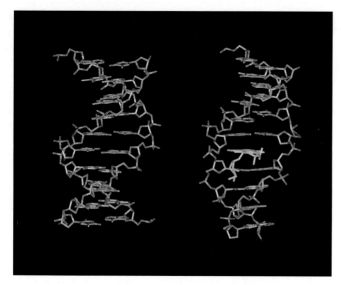

Fig. 2 A representation of the anthracycline intercalation into DNA, with the drug molecule shown in outline.

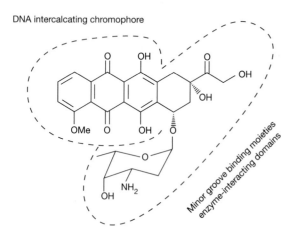

Fig. 3 A schematic representation of the putative functional moieties of the anthracyclines.

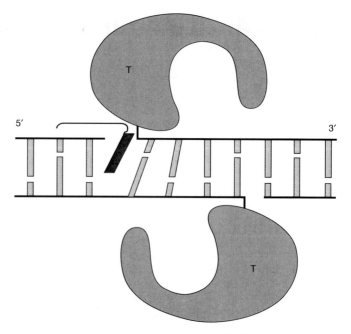

Fig. 4 A schematic model of the ternary DNA–drug–enzyme complex. Intercalated drug is shown in red. T, topoisomerase subunits.

Mechanism of action

Doxorubicin, like other effective anthracycline glycosides, is a well-known DNA intercalating agent. DNA is recognized as being the primary target for the pharmacological action of such agents. The drug–DNA intercalation complex, resulting from the insertion of the planar tetracyclic chromophore between adjacent base pairs, is stabilized by electrostatic interactions between DNA phosphate groups and the positively charged amino group of the sugar moiety. The intercalation site depends not only on the planar chromophore, but also on a variety of intrinsic properties (steric and electronic) that also involve the external binding moieties. However, the cytotoxic activity is not simply related to the drug's ability to bind to DNA, since the mode and the site of binding appear to be more critical than the binding affinity. Although DNA binding is central to the antitumour activity of anthracyclines, available evidence indicates that

it is the inhibition of a specific DNA function that is responsible for their therapeutic effects. The mechanism of cytotoxic and antitumour activity of the compounds, and of other effective intercalating agents, is now ascribed to their interference with the function of topo-isomerase II.[6],[7]

DNA topoisomerases are nuclear enzymes that regulate DNA topology during multiple DNA functions (including transcription, replication, and recombination), and they are essential for the integrity of genetic material.[8] Antitumour inhibitors of topoisomerases function as enzyme poisons by forming a DNA–drug–enzyme ternary complex (Fig. 4), thus stabilizing an intermediate of the enzyme reaction (the so-called cleavable complex) in which DNA strands are broken and enzyme subunits are covalently linked to DNA.[8] A definitive model for the drug interaction in the ternary complex is not available. However, it is likely that the intercalating agent is placed at the interface between the enzyme active site and the DNA cleavage site, thus preventing DNA relegation. Stabilization of the cleavable complex causes specific DNA damage (i.e. double-strand protein-associated DNA breaks), which may be lethal lesions. A large number of other topoisomerase II poisons have been found, including el-lipticines, amsacrines, flavones, and epipodophyllotoxins.[7] Among these poisons, anthracyclines still remain the most effective as anti-tumour agents. The molecular basis of their efficacy and selectivity toward specific tumour types is not understood. The initial DNA lesion—a drug-stabilized cleavable complex—is a potentially re-versible molecular event. The persistence of DNA lesions, as a con-sequence of the strong intercalation, may be recognized as an apoptotic stimulus. Doxorubicin exhibits a unique sequence specificity of stimu-lation of enzyme-mediated DNA cleavage. It is conceivable that the drug's ability to damage critical genomic sites may play a role in antitumour activity and different responsiveness of various tumour types.

In addition to intercalation in DNA, anthracyclines have the structural potential for other molecular interactions. The quinone function can be reduced to a hydroquinone form, with formation of intermediate semiquinone free radicals, which can reduce oxygen to produce superoxide and other reactive oxygen-derived species, including hydrogen peroxide and hydroxyl radicals.[9] A number of studies have suggested that drug-induced free radical formation is a mechanism of antitumour activity of anthracyclines, since the reactive species could induce DNA strand scission and lipid peroxidation. The precise role of free radical formation is still a matter of debate. A major weakness with the free radical hypothesis is related to the difficulty in establishing a quantitative correlation between drug-induced reactive species (and consequent extent of cellular damage) and various parameters of pharmacological activity (i.e. tumour response and organ-specific toxicities). There is limited support for the assumption that free radicals play a significant role in the antitumour activity of anthracyclines.[10] Since the drug accumulates in the nucleus, it is conceivable that intercalated molecules cannot undergo metabolic activation due to inaccessibility by quinone reductase. However, several lines of evidence support that superoxide and hydrogen peroxide may be implicated in influencing cell proliferation or cell death, depending on the extent of oxidative stress.[11] In addition, apoptosis induced by DNA damage may involve the formation of reactive oxygen species and oxidative damage of mitochondrial components.[12] Thus, the possibility that anthracycline-mediated oxidative stress may be a contributing factor to drug-induced cell death cannot be ruled out.

Whereas available information supports that the primary mechanism of antitumour action is related to topoisomerase inhibition, redox metabolism has been implicated in cardiotoxicity.[13] It is thus conceivable that antitumour activity and cardiotoxicity occur through different biochemical mechanisms. The possibility is supported by some indirect evidence: (i) free-radical scavengers or antioxidant agents (e.g. tocopherol, N-acetyl-cysteine) can reduce cardiac toxicity without affecting tumour inhibition in preclinical systems; (ii) 5-imino-daunorubicin, which is markedly less effective in producing reductase-dependent free radicals, lacks cardiac toxicity but retains antitumour activity; and (iii) the biochemical profile of cardiac tissue in terms of ability to protect against oxidative damage (high levels of reductase and low activity of catalase and superoxide dismutase) could account for organ-specific toxicity of anthracyclines.

The cytotoxic effects of superoxide and hydrogen peroxide are substantially enhanced by iron.[9] Doxorubicin may form a complex with iron, which, following reduction, initiates a cascade of free-radical production. Hydrogen peroxide can promote lipid peroxidation through reaction with drug–iron complexes, which yields hydroxyl radicals. The drug itself, or reactive free radicals, may also cause damage to nuclear and mitochondrial DNA, resulting in inhibition of protein synthesis. Identification of the role of iron in mediating reactive oxygen species led to the development of iron-chelating agents (ICRF 159, ICRF 187) as modulators of cardiac toxicity.[14] ICRF 187 (dexrazoxane) was found effective in reducing cardiotoxicity of doxorubicin without interfering with antitumour activity and is registered for clinical use.[15] Recently, a novel mechanism of cardiotoxicity has been proposed, relating intramyocardial formation of doxorubicinol and perturbation of the homeostatic processes involved in iron uptake and sequestration.[16] Other causes of cardiotoxicity may be related to drug effects at the cell membrane

Table 1 Multiple mechanisms of resistance to anthracyclines

Defence factors (implicated in preventing drug–target interaction):
  Overexpression of transport systems (mdr-1, MRP, LRP)
  Subcellular compartmentation
  Drug metabolism

Alterations involving drug–target interaction:
  Reduced expression of the target
  Reduced sensitivity of the target following mutation
  Chromatin changes and accessibility to critical genomic sites
  Stability of the cleavable complex (persistence of topoisomerase-
  mediated DNA breaks)

Cellular response to DNA damage:
  DNA repair
  Defects in apoptosis pathways

LRP, lung resistance protein; mdr-1, multidrug resistance 1; MRP, mutidrug resistance-associated protein.

level. In particular, drug binding to membrane phospholipids can lead to modifications of specific membrane functions (in particular, calcium and electrolyte transport). Again, the pharmacological significance of drug–membrane interactions and possible alterations of membrane function remains unclear.

Mechanisms of resistance

As for several antitumour agents, cellular resistance to anthracyclines is referred to as a multifactorial phenomenon. Intrinsic and acquired resistance to anthacyclines is a major obstacle to the curative efficacy in the treatment of several tumours. It is likely that both types of resistance share common biochemical mechanisms. They include: overexpression of defence factors implicated in reduction of intracellular drug concentration, quantitative or qualitative alterations of the target enzyme topoisomerase II, and changes in cellular response to drug-induced DNA lesions[17] (Table 1).

All these mechanisms result in the phenomenon known as multidrug resistance, since cells that display the multidrug resistance phenotype are resistant to multiple agents. The best studied multidrug resistance phenomenon (also termed typical multidrug resistance) is mediated by overexpression of the *mdr-1* product, a membrane glycoprotein (P-glycoprotein). A large number of natural compounds (including anthracyclines, epipodophyllotoxins, vinca alkaloids, actinomycin D, and taxanes) are substrates for P-glycoprotein, which functions as an energy-dependent drug efflux pump.[18] This protein is not tumour-specific, since it is expressed also in normal tissues, including kidney, liver, colon, and adrenal gland, and might be involved in the transport of hydrophobic metabolites or hormones. Thus, expression of P-glycoprotein in tumours derived from such tissues could account for their natural resistance.

More recently, in lung tumour cells selected *in vitro* for resistance to doxorubicin, a multidrug resistance phenotype was found to be associated with the overexpression of a different transporter protein, **MRP** (multidrug resistance-associated protein, gp180).[19] The cross-resistance pattern of the MRP-mediated phenotype is similar to P-glycoprotein-mediated multidrug resistance but does not involve taxanes.[20] MRP is homologous to the glutathione-*S*-conjugate transporter.[21] In cells overxpressing MRP, cellular glutathione content could thus influence activity of the MRP pump and consequently the intracellular concentration of the cytotoxic drug. Overexpression of transport systems may also play a role in subcellular sequestration of drugs (thus reducing the drug–target interaction). A similar function has been proposed for the human major vault protein LRP (lung resistance protein).[17]

Quantitative and qualitative alterations of the primary target, topoisomerase II, may be responsible for the variable chemosensitivity of tumour cells to anthracyclines. Reduced topoisomerase II expression or specific alterations in enzyme activity or sensitivity (e.g. mutation) may be responsible for a different multidrug resistance phenotype, involving only topoisomerase II poisons. The down-regulation of topoisomerase IIα in quiescent cells may account for the low responsiveness of slowly growing solid tumours.

However, despite adequate drug concentration at the target level, the cellular response to DNA damage may play a critical role in determining chemosensitivity and may account for the heterogeneity of tumour response to drug treatment. A number of molecular alterations associated with malignant transformation and tumour progression are implicated in regulation of cell death pathways and probably in development of drug resistance. In particular, loss of wild-type *p53* function (a critical gene involved in cellular response to DNA damage) may cause resistance to anthracyclines (as well as other DNA-damaging agents) as a consequence of reduced susceptibility of mutant cells to apoptosis.[22] Since impaired regulation of the apoptotic process is a common feature of several human tumours, it is conceivable that apoptosis-related resistance is relevant to clinical manifestations of intrinsic multidrug resistance that may involve most (if not all) cytotoxic drugs.

Clinical pharmacology

Drug administration for systemic treatment with daunorubicin and doxorubicin is only by the intravenous route. Drug extravasation causes severe local tissue necrosis. As a consequence of tissue injury, locoregional treatment (e.g. intraperitoneal administration) has very limited application.

Daunorubicin exhibits a triphasic plasma disappearance with a terminal half-life of 18 h (see Table 2). The main metabolite daunorubicinol is less active than daunorubicin. The drug is excreted mainly in bile and to a lesser extent in urine (less than 25 per cent). The usual dose and schedule for daunorubicin administration is 45 to 60 mg/m^2 per day for 3 consecutive days.

A dose of 60 to 75 mg/m^2 every 3 weeks is used for doxorubicin as a single agent. The dose of doxorubicin is usually reduced to 25 to 30 mg/m^2 in combination with other myelotoxic agents. Since anthracyclines produce a dose-related cumulative myocardial damage, the cumulative dose of doxorubicin should not exceed 450 mg/m^2.[23] Following intravenous bolus injection of doxorubicin, there is a triphasic decay of the drug in plasma, with approximately 10 min, 2 h, and 30 h half-lives, respectively. The initial decay phase reflects redistribution of the drug in the tissues followed by a gradual decay during the elimination phase. Plasma protein binding is around 75 per cent. Tissue distribution is not uniform, with the highest concentrations achieved in the lung, liver, spleen, and bone marrow, probably related to preferential accumulation in the reticuloendothelial system. The pattern of distribution can be altered by the kinetics of drug administration (slow infusion or fractionation). Drug concentration in the heart can be reduced using slow (24 h) infusion

rather than bolus injection.[23] There is evidence that administration by slow infusion, avoiding peak plasma concentrations, may reduce the risk of cardiomyopathy without impairing antitumour efficacy. An improvement in the therapeutic index of doxorubicin with slow (96 h) infusion has been documented in patients with breast cancer treated with high doses (150 mg/m^2 or greater).[24] The primary route of elimination is via the bile; around 50 per cent of the administered dose is eliminated in 7 days. Only a small proportion (5 per cent) is excreted in the urine.

Doxorubicin and daunorubicin do not reach the central nervous system, since they are not able to cross the blood–brain barrier. The two antibiotics follow a similar metabolic pathway. The major metabolites of doxorubicin and daunorubicin are doxorubicinol and daunorubicinol, the products of reduction of the side-chain carbonyl group by aldo-keto reductase. The enzyme has a ubiquitous distribution, the highest activity being present in the liver and kidney. The metabolites still retain antitumour activity with a reduced potency consequent to their hydrophilic nature. A further biotransformation of anthracyclines occurs by a reductive deglycosylation to produce insoluble 7-deoxyaglycones. Such metabolic products are inactive and require conjugation with glucuronic or sulphonic acid in order to be excreted.

Clinical efficacy and toxicity

Daunorubicin is one of the most effective agents in the treatment of acute lymphocytic and myelogenous leukaemias, but it has little, if any, activity against solid tumours. Its primary indication is for the treatment of acute myelogenous leukaemia in combination with cytarabine as induction or consolidation therapy.[5]

In spite of the minor molecular change, doxorubicin exhibits a broad spectrum of activity and remains one of the most effective drugs for the treatment of solid tumours. Breast carcinoma, small-cell lung carcinoma, and ovarian carcinoma are the most doxorubicin-responsive solid tumours. Doxorubicin is recognized as the critical component of a number of effective regimens in the treatment of advanced breast carcinoma. The standard combination includes doxorubicin, cyclophosphamide, and 5-fluorouracil. A promising new combination includes doxorubicin and taxol.[25] Doxorubicin is widely used in combination with cyclophosphamide and etoposide for the treatment of small-cell lung carcinoma. Again, it is used in combination with platinum compounds and alkylating agents for the treatment of advanced ovarian carcinoma. However, the introduction of very effective agents (cisplatin and taxanes) has raised doubts about the use of doxorubicin in first-line therapy of ovarian carcinoma. Doxorubicin exhibits a significant activity also in Wilms' tumour, rhabdomyosarcoma, neuroblastoma, soft tissue sarcomas, and carcinomas of the bladder, stomach, liver, and thyroid. It is also highly effective in leukaemias and lymphomas. In particular, it is an important component of the effective regimen for the treatment of Hodgkin's disease in combination with bleomycin, dacarbazine, and vinblastine. Doxorubicin is usually used in combination regimens.

The most common side-effects of anthracyclines are gastrointestinal toxicity (including mucositis, nausea/vomiting, and diarrhoea), alopecia, and myelosuppression. The white blood cell nadir usually occurs at 1 to 2 weeks after drug administration, with a rapid recovery within the following week. The clinical therapy with anthracyclines is associated with both acute and chronic cardiotoxicity. Acute manifestations of cardiac toxicity may be detected shortly

Table 2 Summary of clinical uses, pharmacological features, and toxic effects of anthracyclines

	Therapeutic indications	Doses and schedules	Pharmacology	Toxicity
Daunorubicin	Acute leukaemias	30–60 mg/m² (days 1–3 every 4 weeks) Cumulative dose*: ≤ 550 mg/m²	$t_{\frac{1}{2}}\gamma$, 18–20 h Primary hepatic metabolism (main metabolite, 13-OH derivative, daunorubicinol) Primary biliary excretion	Myelotoxicity (dose-limiting) Alopecia Gastrointestinal toxicity (stomatosis, nausea/vomiting, diarrhoea) Acute cardiotoxicity (not dose-related) Chronic irreversible cardiomyopathy (dose-related)
Idarubicin	Acute leukaemias Non-Hodgkin's lymphoma	Intravenously: 12 mg/m² (days 1–3 every 4 weeks) Cumulative dose: 150 mg/m² Orally: 15–25 mg/m² (days 1–3 every 4 weeks) Cumulative dose*: ≤ 400 mg/m²	$t_{\frac{1}{2}}\gamma$, 15–25 h Main metabolite: 13-OH derivative, idarubicinol ($t_{\frac{1}{2}}\gamma$, 40–70 h) Oral bioavailability: 20–40%	Toxic effects similar to daunorubicin Increased potency with improved therapeutic index
Doxorubicin	Hodgkin's lymphoma Solid tumours (breast carcinoma, small-cell lung cancer, ovarian carcinoma, soft tissue sarcomas, gastric carcinoma, bladder cancer)	50–75 mg/m² (every 3 weeks) Cumulative dose*: ≤ 450 mg/m²	$t_{\frac{1}{2}}\gamma$, 25–30 h Metabolic and excretion pathways similar to daunorubicin (main metabolite: 13-OH derivative, doxorubicinol)	Myelotoxicity (dose-limiting neutropenia) Alopecia Gastrointestinal toxicity Acute and chronic cardiotoxicity
Epirubicin	Clinical use similar to doxorubicin	Standard-dose therapy: 60–90 mg/m² (every 3 weeks) High-dose therapy: 120–150 mg/m² Cumulative dose*: ≤ 900 mg/m²	$t_{\frac{1}{2}}\gamma$, 30–40 h Extensive liver metabolism (main metabolites: glucuronide by conjugation to glucuronic acid through 4'-OH; epirubicinol)	Toxic effects similar to doxorubicin Improved tolerability for non-haematological toxicity and cardiotoxicity

*Maximum cumulative dose associated with acceptable risk of cardiotoxicity.

after infusion by ECG changes including arrhythmias. Such dose-independent changes are usually not severe and are transient. A relatively rare form of acute toxicity is the pericarditis–myocarditis syndrome. However, the most severe toxic manifestation of anthracyclines is chronic cardiotoxicity. These drugs may induce a cumulative, potentially irreversible cardiomyopathy. The risk of congestive heart failure is increased in combination with other cardiotoxic agents or in patients pretreated with mediastinal irradiation or affected by concomitant heart diseases. The risk of cardiac damage is also dependent on patient age. Congestive heart failure may be predicted by serial measurement of left ventricular function or endomyocardial biopsy. The severity of chronic cardiotoxicity requires adequate monitoring to detect subclinical cardiac dysfunctions and to predict the potential risk of onset of congestive heart failure. The most useful non-invasive test is serial radionuclide angiocardiography. This test provides a reproducible measure of left ventricular ejection fraction and is accepted as a sensitive parameter to detect subclinical cardiotoxicity. Cessation of therapy is indicated if cardiac contractility is impaired (10 per cent or greater decrease of left ventricular ejection fraction). In the absence of risk factors, the cumulative doses of anthracyclines should not exceed the maximum tolerated doses reported in Table 2. Prolonged continuous infusion (over 96 h) or fractionation of the dose on consecutive days are employed to reduce the incidence of cardiotoxicity. The relative success of these strategies

relates to reduction of peak plasma concentration of the anthracycline. However, the most successful approach to prevent cardiac damage is the use of the chelating agent, dexrazoxane.[15],[23] The biochemical protector, used at a dose ratio of 10:1 (dexrazoxane:doxorubicin), is usually administered as a 15- to 30-min infusion before doxorubicin.

Epirubicin (4′-epi-doxorubicin)

Epirubicin is the only doxorubicin analogue available for clinical use. It is characterized by epimerization of the hydroxyl group at position 4 of the amino sugar (Fig. 1). The mechanism of action is the same as for doxorubicin. Its pharmacological interest is related to a somewhat improved therapeutic index. However, antitumour efficacy and spectrum of activity are superimposable to those of the parent drug.[5] Peculiar pharmacological features of epirubicin are increased liver metabolism and plasma clearance, and reduced cardiotoxic potential. Epirubicin undergoes an extensive liver metabolism with formation of glucuronides, which are rapidly excreted. Indeed, 50 per cent of the administered dose is excreted in the bile in 4 days and less than 20 per cent in the urine. The improved toxicological profile of epirubicin over doxorubicin is ascribed not only to increased metabolism but also to a reduced cytotoxic potential and reduced ability to generate free radicals. Thus, whereas acute side-effects are comparable with those of doxorubicin, with an equitoxic dose ratio of 1:1.2 (doxorubicin:epirubicin) for haematological toxicity, the risk of cumulative cardiomyopathy is substantially reduced, allowing a cumulative dose up to 900 mg/m² (i.e. equitoxic dose ratio of 1:1.8). The standard dose of epirubicin as a single agent is 90 mg/m² (every 3 weeks). Without haematological support, the standard dose in combination is usually 75 mg/m². The drug is also used in high-dose regimens at a total dose of 120 to 150 mg/m² administered in 2 days. On the basis of its toxicological profile, epirubicin is preferred to doxorubicin for dose escalation, with the concomitant use of bone marrow protective and cardioprotective agents.[26]

In a standard combination with cyclophosphamide and fluorouracil, epirubicin seems to provide some toxicity advantage over doxorubicin also in terms of nausea/vomiting and mucositis. The analogue has been used as a single agent in the treatment of soft tissue sarcoma and has in part replaced doxorubicin in combination treatment of breast carcinoma, ovarian carcinoma, and small-cell lung cancer. A weekly schedule of epirubicin with paclitaxel has been proposed as an effective and well-tolerated second-line chemotherapy for patients with metastatic breast carcinoma.[27] The drug is widely used for intravesical instillation in the treatment of superficial bladder cancer.

Idarubicin

Idarubicin is the 4-demethoxy derivative of daunorubicin (Fig. 1). Removal of the methoxy group in position 4 of the chromophore resulted in an enhancement of the lipophilic character of the drug. The feature is associated with a significant change in the pharmacological profile. Idarubicin is more potent as a cytotoxic agent as a consequence of an increased intracellular drug accumulation. Idarubicin is able partially to overcome resistance mediated by P-glycoprotein overexpression.[28] The mechanism of action is the same as that of parent anthracyclines, namely DNA intercalation and inhibition of topoisomerase II. However, removal of the methoxy group markedly enhances the drug's ability to induce topoisomerase II-mediated DNA cleavage.[6] It is likely that the removal of the bulky methoxy group in the intercalating moiety allows a more favourable interaction of the drug in the ternary complex. An increased effect at the target level could at least in part contribute to the cytotoxic potential.

The cytotoxic potency of idarubicin is also reflected in antitumour potency, since the drug has comparable or superior antitumour activity at lower dose levels than daunorubicin. The drug lipophilicity allows oral absorption. Oral formulation requires an increase (3.5 times) of the dose to achieve an effect comparable with that obtained with intravenous administration. Such a property represents an additional advantage of idarubicin over daunorubicin, which is completely inactive when administered orally. A major problem with oral idarubicin is the variation in bioavailability, which ranges from 12 to 49 per cent. Idarubicin is extensively metabolized by reduction of the side-chain carbonyl group to a secondary alcoholic group. The 13-hydroxy metabolite, idarubicinol, is still active as an antitumour agent at least in preclinical models, but less cardiotoxic. The terminal half-life of idarubicin is around 15 h, but plasma removal of idarubicinol is slower (40 to 70 h half-life). The drug is excreted, mainly as idarubicinol, in urine (only marginally in bile).

The clinical efficacy of idarubicin is restricted to the treatment of leukaemia. The lack of activity of idarubicin against solid tumours is a common feature of daunorubicin analogues. The pharmacological

basis of this behaviour is still unclear, since the anthracyclines share a common cellular target. The drug is mostly used in the treatment of non-lymphocytic leukaemia, in which it is at least as effective as daunorubicin. Idarubicin is administered intravenously at a dose of 12 mg/m² for 3 consecutive days in combination with cytarabine. In view of the incomplete cross-resistance with daunorubicin, the possibility exists that idarubicin is also useful in patients pretreated with daunorubicin. Idarubicin is also effective against acute lymphocytic leukaemia. Myelotoxicity is the primary acute side-effect of idarubicin. Compared with doxorubicin, idarubicin is characterized by an improved tolerability profile at least in terms of extramedullary toxicity, which allows a safer escalation of the dose. In common with other anthracyclines, idarubicin may have a cardiotoxic potential. However, the risk of cardiotoxicity appears somewhat lower at therapeutic doses than that of daunorubicin.[29] Table 2 shows some relevant pharmacological and toxicological features and clinical use of the currently available anthracyclines.

Novel anthracyclines

Several liposomal formulations of doxorubicin and daunorubicin have been investigated with the aim of improving the drug therapeutic index. Recent studies with doxorubicin encapsulated in pegylated liposomes, doxil, indicated substantial activity in heavily pretreated ovarian cancer[30] and in advanced breast cancer,[31] with mild myelotoxicity. Promising results have been reported even with liposomal daunorubicin (daunoxome) in refractory lymphomas.[32] The altered pharmacological behaviour seems to reduce the risk of myelosuppression and cardiotoxicity.

Methoxymorpholino-doxorubicin (FCE 23762, MMRDX, PNU 152243) is a very potent drug which was originally identified as a new anthracycline with at least a partially novel mode of action and activity against resistant tumours (Fig. 5). Unlike other anthracyclines, MMRDX has been found to act through topoisomerase I-mediated single-strand breaks. A broad phase II study was recently performed in 48 patients with intrinsically resistant tumours.[33] The drug was given by intravenous bolus at 1.5 mg/m², every 4 weeks. A low response rate was observed. Antitumour activity after oral treatment has been reported, but severe gastrointestinal toxicity in phase I studies has hampered its clinical development for oral administration.[34]

MX-2 is a lipid-soluble morpholino anthracycline derivative (Fig. 5) which causes DNA strand breaks through interaction with topoisomerase II.[35] Its pharmacological interest is related to activity against resistant cells with the multidrug resistance phenotype and to reduced cardiotoxicity. MX-2 exhibited a significant activity (overall response rate 43 per cent) in the treatment of recurrent high-grade glioma.[36]

Aclacinomycin A is an anthracycline antibiotic (Fig. 6), first described as a topoisomerase II inhibitor. The drug has been shown to stabilize topoisomerase I covalent complexes efficiently.[37] Clinical use of the drug is mainly in patients with leukaemia or lymphoma, in combination with etoposide or cytosine arabinoside.[38]

A 9-amino-anthracycline (amrubicin, SM-5887) (Fig. 7) was found effective and well tolerated in the treatment of small-cell lung cancer.[39]

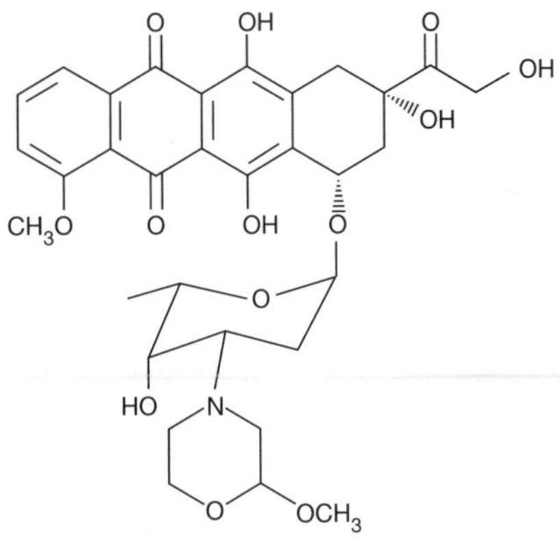

Methoxymorpholino-doxorubicin

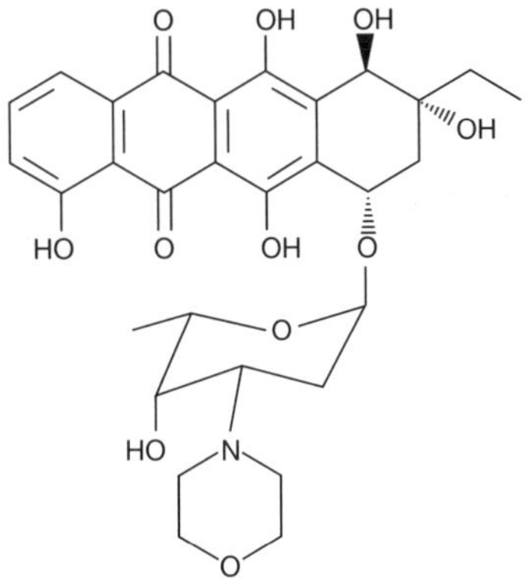

Fig. 7 The chemical structure of amrubicin.

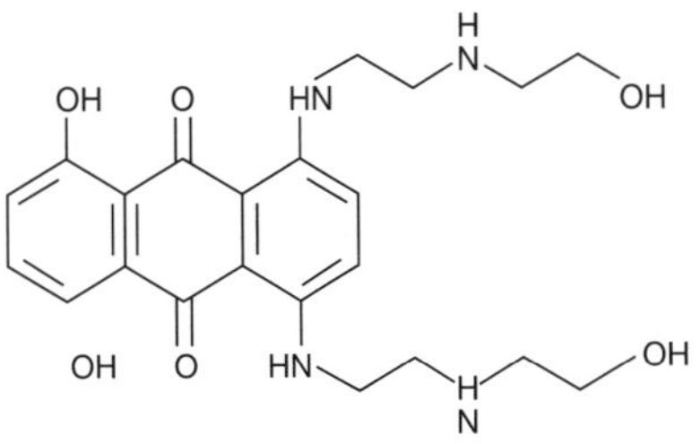

Amrubicin (SM-5887)

Morpholinyloxaunomycin (MX2)

Fig. 5 The chemical structure of morpholino derivatives of anthracyclines.

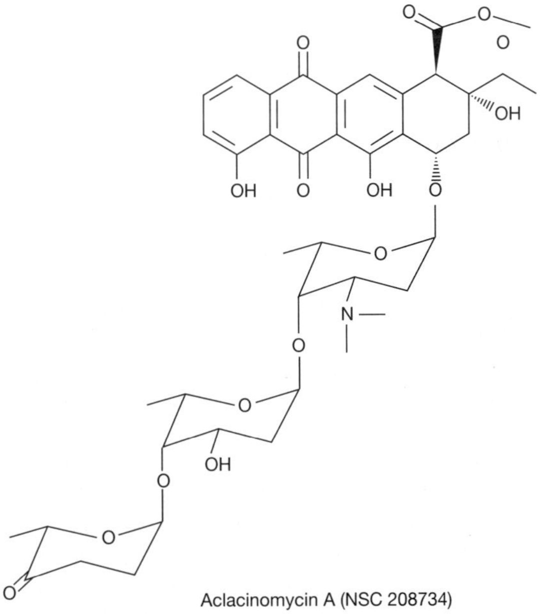

Mitoxantrone

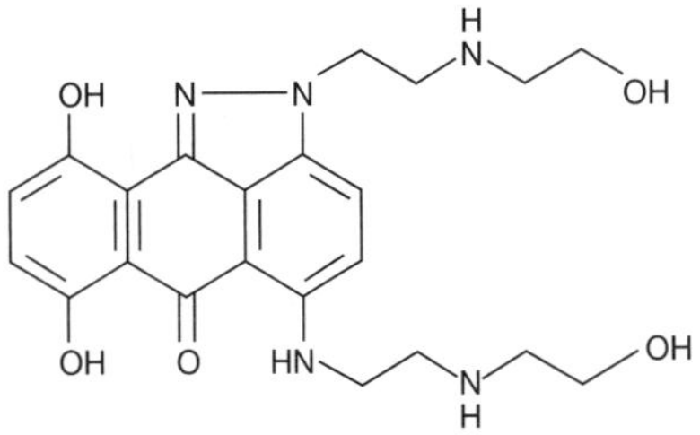

Losoxantrone

Fig. 8 The chemical structure of anthracycline-related synthetic intercalating agents.

Aclacinomycin A (NSC 208734)

Fig. 6 The chemical structure of aclacinomycin A, a trisaccharide anthracycline containing the aklavinone chromophore.

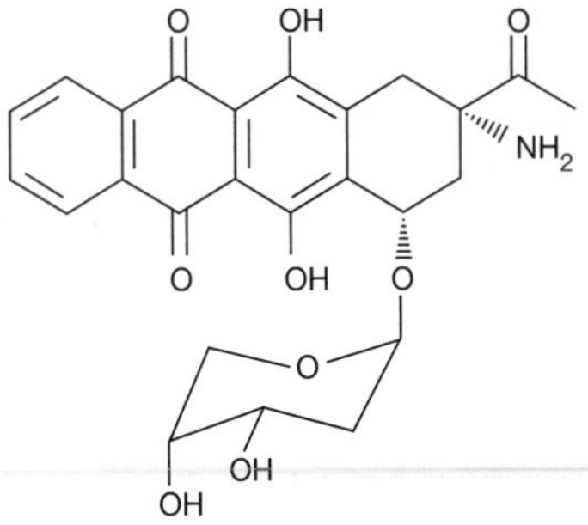

Menogaril is a nogalamycin analogue different from other anthracyclines. This agent is active after oral administration. Its anti-leukaemic activity was found to be comparable with that of other clinically effective anthracyclines.[40]

Anthracycline-related synthetic compounds

Mitoxantrone

Mitoxantrone is the first of a large series of synthetic DNA intercalating agents (anthracenediones) with a significant efficacy in antitumour chemotherapy (Fig. 8).[41] As a synthetic compound, it cannot be grouped among antibiotics. Based on the structural similarities to anthracyclines and on the mechanism of action, mitoxantrone could be regarded as an anthracycline-like agent. However, the structure of mitoxantrone differs significantly from that of naturally occurring anthracyclines (e.g. doxorubicin and daunorubicin), since its chromophore (i.e. the intercalating moiety) is composed of only three aromatic rings and two symmetrical side-chains. Thus, like other intercalators effective as antitumour agents, mitoxantrone has the features of an external binder, since intercalation of the planar chromophore is accompanied by groove binding of the charged side-chains. As in the case of anthracyclines, the external binding moieties are crucial determinants of antitumour activity and of ability to inhibit topoisomerase II function. Anthracyclines and anthracenediones also differ in the sequence specificity of DNA cleavage stimulated by DNA topoisomerase II. In spite of its intercalating properties, mitoxantrone more closely resembles epipodophyllotoxins (e.g. etoposide) in its sequence specificity.[7]

The pharmacological significance of the structural features in drug interaction with the ternary complex remains to be defined. However, it is likely that a specific interaction may be relevant in the different profiles of antitumour activity of various topoisomerase II poisons. As expected on the basis of its mechanism of action, mitoxantrone is most effective in the S-phase of the cell cycle, since expression of DNA topoisomerase II (α-isoform) is increased during DNA synthesis. However, mitoxantrone is cytotoxic to proliferating and non-proliferating cells, thus suggesting the involvement of alternative mechanisms of action. Like other topoisomerase inhibitors, mitoxantrone induces protein-associated DNA strand breaks (i.e. enzyme-mediated DNA cleavage). However, mitoxantrone also induces non-protein-associated DNA damage that has been related to oxidative activation of the drug.[41]

As for other intercalating agents, the development of resistance to mitoxantrone is regarded as multifactorial. Overexpression of P-glycoprotein has been described in some but not in all mitoxantrone-resistant human tumour cell lines. Exposure to mitoxantrone may select cells with an atypical resistance profile, displaying only partial cross-resistance to other intercalating agents and sensitivity to vinca alkaloids.[42] Although the resistant phenotype involves defects in intracellular drug accumulation, it is not related to overexpression of P-glycoprotein.

Clinical pharmacology

Following intravenous administration, mitoxantrone exhibits a rapid tissue distribution with a triphasic plasma disappearance. The terminal half-life is 23 to 42 h. The primary elimination is hepatobiliary. Thus, the dose should be reduced when there is severe liver impairment. Less than 10 per cent of the administered dose can be found in the urine. As a single agent, the standard dose for intravenous administration is 12 to 14 mg/m². The dose is usually reduced to 10 mg/m² in combinations. For the treatment of solid tumours, this dose is repeated every three weeks. For the treatment of leukaemia, the drug is usually administered for 3 consecutive days at a dose of 12 mg/m². The cumulative dose should not exceed 160 mg/m², to avoid cardiotoxicity. The dose should be reduced in the presence of risk factors for cardiotoxicity.

Clinical activity and toxicity

Although mitoxantrone exhibits a limited spectrum of antitumour activity, it is an effective and better tolerated alternative to anthracyclines in haematological malignancies and breast carcinoma.

Comparative studies of mitoxantrone and doxorubicin as monotherapy in patients with advanced breast carcinoma indicated a slightly greater activity of doxorubicin, which is currently considered the most effective agent in the treatment of the disease. For this reason mitoxantrone has been incorporated in a variety of combination regimens for the same indication. As with anthracyclines, a promising combination includes mitoxantrone and taxol.[43] A potential advantage of paclitaxel/mitoxantrone over paclitaxel/doxorubicin is a reduced risk of development of cardiotoxicity. The potential benefit of mitoxantrone-based regimens is probably dependent on the tolerability of a combination rather than on the therapeutic efficacy.

Mitoxantrone is a useful component of induction chemotherapy regimens for the treatment of lymphocytic and non-lymphocytic leukaemia, particularly in combination with cytarabine. The efficacy of mitoxantrone and cytarabine is comparable with that achieved with daunorubicin and cytarabine, but with reduced side-effects. The improved tolerability of mitoxantrone over anthracyclines has allowed the use of very high doses in induction regimens, particularly in aggressive lymphomas.[44] Mitoxantrone is widely used as a component of low-toxicity regimens designed for the treatment of elderly patients. Activity of mitoxantrone has been documented also in the treatment of blast crisis of chronic myelogenous leukaemia. Mitoxantrone in combination with corticosteroids is useful for palliative treatment of hormone-resistant prostate cancer, with an appreciable improvement over corticosteroids alone.[45]

Myelosuppression is a major dose-limiting toxicity which may be more frequent and severe than that produced by doxorubicin. Leucopenia (in particular neutropenia) occurs 10 to 14 days after drug treatment, usually with recovery in a week. However, mitoxantrone displays an improved tolerability profile concerning extramedullary toxicity, with a lower incidence of nausea/vomiting, alopecia, stomatitis, and cardiotoxicity. The toxicity profile and evidence of dose–response effects makes mitoxantrone a drug suitable for use in high-dose therapy regimens.[44] Cardiac monitoring is recommended for patients treated with mitoxantrone, particularly in patients with pre-existing cardiac risk factors. Mitoxantrone may be contraindicated following substantial anthracycline pretreatment and in patients with severe alterations of cardiac function or severe hepatic dysfunction.

Anthrapyrazoles

Like anthracenediones, anthrapyrazoles are synthetic agents with structural similarities to anthracyclines (Fig. 8).[46],[47] The compounds have been designed and developed as potentially less cardiotoxic intercalating agents. Anthrapyrazoles retain the planar structure of anthracyclines and the two side-chains present in effective anthracenediones. Thus, the mechanism of cytotoxic action of anthrapyrazoles has been related to DNA intercalation and topoisomerase II inhibition. However, the addition of a fourth ring to the chromophore modifies the redox properties of the quinone, making it less susceptible to semiquinone reduction and free-radical formation. Indeed, preclinical studies have indicated a minimal superoxide formation and reduced cardiotoxic potential. Losoxantrone (formerly known as CI 941 or DuP 941) is the most widely studied anthrapyrazole. The peculiar pharmacological features of the agent are rapid extensive tissue distribution and a slow rate of elimination with a long-term terminal half-life (greater than 40 h). The activity of losoxantrone as a single agent in metastatic breast carcinoma is

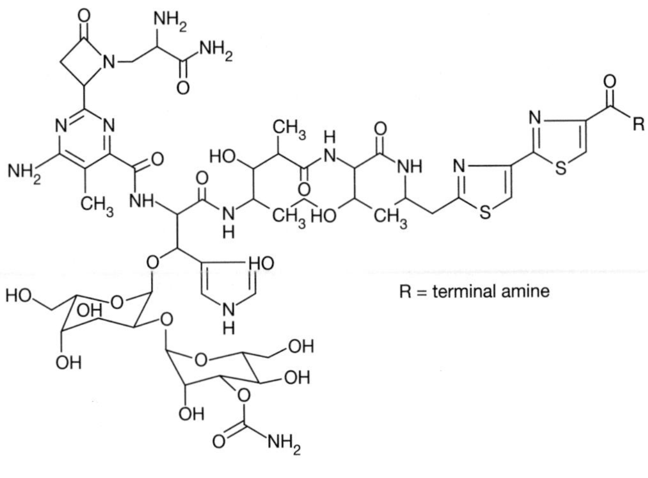

Fig. 9 The chemical structure of bleomycin.

comparable with that of doxorubicin, and the compound may represent a less cardiotoxic alternative to anthracyclines. Combination studies of losoxantrone with other effective agents (in particular, paclitaxel) are planned. A significant activity has been reported in patients with metastatic hormone-refractory prostate carcinoma. As a single agent, the dose of 50 mg/m² every 3 weeks has been used. The major toxicity associated with losoxantrone is neutropenia (grade 3/4 in most treated patients), which occurs around 14 days after treatment with a rapid recovery and no evidence of cumulative toxicity.

Bleomycin

Mechanism of action and resistance

Bleomycin is a glycopeptide antibiotic, originally isolated from *Streptomyces verticillus* as a copper complex (Fig. 9). The antitumour activity of bleomycin is ascribed to its ability to bind to DNA. Although there is evidence that the binding involves a partial intercalation of the bithiazole, the drug induces a type of DNA damage, namely strand scission, different from known intercalators.[48] The effect has been related to the production of reactive oxygen species. The drug forms a co-ordination complex with iron, which is required for the redox reaction. Iron oxidation produces superoxide and other reactive oxygen species, which are responsible for DNA damage associated with deoxyribose degradation and release of damaged base. Bleomycin-induced DNA strand scission shows a sequence specificity. The mode of drug–DNA interaction, involving a partial intercalation and minor groove binding, is responsible for recognition of specific DNA sequences and/or structures. Drug cytotoxicity is enhanced by glutathione, which is involved in recycling of Fe^{3+} to Fe^{2+} required for the redox process. The sensitivity of tumour cells to bleomycin-induced DNA damage is dependent on the intracellular level of Fe^{2+}. Ferritin provides the iron required for drug-induced DNA damage. However, exogenous Fe^{2+} enhances DNA degradation in drug-treated cells. The cytotoxic activity of bleomycin can also be enhanced by

oxygen. Pulmonary toxicity is also potentiated by increasing inhaled oxygen concentration.

Based on the mechanism of action, it is likely that cellular ability to recognize and repair damaged DNA plays an important role in drug resistance. In addition, bleomycin hydrolase activity may represent a relevant factor involved in resistance to the drug, since tumour cell lines selected *in vitro* following drug exposure may express high levels of the bleomycin-inactivating enzyme. The role of the enzyme as a determinant of cellular sensitivity is also suggested by the observation that lung and skin, the normal tissues most susceptible to drug toxicity, exhibit low enzyme levels. Although bleomycin is also toxic to slowly proliferating cells, tumour cells are more susceptible to the drug action during G2 or mitotic phases. Since pharmacokinetic studies have indicated a short half-life of the drug in patients, it is conceivable that continuous infusion should expose a larger fraction of tumour cells during sensitive phases of the cell cycle than bolus administration.

Clinical pharmacology

Following injection of an intravenous bolus, the plasma-clearance curve of bleomycin has two components with half-lives of about 0.5 h and 2 to 4 h, respectively. Since the plasma disappearance may be markedly affected by renal function, as a consequence of altered drug excretion, a dose reduction is necessary in patients with severe renal dysfunction to avoid lung toxicity. Most of the administered drug is excreted unchanged in the urine. Bleomycin may also be given by other routes of administration (subcutaneous or intramuscular), with no obvious differences in clinical antitumour activity associated with different routes. Bleomycin has also been injected into the pleural or peritoneal cavity to control malignant effusions, since high drug levels may be achieved with this route.

The limited drug ability to cross the plasma membrane represents a relevant drawback for its efficacy.[49] Approaches for permeabilization by electric pulses have been attempted to potentiate drug effects at the tumour site.[50],[51]

Clinical activity and toxicity

Bleomycin is used in several combinations for the treatment of Hodgkin's disease, non-Hodgkin's lymphoma, testicular cancer, and several squamous cell carcinomas, including carcinoma of the cervix, vulva, skin, and head and neck. The drug may be useful for intracavitary treatment of malignant effusions. In contrast to most DNA-damaging agents, bleomycin causes only a moderate myelotoxicity. Acute side-effects include fever, chills, flu-like symptoms, and sometimes hypotension and tachypnoea. The most relevant side-effect is pulmonary toxicity, which occurs as a late chronic alteration that may evolve to interstitial fibrosis. The risk of this manifestation is enhanced by concomitant radiation therapy and administration of nephrotoxic drugs causing reduced drug excretion. The occurrence and severity of pulmonary alterations in patients treated with bleomycin-containing regimens depend on risk factors such as age and total dose of bleomycin. Most patients have only subclinical lung damage, which can be detected by specific lung function tests. Pulmonary alterations are common after a cumulative dose of 300 mg. Indirect evidence supports that induction of cytokines following bleomycin treatment may be responsible for acute drug-specific side-effects, including fever and sepsis-like symptoms.[52]

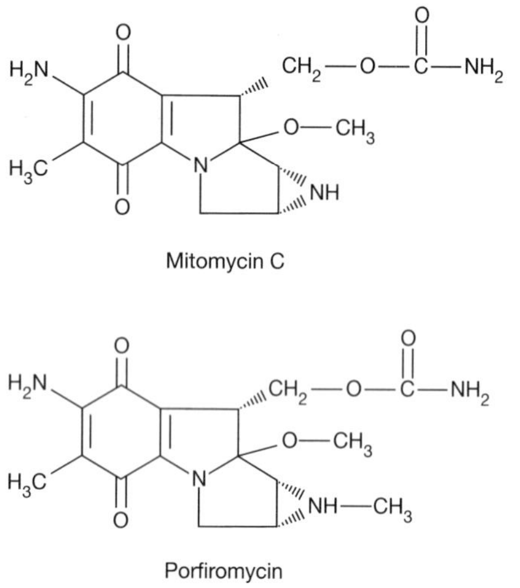

Fig. 10 The chemical structure of mitomycin C and porfiromycin.

Mitomycin C and porfiromycin

Mitomycin

Mechanism of action and resistance

Mitomycin C (Fig. 10), isolated in 1958 from *Streptomyces caespitosus* and originally studied in Japan, belongs to a group of antibiotics with antibacterial and antitumour activity. The previously isolated mitomycin A and B were of no therapeutic interest in spite of minor structural changes. In contrast, mitomycin C displays antitumour activity against some adenocarcinomas and marked activity when administered topically against superficial lesions in transitorial cell carcinoma of the bladder. The antibiotic is relatively inactive in the natural form. A peculiar feature of the agent is its reductive activation to a cytotoxic agent in a hypoxic environment, thus conferring some degree of selectivity toward solid tumours.[53] Following reduction of the quinone to hydroxyquinone, the drug behaves as a bifunctional alkylating agent. In addition to DNA damage by alkylation, oxygen free-radical generation may participate in the antitumour action of the drug. Although mitomycin C is considered the prototype bioreductive agent, selective toxicity toward hypoxic cells is modest. A related compound, porfiromycin, has a somewhat greater hypoxic-selective toxicity than mitomycin C. Whether the effect of mitomycin C on specific tumour types is the result of preferential drug cytotoxicity toward hypoxic cells is still unclear.[54] A DT-diaphorase (NAD(P)H: quinone oxidoreductase) activity has been implicated as a determinant of chemosensitivity in human colon and gastric carcinoma cells. Following metabolic activation, the drug binds covalently to minor groove DNA with preferential alkylation of guanine at the N2 position, resulting in monofunctional and bifunctional adducts. As for other alkylating agents, an association has been reported between cyto-toxicity and interstrand cross-link formation.[55] Drug–DNA in-teraction involves specific DNA sequence recognition, since cross-link formation is selective for minor groove GC sequences.

Information on the mechanisms of resistance to mitomycin has been derived from cell systems selected for resistance *in vitro*. As observed for other natural compounds, resistance to mitomycin C is described as a multifactorial phenomenon. Mitomycin-resistant sublines appear to display accumulation defects, decreased activation, or increased levels of glutathione or glutathione-dependent enzymes. In particular, mitomycin is associated with the multidrug resistance phenotype mediated by overexpression of P-glycoprotein, which is responsible for reduced drug accumulation secondary to enhanced drug efflux. Cells selected for resistance to melphalan (a bifunctional alkylating agent) and characterized by increased repair of interstrand cross-links show cross-resistance to mitomycin.[55] It is thus likely that alkylating agents and mitomycin share common mechanisms of resistance, including increased DNA repair and/or increased tolerance of unrepaired damage.

Clinical pharmacology and toxicity

Following intravenous administration, mitomicin C disappears quickly from the plasma, as a result of tissue distribution and hepatic metabolism (Table 3). Less than 10 per cent of the administered dose is detected in a 24-h urine sample. Most of the administered drug is metabolized, and only a marginal amount is eliminated unchanged by biliary and urinary excretion. Following endovesical instillation, a very low systemic absorption of the drug was detected. The drug is usually administered intravenously at 20 mg/m^2 as a single agent, or at 10 mg/m^2 in combinations. The cumulative dose should not exceed 50 mg/m^2 to avoid relevant toxicity. Care should be taken to avoid extravasation, which may cause severe local tissue injury and necrosis. The main toxic manifestations of mitomycin are delayed cumulative leuco- and thrombocytopenia and cumulative anaemia.[56],[57] Recovery is slow and often incomplete. The drug has been implicated in renal failure, often associated with microangiopathic haemolytic anaemia.[58] The manifestation is rarely reversible. An increased risk of car-diomyopathy has been reported in patients receiving a combination of mitomycin C and doxorubicin. The potentiation of cardiac toxicity is not surprising, since both drugs are implicated in the production of free radicals, which are probably involved in the organ-specific toxicity.

Clinical activity

Mitomycin C is characterized by a wide spectrum of antitumour activity.[56] Significant activity has been documented toward gas-trointestinal tumours (including carcinomas of oesophagus, pancreas, and stomach), breast carcinoma, and bladder carcinoma. The drug is one of the most effective agents for intravesical therapy of superficial bladder cancer and other topical applications.[56],[59] A number of squamous cell carcinomas (e.g. oesophageal, anal, vulvar, and head and neck) are responsive to combination therapy containing mitomycin C. The drug has been used as a radiosensitizer in combination with radiotherapy for the treatment of head and neck cancer and anal squamous cell carcinoma, with a significant therapeutic benefit. Mi-tomycin C has also been proposed for intraperitoneal hyperthermic chemotherapy for the treatment of malignant ascites.[60]

Porfiromycin

Porfiromycin is a closely related analogue of mitomycin C and is characterized by the introduction of an N-methyl group in the aziridine ring (Fig. 10). The antitumour activity profile and the pattern of toxicity of the two compounds are comparable. Porfiromycin was more expensive to manufacture and exhibited a slightly increased

Table 3 Pharmacological and toxicity features of mitomycin C

Clinical use	Doses	Pharmacology	Toxicity
Combination therapy Gastrointestinal tumours (in particular, pancreatic and gastric carcinoma) Breast cancer Squamous cell carcinoma (head and neck, oesophageal, cervical, vulvar, anal)	Intravenous administration: 10–20 mg/m² every 6–8 weeks Intravesical administration: 20–40 mg in 20–40 ml weekly for 8 weeks	$t_{\frac{1}{2}}\alpha$ 8 min $t_{\frac{1}{2}}\beta$ 40–60 min Rapid tissue distribution Primary hepatic metabolism	Delayed leucopenia and thrombocytopenia (cumulative and dose-limiting) Cumulative anaemia Haemolitic-uraemic syndrome* Renal toxicity* Interstitial pneumonitis*
Locoregional therapy Superficial bladder cancer Malignant ascites			

*Low frequency below 50 mg/m².

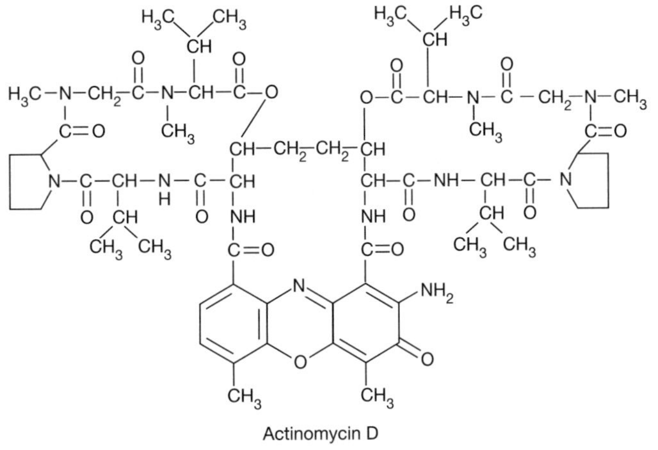

Fig. 11 The chemical structure of actinomycin.

cumulative toxicity. For these reasons, porfiromycin had a limited clinical success. However, preclinical studies have documented an increased preferential toxicity of porfiromycin against hypoxic cells compared with mitomycin C, thus suggesting a therapeutic advantage of porfiromycin over mitomycin C when used in combination with radiation therapy. A recent clinical study suggested the potential interest of the concomitant use of porfiromycin with radiation therapy in the treatment of locally advanced (stage III/IV) squamous cell carcinoma of the head and neck.[61]

Actinomycin D

Actinomycin D (or dactinomycin) is an antibiotic belonging to a large class of compounds produced by *Streptomyces* species. Structurally, the molecule consists of two polypeptide chains linked to a planar three-ring (phenoxazone) chromophore (Fig. 11). Actinomycin is a well-known intercalating agent with specificity for GC-rich sequences. The phenoxazone ring is the intercalating moiety, and the peptide chains bind to the minor groove. As a result of DNA interaction, actinomycin

D is a strong inhibitor of RNA transcription. However, the drug inhibits multiple DNA functions, including DNA synthesis, and is a dual topoisomerase I and II inhibitor.[62] Since a number of more specific topoisomerase poisons are effective antitumour agents, it is likely that drug interference with topoisomerase function is the primary mechanism responsible for antitumour activity. Other (presumably less specific) effects on DNA functions may account for the marked cytotoxic potency and the low therapeutic index of the drug. Actinomycin D is involved in the multidrug resistance phenotype, since it is a substrate of P-glycoprotein.[18] Indeed, the multidrug resistance phenomenon was first described in cell lines selected for resistance to actinomycin D.

Plasma clearance of actinomycin D initially is rapid, reflecting tissue uptake and distribution. A slow release of the drug from the tissues determines a prolonged second phase of drug disappearance with a half-life of 36 h. Most of the drug is excreted unchanged in the urine and bile. Methabolism dose not play a significant role in pharmacological behaviour of the drug.

Clinical activity and toxic effects

Actinomycin has been used mainly in the treatment of choriocarcinoma and of a variety of childhood tumours (Wilms' tumour, Ewing's sarcoma, and embryonal rhabdomyosarcoma). A well-known therapeutic regimen is the combination with vincristine and cyclophosphamide for the treatment of germ cell tumours of the ovary. Testicular cancer is known to be responsive to actinomycin D. Owing to the low therapeutic index of actinomycin D, the drug has been partially replaced by less toxic regimens. Actinomycin D is very potent as a cytotoxic and antitumour agent and is administered intravenously at doses of 0.4 to 0.45 mg/m² daily for 5 days. As for anthracyclines, the drug may cause severe tissue damage following extravasation. Myelosuppression is the dose-limiting toxicity.[63] It may be a severe side-effect beginning within the first week of treatment, but the nadir may be reached later (21 days). Severe vomiting often occurs after a few hours and lasts for up to 24 h. Alopecia, mucositis, and cutaneous alterations (erythema, hyperpigmentation, and desquamation) are common toxicities and are potentiated by previous or concurrent radiation therapy.

References

1. Arcamone F. *Doxorubicin. Anticancer Antibiotics*. Medicinal Chemistry Series, vol. 17. New York: Academic Press, 1981.

2. Zunino F, Capranico G. Sequence-selective groove binders. In: Teicher B, ed. *Cancer Therapeutics: Experimental and Clinical Agents*. Totowa, NJ: Humana Press Inc., 1997: 195–214.

3. Arcamone F, *et al.* Doxorubicin disaccharide analogue: apoptosis-related improvement of efficacy *in vivo*. *Journal of the National Cancer Institute*, 1997; 89: 1217–23.

4. Arcamone F, *et al.* New developments in antitumor anthracyclines. *Pharmacology and Therapeutics*, 1997; 76: 117–24.

5. Weiss RB. The anthracyclines: will we ever find a better doxorubicin? *Seminars in Oncology*, 1992; 19: 670–86.

6. Zunino F, Capranico G. DNA topoisomerase II as the primary target of anti-tumor anthracyclines. *Anticancer-Drug Design*, 1992; 5: 307–17.

7. Capranico G, Zunino F. DNA topoisomerase-trapping antitumor drugs. *European Journal of Cancer*, 1992; 28A: 2055–60.

8. Capranico G, Binaschi M, Borgnetto ME, Zunino F, Palumbo M. A protein-mediated mechanism for the DNA sequence-specific action of topoisomerase II poisons. *Trends in Pharmacological Sciences*, 1997; 18: 323–8.

9. Myers C. Anthracyclines. In: Pinedo HM, Longo DL, Chabner BA, eds. *Cancer Chemotherapy and Biological Response Modifiers Annual 10*. Amsterdam: Elsevier, 1988: 33–9.

10. Alegria AE, Samuni A, Mitchell JB, Riesz P, Russo A. Free radicals induced by adriamycin-sensitive and adriamycin-resistant cells: a spin-trapping study. *Biochemistry*, 1989; 28: 8653–8.

11. Burdon RH. Superoxide and hydrogen peroxide in relation to mammalian cell proliferation. *Free Radical Biology and Medicine*, 1995; 18: 775–94.

12. Polyak K, Xia Y, Zweier JL, Kinzler KW, Vogelstein B. A model for p53-induced apoptosis. *Nature*, 1997; 389: 300–5.

13. Weijl NI, Cleton FJ, Osanto S. Free radicals and antioxidants in chemotherapy-induced toxicity. *Cancer Treatment Reviews*, 1997; 23: 209–40.

14. Hellmann K. Cardioprotection by dexrazoxane (Cardioxane; ICRF 187): progress in supportive care. *Supportive Care in Cancer*, 1996; 4: 305–7.

15. Swain SM, Whaley FS, Gerber MC, Ewer MS, Bianchine JR, Gams RA. Delayed administration of dexrazoxane provides cardioprotection for patients with advanced breast cancer treated with doxorubicin-containing therapy. *Journal of Clinical Oncology*, 1997; 15: 1333–40.

16. Minotti G, *et al.* The secondary alcohol metabolite of doxorubicin irreversibly inactivates aconitase/iron regulatory protein-1 in cytosolic fractions from human myocardium. *FASEB Journal*, 1998; 12: 541–52.

17. Lehnert M. Clinical multidrug resistance in cancer: a multifactorial problem. *European Journal of Cancer*, 1996; 32A: 912–20.

18. Gottesman MM, Pastan I. Biochemistry of multidrug resistance mediated by the multidrug transporter. *Annual Review of Biochemistry*, 1993; 62: 385–427.

19. Cole SPC, *et al.* Overexpression of a transporter gene in a multidrug-resistant human lung cancer cell line. *Science*, 1992; 258: 1650–4.

20. Binaschi M, *et al.* MRP gene overexpression in a human doxorubicin-resistant SCLC cell line: alterations in cellular pharmacokinetics and in pattern of cross-resistance. *International Journal of Cancer*, 1995; 62: 84–9.

21. Zaman GJR, *et al.* The human multidrug resistance-associated protein MRP is a plasma membrane drug-efflux pump. *Proceedings of the National Academy of Sciences (USA)*, 1994; 91: 8822–6.

22. Zunino F, Perego P, Pilotti S, Pratesi G, Supino R. Role of apoptotic response in cellular resistance to cytotoxic agents. *Pharmacology and Therapeutics*, 1997; 76: 177–85.

23. Basser RL, Green MD. Strategies for prevention of anthracycline cardiotoxicity. *Cancer Treatment Reviews*, 1993; 19: 57–77.

24. Synold TW, Doroshow JH. Anthracycline dose intensity: clinical pharmacology and pharmacokinetics of high-dose doxorubicin administered as a 96-hour continuous intravenous infusion. *Journal of Infusional Chemotherapy*, 1996; 6: 69–73.

25. Gianni L, *et al.* Paclitaxel by 3-hour infusion in combination with bolus doxorubicin in women with untreated metastatic breast cancer: high antitumor efficacy and cardiac effects in a dose-findings and sequence-finding study. *Journal of Clinical Oncology*, 1995; 13: 2688–99.

26. Vermorken JB, *et al.* High-dose intensity regimens with epirubicin in ovarian cancer. *Seminars in Oncology*, 1994; 21: 17–22.

27. Kohler U, Olbricht SS, Fuechsel G, Kettner E, Richter B, Ridwelski K. Weekly paclitaxel with epirubicin as second-line therapy of metastatic breast cancer: results of a clinical phase II study. *Seminars in Oncology*, 1997; 24: S17–S40.

28. Animati F, *et al.* Biochemical and pharmacological activity of novel 8-fluoroanthracyclines: influence of stereochemistry and conformation. *Molecular Pharmacology*, 1996; 50: 603–9.

29. Anderlini P, *et al.* Idarubicin cardiotoxicity: a retrospective study in acute myeloid leukemia and myelodysplasia. *Journal of Clinical Oncology*, 1995; 13: 2827–34.

30. Muggia FM, *et al.* Phase II study of liposomal doxorubicin in refractory ovarian cancer: antitumor activity and toxicity modification by liposomal encapsulation. *Journal of Clinical Oncology*, 1997; 15: 987–93.

31. Ranson MR, Carmichael J, O'Byrne K, Stewart S, Smith D, Howell A. Treatment of advanced breast cancer with sterically stabilized liposomal doxorubicin: results of a multicenter phase II trial. *Journal of Clinical Oncology*, 1997; 15: 3185–91.

32. Richardson DS, Kelsey SM, Johnson SA, Tighe M, Cavenagh JD, Newland AC. Early evaluation of liposomal daunorubicin (daunoxome, nexstar) in the treatment of relapsed and refractory lymphoma. *Investigational New Drugs*, 1997; 15: 247–53.

33. Bakker M, *et al.* Broad phase II and pharmacokinetic study of methoxy-morpholino doxorubicin (FCE 23762-MMRDX) in non-small-cell lung cancer, renal cancer and other solid tumour patients. *British Journal of Cancer*, 1998; 77: 139–46.

34. Sessa C, *et al.* Phase I clinical and pharmacokinetic (PK) study of oral (PO) methoxy-morpholino doxorubicin (PNU 152243) on a single intermittent schedule. *Proceedings of the 10th NCI-EORTC Symposium on New Drugs in Cancer Therapy*, Amsterdam, June 16–19, 1998: 118.

35. Duran GE, Lau DH, Lewis AD, Kuhl JS, Bammler TK, Sikic BI. Differential single-versus double-strand DNA breakage produced by doxorubicin and its morpholinyl analogues. *Cancer Chemotherapy and Pharmacology*, 1996; 38: 210–16.

36. Underhill C, *et al.* MX2 (KRN8602), an active new agent with low toxicity in high grade malignant glioma. *Proceedings of the 10th NCI-EORTC Symposium on New Drugs in Cancer Therapy*, Amsterdam, June 16–19, 1998: 170.

37. Nitiss JL, Pourquier P, Pommier Y. Aclacinomycin A stabilizes topoisomerase I covalent complexes. *Cancer Research*, 1997; 57: 4564–9.

38. Rowe JM, Chang AY, Bennett JM. Aclacinomycin A and etoposide (VP-16–213): an effective regimen in previously treated patients with refractory acute myeologenous leukemia. *Blood*, 1988; 71: 992–6.

39. Yana T, Negoro S, Takada Y, Yokota S, Fukuoka M and the West Japan Lung Cancer Group. Phase II study of amrubicin (SM-5887), a 9-amino-anthracycline, in previously untreated patients with extensive stage small-cell lung cancer (ES-SCLC): a West Japan lung cancer group trial. *Proceedings of the American Society for Clinical Oncology*, 1998; 17: 450.

40. Dutcher JP, *et al.* A phase II study of menogaril (7R-O-methylnogarol)

in patients with relapsed/refractory acute myeloid leukemia: a study of the eastern Cooperative Oncology Group. *Leukemia*, 1995; **9**: 1638–42.

41. **Faulds D, Balfour JA, Chrisp P, Langtry HD.** Mitoxantrone. A review of its pharmacodynamic and pharmacokinetic properties, and therapeutic potential in the chemotherapy of cancer. *Drugs*, 1991; **41**: 400–49.

42. **Dalton WS, Cress AE, Alberts DS, Trent JM.** Cytogenetic and phenotypic analysis of a human colon carcinoma cell line resistant to mitoxantrone. *Cancer Research*, 1988; **48**: 1882–8.

43. **Greco FA, Hainsworth JD.** Paclitaxel with mitoxantrone with or without 5-fluorouracil and high-dose leucovorin in the treatment of metastatic breast cancer. *Seminars in Oncology*, 1997; **24**: S17–S61.

44. **LeMaistre CF, Herzig R.** Mitoxantrone: potential for use in intensive therapy. *Seminars in Oncology*, 1990; **17**: 43–8.

45. **Wiseman LR, Spencer CM.** Mitoxantrone. A review of its pharmacology and clinical efficacy in the management of hormone-resistant advanced prostate cancer. *Drugs and Aging*, 1997; **10**: 473–85.

46. **Gogas H, Mansi JL.** The anthrapyrazoles. *Cancer Treatment Reviews*, 1995; **21**: 541–52.

47. **Smith G, Henderson IC.** New treatments for breast cancer. *Seminars in Oncology*, 1996; **23**: 506–28.

48. **Bennett RAO, Swerdlow PS, Povirk LF.** Spontaneous cleavage of bleomycin-induced abasic sites in chromatin and their mutagenicity in mammalian shuttle vectors. *Biochemistry*, 1993; **32**: 3188–95.

49. **Mir LM, Tounekti O, Orlowski S.** Bleomycin: revival of an old drug. *General Pharmacology*, 1996; **27**: 745–8.

50. **Glass LF, Pepine ML, Fenske NA, Jaroszeski M, Reintgen DS, Heller R.** Bleomycin-mediated electrochemotherapy of metastatic melanoma. *Archives of Dermatology*, 1996; **132**: 1353–7.

51. **Glass LF, Jaroszeski M, Gilbert R, Reintgen DS, Heller R.** Intralesional bleomycin-mediated electrochemotherapy in 20 patients with basal cell carcinoma. *Journal of the American Academy of Dermatology*, 1997; **37**: 596–9.

52. **Sleijfer S, Vujaskovic Z, Limburg PC, Koops HS, Mulder NH.** Induction of tumor necrosis factor-α as a cause of bleomycin-related toxicity. *Cancer*, 1998; **82**: 970–4.

53. **Brown JM, Giaccia AJ.** The unique physiology of solid tumors: opportunities (and problems) for cancer therapy. *Cancer Research*, 1998; **58**: 1408–16.

54. **Mikami K, Naito M, Tomida A, Yamada M, Sirakusa T, Tsuruo T.** DT-diaphorase as a critical determinant of sensitivity to mitomycin C in human colon and gastric carcinoma cell lines. *Cancer Research*, 1996; **56**: 2823–6.

55. **Chaney SG, Sancar A.** DNA repair: enzymatic mechanisms and relevance to drug response. *Journal of the National Cancer Institute*, 1996; **88**: 1346–60.

56. **Doll DC, Weiss RB, Issell BF.** Mitomycin: ten years after approval for marketing. *Journal of Clinical Oncology*, 1985; **3**: 276–86.

57. **Cantrell JE, Phillips TM, Schein PS.** Carcinoma-associated hemolytic-uremic syndrome: a complication of mitomycin C chemotherapy. *Journal of Clinical Oncology*, 1985; **3**: 723–34.

58. **Sheldon R, Slaughter D.** A syndrome of microangiopathic hemolytic anemia, renal impairment, and pulmonary edema in chemotherapy-treatment patients with adenocarcinoma. *Cancer*, 1986; **58**: 1428.

59. **Wilson MW, Hungerford JL, George SM, Madreperla SA.** Topical mitomycin C for the treatment of conjunctival and corneal epithelial dysplasia and neoplasia. *American Journal of Ophthalmology*, 1997; **124**: 303–11.

60. **Loggie BW, Perini M, Fleming RA, Russell GB, Geisinger K.** Treatment and prevention of malignant ascites associated with disseminated intraperitoneal malignancies by aggressive combined-modality therapy. *American Surgeon*, 1997; **63**: 137–43.

61. **Haffty BG, et al.** Bioreductive alkylating agent porfiromycin in combination with radiation therapy for the management of squamous cell carcinoma of the head and neck. *Radiation Oncology Investigations*, 1997; **5**: 235–45.

62. **Chen AY, Liu LF.** DNA topoisomerases: essential enzymes and lethal targets. *Annual Review of Pharmacology and Toxicology*, 1994; **34**: 191–218.

63. **Stewart CF, Ratain MJ.** Topoisomerase interactive agents. In: De Vita VT, Hellman S, Rosenberg AS, eds. *Cancer: principles and practice of oncology*, 5th edn, vol. 1. Philadelphia: Lippincott-Raven, 1997: 452–67.

4.18 Vinca alkaloids, taxanes, and podophyllotoxins

Maurizio D'Incalci

Vinca alkaloids

More than 40 years ago alkaloids extracted from the Madagascar periwinkle (*Vinca rosea*) were found to possess marked cytotoxic and antitumour activity.[1] Vinblastine and vincristine, identified as the most active, consist of a catharanthine moiety (a tetracyclic structure) linked to a vindoline ring (a pentacyclic structure), and differ only in a single substitution in the vindoline group (Fig. 1). Subsequently vindesine, a desacetyl carboxyamide derivative of vinblastine possessing good antitumour activity, was synthesized and tested.[2]

In the mid-1970s a new synthetic approach allowed the production of compounds which differed from the natural products in that they had an eight- rather than a nine-member catharanthine. Among these compounds, 5′-noranhydrovinblastine, vinorelbine, was selected because of its marked antitumour activity in preclinical systems.[3],[4]

Mode of action

The molecular target of vinca alkaloids is tubulin, the basic subunit of microtubules. Tubulin is a GTP-binding protein composed of two polypeptide chains, α and β.[5] GTP has to bind to tubulin for microtubule polymerization, but the microtubules are more stable in the presence of some proteins such as microtubule-associated proteins (**MAP**).[6],[7]

Microtubule function depends on tubulin's ability to polymerize or depolymerize. Some compounds act by preventing tubulin assembly—such as colchicine, vinca alkaloids, combretastatins, or dolastatins—while others, such as taxanes or, more recently, epothilones, act by stabilizing microtubule polymers.

The tubulin binding sites of vinca alkaloids are similar to those described for maytansine but are distinct from those of taxanes or other natural products such as colchicine, podophyllotoxin, and combretastatins. There are high-affinity and low-affinity binding sites.[8],[8a] The high-affinity sites of vinca alkaloids ($k_a \sim 50$ μM) are found in low density at the ends of microtubules, and are responsible for the inhibition of microtubule assembly. The low-affinity binding sites ($k_a \sim 4$ mM) are responsible for the microtubules splaying into spiral protofilaments which are stabilized by MAP.

The minimal concentrations of vinca alkaloids required for cell-growth inhibition do not affect microtubule depolymerization. Exposure to vinca alkaloids causes a block in metaphase, due to the inhibition of mitotic spindle function. This is related to the growth

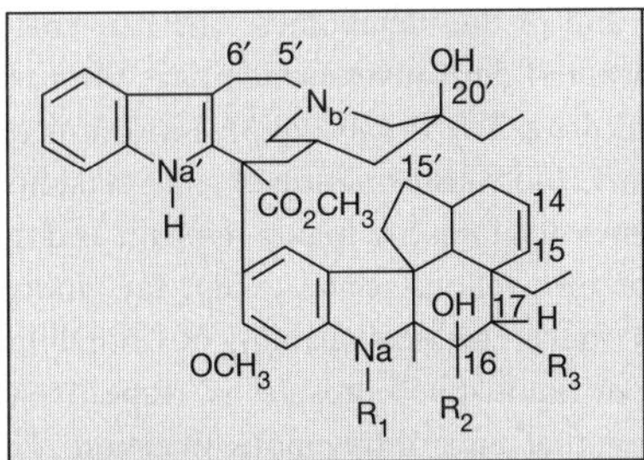

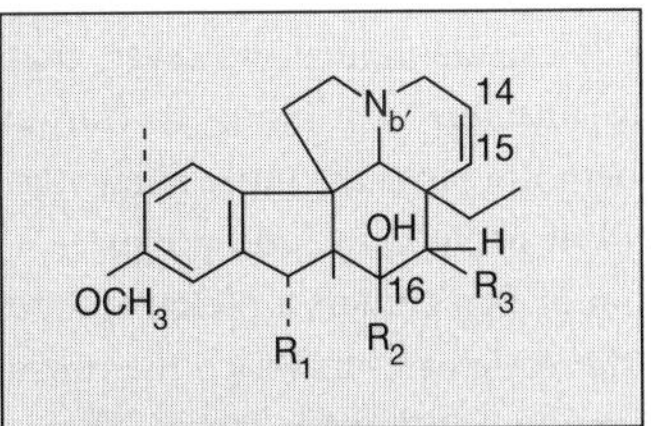

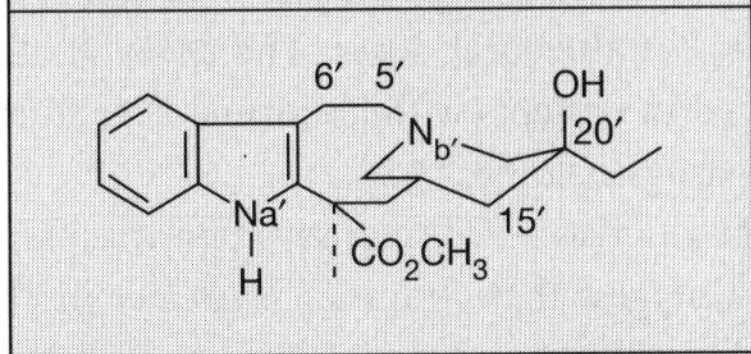

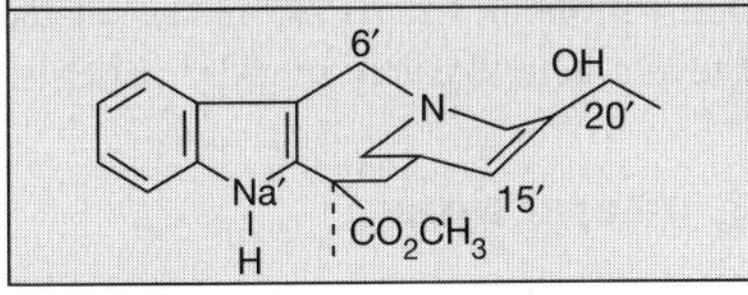

	R$_1$	R$_2$	R$_3$
Vindesine (VDS)	— CH$_3$	— CONH$_2$	— OH
Vincristine (VCR)	— CHO	— CO$_2$CH$_3$	— OCOCH$_3$
Vinblastine (VLB)	— CH$_3$	— CO$_2$CH$_3$	— OCOCH$_3$
17-Desacetyl-vinblastine	— CH$_3$	— CO$_2$CH$_3$	— OH
Vinorelbine	— CH$_3$	— CO$_2$CH$_3$	— OCOCH$_3$

Fig. 1 Structure of the vinca alkaloids vinblastine and vincristine.

inhibition. Like other antimitotic drugs in clinical use, the effects of vinca alkaloids on tubulin results in its loss at the ends of mitotic spindle microtubules. Although the main mechanism of action of vinca alkaloids appears to be related to this effect on the mitotic spindle, there is much current research into the effects of antitubulin drugs on microtubules in interphase, which can affect the adhesion and mobility of cells, possibly resulting in antiangiogenic and antivascular effects (see below 'Mode of action of taxanes').

The mechanism of the selectivity of vinca alkaloids towards some tumours is not understood. No differences in the binding of vinca alkaloids were observed in tubulin extracted from normal and neoplastic tissues. The selectivity of the vinca alkaloids may possibly be related to a different expression of various tubulin isoforms or to differences in intracellular levels of GTP and/or cofactors which can modify the binding of the drug (for example, MAP). The greater susceptibility of some neoplastic tissues might also be related to increased retention of drugs. Cellular pharmacology studies show that the intracellular concentrations of vinca alkaloids vary in different cell lines.[9],[10] Cellular uptake occurs mainly by simple diffusion, although a temperature-dependent process plays a role in the intracellular transport of these alkaloids.[11]

Mechanism of resistance

The most widely investigated mechanism of resistance to vinca alkaloids is overexpression of the *mdr-1* gene leading to a decrease in intracellular drug retention. The increase in the *mdr-1* gene product (p-glycoprotein, **Pgp**) results in a lower intracellular drug concentration because of faster efflux of the drug from the cell.[12],[13] Pgp is a member of a large superfamily of transmembrane transport proteins which utilize ATP to translocate a broad range of structurally different cytotoxic agents, including vinca alkaloids, anthracyclines, podophyllotoxins, and taxanes.[13],[14]

The relevance of *mdr-1* overexpression to clinical resistance to vinca alkaloids and other anticancer drugs is still unproven. The increased percentage of Pgp-positive tumour cells after chemotherapy is only indicative of a potential importance of this protein in the mechanism of resistance. It can be argued, however, that the more advanced and genetically unstable a tumour is (for example in tumours relapsing after chemotherapy) the more likely it is to contain clones expressing any kind of protein, including Pgp.

Although the expression of Pgp confers a pleiotropic resistance to several anticancer drugs, there are cases in which the resistance index is higher for one class of compounds than for others. There is evidence that a Pgp associated with vinca alkaloid resistance has some specific difference in the amino-acid sequence, with consequent changes in the post-translational modifications (that is, *N*-glycosylation and phosphorylation) leading to structural alterations.[15],[16]

The constitutive expression of Pgp in several normal organs including liver, kidney, adrenals, and intestine, suggests that this protein might play a part in limiting the toxicity of vinca alkaloids.[17] Mice not expressing Pgp are more susceptible to the toxicity of several anticancer drugs including the vinca alkaloids.[18] In these mice the drug crosses the blood–brain barrier causing neurotoxicity, whereas in mice expressing Pgp it does not penetrate the CNS in significant amounts, presumably because of the presence of Pgp in the brain capillaries.

Table 1 Elimination half-lives and clearance of the vinca alkaloids in clinical use

Drug	Terminal half-life (h)	Clearance (l/h per m^2)
Vincristine	23–85	5
Vinblastine	20–25	33
Vindesine	20–24	23
Vinorelbine	18–49	35

Pgp is inhibited by a wide range of compounds including calcium-channel blockers (for example, verapamil), cyclosporin, protein kinase inhibitors, hormones, etc. Cells resistant to vinca alkaloids because of overexpression of the *mdr-1* gene can regain their sensitivity if treated simultaneously with Pgp inhibitors. These data have provided a rationale for the clinical testing of Pgp inhibitors with anticancer drugs. However, this approach has been hampered by pharmacokinetic interactions between these drugs (see below 'Clinical Pharmacology'), resulting in increased toxicity requiring dose reductions.

Other mechanisms of resistance to vinca alkaloids involve mutations or changes in post-translational modifications (that is to say, phosphorylation, acetylation) of α- or β-tubulin proteins.[19]–[23] These changes can affect the binding of the drugs or the susceptibility to depolymerization, possibly because of changes in the GTP binding domain. Thus it appears that both structural and dynamic changes of microtubules may affect the sensitivity of tubulin binders.

Clinical pharmacology

The vinca alkaloids currently in clinical use have a large volume of distribution, relatively fast clearance, and a very long terminal half-life (see Table 1).[24],[25] Normally, vinca alkaloids do not cross the blood–brain barrier. Their clearance is mainly due to hepatic metabolism and biliary excretion of the administered drug (in minimal part) and of the metabolites. The best-characterized metabolites are the deacetyl derivatives, which have cytotoxic potency similar to the parent drug. The P-450 cyp 3A isoform is mainly responsible for the oxidative biotransformation of vinca alkaloids used in clinical practice.

Vinca alkaloids are highly resistant and must be administered only by the intravenous route, except for vinorelbine which can also be taken orally. The bioavailability of vinorelbine given orally in powder-filled or liquid-filled capsules is, respectively, 43 per cent and 27 per cent of that after intravenous injection. The peak level is achieved within 2 h after oral doses. The doses of all vinca alkaloids must be reduced in patients with abnormal liver function, whose clearance of these drugs is lower.[25]

For vincristine, comparative pharmacokinetic data in children and adults suggest that clearance is greater in children. The finding that the elimination of vincristine is age-related might account for the more severe neurotoxicity in older patients.

Drug interactions

As discussed in the section on resistance, many drugs inhibit Pgp *in vitro* and some have been used *in vivo* in combination with vinca

Table 2 Dosage schedules and toxicities of vinca alkaloids

Drug (dosage schedule)	Acute toxicity	Delayed toxicity
Vincristine ~1 mg/ m2 IV every 3 weeks	Local tissue damage in case of extravasation	Peripheral neuropathy, paralytic ileus, constipation, mild bone marrow depression
Vinblastine 4–5 mg/m2 IV weekly	Nausea, vomiting, local tissue damage in case of extravasation	Bone marrow depression, peripheral neuropathy, mucositis
Vinorelbine 25 mg/ m² IV weekly	Nausea, vomiting, dyspnoea, erythema, and nel sito phlebitis at the injection site	Bone marrow depression, peripheral neuropathy, mucositis, anorexia

alkaloids to counteract the mechanism of resistance due to overexpression of the *mdr-1* gene. There have been extensive studies in mice on the interactions between vinca alkaloids and Pgp inhibitors. Using several different Pgp inhibitors in combination with vinblastine, very marked effects on drug distribution have been observed.[27] Vinblastine concentrations in the liver and kidney were increased after pretreatment with cyclosporin A or with trifluoroperazine. None of the Pgp inhibitors significantly raised vinblastine levels in the brain or testis. It appears that the changes in the distribution of vinca alkaloids in mice not expressing *mdr* genes cannot be obtained by treatment with Pgp inhibitors. In mice not expressing *mdr* genes, vinblastine penetration in the brain was more than 20 times that in control mice.

Clinical use

The most common dosage schedules and the main acute and delayed toxicity features of vinca alkaloids are listed in Table 2.

Taxanes

Extracted from the bark of *Taxus brevifolia*, taxol (subsequently called paclitaxel) was tested in the National Cancer Institute (NCI) screening system and found to possess cytotoxic properties.[28] Paclitaxel was active as an antitumour drug, but the limited supply of the compound significantly delayed its development. The finding that paclitaxel was not a conventional antimitotic agent, but possessed a mechanism of action distinct from other tubulin binders, stimulated much interest. Paclitaxel can now be obtained by a semisynthetic process from 10-deacetylbaccatin III derived from the needles of more abundant yew species such as the European yew *Taxus baccata*.[29] Both paclitaxel and docetaxel are complex structures with a taxane ring linked to an ester at the C-13 position (see Fig. 2).

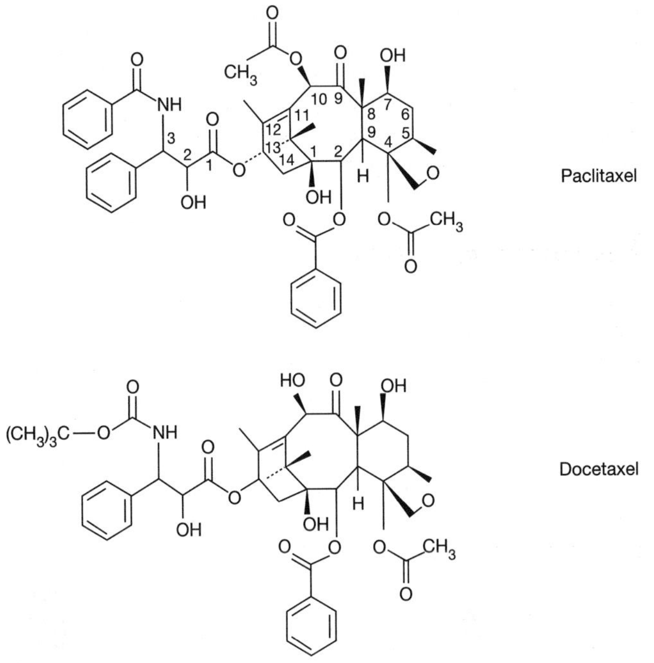

Mode of action

Although the target of taxanes is tubulin, the mechanism of action, as already mentioned, is different from the other tubulin-directed drugs. Paclitaxel or docetaxel stabilize the microtubules,[30]–[33] whereas the conventional antimitotic drugs, such as vinca alkaloids, cause a microtubule depolymerization. Incubation of taxanes with tubulin shortens the lag time to the start of polymerization and induces the assembly of tubulin into stable microtubules. Therefore these drugs act

Fig. 2 Structure of the taxanes paclitaxel and docetaxel.

both as tubulin assembly promoters and as inhibitors of microtubule depolymerization.

The binding sites of these tubulin-directed drugs have not been precisely identified, although it is clear that they do not overlap those of other tubulin binders such as colchicine, vinca alkaloids, or podophyllotoxin.[31],[32] Crystallographic analysis has indicated a possible site of interaction of paclitaxel in the tubulin-αβ heterodimer.[34] However, it is still not known whether the β-tubulin subunit is the exclusive binding site for these drugs. Paclitaxel and docetaxel are believed to bind to the same tubulin sites but the affinity of docetaxel is 1.9 times that of paclitaxel.[33]

The mechanisms of action of the taxanes might be different at different intracellular concentrations. The fact that paclitaxel induces polymerization is associated with stoichiometric binding to microtubules. At low intracellular concentrations (for example, when there is one molecule of paclitaxel for several hundred molecules of tubulin) paclitaxel can suppress microtubule dynamics without significantly modifying the size of microtubule polymers.[35] This might explain why taxanes at a low concentration can affect cellular mobility,[36] a mechanism which might be related to their antiangiogenic properties,[37] while much higher concentrations are required to cause a mitotic block.

Mechanism of resistance

For taxanes, like vinca alkaloids, overexpression of the *mdr-1* gene is one of the mechanisms of resistance reported in cell lines resistant to these drugs.[23] There are cases in which cells overexpressing Pgp are resistant to both vinca alkaloids and taxanes, others in which the resistance is only to vinca alkaloids. However, there is still no convincing evidence that Pgp expression is really involved in clinical resistance to taxanes. The other reported mechanisms of resistance are related to differences in sensitivity to the target, as mentioned for vinca alkaloids.[38]–[40]

Cell lines resistant to tubulin-binders present quantitative or qualitative alterations of tubulin. The KPTA cell line, resistant only to taxanes, has increased expression of the class IVa tubulin isotype.[40] In another tumour cell line resistant to taxanes and vinca alkaloids through a mechanism not related to intracellular drug retention, a reduced amount of total tubulin, a higher percentage of polymerized tubulin, and a higher content of class II tubulin isotype were found.[41] Other reports suggest a relationship between resistance to paclitaxel and an increased class II β-tubulin isotype[42] or overexpression of the class III β-tubulin isotype.[41] Mutations of tubulin isotype genes in paclitaxel-resistant cell lines have also been reported.[43]

Besides these mechanisms of resistance, there might be more general mechanisms related to a low propensity of some cancer cells to activate apoptosis pathways.[23] For example, mutation or inactivation of p53 reduces cell sensitivity to several antineoplastic drugs.[44] However, this does not seem to be the case for paclitaxel. In fact, there are reports that the inactivation of p53 by transfection with the papillomavirus E6 gene or in p53-null mice is associated with an increase in sensitivity to paclitaxel and to other tubulin-directed drugs.[45]–[47] It appears therefore that a p53-independent apoptosis pathway may be activated for this class of drugs.[23] In cells expressing wild-type p53 the increase of p53 after taxane treatment causes a G1 block, preventing the cells reaching the G2–M phase, which is the taxane-sensitive phase. This would explain why, in some cell lines, p53 confers resistance to paclitaxel.[47] On the other hand, in cells in which the increase in p53 causes an increase in bax transcription, paclitaxel treatment induces apoptosis. The importance of bax in the sensitivity to paclitaxel is highlighted by a recent report that this proapoptotic protein is involved in the enhancement of drug intracellular levels.[43]

Clinical pharmacology

The pharmacokinetics of paclitaxel were initially described as linear after prolonged infusion of the drug.[49],[50] Further studies in patients receiving the drug as a 3-h infusion indicated that the disposition is non-linear, with a disproportional increase in the area under the curve (**AUC**) at a higher dose.[51]–[53] The pharmacokinetics of docetaxel are instead linear, with a clearance independent of the dose.[54] (The terminal half-life and clearance rate for paclitaxel and docetaxel are given in Table 3.)

Table 3 Elimination half-lives and clearance of paclitaxel (175 mg/m² in 3-h infusion) and docetaxel (100 mg/m² in 1-h infusion)

Drug	Terminal half-life (h)	Clearance (l/h per m²)
Paclitaxel	18.8	13
Docetaxel	11.2	21

Pharmacodynamic studies indicated a relationship between paclitaxel plasma levels and neutropenia. The absolute neutrophil count is related to the time the plasma paclitaxel level remains above a threshold of 0.1 μmol/l[55] or 0.05 μmol/l.[56] The major elimination mechanism of paclitaxel or docetaxel is hepatic metabolism and biliary excretion.[57]–[59] The two major metabolites of paclitaxel appear to be hydroxytaxol isomers, one (3'-p-hydroxy-paclitaxel) having the hydroxyl group on the *para* position of the phenyl function at position C-3' of the side chain, the other at the C-6 position (6α-hydroxypaclitaxel). Other dihydroxy and monohydroxy series have now been identified by highly sensitive mass spectrometry.[60],[61]

Considering the impact of the hepatic clearance of taxanes it is not surprising that patients with impaired liver function can suffer enhanced toxicity due to altered metabolism and elimination.[26],[62],[63] The doses of paclitaxel probably need to be adjusted in patients with hepatic dysfunction. In the population pharmacokinetic analysis of docetaxel it was found that moderate hepatic impairment increased the drug AUC by about 38 per cent, indicating the need for a significant dose reduction.[59]

Drug interactions

As the cytochrome P-450 cyp 3A is involved in the metabolism of both paclitaxel and docetaxel, an interaction with other drugs that are substrates for these enzymes has been proposed,[50],[63] but more studies are needed before any firm conclusions can be drawn on this point. However, there is convincing preclinical and clinical data showing an interaction between taxanes and anthracyclines. The combination of paclitaxel infused over 3 h with bolus doxorubicin was reported to produce a high rate of complete (41 per cent) and overall (94 per cent) responses, but also a high incidence of congestive heart failure in women with previously untreated metastatic breast cancer.[64] These data stimulated preclinical and clinical pharmacokinetic studies aimed at clarifying what sort of interaction could explain these findings.

Anthracycline levels in different murine tissues, including the heart, are higher when the anthracyclines are given in combination with either paclitaxel or docetaxel.[65],[66] Since the main effect appears to be related to a change in drug distribution, it seems plausible that taxanes inhibit the efflux of anthracyclines from the cells by binding Pgp or other proteins involved in drug transport. *In vitro* data support this hypothesis and indicate that cremophor, the solvent currently used to dissolve the drug, can also act as a Pgp inhibitor and is presumably involved in the complex interaction between anthracyclines and taxanes.[67],[68]

Although it is not possible to investigate drug distribution in patients in the same way, there are indications that a pharmacokinetic

Table 4 Dosage schedules and toxicities of taxanes

Drug (dosage schedule)	Acute toxicity	Delayed toxicity
Paclitaxel 135–225 mg/m² IV every 3 weeks	Hypersensitivity reactions	Bone marrow depression, peripheral neuropathy, mucositis, alopecia
Docetaxel 100–125 mg/m² IV every 3 weeks	Hypersensitivity reactions	Bone marrow depression, peripheral neuropathy, mucositis, alopecia

interaction can also occur in humans. Plasma levels of doxorubicin and doxorubicinol were raised in patients receiving paclitaxel as a 3-h infusion and doxorubicin as an intravenous bolus,[67] thus suggesting that the increased toxicity was due to a pharmacokinetic interaction.

On the basis of the results in mice, a small increase in the plasma levels of doxorubicin may reflect a much larger increase in drug levels in some tissues that are targets for toxicity.

Whether the striking antitumour activity and the unexpected cardiotoxicity of the combinations of taxanes and anthracyclines are related only to pharmacokinetic interactions or whether there are other mechanisms of potentiation is still unclear.

Clinical use

Table 4 shows the commonly used dosage schedules, but these may be different in different protocols. There are several investigations in progress on the use of weekly schedules of the two drugs. The most common acute and delayed toxicity are also shown.

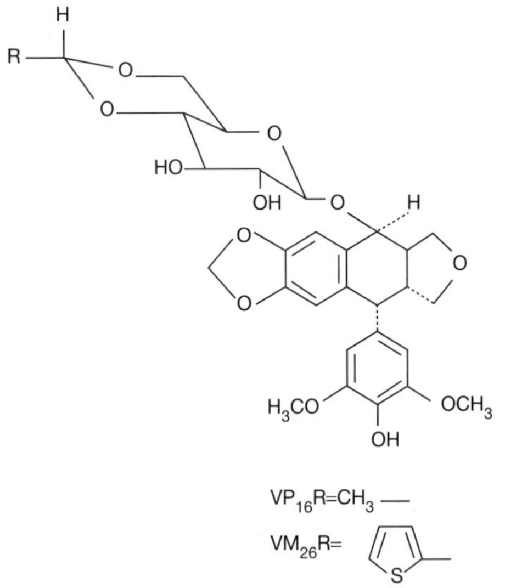

Podophyllotoxins

The American Indians used extracts from the roots of *Podophyllum peltatum* (May apple or mandrake plant) as cathartic and antihelminthic drugs. In 1861 podophyllin by topical administration was reported to be active against venereal warts.[69] Podophyllin and podophyllotoxin are cytotoxic compounds acting as poisons of the mitotic spindle. They showed antitumour activity in experimental animal tumours and in clinical use use,[70]–[72] but their toxicity was too high.

With the aim of identifying other antimitotic podophyllotoxin derivatives with better pharmacological features, the Research Laboratories of Sandoz synthesized and tested several compounds. In 1971 the derivatives VP-16 and VM-26 (Fig. 3) were synthesized by the addition of the carbohydrate moieties β-D-ethylidene or tenylidene to epipodophyllotoxin. These compounds showed promising antitumour activity and a much better therapeutic index than podophyllotoxin.

Mode of action

Whereas podophyllotoxin is a tubulin binder, VP-16 and VM-26 act as DNA topoisomerase II poisons.[73] DNA topoisomerase II regulates DNA topology during transcription, replication, and recombination and is essential for the integrity of the genetic material. Topoisomerases alter DNA conformation by making transient DNA breaks, in which tyrosine residues of the protein are covalently linked to DNA strand termini.[74]

Fig. 3 Structure of the podophyllotoxin derivatives VP-16 and VM-26.

The epipodophyllotoxins etoposide (VP-16) and teniposide (VM-26) act by forming ternary DNA–drug–topoisomerase II complexes in which DNA strands are broken and protein-linked.[73],[75]

Although the mechanism of action of different topoisomerase II poisons such as anthracyclines, ansacrines, and epipodophyllotoxins is similar, epipodophyllotoxins do not intercalate into DNA. In addition, different DNA-topoisomerase II poisons show different DNA sequence-specificities of cleavage that might explain their pharmacological properties.

The mechanism of the partial selective cytotoxicity of topoisomerase II poisons against cancer cells has not been fully elucidated. NIH 3T3 cells transformed with *src1ras* or *raf* oncogenes are more sensitive than control NIH 3T3 cells to VP-16.[76]

The initial event that triggers cell-death pathways after epipodophyllotoxin exposure appears to be double-strand DNA cleavage, and certainly the number of cellular DNA breaks is a major factor in the cytotoxic activity of these drugs. Probably related to the molecular mechanism of action of epipodophyllotoxins, and other related drugs, is the occurrence of secondary leukaemias, characterized by chromosomal translocation at the cytogenetic band 11q23, observed in patients receiving topoisomerase II poisons.[77],[78] The risk of therapy-related acute myeloid leukaemia varies with the treatment schedule: low-dose, prolonged VP-16 regimens seem to involve a lower risk than multiple brief intravenous infusions. This is suggested by laboratory evidence that prolonged exposure of cultured cells to

Table 5 Pharmacokinetic parameters of IV and oral VP-16

Route	Dose	Terminal half-life	Clearance	Bioavailability
	(mg/m^2)	(h)	(ml/min per m^2)	(%)
IV	80–250	4.4–6.5	19–28	100
Oral	100–300	5.5–7.3	—	29–100

Table 6 Dosage schedules and toxicities of podophyllotoxin derivatives

Drug (dosage schedule)	Acute toxicity	Delayed toxicity
Etoposide 80–100 mg IV daily for 3–5 consecutive days every 4 weeks 200 mg orally for 5 consecutive days every 4 weeks	Nausea and vomiting, diarrhoea, hypersensitivity reactions, hypertension, phlebitis at infusion site	Bone marrow depression, mucositis, alopecia, hepatic toxicity with transaminase elevation
Teniposide 60–100 mg IV daily for 3–5 consecutive days every 4 weeks	Nausea and vomiting, diarrhoea, hypersensitivity reactions, hypertension, phlebitis at infusion site	Bone marrow depression, mucositis, alopecia, hepatic toxicity with transaminase elevation

the poison produces less DNA recombination events than equitoxic brief treatment with high doses.

Mechanism of resistance

One of the mechanisms of resistance to VP-16 or VM-26 that has been widely investigated in the last few years is overexpression of the *mdr-1* gene and the multidrug resistance phenotype, which is discussed in more detail elsewhere. As for other drugs, the resistance of cancer cell lines to podophyllotoxins has been associated with an increase in Pgp, MRP, or lung resistance protein (**LRP**). However, it is still debated whether these mechanisms help explain the clinical resistance to these drugs.[79]

There are several mechanisms of resistance related to the quantitative or qualitative alteration of DNA-topoisomerase II and which seem to be responsible for the cytotoxicity and antitumour activity of these drugs.

The levels of expression of topoisomerase II are important for the drug sensitivity. This has been demonstrated by studies in which human brain-cancer cell lines with different degrees of sensitivity to VP-16 were transfected with the human topoisomerase IIα gene. An increase in topoisomerase II expression paralleled an increase in sensitivity to VP-16.[80] The levels of nuclear matrix-associated topoisomerase II appear to be more important for drug sensitivity.[81] The expression of both topoisomerase II isoforms (α and β) was reduced in cell lines from a patient with small-cell lung cancer before and after treatment with VP-16 and doxorubicin-containing chemotherapy, as well as in an *in vitro* selected VP-16-resistant subline.[82]

Several reports have established an association between mutations of topoisomerase IIα and resistance to VP-16 or other topoisomerase II poisons. Topoisomerase II gene alteration can lead to localization of the enzyme only in the cytoplasm.[83] The loss of the proteins' nuclear localization signals was also recently noted in a small-cell

lung cancer cell line resistant to VP-16.[84] Although most studies on resistance mechanism have been performed in cell lines selected for resistance to VP-16 or VM-26, some of these mutations can be detected in fresh tumour cells from cancer patients. However, how these mechanisms are implicated in the clinical resistance to these drugs is still unknown.[79]

Clinical pharmacology

After intravenous injection etoposide disappears from the plasma in a biphasic fashion with a terminal half-life around 6 h (Table 5).[85]–[89] Both peak and AUC values appear to increase proportionally to the dose, but many studies found some interindividual variability. About 30 to 40 per cent of the dose is eliminated by the renal route as unchanged drug. An additional 20 per cent is eliminated in the urine as VP-16 glucouronide. VP-16 clearance was reported to be decreased in patients with abnormal renal function,[86] but not in patients with abnormal liver function.[86],[90]

Similar pharmacokinetic properties have been reported for VM-26, which has a slightly lower rate of elimination and clearance than VP-16.[91]

Both VP-16 and VM-26 penetrate the cerebrospinal fluid poorly, and variable levels of the two drugs have been reported in brain tumours.[92],[93]

The poor water solubility of VP-16 requires the use of solubilizing agents which may contribute to the toxicity. To overcome this problem, etoposide phosphate has now been synthetized and evaluated in phase I clinical trials.[94] Etoposide phosphate is rapidly converted to VP-16 by blood esterases, the toxicity profile of which is virtually identical to that reported for VP-16 with myelosuppression, alopecia, and stomatitis.[95],[96] Since etoposide phosphate is very stable in saline it can be used for very prolonged infusion as a VP-16 prodrug. When given orally, the bioavailability of etoposide phosphate, assessed by determining VP-16, was comparable to or only slightly better than VP-16.[95],[97],[98]

Drug interactions

Several experimental and clinical reports have been published on the combination of inhibitors of DNA-topoisomerase I with DNA-topoisomerase II poisons. Simultaneous administration of topotecan and etoposide was found to be antagonistic in human xenografts.[99] However, the sequential administration of topotecan and etoposide was synergistic, probably because topotecan induced high tumour levels of DNA-topoisomerase II, increasing the responsiveness of xenografts to subsequent doses of VP-16. These findings have prompted clinical studies on the combination of topoisomerase I and topoisomerase II inhibitors, but the results so far are not as encouraging as the preclinical data.[100]

Several studies indicate that modulators of multidrugs, such as cyclosporin given in combination with VP-16 or VM-26, alter the pharmacokinetic and pharmacodynamic properties of these drugs.[101],[102] To avoid severe toxicity, the doses of epipodophyllotoxins should be reduced when the drugs are combined with cyclosporins.

Clinical use

Table 6 indicates some of the dosage schedules which are used and the main acute and delayed toxicities of etoposide and teniposide.

References

1. Johnson IS, Armstrong JG, Gorman M, Burnett JP. The vinca alkaloids: a new class of oncolytic agents. *Cancer Research*, 1963; 23: 1390–1427.

2. Cersosimo RJ, Bromer R, Licciardello JT, Hong WK. Pharmacology, clinical efficacy and adverse effects of vindesine sulfate, a new vinca alkaloid. *Pharmacotherapy*, 1983; 3: 259–74.

3. Mangeney P, Adriamialisoa RZ, Langlois N, Langlois Y, Potier P. A new class of antitumour compounds: 5′ nor 5′, and 6 seco derivatives of vinblastine-type alkaloids. *Journal of Organic Chemistry*, 1979; 44: 3765–8.

4. Maral R, Bourut C, Chenu E, Mathe G. Experimental antitumour activity of 5′-nor-anhydrovinblastine navelbine. *Cancer Letters*, 1984; 22: 49–54.

5. Sullivan KF. Structure and utilization of tubulin isotypes. *Annual Review of Cell Biology*, 1988; 4: 687–716.

6. Olmsted JB. Microtubule-associated proteins. *Annual Review of Cell Biology*, 1986; 2: 421–57.

7. Vallee RB, Bloom GS, Theurkauf WE. Microtubule-associated proteins: subunits of the cytomatrix. *Journal of Cell Biology*, 1984; 99: 38s–44s.

8. Himes RH. Interactions of the catharanthus (Vinca) alkaloids with tubulin and microtubules. *Pharmacology and Therapeutics*, 1991; 51: 257–67.

8a. Bhattacharyya B, Wolff J. Maytansine binding to the vinblastine sites of tubulin. *FEBS Letters*, 1977; 75: 159–62.

9. Ferguson PJ, Phillips JR, Selner M, Cass CE. Differential activity of vincristine and vinblastine against cultured cells. *Cancer Research*, 1984; 44: 3307–12.

10. Bleyer WA, Frisby SA, Oliverio VT. Uptake and binding of vincristine by murine leukemia cells. *Biochemical Pharmacology*, 1975; 24: 633–9.

11. Zhou XJ, Rahmani R. Preclinical and clinical pharmacology of vinca alkaloids. *Drugs*, 1992; 44(Suppl. 4): 1–16. [Discussion]

12. Beck WT. Cellular pharmacology of vinca alkaloid resistance and its circumvention. *Advances in Enzyme Regulation*, 1984; 22: 207–27.

13. Moscow JA, Cowan KH. Multidrug resistance. *Journal of the National Cancer Institute*, 1988; 80: 14–20.

14. Cornwell MM, Tsuruo T, Gottesman MM, Pastan I. ATP-binding properties of P glycoprotein from multidrug-resistant KB cells. *FASEB Journal*, 1987; 1: 51–4.

15. Greenberger LM, Williams SS, Horwitz SB. Biosynthesis of heterogeneous forms of multidrug resistance-associated glycoproteins. *Journal of Biological Chemistry*, 1987; 262: 13685–9.

16. Choi KH, Chen CJ, Kriegler M, Roninson IB. An altered pattern of cross-resistance in multidrug-resistant human cells results from spontaneous mutations in the mdr1 (P-glycoprotein) gene. *Cell*, 1988; 53: 519–29.

17. Fojo AT, Ueda K, Slamon DJ, Poplack DG, Pastan I. Expression of a multidrug-resistance gene in human tumours and tissues. *Proceedings of the National Academy of Sciences of the United States of America*, 1987; 84: 265–9.

18. Schinkel AH, *et al.* Disruption of the mouse mdr1a P-glycoprotein gene leads to a deficiency in the blood–brain barrier and to increased sensitivity to drugs. *Cell*, 1994; 77: 491–502.

19. Houghton JA, Houghton PJ, Hazelton BJ, Douglass EC. In situ selection of a human rhabdomyosarcoma resistant to vincristine with altered beta-tubulins. *Cancer Research*, 1985; 45: 2706–12.

20. Minotti AM, Barlow SB. Resistance to antimitotic drugs in Chinese hamster ovary cells correlates with changes in the level of polymerized tubulin. *Journal of Biological Chemistry*, 1991; 266: 3987–94.

21. Cabral FR, Brady RC, Schibler MJ. A mechanism of cellular resistance to drugs that interfere with microtubule assembly. *Annals of the New York Academy of Sciences*, 1986; 466: 745–56.

22. Cabral F, Barlow SB. Mechanisms by which mammalian cells acquire resistance to drugs that affect microtubule assembly. *FASEB Journal*, 1989; 3: 1593–9.

23. Dumontet C, Sikic BI. Mechanisms of action of and resistance to antitubulin agents: microtubule dynamics, drug transport, and cell death. *Journal of Clinical Oncology*, 1999; 17: 1061–70.

24. Rowinsky EK, Donehower RC. Antimicrotubule agents. In *Cancer chemotherapy and biotherapy: principles and practice* (ed. BA Chabner, DL Longo). Philadelphia, PA: Lippincott-Raven, 1996: 263–96.

25. Rowinsky EK, Donehower RC. The clinical pharmacology and use of antimicrotubule agents in cancer chemotherapeutics. *Pharmacology and Therapeutics*, 1991; 52: 35–84.

26. Donelli MG, Zucchetti M, Munzone E, D'Incalci M. Pharmacokinetics of anticancer agents in patients with impaired liver function. *European Journal of Cancer*, 1998; 34: 33–46.

27. Arboix M, Paz OG, Colombo T, D'Incalci M. Multidrug resistance-reversing agents increase vinblastine distribution in normal tissues expressing the P-glycoprotein but do not enhance drug penetration in brain and testis. *Journal of Pharmacology and Experimental Therapeutics*, 1997; 281: 1226–30.

28. Wani MC, Taylor HL, Wall ME, Coggon P, McPhail AT. Plant antitumour agents: VI. The isolation and structure of Taxol, a novel antileukemic and antitumour agent from *Taxus brevifolia*. *Journal of the American Chemical Society*, 1971; 93: 2325–7.

29. Stierle A, Strobel G, Stierle D. Taxol and taxane production by *Taxomyces andreanae*, an endophytic fungus of Pacific yew. *Science*, 1993; 260: 214–16.

30. Schiff PB, Fant J, Horwitz SB. Promotion of microtubule assembly *in vitro* by taxol. *Nature*, 1979; 277: 665–7.

31. Manfredi JJ, Horwitz SB. Taxol: an antimitotic agent with a new mechanism of action. *Pharmacology and Therapeutics*, 1984; 25: 83–125.

32. Ringel I, Horwitz SB. Studies with RP 56976 (taxotere): a

semisynthetic analogue of taxol. *Journal of the National Cancer Institute*, 1991; **83**: 288–91.

33. Diaz JF, Andreu JM. Assembly of purified GDP-tubulin into microtubules induced by taxol and taxotere: reversibility, ligand stoichiometry, and competition. *Biochemistry*, 1993; **32**: 2747–55.

34. Nogales E, Wolf SG, Khan IA, Luduena RF, Downing KH. Structure of tubulin at 6.5 A and location of the taxol-binding site. *Nature*, 1995; **375**: 424–7.

35. Jordan MA, Toso RJ, Thrower D, Wilson L. Mechanism of mitotic block and inhibition of cell proliferation by taxol at low concentrations. *Proceedings of the National Academy of Sciences of the United States of America*, 1993; **90**: 9552–6.

36. Belotti D, Rieppi M, Nicoletti MI, Casazza AM, Taraboletti G, Giavazzi R. Paclitaxel (Taxol®) inhibits motility of paclitaxel-resistant human ovarian carcinoma cells. *Clinical Cancer Research*, 1996; **2**: 1725–30.

37. Belotti D, *et al.* The microtubule-affecting drug paclitaxel has antiangiogenic activity. *Clinical Cancer Research*, 1996; **2**: 1843–9.

38. Cabral F, Sobel ME, Gottesman MM. CHO mutants resistant to colchicine, colcemid or griseofulvin have an altered beta-tubulin. *Cell*, 1980; **20**: 29–36.

39. Otha S, Nishio K, Ohmori T. Resistance to tubulin interacting agents taxol and vinca alkaloids. In *The mechanism of and new approach to drug resistance of cancer cells* (ed. T Miyazaki, F Takaku, K Sakurada). New York: Elsevier Science, 1993: 209–12.

40. Jaffrezou JP, *et al.* Novel mechanism of resistance to paclitaxel (Taxol) in human K562 leukemia cells by combined selection with PSC 833. *Oncology Research*, 1995; **7**: 517–27.

41. Cabral F, Abraham I, Gottesman MM. Isolation of a taxol-resistant Chinese hamster ovary cell mutant that has an alteration in alpha-tubulin. *Proceedings of the National Academy of Sciences of the United States of America*, 1981; **78**: 4388–91.

42. Haber M, Burkhart CA, Regl DL, Norris MD, Horwitz SB. Altered expression of M beta 2, the class II beta-tubulin isotype, in a murine J774.2 cell line with a high level of taxol resistance. *Journal of Biological Chemistry*, 1995; **270**: 31269–75.

43. Giannakakou P, Sackett DL, Kang YK, Zhan Z, Buters JT, Poruchynsky MS. Paclitaxel-resistant human ovarian cancer cells have mutant beta-tubulins that exhibit impaired paclitaxel-driven polymerization. *Journal of Biological Chemistry*, 1997; **272**: 17118–25.

44. Wu GS, El-Diery WS. p53 and chemosensitivity. *Nature Medicine*, 1996; **2**: 255–6.

45. Wahl AF, Donaldson KL, Fairchild C, Lee FY, Demers GW, Galloway DA. Loss of normal p53 function confers sensitization to Taxol by increasing G2/M arrest and apoptosis. *Nature Medicine*, 1996; **2**: 72–9.

46. Debernardis D, *et al.* p53 status does not affect sensitivity of human ovarian cancer cell lines to paclitaxel. *Cancer Research*, 1997; **57**: 870–4.

47. Vikhanskaya F, *et al.* Inactivation of p53 in a human ovarian cancer cell line increases the sensitivity to paclitaxel by inducing G2/M arrest and apoptosis. *Experimental Cell Research*, 1998; **241**: 96–101.

48. Strobel T, Kraeft SK, Chen LB, Cannistra SA. BAX expression is associated with enhanced intracellular accumulation of paclitaxel: a novel role for BAX during chemotherapy-induced cell death. *Cancer Research*, 1998; **58**: 4776–81.

49. Rowinsky EK, Donehower RC. Paclitaxel (taxol). *New England Journal of Medicine*, 1995; **332**: 1004–14.

50. Huizing MT, *et al.* Taxanes: a new class of antitumour agents. *Cancer Investigation*, 1995; **13**: 381–404.

51. Huizing MT, *et al.* Pharmacokinetics of paclitaxel and metabolites in a randomized comparative study in platinum-pretreated ovarian cancer patients. *Journal of Clinical Oncology*, 1993; **11**: 2127–35.

52. Sonnichsen DS, Hurwitz CA, Pratt CB, Shuster JJ, Relling MV. Saturable pharmacokinetics and paclitaxel pharmacodynamics in children with solid tumours. *Journal of Clinical Oncology*, 1994; **12**: 532–8.

53. Gianni L, *et al.* Nonlinear pharmacokinetics and metabolism of paclitaxel and its pharmacokinetic/pharmacodynamic relationships in humans. *Journal of Clinical Oncology*, 1995; **13**: 180–90.

54. Extra JM, Rousseau F, Bruno R, Clavel M, Le Bail N. Phase I and pharmacokinetic study of Taxotere (RP 56976; NSC 628503) given as a short intravenous infusion. *Cancer Research*, 1993; **53**: 1037–42.

55. Beijnen JH, Huizing MT, ten Bokkel Huinink WW, Veenhof CH, Vermorken JB, Pinedo HM. Bioanalysis, pharmacokinetics, and pharmacodynamics of the novel anticancer drug paclitaxel (Taxol). *Seminars in Oncology*, 1994; **21**: 53–62.

56. Kearns CM, Gianni L, Egorin MJ. Paclitaxel pharmacokinetics and pharmacodynamics. *Seminars in Oncology*, 1995; **22**: 16–23.

57. Huizing MT, *et al.* Pharmacokinetics of paclitaxel and carboplatin in a dose-escalating and dose-sequencing study in patients with non-small-cell lung cancer. The European Cancer Centre. *Journal of Clinical Oncology*, 1997; **15**: 317–29.

58. Walle T, Walle UK, Kumar GN, Bhalla KN. Taxol metabolism and disposition in cancer patients. *Drug Metabolism and Disposition*, 1995; **23**: 506–12.

59. Fulton B, Spencer CM. Docetaxel. A review of its pharmacodynamic and pharmacokinetic properties and therapeutic efficacy in the management of metastatic breast cancer. *Drugs*, 1996; **51**: 1075–92.

60. Sottani C, Minoia C, Colombo A, D'Incalci M, Fanelli R. Structural characterization of mono- and dihydroxylated metabolites of paclitaxel in rat bile using liquid chromatography/ion spray tandem mass spectrometry. *Rapid Communications in Mass Spectrometry*, 1997; **11**: 1025–32.

61. Sottani C, Minoia C, D'Incalci M, Paganini M. High-performance liquid chromatography tandem mass spectrometry procedure with automated solid phase extraction sample preparation for the quantitative determination of paclitaxel (Taxol) in human plasma. *Rapid Communications in Mass Spectrometry*, 1998; **12**: 251–5.

62. Bruno R, Vivler N, Vergniol JC, De Phillips SL, Montay G, Sheiner LB. A population pharmacokinetic model for docetaxel (Taxotere): model building and validation. *Journal of Pharmacokinetics and Biopharmaceutics*, 1996; **24**: 153–72.

63. Nannan Panday VR, *et al.* Hepatic metabolism of paclitaxel and its impact in patients with altered hepatic function. *Seminars in Oncology*, 1997; **24**: S11–S34.

64. Gianni L, *et al.* Paclitaxel by 3-hour infusion in combination with bolus doxorubicin in women with untreated metastatic breast cancer: high antitumour efficacy and cardiac effects in a dose-finding and sequence-finding study. *Journal of Clinical Oncology*, 1995; **13**: 2688–99.

65. Colombo T, *et al.* Paclitaxel induces significant changes in epidoxorubicin distribution in mice. *Annals of Oncology*, 1996; **7**: 801–5.

66. Colombo T, Parisi I, Zucchetti M, Sessa C, Goldhirsch A, D'Incalci M. Pharmacokinetic interactions of paclitaxel, docetaxel and their vehicles with doxorubicin. *Annals of Oncology*, 1999; **10**: 391–5.

67. Gianni L, Vigano L, Locatelli A, Capri G, Giani A, Bonadonna G. Human pharmacokinetic characterization and *in vitro* study of the interaction between doxorubicin and paclitaxel in patients with breast cancer. *Journal of Clinical Oncology*, 1997; **15**: 1906–15.

68. Desai PB, Duan JZ, Zhu YW, Kouzi S. Human liver microsomal metabolism of paclitaxel and drug interactions. *European Journal of Drug Metabolism and Pharmacokinetics*, 1998; **23**: 417–24.

69. Bentley R. New American remedies. I. *Podophillum pelatum*. *Pharmaceutical Journal Translation*, 1861; **3**: 456–64.

70. Newton KA, Westbury G, Wite WF. Intra-arterial administration of 2-ethylhydrazide of podophyllic acid (NSC-72274) in localized malignant disease. *Cancer Chemotherapy Reports*, 1964; **43**: 33–8.

71. Stahelin H, Cerletti A. Experimentelle ergebnisse mit den

podophyllum-cytostatica SP-I und SP-G. *Schweizerische Medizinische Wochenschrift*, 1964; **94**: 1490–502.

72. **Vaitkevicius VK, Reed ML.** Clinical studies with podophyllum compounds SPI-77 (NSC-72274) and SPG-827 (NSC-42076). *Cancer Chemotherapy Reports—Part 1*, 1966; **50**: 565–71.

73. **Liu LF.** DNA topoisomerase poisons as antitumour drugs. *Annual Review of Biochemistry*, 1989; **58**: 351–75.

74. **Osheroff N, Zechiedrich EL, Gale KC.** Catalytic function of DNA topoisomerase II. *Bioessays*, 1991; **13**: 269–73.

75. **Pommier Y.** DNA topoisomerase I and II in cancer chemotherapy: update and perspectives. *Cancer Chemotherapy and Pharmacology*, 1993; **32**: 103–8.

76. **Chen G, Shu J, Stacey DW.** Oncogenic transformation potentiates apoptosis, S-phase arrest and stress-kinase activation by etoposide. *Oncogene*, 1997; **15**: 1643–51.

77. **Nichols CR, Breeden ES, Loehrer PJ, Williams SD, Einhorn LH.** Secondary leukemia associated with a conventional dose of etoposide: review of serial germ cell tumour protocols. *Journal of the National Cancer Institute*, 1993; **85**: 36–40.

78. **Felix CA, Winick NJ, Negrini M, Bowman WP, Croce CM.** Common region of ALL-1 gene disrupted in epipodophyllotoxin-related secondary acute myeloid leukemia. *Cancer Research*, 1993; **53**: 2954–6.

79. **Kaye SB.** Multidrug resistance: clinical relevance in solid tumours and strategies for circumvention. *Current Opinion in Oncology*, 1998; **10**(Suppl. 1): S15–S19.

80. **Asano T, An T, Mayes J, Zwelling LA, Kleinerman ES.** Transfection of human topoisomerase II alpha into etoposide-resistant cells: transient increase in sensitivity followed by down-regulation of the endogenous gene. *Biochemical Journal*, 1996; **319**: 307–13.

81. **Valkov NI, Gump JL, Sullivan DM.** Quantitative immunofluorescence and immunoelectron microscopy of the topoisomerase II alpha associated with nuclear matrices from wild-type and drug-resistant chinese hamster ovary cell lines. *Journal of Cellular Biochemistry*, 1997; **67**: 112–30.

82. **Andoh T, Nishizawa M, Hida T, Ariyoshi Y, Takahashi T.** Reduced expression of DNA topoisomerase II confers resistance to etoposide (VP-16) in small cell lung cancer cell lines established from a refractory tumour of a patient and by *in vitro* selection. *Oncology Research*, 1996; **8**: 229–38.

83. **Yu Q, Mirski SE, Sparks KE, Cole SP.** Two COOH-terminal truncated cytoplasmic forms of topoisomerase II alpha in a VP-16-selected lung cancer cell line result from partial gene deletion and alternative splicing. *Biochemistry*, 1997; **36**: 5868–77.

84. **Wessel I, Jensen PB, Falck J, Mirski SE, Sehested M.** Loss of amino acids 1490Lys–Ser–Lys1492 in the COOH-terminal region of topoisomerase IIalpha in human small cell lung cancer cells selected for resistance to etoposide results in an extranuclear enzyme localization. *Cancer Research*, 1997; **57**: 4451–4.

85. **D'Incalci M, Sessa C, Rossi C, Roviaro G, Mangioni C.** Pharmacokinetics of etoposide in gestochoriocarcinoma. *Cancer Treatment Reports*, 1985; **69**: 69–72.

86. **D'Incalci M, et al.** Pharmacokinetics of etoposide in patients with abnormal renal and hepatic function. *Cancer Research*, 1986; **46**: 2566–71.

87. **Hande KR, Wedlund PJ, Noone RM, Wilkinson GR, Greco FA.** Pharmacokinetics of high-dose etoposide (VP-16–213) administered to cancer patients. *Cancer Research*, 1984; **44**: 379–82.

88. **Evans WE, Sinkule JA, Crom WR, Dow L, Look AT, Rivera G.** Pharmacokinetics of Teniposide (VM26) and etoposide (VP16–213) in children with cancer. *Cancer Chemotherapy and Pharmacology*, 1982; **7**: 147–50.

89. **Hande KR.** Etoposide: four decades of development of a topoisomerase II inhibitor. *European Journal of Cancer*, 1998; **34**: 1514–21.

90. **Joel SP, Shah R, Clark PI, Slevin ML.** Predicting etoposide toxicity: relationship to organ function and protein binding. *Journal of Clinical Oncology*, 1996; **14**: 257–67.

91. **D'Incalci M, Rossi C, Sessa C, Urso R, Zucchetti M, Mangioni C.** Pharmacokinetics of teniposide in patients with ovarian cancer. *Cancer Treatment Reports*, 1985; **69**: 73–7.

92. **Zucchetti M, et al.** Concentrations of VP16 and VM26 in human brain tumours. *Annals of Oncology*, 1991; **2**: 63–6.

93. **Stewart DJ, et al.** Penetration of VP-16 (etoposide) into human intracerebral and extracerebral tumours. *Journal of Neuro-Oncology*, 1984; **2**: 133–9.

94. **Rose WC, Basler GA, Trail PA, Saulnier M, Crosswell AR.** Preclinical antitumour activity of a soluble etoposide analog, BMY-40481–30. *Investigational New Drugs*, 1990; **8**(Suppl. 1): S25–S32.

95. **Sessa C, et al.** Phase I clinical and pharmacokinetic study of oral etoposide phosphate. *Journal of Clinical Oncology*, 1995; **13**: 200–9.

96. **Brooks DJ, et al.** Phase I and pharmacokinetic study of etoposide phosphate. *Anti-Cancer Drugs*, 1995; **6**: 637–44.

97. **D'Incalci M, et al.** Pharmacokinetics of VP16–213 given by different administration methods. *Cancer Chemotherapy and Pharmacology*, 1982; **7**: 141–5.

98. **Hande KR, Krozely MG, Greco FA, Hainsworth JD, Johnson DH.** Bioavailability of low-dose oral etoposide. *Journal of Clinical Oncology*, 1993; **11**: 374–7.

99. **Whitacre CM, Zborowska E, Gordon NH, Mackay W, Berger NA.** Topotecan increases topoisomerase IIalpha levels and sensitivity to treatment with etoposide in schedule-dependent process. *Cancer Research*, 1997; **57**: 1425–8.

100. **Vasey PA, Kaye SB.** Combined inhibition of topoisomerases I and II—is this a worthwhile/feasible strategy? *British Journal of Cancer*, 1997; **76**: 1395–7.

101. **Lum BL, et al.** Clinical trials of modulation of multidrug resistance. Pharmacokinetic and pharmacodynamic considerations. *Cancer*, 1993; **72**: 3502–14.

102. **Gigante M, et al.** Effect of cyclosporine on teniposide pharmacokinetics and pharmacodynamics in patients with renal cell cancer. *Anti-Cancer Drugs*, 1995; **6**: 479–82.

4.19 New anticancer drugs

C. Twelves

Introduction

Although many childhood cancers, and some of the rarer adult tumours, can be cured with chemotherapy, treatment for the common adult solid tumours is usually given with palliative rather than curative intent. For many years drug development in oncology focused largely on the development of analogues of established agents. This led to some modest but useful advances in terms of improved activity, or more often reduced toxicity, but not to major advances. In recent years the pattern of drug development has changed dramatically, driven largely by an improved understanding of the molecular biology of cancer (Fig. 1). We now see an unprecedented number of new agents emerging from the laboratory for testing in the clinic. Many of these new agents have novel mechanisms of action. They do not easily fit into the conventional scheme of drug development and their development offers challenges to scientists based both in the clinic and the laboratory.

The identification of new lead anticancer compounds is increasingly based on rational selection rather than empiricism. A large number of naturally occurring or synthesized chemical entities have been screened by the National Cancer Institute (NCI) over the last 30 years. This process has been refined with the use of human tumour cell lines (see Chapter 4.22). Better characterization of the cell lines

and patterns of differential activity can give indications as to the mechanism of action of a new compound. Molecules with a novel structure or mode of action that can be formulated and tested *in vivo* at an early stage are strong candidates to take to the clinic. Increasingly, however, anticancer drugs are being designed rationally and directed at specific targets identified from molecular studies as characterizing the malignant phenotype. These new agents are often directed at the cell membrane or cytoplasm rather than DNA which has been the traditional target for anticancer drugs. A further change has come from an appreciation of the importance of interactions between the tumour cell and the stroma so that new agents may act on the host tissues rather than the cancer.

Advances in the laboratory are leading to new types of therapeutic molecule and fresh challenges in their clinical evaluation. The development of antisense oligonucleotides represents one such area where molecular biology led to the emergence of a novel therapeutic. The antisense oligonucleotide hybridizes with the complementary base sequence of mRNA which acts as the 'receptor'. This binding prevents translation of the mRNA and reduces expression of the target protein. This approach is a valuable part of rational drug development where structure or function of the target protein are not known but the nucleic acid sequence has been identified. It has also been used to target *ras* and protein kinase C (**PKC**), two important components of intracellular signalling pathways, where several different isoforms of the target protein exist. One of the major challenges in taking this approach to the clinic has been that of delivery. Obtaining adequate cellular uptake has been the first difficulty. Once inside the cell the oligonucleotides are rapidly destroyed by nucleases, but they have been modified with sulphur groups in an attempt to overcome problems of delivery and to prolong their half-life. Despite these obstacles, early trials have demonstrated proof of principle with reduction in target RNA and reports of clinical responses.

There is particular interest in agents directed at specific, new targets. Such agents may be cytostatic rather cytotoxic, challenging preconceptions about killing the cancer cell to achieve a cure—which has been possible for only a few cancers to date. Novel targets such as signal transduction are well defined in the laboratory. However, we do not yet know whether an agent that acts only against tumours transformed by a specific oncogene will be useful clinically where several oncogenic abnormalities are likely to be present in a single tumour cell. In some situations surrogate endpoints of biological activity have been identified clinically. In most cases, however, these new targets remain to be validated in terms of therapeutic utility. In this context the randomized trial of Herceptin, an antibody directed

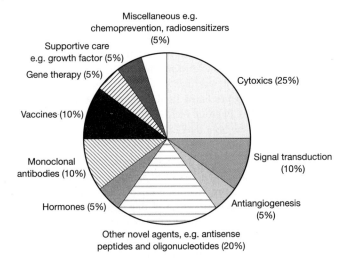

Fig. 1 Approximate proportions of different classes of oncology compounds in preclinical and clinical development (arround 400 in total).

against the growth-factor receptor HER-2, is encouraging. Response rates were higher, and survival prolonged, in women with advanced breast cancer and HER-2-positive tumours who received Herceptin in addition to conventional chemotherapy. Objective responses have also been seen in women treated with Herceptin alone. This offers important 'proof of principle' in the clinic for the development of novel agents.

This chapter describes certain new targets and some of the established targets that point the way ahead for drug development. We will restrict the discussion to areas where compounds are entering the clinic and may make a significant clinical impact over the next few years. The agents to be considered fall into four broad groups:

1. There are 'conventional' cytotoxics directed at DNA and/or other well-recognized targets. Thymidylate synthase, the main target for 5-fluorouracil, is an example where a better understanding of pyrimidine enzymology has led to the introduction of more specific or oral compounds. These are described in detail in the chapter on folate antagonists (see Chapter 4.16). The interactions between cytotoxics and DNA are now being better defined, and new agents that target specific base sequences may inhibit transcription factors in a more specific manner are described below.

2. The second area is cell signalling, the process by which extracellular signals are conveyed from the cell surface to the genome leading to changes in cell growth, differentiation, and death. The concept that these processes are disturbed in cancer has led to the identification of several potential new targets for anticancer drugs. The protein kinases play a central role in signal transduction. They are a large family of enzymes that phosphorylate other proteins, leading to changes in catalytic activity or the ability to bind macromolecules. The importance of these kinases is illustrated by the expectation that they will comprise 2000 of the 100 000 genes in the human genome.

3. The processes of metastasis and angiogenesis, which are recognized as central to the malignant process, are now better understood. Novel targets have been identified and molecules directed at these targets are now in clinical development.

4. Finally, telomerase represents a more speculative, but potentially important, target. This enzyme is required to maintain the ends of chromosomes. It is usually switched off in most somatic cells but reactivated in the majority of cancer cells.

Conventional targets

Enthusiasm for well-characterized 'new targets' should not obscure the fact that established targets such as DNA and tubulin have been productive to date and remain the focus of much research. Our understanding of the nature of interactions between drugs and either DNA or tubulin is increasing, as is our knowledge of the mechanisms underlying drug resistance. Several compounds with promising preclinical activity and encouraging early clinical results are highlighted here.

DNA-interacting drugs

Damaging DNA remains the principal mode of action of most cytotoxics. This damage can, however, take many forms. Some agents inhibit DNA replication or transcription, whilst others may induce the formation of crosslinks or strand breaks, and still others prevent the resolution of torsion or inhibit chromosomal segregation. Although DNA-damaging agents have had important successes, they have limited selectivity for tumour cells, and toxicity is a major drawback. Indeed, the value of investigating DNA-damaging agents has been questioned on this basis.

Nevertheless, new DNA-interacting agents with novel mechanisms of action, or that are not cross-resistant with established agents, are in clinical development and showing promise.

DNA minor-groove binders

The commonly used alkylating cytotoxics such as melphalan and cyclophosphamide form crosslinks with exposed bases in the major groove of DNA. This binding is usually at the 06 or N7 position on guanine and is not highly dependent on the sequence of bases. More recently, several novel alkylating agents have been developed that bind bases in the minor groove of DNA in a highly sequence-specific manner. Typically, those minor-groove binders of clinical interest bind at the N3 position of adenine bases at specific AT-rich regions of DNA.[1]

Distamycin A and derivatives

The parent compound, distamycin A, is an antiviral agent that binds the minor groove of DNA but does not alkylate and is not cytotoxic. Derivatives have been developed that predominantly alkylate adenine bases in the minor groove at the N3 position and are cytotoxic. Tallimustine, the first distamycin A derivative tested clinically, alkylates with strong specificity for 5'-TTTGA sequences and a few other AT-rich hexamers, inhibiting the binding of transcription factors and DNA ligase at these sites. Preclinical studies showed that tallimustine was highly potent against human and murine cell lines as well as transplanted murine solid tumours and human tumour xenografts.[2]

In phase I trials, the major toxicity of intravenous tallimustine was myelosuppression, irrespective of whether a 1- or a 3-day schedule was employed. Initial reports from the phase I trials of activity in both solid tumours and adult myelogenous leukaemia were encouraging.[3] However, phase II trials were disappointing, with no objective responses in small-cell lung cancer or colorectal cancer.

The cyclopropylpyrrolindoles (CPIs)

A second group of compounds, the cyclopropylpyrrolindoles (CPIs), also bind covalently with AT-rich regions of the minor groove. CC-1065 was isolated from the fermentation broth of a soil bacterium, *Streptomyces zelensis*. It was highly active, but murine toxicity at subtherapeutic doses precluded its development. Structure–activity analyses showed the CPI group was the active site, and three analogues of CC-1065 have now been developed clinically.[4]

Adozelesin, which is closely related to CC-1065, is active *in vitro* at picomolar concentrations but has a substantially better toxicity profile. Bizelesin was designed as a CPI analogue capable of forming DNA crosslinks. It is a prodrug that is rapidly converted to the active CPI *in vitro* and possesses two alkylating groups so it can bind adenosine bases on opposite strands of DNA. Carzelesin was developed in an attempt to moderate the very rapid alkylation of DNA by CPI analogues. It is an inactive prodrug that is converted to the active compound intracellularly, where it is more potent than adozelesin *in vivo* against human tumour xenografts.

All three CPI analogues are undergoing clinical evaluation, with results of early clinical trials available. Each has been given as an intravenous infusion with a range of schedules employed. In phase I trials of adozelesin and carzelesin, neutropenia and thrombocytopenia were dose-limiting. Myelosuppression may be delayed, prolonged, and cumulative. A biphasic pattern of myelosuppression has also been seen. This may reflect different populations of progenitor cells being targeted by the CPI or its metabolites. Bizelesin is at an earlier stage of development, but haematological toxicity is again likely to be dose-limiting.

Antitumour activity in phase II trials of the CPIs has been modest to date. Isolated responses have been reported with carzelesin in melanoma, non-Hodgkin's lymphoma, and breast and ovarian cancer. This limited activity may be due to suboptimal dosing since levels of the active metabolite U-76,073 in plasma are often lower than those achieved in mice.[5] Responses were seen in the phase I trials of adozelesin but it had only minimal activity against breast cancer in a phase II trial. It is unclear whether different dose schedules can improve the antitumour activity of the CPIs.

Illudins and related compounds

The illudins are a family of molecules derived from the *Ompholatus illudens* mushroom. They are structurally distinct from other cytotoxics, and, although they bind to DNA, their precise mechanism of action is not known. In contrast to many other DNA-interacting agents, the illudins are more toxic to cells with mutations inactivating the helicase component of nucleotide excision repair (**NER**), suggesting that specific helicases repair the damaged DNA. The illudins also retain their cytotoxicity in multidrug-resistant cell lines, and the related compound MGI-114 induces apoptosis independent of the functional activity of p53 or p21.

Hydroxymethylacylfulvene (HMAF) or MGI-114

The illudins have broad activity *in vitro* at picomolar concentrations, but toxicity precluded their development *in vivo*. A range of better tolerated analogues has been made. There is an encouragingly high single-agent activity of one of these, MGI-114, both *in vitro* and *in vivo* against a range of human tumour models,[6] including the MV522 lung cancer xenograft which is resistant to many cytotoxics. Antitumour activity is retained in MV522 lines overexpressing the *mdr1* gene or the *MRP* gene, thus confirming its activity in drug-resistant models.[7] There may, however, be a particular rationale for using HMI-114 in combination with other cytotoxics since synergy has been identified in combination with 5-fluorouracil (**5-FU**) and irinotecan. This synergy may be mediated through inhibition of helicases, reflecting the greater activity of MGI-114 itself against cells with *RER* mutations.

Preliminary results have been presented for several phase I and II trials of MGI-114 given as an intravenous infusion. A 5-day schedule repeated every 4 weeks caused fatigue and myelosuppression, as well as renal tubular acidosis that was subsequently prevented by intravenous hydration or the use of oral bicarbonate. This schedule has been evaluated in phase II trials at a dose of 11 mg/m^2 in patients with previously treated ovarian, pancreatic, or prostate cancer. Responses have been seen in each tumour type, including women with cisplatin- or paclitaxel-resistant ovarian cancer.

ET-743

ET-743 is a DNA-interacting agent and a member of the family of ecteinascidins, a group of novel compounds extracted from the marine tunicate *Ecteinascidia turbinata* found in Caribbean mangrove swamps. ET-743 is a tetrahydroisoquinolone alkaloid selected for development because of its potency and broad range of antitumour activity *in vitro* and *in vivo*. The mechanism of cytotoxicity of ET-743 is unclear, but it causes prolonged blockade of the cell cycle at G2–M. ET-743 binds to the N2 position of guanine in the minor groove of DNA, and this binding appears to be specific to GC-rich sequences. Structural studies suggest that when ET-743 is bound to DNA, the C ring of the molecule protrudes away from minor groove. This protruding 'arm' of ET-743 may bind proteins, such as transcription factors, that interact with DNA. Function of the general transcription factor NF-Y can be disrupted in this way at clinically relevant concentrations of ET-743.

In preclinical testing ET-743 had both high potency and a broad range of efficacy against human tumour cell lines, with prolonged exposure enhancing this cytotoxicity.[8] This activity was confirmed *in vivo* in several human tumour xenografts, most notably ovarian, breast, non-small-cell lung cancer, and melanoma. Cells deficient in nucleotide excision repair are less sensitive to ET-743, in contrast to their greater sensitivity to other alkylating agents. Sensitivity to ET-743 appears not to be influenced by mismatch repair or the functional state of p53. Although the activity of ET-743 is partially abrogated in cell lines with the Pgp phenotype, ET-743 may retain activity against tumours resistant to other cytotoxics. Many human tumour samples tested *ex vivo* that were resistant to doxorubicin, cisplatin, and paclitaxel retained their sensitivity to ET-743.[9]

In animal models ET-743 caused dose-limiting haematological and hepatic toxicity. The hepatotoxicity was irreversible at the highest doses and appeared to be related to peak blood levels of ET-743 or a metabolite. This led to a number of different intravenous ET-743 schedules being tested in phase I trials. In trials of varying schedules of administration myelosuppression was the major toxicity, but a dose-dependent transient increase in serum transaminases frequently occurred.

ET-743 has demonstrated a striking level of activity against a wide range of tumours including heavily pretreated osteosarcoma, leiomyosarcoma, breast cancer, melanoma, and mesothelioma. The activity against sarcomas has been confirmed by preliminary results of phase II trials, and studies in other types of tumour are underway. Most of these trials use a 3-h intravenous infusion of ET-743 at a dose of 1500 µg/m^2 but an association between abnormal liver biochemistry tests and an increased risk of treatment toxicity has resulted in dose modifications.

It is not yet clear if these new DNA-interactive agents will be a major step forward, but ET-743 and MGI-114 look particularly interesting. These agents interact with DNA in novel ways and may not be substrates for classical mechanisms of resistance. It is very probable that other DNA-interacting agents will emerge as established cytotoxics.

Tubulin inhibitors

The tubulin-interacting agents paclitaxel, docetaxel, and vinorelbine are amongst the most important new drugs to enter routine clinical practice. Recently there has been renewed interest in tubulin as this

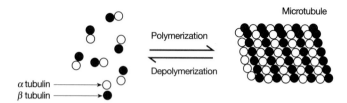

Fig. 2 Formation of microtubules from tubulin: a balance between polymerization (inhibited by vinca alkaloids, cryptophycin S2 and dolastatins and depolymerization inhibited by taxoids, epothilones, and T138067, T138607.

is a validated target (Fig. 2). In particular, compounds have been sought with greater activity than those currently in use or that retain cytotoxicity in resistant cell lines.

T138607 binds irreversibly to β-tubulin to inhibit tubulin depolymerization. It is a synthetic compound and not a substrate for Pgp, retaining activity in cell lines resistant to paclitaxel. A more lipophilic analogue, T138067, and RPR109881 are also active against some taxoid-resistant models but cross the blood–brain barrier. BMS 184476 is another analogue with superior activity to paclitaxel in multidrug-resistant lines, and it is more soluble, thus reducing the need for cremophor. Novel delivery systems such as taxoprexin, where paclitaxel is conjugated to a fatty acid substantially modifying drug distribution, are also being evaluated in the clinic as are orally bioavailable tubulin inhibitors.

The epothilones are bacterial products that have a similar mechanism of action to the taxoids in that they induce tubulin polymerization, but they are structurally distinct from taxoids. Some members of this family of compounds are more active than the taxoids. In particular, BMS-247550 and EPO906 retain activity in taxoid-resistant preclinical models. Both are being evaluated in the clinic, with encouraging signs of antitumour activity in pretreated patients and tumours such as colorectal cancer that are not usually considered sensitive to taxoids.

A second group of compounds, this time targeting tubulin at the vinca binding site, are being evaluated in the clinic. Cryptophycin 52 is a novel marine compound that is much more potent than the current tubulin inhibitors. The fluorinated vinca alkaloid, vinflunine, again has enhanced activity *in vitro* and *in vivo*. TZT-1027, an analogue of dolastatin 10, inhibits microtubule assembly but appears to bind tubulin at neither the vinca nor taxoid sites. TZT-1027 was active in phase I trials, with neutropenia the main toxicity. Cematodin, derived from dolastatin 15, is a similar compound also under development.

Although tubulin has been identified as the target for these agents, the mechanism by which microtubular damage initiates apoptosis has not been defined. This is another potentially important area of investigation that may lead to new therapeutic approaches. Indeed, several tubulin binding agents are toxic to the vascular endothelium and may act as antiangiogenic agents.

Signalling pathways

'Signal transduction' is the term given to the process of transmitting cellular responses from one location in the cell to another. Biological events such as cellular proliferation, adhesion, migration, and apoptosis are mediated by signal transduction. These mechanisms are driven by distinct signalling pathways in different tumours. Signalling pathways offer new rational targets. Several small molecules and monoclonal antibodies acting on signalling pathways are now entering the clinic.

Drugs targeting signal transduction are expected to be largely cytostatic rather than cytotoxic and could have toxicity profiles distinct from cytotoxic chemotherapy agents. Although they may be less toxic than conventional chemotherapeutic agents, the development of these signal-transduction inhibitors raises many challenges. The signalling pathways are complex with 'cross-talk' between different cascades. It is possible that, even if a pathway can be inhibited at one site, this inhibition may be bypassed through other pathways. Moreover, tumours frequently mutate and may easily lose expression of the target protein. In addition, the signalling kinases are present in normal tissues as well as tumours so inhibitors may need to be targeted at specific isoforms in cancer cells. Indeed, it is unclear whether targeting a single molecular abnormality will be as effective in the clinic, where an individual tumour is made up of highly heterogeneous cells, as it is in the laboratory. Clinical trials need to incorporate biological endpoints to confirm proof of principle of mode of action.

Signalling pathways can be broken down into several distinct, but overlapping groups:

- receptor tyrosine kinases that interact with growth-factor ligands to initiate signalling;
- neuropeptide growth factors that lack enzymatic activity also activate signalling pathways;
- protein kinase C and Ca^{2+} channel blockers, and signalling proteins such as ras convey the cytoplasmic signal;
- cyclin-dependent kinases that regulate the cell cycle.

Receptor tyrosine kinases

The receptor tyrosine kinases (**RTKs**) are a group of over 50 transmembrane glycoproteins classified into 18 families. They comprise an extracellular ligand-binding domain, a transmembrane domain, and a cytoplasmic tyrosine-kinase domain. Binding of growth-factor ligands to cell-surface RTKs results in receptor dimerization and phosphorylation of tyrosine residues on the intracellular domain. The phosphotyrosinase groups bind and phosphorylate other molecules. In turn, these activated molecules interact with downstream signalling proteins leading to changes in gene transcription. Hence signals that regulate cell function are transmitted from the cell surface to the nucleus (Fig. 3).

The RTKs are overexpressed or activated in many different tumours including breast cancer (for example, HER), sarcoma (platelet-derived, growth-factor receptor; **PDGFR**), and chronic myelogenous leukaemia (bcr-abl). In many cases the degree of RTK expression correlates with increasing tumour grade and a poorer prognosis. Their biological roles vary widely depending on the receptor and the cell in which it is expressed. Some, such as epithelial growth-factor receptor (**EGFR**), HER-2, and PDGFR promote growth; others such as Flt promote chemotaxis, whereas members of the vascular endothelial growth-factor (**VEGF**) receptor family such as Flk-1/KDR promote angiogenesis.

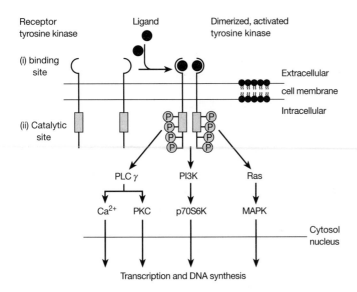

Fig. 3 Schematic diagram of some of the signalling pathways activated by receptor tyrosine kinases. The ligand binds to the RTK which dimerizes, leading to autophosphorylation of the catalytic sites which become active, switching on (i) PLC-γ (an isoform of phospholipase C), Ca²⁺ and PKC (protein kinase C), (ii) PI3K (phosphoinositol-3 kinase) and p7056 kinase, and (iii) Ras and MapK (mitogen-activated protein kinase). These and other pathways transmit signals to the nucleus.

The biological characteristics of RTKs make them important targets for anticancer drug development.[10] Attempts at inhibiting RTKs were initially directed at substrate inhibitors such as the tyrphostins. The first of these to enter the clinic was **quercetin**. It is a naturally occurring flavenoid that inhibits tyrosine kinase, but it has many other actions including inhibition of PKC and phosphatidyl inositol-3 kinase. In preclinical models querciten has antiproliferative activity as a single agent and potentiates the actions of cisplatin *ex vivo*. In clinical trials querciten was nephrotoxic at high doses but plasma concentrations were achieved that are active *in vitro*.[11] Some indication of biological activity came from the observation that lymphocyte tyrosine phosphorylated protein levels fell in patients treated with quercetin.

Subsequently, the main focus has been on targeting the ATP binding site and the rational development of inhibitors directed at specific RTKs. It might be expected that selectivity would be reduced by targeting the ATP binding site rather than the substrate binding site. However, the ATP binding site often lies close to the substrate binding site and has a distinct three-dimensional structure giving it considerable specificity as a target. These approaches use small molecules acting within the cell, but monoclonal antibodies have also been developed to bind specifically the extracellular receptor.

Epithelial growth factor-receptor family inhibitors

The EGF-receptor family comprises HER-1, HER-2, HER-3, and HER-4. They have several ligands including EGF, tumour growth factor-α (**TGF-α**), and amphiregulin. Ligand binding leads to receptor activation and a complex pattern of cell signalling. Members of the EGFR family are overexpressed, or expressed as an autocrine loop, in many different types of tumour including breast, ovarian, colon,

and prostate cancer. Moreover, EGFR is required for growth in experimental tumour models.

The potential impact of RTKs and their inhibitors as therapeutic targets is illustrated by HER-2. Overexpression is detected by the technique of fluorescent *in situ* hybridization (**FISH**) in about 25 per cent of human breast cancers and is associated with a poor prognosis. More important has been the development of **Herceptin**, a humanized, murine monoclonal antibody, as a therapeutic agent. As a single agent, Herceptin achieves responses in at least 15 per cent of women with advanced breast cancer whose tumours overexpress HER-2. In this same group of women, the addition of Herceptin to conventional chemotherapy significantly increases response rates and prolongs survival. These trials vindicate the principle of developing novel agents directed at specific tumours in which that target is relevant. They also emphasize the emerging role of molecular pathology as a part of the therapeutic decision-making process, a role that is likely to increase greatly in coming years.

Several small molecule EGFR inhibitors are also in development. The most advanced is Iressa (ZD1839). Iressa illustrates the therapeutic potential and specificity of molecules directed at the ATP binding site. In experimental models tumour growth is inhibited by Iressa with a fall in mRNA for the downstream mitogenic factor c-*fos*, demonstrating that the desired biological effect has been achieved. Proof of principle in patients comes from the demonstration that EGFR phosphorylation and **MAPK** (mitogen-activated protein kinase) activation are inhibited in skin biopsies from patients treated with oral Iressa in early clinical trials. The principal toxicities seen with Iressa are skin rashes and diarrhoea, which reflect the biological target. Responses to Iressa have been seen in patients with non-small-cell lung cancer over a range of well-tolerated doses.

Cetuximab is a monoclonal antibody directed at the EGF receptor. In contrast to Iressa, Cetuximab binds to the extracellular ligand binding domain, competing with EGF to inhibit tyrosine kinase activity. Cetuximab is given intravenously. Allergic reactions may also occur in addition to cutaneous toxicity. Both Iressa and Cetuximab are in phase II/III trials as single agents and in combination with chemotherapy. Several other EGF-receptor inhibitors are at earlier stages of development.

Platelet-derived, growth factor-receptor family inhibitors

Platelet-derived growth factor (PDGF) is a mitogen and its receptor has been identified in breast cancer, colon cancer, and melanoma cell lines. More importantly, PDGF and its receptor have been detected in human glioblastoma and ovarian cancer biopsies.

Several PDGF receptor inhibitors are under development including SU101 and CEP-2563. SU101 (leflunomide) given as an intravenous infusion showed activity against glioblastoma, prostate, and ovarian cancer in phase I, and further studies are underway.[12]

Abl kinase inhibitors

c-abl is a cytoplasmic proto-oncogene rather than a cell-membrane tyrosine kinase. It is best known for its role in chronic myelogenous leukaemia (**CML**) through the Philadelphia chromosome. Fusion between chromosome 9 (*abl*) and chromosome 22 (*bcr*) creates the Philadelphia chromosome that encodes the bcr/abl fusion protein with activated abl kinase activity which is a prerequisite for transformation (Fig. 4).

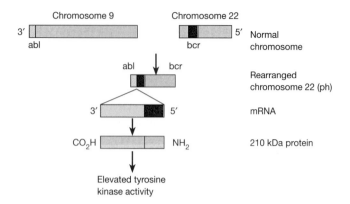

Fig. 4 The bcr/abl or Philadelphia chromosome. Reciprocal translocation between long arms of chromosomes 9 and 22 generates the Philadelphia chromosome encoding an 8.2 kb transcript coding for the bcr/abl protein. Unlike wild type abl, which is located in the nucleus, the frozen protein is cytoplasmic and has increased tyrosine kinase activity.

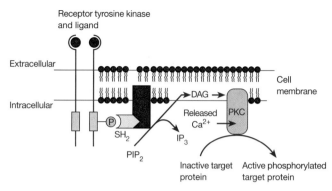

Fig. 5 Activation of protein kinase C. Ligand binding to RTK activates membrane bound phospholipase C via an SH2 binding molecule. PLC-γ then leaves phosphatidyl inositol (PIP$_2$) into diacyl glycerol (DAG) and inositol triphosphate (IP$_3$). IP$_3$ causes release of Ca^{2+} ions which recruit PKC to the cell membrane where it is activated by DAG. Once activated, PKC phosphorylates intracellular receptors and enzymes.

The Philadelphia chromosome is present in almost all cases of CML and about 20 per cent of cases of adult acute lymphoblastic leukaemia. Targeting the abl kinase is a rational approach to the treatment of both diseases. CGP 57148/STI571 is a potent, oral inhibitor of the bcr/abl kinase but also has activity against PDGFR. Both *in vitro* and *in vivo* STI571 has selective antiproliferative activity against bcr/abl-positive cells.[13] The development of STI571 has focused especially on CML, with STI571 being well tolerated and showing dramatic early results. Haematological responses have been reported in CML patients, all either refractory to, or intolerant of, standard treatment with interferon. Many patients also have a cytogenetic response, with the Philadelphia chromosome no longer detectable. STI571 is also showing activity in patients in blast crisis and is being evaluated in solid tumours.

Other RTK inhibitors

Other RTKs such as vascular endothelial growth factor (VEGF), fibroblast growth factor and src have been implicated in human malignancy. VEGF is an attractive target as it stimulates endothelial cell growth and is secreted by human tumour cells. Inhibitors such as SU5416 and CGP 79787 are already in clinical development and other RTKs will follow.

Neuropeptide growth-factor signalling

Neuropeptides bind to receptors that have seven transmembrane domains but lack enzymatic activity. These seven transmembrane domain receptors (**7TMRs**) utilize heterotrimeric G proteins to generate downstream signals. Although their mode of action is different from the RTKs, many of the same pathways are activated by 7TMRs, including MAP kinase, calcium mobilization, and p70 S6 kinase. These pathways are potentially important targets for anticancer drugs. **Rapamycin** is an immunosuppressant drug that binds to cytosolic kinase mTOR, upstream to p70 S6 kinase and inhibits tumour growth in preclinical models. CCI-779 is a derivative of rapamycin that appears not to be immunosuppressive but has shown antitumour activity in phase I trials. A second group of compounds, analogues of substance P, are broader neuropeptide inhibitors that

inhibit small-cell lung cancer both *in vitro* and *in vivo*.[14] Already, one substance-P analogue has entered phase I clinical trials but clinical activity has still to be demonstrated.

Protein kinase C (PKC)

Interactions between RTKs, including EGF, VEGF, and HER-2, and their ligands lead to the generation of the second messengers diacylglycerol (**DAG**) and calcium that activate protein kinase C (PKC) (Fig. 5). This family of serine–threonine kinases phosphorylates downstream proteins. Each PKC comprises a C-terminal catalytic domain and an N-terminal regulatory domain. There are more than 12 PKC isoenzymes that can be divided into three groups according to their dependence on calcium and DAG. PKCs are ubiquitous, but the subtypes differ in their distribution, regulation, and catalytic activity.

There are good reasons to consider PKCs attractive targets for anticancer drugs.[15] Phorbol esters promote tumours by activating PKC over a prolonged period. In many cases PKC activity is increased in tumour cells, and those with the highest PKC activity may have the greatest potential for invasion and metastasis. PKC levels are increased in breast tumours, but no single pattern of PKC expression is as characteristic of malignancy. It is, therefore, unclear which, if any, specific PKC isoenzymes should be targeted to achieve tumour selectivity. Indeed, an important role for PKC inhibitors may be as modulators of MDR in combination with conventional cytotoxics.

PKC has been targeted in different ways. The first group of compounds, of which the bryostatins are the most important, act at the regulatory domain of PKC. Staurosporine is the lead compound amongst those targeting the catalytic site. Finally, the antisense oligonucleotides can hybridize mRNA to reduce PKC expression.

Bryostatin 1 and related compounds

Bryostatin 1 was the first PKC inhibitor to be tested in the clinic. The bryostatins are macrocyclic polylactones derived from marine invertebrates. Bryostatin 1, isolated from *Bugula neritina*, is the most widely studied PKC modulator. It has differential effects on PKC isoenzymes and, according to the circumstances, can act either as an agonist or an antagonist, but is probably best considered a partial agonist. In some preclinical models bryostatin shows antiproliferative activity but it can also induce differentiation.

In phase I trials bryostatin 1 was given as a 1-, 24-, or 72-h infusion. The principal toxicity has been cumulative myalgia. Measurement of surrogate endpoints suggest that bryostatin 1 has significant biological effects at tolerable doses. Increased plasma levels of interleukin-6 (IL-6) and tumour-necrosis factor-α (TNF-α) have been described,[16] as have changes in mononuclear-cell PKC activity and increased lymphokine-activated, killer-cell activity.[17] Tumour responses were reported in these phase I trials. However, early indications of activity against melanoma were not confirmed in phase II trials, and bryostatin 1 may be best used in combination with other agents. For example, resistance to cytosine arabinoside in fresh blast cells from patients with acute myeloid leukaemia can be partially overcome by co-incubation with bryostatin 1. Bryostatin 1 has a complex structure and has been difficult both to synthesize and to formulate. Other members of the bryostatin family and analogues of bryostatin 1 are being evaluated.

Safingol is a sphingosine derivative that also binds to the PKC regulatory domain. Alone, safingol has little anti-tumour activity *in vivo*, but it enhances the activity of cytotoxics and can reverse multidrug resistance in preclinical models. Safingol can be given at potentially effective doses in combination with doxorubicin (45 or 60 mg/m²).[18] At high concentrations tamoxifen also inhibits PKC in cell lines, as can the ether lipids such as edelfosine, but it is unclear whether this is important for their antitumour activity.

Staurosporine and its analogues

Staurosporine is the lead compound amongst the PKC inhibitors acting at the catalytic site. It is one of the most potent PKC inhibitors and is active against several cell lines *in vitro*. Because the catalytic domain is conserved between different kinase families, staurosporine lacks specificity and also inhibits tyrosine and cyclin-dependent kinases. Analogues have been developed seeking greater selectivity and a better therapeutic index.

7-hydroxy-staurosporine (UCN-01) is a more potent PKC inhibitor than staurosporine, which is active as a single agent and can induce apoptosis *in vitro* independent of p53.[19] Downstream effects of UCN-01 include inhibition of specific cyclin-dependent kinases (**CDKs**). This may represent an important mode of action, overcoming the G2 cell-cycle arrest caused by conventional DNA-damaging agents in cells lacking normal p53 function, which may enhance cytotoxicity. In preclinical testing, UCN-01 was active *in vivo* as a single agent against breast and renal cancer. Phase I trials of UCN-01, given as a 3- or 72-hour infusion, were complicated by binding to α-1 acid glycoprotein (**AAG**) which dramatically prolonged the elimination half-life.[20] Nevertheless, free UCN-01 levels in the saliva of around 100 nM were achieved, high enough to inhibit the G2 checkpoint and to have antiproliferative activity *in vitro*. Dose-limiting toxicities were hyperglycaemia, nausea, and vomiting, but there was clear evidence of antitumour activity in patients with melanoma, leiomyosarcoma, non-Hodgkin's lymphoma, and lung cancer.

N-benzoyl-staurosporine (PKC 412A or CGP42151A) is a second staurosporine derivative. PKC 412A preferentially inhibits specific PKCs and can be given orally. It has antiproliferative activity *in vitro* and in xenograft models. PKC 412A also binds strongly to AAG, but changes in the release of TNF-α and IL-6 from whole blood stimulated by the mitogen phytohaemagglutinin (**PHA**) and downregulation of MAP kinase in lymphocytes confirm that PKC 412A affects pathways downstream from PKC.[21] In the phase I study PKC 412A caused some gastrointestinal toxicity but little myelosuppression. This suggests that combinations of PKC 412A with conventional cytotoxics or with radiotherapy should be feasible. PKC 412A is synergistic with conventional cytotoxics and its ability to overcome mdr1-mediated drug resistance at low concentrations emphasizes the potential importance of combination therapy with this and other PKC inhibitors.[22]

PKC antisense

Unlike the other PKC inhibitors, which act on the protein, ISIS 3521 targets mRNA. ISIS 3521 comprises 20 nucleotides linked by a phosphothiorate backbone designed to hybridize PKC-α mRNA. This makes ISIS 3521 potentially a much more specific PKC inhibitor than those that bind the catalytic or regulatory site of the enzyme. ISIS 3521 is a potent inhibitor of PKC-α in human tumour cell lines and inhibition of tumour growth *in vivo* is accompanied by dose-dependent falls in PKC-α protein expression. This compound is in early trials, as are ISIS 2503, directed at H-Ras mRNA, and ISIS 5132, which binds to the mRNA of C-*raf* kinase. The principal toxicities of these oligonucleotides have been fatigue as well as thrombocytopenia and altered coagulation states (both attributed to the phosphothiorate backbone) and fatigue.

Calcium channel blockers

Intracellular calcium is an important component of cell signalling. It can either be mobilized within the cell or enter through either voltage-dependent or receptor-mediated calcium channels. Inhibiting the influx of calcium is, therefore, another way of influencing signal transduction. Carboxyamidotriazole (CAI) is a novel synthetic compound identified in a screen for agents that inhibited cell migration. It inhibits calcium influx and has antiproliferative, antimetastatic, and antiangiogenic properties *in vitro*. In preclinical models, CAI is cytostatic rather than cytotoxic but has relatively few toxicities. Phase I trials using different oral formulations achieved potentially active plasma drug concentrations with reversible neurotoxicity limiting further dose escalation.[23]

Ras protein

Activation of the Ras/Raf1/MEK1/MAPK pathway plays a central role in cell signalling and has been closely implicated in malignancy (Fig. 6). In experimental models constitutively active mutations of *ras* lead to cell transformation, whereas Ras antibody blocks growth factor-induced mitogenesis. The *ras* oncogene is mutated in 30 per cent of human cancers, especially pancreatic (70 to 90 per cent) and colon (40 to 60 per cent) cancers, making it a potentially important therapeutic target.

Ras might be targeted at several points. Before they can function, many important proteins must undergo post-translational prenylation. This modification involves the transfer of a farnesyl or geranylgeranyl group. The Ras proteins H-ras, K-ras, and N-ras undergo post-translational farnesylation and localize in the cell membrane. The rate-limiting step in this process is controlled by the enzyme farnesyl transferase. Once inserted in the membrane the Ras proteins switch between their 'on' (bound to GTP) and 'off' (bound to GDP) forms in response to signals, including those from receptor

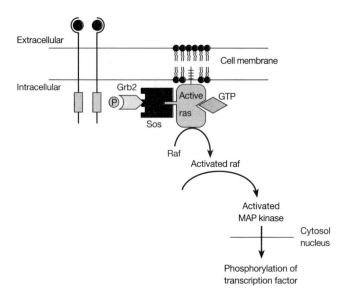

Fig. 6 Activated RTK binds the adaptor protein GRB2 and in turn the exchange factor SOS. Binding of SOS to inactive GDP ras, anchored to cell membrane, stimulates conversion to active GTP ras. In turn, ras acts through rafγ, mitogen activated protein kinase (MAPK kinase), to phosphorylate nuclear transcription factors.

tyrosine kinases. In turn, Ras activates the serine–threonine kinase raf-1, which has downstream effects on cell division through the extracellular regulated kinases (ERKs). Nuclear ERKs regulate gene transcription, the final step in transmitting extracellular signals from the cell membrane to the nucleus.

The conversion of Ras to its functional form has been targeted through both the isoprenoid substrate and the farnesyltransferase enzyme. The isoprenoids are intermediates in the mevalonate pathway for cholesterol biosynthesis. Phenylacetate, lovastatin, and the monoterpenes are inhibitors of this pathway and have antitumour activity *in vitro* and *in vivo*. **Lovastatin** is a cholesterol-lowering agent, and in early trials its biological activity was monitored through changes in the serum concentrations of cholesterol and ubiquinone, both endproducts of the mevalonate pathway. High doses of lovastatin caused a myopathy that could be prevented by the coadministration of ubiquinone.[24] **D-Limonene** is a naturally occurring monoterpene which is a component of many plant oils. It selectively inhibits the post-translational isoprenylation of small GTP-binding proteins, including p21^{ras} which regulates signal transduction. D-Limonene is well absorbed and its metabolites include perillic acid. A second, more potent, monoterpene, perillyl alcohol was identified and found to be tolerable when given orally for prolonged periods.[25] However, the optimal dose and schedule of these compounds are unclear since no pharmacodynamic effect has been demonstrated.

A more promising approach may be inhibition of the farnesyltransferase enzyme itself. Several farnesyltransferase inhibitors (**FTIs**) have been developed which inhibit tumour formation and growth in preclinical models but have little effect on normal tissues. Already the oral agents SCH66336, R115777, and BMS-214662 and the intravenous compound L778,123 are in clinical trials. They have been well tolerated at doses that achieve plasma levels and are active *in vitro*. Reduced prenylation of marker proteins in circulating

mononuclear cells suggest that the desired biological effect can be achieved, and tumour responses have been reported. BMS-214662 appears to be highly cytotoxic to tumour cells and capable of inducing apoptosis *in vitro* at very low concentrations. The FTIs may be more active against resting tumour cells, whereas conventional cytotoxics act principally on the proliferating tumour-cell compartment. Each of these FTIs is being tested in combination with conventional cytotoxics, where perhaps they are more likely to prove useful than as single agents.

These early results are encouraging but many questions remain. In particular, the growth inhibition seen with the FTIs may not be mediated through *ras*. Compounds which inhibit H-*ras* can suppress growth in cells transformed with K-*ras*, the function of which is not affected by FTIs. This suggests that *ras* may not be the primary target, as does the lack of correlation between sensitivity to FTIs and *ras* mutation status. There is increasing evidence that the FTIs may act through the Rho proteins which regulate the cytoskeleton and also require prenylation. FTI treatment *in vitro* can alter RhoB function leading to growth inhibition and induction of the endogenous CDK inhibitor p21^{waf} which may be a biological marker of FTI activity.

Although the mode of action of the FTIs is unclear, *Ras* itself has also been targeted directly. Antisense 20-mer oligonucleotides designed to hybridize with mRNA, have been directed at both *Ras* and *Raf*. ISIS 2503 targets H-*Ras* mRNA and reduces H-*Ras* expression, whereas ISIS 5132 binds to the mRNA of C-*raf* kinase so inhibiting protein synthesis. They are administered as prolonged intravenous infusions and appear to be well tolerated. The reduction in C-*raf* mRNA expression seen in the peripheral leucocytes of patients treated with ISIS 5132 suggests that the desired biological effect is being achieved.

Other components of the phosphorylation cascade are emerging and are potential targets for drug development. One of the most interesting is the heat-shock protein Hsp90, which is one of several intracellular chaperones. These chaperones play a critical role in the assembly, folding, and activity of steroid receptors, tyrosine kinases, and tumour-suppressor genes. These include Raf-1 which can only be fully activated when associated with Hsp90 and the co-chaperone p50^{cdc37}. The antibiotics geldanamycin and radicol disrupt the Hsp90/p50^{cdc37}/Raf-1 complex and downregulate signalling through this pathway. The development of geldanamycin was stopped because of a low therapeutic index and liver toxicity in preclinical testing. 17-AAG is an analogue of geldanamycin which leads to the degradation of c-Raf and other client proteins *in vitro*. It is also active *in vivo*, but it is less toxic than geldanamycin and is now in phase I trials.

Although FTIs were rationally developed against a specific target, it may be that their use in the clinic will not be determined solely by Ras status. Inhibitors of other elements of the Ras/Raf1/MEK1/MAPK pathway, downstream of Ras, are also in development.

Cyclin-dependent kinases (CDK)

The cell cycle is regulated by cyclin-dependent kinases (CDKs), a group of at least nine serine–threonine protein kinases acting with their partner cyclins. For example, the transition from G1 to S is driven by CDK4 and CDK6 acting with cyclin D. This complex then phosphorylates the product of the retinoblastoma (*Rb*) tumour-suppresser gene, releasing E2F which acts as a transcription factor (Fig. 7). E2F switches on genes allowing cells to progress to S phase.

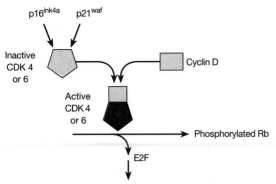

Fig. 7 Regulation of cell cycle by the retinoblastoma gene product (R6).

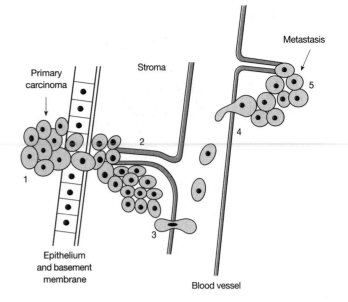

Fig. 8 Tumour invasion and metastasis. (1) Primary carcinoma invades through the basement membrane into the stroma. (2) Tumour induces growth of new vessels (angiogenesis) that grow away from the host vessel into the stroma. Endothelial cells proliferate to form tube-like structures, then canalize. (3) Tumour cells invade the vasculature, circulate, then lodge in capillaries. (4) Tumour cells extravasate and angiogenesis is induced to support growth of the metastasis.

Specific CDK inhibitors such as p21^{waf}, which acts downstream from the tumour-suppresser gene *p53*, and p16^{ink4a} inhibit this process.

Deregulation of the CDKs is seen in many human tumours and it can take many forms. For example, activity of the endogenous CKD inhibitors may be lost due to deletion of *p16* or changes in p53 function. Alternatively, cyclin D may be overexpressed or the *Rb* gene mutated. The CDKs are, therefore, an important target for drug development and inhibitors have entered early clinical trials with encouraging preliminary results.

Flavopiridol, the lead compound of this class, is a flavonoid that acts at the catalytic site and is a potent CDK inhibitor. It has only limited specificity, inhibiting CDK-1, -2, and -4 and, to a lesser extent, other kinases. Its potential was shown in preclinical models where flavopiridol caused cell-cycle arrest and induced apoptosis in lymphoid or head and neck cancers irrespective of BCL-2 or p53 function.[26] In a phase I trial the dose-limiting toxicities of flavopiridol given as a 72-hour infusion were secretory diarrhoea, hypotension, and an inflammatory myalgia. The diarrhoea could be controlled with lo-peramide or cholestyramine, allowing further dose-escalation. Plasma flavopiridol concentrations between 300 and 500 nM were achieved, equivalent to those that inhibit CDKs and are antiproliferative *in vitro*. Antitumour activity was seen in early trials against renal, prostate, and colon cancer and non-Hodgkin's lymphoma.[27] Alternative schedules are being studied and activity against a range of tumours is being investigated.

UCN-01 is another CDK inhibitor, albeit at concentrations several fold higher than required to inhibit PKC. At lower concentrations, however, UCN-01 can influence CDK activity indirectly and block G2 arrest induced by DNA-damaging agents. Early results with both these CDK inhibitors are encouraging, but the optimal schedules of administration are still to be defined.

CDK inhibitors with potentially greater specificity are in preclinical development. Amongst these are purvalanol A and B, olomucine, and roscovitine—purine-based inhibitors that act at the catalytic site but have greater specificity for specific CDKs. Roscovitine, for example, is given orally and is active against CDK2 and CDK1. Rather than administer pharmacological inhibitors, a different approach is to restore the activity of endogenous CDK inhibitors. This might be achieved by restoring p53 function leading to increased expression of the naturally occurring inhibitor p21waf. Alternatively, it may be possible to preserve the inhibitory activity of endogenous inhibitors such as p16ink-4a in a small peptide that could be delivered directly to tumour cells.

Other molecules may inhibit CDKs without it being clear that this is their principal mode of action. Ro 31-7453 is active *in vitro* and *in vivo* against a wide range of human tumours. Its precise molecular target is not known, but Ro 31-7453 is a relatively weak inhibitor of CDK-1, -2, and -4 and of tubulin polymerization in cell-free systems. E7070 is a sulphonamide derivative that inhibits tubulin poly-merization, blocks cell-cycle progression in G1, and is also active preclinically. Myelosuppression, which is more characteristic of conventional antiproliferative agents than of other CDK inhibitors, was seen with both Ro 31-7453 and E7070 in early clinical testing.

Metastasis and angiogenesis

The ability to invade and metastasize is characteristic of cancer cells. These are complex processes, first involving the escape of tumour cells through the basement membrane and into the lymphatic or blood circulation. Tumour cells must survive to be transported to other parts of the body to extravasate and form secondary tumours. Metastasis may, therefore, be targeted at any of these stages (Fig. 8).

Gene transfection can enhance the metastatic potential of cells, but a specific gene that determines the metastatic phenotype has not been identified. Rather, different regulatory genes appear to be responsible for the various stages of the metastatic process. A key feature is the ability to induce proteolysis in order that the tumour can invade adjacent tissues. The matrix metalloproteases (**MMPs**)

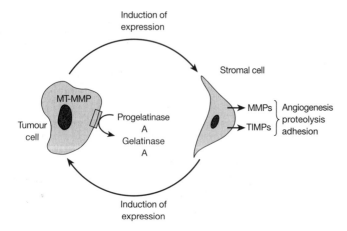

Fig. 9 Interaction of tumour and stromal cells: the balance of MMPs and TIMPs influences tumour invasion and metastasis.

appear to play a key role in this process. MMP inhibitors have clear antitumour activity in preclinical models and have been more extensively tested in clinical trials than most other novel approaches.

Matrix metalloproteases and their inhibitors

The matrix metalloproteases are a family of secreted and transmembrane enzymes whose physiological role is in remodelling connective tissue. However, during tumour progression MMPs break down the extracellular matrix and enhance angiogenesis. The MMPs are, therefore, attractive targets for anticancer drug development (Fig. 9).

More than 20 MMPs have been described to date, each with a highly conserved active site containing a zinc atom. The soluble MMPs are produced as inactive proenzymes, which are activated by cleavage of a 10-kDa amino-terminal domain. The membrane type (**MT-MMPs**) share the same active site but also contain a transmembrane domain. Once activated, the MMPs are regulated by endogenous inhibitors such as α2-macroglobulin and, more specifically, by a family of four tissue inhibitors of metalloproteases (**TIMPs**). Increased expression of MMPs does not, therefore, necessarily imply increased enzymatic activity. Likewise, it was initially assumed that MMPs were produced by tumour cells. Now it is clear that the stroma is a major source of MMPs, emphasizing the importance of interactions between the tumour and its stroma. Some of the MMPs such as MMP1, MMP8, and MMP13, are relatively specific with fibrillar collagens as their substrate. By contrast, the gelatinases A and B (MMP2 and -9, respectively) have a broader spectrum of activity.

There is strong evidence that the MMPs play an important role in malignancy.[28] Intraperitoneal injection of recombinant TIMP-1 in mice reduces lung metastases from B16F10 melanoma cells. By contrast, reducing TIMP-1 levels using antisense RNA enhances metastasis. Synthetic, specific inhibitors of MMPs (**MMPIs**) developed for clinical use also have antimetastatic properties in preclinical models. For example, batimastat (BB-94) reduced both lung colonization and spontaneous B16-BL6 melanoma metastases in mice. Several studies have confirmed a high expression of MMPs, especially MMP2 and MMP9, in human tumours. In general, there is a correlation between tumour progression and MMP expression. Patients with colorectal cancer with more advanced disease, as indicated by Duke's staging, have a higher proportion of cells staining for MMP2. An increased ratio of MMP to TIMP expression is associated with a poor prognosis in cervical cancer. However, in other situations the association of high MMP and low TIMP levels, that might be expected in tumours, has not been seen.

The importance of MMPs extends beyond their role in degrading the basement membrane and extracellular matrix. Expression of MMP2 in human breast cancers correlates with VEGF expression, and synthetic MMP inhibitors can inhibit angiogenesis *in vitro* and in animal models. Recent data that the tumorigenicity of human breast cancer cells is increased by injecting them with fibroblasts transfected with stromolysin-3, suggest that MMPs may act as tumour promoters.[29]

Inhibitors of MMPs have clear potential as anticancer agents and are likely to be quite distinct from conventional cytotoxics. They should be cytostatic rather than cytotoxic although they may be most effective in combination with current treatments. Also, by targeting the processes of invasion and metastasis that characterize the malignant phenotype they may be active against a range of tumours, independent of site and histological type. Since they should not affect cell proliferation, the MMPIs would not be expected to share the toxicities that are characteristic of cytotoxics.

Because of their relatively high molecular weight and poor oral bioavailability, enhancing the activity of naturally occurring TIMPs is unlikely to be effective unless their active domains can be exploited. Most attention has, therefore, focused on the synthetic MMPIs batimastat (BB-94), marimistat (BB-2516), CGS27023A, AG3340, BAY12–9566, and BMS-275291. The clinical development of MMPIs illustrates the complexity of working with drugs that have novel mechanisms of action and new patterns of toxicity.

Batimastat

Batimastat, a potent broad-spectrum MMPI, was the first of these compounds to enter the clinic. In addition to inhibiting metastasis and angiogenesis in preclinical models, batimastat prolonged the survival of mice bearing peritoneal ovarian carcinoma xenografts. There was also evidence of synergy with cisplatin, again using an ovarian xenograft model, emphasizing the rationale for using treatment like this in combination with conventional therapy. Because of its poor oral bioavailability, batimastat was administered into the peritoneal or pleural cavity of patients with pleural effusions and ascites, respectively. Pharmacokinetic studies confirmed potentially therapeutic levels of batimastat and, interestingly, several patients did not reaccumulate ascites.[30]

The development of batimastat was stopped in favour of **marimastat**, which can be taken orally. Marimastat also has a broad spectrum of activity with median inhibitory concentrations (**IC50**) against several MMPs in the nanomolar range. In contrast to conventional anticancer agents, initial studies with marimastat were conducted in healthy volunteers, confirming the absorption of marimastat after oral administration.[31] The first clinical trial of marimastat in cancer patients identified characteristic dose- and duration-dependent joint pains as the principal toxicity. Earlier studies had suggested that MMP levels may be elevated in patients with cancer.[32] As the traditional cytotoxic approach of administering the maximum safe dose may not be appropriate for MMPIs, MMP levels were measured in an attempt to identify a therapeutic dose. Peak concentrations of marimastat were several-fold higher than those required to inhibit MMPs *in vitro*, but no consistent changes in MMP2 or MMP9 were seen to guide dosing.

Subsequently, a large phase I/II trial programme sought to use a change in the rate of increase in tumour markers as an indicator of the activity of marimastat.[33] Patients with rising markers received marimastat at a range of different doses for 4 weeks, after which the tumour markers were again measured. Again, cumulative joint pains were seen, but the key finding was that tumour markers appeared to rise more slowly during the period of marimastat treatment. There are, however, difficulties in interpreting this trial. In particular, the use of tumour markers as a surrogate endpoint in this setting is unproven. The fall in the rate of rise in tumour markers may reflect reduced shedding of the marker rather than alterations in tumour progression. Preliminary results from randomized trials in gastric and pancreatic cancer have failed to establish clearly whether or not marimastat is a useful anticancer agent. In both studies the primary analysis with respect to survival showed trends favouring marimastat, but these did not achieve statistical significance.

Other MMPIs

Several more oral MMPIs, each with distinctive characteristics, have entered clinical trials. CGS27023A is another broad-spectrum MMPI that causes a maculopapular rash in addition to the usual joint pains. AG3340 is a hydroxamic acid derivative but it was designed from analysis of MMP X-ray crystal structures. In contrast to the other MMPIs, AG3340 and BAY12-9566 are more specific with inhibition constant (K_i) values for MMP2 and MMP9 several-fold lower than for other MMPIs. AG3340 causes joint symptoms, but pharmacokinetic studies suggest that a tolerable, potentially effective dose can be administered clinically. By contrast, there is a striking lack of musculoskeletal toxicity with BAY12-9655, although it does cause thrombocytopenia and has non-linear pharmacokinetics.

The future of MMPIs is unclear, with the clinical development of several having been suspended. Preclinical studies established a defined, validated target and clearly demonstrated antitumour activity. However, their clinical development proved difficult with no surrogate marker for activity and no clear evidence that MMPs are a useful target in patients with cancer. The apparently limited activity of MMPIs in the clinic may reflect the difficulty in achieving inhibition of specific MMPs. Alternatively, a high level of selectivity may not be desirable if there is a high level of cross-talk and redundancy within signal-transduction pathways in human tumours. Many of the lessons learnt in the development of MMPIs may be relevant to the clinical evaluation of other non-cytotoxic agents.

Angiogenesis

The concept that angiogenesis, the formation of new vessels, is essential for the growth of solid tumours and a potential therapeutic target was promulgated by Folkman.[34] He proposed that tumours produced a 'tumour angiogenesis factor' leading to the formation of new vessels that delivered oxygen and nutrients to the tumour. The formation of these new vessels is critical to the growth and metastasis of tumours once they become more than 2 mm in diameter. Angiogenesis is a clinically relevant prognostic factor, with the microvessel density in a range of human tumours correlating with the presence of locoregional lymph node metastases, distant metastases, and a poor prognosis.[35]

Over the last decade evidence has accumulated to support these ideas. Targeting the process of angiogenesis has many attractions:

1. If angiogenesis is common to all tumours, this may be a means of attacking cancer cells irrespective of their tissue of origin, site of metastasis, or tumour heterogeneity.

2. By definition, these new vessels are accessible to vascular drug delivery.

3. The tumour vessels have not undergone neoplastic transformation so should be more genetically stable and less liable to develop resistance than tumour cells.

4. Antiangiogenic drugs may again be better tolerated than conventional anticancer drugs.

The process of angiogenesis involves stages, each a potential target for anticancer treatment. First, pericytes retract from the abluminal endothelial surface. Proteases such as urokinase and metalloproteases are then released from the endothelial cells, breaking down the basement membrane and connective tissue stroma. This is followed by migration and proliferation of the endothelial cells which align themselves into tube-like structures. These canalize to form a lumen, then anastamose creating a capillary loop through which blood flows.

Currently, at least 20 angiogenesis inhibitors are in clinical trial, with some entering phase III testing. Since agents directed at angiogenesis are targeting these processes rather than a single molecular species, there is overlap with other aspects of new drug development such as signal transduction and metalloprotease activity that are described above. As with other potentially cytostatic treatments, inhibitors of angiogenesis are likely to be used in combination with conventional cytotoxics, a concept first explored in animal models with the combination of TNP-470, minocycline, and chemotherapy.[36]

Endogenous inhibitors of angiogenesis

Many potential antiangiogenic agents, such as angiostatin, endostatin, interferon-α, and platelet factor 4 (**PF4**), are naturally circulating antiangiogenic molecules. PF4, a naturally occurring protein found in the α-granules of platelets, inhibits angiogenesis *in vivo* and delays tumour growth in mice. In phase I trials it was well tolerated in patients[37] but its short half-life may limit its use.

Angiostatin is a plasminogen fragment that was isolated from the urine of mice bearing Lewis lung carcinoma. So long as the primary tumour was *in situ* it induced the production of angiostatin which suppressed angiogenesis and the growth of metastases.[38] However, when the primary tumour was removed the metastases vascularized and grew rapidly. When tested *in vitro*, angiostatin inhibited the proliferation of endothelial cells but not tumour cell lines. Angiostatin did, however, suppress tumour growth *in vivo*. Difficulties of drug supply initially limited its development, but recombinant angiostatin is now being evaluated in the clinic. Recombinant endostatin, a 20-kDa protein derived from the C terminal portion of collagen XVIII, is also being tested. Preliminary reports indicate that endostatin levels similar to those that are effective in animal models can be achieved in patients. These studies incorporate pharmacodynamic endpoints such as skin biopsy or measurement of tumour blood flow in addition to conventional response criteria, early results of which are encouraging.

Inhibitors of angiogenic cytokines

Since the identification of basic fibroblast growth factor (bFGF) as the first angiogenic growth factor, many others have been described. Perhaps the most important is vascular endothelial growth factor (VEGF), a glycoprotein that binds to the Flk-1/KDR and Flt-1 tyrosine kinase receptors on 'activated' endothelial cells, acting as a potent and specific mitogen. VEGF expression has been described in many solid human tumours, including breast, lung, ovary, kidney, and gastrointestinal malignancies. Overexpression of VEGF correlates with microvessel density and a poor prognosis.

In experimental models anti-VEGF antibodies can suppress tumour growth and metastasis, emphasizing the potential of VEGF as a therapeutic target.[39] There has been most progress with small molecule RTK inhibitors, especially SU5416 that is directed at Flk-1/KDR. SU5416 inhibits metastasis, microvessel formation, and cell proliferation in murine models.[40] The strong expression of both Flk-1/KDR and flt-1 in Kaposi's sarcoma, suggests VEGF has an important role in regulating angiogenesis. Preliminary results with SU5416 in patients with Kaposi's sarcoma are encouraging, with clear evidence of biological activity and no major toxicities. In phase I trials SU5416 also demonstrated activity in patients with lung cancer and colorectal cancer, and is now being evaluated further both alone and in combination with conventional cytotoxics such as 5-fluorouracil with leucovorin.

SU6668 is a second RTK inhibitor with potentially broader anti-angiogenic activity that inhibits the VEGF, bFGF, and PDGF receptors. SU6668 inhibits the growth of implanted xenografts in mice when given orally, a potential advantage for agents that may require long-term, regular administration. Preliminary clinical studies have confirmed the feasibility of chronic daily oral administration with evidence of antitumour activity. Other RTK inhibitors are in clinical development, as are a synthetic ribozyme targeting the Flt-1 receptor for VEGF and HuMV833, an anti-VEGF antibody.

Endothelial cell toxins

Several low molecular weight drugs appear selectively toxic to the vascular endothelium in tumours. Initially, attention focused on flavone acetic acid, but its excellent activity in the laboratory was not reproduced in the clinic. More recently, tubulin-binding agents have shown more promise. Colchicine was first noted to have antivascular effects, but a narrow therapeutic window precluded its development in this setting. The **combretastatins** are a group of compounds structurally similar to colchicine that have been isolated from the *Combretum caffrum* tree. In animal models the prodrug combretastatin A₄ induces vascular shutdown and haemorrhagic necrosis in tumours at doses well below those that are toxic.[41] Combretastatin A₄ is now being tested clinically, with attempts being made to determine whether a significant reduction in tumour blood flow can be achieved in patients at tolerable doses.

Proliferating endothelial cells within tumours are also the target for fumagillin derivatives that are being evaluated in the clinic. TNP-470 (AGM-1470) is a synthetic derivative of fumagillin, a fungal protein. Whereas most phase I trials are done in a heterogeneous patient population, early work with TNP-470 was specifically carried out in patients with Kaposi's sarcoma where angiogenesis is a prominent feature. One-hour infusions of TNP-470 were well tolerated

and therapeutic levels achieved with responses were seen, justifying this patient selection at an early stage in development.[42]

Telomerase

In normal cells, the telomeres, which cap the ends of chromosomes, erode with each cycle of division. This ultimately leads to the senescence and death of normal cells after 20 to 40 divisions. Conversely, cancer cells can maintain their telomeres so they continue to proliferate and are 'immortalized'. Repair of the telomere is carried out by telomerase, a ribonucleoprotein reverse transcriptase. It comprises the RNA subunit hTERC, which acts as a template, and the catalytic hTERT subunit. The telomerase enzyme is switched off in most cells shortly after birth, an important exception being germ-line cells. Telomerase is, however, reactivated in up to 90 per cent of cancers and is a major component of the malignant phenotype. The mechanisms of telomerase reactivation are not fully understood, but loss of transcriptional repressors of the catalytic subunit and upregulation appear to be involved.

There is a correlation between telomerase activity and the malignant characteristics of both established tumour cell lines and fresh tumour tissue from patients. This suggests that, as a target, telomerase may have a greater degree of specificity than conventional targets with a correspondingly better toxicity profile. The therapeutic potential of telomerase has been shown experimentally. Reactivation of telomerase in tumours leads to the telomeres of most cancer cells being longer than somatic cells. Interfering with telomere function, either by the introduction of mutant telomerase into tumour cells or treatment with specific oligomers, causes telomere shortening, growth arrest, and ultimately apoptosis.

Experiments such as these have led to considerable interest in telomerase as a target for anticancer treatment. However, several potential obstacles to telomerase as an anticancer strategy remain. First, up to 20 per cent of human tumours do not have telomerase activity and may use other mechanisms to maintain their telomeres. Advances in molecular pathology techniques should, however, be able to identify those tumours in which telomerase is not an appropriate target. Second, some normal tissues do express telomerase and may be susceptible to toxicity. A third potential criticism is that since tumour cells have well-preserved telomeres, treatment with a telomerase inhibitor would not cause significant telomere shortening until the cell had undergone at least 20 divisions. During that time the tumour may continue to grow, so telomerase inhibition may not be a useful therapeutic approach in patients with advanced disease.

Despite these caveats, telomerase is a particularly appealing target because of the distinction between its expression in tumours and repression in most normal tissues. Several approaches are being pursued: direct inhibition of the enzyme, interference with the telomere itself, or interactions with the transcription factors or other proteins involved in telomere regulation. The introduction of telomerase inhibitors into clinical practice raises many of the issues in trial design for novel agents discussed above. Their evaluation may be limited to patients whose tumours express the telomerase in biopsies. In early trials it will be important to identify biologically effective doses as well as defining both acute and long-term toxicities. Proof of efficacy may come only in randomized trials of conventional chemotherapy with or without telomerase inhibitors.

With telomerase activity largely confined to malignant cells, this may be a marker for the early detection of malignancy. Telomerase expression may also be a valuable prognostic factor since telomerase activity correlates with poor outcome in breast cancer and gastric cancer. In the therapeutic setting, telomerase may be suited to treating patients with low-volume tumours following debulking by surgery, chemotherapy, or radiotherapy.

New challenges in the design of early clinical trials for anticancer drugs

The conventional model for early clinical development comprises initial dose-escalation phase I trials to identify the pattern of toxicities and the maximum tolerated dose (**MTD**). Activity, as reflected by tumour shrinkage, is then investigated in a series of phase II trials. Although familiar and widely used, the shortcomings of this approach are increasingly recognized, especially in relation to testing agents on new targets.

Phase I trial design

Traditionally in phase I trials, successive cohorts of between three and six patients with advanced cancer receive increasing doses of the new drug, the dose increments usually being smaller as the trial progresses (a 'modified Fibonacci' scheme). Once predefined, dose-limiting toxicities (**DLTs**) are identified in a specified proportion of patients (typically 33 per cent), dose escalation ceases at the MTD.

This approach can be criticized for exposing too many patients to low doses of the new agent with no realistic chance of benefit. With starting doses typically based on the dose that is lethal to 10 per cent of animals (**LD10**), and conventional dose escalation, the median number of dose levels is eight. Most responses in phase I trials occur at or close to the MTD, so the majority of patients will be treated at non-toxic but ineffective dose levels, raising serious ethical and practical concerns. Alternative designs have been proposed, such as the modified continual reassessment method which uses Bayesian mathematical modelling of preclinical and accumulating clinical data to guide dose escalation. Pharmacokinetically guided dose escalation exploits the relationship between pharmacokinetic exposure at the animal LD10 and human MTD to allow accelerated dose escalation. Approaches such as these have proved useful, and phase I trial designs for cytotoxics as well as more novel agents are increasingly innovative.

Endpoints in early trials

The second major limitation of traditional phase I trial design is that it is directed principally at identifying toxicities rather than the optimal therapeutic doses. This has proved satisfactory in the development of conventional cytotoxics where antiproliferative toxicities are a 'surrogate' for doses that are potentially cytotoxic. However, for drugs directed at new targets, the identification of appropriate endpoints is a real challenge.

With an unprecedented number of anticancer drugs directed at a range of novel targets emerging from the laboratory, identification of a biological effect confirming inhibition of the target may become a prerequisite in selecting compounds for further development.

Conventional phase I trials of cytotoxics effectively use toxicity as a pharmacodynamic endpoint, in the knowledge that responses are usually seen at doses close to those which are toxic. In addition, most cytotoxics that have succeeded in the clinic achieved responses in phase I trials. These principles are not easy to apply to novel agents which are likely to be taken for prolonged periods, have chronic toxicities, and are cytostatic rather than cytotoxic.

Phase I studies will increasingly seek to identify a safe and potentially active dose of a new anticancer agent. With many new agents we cannot assume that the dose–effect curves for response and toxicity have the same profile, so there is a need to identify surrogate pharmacodynamic markers demonstrating inhibition of the biochemical target *in vivo*. This has already been achieved with some novel therapeutics such as the PKC inhibitor CGP41251.[43] More direct evidence of a therapeutic effect comes from tumour samples, but these are difficult to obtain. Non-invasive techniques such as positron-emission tomography (**PET**) scanning may also contribute to early trials.[44] A new drug can be labelled and administered at tracer levels for preliminary pharmacokinetic studies. Alternatively, fluorodeoxyglucose (**FDG**)-PET scanning may detect early changes in tumour metabolism rather than later reductions in size.[45]

We may need also to reconsider the subjects in whom early trials of novel, non-cytotoxic agents are developed. In some cases, patients with less advanced disease or even healthy volunteers may be appropriate. This would allow more prolonged administration and a clearer assessment of toxicities, which may be difficult to identify in a symptomatic patient with cancer whose disease is likely to progress rapidly. It may also be appropriate to restrict eligibility to patients whose tumours express the molecular target at which the new agent is directed.

With phase I trials increasingly incorporating measures of biological activity, studies of surrogate markers in phase I trials may make it possible to identify a maximum target inhibiting dose (**MTID**) as well as a conventional MTD.[46] These innovations in trial design will reduce the distinction between phase I and phase II trials. Conventional response-rate studies are inappropriate if tumour shrinkage is not anticipated. 'Proof of principle' studies using surrogate markers of biological activity in early clinical trials may be the main requirement before embarking on large, randomized trials. Alternatively, clinical activity may be defined by the absence of progression, which appears to identify 'active' compounds as effectively as response rate.[46]

Rather than the single design for early clinical trials of new anticancer drugs that we have had until recently, it is increasingly likely that these trials will incorporate different elements of novel design tailored to each particular agent and patient population.

Conclusions

We are already witnessing advances in the translation of improved understanding of cancer biology into novel therapeutics. The next 5 to 10 years will see an acceleration in these developments, with a real expectation of major improvements in the drug treatment of cancer.

We can anticipate new cytotoxics that are either more effective against resistant tumours or better tolerated than current chemotherapy. Non-cytotoxic drugs will become as an integral part of the management of other solid tumours as tamoxifen has been for women with breast cancer. However, cytotoxics are likely to remain important, with many of these novel agents likely to be used in combination with chemotherapy rather than as single agents. Finally, as new treatments become more specific, they will increasingly be directed at particular cellular targets identified through molecular pathology.

References

1. D'Incalci M. DNA-minor-groove alkylators, a new class of anticancer agents. *Annals of Oncology*, 1994; **5**: 877–8.

2. Pezzoni G, *et al.* Biological profile of FCE 245517, a novel benzoyl mustard analogue of distamycin A. *British Journal of Cancer*, 1991; **64**: 1047–50.

3. Beran M, *et al.* Tallimustine an effective antileukaemic agent in a severe combined immunodeficient mouse model of adult myelogenous leukaemia, induces remissions in a phase I study. *Clinical Cancer Research*, 1997; **3**: 2377–84.

4. Li LH, *et al.* Structure and activity relationship of several novel CC-1065 analogs. *Investigational New Drugs*, 1987; **5**: 329–37.

5. Van Tellingen O, *et al.* A clinical pharmacokinetics study of carzelesin given by short-term intravenous infusion in a phase I study. *Cancer Chemotherapy and Pharmacology*, 1998; **41**: 377–84.

6. MacDonald JR, *et al.* Preclinical activity of 6-hydroxymethylacylfulvene, a semisynthetic derivative of the mushroom toxin illudin S. *Cancer Research*, 1997; **57**: 279–83.

7. Kelner MJ, McMorris TC, Estes L, Samson KM, Bagnell RD, Taetle R. Efficacy of MGI 114 (6-hydroxymethylacylfulvene, HMAF) against the mdr1/gp 170 metastatic MV522 lung carcinoma xenograft. *European Journal of Cancer*, 1998; **34**: 908–13.

8. Ghielmini M, *et al.* In vitro schedule-dependency of myelotoxicity and cytotoxicity of Ecteinascidin 743 (ET-743). *Annals of Oncology*, 1998; **9**: 989–93.

9. Izbicka E, *et al.* In vitro antitumour activity of the novel marine agent, ecteinascidin-743 (ET-743, NSC-648766) against human tumours explanted from patients. *Annals of Oncology*, 1998, **9**: 981–7.

10. Levitzki A, Gazit A. Tyrosine kinase inhibition: an approach to drug development. *Science*, 1995; **267**: 1782–8.

11. Ferry D, *et al.* Phase I clinical trial of the flavenoid quercetin: pharmacokinetics and evidence for in vivo tyrosine kinase inhibition. *Clinical Cancer Research*, 1996; **2**: 659–68.

12. Eckhardt, *et al.* Phase I and pharmacologic study of the tyrosine kinase inhibitor SU101 in patients with advanced solid tumours. *Journal of Clinical Oncology*, 1999; **17**: 1095–104.

13. Coutre P, *et al.* In vivo eradication of human BCR/ABL positive leukemia cells with an ABL kinase inhibitor. *Journal of the National Cancer Institute*, 1999; **91**: 163–8.

14. Seckl MJ, Higgins T, Widmer F, Rozengurt E. Substance P: a novel inhibitor of signal transduction and growth in vivo and in vitro in small cell lung cancer. *Cancer Research*, 1997; **57**: 51–4.

15. Caponigro F, French R, Kaye SB. Protein kinase C: a worthwhile target for anticancer drugs? *Anti-cancer drugs*, 1997; **8**: 26–33.

16. Philip P, *et al.* Phase I study of Bryostatin 1: assessment of interleukin 6 and tumour necrosis factor-α induction in vivo. *Journal of the National Cancer Institute*, 1993; **85**: 1812–18.

17. Jayson GC, *et al.* A phase I trial of bryostatin 1 in patients with advanced malignancy using a 24 hour intravenous infusion. *British Journal of Cancer*, 1995; **72**: 461–8.

18. Schwartz GK, *et al.* A pilot clinical/pharmacological study of the protein kinase C-specific inhibitor salfingol alone and in combination with doxorubicin. *Clinical Cancer Research*, 1997; **3**: 537–43.

19. Husain A, Yan XJ, Rosales N, Aghajanian C, Schwartz GK, Spriggs DR. UCN-01 in ovary cancer cells: effective as a single agent and in

20. Fuse E, *et al.* Unpredicted clinical pharmacology of UCN-01 caused by specific binding to human alpha1-acid glycoprotein. *Cancer Research*, 1998; **58**: 3248–53.

21. Thavasu P, *et al.* The protein kinase C inhibitor CGP 41251 suppresses cytokine release and extracellular signal-related kinase 2 expression in cancer patients. *Cancer Research*, 1999; **59**: 3980–4.

22. Utz I, *et al.* Reversal of multidrug resistance by the staurosporine derivatives CGP 41251 and CGP 42700. *International Journal of Cancer*, 1998; **77**: 64–9.

23. Kohn EC, *et al.* Phase I trial of micronized formulation carboxyamidotriazole in patients with refractory solid tumors: pharmacokinetics, clinical outcome, and comparison of formulations. *Journal of Clinical Oncology*, 1997; **15**: 1985–93.

24. Thibault A, *et al.* Phase I study of Lovastatin, an inhibitor of the mevalonate pathway in patients with cancer. *Clinical Cancer Research*, 1996; **2**: 483–91.

25. Vigushin DM, *et al.* Phase I and pharmacokinetic study of D-limonene in patients with advanced cancer. *Cancer Chemotherapy and Pharmacology*, 1998; **42**: 111–17.

26. Senderowicz AM, *et al.* Flavopiridol, a novel cyclin-dependent kinase inhibitor, suppresses the growth of head and neck squamous carcinomas by inducing apoptosis. *Journal of Clinical Investigation*, 1998; **102**: 1674–81.

27. Senderowicz AM, *et al.* Phase I trial of continuous infusion flavopiridol, a novel cyclin-dependent kinase inhibitor, in patients with refractory neoplasms. *Journal of Clinical Oncology*, 1998; **16**: 2968–99.

28. Chambers A, Matrisian L. Changing views of the role of matrix metalloproteinases in metastasis. *Journal of the National Cancer Institute*, 1997; **89**: 1260–70.

29. Masson R, *et al.* In vivo evidence that the stromolysin-3 metalloproteinase contributes in a paracrine manner to epithelial cell malignancy. *Journal of Cell Biology*, 1998; **140**: 1535–41.

30. Beattie GJ, Smyth J. Phase I study of intraperitoneal metalloproteinase inhibitor BB94 in patients with malignant ascites. *Clinical Cancer Research*, 1998; **4**: 1899–902.

31. Wajtowicz-Praga, *et al.* Phase I trial of Marimastat, a novel matrix metalloproteinase inhibitor, administered only to patients with advanced lung cancer. *Journal of Clinical Oncology*, 1998; **16**: 2150–6.

32. Zucker S, *et al.* Plasma assay of metalloproteinases (MMPs) and MMP-inhibitor complexes in cancer. Potential use in predicting metastasis and monitoring treatment. *Annals of the New York Academy of Science*, 1994; **732**: 248–62.

33. Nemunaitis J, *et al.* Combined analysis of studies of the effects of the metalloproteinase inhibitor marimastat on serum tumour markers in advanced cancer: selection of a biologically active and tolerable dose for longer term studies. *Clinical Cancer Research*, 1998; **4**: 1101–9.

34. Folkman J. Anti-angiogenesis: new concept for therapy of solid tumours. *Annals of Surgery*, 1972; **175**: 414–20.

35. Gasparini G, Weidner N, Bevilaqua P, Maluta S, Della Palma P, Caffo O. Tumor microvessel density, p53 expression, tumour size and peritumoral lymphatic vessel invasion are relevant prognostic markers in node negative breast carcinoma. *Journal of Clinical Oncology*, 1994; **12**: 454–66.

36. Teicher BA, Emi Y, Kakeji Y, Northey D. TNP-470/minocycline/cytotoxic therapy: a systems approach to cancer therapy. *European Journal of Cancer*, 1996; **32A**: 2461–6.

37. Belman N, Bonnem EM, Harvey HA, Lipton A. Phase I trial of recombinant platelet factor 4 (rPF4) in patients with advanced colorectal cancer. *Investigational New Drugs*, 1996; **14**: 387–89.

38. O'Reilly MS, *et al.* Angiostatin: a novel angiogenesis inhibitor that mediates the suppression of metastases by Lewis lung carcinoma. *Cell*, 1994; **79**: 315–28.

39. Warren RS, Yuan H, Matli MR, Gillett NA, Ferrarra N. Regulation by vesicular endothelial growth factor expression of human colon cancer tumorigenesis in a mouse model of experimental liver metastasis. *Journal of Clinical Investigation*, 1995; **95**: 1789–97.

40. Fong TA, *et al.* SU5416 is a potent and selective inhibitor of the vascular endothelial growth factor receptor (Flk-1/KDR) that inhibits tyrosine kinase catalysis, tumor vascularization and growth of multiple tumour types. *Cancer Research*, 1999; **59**: 99–106.

41. Dark GG, Hill SA, Prise VE, Tozer GM, Pettit GR, Chaplin DJ. Combretastatin A-4, an agent that displays potent and selective toxicity toward tumor vasculature. *Cancer Research*, 1997; **57**: 1829–34.

42. Dezube BJ, *et al.* Fumagillin analog in the treatment of Kaposi's sarcoma: a phase I AIDS Clinical Trials Group study. *Journal of Clinical Oncology*, 1998, **16**: 1444–9.

43. Thavasu P, *et al.* The PKC inhibitor CGP41251 suppresses cytokine release and ERK2 expression in cancer patients. *Cancer Research*, 1999; **59**: 3980–4.

44. Meikle SR, *et al.* Pharmacokinetic assessment of novel anticancer drugs using spectral analysis and positron emission tomography: a feasibility study. *Cancer Chemotherapy and Pharmacology*, 1998; **42**: 183–93.

45. Von Hoff DD. There are no such things as bad anticancer agents, only bad clinical trial designs – twenty-first Richard and Hilda Rosenthal Foundation Award Lecture. *Clinical Cancer Research*, 1998; **4**: 1079–86.

46. Eisenhauer EA. Phase I and II trials of novel anticancer agents: endpoints, efficacy and existentialism. *Annals of Oncology*, 1998, **9**: 1047–52.

4.20 Mechanisms of drug resistance

S. de Jong, N. H. Mulder, and E. G. E. de Vries

Introduction

Drug resistance is the central problem in drug intervention as cancer therapy. Whereas surgery and/or radiotherapy can usually remove or destroy the initial tumour and its outgrowth in surrounding tissues, it is the lack of adequate drug treatment for disseminated forms of cancer or the failing of locoregional control that are responsible for the death of cancer patients.

Resistance to drugs may be primary when the tumour does not respond to drugs from the start (i.e. intrinsic resistance), or secondary, in which case the tumour initially responds but becomes resistant during treatment (i.e. acquired resistance).

Apparent and intrinsic resistance

To kill a cancer cell, a drug must reach it in sufficient amounts. Resistance may only be apparent, because the drug is given in an inadequate dosage, for inadequate times, or via an ineffective route. Inadequate dosing of chemotherapy results in reduced treatment efficacy as has been shown for adjuvant CMF (cyclophosphamide, methotrexate, and 5-fluorouracil) chemotherapy for breast carcinoma.[1] A twofold increment of the standard dose, however, rarely increases efficacy of the drugs. The recent availability of haematopoietic peripheral stem cells allows a 10-fold dose increment of several chemotherapeutic drugs. Studies, including randomized studies, have now shown that high-dose chemotherapy does increase the cure rate for a number of diseases such as subgroups of patients with non-Hodgkin's lymphoma and acute myeloid leukaemia. This shows that dose escalation can circumvent drug resistance to some extent.[2]

Even if a drug is administered at an appropriate dose and schedule, it may still fail to reach the tumour. For example, if the drug does not cross the blood–brain barrier, it will not reach tumour cells behind this barrier. The clinical relevance of these 'sanctuaries' became apparent following the achievement of long-term remissions in chemosensitive tumours such as acute lymphocytic leukaemia and small cell lung cancer. It has become clear that certain drug efflux pumps are not only present in tumour cells but also in the blood–brain barrier, the testicular barrier, and other physiological sites. These drug efflux pumps transport several chemotherapeutic drugs out of the brain and testis into the circulation. This mechanism is further addressed in the section on multidrug resistance.

Biochemical mechanisms can prevent cell kill even if a drug accumulates sufficiently in the proliferating tumour cell. The

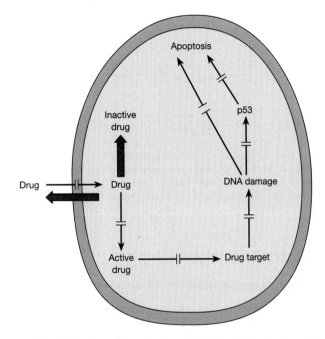

Fig. 1 Simplified scheme illustrating the main biochemical mechanisms of drug resistance. The bold arrow means an upregulated route in drug-resistant cells, while the broken arrow means a downregulated or inactivated route in drug-resistant cells.

biochemical mechanisms of primary drug resistance are largely the same as those of acquired resistance and these will be discussed below (Fig. 1). Many reports over the last years have demonstrated that tumours are resistant despite the fact that the drug does indeed reach the intracellular target. In this case the resistance is due to a deficient intracellular apoptotic (regulated cell death) response after drug-induced damage has occurred in the tumour. Numerous routes and factors are now considered to play a part in the physiological death of a cell. Figure 2 shows a number of prominent factors involved in apoptosis. This knowledge has shed a new light on potential targets and interventions in order to circumvent drug resistance by restoration of this defective route. For example, in the case of mutated p53 expressing tumour cells, gene therapy with wild-type p53 can restore cisplatin sensitivity in *in vitro* and animal models.

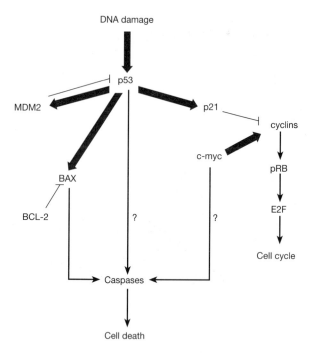

Fig. 2 Simplified scheme illustrating the p53-dependent apoptotic route involved in cell death following chemotherapeutic drugs. The bold arrow indicates activation. The T line indicates inhibition. The arrows with a question mark indicate unknown pathways; see text for explanation.

Acquired resistance

Biochemical mechanisms of acquired drug resistance

Experiments with cell lines incubated with stepwise increasing concentrations of a chemotherapeutic drug allow the development of highly resistant cell lines. These cell lines have provided ideal models to study drug resistance mechanisms. Cells will acquire resistance mechanisms at different cellular levels depending on the mechanism of action of a drug. However, as the mechanisms of action of most drugs are only partially known, many mechanisms of resistance may still be undiscovered. In addition, mechanisms observed, and amplified, in highly resistant cell lines are not necessarily present in human tumours, which may develop low levels of resistance. Therefore, caution is needed in translating these mechanisms to the clinic.

1. As most drugs are effective through the induction of DNA damage, the first and most effective way to prevent DNA damage in a cell is by decreased cellular drug accumulation, which can be due to:

   (a) decreased drug uptake, and

   (b) increased drug efflux.

2. If drugs enter the cell, they sometimes need to be metabolically activated within the cell. Other drugs that are already in an active form can be inactivated by cellular enzymes. Many drugs form a complex with a specific target in the cell. Resistance mechanisms observed in cells are:

   (a) decreased drug activation;

   (b) increased drug inactivation; and

   (c) decreased formation of drug–target complexes.

3. If the drug induces DNA damage, despite the presence of some of the above described mechanisms, the cell has mechanisms to limit or remove the damage. It is known that decreased DNA repair can sensitize cells to DNA damage. In theory we should expect increased DNA repair (which is, however, not frequently observed in resistant cells).

4. After a drug has induced DNA damage, if the cell does not succeed in the repair of DNA damage, due to absence of effective repair or uncontrolled DNA repair, the cell receives a stimulus to die. The tumour suppressor gene product p53 plays a central part in this process. Cells will then go into apoptosis, also known as regulated or programmed cell death. Many proteins are involved in the cascade from DNA damage to cell death. Upregulation of apoptosis-inducing proteins and downregulation of apoptosis-inhibiting proteins will finally result in an apoptotic cell. Various resistance mechanisms that disturb or prevent an apoptotic stimulus have been observed, but they all have the same principle, that is increased tolerance to DNA damage.

Alterations in gene expression resulting in acquired drug resistance

The analysis of drug resistance in tumour cell lines has demonstrated that the high levels of drug resistance induced in cultured cells usually results from genetic alterations. The mutant variants arise spontaneously at a low rate in the population, but this rate can be increased by mutagenic agents, including several clinically used chemotherapeutic drugs.[3] Goldie and Coldman have suggested that drug-resistant mutants appear in solid tumours with a frequency of 10^{-6} per cell division.[3] Hence, a large tumour of more than 10^{10} cells will contain many somatic mutants conferring varying degrees of resistance. Whether all mechanisms of drug resistance are caused by genetic mutations is not known at present. Small changes in protein expression profiles of various members of signal transduction and/or transcription regulating pathways induced by, for example, cell–cell contacts, hypoxia, or growth factors can finally result in either an increased or decreased transcription of specific genes. However, it cannot be excluded that mutations in genes, encoding the proteins involved in these complex pathways, are the initial events leading to the observed mechanism of drug resistance.

Combining different drugs with different modes of action and little shared mechanisms of resistance is one approach to reduce the likelihood of survival of resistant cells in a tumour, and therefore to improve chemotherapeutic efficacy. Unfortunately, many drugs use the same apoptotic pathway to kill a tumour cell despite their different modes of action. This may limit the success of multidrug treatment.

The drug-resistant tumour cell lines demonstrated the following genetic changes that affected a protein (or proteins), such as drug transport proteins, drug metabolizing enzymes and drug targets.

1. *Decreased amount of functional protein.* The most common and drastic alteration is the complete loss of functional protein. This can happen by: (i) gross alterations in DNA (deletions, translocations) that inactivate the gene; (ii) mutations that prevent synthesis of the complete protein; (iii) hypermethylation which inactivates the gene without mutation; (iv) reduced stability

of mRNA; or (v) a reduced level of transcription due to a changed expression of its transcription factors. A drastic decrease in the amount of functional protein can also occur by mutations that result in amino acid substitutions in the protein, which are incompatible with function or stability. Loss of functional protein by recessive mutations, require the inactivation of both gene copies present in a diploid cell with the exception of genes on the X-chromosome. If proteins are active as multimers, mutations in one gene copy can be sufficient. As many tumour cells are not diploid but aneuploid, loss of chromosome copies can also result in a decreased amount of protein.

2. *Production of a protein with an increased affinity for a drug.* These mutations are nearly always due to amino acid substitutions caused by point mutations. Such mutations usually behave in a dominant fashion.

3. *Increased production of a normal protein.* This increase can be mediated by alterations that affect any step in gene expression. The most prevalent are transcriptional activation (an increase in the rate of mRNA synthesis) and gene amplification (an increase in the copy number of the protein-coding gene). The genomic instability observed in most cancer cells promotes such DNA rearrangements.

Drug-specific biochemical and genetic alterations causing acquired resistance in cell lines

The general mechanisms of resistance 1 to 3, outlined above, are illustrated by a detailed consideration of the drug specific mechanisms described in the following section.

Methotrexate (MTX) resistance

This topic has been reviewed by Kinsella *et al.*[4] and Jansen and Pieters.[5] Five distinct mechanisms are now known to result in MTX resistance, which are shown in Fig. 3. Most antifolates, such as MTX, require active transport for their cellular uptake. Two routes have been identified. The first transport route proceeds via a carrier-mediated system, the reduced folate carrier (**RFC**) with a high affinity for MTX. The second transport route is mediated by the membrane-associated folate receptors with a low binding affinity for MTX as compared with folic acid. These proteins can be independently expressed in normal as well as tumour cells. At high-dose schedules with an extracellular concentration of MTX of 5 to 40 mM, the RFC is the major route for MTX uptake and the contribution of membrane-associated folate receptors is negligible. MTX inhibits the target enzyme in folate metabolism, dihydrofolate reductase (**DHFR**), which results in the depletion of reduced folate pools that are required as cofactors in the biosynthesis of purines, thymidylate, and amino acids. Other folate-dependent enzymes in thymidylate synthesis i.e. thymidylate synthase (TS), and purine *de novo* synthesis, i.e. glycinamide ribonucleotide formyltransferase, are also inhibited by MTX. Polyglutamylation of MTX results in an increased efficacy of MTX because rapid efflux is prevented and MTX-polyglutamates are more potent inhibitors of DHFR, TS, and glycinamide ribonucleotide formyltransferase than MTX monoglutamates. Acquired resistance to

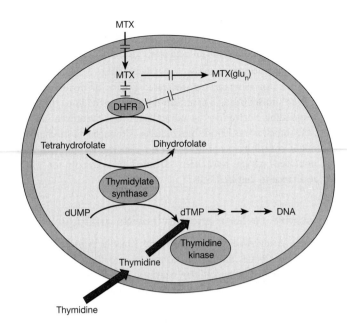

Fig. 3 Simplified scheme illustrating the biochemical mechanisms of MTX resistance (see text for explanation). The bold arrow indicates an upregulated pathway in resistant cells. The broken arrow means a downregulated or inactivated route in resistant cells. The broken T line indicates loss of inhibition in resistant cells. MTX(glu$_n$) means polyglutamated form of MTX.

MTX has been observed at each level of drug delivery and activation.

1. *Decreased MTX uptake as a result of decreased RFC expression or altered transport affinity.* Several mutations have been detected in the RFC gene, which resulted in a non-functional RFC due to an amino acid substitution or a truncated, and thus inactive, RFC protein. A structurally altered RFC with an increased affinity for natural folate co-factors is another mechanism of resistance, as the elevated intracellular folate pool abolishes poly-glutamylation of antifolates. Thirdly, a defective efflux of folic acid results in an increased intracellular folate pool and abolishes RFC activity, which may reflect a response to control folate homeostasis. This will reduce the uptake of antifolates.[5]

2. *Decreased polyglutamylation of MTX.* The polyglutamyl derivatives of MTX formed in the cell have a higher affinity for the target enzyme, DHFR, and are also retained longer in the cell than MTX itself. Hence, decreased polyglutamylation of MTX due to a reduced expression of folylpolyglutamate synthetase can lead to resistance.

3. *Production of an altered DHFR with decreased affinity for MTX.* Several different amino acid substitutions in DHFR are now known that decrease the enzyme's affinity for MTX without seriously decreasing catalytic activity. Each of these altered forms of DHFR is due to a single point mutation in the gene encoding the enzyme.[4]

4. *Increased production of normal DHFR.* Although MTX has a high affinity for DHFR, the drug does not bind irreversibly to this enzyme. Hence, it is difficult to obtain more than 95 per cent enzyme inhibition with the drug concentrations achieved clinically. Overexpression of DHFR will thus result in an absolute

increase in the amount of active enzyme due the incomplete inhibition by MTX. Increased enzyme levels in resistant cells are nearly always the result of gene amplification.[4]

5. *Increased nucleoside salvage.* It has been claimed that MTX resistance can arise through increased uptake of thymidine and purine nucleosides. These can be converted into the corresponding nucleotides by salvage pathways circumventing the MTX block in nucleotide biosynthesis. Although this mechanism might contribute to primary MTX resistance, no mutants with increased salvage have been obtained by selection for MTX resistance in cultured cells.[4]

Resistance to base and nucleoside analogues

This topic is reviewed by Lennard[6] and Kinsella *et al.*[4] Base and nucleoside analogues have to be converted into the corresponding nucleotide analogues by cellular enzymes before they can inhibit their target, which is one of the enzymes required for the normal biosynthesis of nucleotides. One may therefore expect resistance to arise by a decrease in analogue uptake or in its conversion into the active inhibitor, by an alteration in the target enzyme, or by more complex alterations leading to more effective production of normal nucleotides. In practice, each of these resistance mechanisms has been observed in resistant cell lines.

5-Fluorouracil

5-Fluorouracil and its nucleoside analogue are converted into 5-fluoro-deoxyuridine monophosphate (5-FdUMP) by cellular enzymes and this inhibits thymidilate synthase, the key enzyme in the biosynthesis of deoxythymidine monophosphate, essential for DNA synthesis. Although the affinity of 5-FdUMP for TS is approximately 1000-fold higher than that of the natural substrate, deoxyuridine monophosphate, effective inhibition resulting in deoxythymidine triphosphate depletion requires formation of the ternary complex of TS, 5-FdUMP and the folate co-factor 5,10-methylene-tetrahydrofolate. Hence, cell killing by 5-fluorouracil only occurs when the cell contains adequate levels of leucovorin (methylene-tetrahydrofolate), presumably in the polyglutamated form. 5-Fluorouracil is also converted into 5-FUTP (5-fluorouridine triphosphate) and 5-FdUTP (5-fluoro-deoxyuridine triphosphate) and incorporated directly into RNA and DNA, resulting in the production of DNA single-strand breaks. The relative contribution of these mechanisms in cell killing may depend on the specific patterns of 5-fluorouracil metabolism in various tumour cell types. In cultured cells, resistance can arise by one of the following mechanisms as are shown in Fig. 4 (see Kinsella *et al.*[4] and Kamm *et al.*[7]):

1. *Decreased conversion of 5-fluorouracil into 5-FdUMP.* 5-Fluorouracil is enzymatically activated into FdUMP and FUMP by uridine phosphorylase, uridine kinase, orotate phosphoribosyltransferase, thymidine phosphorylase, dihydropyrimidine dehydrogenase and thymidine kinase. A reduced activity of the enzymes was observed in several 5-fluorouracil resistant tumour cell lines.

2. *Lowered levels of the tetrahydrofolate co-factor required for TS function.* Cellular depletion of folates is an important potential source of clinical resistance[8] and, indeed, leucovorin can enhance

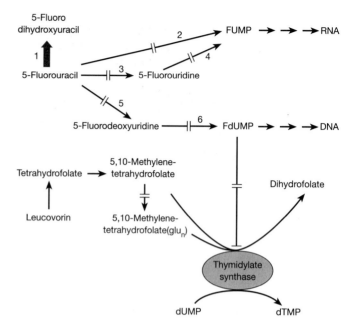

Fig. 4 Simplified scheme illustrating the biochemical mechanisms of 5-fluorouracil resistance (see text for explanation). The bold arrow indicates upregulated conversion in resistant cells. The broken arrow means a downregulated or inactivated route in resistant cells. The broken T line indicate loss of inhibition in resistant cells. 5,10-methylene-tetrahydrofolate(glu_n) means polyglutamated form of 5,10-methylene-tetrahydrofolate. Enzymes indicated with numbers are: (1) dihydropyrimidine dehydrogenase, (2) orotate phosphoribosyltransferase, (3) uridine phosphorylase, (4) uridine kinase, (5) thymidine phosphorylase, (6) thymidine kinase.

the cytotoxicity of 5-fluorouracil in cell lines of various histological origins.[4] A decreased activity of folylpolyglutamate synthase results in a reduced level of the polyglutamated folate co-factor and thus reduced retention of folates in the cell and less efficient inhibition of TS.[7]

3. *Increased levels of TS or increased TS activity due to a mutation.* Resistance in cell lines, associated with elevated TS levels, can be due to amplification of the TS gene.[9] An increased TS activity due to a single amino acid substitution in TS was observed in a naturally occurring genetic variant and resulted in resistance to 5-fluorouracil.[10]

Cytosine arabinoside

In cells, cytosine arabinoside is converted into cytidine arabinoside triphosphate, which acts as a substrate for cellular DNA polymerases in competition with the normal substrate, deoxycytidine triphosphate. The incorporated cytidine arabinoside monophosphate moiety prevents further DNA chain elongation; this block in DNA synthesis eventually kills the cell. Resistance to cytosine arabinoside can arise by one of the following mechanisms as are shown in Figure 5 (see Grant[11]):

1. *Decreased cellular uptake of cytosine arabinoside.* Cellular uptake of nucleosides, like cytosine arabinoside, can occur by an energy-dependent nucleoside transport mechanism. The number of nucleoside-binding sites appears to correlate with the rate

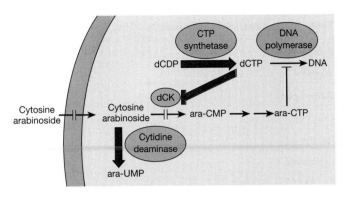

Fig. 5 Simplified scheme illustrating the biochemical mechanisms of cytosine arabinoside resistance (see text for explanation). The bold arrows indicate an upregulated route in resistant cells. The broken arrows mean a downregulated or inactivated route in resistant cells. The bold T line indicates an increased inhibition in resistant cells. Ara means arabinoside.

of transport into leukaemic cells and the sensitivity of these cells to cytosine arabinoside, but this only applies at cytosine arabinoside concentrations below 1 μM. At the higher concentrations (>10 μM), phosphorylation of cytosine arabinoside becomes the rate-limiting step in cytosine arabinoside metabolism.

2. *Decreased expression of deoxycytidine kinase (dCK).* Cytosine arabinoside is converted into cytidine arabinoside monophosphate by dCK, an enzyme deficient in some cytosine arabinoside resistant mutants. Loss of the enzyme can be due to mutations within the dCK gene.

3. *Increased cellular pools of deoxycytidine triphosphate.* Mutations in the cytidine triphosphate (**CTP**) synthetase gene rendered CTP synthetase insensitive to a negative feedback by an increased deoxycytidine triphosphate concentration, leading to higher intracellular deoxycytidine triphosphate concentrations in resistant tumour cells. Increased levels of deoxycytidine triphosphate will compete with cytidine arabinoside triphosphate for DNA polymerases. High deoxycytidine triphosphate also inhibits dCK, leading to a decrease in the conversion of cytosine arabinoside into cytidine arabinoside monophosphate.

4. *Overexpression of cytidine deaminase.* This enzyme causes deamination of cytotoxic analogues of cytidine. Overexpression of cytidine deaminase by transfection of the gene into tumour cells confers resistance to cytosine arabinoside.[12] This mechanism has not yet been observed in cells with acquired resistance.

Alterations in the target enzyme, DNA polymerase, have not been found in cytosine arabinoside-resistant cells. Apparently, a polymerase that discriminates effectively between cytidine arabinoside triphosphate and deoxycytidine triphosphate is not easily obtained by mutation.

Gemcitabine

Gemcitabine (difluorodeoxycytidine) is a deoxycytidine analogue like cytosine arabinoside with promising antitumour activity especially in combination with cisplatin. Interestingly, gemcitabine when compared with cytosine arabinoside has a different mode of action, pharmacokinetics, and antitumour activity. Its spectrum of activity includes

among others tumours with well-known intrinsic drug resistance such as pancreatic cancer, non-small cell lung cancer, ovarian cancer, and bladder cancer. Gemcitabine is, compared with cytosine arabinoside, a better transport substrate, more efficiently phosphorylated and eliminated more slowly. Furthermore, following gemcitabine incorporation in DNA, only one additional deoxynucleotide is incorporated, which prevents detection by the DNA proof-reading system. These effects may explain why gemcitabine is active in solid tumours in contrast to cytosine arabinoside.[13] A few drug-resistant cell lines have been established that showed the same level of resistance for gemcitabine and cytosine arabinoside. The major mechanisms of gemcitabine resistance are:

1. *Decreased expression of dCK.* Gemcitabine is converted into gemcitabine diphosphate and triphosphate by dCK, an enzyme deficient at the protein level but not at the mRNA level in gemcitabine-resistant mutants.[14]

2. *Overexpression of cytidine deaminase.* Gene transfer of the cytidine deaminase gene confers resistance to gemcitabine. In human tumour cell lines and xenografts, cytidine deaminase activity inversely correlated with the sensitivity to gemcitabine.

6-Thioguanine

The purine analogue 6-thioguanine is cytotoxic to proliferating cells. Cytotoxicity requires conversion of 6-thioguanine to 6-thioguanine nucleotides via the purine salvage pathway, followed by incorporation into DNA in place of dGTP (deoxyguanosine triphosphate). The incorporation of 6-thioguanine nucleotides is not toxic but appears to prevent subsequent replication, as this modified DNA is a poor template for human DNA polymerases and ligases. Reported mechanisms of resistance include decreased uptake, increased capacity of *de novo* purine synthesis, or increased degradation of the purine analogue or the purine analogue nucleotide.[15] The main mechanism of resistance to 6-thioguanine and 6-mercaptopurine is decreased activity of hypoxanthine-guanine phosphoribosyl transferase (**HGPRT**). Decreased conversion of 6-thioguanine by the salvage pathway into the corresponding nucleoside monophosphate due to a loss of HGPRT activity results in resistance. The loss of activity is mainly due to the presence of mutations in the *hgprt* gene.[6]

Multidrug resistance

Simultaneous resistance to various structurally unrelated chemotherapeutic drugs is termed pleiotropic drug resistance or multidrug resistance (**MDR**). It is commonly caused by one or more of the following mechanisms namely: (i) increased expression of drug efflux pumps; (ii) increased expression of the lung resistance related protein; (iii) reduced expression of the drug target topoisomerase II (**TopoII**).

Increased expression of drug efflux pumps

Resistance due to P-glycoprotein overexpression

Growth of human tumour cells in the presence of inhibitory concentrations of large hydrophobic drugs, such as doxorubicin or vincristine, can lead to the selection of stable variants that overproduce a cell membrane glycoprotein of 170 kDa. This glycoprotein, discovered by Riordan, Ling and co-workers, was called P-glycoprotein and is the most extensively studied drug resistance pump.[16] P-glycoprotein is encoded by the *mdr1* gene, which is located on chromosome 7q21 in humans. The protein acts as a molecular pump that extrudes a wide variety of drugs, resulting in a decreased intracellular drug concentration at the target and, hence, induces drug resistance. The specificity of the human P-glycoprotein has been studied by introducing and overexpressing the cloned *mdrl* gene in human cells with low P-glycoprotein levels. P-glycoprotein overproduction in human tumour cells results in resistance to anthracyclines, such as doxorubicin, to epipodophyllotoxins, such as etoposide, and to vinca-alkaloids, taxoids, topotecan, and actinomycin D, but not to many of the other clinically important drugs, such as alkylating agents, cisplatin, MTX, and purine and pyrimidine analogues. P-glycoprotein belongs to the superfamily of adenosine triphosphate (ATP)-binding cassette transporters and has six transmembrane loops and an intracellular domain that binds various substrates.

Although P-glycoprotein was discovered in tumour cells, it is also extensively present in normal tissues. In humans, P-glycoprotein expression is known to be present in the epithelia of excretory organs such as the biliary canalicular surface of hepatocytes and the brush border of the proximal tubules of the kidney. It is also present in natural barriers such as the blood–brain barrier and the testicular barrier. Knowledge of its function has been obtained using knockout mice where disruption of the *mdrla* gene made them sensitive to many drugs.[17] In these mice, pharmacokinetic analysis of drugs such as vinblastine, showed reduced faecal excretion and prolonged elimination half-life, while higher vinblastine levels were reached in the brain.

Reversal of P-glycoprotein-mediated multidrug resistance in cultured cells and animal models

Considerable interest has been generated by the discovery that P-glycoprotein-mediated MDR can be reversed by the calcium-channel blocker verapamil. Subsequent work has resulted in a long list of compounds that share this property with verapamil. A selection is presented in Table 1.[18] These 'reversal compounds' are substrates of the P-glycoprotein pump and compete with the drugs for extrusion from the cell. Some of these agents have also prevented the development of P-glycoprotein-mediated drug resistance when used during selections of drug resistant cell lines with P-glycoprotein substrate drugs. The effects of these blockers varies with the model. This is partly due to other mechanisms involved in MDR in the cell lines tested. Reversal compounds have been used with some success to overcome resistance in syngeneic tumour models in mice.

In *mdrla* knock-out mice, it was shown that oral treatment of mice with the P-glycoprotein blocker PSC833 did inhibit the blood–brain barrier P-glycoprotein extensively and the intestinal P-glycoprotein completely. This resulted in, for example, enhanced oral bioavailability of paclitaxel in wild-type mice treated with PSC833. Positron emission scans showed lower [^{11}C]verapamil levels in the brain of wild-type mice compared with those in knock-out mice. Cyclosporin A increased [^{11}C]verapamil accumulation in the brain of wild-type mice to levels comparable with those in knock-out *mdrla* mice. This illustrates that cyclosporin A can fully block the P-glycoprotein function in the blood–brain barrier.[19]

Resistance due to overexpression of multidrug resistance protein (MRP)

The multidrug resistance protein 1 (**MRP1**) is a 190 kDa protein which is another ATP-dependent transport molecule involved in

Table 1 Antagonists of P-glycoprotein (modified from Sandor *et al.*[18])

Antagonists
Verapamil
Dexverapamil
Quinidine
Quinine
Cyclosporin A
PSC 833 (SDZ PSC 833)
Amiodarone
Trifluoperazine
Progesterone
Tamoxifen
Megestrol acetate
VX-710
GF120918
LY335979

MDR. The *mrp1* gene is located on chromosome 16p13. In 1992, Cole *et al.*[20] described the sequence of the *mrp1* gene, which showed 15 per cent homology with the *mdr1* gene. In contrast, there is a high degree of homology between MRP1 and the yeast cadmium factor. Transfection of the *mrp1* gene in tumour cell lines resulted in MDR. We and others demonstrated separately that MRP1 transports glutathione conjugates including leukotriene C$_4$.[21],[22] This pump is now considered to transport neutral or cationic chemotherapeutic drugs, heavy metals, and organic anions including glutathione conjugates and glucuronate conjugates. If the cells are depleted of glutathione, MRP1 activity towards cationic drugs is abrogated but is preserved for organic anions, indicating the important role of glutathione in MRP1 functionality. The spectrum of resistance for chemotherapeutic drugs does not differ much between P-glycoprotein and MRP1. However, cross-resistance to paclitaxel is higher for P-glycoprotein-mediated resistance than for MRP1-mediated resistance.

In *mrp1* knock-out cells, the export of glutathione is reduced compared with wild-type cells. In mice with a complete absence of MRP1 expression, there is hypersensitivity to the toxic effects of etoposide.[23] Etoposide-phosphate administration in these mice results in increased etoposide-induced damage to the oropharyngeal mucosa and to the seminiferous tubules of the testis. The high concentrations of MRP1 protein, normally present in the basal layers of the oropharyngeal mucosa and in the basal membrane of the Sertoli cells in the testis, apparently protect wild-type mice against drug-induced tissue damage.[24] Knock-out mice also have an impaired response to an inflammatory stimulus which can be attributed to a decreased secretion of the MRP1 substrate leukotriene C$_4$ from leukotriene-synthesizing cells.[25] Like P-glycoprotein MRP1 protein expression was first detected in tumour cells, but is also extensively expressed in normal tissues, including stomach, colon, kidney, spleen, pancreas, liver, heart, blood–brain barrier, bronchial epithelium, and haematopoietic cells.[26] The MRP1 protein is localized in the cell cytoplasma and plasma membrane.

Apart from MRP1, other members of the MRP family have been detected. The *mrp2* gene encodes the canalicular multispecific organic anion transporter, cMoat. This transporter was initially found to play a part in an inborn error of bilirubin transport in rat and human. Mutation of this gene results in hyperbilirubinaemia. At present, there is no clear relation between the *mrp2* gene and MDR. Following database searches, four additional MRP genes were detected, designated *mrp3* to *mrp6*. Whether these four genes are involved in MDR is unknown at the moment.[27]

Reversal of MRP-mediated MDR in cultured cells and animal models

In cell lines, the best known agent to reverse MRP-mediated resistance is buthionine sulfoximine which induces glutathione depletion. Much effort is now put in the development of compounds that can increase drug sensitivity by blocking drug efflux. In cell lines, it is shown that probenecid is a specific modulator of MRP. Another active compound is VX-710 also known as a P-glycoprotein modulator (Table 1).

Lung resistance related protein

Lung resistance related protein (LRP) was first detected in MDR cell lines that did not overexpress P-glycoprotein. LRP was identified as the human major vault protein. Vaults are mainly located in the cytoplasm and are considered to play a part in transport between nucleus and cytoplasm. LRP might play a part in the compartmentalization of the chemotherapeutic drug and transport out of the cells, but transfection of the *lrp* cDNA did not result in MDR.[28] Several studies in cell lines and clinical specimens, however, still suggest a role for this protein in MDR. The *lrp* gene is located at chromosome 16p11.2 in human and maps, like *mrp1*, to the short arm of chromosome 16.[29] LRP is extensively present in normal tissues. High expression was seen especially in epithelial cells with excretory function and cells chronically exposed to xenobiotics such as bronchus, digestive tract, renal proximal tubulus, keratinocytes, macrophages, and adrenal cortex.[30]

Resistance due to altered topoisomerase II

Topoisomerase (Topo) IIα and β are homodimeric molecules with a molecular weight of 170 and 180 kDa, respectively. The position of the gene encoding Topo IIα is 17q21–22, while *topoIIb* is positioned at 3p24. The homodimeric molecule changes the topology of DNA by introducing a staggered double strand break into the DNA. The DNA break is held together by the Topo II dimer which is covalently bound to the 5′-end of each nicked strand via a tyrosyl phosphate bond, thus forming an enzyme-gapped bridge through which another DNA duplex can pass. The protein–DNA complex is called the cleavable complex, as denaturation of this complex leads to protein linked DNA breaks. After DNA strand passage the transient DNA break re-ligates rapidly. Topo II binds to DNA at loosely defined consensus sequences, in which the secondary structure of the DNA is also important.

Anthracyclines, (e.g. doxorubicin), epipodophyllotoxins, such as etoposide and teniposide, acridines (e.g. amsacrine (mAMSA)), and anthracenediones (e.g. mitoxantrone) are important examples of cleavable complex stabilizing Topo II inhibitors (Fig. 6). Often, Topo II drugs are divided into a class of drugs which intercalate in DNA

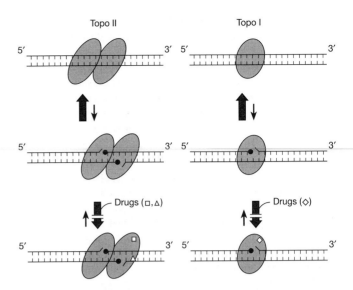

Fig. 6 Induction of cleavable complexes by Topo II and Topo I inhibitors. Normally, the equilibrium between covalently bound and non-covalently bound Topo II or Topo I will be in favour of non-covalently bound Topo. Intercalating (△) and non-intercalating (□ —) Topo II and Topo I inhibitors induce a shift in the equilibrium towards covalently bound Topo–DNA complexes. A reduced affinity of Topo II or Topo I for a drug and thus a reduced formation of cleavable complexes, as indicated by the broken bold arrows, will induce resistance.

(doxorubicin, mAMSA, and mitoxantrone) and a class of non-intercalators (etoposide and teniposide). There is a general relationship between Topo II levels, drug-induced Topo II-mediated DNA breaks and cytotoxicity. However, this relation varies for different types of drugs or cell lines and additional factors are involved such as the level of phosphorylated Topo II, DNA repair and apoptosis induction (see Osheroff *et al.*[31] and Hwang and Hwong[32]).

A major problem in anticancer treatment with Topo II inhibitors, is the emergence of drug resistance. Although many Topo II inhibitors are substrates for such drug efflux pumps, changes in Topo II level induce resistance as well. Additionally, both drug accumulation defects and Topo II changes can be found. Topo II-related drug resistance is sometimes described as at-MDR which stands for *a*-typical-MDR (sometimes also called '*a*ltered *t*opo-MDR'). Some of the characteristics are described below (see Pommier *et al.*[33] and Beck *et al.*[34]).

1. *Decreased Topo IIα expression.* An important cause of the decrease in cleavable complexes is the physiological decrease of Topo IIα in the G_0/G_1 phase of the cell cycle. This decrease and the relative resistance during quiescence has been shown for several cell lines and human tissues. Inactivating rearrangements of the *topoIIα* gene and loss of gene copy numbers, due to the deletion of chromosomal areas where the genes are located, also resulted in a decrease in Topo IIα levels in resistant cells without affecting the cell cycle distribution.[35]

2. *Expression of mutated Topo IIα.* Mutations in the *topoIIα* gene have been linked to resistance. The occurrence of mutations can be due to treatment with Topo II drugs as these are known to cause deletions, mutations, chromosomal aberrations, illegitimate

recombination, and sister chromatid exchanges. Most point mutations in the *topoIIα* gene are located around the consensus B sequence of the ATP-binding site, or near the reactive tyrosine 804, which covalently binds to DNA. These mutations impair ATP binding or drug binding, or binding of Topo IIα to DNA. It has to be realized that single allele mutations do not imply that wild-type Topo IIα is absent, as the other allele may be unchanged. In heterodimers a dominant negative mutation will block the activity of the normal subunit.

3. *A changed cellular localization of Topo IIα.* Several cell lines with deletions in the COOH-terminus of the *topoIIα* gene have been described. This results in deletions of nuclear localization signals causing cytoplasmatic localization of Topo IIα. When Topo IIα is present at low levels in the nucleus, Topo II targeting drugs will induce few cleavable complexes which leads to drug resistance. Either one or both alleles have been found to be mutated.[36],[37]

4. *Decreased Topo IIβ expression.* Few data are available on Topo IIβ-mediated resistance. However, cell lines resistant to mitoxantrone displayed decreased Topo II activities and a reduction in Topo IIβ expression. It has been suggested that Topo IIβ may be specifically targeted by mitoxantrone, as cell lines with acquired mitoxantrone resistance all express no Topo IIβ protein.[36]

Resistance to topoisomerase I inhibitors

Human Topo I is monomeric 100 kDa protein encoded by a single copy gene located on chromosome 20q12–13.2 in human. Topo I is involved in the relaxation of supercoiled DNA, a process important for DNA replication and RNA transcription. Topo I introduces a single-strand nick in the phosphodiester backbone of the DNA and binds covalently to the 3′-phosphate end at the DNA break site. After allowing an intact strand to pass, the nicked strand is re-sealed by Topo I and the enzyme dissociates from the DNA. In general, an extremely low percentage of the Topo I molecules is covalently bound to DNA. Camptothecin and its water soluble analogues including topotecan, irinotecan, lurtotecan, and 9-aminocamptothecin bind covalently to the Topo I–DNA complex and stabilizes it (Fig. 6). The cytotoxicity of camptothecin is highly S-phase specific. This topic has been reviewed by Gerrits *et al.*[38] Several mechanisms of resistance have been observed:

1. *Decreased drug accumulation.* Decreased drug accumulation has not frequently been observed. In a few cell lines, an increased efflux has been observed in P-glycoprotein overexpressing cells as well as P-glycoprotein negative cells for the positively-charged topotecan.[39]

2. *Reduced number of cells in S-phase.* The Topo I level in a cell is not cell cycle dependent. As Topo I inhibitors are predominantly effective in S-phase cells, a low percentage of replicating cells in a tumour will result in intrinsic resistance to the drug.

3. *Decreased Topo I expression and activity.* A decrease in the cellular level of Topo I has been observed in cell lines, which was sometimes compensated by an increase in Topo II levels.[40] The reduced expression can be due to loss of gene copies, because Topo I expression correlates with the *topoI* gene copy number.[41] Increased dephosphorylation of the enzyme also reduces the

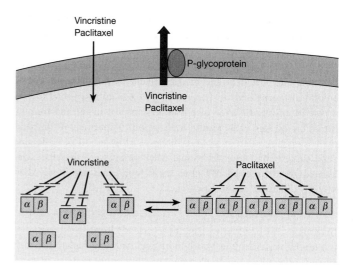

Fig. 7 Simplified scheme illustrating the biochemical mechanisms of vinblastine and paclitaxel resistance (see text for explanation). The bold arrow indicates upregulated transport in resistant cells. The broken T line indicates loss of inhibition in resistant cells.

catalytic activity, as well as drug-induced enzyme–DNA complexes.

4. *Expression of mutated Topo I.* Point mutations in the *topoI* gene results in a very low affinity of Topo I for camptothecin,[42] but may also increase the catalytic activity of the enzyme. Deletions in the *topoI* gene results in an inactivated enzyme.

Resistance to vinca-alkaloids and taxoids

Drugs that have the tubulin proteins as targets for their cytotoxic action are substrates for P-glycoprotein and MRP1. While these mechanisms lead to decreased intracellular drug levels, other mechanisms, based on the mode of action of these drugs, also play a part in resistance without affecting intracellular levels directly. Movement of cell parts, such as chromosomes and membranes, is a function of microtubules and microtubule-associated proteins. Microtubules are assembled from α- and β-tubulin heterodimers through polymerization, an energy-dependent process provided by hydrolysis of guanosine triphosphate (GTP). The polymer end can switch rapidly between a slowly growing and a rapidly shrinking state, known as dynamic instability, and allows the various functions of movement.[43] Human genes encoding α- and β-tubulins constitute a multigene family of 15 to 20 members.

Vinca-alkaloids, such as vincristine and vinblastine, bind to α- and β-tubulin leading to reduced dynamic instability and can, at high concentrations, inhibit polymerization and stabilize the mitotic spindle independently from GTP hydrolysis. The taxoid paclitaxel binds preferentially to the β-tubulin subunit of the microtubule. It is an antimitotic agent that binds to microtubule, and at low concentrations reduces the dynamic instability. At high concentrations paclitaxel induces microtubule polymerization and inhibits the formation of the mitotic spindle independently from GTP hydrolysis. This mechanism of action of these hydrophobic natural products already indicates the mechanisms of resistance to be expected and are shown in Fig. 7:

1. *Reduced drug accumulation.* Overexpression of the P-glycoprotein efflux pump results in an increased efflux of vinca-alkaloids and paclitaxel and thus resistance.[44]

2. *Changed tubulin composition.* Resistance to vinca-alkaloids occur when there are changes in tubulin that affect the binding sites on the α and β subunits.[45] This site is different from the paclitaxel binding site, so no cross-resistance would be expected for that mechanism. Immunofluorescence can distinguish cells with sensitive microtubular networks from unaffected networks.

3. *Changed b-tubulin isotype expression.* Changes in the expression of the classes of β-tubulin isotypes result in drug resistance. The different classes of β-tubulin are differentially sensitive to paclitaxel with the class III and class IV β-tubulin isotypes being less sensitive.[46] The β-tubulin classes, that are less sensitive to paclitaxel, can be glutamylated and phosphorylated, which may regulate *in-vivo* microtubule assembly and thus have an effect on the level of resistance to paclitaxel.[44]

Resistance to cisplatin and alkylating agents

This topic has been reviewed by Van der Zee *et al.*,[47] Crul *et al.* 1997,[48] and Johnson *et al.*[49] Whereas it is relatively easy to select mutant cells highly resistant (more than 1000-fold) to MTX or one of the drugs extruded by P-glycoprotein, resistance to alkylating agents and cisplatin is difficult to obtain and resistance is no more than 10 to 20-fold. This has complicated the analysis of resistance mechanisms.

Cisplatin is one of the most effective chemotherapeutic drugs in the treatment of cancer. In case of the metastatic testicular germ cell tumours, over 70 per cent of the patients can be cured.[50] However, the precise mechanism by which cisplatin is cytotoxic is still not known. Cisplatin reacts with the N7 position of guanine and adenine residues in DNA and forms a variety of monofunctional and bifunctional adducts. The major bifunctional lesions formed in DNA are platinum-GG, platinum-AG, and platinum-GNG intrastrand cross-links (i.e. within one DNA strand). Less than 5 per cent of all platinum-DNA adducts formed are interstrand cross-links (i.e. between two DNA strands). To what extent each of these adducts contributes to the cytotoxicity is not known and may be specific for the various cisplatin analogues.

For most cross-linking alkylating agents, the most frequent site of alkylation is the N7 position of guanine but other nitrogen, sulphur, oxygen, and phosphorus positions, also in other nucleotides, can be the site of covalent binding. Nitrosoureas on the other hand have a predominant site of alkylation, which is the O6 position of guanine.

Cisplatin

Cisplatin and its analogues show precise nucleotide sequence preferences. Nevertheless, a variety of lesions, including interstrand and intrastrand cross-links and monofunctional adducts are formed and the mechanisms of repair have not been fully elucidated. Several mechanisms of resistance are detected in the various *in-vitro* models, but do not consistently correlate with cisplatin resistance in general.[47]–[49]

1. *Reduced drug accumulation.* In several cisplatin-resistant cell lines a decreased drug accumulation has been detected. Reduced facilitated diffusion is one possible explanation as Na$^+$/K$^+$ ATPase inhibition decreased the cisplatin uptake substantially. An

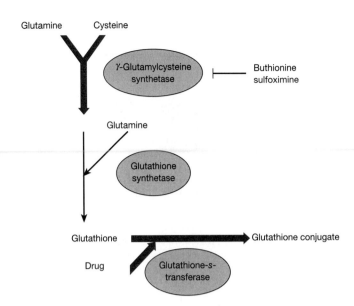

Fig. 8 Simplified scheme of the glutathione synthesis pathway and conjugation of glutathione to drugs catalysed by glutathione-S-transferase. The bold arrow indicates an upregulated route in resistant cells.

increased expression of MRP2 (cMOAT) has been observed in several cisplatin resistant human cancer cell lines.[51] A reduction in MRP2 expression using an anti-sense strategy did indeed increase cisplatin cytotoxicity.[52]

2. *Increased drug inactivation.* The formation of conjugates between glutathione and cisplatin (analogues) may be an important step not only for active drug efflux but also to inactivate the drug by preventing the formation of platinum-DNA adducts (Fig. 8). Conjugation of glutathione to cisplatin is catalysed by glutathione-S-transferases. Elevated glutathione levels correlate with cisplatin resistance. Inhibition of the key enzyme in the glutathione synthesis, γ-glutamylcysteine synthetase, by buthionine sulfoximine lowers glutathione levels strongly, but only moderately potentiates cisplatin cytotoxicity. Overexpression of glutathione-S-transferases did not consistently induce resistance to cisplatin.[47] Inactivation of cisplatin can also occur through binding to metallothionein proteins. Overexpression of metallothionein levels, however, did not exclusively result in cisplatin resistance.[49]

3. *Increased DNA repair.* If cytotoxic platinum-DNA adducts are formed, cells must either repair or tolerate the damage. Increased repair capacity of platinum-DNA adducts has been observed in many cisplatin-resistant cell lines. Repair of platinum-DNA adducts is believed to occur by the process of nucleotide excision repair (Fig. 9). This type of repair may occur preferentially in actively transcribed genes. No components of this type of repair have yet been related to cisplatin resistance. Increased expression of the DNA repair genes ERCC1 and ERCC4, has been found in cisplatin-resistant human ovarian tumours. However, when the nucleotide excision repair deficiency of tumour cells that are hypersensitive to cisplatin, was corrected by the expression of ERCC1 and ERCC4, no effect on platinum-DNA repair and cytotoxicity was observed.[49] The presence of platinum-DNA

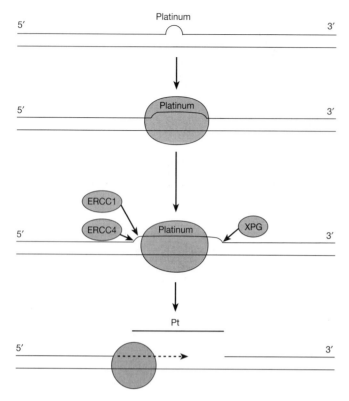

Fig. 9 A highly simplified scheme of the nucleotide excision repair. After the platinum–DNA adduct has been detected by a DNA damage recognizing complex, a DNA helicase complex unwind the DNA strands. ERCC1, ERCC4, and XPG are DNA damage recognizing proteins, which may act as single-strand nicking enzymes to remove a oligodeoxynucleotide. DNA polymerase will then fill in the gap.

recognition proteins may also have an effect on repair activity. These proteins are either high mobility group proteins or proteins that contain one or more high mobility group DNA binding motifs. No correlation between expression of these proteins and cisplatin cytotoxicity has been observed yet.[48]

4. *Decreased DNA repair.* Increased DNA damage tolerance due to dysfunction of the DNA mismatch repair system is a mechanism that may appear in cisplatin-resistant cells. hMSH2, hPMS2, and hMLH1 proteins are possibly involved in the mismatch repair system.[48] Decreased expression of hPMS2 and hMLH1 proteins has been observed in cisplatin-resistant cell lines.[53]

Nitrogen mustard and chlorambucil

Similar mechanisms were identified as described for cisplatin, but nitrogen mustard and chlorambucil are good substrates for the glutathione-transferase-α.[54] An increased expression of Topo II has also been observed in nitrogen mustard resistant human cancer cells suggesting a role in DNA repair.[55]

Increased drug inactivation

The most compelling evidence for a contribution of glutathione-S-transferase to drug resistance has come from the analysis of a chlorambucil-resistant Chinese hamster ovary line studied by Lewis *et al.*[56] This mutant line was 20-fold resistant, cross-resistant to

melphalan, but not to cisplatin. Resistance was associated with a four- to eight-fold amplification of a DNA segment containing a gene for an α(basic)-type glutathione-S-transferase. The corresponding 50-fold elevation of a glutathione-S-transferase coupling of chlorambucil and melphalan to glutathione, would seem to account for the resistance of this mutant cell line.

Cyclophosphamide and ifosfamide

Cyclophosphamide, one of the most widely used drugs in treatment of human tumours, requires bioactivation, catalysed by liver P450 enzymes to become active.[57] Ifosfamide is also bioactivated in the liver but by another type of P450. The formed prodrugs 4-hydroxyl-cyclophophamide or 4-hydroxifosfamide are spontaneously converted into the active bifunctional nitrogen mustards phosphoramide mustard and isophosphoramide mustard, respectively. Potential resistance mechanisms are similar as those described for cisplatin.[58] Mechanisms of resistance have not been studied extensively.

1. *Increased drug inactivation by aldehyde dehydrogenase.* Overexpression of the detoxifying enzyme aldehyde dehydrogenase prevents the formation of the bifunctional nitrogen mustards. In several resistant cell lines elevated levels of aldehyde dehydrogenase have been detected. Even more convincing, transfection of the aldehyde dehydrogenase gene induces resistance in cancer cells.[59]

2. *Glutathione mediated detoxification.* Following formation of active bifunctional nitrogen mustards, glutathione can react with these active mustards in order to prevent the formation of DNA cross-links. Glutathione-S-transferase catalysis the reaction of glutathione with these mustards. Elevated levels of glutathione, glutathione-S-transferase and γ-glutamylcysteine synthetase correlate with cyclophosphamide resistance. Inhibition of γ-glutamylcysteine synthetase by buthionine sulfoximine reduces glutathione levels and potentiates cyclophosphamide cytotoxicity in these cell lines.[60] In assessing the importance of glutathione it should be realized, that the drastic decrease in glutathione levels by buthionine sulfoximine may make the glutathione concentration rate-limiting in cell survival under drug stress, even if resistance is due to another mechanism.

3. *Increased DNA repair.* Decreased initial levels of DNA interstrand cross-links have been observed in several resistant cancer cell lines. This could be mediated by the increased glutathione-mediated detoxification activity observed in these cell lines. However, if similar levels of DNA interstrand cross-links are induced, these lesions are more rapidly removed in the resistant cells. Involvement of ERCC1 and ERCC4 in repair of these lesions has been observed in a few cell lines.[58]

Melphalan

Several mechanisms of resistance, similar to those identified in cisplatin-resistant cells, have been described such as decreased uptake and increased glutathione levels.

1. *Decreased drug uptake.* Two amino acid transporters have been identified, the sodium-dependent carrier with substrate preference for alanine-serine-cysteine (system ASC), and a sodium-independent carrier with preference for leucine (system L). A

fourfold decrease in initial melphalan accumulation has been observed in resistant cells, which was due to a reduced expression sodium independent transport system.[61]

2. *Increased drug inactivation.* Elevated levels of glutathione are probably an important cause for resistance to melphalan. Inhibition of γ-glutamylcysteine synthetase by buthionine sulfoximine lowers glutathione levels and increases the sensitivity of cancer cells to melphalan.[62] In addition, levels of γ-glutamylcysteine synthetase, the rate-limiting enzyme in glutathione synthesis, were increased in resistant cells with elevated levels of glutathione.[63]

Nitrosoureas

The fully characterized O6-alkylguanine-DNA-alkyltransferase (ATase) system in mammalian cells can remove the methyl group from the O^6-position of guanine. O^6-alkylation of guanine appears to be the major lesion induced in tumours by drugs such as the nitrosoureas.

Increased DNA repair

It has been shown that overproduction of ATase can lead to resistance to nitrosoureas, whereas inhibition of ATase by O^6-benzylguanine reverses resistance.[64] Glutathione-transferase may be involved in the denitrosation of these compounds.[65]

Drug resistance mediated by changes in the apoptotic pathway

In a normal cell, when DNA damage is sensed, a cell rapidly increases its p53 level by an increased stability of p53. This increase can lead to the triggering of two different pathways, either a G_1 arrest to allow DNA repair, or apoptosis. In tumour cells, the two pathways are less strictly separated (reviewed by Levine[66] and Agarwal et al.[67]). The exact mechanism that causes a tumour cell to die apoptotically is unknown at present. In general, apoptosis is a faster process in tumour cells which express functional p53 compared with tumour cells expressing mutant p53. In both cases, p53 partly functions as a transcriptional activator. The G_1 arrest pathway has been clarified (at least in part). P53 binds directly to a *p53*-specific sequence in the p21(waf1/cip1) promoter and activates transcription of the *p21* gene. The p21 protein can bind to, and thereby inhibit cyclin-dependent kinases, which are necessary for the phosphorylation of the retinoblastoma (*rb*) gene. When the RB protein phosphorylation is inhibited, the E2F family of transcription factors will not be activated and cells will not enter the S-phase. During this arrest the cell has the opportunity to repair DNA damage. After the DNA has been repaired, MDM2 levels will rise due to transcriptional activation by p53 via *p53*-specific binding sequences. MDM2 will bind to and inactivate p53. This results in a downregulation of *p21* activation abrogating the p53-mediated cell cycle arrest. An increased c-myc protein expression will reduce G_1 arrest and strongly enhance DNA-damage induced apoptosis. The reduced control of the G_1 arrest, which is a characteristic of transformed cells, could be an explanation for the relatively high sensitivity of tumour cells to DNA damage compared with normal cells.

The BAX protein is involved in the p53-mediated apoptotic pathway as well, as p53 transactivates transcription of the *bax* gene. Normally, BCL-2 protects cells from apoptosis by heterodimerizing with the BAX protein, because BAX homodimers give the signal

to apoptosis. BAX activation results in mitochondrial dysfunction, followed by caspases (interleukin-converting enzyme-like proteases) activation. Several members of the bcl-2 family are able to bind to BCL-2, BAX, or to each other either promoting or inhibiting p53-dependent apoptosis.[68]

Whether p53 is directly involved in the activation of caspases is not known. Activation of caspases is the last step in apoptosis. When caspases have been activated by cleavage, proteins will be cleaved resulting in apoptotic morphological changes on cells and nuclei, and often results in DNA fragmentation.[69]

p53, the apoptotic pathway, and drug resistance

Many tumour cell lines express mutant p53 as was also found for human tumours.[70] Mutations in p53 are distributed over a large region of the molecule, especially in the mid-portion where these mutations may alter p53 conformation and the formation of a p53 tetramer, which is the active form.

Evidence for a relation between p53, apoptosis, and drug resistance came from *in vitro* studies using *p53* knock-out cells or mutant p53 expression vectors. Resistance to chemotherapeutic drugs was observed in cells without functional p53 compared with the wild-type p53 expressing parental cells.[71],[72] However, this effect on drug sensitivity was not observed in all tumour cell types. A direct effect of p53 on specific resistance mechanisms has been suggested for P-glycoprotein expression. Studies showed that the *MDR1* promoter could be repressed by the wild-type p53 but not by mutant p53.[73] The presence of a mutated p53 might therefore result in an increased expression of P-glycoprotein and concomitantly drug resistance. At present the importance of this mechanism is not clear.

The appearance of *p53* mutations in tumour cell lines during resistance induction has not frequently been observed. The involvement of p53 in intrinsic resistance is more likely. Cell lines of different origins expressing mutant p53 were resistant to many anticancer agents compared with cell lines expressing wild-type p53. The drugs include DNA cross-linking agents, antimetabolites, and Topo I and Topo II inhibitors.[74] There is a positive correlation between cisplatin resistance and the presence of mutant p53, but not with antimitotic agents such as paclitaxel.[74] Similar findings have been described in human lymphoma cell lines. In contrast, in human ovarian cell lines cisplatin sensitivity did not correlate with the p53 status.[75] These results suggest that *p53* mutations can have an effect on intrinsic drug resistance, which may be drug specific and cell-type specific. Although the presence of mutant p53 does not necessarily have to result in intrinsic drug resistance, it may also increase the chance to acquire drug resistance in a tumour cell population. First, the presence of mutant p53 may increase the genetic variability in cells due to a reduced cell cycle control, less efficient DNA damage detection, and reduced apoptotic capacity. Second, drug treatment of tumour cells expressing mutant p53 instead of inducing cell death can result in a reduced G_1 arrest and a block of the transition of cells from G_2- into M-phase. Cells with damaged DNA showing multiple nuclei and polyploidy will appear, which may increase the genetic variability.[76] This hypothesis has to be proven yet.

BCL-2 and BAX may also be important in drug resistance. Transfection studies using BCL-2 expressing vectors showed a large induction of cisplatin resistance after BCL-2 overexpression in a human ovarian carcinoma cell line.[72] BAX-deficient cells demonstrate less drug-induced apoptosis and display a drug resistance phenotype.[76]

Some results suggest that BCL-2 overexpression is only delaying cell kill without increasing long-term cell survival after drug exposure. In a few tumour cell lines with acquired resistance either an increased level of BCL-2 or a decreased level of BAX protein has been observed. Levels of BCL-2, BAX, and other members of the BCL-2 family may be more predictive for intrinsic resistance.[77]

Clinical analysis of drug resistance

Most of our knowledge of drug efficacy in cancer is empirical. We know that cisplatin is effective in testicular cancer and ovarian carcinoma but not in colon carcinomas. It is only recently that a potential explanation for the exquisite sensitivity of testicular cancer for cisplatin has been considered to be, at least in part, due to the absence of p53 mutations in those tumours.

One of the reasons for the lack of predictability is the fact that the cellular pharmacodynamics of most cytotoxic drugs are not known in sufficient detail. Ideally, one would like to know how every drug is handled in every specialized tissue of the body, what the molecular basis is for the dose-limiting toxicity, and why it kills some tumour cells but not others. Without this knowledge we cannot hope to understand clinical resistance fully.

Even if a resistance mechanism is precisely defined by studies of established tumour cell lines, made resistant in vitro, it will still be very difficult to extrapolate the results to tumours in patients. Tumour cells in tissue culture lack stromal interaction, they are usually much less heterogeneous than a real tumour, they cannot be rescued by metabolic cooperation, and they are homogeneously exposed to drugs in contrast to cells in a tumour. Therefore, within a tumour there is likely to be an enormous heterogeneity in drug resistance mechanisms.

Research on the role of the drug resistance mechanisms in the clinic has been performed along two lines. First, various factors involved in drug resistance in vitro have been determined in tumour samples of patients. The results have been correlated with the response rate of the tumour and survival time. Second, studies have been performed in which patients have been treated according to knowledge about drug resistance mechanisms obtained in the laboratory.

Drug resistance mechanisms in tumour samples from patients and knowledge-based circumvention of drug resistance in the clinic

Resistance mechanisms in clinical samples have either been studied directly or on cultured cells. Direct tests are limited to analyses on surviving, non-replicating cells, such as drug uptake, drug binding to target, inhibition of metabolic pathways, and acute cellular defence reactions, such as induced DNA repair. These tests are hampered by problems in the preparation of representative intact cell suspensions from fresh solid tumours and by the presence of variable amounts of normal tissue and stromal elements in suspension. The analysis of cultured cells is complicated by difficulties in growing a representative fraction of the tumour cells and the potential loss of resistance during growth in vitro. An impressive variety of techniques is now available to perform molecular and functional typing on human tumour samples such as enzyme activity assays, Western blotting, immuno-histochemistry, Northern blotting, reverse transcription–polymerase chain reaction (PCR) and PCR techniques, Southern blotting, gene

display techniques, and fluorescence-activated cell sorting functional assays. It is to be expected that the availability of chip technology will further speed up the genetic analyses of human tumours. A critical step in future will be to combine the results of these studies with chemotherapy response and survival in large groups of equally treated patients.[80]

Knowledge of mechanisms of action has led to attempts to modify resistance mechanisms. Modulation of the P-glycoprotein has received most attention. Clinical studies of modulation of the apoptotic pathway are now receiving great attention.

These two aspects, with emphasis on data obtained over the last years, will be discussed below.

Methotrexate

Dihydrofolate reductase

MTX resistance in cell lines is usually due to an uptake defect or to DHFR overexpression. In nine of 29 patients with a relapse of acute lymphocytic leukaemia, DHFR gene amplifications were associated with increased levels of DHFR mRNA and enzyme activity.[81] Impaired uptake of MTX has not been reported as a cause of resistance in clinical samples.

5-fluorouracil

Thymidylate synthase

TS is currently considered to be the most sensitive predictor of response to 5-fluorouracil. TS can be studied in patient samples with quantitative PCR for RNA detection or with immunohistochemistry. With both techniques it appeared that colon carcinoma patients with low TS tumour levels respond better on 5-fluorouracil treatment and survive longer.[82]

Modulation

Several studies have been performed to modulate the effect of 5-fluorouracil biochemically. Based on randomized studies, the combination of 5-fluorouracil and leucovorin is now considered standard treatment in colorectal cancer.[83]

Cytosine arabinoside

Deoxycytidine kinase

Because cytosine arabinoside is used in the treatment of leukaemia, the mechanism of resistance has been studied extensively in clinical specimens that can be obtained with relative ease. Initial and relapsed childhood acute lymphocytic leukaemia were investigated for mutations and expression levels of dCK. No mutations in the dCK gene were observed, but a low or absent dCK expression was more frequently observed in relapsed acute lymphocytic leukaemia.[84] Several amino acid substitutions were observed in dCK of relapsed acute myeloid leukaemia. Only one mutation resulted in an complete loss of dCK activity, which does not suggest a major role for dCK in clinical resistance to cytosine arabinoside.[85]

6-Thioguanine

Hypoxanthine-guanine phosphoribosyl transferase

The clinical significance of a decreased HGPRT activity was determined in a group of children with untreated acute lymphocytic leukaemia. Although HGPRT activity correlated with a poorer prognosis only in patients with precursor B-lineage acute lymphocytic leukaemia, no relation was observed between HGPRT activity and *in vitro* 6-thio-guanine resistance of acute lymphocytic leukaemia.[86]

Multidrug resistance

P-glycoprotein expression

The mRNA expression of the *mdrI* gene can be measured in tumour samples with Northern blotting, RNase protection and PCR assays and the P-glycoprotein expression with Western blotting and immuno-histochemistry. The results reported in the various studies vary greatly. One of the main reasons for this is the lack of standardization for the techniques used. The clinical relevance of the presence of P-glycoprotein is still unclear. Chan et al.[87],[88] reported that P-glycoprotein expression before treatment may predict the success of therapy for non-localized neuroblastoma and for osteosarcoma. This relation has not been observed in a smaller study of neuroblastoma.[89] In addition, in an ovarian carcinoma study, in which all patients received doxorubicin containing chemotherapy, the determination of P-glycoprotein, glutathione-transferase pi, c-erbB-2, and p53 at diagnosis did not permit more adequate prediction of response to chemotherapy. The higher frequency of P-glycoprotein immunoreactivity in residual ovarian tumours after chemotherapy compared with before treatment pointed to either induction of P-glycoprotein in these tumours or selection of P-glycoprotein overexpressing tumour cells by doxoru-bicin-containing combination chemotherapy.[90] Functional assays for P-glycoprotein in samples using fluorescent substrates are ideal to study efflux in haematological malignancies (see below under MRP expression). Another option to study P-glycoprotein functionality can now be assessed in tumours of patients treated with or without a non-toxic P-glycoprotein blocker and a radioactive labelled substrate for P-glycoprotein such as ^{99m}Tc-Sestamibi and ^{11}C-verapamil.[19] This would allow the study of the functional effect of the addition of a modulator to MDR drugs. Recently, it has been shown that ^{99m}Tc-Sestamibi, as well as being a substrate for P-glycoprotein, is also a substrate for MRP1.

P-glycoprotein modulation

Evidence for clinical effectiveness of modulation of P-glycoprotein has been obtained in phase II studies. In multiple myeloma patients which had progressed during therapy, continuous cyclosporin treatment during vincristine, doxorubicin, dexamethasone therapy induced responses in 33 per cent of the patients.[91] A phase II study with verapamil plus anthracycline demonstrated a partial response in 10 per cent of patients with metastatic breast cancer, whose disease had progressed on an anthracycline regimen.[92]

Several randomized studies have been performed to study the effect of the addition of P-glycoprotein modulators to chemotherapy. In multiple myeloma patients, no beneficial effect of oral verapamil to the vincristine, doxorubicin, dexamethasone regimen was observed. A relatively small study in non-small cell lung cancer patients showed a higher response rate and a longer survival for those who received verapamil in combination with vindesine and ifosfamide. Patients who received verapamil also experienced more neurotoxicity. In a study with small cell lung cancer patients, the addition of verapamil to cyclophosphamide, doxorubicin, vincristine, and etoposide had no effect on response, survival, or toxicity. The addition of another antagonist of P-glycoprotein, quinidine, to epirubicin treatment of breast cancer patients showed no effect on response rate and survival.

Quinidine in relapsed or refractory acute leukaemia patients had no effect on response rate, although there was a trend towards improved response rate for the quinidine arm.[18] No effect was observed of megestrol acetate versus placebo in patients, who received first-line treatment for small cell lung carcinoma.[93] It can be concluded that most randomized studies show no effect of the addition of a P-glycoprotein modulator. Most of these studies, however, did not determine the P-glycoprotein expression in the tumour. It cannot therefore be excluded that a different patient selection might reveal a subgroup that can still benefit from co-treatment with a P-glycoprotein modulator.

MRP expression

Most data on presence and function are available from studies on samples from patients with leukaemia. Uptake and efflux of the MRP probe calcein-AM was tested in fresh samples obtained from 53 acute myeloid leukaemia patients. P-glycoprotein expression and activity and MRP activity, but not MRP1 expression, were prognostic factors for achievement of complete remission. These results suggest that functional testing for the presence of both MRP and P-glycoprotein activities is of prognostic value and that MRP contributes to drug resistance in acute myeloid leukaemia.[94] Others also found a good correlation between MRP1 protein expression and blocking of efflux of the MRP-dependent substrate carboxy fluorescein diacetate by the MRP antagonist MK-571 in acute myeloid leukaemia samples.[95]

In breast cancer *MRP1* mRNA expression can be detected in 70 per cent of the breast cancer tissues and expression levels are increased in tumours compared with benign breast tissues. The MRP1 level is higher in the relapsed patients. The expression of MDR1 and MRP1 in primary breast carcinoma and normal adjacent tissue have been examined using a highly quantitative and reproducible reverse tran-scription–PCR assay. Expression of both genes was observed in tumour and normal adjacent tissue. There was a correlation of MDR1 expression with age and histology. Approximately twice the expression of MDR1 was observed in the under-50 age group compared with the over-50 age group, and lobular carcinoma had four times the expression of MDR1 of other histological types. MRP1 expression was independent of all other clinical parameters.[96]

MRP modulation

There are few data and certainly no randomized studies available on modulation of MRP-mediated resistance. VX-710, an agent that modulates MDR conferred by overexpression of both P-glycoprotein and MRP *in vitro*, is associated with minimal toxicity in combination with paclitaxel in patients.[97]

Lung resistance related protein (LRP) expression

Although the precise role of LRP is unknown, intriguing data on patient samples are available. In untreated acute myeloid leukaemia patients, clinical outcome was shown to be best in the patients lacking both LRP and P-glycoprotein.[98] A study in advanced ovarian carcinoma showed that positive LRP immunostaining was an indicator of poor response to standard platinum or alkylating agents containing chemotherapy.[99]

Topoisomerase expression

Biochemical and molecular data on topoisomerases in solid tumours are relatively rare. Topo II activity has been shown to be reduced in relapsed ovarian tumours compared with untreated ovarian tumours, while Topo I activities are similar. Both Topo I and Topo II extracted from these samples were able to form drug-induced cleavable complexes, the supposed toxic lesions, in an *in-vitro* assay.[100] No mutations were found in Topo IIα in blasts from patients with relapsed acute lymphocytic leukaemia which were previously treated with etoposide or teniposide.[101] In one of 13 small cell lung cancer patients treated with etoposide-containing chemotherapy, a mutation was detected in Topo IIα similar to that previously described for two cell lines selected for amsacrine resistance.[102] Thus, mutations in Topo IIα do not seem to be of major importance for the development of clinical resistance to Topo II inhibitors.

Cisplatin

Glutathione-S-transferase expression

Glutathione-S-transferase subtypes α, μ, and π have been determined especially in ovarian tumours. Less than half the studies indicate a correlation between glutathione-S-transferase π expression and resistance to cisplatin containing chemotherapy.

Platinum-DNA adducts

Clinically, it is often difficult to obtain tumour samples during treatment to quantify the number of platinum-DNA adducts in a tumour. The induction of platinum-DNA adducts has, therefore, been measured in peripheral blood after cisplatin treatment to test whether this could predict response to chemotherapy. Over the last years more sensitive techniques have become available compared with the initially used treatment with atomic absorption spectrometry. Examples of platinum-DNA adduct measurement techniques are a competitive enzyme-linked immunosorbent assay, a ^{32}P-postlabelling assay, and an immunocytochemical analysis.[103]–[105] Several studies have been performed in peripheral blood cells of patients after cisplatin and carboplatin treatment. Apart from cellular factors it is clear that the drug–target interaction also depends on pharmacokinetics. Conflicting results have been obtained in the various studies. Recently, Fisch *et al.* found no correlation between platinum-adduct levels and favourable outcome in patients with advanced germ cell cancer. Platinum-DNA adduct measurements, therefore, are not yet useful in the predictive testing of patients.[106]

Melphalan

Glutathione modulation

In the clinic, the glutathione synthesis inhibitor buthionine sulfoximine has been combined only with melphalan in phase I trials. A reduction in glutathione levels in tumour biopsies after treatment with butathionine sulfoximine has been observed.[107]

Nitrosoureas

ATase expression

In ovarian tumours, which are in general resistant to nitrosourea chemotherapy, high levels of ATase have been detected, whereas in Hodgkin's tumours and blasts from leukaemic patients lower levels of ATase have been found.[108]

ATase modulation

O6-benzylguanine is a potent inactivator of ATase. A phase I trial with O6-benzylguanine for patients undergoing surgery for malignant glioma has been conducted. This study indicates that ATase activities in the tumours are greatly reduced by O6-benzylguanine.[109]

Genes involved in apoptosis

p53

More than 50 per cent of human cancers have *p53* mutations.[70] Greenblatt *et al.* reviewed 2567 mutations in human carcinomas and found that 99 per cent of the mutations could be identified to exons 4, 5, 6, 7, 8, and 10 (95 per cent in exons 5 to 8).[70] Among the frequently mutated amino acids in human cancers, hot-spots are Arg248 with 9.6 per cent of the *p53* mutations, Arg273 with 8.8 per cent and Arg175 with 6.1 per cent. In testicular germ cell tumours, however, no *p53* mutations have been detected, and these tumours are highly sensitive to cisplatin. Although *p53* mutations in most tumours are regarded as homozygous or hemizygous alterations, a recent study in ovarian tumours showed predominantly heterozygous *p53* alterations.[110] Only *p53* mutations located in the DNA binding domains of p53 were associated with tumours refractory to cisplatin treatment of ovarian carcinomas and to doxorubicin treatment in breast cancer.[110],[111]

p53 modulation

Gene transfer of wild-type *p53* can reverse drug resistance and induce apoptosis in *in vitro* and in preclinical *in vivo* models. Phase I studies have shown that wild-type *p53* gene therapy by intratumoural injection is safe and feasible.[112] Its effect appears higher at a higher dose of vector and in combination with cisplatin. At the moment, several *p53* gene therapy studies are ongoing.

BAX/BCL-2

In ovarian carcinoma patients, high BAX levels has been correlated with tumour response and disease-free survival.[113] Similar results have been obtained for metastatic breast cancer. BCL-2 expression could not be correlated to clinical response in ovarian cancer.[114]

BCL-2 modulation

Overexpression of BCL-2 is frequently observed in non-Hodgkin's lymphoma which results in resistance to apoptosis. Using a bcl-2 anti-sense oligonucleotide to downregulate specifically the translation of *bcl-2* mRNA and thus BCL-2 expression, nine patients were treated daily with anti-sense oligonucleotides subcutaneously. Down-regulation of BCL-2 protein was observed in some patients, while a reduction in tumour size was observed in two patients.[115]

Conclusions

Knowledge of mechanisms involved in *in-vitro* acquired drug resistance is rapidly growing. After detection of the mechanisms of resistance, a number of drugs have been identified, which can overcome the resistance mechanism and increase drug sensitivity. In particular, the drug efflux pumps can be effectively modulated *in vitro*. Clinical studies, however, using modulators of the efflux pumps have not been promising. A major problem in the translation of *in vitro* results into a clinical setting is the heterogeneity of the tumour in a patient. Second, patients with cancer are treated with a multidrug regimen, whereas most acquired resistant tumour cell lines have been obtained by single drug incubations. Multiple resistance mechanisms instead of one mechanism can thus be expected in a tumour. Another clinically important mechanism could be intrinsic drug resistance due to a reduced triggering of apoptosis by a multidrug treatment, because many drugs induce cell kill via p53-dependent apoptosis despite the different modes of action. In future, *in vitro* studies have to unravel the apoptotic pathway(s) in order to design highly effective multidrug treatment regimens. Although the apoptotic pathway is largely unknown, introduction of wild-type p53 or inhibition of BCL-2 expression in tumours show promising clinical results.

Until now, the introduction of new or improved chemotherapeutic drugs such as gemcitabine, topotecan, and paclitaxel has been more successful than modulation of resistance mechanisms. The introduction of new drugs against targets, such as angiogenesis, telomerase, mutant p53, and c-erbB2, and the development of techniques, such as gene therapy and anti-sense strategies, may have major implications for the treatment of cancer in future.

References

1. Bonadonna G, Valagussa P. Dose-response effect of adjuvant chemotherapy in breast cancer. *New England Journal of Medicine*, 1981; **304**: 10–15.

2. Savarese DM, Hsieh C, Stewart FM. Clinical impact of chemotherapy dose escalation in patients with hematologic malignancies and solid tumors. *Journal of Clinical Oncology*, 1997; **15**: 2981–95.

3. Goldie JH, Coldman AJ. Mathematic modeling of drug resistance. In: Woolley PV, Tew KD (eds). *Mechanisms of drug resistance in neoplastic cells*. San Diego: Academic Press, 1988: 13–28.

4. Kinsella AR, Smith D, Pickard M. Resistance to chemotherapeutic antimetabolites: a function of salvage pathway involvement and cellular response to DNA damage. *British Journal of Cancer*, 1997; **75**: 935–45.

5. Jansen G, Pieters R. The role of impaired transport in (pre)clinical resistance to methotrexate: insights on new antifolates. *Drug Resistance Updates*, 1998; **1**: 211–18.

6. Lennard L. The clinical pharmacology of 6-mercaptopurine. *European Journal of Clinical Pharmacology*, 1992; **43**: 329–39.

7. Kamm YJL, Wagener DJT, Rietjens IMCM, Punt CJA. 5-Flourouracil in colorectal cancer: rationale and clinical results of frequently used schedules. *Anticancer Drugs*, 1998; **9**: 371–80.

8. Spears CP, Gustavsson BG, Frösing R. Folinic acid modulation of fluorouracil tissue kinetics of bolus administration. *Investigational New Drugs*, 1989; **7**: 27–36.

9. Berger SH, Jenh CH, Johnson LF, Berger FG. Thymidylate synthase overproduction and gene amplification in fluorodeoxyuridine-resistant human cells. *Molecular Pharmacology*, 1985; **28**: 461–7.

10. Barbour KN, Berger SH, Berger FH. Single amino acid substitution defines a naturally occurring genetic variant of human thymidylate synthase. *Biochemical Pharmacology*, 1990; **37**: 515–18.

11. Grant S. Ara-C: cellular and molecular pharmacology. *Advances in Cancer Research*, 1998; **72**: 197–233.

12. Schroder JK, et al. Constitutive overexpression of the cytidine deaminase gene confers resistance to cytosine arabinoside *in vitro*. *Leukemia*, 1996; **10**: 1919–24.

13. Plunkett W, Huang P, Gandhi V. Preclinical characteristics of gemcitabine. *Anticancer Drugs*, 1995; **6**: 7–13.

14. Van Haperen RVW, et al. Development and molecular characterization of a 2′,2′-difluorodeoxycytidine-resistant variant of the human ovarian carcinoma cell line A2780. *Cancer Research*, 1994; **54**: 4138–43.

15. Morgan CJ, Chawdry RN, Smith AR, Siravo-Sagraves G, Trewyn RW. 6-thioguanine-induced growth arrest in 6-mercaptopurine-resistant human leukemia cells. *Cancer Research*, 1994; **54**: 5387–93.

16. Riordan JR, Deuchars K, Kartner N, Alon N, Trent J, Ling V. Amplification of P-glycoprotein genes in multidrug-resistant mammalian cell lines *Nature*, 1985; **316**: 817–19.

17. Borst P, Schinkel AH. Genetic dissection of the function of mammalian P-glycoproteins. *Trends in Genetics*, 1997; **13**: 217–22.

18. Sandor V, Fojo T, Bates SE. Future perspectives for the development of P-glycoprotein modulators. *Drug Resistance Updates* 1998; **1**: 190–200.

19. Hendrikse NH, et al. Complete *in vivo* reversal of P-glycoprotein pump function in the blood-brain barrier visualized with positron emission tomography. *British Journal Pharmacology*, 1998; **124**: 1413–18.

20. Cole SPC, et al. Overexpression of a transporter gene in a multidrug-resistant human lung cancer cell line. *Science*, 1992; **258**: 1650–4.

21. Leier I, Jedlitschky G, Buchholz U, Cole SP, Deeley RG, Keppler D. The MRP gene encodes an ATP-dependent export pump for leukotriene C4 and structurally related conjugates. *Journal of Biological Chemistry*, 1994; **269**: 27807–10.

22. Muller M, et al. Overexpression of the gene encoding the multidrug resistance-associated protein results in increased ATP-dependent glutathione S-conjugate transport. *Proceedings of the National Academy of Science USA*, 1994; **91**: 13033–7.

23. Lorico A, Rappa G, Finch RA, Young D, Flavell RA, Sartorelli NC. Disruption of the murine MRP (multidrug resistance protein) gene leads to increased sensitivity to etoposide (VP-16) and increased levels of glutathione. *Cancer Research*, 1997; **57**: 5238–42.

24. Wijnholds J, et al. Multidrug resistance protein 1 protects the oropharyngeal mucosal layer and the testicular tubules against drug-induced damage. *Journal of Experimental Medicine*, 1998; **188**: 797–808.

25. Wijnholds J, et al. Increased sensitivity to anticancer drugs and decreased inflammatory response in mice lacking the multidrug resistance-associated protein. *Nature Medicine*, 1997; **3**: 1275–9.

26. Flens MJ, et al. Tissue distribution of the multidrug resistance protein. *American Journal of Pathology*, 1996; **148**: 1237–47.

27. Borst P, Kool M, Evers R. Do cMOAT (MRP2), other MRP homologues, and LRP play a role in MDR? *Seminars in Cancer Biology*, 1997; **8**: 205–13.

28. Scheffer GL, et al. The drug resistance-related protein LRP is the human major vault protein. *Nature Medicine*, 1995; **1**: 578–82.

29. Slovak ML, et al. The LRP gene encoding a major vault protein associated with drug resistance maps proximal to MRP on chromosome 16: evidence that chromosome breakage plays a key role in MRP or LRP gene amplification. *Cancer Research*, 1995; **55**: 4214–19.

30. Izquierdo MA, et al. Broad distribution of the multidrug resistance-related vault lung resistance protein in normal human tissues and tumors. *American Journal of Pathology*, 1996; **148**: 877–87.

31. Osheroff N, Corbett AH, Robinson MJ. Mechanism of action of topoisomerase II-targeted antineoplastic drugs. *Advances in Pharmacology*, 1994; **29B**: 105–26.

32. Hwang J, Hwong CL. Cellular regulation of mammalian DNA topoisomerases. *Advances in Pharmacology*, 1994; **29A**: 167–89.

33. Pommier Y, et al. Cellular determinants of sensitivity and resistance to DNA topoisomerase inhibitors. *Cancer Investigation*, 1994; **12**: 530–42.

34. Beck WT, et al. Resistance of mammalian tumor cells to inhibitors of DNA topoisomerase II. *Advances in Pharmacology*, 1994; **29B**: 145–69.

35. Withoff S, et al. Selection of a subpopulation with fewer DNA topoisomerase II alpha gene copies in a doxorubicin-resistant cell line panel. *British Journal of Cancer*, 1996; **74**: 502–7.

36. Harker WG, Slade DL, Parr RL, Feldhoff PW, Sullivan DM, Holguin MH. Alterations in the topoisomerase IIα gene, messenger RNA, and subcellular protein distribution as well as reduced expression of the DNA topoisomerase IIβ enzyme in a mitoxantrone-resistant HL-60 human leukemia cell line. *Cancer Research*, 1995; **55**: 1707–16.

37. Yu Q, Mirski SE, Sparks KE, Cole SP. Two COOH-terminal truncated cytoplasmic forms of topoisomerase II alpha in a VP-16-selected lung cancer cell line result from partial gene deletion and alternative splicing. *Biochemistry*, 1997; **36**: 5868–77.

38. Gerrits CJ, de Jonge MJ, Schellens JH, Stoter G, Verweij J. Topoisomerase I inhibitors: the relevance of prolonged exposure for present clinical development. *British Journal of Cancer*, 1997; **76**: 952–62.

39. Ma J, *et al.* Reduced cellular accumulation of topotecan: a novel mechanism of resistance in a human ovarian cancer cell line. *British Journal of Cancer*, 1998; **77**: 1645–52.

40. Tan KB, Mattern MR, Eng WK, McCabe FL, Johnson RK. Nonreproductive rearrangement of DNA topoisomerase I and II genes: correlation with resistance to topoisomerase inhibitors. *Journal of the National Cancer Institute*, 1989; **81**: 1732–5.

41. McLeod HL, Keith WN. Variation in topoisomerase I gene copy number as a mechanism for intrinsic drug sensitivity. *British Journal of Cancer*, 1996; **74**: 508–12.

42. Wang LF, *et al.* Identification of mutations at DNA topoisomerase I responsible for camptothecin resistance. *Cancer Research*, 1997; **57**: 1516–22.

43. Hunt AJ, McIntosh JR. The dynamic behavior of individual microtubules associated with chromosomes *in vitro*. *Molecular Cellular Biology*, 1998; **9**: 2857–71.

44. Horwitz SB, Cohen D, Rao S, Ringelk I, Shen HJ, Yang CP. Taxol: mechanisms of action and resistance. *Journal of the National Cancer Institute Monographs*, 1993; **15**: 55–61.

45. Cabral F, Barlow SB. Mechanisms by which mammalian cells acquire to drugs that affect microtubule assembly. *FASEB Journal*, 1989; **3**: 1593–9.

46. Kavallaris M, *et al.* Taxol-resistant epithelial ovarian tumors are associated with altered expression of specific beta-tubulin isotypes. *Journal of Clinical Investigation*, 1997; **100**: 1282–93.

47. Van der Zee AGJ, *et al.* Cell biological markers of drug resistance in ovarian carcinoma. *Gynecologic Oncology*, 1995; **58**: 165–78.

48. Crul M, Schellens JHM, Beijnen JH, Maliepaard M. Cisplatin resistance and DNA repair. *Cancer Treatment Reviews*, 1997; **23**: 341–66.

49. Johnson SW, Ferry KV, Hamilton TC. Recent insights into platinum drug resistance in cancer. *Drug Resistance Updates*, 1998; **1**: 243–54.

50. O'Dwyer PJ, Johnson SW, Hamilton TC. Cisplatin and its analogues. In: DeVita VJ Jr (ed.), *Principles and practice of oncology*. Philadelphia: J.B.Lippincott Co., 1997: 418–32.

51. Kool M, *et al.* Analysis of expression of cMOAT (MRP2), MRP3, MRP4, and MRP5, homologues of the multidrug resistance-associated protein gene (MRP1), in human cancer cell lines. *Cancer Research*, 1997; **57**: 3537–47.

52. Koike K, *et al.* A canicular multispecific organic anion transporter (cMOAT) antisense cDNA enhances drug sensitivity in human hepatic cancer cells. *Cancer Research*, 1997; **57**: 5475–9.

53. Brown R, *et al.* HMLH1 expression and cellular responses of ovarian tumor cells to treatment with cytotoxic anticancer agents. *Oncogene*, 1997; **15**: 45–52.

54. Tew KD. Glutathione-associated enzymes in anticancer drug resistance. *Cancer Research*, 1994; **54**: 4313–20.

55. Fan S, *et al.* P53 mutations are associated with decreased activity of human lymphoma cells to DNA damaging agents. *Cancer Research*, 1994; **54**: 5824–30.

56. Lewis AD, *et al.* Amplification and increased expression of alpha class glutathione S-transferase-encoding genes associated with resistance to nitrogen mustards. *Proceedings of the National Academy of Sciences USA*, 1988; **85**: 8511–15.

57. Chang TK, Maurel P, Waxman. Enhanced cyclophosphamide and ifosfamide activation in primary human hepatocyte cultures: response to cytochrome P-450 inducers and autoinduction by oxazaphosphorines. *Cancer Research*, 1997; **57**: 1946–54.

58. Colvin OM. Drug resistance in the treatment of sarcomas. *Seminars in Oncology*, 1997; **24**(5): 580–91.

59. Magni M, Shammah S., Schiro R, Mellado W, Dalla-Favera R, Gianni AM. Induction of cyclophosphamide-resistance by aldehyde-dehydrogenase gene transfer. *Blood*, 1996; **87**: 1097–03.

60. Richardson ME, Siemann DW. DNA damage in cyclophosphamide-resistant tumor cells: the role of glutathione. *Cancer Research*, 1995; **55**: 1691–5.

61. Moscow JA, Swanson CA, Cowan KH. Decreased melphalan accumulation in a human breast cancer cell line selected for resistance to melphalan. *British Journal of Cancer*, 1993; **68**: 732–7.

62. Mistry P, Kelland LR, Abel G, Sidhar S, Harrap KR. The relationships between glutathione, glutathione-S-transferase and cytotoxicity of platinum drugs and melphalan in eight human ovarian carcinoma cell lines. *British Journal of Cancer*, 1991; **64**: 215–20.

63. Mulcahy RT, Untawale S, Gipp JJ. Transcriptional up-regulation of gamma-glutamylcysteine synthetase gene expression in melphalan-resistant hguman prostate carcinoma cells. *Molecular Pharmacology*, 1994; **46**: 909–14.

64. Pegg AE. Mammalian O6-alkylguanine-DNA alkyltransferase: regulation and importance in response to alkylating carcinogenic and therapeutic agents. *Cancer Research*, 1990; **50**: 6119–29.

65. Berhane K, Hao XT, Egyhazi S, Hansson J, Ringborg U, Mannervik B. Contribution of glutathione transferase M3–3 to 1,3-bis(2-chloroethyl)-1-nitrosourea resistance in a human non-small cell lung cancer cell line. *Cancer Research*, 1993; **53**: 4257–61.

66. Levine AJ. p53, the cellular gatekeeper for growth and division. *Cell*, 1997; **88**: 323–31.

67. Agarwal ML, Taylor WR, Chernov MV, Chernova OB, Stark GR. The p53 network. *Journal of Biological Chemistry*, 1998; **273**: 1–4.

68. Chao DT, Korsmeyer SJ. BCL-2 family: regulators of cell death. *Annual Reviews in Immunology*, 1998; **16**: 395–419.

69. Nagata S. Apoptosis by death factor. *Cell*, 1997; **88**: 355–365.

70. Greenblatt MS, Bennett WP, Hollstein M, Harris CC. Mutations in the P53 tumor suppressor gene: Clues to cancer ethiology and molecular pathogenesis. *Cancer Research*, 1994; **54**: 4855–78.

71. Cho Y, Gorina S, Jeffrey PD, Pavletich NP. Crystal structure of a p53 tumor suppressor-DNA complex: understanding tumorigenic mutations. *Science*, 1994; **265**: 346–55.

72. Lowe SW, Ruley HE, Jacks T, Housman DE. p53-dependent apoptosis modulates the cytotoxicity of anti-cancer agents. *Cell*, 1993; **74**: 957–67.

73. Eliopoulos AG, *et al.* The control of apoptosis and drug resistance in ovarian cancer: influence of p53 and Bcl-2. *Oncogene*, 1995; **11**: 1217–28.

74. Chin KV, Ueda K, Pastan I, Gottesman MM. Modulation of activity of the promoter of the human MDR1 gene by Ras and P53. *Science*, 1992; **255**: 459–62.

75. O'Connor PM, *et al.* Characterization of the p53 tumor suppressor pathway in cell lines of the National Cancer Institute anticancer drug screen and correlations with the growth-inhibitory potency of 123 anticancer agents. *Cancer Research*, 1997; **57**: 4285–300.

76. De Freudis P, *et al.* DDP-induced cytotoxicity is not influenced by p53 in nine human ovarian cancer cell lines with different p53 status. *British Journal of Cancer*, 1997; **76**: 474–9.

77. Waldman T, Lengauer C, Kinzler KW, Vogelstein B. Uncoupling of S phase and mitosis induced by anticancer agents in cells lacking p21. *Nature*, 1996; **381**: 713–16.

78. McCurrach ME, Connor TM, Knudson CM, Korsmeyer SJ, Lowe SW. Bax-deficiency promotes drug resistance and oncogenic transformation by attenuating p53-dependent apoptosis. *Proceedings of the National Academy of Science USA*, 1997; **94**: 2345–9.

79. Lock RB, Stribinskiene L. Dual modes of death induced by etoposide in human epithelial tumor cells allow Bcl-2 to inhibit apoptosis without affecting clonogenic survival. *Cancer Research*, 1996; 56: 4006–12.

80. Spriggs DR, Makhija S. Ovarian cancer staging: time for a closer look? *Journal of Clinical Oncology*, 1998; 16: 2577–8.

81. Goker E, *et al.* Amplification of the hydrofolate reductase gene is a mechanism of acquired resistance to methotrexate in patients with acute lymphoblastic leukemia and is correlated with p53 mutations. *Blood*, 1995; 86: 677–84.

82. Leichman CG, *et al.* Quantitation of intratumoral thymidylate synthase expression predicts for disseminated colorectal cancer response and resistance to protracted-infusion fluorouracil and weekly leucovorin. *Journal of Clinical Oncology*, 1997; 15: 3223–9.

83. Advanced Colorectal Cancer Meta-Analysis Project. Modulation of flourouracil by leucovorin in patients with advanced colorectal cancer: evidence in terms of response rate. *Journal of Clinical Oncology*, 1992; 10: 896–903.

84. Stammler G, Zintl F, Sauerbrey A, Volm M. Deoxycytidine kinase mRNA expression in childhood acute lymphoblastic leukemia. *Anticancer Drugs*, 1997; 8: 517–21.

85. Flasshove M, *et al.* Structural analysis of the deoxycytidine kinase gene in patients with acute myeloid leukemia and resistance to cytosine arabinoside. *Leukemia*, 1994; 8: 780–5.

86. Pieters R, *et al.* Hypoxanthine-guanine phosphoribosyl-transferase in childhood leukemia: relation with immunophenotype, *in vitro* drug resistance and clinical prognosis. *International Journal of Cancer*, 1992; 51: 213–17.

87. Chan HS, *et al.* P-glycoprotein expression as a predictor of the outcome of therapy for neuroblastoma. *New England Journal of Medicine*, 1991; 325: 1608–14.

88. Chan HS, Grogan TM, Haddad G, DeBoer G, Ling V. P-glycoprotein expression: critical determinant in the response to osteosarcoma chemotherapy. *Journal of the National Cancer Institute*, 1997; 89: 1706–15.

89. Dhooge CR, De Moerloose BM, Benoit YC, Van Roy N, Philippe S, Laureys GG. Expression of the MDR1 gene product P-glycoprotein in childhood neuroblastoma. *Cancer*, 1997; 80: 1250–7.

90. Van der Zee AGJ, *et al.* The value of P-glycoprotein, glutathione S-transferase pi, c-erbB-2 and p53 as prognostic factors in ovarian carcinomas. *Journal of Clinical Oncology*, 1995; 13: 70–8.

91. Sonneveld P, *et al.* Modulation of multidrug-resistant multiple myeloma by cyclosporin. The Leukaemia Group of the EORTC and the HOVON. *Lancet*, 1992; 340: 255–9.

92. Warner E, *et al.* Phase II study of dexverapamil plus anthracycline in patients with metastatic breast cancer who have progressed on the same anthracycline regimen. *Clinical Cancer Research*, 1998; 4: 1451–7.

93. Wood L, *et al.* Results of a phase III, double-blind, placebo-controlled trial of megestrol acetate modulation of P-glycoprotein-mediated drug resistance in the first-line management of small-cell lung carcinoma. *British Journal of Cancer*, 1998; 77: 627–31.

94. Legrand O, Simonin G, Perrot JY, Zittoun R, Marie JP. Pgp and MRP activities using calcein-AM are prognostic factors in adult acute myeloid leukemia patients. *Blood*, 1998; 91: 4480–8.

95. Van der Kolk DM, De Vries EG, Koning JA, Van den Berg E, Muller M, Vellinga E. Activity and expression of the multidrug resistance proteins MRP1 and MRP2 in acute myeloid leukemia cells, tumor cell lines, and normal hematopoietic CD34 + peripheral blood cells. *Clinical Cancer Research*, 1998; 4: 1727–36.

96. Dexter DW, *et al.* Quantitative reverse transcriptase-polymerase chain reaction measured expression of MDR1 and MRP in primary breast carcinoma. *Clinical Cancer Research*, 1998; 4: 1533–42.

97. Rowinsky EK, *et al.* Phase I and pharmacokinetic study of paclitaxel in combination with biricodar, a novel agent that reverses multidrug resistance conferred by overexpression.

98. Filipits M, *et al.* Expression of the lung resistance protein predicts poor outcome in de novo acute myeloid leukemia. *Blood*, 1998; 91: 1508–13.

99. Izquierdo MA, *et al.* Drug resistance-associated marker Lrp for prediction of response to chemotherapy and prognoses in advanced ovarian carcinoma. *Journal of the National Cancer Institute*, 1995; 87: 1230–7.

100. Van der Zee AGJ, De Jong S, Keith WN, Hollema H, Boonstra H, De Vries EGE. Quantitative and qualitative aspects of topoisomerase I and IIα and β in untreated and platinum/cyclophosphamide treated malignant ovarian tumors. *Cancer Research*, 1994; 54: 749–55.

101. Danks MK, *et al.* Single-strand conformational polymorphism analysis of the M_r 170,000 isoenzyme of DNA topoisomerase II in human tumor cells. *Cancer Research*, 1993; 53: 1373–9.

102. Kubo A, *et al.* Point mutations of the topoisomerase IIalpha gene in patients with small cell lung cancer treated with etoposide. *Cancer Research*, 1996; 56: 1232–6.

103. Peng B, *et al.* Platinum—DNA adduct formation in leucocytes of children in relation to pharmacokinetics after cisplatin and carboplatin therapy. *British Journal of Cancer*, 1997; 76: 1466–73.

104. Welters MJ, *et al.* Improved 32P-postlabelling assay for the quantification of the major platinum—DNA adducts. *Carcinogenesis*, 1997; 18: 1767–74.

105. Meijer C, *et al.* Immunocytochemical analysis of cisplatin-induced platinum-DNA adducts with double fluorescence video microscopy. *British Journal of Cancer*, 1997; 76: 290–8.

106. Fisch MJ, Howard KL, Einhorn LH, Sledge GW. Relationship between platinum-DNA adducts in leukocytes of patients with advanced germ cell cancer and survival. *Clinical Cancer Research*, 1996; 2: 1063–6.

107. O'Dwyer PJ, *et al.* Phase I trial of buthionine sulfoximine in combination with melphalan in patients. *Journal of Clinical Oncology*, 1996; 14: 249–56.

108. Lee SM, *et al.* Expression of O6-alkyl-DNA-alkyltransferase *in situ* in ovarian and Hodgkin's tumours. *European Journal of Cancer*, 1993; 29A: 1306–12.

109. Friedman HS, *et al.* Phase I trial of O6-benzylguanine for patients undergoing surgery for malignant glioma. *Journal of Clinical Oncology*, 1998; 16: 3570–5.

110. Righetti SC, *et al.* A comparative study of p53 gene mutations, protein accumulation, and response to cisplatin-based chemotherapy in advanced ovarian carcinoma. *Cancer Research*, 1996; 56: 689–93.

111. Aas T, *et al.* Specific p53 mutations are associated with *de novo* resistance to doxorubicin in breast cancer patients. *Nature Medicine*, 1996; 2: 811–14.

112. Schuler M, *et al.* A phase I study of adenovirus-mediated wild-type p53 gene transfer in patients with advanced non-small cell lung cancer. *Human Gene Therapy*, 1998; 9: 2075–82.

113. Tai YT, Lee S, Niloff E, Weisman C, Strobel T, Cannistra SA. BAX protein expression and clinical outcome in epithelial ovarian cancer. *Journal of Clinical Oncology*, 1998; 16: 2583–90.

114. Herod JJ, Eliopoulos AG, Warwick J, Niedobitek G, Young LS, Kerr DJ. The prognostic significance of Bcl-2 and p53 expression in ovarian carcinoma. *Cancer Research*, 1996; 56: 2178–84.

115. Webb A, *et al.* BCL-2 antisense therapy in patients with non-Hodgkin lymphoma. *Lancet*, 1997; 349: 1137–41.

4.21 Dose-intensive chemotherapy

John Crown

Introduction: dose and schedule in cancer chemotherapy

Dose–response relationship in cancer chemotherapy

Although some degree of sensitivity to chemotherapy has now been documented for most cancers, drug treatment still produces routine cures in only a handful of generally uncommon tumour types, for example testicular germ cell tumours,[1] Hodgkin's disease,[2] non-Hodgkin's lymphomas,[3] and childhood leukaemias.[4] Other, more common, neoplasms exhibit varying but lesser degrees of chemotherapy sensitivity, with responses, remissions, and, in some diseases, a modest proportion of cures. For instance approximately 50 per cent of patients with small cell lung cancer achieve complete remission, however, only 5 to 10 per cent are cured.[5] Adult acute leukaemia generally responds to treatment, but only a minority of patients are cured.[6] Ovarian cancer is a tumour which has long been a source of particular frustration for oncologists.[7] The impact on survival of agents such as cisplatin and paclitaxel, while real, has been relatively modest, and the disease is seldom cured. Metastatic carcinoma of the breast is a common neoplasm which also exhibits prominent, but partial, chemotherapy sensitivity, with chemotherapy producing objective responses in 60 to 80 per cent of patients. These responses can result in the palliation of the distressing symptoms of cancer, and result in an approximately 1-year prolongation of average survival.[8] However, with the rarest of exceptions, response is temporary, and cure is exceptional.[9] Other solid tumours exhibit lesser degrees of chemotherapy sensitivity.

This frustrating phenomenon of partial chemotherapy sensitivity has prompted a critical evaluation of dose in clinical oncology. Is it possible that meaningful improvements in the therapy of some of these partially sensitive tumours might results from the administration of larger doses of partially active agents? Dose–response relationships are fundamental in pharmacology. Inadequate dosing of medicinal agents compromises their effectiveness. In the case of antibiotics, inadequate dosing can result in the emergence of drug-resistant organisms, a situation which may have parallels in human oncology. For some agents, for example digitalis and anticonvulsants, monitoring of blood levels are used to ensure adequate dosing. Chemotherapeutic dosing is far less precise. Chemotherapy dosage is usually calculated on the basis of the estimated body surface area of the patient or, less commonly, according to the patient's weight. The use of high-dose methotrexate in the therapy of osteogenic sarcoma is one of the few examples in oncology where blood concentrations of chemotherapeutic drugs are monitored. Even here, the levels are not used to determine dose, but to decide on the duration of folinic acid rescue.[10] It is increasingly recognized that dosing based on weight and surface area calculation may fail to take account of all the factors which determine the pharmacokinetics of a drug.[11] Furthermore, the recommended doses of most drugs and regimens were determined in phase I trials which had toxicity as the primary endpoints. Our ability to support patients through toxicity has improved greatly in recent years. As a result, the definitions of standard doses for most older chemotherapeutic agents may have lost some of their meaning.

There is ample experimental evidence that a relationship exists between the concentration of a drug to which a cancer cell is exposed and the likelihood that the cell will be killed. Studies in experimental systems, mainly in non-vascularized tumours, by Skipper and Schabel[12] and by Teicher et al.,[13] demonstrated that there was a relatively steep relationship between dose and cell-kill. In these studies, the degree of dose escalation that was required to eradicate cancers was in general substantial, typically of a log order of magnitude. This situation would be very difficult to replicate in the clinic due to toxicity. It is thus scarcely surprising that in the clinic, as will be discussed, minor degrees of dose escalation within the 'conventional' range (i.e. to levels which do not require haematopoietic support), have a modest and inconsistent effect on antitumour endpoints.[14]–[16]

In recent years, substantial advances in supportive care, in particular in the area of haematopoietic support, have allowed clinical investigation of greatly increased doses of chemotherapy in the clinic,[17] doses of an order of magnitude which appear to mimic those which were necessary for cure in experimental systems. It is important to note that the profound escalation which is achieved with autologous transplantation, which approaches that achieved experimentally, may have a more substantial clinical effect than that which is seen with modest dose variations.[18]

Dose intensity and dose density

Chemotherapy is usually administered in repetitive cycles at fixed treatment intervals and the precise nature of the inter-relationships between dose, schedule, and efficacy remain undefined. The concept of dose intensity, or dose per unit time, has been formulated in an attempt to quantitate these variables, and retrospective studies have suggested that there is a relationship between dose intensity and survival in breast,[19] colon,[20] and ovarian cancers,[21] and in Hodgkin's disease.[22] Other studies, however, have not supported the existence of a major role for dose intensification, and the retrospective studies have methodological difficulties.

Variations in either of the two components of dose intensity, that is dose per cycle or intertreatment interval, can produce identical differences in the dose intensity of a regimen. Thus the dose intensity of a given programme can be doubled by either doubling the dose per cycle, while holding the treatment interval constant, or by halving the treatment interval while holding the dose per cycle constant. The concept of dose density was introduced to emphasize the potential importance of the time component of dose intensity. Total dose is another potentially important variable, and one which is not measured at all in the dose intensity calculation. For example the dose intensities of two regimens consisting of either two or 20 cycles of identically-dosed cycles of treatment administered at identical treatment intervals are identical, even though there is a 10-fold difference in the total dose which is administered.

If dose intensity is the prevailing determinant of cell kill, regardless of how it is achieved or the total dose administered, then either increasing the dose per cycle, or decreasing the intertreatment interval, would be expected to produce an equivalent enhancement of cytotoxicity. Hypotheses concerning the potential clinical impact of dose and schedule could be tested in comparatively simple, randomized trials by altering either variable. The results of such studies in a number of different tumour types have, however, been inconsistent and generally disappointing.[23]–[25]

Alternatively, the antitumour impact of the dose per cycle, treatment interval, and total dose may be mediated by different biological mechanisms. If so, dose intensity, while providing a useful summary for its component parts, is itself essentially an artefact. To test this hypothesis, and to assess the full range of potential dose–schedule–response relationships would require multiarm trials of a degree of complexity far greater than those which have been performed to date, in which simple comparisons of higher versus lower intensity treatments have been carried out. While such a systematic evaluation of these variables seems unlikely to be carried out, another somewhat less rigorous approach might be to study the results of separate two-armed, random assignment trials which had independently addressed the impact of the three variables in a single tumour category. Relevant data of this type are available for ovarian cancer.

The impact of chemotherapy dose escalation or intensification in patients with ovarian cancer has been studied in 12 separate, prospective, random assignment trials. All of these studies involved intensification which was either within the standard range or somewhat beyond it, but which did not require haematopoietic support. They addressed four separate intensification strategies.

Higher dose per cycle and higher total dose

This strategy was studied in five separate trials. In three, the treatment interval was held constant. In one of these the higher dose arm was associated with superior survival.[26] In the other two, non-significantly longer survival was seen.[27],[28] In a fourth study, patients receiving a higher dose of cisplatin, with variable treatment intervals, had superior survival.[29] In the final study in this category, the dose of one drug, in a three-drug combination, was increased with no effect.[30]

Higher dose per cycle, identical total dose

In three trials, the effects of increasing the dose per cycle of one or more agents in a combination, while holding the total dose constant

were studied. In two of these studies, no advantage was associated with higher doses per cycle,[31],[32] although in one, intertreatment interval was also prolonged. In the third, the higher intensity treatment produced superior response and survival.[33]

Schedule intensification

Intensification was achieved through schedule acceleration in two studies. In one, otherwise identical chemotherapy was given in either a standard or accelerated schedule.[34] The accelerated therapy produced a statistically significant survival advantage. In the other study, weekly, lower-dose chemotherapy was administered in the intensified arm, versus three-weekly standard dose treatment. No advantage was seen for the intensified treatment.[35]

Increased total dose

In two studies, in which additional cycles of identically dosed treatment were administered, no advantage was reported.[36],[37]

Taken collectively these data could be interpreted to suggest that dose intensity is a weak and inconsistent determinant of clinical outcome in the treatment of ovarian cancer. If however, dose per cycle, total dose, and treatment interval exert independent influences on cytotoxicity, then a global overview of these studies based simply on their dose intensities might obscure real differences. It must also be pointed out that the degree of dose escalation which was achieved in these studies was relatively modest.

In analysing studies of dose intensity it is also important to differentiate between planned, or ideal dose intensity, and delivered dose intensity. The planned dose intensity is the dose intensity which would have been delivered if all planned treatments were delivered on time and in full dose. The actual dose intensity takes account of unplanned treatment delays and dose reductions due to toxicity and protocol compliance issues.

The term 'treatment intensification' must not be confused with 'dose intensification'. A regimen might be 'intensified' by the addition of other active drugs. For example, in the 1970s and 1980s, increasingly complex multidrug programmes were introduced for the treatment of diffuse non-Hodgkin's lymphoma. These programmes were often described as being more 'intensive' than standard CHOP (cyclophosphamide, hydroxy-daunorubicin, Oncovin (vincristine), prednisolone). However, in a randomized trial, CHOP was demonstrated to be equivalent to the more 'intensive' regimens.[38] It is clear that something other than dose intensity was being tested in this study. The complex regimens frequently delivered lower doses intensities of the most active drugs in order to accommodate the inclusion of other agents.

Hryniuk and colleagues recently developed the dose intensity concept further in an attempt to deal with multidrug regimens. First, they reviewed single agent literature to determine the dose intensity of a single agent that would produce a 30 per cent response rate. This was labelled the unit dose intensity. They next reviewed random assignment trials of dose intensity. The dose intensities of the individual drugs in each arm were expressed as fractions of their unit dose intensities. These were then added together for each arm, and expressed as the summation dose intensity. This in turn was found to be corelated with treatment outcomes in retrospective studies.[39]

Relevance of kinetic models to considerations of dose and schedule

Skipper and Schabel provided a theoretical rationale for much of modern chemotherapy clinical practice. These investigators described growth curves for experimental tumours which were essentially exponential. The growth rate of the tumour was constant throughout its natural history. Their experiments revealed that chemotherapy killed a constant proportion of cells, that there was an inverse relationship between tumour size and curability and that both dose and schedule were important determinants of cell kill and tumour eradication. The clinical importance of these observations was profound.[40]

This 'log kill' model predicted a dramatic impact for adjuvant chemotherapy in the treatment of early stage breast cancer, given the activity of the existing drugs and regimens in the therapy of metastatic disease. This, however, did not prove to be the case. Adjuvant therapy has had an important impact, but the magnitude of the benefit is relatively small.[41] Nevertheless, the demonstration of an important survival benefit for patients with stages I–II breast[42] and colorectal cancer[43] who receive adjuvant chemotherapy, in multiple, large, random assignment trials, can, in the context of the essential incurability of these cancers when metastatic, be taken as firm clinical evidence that there is an inverse relationship between tumour size and chemocurability. This might, however, be related to mechanisms other than the log cell kill hypothesis; for example more homogeneous vascularization of smaller tumours.

Norton and Simon proposed an alternative model for tumour growth kinetics, and one which went some considerable distance to explaining why the impact of adjuvant therapy had not been more substantial. These researchers hypothesized that tumours grew and regressed according to Gompertzian kinetics. The essential feature of Gompertzian growth is that the rate of growth is not constant, as had been predicted in the exponential model but, rather, varied inversely with the size of the tumour. Thus, large tumours had lower growth fractions than did smaller ones, and hence were less sensitive to cytotoxics. According to this model, patients with overt cancer should first be treated with chemotherapy to reduce their tumour burden, which would place them in the more sensitive phase of their growth curve, at which point eradication might be attempted. Paradoxically, the same rapid regrowth that enhances cytotoxicity, could, in the case of very small amounts of residual cancer cells, also make tumour eradication more difficult, in that any small populations of cells which are resistant to a given cycle of treatment would undergo rapid inapparent regrowth prior to the next cycle. They suggested that cell kill induced by a chemotherapy drug was directly related to the size of the dose, and to the growth rate of the unperturbed tumour at that point in its growth curve.[44] Several randomized trials have tested this hypothesis. The Cancer and Leukemia Group B randomized patients with node-positive breast cancer to receive either intensification (i.e. anthracycline-containing chemotherapy) or further CMF (cyclophosphamide, methotrexate, 5-fluorouracil)[45] as cross-over therapy following a phase of CMF induction. The Italian Oncology Group for Clinical Research (GOIRC) performed a similar study in patients with metastases.[46] While both studies showed advantages of the intensified therapy, it can be argued that both, in fact, showed a benefit for anthracycline, rather than validating the kinetic model.

Another theoretical model which had implications for the field of intensified therapy was that of Goldie and Coldman. These investigators hypothesized that the there was a direct relationship between the size of a tumour and the likelihood that it would contain drug-resistant cells. In addition, resistance could actually develop during treatment by a process of clonal selection. Goldie and Coldman argued for the inclusion of as many active drugs as possible in combination regimens, in an attempt to maximize the chance that all subclones would be eradicated. In the event that overlapping toxicity precluded such coadministration, an alternative strategy would be to administer alternating non-cross resistant regimens.[47] The recommendations of the Goldie–Coldman model were thus at variance with those of the Norton–Simon model, which stressed the need to give active agents at their maximum intensity, both in terms of dose and of schedule, and then to cross-over to other active agents, also to be given in maximum dose and intensity.

A trial of these two approaches, and one which indirectly provided evidence for a dose–response effect in the adjuvant chemotherapy of breast cancer was conducted by Buzzoni, Bonadonna, and colleagues. In this study, patients with breast cancer which involved at least four axillary lymph nodes were randomized to receive one of two different schedules of a cross-over regimen, which consisted of doxorubicin and the CMF combination. In one arm, patients received the doxorubicin in four consecutive cycles, followed by eight cycles of CMF. In the other arm, the doxorubicin and CMF were alternated. Although the planned doses were identical, as were the planned dose intensities of the regimens (using the entire duration of the study as the denominator of time), there was a substantial advantage for the sequential arm, as predicted by the Norton–Simon model.[48]

Importance of maintaining standard dose and intensity in cancer chemotherapy

The quantitative nature of the dose–response relationship is unknown in clinical cancer treatment. A linear relationship between dose and effect may exist at the lower part of the curve but the curve may flatten at higher doses. If so, it may be essential to achieve a minimum standard dose or dose intensity in order to achieve clinical benefit, but increasing the dose or intensity beyond this standard range might not greatly improve the response.

Much of the evidence which is used to support the concept that dose and/or dose intensity are important determinants of anticancer effect deal with variations at the lower end of scale, that is they are studying standard versus lower-dose therapy. This evidence is nonetheless important and indeed it can be argued that the earliest and most important conclusion from the dose intensity debate was that it was important to maintain standard dose and intensity in situations where cure is a reasonable expectation.

The Cancer and Leukemia Group B conducted a randomized trial in which patients with node-positive stage II breast cancer were assigned to receive either low, intermediate, or high-dose intensities of CAF (cyclophosphamide, Adriamycin (doxorubicin), 5-fluorouracil) chemotherapy. The high-intensity arm was clearly superior to the low, with a trend towards a separation of all three survival curves. It is apparent that the high-intensity arm is standard therapy, and that the low-intensity arm is considerably less intensive than standard. These data provide firm evidence that reductions in the doses or intensities of adjuvant programmes for the treatment of early stage breast cancer were inadvisable.[49] Similarly, in the treatment of metastatic breast cancer with CMF chemotherapy, Tannock and colleagues demonstrated the superiority of a more intensive programme over a regimen that was of lower than standard intensity.[50]

These studies indicate that in those circumstances where cure is a reasonable possibility, that reductions in dose and intensity should be avoided. In the light of the strong evidence that colony-stimulating factors can facilitate the maintenance of standard dose intensity in situations where it is threatened by neutropenia and its complications, some clinicians now consider the use of these growth factors to be evidence-based in this setting.[51] However, there is still little evidence of survival benefit in the systematic use of haematopoietic growth factors in the chemotherapy of solid tumours.

Impact of moderate increases in dose and intensity in the clinic

Chemotherapy doses can be escalated or intensified with or without haematopoietic support. With exceptions, the colony-stimulating factors facilitate relatively modest increases in dose and intensity. The occurrence of cumulative myelosuppression, and of thrombocytopenia, limit their utility in the intensification of most drugs.[52] For some putatively stem-cell-sparing agents, which can be given without haematopoietic cellular support (prominently cyclophosphamide and etoposide), the colony-stimulating factors do facilitate substantial dose escalation.[53] For the purposes of this section, moderate dose escalation or intensification is defined as increases in dose and/or dose intensity which do not require autograft support, and will include both agents and combinations which are given with, and those which are given without, colony-stimulating factors. A large number of prospective, random assignment trials have now addressed the issue of moderate dose escalation or intensification in the clinic. In general, these studies have produced marginal and inconsistent results. This finding is not entirely surprising, given the results of the preclinical experiments, which suggested that tumour eradication required relatively extreme degrees of intensification.

In a recent study by the German Hodgkin's Disease Study Group, an escalated version of the regimen BEACOPP (bleomycin, etoposide, doxorubicin, cyclophosphamide, vincristine, prednisolone, procarbazine) was compared to standard BEACOPP, and to COPP/ABVD (cyclophosphamide, vincristine, prednisolone, procarbazine/doxorubicin, bleomycin, vinblastine, dacarbazine). Both BEACOPP regimens were superior to COPP/ABVD, and the intensified BEACOPP was superior to the conventional.[54] In acute myeloid leukaemia, high-dose cytosine arabinoside was shown to be superior to a conventional dose.[55] For patients with aggressive non-Hodgkin's lymphoma, modestly intensified regimens have not consistently been shown to be beneficial.[56]

As discussed above in the section on dose intensity, it seems, on the basis of 12 random assignment trials, that modest dose intensification has only a small impact on survival in the treatment of ovarian cancer.

Dose escalation/intensification has been extensively studied in the treatment of metastatic breast cancer.[57]–[59] In most of these studies,

the more intensive regimens produce higher response rates, with a less consistent impact on survival. In view of the essentially palliative nature of chemotherapy in metastatic breast cancer, the use of moderately escalated therapy is still considered investigational.

The use of moderate dose intensification in the adjuvant treatment of early stage breast cancer has also been addressed in randomised trials. In recent years, a Cancer and Leukemia Group B study, in which patients with node-positive disease were randomly assigned to receive one of three dose levels of doxorubicin, failed to reveal any difference in survival between the arms.[60] The National Surgical Adjuvant Breast and Bowel Project randomly allocated patients with node-positive disease to one of three dose levels of cyclophosphamide consolidation following anthracycline-based induction, and again failed to demonstrate any superiority for the intensified regimen.[61] Levine and colleagues randomly assigned patients with stage II breast cancer to receive either conventional chemotherapy or a short, intensive regimen. No advantage was seen for the intensive programme.[62] Bonneterre and colleagues randomly assigned patients with node-positive breast cancer to receive one of two dose levels of FEC (cyclophosphamide, epirubicin, 5-fluorouracil) chemotherapy, and reported superior survival for patients receiving the higher-dose regimen.[63] In view of the inconsistency of these results, the use of modestly dose-escalated or dose-intensified chemotherapy in the adjuvant treatment of breast cancer cannot yet be considered evidence based.

Small cell lung cancer is another tumour type in which dose escalation/intensification has been extensively studied, again without firm evidence that it offers clinical benefits. Some studies have been completely negative, others suggested modest benefits in reponse,[64] and a few have suggested survival benefits.[65] Again, there is not yet a consensus that intensified therapy is of benefit.

Dose escalation has been studied in testicular cancer,[66] transitional cell carcinoma,[67] sarcoma,[68] and other tumours, without proof that it possesses superiority over conventional therapy for any of these tumours.

In summary, with the exception of the use of high-dose cytosar as consolidative treatment for patients with acute leukaemia who are in remission and now, possibly, the use of intensified BEACOPP chemotherapy for patients with advanced Hodgkin's disease, moderate dose escalation/intensification cannot be recommended in routine cancer treatment. However, it will be obvious that the degree of dose escalation or intensification which was achieved in most of these prospective studies fell far short of that which would have been predicted to be necessary for tumour eradication according to the evidence of the preclinical investigations alluded to above. Very-high-dose chemotherapy with haematopoietic autograft support provides a closer approximation of the dose levels which were achieved in these experiments, and this modality has been the subject of extensive investigation. At present, the data from validated, randomized trials do not support the routine use of this treatment in any non-haematological malignancy. However, it is possible that the dominant high-dose strategy which has been investigated to date, namely the use of single-cycle, high-dose treatment as a form of consolidation following conventional chemotherapy, is unsound. The use of multiple cycles of high-dose chemotherapy as the primary treatment for partially chemotherapy-sensitive malignancies appears to have a sounder theoretical rationale,[69] and is the subject of current investigation in both breast[70] and ovarian cancer.[71]

References

1. Einhorn LH, Donohue JP. Cisdiamminedichloroplatinum, vinblastine and bleomycin combination chemotherapy in disseminated testicular cancer. *Annals of Internal Medicine*, 1977; **87**: 293–8.

2. DeVita VT, Serpick AA, Carbone PP. Combination chemotherapy in the treatment of advanced Hodgkin's Disease. *Annals of Internal Medicine*, 1970; **73**: 891–5.

3. DeVita VT Jr, Canellos GP, Chabner BA, *et al.* Advanced diffuse histiocytic lymphoma, a potentially curable disease. *Lancet*, 1975; **1**: 248–50.

4. Poplack DG, Reaman G. Acute lymphoblastic leukaemia in childhood. *Pediatric Clinics of North America*, 1988; **35**: 903–19.

5. Crown J, Chahinian AP, Glidewell OJ, Kaneko M, Holland JF. Predictors of five year survival and curability in small cell lung cancer. *Cancer*, 1990; **66**: 382–6.

6. Rees JKH, Gray RG, Swirsky D, Hayhoe FGJ. Principal results of the Meducal Research Councils 8th acute myeloid leukaemia trial. *Lancet*, 1988; **ii**: 1236–41.

7. McGuire WP, Ozols RF. Chemotherapy of advanced ovarian cancer. *Seminars in Oncology*, 1998; **25**: 340–8.

8. Cold S, Jensen NV, Brincker H, Rose C. The influence of chemotherapy on survival after recurrence in breast cancer-a population-based study of patients treated in the 1950s, 1960s and the 1970s. *European Journal of Cancer*, 1993; **29A**: 1146–52.

9. Greenberg PAC, Hortobagyi GN, Smith TL, *et al.* Long-term follow-up of patients with complete remission following combination chemotherapy for metastatic breast cancer. *Journal of Clinical Oncology*, 1996; **14**: 2197–205.

10. Ackland SP, Schilsky R. High-dose methotrexate: a critical reappraisal. *Journal of Clinical Oncology*, 1987; **5**: 2017–22.

11. Calvert AH, Newell DR, Gumbrell LA, *et al.* Carboplatin dosage: Prospective evaluation of a simple formula based on renal function. *Journal of Clinical Oncology*, 1989; **7**: 1748–56.

12. Skipper HE, Schabel FM. Quantitative and cytokinetic studies in experimental tumor systems. In: Holland J, Frei FE, ed. *Cancer medicine*. Philadelphia: Lea and Febiger, 1988: 663–84.

13. Teicher BA, Holden SA, Cucchi CA, *et al.* Combination thiotepa and cyclophosphamide *in vivo* and *in vitro*. *Cancer Research*, 1988; **48**: 94–100.

14. Tannock IF, Boyd NF, Deborer G, *et al.* A randomized trial of two dose levels of CMF chemotherapy for patients with metastatic breast cancer. *Journal of Clinical Oncology*, 1988; **6**: 1377–87.

15. Ardizzoni A, Venturini M, Sertoli MR, *et al.* Granulocyte-macrophage colony-stimulating factor (GM-CSF) allows acceleration and dose-intensity increase of CEF chemotherapy: a randomized study in patients with advanced breast cancer. *British Journal of Cancer*, 1994; **69**: 385–91.

16. Hortobagyi GN, Buzdar AU, Bodey GP, *et al.* High-dose induction chemotherapy of metastatic breast cancer in protected environment units: A prospective randomized study. *Journal of Clinical Oncology*, 1987; **5**: 178–84.

17. Lazarus H, Reed MD, Spitzer TR, *et al.* High-dose iv thiotepa and cryopreserved autologous bone marrow transplantation for therapy of refractory cancer. *Cancer Treatment Reports*, 1987; **71**: 689–95.

18. Eder JP, Antman K, Peters WP, *et al.* High-dose combination alkylating agent chemotherapy with autologous marrow support for metastatic breast cancer. *Journal of Clinical Oncology*, 1986; **4**: 1592–7.

19. Hryniuk W, Bush H. The importance of dose intensity in chemotherapy of metastatic breast cancer. *Journal of Clinical Oncology*, 1984; **2**: 81–8.

20. Hryniuk WM, Figueredo A, Goodyear M. Applications of dose intensity to problems in chemotherapy of breast and colorectal cancer. *Seminars in Oncology*, 1987; **14** (Suppl. 4):12–19.

21. Levin L, Hryniuk WM. Dose intensity analysis of chemotherapy regimens in ovarian cancer. *Journal of Clinical Oncology*, 1987; **5**: 756–67.

22. Longo DL, Young RC, Wesley M, *et al.* Twenty years of MOPP chemotherapy for Hodgkin's disease. *Journal of Clinical Oncology*, 1986; **4**: 1295–306.

23. Levine MN, Gent M, Hryniuk WM, *et al.* A randomized trial comparing 12 weeks versus 36 weeks of adjuvant chemotherapy in stage II breast cancer. *Journal of Clinical Oncology*, 1990; **8**: 1217–25.

24. Hryniuk W. Randomized trial of escalated versus standard BACOP for intermediate grade lymphoma. *Proceedings of the American Society of Clinical Oncology*, 1991; **10**: 272.

25. McGuire WP. How many more nails to seal the coffin of dose intensity? *Annals of Oncology*, 1997; **8**: 311–3.

26. Kaye SB, Lewis CR, Paul J, *et al.* Randomized study of two doses of cisplatin and cyclphosphamide in epothelial ovarian cancer. *Lancet*, 1992; **340**: 329–33.

27. Gore M, Mainwaring P, A'Hern R, *et al.* for the London Gynaecological Oncology Group. *Journal of Clinical Oncology*, 1998; **16**: 2426–34.

28. Jakobsen A, Bertelsen K, Andersen JE, Havsteen H, Jakobsen P, Moeller KA, *et al.* Dose-effect study of carboplatin in ovarian cancer: a Danish Ovarian Cancer Group study. *Journal of Clinical Oncology*, 1997; **15**: 193–8.

29. Ngan HY, Choo YC, Cheung M, Wong LC, Ma HK, Collins R, Fung C, Ng CS, Wong V, Ho HC, *et al.* A randomized study of high-dose versus low-dose cis-platinum combined with cyclophosphamide in the treatment of advanced ovarian cancer. Hong Kong Ovarian Carcinoma Study Group. *Chemotherapy*, 1989; **35**: 221–7.

30. Conte PF, Bruzzone M, Carnino F. High dose versus low dose cisplatin in combination with epidoxorubicin and cyclophosphamide in suboptimal ovarian cancer: a randomized trial. *Journal of Clinical Oncology*, 1996; **14**: 351–65.

31. McGuire WP, Hoskins WJ, Brady MF, *et al.* Assessment of dose-intensive therapy in suboptimally debulked ovarian cancer: a Gynecologic Oncology Group study. *Journal of Clinical Oncology*, 1995; **13**: 1589–99.

32. Sutton GP, Stehman FB, Einhorn LH, Roth LM, Blessing JA, Ehrlich CE. Ten-year follow-up of patients receiving cisplatin, doxorubicin, and cyclophosphamide chemotherapy for advanced epithelial ovarian carcinoma. *Journal of Clinical Oncology*, 1989; **7**: 223–9.

33. Murphy D, Crowther D, Renninson J, *et al.* A randomised dose intensity study in ovarian carcinoma comparing chemotherapy given at four week intervals for six cycles with half dose chemotherapy given for twelve cycles. *Annals of Oncology*, 1993; **4**: 377–83.

34. Bella M, Cocconi G, Lottici R, *et al.* Mature results of a prospective randomized trial comparing two different dose-intensity regimens of cisplatin in advanced ovarian cancer [abstract]. *Annals of Oncology*, 1994; **5** (Suppl. 8):2.

35. Colombo N, Pittelli PR, Parma G, Marzola M, Torri W, Mangiono C. Cisplatin dose intensity in advanceed ovarian cancer: a randomized study of conventional dose versus dose-intense cisplatin monochemotherapy. *Proceedings of the American Society of Clinical Oncology*, 1993; **12**: 255.

36. Hakes TB, Chalas E, Hoskins WJ, Jones WB, Markman M, Rubin SC, *et al.* Randomized prospective trial of 5 versus 10 cycles of cyclophosphamide, doxorubicin, and cisplatin in advanced ovarian carcinoma. *Gynecologic Oncology*, 1992; **45**: 284–9.

37. Bertelsen K, Jakobsen A, Stroyer J, *et al.* A prospective randomized comparison of 6 and 12 cycles of cyclophosphamide, adriamycin, and

cisplatin in advanced epithelial ovarian cancer: a Danish Ovarian Study Group trial (DACOVA). *Gynecologic Oncology*, 1993; **49**: 30–6.

38. Fisher RI, Gaynor ER, Dahlberg S, *et al.* Comparison of a standard regimen (CHOP) with three intensive chemotherapy regimens for advanced non-Hodgkin's lymphoma. *New England Journal of Medicine*, 1993; **328**: 1002–6.

39. Hryniuk W, Frei III E, Wright FA. Summation of dose intensity a single scale for comparing dose-intensity of all chemotherapy regimens in breast cancer: summation dose-intensity. *Journal of Clinical Oncology*, 1998; **16**: 3137–47.

40. Skipper HE, Schabel FM. Quantitative and cytokinetic studies in experimental tumor systems. In: Holland J, Frei FE, ed. *Cancer medicine*. Philadelphia: Lea and Febiger, 1988: 663–84.

41. Norton L, Simon R. The Norton-Simon hypothesis revisited. *Cancer Treatment Reports*, 1986; **70**: 163–9.

42. Early Breast Cancer Trialist's Collaborative Group. Systemic treatment of early breast cancer by hormonal, cytotoxic or immune therapy: 133 randomized trials involving 31 000 recurrences and 24 000 deaths among 75 000 women. *Lancet*, 1992; **339**: 1–15.

43. Mamounas E, Wieand S, Wolmark N, *et al.* Comparative efficacy of adjuvant chemotherapy in patients with Dukes' B versus Dukes' C colon cancer: results from four national surgical adjuvant breast and bowel project adjuvant studies (C-01, C-02, C-03, and C-04). *Journal of Clinical Oncology*, 1999; **17**: 1339–49.

44. Norton L, Simon R, Brereton HD, *et al.* Predicting the course of Gompertzian growth. *Nature* (London), 1976; **264**: 542–5.

45. Perloff M, Norton L, Korzun AH, *et al.* Post surgical adjuvant chemotherapy of stage II breast carcinoma with or without crossover to a non-cross-resistant regimen: a Cancer and Leukemia Group B study. *Journal of Clinical Oncology*, 1996; **14**: 1589–98.

46. Cocconi G, Bisagni G, Bacchi M, *et al.* A comparison of continuation versus late intensification followed by discontinuation of chemotherapy in advanced breast cancer. A prospective randomized trial of the Italian Oncology Group for Clinical Research (G.O.I.R.C.). *Annals of Oncology*, 1990; **1**: 36–44.

47. Goldie J, Coldman AJ. A mathematical model for relating the drug sensitivity of tumors to their spontaneous mutation rate. *Cancer Treatment Reports*, 1979; **63**: 1727–73.

48. Buzzoni R, Bonnadonna G, Vallagussa P, *et al.* Adjuvant chemotherapy with doxorubicin plus cyclophosphamide, methotrexate, and flurouracil in the treatment of resectable breast cancer with more than 3 positive axillary nodes. *Journal of Clinical Oncology*, 1994; **9**: 2134–40.

49. Wood WC, Budman DR, Korzun AH, *et al.* Dose and dose-intensity of adjuvant chemotherapy for stage II node-positive breast cancer. *New England Journal of Medicine*, 1994; **330**: 1253–9.

50. Tannock IF, Boyd NF, Deborer G, *et al.* A randomized trial of two dose levels of CMF chemotherapy for patients with metastatic breast cancer. *Journal of Clinical Oncology*, 1988; **6**: 1377–87.

51. Ozer H, Miller LL, Schiffer CA, Winn RJ, Smith TJ. American Society of Clinical Oncology update of recommendations for the use of hematopoietic colony-stimulating factors: evidence-based, clinical practice guidelines. *Journal of Clinical Oncology*, 1996; **14**: 1957–60.

52. O'Dwyer PJ, LaCreta FP, Schilder R, *et al.* Phase I trial of thiotepa in combination with recombinant human granulocyte-macrophage colony-stimulating factor. *Journal of Clinical Oncology*, 1992; **10**: 1352–8.

53. Gianni AM, Bregni M, Siena S, *et al.* Granulocyte-macrophage colony-stimulating factor or granulocyte colony-stimulating factor infusion makes high-dose etoposide a safe outpatient regimen that is effective in lymphoma and myeloma patients. *Journal of Clinical Oncology*, 1992; **10**: 1955–62.

54. Diehl V, Franklin J, Hasenclever D, *et al.* BEACOPP: a new regimen for advanced Hodgkin's disease. German Hodgkin's Lymphoma Study Group. *Annals of Oncology*, 1998; **9** (Suppl 5):S67–71.

55. Bishop JF, Matthews JP, Young GA, *et al.* A randomised study of high-dose cytarabine in induction in acute myeloid leukaemia. *Blood*, 1996; **87**: 1710–17.

56. Hryniuk W. Randomized trial of escalated versus standard BACOP for intermediate grade lymphoma. *Proceedings of the American Society of Clinical Oncology*, 1991; **10**: 272a.

57. Bastholt L, Dalmark M, Gjedde S. Dose-response relationship of epirubicin in the treatment of postmenopausal patients with metastatic breast cancer: a randomized study of epirubicin at four different dose levels performed by the Danish Breast Cancer Cooperative Group. *Journal of Clinical Oncology*, 1996; **14**: 1146–55.

58. Hortobagyi GN, Buzdar AU, Bodey GP, *et al.* High-dose induction chemotherapy of metastatic breast cancer in protected environment units: a prospective randomized study. *Journal of Clinical Oncology*, 1987; **5**: 178–84.

59. Ardizzoni A, Venturini M, Sertoli MR, *et al.* Granulocyte-macrophage colony-stimulating factor (GM-CSF) allows acceleration and dose-intensity increase of CEF chemotherapy: a randomized study in patients with advanced breast cancer. *British Journal of Cancer*, 1994; **69**: 385–91.

60. Henderson IC, Berry D, Demetri G, *et al.* Improved disease-free survival and overall survival from the addition of sequential Paclitaxel but not from the escalation of doxorubicin dose in the adjuvant chemotherapy of patients with node-positive primary breast cancer. *Proceedings of the American Society of Clinical Oncology*, 1998; **17**: 101a.

61. Fisher B, Anderson S, Wickerham DL, *et al.* Increased intensification and total dose of cyclophosphamide in a doxorubicin-cyclophosphamide regimen for the treatment of primary breast cancer: Findings from National Surgical Adjuvant Breast and Bowel Project B-22. *Journal of Clinical Oncology*, 1997; **15**: 1858–69.

62. Levine MN, Gent M, Hryniuk WM, *et al.* A randomized trial comparing 12 weeks versus 36 weeks of adjuvant chemotherapy in stage II breast cancer. *Journal of Clinical Oncology*, 1990; **8**: 1217–25.

63. Bonneterre J, Roché H, Bremond A, *et al.* Results of a randomized trial of adjuvant chemotherapy with FEC 50 vs FEC 100 in high-risk node positive breast cancer patients. *Proceedings of the American Society of Clinical Oncology*, 1998; **17**: 124a.

64. Furuse K, Fukuoka M, Nishiwaki Y, *et al.* Phase III study of intensive weekly chemotherapy with recombinant human granulocyte colony-stimulating factor versus standard chemotherapy in extensive-disease small-cell lung cancer. The Japan Clinical Oncology Group. *Journal of Clinical Oncology*, 1998; **16**: 2126–32.

65. Thatcher N, Lee SM, Woll PJ, *et al.* Dose intensity in small cell lung cancer. *Seminars in Oncology*, 1998; **25** (Suppl. 4):12–18.

66. Ozols RF, Ihde DC, Linehan M, *et al.* A randomized trial of standard chemotherapy versus a high-dose chemotherapy regimen in poor prognosis non-seminomatous germ cell tumours. *Journal of Clinical Oncology*, 1988; **6**: 1031–40.

67. Seidman AD, Scher HI, Gabrilove JL, *et al.* Dose-intensification of MVAC with recombinant granulocyte colony-stimulating factor as initial therapy in advanced urothelial cancer. *Journal of Clinical Oncology*, 1993; **11**: 408–14.

68. Seynaeve C, Verweij J. High-dose chemotherapy in adult sarcomas: no standard yet. *Seminars in Oncology*, 1999; **26**: 119–33.

69. Crown J, Norton L. Potential strategies for improving the results of high-dose chemotherapy in patients with metastatic breast cancer. *Annals of Oncology*, 1995; **6** (Suppl. 4):S21–6.

70. Crown J, Raptis G, Vahdat L, *et al.* Rapidly administration of sequential high-dose cyclophosphamide. melphalan, thiotepa supported

by filgrastim and peripheral blood progenitors in patients with metastatic breast cancer: a novel and very active treatment strategy [abstract]. *Proceedings of the American Society of Clinical Oncology*, 1994; **13**: 110.

71. **Crown J, Wasserheit C, Hakes T,** *et al.* Rapid delivery of multiple high-dose chemotherapy courses with G-CSF and peripheral blood-derived haemopoietic progenitor cells. *Journal of the National Cancer Institute*, 1992; **84**: 1935–6.

New drug development

Robert H. Shoemaker and Edward A. Sausville

Introduction

During the last four decades, the process of anticancer drug discovery has evolved from a largely empirical process to one focused on intervening in the fundamental molecular features of malignant disease. This chapter will provide an overview of the process and history of anticancer drug discovery and development and then address aspects of the evolution of this work that have brought us to the current state of the art. Particular emphasis will be placed on research conducted by the US National Cancer Institute (NCI).

The process of drug discovery and development

The steps in preclinical development of an anticancer drug are illustrated in Fig. 1. This is a generic representation of the process that, as indicated below, has changed considerably over the last 40 years. Lead discovery can be the result of serendipitous observations, systematic screening, or drug design efforts. Lead optimization may involve substantial chemical modification of the lead structure to improve pharmaceutical properties, such as metabolic stability or tissue distribution. This may require extensive pharmacokinetic evaluations in concert with formulation efforts. In the case of natural product drug development, a total synthesis may be possible or semisynthetic derivatives may be prepared in an attempt to improve the properties of the lead molecule. Once an acceptable

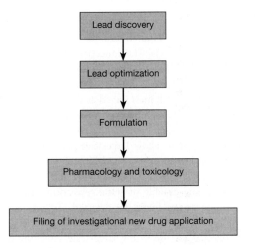

Fig. 1 Steps in preclinical development.

formulation has been obtained, formal pharmacokinetic and toxicology studies are performed to support the filing of an Investigational New Drug Application. A brief discussion of clinical drug development, particularly as it is being impacted by changes in drug discovery strategies, is included at the end of this chapter.

Anticancer drug discovery

Identification and development of the first anticancer drugs

The first approaches to chemotherapy of cancer emerged in the Second World War era. Observations on the lymphosuppressive and myelosuppressive activity of mustard gas suggested a potential role for alkylating agents in treatment of leukaemia.[1],[2] Following the post-war disclosure of clinical therapeutic activity of nitrogen mustard,[3],[4] research on alkylating agents rapidly expanded and led to the approval of several drugs in this class for use in cancer treatment in the late 1940s and early 1950s. Insight into the biochemical mechanisms of action of antibacterial drugs such as sulphonamides stimulated research on antimetabolites as potential antitumour agents. Methotrexate was approved for clinical use in 1953 and four additional antimetabolites were approved in the ensuing decade. The value of natural products as potential sources of new antitumour agents became apparent at about this time. Colchicine, a plant product known as an antimitotic agent, found application in a novel laboratory protocol that made detailed study of lymphocyte cytogenetics possible. The tubulin-binding plant products vinblastine and vincristine were approved for use in cancer treatment in 1961 and 1963, respectively.

In order to access potential antitumour agents that might be present in microbial sources, screening of fermentation broths was pursued in Japan using transplantable rodent tumour models.[5] This work led to the identification of mitomycin C that was approved for use in clinical cancer treatment in 1974, as well as other antitumour antibiotics.

The introduction of transplantable animal tumour models for use in experimental chemotherapy allowed more detailed studies that supported the development of fundamental concepts of the new field of cancer chemotherapy.[6] Insight into tumour growth kinetics, the concept of log cell kill, and combination chemotherapy emerged in the 1950s. By the mid-1950s there was an intense interest in the search for new anticancer drugs: it was being demonstrated that chemotherapy could have clinical therapeutic activity, coupled with the emerging concepts of combination chemotherapy and intensive research on analogues of available alkylating agents, antimetabolites, and the observations that natural sources could be a source for discovery of agents acting by novel mechanisms resulted.

Empirical screening for antitumour activity

The first large-scale effort aimed at anticancer drug discovery was organized by the NCI in 1955 as the Cancer Chemotherapy National Service Center.[7] Transplantable rodent tumour models were used as the primary experimental models for screening. While various models and strategies for use of these models were employed over the lifetime of this programme, the transplantable murine leukaemia models L1210 and P388 were most extensively used for primary screening. These models were relatively rapid and employed lifespan as an objective measure of anticancer effect. While the character of the programme evolved under the influence of a series of peer-reviews, large-scale *in vivo* anticancer drug screening continued under NCI sponsorship up to 1990. During this era, numerous pharmaceutical companies in the United States, Europe, and Japan entered the field of anticancer drug discovery and development. Programmes operated by these companies also relied heavily on the use of transplantable rodent tumour models for the screening and detailed testing of lead drug compounds. Some historical perspective on the use of rodent leukaemia and solid tumour models and the more recent strategies used at Lilly Research Laboratories has been provided by Pearce.[8]

Effectiveness of empirical screens

The impact of the NCI programme on drugs entered into clinical testing and approved for use by the US Food and Drug Administration (FDA) has been summarized by Driscoll in 1984.[9] At the time of that review, 32 drugs (excluding hormonal agents) were approved for use in cancer treatment. Of these, half had been identified prior to initiation of the NCI screening programme. The majority of the newer drugs (11 of 16) were either identified by the NCI screen, or developed with significant input by the NCI. Empirical screening discoveries among this group of new drugs included additional alkylating agents, antimetabolites, antimitotic agents, and antitumour antibiotics. Doxorubicin and cisplatin have been among the most widely used drugs discovered during this period. In the intervening years, the list of FDA drugs has grown to over 50. While additional mechanistic types have been introduced among newer agents, notably paclitaxel and related agents, which promote the polymerization of tubulin and DNA topoisomerase I and II inhibitors, the initial discovery of lead compounds was largely based on empirical screening.

These developments clearly indicated the ability of *in vivo* empirical screens to identify novel compounds with antitumour activity. However, while selected examples could be cited where curative chemotherapy had been enabled by this process, identification of new drugs for treating the most common solid tumours, such as lung, breast, colon, and prostate cancer, remained elusive.[10] For a European perspective on the use and productivity of empirical screens as well as some of the other issues discussed in this chapter see Schwartzman and Workman.[11]

In vitro cytotoxicity testing

Cell culture screens have long played a part in anticancer drug screening. The NCI programme used the KB and P388 cell lines for basic cytotoxicity testing and bioassay-directed isolation of natural products.[12] *In vitro* screening in this application had the advantage of being rapid and amenable to the testing of small amounts of material, including complex mixtures. A retrospective analysis of data from the KB assay, based on response to the positive control compound, demonstrated remarkable stability over a period of more than 20 years.[13] Industrial groups also made use of *in vitro* cell culture screens for natural product drug discovery, sometimes in conjunction with rather ingenious schemes to facilitate dereplication of known compounds.[14]

Application of the human tumour colony-forming assay to new drug screening

The introduction of laboratory methods for cloning human tumour cells from fresh surgical specimens in primary soft-agar culture[15] suggested a new approach to drug screening. Salmon[16] proposed that such cultures, representing tumour stem cell populations with genetic and biochemical features reflecting a variety of solid tumours, might have more relevance to human cancer than transplantable murine tumours or established tumour cell lines. The NCI organized a multicentre project to evaluate this technology for use in new drug screening.[17] Efforts of the group resulted in the development of a standardized protocol that addressed a variety of technical problems associated with processing, culturing, and scoring colony formation[18] and allowed a small-scale pilot screening project to go ahead. While the overall conclusion of this project was that the technology was not appropriate for use in large-scale screening, two novel clinical testing candidates, which demonstrated *in vivo* activity in human tumour xenograft models, emerged from this project.[19]–[21] Dihydrolenperone produced marked sedation at doses associated with plasma concentrations consistent with *in vitro* inhibition of tumour colony formation.[20] Chloroquinoxaline sulphonamide demonstrated some evidence of antitumour activity in a phase I trial that employed a 1 h infusion every 28 days.[22] A subsequent trial of this compound in non-small cell lung cancer using weekly treatment did not show antitumour effects.[23] No mechanism of action has yet been established for the preclinical growth inhibitory activity of either dihydrolenperone or chloroquinoxaline sulphonamide.

Development of the NCI 60 tumour cell line screen

The number of established human tumour cell lines expanded rapidly during the 1970s and 1980s. The concerted effort of investigators at the NCI Navy Medical Oncology Branch produced hundreds of well-characterized lung cancer cell lines representing various histological types.[24] These tumour cell lines served as the nucleus for developing a new approach to *in vitro* antitumour drug screening.[25] Automated assay methodology, compatible with the use of 96-well microculture plates, was developed to allow large-scale screening using disease-oriented panels of human tumour cell lines.[26],[27]

The fundamental hypothesis underlying this screening strategy was that new agents capable of selectively affecting the growth of particular tumour types might be detected. To this end, cell line panels composed of 60 cell lines representing a variety of tumour types were selected for use in the large-scale screening of synthetic compounds and crude natural product extracts.[28],[29] Dose–response screening of each compound or extract against 60 cell lines was found to generate a complex form of data that required specialized treatment. Computerized graphic data display formats and pattern recognition programs, such as COMPARE, rapidly demonstrated the information-rich character of this screen.[30] An unexpected finding was that the screen had remarkable powers in helping identify the mechanism of growth inhibition or cell killing. This was initially observed by simple comparisons of MEAN GRAPH patterns, and COMPARE was subsequently shown to extend to numerous mechanistic groups of antitumour agents (see reference 31 for a review). Biochemical and molecular characterization of the tumour cells with respect to drug resistance and sensitivity phenotypes has helped explain the basis for this phenomenon. Additional approaches to detailed analysis of the data contained in this database, and relating it to the growing body of information on molecular characterization of the tumour cell lines, have been reported.[32],[33] Much of the screening data and analytical tools generated by this program have been made publicly available for access and downloading via the Developmental Therapeutics Program website (http://www.dtp.nci.nih.gov/).

As in the case of previous *in vitro* screens, this cell line panel has operated in concert with *in vivo* testing of lead compounds. In fact, their usefulness as *in vivo* xenografts was a major consideration in selecting cell lines for inclusion in the panel.[34] Special consideration was given to cell lines useful in orthotopic or metastatic models.[35],[36] More recently, Hollingshead *et al.*[37] have developed a novel hollow fibre model that allows testing of multiple tumour cell lines implanted into mice at various anatomical locations. This short-term, relatively inexpensive model has been shown to be useful in generating initial information regarding the pharmaceutical potential of *in vitro* drug screening leads.

Since screening began in 1990, more than 70 000 pure synthetic compounds and a comparable number of crude natural products have been tested. The majority of samples screened either lacked cytotoxicity or affected all cell lines in a similar manner. A few compounds, such as the brain tumour-selective ellipticiniums,[38] have generated patterns associated with particular tumour types. Other compounds have generated novel patterns of activity (patterns shown to be distinct from established anticancer agents) and have been selected for *in vivo* testing. A recent review[39] indicated that approximately 5000 synthetic compounds demonstrated activity of interest in the primary screen. Approximately 1600 of these were selected for *in vivo* studies, 39 had evidence of *in vivo* activity, and five had started phase I clinical testing. These latter compounds incorporate agents that apparently act via novel mechanisms, including antagonism of protein kinase and disruption of glycoprotein processing.

As mentioned above, the power of the cell line screen in identifying mechanisms of cytotoxicity has aided in identifying and prioritizing *in vitro* screening leads for *in vivo* evaluation. The screen has also demonstrated value as a basic research tool. As a recent example of this, Duesbery *et al.*[40] utilized the screening pattern obtained with the anthrax lethal factor to infer action via inhibition of MAP-kinase-kinase. Detailed laboratory studies confirmed this as the mode of action of this toxin molecule. This insight may allow the development of strategies to circumvent the toxic effects of anthrax.

Relative merits of *in vivo* versus *in vitro* screens

As discussed above, primary *in vivo* screens have been effective in identifying clinically useful drugs. Such screens intrinsically incorporate critically important issues of drug distribution, pharmacokinetics, and toxicity to normal tissues. However, this modelling is far from perfect, in that these pharmacological features are represented as they occur in the animal host used for the experiments. Significant departures from human metabolism, pharmacokinetics, and toxicology have been observed for particular compounds. In addition, the logistical and cost considerations in handling, maintaining, and accessioning data from *in vivo* studies limit their use in large-scale screening.

Cell-based *in vitro* screens cannot model drug distribution, pharmacokinetics, or toxicity to normal tissues. Biochemical screens do not even represent cell membrane barriers, which may prevent a potent enzyme inhibitor from affecting an intracellular target. Drug leads emerging from such screens must therefore be further qualified to demonstrate potential for *in vivo* activity and frequently require substantial chemical optimization to identify clinical development candidates with appropriate pharmaceutical properties. As discussed below, recent technological advances have increased the efficiency of *in vitro* screens applicable to anticancer drug discovery.

The scientific mandate for molecular targeted screens

The rapidly emerging data from the Human Genome Project and from private sequencing endeavours are providing an unprecedented opportunity for new drug discovery. Exploiting this opportunity for the development of novel anticancer agents will require the identification and characterization of genes that may serve as targets for these new agents. The Cancer Genome Anatomy Project is already providing information that is useful in this context. Functional and structural characterization of cancer-related gene products will be fundamental to this effort and will enable identification of inhibitors through molecular modelling and screening approaches.

Certain molecular targets have already been selected by industry for screening. Many of these have been apparent for some time[41] and now include genes and proteins involved in cell cycle control, signal transduction, and targets related to the processes of metastasis and angiogenesis. The development of new mouse models of human cancer, created using mutagenesis, gene knockout, transgenic, and xenografting technology, has provided further rationale for focusing on molecular targets in drug discovery. This form of targeted drug discovery has considerable implications for clinical evaluation strategies, as discussed below. Selected examples of the convergence of targeted drug discovery opportunities and availability of novel *in vivo* models are described in the following.

- In the area of cell cycle control, heterozygous mutation of the tumour suppressor Rb gene has been shown to lead to mice that develop pituitary tumours.[42] The Rb gene functions as a negative regulator of the transcription factor E2F and its loss therefore can result in uncontrolled cell proliferation.[43] A targeted screen for antagonists of E2F could potentially yield anti-E2F drugs with activity against tumours lacking functional Rb protein. Candidate anti-E2F drugs could be appropriately evaluated in Rb-mutant mice to verify activity in a model known to present the relevant molecular target *in vivo*.

- The potential importance of tyrosine kinase signalling as a target for anticancer drug development has been recognized.[44] In a transgenic mouse model, Daley *et al.*[45] demonstrated that introduction of the p210bcr/abl gene, with its associated tyrosine kinase activity, resulted in a form of chronic myelogenous leukaemia similar to that observed in patients bearing this gene. Preclinical therapeutic exploitation of this target using a small molecule inhibitor, developed from an empirical screening lead, was recently reported using xenotransplanted human leukaemia cells bearing the Philadelphia chromosome.[46]

- Creation of transgenic mice expressing the E6 and E7 oncoproteins encoded by human papilloma virus type 16 has provided a novel model of human cervical cancer.[47] The invasive cervical tumours that arise when transgenic mice are chronically treated with oestrogen provide an *in vivo* model for the evaluation of new agents targeting processes associated with these oncoproteins.

- Transgenic mice overexpressing N-ras have been used to demonstrate the therapeutic effect of a novel inhibitor (L-744,832) of ras processing.[48] This compound, which was developed as a ras farnesylation inhibitor,[49] has recently been shown to be therapeutic in mouse mammary tumour virus-transforming growth factor transgenic mice, which provide a long latency model of breast cancer with activation of receptor tyrosine kinase signaling.[50] This latter observation illustrates the potential importance of *in vivo* studies in helping to identify additional activities of compounds selected for activity *in vitro*.

The advent of high-throughput screening technology

Continuing advances in laboratory automation and robotics and assay technology have allowed huge increases in screening capacity. During the last 10 years large pharmaceutical companies have invested heavily in this technology for use in many disease areas, including cancer. With relatively modest investments in automation equipment and plate reading instrumentation, throughput in the order of 5000–10 000 samples per day can be achieved in high-throughput (single concentration) mode using the long-standard 96-well plates. Full robotic laboratory operations can substantially exceed this rate.

The nature of the screening assay itself has a major impact on throughput. The current trend is towards 'homogeneous' assays that avoid plate washing or filtration steps. The development of new microplate readers, suitable for use with assay endpoints such as time-resolved fluorescence or fluorescence polarization, has been critical to implementation of such assays. Higher density microculture assay plates and off-the-shelf automation equipment are now available at the 384-well per plate density that allows a considerable reduction in sample and reagent consumption and further increases potential assay throughput. More radical changes in assay format and the reduction of working volumes to the nanolitre scale are currently under development. This requires the development of novel sample handling equipment to be made practical, but may offer quantum increases in screening assay throughput.

Chemical diversity

The advent of high-throughput screening technology has created new opportunities for evaluating very large numbers of chemical compounds. New methods for generating chemical 'libraries' by combinatorial chemistry have been developed during the last 10 years that complement high-throughput screening technology by providing very large numbers of structurally diverse compounds. Combinatorial methods have evolved from an orientation towards generating peptide[51] and oligonucleotide libraries to methods that emphasize small-molecule libraries.[52] Sophisticated computer software has been developed to support the design and synthesis of combinatorial libraries and also to assess the chemical diversity of the libraries.[53] Considerable differences in philosophy have existed regarding the extent of diversity that is desirable in the libraries. Some groups have argued that screening the largest libraries with the maximal structural diversity is the best approach in identifying novel pharmacophores that address molecular targets of interest; whereas others argue that smaller libraries of compounds designed to represent samplings of 'chemical space' are adequate to find initial leads that can be further explored in additional iterations of combinatorial library synthesis.

Natural products have continued to serve as an important source of novel antitumour drug leads.[54] Many natural product molecules identified in various screening programmes have also proven useful as biochemical reagents that have been critical in dissecting cellular processes such as mitosis and protein trafficking and processing. Indeed, the diversity and effectiveness of natural products as inhibitors of enzymatic processes and macromolecular interactions have led some investigators to advocate combinatorial synthesis of 'natural product-like' libraries characterized by the incorporation of rigid three-dimensional backbones.

The NCI has created a repository of more than one hundred thousand natural product extracts based on world-wide collections of plants, lichens, blue–green algae, fungi, marine organisms, and other sources.[55] This repository has yielded antihuman immunodeficiency virus drug leads with clinical potential[56] as well as novel anticancer leads[57] and constitutes a unique source of chemical diversity that complements the NCI's library of several hundred thousand synthetic compounds amassed since the mid-1950s. The application of high-throughput screening technology to these sources of chemical diversity offers a powerful approach to discovery of novel drug leads addressing the growing body of molecular targets relevant to cancer.

Structural biology and molecular modelling

In instances where structural information is available for a particular target, molecular modelling may allow *de novo* design of drug molecules. Alternatively, consideration of structure–activity information may be combined with structural information to guide chemical synthesis. Crystallographic and protein databases are growing at a very rapid pace. New information management tools, including tools for the integration of nucleic acid and protein sequence information with structural and functional information (e.g. the US National Library of Medicine's Pubnet system), make accessing and utilizing key information relatively easy for anyone with access to the Internet. Chemical structure information is increasingly available, including the NCI's chemical database with much of the screening data described above. Existing information on known protein–ligand interactions can give important clues to the basis for structure–activity relations and suggest drug design strategies. Publicly accessible protein-ligand databases with easy to use interfaces are already available via the Internet.

Preclinical anticancer drug development

Lead optimization

Many natural product drug leads are large, complex molecules that are either not amenable to chemical synthesis, or cannot be synthesized in an economically feasible way. While this may prevent optimization of leads using classical medicinal chemistry approaches, semisynthetic modification can, in some instances, improve aqueous solubility or other pharmaceutical properties of the lead molecule.

It may be possible to optimize synthetic leads through the use of combinatorial chemistry or the parallel synthesis of analogues. The objectives of this process are the same as in more classical medicinal chemistry approaches and may focus on improving the potency of the lead molecule or focus on specific problems with the lead molecule, such as metabolic inactivation or unfavourable pharmacokinetics. In the case of target-directed therapy, retention of activity at the target must be monitored throughout the lead optimization process.

Formulation

Once a molecule has been identified for clinical development, a suitable formulation must be defined. This process may blend with optimization of the lead compound whose limiting solubility properties may be the focus for synthesizing analogues. As initial clinical trials of anticancer agents have been traditionally conducted using intravenous formulations, this is generally the focus for the formulation efforts. Useful formulations must have reasonable stability and shelf-life characteristics and be relatively simple to prepare for administration.[58] Characterization of the former properties, as well as characterization of the chemical composition of the product, are essential features of a formulated product. In practice each formulation project requires individualized handling and various strategies are required.[59]

Advances in formulation methodology, such as the use of cyclodextrins and liposomes, have increased the options for formulating difficult molecules. Similarly, developments in drug delivery technology, such as implantable or transdermal devices, may make otherwise intractable molecules available for clinical testing.

The potential for developing novel drugs with a high degree of selectivity for molecular targets uniquely expressed in malignant cells may allow the development of relatively non-toxic drugs consistent with the use of oral dosing forms on chronic schedules of administration. This will introduce issues of oral bioavailability into the lead drug optimization and formulation process.

Pharmacology and toxicology

In developing cytotoxic agents for use in cancer chemotherapy, preclinical toxicology studies have been primarily oriented towards establishing safe starting doses for clinical trials and predicting qualitative and quantitative toxicities that may be encountered when the

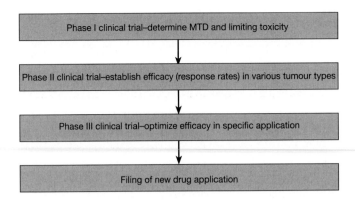

Fig. 2 Steps in 'traditional' clinical development.

agent is used in the clinic. Toxicology protocols developed during the early 1980s have led to the use of one-tenth of the mouse LD_{10} value as the usual dose for the initiation of clinical testing.[60] Testing in an additional species, such as the dog is considered in making predictions about toxicities that may be observed in humans.[61]

Preclinical pharmacokinetic information has provided a useful background to clinical testing in phase I, which has been oriented towards establishing maximally tolerated doses. Indeed, efforts have been made to utilize these data to optimize dosage escalation schemes in phase I testing.[62] With the advent of standardized methods for the culture and assay of relevant bone marrow cell populations,[63] data on susceptibility of these normal cellular elements to the toxic effects of new agents have increasingly been integrated with toxicology work.

The development of agents with a high degree of specificity for molecular targets uniquely expressed in malignant cells will require different handling. In this case the optimal therapeutic dose may be well below the maximal tolerated dose. Pharmacokinetic data from preclinical efficacy studies will have to serve as a guide in conducting toxicology studies oriented towards establishing safe starting doses for clinical trials.

Clinical anticancer drug development

The cytotoxic nature of agents employed for cancer chemotherapy has required the development of specialized strategies for clinical development. Figure 2 illustrates what has come to represent a relatively standard scheme for clinical testing. Phase I clinical trials have been conducted with the objectives of defining the maximum tolerated dose on a particular schedule of administration and defining toxic effects of the treatment. (For a discussion of some of the major issues in phase I testing, see Von Hoff et al.[64]) As mentioned above, pharmacokinetic data from preclinical studies can be integrated with clinical pharmacokinetic data for use as a guide to efficient and appropriate dose escalation. Phase II studies are conducted to establish efficacy on a regimen supported by the phase I results. Testing has generally been conducted in a variety of different tumour types with the aim of identifying tumour types responsive to the agent. Statistical guidelines have been established to determine the minimum number of patients with a particular tumour type that must be studied in order to avoid missing an agent with a potentially useful response

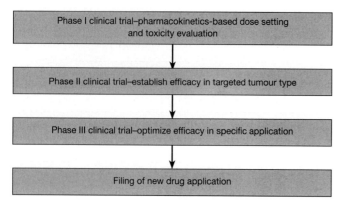

Fig. 3 Steps in 'molecular-targeted' clinical development.

rate.[65] New drugs with demonstrated efficacy are then tested in advanced (phase III) trials to optimize activity and more fully define clinical indications for their use. Registration, or FDA approval, can then be sought for new drugs with proven efficacy for a given indication. This schema for testing drugs, the establishment of a maximal tolerated dose in phase I, and the screening of tumour types to identify clinical target populations in phase II, evolved from experience in developing antiproliferative agents for cancer treatment. The precedent for optimal activity of these agents at, or near, the maximal tolerated dose is based on a large foundation of preclinical and clinical research.

Future pathways for clinical testing may more closely follow the scheme illustrated in Fig. 3. The development of new agents with a high degree of specificity for molecular targets, unique to a particular form of malignancy, will have a clinical target population from the outset. Phase I studies will be required to establish the feasibility of achieving plasma, tissue, and tumour concentrations consistent with achieving a therapeutic effect. This may be based on concentrations of drug attained in specialized animal models of human cancer or from *in vitro* data. Phase I studies will also need to define toxic effects associated with human use of the new agent and phase II studies will be directed towards defining antitumour efficacy and action of the agent at the level of the molecular target. As above, phase III studies will be oriented towards optimizing activity and more fully defining clinical indications.

Conclusions

Advances in understanding cancer at the molecular level are creating new opportunities for developing selective therapies. Application of high-throughput screening assays addressing novel targets and exploiting sources of chemical diversity available from natural products or created through combinatorial chemistry is likely to produce novel drug leads with the potential for a substantially improved therapeutic index. Optimization of these leads through modern medicinal chemistry, use of structural information and molecular modelling approaches, and evaluation of optimized drug candidates in relevant animal models of human cancer may provide substantially improved candidates for clinical trials in the next decade.

References

1. **Marshal EK, Jr.** Historical perspectives in chemotherapy. Goldin A, Hawking IF (eds). *Advances in chemotherapy.* New York: Academic Press, 1964; **1**: 1–8.
2. **DeVita VT.** The evolution of therapeutic research in cancer. *New England Journal of Medicine*, 1978; **298**: 907–10.
3. **Gilman A, Philips FS.** The biological actions and therapeutic applications of the β-chlorethyl amines and sulfides. *Science*, 1946; **1103**: 409–15.
4. **Goodman LS, Wintrobe MM, Dameshek W, Goodman MJ, Gilman A, McLennan MT.** Nitrogen mustard therapy; use of methyl-bis(beta-chloroethyl)amine hydrochloride and tris(betachloroethyl)amine hydrochloride ('nitrogen mustards') in the therapy of Hodgkin's disease, lymphosarcoma, leukemia, and certain allied and miscellaneous disorders. *Journal of the American Medical Association*, 1946; **132**: 126–32.
5. **Umezawa H,** *et al.* Studies on anti-tumor substances produced by microorganisms. III. On sarkomycin produced by a strain resembling *Streptomyces erythrochromogenes. Journal of Antibiotics*, 1953; **A6**: 147–52.
6. **Skipper HE, Schabel FM, Wilcox WS.** Experimental evaluation of potential anticancer agents: XII. On the criteria and kinetics associated with 'curability' of experimental leukemia. *Cancer Chemotherapy Reports*, 1964; **35**: 1–111.
7. **Zubrod CG.** Origins and development of chemotherapy research at the National Cancer Institute. *Cancer Chemotherapy Reports*, 1984; **68**: 9–19.
8. **Pearce HL.** Anticancer drug development at Lilly Research Laboratories. *Annals of Oncology*, 1995; **6**: 55–62.
9. **Driscoll JS.** The preclinical new drug research program of the National Cancer Institute. *Cancer Treatment Reports*, 1984; **68**: 63–76.
10. **Marsoni S, Hoth D, Simon R, Leyland-Jones B, De Rosa M, Wittes R.** Clinical drug development: an analysis of phase II trials,, 1970–1985. *Cancer Treatment Reports*, 1987; **71**: 71–80.
11. **Schwartzman G, Workman P.** Anticancer drug screening and discovery in the, 1990's: a European perspective. *European Journal of Cancer*, 1992; **29A**: 3–14.
12. **Geran RI,** *et al.* Protocols for screening chemical agents and natural products against animal tumors and other biological systems. *Cancer Chemotherapy Reports*, 1972; **3**: 1–103.
13. **Shoemaker RH, Abbott BJ, Macdonald MM, Mayo JG, Venditti JM, Wolpert-DeFilippes MK.** Use of the KB cell line for *in vitro* cytotoxicity assays. *Cancer Treatment Reports*, 1983; **67**: 97.
14. **Hanka LJ, Bhuyan BK, Martin DG, Neil GL, Douros JD.** A multi-end point *in vitro* system for detection of new antitumor drugs. *Antibiotic Chemotherapy*, 1978; **23**: 26–32.
15. **Hamburger AW, Salmon SE.** Primary bioassay of human tumor stem cells. *Science*, 1977; **197**: 461–3.
16. **Salmon SE.** Applications of the human tumor stem cell assay to new drug evaluation and screening. *Progress in Clinical Biology Research*, 1980; **48**: 291–312.
17. **Shoemaker RH,** *et al.* Application of a human tumor colony forming assay to new drug screening. *Cancer Research*, 1985; **45**: 2145–53.
18. **Shoemaker RH, Wolpert-DeFilippes MK, Venditti JM.** Potentials and drawbacks of the human tumor stem cell assay. *Behring Institute Mitteilungen*, 1984; **74**: 262–72.
19. **Shoemaker RH.** New approaches to antitumor drug screening: the human tumor colony forming assay. *Cancer Treatment Reports*, 1986; **70**: 9–11B.
20. **Johnson BE,** *et al.* Phase I trial of dihydrolenperone in lung cancer patients, a novel compound with *in vitro* activity against lung cancer. *Investigational New Drugs*, 1993; **11**: 29–37.

21. Fisherman JS, *et al.* Chloroquinoxaline sulfonamide: a sulfanilamide antitumor agent entering clinical trials. *Investigational New Drugs*, 1993; **11**: 1–9.

22. Rigas JR, Tong WP, Kris MG, Orazem JP, Young CW, Warrell RP, Jr. Phase I clinical and pharmacological study of chloroquinoxaline sulfonamide. *Cancer Research*, 1992; **52**: 6619–23.

23. Miller VA, *et al.* Phase II trial of chloroquinoxaline sulfonamide (CQS) in patients with stage III and IV non-small-cell lung cancer. *Cancer Chemotherapy and Pharmacology*, 1997; **40**: 415–18.

24. Phelps RM, *et al.* NCI-Navy Medical Oncology Branch cell line data base. *Journal of Cellular Biochemistry*, 1996; **24** (Suppl): 32–91.

25. Shoemaker R, *et al.* Development of human tumor cell lines for use in disease-oriented drug screening. *Progress in Clinical Biology Research*, 1988; **276**: 265–86.

26. Alley MC, *et al.* Feasibility of drug screening with panels of human tumor cell lines using a microculture tetrazolium assay. *Cancer Research*, 1988; **48**: 589–601.

27. Skehan P, *et al.* New colorimetric cytotoxicity assay for anticancer-drug screening. *Journal of the National Cancer Institute*, 1990; **82**: 1107–12.

28. Monks A, *et al.* Feasibility of a high-flux anticancer drug screen utilizing a diverse panel of cultured human tumor cell lines. *Journal of the National Cancer Institute*, 1991; **83**: 757–66.

29. Boyd MR. The NCI *in vitro* anticancer drug discovery screen; concept, implementation and operation, 1985–1995. In: Teicher BA (ed.). *Cancer Drug discovery and development, Vol. 2: Drug development: preclinical screening, clinical trial, and approval.* Totowa, NJ: Humana Press, 1997; **2**: 23–42.

30. Paull KD, *et al.* Display and analysis of patterns of differential activity of drugs against human tumor cell lines: development of mean graph and COMPARE algorithm. *Journal of the National Cancer Institute*, 1989; **81**: 1088–92.

31. Boyd MR, Paull KD. Some practical considerations and applications of the National Cancer Institute *in vitro* anticancer drug discovery screen. *Drug Development Research*, 1995; **34**: 91–109.

32. Weinstein JN, *et al.* An information-intensive approach to the molecular pharmacology of cancer. *Science*, 1997; **275**: 343–9.

33. Shi LM, *et al.* Mining the NCI anticancer drug discovery databases: genetic function approximation for the QSAR study of anticancer ellipticine analogues. *Journal of Chemical Information and Computer Science*, 1998; **38**: 189–99.

34. Shoemaker RH, *et al.* Human tumor xenograft models for use with an *in vitro* based, disease-oriented antitumor drug screening program. In: Winograd B, Peckham MG, Pinedo HM (eds). *Human tumor xenografts in anticancer drug development.* European School of Oncology Monograph. Berlin: Springer-Verlag, 1988: 115–20.

35. McLemore TL, *et al.* A novel intrapulmonary model for the orthotopic propagation of human lung cancers in athymic nude mice. *Cancer Research*, 1987; **47**: 5132–40.

36. Shoemaker RH, *et al.* Practical spontaneous metastasis model for *in vivo* therapeutic studies using a human melanoma. *Cancer Research*, 1991; **51**: 2837–41.

37. Hollingshead MG, *et al.* In vivo cultivation of tumor cells in hollow fibers. *Life Science*, 1995; **57**: 131–41.

38. Acton EM, Narayanan VL, Risbood P, Shoemaker RH, Vistica DT, Boyd MR. Anticancer specificity of some ellipticinium salts against human brain tumors *in vitro*. *Journal of Medicinal Chemistry*, 1994; **37**: 2185–9.

39. Monks A, Scudiero DA, Johnson GS, Paull KD, Sausville EA. The NCI anti-cancer drug screen: a smart screen to identify effectors of novel targets. *Anticancer Drug Design*, 1997; **12**(7): 533–41.

40. Duesbery NS, *et al.* Proteolytic inactivation of MAP-kinase-kinase by anthrax lethal factor. *Science*, 1998; **280** (5364): 734–7.

41. Johnson RK. Mechanism-based discovery of anticancer agents. *Annual Reports of Medicinal Chemistry*, 1990; **25**: 129–40.

42. Jacks T, Fazeli A, Schmitt EM, Bronson RT, Goodell MA, Weinberg RA. Effects of an Rb mutation in the mouse. *Nature*, 1992; **359**: 295–300.

43. McCormick F, Meyers P. From genetics to chemistry: tumor suppressor genes and drug discovery. *Chemistry and Biology*, 1994; **1**: 7–9.

44. Levitski A, Gazit A. Tyrosine kinase inhibition: an approach to drug development. *Science*, 1995; **267**: 1782–8.

45. Daley GQ, Van Etten RA, Baltimore D. Induction of chronic myelogenous leukemia in mice by the p210bcr/abl gene of the Philadelphia chromosome. *Science*, 1990; **247**: 824–30.

46. Le Coutre P, *et al.* In vivo eradication of human BRC/ABL-positive leukemia cells with an ABL kinase inhibitor. *Journal of the National Cancer Institute*, 1999; **91**: 163–8.

47. Arbeit JM, Howley PM, Hanahan D. Chronic estrogen-induced cervical and vaginal squamous carcinogenesis in human papillomavirus type 16 transgenic mice. *Proceedings of the National Academy of Sciences USA*, 1996; **93**: 2930–5.

48. Mangues R, *et al.* Antitumor effect of a farnesyl protein transferase inhibitor in mammary and lymphoid tumors overexpressing N-ras in transgenic mice. *Cancer Research*, 1998; **58**: 1253–9.

49. Heimbrook DC, Oliff A. Therapeutic intervention and signaling. *Current Opinion in Cell Biology*, 1998; **10**: 284–8.

50. Norgaard P, *et al.* Treatment with farnesyl-protein transferase inhibitor induces regression of mammary tumors in transforming growth factor (TGF) 'and TGF'/neu transgenic mice by inhibition of mitogenic activity and induction of apoptosis. *Clinical Cancer Research*, 1999; **5**: 35–42.

51. Houghten RA. The broad utility of soluble peptide libraries for drug discovery. *Gene*, 1993; **137**: 7–11.

52. Hoekstra WJ, Poulter BL. Combinatorial chemistry techniques applied to nonpeptide integrin antagonists. *Current Medicinal Chemistry*, 1998; **5**: 195–204.

53. Bures MG, Martin YC. Computational methods in molecular diversity and combinatorial chemistry. *Current Opinion in Chemical Biology*, 1998; **2**: 376–80.

54. Pettit GR. Progress in the discovery of biosynthetic anticancer drugs. *Journal of Natural Products*, 1996; **59**: 812–21.

55. Cragg GM, Newman DJ, Weiss RB. Coral reefs, forests, and thermal vents: the worldwide exploration of nature for novel antitumor agents. *Seminars in Oncology*, 1997; **24**: 156–63.

56. Fuller RW, *et al.* HIV-Inhibitory coumarins from latex of the tropical rainforest tree *Calophyllum teysmannii* var. *inophylloide*. *Bioorganic and Medicinal Chemistry Letters*, 1994; **4**: 1961–4.

57. Beutler JA, *et al.* Antiviral and antitumor plant metabolites. In: Arnason JT, Romeo JT (eds). *Phytochemistry of medicinal plants.* New York: Plenum Press, 1995: 47–64.

58. Davignon JP, Cradock JC. The formulation of anticancer drugs. In: Hellman S, Carter SK (eds). *Fundamentals of cancer chemotherapy.* New York: McGraw-Hill, 1987: 212–27.

59. Beijnen JH, Flora KP, Halbert GW, Henrar RE, Slack JA. CRC/EORTC/NCI Joint Formulation Working Party: experiences in the formulation of investigational cytotoxic drugs. *British Journal of Cancer*, 1995; **72**: 210–18.

60. Grieshaber CK, Marsoni S. Relation of preclinical toxicology to findings in early clinical trials. *Cancer Treatment Reports*, 1986; **70**: 65–72.

61. Greishaber CK. Prediction of human toxicity of new antineoplastic drugs from studies in animals. In: Powis G, Hacker MP (eds). *The toxicity of anticancer drugs.* New York: Pergamon Press, 1991.

62. Collins JM, Greishaber CK, Chabner BA. Pharmacologically guided

phase I clinical trials based upon preclinical drug development. *Journal of the National Cancer Institute*, 1990; **82**: 1321–6.

63. **Parchment RE, Gordon MA, Grieshaber CK, Sessa CA, Volpe D, Ghielmini M.** Predicting hematological toxicity (myelosuppression) of cytotoxic drug therapy from *in vitro* tests. *Annals of Oncology*, 1998; **9**: 357–64.

64. **Von Hoff DD, Kuhn J, Clark GM.** Design and conduct of phase I clincal trials. In: Buyse ME, Staquet MJ, Sylvester RJ (eds). *Cancer clinical trials: methods and practice*. Oxford University Press, 1984: 210–20.

65. **Simon R.** Optimal two-stage designs for phase II clinical trials. *Controlled Clincal Trials*, 1989; **10**: 1–10.

4.23 Regional chemotherapy

Harald J. Hoekstra

Introduction

Regional chemotherapy is the direct infusion of chemotherapy into the arterial supply of a tumour-bearing area or the instillation of chemotherapy into a body cavity, including intraperitoneal, intravesical, and intrathecal chemotherapy. Regional chemotherapy is therefore only appropriate for regionally confined malignancies.

The theory behind regional chemotherapy is that a high drug uptake by the tumour may be achieved with higher doses of antineoplastic agents without increasing systemic toxicity. Intra-arterial infusion may also be combined with radiation treatment, to increase the tumoricidal effect. In this combination treatment the antineoplastic agent may act as a radiation sensitizer.

There is a major difference between intra-arterial infusion and regional perfusion. During intra-arterial infusion the antineoplastic agent is delivered through an intra-arterial catheter to the tumour-bearing area. Placement of the catheter can be performed surgically or non-surgically with percutaneous catheter placement under fluoroscopy. During regional perfusion a part of the body or a whole organ is exclusively perfused. The arterial supply and the venous outflow are connected to an extracorporeal circulation system with a membrane oxygenator, isolating the limb or organ from the systemic circulation (Fig. 1). After the perfusion the normal circulation is restored. Large doses of antineoplastic agents may be delivered, where only low drug concentrations are reached in the systemic circulation. This is attended with minor or no systemic side-effects. Dose limitations in perfusion are dependent only on locoregional toxicity. The major advantages of perfusion over infusion include the potential use of a wider range of perfusion compounds, the ability to control a number of variables such as temperature, oxygen tension and pH, and the reduction in systemic leakage of the perfusate to the general circulation (Table 1).

Renewed interest in regional chemotherapy, especially perfusion and intraperitoneal chemotherapy, is based on the results achieved recently with regional perfusion techniques using tumour necrosis factor (TNF), and on the applicability of adjuvant intraperitoneal chemotherapy after extensive surgical resections for peritonitis carcinomatosis of ovarian or colon cancer.

The development of regional therapy, the pharmacological considerations, and the indications for different types of regional chemotherapy are reviewed in the present chapter.

Development of regional chemotherapy

The first intra-arterial chemotherapy treatment was performed by Klopp in 1950 by injection of nitrogen mustard directly into the arterial supply of a malignant tumour.[1] Sullivan introduced the technique of continuous intra-arterial infusion later that decade.[2] Attempts to reduce the systemic toxicity associated with intra-arterial infusion led Creech and Krementz to develop the technique of isolated limb perfusion for the treatment of limb melanoma and sarcomas with chemotherapy.[3] In the 1960s Cavaliere performed the first hyperthermic isolated regional perfusion, showing selective effects of heat against tumour cells.[4] Hyperthermia was later used in isolated limb perfusion as an adjunct to chemotherapy. In the 1980s the isolated regional perfusion technique, the perfusion equipment (pump and membrane oxygenator), the technique of leakage monitoring, and the formula for the correct dose calculation of the cytostatic agents were developed further.

Since the early 1960s the role of intra-arterial chemotherapy has been investigated extensively in the treatment of liver metastases, bone and soft tissue sarcomas of the limb, and other tumour sites (e.g. ref. 5). Several techniques for the application of intra-arterial infusion were developed, such as the tourniquet infusion technique, the balloon stopflow infusion technique, and the isolated limb infusion technique, with the ultimate goal being to increase the therapeutic effectiveness without increasing the systemic side-effects. Continuous intra-arterial chemotherapy in combination with fractionated external beam radiotherapy was also developed for soft tissue sarcomas of the limb.[6],[7]

There have been few further developments in intraperitoneal, intravesical, or intrathecal chemotherapy, other than the development of the concept of aggressive surgical resection of intraperitoneal metastatic disease of ovarian or colon cancer in combination with intraperitoneal chemotherapy.

Pharmacological considerations

The antineoplastic agents used in regional chemotherapy must have appropriate pharmacokinetic properties, such as a relatively steep dose–response curve, and no required metabolic activation. Antineoplastic agents with a high degree of extraction by the perfused region and a high total body clearance in case of systemic leakage are, therefore, suitable for regional chemotherapy. Antineoplastic

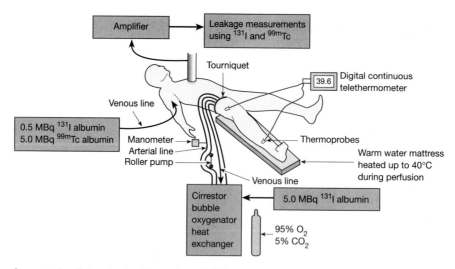

Fig. 1 Schematic drawing of a regional perfusion circuit with membrane bubble oxygenator, heat exchanger, roller pump, and leakage monitoring with radioactive iodine and technetium in the central circulation and the perfusion circuit.[45]

Table 1 Differences between regional perfusion, intra-arterial infusion, and systemic infusion

Treatment	Technique	Appropriate drugs	Concentration (area under the curve)	First pass effect	Applicability to hyperthermia	Toxicity
Regional perfusion	extremely difficult	few	increased	yes	yes	locoregional
Intra-arterial infusion	difficult	few	standard	yes	no	systemic
Systemic infusion	not difficult	all	standard	no	no	systemic

agents that are cleared at a slow rate from the perfused body compartment and at a more rapid rate from the systemic circulation have a pharmacokinetic advantage.

The intra-arterial infusion of chemotherapy especially during regional perfusion results in a markedly higher concentration of cytostatic agents in direct contact with the tumour when concentrations are compared with those achieved by intravenous administration, as measured by the area under the curve The advantage of regional chemotherapy versus systemic chemotherapy is a result of the high intra-arterial concentration compared with the level of concomitant systemic concentration during regional chemotherapy. Collins showed that there was a sigmoid response versus concentration relationship.[8] Each increment in drug concentration produces an increase in drug effect, until the maximal effect is reached (Fig. 2). The real advantage of all regional chemotherapy should be expressed by comparing the area under the curve of the concentration versus time profile using the regional drug application versus the conventional intravenous drug delivery (Fig. 3). The pharmacological benefit of various antineoplastic agents for regional versus systemic chemotherapy, the concentration–response behaviour of these antineoplastic agents and their optimal exposure time are now defined more precisely.[9]

Another advantage of regional perfusion or intra-arterial chemotherapy over systemic chemotherapy could be the so-called 'first pass'

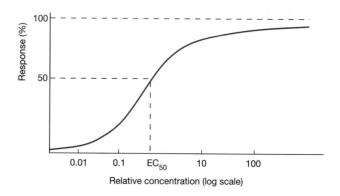

Fig. 2 Pharmacodynamic profile, response versus concentration relationship. The concentration–response curve is steepest around the EC50 level and quite flat at low and high concentrations levels, where a further increase in drug concentrations produces only a minimal increase in response. (Modified from Collins JM. Pharmacological rationale for regional chemotherapy, *Journal of Clinical Oncology* 1984; **2**: 498–504).

effect with an increased drug extraction by the first organ encountered. Additional factors influence the pharmacology of anticancer drugs used in specific types of regional chemotherapy. For example, in limb

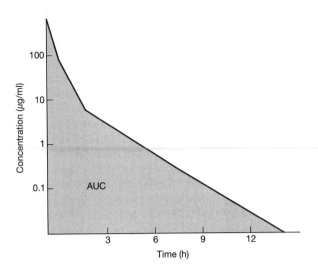

Fig. 3 The pharmacokinetic profile of cytostatic agents in the treatment of cancer is expressed by, the concentration versus time curve, area under the curve (AUC).

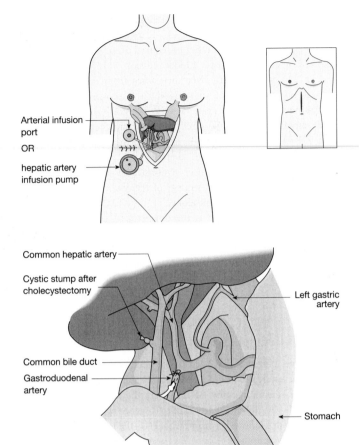

Fig. 4 Intra-arterial chemotherapy of the liver through a subcutaneous port or pump with a catheter placed via the gastroduodenal artery in the hepatic artery.

perfusion the dose calculation should be calculated using the perfused limb volume rather than the body surface area.[10] Hyperthermia may also influence the pharmacology of anticancer drugs (e.g. cisplatin). The pharmacology of intraperitoneal chemotherapy depends on several factors including the timing of the chemotherapy in relation to surgery, the extent of prior surgery, and the peritoneal/plasma ratio.[11] A limited number of antineoplastic agents have been found effective in regional cancer treatment, which are described in the following sections.

Regional chemotherapy of the liver

The treatment of hepatic metastases is related to the underlying malignancy, the previous treatment, the extent of the metastatic disease in the liver and other sites, and the availability of effective systemic treatment. The portal vein drains the entire abdominal viscera, and the liver is the common site of gastrointestinal metastases. When feasible, surgical resection of liver metastases from colorectal cancer may be the treatment of choice. Unfortunately, it is usually not possible because the liver metastases are too numerous and/or the location and size of the liver metastases precludes surgical resection. In addition to the systemic route, there are two alternatives for regional treatment, i.e. intra-arterial hepatic infusion through the gastroduodenal artery to the common hepatic artery or isolated liver perfusion.

Intra-arterial hepatic infusion

The liver parenchyma is supplied predominately by the portal vein, in contrast to the liver metastases which derive their blood supply mainly from the hepatic artery.[12] Most clinical trials have investigated infusion of 5-fluorouracil (**5-FU**) or 5-fluorodeoxyuridine (**FUDR**) into the hepatic artery. During a single pass almost all FUDR is extracted by the liver, while less than 50 per cent of 5-FU is metabolized by liver cells. Therefore, FUDR is an ideal drug for hepatic arterial

infusion achieving higher local drug concentrations and lower systemic drug exposure, than those seen after systemic or portal infusion.[13]

Externally fed catheters resulted in an increased risk of complications, such as catheter migration, arterial thrombosis, infection, gastrointestinal haemorrhage, and bleeding. Therefore, subcutaneous implantable ports and pumps have been developed for (continuous) intra-arterial hepatic infusion. Under general anaesthesia the port or implantable pump and catheter is placed through a right subcostal incision via the gastroduodenal artery into the hepatic artery. A cholecystectomy is routinely performed to prevent drug-induced cholecystitis (Fig. 4)

There are several clinical trials which have evaluated intra-arterial 5-FU or FUDR as treatment of unresectable liver metastases from colorectal cancer. Although higher rates of tumour regression are encountered with regional chemotherapy than with intravenous chemotherapy, a recently performed meta-analysis demonstrated no influence on overall survival.[14] Increased liver toxicity was seen with regional chemotherapy.

Surgical resection of metastatic colorectal liver metastases is the only treatment option with curative potential, resulting in a 20 to 30 per cent long-term survival in highly selected patients and a low morbidity and mortality rate.[15] As a large number of patients recur in the liver after metastectomy, combining the hepatic resection with regional chemotherapy with FUDR may be superior to hepatic resection alone.[16] A recent randomized trial of surgery versus surgery followed by adjuvant hepatic arterial infusion with 5-FU and folinic acid in 226 patients with liver metastases from colorectal cancer showed no improvement in survival.[17] A prospective study investigating the value of hepatic arterial infusion (HAI) with FUDR + dexamethasone (FUDR + D) and systemic chemotherapy (sys) with 5FU + leucovorin (FU + LV) versus systemic chemotherapy (FU + LV) alone as adjuvant therapy after resection of hepatic metastases from colorectal cancer demonstrated an increased survival after the combined adjuvant strategy of regional and systemic treatment over systemic treatment alone.[18]

An interesting approach is the downstaging of liver metastases with preoperative intra-arterial chemotherapy (5-FU, folinic acid, and oxaliplatin) to improve the resectability rate. The survival rate of patients with these unfavourable liver metastases appeared to be similar to that seen with primary liver resection for less extensive disease in one series of 53 patients, but this may be due to patient selection.[19]

Isolated liver perfusion

Isolated liver perfusion has been studied in large animal models, but the clinical application of liver perfusion has been hampered by the complex vascular anatomy of the liver, the ineffective neoplastic agents, and the potential morbidity. Together with the promising reports of isolated limb perfusion with TNF, the technical progress of the perfusion equipment used in liver transplantation has resurrected interest in liver perfusion, as a treatment modality for metastatic cancer of the liver. Hepatic perfusion can be performed with extracorporeal venovenous bypass or with balloon catheter techniques.

The technique of isolated liver perfusion allows for the use of high doses of antineoplastic agents with minimal systemic leakage.[20] Phase I and II trials have been performed with mitomycin C, melphalan, cisplatin, and TNF for unresectable liver metastases from various tumours (e.g. ref. 21). The treatment-related mortality and morbidity, including hepatic toxicity depends on the antineoplastic agents used and the extent of the involvement of the liver with metastatic disease. Multiorgan failure and venocclusive disease are the major causes of treatment-related mortality. For this reason mitomycin C has been abandoned in liver perfusion.

Several phase I and II trials of hyperthermic liver perfusion via the hepatic artery have been conducted with melphalan, TNF, or melphalan and TNF, and have demonstrated that liver perfusion with mild hyperthermia is feasible with an acceptable liver toxicity and minimal systemic toxicity.[22] Trials of TNF with higher doses of melphalan are in progress.

Regional chemotherapy of the limbs

For locally advanced soft tissue or bone sarcoma, or for melanoma with satellite or in transit metastases in the limb, an ablative surgical procedure may be the only treatment option with a chance of cure. Considering the suitability of the anatomy of the limb for regional chemotherapy and the potential for avoiding mutilating procedures, the role of intra-arterial chemotherapy and limb perfusion has been studied.

Intra-arterial chemotherapy for sarcomas

The concept of intra-arterial preoperative chemotherapy for bone and soft tissue sarcoma is to downstage the tumour and to increase the limb salvage rate. Intra-arterial cisplatin has been used as presurgical chemotherapy for bone sarcomas. Although high local drug concentrations were achieved in bone sarcomas, a randomized controlled trial (COSS-86) comparing intra-arterial and intravenous cisplatin in 109 evaluable patients with bone sarcomas found no differences with respect to limb salvage rate, local, and/or distant failures.[23]

Intra-arterial chemotherapy, with or without application of a tourniquet to increase the concentration in the limb, has been used to administer chemotherapy to localized extremity soft tissue sarcomas. The most commonly used antineoplastic agent has been doxorubicin either alone or with other drugs in both intra-arterial and intravenous trials. Intra-arterial doxorubicin has also been combined with fractionated preoperative radiation therapy at dose levels varying from 17.5 to 35 Gy in 5 to 10 consecutive days as presurgical treatment.[6],[7] The potential benefit of intra-arterial chemotherapy for soft tissue sarcomas relies on the 'first pass' effect, or increased drug extraction. However, there are no pharmacokinetic data to indicate an advantage, and there is no apparent difference between the intra-arterial and intravenous route with respect to tumoricidal effect, limb salvage rate, and local control.[6] The combined treatment of preoperative intra-arterial chemotherapy and external beam radiotherapy is not only tumoricidal but also 'toxic', resulting in severe short-term and long-term morbidity to the healthy tissues.[24] To date there is no indication for intra-arterial chemotherapy in the treatment of bone or soft tissue sarcomas of the extremities.

Limb perfusion

Melphalan was the first drug used in isolated limb perfusion (see Fig. 1) for the treatment of recurrent melanoma of the foot.[3] A variety of antineoplastic agents have since been used in limb perfusion for melanoma and sarcoma including melphalan, dacarbazine, actinomycin-D, thiotepa, mitomycin-C, doxorubicin, cisplatin, and carboplatin. One randomized trial compromised of 832 evaluable patients with high-risk primary melanoma (Breslow thickness 1.5 mm) treated with wide local excision with or without adjuvant limb perfusion with melphalan. There was a limited but definite benefit of limb perfusion in terms of local-regional disease control, but no impact on survival.[25] Melphalan is still the most effective antineoplastic agent for regional perfusion of in-transit or satellite metastase of limb melanoma. A phase III trial to evaluate the efficacy of melphalan alone versus the combination of melphalan and TNF in patients with in-transit or satellite metastases of melanoma of the limb has been discontinued in 1999 due to a slow accrual.[26] The major evidence in favour of the limb-saving treatment of locally advanced primarily non-resectable soft tissue sarcoma of the limb was a phase II study in 186 patients, which showed a complete pathological response in 29 per cent, partial pathological response in 53 per cent, no change in 16 per cent, and progressive disease in 2 per cent. This resulted in a limb salvage rate of 82 per cent during a median follow up of 2 years.[27]

The use of extracorporeal circulation allows hyperthermia to be used with regional chemotherapy. Hyperthermia increases tumour blood flow and changes the permeability of the cell membrane. There is a correlation between temperature, blood flow, microcirculation, cell membrane permeability, and drug uptake.[28] Enhanced blood flow due to vasodilatation, enhanced cellular drug uptake, DNA cross-linking, and decreased DNA repair[29] have been postulated to explain the phenomenon of the potentiation of chemotherapy by hyperthermia (see Chapter 4.6). Moderate hyperthermia with temperatures of 39 to 40 °C is used in regional perfusion, as higher temperatures (42 °C) are accompanied by severe treatment morbidity.[30] Hyperthermia may increase the neurotoxicity of cisplatin in isolated limb perfusion.[31]

The biological response modifiers, interferon and TNF were introduced recently in regional perfusion research, and were shown to possess antineoplastic activity. The combination of TNF with antineoplastic agents and hyperthermia seems promising, albeit quite toxic.[32] The optimal dose of TNF is still to be defined, and lower doses are being investigated. The concentration of melphalan in the perfusion circuit is approximately 10 times higher than the maximum tolerable dose (MTD) for systemic administration, and the melphalan peak concentration in the perfusate is about 150 times the systemic peak concentration.[33] Bone marrow toxicity of melphalan most likely results from leakage during the first 10 min after melphalan injection into the perfusion circuit, as the concentration of melphalan in the perfusate declines rapidly. After 30 min almost all melphalan is accumulated in the tissues. Although melphalan leakage of up to 15 per cent is well tolerated, TNF leakage to the systemic circulation should be avoided. Systemic TNF can induce severe toxicity and may lead to hyperdynamic shock syndrome and multi-organ failure.[34]

The treatment of melanoma and sarcoma is discussed in more detail in Chapters 8.1 and 16.1.

Lung perfusion

The majority of patients with metastatic disease to the lungs are not candidates for surgery, and systemic chemotherapy is generally only palliative. Isolated lung perfusion is an experimental procedure that might provide additional treatment for such patients.

More than 80 per cent of pulmonary metastases are supplied by the pulmonary arteries and isolated regional perfusion is feasible. Early experimental work with isolated lung perfusion in a canine model was performed with nitrogen mustard and doxorubicin. More recently, isolated lung perfusions of doxorubicin, TNF, and FUDR were performed in rats at the Memorial Sloan-Kettering Institute and of TNF in swine at the National Cancer Institute.[35],[36] Isolated lung perfusion is associated with an increased pulmonary artery pressure, a decreased cardiac output, and an increased heart rate, although no significant changes in systemic arterial pressure occur. However, when TNF is used in the perfusion setting, release of other cytokines, vasoactive peptides, oxygen free radicals, or nitric oxide may potentiate the haemodynamic instability, and leakage into the systemic circulation should be minimized. The two options in using isolated lung perfusion as a treatment modality of metastatic lung disease are isolated lung perfusion followed by metastasectomies, or isolated single lung perfusion without adjuvant surgery. Phase I/II trials of isolated lung perfusion are in progress using cisplatin and TNF and have demonstrated that the single lung perfusion technique is feasible and safe in selected patients.[37]

Pelvic perfusion and infusion

Regional perfusion for pelvic tumours is a palliative procedure for the treatment of recurrent pelvic cancer. Vascular occlusion of the pelvis is achieved with external tourniquets placed around the limbs and vascular occlusion of the aorta and vena cava with balloon occlusion catheters inserted in the groin and positioned with fluoroscopy. Hyperthermic perfusions have been performed with an extracorporal circuit using the drugs 5-FU or cisplatin.[38] The technique is complex and it is difficult to achieve complete vascular occlusion, resulting in substantial leakage (30 to 40 per cent) to the systemic circulation. Alleviating interventions include additional chemofiltration, that may absorb excess drug after pelvic perfusion and the administration of colony-stimulating factors such as granulocyte-colony-stimulating factor, which may decrease neutropenia. Further clinical research is required to assess the clinical applicability and benefit of pelvic perfusion in the treatment of pelvic malignancies.

Intra-arterial chemotherapy via bilateral percutaneously placed femoral artery catheters threaded up to the common iliac arteries with a variety of single cytostatic agents or combinations of cytostatic agents (e.g. doxorubicin and cisplatin), has been used with or without radiation, and or cystectomy, in the treatment of locally advanced bladder cancer with promising results.[39],[40] These preliminary results require confirmation in randomized studies.

Intraperitoneal chemotherapy

Intraperitoneal administration of antineoplastic agents in a large volume may have a pharmacological advantage as compared with the intravenous route. Also, locally high drug concentrations may lead to improved drug penetration into metastatic nodules on the peritoneum.

Uniform distribution of the drug-containing dialysate within the peritoneal cavity depends on the presence or absence of adhesions caused by the tumour or by previous surgical procedures. Irrigation of the abdominal cavity with antineoplastic agents in the presence of a large tumour volume has no effect. Effectiveness can only be expected if minimal (<0.5 cm) or microscopic disease is left behind on the peritoneal surface, and if uniform distribution of large volumes of dialysate (>2 litres) can be achieved.

A variety of antineoplastic agents has been used including doxorubicin, cisplatin, carboplatin, pactitaxol, mitoxantrone, 5-FU, methotrexate, and mitomycin C, as well as biological response modifiers such as interferon, TNF, and adoptive immunotherapy.[41],[42] Dose-limiting factors for the various agents may be due to local toxic reactions (e.g. chemical peritonitis with doxorubicin and mitomycin C), or to absorption of the antineoplastic agents into the systemic circulation (e.g. neurotoxicity and nephrotoxicity of cisplatin).

For locally advanced ovarian cancer cytoreductive surgery has been combined with intraperitoneal chemotherapy (see also Chapter 12.1). In a prospective randomized study of 654 patients intraperitoneal cisplatin chemotherapy combined with intravenous cyclophosphamide improved survival significantly and had less toxic effects than intravenous cyclophosphamide or intravenous cisplatin and cyclophosphamide.[43] Ongoing trials are evaluating intravenous paclitaxel in combination with intraperitoneal cisplatin, and the value of six cycles of intraperitoneal cisplatin as maintenance therapy after surgically confirmed complete remission. Intraperitoneal chemotherapy with an implantable peritoneal access device is well tolerated with a low complication rate.

Intraperitoneal chemotherapy may be applied to other malignancies with peritoneal implants, other than ovarian cancer, provided that the primary tumour is adequately resected. Intraperitoneal 5-FU chemotherapy has been used for peritoneal carcinomatosis of pseudomyxoma peritonei and may lead to improved local control.[44] Cisplatin has been used as an adjunct to extensive cytoreductive surgical procedures for sarcoma in patients with disease on the peritoneal surface with no progressive cancer at other sites.[44] However, with the exception of pseudomyxoma peritonei and ovarian cancer no advantage of intraperitoneal chemotherapy could be demonstrated with the currently available antineoplastic agents. In a prospective National Cancer Institiute trial of intravenous versus intraperitoneal 5-FU in 66 patients with advanced primary colon and rectal cancer, there was a significant decrease in the progression of disease on the peritoneal surface but no increase in survival.[11] The favourable regional pharmacological profile of the combination of cisplatin and TNF suggests that these agents administered via continuous hyperthermic peritoneal perfusion warrant further evaluation as prophylaxis against or treatment for peritoneal carcinomatosis.

Intravesical chemotherapy

Intravesical chemotherapy may be effective because of a direct tumoricidal effect or because of a non-specific inflammatory reaction. In the treatment of superficial bladder cancer thiotepa, mitomycin C, doxorubicin, or BCG (bacillus Calmette-Guérin), sometimes combined with cytokines, are used frequently to prolong the interval to recurrent disease or to eliminate recurrences. Toxicity of intravesical chemotherapy includes vesical irritability, myelosuppression, and contact dermatitis. The effects of these treatments are described in Chapter 13.2.

Intrathecal chemotherapy

Both haematological malignancies and solid tumours, such as breast cancer, melanoma, small cell lung cancer, and sporadically other solid tumours disseminate into the leptomeninges. The blood–brain barrier prevents most cytostatic agents from reaching therapeutic levels within the central nervous system following systemic administration. If other sites of disease are controlled, intrathecal chemotherapy, usually with methotrexate or cytosine arabinoside, may be given. These treatments are discussed in Chapter 5.5.

Summary

Regional chemotherapy has the potential to deliver high doses of antineoplastic agents to specific tumour-bearing areas or organs. The potential therapeutic effectiveness of regional chemotherapy may be calculated by comparing the areas under the drug concentration–time complexity of the different techniques and the efficacy of the regional chemotherapy differ widely.

There are no established differences in outcome between the intra-arterial and intravenous routes of chemotherapy in the treatment of liver metastases, bone and soft tissue sarcomas, and other malignancies. Currently, the only proven indication for intraperitoneal

chemotherapy is locally advanced ovarian cancer, with possible benefit for pseudomyxoma peritonei. Since the discovery of TNF there may be an indication for its use with hyperthermic isolated limb perfusion for locally advanced soft tissue sarcomas. Intravesical and intrathecal chemotherapy are well established. All other regional treatment should be considered experimental.

References

1. Klopp C, Alford TC, Bateman J, Berry GN, Winship T. Fractionated intra-arterial cancer chemotherapy with methyl bis-amine hydrochloride; a preliminary report. *Annals of Surgery*, 1950; **132**: 811–32.
2. Watkins E, Sullivan RG. Cancer chemotherapy by prolonged arterial infusion. *Surgery Gynecology and Obstetrics*, 1964; **118**: 3–19.
3. Creech O, Krementz ET, Ryan RF, Winblad JN. Chemotherapy of cancer: regional perfusion utilizing an extracorporeal circuit. *Annals of Surgery*, 1958; **148**: 616–32.
4. Cavaliere R, et al. Selective heat sensitivity of cancer cells. Biochemical and clinical studies. *Cancer*, 1967; **20**: 1351–81.
5. Sullivan RD, Norcross JW, Watkins E. Chemotherapy of metastatic liver cancer by prolonged hepatic-artery infusion. *New England Journal of Medicine*, 1964; **270**: 321–7.
6. Eilber FR, Eckhardt JJ, Rosen GR, Shi Fu Y, Seeger LL, Selch MT. Neoadjuvant chemotherapy and radiotherapy in the multidisciplinary management of soft tissue sarcomas of the extremity. *Surgical Oncology Clinics of North America*, 1993; **2**: 611–20.
7. Hoekstra HJ, et al. A combination of intraarterial chemotherapy, preoperative and postoperative radiotherapy, and surgery for primarily unresectable high-grade soft tissue sarcomas of the extremities. *Cancer*, 1989; **63**: 59–62.
8. Collins JM. Pharmacological rationale for drug delivery. *Journal of Clinical Oncology*, 1984; **2**: 498–504.
9. Link KH, et al. In vitro concentration response studies and in vivo phase II tests as the experimental basis for regional chemotherapeutic protocols. *Seminars in Surgical Oncology*, 1998; **14**: 189–201.
10. Van Os J, Schraffordt Koops H, Oldhoff J. Dosimetry of cytostatics in hyperthermic regional; perfusion. *Cancer*, 1985; **55**: 698–701.
11. Sugarbaker PH, et al. Prospective randomized trial of intravenous versus intraperitoneal 5-fluorouracil in patients with advanced primary colon or rectal cancer. *Surgery*, 1985; **98**: 414–22.
12. Ridge JA, Bading JR, Gelbard AS, Benua RS, Daly JM. Perfusion of colorectal hepatic metastases: relative distribution of flow from the hepatic artery and portal vein. *Cancer*, 1987; **59**: 1457–553.
13. Ensmiger WD, et al. A clinical-pharmacological evaluation of hepatic arterial infusions of 5-fluoro-2-—-deoxyuridine and 5-fluorouracil. *Cancer Research*, 1978; **38**: 3784–92.
14. Meta-Analysis Group in Cancer. Reappraisal of hepatic arterial infusion in the treatment of nonresectable liver metastases from colorectal cancer. *Journal of the National Cancer Institute*, 1996; **88**: 252–8.
15. Cromheecke M, de Jong KP, Hoekstra HJ. Current treatment for colorectal metastatic disease to the liver. *European Journal of Surgery Oncology*, 1999; **25**: 451–63.
16. Kemeny MM, Goldberg DA, Browning S, Metter GE, Miner PJ, Terz JJ. Experience with continuous regional chemotherapy and hepatic resection as treatment of hepatic metastases from colorectal primaries: prospective randomized study. *Cancer*, 1985; **55**: 1265–70.
17. Lorenz M, et al. Randomized trial of surgery versus surgery followed by adjuvant hepatic arterial infusion with 5-fluorouracil and folinic acid for liver metastases of colorectal cancer. *Annals of Surgical Oncology*, 1998; **6**: 756–62.

18. Kemeny NE, Cohen A, Huang Y, *et al.* Randomized study of hepatic arterial infusion (HAI) and systemic chemotherapy (SYS) versus SYS alone as adjuvant therapy after resection of hepatic metastases from colorectal cancer. *Journal of Clinical Oncology*, 1999; **18**: 263a (abstract 1011).

19. Bismuth H, *et al.* Resection of non resectable liver metastases from colorectal cancer after neoadjuvant chemotherapy. *Annals of Surgery*, 1996; **224**: 509–22.

20. Vahrmeijer AL, van der Erb MM, Dierendonck JH, Kuppen PJK, van de Velde CJH. Delivery of anticancer drugs via isolated hepatic perfusion: a promising strategy in the treatment of irresectable liver metastases. *Seminars in Surgical Oncology*, 1998; **14**: 262–8.

21. Alexander HR, Bartlett DL, Libutti SK, Fraker DL, Moser T, Rosenberg SA. Isolated hepatic perfusion with tumor necrosis factor and melphalan for unresectable cancers confined to the liver. *Journal of Clinical Oncology*, 1998; **16**: 1479–89.

22. Fraker DL, Alexander H Jr Isolated perfusion of the liver. In: Lotze MT, Rubin JT (eds). *Regional therapy of advanced cancer*. Philadelphia: Lippincott-Raven Publishers, 1997: 141–51.

23. Winkler K, *et al.* Effect of intraarterial versus intravenous cisplatin in addition to systemic doxorubicin, high-dose methotrexate, and ifosfamide on histologic tumor response in osteosarcoma (Study Coss-86). *Cancer*, 1990; **66**: 1703–10.

24. Nijhuis PHA, Pras E, Sleijfer DTH, Molenaar WM, Hoekstra HJ. Longterm results of preoperative intra-arterial doxorubicin combined with neoadjuvant radiotherapy, followed by extensive surgical resection for locally advanced soft tissue sarcomas of the extremities. *Radiotherapy and Oncology*, 1999; **51**: 15–19.

25. Schraffordt Koops H, *et al.* Prophylactic isolated limb perfusion for localized, high-risk limb melanoma: results of a multicenter randomized phase III trial. European Organization for Research and Treatment of Cancer Malignant Melanoma Cooperative group Protocol 18832, the World Health Organization Melanoma Program Trial 15, and the North American Perfusion group South West Oncology Group-8593. *Journal of Clinical Oncology*, 1998; **16**: 2906–12.

26. Lienard D, Eggermont AMM, Kroon BBR, Schraffordt Koops H, Lejeune FJ. Isolated limb perfusion in primary and recurrent melanoma: indications and results. *Seminars in Surgical Oncology*, 1998; **14**: 202–9.

27. Eggermont AMM, *et al.* Isolated limb perfusion with tumor necrosis factor and melphalan for limb salvage in 186 patients with locally advanced soft tissue extremity sarcomas. The cumulative multicenter European experience. *Annals of Surgery*, 1996; **224**: 756–65.

28. Di Filippo FD, *et al.* The application hyperthermia regional chemotherapy. *Seminars in Surgical Oncology*, 1998; **14**: 215–23.

29. Guchelaar HJ, Hoekstra HJ, de Vries EGE, Uges DRA, Oosterhuis JW, Schraffordt Koops H. Cisplatin and platinum pharmacokinetics during hyperthermic isolated limb perfusion for human tumours of the extremities. *British Journal of Cancer*, 1992; **65**: 898–902.

30. Vrouwenraets BC, Klaase JL, Nieweg OC, Kroon BBR. Toxicity and morbidity of isolated limb perfusion. *Seminars in Surgical Oncology*, 1998; **14**: 224–31.

31. Hoekstra HJ, Schraffordt Koops H, de Vries EG, Weerden TW, Oldhoff J. Toxicity of hyperthermic isolated limb perfusion with cisplatin for recurrent melanoma of the lower extremity after previous perfusion treatment. *Cancer*, 1993; **15**: 1224–9.

32. Fraker DL, Alexander HR, Andrich M, Rosenberg SA. Treatment of patients with melanoma of the extremity using hyperthermic isolated limb perfusion with melphalan, tumor necrosis factor, and interferon gamma: results of tumor necrosis factor dose-escalation study. *Journal of Clinical Oncology*, 1996; **14**: 479–89.

33. Scott RN, *et al.* The pharmacokinetic advantage of isolated limb perfusion with melphalan for malignant melanoma. *British Journal of Cancer*, 1992; **66**: 159–66.

34. Zwaveling JH, *et al.* High plasma levels of tumor necrosis factor alpha and shortlived sepsis syndrome in patients undergoing isolated perfusion with recombinant tumor necrosis factor alpha, interferon gamma and melphalan. *Critical Care Medicine*, 1996; **24**: 765–70.

35. Ng B, Lenert TJ, Weksler B, Port JL, Ellis JL, Burt ME. Isolated single lung perfusion with FUDR is an effective treatment for colorectal adenocarcinoma lung metastases in rats. *Annals of Thoracic Surgery*, 1994; **58**: 328–31.

36. Progrebniak HW, *et al.* Isolated lung perfusion with tumor necrosis factor: a swine model in preparation of human trials. *Annals of Thoracic Surgery*, 1994; **57**: 1477–8357.

37. Pass HI, Mew DJ, Kranda KC, Temeck BK, Donington JS, Rosenberg SA. Isolated lung perfusion with tumor necrosis factor for pulmonary metastases. *Annals of Thoracic Surgery*, 1996; **61**: 1609–17.

38. Wanebo HJ, Chung MA, Levy AI, Turk PS, Vezeridis MP, Belliveau JF. Pre-operative therapy for advanced pelvic malignancy by isolated pelvic perfusion with the balloon-occlusion technique. *Annals of Surgical Oncology*, 1996; **3**: 295–303.

39. Eapen L, *et al.* Intraarterial cisplatin and concurrent radiation for locally advanced bladder cancer. *Journal of Clinical Oncology*, 1989; **7**: 230–5.

40. Jacobs SC, Mneashe DS, Mewisen MW, Lipchik EO. Intraarterial cisplatin infusion in the management of transitional cell carcinoma of the bladder. *Cancer*, 1998; **64**: 388–91.

41. Markman M. Intraperitoneal anti-neoplastic agents for tumors principally confined to the peritoneal cavity. *Cancer Treatment Reviews*, 1986; **13**: 219–42.

42. Sugarbaker PH (ed.) *Intraperitoneal chemotherapy and peritoneal carcinomatosis: drugs and diseases.* (*Cancer treatment and research*; Series editor: Freireich EJ). Boston: Kluwer Academic Publishers, 1996.

43. Alberts DS, *et al.* Intraperitoneal cisplatin plus intravenous cyclophosphamide versus intravenous cisplatin plus intravenous cyclophosphamide for stage III ovarian cancer. *New England Journal of Medicine*, 1996; **335**: 1950–5.

44. Sugarbaker PH. Intraperitoneal chemotherapy and cytoreductive surgery for the prevention and treatment of peritoneal carcinomatosis and sarcomatosis. *Seminars in Surgical Oncology*, 1998; **14**: 254–61.

45. Hoekstra HJ, *et al.* Continuous leakage monitoring during hyperthermic isolated regional perfusion of the lower limb: techniques and results. *Regional Cancer Treatment*, 1992; **4**: 301–4.

High-dose chemotherapy and stem cell rescue

C. Irle and T. Philip

Introduction

Rationale for high-dose chemotherapy

The rationale for high-dose chemotherapy resides in the observation that a dose–response curve varying in steepness according to drugs and cell types can be found in a variety of preclinical models. For most drugs a plateau of maximal cell kill is found. Clinical research has shown that there is a narrow window between the dose needed to give a tumour response and that which causes severe damage to normal tissues, most often the bone marrow, and that exploitable dose increments are therefore often limited to less than a 1 log increase. This difference between toxicity to normal and tumour cells is exploited by high-dose chemotherapy. The choice of useful drugs is limited to those with primarily haematological toxicity, which can be overcome by stem cell rescue thereby allowing the use of drugs just below the level that causes severe non-haematological toxicity (Fig. 1). Clinical studies have found that the capacity to induce complete remission of tumours that are sensitive to chemotherapy has often been dependent on dose. However, in the clinical setting the relation between maximum tolerated dose and the desirable dose increment defined in preclinical models for optimal tumour cell kill is often unknown.

An increase in the effective dose of chemotherapy can be achieved either by dose escalation or by more frequent administration of chemotherapy. Hryniuk and his colleagues have analysed treatment outcome in different tumours as a function of the drug dose delivered per unit time, or relative dose intensity, expressed as milligrams per square metre per week, regardless of the schedule or route of administration.[1] In combination chemotherapy, dose intensity may be defined by summation of the dose intensity for individual agents used within a regimen.[2] A positive correlation between relative dose intensity, dose, and response rate has been reported for leukaemias, lymphomas, testicular cancers, and childhood cancers. For ovarian and breast tumours dose increments have generally resulted in better response rates. In haematological malignancies, 3 log dose increments of aracytidine (ARA-C) for consolidation resulted in significantly better survival in a three-dose-level randomized trial.[3] In solid tumours most of the data from comparison of non-randomized series support the benefit of dose-intense chemotherapy with regard to response rates, but randomized trials appear to be inconsistent in demonstrating its benefit for survival. This may be due in part to the selection of patients with better performance status to receive a higher dose intensity.

Increasing the intensity of treatment by drug delivery over a shorter period of time can be a useful way to improve the effectiveness of certain drugs in tumours with steep dose–response curves. Smaller tumours tend to grow faster, and therefore repopulation of tumour cells between treatments is likely to be more rapid when tumour kill is most effective. Thus, shortening the time between treatment cycles may allow less repopulation from surviving cells, and may have a greater impact than dose escalation alone. This concept underlies the use of sequential high-dose therapy, with optimal doses used in dose-dense cycles.

Systemic dose intensity is defined as systemic exposure (given by the area under the concentration versus time curve or 'area under the curve') resulting from the administration of a given dose of drug, and is dependent on the pharmacokinetics of the drug (see Chapter 4.13). Calculation of drug doses based upon body surface area does not account for interpatient variation in pharmacokinetics, since

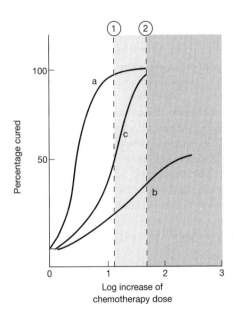

Fig. 1 Dose–effect curve. While chemosensitive tumours (a) may be cured by dose levels attainable within the range of conventional therapy, chemoresistant tumours (b) escape even supralethal doses. A finite number of tumours (c) may be cured by the doses given with high-dose chemotherapy followed by stem cell rescue. 1: Dose level resulting in irreversible haematological toxicity. 2: Dose level resulting in irreversible organ damage.

individuals have a variable ability to metabolize drugs, and a variable area under the curve. The areas under the curve of most drugs used in high-dose chemotherapy have not been studied extensively. Data are available for a few drugs such as carboplatin and methotrexate, but are difficult to obtain for many others because of complex patterns of metabolism and elimination.[4],[5] Pharmacokinetically adjusted drug dose calculation correlates well with toxicity, and increasing use of this method is important in the development of safer high-dose strategies.[4] It correlates with tumour sensitivity, at least in acute leukaemia, lymphoma, myeloma, and testicular cancer. Unfortunately the practical difficulties of therapeutic drug monitoring for most cytotoxic agents make pharmacokinetic drug dosing unfeasible for most patients. Other methods for calculating dose are therefore needed, to avoid the inaccuracies leading to overdosing and excessive systemic toxicity which are magnified by high-dose chemotherapy.

The safety of high-dose chemotherapy programmes has been enhanced over the past decade by the availability of effective supportive therapy including broad-spectrum antibiotics, new antifungal and antiviral agents, a variety of haematopoietic growth factors, improved nutrition, and haematopoietic stem cell support.

Rationale for the use of stem cells

The therapeutic potential of bone marrow transplantation to circumvent the dose-limiting haematological toxicity and mortality of high-dose chemotherapy was established by the finding that spleen cells, and subsequently bone marrow cells, could restore haematopoietic function following otherwise lethal irradiation in experimental animals. In patients, contamination of the transplant by tumour cells was a concern, and initially high-dose chemotherapy was followed by the reinfusion of allogeneic bone marrow obtained from an HLA-matched related donor. This treatment became standard for patients with acute myeloid leukaemia and who had an HLA-matched donor, as immunosuppressive treatments and progress in donor matching improved.

Fewer than 20 per cent of all patients have a suitable related HLA-matched donor. Despite the clinical progress in using transplants from unrelated phenotypically HLA-matched donors and the worldwide development of registries of unrelated volunteer bone marrow donors, donor availability remains a limiting factor in the wider application of allogeneic bone marrow transplantation. Because graft versus host disease is a frequent and severe complication of allogeneic bone marrow transplantation, and inceases with donor HLA incompatibility, age, sex disparity, multiple transfusions, and infections, allogeneic transplantation is limited to younger patients. The development of allogeneic cord blood and procurement of placental blood-derived stem cells may circumvent some of these difficulties in the future.

The cryopreservation and successful reinfusion of bone marrow taken from the same patient has led to the growing use of autologous bone marrow transplantation to overcome the haematological toxicity of high-dose chemotherapy. Autologous bone marrow transplantation has broadened the range of patients who can be treated with high-dose chemotherapy and has stimulated the extension of this method to non-haematopoietic malignancies that are sensitive to chemotherapy.

The quantity of autologous bone marrow which can be harvested from a patient with cancer is limited since prior chemotherapy depletes stem cells, and repeated bone marrow collections are difficult.

The presence of small numbers of circulating pluripotent stem cells in the blood has long been recognized from cross-circulation experiments in lethally irradiated animal models. The first quantitation of pluripotent progenitors from human peripheral blood mononuclear cells was reported in the early 1970s by the *in vitro* growth of erythroid, granulocytic, and monocytic colonies.[6],[7] They were recognized initially by *in vitro* culture techniques, and quantitated by counting of colonies of granulocyte forming units or colony forming units in culture (CFU-C), and represent 0.1 per cent of the bone marrow, and less than 0.01 per cent of peripheral blood mononucleated cells. Immunological methods have been used to identify the subset of cells containing pluripotent stem cells since these are within the mononuclear population expressing the CD34 surface antigen. The important pluripotent stem cells can be found only in the tiny fraction of CD34 +, Thy1 +, LIN–, DR + cells. Recently, the most primitive subsets of CD34 + cells were found to express the human haematopoietic cell antigen huHCA.[8] However, the direct identification of pluripotent stem cells remains elusive. At present, most centres rely on the monitoring of peripheral blood stem cells through quantitation of CD34 + cells using automatic fluorescent cell sorters.

Recognition that the growth and differentiation of haematopoietic precursor cells is regulated by multiple factors released by stromal cells, lymphocytes, and monocytes has led to the discovery of a rapidly increasing number of haematological growth factors (see Chapter 15.1) which are now used to stimulate production of peripheral blood stem cells. The use of peripheral blood stem cells has largely supplanted autologous bone marrow harvesting, and is likely to play an increasing role in allotransplantation. The lack of sufficient stem cells for repeated treatments has been resolved by the harvesting of large numbers of peripheral blood stem cells, and this progress allows further testing of the dose intensity concept by allowing sequential high-dose therapies with stem cell rescue.

Stem cell collection, storage, and reinfusion

Harvesting of bone marrow

Bone marrow is obtained from the anterior and posterior iliac crests under epidural or general anaesthesia by multiple needle aspirations using heparinized syringes to avoid clotting. Marrow suspensions are collected in sterile transfusion sets containing heparin or a mixture of heparin and citrate/phosphate/dextrose. A total volume of 800 to 1000 ml of bone marrow is usually obtained by individual sample aspirations of 2 ml. Larger sample aspirates decrease the number of stem cells per aspirate, and should therefore be avoided. Larger volumes may be collected if the bone marrow is hypocellular, for example following chemotherapy, or in cases of anticipated cell loss, for example by a purging procedure.

The risk of bone marrow harvesting is quite small, and limited in most instances to pelvic discomfort which typically lasts only a short time; in 15 per cent of cases a low-grade temperature develops which resolves rapidly postoperatively. Rarely, bleeding at the sites of puncture may occur, and, very uncommonly, local wound infection. Isolated cases of fatal anaesthesia-related complications have been reported. This may be avoided by taking a careful history and clinical examination before the harvest to rule out cardiovascular risk factors and reduce the risk of allergic reactions.

Acute anaemia resulting from the harvesting should be compensated. Whenever possible, two to four units of autologous blood should be collected and stored in order to avoid unnecessary exposure to blood-borne viral infections if transfusion is required. When cell separators are used for the preparation of marrow cell suspensions, the separated red blood cells can be reinfused to eliminate transfusions.

Harvesting of peripheral blood stem cells

Peripheral blood stem cells are collected by using automated cell separator machines which can process large volumes of blood and separate them into their different components. In children weighing less than 25 kg, priming of the extracorporeal lines with irradiated red blood cells is required. The early clinical use of peripheral blood stem cells harvested without stimulation proved to be a cumbersome and time-consuming process, involving the processing of large volumes of blood (7 to 14 litres), and requiring 10 or more sessions of cytaphaeresis to collect sufficient numbers of stem cells.

The discovery that stem cells migrate from the bone marrow into the peripheral blood following chemotherapy resulted in specific mobilizing schemes that can increase the number of peripheral blood stem cells up to 50-fold over baseline levels. The chemotherapy can be of standard type or designed specifically to stimulate the mobilization of stem cells, such as use of high doses of cyclophosphamide or etoposide. There are several disadvantages to the use of higher-dose chemotherapy for mobilization, including the length of time required, the toxicity of treatment including complications of neutropenic fever and haemorrhagic cystitis, and the lack of increase of peripheral blood stem cells in patients that have undergone repeated cycles of treatment; it can result in difficulties of scheduling the aphaeresis procedure due to variability in the recovery time.

The administration of haematopoietic growth factors increases the number of peripheral blood stem cells. Numerous schedules of growth factors given either individually or in combination have been reported. Granulocyte-macrophage colony stimulating factor (**GM-CSF**) was used initially, starting on the day after chemotherapy until the last leukaphaeresis. GM-CSF, because of its greater toxicity (capillary leak syndrome, flu-like syndome, and first-dose effect), has been gradually replaced by the equally effective granulocyte colony stimulating factor (**G-CSF**); following daily G-CSF at 5 µg or 10 µg sufficient peripheral blood stem cells can be obtained after five or fewer aphaeresis sessions. A pegylated form of G-CSF which may require only a single injection is being explored. Use of growth factors has facilitated the clinical use of peripheral blood stem cells, particularly from allogeneic donors, as a surrogate for bone marrow.

Interleukin 3 (IL-3) has a modest capacity to mobilize stem cells. This may be explained by its stimulation of stromal cell proliferation and consequent enhanced stem cell retention in the bone marrow.[9] The sequential administration during mobilization of IL-3 followed by G-CSF or GM-CSF has been evaluated. There seems to be only a modest effect on CD34 + cell mobilization, but sequential treatment of IL-3 with G-CSF or GM-CSF resulted in an increased number of clonogenic haematopoietic precursors, determined by *in vitro* growth of CFU-GM (GM, containing granulocytes, macrophages) and CFU-GEMM (GEMM, containing granulocytes, erythrocytes, macrophages, and monocytes), and accelerated engraftment.[10],[11]

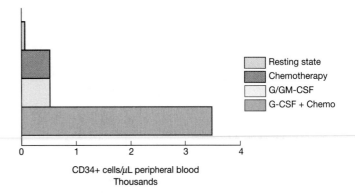

Fig. 2 Mobilization of CD34 + cells following chemotherapy, growth factor, or combination treatments. The numbers of CD34 + cells were estimated by extrapolation from the fluoroscence activated cell sorter (FACS) analysis of the percentage of positively stained cells among mononuclear cell suspensions of cytaphaeresis products to the number of mononucleated cells counted in the peripheral blood. (Personal representative results representing individual patients.)

The combined use of chemotherapy with the administration of G-CSF or GM-CSF has increased the level of circulating CD34 + cells in the early phase of haematological recovery by up to and over 100-fold. Both mobilization-specific and conventional-dose chemotherapy followed by growth factors have been effective.[12]

Stem cell growth factor (SCF), a ligand of c-*kit*, has not been tested alone in mobilization trials, and available data indicate that SCF-mobilized peripheral blood stem cells may result in delayed engraftment. The clinical application of combinations of SCF and G-CSF is being evaluated following experiments in baboons that showed growth factor synergism.[13] A randomized comparison beween G-CSF ± SCF after chemotherapy mobilization demonstrated that the combination increased the levels of circulating progenitors by more than two-fold.[14] In patients who had been previously exposed to extensive therapy, the combination released five times more CD34 + cells.[15]

The optimal timing of harvest differs between the mobilization protocols, but can be determined by monitoring the haematological rebound of CD34 + cells. The mobilization of CD34 + cells appears to correlate with rebound of the white blood cell count to between 3×10^9 and 10×10^9 cells/litre. At this time it is often possible to collect sufficient stem cells with a single aphaeresis when myelotoxic chemotherapy has not been previously administered. Figure 2 summarizes the impact of mobilization protocols on circulating CD34 + cells.

Previous chemotherapy and radiation affect the quality of the progenitor harvests, and in some patients there is insufficient mobilization. Secondary autologous bone marrow harvesting has then generally been performed. There has been concern that the quality of bone marrow harvested in this setting may be poor and might result in slow engraftment and an increased risk of procedure-related complications (in one series five out of 12 patients died after marrow transplants which were obtained following poor mobilization).[16]

Recently the *ex vivo* expansion of as few as 107 peripheral CD34 + cells contained in 100 to 200 ml of peripheral blood obtained at the rebound of white blood cells after mobilization was reported to result

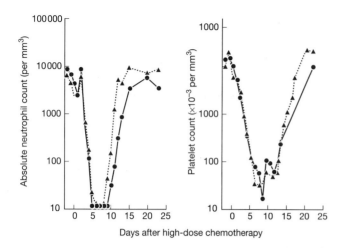

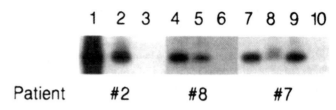

Fig. 3 Haematopoietic recovery in nine patients after treatment with high-dose etoposide, ifosfamide, carboplatin, and epirubucin and transplantation of progenitor cells generated ex vivo. Data are expressed as median absolute neutrophil counts and median platelet counts in the four patients who received both progenitor cells generated ex vivo and uncultured CD34+ cells (dashed lines), and the five patients who received only progenitor cells generated ex vivo (full lines). (By courtesy of Dr W. Brugger et al. and reproduced with permission.[17])

Fig. 4 Polymerase chain reaction analysis showing the detection of transplanted gene-marked (transduced) neuroblastoma cells (GD2+CD45–), cells obtained from the site of relapse of three patients, and from individual G-418-resistant neuroblastoma colonies grown in methylcellulose. Patient 2: lane 1, marrow tumour; lane 2, G418-resistant neuroblastoma colony; lane 3, negative control. Patient 8: lane 4, marrow tumour; lane 5, G418-resistant neuroblastoma colony; lane 6, negative control. Patient 7: lane 7, liver tumour; lanes 8 and 9, G418-resistant liver and marrow-derived colonies, lane 10, negative control The band shown is the 720 base pair neomycin-resitance gene amplification product. (By courtesy of Dr D. Rill and reproduced with permission. For further technical details see Rill et al.[21])

in engraftment (Fig. 3).[17] This technology may allow a further reduction in the inconvenience of stem cell procurement to the patient, and the aphaeresis laboratories.

Tumour cells in stem cell preparations

That the reinfusion of leukaemia cells can contribute to relapse has been demonstrated in gene marker studies following transplantation for acute myeloid and chronic myeloid leukemia.[18],[19] However, syngeneic transplants from identical twins and non-purged autologous transplants have resulted in comparable rates of leukaemic relapse, so most relapses are probably caused by malignant cells that have resisted the conditioning regimen.[20] Pharmacological purging seems to decrease the relapse rate and increase disease-free survival in leukaemias, but the available data are based on retrospective analysis and suffer from problems of patient selection and variability in treatment. In patients with solid tumours and lymphomas, only isolated cases of relapse after autotransplantation due to reinfused tumour cells have been reported. However, in an elegant study using gene-marked bone marrow cells, the presence of the marker in a proportion of resurgent neuroblastoma cells at relapse indicated that reinfused tumour cells can contribute to relapse in patients treated for solid tumours (Fig. 4).[21]

In patients with involvement of the bone marrow by lymphoma, non-randomized studies have reported encouraging results following purging with 4-hydroxy-peroxy-cyclophosphamide. In contrast, a retrospective analysis from the European Bone Marrow Transplant registry of lymphoma patients with known bone marrow contamination was unable to demonstrate a significant advantage in favour of purging for either progression-free or overall survival, suggesting that relapse occurs mainly due to failure of the conditioning regimen (Fig. 5).[22] The benefit of marrow purging has not yet been

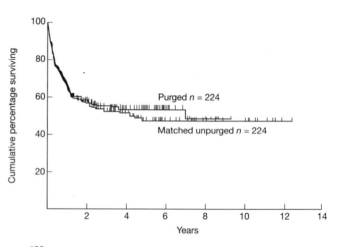

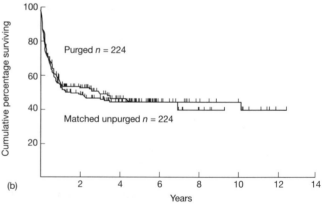

Fig. 5 Effect of lymphoma cell purging on survival: case-matched comparison from the European Bone Marrow Transplant lymphoma registry. The Kaplan–Meier curves shown in (a) represent overall patient survival after autologous bone marrow transplantation of purged and unpurged transplants, those in (b) show progression-free survival. (By courtesy of Dr C. D. Williams and reproduced with permission.[22])

shown in prospective, randomized trials, primarily because of the logistical problems inherent in the design of such studies.

Peripheral blood stem cells were initially thought to represent a better source of stem cells than bone marrow with less likelihood of tumour contamination. However, the development of immunological, tissue culture, and genetic techniques for the detection of minimal residual disease has demonstrated tumour cells in peripheral blood stem cells from patients treated for lymphoma, myeloma, breast cancer, neuroblastoma, and Ewing's sarcoma. For lymphomas, several studies using polymerase chain reaction analysis of the T-cell receptor beta rearrangement, or immunoglobulin gene rearrangement, or of the major breakpoint region t(14;18), or the bcl–2/JH fusion product suggest that autologous stem cells harvested in remission are often contaminated by tumour cells.[23]–[25] For myelomas, tumour-specific immunoglobulin variable-region sequences have been used as markers of clonality. The presence of submicroscopic breast cancer cells in stem cell products has been demonstrated using monoclonal anticytokeratin antibody labelling, clonogenic assays for tumour cells, and polymerase chain reaction detection of cytokeratin 19 mRNA reverse transcriptase and of maspin, a breast cancer-specific protease inhibitor of the serpin family.[26]–[28]

The level of circulating tumour cells appears to increase after repeated courses of mobilization chemotherapy. For neuroblastoma the detection of TRK-A, GAGE, or N-myc in stem cell products, and for Ewing's sarcoma the t(11,22) or t(21,22) translocations, found in 95 per cent of tumours, have been used to detect minimal residual disease.[29],[30] Since the threshold of detection of residual tumour cell DNA is approximately 1 in 10^6 cells, the level of residual tumour cells in a marrow or peripheral blood stem cells harvest may be as high as 10^3 cells even in the case of a negative polymerase chain reaction assay.

The metastatic capability of circulating tumour cells with or without mobilization of peripheral blood stem cells, and of those detected in the resting bone marrow or after purging, is unknown. In a prospectively randomized comparison between autologous bone marrow and chemotherapy-mobilized peripheral blood stem cells, the latter showed more detectable lymphoma cells (47 per cent versus 67 per cent) but there was no apparent difference in clinical outcome.[31] In a non-randomized prospective study, patients with non-Hodgkin's lymphoma who had occult tumour cells in their bone marrow showed a significantly worse 5-year disease-free survival rate than those with tumour-free marrow (Fig. 6).[32] Following high-dose therapy, the reinfusion of bone marrow with lymphoma cells detectable by polymerase chain reaction was followed by the rapid appearance of tumour cells in the circulation, and most but not all patients with grafts contaminated by tumour cells relapsed.[33]

Differences in mobilization of tumour cells into the peripheral blood have been reported and seem to depend on the type of tumour and disease status. In breast cancer patients without marrow involvement, circulating tumour cells precede the peak of haematopoietic stem cells following chemotherapy and growth factor mobilization, while with bone marrow involvement the timing of the appearance of tumour cells in the peripheral blood seems delayed and contemporary with the upswing in CD34 cells (Fig. 7).[34] In patients with multiple myeloma, the use of chemotherapy and growth factors for mobilization also resulted in simultaneous increments of CD34 + peripheral blood stem cells and CD19 + peripheral plasma

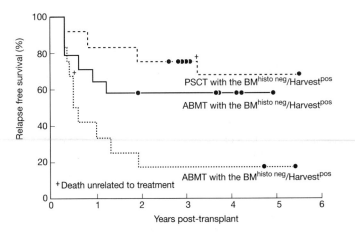

Fig. 6 Influence of tumour cells detected in the marrow or infused haematopoietic harvests on the outcome of high-dose chemotherapy and autologous transplantation. The curves represent the disease-free interval of patients with non-Hodgkin's lymphoma after autologous bone marrow transplantation or peripheral blood stem cell reinfusion performed in complete remission. All patients with peripheral blood stem cell reinfusion were marrow-positive histologically (BM^histo pos), but none of the peripheral blood stem cell harvests contained any tumour cells (Harvest^neg). All patients with autologous bone marrow transplantation were bone marrow-negative, but had either either Harvest^pos or Harvest^neg assessments. (By courtesy of Dr J. G. Sharp and reproduced with permission.[32])

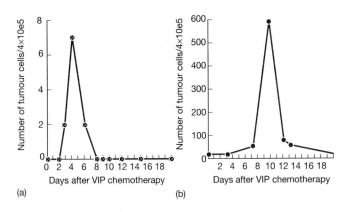

Fig. 7 Effect of mobilization by chemotherapy and growth factor administration on tumour cells in patients with or without bone marrow infiltration. Pattern of recruitment of malignant epithelial tumour cells in patients without (a) or with (b) bone marrow infiltration. The data represent numbers of (cytokeratin positive) tumour cells per 4×10^5 mononuclear cells from two patients. (By courtesy of Dr W. Brugger and reproduced with permission.[34])

cells.[35] These findings are important for choosing the method and timing of stem cell procurement.

Purging methods

In an effort to decrease the number of occult tumour cells in the stem cell product before reinfusion, a number of physical, chemical, and immunological techniques have been employed and are reviewed below.

Physical methods

The discovery that lectins can be used to separate cell populations on the basis of differential levels of terminal saccharide residues on cell surface polysaccharides has been exploited by rosetting and cell aggregation. These approaches have been quite successful for removal of normal T cells, but they have proved less effective for the depletion of neuroblastoma cells, of T- or B-cell lymphoblastic leukaemia cells, and for stem cell enrichment.[36] Density gradient floatation methods have been widely used to separate cell populations, and have subsequently evolved into selection of stem-cell-enriched mononuclear cell suspensions by automated counterflow cell separators. Contamination by tumour cells is significantly reduced in the leukaphaeresis products (by about 3 orders of magnitude) when compared with autologous bone marrow.[26]

Chemical methods

The use of cytotoxic drugs for the *ex vivo* treatment of autologous marrow has been widely adopted in leukaemia. It is based on the hypothesis that *in vitro* chemotherapy can lyse tumour cells while sparing, at least partially, the more resistant resting pluripotent stem cells. However, pharmacological purging is toxic to stem cells and thus increases the overall toxicity of the transplant procedure. Chromosome abnormalities can be detected in dividing bone marrow cells after *in vitro* drug-purged transplantation, but it is not known if *ex vivo* purging with chemical agents induces chromosome abnormalities in normal stem cells. The most popular method uses the *ex vivo* treatment of bone marrow with 4-hydroxy-peroxy-cyclophosphamide or mafosphamide. Other cytotoxic drugs explored in limited studies include etoposide, vincristine, nitrogen mustard, cisplatin, and cytosine arabinoside. Toxicity to stem cells might be circumvented by pretreatment exposure to cytoprotectors such as amifostine which can protect normal haematopoietic precursors from damage by 4-hydroxy-peroxy-cyclophosphamide.

Bacterial, plant, and fungal toxins represent some of the most potent cytotoxic agents, but must be targeted to specific cancer cells. This has severely restricted their development. Shiga-like toxin, an unconjugated native bacterial toxin, binds to the CD77 surface glycoprotein restricted to a subset of activated B cells present in follicular lymphomas, to myeloma cells, and to germ cell tumours It may represent a powerful purging tool.[37]

Incubation with ether lipids, e.g. 1-O-octadecyl-2-methyl-rac-glycero-3-phosphocholine (ET-18-OCH₃), or alkyl-lysophospholipid leads to a significant reduction in tumour cell contamination of stem cell preparations.[38] 6-Hydroxydopamine or phenylalanine methylester also appear to be effective.

Photodynamic purging involves photosensitizers like merocyanin-540, di-haematoporphyrin ether,or benzoporphyrin derivative. They exhibit a preferential retention in malignant cells. Photoactivation-induced tumour cell lysis is obtained after exposure to light (see Chapter 4.29). This approach has been successfully tested in small series to remove leukaemia, neuroblastoma, and lymphoma cells from autografts.

Immunological methods

Monoclonal antibodies are effective purging tools for malignant cells which express specific antigens. In lymphomas and breast cancer, cocktails of antibodies have been used, followed either by complement-mediated lysis or by immunoabsorption with magnetic beads. This procedure can remove all residual tumour cells containing the t(14; 18) breakpoints that are detectable by polymerase chain reaction analysis (see Chapter 1.2 for a description of the polymerase chain reaction method).[23]

Immunotoxins are formed by the conjugation of potent toxins to monoclonal antibodies, for example ricin toxin A chain, diphtheria toxin, or pseudomonas endotoxin, and have been evaluated in the treatment of lymphomas, myeloma, and some solid tumours such as neuroblastoma, small cell lung cancer, and breast cancer (see Chapter 4.26). Their development for solid tumours has been hampered by the difficulty of finding appropriate target antigens and of linking sufficiently potent toxins. Using leucine zippers of Fos and Jun which form preferential heterodimers, toxins can be attached by gene fusion to antibody fragments containing the antigen-specific determinants (Fab fragments), resulting in bispecific monoclonal antibodies.[39] Polymerase chain reaction technology is being applied to the development of new, more potent, immunotoxins consisting of smaller proteins limited to the toxic domain from which non-essential amino acids are deleted. It is too early to determine the efficacy of these new constructs in comparison with older immunotoxins. Immunotoxins can selectively eliminate clonogenic tumour cells without impairing lymphohaematopoietic engraftment, but their clinical impact may be limited by the failure of chemotherapy regimens to reduce residual disease to a level allowing their effective use.

Anti-CD34 monoclonal antibodies and positive selection provide another means to prepare tumour cell depleted stem cell products, resulting in a median tumour cell survival of about 1 in 100 tumour cells.[40] These preparations result in durable engraftment. Their use involves a time-consuming and expensive procedure; in addition the loss of CD34 + cells can be substantial. Despite the high purity and yield of CD34 + cell selection, contaminating tumour cells can still be found. Since the CD34 antigen appears to play an important role in cell traffic to bone marrow by allowing binding to endothelium and extravasation, and since it can also be expressed by leukaemia and myeloma cells, combinations of different techniques for removal of tumour cells may be optimal.

Cryopreservation

Autologous bone marrow and peripheral blood stem cells are stored by cryopreservation following the preparation of a red blood cell depleted cell suspension. Typically this is placed at concentrations of about 5×10^7 cells/ml in a serum albumin-containing culture medium such as RPMI containing 10 per cent dimethysulphoxide, and frozen in the vapour phase of liquid nitrogen by using automatic step freezing equipment. There is an inverse relationship between the rate of freezing and the optimal viability of stem cells. Successful transplants have been reported using cryopreserved stem cells after as long as 5 years. The technique of cryopreservation of peripheral blood stem cells is similar to that of autologous bone marrow. With higher numbers of stem cells, the use of controlled rate freezing may be less important, and bags containing the cells can simply be placed in the vapour phase of liquid nitrogen and frozen to $-80\,°C$. If contamination by neutrophilic granulocytes is excessive, their removal by density floatation prior to freezing may be useful to avoid the clotting of cells which is due to release of DNA by lysed granulocytes. Most often the released DNA can be digested with DNAase, but a variable loss of thawed stem cells may result from cell aggregation during reinfusion.

Bone marrow and stem cell infusion

While freshly harvested allogeneic marrow may be infused without separation of red blood cells in cases of blood group compatibility between the patient and the donor, red cells are otherwise removed to avoid acute haemolysis, either by density floatation over a Ficoll–Hypaque gradient, by buffy coat sedimentation over hydroxyethyl starch, or by elutriation using an automatic cell separator. The latter improves the recovery of stem cells and decreases the risk of bacterial contamination inherent in manual techniques. During the reinfusion special attention to the risk of volume overload is mandatory.

When cryopreserved autologous marrow is needed, the bags containing the frozen cells are thawed rapidly at $37\,°C$ in a water-bath and usually reinfused within 15 minutes to avoid prolonged exposure to toxic levels of dimethysulphoxide. Since any residual red blood cells are haemolysed during the freezing and thawing procedure, care must be taken to avoid renal haemoglobin overload and acute renal failure. The reinfused dimethysulphoxide is mainly eliminated via the airways following hepatic metabolism and does not result in significant tissue damage. Transient fever, abdominal and bone pain, tachycardia, nausea, vomiting, bradycardia, transient dyspnoea, and perspiration are frequently encountered during or immediately after the reinfusion. Appropriate supportive care reduces these side-effects promptly in most instances.

Positively selected CD34 + peripheral blood stem cells and cultured stem cells occupy a very small volume, and their infusion reduces the incidence of postinfusional nausea and emesis related to the larger volume of dimethysulphoxide in standard peripheral blood stem cell preparations, and the frequently observed transient O_2 desaturation.

Engraftment

Early engraftment is thought to be mediated by committed progenitor cells, and long-term engraftment by the most primitive stem cells. In recipients of autologous bone marrow, haematological reconstitution was reportedly delayed in transplants containing fewer than 10^3 CFU-GM/kg or fewer than 10^6 CD34 + cells/kg so that the number of CFU-GM or CD34 + cells can be used to assess the quality of the preparation.[41],[42] Engraftment can be accelerated by pretreating the patient prior to harvest with haematopoietic growth factors. The number of CFU-GM necessary to obtain engraftment with peripheral blood stem cells was found to be at least 5×10^5/kg, significantly higher than for bone marrow.[43]

Both in vitro and engraftment studies indicate that peripheral blood stem cells have a greater number of committed progenitors than bone marrow.[43] There was concern that peripheral blood stem cell preparations might have a low content of long-term repopulating cells and that the long-term haematological engraftment might be tenuous, but subsequent experience has shown that long-term engraftment following reinfusion of peripheral blood stem cells has

generally not been a problem. Autologous bone marrow transplantation and reinfusion of peripheral blood stem cells have been compared in randomized, controlled trials: peripheral blood stem cells demonstrated a substantially accelerated granulocyte recovery and a faster platelet recovery. They have decreased the incidence of infections, the duration of febrile neutropenia, and the length of stay in hospital, and reduced the number of platelet transfusions required and the cost of the procedure. There was no advantage in long-term progression-free survival, or overall survival.[44],[45]

There are differences in expression of surface antigens including cell adhesion molecules (e.g. LFA-3, aLb2, and integrins) which determine the stromal attachment, and are involved in the regulation of migration-associated events.[46] Long-term culture-initiating cells are progenitors able to generate colony forming unit cells and are the best approximation of stem cells, and their quantitation allows an estimate of the frequency of marrow repopulating cells.[47] Stem cells mobilized with chemotherapy and growth factors result in a number of long-term repopulating cells comparable with that in bone marrow mononuclear cell suspensions, suggesting that the different mix of more committed progenitors may explain the differences described above.[48],[49]

Delayed or incomplete engraftment and late graft failures have been reported when using a small graft of peripheral blood stem cells. A clear dose–response has been shown between the number of CD34 + peripheral blood stem cells infused and the timing of neutrophil and platelet recovery. The threshold value for CD34 + cells allowing sustained engraftment has been estimated to be 10^6/kg.[50],[51] The positive selection of CD34 + cells results in purified cell suspensions that appear no different in their ability to generate sustained haematological recovery with unselected marrow or peripheral blood stem cells.[52] In vitro culture of CD34 + cells allows enrichment for CD34 + cells without increasing the number of clonogenic epithelial tumour cells. Ex vivo expansion of as few as 10^7 peripheral CD34 + cells allows engraftment (Fig. 3).[17] This technology may reduce contaminating tumour cells but the long-term reconstitutional capability of cultured cells is not yet known. Gene marking studies will provide definitive answers to this still debated question.

Administration of haematopoietic growth factor after transplantation

Myeloid growth factors are administered routinely after autologous bone marrow transplantation and peripheral blood stem cell reinfusions, following earlier reports of clinical benefit.[53] Differences with regard to the need for posttransplantation growth factor therapy may exist between marrow- or blood-derived stem cells.

Following autologous bone marrow transplantation, randomized controlled trials of posttransplantation GM-CSF accelerated neutrophil recovery and reduced the number of days of neutropenic fever and the length of hospital stay.[41],[54],[55] G-CSF may be equally effective.

Combinations of G-CSF $\pm$ IL-3 accelerated multilineage recovery, and fewer infections and hospital days were found in the combination arm, thereby offering the potential of superiority over single growth factors.[56] The GM-CSF/IL-3 fusion protein PIXY 321 was comparable to GM-CSF in stimulating neutrophil recovery in a randomized trial, but platelets seem to recover faster after PIXY 321.[57] IL-6 and IL-11 alone or with G-CSF or GM-CSF have also been evaluated in small non-randomized trials with no noticeable improvement over G-CSF or GM-CSF alone.

Following peripheral blood stem cell infusion, the benefit of using growth factors until neutrophil recovery is uncertain. Multivariate analyses of parameters which may influence engraftment of neutrophils and platelets indicate that dose of stem cells is the most potent factor. After infusing lower numbers of stem cells, G-CSF appeared to enhance neutrophil engraftment and in a prospective randomized trial the delay of G-CSF until day 5 after reinfusion did not adversely affect engraftment.[51],[58] In randomized studies, no consistent clinical benefit regarding the number of febrile days, septic episodes, and transfusion requirements could be demonstrated, although hospital recovery was shortened.[54],[59],[60] Rigorously controlled prospective randomized trials must document the benefit of growth factors before their clinical use can be recommended in the setting of peripheral blood stem cells rescue.

Engraftment does not seem to depend on growth factors used in the mobilization phase. However, in non-randomized studies with combinations of either G-CSF or GM-CSF and recombinant human stem cell growth factor (huSCF) for mobilization of peripheral blood stem cells, and postreinfusional G-CSF or GM-CSF, the combinations appeared to enhance the recovery of peripheral blood stem cells and to reduce the time to platelet recovery.

Immunotherapy

Autologous stem cell reinfusion circumvents the immunological complications that plague allogeneic transplantation and donor availability, but relapse following high-dose strategies remains the most important problem. The use of syngeneic or allogeneic bone marrow and stem cells avoids the reinfusion of tumour cells. Following allografts, graft versus host disease reduces the relapse rate of acute and chronic myeloid leukaemia. This antitumour effect follows an inverse correlation between the intensity of graft versus host disease and relapse, and is mediated by a subset of T lymphocytes.[61] Following T-cell purging of the graft (reduction of T cells present in the graft by a factor of 10^{-2} or 10^{-3}) graft versus host disease was abolished almost completely, while the rate of relapse increased to almost 80 per cent in chronic myelogenous leukaemia.[62],[63]

Favourable results have been reported following allogeneic bone marrow transplantation for low-grade lymphomas, and in patients failing autologous transplantation. Regression of lymphoma was also reported in isolated patients with recurrent non-Hodgkin's lymphoma after allogeneic bone marrow transplantation, following the transient discontinuation of immunosuppressive therapy and development of graft versus host disease, or following donor leucocyte infusion.[64]

In a retrospective case-matched study of 189 patients with myeloma comparing autologous transplantation with allogeneic transplantation, the progression-free survival was significantly better for the autologous arm (34 months versus 18 months), due to greater toxicity from allogeneic transplantation. However, for those who survived for more than a year, a significant advantage in relapse-free survival of allogeneic over autologous transplantation was observed, indicating a 'graft versus myeloma' effect.[65] In some case reports, graft versus host disease induced by donor-derived leucocyte transfusions following allogeneic transplantation has been associated with a potent 'graft versus myeloma' effect. Phase 1 trials in patients with primary refractory myeloma have shown the feasability of this immune manipulation.

New strategies are exploring whether minimal residual disease after high-dose chemotherapy can be further reduced by the addition of immune interventions via, for example, adoptive immunotherapy, in vivo administration of regulatory cytokines, or antitumour vaccination (see Chapter 1.10).

In a non-randomized trial in lymphoma patients following transplantation comparing interferon-α and IL-2 with no additional treatment, the cytokine combination seemingly resulted in a better disease-free survival (80 per cent after 34 months versus 52 per cent after 23 months) when compared with historical controls.[66] Larger, randomized trials are necessary to determine the contribution of these approaches.

Gene therapy

That peripheral blood stem cells can be used as transfection targets for therapeutic gene transfer has been demonstrated in investigations of gene replacement therapy for single genetic defects (e.g. ADA deficiency, cystic fibrosis, and RevM10 gene transfer in HIV-1 infections).[67]–[69] The transfer of the MDR1 gene into haematopoietic pecursor cells may provide a means to confer resistance to the toxic effects of chemotherapy.[70] Several other genes appear promising for gene transfer to induce drug resistance in haematological precursors, such as the dihydrofolate reductase gene, or the methyl-guanine methyl-transferase gene.[71] Although gene expression in haematological presursors remains a safety concern, the successful use of this technology may soon broaden its clinical application (see also Chapter 4.26).

High-dose chemotherapy and clinical applications

Toxicity

Strategies integrating high-dose chemotherapy and autologous transplantation have been based upon short pretransplant treatments, followed by very high-dose consolidation therapy in patients who have achieved either complete or very good partial responses. The most important element in high-dose chemotherapy is the preparative regimen. It must provide maximal antitumour activity with comparatively low systemic toxicity.

Dose escalations of approximately 10-fold over conventional treatment may be achieved for cyclophosphamide, etoposide, BCNU, melphalan, mitomycin C, and thiotepa, which demonstrate a steep dose–response curve in tumour cell kill. At these doses, which cannot be exceeded due to the excessive non-bone-marrow toxicity, cyclophosphamide and etoposide are not myeloablative, and bone marrow support is not necessary, while after high-dose chemotherapy with thiotepa or BCNU the neutropenic period is significantly shortened by using stem cell rescue.

The role of total body irradiation

Following the demonstration of the feasibility of total body irradiation with bone marrow rescue, total body irradiation alone and subsequently with cyclophosphamide was used primarily for haematological malignancies The impact of total body irradiation varies with dose, dose rate, fractionation, and dose distribution, which may vary between institutions thus rendering comparative analysis of published results difficult. Acute and late toxicities depend on these variables (see Chapter 4.8). Other drugs have subsequently been explored in combination with total body irradiation, but no demonstrable superiority over cyclophosphamide has been reported in preparatory regimens for stem cell transplantation. There is an understandable reluctance to use total body irradiation in children because of its considerable early and delayed impact on growth and development.

Preparative regimens for transplantation

Many candidates for high-dose chemotherapy with lymphomas or solid tumours have already been exposed to drugs that carry a cumulative risk of organ toxicities that can be augmented by radiation therapy, or else have been extensively treated with radiation therapy. Conditioning regimens that avoid radiation exposure have been developed, and are now most commonly used in the setting of autologous marrow rescue. The drugs in these regimens have been evaluated in dose escalation studies and many exhibit a steep dose–response in phase 1 studies, which have established their maximal tolerated dose. Some drugs may be used without stem cell support, particularly with subsequent administration of growth factor. These drugs mainly have myelotoxicity and limited organ toxicity at the levels defined, allowing for drug combinations. Toxicities in combination regimens are often overlapping, and may result in fatal interstitial pneumonitis, veno-occlusive hepatic disease, myocardial necrosis, acute renal failure, haemorrhagic cystitis, and severe mucositis. Therefore, the use of drug combinations has often required dose reductions to avoid such overlapping toxicities. In general, combinations for the treatment of given types of malignancy have been developed by selecting combinations of drugs that are active at conventional doses. Small numbers of patients and the extensive mixture of important variables related to disease and to patients make meaningful comparisons between the many regimens illusory. Some important drugs and their use either alone or in combination regimens are summarized below. The pharmacology of these drugs is described in greater detail in Chapters 4.13 to 4.18.

Cyclophosphamide was the first drug used in conjunction with total body irradiation at 60 mg/m^2 for two consecutive days. It can result in acute myocardial multifocal necrosis and severe haemorrhagic cystitis: the latter can be avoided by using hyperhydration, alkalinization of the urine, and mesna.

Busulphan replaced total body irradiation as an alternative treatment with similar antileukaemic and immunosuppressive effects, and is still in use for both allogeneic and autologous transplants. For Ewing's sarcoma, the use of busulphan was found to be superior to total body irradiation. The dose-limiting toxicities are mucositis, anorexia, and hepatic toxicity, including sometimes fatal hepatovenoocclusive disease, and uncommonly interstitial pulmonary fibrosis which may occur as late as 10 years after treatment.

Melphalan is widely used either alone at 200 to 240 mg/m^2 or in conjunction with other alkylating agents. It is a frequent component of sequential high-dose chemotherapies. The oral formulation shows considerable interpatient variability and parenteral administration is more frequently used. Toxicities include mucositis and diarrhoea, and it can contribute to veno-occlusive disease.

BCNU is widely used in high-dose chemotherapy. Its dose-limiting toxicity is veno-occlusive disease of the liver, which has been observed in 5 per cent to 20 per cent of patients, and pulmonary fibrosis, which can be fatal. It is a component of many popular multidrug regimens used in high-dose chemotherapy. CCNU was used as an alternative in some regimens but was found to produce dose-dependent nephrotoxicity.

Thiotepa has proven to be useful in high-dose chemotherapy for lymphomas, breast cancer, and paediatric solid tumours. Central nervous system toxicity occurs at high doses.

Ifosfamide is an alkylating agent used in combination regimens. Renal and central nervous system toxicity are limiting factors.

Cisplatin has been used in regimens for the treatment of small cell lung cancer, breast, and ovarian carcinomas, but it displays a shallow dose–response relationship above 100 mg/m^2, and the dose cannot be increased above 200 mg/m^2 due to its renal and neurological toxicity.

Carboplatin has a different dose–effect and toxicity profile from cisplatin which allows dose escalation. It is used frequently in combination therapy. Area under the curve values for carboplatin are correlated with mucosal, liver, renal, and neurological toxicities.

Cytosine arabinoside in high dose is a component of several regimens effective for the treatment of leukaemias and lymphoid malignancies. Its main dose-limiting toxicity is to the liver and central nervous system.

Paclitaxel has been used in limited numbers of patients, and dose-escalation studies have shown that it may be given at four- to fivefold increases over conventional doses in combination with other agents. Severe mucosal, neurological, gastrointestinal, and cardiac toxicities have been reported.

Etoposide dose escalation has been explored in a variety of haematological and solid tumours. Its mucosal toxicity is dose limiting.

Mitoxantrone has been escalated six-fold in preparative regimens for the treatment of leukaemias, lymphomas, and breast cancer. Cardiac toxicity limits the total dose that can be used.

Mitomycin C has been tested with autologous bone marrow transplantation, and has resulted in dose-limiting veno-occlusive disease.

High-dose chemotherapy for specific malignancies

In the following brief review of high-dose chemotherapy and stem cell transplantation for specific malignancies, emphasis is placed on the results of randomized clinical trials that have compared the use of high-dose and conventional approaches. There are numerous uncontrolled trials and case series which suggest a higher rate of complete response than after conventional chemotherapy. However, patients are usually selected to receive high-dose chemotherapy on the basis of better performance status, prior response to conventional chemotherapy, or, in the adjuvant setting, after more extensive screening to rule out metastatic disease.[72] For these reasons such trials provide little or no evidence about the value of high-dose chemotherapy and stem cell rescue.

Leukaemias

The utility of high-dose chemotherapy was first explored in leukaemias. Since myelosuppression is the main toxicity of treatments, stem cell transplantation allowed intensification of treatment, regardless of the damage to bone marrow. A prospective trial of patients with acute myeloblastic leukaemia with poor prognostic factors who were in first complete remission following remission-induction compared the outcome of a treatment arm consisting of allogenic HLA-matched bone marrow transplantation for patients with a suitable donor, with the results of a treatment arm in which patients were randomized to receive either autologous bone marrow transplantation or standard chemotherapy. The results showed that both allogeneic and autologous transplantation can achieve a better relapse-free survival than conventional therapy, and that allogeneic transplantation was superior.[73] In many prospective trials comparing allografts and conventional chemotherapy, allogeneic matched donor transplantation results in improved long-term survival. In a randomized trial comparing autologous transplantation in first complete remission as consolidation versus observation the high-dose arm has also shown improved survival.[74] Allogeneic transplantation is the only therapy able to cure acute myeloblastic leukaemia, which does not respond to induction chemotherapy. Following relapse after conventional chemotherapy, some transplants have been carried out without remission reinduction, but most were performed in second complete remission, with comparative survival results. No randomized trials have addressed this approach in comparison with conventional treatment, but analysis of retrospective registry data strongly suggests a benefit for allogeneic transplantation from a matched donor, and possibly unrelated matched donor transplants. Whether autologous stem cell transplantation in second complete remission is superior to the best standard chemotherapy is not known.

In acute lymphoblastic leukaemia, non-responding children or adult patients may be rescued by allogeneic bone marrow transplantation. In first complete remission, data from randomized studies do not support transplantation over standard chemotherapy except for a subgroup of high-risk patients presenting with a positive Philadelphia chromosome, white cell counts of more than 30 000 per mm^3, null cell phenotype, and older patients (over 35 years).[75] Multiple phase 2 studies have shown efficacy of autologous bone marrow transplantation, which is less toxic and more readily performed than allogeneic transplantation. In a randomized trial comparing allogeneic versus autologous transplantation as consolidation treatment of adult acute lymphoblastic leukaemia, the 3-year relapse-free survival was 68 versus 26 per cent.[74] Following relapse, the impact of bone marrow transplantation in second complete remission was compared with maintenance therapy in a small, prospective, comparative study which showed a significant superiority of bone marrow transplantation, regardless of the origin of stem cells (autologous, $N = 7$, allogeneic $N = 11$), resulting in a 2-year event-free survival of 37 per cent ($\pm$ 22 per cent) versus 18 per cent ($\pm$ 13 per cent).[75] For relapsed acute lymphoblastic leukaemia in children, autologous bone marrow transplantation was not associated with any benefit, in contrast to allogeneic bone marrow transplantation, which resulted in a 14 per cent gain in event-free 5-year survival (40.7 versus 26.4 per cent) in the large United Kingdom Medical Research Council Acute Lymphoblastic Leukaemia X Trial.[78]

Lymphomas

Following two decades of phase 2 studies for non-Hodgkin's lymphomas that have resulted in increasingly intense regimens which appeared to approximately double the response rate and survival compared to standard **CHOP** (cyclophosphamide, doxorubicin, vincristine, prednisone) therapy, the concept of dose intensity within the range of conventional chemotherapy has been examined in the phase 3 South West Oncology Group trial comparing the CHOP regimen with the most effective second- and third-generation regimens (see also Chapter 15.11).[79] In contrast to the results obtained in historical and comparative studies that had indicated a survival advantage for the more intense treatments, this study found no difference in survival for any subgroup of disease. The heterogeneity in the historical studies for lymphoma subtypes, differences in risk factors, and the differences in treatment designs misled investigators. This caveat must be kept in mind for the interpretation of, and comparison between, the many non-randomized high-dose chemotherapy studies.

Strategies to increase the cure rate of lymphomas using high-dose chemotherapy with stem cell rescue have been pursued intensively, and a number of conditioning regimens have been explored in phase 2 studies. While mainly autologous stem cell rescue has been utilized in consolidation of first remission, the use of both autologous and allogeneic stem cell products has been explored following high-dose chemotherapy consolidation after relapse. The results of randomized controlled trials that have compared high-dose chemotherapy with conventional chemotherapy for patients with lymphomas or myeloma are summarized in Table 1.

Low-grade lymphomas cannot be cured by standard chemotherapy, and therefore high-dose strategies have been explored in a number of small or non-randomized studies. The role of high-dose chemotherapy in first remission of low-grade lymphomas is not established. One small phase 3 trial (presented only in abstract form) suggests a possible benefit for disease-free survival but no difference in overall survival at 2 years.[80] Due to the long natural history of these lymphomas a survival benefit seems unlikely due to the risks of high-dose chemotherapy and the median age at diagnosis of the patients, but this procedure may benefit younger patients.

For intermediate- and high-grade lymphomas current conventional chemotherapy regimens produce 3-year disease-free survival in only about 50 per cent of the patients. The LNH-87 randomized trial compared sequential conventional chemotherapy with a high-dose consolidation program (Table 1). The initial analysis based on 464 patients showed no advantage for autologous bone marrow transplantation, but subsequent reanalysis stratifying 541 randomized patients for the criteria of the International Prognostic Index demonstrated that high-risk patients who were transplanted in remission had a significantly superior disease-free survival.[81],[82] There is a possibility that the retrospective assignment of International Prognostic Index criteria might have influenced the results. In a follow-up study from the same group of investigators (at present only published in abstract form) which included 301 patients with aggressive lymphomas and two or more International Prognostic Index adverse prognostic factors, high-dose chemotherapy did not increase the rate of complete remission (66 per cent versus 67 per cent), nor prevent relapse (16-month event-free survival 57 per cent versus 48 per cent) (LNH 93–3; 8) (Table 1).[3] This study differed from the earlier one by an abbreviated induction in the high-dose chemotherapy

Table 1 Randomized trials of high-dose chemotherapy and stem cell rescue for hematological malignancies

	Diagnosis/treatment	Number of patients	Percentage survival	Median survival (years)	P log rank	Reference
NHL, after first CR induction:						
	CHOP × 6	24	80	2	NS	Schouten et al.[80]
versus	CHOP × 3 + HD Cyt/TBI without purging	33	73			
versus	Cyt/TBI with purging	32	89			
	IVA/L-asp	273 (111)*	67 (52)	5	NS (0.06)	Haioun et al.[82]
versus	HD CVB + ABMT	268 (86)*	69 (65)			
	MACOP-B	50	55	4	0.09	Gianni et al.[87]
versus	HD sequential	48	81			
	CHOP	35	85	5	NS	Verdonck et al.[86]
versus	CHOP-HD Cyt + TBI	34	56			
	ACVBP × 8	301†	73	3	0.1	Gisselbrecht et al.[83]
versus	ECVP → ECVBP × 2 → HD BEAM		61			
	CHOEP × 5 +IFRT	312†	75	2	NS	Kaiser et al.[84]
versus	CHOEP × 3 → HD BEAM		73			
	CHVmP/BV × 8	184†	75	5	NS	Kluin-Nelemans et al.[85]
versus	CHVmP/BV × 3 +HD BEAC		67			Sweetenham et al.[89]
NHL after relapse :						
	DHAP × 4	54	32	5	0.038	Philip et al.[92]
versus	DHAP × 2 + HD BEAC	55	53			
HD following relapse						
	mini-BEAM	20	10	3	0.025	Linch et al.[97]
versus	BEAM + ABMT	20	53			
	Non-crossresistant	103	47	4	NS	Yuen et al.[98]†
versus	CVB or fTBI + CV	60	54			
	dexaBeam × 4	139	NA	(3)	NS	Schmitz et al.[99]
versus	dexaBeam × 2 + Beam		NA			
Multiple myeloma:						
	VMCP/BVAP × 8	100	12		0.03	Attal et al.[101]
versus	VMCP/BVAC × 2 + ABMT	100	52			
	VMCP → delayed ABMT	92	74.5	3	NS	Fermand et al.[102]
versus	VMCP → early ABMT	90	73.5			
	VAD + interferon	116	39	5	0.01	Barlogie et al.[104]‡
versus	VAD + tandem transplant	123	61			

*Results in parentheses are for IPI 2,3 patients.

†Total number of randomized patients.

‡Comparative, non-randomized study.

HD = high dose; ID = intermediate dose.

Abbreviations for chemotherapy regimens, for doses see in references:

CHO(±E)P: cyclophosphamide, Adriamycin, vincristine, (etoposide), prednisone.

IVA/L-asp: ifosfamide, etoposide, cytarabine, L-asparaginase.

CVB±(P): cyclophosphamide, carmustine, etoposide, (prednisone).

MACOP-B: methotrexate, Adriamycin, cyclophosphamide, vincristine, prednisone, bleomycin.

HD sequential: Adriamycin, vincristine, prednisone → cyclophosphamide HD → peripheral blood stem cell harvest → vincristine, methotrexate HD/ leucovorin rescue → etoposide HD → melphalan HD + total body irradiation → peripheral blood stem cell reinfusion → mitoxantrone HD, melphalan HD → peripheral blood stem cell reinfusion.

ACVBP: Adriamycin, cyclophosphamide, vincristine, bleomycin, prednisone.

ECV(±B)P: epirubicine, cyclophosphamide, vincristine, bleomycin, prednisone.

dexaBEAM: (dexamethasone) carmustine, etoposide, aracytidine, melphalan.

CHVmP/BV: cyclophosphamide, Adriamycin, VM-26, prednisone/bleomycin, vincristine.

BP: carmustine, prednisone.

BEAC: carmustine, etoposide, aracytidine, cyclophosphamide.

DHAP: cisplatin, aracytidine, prednisone.

VMCP: vincristine, melphalan, cyclophosphamide, prednisone.

BVAP: carmustine, vincristine, Adriamycin, prednisone.

VAD: vincristine, Adriamycin, dexamethasone.

Tandem transplant: cyclophosphamide HD → peripheral blood stem cell harvest → etoposide, dexamethasone, cytarabine, cisplatin → melphalan HD → peripheral blood stem cell reinfusion → melphalan HD + total body irradiation → peripheral blood stem cell reinfusion.

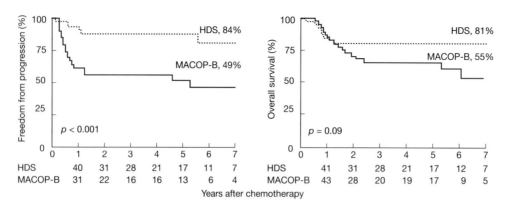

Fig. 8 Kaplan–Meier plot of freedom from disease progression and overall survival for 48 patients assigned to high-dose sequential chemotherapy and 50 patients given MACOP-B. The median follow-up was 55 months. The number of patients at risk is shown below each time point . Percentages are right for each category of survival at 7 years. (By courtesy of Dr M. Gianni and reproduced with permission.[87])

arm, and poorly responding and non-responding patients were included in the high-dose chemotherapy arm since patients were stratified initially to receive or not high-dose chemotherapy. The abbreviated induction therapy might explain the different outcome compared with the earlier trials that treated patients with six courses of dose-intense induction therapy. In two other randomized trials (published in abstract form), no survival advantage could yet be found for patients that were undergoing high-dose chemotherapy (for treatment regimens see Table 1).[84],[85] Longer follow-up is needed. In another small randomized trial, five courses of CHOP and autologous bone marrow transplantation were compared in low-, intermediate-, and high-grade aggressive lymphomas with a slow response after three courses of CHOP. No benefit for high-dose chemotherapy was found for this subset of patients at high risk of relapse, and there was a trend towards a better outcome with conventional chemotherapy.[86] Given the heterogeneity of disease grades, the particular patient selection, and the lack of power of this small trial, these results cannot be directly compared with those of patients that are consolidated in first remission. These studies illustrate the difficulties in study design and the caution that is necessary before conclusions based on comparisons between trials are drawn.

Sequential high-dose chemotherapy protocols have been explored as first-line therapy for patients with a poor prognosis, following the demonstration of its feasibility in several phase 1 to 2 studies. In a phase 3 trial for patients with aggressive lymphoma comparing sequential high-dose chemotherapy treatment followed by myeloablative therapy and bone marrow transplantation to the **MACOP-B** (methotrexate, Adriamycin, cyclophosphamide, vincristine, prednisone, bleomycin) regimen as initial or salvage therapy, a significant improvement in the 5-year disease-free survival was found in the sequential high-dose chemotherapy arm (Fig. 8).[87]

Burkitt's and Burkitt's-like small cleaved-cell lymphomas have poor responses to conventional treatments. A retrospective report from the European Bone Marrow Transplant registry indicated an encouraging 5-year disease-free survival of 72 per cent with high-dose chemotherapy.[88] Multicentre prospective trials are needed to address the question of superiority of high-dose chemotherapy.

Lymphoblastic lymphoma is a distinct entity, biologically closer to acute lymphocytic leukaemia, and is therefore not included in studies of aggressive lymphomas. high-dose chemotherapy with stem cell support as consolidation of first remisson for patients with poor prognostic features has obtained encouraging results with over 60 per cent disease-free survival after 5 years, compared with historical values of 20 per cent in such patents. A randomized European Bone Marrow Transplant/United Kingdom Lymphoma Group trial comparing conventional chemotherapy and high-dose chemotherapy with autologous stem cell rescue produced a 45 per cent decrease in relapse/death risk at 12 months in the high-dose arm.[89] These results do include patients who were treated in chemosensitive relapse. The use of high-dose chemotherapy with stem cell support as consolidation for poor-risk lymphoblastic lymphoma in first complete remission is still under investigation and is not indicated outside prospective trials specifically designed to validate these observations.

Following relapse, retrospective studies in children and adults have shown that only chemotherapy-sensitive disease can benefit from high-dose chemotherapy, and that those with disease progression at the time of high-dose therapy could not usually be cured. While the survival following partial or complete histological remission following conventional salvage therapy resulted in approximately 50 per cent disease-free survival, fewer than 10 per cent of those with drug-resistant relapse were alive after 1 year.[90],[91] These observations led to an international study which randomized 109 relapsed patients who attained complete remission or partial remission after two courses of treatment independently of their initial disease grade to either salvage chemotherapy with the DHAP (cisplatin, aracytidine, prednisolone) regimen (54 patients), or DHAP × 2 followed by consolidation with high-dose chemotherapy (55 patients).[92] Chemosensitivity was predictive for a better 5-year outcome using transplantation. These results demonstrate that high-dose chemotherapy following relapse in patients who are sensitive to chemotherapy is significantly superior to conventional salvage therapy. Since this trial included heterogeneous types of patients with regard to International Prognostic Index criteria, a retrospective stratification according to International Prognostic Index risk factors was applied to the data of this phase 3 trial, and has identified a benefit for high-dose chemotherapy only for the subgroup with poor prognostic factors (Fig. 9).[93]

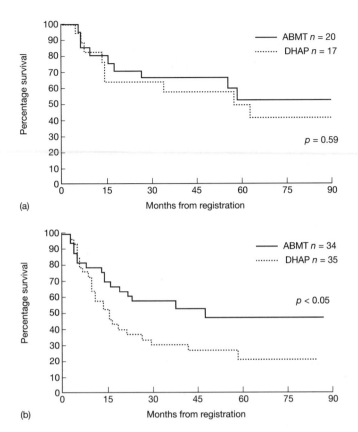

Fig. 9 Overall survival of 106 randomized patients with relapsed non-Hodgkin's lymphoma according to International Prognostic Index at relapse. Survival is calculated from the first day of the first course of DHAP. (a) Patients with International Prognostic Index = 0, DHAP versus autologous bone marrow transplantation arm. (b) Patients with International Prognostic Index = 1–3, DHAP versus autologous bone marrow transplantation arm. (By courtesy of Dr J.-Y. Blay and reproduced with permission.[93])

In relapsed lymphoblastic lymphoma, the randomized European Bone Marrow Transplant/United Kingdom Lymphoma Group trial referred to above showed that relapse/death risk was reduced in the high-dose arm quite comparably with the patients treated in first complete remission or chemosensitive relapse.[89] These results suggest that all relapsed/refractory patients with this subtype who are sensitive to salvage chemotherapy should be offered high-dose chemotherapy consolidation and stem cell transplantation.

A large North-American Intergroup study of high-dose chemotherapy for non-Hodgkin's lymphoma will address the important questions of appropriate timing of high-dose chemotherapy with regard to the length of induction therapy and its timing in relation to remission, and definitively allow the identification of the therapeutic value of this approach.

Hodgkin's disease

In Hodgkin's disease (see Chapter 15.8), the role of high-dose chemotherapy with stem cell rescue has been evaluated in patients who progressed during induction or who relapsed within 12 months of therapy, since these patients have a 5-year survival of 0 to 20 per cent following conventional salvage chemotherapy. Even after prolonged

first remission, survival after relapse is less than 40 per cent with conventional salvage chemotherapy. In multiple uncontrolled series of relapsed patients with a poor prognosis, high-dose chemotherapy with stem cell rescue produced a disease-free survival of between 30 and 80 per cent.[94]–[96]

The wide range of reported survival reflects the heterogeneity of patient populations with regard to important prognostic factors for the outcome of high-dose treatment such as timing, treatment history, sensitivity to chemotherapy, and extent of disease. In a matched case-control study, event-free survival of patients with fewer than 12 months of remission after first-line therapy was superior in the high-dose chemotherapy arm, adding evidence to an earlier small randomized trial performed by the British National Lymphoma Investigation Group which had found a superior progression-free survival of high-dose chemotherapy with marrow support compared with conventional salvage treatment.[97],[98] The results for the more favourable subgroup of patients who relapsed after more than 12 months of remission were less clearcut: the high-dose chemotherapy and stem cell rescue produced no statistically significant survival advantage despite an apparently superior cure rate, thus indicating a lesser additional benefit of the high-dose chemotherapy.[98] This point was investigated in a larger European trial which showed a significantly better progression-free survival in both patient subgroups of early and late relapses, but again no significant overall survival benefit was found, possibly because of the relatively short median follow-up of only 34 months.[99]

For the very unfavourable subset of patients who are not sensitive to induction chemotherapy, or who present with diffuse pulmonary infiltration, high-dose chemotherapy allows salvage of only a minority of patients. Future studies should explore less toxic high-dose chemotherapy for the group of patients with favourable prognosis, and more effective remission-induction for the poorest-risk patients with early progressive/refractory disease.

Myeloma

Following conventional treatment for myeloma, a median survival of approximately 3 years can be expected regardless of the chemotherapy regimen (see Chapter 15.13). In advanced-stage patients, high-dose melphalan ($140 \, mg/m^2$) without any stem cell support resulted in high response rates and good remissions, but they were often short-lived in advanced-stage patients and a plateau of survival was not reached.[100] This prompted attempts to use high-dose chemotherapy without marrow support in untreated patients, with good responses but high haematological toxicity. To reduce toxicity, high-dose chemotherapy with stem cell rescue has been evaluated with promising results in a number of phase 1 to 2 studies after relapse, or in refractory patients. Only one large prospective randomized trial (the IMF-90 trial) has been published; this involved 200 previously untreated patients assigned to conventional alternating chemotherapy for 18 courses or, after four to six courses, switching over to high-dose melphalan with total body irradiation for early intensification.[101] It demonstrated the superiority of the high-dose chemotherapy arm over conventional chemotherapy in induction of remission (38 per cent complete remission versus 14 per cent complete remission), 5-year event-free survival (28 per cent versus 10 per cent), and survival (52 per cent versus 12 per cent).[101] Longer follow-up is necessary, and there is a need for confirmatory studies.

The issue of the best timing for high-dose chemotherapy has been addressed in a prospective randomized trial of 182 patients. Peripheral blood stem cells were harvested after induction of remission with four cycles of VMCP (vincristine, melphalan, cyclophosphamide, prednisone) chemotherapy, and this was then followed by high-dose chemotherapy and reinfusion immediately or at the time of disease progression or relapse, which occurred after a median duration of 53 months on continued chemotherapy. The median survival after transplantation was 18 months, with overall median survival of 58 months. The early high-dose chemotherapy arm showed no survival advantage.[102] This important issue also needs confirmation in larger trials.

Despite the possible benefit of high-dose chemotherapy, only approximately 30 per cent of patients survive for more than 5 years, and new strategies to reduce the rate of relapse are needed. Because bone marrow is generally contaminated by myeloma cells, various purging procedures have been used, and promising results have been obtained in uncontrolled studies; however, this may be due to selection bias. In a study involving patients aged less than 65 years and responding to first-line conventional chemotherapy who would have been candidates for high-dose chemotherapy, the median survival was 5 years, quite comparable with outcomes after high-dose chemotherapy and stem cell rescue.[103]

Sequential high-dose therapies have been explored in myeloma. 'Total therapy', consisting of three cycles of VAD (vincristine, Adriamycin, dexamethasone) chemotherapy, followed by high-dose cyclophosphamide with stem cell collection, and two sequential non-crossresistant conditioning regimens with tandem transplantation was given to 123 patients who were compared with closely matched patients from previous South West Oncology Group trials. The patients included in the high-dose arm were given interferon-α until relapse. The median event-free survival was 49 months and overall survival was more than 62 months, which were prolonged in comparison with the conventionally treated controls as well as with the outcome of the only randomized trial with single autologous transplantation which resulted in event-free survival of 27 months and overall survival of 49 months.[101],[104] A trial comparing single with tandem transplantation is under way.

Since no plateau is observed following high-dose chemotherapy and stem cell rescue, some form of maintenance treatment seems indicated. The use of interferon-α, which has been shown to exhibit a marginal benefit after standard chemotherapy, was not found consistently useful after high-dose chemotherapy. Despite the administration of interferon-α to all patients treated in the IMF trial, there was no plateau of the event-free survival curve, indicating that cure is not achieved with this addition.

Allogeneic transplantation for myeloma has been carried out in a limited number of patients, since it is complicated by serious side-effects in this generally elderly population of patients.

Breast cancer

High-dose chemotherapy with stem cell transplantation has been used in multiple uncontrolled trials for patients with metastatic breast cancer, and is in common use for this indication in the United States. 'Higher than expected' rates of complete remission are often obtained, with a few patients achieving long-term disease-free survival.[105] In the European Bone Marrow Transplant registry 1293 patients with metastatic disease were evaluable as of 1997. While approximately 50 per cent of the patients consolidated in first complete remission ($N = 589$) were alive after 60 months, only 10 per cent survived among patients that have not reached complete remission ($N = 704$). These results may of course be due to selection of patients and are not necessarily superior to those obtained with conventional treatment (see also Chapter 11.8). A small randomized trial including 90 metastatic patients compared six to eight cycles of conventional treatment with tandem cycles of high-dose chemotherapy (Table 2). This trial was subsequently shown to have had serious irregularities invalidating its conclusions. A further trial, published only in abstract form, 98 patients (out of 423 hormone-insensitive treated patients) who reached complete remission after conventional chemotherapy were randomized to immediate or delayed high-dose chemotherapy with stem cell rescue (Table 2).[106] The disease-free survival of the transplanted patients was significantly longer for patients transplanted early (3.2 years versus 1.9 years), but overall survival was superior in the delayed transplant arm, which suggests evidence against its value. In another small randomized trial, 61 metastatic or relapsed patients who had responded to a conventional anthracyclin-based (FEC/FAC) regimen were treated either with the same conventional therapy or with high-dose chemotherapy Although 2-year survival was no different, the authors reported a positive trend for the intensively treated group (Table 2).[107]

The large PBT-1 trial included 553 metastatic patients given four times to six times induction CAF (cyclophosphamide, Adriamycin, 5-fluorouracil) or CMF (cyclophosphamide, methotrexate, 5-fluorouracil). Of 303 patients who responded, only 199 were ultimately randomized to receive either maintenance CMF or high-dose chemotherapy with CTCb (cyclophosphamide, thiotepa, carboplatin) and stem cell rescue, and only 180 were evaluable for the comparison at the time of analysis. The median survival was 24 months after high-dose chemotherapy, and 26 months for the group that received conventional treatment. No survival advantage was found after 3 years for the high-dose chemotherapy arm (32 per cent) versus the conventionally treated arm (38 per cent). Toxicities were more frequently reported for the high-dose chemotherapy arm, but there was no difference in lethal toxicities between arms. No differences were found for progression-free survival, independently of the quality of the response obtained by the treatment.[108]

There has been widespread use of high-dose chemotherapy as adjuvant treatment for selected patients with stage II to III disease and high risk of relapse. An early retrospective matched pair analysis of breast cancer patients with more than 10 positive lymph nodes who were treated in the adjuvant setting found a two-fold increase in the 5-year survival following high-dose as compared with standard chemotherapy.[109] This analysis has been appropriately criticized because the historical population was unmatched for the extensive staging selection criteria applied to the patients undergoing high-dose chemotherapy and inevitably included an unknown number of patients with occult metastatic disease in the control arm. This contention was supported by the results of a study exploring the effect of extensive screening and selection usually applied to candidates for high-dose chemotherapy on the survival of patients with 10 or more positive axillary lymph nodes who qualified for high-dose chemotherapy but who were treated conventionally. The survival of this selected population was significantly better than expected from historical series of unselected patients.[72] The impact of selection

Table 2 High dose chemotherapy with stem cell rescue for breast cancer

	Diagnosis/treatment	Number of patients	Survival*	P log rank	Reference
Breast cancer, metastatic:					
	CNV × 6–8	45	(45 weeks)		
versus	Late HD CPB	98†	(3.2 years)	0.04	Peters et al.[106]
versus	Early HD CPB		(1.9 years)		
	4–6 FEC → FEC	61†	(15.2 months)	NS	Lotz et al.[107]
versus	4–6 FEC → CMA		(26.9 months)		
	CAF × 2→CMF	79	52% at 2 years	NS	Stadtmauer et al.[108]
versus	CAF × 2 → CTCb	101	49%		
Breast cancer, adjuvant					
	FEC × 10	78†	68% at 4 years	NS	Hortobagy et al.[111]
versus	FEC × 4 → 2 HD CVP		60%		
	FEC × 4	40	72% at 4 years	NS	Rodenhuis et al.[112]
versus	FEC × 4 → HD CTCb	41	79%		
	CAF → CPB int.	391	68% at 3 years	NS	Peters et al.[113]
versus	CAF → HD CPB	394	64%		
	FEC × 9 'tailored'	525²	NR	NS	SBCSG[114]
versus	FEC × 2 → HD CTCb				
versus	HD CNV × 2		(>400 weeks)		

*Median survival is indicated in brackets.

†Total number of patients randomized.

SBCSG = Scandinavian Breast Cancer Study Group.

NS = not significant; NR = not reached.

HD: high-dose regimens followed by stem cell rescue.

Abbreviations for chemotherapy regimens, for doses see references:

CMF: cyclophosphamide, methotrexate, 5-fluorouracil.

FEC: 5-fluorouracil, epirubicin, cyclophosphamide.

CAF: cyclophosphamide, Adriamycin, 5-fluorouracil.

CMA: cyclophosphamide, mitoxantrone, L-PAM.

CVP: cyclophosphamide, etoposide, cisplatin.

CNV: cyclophosphamide, mitoxantrone, etoposide.

CPB: cyclophosphamide, cisplatin, carmustine.

CTCb: cyclophosphamide, thiotepa, carboplatin.

CMA: cyclophosphamide, mitoxantrone, Adriamycin.

CVB: cyclophosphamide, etoposide, carmustine.

L-PAM: melphelan.

criteria on survival was also demonstrated in another study. In this analysis 39 patients were transplanted, allowing the authors to compare their outcome with the conventionally treated group of 128 patients who met the same criteria. There was no significant difference in survival.[108]

The contribution of high-dose chemotherapy to adjuvant therapy for high-risk breast cancer has been investigated in a few randomized trials, some of which have been reported recently in abstract form. They generally included patients with more than 10 positive nodes who are known to be at high risk for relapse after conventional therapy. The results of these trials are summarized in Table 2. They cannot be directly compared due to differences in their design. In the two small trials no significant difference was found in relapse-free survival between conventional and high-dose chemotherapy arms.[111],[112] One large study included 874 women given four courses of standard FAC (5-fluorouracil, Adriamycin, cyclophosphamide) chemotherapy followed either by immediate high-dose chemotherapy with stem cell support or intermediate-dose chemotherapy, with a delayed crossover at relapse to high-dose chemotherapy and stem cell rescue. The first 341 patients have been followed for 3 years: there have been fewer relapses in the high-dose chemotherapy arm (22 per cent versus 32 per cent), but the overall survival is no different at 68 per cent versus 64 per cent, with only 60 per cent of the expected events. There were some treatment-related deaths (7 per cent) in the high-dose arm but none in the intermediate-dose arm. The overall outcome in both treatment groups exceeded the results expected from previous studies. Final conclusions cannot be drawn for at least 2 more years.[113]

Another large report from the Scandinavian Breast Cancer Study Group randomized 525 patients to either so-called 'tailored' (adjusted to haematological tolerance), higher-than-conventional dose FEC (5-fluorouracil, epirubicin, cyclophosphamide) chemotherapy for nine courses versus a short, two-course arm of FEC followed by high-dose chemotherapy with stem cell rescue. With a median follow-up of 20 months, no difference was found between the two arms. Toxicity was significantly increased in the high-dose arm. However, an increased risk of secondary leukaemias was reported for the 'tailored' arm, a probable consequence of the increase in anthracycline dose.[114]

None of these trials compared high-dose chemotherapy with the more dose-intense anthracycline- and taxane-containing regimens currently used for high-risk patients in many centres, rather than the less effective 'standard' regimens. The ability to cure breast cancer by high-dose chemotherapy has not yet been established, and therefore high-dose chemotherapy with stem cell rescue for any stage of breast cancer should be performed only in the context of well-designed (randomized) clinical trials, awaiting the timely analysis of these and other ongoing studies.

Germ cell tumours

The probability of survival among patients with germ cell tumours who relapse following optimal platinum-based regimens is less than 25 per cent following rescue therapy with ifosfamide, cisplatin and vinblastine (see Chapter 13.4). High-dose chemotherapy supported by stem cells has been used as a third-line therapy for this subgroup of patients with a poor prognosis, as these tumours retain some chemosensitivity. The best drug combinations appear to be carboplatin and etoposide, with or without cyclophosphamide or ifosfamide. There are no randomized trials, but in a retrospective analysis of 436 patients, 22 per cent were long-term disease-free survivors. Following platinum treatment, fewer than 10 per cent of refractory patients can be expected to attain long-term survival, in contrast to 40 per cent of patients with sensitive disease.[115]

The identification of prognostic factors predictive for poor risk,. such as high serum tumour markers, delayed marker clearance, extragonadal primary disease, and large tumour burden, has led to the definition of prognostic models aimed at optimizing the use of high-dose chemotherapy as a first-line therapy.[116] Results from comparative high-dose chemotherapy trials using historical controls treated with conventional therapy indicated an improved event-free and overall survival.[117],[118] In a preliminary report of a small, randomized trial of 115 patients in first-line therapy for patients with a poor prognosis no benefit was apparent for high-dose therapy after 2 years.[119] Larger prospective randomized studies addressing this important issue are under way.

Ovarian cancer

Fewer than 30 per cent of patients with residual disease at second-look surgery following platinum-containing regimens are alive after 5 years (see Chapter 12.1). Dose escalation with stem cell support has been explored. The most commonly used conditioning regimens have been based on cyclophosphamide and carboplatin, with the addition of etoposide, or mitoxantrone. A number of phase 2 studies have reported promising results with complete response rates of up to 50 per cent in patients treated following debulking surgery, but durations of remission were usually short, and 5-year survival was poor. When patients were given consolidation high-dose chemotherapy following attainment of complete remission, there was a suggestion of improved survival, but no plateau of survival to suggest cure. Predictive factors for outcome were residual tumour bulk (more than 1 cm), response to first-line platinum-containing treatment, and possibly age. Because of selection bias towards younger patients with smaller tumour bulk in high-dose chemotherapy series, their outcome cannot be compared directly with results of conventional salvage therapy.

Small cell lung cancer

Small cell lung cancer is highly sensitive to induction chemotherapy, with complete remission obtained in most patients. However, cure is acheived in fewer than 15 per cent of patients, mainly among those presenting with limited disease. This has led to experimental high-dose strategies in an effort to improve survival (see also Chapter 14.4). Late intensification of patients in remission with high-dose chemotherapy and stem cell transplantation has resulted in generally disappointing results, with little or no evidence of survival benefit. A randomized controlled trial is in progress.

High-dose chemotherapy for paediatric tumours

Rhabdomyosarcoma

Intensive therapy without stem cell support cures more than 70 per cent of patients with non-metastatic disease, but only approximately 20 per cent of patients with primary disseminated disease and unfavourable alveolar histology survive (see Chapter 16.2). Since this is a chemosensitive tumour, dose escalation was viewed as a means to improve results, In a survey of the European Bone Marrow Transplant registry data for 189 rhabdomyosarcomas with poor prognosis, 120 patients were treated between June 1979 and February 1994 in clinical first or second complete remission, and 34 per cent and 26 per cent respectively are alive as of March 1997.[120]

Ewing's sarcoma

While chemotherapy cures most patients with peripheral non-bulky Ewing's sarcoma, large tumours carry a poor prognosis, and in metastatic disease survival is exceptional after 4 years (see Chapter 16.3). In localized Ewing's sarcoma, the response to initial therapy is an important prognostic factor, and high-dose therapy should be restricted to tumours that show more than 30 per cent of viable residual tumour cells. In the European Bone Marrow Transplant Solid Tumour Working Party registry, 497 patients have been reported. In this heterogeneous group, the overall 5-year survival was approximately 40 per cent following single high-dose therapy in remission, in contrast to approximately 20 per cent when residual disease was present at transplantation.[121]

Neuroblastoma

The dose–response relationship for chemotherapy within the conventional treatment range has been well demonstrated in neuroblastoma (see Chapter 17.2). High-dose treatments with stem cell rescue have been investigated and initial results were promising. Between 1978 and 1992, 549 patients were reported to the European Bone Marrow Transplant registry. Approximately 30 per cent were alive in remission after 5 years with bone-marrow-negative and skeleton-negative status before high-dose chemotherapy, and about 20 per cent with bone-marrow-positive but skeleton-negative status. The toxic death rate due to high-dose chemotherapy has been over 10 per cent, with the highest rates being among relapsed/refractory patients (23 per cent), and the lowest in patients in complete remission (7 per cent).[122]

Few studies allow the evaluation of the efficacy of high-dose chemotherapy versus conventional treatment. A comparison between two Pediatric Oncology Group studies evaluating elective high-dose chemotherapy consolidation treatment after attaining first complete remission with conventional therapy has not shown a significant difference between treatment cohorts.[123] Similarly, a non-randomized comparison by the Study Group of Japan showed no statistically significant difference in 5-year event-free survival rates (50 versus 38.8 per cent) between patients who did or did not undergo high-dose chemotherapy consolidation in first complete remission.[124] Since these results do not come from randomized studies they must be regarded with caution. A comparative study by the Children's Cancer Group included 207 stage IV patients over 1 year old who were treated within the same time period either by continued conventional chemotherapy or by high-dose chemotherapy with autologous bone marrow transplantation (67 patients). Four-year overall event-free survival of 19 per cent versus 40 per cent was reported. For the high-risk subset with amplified N-*myc* the event-free survival was 0 versus 67 per cent, and for partial responders to induction therapy event-free survival was 6 versus 29 per cent.[125] To date, only results from a small randomized trial including 67 patients have been reported, and they indicated an improved prognosis following high-dose chemotherapy.[126] A large ongoing Pediatric Oncology Group trial is aimed at resolving the question of high-dose chemotherapy and stem cell rescue in advanced poor-risk neuroblastoma.

Future prospects for high-dose chemotherapy

Although there have been some notable successes with high-dose chemotherapy in haematological malignancies, there are few data from randomized comparisons with conventional treatments for solid tumours. In most settings, the lack of available data does not allow for the widespread use of this approach to treatment. The cost and burden to patients can only be justified if firm data are produced from prospective randomized trials with meaningful numbers of patients allowing for stratification according to important prognostic indicators.

Since relapse remains the most significant problem despite high rates of remission following high-dose chemotherapy, other approaches need to be explored to resolve the problem of refractory residual disease. Contributions from biological therapies such as monoclonal antibodies, graft engineering by positive and negative selection, manipulations of the cellular immune response in minimal residual disease, and various types of gene therapy may result in new treatment strategies.

References

1. Hryniuk W, Bush H. The importance of dose intensity in chemotherapy of metastatic breast cancer. *Journal of Clinical Oncology*, 1984; **2**: 1281–8.

2. Hryniuk W, Frei E, Wright FA. A single scale for comparing dose-intensity of all chemotherapy regimens in breast cancer: Summation dose-intensity. *Journal of Clinical Oncology*, 1998; **16**: 3137–47.

3. Mayer RJ, Davis RB, Schiffer CA. Intensive postremission chemotherapy in adults with acute myeloid leukemia. *New England Journal of Medicine*, 1994; **331**: 896–903.

4. Evans WE, Crom WR, Abromowitch M, *et al.* Clinical pharmacodynamics of high-dose methotrexate in acute lymphocytic leukemia. Identification of a relation between concentration and effect. *New England Journal of Medicine*, 1986; **314**: 471–7.

5. Calvert AH, Newell DR, Gumbrell LA, *et al.* Carboplatin dosage: Prospective evaluation of a simple formula based on renal function. *Journal of Clinical Oncology*, 1989; **7**: 1748–56.

6. Chervenick PA, Boggs DR. *In vitro* growth of granulocytic and mononuclear cell colonies from blood of normal individuals. *Blood*, 1971; **37**: 131–5.

7. McCredie KB, Hersh EM, Freireich EJ. Cells capable of colony formation in the peripheral blood of man. *Science*, 1971; **171**: 293–4.

8. Uchida N, Yang Z, Combs J, *et al.* The characterization, molecular cloning, and expression of a novel hematopoietic cell antigen from CD34 + human bone marrow cells. *Blood*, 1997; **89**: 2706–16.

9. Orazi A, Cattoretti G, Schiro RS, Bregni M, Di Nicola M, Gianni AM. Recombinant human interleukin-3 and recombinant human granulocyte-macrophage colony-stimulating factor administered *in vivo* after high-dose cyclophosphamide cancer chemotherapy: Effect on hematopoiesis and microenvironment in human bone marrow. *Blood*, 1992; **79**: 2610–19.

10. Brugger W, Bross K, Frisch J, *et al.* Mobilization of peripheral blood progenitor cells by sequential administration of interleukin-3 and granulocyte-macrophage colony-stimulating factor following polychemotherapy with etoposide, ifosfamide, and cisplatin. *Blood*, 1992; **79**: 1193–200.

11. Rosenfeld CS, Bolwell B, LeFever A, *et al.* (1996). Comparison of four cytokine regimens for mobilization of peripheral blood stem cells: IL-3 alone and combined with GM-CSF or G-CSF. *Bone Marrow Transplantation*, 1996; **17**: 179–83.

12. Demirer T, Buckner CD, Storer B, *et al.* Effect of different chemotherapy regimens on peripheral-blood stem-cell collections in patients with breast cancer receiving granulocyte colony-stimulating factor. *Journal of Clinical Oncology*, 1997; **15**: 684–90.

13. Andrews RG, Briddell RA, Knitter GH, *et al.* In vivo synergy between recombinant human stem cell factor and recombinant human granulocyte colony-stimulating factor in baboons: Enhanced circulation of progenitor cells. *Blood*, 1994; **84**: 800–10.

14. Weaver A, Chang J, Wrigley E, *et al.* Randomized comparison of progenitor-cell mobilization using chemotherapy, stem-cell factor, and filgrastim or chemotherapy plus filgrastim alone in patients with ovarian cancer. *Journal of Clinical Oncology*, 1998; **16**: 2601–12.

15. Moskowitz CH, Stiff P, Gordon MS, *et al.* Recombinant methionyl human stem cell factor and filgrastim for peripheral blood progenitor cell mobilization and transplantation in non-Hodgkin's lymphoma patients—results of a phase I/II trial. *Blood*, 1997; **89**: 3136–47.

16. Watts MJ, Sullivan AM, Jamieson E, *et al.* Progenitor-cell mobilization after low-dose cyclophosphamide and granulocyte colony-stimulating factor: an analysis of progenitor-cell quantity and quality and factors predicting for these parameters in 101 pretreated patients with malignant lymphoma. *Journal of Clinical Oncology,* 1997; **15**: 535–46.

17. Brugger W, Heimfeld S, Berenson RJ, Mertelsmann R, Kanz L. Reconstitution of hematopoiesis after high-dose chemotherapy by autologous progenitor cells generated *ex vivo. New England Journal of Medicine,* 1995; **333**: 283–7.

18. Brenner MK, Rill DR, Moen RC, *et al.* Gene-marking to trace origin of relapse after autologous bone-marrow transplantation. *The Lancet,* 1993; **341**: 85–6.

19. Deisseroth AB, Zu Z, Claxton D, *et al.* Genetic marking shows that Ph+ cells present in autologous transplants of chronic myelogenous leukemia (CML) contribute to relapse after autologous bone marrow in CML. *Blood,* 1994; **83**: 3068–76.

20. Fefer A, Cheever MA, Thomas ED, *et al.* Bone marrow transplantation for refractory acute leukemia in 34 patients with identical twins. *Blood,* 1981; **57**: 421–30.

21. Rill DR, Santana VM, Roberts WM, *et al.* Direct demonstration that autologous bone marrow transplantation for solid tumors can return a multiplicity of tumorigenic cells. *Blood,* 1994; **84**: 380–3.

22. Williams CD, Goldstone AH, Pearce RM, *et al.* Purging of bone marrow in autologous bone marrow transplantation for non-Hodgkin's lymphoma: A case-matched comparison with unpurged cases by the European blood and marrow transplant lymphoma regisstry. *Journal of Clinical Oncology,* 1996; **14**: 2454–64.

23. Gribben JG, Saporito L, Barber M, *et al.* Bone marrows of non-Hodgkin's lymphoma patients with a bcl-2 translocation can be purged of polymerase chain reaction-detectable lymphoma cells using monoclonal antibodies and immunomagnetic bead depletion. *Blood,* 1992; **80**: 1083–9.

24. Lambrechts AC, Hupkes PE, Dorssers LC, van't Veer MB. Translocation (14;18)-positive cells are present in the circulation of the majority of patients with localized (stage I and II) follicular non-Hodgkin's lymphoma. *Blood,* 1993; **82**: 2510–16.

25. Corradini P, Astolfi M, Cherasco C, *et al.* Molecular monitoring of minimal residual disease in follicular and mantle cell non-Hodgkin's lymphomas treated with high-dose chemotherapy and peripheral blood progenitor cell autografting. *Blood,* 1997; **89**: 724–31.

26. Ross AA, Cooper BW, Lazarus HM, *et al.* Detection and viability of tumor cells in peripheral blood stem cell collections from breast cancer patients using immunocytochemical and clonogenic assay techniques. *Blood,* 1993; **82**: 2605–10.

27. Kruger WH, Stockschlader M, Hennings S, *et al.* Detection of cancer cells in peripheral blood stem cells of women with breast cancer by RT-PCR and cell culture. *Bone Marrow Transplantation,* 1996; **18** (Suppl. 1): S18–S20.

28. Passos-Coelho JL, Ross AA, Kahn DJ, *et al.* Similar breast cancer cell contamination of single-day peripheral-blood progenitor-cell collections obtained after priming with hematopoietic growth factor alone or after cyclophosphamide followed by growth factor. *Journal of Clinical Oncology,* 1996; **14**: 2569–75.

29. Cheung IY, Cheung NKV. Molecular detection of GAGE expression in peripheral blood and bone marrow: Utility as a tumor marker for neuroblastoma. *Clinical Cancer Research,* 1997; **3**: 821–6.

30. Thomson B, Radich J, Hawkins D. Detection of minimal residual disease in Ewing's sarcoma by a quantitative reverse transcription-polymerase chain reaction (RT-PCR). (Meeting abstract). *Proceedings of the Annual Meeting of the American Society of Clinical Oncologists,* 1998; **17**: A2096.

31. Vose JM, Sharp JG, Chan W, *et al.* High-dose chemotherapy (HDC) and autotransplant for non-Hodgkin's lymphoma (NHL): randomized trial of peripheral blood (PSCT) versus bone marrow (ABMT) and evaluation of minimal residual disease (MRD) (Meeting abstract). *Proceedings of the Annual Meeting of the American Society of Clinical Oncologists,* 1997; **16**: A315.

32. Sharp JG, Kessinger A, Mann S, *et al.* Outcome of high-dose therapy and autologous transplantation in non-Hodgkin's lymphoma based on the presence of tumor in the marrow or infused hematopoietic harvest. *Journal of Clinical Oncology,* 1996; **14**: 214–19.

33. Gribben JG, Neuberg D, Barber M, *et al.* Detection of residual lymphoma cells by polymerase chain reaction in peripheral blood is significantly less predictive for relapse than detection in bone marrow. *Blood,* 1994; **83**: 3800–7.

34. Brugger W, Bross KJ, Glatt M, Weber F, Mertelsmann R, Kanz L. Mobilization of tumor cells and hematopoietic progenitor cells into peripheral blood of patients with solid tumors. *Blood,* 1994; **83**: 636–40.

35. Lemoli RM, Fortuna A, Motta MR, *et al.* Concomitant mobilization of plasma cells and hematopoietic progenitors into peripheral blood of multiple myeloma patients: Positive selection and transplantation of enriched CD34+ cells to remove circulating tumor cells. *Blood,* 1996; **87**: 1625–34.

36. Irle C. Rapid purification of peanut agglutinin by sialic acid-less fetuin-sepharose column. *Journal of Immunological Methods,* 1977; **17**: 117–21.

37. LaCasse EC, Saleh MT, Patterson B, Minden MD, Gariepy J. Shiga-like toxin purges human lymphoma from bone marrow of severe combined immunodeficient mice. *Blood,* 1996; **88**: 1561–7.

38. Dietzfelbinger HF, Kuhn D, Zafferani M, Hanauske AR, Rastetter JW, Berdel WE. Removal of breast cancer cells from bone marrow by *in vitro* purging with ether lipids and cryopreservation. *Cancer Research,* 1993; **53**: 3747–51.

39. Kostelny SA, Cole MS, Tso JY. Formation of a bispecific antibody by the use of leucine zippers. *Journal of Immunology,* 1992; **148**: 1547–53.

40. Mapara MY, Korner IJ, Hildebrandt M, *et al.* Monitoring of tumor cell purging after highly efficient immunomagnetic selection of CD34 cells from leukapheresis products in breast cancer patients: Comparison of immunocytochemical tumor cell staining and reverse transcriptase-polymerase chain reaction. *Blood,* 1997; **89**: 337–44.

41. Gorin NC, Coiffier B, Hayat M, *et al.* Recombinant human granulocyte-macrophage colony-stimulating factor after high-dose chemotherapy and autologous bone marrow transplantation with unpurged and purged marrow in non-Hodgkin's lymphoma: A double-blind placebo-controlled trial. *Blood,* 1992; **80**: 1149–57.

42. Bentley SA, Brecher ME, Powell E, Serody JS, Wiley JM, Shea TC. Long-term engraftment failure after marrow ablation and autologous hematopoietic reconstitution: Differences between peripheral blood stem cell and bone marrow recipients. *Bone Marrow Transplantation,* 1997; **19**: 557–63.

43. To LB, Roberts MM, Haylock DN, *et al.* Comparison of haematological recovery times and supportive care requirements of autologous recovery phase peripheral blood stem cell transplants, autologous bone marrow transplants and allogeneic bone marrow transplants. *Bone Marrow Transplantation,* 1992; **9**: 277–84.

44. Beyer J, Schwella N, Zingsem JJ, *et al.* Hematopoietic rescue after high-dose chemotherapy using autologous peripheral-blood progenitor cells or bone marrow: a randomized comparison. *Journal of Clinical Oncology,* 1995; **13**: 1328–1335.

45. Hartmann O, Le Corroller AG, Blaise D, *et al.* Peripheral blood stem cell and bone marrow transplantation for solid tumors and lymphomas: hematologic recovery and costs. A randomized, controlled trial. *Annals of Internal Medicine,* 1997; **126**: 600–7.

46. Bender JG, Williams SF, Myers S, *et al.* Characterization of chemotherapy mobilized peripheral blood progenitor cells for use in autologous stem cell transplantation. *Bone Marrow Transplantation,* 1992; **10**: 281–5.

47. Hao Q-L, Thielmann FT, Petersen D, Smogorzewska EM, Crooks GM. Extended long-term culture reveals a highly quiescent and primitive human hematopietic progenitor population. *Blood*, 1996; **88**: 3306–13.

48. Sutherland HJ, Lansdorp PM, Henkelman DH, Eaves AC, Eaves CJ. Functional characterization of individual human hematopoietic stem cells cultured at limiting dilution on supportive marrow stromal layers. *Proceedings of the National Academy of Sciences of the USA*, 1990; **87**: 3584–8.

49. Pettengell R, Testa NG, Swindell R, et al. Transplantation potential of hematopoietic cells released into the circulation during routine chemotherapy for non-Hodgkin's lymphoma. *Blood*, 1993; **82**: 2239–48.

50. Bensinger WI, Longin K, Appelbaum F, et al. Peripheral blood stem cells (PBSCs) collected after recombinant granulocyte colony stimulating factor (rhG-CSF): An analysis of factors correlating with the tempo of engraftment after transplantation. *British Journal of Haematology*, 1994; **87**: 825–31.

51. Weaver CH, Hazelton B, Birch R, et al. An analysis of engraftment kinetics as a function of the CD34 content of peripheral blood progenitor cell collections in 692 patients after the administration of myeloablative chemotherapy. *Blood*, 1995; **86**: 3961–9.

52. Berenson RJ, Bensinger WI, Hill RS, et al. Engraftment after infusion of CD34 + marrow cells in patients with breast cancer or neuroblastoma. *Blood*, 1991; **77**: 1717–22.

53. Nemunaitis J, Singer JW, Buckner CD, et al. Use of recombinant human granulocyte-macrophage colony-stimulating factor in graft failure after bone marrow transplantation. *Blood*, 1990; **76**: 245–53.

54. Nemunaitis J, Rabinowe SN, Singer JW, et al. Recombinant granulocyte-macrophage colony-stimulating factor after autologous bone marrow transplantation for lymphoid cancer. *New England Journal of Medicine*, 1991; **324**: 1773–8.

55. Link H, Boogaerts MA, Carella AM, et al. A controlled trial of recombinant human granulocyte-macrophage colony-stimulating factor after total body irradiation, high-dose chemotherapy, and autologous bone marrow transplantation for acute lymphoblastic leukemia or malignant lymphoma. *Blood*, 1992; **80**: 2188–95.

56. Lemoli RM, Rosti G, Visani G, et al. Concomitant and sequential administration of recombinant human granulocyte colony-stimulating factor and recombinant human interleukin-3 to accelerate hematopoietic recovery after autologous bone marrow transplantation for malignant lymphoma. *Journal of Clinical Oncology*, 1996; **14**: 3018–25.

57. Vose JM, Pandite AN, Beveridge RA, Geller RB, Schuster MW, Anderson JE. Granulocyte-macrophage colony-stimulating factor/interleukin-3 fusion protein versus granulocyte-macrophage colony-stimulating factor after autologous bone marrow transplantation for non-Hodgkin's lymphoma: Results of a randomized double-blind trial. *Journal of Clinical Oncology*, 1997; **15**: 1617–23.

58. Bolwell BJ, Pohlman B, Andresen S, et al. Delayed G-CSF after autologous progenitor cell transplantation: A prospective randomized trial. *Bone Marrow Transplantation*, 1998; **21**: 369–73.

59. Linch DC, Scarffe H, Proctor S, et al. Randomised vehicle-controlled dose-finding study of glycosylated recombinant human granulocyte colony-stimulating factor after bone marrow transplantation. *Bone Marrow Transplantation*, 1993; **11**: 307–11.

60. Spitzer G, Adkins DR, Spencer V, et al. Randomized study of growth factors post-peripheral-blood stem-cell transplant: Neutrophil recovery is improved with modest clinical benefit. *Journal of Clinical Oncology*, 1994; **12**: 661–70.

61. Weiden PL, Flournoy N, Thomas ED, Prentice R, Fefer A, Buckner CD, Storb R. Antileukemic effect of graft-versus-host disease in human recipients of allogeneic-marrow grafts. *New England Journal of Medicine*, 1979; **300**: 1068–73.

62. Irle C, Kaestli M, Aapro M, Chapuis B, Jeannet M. Quantity and nature of residual bone marrow T cells after treatment of the marrow with Campath-1. *Experimental Hematology*, 1987; **15**: 163–70.

63. Hale G, Waldmann H. Campath-1 monoclonal antibodies in bone marrow transplantation. *Journal of Hematotherapy*, 1994; **3**: 15–31.

64. Kolb HJ, Schattenberg A, Goldman JM, et al. Graft-versus-leukemia effect of donor lymphocyte transfusions in marrow grafted patients. *Blood*, 1993; **86**: 2041–50.

65. Bjorkstrand BB, Ljungman P, Svensson H, et al. Allogeneic bone marrow transplantation versus autologous stem cell transplantation in multiple myeloma: a retrospective case-matched study from the European Group for Blood and Marrow Transplantation. *Blood*, 1996; **88**: 4711–18.

66. Nagler A, Ackerstein A, Or R, Naparstek E, Slavin S. Immunotherapy with recombinant human interleukin-2 and recombinant interferon-alpha in lymphoma patients. *Blood*, 1997; **89**: 3951–9.

67. Anderson WF. Human gene therapy. *Science*, 1992; **256**: 808–13.

68. Alton EW. Towards gene therapy for cystic fibrosis. *Journal of Pharmacy and Pharmacology*, 1995; **47**: 351–4.

69. Su L, Lee R, Bonyhadi M, et al. Hematopoietic stem cell-based gene therapy for acquired immunodeficiency syndrome: efficient transduction and expression of RevM10 in myeloid cells *in vivo* and *in vitro*. *Blood*, 1997; **89**: 2283–90.

70. Hesdorffer C, Ayello J, Ward M, et al. Phase I trial of retroviral-mediated transfer of the human MDR1 gene as marrow chemoprotection in patients undergoing high-dose chemotherapy and autologous stem-cell transplantation. *Journal of Clinical Oncology*, 1998; **16**: 165–72.

71. Koc ON, Allay JA, Lee K, Davis BM, Reese JS, Gerson SL. Transfer of drug resistance genes into hematopoietic progenitors to improve chemotherapy tolerance. *Seminars in Oncology*, 1996; **23**: 46–65.

72. Crump M, Goss PE, Prince M, Girouard C. Outcome of extensive evaluation before adjuvant therapy in women with breast cancer and 10 or more positive axillary lymph nodes. *Journal of Clinical Oncology*, 1996; **14**: 66–9.

73. Zittoun RA, Mandelli F, Willemze R, et al. Autologous or allogeneic bone marrow transplantation compared with intensive chemotherapyy in acute myelogenous leukemia. *New England Journal of Medicine*, 1995; **332**: 217–23.

74. Burnett AK, Goldstone AH, Stevens RMF, et al. Randomised comparison of addition of autologous bone marrow transplantation to intensive chemotherapy for acute myeloid leukaemia in first remission: Results of MRC AML 10. *The Lancet*, 1998; **351**: 700–8.

75. Fiere D, Lepage E, Sebban C, et al. A multicentric randomized trial testing bone marrow transplantation as postremission therapy. *Journal of Clinical Oncology*, 1993; **11**: 1990–2001.

76. Attal M, Blaise D, Marrit G, et al. Consolidation treatment of adult acute lymphoblastic leukemia: A prospective, ramdomized trial comparing allogeneic versus autologous bone marrow transplantation and testing the impact of recombinant interleukin-2 after autologous bone marrow transplantation. *Blood*, 1995; **86**: 1619–28.

77. Feig SA, Harris RE, Sather HH. Bone marrow transplantation versus chemotherapy for maintenance of second remission of childhood acute lymphoblastic leukemia: A study of the Children's Cancer Group. *Medical and Pediatric Oncology*, 1997; **29**: 534–40.

78. Wheeler K, Richards S, Bailey C, Chessells J. Comparison of bone marrow transplant and chemotherapy for relapsed childhood acute lymphoblastic leukaemia: the MRC UK ALL experience. *British Journal of Haematology*, 1998; **101**: 94–103.

79. Fisher RI, Gaynor ER, Dahlberg S, et al. Comparison of a standard regimen (CHOP) with three intensive chemotherapy regimens for advanced non-Hodgkin's lymphoma. *New England Journal of Medicine*, 1993; **328**: 1002–6.

80. Schouten HC, Kvaloy S, Sydes M, Qian W, Fayers PM. The CUP trial: a randomized study analyzing the efficacy of high dose therapy and purging in low-grade non-Hodgkin's lymphoma (NHL). *Annals of Oncology*, 1999; **10** (Suppl. 3): 24, a68.

81. Haioun C, Lepage E, Gisselbrecht C, *et al.* Comparison of autologous bone marrow transplantation with sequential chemotherapy for intermediate-grade and high-grade lymphoma in first remission: A study of 464 patients. *Journal of Clinical Oncology*, 1994; **12**: 2543–51.

82. Haioun C, Lepage E, Gisselbrecht C, *et al.* Benefit of autologous bone marrow transplantation over sequential chemotherapy in poor-risk aggressive non-Hodgkin's lymphoma: updated results of the prospective study LNH87–2. Groupe d'Etude des Lymphomes de l'Adulte. *Journal of Clinical Oncology*, 1997; **15**: 1131–7.

83. Gisselbrecht C, Lepage E, Morel P, *et al.* Intensified induction phase including autologous stem cell transplantation does not improve response rate and survival in lymphoma with at least two adverse prognostic factors when compared to ACVB regimen [abstract]. *Blood*, 1996; **88** (Suppl. 1): A470.

84. Kaiser U, Ueberlacker I, Havemann K. High dose chemotherapy with autologous stem cell transplantation in aggressive NHL: Analysis of a randomized multicenter study. *Annals of Oncology*, 1999; **10**: 76, a262.

85. Kluin-Nelemans JC, Zagonel V, Thomas J, *et al.* Consolidation autologous bone marrow transplantation after standard chemotherapy vs. CHVmP/BV alone for primary intermediate and high grade NHL: a randomized phase 3 EORTC study [meeting abstract]. *Proceedings of the Annual Meeting of the American Society of Clinical Oncologists*, 1999; **18**: A6.

86. Verdonck LF, van Putten WL, Hagenbeek A, *et al.* Comparison of CHOP chemotherapy with autologous bone marrow transplantation for slowly responding patients with aggressive non-Hodgkin's lymphoma. *New England Journal of Medicine*, 1995; **332**: 1045–51.

87. Gianni AM, Bregni M, Siena S, *et al.* High-dose chemotherapy and autologous bone marrow transplantation compared with MACOP-B in aggressive B-cell lymphoma. *New England Journal of Medicine*, 1997; **336**: 1290–7.

88. Sweetenham JW, Pearce R, Taghipour G, Blaise D, Gisselbrecht C, Goldstone AH. Adult Burkitt's and Burkitt-like non-Hodgkin's lymphoma—outcome for patients treated with high-dose therapy and autologous stem-cell transplantation in first remission or at relapse: Results from the European Group for Blood and Marrow Transplantation. *Journal of Clinical Oncology*, 1996; **14**: 2465–72.

89. Sweetenham JW, Santini G, Simnett S, *et al.* Autologous stem cell transplantation in 1st remission improves relapse free survival in adult patients with lymphoblastic lymphoma: Results from a randomised trial of the European Group for Blood and Bone Marrow Transplantation and the UK Lymphoma Group [meeting abstract]. *Proceedings of the Annual Meeting of the American Society of Clinical Oncologists*, 1998; **17**: a63.

90. Philip T, Biron P, Maraninchi D. Role of massive chemotherapy and autologous bone marrow transplantation in non-Hodkin's malignant lymphoma. *Lancet*, 1984; **i**: 391–2.

91. Philip T, Armitage JO, Spitzer G, *et al.* High-dose therapy and autologous bone marrow transplantation after failure of conventional chemotherapy in adults with intermediate-grade or high-grade non-Hodgkin's lymphoma. *New England Journal of Medicine*, 1987; **316**: 1493–8.

92. Philip T, Gugliemi C, Hagenbeck A, *et al.* Autologous bone marrow transplantation as compared with salvage chemotherapy in relapses of chemotherapy-sensitive non-Hodgkin's lymphoma. *New England Journal of Medicine*, 1995; **333**: 1540–5.

93. Blay J-Y, Gomez F, Sebban C, *et al.* The international prognostic index correlates to survival in patients with aggressive lymphoma in relapse: analysis of the PARMA trial. *Blood*, 1999; **92**: 3562–8.

94. Gianni AM, Siena S, Bregni M, *et al.* High-dose sequential chemo-radiotherapy with peripheral blood progenitor cell support for relapsed or refractory Hodgkin's disease—a 6-year update. *Annals of Oncology*, 1993; **4**: 889–91.

95. Reece DE, Connors JM, Spinelli JJ, *et al.* Intensive theraapy with

96. cyclophosphamide, carmustine (BCNU), etoposide (VP16–213), +/– cisplatin (CBV +/– P), and autologous bone marrow transplantation for Hodgkin's disease in first relapse after combination chemotherapy. *Blood*, 1994; **83**: 1193–9.

96. Horning SJ, Chao NJ, Negrin RS, *et al.* High-dose therapy and autologous hematopoietic progenitor cell transplantation for recurrent or refractory Hodgkin's disease: Analysis of the Stanford University results and prognostic indices. *Blood*, 1997; **89**: 801–13.

97. Linch DC, Winfield D, Goldstone AH, *et al.* Dose intensification with autologous bone-marrow transplantation in relapsed and resistant Hodgkin's disease: results of a BNLI randomised trial. *The Lancet*, 1993; **341**: 1051–4.

98. Yuen AR, Rosenberg SA, Hoppe RTJD, Horning SJ. Comparison between conventional salvage therapy and high-dose therapy with autografting for recurrent or refractory Hodgkin's disease. *Blood*, 1997; **89**: 814–22.

99. Schmitz N, Sextro M, Pfistner D, *et al.* High dose therapy followed by hematopoietic stem cell transplantation (HSCT) for relapsed chemosensitive Hodgkin's disease (HD): final results of a randomized GHSG and EBMT trial (HD-R1) [meeting abstract]. *Proceedings of the Annual Meeting of the American Society of Clinical Oncologists*, 1999; **17**: A5.

100. McElwain TJ, Powles RL. High-dose intravenous melphalan for plasma-cell leukaemia and myeloma. *The Lancet*, 1983; **2**: 822–4.

101. Attal M, Harousseau JL, Stoppa AM, *et al.* A prospective, randomized trial of autologous bone marrow transplantation and chemotherapy in multiple myeloma. *New England Journal of Medicine*, 1996; **335**: 91–7.

102. Fermand JP, Ravaud P, Chevret S, *et al.* High-dose therapy and autologous blood stem cell transplantation in multiple myeloma: preliminary results of a randomized trial involving 167 patients. *Stem Cells*, 1995; **13** (Suppl. 2): 156–9.

103. Blade J, San Miguel JF, Fontanillas M, *et al.* Survival of multiple myeloma patients who are potential candidates for early high-dose therapy intensification/autotransplantation and who were conventionally treated. *Journal of Clinical Oncology*, 1996; **14**: 2167–73.

104. Barlogie B, Jagannath S, Vesole DH, *et al.* Superiority of tandem autologous transplantation over standard therapy for previously untreated multiple myeloma. *Blood*, 1997; **89**: 789–93.

105. Antman KH, Rowlings PA, *et al.* High-dose chemotherapy with autologous hematopoietic stem-cell support for breast cancer in North America. *Journal of Clinical Oncology*, 1997; **15**: 1870–9.

106. Peters WP, Jones RB, Vredenburgh J, *et al.* A large, prospective, randomized trial of high dose combination alkylating agents (CBC) with autologous cellular support (ABMS) as consolidation for patients with metastatic breast cancer achieving complete remission qfter intensive doxorubicine based induction therapy (AFM) [abstract 149]. *Proceedings of the American Society of Clinical Oncologists*, 1996; **15**: 121.

107. Lotz JP, Curé H, Janvier M, *et al.* High-dose chemotherapy (HD-CT) with hematopoietic stem cell transplantation (HSCT) for metastatic breast cancer (MBC): Results of the French protocol PEGASE 04. *Proceedings of the Annual Meeting of the American Society of Clinical Oncologists*, 1999; **18**: a161.

108. Stadtmauer EA, O'Neill A, Goldstein LJ, *et al.* Phase 3 trial of high-dose chemotherapy (HDC) and stem cell support (SCT) shows no difference in overall survival or severe toxicity compared to maintenance chemotherapy with cyclophosphamide, methotrexate, and 5-fluorouracil (CMF) for women with metastatic breast cancer who are responding to conventional induction chemotherapy: the 'Philadelphia' intergroup study (PBT-1). *Proceedings of the Annual Meeting of the American Society of Clinical Oncologists*, 1999; **18**: a1.

109. Peters WP, Ross M, Vredenburgh J, *et al.* High-dose chemotherapy and autologous bone marrow support as consolidation after standard-dose adjuvant therapy for high-risk primary breast cancer. *Journal of Clinical Oncology*, 1993; **11**: 1132–43.

110. Garcia-Carbonero R, Hidalgo M, Paz-Ares I, *et al.* Patient selection in high-dose chemotherapy trials: Relevance in high-risk breast cancer. *Journal of Clinical Oncology,* 1997; **15**: 3178–84.

111. Hortobagy GN, Buzdar AU, Champlin R, *et al.* Lack of efficacy of high dose (HD) tandem combination chemotherapy (CT) for high risk primary breast cancer (HRPBC)—a randomized trial [meeting abstract]. *Proceedings of the Annual Meeting of the American Society of Clinical Oncologists,* 1998; **17**: A471.

112. Rodenhuis S, Richel DJ, van der Wall E, *et al.* A randomized trial of hdct and hematopoietic stem cell support in operable breast cancer with extensive axillary lymph node involvement [meeting abstract]. *Proceedings of the Annual Meeting of the American Society of Clinical Oncologists,* 1998; **17**: A470.

113. Peters WP, Rosner G, Vredenburgh J, *et al.* A prospective, randomized comparison of two doses of combination alkylating agents (AA) as consolidation after CAF in high-risk primary breast cancer involving ten or more lymph nodes (LN): Preliminary results of CALGB 9082/ SWOG 9114/NCIC MA-13. *Proceedings of the Annual Meeting of the American Society of Clinical Oncologists,* 1999; **18**: a2.

114. The Scandinavian Breast Cancer Study Group. [meeting abstract]. Results from a randomized adjuvant breast cancer study with high dose chemotherapy with CDC$_b$ supported by autologous bone marrow stem cells versus dose-escalated and tailored FEC therapy. *Proceedings of the Annual Meeting of the American Society of Clinical Oncologists,* 1999; **18**: a3.

115. Droz JP, Culine S, Biron P, Kramar A. High-dose chemotherapy in germ-cell tumors. *Annals of Oncology,* 1996; **7**: 997–1003.

116. Beyer J, Kramar A, Mandanas R, *et al.* High-dose chemotherapy as salvage treatment in germ cell tumors: a multivariate analysis of prognostic variables. *Journal of Clinical Oncology,* 1996; **14**: 2638–45.

117. Motzer RJ, Mazumdar M, Bosl GJ, Bajorin DF, Amsterdam A, Vlamis V. High-dose carboplatin, etoposide, and cyclophosphamide for patients with refractory germ cell tumors: Treatment results and prognostic factors for survival and toxicity. *Journal of Clinical Oncology,* 1996; **14**: 1098–105.

118. Motzer RJ, Mazumdar M, Gulati SC, *et al.* Phase II trial of high-dose carboplatin and etoposide with autologous bone marrow transplantation in first-line therapy for patients with poor-risk germ cell tumors. *Journal of the National Cancer Institute,* 1993; **85**: 1828–35.

119. Chevreau C, Droz JP, Pico JL, *et al.* Early intensified chemotherapy with autologous bone marrow transplantation in first line treatment of poor risk non-seminomatous germ cell tumors. Preliminary results of a French randomized trial. *European Urology,* 1993; **23**: 213–18.

120. Koscielniak E. EBMT rhabdosarcoma. Aix-le-Bains Meeting, March 1997. In: EBMT Solid Tumour Working Party Registry. *Annual Report 1997* (ed. Rosti G, Ferrante P). STWP Registry, 1997.

121. Hartmann O, Ladenstein R. EBMT. STWP Registry 1997.

122. Ladenstein R, Philip T, Lasset C, *et al.* Multivariate analysis of risk factors in stage 4 neuroblastoma over the age of one year treated with megatherapy and stem cell transplantation: A report from the European Bone Marrow Transplantation Solid Tumor Registry. *Journal of Clinical Oncology,* 1998; **15**: 1302–8.

123. Stram DO, Matthay KK, O'Leary M, *et al.* Consolidation chemoradiotherapy and autologous bone marrow transplantation versus continued chemotherapy for metastatic neuroblastoma: A report of two concurrent Children's Cancer Group studies. *Journal of Clinical Oncology,* 1996; **14**: 2417–26.

124. Shuster JJ, Cantor AB, McWilliams N, *et al.* The prognostic significance of autologous bone marrow transplant in advanced neuroblastoma. *Journal of Clinical Oncology,* 1991; **9**: 1045–9.

125. Ohnuma N, Takahashi H, Kaneko M, *et al.* Treatment combined with bone marrow transplantation for advanced neuroblastoma: An analysis of patients who were pretreated intensively with the protocol of the Study Group of Japan. *Medical and Pediatric Oncology,* 1995; **24**: 181–7.

126. Pinkerton CR. ENSG 1-randomised study of high-dose melphalan in neuroblastoma. *Bone Marrow Transplantation,* 1991; **7** (Suppl. 3): 112–13.

4.25 Hormone therapy

M. Dowsett and S. R. D. Johnston

Introduction

The growth and development of normal tissues is critically controlled by hormones. For some tissues, particularly those related to secondary sexual characteristics, the trophic stimuli persist into adult life. Neoplastic growths from these tissues frequently maintain at least some sensitivity to these stimuli, which can be exploited in their treatment. These relationships are particularly well-established for breast and prostate cancer, where tumour growth may be stimulated by oestrogen and androgen, respectively; however, other tumours such as those of the endometrium and ovary may also respond to hormonal therapy.

The earliest advances in hormonal therapy were made through ablative surgery of glands supplying these hormonal stimuli, prior to the stimuli being characterized at a biochemical level, e.g. ovariectomy for breast cancer[1] and orchiectomy for prostate cancer.[2] Over the last 30 years, a large number of different medical agents have become available for hormonal therapy and there are many contemporary developments based on an increasingly detailed knowledge of molecular endocrine relationships. These newer agents are sufficiently well tolerated to be strong candidates for chemoprevention of the respective malignancies as well as for the treatment of established disease.

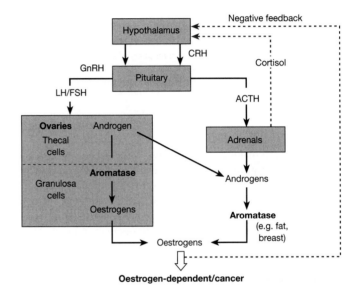

Fig. 1 Oestrogen synthesis in premenopausal women. Ovarian oestrogen synthesis and adrenal androgen synthesis are affected by negative feedback to the hypothalamopituitary axis. In postmenopausal women the ovaries are devoid of aromatase. GnRH, gonadotrophin-releasing hormone; CRH, corticotrophin-releasing hormone; LH, luteinizing hormone; FSH, follicle-stimulating hormone; ACTH, adrenocorticophic hormone.

Breast cancer

Oestrogens

The primary growth stimulant for breast carcinomas is oestrogen and oestrogen deprivation forms the mainstay of hormonal therapy. The sensitivity of breast cancer cells to oestrogen is enhanced markedly by insulin-like growth factor 1 (**IGF1**) *in vitro*.[3] The possibility that somatostatin analogues, which reduce IGFI levels, may be therapeutic in breast cancer is being explored.[3] Prolactin has a strong stimulating influence on both normal and malignant tissues in rodents but, although there are some *in vitro* data supporting a role for prolactin in human breast cancer, clinical data do not support this.

Hormonal therapy has generally been described as cytostatic implying that cell proliferation is suppressed and that tumour regression occurs by the maintenance of apoptosis (programmed cell death), in contrast to cytotoxic chemotherapy, which leads directly to the death of cancer cells. The antiproliferative effect of oestrogen deprivation can be demonstrated in most oestrogen receptor positive breast cancer cell lines, the most widely used of these being the MCF7 line[4] and in xenografts of these lines in immune-deprived mice.

Antioestrogens, such as tamoxifen inhibit cell proliferation by a G_1/G_0 block resulting from decreases in cyclin D1 activation. Apoptosis, however, is also increased by oestrogen deprivation in model systems and in human breast carcinomas *in vivo*. This increased cell death may be due to an induced decrease in the antiapoptotic protein Bcl2.[5]

Oestrogens are synthesized from androgens by the cytochrome P450 enzyme, aromatase (Fig. 1). The richest source of this enzyme is in the ovarian granulosa cells of premenopausal women and the syncytiotrophoblastic layer of the placenta. Aromatase is also present in many other non-glandular, peripheral tissues. Probably most important among these, for the synthesis of plasma oestrogens, are the stromal cells of subcutaneous fat. However, breast tissues, both normal and malignant also synthesize oestrogens from circulating androgen, mainly of adrenal origin and this may provide an important local source of oestrogenic stimulation. In postmenopausal women the ovary is devoid of aromatase. Plasma oestradiol levels fall from mean levels of about 300 to 400 pmol/litre to about 30 pmol/litre. These

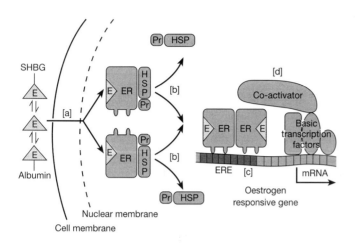

Fig. 2 Transcription activation of an oestrogen responsive gene. The letters in square brackets refer to the description of the process given in the text. E: oestrogen; ER: oestrogen receptor; SHBG: sex hormone binding globulin; HSP: heat shock protein; Pr: associated protein; ERE oestrogen responsive element.

Table 1 Approximate proportions of ER and PgR positivity in primary breast carcinomas and associated response of advanced breast cancer in nearly 2000 patients[7]

	Proportion of total	Response rate
ER + PgR +	58	77
ER + PgR−	23	27
ER−PgR +	4	46
ER−PgR−	15	11

reduced levels are still important for breast cancer growth and remain a target for therapeutic intervention. The major biologically active plasma oestrogens are oestradiol and oestrone, oestradiol being substantially the more potent. Oestrone sulphate has much higher plasma concentrations than the primary oestrogens. Although it has no direct biological activity, it may be hydrolysed to oestrone and thus act as a 'prohormone'.

Oestrogen receptors

Unconjugated oestrogens in plasma are bound to plasma proteins (albumin and sex hormone binding globulin), which restrict their free diffusion across the cell membrane (Fig. 2(a)). The response of cells to oestrogens is via (o)estrogen receptors (**ERs**), which are ligand-activated nuclear transcription factors (Fig. 2). When bound to their cognate ligand, ERs dissociate from heat shock proteins and other associated proteins, homodimerize, are phosphorylated at specific sites and show a conformational change (Fig. 2(b)). The dimer binds to specific palindromic nucleotide sequences, called (o)estrogen response elements (**EREs**) upstream of oestrogen responsive genes (Fig. 2(c)). The degree to which transcription of these genes is activated is determined largely by the presence of protein co-activators and co-repressors that bridge or block the gap, respectively, between the receptor complex and the basal transcriptional machinery (Fig. 2(d)).

Until recently only one oestrogen receptor gene had been identified but a second gene has been discovered.[6] This is termed ERβ with the earlier gene now being termed ERα. As yet there are very few data about the importance of ERβ in breast cancer.

It has been known for about 25 years that the intrinsic response or resistance of breast carcinomas to oestrogen deprivation therapy is strongly dependent on the quantity of ER in the tumour. For the first 15 years of that period almost all analyses of ER content were conducted using the ligand-binding assay or dextrose-coated charcoal assay in which the amount of radioactive oestradiol required to saturate the ER in an homogenate of tumour was calculated. Tumours

with ER levels below a certain threshold, commonly 10 fmol ER/mg protein, were classified as ER negative; this is an unfortunate nomenclature as many have regarded this as indicative of zero levels. Some of the (minor) benefits which accrue to patients with ER 'negative' tumours may be due to these low levels having some biological and/or clinical importance.[8]

The ligand-binding assay/dextrose-coated charcoal assay has largely been superseded by enzyme immunoassays, which use two monoclonal antibodies to measure the concentration of ER in an homogenate, and more recently by immunocytochemical assays, which work in both frozen and formalin-fixed tissues. Immunocytochemical assays are particularly popular as they are less labour intensive, require less tissue, which does not need to be kept frozen, and are substantially cheaper. This type of assay also has the advantage of being able to take account of the heterogeneous expression of ER, which is frequently seen in breast cancer. However, immunocytochemical assays have derived their positive/negative cut-offs by comparison with measurements made with other techniques rather than by directly analysing data on response. A comparison of the methods for ER analysis is shown in Fig. 3.

Table 1 shows typical data indicating that ER + tumours have a much higher response to hormonal therapy than ER negative tumours. However, many ER + tumours do not respond. One possible reason is that there may be molecular defects in the oestrogen–ER–ERE–protein synthesis pathway. The additional measurement of progesterone receptor (**PgR**), which is an oestrogen-dependent protein, addresses this possibility. Response rates are greater for ER + PgR + tumours, but the response rate of 25 to 30 per cent seen in ER + PgR− tumours is generally considered worthwhile, which makes routine, double receptor analyses less valuable. Another possible reason for the non-response of ER + tumours is that in about one-third of patients with ER + primary tumours the metastatic disease may be ER−. This may occur as a result of phenotypic drift or metastatic selection, but whatever the reason, response of the metastatic disease relates better to its ER status than to the ER status of the primary.

The phenotype of PgR positivity in ER− tumours is unexpected. It has been hypothesized that this results from a constitutively active ER variant that is not detectable by conventional ER assays, but experimental evidence does not support this. In some cases the data may indicate a false negative ER assay, but more frequently the PgR positivity is associated with ER that is detectable with modern assays, but is at a concentration below positive/negative cut-off levels.

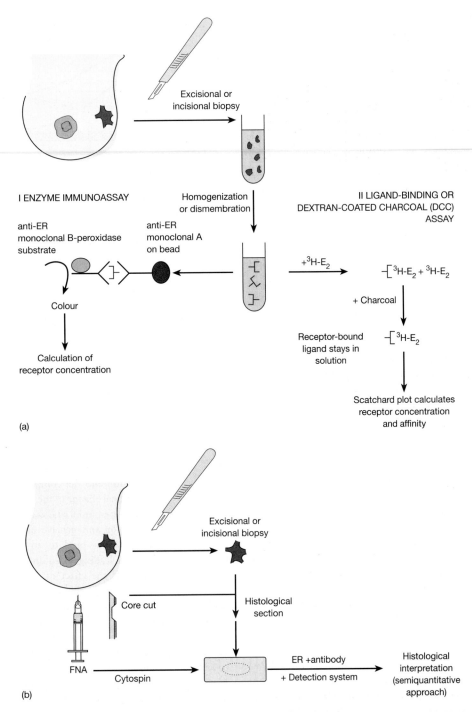

Fig. 3 Diagramatic representation of methods for analysing ER in breast carcinomas. (a) Enzyme immunoassay or ligand binding assay is conducted on homogenates of tissue. (b) Immunocytochemistry can be conducted on sections after excisional, incisional or core-cut biopsy or on cytospins after fine needle aspiration (FNA).

Therapeutic manoeuvres

Ovarian ablation

In premenopausal women the ovary is the obvious target for hormonal intervention. Ovarian ablation can be achieved in three ways—surgical, radiotherapeutic or medical (using gonadotrophin releasing hormone (GnRH) agonists). Overview analysis has confirmed that ovarian ablation by surgical or radiotherapeutic means leads to survival benefits when given as an adjuvant to surgery.[9] The clinical studies in the overview do not include ER status (as most studies were started before ER was discovered), and given that only about 50 per cent of premenopausal women are ER +, the benefit might be doubled by selection of the ER+ population. Ovariectomy yields plasma steroid levels equivalent to or a little lower than those in naturally postmenopausal women.

GnRH agonists are the current treatment of choice for many clinicians wishing to achieve ovarian ablation, as a result of the irreversible nature of ovariectomy and the fact that only a minority of patients respond. There are several GnRH agonists available, each being a stabilized derivative of the natural, rapidly degradable hypothalamic decapeptide. The normal control of gonadotrophin secretion from the pituitary depends on pulses of GnRH from the hypothalamus. GnRH binds to cell surface receptors on the gonadotrophs of the anterior pituitary where the receptor–ligand complexes come together in 'coated-pits' and the complex is internalized. In contrast, GnRH agonists are present at essentially unchanging levels leading to receptor downregulation and a desensitization of the gonadotroph to the normal pulsatile stimulation.

These local molecular events lead to an increase in plasma gonadotrophin levels over the first few days of treatment followed by profound suppression. Luteinizing hormone (**LH**) levels remain low, but follicle-stimulating hormone (**FSH**) levels increase over a period of weeks to near pretreatment levels, possibly due to increased secretion of inhibin, a hormone which is derived in the gonads and specifically suppresses FSH secretion.[10] Depending on the time of the menstrual cycle when therapy is instigated, plasma oestradiol levels may show an initial rise before falling to postmenopausal levels by the end of the first 4 weeks of treatment. However, low-level ovarian folliculogenesis persists during therapy, which leads to mean plasma oestradiol levels above the mean in postmenopausal or ovariectomized women but still in the postmenopausal range. The significance of this for therapeutic efficacy is unknown.

It has been argued that GnRH agonists may have a direct effect on breast tumour growth, i.e. independent of ovarian suppression, but their poor efficacy in postmenopausal women does not support this.

GnRH antagonists have been under development for several years. These have the benefit of no initial stimulatory phase, but given that this is rarely a problem in breast cancer patients, they are unlikely to have a significant role in treatment.

Antioestrogens

Tamoxifen

Tamoxifen is the most widely used drug in the hormonal treatment of breast cancer (see Chapters 11.7 and 11.8). Its use as an adjuvant after surgery increases survival for patients with ER+ disease and when administered to some groups of healthy women at high risk of breast cancer it decreases breast cancer incidence by 50 per cent (at least over the first few years)[11] (see also Chapters 2.5 and 11.1).

Although frequently described as an antioestrogen, tamoxifen has a complex pharmacology, which has been described as that of a partial or mixed agonist. However, the observation that the agonist/antagonist balance of tamoxifen and associated drugs differs substantially between tissues has led to the derivation of the term selective (o)estrogen receptor modulator (**SERM**), which more accurately describes their biological activity.

The partial agonist activity of tamoxifen on a single tissue is well illustrated by its action on the immature rat uterus (Fig. 4). In young female rats, prior to the maturity of the ovaries, the uterus is small,

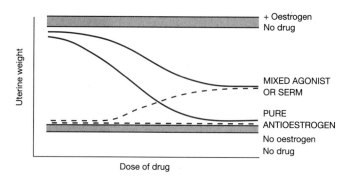

Fig. 4 Immature rat uterine weight model comparing the effect of a pure antioestrogen (e.g. ICI182780) with that of a SERM (e.g. tamoxifen). The dotted and continuous lines show the effect of increasing dose in the absence and presence of oestrogen, respectively.

but is exquisitely sensitive to exogenous oestrogen that can increase the weight about fivefold. In these circumstances tamoxifen acts as an antagonist, inducing a dose-related decrease in uterine weight but not to the level of unoestrogenized animals. In contrast, in the absence of oestrogen tamoxifen induces a dose-related increase in weight, an agonist effect.

The molecular mechanisms underlying these effects depend on tamoxifen competing with oestrogen for the ER and when binding, like oestrogen, causing loss of heat shock protein, dimerization, a ligand-specific conformational change, phosporylation of ER at specific amino acids and binding of the complex to palindromic EREs upstream of oestrogen responsive genes. The incorporation of a co-activator or co-repressor into the complex depends on the ligand-dependent conformational change of the receptor; thus in some cases the changes elicited by oestradiol and tamoxifen may allow binding of the same co-activator and achieve an agonist response, while in others co-activators may bind to an oestradiol–ER but not a tamoxifen–ER complex leading to an antagonist effect.[12] As far as the breast is concerned the effect of tamoxifen is predominantly antagonist, although even in this gland an agonist effect on progesterone receptor expression occurs.

Several pharmacological effects of tamoxifen are described, which may not depend on ER, such as protein kinase C inhibition and calmodulin inhibition. However, these effects generally occur only at concentrations above those found when usual doses of approximately 20 mg/day are given to patients. Recent data from xenografts indicate no more than a minor part for calmodulin inhibition.[13] The increases in transforming growth factor-β which are seen with tamoxifen are probably due to ER antagonism. Tamoxifen also reduces plasma levels of the potent breast cancer mitogen IGFI,[14] and this may have pharmacological importance in synergizing with the direct antioestrogenic effects of tamoxifen.

Much of the pharmacological activity of tamoxifen is exerted by the additive effects of numerous metabolites and the parent drug (Table 2). The most potent of the metabolites is 4-hydroxytamoxifen, which exists as cis- and trans-isomers. The latter has approximately 100 times greater affinity for ER than tamoxifen, but the very much lower plasma levels reduce its influence to approximately three times more than the parent drug. Desmethyltamoxifen has about half the potency but twice the plasma level of the parent drug. Tamoxifen has

Table 2 Relative pharmacological activity of tamoxifen and its major metabolites. Css: Steady-state concentration at a dose of 20 mg/day. RBA: relative binding affinity for ER. The data are derived as mean values from a comprehensive literature search (contact MD for references).

	Css (nmol/l)	RBA	'Activity' (nmol/l × RBA)
Tamoxifen	315	1.0	315
Desmethyl tamoxifen	602	0.78	470
Didesmethyl tamoxifen	99	0.64	63
4-hydroxy tamoxifen	8	70	560
metabolite Y	65	0.11	7

a terminal half-life of about 10 days, but it has been detected in tissues over a year after cessation of therapy.[15]

In premenopausal women, tamoxifen leads to an increase in plasma oestrogen levels of up to fivefold.[16] This seems to be largely due to an antagonist effect at the hypothalamus, leading to increased gonadotrophin secretion, but there may also be direct effects on the ovary. Although sex hormone binding globulin levels are also increased these do not fully compensate for the increase in oestradiol levels. The continued cyclical menstrual activity in most premenopausal women on tamoxifen indicates that the increased oestrogen levels overcome any antagonism by tamoxifen on the endometrium. Despite this, tamoxifen is an effective anti-breast cancer drug in pre-menopausal patients. The possibility that higher dosages of tamoxifen may be more effective has not been subject to large-scale trials.

In contrast to the effects in premenopausal patients, gonadotrophin levels fall in postmenopausal women on administration of tamoxifen, which is another example of a partial agonist activity that depends on prevailing oestrogen levels. Increased plasma levels of oestrone sulphate are seen after starting tamoxifen in postmenopausal women, but this probably has little effect on pharmacological efficacy.

Mechanisms of acquired resistance to tamoxifen are discussed below.

Other SERMs

A series of tamoxifen analogues (Fig. 5) have entered clinical trials and some are available for widespread usage (e.g. toremifene). They vary markedly in their selective modulation of oestrogen regulated pathways.

Toremifene has about one-third the overall potency of tamoxifen, but the balance of agonist and antagonist activity is very similar in most model systems. In advanced breast cancer toremifene has little clinical activity in patients after tamoxifen failure.[17] Droloxifene (3-hydroxytamoxifen) has a shorter half-life than tamoxifen and therefore more rapid achievement of steady state, but this has not translated to improved clinical efficacy. Idoxifene (4-iodopyrrolidinotamoxifen) shows reduced agonism in the gynaecological organs of rodents than tamoxifen.[18] It reduces the growth of tamoxifen-resistant breast cancer cell lines and xenografts but it is not yet known whether this will translate to improved clinical efficacy.

Raloxifene is a near pure antagonist in the rat uterus and unlike tamoxifen has no stimulatory effects on the human endometrium. In a phase II study in advanced breast cancer patients after tamoxifen failure, raloxifene had no significant activity, but in a large trial of

the drug for the prevention of osteoporosis an early reduction of more than 50 per cent in breast cancer incidence has been reported.[19] A close analogue of raloxifene, SERM3, has shown superior anticancer effects over raloxifene and tamoxifen in animal xenograft studies, and is in early clinical trial.

Each of the SERMs described above has been shown to have oestrogen agonist effects on bone. As a result there is major interest in exploiting SERMs as hormone replacement therapy without the disadvantageous effects on breast and endometrium of oestrogen-based hormone replacement therapy. As such, these agents also have promise for breast cancer prevention. However, long-term safety still needs to be demonstrated. It is also disappointing to note that none of the agents has beneficial effects on the neurological symptoms of oestrogen deprivation (e.g. hot flushes and night sweats).

Pure antioestrogens

All of the above compounds have some agonist activity in certain tissues, and may stimulate the growth of breast cells in some circumstances. In contrast, a number of steroidal compounds have been developed (Fig. 5), which elicit a uniformly antagonist response. Pure antagonism appears to be based on two aspects: (i) maintenance of ER in a similar conformation to the unliganded form, and (ii) a markedly reduced stability of ER leading to its near absence in treated breast carcinomas.[20] The result is compounds which remain effective in tamoxifen-resistant breast cancer, both in model systems and in patients. One of these compounds, ICI182780, unlike tamoxifen and toremifene, has been shown not to enhance the growth of endometrial tumours in immune-deprived mice.[21]

Aromatase inhibitors

Inhibition of aromatase was demonstrated to be an effective means of treating breast cancer by the use of aminoglutethimide. This is, however, a relatively non-specific cytochrome P450 inhibitor which interacts with 20,22-desmolase, 11β-hydroxylase, and 21-hydroxylase all of which are involved in synthesis of glucocorticoids, and it also is associated with several significant side-effects. Many new inhibitors have been developed over recent years and phase III clinical trials have established some of these as the preferred second-line hormonal agents to use after tamoxifen in postmenopausal women. None of the aromatase inhibitors is recommended for use in premenopausal women as reproducible suppression of ovarian steroidogenesis is not achieved. It is also questionable whether the drugs would be tolerable

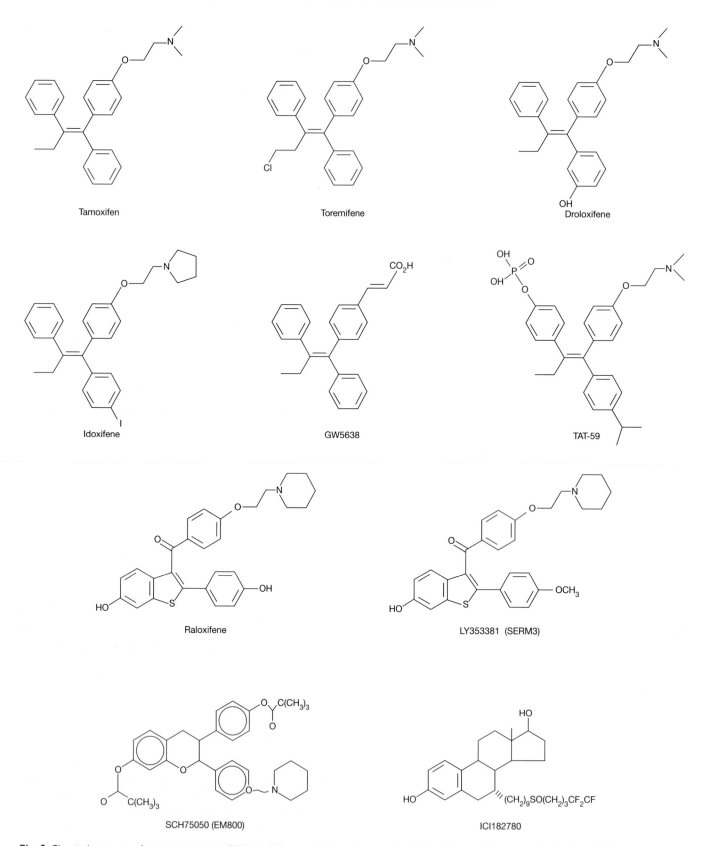

Fig. 5 Chemical structure of antioestrogens and SERMs, which are clinically available or in clinical trial. All of the drugs other than ICI182780 have predominantly agonist activity on some tissues mixed with antagonist activity on others.

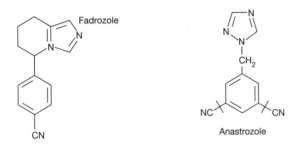

Fig. 6 Chemical structure of aromatase inhibitors which are clinically available or in clinical trial.

in this scenario as preclinical studies indicate that cystic ovaries might result.

The drugs are generally classified as type I, steroidal inhibitors, which act as substrate analogues and may lead to irreversible aromatase inactivation or type II, non-steroidal inhibitors, which bind through a basic nitrogen atom to the prosthetic haem group of aromatase (Fig. 6).

The most prominent steroidal compounds are formestane and exemestane, but only the latter is orally active. The degree of aromatase inhibition achieved by these compounds at clinically used dosages is about 85 per cent and 97 per cent, respectively.[22] The compounds have some intrinsic androgenic activity, but this is only exhibited in short-term studies at doses above those used clinically.

Fadrozole is a highly potent imidazole derivative, but its inhibition of 18-hydroxylase and the consequent suppression of aldosterone

levels has resulted in its dosage being limited to 1 mg twice daily, which achieves about 85 per cent inhibition of aromatase in vivo compared with about 91 per cent with 1000 mg/day amino-glutethimide.[22]

Several triazole compounds have been found to be highly effective in clinical usage and to have minimal non-specific effects or tolerability problems. The compounds which have been evaluated clinically are anastrozole, letrozole, vorozole, and YM511. Anastrozole and letrozole have been shown to inhibit aromatase activity in patients by about 97 per cent and more than 99 per cent, respectively, and thus show a substantially improved pharmacological effectiveness over aminoglutethimide. Although it is unproven that the greater aromatase inhibition achieved by these compounds will translate to greater clinical efficacy, an analysis of the outcome of recent phase III trials supports such a dose relationship.[22]

The clinical response of these compounds is largely restricted, like other hormonal agents, to ER+ tumours, but there is also some evidence that the presence or absence of measurable aromatase activity in the breast carcinoma may predict response to aromatase inhibitors.[23] However, the lack of a ready availability of unfixed tumour tissue in a sufficient quantity (≥ 500 mg) to allow biochemical analysis has limited the conduct of the supporting studies needed to demonstrate clinical utility. Intratumoral studies with anti-aromatase antibodies to detect intratumoral aromatase have unfortunately varied in the populations of cells identified as aromatase positive and have therefore led to doubt in the clinical–pathological relationships derived with them.

The bonding of some inhibitors to the enzyme's active site stabilizes the enzyme.[24] The non-steroidal inhibitors, fadrozole, vorozole, and pentrozole all increased enzyme concentration threefold in vitro, while the steroidal compound, formestane has no effect. It is not known whether this has clinical significance, but it could explain the increase in aromatase activity that was seen in breast carcinomas after 3 months treatment with aminoglutethimide.

The potential for aromatase inhibitors to be used in the prevention of breast cancer has been supported by the observation that fadrozole markedly decreased in a dose-related manner the incidence of spontaneous mammary carcinomas over the lifetime of Sprague–Dawley rats. Similarly, vorozole decreased the incidence of carcinogen-induced rat mammary cancer. However, these experiments used rats with intact ovarian function (equivalent to premenopausal women) and the doses of drug were sufficient to ablate ovarian function. Thus these data are not directly relevant to the application of these drugs in postmenopausal women.

Patients with metastatic breast cancer who respond initially to aromatase inhibitors almost invariably relapse. There are a number of potential resistance mechanisms for which there is a variable amount of supporting data. Relatively minor increases in plasma oestrone but not oestradiol levels at the time of relapse may be important in some patients. As mentioned above, aminoglutethimide treatment is known to enhance the overall aromatase activity of breast carcinomas. In the continued presence of the drug the activity is suppressed but probably not to the same degree as baseline enzyme concentrations. Also the sensitivity of breast cancer cells in vitro to the mitogenic effects of oestrogen is markedly enhanced by long-term oestrogen deprivation: cells which initially are maximally stimulated at 10^{-11} M oestradiol are maximally stimulated by 10^{-14} M after long-term deprivation.[25] The observation that some breast carcinomas will

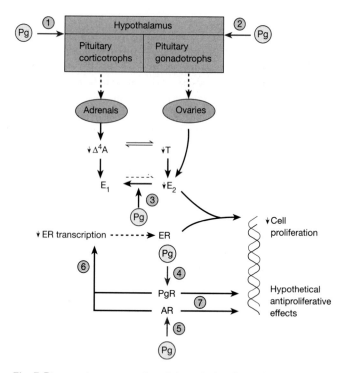

Fig. 7 Diagramatic representation of the multiple effects of progestogens (Pg) on breast cancer cell proliferation. The glucocorticoid (1) and progestogenic (2) activity of Pg reduces adrenal androgen (androstenedione (Δ^4A) and testosterone (T)) and ovarian oestrogen production respectively. The oxidative activity of oestradiol dehydrogenase is increased (3) altering the equilibrium between oestrone (E_1) and oestradiol (E_2). Binding of Pg to PgR (4) or AR (5) reduces ER transcription (6) and oestrogenic stimulation of proliferation and also may have direct antiproliferative effects (7).

respond to a more potent aromatase inhibitor at relapse suggest that this is a clinically relevant mechanism.

Progestins

There are two progestins which are used widely in breast cancer: megestrol acetate and medroxyprogesterone acetate. Their pharmacological mechanism is ill-defined. Many effects which could contribute to an antiproliferative effect have been described and it seems likely that most may play a part (Fig. 7). As well as the direct effect that these agents may exert through the progesterone receptor, they have indirect effects on oestrogen action. In premenopausal women, the high doses used in breast cancer can lead to down-regulation of ovarian steroidogenesis. They also have glucocorticoid effects which reduce adrenal steroidogenesis. In postmenopausal women, in whom oestrogen is derived from androgen precursors largely of adrenal origin, the suppression of oestrogen levels by megestrol acetate can approach that of some aromatase inhibitors.[26] The progestins also suppress the reductive effects of 17β-hydroxysteroid dehydrogenase on oestrone thus increasing the oestrone/oestradiol ratio and decreasing the overall bioactivity of the oestrogens, and lead to reduced ER expression which may contribute to a reduced proliferative response to the prevailing oestrogenic environment.

The relationship between the clinical effectiveness of progestins and steroid receptor expression is stronger for ER than PgR which suggests that the 'antioestrogenic' effects of progestins are more important than direct effects through the progesterone receptor. However, others have reported a stronger relationship with androgen receptor expression, suggesting that the androgenic activity which these compounds possess may be yet more important.[27]

The data on the effect of progestins on the proliferation of breast cancer cells *in vitro* are contradictory with reports of inhibition, stimulation, and no effect according to cell culture conditions; most reports show antiproliferative effects in the presence of oestrogen. Some of the contradictory data from cell culture may result from progesterone's biphasic effect on the cell cycle with an initial transient stimulation followed by inhibition of cycle progression.[28]

Two antiprogestins have been explored in breast cancer: mifepristone and onapristone. An advantage of the latter is reduced antiglucocorticoid activity when compared with mifepristone which leads to increased oestrogen levels in mifepristone-treated postmenopausal women.[29] The mode of action of these agents is poorly understood, but it is notable that the administration of onapristone to mice bearing hormone-dependent MXT mammary tumours, in addition to causing tumour repression also led to progesterone receptor mediated histological changes including increased cell death, which were suggestive of differentiation to a more benign status.[30]

Mechanisms of resistance

In the setting of advanced breast cancer nearly all patients that respond to hormone therapy eventually relapse as do a large proportion of those treated with adjuvant therapy. In many patients, however, the acquisition of resistance to one agent does not lead to resistance to all. Indeed, patients who respond initially to tamoxifen, and then relapse have about a 50 per cent chance of responding to an aromatase inhibitor (Fig. 8). This indicates that a variety of resistance mechanisms may operate according to a tumour's initial genotype/phenotype and the particular selective pressure exerted by therapy. Available clinical laboratory data on resistance mechanisms relate largely to tamoxifen.[31] Mechanisms of relevance to aromatase inhibition have been discussed above.

Loss of functional ER

De novo or intrinsic resistance to hormonal therapy relates strongly to ER status. However, acquired resistance, i.e. relapse after initial response, is not frequently associated with ER loss.[32] Certain experimentally derived point mutations can lead to profound changes in ER function, e.g. reacting to tamoxifen as a full agonist, but very few such mutations occur in human breast carcinomas. Numerous splice variants of ER have been characterized at the level of mRNA, and some of these can be shown to be constitutively active *in vitro*, but these variants also appear to have little clinical importance.[32] Maintained functionality of ER in tamoxifen resistant disease is also supported by the binding of extracted ER to EREs in gel shift assays.

Pharmacokinetic mechanisms.

The pharmacokinetics of tamoxifen are complex, there being numerous biologically active metabolites which are present in plasma in significant concentrations (Table 2). It has been hypothesized that altered tamoxifen metabolism could lead to increased relative concentrations of agonist metabolites, but results from studies in model

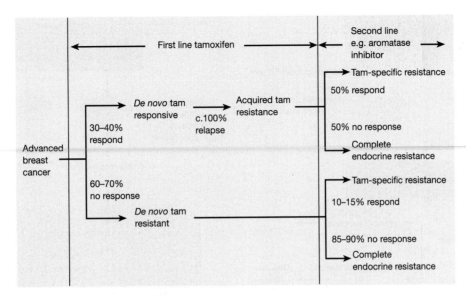

Fig. 8 The approximate response rates to be expected from the application of tamoxifen for first-line therapy and an aromatase inhibitor for second-line therapy in advanced breast cancer.

systems of stabilized forms of these metabolites do not suggest their having a significant role in acquired resistance.

Human MCF7 xenografts in athymic mice which become resistant to tamoxifen have markedly lower intratumoral concentrations of the drug than those in sensitive tumours during regression. Similar findings have been found in a minority of human breast carcinomas with acquired tamoxifen resistance in which drug levels may be decreased 10-fold.[33],[34] The mechanism underlying this effect is unknown, although it is not due to changes in either the concentration or protein binding of the drug in plasma.

Growth factors/receptors/downstream signalling pathways

The growth of breast cancer cells *in vitro* is supported by numerous growth factors. The epidermal growth factor family of ligands (e.g. transforming growth factor-α, amphiregulin, heregulin) and four receptors appear to be particularly important (see Chapter 1.5). Epidermal growth factor receptor (HER1) and c-erbB2 (HER2/neu) expression are inversely correlated with ER and the signalling pathways that these growth factor receptors co-ordinate are probably important in *de novo* hormone-resistant disease.[35] Increased expression of these receptors or ligands has not been found in tamoxifen-relapsed disease indicating that alterations in the signalling pathway at that level are unimportant.

In contrast IGFI receptor levels correlate positively with ER expression and IGFI synergizes with oestrogen as a mitogenic stimulant for breast cancer cells *in vitro*. Some data indicate that enhanced IGF receptor signalling may be a determinant of an increased agonist response to tamoxifen.

More recently it has been noted that the AP-1 transcription factor complex of Fos and Jun dimers has increased transcriptional activity both in xenografts and in human breast carcinomas that have acquired tamoxifen resistance. It is unclear whether this is due to increased interaction of ER with AP1 complexes or increased activity of upstream signalling pathways, such as those related to oxidative stress.

The complexity of these signalling pathways and the potential for multiple aberrations which would result in hormone resistance is emphasized by the observation that MAPkinase, which is activated by growth factor pathways (see Chapter 1.5) can phosphorylate and activate ER in the absence of ligand.

Increased agonist activity

The oestrogen agonist activity of tamoxifen has been the focus of much work on resistance mechanisms as well as providing theoretical support for the development of new drugs. Several lines of evidence support the importance of this mechanism: (i) responses may occur rarely on withdrawal of tamoxifen during disease progression; (ii) premenopausal women have been reported to respond to ovariectomy after tamoxifen relapse but only when tamoxifen is withdrawn concurrently;[36],[37] (iii) breast cancer cells derived from ascitic fluid from advanced breast cancer patients relapsing on tamoxifen in some cases show clonogenic growth on addition of either oestradiol or tamoxifen yet this response is blocked by a pure antioestrogen; and (iv) a xenograft of the MCF-7 human breast cancer cell line has been derived with acquired resistance to tamoxifen—the growth of this is promoted by tamoxifen as well as oestrogen but not by a pure antioestrogen.[38]

The mechanism behind this tamoxifen-stimulated growth is not known but changes in the expression of co-activators and co-repressors of ER are probably involved.[12] In support of this are observations of reduced levels of the co-repressor nCoR-1 in human breast cancer xenografts. The agonist activity may be exacerbated by an increased oestrogenic synergism with the IGF1 pathway, which occurs in some cell lines. An ER mutation, which leads to an increased agonist response to tamoxifen, has been found in a tamoxifen-resistant xenograft, but this has not been detected in human breast carcinomas.

Breast cancer resistance genes

Molecular approaches using retroviral insertion to perturb the genome have revealed a series of genes whose activation is associated with

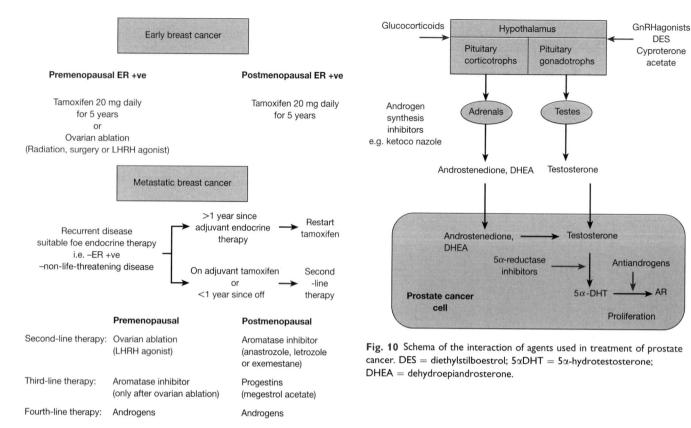

Fig. 9 Schema for endocrine therapy of breast cancer.

Fig. 10 Schema of the interaction of agents used in treatment of prostate cancer. DES = diethylstilboestrol; 5αDHT = 5α-hydrotestosterone; DHEA = dehydroepiandrosterone.

tamoxifen resistance *in vitro*.[39] The function of these and their role in human breast cancer remains to be established. A deficiency in this approach to the discovery of mechanisms of resistance is that any pathways requiring multiple aberrations to have a significant impact are unlikely to be revealed.

An algorithm summarizing the present strategies for the hormonal therapy of premenopausal and postmenopausal breast cancer patients is shown in Fig. 9.

Prostate cancer

Androgen deprivation

Withdrawal of androgens or the peripheral blockade of androgen action are the critical therapeutic options for the medical treatment of prostate cancer (see Chapter 13.1). Given that the majority of testosterone is derived from the testes, orchiectomy or testicular downregulation with GnRH agonists (see above for mechanism) are the first line treatment of choice (Fig. 10). The early stimulatory effect of GnRH agonists can lead to disease flare and this has led to the application of one of a number of antiandrogens during the first few weeks of treatment. High dose oestrogens, primarily in the form of diethylstilboestrol also lead to gonadotrophin suppression and consequent gonadal downregulation.

The adrenal glands are responsible for the synthesis of the remaining androgens in the plasma and the blockade of these androgens has become a target either combined with testicular ablation as in

so-called 'complete androgen blockade' or as second-line therapy after initial testicular ablation alone.[40] The intratissular concentrations of androgens in the prostate, particularly 5α-dihydrotestosterone, which is the predominant androgenic mitogen present in the prostate, are reduced to a much lesser extent than plasma androgens by testicular ablation such that the additional blockade of adrenal androgens might have an importance disproportionate to their plasma concentrations. Geller has estimated that 25 per cent of the intraprostatic 5α-dihydrotestosterone is derived from adrenal androgens and that this proportion persists when castration alone is performed.[41] The correlation between the concentration of residual 5α-dihydrotestosterone and both protein synthesis and prostate specific antigen (PSA) levels supports the biological importance of this androgen. Its clinical significance is underscored by the responses that are seen in some patients to adrenal androgen blockade after their relapse from prior castration.

Despite this rationale for complete (or maximal) androgen blockade and some encouraging early clinical results, overview analysis of 25 trials found no survival advantage for the combination therapy compared with castration alone (surgical or medical).[42] There has been criticism of the methodology of the overview, but even if this is well founded any benefit of complete androgen blockade would appear to be slight.

The most common approach to blocking adrenal androgens is to use an antiandrogen such as the steroidal compound, cyproterone acetate, or one of the non-steroidals flutamide, nilutamide, or bicalutamide which are competitive binders to androgen receptor (AR) (Fig. 11). Cyproterone acetate has affinity for PgR as well as AR, while the non-steroidal compounds bind significantly only to AR. Cyproterone acetate shows some agonism in HeLa cells transfected with wild-type AR and greater agonism with the mutated AR found

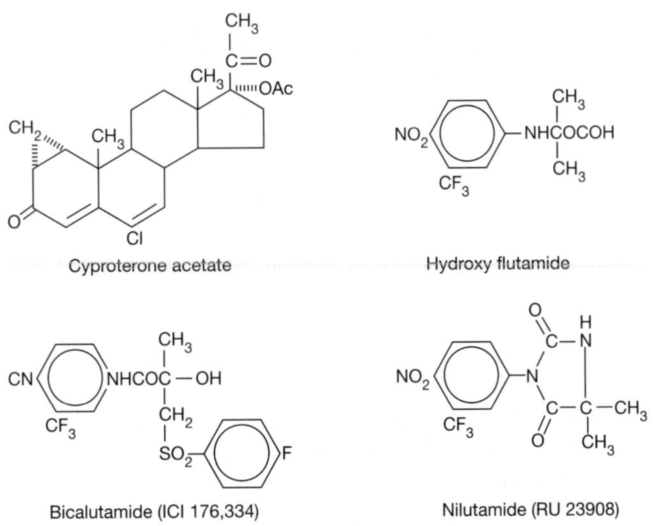

Fig. 11 Chemical structure of antiandrogens which are in clinical use.

in LNCaP prostate cancer cells. Hydroxyflutamide and nilutamide also show some agonism on the LNCaP AR but bicalutamide remains entirely antagonistic as with the wild-type receptor.[43] These data may be significant in the context of withdrawal responses to some of these antiandrogens (see below). Reduced adrenal androgen output can be achieved by glucocorticoid administration which reduces ACTH drive, but so-called replacement dosages do not achieve complete ablation. Inhibition of the 17,20-lyase enzyme has been attempted using agents such as ketoconazole or more promisingly, more specific and potent compounds such as abiraterone. This approach is complicated, however, by 17,20-lyase being a complex with 17α-hydroxylase, which is involved in cortisol synthesis, such that cortisol production is also impeded by these compounds.

There has been some interest in the use of aromatase inhibitors in prostate cancer. This largely resulted from the application of aminoglutethimide to advanced prostate cancer patients under the rationale that this would achieve adrenal suppression. It is clear, however, that aminoglutethimide does not suppress adrenal androgen secretion and any benefit may derive from the adrenal suppressive effects of the concurrently administered glucocorticoid,[44] or from suppression of the drug's main target, aromatase. The application of the more specific aromatase inhibitor, formestane, also yielded some subjective benefit. The mechanism by which oestrogen deprivation may lead to this benefit is unknown, although aromatase has been identified in some prostate cancer cell lines, as has ERβ.

The cellular outcome of androgen ablation in model systems such as PC82 human prostate cancer in nude mice is an elevation of apoptosis accompanied by a decrease in proliferation. Clinical studies, however, have revealed that while decreased proliferation occurred in almost all tumours, increased apoptosis was seen in only a minority. Recurrent prostate cancer has increased proliferation and decreased apoptosis compared with the corresponding untreated primary tumour.[45]

Androgen receptor

The promotion of prostate cancer cell growth by androgens is by its interaction with AR in the cancer cells in an analogous manner to

that with breast cancer and oestrogens (Fig. 2). Much work has been orientated to assessing whether the absence of AR or malfunctioning forms of it may be the cause of the small proportion (about 15 per cent) of patients who are refractory to primary therapy and/or the near 100 per cent of patients that become resistant to such treatment. Quantitative measures of AR have not been helpful in predicting response or time to progression[46] and AR measurements are not routinely conducted in the way that ER measurements are made in breast cancer.

Molecular analyses of the role of AR in tumour recurrence and progression have focused in the vast majority of studies on AR gene mutations, although recent studies suggest that amplification and increased transcriptional activity of a wild-type AR gene may also contribute to the progression of many prostate cancers in the face of continuing therapy.

Aberrations of AR in prostate cancer

Many of the AR mutations found in prostate cancer lead to transcriptional activity on binding to ligands other than androgens, such as oestrogens, progestogens, and of particular significance antiandrogens. In most studies a low frequency of AR mutations has been found in primary disease and even in advanced hormone refractory disease. However, Tilley et al.,[47] who in contrast to most other groups, studied all eight exons, found mutations in 11 of 25 (44 per cent) untreated primary prostate cancers. Another study[48] revealed mutations in the ligand binding domain of AR in distant metastases in five of 10 hormonally treated patients. Certain mutations of AR found in patients with recurrent prostate cancer cause increased transcriptional activity on exposure to the antiandrogens, flutamide and nilutamide, while bicalutamide remains an antagonist for these mutant receptors.[49] This may provide a mechanism for the responses seen on withdrawal of flutamide and also the responses to high-dose bicalutamide in patients progressing on flutamide.[50] Also of significance is the finding that a low number of CAG repeats in a polymorphic region of exon A of the AR gene is correlated with the likelihood of developing high-grade, advanced-stage prostate cancer. The length of the resulting sequence of glutamine residues in the receptor protein is inversely related to transcriptional activity.[51]

It is therefore apparent that AR mutations occur in prostate cancer and their presence may influence hormonal response of the disease. The true frequency remains unclear, but it seems that a large proportion of tumours retain wild-type AR.

The AR gene has been found to be amplified in 28 per cent (15 of 54) of locally recurrent tumours by 2.7 to 28-fold while there was no amplification in primary tumours.[52] These tumours were those which had initially shown the best response to androgen deprivation. It is possible that such recurrences may result from acquired hypersensitivity to androgen rather than from androgen independence (see comments above on oestrogen hypersensitivity in breast cancer). If so these tumours are candidates for second-line hormonal therapy targeted at maximal androgen blockade.

Like other steroid receptors, AR interacts with various co-activators and co-repressors, which not only modify the response to endogenous ligands but also influence the balance in the agonist/antagonist response to mixed-function antiandrogens. Of particular interest is ARA-70 which is a specific co-activator for AR.[53] Changes in the expression and functionality of these proteins may markedly influence the response of prostate cancer to hormonal agents.

There is substantial 'cross-talk' between the AR pathway and the signalling of peptide growth factors. These other signalling pathways may contribute increasingly to overall growth promotion during androgen deprivation and be significant in the emergence of disease which is resistant to hormonal deprivation.

Ovarian cancer

There are both experimental and epidemiological data to suggest that ovarian cancer may be an endocrine-related tumour (see also Chapter 12.1). Chronic oestrogen and progestin administration in animal studies may induce ovarian cancer, and persistent ovulation which may be associated with nulliparity or low number of pregnancies is a known premenopausal risk factor.[54] The ovary represents the major source of oestrogen and progesterone synthesis in premenopausal women, and is also a target organ for these hormones. In post-menopausal women, the high gonadotrophin environment may also confer additional risk. As with breast cancer, any growth stimulatory role of steroid hormones on malignant ovarian cells upon which a rational approach for hormonal therapy could be based requires expression of functional steroid hormone receptors.

ER and PgR expression

Both ERs and PgRs have been identified in clinical studies of primary and recurrent ovarian carcinomas. Initially, using the ligand-binding assay/dextrose-coated charcoal method, oestrogen-binding macromolecules with high specificity and binding affinity consistent with classic cytosolic oestrogen receptors were detected in human epithelial ovarian cancers. A review of several series published in the early 1980s indicated ER positivity in approximately 55 per cent of ovarian cancers (range 35 to 73 per cent; reviewed in ref. 55). The mean receptor content in these series was 43 fmol/mg protein, a value somewhat lower than that seen in breast cancers. Again unlike breast cancer, there appears to be no correlation with tumour differentiation or menopausal status, although ovarian cancers with endometrioid histology often have higher levels of receptors. PgR expression was found in approximately 20 to 40 per cent of ovarian carcinomas, with a mean level of 64 fmol/mg protein.

In vitro studies have investigated more closely the relationship between receptor expression in ovarian cancer and responsiveness to hormonal therapy. Significant and dose-dependent inhibition of colony forming ability was greatest with the antioestrogen tamoxifen in comparison with progestins, although no significant correlation between *in-vitro* responsiveness and level of receptor expression was found in cell cultures derived from 25 patients.[56] Likewise other studies have failed to show a clear relationship between PgR levels and response to medroxyprogesterone acetate.[57] Comparison of human derived ovarian carcinoma cell lines with a rich ER content (>100 fmol/mg protein) confirm that growth of ER+ cells in oestrogen-depleted fetal calf serum can be stimulated by levels of oestradiol as low as 0.1 nmol/litre.[58] Tamoxifen at concentrations of 1 mmol/litre antagonized oestrogenic stimulation, but had no effect on growth in the absence of oestradiol. In the same study ovarian cancer cell lines without any detectable ER were not affected by oestradiol, tamoxifen, or both.

In clinical studies where ER and PgR levels have been measured correlation with response to hormonal therapy has been variable. In a study of 105 patients with advanced ovarian cancer treated with tamoxifen, there was a trend toward correlation, with eight of nine complete responders (89 per cent) having elevated ER levels versus 59 per cent of non-responders.[59] Other studies have failed to see any clear association, suggesting that ER status is less predictive of response in ovarian cancer than in breast or endometrial cancer. Reasons for this are unclear, but may include the lower quantitative level of receptor expression which has been reported. Separate studies have indicated that ER positivity in ovarian cancer is associated with improved prognosis and survival, an effect which was greatest in patients with tumours which co-expressed PgR.[60]

The functional role of steroid hormone receptors has been demonstrated in ovarian cancer, with induction of PgR after oestradiol treatment in ER+ cells. This relationship has been confirmed *in-vivo* by xenograft experiments in which oestradiol regulated the expression of tumour PgR in ER+ ovarian cancer cells.[61] Absence of PgR expression in ER+ ovarian cancers may relate to loss of heterozygosity at chromosome 11q22, close to the PgR gene, and this cytogenetic abnormality has been associated with a poorer clinical prognosis.[62] More recently, it has been confirmed that oestradiol may increase transforming growth factor-α production in ER+ ovarian cancer cells, which in turn may act through epidermal growth factor receptor in an autocrine/paracrine manner.[63]

Hormonal therapeutic options

Progestins have been used as palliative agents in refractory advanced ovarian cancer, although response rates vary enormously between reported trials and in randomized phase III trials the response rates are less than 10 per cent.[64] Tamoxifen has been studied in numerous small series, and in the largest report an objective response rate of 17 per cent was seen with evidence in some patients of a complete response. Review of all the literature suggested a possible trend to a higher response with increasing doses of tamoxifen,[48] but this has never been studied prospectively. There is little evidence of significant clinical activity with oestrogens, androgens, luteinizing hormone-releasing agonists, or aromatase inhibitors.

Endometrial cancer

Progestins are an effective standard form of therapy for advanced endometrial adenocarcinoma, with responses seen in a third of patients treated (see also Chapter 12.4). Both ERs and PgRs are detected in a high proportion (70 to 80 per cent) of endometrial cancers, and levels are higher in well versus poorly differentiated tumours. Receptor expression correlates with improved survival.[65] A review of published series demonstrated a strong relationship between PgR expression and response of recurrent/advanced endometrial adenocarcinoma to progestins; 38 of 44 (86 per cent) responders were PgR-positive compared with only 13 of 83 (16 per cent) non-responders.[66]

Antioestrogens such as tamoxifen have also been shown to be effective in treating endometrial cancer in clinical studies. In experimental tumours a combination of tamoxifen and medroxy-progesterone was found to be superior to the progestin alone. Tamoxifen is known to have oestrogen-like effects on endometrial cells with increased PgR expression in these tumours, which could augment the degree and duration of response to progestins. However, in subsequent experiments such tumours became resistant to combined tamoxifen/progestin therapy, possibly due to subsequent downregulation of PgR expression.[67] Combined endocrine therapy is not used widely in clinical practice.

Tamoxifen is known to stimulate the growth of ER+ EnCa101 endometrial tumours in xenograft studies while at the same time inhibiting the growth of contralateral ER+ MCF-7 breast cancer cells.[68] The basis for this differential tissue-specific response is the subject of numerous current studies, which may relate to altered levels of steroid receptor co-activators/co-repressors as discussed above. Novel antioestrogens, including SERMs (see above, breast cancer section), have been developed in view of concerns about the uterine effects of tamoxifen. The effects of these drugs on endometrial cancer are largely unknown at present, although recent reports have shown a similar stimulatory effect with toremifene (a chlorinated derivative of tamoxifen), but an inhibitory effect with the pure antioestrogen ICI182,780.[69] This raises the possibility that the new generation of antioestrogens may provide an effective new endocrine treatment for endometrial cancer, and clinical trials are ongoing with several of these agents.

Melanoma

There has been a long debate about the possible association of malignant melanoma with steroid hormones, in particular oestrogen (see also Chapter 8.1). Epidemiological evidence suggests that the prognosis in women is better than in men.[70] Other clinical studies have looked at the implications of pregnancy or exogenous hormones on the natural history of melanoma. Primary melanomas which present during pregnancy have been found to be thicker than those in non-pregnant controls, but when corrected for this variable, pregnancy appears to have no adverse affect on outcome.[71] Oral contraceptives do not have an impact on the prognosis of melanoma.

Clinical data which implied a potential role of hormones on the biology of malignant melanoma promoted laboratory studies to examine the influence of hormones on growth. Early experimental studies found that some melanomas may be sensitive to steroid hormones in culture or in animal models, and applied studies suggested that up to 20 per cent of human melanoma biopsies may demonstrate high-affinity intracytoplasmic oestrogen binding.[72] However, reports in the literature are conflicting regarding expression of nuclear ERs, and studies using monoclonal antibodies in human melanomas failed to detect true immunoreactive ER.[73] The previous binding of oestrogen which was noted in early studies may represent non-specific binding, possibly to the enzyme tyrosinase.

Despite the lack of laboratory evidence to support a steroid hormone regulated growth pathway, the epidemiological evidence has prompted clinical studies to investigate the role of tamoxifen. Therapeutic trials of tamoxifen as single agent therapy demonstrate only a 4 to 6 per cent objective response rate.[74] Likewise there appears to be a low clinical response rate in patients who receive megesterol acetate. Tamoxifen has been investigated in combination with chemotherapy for melanoma, based on experimental data suggesting that tamoxifen may synergize with cisplatin in killing melanoma cells in vitro.[75] Only one randomized trial has shown an improvement in clinical response (28 per cent versus 12 per cent) and time to disease progression for the addition of tamoxifen to dacarbazine chemotherapy.[76]

Renal cell cancer

Following early reports that oestrogen-induced renal cell cancer in male Syrian hamsters could be inhibited by progestin therapy,[77] medroxyprogesterone acetate became a 'standard' therapeutic drug for advanced disease. However, critical review of the published clinical studies has suggested that response rates are low (less than 5 per cent) and of short duration[78] (see also Chapter 13.3). There are no reliable data indicating significant steroid hormone receptor expression in human renal cell carcinomas, and no evidence from randomized trials to support a beneficial effect for adjuvant progestin therapy.[79] Indeed a recently reported United Kingdom randomized trial showed a significantly improved clinical benefit for immunotherapy with interferon-α over medroxyprogesterone acetate in advanced renal cell cancer.[80]

Summary

Hormone therapy has become an integral part of the management of several solid cancers. While earlier treatments often involved ablative surgery to remove the source of endogenous growth-stimulating hormones, novel and effective medical therapies are now available. Following successful clinical trials, many of these are becoming standard therapies in the clinic. At the same time there has been an increased understanding of the molecular biology of steroid receptor action, and of adaptive mechanisms of endocrine resistance, which can occur in hormonally treated tumours.

References

1. **Beatson GT.** On the treatment of inoperable cases of carcinoma of the mamma. Suggestions for a new method of treatment with illustrative cases. *The Lancet*, 1896; **ii**: 104–7.

2. **Huggins C, Hodges CV.** Studies on prostatic cancer; effect of castration, estrogen and of androgen injection on serum phosphates in metastatic carcinoma of the prostate. *Cancer Research*, 1941; **1**: 293–97.

3. **Stewart AJ, Westley BR, May FEB.** Modulation of the proliferative response of breast cancer cells to growth factors by oestrogen. *British Journal of Cancer*, 1992; **66**: 640–8.

4. **Lippman M, Monaco ME, Bolan G.** Effects of estrone, estradiol, and estriol on hormone-responsive human breast cancer in long-term tissue culture. *Cancer Research*, 1977; **37**: 1901–7.

5. **Teixeira C, Reed JC, Pratt MAC.** Estrogen promotes chemotherapeutic drug resistance by a mechanism involving bcl-2 proto-oncogene expression in human breast cancer cells. *Cancer Research*, 1995; **55**: 3902–7.

6. **Kuiper GG, Enmark E, Pelto-Huikko M, Nilsson S, Gustaffson J-A.** Cloning of a novel receptor expressed in rat prostate and ovary. *Proceedings of the National Academy of Science USA*, 1996; **93**: 5925–30.

7. **McGuire WL, Chamness GC, Fuqua FAW.** Mini-review: estrogen receptor variants in clinical breast cancer. *Molecular Endocrinology*, 1991; **5**: 1571–7.

8. **Elledge RM, Osborne CK.** Oestrogen receptors and breast cancer. *British Medical Journal*, 1997; **314**: 1843–4.

9. Early Breast Cancer Trialists Collaborative Group. Ovarian ablation in early breast cancer: overview of the randomized trials. *The Lancet,* 1996; **348**: 1189–96.

10. Dowsett M, Mehta A, Mansi J, Smith IE. A dose-comparative endocrine-clinical study of Leuprorelin in premenopausal breast cancer patients. *British Journal of Cancer,* 1990; **62**: 834–7.

11. Fisher B, *et al.* Tamoxifen for prevention of breast cancer; report of the National Surgical Adjuvant Breast and Bowel Project P-1 Study. *Journal of the National Cancer Institute,* 1998; **90**: 1371–88.

12. Smith CL, Nawaz Z, O'Malley BW. Coactivator and corepressor regulation of the agonist/antagonist activity of the mixed antiestrogen, 4-hydoxytamoxifen. *Molecular Endocrinology,* 1997; **11**: 657–66.

13. Johnston SRD, *et al.* Increased activator protein-1 DNA binding and c-Jun NH₂ terminal kinase activity in human breast tumours with acquired tamoxifen resistance. *Clinical Cancer Research,* 1999; 5: 251–6.

14. Pollack M, Constantino J, Polychronakos C. Effect of tamoxifen on serum insulin-like growth factor 1 levels in stage 1 breast cancer patients. *Journal of the National Cancer Institute,* 1990; **82**: 1693–7.

15. Lien EA, Solheim E, Ueland PM. Distribution of tamoxifen and its metabolites in rat and human tissues during steady-state treatment. *Cancer Research,* 1991; **51**: 4837–44.

16. Ravdin PM, Fritz NF, Torney DC, Jordan C. Endocrine status of premenopausal node-positive breast cancer patients following adjuvant chemotherapy and long-term tamoxifen. *Cancer Research,* 1988; **48**: 1026–9.

17. Stenbygaard LE, Herrstedt J, Thomsen JF, Svendsen KR, Engelholm SAS, Dombernowsky P. Torimefene and tamoxifen in advanced breast cancer—a double-blind cross-over trial. *Breast Cancer Research and Treatment,* 1993; **25**: 57–63.

18. Chander SK, Newton C, McCague R, Dowsett M, Luqmano Y, Coombes RC. Pyrrolodine-4-iodotamoxifen and 4-iodotamoxifen, new analogues of the antioestrogen tamoxifen for the treatment of breast cancer. *Cancer Research,* 1991; **51**: 5851–8.

19. Jordan VC, *et al.* Raloxifene reduces incident primary breast cancers: integrated data from multicentre, double-blind, placebo-controlled, randomized trials in postmenopausal women. *Breast Cancer Research and Treatment,* 1998; **50**: 227.

20. DeFriend DJ, *et al.* Investigation of a new pure antiestrogen (ICI 182780) in women with primary breast cancer. *Cancer Research,* 1994; **54**: 408–14.

21. Hayes DF, *et al.* Randomized comparison of tamoxifen and 2 separate doses of toremifene in postmenopausal patients with breast cancer. *Journal of Clinical Oncology,* 1995; **13**: 2556–66.

22. Dowsett M. Theoretical considerations for the ideal aromatase inhibitor. *Breast Cancer Research and Treatment,* 1998; **49**: S39–44.

23. Miller WR, O'Neill J. The significance of local synthesis of estrogen within the breast. *Steroids,* 1987; **50**: 537–48.

24. Harada N, Hatano O. Inhibitors of aromatase prevent degradation of the enzyme in cultured human cells. *British Journal of Cancer,* 1998; 77: 567–72.

25. Masamura S, Santner SJ, Heitjan DF, Santen RJ. Estrogen deprivation causes estradiol hypersensitivity in human breast cancer cells. *Journal of Clinical Endocrinology and Metabolism,* 1995; **80**: 2918–25.

26. Lundgren S, Helle SL, Lonning PE. Profound suppression of plasma estrogens by megestrol acetate in postmenopausal breast cancer patients. *Clinical Cancer Research,* 1996; **2**: 1515–21.

27. Birrell SN, Roder DM, Horsfall DJ, Bentel JM, Tilley WD. Medroxyprogesterone acetate therapy in advanced breast cancer: the predictive value of androgen receptor expression. *Journal of Clinical Oncology,* 1995; **13**(7): 1572–7.

28. Sutherland RL, Watts CKW, Musgrove EA. Cell cycle control by steroid hormones in breast cancer: implications for endocrine resistance. *Endocrine Related Cancer,* 1995; **2**: 87–96.

29. Klijn JG, de-Jong FH, Bakker GH, Lamberts SW, Rodenburg CJ,

30. Alexieva-Figureusch J. Antiprogestins, a new form of endocrine therapy for human breast cancer. *Cancer Research,* 1989; **49**: 2851–6.

30. Schneider MR, Michna H, Nishino Y, Neef G, el-Etreby MF. Tumor-inhibiting potential of ZK 112.993, a new progesterone antagonist, in hormone-sensitive, experimental rodent and human mammary tumors. *Anticancer Research,* 1990; **10**: 683–7.

31. Johnston SRD, Dowsett M, Smith IE. Towards a molecular basis for tamoxifen resistance in breast cancer. *Annals of Oncology,* 1992; **3**: 503–11.

32. Dowsett M, Daffada A, Chan CMW, Johnston SRD. Oestrogen receptor mutants and variants in breast cancer. *European Journal of Cancer,* 1997; **33**: 1177–83.

33. Osborne CK, Coronado E, Allred DC, Wiebe V, DeGregorio M. Acquired tamoxifen resistance: correlation with reduced breast tumor levels of tamoxifen and isomerization of trans-4-hydroxytamoxifen. *Journal of the National Cancer Institute,* 1991; **83**: 1477–82.

34. Johnston SRD, *et al.* Acquired tamoxifen resistance in human breast cancer and reduced intratumoral drug concentration. *The Lancet,* 1993; **342**: 1521–2.

35. Newby JC, Johnston SRD, Smith IE, Dowsett M. Expression of epidermal growth factor receptor and c-erbB2 during the development of tamoxifen resistance in human breast cancer. *Clinical Cancer Research,* 1997; **3**: 1643–51.

36. Pritchard KI, Thomson DB, Myers RE, Sutherland DJA, Mobbs BG, Meakin JW. Tamoxifen therapy in premenopausal patients with metastatic breast cancer. *Cancer Treatment Reports,* 1980; **64**: 787–96.

37. Hoogstraten B, *et al.* Combined modality therapy for first recurrence of breast cancer. A Southwest Oncology Group Study. *Cancer,* 1984; **54**: 2248–56.

38. Gottardis MM, Jiang SY, Jeng MH, Jordan VC. Inhibition of tamoxifen-stimulated growth of an MCF-7 tumor variant in athymic mice by novel steroidal antiestrogens. *Cancer Research,* 1989; **49**(15): 4090–3.

39. van-Agthoven T, van-Agthoven TL, Dekker A, van-der-Spek PJ, Vreede L, Dorssers LC. Identification of BCAR3 by a random search for genes involved in antiestrogen resistance of human breast cancer cells. *EMBO Journal,* 1998; **17**: 2799–808.

40. Labrie F, *et al.* Advantages of combination therapy in previously untreated and treated patients with advanced prostate cancer. *Journal of Steroid Biochemistry,* 1986; **25**: 877–83.

41. Geller J. The role of adrenal androgens in prostate cancer. In: Pasqualini JR, Katzenellenbagen BS (eds). *Hormone dependent cancer.* New York: Marcel Dekker, 1996: 289–305.

42. Prostate Cancer Trialists' Collaborative Group. Maximum androgen blockade in advanced prostate cancer: an overview of 22 randomized trials with 3283 deaths in 5710 patients. *The Lancet,* 1995; **346**: 265–9.

43. Mulder E, Veldscholte J, Kuil CW. Molecular mechanisms of androgen antagonists. In: Pasqualini JR, Katzenellenbagen BS (eds). *Hormone dependent cancer.* New York: Marcel Dekker, 1996: 357–72.

44. Dowsett M, Shearer RJ, Ponder B, Malone P, Jeffcoate SL. The effects of aminoglutethimide and hydrocortisone, alone and combined on androgen levels in postorchiectomy prostatic cancer patients. *British Journal of Cancer,* 1988; **57**: 190–2.

45. Koivisto P, Visakorpi T, Rantala I, Isola J. Increased cell proliferation activity and decreased cell death are associated with the emergence of hormone-refractory recurrent prostate cancer. *Journal of Pathology,* 1997; **183**: 51–6.

46. Sadi MV, Barrack ER. Androgen receptors and growth fraction in metastatic prostate cancer as predictors of time to tumour progression after hormonal therapy. In: Isaacs J (ed.). *Cancer surveys. Prostate cancer cell and molecular mechanisms in diagnosis and treatment.* New York: Cold Spring Harbor Press, 1991: 195–215.

47. Tilley WD, Buchanan G, Hickey TE, Bentel JM. Mutations in the androgen receptor gene are associated with progression of human

prostate cancer to androgen independence. *Clinical Cancer Research*, 1996; **2**: 277–85.

48. Taplin ME, *et al.* Mutation of the androgen-receptor gene in metastatic androgen-independent prostate cancer. *New England Journal of Medicine*, 1995; **332**: 1393–8.

49. Fenton MA, *et al.* Functional characterization of mutant androgen receptors from androgen-independent prostate cancer. *Clinical Cancer Research*, 1997; **3**: 1383–8.

50. Scher HI, Zhang ZF, Nanus D, Kelly WK. Hormone and antihormone withdrawal: implications for the management of androgen-independent prostate cancer. *Urology*, 1996; **47** (Suppl.): 61–9.

51. Giovannucci E, *et al.* The CAG repeat within the androgen receptor gene and its relationship to prostate cancer. *Proceedings of the National Academy of Sciences USA*, 1997; **94**: 3320–3.

52. Koivisto P, *et al.* Androgen receptor gene amplification: a possible molecular mechanism for androgen deprivation therapy failure in prostate cancer. *Cancer Research*, 1997; **57**: 314–19.

53. Miyamoto H, Yeh S, Wilding G, Chang C. Promotion of agonist activity of antiandrogens by the androgen receptor coactivator, ARA70, in human prostate cancer DU145 cells. *Proceedings of the National Academy of Science USA*, 1998; **95**: 7379–84.

54. Cramer DW, Hutchinson GB, Welch WR, Scully RE, Ryan KJ. Determinants of ovarian cancer risk. *Journal of the National Cancer Institute*, 1983; **71**: 711–21.

55. Ahlgren JD, *et al.* Hormonal palliation of chemoresistant ovarian cancer: three consecutive phase II trials of the mid-Atlantic Oncology Program. *Journal of Clinical Oncology*, 1993; **11**: 1957–68.

56. Runge HM, Teufel G, Neulen J, Geyer H, Pfleiderer A. *In vitro* responsiveness of ovarian epithelial carcinomas to endocrine therapy. *Cancer Chemotherapy and Pharmacology*, 1986; **16**: 58–63.

57. Grongroos M, *et al.* Steroid receptors and response of ovarian cancer to hormones *in vitro. British Journal of Obstetrics and Gynaecology*, 1984; **91**: 472–8.

58. Langdon SP, *et al.* Oestrogen receptor expression and the effects of oestrogen and tamoxifen on the growth of human ovarian carcinoma cell lines. *British Journal of Cancer*, 1990; **62**: 213–16.

59. Hatch KD, Beecham JB, Blessing JA, Creasman WT. Responsiveness of patients with advanced ovarian carcinoma to tamoxifen. *Cancer*, 1991; **68**: 269–71.

60. Iverson OE, Skaarland E, Utaaker E. Steroid receptor content in human ovarian tumours; survival of patients with ovarian carcinoma related to steroid receptor content. *Gynaecological Oncology*, 1986; **23**: 65–76.

61. Langdon SP, *et al.* Functionality of the progesterone receptor in ovarian cancer and its regulation by estrogen. *Clinical Cancer Research*, 1998; **4**: 2245–51.

62. Gabra H, *et al.* Loss of heterozygosity a 11q22 correlates with low progesterone receptor content in epithelial ovarian cancer. *Clinical Cancer Research*, 1995; **1**; 945–53.

63. Simpson BJB, *et al.* Estrogen regulation of transforming growth factor alpha in ovarian cancer. *Journal of Steroid Biochemistry Molecular Biology*, 1998; **64**: 137–45.

64. Slayton R, Ragano M, Creech R. Progestin therapy for advanced ovarian cancer: a phase III Eastern Cooperative Oncology Group Trial. *Cancer Treatment Reports*, 1981; **65**: 895.

65. Creasman WT, Soper JT, McArthy KS, Hinshaw W, Clarke-Pearson DL. Influence of cytoplasmic steroid receptor content on prognosis or early stage endometrial carcinoma. *American Journal of Obstetrics and Gynecology*, 1985; **151**: 922–32.

66. Ehrlich CE. Current status of steroid hormone therapy for endometrial cancer. In: Rutledge FN, Freedman RS, Gershenson DM (eds). *Gynecologic cancer: diagnosis and treatment strategies*. Austin, TX: University of Texas Press, 1987: 335–43.

67. Satyaswaroop PG, Clarke CL, Zaino RJ, Mortel R. Apparent resistance in human endometrial carcinoma during combination treatment with tamoxifen and progestin may result from desensitization following downregulation of tumour progesterone receptor. *Cancer Letters*, 1992; **62**: 107–14.

68. Gottardis MM, Robinson SP, Satyaswaroop PG, Jordan VC. Contrasting actions of tamoxifen on endometrial and breast tumour growth in the athymic mouse. *Cancer Research*, 1988; **48**: 812–15.

69. O'Regan RM, *et al.* Effects of the antiestrogens tamoxifen, toremifine and ICI 182,780 on endometrial cancer cell growth. *Journal of the National Cancer Institute*, 1998; **90**: 1552–8.

70. Stidham KR, Johnson JL, Seigler HF. Survival superiority of females with melanoma. *Archives of Surgery*, 1994; **129**: 316–24.

71. Mackie RM, Bufalino R, Morabito A, Sutherland C, Cascinelli N. Lack of effect on pregnancy on outcome of melanoma. *The Lancet*, 1991; **337**: 653–5.

72. Singluff CL, Reintgen D. Malignant melanoma and the prognostic implications of pregnancy, oral contraceptives and exogenous hormones. *Seminars in Surgical Oncology*, 1993; **9**: 228–31.

73. Flowers JL, Seigler HF, McCarthy KS, Konrath J, McCarthy KS. Absence of oestrogen receptor in human melanoma as evaluated by a monoclonal anti-oestrogen receptor antibody. *Archives of Dermatology*, 1987; **123**: 764–5.

74. Wagstaff J, Thacher N, Rankin E, Crowther D. Tamoxifen in the treatment of metastatic malignant melanoma. *Cancer Treatment Reports*, 1982; **66**: 1771.

75. McClay EF, *et al.* Tamoxifen modulation of cisplatin sensitivity in human malignant melanoma cells. *Cancer Research*, 1993; **53**: 1571–6.

76. Cocconi G, *et al.* Treatment of metastatic melanoma with dacarbazine plus tamoxifen. *New England Journal of Medicine*, 1992; **327**: 516–23.

77. Bloom HJG, Baker WH, Dukes CE, Mitchley BCV. Hormone-dependent tumours of the kidney: I. The oestrogen-induced renal tumour of the Syrian hamster—hormone treatment and possible relationship to carcinoma of the kidney in man. *British Journal of Cancer*, 1963; **17**: 611–46.

78. Kjaer M. The role of medroxyprogesterone acetate in the treatment of renal adenocarcinoma. *Cancer Treatment Reviews*, 1988; **15**: 195–209.

79. Pizzocaro G, *et al.* Adjuvant medroxyprogesterone acetate to radical nephrectomy in renal cancer: 5 year results of a prospective randomised study. *Journal of Urology*, 1987; **138**: 1379.

80. Medical Research Council Renal Cell Cancer Collaborators. Interferon-alpha and survival in metastatic renal carcinoma; early results of a randomised controlled trial. *The Lancet*, 1999; **352**: 14–17.

Biologically based therapies

D. W. Miles and T. A. Plunkett

Introduction

Biologically based therapies are mechanistically dependent on the tumour–host interaction. They exploit our understanding of the malignant process and the host response to it. The increasing use of molecular biological techniques continues to improve our understanding of the pathophysiology of cancer, with the associated definition of potential therapeutic targets. Biologically based therapy can reasonably be divided into immunomodulation, inhibition of metastasis, the promotion of differentiation, and finally, direct antiproliferative or cytotoxic mechanisms. There is obviously considerable overlap with other treatment modalities, such as endocrine therapy for the treatment of cancer.

This chapter will outline the immunomodulatory approaches to the treatment of cancer and will also summarize the principles of gene therapy, a method to modify tumour cell behaviour, or the host response to it, by the introduction of specific genes.

Immunomodulatory therapy

The immune system has frequently been invoked as a mechanism by which 'mutant' tumour cells might be targeted and killed. The 'immune surveillance' hypothesis has many attractions and may be used as an explanation for several clinical observations. For example, it is well known that most solid tumours develop over many years; part of this period may reflect the time needed to acquire growth-promoting mutations, but may also reflect the time required to develop a population of cells lacking immunogenic determinants. Also, in diseases such as melanoma and renal cell carcinoma, spontaneous regressions have been noted. In patients with melanoma, paraneoplastic depigmentation noted at the time of spontaneous regression supports the view that a specific immune response to melanin-producing cells might be responsible (see also Chapters 1.9, 8.1, and 13.3).

However, prolonged immunosuppression, either in the context of organ transplantation or congenital/acquired immune deficiency syndromes, is associated not with the common epithelial malignancies, but rather with those which are assumed to be virally induced.[1] Therefore, it seems that immune surveillance as originally envisaged does not act as the primary defence against most common cancers. It is likely that most tumours express determinants that are at least potentially capable of immune recognition, but fail to elicit an immune response, that is, they are not immunogenic. The aim of immunomodulatory therapy is to increase the host response to tumour.

Immunomodulatory approaches to the treatment of cancer can be divided into non-specific and specific therapies. Non-specific therapy includes administration of cytokines, the signalling molecules between cells of the immune system, in an attempt to induce or augment an immune response to the tumour. Specific approaches to immunotherapy have included the use of antibodies to tumour-associated antigens and injection of allogeneic tumour cell lines (which are presumed to bear antigens shared with the host tumour) or autologous tumour cells modified to increase their immunogenicity or given with immunological adjuvants. Antigen-specific cancer vaccines may be in the form of peptides, DNA encoding tumour-associated antigens, and latterly, with the recognition of the importance of costimulatory molecules in inducing appropriate and effective T-cell responses, vaccines based on antigen-presenting cells, such as dendritic cells. The putative mechanisms underlying specific and non-specific antitumour immune effector responses are illustrated in Fig. 1.

Non-specific biologically based therapy

Non-specific immune stimulation as a potential therapy for cancer probably started in the nineteenth century when a French practitioner named Tanchou 'treated' patients with breast cancer with soiled dressings. These cases led to the use of what was termed 'laudable pus'.[2] Subsequently, Coley noted spontaneous regression of tumour in some patients with advanced sarcoma who had coincidentally developed severe infections, such as erysipelas. Following this observation, bacterial 'toxins' derived from *Streptococcus pyogenes* were tested in patients with a variety of malignancies and instances of tumour regression were reported.[3] Coley recognized the importance of a 'biologically effective dose' in that his strategy was to increase the dose of bacterial toxin until the patient became pyrexial. The tumour regressions were probably attributable to cytokines released in response to bacterial products, particularly lipopolysaccharide. Whilst the subsequent identification and cloning of genes which encode such cytokines have led to their administration in purer form, bacterial products have been licensed for use in specific cancers, for example bacille Calmete–Guérin (**BCG**) for bladder cancer, and bacterial components are an integral part of many immunological adjuvants.

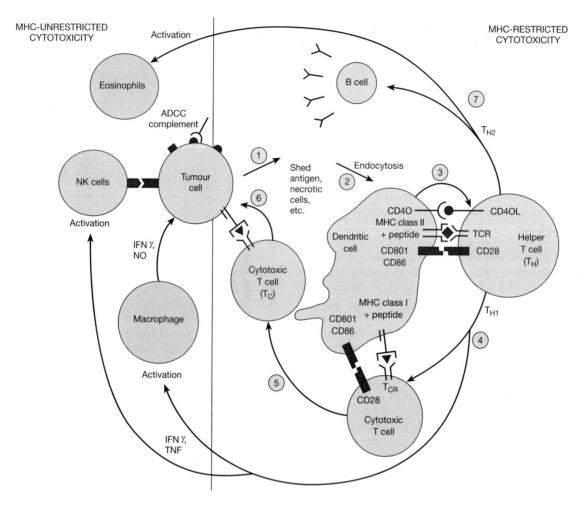

Fig. 1 The diagram demonstrates, in a simplified form, MHC-restricted and MHC-unrestricted tumour cell recognition. Tumour cells may evade many or all of these processes *in vivo*, e.g. loss of MHC expression, secretion of immunosuppressive cytokines. (1) Tumour antigens shed from tumour cells or necrotic cells are (2) endocytosed by dendritic cells. These antigens are processed by the dendritic cells and peptides are presented at the cell surface in association with MHC. In the presence of inflammatory signals, the dendritic cell is activated and migrates to the draining lymph node. The activated dendritic cell expresses large amounts of MHC class I and II, as well as the important co-stimulatory molecules CD40, CD80, and CD86. In the lymph node, the activated dendritic cells interact with antigen-specific T cells. Helper T cells (T$_H$) recognize specific peptide antigen plus MHC class II via their T cell receptor (TCR). (3) Peptide recognition, in association with binding of CD40 to CD40 ligand and CD80/CD86 to CD28, results in T$_H$ activation. T$_H$ cells can stimulate either cellular (T$_{H1}$) or humoral (T$_{H2}$) responses. (4) T$_{H1}$ helper T cells activate cytotoxic T cells (which recognize specific peptide antigen in association with MHC class 1) and also activate macrophages (MHC-unrestricted). (5) The CTL traffic to tumour sites and (6) lyse cells with the specific peptide/MHC class I complex on the cell surface. (7) T$_{H2}$ cells activate antigen-specific B cells to secrete antibody. Antibody can bind to tumour cells and activate antibody-dependent cell-mediated cytotoxicity (ADCC), complement-mediated lysis, and opsonization. These processes are MHC-unrestricted. T$_{H2}$ cells also activate eosinophils. Natural killer (NK) cells lyse tumour cells that do not express MHC at the cell surface.

BCG

Recent studies have demonstrated that intravesical installation of BCG for superficial bladder cancer is associated with objective reduction in tumour burden and prolongation of disease-free survival[4] (and see Chapter 13.2). The mechanism of action of BCG is unknown, but presumed to be related to non-specific inflammatory responses. Correlations have been made between tumour regression and induction of a variety of cytokines.

Polynucleotides

The induction of interferons after viral infection is correlated with the presence of double-stranded RNA. Following this observation, double-stranded polynucleotides were synthesized and tested. Polyadenylic-polyuridilic acid has been shown to have immunomodulatory properties *in vitro* and antitumour activity in preclinical models. In a randomized trial of 300 patients with early breast cancer, polyadenylic-polyuridilic acid significantly improved the overall survival of patients, with an 8-year survival of 71 per cent in the group given adjuvant treatment and 57 per cent in controls ($P < 0.05$).[5] With the advent of recombinant cytokines, interest in polynucleotides has waned and this work has not been repeated.

Cytokine therapy

Many of the signalling molecules which mediate the interactions between cells of the immune system have been identified, and the genes which encode them have been cloned and sequenced. These molecules are referred to collectively as cytokines. Cytokines are proteins of low molecular weight (< 80 kDa) which act via autocrine or paracrine pathways to regulate cell behaviour. They bind to high-affinity cell surface receptors specific for each cytokine, or each cytokine subgroup. Cytokines have overlapping and pleiotropic regulatory activities and interact as part of a network with other cytokines and growth factors. Perhaps the most widely used cytokines currently in cancer therapy are the colony-stimulating factors, such as granulocyte colony-stimulating factor (**G-CSF**) and granulocyte–macrophage colony-stimulating factor (**GM-CSF**). These agents are used to stimulate haematopoiesis following chemotherapy or radiotherapy (see Chapter 15.1).

The main immunoregulatory consequences of cytokines, excluding colony-stimulating factors, are summarized in Table 1. The observations that they are direct regulators of cell growth and differentiation and that some of them are toxic to tumours, either directly or by stimulating the host immune response, have led to their use in cancer therapy.

Clinical assessment of cytokine therapy is more complex than for conventional cytotoxic agents because, as with other biological therapies, a simple dose–response relationship may not always occur. Also, unlike conventional therapy, use of cytokines may promote differentiation and lead to tumour stasis rather than measurable reduction in tumour burden, rendering assessment of efficacy by standard criteria difficult. In addition, owing to the complex interaction of cytokines, particularly at the local level, administration of one agent may influence production of cytokines elsewhere which may themselves also mediate antitumour effects.

The interferons

Interferons have stimulatory effects on macrophages, natural killer (**NK**) cells, T lymphocytes, and neutrophils (Fig. 2). They upregulate the expression of major histocompatibility complex (**MHC**) class I and II on several cell types required for antigen presentation. Interferons also have direct growth inhibitory effects on certain tumour cell lines and may induce differentiation through regulation of oncogene expression.

Hairy cell leukaemia was perhaps the archetypal example of the role of cytokine therapy in the treatment of malignancy. Responses to interferons were first noted in the mid-1980s[6] and subsequent studies demonstrated that about 75 per cent of patients treated with interferon-α experienced clinical responses lasting 12 to 24 months. Further studies demonstrated that only 5 to 10 per cent of patients achieved a complete remission and newer agents such as the adenosine deaminase inhibitor, pentostatin, have been demonstrated to prolong relapse-free survival compared with interferon-α.[7]

Objective responses to interferon-α have been noted in previously untreated patients with mulitple myeloma and in those who have relapsed following chemotherapy. Although studies have generally failed to show any benefit from the addition of interferon-α to chemotherapeutic regimens for remission induction, there is some evidence from randomized studies of the benefit from maintenance interferon-α following remission induction[8] (see also Chapter 15.3).

In non-Hodgkin's lymphoma, single-agent activity with interferon-α was demonstrated in the 1970s. Studies of maintenance treatment following response to chemotherapy have been associated with prolonged time to progression, but its influence on survival remains uncertain (see also Chapter 15.1). In chronic myeloid leukaemia, interferon-α has a direct antiproliferative effect on the leukaemic clone and has been shown to reduce the number of Philadelphia chromosome-positive cells in more than half of treated patients, with a minority converting to cytogenetically normal marrow.[9] In a randomized comparison of interferon-α and chemotherapy with hydroxyurea or busulphan, time to disease progression and overall survival were better in the group treated with interferon-α,[10] although at the expense of considerable toxicity (see also Chapter 15.5).

There are considerable data on the use of interferon-α in the treatment of AIDS-associated Kaposi's sarcoma.[11] Mean objective response rates of approximately 30 per cent have been reported although the duration of response was short, at approximately 6 months (and see Chapter 15.15).

Studies of interferon-α have also been performed in patients with malignant melanoma. Early reports showed evidence of activity for interferon-α in the treatment of metastatic disease.[12] However, the overall response rates were no better than those for most active single-agent chemotherapy drugs. Some studies have suggested a benefit for combination therapy using standard chemotherapy and cytokines in the treatment of metastatic disease, but a lack of well-designed, prospective randomized trials precludes definite recommendations.

The North Central Cancer Treatment Group investigated high doses of interferon-α given intramuscularly for 3 months in patients with intermediate-risk or high-risk, node-positive resected melanoma.[13] This study showed a benefit in relapse-free interval in node-positive patients, but the trial results were not significant overall, perhaps because only 160 of 262 patients were node positive and at high risk of relapse.

Recent evidence suggests a possible benefit for high-dose interferon-α as an adjuvant therapy in patients with resected high-risk malignant melanoma. In a randomized controlled trial, compared with observation alone, adjuvant therapy with interferon-α significantly increased 5-year disease-free survival (26 compared with 37 per cent) and median overall survival (2.8 compared with 3.8 years).[14] The toxicity from the high-dose interferon-α was considerable. More than two-thirds of patients required a dose reduction or delay and two patients died from liver failure. Notably, when the original study data were reanalysed taking into account toxicity, overall survival adjusted for quality of life was no longer statistically significant using a two-tailed t-test.[15] The results of a confirmatory study of high-dose interferon-α are awaited with interest; preliminary results suggest that there is a benefit in relapse-free but not overall survival. The apparent discrepancy between the two trials could result from the fact that many patients in the observation arm of the later trial were treated with high-dose interferon-α at relapse.

Studies of lower doses of interferon-α in patients with intermediate-risk melanoma demonstrated a prolongation of relapse-free survival, but this effect was gradually lost following discontinuation

Table 1 The main immunoregulatory consequences of cytokines

Cytokine	Molecular mass (kDa)	Effects
Interferons		
Type 1: interferon-α	17–23	Antiviral; cytostatic; immunoregulatory ($\uparrow$ MHC class I, $\uparrow$ NK activity)
Type 1: interferon-β	20	
Type 2: interferon-γ	20	Immunoregulatory ($\uparrow$ MHC class I and II, $\uparrow$ T-cell proliferation, $\uparrow$ NK activity, activates macrophages, $\uparrow$ B-cell differentiation); antiviral; growth inhibitory for tumour and endothelial cells; inhibitory to CD4 T_{H2} cells
TNF	17	Cytotoxic for tumour/endothelial cells; $\uparrow$ cytotoxicity of LAK, TIL, and macrophages; $\uparrow$ growth and differentiation; $\uparrow$ MHC class I; $\uparrow$ osteoclastic resorption of bone
IL-1	17	Macrophage activation; $\uparrow$ T- and B-cell growth, differentiation, chemotaxis, and LAK induction (with IL-2); $\uparrow$ NK activity (with interferon); $\uparrow$ acute-phase proteins; $\uparrow$ IL-6; $\uparrow$ TNF; $\uparrow$ proliferation and differentiation of stem cells; $\uparrow$ osteoclastic resorption of bone
IL-2	15.5	$\uparrow$ T- and B-cell proliferation and differentiation; $\uparrow$ NK, LAK, TIL, and T_C activity; macrophage activation
IL-3	28	Growth factor for multipotential progenitor cells, megakaryocytes, erythrocyte precursors, NK cells, and T cells (with IL-2)
IL-4	20	$\uparrow$ Proliferation and immunoglobulin secretion of B lymphocytes; $\uparrow$ differentiation of T_{H2} cells; $\uparrow$ activation of LAK cells and dendritic cells; $\uparrow$ class II MHC
IL-5	12–18	$\uparrow$ Growth and differentiation of eosinophils; $\uparrow$ growth and Ig secretion of B cells; differentiation of T cells (with IL-2); activation of LAK and NK cells (with IL-2)
IL-6	25	$\uparrow$ Differentiation and Ig secretion of B cells; $\uparrow$ differentiation and activation of T cells (with IL-2); $\uparrow$ acute-phase proteins
IL-7	25	$\uparrow$ Growth and differentiation of precursor T and B cells; growth and activation of monocytes and macrophages; activation of NK, LAK, and TIL; $\uparrow$ growth and antigen presentation of dendritic cells
IL-8	8	Chemotactic for T cells, neutrophils, mast cells, endothelial cells, eosinophils, and NK cells
IL-9	32–39	Costimulatory factor for platelets (with IL-3 and GM-CSF), erythoid precursors (with erythropoietin), and T cells (with IL-2)
IL-10	17	$\downarrow$ Cellular immunity (decreased Ag presentation, $\downarrow$ macrophage activation, $\downarrow$ IL-12 production and T-cell stimulation); $\uparrow$ humoral immunity ($\uparrow$ growth and differentiation of B cells)
IL-11	22	$\uparrow$ Growth of haemopoietic progenitors; $\uparrow$ Ig production by B cells; $\uparrow$ cytokine production by T cells
IL-12	70	$\uparrow$ Growth and cytotoxicity of NK cells; $\uparrow$ LAK activity; $\uparrow$ growth and cytotoxicity of CD8 T cells; $\uparrow$ growth of CD4 T_{H1} cells; $\downarrow$ growth of CD4 T_{H2} cells.
IL-13	14	$\downarrow$ Macrophage function; $\downarrow$ T-cell chemotaxis; $\uparrow$ neutrophil production of anti-inflammatory factor
IL-14	53–65	$\uparrow$ Growth and differentiation of B cells
IL-15	14–15	Proliferation and Ig secretion by B cells; $\uparrow$ NK and LAK activity

GM-CSF, granulocyte–macrophage colony-stimulating factor; LAK, lymphokine-activated killer cell; NK, natural killer cell; T_C, cytotoxic T lymphocyte; TIL, tumour-infiltrating lymphocyte; TNF, tumour necrosis factor.

of therapy and there was no benefit in overall survival.[16],[17] Further studies are required to determine the most effective schedule.

In patients with renal cancer, prolonged stabilization of advanced disease and rare spontaneous regressions in the absence of systemic treatment suggest that host immune responses are important in regulating tumour growth and have led to the study of immunotherapy for this malignancy. The overall proportion of responses to interferon-α in over 1000 patients with metastatic renal cancer was 12 per cent,[18] although in patients whose predominant site of metastatic disease was pulmonary, the response rate has been reported to be as high as 30 per cent.[19]

A recent study compared interferon-α with medroxyprogesterone acetate in 335 patients with metastatic renal cell cancer.[20] The results demonstrated a 28 per cent reduction in the risk of death, a 12 per cent improvement in 1-year survival, and a 2.5 month improvement in median survival for patients treated with interferon-α. However, there was considerable early toxicity from interferon-α treatment which, although less apparent by the end of treatment, should be set against the survival benefits. The use of interferon-α in the management of early renal cell cancer, and in combination with other agents such as interleukin 2 (IL-2) and 5-fluorouracil, require further investigation. A study of patients with progressive metastatic disease

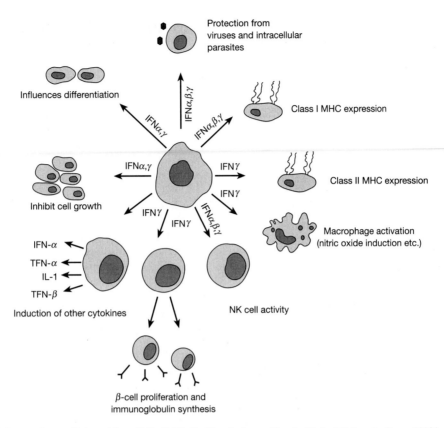

Fig. 2 Regulatory roles of the interferons. (Adapted from Balkwill FR. *Cytokines in Cancer Therapy.* Oxford University Press, 1989.)

suggested a benefit for combination therapy with IL-2 and interferon-α.[21] However, the benefits were achieved at the cost of substantial toxicity (see also Chapter 13.3). A placebo-controlled trial of interferon-γ revealed no benefit in patients with metastatic renal cell cancer.[22]

Tumour necrosis factor (TNF)

Tumour necrosis factor-α was named originally for its ability to induce haemorrhagic necrosis in tumours and is produced by cells of the monocyte and macrophage lineage. It has 30 per cent amino acid sequence homology with lymphotoxin (**TNF-β**), which is produced by activated T lymphocytes. TNF-α has many effects, including induction of secretion of other cytokines, collagenases, and plasminogen activators. TNF-α also inhibits the growth of some tumour cell lines and mediates cytotoxicity in combination with interferon-γ. In animal models, TNF-α mediates much of its antitumour effect through effects on the vascular endothelium and procoagulation. TNF-α has immunomodulatory properties through increased antigen expression, and augmentation of lymphokine-activated killer (**LAK**) cell and NK cell activity (Fig. 1). TNF-α also has properties that are deleterious to the host, including osteoclastic resorption of bone and cachexia.

The clinical use of TNF-α, and other cytokines which induce its release, such as IL-2, has been limited by hypotension through induction of reactive nitrogen species, for example nitric oxide, as well as by its effects on endothelium leading to a 'capillary leak syndrome'. Attempts to abrogate the systemic effects of TNF-α have included regional perfusion[23] (and see also Chapter 4.23) and the induction of local TNF-α expression through targeted gene therapy. Recent work has suggested a role for TNF in tumour development, and is the subject of further investigation.[24]

Interleukin 1 (IL-1)

IL-1 stimulates haematopoiesis causing the proliferation and differentiation of early stem cells. It also has stimulatory effects on T and B lymphocytes. As with TNF-α, it has effects on adhesion molecules and vascular endothelium. IL-1 has little antitumour activity in clinical studies. It reduces the activity of cytochrome p450 and so may delay the metabolism of some cytotoxic agents.

Interleukin 2 (IL-2)

IL-2 has no direct effect on tumour growth but is a critical cytokine in the activation of cellular and humoral immune responses. As well as stimulating the proliferation and activation of T lymphocytes, it activates and increases the cytotoxic potential of NK cells and LAK cells. IL-2 stimulates secretion of other cytokines, such as TNF-α and interferon-γ.

Early studies used bolus intravenous doses of IL-2. Objective responses were seen in about 15 per cent of patients with melanoma or renal cell cancer[25] (and see Chapters 8.1 and 13.3). Dose-limiting toxicities included fever, hypotension, dyspnoea, and peripheral oedema. In a multicentre study, 255 patients with metastatic renal cell cancer were treated with high-dose IL-2: 14 per cent of patients had complete or partial responses lasting for a median of 23 months.[26]

In order to limit systemic exposure to IL-2, attempts have been made to culture lymphocytes with the cytokine *ex vivo*. The adoptive transfer of IL-2-stimulated lymphocytes derived from peripheral blood (LAK cells) and from tumour-infiltrating lymphocytes (TILs) has been shown to be feasible. While LAK cells have a broad range of cytotoxicity, they are also capable of lysing normal endothelial cells, contributing to the toxicity of this approach. Expansion of TILs may augment a pre-existing immune response, but is practically more difficult. Several studies have attempted to define the additional benefit of LAK cell[27] or TIL[28] infusions with IL-2, but there have been no consistent survival benefits. Subsequently, lower doses of IL-2, which maintain immunomodulatory effects, but with less toxicity, have been tested and shown to produce comparable response rates, although their duration is not yet known.[29]

Combinations of IL-2 with other cytokines, and with chemotherapeutic agents, continue to be the subject of phase II studies, but few data are available from randomized studies to examine the attributable benefit of IL-2.

Interleukin 3 (IL-3)

IL-3 is a haemopoietic growth factor which acts on pluripotent progenitor cells and has been tested in combination with other growth factors to accelerate recovery of neutrophils and platelets following cytotoxic chemotherapy (see also Chapter 15.1). Phase II studies have suggested that IL-3 may reduce myelosuppression following chemotherapy, although recent data from randomized studies suggest that single-agent IL-3 does not reduce thrombocytopenia.[30]

Interleukin 4 (IL-4)

IL-4 is generally associated with augmentation of humoral responses, and acts by stimulating B-cell proliferation and immunoglobulin secretion as well as by increasing the growth and differentiation of CD4 + T-helper cells which contribute to the humoral response (TH2). IL-4 is also important in antigen presentation, because it stimulates antigen-presenting cell growth and capacity to present antigen. IL-4 also directly inhibits the growth of some tumour cell lines. Phase I and phase II studies in advanced malignancy have, however, been disappointing[31] and as with other cytokines, its effects may be better exploited through local expression by genetically engineered tumour cells used as cancer vaccines (see below: gene therapy).

Other interleukins

Interleukins 6 (IL-6) and 11 (IL-11) are being examined for their potential as haemopoietic growth factors. It is noteworthy that IL-6 has been cited as a growth factor for renal cancer and myeloma *in vitro*, raising the possibility of anticytokine therapy as a potential antitumour therapeutic modality. Phase II data[32] suggest that IL-11 in combination with G-CSF may accelerate haematological recovery following chemotherapy. Interleukin 12 (IL-12) has widespread effects to augment the immune response; it stimulates NK cells, induces LAK cells, and increases the cellular arm of the immune response through stimulating growth of T_{H1} CD4 + T cells and CD8 + T cells. Preclinical data suggest a central role for IL-12 in the cellular immune response; phase II studies using a subcutaneous regimen have suggested some activity in patients with metastatic melanoma.[33]

Tumour-specific therapy

The objective of tumour-specific immunotherapy is to produce tumour-specific immunity by combining tumour-associated antigens with a non-specific immune adjuvant. Antigen-specific cellular immune responses depend upon interaction between T cells and antigen-presenting cells. T cells can be broadly divided into two classes: helper T cells (T_H; usually CD4 +) which secrete cytokines to expand antigen-specific T- (T_{H1}) and B-cell (T_{H2}) responses, and cytotoxic T cells (TC; usually CD8 +) which destroy the target cell (Fig. 1 see also Chapter 1.9).

T cells do not recognize antigen directly. Instead, each T cell recognizes a specific short peptide sequence (epitope) bound to MHC class I (for CD8 + T cells) or MHC class II (for CD4 + T cells) on the surface of antigen-presenting cells (Fig. 3(a and b)). Dissection of the cellular interactions involved in T_C-cell priming revealed that helper cells must recognize antigen on the same antigen-presenting cell that cross-presents antigen to the T_C cells (Fig. 1).

It was recently demonstrated that T-cell help for T_C-cell priming necessitates interaction between CD40L (CD156) on the T_H cell and CD40 on the antigen-presenting cell.[34]–[36] The interaction most likely 'empowers' the antigen-presenting cells to prime the antigen-specific T_C cells. CD40-induced activation of the antigen-presenting cells also upregulates expression of CD80 (B7.1) and CD86 (B7.2). These so-called costimulatory molecules are vital for effective T-cell activation. Costimulation via CD80 and CD86, in the presence of a suboptimal T-cell receptor signal, results in increased transcription and translation of multiple cytokines as well as clonal expansion of T cells and enhancement of their effector function.

In the absence of costimulatory signals, antigen presented by antigen-presenting cells to T cells may lead to immune tolerance rather than activation. This scenario may occur in many tumours, since they are rarely accompanied by an inflammatory infiltrate. The ability of tumour cells to induce antigen-specific T-cell tolerance has been demonstrated.[37] Such findings emphasize that the development of effective specific immunotherapies depends not only on the identification of tumour-associated antigens, but also on an understanding of how the immune system is subverted by malignancy. Several other mechanisms have been implicated in the avoidance of the immune response by tumour cells, including failure to express appropriate antigens (so-called antigen-loss tumour variants),[38] loss of expression of the MHC molecules required for antigen presentation,[39] and failure of antigen processing machinery,[40] as well as local production of inhibitory molecules such as transforming growth factor-β (TGF-β) and Fas ligand,[41] which may lead to apoptosis of infiltrating T cells (see also Chapter 1.9).

Sources of tumour-associated antigens for clinical study have included autologous tumour, or allogeneic tumour cell lines which are known or assumed to bear relevant antigens. An alternative is to employ defined tumour-associated antigens which by virtue of their preferential or exclusive expression in tumour tissue may represent appropriate targets for immunotherapy (Table 2). These include viral antigens, mutated proteins, and oncogene products (see also Chapter 1.9).

Tumour cell-based immunogens

Autologous tumour cell vaccines have the potential advantage that, by definition, they are MHC-matched with the recipient. However,

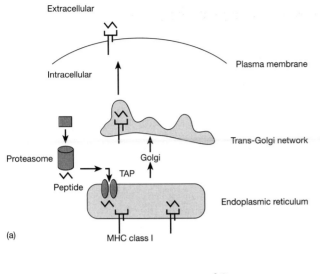

(a)

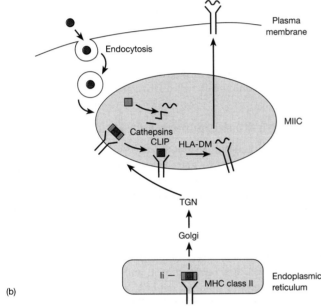

(b)

Fig. 3 (a) MHC class I antigen processing and presentation. The proteasome generates peptides from cytosolic proteins. These are translocated into the endoplasmic reticulum via the transporter-associated with antigen processing (TAP) molecules. Some peptides bind MHC class I with high affinity; the MHC class I–peptide complex is transported through the Golgi to the trans-Golgi network (TGN) for export to the cell surface. (b) MHC class II antigen processing and presentation. MHC class II molecules are synthesized in the endoplasmic reticulum with invariant chain (Ii) The Ii ensures correct MHC class II folding, prevents peptide binding prematurely, and targets the complex to the MHC class II compartment (M II C), part of the endocytic pathway where MHC class II loading occurs. In the MHC, the Ii is degraded until only the class I invariant peptide (CLIP) remains bound to the peptide binding site of MHC class II. HLA DM catalyses the removal of CLIP and its replacement by peptide. Peptide-loaded MHC class II is then transported to the cell surface.

they require the patient to have surgically accessible disease that will yield sufficient cells to prepare vaccine (50 to 100 × 10⁶ cells, generally requiring a sample of about 2.5 cm in diameter). A recent trial of autologous tumour cell vaccination was reported in patients with colon cancer.[42] In this trial, 254 patients were randomized to receive vaccination or no further treatment. The vaccine consisted of intra-dermal injection with irradiated autologous tumour cells using BCG as the adjuvant. At a median follow-up of 5 years there were no significant benefits in terms of disease-free or overall survival, although in a subgroup analysis of patients with node-positive disease, there was a significant increase in recurrence-free survival. Although further studies are required, preparation of the tumour cells is technically difficult.

A simpler approach is the use of multiple allogeneic tumour cell lines which express many potential tumour-associated antigens and a broad range of MHC expression. Allogeneic vaccines are also more immunogenic, possibly due to the induction of a strong T_H cell immune response against foreign MHC antigens. A combination of three allogeneic melanoma cell lines, chosen for their expression of immunogenic antigens and which provide an MHC haplotype match with 95 per cent of patients with melanoma, has been used in a phase II study of patients with advanced melanoma.[43] Immune responsiveness appeared to correlate with clinical response and the 5-year survival rate of 26 per cent compared favourably with historical controls (5-year survival of 6 per cent). A randomized study examining this approach is in progress. Other groups have compared allogeneic cell lysates given with an adjuvant to combination chemotherapy in patients with advanced melanoma. Survival was comparable in the two treatment arms, although more toxicity was noted with chemo-therapy.[44] Results are awaited from trials comparing such vaccines with no further treatment or interferon-α in patients with resected melanoma at high risk of relapse.

Other studies using different vaccines have been reported. A polyvalent shed antigen vaccine has been prepared from melanoma cell lines.[45] Use of the vaccine conferred a survival benefit compared with historical controls. Preliminary results from a phase III study demonstrated that mortality at 2 years in the vaccine-treated group was half that of the placebo-treated group.[46] The trial was interrupted early because of slow patient accrual and the data are based on a total of only 38 patients. Further trials of this vaccine are awaited.

Expression of xenogeneic proteins by cellular vaccines leads to expression of 'helper' epitopes that augment the T-cell response. This process, termed antigen supplementation, is often achieved using virus, usually vaccinia virus. While there is some evidence of activity in phase II studies of patients with metastatic melanoma,[47] no impact on survival was noted in the adjuvant setting.[48]

Transfer of genes encoding cytokines into tumour cells has been employed to activate or bypass T_H cell function. In animal studies, such cellular vaccines have eradicated established tumours,[49] and are now being employed in humans (see below: gene therapy).

Dendritic cell vaccines

Recent work in immunotherapy has focused on the role of the antigen-presenting cells and, in particular, dendritic cells. Studies in humans have shown that autologous dendritic cells exposed to, or pulsed with, antigen *in vitro* and then reinfused can induce immune responses that lead to inhibition of tumour growth *in vivo*.[50] A previous limitation to these studies had been the generation of sufficient dendritic cells, but it is now possible to generate dendritic cells from peripheral blood *ex vivo* by using GM-CSF and IL-4.[51],[52]

Table 2 Potential specific immunogens

Cell based	Autologous tumour cells ± adjuvant
	Allogeneic cell lines ± adjuvant
	Viral oncolysates
	Genetically modified autologous tumour cells or allogeneic tumour cell lines
	Dendritic cell based vaccines:
	Fused with tumour cell lines
	Pulsed with defined antigens/tumour cell lysates
	Transfected with tumour antigens
Defined antigens	Peptide, e.g. MAGE, gp100
	Carbohydrate, e.g. gangliosides (GM2), sialyl-Tn
	DNA vaccines
	Viral vaccines
Antibodies	Mouse monoclonal, e.g. anti-17–1A
	Chimeric monoclonal, e.g. anti-CD20 (rhituximab)
	Humanized monoclonal, e.g. anti-erbB-2 (trastuzumab)

More recent data have shown this to be a feasible approach in melanoma, where injection of peptide- or tumour lysate-pulsed dendritic cells led to regression of tumour in one-third of cases.[53] Other workers have fused tumour cells with dendritic cells, or transfected dendritic cells with tumour-associated antigens, in an effort to increase the effectiveness of antigen presentation (see below: gene therapy). Recent clinical trials using renal cancer/dendritic cell fusions produced impressive results.[54]

Peptide vaccines

The genes encoding many tumour-associated antigens have been cloned. The elucidation of the structure of class I and II MHC molecules has made it possible to identify putative MHC-binding regions from the DNA sequences of known tumour-associated antigens. As a result, peptide sequences likely to bind to MHC can be identified in tumour associated antigens. These peptides, given with an appropriate adjuvant, may be used as a basis for tumour vaccine development.

Phase I clinical studies of peptide vaccines have been reported in patients with melanoma. These have included, for example, an HLA A1-restricted MAGE3 peptide,[55] a combination of three melanoma-associated HLA A2-restricted peptides,[56] and an HLA A2-restricted gp100 peptide analogue, modified to increase the binding affinity to HLA A2.[57] In all the studies, toxicity was minimal, and immunological and clinical responses were detected.

Recently, the modified gp100 peptide was used either alone or followed by high-dose IL-2.[58] The modified peptide induced T-cell responses in 91 per cent of patients. The administration of high-dose IL-2 reduced the frequency of T-cell responses to 16 per cent, yet in these patients a clinical response rate of 42 per cent was observed, with no responses seen in the patients receiving modified peptide alone. As an IL-2 treatment alone arm was not included, it is not clear whether the modified peptide contributed to the responses seen. However, the results demonstrate the difficulty of equating immunological responses with clinical responses.

Single-peptide vaccines are by definition restricted to use in patients with the appropriate MHC haplotype. Also, at least in animal models, altering the dose, schedule, or route of administration can result in tolerance rather than immunity.[59] Alternatives to the use of peptide include viral vectors engineered to express tumour-associated antigens, or injection with naked DNA (see below: gene therapy).

Carbohydrate antigen-based vaccines

Carbohydrate antigens aberrantly expressed or overexpressed on tumour cells are further targets for immunotherapy. Gangliosides, such as GM2, have been used as immunogens in patients with cancer.[51] Randomized trials are currently underway comparing high-dose interferon-α to immunization with a GM2 conjugate in patients with high-risk melanoma.

Expression of the disaccharide sialyl-Tn (**STn**) is associated with a poor prognosis in a variety of malignancies.[60] In phase II studies of STn coupled to a carrier protein and given with adjuvant, the ability to generate a humoral response to STn but not the carrier appeared to correlate with survival.[61] A prospective randomized study with this immunogen is currently in progress.

Antibody therapy

Monoclonal antibodies against tumour-associated antigens are being tested in a variety of forms in different clinical settings. Initial studies were hampered by the development of human antibody against the constant regions of xenogeneic monoclonal antibodies. Human and humanized monoclonal antibodies are now available, and these as well as murine antibodies have been used (see also Chapter 4.27).

Antibodies to tumour-associated antigens can activate immune effector functions by complement fixation, opsonization, or antibody-dependent cell-mediated cytotoxicity (ADCC) in which 'killer cell' and tumour cell are conjugated by antibody (Fig. 1). Antibodies may also act as specific immunogens which elicit a response against tumour-associated antigens, as in Fig. 4.

As well as mediating immunological effects, antibodies may also bind to growth factor receptors and thereby inhibit the effects of growth factors on cells. They may be conjugated with radioisotopes, anticancer drugs, and toxins to target these agents to cancer cells (see

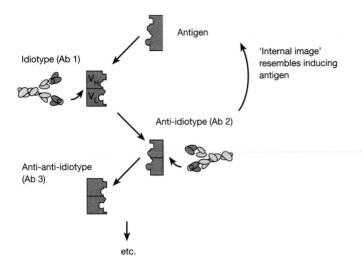

Fig. 4 Anti-idiotype responses. Antibodies may also act as specific immunogens which elicit a response against tumour-associated antigens. A monoclonal antibody specific for a known tumour-associated antigen (Ab1) may induce a host immune response with generation of antibodies to Ab1, including so-called anti-idiotype antibodies against its variable region (termed Ab2). The anti-idiotype antibody (Ab2), if properly selected, would have a three-dimensional conformation similar to the tumour-associated antigens and may therefore act as an immunogen inducing antibodies (Ab3) that bind to the original antigen.

Chapter 4.27). There is evidence for the effectiveness of antibody therapy in several tumour types.

In a randomized trial, 189 patients with colorectal cancer who had undergone curative resection for Dukes C cancer received either the 17–1A murine antibody which recognizes a 34-kDa glycoprotein on the cell membrane of epithelial cells or were assigned to an observation arm.[62] At a median follow-up of 5 years the mortality and recurrence rates were reduced by 30 and 27 per cent, respectively, in the treatment group compared with controls. These benefits were maintained at 7 years of follow-up.[63] The effects were greatest in reducing distant rather than local recurrence, suggesting that the antibody therapy inhibited growth of distant occult metastases. The overall survival benefit was comparable with that of adjuvant leucovorin-primed 5-fluorouracil, but was associated with minimal toxicity. The two treatments alone or in combination are now being tested in randomized trials.

Encouraging results have also been demonstrated with antibody-based therapy in leukaemias and lymphomas.[64] An unconjugated chimeric monoclonal antibody to CD20 was recently licensed for use in relapsed low-grade or follicular non-Hodgkin's B-cell lymphoma.[65]

In patients with metastatic breast cancer whose tumours over-expressed the oncogene *HER2*, and who had received extensive prior anticancer therapy, treatment with HER2-specific antibody (trastuzumab) produced response rates comparable with third- or fourth-line chemotherapy, but with minimal toxicity.[66] In a multicentre, controlled trial, 469 women with HER2-positive metastatic breast cancer were randomized to receive chemotherapy with or without trastuzumab. At a median follow-up of 25 months there was a significant survival benefit for women receiving concurrent trastuzumab (25.4 months compared with 20.9 months).[67] Since

there was considerable crossover to trastuzumab treatment from the control arm of the study, the benefits may have been underestimated. Further study is required, but the results to date are encouraging.

The interaction between CD40 and CD40L is essential for effective T_C-cell priming. There is evidence that this interaction can be mimicked by the use of anti-CD40 antibody. As stated earlier, peptide vaccines can sometimes induce tolerance rather than an effective immune response. In recent studies, the use of antibody to CD40 converted a tolerizing peptide vaccine into a strong T_C-cell priming vaccine, with antitumour efficacy.[68] Antibody to CD40 was also able to overcome tumour-specific T-cell tolerance in tumour-bearing animals.[69] These promising results need further investigation, but as our understanding of the immune response grows so too may opportunities to employ antibodies that mimic or inhibit molecular interactions.

Principles of gene therapy

Gene therapy is the incorporation of specific nucleotide sequences into cells with the aim of correcting genetic defects which contribute to malignancy or with the aim of modifying the host–tumour interaction. Gene therapy is being investigated intensively outside the field of oncology, particularly for single-gene disorders such as cystic fibrosis and Fanconi's anaemia. The correction of germline genetic defects, including mutations in cancer susceptibility genes, has been demonstrated in animal models, but the transfer of such technology to humans will be limited by practical and ethical considerations, as well as the absence of data on its long-term effects. The transfer of genes into somatic cells in humans is more feasible.

Gene transfer

The main impediment to progress in gene therapy is the delivery of genes to the cell of interest. Vectors are the vehicles which deliver the gene of interest (transgene) to the target cell. The ideal vector would be mass produced in a concentrated form, be able to accommodate any gene or genes of interest, be non-toxic, non-immunogenic, and target the cell of interest. No currently available vectors fulfil all these criteria, but the different properties of available vectors may lend themselves to particular applications (Table 3). Gene therapy strategies can be divided according to the site of gene transfer. Many clinical trials have utilized *ex vivo* transfer in which the target cells are removed, transfected with the gene of interest, and subsequently returned to the patient. *In vivo* gene transfer, usually by direct injection of vectors into tumour or normal tissue, is an easier but less efficient approach.

Viral vectors

Viruses have been used as gene vectors because of their ability to infect cells and to exploit their replicative machinery. Vectors currently available differ in their properties with respect to persistence of gene expression, immunogenicity, and possible toxicities.

Retroviral vectors are produced by replacing essential viral replication genes (*gag, pol*, and *env*) with the gene of interest. The retroviral vector sequence is introduced into 'packaging' cell lines, which themselves provide the genes for viral replication. This allows the production of viral particles which can transfer the gene of interest

Table 3 Vectors for gene therapy

Vector	Advantages	Disadvantages
Viral		
Retrovirus	Integration into host genome Prolonged expression High level of gene expression	Infects only dividing cells Unstable *in vivo* Random integration into genome Risk of insertional mutagenesis Limited transgene size
Adenovirus	Infect non-dividing cells Efficient *in vivo* Not integrated into host genome	Transient expression Immunogenic Limited transgene size
Adeno-associated	Infect non-dividing cells Prolonged gene expression Integrate into chromosome 19 Reduced immunogenicity	Limited transgene size
Poxvirus (vaccinia)	Accommodates large transgene Experience with parent virus	Transient expression Replication competent Immunogenic
Herpes simplex	Efficient *in vivo* Accommodates large transgene Neurotropic Vector itself is cytotoxic	
Non-viral		
Liposomes	Repeated administration is safe and feasible	Inefficient delivery Transient expression
Naked DNA	Ease of preparation Repeated administration is safe and feasible	Transient expression

uncontaminated by replication-competent virus. Retroviral vectors are incorporated into the genome of the host cell only during cell division and the integration into the genome at random leads to the risk of mutagenesis. Incorporation is, however, stable and leads to high-level gene expression. High-titre retroviral preparations are available and since much of the viral genome is removed, such vectors are less liable to inactivation by the host immune system. However, retroviruses are relatively unstable *in vivo* and clinical experience with them has largely been restricted to *ex vivo* modification of target cells.

Adenoviral vectors are able to infect non-dividing cells and are produced by replacing the essential viral gene, *E1*, with the gene of interest. High titres of adenoviral vectors can be produced by packaging cell lines enabling highly efficient transfer and integration into the target cell. Adenoviruses do not integrate into the host genome so the construct exists as an episome. Consequently, expression of the transgene is transient. In addition, adenoviral constructs still encode viral proteins and can therefore be targeted by the host immune system.

Adeno-associated viruses are also able to infect non-replicating cells. They integrate selectively into chromosome 19, thereby reducing the risk of insertional mutagenesis. Prolonged gene expression has been achieved and since few viral genes are retained in the construct, immunogenicity is reduced.

The size of transgene which retroviral and adenoviral vectors can accommodate is limited, being typically less that 10 kb. Vaccinia virus can accommodate larger genes but is replication competent. The safety profile of vaccinia is, however, well defined following its global use in vaccination against smallpox. A limitation of vaccinia is that it induces a potent inflammatory response which may lead to inactivation of the construct following repeated administration. Related viruses, including fowlpox and canarypox, are unable to replicate in mammalian cells and may therefore have a better safety profile in immunocompromised patients.

Other viruses are being studied for their ability to act as vectors. The herpes simplex virus is highly efficient *in vivo* and can carry large transgenes. The neurotropism of herpes simplex may make it effective for use in the central nervous system. Lentiviruses are retroviruses which are capable of infecting both dividing and non-dividing cells, but technical problems have so far prevented their clinical development.

Liposomal vectors

Concerns about the production of adequate titres of virus and, in particular, safety issues have led to the development of non-viral vectors. DNA sequences can be incorporated into liposomes. Repeated administration is safe and the liposome itself is non-immunogenic.

Direct injection of DNA

The simplest method of gene transfer is the direct injection of plasmid DNA encoding the sequences of interest (naked DNA). This method is effective at inducing cellular and humoral immune responses due to efficient processing of DNA by antigen-presenting cells. A modification of this approach is the use of DNA-coated gold particles which are used in a high-velocity 'gene gun' to deliver complexes transcutaneously to dendritic cells in underlying tissues. DNA sequences have also been linked to proteins or cationic molecules in order to facilitate endocytosis into cells. The use of DNA coupled to specific ligands may allow gene transfer to defined, receptor-bearing cell populations.

In general, although non-viral vector systems are safer, gene delivery is relatively inefficient and because the DNA sequences of interest are not incorporated into the host genome, expression is necessarily transient.

Targeting transgene delivery

In many studies of gene therapy, delivery of high titres of vector to the target cell has been achieved either by infecting cells *ex vivo* or by direct injection into sites of tumour. Such approaches limit the potential applications of gene therapy. Considerable effort is being directed at methods of expressing systemically administered vectors selectively in target cells. Such methods have included the use of mutated viruses which replicate only under certain conditions (conditionally replication-competent vectors), delivery of vectors into specific cell types (transductional targeting), and expression of vectors in certain cell types (transcriptional targeting).

Conditionally replication-competent vectors

Expression of the adenovirus *E1B* gene inactivates p53 in the host cell and thereby allows replication and cell lysis. Mutant adenoviruses have been designed which lack *E1B* and can therefore replicate in p53-deficient tumour cells but not in normal cells.[70] This construct is being tested in clinical trials. Conditional replication has also been noted in the human reovirus which replicates selectively in cells with intact Ras signalling pathways.[71]

Transductional targeting

Entry of adenoviral particles into mammalian cells is dependent upon binding of capsid proteins to a specific cell surface receptor, followed by membrane fusion mediated by binding of the tripeptide sequence, RGD, to integrins on the host cell. Constructs expressing antibodies to capsid proteins which are then conjugated to specific ligands, such as epidermal growth factor, are capable of targeting entry of virus to specific receptor-bearing cells.[72] Other methods of targeting include development of bispecific antibodies recognizing epitopes in the capsid and structures on the cell surface.[73] These methods depend on the continued association of vector with antibody–ligand constructs or bispecific antibodies. The difficulties associated with the use of bispecific conjugates may be avoided by genetic modification of the viral capsid proteins to contain ligands which will target specific cell surface receptors.[74]

Modification of retroviruses has proved more difficult. Entry of retrovirus into mammalian cells is mediated by an envelope glycoprotein. Although attempts have been made to modify this by, for example, expression of single-chain antibodies and growth factors, they have failed to mediate specific uptake of vector.

Transcriptional targeting

Gene transcription depends upon the binding of transcription factors to regions of DNA known as promoters. The promoter is upstream of the gene to be transcribed. A variety of genes have been identified that are overexpressed in cancer, such as *MUC-1* in breast, ovarian, and pancreatic cancer,[75] *HER2* in breast and ovarian cancer,[76] and α-fetoprotein in hepatoma.[77] Targeted expression of transgenes has been achieved by the incorporation of the promoter sequences from such genes into the vector (Fig. 5). Transcription of the transgene will therefore be restricted to tissues in which the appropriate transcription factor is present.

Tumour physiology

The previous attempts to target gene delivery depend on the ability to exploit differences in tumour cells at the DNA or protein level. Differences in the tumour microenvironment may also provide a level of selectivity. For example, transcriptional control could be provided by using the promoter sequences of genes which are expressed, under hypoxic conditions.

Use of gene therapy in cancer

A number of approaches have been adopted to exploit the potential of gene therapy (Table 4).

Restoration of phenotype

Altered expression of genes which contribute to the malignant phenotype (oncogenes) has been documented in many tumour types. One method by which the malignant phenotype could be reversed is by inhibition of oncogene expression.

Inhibition of oncogene transcription

This can be achieved by using nucleotide sequences which bind to promoters of known oncogenes. An example of this is the use of the adenoviral gene *E1A*, which inhibits transcription of the *HER-2* promoter and therefore reduces expression of the *HER-2* oncogene, leading to suppression of tumorigenicity.[78] A clinical trial of the *E1A* gene in a liposomal vector is underway in patients with breast or ovarian cancer overexpressing *HER-2*.

Inhibition of oncogene translation (antisense oligonucleotides)

Inhibition of oncogene expression has also been achieved at the level of translation.[79] Nucleotide sequences complementary to the relevant mRNA (antisense oligonucleotides) prevent translation and promote mRNA degradation (Fig. 6). Antisense strategies have targeted insulin-like growth factor in primary liver cancer, *k-ras* in non-small cell lung cancer, *c-myc* and *c-fos* in breast and prostate cancer, and TGF-β in glioblastoma. The feasibility of this approach in humans has been demonstrated in a phase I study which targeted the *bcl-2* oncogene in lymphoma.[80] Vectors which encode intracellular antibodies capable of blocking the oncogene protein product have been

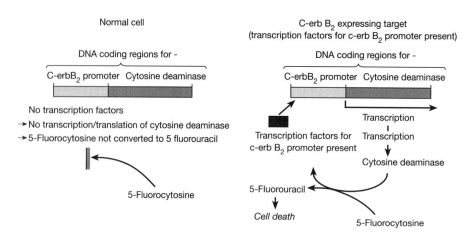

Fig. 5 Targeted gene expression. The pro-drug 5-fluorocytosine is converted to the cytotoxic agent 5-fluorouracil by the enzyme cytosine deaminase. The DNA encoding the enzyme has been transfected into cells and expression is controlled by the c-erb B_2 promoter. As only tumour cells produce transcription factors for this promoter, only tumour cells synthesize the enzyme and therefore only tumour cells convert the pro-drug to its toxic metabolite.

Table 4 Strategies for gene therapy

Aim	Target	Strategy	Examples
Restoration of phenotype	Tumour cell	Inhibition of oncogene expression Replacement of tumour suppressor genes	E1A (HER2), bcl-2, IGF-1, k-ras, c-myc, c-fos, TGF-β p53, RB, BRCA-1
Enhance cytotoxicity	Tumour cell	Delivery of enzymes to activate prodrugs Restoration of tumour cell sensitivity	HSV-TK, cytosine deaminase, cytochrome p450 p53
Cytoprotection	Stem cell	Delivery of drug resistance genes	MDR, MRP, GST, MnSOD, DHFR
Immunomodulation (ex vivo)	Tumour cells	Increase immunogenicity (cytokines/costimlatory molecules)	IL-2, GM-CSF, CD80
(in vivo)	Tumour cells	Increase immunogenicity	MHC
(ex vivo)	Immune cells	Transfection of APCs with cDNA of tumour-associated antigens	
(in vivo)	Immune cells	Immunization with genes encoding tumour-associated antigens	CEA, gp100, MART-1, MUC1, PSA

APC, antigen-presenting cells; CEA, carcinoembryonic antigen; DHFR, dihydrofolate reductase; GST, glutathione-S-transferase; MnSOD, manganese superoxide dismutase; MDR, multidrug resistance gene; MRP, multidrug resistance protein; PSA, prostate-specific antigen.

shown to be feasible in preclinical studies and are in early clinical trial.

Restoration of tumour suppressor gene expression

Loss of function mutations in tumour suppressor genes contribute to the malignant phenotype by abolishing cell-cycle checkpoints, interfering with apoptotic pathways, and inhibiting DNA repair mechanisms. Mutations in tumour suppressor genes have been described in many tumour types. Restoration of suppressor gene function in tumour cells *in vitro*, by transduction with the wild-type gene, causes reversion of the malignant phenotype and often apoptosis. *p53* is the most commonly mutated tumour suppressor gene in solid tumours and restoration of function has been shown in non-small cell lung cancer using adenovirus which selectively infects *p53*-deficient cells.[81] Replacement of *p53* is also being investigated in other solid tumours including breast, prostate, colon, and head and neck tumours. Replacement of other candidate tumour suppressor genes being

investigated clinically includes *RB* in bladder cancer and *BRCA-1* in breast and ovarian cancer.

Potentiation of cytotoxicity

Some gene therapy strategies are directed at enhancing the selectivity of cytotoxic therapy or restoring tumour cell sensitivity to cytotoxic agents. Prodrug activation involves the delivery to tumour cells of a transgene which encodes an enzyme capable of activating a relatively non-toxic prodrug to its toxic metabolites. This approach is exemplified by the use of the gene encoding herpes simplex virus thymidine kinase (**HSV-TK**). Unlike mammalian TK, HSV-TK preferentially monophosphorylates ganciclovir to toxic metabolites and induces cell death. This approach also has the advantage that not all tumour cells need to be transduced with the HSV-TK gene, since toxic metabolites may be transferred through gap junctions to neighbouring cells ('bystander' effect). Another potentially important consequence

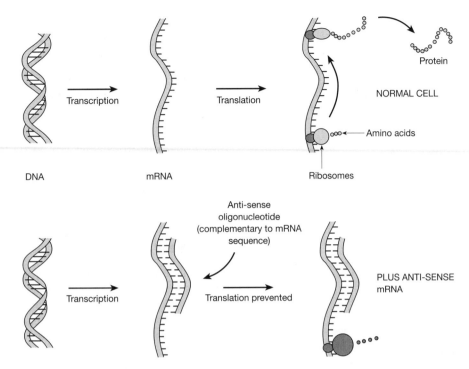

Fig. 6 Antisense oligonucleotides. The antisense oligonucleotide binds to the complementary specific mRNA sequence and prevents mRNA translation. Therefore, synthesis of the specific protein product is prevented.

of this approach, namely induction of systemic immunity following cell death, has been confirmed in animal models. Until expression of prodrug-activating enzymes can be restricted to tumour cells, clinical trials of the HSV-TK/ganciclovir approach are limited to situations where high levels of vector can be achieved by direct injection into tumour sites. The first studies examining its role were in glioma.[82] Other sites where such injection is feasible include recurrent prostate cancer and malignant mesothelioma.[83],[84]

Other enzyme/prodrug combinations being investigated include bacterial cytosine deaminase, which converts the relatively non-toxic 5-fluorocytosine to 5-fluorouracil. Preclinical studies suggest that only a small proportion of tumour cells need to be transduced, possibly because unlike the TK/gancyclovir system, the bystander effect of 5-fluorouracil is not dependent on the presence of gap junctions between target cells. Transduction of tumour with genes encoding enzymes of the cytochrome p450 complex which activate cyclophosphamide have also shown encouraging results in preclinical studies.

Tumour cell resistance to chemotherapy and radiotherapy is in part due to alterations in apoptotic pathways which allow DNA damage to accumulate without causing cell death. Restoration of pro-apoptotic capacity by correction of *p53* function has led to increased tumour cell chemosensitivity in preclinical studies. Local delivery of adenoviral vectors containing *p53* in non-small cell lung cancer has shown antitumour effects in a phase I study, although the exact nature of the interaction between gene transfer and chemosensitivity has yet to be clarified. Downregulation of *bcl-2* has been shown to increase chemosensitivity *in vitro* and this is a potential target for clinical development.

Cytoprotection

Reducing sensitivity of stem cells in bone marrow to cytotoxic agents could increase tolerance to higher doses of chemotherapy. Preclinical studies have shown this approach to be possible using retroviral transfer of human *MDR1*.[85] Transfer of genes encoding other drug resistance molecules is also being investigated, including multidrug resistance protein, glutathione-*S*-transferase, manganese superoxide dismutase, and dihydrofolate reductase.

Immunomodulation

The majority of clinical trials utilizing gene therapy have had the goal of inducing or augmenting immunologically mediated tumour rejection. Initial attempts at augmenting the host immune response to tumour aimed to increase the cytotoxic ability of tumour-infiltrating lymphocytes (TILs) by *ex vivo* transfection with IL-2. Modified TILs accumulated in liver and spleen rather than in tumour and although transfection of TILs with other cytokines has been investigated, most immunotherapuetic approaches are now focused on the induction of a specific immune response to tumour.

Genetic modification of tumour cells

Strategies to augment the immune response to tumour have included attempts to increase the immungenicity of tumour cells. Irradiated tumour cells have been used with conventional immunological adjuvants in an attempt to induce an immune response to tumour. Tumour cells transfected with cytokine genes, such as IL-2, IL-12, and GM-CSF, can induce a greater antitumour response and have caused regression in animal models. Similar effects have been described following introduction of genes expressing costimulatory molecules, such as CD80. Clinical studies using genetically modified allogeneic tumour cell vaccines have begun and early results using IL-2-transfected melanoma cells demonstrated the development of inflammatory infiltrates in distant metastases, suggesting induction of an immune response.[86]

The use of allogeneic cell lines assumes that relevant tumour antigens are present. An alternative strategy is to use genetically modified autologous tumour cells. Following vaccination with irradiated, GM-CSF-transfected autologous tumour cells, regressions have been noted in renal cell carcinoma and melanoma.[87],[88] However, as noted earlier, there are considerable practical difficulties in preparing autologous tumour cell vaccines.

Genetic modification of immune cells

Whilst some groups have utilized modified tumour cells, others have focused on modification of immune cells, such as dendritic cells. Although antigen presentation by dendritic cells has been investigated by pulsing them with peptide or tumour cell lysates, or by fusing them with tumour cells, a promising approach involves transfection of dendritic cells with the cDNA for tumour-associated antigens. The aim of this strategy is to harness the endogenous antigen-presenting machinery of the dendritic cell and allow it to identify epitopes within tumour-associated antigens that bind to host MHC. These epitopes may then be presented to T cells to induce a specific immune response.

Recombinant virus vaccines

Parenteral administration of vectors engineered to express tumour-associated antigens is being investigated in an attempt to overcome the requirement for *ex vivo* manipulation of tumour or cells of the immune system. The viral vector acts as an adjuvant by altering the intra- and extracellular trafficking of antigen, and provides an additional substrate for specific and non-specific immune recognition. In animal models, vaccination with tumour cells expressing a model antigen resulted in a negligible immune response. Vaccination with recombinant viral vectors expressing the same antigen resulted in specific cell-mediated immunity and caused tumour regression.[89] It is also possible to engineer vectors that express costimulatory molecules or cytokines as well as tumour-associated antigens.[90],[91]

In clinical studies, T_C-cell responses have been noted following immunization with a vaccinia virus encoding carcinoembryonic antigen.[92] A recombinant HPV16 and 18 E6- and E7-expressing vaccinia virus has been tested in eight patients with metastatic cervical cancer.[93] There was no significant toxicity, but no significant clinical response either. All patients developed an antivaccinia antibody response. Clinical testing of other candidate antigens including gp100, MART-1, MUC-1, and prostate-specific antigen are in progress.

Immunization and repetitive boosting with the same recombinant virus can induce a strong immune response to the viral vector itself. These responses limit the immunogenicity of tumour-associated antigens, perhaps by rapidly eliminating the recombinant virus. Alternatively, the response to immunodominant epitopes on the vector may suppress those to the weaker determinants of the tumour-associated antigens. These problems may be overcome by using different viral vectors that express the same tumour-associated antigens to prime and then to boost the response.

DNA vaccines

Naked plasmid DNA encoding tumour-associated antigens has also been used as a gene therapy. Both methylation and the high proportion of CpG motifs within bacterial DNA may stimulate a local inflammatory infiltrate. T_C-cell priming following DNA injection involves antigen-presenting cells derived from bone marrow.[94] The use of MUC1 DNA vaccines was partially protective in murine tumour models[95] and other examples have been reported. A combination of DNA followed by recombinant viral vaccination has proved very effective in protecting non-human primates against infectious diseases,[96],[97] and similar strategies are being investigated for treatment of cancer.

Summary

Biologically based therapies for cancer are beginning to deliver clinical benefits. Although toxicity from treatment is considerable, interferon-α may have a role in the treatment of some haematological malignancies, malignant melanoma, and renal cancer, and IL-2 is licensed for use in patients with metastatic renal cancer. The use of colony-stimulating factors has had a major impact in bone marrow transplantation and may allow the delivery of standard chemotherapy of adequate dose-intensity. Monoclonal antibodies, which have revolutionized many aspects of medicine, have also entered oncological practice with the use of anti-CD20 and anti-HER2 antibodies.

These advances have taken decades of preclinical and clinical research. In comparison with cytokine and monoclonal antibody technology, gene therapy and tumour-specific immunotherapy are in their infancy. Nevertheless, the dramatic pace of discovery in molecular biology and immunology has resulted in their rapid translation into the clinic, and some clinical trials are already showing promising results.

These treatments may not be relevant to every tumour type or perhaps to every patient with a particular cancer. In the future, it is likely that we will identify tumour or patient characteristics that predict for potential benefit. Until then, progress depends on continued basic research and well-designed clinical trials.

References

1. Penn I. Cancers complicating organ transplantation. *New England Journal of Medicine*, 1990; **323**: 1767–9.

2. Hall S. *A Commotion in the Blood*. UK: Little, Brown and Company, 1998: 44.

3. Coley-Nauts HC, Fowler GA, Bogatko FN. A review of the influence of bacterial infection and of bacterial products (Coley's toxins) on malignant tumours in man. *Acta Medica Scandinavica Supplementum*, 1953; **274-7**: 29–97.

4. Herr HW, Frader Y, Klein FA. Summary of effect of intravesical bacillus Calmette–Guérin (BCG) on carcinoma *in situ* of the bladder. *Seminars in Urologic Oncology*, 1997; **15**: 80–5.

5. Lacour J, *et al.* Adjuvant treatment with polyadenylic-polyuridylic acid in operable breast cancer: updated results of a randomised tiral. *British Medical Journal*, 1984; **288**: 589–92.

6. Quesada J, Reuben J, Manning J, Hersh E, Gutterman J. α-Interferon for induction of remission in hairy cell leukaemia. *New England Journal of Medicine*, 1984; **310**: 510–18.

7. Grever M, *et al.* Randomised comparison of pentostatin versus interferon α-2 in previously untreated patients with hairy cell leukaemia: an intergroup study. *Journal of Clinical Oncology*, 1995; **13**: 974–9.

8. Ludwig H, *et al.* Interferon-α for induction and maintenance in multiple myeloma: results of two multicenter randomised trials and summary of other studies. *Annals of Oncology*, 1995; **6**: 467–76.

9. Kantarjian HM, O'Brien S, Anderlini P, Talpaz M. Treatment of myelogenous leukaemia: current status and investigational options. *Blood*, 1996; **87**: 3069–81.

10. Tura S, *et al.* for the Italian Cooperative Study Group on Chronic Myeloid Leukaemia. Interferon α-2a as compared with conventional chemotherapy for the treatment of myeloid leukaemia. *New England Journal of Medicine*, 1994; **330**: 820–5.

11. Krown SE. Interferon-α: evolving therapy for AIDS-associated Kaposi's sarcoma. *Journal of Interferon and Cytokine Research*, 1998; **18**: 209–14.

12. Nethersell A, Sikora K. Interferons and malignant disease. In: Taylor-Papadimitriou J, ed. *Interferons: their Impact in Biology and Medicine.* Oxford: Oxford University Press, 1985: 127–44.

13. Creagan E, *et al.* Randomised, surgical adjuvant clinical trial of recombinant interferon α-2a in selected patients with malignant melanoma. *Journal of Clinical Oncology*, 1995; **13**: 2776–83.

14. Kirkwood J, Strawdermann M, Ernstoff M, Smith T, Borden E, Blum R. Interferon α-2b adjuvant therapy of high-risk resected cutaneous melanoma: the Eastern Cooperative Oncology Group Trial EST 1684. *Journal of Clinical Oncology*, 1996, **14**: 7–17.

15. Cole B, Gelber R, Kirkwood J, Goldhirsch A, Barylak E, Borden E. Quality of life adjusted survival analysis of interferon α-2b adjuvant treatment of high risk resected cutaneous melanoma: an Eastern Cooperative Oncology Group study. *Journal of Clinical Oncology*, 1996; **14**: 2666–773.

16. Grob J, *et al.* Randomised trial of interferon α-2a as adjuvant therapy in resected primary melanoma thicker than 1.5 mm without clinically detectable lymph node metastases. *Lancet*, 1998; **351**: 1905–10.

17. Pehamberger H, *et al.* Adjuvant interferon α-2a treatment in resected primary stage II cutaneous melanoma. *Journal of Clinical Oncology*, 1998; **16**: 1425–9.

18. Wirth M. Immunotherapy for metastatic renal cell carcinoma. *Urologic Clinics of North America*, 1993; **20**: 283–95.

19. Neidhart J, *et al.* Vinblastine fails to improve response of renal cancer to interferon α-n1: high response rate in patients with pulmonary metastases. *Journal of Clinical Oncology*, 1991; **9**: 832–6.

20. MRC Collaborators. Interferon-α and survival in metastatic renal carcinoma: early results of a randomised controlled trial. *Lancet*, 1999; **353**: 14–17.

21. Negrier S, *et al.* Recombinant human interleukin-2, recombinant human interferon α-2a, or both in metastatic renal cell cancer. *New England Journal of Medicine*, 1998; **338**: 1272–8.

22. Gleave M, *et al.* Interferon γ-1b compared with placebo in metastatic renal cell carcinoma. *New England Journal of Medicine*, 1998; **338**: 1265–71.

23. Eggermont AM, *et al.* Isolated limb perfusion with high-dose tumour necrosis factor-α in combination with interferon-γ and melphalan for nonresectable extremity soft tissue sarcomas: a multicenter trial. *Journal of Clinical Oncology*, 1996; **14**: 2653–65.

24. Moore RJ, Owens DM, Stamp G, *et al.* Mice deficient in tumour necrosis factor-alpha are resistant to skin carcinogenesis. *Nature Medicine* 1999; **5**: 828–31.

25. Fyfe G, *et al.* Results of treatment of 255 patients with metastatic renal cell carcinoma who received high-dose recombinant interleukin-2 therapy. *Journal of Clinical Oncology*, 1995; **13**: 688–96.

26. Fyfe G, *et al.* Long-term response data for 255 patients with metastatic renal cell carcinoma treated with high-dose recombinant interleukin-2 therapy. *Journal of Clinical Oncology*, 1996; **14**: 2410–11.

27. Rosenberg SA, *et al.* Prospective randomised trial of high dose interleukin-2 alone or in conjunction with lymphokine-activated killer cells for the treatment of patients with advanced cancer. *Journal of the National Cancer Institute*, 1994; **85**: 622–32.

28. Figlin RA, *et al.* Multicenter, randomised, phase III trial of CD8 + tumour-infiltrating lymphocytes in combination with recombinant interleukin-2 in metastatic renal cell carcinoma. *Journal of Clinical Oncology*, 1999; **17**: 2521–9.

29. Yang YC, Topalian SL, Parkinson D, *et al.* Randomized comparison of high dose and low dose intravenous IL-2 for therapy of metastatic renal cell carcinoma: an interim report. *Journal of Clinical Oncology*, 1994; **12**: 1572–6.

30. Toner GC, *et al.* Interleukin-3 fails to reduce thrombocytopenia after carboplatin and etoposide chemotherapy: a randomised, placebo-controlled trial. *Proceedings of the American Society of Clinical Oncology*, 1998; **17**: 85a.

31. Margolin K, *et al.* Phase II studies of recombinant human interleukin-4 in advanced renal cancer and malignant melanoma. *Journal of Immunotherapy*, 1994; **15**: 147–53.

32. Cairo MS, *et al.* Recombinant human interleukin-11 enhances haematologic recovery following ICE chemotherapy in children with solid tumours or lymphoma: analysis of haematopoietic responses, cytokine induction, pharmacokinetics and stem cell mobilisation. *Proceedings of the American Society of Clinical Oncology*, 1998; **17**: 538a.

33. Bajetta E, *et al.* Pilot study of subcutaneous recombinant human interleukin-12 in metastatic melanoma. *Clinical Cancer Research*, 1998; **4**: 75–85.

34. Schoenberger S, Toes R, van der Voort E, Offringa R, Melief C. T-cell help for cytotoxic T lymphocytes is mediated by CD40–CD40L interactions. *Nature*, 1998; **398**: 480–3.

35. Ridge J, Di Rosa F, Matzinger P. A conditioned dendritic cell can be a temporal bridge between a CD4 + T-helper and a T-killer cell. *Nature*, 1998; **393**: 474–8.

36. Bennett S, *et al.* Help for cytotoxic T-cell responses is mediated by CD40 signalling. *Nature*, 1998; **393**: 478–80.

37. Staveley-O'Carroll K, *et al.* Induction of antigen-specific T cell anergy: an early event in the course of tumour progression. *Proceedings of the National Academy of Sciences (USA)*, 1998; **95**: 1178–83.

38. Urban JL, Burton RC, Holland JM, Kripke ML, Schreiber H. Mechanisms of syngeneic tumour rejection. Susceptibility of host-selected progressor variants to various immunological effector cells. *Journal of Experimental Medicine*, 1982; **155**: 557–73.

39. Trowsdale J, Travers P, Bodmer WF, Patillo RA. Expression of HLA-A, -B and -C and β₂-microglobulin antigens in human choriocarcinoma cell lines. *Journal of Experimental Medicine*, 1980; **152**: 11s–17s.

40. Restifo NP, *et al.* Defective presentation of endogenous antigens by a murine sarcoma. Implications for the failure of an anti-tumour immune response. *Journal of Immunology*, 1991; **147**: 1453–9.

41. Hahne M, *et al.* Melanoma cell expression of Fas(Apo-1/CD95) ligand: implications for tumour immune escape. *Science*, 1996; **274**: 1363–6.

42. Vermorken JB, *et al.* Active specific immunotherapy for stage II and stage III human colon cancer: a randomised trial. *Lancet*, 1999; **353**: 345–50.

43. Chan A, Morton D. Active immunotherapy with allogeneic tumour cell vaccines: present status. *Seminars in Oncology*, 1998; **25**: 611–22.

44. Mitchell MS. Perspective on allogeneic melanoma lysates in active specific immunotherapy. *Seminars in Oncology*, 1998; **25**: 623–35.

45. Bystryn J, *et al.* Preparation and characterisation of a polyvalent human melanoma antigen vaccine. *Journal of Biological Response Modifiers*, 1986; **5**: 211–24.

46. Bystryn J, *et al.* Phase III, double-blind, trial of a shed polyvalent melanoma vaccine in stage III melanoma. *Proceedings of the American Society of Clinical Oncology*, 1998; **17**: 434a.

47. **Murray DR, et al.** Viral oncolysates in the management of malignant melanoma. *Cancer*, 1977; **40**: 680–6.

48. **Wallack MK, et al.** A phase III randomised, double-blind, multiinstitutional trial of vaccinia melanoma oncolysate-active specific immunotherapy for patients with stage II melanoma. *Cancer*, 1995; **75**: 34–42.

49. **Dranoff G, et al.** Vaccination with irradiated tumour cells engineered to secrete murine granulocyte–macrophage colony-stimulating factor stimulates potent, specific, and long-lasting anti-tumour immunity. *Proceedings of the National Academy of Sciences (USA)*, 1993; **90**: 3539–43.

50. **Hsu F, et al.** Vaccination of patients with B cell lymphoma using autologous antigen-pulsed dendritic cells. *Nature Medicine*, 1996; **2**: 52–8.

51. **Livingstone P.** Ganglioside vaccines with emphasis on GM2. *Seminars in Oncology*, 1998; **25**: 636–45.

52. **Itzkowitz S, et al.** Sialosyl-Tn: a novel mucin antigen associated with prognosis in colorectal cancer patients. *British Journal of Cancer*, 1990; **66**: 1960–6.

53. **Nestle FO, et al.** Vaccination of melanoma patients with peptide- or tumour lysate-pulsed dendritic cells. *Nature Medicine*, 1998; **4**: 328–32.

54. **Kugler A, et al.** Regression of human metastatic renal cell carcinoma after vaccination with tumor cell–dendritic cell hybrids. *Nature Medicine*, 2000; **6**: 332–6.

55. **Marchand M, et al.** Tumour regression responses in melanoma patients treated with a peptide encoded by MAGE3. *International Journal of Cancer*, 1995; **63**: 883–5.

56. **Jager E, et al.** GM-CSF enhances immune responses to melanoma peptides *in vivo*. *International Journal of Cancer*, 1996; **67**: 54–62.

57. **Parkhurst M, et al.** Improved induction of melanoma-reactive CTL with peptides from the melanoma antigen gp100 modified at HLA-A*0201-binding residues. *Journal of Immunology*, 1996; **157**: 2539–48.

58. **Rosenberg S, et al.** Immunologic and therapeutic evaluation of a synthetic peptide vaccine for the treatment of patients with metastatic melanoma. *Nature Medicine*, 1998; **4**: 321–7.

59. **Toes R, Blom R, Offringa R, Kast W, Melief C.** Functional deletion of tumour-specific CTLs induced by peptide vaccination can lead to the inability to reject tumours. *Journal of Immunology*, 1996; **156**: 3911–18.

60. **Plunkett TA, Miles DW.** Immunotherapy of breast cancer. *Cancer Treatment Reviews*, 1998; **24**: 55–67.

61. **MacLean G, Miles D, Rubens R, Reddish M, Longenecker B.** Enhancing the effect of THERATOPE STn-KLH cancer vaccine patients with metastatic breast cancer by pre-treatment with low-dose intravenous cyclophosphamide. *Journal of Immunotherapy*, 1996; **19**: 309–16.

62. **Riethmuller G, et al.** Randomised trial of monclonal antibody for adjuvant therapy of resected Dukes' C colorectal carcinoma. *Lancet*, 1994; **343**: 1177–83.

63. **Riethmuller G, et al.** Monoclonal antibody therapy for resected Dukes C colorectal cancer: seven year outcome of a multicentre randomised trial. *Journal of Clinical Oncology*, 1998; **16**: 1788–94.

64. **Kaminski M, et al.** Iodine-131-anti-B1 radioimmunotherapy for B-cell lymphoma. *Journal of Clinical Oncology*, 1996; **14**: 1974–81.

65. **Maloney D, Press O.** New treatments for non-Hodgkin's lymphoma: monoclonal antibodies. *Oncology*, 1998; **12**: 63–76.

66. **Baselga, J, et al.** Phase II study of weekly intravenous recombinant humanised anti-p185HER2 monoclonal antibody in patients with HER2/neu-overexpressing metastatic breast cancer. *Journal of Clinical Oncology*, 1996; **14**: 737–44.

67. **Norton L, et al.** Overall survival (OS) advantage to simultaneous chemotherapy (CRx) plus the humanised anti-HER2 monoclonal antibody herception (H) in HER2-overexpressing (HER2+) metastatic breast cancer (MBC). *Proceedings of the American Society of Clinical Oncology*, 1999; **18**: 127a.

68. **Diehl L, et al.** CD40 activation *in vivo* overcomes peptide-induced peripheral cytotoxic T-lymphocyte tolerance and augments anti-tumour vaccine efficacy. *Nature Medicine*, 1999; **5**: 774–9.

69. **Sotomayor EM, et al.** Conversion of tumour-specific CD4+ T-cell tolerance to T-cell priming in rough *in vivo* ligation of CD40. *Nature Medicine*, 1996; **2**: 780–9.

70. **Bischoff JR, et al.** An adenovirus mutant that replicates selectively in p53-deficient human tumour cells. *Science*, 1996; **274**: 373–6.

71. **Coffey MC, Strong JE, Forsyth PA, Lee PWK.** Reovirus therapy of tumours with activated Ras pathway. *Science*, 1998, **282**: 1332–1334.

72. **Miller CR, et al.** Differential susceptibility of primary and established human glioma cells to adenovirus infection: targeting via the epidermal growth factor receptor achieves fibre receptor-independent gene transfer. *Cancer Research*, 1998; **58**: 5738–48.

73. **Wickham TJ, et al.** Targeted adenovirus-mediated gene delivery to T cells via CD3. *Journal of Virology*, 1997; **71**: 7663–9.

74. **Yoshida Y, Sadata A, Zhang W, Saito K, Shinoura N, Hamada H.** Generation of fiber-mutant recombinant adenoviruses for gene therapy of malignant glioma. *Human Gene Therapy*, 1998; **9**: 2503–15.

75. **Chen L, et al.** Breast cancer selective gene expression and therapy mediated by recombinant adenoviruses containing the DF3/MUC1 promoter. *Journal of Clinical Investigations*, 1995; **96**: 2775–82.

76. **Pandha HS, et al.** Genetic prodrug activation therapy for breast cancer: a phase I clinical trial of erbB-2-directed suicide gene expression. *Journal of Clinical Oncology*,1999; **17**: 2180–9.

77. **Ido A, et al.** Gene therapy for hepatoma cells using a retrovirus vector carrying herpes simplex virus thymidine kinase gene under the control of human α-phetoprotein gene promoter. *Cancer Research*, 1995; **55**: 3105–9.

78. **Yu D, Matin A, Xia W, Sorgi E, Huang L, Hung MC.** Liposome-mediated *in vivo* E1A gene transfer suppressed dissemination of ovarian cancer cells that overexpress HER-2/neu. *Oncogene*, 1995; **11**: 1383–8.

79. **Anthony DD, Pan YX, Wu SG, Shen F, Guo YJ.** Ex vivo and *in vivo* IGF-1 antisense RNA strategies for treatment of cancer in humans. *Advances in Experimental Medicine and Biology*, 1998; **451**: 27–34.

80. **Webb A, et al.** BCL-2 antisense therapy in patients with non-Hodgkin lymphoma. *Lancet*, 1997; **349**: 1137–41.

81. **Roth JA, et al.** Retrovirus-mediated wild-type p53 gene transfer to tumours of patients with lung cancer. *Nature Medicine*, 1996; **2**: 985–91.

82. **Ram Z, et al.** Therapy of malignant brain tumours by intratumoral implantation of retroviral vector-prodrug cells. *Nature Medicine*, 1997; **3**: 1354–61.

83. **Herman JR, et al.** Preliminary report of phase I dose escalation study of *in situ* gene therapy (HSV-tk+GCV) for locally recurrent prostate cancer: absence of toxicity. *Proceedings of the American Soceity of Clinical Oncology*, 1997; **16**: 440a.

84. **Treat J, et al.** Adenoviral-mediated intrapleural HSVtk gene therapy (AdRSVtk) for malignant mesothelioma: a phase I clinical trial. *Proceedings of the American Society of Clinical Oncology*, 1997; **16**: 433a.

85. **Sorrentino BP, et al.** Selection of drug-resistant bone marrow cells *in vivo* after retroviral transfer of human MDR1. *Science*,1992; **257**: 99–103.

86. **Belli F, et al.** Active immunisation of metastatic melanoma patients with interleukin-2-transduced allogeneic melanoma cells: evaluation of efficacy and tolerability. *Cancer Immunology, Immunotherapy*,1997; **44**: 197–203.

87. **Ellem KA, et al.** A case report: immune responses and clinical course of the first human use of granulocyte/macrophage-colony-stimulating-factor-transduced autologous melanoma cells for immunotherapy. *Cancer Immunology, Immunotherapy*, 1997; **44**: 10–20.

88. **Simons JW, et al.** Bioactivity of autologous irradiated renal cell carcinoma vaccines generated by *ex vivo* granulocyte–macrophage

colony-stimulating factor gene transfer. *Cancer Research*, 1997; **57**: 1537–46.

89. **Wang M,** *et al.* Active immunotherapy of cancer with a nonreplicating recombinant fowlpox virus encoding a model tumour associated antigen. *Journal of Immunology*, 1995; **154**: 4685–92.

90. **Bronte V,** *et al.* IL-2 enhances the function of recombinant poxvirus-based vaccines in the treatment of established pulmonary metastases. *Journal of Immunology*, 1995; **154**: 5482–92.

91. **Chamberlain R,** *et al.* Costimulation enhances the active immunotherapy effect of recombinant anti-cancer vacines. *Cancer Research*, 1996; **56**: 2832–6.

92. **Tsang KY,** *et al.* Generation of human cytotoxic T cells specific for human carcinoembryonic antigen epitopes from patients immunised with recombinant vaccinia-CEA vaccine. *Journal of the National Cancer Institute*, 1995; **87**: 982–90.

93. **Borysiewicz L,** *et al.* A recombinant vaccinia virus encoding human papillomavirus types 16 and 18, E6 and E7 proteins as immunotherapy for cervical cancer. *Lancet*, 1996; **347**: 1523–7.

94. **Corr M, Lee D, Carson D, Tighe H.** Gene vaccination with naked plasmid DNA: mechanism of CTL priming. *Journal of Experimental Medicine*, 1996; **184**: 1555–9.

95. **Graham R, Stewart L, Peat N, Beverley P, Taylor-Papadimitriou J.** MUC1-based immunogens for tumour therapy: development of murine model systems. *Tumour Targeting*, 1995; **1**: 211–21.

96. **Schneider J,** *et al.* Enhanced immunogenicity for CD8 + T cell induction and complete protective efficacy of malaria DNA vaccination by boosting with modified vaccinia virus Ankara. *Nature Medicine*, 1998; **4**: 387–402.

97. **Robinson H,** *et al.* Neutralising antibody-independent containment of immunodeficiency virus challenges by DNA priming and recombinant post virus booster immunisation. *Nature Medicine*, 1999; **5**: 526–34.

4.27 Targeted cancer therapy

Richard Begent

Introduction

Selective delivery of therapy to cancer can overcome the limitations of conventional therapy by achieving high potency in tumours with minimal normal tissue toxicity. Several targeting and therapeutic systems have been devised. There is growing clinical evidence of efficacy and much experimental work on novel systems.

History

In 1895, Hericourt and Richet[1] immunized animals with human tumour extracts and gave the serum to patients with cancer. They reported tumour responses and some of the adverse effects associated with modern antibody targeted therapy. From the 1940s, polyclonal antibodies reactive with defined tumour antigens[2] were used to show the specificity of targeting. Monoclonal antibodies were reported in 1975[3] giving defined and reproducible reagents which were amenable to genetic modification. Other targeting systems have emerged depending on metabolic pathways exclusive to the tissue of origin of the tumour. [131]Iodine therapy is the prime example, and has been used for treatment of thyroid carcinoma since the 1940s.

A growing knowledge of the normal human genome leads to a corresponding identification of the mutations that define cancer. The abnormal spectrum of proteins (proteome) that results includes products of mutant genes as well as over or under expression of protein products of unmutated genes which contribute to the phenotype of a cancer cell. Both mutant and non-mutant cancer-associated proteins may serve as targets for therapy. The proteome is more complex than the genome because of post-translational modifications of proteins and aberrations in folding. Developments in protein chemistry, protein engineering, cellular and structural biology, and tumour biology have been applied in the last three decades to make many targeted therapy systems for cancer.

I am grateful to the Cancer Research Campaign who support targeted therapy research at the Royal Free and University College Medical School which made this review possible. I thank colleagues in the Department of Oncology for their many contributions to the work described.

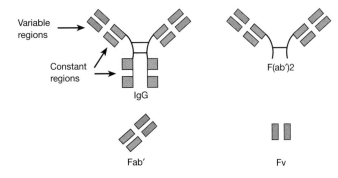

Fig. 1 Antibodies and their fragments.

Targeting molecules

Antibodies

Antibodies have a complex antigen-binding region and potential for great diversity of structure. They can bind with high affinity to diverse proteins and carbohydrate structures found in malignant cells. Antibodies can be generated against antigens that are expressed by most common cancers and this makes them practical reagents. They can be modified by genetic engineering or protein chemistry into a range of different antibody structures and molecular weights (Fig. 1). For a review see Chester and Hawkins, 1995.[4]

Peptides

Peptides have smaller molecular weight and less complexity than antibodies, and thus diffuse through tumour masses more uniformly than whole antibodies. Where high affinity of binding, for instance to a tumour-selective cell surface receptor, can be achieved they make effective targeting agents. [90]yttrium-labelled octreotide, which binds to somatostatin receptors, for treatment of carcinoid tumours, is a good example. However, it causes dose-limiting myelosuppression and renal toxicity. The ability to produce peptide libraries with very large numbers of peptides means that it is possible to select tumour-binding peptides from this diversity.[5]

Macromolecular targeting agents

Non-tumour-specific proteins are retained in cancers. This is characterized by retention of the protein in poorly vascularized or necrotic tumour areas.[6] Large molecules given into the bloodstream penetrate tumour vasculature through the large fenestrations present in most tumour vessels. They are not found in well vascularized parts of tumour but are retained in poorly vascularized tumour areas from which there is no organized lymphatic drainage system. It is probable that liposomes, synthetic polymers, and large or aggregated proteins localize in tumours by this mechanism.

Liposomally-entrapped doxorubicin has been shown to have antitumour activity in Kaposi's sarcoma and appears to give higher response rates than regimens including conventional doxorubicin.[7] Doxorubicin is probably concentrated in the tumour by liposomes and released over a period of days. Plasma half-life is often extended compared with more conventional ways of administering the drug, and changes in response rate and adverse effects might be caused by either tumour entrapment or by prolonged residence in plasma.

Substrates of metabolic pathways in tumours

[131]Iodine uptake into thyroxine is an excellent example of the principle of using specific substrates of metabolic pathways for treatment of tumours. ^{131}I-meta-iodobenzylguanidine (MIBG), a substrate for catecholamine synthesis, as used for treatment of phaeochromocytoma, neuroblastoma, and some other tumours, is a further example.

The target metabolic pathways are features of the normal tissue from which the tumour arises. The function of the tissue of origin of the tumour must not be essential or should be replaceable. Whilst this is so for the examples given, it is doubtful whether the approach could be used in treatment of common epithelial tumours.

Antitumour antibodies

Monoclonal antibodies derived from hybridomas[3] are clonal and their specificity can be defined. They are amenable to genetic engineering (i.e. to the introduction or deletion of specific DNA sequences in the genes that encode them, see Chapter 1.2) and to studies of their molecular structure. However, only a small part of the antibody repertoire can be examined because each clone must be individually studied for its specificity.

The ability to purify antibody genes by PCR from populations of B cells has made it possible to examine very large numbers of antibody clones (>10[11]) derived from cDNA libraries and to explore the antibody specificity contained in the germline or in an immunized host (Fig. 2).[8]–[10] A population of B cells large enough to contain the required antibody diversity is used as a source of RNA from which a cDNA library is constructed. Antibody variable regions are amplified from the cDNA with specific primers and cloned as a single chain Fv (scFv) (variable heavy and variable light (VH and VL) joined by a flexible linker) into filamentous bacteriophage, producing an antibody library. Each phage contains the gene for the scFv and expresses the scFv antibody on its surface. Selection for a defined specificity can be achieved by reacting the library with the relevant antigen on a solid support. The conditions in which the selection is done can be varied, for instance by performing the selection in low antigen concentration to favour retrieval of high affinity antibodies. Phage antibody library technology appears set to take over from monoclonal antibodies made by the hybridoma technique for the reasons given in Table 1.

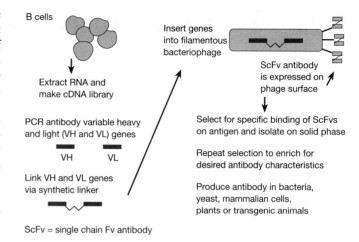

Fig. 2 Phage libraries and antibody selection.

Immunoglobulin G (IgG) is the basis for most cancer therapies based on antibodies but this has been adapted for different types of therapeutic use; common variants are shown in Fig. 3. Immunoglobulin purification, classification, definition of the fragments of the molecules, their structure and function have been elucidated.

Control of antibody targeting performance

Design of a targeting system requires appropriate tumour and normal tissue pharmacokinetics. These are substantially controllable by the choice of targeting molecule.[11]

The rate of clearance of antibodies from the blood stream is related principally to the molecular mass. Thus a whole IgG will clear more slowly than an Fv (see Fig. 1). Fvs are the smallest antibody fragments retaining full antigen specificity but they are unstable unless the variable heavy and variable light components are linked. This is most effectively achieved by genetically inserting a synthetic peptide linker to form a single chain Fv (scFv) (Figs 2 and 3).[12] These molecules have a molecular weight of about 27 kDa and are filtered by the kidney as well as undergoing proteolysis, mostly in the liver.[13] Human antibodies generally clear more slowly in man than those of murine origin. The slower the clearance from the circulation, the greater the availability of antibody for tumour binding and the absolute tumour antibody level but the lower the tumour to normal tissue ratio. Systems which accelerate clearance of antibody from the circulation increase tumour to normal tissue ratio.[14],[15]

Binding of antibody to antigen depends on an adequate on rate and slow off rate. High affinity is particularly important when antigen concentration is low. For any given antigen concentration there is a level of affinity beyond which no further increase will result in further tumour uptake.

The number of binding sites of an antibody for antigen determines functional affinity. Generally, tumour localization is superior with divalent rather than monovalent antibodies.[16] Where trivalent antibodies have been constructed (Fig. 3) and studied in animal models, they probably have an advantage over divalent versions. Genetic fusions of antibody and a therapeutic molecule, such as an enzyme

Table 1 Comparison of phage library and hybridoma technology for antibody production

Phage libraries	Hybridomas
< 10^{12} antibody clones cane be studied	<10^{3} clones can practically be studied
Selection for desired function from whole library—potential for superior product	Screening for function clone by clone
Cloned product amenable for engineering	–
Amenable to affinity maturation strategies	–
Bacterial or yeast production	Mammalian cell
Low cost production	–
Freedom from mammalian virus and DNA contamination	–
Ability to use human libraries producing human antibodies	Usually murine; large human repertoire not accessible

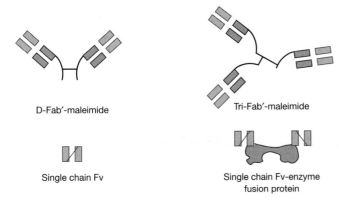

D-Fab'-maleimide

Tri-Fab'-maleimide

Single chain Fv

Single chain Fv-enzyme fusion protein

Fig. 3 Examples of engineered antibodies.

for ADEPT (see below), should generally be constructed to be divalent (see example in Fig. 3).

Stability of an antibody in storage, in the circulation, and in the tumour environment are critical factors for good performance. There is still much work to be done before chemically conjugated and genetically engineered products can reliably meet the necessary standards of stability.

Glycosylation of antibodies can help maintain stability and/or accelerate clearance. When antibodies are produced in yeasts or plant systems the glycosylation will usually differ from that of mammalian cells. The introduction of galactose by chemical linkage or by engineering of glycosylation sites into the antibodies will accelerate clearance from the liver via galactose receptors on hepatocytes. The yeast *Pichea pastoris* can produce branched mannose glycosylation whose extent depends on culture conditions but in some forms may induce adverse reactions.

Conjugation, radiolabelling, and genetic fusion

Chemical conjugation of antibodies with other proteins often produces a heterogeneous population while genetic fusions give a homogeneous and reproducible product. Production of a sufficient quantity of the final purified product often causes technical problems; these are improving with advances in production technology, which is allowing selection for high yield.

Antibodies labelled with iodine isotopes by attachment to tyrosine have been used successfully in patients. The process of radiolabelling may, however, damage the antigen-binding site if this contains tyrosine. Site-specific labelling, in which the antibody incorporates a macrocycle (a cage-like structure used for binding radionuclides such as ^{90}yttrium or indium isotopes) or a peptide which binds a radionuclide, can overcome this. 131-Iodine has many advantages for radioimmunotherapy with rapid clearance from normal tissues and a suitable energy β emission for treating small or medium sized tumour deposits. The high energy γ emission is usable for imaging but presents radiation protection problems. ^{90}Yttrium is a pure β-emitter but has a long path length making it inefficient for treating micrometastases because most of the targeted activity will be deposited outside such lesions. It is also retained in normal tissues to a greater extent than iodine isotopes. Other radionuclides, such as ^{67}copper and ^{188}rhenium and ^{186}rhenium may overcome these problems.

Tumour heterogeneity

Carcinomas begin to outgrow their blood supply after reaching about 1 mm diameter (see also Chapter 1.8). Although they stimulate vascular growth, this is disorderly, resulting in poorly nourished and necrotic areas. Delivery of any drug to poorly vasularized areas is reduced but access of large molecules such as whole antibodies is even more limited. Small antibody fragments such as scFvs penetrate better than whole IgG but do not completely overcome the problem. Figure 4 shows the heterogeneity of a human colon carcinoma xenograft. There is a viable peripheral area of tumour with a necrotic centre and an intermediate, poorly vascularized region (Fig. 4(b)). Following intravenous injection the distribution of radiolabelled antibody to the tumour is shown by the accompanying phosphor image (Fig. 4(a)). Antibody localizes well in the vascularized areas but not elsewhere. By contrast, non-specific proteins do not localize in the well vascularized areas, and are only retained in necrotic areas.[6]

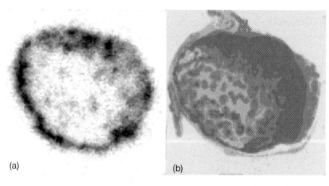

Fig. 4 Heterogeneity of antibody distribution in partially necrotic carcinoma.

Thus, antibody localization in well vascularized tumour areas is better than appreciated from studies of antibody concentration in the whole tumour. The underestimate is about three-fold in the anti-CEA antibody/colon carcinoma.[6] This is one reason why responses to radioimmunotherapy have been better than expected from radiation dose estimates based on macroscopic studies. However, radioimmunotherapy is relatively ineffective in poorly vascularized areas in which cells are resistant also to radiation and many drugs.

Strategies to address the resistance of cells in poorly nourished regions of tumours include the use of isotopes which emit radiation of sufficient range and potency to eradicate the poorly targeted cells or destruction of tumour vasculature. The latter might be achieved by use of dimethyl xanthenone acetic acid (DMXAA) which causes thrombosis and occlusion of tumour blood vessels, thus destroying poorly vascularized tumour areas in human tumour xenografts. A rim of viable tumour remains which can be eradicated by antibody-targeted therapy in this model.[17]

The need for non-immunogenic antibodies

Murine monoclonal antibodies are immunogenic in patients with intact immune systems, restricting their repeated use unless immunosuppressive therapy is given. Protein engineering has been used to replace xenogeneic-antibody-constant regions with those of human antibody in which only the mouse complementarity determining regions (CDRs) are grafted on to a human variable region framework linked to human constant regions.[18] Immunogenicity is low in these 'humanized' antibodies although human CDRs can be immunogenic themselves in some cases. The use of human constant regions has the benefit that effector functions of the constant regions are human, thus optimizing activation (Fig. 5).

Therapeutic strategies

Natural effector mechanisms have been employed in the earliest studies of antibody therapy[1] although little was then known about mechanisms. Antitumour effects may be achieved by direct cytotoxicity, activation of antibody-dependent cellular cytotoxicity, activation of the complement cascade, anti-idiotype effects (see below),

and growth control via effects on membrane-mediated signal transduction following binding of antibodies to receptors. At the time of writing, three antibodies are licensed for therapy of human cancer. Others are in clinical trials.

Anti-c-erbB2 (Herceptin) in breast carcinoma

This humanized antibody, directed against the c-erbB2 growth factor receptor, down regulates c-erbB2-induced intracellular signalling causing apoptosis as well as stimulating antibody-dependent cellular cytotoxicity. It is not clear which of these mechanisms dominates in the clinic.

Treatment with the antibody alone has been reported to produce responses (11 per cent complete or partial response) in previously heavily treated patients with breast cancer whose cells express c-erbB2.[19] When combined with cisplatin, response rates of 24 per cent were reported.[20] There is also evidence that Herceptin prolongs survival in advanced breast cancer when given in combination with paclitaxel (unpublished). Relapse is delayed when Herceptin is given with doxorubicin. Cardiotoxicity has been reported and further trials will elucidate its importance. Herceptin has been approved for use in the United States in patients with advanced breast cancer whose tumours express c-erbB2.

Antibodies to growth factor receptors such as that for c-erbB3 and for epithelial growth factor are being investigated, as well as antibodies to growth factors such as vascular endothelial growth factor.

17–1A antibody in colorectal carcinoma

The 17–1A antibody (Panorex) is a murine antibody directed against the EpCam antigen expressed on gastrointestinal and other carcinomas. It was largely ineffective against measurable metastatic colon carcinoma. In adjuvant therapy of Dukes stage C carcinoma[21] it produced 32 per cent reduction in mortality ($p = <0.01$ by log rank) compared to no treatment in a randomized trial that included 189 patients. This effect is comparable to that with cytotoxic chemotherapy but with less toxicity. Distant metastases were significantly reduced in the treated group whereas local recurrences were not. The probable reason is that distant metastases develop from smaller tumour deposits that are more effectively treated by antibody. As a result, 17–1A is licensed for adjuvant therapy of colorectal carcinoma in Germany and is in multinational clinical trials comparing it with conventional adjuvant chemotherapy.

Anti-CD20 (Mabthera, Rituximab) in B cell lymphoma

CD20 antigen, expressed on the cells of well differentiated and follicular B cell lymphomas, is the target of this chimeric antibody. Responses occur in patients whose lymphomas relapse after cytotoxic and radiation therapy.[22] In a pivotal study of 166 patients receiving 375 mg/m² intravenous infusion weekly times 4, complete responses occurred in 6 per cent and partial responses in 42 per cent of patients (overall response rate = 48 per cent). The median duration of response was 11+ months.

Toxicity is generally mild and short lasting with fever, nausea, pruritus, fatigue, mild hypotension, tumour-related pain, and bronchospasm. However, deaths have occurred due to an early

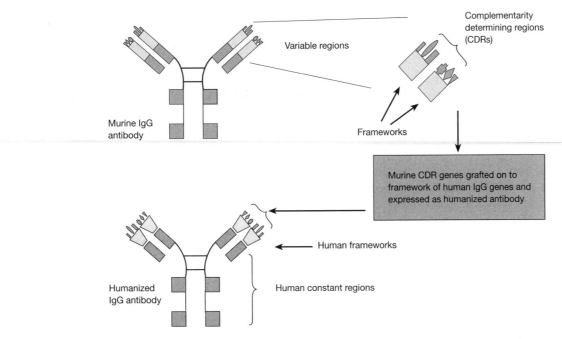

Fig. 5 Humanizing murine antibodies.

tumour lysis-like reaction in patients with bulky tumour. Mabthera is an important advance in the management of low grade and follicular lymphoma and the antibody is licensed as therapy for this indication in the United States and Europe.

Anti-idiotype antibodies

Anti-idiotype antibodies have been investigated clinically in melanoma and colorectal carcinoma (see also Chapter 4.26). The principal of action is that an antibody is made against the idiotype of an antitumour antibody (i.e. the part of the antibody that binds to the antigen) and may thus contain a structure that can mimic a tumour antigen. When the anti-idiotype antibody is given to a patient an antitumour immune response is elucidated. Evidence of tumour recognition has been found in melanoma and colorectal carcinoma. Possible clinical benefit is being investigated.

Combination therapies

Combination with other therapies is promising, particularly of Herceptin with paclitaxel and doxorubicin.[23] Trials are in progress of Mabthera in combination with chemotherapy in previously untreated patients with lymphoma and of anti-EGF antibodies in combination with external beam radiotherapy in head and neck cancer.

Radioimmunotherapy

Principles

Radioimmunotherapy uses an antitumour antibody to target a radionuclide to the tumour after intravenous, intra-arterial, or intracavitary administration. The targeted radionuclide usually has a β emission although α emitters are also being investigated. The range of the emission allows a bystander effect so that cells neighbouring

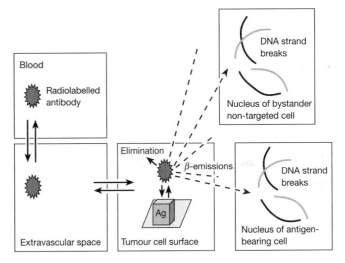

Fig. 6 Radioimmunotherapy and the bystander effect.

the one targeted can also receive a lethal radiation dose. The concept of radioimmunotherapy is illustrated in the simplified compartmental model shown in Fig. 6.

Toxicity to the bone marrow, lungs, and heart can be caused by circulating radionuclide. Prolonged exposure from circulating radiolabelled antibody permits equilibration between tumour extracellular spaces and blood and drives the antigen binding reaction on the tumour cell surface. Antibody is broken down in the tumour environment and radionuclide is released. Iodine isotopes tend to be released rapidly into the circulation and excreted while others such as yttrium are retained in tumour or normal cells. Therapeutic effect depends on production of DNA strand breaks, on the rate of DNA repair (which influences the balance of cell survival and cell death), and on the rate of tumour cell proliferation.

Clinical trials in lymphoma

Press et al.[24] treated 21 patients with refractory B cell lymphomas with maximal doses of ^{131}I anti-CD20 antibody and gave autologous stem cell support for the resulting bone marrow suppression; 18 patients responded and 16 had complete responses. Progression-free survival was 62 per cent after a median of 2 years. This raises the possibility that some of the patients are cured. The results are remarkable considering that the patients' tumours had progressed after multiple conventional therapies, and illustrate the potential of radioimmunotherapy.

DeNardo and colleagues[25] used ^{131}I-labelled, and later [67]Cu-labelled, Lym-1 antibody to produce responses in more than 50 per cent of patients without the high levels of radioactivity administered by Press,[24] thus avoiding stem cell or bone marrow transplantation. Similar results have been reported by other groups using anti-CD20 antibody in B cell lymphomas,[26] anti-CD25 (Il2 receptor) in T cell tumours,[27] and antiferritin antibody in Hodgkin's disease.[28] Sustained, complete responses were less frequent than with the high-dose approach of Press.

Clinical trials in common carcinomas

Tumour localization of radiolabelled antitumour antibodies is readily shown in common epithelial malignancies. Responses in phase I and II trials are reported in colorectal carcinoma,[29] breast carcinoma,[30] hepatocellular carcinoma,[31] and melanoma.[32] Response rates for radioimmunotherapy alone are in the range of 5 to 40 per cent, justifying further studies.

Intraperitoneal therapy for ovarian carcinoma delivers higher local doses than systemic therapy. A case–control study showed survival benefit in patients with minimal tumour bulk given ^{90}Y antibody to MUC-1 mucin.[33] Bias may affect this trial design and a randomized phase III trial is in progress. Therapy of gliomas by injection of radiolabelled antibody into the cavity formed after surgery has given about 20 per cent responses in phase II studies.[34]

Immunotoxins

Plant or bacterial toxins such as ricin and pseudomonas exotoxin have great potency, causing cell death through inhibition of ribosomal elongation and, thereby, inhibiting protein synthesis. These toxins possess cell binding and internalization domains, which are replaced in immunotoxins by antibodies causing internalization selectively in tumour cells. High levels of selectivity between target-bearing tumour cells and other cells are seen in tissue culture systems. The great potency of toxins means that only a few molecules of immunotoxin need to be internalized in each tumour cell. However, there is no bystander effect, and high specificity is required to avoid toxicity to normal tissues.

Amlot et al.[35] reported 25 per cent responses to anti-CD19-ricin A chain immunoconjugate in patients with lymphoma resistant to conventional therapy. This and other studies with the first generation of immunotoxins produced toxicity which inhibited their further use.[36] The vascular leak syndrome is a serious, and occasionally fatal, complication putatively caused by internalization of immunotoxins in vascular endothelial cells.

Recombinant immunotoxins[37] appear to have greater promise. Studies of the molecular structure of pseudomonas exotoxin have made it possible to select those parts concerned with intracellular translocation to ribosomes and with inhibition of protein synthesis. Whole antibodies have been replaced by disulphide-linked Fv (dsFv) antibodies to generate a genetic fusion protein incorporating antibody and toxin functions. Clinical trials of these agents are in progress.

The immunogenicity of plant or bacterial toxins limits their potential for repeated therapy. Human ribonucleases provide a possible alternative to plant toxins; they have high potency and are probably less immunogenic.[38]

Antibody–cytotoxic drug conjugates

Initial attempts to improve the therapeutic ratio of cytotoxic drugs in general use by linking them to antitumour antibodies were unsuccessful because of the low potency of cytotoxic drugs and the limited number of drug molecules that could be targeted to a cancer cell.

Calicheamicin $\gamma 1$, an ene-diyne antibiotic, binds in the minor groove of DNA and has potency comparable to plant toxins.[39],[40] Phase II and III trials are in progress of calicheamicin linked to humanised anti-CD33 antibody for treatment of acute myeloid leukaemia and anti-MUC-1 antibody for treatment of ovarian cancer.

Potential for cure of established cancer

To have a prospect of eradicating human cancer, therapy should destroy all cancer cells capable of replicating. The activation of natural effector mechanisms at the site of antigen/antibody interaction appears to have this potential. Although antibodies with good levels of specificity have been investigated, it is only in the adjuvant setting that cures have been achieved. More potent therapy is needed for established tumours. Targeted toxins, enzymes, and cytotoxic drugs have the potency and potential for high selectivity because they are only effective against cells in which they are internalized. This is, however, a limitation because internalization into a whole population of tumour cells is rarely, if ever, possible due to variations in tumour antigen expression and in penetration within tumour masses.

Clinical experience is consistent with these concepts. 17–1A antibody (Panorex) appears to be effective in adjuvant therapy of colorectal cancer, but has minimal effects against overt metastatic disease. Mabthera produces remissions but not cures in B cell lymphomas and preliminary data with anti-CD33-calicheamicin suggests that it will reduce the tumour burden in acute myeloid leukaemia without cure.

As described in above, a bystander effect whereby antibody-targeted therapy could kill cells in the immediate neighbourhood of those targeted might also cure cancer.

Pretargeting systems

Systemic targeted therapy is often limited by toxicity, thus preventing sufficient therapeutic agent from being delivered to the tumour to cure it. Antibody fragments achieve higher ratios in tumour as compared to normal tissue than whole antibody, but with lower absolute tumour levels. Two-stage or pretargeting systems give higher relative concentrations in tumour than single-step targeting, making this a promising strategy for improving therapeutic ratio.

The first component, typically an antibody linked to a molecule which is not toxic in its own right, is given intravenously and concentrates in the tumour. This first component clears from the circulation, sometimes accelerated by a clearing agent. When tumour to normal tissue ratios of the first component are high, a therapeutic component is given which is bound or activated by reaction with the first component. This gives a high concentration of the therapeutic agent in the tumour with lower levels in normal tissues.

Avidin–biotin systems

Magnani et al.[41] compared direct antibody targeting with a three-phase pretargeting system based on an antitumour antibody linked to biotin, followed by administration of avidin which binds strongly to biotin, with radiolabelled biotin providing the third and therapeutic step. In patients having enucleation of the eye for uveal melanoma, they showed a mean tumour to normal tissue ratio of 3.1:1 with the pretargeting system and 1.5:1 with the direct targeting system. For a review of avidin/biotin pretargeting see Stoldt et al.[42]

Radionuclide capture

Antibodies targeting agents which are reactive with therapeutic radionuclides such as [90]yttrium, given as a second step, and antibodies targeting oligonucleotides with no tumour specificity, with complementary antisense oligonucleotides labelled with [125]iodine as the second step, are examples of radionuclide capture systems (reviewed by Goodwin and Meares).[43]

Antibody-directed enzyme prodrug therapy (ADEPT)

ADEPT uses the principle of pretargeting but augments the therapeutic effect by targeting an enzyme. Each molecule of enzyme then has the ability to activate many molecules of cytotoxic drug in the cancer[44],[45] (Fig. 7).

An antibody directed against a tumour-associated antigen is linked to an enzyme and given intravenously, resulting in selective accumulation of enzyme in the tumour. When the discrimination between tumour and normal tissue enzyme levels is sufficient, a prodrug is given intravenously which is converted to an active cytotoxic drug by enzyme within the tumour. This gives higher tumour to normal tissue ratios at the time when therapy is given than can be achieved with direct tumour targeting. Several enzyme and prodrug systems have been investigated (for review see Bagshawe).[46]

Demonstration that such a complex system can be developed for clinical use requires evidence that each of the components of ADEPT functions by the mechanisms proposed. This can be provided by measuring antibody–enzyme conjugate concentration, enzyme activity, and prodrug and drug levels in the tumour and in normal tissues.[47] Patients with colorectal carcinoma expressing carcinoembryonic antigen (CEA) received ADEPT with antibody to CEA conjugated to the enzyme carboxypeptidase G2 (CPG2). A galactosylated antibody directed against the active site of CPG2 was then used to clear and inactivate circulating enzyme. A benzoic acid

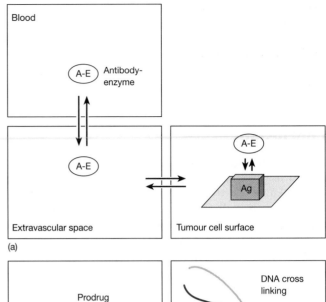

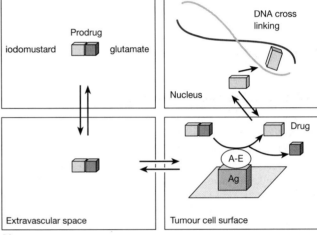

Fig. 7 ADEPT. (a) First phase; (b) second phase; compartment model for tumour.

mustard–glutamate prodrug was given when plasma enzyme levels had fallen to a predetermined safe level and this was converted by CPG2 in the tumour into a cytotoxic benzoic acid mustard.

Tumour selectivity was shown with high tumour to blood ratio of enzyme at the time of prodrug administration. Enzyme concentrations in tumour were sufficient to generate cytotoxic levels of active drug. Prodrug was present at levels necessary for activation to generate cytotoxic levels of active drug.[48] There was evidence of tumour response in colorectal cancer.[45] An improved prodrug[49] and a genetic fusion protein of a single chain Fv and carboxypeptidase are being investigated.[50]

Bispecific antibodies

Bispecific antibodies with specificities for two different antigens, such as a tumour antigen and an effector molecule, have been produced.[51],[52] These may recruit natural effector mechanisms such as cytotoxic or phagocytosing cells, complement components, and cytokines as well as artificial effector functions such as toxins, prodrug converting enzymes, and radionuclides.[53]–[55] Bispecific diabodies are composed of two ScFvs each bearing the variable heavy chain specific for one antigen and the variable light chain for another; together the two ScFvs exhibit both specificities. These are produced in bacteria and can recruit a variety of effector functions such as immunoglobulins, C1q complement, and effector cells such as cytotoxic T cells to tumour cells.[56]–[60]

Conclusions

Lymphoma, breast, and colon cancer can be treated effectively by targeted therapies in some circumstances. Effective cell killing has been shown with targeted activation of natural effector mechanisms, with actions on cell growth control, and with toxicity from radionuclides, toxins, and cytotoxic drugs. Eradication of common cancers remains a challenge but the high specificity and potency of pretargeting and multiple phase treatments gives a prospect of more effective therapies than those in routine use.

References

1. Hericourt J, Richet C. De la serotherapie dans le traitment du cancer. *Comptes Rendus de l'Academie des Sciences (Paris)*, 1895; **121**: 567–9.

2. Boshoff C, Begent RHJ. Tumour markers. In: Taylor I, Cooke TG, Guillou P, eds. *Essential general surgical oncology*. Edinburgh: Churchill Livingstone, 1996: 131–40.

3. Kohler G, Milstein C. Continuous cultures of fused cells secreting antibody of predefined specificity. *Nature*, 1975; **256**: 495–7.

4. Chester KA, Hawkins RE. Clinical issues in antibody design. *Trends in Biotechnology*, 1995; **13**: 294–300.

5. Lane DP, Stephen CW. Epitope mapping using bacteriophage peptide libraries. *Current Opinion in Immunology*, 1993; **5**: 268–71.

6. Flynn AA, Green AJ, Boxer GM, Casey JL, Pedley RB, Begent RHJ. A novel technique, using radioluminography, for the measurement of uniformity of radiolabelled antibody distribution in a colorectal cancer xenograft model. *International Journal of Radiation Oncology Biology Physics*, 1999; **43**: 183–9.

7. Harrison M, Tomlinson D, Stewart S. Liposomal-entrapped doxorubicin: an active agent in AIDS-related Kaposi's sarcoma. *Journal of Clinical Oncology*, 1995; **13**: 914–20.

8. Huse W, *et al.* Generation of a large combinatorial library of the immunological repertoire in phage lambda. *Science*, 1989; **246**: 1275–81.

9. McCafferty J, Griffiths AD, Winter G, Chiswell DJ. Phage antibodies: filamentous phage displaying antibody variable domains. *Nature*, 1990; **348**: 552–4.

10. Chester KA, *et al.* Phage libraries for generation of clinically useful antibodies. *Lancet*, 1994; **343**: 455–6.

11. Pedley RB. Pharmacokinetics of monoclonal antibodies. Implications for their use in cancer therapy. *Clinical Immunotherapy*, 1996; **6**: 54–67.

12. Huston JS, *et al.* Protein engineering of antibody binding sites: recovery of specific activity in an anti-digoxin single chain Fv analogue produced in Eschericia coli. *Proceedings of the National Academy of Science, USA.* 1988; **85**: 5879–83.

13. Begent RHJ, *et al.* Clinical evidence of efficient tumor targeting based on single-chain Fv antibody selected from a combinatorial library. *Nature Medicine*, 1996; **2**: 979–84.

14. Begent RHJ, *et al.* Liposomally entrapped second antibody improves tumour imaging with radiolabelled (first) antitumour antibody. *Lancet*, 1982; **ii**: 739–42.

15. Begent RHJ, *et al.* Antibody distribution and dosimetry in patients receiving radiolabelled antibody therapy for colorectal cancer. *British Journal of Cancer*, 1989; **60**: 406–12.

16. King DJ, *et al.* Improved tumour targeting with chemically cross-linked recombinant antibody fragments. *Cancer Research*, 1994; **54**: 6176–85.

17. Pedley RB, Boden JA, Boden R, Begent RHJ. Ablation of colorectal xenografts with combined radioimmunotherapy and tumor blood flow-modifying agents. *Cancer Research*, 1996; **56**: 3293–300.

18. Riechmann L, Clark M, Waldman H, Winter G. Reshaping human antibodies for therapy. *Nature*, 1988; **332**: 323–7.

19. Baselga J, *et al.* Phase II study of weekly intravenous recombinant humanised anti-p185HER2 monoclonal antibody in patients with HER2/neu overexpressing metastatic breast cancer. *Journal of Clinical Oncology*, 1996; **14**: 737–44.

20. Pegram MD, *et al.* Phase II study of receptor-enhanced chemosensitivity using recombinant humanised anti-p185HER2/new monoclonal antibody plus cisplatin in patients. *Journal of Clinical Oncology*, 1998; **16**: 2659–71.

21. Riethmuller G, *et al.* Monoclonal antibody therapy for resected Duke's C colorectal cancer: Seven year outcome of a randomised controlled trial. *Journal of Clinical Oncology*, 1998; **16**: 1788–94.

22. Maloney DG, *et al.* IDEC-C2B8 (Rituximab)anti-CD20 monoclonal antibody therapy in patients with relapsed low grade non-Hodgkin's lymphoma. *Blood*, 1997; **90**: 2188–95.

23. Baselga J, Norton L, Albanell J, Kim YM, Mandelson J. Recombinant humanized antiHER2 antibody (Herceptin) enhances the antitumour activity of paclitaxel and doxirubicin against HER2-neu overexpressing human breast cancer xenografts. *Cancer Research*, 1998; **58**: 2825–31.

24. Press OW, *et al.* Phase II trial of 131I-1-B1 (anti-CD20) antibody therapy with autologous stem cell transplantation for relapsed B cell lymphomas. *Lancet*, 1995; **346**: 336–40.

25. Lewis JP, DeNardo GL, DeNardo SJ. Radioimmunotherapy of lymphoma: a UC Davis experience. *Hybridoma*, 1995; **14**: 115–20.

26. Kaminski MS, *et al.* Iodine-131-anti-B1 radioimmunotherapy for B cell lymphoma. *Journal of Oncology*, 1996; **14**: 1974–81.

27. Waldmann TA, White JD, Carrasquillo JA, Radioimmunotherapy of interleukin2 Rx-expressing adult T-cell leukaemia with yttrium-90 labelled anti-tac. *Blood*, 1995; **86**: 4063–75.

28. Vriesendorp HM, Herpst JM, Germack MA. Phase I-II studies of yttrium-labelled anti-ferritin treatment for advanced Hodgkin's disease including radiation therapy oncology group 87–01. *Journal of Clinical Oncology*, 1991; **9**: 918–28.

29. Lane DM, *et al.* Radioimmunotherapy of metastatic colorectal tumours with iodine-131-labelled antibody to carcinoembryonic antigen: phase i/ii study with comparative biodistribution of intact and f(ab')-2 antibodies. *British Journal of Cancer*, 1994; **70**: 521–5.

30. DeNardo SJ, Mirick JR, Kroger LA. The biologic window of chimeric L.6 radioimmunotherapy. *Cancer*, 1994; **73**: 1023–32.

31. Order SE, *et al.* A randomised prospective trial comparing full dose chemotherapy to 131-I antiferritin: an RTOG study. *International Journal of Radiation, Biology, Physics*, 1991; **20**: 953–63.

32. Carrasquillo JA, Krohn KA, Beumier P. Diagnosis and therapy for solid tumours with radiolabelled antibodies and immune fragments. *Cancer Treatment Reports*, 1984; **68**: 317–28.

33. Hird V, Maraveyas A, Snook D, Epenetos AA. Adjuvant therapy of ovarian cancer with radioactive monoclonal antibody. *British Journal of Cancer*, 1991; **68**: 403–6.

34. Riva P, Fanceschi G, Arista A, Fraterelli M, Riva N, Cremonini A-M, Giuliani G, Casi M. Local application of radiolabelled monoclonal antibodies in the treatment of high grade malignant gliomas: A six year clinical experience. *Cancer*, 1997; **80** (Suppl.12): 2733–42.

35. Amlot PL, *et al.* A phase I study of an anti-CD22-deglycosylated A

chain immunotoxin in the treatment of B cell lymphomas resistant to conventional therapy. *Blood*, 1993; **82**: 2624–33.

36. Vitetta ES. From the basic science of B cells to biological missiles at the bedside. *Journal of Immunology*, 1994; **153**: 1407–20.

37. Reiter Y, Pastan I. Recombinant Fv immunotoxins and Fv fragments as novel agents for cancer therapy and diagnosis. *Trends in Biotechnology*, 1998; **16**: 513–20.

38. Zewe E, *et al.* Cloning and cytotoxicity of a human pancreatic RNase immunofusion. *Immunotechnology*, 1997; **3**: 127–36.

39. Lee MD, Dunne TM, Chang CC, Morton TO, Borders DB. Calicheamicins, a novel family of antibiotics. 1. Chemistry and partial characterisation. *Journal of the American Chemical Society*, 1987; **109**: 3464–6.

40. Zein N, Poncin M, Nilakantan R, Ellestad G. Calicheamicin γ1 and DNA: molecular recognition process responsible for site-specificity. *Science*, 1989; **244**: 697–9.

41. Magnani P, *et al.* Quantitative comparison of direct antibody labelling, and tumour pretargeting in uveal melanoma. *Journal of Nuclear Medicine*, 1996; **37**: 967–71.

42. Stoldt HS, *et al.* Pretargeting strategies for radioimmunoguided tumour localisation and therapy. *European Journal of Cancer*, 1997; **33**: 186–92.

43. Goodwin DA, Meares CF. Pretargeting. *Cancer, Supplement*, 1997; **80** (Suppl. 12):2675–80.

44. Bagshawe KD, *et al.* A cytotoxic agent can be generated selectively at cancer sites. *British Journal of Cancer*, 1988; **58**: 700.

45. Bagshawe KD, Sharma SK, Springer CJ, Antoniw P. Antibody directed enzyme prodrug therapy: a pilot-scale clinical trial. *Tumour Targeting*, 1995; **1**: 17–30.

46. Bagshawe KD. Developments with targeted enzymes. *Tumour Targeting*, 1998; **3**: 21–4.

47. Begent RHJ, Bagshawe KD. Biodistribution studies. *Advanced Drug Delivery Reviews*, 1996; **22**: 325–9.

48. Martin J, *et al.* Antibody-directed enzyme prodrug therapy: pharmacokinetics and plasma levels of prodrug and drug in a phase 1 clinical trial. *Cancer Chemotherapy and Pharmacology*, 1997; **40**: 189–201.

49. Blakey DC, *et al.* ZD2767, an improved system for antibody-directed enzyme prodrug therapy that results in tumor regressions in human colorectal tumor xenografts. *Cancer Research*, 1996; **56**: 3287–92.

50. Michael NP, *et al.* In vitro and *in vivo* characterisation of a recombinant carboxypeptidase G$_2$::anti-CEA scFv fusion protein. *Immunotechnology*, 1996; **2**: 47–57.

51. Fanger MW, Morganelli PM, Guyre PM. Bispecific antibodies. *Critical Reviews in Immunology*, 1992; **12**: 101–24.

52. van der Winkel JGJ, Bast B, deGast GC. Immunotherapeutic potential of bispecific antibodies. *Immunology Today*, 1997; **18**: 562–4.

53. Konterman RE, Wing MG, Winter G. Complement recruitment using bispecific antibodies. *Nature Biotechnology*, 1997; **15**: 629–32.

54. Bonardi MA, *et al.* Delivery of saporin to human B-cell lymphoma using bispecific antibody: targeting via CD22, but not CD19, CD37 or immunoglobulin, results in efficient killing. *Cancer Research*, 1993; **53**: 3015–21.

55. Le Doussal JM, *et al.* Targeting of 111-labelled bivalent hapten to human melanoma mediated by bispecific monoclonal antibody conjugates: imaging of tumours hosted in nude mice. *Cancer Research*, 1990; **50**: 3445–52.

56. Holliger P, Prospero TD, Winter G. Diabodies, small bivalent and bispecific antibody fragments. *Proceedings of the National Academy of Science, USA*, 1993; **90**: 6444–8.

57. Holliger P. Specific killing of lymphoma cells by cytotoxic T-cells mediated by bispecific diabody. *Protein Engineering*, 1996; **9**: 299–305.

58. Holliger P. Pretargeting serum immunoglobulins with bispecific antibodies. *Nature Biotechnology*, 1997; **14**: 192–6.

59. Fitzgerald, Holliger P, Winter G. Improved tumour targeting by disulphide stabilised diabodies expressed in Pichea pastoris. *Protein Engineering*, 1997; **10**: 1221–5.

60. Krebs B, *et al.* Recombinant human single chain Fv antibodies: recognising human interleukin-6. Specific targeting of cytokine secreting cells. *Journal of Biological Chemistry*, 1998; **273**: 2858–65.

4.28 Cancer in the elderly: principles of treatment

D. Raghavan, Jonathan Weiner, and Loren Lipson

Introduction

During the twentieth century, the proportion of the population older than 65 to 70 years has increased dramatically, the so-called 'ageing imperative'. For example, in 1900, there were 3.1 million Americans over the age of 65 years, representing 4 per cent of the population. By contrast, in 1994, 33.2 million people were aged more than 65 years, representing more than 12 per cent of the community, and figures in excess of 15 per cent of the community have been projected.[1]–[3] Moreover, nearly 30 per cent of health resources are consumed by this group.

As the aged population is increasing and because the prevalence of malignancy rises with age, it is clear that the management of cancer in the elderly will occupy a much greater proportion of health expenditure in the future. The active life expectancy of the elderly, a figure representing the period during which the older population can expect to lead self-caring, active, and relatively normal lives, has increased this century. Patients aged 65 and 70 years can expect an active life of more than 10 and 8 years, respectively,[4],[5] and this figure appears to be increasing. In patients aged 80 years and above, cancer is the second most common cause of death in both men and women, exceeded only by heart disease.[6] Thus the potential benefits of a rational and carefully planned approach to cancer care in the elderly are self-evident. It is becoming increasingly important to define clearly the extent of clinical activity or aggression that should be employed in this group of patients, the level of health resources that should be expended in their care, and the philosophical and ethical considerations that will govern such approaches.

The ageing human body undergoes many physiological changes and functions of all organ systems are irreversibly altered. It appears that organ dysfunction occurs via two pathways. There is a slowly evolving dysfunction related to an independent biological clock, and a second impairment of function that relates to specific organic disease. Ageing alters the ability of the human body to adapt to illness as well as to any treatment. This has direct relevance to the development of cancer as well as in the complexity of treatment.

Biology of ageing

Theories of ageing

There are many causes for the ageing process and many theories to explain why we age. With the advent of molecular biology, many scientific theories have been rationalized, but also relevance to cancer development and treatment has been established, reflecting the interplay of stimuli that lead to genetic instability, finite replicative function, telomeric stabilization, and the expression/ deletion of suppressor genes, such as p53. It is likely that no sole theory will define the basis for ageing and the inter-relationship with carcinogenesis, although these issues have been reviewed in detail elsewhere.[7]

The error theory

Orgel proposed the 'error theory' in 1963, based on the genetic code. As transcription takes place and proteins are created, small errors take place at every step. For example in a healthy cellular system, if tRNA produces an incorrect amino acid sequence, corrections are made. If not properly corrected, the resulting protein may have minor changes in function. If this protein aids in the production of other proteins, the errors can become compounded. In addition, as a cell ages, the chances of error increase and the erroneous proteins will eventually result in permanent alterations in the intracellular and extracellular function of the protein. This may even cause cell death.[8],[9] It has since been shown that ageing cells do not necessarily contain erroneous proteins, and if erroneous proteins are introduced into a cell, the cell does not age prematurely. Other theories on ageing are built around the genetic code. For example Von Hahn (1970) suggested that errors at the DNA level might cause ageing in a way similar to the 'error theory'.[10]

The free radical theory

During a chemical reaction, there may be a transient presence of a highly reactive intermediate (a free radical) with an unpaired electron.[10] Free radicals originate mainly from oxidation and can accumulate over time.[11] Harman, in 1956,[12] proposed that free radicals are involved in the process of ageing—as a result of free radical accumulation cellular function decreases and cell death eventually follows. Collagen and elastin are two major tissue proteins affected by free radical formation during ageing. Studies involving the addition of antioxidants either to animals or to cells in culture, however, have not shown decreases in mortality.[13]

The Hayflick model of ageing

Based on the observation that human diploid fibroblasts would double only a finite number of times, a third theory of ageing has developed. Despite an ability of the remaining cells to continue to survive for several months, they will not continue to divide beyond approximately 50 doublings.[14] It is still believed that if the reason for this cessation of cellular turnover is understood, the basis of ageing may be clarified.

Later research by Hayflick and others has continued to support this finding. Hybrids between elderly human diploid fibroblasts and immortalized cell lines still have shown a finite division potential.[15] The manipulation of DNA synthesis and mitogenic growth was successful in altering this finite potential, but no true mechanism was identified.

More recently, the clarification of the role of telomeres in ageing have cast further light on this intriguing issue, supporting the concepts of Hayflick. The ends of eukaryotic chromosomes have repetitive DNA sequences ('telomeres') which function to maintain stability of the chromosomes. Chromosomes without telomeres are unstable and can break and fuse,[16] with consequent loss of genetic material. If this cycle is repeated, there would be a progressive shortening of the chromosomes in replication. Telomerase is an enzyme that adds new telomeric sequences to chromosomal ends, overcoming the problem.[17] There is considerable evidence that telomeres may be involved in the process of ageing, via sequential loss of chromosomal material with replication.[18] Human somatic cells show loss of telomeres and have low telomerase activity with ageing,[17] whereas immortalized cells and cancer cells often have high telomerase activity and do not show shortening of telomeric structures.[19]

Specific organ systems

The elderly undergo age-related changes in their physiology, which may result in altered tolerance to disease and to the requirements of the management of illness. One of the most important physiological changes to occur with ageing is a diminution of physiological reserves, characterized by a generalized decline in the ability to respond to physiological insults and a slower recovery from them.[20] These alterations in physiology occur in the absence of disease and simply reflect the phenomenon of ageing, although they may be substantially exacerbated by intercurrent illness. Accordingly, it is relevant to discuss the specifics of ageing as they relate to function of the various organ systems.

Cardiovascular system

Cardiovascular disease is the most common cause of death in the elderly population, either because of the natural process of ageing or because of disease. Ageing may be associated with loss of cardiac muscle fibres from ischaemia or degenerative disorders or with ventricular hypertrophy. Cardiac output reduces by approximately 1 per cent each year between the ages of 25 and 80 years.[21] With increasing age, the heart rate decreases. Peripheral factors such as the decrease in muscle mass and the increase in body fat contribute to a decrease in tissue oxygen delivery. As a result, there is a reduction in the perfusion of the kidneys, liver, lungs, gastrointestinal tract, and skeletal muscle, although compensatory mechanisms retain blood flow to the brain and heart.

In addition, as the elderly body exercises, responses in cardiac output occur more slowly and the demand on the heart is tolerated less well. Although many studies have shown a decrease in left ventricular compliance with ageing, there has been scanty comparable information from healthy seniors. Arterial stiffening has been shown to occur in ageing, irrespective of disease, and has been associated with the elevations in peripheral vascular resistance seen in the elderly. At rest, the ejection fraction of the heart, and thus the cardiac output, is not altered in ageing of healthy adults. These issues are of particular

importance when the elderly body is stressed by cancer therapy, such as the added physiological requirements for surgery, or if cardiotoxic agents, such as the anthracyclines or anthraquinones, are used. Furthermore, the recent introduction of the taxanes, which may be associated with cardiac rhythm disorders, may stress the aged heart sufficiently to cause cardiac decompensation unexpectedly, sometimes when the resting ejection fraction appears normal. Cardiac failure may even be precipitated by a fluid load, such as that required for the use of cisplatin.

Renal function

As people age, their renal mass shrinks. A normal kidney weighs 150 to 200 g at age 30, while by age 90, the average is 110 to 150 g.[22] There is an associated reduction in glomerular number, number of functioning nephrons, and cortical volume.[23]

The renal blood flow is reduced to a greater extent than would be predicted solely on the basis of reduced cardiac output[24] and probably reflects glomerular sclerosis. A young adult may have renal blood flow of 600 ml/min, while an octogenarian will have half that rate.[25] The glomerular filtration rate consequently decreases with advancing age.[26] With increased age, the kidney is less able to concentrate urine maximally[27] and the consequent increased flow of dilute urine may, in fact, decrease the contact time of potential tubular toxins.[28] Furthermore, in the elderly, a substantial decrease in lean muscle mass results in reduced creatinine excretion. This reduction, and the decrease in creatinine clearance with ageing, may not necessarily be reflected by a rise of serum creatinine, which may thus be a misleading index of renal function in the aged,[29] particularly important when considering the use of potentially nephrotoxic agents, such as cisplatin and methotrexate.

In addition, parenchymal functions, such as acid–base regulation, electrolyte balance, and water homeostasis, are similarly hampered,[30] and the situation may be exacerbated by age-related intercurrent disease. In the medical management of this age group, renal function and drug levels of medications must be followed closely. In addition, chemotherapy must be tailored with these limitations in mind.

Hepatic and gastrointestinal function

The gastrointestinal tract undergoes many age-related changes. Age related disease in the autonomic nervous system reduces the motility of the entire gastrointestinal tract.[31] Oesophageal peristalsis is impaired in old age,[32] gastric emptying is slowed,[33] and there is a reduction in gastric acid secretion and in the number of functional absorbing cells. As a result, there are significant changes in absorption of many orally administered agents (e.g. methotrexate), and there may be an exacerbation of the complications (e.g. constipation) of analgesics.

The liver gradually decreases in size with ageing. Before age 50, the liver accounts for about 2.5 per cent of total body weight, but by age 90, it accounts for about 1.6 per cent of total body weight.[34] Liver blood flow also appears to decrease.[23] In addition, there may be a reduced capacity for repair of hepatic damage.[35] As a result, there are significant changes in hepatic enzyme function, with consequent reduction in the metabolism of many medications, including cytotoxics that may require activation or breakdown in the liver. However, these changes are somewhat unpredictable and are heavily influenced by intercurrent disease. For example the functions of acetylation and conjugation do not usually change with age, whereas the function of the microsomal oxidative enzymes is reduced in the aged.

Respiratory system

There are several age-related changes in pulmonary function, which contribute to ventilation–perfusion mismatch and a consequent reduction in respiratory function. The most important disorder in the lung, related to ageing, is a decrease in arterial partial pressure of oxygen (PaO_2). As humans age, elastic recoil of the lung decreases, the chest wall becomes stiffer, the inspiratory muscles lose strength, the respiratory centre in the brain becomes less sensitive to $PaCO_2$, and the blood flow to the lungs falls due to an overall decrease in cardiac output. The result is an increase in residual volume, residual capacity, and a decrease in vital capacity and FEV_1.[36] The pulmonary diffusing capacity decreases with age because of a loss of capillary segments in the lung, deranged ventilation-perfusion ratios, and a reduced cardiac output.

In addition to these normal accommodations of age, a large percentage of the elderly suffer from chronic obstructive airways disease and asthma, adding to the aged-related changes. Compounded by decreases in immune function, blood flow, and ventilation, patients with mild pulmonary insults in the older age groups often have poor clinical outcomes when subjected to physiological stresses. Particular caution must thus be exercised when considering the use of chemotherapy with known pulmonary toxicity, such as bleomycin or busulfan.

Haemopoiesis and immunity

Although it has been reported that the bone marrow progressively involutes in distribution and cellularity with increasing age,[37] this issue remains controversial. It is not clear whether age-related changes are a function of normal physiology, or are due to maturity-onset disease processes. In mice, a range of haematopoietic alterations occur with ageing, including reduced marrow reserve, decreased cytokine production, increased chromosomal abnormalities, and increased differentiation of stem cells. Much of the published literature is somewhat unclear, with overlap of murine and human data, and with a relative paucity of specific human studies.

The elderly population responds less well to haematological stressors. Anaemia occurs commonly in elderly males,[38] although much of this may be due to a dilutional effect from the increasing proportion of extracellular fluid[39] or may be from a nutritional deficit. However, there is also a slight reduction in stem cell function with a consequent decline in the circulating haemoglobin level after 70 years of age.[40]

In the elderly, both the neutrophil count and neutrophil function remain stable,[41] but there is a reduction in the number of peripheral blood lymphocytes,[42] which may contribute to the reduced immune function of the aged. There is an overall reduction of cell-mediated and humoral immune responses to foreign antigens in the aged, while the responses to self-antigens are increased.[43] The reduced cell-mediated immunity is partly a result of the thymic involution of ageing, but may be influenced by the poor nutrition that is often characteristic of the elderly. There is also a reduction in the antibody response to antigenic stimulation in the elderly.[44] An age-specific decline observed in T-cell function has been attributed to defective interleukin-2 (IL-2) production and responsiveness.

Ershler[45] has suggested that IL-6, a multifunctional protein that acts on haemopoietic, lymphopoietic, and bone tissue, may be one of the most important cytokines among aged populations. He has proposed that, in view of its protean effects on several organ systems, as well as its increased circulating levels with ageing, this protein may be fundamental to ageing.

Nervous system

Natural changes occur in ageing which affect cognition, language, speech, and general conceptual thought.[46] After the age of approximately 25 years, there is progressive loss of neuronal tissue in the central nervous system. Although the consumption of glucose and oxygen is not reduced at rest in the aged brain, sensory stimulation results in smaller increments in metabolic activity with advancing age, suggesting a limited ability of the central nervous system to adapt to stress in old age.[47] As this increases, there are progressive changes in behavioural patterns and reductions in cognitive function. These changes can affect the patient's ability to process information as well as to communicate. If these changes are substantial, they can result in feelings of detachment and isolation. In addition to these changes, patients can develop dementia and delirium, and it has been estimated that up to one-third of patients over the age of 85 years have some degree of dementia.[48]

Acute neurological insult can often affect cognitive ability, but in seniors this change can result from a minor insult. Minor insults such as sleep loss, psychological stress, and sensory changes have all been shown to cause delirium in seniors.[49] Delirium resulting from medications is often missed as a diagnosis, despite the frequency of cognitive changes in the hospital setting. Lastly, it is not uncommon for the only manifestation of electrolyte abnormalities, central nervous system infection, or neoplasm to be delirium.[50] It is crucial for optimal cancer management in the elderly to include neuropsychiatric monitoring and sensitivity to changes in mental status.

Depression, which can be found in all age groups, can cause change in cognition and functional status. The predominant form found in younger patients, however, is major depression. The elderly more commonly have situational depression, which can be present due to concern over impending death, affects of chronic illness or chronic pain, bereavement, loss of autonomy or control, and financial problems (see Chapter 6.1); it thus has a particular impact in the context of the elderly patient with cancer. In addition, suicide rates have been correlated with age, although there is little specific information regarding suicide in elderly patients with cancer. As the specific mechanisms for depression in the elderly are unknown, the interactions with the pathophysiology and treatment of cancer have not yet been well defined.

In addition to the central nervous system changes, there is a progressive reduction in peripheral neuronal function with increased age, a situation which is often compounded by intercurrent disorders such as malnutrition, diabetes, or alcohol abuse. This can be of particular importance in cancer management as many chemotherapeutic agents cause peripheral nerve damage, and these problems can be compounded in the healthy senior, and may be even worse in the older patient with intercurrent disease.

Metabolic and nutritional changes

A broad range of other biochemical and physiological changes occur as part of the ageing process. The ageing process is characterized by a slowing of protein synthesis and degradation, sometimes with an accumulation of altered proteins that may be a function of reduced transcriptional or translational accuracy.[51] For example there is impairment in the induction of glucose-metabolizing enzymes with age, accompanied by increased peripheral insulin resistance. There is a progressive reduction of lean body mass, with replacement by fat or adipose tissue with increasing age.[52] These issues may be compounded by the nutritional state of the patient as malnutrition is a frequent concomitant of ageing for a range of reasons,[53] in association with poverty and depression.

An understanding of nutritional requirements is crucial for treating the elderly with cancer. Up to 15 per cent of ambulant geriatric patients and 35 to 65 per cent of elderly inpatients show evidence of malnutrition.[50] For example the loss of lean body mass may result in a decline of energy requirements. Fat soluble vitamins, such as vitamin A, are taken up by peripheral tissues in older persons at a slower rate. Therefore tissues can be damaged by vitamin A deficiency, despite elevated serum levels. Vitamin D levels can also be low due to decreases in renal plasma blood flow as well as due to a decreased ability of the skin in the elderly to convert vitamin D.[54] Many vitamins can be lacking in the elderly and can result in a broad range of specific syndromes. There is a misconception that the aged have lower nutritional requirements than younger populations, but it is important to note that current recommended dietary allowances do not acknowledge any such difference, recommending common dietary intake for all patients over the age of 51 years.[55] Although the details are beyond the scope of this chapter, it is clear that the elderly patient with cancer presents important nutritional challenges, and optimal management requires specific attention to nutritional assessment and replacement of deficient nutrients, especially for the cancer patient on active treatment. This can best be achieved by the provision of multidisciplinary specialist care for the elderly cancer patient, involving careful interaction of oncologists, geriatricians, and nursing, nutritional, and social service professionals.

The biology of cancer in the elderly

Epidemiological aspects

In Western society, more than 50 per cent of cancer occurs in only 15 per cent of the community, those over 65 to 70 years of age.[55]–[57] It has been estimated that a man aged 65 years has 50 times the probability of developing cancer in the next 5 years as a man aged 25 years.[58] As shown in Table 1, there is an illusion that cancer is predominantly a disease of late middle age and not of the elderly. However, if reduced population numbers over the age of 70 years are taken into consideration, it is clear that the absolute age-specific cancer incidence and mortality continue to rise as a function of age[57],[58] (see also Chapter 2.4). This, in turn, explains why this issue is of such importance to future health planning, with the evolution of ageing 'baby boomers' into a dominant section of the population in the early twenty-first century.

Associations between cancer and ageing

The basis of the association between malignancy and ageing remains unclear.[58],[59] Possible reasons for the increased prevalence of cancer in the elderly may include: a longer potential duration of exposure to carcinogens, a longer period for expression of outcome from such exposure (e.g. mutations contributing to carcinogenesis), increased susceptibility of aged cells to the effects of carcinogens, reduced ability to repair DNA, reduced host defences, and programmed changes of gene expression during ageing which increase the probability of development of cancer.

Tumour aggression and age

A controversial issue is whether the activity or aggression of malignancy changes with age. Conflicting data have been produced from experimental models[59],[60] and from clinical studies.[60]–[62] In many tumours occurring in older animals, longer survival is seen for those that arise spontaneously, those which are weakly immunogenic, and those under endocrine control.[60] In highly immunogenic tumours (for example sarcomas induced by methylcholanthrene or by ultraviolet irradiation), older animals have a shorter survival.

The optimal index of tumour aggression in the elderly has not been defined. Potential parameters include stage at presentation, histological grade, duration of survival after diagnosis, and anatomical distribution of malignancy at death. However, each of these can be strongly influenced by unrelated factors that cause delayed presentation, altered diagnosis or sampling of sites of disease, and differences in completed therapies.

Some tumours are more advanced at presentation in the elderly. Whether this is a function of increased tumour aggressiveness or is simply a reflection of delayed clinical presentation in the elderly is not clear. Several other factors may influence the duration of survival:[62]–[64] there may be differences in the biology of the tumour, the prevalence of other medical diseases, physical fitness and the ability to withstand treatment, biases among clinicians which influence the treatment actually prescribed, conservatism of the patients with respect to seeking medical care for cancer, and available facilities for treatment.

Data culled from large series of autopsies contrast with much of the published clinical experience. For example, in such studies, cancers of bladder, breast, colorectum, kidney, lung, pancreas, prostate, and uterus have been documented to metastasize less often in the elderly.[65]–[67] However, the apparent distribution of metastases at autopsy may also reflect the aggression of clinical management before death. For example early referral for terminal care (without active intervention) in an elderly patient may be associated with early death from a primary bronchogenic malignancy with insufficient time to develop clinically or histologically evident metastases.

Histological evidence of tumour aggression or indolence *per se* does not generally appear to be a function of age.[68] It has been suggested that indolent patterns of ovarian cancer may be more common in the young, and that more aggressive, and less differentiated mammary carcinomas are a feature of the old. In contrast, there is a trend towards reduced differentiation with increasing age for cancers of the lung, prostate, bladder, and colorectum.[69] It is generally agreed that Hodgkin's disease is more aggressive in the elderly, based upon a more advanced pattern of presentation, a predominance of mixed cellularity histology, and the results of treatment. More recently, sophisticated indices of tumour aggression have been assessed in the elderly, including the measurement of ploidy, S-phase fraction, expression of oncogenes, and growth factors, but without a consistent pattern of age-dependent prognostic implication.[70]

Perhaps the most important ultimate index is survival. However, many of the factors noted above can cause artefacts in the outcome:

Table 1 Age-specific incidence of common cancers in the elderly

Type	Age-specific incidence (per 100 000 population in age group)			
	65–69 years	70–74 years	75–79 years	80+ years
Male				
All sites	1530	2083	2526	3080
Lung	374	485	460	450
Prostate	221	378	558	788
Colon	119	187	235	307
Bladder	117	140	209	241
Rectum	106	111	122	185
Pancreas	48	82	83	105
Stomach	51	114	160	171
Oesophagus	37	33	49	21
Melanoma	58	71	67	87
Lymphoma[a]	34	53	52	56
Female				
All sites	936	1003	1198	1392
Breast	196	183	226	223
Colon	87	139	199	267
Lung	97	103	84	35
Rectum	47	53	70	80
Stomach	30	28	67	120
Pancreas	36	31	50	58
Bladder	35	35	41	47
Ovary	34	44	26	35
Melanoma	42	31	34	35
Uterus body	38	43	41	40
cervix	32	20	14	17

[a] Lymphoma, ICD 200 including lymphosarcoma and reticulum cell sarcoma.

Data from New South Wales Cancer Registry (1986).

death from other comorbid diseases, selection factors of patients and treatment, inaccurate data from death certificates, and changing demographic patterns among the elderly. Although there is no real concordance of published data, it appears that, at least in the context of definitive surgery, there is no difference in outcome between young and old patients treated for bronchogenic or colonic cancer, provided that appropriate surgical precautions for the elderly are applied.[71],[72] In contrast, the Surveillance, Epidemiology, and End Results (SEER) data show a decline in observed 5-year survival for most tumour sites and stages with increasing age in both sexes, although this situation is substantially different if deaths from intercurrent disease are excluded.[73]

Problems of active treatment of cancer in the elderly

Surgical considerations

The major roles for surgical intervention in the elderly patient with cancer include the establishment of a diagnosis and the definitive or palliative treatment of the malignancy. A limited surgical procedure, by establishing the diagnosis quickly, may reduce the length of a hospital stay and its attendant morbidity, in contrast to a prolonged schedule of 'non-invasive' (but often morbid) investigations.

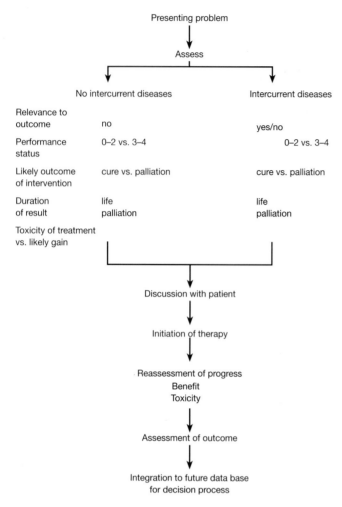

Fig. 1 Flow diagram of decision process in management of cancer in old age.

The decision to operate on the older-aged patient represents a balance between cost and benefit in the clinical context, and these issues are compounded by the implications of the specific cancer under consideration (Fig. 1). As already detailed, patients over the age of 65 years have significant differences in physiological function, characterized most importantly by a reduced reserve against physiological or pathological stress. Such factors as reduced cardiorespiratory function will present increased hazards to the elderly candidate for surgery. Many drugs applied in the perioperative period will be metabolized differently in the aged patient, especially due to changes in hepatic and renal function and altered fat stores. For example there may be significant differences in the disposition of anaesthetic agents,[74],[75] and in the efficacy and toxicity of the techniques of analgesic management.[76]

When planning surgery for the elderly, it should not be forgotten that most elderly patients have a substantial fear of any such procedure and may entertain the misconception that surgery will cause cancer to spread.[77] Thus, care should be taken to explain the details of the planned procedure and to resolve such concerns with both the patient and the family.

Preoperative assessment

Before surgery is undertaken, the clinical team must consider several issues:

(1) the anticipated life expectancy of the patient;

(2) the physiological status of the patient and ability to withstand the stress of the planned procedures;

(3) the influence of the surgical procedure on quality of life and life expectancy;

(4) the morbidity of the procedure;

(5) alternatives to surgery (for example percutaneous bypass rather than surgical bypass of an obstruction, radiotherapy versus surgery to achieve local tumour control);

(6) the competence of the patient to give informed consent regarding the procedure and its implications;

(7) the intellectual and physical ability of the patient to cope with the sequelae of the surgery (for example a colostomy or ileostomy).

In general, elective surgery can be performed safely on geriatric patients, provided that care is taken to manage their specific physiological problems.[75],[78],[79] As discussed above, a range of changes occur with ageing, which contribute to a reduced ability of the elderly to withstand physiological or surgical stress. For example Del Guerico and Cohn[80] reported that only 13.5 per cent of a series of preoperative patients aged at least 65 years had normal physiological function and 23 per cent had abnormalities that could not be corrected before operation. Elective surgery is clearly preferable to an emergency procedure. A planned operation allows preoperative assessment and correction of common medical problems in this age group (for example cardiac failure, dehydration, hypertension, infection, or malnutrition) and attention to prophylactic manoeuvres to reduce intra- and postoperative complications (cessation of smoking for the preoperative period, chest physiotherapy, bowel care).

The clinician evaluating such a patient should be experienced in the care of the aged to avoid common traps in management. Specific physical characteristics of the elderly must be recognized: for example lack of periorbital fat and reduced skin elasticity may be mistaken for dehydration; peripheral oedema may be due to vascular insufficiency or lymphatic obstruction, rather than cardiac failure; trivial cardiac murmurs may mistakenly be interpreted to represent significant valve lesions in the elderly; and cursory clinical examination may not reveal the subtle signs of dementia.

The most appropriate operation and anaesthetic should be planned. In general, a curative procedure should not be compromised solely because of the age of the patient. However, common sense and experience will dictate the ability of the patient to withstand radical surgery and the balance between the probable benefits and drawbacks of such a procedure. For example there is a higher perioperative mortality rate among elderly patients with lung cancer who undergo pneumonectomy compared with those who undergo a lesser procedure such as lobectomy.[81] In that situation, the potential for cure from each procedure must be balanced by the risks of operative death. These considerations are of particular relevance in patients with smoking-related malignancies, in view of their increased cardiac and respiratory risk status.

In some instances, where cardiorespiratory function is of concern, local anaesthesia may offer a useful alternative, although the patient must not be subjected to unnecessary pain or the discomfort of a prolonged procedure without appropriate sedation and analgesia. Formal preoperative anaesthetic consultation is essential to ensure the optimal preparation of the elderly patient for surgery, and to avoid unnecessary complications. Of specific importance, consideration should be given to the choice of anaesthetic agents, in the context of potential physiological dysfunction and the possibility of drug interactions and age-related toxicities, as well as the mode of anaesthesia (general versus regional or epidural) and the likely postoperative anaesthetic complications.[75]

Intraoperative care

An anaesthetic plan of management should be developed preoperatively, and particular care must be taken in the intraoperative monitoring of an aged patient. Attention must be paid to replacement of fluids and blood products, with regard to both overload and under-replacement. Aged tissues (teeth, skin) are more liable to inadvertent trauma and particular care should be taken in the insertion of the endotracheal tube, positioning on the operating table, and insertion of cannulae. Of importance, there is an increased risk of osteoporosis with increased age in both men and women, and thus the elderly are at increased risk of fractures on the operating table. It is often helpful to position the aged patient on the operating table while they are still awake, to reduce the risk of inadvertent soft tissue or bony damage. Care must also be taken to avoid hyperextension of the aged neck during anaesthetic intubation to avoid cerebrovascular insufficiency and the problems associated with compression of neurovascular structures by large osteophytes.

In major procedures or with an unusually frail patient, there should be facilities for continuous intraoperative monitoring of cardiorespiratory function (electrocardiography, blood oxygenation, etc.); in prolonged procedures, changes in electrolytes, renal function, blood glucose, haematological indices, and coagulation should be assessed serially. Older patients are more sensitive to fluctuations in body temperature, and are at particular risk of the complications of hypothermia. Pragmatic considerations, such as the cost-effectiveness of interventions, are also of importance; for example, intensive monitoring is usually not necessary for a simple biopsy in a fit elderly patient and many such procedures can be performed safely in a day-surgery unit with less disruption to the aged patient's routine and less risk of hospital-based complications, such as infection.

Postoperative management

The principles of postoperative management simply reflect the practice of good general surgical care. A continuing awareness of the aged patient's diminished capacity to respond to stress is essential and there should be careful monitoring of the same indices that are assessed during the procedure. In addition, attention should be given to the provision of adequate analgesia to ensure that the patient is able to move freely and to perform the necessary breathing exercises. Care should be taken to avoid thromboembolism, with measures such as anticoagulation, the use of support stockings, etc. Attention must be directed to skin care, the avoidance of pressure sores, and active management of the operative wound. Wound infection is of particular importance in the older patient, both in the context of the increased friability of tissues, compromised vascularity, and reduced immune function.

The postoperative routine is important in the care of the elderly. A diurnal rhythm should be maintained and the potential loss of such a rhythm in prolonged admission to an intensive care facility should be avoided if possible. The elderly are at particular risk of nocturnal disorientation in reduced light.

Palliative surgery

A simple surgical procedure can be effective in palliating an incurable, locally advanced malignancy. The elderly patient may benefit greatly, both in a reduction of symptoms and in the duration of hospitalization, from surgical resection or bypass of an obstructing gastrointestinal malignancy, the removal of a fungating skin cancer, or even surgical attention to a locally advanced breast cancer. As noted previously, consideration of appropriate alternatives is of great importance in this context. For example in the context of palliative treatment of advanced breast cancer, it has been proposed that simple hormonal manipulation (tamoxifen, progestational drugs) may control a locally advanced tumour with less morbidity and equal efficacy to a surgical procedure.[82] However, there are emerging data that an increasing population of aged women are surviving initial hormonal therapy to suffer the morbidity and potential mortality of locoregional relapse after definitive local treatment has been withheld in the anticipation of short survival from intercurrent disease.[83],[84]

Preventative surgery

Another aspect of the care of the elderly is the attention to pre-malignant and early malignant conditions. The aged are at particular risk of developing malignant degeneration of adenomatous polyps and changes in skin lesions (for example solar keratosis, Hutchinson's melanotic freckle). Such conditions can often best be managed by early surgical intervention, thus limiting the extent of required dissection and increasing the chances of cure. The issues of prevention and screening for malignancy in the elderly are beyond the scope of this chapter, but are reviewed elsewhere.[79]

Radiotherapy in the aged

Analogous to the practice of surgery in the aged, the optimal delivery of radiotherapy to such patients requires careful planning. The specific considerations vary widely, depending upon the organ to be treated. However, some general principles apply, although little has been published regarding the specific problems that pertain to radiotherapy in the elderly.[85]–[87] Most of the data that relate radiobiological indices to age have been obtained either from animal models or from detailed studies of paediatric populations.[87] One potentially important observation from a murine model is that there is a higher hypoxic fraction in tumours grown in older animals, as compared to equivalent numbers of tumour cells implanted into young animals.[88] As hypoxia is associated with radioresistance, this could have important implications for the design of radiation schedules for elderly patients, if confirmed in human studies.

Elderly tissues (particularly skin and mucosae) are less resilient and are repaired less rapidly. Thus, the elderly patient will often tolerate standard radiation treatment protocols less well.[86] This should be taken into consideration when planning the dosage, field size, and fractionation of radiotherapy of tumours arising in the oral cavity, larynx, lung, oesophagus, rectum, and genitourinary tract because of the risks of severe normal tissue toxicity with significant discomfort for the patient. The probable potential for cure or long-term local control must be balanced against the toxicity of radical treatment doses. Conversely, the improvement in quality of life due to reduced doses or interruption of treatment may be offset by a reduction in survival. For example the technique of split-course irradiation (in which the planned dose is delivered in two parts, separated by a gap of 2 to 3 weeks to reduce toxicity) achieves a lower rate of local control in some forms of head and neck cancer.[89] Similarly, there is clear evidence of reduced local control and cure rates when radiation dosage is compromised for tumours of the bladder, prostate, and rectum.

Other practical problems may require attention. One of the most common problems for aged patients receiving cancer therapy is the inconvenience and physical or financial problems posed by commuting to the treatment centre. This may apply particularly to the patient faced with daily radiotherapy appointments for periods of 4 to 8 weeks, and steps must be taken to assist the patient with the resolution of these issues. Furthermore, the elderly patient with severe arthritis may experience substantial difficulty or pain when being positioned for radiotherapy, particularly when prone. Chronic airway limitation or cardiac failure, with associated orthopnoea, may also cause problems. The elderly male with severe prostatism or with an extensive pelvic malignancy may not be able to remain comfortably in the correct position for prolonged periods during definitive treatment. Elderly patients suffering severe radiation-induced nausea or diarrhoea may develop substantial iatrogenic complications from antinauseant or antidiarrhoeal medications (discussed below in the context of chemotherapy) or from dehydration.

The radiotherapy treatment bunker, often colourless and isolated, may frighten the elderly patient, particularly if confused or demented, and great care should be taken to explain the nature of treatment and to reassure the patient. In some instances, prophylactic gentle sedation may be used effectively to minimize the distress of the geriatric patient, although this can cause additional problems in the aged patient with borderline or established dementia or delirium.

The major problem that is posed by aged patients with localized tumours is to establish a realistic and accurate balance between the potential for cure and the toxicity of the requisite treatment. With an increasing population of elderly patients with good general physical status, a particularly important error of judgement is to miss the potential for cure, based on an inaccurate assumption of a short life expectancy, with consequent inappropriate dose reduction or failure to use optimal therapy. It is also important to identify clearly the goals of purely palliative therapy, avoiding prolonged schedules of radiation that may be debilitating and inconvenient. The specific application of these principles has been covered in chapters describing the oncological management of individual tumour types.

Pharmacology of anticancer drugs in the elderly

Many of the physiological changes of old age, discussed previously, may alter the pharmacological disposition of drugs, including cytotoxics (Table 2). The changes of organ function in the aged, as discussed above, may cause changes in absorption, distribution, and elimination of many drugs, as reviewed elsewhere.[24],[26],[90],[91] As many of the cytotoxic drugs have a relatively narrow therapeutic index, any factors that potentially alter the pharmacokinetics in the elderly may be of great importance with regard to efficacy and toxicity. In recent times, the prevalence of the 'fit' elderly in the community has increased, consequent upon improved nutrition and community health practices

Table 2 Examples of predisposing factors to toxicity of cytotoxic drugs in the elderly

Side-effect	Predisposing factors	Cytotoxic drugs potentially affected
Cardiac failure	Reduced cardiac output Ischaemic heart disease Cardiac valve disorder Impaired hepatic function	Doxorubicin Daunorubicin Mitoxantrone Epirubicin
Pneumonitis	Reduced density of lung Reduced renal function Chronic bronchitis/airways limitation	Bleomycin
Myelosuppression	Reduced plasma protein binding Reduced renal function Reduced hepatic function Age-related changes in fat stores and marrow reserves	Methotrexate Doxorubicin Epirubicin Mitoxantrone Nitrosoureas
Mucositis	Reduced renal function Age-related changes in mucosae Reduced plasma protein binding Reduced hepatic function	Methotrexate Fluorouracil Doxorubicin Epirubicin
Peripheral neuropathy	Age-related changes in nerves Diabetes mellitus Chronic alcohol abuse Peripheral vascular disease	Vinca alkaloids Cisplatin
Deafness	Noise-induced hearing loss Age-related hearing loss[a] Reduced renal function?	Cisplatin
Haemorrhagic cystitis	Prostatism	Cyclophosphamide[b]
Constipation	Age-related changes in nerves and bowel function	Vinca alkaloids

[a] No obvious increment noted in elderly patients with bladder cancer (Raghavan et al. 1998).[100]

[b] Theoretical consideration; not observed in a series of 60 cases treated with oral cyclophosphamide.

and health care. It is not yet clear whether these patients tolerate cytotoxic chemotherapy better than the older aged population of previous eras, and this important issue is the object of extensive ongoing investigation. For example a substantial programme at the University of Southern California is specifically addressing the level of comorbidity in cancer patients aged 75 years and above, and comparing the pharmacokinetics of cytotoxic agents in cohorts of patients with few and many intercurrent diseases, and with varying levels of performance status.

The prediction of these changes is complex for many reasons. Dose–response relationships may be different in the aged.[1],[24],[26],[90],[92] Moreover, it has been estimated that 80 per cent of such patients have one or more chronic disorders[2] and that they are treated with a mean of 3 to 12 concomitant medications.[93] Thus, in addition to changes in metabolism and organ function, polypharmacy is a significant cause of pharmacological complication in the elderly. Ninety per cent of Americans older than 65 years of age take at least one prescription medication daily, and most take two or more.[94] The elderly population most commonly use cardiovascular drugs, anti-inflammatory drugs, sedatives, analgesics, and agents that affect gastrointestinal function.

Absorption

Most cytotoxics are administered parenterally, although cyclophosphamide, methotrexate, busulfan, etoposide, demethoxydaunorubicin, JM-216, uracil-ftorafur (UFT), captecitabine, and chlorambucil may be used orally and are thus subject to variable absorption. To avoid the problems of repeated parenteral therapy, there is an increasing tendency to prescribe orally-active cytotoxics for elderly patients. Many ancillary medications, such as analgesics, antiemetics, laxatives, steroids, and folinic acid, are administered by mouth. The major factors that determine the bioavailability of most of these drugs include the absorption process itself and initial elimination (first-pass hepatic metabolism or degradation in the small bowel).[95] The age-related reduction in gastric acid secretion and in gastrointestinal motility may affect the absorption of basic and poorly lipid soluble drugs in particular.[95],[96] The changes in hepatic blood flow can either increase or reduce bioavailability. In a patient with cancer, the metabolic implications of hepatic metastases are variable and poorly understood.

Drug distribution

The distribution of a drug is a function of its relative lipid–water partition characteristics, the degree of binding to plasma proteins and other tissues, and the overall patterns of blood flow.[92] Because of the reduction in lean body mass, increase in lipid composition of the body, and reduction in total body water, the distribution of lipid-soluble drugs (for example diazepam or the nitrosoureas) changes markedly in the elderly.[23],[26] Plasma protein binding is also reduced in the elderly, with a concomitant rise in the level of free drug. In patients with substantial third spaces (such as ascites or pleural effusions from malignancy or cardiac failure), the distribution of water-soluble drugs is further distorted and toxicity can be significantly increased.

Metabolism

Hepatic and extra-hepatic enzyme systems contribute to the metabolism of many cytotoxic drugs. The rate of drug metabolism is influenced by the state of nutrition, hepatic function, drug interactions, other diseases, the presence of metastases, smoking, and plasma protein levels.[90],[95] There are no simple indices of drug metabolism and standard liver function tests are an unreliable guide. This variability of function is a particular hazard for the use of antinauseants, analgesics, and sedatives in the elderly. Of importance, not all drug metabolism relates to inactivation of these agents—for example cyclophosphamide requires hepatic microsomal function for activation to its clinically useful state.

Excretion

The kidneys provide the major route of excretion for many cytotoxic drugs, including methotrexate, bleomycin, ifosfamide, cyclophosphamide, carboplatin, and cisplatin. If renal function is impaired, the drugs that are predominantly excreted by this route have prolonged half-lives, with increased plasma concentrations and the concomitant risk of increased toxicity. In elderly patients with tumours of the urothelium, the nature of the malignancy can be of particular importance. For example the association of analgesic nephropathy, chronic renal failure, and multifocal bladder cancer, complicated by hydronephrosis or antecedent nephrectomy,[91] may have a significant influence on excretion of the drug. In the elderly patient, the ability of a solitary kidney to compensate after nephrectomy is reduced by approximately 50 per cent. Most other cytotoxics are excreted via the biliary tract and toxicity is thus dependent upon the changes in hepatic function outlined above. Chronic alcohol abuse and the presence of congestive cardiac failure, as well as the reduction in hepatic perfusion consequent upon the normal decline in cardiac output, are of particular importance in the elderly.

General applications

A general dictum, not really supported by objective evidence, is that increased toxicity of chemotherapy is a function of advanced age *per se*, irrespective of the general physiological state of the patient. Early studies reflected experience gained from only small numbers of cases. For example methotrexate was noted to cause increased haematological side-effects,[97] and bleomycin was said to be associated with increased lung damage in the elderly.[98] However, Begg and Carbone,[99] in a detailed review of more than 5000 patients from studies by the Eastern Cooperative Oncology Group, noted that the extent and severity of side-effects were functions of the agents and doses employed, rather than being due to the ages of the patients *per se*. Although age-related toxicity occurred with methotrexate and methyl-CCNU, this did not appear to be the case for doxorubicin, cyclophosphamide, the vinca alkaloids, or mitomycin C. Although this is an important study, it should not be forgotten that there may have been significant selection of patients as the data were obtained only from cases entered into randomized trials. Similarly, in selected elderly patients with bladder cancer[100] and other malignancies,[28] the toxicity of cisplatin is not a function of age.

There have been conflicting views on the topic of dose modification in the elderly and the balance between reduced toxicity (from dose reduction) compared with the potential for reduced antitumour efficacy.[101],[102] In general, decisions regarding the dosing of cytotoxic agents should represent a balance between the likelihood of cure, details of dose–response relationships, and the overall physical condition and prognosis of the patient. For patients who are likely to achieve cure or prolonged palliation, and who have few intercurrent disorders and a good performance status, we believe that optimal results are achieved by the maintenance of standard dosing of chemotherapy, modified for specific changes in renal or hepatic function if indicated. By contrast, it is inappropriate to pursue dose-intensive, toxic therapy when the potential for cure is small, and short-term palliation is the goal.

Psychosocial factors

When planning active management of cancer in the elderly, whatever modality of treatment is intended, the unique psychosocial context of these patients must be considered if optimal care is to be achieved. A range of factors can have an important impact on the presentation and management of cancer in elderly patients. In Western society, the older patient who develops cancer must face the dual social stigmata of advanced age and cancer.

The ageing process is heavily influenced by a changing psychological profile in addition to physical change. In addition to changes in cognitive function, health behaviour and attitudes are likely to alter as a function of ageing.[103] There is a greater acceptance of ill health, accompanied by less awareness of current or evolving trends in optimal health care. In addition, increases in patterns of smoking and alcohol intake, and a reduction in the level of personal interactions with medical attendants often evolve with advancing age. Other important factors include a reduced level of social integration (fewer friends and family, reduced family or social support, fewer incentives, poverty), evolving physical weakness and problems with sight and hearing, and reduced coping mechanisms. Changing patterns of acceptance of the elderly in society will often influence the quality, variability, and use of health care for the aged. All of these factors will frequently contribute to an underlying, but dominant, clinical depression (situational depression), which may have a very dramatic impact on cancer therapy.

Although the elderly receive medical attention more frequently than the young (and thus could benefit from earlier medical diagnosis), several factors may contribute to delayed presentation. For example elderly patients may procrastinate (due to misconceptions regarding likely outcome of treatment, greater acceptance of ill health, fear, depression, or poverty). In some cases, the medical profession will be reluctant to seek out problems in elderly patients, taking a nihilistic view of the role of cancer therapy in the aged, or viewing the anticipated life expectancy of a geriatric patient as being too short to justify active intervention. These issues must be taken into consideration when devising strategies for cancer management in this group.

However, some studies suggest that the elderly often have a better psychosocial adaptation to established illness than do the young.[104] Using the Cancer Inventory of Problem Situations, a self-administered survey of physical and psychosocial problems associated with cancer, Ganz et al.[105] compared 158 men aged 65 years or less with 82 men older than 65 years. They showed that the older cohort had a similar spectrum of problems to their younger counterparts, despite a higher prevalence of chronic illness. However, the younger group experienced more psychosocial problems, particularly in coping with the health-care environment, chemotherapy, and work-related problems.

When establishing a plan of active management, in addition to considering the balance between the toxicity of treatment and the likely prognosis, psychosocial issues must be considered and incorporated into the programme of treatment. When planning the overall campaign of management, the clinician should muster the appropriate social resources (district nursing, occupational therapy, social work, psychogeriatric support, etc.) to ensure optimal management of the elderly patient with cancer.

Future considerations

Within 30 years, the problems of geriatric patients will dominate the pattern of care in internal medicine, with a large component of expenditure of resources being allocated to the management of cancer. The 'baby boomers', born in the period after the Second World War, will become the 'elder boomers', with a projected census of 51.4 million in the United States by the year 2020.[106] The management of the increasing population of geriatric patients, with an increased active life expectancy and an increased potential prevalence of malignancy, will require careful planning. Adequate allocation of resources will be necessary, particularly as the costs of new treatment programmes are increasing and the proportional financial burdens on the young are likely to become insupportable.

In order to cope effectively with this problem, we must address these issues now. Large, co-operative cancer trial groups should be encouraged to deal specifically with the management of common cancers in the elderly, emphasizing the balance between costs (financial, toxicity) and benefits of the treatments under consideration. Patterns of response and toxicity must be defined with increasing precision to facilitate the modification of standard treatment approaches and the development of new management strategies for the unique characteristics of the aged. It is encouraging to note that several large, multicentre, co-operative research groups, such as the Southwest Oncology Group and the Cancer and Acute Leukaemia Group B, have established committees to define research agendas for elderly patients with cancer, and specific grants for research in this domain have been made available from national scientific administrations.

The specific problems of health screening in the elderly must be addressed and public health education campaigns should be tailored to the characteristics and prejudices of the elderly if they are to be effective. If these issues are not addressed now, we shall be faced with a problem of epidemic proportions in the early part of the next century and it is us who will be the likely victims of a system that cannot cope with the onslaught.

References

1. **Vestal RE.** Drug use in the elderly: a review of problems and special considerations. *Drugs*, 1978; **16**: 358–82.

2. **WHO (World Health Organization).** Health care in the elderly: a report of the technical group on use of medicaments by the elderly. *Drugs*, 1981; **22**: 279–94.

3. **Yancik R, Ries LA.** Cancer in older persons. Magnitude of the problem—how do we apply what we know? *Cancer*, 1994; **74**: 1995–2003.

4. **Katz S, et al.** Active life expectancy. *New England Journal of Medicine*, 1983; **309**: 1218–24.

5. **Fentiman IS, et al.** Cancer in the elderly: why so badly treated? *Lancet*, 1990; **335**: 1020–2.

6. **Landis SH, Murray T, Bolden S, Wingo PA.** Cancer statistics, 1999. *CA: A Cancer Journal for Clinicians*, 1999; **49**: 8–31.

7. **Kim, S, Jiang JC, Kirchman PA, et al.** Cellular and molecular ageing. In: Balducci L, Lyman GH, Ershler WB, eds. *Comprehensive geriatric oncology*. Amsterdam: Harwood Academic, 1998: 123–55.

8. **Orgel LE.** Aging of clones of mammalian cells. *Nature*, 1963; **243**: 441–5.

9. **Orgel LE.** The maintenance of the accuracy of protein synthesis and its relevance to ageing. *Proceedings of the National Academy of Science, USA*, 1963; **49**: 517–21.

10. **Von Hahn HP.** The regulation of protein synthesis in the ageing cell. *Experimental Gerontology*, 1970; **5**: 323–34.

11. Nohebel DC, Walton JC. *Free radical chemistry*. Cambidge, MA: University Press, 1974.

12. Harman D. A theory based on free radical and radiation chemistry. *Journal of Gerontology*, 1956; **11**: 298–300.

13. Cutler RG. Antioxidants and longevity of mammalian species. In: Woodhead AD, Blackett AD, Hollaender A, eds. *Molecular biology of ageing*. New York: Plenum, 1985: 15–73.

14. Hayflick L, Moorhead PS. The serial cultivation of human diploid cell strains. *Experimental Cell Research*, 1961; **25**: 585.

15. Stein GH, Namba M, Corsaro CM. Relationship of finite proliferative life span, senescence, and quiescence in human cells. *Journal of Cellular Physiology*, 1985; **122**: 343–9.

16. Zakian VA. Structure and function of telomeres. *Annual Review of Genetics*, 1989; **23**: 579–604.

17. Harley CB. Telomerases. *Pathology and Biology*, 1994; **42**: 342–6.

18. Harley CB, Futcher AB, Greider CW. Telomeres shorten during ageing of human fibroblasts. *Nature*, 1990; **345**: 458–60.

19. Counter CM, Hirte HW, Bacchetti S, Harley CB. Telomerase activity in human ovarian carcinoma. *Proceedings of the National Academy of Science, USA*, 1994; **91**: 2900–5.

20. Leventhal EA. The dillemma of cancer in the elderly. In: Vaeth JM, Meyer J, eds. *Cancer and the elderly*. Basel: Karger, 1986: 1–13.

21. Bender AD. The effects of increasing age on the distribution of peripheral blood flow in man. *Journal of the American Geriatric Society*, 1965; **13**: 192–8.

22. McLauchlan M. Anatomic structural and vascular changes in the ageing kidney. In Nunez JFM, Cameron JS, eds. *Renal function and disease in the elderly*. London, Butterworths, 1987: 3–26.

23. McLachlan MSF. The ageing kidney. *Lancet*, 1978; **ii**: 143–6.

24. Triggs EJ, Nation RLL. Pharmacokinetics in the aged: a review. *Journal of Pharmacokinetics and Biopharmacology*, 1975; **3**: 387–418.

25. Davies DF, Shock NW. Age changes in glomerular filtration rate, effective renal plasma flow, and tubular excretory capacity in adult males. *Journal of Clinical Investigation*, 1950; **29**: 496.

26. Greenblatt DJ, Sellers EM, Shader RI. Drug disposition in old age. *New England Journal of Medicine*, 1982; **306**: 1081–8.

27. Dontas AS, Marketos S, Papanayiotou P. Mechanisms of renal tubular defects in old age. *Postgraduate Medical Journal*, 1972; **48**: 295.

28. Hrushesky WJ, Shimp W, Kennedy BJ. Lack of age-dependent cisplatin nephrotoxicity. *American Journal of Medicine*, 1974; **76**: 579–84.

29. Rowe JW, *et al*. The effect of age on creatinine clearance in man: a cross sectional and longitudinal study. *Journal of Gerontology*, 1976; **31**: 155–63.

30. Schuck O, *et al*. Acidification capacity of the kidneys and ageing. *Physiology and Biochemistry*, 1989; **38**: 117.

31. Kupfer RM, *et al*. Gastric emptying and small bowel transit rate in the elderly. *Journal of the American Geriatrics Society*, 1985; **33**: 340.

32. Khan TA, *et al*. Esophageal motility in the elderly. *American Journal of Digestive Diseases*, 1977; **22**: 1049–54.

33. Evans MA, *et al*. Gastric emptying rate in the elderly: implications for drug therapy. *Journal of the American Geriatrics Society*, 1981; **29**: 201–5.

34. Calloway NC, *et al*. Uncertainties in geriatric data: II. Organ size. *Journal of the American Geriatrics Society*, 1965; **13**: 20.

35. Popper H. Aging and the liver. *Progress in Liver Diseases*, 1986; **8**: 659–83.

36. Brandsteller RD, Kazemi H. Aging and the respiratory system. *Medical Clinics of North America*, 1983; **67**: 419–31.

37. Hartstock RJ, Smith EB, Petty ES. Normal variations with ageing on the amount of hematopoietic tissue in bone marrow from the anterior iliac crest. *American Journal of Clinical Pathology*, 1965; **43**: 326–31.

38. Timiras ML, Brownstein H. Prevalence of anemia and correlation of hemoglobin with age in a geriatric screening clinic population. *Journal of the American Geriatrics Society*, 1987; **35**: 639–43.

39. Piomelli S, Nathan DG, Cummins JF, Gardner FH. The relationship of total red cell volume to total body water in octogenarian males. *Blood*, 1962; **19**: 89–98.

40. Lipschitz DG, Udupa KB. Age and the hematopoietic system. *Journal of the American Geriatrics Society*, 1986; **34**: 448–54.

41. Zauber NP, Zauber AG. Hematologic data of healthy very old people. *Journal of the American Medical Association*, 1987; **257**: 2181–4.

42. Bender BS, *et al*. Absolute peripheral blood lymphocyte count and subsequent mortality of elderly men. *Journal of the American Geriatric Society*, 1986; **34**: 649–54.

43. Schwab R, Walters CA, Weksler ME. Host defence mechanisms and ageing. *Seminars in Oncology*, 1989; **16**: 20–7.

44. Ershler WB, Moore AL, Socinski MA. Influenza and ageing: age-realted changes and the effects of thymosin on the antibody response in influenza vaccine. *Journal Clinical Immunology*, 1984; **4**: 445.

45. Ershler WB. Interleukin-6: A cytokine for gerontologists. *Journal of the American Geriatrics Society*, 1993; **41**: 176–81.

46. Albert MS. Cognitive function. In: Albert MS, Moss MB, eds. *Geriatric neuropsychology*. New York: Guilford, 1988: 33.

47. Rapaport SI. Positron emission tomography in normal ageing and Alzheimer's disease. *Gerontology*, 1986; **32**: 6–13.

48. Skoog I, Nilsson L, Palmertz B, Andreasson LA, Svanborg A. A population based study of dementia in 85 year olds. *New England Journal of Medicine*, 1993; **328**: 153–7.

49. Lindesay J, *et al*. *Delirium in the elderly*. Oxford University Press, 1990.

50. Silver AJ. Malnutrition. In: Beck JC, ed. *Geriatrics review syllabus. A core curriculum in geriatric medicine*. Book 1. New York: American Geriatrics Society, 1991.

51. Tolefsbol TO, Cohen HJ. Role of protein molecular and metabolic aberrations in ageing in the physiologic decline of the aged, and in age-associated diseases. *Journal of the American Geriatrics Society*, 1986; **34**: 282–94.

52. Rossman I. Anatomic and body composition changes with ageing. In: Finch CF, Hayflick L, eds. *Handbook of the biology of ageing*. New York: van Nostrand Reinhold, 1980: 189.

53. Baker H, *et al*. Vitamin profiles in elderly persons living at home or in nursing homes versus profiles in healthy subjects. *Journal of the American Geriatrics Society*, 1979; **29**: 444.

54. Tsai KS, *et al*. Effect of ageing on vitamin D stores and bone density in women. *Calcified Tissue International*, 1987; **40**: 241.

55. *Recommended daily allowances*. 10th edn. Washington, DC: National Academy Press, 1989.

56. Ries LG, Pollack ES, Young JL. Cancer patient survival: surveillance, epidemiology, and end results. *Journal of the National Cancer Institute*, 1983; **70**: 693–707.

57. Crawford J, Cohen HJ. Relationship of cancer and ageing. *Clinics in Geriatric Medicine*, 1987; **3**: 419–31.

58. Peto R, *et al*. Cancer and ageing in mice and men. *British Journal of Cancer*, 1975; **32**: 411–26.

59. Anisimov VN. *Carcinogenesis and ageing*, Vol 1. Boca Raton: CRC Press, 1987: 1–47.

60. Kaesberg PR, Ershler WB. The change in tumor aggressiveness with age: lessons from experimental animals. *Seminars in Oncology*, 1989; **16**: 28–33.

61. Holmes FF, Hearne E. Cancer stage-to-age relationship: Implications for cancer screening in the elderly. *Journal of the American Geriatrics Society*, 1981; **29**: 55–7.

62. Lipschitz DA, *et al*. Cancer in the elderly: basic science and clinical aspects. *Annals of Internal Medicine*, 1985; **102**: 218–28.

63. Goodwin JS, *et al*. Stage at diagnosis of cancer varies with the age of the patient. *Journal of the American Geriatrics Society*, 1986; **34**: 20–6.

64. Mor V, *et al.* Relationship between age at diagnosis and treatment received by cancer patients. *Journal of the American Geriatrics Society,* 1985; **33**: 585–9.

65. Suen KC, Lau LL, Yermakov V. Cancer and old age. An autopsy study of 3535 patients over 65 years old. *Cancer,* 1974; **33**: 1164–8.

66. Saitoh H, Shiramizu T, Hida M. Age changes in metastatic patterns in renal adenocarcinoma. *Cancer,* 1982; **50**: 1646–8.

67. O'Rourke MA, Crawford J. Lung cancer in the elderly. *Clinics in Geriatric Medicine,* 1987; **3**: 595–623.

68. Lees JC, Park WW. The malignancy of cancer at different ages: a histological study. *British Journal of Cancer,* 1950; **3**: 186–97.

69. Holmes FF. Clinical evidence for changes in tumor aggressiveness with age. In: Balducci L, Lyman GH, Ershler WB, eds. *Comprehensive geriatric oncology.* Amsterdam: Harwood Academic, 1998: 223–6.

70. Fernandez-Pol JA. Growth factors, oncogenes and ageing. In: Balducci L, Lyman GH, Ershler WB, eds. *Comprehensive geriatric oncology.* Amsterdam: Harwood Academic Publishers, 1998: 179–96.

71. Calabrese CT, Adam YG, Volk H. Geriatric colon cancer. *American Journal of Surgery,* 1973; **125**: 181–4.

72. Kirsh MM, *et al.* Major pulmonary resection for bronchogenic carcinoma in the elderly. *Annals of Thoracic Surgery,* 1976; **22**: 369–73.

73. Sondik EJ, Young JL, Horn JW. *1986 Annual cancer statistics review.* NIH Publication 87–2789. Bethesda, MD: Department of Health and Human Services, 1987.

74. Djokovic JL, Hedley-Whyte J. Prediction of outcome of surgery and anesthesia in patients over 80. *Journal of the American Medical Association,* 1979; **242**: 2301.

75. Kreehel SW. Anesthesia for surgical care of the elderly. In: Meakins JL, McClaren JC, eds. *Surgical care of the elderly.* Chicago: Year Book Medical Publishers, 1988: 276–87.

76. Moore AK, Vilderman S, Lubensky W, *et al.* Differences in epidural morphine requirements between elderly and young patients after abdominal surery. *Anesthesia and Analgesia,* 1990; **70**: 316.

77. Stults BM. Preventive care for the elderly. In: Vaeth JM, Meyer J, eds. *Cancer and the elderly.* Basel: Karger, 1983: 182–91.

78. Bowles LT. Surgical essentials in the care of the elderly cancer patient. In: Yancik R *et al.*, eds. *Perspectives on prevention and treatment of cancer in the elderly.* Raven Press, New York, 1983: 57–61.

79. Patterson WB. Oncology perspective on colorectal cancer in the geriatric patient. In: Yancik R *et al.*, eds. *Perspectives on prevention and treatment of cancer in the elderly.* New York: Raven Press, 1983: 105–20.

80. Del Guerico LRM, Cohn JD. Monitoring operative risk in the elderly. *Journal of the American Medical Association,* 1980; **243**: 1350–5.

81. Martini N. Lung cancer in the elderly. In: Vaeth JM, Meyer J, eds. *Cancer and the elderly.* Basel: Karger, 1986: 125–32.

82. Gazet J-C, *et al.* Prospective randomised trial of tamoxifen versus surgery in elderly patients with breast cancer. *Lancet,* 1988; **i**: 679–81.

83. Balducci L, Silliman RA, Baekey. Breast cancer: An oncological perspective – part 1. In: Balducci L, Lyman GH, Ershler WB, eds. *Comprehensive geriatric oncology.* Amsterdam: Harwood Academic Publishers, 1998: 629–60.

84. Silliman RA, Balducci L. Breast cancer: A geriatric perspective – part 2. In: Balducci L, Lyman GH, Ershler WB, eds. *Comprehensive geriatric oncology.* Amsterdam: Harwood Academic Publishers, 1998: 661–4.

85. Gunn WG. Radiation therapy for the ageing patient. *CA: A Cancer Journal for Clinicians,* 1980; **30**: 337–47.

86. Crocker I, Prosnitz L. Radiation therapy of the elderly. *Clinics in Geriatric Medicine,* 1987; **3**: 473–81.

87. Scalliet P. Radiotherapy in the elderly. *European Journal of Cancer,* 1991; **27**: 3–5.

88. Rockwell S, Hughes CS, Kennedy KA. Effect of host age on microenvironmental heterogeneity and efficacy of combined modality therapy in solid tumors. *International Journal of Radiation Oncology, Biology, Physics,* 1991; **20**: 259–63.

89. Parsons J, Bova F, Million R. A reevaluation of split-course technique for squamous cell carcinnoma of the head and neck. *International Journal of Radiation Oncology, Biology, Physics,* 1980; **6**: 1645–52.

90. Ho PC, Triggs EJ. Drug therapy in the elderly. *Australian and New Zealand Journal of Medicine,* 1984; **14**: 179–90.

91. Skinner EC, Skinner DG, Kim S, Raghavan D. Management of bladder cancer in the elderly. In: Raghavan D, Scher HI, Leibel SA, Lange PH, eds. *Principles and practice of genitourinary cancer.* Philadelphia: Lippincott-Raven, 1997.

92. Vestal RE. Aging and pharmacology. *Cancer,* 1997; **80** (Suppl. 7): 1302–10.

93. Shaw PG. Common pitfalls in geriatric drug prescribing. *Drugs,* 1982; **23**: 324–8.

94. Moellar JF, *et al. Prescribed medicine: a summary of use and expenditures by medicare beneficiaries.* Rockville, MD: US Department of Health and Human Services, 1989.

95. Cohen HJ. Clinical aspects of cancer in the elderly. In: Pullman B, Ts'o POP, Schneider EL, eds. *Interrelationship among ageing, cancer and differentiation.* Dordrecht: Reidel, 1985: 15–21.

96. Hutchins LF, Lipschitz DA. Cancer, clinical pharmacology and ageing. *Clinics in Geriatric Medicine,* 1987; **3**: 483–503.

97. Hansen HH, Selawry OS, Holland JF, McCall CB. the variability of individual tolerance to methotrexate in cancer patients. *British Journal of Cancer,* 1971; **25**: 298–305.

98. Ginsberg SI, Comis RL. The pulmonary toxicity of antineoplastic agents. *Seminars in Oncology,* 1982; **9**: 34–51.

99. Begg CB, Carbone PP. Clinical trials and drug toxicity in the elderly: the experience of Eastern Cooperative Oncology Group. *Cancer,* 1983; **52**: 1986–92.

100. Raghavan D, *et al.* Pre-emptive (neo-adjuvant) chemotherapy prior to radical radiotherapy for fit septuagenarians with bladder cancer: age itself is not a contraindication. *British Journal of Urology,* 1988; **62**: 154–9.

101. Armitage JO, Potter JF. Aggressive chemotherapy for diffuse histiocytic lymphoma in the elderly: increased complications with advancing age. *Journal of the American Geriatrics Society,* 1984; **32**: 269–73.

102. Gelman RS, Taylor SG. CMF chemotherapy in women more than 65 years old with advanced breast cancer: the elimination of age trends in toxicity by using doses based on creatinine clearance. *Journal Clinical Oncology,* 1984; **2**: 1404–13.

103. Yancik R. Cancer burden in the aged. An epidemiologic and demographic overview. *Cancer,* 1997; **80** (Suppl. 7):1273–83.

104. Holland JC, Massie MJ. Psychosocial aspects of cancer in the elderly. *Clinics in Geriatric Medicine,* 1987; **3**: 533–8.

105. Ganz PA, Schag CC, Heinrich RI. The psychosocial impact of cancer on the elderly: a comparison with younger patients. *Journal of the American Geriatrics Society,* 1985; **33**: 429–35.

106. Kennedy BJ. Presidential address: ageing and cancer. *Journal of Clinical Oncology,* 1988; **6**: 1903–11.

4.29 Photodynamic therapy and lasers in oncology

Stephen G. Bown

From the medical point of view, lasers are a convenient but sophisticated source of light in the visible, ultraviolet, and infrared parts of the spectrum. They are easy to control and the light beam (of a single colour) can be focused to a small spot. This makes it feasible to transmit most beams via thin, flexible fibres so treatment can be delivered to any site accessible to such a fibre directly, through a puncture site or surgical incision, or in conjunction with a flexible endoscope. All the light transmitted via a fibre is emitted from the distal end and has no effect on the tissues through which the fibre passes. Thus it is possible to produce precise, localized biological effects at sites deep within the body with little or no trauma to overlying, normal tissues. The predictability of both the nature and extent of the biological changes is better than for most other means of producing localized tissue necrosis and, unlike radiotherapy, there is no chronic, cumulative toxicity as the photon energies used are too low to cause ionization, so treatment can be repeated at the same site, if necessary. Thus lasers provide a powerful technique for local destruction of diseased tissue (Table 1). To be clinically useful, the keys are to match the extent of laser damage to the extent of the neoplasm being treated and to be sure that all treated areas will heal safely. Laser treatments are local treatments. In the management of disseminated disease, they can only provide local palliation.

Interaction of laser light with living tissue

The most important effects of laser light used in oncology are thermal and photochemical. The thermal applications are simplest to understand, the effect depending on how much heat is delivered, how fast it is delivered, and the volume of tissue in which it is absorbed. The most important photochemical application is photodynamic therapy (PDT). This involves local or systemic administration of a photosensitizing drug and subsequent activation of the drug by low power red light, usually from a laser. There is no increase in tissue temperature during treatment. These effects are summarized in Table 2. The types of laser used most frequently in oncology are shown in Table 3.

Thermal laser therapy

The first laser to be used in oncological surgery was the carbon dioxide laser with a beam which is strongly absorbed in water. This can cut or vaporize tissue with little damage to underlying layers. It is well established as a non-contact knife in relatively inaccessible areas such as the brain and upper airways and for ablating small lesions on sites such as the skin or cervix.[1] However, the beam cannot be transmitted via flexible fibres and can only produce haemostasis in vessels below about 0.2 mm in diameter.

Near infrared light, as from a NdYAG (neodymium yttrium aluminium garnet) or a semiconductor diode laser (Table 3), penetrates tissue much better, producing effects through up to 10 mm of tissue, and can be transmitted via flexible fibres. As tissue is heated it shrinks, which provides good haemostasis in soft tissue as it seals small blood vessels. The effects depend on the laser power, target area, and exposure time. The range of changes seen is shown in Table 4.

NdYAG laser and flexible endoscopy

Gastroenterologists were the first specialists to use lasers in conjunction with flexible endoscopes, for the control of haemorrhage from peptic ulcers. This was effective but it has been superseded by injection sclerotherapy. The best established application now is for palliation of advanced malignant disease.

Upper gastrointestinal tract cancers

Most patients with carcinomas of the oesophagus and gastric cardia have no prospect of cure at the time of presentation due to the extent of their disease (see Chapters 10.1 and 10.2). The dominant symptom is usually dysphagia and the therapeutic challenge is to relieve the dysphagia with the minimum upset to the patient. For those unsuitable for surgery or radical radiotherapy, one is left with the endoscopic options, the most important of which are laser therapy and stent insertion.

Table 1 Attractions of laser therapy

Precise, localized treatment
Fibreoptic light delivery
Predictable biological response
Suitable for minimally invasive, image guided therapy
No cumulative toxicity

Table 2 Laser effects used in oncology

High power thermal	cutting or debulking of tissue by vaporization and coagulation
Low power thermal(interstitial laser photocoagulation, ILP)	gentle coagulation of lesions within solid organs
Photochemical (photodynamic therapy, PDT)	non-thermal destruction of tissue by activation of a previously administered photosensitizing drug

Table 3 Lasers used most frequently in oncology

	Wavelength (nm)	Fibre transmission	Comment
Carbon dioxide (CO_2)	10 600	no	Precise, no contact incision but only moderate haemostasis
Neodymium YAG (NdYAG)	1064	yes	Vaporization, deep coagulation, good haemostasis
Copper vapour or KTP pumped dye	630–750	yes	Tuneable wavelength to match photosensitizer absorption
Diode	630–900	yes	Simple, reliable, range of wavelengths, but not tuneable

Table 4 Thermal effects of lasers on biological tissue

Total destruction	immediate vaporization necrosis with later sloughing
Destruction with reconstruction	necrosis with healing by scarring necrosis with healing by regeneration
Reversible	oedema and inflammation local warming only

Endoscopic NdYAG laser recanalization of advanced oesophageal cancers was first reported in 1982.[2] The aim is to reduce the intraluminal tumour bulk, concentrating on those parts causing the worst obstruction. Prominent nodules can be vaporized. Smaller nodules can be coagulated and the dead tissue sloughs over a few days. The deep penetration of the NdYAG laser beam ensures haemostasis in the underlying tissues. Endoscopic views of an oesophageal cancer before and after laser recanalization are shown in Fig. 1. A barium swallow of the same patient before and after laser therapy is shown in Fig. 2.

An international inquiry soon after the introduction of this technique reported results in 1184 patients in 20 centres.[3] This reported 83 per cent of patients could swallow at least some solids after a mean of three laser treatments. Major complications (perforation and fistulation) were seen in 4.1 per cent with a 1 per cent treatment-related mortality. The main problem is the need to repeat laser treatment every 4 to 6 weeks to maintain good palliation, which has led to studies of adjuvant radiotherapy to slow down local tumour regrowth. Options include palliative external beam irradiation and brachytherapy (intraluminal radiotherapy).[4] The simplest, and probably the most effective option, is brachytherapy which can increase the duration of palliation of dysphagia from an average of 5 weeks using laser alone to 19 weeks in those also receiving a single dose of

10 Gy brachytherapy, although it does not change the median survival (32 weeks).

Lasers are compared with conventional and expanding metal stents in Table 5. Conventional, silicon rubber stents can be inserted endoscopically, and enable most patients to swallow at least semisolids, but there is a risk of perforation of about 10 per cent. Over the last few years, several types of expanding metal stents have become available. They are simpler and safer to insert as much less dilatation is required, but once in are difficult to adjust and may have as many long-term problems as the old type of stent. Laser therapy and stenting are complimentary, and the best management requires access to both.

Haemorrhage or obstruction due to advanced cancers of the distal stomach and duodenum can be treated with endoscopic laser therapy, but the results are often less satisfactory than with lesions of the oesophagus and gastric cardia.

Lower gastrointestinal tract cancers

Most colorectal cancers are best treated surgically (see Chapter 10.4), but 5 to 10 per cent are unsuitable for resection due to the general condition of the patient or the extent of local or metastatic disease. A defunctioning colostomy palliates obstruction, but does not relieve bleeding or mucus discharge from advanced rectal cancers. A range of non-surgical options has been explored to relieve symptoms due to tumour bulk in the rectum, including radiotherapy, cryotherapy, electrocoagulation, and laser sigmoidoscopy. Laser therapy has the advantages of being applied under direct vision (so it can be applied safely above the peritoneal reflection), it can be carried out as a day case procedure with little or no sedation, and repeated as necessary. Adjuvant, palliative radiotherapy may enhance the effect. Initial palliation of obstruction, tenesmus, bleeding, mucus discharge, and diarrhoea can be achieved in up to 90 per cent of patients and maintained for the remainder of the patients' life in up to 80 per cent.[5] Laser therapy can do nothing to help pain or obstruction due to tumour that has spread beyond the lumen.

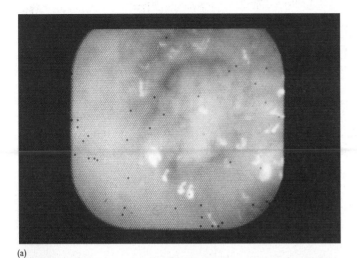

(a)

(b)

Fig. 1 Endoscopic view of an advanced oesophageal cancer (a) before and (b) after laser recanalization.

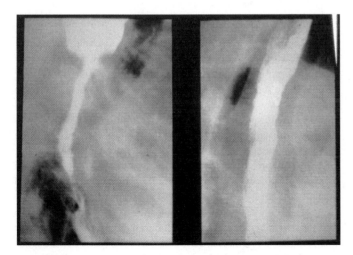

Fig. 2 Barium swallow of a patient with an obstructing oesophageal cancer before (left) and after (right) endoscopic laser therapy (same patient as Fig. 1).

Some patients with small cancers which have not metastasized, and who are unfit for surgery because of their general condition, can justifiably be treated just with laser endoscopy, but PDT, as discussed below, is more appropriate than thermal laser treatment.

Cancers of the major airways

Endoscopic laser palliation of advanced bronchial cancers has developed in parallel to applications in the gastrointestinal tract. As many as 50 per cent of patients with inoperable lung cancer have haemoptysis at some stage of their illness and about 60 per cent become dyspnoeic from tumour obstruction of a major airway. For patients with symptoms due primarily to endoscopically accessible, intraluminal tumour, perhaps up to 10 per cent of all lung cancers, NdYAG laser therapy can play a useful palliative role.[6]

The procedure is technically more difficult and potentially more hazardous than in the gastrointestinal tract. Temporary total occlusion of the oesophagus is tolerable, but of the trachea is not! Further, the gastrointestinal tract has a convenient route for disposing of necrotic debris, which the airways do not. Procedures in the gastrointestinal tract are usually performed under sedation, but bronchoscopic laser treatments require general anaesthesia using an intravenous regimen. This has proved remarkably safe despite the frequent coexistence of other major smoking-related diseases. Insertion of a rigid bronchoscope gives access for ventilation, aspirating blood, and secretions and clearing debris. Laser therapy is undertaken with a flexible bronchoscope inserted through the rigid one. Necrosed tissue is removed immediately with large biopsy forceps.

Response to therapy is immediate and treatment can be repeated if necessary. In a group of 116 patients treated at the Mayo clinic, improvement in the calibre of the airway was documented in 80 per cent after the first treatment and 58 per cent of completely obstructed airways could be opened.[7] Best results are achieved with tumours in the proximal tracheobronchial tree with viable lung beyond the obstruction. An example of the functional response to laser therapy of a patient with a cancer at the carina is shown in Fig. 3. The commonest cause of treatment-related death is haemorrhage, but the incidence is surprisingly low, only 2 to 3 per cent. Occasionally, resuscitative treatment of an obstructing tracheal tumour can pave the way for potentially curative surgery.

Urology

The carbon dioxide and NdYAG lasers have been used to treat lesions of the external genitalia such as warts, balanitis xerotica obliterans, erythroplasia of Queyrat, and superficial penile cancer. Endoscopically, the main target is bladder tumours. The NdYAG and near infrared diode lasers have a role in the management of benign prostatic hypertrophy, but photodynamic therapy has much greater potential in the management of prostate cancer, as discussed below.

Bladder tumours often cause haematuria at an early stage and so are detected when still small and suitable for definitive local treatment (see Chapter 13.2). This has been done with diathermy for many years, but is most effective with rigid cystoscopy under general anaesthesia. Diagnostic flexible cystoscopy under local anaesthesia is now routine. The greater control and precision of laser treatment makes it an attractive option compared with diathermy for ablation of small tumours under local anaesthesia,[8] although it is not widely used. It may also have a palliative role in controlling haemorrhage from advanced bladder cancers.

Table 5 Laser versus stent for palliation of malignant dysphagia

	Laser	Conventional stent	Expanding metal stent
Technique	Basically safe (risk of perforation if dilatation also needed)	10% risk of perforation on insertion	Usually safe and easy to insert
Contraindications	Fistula No endoscopic target	High lesion Tracheal compression	High lesion Tracheal compression Care with lesions crossing cardia
Dysphagia post therapy	Variable, can be close to normal	Semisolids, some solids	Variable, can be close to normal
Enhancement of dysphagia relief with radiotherapy	Yes	No	No
Follow-up	Therapy can be repeated	Stent can be adjusted	Difficult to adjust once inserted
Cost	High to set up, low per patient	Low per patient	High per patient

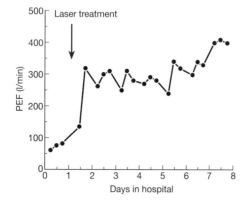

Fig. 3 PEF (peak expiratory flow) measurements on a patient with an obstructing carcinoma at the carina before and after bronchoscopic laser therapy. (Reproduced by courtesy of Dr M.R. Hetzel.)

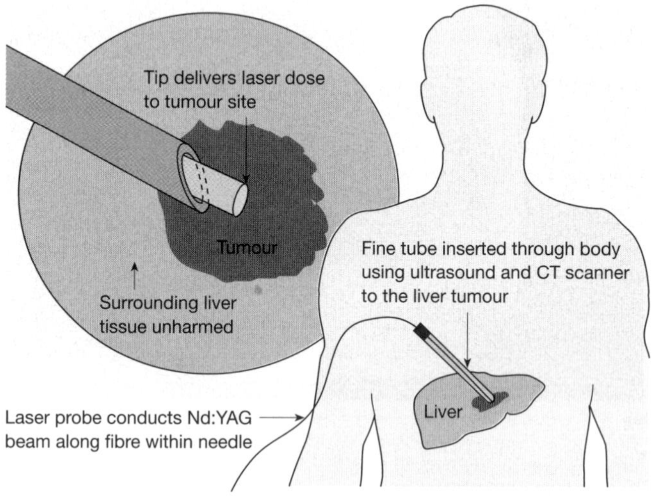

Fig. 4 Technique for percutaneous treatment of liver tumours with ILP (sketch).

Interstitial laser photocoagulation

The thermal applications of lasers described in the first part of this chapter use high powers (60–80 W) and, although effective, are relatively crude, as in the endoscopic palliation of advanced cancers of the aerodigestive tract. The concept of interstitial laser photocoagulation (ILP) is quite different. One or more laser fibres are inserted through needles directly into a lesion in the centre of a solid organ. The laser is then activated to deliver a low power beam, typically 2 to 3 W per fibre for 300 to 500 s. This causes gentle thermal coagulation without vaporization, centred around each fibre tip, with no more damage to the overlying normal tissues than the minimal trauma of inserting the needles. The technique was first described in 1983.[9] Subsequently, a series of *in vivo* experiments showed that it was possible to produce an area of necrosis about 1.5 cm in diameter around each fibre site in normal liver, and that these lesions healed safely, mainly by regeneration of normal liver. This led to the first clinical report of the percutaneous treatment of small hepatic secondary tumours in 1989.[10] The arrangement for percutaneous ILP is illustrated in Fig. 4.

As the purpose of ILP is to treat lesions within solid organs, it is essential that good imaging is available to position fibres correctly and to assess the results both at the time of treatment and during follow-up. It must be possible to define the limits of the target lesion and to match the treatment to these limits to maximize the prospects of destroying the entire lesion and minimize the risk of unacceptable damage to adjacent normal tissues. Most clinical experience has been with the treatment of small tumours of the liver in patients unsuitable for surgery (particularly isolated secondary tumours after previous resection of primary colorectal cancers). Ultrasound has proved valuable for inserting fibres but is poor at documenting the tissue response. Contrast enhanced CT scans are useful, but only give a true picture of the extent of laser-induced necrosis 24 h or longer after treatment.[11] CT scans before and after ILP for a small hepatic secondary tumour are shown in Fig. 5. A series using MR guidance reported 1048 laser applications in 383 hepatic metastases (mostly from previously resected colorectal primary tumours) in 134 patients.

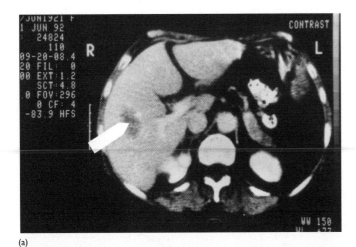

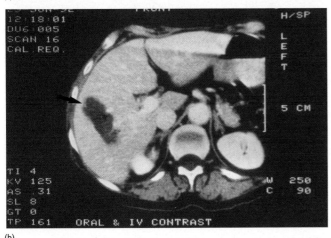

Fig. 5 Contrast enhanced CT scans of a liver showing in the right lobe, a 3.5 × 2.0 cm isolated metastasis from a previously resected carcinoma of the colon (arrow): (a) at presentation, (b) 24 h after interstitial laser photocoagulation (ILP). The laser-induced necrosis is shown as the newly devascularized black area. (Reproduced with permission from Amin Z, et al., *Radiology* 1993; **187**: 339–47.)[13]

There were no major complications and the mean survival time was 35 months.[12]

Recently, laser induced thermal changes have been monitored in real time with dynamic magnetic resonance imaging (MRI), as optical fibres do not cause artefacts on MR scans.[14] The MRI indicates temperature changes in the area being treated which can be correlated with the final extent of laser induced necrosis.

An increasing number of therapeutic options are being considered for the localized destruction of diseased tissue within solid organs. In addition to ILP, these include injection of alcohol or chemotherapeutic agents, heating by microwaves, radiofrequency waves or high intensity focused ultrasound (see Chapter 4.6), cryotherapy, brachytherapy, or photodynamic therapy. ILP and PDT have the advantage that the fibres are thin and can be inserted percutaneously through needles, so they can be positioned relatively easily within firm tissue, such as in secondary tumours. Further, the area of necrosis produced is well defined, roughly ellipsoidal, and does not depend on the physical properties of the tissue as much as with the other techniques.

Radiofrequency heating may give comparable results, but the necrosis produced is more dependent on the electrical properties of the target tissue. It is difficult to inject alcohol into hard tissue, although this is a much cheaper option and works reasonably well for softer lesions such as primary hepatomas. Focused ultrasound is totally non-invasive, but is more difficult to use on deeper lesions.

Recent interest has centred on whether ILP could have any role in the management of small, localized breast cancers, as an alternative to lumpectomy. The attractions would be that treatment would leave no scar or change in the shape of the breast and could be carried out just with sedation and local anaesthetic under image guidance as a day-case procedure. Studies treating small breast cancers with ILP prior to conventional surgical excision have shown that contrast enhanced MRI can define both the tumour limits and the limits of laser-induced necrosis remarkably accurately (Figs 6 and 7).[15] However, a lot more work is required to clarify whether ILP could be used as an alternative to lumpectomy.

ILP has the potential to treat lesions within any solid organ that are not suitable for surgical excision and which are accessible for image-guided needle insertion. There are isolated reports of its application to peripheral lung tumours and to intracranial lesions.[16] It is under assessment for fibroadenomas of the breast, fibroids of the uterus, and benign prostatic hypertrophy, but, in principle, it could be used to treat any tumour of a solid organ where the limits of the lesion can be accurately defined and the surrounding normal tissue can tolerate a small amount of localized thermal necrosis.

ILP is a technique still in the evolutionary stage and there are few large studies with long-term follow-up, but it does appear safe, effective, and relatively simple.

Photodynamic therapy (PDT)

Photodynamic therapy (PDT) is a way of producing localized tissue necrosis with light after prior administration of a photosensitizing agent.[17] It attracted considerable interest initially as many photosensitizing agents are retained slightly more in cancers than in the adjacent normal tissue in which the tumour arose, which raised the possibility of truly selective destruction of cancers. Regrettably, the selectivity of uptake of photosensitizers is rarely enough to produce selective necrosis when both tumour and normal tissue are exposed to the same light dose. The real attraction of PDT is the nature of the biological effects produced.

Enthusiasts started clinical studies of PDT using the first photosensitizer available, haematoporphyrin derivative (HpD), in the late 1970s and the 1980s. Unfortunately, patients were treated without an adequate understanding of the biology of PDT. As a result, serious problems were encountered. It worked reasonably for cutaneous secondaries from breast cancers and small skin cancers, but when it was used, for example, for widespread carcinoma *in situ* of the bladder, necrosis and subsequent scarring of the muscle layer left some patients with such irritable and contracted bladders that a cystectomy was necessary, even though there was no remaining neoplastic tissue.[18] After such experiences, more effort was put into understanding what PDT did to both normal and neoplastic tissue. As a result, PDT is now being applied in more appropriate clinical situations and is beginning to establish an important therapeutic role.

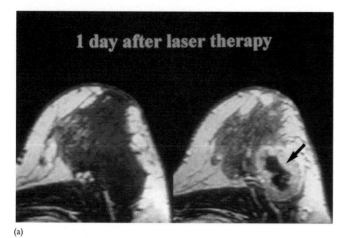

(a)

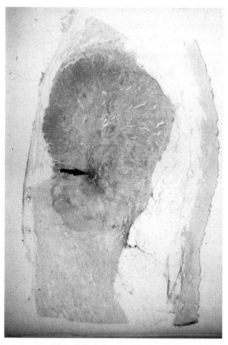

(b)

Fig. 6 (a) Transverse T1-weighted MR image of a breast (left) without contrast and (right) with gadolinium enhancement, 1 day after interstitial laser photocoagulation (ILP) to a small cancer. The outer half of the tumour (arrow) enhances whereas the centre has been devascularized and remains dark. (b) Histological section of the same tumour after surgical removal. The outer rim of the tumour is viable. Within the tumour, there is an upper area of spontaneous tumour necrosis and, below this, an area of laser-induced coagulative necrosis. The position of the tip of the laser fibre is indicated by an arrow. (Reproduced, with permission, from Mumtaz H, *et al. Radiology* 1996; **200**: 651–8.)[15]

The biology of PDT

In contrast to the laser applications discussed above, no heat is involved, and there is only an effect in oxygenated tissue. Red light activates the photosensitizer, which then interacts with molecular oxygen to produce singlet oxygen, which is the mediator of cytotoxicity. Different photosensitizers locate at different sites within cells, but the main targets are probably mitochondria and cell membranes.

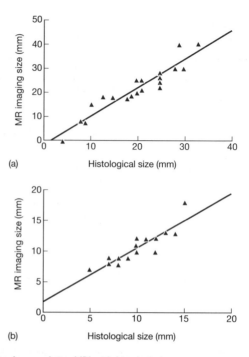

(a)

(b)

Fig. 7 Graphs correlating MRI with histological measurements on small breast cancers treated with interstitial laser photocoagulation (ILP) and excised a few days later. (a) overall tumour size, (b) extent of laser-induced necrosis. (Reproduced, with permission, from *Radiology* 1996; **200**: 651–8.)[15]

There is also considerable variation in which cells retain photosensitizer. Many photosensitizers localize predominantly in the microvasculature, whereas others go to normal and neoplastic glandular cells.[17] These differences can be exploited to match the biological effect to the disease being treated.

One of the most striking aspects of PDT-induced necrosis is that connective tissues such as collagen and elastin are largely unaffected.[19] Thus the mechanical integrity of hollow organs can be maintained, even in the presence of full thickness necrosis, as long as the tissue contains enough connective tissue. Also, many PDT-necrosed tissues heal with more regeneration and less scarring than after other local insults such as heat. Although it is difficult to obtain selective necrosis of tumours compared with the adjacent normal tissue in which the tumour arose, it is possible to obtain selectivity between different normal tissues, and sometimes between different layers of the same tissue.[20] PDT is compared with ILP in Table 6.

Clinical applications of PDT

Like all laser treatments, PDT is a local treatment. Even if the photosensitizer is given systemically, there will only be a biological effect in areas that contain enough photosensitizer and receive an adequate light dose. Neither photosensitizer alone nor light alone will produce any effect. Thus for there to be any prospect of local control, it must be possible to define the limits of a lesion being treated and deliver an adequate light dose to all relevant areas. Nevertheless, even though red light, usually from a laser, is used to activate photosensitizing drugs therapeutically, ambient light may activate drug in the skin, and care must be taken to avoid this sunburn-like

Table 6 Comparison of interstitial laser photocoagulation (ILP) and photodynamic therapy (PDT)

	ILP	PDT
Nature of biological effect	Thermal	Photochemical
Effect on connective tissue	Destroyed	Mainly unaffected
Healing	Resorption and scarring, some regeneration	Regeneration, sometimes with scarring
Selectivity of necrosis between tumour and tissue of origin of tumour	None	Minimal
Selectivity of necrosis between tissue of tumour and other adjacent tissues	None	Possible between mucosa and underlying muscle in hollow organs
Cumulative toxicity	None	None
Wavelength of light used	Infrared (805–1064 nm)	Red (630–760 nm)
Typical laser power per fibre	3–5 W	0.1–0.3 W (higher for illuminating hollow organs)

Table 7 Potential targets for photodynamic therapy in oncology

Small tumours in the wall of hollow organs
Areas of dysplasia in hollow organs
Skin tumours
Localized tumours in solid organs
As an adjunct to surgery

reaction. Using the photosensitizer porfimer sodium (Photofrin), skin sensitivity to bright sunlight can last for up to 3 months. For meso-tetrahydroxyphenyl chlorin (mTHPC, Foscan), the period is 2 to 3 weeks and for 5-amino laevulinic acid (ALA, Levulan) it is only 1 to 2 days. The range of potential targets for PDT in oncology is shown in Table 7.

Tumours of hollow organs

The gentle nature of PDT necrosis and its relative sparing of connective tissue make it suitable for treating small lesions of hollow organs that have not spread beyond the wall of the organ in which they arose. This is of particular value in patients who are not fit for surgery or in whom the cosmetic or functional impairment left after other treatments may be unacceptable, as for example with premalignant and early malignant lesions of the mouth. An early invasive squamous carcinoma of the tongue is shown before and after PDT in Fig. 8.

Most work on localized cancers of the oral cavity has been undertaken with the photosensitisers porfimer sodium and mTHPC. These show no selectivity of necrosis either between normal and neoplastic tissue or between mucosa and the underlying layers, but necrosis can be produced down to a depth of about 4 mm.[22] mTHPC has the advantage that the light doses required are much lower, so the treatment time is shorter.

Normal bone seems remarkably resistant to PDT, so it may prove feasible to treat cancers that invade the maxilla or mandible. Mucosa, submucosa, and salivary glands heal mainly by regeneration. Muscle

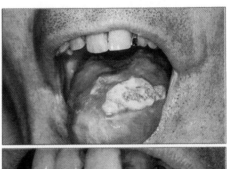
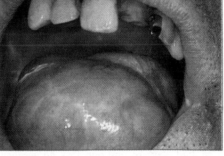

Fig. 8 A small cancer of the tongue before (upper) and after (lower) photodynamic therapy using mTHPC. (Reproduced, with permission, from Bown SG. *British Medical Journal*, 1998; **316**: 754–7.)[21]

regeneration is only partial and there is usually some scarring, but this is acceptable if the area of muscle necrosis is small. Regeneration may continue over a period of several months.

Most small, localized cancers of the gastrointestinal tract and major airways are best treated with surgery, but for unfit patients PDT is an attractive alternative. The preservation of collagen means that it is safe to produce full thickness PDT necrosis with little risk of perforation, even if the cancer involves the muscle layer as histological studies have shown that most early cancers in these organs have as much, if not more, collagen in them as the normal tissue. In a series of 123 patients with early oesophageal cancers treated with PDT using porfimer sodium, the complete response rate at 6 months (no disease detectable on endoscopy and biopsy) was 87 per cent. Although the overall 5-year survival was only 25 per cent, the disease-specific 5-year survival was 74 per cent, so effectively, half the patients died of the underlying cardiorespiratory problems that made them unfit for surgery without major problems from their cancer.[23]

PDT has been proposed as an option for palliating advanced cancers of the aerodigestive tract, particularly obstructing oesophageal cancers. It is questionable whether PDT can offer more than endoscopic thermal laser recanalization or stent insertion, and it has the major disadvantage of making these patients sensitive to bright lights for much of their remaining life;[24] nevertheless, using porfimer sodium, this was the first application of PDT to be licensed by the Food and Drug Administration in the United States. It is understandable that the first approval should be for patients with advanced, incurable disease, but PDT is far more likely to establish a significant role in the treatment of early disease.

5-Amino laevulinic acid (ALA) is a naturally occurring substance that *in vivo* is converted, through a series of intermediates, to protoporphyrin IX (PPIX), which is a photosensitiser, and haem.[17] ALA is an important photosensitizing agent as it can be given by mouth, produces clinically useful levels of PPIX in target tissues in 3 to 6 h and is cleared from the body in 24 to 48 h. After systemic administration, PPIX is produced predominantly in the mucosa of the aerodigestive and urogenital tracts, with very little in the underlying layers. This makes it possible to achieve mucosal necrosis with essentially no effect in deeper layers, particularly muscle, which is difficult with any of the other photosensitisers.[20] The potential value of this property is in treating large areas of abnormal mucosa, such as those showing dysplasia or carcinoma *in situ*. This is useful in the mouth, but the indication that is attracting most attention is for Barrett's oesophagus where it may be possible to destroy areas of mucosa circumferentially (with or without dysplasia) without the risk of strictures (which can be as high as 50 per cent using other photosensitisers such as porfimer sodium). In a recent report using ALA PDT in patients with Barrett's oesophagus, high grade dysplasia was cleared in 10 out of 10 and mucosal carcinoma was cleared in 17 out of 22 patients, and there were no oesophageal strictures.[25] However, mucosal ablation is not always complete and further research is required to find ways of ensuring that no residual columnar epithelium remains under regenerated squamous epithelium. Surgery is still the treatment of choice for Barrett's oesophagus with high grade dysplasia, but for those who are unfit for surgery, PDT is a worthwhile alternative.

In the bladder, intravesical instillation of ALA is proving a valuable aid to diagnosis as there is sufficient selectivity of synthesis of PPIX in dysplastic tissue to identify these areas using fluorescence endoscopy. The sensitivity for detecting neoplastic areas can be increased from 73 per cent with conventional white light cystoscopy to 97 per cent with PPIX fluorescence, although there was no improvement in specificity.[26]

Superficial skin tumours, particularly basal cell carcinomas, are well suited to PDT with ALA, as the ALA can be applied topically under an occlusive dressing. This avoids any generalized photosensitivity, the cosmetic results are usually excellent and the complete response rate can be over 90 per cent. Nevertheless, it is appropriate only for lesions no more than 1 to 2 mm thick.[27]

Tumours of solid organs

Most PDT research has centred on treating tumours of hollow organs and the skin, but there is more recent interest in its potential for lesions of solid organs. Most primary cerebral tumours take up much more of many photosensitizers than adjacent normal brain but, unfortunately, normal brain is very sensitive to PDT. Nevertheless, PDT with porfimer sodium has been tried as a way of sterilizing the tumour bed after excision of intracranial gliomas for some years. The data are limited, but one series of 56 cases reports encouraging results using PDT after resection of recurrent tumours.[28]

The relative sparing of connective tissues exposed to PDT[19] has stimulated research on its application to three much commoner cancers, those of the prostate, pancreas, and lung. Small tumours of the major airways can be treated with PDT bronchoscopically, but inoperable, peripheral lung cancers may be suitable for interstitial PDT. Animal studies on all three of these organs[29] have shown that although PDT affects them and the surrounding tissues, these changes can be tolerated, so justifying pilot clinical studies. Clinical studies have not yet started for peripheral lung tumours, but for the prostate and pancreas preliminary results have been reported using mTHPC. In the prostate study, 12 patients with locally recurrent cancers (detected by increasing levels of PSA, prostate specific antigen, after previous radical radiotherapy) were treated.[30] Light was delivered to the tumour areas in the prostate using fibres passed through needles positioned through the perineal skin under transrectal ultrasound or interventional magnetic resonance guidance. The PSA level came down in seven patients. There were some complications (stress incontinence in two, which improved, and impotence in two which did not improve), but these problems were less than would have been anticipated from other salvage treatments such as cryotherapy or radical prostatectomy. The pancreas study reported treatment of 12 patients with localized but inoperable cancers.[31] Light was delivered via fibres inserted through needles positioned in the tumours through the anterior abdominal wall under CT guidance. There were no major complications and zones of necrosis up to 5 cm in diameter were demonstrated on contrast enhanced CT scans taken a few days after PDT. One patient lived for 16 months and two more were still alive more than a year after treatment.

Interstitial PDT for small, localized tumours of solid organs is in its infancy, but appears to have considerable potential as it is well tolerated. Yet another application is to use PDT as adjunctive therapy in association with conventional surgery to destroy small tumour deposits that may not be visible to the surgeon or that involve vital structures that cannot be excised. This was discussed above in relation to intracranial tumours, but could be applied in many other areas, as for example with radical dissections of the neck.

Conclusions

Early clinical uses of lasers in oncology were crude and the equipment was large, expensive, unreliable and difficult to use. Many clinical lasers are now the size of a briefcase, can be plugged into a standard power socket, and are rugged enough to be moved easily between different sites. The applications are becoming more sophisticated as the biological effects are better understood. The basic principles of both thermal and photochemical effects can be applied to disease processes in a wide range of organs. The challenge is to define the true extent of the neoplastic disease being treated and then match the extent of the treatment such that the disease process is controlled and all treated tissue maintains adequate structure and function during healing.

References

1. Ambrosch P, Kron M, Steiner W. Carbon dioxide laser microsurgery for early supraglottic carcinoma. *Annals of Otology Rhinology and Laryngology*, 1998; **107**: 680–8.

2. Fleischer D, Kessler F, Haye O. Endoscopic NdYAG laser therapy for carcinoma of the oesophagus. A new palliative approach. *American Journal of Surgery*, 1982; **143**: 280–3.

3. Ell C, Riemann JF, Lux G, Demling L. Palliative laser treatment of malignant stenoses in the upper gastrointestinal tract. *Endoscopy*, 1986; **18** (Suppl. 1):21–6.

4. Bown SG. Palliation of malignant dysphagia: surgery, radiotherapy, laser, intubation—alone or in combination? *Gut*, 1991; **32**: 841–4.

5. Brunetaud JM, Manoury V, Ducrotte P, Cochelard D, Cortot A, Paris JC. Palliative treatment of rectosigmoid carcinomas by laser endoscopic photoablation. *Gastroenterology*, 1987; **92**: 663–8.

6. Hetzel MR, Smith SGT. Endoscopic palliation of tracheobronchial malignancies. *Thorax*, 1991; **46**: 325–33.

7. Brutinel WM, Cortese DA, McDougall JC, Gillio RG, Bergstralh EJ. A two year experience with the neodymium-YAG laser in endobronchial obstruction. *Chest*, 1987; **91**: 159–65.

8. Beisland HO, Seland P. A prospective, randomised study on NdYAG laser irradiation versus TUR in the treatment of urinary bladder cancer. *Scandinavian Journal of Urology and Nephrology*, 1986; **20**: 209–12.

9. Bown SG. Phototherapy of tumours. *World Journal of Surgery*, 1983; **7**: 700–9.

10. Steger AC, Lees WR, Walmesely K, Bown SG. Interstitial laser hyperthermia: a new approach to local destruction of tumours. *British Medical Journal*, 1989; **299**: 362–5.

11. Amin Z, Bown SG, Lees WR. Liver tumour ablation by interstitial laser photocoagulation—review of experimental and clinical studies. *Seminars in Interventional Radiology*, 1993; **10**: 88–100.

12. Vogl TJ, Mack MG, Straub R, Roggan A, Felix R. Magnetic resonance imaging guided abdominal interventional radiology: laser induced thermotherapy of liver metastases. *Endoscopy*, 1997; **29**: 577–83.

13. Amin Z, Donald JJ, Masters A, *et al.* Hepatic metastases: interstitial laser photocoagulation with real-time US monitoring and dynamic CT evaluation of treatment. *Radiology*, 1993; **187**: 339–47.

14. Kettenbach J, Silverman SG, Hata N, *et al.* Monitoring and visualisation techniques for MR guided laser ablation in an open MR system. *Journal of Magnetic Resonance Imaging*, 1998; **8**: 933–43.

15. Mumtaz H, Hall-Craggs MA, Wotherspoon A, Paley M, Buonaccorsi G, Amin Z, *et al.* Laser therapy for breast cancer: MR imaging and histopathologic correlation. *Radiology*, 1996; **200**: 651–8.

16. Menovsky T, Beek JF, van Gemert MJ, Roux FX. Interstitial laser thermotherapy in neurosurgery: a review. *Acta Neurochirurgica*, 1996; **138**: 1019–26.

17. Dougherty TJ, Gomer CJ, Henderson BW, *et al.* Photodynamic therapy. *Journal of the National Cancer Institute*, 1998; **90**: 889–905.

18. Harty JI, Amin M, Wieman TJ, Tseng MT, Ackerman D, Broghamer W. Complications of whole bladder dihematoporphyrin ether photodynamic therapy. *Journal of Urology*, 1989; **141**: 1341.

19. Barr H, Tralau CJ, Boulos PB, MacRobert AJ, Tilly R, Bown SG. The contrasting mechanisms of colonic damage between photodynamic therapy and thermal injury. *Photochemistry and Photobiology*, 1987; **46**: 795–800.

20. Loh CS, MacRobert AJ, Buonaccorsi G, Krasner N, Bown SG. Mucosal ablation using photodynamic therapy for the treatment of dysplasia—an experimental study in the normal rat stomach. *Gut*, 1996; **38**: 71–8.

21. Bown SG. Science, medicine and the future. New techniques in laser therapy. *British Medical Journal* 1998; **316**: 754–7.

22. Grant WE, Speight PM, Hopper C, Bown SG. Photodynamic therapy—an effective but non–selective treatment for superficial cancers of the oral cavity. *International Journal of Cancer*, 1997; **71**: 937–42.

23. Sibille A, Lambert R, Souquet JC, Sabben G, Descos F. Long term survival after photodynamic therapy for esophageal cancer. *Gastroenterology*, 1995; **108**: 337–44.

24. Bown SG, Millson CE. Photodynamic therapy in gastroenterology. *Gut*, 1997; **41**: 5–7.

25. Gossner L, Stolte M, Sroka R, *et al.* Photodynamic ablation of high grade dysplasia in Barrett's esophagus by means of 5-amino levulinic acid. *Gastroenterology*, 1998; **114**: 448–55.

26. Kriegmair M, Baumgartner R, Knochel R, Stepp H, Hofstadter F, Hofstetter A. Detection of early bladder cancer by 5-aminolevulinic acid induced porphyrin fluorescence. *Journal of Urology*, 1996; **155**: 105–10.

27. Fritsch C, Goerz G, Ruzicka T. Photodynamic therapy in dermatology. *Archives of Dermatology*, 1998; **134**: 207–14.

28. Muller PJ, Wilson BC. Photodynamic therapy for recurrent supratentorial gliomas. *Seminars in Surgery and Oncology*, 1995; **11**: 346–54.

29. Chang SC, Buonaccorsi G, MacRobert AJ, Bown SG. Interstitial and transurethral photodynamic therapy of the canine prostate with meso-tetra hydoxyphenyl chlorin. *International Journal of Cancer*, 1996; **67**: 555–62.

30. Nathan TR, Whitelaw DE, Lees WR, *et al.* Photodynamic therapy for prostate cancer: a phase I study treating recurrence after radiotherapy. *Journal of Urology*, 1999; **161**: 340 (suppl.).

31. Rogowska AZ, Whitelaw DE, Lees WR, *et al.* Photodynamic therapy for palliation of unresectable pancreatic cancer. *Gut*, 1999; **44**: A.48 (suppl. 1).

5

Complications
of cancer

5.1 Serous effusions

Ian S. Fentiman

Introduction

Serous effusions can produce severe yet reversible symptoms which, if inadequately treated, result in prolonged morbidity and multiple hospital admissions. Effective local procedures may improve quality of life and postpone requirement for systemic palliative therapy. Treatment decisions and procedures are often made by the least experienced team members whereas involvement of senior staff in management of effusions will improve results. Ample evidence from clinical trials is available on malignant pleural effusions but treatments for ascites and pericardial effusions have not been subjected to randomized study.

Pathophysiology

The pleural space contains only 5 to 10 ml, and the peritoneal cavity less than 100 ml, of fluid in an unobstructed state, despite a normal diurnal flow of 5 to 10 litres from the parietal to the visceral surface.[1] Fluid enters the serosal space as a result of high hydrostatic pressure and capillary permeability of the parietal surface. Resorption occurs on the visceral surface which has a relatively large capillary network draining into the low pressure pulmonary or hepatic portal systems. Capillary permeability leads to small losses of protein into serous cavities, with larger molecules being absorbed by lymphatics. This maintains a low colloid osmotic pressure within the space so that egress of fluid is facilitated.

Either singly or jointly, any of the factors modulating fluid flux can be disturbed in patients with malignancy. The most frequent is altered capillary permeability arising from tumour deposits on the serosal surface. Obstruction of lymphatics resulting from either tumour or radiation can lead to a failure of absorption of protein which in turn increases the colloid osmotic pressure within the serous cavity. These causes lead to the production of an exudate (protein >3 g/l00 ml). Rarely, patients with malignancy may develop congestive cardiac failure leading to bilateral pleural effusion which are transudates (protein <3 g/l00 ml). Transudates also occur in patients with hypoproteinaemia resulting from malignant cachexia.

Pleural effusions

Aetiology

From an oncological rather than a general thoracic viewpoint, the commonest cause of malignant pleural effusions is lung cancer in males and breast cancer in females. A review of primary histology from patients with cytologically-verified malignant pleural effusions is summarized in Table 1.[2]

Most commonly, these effusions result from increased production of fluid due to alteration in capillary permeability at the site of parietal pleural metastases. Under these circumstances pleural fluid will most likely contain malignant cells, which may also be detectable on blind pleural biopsy. Patients with pulmonary metastases and visceral pleural involvement may also shed cells into the pleural fluid, but in those with lymphatic obstruction malignant cells are least likely to be present.

Presenting features

The commonest symptom is dyspnoea, which may or may not be associated with dull or pleuritic pain. Often patients complain of an irritating, dry cough. Depending upon the volume of fluid, there may be dullness to percussion over the lung base(s) with decreased breath sounds. Confirmation of clinical suspicion is by chest radiograph. A posteroanterior view will show basal opacity which shifts to lie inferiorly on the lateral decubitus view. Having verified that an effusion is present in a patient with known malignancy, further evaluation will be necessary to determine whether cancer relapse is responsible. This may pose problems when the effusion is the first evidence of possible recurrence.

Table 1 Primary tumours of patients with proven malignant pleural effusions (Johnston, 1985)[2]

Male	%	Female	%
Lung	49	Breast	39
Lymphoma/leukaemia	21	Genitourinary	21
Gastrointestinal	7	Lung	15
Genitourinary	6	Lymphoma/leukaemia	8
Melanoma	1	Gastrointestinal	4
Mesothelioma	1	Melanoma	3
Other	4	Other	2
Unknown	11	Unknown	9

Definitive diagnostic procedures

Thoracentesis

The first invasive step should be a diagnostic thoracentesis, taking a small volume of pleural fluid (10–20 ml) for cytological examination. Contraindications to this procedure are the presence of a clotting abnormality or a low platelet count which might predispose to a haemothorax. The colour of pleural fluid is variable but is most commonly yellow or amber and less often bloodstained. Rare cases with thoracic duct infiltration have a milky chylothorax. Cytologically-identifiable malignant cells are present in approximately 50 per cent of cases with proven malignant effusions,[3],[4] with atypical cells reported in 12 per cent of such cases.[4] Because of the low specificity of cytology, other techniques have been used in an attempt to reduce the number of false negative reports in patients with metastatic effusions.

Cell culture has been examined as an adjunct to cytology, but the results were not encouraging.[5] Hostmark et al. used flow cytometry to examine cells in effusions from 37 patients with malignancy, of which 13 effusions contained malignant cells (nine aneuploid and four diploid).[6] Of the 24 cytologically-negative cases, 21 contained diploid and three contained aneuploid cells. The accuracy of cytology was not improved by flow cytometry among patients with primary tumours of lung, breast, pancreas, and ovary. As a different approach, fluorescence in situ hybridization (FISH) was used to identify changes in chromosome number in cells from 41 breast cancer patients with pleural effusions.[7] Aneuploid cells were present in 94 per cent of effusions which were cytologically positive and in 48 per cent of those that were negative.

Pleural biopsy

In patients with negative cytology, attempts have been made to increase the diagnostic yield by blind biopsy of the parietal pleura using either an Abram's or a Cope's needle. Because of the patchy nature of parietal nodules or the location of tumour on the visceral surface, the additional histological yield has been variable. In three series comprising 428 cases, the overall positivity rate was 50 per cent.[8]–[10] It was reported that when parietal pleural biopsies were positive, 11 per cent of such cases had negative effusion cytology.[8] The diagnostic yield of pleural biopsy may be increased slightly by altering the needle angle, thereby taking a larger area of parietal pleura.[11] Because of the hit and miss nature of blind biopsy, the assessment of patients with suspected malignant effusions can be improved when thoracoscopy is included within the diagnostic work-up. This may also have therapeutic implications when pleurodesis is being considered.

Thoracoscopy

This procedure can be performed using either regional or general anaesthesia, the latter being preferred if it is planned to proceed to a pleurodesis. The diagnostic yield of thoracoscopy in patients with suspected malignant effusions, in three series, was 95 per cent and in the majority a histological diagnosis was made.[12]–[14] Morbidity from parietal pleural biopsy is minimal although occasionally it may be necessary to diathermy bleeding vessels.

Prognosis

Determination of the prognosis, and thus the need for aggressive local therapy, can be difficult. There are wide ranges of survival for patients with particular primary tumours. Median survival after development of a pleural effusion in patients with breast cancer is 15 months.[15] For patients with lung primaries, median survival is 6 months, falling to 3 months in those with gastric cancer.[16] Like breast cancer, mesothelioma has a relatively prolonged survival of 18 months after presentation with an effusion.[17] Patients who have lymphoma and pleural effusions are treated by systemic rather than local therapy, and their prognosis relates to the response of the effusion.[18] Non-responders had a median survival of 6 months, compared with greater than 40 months for those whose effusion disappeared after systemic therapy.

It is an indication of the imprecision of prognostic factors that almost one in five of patients entered into clinical trials of different pleurodesis methods died within 2 months of treatment.[19] Until more reliable techniques of determining prognosis are found, whenever possible patients should be offered definitive treatment for malignant pleural effusion.

Direct approaches

Decortication of entrapped lung and stripping of parietal pleural will lead to a very successful pleurodesis but with an associated mortality of up to12.5 per cent.[20] Partial pleurectomy can be performed as a video-assisted thoracoscopic procedure using hydrodissection but still carries a mortality rate of 9 per cent.[21] These approaches should be reserved for patients who have had previous unsuccessful attempts at pleurodesis.

A direct drainage approach has been used whereby an implanted Leveen or Denver shunt connects the pleural and peritoneal cavities.[22]–[24] Such shunts do not drain spontaneously because of the similar intrapleural and intraperitoneal pressures, and patients have to compress the pump up to 80 times daily. Although shunts carry the theoretical risk of transforming a malignant pleural effusion into a malignant peritoneal effusion, this has not been encountered. The need for regular pumping may be problematic in patients becoming incapacitated by other problems of metastatic malignancy.

Pleurodesis

Despite intensive efforts, there will be 5 to 10 per cent of patients with pleural effusions due to malignancy in whom proof of recurrence of disease cannot be obtained. Provided that other causes of effusions have been excluded by appropriate tests, if the patient is dyspnoeic, pleurodesis should be performed. The object of treatment is to achieve palliation as simply and as effectively as possible without compromising the use of subsequent systemic therapy. Although hospitalization may be required at the time of pleurodesis, if this is successful this will substantially reduce subsequent hospital visits since repeated thoracenteses will be unnecessary. It is important that appropriate therapy is given at the time of first diagnosis. Unsuccessful pleurodesis will lead to loculation and pleural entrapment which can be difficult to treat by means other than pleurectomy.

Despite there being a plethora of agents which have been used, and sometimes tested, they may be divided into four main groups—radioactive isotopes, cytotoxic agents, biological response modifiers, and sclerosants. Although there are theoretical reasons for particular approaches having a greater or lesser tumouricidal effect, the success of any of these techniques depends upon the ability of the agent to excite a pleural reaction whereby the parietal and visceral layers of pleura fuse. In order to achieve this, the pleural space needs to be drained of fluid, and the parietal and visceral layer of pleura must be apposed so that they are joined by the resulting inflammatory response engendered by the intracavitary agent. Even the most effective agents will not achieve pleural fusion in the presence of undrained effusions, or where the lung has not re-expanded because of a persistent pneumothorax.

Assessment of response

The major problem in the interpretation of results of studies using intracavitary agents is the absence of any agreed system of measuring response to treatment. A variety of methods have been used ranging from subjective endpoints, such as relief of dyspnoea, to objective measurements, such as presence or absence of fluid in subsequent radiographs or the need for subsequent aspirations. Often, no defined length of follow-up is given. A simple system has been proposed which includes both an objective and a subjective element.[19] There are three categories, each based on chest radiograph and symptoms. The post-aspirational chest radiograph is used as the baseline. The complete response category comprises those who have no recurrence of fluid from the time of pleurodesis until death, or date of last follow-up. A minimum of 4 weeks should elapse between treatment and follow-up chest radiograph. Partial responders have recurrence of fluid but without a need for further treatment. The failure category means that there has been symptomatic reaccumulation of pleural fluid, confirmed by chest radiograph.

Controlled trials of agents for pleurodesis

Representatives of each of the four classes of agents have been tested in prospective, randomized trials. Only one study examined the use of a radioisotope and this compared intrapleural instillation of ^{32}P with drainage alone.[25] There were 68 evaluable cases and control was achieved in 19/31 (60 per cent) of those treated with ^{32}P and 16/37 (34 per cent) of those who had drainage alone.

Three trials have examined the efficacy of mustine which has been compared with *Corynebacterium parvum*, Adriamycin/ tetracycline, and talc.[26]–[28] The overall success rate was 47 per cent (95 per cent CI 43–54). One explanation for the relative inefficacy is the rapid transpleural flux, as witnessed by early production of nausea after instillation so that there is insufficient retained drug within the pleural space to elicit an inflammatory response. The rapid hydrolysis of mustine in aqueous solution also limits its vesicant effect. Bleomycin has been used as an intracavitary agent in three trials.[29]–[31] With the exception of the trial of Ostrowski *et al.*, the other studies found that less than half the patients treated had successful control of their effusions.

Thiotepa has been tested against quinacrine and against drainage alone.[32] Control was achieved in only 27 per cent of those treated with thiotepa, in 11 per cent of those having drainage alone, and in 64 per cent of cases in which quinacrine was instilled. Only one published trial used intracavitary Adriamycin and achieved a control rate of 80 per cent.[27] In a trial from Hong Kong, intracavitary mitomycin-C and *C. parvum* were compared.[33] Thirty patients were

Table 2 Ranking of efficacy of agents for pleurodesis tested in clinical trials

Agent	Percentage control (95% CI)
Talc	96 (93.5–98.5)
Quinacrine	82 (76–85)
C. parvum	72 (52–87)
Tetracycline	65 (58–72)
Mustine	48 (43–54)
Drainage alone	46 (38–54)
Bleomycin	39 (24–53)

treated and control of the effusion was achieved in only 5/15 (33 per cent) of cases in each group.

C. parvum is the only biological agent which has been used in randomized trials of intracavitary therapy and five studies have been carried out.[29],[30],[33]–[35] The early trials were very promising and reported high control rates, but more recently effusion control has been unexpectedly disappointing. Overall effusion control was achieved in 72 per cent (95 per cent CI 57–87).

Of the sclerosing agents, tetracycline has been the most extensively studied in controlled trials.[27],[35]–[39] The overall rate of control was 65 per cent (95 per cent CI 58–72). Despite this low rate of success, tetracycline is still regarded by many as the ideal agent for pleurodesis. When tetracycline instillation was compared with dilute hydrochloric acid, at a similar pH of 2.8, the latter had a very low success rate suggesting that the mechanism of sclerosis is unrelated to the low pH of tetracycline solution.[37] In a small trial, Evans *et al.* compared medical pleurodesis using tetracycline 500 mg (17 cases) with surgical drainage followed by instillation of tetracycline 500 mg (17 cases). There was recurrence of effusion in eight (47 per cent) of the medical cases and in six (35 per cent) of those treated surgically.

Three studies have tested intracavitary quinacrine.[32],[36],[40] The overall success rate was 82 per cent (95 per cent CI 76–88). Stiksa *et al.* compared two methods of administering quinacrine, with and without an intercostal drain, and achieved similar rates of control after repeated thoracentesis or continuous drainage.

There have been four trials of talc poudrage.[28],[31],[38],[41] There is a consistently high rate of effusion control in 96 per cent (95 per cent CI 93.5–98.5). When agents are ranked in terms of success rates derived from clinical trials (Table 2), it is apparent that the best control of pleural effusions is obtained after talc poudrage. The majority of trials used simple rather than iodized talc. Hence insufflation of simple talc should be regarded as the treatment of choice for patients with malignant pleural effusions who are fit enough for a general anaesthetic. The agent can be instilled under local or general anaesthesia. The latter enables a complete drainage of pleural fluid and permits thoracoscopy to be performed, with the opportunity to biopsy pleural lesions and obtain tissue confirmation of relapse.[42] It should be stressed that an experienced anaesthetist is required to administer the anaesthetic.

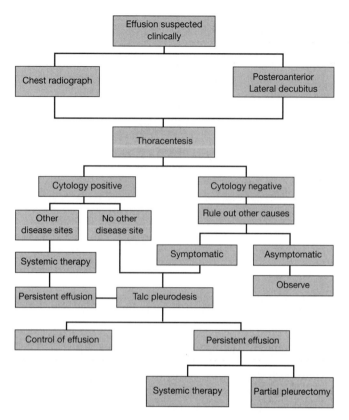

Fig. 1 Scheme of management for patients with cancer and pleural effusions.

Plan of treatment

A scheme of management for patients with malignancy and who have developed pleural effusions is shown in Fig. 1. For a patient with a symptomatic effusion, in whom no non-malignant cause is present, the decision to perform a talc pleurodesis should be made as soon as the effusion is symptomatic, irrespective of effusion cytology. The procedure, which may appear deceptively simple, needs to be performed by an experienced team. The effusion is drained to dryness, and then 10 to 15 g of simple talc is insufflated. One intercostal drain is sufficient, provided that there have not been previously unsuccessful attempts at pleurodesis using inferior techniques.

Postoperatively the drain remains *in situ* for 5 days, with applied negative pressure and physiotherapy if there is a persistent pneumothorax. Premature drain removal may lead to further fluid accumulation so that the parietal and visceral pleural surfaces become separated. Retention of intercostal drains beyond 5 days leads to an increased risk of empyema. Talc pleurodesis has an undeserved reputation for producing severe postoperative pain. Opiate analgesics may be required for 24 h postoperatively, and occasionally prior to physiotherapy. Thereafter only moderate analgesics are required. Now that talc poudrage is becoming accepted as first line therapy, it is important that better prognostic indices are developed in order that effective local treatment is given to those who will benefit and that simple palliation (thoracentesis) is used for patients in a terminal state.

Pericardial effusions

Aetiology

Excess fluid within the pericardial space of patients with cancer may arise either as a result of altered capillary permeability associated with visceral or parietal tumour nodules, or alternatively from lymphatic obstruction due to infiltration of mediastinal lymphatics.[26] Additionally, the effusion may be non-neoplastic in origin from causes such as trauma, infection, or connective tissue disease. Finally, pericardial effusions may follow radiotherapy, or be mimicked by the pericardial fibrosis resulting from such treatment. In one series, approximately 60 per cent had malignant infiltration of the pericardium, 32 per cent had idiopathic pericarditis, and 10 per cent had radiation-induced effusions.[43]

Presenting features

Some pericardial effusions are asymptomatic and are detected as a result of routine chest radiographs or echocardiogram. In other patients the effusion produces cardiac tamponade and presents as an acute medical emergency. The commonest symptom in patients with pericardial effusions is dyspnoea, either on exertion, at night, or in the form of orthopnoea. A cough may be associated and chest pain may be present. In a large series of 66 cases, dyspnoea was present in 97 per cent, cough in 26 per cent, orthopnoea in 21 per cent, and chest pain in 18 per cent.[44] The most frequent clinical signs are pulsus paradoxus (50 per cent), jugular venous distension (42 per cent), peripheral oedema (36 per cent), and hypotension (33 per cent). Heart sounds may be distant and a pericardial rub and hepatomegaly are present in up to one-quarter of cases. More rarely, there may be splenomegaly, pleural effusions, a gallop rhythm, or rales. Patients with idiopathic effusions are more likely to be pyrexial and have an associated pericardial friction rub.[43] The key to diagnosis is a high index of suspicion in cancer patients who suddenly deteriorates with shortness of breath and chest pain. Asymptomatic patients are best managed conservatively since they are the group with the best long-term survival.[45]

Investigations

A plain chest radiograph will show evidence of cardiomegaly, possibly with associated bilateral effusions. Presence of fluid can be confirmed by echocardiography, with a pericardial echo distinct from the posterior cardiac border. More complex techniques include simultaneous cardiac/lung isotopic scans, or CT scan of the chest. Electrocardiographic changes are usually non-specific, showing low voltage activity and occasional T-wave abnormalities with alterations in the ST segment.[46]

Pericardiocentesis

Confirmation of the presence of an effusion is by pericardial aspiration, which may be both diagnostic and therapeutic. The standard approach to the pericardium is subxiphoid. A 14-gauge needle is used and inserted midway between the xiphoid process and the left costal margin.[47] It is angled at 45 degrees to the chest wall and aimed in the direction of the right sternoclavicular joint. Once the pericardial space has been entered, fluid is withdrawn, after which a fine catheter (SF) can be inserted for drainage and, if necessary, for instillation of

Table 3 Results of pericardiocentesis (with or without drainage) for malignant pericardial effusions

Author	Method	Success rate
Flannery et al. 1975[47]	Tap	2/2
	Catheter drainage	4/4
Reynolds and Byrne 1977[48]	Tap	3/3
Posner et al. 1981[43]	Catheter drainage	4/9
Woll et al. 1987[49]	Tap	18/22
Buck et al. 1987[50]	Tap	1/4
Moores et al. 1995[51]	Tap	80/82
Total		112/123 (91%)

Table 4 Results of intracavitary agents for control of malignant pericardial effusions

Author	Agent	Success rate
Weisberger et al. 1955[53]	Mustine	3/3
Suhrland and Weisberger 1965[54]	Fluorouracil	3/3
Smith et al. 1974[55]	Mustine	0/1
	Thiotepa	2/4
	Quinacrine	2/2
Davies et al. 1984[52]	Tetracycline	30/32
Lentzsch et al. 1994[56]	Mitoxantrone	5/6
Overall		45/49

Table 5 Pericardial window formation and control of malignant pericardial effusions

Author	Success rate
Hawkins et al. 1980[57]	17/17
Pichler et al. 1985[58]	13/16
Osuch et al. 1985[59]	12/12
Buck et al. 1987[50]	10/10
Overall	52/55 (95%)

sclerosants. During the procedure, continuous ECG monitoring is used to give warning of the needle abutting against the ventricle and avoid myocardial puncture with risk of ventricular fibrillation or haemorrhage.

Treatment

Pericardial aspirations may serve as definitive therapy for some patients. Series reporting results of aspiration, with or without catheter drainage, are summarized in Table 3. Overall, this relatively simple procedure achieved control of the effusion and prevented recurrence in 91 per cent of cases.

Because of the success of intrapleural agents in producing pleurodesis and thereby preventing recurrent pleural effusions, similar procedures have been used in patients with pericardial effusion. The results obtained with a variety of agents are summarized in Table 4. With the exception of one study, which indicated control of effusions by intracavitary tetracycline in 30/32 (94 per cent),[52] all the other reports comprised small numbers of cases.[53]–[56] Overall, control of the pericardial effusion was achieved in 93 per cent. There is minimal gain from intracavitary instillation of sclerosants in patients with

malignant pericardial effusions, and no evidence that there is subsequent difficulty in controlling effusions which do not respond to drainage alone.

Formation of pericardial window

This procedure may be performed as an emergency, if necessary under local anaesthesia, to achieve relief of tamponade and prevent recurrence of the pericardial effusion. Usually the surgical approach is subxiphoid, but a thoracic approach may be used in patients in whom pulmonary resection is contemplated. The xiphoid process is resected, and the pericardium displayed after splitting the sternal attachment of the diaphragm. After insertion of stay sutures, a 2-cm pericardial window is made and one of the drains inserted into the pericardial cavity. These remain *in situ* until drainage of fluid has ceased, usually 4 to 7 days. Almost universally good results have been reported, as shown in Table 5.[50],[57]–[59] An overall control rate of 95 per cent was achieved. For those few patients in whom recurrent fluid develops, or when pericardial fibrosis produces tamponade, a pericardiectomy may be necessary, but this will be a rare event.

Treatment scheme

Figure 2 is a suggested management scheme for patients with malignant pericardial effusions. Unless the patient has non-life-threatening disease, and has lymphoma where systemic therapy would be first-line treatment, a local approach should be used. Among patients in

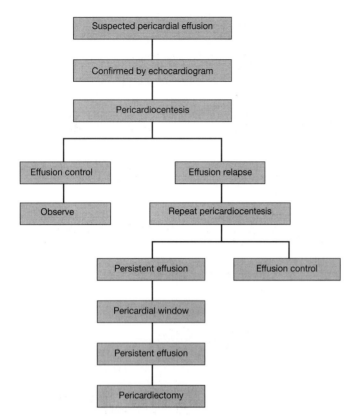

Fig. 2 Management scheme for patients with malignant pericardial effusions.

whom effusion control cannot be achieved after two attempts at drainage, surgical formation of a pericardial window should be considered since this will almost invariably lead to control of symptoms and prevention of recurrence of pericardial fluid.

Peritoneal effusions

Aetiology

Malignant ascites commonly results from the presence of peritoneal metastatic nodules which both increase the production and inhibit the absorption of peritoneal fluid. In ovarian carcinoma, ascites is the presenting feature in one-third of cases and occurs during the course of the disease in two-thirds.[60] Alternatively, ascites may arise in the terminal stages of liver metastases from almost any primary source. The different causes have important prognostic implications. Patients with breast cancer who have malignant ascites associated with hepatomegaly or jaundice have a poor prognosis with 90 per cent dying within 3 months.[61]

Diagnosis

The usual presenting symptom is abdominal swelling which is uncomfortable and may be associated with an unpleasant feeling of fullness and consequent diminution of appetite. Patients may also complain of weight gain despite eating very little. Clinically, the abdomen is tensely distended with a dull percussion note which may become tympanitic in the flank on shifting the patient from supine to a lateral position. The diagnosis may be backed up by an ultrasound and can be confirmed by needle aspiration. In a patient who has not relapsed previously and who has no other evidence of metastatic disease, proof that the ascites is malignant in origin may be more difficult. Cytological confirmation of the presence of malignant cells is possible in approximately 50 per cent of cases, but it may be difficult to distinguish between atypical mesothelium and malignant cells.

Treatment

First-line therapy in malignant ascites is medical with surgical intervention being reserved for refractory cases. For those patients with other sites of metastatic disease, systemic cytotoxic or endocrine therapy will be required as this may in itself produce regression of ascites. If this does not achieve control, or in patients with isolated ascites, diuretic therapy should be instituted to palliate the problem. Unless the patient is severely distressed by massive ascites, aspiration of large volumes should be avoided because of rapid refilling and large protein losses.

Diuretic therapy

Just as with ascites of non-malignant origin, so it is possible in some cases to achieve control of ascites with appropriate use of diuretics. Seventeen patients with malignant ascites resulting from a variety of primaries were treated with spironolactone at an initial dosage of 150 mg daily, in divided doses, increasing by 50 mg if the weight loss was less than 0.5 kg daily.[62] Two patients died within 1 week. Control of the effusion was achieved in 13/15 (87 per cent) of the others. In another study of patients with malignant ascites, frusemide was used at a dosage of 100 mg/24 h and control was achieved in 4/4 (100 per cent).[63]

Instillation of intraperitoneal agents

Because of the success of intracavitary isotopes, cytotoxics, sclerosants, and biological agents in controlling pleural effusions, they have been similarly employed in attempts to control malignant ascites. Intracavitary bleomycin has been used in four series comprising a total of 79 cases; control of ascites was achieved in 39 (49 per cent).[64]–[67] Better results have been reported for intracavitary quinacrine where an overall rate of control of 68 per cent (44/65) was achieved.[68]–[71]

Various biological agents have been used for intracavitary treatment of malignant ascites. Using *C. parvum*, control of ascites occurred in 7/11 cases (64 per cent).[72] Intraperitoneal OK-432, an extract from *Steptococcus pyogenes*, was given to 134 Japanese patients with malignant ascites and the effusion disappeared in 76 (57 per cent) and was reduced in volume in a further eight (6 per cent).[73] Recombinant tumour necrosis factor was administered intraperitoneally to 13 women with refractory ascites and production of ascitic fluid ceased in all cases.[74] Using a combination of intraperitoneal interferon-α-2b interferon (20–50 MU) and mitoxantrone (20–50 mg) control of malignant ascites was achieved in 8/16 (50 per cent) but with half the patients suffering side-effects including flu-like symptoms, abdominal pain, vomiting, diarrhoea, and bowel obstruction.[75]

Table 6 Results of peritoneovenous shunts for palliation of malignant ascites

Author	Success rate	
	LeVeen shunt	**Denver shunt**
Kudsk *et al.* 1978[77]	6/8 (75%)	
Strauss *et al.* 1979[78]	27/35 (77%)	
Oosterlee 1980[79]	5/13 (38%)	7/8 (88%)
Lokich *et al.* 1980[80]	6/8 (75%)	
Holman and Albo 1981[81]		5/6 (83%)
Gough 1982[82]	9/11 (82%)	
Souter *et al.* 1985[83]	5/16 (31%)	14/27 (52%)
Overall	62/98 (63%)	26/41 (63%)

Only one prospective, randomized trial has evaluated the role of intracavitary agents in control of ascites.[27] Three agents were compared; adriamycin, mustine, and tetracycline, and 15 patients were treated. A complete response was achieved in 2/4 given adriamycin and in none of those given either mustine or tetracycline. A partial response to therapy was seen in 2/4 receiving adriamycin, 2/8 given tetracycline, and none of those given tetracycline. None of the studies of intracavitary agents provides unequivocal proof that they are better than diuretics in achieving control of ascites.

Peritoneovenous shunts

These devices offer a mechanical approach to the long-term control of ascites without the loss of protein associated with repeated paracenteses. They comprise a distal perforated catheter which is placed in the peritoneal cavity, a valve chamber, with or without a valve located subcutaneously just above the costal margin, and a proximal catheter which is tunnelled subcutaneously and placed via the external or internal jugular vein with its tip in the superior vena cava. Originally, a Holster shunt was implanted to treat patients with both peritoneal and pleural effusions.[76] Subsequently, the Leveen and Denver shunts have been employed and the results of series reporting their use are given in Table 6.[77]–[83] Overall, control was achieved in 63 per cent of patients treated with Leveen shunts and in 63 per cent of those given Denver devices. The latter shunts carries the theoretical advantage of a compressible chamber associated with the valve which enables external compression to increase flow through the catheter and reduce blockage resulting from stasis of ascitic fluid. Despite similar rates of control, the Denver shunt is becoming used more frequently. It has been reported that peritoneovenous shunts function for longer periods in patients with negative effusion cytology.[84] The median shunt survival time was 140 days in cases with cytologically-negative effusion compared with only 26 days for those with positive effusion.

Although shunts can be effective, there are several problems which can be associated with their use. The complications have been assigned to five categories: wound problems, mechanical pump problems, biological/functional metastasis, and long-term failure.[85] In a series

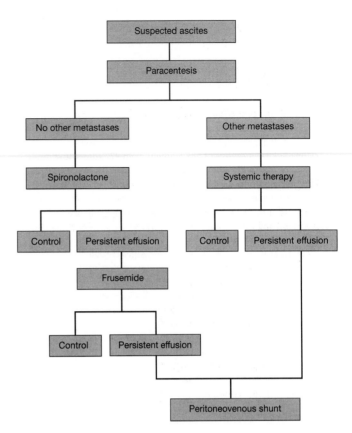

Fig. 3 Treatment plan for patients with malignant ascites.

of 86 cases, the commonest problem was pyrexia (29 per cent), followed by shunt failure in the medium term, that is between 1 and 3 months after implantation. Disseminated intravascular coagulopathy (DIC) due to probable activation of factor X in ascitic fluid was less common in patients with ascites of malignant origin compared with those with cirrhosis. Long-term function was maintained in only 25 (29 per cent).

Because malignant ascites is usually an end-stage of malignancy, intravenous perfusion of tumour containing ascitic fluid has not been found significantly to affect prognosis although shunt-related metastases have been reported. Many of the problems associated with shunt placement are technical and relate to surgical technique so that problems diminish with increasing experience. Perioperative monitoring of the location of the shunt catheter tip can help to ensure that it is located in the superior vena cava and has not become unintentionally located in the axillary vein.

Management scheme

Figure 3 is a suggested scheme for the management of patients with suspected malignant ascites. Unless cytotoxics are indicated for other symptomatic metastases, diuretic therapy should be given as first-line treatment. Only for the few patients with refractory ascites in whom it is anticipated that their survival will be more than 3 months should a shunt be inserted. Many patients with malignant ascites are preterminal and require simple palliative procedures rather than aggressive therapy.

References

1. Black LF. The pleural space and pleural fluid. *Mayo Clinic Proceedings*, 1972; **47**: 493–506.

2. Johnston WW. The malignant pleural effusion. A review of cytopathologic diagnosis of 584 effusions from 472 consecutive patients. *Cancer*, 1985; **58**: 905–9.

3. Broghamer WL, Richardson ME, Faurest SE. Malignancy-associated sero-sanguinous pleural effusions. *Acta Cytologica*, 1984; **28**: 46–50.

4. Martensson G, Petterson K, Thringer G. Differentiation between malignant and non-malignant pleural effusion. *Journal of Respiratory Diseases*, 1985; **67**: 326–34.

5. Singh G, Dekker A, Ladoulis CT. Tissue culture of cells in serous effusions. Evaluation as an adjunct to cytology. *Acta Cytologica*, 1978; **22**: 487–9.

6. Hostmark J, Vigander T, Skaarland E. Characterisation of pleural effusions by flow-cytometric DNA analysis. *European Journal of Respiratory Diseases*, 1985; **66**: 315–9.

7. Zojer N, Fiegl M, Angerler J, et al. Interphase fluorescence *in-situ* hybridisation improves the detection of malignant cells in effusions from breast cancer patients. *British Journal of Cancer*, 1997; **75**: 403–7.

8. Winkelmann M, Pfitzer P. Blind pleural biopsy in combination with cytology of pleural effusions. *Acta Cytologica*, 1984; **25**: 373–6.

9. Poe RH, et al. Sensitivity, specificity, and predictive values of closed pleural biopsy. *Archives of Internal Medicine*, 1984; **144**: 325–9.

10. Prakash UBS, Reiman HM. Comparison of needle biopsy with cytologic analysis for the evaluation of pleural effusion: analysis of 414 cases. *Mayo Clinic Proceedings*, 1985; **60**: 158–64.

11. Raja OG, Lalor AJ. Modification to the technique of percutaneous pleural biopsy using Abram's needle. *British Journal of Diseases of the Chest*, 1980; **74**: 285–6.

12. DeCamp PT, Moseley PW, Scott ML, Haton HB. Diagnostic thoracoscopy. *Annals of Thoracic Surgery*, 1973; **16**: 79–84.

13. Boutin C, Cargnino P, Viallat JR. Thoracoscopy in the early diagnosis of malignant pleural effusions. *Endoscopy*, 1980; **12**: 155–60.

14. Wu M-H, Hsive R-H, Tseng K-H. Thoracoscopy in the diagnosis of pleural effusions. *Japanese Journal of Clinical Oncology*, 1989; **19**: 116–9.

15. Fentiman IS, Millis RR, Sexton S, Hayward JL. Pleural effusion in breast cancer: a review of 105 cases. *Cancer*, 1981; **47**: 2087–92.

16. Yamada S, Takeda T, Matsumoto K. Prognostic analysis of malignant pleural and peritoneal effusion. *Cancer*, 1983; **51**: 136–40.

17. Martini N, Bains MS, Beattie EJ. Indications for pleurectomy in malignant effusions. *Cancer*, 1975; **35**: 734–8.

18. Xaubet A, et al. Characteristics and prognostic value of pleural effusions in non-Hodgkin's lymphomas. *European Journal of Respiratory Diseases*, 1985; **66**: 135–40.

19. Fentiman IS. Diagnosis and treatment of malignant pleural effusions. *Cancer Treatment Reviews*, 1987; **14**: 107–18.

20. Fry WA, Khandekar JD. Partial pleurectomy for malignant pleural effusion. *Annals of Surgical Oncology*, 1995; **2**: 160–4.

21. Harvey JC, Erdman CB, Beattie EJ. Early experience with videothoracoscopic hydrodissection pleurectomy in the treatment of malignant pleural effusion. *Journal of Surgical Oncology*, 1995; **59**: 243–5.

22. Dorsey JS, Cogordan JA. Pleuroperitoneal shunt for intractable pleural effusion. *Canadian Journal of Surgery*, 1984; **27**: 598–9.

23. Cimochowski GE, et al. Pleuroperitoneal shunting for recalcitrant pleural effusions. *Journal of Thoracic and Cardiovascular Surgery*, 1986; **92**: 866–70.

24. Little AG, et al. Pleuroperitoneal shunting. Alternative therapy for pleural effusions. *Annals of Surgery*, 1988; **208**: 443–50.

25. Izbicki R, Weyhing BT, Baker C. Pleural effusion in cancer patients. A prospective randomised study of pleural drainage with the addition of radioactive phosphorus to the pleural space versus pleural drainage alone. *Cancer*, 1975; **36**: 1511–8.

26. Miller AJ. Some observations concerning pericardial effusions and their relationship to the venous and lymphatic circulation of the heart. *Lymphology*, 1970; **2**: 76–8.

27. Kefford RF, et al. Intracavitary adriamycin nitrogen mustard and tetracycline in the control of malignant effusions. *Medical Journal of Australia*, 1980; **2**: 447–8.

28. Fentiman IS, Rubens RD, Hayward JL. Control of pleural effusions in patients with breast cancer. A randomised trial. *Cancer*, 1983; **52**: 737–9.

29. Hillerdal G, et al. Corynebacterium parvum in malignant pleural effusion. A randomised prospective study. *European Journal of Respiratory Diseases*, 1986; **69**: 204–6.

30. Ostrowski MJ, et al. A randomised trial of intracavitary bleomycin and Corynebacterium parvum in the control of malignant pleural effusions. *Radiation Oncology*, 1989; **14**: 19–26.

31. Hamed H, Fentiman IS, Chaudary MA, Rubens RD. Comparison of intracavitary bleomycin and talc for control of pleural effusions secondary to carcinoma of the breast. *British Journal of Surgery*, 1989; **76**: 1266–7.

32. Mejer J, Mortensen KM, Hansen HH. Mepacrine hydrochloride in the treatment of malignant pleural effusion. A controlled randomised trial. *Scandinavian Journal of Respiratory Diseases*, 1977; **58**: 319–23.

33. Yew WW, Chan SL, Kwan SYL. Comparison of efficacy of mitomycin-C and Corynebacterium parvum in the management of malignant pleural effusion. *Chinese Medical Journal*, 1988; **101**: 737–9.

34. Millar JW, Hunter AM, Horne NW. Intrapleural immunotherapy with Corynebacterium parvum in recurrent malignant pleural effusions. *Thorax*, 1979; **35**: 856–8.

35. Leahy BC, et al. Treatment of malignant pleural effusions with intrapleural Corynebacterium parvum or tetracycline. *European Journal of Respiratory Diseases*, 1985; **66**: 50–4.

36. Bayly TC, et al. Tetracycline and quinacrine in the control of malignant pleural effusions. A randomised trial. *Cancer*, 1978; **41**: 1188–92.

37. Zaloznik AJ, Oswald SG, Langin M. Intrapleural tetracycline in malignant pleural effusions. A randomized study. *Cancer*, 1983; **51**: 752–5.

38. Fentiman IS, Rubens RD, Hayward JL. A comparison of intracavitary talc and tetracycline for the control of pleural effusions secondary to breast cancer. *European Journal of Cancer and Clinical Oncology*, 1986; **22**: 1079–81.

39. Evans TRJ, et al. A randomised prospective trial of surgical against medical tetracycline pleurodesis in the management of malignant pleural effusions secondary to breast cancer. *European Journal of Cancer*, 1993; **29A**: 316–9.

40. Stiksa G, Korsgaard R, Simonsson BG. Treatment of recurrent pleural effusion by pleurodesis with quinacrine. Comparison between instillation by repeated thoracentesis and by tube drainage. *Scandinavian Journal of Respiratory Diseases*, 1979; **60**: 197–205.

41. Sorensen PG, Svendsen TL, Erik B. Treatment of malignant pleural effusion with drainage, with and without instillation of talc. *European Journal of Respiratory Diseases*, 1984; **65**: 131–5.

42. Fentiman IS, Rubens RD, Hayward JL. The pattern of metastatic disease in patients with pleural effusions secondary to breast cancer. *British Journal of Surgery*, 1982; **69**: 193–4.

43. Posner MR, Cohen GI, Skarin AT. Pericardial disease in patients with cancer. *American Journal of Medicine*, 1981; **71**: 407–13.

44. Reitknecht F, *et al.* Management of cardiac tamponade in patients with malignancy. *Journal of Surgical Oncology*, 1985; **30**: 19–22.

45. Laham RJ, *et al.* Pericardial effusion in patients with cancer—outcome with contemporary management strategies. *Heart*, 1996; **75**: 67–71.

46. Cham WC, *et al.* Radiation therapy of cardiac and pericardial metastases. *Radiology*, 1975; **114**: 701–4.

47. Flannery EP, Gregoratos G, Corder MP. Pericardial effusions in patients with malignant disease. *Archives of Internal Medicine*, 1975; **135**: 976–7.

48. Reynolds PM, Byrne J. The treatment of malignant pericardial effusion in carcinoma of the breast. *Australian and New Zealand Journal of Medicine*, 1977; **7**: 169–71.

49. Woll PJ, Knight RK, Rubens RD. Pericardial effusion complicating breast cancer. *Journal of the Royal Society of Medicine*, 1987; **80**: 490–1.

50. Buck M, *et al.* Pericardial effusion in women with breast cancer. *Cancer*, 1987; **60**: 263–9.

51. Moores DWO, *et al.* Subxiphoid pericardial drainage for pericardial tamponade. *Journal of Thoracic and Cardiovascular Surgery*, 1995; **109**: 546–52.

52. Davies S, Rambotti P, Grifnani F. Intra-pericardial tetracycline sclerosis in the treatment of malignant pericardial effusion: an analysis of thirty-three cases. *Journal Clinical Oncology*, 1984; **2**: 631–4.

53. Weisberger AS, Levine B, Storaasli JP. Use of nitrogen mustard in treatment of serous effusions of neoplastic origin. *Journal of the American Medical Association*, 1955; **159**: 1704–7.

54. Suhrland LG, Weisberger AS. Intracavitary 5-fluorouracil in malignant effusions. *Archives of Internal Medicine*, 1965; **116**: 431–3.

55. Smith FE, Lane M, Hudgins PT. Conservative management of malignant pericardial effusion. *Cancer*, 1974; **33**: 47–57.

56. Lentzsch S, Reichardt P, Gurtler R, Dorken B. Intrapericardial application of mitoxantrone for treatment of malignant pericardial effusion. *Onkologie*, 1994; **17**: 504–7.

57. Hawkins JR, *et al.* Pericardial window for malignant pericardial effusion. *Annals of Thoracic Surgery*, 1980; **30**: 465–71.

58. Pichler JM, *et al.* Surgical management of effusive pericardial disease. *Journal of Thoracic Cardiovascular Surgery*, 1985; **90**: 506–16.

59. Osuch JR, Khandekar JD, Fry WA. Emergency subxiphoid pericardial decompression for malignant pericardial effusion. *Annals of Surgery*, 1985; **51**: 298–300.

60. Lifshitz S. Ascites, pathophysiology and control measures. *International Journal of Radiation Oncology Biology Physics*, 1982; **8**: 1423–6.

61. Fentiman IS, Rubens RD, Hayward JL. Ascites in breast cancer. *British Medical Journal*, 1983; **287**: 1023.

62. Greenway B, Johnson PJ, Williams R. Control of malignant ascites with spironolactone. *British Journal of Surgery*, 1982; **69**: 441–2.

63. Amiel SA, Blackburn AM, Rubens RD. Intravenous infusion of frusemide as treatment for ascites in malignant disease. *British Medical Journal*, 1984; **288**: 1041.

64. Paladine W, *et al.* Intracavitary bleomycin in the management of malignant effusions. *Cancer*, 1976; **38**: 1903–8.

65. Bitran JD, Evans R, Brown C. The management of cardiac tamponade in patients with breast cancer. *Journal of Surgical Oncology*, 1984; **27**: 42–4.

66. Ostrowski MJ, Halsall GM. Intracavitary bleomycin in the management of malignant effusions: a multicentre study. *Cancer Treatment Reports*, 1982; **66**: 1903–7.

67. Ostrowski MJ. An assessment of long-term results of controlling the accumulation of malignant effusions using bleomycin. *Cancer*, 1986; **57**: 721–7.

68. Ultmann JE, *et al.* The effect of quinacrine on neoplastic effusions and certain of their enzymes. *Cancer*, 1963; **16**: 283–8.

69. Gellhorn A, *et al.* The use of Atabrine (quinacrine) in the control of recurrent neoplastic effusions. *Diseases of the Chest*, 1961; **39**: 165–76.

70. Rochlin DB, Smart CR, Wagner DE, Silver ARM. The control of recurrent malignant effusions using quinacrine hydrochloride. *Surgery Gynecology and Obstetrics*, 1964; **118**: 991–4.

71. Dollinger MR, Krakoff IH, Karnofsky DA. Quinacrine (Atabrine) in the treatment of neoplastic effusions. *Annals of Internal Medicine*, 1967; **66**: 249–57.

72. Currie JL, *et al.* Intracavitary corynebacterium parvum for treatment of malignant effusions. *Gynecologic Oncology*, 1983; **16**: 6–14.

73. Torisu M, *et al.* New approach to management of malignant ascites with a streptococcal preparation OK-432. 1. Improvement of host immunity and prolongation of survival. *Surgery*, 1983; **93**: 357–64.

74. Sistermanns J, Hoffmanns HW, Dux A. Intraperitoneal infusion of recombinant tumour necrosis factor for palliative therapy of terminally ill patients with refractory malignant ascites. *Onkologie*, 1993; **16**: 111–3.

75. Maenpaa J, *et al.* Combined intraperitoneal interferon-alpha-2b and mitoxantrone in refractory ovarian cancer. *Annales Chirurgiae et Gynaecology*, 1994; **83**: 35–7.

76. Pollock AV. The treatment of resistant malignant ascites by insertion of a peritoneo-atrial Hotter valve. *British Journal of Surgery*, 1978; **62**: 104–7.

77. Kudsk KA, *et al.* Leveen shunts. *Lancet*, 1978; i: 881.

78. Straus AK, Roseman DL, Shapiro TM. Peritoneo-venous shunting in the management of malignant ascites. *Archives of Surgery*, 1978; **114**: 489–91.

79. Oosterlee J. Peritoneovenous shunting for ascites in cancer patients. *British Journal of Surgery*, 1980; **67**: 663–6.

80. Lokich J, *et al.* Complications of peritoneovenous shunt for malignant ascites. *Cancer Treatment Reports*, 1980; **64**: 305–9.

81. Holman JM, Albo D. Peritoneovenous shunts in patients with malignant ascites. *American Journal of Surgery*, 1981; **142**: 774–6.

82. Gough IR. Peritoneo-venous shunts for malignant ascites. *Australian and New Zealand Journal of Medicine*, 1982; **52**: 47–9.

83. Souter RG, *et al.* Surgical and pathologic complications associated with peritoneovenous shunts in management of malignant ascites. *Cancer*, 1985; **55**: 1973–8.

84. Cheung DK, Raaf JH. Selection of patients with malignant ascites for a peritoneovenous shunt. *Cancer*, 1982; **50**: 1204–9.

85. Vo NM, *et al.* Complications of peritoneovenous shunting for malignant ascites. A collective review. *Connecticut Medicine*, 1981; **45**: 1–4.

5.2 **Metabolic complications**

Luc Y. Dirix and Allan T. van Oosterom

Hypercalcaemia

Introduction

Calcium is essential to man for both his biochemical and his structural integrity. The role of calcium varies from an intracellular second messenger to that of a major component of the skeleton. Major gradients in calcium exist over cellular membranes and between different intracellular compartments, and rapid transmembrane fluxes accompany processes such as neurotransmission and contractile phenomena. Many different enzyme systems are dependent on calcium as a cofactor, for example the coagulation system, the complement system, and enzymes involved in intracellular transduction processes. This highlights the importance of an efficient homeostatic system to control intra- and extracellular calcium concentrations.

Calcium circulates in the extracellular fluid in three distinct fractions: some 50 per cent is the biologically important, free ionized fraction, 40 per cent is protein-bound and is not filterable by the kidney, and a remaining 10 per cent is a diffusible but non-ionized fraction, complexed to different anions such as bicarbonate, phosphate, and lactate. The majority of the protein-bound calcium is bound to albumin and the remainder to globulins. Total serum calcium fluctuates with changes in serum protein concentration, although the ionized calcium will be relatively unaffected. Several formulas for correcting measured serum calcium to the existing serum protein and albumin concentration are available. Total serum calcium level is decreased by 0.8 mg/dl (0.2 mmol/l) for every 1.0 g/dl decrease in serum albumin below 4.6 g/dl. Serum calcium levels should always be given in relation to the prevailing serum albumin levels.[1] In patients with hyperproteinaemia and elevated serum calcium, a reliable assessment of free calcium will depend on its measurement by ion-specific electrodes. Calcium binding to albumin is strongly pH dependent between pH 7.0 and 8.0. Acute acidosis decreases protein binding, resulting in an increase in free, ionized calcium, whereas alkalosis has the opposite effect. For each 0.1 decrease in pH, ionized calcium rises by about 0.05 mmol/l. The extracellular fluid calcium concentration is result of the effects of three different endocrine effectors: parathyroid hormone (PTH), calcitriol (1,25-dihydroxyvitamin D or 1,25 $[OH]_2 D$), and calcitonin. Maintenance of the normal serum calcium is the result of tightly regulated ion transport by the kidney, intestinal tract, and bone. These three target organs are susceptible to the influence of these calciotropic hormones.[2]

The first component of the homeostatic control resides in the presence of calcium-ion sensors on cells that recognize and respond to small changes in the extracellular fluid ionized calcium. This receptor was identified through functional screening of a complementary-DNA library prepared from messenger RNA from parathyroid glands.[3] Transcripts for this receptor have been identified in cell types involved in calcium homeostasis (parathyroid, kidney, C cells). The receptor functions as a calcium sensing element, which, upon stimulation, decreases PTH secretion and increases calcitonin secretion. Mutations that inactivate the calcium-ion sensing receptor have been found to be responsible for rare disorders such as familial hypocalciuric hypercalcaemia.[4] Agonists of these receptors are being developed as a potential therapy for primary hyperparathyroidism.

The second component of the calcium homeostatic system is the effector tissues (intestine, bone, kidney) through which calcium ions move in response to the three calciotropic hormones (Fig. 1).[5]

PTH is synthesized in the chief cells of the parathyroid gland, and its concentration is highly dependent on the ionized calcium concentration in the extracellular compartment. Serum PTH increases as serum calcium decreases representing a simple negative feedback loop. The biological actions of PTH include the stimulation of osteoclastic bone resorption with release of calcium and phosphate,

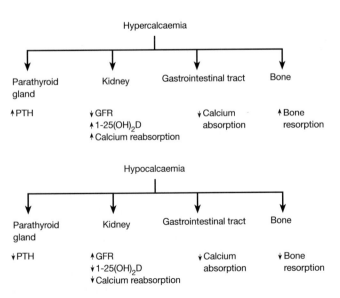

Fig. 1 Regulation of extracellular calcium concentration.

the stimulation of calcium reabsorption in the kidney, and increased 1-α-hydroxylase activity leading to increased formation of calcitriol. The effects of PTH on the renal tubular cells are mediated by adenylate cyclase activity which increases intracellular cyclic AMP concentration. Increased urinary cAMP levels under conditions of tumour-induced hypercalcaemia have therefore been considered as suggestive for a role for a PTH-like factor. Calcitriol or $1,25 [OH]_2 D$ is the active metabolite of vitamin D. $1,25 [OH]_2 D$ increases plasma calcium and phosphate concentration by increasing the absorption of calcium and phosphate. It also increases bone resorption and enhances the capacity of PTH to enhance renal tubular calcium reabsorption. Calcitonin is increasingly secreted if plasma-ionized calcium levels decrease. Calcitonin protects to some extent against hypercalcaemia, although its actual contribution should not be overestimated.

Dietary calcium intake averages 20 mmol/day (range 15–30 mmol/day) of which some 30 to 40 per cent is absorbed. The active part of this process is under control of $1,25 [OH]_2 D$. This implies an indirect control by PTH on gastrointestinal absorption, as this hormone modulates the 1-α hydroxylation of 25-hydroxyvitamin D in the kidney. Although increased intestinal uptake can contribute significantly to the emergence of hypercalcaemia, the gastrointestinal tract is not a major regulator of calcium excretion. Under normal conditions, 98 per cent of the body calcium content (1000 g) is present as skeletal calcium of which only 1 per cent appears to be freely exchangeable with the extracellular fluid. In normal adult life no net calcium uptake occurs and bone formation is balanced by continuous bone degradation.

Hypercalcaemia in primary hyperparathyroidism is characterized by increased bone resorption and increased gastrointestinal calcium absorption due to the increased $1,25 [OH]_2 D$ levels, increased renal calcium resorption, increased levels of nephrogenous cyclic-AMP, a reduction in tubular phosphate reabsorption, and moderately increased calciuria.

This balance in bony remodelling is shifted towards increased bone degradation in patients with tumour-induced hypercalcaemia (TIH). Although the major mechanism of TIH is calcium release from bone, there is nearly always a concomitant impairment of the renal mechanisms of calcium clearance from the extracellular fluid compartment. Renal excretion is the only important way of removing excess calcium from the body and of protecting against hypercalcaemia. Normal adults filter approximately 270 mmol calcium every day. Under these conditions urinary calcium excretion is 4 to 6 mmol/day, implying that 97 per cent of the filtered amount is being reabsorbed by the renal tubuli. The majority of this reabsorptive activity takes place in the more proximal portion of the nephron. Calcium reabsorption in the proximal convolute tubule accounts for some 60 per cent of the filtered load. Reabsorption is enhanced by extracellular fluid contraction and diminished by extracellular volume expansion . The thick ascending limb of Henle loop reabsorbs some 20 per cent of the filtered load. The absorption in the medullary portion is passive, sensitive to furosemide, and driven by a positive luminal potential. In the distal convolute tubule some 10 per cent more is reabsorbed and it is here that PTH increases calcium reabsorption independent of changes in sodium reabsorption or luminal potential. It is assumed that the fine regulation of renal calcium excretion takes place at this level. The regulatory factors of calcium homeostasis probably interact at different levels.

Table 1 Aetiology of hypercalcaemia according to the major underlying mechanism

I. Increased bone resorption
a. Malignancy
b. Primary hyperparathyroidism
c. Immobilization
d. Hyperthyroidism
e. Vitamin A intoxication
f. Post-transplantation hypercalcaemia

II. Increased intestinal absorption
a. Vitamin D intoxication
b. Sarcoidosis
c. Granulomatous diseases
d. Milk-alkali syndrome
e. Idiopathic hypercalcaemia of infancy

III. Other causes
a. Recovery from acute renal failure
b. Familial hypocalciuric hypercalcaemia
c. Addison's disease
d. Pheochromocytoma
e. Acromegaly
f. Thiazide diuretics
g. Lithium treatment

As already mentioned, the amount of $1,25 [OH]_2 D$ depends upon the PTH level. In the same way, $1,25 [OH]_2 D$ potentiates the effect of PTH on the tubular reabsorption. The most important factor determining serum calcium concentration is bone turnover. The balance between bone formation and bone accretion is the determining factor of net calcium flux into the extracellular fluid. The kidney has considerable, albeit finite, capacity to protect against the occurrence of hypercalcaemia, by increasing calcium excretion up to five times the normal amount; however urinary excretion seldom exceeds 15 mmol/day. If the amount released from the bone is in excess of this, hypercalcaemia is likely to occur.

Pathophysiology of malignancy-associated hypercalcaemia

In the hospital population, an underlying malignancy is the most frequent cause of hypercalcaemia (Table 1). In a study on 7610 patients with different neoplasms, 1.5 per cent had hypercalcaemia.[6] Breast, lung, head and neck, and kidney cancer are the leading causes among solid tumours (Table 2).[6],[7] The pathophysiology of hypercalcaemia is probably somewhat different according to the underlying malignancy. In patients with bronchial carcinoma, hypercalcaemia is frequent in squamous cell carcinoma and rare in small-cell anaplastic carcinoma. In patients with breast cancer, hypercalcaemia nearly invariably occurs in patients with bone metastases.

Mediators of malignancy-associated hypercalcaemia

Parathyroid hormone (PTH)

In 1941, Albright suggested that tumour-induced hypercalcaemia (TIH) was caused by tumoural production of PTH. Although many of the biochemical abnormalities seen in this syndrome resemble those

Table 2 Frequency of tumour types in 219 patients with tumour-induced hypercalcaemia (TIH)

Primary site	Number of cases
Bronchus	54
Breast	44
Ear, nose, or throat	15
Ureters, bladder, or urethra	15
Myeloma	14
Female genital tract	14
Oesophagus	13
Unknown primary	10
Lymphoma	9
Renal	7
Large bowel	5
Thyroid	4
Prostate	3
Others	12

(Fisken et al. 1980.[7])

known from primary hyperparathyroidism, it remains impossible to explain the many biochemical characteristics of tumour-related hypercalcaemia exclusively on the basis of tumoural-related PTH production.[8] Osteoclastic bone resorption is much more prominent in cancer patients with hypercalcaemia and the treatment with bisphosphonates, inhibiting osteoclast-mediated bone resorption, is much more efficient than in patients with primary hyperparathyroidism. The latter patients have increased levels of 1,25 [OH]$_2$ D, whereas the majority of patients with cancer-related hypercalcaemia have suppressed levels of the active vitamin D metabolites. Patients with primary hyperparathyroidism tend to be hyperchloraemic and mildly acidotic, whereas those with tumour-related hypercalcaemia are more frequently alkalotic. In a biochemical comparison of 41 patients with tumour-associated hypercalcaemia and increased urinary cyclic AMP levels and 15 patients with primary hyperparathyroidism, a similar increase in the production of renal cyclic AMP was observed, but urinary calcium excretion was higher in the cancer patient group, 1,25-OH-vitamin D levels were much lower, and PTH levels were suppressed in patients with tumour-related hypercalcaemia.[9] Northern blot analysis of messenger RNA extracted from human tumours associated with hypercalcaemia failed to detect parathyroid hormone transcript in any of the 13 human tumours that were investigated.[10] Interestingly, in the patients with TIH and increased urinary cyclic AMP, renal phosphate wasting was much more elevated than in those patients with hypercalcaemia and normal levels of urinary cyclic AMP. This biochemical analysis suggested that patients in the high cyclic AMP group, have a circulating renotropic factor that resembles native PTH in its ability to stimulate proximal-tubular adenylate cyclase and to inhibit proximal-tubular phosphate reabsorption. However, this factor differed from native PTH in its relative inability to stimulate distal-tubular calcium reabsorption, its inability to stimulate 25-vitamin D 1-α-hydroxylase, and its diminished or absent reactivity with a variety of region-specific parathyroid-hormone antiserums. With the exception of parathyroid carcinoma, increased PTH production is rarely responsible for hypercalcaemia in cancer.

Parathyroid hormone-related protein (PTHrP)

Although no clear evidence existed for the role of parathyroid hormone itself in the pathogenesis of tumour-induced hypercalcaemia, biochemical characteristics suggested at least the presence of a humoral factor with functional properties resembling, in part, those of native PTH.[11] These biochemical studies led to a clear distinction between two different types of TIH, with accompanying differences in the mechanisms involved. The first type occurred in the absence of bone metastases whereby humoral factors secreted by the tumour act on bone, kidney, and intestine and disrupt calcium homeostasis. The second phenotype of tumour-induced hypercalcaemia occurred in the presence of multiple bone metastases and, due to locally acting factors, these tumour deposits released calcium from bone by their local action on bone or on osteoclasts. It is becoming apparent that these two situations reflect the extremes of a continuous spectrum rather than discrete entities. One very important mediator involved in both these conditions is the parathyroid hormone-related protein (PTHrP). This protein was isolated from different cell lines (squamous lung, breast, and renal carcinoma). It is a 139- to 173-amino-acid protein with amino terminal homology to parathyroid hormone (PTH). As with PTH, the amino-terminal peptides comprising the 1 to 34 sequence of PTHrP are fully active at the PTH receptor.[12] In humans, PTHrP was shown equipotent to PTH *in vivo*.[13] PTHrP stimulates adenylate cyclase in kidney and bone, increases tubular reabsorption of calcium, and increases osteoclastic bone resorption, decreases renal phosphate uptake, and stimulates 1-α-hydroxylase activity. Initially, this protein was isolated from tumours from patients with tumour-induced hypercalcaemia, but later it was shown to have a multitude of physiological functions. The human gene for PTHrP is much larger and more complex than the human PTH gene. Cell-line specific utilization of promoters and of the alternative splicing pathways have been demonstrated.[14] Like other endocrine peptides, PTHrP undergoes endoproteolytic post-translational processing and glycosylation that results in several secretory forms.[15] PTHrP has an important role in normal physiology, including normal breast physiology. PTHrP is expressed in lactating mammary tissue and secreted in milk at concentrations 10 000 to 100 000 times greater than plasma concentrations of humans with hypercalcaemia. These observations underscore the primary role in TIH in patients with breast cancer. Approximately 70 to 80 per cent of patients with TIH have detectable increased plasma PTHrP concentrations.[16]

This percentage is more dependent on tumour type than on the presence or absence of bony metastases. In patients without bone metastases and with TIH, PTHrP levels are nearly invariably elevated. In one study on PTH and PTHrP levels in a hypercalcaemic population, coexistence of hyperparathyroidism and TIH was observed in seven out of a total of 121 hypercalcaemic patients.[17] There is some relationship between the plasma levels of PTHrP and serum calcium, however increased PTHrP levels are predictive for an inferior control rate of hypercalcaemia after treatment with bisphosphonates.[18],[19] Treatment with bisphosphonates does not seem to influence plasma PTHrP levels.[18],[20]

Prostaglandins

Tashjian suggested a role for prostaglandins of the E-series in the pathogenesis of TIH on the basis of experimental work with a mouse fibrosarcoma model.[21] In the study by Seybert et al., the common urinary metabolites of PGE_1 and PGE_2, were found to be strikingly elevated in 12 out of 14 patients with solid tumours and hypercalcaemia.[22] Treatment with indomethacin in six of these patients resulted in a marked decrease in urinary prostaglandin excretion and some decrease of the hypercalcaemia. Other investigators failed, however, to observe a beneficial effect of these drugs. In view of the general physiological role of prostaglandins, it seems more likely that their role is confined to one of a local mediator of bone resorption, rather than a tumoral product stimulating calcium release from bone. Indomethacin has been shown to block part of the osteoclast-stimulating effects of interleukin-1 in vivo.[23]

Growth factors

Transforming growth factors are produced by human tumours and are polypeptide stimulators of cell replication.[24] Transforming growth factor-α (TGF-α) is a 5.6-kDa single chain, 50-aminoacid polypeptide which shares considerable identity with epidermal growth factor (EGF) and competes for binding to the epidermal growth factor receptor. Several studies in the rat Leydig cell tumour, which rapidly induces severe hypercalcaemia, have demonstrated the bone resorbing capacity of TGF-α and its blocking by neutralizing antibodies to the EGF receptor.[25]

In an in-vitro model for bone resorption, both TGF-α and EGF stimulate bone resorption in neonatal mouse calvaria, with TGF-α being the more potent one.[26],[27] Several human tumours associated with the emergence of TIH are known to express TGF-α. TGF-α has been shown to potentiate the activity of PTHrP in inducing TIH, an effect at least in part due to enhanced bone resorption by PTHrP.[28] The exact contribution of TGF-α in the pathogenesis of TIH remains unclear.

Transforming growth factor-β (TGF-β) is a member of a larger superfamily of proteins that are important regulators of bone cell activity. Multiple isoforms of TGF-β exist and these appear to control proliferation and differentiation in many human cell types. The prototype of these is $TGF-\beta_1$ which is highly expressed by bone cells and is released during osteoclastic bone resorption. TGF-β has also been shown to increase bone resorption in mouse calvaria, which can be blocked by indomethacin suggesting prostaglandins as second messenger of this effect. TGF-β is present in high concentrations in the bone microenvironment and is expressed in breast cancer both in tumour cells and in associated stromal cells. TGF-β is the only growth factor known to increase secretion of PTHrP and to stabilize mRNA for PTHrP in different human cancers (Fig. 2).[29] These characteristics make TGF-β an important candidate factor in the establishment and progression of breast cancer metastases to bone. This critical paracrine interaction, between bone and tumour TGF-β and tumour derived PTHrP in the progression of bone metastases, underscores a common final pathway with a central role of PTHrP in tumoural hypercalcaemia, both in patients with and without bone metastases. In patients without important bone metastases, PTHrP is produced by tumour cells and acts as an endocrine messenger overruling other mechanisms of calcium homeostasis. In this subset of patients the contribution of renal calcium reabsorption might be more important. In patients with extensive bone metastases, PTHrP

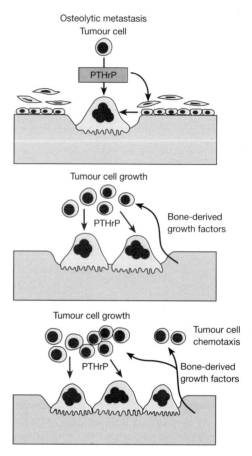

Fig. 2 Autocrine, paracrine and endocrine effect of PTHrP. In the top panel, tumour cell arrives in bone and stimulates osteoclastic bone resorption via secretion of PTHrP, an effect that is mediated through the osteoblast and stromal cells. In the middle panel, osteoclastic bone resorption results in release and activation of growth factors present in bone matrix, such as TGF-β, IGF-I, and -II, etc. Such factors may increase tumour production of PTHrP (in the case of TGF-β) and/or increase tumour cell growth (in the case of IGFs). The lower panel illustrates the end result of this cycle in which increased tumour-stimulated osteoclastic bone resorption results in increased local concentration of bone-derived growth factors. Such factors increase PTHrP production, tumour cell growth, and chemotaxis. From Guise TA, Mundy GR (1998). Cancer and Bone. Endocrine Reviews, 1998; **19**: 18–54.[30]

acts as a paracrine and autocrine factor resulting mainly in releasing large quantities of calcium from bone into the extracellular compartment. In these patients, serum PTHrP is probably less elevated and this syndrome has none or only moderately elevated serum levels of PTHrP.

Interleukins

Solid tumours may produce other factors that can stimulated osteoclastic bone resorption. These include interleukin-1 (IL-1), IL-6, and tumour necrosis factor-α (TNF-α). Most of these factors are also capable of modulating the end-organ effects of PTHrP on bone and kidney. These different modulations, together with different processing of the message of PTHrP, are probably the reason for the biochemical differences between TIH and primary hyperparathyroidism.

Calcitriol (1,25 [OH]$_2$ D)

Under conditions of hypercalcaemia serum concentrations of 1,25 [OH]$_2$ D are expected to be either normal or suppressed as is the case for serum PTH levels. Lack of suppression of 1,25 [OH]$_2$ D synthesis suggests disordered regulation and production of active vitamin D outside the kidney as is the case in granulomatous diseases. Increased 1,25 [OH]$_2$ D concentrations have been demonstrated in a majority of non-Hodgkin's lymphoma patients.[31],[32]

Other mediators

Granulocyte–macrophage colony stimulating factor (GM-CSF) is a cytokine with specific stimulatory and differentiating capacities on specific precursor cells of the bone marrow. It might contribute to the differentiation of osteoclasts cells. In clinical studies with GM-CSF, no hypercalcaemia has as yet been observed. An association of leucocytosis and hypercalcaemia has been observed in head and neck and lung cancers. A human tumour cell xenograft producing both PTHrP and GM-CSF suggests a possible explanation for this association.[33]

Malignancy-associated hypercalcaemia with extensive bone metastases In breast cancer with hypercalcaemia most patients have extensive skeletal disease and hypercalcaemia is often a terminal event. In the majority of breast cancer patients with skeletal metastasis, an increased urinary calcium excretion is present even in the absence of hypercalcaemia.[34] The principal mechanism of TIH in these patients is release of calcium from bone. Initially, this calcium efflux was thought to be the result of a direct effect of tumour cells on bony tissue. Detailed morphological studies have shown that osteoclasts are the principal bone-destroying cells.[35] In patients with bone metastasis, a stimulating effect of tumour cells on osteoclasts is the major mechanism of osteolysis.[36] The mechanism of TIH in these patients is, however, not only the result of locally acting mechanisms. Some 50 per cent of patients with TIH in this setting have raised PTHrP levels and/or increased urinary cAMP production, suggestive of systemic influences on bone resorption and renal calcium reabsorption as contributing mechanisms in the genesis of hypercalcaemia. The role of PTHrP is important in mediating both the local mechanisms and the systemic influence of tumour cells on calcium metabolism. The importance of PTHrP in normal breast physiology has already been mentioned. PTHrP and its receptor are expressed both in normal breast epithelium and in breast carcinomas. A positive relationship between breast cancer labelling indices and PTHrP expression has been observed.[37] Positive staining for PTHrP in primary breast cancer has been shown to be predictive for the development of bone metastases.[38] In addition, breast carcinoma metastatic to bone expresses PTHrP in greater than 90 per cent of cases, compared to only 17 per cent of metastasis to non-osseous sites. These observations suggest that PTHrP is not only a potential autocrine growth factor in primary breast cancer, but that PTHrP expression may represent a selective growth advantage in bone due to its ability to stimulate bone resorption. This process might then be held responsible for releasing and activation of bone matrix growth factors such as TGF-β. In an *in vivo* model of osteolytic bone metastases using a human breast cancer cell line, treatment with a monoclonal antibody against PTHrP resulted in marked inhibition of osteolysis. In patients with breast cancer and TIH, elevated circulating PTHrP levels were observed in 65 per cent of patients.[39] Different studies have shown a lower efficacy of bisphosphonates in patients with increased PTHrP levels, and this was related to the increased tubular calcium reabsorption in these patients, an effect not influenced by bisphosphonate therapy.

Tamoxifen-induced hypercalcaemia A specific condition is the hypercalcaemia in patients with hormone-sensitive breast cancer treated with tamoxifen. In a series of 470 patients with metastatic breast cancer treated with tamoxifen, 10 (2.3 per cent) developed hypercalcaemia.[40] Hypercalcaemia occurs after a median period of 7 days (4–11 $\pm$ days). Patients with extensive lytic bone metastasis are more prone to this complication. In an oestrogen-receptor-positive cell line with *in vitro* increased PTHrP secretion, isolated from a patient with TIH, oestrogen was shown to inhibit PTHrP production, whereas anti-oestrogens (both tamoxifen and a pure anti-oestrogen) stimulated PTHrP secretion. This stimulatory influence by anti-oestrogens on PTHrP secretion occurred simultaneously with their growth inhibitory effects on this cell line.[41] This type of hypercalcaemia should not lead to interruption of treatment as it is often predictive of tumour response. Patients with metastatic, hormone-sensitive breast carcinoma and extensive lytic bone metastasis should have regular monitoring of serum calcium during the first weeks after starting tamoxifen.

Malignancy-associated hypercalcaemia without bone metastasis (HHM) Although only a minority in comparison with the patients with bone metastasis and hypercalcaemia, this group has received great interest by both clinicians and researchers. This group has been termed paraneoplastic hypercalcaemia, pseudohyperparathyroidism, or humoral hypercalcaemia of malignancy (HHM). It occurs typically in patients with head and neck cancer and non-small cell lung cancer. Whereas local destruction is relatively easy to conceive as the mechanism of bone resorption and subsequent calcium release into the extracellular compartment in patients with bone metastasis, this is not the case in this group of patients. It is now recognized that PTHrP secretion by tumour cells is critical for the genesis of HHM. This is substantiated by the observations that most, if not all, patients with HHM have increased levels of circulating PTHrP. However, HHM remains somewhat heterogeneous, making it impossible to explain all biochemical abnormalities by the secretion of a single bone resorbing peptide. PTHrP probably acts in concert with other factors such as TGFs and interleukins. In this syndrome, the importance of renal mechanisms is probably of greater importance. The stimulation of renal calcium reabsorption is due to a diminished circulating volume and thus a decrease in glomerular filtration rate combined with a specific tubular effect of circulating peptides. This leads to a relative hypocalciuria in the presence of hypercalcaemia. Nonetheless, bone resorption is taking place in patients with HHM, and this is most certainly the basic mechanism for the emergence of hypercalcaemia.

Hypercalcaemia associate with multiple myeloma Multiple myeloma is a haematological malignancy of the β-cell lineage characterized by extensive lytic bone disease with moderate or even absent osteoblastic bone remodelling.[42] Hypercalcaemia and skeletal disease are major problems in patients with myelomatosis. The bony lesions in multiple myeloma are mainly localized or diffuse osteolytic; in some it is so generalized that patients present with an osteoporosis-like picture. A rare syndrome is that of diffuse osteosclerosis which most often occurs as part of the POEMs syndrome. Hypercalcaemia is a frequent complication in advanced disease. The bone resorption is characterized by the activation of osteoclasts due to the production of osteoclastic activating factors. Myeloma cells *in vitro* produce such factors in large amounts. The number of potential mediators that could fulfil the osteoclastic activating factor role is large. Interleukin-1β, IL-6, and TNF-β all have been implicated. Lymphotoxin or TNF-β might also be a mediator of bone resorption in multiple myeloma.

The bone resorbing activity of culture media from five cultured myeloma cell lines was inhibited by antibodies against TNF-β.[43] Interleukin-1β (IL-1β) is one of the most potent bone resorbing substances of β origin. In 11 human cell lines of human myeloma, however, no spontaneous production of IL-1β was observed. Interleukin-6 is a central cytokine in patients with multiple myeloma. Although endogenous IL-6 production is very high, IL-6 is not a powerful bone-resorbing factor. It is, however, capable of potentiating the effects of PTHrP. In fact, recent data from different centres suggest that PTHrP may also be important in the development of hypercalcaemia in multiple myeloma. Levels of PTHrP were positively related to serum calcium levels.[44] The often impaired renal function in patients with multiple myeloma further increases their susceptibility to hypercalcaemia. PTH levels are suppressed in these cases and increased urinary calcium reabsorption is now present. Hypercalcaemia can even occur in patients with non-secreting myeloma.

Hypercalcaemia associated with lymphoma In 1977, a rapidly fatal, T-cell lymphoproliferative syndrome was described in adults born in the south-western Japanese archipelago. The syndrome is characterized by pleomorphic neoplastic T-cells, lymphadenopathy, splenomegaly, hepatomegaly, cutaneous infiltration, hypercalcaemia, and interstitial pulmonary infiltrates. In a study on the first 10 patients identified with this syndrome in the United States, nine of them suffered from hypercalcaemia.[45] The HTLV-I virus was identified as the cause of this disease. These patients show evidence of increased osteoclasts activation with increased bone turnover with lytic bone lesions. Parathyroid hormone levels are appropriately low, suggesting normal parathyroid function. One of the cytokines resembling the osteoclastic activating factors of multiple myeloma, interleukin-1α is one of the possible candidates of mediating osteolytic activity in these patients.[46] In this disease an important role for PTHrP is also suggested.[47] In patients with Hodgkin's disease hypercalcaemia is rare. In a report on three patients with symptomatic hypercalcaemia without skeletal involvement and bulky abdominal disease, serum 1, 25-dihydroxyvitamin D was found to be elevated.[48] Increased levels of 1,25 [OH]₂ D were noted in 12 of 22 hypercalcaemic patients with non-Hodgkin's lymphoma. In addition, 71 per cent of 22 normocalcaemic patients with non-Hodgkin's lymphoma were hypocalciuric, and 18 per cent of these had increased serum 1,25 [OH]₂ D concentrations.[32] In spite of these elevated levels of the active vitamin D metabolites, another factor has to be responsible for the increased bone resorption in lymphoma-associated hypercalcaemia. In non-Hodgkin's lymphoma patients with hypercalcaemia serum levels of 1,25 [OH]₂ D were suppressed in the majority of those with increased PTHrP levels.[49],[50]

Clinical presentation

The clinical manifestations of hypercalcaemia are dependent on the degree and rate of progression of hypercalcaemia and the underlying aetiology. Other associated diseases or metabolic abnormalities can influence clinical presentation. The clinical spectrum can vary from asymptomatic to deep coma. The major clinical features can be categorized according to the four major target organs of hypercalcaemia.

Central nervous system

The neurological features of hypercalcaemia can be very subtle with only discrete changes in affect or mild headache. Delusions and changes in personality are most often present. Episodes of depression and memory impairment are sometimes prominent in patients with extensive solid tumours, but although these symptoms can be explained otherwise, hypercalcaemia should always be excluded. Agitation or even frank psychosis can be seen, but in general severe hypercalcaemia is more often associated with decreased central nervous activity eventually leading to stupor or coma. Focal or generalized seizures are rare. Muscular weakness is also a prominent feature.

Cardiovascular effects

Hypercalcaemia leads to shortening of the systolic time intervals, which is seen on the ECG as a shortening of the QT-interval. Major arrhythmias do not tend to occur with mild hypercalcaemia. At high levels of hypercalcaemia; that is above 4 mmol/l, paradoxical slowing of conduction occurs with QT-time and PR-time prolongation. Different degrees of heart block can occur and this can lead to ventricular fibrillation in patients with hypercalcaemia of rapid onset. Digitalis and all other antiarrhythmic drugs should be used with great care in these patients. Hypertension is another manifestation of hypercalcaemia. The positive influence on peripheral vascular tone can be explained in part by the direct effect of increased ionized calcium, but an indirect effect on the renin–angiotensin axis has also been suggested.

Renal manifestations

One of the earliest clinical manifestations of hypercalcaemia is increased diuresis and thirst. Impairment of sodium reabsorption in the thick ascending limb, of Henle's loop and in the distal tubules, leads to the loss of the medullary concentration gradient and the emergence of a nephrogenic, vasopressin-resistant form of diabetes insipidus. Calcium can inhibit adenylate cyclase and directly oppose the effect of antidiuretic hormone on the collecting ducts. This fluid loss will lead to a volume contraction, thus limiting the renal excretory capacity for calcium and aggravating the hypercalcaemia. Loss of tubular reabsorption will lead in a later phase to hypomagnesaemia, hypokalaemia, glycosuria, aminoaciduria, and hyperuricaemia. Although some degree of calcium phosphate precipitation occurs in the kidney, nephrolithiasis is very uncommon in comparison with patients suffering from primary hyperparathyroidism.

Gastrointestinal effects

Diminished motility in the gastrointestinal tract will lead to constipation, and will contribute to anorexia, nausea, and vomiting. Calcium has a direct stimulatory effect on gastric acid secretion and

Table 3 Drugs used in the treatment of tumour-associated hypercalcaemia

Drugs	Mechanism of action	Standard dose	Success rate (%)	Time-effect	Side-effects
Bisphosphonates	Inhibit osteociast-mediated calcium release from bone			normalization after 3–4 days	
Etidronate		7.5 mg/kg/day d1–d3–(d5)	30		
Clodronate		300–1500 mg/6 h d1–d10	80		
Pamidronate		60 (90) mg/2 h d1	80		mild fever hypocalcaemia
Alendronate		10–15 mg/2 h d1	80		
Ibandronate		4 mg IV bolus d1	80		
Zolendronate		1–3mg/ IV bolus d1	90		
Calcitonin	Inhibits bone resorption Inhibits renal calcium reabsorption	5–10 U/kg/6 h in 500 ml saline (can be repeated)	30	24 h	nausea, hypersensitivity
Mitramycin	Inhibits bone resorption	15–25 µg/kg IV bolus or in 1l 5% glucose/4 h		6–48 h	marrow suppression liver toxicity renal toxicity coagulopathy
Gallium nitrate	Inhibits bone resorption	200 mg/m^2/24 h d1–d5	75		renal toxicity hypophosphataemia
Haemodialysis	Removes calcium directly from serum		100	2–4 hours short lasting	hypotension

an indirect effect via the stimulation of gastric secretion. Duodenal ulcers are a frequent complication of hypercalcaemia.

Treatment (Table 3)

Fluid repletion

The renal concentration defect and the neurological and gastrointestinal symptoms all lead to extracellular volume contraction, leading to further aggravation of the hypercalcaemia. The institution of intravenous fluid repletion with normal saline solution is important. Careful monitoring of the patients fluid balance is mandatory especially in patients with severe cardiac or renal insufficiency. This fluid re-expansion is effective in both ameliorating the general condition and in increasing urinary calcium excretion. Frequent monitoring of serum potassium and magnesium is needed. The measurement of calcium excretion per unit of glomerular filtration (CaE) is useful in predicting the effect on calcaemia.[51] With aggressive fluid repletion a fall in serum calcium of 0.5 to 0.75 mmol/l can be expected within 36 h in a majority of patients. The emergence of hypernatraemia and fluid overload remain major limitations. With the availability of potent bisphosphonates the heroic rehydration schedules are no longer indicated.

Bisphosphonates

Bisphosphonates constitute the most efficient tool in the treatment of tumour-related hypercalcaemia. These compounds are characterized by P–C–P links and are analogues of pyrophosphate,

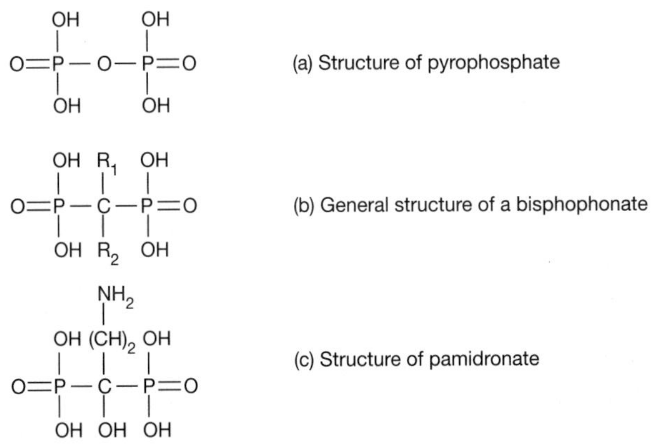

Fig. 3 Structure of pyrophosphate and bisphosphonates.

containing an oxygen instead of a carbon atom (Fig. 3). The bisphosphonates have two fundamental biological effects: inhibition of calcification at high doses and inhibition of bone resorption. This last activity is the one sought after in oncological practice. The most important mechanism of their antiresorptive activity resides not in a physicochemical action, but rather in a cellular mechanism resulting in the inhibition of the activity of osteoclasts on bone.

Many different bisphosphonates are currently in clinical practice or in development with different degrees of activity. Some insight exists into the structure–activity relationship. Adding an hydroxyl group to the carbon atom at position 1 increases potency. Derivatives with an amino group at the end of the side chain are very active. The optimal length of the aliphatic side-chain is also important with the highest activity where there is a backbone of four carbons. Activity is further increased when other groups are added to the nitrogen, as in ibandronate.

Etidronate disodium (ethane-1-hydroxy-1-diphosphonate or EHPD) not only inhibits bone resorption it also impairs bone mineralization. It is administered intravenous at 7.5 mg/kg per day for 3 to 5 days. In a large, multicentre, randomized trial including 202 patients with hypercalcaemia, etidronate was compared to saline infusion with efficacy rates of 63 per cent versus 33 per cent.[52] However, when serum calcium levels were corrected for the prevailing albumin level, response rates dropped to 24 per cent and 7 per cent respectively.

Dichloromethylene diphosphonate (Cl2MDP) has been administered at doses of 300 to 1000 mg/day for a variable number of consecutive days. In a randomized comparison between the 3-day etidronate regimen, a single intravenous infusion of 600 mg clodronate over 6 h, and a single infusion of 30 mg pamidronate over 4 h, the first two bisphosphonates were equally effective with roughly one-third of patients being normocalcaemic after 6 days versus 85 per cent in the pamidronate group.[53]

The first derivative with an amino group at the C1 side chain was pamidronate. It is currently the most effective available compound with response rates of some 90 per cent. Initially, pamidronate was administered as a daily 15 mg 2-h infusion.[54] A similar efficacy with a single 24-hour infusion was demonstrated.[55] In another randomized study 60 mg of pamidronate administered over 4 h or as a 24-h infusion were both equally effective and safe.[56] Dose–response studies have shown that a single intravenous doses of 15 to 45 mg administered in 500 ml of normal saline over 2 h is efficient.[57] In hypercalcaemic patients with breast carcinoma, 15 out of 23 became normocalcaemic after a single dose of less than 15 mg, whilst three patients needed a higher dose.[58] Other dose–response studies have confirmed these findings[59] with the suggestion of dose–response relationships in patients with more severe hypercalcaemia. When given as a single 24-h infusion, pamidronate resulted in a normalized serum calcium in 30 per cent of patients who received 30 mg, 61 per cent of patients who received 60 mg, and 100 per cent of patients who received 90 mg.[60] A single 60 or 90-mg infusion over 2 h is currently considered standard therapy.

A clear fall in serum calcaemia occurs within 48 h after administration. Normalization of serum calcaemia usually takes from 2 to 5 days, with a mean time of approximately 4 days. The combination of pamidronate and calcitonin may be considered if a more rapid normalization of serum calcium is sought. The mean duration of this effect is 28 days. Successful treatment results in a decrease in the biochemical markers of bone resorption and an increase in plasma PTH and 1,25 [OH]$_2$ D. The efficacy of pamidronate relates positively to the presence of bone metastases and negatively to both an increased renal calcium and/or a lower renal phosphate threshold.[61] These last effects is probably explained by the negative correlation between response to bisphosphonates and plasma PTHrP levels.[18],[62] In a direct comparison pamidronate was shown to be more effective

than etidronate or clodronate.[53],[63] In a comparative study between pamidronate, mitramycin, and the corticosteroid–calcitonin combination, pamidronate was the slowest in normalizing calcaemia, but its effect was long lasting.[64] Side-effects are mild and include nausea and diarrhoea; fever and hypotension were only reported when higher doses (>3 mg/kg) were used.[59]

Newer bisphosphonates are being developed all of which are milligram per milligram more potent than pamidronate. Whether this will translate into improved clinical efficacy in hypercalcaemia remains unclear. Hopefully, one of these compounds will be more effective as an oral drug in the prevention and treatment of osteoporosis. Alendronate is such a compound, used orally in prevention postmenopausal bone loss. Alendronate has been shown to be more active than etidronate in the treatment of hypercalcaemia, with response rates of 79 per cent versus 33 per cent. Ibandronate is a new bisphosphonate characterized by methyl groups being added to the amino group. It is approximately 50 times more potent than pamidronate in inhibiting bone resorption in animal models. Treatment with 4 mg as a single infusion resulted a 75.6 per cent response rate with excellent tolerance.[65] Zolendronate belongs to this group achieving a normalization rate in excess of 90 per cent with a dose range of 1 to 3 mg.[66]

Diuretics

The loop diuretics, frusemide or ethacrynic acid, will inhibit renal tubular calcium reabsorption. Frusemide has to be used in high doses (up to 100 mg intravenously given every 1 or 2 h) until serum calcium begins to drop.[67] Frusemide (40 mg every 6 h) can be used once adequate rehydration has been established. Careful management of fluid balance and serum electrolytes is essential if these high doses of potent diuretics are given. The role for diuretics in the management of hypercalcaemia should be restricted to the balancing of fluid intake and urinary output after adequate rehydration.

Corticosteroids

Glucocorticosteroids lower serum calcium by decreasing gastro-intestinal calcium absorption, as well as by inhibiting osteoclastic bone resorption and by increasing calciuria. In view of the possible role of prostaglandins and the different cytokines in the mediation of bone resorption, corticosteroids might inhibit any of these factors. Their efficacy is mainly limited to hypercalcaemia associated with haematological malignancies, for example leukaemia, myeloma, lymphoma, and in breast cancer. In other solid tumours their efficacy is, in general, disappointing and unpredictable and is no longer recommended.[68]

Calcitonin

Calcitonin decreases serum calcium by inhibiting both osteoclasts bone resorption and renal calcium reabsorption.[69] Calcitonin has the major advantages of both being without any serious side-effect and able to induce a rapid decrease (within 2 to 4 h) of serum calcium. Because of this, and although bisphosphonates are much more effective compounds, there remains a role for calcitonin in the acute management of hypercalcaemia. Although it is a compound with a rapid action, normalization of serum calcium is rarely achieved with calcitonin alone. Its current role in the management of tumour-induced hypercalcaemia is in combination with potent antiosteoclast compounds, such as the bisphosphonates or gallium nitrate, to lower calcium in severely sick patients with extreme hypercalcaemia. Its major disadvantage when used as a single agent is the occurrence of an 'escape' phenomenon after 2 to 4 days. In combination with 60 mg of prednisolone this escape might be alleviated.[70] This combination is probably only effective in patients with steroid responsive diseases such as myeloma.

Calcitonin can be applied intravenously, intramuscularly, or subcutaneously; 5 to 10 MRC U/kg per 24 h divided in four doses, each in 250 ml normal saline to be given in 1 h may be recommended. A continuous infusion in 500 ml of normal saline over 6 h is reported to be equally efficient. As an alternative route 2 to 4 MRC U/kg can be given subcutaneously or intramuscularly ever 12 h. Minor side-effects include some nausea and flushing; allergic phenomena occur rarely.

Mithramycin

This cytostatic antibiotic inhibits DNA-dependent RNA synthesis. It lowers serum calcium by inhibition of osteoclastic bone resorption. It can be given as 4-hourly infusion in 1l of 5 per cent glucose or as a bolus injection at a dose of 15 to 25 mg/kg body weight. It is a very efficient therapy, lowering serum calcium within 6 to 48 h. If no response has occurred by then a second dose can still be efficient. Relapse, however, frequently occurs.[64] Toxicity can be important with bone marrow suppression, liver and kidney toxicity, and coagulopathy as the most prominent features. Extravasation leads to severe ulceration and subsequent fibrosis. In a recent, randomized study the efficacy of mithramycin was shown to be inferior to pamidronate, which normalized serum calcium in 88 per cent of patients compared to 45 per cent for mithramycin.[71]

Gallium nitrate

Gallium nitrate was originally developed as an anticancer agent. During early clinical trials it was found to possess hypocalcaemic properties.[72],[73] The mechanism whereby gallium perturbs calcium homeostasis is incompletely understood. Elemental gallium has been shown to localize preferentially to bone and is known to make hydroxyapatite less soluble to cell-mediated resorption. Clinical treatment with gallium nitrate reduces parameters indicative of increased bone turnover such as urinary calcium and hydroxyproline excretion, whilst also exerting a favourable effect on bone formation. Unlike mithramycin, gallium nitrate does not, however, induce lethal effects on osteoclasts.

During sequential phase 2 studies gallium nitrate was found to be safe and effective treatment for patients with moderate and severe hypercalcaemia. Administration of gallium nitrate in a dose of 200 mg/m² per day as a 24-h infusion for 5 days results in normalization of serum calcium in some 70 per cent of patients.

Compared to calcitonin, gallium nitrate was clearly more effective with normocalcaemia obtained in 75 per cent of gallium-treated patients versus 27 per cent of patients treated with calcitonin.[74] In other studies gallium nitrate was compared in randomized fashion with a first-generation bisphosphonate, etidronate.[75] Normocalcaemia was obtained in 82 per cent of patients given gallium nitrate and in 43 per cent of etidronate-treated subjects. Furthermore, the median duration of normocalcaemia was significantly longer with gallium nitrate. In a double-blind, randomized study, gallium nitrate 200 mg/m² per day as a 24-h infusion for 5 days was compared to a single infusion of pamidronate of either 60 or 90 mg, depending on the severity of hypercalcaemia.[76] The gallium treatment achieved normocalcaemia in 23 of 32 patients (72 per cent) compared to 19 out of 32 (59 per cent) patients in the pamidronate arm.

Gallium nitrate is relative slow in decreasing serum calcium, with a continued drop in calcaemia after the infusion has been interrupted. Initially, gallium nitrate was administered in dose-finding studies as an once every 3 weeks brief infusion regimen. The nephrotoxicity was dose limiting. Pharmacokinetics have shown that the drug has an apparent volume of distribution of 670 l/m² with a mean post-infusional half-life of 105 h. The renal toxicity has been reduced by prolonging the infusion time, however patients should be rehydrated before the start of infusion and the use of concomitant nephrotoxic agents should be avoided.

Dialysis

In patients with renal failure, both haemo- and peritoneal dialysis are effective means of lowering serum calcium. This can be particular useful in the management of hypercalcaemia in the setting of renal failure which precludes the administration of large volumes of fluids and is a contraindication to the use of bisphosphonates. With a calcium-free haemodialysis it is possible to normalize serum calcium with 2 to 3 h of dialysis.[77]

Antitumour treatment

All therapy for hypercalcaemia can only be judged to be meaningful if it is accompanied by a general oncological treatment strategy to prevent its recurrence.

Hypocalcaemia in malignancy

Introduction

Generally, the aetiology of hypocalcaemia can be traced back to some defect in either PTH or vitamin D function. Both PTH and 1,25 [OH]₂ D act on three target organs: the gastrointestinal tract, the kidney, and bone tissue. Whenever calcaemia tends to decrease, PTH secretion will be stimulated and, in a concerted action with 1,25 [OH]₂, will increase gastrointestinal absorption, renal tubular reabsorption, and release of calcium from the skeletal reservoir. Calcitonin, a hormone produced by the parafollicular C-cells in the thyroid gland, has a calcium lowering effect. Increased calcitonin secretion as in medullary thyroid cancer very rarely results in hypocalcaemia. This demonstrates the efficacy of the PTH–1,25 [OH]₂ D axis in the prevention of hypocalcaemia. The discussion will be limited to hypocalcaemia where the cause is more or less specific or frequently occurs in patients with cancer.

Pathophysiology

Although in post-mortem studies malignant infiltration of the parathyroid glands in patients with widespread metastatic disease has been reported to by as high as 5 to 15 per cent, clinical hypoparathyroidism is very rare in patients with cancer. Sporadic cases of hypoparathyroidism have been reported after treatment with external radiotherapy to the neck and mediastinum or high doses of radioactive iodine (¹³¹I). Transient hypocalcaemia occurring within a few days after total or subtotal thyroidectomy is not exceptional, but permanent hypoparathyroidism occurs in probably less than 1 per cent of patients.

One of the most frequent causes of hypocalcaemia in cancer patients is related to cisplatin-based chemotherapy. This type of hypocalcaemia is secondary to magnesium wasting resulting from renal tubular damage by cisplatin and is usually accompanied by hypokalaemia.[78] Magnesium depletion may lead to an impaired release of PTH, and end-organ resistance of bone and renal tissue to the effects of PTH. Hypermagnesaemia could also lead to an impairment of PTH release in response to hypocalcaemia. Other metabolic causes of hypocalcaemia are multiple blood transfusions, hyperventilation, osteoblastic bone metastases,[79] and oncogenical osteomalacia. Hypocalcaemia associated with the tumour lysis syndrome will be discussed below.[80]

Clinical presentation

Clinical symptomatology consists of increased neuromuscular irritability. Early findings may be feelings of numbness or paraesthesia involving fingers, toes, or perioral region. Tetany of facial muscles in response to stimulation of the facial nerve (Chvostek's sign) and carpopedal spasm after inflation of a blood pressure cuff (Trousseau's sign) are classic signs of this increased irritability. Central nervous system abnormalities vary from grand to petit mal seizures, impairment of cognitive function, and emotional disturbances. Extrapiramidal signs may occur. In severe or acute onset hypocalcaemia laryngospasm or bronchospasm may be life-threatening. Hypocalcaemia results in a moderate slowing of atrioventricular and intraventricular conduction during cardiac depolarization. Electrocardiographically, QT prolongation can be observed, thus increasing the vulnerability period for the emergence of Q on T extrasystoles. Certainly in the presence of hypokalaemia and hypomagnesaemia, this can lead to a special type of ventricular fibrillation, the so-called torsades de pointe. Isolated hypocalcaemia will rarely lead to arrhythmias.

Diagnosis and treatment

A decreased serum calcium after correction for existing serum albumin concentration will confirm the diagnosis. Measurement of ionized calcium may be helpful in complex situations, such as concurrent acid–base disturbances. Assessment of circulating parathyroid hormone, serum phosphate, and eventually vitamin D metabolites will lead to a diagnosis in the majority of cases.

Acute severe hypocalcaemia has to be treated with intravenous calcium administration. This can best by done with ECG monitoring, especially in digitalized patients who are sensitive to arrhythmias that may arise from temporary hypocalcaemia. Intravenous calcium salts exist in two forms:

(1) calcium chloride 10 per cent containing 9 mmol of elemental calcium in ampoules of 10 ml; or

(2) calcium gluconate 10 per cent containing 2.25 mmol of calcium in a 10 ml ampoule.

Ampoules should be diluted with 50 to 100 ml of glucose solution 5 per cent. Solutions of more than 50 mmol/l (1 mmol per 20 ml) should be avoided as these are irritating to veins.

In patients with chronic hypocalcaemia due to irreversible hypoparathyroidism, treatment is aimed at maintaining serum calcium levels in the low normal range.

Oral calcium supplementation will consist of 2 to 4 g of elemental calcium in combination with a vitamin D metabolite. The biological potency of these metabolites differs widely, for example 1,25 [OH]$_2$ D (rocalcitrol) is 1000 times more potent than ergocalciferol (vitamin D$_2$). In practice this means that virtually no extra oral calcium intake is needed with rocalcitrol (0.5–2.0 mg daily) and the time needed to obtain normocalcaemia is shortened compared to when ergocalciferol is used. Ergocalciferol is much cheaper and the daily dose is 750 to 3000 mg.

Oncogenic osteomalacia

Osteogenic osteomalacia is a tumour-associated form of osteomalacia characterized by renal wasting of phosphorus and markedly reduced levels of 1,25 [OH]$_2$ D. Symptoms consist of bone pain, muscle weakness, and occasionally fractures of bone or gait disturbances. Biochemical alterations include hypophosphataemia with increased phosphaturia, normocalcaemia or only moderate hypocalcaemia, increased alkaline phosphatase levels, low or unmeasurable 1,25 [OH]$_2$ D levels with normal values for 25[OH] D and PTH.[81],[82] Radiological appearance is that of osteomalacia. Histological examination of bone biopsies shows the presence of increased amounts of unmineralized osteoid covering the trabecular bone surface. There is no evidence for increased bone resorption. Removal of the tumour leads to return of serum phosphate levels to normal within 1 week and the healing of bone lesions within months. Most frequently the syndrome has been found in association with benign or malignant tumours of mesenchymal origin, which are small and difficult to locate, but is has also been described in association with carcinoma of the prostate,[83] oat cell lung cancer,[84] and breast cancer.[82] The pathophysiology of the altered phosphate transport remain unclear, but the disappearance after all manifestations of the syndrome after removal of the tumour suggests the production of a humoral factor that may affect multiple functions of the proximal renal tubule, including inhibition of phosphate resorption and synthesis of 1,25 [OH]$_2$ D. Both the phosphaturia and the decrease in plasma 1,25 [OH]$_2$ D might contribute to a diminished bone mineralization. Different studies with conditioned medium from cell cultures of oncogenic osteomalacia tumours resulted in inhibition of renal phosphate uptake in cultured kidney cells.[85]–[87] The presence of this phosphaturic factor, should normally lead to increased 1,25 [OH]$_2$ D levels, because hypophosphataemia upregulates 1α-hydroxylase. Transplantation of a haemangioperytoma associated with osteomalacia in nude mice induced hyperphosphaturia, hypophosphataemia, and high serum alkaline phosphatase levels in tumour-bearing animals. Tumour extracts added to cultured mouse renal tubular cells reduced 1,25 [OH]$_2$ D formation, again pointing to humoral factor(s) leading to both decreased phosphate reabsorption and decreased 1α-hydroxylase activity.[87],[88]

Treatment preferably consist of removal of the tumour. However, when this is not feasible, administration of high-dose 1,25 [OH]$_2$ D and moderate oral phosphate administration may heal bone lesions. A suggested regimen is 3 mg 1,25 [OH]$_2$ D and 2 mmol of phosphate daily. It is important to be aware of this syndrome in prostate cancer patients who present with hypophosphataemia and bone pains.

Magnesium disturbances in malignancy

Introduction

Magnesium is the fourth most abundant cation in the body and, after potassium, the second most prevalent intracellular cation. Liver and muscle cells have an intracellular concentration around 7.5 to 10 mmol/l and red blood cell magnesium is 2.5 mmol/l. Normal serum magnesium ranges between 0.75 and 1.05 mmol/l (1.7–2.4 mg/dl; 1.5–2.1 meq/l). Total body magnesium depends on gastrointestinal absorption and renal elimination. Gastrointestinal absorption is situated in the upper gastrointestinal tract. An average diet will contain some 12.5 mmol, nearly 300 mg of magnesium per day. Approximately 30 to 40 per cent of this will be absorbed. Under conditions of magnesium balance nearly all of this will by found in the urine. Tubular reabsorption takes place in the proximal tubule and in the ascending loop of Henle. In the distal tubule some 10 per cent of filtered magnesium is reabsorbed. These are the sites of magnesium regulation. Extracellular fluid status, parathyroid hormone, serum magnesium, and calcium are the major factors determining tubular magnesium reabsorption.

Magnesium is an essential cofactor for a number of critical enzymes involved in DNA replication and transcription. Various phosphokinases and phosphatases are critically dependent on magnesium. Among these are the different ATPases regulating cellular calcium, hydrogen, sodium, and potassium pumps. Magnesium is also a cofactor in the phosphorylation of glucose and in the oxidative metabolism in mitochondria.

Pathophysiology

Cisplatin

The occurrence of hypomagnesaemia and hypermagnesuria in 21 out of 37 patients treated with cisplatin was first described by Schilsky and Anderson in 1979.[89] These observations suggested a primary tubular lesion responsible for the increased urinary loss in face of the hypomagnesaemia. Other studies have confirmed this finding and this reversible complication may develop in 50 to 90 per cent of patients within 14 days of cisplatin administration.[90] The cisplatin-induced renal wasting of magnesium increases with the applied cisplatin dose and is of concern in regimens using high-dose cisplatin administration. Simple supplementation with intravenous and later oral magnesium ameliorates hypomagnesaemia, but does not prevent the renal magnesium wasting.[90],[91] The hypomagnesaemia will frequently cause hypokalaemia and hypocalcaemia. Despite hypokalaemia and hypocalcaemia these patients exhibit renal calcium and potassium wasting. This will not be corrected until the hypomagnesaemia itself has been resolved.[78] In most cases, hypomagnesaemia will resolve spontaneously after interruption of treatment; in a minority of cases, however it can persist for long periods.

The use of diuretics, volume expansion with saline infusion, and mannitol diuresis will further aggravate renal magnesium wasting. Carbenicillin and ticarcillin also cause a solute diuresis and thus increase magnesuria.[92] Aminoglycosides and amphotericin B can potentiate the cisplatin nephrotoxicity and increase of renal magnesium wasting in patients receiving cisplatin.

Other causes

The syndrome of inappropriate antidiuretic hormone secretion and hyperaldosteronism, will cause renal magnesium wasting by increasing extracellular fluid volume. Hypercalcaemia will also lead to an increased urinary magnesium loss. Hypokalaemia can be caused by, and also be the result of, hypomagnesaemia. Massive blood transfusion can also lead to hypomagnesaemia.[93]

Clinical presentation

It is important to be aware of the consequences of other electrolyte deficiencies due to the function of magnesium on ion distribution pumps. The effect of magnesium deficiency on the appearance of hypocalcaemia has been discussed previously. The interaction between potassium and magnesium are many fold and complicated. Hypomagnesaemia is accompanied by hypokalaemia in approximately 40 per cent of cases. Intracellular potassium depletion is often pronounced due to the effect on the sodium–potassium ATPase pump. Hypokalaemia, refractory to even parenteral substitution, should always raise the suspicion of underlying magnesium deficiency. Hypophosphataemia is also frequently associated with hypomagnesaemia.

Electrocardiographic abnormalities are difficult to define as in the majority of cases other electrolyte disturbances are also present. Most important is the QT interval prolongation as a reflection of slower diastolic depolarization. These patients are at risk for sudden death due to torsade de pointe-type ventricular fibrillation. The inhibition of the Na/K ATPase pump by both hypomagnesaemia and digitalis implies that this drug should never be used in hypomagnesaemia. Digitalis will also slow cardiac conduction with a resultant further increment in QT-interval. Neuromuscular and central nervous symptomatology is comparable with those of hypocalcaemia. Seizures and even coma have been described in patients with cisplatin-induced hypomagnesaemia. Raynaud's phenomenon developed in 13 out of 30 patients treated with cisplatin, vinblastine, and bleomycin (PVB) for testicular cancer and the severity of prior hypomagnesaemia had a predictive value.[94]

Treatment

Symptomatic patients with neuromuscular irritability or cardiac conduction disturbances should receive 25 mmol magnesium intravenously over 12 to 24 h. In case of seizure or acute arrhythmia 4 to 8 mmol should be administered intravenously as a rapid infusion over 10 min. Patients with chronic hypomagnesaemia should receive oral magnesium supplementation. One gram of the most commonly used salt, $MgSO_4 \cdot 7H_2O$, provides 4.0 mmol or 8 meq or 97.6 mg of elemental magnesium. One mmol constitutes 24 mg of magnesium. Regular tablets contain between 50 and 100 mg of magnesium.

Hyponatraemia

Introduction

Sodium is the major cation in the plasma and extracellular fluid. The plasma sodium concentration (normal 137–145 mmol/l) is regulated indirectly by alterations in total body water content. This is accomplished by sensors that either promote the uptake of water or the excretion of urine. Total body water constitutes approximately 60 per cent of the lean body weight in men and 50 per cent in women. Approximately 60 per cent of total body water is in the intracellular compartment and 40 per cent in the extracellular compartment. Approximately one-quarter to one-fifth of the total extracellular fluid is contained in the plasma compartment. The distribution of total body water between the intracellular and extracellular compartment is governed by the osmolality of the fluids on both sides of the cell membrane. The osmolality of a solution refers to the absolute number of solute particles per kilogram of water. The major determinants of extracellular solute content are sodium salts, which account for 95 per cent of the plasma osmotic pressure, whereas glucose, potassium, and urea under normal circumstances play only a minor role.

Sodium is actively extruded from all cells and has only limited permeability over most cellular membranes making it the major determinant of serum tonicity. Clinically, osmolality in expressed as the solute concentration per litre of solution (molar or per kilo gram solution (molal)).

Plasma osmolality can be measured directly, or it can be estimated by the equation:

$$\text{plasma osmolality (mosm/l)} = 2 \times \text{sodium (mmol/l)} +$$
$$\text{glucose concentration (mmol/l)} + \text{urea concentration (mmol/l)}$$

The normal value of plasma osmolality varies between 285 and 295 mosm/l. It is useful to compare the measured osmolality with the calculated estimation in order to detect the presence of unknown osmotic active particles. Since the cell membrane is in general freely permeable to water, any gradient between intracellular and extracellular osmolality will result in a movement of water from the compartment with the lower to the one with the higher osmolality until equilibrium has been reached. Only the 'effective osmolality' or tonicity will affect the distribution of water. The 'effective osmolality' is expressed by the tonicity of the solution. As urea can permeate cells freely it does not contribute to the tonicity.[95] Only a difference in tonicity across a membrane will cause water movements to occur.

Sodium and mannitol are both impermeable solutes and their distribution causes fluid movements. Acute lowering of serum sodium will lead to intracellular water accumulation with cellular swelling. This can cause brain oedema with, eventually, dramatic consequences. This constitutes the major problem when confronted with a patient with hyponatraemia.

The occurrence of hyponatraemia in patients with an underlying malignancy often leads to the diagnosis of the syndrome of inappropriate antidiuretic hormone secretion (SIADH). The water balance of the body is regulated by a system of osmoreceptors that affect the release of antidiuretic hormone (ADH) and the feeling of thirst. The nonapeptide arginine vasopressin is synthesized as part of a much larger precursor molecule, arginine vasopressin-neurophysin, in the neurones of the supraoptic and paraventricular nuclei of the hypothalamus. The vasopressin precursor gene comprises three exons coding for three major protein components: arginine vasopressin, neurophysin II, and a C-terminal glycopeptide.[96] It is believed that this large precursor molecule is cleaved to its constituents along the axonal transport towards the neurohypophysis. The synthesis of arginine vasopressin is not restricted to the to the hypothalamic

region. The presence of vasopressin and its associated neurophysin has been identified in many different organs, for example the ovaries, the uterus, the testis, the adrenal glands, the thymus, and both central and peripheral nervous tissue. The physiological implications of these observations are not obvious,[97] but a paracrine role for these peptides has been suggested. ADH promotes the back-diffusion of free water in the collecting tubules of the nephrons, thus decreasing the urinary volume and increasing the concentration of urinary solutes. Vasopressin exerts its effect on water permeability in the collecting duct cells by interaction with a specific receptor—the arginine-vasopressin type-2 or V_2 receptor. This binding will trigger a cyclic-AMP-dependent chain of events leading to the insertion of aquaporin-2-containing vesicles into the normally watertight luminal membrane of these duct cells.[98] The aquaporins are family of water-channel proteins. Urinary excretion of aquaporin-2 can be regarded as an index of the action of vasopressin in the kidney.[99] In healthy adults, plasma ADH will be undetectable when plasma osmolality is below 280 mosm/kg. In these circumstances diuresis will be maximal, allowing the excretion of large volumes of diluted urine (>10 l/day) (low urine osmolality and specific gravity).

Within the physiological range of plasma osmolality, plasma ADH concentration increases linearly with increases in osmolality and maximal antidiuresis is achieved with plasma ADH levels of 5 pmol/l, a level that is usually reached when plasma osmolality approaches 295 mosm/kg. At this time a concentrated urine will be produced and urinary volume may be as low as 20 ml/h. This corresponds with the activation of specialized receptors located in the supraoptic nucleus that induce thirst. The set point of these receptors is approximately 10 to 15 mosmo/kg above the set point of the osmoreceptors that influence the secretion of ADH.[100] The ADH thirst system regulating water balance is closely connected to the volume regulatory system that is responsible for the maintenance of adequate tissue perfusion. The latter system contains baroreceptors located in the arterial wall, the atria, and the venous system and governs urinary sodium excretion. Effectors of this baroreceptor system, the renin–angiotensin II–aldosterone axis and atrial natriuretic peptide, modulate the sensitivity and the set point of the receptors governing the release of ADH. In addition to antidiuresis, ADH also exerts vasopressor effects and in some instances, such as cardiac failure of hypovolaemic shock, the secretion of ADH may be stimulated in order to maintain the effective circulating volume although this might lead to hypotonicity.[101] However, the discussion of hyponatraemia will be limited to those causes judged to be frequent and more or less specific to patients with malignant disease (Table 4).

Routine clinical evaluation of hyponatraemia, including evaluation of fluid status, recent changes in body weight, skin turgor, mucosal dryness, central venous pressure, peripheral oedema, tachycardia, postural hypotension, together with an anamnesis of recent drug and fluid intake (oral and intravenous) determination of serum electrolytes, glucose, urea and creatinine, albumin and total protein, serum osmolality, urinary electrolyte concentration, and urinary osmolality normally enables the clinician to determine which type of hyponatraemia is present.[102]

Pathophysiology

Syndrome of inappropriate antidiuretic hormone secretion

The syndrome of inappropriate ADH secretion was first described by Schwartz and Bartter in two patients with bronchogenic carcinoma

Table 4 Conditions associated with hyponatraemia

Isotonic and hypertonic hyponatraemia	
Presence of increased concentrations of glucose, mannitol, or non-sodium solutes	
Hypotonic hyponatraemia	
Hypervolaemic	Cardiac failure, liver cirrhosis, inferior vena cava obstruction, nephrotic syndrome
Hypovolaemic	Diuretics, Addison's disease, salt-losing, osmotic diuresis, diarrhoea, vomiting
Euvolaemic	SIADH, water intoxication, reset osmostat, hypothyroidism, glucocorticoid deficiency

who continued to produce hypotonic urine in the presence of serum hyponatraemia.[103] The initial explanation for this syndrome was a suspected stimulation, by the primary tumour, on the neurohypophysis to secrete an excess of ADH. It took several years before the actual production of ADH by the tumour could be demonstrated.[104] Afterwards *in vitro* cultures of cell lines producing ADH gave further insight into the syndrome.[105]

Arginine vasopressin has a prime role in modulating urinary water excretion. In response to many stimuli, most of all from the osmoreceptors, arginine vasopressin secretion will increase the permeability of the renal collecting system, thus allowing water reabsorption in relation to the prevailing interstitial concentration of the renal medulla. In the presence of an hypertonic medulla, arginine vasopressin will cause the production of concentrated urine and thus result in a negative free water clearance. This condition is judged appropriate if it occurs in the presence of an increased serum osmolality.[100] Apart from the condition of underlying malignancy, a wide variety of stimuli other than osmolality can influence ADH secretion and the response of the kidney to ADH.

The basic abnormality underlying the Schartz–Bartter syndrome is the failure to suppress arginine vasopressin secretion when plasma osmolality drops below the normal threshold value of 275 to 285 mosm/kg. Patients with this syndrome should however always be suspected of an underlying malignancy as its cause. Patients with the Schwartz–Bartter syndrome produce a hypotonic urine, but the urinary volume is related to fluid intake. Serum sodium concentration can be as low as 105 meq/l.[106] Hypouricaemia is a frequent feature of SIADH of any type.[107]–[109] Urinary salt loss can be normal in absolute terms, that is in balance with the intake. Urinary sodium concentration is, however, nearly always in excess of 20 meq/l. This increased loss of sodium with its negative free water clearance will lead to hyponatraemia when hypotonic fluids are taken in order to maintain euvolaemia. Once a new steady state has been reached, the balance for water and sodium losses and intake will be matched. In patients with euvolaemic, hypotonic hyponatraemia, and urinary osmolality above 100 mosm/kg, the diagnosis of SIADH is almost certain.

In patients with a urinary osmolality below 100 mosm/kg a dehydration test is the only diagnostic test to determine the presence of a reset osmostat.[110]

The tumour type most often associated with SIADH is small-cell carcinoma of bronchogenic or extrapulmonary origin, but this syndrome is not restricted to patients with malignancies. Overt SIADH has been reported in 7 to 14 per cent of patients with extensive compared to limited disease (20 versus 11 per cent).[111],[112] An abnormal response to water loading was found in up to 47 per cent of patients with small-cell lung cancer.[113] Others have confirmed this high prevalence of subclinical disturbed ADH secretion.[114] In patients with small-cell carcinoma and central nervous system metastasis, the prevalence of SIADH is even higher.[115] No clear significance regarding prognosis can be given to the presence or absence of SIADH in small-cell carcinoma, unless brain metastasis are being diagnosed. Small-cell lung cancer patients with hyponatraemia have been identified who have no detectable arginine vasopressin in their tumours or plasma. Recent studies suggest that ectopic production of atrial natriuretic factor might be involved.[116] Molecular studies on small-cell lung cancer cell lines showed frequent increased mRNA and protein expression of atrial natriuretic factor. In patients with hyponatraemia, either atrial natriuretic factor and/or arginine vasopressin mRNA could be demonstrated.[117] As a preliminary conclusion it seems that in the majority of patients with lung cancer and hyponatraemia, arginine vasopressin levels correlate best with the presence or absence of hyponatraemia, but atrial natriuretic factor might, however, prove to be a contributing factor.[118]

Drug-related SIADH

A variety of chemotherapeutic drugs have also been implicated in the aetiology of hyponatraemia due to SIADH (Table 5).

A well-known example is vincristine.[119] The emergency of hyponatraemia was first reported in children with leukaemia, while case reports in adults confirmed the association of SIADH with vincristine therapy.[120] No clear dose was ever observed with regard to this toxicity.

Cyclophosphamide, its analogue ifosfamide, and melphalan have all been reported to cause severe hyponatraemia due to SIADH.[121],[122]

Cisplatin is associated with renal tubular damage and may cause severe perturbations in electrolyte and water balance. Most prominent are urinary magnesium wasting and, eventually, hypokalaemia and hypocalcaemia, and even hyponatraemia due to salt-loosing nephropathy.[123] Treatment with short-acting intravenous somatostatin can also result in severe hyponatraemia.[124]

Clinical manifestations

Symptoms of acute hyponatraemia, occurring within 48 h, are mainly gastrointestinal and neuropsychiatric. Initial symptoms with hyponatraemia above 125 mmol/l consist of headache, nausea, vomiting, and muscular weakness. Once sodium falls below 125 mmol/l mental changes predominate with lethargy, apathy, or agitation, seizures, coma, and, ultimately, cerebral anoxia and death.

The symptomatology of hyponatraemia primarily results from cellular overhydration of brain cells and its severity is strongly dependent on the rapidity of onset and the degree of hyponatraemia. Acute hyponatraemia may cause severe neurological symptoms, whereas a long-standing hyponatraemia may be asymptomatic. This is thought to be due to defence mechanisms of the brain against overhydration, diverting excess interstitial fluid into the liquor and lowering the intracellular osmotic pressure by extrusion of amino acids. This mechanism is both a major protection against cerebral

Table 5 Differential diagnosis of SIADH

I. Malignancies
Bronchogenic carcinoma (small-cell type)
Carcinoid tumour (bronchial, foregut type)
Pancreas carcinoma
Duodenal carcinoma
Hodgkin and non-Hodgkin lymphoma
Leukaemia
Prostate cancer
Ewing's sarcoma
Thymoma
Ureteral carcinoma
Neuroblastoma
Nasopharyngeal carcinoma

II. Chest diseases
Tuberculosis
Pneumonia
Lung abscess
Cystic fibrosis
Aspergillus infection
Acute respiratory failure
Chronic obstructive airway disease
Pneumothorax
Positive pressure breathing

III. Central nervous system diseases
Trauma
Meningitis
Brain abscess
Encephalitis
Subdural haematoma
Subarachnoidal bleeding
Cerebral thrombosis
Sinus cavernosus thrombosis
Acute psychosis
Guillain–Barré syndrome
Primary brain tumour
Brain metastasis
Multiple sclerosis
Rocky Mountain spotted fever
Acute intermittent porphyria
Wernicke encephalopathy
Seizures

IV. Drug related
Vasopressin, oxytocin, desmopressin
Vincristine, vinblastine
Cisplatin
Cyclophosphamide, high-dose melphalan
Somatostatin
Thiazide diuretics, sulphonylureas
Phenothiazines
Carbamazepine
Nicotine, ethanol
Clofibrate

V. Idiopathic

oedema in acute hyponatraemia, but these patients are also at increased risk of osmotic demyelinization syndrome if the hyponatraemia is corrected too rapidly.

Treatment

The therapy of hyponatraemia will differ depending on the underlying disorder, the presence of symptoms, and the rapidity of its onset. Hypovolaemia, hypotension, and vomiting, if present, need correction. There are conflicting opinions, however, with regard to the administration of sodium. Correction of hyponatraemia will lead to the movement of water out of the cells. The degree to which this occurs is dependent upon the duration of the hyponatraemia and the presence of specific adaptation mechanisms to hypo-osmolality in the brain. After 48 h the neurones have reconstituted their cellular osmolality in accordance with the prevailing extracellular osmolality by extruding osmotically active particles. If under these circumstances hypertonic saline is administered, a specific syndrome, known as central pontine myelinolysis, may develop, characterized by seizures, limb paralysis, a persistent vegetative state, or even death.[125] To prevent this syndrome the following guidelines have been developed with regard to the correction of hyponatraemia and the associated hypo-osmolality.

Acute onset severe hyponatraemia should be treated promptly using hypertonic saline and frusemide, aiming at an increase of 1 mmol/h.[126] The rate of correction in patients who have a severe symptomatic hyponatraemia of a more chronic duration should be below 0.5 mmol/h, as severe morbidity and even mortality have been associated with a more aggressive approach.[127],[128] In patients with severe but asymptomatic hyponatraemia treatment must be directed to prevent further decline of serum sodium and active intervention should be performed very carefully.

Treatment of patients with SIADH consists of fluid restriction to 500 ml/day. This restriction will further limit urine production, and thus limit the negative free water clearance. Under these conditions urinary sodium concentration can be decreased to less than 10 meq/litre. This will limit urinary production and sodium losses and prevents the dilution of the extracellular fluid caused by hypotonic fluid intake. This therapy is often very difficult to manage outside the hospital. Demeclocycline, a tetracycline derivative, in a dose up to 1200 mg/day, causes a form of transient nephrogenic diabetes insipidus and is superior to lithium.[129] The effect on hyponatraemia becomes apparent within 5 to 7 days and serum sodium returns to normal values within 5 to 14 days.

Oral urea in a dose of 30 g will cause osmotic diuresis and alleviate the need for fluid restriction, but one of its the major drawbacks is its bad taste. Loop diuretics, such as frusemide and ethacrynic, acid will increase diuresis and decrease the concentrating capacity of the kidney. Thiazide diuretics, on the contrary, will worsen the hyponatraemia in SIADH. Treatment of the underlying neoplasm is the best and only lasting therapy.

Hypernatraemia

Introduction

Sodium is the major determinant of serum osmolality and tonicity. Rapid changes in serum sodium levels will lead to parallel changes in tonicity and will cause water movement across cellular membranes. In the case of hypernatraemia this would result in cellular dehydration. Because sodium and water intake are very variable, a major feedback control mechanism exists to provide protection from too drastic

Table 6 Diagnostic approach to hypernatraemia

I. Loss of water in excess of sodium loss: hypovolaemic hypernatraemia

a. gastrointestinal: diarrhoea, vomiting, hypertonic enemas

b. renal: diuretics, glycosuria, osmotic diuresis e.g. mannitol, iv contrast, acute and chronic renal failure, partial obstruction

c. skin: fever, heat stroke

d. lung: hyperventilation

e. other: impossibility or unavailability to drink

II. Excessive sodium intake or retention: hypervolaemic hypernataemia

a. hyperaldosteronism

b. excessive sodium administration oral or intravenous e.g. sodium bicarbonate, fresh frozen plasma

III. Isovolaemic hypernatraemia

a. diabetes insipidus central and nephrogenic

b. reset osmostat

c. skin loss

d. iatrogenic

changes in tonicity. This is accomplished by the integration of the two major osmoregulatory systems.

The first line of defence against water depletion and hyperosmolality consists of the renal concentrating mechanism. The neurohypophyseal antidiuretic hormone (ADH; arginine vasopressin) is an nonapeptide synthesized in the supraoptic and paraventricular nuclei of the hypothalamus and secreted by the posterior pituitary. When plasma osmolality is less than 280 mosm/kg, ADH is undetectable and urinary osmolality is less than 150 mosm/kg. Once plasma osmolality rises above 280 mosm/kg both plasma ADH and urinary osmolality rise sharply in a linear fashion. The mechanism of action of ADH is primarily mediated by stimulation of adenylate cyclase via the interaction with the V_2 receptor on the serosal surface of the epithelial cells of the renal collecting tubules. This receptor stimulation will lead to an increased expression of aquaporin-2 on the apical membrane of the renal collecting ducts. This will ultimately lead to an increased permeability of this collecting tubular cells. The high tonicity in the renal medulla will force water out of the tubular lumen into the renal medulla. This will lead, in the presence of a high plasma ADH, to the excretion of a very concentrated urine with a 'negative' free water clearance. Thus, an excess of sodium to water will be lost from the body in an attempt to counterbalance serum hyperosmolality.

The second line of defence against hypernatraemia is the thirst centre in the hypothalamus with cortical extensions, leading to increased fluid intake whenever tonicity threatens to increase. Due to the integrated action of thirst and arginine vasopressin secretion, an increased intake of largely hypotonic solutes will lead to a further fall in serum osmolality.[110]

Hypernatraemia is therefore infrequent in adult patients who are mentally alert. Although other reasons can be responsible for the occurrence of hypernatraemia in patients with malignancy, we will concentrate on both central and nephrogenous diabetes insipidus (Table 6).

Pathophysiology

In both central and nephrogenic diabetes insipidus the patient presents with polyuria and polydipsia. These entities can be differentiated by

Table 7 Aetiology of central diabetes insipidus

Posthypophysectomy

Post trauma

Primary tumours:
craniopharyngioma
pinealoma
pituitary adenoma
germ cell tumours
pituitary carcinoma

Secondary tumours:
breast carcinoma
bronchogenic carcinoma
leukaemia
lymphoma

Infections

Vascular disorders

Granulomas

Drug related:
Clonidine
Phencyclidine

Idiopathic

Hereditary

measurement of vasopressin and the response to water deprivation followed by vasopressin.

Central diabetes insipidus

Central diabetes insipidus can result from either partial or complete deficiency of ADH secretion. Some 50 per cent of cases of central diabetes insipidus are idiopathic, the rest are caused by a variety of reasons (Table 7). The different anatomical parts of the osmostat, ADH-producing neurones, neurohypophysis, and their interconnections can be destroyed by any space-occupying lesion. Although primary tumours can be responsible for this syndrome, discussion here will be limited to secondary localizations. In a survey from the Mayo Clinic,[130] 14 patients out of 100 consecutive, newly-diagnosed cases of diabetes insipidus were due to metastatic disease. In the majority of cases, diabetes insipidus emerges at a late stage of the disease. In the Mayo clinic series however, 11 out of 25 patients with diabetes insipidus as a complication of malignancy presented with diabetes insipidus as the initial manifestation of their malignancy. Three of these had myeloid leukaemia, two had a carcinoma of unknown primary, one had a breast carcinoma, and two other patients suffered from small-cell lung cancer. The posterior lobe is twice as frequently involved in comparison with the adenohypophysis. This relative high incidence of metastatic disease in the neurohypophysis is only rarely translated into clinical symptomatology.[131] Even if symptomatic pituitary metastasis is an uncommon clinical problem, diabetes insipidus is present in every case with visual symptoms and anterior pituitary symptoms present in only 25 per cent of cases.[132] The reverse is true for primary pituitary carcinomas. These rare adenohypophyseal neoplasms have an increased propensity of systemic metastases and rarely, if ever, are associated with central diabetes insipidus. The majority of cases are either adrenocorticotropic hormone- or prolactin-producing tumours.[133]

Of the solid tumours, breast cancer and lung carcinoma are most frequently responsible for metastatic diabetes insipidus. A survey studied 39 cases of diabetes insipidus due to metastatic involvement in patients with breast carcinoma.[134] All patients had widely metastatic disease at the time of diagnosis of diabetes insipidus. Many of them had either other central nervous system metastasis or meningeal carcinomatosis. Although lung cancer is complicated with a high incidence of central nervous system metastasis, diabetes insipidus is rare.[135] Haematological malignancies of the leukaemia/lymphoma group are more frequently complicated with diabetes insipidus.[130],[136]–[139] Diabetes insipidus can be caused both by direct infiltration, by vascular complications such as bleeding or infarction, or even due to extramedullary haematopoiesis.

Treatment of cancer is an increasing cause of central diabetes insipidus. In a national survey on the complications of trans-sphenoidal surgery, endocrine abnormalities had the highest incidence with central diabetes insipidus occurring in 17 per cent of cases.[140] In long-term survivors of childhood low-grade hypothalamic/chiasmatic glioma, treated with surgery, radiotherapy, or both, central diabetes insipidus occurs in nearly 12 per cent of patients.[141]

Nephrogenic diabetes insipidus

Several diseases, metabolic abnormalities, and drugs can interfere with the normal capacity of the kidney to produce concentrated urine. Some of these are of particular interest in oncological patients. Kidney infiltration by multiple myeloma as well as amyloidosis can lead to decreased responsiveness of the kidney to ADH. Prolonged use of diuretics and mannitol can impair the build-up of a significant osmotic gradient in the renal medulla. Lithium, colchicine, amphotericin B, and foscarnet (Foscavir) all lead to a decreased efficacy of ADH on the kidney. Ifosfamide has been reported to cause nephrogenic diabetes insipidus as a correlate of its distal tubular toxicity.

Demeclocycline inhibits the formation of, and action of, cAMP in the renal collecting ducts. It acts as a transduction pathway inhibitor after the arginine vasopressin–V$_2$ receptor interaction. Both

Table 8 Symptoms due to hypertonicity

Muscular weakness
Restlessness, irritability, disorientation
Depression, lethargy
Low grade fever
Intracranial bleeding
Convulsions
Stupor, coma

hypokalaemia and hypercalcaemia both result in a reversible abnormality in urinary concentration.

Clinical symptomatology

Hypernatraemia is far less common than hyponatraemia. It always reflects hyperosmolality and hypertonicity. This implies the presence of neurological symptoms and signs. Clinical symptoms consist mainly of pronounced polyuria and polydipsia. Patients drink up to 15 to 20 l, often very cold drinks per day. This intact thirst mechanism, although often very bothersome, protects patients against more pronounced hypertonicity and the ensuing cellular dehydration. Symptoms due to hypertonicity are listed in Table 8.

Diagnosis and treatment

Signs of dehydration, thirst, rapid weight loss, recent infusions and drugs, serum sodium and osmolality, and urine volume and osmolality often are enough to make a correct diagnosis of the pathophysiology of the hypernatraemia (Table 6). CT scan and MRI may assist in the diagnosis of metastatic diabetes insipidus. The measurement of urinary osmolality, plasma vasopressin, both before and after water deprivation, and the effect of urinary osmolality after exogenous arginine vasopressin enable a differentiation between central diabetes insipidus, nephrogenic diabetes insipidus, and primary polydipsia (Table 9).

The primary goal in the management of hypernatraemia is the restoration of serum tonicity. The brain is particular vulnerable to cellular dehydration. This can lead to rupture of blood vessels connected to the calvarium. To protect itself from these harmful consequences, brain cells generate new intracellular solute, so called 'idiogenic osmoles'. This of course takes some time to occur and it will not prevent severe brain dehydration in rapidly emerging hypernatraemia. On the other hand treatment, of a more subacute hypernatraemia with hypotonic fluids may lead to severe brain oedema. A discriminant time interval seems to be between 6 and 12 h before these protective mechanisms come into action.

It is important to estimate the probable fluid deficit from the equation:

$$\text{Body weight} \times 65 = \frac{\text{Normal serum sodium-actual serum sodium}}{\text{Normal serum sodium}}$$

This fluid deficit can be repleted with glucose 5 per cent solutions in alternation with 0.45 per cent NaCl solution. The hypernatraemia should be corrected over 2 to 3 days. Too rapid correction can lead

Table 9 Differential diagnosis of diabetes insipidus

Diagnosis	Plasma vasopressin deprivation	Urinary osmolality deprivation	Urinary osmolality after DDAVP
Normal	>2 pg/ml	>800	unchanged
Central diabetes insipidus	–	<300	substantial
Partial diabetes insipidus	<1.5 pg/ml	300–800	>10% increase
Nephrogenous diabetes insipidus	>5 pg/ml	<300–500	unchanged
Primary polydipsia	<5 pg/ml	>500	unchanged

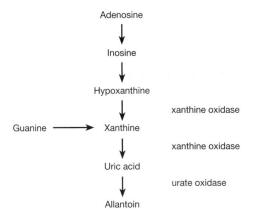

Fig. 4 Metabolic generation of uric acid from the purine bases.

to brain oedema and should only be undertaken if there is rapid-onset hypernatraemia in the presence of neurological symptoms. The treatment will depend of the degree of hypernatraemia, the volume status, and the acute or chronic nature of the hypertonicity. In a state of hypovolaemia it is appropriate to correct the volume deficit with isotonic saline and to correct the water deficit with 0.45 per cent saline or glucose solutions.

Hyperuricaemia

Introduction

Uric acid is the main end-product of the catabolic pathway of the purine bases adenine and guanine. Purines are part of many cellular components, such as DNA, RNA, and nucleosides, being critical to cellular function, either as energy sources or as secondary messengers, such as ATP and GTP. Normal metabolism of purine bases leads to the formation of inosinic acid, which is converted to inosine by the enzyme 5'-nucleotidase or to adenylic acid or guanylic acid, both compounds being substrates for nucleic acid and deoxynucleic acid synthesis. Further catabolism of inosine consist of two consecutive oxidations, both dependent on xantine oxidase, a flavoprotein that will convert hypoxanthine to xanthine and further to uric acid (Fig. 4).

Normal serum urate concentrations vary between 0.24 and 0.48 mmol/l and are higher in men than in women. Increased levels are positively correlated with protein intake, alcohol consumption,

weight, body mass, and social class. At physiological pH of 7.4, uric acid exists for 98 per cent of the time in its monovalent sodium salt. Serum is saturated with monosodium urate at a concentration of 0.42 mmol/l, but higher levels may remain stable in a supersaturated solution for long periods of time and the majority of individuals with hyperuricaemia are asymptomatic.

The total body uric acid pool is around 200 mmol (1200 mg).[142] Approximately 60 per cent of the total body pool turns over every day. Two-thirds of the urate formed each day is excreted by the kidney and the remainder is eliminated via the gastrointestinal tract. Gut bacteria metabolize uric acid further to form carbon dioxide and ammonia. The average man, on a purine free diet, will dispose of 600 to 700 mg of uric acid.

The renal handling of uric acid consists of glomerular filtration, proximal renal tubular reabsorption, active tubular secretion, and postsecretory reabsorption. A variety of factors modify the final uric acid excretion. Expansion of the volume will promote uric acid clearance, whilst volume contraction will have the opposite effect. Acidosis also reduces uric acid secretion, most probably by competitive interaction between different organic acids. Several drugs can influence any of these steps and lead to a change in uricosuria and uricaemia.

Urinary pH markedly influences the solubility of uric acid. At pH of 5.5 or less, uric acid is present in its free acidic form, whereas at higher pH more uric acid is present as urate. This change in ionization has dramatic consequences on solubility, being 20 mmol/l for the salt and 1.1 mmol/l for the acid.[143] In the distal portion of the nephron, the high urinary concentration of uric acid and the low pH may lead to supersaturation of urine, promoting the formation of uric acid crystals. Hypoxantine and xanthine, earlier products of purine catabolism, are more soluble in an aqueous medium and the beneficial effect of allopurinol, an inhibitor of xanthine oxidase, in patients with hyperuricaemia is explained by the inhibition of the further breakdown of these compounds to uric acid.

Pathophysiology

Hyperuricaemic nephropathy

Elevated serum uric acid and hyperuricosuria were first observed in patients with haematological malignancies. In 1853, Virchow mentioned uric acid crystal deposits in the renal pelvis on obduction of patients with leukaemia. Serum urate concentration depends on the balance between purine ingestion, endogenous purine metabolism, and urine elimination. The mechanisms of hyperuricaemia and/or hyperuricosuria in malignancy are due to increased production with the eventual aggravating presence of diminished renal excretory capacity, the hyperuricaemia being the consequence of increased cellular turnover. This may result in hyperuricaemic nephropathy and acute renal failure, and, only rarely, in acute arthritis. Hyperuricaemic nephropathy is caused by intratubular precipitation of uric acid crystals in the urine oversaturated with uric acid. This obstruction is the principal mechanism of renal failure. Experiments in rats, pretreated with oxinic acid in order to inhibit urate oxidase, and given an oral uric acid loading, are supportive of this intrarenal obstructive hypothesis.[144] Some degree of interstitial nephritis may be present. This form of acute renal failure may be part of the tumour lysis syndrome and occurs mainly, although not exclusively, after institution of an effective treatment regimen in patients with haematological malignancies.[145],[146] Sporadic cases have been reported in patients with solid tumours.

The uric acid load to be disposed of by the kidneys is dependent on the growth fraction of the tumour, the tumour burden, and the sensitivity of the malignancy to the treatment.[147] Some chemotherapeutic agents, such as the folic acid antagonists, interfere with purine metabolism at a stage before that of uric acid formation, their use more often leads to a decrease in uricosuria. Studies of uric acid metabolism in untreated patients with haematological malignancies disclosed that uricosuria is markedly increased in virtually all patients with acute lymphoblastic leukaemia, and moderately so in acute myeloid leukaemia and chronic leukaemia.[148] In acute lymphoblastic leukaemia the hyperuricosuria a has a direct correlation with the peripheral cell count. In patients with chronic lymphocytic leukaemia, a disease with a much slower cellular turnover, uricosuria has been found to be normal in most instances. Among myeloproliferative disorders, idiopathic myelofibrosis is associated with the most pronounced hyperuricosuria, polycythaemia vera being second. In multiple myeloma, impairment of renal function often leads to hyperuricaemia. In solid tumours, this complication is limited to patients suffering from fast growing and bulky tumours such as testicular teratomas, small-cell lung cancer, and small round and blue cell tumours (Ewing's sarcoma and peripheral neuroectodermal tumour (PNET)).

Acute arthritis

Secondary gout refers to patients in whom hyperuricaemia is part of a known metabolic abnormality as a cause for uric acid overproduction. This most frequently occurs in patients with myeloproliferative disorders, but it is infrequent in patients with underlying non-haematological malignancies.

Clinical manifestations

Hyperuricaemic nephropathy

The acute renal failure due to hyperuricaemia nephropathy is most often of the oliguric or anuric type. Patients usually present with symptoms of uraemia. Most of them have, at the time of diagnosis, an uricaemia in excess of 330 mmol/l. Sometimes flank pain suggestive of ureteral colic is present and voiding of concrement or haematuria may occur. The onset of acute renal failure in a patient with cancer and an elevated serum uric acid should always lead to a suspicion of hyperuricaemic nephropathy. A positive diagnosis of uric acid-induced renal failure is, however, not straightforward once uraemia has already been established, as renal failure in itself will produce elevated uric

acid levels. In this respect the clinical context of a therapy-sensitive malignancy with a large tumour load and the recent onset of chemo- and/or radiotherapy is important. Kjellstrand *et al.*, however, described five patients out of a total of 16 with haematological malignancies who developed acute renal failure without prior treatment.[145] Urine analysis may reveal the presence of uric acid crystals and concentration of uric acid in the urine may exceed 25 mmol/l. A urinary uric acid to creatinine ratio above 0.66 is suggestive of hyperuricaemic nephropathy.[149] Ultrasound of the kidney may show distension of the renal pelvis.

Treatment

With the insights into the physiopathology of this condition and the availability of allopurinol, most cases of hyperuricaemic nephropathy can be prevented. Vigorous hydration is important in order to prevent dehydration with its associated impairment of uric acid excretion and to stimulate glomerular filtration. A standard infusion of 3 to 4 l over 24 h in order to keep urinary output above 100 ml/h is recommended to prevent urinary saturation with uric acid[150] and urinary pH should be kept above 7.0 to improve solubility. Frequent measurement of urinary pH should be performed at the bedside. Acetazolamide, carboxyanhydrase inhibitor, will also lead to alkalinization of the urine and can be administered either orally at a dose of 500 mg daily or intravenously (2 to 3 × 250 mg). The presence of metabolic acidosis precludes the use of this drug.

Allopurinol, and its major oxidation product oxypurinol, are inhibitors of xanthine oxidase, the enzyme that catalyses the breakdown of hypoxanthine via xanthine to uric acid. Consequently, more hypoxanthine and xanthine is excreted in the urine and the formation of uric acid is reduced. This is beneficial as hypoxanthine and xanthine have a higher solubility in aqueous media than uric acid. Allopurinol was originally developed in an attempt to inhibit the degradation of 6-mercaptopurine. Different trials it the mid-1960s established the role of allopurinol in the prevention of hyperuricaemia and hyperuricaemic nephropathy.[80],[151],[152] The usual starting dose is 300 mg daily. The long half-life of oxipurinol (18–30 h), makes multiple daily dosing unnecessary. After oral administration in hyperuricaemic patients, a decline in serum uric acid is observed within 24 to 48 h, although it can take up to 14 days before its maximal effect is reached. A dose–response relationship for allopurinol is present. Patients treated with doses up to 800 mg daily had a more rapid decline in serum uric acid compared to those who received 200 mg daily. Allopurinol and oxypurinol elimination is decreased in renal failure, necessitating dose adjustments depending on the prevailing creatinine clearance.[153] The prolonged half-life of oxypurinol can lead to severe toxicity. Haemodialysis is an effective way of clearing oxypurinol.[145] The use of uricosuric drugs is not advisable in patients with an increased production. Inhibition of production constitutes a more rational approach. Side-effects of allopurinol are fever, gastrointestinal discomfort, and dermatitis. Although skin rash is frequent, a generalized hypersensitivity reaction with toxic epidermolysis is rare. Some drug interactions of allopurinol are relevant to patients with malignancies. The biological activity of both azathioprine and 6-mercaptopurine is prolonged by allopurinol. Only one-quarter of the scheduled dose should be administered in the presence of allopurinol. Cyclophosphamide is also potentiated by allopurinol. Oral anticoagulative drugs of the coumarine series also have a prolonged half-life, which often makes dose reduction of these drugs necessary.

Once hyperuricaemia nephropathy is established, allopurinol can at best impair further uric acid production, but whether by itself it will reverse renal failure is doubtful.[154] Other measures can be tried, such as mannitol diuresis and urinary alkalinization. Early use of dialysis is, however, the treatment of choice. Haemodialysis is 10 to 20 times more efficient than peritoneal dialysis in removing uric acid. A 6-h dialysis session reduces serum uric acid levels by 50 per cent.[145] The ominous prognosis of this form of acute renal failure has changed dramatically for the better due to early institution of haemodialysis.

Recently, a recombinant urate oxidase was isolated as a cDNA clone from *Aspergillus* and expressed in yeast. The naturally occurring proteolytic enzyme urate oxidase converts uric acid to allantoins, which are 10 times more soluble than uric acid. The recombinant form of this enzyme, known as SR29142, has shown promising preliminary results in clinical trials. Apparently it lowers uric acid more rapidly and more potently than allopurinol.[155]

Treatment of gouty arthritis associated with malignancy is similar to primary gout. Non-steroidal anti-inflammatory agents are very effective in reducing the inflammatory component, whereas allopurinol is used if recurrent attacks occur. In these circumstances the dose of allopurinol is carefully adjusted to keep serum uric acid levels within the normal range.

Tumour lysis syndrome

Introduction

Tumour lysis syndrome is a potential consequence of antitumour therapy, causing metabolic disturbances that, if left untreated, may result in potentially fatal renal, cardiac, and neurological complications. Tumour lysis syndrome is characterized by the development of hyperphosphataemia, hypocalcaemia, hyperkalaemia, hyperuricaemia, and often renal failure, as the result of the destruction of a large amount of rapidly proliferating neoplastic cells. The release of potassium, phosphate, and purine bases can occur to such an extent that it can both overwhelm and further limit the available renal excretory capacity resulting in a life-threatening metabolic emergency. This syndrome has been reported to occur in association with the treatment of high-grade non-Hodgkin's lymphomas, in particular with Burkitt's lymphoma, with acute lymphoblastic leukaemia, and in some myeloproliferative syndromes, most notably in patients with chronic myelocytic leukaemia in the accelerated phase.[80],[147],[156]–[161] More recently, tumour lysis syndrome has also been reported in patients with chronic lymphocytic leukaemia.[162],[163] It is less frequent in the treatment of solid tumours, but it has been reported in patients with small-cell lung carcinoma, breast cancer, Merckel cell carcinoma, colorectal cancer, and germ cell tumours.[164]–[168]

Tumour lysis syndrome is usually associated with the initiation of chemotherapy, but is can occur after surgery, radiotherapy, hormonal treatment, biological response modifiers, intrathecal chemotherapy, or spontaneously.[169],[170] With the introduction of high-dose chemotherapy regimens there is an increased risk for the development of this syndrome.[171]

Pathophysiology

Tumour lysis syndrome is characterized by the emergency of hyperphosphataemia, hypocalcaemia, hyperkalaemia, hyperuricaemia, and acute renal failure, which typically occurs 1 to 2 days, after initiation of chemotherapy. Whether tumour lysis syndrome will emerge as a result of the treatment of a tumour will be dependent on both characteristics of the tumour and the patient.

Phosphate is the major intracellular anion in any cell, but in lymphoblasts the level of phosphorus is four times that of mature lymphocytes.[172] The massive tumour cell death with release of phosphate will lead to an acute onset hyperphosphataemia, this being more severe in direct correlation with the prevailing serum creatinine. When the ion solubility product of phosphate × calcium concentration is exceeded, calcium phosphate will precipitate in extraskeletal tissues, including the kidney, with concomitant decrease of serum calcium. The risk occurs if the calcium × phosphate concentration reaches 4.6 mmol/l.[173] This leads to renal interstitial inflammation and later tubular atrophy. Kidney ultrasound scans have shown the transient development of renal calculi under these conditions.[174] The nephrocalcinosis will compromise renal function, limiting further the excretory capacity for phosphate. This implies that both overzealous alkalinization (urinary pH should be not above 7.5) and administration of intravenous calcium salts as a treatment for hyperphosphataemia and/or hypocalcaemia should be disregarded.

Hypocalcaemia has early been recognized as a feature of the tumour lysis syndrome.[175] It has always been thought to be the consequence of the massive phosphate release into the extracellular compartment. This would be followed by extracellular calcium phosphate deposition.[176] Although this appears an adequate explanation for the acute hypocalcaemia, it seems insufficient to explain the often prolonged hypocalcaemia seen in this syndrome. Massive rhabdomyolysis most closely resembles tumour lysis syndrome. Just as in tumour lysis syndrome, an augmented parathyroid hormone secretion is observed, both for increasing phosphate excretion and mobilizing calcium from the bone as a homeostatic protection against hypocalcaemia. In patients with rhabdomyolysis, PTH levels were appropriately elevated, but 1,25 [OH]$_2$ D levels were very low. In a recent report on tumour lysis syndrome in a patient with Burkitt's lymphoma with prolonged and clinically severely symptomatic hypocalcaemia, 1,25 [OH]$_2$ D levels were extremely low, only after treatment with vitamin D did hypocalcaemia subside.[177] It has been postulated that phosphate retention leads to an altered hydroxylation of vitamin D by the proximal renal tubular cells. As mentioned previously, 1,25 [OH]$_2$ D has a potentiating role on the different effects of PTH.

The release of intracellular potassium will lead rapidly to hyperkalaemia when renal function is impaired.[157],[147] This may be life-threatening, as the simultaneous occurrence of hypocalcaemia may increase the susceptibility to ventricular fibrillation and sudden death. Intravenous calcium remains the most effective treatment for the electrophysiological abnormalities caused by hyperkalaemia even at the risk of causing some increment in calcium phosphate precipitation.

It has become more and more apparent from recent clinical studies that patients suffering from a wide variety of haematological malignancies have pre-existing but often subclinical renal abnormalities.[147] Most patients who develop tumour lysis syndrome have elevated serum uric acid concentrations prior to treatment. The rapidly rising hyperuricaemia in this syndrome is the major threat to

Table 10 Preventive measures for patients at risk of tumour lysis syndrome

1. Initiate treatment with allopurinol at least at 300 mg/24 h
2. Hydration with at least 3 litre/ 24 h
3. Postpone chemotherapy if possible, until dehydration and/or hyperuricaemia have been corrected
4. Start chemotherapy not before 48 h on this regimen
5. Monitor central filling pressure, pulse, blood pressure, urine output 4-hourly
6. Alkalinize with intravenous bicarbonate until urine pH is >7.0

kidney function.[150] The development of hyperuricaemia nephropathy will result in the initiation of a vicious cycle leading to further increases in hyperkalaemia, hyperphosphataemia, and hyperuricaemia. Once this stage has been reached, dialysis is the only effective treatment.

Clinical manifestations

Tumour lysis syndrome usually emerges within 1 to 2 days after the administration of effective chemotherapy. Clinical symptomatology is initially limited to non-specific complaints such as general weakness, anorexia, and vomiting. Later on muscle weakness and cramps, convulsions and mental disturbances, cardiac dysrhythmias, and, eventually ventricular fibrillation and sudden death arise as a consequence of hyperkalaemia and hypocalcaemia. Renal failure is often of the anuric or oliguric type with rapidly raising blood urea nitrogen and serum creatinine levels.

Prevention and treatment

The need for preventive measures is dependent on both patient and tumour characteristics. Pre-existing renal function impairment and hyperuricaemia, bulky disease, and increased LDH levels are risk factors for the development of tumour lysis syndrome.

Preventive measures (Table 10) should include vigorous intravenous hydration with normal saline (4–5 l over 24 h) provided that kidney and cardiac function allow this. Allopurinol (300 mg/24 h) should be started 2 to 3 days prior to the initiation of chemotherapy in order to return serum uric acid levels to normal. Intensive hydration and allopurinol administration should be continued for 3 to 4 days after the start of chemotherapy. Urine alkalinization is efficient in promoting renal uric acid secretion. Urinary pH should be kept above 7 with intravenous sodium bicarbonate, but too high levels should be avoided as these are associated with the risk of phosphate precipitation. Measurement of urinary pH at every micturition and of serum electrolytes, calcium, magnesium, uric acid, and albumin at least daily is recommended. Close monitoring of fluid balance is essential especially in patients with reduced cardiac reserve or renal function. The use of methotrexate in these conditions may pose an increased risk for unanticipated toxicity due to diminished renal excretion.

If, in spite of the above mentioned measures, metabolic abnormalities emerge these should be treated vigorously. Patients should be transferred to intensive care units early on. Hyperkalaemia should be treated actively with intravenous glucose combined with insulin (50 ml of 50 per cent glucose solution with 15 IU rapid acting insulin/1 h), or intravenous 10 ml calcium gluconate (10 per cent), aggressive intravenous fluid administration and diuretics. Hypocalcaemia should

Table 11 Criteria for haemodialysis in the tumour lysis syndrome

Serum potassium	>6 mmol/l
Serum uric acid	>600 μmol/l
Serum creatinine	>880 μmol/l
Serum phosphorus	>3.33 μmol/l
Fluid overload	
Symptomatic hypocalcaemia	

(Cohen *et al.* 1980.[159])

be treated with intravenous calcium gluconate when very profound and/or symptomatic. Treatment with intermittent or continuous haemodialysis should be instituted early on (Table 11).[178]

Lactic acidosis

Introduction

At physiological pH lactic acid is completely dissociated into lactate and hydrogen ions and under normal conditions its concentration in venous blood is maintained between 0.6 and 1.2 mmol/l. Lactate is formed in the cytosol from pyruvate, which is an important intermediate component of glucose metabolism via the Embden Meyerhof pathway. During this process the coenzyme nicotinamide adenine dinucleotide (NAD^+) is reduced, thereby increasing the redox state (the ratio of $NADH/NAD^+$) of the cell. Pyruvate is the end point of this cycle. Only in the presence of pyruvate dehydrogenase, mitochondria and oxygen, is pyruvate completely oxidized to carbondioxide and water. The other metabolic alternative for pyruvate metabolism is its reduction to lactate. This enables reoxidation of NADH to NAD^+. Lactate has been called a metabolic 'dead-end' as pyruvate is its only precursor and at the same time its only route for metabolic transformation. The relative amounts of lactate to pyruvate are determined by the redox state of the cell. The conversion of pyruvate to lactate is catalysed by lactate dehydrogenase and is affected by the intracellular oxygenation and pH. The reaction kinetics are such that the concentration of lactate is approximately 10 times higher than that of pyruvate. Most of the lactate is produced in muscles, erythrocytes, brain, skin, and renal medulla. The liver and renal cortex are the organs which remove lactate from the blood by utilizing it as

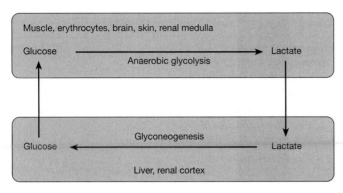

Fig. 5 The Cori cycle.

Table 12 Aetiology of lactic acidosis

Type A: with tissue hypoxia
Cardiac failure
Respiratory failure with PaO_2 <4.6 kPa
Shock from any cause, for example septicaemia
Severe anaemia
Strong muscular exercise
Generalized convulsions

Type B: without tissue hypoxia
Sepsis
Diabetes mellitus
Malignant disease
Renal failure
Liver failure
Drugs e.g. biguanides
Intoxications e.g. ethylene glycol, salicylates
Catecholamines excess e.g. pheochromocytoma
Congenital enzymatic defects in glucose metabolism

a substrate for glyconeogenesis. This succession of events is called the Cori cycle (Fig. 5). Production of lactic acid is to some extent also part of normal acid–base balance. Manipulations of acid–base homeostasis have shown that plasma lactate concentrations are usually increased during alkalaemia and decreased during acidaemia.[179] Lactic acidosis arises when the buffer system of the blood is not capable of maintaining pH within the physiological limits of 7.36 to 7.42. During strong exercise or tissue hypoxia excess lactate is generated, but the large reserve capacity of the liver to extract lactate from the blood will usually prevent overt acidosis, unless utilization of lactate is also compromised. A reduction in hepatic blood flow to less than 30 per cent or severe hypoxia markedly depresses lactate uptake by the liver and more severe alterations may even lead to net lactate production. Lactate acidosis, therefore, results from both increased production and decreased utilization. Lactic acidosis only occurs when the serum lactate exceeds 4 to 5 mmol/l.

Pathophysiology

Lactic acidosis is commonly divided into types A and B, according to the presence or absence of tissue hypoxia (Table 12). Lactic acidosis may be suspected if the anion gap exceeds 18 meq/l; the anion gap is the amount of anions that escape routine detection and is derived from the equation:

$$\text{anion gap} = [Na^+] + [K^+] - [Cl^-] - [HCO_3^-]$$

Proof of the presence of lactate acidosis will only be obtained by direct measurement of serum pH and lactate, as excess quantities of other organic anions, for example 3-hydroxybutyrate and acetoacetate, will also increase the anion gap. Elevated concentration of the latter compounds are often present in diabetic ketoacidosis.

Type A lactic acidosis is the most common type, and may be accompanied by signs of tissue hypoxia or poor perfusion. Examples are cardiorespiratory failure and septicaemia. Both increased production and decreased utilization of lactate are thought to be responsible for the hyperlactaemia in these circumstances.

However, a type B lactic acidosis has been described in association with malignant disease. Most often this is observed in acute lymphoblastic leukaemia, acute myeloid leukaemia, high-grade non-Hodgkin's lymphomas, and Hodgkin's disease.[159],[180]–[182] Reports of the same phenomenon in patients with solid tumours are ever scarcer; however, type B lactic acidosis has been reported in breast carcinoma, colon cancer, small-cell lung carcinoma, osteosarcoma, soft tissue sarcoma, and phaeochromocytoma.[183]–[188]

The pathophysiological derangements underlying this condition are incompletely understood, but the high glycolytic capacity of malignant tissue is probably important. Massive, near complete replacement of normal liver by metastatic infiltration was also present in the majority of patients.[180]

Several metabolic studies in cancer patients have demonstrated increased glucose uptake and an increased Cori cycle activity.[184],[189] In a lymphoma patient presenting with lactic acidosis and hypoglycaemia, enhanced intratumoural glucose metabolism was visualized by positron emission tomography employing 2-fluoro-2-deoxy-D-glucose.[182] The disappearance of severe lactic acidosis with successful chemotherapy in patients with lymphomas lends further support to the concept of tumoural lactate production.[182],[186]

Higher than normal rates of glucose uptake and lactic acid production are considered characteristic features of the neoplastic cell.[184] This increased Cori cycle activity might even contribute to the cachexia in cancer patients because lactic acid metabolism is an energy consuming process. In patients with phaeochromocytoma, lactic acidosis is probably caused by a combination of peripheral vasoconstriction, leading to some degree of hypoxia, and the effects of catecholamines on intermediary metabolism.[188] In patients with soft tissue tumours and paraneoplastic hypoglycaemia, the lactic acidosis observed might well be explained by the combination of reactive hypercatecholaemia and the decreased liver function due to the hypoglycaemia, the first causing an increased production of lactic acid the second decreased liver uptake of lactic acid.[183]

Regions of local hypoxia are present in nearly all solid tumours and the most hypoxic tumours have been shown to be both biologically more aggressive and more resistant to treatment.[190],[191] Increased intratumoural lactate production is a frequent observation in head and neck tumours and cervical carcinomas and seems to be correlated with the incidence of metastasis.[192],[193] These observations suggest that even in the presence of seemingly normal tissue perfusion, local hypoxia is responsible for tumoural lactate production.

Several case reports mention the occurrence of lactic acidosis in patients with AIDS treated with zidovudine. Direct mitochondrial toxicity is suspected to be responsible both for the lactic acidosis and the zidovudine-associated myopathy.[194]

Clinical symptomatology

Symptoms of lactic acidosis are heavily influenced by the underlying condition. General malaise, anorexia, vomiting, disorientation, cardiac instability, hypotension, and hyperventilation are symptoms that should alert the clinician to the presence of acidosis. Hypobicarbonataemia and an increased anion gap further support the diagnosis. This should lead to a thorough search for any active infection or other cause of type A lactic acidosis. Only after exclusion of these more common causes of hyperlactataemia should tumour-associated hyperlactataemia be considered.

Treatment

Treatment of lactic acidosis should be directed towards the underlying aetiology. Lactic acidosis carries a poor prognosis and vigorous treatment is necessary, preventing tissue hypoxia and circulatory collapse.

The role of bicarbonate administration, aimed at the reduction in the degree of acidosis and an improvement of cardiac function is controversial, the only exception being the correction of acidosis accompanying cardiac arrest. Bicarbonate administration may adversely affect tissue oxygenation by diminishing arterial vasodilatation, oxygen delivery, myocardial contractility, and intracellular pH.[195],[196] Sodium dichloroacetate ameliorates lactic acidosis by inhibiting lactate production and increasing lactate uptake in peripheral tissues and stimulates myocardial contractility. The potential advantage of this compound did not translate, however, in improved survival of patients being treated with this agent in intensive care setting.[197] In 'paraneoplastic' lactic acidosis bicarbonate administration may actually increase lactate concentration.[198] The explanation for this paradoxical effect may be that acidosis in itself inhibits lactate production.[180] In spite of these controversies, it is reasonable to administer bicarbonate in order to allow for a blood pH greater than 7.2. Below that value acidosis exerts adverse heamodynamic effects. Only institution of antitumour-directed treatment will have a long-lasting effect.

Hypoglycaemia in malignancy

Introduction

Tumour-associated hypoglycaemia is a rare disorder in which low insulin levels are found in the presence of severe hypoglycaemia. Its occurrence has been described in non-β-cell tumours of mesenchymal, epithelial, or haematological origin (Table 13). Usually these tumours are slowly growing and bulky (>1 kg) neoplasms located in the retroperitoneum, abdomen, or thorax.[199] The tumour types most often associated with hypoglycaemia are fibrosarcoma, mesothelioma, haemangiopericytoma, malignant hepatoma, and adrenocortical carcinoma. Other causes of hypoglycaemia which must be excluded are pancreatic β-cell tumours, drugs (especially insulin, suphonylureas,

Table 13 Non-β-cell tumours associated with hypoglycaemia

I. Mesenchymal tumours:	50%
fibrosarcoma, mesothelioma, neurofibroma, leiomyosarcomas, rhabdomyosarcoma, haemangiopericytoma, spindle cell sarcoma	
II. Hepatocellular carcinomas:	25%
poorly differentiated (type A) 87% moderately differentiated (type B) 13%	
III. Adrenocortical carcinomas:	5–10%
IV. Gastrointestinal carcinomas:	5–10%
pancreatic and biliary carcinomas	
V. Lymphomas	5–10%
VI. Other tumours:	
kidney, anaplastic lung tumours, carcinoid, Wilms' tumour, phaeochromocytoma, ovarian carcinoma, neuroblastoma	

Table 14 Differential diagnosis of fasting hypoglycaemia

Disorder	Plasma insulin	C peptide
Insulinoma	↑	↑
Factitious hypoglycaemia:		
sulphonylurea	↑	↑
exogenous insulin	↑	↓
Low-affinity insulin antibodies	↑	↓
Tumour-associated hypoglycaemia	↓	↓

alcohol) hepatic, renal, and cardiac disease, sepsis hormonal deficiencies (cortisol, growth hormone, glucagon), and congenital deficiencies of glycolytic enzymes.

Pathophysiology of non-islet cell tumour hypoglycaemia

Normal fasting blood glucose concentration is maintained between 4 and 5 mmol/l and whenever the blood glucose falls below this level, the liver produces glucose either from glycogen stores (glycogenolysis) or through new synthesis (glyconeogenesis).

Hypoglycaemia in the fed state is well known to occur in patients with insulinomas. In patients with other malignancies hypoglycaemia is rare, both with respect to the type of associated neoplasms and its actual prevalence. A low or undetectable insulin concentration when blood glucose is below 2.5 mmol/l will rule out an insulinoma and points to tumour-associated hypoglycaemia (Table 14).

Investigators have long been puzzled by the mechanism of tumour-associated hypoglycaemia, as it had been calculated that increased glucose consumption by the tumour could not be the sole explanation.[200] Several mechanisms have been proposed to be involved, including increased glucose utilization by tumour, suppression of hepatic glucose production, and enhanced peripheral glucose utilization. Ectopic secretion of insulin has never been convincingly

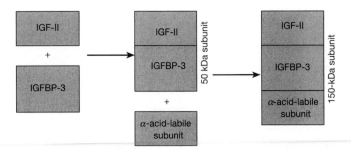

Fig. 6 Generation of the 150-kDa complex consisting of IGF-II, IGFBO-3, and α-subunit.

demonstrated in any of these patients; on the contrary, insulin and C-peptide levels are usually appropriately suppressed. The currently most accepted mechanism of tumour-associated hypoglycaemia suggests a primary role for the secretion of insulin-like growth factor II by the tumour.[201]

The insulin-like growth factor (IGF) family consists of three members: insulin, IGF-I, and IGF-II.[202] They share approximately 50 per cent amino acid similarity. Insulin is produced in the pancreas as proinsulin, which is cleaved into insulin and C-peptide. Insulin circulates at picomolar concentrations and has a short half-life. The IGFs and their binding proteins are primarily synthesized in the liver, they retain the C-peptide, have an extended carboxy terminus, and circulate at much higher concentration, largely bound to one of six IGF-binding proteins (IGFBPs). IGFs and IGFBPs are also synthesized locally in most tissues where they exert autocrine or paracrine activity.[203] Insulin, IGF-I, and IGF-II bind specifically to at least two high-affinity membrane-associated tyrosine kinase receptors. The binding to the insulin receptor has primarily metabolic effects, the interaction with the IGF-I receptor has primarily mitogenic and differentiation effects.

In the circulation, the IGFs are extensively bound to IGFBPs and consequently plasma levels are very low. Of the six known IGFBPs, IGFBP-3, binds more than 95 per cent of IGFs in serum. The IGF–IGFBP-3 dimer forms a complex with another protein subunit, the acid-labile subunit (ALS) (Fig. 6). This forms a 150-kDa heterotrimeric complex which effectively retains IGF activity within the capillary barrier. This ternary complex, also called the 'inactive' form, binds most of the serum IGFs. Once released from this complex, the IGFs leave the circulation and enter target tissues. Growth hormone increases the serum concentration of both the ALS and the IGFBP-3. Although IGFs have a mitogenic activity, both IGF-I and IGF-II lead to acute hypoglycaemia after short-term intravenous infusion.[204] A number of tumours express IGF-I and II, the IGF-I receptor, and various binding proteins.[202],[203],[205],[206]

In tumour-associated hypoglycaemia, excessive amounts of a prohormone form of IGF-II are produced and released ('big IGF-II').[207]–[209] The oversecretion of 'big IGF-II' leads to a suppression of growth hormone. As a consequence, the formation of a growth hormone-dependent 150-kDa IGF binding protein complex is impaired, which normally carries the majority of total IGF-II and restricts its bioavailibity. This impaired formation of the 150-kDa complex leads to a shift of IGF-II to a 50-kDa IGFBP complex, resulting in a 30-fold shorter half-life, increased turnover, and enhanced bioavailability. These increased levels of free IGFs lead to a further inhibition in the secretion of growth hormone, which by itself decreases the concentration of both the ALS and the IGFBP-3, of insulin, and IGF-I. Metabolic studies in tumour-associated hypoglycaemia using clamp techniques show that the glucose output by the liver is considerably suppressed.

Thus, tumour-associated hypoglycaemia is characterized by increased peripheral glucose uptake by muscle, increased glycogen stores in the liver, and inhibition of hepatic glucose production and inhibition of lipid mobilization from adipose tissue. Biochemically, this results in low levels of insulin and growth hormone, increased levels of glucagon and cortisol, normal or increased total IGF-II, and increased free IGF-II.

The hypoglycaemia is thus thought to arise through interaction of 'big IGF-II' with the receptors for insulin and IGF-I, leading to stimulation of glucose uptake by muscles and fat and potentially also by tumour cells, while hepatic glucose output is suppressed.

Clinical manifestations

Symptoms of hypoglycaemia usually occur when blood glucose is below 2.5 mmol/l, but the set point varies from person to person. In patients with frequent attacks, the set point before symptoms arise may become considerably lower, whereas the reverse is true for patients with poorly controlled diabetes mellitus.

Symptomatology of tumour-associated hypoglycaemia is similar to that of insulinoma and many other causes of hypoglycaemia and consists of pallor, sweating, behavioural changes, drowsiness, seizures, and coma. The attacks in tumour-associated hypoglycaemia occur most often at night or at waking. The onset may be insidious and initially rapid relieved by food or administration of glucose. Unlike patients with insulinoma, patients with tumour-associated hypoglycaemia frequently loose weight, despite their increased intake of food.

Treatment

The only effective therapy of tumour-associated hypoglycaemia is removal of the tumour. If this is not feasible, resection of tumour bulk will alleviate symptoms. Regular meals, divided over the day and at night, are recommended. When effective antitumour treatment becomes more problematic, the severity and frequency of the attacks will increase. Sometimes glucocorticoids are temporarily beneficial, but eventually patients have to be kept on continuous administration of glucose. Unlike the situation in insulinoma, long-acting analogues of somatostatin are not particularly helpful.[175],[210] Studies have shown that somatostatin can reduce the elevated levels of IGF-II and the glucose uptake by muscle, but fail to control hypoglycaemia. This might be due to the concomitant inhibition of pancreatic glucagon secretion by somatostatin.

However, alleviation of hypoglycaemia has been noticed incidentally in patients being treated with growth hormone.[211] Growth hormone is a glucose counter regulatory hormone, but its primary beneficial effect in tumour-associated hypoglycaemia is probably mediated though its ability to decrease the IGFBP-2 levels, increase the production of ALS and IGFBP-3, and thus restoring the formation of the 150-kDa ternary complex.

Table 15 Prevalence of the different aetiologies of Cushing's syndrome

ACTH dependent 79%:	Pituitary 80%
	Ectopic 15%
	Indeterminate 5%
ACTH independent 21%:	Adrenal adenoma 80%
	Adrenal carcinoma 20%

Data from Trainer and Grossman, 1991.[213]

Table 16 Pathogenetic mechanisms of Cushing's syndrome

Cushing's disease (pituitary adenoma secreting ACTH)
Ectopic corticotropin syndrome
Ectopic corticotropin-releasing hormone syndrome
Adrenal Cushing's syndrome
Adrenal carcinoma
Adrenal adenoma
Bilateral nodular hyperplasia
Pseudo-Cushing's syndrome
Alcoholism
Obesity
Depression
Drug-related Cushing's syndrome

Recent studies suggest a potential role for glucagon because the majority, but not all, of patients with tumour-associated hypoglycaemia have sufficient hepatic glycogen reserves. Continuous intravenous infusion of glucagon at a dose of 0.06 to 0.3 mg/h might be effective in mobilizing these stores.[212]

Hypercortisolism in malignancy

Introduction

Symptomatic hypercortisolism (Cushing's syndrome) is a rare disorder. It mainly results from increased production of adrenocorticotropic hormone (ACTH), either in pituitary or in nonpituitary (ectopic) tumours. Increased production of cortisol by the adrenal gland is the central feature of endogeneous Cushing's syndrome (Table 15). In normal subjects cortisol is secreted in a circadian rhythm; levels peak early in the morning and are lowest around midnight. This adrenal cortisol secretion pattern is under direct control of the parallel diurnal variation in secretion of the ACTH by the basophylic cells of the pituitary. Cortisol is a glucocorticoid because it stimulates the catabolism of peripheral fat and protein to provide substrates for hepatic glucose production. Cortisol is the major glucocorticoid in humans and up to 90 per cent is bound to cortisol binding globulin. The unbound fraction is presumably the biologically important one. This free cortisol is filtered by the glomeruli and is the principal determinant of cortisoluria. Urinary cortisol excretion will increase exponentially as the binding capacity of cortisol binding globulin is exceeded. As conventional plasma cortisol assays measure total cortisol, conditions that increase cortisol binding globulin content, for example oestrogen treatment, pregnancy, and oral contraceptive use, may falsely suggest hypercortisolism. However, the unbound, biologically-active fraction will be normal and urinary-free cortisol concentration will not be elevated. Plasma cortisol has a double negative feedback influence on its own secretion by inhibiting hypothalamic cortisol releasing hormone secretion and pituitary ACTH production.

ACTH is derived from a larger precursor molecule, pro-opiomelanocortin. Processing of pro-opiomelanocortin to smaller peptides yields pro-ACTH, b-lipotrophin and further cleavage leads to the formation of ACTH, melanocyte stimulating hormone, b-endorphin, and several related peptides.[214] Under normal conditions the synthesis and release of ACTH at the pituitary level is regulated by cortisol releasing hormone, arginine vasopressin, oxytocin, catecholamines, glucocorticoids, and a number of other hormones. These provide for the circadian rhythm of ACTH and the acute stress-related ACTH response. Transcription of the pro-opiomelanocortin gene, a process which is stimulated by cortisol releasing hormone, and inhibited by cortisol, occurs predominantly, but not exclusively, in the pituitary gland. Low levels of expression of pro-opiomelanocortin gene has been found in a variety of tissues, including adrenal, testis, spleen, kidney, ovary, lung, thyroid, liver, colon, and duodenum. The size of the pro-opiomelanocortin mRNA isolated from these sources is usually significantly shorter than that in the pituitary and it is uncertain to what extent these pro-opiomelanocortin-derived products reach the circulation.[214]

Pathophysiology

The pathophysiology mechanisms of Cushing's syndrome are summarized in Table 16 and Fig. 7. Several reviews have indicated the clinical and biological differences between pituitary adenoma versus ectopic ACTH-producing tumours.[215]–[217] In pituitary Cushing's disease, circadian rhythmicity of ACTH secretion is usually absent, but the oversecretion of ACTH remains suppressible by exogenous corticosteroids and can be stimulated by cortisol releasing hormone. Pro-opiomelanocortin gene expression and transcription are usually qualitatively unaltered.[218],[219] This contrasts with non-pituitary ACTH-producing tumours, in which pro-opiomelanocortin gene expression and the enzymatic cleavage of pro-opiomelanocortin are frequently altered and the response to exogenous steroids or cortisol releasing hormone is absent or impaired.

It remains an enigma as to why tumours derived from non-endocrine tissues may become secretors of hormones such as ACTH, although it has become evident that many different types of tumours contain immunoreactive ACTH, b-endorphin, and other pro-opiomelanocortin-derived peptides. Apart from small quantities of the normal pituitary pro-opiomelanocortin mRNA transcript, many tumours also contain a larger species of pro-opiomelanocortin mRNA.[218],[219] In addition, short transcripts have been found, probably identical to the short transcripts found in normal tissues. This indicates that many tumours, apparently, are able to synthesize pro-opiomelanocortin peptides, although only a minority of them give

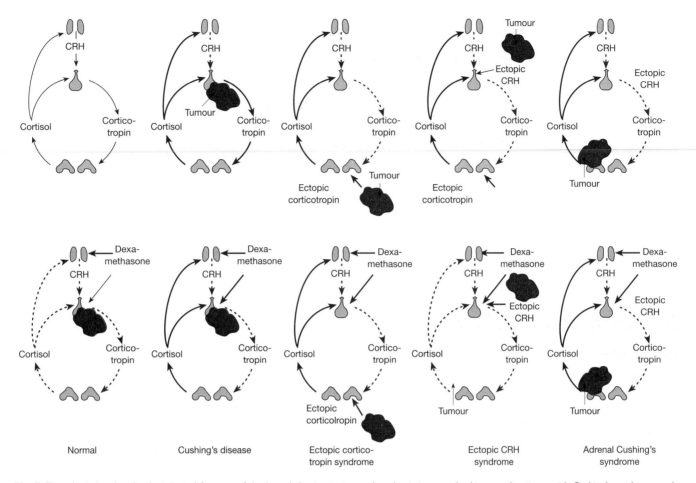

Fig. 7 Physiological and pathophysiological features of the hypothalamic–pituitary–adrenal axis in normal subjects and patients with Cushing's syndrome and the effect of dexamethasone. Stimulation of the hypothalamus by other central nervous system centres, such as the locus caeruleus, regulates the secretion of cortisol releasing hormone (CRH); corticotrophin stimulates adrenal secretion of cortisol; and cortisol inhibits the secretion of both CRH and corticotrophin. Adrenal (i.e. corticotrophin-independent) Cushing's syndrome is caused by adrenal tumours and corticotrophin-independent bilateral micronodular and macronodular adrenal hyperplasia. Low doses of dexamethasone are shown by thin black arrows, and high doses by thick black arrows. Normal hormone secretion is shown by thin black lines, suppressed secretion by dotted lines, and hypersecretion by thick black lines. (Orth DN. Cushing's syndrome. *New England Journal of Medicine*, 1995; **332**: 791–803.)[220]

rise to symptoms of hormonal overproduction. Thus, it is unclear whether 'ectopic' secretion of ACTH is merely inappropriate secretion or truly ectopic. Tentatively, it has been suggested that the tumour products transcribed from short pro-opiomelanocortin mRNA may not be in a form that can be secreted by the cell, or that high molecular weight ACTH precursor molecules have reduced bioactivity.[221] While this could explain the presence of increased levels of ACTH precursor and b-lipotrophin in the blood of 50 per cent of patients with lung cancer without causing symptoms of Cushing's syndrome, many questions remain.[221] Interestingly, ectopic ACTH syndrome may be confined to tumours capable of generating high amounts of a precursor transcript similar to that found in the pituitary, a phenomenon that seems to be restricted to an occasional tumour with features of neuroendocrine differentiation.[222] Cushing's syndrome can even be caused by secretion of corticotrophin by diffuse pulmonary tumourlets, supposedly consisting of a state of diffuse hyperplasia of the neuroendocrine cell system of the lung.[223]

In the ectopic corticotrophin syndrome the tumour produces ACTH in large quantities and often other peptides.[224],[225] The secreted

ACTH will force the adrenal glands to increase the production of cortisol. The high levels of ACTH, and the increased levels of cortisol together with the inability to suppress ACTH production by exogenous steroids are the key diagnostic elements. This is, however, somewhat simplified; not all patients with an ectopic corticotrophin syndrome exhibit lack of suppressibility which leads to some diagnostic difficulty in discriminating these patients from those with Cushing's disease. Secondly, observations of tumoural production of cortisol releasing hormone and only secondary increase in ACTH and cortisol secretion, makes the differential diagnosis even more challenging.[217],[226]

The tumour types most commonly associated with ectopic ACTH secretion are small-cell lung cancer and bronchial carcinoids. Small-cell lung cancer accounts for about three-quarters of all cases of ectopic-corticotrophin-induced Cushing's syndrome (Table 17).

Clinical symptomatology

The overall incidence of ectopic ACTH-secreting tumours is low. Based on retrospective surveys, ectopic ACTH secretion had been

Table 17 Distribution of underlying tumours in 51 patients with ectopic ACTH secretion

Bronchogenic carcinoma:	25	
small-cell		19
large-cell		2
adenocarcinoma		3
squamous cell		1
Carcinoid tumours:	8	
bronchus		4
thymus		1
oesophagus		1
stomach		1
duodenum		1
Malignant thymoma	5	
Pancreatic islet cell carcinoma	3	
Medullary thyroid carcinoma	3	
Oesophageal oat-cell carcinoma	3	
Squamous laryngeal carcinoma	1	
Pheochromocytoma	1	
Plasmacytoma	1	
Small-cell, primary unknown	1	

Data from Imura, 1980.[225]

diagnosed in less than 5 per cent of patients of small-cell lung cancer.[227]–[229] Similarly, only 15 cases of ectopic Cushing's syndrome associated with bronchial carcinoids were identified over a 40-year period during which 626 patients were evaluated for bronchial carcinoid tumours.[230] In only approximately half of the patients with small-cell lung cancer was Cushing's syndrome found at the initial diagnosis; in the remainder this was associated with recurrent disease.

Ectopic ACTH production is often completely asymptomatic. In a study on 280 consecutive patients with bronchogenic carcinoma, clinical hypercortisolism was diagnosed in only one patient.[227] In 15 patients with lung cancer and without clinical evidence of Cushing's syndrome, nearly all (14/15) had positive immunostaining for ACTH and a majority of patients had increased plasma ACTH levels; all were without clinical features of Cushing's syndrome.[231]

In patients with slowly growing tumour such as carcinoids, the clinical expression may be much more complete due to the longer natural history of the underlying disease in comparison with bronchogenic carcinomas, and symptoms of Cushing's syndrome may even precede the clinical diagnosis by many years in 'occult' tumours that are nowadays more often detected (Table 18). Hypertension, a nearly constant feature in the other aetiological groups of Cushing's syndrome, is present in only one-third of ectopic cases. Oedema, on the contrary, is more frequent in the rapid-onset Cushing's syndrome associated with small-cell lung cancer. The other physical signs, such as weight gain, moon facies, 'buffalo hump', truncal obesity, and a florid complexion are observed in a small minority of patients, most notably patients with indolent tumours. Cutaneous hyperpigmentation is unusual except in patients with the ectopic ACTH syndrome in whom plasma corticotrophin levels are markedly elevated. Metabolic abnormalities may be the only clue to the diagnosis

of ectopic ACTH production. Hypokalaemia, sometimes associated with metabolic alkalosis, is present in more than 90 per cent of patients with ectopic ACTH syndrome, compared to only 10 per cent in Cushing's disease of other aetiologies.[232]

Diagnosis and treatment

A suggestive clinical presentation will usually be the stimulus for further investigation. The laboratory diagnosis of Cushing's syndrome requires the demonstration of sustained cortisol overproduction, with at least a certain degree of autonomy. As an initial screening test the measurement of the excretion of free cortisol in 24-h urine sample is superior to the urinary 17-keto- and 17-hydroxycorticosteroids. This test is not influenced by alterations in plasma cortisol binding globulin content, as the kidneys only filter unbound cortisol and smooth out the variations in cortisol during the day. In normal subjects urinary free cortisol excretion is below 270 mmol/day.[233] The false negative rate is approximately 5 per cent, but in 11 per cent of patients with proven Cushing's syndrome at least one out of four samples was in the normal range. Repeated sampling over 3 to 4 days will thus increase the sensitivity of the test and a normal result makes the diagnosis of Cushing's syndrome extremely unlikely. If the result is ambiguous, plasma cortisol levels are indicated. Single plasma cortisol measurements are of little use, as cortisol levels fluctuate during the day and are subject to stress-like conditions. Measured cortisol values may also be elevated in conditions associated with increases in cortisol binding globulin, while free cortisol will be normal. Sampling of cortisol values at 9.00 a.m. and at midnight may reveal the absence of circadian rhythmicity, but in general dynamic tests have to be preferred.

Dexamethasone, which does not cross-react in most radioimmunoassays for cortisol, is commonly used for the assessment of the integrity of the hypothalamic–pituitary–adrenal axis and in the differential diagnosis of Cushing's syndrome. A dose of 0.5 to 1.0 mg of dexamethasone administered to normal subjects a bedtime will suppress morning plasma cortisol levels to below 50 nmol/l, depending on laboratory conditions, and can be conveniently performed in the outpatient clinic. Reportedly, the 1-mg overnight dexamethasone suppression test has a false negative rate of 2 per cent or less, but the false positive rate is 12.5 per cent. Plasma cortisol and urinary free cortisol measurements after administering 2 to 8 mg dexamethasone for 48 h and cortisol measurements during deliberately invoked hypoglycaemia may be required to differentiate between Cushing's syndrome and other conditions mimicking this disorder, notably obesity, depression, and alcoholism and to distinguish Cushing's disease from ectopic ACTH syndrome.

Plasma ACTH measurements are most useful in differentiating adrenal overproduction from other causes of Cushing's syndrome. In the absence of exogenous corticosteroid administration, a low or undetectable ACTH concentration is a strong indication that the adrenals are the source of the increased cortisol production. Plasma ACTH levels are usually unhelpful in the differentiation between Cushing's syndrome and pituitary disease. Greatly increased plasma levels, however, are usually associated with ectopic production, but levels do overlap. Observation of ectopic production of cortisol releasing hormone, with only secondary increases in ACTH and cortisol, makes the diagnosis even more challenging. Moreover, co-secretion of other hormones, such as bombesin, calcitonin, antidiuretic

Table 18 Clinical symptoms in Cushing's disease and in ectopic ACTH syndrome

Classical Cushing's syndrome[a]		Ectopic ACTH syndrome			
		Small-cell lung cancer[b]		Occult tumours[c]	
Symptom	%	Symptom	%	Symptom	%
Obesity	88	Peripheral oedema	83	Centripetal obesity	100
Moon face	75	Proximal myopathy	61	Proximal myopathy	100
Hypertension	74	Moon face	52	Moon face	100
Hirsutism	64	Truncal obesity	35	Polydipsia/polyuria	100
Muscle weakness	61	Hyperpigmentation	22	Mental disorders	100
Menstrual disorders	60	Psychosis	22	Hirsutism in women	100
Acne	45	Hypertension	22	Hypertension	70
Ecchymoses	42	Ecchymoses	17	Ecchymoses	50
Mental disorders	42	Hirsutism	4	Acne	50
Backache (osteoporosis)	40	Striae	4	Oedema	50
				Striae	40
				Pigmentation	30

Derived from data of [a]Gold, 1979: [b]Shepherd *et al.*, 1992; [c]Howlett *et al.*, 1986.[215],[228],[232]

hormone, and gastrin, may complicate the clinical presentation. The measurement of circulating ACTH precursor molecules has been reported to improve differential diagnosis between ectopic ACTH secretion and other forms of Cushing's disease.

Imaging procedures usually will provide the necessary additional information for a correct diagnosis and treatment plan. MRI appears superior to CT scanning in localizing small pituitary adenomas. CT scanning of the chest will be helpful in localizing ectopic ACTH-producing tumours and for detecting metastases. Octreotide scanning can also be considered in localizing obscure neuroendocrine tumours.[234]

Pituitary tumours, adrenal tumours, and carcinoids are preferably treated with surgical resection. Ectopic ACTH syndrome associated with small-cell lung cancer must be treated with chemotherapy. Results of treatment are poor. The median survival of these patients is less than that of patients with small-cell lung cancer without this syndrome due to a high incidence of infectious complications and gastrointestinal bleeding and ulceration.[228],[229]

If tumour reduction is not feasible or the cause of hypercortisolism remains obscure, medical treatment is indicated. Mitotane, metyrapone, and ketoconazole have all been used to interfere with adrenal steroid production.[217],[235],[236] Perhaps ketoconazole is the drug of choice, because of its toxicity it compares favourably with that of the other compounds. Doses of 400 to 1200 mg rapidly blocked corticosteroid synthesis in Cushing's disease, but in some patients with ectopic ACTH syndrome the effect was only temporary or incomplete.

Adrenocortical insufficiency

Introduction

The most frequent cause of adrenal dysfunction in cancer patients is glucocorticoid treatment. Secondary adrenal insufficiency may develop upon discontinuation of pharmacological dose of glucocorticoids and may persist for months. Adrenocortical failure is a rare disorder in the general population, but may be more frequently encountered in a population of cancer patients. The recognition of the syndrome is important because it affects a patient's well-being and may present as a life-threatening disease, yet proper treatment will reverse the condition rapidly. The clinical manifestations mainly result from deficiency of glucocorticoid and mineralocorticoid activity, although other deficiencies might also be present.

Pathophysiology

Both diseases of the adrenocortex and the hypothalamic–pituitary disorders may lead to adrenocortical failure, the clinical presentation depending on the underlying cause and the rapidity of its onset.

Secondary adrenal insufficiency is the result of inadequate stimulation of the adrenal by a failing hypothalamic–pituitary system. Acute pituitary insufficiency can result from sudden haemorrhage in a large pituitary tumour and constitutes a medical emergency. Patients will experience severe headache, vomiting, and frequently acute visual field loss. Radiographs of the sella region, CT scanning, or MRI will reveal the presence of a mass lesion.[237] Treatment consists of immediate trans-sphenoidal decompression of the optic chiasma and institution of corticosteroid administration, after blood samples have been taken for hormonal assays. Chronic hypopituitarism may result from pituitary tumours, craniopharyngioma, autoimmune disease, amyloidosis, granulomatous disease, irradiation, and extensive metastasis, causing either isolated ACTH deficiency or, more commonly, multiple alterations in the secretion of pituitary hormones.[238] The majority of symptomatic pituitary metastasis originate from primary breast or lung cancer.[239]

The differing aetiologies of primary adrenocortical failure are summarized in Table 19. Acute primary adrenal insufficiency may result from adrenal haemorrhage, but more frequently the condition is precipitated by stress-like conditions, for example surgery or an intercurrent infection, in a patient in whom subclinical Addison's disease has been present. Although the majority of cancer patients with adrenal metastases present with slow-onset adrenocortical

Table 19 Aetiology of adrenal cortical insufficiency

Autoimmune disease:
    adrenal cytoplasmatic antibodies
    ACTH receptor-blocking antibodies

Infection:
    tuberculosis, histoplasmosis, blastomycosis, AIDS related

Bilateral adrenal metastases:
    lung and breast carcinoma, malignant melanoma
    non-Hodgkin's lymphoma

Haemorrhage:
    anticoagulation
    postoperative
    sepsis (Waterhouse–Friedrichsen syndrome)
    antiphospholipid syndrome

Drugs interfering with steroidogenesis:
    imidazole derivates (ketoconazole, etomidate)
    aminoglutethimide, o,p, DDD (mitotane)
    suramin
    medroxyprogesterone acetate

Recent corticosteroid withdrawal

failure, abrupt-onset Addisonian crisis has been reported at presentation.[240],[241]

The adrenal glands are a common site for metastases. At autopsy malignant infiltration of the adrenal glands has been found in 8.6 to 27 per cent.[242] The incidence of adrenal metastases is particularly high in breast cancer (58 per cent), malignant melanoma (50 per cent), lung cancer (42 per cent), and non-Hodgkin's lymphoma (25 per cent).[243],[244]

Primary non-Hodgkin's lymphoma presenting as an Addisonian crisis

The general opinion is that these metastases rarely give rise to adrenocortical failure, unless more than 75 to 90 per cent of adrenocortical tissue has been destroyed. However, this does not take into account the limited adrenal reserve that may remain subclinical unless severe stress is induced.

Several authors have reported that symptoms of adrenocortical failure in patients with bilateral adrenal metastases on CT scanning occurred at a higher than expected incidence and have recommended assessment of adrenocortical function in these circumstances.[243],[245],[246] The relatively rare occurrence of Addison's disease due to malignant infiltration in comparison with the high frequency of metastases in the adrenal glands is remarkable.[247] There might be some over diagnosis of inappropriate antidiuretic hormone secretion when confronted with a patient with bronchogenic carcinoma and hypotonic hyponatraemia.

A number of drugs used in the treatment of cancer are associated with risk for adrenal failure. Aminoglutethimide was originally introduced as a medical adrenalectomy for breast cancer patients,[248] although inhibition of steroidogenesis most probably is not of clinical relevance at the currently used dosage of approximately 500 mg

daily.[249] Mitotane (o',p'-DDD) is structurally related to dichlorodiphenyltrichloroethane (DDT), and has selective toxicity for normal and neoplastic adrenocortical cells. Adrenal failure is frequently observed at doses used to treat adrenal cancer, making substitution therapy mandatory.[250]

Suramin was considered for the treatment of adrenocortical carcinoma because of its ability to produce adrenal cortical necrosis.[251] At present, suramin is being investigated for the treatment of prostate cancer. Suramin causes both primary mineralocorticoid and primary glucocorticoid insufficiency. This effect seems to be dose-dependent. Both mineralocorticoid and glucocorticoid replacement are mandatory in patients receiving high-dose suramin therapy.

Similarly, high-dose ketoconazole (800–1200 mg) has been used for the treatment of prostate carcinoma and Cushing's syndrome after it was demonstrated that the drug could inhibit cytochrome P450-dependent steps in steroidogenesis.[236] More recently, the abrupt onset of adrenal failure after withdrawal of medroxyprogesterone acetate has been observed in breast cancer patients who had received treatment with this agent for more than 2 years.[252] Temporary suppression of adrenocortical function should be considered in patient who receive high-dose corticosteroids.

Clinical manifestations

Symptomatology due to adrenal failure is very similar to that of patients suffering from advanced malignant disease. Most symptoms are non-specific and usually occur insidiously. Severe weakness often makes patients bedridden, and anorexia, nausea, and vomiting cause severe weight loss. Some form of dehydration with orthostatic hypotension is due to renal salt wasting in the typical form of adrenal failure.

In acute primary adrenocortical failure (addisonian crisis), unexplained hypovolaemic shock, fever, and tachycardia may dominate the clinical presentation. This suspicion for underlying Addison's crisis is especially justified in the presence of hyperpigmentation and hyponatraemia or hyperkalaemia. Chronic adrenal failure usually presents with general weakness, fatigue, nausea, and (orthostatic) hypotension. Other symptoms include anorexia, nausea and vomiting, myalgias, and abdominal cramping.

The most specific sign of primary adrenal failure is hyperpigmentation of the skin and mucosal surfaces. It is characteristically present around recent scars and in the creases of the palms of the hands; in all races patchy pigmentation on the buccal mucosa is seen. This ACTH-related hyperpigmentation is not a feature of secondary adrenal failure.

Diagnosis

In primary adrenal insufficiency the biochemical findings are related to glucocorticoid and mineralocorticoid deficiencies. Hypovolemic, hypotonic, hyponatraemia, with elevated urea and an increased urinary sodium concentration occurs in over 90 per cent of patients, whereas hyperkalaemia is present in approximately 60 per cent of cases. Occasionally, mild hypercalcaemia and hypoglycaemia are observed. Due to some degree of circulating volume depletion, increased antidiuretic hormone secretion will lead to increased urinary tonicity and some elevation of blood urea. Inappropriately elevated ADH levels in glucocorticoid deficiency will impair free water clearance, but this will rapidly be corrected after glucocorticoid replacement therapy.[253] In secondary adrenal failure, mineralocorticoid activity is usually better preserved. Hyponatraemia is present, but patients appear water intoxicated and serum potassium levels are often less increased.

Confirmation of diagnosis is obtained by assessment of free cortisol excretion in a 24-h urine collection and the demonstration of functional impairment of cortisol secretion in response to a test dose of 0.25 mg synthetic ACTH. Plasma ACTH will discriminate between primary and secondary adrenal failure, low levels being found in secondary failure.

Treatment

When adrenocortical failure is suspected in an emergency, 100 mg of hydrocortisone should be administered intravenously, after blood has been taken for glucose, electrolyte, cortisol, and aldosterone assessments. Parenteral fluid administration should be carefully monitored because of the relative inability of these patients to excrete free water. Long-term treatment consists of replacement doses of corticosteroids, preferably hydrocortisone (20 mg in the morning and 10 mg in the evening). Alternatively, cortisone acetate (25 mg) or prednisone (5 mg in the morning and half the dose in the evening) may be used.

Patients with primary adrenal failure will usually need exogenous substitution of mineralocorticoid activity. This is supplied with fludrocortisone (0.05–0.15 mg daily). While the recommended hydrocortisone dosages will usually suffice in uncomplicated adrenocortical failure, higher dosages may be required in patients treated with mitotane and suramin. Under conditions of stress, such as surgery and infections, dosages should be increased, for example hydrocortisone 50 to 100 mg orally or intravenously three times daily.

References

1. Berry EM, *et al.* Variations in plasma calcium with induced changes in plasma specific gravity, total protein and albumin. *British Medical Journal*, 1973; **4**: 640–3.

2. Bushinsky DA, Monk RD. Calcium. *Lancet*, 1998; **352**: 306–11.

3. Brown EM, *et al.* Cloning and characterization of an extracellular Ca +2 -sensing receptor from bovine parathyroid. *Nature*, 1993; **366**: 575–80.

4. Brown EM, *et al.* Calcium-ion-sensing cell-surface receptors. *New England Journal of Medicine*, 1995; **333**: 234–40.

5. Mundy GR, Guise AT. Hypercalcemia of malignancy. *American Journal of Medicine*, 1997; **103**: 134–45.

6. Blomqvist CP. Malignant hypercalcemia—a hospital survey. *Acta Medica Scandinavica*, 1986; **220**: 455–63.

7. Fisken RA, Heath DA, Bold AM. Hypercalcemia—a hospital survey. *Quaterly Journal of Medicine*, 1980; **196**: 405–18.

8. Skrabanek P, McPartlin J, Powell D. Tumor hypercalcemia and ectopic hyperparathyroidism. *Medicine*, 1980; **59**: 262–82.

9. Stewart AF, *et al.* Biochemical evaluation of patients with cancer-associated hypercalcemia. *New England Journalof Medicine*, 1980; **303**: 1377–83.

10. Simpson EL, *et al.* Absence of parathyroid hormone messenger RNA in non parathyroid tumors associated with hypercalcemia. *New England Journal of Medicine*, 1983; **309**: 325–30.

11. Stewart AF, *et al.* Synthetic human parathyroid hormone-like protein stimulates bone resorption and causes hypercalcemia. *Journal of Clinical Investigation*, 1988; **81**: 596–600.

12. Abou-Samra AB, *et al.* Expression cloning of a common receptor for parathyroid hormone and parathyroid hormone-related peptide from rat osteoblast-like cells: a single receptor stimulates intracellular accumulation of both cAMP and inositol trisphosphates and increases intracellular free calcium. *Proceedings of the National Academy of Sciences USA*, 1992; **89**: 2732–6.

13. Everhart-Caye M, Inzucchi SE, Guiness-Henry J, Mitnick MA, Stewart AF. Parathyroid hormone (PTH)-related protein (1–36) is equipotent to PTH(1–34) in humans. *Journal of Endocrinology and Metabolism*, 1996; **81**: 199–208

14. Brandt DW, Wachsman W, Deftos LJ. Parathyroid hormone-like protein: alternative messenger RNA splicing pathways in human cancer cell lines. *Cancer Research*, 1994; **54**: 850–3.

15. Yang KH, *et al.* Parathyroid hormone-related protein: evidence for isoform- and tissue-specific posttranslational processing. *Biochemistry*, 1994; **33**: 7460–9.

16. Walls J, Ratcliffe WA, Howel A, Bundred NJ. Parathyroid hormone and parathyroid hormone-related protein in the investigation of hypercalcaemia in two hospital populations. *Clinical Endocrinology*, 1994; **41**: 407–13.

17. Ratcliffe WA, Hutchesson ACJ, Bundred NJ, Ratcliffe JG. Role of assays for parathyroid-hormone related protein in investigation of hypercalcaemia. *Lancet*, 1992; **339**: 164–7.

18. Walls J, Ratcliffe WA, Howel A, Bundred NJ. Response to intravenous bisphosphonate therapy in hypercalcaemic patients with and without bone metastases: the role of parathyroid hormone-related protein. *British Journal of Cancer*, 1994; **70**: 169–72.

19. Lee JK, *et al.* Parathyroid hormone and parathyroid hormone related protein assays in the investigation of hypercalcaemic patients in hospital in a Chinese population. *Journal of Endocrinological Investigation*, 1997; **20**: 404–9.

20. Budayr AA, *et al.* Effect of treatment of malignancy-associated hypercalcaemia on serum parathyroid hormone-related protein. *Journal of Bone and Mineral Research*, 1994; **9**: 521–6.

21. Tashjian AH Jr, *et al.* Succesful treatment of hypercalcaemia by indomethacin in mice bearing a prostaglandin-producing fibrosarcoma. *Prostaglandins*, 1973; **3**: 515–24.

22. Seyberth HW, *et al.* Prostaglandins as mediators of hypercalcemia associated with certain types of cancer. *New England Journal of Medicine*, 1975; **293**: 1278–83.

23. Boyce BF, Aufdemorte TB, Garett IR, Yates AJ, Mundy GR. Effects of interleukin-1 on bone turnover in normal mice. *Endocrinology*, 1989; **125**: 1142–52.

24. Malden LT, Novak U, Burgess AW. Expression of transforming growth factor alpha messenger RNA in the normal and neoplastic gastrointestinal tract. *International Journal of Cancer*, 1989; **43**: 380–4.

25. Ibbotson KJ, *et al.* Tumor-derived growth factor increases bone resorption in a tumor associated with humoral hypercalcemia of malignancy. *Science*, 1983; **221**: 1292–4.

26. Ibbotson KJ, *et al.* Stimulation of bone resorption *in vitro* by synthetic transforming growth factor-alpha. *Science*, 1985; **228**: 1007–9.

27. Stern PH, *et al.* Human transforming growth factor-alpha stimulates bone resorption *in vitro*. *Journal of Clinical Investigation*, 1985; **76**: 2016–9.

28. Guise TA, Yoneda T, Yates AJ, Mundy GR. The combined effect of tumor-produced parathyroid hormone-trelated ptotein and transforming growth factor alpha enhance hypercalcaemia *in vivo* and bone resorption *in vitro*. *Journal of Endocrinology and Metabolism*, 1993; **77**: 40–5.

29. Merryman JI, DeWille JW, Werkmeister JR, Capen CC, Rosol TJ. Effects of transforming growth factor-beta on parathyroid hormone-related protein production and ribonucleic acid expression by a squamous carcinoma cell line *in vitro*. *Endocrinology*, 1994; **134**: 2424–30.

30. Guise TA, Mundy GR. Cancer and bone. *Endocrine Reviews* 1998; **19**: 18–54.

31. Davies M, Haeyes ME, Yin JA, Berry JL, Mawer EB. Abnormal synthesis of 1,25-dihydroxyvitamin D in patients with malignant lymphoma. *Journal of Clinical Endocrinology and Metabolism*, 1994; **78**: 1202–7.

32. Seymour JF, Gagel RF, Hagemeister TJ, Dimopoulos MA, Cabanillas F. Calcitriol production in hypercalcemic and normocalcemic patients with non-Hodgkin's lymphoma. *Annals of Internal Medicine*, 1994; **121**: 633–40.

33. Oshika Y, *et al.* A human lung cancer xenograft producing both granulocyte-colony stimulating factor and parathyroid hormone-related protein. *Oncology Reports*, 1998; **5**: 359–62.

34. Coleman RE, Rubens RD. The clinical course of bone metastases from breast cancer. *British Journal of Cancer*, 1987; **55**: 61–6.

35. Taube T, Elomaa I, Blomqvist C, Benneton MNC, Kanis JA. Histomorphometric evidence for osteoclast-mediated bone resorption in metastatic breast cancer. *Bone*, 1994; **15**: 161–6.

36. Athanasou NA, *et al.* The origin and nature of stromal osteoclast-like multinucleated giant cells in breast carcinoma implications for tumour osteolysis and macrophage biology. *British Journal of Cancer*, 1989; **59**: 491–8.

37. Dowsey SE, Hoyland J, Freemont AJ, Knox F, Walls J, Bundred NJ. Expression of the receptor for parathyroid hormone-related protein in normal and malignant breast tissue. *Journal of Pathology*, 1997; **183**: 212–7.

38. Bundred NJ, *et al.* Parathyroid hormone-related protein and skeletal morbidity in breast cancer. *European Journal of Cancer*, 1992; **28**: 690–2.

39. Grill V, Ho P, Body JJ, *et al.* Parathyroid hormone-related protein: elevated levels in both humoral hypercalcemia of malignancy and hypercalcemia complicating metastatic breast cancer. *Journal of Clinical Endocrinology and Metabolism*, 1991; **73**: 1309–15.

40. Legha SS, *et al.* Tamoxifen-induced hypercalcemia in breast cancer. *Cancer*, 1981; **47**: 2803–6.

41. Kurabayashi J, Sonoo H. Parathyroid hormone-related protein secretion is inhibited by oestradiol and stimulated by antioestrogens in KPL-3C human breast cancer cells. *British Journal of Cancer*, 1997; **75**: 1819–25.

42. Kanis JA, *et al.* Calcium metabolism and myeloma and the treatment of hypercalcemia. *Hematology and Oncology*, 1988; **6**: 115–7.

43. Garret IR, *et al.* Production of lymphotoxin, a bone-resorbing cytokine, by cultured human myeloma cells. *New England Journal of Medicine*, 1987; **317**: 526–32.

44. Horiuchi T, Miyachi T, Arai T, Nakamura T, Mori M, Ito H. Raised plasma concentrations of parathyroid hormone related peptide in hypercalcaemic multiple myeloma. *Hormone and Metabolic Research*, 1997; **29**: 469–71.

45. Broder S. T-cell lymphoproliferative syndrome associated with human T-cell leukemia/lymphoma virus. *Annal of Internal Medicine*, 1984; **100**: 543–57.

46. Shirakawa F, *et al.* Production of bone-resorbing activity corresponding to interleukin-1a by adult T-cell leukemia cells in humans. *Cancer Research*, 1988; **48**: 4284–7.

47. Ikeda K, *et al.* Development of a sensitive two-site immunoradiometric assay for parathyroid hormone-related peptide: evidence for elevated lezvels in plasma from patients with adult T-cell leukemia/lymphoma and B-cell lymphoma. *Journal of Clinical Endocrinology and Metabolism*, 1994; **79**: 1322–7.

48. Jacobson JO, *et al.* Humoral hypercalcemia in Hodgkin's disease. *Cancer*, 1989; **63**: 917–23.

49. Firkin F, Seymour JF, Watson AM, Grill V, Martin TJ. Parathyroid hormone-related protein in hypercalcaemia associated with haematological malignancy. *British Journal of Haematology*, 1996; **94**: 486–92.

50. Kremer R, Shustik C, Tabak T, Papavasiliou V, Goltzman D. Parathyroid-hormone related peptide in hematologic malignancies. *American Journal of Medicine*, 1996; **100**: 406–11.

51. Hosking DJ, Cowley A, Bucknall CA. Rehydration in the treatment of severe hypercalcemia. *Quarterly Journal of Medicine*, 1981; **200**: 473–81.

52. Singer FR, *et al.* Treatment of hypercalcaemia of malignancy with intravenous etidronate: a controlled multicenter study. *Archives of Internal Medicine*, 1991; **151**: 471–6.

53. Ralston SH, *et al.* Comparison of three intravenous bisphosphonates in cancer-related hypercalcaemia. *Lancet*, 1989; **ii**: 1180–2.

54. Sleeboom HP, Bijvoet OLM, Van Oosterom AT, Gleed JH, O'Riordan JLH. Comparison of intravenous (3-amino-1-hydropropylidene)-1,1-bisphosphonate and volume repletion in tumour induced hypercalcaemia. *Lancet*, 1983; **ii**: 239–43.

55. Body JJ, *et al.* Amino-hydroxypropylidene bisphosphonate (APD) treatment for tumor-associated hypercalcaemia: a randomized comparison between a 3-day treatment and a single 24 h infusion. *Journal of Bone and Mineral Research*, 1989; **4**: 923–8.

56. Gucalp R, *et al.* Treatment of cancer-associated hypercalcemia. Double-blind comparison of rapid and slow intravenous infusion regimens of pamidronate disodium and saline alone. *Archives of Internal Medicine*, 1994; **154**: 1935–44.

57. Ralston SH, *et al.* Treatment of severe hypercalcaemia with mithramycin and aminohydroxypropylidene bisphosphonate. *Lancet*, 1988; **ii**: 277.

58. Coleman RE, Rubens RD. 3-(Amino-1,1-hydroxypropylidene) bisphosphonate (APD) for hypercalcemia of breast cancer. *British Journal of Cancer*, 1987; **56**: 465–9.

59. Body JJ, *et al.* Dose/response study on aminohydroxypropylidene bisphosphonate in tumor-associated hypercalcaemia. *American Journal of Medicine*, 1987; **82**: 957–63.

60. Nussbaum SR, *et al.* Single-dose intravenous therapy with pamidronate for the treatment of hypercalcaemia of malignancy: comparison between 30-, 60-, and 90-mg dosages. *American Journal of Medicine*, 1993; **95**: 297–304.

61. Gurney H, Kefford R, Stuart-Harris R. Renal phosphate threshold and response to pamidronate in humoral hypercalcaemia of malignancy. *Lancet*, 1989; **ii**: 241–4.

62. Gurney H, Grill V, Martin RJ. Parathyroid hormone-related protein and response to pamidronate in tumour-induced hypercalcaemia. *Lancet*, 1993; **341**: 1611–3.

63. Gucalp R, *et al.* Comparative study of pamidronate disodium and etidronate disodium in the treatment of cancer-related hypercalcemia. *Journal of Clinical Oncology*, 1992; **10**: 134–42.

64. Ralston SH, *et al.* Comparison of aminohydroxypropylidene diphosphonate, mithramycin and corticosteroids/calcitonin in treatment of cancer-associated hypercalcaemia. *Lancet*, 1985; **ii**: 907–10.

65. Ralston SH, *et al.* Dose-response study of ibandronate in the treatment of cancer associated hypercalcaemia. *British Journal of Cancer*, 1997; **75**: 295–300.

66. Berenson R, *et al.* Phase I clinical study of a new bisphosphonate, zoledronate (CGP-42446), in patients with osteolytic bone metastases. *Blood*, 1997; **88** (Suppl.1):586.

67. Suki WN, *et al.* Acute treatment of hypercalcemia with furosemide. *New England Journal of Medicine*, 1970; **283**: 836–40.

68. Percival RC, *et al.* Role of glucocorticoids in management of malignant hypercalcemia. *British Medical Journal*, 1984; **289**: 287.

69. Hosking DJ, Gilson D. Comparison of the renal and skeletal actions of calcitonin in the treatment of severe hypercalcemia of malignancy. *Quarterly Journal of Medicine*, 1984; **211**: 359–68.

70. Binstock ML, Mundy GR. Effect of calcitonin and glucocorticoids in

combination on the hypercalcemia of malignancy. *Annals of Internal Medicine*, 1980; **93**: 269–72.

71. **Thurlimann B, Waldburger R, Senn HJ, Thiebaud D.** Plicamycin and pamidronate in symptomatic tumor-related hypercalcaemia: a prospective randomized cross-over trial. *Annals of Oncology*, 1992; **3**: 619–23.

72. **Warrel RP Jr, et al.** Gallium nitrate inhibits calcium resorption from bone and is effective treatment for cancer-related hypercalcaemia. *Journal of Clinical Investigation*, 1984; **73**: 1487–90.

73. **Guidon PT Jr, Salvatori R, Bockman RS.** Gallium nitrate regulates rat osteoblast expression of osteocalcin protein and mRNA levels. *Journal of Bone and Mineral Research*, 1993; **8**: 103–12.

74. **Warrel RP Jr, et al.** Gallium nitrate for acute treatment of cancer-related hypercalcaemia: a randomized, double blind comparison to calcitonin. *Annals of Internal Medicine*, 1988; **108**: 669–74.

75. **Warrel RP, et al.** A randomized double-blind study of gallium nitrate compared to etidronate for acute control of cancer-related hypercalcaemia. *Journal of Clinical Oncology*, 1991; **9**: 1467–75.

76. **Bertheault-Cvitkovic F, Armand J-P, Tubiana-Hulin M, Chevalier B, Rossi J-F, Warrel RP.** Randomized, double-blind comparison of pamidronate vs. gallium nitrate for acute control of cancer-related hypercalcemia. *Annals of Oncology*, 1996; **7**(S1):140 (Abstr. 499).

77. **Koo WS, Jeon DS, Ahn SJ, Kim YS, Yoon YS, Bang BK.** Calcium-free hemodialysis for the management of hypercalcemia. *Nephron*, 1996; **72**: 424–8.

78. **Blachley JD, Hill JB.** Renal and electrolyte disturbances associated with cisplatin. *Annals of Internal Medicine*, 1981; **95**: 628–32.

79. **Hall TC, Griffiths CT, Petranek JR.** Hypocalcemia—an unusual metabolic complication of breast cancer. *New England Journal of Medicine*, 1966; **275**: 1474–7.

80. **Muggia FM, Chia GA, Mickley DW.** Hyperphosphatemia and hypocalcemia in neoplastic disorders. *New England Journal of Medicine*, 1974; **299**: 857–8.

81. **Olefsky J, et al.** Tertiary hyperparathyroidism and apparent cure of vitamin-D-resistant rickets after removal of an ossifying mesenchymal tumor of the pharynx. *New England Journal of Medicine*, 1972; **286**: 740–5.

82. **Agus ZS.** Oncogenic hypophosphatemic osteomalacia. *Kidney International*, 1983; **24**: 113–23.

83. **Lyles KW, et al.** Hypophosphatemic osteomalacia: association with prostatic carcinoma. *Annals of Internal Medicine*, 1980; **93**: 275–8.

84. **Taylor HC, Fallon MD, Velasco ME.** Oncogenic osteomalacia and inappropriate antidiuretic hormone secretion due to oat-cell carcinoma. *Annals of Internal Medicine*, 1984; **101**: 786–8.

85. **Cai Q, et al.** Brief report: inhibition of renal phosphate transport by a tumor product in a patient with oncogenic osteomalacia. *New England Journal of Medicine*, 1994; **330**: 1645–9.

86. **Wilkins GE, et al.** Oncogenic osteomalacia: evidence for a humoral phosphaturic factor. *Journal of Clinical Endocrinology and Metabolism*, 1995; **80**: 1628–34.

87. **Rowe PSN, Ong ACM, Cockerill FJ, Goulding JN, Hewison M.** Candidate 56 and 58 kDa protein(s) responsible for mediating the renal defects in oncogenic hypophosphatemic osteomalacia. *Bone*, 1996; **18**: 159–69.

88. **Miyauchi A, Fukase M, Tsutsumi M, Fujita T.** Hemangiopericytoma-induced osteomalacia: tumor transplantation in nude mice causes hypophosphatemia and tumor extracts inhibit renal 25-hydroxyvitamin D 1-hydroxylase activity. *Journal of Clinical Endocrinology and Metabolism*, 1988; **67**: 46–53.

89. **Schilsky RL, Anderson T.** Hypomagnesemia and renal magnesium wasting in patients receiving cisplatin. *Annals of Internal Medicine*, 1979; **90**: 929–31.

90. **Evans TRJ, Harper CL, Beveridge IG, Wastnage R, Mansi JL.** A randomized study to determine whether routine magnesium supplements are necessary in patients receiving cisplatin chemotherapy with continuous infusion 5-fluorouracil. *European Journal of Cancer*, 1995; **31A**: 174–8.

91. **Willox JC, et al.** Effect of magnesium supplementation in testicular cancer patients receiving cis-platin: randomised trial. *British Journal of Cancer*, 1986; **54**: 19–23.

92. **Flombaum CD.** Hypomagnesemia associated with cisplatin combination chemotherapy. *Archives of Internal Medicine*, 1984; **144**: 2336–7.

93. **McLellan BA, Reid SR, Lane PL.** Massive blood transfusion causing hypomagnesemia. *Critical Care Medicine*, 1984; **12**: 146–7.

94. **Vogelzang NJ, Torkelson JL, Kennedy BJ.** Hypomagnesemia, renal dysfunction, and Raynaud's phenomenon in patients treated with cisplatin, vinblastine, and bleomycin. *Cancer*, 1985; **56**: 2765–70.

95. **Rose BD.** New approach to disturbances in the plasma sodium concentration. *American Journal of Medicine*, 1986; **81**: 1033–40.

96. **Schmale H, Fehr S, Richter D.** Vasopressin biosynthesis- from gene to peptide hormone. *Kidney International*, 1987; **32**(Suppl. 21):S8–S13.

97. **Clements JA, Funder JW.** Arginine vasopressin (AVP) and AVP-like immunoreactivity in peripheral tissues. *Endocrine Reviews*, 1986; **7**: 449–65.

98. **Deen PM, et al.** Requirement of human renal water channel aquaporin-2 for for vasopressin-dependent concentration of urine. *Science*, 1994; **264**: 92–5.

99. **Kanno K, et al.** Urinary excretion of aquaporin-2 in patients with diabetes insipidus. *New England Journal of Medicine*, 1995; **332**: 1540–5.

100. **Robertson GL, Aycinen P, Zerbe RL.** Neurogenic disorder of osmoregulation. *American Journal Medicine*, 1982; **72**: 339–53.

101. **Gross PA, Ketteler M, Hausmann C, Ritz E.** The charted and uncharted waters of hyponatraemia. *Kidney International*, 1987; **32**(suppl. 2): S67–S75.

102. **Narins RG, et al.** Diagnostic strategies in disorders of fluid, electrolyte and acid-base homeostasis. *American Journal of Medicine*, 1982; **72**: 496–520.

103. **Schwartz WB, et al.** Syndrome of renal sodium loss and hyponatremia probably resulting from inappropriate secretion of antidiuretic hormone. *American Journal of Medicine*, 1957; **23**: 529–42.

104. **Amatruda TT, et al.** Carcinoma of the lung with inappropriate antidiuresis. Demonstration of antidiuretic-hormone-like activity in tumor extract. *New England Journal of Medicine*, 1963; **269**: 544–9.

105. **Pettengill OS, et al.** Isolation and characterization of a hormone-producing cell line from human small cell anaplastic carcinoma of the lung. *Journal of the National Cancer Institute*, 1977; **58**: 511–8.

106. **De Troyer A, Demanet JC.** Clinical, biological and pathogenetic features of the syndrome of inappropriate sectretion of antidiuretic hormone. *Quarterly Journal of Medicine*, 1976; **180**: 521–31.

107. **Passamonte PM.** Hypouricemia, inappropriate secretion of antidiuretic hormone, and small cell carcinoma of the lung. *Archives of Internal Medicine*, 1984; **144**: 1569–70.

108. **Decaux G, et al.** Mechanisms of hypouricemia in the syndrome of inappropriate secretion of antidiuretic hormone. *Nephron*, 1985; **39**: 164–8.

109. **Sorensen JB, et al.** Hypouricemia and urate excretion in small cell lung carcinoma patients with syndrome of inappropriate antidiuresis. *Acta Oncologica*, 1988; **27**: 351–5.

110. **Vokes TJ, Robertson GL.** Disorders of antidiuretic hormone. *Endocrinology and Metabolism Clinics of North America*, 1988; **17**: 281–99.

111. **Hainsworth JD, Workman R, Greco A.** Management of the syndrome of inappropriate antidiuretic hormone secretion in small cell lung cancer. *Cancer*, 1983; **51**: 161–5.

112. **Lockton JA, Thatcher NA.** A retrospective study of thirty-two patients

with small cell bronchogenic carcinoma and inappropriate secretion of antidiuretic hormone. *Clinical Radiology*, 1986; **37**: 47–50.

113. Comis RL, Miller M, Ginsberg SJ. Abnormalities in water homeostasis in small cell anaplastic lung cancer. *Cancer*, 1980; **45**: 2414–21.

114. Gilby ED, Bondy PK, Fosling M. Impaired water excretion in oat cell lung cancer. *British Journal of Cancer*, 1976; **34**: 323–4.

115. Lokich JJ. The frequency and clinical biology of the ectopic hormone syndromes of small cell carcinoma. *Cancer*, 1982; **50**: 2111–14.

116. Bliss DP, Battey JF, Linnoila RI, Birrer MJ, Gazdar AF, Johnson BE. Expression of the atrial natriuretic factor gene in small cell lung cancer tumors and tumor cell lines. *Journal of the National Cancer Institute*, 1990; **82**: 305–10.

117. Gross AJ, *et al.* Atrial natriuretic factor and arginine vasopressin production in tumor cell lines from patients with lung cancer and their relationship to serum sodium. *Cancer Research*, 1993; **53**: 67–74.

118. Johnson BE, *et al.* A prospective study of patients with lung cancer and hyponatremia of malignancy. *American Journal of Respiratory and Critical Care Medicine*, 1997; **156**: 1669–78.

119. Rosenthal S, Kaufman S. Vincristine neurotoxicity. *Annals of Internal Medicine*, 1974; **80**: 733–7.

120. Cutting HO. Inappropriate secretion of antidiuretic hormone secondary to vincristine therapy. *American Journal of Medicine*, 1971; **51**: 269–71.

121. Harlow PJ, DeClerck YA, Shore NA, Ortega JA, Carranza A, Heuser E. A fatal case of inappropriate ADH secretion induced by cyclophosphamide therapy. *Cancer*, 1979; **44**: 896–8.

122. Greenbaum-Lefkoe B, Rosenstock JG, Belasco JB, Rohrbaugh TM, Meadows AT. Syndrome of inappropriate antidiuretic hormone secretion: a complication of high-dose intravenous melphalan. *Cancer*, 1985; **55**: 44–6.

123. Hutchinson FN, *et al.* Renal salt wasting in patients treated with cisplatin. *Annals of Internal Medicine*, 1988; **108**: 21–5.

124. Halma C, Jansen JBMJ, Janssens R, *et al.* Life-threatening water intoxication during somatostatin therapy. *Annals of Internal Medicine*, 1987; **107**: 518–20.

125. Tomlinson BE, Pierides AM, Bradle WG. Central pontine myelinolysis. *Quarterly Journal of Medicine*, 1976; **179**: 373–86.

126. Cluitmans FHM, Meinders AE. Management of severe hyponatraemia: rapid or slow correction? *American Journal of Medicine*, 1990; **88**: 161–6.

127. Sterns RH, Riggs JE, Schochet SS. Osmotic demyelination syndrome following correction of hyponatremia. *New England Journal of Medicine*, 1986; **314**: 1535–42.

128. Sterns RH. Severe symptomatic hyponatremia: treatment and outcome. A study of 64 cases. *Annals of Internal Medicine*, 1987; **107**: 656–64.

129. Forrest JN, *et al.* Superiority of demeclocycline over lithium in the treatment of chronic syndrome of inappropriate secretion of antidiuretic hormone. *New England Journal of Medicine*, 1978; **298**: 173–7.

130. Kimmel DW, O'Neill BP. Systemic cancer presenting as diabetes insipidus. *Cancer*, 1983; **52**: 2355–8.

131. Teears RJ, Silverman EM. Clinicopathologic review of 88 cases of carcinoma metastatic to the pituitary gland. *Cancer* 1975; **36**: 216–20.

132. Sioutos P, Yen V, Arbit E. Pituitary gland metastases. *Annals of Surgical Oncology*, 1996; **3**: 94–9.

133. Pernicone PJ, *et al.* Pituitary carcinoma: a clinicopathological study of 15 cases. *Cancer*, 1996; **79**: 804–12.

134. Yap HY, *et al.* Diabetes insipidus and breast cancer. *Archives of Internal Medicine*, 1979; **139**: 1009–1.

135. Krol TC, Wood WS. Bronchogenic carcinoma and diabetes insipidus: a case report and review. *Cancer*, 1982; **49**: 596–9.

136. Kornberg A, *et al.* Acute lymphoblastic leukemia. Association with

vasopressin-responsive diabetes insipidus. *Archives of Internal Medicine*, 1980; **140**: 1236.

137. Juan D, Hsu SD, Hunter J. Case report of vasopressin-responsive diabetes insipidus associated with chronic myelogeneous leukemia. *Cancer*, 1985; **56**: 1468–9.

138. Badon SJ, *et al.* Diabetes insipidus caused by extra medullary hematopoiesis. *American Journal of Clinical Pathology*, 1985; **83**: 509–12.

139. Smits P, *et al.* Diabetes insipidus associated with leukemia. *The Netherlands Journal of Medicine*, 1989; **34**: 264–9.

140. Ciric I, Ragin A, Baumgartner C, Pierce D. Complications of transsphenoidsal surgery: results of a national survey, review of the literature, and personal experience. *Neurosurgery*, 1997; **40**: 225–36.

141. Collett-Solberg PF, *et al.* Endocrine outcome in long-term survivors of low-grade hypothalamic/chiasmatic glioma. *Clinical Endocrinology*, 1997; **47**: 79–85.

142. Boss GR, Seegmiller JE. Hyperuricemia and gout. *New England Journal of Medicine*, 1979; **300**: 59–68.

143. Seegmiller JE, Laster L, Howell RR. Biochemistry of uric acid and its relation to gout. *New England Journal of Medicine*, 1963; **268**: 712–6.

144. Spencer HW, Yarger WE, Robinson RR. Alterations in renal function during dietary -induced hyperuricemia in the rat. *Kidney International*, 1976; **9**: 489–500.

145. Kjelstrand CM, *et al.* Hyperuricemic acute renal failure. *Archives of Internal Medicine*, 1974; **133**: 49–59.

146. Crittenden DR, Ackerman GL. Hyperuricemic acute renal failure in disseminated carcinoma. *Archives of Internal Medicine*, 1977; **137**: 97–9.

147. Tsokos GC, Balow JE, Spiegel RJ, Magrath IT. Renal and metabolic complications of undifferentiated and lymphoblastic lymphomas. *Medicine*, 1981; **60**: 218–29.

148. Lynch EC. Uric acid metabolism in proliferative disease of the marrow. *Archives of Internal Medicine*, 1962; **109**: 639–53.

149. Kelton JG, Kelley WN, Holmes EW. A rapid method for the diagnosis of acute uric acid nephropathy. *Archives of Internal Medicine*, 1978; **138**: 612–5.

150. Schilsky RL. Renal and metabolic toxicities of cancer chemotherapy. *Seminars in Oncology*, 1982; **9**: 75–83.

151. Krakoff IH, Meyer RL. Prevention of hyperuricemia in leukemia and lymphoma. *Journal of the American Medical Association*, 1965; **193**: 1–6.

152. DeConti RC, Calabresi P. Use of allopurinol for prevention and control of hyperuricemia in patients with neoplastic disease. *New England Journal of Medicine*, 1966; **274**: 481–6.

153. Hande KE, Noone RM, Stone WJ. Severe allopurinol toxicity. *American Journal of Medicine*, 1984; **76**: 47–56.

154. Watts RWE, *et al.* Allopurinol and acute uric acid nephropathy. *British Medical Journal*, 1966; **1**: 205–8.

155. Mahmoud HH, Leverger G, Patte C, Harvey E, Lascombes F. Advances in the management of malignancy-associated hyperuricaemia. *British Journal of Cancer*, 1998; **77**(Suppl. 4):18–20.

156. Arseneay JC, Bagley CM, Anderson T, Canellos GP. Hyperkalaemia, a sequel to chemotherapy of Burkitt's lymphoma. *Lancet*, 1973; **i**: 10–4.

157. Fenneley JJ, Smyth H, Muldowney FP. Extreme hyperkalemia due to rapid lysis of leukemic cells. *Lancet*, 1974; **i**: 27.

158. Meyers AM, Jowsey J. Hyperphosphatemia and hypocalcemia in neoplastic disorders. *New England Journal of Medicine*, 1974; **299**: 858–9.

159. Cohen LF, Balow JE, Magrath IT, Poplack DG, Ziegler JL. Acute tumor lysis syndrome. A review of 37 patients with Burkitt's lymphoma. *American Journal Medicine*, 1980; **68**: 486–91.

160. Cervantes F, Ribera JM, Granena A, Montserrat E, Rozman C. Tumour lysis syndrome with hypocalcemia in accelerated chronic granulocytic leukemia. *Acta Haematologica*, 1982; **68**: 157–9.

161. Hande KR, Garrow GC. Acute tumor lysis syndrome in patients with

high-grade non-Hodgkin's lymphoma. *American Journal of Medicine*, 1993; **94**: 133–9.

162. List AF, Kummet TD, Adams JD, Chun HG. Tumor lysis syndrome complicating treatment of chronic lymphocytic leukemia with fludarabine phosphate. *American Journal of Medicine*, 1990; **89**: 388–90.

163. Dann EJ, Gillis S, Polliack A, Okon E, Rund D, Rachmilewitz EA. Brief report: tumor lysis syndrome following treatment with 2-chlorodeoxyadenosine for refractory chronic lymphocytic leukemia. *New England Journal of Medicine*, 1993; **329**: 1547–8.

164. Vogelzang NJ, Nelimark RA, Nath KA. Tumor lysis syndrome after induction chemotherapy of small-cell bronchogenic carcinoma. *Journal of the American Medical Association*, 1983; **249**: 513–4.

165. Stark ME, Dyer MCD, Coonley CJ. Fatal acute tumor lysis syndrome with metastatic breast cancer. *Cancer*, 1987; **60**: 762–4.

166. Dirix LY, Prove A, Becquart D, Wouters E, Vermeulen P, Van Oosterom AT. Tumour lysis syndrome with acute renal failure in a patient with Merckel cell carcinoma. *Cancer*, 1991; **67**: 2207–10.

167. Boisseau M, Bugat R, Mahjoubi M. Rapid tumor lysis syndrome in a metastatic colorectal cancer increased by treatment with irinotecan (CPT-11). *European Journal of Cancer*, 1996; **32**: 737–8.

168. Kalemkerian GP, Darwish B, Varterasian ML. Tumor lysis syndrome in small cell carcinoma and other solid tumors. *American Journal of Medicine*, 1997; **103**: 363–7.

169. Benekli M, *et al.* Acute tumor lysis syndrome following intrathecal methotrexate. *Leukemia Lymphoma*, 1996; **22**: 361–3.

170. Levin M, Cho S. Acute tumor lysis syndrome in high grade lymphoblastic lymphoma after a prolonged episode of fever. *Medical and Pediatric Oncology*, 1996; **26**: 417–8.

171. Nomdedeu J, Martino R, Sureda A, Huidobro G, Lopez R, Brunet S. Acute tumor lysis syndrome complicating conditioning therapy for bone marrow transplantation in a patient with chronic lymphocytic leukemia. *Bone Marrow Transplantation*, 1994; **13**: 659–60.

172. Zusman J, Brown DM, Nesbit ME. Hyperphosphatemia, hyperphosphaturia and hypocalcemia in acute lymphoblastic leukemia. *New England Journal of Medicine*, 1973; **289**: 1335–40.

173. Herbert LA, Leman J, Petersen JR, Lennon EJ. Studies on the mechanism by which phosphate infusion lowers serum calcium concentration. *Journal of Clinical Investigation*, 1966; **45**: 277–81.

174. Ettinger DS, Harker WG, Gerry HW, Sanders RC, Saral R. Hyperphosphatemia, hypocalcemia and transient renal failure. *Journal of the American Medical Association*, 1978; **239**: 2472–4.

175. Joffe BI, Kew MC, Panz VR, *et al.* Evaluation of the synthetic somatostatin analogue SMS 201–995 in patients with hypoglycaemia associated with hepatocellular carcinoma. *British Journal of Cancer*, 1988; **58**: 91–2.

176. Cadman EC, Lundberg WB, Bertino JR. Hyperphosphatemia and hypocalcemia accompanying rapid cell lysis in patient with Burkitt's lymphoma and Burkitt cell leukemia. *American Journal of Medicine*, 1977; **62**: 283–90.

177. Dunlay RW, Camp MA, Allon M, Fanti P, Malluche HH, Llach F. Calcitriol in prolonged hypocalcemia due to tumor lysis syndrome. *Annals of Internal Medicine*, 1989; **110**: 162–4.

178. Pichette V, Leblanc M, Bonnardeaux A, Ouimet D, Geadah D, Cardinal J. High dialysate flow rate continuous artiovenous hemodialysis: a new approach for the treatment of acute renal failure and tumor lysis syndrome. *American Journal of Kidney Disease*, 1994; **23**: 591–6.

179. Hood VL, Tannen RL. Protection of acid-base balance by pH regulation of acid production. *New England Journal of Medicine*, 1998; **339**: 819–26.

180. Sculier JP, Nicaise C, Klastersky J. Lactic acidosis : a metabolic complication of extensive metastatic cancer. *European Journal of Cancer and Clinical Oncology*, 1983; **19**: 597–601.

181. Doolittle GC, Wurster MW, Rosenfeld GS, Bodensteiner DC. Malignancy-induced lactic acidosis. *Southern Medical Journal*, 1988; **81**: 533–6.

182. During J, Fiedler W, De Wit M, Steffen M, Hossfeld DK. Lactic acidosis and hypoglycemia in a patient with high-grade non-Hodgkin's lymphoma and elevated circulating TNF-alpha. *Annals of Hematology*, 1996; **72**: 97–9.

183. Medalle R, Webb R, Waterhouse C. Lactic acidosis and associated hypoglycemia. *Archives of Internal Medicine*, 1971; **128**: 273–8.

184. Holroyde CP, *et al.* Altered glucose metabolism in metastatic carcinoma. *Cancer Research*, 1975; **35**: 3710–4.

185. Spechler SJ, *et al.* Lactic acidosis in oat cell carcinoma with extensive hepatic metastasis. *Archives of Internal Medicine*, 1978; **138**: 1663–4.

186. Nadiminti Y, *et al.* Lactic acidosis associated with Hodgkin's disease. *New England Journal of Medicine*, 1980; **303**: 15–7.

187. Madias NE. Lactic acidosis. *Kidney International*, 1986; **29**: 752–74.

188. Bornemann M, Hill SC, Kid II GS. Lactic acidosis in pheochromocytoma. *Annals of Internal Medicine*, 1986; **105**: 880–2.

189. Waterhouse C. Lactate metabolism in patients with cancer. *Cancer*, 1974; **33**: 66–71.

190. Lyng H, Sundfor K, Tropé C, Rofstad EK. Oxygen tension and vascular density in human cervix carcinoma. *British Journal of Cancer*, 1996; **74**: 1559–63.

191. Brizel DM, *et al.* Tumor oxygenation predicts for the likelihood of distant metastases in human soft tissue sarcoma. *Cancer Research*, 1997; **56**: 941–3.

192. Schwickert G, Walenta S, Sundfor K, Rofstand EK, Mueller-Klieser W. Correlation of high lactate levels in human cervical cancer with incidence of metastasis. *Cancer Research*, 1995; **55**: 4757–9.

193. Walenta S, *et al.* Correlation of high lactate levels in head and neck tumors with incidence of metastasis. *American Journal of Pathology*, 1997; **150**: 409–15.

194. Olano JP, Borucki MJ, Wen JW, Haque AK. Massive hepatic steatosis and lactic acidosis in a patient with AIDS who was receiving zidovudine. *Clinical Infectious Diseases*, 1995; **21**: 973–6.

195. Stacpoole PW. Lactic acidosis : the case against bicarbonate therapy. *Annals of Internal Medicine*, 1986; **105**: 276–9.

196. Ritter JM, Doktor HS, Benjamin N. Paradoxical effect of bicarbonate on cytoplasmatic pH. *Lancet*, 1990; **335**: 1243–6.

197. Stacpoole PW, *et al.* and the dichloroactetate-lactate acidosis study group. A controlled trial of dichloroacetate for the treatment of lactic acidosis in adults. *New England Journal of Medicine*, 1992; **327**: 1564–9.

198. Fraley DS, *et al.* Stimulation of lactate production by administration of bicarbonate in a patient with a solid neoplasm and lactic acidosis. *New England Journal of Medicine*, 1980; **303**: 1100–2.

199. Gorden P, Hendricks CM, Kahn CR, Megyesi K, Roth J. Hypoglycemia associated with non-islet-cell tumor and insuline-like growth factors. *New England Journal of Medicine*, 1981; **305**: 1452–5.

200. Kahn RC. The riddle of tumor hypoglycemia revisited. *Clinics in Endocrinology and Metabolism*, 1980; **9**: 335–60.

201. Zapf J. Role of insulin like growth factor II and IGF binding proteins in extrapancreatic tumor hypoglycemia. *Hormone Research*, 1994; **42**: 20–6.

202. Le Roith D. Insuline-like growth factors. *New England Journal of Medicine*, 1997; **336**: 633–40.

203. Minuto F, Del MonteP, Barreca A, *et al.* Evidence for autocrine mitogenic stimulation by somatomedin-C/insuline-like growth factor I on an established human lung cancer cell line. *Cancer Research*, 1988; **48**: 3716–9.

204. Zapf J, Hauri C, Waldvogel M, Froesch ER. Acute metabolic effects and half-lives of intravenously administered insulinelike growth factors I and II in normal and hypophysectomized rats. *Journal of Clinical Investigation*, 1986; **77**: 1768–75.

205. Tricoli JV, Rall LB, Karakousis CP, *et al*. Enhanced levels of insuline-like growth factor messenger RNA in human colon carcinomas and liposarcomas. *Cancer Research*, 1986; **46**: 6169–73.

206. Macauly VM, Teale JD, Everard MJ, *et al*. Somatomedin-C/insulin-like growth factor-I is a mitogen for human small cell lung cancer. *British Journal of Cancer*, 1988; **57**: 91–3.

207. Daughaday WH, *et al*. Synthesis and secretion of insulin-like growth factor II by a leiomyosarcoma with associated hypoglycemia. *New England Journal of Medicine*, 1988; **319**: 1434–40.

208. Shapiro ET, Bell GI, Polonsky KS, Rubenstein AH, Kew MC, Tager HS. Tumor hypoglycemia: relationship to high molecular weight insulin-like growth factor-II. *Journal of Clinical Investigation*, 1990; **85**: 1672–9.

209. Zapf J, Futo E, Peter M, Froesh ER. Can 'big' insulin-like growth factor II in serum of tumor patients account for the development of extrapancreatic hypoglycaemia? *Journal of Clinical Investigation*, 1992; **90**: 2574–84.

210. Chung J, Henry RR. Mechanisms of tumour-induced hypoglycemia with intraabdominal hemangiopericytoma. *Journal of Clinical Endocrinology and Metabolism*, 1996; **81**: 919–25.

211. Teale JD, Blum WF, Marks V. Alleviation of non-islet cell tumour hypoglycemia by growth hormone therapy is associated with changes in IGF binding protein-3. *Annals of Clinical Biochemistry*, 1992; **29**: 314–4.

212. Hoff AO, R Vassilopoulou-Sellin R. The role of glucagon administration in the diagnosis and treatment of patients with tumor hypoglycemia. *Cancer*, 1998; **82**: 1585–92.

213. Trainer PJ, Grossman A. The diagnosis and differential diagnosis of Cushing's syndrome. *Clinical Endocrinology*, 1991; **34**: 317–30.

214. White A, Clark AJL, Stewart MF. The synthesis of ACTH and related peptides by tumours. *Ballière's Clinical Endocrinology and Metabolism*, 1990; **4**: 1–27.

215. Gold EM. The Cushing syndrome: changing views of diagnosis and treatment. *Annals of Internal Medicine*, 1979; **90**: 829–44.

216. White A, Clarck AJL. The cellular and molecular basis of the ectopic ACTH syndrome. *Clinical Endocrinology*, 1993; **39**: 131–41.

217. Orth DN, Liddle GW. Results of treatment in 108 patients with Cushing's syndrome. *New England Journal of Medicine*, 1971; **285**: 243–7.

218. De Keyzer Y, Beragna X, Lenne F, Girard F, Luton J-P, Kahn A. Altered proopiomelanocortin gene expression in adrenocorticotropin-producing nonpituitary tumors. *Journal of Clinical Investigation*, 1985; **76**: 1892–8.

219. Clark AJL, Lavender PM, Besser GM, Rees LH. Pro-opiomelanocortin in ACTH-dependent Cushing's syndrome. *Journal of Molecular Endocrinology*, 1989; **2**: 3–9.

220. Orth D. Cushing's syndrome. *New England Journal of Medicine*, 1995; **332**: 791–803.

221. Odell WD. Ectopic ACTH secretion: a misnomer. *Endocrinology and Metabolism Clinics of North America*, 1991; **20**: 371–9.

222. Texier P-L, *et al*. Proopiomelanocortin gene expression in normal and tumor human lung. *Journal of Clinical Endocrinology and Metabolism*, 1991; **73**: 414–20.

223. Arioglu E, *et al*. Cushing's syndrome caused by corticotropin secretion by pulmonary tumorlets. *New England Journal of Medicine*, 1998; **339**: 883–6.

224. Hattori M, *et al*. Multiple-hormone producing lung carcinoma. *Cancer*, 1979; **43**: 2429–37.

225. Imura H. Ectopic hormone syndromes. *Clinics in Endocrinology and Metabolism*, 1980; **9**: 235–60.

226. Carey RM, *et al*. Ectopic secretion of corticotropin-releasing factor as a cause of Cushing's syndrome. *New England Journal of Medicine*, 1984; **311**: 13–20.

227. Rassam JW, Anderson G. Incidence of paramalignant disorders in bronchogenic carcinoma. *Thorax*, 1975; **30**: 86–90.

228. Shepherd FA, Laskey J, Evans WK, Goss PE, Johansen E, Khamsi F. Cushing's syndrome associated with ectopic corticotropin production and small-cell lung cancer. *Journal of Clinical Oncology*, 1992; **10**: 21–7.

229. Delisle L, *et al*. Ectopic corticotropin syndrome and small-cell carcinoma of the lung. *Archives of Internal Medicine*, 1993; **153**: 746–52.

230. Limper AH, Carpenter PC, Scheithauer B, Staas BA. The Cushing syndrome induced by bronchial carcinoid tumors. *Annals of Internal Medicine*, 1992; **117**: 209–14.

231. Gewirtz G, Yalow RS. Ectopic production in carcinoma of the lung. *Journal of Clinical Investigation*, 1974; **53**: 1022–32.

232. Howlett TA, Drury PL, Doniach PI, Rees LH, Besser GM. Diagnosis and management of ACTH-dependent Cushing's syndrome: comparison of features in ectopic and pituitary ACTH production. *Clinical Endocrinology*, 1986; **24**: 699–713.

233. Blunt SB, Sandler LM, Burrin JM, Joplin GF. An evaluation of the distinction of ectopic and pituitary ACTH dependent Cushing's syndrome by clinical features, biochemical tests, and radiological findings. *Quarterly Journal of Medicine*, 1990; **77**: 1113–33.

234. Mansi L, Rambaldi PF, Panza N, Esposito D, Esposito V, Pastore V. Diagnosis and radioguided surgery with (111)In-pentetreotide in a patient with paraneoplastic Cushing's syndrome due to a bronchial carcinoid. *European Journal of Endocrinology*, 1997; **137**: 688–90.

235. Carey RM, Orth DN, Hartmann WH. Malignant melanoma with ectopic production of adrenocorticotropic hormone: palliative treatment with inhibitors of adrenal steroid biosynthesis. *Journal of Clinical Endocrinology and Metabolism*, 1973; **36**: 482–7.

236. Feldman D. Ketoconazole and other imidazole derivatives as inhibitors of steroidogenesis. *Endocrine Reviews*, 1986; **7**: 409–20.

237. Kyle CA, Laster RA, Burton EM, Sanford RA. Subacute pituitary apoplexy: MR and CT appearance. *Journal of Computer Assisted Tomography*, 1990; **14**: 40–4.

238. Constine LS, *et al*. Hypothalamic-pituitary dysfunction after radiation for brain tumors. *New England Jounal of Medicine*, 1993; **328**: 87–94.

239. Morita A, Meyer FB, Laws ER. Symptomatic pituitary metastases. *Journal of Neurosurgery*, 1998; **89**: 69–73.

240. Kung AWC, Pun KK, Lam K, Wang C, Leung CY. Addisonian crisis as presenting feature in malignancies. *Cancer*, 1990; **65**: 177–9.

241. Serrano S, Tejedor L, Garcia B, Hallal H, Polo JAZ, Alguacil G. Addisonian crisis as the presenting feature of bilateral primary adrenal lymphoma. *Cancer*, 1993; **71**: 4030–3.

242. Mor F, Lahaw M, Kipper E, Wysenbeek AJ. Addison's disease due to metastases to the adrenal glands. *Postgraduate Medical Journal*, 1985; **61**;637–9.

243. Seidenwurm DJ, Elmer EB, Kaplan LM, Williams EK, Morris DG, Hoffman AR. Metastases to the adrenal glands and the development of Addison's disease. *Cancer*, 1984; **54**: 552–7.

244. Kannan CR. *The adrenal gland*. New York: Plenum, 1988: 31–96.

245. Redman DG, Pazdur R, Zingas AP, Loredo R. Prospective evaluation of adrenal insufficiency in patients with adrenal metastasis. *Cancer*, 1987; **60**: 103–8.

246. Gamelin E, *et al*. Non-Hodgkin's lymphoma presenting with primary adrenal insufficiency. A disease with underestimated frequency? *Cancer*, 1992; **69**: 2333–6.

247. Guttman PH. Addison's disease. A statistical analysis of 566 cases and a study of pathology. *Archives of Pathology*, 1930; **10**: 742–785;895–935.

248. Hughes SWM, Burley DM. Aminoglutethimide. A 'side-effect' turned to therapeutic advantage. *Postgraduate Medical Journal*, 1970; **46**: 409–16.

249. Hofken K, *et al*. Aminoglutethimide without hydrocortisone in the

treatment of postmenopausal patients with advanced breast cancer. *Cancer Treatment Reports*, 1986; **70**: 1153–7.

250. **Gutierrez ML, Crooke ST**. Mitotane (o′,p′-DDD). *Cancer Treatment Reports*, 1990; **7**: 49–55.

251. **Feuillan P, *et al***. Effects of suramin on the function and structure of the adrenal cortex in the cynomolgus monkey. *Journal of Clinical Endocrinology and Metabolism*, 1987; **65**: 153–8.

252. **Hug V, Kau S, Hortobagyi GN, Jones L**. Adrenal failure in patients with breast carcinoma after long-term treatment of cyclic alternating oestrogen progesterone.*British Journal of Cancer*, 1991; **63**: 454–6.

253. **Kamoi K, Tamura T, Tanaka K, Ishibashi M, Yamaji T**. Hyponatremia and osmoregulation of thirst and vasopressin secretion in patients with adrenal insufficiency. *Clinical Endocrinology and Metabolism*, 1993; **77**: 1584–8.

5.3 Paraneoplastic syndromes other than metabolic

Ian E. Smith and Richard H. de Boer

Introduction

Paraneoplastic syndromes are a group of pathological conditions that are caused by a cancer but not brought about directly by local infiltration or metastatic spread. They are estimated to occur in 5 to 10 per cent of patients with cancer, but their incidence varies markedly with different tumours and with tumour stage. Paraneoplastic syndromes are clinically important because:

(i) They may be the presenting feature of a tumour and lead to diagnosis.

(ii) They can cause significant symptoms, which may be treatable leading to an improved quality of life.

(iii) They may act as a marker of disease activity or of the response of a tumour to treatment.

(iv) They may provide prognostic information.

(v) Research into their cause may provide greater knowledge of basic tumour biology, or shed light on similar diseases of unknown aetiology (e.g. arthritis).

An outline for the investigation and management of paraneoplastic syndromes is shown in Fig. 1. To be classified as a true neoplastic syndrome, a number of criteria need to be fulfilled:

(i) Direct association between the syndrome and the presence of a tumour, particularly with the syndrome antedating tumour diagnosis.

(ii) Presence of an agent, for example a hormone or antibody, that can be detected in the tumour, in the circulation, and in the affected organ.

(iii) *In vitro* production of the agent by tumour cells.

(iv) An effect on the levels of the agent by removal/treatment of the tumour.

Resolution or improvement of the paraneoplastic syndrome following effective antitumour therapy is further supportive evidence, although this is difficult to demonstrate in many tumour types where effective treatment is not available.

Underlying mechanisms

The causes of paraneoplastic disease are not fully understood, but two main mechanisms have been identified. The first is inappropriate

Our thanks are due to Dr Mark Paine for his review of the section on neurological syndromes.

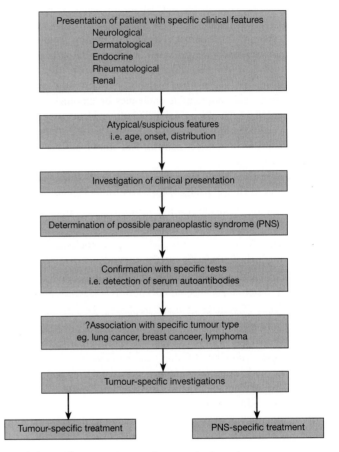

Fig. 1 Approach to management of paraneoplastic syndromes.

secretion of hormones or growth factors, and the second is the production of antitumour antibodies that cross-react with components of normal tissues.

Inappropriate hormone secretion occurs through excessive or unregulated secretion by the normal source of the hormone ('eutopic' secretion) or through synthesis by an organ or tissue not normally associated with that hormone ('ectopic' secretion). Well-recognized examples include the syndrome of inappropriate antidiuretic hormone secretion, Cushing's syndrome (excess secretion of ACTH), and humoral hypercalcaemia of malignancy (secondary to excess secretion of parathyroid hormone-related peptide); the same process is increasingly also recognized as a probable cause of some of the paraneoplastic haematological and dermatological conditions, and of fever and cachexia.

The production of antitumour antibodies which cross-react with epitopes on normal tissues is the likely cause of many syndromes affecting the nervous system and of some of the haematological paraneoplastic conditions. As an extension of this mechanism, formation of immune complexes between antitumour antibodies and cross-reacting normal cellular epitopes may be the cause of paraneoplastic glomerulonephritis and arthritis.[1],[2] In order to cause a clinical paraneoplastic syndrome, the immune mediator must first gain access to the target, which in the case of the nervous system may require increased permeability of the blood–brain or blood–retinal barrier, and then interact with the target and impair its function. The demonstration of antineuronal antibodies or immune complexes is, in itself, not sufficient evidence to implicate these in the pathogenesis of a paraneoplastic syndrome; it is possible that an alternative mechanism causes tissue damage, and the immune response is a secondary phenomenon. Also, antitumour antibodies or immune complexes may be found in the absence of a clinically evident paraneoplastic syndrome; antineuronal antibody expression has been shown in a small proportion of normal controls and cancer patients without paraneoplastic syndromes.[3]

Criteria for assessing the role of immune mechanisms in the pathogenesis of clinical paraneoplastic syndromes include:[4]

(i) A clinical/epidemiological link between specific tumour(s) and defined paraneoplastic syndrome.

(ii) Patients with the tumour and the paraneoplastic syndrome having high-titre specific reactive antibodies.

(iii) Evidence that a specific immune mechanism is active at the site of the lesion in patients but not controls (i.e. access to a target).

(iv) Evidence of damage of tissue displaying the relevant antigen (i.e. immunoablation).

(v) Evidence from passive transfer experiments that the same pathological and clinical features can be induced by specific immune mechanisms (autoantibodies extracted from patients' sera or antibodies raised experimentally against the same or similar antigenic determinants).

(vi) Clinical response to removing or lowering the titre of autoantibodies. In the metabolic paraneoplastic syndromes the tumour and the syndrome often run a parallel clinical course. This is not as common in syndromes secondary to antibodies, probably due to persistence of immune mediators even after effective treatment of the tumour, and the limited ability of target tissue (i.e. neural) to repair damage.

Patients with paraneoplastic syndromes often have a protracted clinical course and have small occult tumours which may be diagnosed only at post-mortem examination. It has been hypothesized that the cross-reacting antitumour antibodies which are responsible for some paraneoplastic syndromes may also function to keep tumour growth under control. Identification of the antigen recognized by anti-Purkinje cell antibodies in paraneoplastic cerebellar degeneration has revealed homology with two protease inhibitors, α_2-macroglobulin and α_1-antitrypsin. High-titre autoantibodies against these proteins might reduce protease inhibitor activity and thus enhance protease activity, altering the turnover of the pulmonary connective tissue

matrix. This in turn may decrease the potential for local and metastatic tumour growth.[5] Further support for this hypothesis comes from a number of clinical studies. A retrospective study of patients with small cell lung cancer found that patients with clinical evidence of a paraneoplastic syndrome survived for significantly longer (10.5 months versus 7.4 months) than patients without a paraneoplastic syndrome, and had significantly fewer cerebral metastases.[6] A second study reported that gynaecological tumours associated with the presence of anti-Yo antibodies and paraneoplastic cerebellar degeneration were more indolent than tumours of a similar histological grade in patients without antibodies present.[7] Verschuuren et al. examined the toxic effects of serum from patients with small cell lung cancer, with or without anti-Hu antibodies, on human tumour cell lines and found that a higher percentage of anti-Hu-positive sera were toxic to tumour cells compared with anti-Hu-negative sera.[8] However, this effect did not appear to be related to the antibody titre. In addition, purified anti-Hu antibodies alone were not toxic, while serum depleted of anti-Hu antibodies was. Thus, the presence of antibodies alone cannot fully explain the findings of de la Monte et al. or Hetzel et al.[6],[7]

Constitutional symptoms

Fever

Fever in cancer patients is most commonly due to infection, particularly in immunocompromised patients, but can be the presenting symptom of malignancies such as Hodgkin's disease, non-Hodgkin's lymphoma, the acute and chronic leukaemias, renal cell carcinoma, and hepatoma. More rarely, paraneoplastic fever is found in patients with osteosarcoma, multiple myeloma, ovarian tumours, and atrial myxoma. It can also occur in metastatic malignancy from any cause, especially when there is hepatic involvement.

Paraneoplastic fever can be secondary to the release of endogenous pyrogens by the tumour cells. Following release the pyrogens act on the hypothalamus, the area of the central nervous system where temperature regulation occurs. The pyrogens enhance the synthesis and release of prostaglandin E_2 from brain microvessel endothelium, which then elevates the hypothalamic temperature set point. The elevated temperature set point then initiates an increase in the body's core temperature through shivering (production of heat) or non-shivering (vasoconstriction—conservation of heat) mechanisms. This continues until the hypothalamus senses that the body's core temperature has reached the level of the new set point. These endogenous pyrogens have been shown to be various cytokines. The first to be determined was interleukin 1 (IL-1) which was initially known as 'endogenous pyrogen'. Other cytokines have since been discovered and have been found to be produced by various tumour cell types (Table 1).

IL-1 has been shown to be synthesized by Hodgkin's cell lines in vitro, and has been detected by immunohistochemistry in 50 per cent of biopsies of Hodgkin's disease, although there is poor correlation between the degree of staining and the presence of type-B symptoms. Xerri et al. found IL-1 gene expression in Reed–Sternberg cells in 12 out of 19 Hodgkin's disease specimens examined.[9]

IL-1 gene expression has also been found in acute myeloid leukaemia blast cells and there is some evidence to suggest an inverse

Table 1 Pyrogenic cytokines

Cytokine	Tumour associations
IL-1	Hodgkin's disease, NHL, AML, ALL, CLL, HCL, MM, renal, ovarian, sarcoma, melanoma
IL-6	Myeloma, CLL, lung, renal, NHL, hepatocellular carcinoma
Tumour necrosis factor	NHL, AML, melanoma, hepatocellular carcinoma
Interferon-α	HCL
Interferon-β	AML, colon, embryonal carcinoma
Interferon-γ	NHL, AML, melanoma, bladder, hepatocellular carcinoma

NHL, non-Hodgkin's lymphoma; AML, acute myeloid leukaemia; ALL, acute lymphocytic leukemia; CLL, chronic lymphocytic leukaemia; HCL, hairy cell leukaemia; MM, multiple myeloma.

relationship between *IL-1* mRNA levels and duration of disease remission.[10] In addition to being pyrogenic, IL-1 may act as an actual growth factor for leukaemic blast cells. *IL-1* mRNA has also been detected in human non-Hodgkin's lymphoma cells, and IL-1 pyrogenic bioactivity has been found in other types of leukaemic cells, in multiple myeloma cells, and in tumour cells from certain solid tumours, namely melanoma, sarcoma, and ovarian cancer. IL-1 is additionally involved in complex interactions between tumour cells and cells of the surrounding environment, which may have an impact on tumour growth and metastases.

Other cytokines shown to be pyrogenic include IL-6, IL-11, tumour necrosis factor-α and -β, and members of the interferon family— interferon-α, -β, and -γ. IL-6 has been shown to be produced by malignancies such as multiple myeloma, chronic lymphocytic leukaemia, renal cell carcinoma, lung cancer, atrial myxoma, and sarcoma. In some cases, production of IL-6 is determined by IL-1 production, resulting in a cascade of cytokine responses and the development of pyrexia and tumour growth.

The diagnosis of tumour-associated fever is essentially one of exclusion, and patients should be carefully evaluated for the possibility of infections. Tumour necrosis, haematomas, or drug reactions may also cause fever in these patients. One diagnostic test is the response of pyrexia to antitumour therapy. Response of a fever to non-steroidal anti-inflammatory drugs can also be used to help distinguish between an infective cause and a paraneoplastic cause. Non-steroidal anti-inflammatory drugs (i.e. aspirin and ibuprofen) work by blocking brain cyclo-oxygenase and thus inhibiting synthesis of prostaglandin E_2. Corticosteroids suppress most types of fever and can be used as a short-term treatment, but may be dangerous if infection has not been definitely excluded. Corticosteroids work at two levels: blocking synthesis of prostaglandin E_2 in the hypothalamus as well as blocking transcription of pyrogenic cytokine mRNA at the cellular level.

Cancer cachexia

Up to 80 per cent of cancer patients experience weight loss to some degree.[11] Significant weight loss (more than 10 per cent of pre-illness weight) has an adverse effect on prognosis as patients suffer from increased rates of infection, other complications, and a lowered ability to tolerate full doses of antitumour treatment. Patients with cancer may experience anorexia and weight loss due to identifiable complications of the tumour (oral ulceration, intestinal obstruction, abdominal distension, depression, anxiety) or due to antitumour treatment.

Patients with no clear cause for weight loss are said to have cancer cachexia, which is a complex metabolic syndrome probably secondary to an endogenous host response to the tumour (Fig. 2). Apart from anorexia and significant weight loss, the syndrome is characterized by lethargy, altered taste, muscle wasting, hypoproteinaemia, anaemia, glucose intolerance, and oedema. Most of the lost weight is fat and skeletal muscle, and it has been reported that patients who lose 30 per cent of their pre-illness stable weight lose over 70 per cent of their body fat and skeletal muscle.

The incidence of cancer cachexia varies with tumour type, stage, bulk, and performance status. Significant weight loss (more than 10 per cent of premorbid weight) occurs in 70 to 80 per cent of patients with cancer of the pancreas or stomach, and in 50 to 60 per cent of patients with lung or colon cancer.

There is some evidence to suggest that there is abnormal appetite control in cancer patients. This is possibly related to changes in blood glucose, free fatty acid, and amino acid kinetics or may also be due to changes in the neural or hormonal (insulin, glucagon, bombesin, cholecystokinin) regulation of the gastrointestinal tract. Another possible factor is decreased binding of tryptophan to albumin which may increase synthesis or turnover of serotonin in the brain, which in turn leads to decreased appetite and food intake.[13]

A third of cancer patients have been shown to be hypermetabolic, possibly due to enhanced activity of energy-dependent metabolic cycles. There are reports of increased protein turnover with increased proteolysis in skeletal muscle, and increased Cori cycle activity, in cancer patients with weight loss. There is also abnormal glucose metabolism with decreased insulin secretion by the pancreas and increased gluconeogenesis in the liver (Fig. 2). A loss of lipid stores occurs secondary to increased lipolysis and fatty acid oxidation. This may be partially due to tumour production of a proteoglycan with lipolytic properties.[14] The catabolic response to cancer is mediated, at least in part, by production of various inflammatory cytokines, i.e. tumour necrosis factor-α (cachectin), IL-6, IL-1, and interferon-γ. These cytokines can be produced by the tumour itself, or by host cells in response to the tumour. *In vitro* treatment with cachectin has

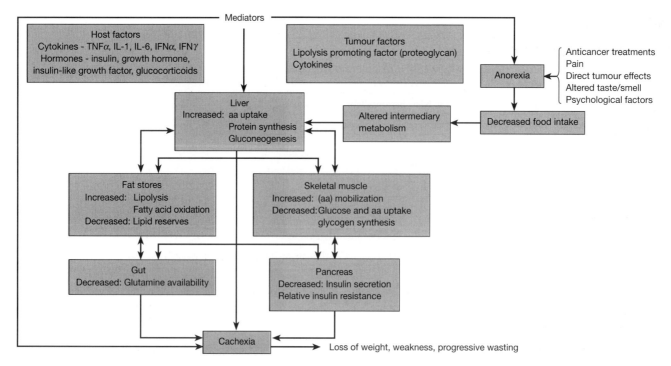

Fig. 2 Mechanisms of cancer cachexia. (TNF, tumour necrosis factor; IL, interleukin; IFN, interferon; aa, amino acid.) (Adapted with permission from Lind *et al.*[12])

been shown to cause metabolic abnormalities including loss of cell lipid in adipocytes, and mice inoculated with a cell line secreting cachectin develop a profound wasting syndrome, in large part due to anorexia. In addition, antibodies to tumour necrosis factor-α have been shown to attenuate the development of anorexia and cachexia in tumour models. Patients with non-small-cell lung cancer who were hypermetabolic had significantly increased levels of inflammatory cytokines such as soluble tumour necrosis factor receptor 55, lipopolysaccharide-binding protein and C-reactive protein.[15] Patients with a weight loss of greater than 10 per cent had increased levels of soluble tumour necrosis factor receptors, IL-6, and C-reactive protein. An acute phase response (measured by elevations in levels of C-reactive protein) in patients with pancreatic cancer correlated with a hypermetabolic state and increased expenditure of resting energy.[16] There was no correlation with serum levels of tumour necrosis factor or IL-6, but spontaneous production of tumour necrosis factor and IL-6 by peripheral blood monoclonal cells was increased, suggesting that local cytokine production may play a key role in the acute phase response to cancer.

Management of cancer cachexia is complex. It is important to first determine the degree of weight loss, history of food intake, and any complicating factors. Assessment of plasma proteins produced by the liver, such as albumin and transferrin, can be done. The most important assessment to determine adequate nutritional input is the nitrogen balance. Treatment is based upon adequate intake of calories, preferably enterally rather that parentally.

Fatigue

Fatigue is one of the most common symptoms experienced by cancer patients. Depending upon the definition used, up to 80 per cent of patients experience fatigue (defined as a loss of energy or debilitating tiredness at least once per week).[17] Despite being such a common, often severe, symptom, there has been little research on its causes, effects, relationships, and treatment; even its definition varies greatly.[18] In a patient with cancer, there are many possible contributing factors to the development of fatigue, apart from the malignancy itself (Table 2).

The causes of paraneoplastic fatigue are not known. Possible mechanisms include abnormal energy metabolism, i.e. a hypermetabolic state secondary to tumour growth, or the release of cytokines such as tumour necrosis factor. Other paraneoplastic phenomena such as myopathy, peripheral neuropathy, and cancer cachexia may also contribute to the development of fatigue.

Management of cancer-related fatigue requires a comprehensive assessment of the contributing factors. As a first step, correction of treatment-related side-effects such as anaemia, metabolic disturbances, infection, etc. is required. Proper psychological and nutritional assessment enables treatment of these important cofactors, especially depression. Although specific treatments for fatigue have not been studied in large trials, there is evidence to support the use of certain agents such as psychostimulants, for example premoline and methylphenidate, and corticosteroids. Diet, rest patterns, adequate exercise, and support/counselling can also play an important therapeutic role.

Neurological syndromes

Neurological paraneoplastic syndromes have been reported to occur in significant numbers of patients with malignant disease, including up to 50 per cent of patients with carcinomas of the lung.[19] However,

Table 2 Causative factors of cancer fatigue

Cancer-related paraneoplastic phenomena

Metabolic disturbances
   Hypermetabolic state
   Abnormal lactate production
   Cachexia
   Renal insufficiency, electrolyte abnormalities

Neurological disturbance
   Peripheral neuropathy
   Neuromuscular
   Myopathy

Anaemia of chronic disease

Direct tumour effects

Organ failure
   Pulmonary
   Hepatic
   Cerebral

Pain syndromes

Treatment-associated conditions

Infection

Anaemia

Chemotherapy

Radiation

Biological response modifiers
   IL-2, interferon

Supportive drugs
   Opioids

Psychological

Anxiety

Depression

Sleep disturbance

---

most cases involve mild proximal myopathy or mild peripheral neuropathy. Other, more clinically significant, neurological syndromes are rare, occurring in fewer than 4 per cent of patients.[20],[21] Neurological paraneoplastic syndromes can arise from any part of the neurological system, and can reflect either widespread cellular dysfunction, for example paraneoplastic encephalomyelitis, or more focal involvement, for example the cancer-associated retinopathy syndrome and paraneoplastic cerebellar degeneration. The main syndromes and their tumour associations are listed in Table 3. The Lambert–Eaton myasthenic syndrome, described in more detail below, is a classic example of a neurological paraneoplastic syndrome mediated by humoral immunity. There is a clear association with a specific tumour (small cell lung cancer), target-specific autoantibodies are almost invariably detected, the condition often improves in response to treatment designed to reduce antibody titres, and clinical and pathological features of the disease can be induced in passive transfer experiments.[4] There is increasing evidence for an autoimmune mechanism in other neurological syndromes, including encephalomyelitis, subacute sensory neuropathy, paraneoplastic cerebellar degeneration,

cancer-associated retinopathy, and peripheral neuropathies associated with IgM paraproteinaemia.[22] Figure 3 illustrates possible autoimmune mechanisms of neuronal damage.

It remains unclear why only such a small percentage of patients with cancers such as small cell lung cancer actually develop a clinically significant paraneoplastic syndrome, when tumoral expression of neuronal antigens such as the Hu antigen is widespread. One hypothesis is that certain patients have a genetic susceptibility to the development of autoimmune reactivity, and when these patients are exposed to tumour antigens they are more likely to develop neuronal cross-reacting antibodies.[23] Table 4 lists the currently identified autoantibodies and their tumour associations and neurological syndromes.[24]

Syndromes involving the brain

Paraneoplastic encephalomyelitis

Paraneoplastic encephalomyelitis refers to an inflammatory disorder affecting several levels of the nervous system including the brain, spinal cord, peripheral nerves, and autonomic system.[25] The potential involvement of several neurological levels, when combined with various neuronal cell types, leads to a variety of possible clinical manifestations. The most common clinical presentation is a disabling subacute sensory neuronopathy due to involvement of the dorsal root ganglia.[26],[27] Other common presentations of paraneoplastic encephalomyelitis include cerebellar degeneration with ataxia and motor inco-ordination, 'limbic encephalitis' with amnestic dementia and seizures, 'brainstem encephalitis' with vertigo, hearing loss, and ocular palsies, and autonomic failure with urinary retention, intestinal pseudo-obstruction, and orthostatic hypotension. The most common tumour association is with small cell lung cancer, with occasional reports of other tumour types.[25] Pathologically there is patchy, multifocal neuronal loss in multiple levels of the nervous system, with some degree of perivascular infiltration by lymphocytes and plasma cells (Fig. 4).

There is a clear association between paraneoplastic encephalomyelitis, small cell lung cancer, and an autoimmune aetiology. The antibody associated with paraneoplastic encephalomyelitis is the anti-Hu antibody—a polyclonal group of IgG type 1 antineuronal nuclear antibodies that are usually found at a higher titre in the cerebrospinal fluid than in the serum, indicating localized production in the central nervous system. The antibodies react against a number of proteins that belong to a family of RNA-binding proteins that have been found to be expressed both by neuronal cells and by small cell lung cancer cells. Paraneoplastic encephalomyelitis usually precedes tumour diagnosis, and in most cases evolves from its initial presentation into a widespread encephalomyelopathy. Specific treatments such as plasma exchange, corticosteroids, and intravenous gammaglobulin have not proved successful.[27] Spontaneous remission may occasionally occur. There is evidence to suggest that patients with small cell lung cancer who have positive serology for anti-Hu antibodies have more limited disease at diagnosis, have a greater chance of having a complete response to therapy, and have a longer survival.[28]

Paraneoplastic limbic encephalitis can occur as part of the paraneoplastic encephalomyelitis syndrome or as an isolated entity. It is usually associated with small cell lung cancer, although it has been reported with other tumour types. It is characterized clinically by

Table 3 Main neurological syndromes and tumour associations

Syndromes	Associated tumours
Syndromes involving the brain	
Dementia	
Paraneoplastic encephalomyelitis	SCLC, breast, NSCLC, ovary
Paraneoplastic cerebellar degeneration	SCLC, ovary, HD, breast
Visual paraneoplastic syndromes	SCLC, ovary, melanoma
Opsoclonus–myoclonus	CNS, SCLC, breast, renal
Syndromes involving the spinal cord	
Myelitis	SCLC, HD
Necrotizing myelopathy	NHL, leukaemia, SCLC, renal
Stiff-man syndrome	SCLC, breast, HD
Motor neurone disease	Breast, SCLC, prostate, NHL
Subacute motor neuronopathy	NHL, SCLC
Peripheral neuropathy	
Subacute sensory neuronopathy	SCLC, breast
Paraprotein neuropathy	Multiple myeloma
Autonomic neuropathy	SCLC, GIT, HD, NHL
Acute neuropathy	HD
Disorders of neuromuscular transmission	
Lambert–Eaton myasthenic syndrome	SCLC, breast, prostate, NHL
Myasthenia gravis	Thymoma, HD
Syndromes involving muscle	
Dermatomyositis and polymyositis	Breast, SCLC, GIT, renal

SCLC, small cell lung cancer; NSCLC, non-small-cell lung cancer; HD, Hodgkin's disease; CNS, central nervous system; NHL, non-Hodgkin's lymphoma; GIT, gastrointestinal tract.

subacute cognitive dysfunction with severe impairment of short-term memory, mood changes, depression, and hallucinations. Electro-encephalography and magnetic resonance imaging changes are usually found in the temporal lobes, and pathological changes such as extensive loss of neurones and perivascular lymphocyte cuffing are seen in the limbic structures such as the amygdala. The syndrome is often associated with the presence of anti-Hu antibodies, but sometimes these can be absent; there is evidence to suggest that patients with anti-Hu-negative paraneoplastic limbic encephalitis are less likely to develop paraneoplastic encephalomyelitis and appear more likely to improve neurologically with anticancer therapy than patients with anti-Hu-positive paraneoplastic limbic encephalitis.[29]

Paraneoplastic cerebellar degeneration

Paraneoplastic cerebellar degeneration is a rare condition characterized by the rapid onset of cerebellar dysfunction, manifested clinically by disturbance of gait, truncal and limb ataxia, dysarthria, dysphagia, and ocular disturbances. Paraneoplastic cerebellar degeneration can be classified in a number of ways. The first classifies paraneoplastic cerebellar degeneration on the basis of whether inflammatory infiltrates are present or not. If an inflammatory infiltrate is present, then the paraneoplastic cerebellar degeneration is more likely to be a part of the paraneoplastic encephalomyelitis syndrome than to be an isolated paraneoplastic entity. Posner classified paraneoplastic cerebellar degeneration according to the presence or absence of specific antibodies.[20] The classic pathological lesion is a diffuse loss of Purkinje cells with associated degeneration of deep cerebellar nuclei and long tracts in the spinal cord. The most common

tumour associations are with gynaecological tumours, especially ovarian, small cell lung cancer, Hodgkin's disease, and breast cancer.

A number of different autoantibodies have been detected in patients with paraneoplastic cerebellar degeneration, supporting its classification as a paraneoplastic condition, although there are cases where no autoantibodies have been found. The different antibodies that have been detected are associated with specific and distinct clinical and pathological variants of paraneoplastic cerebellar degeneration. The anti-Yo antibodies are a group of polyclonal IgG anti-Purkinje cell antibodies. Anti-Yo antibody-associated paraneoplastic cerebellar degeneration is almost exclusively found in females with breast or ovarian cancer who commonly die due to the effects of their underlying malignancy. The paraneoplastic cerebellar degeneration precedes the diagnosis of tumour in most cases. Patients develop severe neurological disability with a near total loss of Purkinje cells with little neurological inflammation.[30] It has been reported that the tumours themselves are more indolent than tumours of a similar histological grade in patients without associated anti-Yo antibodies.[7] Because of the strong association between anti-Yo antibodies and these tumour types, it has been recommended that all patients with anti-Yo-associated paraneoplastic cerebellar degeneration should be investigated for breast and gynaecological malignancies, including surgical exploration if required. Only a couple of cases of male patients with paraneoplastic cerebellar degeneration and anti-Yo antibodies have been reported.

Anti-Hu antibody-associated paraneoplastic cerebellar degeneration is nearly always found in association with small cell lung cancer, and patients often die as a direct result of their neurological

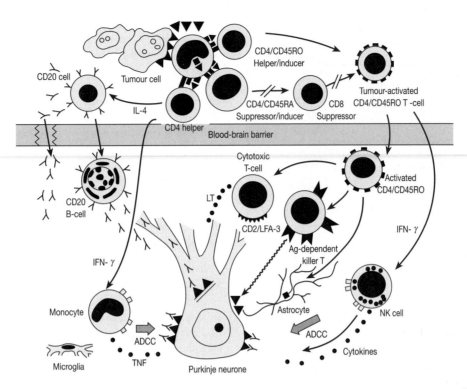

Fig. 3 Postulated action of autoimmune mechanisms in paraneoplastic neurological conditions. Secreted or cell membrane antigens (▽) are processed by the antigen-presenting cell and re-expressed with a class II gene product (↑) allowing recognition by CD4 T cells. Up-regulation of CD4 helper-inducer cells, or down-regulation of CD4 suppressor-inducer and CD8 suppressor T-cell phenotypes (top right), could potentially result in the migration of tumour antigen-activated T cells through the blood–brain barrier, promoting antigen-dependent killer T-cell cytolysis or cytokine release (bottom right). Alternatively, activated CD20+ B cells could migrate through the barrier or secrete antibody which reaches neurones by retrograde axoplasmic transport or via the cerebrospinal fluid (left). Antibody could bind to similar membranous or intracytoplasmic antigenic epitopes providing a mechanism for lysis by complement or via cell-mediated cytotoxicity mediated by natural killer cells, monocytes, or antigen-dependent T cells. (Reprinted with permission from Jaeckle.[22])

dysfunction. It is often part of a more general neurological condition with widespread inflammation and loss of neuronal cells (see above). Antivoltage gated calcium channel antibodies have also been found in a subset of patients with paraneoplastic cerebellar degeneration,

and these patients all go on to develop Lambert–Eaton myasthenic syndrome (see below). Finally, anti-Tr antibodies have been found in association with paraneoplastic cerebellar degeneration and Hodgkin's disease; in these case there is usually specific Purkinje cell loss.[31]

Table 4 Antineuronal antibodies in paraneoplastic neurological syndromes

Antibody	Target cell	Main tumour association	Neurological syndrome
Anti-Hu	All CNS neurones	SCLC, breast	PEM, PCD, PSN
Anti-Yo	Purkinje cells	Ovarian, Hodgkin's disease	PCD
Anti-Tr	Purkinje cells	Hodgkin's disease	PCD
Anti-Ri	All CNS neurones	Breast, SCLC	Opsoclonus–myoclonus
Antiretinal	Photoreceptor cells	SCLC, melanoma	Cancer-associated retinopathy
Antiamphiphysin	Neural synapse	Breast, SCLC	Stiff-man syndrome
Anti-MAG	Myelin	Paraproteinaemias, e.g. MGUS, multiple myeloma, Waldenström's macroglobulinaemia, osteosclerotic myeloma	Peripheral neuropathy
Anti-VGCC	Presynaptic neuromuscular junction	SCLC	Lambert–Eaton myasthenic syndrome.

CNS, central nervous system. SCLC, small cell lung cancer. PEM, paraneoplastic encephalomyelitis. PCD, paraneoplastic cerebellar degeneration. PSN, paraneoplastic sensory neuropathy. MGUS, monoclonal gammopathy of unknown significance. Anti-MAG, antimyelin-associated glycoprotein. Anti-VGCC, antivoltage gated calcium channels.

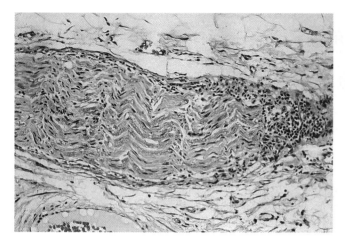

Fig. 4 Histological appearance of a paraneoplastic lesion in the central nervous system.

There is some evidence that patients with paraneoplastic cerebellar degeneration who are antibody positive differ from those patients whose paraneoplastic cerebellar degeneration is not associated with detectable antibodies; antibody-positive patients are more likely to be female, have multifocal neurological disease, and to be severely disabled.

Paraneoplastic cerebellar degeneration may present during the clinical course of the cancer, or precede the diagnosis by up to 3 years. Although the condition is very rare, the subacute development of a pancerebellar syndrome is indicative of a paraneoplastic phenomenon in about 50 per cent of cases.[25] Cerebellar signs usually proceed relentlessly, and patients have a poor prognosis. Treatment of paraneoplastic cerebellar degeneration has been disappointing, no significant benefit having been shown with the use of high-dose steroids, cyclophosphamide, or azathioprine, although there have been case reports of response to treatments such as immunoglobulin and plasmapheresis, and improvement has also occasionally been reported with effective antitumour therapy in Hodgkin's disease and carcinomas of the lung and breast.[30] Spontaneous remissions occasionally occur, primarily in patients with Hodgkin's disease.

Visual paraneoplastic syndromes

Cancer-associated retinopathy syndrome

Rapid loss of visual acuity or visual field was first described in 1976 as a paraneoplastic syndrome in patients with small cell lung cancer. The cancer-associated retinopathy syndrome is now described as a retinopathy characterized by subacute visual loss with night blindness, photosensitivity, and impaired colour vision. The majority of cases have been described in association with small cell lung cancer, but there are reports of association with other solid tumours, including gynaecological malignancies.

The cancer-associated retinopathy syndrome is associated with the presence of an antibody directed against a 21 kDa calcium-binding protein present in retinal photoreceptor cells which has also been demonstrated to be expressed by tumours.[32] These cells play a key role in light–dark adaptation. Visual symptoms usually precede diagnosis of the tumour, and patients develop blurred vision, photopsias, scotomata (often with bizarre episodic visual defects), and sometimes impaired colour vision; this is followed by rapidly progressive painless loss of vision. Retinal arterioles are narrowed, and there are changes in vitreous cells and retinal pigment epithelium. Electroretinography is abnormal, indicating widespread damage to rods and cones, and establishes the diagnosis. Pathological examination demonstrates loss of photoreceptor cells, together with loss of the outer nuclear layer of the retina (specifically the ganglion cells) and the presence of IgG or IgM in the retinal ganglion layer. This suggests that antiretinal autoantibodies are able to cross the blood–retinal barrier to gain access to the target cells. Stabilization of visual loss and subsequent improvement has been reported with the use of oral corticosteroids and plasmapheresis, in combination with antitumour therapy.[33]

Melanoma-associated retinopathy syndrome

Melanoma-associated retinopathy is a distinct clinicopathological syndrome with clinical features such as photopsias and night blindness, although night blindness may not be a universal finding. Full-field electroretinography classically shows attenuation of the b-wave amplitude, and autoantibodies can usually be detected. These autoantibodies have been shown to be directed against the bipolar cells in the retina.[34] Use of corticosteroids may be beneficial in some cases.

Other visual syndromes

There are isolated reports of optic neuritis as the major manifestation of paraneoplastic encephalomyelitis in patients with lung cancer and non-Hodgkin's lymphoma. However, this may be a chance association, or may be related to meningeal metastases which can be difficult to diagnose except at autopsy.

Opsoclonus–myoclonus

Opsoclonus is an ocular dyskinesia occurring when there is loss of inhibitory control over ocular saccades. These are reflex or voluntary, brief, rapid, conjugate eye movements necessary for the refixation of a visual target of interest on the fovea. Loss of control leads to a clinical picture of involuntary, rapid, repetitive conjugate movements that are irregular in frequency and amplitude occurring in vertical, horizontal, and oblique planes. The eye movements are described as 'chaotic'. These are usually accompanied by ataxia and myoclonus, involving the trunk, limbs, head, diaphragm, larynx, pharynx, and palate.

Opsoclonus can be idiopathic or can be a complication of a number of conditions including trauma, brain tumours, and encephalitis. Paraneoplastic opsoclonus has been a recognized entity for many years, and is most commonly associated with neuroblastoma in children. In adults, it has been associated with a number of tumour types including small cell lung cancer, breast cancer, ovarian cancer, pancreatic cancer, and renal cell cancer. There is often a paucity of pathological findings (perivascular lymphocyte cuffing with some gliosis), despite significant neurological deficits.

There are several strands of evidence supporting opsoclonus as a paraneoplastic disorder. The condition usually precedes the tumour diagnosis, often by up to a year. The clinical course of the opsoclonus and the tumour can be linked. There is increasing evidence that the neurological dysfunction is immune mediated, with reports of anti-Ri antibodies and anti-Hu antibodies in association with cancer and opsoclonus.[35],[36] Initial treatment with steroids can be effective, followed with specific antitumour therapy. The impact of treatment on paraneoplastic opsoclonus can be difficult to determine because the condition often follows a relapsing and remitting course. Investigation for an underlying malignancy is recommended in all patients presenting with opsoclonus over the age of 40 years.

Spinal cord syndromes

The spinal cord is primarily involved in around 10 per cent of all paraneoplastic neurological syndromes.

Myelitis

Patients with paraneoplastic encephalomyelitis may present with predominant spinal cord involvement and thus be diagnosed with a myelopathy. Paraneoplastic myelitis is particularly associated with small cell lung cancer and Hodgkin's disease.[37] Patients with myelopathy and small cell lung cancer, like those with paraneoplastic encephalomyelitis, have been shown to have circulating anti-Hu antineuronal IgG antibodies which bind to antigens in normal human spinal cord, cerebral grey matter, retina, and tumour. The pathological signs are intense inflammation and loss of neurones in the anterior and posterior horns, affecting either a few segments (usually cervical or lumbar) or the entire spinal cord. Destruction of anterior horn cells often predominates, leading to degeneration of the anterior roots, with motor neuropathy and neurogenic muscle atrophy.[38]

Necrotizing myelopathy

This is a very rare complication of lymphoma, leukaemia, lung cancer (especially small cell lung cancer), and renal cell cancer. There have also been case reports of other tumour associations including thyroid cancer and multiple myeloma. Patients can present with a variety of clinical features depending upon the major area of spinal cord necrosis, and often appear to have a subacute transverse myelitis. Clinical findings include leg and arm paralysis, sensory changes, and loss of sphincter control. The pathological signs are usually those of patchy multifocal necrotic degeneration throughout the whole spinal cord (particularly in the white matter of the posterior and lateral columns), or there can be massive necrosis of the thoracic cord.

Necrotizing myelopathy is considered to be a true paraneoplastic phenomenon, although autoantibodies have not yet been identified.[39] There have been pathological reports of the presence of herpes simplex virus type 2 infection in conjunction with necrotizing myelopathy, suggesting that there may be two possible pathogenic mechanisms, autoimmune or infective.[40]

Stiff-man syndrome

Stiff-man syndrome describes a condition of skeletal muscle rigidity, especially of muscles of the lower limbs, associated with painful muscle spasm. There are both paraneoplastic and non-paraneoplastic variants of the condition, and each can be associated with different autoantibodies: antiamphiphysin 1 autoantibodies (directed against amphiphysin, a protein located in the presynaptic compartment of neurones) are most commonly found in the paraneoplastic condition, while antibodies against glutamic acid carboxylase have been found in the non-paraneoplastic type.[41] There appears to be some crossover, with glutamic acid carboxylase antibodies having been detected in a patient with breast cancer and stiff-man syndrome. Stiff-man syndrome is associated with a number of tumour types including small cell lung cancer, breast cancer, and Hodgkin's disease.[42] The neurological condition can improve following a combination of corticosteroids and antitumour therapy.

Motor neurone disease

Although some early studies reported a significant association between amyotrophic lateral sclerosis and malignancy, subsequent reviews suggested that the incidence was no greater than in the general population. Thus, the existence of motor neurone disease as a paraneoplastic syndrome remains controversial. Nevertheless, with reports of the detection of anti-Hu antibodies in patients with motor neurone disease, and of cases where the clinical course of the motor neurone disease parallels the course of the tumour, it is likely that in some cases motor neurone disease does represent a paraneoplastic process.[43] Further supportive evidence came from a study by Forsyth et al. which reported on 14 patients with both cancer and motor neurone disease who they were able to divide into three distinct groups:[44]

(i) Patients with rapidly progressive motor neurone disease, cancer, and the presence of anti-Hu antibodies.

(ii) Patients with motor neurone disease with predominantly upper motor neurone dysfunction (resembling primary lateral sclerosis) and breast cancer.

(iii) Patients with motor neurone disease resembling amyotrophic lateral sclerosis developing within a 4-year period before or after cancer diagnosis.

The authors concluded that on the basis of the clinical picture and the presence of autoantibodies, the patients in the first group definitely had a paraneoplastic syndrome, while those in the second group were likely to have one. Thus, although in most cases motor neurone disease is not a paraneoplastic phenomenon, patients presenting in a similar fashion to those in groups (i) and (ii) above require investigation for a possible underlying malignancy. Key sites to be investigated are breast, lung, and prostate. There have also been reports of an increased incidence of lymphoma in patients with motor neurone disease, especially those presenting with amyotrophic lateral sclerosis, and so investigations for haematological malignancy may be warranted in such patients.

Subacute motor neuronopathy

This very rare condition is associated primarily with the lymphomas and with small cell lung cancer. It is basically the motor counterpart of subacute sensory neuronopathy (see below) and presents with progressive motor weakness over weeks to months. Patients have flaccid weakness and develop significant muscle atrophy. The lower limbs tend to be more affected than the arms, and bulbar muscles are not affected. Pathology shows a loss of motor neurones in the anterolateral grey matter of the spinal cord with some surrounding gliosis. Patients with subacute motor neuronopathy in association with small cell lung cancer often have detectable anti-Hu antibodies.[45]

Peripheral neuropathy

Most cases of peripheral neuropathy in patients with cancer are due to causes other than paraneoplastic: these include direct neoplastic involvement either by compression or by infiltration, induction by chemotherapy, for example by cisplatinum, taxoids, and vinca alkaloid drugs, and nutritional/metabolic causes. Symptomatic paraneoplastic peripheral neuropathy occurs in approximately 2.5 to 5.5 per cent of patients with lung or breast carcinoma, Hodgkin's disease, and myeloma.[46] However, asymptomatic electromyographic abnormalities are much commoner and occur in 35 to 50 per cent of patients with lung cancer, 25 per cent with Hodgkin's disease, and 13 per cent with myeloma. Previously undiagnosed cancer is a relatively rare cause of progressive peripheral neuropathy.

In contrast to the neuropathies described in previous sections, where the key lesion is neuronal degeneration, paraneoplastic peripheral neuropathies are usually caused by axonal degeneration or demyelination. Electromyography is useful in pinpointing the anatomical site of the lesion, and in differentiating axonal and demyelinating pathology. There are many different classifications of paraneoplastic peripheral neuropathy. The most common clinical syndromes are as follows.

Sensory peripheral neuropathy

Subacute sensory neuronopathy

Subacute sensory neuronopathy, also known as ganglioradiculitis, was first recognized as a paraneoplastic syndrome in 1948. It is a rare neurological paraneoplastic syndrome and is more commonly diagnosed in patients with Sjögren's syndrome with no evidence of malignancy. Patients present clinically with a rapidly developing severe sensory loss, often affecting all four limbs, and usually beginning peripherally. There may be associated areflexia, pain, and incoordination. A sensory ataxia due to loss of proprioception is typical and can be severe. In most patients the neuronopathy precedes tumour diagnosis, sometimes by many years, and the tumour may be diagnosed only at post-mortem examination.

Small cell lung cancer is the most common tumour association, an association with breast cancer having also been reported. Nerve conduction studies show markedly decreased or absent sensory potentials, whilst motor conduction is often normal. Pathologically, the dorsal root ganglia are infiltrated by lymphocytes (such as CD8+ T cells) and macrophages, leading to destruction of the neurones of the dorsal root ganglia and secondary wallerian degeneration of the posterior nerve roots, peripheral sensory nerves, and posterior columns (ascending sensory long tracts) of the cord. Around 50 per cent of patients have evidence of paraneoplastic encephalomyelitis elsewhere in the spinal cord and brain.

Patients with subacute sensory neuronopathy and small cell lung cancer usually have anti-Hu antibodies which recognize basic nuclear protein(s) of molecular weight 35 to 40 kDa present in the neuronal nuclei of dorsal root ganglia, trigeminal ganglia, and the central nervous system as well as in primary and metastatic small cell lung cancer.[25] Because of the strong association between small cell lung cancer, subacute sensory neuronopathy, and anti-Hu antibodies, it is recommended that any patient with a rapid onset of subacute sensory neuronopathy should be tested for the presence of anti-Hu antibodies, and if positive, a search for an underlying lung cancer should be undertaken. Importantly, not all cases of autoantibody-associated subacute sensory neuronopathy are associated with a detectable malignancy.[47]

There have also been reports of an association between paraneoplastic subacute sensory neuronopathy and another type of autoantibody, antiamphiphysin 1.[42] Amphiphysin 1 is a protein present in nerve terminals, where it has a possible role in endocytosis, and has been detected in breast cancer and small cell lung cancer tissues. Antiamphiphysin 1 antibodies have also been detected in paraneoplastic stiff-man syndrome (see above).

It is generally reported that paraneoplastic subacute sensory neuronopathy is resistant to treatment.[48] However, there are reports of sustained clinical improvement following the use of high-dose intravenous immunoglobulin, and successful antitumour treatment may halt progression of neurological dysfunction.[49]

Paraprotein neuropathy

Patients investigated for peripheral neuropathy are frequently found to have an excess of abnormal circulating immunoglobulins which are usually monoclonal and are referred to as M protein.[50],[51] The paraprotein can be either IgM, IgG, or IgA, and be either κ or λ. In this group of patients the neuropathy is usually of a sensorimotor type and is often classified as a chronic inflammatory demyelinating polyradiculopathy, with symmetrical sensory and motor loss affecting all four limbs, often associated with tremor. Electrophysiological studies show marked slowing of conduction velocity and conduction block. Sural nerve biopsies demonstrate a loss of myelinated fibres, focal axonal degeneration, widespread demyelination and remyelination with 'onion-skin' formation, and widening of myelin lamallae in myelinated fibres.

Paraprotein neuropathy is estimated to occur in up to 13 per cent of patients with multiple myeloma, and is also found in patients with Waldenström's macroglobulinaemia, monoclonal gammopathy of undetermined significance, and plasmacytoma. Osteosclerotic myeloma, seen in association with the so-called POEMS syndrome (polyneuropathy, organomegaly, endocrinopathy, monoclonal gammopathy, and skin changes) is typically associated with paraneoplastic peripheral neuropathy.[52]

The circulating M protein often recognizes myelin-associated glycoprotein, and an antibody binding to myelin-associated glycoprotein is postulated to be the mechanism for the polyneuropathy associated with the paraproteinaemia. Electron microscopy can demonstrate selective deposition of IgM gammaglobulin in areas of myelin where pathological changes have occurred. Further support for this proposed mechanism comes from experiments involving the passive transfer of human IgM antimyelin-associated glycoprotein antibodies to animals. Following transfer, the animals developed a peripheral demyelination highly characteristic of the human syndrome. It has also been shown that in certain cases the paraprotein, in addition to binding to myelin-associated glycoprotein, acts as a cold agglutinin recognizing a red blood cell membrane-associated antigen. This may play a causative role in the development of myelin damage.

In most cases paraprotein neuropathy responds poorly to treatment, although surgical/radiation treatment of osteosclerotic myeloma can lead to an improvement in the associated neuropathy. The neuropathy associated with monoclonal gammopathy of undetermined significance has been successfully treated with a number of therapies including high-dose intravenous immunoglobulin, plasma exchange, and corticosteroids, although there is trial evidence supporting plasma exchange only. The addition of chorambucil, melphalan, prednisolone, or cyclophosphamide may also lead to improvement in certain cases by reducing the amount of M protein in circulation.

Autonomic neuropathy

So called 'pseudo-obstruction' was first described in 1948 in a patient with carcinoma and metastases outside the gastrointestinal tract. This, and other manifestations of autonomic neuropathy, is associated especially with small cell lung cancer, but can also occur in other malignancies including pancreatic cancer, colon cancer, and lymphoma. Paraneoplastic autonomic neuropathy can occur as part of a more widespread paraneoplastic neurological syndrome, i.e. anti-Hu antibody-associated paraneoplastic encephalomyelitis, or as an isolated disorder. It can affect specific components, or all, of the autonomic nervous system.

Clinical presentations include orthostatic hypotension, pseudo-obstruction with abdominal distension and constipation, urinary incontinence, and impotence. It has been reported that subclinical paraneoplastic autonomic dysfunction is common in patients with lymphoma.[53] In the gastrointestinal tract there is a visceral neuropathy of the myenteric plexus, with infiltration by lymphocytes and plasma cells. Later there is widespread degeneration of axons and neurones, and glial proliferation in the myenteric plexus. Studies attempting to demonstrate serum autoantibodies cross-reacting with the patient's tumour and the gastrointestinal tract have not been successful. Thus there is no clear evidence of autoimmune aetiology, although the pathology is very similar to the changes seen in the paraneoplastic encephalomyelopathies. Autonomic neuropathy also occurs in Lambert–Eaton myasthenic syndrome, although only a small percentage of cases are paraneoplastic. The main symptoms are dry mouth and impotence. Anti-Hu antibodies have been detected and the mechanism is thought to be autoimmune in type.

Acute neuropathy

Guillain–Barré syndrome

Guillain–Barré syndrome is characterized by subacute ascending paralysis with associated areflexia and some degree of sensory loss. Typical Guillain–Barré syndrome is a very uncommon paraneoplastic complication, but it has been reported to be associated with Hodgkin's disease. Pathologically, there is a neuronal inflammatory infiltrate, and segmental demyelination with relative axonal sparing.

Other neurological syndromes

Chronic inflammatory demyelinating polyneuropathy

This is a sensorimotor neuropathy usually affecting all four limbs with a graded distal to proximal distribution, with diffuse areflexia, high levels of protein in the cerebrospinal fluid, and a demyelinating pattern on electromyography. It is usually idiopathic, but has been reported in association with paraproteinaemias (see above) and with gastrointestinal adenocarcinomas, seminoma, and lymphoma. Pathologically there is a mixed picture of axonal degeneration with evidence of demyelination and remyelination. An immune mechanism has been postulated with coexpression of antigens by the tumour and by Schwann cells. Successful treatment has been reported with intravenous gammaglobulin and/or corticosteroids.

Mononeuritis and mononeuritis multiplex

Mononeuritis occurs in patients with carcinoma and lymphoma, as an isolated lesion, or in the setting of an underlying symmetrical peripheral neuropathy, particularly in small cell lung cancer. Paraneoplastic mononeuritis multiplex is due to vasculitis of the vasa nervorum of unknown cause.

Disorders affecting neuromuscular transmission

There are two important paraneoplastic disorders of the neuromuscular junction. Lambert–Eaton myasthenic syndrome is a presynaptic disorder characterized by impaired release of acetylcholine. Myasthenia gravis is a postsynaptic disorder affecting the acetylcholine receptor.

Lambert–Eaton myasthenic syndrome

A myasthenic syndrome associated with lung cancer was first described in 1953. In 1956, Lambert and colleagues recognized the distinctive electrophysiological features of this condition, distinct from myasthenia gravis.[54] This is now recognized as a presynaptic disorder of peripheral cholinergic neurotransmission in which calcium-dependent acetylcholine release is reduced both in the resting state and in response to motor nerve stimulation.[55] Approximately 50 to 60 per cent of patients with Lambert–Eaton myasthenic syndrome have an underlying malignancy, nearly always small cell lung cancer, with a few other tumour types (see Table 1).[56] In patients without cancer, Lambert–Eaton myasthenic syndrome occurs in association with autoimmune conditions such as rheumatoid arthritis, thyroid disease, and pernicious anaemia.

Proximal muscle weakness occurs in all patients and is the presenting symptom in 60 per cent of cases. This may be demonstrable clinically, or conversely may be difficult to detect as strength is augmented during the course of maximal effort. Reflexes may be depressed or absent, but are similarly enhanced after voluntary muscle contraction. Bulbar muscles are not usually involved, but if they are, the clinical features are mild. Cholinergic symptoms including impotence, blurred vision, and dry mouth are common. The diagnostic electromyographic feature is reduced amplitude of the compound muscle action potential evoked by supramaximal nerve stimulation, with enhancement (by more than 200 per cent) immediately after 10 to 15 s of maximal voluntary contraction or during high-frequency nerve stimulation. There is minimal or no improvement after administration of the short-acting anticholinesterase edrophonium (the Tensilon test), distinguishing Lambert–Eaton myasthenic syndrome from myasthenia gravis. Single-fibre electromyography may also demonstrate impairment of neuromuscular transmission. Lambert–Eaton myasthenic syndrome occurs over the age of 45 and is four times more common in men than women. The tumour usually presents soon after diagnosis of Lambert–Eaton myasthenic syndrome but sometimes up to 2 years later.

There is strong evidence for an autoimmune aetiology. The clinical, ultrastructural, and electrophysiological features of Lambert–Eaton myasthenic syndrome are thought to be due to an autoimmune attack directed against the voltage gated calcium channels on the presynaptic motor terminals. Antibodies against various subtypes of the voltage gated calcium channels have been identified, and are present in up to 85 per cent of patients.[56] It has been found that a positive result for antivoltage gated calcium channel antibodies by radioimmunoassay is highly specific for Lambert–Eaton myasthenic syndrome, and Lambert–Eaton myasthenic syndrome has been induced in animals by passive transfer of IgG from patients with the condition. Functional voltage gated calcium channels have been detected in small cell lung cancer cell lines.

There are reports of patients developing paraneoplastic Lambert–Eaton myasthenic syndrome in the absence of detectable antivoltage gated calcium channel antibodies, thus suggesting the presence of antibodies directed against different epitopes.[57] These may include the anti-Hu antibody, and an antisynaptotagmin antibody, which is directed against a synaptic vesicle protein.[58]

Therapy for Lambert–Eaton myasthenic syndrome should be individually determined, depending upon the severity of the disorder, the type of underlying malignancy, and the life expectancy of the patient. Most patients show improvement in parallel with the response of the tumour to effective antitumour therapy. In addition, corticosteroids, daily plasma exchange, and intravenous gammaglobulin can produce clinical and electrophysiological improvement. This probably occurs via an induced reduction in calcium channel antibodies, although the exact mechanism remains unclear. Oral 4-aminopyridine can be used to improve motor function. It stimulates release of acetylcholine at the neuromuscular junction, probably by increasing calcium influx during depolarization, but it does cross the blood–brain barrier and has a significant toxic effect on the central nervous system, causing confusion and fits. Oral 3,4-diaminopyridine improves motor and autonomic symptoms and electrophysiological abnormalities and appears to be less toxic.

Myasthenia gravis

Most patients with myasthenia gravis do not have an underlying neoplasm. About 10 per cent, however, have a thymoma and 30 per cent of patients presenting with thymoma have myasthenia gravis. There is no specific association with any other tumour type, although myasthenia gravis with Hodgkin's disease and resolution of myasthenic symptoms following treatment for Hodgkin's disease has been reported.

Ninety per cent of patients with myasthenia gravis and thymoma have detectable antibodies against titan, a non-acetylcholine receptor protein of striated muscle, and titan mRNA has also been identified in thymoma cells.[59]

Myasthenia gravis usually precedes diagnosis of thymoma. The diagnosis is confirmed by the Tensilon test. The administration of the short-acting anticholinesterase edrophonium (Tensilon) provokes a short-lived (2 to 10 min) increase in muscle strength, and electromyography shows a decremental motor response to repetitive nerve stimulation. Tumour resection rarely improves the symptoms of myasthenia gravis, and patients usually need treatment with long-acting anticholinesterases and steroids. Patients with myasthenia gravis and thymoma tend to be more difficult to manage than those with isolated myasthenia gravis, and may require plasmapheresis for rapidly progressive or chronic profound weakness. Survival is shorter than if there is no associated thymoma, and myasthenia gravis is the usual cause of death.

Syndromes involving muscle

Dermatomyositis and polymyositis

Dermatomyositis and polymyositis are acquired inflammatory myopathies which affect all ages. The classical clinical picture is that of the subacute development of symmetrical proximal muscle weakness with or without pain. In dermatomyositis there are also skin changes

of periorbital oedema and erythema (heliotrope rash), erythema/telangiectasia over the phalangeal joints, and erythema over the chest. The diagnosis is based upon the clinical and laboratory findings, including elevated serum muscle enzymes, i.e. creatanine kinase, lactate dehydrogenase, and aldolase, a myopathic picture on electromyography (fibrillation, insertion irritability, short polyphasic motor units), and muscle biopsy showing inflammatory degeneration of muscle.

A possible link between cancer and dermatomyositis/polymyositis has been reported since the early 1900s. However, the strength of this association remains unclear, and whether dermatomyositis/polymyositis are true paraneoplastic syndromes remains controversial. Zantos et al. analysed all published case control and cohort studies to evaluate the association of myositis and cancer.[60] They showed that there does appear to be an association of both polymyositis and dermatomyositis with cancer. The overall odds ratio for cancer associated with dermatomyositis was 4.4 (95 per cent confidence interval 3.0–6.6) and for polymyositis was 2.1 (95 per cent confidence interval 1.4–3.3). In patients with dermatomyositis the risk of cancer was high both before and after the diagnosis of cancer, thus suggesting that dermatomyositis is a true paraneoplastic syndrome, whilst in polymyositis the cancer risk was only high after the diagnosis of myositis. This suggests that polymyositis may not necessarily be a paraneoplastic disorder, but may occur in patients with an increased susceptibility to both myositis and to cancer.

The most common cancers associated with dermatomyositis/polymyositis are breast, lung, ovarian, and stomach. In females with dermatomyositis, ovarian cancer is the most overrepresented malignancy. The cancer often presents late, at an advanced stage, and has a poor prognosis. There have also been a number of reports of an association between dermatomyositis and melanoma and the development of dermatomyositis in patients with previously diagnosed melanoma may indicate the presence of metastatic disease.

Therefore, patients over 40 who present with dermatomyositis should be investigated for an underlying malignancy. The degree of investigation remains controversial, but should at least include chest radiography, mammography, pelvic assessment and carcinoembryonic antigen 125 (CA125) in women, and stool analysis for occult blood. Steroids are the generally recommended treatment, although there have been no controlled trials of their effects. Azathioprine has been used where steroids are ineffective, or to spare the steroid dose. Dermatomyositis/polymyositis may go into remission with effective antitumour treatment, and may worsen with progressive disease. However, inflammatory myopathies can fluctuate spontaneously, and in general the clinical course of dermatomyositis/polymyositis does not run parallel to that of the tumour.

Other paraneoplastic disorders of muscle

Polymyalgia rheumatica

Polymyalgia rheumatica occurs in elderly patients. This population group is also at increased risk of developing cancer; thus it is not clear if these two conditions are specifically associated. There have been reports of a polymyalgia rheumatica-like syndrome preceding either the initial diagnosis of cancer or the discovery of recurrence.[61]

Myopathy

Myopathy may develop in patients with Cushing's syndrome, hypercalcaemia, hyponatraemia, and, rarely, carcinoid syndrome. Carcinoid myopathy usually presents several years after the onset of carcinoid syndrome, with progressive proximal weakness. It is thought possibly to be due to the myopathic effects of secretion of serotonin or other substances by the tumour, and can respond to a serotonin antagonist such as cyproheptadine.

Acute necrotizing myopathy

Acute necrotizing myopathy is a rare complication of carcinoma. The myopathy is proximal, symmetrical, and painful. It initially involves the limbs and later the bulbar and respiratory muscles and is usually fatal. Creatinine kinase levels can be elevated, and electromyography demonstrates myopathic changes. Widespread necrosis of skeletal muscle with little or no inflammation can be seen on muscle biopsy. It can be found in association with a variety of tumour types including gastrointestinal adenocarcinoma, prostate cancer, bladder cancer, and non-small-cell lung cancer. Levin *et al.* reported on two out of four cases responding to of tumour resection and corticosteroids.[62] The cause is unknown, although an autoimmune pathogenesis has been postulated.[63]

Neuromyotonia

Neuromyotonia is a rare paraneoplastic complication presenting with muscle stiffness, cramping, and excessive sweating. There are both idiopathic and paraneoplastic forms of the disorder. Associations with lung cancer, Hodgkin's disease, and rectal cancer have been reported. Electrophysiological studies show abnormal high-frequency bursts of motor unit discharges. It may remit spontaneously or in response to anticonvulsants, or plasma exchange.

Haematological syndromes

Paraneoplastic syndromes involving either haematopoietic cells or the haemostatic system are common. The syndromes and their tumour associations are listed in Table 5.

Red cell disorders

Anaemia of chronic disease

The anaemia of chronic disease is one of the commonest paraneoplastic manifestations of cancer and accounts for approximately 15 per cent of all cases of anaemia. The cause of the anaemia is thought to be multifactorial, with potential mechanisms including:

- possible impairment of erythropoietin synthesis, or of the response of erythroblasts to erythropoietin;
- abnormal iron metabolism, with either a block in the transfer of iron from macrophages to developing erythroblasts or the induction of lactoferrin synthesis by granulocytes interfering with iron transport;
- decreased erythrocyte survival time.

Some of these effects may be mediated by cytokines secreted by activated macrophages such as IL-1 or tumour necrosis factor. Laboratory investigations show that plasma iron and saturation of iron-binding protein are both low, but ferritin levels are high. The diagnosis is one of exclusion, and it is important not to overlook correctable causes of anaemia, for example those secondary to the effects of tumour treatment, infiltration of marrow by tumour cells,

and iron-deficiency anaemia. Treatment, if required, is either with blood transfusions or with recombinant human erythropoietin.[64]

Haemolytic anaemia

Two types of haemolytic anaemia occur as paraneoplastic complications of cancer: autoimmune haemolytic anaemia and microangiopathic haemolytic anaemia (see below). Autoimmune haemolytic anaemia may be of warm or of cold antibody type.

Warm autoimmune haemolytic anaemia is associated with B-cell chronic lymphocytic leukaemia, B-cell non-Hodgkin's lymphoma, and Hodgkin's disease. The autoantibodies are usually polyclonal IgG, probably synthesized as a result of immune deregulation rather than antibody production by the malignant clone. The antibodies often react with membrane epitopes on all erythrocytes, but are occasionally of limited specificity. Some patients with warm autoimmune haemolytic anaemia also develop immune thrombocytopenia (Evans' syndrome), neutropenia, or pancytopenia. Serum autoantibody is detectable by the indirect antiglobulin test at 37 °C.

Cold-type autoimmune haemolytic anaemia is associated with B-cell lymphomas and chronic lymphocytic leukaemia. The autoantibody is usually complement-fixing IgM, a monoclonal product of the malignant clone, and is detected by agglutination of normal red cells at 4 °C. These autoantibodies often have specific reactivity, and unlike autoimmune haemolytic anaemia may be associated with intravascular haemolysis. Patients complain of purplish skin discoloration occurring particularly in the extremities (acrocyanosis). This is secondary to stasis in the peripheral circulation caused by red cell agglutination. Treatment is with steroids, although in refractory cases splenectomy may be required.

Red cell aplasia

Anaemia may be due to red cell aplasia, with failure of marrow erythropoiesis, and is a rare condition. One-third to one-half of patients with acquired pure red cell aplasia have an underlying malignancy and in nearly all cases this is a thymoma. There have been case reports of red cell aplasia associated with other malignancies, mainly the lymphoproliferative disorders. In patients with thymoma, the red cell aplasia is often associated with other paraneoplastic syndromes including hypogammaglobulinaemia and myasthenia gravis.[65] Around 50 per cent of patients respond to thymectomy, but often relapse later.

Erythrocytosis

Erythrocytosis is diagnosed in the presence of a raised haemoglobin, packed cell volume, and red cell mass (more than 55 per cent in men, 50 per cent in women). Erythrocytosis due to eutopic secretion of erythropoietin occurs in about 3 per cent of patients with renal cell carcinoma, although serum immunoreactive erythropoietin is elevated in up to 33 per cent of patients with this tumour, with no apparent haematological manifestations.[66] This suggests that in the majority of patients either erythropoietin is secreted as an inactive precursor, or there is a concurrent block in erythrocyte production. Erythropoietin mRNA has been demonstrated in tumour tissues, and erythropoietin has shown to be constitutively produced by tumour cells.[67] Erythropoietin can be detected immunohistochemically in paraffin-embedded tumour tissue using an antigen retrieval method, suggesting that this may be useful in confirming renal cell carcinomas.

Table 5 Main haematological syndromes and tumour associations

Syndromes	Associated tumours
Red cell disorders	
Autoimmune haemolytic anaemia	CLL, NHL, Hodgkin's disease
Red cell aplasia	Thymoma
Erythrocytosis	Renal, hepatoma, CNS, SCLC
White cell disorders	
Neutrophilia	Bladder, thyroid, NSCLC, SCLC
Eosinophilia	Hodgkin's disease
Platelet disorders	
Thrombocytopenia	CLL, Hodgkin's disease, NHL
Thrombocytosis	Hodgkin's disease, NHL, breast, SCLC, NSCLC, renal
Disorders of haemostasis	
Thromboembolic disease	Gastrointestinal tract, SCLC, NSCLC, prostate
Disseminated intravascular coagulation	Gastrointestinal tract, NSCLC, SCLC, prostate
Microangiopathic haemolytic anaemia	Gastrointestinal tract, prostate, NSCLC, SCLC
Non-bacterial thrombotic endocarditis	Gastrointestinal tract, NSCLC

CLL, chronic lymphocytic leukaemia. NHL, non-Hodgkin's lymphoma. CNS, central nervous system. SCLC, small cell lung cancer. NSCLC, non-small-cell lung cancer.

Excessive erythropoietin production also causes erythrocytosis in 3 to 12 per cent of patients with hepatoma and cerebellar haemangioblastomas, and has also been reported in association with Wilms' tumour, small cell lung cancer, thymic or adrenal carcinoid, benign renal tumours and cysts, uterine fibroids, and phaeochromocytoma. Secretion of beta adrenergic agonists by phaeochromocytomas, androgenic steroids by adrenal or ovarian tumours, or prostaglandins by uterine fibroids, may enhance normal erythropoietin secretion from the liver or kidney or increase the sensitivity to erythropoietin of responsive marrow precursor cells.

The degree of erythrocytosis caused by paraneoplastic syndromes is not usually high enough to cause symptoms and to require treatment. Phlebotomy is the treatment of choice. Control of the tumour will often control erythrocytosis.

White cell disorders

Neutropenia

Neutropenia (neutrophils $<1.0 \times 10^9$/litre) in cancer patients is most commonly due to infiltration of the marrow by malignant cells, or due to the myelosuppressive effects of treatment. Cases of paraneoplastic neutropenia have been reported, however, probably caused by interference with the effects of the haemopoietic colony stimulating factors.

Neutrophilia

Neutrophilia (neutrophils $>7.5 \times 10^9$/litre) is common and is most often due to tumour cell production of haemopoietic colony stimulating factors. This has been reported in patients with tumours of the bladder, thyroid, lung, and with lymphomas, as well as being a common feature of hepatic metastases. Tumour cells often produce a number of haemopoietic colony stimulating factors. Patients with lung cancer and neutrophilia show constitutive expression of granulocyte, macrophage, and granulocyte–macrophage colony stimulating factor genes in tumour cells, as well as increased plasma levels

of these haemopoietic colony stimulating factors. These levels return to normal upon removal of the tumour.[68]

Eosinophilia

Eosinophilia (eosinophils $>440 \times 10^9$/litre) occurs in 5 per cent of patients with Hodgkin's disease, and in occasional patients with solid tumours such as melanoma and hepatocellular carcinoma. In patients with Hodgkin's disease the eosinophil count may be as high as $(20–40) \times 10^9$/litre, possibly due to excess tumour cell production of an eosinophil growth factor such as IL-5.

Platelet disorders

Thrombocytopenia

Thrombocytopenia (platelets $<100 \times 10^9$/litre) in cancer patients is usually due to treatment-induced myelosuppression, marrow infiltration, or disseminated intravascular coagulation (see below) with increased peripheral platelet destruction. Idiopathic thrombocytopenia is a frequent complication of chronic lymphocytic leukaemia, and has also been reported in Hodgkin's disease and non-Hodgkin's lymphomas. It is associated with raised levels of platelet-associated IgG autoantibodies. Paraneoplastic idiopathic thrombocytopenia is a rare finding in solid tumours such as those of the lung, gut, or ovary.

Thrombocytosis

Thrombocytosis (platelets $>400 \times 10^9$/litre) is found in up to 30 per cent of patients with untreated cancer, and especially in those with Hodgkin's or non-Hodgkin's lymphoma and cancers of the lung, breast, and kidney. This secondary thrombocytosis is generally mild (platelet count $(400–700) \times 10^9$/litre), asymptomatic, and does not require specific treatment. The cause of paraneoplastic thrombocytosis is thought to be production by the tumour of thrombopoietic cytokines such as IL-6 and granulocyte–macrophage colony stimulating factor.[69],[70] In a prospective study of 663 children (less than 16 years of age) presenting with thrombocytosis there was a 2 per cent incidence of undiagnosed malignancy; a study of 777 adults found to have thrombocytosis on presentation to hospital found a 5.9 per cent incidence of underlying malignancy. These results suggest that a search for an underlying malignancy may be warranted in patients presenting with thrombocytosis.[71],[72]

Pancytopenia

Hasle *et al.* reported eight children with pancytopenia who went on to develop acute lymphoblastic leukaemia, and suggested that the pancytopenia represented a possible paraneoplastic manifestation early in the development of acute lymphoblastic leukaemia.[73] The pancytopenia may be mediated by inhibition of normal marrow development by clonally expanding cells. Possible paraneoplastic pancytopenia has also been reported associated with carcinoma of the lung. Antitumour treatment may lead to improvement in blood counts.

Disorders of haemostasis

Armand Trousseau was the first to report of an association between cancer and an increased incidence of venous thrombosis.[74] Patients with cancer commonly harbour many abnormalities of the haemostatic system. These abnormalities can be multifaceted and require careful investigation to permit appropriate management.[75] The most common abnormality is thrombocytopenia (see above). Abnormalities associated with hypercoagulability and haemorrhage present in variable numbers of patients, depending upon the type of tumour and the anticancer treatment given. Edwards *et al.* found that prior to antitumour treatment, 8 per cent of patients had elevated levels of fibrinogen degradation products, and 48 per cent had elevated levels of fibrinogen; 14 per cent had abnormal prothrombin times.[76]

The pathophysiology of paraneoplastic haemostatic disorders is complex. They appear to be brought about by a number of different mechanisms, including platelet activation by cancer cells, interaction between vascular endothelium and tumour cells, and tumour cell activation of the clotting cascade.[77] Tumour cells can aggregate on both normal and damaged vascular endothelium, and can also damage endothelium directly. Following this, interaction with platelets and the coagulation system can lead to thrombus formation. With respect to the coagulation system, tumour cells can either directly or indirectly cause the breakdown of fibrinogen to fibrin and fibrinopeptides. They can also produce a number of different factors which stimulate the system:

- tissue factor molecules that bind to factor VII and stimulate the extrinsic coagulation pathway;
- a cysteine proteinase which activates factor X; and
- a tissue factor on microvesicles shed by the tumour cells which binds to factor VII.

In addition to the activation of a prothrombotic state, there is an associated down-regulation of antithrombotic mechanisms including reduced antithrombin III levels, and thrombomodulin levels.

Alterations in the fibrinolytic system may also play a role in tumour growth and production of metastases.[78] Fibrinolysis has an important role in providing nutrition for growth of cancer cells and in enabling movement of cells from their site of origin. Excessive expression of urokinase-type plasminogen activator, and tissue plasminogen activator by tumour cells can increase the degradation of extracellular matrix proteins and lead to more rapid growth and spread. Increased expression of urokinase-type plasminogen activator has been associated with decreased survival in a number of different cancer types.

Although nearly all patients with cancer have some degree of activation of the coagulation system, it is usually asymptomatic. Approximately 15 per cent of patients will have clinical manifestations with bleeding, thrombosis, or embolism. There are several defined clinical syndromes described below.

Thromboembolic disease

Thromboembolic disease is a common complication of cancers, presenting either as a deep venous thrombosis/pulmonary embolus or as migratory thrombophlebitis. A syndrome of progressive arterial occlusion with symptoms of intermittent claudication or ischaemic heart disease has also been described.[79] Thromboembolic disease is classically associated with mucin-secreting tumours of the gastrointestinal tract, including the pancreas, stomach, and colon, and also with adenocarcinomas of the lung and prostate cancer. Vitamin K antagonists such as warfarin are ineffective, and intravenous heparin should be used for at least 3 to 4 days. Continuous intravenous treatment may achieve the best control, but subcutaneous heparin may be substituted, aiming to keep the partial thromboplastin time at least one and a half times the normal value. If effective antitumour treatment is available, it may be possible to stop heparin, but otherwise anticoagulation should be continued to avoid severe thromboembolism. Arterial thrombosis can be treated with embolectomy and intravenous anticoagulation, although the condition is often resistant to treatment and is progressive.

Thrombotic episodes may precede the diagnosis of cancer. It has been reported that up to 10 per cent of patients presenting with thromboembolic disease will have occult malignancy, with the possibility of an occult malignancy increasing if the patient presenting with thromboembolic disease is over 50 years of age.[80] Whether an extensive search for an underlying malignancy is appropriate in a patient presenting with primary thromboembolic disease is controversial. Sorensen *et al.* reported a case control study of patients with primary deep vein thrombosis/pulmonary embolus in Denmark.[81] They concluded that although there was an increased risk of several types of cancers in these patients, an aggressive search for a hidden primary cancer was not warranted. This conclusion was based upon the number of patients that would be needed to be screened to pick up the cancers, the cost of such screening, and the lack of impact on the management of the cancer. However, other authors have found that extensive testing may be appropriate in certain situations.[82] A limited investigation with chest radiography, mammogram, CA125, and pelvic ultrasound (women), and prostate specific antigen (PSA) (men) has been recommended.[83]

Disseminated intravascular coagulation

Disseminated intravascular coagulation is characterized by inappropriate and excessive activation of haemostasis.[84] Approximately 60 per cent of clinical cases of disseminated intravascular coagulation are associated with septicaemia. There are two common paraneoplastic associations:

(i) Most patients with acute promyelocytic leukaemia have disseminated intravascular coagulation, particularly following chemotherapy when rapid killing of tumour cells leads to the release of procoagulant(s) from cytoplasmic granules.

(ii) Disseminated intravascular coagulation may complicate mucin-secreting adenocarcinomas, especially cancer of the pancreas, lung, stomach, and prostate.

The major abnormalities in patients with disseminated intravascular coagulation are a prolonged prothrombin time, a low fibrinogen level (<1.0 g/litre, normal 1.5–4 g/litre), and thrombocytopenia (<100×10^9/litre, normal >250×10^9/litre). Patients with acute disseminated intravascular coagulation usually have levels of fibrinogen degradation product above 100 μg/ml (normal <10 μg/ml). An elevated level of fibrinogen degradation product and a platelet count below 100×10^9/litre are virtually diagnostic of disseminated intravascular coagulation, especially if associated with a generalized bleeding diathesis.[85]

Disseminated intravascular coagulation may be low grade and asymptomatic, or overt and acute with bleeding and/or thrombosis. Asymptomatic patients with abnormal clotting tests probably need no treatment, although persistence of low-grade coagulopathy may be related to progression of the tumour. The most important aspects of treatment are effective treatment of precipitating factors, i.e. antitumour therapy and treatment of infection. Bleeding should be treated with vigorous replacement therapy with fresh frozen plasma, cryoprecipitate (factor VIII), and platelets. The use of heparin is controversial; at low dose (100 to 200 units per hour intravenously) it may be beneficial in patients with acute promyelocytic leukaemia. All-*trans* retinoic acid has been shown to be the tumour treatment of choice in acute promyelocytic leukaemia.

Microangiopathic haemolytic anaemia

Microangiopathic haemolytic anaemia occurs:[86],[87]

(i) With vascular tumours, including giant haemangioma and haemangioendothelioma.

(ii) In association with disseminated intravascular coagulation complicating acute promyelocytic leukaemia or carcinoma.

(iii) In rare cases in association with widespread metastatic adenocarcinoma, especially of the gastrointestinal tract, lung, and prostate.

Intravascular tumour cells can damage red cells directly, and can stimulate the formation of fibrin microthrombi which cause fragmentation of red cells. Clinically, microangiopathic haemolytic anaemia is characterized by acute, severe haemolytic anaemia, often accompanied by a bleeding diathesis. The peripheral blood film shows fragmented red cells, nucleated red cells, and a marked reticulocytosis. The total white cell count is often elevated, with a leucoerythroblastic picture, and thrombocytopenia may be present. Up to 60 per cent of patients show involvement of tumour cells in the marrow, but uninvolved marrow shows erythroid hyperplasia and normal or increased levels of megakaryocytes. Heparin and transfusions of blood and plasma may lead to transient improvement in coagulopathy, bleeding diathesis, and anaemia, but most patients die within a few weeks. Effective tumour treatment may help in controlling the microangiopathic haemolytic anaemia.

Non-bacterial thrombotic endocarditis

Non-bacterial thrombotic endocarditis (sometimes called marantic endocarditis) is found in around 1 per cent of patients with advanced cancer. Sterile platelet/fibrin vegetation is found on the mitral and/or aortic valves, which can be demonstrated by echocardiography. The common tumour associations are adenocarcinoma of the lung and adenocarcinoma of the gastrointestinal tract, especially the colon. The typical clinical features are caused by systemic emboli and include acute focal neurological symptoms or diffuse encephalopathy secondary to cerebral emboli. Therapy is to treat the underlying malignancy.

Vasculitic conditions

Vasculitic syndromes associated with malignancy include temporal arteritis, Raynaud's phenomenon, polyarteritis nodosa, leucocytoclastic vasculitis, systemic lupus erythematosus, and others. These are discussed below under rheumatic disorders.

Paraneoplastic conditions of the skin

There are many different paraneoplastic conditions associated with the skin. The major conditions and their tumour associations are listed in Table 6 and examples are illustrated in Fig. 5 (and see Plate 1). The mechanism in most cases is unknown.

Disorders of pigmentation

Acanthosis nigricans

The association of acanthosis nigricans with internal malignancy was first recognized in the late nineteenth century. The symptoms of this disorder are itchy, brown, hyperkeratotic plaques principally affecting the flexures including the axilla. Occasionally there is generalized skin thickening and hyperpigmentation.[88] Acanthosis nigricans is associated with endocrine abnormalities (obesity, polycystic ovaries, acromegaly, hypothyroidism) and with malignancies, or it can be inherited or idiopathic. In a review of tumour-associated cases, approximately three-quarters of patients had intra-abdominal tumours, with gastric adenocarcinoma making up the majority of these.[89] The appearance of skin lesions may precede the diagnosis of malignancy by up to 16 years. The tumour at diagnosis is often highly malignant, metastatic, and is associated with a poor prognosis.

'Tripe palms' describes thickened, velvety palms with pronounced dermatoglyphics which can occur with acanthosis nigricans, especially in patients with lung or gastric cancer.[90] The cause of acanthosis nigricans as a paraneoplastic disorder is unclear, but it may involve an endocrine effect of secretion of transforming growth factor-α by the tumour. The mucocutaneous lesions seen in acanthosis nigricans have been treated with radiotherapy.

The sign of Leser-Trelat

This sign describes the sudden appearance of, or increase in number and size of, seborrhoeic keratoses.[91] There is a frequent association with pruritus and acanthosis nigricans. The sign is usually seen in patients with advanced metastatic malignancy, mainly of the gastrointestinal tract. This condition may also be associated with

Table 6 Main dermatological syndromes and tumour associations

Syndromes	Associated tumours
Disorders of pigmentation	
Acanthosis nigricans	Gastrointestinal tract, NSCLC, SCLC
The sign of Leser-Trelat	Gastrointestinal tract
Sweet's syndrome	AML, myeloproliferative diseases
Paget's disease	Breast
Erythematous conditions	
Erythromelalgia	Myeloproliferative diseases
Necrolytic migratory erythema	Glucagonoma—pancreatic islet alpha-cell tumour
Erythema annulare centrifugum	Hodgkin's disease, NSCLC, SCLC, prostate
Erythema gyratum repens	Breast, NSCLC, SCLC, GIT
Flushing	Carcinoid, medullary carcinoma of the thyroid
Pyoderma gangrenosum	Monoclonal gammopathy, myeloma, NHL, leukaemia
Bullous conditions	
Bullous pemphigoid	CLL, NHL
Dermatitis herpetiformis	NHL
Pemphigus vulgaris	NHL, thymoma, Kaposi's sarcoma
Conditions characterized by hypertrichosis	
Acquired ichthyosis	Hodgkin's disease, NHL, testis, ovary, SCLC
Tylosis	Oesophageal
Bazex's paraneoplastic acrokeratosis	Squamous cell carcinoma of larynx/pharynx
Acquired hypertrichosis	NSCLC, gastrointestinal tract
Pruritus	NHL, Hodgkin's disease, leukaemia, CNS

NSCLC, non-small-cell lung cancer. SCLC, small cell lung cancer. AML, acute myeloid leukaemia. NHL, non-Hodgkin's lymphoma. CLL, chronic lymphocytic leukaemia. CNS, central nervous system.

overexpression of transforming growth factor-α by the tumour and epidermal growth factor receptor by the target skin lesions. Because keratosis and cancer are both common in the elderly, it is not always easy to determine if the sign is present, and controversy still exists whether in fact such a paraneoplastic relationship exists.

Sweet's syndrome

Sweet's syndrome presents clinically with erythematous raised plaques associated with fever and neutrophilia, and occasionally with pulmonary infiltrates. It occurs primarily on the face and upper limbs, and in up to 20 per cent of cases is associated with an underlying malignancy, mainly haematological: acute myeloid leukemia, myeloproliferative disorders, and lymphoproliferative disorders. Histology of the lesions demonstrates a superficial dermis infiltrated primarily by mature neutrophils; vasculitis is not present. It can precede or present concurrently with the tumour, and treatment is with corticosteroids.[92]

Paget's disease of the nipple

Paget's disease can be associated with breast cancer, affecting the breast by causing erythematous keratotic patches over the areolae. It can also be extramammary with erythematous exudative lesions in the anogenital region. Diagnosis is often late as the lesion can appear very similar to candidiasis. Histological examination shows classic Paget's cells within the epidermis. In approximately half the cases there is an underlying malignancy, usually of the affected area, i.e. rectum, anus, or vagina.[93] Treatment is local with resection and/or radiotherapy.

Erythematous conditions

There are several rare cutaneous markers of malignancy in which erythema is the main skin manifestation. The most common paraneoplastic erythematous conditions are erythromelalgia, necrolytic migratory erythema, erythema annulare centrifugum, erythema gyratum repens, flushing, and pyoderma gangrenosum.[94]–[97] These are summarized in Table 7.

Bullous conditions

Bullous pemphigoid

Bullous pemphigoid occurs in elderly patients and may be associated with tumours such as lymphoma and chronic lymphocytic leukaemia simply by chance. Nevertheless, an increasing number of cases are described in the literature, supporting a paraneoplastic entity characterized by distinctive clinical, histopathological, and immunological features.[98] Clinically, there are mucocutaneous erosive and bullous eruptions, histological examination of which shows suprabasilar acantholysis and the presence of necrotic keratinocytes. Immunoflouresence reveals circulating autoantibodies in the intracellular spaces of different types of epithelia. These antibodies immunoprecipitate a number of proteins: desmoplakin I and II, bullous pemphigoid antigen, and a specific 190 kDa antigen.[99] The condition has a poor prognosis.

Dermatitis herpetiformis

Dermatitis herpetiformis is a lifelong, gluten-sensitive skin disorder characterized by chronic, intensely itchy vesicles (subepidermal bullae)

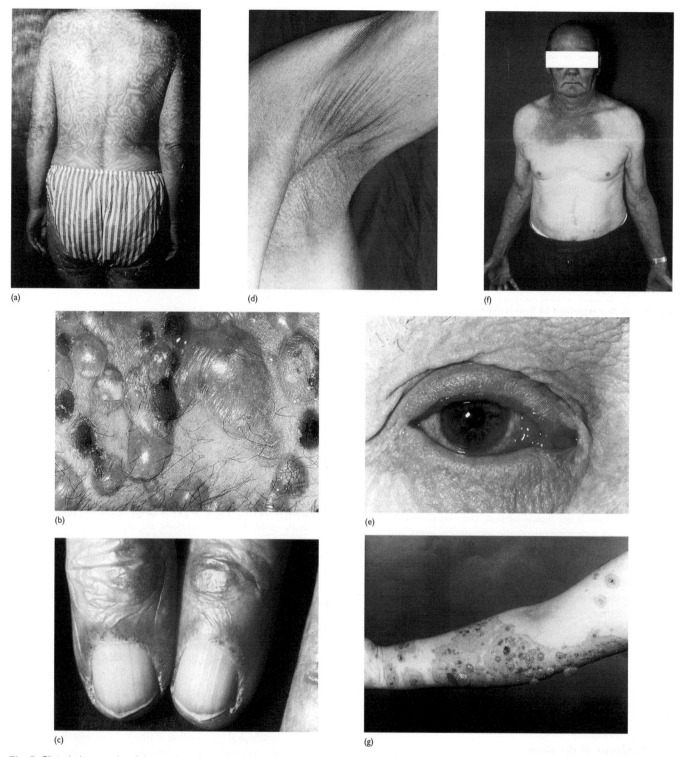

(a)

(d)

(f)

(b)

(e)

(c)

(g)

Fig. 5 Clinical photographs of dermatological paraneoplastic conditions. (See also Plate 1.)

over the elbows, knees, and lumbosacral region. Histological features include subepidermal blisters and neutrophilic abscesses. Most patients also have a degree of villous atrophy on jejunal biopsy, although clinical malabsorption is rare. Granular IgA can be detected at the dermoepidermal junction by direct immunofluorescence. The major tumour association is with non-Hodgkin's lymphoma, particularly arising in the jejunum, although association with other malignancies has been reported, including lung cancer and bladder

Table 7 Paraneoplastic erythematous skin conditions

Condition	Rash	Pathological findings	Other features	Treatment
Erythromelalgia	Episodes of painful erythema of the extremities. Precipitated by exposure to heat, exercise	Platelet thrombi in arterioles	Can be secondary to rheumatoid arthritis, systemic lupus erythematosus, diabetes, pregnancy. Often greatly precedes malignancy	Elevation of affected region, exposure to cold
Necrolytic migratory erythema	Ring-like areas of erythema→ vesicles/bullae→burst→crust→ scaling and hyperpigmentation. On face, vulva, lower limbs	Superficial epidermal necrosis, neutrophil infiltration and vacuolated keratinocytes	Typical in middle-aged diabetic females. Stomatitis, anaemia, weight loss, serum glucagon 1000–5000 pg/ml (n = <200)	Long-acting somatostatin analogues
Erythema annulare centrifugum	Annular erythematous lesions with raised edges, slowly migrate	Perivascular infiltrate, mainly lymphocytic	Can be secondary to infection	
Erythema gyratum repens	Parallel curving red bands with scaly edge—'woodgrain' pattern. Moves daily; trunk and limbs	Perivascular lymphocytic infiltration	Pruritus may be severe	Antitumour treatment, oral corticosteroids
Flushing	Sudden reddening of face, neck and upper trunk		Related to serotonin release	
Pyoderma gangrenosum	Painful ulcerating nodules/ vesicopustules. Swollen red/blue edge, heals with scarring. Painful concentric superficial bullae with blue/grey haloes	Heavy neutrophilic infiltrate, fibrinoid necrosis, haemorrhage and capillary engorgement	Associated with ulcerative colitis, Crohn's disease, rheumatoid arthritis. No cause found in over a third of patients	Oral corticosteroids and antitumour treatment

cancer. There may be a long time lag between the diagnosis of dermatitis herpetiformis and a subsequently diagnosed malignancy. It is not yet clear if a gluten-free diet will reduce the risk of malignancy in dermatitis herpetiformis, and the issue is controversial.[100]

Pemphigus vulgaris

Pemphigus vulgaris consists of intraepidermal bullae with erosions, and histology shows suprabasal acantholysis and a perivascular lymphocytic infiltrate. Indirect immunofluorescence reveals detectable levels of circulating antibodies directed against the keratinocyte cell surface. It is associated with lymphoma, Kaposi's sarcoma, and thymoma.

Conditions characterized by scaling or hypertrichosis

Acquired ichthyosis

Acquired ichthyosis describes generalized scaliness of the skin, particularly of the face and trunk, due to thickening of the stratum corneum. Hodgkin's disease is the commonest malignant association, and the skin abnormality usually appears weeks or months after other manifestations of the disease. Other tumour associations include non-Hodgkin's lymphoma, carcinomas of the lung, testis, and ovary, Kaposi's sarcoma (with or without AIDS), and mycosis fungoides. The skin condition and the malignancy may run a parallel course and the cause is unknown. Acquired ichthyosis can complicate non-malignant conditions including sarcoidosis, AIDS, systemic lupus erythematosus and is a side-effect of drugs such as clofazimine and nicotinic acid.[101]

Non-epidermolytic palmoplantar keratoderma (tylosis)

This condition is characterized by massive thickening of the skin of the palms and soles. It can be isolated, but in certain families has been associated with oesophageal carcinoma.[102] In these families, the tylosis is inherited as an autosomal dominant defect of keratinization with a late onset, usually becoming apparent at 7 to 8 years of age. The disease locus has been mapped to chromosome 17.

Bazex's paraneoplastic acrokeratosis

This condition consists of erythematous scaly involvement of the hands, feet, ears, and bridge of the nose. It is strongly associated with cancer, and is particularly associated with squamous tumours of the laryngopharyngeal region, including metastatic squamous carcinoma in cervical lymph nodes without an identifiable primary. The course of the skin lesions often parallels the course of the tumour.[103] If the cancer is untreatable, then oral retinoids have been proposed as a treatment strategy.

Acquired hypertrichosis

This is usually a side-effect of drugs including spironolactone, phenytoin, and minoxidil. 'Hypertrichosis lanuginosa acquisita' describes the acquired generalized growth of fair, downy hair without signs of virilization. It has been associated in around 30 patients with an underlying carcinoma of the lung or colon.

Other dermatological conditions

Pruritus

Pruritus is one of the commonest skin symptoms of patients with underlying tumours, and an associated malignancy can be found in up to 11 per cent of patients presenting with pruritus.[101] It is a characteristic complaint (B symptom) in lymphomas, and is also common in other haematological malignancies (leukaemias, multiple myeloma etc.). It can also occur in patients with brain tumours, where it may be associated with hyperkeratosis and vitiligo or hyperpigmentation.[104]

Calcinosis cutis

Calcinosis cutis consists of dermal/subcutaneous deposition of calcium phosphate and carbonate which can occur in association with destruction of bone secondary to metastatic carcinoma, multiple myeloma, and leukaemia. This condition is characterized by the slow development of hard nodules under the skin, which ultimately ulcerate.

Porphyria

Porphyria is a rare paraneoplastic complication of liver tumours. A clinical picture resembling porphyria cutania tarda (photosensitivity, increased skin fragility, hypertrichosis, and hyperpigmentation) has been described in around 10 cases of malignant hepatoma and a few cases with liver metastases or benign hepatoma.[105] Porphyrin fluorescence has been shown in a biopsy specimen of liver tumour but not in normal hepatocytes or erythrocytes, suggesting porphyrin synthesis by the tumour. The biochemical abnormality lies in hepatic uroporphyrinogen decarboxylase. The definitive treatment is resection, but where complete resection is not feasible, local arterial perfusion with cytotoxic drugs may reduce tumour bulk and symptoms of porphyria.

Dermatomyositis

This is discussed above.

Paraneoplastic rheumatic disorders

Paraneoplastic rheumatic disorders can present with predominant articular or systemic involvement.[1] The incidence of occult cancer in patients presenting with a rheumatic disorder of new onset has been found to be up to 23 per cent.[106] The main syndromes and their tumour associations are listed in Table 8.

Articular

Arthritis

Although many patients with cancer may coincidentally have arthritis, there is a specific association between cancer, particularly lung cancer and the haematological malignancies, and a seronegative polyarthritis.[107] The condition may be clinically indistinguishable from rheumatoid arthritis but some patients have atypical features, including very acute onset, monoarticular or asymmetrical involvement, or unusual distribution favouring the lower limbs. Most patients lack circulating rheumatoid factor or radiological evidence of joint erosion.

In some cases the arthritis clearly parallels the clinical course of the tumour, with remission induced by effective antitumour treatment, and exacerbation of arthritis with tumour relapse. Apart from specific antitumour treatment, joint symptoms can be treated with analgesics and anti-inflammatory drugs. Possible mechanisms include the production of antitumour antibodies cross-reacting with determinants expressed on normal cartilage. There is conflicting evidence that immune complexes formed between tumour antigens and host antitumour antibodies may be deposited within the joints in these patients.[1]

Finger clubbing and hypertrophic osteoarthropathy

Hypertrophic osteoarthropathy is characterized by finger clubbing and new periosteal bone formation. It can be classified as primary (usually hereditary) or secondary (generalized or localized). Secondary causes include pulmonary and cardiac diseases, hepatic disease, and mediastinal disease. In all of these secondary disease groupings there are both malignant and non-malignant conditions. The most common tumour type is non-small-cell lung cancer, where finger clubbing/hypertrophic osteoarthropathy is the presenting feature in 1 per cent of patients. However, on close review, 10 to 20 per cent of patients with non-small-cell lung cancer have clinical features of the condition.[108] Other associated tumour types include liver, breast, oesophageal, and thymoma. It is extremely rare in children, although it has been reported in association with childhood Hodgkin's disease.

Patients with hypertrophic osteoarthropathy complain of pain and swelling, affecting the metacarpophalangeal joints in particular; the knees, ankles, wrists, and occasionally the elbows and shoulders may also be involved. Physical examination shows finger clubbing (enlargement of the paronychial soft tissue with loss of the angle between the nail and the skin) and tenderness over the adjacent long bones (periostitis). Radiographs show periosteal shadowing due to new bone formation and a bone scan may show increased uptake over the shafts of affected bones.

The pathogenesis of this condition is unclear, but a number of hypotheses have been formulated. These include abnormalities in the 'endothelium/platelet unit'; abnormal levels of hepatocyte growth factor, or increased levels of transforming growth factor-β1. Measures which reportedly cause symptomatic improvement include nonsteroidal anti-inflammatory agents, corticosteroids, intercostal nerve section, local radiotherapy, and pamidronate. The symptoms, signs, and radiographic and radionuclide imaging abnormalities improve within 2 to 6 months of effective antitumour treatment.[108]

Systemic disorders

There are a number of systemic rheumatological conditions associated with cancer. These include connective tissue diseases such as Sjögrens syndrome, systemic lupus erythematosus, and scleroderma and vasculitides such as polyarteritis nodosa and Sweet's syndrome.

Connective tissue diseases

Systemic lupus erythematosus

There is controversy about whether systemic lupus erythematosus can be a paraneoplastic manifestation of malignancy. Sweeney *et al.* found no increased incidence of malignancy in patients with systemic lupus erythematosus, whilst Mallemkjaer *et al.* did find an relationship between systemic lupus erythematosus and non-Hodgkin's lymphoma,

Table 8 Main rheumatological syndromes and tumour associations

Syndromes	Associated tumours
Articular syndromes	
Arthritis	NSCLC, SCLC, leukaemia, NHL
Finger clubbing and hypertrophic osteoarthropathy	NSCLC, hepatic, thymoma, oesophageal
Systemic syndromes	
Connective tissue disorders	
Systemic lupus erythematosus	NHL, hepatic, NSCLC, genitourinary tract
Sjögren's syndrome	NHL
Reflex sympathetic dystrophy	CNS, ovary, breast, lung
Scleroderma	Lung
Raynaud's phenomenon	Renal, gastrointestinal tract, lung, ovary
Vasculitis	HCL, NHL, Hodgkin's disease, lung, gastrointestinal tract, renal

NSCLC, non-small-cell lung cancer. SCLC, small cell lung cancer. NHL, non-Hodgkin's lymphoma. CNS, central nervous system. HCL, hairy cell leukaemia.

lung cancer, liver cancer, and cancer of the lower female genital tract.[109],[110] In cases of malignancy developing after the diagnosis of systemic lupus erythematosus, it can be difficult to distinguish between a true paraneoplastic effect and the possible predisposing effect of chronic use of immunosuppressive agents.

Sjögren's syndrome

Sjögren's syndrome is a chronic autoimmune inflammatory disease which is characterized by progressive proliferation of lymphocytes in exocrine glands which eventually leads to destruction of the gland. Sjögren's syndrome can be primary or secondary (developing in association with a connective tissue disease such as rheumatoid arthritis). Patients present clinically with lymph node enlargement in the parotid and cervical regions with associated xerostomia. The proliferating lymphocytes (primarily CD4+ T cells) can also invade other organs, i.e. lungs, spleen, and kidney, to cause pathological effects. In addition, there is a strong association between Sjögren's syndrome and lymphoproliferative malignancies, in particular B-cell non-Hodgkin's lymphoma. The proposed mechanism is chronic overstimulation of B lymphocytes leading to clonal transformation and development of lymphoma. The involvement of Epstein–Barr virus has been postulated, but recent studies have not supported this.[111] The majority of lymphomas are of low-grade marginal zone type. In view of the high risk of developing lymphoma (a 44-times greater risk compared with the normal population), early detection of malignant transformation is important.[112] Predictive factors include clinical features such as rapid lymph node and parotid enlargement; and laboratory factors such as the presence of mixed monoclonal cryoglobulinaemia, and detection of immunoglobulins with the cross-reactive idiotypes 17109 and G-6.[112]

Reflex sympathetic dystrophy syndrome

Reflex sympathetic dystrophy syndrome is characterized by non-segmental pain and swelling in the extremities, trophic skin changes, vasomotor instability, and localized osteoporosis. It has been described as a paraneoplastic effect of tumours of the brain, lung, ovary, and breast. The shoulder–hand variant of reflex sympathetic dystrophy syndrome has been particularly described in association with carcinoma of the ovary.

Scleroderma (systemic sclerosis)

This is a condition affecting multiple organ systems and is characterized by fibrosis of the skin, lungs, gastrointestinal tract, heart, and blood vessels. There is no obvious causative agent, although numerous immunological abnormalities have been found in patients with the disorder. There have been a number of studies suggesting an association between cancer and scleroderma.[113] The strongest association appears to be with lung cancer.

Raynaud's phenomenon

Raynaud's phenomenon is characterized by episodic digital ischaemia. Clinically, there is a triphasic colour response (blanching, cyanosis, and rubor) of the affected digit in response to exposure to the cold and subsequent rewarming. Raynaud's phenomenon can be idiopathic, or can be secondary, when it is associated with diseases such as the connective tissue disorders, blood dyscrasias, trauma, and arterial occlusive disease. It is associated with a number of solid tumours including kidney, lung, gastrointestinal tract, and ovary.[114] It can also occur secondary to the hyperviscosity caused by paraproteinaemia in diseases such as Waldenström's macroglobulinaemia.

Palmar fasciitis

This condition is characterized by a rapidly progressive fasciitis of the palmar area with associated inflammatory arthritis. It has been associated with ovarian adenocarcinoma and often precedes the diagnosis of malignancy. The condition often parallels the course of the tumour.

Vasculitis

The vasculitides are a broad group of disorders characterized by inflammation of blood vessels resulting in organ damage and dysfunction. They include Henoch–Schonlein purpura, cryoglobulinaemia, granulomatous vasculitis, polyarteritis nodosa, and leucocytoclastic vasculitis.[115] Up to 5 per cent of patients with a vasculitic condition will be found to have an underlying malignancy. The most common associated malignancies are hairy cell leukaemia, myelodysplastic syndrome, the lymphomas, and lung, colon, and renal cell carcinoma. Immune complex deposition or activation of T cells by tumour-derived antigens appears to be the most likely mechanism.

The most common malignancy associated with a paraneoplastic vasculitis is hairy cell leukaemia, which is associated primarily with a cutaneous leucocytoclastic vasculitis or with polyarteritis nodosa.[116] The leucocytoclastic vasculitis commonly precedes the diagnosis of hairy cell leukaemia. A lymphocytic vasculitis with perivascular invasion by non-malignant T lymphocytes has also been reported to be a relatively common paraneoplastic condition in non-Hodgkin's lymphoma and chronic lymphocytic leukaemia. Sweet's syndrome (acute febrile neutrophilic dermatosis) is a vasculitic-type disorder characterized by fever, neutrophilia, and an erythematous papular rash over the upper part of the body and head. It has been reported that up to 16 per cent of patients with Sweet's syndrome have an underlying malignancy, predominantly haematological.[92] It is further described above in the section on paraneoplastic conditions of the skin.

Whether to search for an occult malignancy in a patient presenting with a rheumatological disorder, and to what extent, is controversial. Naschitz *et al.* proposed a series of clinical groups in which a thorough malignant work-up could be justified:[107]

(i) Asymmetric Raynaud's disease presenting at an age of more than 50 years.

(ii) Cutaneous leucocytoclastic vasculitis presenting at an age of more than 50 years.

(iii) Palmer fasciitis and arthritis, or eosinophilic fasciitis unresponsive to steroids.

(iv) Monoclonal gammopathy in a patient with rheumatoid arthritis.

(v) Sudden onset of an asymmetrical polyarthritis, especially of the lower limbs, in a patient aged over 50 years, without circulating rheumatoid factor.

Renal syndromes

Non-renal malignancies can involve the kidneys in many ways. The kidneys are often affected by cancer treatments, i.e. cisplatin-induced nephropathy, and can also be affected by the infiltration of tumour cells as seen in acute leukaemia. Common paraneoplastic syndromes occur secondary to endocrine abnormalities (e.g. inappropriate antidiuretic hormone secretion, which leads to renal sodium loss and hyponatraemia; this and other endocrine-related paraneoplastic syndromes are discussed elsewhere. The other renal paraneoplastic syndromes can be grouped into those affecting the glomerulus, i.e. the glomerular nephropathies, and those affecting the renal tubular system.

Glomerular disorders

Glomerular disease develops in 6 to 10 per cent of patients with cancer.[117] The strongest association has been described between carcinomas, usually lung, breast, and gastrointestinal tract cancer, and the development of membranous nephropathy. Membranous

nephropathy usually presents with hypertension, microscopic haematuria, and nephrotic syndrome (proteinuria, oedema, and hyperlipidaemia), and its clinical course is variable, ranging from spontaneous remission to end-stage renal failure. The incidence of an underlying malignancy in patients presenting with membranous nephropathy has been reported to range from 5.8 per cent to 22 per cent.[118] The malignancy can present before, after, or simultaneously with the renal disease, although it tends to present either before or concurrently, thus supporting the paraneoplastic nature of the membranous nephropathy. There have also been reports of membranous nephropathy paralleling the clinical course of the tumour.

The mechanism by which a tumour causes membranous nephropathy is uncertain, although there have been reports of circulating immune complexes containing tumour antigens which may then lodge in the glomerular basement membrane leading to the development of membranous nephropathy. There is controversy over whether to investigate all patients presenting with membranous nephropathy for an underlying malignancy, although there appears to be support for investigating patients presenting over the age of 40, in particular for lung, breast, and gastrointestinal tract tumours.[119] Treatment of the condition is a combination of specific anticancer therapy with specific treatment for membranous nephropathy, i.e. diuretics for oedema. It is important to be vigilant regarding thromboembolic events, as both membranous nephropathy and cancer predispose to thromboembolic disease.

Minimal change nephropathy presents clinically with nephrotic syndrome and is primarily associated with Hodgkin's disease.[2] Minimal change nephropathy is a rare association of solid tumours. Hodgkin's disease and minimal change nephropathy usually present concurrently or within a few months of one another, and there is a close temporal relationship between improvement in minimal change nephropathy and nephrotic syndrome and response to tumour treatment, and with exacerbation of the minimal change nephropathy on relapse of disease. The pathogenesis of this condition is not known, and renal biopsy shows a normal light microscopic appearance with no deposits of immunoglobulin or complement on the glomerular basement membrane. The mechanism by which the Hodgkin's disease and the minimal change nephropathy are linked is also unclear.

There are other glomerular disorders which occur as a paraneoplastic manifestation.[120] These include IgA nephropathy, which is the most common form of glomerulonephritis, and which presents with haematuria with or without proteinuria. IgA nephropathy has been associated with a variety of tumours including lung cancer, gastrointestinal tract adenocarcinomas, and non-Hodgkin's lymphoma. Membranoproliferative glomerulonephritis has been reported to be associated mainly with haematological malignancies such as hairy cell leukaemia and chronic lymphocytic leukaemia. Patients usually present with nephrotic syndrome, and treatment of the underlying malignancy (i.e. chronic lymphocytic leukaemia with chlorambucil) often induces complete remission of the nephrotic syndrome.

Renal tubular disorders

These occur most commonly in the setting of multiple myeloma, where immunoglobulin light chains produced by the myeloma can affect the renal tubules in a number of ways, for example proximal tubule damage due to direct toxicity of light chains, distal tubular blockage by cast formation (combinations of light chains with Tamm–Horsfall proteins), and amyloid light-chain-related amyloidosis.[121],[122]

The amyloid light chain in monoclonal gammopathy

Amyloidosis complicates up to 15 per cent of cases of myeloma and around 5 per cent of cases of 'benign' monoclonal gammopathy. Amyloid light chain protein is made up of two components, fibrillar and non-fibrillar. The fibrils in monoclonal gammopathy have been identified as light chains, hence they are called amyloid light-chain fibrils. The light chains can either be λ or κ and may be whole molecules, fragments, or a mixture thereof, with molecular weights of 8 to 30 kDa. Amyloid light-chain amyloidosis typically affects patients over the age of 50 and causes amyloid deposits in mesenchymal tissues, although it can affect any organ system and renal and gut involvement are common. The clinical features of systemic amyloidosis vary depending upon the organ system involved. The prognosis in amyloid light-chain complicating myeloma is poor with a median survival of less than 6 months.

Amyloid A protein in other malignancies

Amyloidosis occasionally complicates Hodgkin's disease, renal carcinoma, cancer of the lung, cancer of the genitourinary tract, malignant melanoma, basal cell carcinoma, and hairy cell leukaemia. In these patients the fibrillar component of amyloid is amyloid A protein. This protein contains 76 amino acids and has a molecular weight of 8 kDa. It is derived from a circulating precursor serum amyloid A which is an acute phase protein. Amyloid A amyloidosis is therefore found in any condition associated with sustained elevation of circulating serum amyloid A levels, principally chronic infections, inflammation, and the tumours listed above. The non-fibrillar component is derived from SAP, as in other forms of amyloid.

The clinical picture is known as reactive systemic amyloidosis and is characterized by involvement of parenchymal organs, particularly the liver, spleen, kidney, and adrenal. Patients may be asymptomatic from amyloidosis, but the commonest clinical presentation is with proteinuria, nephrotic syndrome, and hepatosplenomegaly. Infiltration of the gut is common and rectal biopsy is nearly always positive; 50 to 60 per cent of patients have cardiac involvement, but these are often asymptomatic. If specific antitumour treatment succeeds in lowering the circulating paraprotein, it may be possible to slow the rate of amyloid deposition. However, there is no other effective treatment to stop the accumulation of fibrils or to encourage resorption of fibrils already laid down, and the prognosis for patients with amyloidosis in the setting of malignant disease is very poor.

References

1. Butler RC, Thompson JM, Keat ACS. Paraneoplastic rheumatic disorders: a review. *Journal of the Royal Society of Medicine*, 1987; **80**: 168–72.

2. Boulton-Jones JM. Renal complications of malignant disease. In: Kaye SB, Rankin EM (ed.) *Balliere's Clinical Oncology*, vol. 2. London: Bailliere Tindall, 1988: 347–74.

3. Mason WP, *et al*. Small-cell lung cancer, paraneoplastic cerebellar degeneration and the Lambert–Eaton myasthenic syndrome. *Brain*, 1997; **120**: 1279–300.

4. Antel JP, Moumdjian R. Paraneoplastic syndromes: a role for the immune system. *Journal of Neurology*, 1989; **236**: 1–3.

5. Kornguth SE. Neuronal proteins and paraneoplastic syndromes. *New England Journal of Medicine*, 1989; **321**: 1607–8.

6. De la Monte S. Hutchins GM, Moore GW. Paraneoplastic syndromes and constitutional symptoms in prediction of metastatic behaviour of small cell carcinoma of the lung. *American Journal of Medicine*, 1984; 77: 851–7.

7. Hetzel DJ, Stanhope CR, O'Nell BP, Lennon VA. Gynecologic cancer in patients with subacute cerebellar degeneration predicted by anti-Purkinje cell antibodies and limited in metastatic volume. *Mayo Clinic Proceedings*, 1990; **65**: 1558–63.

8. Verschuuren JJ, Dalmau J, Hoard R, Posner JB. Paraneoplastic anti-Hu serum: studies on human tumor cell lines. *Journal of Neuroimmunology*, 1997; **79**: 202–10.

9. Xerri L, Birg F, Guigou V, Bouabdallah R, Poizot-Martin I, Hassoun J. *In situ* expression of the IL-a alpha and TNF alpha genes by Reed–Sternberg cells in Hodgkin's disease. *International Journal of Cancer*, 1992; **50**: 689–93.

10. Preisler HD, Raza A, Kukla C, Larson R, Goldberg J, Browman G. Interleukin-1β expression and treatment outcome in acute myelogenous leukemia. *Blood*, 1991; **78**: 849–50.

11. Albrecht JT, Canada TW. Cachexia and anorexia in malignancy. *Hematology and Oncology Clinics of North America*, 1996; **10**: 791–800.

12. Lind DS, Souba WW, Copeland EM. Weight loss and cachexia. In: Abeloff MD, Armitage JO, Lichter AS, Neiderhuber JE, eds. *Clinical Oncology*. Churchill Livingstone, New York; 1995: 393–407.

13. Cangiano C, Laviano A, Muscaritoli M, Meguid MM, Cascino A, Fanelli FR. Cancer anorexia: new pathogenic and therapeutic insights. *Nutrition*, 1996; **12** (suppl.): S48–S51.

14. Todorov P, Cariuk P, Mecdevitt T, Coles B, Fearon K, Tisdale M . Characterisation of a cancer cachetic factor. *Nature*, 1996; **379**: 739–42.

15. Staal Van den Brekel AJ, Dentener MA, Schols AMWJ, Buurman WA, Wouters EFM. Increased resting energy expenditure and weight loss are related to a systemic inflammatory response in lung cancer patients. *Journal of Clinical Oncology*, 1995; **13**: 2600–5.

16. Falconer JS, Fearon KCH, Plestes CE, Ross JA, Carter DC. Cytokines, the acute phase response, and resting energy expenditure in cachectic patients with pancreatic cancer. *Annals of Surgery*, 1994; **219**: 325–31.

17. Vogelzang N, *et al*. Patients, caregivers, and oncologist perceptions of cancer related fatigue: results of a tripart assessment survey (abstract). *Proceedings of the American Society of Clinical Oncology*, 1997; **16**: 53.

18. Portenoy RK, Miaskowski C. Assessment and management of cancer-related fatigue. In: Berger AM, Portenoy RK, Weissman DE (ed.) *Principles and Practice of Supportive Oncology*. Philadelphia: Lippincott-Raven, 1998: 109–18.

19. Elrington GM, Murray NM, Spiro SG, Newsom-Davis J. Neurological paraneoplastic syndromes in patients with small cell lung cancer. A prospective survey of 150 patients. *Journal of Neurology, Neurosurgery and Psychiatry*, 1991; **54**: 764–7.

20. Posner JB. *Neurologic complications of cancer*. Philadelphia: FA Davis, 1995.

21. Van Oosterhout AGM, Van de Pol M, Ten Velde GPM, Twijnstra A. Neurologic disorders in 203 consecutive patients with small cell lung cancer. *Cancer*, 1996; **77**: 1434–40.

22. Jaeckle KA. Autoimmune mechanisms in the pathogenesis of paraneoplastic nervous system disease. *Clinical Neurology and Neurosurgery*, 1995; **97**: 82–8.

23. Moll JWB, Hooijkaas H, van Goorbergh BCM, Roos LGE, Henzen-Logmans SC, Vecht CJ. Systemic and anti-neuronal auto-antibodies in patients with paraneoplastic neurological disease. *Journal of Neurology*, 1996; **243**: 51–6.

24. Jaeckle KA. Paraneoplastic nervous system syndromes. *Current Opinion in Oncology*, 1996; **8**: 204–8.

25. Dalmau J, Posner JB. Paraneoplastic syndromes affecting the nervous system. *Seminars in Oncology*, 1997; **24**: 318–28.

26. Dropcho EJ. Autoimmune central nervous system paraneoplastic disorders: Mechanisms, diagnosis, and therapeutic options. *Annals of Neurology*, 1995; 37 (suppl. 1): S102–S13.

27. Voltz RD, Graus F, Posner JB, Dalmau J. Paraneoplastic encephalomyelitis: an update of the effects of the anti-Hu immune response on the nervous system and tumour (editorial). *Journal of Neurology Neurosurgery and Psychiatry*, 1997; **63**: 133–6.

28. Graus F, *et al.* Anti-Hu antibodies in patients with small-cell lung cancer: Association with complete response to therapy and improved survival. *Journal of Clinical Oncology*, 1997; **15**: 2866–72.

29. Alamowitch S, Graus F, Uchuya M, Rene R, Bescansa E, Delattre JY. Limbic encephalitis and small cell lung cancer: Clinical and immunological features. *Brain*, 1997; **120**: 923–8.

30. Peterson K, Rosenblum MK, Kotanides H, Posner JB. Paraneoplastic cerebellar degeneration: a clinical analysis of 55 anti-Yo antibody-positive patients. *Neurology*, 1992; **42**: 1931–7.

31. Graus F, *et al.* Immunological characterisation of a neuronal antibody (anti-Tr) associated with paraneoplastic cerebellar degeneration and Hodgkin's disease. *Journal of Neuroimmunology*, 1997; **74**: 55–61.

32. Polans AS, Witkowska D, Haley TL, Amundson D, Baizer L, Adamus G. Recoverin, a photoreceptor-specific calcium-binding protein, is expressed by the tumour of a patient with cancer-associated retinopathy. *Proceedings of the National Academy of Sciences of the USA*, 1995; **92**: 9176–80.

33. Murphy MA, Thirkill CE, Hart WM Jr. Paraneoplastic retinopathy: A novel autoantibody reaction associated with small-cell lung carcinoma. *Journal of Neuro-opthalmology*, 1997; **17**: 77–83.

34. Boeck K, Hofmann S, Klopfer M, Ian U, Schmidt T, Engst R, Thirkill CE, Ring J. Melanoma-associated paraneoplastic retinopathy: case report and review of the literature. *British Journal of Dermatology*, 1997; **137**: 457–60.

35. Luque FA, *et al.* Anti-Ri: an antibody associated with paraneoplastic opsoclonus and breast cancer. *Annals of Neurology*, 1991; **29**: 241–51.

36. Hersh B, Dalmau J, Dangond F, Gultekin S, Geller E, Wen PY. Paraneoplastic opsoclonus-myoclonus associated with anti-Hu antibody. *Neurology*, 1994; **44**: 1754–5.

37. Hughes M, Ahern V, Kefford R, Boyages J. Paraneoplastic myelopathy at diagnosis in a patient with pathologic stage 1A Hodgkin disease. *Cancer*, 1992; **70**: 1598–600.

38. Babikian VL, Stefansson K, Dieperink ME, Arnason BGW, Marton LS, Levy BE. Paraneoplastic myelopathy: antibodies against protein in normal spinal cord and underlying neoplasm. *The Lancet*, 1985; **ii**: 49–50.

39. Nath U, Grant R. Neurological paraneoplastic syndromes. *Journal of Clinical Pathology*, 1997; **50**: 975–80.

40. Iwamasa T, Utsumi Y, Sakuda H, *et al.* Two cases of necrotizing myelopathy associated with malignancy caused by herpes simplex virus type 2. *Acta Neuropathologica*, 1989; **78**: 252–7.

41. Folli F, *et al.* Autoantibodies to a 128-kd synaptic protein in three women with the stiff-man syndrome and breast cancer. *New England Journal of Medicine*, 1993; **328**: 546–51.

42. Floyd S, *et al.* Expression of amphiphysin 1, an autoantigen of paraneoplastic neurological syndromes, in breast cancer. *Molecular Medicine*, 1998; **4**: 29–39.

43. Verma A, Berger JR, Snodgrass S, Petito C. Motor neurone disease: a paraneoplastic process associated with anti-Hu antibody and small cell lung carcinoma. *Annals of Neurology*, 40: 112–16.

44. Forsyth PA, Dalmau J, Graus F, Cwik V, Rosenblum MK, Posner JB. Motor neurone syndromes in cancer patients. *Annals of Neurology*, 1997; **41**: 722–30.

45. Lucchinetti CF, Kimmel DW, Lennon VA. Paraneoplastic and oncologic profiles of patients seropositive for type 1 antineuronal nuclear antibodies. *Neurology*, 1998; **50**: 652–7.

46. Hughes RAC, Sharrack B, Rubens RD. Carcinoma and the peripheral nervous system. *Journal of Neurology*, 1996; **243**: 371–6.

47. Briellmann RS, Sturzenegger M, Gerber HA, Schaffner T, Hess CW. Autoantibody-associated sensory neuronopathy and intestinal pseudo-obstruction without detectable neoplasia. *European Neurology*, 1996; **36**: 369–73.

48. Dalmau J, Graus F, Rosenblum MK, Posner JB. Anti-Hu associated paraneoplastic encephalomyelitis/sensory neuronopathy. A clinical study of 71 patients. *Medicine*, 1992; **71**: 59–72.

49. Uchuya M, Graus F, Vega F, Rene R, Delattre JY. Intravenous immunoglobulin therapy in paraneoplastic neurologic syndromes with antineuronal autoantibodies. *Journal of Neurology, Neurosurgery and Psychiatry*, 1996; **60**: 388–92.

50. Yeung KB, *et al.* The clinical spectrum of peripheral neuropathies associated with benign monoclonal IgM, IgG and IgA paraproteinaemia. Comparative clinical, immunological and nerve biopsy findings. *Journal of Neurology*, 1991; **238**: 383–91.

51. Ropper AH, Gorson KC. Neuropathies associated with paraproteinemia. *New England Journal of Medicine*, 1998; **338**: 1601–7.

52. Soubrier MJ, Dubost JJ, Sauvezie BJ. POEMS syndrome: a study of 25 cases and a review of the literature. French study group on POEMS Syndrome. *American Journal of Medicine*, 1994; **97**: 543–53.

53. Turner ML, Boland OM, Parker AC, Ewing DJ. Subclinical autonomic dysfunction in patients with Hodgkin's disease and non-Hodgkin's lymphoma. *British Journal of Haematology*, 1993; **84**: 623–6.

54. Lambert EH, Eaton LM, Wrooke ED. Defects of neuromuscular conduction associated with malignant neoplasms. *American Journal of Physiology*, 1956; **187**: 612–13.

55. Sanders DB. Lambert–Eaton myasthenic syndrome: Clinical diagnosis, immune-mediated mechanisms, and update on therapies. *Annals of Neurology*, 1995; 37 (suppl. 1): S63–S73.

56. Lang B, Newsom-Davis J. Immunopathology of the Lambert–Eaton myasthenic syndrome. *Springer Seminars in Immunopathology*, 1995; **17**: 3–15.

57. Lennon VA, *et al.* Calcium-channel antibodies in the Lambert-Eaton syndrome and other paraneoplastic syndromes. *New England Journal of Medicine*, 1995; **332**: 1467–74.

58. Takamori M, *et al.* Antibodies to recombinant synaptotagmin and calcium channel subtypes in Lambert–Eaton myasthenic syndrome. *Journal of Neurological Science*, 1995; **133**: 95–101.

59. Voltz RD, *et al.* Paraneoplastic myasthenia gravis: Detection of anti-MGT30 (titin) antibodies predicts thymic epithelial tumor. *Neurology*, 1997; **49**: 1454–7.

60. Zantos D, Zhang Y, Felson D. The overall and temporal association of cancer with polymyositis and dermatomyositis. *Journal of Rheumatology*, 1994; **21**: 1855–9.

61. Naschitz JE, Slobodin G, Yeshurun D, Rozenbaum M, Rosner I. A polymyalgia rheumatica-like syndrome as a presentation of metastatic cancer. *Journal of Clinical Rheumatology*, 1996; **2**: 305–8.

62. Levin MI, Mozaffar T, Al-Lozi MT, Pestronk A. Paraneoplastic necrotizing myopathy: clinical and pathological features. *Neurology*, 1998; **50**: 764–7.

63. Grignani G, Gobbi PG, Piccolo G, *et al.* Progressive necrotic myelopathy as a paraneoplastic syndrome: report of a case and some pathogenetic considerations. *Journal of Internal Medicine*, 1992; **231**: 81–5.

64. Henry DH. Recombinant human erythropoietin for the treatment of anaemia in patients with advanced cancer. *Seminars in Hematology*, 1993; 30 (suppl. 6): 12–16.

65. Morgenthaler TI, Brown LR, Colby TV, Harper CM Jr, Coles DT. Thymoma. *Mayo Clinic Proceedings*, 1993; **68**: 1110–23.

66. Ljungberg B, Rasmuson T, Grankvist K. Erythropoietin in renal cell carcinoma: evaluation of its usefulness as a tumour marker. *European Urology*, 1992; **21**: 160–3.

67. Shiramizu M, *et al.* Constitutive secretion of erythropoietin by human renal adenocarcinoma cells *in vivo* and *in vitro. Experimental Cell Research*, 1994; **215**: 249–56.

68. Adachi N, Yamaguchi K, Morikawa T, Suzuki M, Matsuda I, Abe K. Constitutive production of multiple colony-stimulating factors in patients with lung cancer associated with neutrophilia. *British Journal of Cancer*, 1994; **69**: 125–9.

69. Blay JY, Favrot M, Rossi JF, Wijdenes J. Role of interleukin-6 in paraneoplastic thrombocytosis. *Blood*, 1993; **82**: 2261–2.

70. Estrov Z, Talpaz M, Mavligit G, Pazdur R, Harris D, Greenberg SM, Kurzrock R. Elevated plasma thrombopoietic activity in patients with metastatic cancer-related thrombocytosis. *American Journal of Medicine*, 1995; **98**: 551–8.

71. Yohannan MD, Higgy KE, Al-Mashhadani SA, Santhosh-Kumar CR. Thrombocytosis: Etiologic analysis of 663 patients. *Clinical Pediatrics*, 1994; **33**: 340–3.

72. Santhosh-Kumar CR, Yohannan MD, Higgy KL, al Mashhadani SA. Thrombocytosis in adults: Analysis of 777 patients. *Journal of Internal Medicine*, 1991; **229**: 493–5.

73. Hasle H, Heim S, Schroeder H, Schmiegelow K, Ostergaard L, Kerndrup G. Transient pancytopenia preceding acute lymphoblastic leukemia (pre-ALL). *Leukemia*, 1995; **9**: 605–8.

74. Trousseau A. Phlegmasia alba dolens. *Clinique Medicale de Hotel-Dieu de Paris*, vol. 3. London: New Sydenham Society, 1868: 695–727.

75. Glassman AB. Hemostatic abnormalities associated with cancer and its therapy. *Annals of Clinical Laboratory Science*, 1997; **27**: 391–5.

76. Edwards RL, *et al.* Abnormalities of blood coagulation tests in patients with cancer. *American Journal of Clinical Pathology*, 1987; **88**: 596–602.

77. Naschitz JE, Yeshurun D, Eldar S, Lev LM. Diagnosis of cancer-associated vascular disorders. *Cancer*, 1996; **77**: 1759–67.

78. Bell WR. The fibrinolytic system in neoplasia. *Seminars in Thrombosis and Hemostasis*, 1996; **22**: 459–78.

79. Naschitz JE, Yeshurun D, Abrahamson J. Arterial occlusive disease in occult cancer. *American Heart Journal*, 1992; **124**: 738–45.

80. Bick RL, Ancypa D. Prevalence of deep venous thrombosis as the presenting clinical finding in occult malignancy. *Procedures of the Annual Meeting of the American Society of Clinical Oncology*, 1994; **13**: A269.

81. Sorensen HT, Mellemkjaer L, Steffensen FH, Olsen JH, Nielsen GL. The risk of a diagnosis of cancer after primary deep venous thrombosis or pulmonary embolism. *New England Journal of Medicine*, 1998; **338**: 1169–73.

82. Barosi G, Marchetti M, Dazzi L, Quaglini S. Testing for occult cancer in patients with idiopathic deep vein thrombosis—a decision analysis. *Thrombosis and Haemostasis*, 1997; **78**: 1319–26.

83. Buller H, Wouter Ten Cate J. Primary venous thromboembolism and cancer screening. *New England Journal of Medicine*, 1998; **338**: 1221–2.

84. Carey MJ, Rodgers GM. Disseminated intravascular coagulation: clinical and laboratory aspects. *American Journal of Hematology*, 1998; **59**: 65–73.

85. Bick RL. Disseminated intravascular coagulation: objective clinical and laboratory diagnosis, treatment and assessment of therapeutic response. *Seminars in Thrombosis and Haemostasis*, 1996; **22**: 69–88.

86. Gorden-Smith EG, Contreras M. Acquired haemolytic anaemia. In: Weatherall DJ, Ledingham JGG, Warrell DA (ed.) *Oxford Textbook of Medicine*, vol.3. Oxford: Oxford University Press, 1996: 3547–8.

87. Nordstrom B, Strang P. Microangiopathic hemolytic anemias (MAHA) in cancer. A case report and review. *Anticancer Research*, 1993;13: 1845–9.

88. Finlay AY. Dermatological complications of malignant disease. In: Kaye SB, Rankin EM (ed.) *Balliere's Clinical Oncology*, vol. 2. London: Bailliere Tindall, 1988: 479–98.

89. Rigel DS, Jacobs MI. Malignant acanthosis nigricans: a review. *Journal of Dermatology and Surgical Oncology*, 1980; **6**: 923–7.

90. Requena L, Aguilar A, Renedo G, Martin L, Pique E, Farina MC, Escalonilla P. Tripe palms: a cutaneous marker of internal malignancy. *Journal of Dermatology*, 1995; **22**: 492–5.

91. Schwartz RA. Sign of Leser-Trelat. *Journal of the American Academy of Dermatology*, 1996; **35**: 88–95.

92. Bourke JF, *et al.* Sweet's syndrome and malignancy in the UK. *British Journal of Dermatology*, 1997; **137**: 609–13.

93. Geisler JP, *et al.* Extramammary Paget's disease with diffuse involvement of the lower female genito-urinary system. *International Journal of Gynecological Cancer*, 1997; **7**: 84–7.

94. Kurzrock R, Cohen PR. Paraneoplastic erythromelalgia. *Clinics in Dermatology*, 1993; **11**: 73–82.

95. Jones SAV, *et al.* Necrolytic migratory erythema: A classical cutaneous presentation of the glucagonoma syndrome. *Journal of the European Academy of Dermatology and Venereology*, 1997; **9**: 68–73.

96. Greaves MW, Burova EP. Flushing: Causes, investigation and clinical consequences. *Journal of the European Academy of Dermatology and Venereology*, 1997; **8**: 91–100.

97. Lear JT, Atherton MT, Byrne JPH. Neutrophilic dermatoses: Pyoderma gangrenosum and Sweet's syndrome. *Postgraduate Medical Journal*, 1997; **73**: 65–8.

98. Helm TN, Camisa C, Valenzuela R, Allen CM. Paraneoplastic pemphigus: A distinct autoimmune vesiculobullous disorder associated with neoplasia. *Oral Surgery, Oral Medicine, Oral Pathology, Oral Radiology and Endodontics*, 1993; **75**: 209–13.

99. Mascaro JM Jr, Sole T, Ferrando J. Paraneoplastic pemphigus. A review. *Skin Cancer*, 1995; **10**: 283–90.

100. Egan CA, O'Loughlin S, Gormally S, Powell FC. Dermatitis herpetiformis: A review of fifty-four patients. *Irish Journal of Medical Science*, 1997; **166**: 241–7.

101. Cohen PR, Kurzrock R. Mucocutaneous paraneoplastic syndromes. *Seminars in Oncology*, 1997; **24**: 334–59.

102. Stevens HP, *et al.* Linkage of an American pedigree with palmoplantar keratoderma and malignancy (palmoplantar ectodermal dysplasia type III) to 17q24: Literature survey and proposed updated classification of the keratodermas. *Archives of Dermatology*, 1996; **132**: 640–51.

103. Bolognia JL. Bazex syndrome: Acrokeratosis paraneoplastica. *Seminars in Dermatology*, 1995; **14**: 84–9.

104. Lober CW. Pruritus and malignancy. *Clinics in Dermatology*, 1993; **11**: 125–8.

105. Ochiai T, Morishima T, Kondo M. Symptomatic porphyria secondary to hepatocellular carcinoma. *British Journal of Dermatology*, 1997; **136**: 129–31.

106. Naschitz JE, Yeshurun D, Rosner I. Rheumatic manifestations of occult cancer. *Cancer*, 1995; **75**: 2954–8.

107. Mellemkjaer L, Linnet MS, Gridley G, Frisch M, Moller H, Olsen JH. Rheumatoid arthritis and cancer risk. *European Journal of Cancer*, 1991; **32**: 1753–7.

108. Burstein HJ, Janicek MJ, Skarin AT. Hypertrophic osteoarthropathy. *Journal of Clinical Oncology*, 1997; **15**: 2759–60.

109. Sweeney DM. Risk of malignancy in women with systemic lupus erythematosus. *Journal of Rheumatology*, 1995; **22**: 1478–82.

110. Mellemkjaer L, Anderson V, Linnet MS, Gridley G, Hoover R, Olsen JH. Non-Hodgkin's lymphoma and other cancers among a cohort of patients with systemic lupus erythematosus. *Arthritis and Rheumatism*, 1997; **40**: 761–8.

111. Royer B, *et al.* Lymphomas in patients with Sjögren's syndrome are marginal zone B-cell neoplasms, arise in diverse extranodal and nodal sites, and are not associated with viruses. *Blood*, 1997; **90**: 766–75.

112. **Tzioufas AG.** B-cell lymphoproliferation in primary Sjögren's syndrome. *Clinical Experimental Rheumatology,* 1996; **14** (suppl.): S65–S70.

113. **Rosenthal AK, McLaughlin JK, Linet MS, Persson I.** Scleroderma and malignancy: An epidemiologic study. *Annals of the Rheumatic Diseases,* 1993; **52**: 531–3.

114. **Carsons S.** The association of malignancy with rheumatic and connective tissue diseases. *Seminars in Oncology,* 1997; **24**: 360–72.

115. **Kurzrock R, Cohen PR.** Vasculitis and cancer. *Clinical Dermatology,* 1993; **11**: 175–87.

116. **Hasler P, Kistler H, Gerber H.** Vasculidities in hairy cell leukemia. *Seminars in Arthritis and Rheumatism,* 1995; **25**: 134–42.

117. **John WJ, Foon KA, Patchell RA.** Paraneoplastic syndromes. In: DeVita VT, Hellman S, Rosenberg SA (ed.) *Cancer: Principles and Practice of Oncology,* 5th edn. Philadelphia: Lippincott-Raven, 1997: 2397–422.

118. **Burstein DM, Korbet SM, Schwartz MM.** Membranous glomerulonephritis and malignancy. *American Journal of Kidney Disease,* 1993: **22**: 5–10.

119. **Maesaka JK, Mittal SK, Fishbane S.** Paraneoplastic syndromes of the kidney. *Seminars in Oncology,* 1997; **24**: 373–81.

120. **Norris SH.** Paraneoplastic glomerulopathies. *Seminars in Nephrology,* 1993; **13**: 258–72.

121. **Sanders PW.** Myeloma kidney. *Kidney,* 1993; **25**: 1–7.

122. **Sanders PW, Herrera GA.** Monoclonal immunoglobulin light chain-related renal diseases. *Seminars in Nephrology,* 1993; **3**: 324–41.

5.4 Immunohaematological complications of cancer

P. L. Amlot and R. Pawson

Introduction

Haematological problems occur in at least half of all patients with non-haematological malignancy and are a significant cause of morbidity and mortality. Disorders of erythrocytes, leucocytes, platelets, and coagulation all occur regularly in patients with cancer. Cancer decreases the number of erythrocytes by various mechanisms, so producing anaemia. Although anaemia is common in cancer and causes considerable morbidity, it seldom causes death. Cancer leads to the activation of platelets and coagulation and is the second most common contributory cause of death in cancer. Lastly, immunodeficiency is the outcome of the many ways in which cancer can affect the leucocytes:

1. It may depress immunity through the direct physical invasion and replacement of normal myeloid and lymphoid tissue (particularly evident in lymphomas, myelomas, and leukaemia) or through the production of proteins, which interfere with immune function.

2. If the cancer is not controlled by treatment but grows and disseminates, the patient becomes cachectic and malnourished, which increase the severity of the immunodeficiency.

3. The integrity of mucosal or epidermal surfaces is often breached, either directly by the cancer or indirectly because of surgical and medical intervention (e.g. operations, indwelling venous lines, intubation, etc.), which breaks down natural defence barriers to invasion by micro-organisms.

4. All modes of cancer therapy impair immunity, whether as a result of surgery and anaesthesia, radiotherapy, cytotoxic chemotherapy, corticosteroids, or antimicrobial chemotherapy.

5. Pre-existing immunodeficiency may contribute to the development of cancer.

6. Associated with immunodeficiency, some patients make abnormal or autoimmune responses.

7. The psychological characteristics and attitudes of patients have been correlated with their ability to survive with cancer.

Immunological effector mechanisms have been invoked to explain why patients with beneficial attitudes towards their cancer may survive longer. Depression is the only psychological state that consistently produces immunological deficiency,[1] and a reactive depression to cancer may contribute in its turn to the cascade of immunosuppressive effects induced by this disease.

It is hardly surprising that cancer patients are prone not only to common infections but also occasionally to organisms which are not normally pathogenic. Serious and life-threatening infection occurs most often when the immunosuppressive effects are multiple, especially where there is progressive tumour growth despite cytotoxic chemotherapy or radiotherapy. Infection is the major contributory cause of mortality in cancer.

Red cells

Anaemia

Anaemia is the commonest haematological manifestation in cancer and occurs in over half the patients at some stage of their disease. Fatigue has been identified as one of the most distressing symptoms for cancer patients[2] and anaemia is a major contributory factor. The different causes of anaemia in cancer are listed in Table 1. Since anaemia can cause significant morbidity, identification of the cause is important for appropriate treatment. However, the anaemia is often multifactorial and can be difficult to correct.

Anaemia of chronic diseases (ACD)

This is the commonest cause of anaemia in cancer patients; it is usually mild, with a haemoglobin of between 8 and 11 g/dl, and is normochromic normocytic or mildly hypochromic microcytic. The reticulocyte count is low for the degree of anaemia and serum iron and iron-binding capacity are low. Differentiating ACD from iron deficiency in patients with malignant disease may be difficult (see below). Occasionally, bone-marrow aspiration is required to confirm ACD, which shows abundant storage iron in macrophages but a marked reduction in iron-containing erythroblasts.

Table 1 Causes of anaemia in cancer

Mechanism	
Decreased erythropoiesis	Anaemia of chronic disease
	Haematinic deficiency—iron, folate, vitamin B_{12}
	Bone-marrow infiltration
	Red-cell aplasia
	Iatrogenic—drug related
Increased loss/destruction	Blood loss
	Anaemia of chronic disease
	Haemolysis—immune or non-immune
	Iatrogenic—drug related or surgery

Reduced erythropoiesis, disordered maturation, and shortened red-cell survival appear to contribute to the ACD, although its pathogenesis is not fully understood. Depressed erythropoiesis is associated with:[3]

(1) impaired availability of storage iron;

(2) inadequate erythropoietin response to anaemia; and/or

(3) overproduction of deleterious cytokines.

Altered cellular iron metabolism results from a complex network of events at the transcriptional and translational levels, with decreased synthesis of proteins involved in the uptake, storage, and utilization of iron. Nitric oxide may be involved in iron homeostasis and ACD.[4]

Normally the chronic hypoxia of anaemia or a low haematocrit leads to increased erythropoietin production, but erythropoietin levels in patients with cancer are often inappropriately low for the degree of anaemia even with normal renal function. About half the patients with cancer and ACD will benefit from treatment with human recombinant erythropoietin (rEpo)[5] and show improved quality-of-life scores,[6],[7] apart from those concurrently treated with cytotoxic chemotherapy.[8],[9] Treatment with rEpo costs between three and five times that of blood transfusion,[10],[11] and consequently prediction of responders or non-responders becomes economically important. Severe bone-marrow infiltration and haematinic deficiency are unresponsive to rEpo therapy, and therefore other forms of correctable anaemia (Table 1) should be excluded before considering rEpo therapy. Patients with inappropriately low erythropoietin blood levels (< 200 mU/ml) will benefit most. A 2-week trial of rEpo treatment can identify responders who show: (1) a haemoglobin increase of more than 0.5 g/dl, or (2) more than a 25 per cent increase in transferrin levels, or (3) an early rise in reticulocyte count, and who are likely to benefit with persistent haemoglobin increases of more than 2 g/dl.[5],[12] Erythropoietin only has an 8-h half-life after intravenous administration and it is more cost-effective to give it subcutaneously once-weekly.

An impaired marrow response to erythropoietin has been associated with the cytokines tumour necrosis factor-α (TNF-α), interleukin-1 (IL-1), and IL-6, which may exert direct inhibitory effects on erythroid precursors.[13] These cytokines are also involved in the retention of iron in the reticuloendothelial system, gastrointestinal tract, and hepatocytes and may interfere with erythropoietin production by the kidney. IL-1 inhibition of erythropoietin can be overcome if sufficiently high doses of rEpo are given,[14] similar to its effects in chronic renal failure and in the presence of uraemic toxins. The *in vivo* administration of monoclonal antibodies against TNF-α has led to an increase in haemoglobin in patients with ACD associated with rheumatoid arthritis.[15] Apart from such experimental approaches and the administration of erythropoietin, the management of patients with ACD is generally based on treatment of the underlying malignancy and supportive therapy with blood transfusions. The latter are only occasionally required because of the generally mild degree of anaemia.

Haematinic deficiency

Folic acid deficiency may occur in cancer patients due to a combination of reduced absorption, increased utilization (from rapidly proliferating cells or prolonged cytotoxic therapy), and occasionally by direct antagonism (methotrexate administration). Vitamin B₁₂ deficiency may occur in patients who have undergone gastric surgery, thereby

Table 2 Causes of leucoerythroblastic anaemia

Mechanism	
Marrow infiltration	Metastatic carcinoma
	Lymphoma
	Myeloma
	Myelofibrosis
Others	Severe haemolysis
	Severe haemorrhage
	Severe sepsis
	Megaloblastic anaemia
	Thrombotic thrombocytopenic purpura
	Burns
	Eclampsia

reducing intrinsic factor production, resection, and bypass procedures involving the terminal ileum, the major site of vitamin B₁₂ absorption. As it may take up to 4 years to deplete body stores, frank B₁₂ deficiency is unusual in cancer patients. Deficiencies of vitamin B₁₂ and folate manifest as megaloblastic anaemia with macrocytosis, hypersegmented neutrophils (> five nuclear lobes), and characteristic bone-marrow morphology with nucleocytoplasmic asynchrony. Diagnosis is established by serum vitamin B₁₂ and by serum and red-cell folate levels. Measurement of homocysteine and methylmalonic acid levels provides a more sensitive index of haematinic deficiency, but the exact role of these assays is unclear.[16] Treatment is by intramuscular injection of vitamin B₁₂ and/or oral folic acid.

Bone-marrow infiltration

Bone-marrow infiltration with metastatic carcinoma is usually associated with a leucoerythroblastic blood film, in other words with circulating immature white cells and nucleated red cells. Causes of a leucoerythroblastic picture are shown in Table 2. Bone-marrow aspiration and biopsy may be performed for diagnostic or staging purposes. Malignant cells often occur in clumps and are usually larger than most haemopoietic cells. It is generally not possible to determine the tissue of origin of the malignant cells, although melanoma cells may be recognized by the presence of pigment and adenocarcinoma may be suspected if gland formation is seen. Mucin can be detected with the Periodic acid–Schiff (PAS) stain. Immunocytochemistry can also be performed using monoclonal antibodies against epithelial markers such as cytokeratin.[17] A variety of immunological and molecular methods are available for detecting circulating tumour cells in peripheral blood and micrometastases from solid tumours, and are capable of identifying one carcinoma cell in up to one million haemopoietic cells.[18],[19]

Acquired red-cell aplasia

The malignancy most commonly associated with pure red-cell aplasia (PRCA) is thymoma. Approximately 5 per cent of patients with thymoma have PRCA, whereas up to 10 to 15 per cent of patients with PRCA have thymomas that are usually benign.[20] PRCA also occurs in association with haematological malignancies such as chronic lymphocytic leukaemia, large granular lymphocytosis (LGL),[21] and acute lymphoblastic leukaemia.[22] A reduction or absence of red-cell precursors in the bone marrow accompanies anaemia and reticulocytopenia. The aetiology is thought to be autoimmune, with antibodies to erythroid precursors in some cases[23] or plasma factors blocking the differentiation of erythroblastic colonies (colony-forming units—erythroid (CFU-E) or burst-forming units— erythroid (BFU-E)).[24] The presence of serum inhibitors against erythropoietin has also been reported.[25],[26] In one patient with PRCA, antibodies inhibited the binding of erythropoietin to its receptor and blocked the differentiation of erythroid precursors *in vitro*.[25]

Clonal, T-cell receptor gene rearrangement of blood and thymoma tissue from a patient with PRCA whose anaemia responded to treatment with cyclosporin A, suggested that a neoplastic population of T cells may mediate the suppression of erythropoiesis.[27] Thymectomy gives remission rates of 25 to 30 per cent,[28] but a significant number of these patients will relapse. Occasionally, PRCA may develop after thymectomy. Immunosuppression with conventional agents such as corticosteroids, cyclophosphamide, and azathioprine has been disappointing and other immunomodulatory drugs such as cyclosporin and antilymphocyte globulin have been used with variable success. Resolution of PRCA with cyclosporin has been reported in LGL leukaemia[29] and chronic lymphocytic leukaemia (CLL).[30]

Acquired red-cell aplasia in cancer patients may also be associated with viral infections. Persistent infection with parvovirus B19 can result in PRCA in a wide variety of immunosuppressed states, most commonly in congenital and acquired immunodeficiency states but also in lymphoproliferative disorders[31] and after bone marrow and other organ transplantation.[32] Human herpesvirus-6 is a ubiquitous herpesvirus than can cause myelosuppression and haemophagocytosis in bone-marrow transplant recipients.[33],[34] Its relevance in less heavily immunosuppressed cancer patients is not yet known.

Blood loss and iron deficiency

Blood loss is the second most common cause of anaemia in patients with malignant disease. Chronic blood loss as low as 3 to 4 ml per day can result in iron deficiency and may be associated with tumours of the gastrointestinal and genitourinary tracts and lung. As many as one-quarter of patients presenting with iron deficiency may be harbouring a gastrointestinal neoplasm,[35] rising to half of all elderly patients with severe iron deficiency anaemia.[36] The finding of iron deficiency anaemia (IDA) in any male and all post-menopausal female patients should prompt a thorough search for a source of blood loss and occult malignancy.[37]

In iron deficiency, examination of the blood film reveals hypochromic, microcytic red cells with 'pencil cells' or elliptocytes. Serum iron is decreased in iron deficiency as well as in ACD. Determination of the total iron-binding capacity (TIBC), a reflection of serum transferrin concentration, helps to distinguish the two conditions. A raised TIBC generally indicates iron deficiency (but it also occurs in pregnancy and with oral contraceptive use), whereas malignant, infective and inflammatory conditions, and liver disease are associated with a lower TIBC. The saturation of iron-binding capacity is reduced in iron deficiency, usually to less than 16 per cent. Serum ferritin is an indicator of storage iron and a low level usually indicates iron deficiency. However, it is also an acute-phase protein that rises in malignant and inflammatory conditions to give spuriously normal values in patients with true iron deficiency. A confident diagnosis of IDA can be made when the serum ferritin is low (< 12 µg/l). Indicators

that distinguish IDA from ACD in patients with malignant disease include the concomitant measurement of parameters of inflammation independent of iron metabolism such as the erythrocyte sedimentation rate (ESR) or C-reactive protein,[38] measurement of free erythrocyte protoporphyrin, and therapeutic trials of oral iron. For example, if the ferritin is in the low to normal range (13 to 100 µg/l) in patients suspected to have ACD, oral ferrous sulphate 200 mg three-times daily for 1 month can be tried. Newer techniques include determining the hypochromic red-cell index and the serum soluble transferrin receptor (sTfR) assay. Perl's stain of bone-marrow aspirates to demonstrate iron stores remains the reference standard for the assessment of these newer methods. Some automated red-cell counters generate percentages of hypochromic or microcytic red cells. A finding of more than 11 per cent hypochromic cells may be relatively specific for iron deficiency, but it is insensitive.[38] Soluble transferrin receptors are truncated forms of the tissue TfR. All cells have TfR on their surface, but 80 per cent of them are in the erythroid marrow.[38] The number of TfRs on a cell surface reflects its iron requirement, and iron deprivation results in rapid induction of TfR synthesis.[39] Serum sTfR levels appear to reflect the total body mass of the tissue receptor, and increased concentrations occur in patients with erythroid hyperplasia and in iron deficiency. However, the value of a raised sTfR concentration in discriminating between iron deficiency and ACD[39] has not been uniformly corroborated.[38] sTfR measurement by an enzyme-linked immunosorbent assay (ELISA) remains expensive and its further evaluation in large numbers of patients is required.

Autoimmune haemolysis

Autoimmune haemolytic anaemia (AIHA) is a recognized complication of haematological malignancies such as non-Hodgkin's lymphoma and chronic lymphocytic leukaemia, but it is a rare complication of most other solid tumours. AIHA is due to antibody production by the body against its own red blood cells, and is divided into 'warm' (IgG autoantibody) and 'cold' (IgM antibody) types according to whether the antibody reacts better with red cells at 37 °C or 4 °C, respectively. IgM antibodies (cold agglutinins) can cause intravascular haemolysis, but the severity of the associated clinical picture depends on the activity of the antibody at 37 °C. Red-cell agglutination is seen on blood films made at room temperature. Clinically, acrocyanosis or chronic mild haemolysis can occur. IgG antibodies mediate extravascular haemolysis with red-cell destruction in the reticuloendothelial system, predominantly the spleen. Severe anaemia and jaundice may occur with polychromasia, spherocytes, and nucleated red cells in the peripheral blood and a positive direct Coombs' or antiglobulin test. If no underlying cause for AIHA is obvious, investigation for an underlying lymphoma should be undertaken before the haemolytic anaemia is labelled idiopathic. Ovarian, breast, colon, and prostate cancers have been associated with AIHA.[40],[41] Treatment of patients with CLL or lymphoma may trigger AIHA. This phenomenon has been especially associated with chlorambucil and fludarabine.[42] Treatment of AIHA is aimed at removing the cause and suppressing haemolysis. Steroids are standard therapy but, occasionally, additional immunosuppressive drugs may be required. Autoimmunity in cancer is dealt with more extensively below.

Non-immune haemolysis

Microangiopathic haemolytic anaemia (**MAHA**) is a clinical syndrome characterized by intravascular haemolysis with fragmentation of red blood cells as they pass through fibrin deposited in abnormal blood vessels. In cancer, the causes of MAHA include disseminated intravascular coagulation and thrombotic thrombocytopenic purpura/haemolytic uraemic syndrome which are considered below, as well as a direct effect of red-cell fragmentation in the abnormal vessels of the primary tumour or in metastatic tumour thrombi. The anaemia is often severe. Features of intravascular haemolysis include raised serum levels of bilirubin and lactate dehydrogenase, reduced haptoglobins, haemosiderinuria, and a negative direct antiglobulin test. Treatment is aimed at removing the cause and giving supportive therapy with red-cell transfusions.

Erythrocytosis

Erythrocytosis, or polycythaemia, is characterized by an increase in red-cell mass and elevation of haemoglobin (> 17.5 g/dl in males, more than 15.5 g/dl in females) with an accompanying increase in haematocrit (> 0.55 in males and more than 0.47 in females). When associated with malignancy it is due to the inappropriate production of erythropoietin or erythropoietin-like peptides by the tumour, most commonly renal-cell[43] and hepatocellular carcinoma.[44] Rarer associations include cerebellar haemangioblastoma, phaeochromocytoma, and androgen-secreting ovarian tumours. Investigation must exclude other causes of erythrocytosis such as polycythaemia rubra vera, tissue hypoxia, and reduced plasma volume (relative polycythaemia). If the patient is symptomatic and/or the haematocrit is greater than 0.55, venesection should be performed. Myelosuppressive agents are rarely required in tumour-associated erythrocytosis.

Transfusion in cancer patients

Important issues in the transfusion of patients with cancer include possible immunosuppressive effects of transfusion, transfusion-associated graft-versus-host disease (GVHD) and the prevention of HLA alloimmunization, and cytomegalovirus infection. The latter two features are important mainly in patients who may be considered for high-dose chemotherapy and stem-cell transplantation.

An immunomodulatory effect of blood transfusion was first suspected in the 1970s when allogeneic blood transfusion improved the survival of renal allografts.[45] In the early 1980s, a dramatic epidemiological association between the increased recurrence of colorectal and lung cancer and perioperative blood transfusion was reported.[46],[47] Since then nearly 100 studies have been conducted to investigate this observation but the issue remains controversial. In a prospective study of 339 patients with colorectal cancer undergoing elective surgery, patients receiving allogeneic transfusion had a significantly greater recurrence of cancer than patients who were not transfused.[47] Such non-randomized studies are prone to confounding factors such as tumour stage. Advanced tumours are associated with more blood loss, a lower preoperative haemoglobin level, and more extensive surgery, all of which lead to a higher incidence of transfusion. Unless carefully controlled studies are conducted, increased cancer recurrence in transfused patients may just reflect the more advanced nature of their presenting tumour. Immunomodulatory effects of transfusion are demonstrable *in vitro* and *in vivo*. Decreased natural killer-cell function, macrophage migration to sites of injury, and reduced lymphocyte proliferation occur *in vitro*[48] and impaired delayed-type hypersensitivity skin responses, low helper to suppressor T-cell ratios, and reduced interleukin-2 production have been reported *in vivo*.[48] Experimental evidence suggests that these immunomodulatory effects of allogeneic transfusion are leucocyte-mediated[48] and that the immunomodulatory effects of transfusion are abrogated by using leucocyte-depleted or autologous products.[48],[50] However, a recent meta-analysis of eight unconfounded studies with 2532 patients concluded that there is no evidence that allogeneic blood transfusion increases the risk of clinically important adverse sequelae in patients with cancer undergoing surgery.[49] The issue thus remains controversial. Transfusion services in the United Kingdom are moving towards universal leucocyte depletion of blood products because of the theoretical risk of transmitting new-variant Creutzfeld–Jakob disease (vCJD).

GVHD is a potential problem in certain groups of patients with cancer and results when there is a degree of disparity in histocompatibility antigens between donor and patient. Under certain circumstances viable donor (transfused) T lymphocytes engraft and proliferate in the recipient. Interaction between donor T lymphocytes and recipient cells carrying either class I or class II HLA antigens results in cellular damage, which may be natural killer cell-mediated. Major target tissues include the skin, liver, gut, and bone marrow leading to aplasia identical to transplant-associated GVHD. Transfusion-associated GVHD is almost universally fatal. This complication can be prevented by gamma irradiation of cellular blood components with a minimum irradiation dose of 25 Gy.[51] Risks of GVHD are highest in patients with immunodeficiency or significant immune suppression, such as patients receiving autologous or allogeneic bone-marrow transplantation, patients with Hodgkin's disease, or patients receiving purine analogues such as fludarabine, deoxycoformycin, and chlorodeoxyadenosine. Irradiated blood products should always be given to these patients. Transfusion-associated GVHD rarely occurs and its rarity in patients with non-haemopoietic tumours, for example neuroblastoma,[52] means that irradiation of blood products is not currently recommended for such patients.[51]

White cells

Leucocytosis

A neutrophil leucocytosis is common in all types of malignant disease. If the leucocytosis is excessive and associated with immature cells (myeloblasts, promyelocytes, and myelocytes) in the peripheral blood, a leukaemoid reaction is said to be present. This usually signifies metastatic or necrotic tumours or coexistent severe infection and may be mediated by neutrophil growth factors secreted by the underlying tumour. The white cell count may be as high as 100 × 10⁹/l and it is important to distinguish a leukaemoid reaction from a primary myeloproliferative disorder. Granulocyte changes such as toxic granulation, Dohle bodies, a high neutrophil alkaline phosphatase score, and absence of the Philadelphia chromosome help to differentiate leukaemoid reactions from chronic myeloid leukaemia.

Eosinophilia occurs in all types of malignancies but is commonest in Hodgkin's disease and some T-cell lymphomas.

Splenectomy and functional hyposplenia

The loss of the spleen is infrequently followed by overwhelming postsplenectomy infections (OPSI), with the frequency of their occurrence determined by the patient's age and the underlying disease process which led to the splenectomy. Splenectomy performed as part of the staging laparotomy for Hodgkin's disease (now a rare procedure) precedes OPSI in 2 to 4 per cent of adults and 6 to 9 per cent of children. On the other hand, the same operation performed for patients with hypersplenism or idiopathic thrombocytopenic purpura leads to a 5 per cent and 14 per cent incidence of OPSI, respectively. Identical overwhelming infections may arise in patients with chronic leukaemias, lymphomas, or following bone-marrow transplantation (BMT) without splenectomy as a result of hypogammaglobulinaemia and/or functional asplenia. The pathogenesis of OPSI is linked to the loss of both the special phagocytic and antibody-producing properties of the spleen.[53] This will occur despite normal to high blood leucocyte counts.

The major pathogenic organisms in all these conditions, in the order of their frequency, are *Streptococcus pneumoniae*, *Haemophilus influenzae*, *Neisseria meningitidis*, *Escherichia coli*, and *Pseudomonas aeruginosa*. Other infections include severe malaria, babesiosis, and *Capnocytophaga canimorsus* associated with dog bites. Functional asplenia is detected from blood films showing Heinz and Howell–Jolly bodies, thrombocytosis, and monocytosis. *Pseudomonas aeruginosa* is the most frequent infecting organism in patients with chronic leukaemias.[54] Most of these infections are readily treated with the penicillin group of antibiotics. Guidelines recommend long-term prophylactic penicillin therapy in splenectomized children and for at least 2 years in adults, since the highest risk of OPSI occurs during that time.[55] A polyvalent pneumococcal vaccine should be administered at least 2 weeks before an elective splenectomy is performed, and in other circumstances as soon as the patient has recovered from the operation. Vaccination should be delayed for at least 6 months after cytotoxic chemotherapy or other immunosuppressive therapy. Immunization against pneumococcal antigens should not lead to complacency—first, the benefit of immunization for splenectomized patients has not been unequivocally established and, secondly, it will not protect against organisms not contained within the vaccine. All patients should be: (1) educated on the dangers of infection; (2) encouraged to wear a Medic-alert disc; and (3) have a supply of antibiotics—amoxicillin or erythromycin—to be taken if a febrile or infective illness develops and there is even a minor delay in seeing a doctor.[55]

Hypogammaglobulinaemia occurring in chronic lymphocytic leukaemia and low-grade lymphomas which leads to recurrent infection should be treated with replacement intravenous or intramuscular gammaglobulin. The dose and frequency should be adjusted to the individual, aiming to maintain the serum IgG level above the lower limit of normal (7 to 8 g/litre).

Leucopenia

Neutropenia is usually seen as part of pancytopenia in association with bone-marrow infiltration or myelosuppression secondary to cancer chemo- or radiotherapy. A low granulocyte count is widely used as an indicator of acute susceptibility to bacterial infection. This can occur spontaneously in leukaemias and more rarely in other cancers, but overwhelmingly it follows cancer treated by cytotoxic drugs. Neutropenia predisposes the patient to a variety of bacterial infections. The commonly encountered infections are from Gram-negative aerobic organisms (*E. coli*, *Pseudomonas aeruginosa*, and *Klebsiella* and *Proteus* spp.), which usually arise from the patient's own gastrointestinal tract, mucosal or cutaneous flora. Patients with granulocytopenia are also susceptible to certain types of fungi (*Candida albicans* and *Aspergillus* spp.). Neutropenia in cancer is rarely due to autoimmunity; however, an example has been reported of a patient with thymoma, hypogammaglobulinaemia, and absent B cells due to an inhibitor of granulocyte–macrophage colony-forming units (CFU-GM).[56]

Neutrophil function is usually normal in untreated malignant disease; although *in vitro* studies have occasionally shown decreased chemotaxis,[57] it is not clinically significant.

Lymphocytopenia and cell-mediated anergy

Although many sophisticated tests can be performed to examine lymphocyte function, the simple lymphocyte count is almost as good an index of susceptibility to infection as any other. Less attention is paid to the lymphocyte count in patient monitoring (compared with neutrophils) because of the variable and often prolonged delay between a fall in lymphocyte number and any evidence of infection. None the less, an individual with persistently low lymphocyte counts is more susceptible to viral, fungal, and opportunistic infection.[58] In comparison with the total lymphocyte count, clinical testing of delayed cutaneous hypersensitivity (DCH) has to be performed with a battery of recall DCH antigens if it is to be of any value in grading the strength of cell-mediated immunity (CMI), and for monitoring it would have to be performed repeatedly. There are methodological problems with repeated DCH testing, both of interpretation and convenience. Lymphocyte-subset determinations of T-helper (CD4) and T-cytotoxic/suppressor cells (CD8) have been of value in monitoring patients with the acquired immunodeficiency syndrome (AIDS). But these have not been widely used in patients with cancer, even though an inversion in the CD4/CD8 ratio often occurs.

Anergy to several DCH inducing antigens (for instance, tuberculin, candida, trichophyton, mumps, and streptokinase–streptodornase) is associated with a greater risk of postoperative infection.[59],[60] Anergy is often a manifestation of the patient's state of health, degree of cachexia, and the stage of malignant dissemination. Cellular immunity appears to be normal in the early stages of cancer and then becomes impaired as the cancer spreads. Impairment of cell-mediated immunity may appear early in the course of some cancers (for example, in Hodgkin's disease) and later in others, but the trend is the same. *In vitro* lymphocyte responses to phytohaemagglutinin in both cancer of the lung and Hodgkin's disease become more and more depressed as the cancer spreads, but the lymphocyte impairment is more marked in the latter (Fig. 1). Immune responses may be heightened in the early stages of cancer and then decline as the disease disseminates. An animal model, using *Listeria monocytogenes* as an infective organism, showed augmented resistance to *Listeria* after implantation of a methylcholanthrene-induced tumour, but with progression of the tumour the resistance diminished and became subnormal.[61] Measurement of immunocompetence in women with breast cancer at diagnosis did not correlate with their survival or relapse-free survival,[62] impaired cellular immunity was associated with low lymphocyte counts.

The most severe expression of cellular immunodeficiency is in graft-versus-host disease. Fatal GVHD from a blood transfusion can

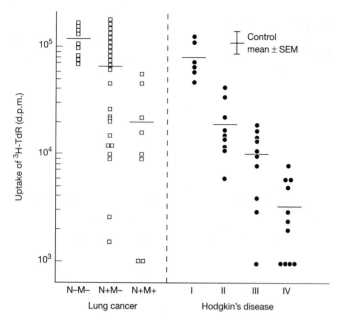

Fig. 1 Non-specific impairment of immunity with advancing cancer as shown by decreasing lymphocyte responsiveness to phytohaemagglutinin.

occur in untreated patients with malignant disease. Although very rare, this is most likely to affect patients with leukaemias or lymphomas and only occasionally with other cancers such as neuroblastoma.[52]

Bacterial and fungal infections

Patients with impaired CMI are particularly susceptible to infection by intracellular pathogens (*Listeria monocytogenes*, *Brucella* and *Mycobacteria* spp.), protozoa (*Pneumocystis carinii* and *Toxoplasma gondii*), fungi (*Candida albicans*, *Nocardia asteroides*, *Aspergillus* and *Cryptococcus* spp.), and viral infections (herpesviruses, measles, and vaccinia). Infection with *Salmonella* spp., *Pseudomonas aeruginosa*, and *Staphylococci* spp. is also more frequent than would be expected.[63] *Pneumocystis carinii* is a frequent and dangerous infection developing in the immunocompromised host. A review at the Mayo clinic of 53 patients developing pneumocystis infection illustrated its predilection for patients with cancer: 28 per cent of whom had leukaemia, 16 per cent lymphoma, 9 per cent non-haematological malignancy, while the remainder had inflammatory diseases treated by corticosteroids. Over half of their patients died within a month of admission to hospital.[64] Patients treated with corticosteroids are not only prone to infection with *Pneumocystis carinii* but also *Candida albicans* and *Cytomegalovirus* spp. The diagnosis of toxoplasmosis is often missed in immunocompromised patients, with most cases being diagnosed at postmortem. Therapy with pyrimethamine and sulphonamide can be successful in about three-quarters of the cases,[65] reinforcing the importance of considering this diagnosis. Tuberculosis occurs in about 1.5 per cent of all patients dying of cancer, and shows florid growth with elongated and numerous bacteria in immunocompromised patients.[66]

Fungi are the most common organisms infecting the CNS in anergic patients, usually originating in the lung and often with associated lung lesions: *Nocardia asteroides* causes brain abscesses; *Cryptococcus neoformans* causes meningitis, meningoencephalitis, and

focal masses; *Candida* spp. infecting the CNS can lead to multiple small abscesses, especially when there is an associated neutropenia, but unlike the other fungal infections it usually arises from the gastrointestinal tract or infected cannulas; *Aspergillus* spp. causes abscesses, infarction, and focal meningitis.[67]

The presentation of certain infecting organisms will vary depending upon which effector arm of the immune system is impaired. Thus systemic candidiasis is the more usual manifestation in neutropenic patients, but it is often limited to oesophageal candidiasis in patients with cell-mediated immunodeficiency and normal neutrophil counts.[68] Although much more frequently seen in treated patients, candidal infection can be a presenting manifestation in patients with acute leukaemia or lymphoma *ab initio*[69] and may present primarily as a pulmonary infection.[70] Hepatic candidiasis is a severe complication in such patients and is frequently fatal (34 per cent), which may prompt the use of more costly therapies with liposomal forms of amphotericin B.[71]

Viral infections

Primary infection with human herpesviruses (**HHV**)—herpes simplex type 1 (HHV-1), herpes simplex type 2 (HHV-2), varicella zoster (HHV-3), Epstein–Barr (HHV-4), cytomegalovirus (HHV-5), or Kaposi's sarcoma virus (HHV-8)—leads to persistent infection of the host. Reactivation may occur because of impairment or deficiency of either specific, cytotoxic T cells (CD8 +) or non-specific, natural-killer cells (**NK**). It is debatable whether HHV-1 and HHV-2 reactivation is increased in patients with depressed CMI, but these patients are definitely more susceptible to viral warts and HHV-3 infection.[72] Rarely, chronic herpesvirus infections can occur in areas of skin infiltrated by CLL or lymphoma, accompanied by hypogammaglobulinaemia.[73]

Herpes zoster or shingles ensues from the reactivation of HHV-3 in 36 per cent of BMT patients; 25 per cent of patients with Hodgkin's disease, where it will often affect X-irradiated dermatomes, and in up to 50 per cent of such patients who have undergone splenectomy as well; in 5 per cent of leukaemic patients; and subclinical reactivation, detected by antibody responses and proliferation to HHV-3 *in vitro*, occurs in equal number to those with clinical disease.[74],[75] Lesions from HHV-3 may become generalized, but visceral involvement is rare.

HHV-5 reactivation occurs in immunocompromised hosts. The presence of HHV-5 antibody has little significance and usually implies viral shedding which can continue for months. As immunosuppression becomes more severe viral shedding can progress to HHV-5 dissemination and multiorgan infection.[76] Interestingly, a relationship exists between alloreactivity (GVHD in BMT or allograft rejection in solid-organ transplants) and CMV infection.

Children with malignant disease are particularly susceptible to measles. Interstitial pneumonitis due to measles is a severe and often fatal infection in children with cancer:[77] 29 per cent of all deaths while in first remission from childhood acute lymphoblastic leukaemia were due to measles or its complications.[78]

Acyclovir and possibly interferon have helped greatly in treating herpesvirus infections.[79] Acyclovir can shorten the infection, restrict dissemination, and accelerate healing of lesions if given within the first 3 days of infection; and it is superior to vidarabine.[80] For HHV-3 infections, immune globulin can confer protection if given within the first 3 days of exposure. For prophylactic treatment of HHV-3, there is an attenuated varicella vaccine (Oka strain) which induces a more than 90 per cent antibody response. Side-effects include rashes and fever and these are increased in high-risk groups and can be severe in immunocompromised patients.[81] Live attenuated vaccine, given to children in remission from leukaemia, induced immunity in about 80 per cent of patients.[82]

Note that antibody-based diagnostic tests for infection in immunocompromised patients may be unreliable because the patient may be unable to make antibody.

Vaccination

Attenuated live vaccines should be avoided in immunocompromised patients. Bacille Calmette–Guérin (BCG) or *Corynebacterium parvum* have been used to augment immune responses non-specifically. Both these bacteria can activate macrophages, which are then capable of causing tumour-cell destruction as a bystander effect. Injection of the BCG at a remote site from the tumour is not effective.[83] This mode of therapy has become the treatment of choice for transitional-cell cancer of the bladder because these are superficial and amenable to repeated intravesical instillation of BCG.[84] Use of these attenuated micro-organisms in immunocompromised patients with malignant disease runs the risk of producing an iatrogenic illness from persistent and disseminated BCG infection with hepatitis, activation of old tuberculosis and possible hypersensitivity reactions,[85] or dysuria in bladder cancer.[86] Disseminated BCG infection can be treated with antituberculous drugs. In certain instances, the opposite to the intended effect can follow the use of immunomodulatory substances, such as BCG or even cytokines like tumour-necrosis factor (TNF), whereby metastasis of tumours is facilitated.[87]

Platelets

Thrombocytosis

High platelet counts ($> 400 \times 10^{(9)}/l$) are frequently seen in patients with non-haematological malignant conditions and termed 'reactive' thrombocytosis. The aetiology is unknown but may involve thrombopoietin or unidentified platelet growth factors.[88] Reactive thrombocytosis rarely requires therapeutic intervention, except for treatment of the underlying disease. The degree of thrombocytosis may be an independent prognostic factor for survival in some patients with primary lung cancer.[89]

Thrombocytopenia

Thrombocytopenia is a common complication of solid tumours. The severity and duration of the thrombocytopenia are usually less than that seen in bone-marrow failure due to leukaemia or bone-marrow aplasia.[90] Decreased production secondary to bone-marrow infiltration or myelotoxic drugs are the commonest cause of thrombocytopenia, but other mechanisms can operate which lead to increased platelet destruction (Table 3). The incidence of thrombocytopenia in cancer patients has increased over the past 15 years due to the use of more intensive myelotoxic chemo- or radiotherapeutic regimens. Generally, patients with solid tumours have enough marrow reserve following myelotoxic chemotherapy to maintain an adequate platelet count. Infection, especially gram negative bacteraemia, will increase

Table 3 Causes of thrombocytopenia in cancer patients

Mechanism	
Decreased platelet prodution	Marrow infiltration
	Haematinic deficiency (vitamin B$_{12}$ and folate)
	Iatrogenic—chemotherapy/radiotherapy
Increased platelet consumption	Disseminated intravascular coagulation
	Microangiopathic haemolytic anaemia
	Thrombotic thrombocytopenic purpura
	Idiopathic–immune, alloimmune
	Post-transfusion purpura
	Heparin
Abnormal distribution	Splenomegaly
Dilutional loss	Massive transfusion

platelet consumption. The mechanisms underlying this include: subclinical or overt disseminated intravascular coagulopathy, microangiopathic haemolytic anaemia, or splenomegaly. Clinically significant dilutional thrombocytopenia only occurs with a transfusion of more than 1.5 times the blood volume of the recipient. 'Formula' replacement should be avoided, but the platelet count should be maintained above $50 \times 10^{9}/l$ in massive transfusion in bleeding patients.[91] Amongst the many causes of thrombocytopenia in cancer patients it is very important to recognize those cases related to heparin therapy. Heparin-induced thrombocytopenia (HIT) occurs in a small but significant proportion (1 to 3 per cent) of individuals receiving heparin; it may also occur in patients receiving only heparin-based flushes of indwelling catheters.[92] In type I HIT the thrombocytopenia is early and mild, rarely less than $100 \times 10^{(9)}/l$, and has no clinical sequelae. Type II HIT is a severe thrombocytopenia with a delayed onset usually starting 4 to 14 days after commencing heparin, but sooner if there has been previous exposure to the drug. The platelet count drops below $100 \times 10^{9}/l$, often below $60 \times 10^{9}/l$. Haemorrhage is unusual, but new thrombosis, arterial and venous, is common and may be devastating. A mortality rate of 30 per cent in patients with HIT and thrombosis has been estimated.[92] Type II HIT is mediated by the production of an antibody against heparin complexed to platelet factor 4 to form an immune complex, which binds to platelet Fcγ receptors and causes platelet activation and aggregation.[93] The diagnosis of HIT is clinical, and therapy should be stopped or substituted as soon as this complication is suspected. Alternative agents include Orgaran (a synthetic heparinoid), Ancrod (a defibrinating agent) and direct thrombin inhibitors such as hirudins and argatroban.[92] Tests for the heparin-dependent platelet antibody assay may be performed as confirmation. The ^{14}C-serotonin release assay is the reference method but more rapid methods such as ELISA have been described.[94]

Prophylactic platelet transfusion reduces the risk of haemorrhage in patients with thrombocytopenia. The threshold at which prophylactic transfusions should be given remains controversial and varies with the clinical context. Recent studies in patients with leukaemic suggest that significant haemorrhage can be prevented using a threshold platelet count of $10 \times 10^{9}/l$ but that an even lower trigger of $5 \times 10^{9}/l$ is safe in patients without fever or bleeding manifestations.[95]–[97] In the presence of coagulopathy, heparin therapy, or anatomical lesions such as recent peptic ulceration or brain tumour, the threshold should be at least $20 \times 10^9/l$. For elective minor and surgical procedures such as lumbar puncture, insertion of indwelling lines, transbronchial biopsy, liver biopsy, or laparotomy, the platelet count should be raised to at least $50 \times 10^9/l$ and $100 \times 10^9/l$ for operations in critical sites such as ophthalmic and neurosurgery.[98]

Defects of platelet function in cancer patients can occur secondary to uraemia, paraproteinaemia, or drug therapy (melphalan, cytosine arabinoside, non-steroidal anti-inflammatory agents). Platelet transfusion in these situations is often ineffective, whereas treatment of the underlying disease offers the best approach to reverse the abnormality of platelet function. Correcting the haematocrit in uraemia to more than 0.30 or the use of **DDAVP** (deamino-*d*-arginine vasopressin) may help correct the haemorrhagic diathesis.[98],[99]

The problems encountered following regular platelet transfusion in patients with primary bone-marrow failure (aplastic anaemia or acute leukaemia) who undergo myeloablative chemo- or radiotherapy and bone-marrow transplantation for their disease can occur in patients with solid tumours but fortunately are rare. The most frequent are transfusion reactions (chills, fevers, rigors) reflecting sensitization to HLA, red-cell antigens, or plasma proteins. The use of antihistamines and corticosteroids prior to platelet transfusion in patients with troublesome side-effects is usually effective in controlling symptoms, but leucocyte-depleted platelets can be given if these reactions are recurrent. Contamination with infectious agents (especially bacteria) is another important cause of chills, fevers and rigors and, although rare, occurs more commonly with transfusion of platelets than with red cells because platelets are stored at $4\,^\circ C$. Platelet refractoriness, the repeated failure to obtain satisfactory responses (clinical or increment in platelet count) to transfusion of platelet concentrates, is a common problem in patients with prolonged therapy-induced thrombocytopenia. The commonest causes are non-immune—such as sepsis, fevers, disseminated intravascular coagulation (DIC), and splenomegaly—but some cases are due to HLA alloimmunization. Alloimmunization against HLA class I antigens on platelet membranes occurs in approximately 70 per cent of patients receiving multiple platelet transfusions, although not all will become refractory.[100] There are two approaches to managing immune refractoriness: (1) taking no preventive methods and using HLA-matched platelet transfusions in the presence of HLA-specific antibodies, or (2) taking measures to prevent HLA alloimmunization from the start of transfusion therapy. A recent study suggests that reduction of viable lymphocytes in transfused products by ultraviolet-B irradiation is as effective as the conventional approach of leucocyte depletion via white-cell filters.[100],[101]

Coagulation

Hypercoagulability (thrombosis)

An association between hypercoagulability and cancer has been recognized for more than 130 years. Trousseau's observations, of the frequent occurrence of lower-limb, deep-vein thrombosis in patients with visceral cancer,[102] have subsequently been corroborated by a wealth of clinicopathological data indicating systemic activation of the coagulation cascade in patients with malignant disease. Postmortem studies have shown a marked increase in the incidence of thromboembolism in patients who have died of cancer, especially of mucinous carcinomas of the pancreas, gastrointestinal tract, and the lung. Histological analysis shows fibrin or platelet plugs in and around many tumours.[103] Thromboembolic disease is second to infection as the commonest cause of death in patients with solid tumours.[104] It may also be the earliest recognizable clinical manifestation of cancer. Studies show that between 10.5 per cent and 23 per cent of patients with lower limb, deep-vein thrombosis (DVT) without obvious predisposing factors have malignant disease or develop it within a short time.[105]–[107] Prandoni *et al.* used a simple diagnostic approach including physical examination, routine blood tests, erythrocyte sedimentation rate, and chest radiography in a prospective study of 250 patients with DVT.[107] They diagnosed cancer in 16 out of 153 (10.5 per cent) patients with 'idiopathic' thrombosis within a 2-year follow-up period.[107] Of the 16 diagnoses of cancer, five were made at the time of initial presentation and six were made within the next 6 months. The incidence of cancer in patients who had recurrent DVT during the 2-year follow-up period was even higher at 17 per cent, confirming that thromboembolic disease refractory to anticoagulant therapy is particularly suggestive of underlying malignancy.[107]

The issue of screening for malignancy in patients with thromboembolic disease is controversial.[103] Without prospective studies it cannot yet be concluded that aggressive diagnostic screening will lead to improved survival. However, it seems reasonable to carefully evaluate patients who present with DVT with no identifiable risk factors. In addition to careful history taking and examination, most physicians advocate at least faecal occult-blood testing and the measurement of carcinoembryonic antigen, prostate-specific antigen in men, and mammography in women. More complex and invasive testing such as abdominopelvic computed tomography (CT) and gastrointestinal endoscopy may further increase the diagnosis of malignancy,[106] but such an approach is expensive and may place excessive demands on resources.

The pathogenic mechanisms responsible for the hypercoagulable state in cancer are numerous and can be considered as disturbances of the blood-vessel wall, disturbances of blood flow, and abnormalities of the blood constituents. Tumour invasion of the blood-vessel wall leads to damage, as a result of their interaction with platelets and endothelial cells leading to platelet aggregation and endothelial activation. Even without invasion of the vascular wall, tumours obstruct and slow the rate of venous blood flow. The presence of cancer is often associated with inappropriate activation of the coagulation and fibrinolytic systems. Tumour cells express procoagulant factors, many of which activate factor X and so lead to the generation of thrombin and fibrin formation. These include tissue factor (which works with factor VII), mucin, and a vitamin K-dependent cysteine protease with direct factor X-activating activity.[108],[109] Tumour cells may also secrete plasminogen-activator inhibitor which reduces fibrinolysis and contributes to the procoagulant state. Tumour interactions with leucocytes may lead to the generation of inflammatory cytokines, which, in turn, further augments the induction of endothelial and monocytic procoagulant activities.

The risk of thromboembolic disease in patients with malignancy is compounded by cancer therapies. For example, postoperative thrombosis occurs three to five times more frequently in patients with malignancy than in patients without.[110] The mechanisms by which hormone therapy can contribute to thrombotic risk are complex and poorly understood.[111] Chemotherapy may also increase thrombotic risk by three main mechanisms. First, procoagulants and cytokines may be released from damaged tumour cells. Second, drugs may be toxic to the vascular endothelium (see the section on thrombotic thrombocytopenic purpura below). Third, the levels of naturally occurring anticoagulants, such as protein C, protein S, and antithrombin, are reduced by some chemotherapeutic agents. Doxorubicin and daunorubicin can promote primary fibrinolysis and l-asparaginase causes the production of abnormal fibrinogens. One randomized trial in 700 women with breast cancer found a fivefold increase in thromboembolic events in patients treated with tamoxifen plus chemotherapy (cyclophosphamide, methotrexate, and 5-fluorouracil) compared with tamoxifen alone.[112] Long-term treatment with tamoxifen alone is associated with an increased incidence of thromboembolic events.[113]

The diagnosis of DVT is provisionally made by clinical examination and confirmed either by venography, Doppler or β-mode ultrasound, impedance plethysmography, or radiolabelled fibrinogen scanning. Venography remains the only reliable method for detecting calf-vein thromboses. The gold standard method of diagnosing pulmonary emboli is pulmonary angiography, but this test is not readily available in many institutions and is associated with a small but significant mortality.[114] Ventilation-perfusion scanning is safer and more accessible but is less accurate. The recently introduced technique of spiral CT is an accurate and non-invasive tool for diagnosing pulmonary embolism.[115]

The treatment of thrombosis in cancer patients is problematic. A relatively high INR (International normalized ratio) with warfarin anticoagulation may be needed to prevent recurrent thrombosis, but then the risks of bleeding from the site of malignancy are increased. Low molecular weight (LMW) heparin may provide increased efficacy in treating and preventing recurrent thromboses in cancer patients.[116],[117] Any patient with cancer should be considered for antithrombotic prophylaxis with standard unfractionated or LMW heparin during times of high risk such as major surgery or immobilization. The incidence of venous thromboembolism is reduced with low-dose warfarin in women receiving chemotherapy for metastatic breast cancer.[118] If the risks of bleeding from the primary malignancy are felt to be high, graduated compression stockings and early immobilization without anticoagulants may be employed.

Thrombotic thrombocytopenic purpura

Thrombotic thrombocytopenic purpura (TTP) is characterized by microangiopathic haemolytic anaemia (red-cell fragmentation), thrombocytopenia, fever, and ischaemic organ damage. In TTP, the main organ affected is the brain, whereas in the closely related haemolytic–uraemic syndrome (HUS) it is the kidney. Histologically, hyaline thrombi rich in platelets are present in capillaries and arterioles, and platelet and endothelial abnormalities are thought to be pivotal in the pathogenesis of TTP. Endothelial damage is manifest in altered endothelial-cell functions such as impaired prostacyclin production and reduced fibrinolytic activity.[96] Sera from patients with TTP stimulate tissue-factor production by human endothelial cells in culture.[119] Electron-microscopic studies of microvascular endothelial cells in HUS show apoptosis in the endothelial cells of involved tissues and plasma from patients with TTP, and HUS can induce apoptosis and the expression of the apoptosis-associated

molecule Fas (CD95) in microvascular endothelial cells.[120] In HUS, the E. coli-associated verocytotoxin may be the cause of endothelial damage as it can induce apoptosis in cultured endothelial cells.[121] Autoantibodies against endothelial-cell and platelet-glycoprotein IV have been detected in the plasma of patients with TTP.[122] Further support for an immunological mechanism of endothelial-cell dysfunction in TTP comes from studies suggesting that macrophages and lymphocytes are activated in TTP. Increased levels of IL-1, IL-6, the soluble IL-2 receptor, TNF, and transforming growth factor-β (TGF-β) occur.[123],[124] Preliminary evidence suggests that individuals lacking the human leucocyte antigen DR53 may be more susceptible to TTP.[125]

The agents responsible for platelet aggregation in TTP/HUS are unknown. Unidentified proteins of 37 and 59 kDa and a calcium-dependent protease (calpain) have been implicated.[126] Absence or defective binding of platelet-aggregation inhibitors, such as prostacyclin, may also play a role as well as von Willebrand factor (vWF).[119] vWF crosslinks platelets to other platelets or endothelial cells. High levels of vWF are found in TTP thrombi and unusually large vWF multimers (ULvWF) are found in the plasma of TTP patients, which may reflect the release of ULvWF multimers from damaged endothelial cells. ULvWF multimers may be more effective than normal vWF multimers at binding platelets under conditions of shear stress. Persistence of ULvWF multimers in a patient's plasma after recovery from TTP predicts recurrent disease.[127],[128] Recently, a specific vWF-cleaving metalloprotease has been isolated from human plasma[129] and a deficiency of this protease has been found in patients with familial forms of TTP.[130] In acquired forms of the disease there is an inhibitor or autoantibody against this vWF-cleaving protease.[130],[131] There is no defect in the activity of this protease in patients with HUS.[130]

TTP is associated with cancer and cancer therapies and it is often difficult to establish the relative contribution of treatment and disease in an individual case. TTP is most often associated with adenocarcinoma, but it also occurs with small-cell lung cancer, squamous cancers, thymoma, Hodgkin's disease, and non-Hodgkin's lymphomas.[96] It is caused by chemotherapeutic agents including mitomycin C, bleomycin, cytosine arabinoside, daunorubicin, deoxycoformycin, and tamoxifen in addition to other drugs used in the treatment of cancer, such as cyclosporin A and tacrolimus.[96]

The main differential diagnosis of TTP is disseminated intravascular coagulation. The distinction between DIC and TTP in patients with cancer can be difficult as a low level of coagulation-factor activation and consumption is common in patients with metastatic disease. However, the presence of significant coagulopathy suggests underlying DIC. The treatment of TTP involves the removal of the precipitating agent where possible, for example stopping the implicated drug or resecting tumour. Plasma exchange (40 to 80 ml/kg body mass) with cryodepleted fresh-frozen plasma (FFP) is more effective than with whole FFP, and may operate via the removal of endothelial toxins or proapoptotic factors and/or replacement of antiapoptotic factors.[121],[132] A substance in cryodepleted FFP is capable of reducing the size of ULvWF multimers released by human endothelial cells in culture.[133] Platelet transfusions should be avoided as they may aggravate ischaemic organ damage.[134] Other therapeutic approaches include prostacyclin, vincristine, steroids, and immunoadsorption with staphylococcal protein A columns.[132] Defibrotide is a novel, mammalian tissue-derived, polydeoxyribonucleotide adenosine-receptor agonist with antithrombotic, anti-ischaemic, and thrombolytic properties which appears to be effective in preliminary studies of patients with refractory TTP.[135]

Disseminated intravascular coagulation (DIC)

DIC frequently occurs in patients with metastatic malignancy. It arises from the inappropriate and continued activation of clotting pathways that lead to excessive thrombin generation, coagulation factor consumption, platelet aggregation with secondary fibrinolysis, and the formation of fibrin/fibrinogen degradation products (**FDPs**) which themselves act as anticoagulants. There are acute and chronic forms of DIC. The chronic form is more common in patients with solid tumours, and haemorrhage is rare as the haemostatic defect is compensated for by the increased synthesis of coagulation factors. The acute form is severe and may result in catastrophic haemorrhage from surgical and venepuncture sites, gastrointestinal or genitourinary tracts. Acute DIC is usually seen in acute promyelocytic leukaemia (**APL**) or following surgery for prostatic carcinoma. Patients may present with or have coexistent thrombotic complications such as digital gangrene, renal failure, or purpura fulminans.

The diagnosis of acute DIC rests on establishing prolongation of prothrombin, activated partial thromboplastin, and thrombin times with hypofibrinogenaemia (fibrinogen level of less than 1 g/l), raised FDPs, and thrombocytopenia. Red-cell fragmentation may be seen on a blood film but is generally not as pronounced as in TTP/HUS. Signs of infection should be sought as septicaemia may precipitate acute DIC in immunocompromised cancer patients. Management remains controversial, but the precipitating factor, for instance a concurrent infection, should be treated where possible and supportive care given. If bleeding occurs, FFP should be administered (10 to 15 ml/kg initially) to replace all clotting factors with cryoprecipitate (1 unit/5 kg) when fibrinogen replacement is required, and platelet transfusions to keep a platelet count of more than $50 \times 10^9/l$.[98],[99] All-*trans*-retinoic acid is critical in reversing DIC associated with APL.[136] Bleeding is unusual in chronic DIC and therapy (other than controlling the underlying tumour) is generally unwarranted.[99]

Acquired coagulation-factor inhibitors

Acquired inhibitors of coagulation factors are antibodies that partially or completely neutralize the activation or function of a specific clotting factor, or that interfere with interactions between coagulation-factor proteins. As well as occurring in patients with inherited coagulation-factor deficiencies, such inhibitors may be idiopathic or occur in association with malignancy or autoimmune diseases. Inhibitors have been identified in patients with solid tumours such as prostate, kidney, lung, colon, head and neck cancers and in association with chronic lymphocytic leukaemia, lymphomas, and myeloma.[137] Specific inhibitory activity is most commonly directed at factor VIII, but it may affect von Willebrand factor or other clotting proteins. Patients often present with dramatic haemorrhage into soft tissues, muscles, or retroperitoneal structures and can be the first manifestation of an otherwise occult malignancy. Management of acquired inhibitors is problematic and specialist referral is advised.[138]

Table 4 Relative risk of cancer in immunodeficient patients compared with the general population

Immunodeficiency	Relative risk*
Congenital or primary	100–1000
Transplant recipient	80
AIDS	60

*Age may play an important role—see text. See references 140, 141.

Table 5 Estimated frequency of cancer in specific immunodeficient states

Immunodeficiency	Frequency (%)
Congenital	
Selective IgA	1
X-linked agammaglobulinaemia	4
Severe combined immunodeficiency	9
Wiskott–Aldrich syndrome	14
Ataxia telangiectasia	29
X-linked lymphoproliferative syndrome	40
Acquired	
Common variable immunodeficiency	11
Organ transplantation	10
AIDS	
Lymphoma	3
Kaposi's sarcoma	16

*Chromosomal instability. See references 147–150.

Immunodeficiency, immunosuppression, and cancer

Cancer is more frequent in patients who are chronically immunodeficient (Table 4). Even with minor immunodeficiency states, such as the hyper IgE syndrome, lymphomas are more frequent.[139] Estimates of the relative risk of developing cancer are fairly consistent for the major different categories of immunodeficiency (Table 4), but some calculate the risk as being much higher (up to 1000-fold normal) in congenitally immunodeficient patients. This may be because the early onset of immunodeficiency increases the risk of developing cancer. As an example, the risk of developing a lymphoma in all AIDS patients is 60-fold that of normal but this risk rises to 360-fold for patients aged 20 years or less.[140]

The frequency of cancer in specific immunodeficiency states is given in Table 5. The very high incidence of malignancy (mostly lymphomas) in ataxia–telangiectasia is attributed as much to its mild immunodeficiency as to its associated susceptibility to chromosomal breakage and translocation which selectively involve genes of the immune system, namely the immunoglobulin genes at 2p12, 14q32, and 22q11 and the T-cell receptor genes at 7p13, 7q35, and 14q11.[142] There is also an unusually high frequency of lymphoma (as the only malignancy) in the rare X-linked lymphoproliferative syndrome (**XLPS**).[143] XLPS is associated with a defective gene affecting an SH2 domain coding for a protein called SAP.[144],[145] Its relationship to lymphoproliferation is unknown, but it is triggered exclusively by infection with the Epstein–Barr virus (HHV-4) and leads to a range of diseases including hypogammaglobulinaemia, rapidly fatal infectious mononucleosis, or high-grade, disseminated B-cell lymphoma.

Chronic immunosuppression associated with all forms of transplantation is associated with increased malignancy including allogeneic bone-marrow grafts.[146]

Characteristics of cancer in immunodeficiency states

The incidence of cancers in immunocompromised patients is not that seen in the general population (for example, lung, prostate, breast, colon) but consists of an excess of lymphomas, cancers of the skin and lips, vulva, or perineum, and Kaposi's sarcoma. For example, 67 per cent of all cancers arising in congenital immunodeficiency are lymphomas compared with 8 per cent in 'normal' children. The known or suspected association of the cancers arising in immunodeficiency with a viral aetiology (for instance, HHV-4 with lymphomas or HHV-8 with Kaposi's sarcoma) is the distinctive component. For example, the association of HHV-4 and B-cell lymphomas is widely known. However, HHV-4 has also been implicated in T-cell lymphomas and leiomyosarcoma.[151]

The length of time between the onset of immunodeficiency and the diagnosis of cancer varies according to the type of cancer. This incubation time is based mostly on transplant statistics because of the clearly defined start of immunodeficiency with transplant immunosuppression, so that the average delay before Kaposi's sarcoma, lymphoma, or carcinoma is 20, 33, and 107 months, respectively. However, the time to oncogenesis is affected by the intensity and duration of immunosuppression.[152] Both the frequency and the speed of oncogenesis increase proportionally to the intensity of immunosuppression. This is most evident from examining transplantation data. The frequency of cancer differs according to the grafted organ, reflecting the intensity of immunosuppressive therapy required to prevent graft rejection (Table 5). The prolonged use of excessive non-specific immunosuppression increases the risk of cancer. This was seen in early clinical studies of cyclosporin where it was combined with steroids and azathioprine at excessive dosage. Recently the use of the monoclonal antibody OKT3, which suppresses virtually all T-cell function, has been associated with a striking increase in lymphomas. OKT3 at a cumulative dosage above 75 mg has been associated with a sharp rise (36 per cent) in lymphomagenesis.[153]

The treatment of cancers arising in immunodeficient patients is conventional, but it may have to be modified because of the type of immunodeficiency or because of past therapy and bone-marrow suppression. Where possible, the immunosuppression must be reduced and this on its own can lead to resolution of the lymphomas. The role of acyclovir in EBV-driven proliferation is controversial, but no benefit has been seen in XLPS in which there is an 85 per cent mortality from fulminant infectious mononucleosis or lymphoma. Attempts to provide prophylaxis for XLPS patients with immunoglobulin containing EBV-specific antibodies are underway, which is based on the observation that the syndrome does not occur while maternal antibodies are still present.[150] There is the prospect of an EBV vaccine which has successfully been used to immunize tamarin cottontops against the development of lymphomas.[154]

Lymphomas in immunodeficient and immunocompetent individuals

The lymphomas in immunodeficient patients are commonly associated with the Epstein–Barr virus (HHV-4), meaning that the EBV genome is incorporated into the lymphoma cells detected by the Epstein–Barr nuclear antigen (EBNA1–6) or other HHV-3 antigens (LMP1–2, late membrane protein). They are usually high grade (immunoblastic) and in AIDS are often classified as 'Burkitt-like' (estimated as 1000-fold the frequency in the general population). However, a wide variety of histopathological types can be seen including multiple myeloma.[155] Extranodal involvement is commoner in immunodeficient patients (69 per cent compared with 30 per cent normally), and there is frequent involvement of the allograft (18 per cent) in transplanted patients. Primary brain lymphomas are common (28 per cent) at a 1000-fold increase over the normal risk. Some two-thirds of brain lymphomas arising in immunodeficiency are primary and solitary tumours, unlike the brain lymphomas that usually arise late in the course of the disease after disseminating from lymph-node sites. Isolated CNS lymphomas in immunocompromised patients are similar to their peripheral lymphomas in incorporating HHV-4, unlike CNS lymphomas from immunocompetent patients which are usually HHV-3-negative.[156] Patients may show evidence of chronic EBV infection.[157] Many immunodeficient patients with lymphoma have elevated IgG antibody titres to the viral capsid antigen (VCA) and the early antigen (EA). Although IgA antibodies to VCA and EA characterize nasopharyngeal carcinoma (NPC), these can be found in approximately 40 per cent of patients with CLL but at a 10-fold lower titre than in NPC.[158] In immunodeficient patients, the lymphoproliferation may show progression from polyclonal to monoclonal phenotypes, and they are less likely to have chromosomal mutations associated with lymphomas than immunocompetent individuals.[155] Finally, where the immunodeficiency can be corrected rapidly, such as in transplant patients on immunosuppression, the lymphoproliferation can resolve spontaneously (no matter how advanced the stage or histological type) because the HHV-3 antigens provide a potent target for cytotoxic T-cell control of the tumour.[159]

Autoimmunity in cancer

There are three situations in which autoantibodies arise in cancer: (1) as a product of malignant B cells; (2) because of dysregulation by malignant T cells; or (3) where degraded or altered self-proteins released by a tumour are immunogenic to the host. Table 6 summarizes the wide range of autoantibodies occurring in patients with cancer.

Autoantibodies produced by lymphomas

Coomb's-positive, warm antibody haemolytic anaemia (AIHA) occurs in about 15 per cent and idiopathic thrombocytopenia (ITP) in about 10 per cent of chronic lymphocytic leukaemias (CLL) and well-differentiated lymphocytic lymphomas (ML lymphocytic, Kiel), as well as a variety of haemolytic anaemias in Waldenstrom's macroglobulinaemia (ML lymphoplasmacytoid, Kiel). Autoantibody production by malignant plasma cells was easily understood for Waldenstrom's disease but not for CLL. An unusual lineage of normal B cells known as the CD5 + B cell, because they share a membrane

Table 6 Autoantibodies and autoimmunity in cancer

Tissue and syndrome	Autoantibody targets	
	Major	Minor
Haemopoietic tissue:		
Pure red-cell aplasia	CFU-E or BFU-E	
Haemolytic anaemia	Rh I, etc.	
Idiopathic thrombocytopenia	gpIIb/IIIa, gpIb	
Neutropenia	CFU-GM	
Brain and cranial nerves:		
Limbic encephalitis	ANNA-1 (Hu)Ta	CV2
Encephalomyelitis	ANNA-1 (Hu)	CV2 Amphyphysin VGCC
Cerebellar degeneration	PCA-1 (Yo)TrTa	CV2 Amphyphysin VGCCMa
Opsoclonus—myoclonus	ANNA-2 (Ri)	Amphyphysin
Cancer-associated retinopathy	Recoverin	
Optic neuritis	CV2	
Neuromuscular junction:		
Lambert–Eaton myasthenic syndrome	VGCC (P/Q type)	CV2
	ANNA-2 (Ri)	
Myasthenia gravis	Acetylcholine receptor	
Neuromyotonia	VGKC	
Peripheral neuropathy:		
Autonomic	Acetylcholine receptor (muscle)	
Motor	GD1	
Sensory	ANNA-1 (Hu) MAG	CV2
Multiple neural sites:		
Stiff person syndrome	Amphiphysin	
Chronic pseudo-obstruction	ANNA-1 (Hu)	Amphyphysin
Skin:		
Pemphigus	Desmoplakin	
Acanthosis nigricans	Insulin receptor	

Abbreviations: CFU-E, erythroid colony-forming units; BFU-E, erythroid burst-forming units; CFU-GM, granulocyte–macrophage colony-forming units; gp, glycoprotein; ANNA, antineuronal nuclear antibody; PCA, Purkinje-cell antibody; VGCC, voltage-gated calcium channel; VGKC, voltage-gated potassium channel; MAG, myelin associated glycoprotein.

antigen normally found on T cells (CD5), has been identified. These CD5+ B cells are increased in autoimmune diseases, such as rheumatoid arthritis, have a propensity to produce autoantibodies, differentiate independently of other B cells, and have CLL and lymphoplasmacytoid lymphomas as their malignant counterparts.[160],[161] Small amounts of monoclonal paraprotein can be detected in the serum of patients with CLL using sensitive techniques, and this can produce disease if the monoclonal antibody reacts with erythrocyte or platelet antigens. Far greater quantities of paraprotein are produced in lymphoplasmacytoid lymphomas where the hyperviscosity syndrome, impairment of coagulation or platelet function, neurological symptoms, cold sensitivity (cryoglobulins), haemolysis (cold agglutinins), or pseudohyponatraemia may occur. Conversely, the incidence of lymphomas is increased in autoimmune diseases, particularly in rheumatoid arthritis. Chronic T-cell immunodeficiency, immunosuppressive therapy, and EBV infection may combine to cause this increased susceptibility.[162]

Rarely, Waldenstrom's macroglobulinaemia is associated with multiple mononeuropathy, but IgM monoclonal gammopathies of unknown significance (**MGUS**) are more frequently associated with distal sensory neuropathies. The neuropathy is associated with monoclonal antibody recognizing myelin-associated glycoprotein (**MAG**). The anti-MAG antibodies are associated with marked reduction in motor nerve conduction, segmental demyelination, and IgM deposits in the peripheral nerves.[163] In addition to reactivities with MAG, anti-sulphatide, -ganglioside, -GM1, -chondroitin sulphate, -neurofilament, and -tubulin reactivity has been described.[164] Most are associated with sensory neuropathies, but anti-GM1 at high titres may have motor neuropathies or a motor neurone-like disease. The reactivity of anti-MAG antibodies overlaps with HNK1, a natural killer-cell antibody that also detects neuroendocrine tissue. Passive transfer of anti-MAG antibodies induces the same neuropathies in animals. There is massive accumulation of antibody at the nodes of Ranvier leading to paranodal degeneration. **POEMS**—polyneuropathy, organomegaly, endocrinopathy, M-protein, and skin changes—are associated with IgG and IgA paraproteins and are similar to chronic inflammatory demyelinating polyneuropathy.[165] An autoimmune bullous disease, paraneoplastic pemphigus, is associated with lymphomas (non-Hodgkin's lymphoma, CLL, Waldenstrom's macroglobulinaemia, and Castleman's disease) and less frequently with thymomas, small-cell lung cancers (**SCLC**), and sarcomas.[166] This polymorphous skin eruption with mucositis is caused by the deposition of IgG and complement in the intercellular spaces of the epidermis due to reactivity of the autoantibodies with desmoplakins. The complement-mediated damage leads to suprabasilar acantholysis and blister formation.[167] Autoantibodies precipitate five different proteins from keratinocytes, of which the two major components are desmoplakins I and II, one is the bullous pemphigoid antigen occurring in non-neoplastic pemphigus, and the other two are unknown proteins of 170 and 190 kDa. These autoantibodies can be detected in the sera of patients by immunofluorescent tests on rat bladder epithelium, by complement fixation, or immunoprecipitation techniques. The rat-bladder technique alone has a specificity of 83 per cent and a sensitivity of 75 per cent. Performing the complement-fixation test increases the specificity. Passive transfer of these autoantibodies into mice produces intraepidermal vesiculation, which supports their pathogenic role. Desmoplakins and the bullous pemphigoid antigen are intracellular, so the 170 and 190 kDa antigens are likely to be the pathogenic targets.

T-cell dysregulation in T-cell lymphomas

Angioimmunoblastic lymphadenopathy with dysproteinaemia (**AILD**), a T-cell lymphoma, is characterized by hypergammaglobulinaemia, Coomb's positivity, and high titres of smooth muscle antibody (**SMA**, binding to intermediate filaments) that occurs in 75 per cent of cases. The SMA may relate to endothelial antigens, because there is marked vascular endothelial proliferation in this disease, or to viral antigens crossreacting with intermediate filaments, because there is often a preceding viral infection in AILD.[168] The antibodies are polyclonal and consist of IgM, IgG, and IgA classes at titres of 1/64 to 1/512. They react with determinants shared by vimentin, desmin, and keratin. This 'multiple determinant reactivity' or polyspecificity is characteristic of CD5 + B cells, raising the question as to whether cytokines produced by the malignant T cells encourage their differentiation and antibody production. Rare patients have been described with T-cell lymphocytic leukaemia, immunodeficiency, and hyper IgM. The leukaemic T cells have been reported to provide selective helper function for IgM but to suppress IgG and IgA.[169]

Autoantibodies to altered or crossreactive self-proteins

While Chapter 5.3 describes the clinical aspects of paraneoplastic disease (PND), the immunological aspects will be covered here. In 1951, Russell Brain first suggested that PND might be related to immune responses triggered by the tumour crossreacting with proteins expressed by the nervous system, thus leading to nervous damage. The detection of autoantibodies reacting with neuronal tissue in both the serum and CSF supported this original hypothesis. It is now known that tumours and nervous tissue share antigens involved in the autoantibody responses. These antibodies have been detected by immunofluorescence, immunoenzyme, and Western blotting (where the antigen has been purified or recombinant protein is available). Many autoantibodies have now been described and antibody assays to the most frequent autoantigens involved in PND (antineuronal nuclear antibodies (ANNA)-1 and -2, and Purkinje cell antibodies (PCA-1)) are commercially available.

Pathogenesis and antibodies in PND

A pathogenic mechanism of autoantibodies has been established in Lambert–Eaton myasthenic syndrome (LEMS), myasthenia gravis, and neuromyotonia.[170],[171] The antibodies react against voltage-gated calcium channels (VGCC) in the presynaptic active zones of the neuromuscular junction so altering acetylcholine release. Plasma exchange improves the condition and passive transfer into animals provokes it.[172] On the other hand, passive transfer with antineuronal nuclear antibodies (ANNA-1 and -2; see below) or Purkinje cell antibodies (PCA-1; see below) or immunization of animals with the corresponding antigens have failed to induce neurological damage.[173],[174] Even disturbance of the blood–brain barrier and direct intraventricular injection of antibody have failed to produce evidence of neurological toxicity. Since these antigens are intracellular, antibody access is limited. Hence, the antibodies may develop as a result of neuronal damage and release of sequestered antigen following a separate pathogenic effect. However, there is recent evidence that antibodies may penetrate cells and could give rise to tissue damage. Many patients with PND have small, localized tumours that do not progress or metastasize as rapidly as tumours in patients without PND.[175] This raises the question whether the immune response, despite causing distressing clinical disease, is not involved in the control of tumour spread.

The autoantibodies causing functional neurological impairment such as LEMS and opsoclonus–myoclonus can be removed by plasma exchange, immunosuppression, or treatment of the tumour so as to reverse the PND. However, this is not the case for the other PND in which no pathogenic role for autoantibodies has been established. It is possible that these syndromes have already caused irreversible neurological damage. T-cell mediated disease may cause the neurological damage seen in some PND, in which autoantibody production may be a secondary event. Extensive infiltration of the nervous system by small lymphocytes has been seen in patients with ANNA-1 and ANNA-2.[176],[177]

Antibody specificities in PND

Antineuronal nuclear antibodies (ANNA)

There are two major types of these antibodies. ANNA-1 (anti-Hu) binds to three proteins, ranging in size from 38 to 40 kDa, in CNS neuronal nuclei and SCLC (recombinant cloned proteins are HuD, HuC, Hel-N1/N2). ANNA-1 strongly stains all neuronal nuclei (CNS as well as peripheral) with weaker cytoplasmic staining. Antibodies react with two RNA-binding sites on HuD and crossreact with HuC and Hel-N1. HuD is located on chromosome 1p34. The antigens are neurone-specific RNA/DNA-binding proteins involved in the RNA processing of neurones. Polyclonal IgG, complement-fixing antibodies are found in the serum and CSF of affected patients. At high titres (> 1:500), the paraneoplastic disorder precedes the diagnosis of the cancer by 4 months on average. Low titres can be detected in 15 per cent of patients with SCLC without neurological symptoms. No tumour was found in 12 per cent of ANNA-1-positive patients.[178] Antibody responders often express MHC class I antigen on neurones, whereas antibody-negative individuals do not. Immune attack may lead to the upregulation of MHC I.

ANNA-2 (anti-Ri) recognizes 55 and 80 kDa neuronal proteins (the 55-kDa antigen is a recombinant protein known as NOVA, homologous to the RNA-binding protein hnRNPK). These RNA-binding proteins regulate metabolism in a subset of developing motor neurones. In vitro, ANNA-2 inhibits the RNA-binding activity of NOVA. ANNA-2 stains all neuronal nuclei of the CNS except dorsal root ganglia.[179]

Purkinje-cell antibodies

PCA-1 or anti-Yo (discovered in patients with gynaecological tumours) are polyclonal IgG, complement-fixing antibodies that recognize a 34-kDa protein (CDR34; CDR, calcium-dependent regulator protein) and a 62-kDa antigen (CDR62) shared by tumour- and Purkinje-cell cytoplasm and neurones of the cerebellum and gut mucosa. The gene encoding CDR34 contains a leucine-zipper motif and marks the upper boundary of the FRAX marker for the fragile X gene, while the gene for CDR62 has been mapped to the short arm of chromosome 16 and codes for DNA-binding, gene-transcription regulators carrying zinc-finger motifs. PCA-1 produces coarse granular staining of Purkinje-cell cytoplasm and proximal dendrites sparing the nucleus. It binds to clusters of ribosomes, the Golgi apparatus, and granular endoplasmic reticulum in Purkinje cells. Cancers could be found in 52 out of 55 (95 per cent) patients with PCA-1 antibodies.[180]

Anti-Tr is found in the serum and CSF of patients with Hodgkin's disease either following diagnosis, or in relapse or remission. It has no identified protein antigen to date. It reacts with Purkinje-cell cytoplasm with a characteristic fine granular staining in the molecular layer. It occurs in more slowly developing cerebellar syndromes associated with Hodgkin's disease.

Other autoantibodies

Antiamphiphysin reacts with a 128-kDa protein present in neuronal extracts. It stains the neuropil of rat cerebellum, sparing the neuronal nuclei and cytoplasm. It reacts with a synaptic vesicle in the CNS whose function is unknown.[181]

Anti-VGCC reacts with VGCC in a presynaptic state and prevents acetylcholine release. SCLC also express Ca^{2+} channel antigens that crossreact with the anti-VGCC. In LEMS, the antibody response is against the P/Q type of VGCC.[182],[183]

Anti-Ta reacts with a 40-kDa neuronal protein whose function is unknown. It stains discrete granules in the nucleus or perkarion of rat neurones and stains the nucleus in human cortex. The cloned protein, Ma2, is expressed in brain and testicular tumours. Ma2 is homologous with Ma1, also found in PND, and is expressed by brain and testes, but with no known function.

Anti-CV2 is an IgG antibody that stains the cytoplasm of oligodendrocytes, and is a 66-kDa protein found in the brains of newborn rats. It is always associated with cancers.

References

1. Dorian B, Garfinkel PE. Stress, immunity and illness—a review. *Psychological Medicine*, 1987; **17**(2): 393–407.

2. Vogelzang NJ, *et al.* Patient, caregiver and oncologist perceptions of cancer-related fatigue: results of a tripartite assessment survey. The fatigue coalition. *Seminars in Hematology*, 1997; **34**: 4–12.

3. Means RT, Krantz SB. Progress in understanding the pathogenesis of the anaemia of chronic disease. *Blood*, 1992; **80**: 1639–47.

4. Domachowske JB. The role of nitric oxide in the regulation of cellular iron metabolism. *Biochemistry and Molecular Medicine*, 1997; **60**(1): 1–7.

5. Beguin Y. Prediction of response to optimize outcome of treatment with erythropoietin. *Seminars in Oncology*, 1998; **25**: 27–34.

6. Ludwig H, *et al.* Recombinant human erythropoietin for the correction of cancer associated anemia with and without concomitant cytotoxic chemotherapy. *Cancer*, 1995; **76**: 2319–29.

7. Glaspy J. The impact of epoetin alfa on quality of life during cancer chemotherapy: a fresh look at an old problem. *Seminars in Hematology*, 1997; **34**: 20–6.

8. Beguin Y. Erythropoiesis and erythropoietin in multiple myeloma. *Leukemia and Lymphoma*, 1995; **18**(5–6): 413–21.

9. Krantz SB. Erythropoietin and the anaemia of chronic disease. *Nephrology, Dialysis, and Transplantation*, 1995; **10**(Suppl. 2): 10–17.

10. Goodnough LT, Monk TG, Andriole GL. Erythropoietin therapy. *New England Journal of Medicine*, 1997; **336**: 933–8.

11. Sheffield R, Sullivan SD, Saltiel E, Nishimura L. Cost comparison of recombinant human erythropoietin and blood transfusion in cancer chemotherapy-induced anemia. *Annals of Pharmacotherapy*, 1997; **31**: 15–22.

12. Adamson JW, Ludwig H. Predicting the hematopoietic response to recombinant erythropoietin (Epoetin alfa) in the treatment of the anemia of cancer. *Oncology*, 1999; **56**: 46–53.

13. Schooley JC, Kullgren B, Allison AC. Inhibition by interleukin-1 of the action of erythropoietin on erythroid precursors and its possible role in the pathogenesis of hypoplastic anaemias. *British Journal of Haematology*, 1987; **67**: 11–17.

14. Henry DH. Clinical application of recombinant erythropoietin in anemic cancer patients. *Hematology/Oncology Clinics of North America*, 1994; **8**: 961–73.

15. Davis D, Charles PJ, Potter A, Feldmann M, Maini RN, Elliott MJ. Anaemia of chronic disease in rheumatoid arthritis: *in vivo* effects of tumour necrosis factor alpha blockade. *British Journal of Rheumatology*, 1997; **36**(9): 950–6.

16. Chanarin I, Metz J. Diagnosis of cobalamin deficiency: the old and the new. *British Journal of Haematology*, 1997; **97**(4): 695–700. [See Comments]

17. Bain BJ, Clark DM, Lampert IA. Metastatic tumour. In *Bone marrow pathology* (ed. BJ Bain, DM Clark, IA Lampert). Oxford: Blackwell Scientific, 1992: 000–00.

18. Pelkey TJ, Frierson HFJ, Bruns DE. Molecular and immunological detection of circulating tumor cells and micrometastases from solid tumors. *Clinical Chemistry*, 1996; **42**(9): 1369–81.

19. Theocharous P, Lowdell MW, Jones AL, Prentice HG. Immunocytochemical detection of breast cancer cells: a comparison of three attachment factors. *Journal of Hematotherapy*, 1997; **6**(1): 21–9.

20. Dessypris EN. The biology of pure red cell aplasia. *Seminars in Hematology*, 1991; **28**(4): 275–84.

21. Lacy MQ, Kurtin PJ, Tefferi A. Pure red cell aplasia: association with large granular lymphocyte leukemia and the prognostic value of cytogenetic abnormalities. *Blood*, 1996; **87**(7): 3000–6. [See Comments]

22. Nishioka R, Nakajima S, Morimoto Y, Suzuki H, Nakamura H, Suzuki M. T-cell acute lymphoblastic leukemia with transient pure red cell aplasia associated with myasthenia gravis and invasive thymoma. *Internal Medicine*, 1995; **34**(2): 127–30.

23. Marmont A, Peschle C, Sanguineti M, Condorelli M. Pure red cell aplasia (PRCA): response of three patients of cyclophosphamide and/or antilymphocyte globulin (ALG) and demonstration of two types of serum IgG inhibitors to erythropoiesis. *Blood*, 1975; **45**(2): 247–61.

24. Messner HA, Fauser AA, Curtis JE, Dotten D. Control of antibody-mediated pure red-cell aplasia by plasmapheresis. *New England Journal of Medicine*, 1981; **304**(22): 1334–8.

25. Casadevall N, Dupuy E, Molho-Sabatier P, Tobelem G, Varet B, Mayeux P. Autoantibodies against erythropoietin in a patient with pure red-cell aplasia. *New England Journal of Medicine*, 1996; **334**(10): 630–3. [See Comments]

26. Peschle C, Marmont AM, Marone G, Genovese A, Sasso GF, Condorelli M. Pure red cell aplasia: studies on an IgG serum inhibitor neutralizing erythropoietin. *British Journal of Haematology*, 1975; **30**(4): 411–17.

27. Masuda M, Arai Y, Okamura T, Mizoguchi H. Pure red cell aplasia with thymoma: evidence of T-cell clonal disorder. *American Journal of Hematology*, 1997; **54**(4): 324–8.

28. Krantz SB. Pure red-cell aplasia. *New England Journal of Medicine*, 1974; **291**(7): 345–50.

29. Bible KC, Tefferi A. Cyclosporine A alleviates severe anaemia associated with refractory large granular lymphocytic leukaemia and chronic natural killer cell lymphocytosis. *British Journal of Haematology*, 1996; **93**(2): 406–8.

30. Tura S, Finelli C, Bandini G, Cavo M, Gobbi M. Cyclosporin A in the treatment of CLL associated PRCA and bone marrow hypoplasia. *Nouvelle Revue Francaise d'Hematologie*, 1988; **30**(5–6): 479–81.

31. Kurtzman GJ, Cohen B, Meyers P, Amunullah A, Young NS. Persistent B19 parvovirus infection as a cause of severe chronic anaemia in children with acute lymphocytic leukaemia. *Lancet*, 1988; **2**(8621): 1159–62.

32. Brown KE, Young NS. Parvovirus B19 infection and hematopoiesis. *Blood Reviews*, 1995; **9**(3): 176–82.

33. Carrigan DR, Knox KK. Bone marrow suppression by human herpesvirus-6: comparison of the A and B variants of the virus. *Blood*, 1995; **86**(2): 835–6. [Letter; Comment]

34. Singh N, Carrigan DR. Human herpesvirus-6 in transplantation: an emerging pathogen. *Annals of Internal Medicine*, 1996; **124**(12): 1065–71.

35. Cook IJ, Pavli P, Riley JW, Goulston KJ, Dent OF. Gastrointestinal

investigation of iron deficiency anaemia. *British Medical Journal (Clinical Research edn)*, 1986; **292**(6532): 1380–2.

36. Croker JR, Beynon G. Gastro-intestinal bleeding—a major cause of iron deficiency in the elderly. *Age and Ageing*, 1981; **10**(1): 40–3.

37. Pawson R, Mehta A. Review article: the diagnosis and treatment of haematinic deficiency in gastrointestinal disease. *Alimentary Pharmacology and Therapeutics*, 1998; **12**(8): 687–98.

38. Baumann KS, Seifert B, Michel B, Ruegg R, Fehr J. Prediction of iron deficiency in chronic inflammatory rheumatic disease anaemia. *British Journal of Haematology*, 1995; **91**(4): 820–6.

39. Punnonen K, Irjala K, Rajamaki A. Serum transferrin receptor and its ratio to serum ferritin in the diagnosis of iron deficiency. *Blood*, 1997; **89**(3): 1052–7.

40. Rytting M, Worth L, Jaffe N. Hemolytic disorders associated with cancer. *Hematology/Oncology Clinics of North America*, 1996; **10**(2): 365–76.

41. Sokol RJ, Booker DJ, Stamps R. Erythrocyte autoantibodies, autoimmune haemolysis, and carcinoma. *Journal of Clinical Pathology*, 1994; **47**(4): 340–3.

42. Myint H, *et al*. Fludarabine-related autoimmune haemolytic anaemia in patients with chronic lymphocytic leukaemia. *British Journal of Haematology*, 1995; **91**(2): 341–4.

43. Damon A, Hollut DA, Melicon MM, Ucon AC. Polycythemia and renal cell carcinoma. *American Journal of Medicine*, 1958; **25**: 182–97.

44. Brownstein MH, Ballard HS. Hepatoma associated with erythrocytosis. *American Journal of Medicine*, 1966; **40**(2): 204–10.

45. Opelz G, Sengar DP, Mickey MR, Terasaki PI. Effect of blood transfusions on subsequent kidney transplants. *Transplantation Proceedings*, 1973; **5**(1): 253–9.

46. Tartter PI, Burrows L, Kirschner P. Perioperative blood transfusion adversely affects prognosis after resection of Stage I (subset N0) non-oat cell lung cancer. *Journal of Thoracic and Cardiovascular Surgery*, 1984; **88**(5, Pt 1): 659–62.

47. Tartter PI. The association of perioperative blood transfusion with colorectal cancer recurrence. *Annals of Surgery*, 1992; **216**(6): 633–8.

48. Blumberg N. Allogeneic transfusion and infection: economic and clinical implications. *Seminars in Hematology*, 1997; **34**(3, Suppl. 2): 34–40.

49. Blajchman MA, Bardossy L, Carmen R, Sastry A, Singal DP. Allogeneic blood transfusion-induced enhancement of tumor growth: two animal models showing amelioration by leukodepletion and passive transfer using spleen cells. *Blood*, 1993; **81**(7): 1880–2. [See Comments]

50. McAlister FA, Clark HD, Wells PS, Laupacis A. Perioperative allogeneic blood transfusion does not cause adverse sequelae in patients with cancer: a meta-analysis of unconfounded studies. *British Journal of Surgery*, 1998; **85**(2): 171–8. [See Comments]

51. Guidelines on gamma irradiation of blood components for the prevention of transfusion-associated graft-versus-host disease. BCSH Blood Transfusion Task Force. *Transfusion Medicine*, 1996; **6**(3): 261–71. [See Comments]

52. Kennedy JS, Ricketts RR. Fatal graft v host disease in a child with neuroblastoma following a blood transfusion. *Journal of Pediatric Surgery*, 1986; **21**(12): 1108–9.

53. Amlot PL, Hayes AE. Impaired human antibody response to the thymus-independent antigen, DNP-Ficoll, after splenectomy. Implications for post-splenectomy infections. *Lancet*, 1985; **1**(8436): 1008–11.

54. Mower WR, Hawkins JA, Nelson EW. Postsplenectomy infection in patients with chronic leukemia. *American Journal of Surgery*, 1986; **152**(6): 583–6.

55. Working Party of the British Committee for Standards in Haematology Clinical Haematology Task Force. Guidelines for the prevention and treatment of infection in patients with an absent or dysfunctional spleen. *British Medical Journal*, 1996; **312**: 430–4.

56. Degos L, Faille A, Housset M, Boumsell L, Rabian C, Parames T. Syndrome of neutrophil agranulocytosis, hypogammaglobulinemia, and thymoma. *Blood*, 1982; **60**(4): 968–72.

57. McCormack RT, Nelson RD, Bloomfield CD, Quie PG, Brunning RD. Neutrophil function in lymphoreticular malignancy. *Cancer*, 1979; **44**(3): 920–6.

58. Oizumi K. [Infectious complications of lung cancer and its management.] *Gan No Rinsho*, 1985; **31**(9, Suppl.): 1203–10. [In Japanese]

59. Belghiti J, Champault G, Fabre F, Patel JC. [Assessment of postoperative infective risk by delayed hypersensitivity tests. The influence of deficient nutrition and its correction.] (author's translation) *Nouvelle Presse Medicale*, 1978; **7**(37): 3337–41. [In French]

60. Perramant M, Perramant-Creach Y, Delalande JP, Miossec A, Egreteau JP. [Significance of skin tests in pre-operative assessment.] *Annales de l'Anesthesiologie Francaise*, 1981; **22**(3): 279–84. [In French]

61. Nomoto K, Mitsuyama M, Miake S, Yokokura T. Augmented nonspecific resistance and simultaneous impairment of specific immunity to *Listeria monocytogenes* in tumor-bearing mice. *Journal of Clinical and Laboratory Immunology*, 1987; **24**(2): 75–9.

62. Shukla HS, Hughes LE, Whitehead RH, Newcombe RG. Long-term (5–11 years) follow-up of general immune competence in breast cancer. I. Pre-treatment levels with reference to micrometastasis. *Cancer Immunology and Immunotherapy*, 1986; **21**(1): 1–5.

63. Klastersky J. Infections in cancer patients with suppressed cellular immunity. *Recent Results in Cancer Research*, 1993; **132**: 147–54.

64. Peters SG, Prakash UB. *Pneumocystis carinii* pneumonia. Review of 53 cases. *American Journal of Medicine*, 1987; **82**(1): 73–8.

65. Ruskin J, Remington JS. Toxoplasmosis in the compromised host. *Annals of Internal Medicine*, 1976; **84**(2): 193–9.

66. Fukushige J, Maruyama K, Kawakami H, Kihara M. [Tuberculosis in patients with malignant neoplasms.] *Gan No Rinsho*, 1986; **32**(3): 234–40. [In Japanese]

67. Escudier E, Cordonnier C, Poirier J. [Infections of the central nervous system in malignant hemopathies.] *Revue Neurologie (Paris)*, 1986; **142**(2): 116–25. [In French]

68. Rex JH, Walsh TJ, Anaissie EJ. Fungal infections in iatrogenically compromised hosts. *Advances in Internal Medicine*, 1998; **43**: 321–71.

69. Cole S, Zawin M, Lundberg B, Hoffman J, Bailey L, Ernstoff MS. Candida epiglottitis in an adult with acute nonlymphocytic leukemia. *American Journal of Medicine*, 1987; **82**(3, Spec. No): 662–4.

70. Haron E, Vartivarian S, Anaissie E, Dekmezian R, Bodey GP. Primary Candida pneumonia. Experience at a large cancer center and review of the literature. *Medicine (Baltimore)*, 1993; **72**(3): 137–42.

71. Haron E, Feld R, Tuffnell P, Patterson B, Hasselback R, Matlow A. Hepatic candidiasis: an increasing problem in immunocompromised patients. *American Journal of Medicine*, 1987; **83**(1): 17–26.

72. Penn I. Kaposi's sarcoma in transplant recipients. *Transplantation*, 1997; **64**(5): 669–73.

73. Meunier L, Guillot B, Lavabre-Bertrand T, Barneon G, Izarn P, Meynadier J. [Chronic herpes of the pyodermatitis vegetans type in chronic cutaneous lymphoid leukemia.] *Annales de Dermatologie et de Venereologie*, 1986; **113**(12): 1199–204. [In French]

74. Ljungman P, Lonnqvist B, Gahrton G, Ringden O, Sundqvist VA, Wahren B. Clinical and subclinical reactivations of varicella-zoster virus in immunocompromised patients. *Journal of Infectious Diseases*, 1986; **153**(5): 840–7.

75. Ljungman P. Herpes virus infections in immunocompromised patients: problems and therapeutic interventions. *Annals of Medicine*, 1993; **25**(4): 329–33.

76. Betts RF, Hanshaw JB. Cytomegalovirus (CMV) in the compromised host(s). *Annual Review of Medicine*, 1977; **28**: 103–10.

77. Lemerle J, Backes C, Lallemand D, Lejeune JA, Reinert P. [Interstitial pneumopathies in children treated for malignant diseases.] *Archives Francaises de Pediatrie*, 1976; **33**(6): 569–98. [In French]

78. Gray MM, Hann IM, Glass S, Eden OB, Jones PM, Stevens RF. Mortality and morbidity caused by measles in children with malignant disease attending four major treatment centres: a retrospective review. *British Medical Journal (Clinical Research edn)*, 1987; **295**(6589): 19–22.

79. Abb J. [Prevention and therapy of herpesvirus infections.] *Zentralblatt fur Bakteriologie, Mikrobiologie und Hygiene. Serie B, Umwelthygiene, Krankenhaushygiene, Arbeitshygiene, Praventi Medizin*, 1985; **180**(2–3): 107–20.

80. Shepp DH, Dandliker PS, Meyers JD. Treatment of varicella-zoster virus infection in severely immunocompromised patients. A randomized comparison of acyclovir and vidarabine. *New England Journal of Medicine*, 1986; **314**(4): 208–12.

81. Katsushima N, Yazaki N, Sakamoto M. Effect and follow-up study on varicella vaccine. *Biken Journal*, 1984; **27**(2–3): 51–8.

82. Gershon AA, Steinberg SP, Gelb L. Live attenuated varicella vaccine use in immunocompromised children and adults. *Pediatrics*, 1986; **78**(4, Pt 2): 757–62.

83. Zbar B. Tumor regression mediated by *Mycobacterium bovis* (strain BCG). *National Cancer Institute Monographs*, 1972; **35**: 341–4.

84. Morales A. Intravesical therapy of bladder cancer: an immunotherapy success story. *International Journal of Urology*, 1996; **3**(5): 329–33.

85. Aungst CW, Sokal JE, Jager BV. Complications of BCG vaccination in neoplastic disease. *Annals of Internal Medicine*, 1975; **82**(5): 666–9.

86. Lamm DL, Stogdill VD, Stogdill BJ, Crispen RG. Complications of bacillus Calmette–Guerin immunotherapy in 1,278 patients with bladder cancer. *Journal of Urology*, 1986; **135**(2): 272–4.

87. Ishibashi T, *et al.* Distant metastasis facilitated by BCG: spread of tumour cells injected in the BCG-primed site. *British Journal of Cancer*, 1980; **41**(4): 553–61.

88. Estrov Z, *et al.* Elevated plasma thrombopoietic activity in patients with metastatic cancer-related thrombocytosis. *American Journal of Medicine*, 1995; **98**(6): 551–8.

89. Pedersen LM, Milman N. Prognostic significance of thrombocytosis in patients with primary lung cancer. *European Respiratory Journal*, 1996; **9**(9): 1826–30.

90. Dutcher JP, *et al.* Incidence of thrombocytopenia and serious hemorrhage among patients with solid tumors. *Cancer*, 1984; **53**(3): 557–62.

91. British Committee for Standardization in Haematology Blood Transfusion Task Force. Guidelines for transfusion for massive blood loss. A publication of the British Society for Haematology. *Clinical and Laboratory Haematology*, 1988; **10**(3): 265–73.

92. Chong BH. Heparin-induced thrombocytopenia. *British Journal of Haematology*, 1995; **89**(3): 431–9. [See Comments]

93. Amiral J, *et al.* Platelet factor 4 complexed to heparin is the target for antibodies generated in heparin-induced thrombocytopenia. *Thrombosis and Haemostasis*, 1992; **68**(1): 95–6. [Letter] [See Comments]

94. Gruel Y, *et al.* Specific quantification of heparin-dependent antibodies for the diagnosis of heparin-associated thrombocytopenia using an enzyme-linked immunosorbent assay. *Thrombosis Research*, 1991; **62**(5): 377–87.

95. Gmur J, Burger J, Schanz U, Fehr J, Schaffner A. Safety of stringent prophylactic platelet transfusion policy for patients with acute leukaemia. *Lancet*, 1991; **338**(8777): 1223–6. [See Comments]

96. Gordon LI, Kwaan HC. Cancer- and drug-associated thrombotic thrombocytopenic purpura and hemolytic uremic syndrome. *Seminars in Hematology*, 1997; **34**(2): 140–7.

97. Rebulla P, *et al.* A multicenter randomized study of the threshold for prophylactic platelet transfusions in adults with acute myeloid leukemia. Gruppo Italiano Malattie Ematologiche Maligne dell'Adulto.

98. Murphy MF, Brozovic B, Murphy W, Ouwehand W, Waters AH. Guidelines for platelet transfusions. British Committee for Standards in Haematology, Working Party of the Blood Transfusion Task Force. *Transfusion Medicine*, 1992; **2**(4): 311–18.

99. Contreras M, *et al.* Guidelines for the use of fresh frozen plasma. British Committee for Standards in Haematology, Working Party of the Blood Transfusion Task Force. *Transfusion Medicine*, 1992; **2**(1): 57–63. [See Comments]

100. Kruskall MS. The perils of platelet transfusions. *New England Journal of Medicine*, 1997; **337**(26):, 1914–15. [Editorial] [See Comments]

101. Leukocyte reduction and ultraviolet B irradiation of platelets to prevent alloimmunization and refractoriness to platelet transfusions. The Trial to Reduce Alloimmunization to Platelets Study Group. *New England Journal of Medicine*, 1997; **337**(26): 1861–9. [See Comments]

102. Trousseau A. *Phlegmasia alba dolens*. Clinique Medicale de l'Hotel Dieu de Paris. Paris: Baillière, 1872.

103. Silverstein RL, Nachman RL. Cancer and clotting—Trousseau's warning. *New England Journal of Medicine*, 1992; **327**(16): 1163–4. [Editorial] [See Comments]

104. Ambrus JL, Ambrus CM, Mink IB, Pickren JW. Causes of death in cancer patients. *Journal of Medicine*, 1975; **6**(1): 61–4.

105. Aderka D, Brown A, Zelikovski A, Pinkhas J. Idiopathic deep vein thrombosis in an apparently healthy patient as a premonitory sign of occult cancer. *Cancer*, 1986; **57**(9): 1846–9.

106. Monreal M, *et al.* Occult cancer in patients with deep venous thrombosis. A systematic approach. *Cancer*, 1991; **67**(2): 541–5.

107. Prandoni P, *et al.* Deep-vein thrombosis and the incidence of subsequent symptomatic cancer. *New England Journal of Medicine*, 1992; **327**(16): 1128–33. [See Comments]

108. Colucci M, *et al.* Warfarin inhibits both procoagulant activity and metastatic capacity of Lewis lung carcinoma cells. Role of vitamin K deficiency. *Biochemical Pharmacology*, 1983; **32**(11): 1689–91.

109. Sloane BF, Rozhin J, Johnson K, Taylor H, Crissman JD, Honn KV. Cathepsin B: association with plasma membrane in metastatic tumors. *Proceedings of the National Academy of Sciences, USA*, 1986; **83**(8): 2483–7.

110. Falanga A, *et al.* Preliminary study to identify cancer patients at high risk of venous thrombosis following major surgery. *British Journal of Haematology*, 1993; **85**(4): 745–50.

111. Vandenbroucke JP, Helmerhorst FM. Risk of venous thrombosis with hormone-replacement therapy. *Lancet*, 1996; **348**(9033): 972. [See Comments]

112. Pritchard KI, Paterson AH, Paul NA, Zee B, Fine S, Pater J. Increased thromboembolic complications with concurrent tamoxifen and chemotherapy in a randomized trial of adjuvant therapy for women with breast cancer. National Cancer Institute of Canada Clinical Trials Group Breast Cancer Site Group. *Journal of Clinical Oncology*, 1996; **14**(10): 2731–7.

113. McDonald CC, Alexander FE, Whyte BW, Forrest AP, Stewart HJ. Cardiac and vascular morbidity in women receiving adjuvant tamoxifen for breast cancer in a randomised trial. The Scottish Cancer Trials Breast Group. *British Medical Journal*, 1995; **311**(7011): 977–80.

114. Hudson ER, *et al.* Pulmonary angiography performed with iopamidol: complications in 1,434 patients. *Radiology*, 1996; **198**(1): 61–5.

115. Remy-Jardin M, *et al.* Diagnosis of pulmonary embolism with spiral CT: comparison with pulmonary angiography and scintigraphy. *Radiology*, 1996; **200**(3): 699–706.

116. Prandoni P. Antithrombotic strategies in patients with cancer. *Thrombosis and Haemostasis*, 1997; **78**(1): 141–4.

117. Walsh-McMonagle D, Green D. Low-molecular-weight heparin in the management of Trousseau's syndrome. *Cancer*, 1997; **80**(4): 649–55.

118. Rajan R, Gafni A, Levine M, Hirsh J, Gent M. Very low-dose warfarin prophylaxis to prevent thromboembolism in women with metastatic breast cancer receiving chemotherapy: an economic evaluation. *Journal of Clinical Oncology*, 1995; **13**(1): 42–6.

119. Moake JL. Studies on the pathophysiology of thrombotic thrombocytopenic purpura. *Seminars in Hematology*, 1997; **34**(2): 83–9.

120. Mitra D, Jaffe EA, Weksler B, Hajjar KA, Soderland C, Laurence J. Thrombotic thrombocytopenic purpura and sporadic hemolytic–uremic syndrome plasmas induce apoptosis in restricted lineages of human microvascular endothelial cells. *Blood*, 1997; **89**(4): 1224–34.

121. Chant I, Rose P. *E. coli*, verocytotoxins and HUS. *Thrombus*, 1997; **1**: 1–4.

122. Tandon NN, Rock G, Jamieson GA. Anti-CD36 antibodies in thrombotic thrombocytopenic purpura. *British Journal of Haematology*, 1994; **88**(4): 816–25.

123. Wada H, *et al.* Plasma cytokine levels in thrombotic thrombocytopenic purpura. *American Journal of Hematology*, 1992; **40**(3): 167–70.

124. Zauli G, *et al.* Increased serum levels of transforming growth factor beta-1 in patients affected by thrombotic thrombocytopenic purpura (TTP): its implications on bone marrow haematopoiesis. *British Journal of Haematology*, 1993; **84**(3): 381–6.

125. Joseph G, *et al.* HLA-DR53 protects against thrombotic thrombocytopenic purpura/adult hemolytic uremic syndrome. *American Journal of Hematology*, 1994; **47**(3): 189–93.

126. Schriber JR, Herzig GP. Transplantation-associated thrombotic thrombocytopenic purpura and hemolytic uremic syndrome. *Seminars in Hematology*, 1997; **34**(2): 126–33.

127. Chintagumpala MM, Hurwitz RL, Moake JL, Mahoney DH, Steuber CP. Chronic relapsing thrombotic thrombocytopenic purpura in infants with large von Willebrand factor multimers during remission. *Journal of Pediatrics*, 1992; **120**(1): 49–53. [See Comments]

128. Moake J, *et al.* Solvent/detergent-treated plasma suppresses shear-induced platelet aggregation and prevents episodes of thrombotic thrombocytopenic purpura. *Blood*, 1994; **84**(2): 490–7.

129. Furlan M, Robles R, Solenthaler M, Wassmer M, Sandoz P, Lammle B. Deficient activity of von Willebrand factor-cleaving protease in chronic relapsing thrombotic thrombocytopenic purpura. *Blood*, 1997; **89**(9): 3097–103.

130. Furlan M, *et al.* von Willebrand factor-cleaving protease in thrombotic thrombocytopenic purpura and the hemolytic–uremic syndrome. *New England Journal of Medicine*, 1998; **339**(22): 1578–84. [See Comments]

131. Tsai HM, Lian EC. Antibodies to von Willebrand factor-cleaving protease in acute thrombotic thrombocytopenic purpura. *New England Journal of Medicine*, 1998; **339**(22): 1585–94. [See Comments]

132. Kwaan HC, Soff GA. Management of thrombotic thrombocytopenic purpura and hemolytic uremic syndrome. *Seminars in Hematology*, 1997; **34**(2): 159–66.

133. Frangos JA, Moake JL, Nolasco L, Phillips MD, McIntire LV. Cryosupernatant regulates accumulation of unusually large vWF multimers from endothelial cells. *American Journal of Physiology*, 1989; **256**(6, Pt 2): H1635–44.

134. Gordon LI, Kwaan HC, Rossi EC. Deleterious effects of platelet transfusions and recovery thrombocytosis in patients with thrombotic microangiopathy. *Seminars in Hematology*, 1987; **24**(3): 194–201.

135. Richardson PG, *et al.* Treatment of severe veno-occlusive disease with defibrotide: compassionate use results in response without significant toxicity in a high-risk population. *Blood*, 1998; **92**(3): 737–44.

136. Barbui T, Finazzi G, Falanga A. The impact of all-trans-retinoic acid on the coagulopathy of acute promyelocytic leukemia. *Blood*, 1998; **91**(9): 3093–102.

137. Cohen AJ, Kessler CM. Acquired inhibitors. *Baillières Clinical Haematology*, 1996; **9**(2): 331–54.

138. Morrison AE, Ludlam CA. Acquired haemophilia and its management. *British Journal of Haematology*, 1995; **89**(2): 231–6. [See Comments]

139. Gorin LJ, Jeha SC, Sullivan MP, Rosenblatt HM, Shearer WT. Burkitt's lymphoma developing in a 7-year-old boy with hyper-IgE syndrome. *Journal of Allergy and Clinical Immunology*, 1989; **83**(1): 5–10.

140. Beral V, Peterman T, Berkelman R, Jaffe H. AIDS-associated non-Hodgkin lymphoma. *Lancet*, 1991; **337**(8745): 805–9. [See Comments]

141. Penn I. Occurrence of cancers in immunosuppressed organ transplant recipients. *Clinical Transplantation*, 1994; 99–109.

142. Hecht F, Hecht BK. Chromosome changes connect immunodeficiency and cancer in ataxia–telangiectasia. *American Journal of Pediatric Hematology and Oncology*, 1987; **9**(2): 185–8.

143. Grierson H, Purtilo DT. Epstein-Barr virus infections in males with the X-linked lymphoproliferative syndrome. *Annals of Internal Medicine*, 1987: **106**: 538–45.

144. Sayos J, Wu C, Morra M, *et al.* The X-linked lymphoproliferative-disease gene product SAP regulates signals induced through the co-receptor SLAM [see comments]. *Nature*, 1998; **395**: 462–9.

145. Coffey AJ, Brooksbank RA, Brandau O, *et al.* Host response to EBV infection in X-linked lymphoprotiferative disease results from mutations in an SH2-domain encoding gene [see comments]. *Nature Genetics*, 1998: **20**: 129–35.

146. Kersey JH, Shapiro RS, Filipovich AH. Relationship of immunodeficiency to lymphoid malignancy. *Pediatric Infectious Disease Journal*, 1988; **7**(5, Suppl.): S10–S12.

147. Cunningham-Rundles C, Siegal FP, Cunningham-Rundles S, Lieberman P. Incidence of cancer in 98 patients with common varied immunodeficiency. *Journal of Clinical Immunology*, 1987; **7**(4): 294–9.

148. Kersey JH, Spector BD, Good RA. Cancer in children with primary immunodeficiency diseases. *Journal of Pediatrics*, 1974; **84**(2): 263–4.

149. Nalesnik MA. Clinicopathologic features of posttransplant lymphoproliferative disorders. *Annals of Transplantation*, 1997; **2**(4): 33–40.

150. Purtilo DT. Prevention and treatment of Epstein–Barr virus (EBV)-associated lymphoproliferative diseases in immune deficient patients. *AIDS Research*, 1986; **2**(Suppl. 1): S177–81.

151. Lee ES, *et al.* The association of Epstein–Barr virus with smooth-muscle tumours occurring after organ transplantation. *New England Journal of Medicine*, 1995; **332**(1): 19–25.

152. Opelz G, Schwarz V, Wujciak T, Schnobel R, Henderson R, Grayson H. Analysis of non-Hodgkin's lymphomas in organ transplant recipients. *Transplantation Reviews*, 1995; **9**(4): 231–40.

153. Swinnen LJ, *et al.* Increased incidence of lymphoproliferative disorder after immunosuppression with the monoclonal antibody OKT3 in cardiac-transplant recipients. *New England Journal of Medicine*, 1990; **323**(25): 1723–8. [See Comments]

154. Morgan AJ. Epstein-Barr virus vaccines. *Vaccine*, 1992; **10**(9): 563–71.

155. Knowles DM, *et al.* Correlative morphologic and molecular genetic analysis demonstrates three distinct categories of posttransplantation lymphoproliferative disorders. *Blood*, 1995; **85**(2): 552–65.

156. Bashir RM, Harris NL, Hochberg FH, Singer RM. Detection of Epstein–Barr virus in CNS lymphomas by *in-situ* hybridization. *Neurology*, 1989; **39**(6): 813–17.

157. Okano M, *et al.* Epstein–Barr virus infection and oncogenesis in primary immunodeficiency. *AIDS Research*, 1986; **2**(Suppl.): S115–19.

158. Dolken G, Bross KJ, Hecht T, Brugger W, Lohr GW, Hirsch FW. Increased incidence of IgA antibodies to the Epstein–Barr virus-associated viral capsid antigen and early antigens in patients with chronic lymphocytic leukemia. *International Journal of Cancer*, 1986; **38**(1): 55–9.

159. Rees L, Thomas JA, Amlot PL. Disappearance of an EBV + posttransplant plasmacytoma with controlled reduction of immunosuppression. *Lancet*, 1998; **352**(9130): 789–789.

160. Hardy RR, Hayakawa K, Shimizu M, Yamasaki K, Kishimoto T. Rheumatoid factor secretion from human Leu-1+ B cells. *Science*, 1987; 236(4797): 81–3.

161. Youinou P, Mackenzie LE, Lamour A, Mageed RA, Lydyard PM. Human CD5-positive B cells in lymphoid malignancy and connective tissue diseases. *European Journal of Clinical Investigation*, 1993; 23(3): 139–50.

162. Weir AB III, Herrod HG, Lester EP, Holbert J. Diffuse large-cell lymphoma of B-cell origin and deficient T-cell function in a patient with rheumatoid arthritis. *Archives of Internal Medicine*, 1989; 149(7): 1688–90.

163. Nobile-Orazio E, *et al.* Frequency and clinical correlates of anti-neural IgM antibodies in neuropathy associated with IgM monoclonal gammopathy. *Annals of Neurology*, 1994; 36: 416–24.

164. Nobile-Orazio E, *et al.* Peripheral neuropathy in macroglobulinemia: incidence and antigen-specificity of M proteins. *Annals of Neurology*, 1987; 37: 1506–14.

165. Bromberg MB, Feldman EL, Albers JW. Chronic inflammatory demyelinating polyradiculoneuropathy: comparison of patients with and without an associated monoclonal gammopathy. *Neurology*, 1992; 42: 1157–63.

166. Anhalt GJ, *et al.* Paraneoplastic pemphigus. An autoimmune mucocutaneous disease associated with neoplasia. *New England Journal of Medicine*, 1990; 323(25): 1729–35.

167. Horn TD, Anhalt GJ. Histologic features of paraneoplastic pemphigus. *Archives of Dermatology*, 1992; 128: 1091–5.

168. Dellagi K, Brouet JC, Seligmann M. Antivimentin autoantibodies in angioimmunoblastic lymphadenopathy. *New England Journal of Medicine*, 1984; 310(4): 215–18.

169. Raziuddin S, Assaf HM, Teklu B. T cell malignancy in Richter's syndrome presenting as hyper IgM. Induction and characterization of a novel CD3+, CD4–, CD8+ T cell subset from phytohemagglutinin-stimulated patient's CD3+, CD4+, CD8+ leukemic T cells. *European Journal of Immunology*, 1989; 19(3): 469–74.

170. Altman AJ, Baehner RL. Favorable prognosis for survival in children with coincident opso-myoclonus and neuroblastoma. *Cancer*, 1976; 37: 846–52.

171. Sinha S, Newsom-Davis J, Mills K, Byrne N, Lang B, Vincent A. Autoimmune aetiology for acquired neuromyotonia (Isaacs' syndrome). *Lancet*, 1991; 338(8759): 75–7.

172. Mason WP, *et al.* Small-cell lung cancer, paraneoplastic cerebellar degeneration and the Lambert–Eaton myasthenic syndrome. *Brain*, 1997; 120(Pt 8): 1279–300.

173. Tanaka M, Tanaka K, Onodera O, Tsuji S. Trial to establish an animal model of paraneoplastic cerebellar degeneration with anti-Yo antibody. 1. Mouse strains bearing different MHC molecules produce antibodies on immunization with recombinant Yo protein, but do not cause Purkinje cell loss. *Clinical Neurology and Neurosurgery*, 1995; 97(1): 95–100.

174. Tanaka K, Tanaka M, Igarashi S, Onodera O, Miyatake T, Tsuji S. Trial to establish an animal model of paraneoplastic cerebellar degeneration with anti-Yo antibody. 2. Passive transfer of murine mononuclear cells activated with recombinant Yo protein to paraneoplastic cerebellar degeneration lymphocytes in severe combined immunodeficiency mice. *Clinical Neurology and Neurosurgery*, 1995; 97(1): 101–5.

175. Vincent A, Honnorat J, Antoine JC, Giometto B, Dalmau J, Lang B. Autoimmunity in paraneoplastic neurological disorders. *Journal of Neuroimmunology*, 1998; 84(1): 105–9.

176. Jean WC, Dalmau J, Ho A, Posner JB. Analysis of the IgG subclass distribution and inflammatory infiltrates in patients with anti-Hu-associated paraneoplastic encephalomyelitis. *Neurology*, 1994; 44(1): 140–7.

177. Hormigo A, Dalmau J, Rosenblum MK, River ME, Posner JB. Immunological and pathological study of anti-Ri-associated encephalopathy. *Annals of Neurology*, 1994; 36(6): 896–902.

178. Lucchinetti CF, Kimmel DW, Lennon VA. Paraneoplastic and oncologic profiles of patients seropositive for type 1 antineuronal nuclear autoantibodies. *Neurology*, 1998: 50: 652–7.

179. Dropcho EJ. Autoimmune central nervous system paraneoplastic disorders: mechanisms, diagnosis, and therapeutic options. *Annals of Neurology*, 1995: 37 (Suppl. 1): S102–13: S102–S113.

180. Posner JB, Dalmau JO. Paraneoplastic syndromes affecting the central nervous system. *Annual Reviews of Medicine*, 1997; 48: 157–66.

181. De Camilli P, Thomas A, Cofiell R, *et al.* The synaptic vesicle-associated protein amphiphysin is the 128-kD autoantigen of Stiff-Man syndrome with breast cancer. *Journal of Experimental Medicine*, 1993; 178: 2219–23.

182. Lennon VA, Kryzer TJ, Griesmann GE, *et al.* Calcium-channel antibodies in the Lambert-Eaton syndrome and other paraneoplastic syndromes. *New England Journal of Medicine*, 1995; 332: 1467–74.

183. Graus F, Dalmou J, Rene R, *et al.* Anti-Hu antibodies in patients with small-cell lung cancer: association with complete response to therapy and improved survival. *Journal of Clinical Oncology*, 1997; 15: 2866–72.

5.5   Spinal metastatic disease

Tali Siegal, Tzony Siegal, and Michael Brada

The management of malignant tumours causing neurological deficit due to involvement of the spinal column and the epidural space has witnessed significant changes in the past two decades. These range from urgent laminectomy to a combination of decompressive surgery and radiotherapy and to non-surgical treatment by radiotherapy alone. More recently, attention has been directed towards primary radiotherapy and to new surgical decompressive techniques as preferred treatment modalities.[1],[2] Some attempts have been made to compare various management methods, but the absence of satisfactory controlled trials means that there is no clear consensus on management. A synopsis of the current knowledge and concepts related to various therapeutic measures and prognostic factors is presented.

Incidence

Metastatic tumours of the spine occur three to four times more frequently than primary malignant spinal tumours, and even apparently solitary vertebral lesions are often metastatic.[2],[3] Among skeletal metastases, the vertebral column is the commonest site for neoplastic deposits.[4]–[6] In autopsy series, between 30 and 60 per cent of patients dying of neoplasia have spinal and epidural metastases.[2],[6],[7] Approximately 50 per cent of cases of metastatic epidural compression in adults arise from breast, lung, or prostatic cancer.[1],[2],[8]–[10] Other common primary cancers include lymphoma, renal cancer, sarcoma, and multiple myeloma,[1],[2],[8]–[11] but the origin of the metastases cannot be identified in 9 per cent of cases. The tendency of some tumour types to metastasize to the spine is relatively high: in an autopsy series of 704 cancer patients, multiple myeloma had the highest propensity to spinal metastases, followed by prostatic carcinoma.[12] In patients with breast cancer, the spine is the commonest site of bony metastases.[5]

All patients with vertebral metastases are at potential risk of developing spinal cord compression (**SCC**; the term SCC includes cauda equina compression, unless otherwise noted), but its frequency is unknown. Retrospective clinical studies suggest that between 2 per cent and 20 per cent of patients with vertebral metastases develop myelopathy secondary to SCC.[6],[13] An autopsy study estimated that 5 per cent of cancer patients develop spinal epidural tumour deposits,[12] but a proportion may remain clinically silent. Although spinal metastases generally occur in patients with known malignancy, in 8 to 20 per cent of patients with SCC this is the initial manifestation of malignant disease.[10],[11],[14]

The incidence of SCC secondary to lymphoma, breast, and prostatic cancer has decreased over the years.[2] Declining incidence probably reflects a shift in oncological treatment policies towards the early use of radiotherapy. The routine use of advanced imaging techniques (CT and MRI) also contributes by the early detection and treatment of spinal metastases.[15] (Fig. 1)

The incidence of clinical SCC in children is approximately 5 per cent. The tumour types are different from those encountered in adults and include sarcoma, neuroblastoma, and lymphoma.[1],[16]–[18] Sarcoma and neuroblastoma comprise more than 80 per cent of all cases of paediatric SCC. Most paediatric tumours invade the spinal canal via the neural foramen rather than from bony vertebral metastases.

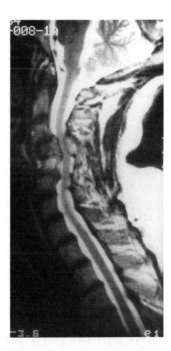

Fig. 1 Unexpected findings of cervical, spinal cord compression detected by MRI. A 57-year-old female with a known breast carcinoma metastatic to the right sacroiliac joint, presented with pain in the area of the cervicothoracic region. Neurological examination was normal apart for mild pain on neck flexion. MRI revealed an unexpected finding of cervical cord compression with anterior and posterior tumour masses compressing the spinal cord at the C4–C5 level. Treatment with radiotherapy yielded resolution of pain and sustained normal neurological status.

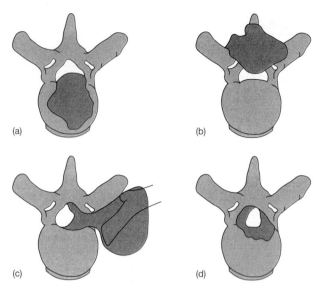

Fig. 2 Location of epidural tumour in relation to the spinal cord. Epidural metastases usually arise from extension of metastases located in the adjacent vertebral column into the spinal canal (a) and (b) or from paravertebral masses penetrating through the intervertebral foramina (c). The extension of the tumour into the spinal canal produces variable involvement of the anterior (ventral) compartment (A), the posterior compartment (b), the lateral gutter (c), or any combination of these conditions (d).

Tumour location

Level of spinal cord compression

The thoracic spine is the commonest site of SCC.[11] The involvement of a specific region of the spine by metastatic deposits is thought to relate to the number of vertebrae contained therein.[11] In a review of 2977 cases of SCC, cervical region involvement occurred at a lower than expected rate (11–13 per cent versus 27 per cent), whereas involvement in the lumbar and thoracic areas was close to the predicted figures.[19] The lower incidence of SCC in the cervical spine may be related to two factors. The bone volume of the cervical spine is smaller than that of other regions, and therefore haematogenous vertebral colonization by a metastatic tumour is less likely to occur. The spinal canal is more capacious in the upper cervical relative to the thoracic region, allowing more space for an expanding epidural tumour and thus a lesser likelihood of epidural deposits becoming clinically evident.

Location of epidural tumours in relation to the spinal cord and the yield of diagnostic imaging

Epidural SCC usually results from metastases to one of three sites: the vertebrae, the paravertebral tissue, or the epidural space itself. Extension of the tumour into the spinal canal may produce variable involvement of the anterior (ventral) compartment, the lateral gutters, the posterior compartment, or any combination of these sites (Fig. 2).

The vertebral column is the commonest site from which metastases may cause epidural SCC. Plain spinal radiographs are therefore frequently predictive of epidural disease[20] and an epidural mass is identified at 86 per cent of symptomatic spinal segments. However, 30 to 70 per cent bony destruction is necessary for radiographic changes to become evident.[21] Although an absent pedicle is often the first radiographic sign of metastatic disease, the pedicle is involved by direct extension from either the vertebral body or the posterior elements and therefore occurs late in the disease process.[22] The region of the vertebral column most often involved is the vertebral body, probably because of its extensive vascular supply. Most epidural tumours therefore arise in a vertebral body and invade the anterior part of the epidural space.[12],[19],[23]

Normal spinal radiographs seen in 6 per cent of SCC do not exclude epidural metastases.[24] In lymphoma, normal radiographs may be found in 89 per cent of patients with epidural compression.[25] A paravertebral tumour mass usually invades the epidural space through the intervertebral foramina rather than by vertebral extension. This mode of epidural invasion is also seen in patients with renal-cell cancer, superior sulcus tumours (Pancoast's syndrome), and neuroblastoma and accounts for approximately 10 per cent of all SCC.[26] In patients with a paraspinal tumour up to 36 per cent have epidural metastases on myelography.[27] With the advent of CT scanning and MRI, which adequately demonstrate the paravertebral soft tissues, these lesions are more frequently recognized. Pure epidural lesions alone are rare, and their incidence is about 5 per cent.[8]

The location of extradural metastases within the vertebral canal has important surgical implications. An accurate definition of the epidural mass as posterior, lateral, cuff, or anterior requires either a non-invasive MRI study or the combination of CT and myelography. The availability of MRI clearly delineating the vertebral column and the spinal cord usually eliminates the need for myelography and CT scans, as well as bone scans and plain radiographs. MRI is equivalent to myelography in detecting epidural disease and superior in detecting vertebral metastases and paravertebral masses.[1],[28],[29] MRI is the imaging method of choice both as a screening tool and as the ultimate diagnostic test to evaluate SCC.[15],[30],[31] MRI also has an impact on management. It detects unexpected vertebral and epidural lesions which lead to a change in treatment in up to 50 per cent of patients.[15],[30],[31] Its use for the diagnosis of SCC is also associated with significant economic benefits.[32] Myelography (combined with CT) should be performed when diagnosis and treatment are delayed by the inability to perform an urgent MRI, when patients are unable to undergo MRI (because of pacemakers or claustrophobia), or when a technically adequate MRI cannot be obtained (e.g. in the presence of spinal instrumentation at the investigated level or extreme obesity).

Symptoms and signs

The onset of SCC symptoms may be acute or insidious, and the duration of symptoms varies widely. Pain is the initial symptom in 96 per cent of cases, preceding other symptoms by 5 days to 2 years (median, 7 weeks).[11],[24],[33] Pain can be localized close to the site of the lesion or it can be radicular. It is considered to be due to nerve root compression or infiltration, compression fractures, segmental instability, displacement of the dura, or dural invasion. In cancer patients with symptoms and signs of spinal metastases, it is difficult to distinguish those with vertebral metastases alone from those with SCC on clinical grounds.[34] All patients with symptomatic spinal metastases must be considered at risk for SCC.

Although pain should alert the clinician to the diagnosis, it may be non-specific or referred to other sites and so frequently leads to a delay in diagnosis. This is especially true in patients without a previous history of cancer. At the time of diagnosis, neurological signs are common[1],[11],[24] and include muscle weakness in 76 per cent, bladder and bowel dysfunction in over than 50 per cent, and sensory deficit in about 50 per cent of cases. The typical neurological deficit is pyramidal weakness with sensory impairment up to a defined segmental level. Nearly half of severely affected patients have no residual spinal cord function at diagnosis before undergoing treatment. Of the paraparetic patients with some residual function, 28 per cent become paraplegic in less than 24 h.[35] SCC should therefore be treated as soon as possible, and early diagnosis is critical as functional outcome largely depends on the neurological function before treatment.[11],[24],[35]–[37]

Patients with SCC may also present with an atypical facial pain and numbness, with Brown–Sequard syndrome, with ataxia secondary to posterior column dysfunction, or with a herpetic rash along the affected dermatomes.[1],[24],[38]

Pathophysiology

The pathophysiological mechanisms involved in neoplastic SCC were investigated in experimental animal tumour models.[39]–[52] The mechanism of spinal cord injury induced by the expanding extradural tumours is complex and probably multifactorial (Fig. 3). The enlarging extradural tumour causes early obstruction of the spinal epidural venous plexus and enhances production of a vasogenic type of oedema. The oedema initially involves the white matter and in the late stage of compression the grey matter. In the endstage, a rapid decrease in spinal cord blood flow occurs at the site of compression. Ischaemia may play the final deleterious role, leading to irreversible loss of function if the compression is not promptly alleviated. In an animal model, abnormalities in spinal somatosensory evoked responses preceded neurological signs of myelopathy.[43] The conduction block may be related to myelin destruction as demonstrated by electron microscopy.[43] The disruption of myelin is probably caused by both mechanical compression and ischaemia. Although demyelination can occur at sites of spinal compression,[53],[54] remyelination may take place after transient compression,[55] thereby providing a possible morphological correlate for recovery of function after prompt decompression.

Local production of cytokines such as prostaglandins, interleukin (IL)-1, and IL-6, may promote an inflammatory response with its associated physiological changes of vasodilation, plasma exudation, and oedema formation.[56],[57] Elevation in prostaglandin E_2 (PGE$_2$) synthesis is demonstrated in the compressed segments concomitantly with the development of spinal cord oedema. In keeping with this concept, a rapid antioedema effect is achieved only when a partial or marked reduction of PGE$_2$ synthesis is accomplished, either by steroidal or by non-steroidal anti-inflammatory drugs (e.g. indomethacin),[44]–[47] or by inhibitors of phagocytic activity.[56],[57] The possible role of microglia and their phagocytic activity was investigated in recent studies. In tumour-bearing paraplegic rats, the normal population of resting microglia is replaced by activated amoeboid cells, which are probably engaged in phagocytosis.[52] The normal neurofilament cytoarchitecture is disrupted at the onset of paraplegia. In vivo pharmacological inhibition of phagocytosis (using chloroquine and colchicine) blocks lysosomal activity and cell migration with a reduction in amoeboid microglia, preservation of neurofilament structure, and inhibition of cytokine (PGE$_2$, IL-1, IL-6) synthesis. This results in attenuation of spinal cord oedema. Starting treatment at the first sign of neurological dysfunction significantly delayed the onset of paraplegia and prolonged the course of neurological deterioration toward paraplegia. These results suggest that inhibition of phagocytosis may delay structural damage and thus enhance the chances of recovery following decompression by antitumour therapy. It provides the scientific background for the clinical use of steroids, and it also explains the favourable neurological outcome in patients with neoplastic SCC treated by radiotherapy who are given high-dose dexamethasone.[58] Although dexamethasone is incapable of blocking phagocytosis, it does inhibit the associated inflammatory responses and the production of some cytokines in the phagocytic cascade.

In addition to phagocytosis, there is a marked increase in the utilization of serotonin in the compressed cord segments. Inhibition of serotonin receptors results in attenuated vascular permeability and a protracted clinical course toward paraplegia, similar to the favourable effect produced by steroids or non-steroidal anti-inflammatory agents.[50],[51],[56],[57] Receptor-activated serotonergic mechanisms, distinct from the mechanism associated with inflammatory responses, probably participate in the disruption of the blood–spinal cord barrier in the subacute phase of compression injury. Both mechanisms can be pharmacologically separately manipulated to yield measurable effects in the experimental model. However, it is unclear whether a combined pharmacological regimen will result in an additive effect.

In endstage SCC, when conduction block and ischaemia are present, cytotoxic oedema may also develop. The glutamate receptor antagonists ketamine and MK-801 produce an antioedema effect in SCC, which is not associated with either inhibition of the inflammatory cytokines (PGE$_2$) nor with the reduction of vascular permeability. Cytotoxic oedema may therefore be present and excitotoxins (such as glutamate) probably mediate its evolution.[48],[49]

The experimental findings indicate that early pharmacological intervention may offer the potential to delay neurological deterioration and may attenuate neuronal damage. However, in face of the complexity of the pathophysiological mechanisms, pharmacological manipulation should first be carefully assessed in animal models before their extrapolation to human clinical studies.

Survival and spinal cord compression

The magnitude of the clinical problem of spinal epidural metastases is usually underestimated. The annual incidence of cancer-induced spinal injury in the United States is 8.5 per 100 000[59] and exceeds the annual incidence of traumatic spinal cord injury (3–5 per 100 000). However, because of the relatively high mortality (50 to 70 per cent at 1 year) the socioeconomic impact of neoplastic SCC is less than that of the traumatic injury. In spite of the poor prognosis of the disease, most patients should receive active treatment[1],[11],[60] to preserve or restore mobility and continence, and to alleviate intractable pain. SCC in itself is usually not the direct cause of death, except

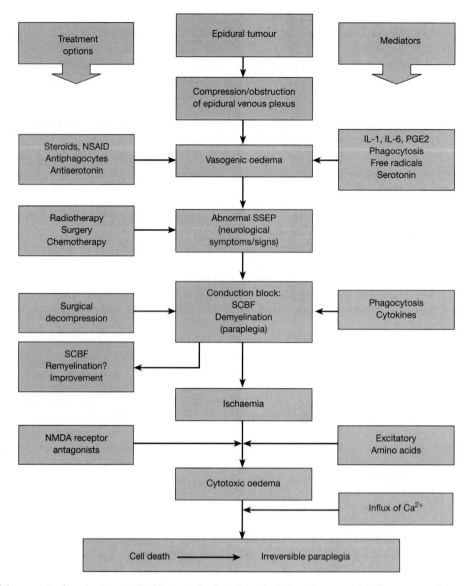

Fig. 3 An algorithm of the recognized mechanisms involved in the pathophysiology of spinal cord compression. Treatment options represent possible pharmacological interventions that may reduce neural tissue damage. Data related to pharmacological manipulations are derived from the investigation of animal models of neoplastic SCC. The relationship of the currently used therapeutic modalities in humans (corticosteroids, radiotherapy, surgery, and chemotherapy) to the specific stage of spinal cord injury is also demonstrated.

when it occurs in the upper cervical spine. The survival in SCC is related to the natural history of the systemic malignancy. Only 30 per cent of patients are expected to survive beyond 1 year, and few as long as 4 to 9 years.[10],[61]–[63]

therapy, and overall survival.[35],[64],[65] Patients with myeloma, lymphoma, Ewing's sarcoma, neuroblastoma, and carcinoma of the breast have a favourable prognosis for recovery of function. The outlook for patients with metastatic bronchogenic carcinoma is generally poor. Overall, high tumour radiosensitivity is associated with a more favourable functional outcome.[11],[23],[33],[35]

Factors influencing recovery of function

Tumour biology and cell type

The biological activity of the primary neoplasm determines the aggressiveness of both local and systemic disease, the success of

Response to high-dose dexamethasone administration

The use of corticosteroids in the treatment of SCC is widely accepted.[11],[23],[33],[35],[37],[58],[66]–[68] The scientific basis for steroid use stems from animal models of SCC, in which reduction of spinal cord oedema and delayed onset of paraplegia were observed after treatment with dexamethasone.[39],[40],[42],[45],[52] The use of high-dose steroids is based on the rapid symptom relief noted in some patients receiving initial doses of 100 mg of dexamethasone,[33] although the outcome was not superior compared to a historical cohort who received lower doses of steroids. In a prospective study, patients with SCC were randomly assigned to receive initial treatment with either high-dose (100 mg) or a conventional dose (10 mg) of dexamethasone intravenous bolus, followed by 16 mg/day orally.[68] No dose effect was observed on neurological outcome, but a substantial effect on pain was noted within 24 h. There is only one well-designed, randomized, controlled trial that compared high-dose dexamethasone to no steroids in patients treated with radiotherapy alone.[58] Of patients receiving steroids 81 per cent were ambulatory compared to only 63 per cent of patients in the control arm. However, steroid treatment was associated with significant side-effects.

Several investigators observed a dramatic resolution of symptoms after treatment with steroids alone.[66],[69],[70] Such steroid-related improvement is related to the type of tumour and probably represents a direct oncolytic effect,[66] as occurs in lymphoma and leukaemia.

Pretreatment neurological status

The outcome of SCC relates to the patient's neurological status at the time of treatment; a positive correlation exists between pretreatment mobility and functional outcome.[1],[5],[8],[11],[23],[35],[65],[71]–[74] Between 80 and 90 per cent of the patients who can walk at the time of diagnosis remain ambulant after treatment, 35 to 45 per cent of those who are initially paraparetic become ambulatory, and only 5 to 7 per cent of paraplegic patients regain the ability to walk. The success of therapy in paraplegic patients depends on the extent of functional-cord transection and the extent of residual neurological function. Only 2 per cent of patients with complete transection recover, compared to 20 per cent of patients with residual neurological function. Regardless of the mode of therapy, complete paraplegia rarely recovers. The value of early diagnosis when mobility is retained is clear. With modern imaging methods the proportion of patients diagnosed while still able to walk is steadily increasing.[11],[23],[33],[36],[58],[67],[73]–[75] Nevertheless, an unacceptable delay in diagnosis, investigation, and referral occurs in most patients with malignant SCC, with a median delay from the onset of symptoms of 14 days. This delay results in the preventable loss of function before treatment.[76], [77]

Progression rate of symptoms

It has been suggested that a rapid onset and progression of neurological symptoms are associated with a worse prognosis.[23],[64] If the degree of spinal cord damage is taken into account, then, in patients with rapidly developing symptoms (less than 24 h), the neurological grade has a greater influence on prognosis than the rate of symptom progression.[35] Thus in patients with a rapidly evolving deficit only 20 per cent of paraparetic patients recover compared with none of paraplegic patients. The importance of the rate of symptom progression was emphasized in a study of 15 paraplegic patients treated with radiotherapy,[78] where five patients regained their mobility after a delay of 3 months or more. The median time from the initial motor symptoms to total paralysis was longer (45 days) in patients who recovered than in those who remained paralysed (9 days). Residual cord function should be taken into account as an important prognostic variable in patients with a rapidly evolving deficit. Once paraplegia

has set in, the duration of paralysis does have prognostic significance, although anecdotal recovery has been reported even after periods of 4 to 8 weeks.[78] The speed of neurological deterioration may be related to other factors, such as tumour biology or topography within the spinal canal.

Location of a tumour within the spinal canal

It has been suggested that the tumour position within the spinal canal carries a prognostic significance because of a correlation between the tumour location and the response to surgical treatment.[8],[64],[79] In addition, the presence of vertebral collapse has been associated with reduced chances of neurological recovery.[36],[64] This information is based on success rates obtained by the indiscriminate use of laminectomy performed in patients with ventrally located tumours. After laminectomy, only 9 to 16 per cent of the patients maintain ambulation, which is considerably less than the overall rates of about 50 per cent ambulation in patients with posterolateral tumours.[35],[36],[79]

When an epidural tumour is situated anterior to the spinal cord, the accessibility to surgical removal by laminectomy is limited. It is possible to employ an alternative approach to the spine by way of an anterolateral route,[67],[71],[74],[80]–[85] which results in 70 to 80 per cent of the patients regaining or maintaining ambulation. In only a few studies was the surgical approach for decompression selected prospectively according to tumour topography in the spinal canal.[67],[74],[83],[84] The success rate, when reported according to tumour location,[67],[83] was 80 per cent for ventrally located tumours when they were decompressed by an anterior approach and only 39 per cent for posteriorly located tumours decompressed by laminectomy.[67] Although the figure for posterior compartment tumours seems inferior, the results should not be considered discouraging because only 8 per cent of the patients with posterior compression were ambulatory at presentation. With appropriate tailoring of the operative approach, there is no evidence that tumour position within the spinal canal is an important or an independent predictor of outcome.

Principles of management

Although spinal canal compression due to metastatic malignancy is relatively common, the management of SCC remains controversial.[11],[35]–[37],[60],[86] Controversy stems from the lack of prospective, well-designed, controlled, clinical studies comparing various treatment modalities, compounded by the absence of standard criteria for evaluating the response. Patients with metastatic SCC have, by definition, tumours that have spread from a primary site and thus are no longer curable by local measures. The therapeutic modalities of surgery and radiotherapy are palliative, and preservation or restoration of ambulation and bladder control are the criteria of successful therapy. Pain relief is also an important, but secondary goal. Because the treatment is not curative, its effect on the quality of further survival is particularly important. The therapeutic modalities currently available for the treatment of patients with epidural SCC are listed in Table 1. An algorithm for treatment selection of the various categories of SCC is shown in Fig. 4.

Table 1 Therapeutic modalities in spinal epidural metastases

Pharmacotherapy
Specific (antineoplastic, combination chemotherapy)
Non-specific (antioedema, analgesia)

Radiation therapy
External—conventional fields
Conformal radiotherapy

Surgery
Laminectomy (posterior decompression) ± spinal stabilization
Vertebral body resection (anterior decompression) + spinal stabilization
Combined anterior and posterior decompression + spinal stabilization (may be staged as sequential procedures)

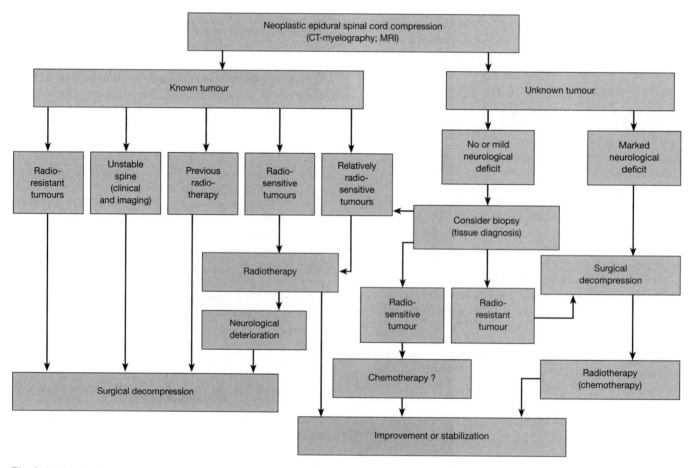

Fig. 4 An algorithm for evaluating and selecting the preferred therapeutic approach in patients with neoplastic SCC.

Pharmacotherapy

Specific chemotherapy

Epidural metastases arising from chemoresponsive primary tumours are likely to respond to chemotherapy, particularly early in the course of the disease. Spinal lymphomas may respond to corticosteroid treatment[66] as well as to chemotherapy.[87] Because corticosteroids are used in almost all patients as non-specific chemotherapy, their occasional specific effect may be indistinguishable from the effect of radiotherapy.

The usual policy is not to use specific chemotherapy alone as the primary treatment of SCC in patients with malignancy with limited chemoresponsiveness, because of the uncertainty of response and the irreversibility of severe, spinal cord dysfunction. Specific chemotherapy is usually combined with other therapeutic modalities.

However, several reports suggest that good recovery of neurological function can be obtained by chemotherapy alone in chemosensitive neoplasms, such as lymphoma,[87] myeloma, Ewing's sarcoma, germ-cell tumours, and neuroblastoma.[88]–[92] The published experience of chemotherapy alone is limited and large-scale studies are not available.

Chemotherapy should be considered for treating spinal metastases with epidural components in the following settings:

1. It could be used in some patients with lymphoma, germ cell tumours, neuroblastoma, or Ewing's sarcoma with SCC as the presenting manifestation of malignancy, or when recognized during evaluation of the extent of disease. When SCC is diagnosed in these chemosensitive tumours early in the course of the disease, with mild neurological dysfunction and no sign of rapid deterioration, chemotherapy should be used first.

2. Patients with SCC of previously irradiated chemoresponsive tumours who are not candidates for further radiation or surgical therapy could be considered for chemotherapy.

3. Chemotherapy could be used in chemosensitive tumours in conjunction with either surgery or radiotherapy in the acute treatment of symptomatic SCC.

Non-specific pharmacotherapy

Corticosteroids

Glucocorticoids rarely, if ever, achieve the dramatic relief of neurological disability seen in patients with brain metastases. When high doses of corticosteroids are used in the treatment of SCC, most patients experience dramatic pain relief.[33],[68] Some experience an arrest of progressively deteriorating neurological function, and few may improve with corticosteroids alone. Although high doses of steroids are frequently used in SCC, no clear advantage over conventional doses has been demonstrated[33],[37],[68] and the side-effects of corticosteroids should be an important consideration.

The incidence of serious steroid-related complications in neuro-oncology patients has been the subject of recent studies.[93]–[95] At least one steroid-related side-effect was seen in 51 per cent of the patients, and 19 per cent required hospital admission. Both the duration and the total dose of steroid therapy predicted toxicity. A significant increase in severe complications, including fatal sepsis, was noted when dexamethasone was used for more than 40 days to treat SCC.[96] In addition, intestinal perforation occurred as frequently as gastrointestinal bleeding, and significantly more rectosigmoid perforation occurred in neurological (non-oncological) patients manifesting steroid toxicity.[93],[95] Patients with SCC present fewer signs and symptoms of peritonitis than patients with an intestinal perforation who are treated with non-steroidal agents. Because major complications occur in patients who receive steroids for more than 1 month, they must be used judiciously, and should be discontinued as quickly as possible or tapered down to the lowest possible level that is compatible with clinical benefit.

The following recommendations apply for the use of steroids:

1. For patients with imaging evidence of SCC, but without signs of myelopathy, dexamethasone does not need to be given during radiotherapy.[37],[97]

2. Patients with SCC and moderate pain, but without myelopathy, may be treated with standard dose (16 mg/d) of dexamethasone for pain relief.

3. Symptomatic patients with SCC should be treated initially with high-dose dexamethasone to increase their chance for post-treatment ambulation.[59]

This comes with a moderate risk of serious toxicity which has to be accepted in view of the expected benefit. The drug should be tapered off as soon as treatment with definitive modalities has been initiated.

Analgesia

Because pain is the presenting symptom in over 95 per cent of patients with epidural SCC,[2],[11],[23],[33] the principles of good analgesic management must be applied. In most patients, treatment with either radiotherapy alone or resection of the tumour and restoration of stability frequently results in pain relief.[1],[2],[19] Exceptionally, neurosurgical procedures directed at pain control (e.g. cordotomy, rhizotomy) may be considered in patients with intractable pain either from a plexus or nerve root invasion, and especially in those patients with limited life expectancy.[98]

Radiation therapy

The results of radiation therapy in patients with a variety of metastatic tumours are summarized in Table 2. Between 28 and 50 per cent of irradiated patients either regain or maintain ambulation at the end of therapy, and of those who survive 1 year, 50 per cent maintain that improvement.[23],[33] The proportion of ambulatory patients at diagnosis is increasing, and they comprise 42 to 64 per cent of diagnosed patients with SCC.[2],[58],[73],[75] Between 80 and 96 per cent of ambulatory patients at diagnosis are likely to maintain mobility. However, 4 to 20 per cent of patients who can walk at the start of treatment will deteriorate and become immobile during or soon after completion of radiotherapy. Radiation therapy also results in pain relief in 50 to 80 per cent of patients.[1],[2],[19],[65],[72],[73]

The efficacy of radiation therapy depends on the radiosensitivity of the tumour, the patient's neurological status at the time that radiation therapy is undertaken, and on the maintenance of spinal stability. Patients with highly radiosensitive tumours (such as lymphoma, Ewing's sarcoma, neuroblastoma, seminoma, and myeloma) are more likely to regain or maintain ambulation than those with less-radiosensitive tumours (overall 60 to 80 per cent versus 40 per cent).[19],[23],[35],[67],[70],[87] It takes a few days before improvements may be seen after the initiation of radiotherapy, even in patients with a radiosensitive tumour. This is of some concern, because 28 per cent of severely paraparetic patients are expected to become paraplegic within 24 h.[35] Radiotherapy should also be considered as primary therapy for moderately radioresponsive neoplasms, such as breast carcinoma. However, the need for surgical intervention should be critically reviewed for each patient. Stable patients who are ambulatory or paraparetic at presentation should be considered for radiotherapy as the treatment of first choice. In severely paraparetic patients, surgical decompression should be considered because radiotherapy may cause a delay in the reduction of spinal cord damage. Radiotherapy alone should be employed if surgery is contraindicated because of the patient's poor general condition, multiple compression levels, or long-standing paraplegia.

The indications for radiotherapy are less clear for tumours generally regarded as poorly radioresponsive. Nevertheless, radiotherapy should be tried as the primary modality if the patient's neurological deficit

Table 2 Results of treatment for spinal cord compression: radiotherapy alone

First authors	Year	Patients (n)	Improved (%)*	Worse (%)
Brady[112]	1975	19	47	—
Mones[113]	1966	41	41	—
Khan[114]	1967	82	42	—
Cobb[13]	1977	18	50	22
Marshall[70]	1977	29	41	—
Gilbert[23]	1978	130	49	—
Greenberg[33]	1980	83	57	7
Stark[115]	1982	31	35	—
Constans[8]	1983	108	39	26
Obbens[114]	1984	83	28	23
Harrison[117]	1985	33	27	36
Bach[10]	1990	149	35	18
Sorensen[58]	1994	27 (dexamethasone)	50	0
		30 (no dexamethasone)	18	12
Posner[2]	1995	54 (non-ambulatory)	28	—
		96 (ambulatory)	—	10
Maranzano[65]	1995	209		
Helweg-Larsen[73]	1996	74 (non-ambulatory)	28	—
		79 (ambulatory)		
Huddart[75]	1997	69	52	—
Maranzano[118]	1997	41	38	8
Mean		—	39	16
Total		1485	—	—

*Improvement was judged by criteria of motor function.

is not severe and if the rate of progression of the deficit is such that there would be time to resort to surgical decompression should radiotherapy fail. Where surgery is the primary therapy, postoperative radiation is traditionally employed to prevent the regrowth of residual tumours and to contribute to pain relief.

No controlled studies have compared the various dose and fractionation schedules of radiation therapy.[99] Single-arm studies (Table 2) suggest that neither the dose nor the fractionation schedule have a major impact on outcome. The chosen treatment schedule should be a short palliative regimen at doses below spinal cord tolerance. The frequently used schedules are 20 Gy in five fractions, 28 Gy in seven fractions and 30 Gy in ten fractions prescribed to a depth of 5 to 8 cm using 4 to 8 megavolt (MV) photons. The treatment is given by single posterior field. The PTV should encompass the site of compression and the tumour causing it (GTV) and a 2 to 4 cm margin.

Surgery

The surgical treatment of SCC is still a subject of debate as there is a lack of prospective randomized trials and surgical series only report

selected subgroups of patients. Some of the surgical studies report a high proportion of non-ambulatory patients regaining ambulation.[67],[74],[80],[82],[100],[101] There is a suggestion that surgery provides better ambulation outcomes than radiation for the severely paretic and paraplegic patients. However, the risk of operative morbidity and mortality should be carefully weighed against the expected gain from surgery.

The traditional approach to the treatment of neoplastic SCC has been decompressive laminectomy, with or without postoperative radiation therapy. Ambulation is maintained or regained in 35 to 50 per cent of treated patients (Table 3), a result similar to that achieved with radiation therapy (Table 2). Pain is improved in 50–70 per cent of patients after laminectomy, which is also similar to radiation therapy. Patients treated by radiotherapy can deteriorate (Table 2) and this is also true following surgery (Table 3). However irradiated patients are spared the operative morbidity and mortality of surgery. Approximately 10 to 20 per cent of patients who are ambulatory at presentation deteriorate neurologically; and of those paraparetic before surgery, about 20 per cent deteriorate. The current consensus in the oncological literature favours initial radiotherapy in the majority of patients, reserving surgery for salvage or diagnosis.

Table 3 Results of treatment for spinal cord compression: laminectomy and radiotherapy

First author	Year	Patients (n)	Improved* (%)	Worse (%)	Operative mortality (%)
Hall[79]	1973	129	30	—	—
Brady[112]	1975	90	61	—	—
Merrin[119]	1976	22	22	0	0
Cobb[13]	1977	26	46	23	—
Marshall[70]	1977	17	29	—	—
Gilbert[23]	1978	65	45	—	—
Gianotta[120]	1978	33	30	18	12
Kleinman[121]	1978	20	15	5	15
Livingston[122]	1978	100	58	—	0
Gorter[124]	1978	31	39	—	13
Baldini[123]	1979	140	30	19	0
Dunn[125]	1980	104	33	23	10
Levy[126]	1982	39	82	15	8
Stark[115]	1982	84	37	—	—
Constans[8]	1983	465	46	13	—
Klein[127]	1984	194	54	16	—
Kollmann[128]	1984	103	56	—	—
Garcia-Picazo[129]	1990	53	41	—	—
Bach[10]	1990	91	59	11	—
Landmann[9]	1992	127	58	2	—
Posner[2]	1995	26	13	30	19
Mean			42	14.5	8.5
Total		1959	—	—	—

*Improvement was judged by criteria of motor function.

Laminectomy, the midline posterior approach, is technically easy and safe and allows for tissue diagnosis, but provides adequate decompression only when the tumour mass lies dorsolateral to the dura. Laminectomy also destabilizes the spine if the vertebral body and the pedicles are destroyed by a tumour and only allows limited access to a tumour lying ventral to the cord. The reasons for surgical failures in the past were: (1) non-selective use of one surgical approach; (2) inadequate tumour resection; (3) ineffective stabilization; and (4) poor patient selection.

Indications for surgical intervention

Some trends have emerged regarding surgical indications. Figure 4 specifies the circumstances in which surgery should be considered, and although some of them are clear-cut, others need further evaluation.

Diagnosis in doubt

In 8 per cent of patients with neoplastic SCC, spinal involvement is the initial presentation of malignancy.[11],[14],[23] When the aetiology of

the spinal lesion is in doubt, surgical decompression should be considered to establish a tissue diagnosis and to achieve rapid decompression. Current, image-assisted, percutaneous needle biopsy of vertebral lesions is diagnostic in 95 per cent of patients with no previous history of malignancy,[14],[102] and has a reported complication rate of less then 1 per cent. Therefore, surgery is rarely needed simply to establish the diagnosis of malignancy. If the biopsy results are not diagnostic, or if the neurological status is unstable with rapidly evolving signs, surgical decompression is advisable to achieve an accurate and prompt diagnosis and to initiate treatment without delay.

Spinal instability or bone compression

A major goal of treatment is the restoration or maintenance of spinal stability. The determination of spinal instability is of paramount importance in choosing the appropriate form of management for patients with metastatic disease of the spine. Unfortunately, no validated system exists for making this assessment.

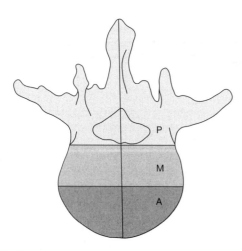

Fig. 5 Classification system for the evaluation of spinal stability. The three-column system of Denis[103] has been devised for the assessment of spinal cord stability in trauma and divides the spine into the anterior (A), middle (M), and posterior (P) columns. The spine is considered unstable if two of the three columns are disrupted. The six-column system of Kostuik and Errico[104] was devised for evaluating stability in connection with spinal tumours. Here, the three columns, as defined by Denis, are subdivided into left (L) and right (R) halves. The spine is unstable if three to four of the columns are destroyed.

Criteria for spinal stability in neoplastic disease

In trauma, the accepted biomechanical model for thoracolumbar fractures is the three-column concept of the spine (Fig. 5):[103]

- the anterior column—consists of the anterior half of the vertebral body, the anterior longitudinal ligament, and the anterior annulus fibrosus;
- the middle column—includes the posterior longitudinal ligament, the posterior half of the vertebral body, and the posterior annulus;
- the posterior column—consists of the neural arch (laminae and pedicles) facets, the ligamentum flavum, and the supraspinous and interspinous ligaments.

The spine is considered unstable if two of the three columns are disrupted. Spinal fractures are classified according to the mechanism of injury and involvement of the columns. In neoplastic destruction of the spine, these concepts may not always be applicable, because trauma and tumours are quite different conditions in terms of the disruption of bone, disc, and ligament; the quality of surrounding bone stock; and the ability of the spine to heal.

A set of criteria, which requires validation, has been developed for spinal tumours.[104] The spine is divided into six columns: the three columns (defined above[103]) subdivided into left and right halves (Fig. 5). The spine is considered to be stable if fewer than three of the six columns are destroyed, is unstable if three to four of the columns are destroyed, and is markedly unstable if five to six of the columns are involved. Angulation of 20 degrees or more adds to the consideration of instability.

Instability does not usually occur when involvement is limited to the vertebral spongy bone core or to the anterior column. When the posterior half (middle column) of the vertebral body is also involved (cortical bone included), a pathological compression fracture can occur, producing kyphosis and extrusion of bone, tumour, or disc into the spinal canal with neural compromise. Tumour involvement of the middle and posterior column may produce a forward shearing deformity. In addition, segmental instability is assumed to be present when the clinical syndrome is characterized by pain aggravated by movement (in the absence of significant neural encroachment) that is associated with progressive collapse of vertebral bodies or localized kyphosis on imaging studies.

A systematic approach to determining the clinical instability of the spine should include anatomical, biomechanical, clinical, and therapeutic considerations.[105],[106] Apart from the neuroimaging studies that define anatomical details used in the three-column spinal model (Fig. 5), the concept of clinical instability should also be taken into account. Clinical instability is defined as 'loss of the ability of the spine under physiological loads to maintain relationships between vertebrae in such a way that there is either damage or subsequent irritation to the spinal cord or nerve roots, and in addition there is development of incapacitating deformity or pain due to structural changes'.[106] Thus, symptoms and signs should direct therapeutic consideration. Patients with fracture-dislocation, localized kyphosis, collapsed vertebra with retropulsion of a bone fragment, or segmental instability may require surgical decompression and stabilization if either pain or neurological symptomatology are present. Not every case defined by the criteria for an unstable spine requires surgical intervention. If the tumour is relatively radiosensitive, a course of radiotherapy may result in satisfactory axial settling and pain relief over a period of weeks or months. These patients should be carefully followed because they are potentially unstable. Surgery is reserved only for symptomatic cases because preventive surgery is not justified in the management of metastatic disease of the spine.

When the anterior and middle columns are destroyed by a tumour, treatment considerations should include decompression by the anterior approach to the spine as well as restoration of stability by vertebral-body replacement constructs. If the posterior column structures are involved, then the treatment plan is to replace (or substitute) for the support role of these structures by posterior decompression combined with posterior instrumentation for the maintenance of stability. The results of surgical treatment where decompression is combined with spinal stabilization are summarized in Tables 4, 5, and 6. The criteria for patient selection and the methods of stabilization vary. Current recommendations for the selection of patients and the optimal methods of decompression and stabilization are undergoing constant development. The criteria of spinal instability that should bring about consideration for spinal stabilization are summarized in Table 7.

Previous radiation exposure

When radiotherapy cannot be used because of previous irradiation, surgical decompression is indicated as the primary therapeutic modality, even in highly radiosensitive tumours, because of the risk of exceeding spinal cord tolerance by further irradiation. Surgery is warranted for a relapse occurring months or even years after a successful previous treatment, in the hope of preserving neurological function. In many patients, however, life expectancy at the time of relapse of SCC is short, but retreatment with radiotherapy often preserves ambulation, with a low risk of radiation myelopathy during the remaining lifespan.[107]

Table 4 Results of treatment for spinal cord compression: laminectomy (posterior decompression) and stabilization*

First authors	Year	Patients (n)	Improved† (%)	Improved pain (%)	Morbidity (%)	Operative mortality (%)
Brunon[130]	1975	20	—	100	—	—
Hansebout[131]	1980	82	84 amb	100	1	—
Miles[132]	1984	23	65	100	—	—
DeWald[133]	1985	17	45	65	12	6
Overby[134]	1985	12	75	—	—	—
Solini[135]	1985	33	73	—	3	3
Heller[136]	1986	33	70	79	21	—
Sherman[137]	1986	23	92 amb	55	13	—
Perrin[138]	1987	200	65 amb	80	4	8
Bauer[63]	1995	67	76	—	20	—
Mean	—		72	83	11	6
Total		510	—	—	—	—

amb = ambulatory.

*Before or after radiotherapy.

†Improvement was judged by criteria of motor function.

Table 5 Results of treatment for spinal cord compression: Vertebral body resection and stabilization*

First author	Year	Patients (n)	Improved† (%)	Improved pain (%)	Morbidity (%)	Operative mortality (%)
Slatkin[110]	1982	29	56	60	41	7
Harrington[80]	1984	52	55	77	8	4
Siegal[67]	1985	61	80 ambulatory	91	11	6
Sundaresan[71]	1985	101	80 ambulatory	80	10	6
Fidler[139]	1986	18	93	94	—	6
Ominus[81]	1986	36	72	97	—	6
Perrin[138]	1987	21	76	90		5
Posner[2]	1995	71	50 83 ambulatory	—	39	8
Walsh[85]	1997	61	75	90	30	8
Mean		—	71	85	23	6
Total		450	—	—	—	—

*Before or after radiotherapy.

†Improvement was judged by criteria of motor function.

Radioresistant tumours

In radioresistant tumours (e.g. renal), decompressive surgery might be considered as the primary mode of therapy. Postoperative radiotherapy is administered with the hope of retarding tumour regrowth. However, this indication is not generally accepted, and sometimes, especially in neurologically stable patients, radiotherapy may be tried first.

Neurological deterioration during radiotherapy

Neurological deterioration occurring during radiotherapy of a relatively radiosensitive tumour should prompt an early consideration of surgical decompression. The decline in neurological function may reflect radioresistance, progressive spinal instability, or bone compression secondary to vertebral collapse, all of which

Table 6 Results of treatment for spinal cord compression: case-dependent approach—vertebral body resection, posterior decompression, and combined approach with stabilization*

First author	Year	Patients (n)	Improved† (%)	Improved pain (%)	Morbidity (%)	Operative mortality (%)
Cooper[100]	1993	33	88 ambulatory	97	42	0
		6 VBR + P				
		27 VBR				
Sundaresan[74]	1996	110	82	90	48	5
		53 VBR + P				
		51 VBR				
		6 P				
Ominus[101]	1996	100	79	62	—	—
		9 VBR + P				
		58 VBR				
		33 P				
Sapkas[140]	1997	20	80	—	25	—
		8 VBR + P				
		2 VBR				
		10 P				
Gokaslan[141]	1998	72	76	92	33	3
		7 VBR + P				
		65 VBR				
Mean		—	81	85	37	2.6
Total		335	—	—		

VBR = vertebral body resection; P = posterior decompression.

*Before or after radiotherapy.

†Improvement was judged by criteria of motor function.

Table 7 Categories of spinal instability in metastatic disease that require consideration for spinal stabilization*

- Anterior + middle column involvement or >50% collapse of vertebral-body height
- Middle + posterior column involvement or shearing deformity
- Three-column involvement
- Involvement of same column in two or more adjacent vertebrae
- Iatrogenic
  Laminectomy in face of anterior and/or middle column disease
  Resection of >50% of cut surface of the vertebral body

*Definition of potential instability relies on imaging studies and is valid only if the vertebral cortical shell is involved.

may be most effectively treated by spinal decompression and stabilization.

There has been concern that radiation therapy may result in neurological deterioration, presumably by inducing radiation oedema in the tumour, spinal cord, or both. So far, experimental studies do not support this concept;[60] therefore, deterioration represents treatment failure, prompting consideration of surgery as the alternative treatment.

Selection of surgical approach

The goal of surgery is the optimal removal of the compressing epidural mass and restoration and maintenance of spinal stability. Therefore the selection of the surgical approach should be determined by variables such as the location of the tumour inside and outside the spinal canal, the main cause of the instability, and the feasible options for stabilization. Table 8 details the preoperative assessment required

Table 8 Pretreatment or preoperative assessment of tumour location and extent of pathology in tumours of the spine

---

- **Bone involvement** (CT, MRI)
  Vertebral body and pedicles, posterior elements, or a combination of both
  Number of vertebrae involved
  Percentage of bone mass loss of the vertebral cut surface

- **Epidural mass** (CT myelography, MRI)
  Epidural mass related or unrelated to the bone lesion
  Number of spinal levels involved
  Position of the epidural mass: anterior, lateral, posterior, and/or encircling

- **Spinal stability** (spinal radiography + CT and/or MRI)
  Involvement of two or more adjacent vertebrae
  Involvement of two or more spinal columns as well as the vertebral cortical shell
  Loss of more than 50% of the vertebral width
  Shearing deformity
  Any combination of the above

- **Retroperitoneal and/or paravertebral mass** (CT, MRI)
  Location
  Extent
  Involvement of adjacent structures or organs (kidneys, uterus, large vessels)
  Involvement of posterior chest or abdominal wall

CT = computed tomography; MRI = magnetic resonance imaging.

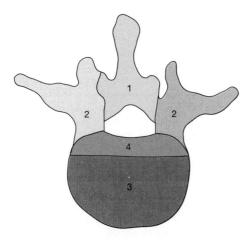

Fig. 6 Classification system of McLain and Weinstein[108] suggested for determining the optimal surgical approach for resecting spinal tumours. The spine is divided into four zones of possible tumour involvement. Zone 1 is best approached posteriorly. Zone 2 tumours may be resected via a posterior or posterolateral approach. Zone 3 tumours are best approached anteriorly. Zone 4 is the most inaccessible region for which a combined anterior and posterior approach may be recommended.

- Zone 1—includes the spinous process to the pars interarticularis and inferior facets and is best approached posteriorly.
- Zone 2—involves the superior articular facets, transverse process, and pedicle; tumours may be resected via a posterior or posterolateral approach.
- Zone 3—the anterior three-quarters of the vertebral body; tumours here are best approached anteriorly.
- Zone 4—the posterior fourth of the body, is the most inaccessible region of the spine; a combined anterior and posterior approach is recommended.

However, in patients with metastatic spine disease and a limited life expectancy, radical excision of the vertebral tumour is not always the main goal; therefore selection of the surgical approach also requires other considerations. In patients with progressive kyphosis without anterior cord compression or in patients with thoracic or lumbar pathological fracture or dislocation without significant soft tissue or bony neural compromise, posterior realignment and stabilization may relieve most cord impingement. In patients in whom the anterior approach is not feasible for technical reasons, poor medical status, or widespread disease, partial decompression (via a posterior approach) and stabilization may be a useful palliative procedure.[109]

for determining the surgical approach. The location of epidural compression should dictate the approach for decompression. Based on the tumour location, primary spinal tumours are classified according to the zones of involvement[108] and this information is used to determine the optimal surgical approach (Fig. 6); these guidelines are also applicable to metastatic spine lesions:

Complications

Radiotherapy

Palliative radiotherapy to the spine is not a known cause of mortality. Death in the first month after radiotherapy is most likely the result of active primary or metastatic disease. The main determinants of

Table 9 Non-neurological, surgical-related morbidity in neoplatic spinal cord compression

Surgical procedure	Morbidity (%)	
	Range	Average
Laminectomy	8–54	15
Laminectomy and stabilization	1–21	11
Vertebral body resection and stabilization	8–41	23
Patient-specific approach (anterior, posterior, or both) and stabilization	25–48	37

survival are performance status and tumour burden; 70 per cent of patients considered severely ill at the time of diagnosis of SCC were reported to die within 30 days after diagnosis.[67] The risk of radiation myelopathy is related to dose/fractionation parameters which, in palliative treatment, are below the level of spinal cord tolerance.

Surgical complications

Mortality

The incidence of death within the first month after decompressive laminectomy ranges from 3 to 19 per cent, with an average mortality rate of 8 per cent (Tables 3 and 4). The surgical mortality rate after vertebral body resection ranges from 4 to 8 per cent (Table 5).

Morbidity

The risk of neurological deterioration as a result of surgery is a major concern in patients who present while they are still able to walk. It occurred in 0 to 30 per cent of patients undergoing laminectomy, (mean of 14 per cent) (Table 3). After vertebral body resection, neurological worsening is rare and occurs in only 2 to 6 per cent of patients.[67],[71],[80],[110]

In patients undergoing laminectomy combined with radiotherapy, non-neurological complications include wound infection, wound dehiscence, spinal epidural haematoma, cerebrospinal fluid leak, and spinal instability. The frequency of these complications ranges from 8 to 54 per cent, with a mean of 12 per cent.[2],[11],[36] Only a few authors mention the problem of instability,[23],[64] which amounts to about 9 per cent of cases.

With the more frequent use of instrumentation the incidence of non-neurological complications (e.g. dislodgement, infections, etc.) is increasing (Table 9). Preoperative protein depletion and perioperative administration of corticosteroids are risk factors for wound infection in patients undergoing surgery for spine metastases.[111] A tailored, patient-specific approach (including vertebral body resection and spinal instrumentation techniques) requires considerable expertise, and should only be undertaken by a surgeon familiar with the techniques and the options to suit specific levels along the spine.

Summary

This chapter is a plea for the early diagnosis and treatment of neoplastic SCC. A high index of suspicion is essential, especially in patients known to harbour malignant disease. Corticosteroids and radiotherapy are the primary treatment in the majority of patients. However, wider acceptance and the judicious use of modern and novel surgical techniques for spinal decompression and stabilization may improve the quality of life of subgroups of patients. Prospective, randomized clinical trials are urgently needed to identify those patients most likely to benefit from different treatment modalities.

References

1. Byrne NT. Spinal cord compression from epidural metastases. *New England Journal of Medicine*, 1992; **327**: 614–19.

2. Posner JB. Spinal metastases. In *Neurologic complications of cancer* (ed. JB Posner). Philadelphia, PA: FA Davis, 1995: 111–42.

3. Paillas J-E, Alliez B, Pellet W. Primary and secondary tumors of the spine. In *Handbook of clinical neurology*, Vol. 20 (ed. PJ Vinken, GW Brnyn). Amsterdam: North-Holland Publishing, 1976: 19–54.

4. Galasko CSB. The anatomy and pathways of skeletal metastases. In *Bone metastases* (ed. L Weiss, HA Gilbert). Boston: GK Hall, 1981: 49–63.

5. Miller F, Whitehall R. Carcinoma of the breast metastatic to skeleton. *Clinical Orthopedics*, 1984; **184**: 121–7.

6. Schaberg J, Gainor BJ. A profile of metastatic carcinoma of the spine. *Spine*, 1985; **10**: 19–20.

7. Abrams HL, Spiro R, Goldstein N. Metastases in carcinoma. Analysis of 1000 autopsied cases. *Cancer*, 1950; **3**: 74–85.

8. Constans JP, *et al.* Spinal metastases with neurological manifestations: review of 600 cases. *Journal of Neurosurgery*, 1983; **59**: 111–18.

9. Landmann C, Hunig R, Gratzi O. The role of laminectomy in the combined treatment of metastatic spinal cord compression. *International Journal of Radiation Oncology, Biology, and Physics*, 1992; **24**: 627–31.

10. Bach F, *et al.* Metastatic spinal cord compression. Occurrence, symptoms, clinical presentations and prognosis in 398 patients with spinal cord compression. *Acta Neurochirugica (Wien)*, 1990; **107**: 37–43.

11. Black P. Spinal metastases: current status and recommended guidelines for management. *Neurosurgery*, 1979; **5**: 726–46.

12. Barron KD, Hirano A, Araki S, Terry RD. Experiences with metastatic neoplasms involving the spinal cord. *Neurology*, 1959; **9**: 91–106.

13. Cobb CA III, Leavens ME, Eckles N. Indications for nonoperative treatment of spinal cord compression due to breast cancer. *Journal of Neurosurgery*, 1977; **47**: 653–8.

14. Schiff D, O'Neill BP, Suman VJ. Spinal epidural metastasis as the initial manifestation of malignancy: clinical features and diagnostic approach. *Neurology*, 1997; **49**: 452–56.

15. Cook AM, Lau TN, Tomlinson MJ, Vaidya M, Wakeley CJ, Goddard P. Magnetic resonance imaging of the whole spine in suspected malignant spinal cord compression: impact on management. *Clinical Oncology*, 1998; **10**: 39–43.

16. Raffel C, Neave VCD, Lavine S, McComb JG. Treatment of spinal cord compression by epidural malignancy in childhood. *Neurosurgery*, 1991; **28**: 349–52.

17. Klein SL, Sanford RA, Muhlbauer MS. Pediatric spinal epidural metastases. *Journal of Neurosurgery*, 1991; **74**: 70–5.

18. Bouffet E, *et al.* Spinal cord compression by secondary epi- and intradural metastases in childhood. *Childs Nervous System*, 1997; **13**: 383–7.

19. Siegal T, Siegal T. Spinal epidural metastases from solid tumors. Clinical diagnosis and management. In *Neuro-oncology. Primary tumors and neurological complications of cancer* (ed. A Twijnstra, A Keyser, BW Onger-boer de Visser). The Netherlands: Elsevier Science, 1993: 283–305.

20. Portenoy RK, *et al.* Identification of epidural neoplasm. Radiography and bone scintigraphy in the symptomatic and asymptomatic spine. *Cancer*, 1989; **64**: 2207–13.

21. Edelstyn GA, Gillespie PJ, Grebbel FS. The radiological demonstration of osseous metastases: experimental observations. *Clinical Radiology*, 1967; **18**: 158–63.

22. Asdourian PL, *et al.* The pattern of vertebral involvement in metastatic vertebral breast cancer. *Clinical Orthopedics*, 1990; **250**: 164–70.

23. Gilbert RW, Kim JH, Posner JB. Epidural spinal cord compression from metastatic tumor: diagnosis and treatment. *Annals of Neurology*, 1978; **3**: 40–51.

24. Graus F, Krol G, Foley KM. Early diagnosis of spinal epidural metastasis: correlation with clinical and radiological findings. Abstract No. C-1047, *Program/Proceedings of the American Society of Clinical Oncology*, 1985; **4**: 269.

25. Perry JR, Deodhare SS, Bilbao JM, Murray D, Muller P. The significance of spinal cord compression as the initial manifestation of lymphoma. *Neurosurgery*, 1993; **32**: 157–62.

26. Posner JB. Spinal metastases: diagnosis and treatment. In *Neuro-oncology course at Memorial Sloan-Kettering Cancer Center* (ed. JB Posner). New York: Sloan-Kettering Cancer Center, 1981, 42–54.

27. Graus F, Krol G, Foley KM. Early diagnosis of spinal epidural metastases: correlation with clinical and radiological findings. *Proceedings of the American Society of Clinical Oncology*, 1985; **4**: 269.

28. Carmody RF, *et al.* Spinal cord compression due to metastatic disease: diagnosis with MR imaging versus myelography. *Radiology*, 1989; **173**: 225–9.

29. Colletti PM, *et al.* Spinal MR imaging in suspected metastases: correlation with skeletal scintigraphy. *Magnetic Resonance Imaging*, 1991; **9**: 345–55.

30. Heldmann U, Myschetzky PS, Thomsen HS. Frequency of unexpected multifocal metastasis in patients with acute spinal cord compression. Evaluation by low-field MR imaging in cancer patients. *Acta Radiologica*, 1997; **38**: 372–5.

31. Colletti PM, Siegel HJ, Woo MY, Young HY, Terk MR. The impact on treatment planning of MRI of the spine in patients suspected of vertebral metastasis: an efficacy study. *Computerized Medical Imaging and Graphics*, 1996; **20**: 159–62.

32. Jordan JE, Donaldson SS, Enzmann DR. Cost effectiveness and outcome assessment of magnetic resonance imaging in diagnosing cord compression. *Cancer*, 1995; **75**: 2579–86.

33. Greenberg HS, Kim J-H, Posner JB. Epidural spinal cord compression from metastatic tumor: results with a new treatment protocol. *Annals of Neurology*, 1980; **8**: 361–6.

34. Bernat JL, Greenberg ER, Barret J. Suspected epidural compression of the spinal cord and cauda equina by metastatic carcinoma. *Cancer*, 1983; **51**: 1953–7.

35. Barcena A, *et al.* Spinal metastatic disease: analysis of factors determining functional prognosis and the choice of treatment. *Neurosurgery*, 1984; **15**: 820–7.

36. Findlay GFG. Adverse effects of the management of malignant spinal cord compression. *Journal of Neurology, Neurosurgery and Psychiatry*, 1984; **47**: 761–8.

37. Loblaw DA, Laperrier NJ. Emergency treatment of malignant extradural spinal cord compression: an evidence-based guideline. *Journal of Clinical Oncology*, 1998; **16**: 1613–24.

38. Hainline B, Tuszynski MH, Posner JB. Ataxia in epidural spinal cord compression. *Neurology*, 1992; **42**: 2193–5.

39. Ushio Y, Posner R, Posner JB, Shapiro WR. Experimental spinal cord compression by epidural neoplasms. *Neurology*, 1977; **27**: 422–9.

40. Ikeda H, *et al.* Edema and circulatory disturbance in the spinal cord compressed by epidural neoplasms. *Journal of Neurosurgery*, 1980; **52**: 203–9.

41. Karo M, *et al.* Circulatory disturbance of the spinal cord with epidural neoplasm in rats. *Journal of Neurosurgery*, 1985; **63**: 260–5.

42. Delattre JY, Arbit E, Thaler HT. A dose-response study of dexamethasone in a model of spinal cord compression caused by epidural tumor. *Journal of Neurosurgery*, 1989; **70**: 920–5.

43. Siegal T, *et al.* Experimental spinal cord compression: evoked potentials, edema, prostaglandins, light and electron microscopy. *Spine*, 1987; **12**: 440–8.

44. Siegal T, *et al.* Indomethacin and dexamethasone in experimental neoplastic spinal cord compression: Part I. Effect on water content and specific gravity. *Neurosurgery*, 1988; **22**: 328–33.

45. Siegal T, Shohami E, Shapira Y, Siegal Tz. Indomethacin and dexamethasone in experimental neoplastic spinal cord compression: Part II. Effect on edema and prostaglandin synthesis. *Neurosurgery*, 1988; **22**: 334–9.

46. Siegal T, Siegal Tz, Shohami E, Shapira Y. Comparison of soluble dexamethasone sodium phosphate with free dexamethasone and indomethacin in the treatment of experimental neoplastic spinal cord compression. *Spine*, 1988; **13**: 1171–6.

47. Siegal T, Siegal Tz, Shapira Y, Shohami E. The early effect of steroidal and non-steroidal anti-inflammatory agents on neoplastic epidural cord compression. *Annals of the New York Academy of Sciences*, 1989; **559**: 488–90.

48. Siegal T, Siegal Tz, Shohami E, Lossos F. Experimental neoplastic spinal cord compression: effect of ketamine and MK-801 on edema and prostaglandins. *Neurosurgery*, 1990; **26**: 963–6.

49. Siegal T, Siegal Tz. Experimental neoplastic spinal cord compression: effect of anti-inflammatory agents and glutamate receptor antagonists on vascular permeability. *Neurosurgery*, 1990; **26**: 967–70.

50. Siegal T, Siegal Tz. Participation of serotonergic mechanisms in the pathophysiology of experimental neoplastic spinal cord compression. *Neurology*, 1991; **41**: 574–80.

51. Siegal T, Siegal Tz. Serotonergic manipulations in experimental neoplastic spinal cord compression. *Journal of Neurosurgery*, 1993; **78**: 929–37.

52. Siegal T. Spinal cord compression: from laboratory to clinic. *European Journal of Cancer*, 1995; **31A**: 1748–53.

53. Blight A. Morphometric analysis of experimental spinal cord injury in the cat: relationship of injury intensity to survival of myelinated axons. *Neuroscience*, 1986; **19**: 321–41.

54. Waxman SG. Demyelination in spinal cord injury. *Journal of Neurological Sciences*, 1989; **91**: 1–14.

55. Gledhill RF, McDonald WI. Morphological characteristics of central demyelination and remyelination: a single-fibre study. *Annals of Neurology*, 1977; **1**: 552–60.

56. Siegal T, Shezen E, Siegal Tz. The effect of *in-vivo* inhibition of phagocytic activity in experimental neoplastic spinal cord compression: immunohistochemistry, vascular permeability and neurologic function. *Journal of Neuro-Oncology*, 1994; **21**: 68.

57. Siegal T, Shezen E, Barak V, Siegal Tz. *In-vivo* inhibition of phagocytic activity in experimental neoplastic spinal cord compression: immunohistochemistry, cytokine production, vascular permeability and neurologic function. *Neurology*, 1995; **45**: 193A.

58. Sorensen PS, Helweg-Larsen S, Mouridsen H, Hansen HH. Effect of high-dose dexamethasone in carcinomatous metastatic spinal cord compression treated with radiotherapy: a randomized trial. *European Journal of Cancer*, 1994; **30A**: 22–7.

59. Murray PK. Functional outcome and survival in spinal cord injury secondary to neoplasia. *Cancer*, 1985; **55**: 197–201.

60. Siegal T, Siegal Tz. Current considerations in the management of neoplastic spinal cord compression. *Spine*, 1989; **14**: 223–8.

61. Podd TJ, *et al.* Spinal cord compression: prognosis and implications for treatment fractionations. *Clinical Oncology*, 1992; **4**: 341–4.

62. Tatsui H, Onomura T, Morishita S, Oketa M, Inoue T. Survival rates of patients with metastatic spinal cancer after scintigraphic detection of abnormal radioactive accumulation. *Spine*, 1996; 21: 2143–8.

63. Bauer HC, Wedin R. Survival after surgery for spinal and extremity metastases. Prognostication in 241 patients. *Acta Orthopaedica Scandinavica*, 1995; 66: 143–6.

64. Brice J, McKissock W. Surgical treatment of malignant extradural spinal tumors. *British Medical Journal*, 1965; 2: 1341–4.

65. Maranzano E, Latini P. Effectiveness of radiation therapy without surgery in metastatic spinal cord compression: final results from a prospective trial *International Journal of Radiation Oncology, Biology and Physics*, 1995; 32: 1259–60.

66. Posner JB, Howieson J, Cvitkovic E. 'Disappearing' spinal cord compression: oncolytic effect of glucocorticoids (and other chemotherapeutic agents) on epidural metastases. *Annals of Neurology*, 1977; 2: 409–13.

67. Siegal T, Siegal T. Surgical decompression of anterior and posterior malignant epidural tumors compressing the spinal cord: a prospective study. *Neurosurgery*, 1985; 17: 424–32.

68. Vecht CHJ, et al. Initial bolus of conventional versus high-dose dexamethasone in metastatic spinal cord compression. *Neurology*, 1989; 39: 1255–7.

69. Clarke P, Saunders M. Steroid-induced remission in spinal canal reticulum cell sarcoma. Report of two cases. *Journal of Neurosurgery*, 1975; 42: 346–8.

70. Marshall LF, Langfitt TW. Combined therapy for metastatic extradural tumors of the spine. *Cancer*, 1977; 40: 2067–70.

71. Sundaresan N, et al. Treatment of neoplastic epidural cord compression by vertebral body resection and stabilization. *Journal of Neurosurgery*, 1985; 63: 676–84.

72. Turner S, Marosszeky B, Timms I, Boyages J. Malignant spinal cord compression: a prospective evaluation. *International Journal of Radiation Oncology, Biology and Physics*, 1993; 26: 141–6.

73. Helweg-Larsen S. Clinical outcome in metastatic spinal cord compression. A prospective study of 153 patients. *Acta Neurologica Scandinavica*, 1996; 94: 269–75.

74. Sundaresan N, et al. Indication and results of combined anterior–posterior approach for spine tumor surgery. *Journal of Neurosurgery*, 1996; 85: 438–46.

75. Huddart RA, Rajan B, Law M, Meyer L, Dearnaley DP. Spinal cord compression in prostate cancer: Treatment outcome and prognostic factors. *Radiotherapy and Oncology*, 1997; 44: 229–36.

76. Husband DJ. Malignant spinal cord compression: prospective study of delays in referral and treatment. *British Medical Journal*, 1998; 317: 18–21.

77. Helweg-Larsen S, Sorensen PS. Symptoms and signs in metastatic spinal cord compression: a study of progression from first symptom until diagnosis in 153 patients. *European Journal of Cancer*, 1994; 30A: 396–8.

78. Helweg-Larsen S, Rasmusson B, Sorensen PS. Recovery of gait after radiotherapy in paralytic patients with metastatic epidural spinal cord compression. *Neurology*, 1990; 40: 1234–6.

79. Hall AJ, Mackay NNS. The results of laminectomy for compression of the cord or cauda equina by extradural malignant tumors. *Journal of Bone and Joint Surgery*, 1973; 55B: 497–505.

80. Harrington KD. Anterior cord decompression and spinal stabilization for patients with metastatic lesions of the spine. *Journal of Neurosurgery*, 1984; 61: 107–17.

81. Ominus M, et al. Surgical treatment of vertebral metastases. *Spine*, 1986; 11: 883–91.

82. Siegal T, Siegal Tz. Vertebral body resection for epidural compression by malignant tumors. Results of forty-seven consecutive operative procedures. *Journal of Bone and Joint Surgery*, 1985; 67A: 375–82.

83. Sundaresan N, et al. Treatment of neoplastic spinal cord compression: results of a prospective study. *Neurosurgery*, 1991; 29: 645–50.

84. Ominus M, Papin P, Gangloff S. Results of surgical treatment of spinal thoracic and lumbar metastases. *European Spine Journal*, 1996; 5: 407–11.

85. Walsh GL, et al. Anterior approaches to the thoracic spine in patients with cancer: indications and results. *Annals of Thoracic Surgery*, 1997; 64: 1611–18.

86. Cybulski GR. Methods of surgical stabilization for metastatic disease of the spine. *Neurosurgery*, 1989; 25: 240–52.

87. Eeles RA, O'Brien P, Horwich A, Brada M. Non-Hodgkin's lymphoma presenting with extradural spinal cord compression: functional outcome and survival. *British Journal of Cancer*, 1991; 63(1): 126–9.

88. Siegal T, Siegal Tz. Spinal epidural involvement in haematological tumors: clinical features and therapeutic options. *Leukemia and Lymphoma*, 1991; 5: 101–10.

89. Wong ET, Portlock CS, O'Brien JP, DeAngelis LM. Chemosensitive epidural spinal cord disease in non-Hodgkins lymphoma. *Neurology*, 1996; 46: 1543–7.

90. Cooper K, Bajorin D, Shapiro W, Krol G, Sze G, Bosl GJ. Decompression of epidural metastases from germ cell tumors with chemotherapy. *Journal of Neuro-Oncology*, 1990; 8: 275–80.

91. Gale GB, O'Connor DM, Chu JY, Tantana S, Weber TR. Successful chemotherapeutic decompression of epidural malignant germ cell tumor. *Medical Pediatric Oncology*, 1986; 14: 97–9.

92. Hayes FA, Thompson EI, Hvizdala E, O'Connor D, Green AA. Chemotherapy as an alternative to laminectomy and radiation in the management of epidural tumor. *Journal of Pediatrics*, 1984; 104: 221–4.

93. Fadul CE, Lemann W, Thaler HT, Posner JB. Perforation of the gastrointestinal tract in patients receiving steroids for neurologic disease. *Neurology*, 1988; 38: 348–52.

94. Weissman DE. Glucocorticoid treatment for brain metastases and epidural cord compression: a review. *Journal of Clinical Oncology*, 1988; 6: 543–51.

95. Weiner HL, Rezai AR, Cooper PR. Sigmoid diverticular perforation in neurosurgical patients receiving high-dose corticosteroids. *Neurosurgery*, 1993; 33: 40–3.

96. Martenson JA, et al. Treatment outcome and complications in patients treated for malignant epidural spinal cord compression. *Journal of Neuro-oncology*, 1985; 3: 77–84.

97. Maranzano E, et al. Radiotherapy without steroids in selected metastatic spinal cord compression patients. A phase II trial. *American Journal of Clinical Oncology*, 1996; 19: 179–83.

98. Sundaresan N, DiGiacinto GV. Antitumor and antinociceptive approaches to control cancer pain. *Medical Clinics of North America*, 1987; 71: 329–48.

99. Loblaw DA, Laperriere NJ. Emergency treatment of malignant extradural spinal cord compression: an evidence-based guideline. *Journal of Clinical Oncology*, 1998; 16(4): 1613–24.

100. Cooper PR, Errico TJ, Martin R, Crawford B, DiBartolo T. A systematic approach to spinal reconstruction after anterior decompression for neoplastic disease of the thoracic and lumbar spine. *Neurosurgery*, 1993; 32: 1–8.

101. Ominus M, Papin P, Gangloff S. Results of surgical treatment of spinal thoracic and lumbar metastases. *European Spine Journal*, 1996; 5: 407–11.

102. Fyfe I, Henry APJ, Mulholland RC. Closed vertebral biopsy. *Journal of Bone and Joint Surgery*, 1983; 65B: 140–3.

103. Denis F. Spinal instability as defined by the three-column spine concept in acute spinal trauma. *Clinical Orthopedics*, 1984; 189: 65–76.

104. Kostuik JP, Errico JN. Differential diagnosis and surgical treatment of metastatic spine tumors. In *The adult spine: principles and practice*, Vol. 1 (ed. JW Frymoyer). New York: Raven Press, 1991: 861–88.

105. Bradford DS. Spinal instability: orthopedic perspective and prevention. *Clinical Neurosurgery*, 1980; **27**: 591–610.

106. White AA III, Panjabi MM. *Clinical Biomechanics of the Spine.* Philadelphia, PA: JB Lippincott, 1987: 191–276.

107. Schiff D, Shaw EG, Cascino TL. Outcome after spinal reirradiation for malignant epidural cord compression. *Annals of Neurology*, 1995; **37**: 583–9.

108. McLain RF, Weinstein JN. Tumors of the spine. *Seminars in Spine Surgery*, 1990; **2**: 157–80.

109. Shimizu K, *et al.* Posterior decompression and stabilization for multiple metastatic tumors of the spine. *Spine*, 1992; **17**: 1400–4.

110. Slatkin NE, Posner JB. Management of spinal epidural metastases. *Clinical Neurosurgery*, 1982; **30**: 698–716.

111. McPhee IB, Williams RP, Swanson CE. Factors influencing wound healing after surgery for metastatic disease of the spine. *Spine*, 1998; **23**: 726–32.

112. Brady LW, *et al.* The treatment of metastatic disease of the nervous system by radiation therapy. In *Tumors of the nervous system* (ed. HG Sey-del). New York: Wiley, 1975: 176–89.

113. Mones RJ, Dozier D, Berrett A. Analysis of medical treatment of malignant extradural spinal cord tumors. *Cancer*, 1966; **19**: 1842–53.

114. Khan FR, Glicksman AS, Chu FC, Nickson JJ. Treatment by radiotherapy of spinal cord compression due to extradural metastases. *Radiology*, 1967; **89**: 495–500.

115. Stark RJ, Henson RA, Evans SJW. Spinal metastases: a retrospective survey from a general hospital. *Brain*, 1982; **105**: 189–213.

116. Obbens EAMT, *et al.* Metronidazole as a radiation enhancer in the treatment of metastatic epidural spinal cord compression. *Journal Neuro-oncology*, 1984; **2**: 99–104.

117. Harrison KM, *et al.* Spinal cord compression in breast cancer. *Cancer,* 1985; **55**: 2839–44.

118. Maranzano E, Latini P, Perruci E, Benenenti S, Lupattelli M, Corgna E. Short-course radiotherapy (8 Gy × 2) in metastatic spinal cord compression: an effective and feasible treatment. *International Journal of Radiation Oncology, Biology, Physics*, 1997; **38**: 1037–44.

119. Merrin C, *et al.* The value of palliative spinal surgery in metastatic urogenital tumors. *Journal of Urology*, 1976; **115**: 712–13.

120. Gianotta SL, Kindt GW. Metastatic spinal cord tumors. *Clinical Neurosurgery*, 1978; **25**: 495–503.

121. Kleinman WB, Kiernan HA, Michelsen WJ. Metastatic cancer of the spinal column. *Clinical Orthopedics*, 1978; **136**: 166–72.

122. Livingston KE, Perrin RG. The neurosurgical management of spinal metastases causing cord and cauda equina compression. *Journal of Neurosurgery*, 1978; **49**: 839–43.

123. Baldini M, *et al.* Neurological results in spinal cord metastases. *Neurochirurgia (Stuttg)*, 1979; **22**: 159–65.

124. Gorter K. Results of laminectomy in spinal cord compression due to tumors. *Acta Neurochirogica (Wien)*, 1978; **42**: 177–8.

125. Dunn RC, Kelly WA, Wohns RNW, Howe JF. Spinal epidural neoplasia. A 15-year review of the results of surgical therapy. *Journal Neurosurgery*, 1980; **52**: 47–51.

126. Levy WJ, Latchaw JP, Hardy RW, Hahn JP. Encouraging surgical results in walking patients with epidural metastases. *Neurosurgery*, 1982; **11**: 229–33.

127. Klein HJ, Richter HP, Schafer M. Extradural spinal metastases. A retrospective study of 197 patients. *Advances in Neurosurgery*, 1984; **12**: 36–43.

128. Kollmann H, Diemath HE, Strohecker J, Spatz H. Spinal metastases as the first manifestation. *Advances in Neurosurgery*, 1984; **12**: 44–6.

129. Garcia-Picazo A, Ramirez PC, Rivas PP, Garcia de Sola R. Utility of surgery in the treatment of epidural vertebral metastases. *Acta Neurologica*, 1990; **103**: 131–8.

130. Brunon J, Sautreaux JL, Sindau M, Fischer G. Posterior osteosynthesis in the treatment of spinal cord tumors. *Neurochirurgie*, 1975; **21**: 435–46.

131. Hansebout RR, Blomquist GA Jr. Acrylic spinal fusion. A 20-year clinical series and technical note. *Journal Neurosurgery*, 1980; **53**: 606–12.

132. Miles J, Banks AJ, Dervin E, Noori Z. Stabilization of the spine affected by malignancy. *Journal of Neurology, Neurosurgery and Psychiatry*, 1984; **47**: 897–904.

133. DeWald RL, Bridwell KH, Prodromas C, Rodts MF. Reconstructive spinal surgery as palliation for metastatic malignancies of the spine. *Spine*, 1985; **10**: 21–6.

134. Overby MC, Rothman AS. Anterolateral decompression for metastatic epidural spinal cord tumors. Results of a modified costotransversectomy approach. *Journal of Neurosurgery*, 1985; **62**: 344–8.

135. Solini A, Paschero B, Orsini G, Guercio N. The surgical treatment of metastatic tumors of the lumbar spine. *Italian Journal of Orthopedics and Traumatology*, 1985; **11**: 427–42.

136. Heller M, McBroom RJ, MacNab T, Perfin R. Treatment of metastatic disease of the spine with posterolateral decompression and Luque instrumentation. *Neuroorthopedics*, 1986; **2**: 70–4.

137. Sherman RPM, Waddell JP. Laminectomy for metastatic epidural spinal tumors. Posterior stabilization, radiotherapy and postoperative assessment. *Clinical Orthopedics*, 1986; **207**: 55–63.

138. Perrin RG, McBroom RJ. Anterior versus posterior decompression for symptomatic spinal metastases. *Canadian Journal of Neurological Sciences*, 1987; **14**: 75–80.

139. Fidler MW. Posterior instrumentation of the spine. An experimental comparison of various possible techniques. *Spine*, 1986; **11**: 367–72.

140. Sapkas G, Kyratzoulis J, Papaioannou N, Babis G, Rologis D, Tzanis S. Spinal cord decompression and stabilization in malignant lesions of the spine. *Acta Orthopaedica Scandinavica (Suppl.)*, 1997; **275**: 97–100.

141. Gokaslan ZL, *et al.* Transthoracic vertebrectomy for metastatic spinal tumors. *Journal of Neurosurgery*, 1998; **89**: 599–609.

5.6 Pathological fracture

A. H. M. Taminiau

Introduction

The most common neoplastic tumours of bones are metastases, more than 80 per cent of which are due to carcinoma of the breast, prostate, lung, or kidney. The majority of these metastases are predominantly found in the axial skeleton. Bone metastases are often asymptomatic unless soft tissues are involved or fracture occurs. Involvement of the long bones frequently results in fractures and is therefore more disabling. Stabilization of impending and pathological fractures is the treatment of choice, which effects pain relief, restoration of limb function, early mobilization, and an improvement in the patients' quality of life.

Epidemiology

The risk (calculated according to the Life-table method) of developing cancer in The Netherlands before the age of 75 years is 22.5 per cent for females and 25.5 per cent for males, based on the incidence patterns of 1994.[1] If this incidence pattern is maintained, nearly 4 out of 10 men and 3.5 out of 10 women will develop cancer at some time. The majority of these patients are over 45 years of age; fewer than 10 per cent of all new cancer patients are under 45 years of age—children seldom develop cancer. The incidence of bone metastases is reported to be between 30 and 70 per cent, the metastases being mainly derived (> 80 per cent) from carcinoma of the breast, prostate, lung, or kidney.[2] However, a significant proportion of other cancers, for example colorectal cancer, may also give rise to bone metastases.[3] The majority of these metastases are found in the axial skeleton and in the major long bones: femur, humerus, and tibia.

The overall incidence of fractures due to bone metastases is between 5 and 10 per cent.[4] In skeletal metastases, the risk of progression to fracture is related primarily to the degree of tumour extension and the amount of bone loading, resulting in a higher incidence of pathological fractures in the long bones.

Aetiology and pathogenesis

A limited proportion of the neoplastic cells that enter the vascular system survive. Those that do establish metastatic foci show an affinity for certain areas, particularly those areas of the skeleton involved in blood cell formation.[5] As a result, skeletal metastases are more often found in the axial skeleton (vertebra, pelvis, rib, scapula) than in the long bones. Spread to the vertebrae may occur by way of Batson vena (venous vertebral system without valves) or, as in other areas, directly by arterial infusion through the sinusoids and capillary system of the red bone marrow. A cellular mechanism through which metastases weaken bone has recently been reported. Local osteoclastic activity and bone resorption has been shown to be increased by factors produced by the cancer cells.[6] This resorptive activity is responsible for the decrease in bone strength. Consequently, therapeutic regimens are focused on inhibiting osteoclastic activity. Results of treatment regimens using biphosphonates and various radiopharmaceuticals are promising.[7]

Metastases of the long bones progress to pathological fractures in about 25 per cent of cases, but this risk is much higher in the proximal femur (40 to 60 per cent) where mechanical load is high.[8]

In primary bone tumours, both benign and malignant, pathological fractures occur due to the same mechanical weakening. However, some primary bone tumours produce a matrix (osteosarcoma, chondrosarcoma) that decreases the risk of fractures, whereas fractures occur more frequently where tumours do not produce a matrix (for example, giant-cell tumour, Ewing's sarcoma). The probability for osteolytic lesions to fracture is higher than osteoblastic or mixed osteolytic/-blastic defects.[9]

In metastatic bone disease, the pattern of bone destruction is related to the aggressiveness of tumour growth. Slow-growing metastases have well-defined lytic areas of geographic destruction, whereas aggressive lesions show a more permeative or moth-eaten destructive pattern.

Pathology

In patients with known primary tumours and where there is a suspicion of bone metastasis the diagnosis can often be confirmed by cytology from a core or open biopsy. In skeletal lesions without a known primary tumour, oncological work-up (scintigraphy/MRI) should precede the biopsy. A number of additional techniques have been developed over the last few years (immunohistochemistry, cytogenetics, and molecular genetic techniques) that can unravel tumour-specific features and are helpful in confirming the diagnosis.

Clinical presentation

The majority of skeletal metastases are asymptomatic and are only diagnosed when patients are screened at follow-up for their primary cancer. However, they may become symptomatic when a fracture occurs or soft tissue is involved. Skeletal metastases are suspected when patients with a history of cancer present with pain and/or hypercalcaemia.[10] Bone pain can be localized or general, but this does not necessarily reflect the presence of metastases. Back pain might be due to metastases producing impending or pathological fractures, spinal instability, or cord or cauda equina compression. The mechanism of the bone pain is not fully understood, but is probably due to periosteal irritation or microfractures and may be associated with infraction of the surrounding bone. Not infrequently patients present with fracture as the first symptom of a tumoural process or a metastatic pathological fracture. Although the incidence of metastasis in bone lesions is high, especially in elderly patients, the possibility of a primary bone tumour should be carefully considered, especially in pathological fractures associated with an unknown primary.

Screening and diagnosis

Skeletal metastases may present as osteolytic, osteoblastic, or mixed osteolytic/osteoblastic lesions.

Radiographs

These may deliver useful information about the site, extension, periosteal reaction, and the presence or absence of mineralization. It is helpful in a symptomatic patient but ineffective as a screening method, because a normal radiograph does not exclude the presence of metastases. To detect metastases by plain radiographs, a more than 50 per cent destruction of the trabecular bone is needed.[11] However, less destruction is needed to detect cortical metastases.

Scintigraphy ($^{99}Tc^m$ HDP)[2],[12]

This is the optimal modality for detecting occult metastases before radiological changes and symptoms occur. Although the sensitivity of scintigraphy is high (95 per cent), the specificity is limited and therefore confirmatory radiographs are often needed. Other causes for increased activity seen on scintigraphy (arthrosis, infection) are not excluded; it must be borne in mind that aggressive osteolytic lesions may not produce increased activity. Comparing scintigraphic changes with prior imaging investigations might be helpful. Single-photon emission computed tomography (SPECT) can be useful for improving lesion detection in difficult anatomical sites (for example, the pelvis, skull, and spine). In general, a suspicion of metastases on scintigraphy occurs if: (1) there are more than five new lesions since the previous investigation; (b) there is increased scintigraphic activity, with radiological changes; (c) there is increased activity in the thoracic spine, without radiological changes. Solitary rib lesions are generally not metastases, although a 'hot spot' in the sternum has a 50 per cent chance of being a metastatic lesion. Several benign multifocal diseases may simulate metastatic lesions (for instance, hyperparathyroidism, Paget's disease, osteoporosis, and osteonecrosis after radiotherapy or chemotherapy) and these should be excluded.

Magnetic resonance imaging (MRI)

MRI[13] is the modality of choice for evaluating skeletal metastases in the spine, especially when compression of the spinal cord is suspected. Due to its multidimensional imaging properties, MRI best shows the presence of multiple metastases, extension into the spinal canal or soft tissues, spinal cord compression, and secondary fractures. MRI is more sensitive than scintigraphy in differentiating osteoporotic fractures from metastases of the spine, and is indicated in clinically suspected cases of metastases, albeit with a negative scintigram.

Computed tomography (CT)

CT-scanning is recommended for identifying bone destruction due to metastases in the spine. CT shows the bone structure better than MRI, but is less accurate in detecting lesions without bone destruction and soft tissue extension.

In a patient with a known primary carcinoma and local skeletal pain, normal radiographs should be followed by scintigraphy; if these are still inconclusive then MRI should be used.[13] However, if the same patient has diffuse pain then scintigraphy comes first.

Impending fractures

Such fractures present with pain and are usually visible as lytic lesions on the radiograph. Primary internal stabilization of a weakened bone which has a significant risk of fracture has certain advantages over treatment after fracture. While the bone is still intact, adequate fixation is much easier to achieve and reduces the length of surgery, rehabilitation period, and convalescence. Where feasible, closed intra-medullary nailing is preferable. Because of the weakened bone, particular care must be taken to avoid producing a fracture both when positioning the anaesthetized patient and during the procedure itself.

By the time a large lytic metastasis has developed there is considerable bone destruction, the cortex is involved, and the risk of fracture is high. Fidler[14] found that this risk of fracture correlated with the degree of cortical destruction. If less than 25 per cent of the circumferential cortex was destroyed then the risk of fracture was virtually negligible. If more than 50 per cent of the cortex of a long bone was involved there was a sudden rise in fracture incidence. Fidler reported a fracture incidence of 3.7 per cent when 25 to 50 per cent of the cortex was involved and 61 per cent when the degree of involvement ranged from 50 to 75 per cent. CT imaging may be helpful in assessing the degree of bone destruction. Internal fixation for stabilizing impending and pathological fractures is the treatment of choice, and will provide pain relief, restoration of limb function, early mobilization, and improve the patient's quality of life.[15]–[17] Prophylactic stabilization of impending pathological fractures might be indicated in large lytic lesions, persistent pain after radiotherapy, or when on a radiograph and CT scan the transcortical defect ratio of the height of the lesion to its outer diameter becomes more than 1.[14],[16] The latter was studied by Dijkstra et al. in a finite-element analysis (FEM) model, from which they concluded that the height of a transcortical destructive lesion in relation to the bone diameter is an important estimate of the risk factor of fracture. However, analysis of the diagnostic tools shows significant intraobserver variability in radiographic and CT measurements of cortical defects in long bones (25 per cent errors).[18] An alternative screening system can be used, as reported by Mirels, where there is doubt in diagnosing an impending pathological fracture.[19] This predictive method analyses each risk factor contributing to an actual fracture in the long bones. In cases where primary sarcomas can not be excluded, the work-up should be performed first. This should include proper staging (always metastatic screening in the case of malignancy: chest radiography/CT), followed

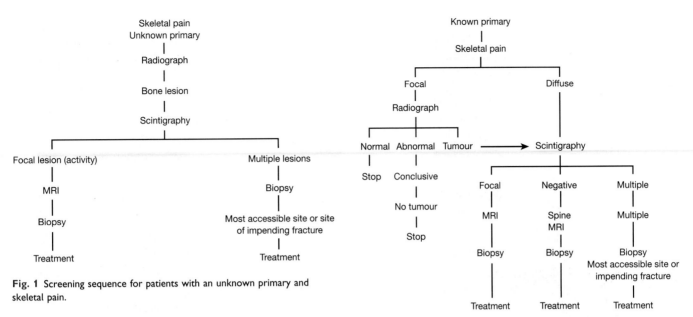

Fig. 1 Screening sequence for patients with an unknown primary and skeletal pain.

Fig. 2 Screening sequence for patients with a known primary and skeletal pain.

by the appropriate biopsy for the lesion, according to oncological rules, to prevent inadequate treatment. It must be kept in mind that several polyostotic diseases are active on bone scintigraphy. These can be benign or malignant as well as non-tumoral, for example: fibrous dysplasia, multiple exostosis, Paget's disease of bone, multiple myeloma, polyostotic osteosarcomas, Ewing's sarcoma, and polyarthropathy and osteomyelitis.

Patients can be divided into two groups for the purpose of screening for suspected skeletal metastases:[13]

(1) patients with a unknown primary and skeletal pain;

(2) patients with a known primary and skeletal pain.

Figures 1 and 2 show the sequences used for screening these two groups of patients.

Management and prognosis

Radiotherapy is the treatment of choice for patients with localized pain due to proven metastases. The response to irradiation in terms of pain relief, decrease in the size of metastases, and bone-remodelling was studied in 1016 patients of which 759 had bone metastases.[7] After 20 to 40 Gray of radiation, pain relief was reported by 90 per cent (680) of the 759 patients: complete pain relief in 54 per cent (408) of these and slight pain relief in the other 36 per cent. The effect of radiotherapy on preventing fracture is uncertain, but it is dependent on several factors, such as metastasis site and life expectancy. The administration of radiation (single or fractionated dose) and the expected responses to radiotherapy remain unclear, these aspects are not discussed in this chapter. The systemic administration of strontium-89 as a first-line therapy should be considered in patients without a predominantly painful site.[20] It can also be used in patients with widely metastatic disease, as an adjuvant to external-beam radiotherapy and in situations when external-beam therapy options have been exhausted, and when normal tissue tolerance has been reached.[21]

Excluding criteria for radionuclide therapy include a life expectancy of less than at least 3 months, no evidence of imminent epidural cord compression, pathological fracture or mechanical instability, and good renal function and marrow reserve.

The evaluation of a patient with a pathological or impending fracture includes an assessment of the general fitness of the patient, the degree of tumour dissemination, the diagnosis of the primary carcinoma if not already known, and the presence of other complications. Since the survival time of patients with pathological fractures has been extended by improvements in management, the treatment of such fractures becomes increasingly important to improve the patient's remaining quality of life. It is important that stabilization results in rigid fixation. This can often be achieved by devices used in the treatment of general fractures such as plates, intramedullary nails, or endoprosthetic replacements. The selection of the type of implant is dependent on: the site, size, type, and extent of the fracture; the quality of the bone stock; and the presence of other metastases in the same or adjacent bones. In the proximal femur and hip region, for example, different kinds of fixation devices are used related to the exact site of the fracture. The available options are plates and screws, intramedullary nails, Gamma nails, Dynamic hip screws, and endoprostheses. Due care should be exercised when choosing the fixation device since inappropriate devices can lead to a loss of rigidity or fractures below the implant, which, of course, can influence the prognosis. It is essential that the internal stabilization of the lesion provides sufficient strength to, at the least, allow unsupported use of the limb. Because the treatment of pathological fractures is different from an intended curative treatment of the lesion, it is classified as an intralesional procedure and local tumour control will be seldom achieved. Here, fracture healing is different from standard non-pathological fracture healing, and it is prolonged by the presence of a tumour and adjuvant treatment (irradiation or

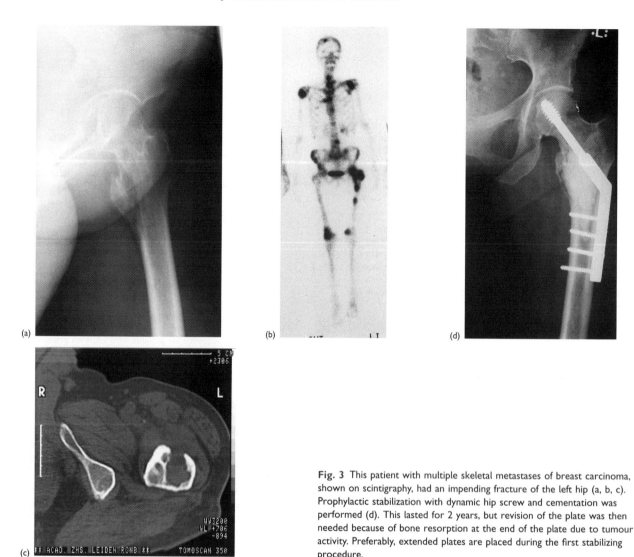

Fig. 3 This patient with multiple skeletal metastases of breast carcinoma, shown on scintigraphy, had an impending fracture of the left hip (a, b, c). Prophylactic stabilization with dynamic hip screw and cementation was performed (d). This lasted for 2 years, but revision of the plate was then needed because of bone resorption at the end of the plate due to tumour activity. Preferably, extended plates are placed during the first stabilizing procedure.

chemotherapy). Therefore satisfactory internal fixation should not simply depend on fracture healing but should provide adequate stability by itself. This often requires supplementary techniques. In many cases, the implant alone is unable to provide adequate stabilization because of extensive bone loss. Augmentation by methylmethacrylate (**PMMA**) or other more complex types of reconstruction (allograft, endoprosthesis) may be used to restore these defects and improve the stabilization. Screws for plate-and-nail devices can be fixed through the methylmethacrylate when it is still soft, and also through the normal bone above and below the lesion. Intramedullary rod fixation can be augmented by methylmethacrylate, although the pressure of the cementation may increase the risk of fat embolism.[12] Often, irradiation is an essential part of the treatment aimed at inhibiting further tumour growth, since the latter will result in progressive bone destruction thereby loosening the stabilization and increasing the risk of re-fracture. If postoperative irradiation is less than 30 Gy, bone healing is expected in about 60 to 90 per cent of patients who survive for more than 3 months.[2] Nevertheless, the risk of fatigue breakdown of the device, loosening, and re-fracture might necessitate replacement of the plate or additional plating if the patient survives for a long time (Fig. 3). Bauer and Wedin[22] showed that the 1-year overall survival rate after treatment of skeletal pathological fractures in patients with metastases was 33 per cent. Depending upon the tumour type of lesion, hormonal therapy or chemotherapy may also be required. The use of hormonal treatment (breast, prostrate) can have an advantageous significant effect on bone healing (Fig. 4).

Highly vascular lesions

Occasional metastases, particular those from renal carcinomas and myelomas, may be highly vascular and surgery may be associated with excessive blood loss. In cases of renal-cell carcinoma or myeloma, preoperative angiography or MRI with gadolinium-enhancement to establish the vascularity of the lesion is advised. Preoperative embolization of the lesion will facilitate surgery and decrease the risk of extensive blood loss[23] (Fig. 5).

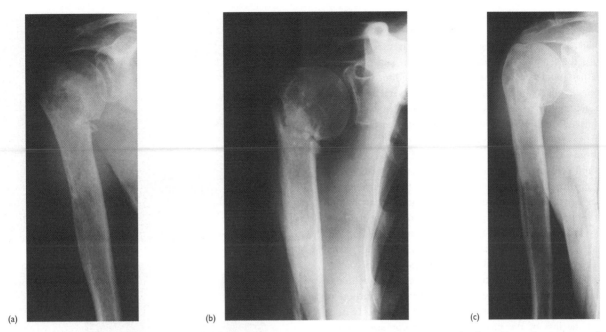

Fig. 4 (a) This 46-year-old man was referred for a pathological fracture of the right proximal humerus, suspected to be a primary bone tumour. Oncological work-up revealed no other lesion. The lesion turned out to be a bone lymphoma. (b) and (c) The fracture was treated conservatively and after chemotherapy healed without any instrumentation, resulting in only a modest limitation of abduction.

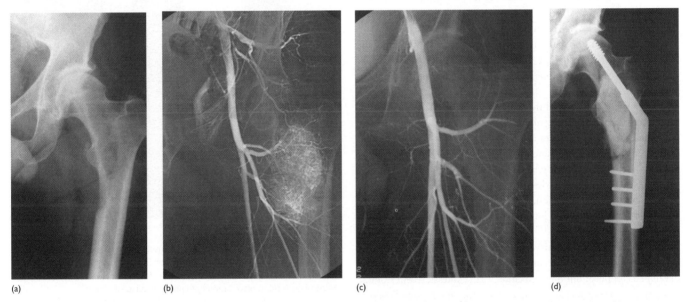

Fig. 5 This 46-year-old man reported some discomfort of several weeks' duration in his upper left leg; otherwise he felt completely normal. Plain radiographs revealed a lytic lesion in the medial cortex of the subtrochanteric region of the left proximal femur, which on MRI turned out to be a highly vascular lesion with an obvious soft tissue component. (a). CT and ultrasound study of the kidney proved the suspicion of a renal-cell carcinoma. The lesion in the femur was proven to be a metastasis. A nephrectomy was performed. Following embolization of the lesion ((b) before and (c) after embolization), the impending fracture of the proximal femur was stabilized by dynamic hip screw fixation augmented with methylmethacrylate (d).

Lower extremity lesion

Pathological fractures of the femoral neck have a high risk of non-union, irrespective of the method of treatment.[12] A failure-of-fixation incidence of between 12 and 33 per cent has been reported after internal fixation of the femoral neck.[24] Endoprosthetic replacement is usually the treatment of choice regardless of the degree of head displacement. It is also prudent to treat this fracture with a long-stemmed, total hip replacement as there is a significant risk of acetabular or more distal femoral metastases which are not revealed by radiological investigations. The advantages of cementation of the femoral stem and acetabulum in patients with a limited lifespan render non-cemented devices of little use. Total hip replacement gives good results, providing several factors are taken into account: the degree of tumour involvement, acetabular involvement, and the presence of more distal lesions in the femoral shaft. In the case of a large metastatic involvement of the proximal femur, custom-made or modular devices can be used to bridge the defect and restore hip function.[25]–[28] Hemiarthroplasty with a double or floating cup is prudent only when the acetabulum is intact, or where there is involvement of the acetabulum but an intact subchondral plate (Fig. 6). Acetabular involvement has been classified by Harrington: class I—intact lateral cortex and superior and medial acetabular walls; class II—deficiences in the medial wall; and class III—deficiences of the medial and superior wall.[29] If stable cup fixation is impossible due to tumour destruction of the acetabulum (Harrington class II–III), prior reconstruction of the pelvis is necessary to restore the acetabular fixation. In such situations (bone loss of the proximal femur and/or acetabulum), custom-made or modular prosthetic replacement devices can be used to bridge the defect and restore hip function, as above.[25],[26] In isolated acetabular metastasis with an intact subchondral plate (Harrington class I),[15] the tumour may be curetted and the defect filled with methylmethacrylate. If there is more extensive involvement of the acetabulum, pelvic reconstruction may be required at the time of arthroplasty. In cases where restoration is inappropriate, special devices for the pelvis can be employed that make use of allografts, methylmethacrylate, rods, custom-built devices, or saddle prosthesis, to solve the problem of the loss of bone stock[25],[26],[30] (Fig. 7).

Intertrochanteric and subtrochanteric fractures may demand the same approach as fractures of the femoral neck.[31] However, conventional stabilization devices can be used if there is limited tumour extension (Zickel nail,[32] Gamma nail or Dynamic hip screw) augmented with methylmethacrylate (Fig. 8). A long-stemmed endoprosthesis is recommended where there is more extensive involvement of the intertrochanteric region.[25] The current generation of devices are available with extended long femoral stems, enabling protection of the entire femoral shaft.[33] Proper proximal and distal locking should be performed to achieve rigid internal fixation. Enders' nails are not recommended because more than one-third of patients developed complications due to fixation.[34] In contrast, recent studies, albeit with a rather short follow-up period, reported no complications after reconstruction with nail fixation.[35]

With femoral and tibial fractures of the meta- and diaphysis, the long bones are better treated by internal fixation. Interlocking nailing is advised for diaphysial lesions and augmentation with methylmethacrylate may restore immediate weight-bearing ability. In patients who survive for more than 3 months, the majority of pathological fractures involving the metaphysis of the femur or tibia often unite with conservative care (Fig. 9).[2],[7],[12] However, internal fixation is indicated if non-operative care severely impairs the patient's quality of life (for example, pain, need for nursing care, pressure sores, immobilization, and lengthy hospital admission). Diaphysial fractures are better fixed by intramedullary nailing, whereas

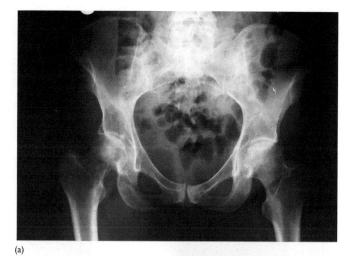

(a)

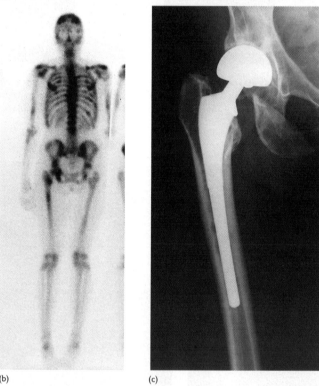

(b)   (c)

Fig. 6 This 49-year-old woman with diffusely metastatic breast carcinoma sustained a pathological fracture of the left femoral neck (a, b). Prosthetic hip replacement with a double cup was performed, required because of the intact subchondral plate in multiple pelvic metastases (c).

fractures in the metaphysis often require fixation with a plate, Dynamic screw devices, or interlocking nails.

Upper extremity lesions

Pathological fractures of the humerus are better managed with a functional cast brace if the patient has a limited life expectancy.[36] Poor results of non-operative treatment of pathological fractures of

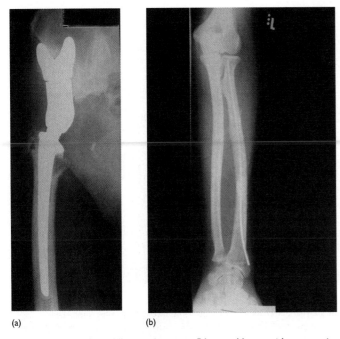

(a)   (b)

Fig. 7 Example of a saddle prosthesis in a 54-year-old man with metastasis from a renal-cell carcinoma to the acetabular region. The acetabulum and hip joint were removed *en-bloc* and the defect was reconstructed with a saddle prosthesis allowing full weight-bearing. (a) During remobilization. During his rehabilitation an impending pathological fracture of his forearm, which was disabling when he used crutches, was stabilized with methylmethacrylate and K-wire (b).

the humerus have been reported.[37] Patients who are expected to survive for longer than 3 months, and/or patients who depend on the support of their arms for walking, or patients with bilateral involvement of the upper extremities require internal fixation to ensure pain relief, restore function, or to avoid subsequent fracture.[25] The vast majority of pathological fractures of the humerus, radius, or ulna are better fixed by intramedullary nailing to provide mobility and rapid pain relief.[38],[39] The advantage of nailing is a decrease in blood loss, a lower complication rate in soft tissues, and improved stability. Subacromial impingement by the protruding tip of the nail should be avoided, as should hyperthermia around the radial nerve caused by polymerization of the methylmethacrylate (PMMA).[38] Adequate stabilization will result in good restoration of function in 90 per cent of cases. Extended fractures or tumour involvement of the proximal humerus may require replacement arthroplasty with a long-stemmed prosthesis or even reconstruction by a special tumour-endoprosthesis.[27] Unstable fixation requires PMMA augmentation. The technique of retrograde humeral nailing by a distal entrance portal in the humerus avoids complications to the rotator cuff region and will achieve adequate fixation. Curettage and cementation of the metastasis can be performed through a separate incision. A closed, reamed, nailing technique with low-viscosity PMMA has been suggested for treating an impending fracture with extended destruction of the humerus[40] (Fig. 10).

Metastases in the ulna and radius are rare. Occasionally, these can be handled by intramedullary rodding (Rush rods) or plate osteosynthesis with or without cementation.[41]

Metastatic disease of the spine

Approximately 50 per cent of the patients with skeletal metastases will have spinal involvement. Back pain is a frequent symptom in

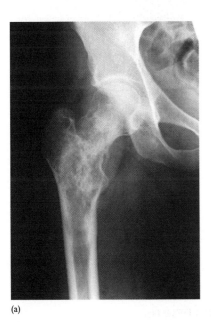 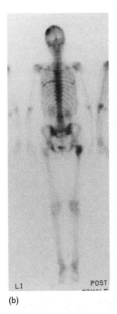 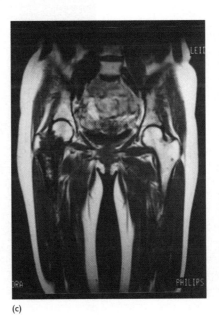 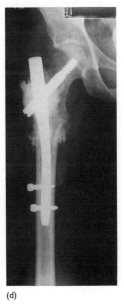

(a)   (b)   (c)   (d)

Fig. 8 This 30-year-old woman with breast carcinoma had metastases to multiple skeletal areas (skull, spine, right hip) and received radiotherapy for the palliation of hip pain due to metastases (a, b). Increasing pain and bone resorption of the femur were suggestive of active metastases and an impending fracture (c). Stabilization was achieved with Gamma nail fixation and methylmethacrylate augmentation (d). The pain decreased and the stability of the hip made full weight-bearing possible. MRI showed an intact joint and no involvement of the acetabulum (c).

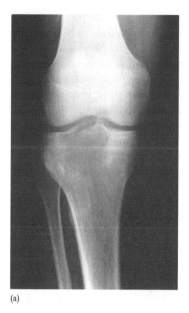
(a)

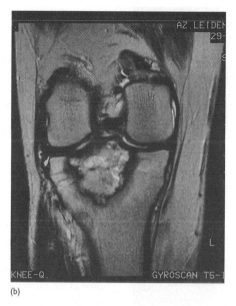
(b)

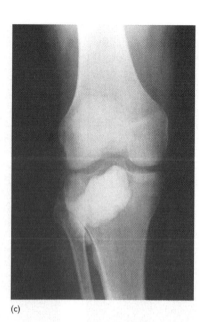
(c)

Fig. 9 This 50-year-old male had undergone nephrectomy for a renal-cell carcinoma, 2 years later he experienced some discomfort in his knee. The radiograph showed a defect in the proximal tibia extending into the intracondylar notch (a). An MRI T_2 weighted image showed a circumscript intraosseous defect with an intact subchondral plate (b). The diagnosis was a renal-cell carcinoma metastasis. After embolization, the lesion was curetted, using an extra-articular approach, and filled with methylmethacrylate (c) leaving the subchondral plate intact. Full weight-bearing was allowed 1 week after surgery.

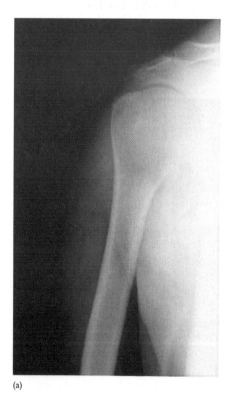
(a)

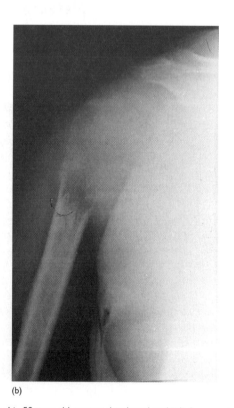
(b)

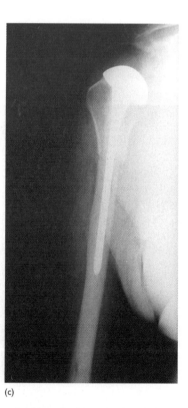
(c)

Fig. 10 Four years after the first event of breast cancer this 59-year-old woman developed multiple bone metastases; shoulder pain due to metastases was treated by irradiation (a). Three years later the proximal humerus showed progressive destruction (b). Because of pain and disability in the dominant arm, resection of the proximal humerus and allograft prosthetic reconstruction was performed resulting in pain relief and acceptable stability and arm control (c).

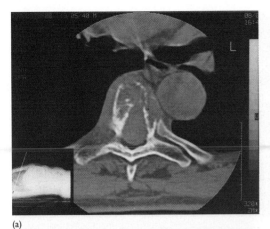

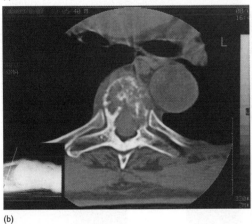

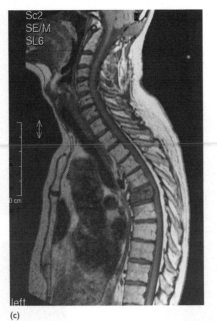

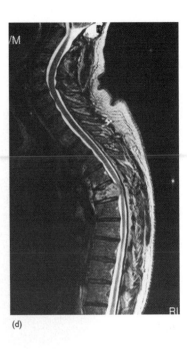

Fig. 11 This 57-year-old male has a progressive neurological deficit due to renal-cell carcinoma metastasis of the spine. The compression of the spinal cord expected by the neurological symptoms is appreciated on CT scan (a, b), but its extension is better seen by MRI (c, d). Furthermore, no other metastases are shown on MRI. Anterior decompression and stabilization was performed.

patients with disseminated carcinoma and can be caused by spinal instability or direct neural compression. Asymptomatic patients should be followed radiologically to determine whether radiotherapy is needed. Radiotherapy is indicated and recommended if the destruction exceeds 50 per cent of the vertebral body, especially in radiosensitive tumours. If the patient presents with local pain without neurological symptoms, plain radiographs should help to determine whether the pain is due to neural compression, bone destruction, fracture, or instability. CT scan and MRI of the affected area should be performed to rule out fracture of the vertebral body (CT) and soft tissue compression of the neural system (MRI). Radiotherapy is recommended in cases of less than 50 per cent destruction and where there is no risk of neural system involvement. If there is more than 50 per cent destruction with instability or with canal compromise, surgery is advocated. In patients with symptoms and a neurological deficit, MRI and CT are used to delineate the affected area, whether the compression occurs anteriorly (75 per cent) or posteriorly (15 per cent), and to establish the amount of vertebral body involvement (Fig. 11). Surgical procedures may be performed anteriorly (corpectomy) or posteriorly (laminectomy) according to the location of the tumour extension. In both situations, subsequent stabilization is required. Surgery may be compromised by multiple non-adjacent metastases, poor bone quality, short life expectancy, or complete paraplegia lasting for more than 2 days.[42],[43] These patients should be irradiated if the tumour is radiosensitive.

Galasko[43] treated 54 patients with spinal instability secondary to spinal metastases. He prefers the use of a posterior implant that can be fixed to the spine at multiple levels either by screws or sublaminal wires (Fig. 12). Several methods of spinal stabilization are available. The implant must be fixed to at least two, but preferably three, vertebrae above the unstable segment and to two vertebrae below it. (Preoperative radiographs and skeletal scintigrams are important.) If there are two areas of instability the stabilizer should support both areas. When posterior stabilization is unlikely to provide sufficient support (for example, instability at the fifth lumbar level) or when decompression has to be performed anteriorly, an anterior or combined anterior and posterior approach should be used, followed by stabilization. If the stabilization extends to the sacrum, a lumbar lordosis must be moulded into the implant to prevent a postoperative flat back, which will interfere with sitting.

Spinal instability can occur in the cervical spine as well as the dorsal or lumbar spine. Anterior and/or posterior spinal stabilization may be required for the cervical spine.[43],[44] Minor degrees of cervical instability can usually be controlled by a surgical collar.

The alternative method of spinal decompression and stabilization is by an anterior approach with excision of the affected vertebral body, decompression of the dural sheath from the front, and subsequent anterior stabilization of the spine by recently developed vertebral implants with or without bone grafting or cementation.[45] As with pathological fractures of the long bones, postoperative irradiation

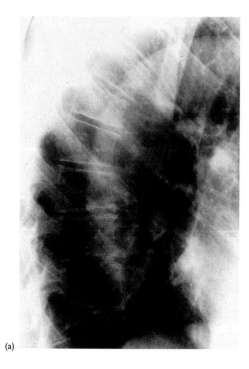

(a)

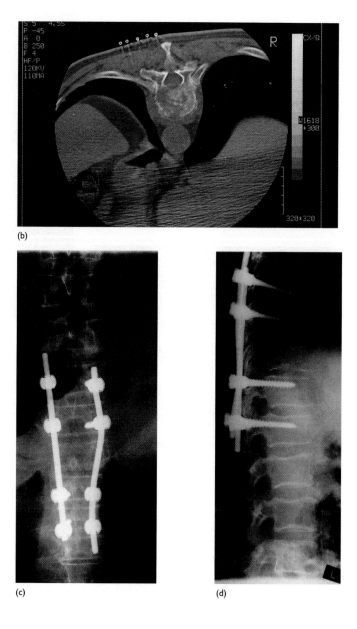

(b)

(c)

(d)

Fig. 12 This 73-year-old man had back pain for some months and was admitted because of increasing neurological deficit. His medical history showed no primary tumour. Plain radiographs at that time showed a lytic lesion of the eleventh thoracic vertebra with a pathological fracture (a). The extension of the lesion from the vertebral body towards the spinal cord causing compression of the spinal cord is shown on CT scan (b). A CT-guided needle biopsy of T11 brought the diagnosis of a leiomyosarcoma. The indication for spinal decompression was stated by the severe neurological symptoms. A posterior decompression was performed and the spine was stabilized by a transpedicular screw fixation (CCD system) and a posterolateral spondylodesis (c,d). A few months later he developed multiple vertebral metastases and died.

may be an essential part of the treatment of spinal metastases. Preoperative irradiation should be avoided as it may be associated with delayed wound healing, wound breakdown, and infection.

Summary

The development of an impending fracture, pathological fracture, or spinal metastases is not necessarily a terminal event. Since the lifespan of these patients has been extended, reduction of the consequences of pathological fractures will improve the quality of life of these patients. Stabilization of pathological fractures is the treatment of choice and will result in pain relief, restoration of function, early mobilization, and a shorter stay in hospital.

Internal stabilization is recommended. The type of stabilization depends on the site and extension of the lesion and the amount of bone loss. Fractures of the femoral neck usually require replacement hip arthroplasty. Metastases in long bones are preferably treated by intramedullary nailing. The supplementary use of methylmethacrylate is advocated if the stabilization is inadequate. It is important that radiographs, scintigrams, and MRI visualize the whole affected bone to minimize postoperative complications caused by fractures at the end of the implant. Postoperative radiotherapy is an essential part of treatment, as is chemotherapy and hormonal therapy, in sensitive carcinomas. Indications for treatment are limited by the life expectancy and the general condition of the patient. Spinal decompression and stabilization in metastatic disease become increasingly important. Better imaging techniques (MRI) and improved reconstruction devices will provide the indication for surgery of the spine in patients with metastases, especially in those with a neurological deficit.

References

1. Visser O, Coebergh JWW, Schouten LJ, van Dijck JAAM. Sixth Report of The Netherlands Cancer Registry. *Incidence of cancer in the Netherlands 1994.* Utrecht: Vereniging van Integrale Kankercentra 1997. ISBN 90–72175–17–4.

2. Galasko C. Pathological fracture. In *Oxford textbook of oncology* (1st edn) (ed. M Peckham, H Pinedo, U Veronesi). Oxford: OUP, 1995; 19.7: 2286–95.

3. Katoh M, Unakami M, Hara M, Fukuchi S. Bone metastasis from colorectal cancer in autopsy cases. *Journal of Gastroenterology*, 1995; **30**: 615–18.

4. Johnston AD. Pathology of metastatic tumors in bone. *Clinical Orthopaedics*, 1970; **73**: 8–12.

5. Springfield DS. Mechanism of metastasis. *Clinical Orthopaedics*, 1982; **169**: 15–19.

6. Clohishy D, Palkert D, Ramnaraine M, Pekurovsky I, Oursler M. Human breast cancer induces osteoclast activation and increases the number of osteoclasts at sites of tumor osteolysis. *Journal of Orthopaedic Research*, 1996; **14**: 396–402.

7. Paebody T. Evaluation and management of carcinoma metastatic to bone. *Current Opinion in Orthopaedics*, 1996; 7, VI: 75–9.

8. Yazawa Y, *et al.* Metastatic bone disease: a study of surgical treatment of 166 pathological humeral and femoral fractures. *Clinical Orthopaedics*, 1990; **251**: 213–19.

9. Bunting R., Lamont-Havers W, Schweon D, Kliman A. Pathological fracture risk in rehabilitation of patients with bon metastases. *Clinical Orthopaedics and Related Research*, 1985; **192**: 222–7.

10. Front D, Schenck SO, Frankel A, Robinson E. Bone metastases and bone pain in breast cancer. Are they closely associated ? *Journal of the American Medical Association*, 242: 1747–8.

11. Edelstyn GA, Gillespie PJ, Grebbel FS. The radiological demonstration of osseous metastases. Experimental obeservations. *Clinical Radiology*, 1967; **18**: 158–62.

12. Levine A. Pathological fractures. In *Skeletal trauma: fractures, dislocations, and ligamentous injuries* (ed. B Browne, J Jupiter). Philadelphia: Saunders, 1992: 401–41.

13. Algra P, Bloem J. Magnetic resonance imaging in metastatic disease and multiple myeloma. In *MRI and CT of the musculoskeletal system* (ed. JL Bloem, DJ Sartorius). Baltimore, MD: Williams and Wilkins, 1992; 218–35.

14. Fidler M. Incidence of fracture through metastases in long bones. *Acta Orthopaedica Scandinavica*, 1981; **52**: 623–7.

15. Harrington K. Impending pathologic fractures from metastatic malignancy; evaluation and management. In *American Association of Orthopaedic Surgeons. Instructional Course Lectures.* American Academy of Orthopaedic Surgeons, 1986; **35**: 357–81.

16. Dijkstra PDS, Wiggers T, Geel AN van, Boxma H. Treatment of impending and actual pathological fractures in patients with bone metastases of the long bones. *European Journal of Surgery*, 1994; **160**: 535–42.

17. Fidler M. Prophylactic internal fixation of secondary neoplastic deposits in long bones. *British Medical Journal*, 1973; **1**: 341–3.

18. Dijkstra P, Zwaag van der H, Mulder P, Snijder C, Oudkerk M, Wiggers T. Comparison of torsional strength reduction of cortical defects in femora estimated by surgeons using radiographs and computed tomography and measured by *in vitro* experiments. Erasmus University Rotterdam, Thesis, 1997.

19. Mirels H. Metastatc disease in long bones: a proposed scoring system

20. for diagnosing impending pathologic fractures *Clinical Orthopaedics*, 1989; **14**: 513–25.

20. Porter AT, Reddy SM. Strontium 89 in the treatment of metastatic prostate cancer. *Advances in Oncology*, 1995; **18**: 19–22.

21. Tong D, Gillick L, Hendrickson FR. The palliation of symptomatic osseous metastases: final results of the study by the Radiation Therapy Oncology Group. *Cancer*, 1982; **50**: 893–9.

22. Bauer H, Wedin R. Survival after surgery for spinal and extremity metastases: prognostification in 214 patients. *Acta Orthopaedica Scandinavica*, 1995; **66**: 143–6.

23. Roscoe M, McBroom R, St Louis E, Grossman H, Perrin R. Preoperative embolization in the treatment of osseous metastases from renal cell carcinoma. *Clinical Orthopaedics and Related Research*, 1989; **238**: 302–7.

24. Menck H, Schulze S, Larsen E. Metastasis size in pathological femoral fractures. *Acta Orthopaedica Scandinavica*, 1988; **59**: 151–4.

25. Aaron AD. Treatment of metastatic adenocarcinoma of the pelvis and the extremities. *Journal of Bone and Joint Surgery*, 1997; **79A**: 917–32.

26. Allan D, Bell R, Davis A, Langer F. Complex acetabular reconstruction for metastatic tumor. *Journal of Arthoplasty*, 1995; **10**: 301–6.

27. Sim FH. Orthopaedic management using new devices and prosthesis. *Clinical Orthopaedics*, 1995; **312**: 160–72.

28. Lane JM, Sculo TP, Zolan S. Treatment of pathological fractures of the hip by endoprosthetic replacement. *Journal of Bone and Joint Surgery*, 1980; **64A**: 954–9.

29. Harrington KD. *Orthopaedic management of metastatic bone disease.* St Louis, MO: Mosby, 1988: 92.

30. Abouliafa A, Buch R, Matthews J, Li W, Malawar M. Reconstruction using the saddle prosthesis following excision of primary and metastatic acetabular tumors. *Clinical Orthopaedics and Related Research*, 1995; **314**: 203–13.

31. Rompe J, Eysel P, Hopf C, Heine J. Metastatic instability at the proximal end of the femur: Comparison of endoprosthetic replacement and plate osteosynthesis. *Archives of Orthopaedic and Trauma Surgery*, 1994; **113**: 260–4.

32. Zickel R, Mouradian W. Intramedullary fixation of pathologic fractures and lesions of the subtrochanteric region of the femur. *Journal of Bone and Joint Surgery*, 1976; **58A**: 1061–6.

33. Karachalios T, Atkins RM, Sarangi PP, Crichlow TPKR, Solomon L. Reconstruction nailing for pathological subtrochanteric fractures with coexisting femoral shaft metastasis. *Journal of Bone and Joint Surgery*, 1993; **75B**: 119–22.

34. Behr JT, Dobozi WR, Badrinath K. The treatment of pathological and impending pathological fractures of the proximal femur in the elderly. *Clinical Orthopaedics*, 1985; **198**: 173–8.

35. Weikert DR, Schwartz HS. Intramedullary nailing for impending pathological subtrochanteric fractures. *Journal of Bone and Joint Surgery*, 1991; **73B**: 668–70.

36. McCormack R, Glass D, Lane J. Functional cast bracing of metastatic humeral shaft lesion. *Orthopaedic Transactions*, 1985; **9**: 50–1.

37. Fleming JE. Pathological fractures of the humerus. *Clinical Orthopaedics*, 1996; **203**: 258–60.

38. Dijkstra P, Stapert J, Boxma H, Wiggers T. Treatment of pathological fractures of the humeral shaft. *European Journal of Surgery*, 1996; **22**: 621–6.

39. Redmond B, Biermann J, Blaser R. Interlocking intra medullary nailing of pathological fractures of the shaft of the humerus. *Journal of Bone and Joint Surgery*, 1996; **78A**: 891–6.

40. Vandeweyer E, Gebhart M. Treatment of humeral pathological fractures by internal fixation and methylmethacrylate injection. *European Journal of Surgical Oncology*, 1997; **23**: 238–42.

41. Leeson MC, Makley JT, Carter JR. Metastatic skeletal disease: distal to

the elbow and knee. *Clinical Orthopaedics and Related Research*, 1986; **206**: 94–9.

42. **Fidler M.** Pathological fractures of the spine including those causing anterior spinal cord compression. In *Recent developments in orthopaedic surgery* (ed. J Noble, CSB Galasko). Manchester: Manchester University Press, 1987: 94–103.

43. **Galasko C.** Spinal instability secondary to metastatic cancer. *Journal of Bone and Joint Surgery*, 1991; **73B**: 104–8.

44. **De Wald R, Bridwell K, Prodromas C, Rodts M.** Reconstructive spinal surgery as palliation for metastatic malignancies of the spine. *Spine*, 1985; **10**: 21–6.

45. **Hosono N, Yonenobu K, Fuyi T, Ebara S, Yamashita K, Ono K.** Vertebral body replacement with ceramic prosthesis for metastatic spinal tumors. *Spine*, 1994; **20**: 2454–62.

5.7 Therapeutic aspects of nutrition in cancer patients

Clare Shaw

Nutritional problems are common in cancer patients before, during, and after treatment. Nutritional intake may be reduced due to the physiological effects of the tumour and the nutritional requirements may be increased due to the presence of malignant disease. Side-effects of treatment, such as anorexia, mucositis, nausea, vomiting, and diarrhoea, may further impair nutritional intake.

Eating and drinking is part of life; food not only sustains life but also has cultural, emotional, and social meaning in all societies. Therefore, symptoms that affect this essential part of day-to-day living can be very socially isolating and the impact of a reduced food intake upon both the individual and concerned carers cannot be underestimated.

Cancer cachexia

Some patients may develop the syndrome of cancer cachexia, the features of which are: weight loss, muscle weakness, lethargy, anorexia, early satiety, changes in taste, anaemia, and altered host metabolism. The risk of developing cancer cachexia is higher in particular diagnoses, for example lung cancer and gastrointestinal and pancreatic cancer with up to 85 per cent of patients experiencing unintentional weight loss at the time of diagnosis.[1] More advanced malignant disease also predisposes patients to developing cachexia.

The development of cancer cachexia is multifactorial and may be due to a combination of reduced food intake and increased energy expenditure.[2] Changes in digestion and absorption of food may also influence the rate of weight loss and the development of other nutritional deficiencies (Table 1).

Reduced nutrient intake

Reduced food intake may arise due to tumour-induced anorexia, the mechanism of which is not completely understood although several theories have been proposed. It is thought that alterations in circulating plasma nutrients, such as the amino acid tryptophan, and their effect on neurotransmitters such as serotonin may have a role to play in anorexia. This may be in addition to the potential anorexic effect of increased circulating cytokines which has been detected in cancer patients.[3] Food intake may also be reduced due to physical problems created by the presence of the tumour, for example swallowing problems in oesophageal cancer or cancer of the head and neck or the development of ascites in gynaecological cancer.

Alterations in metabolism

Increased energy expenditure due to altered metabolism may occur in some cancer patients. Some studies have suggested that 50 to 60 per cent of cancer patients in hospital have abnormal resting energy expenditure although not all studies support this finding.[4] Metabolic pathways which may contribute to increased energy expenditure include increased glucose turnover, increased Cori cycle activity, increased protein turnover, and mobilization of body fat.[5] Cancer patients often display an acute phase protein response. This is an alteration in the balance of protein production. It is characterized by a reduction in albumin production and an increase in serum C-reactive protein levels. During normal conditions of reduced food intake the body adapts to starvation to preserve body stores and reduce energy expenditure. This adaptation appears to be absent in weight-losing cancer patients who continue to lose protein and fat stores from the body (Fig. 1).

The role of cytokines in cancer cachexia

Cytokines, polypeptides produced by cells of the immune system in response to malignant disease, may be mediators of cachexia. Cytokines which have been implicated in the development of cachexia include tumour necrosis factor, interleukin-1 and -6; elevated levels have been detected in cancer patients.[5] The protein leptin, produced by adipocytes which helps regulate food intake and body weight, may be modulated by cytokines.[6] Eicosapentaenoic acid, a n-3 polyunsaturated fatty acid present in fish oils, may be effective at reducing the enhanced proinflammatory cytokine release, thereby reducing the magnitude of cachexia.[7] Studies on other types of medication to control cachexia, such as hydrazine sulphate, have failed to show that these can be used successfully in the clinical setting.

Side-effects of treatment and effect on nutritional status

All types of treatment used for cancer, whether curative or palliative, may potentially affect nutritional status. The magnitude of the impact of treatment on nutritional intake will vary and depends on the nature and extent of surgery, the side-effects of chemotherapy and radiotherapy, and effective symptom control. Multimodality treatment which may result in patients undergoing treatment for long periods of time may further increase the risk of reduced food intake. Some patients are at particularly high risk of developing nutritional problems due to the site of their disease and the treatment undertaken (Table 2).

Table 1 Causes of cancer cachexia

Causes of cachexia	Examples
Reduced food intake	Presence of malignant disease inducing anorexia
	Side-effects of treatment, e.g. mucositis, nausea, vomiting, taste changes
	Social and psychological factors, e.g. anxiety, depression
Reduced digestion or absorption of nutrients	Surgery to gastrointestinal tract or pancreas leading to short bowel syndrome or pancreatic insufficiency
	Chemotherapy-induced gut toxicity
	Early or late radiation enteritis
	Subacute or total bowel obstruction caused by disease or treatment
Physiological alterations in metabolism	Increased whole body protein turnover, synthesis, and catabolism
	Reduced synthesis of albumin and skeletal muscle protein
	High glucose turnover with increased Cori cycle activity
	Increased breakdown of fat stores
	Increased energy expenditure

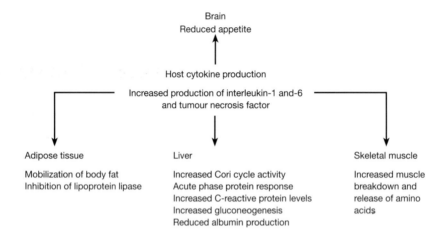

Fig. 1 Alterations in metabolism.

Surgery

After trauma or surgery, hormonal changes cause a prolonged increase in metabolic rate which can lead to a rapid depletion of body tissues.[8] Repeated surgical procedures with the associated periods of reduced oral intake and hypermetabolism may lead to weight loss and extensive depletion of body stores. Surgical resection of head and neck cancer and gastrointestinal cancer probably have the greatest impact on nutritional intake (Table 3). Resection of the mandible, tongue, maxilla, or pharynx may lead to difficulties with chewing or swallowing. There may be an increased risk of aspiration due to poor oral control of food and fluids or because of an alteration in the anatomy or cranial nerves required for swallowing. Resection of the gastrointestinal tract may produce long-term nutritional problems depending on the site and extent of surgery. Some patients may undergo gastrointestinal surgery for strictures and adhesions caused by treatment such as radiotherapy.

Radiotherapy

Radiotherapy affects nutritional intake primarily by the side-effects on the oral cavity and gastrointestinal tract. Side-effects may be both early, whilst treatment is taking place, or late, developing months or years after treatment. The generalized effects of treatment such as tiredness and somnolence may further contribute to a reduced desire to eat (Table 4). Good symptom control is essential to minimize the impact on the intake of food and fluids.

Chemotherapy

Reduced food intake is common with many chemotherapeutic agents due to their effect on the gastrointestinal tract (Table 5). Common side-effects that influence intake include nausea and vomiting, taste changes, learned food aversions, mucositis, tiredness, and lethargy. Chemotherapy may induce periods of neutropenic sepsis which increase patients nutritional and fluid requirements. The impact of

Table 2 Site of disease with a high risk of developing a poor nutritional status

Site of disease	Nutritional problems arising due to disease or treatment
Gastrointestinal cancer	Dysphagia Anorexia Early satiety Nausea and vomiting Dumping syndrome Chronic malabsorption and steatorrhoea Reduced bile salt reabsorption Anaemia caused by reduced or absent vitamin B_{12} absorption Short bowel syndrome
Head and neck cancer	Dysphagia Increased risk of aspiration Mucositis and stomatitis Xerostomia Nausea and vomiting Taste changes and mouth blindness
Leukaemia and lymphoma	Severe mucositis, nausea, and vomiting Risk of sepsis Graft-versus-host disease on allogenic bone marrow transplantation may lead to severe diarrhoea, loss of blood, mucus, and tissue via gastrointestinal tract Anorexia, xerostomia, taste changes Altered liver function
Gynaecological cancer	Early satiety due to presence of tumour Subacute or total bowel obstruction Severe nausea and vomiting Radiation enteritis—early or late Short bowel syndrome
Cancer in children	Mechanical gastrointestinal problems, e.g. neuroblastoma Nausea, vomiting, mucositis, diarrhoea from prolonged aggressive multimodality treatments, particularly in Ewing's sarcoma, Wilms' tumour, head and neck tumours, and advanced lymphomas

chemotherapy on nutritional status will depend on the intensity and duration of chemotherapy and the effective control of side-effects of therapy such as emesis and mucositis. Biological therapies such as interleukin and interferon often produce anorexia.

Identification of malnourished patients

Up to 85 per cent of cancer patients may be malnourished and early identification of patients at risk of malnutrition is essential to enable appropriate support to be initiated as early as possible in the course of treatment. The identification of malnourished patients is often overlooked and studies show that it is not uncommon for malnourished patients to have no nutritional information recorded in their medical notes.[9] In the context of cancer patients, malnutrition often refers to unintentional weight loss with nutrient deficiency which may impair organ function and may occur in patients who are obese or of normal body weight. A simple screening tool may include questions about the normal weight, unintentional weight loss, and impaired appetite supported by the objective measurements of weight and height.[10] Some patients may be oedematous and this should be taken into account in the initial assessment. The following assessment should be carried out on all patients and recorded in the medical or nursing record:

- What is your normal weight?
- What is your current weight?
- What is your height?
- Do you have any difficulties with appetite or food intake?

Patients who have an unintentional weight loss of more than 10 per cent, irrespective of their initial weight or who are experiencing difficulties with eating should be referred to the dietitian for appropriate advice on nutritional intake. Additional measurements of body composition by anthropometry or bioelectrical impedance are inappropriate to use in an initial screening tool and may be used for monitoring patients or in research.

Consequences of malnutrition

Malnutrition may have a profound effect on the physiology and function of the patient. Weight loss, along with the associated loss of lean body mass, can affect muscle strength, both of skeletal and respiratory muscles, and adversely affect organ function. It may impair wound healing, cause an increased susceptibility to infection, and is associated with a poor quality of life. Malnourished patients have a higher morbidity and mortality associated with treatment. In chemotherapy patients weight loss is associated with delays in treatment due to the poor recovery of the immune system and in radiotherapy it is associated with poor tolerance to treatment with an increase in the number of breaks given during the course of radiotherapy.[11]

Rationale and benefits of nutritional support

The aim of nutritional support is to increase the tolerance to treatment and enable the patient to have the optimal chance of completing the proposed course of treatment. Patients referred for nutritional support have been shown to maintain or improve their nutritional status whilst patients not receiving nutritional support show a decline in their nutritional status.[9] Whilst nutritional support may be able to maintain or improve body weight, body fat, and lean body mass, the effect may not be as great as in those who do not have underlying malignant disease.[11]

Perioperative nutritional support may reduce both morbidity and mortality.[12] In malnourished patients both enteral and parenteral nutritional support has been shown to reduce the incidence of major and septic complications in surgical patients, reduced hospital stay, and improvement quality of life indices.[13] Studies that have failed to show the benefit of perioperative nutritional support have often not distinguished between patients with a good nutritional status and

Table 3 Impact of surgery to head, neck, and gastrointestinal tract on nutritional status

Site of surgery	Impact on nutritional status
Oral cavity, tongue, maxilla, or pharynx	Dysphagia Problems with mastication Aspiration of fluids or food
Oesophagus	Dysphagia due to stricture at anastomosis Reduced gastric motility due to vagotomy Intestinal hurry leading to malabsorption and diarrhoea Dumping syndrome (early or late)
Stomach	Early satiety Dumping syndrome (early or late) Intestinal hurry leading to malabsorption and diarrhoea Anaemia—vitamin B_{12} deficiency due to lack of intrinsic factor
Small intestine	General malabsorption Diarrhoea Risk of obstruction and slow transit time if strictures develop
Terminal ileum	Short bowel syndrome Fat malabsorption Decreased absorption of bile salts Anaemia—vitamin B_{12} deficiency
Colon	Diarrhoea Malabsorption of water and electrolytes (particularly if ileocaecal valve removed)

Table 4 Impact of radiotherapy on nutritional status

Site of radiotherapy	Side-effects which affect nutritional intake
Head and neck	Mucositis (inflammation of the mucosa) Stomatitis Dysphagia Xerostomia (dry mouth) Increased viscosity of saliva Anorexia Poor dentition due to dental extractions pretreatment Dental caries Taste changes and mouth blindness Loss of smell Trismus Stenosis Poor wound healing Oesteoradionecrosis Fistula
Oesophagus	Anorexia Mucositis Dysphagia Fibrosis leading to dysphagia
Stomach	Anorexia Nausea and vomiting
Abdomen and pelvis	Anorexia Nausea and vomiting Diarrhoea Early and chronic radiation enteritis Short bowel syndrome Radiation damage leading to strictures and subacute or total bowel obstruction

Table 5 Side-effects of some chemotherapeutic agents which may affect nutritional status

Agent	Side-effects
Methotrexate	Nausea—dose dependent
	Vomiting
	Severe mucositis
Cisplatin	Anorexia
	Severe prolonged nausea
	Nausea and vomiting
	Taste changes (particularly a metallic taste)
	Diarrhoea (high doses)
Doxorubicin	Nausea
	Some vomiting
	Mucositis throughout gastrointestinal tract
Fluorouracil	Diarrhoea
	Occasional nausea
Vincristine	Paralytic ileus

those who are malnourished. For preoperative nutritional support to be effective in influencing clinical outcome it should be given to malnourished patients for 7 to 15 days before surgery.[14] Preoperative enteral nutrition is as effective as parenteral nutrition and should always be the method of choice when there is a functioning gastrointestinal tract. Postoperative parenteral nutrition, enteral nutrition, or adequate oral nutrition is equally effective in reducing nutrition-related postoperative complications.

Studies of the nutritional support of patients undergoing treatment have provided varying results. Some studies, but not all, have shown the benefits of nutritional support with respect to chemotherapy or radiotherapy toxicity in patients.[11] The benefits included a decrease in medications given for symptom control, a reduction in the duration of chemotherapy-induced nausea and vomiting, better tolerance of chemotherapy, and fewer treatment delays. This may have an impact in terms of control of disease as it is recognized that delays in treatment may contribute to a poorer outcome for the patient. Intensive nutritional support may also help patients maintain quality of life during treatment.[15]

Nutritional management of cancer patients

Most cancer patients will require some form of nutritional support during the course of their disease and treatment. A dietitian should assess the patient's nutritional intake and advise on the most appropriate method of nutritional support to meet the patient's nutritional requirement (Table 6). Basal energy requirements may be calculated using the Schofield equation and should be reviewed on a regular basis depending on the patient's clinical condition.[16] Nitrogen requirements are dependent on the patient's clinical condition and nutritional status. They may range from 0.14 to 0.4 g/kg per day.[17] Nutritional management of patients should aim to meet vitamin and

mineral requirements although these too may be altered in patients with cancer.[18] When planning nutritional support the gastrointestinal tract should always be used when possible as this provides the safest route to feed the patient.

Oral intake

Patients require practical ideas to enable them to improve their nutritional intake and overcome eating difficulties. Oral intake may be improved with control of symptoms such as nausea, vomiting, pain, constipation and mucositis.

Anorexia

Anorexia is a common feature of cancer cachexia and may occur in up to 80 per cent of patients. Dietary advice is aimed at increasing energy intake to prevent weight loss and to help the patient enjoy eating and drinking. Patients with severe anorexia may require an appetite stimulant such as medroxyprogesterone acetate, megestrol acetate, or dexamethasone.[19]–[21]

Dietary management of anorexia

- encourage small portions at mealtimes and snacks between meals;
- increase frequency of eating;
- encourage foods which are enjoyed;
- make use of the best meal of the day, e.g. this may be breakfast;
- encourage high energy foods such as those high in fat and sugar;
- fortify food to increase energy intake, e.g. use full cream milk, use extra butter, cheese, and cream;
- use alcohol as an appetite stimulant.

Dysphagia

Problems with swallowing may arise due to disease or treatment. Nutritional management of dysphagic patients is essential to avoid weight loss and malnutrition. Whatever the cause, the consequent effect on the ability to eat and drink often requires a change in the consistency of food to a soft or liquidized diet. For some who are unable to take sufficient or who are at risk of aspiration the safest option may be to rely solely on an enteral tube feed. All patients with dysphagia require an assessment by a speech and language therapist[22] to determine whether the patient is safe to continue with food and fluids orally or whether there is a risk of aspiration.

Nutritional management of dysphagia

- small frequent meals;
- modify consistency of food so all food is soft—food may need to be pureed or liquidized;
- fortify food to increase energy intake;
- may require additional nutritional supplements;
- may need to use commercial thickening agent for thin liquids if there is a risk of aspiration—needs assessment from speech and language therapist;
- may require enteral tube feeding e.g. nasogastric or percutaneous endoscopically-guided gastrostomy (PEG).

Mucositis

Mucositis may severely impair nutritional intake and may necessitate enteral tube feeding if prolonged, for example during and after

Table 6 Methods of nutritional support

Route	Indications	Facilitation of nutritional intake
Oral	Functional gastrointestinal tract Patient is able to take food and fluids orally without aspiration	Alter consistency of food or drink Alter timings of meals and snacks Fortify food and drinks with protein and energy Choose the flavour of food to suit individual taste Use sip feeds and dietary supplements Adequate symptom control e.g. of nausea, mucositis
Enteral tube feeding	Functional gastrointestinal tract Patient is unable to take sufficient food and fluids orally e.g. due to dysphagia or anorexia Patient is required to be nil by mouth e.g. after oral surgery or upper gastrointestinal surgery	Nasogastric or nasojejunal tube Gastrostomy tube Jejunostomy tube
Parenteral nutrition	Non-functioning gastrointestinal tract e.g. total bowel obstruction gastrointestinal failure due to chemotherapy small bowel of less than 1.0 m intractable vomiting	Central line Peripheral line

radiotherapy to the head and neck. Good symptom management can promote an improved intake of food and fluids.

Nutritional management of mucositis

- modify consistency of food so all food is soft;
- avoid rough, coarse, or dry food;
- avoid acidic, salty, or highly spiced food;
- avoid alcohol;
- avoid hot food—foods which are cold or at room temperature may be better tolerated;
- may require additional nutritional supplements;
- take food after taking analgesia.

Early satiety

The aetiology of early satiety in cancer patients is unclear. It may be due to tumour presence near the gastrointestinal tract, a side-effect of cytokine production, atrophic changes in the mucosa and muscles of the gastrointestinal tract, or a reduction in the secretion or activity of gastrointestinal enzymes.[23] It is often overlooked in patient assessment and may be mistaken for loss of appetite.

Nutritional management of early satiety

- small, frequent meals;
- avoid high fat foods which delay gastric emptying;
- avoid drinking large quantities whilst eating;
- use prokinetics to encourage gastric emptying, e.g. metoclopramide.

Nausea and vomiting

Severe vomiting must be controlled with antiemetic drugs. Nausea may be reduced by dietary intervention but an antiemetic should be considered.

Nutritional management of nausea

- choose cold food and drink in preference to hot as these have less odour;
- sip fizzy drinks;
- drink through a straw;
- try ginger flavours, e.g. ginger ale, ginger biscuits;
- eat small, frequent snacks to avoid the stomach being completely empty or too full.

Constipation

The cause of constipation must be considered in the management of this condition. Often a high fibre diet is recommended for constipation but this is only appropriate for patients who do not have tumour pressing on the bowel, for example cancer of the ovary or colon, and have an appetite sufficient to be able to consume a bulky high fibre (non-starch polysaccharide) diet. Many anorexic patients are unable to consume sufficient wholemeal cereals, fruit, and vegetables. A good fluid intake, of approximately 2 litres daily, should be encouraged. Laxatives are often needed to manage constipation. When subacute obstruction is suspected a low fibre diet may be appropriate in symptom relief.

Diarrhoea

Adequate fluid balance is essential and when diarrhoea is severe it is important to replace fluid losses. Oral rehydration solutions may be helpful as these generally provide 50 to 60 mmol/l of sodium and 20 to 25 mmol/l of potassium. Management of diarrhoea will depend on the cause and these should be investigated fully to determine the contribution of antibiotics, bacterial infection, hypoalbuminaemia, chemotherapy, drugs (e.g. magnesium salts), overuse of laxatives, or pelvic or abdominal radiotherapy. Some patients may benefit from a reduction in dietary fibre (non-starch polysaccharides) intake during an acute episode although this has not been shown to be effective in controlling diarrhoea induced by radiotherapy.

Bowel obstruction

Bowel obstruction may be total or subacute. In cases of complete bowel obstruction the clinical condition of the patient must be considered. If the patient is receiving aggressive treatment such as surgery then parenteral nutrition should be provided to support the patient. When the patient's prognosis is poor and no treatment is possible then it may be inappropriate to commence parenteral nutrition. Opinion on the use of such nutritional support in bowel obstruction varies between European countries with some being more likely to instigate parenteral nutrition.[24] In subacute obstruction some patients may benefit from a diet that is low in fibre (non-starch polysaccharides) although there is little research evidence to support their use. If weight loss occurs then high energy drinks and nutritional supplements may help promote energy intake.

Short bowel syndrome

A side-effect of pelvic or abdominal radiotherapy may be radiation enteritis resulting in short bowel syndrome. It may also arise after surgery to the small intestine, particularly after the formation of an ileostomy. Patient with a small intestine of less than 1 to 1.5 m may require long-term parenteral nutrition. Dietary manipulation may alleviate some of the symptoms such as thirst, dehydration, and high stoma losses or large volumes of diarrhoea.[25] Drugs are required to increase transit time and reduce gastrointestinal losses. These include codeine phosphate, loperamide, cimetidine, ranitidine, and octreotide.

Nutritional management of short bowel syndrome

* restrict fluids to 500 ml daily increasing to 1500 ml;
* avoid drinks for 45 min before and after meals;
* sprinkle salt liberally on food (patients with an ileostomy);
* if gut losses are 1000 ml or more, part or all of fluid intake should consist of WHO oral rehydration solution (sodium content 90 mmol/l);
* multivitamin and mineral supplement;
* oral magnesium supplements;
* consider restricting nutrients that increase gastrointestinal output e.g. fat in patients with an intact colon;
* vitamin B_{12} injections when terminal ileum is absent.

Neutropenia

Food restrictions may be used in patients who are neutropenic to reduce the incidence of food-borne infection. Patients should be advised on food hygiene and avoiding foods that carry a risk of transmitting the pathogenic organisms salmonella and *Listeria monocytogenes*, such as raw eggs, cheese from unpasteurized milk, and liver pate. Low microbial diets may be used for patients undergoing high-dose chemotherapy in the hospital setting although there is no consensus between different centres as to which foods should be restricted.[26],[27]

Weight gain

Breast cancer patients may gain weight during treatment. This is often as a result of a change in lifestyle, a relaxation of normal eating habits, and the influence of drugs such as medroxyprogesterone acetate, megestrol acetate, or tamoxifen.[28] Patients receiving high-dose steriods, for example neuro-oncology patients, may also gain weight, have an increased appetite, and are at increased risk of developing steroid-induced diabetes mellitus which may require a reduced sugar diet. Patients who have gained weight may require specific advice on weight reduction, although it is prudent to wait until treatment has finished before starting to reduce dietary intake.

Enteral tube feeding

If patients are unable to swallow enough nourishment to maintain their weight, an enteral tube feed should be considered. The choice of tube will depend on:

* The anticipated length of time the feed will be required as a nasogastric tube may be appropriate for periods of less than 4 weeks whilst a gastrostomy tube is appropriate for longer periods of feeding.
* Placement of the tube may be influenced by the patient's physical condition, e.g. it may not be possible to pass a nasogastric tube in complete oesophageal obstruction. A jejunostomy tube may be preferred following upper gastrointestinal surgery.
* The wishes of the patient concerning the physical appearance of the tube and the invasive nature of the tube placement.

Enteral tube feeding may be undertaken in the hospital or home setting. Many pre-prepared commercial brands of feeds are available and the majority of cancer patients will require complete, whole-protein feeds which provide 4 to 6 kJ/ml (1.0–1.5 kcal/ml). Elemental, peptide, or low fat feeds may be necessary in patients with severe malabsorption. Feed may be delivered via a continuos pump, intermittent feeds, or by bolus. The regimen chosen for the patient must reflect their gastrointestinal tolerance, mobility, treatment regimens, ability to administer feeds, and lifestyle. For patients being discharged home with an enteral tube feed, good communication between acute and community teams helps to ensure continuity and a high standard of care for such patients.

Parenteral nutrition

Parenteral nutrition should only be used when it is not possible to feed patients via the enteral route. Its use carries the risk of life-threatening complications, such as sepsis and metabolic disorders, and therefore must be administered and monitored correctly.

It may be considered for the following patients:[29]

* when all methods and routes of enteral nutrition have been considered but are not deemed appropriate, e.g. bowel obstruction, uncontrollable diarrhoea;
* when the gastrointestinal tract is inaccessible and it is not possible to insert an enteral feeding tube, e.g. due to the presence of tumour;
* when complete rest of the gastrointestinal tract is required, e.g. enterocutaneous fistula.

The use of parenteral nutrition should be considered carefully. It may inappropriate to use parenteral nutrition in cases where the patient's prognosis is poor and no treatment is possible.[30]

Therapeutic diets

Some patients may be following previously prescribed therapeutic diets at the start of anticancer treatment, such as low fat diet for hypercholesterolaemia or a strict weight reducing diabetic diet in the overweight non-insulin dependent diabetic. These may be unnecessarily restrictive and further limit dietary intake. Their use should be considered in the context of diagnosis, treatment, and prognosis and often it is appropriate to review and relax such therapeutic diets.

Alternative and complementary diets

Alternative and complementary diets are often modified diets that claim to cure or treat cancer. There are a number of similarities between these diets as they are often mainly vegetarian or vegan, rely primarily on organic foods, and avoid manufactured or processed foods. The diets are often low in salt, sugar, and fat and high in wholegrains, fruit, and vegetables and may include fruit and vegetable juice. Often high-dose vitamin and minerals are taken in addition to the diet, for example vitamin C, zinc, selenium, and β-carotene. Nutritional imbalances and inadequacies may occur in patients who have a poor appetite or a limited ability to prepare the necessary food.

These diets are often followed for the anticipated antitumour effect, although often they have not been tested or demonstrated to be effective in scientifically acceptable clinical trials. To date, studies appear to show no difference in survival rates between patients following complementary therapies and those receiving conventional treatment alone. Some patients may report psychological benefits of such diets whilst others may find that they are difficult to follow.[31] Some patients who are keen to try certain aspects of complementary therapies may compromise and adapt the regimen to suit themselves.

Palliative care

Patients undergoing palliative care are likely to experience difficulties with their intake of food and fluids. Management of nutritional problems should be a high priority in symptom control for those patients who are concerned about their intake. Many of the dietary strategies that are mentioned in this chapter continue to be relevant to palliative care patients. Loss of appetite and food intake can be a source of anxiety and conflict for patient and carers. The amount of food and fluid taken is often used as an indication of the patient's overall condition.[32] Discussion of dietary intake and appetite needs to be approached in an open and sensitive manner to avoid it becoming an area of conflict. Often, aggressive conventional nutritional support is considered to be inappropriate but they may be quality of life benefits in paying attention to the promotion of oral nutrition with symptom control and dietary strategies.[33],[34]

References

1. Wigmore SJ, Plester CE, Richardson RA, Fearon KCH. Changes in nutritional status associated with unresectable pancreatic cancer. *British Journal of Cancer*, 1997; **75**: 106–9.

2. O'Gorman P, McMillan DC, McArdle CS. Impact of weight loss, appetite and the inflammatory response on quality of life in gastrointestinal cancer patients. *Nutrition and Cancer*, 1998; **32**: 76–80.

3. Wigmore SJ, Plester CE, Ross JA, Fearon KCH. Contribution of anorexia and hypermetabolism to weight loss in anicteric patients with pancreatic cancer. *British Journal of Surgery*, 1997; **84**: 196–7.

4. Macfie J, Burkinshaw L, Oxby C, Holmfield JHM, Hill GL. The effect of gastrointestinal malignancy on resting metabolic expenditure. *British Journal of Surgery*, 1982; **69**: 443–6.

5. Tisdale MJ. Isolation of a novel cancer cachectic factor. *Proceedings of the Nutrition Society*, 1997; **56**: 777–83.

6. Schwartz MW, Seeley RJ, Woods SC. Wasting illness as a disorder of body weight regulation. *Proceedings of the Nutrition Society*, 1997; **56**: 785–91.

7. Barber M, Ross JA, Feraron CH. The anti-cachetic effect of fatty acids. *Proceedings of the Nutrition Society*, 1998; **57**: 571–6.

8. Broom J. Sepsis and trauma. In: Garrow JS, James WPT, ed. *Human nutrition and dietetics*. 9th edn. Edinburgh: Churchill Livingstone, 1994: 456–64.

9. McWhirter JP, Pennington CR. The incidence and recognition of malnutrition in hospital *British Medical Journal*, 1994; **308**: 945–8.

10. Lennard-Jones JE, Arrowsmith H, Davison C, Denham AF, Micklewright A. Screening by nurses and junior doctors to detect malnutrition when patients are first assessed in hospital. *Clinical Nutrition*, 1995; **14**: 336–40.

11. Bozzetti F. Nutrition support in patients with cancer. In: Payne-James J, Grimble G, Silk D, ed. *Artificial nutrition support in clinical practice*. London: Edward Arnold, 1995: 511–33.

12. Heys SD, Park KGM, Garlick PJ, Eremin O. Nutrition and malignant disease: implications for surgical practice. *British Journal of Surgery*, 1992; **79**: 614–23.

13. Pennington C. Disease and malnutrition in British hospitals. *Proceedings of the Nutrition Society*, 1997; **56**: 393–407.

14. Campos ACL, Meguid MM. A critical appraisal of the usefulness of perioperative nutritional support. *American Journal of Clinical Nutrition*, 1992; **55**: 117–30.

15. Fietkau R, Iro H, Sailer D, Sauer R. Percutaneous endoscopically guided gastrostomy in patients with head and neck cancer. *Recent Results in Cancer Research*, 1991; **121**: 269–82.

16. Schofield WN, Schofield C, James WPT. Basal metabolic rate—review and prediction. *Human Nutrition: Clinical Nutrition*, 1985; **39c** (Supp. 1):5–96.

17. Elia M. Artificial nutritional support. *Medicine International*, 1990; **82**: 3392–6.

18. **Committee on Medical Aspects of Food Policy.** *Dietary reference values for food energy and nutrients in the United Kingdom*. Department of Health Report on Health and Social Subjects, Report No. **41**, 1991.

19. Tchekmedyian NS, Hickman M, Siau J, Greco FA, Keller J, Browder H, Aisner J. Megestrol acetate in cancer anorexia and weight loss. *Cancer*, 1992; **69**: 1268–74.

20. Rimmer T. Treating the anorexia of cancer. *European Journal of Palliative Care*, 1998; **5**: 179–81.

21. Fietkau R, Riepl M, Kettner H, Hink A, Sauer R. Supportive use of megestrol acetate in patients with head and neck cancer during radio(chemo)therapy. *European Journal of Cancer*, 1997; **33**: 75–9.

22. Appleton J, Machin J. *Working with oral cancer*. 2nd edn. Oxon: Winslow Press, 1998.

23. Armes PJ, Plant HJ, Allbright A, Silverstone T, Slevin M. A study to investigate the incidence of early satiety in patients with advanced cancer. *British Journal of Cancer*, 1992; **65**: 481–4.

24. Pironi L, Ruggeri E, Tanneberger S, Goirdani S, Pannuti F, Miglioli M. Home artificial nutrition in advanced cancer. *Journal of the Royal Society of Medicine* 1997; **90**: 592.

25. Lennard-Jones JE. Nutrition support in the short-bowel syndrome. In: Payne-James J, Grimble G, Silk D, ed. *Artificial nutrition support in clinical practice*. London: Edward Arnold, 1995: 545–54.

26. Henry L. Immunocompromised patients and nutrition. *Professional Nurse*, 1997; **12**: 655–9.

27. Henry L, Souchon V. Nutritional support. In: Barrett J, Treleaven J, ed. *The clinical practice of stem-cell transplantation*. Oxford: ISIS Medical Media, Vol. 2. 1998.

28. Bishop JF, Smith JG, Jeal PN, Murray R, Drummond RM, Pitt P,

Oliver IN, Showal AK. The effect of danzol on tumour control and weight loss in patients on tamoxifen therapy for advanced breast cancer: a randomised double-blind placebo controlled trial. *European Journal of Cancer*, 1993; **29A**: 814–18.

29. **Parenteral nutrition.** In: Thomas B, ed. *Manual of dietetic practice*. British Dietetic Association. Oxford: Blackwell Scientific Publications, 1994: 80–92.

30. **Lennard-Jones JE.** *Ethical and legal aspects of clinical hydration and nutritional support.* A report for the British Association for Parenteral and Enteral Nutrition, 1998. PO Box 922, Maidenhead, Berks, SL6 4SH.

31. **Downer SM, Cody MM, McCluskey P, Wilson PD, Arnott ST, Lister TA, Slevin ML.** Pursuit and practice of complementary therapies by cancer patients receiving conventional treatment. *British Medical Journal*, 1994; **309**: 86–9.

32. **Holden CM.** Anorexia in the terminally ill. *Hospice Journal*, 1991; 7: 73–84.

33. **Barber MD, Fearon KCH.** Should cancer patients with incurable disease receive parenteral or enteral nutritional support. *European Journal of Cancer*, 1998; **34**: 279–85.

34. **Gallagher-Allred CR.** *Nutritional care of the terminally ill.* Maryland: Aspen Publishers, 1989.

5.8 Cancer pain and its relief

P. J. Hoskin and G. W. Hanks

Introduction

Whilst pain is a concept common to most of us a formal definition is somewhat elusive. The International Association for the Study of Pain has defined this as 'an unpleasant sensory and emotional experience associated with acute or potential tissue damage or described in terms of such damage'.[1] The cancer patient may have many experiences of pain in their journey with the disease. Surveys suggest that independent of the primary site, fewer than 25 per cent of patients with advanced disease will deny the experience of pain.[2] Indeed 'for many patients the fear of cancer is the fear of pain'.[3] The overall incidence of pain in patients with advanced cancer is 60 to 70 per cent of which 75 per cent will be directly attributable to the malignancy.[4]

Considerable progress has been made in our knowledge regarding the use of appropriate drugs and other treatments for pain relief, and for most instances the means and knowledge to relieve pain effectively are available. There is now increasing success in the dissemination and application of this knowledge world-wide.[5] The fundamentals of pain management are no different to those of any medical intervention:

(1) careful and full assessment;

(2) diagnosis of the underlying cause;

(3) identification of both general and specific treatments;

(4) review and reassessment after initiation of treatment.

Data assessing the impact of intervention varies. Overall, simple application of the WHO pain guidelines can be expected to achieve pain relief in 80 per cent of patients presenting with pain secondary to advanced cancer.[6] In other patients, the situation can be more difficult and more specialized pain treatments are indicated.

Different health-care systems and individual centres will develop their own structures for the delivery of symptom control in advanced cancer. In the United Kingdom, there is widespread access to specialist palliative care physicians working within hospital-based continuing care units or local hospices alongside community-based general practitioners. In other parts of the world, management may be led by oncologists, general physicians, or anaesthetists with specific interests in the treatment of pain and other symptoms. Many large hospitals have now established symptom control teams which may be led by specialist nurses working through general medical and surgical teams. Specialist nurses, such as the MacMillan nurse network in the United Kingdom, have an invaluable role in the community care of patients with advanced cancer working through general practitioners or local hospices. Regardless of local structure, the important principle to be adopted is that the management of cancer pain is a team approach incorporating not only physicians with specialist skills in palliative medicine, oncology, surgery, and anaesthesia but also specialist nurses, physiotherapists, occupational therapists, and psychologists.

Pathophysiology of cancer pain

Pain is not a simple sensation: it has both a cognitive and an affective component and the perception of pain stimuli is always modified by an emotional response to that perception. Changes in mood may considerably alter the experience of pain. The successful treatment of cancer pain cannot ever rely merely on analgesics or nerve blocks. Pain associated with advanced cancer will for the patient have sinister implications not only reminding them of their disease but implying spread and progression. This results in a complex response varying between individuals including anxiety, anger, depression, guilt, despair, and fear. This, often combined with other debilitating symptoms such as nausea, anorexia, insomnia, and constipation results in a complex phenomenon loosely termed cancer pain. This may then be complicated further by intermittent episodes of acute pain, for example due to a pathological fracture or an incidental problem such as a migraine attack or tooth abscess.

Three broad categories of pain have been defined: somatic, visceral, and neuropathic.[7] The typical features and examples of these are shown in Table 1. The importance of this classification is not only in relation to identifying the underlying mechanisms but also in enabling treatment selection for specific types of pain.

An alternative classification of pain in cancer relates to the underlying cause, which may be acute or chronic and either directly related to the malignancy and its process of invasion and metastasis or due to accompanying problems either pre-existing or relating to medical intervention for the cancer. This is shown in Table 2. Whilst this is a valuable guide to seeking out the physical cause of pain, a simple analytical approach based on these factors will not always provide the best approach to the patient with advanced cancer. An alternative and complementary classification has been described [2] taking into account the patient's experience at the time of pain assessment defining five groups as shown in Table 3. Again this has important implications with regard to the management of pain in each particular patient group.

Pain assessment

Pain is by definition a subjective phenomenon. It cannot be determined by radiological or serological estimations and for each

Table 1 Categories of cancer pain

Type	Features	Common examples
Somatic	Localized, persistent, associated tenderness	Bone metastases, cellulitis, myositis
Visceral	Poorly localized, variable, associated symptoms e.g. nausea	Hepatomegaly carcinoma of pancreas, para-aortic nodes
Neuropathic	Follows nerve distribution, exacerbations of shooting pain or paraesthesia, associated neurological symptoms	Brachial plexopathy, lumbosacral plexopathy, spinal nerve root compression

Table 2 Classification of cancer pain according to underlying pathology

Pathology	Acute pain	Chronic pain
Malignancy direct cause	Pathological fracture Perforated viscus Acute haemorrhage into cystic tumour	Bone metastases Soft tissue invasion or infiltration Nerve infiltration Raised intracranial pressure Paraneoplastic syndromes Bone marrow pain
Treatment direct cause	Postoperative pain Cannula placement Radiation mucositis	Radiation fibrosis Chemotherapy neuropathy
Related medical conditions	Local infection	Constipation Pressure sores Catheter pain
Coexisting medical conditions	Tooth abscess Ischaemic heart disease Peripheral vascular disease Unrelated trauma	Osteoarthritis Migraine Tension headache Dyspepsia

Table 3 Pain related to past and current pain experience[8]

1. *Acute pain* predominates:	(a) related to cancer directly (b) related to treatment (c) related to coexisting condition
2. *Chronic pain* predominates: (i) physical cause major component:	(a) related to cancer directly (b) related to treatment (c) related to coexisting condition
(ii) emotional response the major component (iii) pre-existing history of drug abuse with (i) or (ii)	
3. Acute and/or chronic cancer pain in the final days of life	

patient its perception is a unique event. Measurement of pain therefore has to rely on the concept that 'pain is what the patient tells you'. The challenge is to unravel the individual components of pain for a particular patient and to rank their severity and likelihood of response to treatment on the basis of which a rational treatment programme may be devised. One of the more important observations in the field of cancer pain management is that rarely does a patient complain of a single pain; in an unselected series of cancer patients only 20 per

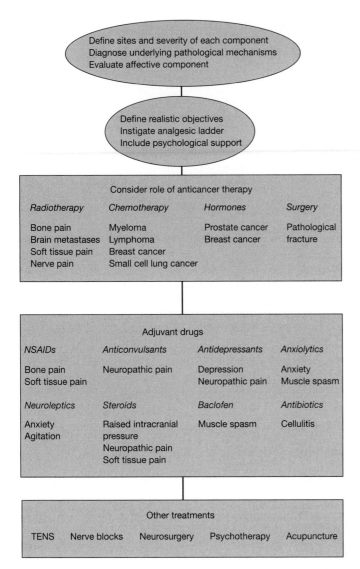

Fig. 1 Approach to the management of cancer pain.

pain in a limb. Such charts are now commonly available on many wards and in many clinics but can readily be improvised with a simple diagram.

Severity of pain

Measurement of the severity of pain can be broadly divided into either categorical or continuous scales. The categorical scale incorporates typically a 4 or 5 point scale, for example none, mild, moderate, severe, whilst a continuous scale is typically a visual analogue composed of a 100-mm line, one extreme of which defines 'no pain' and the other extreme very severe pain within which limits the patient will then define their pain by a mark on the line. Whilst the latter is potentially more sensitive, it may also be far more difficult for the patient to understand and use accurately. The former gives a broad classification of the pain and is often a more practical approach in busy clinical practice. In clinical trials both assessments may be used alongside data on analgesic use.

Assessment of the psychological state of the patient is also important in evaluating the affective component of pain. Formal scales such as the Hospital Anxiety and Depression (HAD) score or the Rotterdam symptom checklist may be used to provide an objective measure of these symptoms.

A review of the oncology literature suggests that, in general, pain is both measured and reported badly. Even studies looking at palliative treatment have only in recent years used formal, validated pain scores. The incorporation of a simple pain chart alongside a quality of life scale is to be recommended in all studies where this is relevant and an example of a simple pain chart used for fractionation trials in metastatic bone pain is shown in Fig. 2.

Treatment of cancer pain

Objectives

Having obtained a full assessment of the pain, the first step in treatment is to set realistic objectives with the patient. In this way trust can be built up with the patient without raising inappropriate expectations of complete pain relief in all situations. In general, it is possible to set three stages of pain relief:

- pain free at night;
- pain free at rest;
- pain free on movement.

Whilst nearly all patients should expect the former and the majority can be pain free at rest in the day also, pain on movement is often more difficult to address particularly when associated with weight bearing. Adequate analgesia for intermittent pain will result in excessive toxicity during the periods of non-movement which is usually unacceptable. Alterations in lifestyle may be a more pragmatic approach for this 'incident' pain. It is also important at the outset to make it clear to the patient that with an underlying cause of pain which is unlikely in the absence of effective chemotherapy or radiotherapy to disappear, continuous and possibly complex medication schedules will be necessary.

Pharmacological pain relief

The drugs available for pain relief can be classified broadly into those with analgesic activity and so-called 'adjuvant analgesics' which refers

cent had a single identifiable cause of pain and 20 per cent had four or more individual pains contributing to their overall pain experience.[4] Thus a careful history and examination is vital and even in patients with advanced disease specific investigations should be undertaken if these will help define an underlying cause of pain. Pain can then be classified according to its physical and non-physical components and the physical components can be further subclassified according to their acute and chronic nature on the basis of which individualized therapy can be devised. This is shown in the flow chart Fig. 1.

Various tools to aid in the assessment of pain have been described. These seek to define two distinct parameters

Distribution of pain

The use of a body chart is often of value in separating individual pains and considering inter-relationships between individual sites of pain, for example a spinal bone metastasis and associated neuropathic

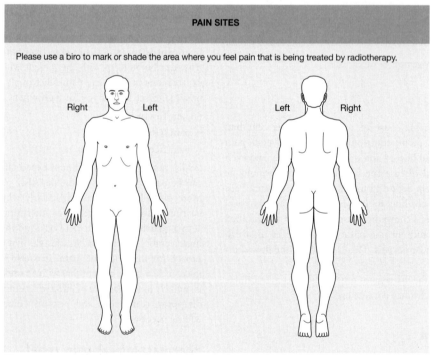

RADIOTHERAPY BONE PAIN TRIA L

A MULTICENTRE COLLABORATION

Name of patient ....   Hospital No. ....

Thank you very much for helping me with this study. We should be very grateful if you would fill in this chart today ....
by putting a tick in the appropriate box.

How is the pain today that is being treated by radiotherapy?	None	☐
	Mild	☐
	Moderate	☐
	Severe	☐

To help us record your pain, please mark or shade the area of pain on the diagrams in part (b)

| Did you take painkillers for this pain today? | Yes | ☐ |
| | No | ☐ |

Please write the names of your painkillers below: How many tablets or liquid doses have you taken in the last 24 hours?

1) ....

2) ....

3) ....

| Have you experienced any nausea today? (nausea is actually **feeling** sick) | None | ☐ | Quite a bit | ☐ |
| | A little | | Very much | |

| Have you experienced any vomiting today? (vomiting is actually **being** sick) | None | ☐ | Quite a bit | ☐ |
| | A little | | Very much | |

(a)

PAIN SITES

Please use a biro to mark or shade the area where you feel pain that is being treated by radiotherapy.

Right   Left   Left   Right

(b)

Fig. 2 Example of a pain chart.

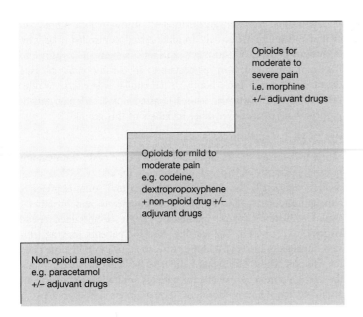

Fig. 3 WHO analgesic ladder.

to 'any drug that has a primary indication other than pain, but is analgesic in some painful conditions'[9] (also sometimes referred to as coanalgesics).

A number of important principles underlie the use of drugs in advanced cancer pain:

1. Regular medication is required to prevent pain rather than deal with pain intermittently.

2. The patient should have ready access to breakthrough or top-up medication if pain occurs between regular doses.

3. Initial treatment and titration is usually easier with immediate release formulations rather than sustained release formulations but the latter are invaluable for maintenance therapy once dose and drug schedules have been defined.

4. Monotherapy is not usually successful and patients are likely to require a combination of analgesics, adjuvant analgesics, and drugs addressing the inevitable side-effects of these, for example laxatives and antiemetics. Again the principle that these should be given on a regular basis is fundamental.

5. Any change in medication, whether the introduction of a new drug or dose escalation of an existing drug, should be carefully monitored and if unsuccessful the drug should be withdrawn or dose reduced and an alternative manoeuvre instigated. Each drug on a patient's drug schedule should have clear justification for its use.

Analgesics

The basis of analgesic use in cancer pain remains that of the WHO analgesic ladder as described in its cancer pain relief programme.[8] This depicts a simple, stepwise escalation of analgesics until pain relief is achieved from non-opioid analgesics such as paracetamol through opioids for mild to moderate pain, typically codeine-based, to opioids for moderate to severe pain of which morphine remains the drug of choice. The ladder concept is illustrated in Fig. 3. Whilst

there is no randomized trial data, there is validation of this approach demonstrated in several large, descriptive studies providing level 2 evidence; in one series of 1229 patients 871 were successfully treated for their cancer pain using only the WHO three-step ladder,[6] the remainder requiring additional measures such as neurolytic procedures; 11 per cent were treated only with step 1, 24 per cent only with step 2, 26.5 per cent with only step 3, and 33.6 per cent moved through all three steps of the ladder.

The advantage of the WHO analgesic ladder lies in its simplicity and its universal application despite persisting difficulties in some countries over the availability and use of strong opioids. This approach has been widely adopted but there has been recent criticism of the strength of evidence to support its use and in particular the lack of randomized, controlled trials.[10] However, the WHO method was never intended to be used in isolation or to exclude other treatment modalities and is more a statement of principles rather than a rigid framework. Thus, as new drugs or new formulations of old drugs are introduced they may find a place in the ladder used according to the principles of:

- simplicity in choice of drug and route of administration;
- individualization of dose;
- treatment of drug-induced adverse effects to allow maximum dose titration;
- continuous medication for continuous pain.

The WHO ladder should be interpreted as more pragmatic than prescriptive.

Non-opioid analgesics

The most common drug in this group is paracetamol; alternatives include aspirin and other non-steroidal anti-inflammatory drugs (NSAIDs). Paracetamol remains the simplest choice associated with the least side-effects. Patients who have not received regular analgesia should be given the opportunity of a trial of regular paracetamol when first treated for their pain. Severity may not be a guide to the strength of analgesia required and indeed paracetamol may be more appropriate than an opioid for some pain conditions where peripheral pain predominates. It is not only analgesic but also antipyretic and has both a central and peripheral non-opioid effect on pain pathways, though its precise mode of action remains unclear. Adverse reactions are rare which is a major advantage in a patient who may be taking many medications. The only significant consideration is the high mortality of overdose due to hepatic necrosis caused by an intermediate metabolite which in therapeutic doses is metabolized to a safe glucuronide or sulphate conjugate.

Paracetamol may also be of value in combination with an opioid such as morphine because of its peripheral activity, for example in controlling musculoskeletal pain whilst the strong opioid may be required for visceral pain. Aspirin is a satisfactory alternative to paracetamol if this is unavailable or in the very rare patient in whom paracetamol is not tolerated. In general, however, aspirin is associated with a far higher incidence of side-effects, in particular gastrointestinal symptoms and haemorrhage. Newer, better tolerated NSAIDs are usually preferred[11] many of which have both anti-inflammatory and potent analgesic effects.

Opioids for mild to moderate pain

This group includes codeine, dihydrocodeine, dextropropoxyphene, and tramadol. Invariably, these drugs are used in combination with

Table 4 Moderate analgesics in cancer pain (WHO ladder step 2)

Codeine phosphate 60 mg 4 hourly

Dihydrocodeine 60 mg 4 hourly

Coproxamol 2 tabs 4–6 hourly

(Dextropropoxyphene 32.5 mg + paracetamol 325 mg)

Cocodamol 2 tabs 4–6 hourly

(Codeine phosphate 30 mg + paracetamol 500 mg)
NB also available as codeine phosphate 8 mg/paracetamol 500 mg

Tramadol 100 mg 4–6 hourly

Meptazinol 200 mg 4–6 hourly

a non-opioid and common combination formulations are shown in Table 4.

Codeine chemically is methyl morphine and has similar actions to morphine in terms of analgesia, smooth muscle relaxation, of particular relevance to the gastrointestinal tract, causing constipation, and cough suppression. It is typically given orally although dihydrocodeine is available as a parenteral formulation. After oral administration absorption is quite variable and this may, in part, account for its lack of efficacy in certain patients. Metabolism is similar to that of morphine and indeed demethylation to morphine occurs and has been postulated as one of the mechanisms for its pharmacological activity.

Its usual analgesic dose is 60 mg, 4- to 6-hourly, and there is controversy as to whether any dose response for analgesia exists above this point. In general, patients who do not have good pain control at this level should switch to a 'step 3' opioid and the equivalent morphine dose from this level is 10 mg, 4-hourly. Dihydrocodeine is a semisynthetic derivative of codeine which by mouth is roughly equipotent. It does not appear to have any particular advantages over codeine.

Dextropropoxyphene has similar analgesic activity to codeine and is most frequently used as part of a combination preparation with paracetamol ('coproxamol' in the United Kingdom).

Codeine and dihydrocodeine are available as controlled-release formulations for twice daily administration, which may have advantages for those patients whose pain is controlled at this level of analgesia and who require regular medication on a long-term basis.

Tramadol has weak opioid agonist activity and also effects on noradrenaline and serotonin uptake in the spinal cord. Single oral doses of 150 mg tramadol were more effective than dextropropoxyphene/paracetamol or codeine in a double blind, randomized, single dose study of postoperative pain relief in 250 patients.[12] In chronic use, however, it is probably similar in potency to other step 2 opioids and may be considered where this level of analgesia is effective but there are limiting side-effects. Whilst tramadol can be given parenterally this is not usually indicated in the patient whose pain is controlled at this level of analgesia. Patients who are not controlled on a dose of 100 mg 6 hourly, regularly, should switch to morphine and again the typical starting dose will be to 10 mg of morphine, 4 hourly.

Meptazinol exerts an analgesic effect through both opioid and central anticholinergic activity. In randomized, controlled trials it has been shown to have equivalent analgesic activity to coproxamol (dextropropoxyphene with paracetamol) in chronic pain, its usual dose being 200 mg, 4 to 6 hourly. It has similar side-effects to other opioid drugs, in particular nausea, dizziness, and sedation and no particular advantages over other members of this group.[13]

Opioids for moderate to severe pain

Morphine remains the strong opioid of choice for oral administration in cancer pain. Its widespread availability, cost, and wide dose range make it universally the drug of choice. The oral route is preferred although alternatives include rectal, subcutaneous, and intrathecal. Oral formulations may be immediate release or sustained release lasting 8, 12, or 24 h. The starting dose for patients moving from step 2 analgesics is 10 mg, 4 hourly, with an almost infinite dose range for titration whilst improving pain relief is being achieved. Whilst the average dose requirements for patients with advanced cancer are 30 to 40 mg, 4 hourly, doses of several grams 4 hourly may, on occasions, be required to achieve pain relief, which should not be denied on the basis of dose alone in the patient responding to continued dose titration.

Morphine pharmacokinetics have been widely studied in recent years leading to an increased understanding of drug use and its mode of action. It is readily absorbed after oral administration predominantly in the upper small bowel and undergoes extensive first pass metabolism in the liver where it is converted predominantly to its two major metabolites, morphine-3-glucuronide and morphine-6-glucuronide, with small amounts of other metabolites including normorphine, morphine ethereal sulphate, and codeine.[14] It has a plasma half-life of 2 to 3 h, its metabolites being excreted through the kidney predominantly although small amounts have also been demonstrated in bile probably contributing to an enterohepatic circulation. Many of the actions of morphine, including its analgesic activity, arise from its interaction with opioid receptors in the central nervous system. It is, however, not highly lipophilic and once within the central nervous system extensive redistribution has been demonstrated.[15] There is a linear relationship between dose and plasma levels of the parent drug but there is poor correlation between blood level and analgesic activity.[16] This is probably partly related to the potent analgesic activity of its metabolite morphine-6-glucuronide and indeed a major component of the analgesic effect of chronic oral morphine is probably due to this glucuronide.[17] Renal failure results in accumulation of the glucuronide with consequently enhanced toxicity of morphine[18] and dose scheduling must therefore be carefully considered and modified in patients with significant renal impairment.

Clinical use of morphine—formulation In the patient who is able to take oral medication this should be the route of choice. A simple oral morphine solution (morphine sulphate, morphine hydrochloride, or morphine tartrate) or immediate release morphine tablets, according to preference and availability, should be used starting with a dose of 5 to 10 mg, 4 hourly, and titrating the dose upwards according to requirements until analgesia is achieved. The simplest method of dose titration is with a dose of immediate release morphine given every 4 h and the same dose for breakthrough pain. This rescue dose may be given as often as required and the total daily dose of morphine can be reviewed every 24 h. The regular dose can then be adjusted according to how many rescue doses have been given.[19] It should be noted that the median morphine dose requirement is around 40 mg, 4 hourly, in patients with advanced cancer[20] and therefore patients requiring doses much above this should be carefully reviewed and consideration given to alternative methods of treatment of their pain. Some types of pain are poorly responsive to opioids and continued dose escalation of morphine merely results in increasing side-effects without greater efficacy.

Controlled release formulations should be substituted if desired for the immediate release morphine once the dose requirements have been established. A simple dose-for-dose conversion is all that is required and there is no need for a loading dose when switching to 12-hourly controlled release formulations despite the lag in absorption from the first dose of controlled release drug.[21] Formulations are available which last for 8, 12, and 24 h and should be chosen according to convenience, availability, and cost. Each of these have been validated in randomized trials and shown to be equally effective as the 4-hourly use of morphine in the patient with stable analgesic requirements.[22] An important principle when using controlled release formulations is that the patient should have access to immediate release morphine for breakthrough pain. Longitudinal studies demonstrate that most patients require a slow increase in their morphine dose during their cancer journey. This can be achieved smoothly by allowing the patient access to breakthrough doses of morphine to be taken as required and, once a regular pattern has been established, for that dose of breakthrough morphine to be included in the regular controlled release formulation dose. The breakthrough dose should be equivalent to the 4-hourly dose based on the daily morphine requirements. Thus a patient on 60 mg twice daily of 12-hourly morphine who required an extra 20 mg of morphine solution each day for breakthrough pain should be switched to a 12-hourly dose of 70 mg twice daily whilst maintaining their access to breakthrough morphine for further adjustments.

Parenteral morphine should only be necessary in the patient who is unable to take oral medication although it is common practice to use the parenteral route in patients whose pain is not being readily controlled with oral morphine. There is in fact no reason why oral morphine should be less effective than parenteral morphine provided consideration is given to the difference in potency through the two routes. The oral bioavailability of morphine is only around 30 per cent and thus the efficacy of a 10 mg dose of morphine given by mouth is less than 10 mg of morphine given intravenously or subcutaneously. Whilst there remains some debate, the oral to parenteral potency ratio ranges between 1:3 and 1:2.[23] In other words, 20 to 30 mg of oral morphine are required to have the same analgesic effect as 10 mg of parenteral morphine. These are important considerations not only to understand the rationale for continuing oral morphine wherever possible, but also in the patient who has to switch from one route to another. As a general rule of thumb, the dose should be halved in the patient switching from oral to parenteral morphine and doubled in the patient switching from parenteral to oral morphine.

When given parenterally, the subcutaneous route is generally preferred. There is some evidence that given by intermittent intravenous bolus injections, rapid tolerance to morphine is acquired resulting in significant dose escalation, an effect which is not seen by the subcutaneous route. For patients requiring short-term parenteral morphine, intermittent injections may be satisfactory but for the majority a continuous subcutaneous infusion is preferred using a proprietary syringe driver. These will be ideal for the patient with intestinal obstruction, severe nausea and vomiting from metabolic causes or raised intracranial pressure, the patient with impaired consciousness, and those with oropharyngeal or oesophageal disease causing dysphagia.

Rectal morphine is an appropriate alternative to oral morphine. Given by this route morphine is equipotent with the oral formulation.

Common adverse effects should always be anticipated when a strong opioid such as morphine is started. In particular all patients will become constipated and therefore regular laxatives should be the rule. This should be adjusted according to patient preference. The combination of a faecal softener and stimulant, as in co-danthramer, is usually effective. Nausea with or without vomiting is reported in between one-third and two-thirds of patients receiving regular morphine[24] and a regular antiemetic should be available on demand or given prophylactically.

Alternative opioids for moderate to severe pain

Diamorphine Diamorphine is a synthetic derivative of morphine and chemically is diacetylmorphine. When taken by mouth diamorphine is deacetylated during the first pass through the liver and the main active form is morphine and its major metabolites. By mouth, therefore, there is no advantage of diamorphine over morphine since it acts simply as a prodrug. It does, however, have some advantages when used parenterally and is the opioid of choice for spinal administration, having greater lipid solubility and also greater water solubility which means that a given amount of strong opioid drug can be given in a smaller volume with diamorphine than with morphine. In countries where diamorphine is not available, however, morphine is entirely suitable for parenteral administration but will require larger infusion volumes.

Fentanyl Fentanyl is a semisynthetic opioid which is considerably more potent than morphine. When given parenterally it is approximately 80 times more potent dose-for-dose than morphine and also has much greater lipid solubility resulting in more rapid and extensive distribution. It has an elimination half-life of up to 12 h and is suitable therefore for maintenance therapy. The common formulation is that of a skin patch taking advantage of its transdermal absorption when a dose of 25 μg/h is approximately equivalent to a dose of 10 to 20 mg of morphine 4 hourly.[25] The major disadvantages of fentanyl using this formulation are in its relative inflexibility for dose titration and many patients require breakthrough doses of morphine to permit dose titration, subsequently moving to additional or stronger patches. Plateau serum levels are reached up to 24 h after a patch is placed on the skin and may take 18 to 24 h for the serum concentration to fall by 50 per cent after removal of the patch.[26] This is subject to considerable individual variation which increases the need for breakthrough analgesia in some patients. It has also been observed that the absorption from the fentanyl patch is temperature-dependent and in patients who have febrile illnesses absorption may be increased.[27] This can result in unexpected side-effects appearing during such episodes.

The transdermal route, however, has clear advantages for patients who have difficulty taking oral medication and in those where nausea and vomiting related to opioid therapy is prominent. A randomized, cross-over study in 202 cancer patients[28] has shown equivalent pain relief to oral sustained release morphine tablets. The side-effect profile of fentanyl suggests that it may be relatively less constipating than morphine.[28] It should therefore be seen as a strong opioid alternative to morphine and a useful option in patients who cannot take oral formulations and who have stable opioid requirements. Up to 10 per cent of patients may experience a morphine withdrawal reaction if switched directly to fentanyl and some have suggested that morphine should be continued for 24 h after starting fentanyl.[29]

Hydromorphone Hydromorphone is chemically and pharmacokinetically very similar to morphine. It is available in comparable oral, rectal, and parenteral formulations and may also be considered a useful substitute for morphine, where available, in patients who find morphine produces unacceptable side-effects. There is no good evidence that its side-effect profile is necessarily different to morphine although it is considerably more potent. Equivalent analgesia is achieved by approximately one-fifth of the dose of morphine and so it may have particular value in patients requiring high morphine doses, particularly where infusions are required allowing a smaller dose and hence infusion volume to be chosen.[30] As with morphine it is important to realise that because its bioavailability is around 30 per cent the parenteral dose needs to be reduced to get equivalent analgesia to an oral dose and the quoted ratio of dose reduction for hydromorphone is 1:5.[31]

Phenazocine Phenazocine is a synthetic opioid which may also be used as an alternative to morphine, particularly where side-effects with the latter are prominent. Its major disadvantage is limited dose flexibility. It is again more potent than morphine with a ratio of around 5:1. It is commonly available in 5-mg tablets which are equivalent to 25 mg of morphine by mouth. This, therefore, introduces less flexibility in dose increments when using phenazocine. Sublingual administration has also been described but is not common practice. The side-effect profile of phenazocine is similar to morphine but psychotomimetic effects are said to be less.[32]

Methadone Methadone is an alternative strong opioid to morphine and its use for cancer pain is increasing. One potential problem which has been highlighted is its variable pharmacokinetics with, in particular, a wide range of elimination half-life values between individuals. Extreme values of more than 5 days are seen, particularly in the elderly. This raises theoretical concerns with regard to the appropriate dosing interval since the standard 8-hourly oral regimen may lead to drug accumulation and toxicity in some individuals. In experienced hands, the side-effect and safety profile of methadone is similar to morphine with constipation and drowsiness predominating. Whilst in single doses methadone is equianalgesic with morphine, in chronic use it may be much more potent and one of the difficulties with this drug in practice is in calculating its relative analgesic potency when switching between opioids.[33]

Other strong opioids not recommended in cancer pain

Pethidine is a synthetic strong opioid drug commonly used for acute pain in the surgical setting. Its major disadvantage is its short half-life of around 2 h and in chronic use the accumulation of a central nervous system-toxic metabolite norpethidine.[34] It is therefore not recommended for regular administration to the cancer patient.

Dextromoramide also has a short half-life of around 2 h and exhibits tachyphyllaxis with a diminished duration of action with repeated doses. It is therefore of little value as a strong analgesic in regular use for cancer pain.

Buprenorphine is a synthetic partial opioid agonist. This results in a theoretical ceiling effect for analgesia beyond which no additional pain relief is seen. Whilst this level has not been clearly established in man, there is in addition a more practical limitation because its mode of administration is sublingual. The number of tablets which can be comfortably held under the tongue limits doses to 800 µg (two tablets). When this dose is given 8 hourly it is equivalent to a morphine dose of 10 to 20 mg given 4 hourly. It may therefore be considered in patients failing moderate strength analgesics requiring a strong opioid for whom the sublingual route may have advantages, for example those with oesophageal or mediastinal tumours affecting swallowing.

Dipipanone has no significant advantage over morphine being approximately half as potent and in its standard formulation combined with cyclizine in a tablet containing 30 mg cyclizine and 10 mg dipipanone. This increases its toxicity profile in the combined formulation with side-effects from the cyclizine including dry mouth and sedation adding to those of the opioid and limiting the flexibility of dose titration.

Nalbuphine is a synthetic drug with both agonist and antagonist activity at the opioid receptor. It is similar in potency to morphine with a similar toxicity profile and has no major advantages. An additional practical disadvantage is that it is not available for oral administration but only in an injectable formulation.

Butorphanol is also a synthetic drug with mixed agonist and antagonist activity at the opioid receptor. It is more potent than morphine but has a similar toxicity profile and only limited availability. It therefore has no significant advantages in this setting.

Spinal opioids

The main indications for delivery of strong opioid drugs through the spinal route are patients in whom systemic opioids provide effective pain relief but severe side-effects and in some patients with movement-related 'incident' pain. Administration may be either epidural, intrathecal, or subarachnoid and by direct delivery of the drug into the central nervous system more efficient and selective delivery to the opioid receptors involved in pain mediation is achieved. Morphine, hydromorphone, and diamorphine may all be used in this setting. Chronic administration is possible but the technique is potentially hazardous and should only be undertaken by a skilled person experienced in its use.

Despite the theoretical advantages, systemic side-effects including nausea, vomiting, and psychotomimetic effects may occur and urinary retention and pruritis, although unusual, are relatively more common. There have been reports of both delayed respiratory depression due to cranial migration of opioid and withdrawal symptoms in patients on high doses of oral or parenteral morphine.[35]

Morphine toxicity

The most common side-effects with morphine are drowsiness, constipation, nausea and vomiting, and dry mouth.

Drowsiness is usually only a problem when first starting morphine or when the dose is increased. Patients can generally be reassured that it will improve within a few days although in some it may become persistent and dose-limiting. It should not, however, be an indication to reduce or stop therapy and is best dealt with by careful explanation and reassurance to both the patient and relatives and if persistent switching to an alternative strong opioid. Stimulant drugs have been recommended in the past but have the potential to cause hallucinations and occasional bizarre psychological reactions.

Constipation and nausea and vomiting have been discussed above and the need for proactive prophylaxis using regular laxatives and either regular or immediate access to antiemetics is intrinsic to the use of morphine in cancer pain.

Respiratory depression is not a problem in cancer patients receiving oral opioid analgesics. Pain acts a physiological antagonist of the depressant effect of morphine on the central nervous system so that as long as a patient has pain the dose of morphine can be safely titrated upwards without fear of respiratory depression.[36] There is always a separation between the dose that will relieve the patient's pain and the dose that will cause significant depression of respiratory function. The only times problems arise is when the dose is allowed to rise above the threshold required for pain relief or else it is not appropriately reduced after a pain-relieving manoeuvre such as radiotherapy. The other area to be approached with caution is the patient with renal failure in whom accumulation of active metabolites can readily occur.[18]

Addiction does not occur in patients receiving strong opioid analgesics[37] for cancer pain because they do not become psychologically dependent or develop 'drug craving'. Both tolerance and physical dependence can occur but these are not problems in clinical practice. Tolerance is relatively uncommon but if it does develop can easily be coped with by appropriate dose adjustment or the careful use of adjuvant analgesic drugs. Physical dependence probably develops in the majority of patients receiving regular opioid analgesics for more than a week or two. However, this does not prevent reduction in dose in patients whose pain ameliorates for whatever reason or discontinuation of opioid in those patients whose pain completely resolves. The patient is weaned off the opioid over 2 to 3 weeks or more quickly if the treatment with the opioid has been relatively short. No special measures are required. It is, however, important to appreciate that because of physical dependence administration of opioid antagonists such as naloxone may result in a severe and acute withdrawal reaction and should be avoided wherever possible.

Pain poorly responsive to opioids

Whilst the above strategy is successful for most patients, there is undoubtedly a small group of patients whose pain responds poorly to opioid medication even in escalating doses. These pains are sometimes termed 'opioid-resistant' although true opioid-resistance is rare. Patients who are requiring dose escalation beyond 110 mg of morphine 4 hourly will be within the top 10 per cent of morphine dose requirements.[19] As these levels are reached it is important to consider the possibility that this patient may have opioid poorly-responsive pain and look towards alternative strategies.

In the patient who has developed intolerable adverse effects or has inadequate analgesia, or both, it is important in the first instance to review and optimize the use of adjuvant analgesics such as antidepressants and anticonvulsants. As far as the opioids are concerned there are two potential manoeuvres which may improve analgesia and reduce adverse effects.[38] The first is to consider the use of an alternative opioid agonist. It has been established empirically that switching to an alternative opioid may, in these circumstances, both allow pain control to be achieved and disabling effects associated with the previous drug to be reduced. Practice varies and some have recommended that switching between several drugs ('opioid rotation')

may be required in a substantial proportion of patients. This is not a strategy to be regarded as standard practice outside specialist units, but there is no doubt that increasing availability of alternatives to morphine, such as fentanyl and hydromorphone, will allow greater flexibility in the management of these most difficult pain problems.

An important component of opioid-resistant pain is the 'wind-up' phenomenon in which there is a change in the setting of sensitivity of central neurones to pain with relatively minor pain stimuli being perceived as severe pain.[39] This is known as allodynia and is mediated through N-methyl-D-aspartate (NMDA) receptors. On this basis, there is increasing interest in the use of NMDA receptor antagonists for difficult pains which are opioid poorly responsive.

Ketamine is the most widely available NMDA antagonist and within a controlled setting may be of value.[40] It allows resetting of the NMDA receptors restoring the normal sensitivity to pain and opioid analgesia. Ketamine needs careful monitoring and is administered by continuous subcutaneous infusion using an initial dose of 0.1 to 0.6 mg/kg per h. Side-effects may include hypotension and psychotomimetic disturbances although these are relatively rare when titrated carefully from a low starting dose.

Because NMDA antagonists work in part through resetting of opioid tolerance, in general a combination of an NMDA antagonist with morphine provides the best approach. It should be emphasized, however, that such difficult pain problems should only be managed in specialized units with expertise in the use of such drug combinations and monitoring of their response. The other important area to consider in patients with opioid poorly-responsive pain is the role of non-pharmacological manoeuvres which would include radiotherapy or chemotherapy, surgery, or anaesthetic interventions.

Neuropathic pain

Neuropathic pain is the commonest type of pain in cancer patients which is poorly-responsive to opioids. Early concurrent use of adjuvant analgesics is particularly indicated in the management of this type of pain. The tricyclic antidepressant amitriptyline and anticonvulsants, such as carbamazepine, are most likely to be effective against a background of regular opioid analgesia.

Opioid-irrelevant pain

This is a term which has been used to describe pain which is not responsive to opioids where the main components are social, psychological, or spiritual rather than physical. This reflects the extreme end of the chronic cancer pain model in which the emotional or affective component predominates to such a degree that it overwhelms any underlying physical pain. Clearly the treatment for such pain will rest with appropriate psychological support and the judicious use of psychotropic drugs rather than opioids.

Adjuvant drugs in the management of cancer pain

Alongside the use of analgesics governed by an escalation through the analgesic ladder additional drugs, the 'adjuvant analgesics', should be considered throughout. These will be drugs which may modify the underlying pain process and their choice therefore depends critically upon careful assessment and diagnosis of the cause of pain at the outset. Such agents should be introduced with the lower levels of the analgesic ladder and maintained through the escalation of analgesia unless there is clear evidence that they have no efficacy.

Non-steroidal anti-inflammatory drugs (NSAIDs)

NSAIDs are primarily utilized for their anti-inflammatory action although they do have both intrinsic analgesic and antipyretic action also. Their mode of action is through blocking cyclo-oxygenase activity which inhibits the production of prostaglandins from arachidonic acid. Prostaglandins are major mediators of the inflammatory response, the sensation of pain through pain fibres and fever.

NSAIDs may be used as alternative analgesics at step 1 and step 2 of the WHO analgesic ladder, and also as adjuvants in certain indications.

NSAIDs were found empirically to relieve bone pain in metastatic breast cancer and haematological malignancies but, as in the treatment of rheumatic disorders, the action of NSAIDs in bone pain is not predictable or consistent.[41] In practice, different drugs within this class may be effective in one patient but not another although there is insufficient data to indicate why this should be. NSAIDs do possess analgesic activity independent of their anti-inflammatory properties and are indicated in any patient with musculoskeletal pain with the option of switching from one drug to an alternative if there is no documented response after a short therapeutic trial. With this in mind, it is important to realise that NSAIDs have varying half-lives and can be classified broadly into those with short half-lives, including aspirin, indomethacin, diclofenac, and ketorolac, and those with long half-lives (greater than 10 h) such as naproxen and piroxicam. Thus, whilst a short half-life NSAID may be assessed within a few days having rapidly reached therapeutic equilibrium, a longer half-life drug may need a week or more to reach steady state levels.

NSAIDs are associated with gastrointestinal upset with a significant incidence of dyspepsia, gastritis, peptic ulceration, and haemorrhage; population-based data from hospital inpatients over 60 years of age reports a relative risk of peptic ulcer bleeding from NSAIDs ranging from 2.0 with ibuprofen to 23.7 with ketoprofen.[42] For patients with a previous history of gastric symptoms or pathology and in those who develop troublesome dyspeptic symptoms an H_2 antagonist or misoprostol[43] should be added to allow continued use of the drug if it is shown to be effective. A reduction in NSAID-related gastric ulceration from 21.7 per cent in controls to 1.4 per cent in patients receiving 100 µg of misoprostol has been shown in a multicentre, randomized, double blind trial in 420 patients receiving ibuprofen, piroxicam, or naproxen. Two combined formulations containing either naproxen or diclofenac with misoprostol are now available and may improve compliance. Other potential side-effects include fluid retention and bronchospasm, as a consequence of which in patients with proven asthma NSAIDs should be used with close supervision of their respiratory function.

Conventional use is by mouth. However, continuous subcutaneous infusions of ketorolac have been reported as an effective manoeuvre in a small series of patients with otherwise unresponsive musculo-skeletal pain but there is no randomized evaluation of this approach against oral NSAIDs; misoprostol prophylaxis is recommended with subcutaneous ketorolac in view of the risk of gastric complications.[44]

Recently, topical formulations of NSAIDs in a gel have been available. Theoretically, these have the advantage of avoiding systemic side-effects and there is some evidence that for superficial pain related to joints they can produce a modest reduction in pain. There are no published data on the use of topical NSAIDs in cancer pain.

Corticosteroids

Corticosteroids have an important role in the management of patients with advanced cancer and a frequent indication is as an adjuvant analgesic. They may be helpful wherever the local pressure associated with a tumour mass is causing pain, for example nerve compression, raised intracranial pressure, hepatomegaly, pelvic or intra-abdominal masses, and head and neck tumours. The mode of action of corticosteroids in this setting is presumed to be related to their anti-inflammatory effect. Corticosteroids inhibit the production of prostaglandins and leucotrienes in the latter case by blocking the action of lipo-oxygenase. The reduction of inflammatory oedema and hyperaemia surrounding a tumour mass or involved bone may reduce the pressure and relieve the pain.

Side-effects from steroid use are well known and their risk and severity depends upon steroid formulation, dose, and duration of therapy. Short-term steroid administration is usually well tolerated. The association of cortoicosteroids and gastrointestinal toxicity is controversial but use of these drugs in combination with NSAIDs results in a definite increase in risk. Fluid overload may occur particularly in patients who already have borderline heart failure in whom this may have potentially serious consequences. Patients with borderline glucose tolerance or established diabetes will have further impairment of glucose tolerance and occasionally severe diabetic ketoacidosis may be precipitated. Established diabetics should not be denied the advantages of steroids but careful monitoring and adjustment of hypoglycaemic medication may be required. Acute psychological disturbance may occur in susceptible individuals and many patients report restlessness, insomnia, and vivid dreams. Proximal myopathy may also develop within only a few weeks of use and in occasional patients may become disabling. Recovery on withdrawal of steroids will occur but can be slow and alongside the process of progressive malignancy may cause prolonged difficulties in mobility.

Steroid withdrawal is often not appropriate in patients with severe cancer pain who achieve good control by the addition of steroids to their treatment schedule. As a general principle, however, the lowest possible dose compatible with efficacy should be sought by slowly reducing doses to a maintenance level wherever possible.

Two corticosteroid drugs are generally available and used in this situation, dexamethasone or prednisolone. Dexamethasone is often preferred being more potent (4 mg is approximately equal to 30 mg prednisolone) so that fewer tablets are needed. It is also said to have fewer mineralocorticoid effects so that less oedema and weight gain occurs although it may be associated with a higher prevalence of psychological side-effects. In general, patients should start with an initial high dose, for example 8 to 16 mg dexamethasone or 60 to 90 mg prednisolone daily, for a few days followed by a slow reduction in dose to a maintenance of around 4 mg dexamethasone or 20 to 30 mg prednisolone.

Psychotropic drugs

Anxiety, depression, fear, restlessness, and sleeplessness may significantly lower a patient's pain threshold and exacerbate the perception of pain. All of these symptoms may respond to psychotropic medication with a consequent reduction in pain or a greater ability to tolerate or cope with it.

Benzodiazepines are the most useful group of drugs for the management of these symptoms in cancer pain because of their wide therapeutic index and small potential for interacting with other agents.

Benzodiazepines can be classified according to their duration of action, short-acting drugs such as temazepam with a duration of effect of 6 to 10 h being most appropriate for the treatment of insomnia with only minimal residual effect the following day. Intermediate acting drugs will work into the following day and include nitrazepam and lorazepam. These may be helpful in patients with both insomnia and mild anxiety. For patients with more severe anxiety and agitation long-acting benzodiazepines such as diazepam may be more appropriate. In the cancer patient ,diazepam has the advantage of needing only once-daily administration in many situations and in patients having difficulty with oral medication the rectal route is also available.

Midazolam is a useful alternative for the treatment of anxiety and terminal restlessness in patients requiring a syringe driver. It is compatible with diamorphine and the usual starting dose is 10 to 20 mg over 24 h.

Neuroleptic drugs include the phenothiazines such as chlorpromazine and methotrimeprazine and the butyrophenones such as haloperidol. These drugs are commonly used for their antiemetic and sedative effects and an opioid-sparing effect possibly due to intrinsic analgesic activity has also been described for methotrimeprazine.[45] In acute pain methotrimeprazine appears to have equivalent analgesic potency to morphine in patients having postoperative pain or myocardial infarction.[46] The evidence for chlorpromazine or haloperidol having intrinsic analgesic activity, however, is generally unconvincing. They may be of particular value in patients with severe anxiety and restlessness and those having hallucinations related to opioid use. Methotrimeprazine can be given by subcutaneous infusion and is compatible with morphine or diamorphine in a syringe driver. It is therefore of particular value in patients with advanced disease who require some sedation for terminal restlessness and agitation. Methotrimeprazine is given in a dose of 25 mg over 24 h initially with dose escalation as required.

The main limiting feature of this group of drugs are their associated side-effects which are predominantly anticholinergic and parkinsonian. Extrapyramidal reactions are more common with haloperidol than the other drugs of this group while anticholinergic effects, such as dry mouth, constipation, and urinary hesitancy, are more common with phenothiazines.

Antidepressants are widely used in the management of chronic pain both in those patients who have associated depression and in the absence of depression with a particular indication for neuropathic-type pains. The greatest body of evidence rests with older tricyclic antidepressants, in particular amitriptyline, one randomized trial reporting a mean reduction in visual analogue pain scores of 40 (out of 100 total) points after 15 days of amitriptylline in 45 patients with chronic deafferentation pain.[47] There is less evidence to support the use of monoamine oxidase inhibitors and in view of their widespread potential for interaction they are probably best avoided in patients with advanced cancer on multiple treatments. The newer antidepressants with more specific serotonin uptake inhibitory action, such as fluoxetine and paroxetine, have been less widely evaluated for pain relief. They may, however, be the drugs of choice for the patient who has clinical depression alongside or as a component of chronic pain. In general, low doses of amitriptyline starting with 25 to 50 mg daily are sufficient for pain relief. This may be lower than the doses used for treating depression and will avoid most of the usual side-effects although drowsiness and anticholinergic effects, in particular dry mouth, can still be troublesome.

Anticonvulsants

Anticonvulsants may be helpful in the management of lancinating or stabbing dysaesthetic pains associated with nerve infiltration or compression, postsurgical neuralgia, postherpetic neuralgia, or other forms of neuropathic pain. Burning dysaesthesia may also respond. There is no convincing evidence that any one anticonvulsant drug is better than another; a non-randomized, sequential study comparing carbamazepine, clonazepam, phenytoin, and sodium valproate found response rates to initial exposure varying from 30 to 66 per cent with no significant difference seen between the individual drugs.[48] The choice will, therefore, usually be influenced by potential side-effects. Carbamazepine is often chosen initially. If this is not effective, switching to an alternative such as clonazepam or sodium valproate may be of value. There is increasing evidence supporting the use of some of the newer anticonvulsants, particularly gabapentin, but comparative data against the older drugs is still required to establish their role in pain management.

Muscle relaxants

Painful muscle spasm frequently occurs, particularly in association with metastatic bone disease in the axial skeleton. Baclofen and diazepam are equally effective; diazepam is more sedative whilst baclofen causes gastrointestinal disturbance more frequently.[49] Muscle spasm may also respond to acupuncture, massage, or heat.

Bisphosphonates

Bisphosphonates are analogues of pyrophosphate and are potent inhibitors of osteoclastic bone reabsorption. Their use in metastatic bone pain is becoming widely established. Both oral clodronate and intravenous pamidronate have been shown in multicentre, randomized trials to have an impact on morbidity from bone metastases when given prophylactically to asymptomatic disease in the setting of myeloma[50] and breast cancer.[51] Fewer instances of vertebral fracture and less bone pain with better performance status is reported in myeloma and a reduction in the number of patients developing bone metastases from 17 to 8 per cent was seen in breast cancer. Anecdotally, bisphosphonates are also effective in established bone pain, particularly in patients with widespread sites of pain which may be difficult to address with local radiotherapy. Data are accumulating in support of the use of either intravenous clodronate 1600 mg, or intravenous pamidronate 60 to 90 mg which can be repeated at 2 to 3-weekly intervals. Single arm studies have documented pain relief[52] and one placebo-controlled trial[53] has shown a statistically significant (p<0.03) reduction in pain scores measured by linear analogue scales in patients receiving oral clodronate for metastatic bone pain.

Anticancer therapy

Whilst cancer pain may be related to pre-existing painful conditions, treatment-related morbidity and other related conditions, such as herpes zoster, by far the majority of causes relate to the progressive invasion and metastatic spread of an underlying malignancy. It follows, therefore, that treatment directed at suppressing this process has a major role in the treatment of cancer pain. Unfortunately for many patients, presentation with metastatic disease heralds rapid decline with disease which is relatively resistant to systemic therapy. It is, however, of vital importance that those patients in whom specific measures are indicated can be identified and treated appropriately.

Systemic chemotherapy for cancer pain

The role of systemic chemotherapy in individual cancer sites will have been discussed in detail in other chapters. Certain scenarios however warrant highlighting where systemic chemotherapy may well have an important role in achieving pain relief despite otherwise incurable disease. In particular the following should be considered:

* Myeloma can cause severe bone pain due to widespread osteolytic disease. Systemic chemotherapy is often the most effective way to control this using alkylating agents or combination chemotherapy.
* Small-cell lung cancer is also commonly associated with widespread bone marrow and bone metastasis. It is typically very sensitive to first line and often second line chemotherapy and these should be considered as the optimal means of achieving relief from generalized bone pain in these patients.
* Breast cancer also accounts for a high proportion of patients presenting with generalized bone pain and soft tissue pain due to hepatic or nodal metastasis. Many patients will have received first line chemotherapy as adjuvant but second or third line chemotherapy is often worth considering for severe symptoms.
* Haematological malignancies, including Hodgkin's disease, non-Hodgkin's lymphoma, and the leukaemias, will often respond to chemotherapy even in advanced stages of the disease after previous treatment.

Hormone therapy for cancer pain

Prostate cancer is perhaps the most common cause of widespread bone pain from metastatic disease. It is also the most satisfactory to treat with first line hormone treatment using antiandrogen therapy with the vast majority of patients showing an excellent response in terms of pain control. Second line antiandrogen therapy may also give symptomatic relief even if objective responses cannot be demonstrated in more advanced disease.

Breast cancer is hormone-sensitive. Many patients will have received adjuvant tamoxifen but second and third line hormone therapy is commonly undertaken with good responses in a substantial minority.

Endometrial cancer is also hormone-sensitive, responding to progestogens or gonadotrophin-releasing hormone analogues. Whilst metastatic disease and even pelvic recurrence is relatively unusual, systemic treatment should be considered in those patients presenting with these problems.

Radiotherapy

Radiotherapy is one of the most effective treatments for localized pain directly related to tumour pressure and infiltration. Even relatively small doses of radiation will result in considerable cell kill within a tumour mass and small degrees of regression where pressure and infiltration is a cause of pain can be highly effective in achieving pain relief. Specific areas where radiotherapy has a major role are shown in Table 5.

Bone pain is perhaps the most common indication for palliative radiotherapy and this is the most effective means of dealing with localized pain related to bone metastasis, confirmed in both randomized trials and a meta-analysis.[54] A considerable body of evidence

Table 5 Indications for radiotherapy in cancer pain

Metastatic bone pain	
Raised intracranial pressure	Primary brain tumour
	Intracranial metastases
Pelvic pain	Presacral rectal recurrence
	Recurrent uterine or ovarian tumour
Retroperitoneal pain	Advanced renal tumours
	Primary soft tissue sarcoma
Hepatic pain	Primary hepatocellular carcinoma
	Liver metastases
Splenic pain	Leukaemias
	Lymphomas
	Myelodysplastic syndrome
Brachial plexopathy	Apical lung tumour
	Recurrent breast cancer

supports the use of single doses of 8 to 10 Gy delivered to the site of pain using external beam radiotherapy from which 80 per cent of patients can expect pain relief with complete pain relief seen in up to 60 per cent of patients.[55] This may be maintained for many months and since the median survival of most patients with metastatic bone pain is of the order of 6 months in the majority the response will be sustained for their life span. In a large, prospective, randomized trial of over 700 patients a single dose of 8 Gy has been shown to be equivalent to multifraction treatment for up to 1 year after treatment.[56] Recurrent bone pain after single-dose radiotherapy can be retreated with a similar expectation of response.[57] Side-effects from this form of radiotherapy are relatively few but around one-third of patients will have some degree of self-limiting nausea particularly when the lumbar spine and pelvis is treated. Appropriate prophylaxis should be considered in these patients.

Since many patients will have multiple metastases and require multiple treatments, careful localization and documentation of treatments is important with accurate simulation whenever possible to avoid potentially hazardous areas of overlap.

Local radiotherapy should also be considered for pathological fracture which cannot be operated on particularly when it affects ribs or pelvic bones or where there is vertebral collapse without spinal cord compression. It is also indicated postoperatively after internal fixation for pathological fracture when doses of 20 to 30 Gy over 1 to 2 weeks will be given.

Where there are multiple sites of bone pain then these may be encompassed in a wide field radiotherapy technique in which an area approximating to a 'half body' will be encompassed delivering a single dose of 6 Gy to the upper half body when the lungs are included in the treatment volume or 8 Gy to other areas in the lower half body. Again around 80 per cent of patients can expect pain relief which for the majority will last until death and after this technique pain relief may be seen more rapidly with an onset within 24 to 48 h distinct from the delay of 2 to 4 weeks after localized external beam treatment.[57] Because a larger volume is irradiated more side-effects may ensue with gastrointestinal upsets seen in around two-thirds of patients and detectable, but usually asymptomatic, bone marrow depression occurring, with spontaneous recovery over a period of 4 to 6 weeks provided there is not extensive bone marrow infiltration by malignancy.

Radioisotopes offer an attractive alternative means of delivering radiotherapy to the patient with widespread bone metastasis. Currently strontium (^{89}Sr) or samarium (^{153}Sm) chelated to ethylenediamine tetramethylene phosphoric acid (Sm-EDMP) are available commercially. Strontium is distributed in the same pattern as calcium and therefore actively taken up at sites of bone mineralization and incorporated into hydroxyapatite. EDMP is also taken up at sites of bone mineralization and hence samarium can also be concentrated in these sites. Rhenium (^{186}Re) has also been developed chelated to EDMP in this way. All bone metastases have an associated osteoblastic reaction, even those where there is a predominant lytic picture on radiographs. These isotopes will therefore be selectively taken up at sites of bone metastases following the pattern of technecium uptake on an isotope bone scan. The advantage is that they may be delivered by a single intravenous injection within the confines of radioprotection precautions. This can usually be undertaken on an outpatient basis. Their principle radiation is beta particle radiation which has a short range of a few millimetres in tissue and hence the main energy deposition is within the bone metastasis. They are excreted in the urine and so special precautions regarding urinary disposal are required and they are relatively contra-indicated in the incontinent patient unless catheterization is secure. They are, however, highly effective at treating widespread bone pain. The greatest body of data relates to carcinoma of the prostate in which these compounds were first developed and evaluated. Around 80 per cent of patients can again expect pain relief with side-effects being negligible.[58] Transient falls in blood count are seen but these rarely are of clinical significance and recover spontaneously. Radioisotope therapy therefore offers an attractive means of treating generalized metastatic bone pain with a single outpatient visit for their intravenous administration and less systemic toxicity. However, a randomized, controlled trial comparing external beam treatment to isotope therapy has shown no difference in incidence or quality of pain relief with 64 per cent of patients reporting response as measured by patient questionnaire scores.[59]

Intracranial tumour

Pain due to rising intracranial pressure secondary to tumour growth within the skull is seen with both progressive primary central nervous system tumours and cerebral metastasis. In both instances high dose steroids may cause temporary respite where oedema is prominent but further tumour progression will result in intractable headache. Radiotherapy will relieve headache in 70 to 80 per cent of patients where this is related to cerebral metastasis. Randomized, controlled trials have compared various dose-fractionation schedules; the RTOG trials,[60] performed between 1976 and 1982, evaluated doses ranging from 40 Gy in 20 fractions to 20 Gy in five fractions and also included two small subgroups who received 12 Gy in two fractions or a single dose of 10 Gy, and a more recent trial from the United Kingdom Royal College of Radiologists compared doses of 12 Gy in two[61] fractions with 30 Gy in 10 fractions. Overall, no advantage for prolonged fractionation has been identified and doses of 12 Gy in two fractions or 20 Gy in five fractions are recommended. For primary intracranial tumours the results are less successful but where symptoms are not readily controlled, even in the patient with poor performance status, local radiotherapy in similar doses to control rising intracranial pressure may be of value in pain control.

Leptomeningeal disease may also cause persistent headache due either to rising intracranial pressure or obstructive hydrocephalus. Again, whole brain irradiation using similar doses to those for cerebral metastasis is indicated for symptom control.

Pelvic pain may arise from uncontrolled growth of intrapelvic tumour, typically presacral recurrence from colorectal cancer or recurrent uterine cancer. Local radiotherapy is effective in these patients achieving pain control in around 70 per cent and single doses of 10 Gy appear as effective as 30 Gy in 10 fractions in one small series.[62]

Hepatic pain

Pain due to rapid expansion of the liver secondary to metastasis may initially respond to steroids and where the tumour is chemosensitive then cytotoxic chemotherapy will be indicated. In many cases, however, this will not be appropriate and single arm studies have shown that radiation doses of 20 to 30 Gy delivered over 2 to 3 weeks to a rapidly enlarging liver mass are effective at controlling pain in around 70 per cent of patients.[63] This may be associated with some nausea which is more profound when large volumes of the liver are included in the treatment area.

Splenic pain

Progressive splenomegaly may be a feature of haematological malignancies, characteristically chronic myeloid leukaemia or myelodysplasia. These are typically exquisitely sensitive to low-dose radiation and doses of 5 to 10 Gy over 1 to 2 weeks will be effective in controlling the painful splenic enlargement.

Brachial plexus neuropathy

This may cause severe pain due to tumour infiltration into the brachial plexus either secondary to an apical lung cancer (superior sulcus syndrome) or recurrent breast cancer in the axilla. Local radiotherapy is again indicated in these circumstances where previous irradiation has not been delivered. Relatively high doses are often recommended in the hope of achieving good tumour regression and control, and indeed in the case of an apical carcinoma of the bronchus the presence of pain is not a contraindication to a radical course of radiotherapy. However, published outcome data is less optimistic with good pain control reported in less than 30 per cent of patients with Pancoast's tumour and no relation to radiation dose seen in one retrospective series.[64]

Surgery

In selected cases surgery has an important role in pain relief.

Pathological fracture

The management of a painful pathological fracture in a long bone is by means of internal surgical fixation. This will allow early stabilization of the fractured bone and mobilization of the patient. Postoperative radiotherapy may be indicated to improve local tumour control around the fracture site but should not be seen as a substitute for primary surgical treatment.

Hydrocephalus

Hydrocephalus due to malignant obstruction of the cerebrospinal fluid channels in the brain may cause persistent headache and is best managed by insertion of a surgical shunt.

Ablative neurosurgical procedures

Relatively few patients with cancer will require ablative neurosurgery for intractable pain as appropriate use of pharmacological methods of pain relief alongside anaesthetic blocks and TENS will result in adequate pain control for most patients. However, a small number may continue to have severe pain despite skilled attention and in these patients neurosurgery may have a role. Cordotomy is perhaps the most common procedure undertaken in which the anterior spinothalamic tract is destroyed, usually by introduction of a diathermy needle under fluoroscopic control. Typically, this will be selected for intractable unilateral pain, although occasionally bilateral cordotomy may be attempted. In single-arm studies high initial response rates are reported but recurrence of pain over subsequent months is common with response rates falling from over 90 per cent immediately after the procedure to under 50 per cent a year later.[65] Hypophysectomy has been described as a means of obtaining pain relief in severe intractable cases as has thalamotomy or cingulotomy.

Peripheral and autonomic nerve blocks

Selected patients may benefit from local anaesthetic or neurolytic blocking of peripheral nerves.

Intercostal nerve blocks are perhaps the most common example in palliative care but other nerves, including the brachial plexus, lumbar sacral plexus, and trigeminal nerve, are amenable to this technique if intractable pain associated with their distribution is a problem.

Coeliac plexus block is indicated in severe abdominal pain characteristically from pancreatic carcinoma but which can be related to any progressive intra-abdominal malignancy. This is one of the few scenarios which has been subject to randomized, controlled trial evaluation in which neurolytic coeliac plexus block has been found to be highly effective in the management of pain from advanced pancreatic cancer.[66]

Stellate ganglia block may be considered for pain arising in the upper limb and both lumbar sympathectomy and superior hypergastric plexus block may be of value in pain in the lower limb and pelvis.

Transcutaneous electrical nerve stimulation (TENS)

TENS is now widely available but still in many circumstances underused, particularly in the patient with advanced cancer. TENS relies upon active stimulation of large-diameter nerve fibres in the skin and subcutaneous tissues. Its use is based on the gate control theory of pain using an electrical stimulus through electrodes attached to the skin, which may be either continuous or pulsed to inhibit afferent pain pathways. A large number of commercial TENS machines are available with varying characteristics but all work on the same basic principle. The main indications for TENS are neuropathic pain either due to nerve compression or associated conditions such as herpes zoster. Occasionally, TENS may be of value for other visceral pain and pain from bone metastases. It is often reserved for intractable pain but there is no reason not to consider TENS as an important adjunct to early pain management while adjusting analgesic therapy where resources are available to provide nerve stimulators.[67]

Psychological pain treatment

As described in the early parts of this chapter, cancer pain has a major emotional component to it. Treatments which can address

this, therefore, are likely to have a significant impact upon pain control. Psychotherapy and cognitive behavioural techniques, such as relaxation therapy, allow the patient to participate in their treatment programme and may have a valuable role in enabling the pharmacological and other antinociceptive treatment to result in good pain control.

Other non-drug treatment

Acupuncture may have striking results in otherwise intractable pain.[67] It is particularly indicated where there is a neuropathic component to the pain and where there is muscle spasm.

Chronic lymphoedema of both upper and lower limbs may be due to surgery, radiotherapy, or recurrent disease. It is a difficult problem to treat and often produces considerable pain and discomfort. In the first instance an elastic stocking or sleeve should be used in conjunction with other measures including massage, limb exercises, compression bandaging, and the use of intermittent compression sleeve devices. Infection should be treated aggressively and some patients benefit from prophylactic antibiotics.

Local massage and the use of local heat or ice pack can also be of value for local painful sites where there may be soft tissue infiltration from tumour or bone metastasis.

Conclusions

Much can be done to alleviate pain associated with advanced and terminal cancer. The principles of pain management are to make a careful evaluation of the pain, identifying individual components and their cause, on the basis of which treatment can be tailored to the individual patient. An additional important principle is to keep treatment regimens as simple as possible within the confines of efficacy.

Cancer pain is but one component of the process of advanced and progressive malignancy. Its treatment should enable the patient to return to as normal a life as possible and will involve not only active pain management as described in this chapter but also physical, emotional, and practical support. A logical and integrated approach is required with co-ordination and co-operation from the various disciplines which may be involved.

Realistic goals are important and continuity of care, support, and follow-up are vital components of the overall pain management philosophy integrated within the wider field of palliative oncology and supporting palliative care services.

References

1. **International Association for the Study of Pain.** Classification of chronic pain. *Pain*, 1986; **Suppl. 3:** 51–226.
2. **Foley KM.** Pain assessment and cancer pain syndromes. In: Doyle D, Hanks GW, MacDonald N, eds. *Oxford textbook of palliative medicine.* 2nd edn. Oxford: Oxford University Press, 1998.
3. **Morris JN, Mor V, Goldberg RJ, Sherwood S, Greer DS, Hiris J.** The effect of treatment setting and patient characteristics on pain in terminal cancer patients: a report from the national hospice study. *Journal of Chronic Disease*, 1986; **39:** 27–35.
4. **Twycross RG, Fairfield S.** Pain in far-advanced cancer. *Pain*, 1982; **14:** 303–10.

5. World Health Organization. *Cancer pain relief and palliative care.* Geneva: World Health Organization, 1990.

6. Ventafridda V, Tamburini M, Caraceni A, DeConno F, Naldi F. A validation study of the WHO method for cancer pain relief. *Cancer*, 1987; **59**: 851–6.

7. Payne R. Cancer pain: anatomy, physiology and pharmacology. *Cancer*, 1989; **63**: 2266–74.

8. World Health Organization. *Cancer pain relief.* 2nd edn. Geneva: World Health Organization, 1996.

9. Portenoy CK. Adjuvant analgesics in pain management. In: Doyle D, Hanks GW, MacDonald N, eds. *Oxford textbook of palliative medicine.* 2nd edn. Oxford: Oxford University Press, 1998: 361–90.

10. Jadad AR, Browman GP. The WHO analgesic ladder for cancer pain management. *Journal of the American Medical Association*, 1995; **274**: 1870–3.

11. Sykes JV, Hanks GW. Non-opioid analgesics in the treatment of pain due to malignant disease. *Pain Reviews*, 1998; **5**: 32–50.

12. Brown P, Mehlisch DR, Minn F. Tramadol hydrochloride: efficacy compared to codeine sulfate, acetaminophen with dextropoxyphene and placebo in dental-extraction pain. *British Journal of Pharmacology*, 1989; **98**: 441.

13. Hoskin PJ, Hanks GW. Opioid agonist-antagonist drugs in acute and chronic pain states. *Drugs*, 1991; **46**: 326–44.

14. Boerner U, Abbott S, Roe RL. The metabolism of morphine and heroin in man. *Drug Metabolism Reviews*, 1975; **4**: 39–73.

15. Max MB, Inturrisi CE, Kaiko RF, Grabinski PY, Li CH, Foley KM. Epidural and intrathecal opiates: cerebrospinal fluid and plasma profiles in patients with chronic cancer pain. *Clinical Pharmacology and Therapeutics*, 1985; **38**: 631–41.

16. Sawe J, Dahlstrom B, Rane A. Steady state kinetics and analgesic effect of oral morphine in cancer patients. *European Journal of Clinical Pharmacology*, 1983; **24**: 537–42.

17. Hanks GW, Hoskin PJ, Aherne GW, Turner P, Poulain P. Explanation for potency of repeated oral doses of morphine. *Lancet*, 1987; **ii**: 723–5.

18. Osborne JR, Joel SP, Slevin ML. Morphine intoxication in renal failure: the role of morphine-6-glucuronide. *British Medical Journal*, 1986; **292**: 1548–9.

19. Expert Working Group of the European Association for Palliative Care. Morphine in cancer pain: modes of administration. *British Medical Journal*, 1996; **312**: 823–6.

20. Hoskin PJ, Hanks GW. The management of symptoms in advanced cancer: experience in a hospital-based continuing care unit. *Journal of the Royal Society of Medicine*, 1988; **81**: 341–4.

21. Hoskin PJ, Poulain P, Hanks GW. Controlled-release morphine in cancer pain: is a loading dose required when the formulation is changed? *Anaesthesia*, 1989; **44**: 897–901.

22. Hanks GW, Cherny N. Opioid analgesic therapy. In: Doyle D, Hanks GW, MacDonald N, eds. *Oxford textbook of palliative medicine.* 2nd edn. Oxford: Oxford University Press, 1998: 331–55.

23. Twycross RG. The therapeutic equivalence of oral and subcutaneous/intramuscular morphine sulphate in cancer patients. *Journal of Palliative Care*, 1988; **2**: 67–8.

24. Hanks GW. Antiemetics for terminal cancer patients. *Lancet*, 1982; **i**: 1410.

25. Hanks GW, Fallon MT. Transdermyl fentanyl in cancer pain: conversion from oral morphine. *Journal of Pain and Symptom Management*, 1995; **10**: 87.

26. Portenoy RK, Southam MA, Gupta SK, et al. Transdermal fentanyl for cancer pain: repeated dose pharmocokinetics. *Anaethesiology*, 1993; **78**: 36–43.

27. Southam MA. Transdermal fentanyl therapy: system design, pharmacokinetics and efficacy. *Anti-Cancer Drugs*, 1995; **6** (Suppl. 3): 26–34.

28. Ahmedzai S, Brooks D. Transdermal fentanyl versus sustained release oral morphine in cancer pain: preference, efficacy, and quality of life. The TTS-Fentanyl Comparative Trial Group. *Journal of Pain and Symptom Management*, 1997; **13**: 254–61.

29. Zenz M, Donner B, Strumpf M. Withdrawal symptoms during therapy with transdermal fentanyl (fentanyl TTS)? *Journal of Pain and Symptom Management*, 1994; **9**: 54–5.

30. Moulin DE, Kreeft JH, Murray PN, Bouquillon AI. Comparison of continuous subcutaneous and intravenous hydromorphone infusions for management of cancer pain. *Lancet*, 1991; **337**: 465–8.

31. Houde RW. Clinical analgesic studies of hydromorphone. In: Foley KM, Inturrisi CE, eds. *Advances in Pain Research and Therapy*, Vol. 8. New York: Raven Press, 1986: 129–36.

32. Anonymous. Phenazocine. *Drug Therapy Bulletin*, 1979; **18**: 70.

33. Ripamonti C, Groff L, Brunelli C, Polastri D, Stavrakis A, DeConno F. Switching from morphine to oral methadone in treating cancer pain: what is the equianalgesic dose ratio? *Journal of Clinical Oncology*, 1998; **16**: 3216–21.

34. Szeto HH, Inturrisi CE, Houde R, Saal R, Cheigh J, Reidenberg MM. Accumulation of normeperidine an active metabolite of meperidine, in patients with renal failure or cancer. *Annals of Internal Medicine*, 1977; **86**: 738–41.

35. Swann RA, Cousins MJ. Anaesthetic techniques for pain control. In: Doyle D, Hanks GW, MacDonald N, eds. *Oxford textbook of palliative medicine.* 2nd edn. Oxford: Oxford University Press, 1998.

36. Hanks GW, Twycross RG. Pain the physiological antagonist of morphine. *Lancet*, 1984; **i**: 1477–8.

37. Porter J, Jick H. Addiction rare in patients treated with narcotics. *New England Journal of Medicine*, 1980; **302**: 123.

38. Hanks GW, Forbes K. Opioid responsiveness. *Acta Anaesthesiologica Scandinavica*, 1997; **41**: 154–8.

39. Woolf CJ, Thompson SWN. The induction and maintenance of central sensitization is dependent on N-methyl-D-aspartic acid receptor activation: implications for the treatment of post-injury pain hypersensitivity states. *Pain*, 1991; **44**: 293–9.

40. Mercadante S. Ketamine in cancer pain: an update. *Palliative Medicine*, 1996; **10**: 225–30.

41. Coombes RC, Munro Neville A, Gazet J-C, et al. Agents affecting osteolysis in patients with breast cancer. *Cancer Chemotherapy and Pharmacology*, 1979; **3**: 41–4.

42. Langman MJS, Weil J, Wainwright P, et al. Risks of bleeding peptic ulcer associated with individual non-steroidal anti-inflammatory drugs. *Lancet*, 1994; **343**: 1075–8.

43. Graham DY, Agrawal NM, Roth SH. Prevention of NSAID-induced gastric ulcer with misprostol: a multicentre, double-blind placebo-controlled trial. *Lancet*, 1988; **ii**: 1277–80.

44. Blackwell N, Bangham L, Hughes M, Melzack S, Trotman I. Subcutaneous ketorolac—a new development in pain control. *Palliative Medicine*, 1993; **7**: 63–5.

45. Lasagna L, DeKornfeld TJ. Methotrimeprazine, a new phenothiazine derivative with analgesic properties. *Journal of the American Medical Association*, 1961; **178**: 887–90.

46. Davidson O, Lindenberg O, Walsh M. Analgesic treatment with levomepromazine in acute myocardial infarction. *Acta Medica Scandinavia*, 1979; **205**: 191–4.

47. Ventafridda V, Bonezzi C, Caraceni A, et al. Antidepressants for cancer pain and other painful syndromes with differentiation component: comparison of amitriptyline and trazadone. *Italian Journal of Neurological Science*, 1987; **8**: 579–87.

48. Swerdlow M, Cundill JG. Anticonvulsant drugs used in the treatment of lancinating pains. A comparison. *Anaesthesia*, 1981; **36**: 1129–32.

49. **Young RR, Delwaide PJ.** Spasticity. *New England Journal of Medicine,* 1981; **304**: 96–9.

50. **McCloskey EV, MacLennan ICM, Drayson MT, Chapman C, Dunn J, Kanis JA, for the MRC Working Party on Leukaemia in Adults.** A randomized trial of the effect of clodronate on skeletal morbidity in multiple myeloma. *British Journal of Haematology,* 1998; **100**: 317–25.

51. **Diel IJ, Solomayer E-F, Costa SD, *et al.*** Reduction in new metastases in breast cancer with adjuvant clodronate treatment. *New England Journal of Medicine,* 1998; **339**: 357–63.

52. **Tyrrell CT, Bruning PF, May-Levin P, *et al.*** Pamidronate infusions as single-agent therapy for bone metastases: A Phase II trial in patients with breast cancer. *European Journal of Cancer,* 1995; **31A**: 1976–80.

53. **Robertson AG, Reed NS, Ralston SH.** Effect of oral clodronate on metastatic bone pain: A double-blind, placebo-controlled study. *Journal of Clinical Oncology,* 1995; **13**: 2427–30.

54. **McQuay H, Carroll D, Moore RA.** Radiotherapy for painful bone metastases: a systematic review. *Clinical Oncology,* 1997; **9**: 150–4.

55. **Hoskin PJ.** Radiotherapy for bone pain. *Pain,* 1995; **63**: 137–9.

56. **UK Bone Pain Trial Working Party.** 8Gy single fraction radiotherapy for the treatment of metastatic skeletal pain: a comparison with a multifraction schedule over 12 months of patient follow up. *Radiotherapy and Oncology,* 1999, **52**: 111–21.

57. **Mithal NP, Needham PR, Hoskin PJ.** Retreatment with radiotherapy for painful bone metastases. *International Journal of Radiation Oncology Biology Physics,* 1994; **29**: 1011–14.

58. **Hoskin PJ.** Using radioisotopes for bone metastases. *European Journal of Palliative Care,* 1994; **1**: 78–82.

59. **Quilty PM, Kirk D, Bolger JJ, Dearnaley DP, Lewington V, Mason MD.** A comparison of the palliative effects of strontium 89 and external beam radiotherapy in metastatic prostate cancer. *Radiotherapy and Oncology,* 1994; **31**: 33–40.

60. **Priestman TJ, Dunn J, Brada M, Rampling R, Baker PG.** Final results of the Royal College of Radiologists' trial comparing two different radiotherapy schedules in the treatment of cerebral metastases. *Clinical Oncology,* 1996; **8**: 308–15.

61. **Borgelt B, Gelber R, Kramer S, *et al.*** The palliation of brain metastases: final results of the first two studies by the Radiation Therapy Oncology Group. *International Journal of Radiation Oncology Biology Physics,* 1980; **6**: 1–9.

62. **Allum WH, Mack P, Priestman TJ, Fielding JWL.** Radiotherapy for pain relief in locally recurrent colorectal cancer. *Annals of the Royal College of Surgeons of England,* 1987; **69**: 220–1.

63. **Borgelt B, Gelber R, Brady LW, Griffin T, Hendrickson FR.** The palliation of hepatic metastases: Results of the Radiation Therapy Oncology Group pilot study. *International Journal of Radiation Oncology Biology Physics,* 1981; 7: 587–91.

64. **Watson PN, Evans RJ.** Intractable pain with lung cancer. *Pain,* 1987; **29**: 163–73.

65. **Arbit E, Bilsky MH.** Neurosurgical approaches in palliative care. In: Doyle D, Hanks GW, MacDonald N, eds. *Oxford textbook of palliative medicine.* 2nd edn. Oxford: Oxford University Press, 1998: 414–20.

66. **Mercadante S.** Celiac plexus block versus analgesics in pancreatic cancer pain. *Pain,* 1993; **52**: 187–92.

67. **Thompson JW, Filshie J.** Transcutaneous electrical nerve stimulation (TENS) and acupuncture. In: Doyle D, Hanks GW, MacDonald N, eds. *Oxford textbook of palliative medicine.* 2nd edn. Oxford: Oxford University Press, 1998: 421–36.

6

Quality of life and psychosocial issues

Psychological sequelae of adult cancer and its treatment

Peter Maguire

Psychological morbidity in adult cancer patients

In the 1980s studies which used rigorous, standardized psychiatric assessments confirmed that the diagnosis and treatment of cancer in adults was associated with a substantial morbidity.[1] Major depressive illness, generalized anxiety disorder, and adjustment disorders were found in up to a third of patients. This represented an increased relative risk of three times the prevalence of affective disorders in the general population. Body image problems and sexual difficulties were also found to be more common in cancer patients.[2] Organic confusional states were evident in up to 10 per cent. Even when cancer patients were free of disease and no longer on treatment, a substantial minority failed to return to their former level of psychological, social, and occupational adjustment and experienced a persistent impairment in their quality of life.

This knowledge should have led to effective ways of reducing this morbidity. However, Fallowfield *et al.* (1990)[3] found that a quarter of patients still developed affective disorders after surgery for breast cancer. Parle, Jones, and Maguire (1996), in a 2-year prospective study of 600 cancer patients with heterogeneous diagnoses, found a prevalence of affective disorder of 20 per cent.[4] Zabora *et al.* (1997)[5] found that 35 per cent of a sample of 386 adult cancer patients selected at random from 12 oncology outpatient departments across the United States obtained scores on the Brief Symptom Inventory consistent with a psychiatric disorder.

Thus, most cancer patients and relatives cope well psychologically but a substantial minority do not. A key question is what factors make them vulnerable to affective disorders. If there are factors that could be modified, effective interventions could be developed.

Aetiological factors in affective disorders

Impact of diagnosis

Uncertainty

In some patients, anxiety and/or depression develops because they fail to come to terms with the knowledge that they have cancer. They fear that the cancer will return, cause physical and mental suffering, and a premature death. They are unable to control these fears despite their best efforts. Reminders that they have cancer, such as reading a magazine article or watching a television programme, intensifies their fears. Their worries will be particularly intense if they have had bad experiences of cancer in a close friend or relative.

Search for meaning

People faced with a serious, life-threatening illness try to find a satisfactory explanation for why they have developed it. They are more likely to adapt psychologically if they can find one. With coronary heart disease this is relatively easy since risk factors have been identified, such as a strong family history, faulty diet, lack of exercise, or heavy smoking. No such explanations are available for most cancers. This leaves a vacuum into which patients and relatives project non-scientific theories. Popular lay theories include the notion that cancer is due to a flaw in personality such as an inability to cope with stress or difficulty in expressing emotions such as anger. Patients accepting these theories then blame themselves for their predicament, and experience lowered self-esteem and demoralization. Patients may blame key relatives or employers because they judge them to be a major source of stress. The resultant bitterness hinders their ability to adapt to their diagnosis and may cause problems in their personal relationships.

Stigma

Some patients feel stigmatized by their disease. They use words such as 'unclean', 'contagious', or 'leprosy' to describe this. Feelings of stigma are likely when the cancer has been linked with undesirable behaviours, as in women with cervical cancer where it is alleged that it can be due to sexual promiscuity. Stigma is also evident when the cancer has been linked with viruses, as in leukaemia. Their embarrassment may cause them to avoid others and become isolated. Such stigma is strongly linked to later affective disorders.

Being secretive

When patients worry about the acceptability of their diagnosis and treatment to close friends, relatives, or employers they may keep their diagnosis secret. They may also keep it hidden because they wish to protect a loved one from anguish. Secretiveness is associated with a poorer psychological adaptation because it prevents them receiving emotional and practical support from family and friends.

Loss of control

Patients cope better with life-threatening illnesses if they believe that they can contribute something positive towards the outcome whether this is realistic or not. In coronary heart disease there are obvious risk factors that patients can modify, such as weight, diet, and exercise.

Patients with cancer have no strong risk factors they can modify apart from smoking. They may then feel helpless and helplessness is associated with later depressive illness. Helplessness is also probable when patients believe they have done their best to preserve their health through adopting a healthy lifestyle but then discover that they have developed cancer. It is also likely if they believe their cancer was caused by stress and the stress is ongoing.

Some patients try to improve their chances of survival by modifying their diet and level of exercise. They will generally cope well unless they become obsessed about changes in their lifestyle and this causes friction within their families.

Patients may also seek to improve their mental well being and sense of mastery by using relaxation, visualization, yoga, or meditation. While relaxation with guided imagery or relaxation alone reduces distress[6] the impact of the other methods is unclear.

Receiving medical and nursing support

Patients who feel that their concerns have not been understood and responded to appropriately by the doctors and nurses providing their care are more vulnerable to affective disorders. They may contribute to this by not disclosing their concerns.

Treatment

Loss of a body part

Treatment may involve the surgical removal of a body part such as a breast or limb. The patient then has to come to terms with the change in body image. This will be difficult if the body part was important to their sense of psychological well being. For example up to 25 per cent of women fail to adapt to the loss of a breast despite being given an adequate external breast prosthesis.[7] Three types of problems may develop singly or in combination. The patient cannot accept that she is no longer physically whole. This loss of physical integrity makes her more vulnerable psychologically. She finds it harder to adapt to other stressful life events. Another patient may feel a heightened self-consciousness and worry that people have only to look at her to realize she has lost a breast even when she conceals her shape by wearing baggy clothes. Some women feel less attractive and feminine and are not reassured by their partners' claims that they love them as much as before surgery. Continued inability to adapt to the loss of a body part or mutilation, whether due to loss of a breast, surgery to the head and neck, or amputation of a limb, is highly correlated with subsequent affective disorders.[8]

When surgery results in complications such as pain, impairment of movement, and swelling levels of psychological morbidity are greater[9] since they hinder physical recovery and provide frequent reminders of the cancer diagnosis.

Loss of body function

Up to 32 per cent of patients who have a stoma after a cancer of the large bowel is removed become morbidly anxious and/or depressed.[10],[11] Bekkers et al. (1995)[12] recently confirmed that these problems remain prevalent despite the advent of stoma nurses. Patients cannot accept the stoma because it represents an 'obscene' part of themselves and/or may be unable to accept the bag because they fear it will bulge, leak, smell, burst, or make inappropriate noises. They worry that it could have serious adverse effects on their personal

relationships and employment. Those who have yet to form a close personal relationship and/or are homosexual face a difficult dilemma. Should they mention their stoma to a potential partner and at what point? While fears associated with the bag and fears of personal rejection contribute to these sexual difficulties, surgical destruction of the nerve supply to the genital organs can result in difficulties in ejaculation, frigidity, or inability to have an orgasm. Loss of other bodily functions, such as the loss of a voice after laryngectomy[8] or problems with eating and drinking after surgery for oral cancers,[13] also increase vulnerability to anxiety and depression.

Radiotherapy

Radiotherapy is explained to patients on the basis that it will destroy any residual cancer cells. This can have a paradoxical effect when patients were led to believe that they had a good prognosis ('They said all they needed was to remove the lump. I thought I was clear. Then they said I needed radiotherapy as an insurance. How do I square the two? I am worried that the cancer is still there'). Radiotherapy may also increase the risk of depression via a fatigue syndrome where patients complain of feeling increasingly exhausted towards the end of treatment. Their fatigue fails to lift and biological symptoms of depression develop (see later). These indirect and direct effects of radiotherapy may explain why women undergoing breast conservation followed by radiotherapy experience slightly more psychiatric morbidity than those undergoing mastectomy.[14],[15]

Radiotherapy can also cause morbidity through direct physical damage. Women with cancer of the cervix given radiotherapy via internal sources may develop anatomical damage in the vagina including stenosis and fibrosis. This may cause profound sexual problems, anxiety, and depression.[16],[17] A strong relationship has been found between adverse effects caused by radiotherapy and subsequent psychiatric morbidity.[18]

Chemotherapy

Chemotherapy also increases psychological morbidity and sexual problems, particularly when given in combination. Psychiatric morbidity is linked to adverse side-effects, notably gastrointestinal effects such as nausea, vomiting, and diarrhoea,[18] and to treatment given for longer than 6 months.[19] Conditioned nausea and vomiting also increases the risk of anxiety and depression. Characteristically, patients experience nausea and vomiting during the first two courses of treatment. Then they find that any sound, sight, or smell which reminds them of treatment provokes the same adverse effects reflexively. This leads to phobic avoidance of treatment.

Prior to the advent of $5HT_3$ serotonin antagonists such as odansetron, granisetron, and tropisetron, anticipatory nausea and vomiting occurred in 25 per cent of patients on chemotherapy. Even after their introduction and use in 14 per cent of an outpatient sample of 95 chemotherapy patients, the prevalence of anticipating nausea and vomiting appeared no different (23 per cent).[20] While clinical practice suggests that these conditioned responses have lessened with better antiemetic agents this requires to be proven.

In other patients on chemotherapy, the mood disturbance is better explained in terms of direct effects on the brain. Some patients become acutely depressed within a few hours of an infusion. Others find it hard to cope with cognitive impairments.

In a rigorous assessment of 28 breast cancer patients who had completed chemotherapy 0.5 to 12 months previously, 75 per cent

Plate for Chapter 1.1

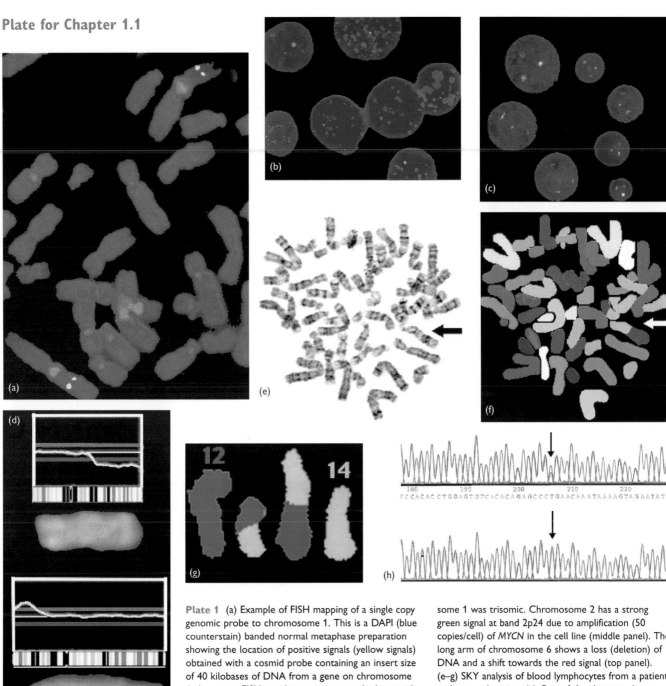

Plate 1 (a) Example of FISH mapping of a single copy genomic probe to chromosome 1. This is a DAPI (blue counterstain) banded normal metaphase preparation showing the location of positive signals (yellow signals) obtained with a cosmid probe containing an insert size of 40 kilobases of DNA from a gene on chromosome 1. A positive FISH signal is present on each chromatid of both pairs of chromosome 1 at band 1q25. (b) *MYCN* amplification in nuclei from neuroblastoma detected by FISH with a *MYCN* probe (magenta speckling) and a deletion of the short arm of chromosome 1. The signal (pale blue/green) from the remaining normal chromosome 1 is seen as a single spot in each nucleus. (c) Detection of a Philadelphia chromosome in interphase nuclei of leukaemia cells. All nuclei contain one green signal (BCR gene), one pink signal (ABL gene), and an intermediate fusion yellow signal because of the 9;22 chromosome translocation. (d) The comparative genomic hybridization analysis profile from a neuroblastoma cell line. Chromosome 1 shows an overall gain of DNA indicated by an increase in the level of green signal (bottom panel). In this cell line most of chromo-

some 1 was trisomic. Chromosome 2 has a strong green signal at band 2p24 due to amplification (50 copies/cell) of *MYCN* in the cell line (middle panel). The long arm of chromosome 6 shows a loss (deletion) of DNA and a shift towards the red signal (top panel). (e–g) SKY analysis of blood lymphocytes from a patient with a translocation. (e) One of the aberrant chromosomes can be seen by classical G-banding; (f) the same metaphase spread has been subjected to SKY; and (g) the 12;14 reciprocal translocation is identified. (h) Automated sequencing of BRCA2, the hereditary breast cancer predisposition gene. Each coloured peak represents a different nucleotide. The lower panel is a sequence of a wild-type DNA sample. The sequence of a mutation carrier in the upper panel contains a double peak (indicated by an arrow) in which the nucleotide 'T' in intron 17 located at 2 bp downstream of the 5' end of exon 18 is converted to a 'C'. This mutation results in aberrant splicing of exon 18 of the BRCA2 gene. The presence of a 'T' nucleotide in addition to the mutant 'C' implies that only one copy of the two BRCA2 genes is mutated in this sample.

Plate for Chapter 2.1

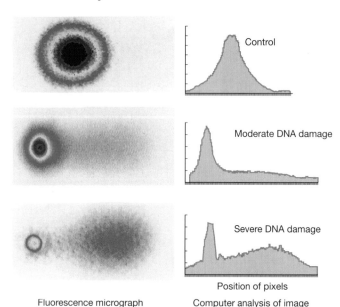

Fluorescence micrograph   Computer analysis of image

Plate 1 Measurement of DNA damage by the single cell gel electrophoresis 'Comet' assay. Individual cells from chemical agent-treated cultures or animals are embedded in agarose gels, lysed, and subjected to electrophoresis under neutral or alkaline conditions. DNA strand breaks allow the DNA to migrate into the gel to an extent that is proportional to the number of strand breaks and this can be quantitated by computerized image analysis of individual cells in the gel (located by eye). The Y-axes indicate the integrated fluorescence intensity of the pixels on the corresponding micrographs.

Plate for Chapter 3.3

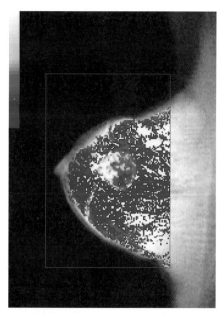

Plate 1 Transfer constant map shows the permeability surface area product of the vasculature, displayed as a pixel map superimposed on the anatomical image (maximum transfer constant displayed is 2 min^{-1}). Highly heterogeneous enhancement is also typical of cancer.

Plates for Chapter 3.1

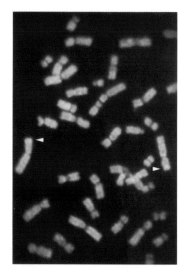

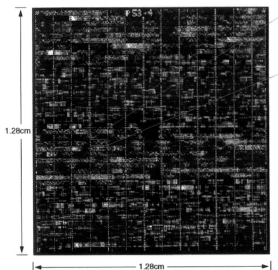

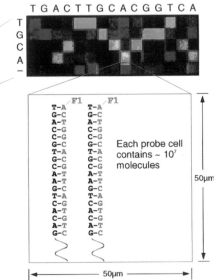

Plate 1 Example of CGH analysis. The DNA from a neuroblastoma cell line was labelled in green and normal DNA was labelled in red and these were co-hybridized to normal metaphase chromosomes. Then greener areas correspond to over-representation and the redder areas, under-representation in the sample. The arrows indicate an amplicon on chromosome 2 corresponding to genomic amplification (multiple gene copies) of the NMYC gene.

Plate 2 This is an Affymetrix Gene Chip for the entire coding region of the human p53 tumour suppressor gene (exons 2–11). Probes on the array are arranged in sets of five. Each probe in the set is perfectly complementary to the reference sequence except for a mismatch position, called the 'substitution position'. At the substitution position, each of the four possible nucleotides (A,C,G,T) and a single base deletion are represented in the probe set.

Assay conditions optimize hybridization of the fluorescently labelled DNA target to the probe that best matches its sequence. This hybrid yields a higher fluorescence intensity relative to the four target:probe hybrid set. There are probe sets complementary to every base in the target gene, so each base along the gene is examined for the presence of mutant sequence (both missense and single base deletions).

Plate for Chapter 3.5

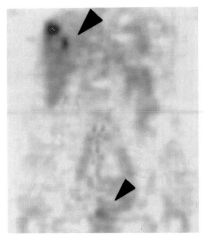

Plate 1 Positron emission tomograph for a patient with colorectal cancer treated by hemicolectomy 2 years previously. Metastatic tumour masses in the liver (above) and a mass in the proximity of the bladder (below) can be seen, suspected to be a local recurrence (by courtesy of Dr W. Weber).

Plates for Chapter 4.3

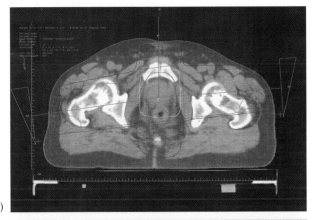

(a)

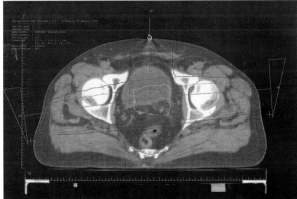

(b)

Plate 1 Two transverse cross-sections of the pelvis generated by X-ray computer tomography in a patient with prostate cancer. The tomograms are used to define and outline the planning target volume. The non-target rectum is also outlined on contiguous anatomical sections, here shown through the centre (a) and upper (b) levels of the radiotherapy volume. X-ray absorption data derived from X-ray computer tomography have been used directly to calculate the radiotherapy isodose distributions. These are shown as dark lines in the figures, based on the intersection of one anterior and two wedged lateral radiotherapy fields. The white 95 per cent isodose encompasses the target volume at both levels (black outline inside 95 per cent isodose).

Plate for Chapter 4.6

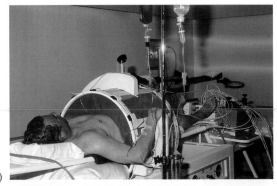

(a)

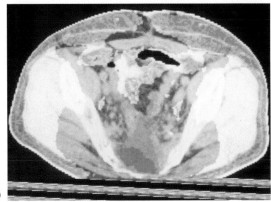

(b)

Plate 1 (a) A patient undergoing deep microwave hyperthermia for locally advanced rectal cancer using a phase array system. (b) Heat distribution shown following invasive thermometry. (Illustration provided by Professor P. Wust, Department of Diagnostic Radiology and Radiation Oncology, Chatité, Humboldt University of Berlin, Germany.)

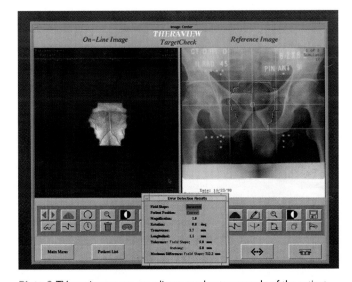

Plate 2 TV monitor screen on a linear accelerator console of the patient represented in Figs 11 and 12 (Chapter 4.3). On the right, the reference image generated by a simulator show a 'beam's eye view' of the anterior field, shaped using a multileaf collimator. The bony outline of the pubis is used to verify the accuracy of field replacement during therapy by imaging the exit beam of the linear accelerator, shown in the on-line image on the left. These two views are compared and verified on a daily basis, with adjustments if defined tolerance limits are not met.

Plate for Chapter 5.3

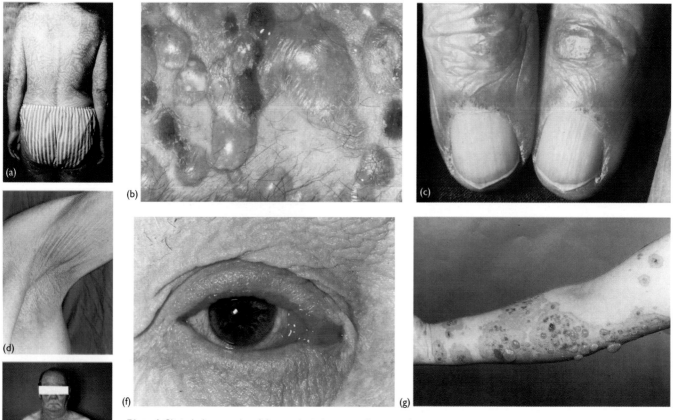

Plate 1 Clinical photographs of dermatological paraneoplastic conditions.

Plates for Chapter 8.1

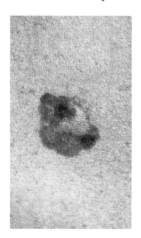

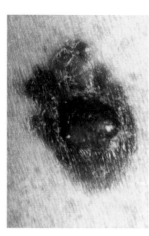

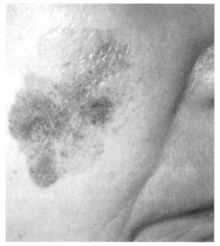

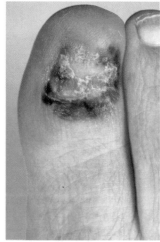

Plate 1 Superficial spreading melanomas. Note irregular border, variations in colour, and area of partial regression.

Plate 2 Nodular melanoma in pre-existing naevus.

Plate 3 Lentigo maligna melanoma with hypopigmented areas in the lesion representing regression.

Plate 4 Acral lentiginous melanoma: subungual melanoma of the big toe.

Plates for Chapter 9.1.4

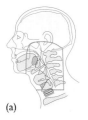 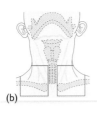

(a)　　　　　(b)

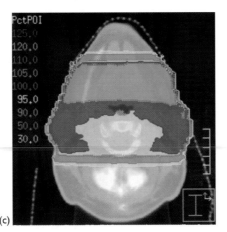 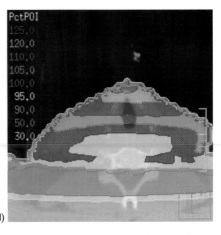

(c)　　　　　(d)

Plate 1 Carcinoma of the base of tongue: large radiation portals. (a) Parallel-opposed lateral portals include the primary lesion, larynx, hypopharynx, most of the cervical spinal cord, and the upper portion of the trachea and cervical oesophagus. Treatment through this portal tangentially irradiates the skin of the anterior neck unnecessarily. If an anterior field is not used to irradiate the low neck, the inferior border of the lateral field may be placed near the clavicle (dashed line). (b) Anterior low-neck portal. The wide midline tracheal block partially shields the low internal jugular lymph nodes, which are located adjacent to the trachea. The supraclavicular lymph nodes, which are less likely to be involved with tumour than the low jugular nodes, are adequately covered. (c) Central axis dosimetry at the level of the base-of-tongue primary lesion. The dose distribution was obtained using parallel-opposed 6-MV X-ray fields weighted equally.

(d) Off-axis contour through larynx. The minimum dose to most of the larynx is 5 per cent higher than the minimum tumour dose specified at the central axis, and a small amount of the anterior larynx receives approximately 25 per cent more irradiation. If the base-of-tongue tumour dose is specified as 50 Gy at 2 Gy per fraction, the maximum larynx dose will be in excess of 62.5 Gy at 2.5 Gy per fraction. (a) and (b) from Mendenhall WM, Parsons JT, Million RR. Unnecessary irradiation of the normal larynx (Editorial). *International Journal of Radiation Oncology Biology Physics*, 1990; **18**:1531–3.

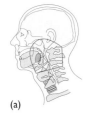 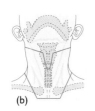

(a)　　　　　(b)

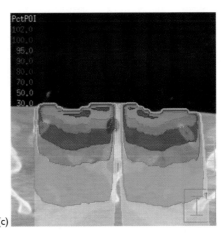 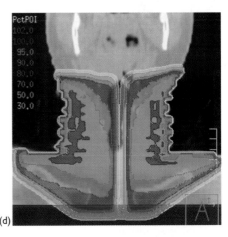

(c)　　　　　(d)

Plate 2 Carcinoma of the base of tongue: radiation portals sparing the larynx. (a) Parallel-opposed fields include the primary lesion with a 2 to 3 cm inferior margin. The lower border of the field is placed at the thyroid notch and slants superiorly as the junction line proceeds posteriorly. This substantially reduces the amount of mucosa, larynx, and spinal cord included in the primary treatment portals. (b) *En face* low portal with tapered midline larynx block. It is not necessary to treat the supraclavicular fossa unless clinically positive nodes are found in that particular hemineck. A 5-mm midline tracheal block may be placed in the low-neck portal (dashed line). (c) Axial and (d) sagittal. Dose distribution under a 5-mm midline tracheal block with an anterior 6-MV X-ray field. (a) and (b) from Mendenhall WM, Parsons JT, Million RR. Unnecessary irradiation of the normal larynx (Editorial). *International Journal of Radiation Oncology Biology Physics*, 1990; **18**:1531–3.

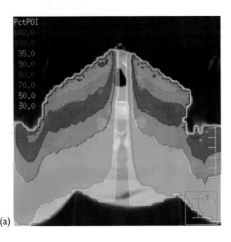 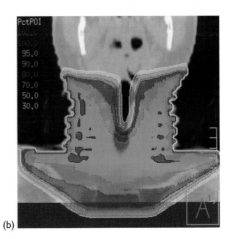

(a)　　　　　(b)

Plate 3 Dose distribution for an anterior 6-MV X-ray field to the lower neck. (a) Axial contour through the level of the thyroid notch. (b) Sagittal contour. The source-to-skin distance (SSD) marker is placed on the anterior surface of the sternocleidomastoid opposite the cricoid cartilage. The internal jugular chain lymph nodes receive a minimum dose that is 80 to 85 per cent of the maximum dose. When 50 Gy is administered to the depth of maximum dose (Dmax), these nodes receive more than 40 Gy. The larynx and spinal cord are shielded by an anterior lead block.

Plates for Chapter 9.1.4 *(continued)*

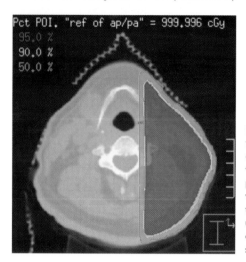

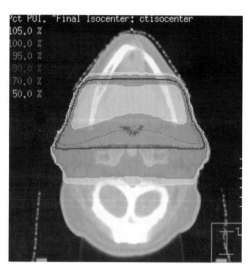

Plate 4 Dose distribution for anterior and posterior wedge 6-MV X-ray portals, both fields weighted 1.0. This technique can be used to boost the dose to one or both sides of the neck.

Plate 5 Dose distribution for parallel-opposed ^{60}Co portals, each weighted 1.0, with reduced 6-MV X-ray portals, each weighted 0.4.

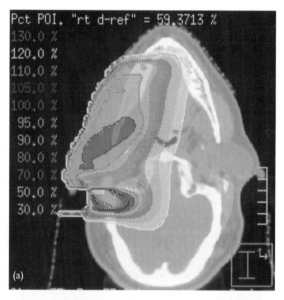

(a)

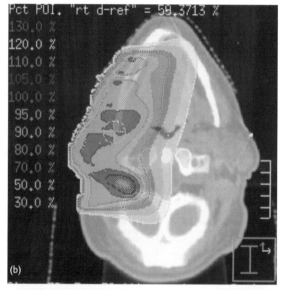

(b)

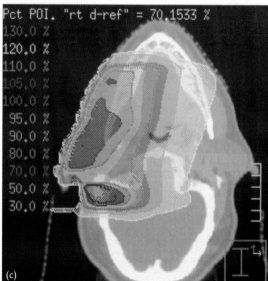

(c)

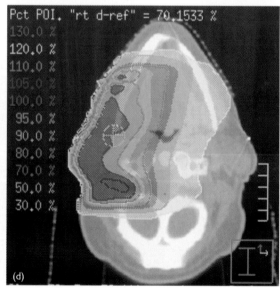

(d)

Plate 6 (a) and (b). Two axial CT slices through the oropharynx showing the dose distribution for 20-MeV electrons, source-to-skin distance 100 cm. (c) and (d) The same two axial CT slices showing the dose distribution for 20-MeV electrons and 6-MV X-rays, source-to-skin distance 100 cm for both. The given doses are weighted 3:2. The addition of the 6-MV X-ray beam reduces the surface dose and gives a dose distribution that is affected less by bone with a minimally increased exit dose to the contralateral side.

Plates for Chapter 9.3

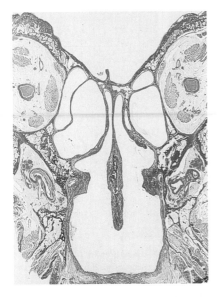

Plate 1 Coronal midfacial section showing pathways of spread from the nose and paranasal sinuses to the orbit, cribriform plate, and anterior cranial fossa.

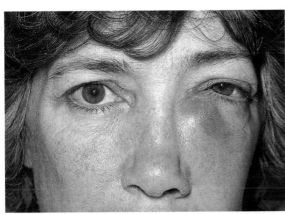

Plate 2 Clinical photograph showing squamous cell carcinoma of left maxilla involving anterior soft tissues of cheek and medial canthus with extension into the inferomedial orbit.

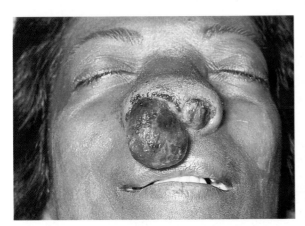

Plate 3 Clinical photograph showing a poorly differentiated squamous-cell carcinoma occupying both nasal cavities.

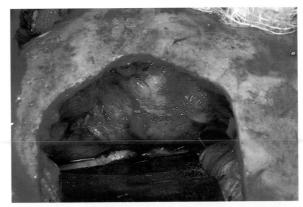

Plate 4 Intraoperative photograph of an anterior craniotomy showing a chondrosarcoma extending through the cribriform plate and ethmoid sinus to involve the dura.

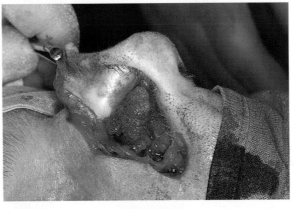

Plate 5 Intraoperative photograph showing the exposure obtained by lateral rhinotomy to reveal a primary mucosal malignant melanoma.

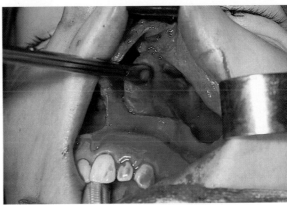

Plate 6 Intraoperative photograph showing mobilization of an angiofibroma from the left nasal cavity, nasopharynx, and left pterygomaxillary region via a midfacial degloving approach.

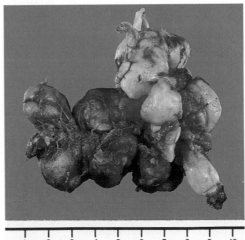

Plate 7 Operative specimen showing an extensive angiofibroma with components that occupied the posterior nasal cavity, nasopharynx, sphenoid, pterygomaxillary, and infratemporal fossa regions.

Plates for Chapter 9.3 *(continued)*

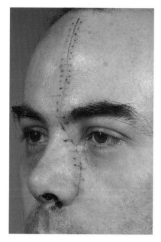

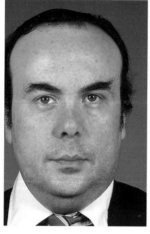

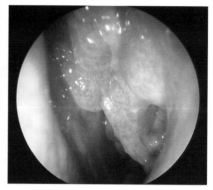

Plate 12 Endoscopic photograph of an inverted papilloma in the middle meatus.

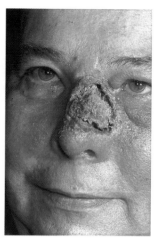

Plate 8 Postoperative photograph 10 days following craniofacial resection.

Plate 9 Photograph of the same patient 22 months later.

Plate 13 Clinical photograph showing a T-cell lymphoma of the nose.

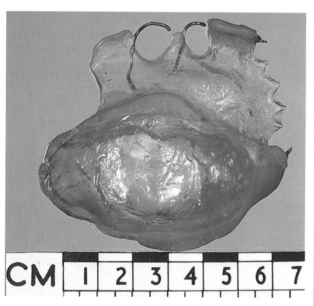

Plate 10 Lightweight acrylic maxillary obturator.

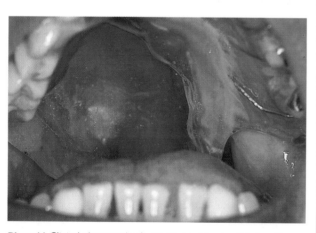

Plate 11 Clinical photograph of a maxillary obturator fitted orally.

Plate for Chapter 9.4

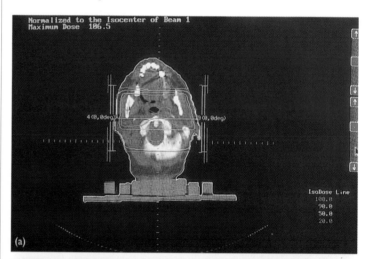

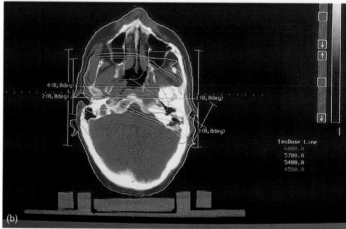

Plate 1 (a) and (b) Examples of dose distribution for lateral portals with 6 MV photons to deliver definitive irradiation to a nasopharyngeal carcinoma. A total dose to 70 Gy can be given to the target with reducing fields.

exhibited moderate cognitive impairments. The impairments were evident in verbal and visual memory, mental flexibility and speed of processing, attention and concentration, visuospatial ability, and motor function.[21] They were related to the length of chemotherapy. Van Dam et al.[22] also subjected breast cancer patients to a battery of neuropsychological tests 2 years after chemotherapy; 32 per cent of those randomized to high-dose chemotherapy had cognitive impairment compared with 17 per cent of those given standard dose treatment and 9 per cent of controls.

Body image problems such as hair loss are usually temporary and have little effect on psychological morbidity. However, chemotherapy can depress oestrogen levels and elevate follicular stimulating and luteinizing hormones. This causes infertility and a premature menopause in premenopausal women. Such effects are most likely when chemotherapy is used as an adjuvant. There is uncertainty about the extent to which these changes are reversible after chemotherapy. In women treated with chemotherapy for Hodgkin's disease and non-Hodgkin's lymphoma, persistent sexual problems were found in over a third of those patients who had a good sexual relationship beforehand.[18]

Chemotherapy in men mainly affects the germinal epithelium of the testis. It can lead to reduced ability to produce sperm and to infertility. Chemotherapy may also reduce Leydig cell function. The risk of permanent gonadal dysfunction appears minimal in patients with normal function before treatment.[23] While persistent sexual problems were found in one-quarter of the men treated with combination chemotherapy for Hodgkin's disease and non-Hodgkin's lymphoma,[18] sexual problems were more temporary in men treated for testicular cancer.[24] Alkylating agents are most likely to cause sexual problems.[25] The use of interferon is associated with greater fatigue, depression, anxiety, and hallucinatory experiences.[26]

Other treatments

Steroids can cause depression, mania, confusional states, a paranoid reaction, or a combination of these. Studies of bone marrow transplantation have suggested that fears about treatment-related mortality, concerns about the donor, and the experience of prolonged isolation all serve to increase psychiatric morbidity in the short and longer term. High levels of psychological morbidity are evident prior to the transplant and persist afterwards.[27] Autologous bone marrow transplantation is less toxic. Patients do not become as sick, graft-versus-host disease is not a danger, and neutropenia is brief. Even so, a third of patients develop affective disorders.

Disease status

Fallowfield et al. (1990)[3] found anxiety and depression in 25 per cent of women in the first year after diagnosis. Hall et al. (1996)[28] using a similar methodology found that 50 per cent of women with a recurrence of breast cancer were clinically depressed. This suggests that the incidence of affective disorders is greater in patients with advanced disease.

Patients' concerns

Weisman and Worden (1977) found that the number of concerns patients had about their predicament after diagnosis predicted high levels of emotional distress.[29] Recent work has confirmed that the number and severity of patients' concerns after diagnosis predicts the later development of anxiety and depression.[4] Patients who perceive they were given too much or too little information and insufficient opportunity to consider treatment options are also more vulnerable to affective disorders.[3]

Aetiology of organic confusional states

These disorders are more likely to occur as the cancer progresses. A confusional state may herald a recurrence of cancer or metastatic spread, particularly to the brain. It may also be due to metabolic changes such as hypercalcaemia, liver failure, hyponatraemia, and hypomagnasaemia caused by the tumour or secretion of atopic hormones and other substances. Less exotic but important causes include the withdrawal of hypnotics, drug and alcohol abuse, infections, trauma to the brain, and other electrolyte and fluid disturbances.

Failure to elicit problems

Unfortunately, the key concerns of cancer patients and psychological morbidity tend to go unrecognized by those involved in their care. Early studies in the 1970s found that doctors seriously underestimated the presence of depression and tended to be unduly affected by patients reports of personal inadequacy, self-depreciation, and anxiety. Hardman et al. (1989) assessed psychiatric morbidity in 126 medical oncology patients using rigorous assessment methods and then asked the doctors and nurses looking after them to make a judgement about these patients' mental state.[30] Less than half of those found to have a depressive illness were detected by the medical and nursing staff. Anxiety was diagnosed correctly in 79 per cent of patients affected but only at the cost of wrongly labelling as morbidly anxious 40 per cent of those who had a normal mental state. This represents a general problem in medical practice.

Similarly, oncologists working in outpatient clinics show a poor ability to recognize which of their patients are distressed.[31] Even in a hospice setting only 40 per cent of patients' concerns are elicited.[32] So, the reasons for this poor recognition need to be understood if the psychological care of patients is to be improved. Both patients and health-care professionals contribute to this.

Patient-led barriers

Patients believe that psychological and social problems are an inevitable consequence of having cancer and cancer treatment. Therefore, nothing can be done to alleviate these problems and there is no point in mentioning them. If they disclose psychological concerns this will detract from the time spent on their physical care and could compromise their physical survival. They also worry that they could be viewed as ungrateful, inadequate, or uncooperative by the clinician responsible for their care. They notice that doctors and nurses are busy and have many patients to look after. Hence, they do not want to burden them further, particularly if they have grown to like them and respect them. Just as they try to protect their close relatives from distress, they pretend that they are coping much better than they are lest health professionals are upset at learning of their true suffering.

Through their interactions with doctors and nurses, patients perceive that few doctors and nurses ask them directly about their concerns, particularly those related to psychological and social aspects. Objective scrutiny of consultations between doctors and patients[33] and between nurses and patients[34] has confirmed that little of the interaction focuses on psychosocial concerns. Instead, it is doctor-led and centres on physical issues (see also Chapter 6.2).

Faced with this lack of active enquiry, patients try to give verbal or non-verbal cues about their concerns. Such cues may include a statement about change in mood ('Since my operation I have felt increasingly low, I can't seem to snap out of it'), body image problems ('I can't bear to look at my stoma, I find it very difficult to manage') or sexual difficulties ('Things are no longer the same between us'). These are either ignored by the doctor or dealt with superficially.

Patients also claim that doctors and nurses respond in a way which makes them unwilling to disclose further information. No attempt is made to acknowledge and explore why they are distressed. So, they learn that it is only legitimate to mention physical aspects.

Professional-led barriers

In-depth interviews with doctors and nurses and direct observations of their consultations with cancer patients and relatives through audio and video recordings have confirmed that patients' perceptions are correct.[34] Questions which focus directly on psychological aspects such as 'How have you been feeling about your illness'? 'How have you felt about losing a breast'? or 'Has your operation had any affect on your relationship with your partner'? are asked rarely (see also Chapter 6.2).

When patients and relatives signal they have major concerns by giving verbal and/or non-verbal cues such as 'I am worried about the future, I don't think I am going to make it', doctors and nurses move the dialogue into emotionally safer areas by using distancing strategies.

Distancing tactics

Premature reassurance and advice

When doctors and nurses hear patients' concerns they tend to offer reassurance immediately before they have checked if the patient has other important concerns. This strong temptation to move into an information and advice mode arises from a genuine belief that this reassures the patient. In practice this is not the case.

Doctor	I have explained to you that you have a form of cancer of the lymph glands, that is a lymphoma. I am confident that it will respond to treatment with strong drugs, that is chemotherapy.
Patient	Yes, but . . .
Doctor	I think we should get on with chemotherapy straight away so that we can get the best response. Is that all right?
Patient	I am not . . .
Doctor	Let me tell you exactly what this chemotherapy will involve.

This patient did not register what was being said because he was terrified chemotherapy would make him sterile. The doctor should have checked how the patient felt about what he was being told and what his concerns were.

Switching

When a patient signals that he wishes to discuss a potentially distressing problem the doctor or nurse may deliberately or unwittingly switch the topic.

Doctor	How have you been getting on since your mastectomy?
Patient	Getting on, I haven't. It has been awful. I just can't bear to look at myself.
Doctor	How has the pain in your arm been?

False reassurance

When doctors and nurses realize that patients are worried about their prognosis they offer false reassurance to ease the patient's distress.

Patient	I am not going to get any better, am I?
Doctor	Of course, you are. You must stop being so pessimistic.

Selective attention to physical aspects

Here, the doctor or nurse pays heed only to physical aspects.

Doctor	How have you been getting on since your chemotherapy started?
Patient	I have felt less tired and I have begun to put weight on but my hair has begun to fall out. I feel so embarrassed. I'm reluctant to go out.
Doctor	You are less tired, you have put weight on, that sounds good. How else have you been physically?

Normalization

When doctors and nurses face distressed patients every day they tend to habituate to it and explain it away as normal.

Patient	I'm so upset it has got to this stage. I wanted to stay at home (begins to cry and looks very distressed).
Doctor	Of course you are upset. You're bound to be. Everybody is when they come into the hospice.

Jollying along

When doctors or nurses notice a patient is looking miserable, for example on a ward round, they seek to jolly them along by saying 'Come on Mr Smith, there is no need to look so glum'.

Recent research has confirmed that these behaviours inhibit patient disclosure of their major concerns.[36] So, it is important to consider why doctors and nurses dedicated to cancer care use these strategies.

Reasons for distancing

In-depth interviews with doctors and nurses[35],[36] have revealed clear reasons.

Fear of probing

Doctors and nurses consider that their professional training has not equipped them to deal with psychological aspects of care. They fear that probing psychologically to check how patients view their futures ('How do you see things working out') will raise patients' anxieties and unleash strong emotions which they would not be able to contain. This might cause irrevocable psychological harm. Similarly, questions like 'How have you felt about having a stoma'? or 'How is chemo-therapy going'? might also unleash such strong emotions that they would not know what to do next. Therefore, it is better to 'keep the lid on'. Behind these views is a belief that patients are psychologically fragile. Saying one wrong thing could cause lasting damage.

Fear of difficult questions

They fear that getting into effective dialogue with patients about their concerns might encourage patients to ask them difficult questions such as 'Am I going to get better, am I dying, or why didn't you diagnose it sooner'. They do not know how to respond.

Adverse emotional consequences

If doctors and nurses interview more effectively and establish the true nature of their patients' suffering, and its impact on their daily lives and their families, it will bring them close to unpleasant realities. If they confront these too often it could adversely affect their own emotional survival. They find deaths of younger patients and/or of those who remind them of people in their own lives especially painful. They worry that getting close to patients and relatives will lead them to question the value of medicine in general and their own role in particular if these patients die despite their best efforts. So, it is preferable to use distancing tactics to prevent themselves getting too close emotionally to patients' experiences. They do not believe that it is possible to promote greater disclosure of patients' problems within their daily practice and survive themselves.

It will take up too much time

They fear it will take up too much time and they will not be able to get through their clinics.

Overcoming barriers to disclosure

Behaviours which promote disclosure

Disclosure of key concerns is promoted by doctors and nurses asking open directive questions about patients' perceptions of their predicament, their reactions to key illness and treatment events, the impact on their daily lives, mood, and personal relationships.[36] When the doctor or nurse reflects back to the patient what they have already heard (summarizing) and checks if this is correct before continuing, patients realize they are being listened to but can also correct what has been understood. Showing a willingness to clarify cues that patients have offered about both physical and psychological aspects is crucial. It indicates that the doctor or nurse wishes to understand their experiences. The use of empathy where the doctor or nurse indicates that they have some idea how the patient is feeling ('It sounds horrendous that your cancer came back so quickly'?) and the use of educated guesses ('As I talk to you I get the feeling you are much more distressed than you are letting on') also communicate a wish to 'get alongside' what patients are going through. The key is to use these techniques from the first assessment of patients so they are educated that the doctor or nurse is interested in them as persons, their perceptions and reactions. They will then be more likely to disclose their key concerns whether these are physical, social, psychological, or spiritual in nature.

Taking an initial history

Surgeon	Your doctor tells me that you found a lump in your left breast. Is that right?
Patient	Yes I did.
Surgeon	How did you come to notice it?
Patient	When I was having a bath. I examined my breast to check that I was OK.
Surgeon	And?
Patient	I felt this lump, it was hard, like a brazil nut.
Surgeon	What did you think it was? (**Asks about perceptions**)
Patient	What does any sensible woman think these days? I thought it was cancer, that's why I went to my doctor. He agreed it might be a cancer and sent me here to see you.
Surgeon	How did you feel when you thought you had cancer? (**Question about patient's feelings**)
Patient	Very worried.
Surgeon	You say that you have been very worried (**Acknowledging cue**) Just how worried have you been? (**Clarifying cue**)
Patient	I can't stop thinking it could be cancer.
Surgeon	What state of mind do you get into when you think that it could be cancer? (**Checking patient's mental state**)
Patient	I get extremely tense and anxious. I am having difficulty getting off to sleep and I am not functioning as well as I should.
Surgeon	Why are you so anxious? (**Exploring reasons for distress**)
Patient	My mother had cancer. She wasted away, had horrendous pain and died a horrible death.
Surgeon	Any other reasons for feeling anxious? (**Screening question**)
Patient	She became confused towards the end and lost her mind. I can't bear to think I would go like that.
Surgeon	Any other reasons? (**Screening question**)
Patient	No.

Monitoring progress

In checking the patient's progress at follow-up it is important to enquire how the illness and treatment has affected the patient's daily life, mood, and relationships unless this has been volunteered.

Oncologist	Has your illness and treatment affected your ability to function day to day? (**Impact on daily functioning**)
Patient	I still try to keep going but it has been an increasing strain.
Oncologist	In what way? (**Clarification**)
Patient	It is increasingly hard to get up in the morning and face work. I have lost interest in doing my chores. My concentration isn't what it should be. I cannot stop thinking that I am going to die from this cancer.
Oncologist	Any other effects? (**Screening question**)
Patient	Yes, I have been much more irritable. I have gone on at my husband for no reason. I blow up at the children as well.
Oncologist	Any other changes? (**Screening question**)
Patient	No, I don't think so.

Through the oncologist establishing her perceptions, feelings, and the impact of her illness she realizes that the oncologist is interested in her as a whole person and is more likely to disclose her key concerns.

Doctors and nurses have to decide whether or not to explore areas that are potentially distressing. It is, therefore, important to negotiate with patients if they are willing to talk about potentially unpleasant events. When they are willing to talk about their experiences it is still necessary to use precision to help them connect with their true experiences and feelings. Otherwise, they may be vague and give misleading information.

Medical oncologist	You said that your sister died of a melanoma, can you bear to tell me more about it? (**Negotiation**)
Patient	It will be hard, but I realize it might help me.
Medical oncologist	Can you try. It would help me to know when exactly she died.
Patient	She died last summer.
Medical oncologist	When exactly? (**Precision**)
Patient	First week in August.
Medical oncologist	Can you remember the exact day? (**Further precision**)
Patient	August 3rd.
Medical oncologist	Can you bear to tell me what happened? (**Negotiation**)
Patient	The cancer had gone to her brain. For a few days before she died she became very confused. She went into a coma. I couldn't bear to see her, it was so distressing. It still upsets me to think about it.
Medical oncologist	In view of what you say I guess you have been worrying you could go the same way? (**Educated guess**)
Patient	Yes I have. I can't get the images of her death out of my mind.

The oncologist has invited his patient to share her experiences of how her sister died. This sheds light on the patient's fears about her future. His use of 'precision' helped the patient to connect with and express painful memories. Even when patients are willing to discuss painful feelings it is important to check if it is safe to continue.

Radiotherapist	I know that you have been told you were referred here because you have cancer of the cervix. When we started discussing your cancer you became upset and tearful. I would like to talk to you about this further but I need to check if you can bear to do so. (**Negotiation**)
Patient	I am not sure. It's so painful to think about.
Radiotherapist	Can you bear to say why? (**Negotiation**)
Patient	Life was going so well. I had just got married and we had a child. I can't believe I've got cancer.
Radiotherapist	I can understand why it is so upsetting. Can you bear to talk about this any further? (**Negotiation**)
Patient	I am terrified you will not be able to get me better.

| Radiotherapist | That's what I am here for. I want to discuss with you what we might be able to do. |

Doctors and nurses often have strong intuitions about what patients or relatives are feeling during the consultation. They keep their intuitions private for fear that if they voice them and get them wrong this will damage their relationship with the patient or relative. Paradoxically, patients and relatives perceive such efforts as helpful since they realize doctors and nurses are seeking to further their doctors understanding, even if the intuition (**educated guess**) is wrong.

Medical oncologist	I get the feeling you are not keen on more drug chemotherapy.
Patient	You are right, I am terrified. I don't think I could cope with it. (**Confirmation**)
Medical oncologist	Why not?
Patient	I dread being sick again. I used to get terrible panics and had to be dragged into the car before coming to the hospital for treatment.

Many doctors and nurses say they avoid focusing on psychological aspects because they have insufficient time available. Observation of consultations has indicated that much time is wasted through ineffective communication. For example when patients are asked to give a history of their presenting problems they may wander off the point and talk about experiences unrelated to the present illness or discuss why they have become ill. It is important that they are brought back to the point.

Medical oncologist	When did you first notice there was anything wrong with you?
Patient	I started having these sweats last October. My pyjamas were saturated. It reminded me of the time I had glandular fever. I was studying architecture and it came on just before finals. The doctor said it was all due to worry about my exams.
Medical oncologist	What you say about having glandular fever is helpful but can I focus on this latest episode of sweating. What exactly are your sweats like. (**Focusing back on current problems**)

Diagnosis and management

Anxiety

Anxious mood should be diagnosed when a patient complains of persistent inability to relax or stop worrying and this represents a significant change both qualitatively and quantitatively from the patient's normal mood and the patient cannot distract himself or be distracted by others. A generalized anxiety disorder should be diagnosed if there are four or more other symptoms including initial insomnia, irritability, sweating, tremor or nausea, impaired concentration, indecisiveness, and spontaneous panic attacks. Patients with such generalized anxiety may also have irrational fears of specific situations such as meeting people (social phobia) or leaving the house because they are afraid they might collapse (agoraphobia).

If the patient is unable to cope from day to day or comply with cancer treatment, an anxiolytic drug (such as lorazepam) is necessary. To forestall dependency in patients with early disease it should be given for only 3 to 4 weeks and taken only when necessary. In those with advanced disease, it can be given regularly. Thus, to cover each infusion of chemotherapy a patient may be advised to take it for 2 days beforehand. If this is not sufficient, a major tranquilliser (such as thioridazine) or a tricyclic antidepressant (such as prothiaden) is indicated. β-blockers (such as propanalol) are indicated when somatic symptoms of anxiety predominate.

Once anxiety is controlled the patient should be taught anxiety management techniques. These involve training in progressive muscular relaxation and positive imaging. These techniques can be taught as soon as the anxiety ceases to be disorganizing. If the anxiety is provoked by irrational fears of recurrence or concerns about body image, cognitive therapy may be used. The antecedents of these irrational beliefs and their consequences are analysed critically and challenged.

When anxiety is being maintained by realistic uncertainty about prognosis, the uncertainty should be acknowledged and patients asked whether they wish to be given markers of what signs and symptoms might herald deterioration in their disease. They should also be asked how often they would like to be monitored physically. Few patients abuse this offer. Those who elect to be given indications of their progress must be given the results of tests when they request them. They will adapt psychologically even if the news is bad. Those who say they prefer not to know the indicators of disease progression should not have them imposed on them.

Depression

Depressed mood should be diagnosed when a patient complains of persistent low mood for 2 to 4 weeks, which is significantly greater quantitatively and qualitatively compared with periods when the patient has been unhappy, and the patient cannot banish it. Depressive illness should be diagnosed when this is accompanied by four or more other symptoms including sleep disturbance (repeated or early morning waking, excessive sleep), irritability, impairment of attention and concentration, restlessness or retardation, loss of energy, social withdrawal, negative ideation (ideas of hopelessness, self blame, guilt, worthlessness, feeling a burden, seeing no future, feeling life is pointless), suicidal ideation, diurnal variation of mood where the mood is worse at some particular time of day, loss of appetite, weight loss, and constipation.

Allowance should be made for the possibility that some symptoms, such as loss of energy, appetite, and weight, are due to progression or recurrence of cancer rather than depression. In practice, even when these symptoms are attributed to cancer they often disappear when the depression is treated. Most depression in cancer patients is understandable in terms of the stressors they are experiencing but this should not be used as an argument against effective treatment when the relevant signs and symptoms are present.

Major depressive disorders should be treated with antidepressants. In prescribing antidepressant medication it is important to emphasize several points to the patient and the relatives. Antidepressants do not cause physical or psychological dependence. They are necessary because the depression has been caused by changes in brain chemistry which were triggered by the stress of the cancer or treatment. Antidepressants encourage the brain to start producing the necessary chemicals again and must be continued for 4 to 6 months to forestall relapse. Medication is only the first step in helping patients and relatives. Once their mood has begun to lift there will be opportunities to talk about any residual problems, such as body image difficulties or problems within the family. They must take the antidepressant medication as prescribed and not just when they feel low. Improvement is not likely to occur for 10 to 14 days and may take longer.

Tricylic antidepressants cause sedation, postural hypotension, and anticholinergic effects (dry mouth, blurred vision, difficulty with micturition, and constipation). They are contraindicated in patients with glaucoma, prostatism, and cardiac arrythmias. They should be used with caution in patients with heart disease. The sedative effects of amitriptyline and dothiepin are useful in patients with insomnia and/or agitation but they are lethal in overdose. Dothiepin causes fewer anticholinergic effects and is well tolerated by cancer patients.[37] Imipramine is more alerting and helps patients who are retarded. Lofepramine is non-sedative and has the least anticholinergic effects.

The serotonin specific reuptake inhibitors (SSRIs) are newer and more expensive and the main side-effects are nausea and diarrhoea. They are not sedating, have no use as hypnotics, but are safe in overdose. Fluoxetine is a good first choice but can increase arousal and agitation in the short term. Paroxetine, paradoxically, may alleviate anxiety. Citalopram and sertraline have fewer drug interactions than the other SSRIs and are less metabolized by the liver. So, they may be useful in patients on multiple drug regimes.

Most patients with major depressive disorder respond well to antidepressant medication and the chance to talk about their concerns. Maintaining factors such as inappropriately negative views of prognosis or persistent body image problems can be dealt with using specific therapies such as cognitive therapy or brief psychotherapy.

Adjustment disorders

These should be diagnosed when anxious and/or depressed mood are present but there are too few other symptoms to justify a diagnosis of major depressive illness or generalized anxiety disorder.

The patients' concerns should be elicited and they should be encouraged to express the associated feelings. Ways of helping them resolve these concerns should then be discussed. They should be encouraged to share their concerns with partners or close relatives. Their progress should be monitored to see if they develop a full disorder although most will recover.

Confusional states

Patients so affected will tend to have a poor attention span and be distractible. Their mood will be labile and they may appear agitated and frightened. They find it hard to concentrate and register what you are saying. You should check if they are orientated to time, place, and date; assess short-term memory by giving them a name and address to remember, and checking it immediately, and 2 and 5 min later. Concentration can be tested by asking them to subtract seven from 100 and taking seven away from the number obtained. They should be asked if they are experiencing any unusual experiences (illusions, misinterpretations, and hallucinations) including false beliefs such as being convinced staff are out to harm them.

Once the diagnosis is confirmed the priority is to determine the underlying causes. Meanwhile, they should be nursed in a quiet, well-lit room with regular staff attending to them. Any problems with fluid and electrolyte balance and nutrition should be corrected. If agitated, delusional, or hallucinating, haloperidol is the drug of choice, with or without lorazepam as an adjuvant.

Body image problems

Behavioural treatments may be effective when patients are taught to manage their anxiety through the use of relaxation and imagery. Graded exposure is then used to help them spend increasing amounts of time looking at the affected part of the body after a period of relaxation. When patients have irrational views of their body image and its impact on people close to them (for example they insist that since they cannot accept how they look their partner cannot, yet the partners are accepting of the body image change) cognitive therapy should be tried.

When surgical reconstruction is possible it can have a beneficial effect providing the patient understands the possible complications, wants surgery for him or herself, and there is evidence of visual avoidance of the affected body part.

Sexual problems

Patients with cancers which are not hormone dependent can be helped by hormone replacement when this is indicated. Those with hormone-dependent tumours or sexual problems due to anatomical damage through surgery or radiotherapy may benefit from practical aids such as dilators, lubricating creams, prostheses, or discussion of alternative modes of pleasuring (as advised in the early stages of Masters and Johnson's therapy).

In Masters and Johnson therapy[38] the underlying premise is that sexual intercourse has come to be associated with anxiety. Therefore, they begin by advising a couple to ban sexual intercourse and educate each other about the kinds of caressing, other than that of genital areas, which gives them most pleasure. Once this is achieved, the couple are advised to proceed to caressing genital areas before proceeding to full intercourse.

Illness behaviour

A substantial proportion of patients fail to return to their former level of adjustment and employment despite being free of disease and off treatment.[17] Chaturvedi et al., 1998[39] found that somatization is a common problem in cancer patients. Despite being disease free and off treatment patients continue to complain of somatic symptoms. While this is often due to unresolved anxiety and depression, it may represent true somatization.

When to seek a psychiatric or psychology opinion

Affective disorders

Specialists in oncology are becoming more competent in diagnosing and managing affective disorders. They may have a reasonable working knowledge of the relative merits of different medications and be prepared to undertake treatment. Referral is indicated, at the outset, if there is evidence of suicidal ideation, agitation, or doubt about the

diagnosis or the most appropriate treatment. Failure of the patient to respond to initial treatment should also lead to referral.

When the affective disorder appears multifactorial in origin (for example the diagnosis of cancer, recent bereavement, problems with body image) a psychiatric assessment should be sought early.

Confusional states

Doubts about diagnosis, causation, or management should lead to early referral. Otherwise, the associated behavioural problems can escalate and create major problems for the patient and staff.

Other problems

When patients present with persistent body image problems referral to a psychiatrist or clinical psychologist should be considered. They can then determine if behavioural cognitive therapy or a psychotherapeutic approach is indicated. It is also worth asking a psychiatrist or clinical psychologist to vet patients seeking surgical reconstruction as a solution to their body image problems.

Referral to a clinic specializing in sexual problems is indicated for persisting problems which have no hormonal basis.

Patients who continue to complain of physical symptoms when free of disease, off treatment, and free of affective disorder merit assessment by a psychiatrist or clinical psychologist to determine if they are 'somatizers' and warrant cognitive therapy.

Preventing psychological morbidity

By the way bad news is broken

Two factors relating to communication influence later anxiety and depression (see also Chapter 6.2). Patients who perceive they were given too much or too little information about their illness, treatment, and prognosis are more at risk.[3] Those who end up with a greater number of concerns of a greater magnitude after their cancer diagnosis are also more vulnerable.[4]

Checking awareness

The key is to determine how much patients want to know about their illness, treatment, and prognosis. The initial history should have elicited their views of what might be wrong with them. Between 80 and 90 per cent of patients are aware of their likely diagnosis. The task for the doctor then is to confirm that their perceptions are correct.

When patients are not aware

When patients do not know that they have a serious illness or prefer to deny it, the task is to break the bad news without pushing them into more denial or overwhelming distress. First, a warning shot should be fired ('You remember I thought the pain in your abdomen was due to an infection. As a result of the tests I have done, I think it is more serious'). It is then most important to pause to allow the patient time to assimilate in this information and respond. This pause need only take a few seconds. Their response will indicate if they wish to know more ('What do you mean you think it is more serious?') or prefer to remain in denial ('That's up to you, you're the expert'). When patients signal they want further information another cue should be provided ('You know we x-rayed your bowel. Some areas looked abnormal'). The patient can still pull out ('That's all right, that's up to you') or pursue it ('What do you mean abnormal'?). Failure to tailor information in this way can have catastrophic consequences.

A woman developed a recurrence of cervical cancer and was seen by an oncologist for consideration of chemotherapy. She was aware of her diagnosis but indicated early on that she did not want to hear the details. She just wished to know if anything could be done. The oncologist insisted on giving her details about the sites and the extent of her disease. Within 24 h she became depressed and agitated and required an urgent psychiatric opinion because she was experiencing strong intrusive thoughts about her cancer spreading throughout her body and causing death and felt suicidal.

Handling distress and identifying concerns

If bad news is being broken effectively patients will become distressed and give verbal and non-verbal cues about this. It might seem banal but it is crucial that the doctor acknowledges the patient's distress to give patients permission to talk about their distress and the reasons for it. ('I can see that what I have told you has upset you. Would you mind telling me just what is upsetting you'?).

Patients may feel this is a stupid question ('Isn't it obvious') but the doctor should explain why the question was asked ('I can appreciate you think I ought to know what is upsetting you. But everybody is individual and I want to know what your concerns are so I can try and help you).

Doctor	You seem very upset? (**Acknowledgement**)
Patient	I am.
Doctor	Can you bear to say what is distressing you? (**Negotiation**)
Patient	I am shattered. I have heard that melanoma can spread and cause havoc.
Doctor	How did you hear this? (**Exploration**)
Patient	I had a neighbour who had it and died. It went to her brain and she ended up in a coma.
Doctor	No wonder you are so upset. Are there any other concerns before we deal with that? (**Screening question**)
Patient	No, it was just the thought it will get me quickly and horribly.

By actively acknowledging her distress and inviting her to talk about the concerns that are provoking it, her distress decreased and became more manageable. The doctor can now reassure the patient that the melanoma is likely to be more controllable than it was in her neighbour and that every effort will be made to prevent such complications.

It is imperative to avoid moving into an information and advice mode until each key concern has been elicited. Once key concerns have been elicited the patient should be asked to prioritize them so the most important is dealt with first.

When the doctor moves into a problem solving mode, reassurance or advice should be pitched at an appropriate level. Thus, the doctor might talk in terms of curing the disease, controlling it, or being able to offer symptom control.

Preventing collusion

Collusion, where relatives pressure the doctor not to tell the patient the true diagnosis results in an even higher incidence of psychological morbidity. It also hinders the resolution of the grief of the relatives. It is, therefore, important to avoid this by asking patients what they want to know about their predicament rather than relying on their relatives' opinions. Having a relative or close friend accompany the patient appears to facilitate adaptation when bad news is broken providing the patient wishes this to occur. They can discuss what was communicated about the nature of the illness and treatment and correct any misconceptions. While giving patients audio tapes of bad news consultations may facilitate adaption, if the consultation conveyed news of a poor prognosis it may prove more distressing.[38]

Establishing needs for further information

Once the patients main concerns have been dealt with, and providing discussion has not already covered further investigations and treatment, it is important to check if the patient wants specific information. This can be done by asking, for example, 'Would you like me to explain the tests that we need to do'? The doctor should be honest about possible adverse effects of treatment rather than minimizing them. If adverse effects then develop patients may feel let down and distrust subsequent advice and treatment. If they have serious worries about treatments their reasons should be explored and respected. They are often rooted in adverse experiences of cancer in other people.

Involving patients in choices

Most patients wish to be involved in decisions about treatment when genuine options are available but a substantial minority do not want the responsibility and prefer to leave it with the doctor.[41] Offering patients choice appears to reduce psychiatric morbidity providing they want to take part in that choice.[42] However, physicians regularly underestimate patients' preferences for involvement.[43]

Giving general information

It has been suggested that all patients should be given a 'package of information' about their illness, investigation procedures, and treatment in the form of a booklet, audio tape, or video tape.[40] This ignores variations between individual patients in their needs for information and how they like it to be presented. It is important to negotiate with each patient 'Would you like me to give you more information in the form of a booklet, audio tape, or video tape which tells you more about the tests we need to do, the treatments, and the possible side-effects'?

Training in communication skills

Prevention through more effective communication with patients will only be possible if health professionals involved in cancer are given opportunities to improve their interviewing, assessment, and counselling skills (see Chapter 6.2). Without such training they tend to use more inhibitory behaviours than positive behaviours which promote disclosure.[34] Short, intensive, residential, multidisciplinary workshops, which utilize video tape demonstrations and allow participants to practice key skills through role play under controlled conditions, help them acquire the positive skills and reduce the inhibitory ones.[44] It is likely that longer courses or individual training will be needed to ensure that the learning from brief workshops is maintained over time and transferred to the workplace. Workshops also need to focus on attitudes to psychological aspects of care.[45],[46]

Doctors and nurses might learn more effectively if they trained in small groups within their own discipline.[47] The relative merits of multidisciplinary and unidisciplinary courses have still to be compared. Without training in communication skills the use of inhibitory behaviours will continue to outweigh the use of positive ones and the majority of patients' concerns and psychological morbidity will not be disclosed.

Other methods of prevention

Use of volunteers

Other patients are an important source of information, advice, and practical and emotional support. If they are to facilitate rather than hinder psychological adaptation, they need to belong to a credible volunteer organization. Credibility should be judged on the organization's willingness to select and train volunteers, audit their work over time, and co-operate with professionals in cancer care. Training should focus on basic listening and responding skills but avoid the trap of changing volunteers into 'professionals'. Fortunately, most major volunteer organizations now meet these criteria and have mechanisms for good quality control in place. Although there are many anecdotal reports of the values of face-to-face contact between patients and volunteers there has been little study of their effectiveness.

Support groups

Only 10 to 20 per cent of patients with cancer utilize self-help groups. Groups have an important role in facilitating the sharing of experiences and concerns, giving support both practically and emotionally, and reducing isolation. When they are led by, or are in co-operation with, people who have a professional knowledge of group dynamics, they appear effective in alleviating distress. Such leaders are able to facilitate discussion even when it is between people with varying prognoses.[48],[49] They are also able to maintain discussion at a safe but constructive level.[50]

Psychoeducational groups

Fawzy et al. (1993) have advocated the use of more structured psychoeducational groups.[51] Patients with malignant melanoma were given health education, learned about stress management and coping strategies, and focused on solving their problems. They showed a greater reduction in depression and fatigue scores than control subjects but both groups of patients were free of psychological morbidity to begin with.

The use of specialist workers

Many cancer units have appointed specialist nurses or social workers to provide information, advice, and practical and emotional support to individual patients or groups. It was hoped that this would reduce psychological and social morbidity. It reduces emotional distress and anxiety but does not have similar effects on depressive illness. However, specialist workers can achieve a marked reduction in morbidity through the early recognition and psychiatric referral of those they detect as having problems. This can only be achieved if they are trained in the relevant interviewing and assessment skills.[52]

Ongoing support from a nurse manager, with supervision and clinical backup by a clinical psychologist or a psychiatrist, are necessary if these schemes are to be effective. Unfortunately, specialist workers are still being appointed without the relevant training, support, or supervision. They then retreat to using distancing tactics and focus selectively on physical issues such as the provision of breast prostheses or stoma bags. Alternatively, they become over-involved, carry too large a case load, and become psychological casualties. Some become too autonomous and give little feedback to the treating clinician about psychological aspects. They hang on to their patients and resist the involvement of others. There is also a danger that in employing specialist workers to deal with psychological care clinicians leave all this care to them and increase the risk of burnout.

In healthy systems, specialist workers give regular feedback to the clinical team about problems that patients are experiencing and discuss what action might be taken. The clinical psychologist, psychiatrist, and/or general practitioner should be involved when appropriate. Specialist workers can also make effective links with, and encourage the development of, volunteer organizations and self-help groups. They can play a vital role in upgrading the psychological assessment and counselling skills of non-specialist nurses involved in cancer care. This can free them to concentrate on those patients and relatives who have more complex problems.

Limited contact

It is only necessary to assess cancer patients once after discharge from hospital to determine whether they have developed social or psychological problems. After a systematic psychosocial assessment has been conducted, patients realize there is a member of the treating team who is prepared to deal with their problems. Up to 90 per cent of patients who develop problems after such an assessment can be relied on to contact a specialist worker. There is no need to continue the time-consuming practice of monitoring every patient regularly.[53] Specialist workers could use their time more efficiently if those at risk of psychosocial morbidity could be identified and helped appropriately.

Preoperative interviews

Burton et al. (1995) assessed the value of a 45-min interview conducted by a clinical psychologist on the afternoon before breast cancer surgery.[54] Some patients then had a 30-min psychotherapy intervention or chat with a surgeon trained in Rogerian client-centred methods. He invited patients to talk about their concerns and feelings by appearing interested, calm, and non-judgmental. He did not interrupt to clarify verbal and non-verbal cues given by patients. Instead he trusted them to elaborate. The preoperative interview focused on eliciting the woman's illness history, her perceptions of her disease and treatment, her concerns, feelings, and mood. Subjects given the preoperative interview showed a reduction in distress about body image and lower caseness rates for anxiety and depression.

Identifying those at risk

Worden and Weisman (1984) pioneered an approach to identifying those at risk.[55] They used questionnaires to identify patients likely to develop high levels of emotional distress. 'At risk' patients were characterized by suppression of feelings, passivity, stoic acceptance, reducing tension through cigarette smoking or alcohol consumption, social withdrawal, blaming themselves or others for their predicament, and being unduly irritable. When they tested this predictive model prospectively, 80 per cent of the 'at risk' group were identified. However, only a minority of patients accepted and completed the offered interventions.

Greer et al. (1992) developed a similar intervention which they named Adjuvant Psychological Therapy.[56] Patients screened out as having psychological morbidity were helped over 6 to 12-hourly sessions to identify their problems, learn new cognitive and behavioural strategies, and adopt a fighting spirit. There were fewer probable cases of anxiety at follow-up in those receiving this intervention compared with control subjects but no significant difference in the prevalence of 'probable' cases of depression. As in the Worden and Weisman study, many of those deemed 'at risk' did not accept the help offered. When limited to cancer patients who accepted referral for psychological help, it appeared superior to non-directive, supportive counselling.[57]

Parle et al. (1996) have suggested that patients who are not clinically depressed but have four or more concerns, high scores on the Hospital Anxiety and Depression Scale, and/or a past psychiatric history should be targeted for cognitive behavioural intervention since their negative appraisals make them vulnerable to affective disorders.[4]

Other possible markers include perceiving that friends and relatives are not supportive, finding it difficult to accept the loss of a body part or function, struggling to tolerate adverse effects of treatment, and failing to handle the key hurdles discussed earlier.

Failure to adapt to these key hurdles after diagnosis leads to high levels of emotional distress and affective disorders. So, it is worth checking how patients are adapting. Unless patients volunteer concerns about these hurdles they should be asked specific questions.

- Uncertainty ('How do you see your illness working out?').
- Search for meaning ('Have you been able to come up with any explanation for why you have developed your illness at this time?').
- Stigma ('Has your illness and treatment changed how you feel about yourself as a person? If so, in what way?').
- Being secretive ('Have you felt able to tell people close to you about your illness and treatment?').
- Loss of control ('Do you feel there are things you can do to contribute towards your own survival?').
- Receiving support ('How do you feel about the level of support you are getting from the doctors and nurses?').

When patients are failing to adapt to any of these hurdles the possibility of anxiety and depression should be explored.

Screening for affective disorders

Several self-rating questionnaires have been developed with the aim of identifying people with affective disorders. The Hospital Anxiety and Depression Scale and Rotterdam Symptom Checklist were developed for use in physically ill patients and cancer patients respectively. They have a high sensitivity but low specificity.[58]–[60] For every five patients scoring above the threshold score for clinically relevant problems only two will be genuine cases. Moreover, the

optimal questionnaire and threshold chosen should vary by disease state and treatment.[59] Although developed for use in the general population, the Centre for Epidemiological Studies Depression Scale[61] has been reported to have similar sensitivity in cancer patients.

In clinical practice, all high scorers must be assessed by an appropriately trained person to determine if they are true cases and warrant psychiatric intervention. There is a real danger that clinicians will use these questionnaires as a quick way of identifying those with mood disorder and disregard the need for a second-line assessment.

Psychological factors and cancer

Onset

Claims that stressful life events cause cancer find a ready audience in lay people but most studies reporting links suffer from methodological weaknesses.[62] A clear demonstration is needed that psychosocial variables are related to cancer onset and the hypotheses under test must be biologically plausible. Studies must test predictive models by evaluating biological, psychological and social variables concurrently if they are to be of value.

Survival

Spiegel et al.[63] found, in a very influential study, that the provision of practical and emotional support to patients with advanced breast cancer through weekly group meetings led to prolonged survival by about 18 months (see also Chapter 6.5). Fawzy et al. found that attendance at psychoeducational groups seemed to lengthen the survival of melanoma patients.[51] A review by Gwikel et al. (1997)[64] concluded that the evidence that psychosocial variables affect progression of early disease is inconsistent, while in advanced disease biological factors were paramount. They did not consider the intriguing finding by Ramirez et al. (1989) of a link between the experiencing of adverse life events and relapse of breast cancer.[65]

However, the work by Spiegel et al. has been criticized. There was no attempt to stratify by prognostic variables before randomization, and those in the control group had a much poorer survival compared with the universe of similar cancer patients. Moreover, the findings were post hoc and not predicted at the outset of the initial study. Attempts to replicate these findings have not yet proved successful. Cunningham et al. (1998)[66] found that regular group support did not influence the survival of patients with metastatic disease when prognostic variables were allowed for. Moreover, only 25 per cent of eligible patients accepted the offered group support.

Longer-term, multicentre trials of psychological interventions are needed which take adequate account of the biological and social variables that may influence survival and test if the hypothesized mediating mechanisms change in the predicted directions.

Support for health-care professionals

If doctors and nurses improve their communication skills (see Chapter 6.2) they will elicit more problems and get closer to the real suffering of their patients and families. They will, therefore, need opportunities to discuss the problems they encounter and the associated feelings. They will need advice and support so they can further improve their knowledge and skills. It is not clear what methods of support are best. Is it better offered informally or through support groups? Current thinking suggests that it is best offered on an *ad hoc* basis, that is as problems arise or by regular supervision in small groups.

Support groups for staff can be helpful providing certain conditions are met.[67] The leader should have a good knowledge of group dynamics and give guidance about the nature and function of the group. The importance of regular attendance and confidentiality should be emphasized. The leader should be able to facilitate discussion, maintain the focus on work-related problems, and prevent disclosure of personal problems, for staff are not patients and support groups should not be turned into therapy groups.

There has been little evaluation of such groups and they can have a negative effect where staff become more aware of the suffering of patients and families and feel they are achieving less.[68] The high levels of burnout (25 per cent) found in cancer clinicians emphasizes the need to develop effective modes of support.[69]

References

1. **Greer S.** Cancer: psychiatric aspects. In: K Granville-Grossman, ed. *Recent advances in clinical psychiatry.* London: Churchill Livingstone, 1985: 87–104.

2. **Anderson BL.** Sexual functioning morbidity among cancer survivors. *Cancer*, 1985; **55**: 1835–42.

3. **Fallowfield LJ, Hall A, Maguire GP, Baum M.** Psychological outcomes of different treatment policies in women with early breast cancer outside a clinical trial. *British Medical Journal*, 1990; **301**: 575–80.

4. **Parle M, Jones B, Maguire P.** Maladaptive coping and affective disorders in cancer patients. *Psychological Medicine*, 1996; **26**: 735–44.

5. **Zabora JR, Blanchard CG, Smith ED, et al.** Prevalence of psychological distress among cancer patients across the disease continuim. *Journal of Psychosocial Oncology*, 1997; **15**: 73–87.

6. **Bridge LR, Benson P, Pietroni PC, Priest RG.** Relaxation and imagery in the treatment of breast cancer. *British Medical Journal*, 1998; **297**: 1169–72.

7. **Maguire P, Brooke M, Tait A, Thomas C, Sellwood R.** Effect of counselling on physical disability and social recovery after mastectomy. *Clinical Oncology*, 1983; **9**: 319–24.

8. **Maguire P, Murray Parkes C.** Coping with loss: surgery and loss of body parts. *British Medical Journal*, 1998; **316**: 1086–8.

9. **Passik SD, Newman ML, Brennan B, Tunkel R.** Predictors of psychological distress, sexual dysfunction and physical functioning among women with upper extremity lymphoedema related to breast cancer. *Psycho-Oncology*, 1995; **4**: 255–63.

10. **Williams NS, Johnson D.** The quality of life after rectal excision for low rectal cancer. *British Journal of Surgery*, 1983; **70**: 460–2.

11. **Thomas C, Madden F, John D.** Psychological effects of stomas. 1. Psychosocial morbidity one year after surgery. *Journal of Psychosomatic Research*, 1987; **31**: 311–16.

12. **Bekkers MJTM, Van-Kippenberg FCE, Van den Borne HW, Poen H, Bergsma J, Van Berge Henegouwen GP.** Psychosocial adaptation to stoma surgery: A review. *Journal of Behaviour Medicine*, 1995; **18**: 1–31.

13. **Chaturvedi SK, Shenoy A, Prasad KMR, Senthilnathan SM, Premakumari BS.** Concerns. Coping and quality of life in head and neck cancer patients. *Supportive Care in Cancer*, 1996; **4**: 32–6.

14. **Fallowfield LJ, Baum M, Maguire GP.** Effects of breast conservation on psychological morbidity associated with diagnoses and treatment of early breast cancer. *British Medical Journal*, 1986; **293**: 1331–4.

15. **Maunsell E, Brisson J, Deschenes L.** Psychological distress after initial treatment for breast cancer: A comparison of partial and total mastectomy. *Journal of Clinical Epidemiology*, 1989; **42**: 765–71.

16. **Bos-Branolte G, Rijshouwer YM, Zielstra EM, Duivenvoorden HJ.** Psychological morbidity in survivors of gynaecological cancers. *International Journal of Gynacological Oncology*, 1988; **9**: 61–76.

17. **Cull A, Cowie V, Farquharson DIM, Livingston JRB, Smart GE, Elton RA.** Early stage cervical cancer: Psychosocial and sexual outcome of treatment. *British Journal of Cancer*, 1993; **68**: 1216–20.

18. **Devlen J, Maguire P, Phillips P, Crowther D, Chambers H.** Psychological problems associated with diagnosis and treatment of lymphomas. II: Prospective Study. *British Medical Journal*, 1987; **293**: 955–7.

19. **Hughson AVM, Cooper AF, McArdle CS, Smith DC.** Psychological impact of adjuvant chemotherapy in the first two years after mastectomy. *British Medical Journal (Clinical Research)*, 1986; **293**: 1268–71.

20. **Watson M, McCarron J, Law M.** Anticipatory nausea and emesis, and psychological morbidity: assessment of prevalence among out-patients on mild to moderate chemotherapy regimens. *British Journal of Cancer*, 1992; **66**: 862–6.

21. **Wieneke MH, Dienst ET.** Neuropsychological assessment of cognitive functioning following chemotherapy for breast cancer. *Psycho-Oncology*, 1995; **4**: 61–6.

22. **Van Dam FS, Schagen SB, Muller MJ, et al.** Impairment of cognitive function in women receiving adjuvant treatment for high-risk breast cancer: high-dose versus standard dose chemotherapy. *Journal of the National Cancer Institute*, 1998; **90**: 210–18.

23. **Aass N, Fossa SD, Theodorson L, Norman N.** Prediction of long term gonadal toxicity after standard treatment for testicular cancer. *European Journal of Cancer*, 1991; **27**: 1087–91.

24. **Moynihan C.** The psychosocial effects of the diagnosis and treatment of testicular cancer: a retrospective study. *Cancer Topics*, 1988; **198**: 18–20.

25. **Whitehead E, Shalet SM, Blackledge G, Todd I, Crowther D, Beardwell C.** The effects of Hodgkin's disease and combination of chemotherapy on gondal function in the adult male. *Cancer*, 1982; **49**: 418–22.

26. **Smith MJ, Mouawad R, Vuillemin E, Benhammouda A, Soubrane C, Khayat D.** Psychological side effects induced by interleukin 2 and interferon treatment. *Psycho-Oncology*, 1994; **3**: 289–98.

27. **Molassiotis A, Van Den Akker OBA, Milligan DW, Goldman JM, Boughton BJ.** Psychological adaptation and symptom distress in bone marrow transplant recipients. *Psycho-Oncology*, 1996; **5**: 9–22.

28. **Hall A, Fallowfield LJ, Hern R.** When brease cancer recurs: A 3 year prospective study of psychological morbidity. *Breast*, 1996; **2**: 197–203.

29. **Weisman A, Worden JW.** *Coping and vulnerability in cancer patients.* Research report, Project Omega. Department of Psychiatry, Harvard Medical School, 1977.

30. **Hardman A, Maguire P, Crowther D.** The recognition of psychological morbidity on a medical oncology ward. *Journal of Psychosomatic Research*, 1989; **33**: 235–7.

31. **Ford S, Fallowfield L, Lewis S.** Can oncologists detect distress in their outpatients? *British Journal of Cancer*, 1994; **70**: 767–70.

32. **Heaven CM, Maguire P.** Training hospice nurses to elicit patients' concerns. *Journal of Advanced Nursing Studies*, 1996; **23**: 280–6.

33. **Ford S, Fallowfield L, Lewis S.** Doctor-patient interactions in oncology. *Social Science and Medicine*, 1996; **42**: 1511–19.

34. **Wilkinson S.** Factors which influence how nurses communicate with cancer patients. *Journal of Advanced Nursing*, 1991; **16**: 677–88.

35. **Maguire P.** Barriers to psychological care of the dying. *British Medical Journal*, 1985; **291**: 1711–13.

36. **Maguire P, Faulkner A, Booth K, Elliott C, Hillier V.** Helping cancer

patients disclose their concerns. *European Journal of Cancer*, 1996; **32A**: 78–81.

37. Chaturvedi SK, Maguire P, Hopwood P. Antidepressant medications in cancer patients. *Psycho-Oncology*, 1994; **3**: 57–60.

38. Masters WH, Johnson VE. *Human sexual inadequacy*. London: Churchill Livingstone, 1970.

39. Chaturvedi SK, Maguire GP. Persistent somatisation in cancer: A controlled follow-up study. *Journal of Psychosomatic Research*, 1988; **45**: 249–56.

40. Hogbin B, Jenkins VA, Parkin AJ. Remembering 'bad news' consultations. *Psycho-Oncology*, 1992; **1**: 147–54.

41. Degner L, Sloan J. Decision making during serious illness: What role do patients want to play? *Journal of Clinical Epidemiology*, 1992; **45**: 942–50.

42. Morris J, Royle GT. Offering patients a choice of surgery for early breast cancer: a reduction in anxiety and depression in patients and their husbands. *Social Science and Medicine*, 1988; **26**: 583–5.

43. Ganz PA. Understanding patient preferences for involvement in care. *European Journal of Cancer*, 1997; **33**: 1169–70.

44. Maguire P, Booth K, Elliott C, Jones B. Helping health professionals involved in cancer care acquire key interviewing skills—the impact of workshops. *European Journal of Cancer*, 1996; **32A**: 1486–9.

45. Razavi D, Delvaux N, Marchal S, Bredart A, Farvacques C, Paesmans M. Effects of a 24 h psychological training programme on attitudes, communication skills and occupational stress in oncology: A randomised study. *European Journal of Cancer*, 1993; **29A**, 1858–63.

46. Parle M, Maguire P, Heaven C. The development of a training model to improve health professionals' skills, self-efficacy and outcome expectancies when communicating with cancer patients. *Social Science and Medicine*, 1996; **44**: 231–40.

47. Fallowfield L, Lipkin M, Hall A. Teaching senior oncologists communication skills. *Journal of Clinical Oncology*, 1998; **16**: 1961–8.

48. Yalom Ed, Grieves C. Group therapy with the terminally ill. *American Journal of Psychiatry*,1977; **134**: 396–400.

49. Speigel D, Bloom JR, Yalom I. Group support for patients with metastatic cancer. *Archives of General Psychiatry*, 1981; **38**: 527–33.

50. Van den Borne HW, Pruyn JFA, van dam de Mey K. Self-help in cancer patients: A review of studies on the effects of contacts between fellow patients. *Patient Education and Counselling*, 1986; **8**: 367–85.

51. Fawzy IF, Fawzy NW, Hyun CS, Eloshoff R, Guthrie D, Fahey JL, Morton DL. Effects of an early structured psychiatric intervention, coping and affective state on recurrence and survival 6 years later. *Archives of General Psychiatry*, 1993; **50**: 681–9.

52. Maguire P, Tait A, Brooke M, Thomas C, Sellwood RA. The effect of counselling on the psychiatric morbidity associated with mastectomy. *British Medical Journal*, 1980; **281**: 454–6.

53. Wilkinson S, Maguire P, Tait A. Life after breast cancer. *Nursing Times*, 1988; **84**: 34–37.

54. Burton MV, Parker RW. A randomised controlled trial of preoperative psychological preparation for mastectomy. *Psycho-Oncology*, 1995; **4**: 1–20.

55. Worden JW, Weisman AD. Psychosocial intervention with newly diagnosed cancer patients. *General Hospital Psychiatry*, 1984; **6**: 243–9.

56. Greer S, Moorey S, Baruch JK, *et al.* Adjuvant psychological therapy for patients with cancer: A prospective randomised trial. *British Medical Journal*, 1992; **304**: 675–80.

57. Moorey S, Greer S, Bliss J, Law M. A comparison of adjuvant psychological therapy and supportive counselling in patients with cancer. *Psycho-Oncology*, 1988; **7**: 218–28.

58. Razavi D, Delvaux N, Farvacques C, Robaye E. Screening for adjustment disorder and major depressive disorders in cancer patients. *British Journal of Psychiatry*, 1990; **156**: 79–83.

59. Ibbotson T, Maguire P, Selby P, Priestman T, Wallace L. Screening for anxiety and depression in cancer patients. Effects of disease and treatment. *European Journal of Cancer*, 1994; **30A**: 37–40.

60. Watson M, Lae M, Maguire GP, *et al.* Further development of a quality of life measure for cancer patients: The Rotterdam Symptom Checklist (Revised). *Journal of Psycho-Oncology*, 1992; **1**: 35–44.

61. Beeber LS, Shea J, McCorkle R. The centre for epidemiological studies depression scale as a measure of depressive symptoms in newly diagnosed patients. *Journal of Psychosocial Oncology*, 1998; **16**: 1–20.

62. McGee R, Williams S, Elwood M. Are life events related to the onset of breast cancer? *Psychological Medicine*, 1996; **26**: 441–7.

63. Spiegel D, Bloom JR, Kramer HC, Gotheil E. Effects of psychological treatment on survival of patients with metastatic breast disease. *Lancet*, 1989; **ii**: 888–91.

64. Gwikel JG, Behar LC, Zabora JR. Psychosocial factors that affect the survival of adult cancer patients: A Review of research. *Journal of Psychosocial Oncology*, 1997; **15**: 1–34.

65. Ramirez A, Craig TK, Watson JP. Stress and relapse of breast cancer. *British Medical Journal*, 1989; **298**: 291–3.

66. Cunningham AJ, Edmonds CVI, Jenkins GP, Pollack H, Lockwood GA, Warr D. A randomised controlled trial of the effects of group psychological therapy on survival in women with metastatic breast cancer. *Psycho-Oncology*, 1998; **7**: 508–17.

67. Moynihan RT, Outlaw E. Nursing support groups in a cancer centre. *Journal of Psychosocial Oncology*, 1984; **2**: 33–47.

68. Silberfarb PM, Levine P. Psychosocial aspects of neoplastic disease III. Group support for the oncology nurse. *General Psychiatry*, 1980; **3**: 192–7.

69. Ramirez AJ, Graham J, Richards MA, *et al.* Burnout and psychiatric disorder among cancer clinicians. *British Journal of Cancer*, 1995; **71**: 1263–9.

6.2 Communication

Lesley Fallowfield and Valerie Jenkins

Introduction

In the course of a clinical career an oncologist is likely to conduct between 150 000 and 200 000 consultations with patients and their families. Doctors talk and listen to patients more often than they perform any other task or medical procedure. Therefore communication is a core clinical skill but one in which few clinicians have received any formal education.[1] This is an important omission, as good communication has many positive effects on patients' adjustment to cancer and its treatment, whereas poor communication has negative consequences for both doctors[2] and patients.[3]

An effective consultation is a major determinant of the accuracy and completeness of data, it dictates the range and number of problems elicited, permits a more precise assessment of the efficacy of therapy, affects adherence to treatment recommendations, influences emotional and physical well being, and contributes to both patient and physician satisfaction. There is compelling evidence from an authoritative literature review that good patient-centred communication is associated with meaningful health outcomes, including adherence to drug regimens and diets, pain control, resolution of physical and functional symptoms, improvements to physiological measures such as control of blood sugar and hypertension, and good psychological functioning of patients.[4]

Given the substantial clinical benefits, it is disappointing that many patients with cancer are unhappy with much of the communication that takes place between themselves and their doctors.[5] The omission of adequate information about the diagnosis, prognosis, and potential therapeutic options can increase anxiety and uncertainty and can lead to dissatisfaction with healthcare in general. Poor communication can create misunderstandings about the importance of diagnostic tests, lead to an under-reporting of side-effects and symptoms, and may exert a negative influence on a patient's motivation and willingness to accept advice about life-style change or treatment.[6]

Many of the complaints received each year by the British National Health Service Ombudsman, have failures of communication at their core rather than technically negligent medical practice.[7] Litigation is more likely if doctor—patient communication has been poor.[8] This unsatisfactory situation is disturbing enough for patients and their families, but it is also professionally and personally unrewarding for the doctors.[2] (Fig. 1)

The basic requirements for establishing the success of any interaction between doctors and patients are that the information relayed is at least adequate, understood, believed, remembered, and,

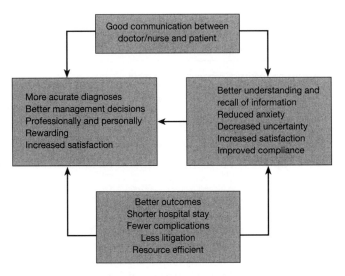

Fig. 1 The benefits for doctors, patients, and healthcare systems if communication skills are good.

hopefully, acted upon. Unfortunately many studies show that these criteria are seldom achieved.

The reasons for poor communication are complex and include certain personality and attitudinal characteristics of both patients and doctors, as well as difficulties created by the system of cancer care delivery.

Communication problems of patients

Many patients have very much lower levels of knowledge than doctors realize about biology, physiology, or anatomy and medical terminology, so they have genuine difficulty in understanding what is wrong with them.[9] Furthermore, anxiety can make interpretation and comprehension of complex information even more difficult. There are several factors contributing to patients' apprehension shown in Table 1, many of which the doctor is powerless to alter. However attempts to minimize anxiety are necessary and worthwhile.[10]

There is experimental evidence from cognitive psychology that anxious individuals attend selectively to information about life-threat, recall more information related to life-threat than neutral information, and impose life-threatening interpretations on any ambiguous statements made by the doctor.[11],[12]

Table 1 Things about which patients might be apprehensive

Diagnosis	Being hospitalized
Prognosis	Talking to staff
Being examined	Competence of staff
Further tests	Effect on family
Treatment	Time off work
Side-effects	Financial implications
Blood/injections	Dying

Table 2 Summary of patient characteristics that influence recall

* Age has no consistent relationship with recall

* Intelligence shows a small but consistent relationship

* Higher baseline medical knowledge produces better recall

* Anxiety usually related to poorer recall, but some evidence that highly anxious patients recall more

Patients are exposed repeatedly to television programmes and other media about cancer; this could be useful means of improving patient education and relieving some of the anxiety. However, much harm is created by the misinformation arising from these sources, who frequently portray misleading, inaccurate images of cancer and its treatment. We await a systematic review of the effects on patients who access some of the strange claims, specious articles, and advertisements for miracle cures posted on the Internet.

Whatever the source of a patient's prior knowledge, doctors need to assess an individual's basic understanding of cancer, their expectations of what lies ahead, and their information needs, if further communication is going to be successful.[13] Recall for medical information is generally poor, with studies of hospital patients showing a mean recall of around 54 per cent.[14] For consultations about cancer, recall is approximately 25 per cent.[15] In one study where oncologists felt that they had provided their patients with good information, patients failed to recall important details about their diagnosis, treatment, therapeutic intent of treatment, and prognosis.[16]

There is some controversy in the literature about the characteristics of patients (see Table 2) that may influence their ability to recall information.[10] Age appears to have no consistent relationship[14],[17] and intelligence shows a weak but consistent relationship[14] with information recall. Social class has little effect,[17] despite the fact that doctors typically spend more time with, and give more information to patients perceived to be from higher socioeconomic backgrounds.[18]

The influence of mood state on information recall is complicated. Although anxiety and depression affect the recall and subjective comprehensibility of medical information in non-patient volunteers,[10] other research in both patient and non-patient samples suggests that moderately high levels of anxiety may actually increase recall by motivating people to attend more actively.[19]

A comprehensive review of the literature[19] revealed good evidence that the structure and content of the consultation influences the patient's ability to remember what has been said in the following ways (Table 3):

1. Patients tend to recall facts given to them at the beginning of a consultation more readily than those provided later.

2. Topics deemed most relevant and important to the patient, which might be quite different to those considered most pertinent to the doctor, are recalled most accurately.

3. The greater the number of statements made by a doctor, the smaller the mean percentage recalled by the patient.

4. Finally, items that patients recall do not decay over time as other memories, in fact many patients have verbatim recall of what they believe was said.

Few doctors recognize the different preferences that their patients have for both the type and amount of information; frequently, a desire for more information is confused with a desire to participate in clinical decision-making.[20] Research with women who have breast cancer shows that the majority prefer a relatively passive role in decision-making but require large amounts of information as to why a doctor may be recommending one treatment over another.[21]–[23]

Several studies conducted on both sides of the Atlantic,[24]–[26] have shown that the overwhelming majority of patients want to know if they have cancer, their chances of cure, and all the possible side-effects of treatment. Fewer doctors these days are reluctant to use the word cancer,[27] but many still believe that disclosure should only be made to those who actively seek it.[28] Unfortunately, unless invited to ask directly, patients rarely ask important questions.[29] Many assume that the doctor would have told them everything relevant, others worry that they will appear foolish if they reveal their ignorance by asking questions, and some feel that they have already taken up too much of the busy doctor's time. In a study examining the structure and content of consultations with 117 patients who were either having their diagnosis of cancer confirmed or news of recurrence given, patients were given few opportunities to ask questions or to respond when asked if they had understood the information conveyed to them.[30] Just as disappointing was the minimal attention paid to patients' psychosocial concerns during these 'bad news' interviews.

Some doctors acknowledge that their own communication skills are limited and abrogate much of the responsibility for the giving of information to specialist nurses. There is no evidence that nurses' skills are any better than those of doctors. Nurses often display similar distancing tactics and inappropriate interviewing behaviours.[31] Furthermore, contrary to popular belief, patients want to receive their diagnosis and information from the most senior hospital doctor, not a nurse.[26]

Communication problems of doctors

A successful consultation with a patient demands not only good communication skills from the doctor, but also personal awareness of the likely barriers to effective communication.[32],[33] The context and content of communication in oncology can generate challenging and highly charged emotions. Faced with a distressed patient and communication about difficult issues, some doctors develop a cold, professional detachment as a means of preserving their own emotional survival. Such distancing tactics are profoundly damaging to patients

Table 3 Effect of content and structure of communication on memory

* Recall shows a primacy effect, i.e what is said first is remembered more frequently
* Information perceived as important to the patient is recalled better
* The greater the number of statements the smaller the mean percentage recalled
* There is no evidence for forgetting over time

and their families. Furthermore, these strategies do not allow doctors to establish satisfying therapeutic relationships that can make medicine so worthwhile.[33] Far too many oncologists become disillusioned with their work and show signs of burnout.[34] Research by Ramirez and her colleagues showed that clinicians specializing in cancer acknowledge that insufficient training in communication and management skills is a major factor contributing to stress, lack of job satisfaction, and burnout.[35],[36]

We know that doctors tend to underestimate the amount of information that patients require[37] and censor their information-giving to patients on an intuitive basis. Talking about cancer is stressful for both patients and doctors, but failing to talk openly due to a misguided notion that no news is good news, or by using euphemisms, only reinforces misunderstandings. As Smith, a former editor of the *British Medical Journal* observed, 'The malignant reputation of cancer is enhanced by the secrecy surrounding it'.[38] Many lay people still assume that the diagnosis heralds a universally gloomy outcome that will be preceded by unpleasant treatment. Failure to be honest about the diagnosis not only impedes acceptance and adaptation but also fuels patients' fears that they have an unspeakably horrible disease and future—'what is unspoken is unspeakable'.[39] There are other problems with an approach of non-disclosure; if for example, as is common practice in many parts of Europe,[28] diagnosis of an abdominal cancer is evaded with euphemistic talk of abnormal cells, ulcers, growths, or blockages, then the only form of abdominal cancers that become known to lay populations are fatal, since the true diagnosis only emerges later when metastases appear. Those patients with cancer who survive, do not contribute the concept of successful surgical resection to public knowledge. Thus the newly diagnosed patient would be even more apprehensive, as their only awareness of such cancers would be from people who had died of the disease.[40]

The manner in which a doctor gives information has just as important an impact on patient recall and understanding as the content. For example, an oncologist gave 40 women at high risk of breast cancer the results that their mammograms were clear. For half the group the oncologist assumed a worried affect and for the others, a non-worried affect. The results showed that those women in the worried affect group recalled less information, thought that the situation was more serious, had significantly higher anxiety-state scores and significantly higher pulse rates.[41]

Attention to non-verbal communication, such as facial expression and tone of voice, are important if the correct message is to be

Table 4 Ways to increase patient recall

* Tell patients the most important information first
* Signpost information topics
* Stress key points
* Simplify with shorter words and sentences
* Use specific, concrete statements not abstract
* Repeat important information
* Back up with written or taped material

conveyed. Several other things that a doctor can do to try and improve patient recall and comprehension are shown in Table 4.

Giving taped or written supplementary information

Butt[41] suggested giving patients a personal record of their consultation in the form of audiotapes, and early descriptive studies reported that patients found these recordings very valuable both for themselves and their family.[42] Personal recordings allowed patients to remind themselves of what was said and, furthermore, helped inform family and friends about treatments and diagnosis. It is also a simple, unobtrusive, and fairly inexpensive practical intervention to help patients make sense of their situation.

However, few studies have examined the value of providing personalized information to patients in a systematic way. A comprehensive review of the area found only eight published randomized studies examining the effectiveness of providing audiotapes or consultancy letters to patients.[43] The studies involved were single-centre trials and the number of participants recruited ranged from 34 to 182 patients with cancer. Most of the studies examined the effect of either providing or not providing patients with a taped recording of their consultation, apart from one[44] where patients were randomized to either receive or not receive a written summary of their consultation. A more recent study compared the use and effect of a computer-based information system for 438 patients receiving radical radiotherapy treatment.[45]

Table 5 Randomized information intervention studies—summary table

Study	Patients	Intervention	Primary findings
Damien and Tattersall (1991)[44]	96 pts; mixed cancer sites	Individual summary letter vs. no letter	• No significant differences in recall of information • Higher satisfaction in the intervention group • Useful and valuable tool
Davison and Degner (1997)[48]	60 pts; male, early prostate cancer	Written information pack and tape vs. no tape	• No significant differences in anxiety or depression • Helped in decision-making about treatments • Useful and valuable tool
Dunn, et al. (1993)[15]	142 pts; mixed cancer sites	Consultation tape vs. general tape vs. no tape	• No significant differences in anxiety or depression • No significant differences in recall of information • Higher satisfaction in the intervention
Ford, et al. (1995)[50]	117 pts; mixed cancer sites	Consultation tape vs. no tape	• No significant differences in anxiety or depression • No significant difference between the groups in the mean number of questions asked in consultation
Hogbin, et al. (1992)[49]	83 pts; female, early breast cancer	Consultation tape vs. no tape	• No significant differences in anxiety or depression • No significant differences in recall of information • Useful and valuable tool
Jones, et al. (1999)[45]	438 pts; mixed sites	Personal vs. general information from computer	• Anxiety significantly higher 3 months later in group that received general information • Greater satisfaction in those patients receiving personal information via the computer
McHugh, et al. (1995)[51]	see Ford et al.		• No significant differences in anxiety or depression • Significant difference in recall of information • Useful and valuable tool
North, et al. (1992)[46]	34 pts; mixed cancer sites	Consultation tape vs. no tape	• No significant differences in anxiety or depression • Significant difference in recall of information • Useful and valuable tool
Reynolds, et al. (1981)[47]	pt number unclear; mixed sites	Consultation tape and information pack vs. no tape	• No significant differences in satisfaction • No significant differences in recall of information • Useful and valuable tool
Tattersall et al. (1994)[89]	182 pts; mixed sites	Cross-over design of consultation tape first, followed by summary letter, and vice versa	• No significant differences in anxiety or depression • No significant differences in recall of information • Both interventions considered useful

Patients in the studies were receiving information at different treatment time points. Some patients were attending clinics concerning treatments,[15],[45]–[48] some consultations involved 'breaking bad news',[49]–[51] others included patients who were attending follow-up clinics.[44] Most studies involved a single clinician, apart from one[50],[51] that included five clinicians.

Each study had a number of outcome variables: these included the usefulness of the intervention, changes in patients' recall and understanding, satisfaction with the consultation, and alterations in the psychological status between the intervention and control groups. The main findings from the studies are summarized in Table 5.

Usefulness

Results from the studies provided overwhelming evidence that both patients and their families found the audiotapes and summary letters

to be very valuable. Few patients found that listening to the consultation again was distressing, despite the fact that a number of them contained 'bad news', although one study[50] suggested that some patients with recurrence of their disease did not wish to listen to the news a second time. Many patients listened to the tape at least twice, often with other family members present and some even played it to their general practitioner.[49] Between 83 and 90 per cent of patients receiving tapes and letters found them useful as a reminder of what was said during the consultation and others indicated that it had aided their decision-making regarding treatments.[46],[48]

Satisfaction

Patient satisfaction with communication is an important parameter in the evaluation and improvement of the quality of healthcare services and may have an influential impact on medical outcomes.[3],[52] Although satisfaction data is normally positively skewed and tends to increase with the severity of the illness,[53],[54] it can decline as a patient's level of psychological morbidity increases. This may be the reason that only two of the four studies that measured patient satisfaction produced evidence that patients who received the intervention were more satisfied with the consultation.[44],[45]

Recall and understanding

There have been six studies examining whether or not the intervention improved patients' recall and understanding. Results are conflicting with only two studies[46],[50] reporting a positive effect. Hogbin and colleagues[49] (1992) noted a difference between the groups in the immediate preoperative period, but this cancelled out at 6 weeks' post-operatively, probably because the control patients had acquired information from other sources. The difference found in the results between the studies probably reflects the mode and time points at which the patients' recall was measured. Sometimes patients were interviewed at regular time points and in other cases patients were seen at intervals ranging from 3 days to 6 weeks.

Psychological status

It could be argued that patients would find it distressing to listen to or read about their consultation a second time, especially if it contained 'bad news'. However, that was not reported in any of the studies that provided personally relevant information to the patient. Only in one study that examined the effect of providing information to patients via a computer was there a difference in anxiety levels. At 3 months, 37 per cent of patients who received general information about cancer were still anxious compared with 19 per cent who had received personal information.

The absence of a significant difference in psychological distress between the groups may also be due to the lack of sensitivity of the test chosen to measure changes in levels of anxiety and depression.

Communication difficulties due to system constraints

Many consultations between doctors and their patients take place in environments that militate against the practice of good skills. Some hospital departments provide less privacy for intimate or distressing consultations than one would find in the office of an accountant, bank manager, or veterinary surgeon, and there are constant interruptions. During a research project measuring the effect of providing patients with tape-recordings of their consultations, one doctor commented that he had no idea just how often his consultations were disrupted by the telephone ringing or by other healthcare professionals entering the room.[42] Doctors may become inured to such things over time, but for patients it can be humiliating to be overheard, and frightening or embarrassing to witness the private conversations of others. This lack of privacy is a major contribution to patient unease, and may lead to an increased inability to either comprehend or contribute to the consultation.

With throughput and waiting lists uppermost in the minds of management, some clinics are so pressured for time that much important two-way communication between the patient and doctor is sacrificed in favour of physical examination and a doctor-centred monologue.

Finally, the lack of communication between different specialists and departments can cause further confusion about the diagnosis, test results, and management. Improvements in communication provided by a multidisciplinary team may be shown, but such approaches are alien to many healthcare professionals[55] who have been educated within a hierarchical system. Unless old practices are abandoned and different patterns of communication between healthcare professionals become established, benefits will not occur. Too often, important information for the patient is omitted on the assumption that someone else must have relayed relevant facts at appropriate times. This can be confusing and cause a loss of confidence in the team, provoking needless anxiety for patients; it is also frustrating for clinicians who may have to spend extra time communicating bad news or quite basic information to an unprepared patient.

Specific problems in communication

Talking about trials

Accrual of patients in clinical trials is very low, impeding progress in research and the introduction of new cancer treatments. Recruitment difficulties arise from: the system of healthcare delivery; concern about ethical and medicolegal issues; and the personality factors and attitudes of both patients[56] and doctors.[57],[58]

The reluctance of doctors to approach eligible patients about clinical trials is probably more important than the patients' reluctance to participate.[59],[60] Some doctors perceive conflicts between the role of clinician and scientist and many express anxiety about the impact that the necessary disclosure of uncertainty might have on the doctor–patient relationship.[57],[58],[61]

Demands for high throughput and cost-containment result in too many patients being seen in busy clinics, with inadequate consultation time and insufficient support to explain trial details and to allow properly informed consent to be given.[58] Also some hospitals do not reward or encourage clinicians who wish to join collaborative trials. However, a fundamental factor in poor recruitment into trials, and the unacceptably low understanding exhibited by patients about the trials they join, is the inadequate communication skills of doctors.

Explaining randomization, giving complex information, and obtaining informed consent were acknowledged by 178 senior oncologists attending courses on communication skills to be their primary problem areas.[1] Discussing trials is extremely difficult and doctors need more education and understanding about patient attitudes, as well as help with their communication skills, if the situation is to improve. Some of the specific communication difficulties are shown in Table 6.

The primary reasons why patients may decline entry into a clinical trial include: uncertainty about personal benefit;[62] concerns as to whether or not the best available treatment would be given (even though trial participation usually leads to better health outcomes);[63] overestimation of the likely therapeutic benefits of standard therapy;[64] and wanting to choose a specific treatment arm rather than be randomized. Poor understanding about the purpose and value of clinical trials has led to suspicion and confusion among the general population.[65],[66] Also considerable ignorance abounds

Table 6 Some of the difficulties, when talking about clinical trials, expressed by senior oncologists attending communication skills' courses in the UK

Communication problems when talking about trials
• Having to give much complex information in a short space of time
• Putting complex information into layman's terms
• Discussing phase I clinical trials
• 'Selling' a trial or treatment I wouldn't really want myself
• Conveying the uncertainty about treatments whilst being reassuring that we are a competent unit
• Genuinely believing that my patients are giving fully informed consent
• Explaining trials with a surveillance arm or watch policy
• Discussing trials with markedly different toxicities in one arm
• Explaining why randomization is necessary

concerning the meaning of randomization; some patients are worried about the process, preferring the doctor, whom they trust, to make treatment decisions rather than to leave this to a computer and the play of chance.[67] In a recent survey, lay people were given seven different statements explaining randomization; favour was found for the less explicit explanations which played down the role of chance.[68] These opinions were from a non-sick population, whether they apply to patients with cancer has yet to be formally tested. Aversion to randomization was the reason given by 63 per cent of patients who refused to participate in one trial.[62] Doctors need to be aware of these issues and to ascertain their patients' understanding about trials.

When patients have agreed to participate in a clinical trial, there is evidence that consent is not always as informed as it ought to be.[69] Many patients do not even recall that they are receiving experimental treatment.[70] This suggests that either the information was inadequate, given in an incomprehensible manner, or that patients' understanding was not checked sufficiently. In our analysis of doctor–patient interactions, despite protocol and ethical requirements exemplified in good clinical practice guidelines, clinicians adopted somewhat idiosyncratic behaviours when providing information and eliciting consent to trials.

Particularly contentious is deciding just how much information needs to be given for consent to be informed.[71] Much has been written about patients' 'right to know', but less about patients' 'right not to know'. Several have questioned the ethics of overburdening patients with unwanted information. Logically, true autonomy should include patients' preferences for less as well as more information. Examination of taped recordings of consultations shows that when information about prognosis and the expected therapeutic benefits from the different treatment arms of a trial is withheld, this is usually an intuitive decision made by the doctor. It is rarely done as a result of enquiry into the patient's own stated preferences for information. A more rational basis for determining how much and what sort of information needs to be given to an individual patient who is eligible for entry into a clinical trial is required.

Some attempts to do this have been published. In one such study 57 patients were randomized either to total disclosure of all possible relevant information or to an individual approach based on the doctors' intuition as to what patients wanted. The main findings suggested that total disclosure led to a better understanding of the research aspects of treatment and side-effects, but less willingness to agree to randomized treatment and increased anxiety.[72]

Problems when talking to relatives

Talking with relatives was the second most problematic communication area cited by senior oncologists during the communication skills courses (1). Some typical problem areas are shown in Table 7.

The primary sources of support for patients throughout the course of their disease and treatment, are likely to be other family members. The relatives of newly diagnosed patients report high levels of concerns and distress that warrant more attention than is commonly available.[73],[74] Brewin has pointed out that '... the nearest relative may be thought of not only as someone who needs information from us, who can advise us and who may play a leading part in caring for the patient, but also as a victim needing our help'.[75]

Interactions between a doctor, the patient, and relatives is difficult, especially when the relative appears to be driving the interview at a rate, or in a direction, that the doctor does not feel is in the patient's best interests.

Some families try to protect their relatives from bad news by insisting that the doctor colludes with them in the pretence that all is well. Such families offer a convenient, beguiling avenue of evasion for busy doctors and nurses, but there is much to argue against this. The rights of a competent patient should override those of family members who wish to be the gatekeepers of information exchange unless the patient has given explicit permission for relatives to intervene in this way.[76]

It is always distressing to witness the desperation of relatives who cannot accept that their loved one has cancer that will not respond to conventional therapy, and who wish to engage the sometimes reluctant patient in a futile quest for a miracle cure. The doctor has a crucial role here in helping the whole family readjust their aims to the more achievable, realistic goals of good-quality palliation and

Table 7 Some of the difficult communication areas cited by senior oncologists in the UK attending communication skills' courses

Communication problems with relatives
• Relatives who break down when I'm trying to support the patient
• Dealing with relatives who try to prevent disclosure of the diagnosis
• Relatives who ask questions about prognosis in front of patient who does not wish to confront that situation yet
• Relatives insisting on further inappropriate treatment
• Angry, abusive, relatives who embarrass or distress the patient
• Parents with conflicting views about their child's treatment
• Divorced parents who use the consultation as a battleground
• Relatives who believe in the power of positive thought
• Relatives who want the patient to try alternative remedies
• Large family groups, especially those from different cultural backgrounds who do not let the patient express his/own views

acceptance of the inevitable without destroying hope. Many complementary treatments such as relaxation, aromatherapy, and therapeutic massage can be supported enthusiastically if they are acceptable to the patient and likely to improve their quality of life.

Some relatives will not be happy until every possible avenue for further treatment has been explored; a second opinion offered early on in the discussion can be valuable and helps to promote trust and confidence in the doctor's openness and objectivity. Family dynamics are difficult and sometimes dangerous to alter, but gentle support from the doctor and encouragement for the patient to express candidly their own preferences has a vital role in these situations.

Talking to children and to adolescents with cancer

Talking with minors about cancer poses several dilemmas. Many clinicians are uncertain about: whose needs to focus upon, those of the parents or of the child; how to handle parents who disagree about management; whether or not the child should have a voice in decision-making; and whether or not doctors and nurses should talk about the diagnosis and prognosis without the parents present or without parental consent.

Many parents and doctors feel instinctively that they should protect children from the knowledge that they have cancer. This is not supported by the controlled studies that have compared the effects of open disclosure with those of withholding the diagnosis.[77] Parents usually opt for telling less about the diagnosis, treatment, and prognosis to younger children. In one study, 43 children discussed with interviewers the information that had been given to them, their causal attributions, illness-related stress, and coping strategies. Children under 9 years were told less than those aged between 9 and 14, who in turn were told less than adolescents. Despite being told much less, younger children reported similar levels of distress to those of the older groups, suggesting that such shielding did not protect them from fears and anxieties about the disease.[78]

Despite overt attempts by adults to maintain a cheerful front, children with cancer can sense the despair and distress of their parents. Consequently the children may harbour frightening fantasies, or feel isolated and mistrustful of their adult carers and parents, assuming that their diagnosis and prognosis are too awful for anyone to discuss with them. Good psychosocial adjustment in 116 long-term survivors of childhood malignancies was associated with patients' early knowledge of their diagnosis, but this was worse in those who had been misled or who had later learned the truth about their illness.[79]

Such information has been available for some time, but Claflin and Barbarin's study[78] showed that 63 per cent of children were given no information about their likely prognoses, despite the fact that this is what they had wanted. In another study conducted with 50 children aged between 8 and 17 years and with 60 accompanying parents, the authors found that despite parental reluctance for full disclosure, the children wanted information about all aspects of their disease, all possible treatments, and the likely outcome. In contrast to the 76 per cent of children who said that they wanted to know their chances of cure, even if the outlook was bleak, only 38 per cent of their parents thought that this information should be disclosed.[80] Most children (82 per cent) did not approve of their parents having private discussions with doctors about their condition, but 13 per cent of younger patients and 42 per cent of older patients said that they wanted the right to have private discussions with the doctor without their parents present.

Talking to adolescents can be difficult even if they do not have cancer, but many doctors misunderstand both the amount and the sorts of information that adolescents require.[80],[81] For example, Pfefferbaum *et al.* surveyed the informational items thought most important to discuss by adolescents compared with those thought most important by their doctors, and found very little agreement. Top of the adolescents' list was 'what to expect if the cancer spreads' (84 per cent), whereas only 19 per cent of doctors thought this important to describe. More than half the adolescents wanted statistics about recurrence, in contrast to the 10 per cent of doctors who deemed this desirable information to impart. There is no evidence that adolescents require less information than that desired by adult cancer patients.

Perhaps the trend for adolescents to be treated in specialist units will allow for more research and training in appropriate communication for healthcare professionals.[82] The guidelines produced by the SIOP (**International Society of Paediatric Oncology**) working party on communication of the diagnosis concluded that the goal should be to produce a knowledgeable family able to talk openly with its members and with oncology staff.[83] It is time that these guidelines influenced practice.

Talking about psychosocial issues

Although awareness of the psychosocial problems experienced by patients with cancer has increased, clinicians still appear reluctant to enquire directly about patients' concerns and feelings. Some lack the skills to probe effectively, while others worry that such probing will damage their patients psychologically and release strong emotions that the clinician will then be unable to address effectively.[84] Patients rarely disclose their concerns, unless encouraged to do so, in the mistaken belief that such difficulties are inevitable consequences of cancer. They also assume that nothing can be done to help, and that their doctors may not be interested in such issues.[85]

Even when patients do make disclosures recognition of psychological morbidity is low. Oncologists fail to detect general distress and do not correctly identify those patients with psychological disorders that merit intervention Psychological interventions can prevent and ameliorate the anxiety and/or depression experienced by approximately 25 to 30 per cent patients.[86]

Clinicians who are unskilled at identifying psychosocial problems tend to avoid eye contact with the patient, and ask many closed questions concerned primarily with physical symptoms. Some fail to recognize their inability to deal well with these types of consultations; others freely admit that they need further training in eliciting psychosocial concerns and handling emotional situations such as dealing with angry patients and relatives, those who are very withdrawn or expressing denial.

What can be done to help ?

Although the old 'learn as you go' apprenticeship model of acquiring communication skills has produced some excellent doctors, the system has failed the majority, to the detriment of both their own[34] and their patients' well being.[4]

Communication skills are critical to the practice of medicine but there is little consensus on criteria for adequate performance.[87] Relatively little attention has been paid to the development of standardized methodologies for the assessment of medical dialogue, and the oncology consultation has remained largely outside the recent emphasis on quality of care and subsequent changes in delivery of cancer services. Few oncologists have systematically analysed their

All consultations have the following functions:

collect	**D**ATA
establish	**R**APPORT
provide	**E**DUCATION
give	**A**DVICE
stimulate	**M**OTIVATION

Fig. 2 The DREAM medical consultation.

own communication skills and they are unaware of what might constitute ideal practice. Although there are, as yet, few rigorously evaluated clinical trials which demonstrate that interventions to improve communication skills results in improved health outcomes in cancer, there is evidence accruing that effective skills can be taught, and when taught well changes are maintained and expand.[1],[88]

Methods to teach skills that produce demonstrable change, adopt approaches incorporating cognitive, affective, and behavioural components, and are learner-centred.[88] One such model, sponsored by the Cancer Research Campaign in the United Kingdom resulted in considerable changes in the skills of senior oncologists and in their attitudes and willingness to teach communication skills to junior staff. Clinicians worked in small groups of four participants with one experienced facilitator on residential courses lasting either $1\frac{1}{2}$ or 3 days.

The courses integrated exercises and activities designed to create simultaneously the development of skills, knowledge acquisition, and personal awareness of how these impact on both the doctor and the patient. Participants defined their own difficulties and directed their own learning needs, which helps to circumvent physician defensiveness and rendered the work relevant and interesting. Groups were led by trained facilitators who were able to create a safe and constructive environment for participants. Groups worked on specific skills with trained actors (simulated patients) followed by video review of their interviews. Small group discussion, interactive group demonstrations, and the provision of published literature led to significant gains in conceptual frameworks. Time was set aside for discussion of emotional responses and personal awareness of communication barriers. If confidentiality is assured, participants are usually surprisingly frank about their own emotional difficulties.

This course revealed many of the communication difficulties experienced by oncologists, some of which have been described in earlier parts of this chapter. The courses produced greater confidence in participants' perceived ability to cope with these problems and the model is now being tested in a large randomized trial in cancer centres throughout the United Kingdom.

Medical education does not develop doctors' ability to critique their own interviewing skills, nor does it provide a conceptual framework for analysing their interviews with patients. Figure 2 shows an example of a framework based on a deliberately ambiguous acronym, the DREAM consultation.[3] To maximize the likelihood of a favourable outcome, oncology consultations should fulfil the primary functions shown in Fig. 2. Obviously different emphasis will be placed on different functions depending on the content and context of the consultation, for example an interview with a new patient would probably be rather different than a follow-up one in terms of building rapport. Elements of all functions are usually present and skilled communicators are adept at integrating them. Doctors should be able to develop styles and techniques that facilitate accurate collection of data concerning a patient's medical history and own concerns. This can be facilitated by establishing at the outset a favourable **rapport** which will enhance the **education** and understanding of the patient about the disease, treatment plan, and prognosis. The patient is then more likely to accept **advice** and is more **motivated** to act upon it. When teaching doctors to acquire better self-critique abilities, frameworks such as the **DREAM** are useful for establishing strengths and weaknesses, and permitting assessment of improvement following training initiatives.

We have extraordinary expectations of oncologists; they have to be scientifically adept; cognisant of and able to implement advances in diagnostic and therapeutic techniques; practically competent, efficient business managers, inspiring teachers of junior staff; empathic and effective communicators with people from a wide range of social and educational backgrounds all of whom have different informational needs, personality styles, and reactions to news of a cancer diagnosis. It is not surprising that such demands make doctors vulnerable to psychiatric disorders, emotional exhaustion, etc. The acquisition of good communication and management skills during undergraduate and postgraduate training with regular opportunities to update these skills is a fundamental requirement if oncologists are to be effective communicators.

References

1. **Fallowfield LJ, Lipkin M, Hall A.** Teaching senior oncologists communication skills: results from phase 1 of a comprehensive longitudinal program in the UK. *Journal of Clinical Oncology,* 1998; **16:** 1961–8.

2. **Fallowfield LJ.** Can we improve the professional and personal fulfilment of doctors in cancer medicine? *British Journal of Cancer,* 1995; **71:** 1132–3.

3. **Fallowfield LJ.** The ideal consultation. *British Journal of Hospital Medicine,* 1992; **47**(5): 364–7.

4. **Stewart MA.** Effective physician–patient communication and health outcomes: a review. *Canadian Medical Association Journal,* 1996; **152:** 1423–33.

5. **Fallowfield LJ, Hall A, Maguire GP, Baum M.** Psychological outcomes of different treatment policies in women with early breast cancer outside a clinical trial. *British Medical Journal,* 1990; **301:** 575–80.

6. **Audit Commission.** *What seems to be the matter? Communication between hospitals and patients.* London: HMSO, 1993.

7. **Reid W.** *Health Service Commission Fourth Report, Session 1992/93.* London: HMSO, 1993.

8. **Levinson W.** Physician–patient communication: a key to malpractice prevention. *Journal of the American Medical Association,* 1994; **273:** 1619–20.

9. **Boyle C.** Differences between patients' and doctors' interpretation of some common medical terms. *British Medical Journal,* 1970; **2:** 286–9.

10. **Pickersgill MJ, Owen A.** Mood-states, recall and subjective comprehensibility of medical information in non-patient volunteers. *Personality and Individual Differences,* 1992; **13**(12): 1299–305.

11. **Beck AT, Clark DA.** Anxiety and depression: an information processing perspective. *Anxiety Research,* 1988; **1:** 23–36,

12. **MacLeod C, Cohen IL.** Anxiety and the interpretation of ambiguity: a text comprehension study. *Journal of Abnormal Psychology,* 1993; **102**(2): 238–47.

13. **Armstrong D.** What do patients want ? Someone who will hear their questions. *British Medical Journal,* 1991; **303:** 261–2.

14. **Ley P.** *Communicating with patients: improving communication,* satisfaction and compliance. (Marcer D, ed. Psychology and Medicine Series.) London: Croom Helm, 1988.

15. **Dunn SM, *et al.*** General information tapes inhibit recall of the cancer consultation. *Journal of Clinical Oncology,* 1993; **11**(11): 2279–85.

16. **Mackillop WJ, Stewart WE, Ginsburg AD, Stewart SS.** Cancer patients' perceptions of their disease and its treatment. *British Journal of Cancer,* 1988; **58:** 355–8.

17. **Anderson JL, Dodmas S, Kopelman M, Fleming A.** Patient information recall in a rheumatology clinic. *Rheumatology and Rehabilitation,* 1979; **18:** 18–22.

18. **Helman CG.** Communication in primary care: the role of patient and practitioner explanatory models. *Social Science and Medicine,* 1985; **20**(9): 923–31.

19. **Ley P.** Recall by patients. In *Cambridge handbook of psychology, health and medicine* (ed. A Baum, S Newman, J Weinman, R West, C McManus). Cambridge: Cambridge University Press, 1997: 315–17.

20. **Hack TF, Degner LF, Dyck DG.** Relationship between preferences for decisional control and illness information among women with breast cancer: a quantitative and qualitative analysis. *Social Science and Medicine,* 1994; **39:** 279–89.

21. **Degner LF, Sloan JA.** Decision-making during serious illness: what role do patients really want to play? *Journal of Clinical Epidemiology,* 1992; **45**(9): 941–50.

22. **Fallowfield LJ, Hall A.** Psychological effects of being offered choice of surgery for breast cancer. *British Medical Journal,* 1994; **309:** 448.

23. **Beaver K, Luker KA, Owens RG, Leinster SJ, Degner LF, Sloan JA.** Treatment decision making in women newly diagnosed with breast cancer. *Cancer Nursing,* 1996; **19**(1): 8–19.

24. **Cassileth BR, Zupkis RV, Sutton-Smith K, March V.** Information and participation preferences among cancer patients. *Annals of Internal Medicine,* 1980; **92:** 832–6.

25. **Fallowfield LJ, Ford S, Lewis S.** No news is not good news: information preferences of patients with cancer. *Psycho-oncology,* 1995; **4:** 197–202.

26. **Meredith C, *et al.*** Information needs of cancer patients in the West of Scotland. *British Medical Journal,* 1996; **313:** 724–6.

27. **Holland JC, Geary N, Marchini A, Tross S.** An international survey of physician attitudes and practice in regard to revealing the diagnosis of cancer. *Cancer Investigation,* 1987; **5**(2): 151–4.

28. **Thomsen O, Wulff HR, Martin A.** What do gastroenterologists in Europe tell cancer patients? *Lancet,* 1993; **341:** 472–6.

29. **Ford S, Fallowfield LJ, Lewis S.** Doctor–patient interactions in oncology. *Social Science and Medicine,* 1996; **42**(11): 1511–19.

30. **Wilkinson S.** Factors which influence how nurses communicate with cancer patients. *Journal of Cancer Nursing,* 1991; **16:** 677–88.

31. **Maguire P.** Barriers to psychological care of the dying. *British Medical Journal,* 1985; **291:** 1711–13.

32. **Fallowfield LJ.** Giving sad and bad news. *Lancet,* 1993; **341:** 476–8.

33. **Whippen DA, Canellos GP.** Burnout syndrome in the practice of oncology: results of a random survey of 1000 oncologists. *Journal of Clinical Oncology,* 1991; **9**(10): 1916–20.

34. **Ramirez AJ, *et al.*** Burnout and psychiatric disorder among cancer clinicians. *British Journal of Cancer,* 1995; **71**(6): 1263–9.

35. **Ramirez AJ, Graham J, Richards MA, Cull A, Gregory WM.** Mental health of hospital consultants: the effects of stress and satisfaction at work. *Lancet,* 1996; **347:** 724–8.

36. **Fallowfield LJ, Ford S, Lewis S.** Information preferences of patients with cancer. *Lancet,* 1994; **344**(3 Dec): 1576.

37. **Smith A.** Should a doctor tell the truth when a patient has cancer? *The Times,* 1976; March 31.

38. **Simpson MA.** Therapeutic uses of truth. In *The dying patient* (ed. E Wilkes) Lancaster: MTP Press, 1982: 255–62.

39. Fallowfield LJ, Clark AW. Delivering bad news in gastroenterology. *American Journal of Gastroenterology*, 1994; **89**(4): 473–9.

40. Shapiro DE, Boggs SR, Melamed BG, Graham-Pole J. The effect of varied physician affect on recall, anxiety, and perceptions in women at risk for breast cancer: an analogue study. *Health Psychology*, 1992; **11**(1): 61–6.

41. Butt, HR. A method for better physician–patient communication. *Annals of Internal Medicine*, 1977; **86**: 478–80.

42. Hogbin B, Fallowfield LJ. Getting it taped: the 'bad news' consultation with cancer patients in a general surgical out-patient department. *British Journal of Hospital Medicine*, 1989; **41**(4): 330–3.

43. Scott, JT, Entwistle, VE, Sowden, AJ, Watt I. Recordings or summaries of consultations for people with cancer (Cochrane Review). *The Cochrane Library*, 1999, 4.

44. Damian, D, Tattersall, MHN. Letters to patients: improving communication in cancer care. *Lancet*, 1991; **338**: 923–5.

45. Jones, R, *et al.* Randomised trial of personalised computer based information for cancer patients. *British Medical Journal*, 1999; **319**: 1241–7.

46. North, N, Cornbleet, MA, Knowles G, Leonard CF. Information giving in oncology: a preliminary study of tape-recorder use. *British Journal of Clinical Psychology*, 1992; **31**: 357–9.

47. Reynolds, PM, Sanson-Fisher RW, Desmond-Poole A, Harker J, Byrne MJ. Cancer and communication: information giving in oncology: a preliminary study of tape-recorder use. *British Medical Journal*, 1981; **282**: 1449–51.

48. Davison, BJ, Degner L. Empowerment of men newly diagnosed with prostate cancer. *Cancer Nursing*, 1997; **20**: 187–96.

49. Hogbin, B, Jenkins VA, Parkin AJ. Remembering 'bad news' consultations: an evaluation of tape-recorded consultations. *Psychooncology*, 1992; **1**: 147–54.

50. Ford, S, Fallowfield, Lewis, S. The influence of audiotapes on patient participation in the cancer consultation. *European Journal of Cancer*, 1995; **31A**: 2264–9.

51. McHugh, P, *et al.* The efficacy of audiotapes in promoting psychological wellbeing in cancer patients: a randomised, controlled trial. *British Journal of Cancer*, 1995; **71**: 388–92.

52. Kaplan, SH, Greenfield, S, Ware, JE. Assessing the effects of physician–patient interactions on the outcome of chronic disease. *Medical Care*, 1989; **27**: S110–S127.

53. Fitzpatrick, R. Surveys of patient satisfaction: I— important general considerations. *British Medical Journal*, 1991; **302**: 887–9.

54. Ben-Sira, Z. Affective and instrumental components in the physician–patient relationship: an additional dimension of interaction theory. *Journal of Health and Social Behaviour*, 1980; **21**: 170–80.

55. Busby A, Gilchrist B. The role of the nurse in the medical ward round. *Journal of Advanced Nursing*, 1992; **17**(3): 339–46.

56. Fallowfield LJ, Jenkins V, Brennan C, Sawtell M, Moynihan C, Souhami RL. Attitudes of patients to randomised clinical trials of cancer therapy. *European Journal of Cancer*, 1998; **34**(10): 1554–9.

57. Taylor KM, Feldstein ML, Skeel RT, Pandya KJ, Ng P, Carbone PP. Fundamental dilemmas of the randomised clinical trial process: results of the 1,737 Eastern cooperative oncology group investigators. *Journal of Clinical Oncology*, 1994; **12**(9): 1796–805.

58. Fallowfield LJ, Ratcliffe D, Souhami RL. Clinicians' attitudes to clinical trials of cancer therapy. *European Journal of Cancer*, 1997; **33**(13): 2221–9.

59. Mackillop WE, Palmer MJ, O'Sullivan B, Ward GK, Steele R, Dotsikas G. Clinical trials in cancer: the role of surrogate patients in defining what constitutes an ethically acceptable clinical experiment. *British Journal of Cancer*, 1989; **59**: 388–95.

60. Tannock, IF. The recruitment of patients into clinical trials. *British Journal of Cancer*, 1995; **71**: 1134–5.

61. Taylor KM, Kelner MJ. Interpreting physician participation in randomised clinical trials: the Physician Orientation Profile. *Journal of Health and Social Behavior*, 1987; **28**: 389–400.

62. Llewellyn-Thomas HA, McGreal MJ, Theil EC, Fine S, Erlichman C. Patients' willingness to enter clinical trials: measuring the association with perceived benefit and preference for decision participation. *Social Science and Medicine*, 1991; **32**(1): 35–42.

63. Van Dongen JA, van de Velde CJ. The benefits of participation in clinical trials. *European Journal of Surgical Oncology*, 1996; **22**(6): 561–2.

64. Sheldon JM, Fetting JH, Siminoff LA. Offering the option of randomised clinical trials to cancer patients who overestimate their prognoses with standard therapies. *Cancer-Investigation*, 1993; **11**: 57–62.

65. Raphael A. How doctors' secret trials abused me. *The Observer*, 1988; 9th October.

66. Toynbee P. Random clinical trials are one of life's biggest gambles. *BMA News Review*, 1997; March 12th: 50.

67. Gotay CC. Accrual to cancer clinical trials: directions from the research literature. *Social Science and Medicine*, 1991; **33**: 569–77.

68. Corbett F, Oldham J, Lilford R. Offering patients entry in clinical trials: preliminary study of the views of prospective participants. *Journal of Medical Ethics*, 1996; **22**(4): 227–31.

69. Montgomery C, Lydon A, Lloyd K. Patients may not understand enough to give their informed consent. *British Medical Journal*, 1997; **314**: 1482.

70. Sutherland HJ, Lockwood GA, Till J. Are we getting informed consent from patients with cancer. *Journal of the Royal Society of Medicine*, 1990; **83**: 439–43.

71. Tobias JS. Informed consent in medical research. Changing the BMJ's position on informed consent would be counterproductive. *British Medical Journal*, 1998; **316**: 1001–2.

72. Simes RJ, Tattersall HHN, Coates AS, Raghavan D, Solomon HJ, Smartt H. Randomised comparison of procedures for obtaining informed consent in clinical trials of treatment for cancer. *British Medical Journal*, 1986; **293**: 1065–8.

73. Harrison J, Haddad P, Maguire P. The impact of cancer on key relatives: a comparison of relative and patient concerns. *European Journal of Cancer*, 1995; **31A**(11): 1736–40. [See comments.]

74. Fallowfield LJ. Helping the relatives of patients with cancer. *European Journal of Cancer*, 1995; **31A**(11): 1731–2.

75. Brewin T, Sparshott M. *Relating to the relatives.* Abingdon, Oxon: Radcliffe Medical Press, 1996.

76. Fallowfield LJ. Truth sometimes hurts but deceit hurts more. In *Communication with the cancer patient: information and truth* (ed. AMZ Surbone). New York: Annals of the New York Academy of Sciences, 1997; **809**: 525–36.

77. Spinetta JJ. The dying child's awareness of death: a review. *Psychological Bulletin*, 1974; **81**(4): 256–60.

78. Claflin CJ, Barbarin OA. Does 'telling' less protect more? Relationships among age, information disclosure, and what children with cancer see and feel. *Journal of Pediatric Psychology*, 1991; **16**(2): 169–91.

79. Slavin L, O'Malley JE, Koocher GP, Foster DJ. Communication of the cancer diagnosis to pediatric patients: impact on long-term adjustment. *American Journal of Psychiatry*, 1982; **139**(2): 179–83.

80. Ellis R, Leventhal B. Information needs and decision-making preferences of children with cancer. *Psycho-oncology*, 1993; **2**(4): 277–84.

81. Pfefferbaum B, Levenson P. Adolescent cancer patient and physician responses to a questionnaire on patient concerns. *American Journal of Psychiatry*, 1982; **139**(3): 348–51.

82. Souhami R. Care for the adolescent with cancer. *European Journal of Cancer*, 1993; **29A**(16): 2215–16.

83. **Masera G,** *et al.* SIOP Working Committee on psychosocial issues in pediatric oncology: guidelines for communication of the diagnosis. *Medical and Pediatric Oncology,* 1997; **28**(5): 382–5.

84. **Buckman R.** Breaking bad news: why is it still so difficult? *British Medical Journal,* 1984; **288**(6430): 1597–9.

85. **Maguire P, Faulkner A, Booth K, Elliott C, Hillier V.** Helping cancer patients disclose their concerns. *European Journal of Cancer,* 1996; **32A**(1 Jan): 78–81.

86. **Fallowfield LJ.** Psychosocial interventions in cancer. *British Medical Journal,* 1995; **311**: 1316–17.

87. **Roter D, Fallowfield L.** Principles of training medical staff in psychosocial and communication skills. In *Psycho-oncology* (ed. JC Holland). New York: Oxford University Press, 1998: 1074–82.

88. **Parle M, Maguire P, Heaven C.** The development of a training model to improve health care professionals' skills, self-efficacy, and outcome expectations when communicating with cancer patients. *Social Science and Medicine,* 1997; **44**(2): 231–40.

89. **Tattersall MH, Bulow PN, Griffin A, Dunn SH.** The take home message: patients prefer consultation audiotapes to summary letters. *Journal of Clinical Oncology,* 1994; **6**: 1305–11.

6.3 Quality of life

Neil Aaronson and Peter Fayers

In the medical context, the question: 'How are you?' represents more than a simple social ritual. It is usually the first question that is asked by the doctor in the consulting room. It represents an informal invitation to the patient to talk about his or her health; for example, whether the pain has improved or worsened since the last visit. At the same time, the patient may be uncertain about the rules of the game. Is it appropriate to talk about his feelings, or how his health is affecting his work or family life? This uncertainty may be shared by the doctor. Do I want to know if the patient is depressed? Should I ask him whether the treatment is affecting his relationship with his wife? Typically, these issues are negotiated and communicated implicitly, often without either the patient or the doctor being aware that they may be setting limits.

In clinical research we cannot afford to be so casual in establishing the rules of conduct. In formally evaluating the effect of a treatment we need to state, up-front, what we consider to be the most important outcomes of interest. In clinical oncology, these have traditionally been objective outcomes, including tumour response, disease-free survival, and overall survival. In other words, the question 'How are you?' has usually been posed in purely biological terms.

There has been a growing recognition that these traditional markers of therapeutic success are often insufficient for evaluating the effect of cancer treatment; that it may be appropriate, and even essential, to broaden our focus to include formal and systematic assessments of the extent to which cancer and its treatment impact on the quality of life (**QoL**) of the patient.

What lies behind this shift of focus? In part, it reflects general trends in the distribution of disease in the modern, industrialized world from acute towards chronic health conditions. In contrast to the infectious diseases, where cure is often a realistic goal of treatment, chronic diseases typically require a moderation of both patients' and physicians' expectations. While slowing of the disease process may be possible, the patient must often learn to adjust to long-term functional limitations. The primary goals of treatment become the relief of symptoms and minimization of the impact of the disease on the patients' physical and psychosocial functioning.

More specific to oncology, although treatment is often directed initially towards cure, a substantial percentage of patients will eventually receive treatment with a palliative intent. The term 'palliation' is used to describe both efforts aimed at controlling the growth of the tumour and thus prolonging life, and those aimed at symptom control. In the former case, it may be important to weigh any gains in survival time against the morbidity caused by the treatment. Many treatments aimed at tumour control are quite aggressive, and thus carry with them a range of short-term and long-term side-effects. The introduction of formal QoL evaluations in such situations can be seen as a means of refining our assessment of treatment costs and benefits. Where the palliation of symptoms is the primary objective, the assessment of QoL in evaluating the effectiveness of treatment is self-evident.

Even where cure is possible, QoL considerations remain important. Most patients are willing to undergo very aggressive forms of treatment—bone marrow transplantation, intensive chemotherapy, or mutilating surgery—in order to be cured of their disease. Yet every clinical advance that diminishes the burden of treatment is welcome. Lumpectomy versus mastectomy in early-stage breast cancer, limb-sparing procedures versus amputation in soft-tissue sarcoma, sphincter-preserving resection versus total rectal excision in colorectal cancer are all examples where the goal of treatment has been to achieve better functional and cosmetic results, and thus presumably a better QoL. While formal QoL studies may not be essential in such cases, they can sometimes yield unexpected and revealing results. Finally, even where it is impossible to reduce the aggressiveness of the treatment, QoL studies can aid in identifying the residual psychosocial problems of long-term survivors of cancer, and can assist in the planning of appropriate rehabilitation services.

Many of the most vocal advocates for including QoL outcomes in clinical research and clinical practice have not come from the social sciences, but rather from within the clinical oncology and larger medical community itself. The 1985 call to include QoL outcomes as part of the drug approval process came from the Oncology Division of the Food and Drug Administration (**FDA**) in the United States.[1] More recently, the National Cancer Institute of Canada has incorporated QoL assessments as an integral part of its phase III clinical trials programme, and the American Society of Clinical Oncology (**ASCO**) has recommended inclusion of QoL outcomes in technology assessment and in developing treatment guidelines in oncology.[2]

The primary role of social scientists has been to develop and test methods for incorporating QoL outcomes in clinical research on the basis of sound scientific principles and feasible practice guidelines. To accomplish this objective, three basic methodological questions need to be addressed: **Who** should assess the QoL of cancer patients? **What** should be assessed? and '**How** can we standardize QoL assessment?

Who should assess the QoL of patients with cancer?

Given the inherently subjective nature of QoL, one would think that the answer to this question is so self-evident as to render it almost trivial. Consensus on this issue, however, was slower in coming than one might expect. Historically, it has most often been the doctor, rather than the patient, who has been asked to assess aspects of QoL, albeit in a limited way. For example, in most clinical studies in oncology, the clinical investigator is asked to assess the patient's performance status, using a rating scale that summarizes the patient's symptom levels and ability to perform normal, everyday activities at home and at work. Such physician-based ratings would seem to offer a simple and efficient means of assessing at least certain aspects of patients' QoL, but any practical advantages may be outweighed by the conceptual and methodological limitations of these scales. From a conceptual standpoint, performance status measures such as the Karnofsky, Eastern Cooperative Oncology Group (**ECOG**), and WHO scales assess only a limited spectrum of issues related to physical health and activities of daily living, and exclude issues relating to psychosocial health. Methodologically, inconsistencies have been noted in performance status ratings provided by different physicians for the same patient, and in ratings of physicians versus patients.[3],[4] While physician-based, performance status ratings provide valuable prognostic information in clinical trials, they cannot substitute for more direct measures of patients' QoL.

Today, it is widely accepted that the patient should be the primary source of information about his or her QoL. This is clearly the case for subjective experiences such as pain, fatigue, or emotional distress. Yet, even for more readily observable symptoms, direct patient feedback can provide a better understanding of their meaning and impact on daily living. For example, alopecia resulting from chemotherapy may have very different emotional and social consequences for a 45-year-old woman than for a 75-year-old man.

There are, however, several patient subgroups for whom the use of observer or so-called 'proxy' QoL ratings may be necessary. Young children with cancer may not have the requisite language skills to express their experiences and feelings in words. Adult patients with brain tumours or brain metastases may, over time, develop such serious cognitive deficits that they are unable to understand or respond to our questions. In the palliative care setting, patients with far advanced cancer may become too ill to complete a questionnaire. Yet, to exclude such patients from our QoL studies, something which is frequently done, is not only inherently unfair, but can also seriously bias our study results. In these situations, information provided by doctors, nurses, and family members may be the only means of obtaining insight into the patients' level of functioning and well being.

Even in those situations where the patient is able to answer questions directly, input from others may provide additional insights into the situation. For example, both patients with prostate cancer and their partners may tell us the patient is impotent due to the treatment. However, if we ask the patient and his partner how **troubled** the patient is by his impotence, real differences may start to emerge. Even if we take the patient's answers as the 'gold standard' against which those of the partner need to be interpreted, awareness of such discrepancies can help us better understand the impact of cancer on the patient–partner relationship.

A 1992 review of 35 published reports comparing QoL ratings provided by patients with those provided by healthcare professionals or informal caregivers, indicated that levels of concordance were far from ideal.[5] However, most of the studies were based on small samples and employed non-standardized QoL measures. More recently, three studies, employing larger samples and standardized measures, have reported moderate to high levels of agreement between cancer patients' ratings of their QoL and those provided by either physicians, nurses, or family members (most typically the patients' partners).[6]–[8] Importantly, Stephens *et al.* were able to demonstrate that the substantive findings relating to treatment-group differences in QoL outcomes were essentially the same regardless of whether the patients' or physicians' ratings were employed in the analysis.[8] These studies have also documented relatively high levels of proxy–patient agreement at the level of the individual patient (exact agreement ranging from 60 per cent to 80 per cent).

How do we define QoL?

Although most of us have some intuitive sense of what QoL means, a precise definition of the term remains elusive. Just as cancer is a collective term for some 100 different diseases, so is QoL an omnibus term summarizing a broad range of issues. As Alvan Feinstein, one of the early advocates of a patient-centred approach to clinical medicine, once put it: '. . . the idea has become a kind of umbrella under which are placed many different indexes dealing with whatever the user wants to focus on.'[9]

One way of avoiding this problem of definition is to view QoL as a Gestalt that can best be measured at a global level. Some years ago, Ian Gough and his colleagues suggested that one need only ask a single question to evaluate the QoL of patients with cancer: 'How would you rate your QoL today?'[10] They supported their position by demonstrating a relatively strong correlation between answers to this single question and scores derived from a more extensive battery of questionnaires. HL Mencken, the American author and pundit, once said: 'There is an easy solution to every human problem—neat, plausible—and wrong.' What then is wrong with this approach?

In choosing an appropriate therapy for an individual patient, or in developing treatment guidelines for a specific diagnostic group, physicians require very specific information on which to base their decisions. For example, it is expected that results of a blood test will be reported in appropriate detail (including calcium, iron, pH, and cholesterol levels), and not as a single value representing a summary of the findings.

The same holds true for evaluation of the QoL of patients. How are we to interpret a patient reporting a low overall QoL? Is the patient in pain? Is he so tired that he can no longer carry out his normal daily activities? Is he very anxious or depressed? Or, more likely, is it a combination of such factors? For this reason, it is today widely accepted that QoL assessment should be approached from a multidimensional perspective. A major advantage of such an approach is that it allows us to disentangle the positive and negative effects of a given treatment. For example, a treatment that effectively reduces pain may do so at the cost of increased fatigue and mood disturbance. It is seldom the case that one treatment offers clear and consistent QoL advantages over its alternatives. Rather, we are often confronted with a series of trade-offs.

The QoL of patients may also be affected in different ways at different points along the disease and treatment trajectory. The side-effects of chemotherapy may be quite severe and distressing, but are often short-lived. Conversely, problems caused by radiotherapy may diminish more slowly, or may emerge only months or even years after treatment. Global measures of QoL may fail to detect such changing patterns of symptoms over time.

Finally, because we do not have a clear picture of the range of physical and psychosocial consequences associated with many forms of cancer and cancer treatment, the assessment of multiple QoL outcomes facilitates the detection of not only anticipated, but also unexpected effects.

This still leaves the question of what should be measured. An important limiting factor is that the focus is on issues that are related to health. It is for this reason that the terms 'health-related QoL' or 'health status assessment' are often used.

Within such a health-oriented framework, two key historical sources provided the basis for the current taxonomy widely used in the field of QoL assessment. The first was the 1948 constitution of the World Health Organization which defined health as: 'a state of complete physical, mental and social well-being, and not merely the absence of disease and infirmity'. While perhaps primarily ideological in its intent, this definition offers a more holistic alternative to the classic medical model in which disease and illness are defined in strictly biological terms. The second source, also from 1948, was a paper in the first volume of *Cancer* by Karnofsky, Abelman, Carver, and Burchenal of the Memorial Hospital in New York.[11] They were investigating a new class of chemotherapy agents—the nitrogen mustards—in the palliative treatment of patients with lung cancer. They identified four sets of criteria necessary to establish the therapeutic value of anticancer treatment. The first of these was what they termed 'subjective improvement', described as: 'The patient's subjective improvement ... in his mood and attitude, his general feelings of well-being, his activity, appetite, and the alleviation of distressing symptoms such as pain, weakness and dyspnoea'.

Taken together, the WHO definition of health and Karnofsky *et al.*'s subjective improvement criteria provided the elements that today, some 50 years later, form the core of QoL measurement in oncology. These include: (1) common disease-related and treatment-related symptoms; and (2) the patients' level of functioning, defined in physical, psychological, and social terms.[12] Beyond this core set of domains, there are many additional issues that may be of importance when studying specific groups of patients. Body image may be of particular relevance in studies of patients with breast cancer, head and neck cancer, and other forms of cancer where treatment often involves mutilating surgery. Sexual functioning may be at issue in gynaecological and genitourinary tract cancers. Cognitive functioning may be of particular concern in studies of childhood cancer or of adults with brain tumours. Ultimately, the QoL issues that should be assessed in a given study depend on the patient population, the nature of the applied treatments, and the specific research questions (for example, whether we are interested in short-term or long-term effects).

Such a simple QoL taxonomy, while useful in promoting a common orientation, is notably lacking in theory. In fact, one of the more troubling aspects of QoL research is the general lack of theory development. Should the individual QoL domains be viewed as relatively independent of one another, or do they interact in predictable ways? Should we assume that each domain contributes equally to overall QoL, or should some sort of weighting be used? Does the relative importance of each domain vary predictably with the age or sex of the patient, or as a function of the stage of disease or phase of treatment? Are there significant cross-cultural differences in the meaning or relative importance attached to different QoL domains? How do patients' coping skills and social support networks factor into the picture? These are questions that have received relatively little attention.

How should QoL be measured?

Ironically, recognition of the need to rely on patients' own ratings of their functional capacity and symptom experience has represented one of the major barriers to incorporating QoL measures in clinical studies in oncology. Medical researchers tend to be distrustful of such subjective ratings, often equating them with 'soft' science. Much of the recent effort in the QoL field has been directed at dispelling this concern; at demonstrating that QoL questionnaires can be developed which meet, or even exceed, the standards of scientific rigor applied to other outcome measures such as tumour response.

QoL instruments used in clinical oncology can be placed along a continuum reflecting their intended spectrum of application: (1) generic instruments designed for both the general population and for a wide range of patient populations; (2) disease-specific measures designed for use with cancer patients, in general; and (3) diagnosis-specific measures (for example, for use with patients with breast cancer, prostate cancer, etc.).

Generic QoL instruments

A major advantage associated with the generic QoL measures is that they allow for comparison of results across studies of different patient populations, and facilitate comparison of patient groups with normative data from the general population. This is particularly relevant for issues of health policy and resource allocation. While there are a number of well-known, generic QoL measures, including the Sickness Impact Profile (SIP),[13] the Nottingham Health Profile,[14] and the World Health Organization QoL Questionnaire,[15] the Medical Outcomes Study Short-Form Health Survey (SF-36)[16] has achieved a dominant position in the health-outcomes field.

The SF-36, developed in the late 1980s for use in a large-scale investigation of the self-reported health status of patients with a range of chronic conditions, is a 36-item questionnaire organized into eight subscales assessing: physical functioning, role limitations due to physical health problems, pain, general health perceptions, vitality, social functioning, role limitations due to emotional problems, and general mental health. Two higher order summary scores for physical and mental health can also be calculated. Both a 'standard' and 'acute' version of the questionnaire (the former employing a 4-week, the latter a 1-week time frame) are available. The questionnaire employs categorical responses, with raw scores converted linearly to a 0 to 100 scale. Extensive background information on the SF-36, as well as standard scoring algorithms and interpretation guides are available elsewhere.[17] The SF-36 has been employed successfully in studies of patients with head-and-neck cancer,[18] lung cancer,[19] breast cancer,[20] metastatic prostate cancer,[21] soft-tissue sarcoma,[22] and Hodgkin's disease.[23] It is available in a wide range of European and

Asian languages, and has been validated extensively in cross-cultural settings.[24]

Cancer-specific QoL instruments

In clinical research in oncology we are most often interested in comparing treatments within well-defined, relatively homogenous patient populations, rather than across populations. For this purpose, generic instruments may be limited in their ability to detect small, yet clinically meaningful group differences in QoL, or in detecting changes in QoL over time. For this reason, substantial efforts have been devoted to developing QoL questionnaires specific for patients with cancer. These include the Functional Living Index—Cancer (**FLIC**), the Rotterdam Symptom Checklist (**RSCL**), the Cancer Rehabilitation Evaluation System (**CARES**), the European Organization for Research and Treatment of Cancer Core QoL Questionnaire (**EORTC QLQ-C30**), and the Functional Assessment of Cancer Therapy—General (**FACT-G**). The majority of these instruments have companion user's guides which include detailed information about their history, structure, scoring, and interpretation. The following paragraphs provide a brief description of their content.

The Functional Living Index—Cancer[25]

The FLIC, developed in the mid-1980s by Schipper and colleagues in Canada, is a 22-item questionnaire assessing physical and occupational functioning, psychological state, sociability, and somatic complaints. Although originally designed to yield a single, overall score, subsequent factor analytical studies have suggested that the questionnaire can be organized into a number of subscales assessing: physical, psychological, and social functioning; hardship due to cancer; and disease symptoms. Questions refer to the previous 3 days, and responses are made on a seven-point, modified visual analogue scale. The FLIC is available in a number of European and Asian languages.

The Rotterdam Symptom Checklist[26]

The RSCL, developed by de Haes and colleagues in the Netherlands, is a 38-item questionnaire assessing physical symptoms, physical activity levels, psychological symptoms, and social functioning. It yields two summary scores for physical and psychological functioning. The questionnaire employs a 3-day time frame, and four-point categorical response choices. It has been used primarily in Europe, and for a number of years was the primary QoL instrument used in clinical trials conducted by the Medical Research Council in the United Kingdom.

The Cancer Rehabilitation Evaluation System[27],[28]

The CARES, developed by Schag and colleagues in Los Angeles, was originally designed to provide a comprehensive picture of the physical and psychosocial rehabilitation needs of cancer patients. The full-length version of the questionnaire is composed of 139 items, of which 93 apply to all patients, The remaining 46 items are relevant to specific patient subgroups (for instance, those undergoing chemotherapy, patients with a prosthesis, etc.). The CARES is organized into five major scales assessing:

(1) physical problems in carrying out daily activities due to the disease;

(2) psychosocial problems (e.g. emotional distress, disrupted social relationships);

(3) problems in interacting and communicating with healthcare professionals;

(4) problems in marital communication and support; and

(5) problems related to sexual interest and performance.

An overall score can also be calculated. The CARES employs a 1-month time frame, and uses five-point categorical responses.

To facilitate its use in cancer clinical trials, an abbreviated version of the parent instrument was developed, the CARES-SF, which contains 59 items grouped into the same five scales as indicated above. All patients complete a minimum of 36 questions, with the remaining items applying to specific subgroups of patients. Both the CARES and the CARES-SF are available in a limited number of European languages.

The European Organization for Research and Treatment of Cancer QLQ-C30[29]

The QLQ-C30 was developed by the EORTC QoL Study Group specifically for use in international clinical trials in oncology. Originally published in 1993, it is now in its fourth revision. The current version of the questionnaire (version 3.0; see Fig. 1) contains 30 items organized into five functional scales (physical, role, emotional, cognitive, and social), three symptom scales (fatigue, nausea and vomiting, and pain), and an overall QoL scale. Additional single items assess other common symptoms of cancer and its treatment (for example, dyspnoea, loss of appetite, constipation and diarrhoea, etc.). The questionnaire employs a 1-week time frame, and four-point categorical response choices. It is the standard instrument employed in all EORTC clinical trials, and is also used widely by other clinical trials' groups in Europe and North America (for instance, the Medical Research Council in the United Kingdom and the National Cancer Institute of Canada). It has been translated into more than 30 languages and has been tested extensively in multinational research settings.

The Functional Assessment of Cancer Therapy—General[30]

The FACT-G, originally published by Cella and colleagues in 1993, is also designed primarily for use in clinical trials. The current version of the questionnaire (version 4; see Fig. 2) contains 27 items grouped into four primary domains: physical well being; social/family well being; emotional well being; and functional well being. A total summary score can also be generated. The questionnaire employs a 1-week time frame, and five-point categorical response choices. To date, the FACT-G has been employed most widely in the United States, including clinical trials of the major cancer clinical trials' groups. It has now been translated into a range of languages, which should facilitate its use in future multinational clinical trials.

Condition-specific and treatment-specific instruments

Both the EORTC and the FACT measurement systems employ a 'modular approach' to QoL assessment, whereby supplemental questionnaire modules are developed to assess condition-specific or treatment-specific issues not (sufficiently) addressed by their core instruments. The EORTC currently has modules available or under development for: breast, lung, colorectal, head-and-neck, bladder,

EORTC QLQ-C30 (version 3)

We are interested in some things about you and your health. Please answer all of the questions yourself by circling the number that best applies to you. There are no 'right' or 'wrong' answers. The information that you provide will remain strictly confidential.

Please fill in your initials: _____

Your birthdate (Day, Month, Year): _____

Today's date (Day, Month, Year): _____

		Not at all	A little	Quite a bit	Very much
1.	Do you have any trouble doing strenuous activities, like carrying a heavy shopping bag or a suitcase?	1	2	3	4
2.	Do you have any trouble taking a *long* walk?	1	2	3	4
3.	Do you have any trouble taking a *short* walk outside of the house?	1	2	3	4
4.	Do you need to stay in bed or a chair during the day?	1	2	3	4
5.	Do you need help with eating, dressing, washing yourself or using the toilet?	1	2	3	4

During the past week:

		Not at all	A little	Quite a bit	Very much
6.	Were you limited in doing either your work or other daily activities?	1	2	3	4
7.	Were you limited in pursuing your hobbies or other leisure time activities?	1	2	3	4
8.	Were you short of breath?	1	2	3	4
9.	Have you had pain?	1	2	3	4
10.	Did you need to rest?	1	2	3	4
11.	Have you had trouble sleeping?	1	2	3	4
12.	Have you felt weak?	1	2	3	4
13.	Have you lacked appetite?	1	2	3	4
14.	Have you felt nauseated?	1	2	3	4
15.	Have you vomited?	1	2	3	4
16.	Have you been constipated?	1	2	3	4
17.	Have you had diarrhoea?	1	2	3	4
18.	Were you tired?	1	2	3	4
19.	Did pain interfere with your daily activities?	1	2	3	4
20.	Have you had difficulty in concentrating on things, like reading a newspaper or watching television?	1	2	3	4
21.	Did you feel tense?	1	2	3	4
22.	Did you worry?	1	2	3	4
23.	Did you feel irritable?	1	2	3	4
24.	Did you feel depressed?	1	2	3	4
25.	Have you had difficulty remembering things?	1	2	3	4
26.	Has your physical condition or medical treatment interfered with your *family* life?	1	2	3	4
27.	Has your physical condition or medical treatment interfered with your *social* activities?	1	2	3	4
28.	Has your physical condition or medical treatment caused you financial difficulties?	1	2	3	4

For the following questions please circle the number between 1 and 7 that best applies to you

29. How would you rate your overall health during the past week?

1 (Very poor) 2 3 4 5 6 (Excellent) 7

30. How would you rate your overall quality of life during the past week?

1 (Very poor) 2 3 4 5 6 (Excellent) 7

© Copyright 1995 EORTC Study Group on Quality of Life. All rights reserved. Version 3.0

Fig. 1 EORTC QLQ-C30 (version 3) (reproduced by permission of the EORTC Study Group on Quality of Life).

FACT-G (Version 4)

Below is a list of statements that other people with your illness have said are important. **By circling one (1) number per line, please indicate how true each statement has been for you during the past 7 days.**

	PHYSICAL WELL-BEING	Not at all	A little bit	Somewhat	Quite a bit	Very much
GP1	I have a lack of energy	0	1	2	3	4
GP2	I have nausea	0	1	2	3	4
GP3	Because of my physical condition, I have trouble meeting the needs of my family	0	1	2	3	4
GP4	I have pain	0	1	2	3	4
GP5	I am bothered by side effects of treatment	0	1	2	3	4
GP6	I feel ill	0	1	2	3	4
GP7	I am forced to spend time in bed	0	1	2	3	4

	SOCIAL/FAMILY WELL-BEING					
GS1	I feel close to my friends	0	1	2	3	4
GS2	I get emotional support from my family	0	1	2	3	4
GS3	I get support from my friends	0	1	2	3	4
GS4	My family has accepted my illness	0	1	2	3	4
GS5	I am satisfied with family communication about my illness	0	1	2	3	4
GS6	I feel close to my partner (or the person who is my main support)	0	1	2	3	4
Q1	*Regardless of your current level of sexual activity, please answer the following question. If you prefer not to answer it, please check this box* ☐ *and go to the next section.*					
	I am satisfied with my sex life	0	1	2	3	4

	EMOTIONAL WELL-BEING					
GE1	I feel sad	0	1	2	3	4
GE2	I am satisfied with how I am coping with my illness	0	1	2	3	4
GE3	I am losing hope in the fight against my illness	0	1	2	3	4
GE4	I feel nervous	0	1	2	3	4
GE5	I worry about dying	0	1	2	3	4
GE6	I worry that my condition will get worse	0	1	2	3	4

	FUNCTIONAL WELL-BEING					
GF1	I am able to work (include work at home)	0	1	2	3	4
GF2	My work (include work at home) is fulfilling	0	1	2	3	4
GF3	I am able to enjoy life	0	1	2	3	4
GF4	I have accepted my illness	0	1	2	3	4
GF5	I am sleeping well	0	1	2	3	4
GF6	I am enjoying the things I usually do for fun	0	1	2	3	4
GF7	I am content with the quality of my life right now	0	1	2	3	4

Fig. 2 FACT-G (version 4).

Table 1 Attributes of five cancer-specific quality-of-life measures

	FLIC	RSCL	CARES-SF (SF)	EORTC QLC-C30	FACT-G
Measurement model					
Conceptual	●	●	●	●	●
Empirical	○	●	●	●	●
Burden	●	●	●	●	●
Reliability					
Internal consistency	●	●	●	●	●
Test–retest	●	○	●	●	●
Validity					
Content	●	●	●	●	●
Construct	●	●	●	●	●
Responsiveness	●	●	●	●	●
Interpretability	○	○	○	○	○
Cultural adaptations					
Translations	●	●	●	●	●
Psychometrics	●	●	●	●	●

FLIC, Functional Living Index Cancer; RSCL, Rotterdam Symptom Checklist; CARES-SF, Cancer Rehabilitation Evaluation System—Short Form; EORTC QLQ-C30, European Organization for Research and Treatment of Cancer Core Quality of Life Questionnaire; FACT-G, Functional Assessment of Cancer Therapy—General; ●, meets criteria; ○, does not meet criteria.

prostate, brain, ovarian, oesophageal, and pancreatic cancer; multiple myeloma; palliative care; and peripheral neuropathy. The FACT group has developed a similar stable of modules to that of the EORTC, but also including measures specific to bone marrow transplantation, anorexia/cachexia, anaemia, fatigue, urinary symptoms, and endocrine symptoms. Both groups provide timely updates of their instrument development activities via their respective Internet sites.

Other groups are also actively contributing to the development of condition-specific questionnaires. Thus, for example, in the area of prostate cancer, at least three instruments, in addition to those developed by the EORTC and FACT groups, have been recently published.[31]–[33]

Selecting the 'best' QoL instrument

Although some published reviews of QoL questionnaires have attempted to identify a 'best bet' for use in oncology research,[34] systematic evaluation of the measurement properties of these instruments suggests that this may not be appropriate. Table 1 summarizes the empirical evidence relating to the performance characteristics of the five QoL instruments described briefly above. Each instrument was evaluated using a set of criteria recommended by the Scientific Advisory Committee of the Medical Outcomes Trust (**MOT**), a Boston-based, non-profit organization whose mission is to identify and disseminate high-quality health status and QoL instruments to the larger research community.[35] These criteria relate to the following measurement properties of an instrument:

(1) the underlying measurement model used to create the subscale structure of a questionnaire (typically evaluated with structural equation modelling or item-response theory);

(2) reliability (i.e. internal consistency and test–retest);

(3) validity (primarily content and construct validity);

(4) responsiveness (i.e. sensitivity to change);

(5) interpretability (i.e. the degree to which one can assign qualitative meaning to an instrument's quantitative scores);

(6) respondent burden (i.e. the time, energy, and other demands placed on patients in completing a questionnaire); and

(7) cultural and language adaptations (i.e. conceptual and linguistic equivalence, comparability of psychometric properties).

All five of the instruments reviewed meet or exceed the large majority of criteria established by the MOT. They are brief and easy to complete, there is evidence supporting their scale structure, and they have proven to be reliable, valid, and responsive when used at the level of group comparisons. Of particular importance is their ability to distinguish clearly between groups of patients formed on the basis of known clinical characteristics (for instance, stage of disease, performance status, treatment status), and their statistical responsiveness to changes in clinical parameters over time (for instance, tumour response, changes in performance status, etc.).

If the most widely used QoL questionnaires exhibit very similar measurement properties, how then can one choose among them when planning a study? The most practical approach is non-technical, involving an examination of the specific content and wording of each candidate instrument. Although all these questionnaires assess similar content areas, the relative emphasis placed on any given QoL domain, and the specific way in which questions are posed vary considerably. For example, in comparison to the other instruments, the RSCL and the EORTC QLQ-C30 include a relatively larger number of questions addressing physical symptoms. Conversely, the CARES places more emphasis on issues surrounding interpersonal relationships (both communication and sexuality).

There is also considerable variation in the way in which questions are posed. For example, both the FLIC and the CARES make specific reference to cancer in the wording of some of their questions. This may be problematic if these questionnaires are used in cultures where it is uncommon to refer to the disease so explicitly.

Other semantic and stylistic differences can be more subtle. For example, in assessing symptoms of depression the SF-36, the FACT-G, and the QLQ-C30 use the following item-phrasing, respectively:

1. 'Have you felt so down in the dumps that nothing could cheer you up?' and 'Have you felt downhearted and blue?'
2. 'I feel sad.'
3. 'Did you feel depressed?'

These items differ in both the degree to which they rely on idiomatic expressions and in the directness with which the questions are posed.

A final example is provided by the questions used to assess future perspective. The following item-wording is employed in the SF-36, the CARES, and the FACT-G, respectively:

1. 'I expect my health to get worse.'
2. 'I worry about not being able to care for myself.' 'I worry about whether the cancer will progress.'
3. 'I am losing hope in the fight against my illness.' 'I worry about dying.' 'I worry that my condition will get worse.'

Again, while all three questionnaires address the same general issues, they do so in ways which may be more or less appropriate for any given patient population. Interestingly, the EORTC, while acknowledging their relevance, decided not to include questions about future perspective in the QLQ-C30. Feedback from patients (particularly those with advanced disease) indicated that they could be upsetting, particularly when posed in a written form.

One choice of item-content or -wording is not, *a priori*, superior to another. Ultimately, it is the task of the investigator to decide which questionnaire is most relevant for a given study, and is most congruent with the cultural norms of the target patient population.

Utility-based assessments

The questionnaires described thus far are typically referred to as 'profile' instruments because they provide a descriptive profile of the patient's functional health and symptom experience. For medical decision-making purposes, therapeutic benefits have to be contrasted against changes in QoL: if more efficacious therapy is associated with poorer QoL outcomes, is it worthwhile? Answering this involves weighing QoL against survival and combining them into a single summary score, most commonly by determining patient 'preference ratings' or 'utilities.' Overall benefits of treatment or management policies can then be contrasted.

Visual analogue rating scales (VAS)

The simplest form of establishing preference ratings is by means of a visual analogue rating scale, in which the patient is presented with a 10-cm line with ends labelled 'best possible QoL' and 'worst possible QoL', or some equivalent wording. The patient is asked to indicate the position of their current state on the line, and also to mark positions corresponding to various scenarios such as their likely condition during or following therapy. This method is efficient and easy to use, and appears to provide meaningful values of relative preference for various states of health and treatment.[36]

Standard gamble (SG)

The standard gamble method involves decisions in the face of uncertainty, in this case the risk of death or some other adverse outcome. Typically, the patient is asked to choose between life in his or her current state of health, and a 'gamble' between death and perfect health. The probability of death is varied systematically until the respondent can no longer choose between the gamble and the certain, albeit compromised state of health. This classical approach to determining patients' preferences is conceptually complex, and may also be confounded by the individual's tolerance for risk-taking.[37]

Time trade-off (TTO)

The time trade-off method contrasts QoL against length of survival. Patients are presented with a scenario in which health is impaired by specific disabilities or symptoms, and are asked whether they would choose 1 year in perfect health or 1 year with impaired health; presumably, the healthy year would be selected. Subsequently, the duration of the healthy period is gradually reduced: 'Would you choose 11 months in perfect health, or 1 year with impaired health?' This iterative process is continued until a state of equilibrium is reached, indicating the value of impaired life that is equivalent to a certain period in a healthy state. While avoiding some of the problems associated with the SG approach (namely, the influence of attitudes toward risk-taking), the TTO is also difficult for some patients to comprehend without extensive interviewer assistance, and thus may not be particularly suitable for use in clinical trials.[38]

Willingness to pay (WTP)

Whereas SG involves a gamble and the element of risk to compare the value of different health states, and TTO uses varying periods, willingness to pay introduces the concept of monetary value. The amount an individual is willing to pay is assumed to be an indicator of the utility or satisfaction that he or she expects to gain from the particular commodity (in this case, health). WTP values can be elicited by questions such as: 'What is the most that you would be willing to pay for …', or by presenting a list of options or a set of cards containing 'bids' of increasing amounts, from which the patient selects the amount they would be willing to pay.

Quality-adjusted life years (QALYs)

Having estimated utilities or preference ratings using VAS, SG, TTO, or WTP, a score for each patient can be obtained by combining their preference rating with their survival. Quality-adjusted life years do this by allowing for varying times spent in different health states, and calculating an overall score for each patient. In broad terms, if the state of health during disease or treatment has been assigned a utility of 60 per cent, then 1 year spent in this state is considered equivalent to 0.6 of a year in perfect health. The scores in each state are then summed, giving a QALY value for each patient.

Q-TWiST

The Quality-adjusted Time Without Symptoms-of-disease and Toxicity-of-treatment (Q-TWiST) approach is conceptually similar to

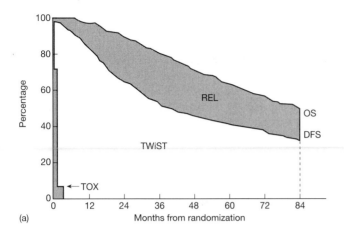

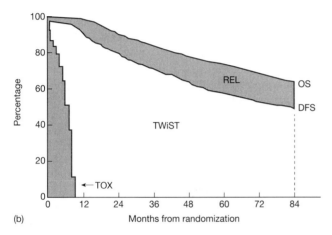

Fig. 3 Partitioned survival plots. Partitioned survival for the long-duration treatment (a) and for the short-duration treatment (b) for IBCSG Trial V at 7 years of median follow-up. In each graph the area under the overall survival curve (OS) is partitioned by the survival curves for disease-free survival (DFS) and time with treatment toxicity (TOX). The areas between the survival curves give the average months spent in TOX, TWiST, and relapse (REL) as indicated.

QALYs, and uses utility scores to adjust (downward) the value of the years survived when health is impaired. However, Q-TWiST can also be applied to censored survival data and is therefore particularly appropriate for use in clinical trials. The overall survival curve for a group of patients is partitioned into a few—typically three—regions that define the time spent in particular clinical states. For example, Fig. 3 shows the time with toxicity (TOX), without toxicity or symptoms (TwiST), and in relapse (REL) for two groups of patients.[39] The areas of these regions then provide scores that are weighted according to their utilities.

Multidimensional health-state classification indices

A final type of utility measure is the health-state classification index. Such an index resembles more classical QoL questionnaires, with the major difference being that scores are weighted on the basis of preferences (or utilities) for discrete health states or combinations of health states derived from a reference sample. The reference sample can be drawn from relevant patient populations or from the general community population. Examples of widely used health-state classification indices include the Quality of Well-Being Scale,[40] the Health Utility Index,[41] the Q-tility Index,[42] and the EuroQol.[43] The major advantage associated with this type of utility measure is that it does not require that preferences be obtained from each individual patient participating in a study. However, questions have been raised about the appropriateness of employing preference weights based on reference populations, and particularly on non-patient populations.[44]

Cost-effectiveness and cost-utility analysis

Methods for combining QoL with outcomes such as survival remain controversial, and even more controversial is the use of QALYs in health–economic analysis when a third dimension (cost) is included. There are logical difficulties in declaring one treatment to be 'better' than another when gains in some dimensions are offset by losses in others; the comparison depends heavily upon the trade-off across the disparate dimensions. Not only will different people have different opinions as to the relative values, but these opinions may change over time according to circumstances, contexts, and experiences.[45] Different patients have different priorities, and average opinions may only reflect the views of a few central individuals. On the other hand, some argue that utility values derived from the general population should be used, since those are the payers for the services used. A single summary index such as cost per QALY may be a convenient aid for healthcare policy decisions, but when presented in a league table all the implicit assumptions regarding value judgements can too easily become obscured or disguised.

Because of the uncertainties and problems of assessing and applying utilities, any cost-effectiveness analysis should be accompanied by a sensitivity or threshold analysis. This considers the impact of a range of alternative utilities, to confirm whether the conclusions regarding treatment superiority would hold over a wide range of other values; if it does, the conclusions may be regarded as relatively robust.

In many situations, such as clinical trials, it would seem preferable to report the observed QoL, the overall survival differences, and the cost, letting the individual—whether it be a patient, clinician, or healthcare planner—decide what relative importance to attach to the separate dimensions. By presenting sufficient information, each individual can apply their own set of utilities.

Application of QoL assessments in clinical oncology research and practice

The substantial investment of time, energy and resources in developing reliable, valid, and practical tools for assessing the QoL of patients with cancer can only be justified if these measures are put to good use. Have QoL studies advanced our understanding of the burden of disease and the impact of treatment on patients' lives? Have they contributed to evaluating the effectiveness of anticancer treatments? Can they be used in the day-to-day care of our patients? How can they contribute to establishing clinical practice guidelines?

Descriptive QoL studies

A recent Norwegian survey compared the self-reported QoL, as assessed by the SF-36, of 459 long-term survivors of Hodgkin's disease with that of an age- and gender-adjusted normative sample drawn from the general population.[46] The results indicated significant deficits among the survivors of Hodgkin's disease in physical functioning, role functioning, vitality, and general health perceptions. Time since diagnosis, the nature of the primary treatment, and whether the patient had experienced a relapse following initial treatment were not associated significantly with SF-36 scores.

Conversely, in a recent survey of 864 long-term survivors of breast cancer,[47] no significant differences in SF-36 scores were found when compared with an age-matched sample from the general population, or in scores on measures of sexuality, marital functioning, or depression. The survivors of breast cancer did report higher rates of physical symptoms, including joint pains, headaches, and hot flushes. Sexual dysfunction was found to be more prevalent in women who had received chemotherapy, regardless of age, and in younger women who were no longer menstruating.

It is increasingly difficult to obtain funding for descriptive epidemiological studies. It is argued that the time has come to intervene, rather than simply point to where the problems lie. It is true that certain patient groups, for example women with primary breast cancer, have been well-studied. For many patient groups, however, we still know very little about the short- and long-term effects of the disease and its treatment. Only by carrying out well-designed, descriptive studies can we identify areas where support and rehabilitation services are most needed.

It is important to look beyond average effects: the 'average' patient is a statistical convenience; not someone seen in the doctor's office. Descriptive studies should aim to identify subgroups of patients who are particularly 'at risk' for psychosocial morbidity. Conversely, there may be much to learn from those patients who do well; who successfully overcome the crisis of cancer without the need for formal interventions.

Evaluative QoL studies—phase III clinical trials

An important application of QoL measures is in comparing the effects of two or more cancer treatments. QoL measures have sometimes been useful in confirming clinical impressions or expectations about the psychosocial benefits of one treatment over another. This has been the case, for example, in trials comparing breast-conserving therapy with mastectomy in the treatment of early-stage breast cancer. The expectation that saving a woman's breast will help her maintain a sense of femininity and preserve a positive body image has been confirmed in a number of studies.[48]

The useful half-life of QoL studies would probably be very short if they merely confirmed clinical expectations. It is the fact that the results of such studies sometimes challenge widely held beliefs that explains, in part, the growing enthusiasm for their use. Drawing again on the example of operable breast cancer, it has often been suggested that breast-conserving therapy, while holding certain psychosocial advantages over mastectomy, might increase a woman's fear that the cancer will recur. Yet, empirical investigations have not supported this hypothesis.[49]

A second example is a clinical trial in metastatic breast cancer in which patients received chemotherapy either continuously (that is, every 3 weeks until the disease progressed) or intermittently (where the treatment was stopped after three cycles and repeated only at disease progression).[50] It was hypothesized that the intermittent treatment schedule would result in fewer side-effects, and thus a better QoL. As expected, women whose chemotherapy was intermittent reported less treatment toxicity. However, over the course of the trial, they reported more mood disturbance, less appetite, and a more rapid deterioration in their physical condition and overall QoL than women receiving continuous chemotherapy. In part, this could be explained by the better tumour response and longer time to disease progression observed in the continuous chemotherapy group. This study illustrates nicely how the QoL trade-offs associated with treatment toxicity, on the one hand, and tumour response, on the other, can be brought into sharper focus with formal QoL assessments.

A final example is a clinical trial which compared medroxyprogesterone acetate (**MPA**) to a placebo in increasing appetite and promoting weight gain in patients with advanced-stage cancer.[51] This study showed that MPA had a significant, albeit modest, beneficial effect on both endpoints. However, these gains in appetite and weight did not translate into improvement in QoL, as measured by the QLQ-C30. Rather, a decline in the mean QoL scores of both the MPA and placebo groups was observed over the 12-week study period. Because weight loss can represent a distressing signal to the patient and his family that the battle against the disease is being lost, it was hypothesized that patients on MPA would report less distress and an improved sense of well being. They did not. This illustrates that direct indicators of treatment success do not necessarily translate into improved functioning or a sense of well being.

An intriguing by-product of QoL investigations in clinical trials is the finding that patients' ratings of their functioning, symptoms, and overall well being obtained prior to the start of treatment are significant, independent predictors of survival. To date, this has been demonstrated in studies of patients with lung cancer,[52] advanced breast cancer,[53] melanoma,[54] metastatic colon cancer,[55] and multiple myeloma.[56] These results should not be overinterpreted; they do not indicate that the emotional state or personality of patients can affect the course of the disease. They do suggest that our current health status is one of the best predictors of future morbidity and mortality, and that patients can be quite accurate in rating their current health. These findings may prove useful in designing future clinical trials. For example, we may be able to employ baseline QoL scores, just as we do tumour stage, performance status, and other prognostic variables, as eligibility criteria for clinical-trial participation, or in stratifying patients prior to randomization to treatment.

Guidelines for incorporating QoL assessment in clinical trials

Quality-of-life assessment is only relevant to some types of clinical trials. It is rarely necessary in phase I or phase II trials, where the primary aim is to determine tumour response and toxicity, although it may sometimes be useful in such trials to pilot the instruments and to test the administrative procedures. The main role for QoL instruments lies in phase III trials. There are four settings in which QoL assessment is particularly relevant:

1. Palliative studies, in which improved QoL may be the principal aim of the intervention and thus QoL assessment may provide the principal endpoint.

2. Equivalence trials, in which little difference is anticipated in terms of improved survival or cure, but where there may be differences in side effects, symptomatology or morbidity.

3. Trials in which a difference in survival or cure-rate might be anticipated, but where the improvement may be small and accompanied by major toxicity or side-effects.

4. Studies involving health economic cost-effectiveness.

When and how often to measure QoL

There will usually be a 'baseline' assessment before randomization, against which a patient's subsequent changes can be compared. This also enables a comparison between the pretreatment scores of the randomized study groups, and if differences are substantial it may be necessary to make compensatory statistical adjustments to later QoL measurements. When analysing the study, baseline information can also be used to explore whether there is systematic bias due to missing forms or incomplete data.

The baseline assessment should be made before the patient has been informed of the randomized treatment allocation; otherwise, knowledge of the treatment assignment may cause different levels of, for example, anxiety between the two treatment groups. Furthermore, by ensuring that QoL is assessed before randomization and made an eligibility criterion, we can ensure that initial compliance is 100 per cent.

It is desirable to limit the number and frequency of questionnaires, so as to avoid imposing an unnecessary burden on patients. Frequently, assessment times during treatment will be chosen to coincide with visits to the clinic. For treatments such as long-term hormonal treatment of breast cancer, the patients' condition may be relatively stable and so the time at which questionnaires are completed may not be critical. For other treatments, such as cytotoxic chemotherapy, patients commonly attend at the start of each course or cycle and can complete the QoL questionnaire while waiting to be reassessed by the clinician. However, some QoL instruments specify a time frame of 'during the last week . . .', and will therefore only collect information about how the patient recalls feeling during the week preceding the next course of therapy. If treatment courses are given at intervals of 3 to 4 weeks, the impact of transient toxicity might remain undetected. In this situation, the investigators will have to decide whether the temporary toxicity-related reductions in QoL or the longer term effects, as seen later during each cycle, are more important. Sometimes it may be appropriate to assess QoL at 1 week after each course of therapy. Sometimes treatment may be delayed because of toxicity, and if assessments are made immediately preceding the next (delayed) course of treatment, the impact of the toxicity upon QoL may remain undetected.

In principle, it is desirable to use the same data collection schedule in all treatment arms, with QoL assessments being made at times relative to the date of randomization. In practice, this may be difficult in trials comparing different modalities of treatment or where the timing of therapy and follow-up differs between the randomized groups. Differences in the timing of assessments within the arms of the study can make the interpretation of results difficult if the patients are deteriorating as a consequence of their disease progressing from the time of randomization.

In summary, there are compromises to be made in those studies that investigate QoL during and after treatments such as surgery and intermittent courses of chemotherapy and radiotherapy. Assessments may be made relative to the treatment events, or relative to the randomization date. Clearly, the general timing of the assessments must be specified—for example, 2 weeks after surgery—and it is often appropriate to define a time interval within which assessments are valid—for example, at least 2, but not more than 3, weeks after surgery.

There may also be follow-up assessments after completion of treatment. If the primary scientific question concerns QoL during therapy, one post-treatment assessment may suffice. Sometimes it is relevant to continue assessment until and after relapses may have occurred, and in some studies, such as those of palliative care, assessments may continue until death. To eliminate bias, long-term assessments in both treatment groups should normally be at similar times relative to the date of randomization.

Administering the questionnaires

Generally, it is advisable for QoL to be assessed before the clinician sees the patient, to avoid influencing the responses by anything occurring during the consultation. It is important that patients complete the QoL questionnaire by themselves, if they are able. Patients may be influenced by the opinions of others when completing questionnaires, and it is advisable that they only receive help when it is absolutely necessary. The study forms should collect details of any assistance or the use of proxies.

Compliance

Many clinical trials have reported problems of compliance. In some trials only 60 per cent or fewer of the anticipated patient-completed QoL forms are returned. This leads to serious questions regarding the validity of the analyses of the trial results. In particular, how do we know whether patients who return forms are representative of the whole study group? For example, perhaps the non-responders are those who are most ill, in which case we could be underestimating the severity of impact of therapy. Although there are statistical methods to allow for missing data, it is impossible to be confident that the analyses remain unbiased. Therefore it is crucial to ensure high compliance.

Missing data, and hence low compliance, may arise from many causes, including clinicians or nurses forgetting to ask patients to complete QoL questionnaires, and patients refusing, feeling too ill, or forgetting. Compliance varies greatly from hospital to hospital, with some centres reporting that their patients have no difficulty completing all their forms. This suggests that perhaps institution-related rather than patient-related factors are most important. These might include availability of local resources for supporting the clinical trial, and the perception of the staff as to the relevance and importance of QoL assessment. For the clinical trial to be successful, both these issues must be addressed.

Methods for improving compliance involve training and communication for both patients and medical staff. Most patients are willing to complete QoL questionnaires, especially if they are assured that the data will be useful for medical research and will benefit future patients. Therefore they should be given a clear explanation of the reasons for collecting the QoL data, with information sheets to supplement verbal information. Similarly, the medical team must receive a convincing explanation of the value of QoL assessment in the particular study; sceptical staff make less effort, and will experience greater difficulty in persuading patients to complete questionnaires. The greater success in collecting QoL data in European and Canadian studies compared to trials in the United States may reflect differences of opinion regarding the importance of QoL endpoints.

Specific strategies to improve compliance have been successfully adopted by several trials' groups. Sadura *et al.*[57] developed and implemented a comprehensive programme specifically aimed at encouraging compliance, and reported overall compliance of above 95 per cent in three Canadian cancer trials using the EORTC QLQ-C30. However, they used a level of resources that might not be available to others: in one study, nurses called the patients at home on the appropriate day to remind them to complete the questionnaire.

Sample size

There are no major differences between planning a clinical trial in which QoL assessment is the primary outcome compared to those in which it is survival or response to therapy. Studies that are too small will rarely be able to detect even important changes in QoL, while studies that are too large will involve a waste of resources. Thus an estimation of sample size is one of the most fundamental aspects of study design. Justification for the chosen study size will be required by funding bodies and ethical review boards, and many medical journals stipulate that authors provide details of the prestudy sample size calculation.

One problem when estimating sample size for QoL scales is that there are frequently many outcome measures of interest. This presents problems of analysis, too, since multiple testing will distort the nominal *p*-values. Thus it is recommended that investigators define one or two outcome measures as being of primary interest, and then design their study so that they have reasonable power for detecting relevant changes in these chosen outcomes. Estimates of sample-size requirements should be increased to allow for missing or incomplete forms, for deaths, and for any other forms of dropout.

Sample-size estimation should reflect the intended analysis at the end of the study. For example, if it is planned to carry out *t*-tests, the sample-size calculation is based upon the properties of the *t*-statistic. When calculating the sample-size requirements for a study that aims to detect a change in QoL, we need to specify the size of the target difference that we wish to be able to detect (which is discussed under interpretation), we need to have an estimate of the variability of the test-statistic (such as the standard deviation), and we may typically assume a (two-sided) significance level of $\alpha = 0.05$ or possibly 0.01, and a power of 80 per cent ($\beta = 0.20$) or 90 per cent ($\beta = 0.10$). Then standard tables or computer programs can be used to perform the calculations. For equivalence studies, in which the objective is to demonstrate that two treatments are associated with approximately equal QoL levels, different considerations apply. In general, the demonstration of equivalence requires a large sample size. Detailed discussions of issues in sample-size estimation, as well as extensive tables and software for performing the calculations are available elsewhere.[58]

Data analysis

In analysing QoL data one can compare groups of patients at a particular timepoint (for example, at 6 months after randomization) using standard methods. Sometimes simple comparison of means

with *t*-tests may be appropriate (for example, when comparing mean global health status across two treatment arms). Often non-parametric tests, such as the Wilcoxon or Mann–Whitney tests, may be more appropriate because many of the QoL items and functioning scales have asymmetrical distributions that are clearly not of a 'normal distribution' form.

An alternative approach, which may be especially suitable for single items, is to consider percentages rather than means or averages. For example, one can calculate the percentage of patients in each group who report 'quite a bit' or 'very much' vomiting; or the percentage who report a large change in scores. Many readers may find percentages more intuitive and easier to understand than average levels. For example, the statement '34 per cent of patients reported vomiting at least quite a bit' has a more obvious interpretation than reports such as 'the average level of vomiting was 45.5'. When percentages are used, the analyses often reduce to comparisons of binomial proportions or possibly Chi-squared tests.

Percentages can also be used for scores from multi-item scales, by defining a 'QoL responder' as a patient who shows a prespecified improvement in a QoL scale—for example, a specified increase in overall QoL, or a particular decrease in pain. The analysis then becomes analogous to analysing the proportion of patients who have a tumour response, with dropouts treated as 'non-responders'.

However, the characteristics of QoL data raise particular problems for analysis: there are usually multiple QoL endpoints, patients are followed-up during and after treatment, a proportion of data is usually missing, and some patients die or withdraw during the follow-up.

Multiplicity of outcomes

Most QoL instruments contain a number of scales and single items, and there are potentially many pairwise statistical comparisons that might be made. As is well known, for every 100 independent statistical tests that are carried out, even if we assume there is no true treatment effect, we would expect approximately 5 comparisons to be statistically significant, $p < 0.05$. Therefore, when performing multiple significance tests the multiplicity of outcomes can invalidate the *p*-values. The analysis of clinical trial data will always be more convincing if one or two principal hypotheses have been specified at the start, and if they are clearly stated in the study protocol. These few outcomes (which could include a summary score) will then become the main focus of the analysis, and the problems of multiple testing will be largely eliminated. After testing differences between the prespecified primary outcomes, the rest of the data may be explored to generate new hypotheses for confirmation or investigation in future studies.

When a larger number of distinct QoL outcomes are of interest, 'conservative *p*-values' may be adopted. Thus if many statistical tests are being performed, $p < 0.01$ can be used as indicating statistical significance, thereby reducing the rate of false-positives. Alternatively, so-called 'Bonferroni corrections' adjust for the total number of statistical tests. If it is planned to make *n* statistical tests, the equivalent *p*-value that will maintain overall significance at, say, 5 per cent is $0.05/n$ for the individual tests. This method is described by Bland and Altman,[59] who note that it tends to be overly cautious.

Repeated measurements

Studies that measure QoL usually assess each patient at multiple timepoints, such as before, during, and after treatment. There are various methods available for data description and statistical significance testing when repeated measurements, or longitudinal data, are available for the comparison of two or more treatments.

One of the simplest approaches is to use graphical displays and accompany these by cross-sectional analyses at a few specific timepoints. Ideally, the study protocol will have prespecified that the analysis will focus upon QoL at these particular timepoints, with the additional measurements being regarded as of secondary importance. For example, a chemotherapy protocol might specify that differences in QoL at the time of the third course, and also at 1 month after completion of chemotherapy will be tested for statistical significance. These tests could be accompanied by graphical displays showing the average levels of QoL for the treatment arms or for various patient subgroups.

A second approach is to condense the repeated measurements for each individual into a few summary statistics. For example, the repeated 'on-treatment' measurements for each patient could be reduced to a single score by calculating the average level during the 'on-treatment' period. The summary statistics that are frequently employed include:

(1) the overall average QoL for each patient;

(2) the average QoL for some specified period, such as during treatment, or after completion of therapy;

(3) the worst QoL experienced during therapy (or highest levels of toxicity); and

(4) the 'area under the curve', or **AUC**, which is equivalent to the average if the timepoints are at equal intervals.

The analyses can then compare and test the summary statistics.[60]

Analysis can also be based upon the 'QoL responder' concept as described briefly above. This again reduces the data to a single summary statistic for each patient, allowing comparison of the proportion of responders in each treatment arm. Alternatively, the analysis can be based on time-to-response ('response' is the 'event' for analysis, instead of death) and survival analysis techniques can be used. Duration of response can also be evaluated; for example, Osoba et al.[61] showed that mitoxantrone added to prednisone for the treatment of metastatic prostate cancer not only resulted in improved QoL but in addition the duration of response was longer.

Finally, some sophisticated statistical methods are available, involving the fitting of mathematical models to the data and thereby enabling a more precise estimate of the treatment effect. Since repeated measurements on any one individual are likely to be correlated, these models allow for this 'auto-correlation'. The main methods are repeated measures of analysis of variance (**ANOVA**), hierarchical models (or multilevel models), and generalized estimating equations (**GEE**). These methods are discussed in detail in ref. 60.

Missing data

Curran et al.[62] present an example using the physical functioning (**PF**) scale of the EORTC QLQ-C30. The first (baseline) assessment was completed by 86 patients, but at each subsequent assessment increasing numbers of patients dropped out through non-compliance or death. Figure 4 shows the mean PF score by time of dropout either by death or failure to complete the QoL assessment. Each profile includes those patients completing all QoL assessments up to the specified number of months. Patients who provide information on all five PF assessments tend to have a higher mean baseline PF score

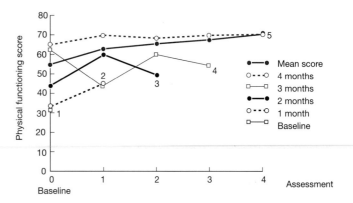

Fig. 4 Physical functioning score by time of dropout.

than the other groups of patients. Thus analysis at later timepoints tends to include only the better patients.

This example illustrates the problems of missing data: there is a potential for bias. How do we know whether the responses of those patients who completed assessments can be assumed to be representative of the whole sample, including the non-responders? Would we have obtained materially different conclusions had we been able to collect all the data? In a randomized trial, can we be confident that any observed treatment effect would still have been found if no data had been missing, or are the results attributable to bias?

A number of statistical methods have been developed to 'impute' the most likely values for missing data when QoL forms are missing. These methods are based upon the assumption that it is better to make an informed guess as to the most likely QoL of patients rather than simply ignore patients if their data are missing. For example, if a patient fails to complete one QoL questionnaire in the middle of the follow-up period but has consistently reported much poorer than average QoL both before and after this occasion, it would seem better to 'impute' a low score rather than omit the data as 'missing.' If omitted, we would in effect be accepting a higher overall mean score across all patients than seems likely given our knowledge of this particular patient's past and future responses. Imputation procedures may draw upon information from many sources, including characteristics of the patient such as performance status. Fayers and Machin[60] describe various methods for analysing QoL data when either whole forms or just a few items on a form are missing.

Interpretation and clinical significance

Typical conclusions from a clinical trial might be that one treatment resulted in a 'statistically significant' reduction (or increase) in a QoL scale. But what does such a statement mean? Statistical significance tests only examine whether the differences observed in a clinical trial might be due to chance fluctuations, and tell us nothing about the clinical importance of the results. A large-sized trial will be able to detect trivially small differences in QoL, and might declare the results as being (statistically) highly significant even though such small differences could be regarded as clinically unimportant. How, therefore, can we decide what is clinically important?

Clinicians have a long experience of working with measurements such as blood pressure, and most clinicians have a feel for the consequences of a reduction of, say, 20 mmHg in systolic blood pressure. However, this 'feel' for the measurements is largely lacking when dealing with QoL assessments. Suppose there is a statistically significant difference of 11 points on a QoL scale such as those in the QLQ-C30, how do we interpret this result? Is 11 points a small and clinically unimportant difference, or is it a very important difference? What differences are discernible by patients, and what magnitude of differences are important to patients? Also, is an Emotional Function score of 60 equally good or bad as a score of 60 on the other functioning scales?

Percentage of 'cases'

Perhaps the simplest method is to report the percentage (or proportion) of patients with particular QoL scores. Many people find it relatively easy to obtain a feeling for percentages (for example, '30 per cent of patients reported quite a bit of problem with tiredness'), but it is more difficult to use this approach for multi-item scales such as those that summate several items and produce a scale-score between, say, 0 and 100.

Reference against normative data from healthy subjects

For many of the more widely used instruments, **normative** data are available, showing the results that may be expected in a random sample of the general population. For example, Ware et al. have provided norm-based interpretations of SF-36 scores based on percentile rankings obtained from large, representative samples from the general population in the United States.[17] Similarly, Hjermstad et al.[63] report normative data for the QLQ-C30 in a randomly selected sample of 3000 people aged between 18 and 93 from the Norwegian population. The results are tabulated by age and sex. These normative data may serve as a guideline when interpreting QoL in groups of patients with cancer.

Contrast with reference data from patient groups

Reference values are often available for groups of patients with different cancer diagnoses. For example, the EORTC Quality of Life Study Group has produced a manual of reference data,[64] based upon pooled data from many clinical trials and observational studies. The manual tabulates age- and gender-specific values for the QLQ-C30 and its scales, according to the main cancer sites divided by stage of disease (early or limited, versus advanced or extensive). Thus investigators can contrast their results against those found in comparable groups of patients.

Measurement of minimal changes that are important to patients

Osoba and colleagues have suggested guidelines for interpreting the 'subjective significance' of change scores on the EORTC QLQ-C30, based on a comparison with direct estimates of change provided by patients retrospectively using so-called 'health transition' questions.[65] In their study, patients were asked to complete the QLQ-C30 on two occasions. At the time of the second administration, they were also asked to complete a Subjective Significance Questionnaire, which inquired about perceived changes in physical, emotional, and social functioning and in global QL, using a seven-point scale ranging from 'much worse' to 'no change' to 'much better'. Patients who reported 'a little' change for better or worse on a particular SSQ scale had

corresponding pretest–post-test QLQ-C30 changes of about 5 to 10 points. Those reporting 'moderate' change on the SSQ had QLQ-C30 changes of about 10 to 20 points, and those reporting 'very much' change on the SSQ had QLQ-C30 changes of more than 20 points. Other studies, including those of Tannock et al. in hormone-resistant prostate cancer,[66] Stephens et al. in small-cell lung cancer,[67] and Rothenberg et al. in advanced pancreatic cancer[68] have employed related strategies for defining a palliative response or 'clinical response benefit' based, in part, on patients' self-reported changes in symptom burden.

Anchor-based interpretations

Anchor-based interpretations compare the changes seen in QoL scores ('anchored') against other clinical changes. In the study of King,[69] 'known groups' of patients who were expected to differ in terms of QoL scores were compared. For example, patients with limited disease were compared to those with advanced disease. Data were collated from 14 published studies, and King concluded that for most scales a difference of 5 or less is a 'small' difference, but the definition of a 'large' difference varied for each scale: for example, large differences were 16 for global QoL, 27 for physical functioning, and 7 for emotional functioning.

Distribution-based interpretations

Distribution-based interpretations are based on the statistical distributions of results. The most commonly used statistics are effect size (**ES**), which relates the observed change to the baseline standard deviation,[70] or the standardized response mean (**SRM**), which uses the standard deviation of the change. In the papers by both Osoba and King, effect sizes were found to correspond to changes in QLQ-C30 scores and SSQ ratings.

In summary, the interpretation of results remains essentially qualitative. Clinical significance is subjective, and is a matter of opinion. The values and opinions of individual patients will differ, as will the opinions of the treating clinician and those of society in general. For a QoL measurement scale, it is unlikely that a single threshold value will be universally accepted as a cut point that separates clinically important changes from trivial and unimportant ones. However, many investigators are finding that, for a variety of scales assessing overall QoL and some of its dimensions, changes of between 5 per cent and 10 per cent (that is, between 5 and 10 points on a 1 to 100 scale) are noticed by patients and are regarded by them as 'significant' changes.

QoL assessment in daily clinical practice

Only a small percentage of patients with cancer are treated in clinical trials. Even in specialized cancer hospitals, the large majority of patients receive standard treatment and care. Is there a place for QoL assessment in daily clinical practice?

At the first major conference on this topic held in Washington, DC in 1993, a range of possibilities was identified,[71] including:

(1) routine screening of patients for functional problems;

(2) monitoring disease progression and treatment effects;

(3) assessing the quality of care; and

(4) facilitating doctor–patient communication.

None of the current QoL questionnaires has been designed specifically for interpretation at the level of the individual patient, and they do not exhibit the very high levels of reliability typically required of a diagnostic or screening instrument. Thus, some of the applications suggested above await further refinements in the precision of QoL measures.

Perhaps the most promising area of clinical application is in promoting better communication between doctors and their patients. Doctors vary in their ability to elicit relevant information from their patients, and patients vary in their ability to articulate their problems and concerns.[72] Time constraints in the typical outpatient clinic setting add to problems of communication. The introduction of standardized QoL assessments in daily clinical practice might represent a useful tool for structuring and facilitating the efficient exchange of information.

While empirical research in this area of application is scarce, a small pilot study conducted in an outpatient clinic has yielded promising results.[73] In this study, a consecutive series of patients receiving palliative chemotherapy was asked to complete the QLQ-C30 while waiting to see their oncologist. The patients' responses were optically scanned into a portable computer, and a graphic summary of the results was generated, a copy of which was provided to both the patient and the oncologist just prior to the medical consultation. At each subsequent outpatient visit, this procedure was repeated, with the QoL summary including both the patients' current scores and those from previous visits. An increase over time was observed in the average number of QoL issues discussed per consultation, and in the active role played by the physicians in initiating such discussions. Importantly, the availability of the QoL summary did not lengthen the average consultation time. This intervention is being tested more rigorously in a large-scale, randomized study in which, in addition to doctor–patient communication, outcomes of interest include physicians' awareness of their patients' physical and psychosocial health problems, patients' and physicians' satisfaction with their medical encounters, and improvement in patients' QoL over time. Parallel efforts are directed to increasing the efficiency with which QoL data can be collected through the use of computer touch-screen technology.[74]

QoL assessment in establishing clinical practice guidelines

One of the most controversial areas of application of QoL data is as an aid in establishing clinical practice guidelines. Seldom does any single clinical trial provide a clear, unequivocal answer to the question of which treatment is best for a given patient population. Typically, we need to synthesize data from many clinical trials. This can be done by indirect comparison of the results of different studies, but formal 'meta-analysis' techniques are preferred. Until now, such meta-analyses in clinical oncology have relied exclusively on objective indicators of treatment success such as disease-free and overall survival. There have been too few clinical trials which have included QoL assessments to be able to incorporate these more subjective types of data into the decision-making process. As QoL assessments become a more common and accepted part of clinical trials, this situation should change.

A meta-analysis of clinical trial data on the adjuvant treatment of breast cancer illustrates the potential impact of including QoL considerations in our calculations. In 1992, a meta-analysis was published in the *Lancet*, using data from nearly 4000 patients aged 50 years or older with node-positive breast cancer, in which tamoxifen alone was compared with tamoxifen plus chemotherapy.[75] The results indicated that the addition of chemotherapy provided a significant advantage in terms of disease-free survival, although not in overall survival. In this original meta-analysis, however, no consideration was given to the toxicity of chemotherapy, which can be substantial.

In 1996, Gelber and colleagues published the results of a reanalysis of the data from the original meta-analysis, using a TWiST analysis.[76] They divided overall survival time into three periods: that spent on treatment, that during which the disease was in remission, and the time after the disease had recurred. They then employed a series of weights (or 'utilities') to discount the time spent on treatment and after disease recurrence, relative to that spent in a disease-free state. In this way they adjusted overall survival for the compromised quality of that survival caused either by the toxicity of treatment or by the symptoms due to the disease. The results indicated that the combination of chemotherapy and tamoxifen did not provide more quality-adjusted survival time than tamoxifen alone; that any advantage of chemotherapy in terms of longer disease-free survival was cancelled out by the side-effects of the treatment.

This latter analysis is open to a number of criticisms, the most important being that the weights used to adjust the survival time were based on a restrictive definition of QoL, and were not derived from patients, but rather were generated by the researchers themselves. Other methods are available for obtaining such weights directly from patients, as well as from the general population, although they too are the subject of much debate. Nevertheless, the general principle underlying this utility approach remains intact. By integrating objective and subjective outcome criteria it may be possible to generate clinical practice guidelines that reflect a more balanced picture of the relative costs and benefits, in both human and economic terms, of cancer therapies.

Future directions

After 20 years of effort in developing the science of QoL assessment, it is now bearing fruit. What are the important questions for future research? In the area of measurement, there are a number of methodological challenges:

1. We need well-designed comparisons of the most promising of the currently available QoL measures. Only by documenting their **relative** strengths and weaknesses, can we make informed recommendations about which instrument to use in a given study. It would also be useful to compare directly (in other words, to calibrate) the scores derived from different QoL measures.

2. Efforts should be intensified to develop supplemental questionnaires for use with specific groups of patients. There is increasing evidence that more specific instruments are best able to detect treatment effects in clinical studies. Such efforts should preferably be characterized by intergroup collaboration to avoid

flooding the market with a large number of competing instruments.

3. We need to develop a much better understanding of the clinical significance of QoL scores. Understanding of such scores will undoubtedly increase as we gain experience with their use, but we can accelerate our learning curve by generating normative or reference data for groups of patients with different diagnoses, stages of disease, and treatment experiences. Use of 'health transition' questions and related methods can also assist in defining clinically important changes in QoL scores over time.

4. Because interest in QoL research has increased worldwide, there is a continued need to evaluate the performance of questionnaires in diverse cultural settings, including among ethnic and cultural minorities within countries. All too often, QoL studies exclude migrant groups simply because they do not speak the dominant language of their host country.

5. We need to re-examine the prevailing assumptions about the (in)ability of children to provide us with direct feedback on their health status and QoL. Historically, studies of the QoL of children with cancer have relied exclusively on ratings provided by proxies (for example, parents, teachers, healthcare providers). Recent efforts have been successful in constructing questionnaires that can be completed reliably by adolescents and even younger children.[77]

Research is also needed to develop QoL instruments with very high degrees of precision for use at the level of the individual patient (that is to say, in daily clinical practice). A particularly exciting possibility in this regard is the use of item-response theory and computer-adaptive testing (CAT) to develop dynamically tailored questionnaires whose length and content can be varied, depending on the intended use, the desired level of measurement precision, and the specific responses to questions provided by each patient.[78] For example, when assessing physical functioning, if we establish that a patient cannot manage a short walk, it would be largely irrelevant to then ask whether (s)he can manage long walks or running; instead, it would more efficient and informative to focus subsequent questions upon less-demanding levels of physical activity. The result is that the patient is required to answer fewer questions, and those questions that are asked are relevant to the patient's current situation. Additionally, with these methods, scale scores can potentially be estimated far more precisely than with questionnaires based on classical test theory.

In the realm of clinical trials, we run the risk of becoming the victims of our own success. Only a few years ago, it was quite uncommon for a clinical trial to include a formal QoL component. Today, there are hundreds of such studies being conducted throughout the world. While this is a positive trend, funding agencies and review committees should require that clinical investigators provide an explicit, well-argued rationale for including QoL outcomes in their trial protocols. When such a rationale is provided, sufficient funding should be made available to facilitate the additional data collection. The most expensive study is that which fails to meet its objectives because of an inadequate research infrastructure.

In the area of daily clinical practice, the need for QoL measures appropriate for use at the level of the individual patient has already been indicated. A related challenge is to find ways of communicating the results of QoL studies so that they can be used effectively in clinical decision-making. This includes not only presenting results in such a way that doctors can interpret and use them in counselling their patients, but also such that patients can draw on such information to make more informed choices.

Finally, there is much to learn about how QoL data might be used in setting health care policy. Legitimate concerns have been expressed that decisions regarding the allocation of our scarce health care resources are based on too restrictive a definition of therapeutic benefit, namely, the number of years of life saved. This has led to attempts to merge QoL and survival data, yielding quality-adjusted life years or QALYs. Such an approach, while representing a potentially powerful analytical tool, carries with it the risk of oversimplifying a very heterogeneous set of considerations.

The process of deciding which medical treatments society is willing to pay for, and which it is not, is rather complex. Those working in the QoL field can perhaps best inform the public debate over health care financing by generating high-quality data on the full range of effects that our medical technologies have on patients' functioning and well being. This will ensure that the patients' perspective is represented in health care policy decisions.

References

1. Johnson JR, Temple R. Food and Drug Administration requirements for approval of new anticancer drugs. *Cancer Treatment Reports*, 1985; **69**: 1155–9.

2. American Society of Clinical Oncology. Outcomes of cancer treatment for technology assessment and cancer treatment guidelines. *Journal of Clinical Oncology*, 1996; **14**: 671–9.

3. Hutchinson TA, Boyd NF, Feinstein AR. Scientific problems in clinical scales, as demonstrated in the Karnofsky index of performance status. *Journal of Chronic Diseases*, 1979; **32**: 661–6.

4. Taylor AE, Olver IN, Sivanthan T, Chi M, Purnell C. Observer error in grading performance status in cancer patients. *Support Care Cancer*, 1999; **7**: 332–5.

5. Sprangers MA, Aaronson NK. The role of health care providers and significant others in evaluating the quality of life of patients with chronic disease: a review. *Journal of Clinical Epidemiology*, 1992; **45**: 743–60.

6. Sneeuw KCA, Aaronson NK, Sprangers MAG, Detmar SB, Wever LDV, Schornagel JH. Evaluating the quality of life of cancer patients: assessments by patients, significant others, physicians and nurses. *British Journal of Cancer*, 1999; **81**: 87–94.

7. Sneeuw KCA, Aaronson NK, Sprangers MAG, Detmar SB, Wever LDV, Schornagel JH. Value of caregiver ratings in evaluating the quality of life of patients with cancer. *Journal of Clinical Oncology*, 1997; **15**: 1206–17.

8. Stephens RJ, Hopwood P, Girling DJ, Machin D. Randomised trials with quality of life endpoints: are doctors' ratings of patients' physical symptoms interchangeable with patients' self-ratings? *Quality of Life Research*, 1997; **6**: 225–36.

9. Feinstein AR. Clinimetric perspectives. *Journal of Chronic Diseases*, 1987; **40**: 635–40.

10. Gough IR, *et al.* Assessment of the quality of life of patients with advanced cancer. *European Journal of Cancer*, 1983; **19**: 1161–5.

11. Karnofsky DA, Abelmann WH, Carver LF, Burchenal JH. The use of nitrogen mustards in the palliative treatment of carcinoma. *Cancer*, 1948; **1**: 634–56.

12. Aaronson NK. Quality of life: What is it? How do we measure it? *Oncology*, 1988; **2**: 69–74.

13. **Bergner M,** *et al.* The Sickness Impact Profile: development and final revision of a health status measure. *Medical Care,* 1981; **19**: 787–805.

14. **Hunt SM, McEwan J, McKenna SP.** *Measuring health status.* Beckenham: Croom Helm, 1986.

15. **The WHOQOL Group.** Development of the World Health Organization WHOQOL-BREF quality of life assessment. *Psychological Medicine,* 1998; **28**: 551–8.

16. **McHorney CA, Ware JE, Raczek AE.** The MOS 36-Item Short-Form Health Survey (SF-36): II. Psychometric and clinical tests of validity in measuring physical and mental health constructs. *Medical Care,* 1993; **31**: 247–63.

17. **Ware JE, Snow KK, Kosinski M, Gandek B.** *SF-36 health survey manual and interpretation guide.* Boston, MA: New England Medical Center, The Health Institute, 1993.

18. **Terrell JE, Nanavati K, Esclamado RM, Bradford CR, Wolf GT.** Health impact of head and neck cancer. *Otolaryngology—Head and Neck Surgery,* 1999; **120**: 852–9.

19. **Kurtz ME, Kurtz JC, Stommel M, Given CW, Given B.** Loss of physical functioning among geriatric cancer patients: relationships to cancer site, treatment, comorbidity and age. *European Journal of Cancer,* 1997; **33**: 2352–8.

20. **Velanovich V, Szymanski W.** Quality of life of breast cancer patients with lymphedema. *American Journal of Surgery,* 1999; **177**: 184–7.

21. **Albertsen PC, Aaronson NK, Muller MJ, Keller SD, Ware JE.** Health-related quality of life among patients with metastatic prostate cancer. *Urology,* 1997; **49**: 207–16.

22. **Davis AM, Devlin M, Griffin AM, Wunder JS, Bell RS.** Functional outcome in amputation versus limb sparing of patients with lower extremity sarcoma: a matched case-control study. *Archives of Physical Medicine and Rehabilitation,* 1999; **80**: 615–18.

23. **Loge JH, Abrahamsen AF, Ekeberg O, Kaasa S.** Reduced health-related quality of life among Hodgkin's disease survivors: a comparative study with general population norms. *Annals of Oncology,* 1999; **10**: 71–7.

24. **Gandek B, Ware JE (ed.)** Translating functional health and well-being: international quality of life assessment (ISOQOL) project studies of the SF-36 health survey. *Journal of Clinical Epidemiology,* 1998; **51**: 891–1214.

25. **Schipper H, Clinch J, McMurray A, Levitt M.** Measuring the quality of life of cancer patients: the functional living index-cancer: development and validation. *Journal of Clinical Oncology,* 1984; **2**: 472–83.

26. **de Haes JCJM, van Knippenberg FC, Neijt JP.** Measuring psychological and physical distress in cancer patients: structure and application of the Rotterdam Symptom Checklist. *British Journal of Cancer,* 1990; **62**: 1034–8.

27. **Ganz PA, Schag CA, Lee JJ, Sims MS.** The CARES: a generic measure of health-related quality of life for patients with cancer. *Quality of Life Research,* 1992; **1**: 19–29.

28. **Schag CA, Ganz PA, Heinrich RL.** Cancer Rehabilitation Evaluation System—Short Form (CARES-SF). A cancer specific rehabilitation and quality of life instrument. *Cancer,* 1991; **68**: 1406–13.

29. **Aaronson NK,** *et al.* The European Organization for Research and Treatment of Cancer QLQ-C30: A quality-of-life instrument for use in international clinical trials in oncology. *Journal of the National Cancer Institute,* 1993; **85**: 365–76.

30. **Cella DF,** *et al.* The functional assessment of cancer therapy scale: development and validation of the general measure. *Journal of Clinical Oncology,* 1993; **11**: 570–9.

31. **Stockler MR,** *et al.* Responsiveness to change in health-related quality of life: a comparison of the Prostate Cancer Specific Quality of Life Instrument (PROSQOLI) with analogous scales of the EORTC QLQ-C30 and a trial specific module. *Journal of Clinical Epidemiology,* 1998; **51**: 37–45.

32. **Litwin MS,** *et al.* The UCLA Prostate Cancer Index: development,

reliability and validity of a health-related quality of life measure. *Medical Care,* 1998; **36**: 1002–12.

33. **Sommers SD, Ramsey SD.** A review of quality-of-life evaluations in prostate cancer. *Pharmacoeconomics,* 1999; **16**: 127–40.

34. **Maguire P, Selby P.** Assessing quality of life in cancer patients. *British Journal of Cancer,* 1989; **60**: 437–40.

35. **Lohr KN,** *et al.* Evaluating quality-of-life and health status instruments: development of scientific review criteria. *Clinical Therapeutics,* 1996; **18**: 979–92.

36. **Andersen NH.** *Contributions to information integration theory.* Hillsdale, NJ: Lawrence Erlbaum, 1991.

37. **Torrance GW.** Measurement of health state utilities for economic appraisal: a review. *Journal of Health Economics,* 1985; **5**: 1–30.

38. **Stiggelbout AM, Kiebert GM, Kievit J, Leer JW, Habbema JD, de Haes JC.** The 'utility' of the time trade-off method in cancer patients: feasibility and proportional trade-off. *Journal of Clinical Epidemiology,* 1995; **48**: 1207–14.

39. **Gelber RD, Cole BF, Gelber S, Goldhirsch A.** Comparing treatments using quality-adjusted survival: the Q-TwiST method. *American Statistician,* 1995; **49**: 161–9.

40. **Kaplan RM, Bush JW, Berry CC.** Health status index: category rating versus magnitude estimation for measuring levels of well-being. *Medical Care,* 1979; **17**: 501–25.

41. **Torrance GW, Feeny DH, Furlong WJ, Barr RD, Zhang Y, Wang Q.** Multi-attribute health status classification systems: health utilities index mark 2. *Medical Care,* 1996; **34**: 702–22.

42. **Weeks J, O'Leary J, Fairclough D, Paltiel D, Weinstein M.** The 'Q-tility Index': a new tool for assessing health-related quality of life and utilities in clinical trials and clinical practice. *Proceedings of the American Society of Clinical Oncology (ASCO),* 1994; **13**: 436.

43. **Brazier J, Jones N, Kind P.** Testing the validity of the EuroQol and comparing it with the SF-36 health survey questionnaire. *Quality of Life Research,* 1993; **2**: 169–80.

44. **Weeks J.** Taking quality of life into account in health economic analyses. *Journal of the National Cancer Institute Monograph,* 1996; **20**: 23–7.

45. **Fayers P, Hand DJ.** Generalisation from phase III clinical trials: survival, quality of life, and health economics. *Lancet,* 1997; **350**: 1025–7.

46. **Loge JH, Abrahamsen AF, Ekeberg O, Kaasa S.** Reduced health-related quality of life among Hodgkin's disease survivors: a comparative study with general population norms. *Annals of Oncology,* 1999; **10**: 71–7.

47. **Ganz PA, Rowland JH, Desmond K, Meyerowitz BE, Wyatt Ge.** Life after breast cancer: understanding women's health-related quality of life and sexual functioning. *Journal of Clinical Oncology,* 1998; **16**: 501–14.

48. **Irwig L, Bennetts A.** Quality of life after breast conservation or mastectomy: a systematic review. *Australian and New Zealand Journal of Surgery,* 1997; **67**: 750–4.

49. **Lasry JC, Margolese RG.** Fear of recurrence, breast-conserving surgery, and the trade-off hypothesis. *Cancer,* 1992; **69**: 2111–15.

50. **Coates A,** *et al.* Improving the quality of life during chemotherapy for advanced breast cancer: a comparison of intermittent and continuous treatment strategies. *New England Journal of Medicine,* 1987; **317**: 1490–5.

51. **Simons JP,** *et al.* Effects of medroxyprogesterone acetate on appetite, weight, and quality of life in advanced-stage, non-hormone-sensitive cancer: a placebo-controlled multicenter study. *Journal of Clinical Oncology,* 1996; **14**: 1077–84.

52. **Dancy J,** *et al.* Quality of life scores: an independent prognostic variable in a general population of cancer patients receiving chemotherapy. *Quality of Life Research,* 1997; **6**: 151–8.

53. **Coates A,** *et al.* Prognostic value of quality-of-life scores during

chemotherapy for advanced breast cancer. *Journal of Clinical Oncology*, 1992; **10**: 1833–8.

54. Coates A, *et al.* Prognostic value of quality of life scores in a trial of chemotherapy with or without interferon in patients with metastatic malignant melanoma. *European Journal of Cancer*, 1993; **29A**: 1731–4.

55. Earlam S, Glover C, Fordy C, Burke D, Allen-Mersh TG. Relation between tumor size, quality of life, and survival in patients with colorectal liver metastases. *Journal of Clinical Oncology*, 1996; **14**: 171–5.

56. Wisløff F, Hjorth M. Health-related quality of life assessed before and during chemotherapy predicts survival in multiple myeloma. *British Journal of Haematology*, 1997; **97**: 29–37.

57. Sadura A, *et al.* Quality-of-life assessment: patient compliance with questionnaire completion. *Journal of the National Cancer Institute*, 1992; **84**: 1023–6.

58. Machin D, Campbell MJ, Fayers PM, Pinol A. *Sample size tables for clinical studies* (2nd edn). Oxford: Blackwell Science, 1997.

59. Bland JM, Altman DG. Multiple significance tests: the Bonferroni method. *British Medical Journal*, 1995; **310**: 170.

60. Fayers P, Machin D. *Quality of life assessment, analysis and interpretation.* Chichester: John Wiley, 2000.

61. Osoba D, Tannock IF, Ernst DS, Neville AJ. Health-related quality of life in men with metastatic prostate cancer treated with prednisone alone or mitoxantrone and prednisone. *Journal of Clinical Oncology*, 1999; **17**: 1654–63.

62. Curran D, Molenberghs G, Fayers PM, Machin D. Incomplete quality of life data in randomized trials: missing forms. *Statistics in Medicine*, 1998; **17**: 697–709.

63. Hjermstad MJ, Fayers PM, Bjordal K, Kaasa S. Health-related quality of life in the general Norwegian population assessed by the European Organization for Research and Treatment of Cancer Core Quality-of-Life Questionnaire: the QLQ-C30 (+3). *Journal of Clinical Oncology*, 1998; **16**: 1188–96.

64. Fayers PM, Weeden S, Curran D. *EORTC QLQ-C30 reference values.* Brussels: EORTC, 1998.

65. Osoba D, Rodrigues G, Myles J, Zee B, Pater J. Interpreting the significance of changes in health-related quality-of-life scores. *Journal of Clinical Oncology*, 1998; **16**: 139–44.

66. Tannock IF, *et al.* Chemotherapy with mitoxantrone plus prednisone alone for symptomatic hormone-resistant prostate cancer: a Canadian randomized trial with palliative end points. *Journal of Clinical Oncology*, 1996; **14**: 1756–64.

67. Stephens RJ, Hopwood P, Girling DJ. Defining and analyzing symptom palliation in cancer clinical trials: a deceptively difficult exercise. *British Journal of Cancer*, 1999; **79**: 538–44.

68. Rothenberg ML, *et al.* A phase II trial of gemcitabine in patients with 5-FU-refractory pancreas cancer. *Annals of Oncology*, 1996; **7**: 347–53.

69. King MT. The interpretation of scores from the EORTC quality of life questionnaire QLQ-C30. *Quality of Life Research*, 1996; **5**: 555–67.

70. Cohen J. *Statistical power analysis for the behavioral sciences* (2nd edn). Hillsdale, NJ: Lawrence Erlbaum, 1988.

71. Lohr KN. Application of health status assessment measures in clinical practice: overview of the Third Conference on Advances in Health Status Assessment. *Medical Care*, 1992; **30**: MS1–MS14.

72. Roter DL, Hall JA. *Doctors talking with patients/patients talking with doctors: Improving communication in medical settings.* London: Auburn House, 1992.

73. Detmar SB, Aaronson NK. Quality of life assessment in daily clinical oncology practice: a feasibility study. *European Journal of Cancer*, 1998; **34**: 1181–6.

74. Velikova G, *et al.* Automated collection of quality-of-life data: a comparison of paper and computer touch-screen questionnaires. *Journal of Clinical Oncology*, 1999; **17**: 998–1007.

75. Early Breast Cancer Trialists' Collaborative Group. Systemic treatment of early breast cancer by hormonal, cytotoxic, or immune therapy. 133 randomised trials involved 31,000 recurrences and 24,000 deaths among 75,000 women. *Lancet*, 1992; **339**: 1–15.

76. Gelber RD, *et al.* Adjuvant chemotherapy plus tamoxifen compared with tamoxifen alone for postmenopausal breast cancer: meta-analysis of quality-adjusted survival. *Lancet*, 1996; **347**: 1066–71.

77. Varni JW, Seid M, Rode CA. The PedsQL: measurement model for the pediatric quality of life inventory. *Medical Care*, 1999; **37**: 126–39.

78. Wainer H, *et al. Computerized adaptive testing: a primer.* Hillsdale, NJ: Lawrence Erlbaum, 1990.

6.4 Support services for cancer patients

Mary M. H. Cody and Maurice L. Slevin

Introduction

For most patients and their families, the experience of cancer is intensely stressful. Maguire[1] summarized it well when he commented that cancer patients 'face the threats that they may lose their health, role, and life. They also have to live with the uncertainty as to whether and when those losses will occur'. Clinical research supports the idea that the diagnosis and treatment of cancer carries with it considerable psychological morbidity. Studies consistently report that 25 to 30 per cent of patients have significant emotional problems and that many of these could be alleviated through some form of intervention (see Chapter 6.1). Indeed, a recent editorial suggests that psychosocial interventions should be an integral part of every patients' management plan[2] (see also Chapter 6.2). Psychosocial studies, which highlight patients' perceptions of their illness, have helped to shape the development of a wide variety of psychological and social support services for cancer patients. In practice, support services are limited by the human and financial resources available.

Our aim in this chapter is to describe the types of cancer support and information services that are available to patients, and to summarize evidence (where available) that these support organizations provide benefit to patients. We will use examples of support services from the United Kingdom, but wherever possible will indicate the availability of parallel services in other countries.

What constitutes support and what do patients want?

Most authors agree that support is a multidimensional construct encompassing provision of information, emotional support, material aid, and services.[3],[4] Analyses of calls to cancer telephone helplines tend to support this all-embracing definition. During 1998, Cancer-BACUP, the British national cancer information service, received over 45 000 enquiries (J. Mossman, personal communication). Fifty per cent of the callers requested specific medical information while 40 per cent per cent of enquiries concerned topics related to emotional support. In a similar survey in the United States, 50 per cent of the telephone calls concerned psychosocial issues, with requests for referral to support groups, anxiety/depression about the diagnosis, family problems, doctor–patient communication problems, and the financial demands of the illness being the most frequent topics of conversation.[5] These data and other studies[6],[7] suggest that a range of services and expertise is necessary if the needs of cancer patients and

their families are to be met adequately. In this chapter psychosocial support, informational support, and financial support are considered separately.

Psychosocial support

The role of the cancer doctor in providing support

The majority of patients with cancer today expect to be well informed about their illness and the treatment options that are available (see Chapter 6.2). Increasingly, patients are looking not just for technical and medical expertise from their doctors, but for someone with whom they can also discuss their psychosocial concerns.[8] A recent study highlighted the central role of cancer doctors in providing emotional support to their patients.[7]

How the initial consultation interview is handled is crucial and may well determine the patient's future adjustment to his or her illness. This is the ideal opportunity for the cancer doctor to commence a supportive relationship built on trust and openness. Information-giving that is accurately timed and appropriately pitched can be extremely supportive. Information should be tailored to the needs of the individual patient and sensitively imparted at a rate that the patient can manage.[9] It needs to be consistent and repeated frequently as recall by patients is notoriously poor.[10] Provision of audiotapes of the clinical consultation has been found to aid recall but does not always reduce distress and may be unhelpful in patients with a poor prognosis.[11]

Plans of action need to be discussed with the patient and every effort should be made to involve the patient in all aspects of care. It is important, though, to take into account individual preferences for the degree of involvement. For example giving an anxious patient responsibility for decisions regarding choices of treatment may only heighten their anxiety. Studies suggest that most patients want specific information about chances of cure with treatment,[12] although some authorities suggest that fewer patients want specific information about their prognosis.[13] Patients in the elderly age group may have less need for specific information.[14]

Enquiries about the emotional, social, and financial impact of the disease reassure the patient that the doctor is interested in them as an individual and not as just another case. Informational support which is not reinforced by emotional support is considered 'unhelpful' by patients.[15]

Relapses are particularly difficult for patients and they often fear that they will be abandoned by their doctors. However, even in advanced cases there is nearly always something that can be done. Focusing on plans for symptom relief and continuing care, even if it is of a palliative nature, can be very reassuring. (For useful articles on doctor–patient communications see reference list.[9],[16]–[18]) Courses and workshops are available to help doctors and nurses improve their communication skills with patients[19] (see also Chapter 6.2) and the topic is becoming an important aspect of the undergraduate curriculum.

The role of counselling

With the increasing recognition of the emotional burden of cancer patients, it is becoming customary for cancer treatment centres to provide counselling services. Designated nurse specialist/ nurse counsellors have extensive knowledge of cancer and its treatment and are thus well equipped to deal with the practical worries and concerns of cancer patients. They are usually trained in communication skills and in eliciting symptoms of psychological distress. Nurse counsellors are not intended to absolve physicians of their responsibility to communicate with their patients. However, within the constraints of a busy practice, it may be impossible to spend as much time as is optimally desirable with the patient and his or her relatives. Furthermore, patients are frequently in such turmoil on hearing their diagnosis that they retain little of the initial information imparted to them. Nurse counsellors reinforce diagnostic and prognostic information from the physician. Misconceptions about cancer and its treatment are readily identified by nurse counsellors and methods of solving both practical and emotional problems are explored with the patient.

Structured psychoeducational interventions have been advocated in the United States for newly diagnosed patients with cancer. They combine a counselling approach with an educational approach and have been shown to be effective in reducing anxiety and depressive symptoms and promoting a greater return to activities of daily living. Education alone did not show the same benefits.[20] Other, more recent studies support the efficacy of nurse-led psychoeducational programmes based on health education, stress management, and coping skills training.[21] A detailed psychoeducational model has been outlined by Fawzy[22] and a randomized, controlled trial in patients with malignant melanoma revealed reduced psychological distress and more adaptive coping methods at 6-weeks, at 6-months, and at 5-years follow-up.[22]

A broader counselling approach may also be undertaken by social workers, hospital chaplains, or indeed lay people with a training in counselling. Since these people have less specific knowledge of cancer and its treatment, this approach is more suitable for patients with interpersonal or emotional problems which may have predated or been exacerbated by the diagnosis. The British Association for Counselling has a large membership nation-wide and can provide the names of counsellors working locally.

It has been suggested that the counselling approach is more suited to alleviating acute, transient mood states than more severe, protracted disturbance. For example counselling failed to prevent psychiatric morbidity in mastectomy patients but led to increased recognition and early psychiatric referral, thus reducing the overall level of morbidity 12 to 18 months later.[23]

Many patients have sufficient personal or social resources to buffer the stressful effects of cancer and therefore have no need for professional counselling. Furthermore, not all of those who are distressed will elect to discuss their problems with a counsellor. In one study of newly diagnosed patients, the acceptance of counselling services among those deemed to be at risk of psychological problems was only 60 per cent.[24] On the evidence of present data, there appears to be little to support the provision of counselling services for all. More research is needed to identify who should receive counselling, who should provide it, when it should occur, and the most effective form of intervention.

Psychotherapy

Psychotherapy may be indicated when the emotional reaction to cancer is intense and protracted. Psychotherapy aims to bring about enduring changes in the patient's way of dealing with stressful situations. Many cancer patients are unable to benefit from in-depth psychoanalytic therapies because they are lengthy and emotionally demanding. However, brief forms of psychotherapy focusing on immediate problems and aimed at improving the patient's quality of life can be very helpful. Spouses and partners are frequently included in these sessions because of the far-reaching effects that the disease and its treatment have on people around the patient. In some cases, the added emotional burden of the illness may highlight and exacerbate pre-existing deficiencies in relationships. Psychiatrists and psychologists with a special interest in the emotional aspects of cancer are increasingly available in general hospitals to provide psychotherapeutic services[25] (see also Chapter 6.1).

Adjuvant psychological therapy is a form of cognitive psychotherapy specifically adapted for cancer patients by psychiatrists at the Royal Marsden Hospital, London. In psychiatry, cognitive therapy has been shown to be effective in reducing depression.[26] In adjuvant psychological therapy, principles of cognitive therapy have been applied to patients with cancer to enable them to overcome negative attitudes and to adopt more positive coping strategies. Patients become familiar with techniques such as calming self-instruction, positive self-statements, methods of distraction, reality testing, and cognitive rehearsal. Behavioural techniques, such as relaxation and activity scheduling, are also employed. The therapy is carried out over six to 12 sessions and the aim is to maximize the patient's involvement in the rewarding aspects of life.[27] Scientific evaluation of adjuvant psychological therapy has demonstrated its effectiveness in reducing anxiety and depression and improving coping responses in patients with cancer.[28] A subsequent, randomized trial revealed the superiority of adjuvant psychological therapy over non-directive supportive counselling.[29] Adjuvant psychological therapy has the advantage that, with some training, it can be practised by health professionals with diverse backgrounds and not just by psychiatrists and psychologists.

Support groups

Oncology support groups are rapidly gaining in popularity. There are at least 600 cancer support or self-help groups throughout the United Kingdom. Information is available from CancerLink and CancerBACUP. CancerBACUP also has a searchable database of all United Kingdom support groups and cancer organizations on its website (www.cancerbacup.org.uk). An up-to-date directory listing the various support groups in the United Kingdom is available through CancerLink. The Groups Support Service set up by CancerLink provides training, finances, and support to those who are in the process of setting up new groups.

Support groups help to reduce the sense of alienation and isolation often engendered by the diagnosis of cancer and its treatment. They differ in the range and type of service offered, depending on the needs and resources of the local community. Some support groups are hospital based, led by doctors and nurses. These are educational as well as supportive.[30],[31] Others are true self-help groups set up in the community, often by people who have experience of cancer personally or in family members or friends. Self-help groups tend to emphasize self-reliance and self-care. Finally, there are the rarer psychotherapeutic groups run by a mental health professional with a training in group dynamics. These explore the wider psychodynamic implications of the illness.[32] It is not a question of which system, self-help or professional, is better. Both have a role to play in helping patients with the psychosocial problems related to cancer. Choice will depend largely on the preference of the individual and the available hospital and community resources. Some groups are limited to those with a specific type of experience (for example laryngectomy, colostomy, or mastectomy groups), while others welcome patients with a variety of cancer types.

The potential benefits of a support group include opportunities for sharing experiences, the ventilation of feelings in a supportive atmosphere, and the exchange of information about the physical, psychological, and social consequences of cancer and its treatment.

In the United States, Spiegel and colleagues carried out a randomized, controlled study of women with advanced breast cancer and demonstrated that participation in an expressive–supportive group weekly for 1 year was associated with improved mood, reduced pain, and reduced maladaptive coping responses.[33] Bottomly and colleagues[34] showed that group cognitive behavioural therapy was associated with a significant reduction in anxiety and an increase in fighting spirit responses in a study of psychologically distressed patients who were consecutively allocated to a cognitive behavioural group, a social support group, and a standard care non-interventional group. No significant changes were found in the social support and non-interventional group on any of the measures. Psychoeducational approaches have also demonstrable efficacy in group settings.[22]

Few patients report feeling more depressed as a result of attending a group, even when a group member dies. This may be because those who attend them are a self-selected, highly motivated minority of cancer patients.[30]

Psychosocial support—conclusion

There is a growing awareness of the importance of providing the cancer patient with emotional support. Medical and nursing staff all have an important role to play in the provision of this support. Counselling and psychotherapy services have also developed to meet the demand, operating both within and outside the hospital setting. Important questions have been asked about the efficacy of this support. Recently, a number of critical reviews of studies have been published which suggest that, despite methodological difficulties, psychosocial interventions have positive benefits for patients. Meyer and Mark,[35] for example, published the results of a meta-analysis of 45 psychosocial intervention studies which used treatment-controlled comparisons and demonstrated significant beneficial effects. Fawzy et

al.[31] has produced an exhaustive review of psychosocial interventions. For a summary see Fallowfield et al.[14]

Informational support

Cancer information and related support services

One of the most frequent sources of dissatisfaction for medical patients is the lack of information provided about their illness[36] (see also Chapter 6.2). Cancer information services were developed specifically to redress this situation. They act as an adjunctive support system but they do not replace a doctor's professional advice to the individual patient. Evaluations of telephone cancer information services suggest that they are effective means of conveying information about cancer and are associated with high levels of patient satisfaction.[37],[38] Patient satisfaction with booklets provided by cancer information services is also high.[7],[39]

CancerBACUP

The British Association for Cancer United Patients (BACUP) was founded in 1984 by Vicky Clement-Jones, a medical practitioner who developed cancer and subsequently recognized that there was little in the way of support and information for cancer patients.[40] Cancer-BACUP, as it is now known, is a national cancer information service which provides up-to-date information on all types of cancer by telephone or letter from a team of specially trained oncology nurses. The staff are supported by a medical and specialist advisory board which they can consult for specialized information. Confidential information is given on every aspect of cancer including treatment and care, support groups, and other services. The telephone service is free.

CancerBACUP also produces leaflets and booklets on different types of cancer and cancer treatments and how to cope with them. Booklets are also available which deal with symptom control, sexuality, diet, complementary therapies, communicating about cancer, and living with cancer. CancerBACUP publishes a newsletter three times a year which focuses on new developments in cancer care. The newsletter acts as an important communication link for cancer patients and their families. Doctors and other health-care professionals are invited to use the information and resources which are maintained on a computerized database.

CancerLink

CancerLink, a United Kingdom-based organization, was founded by a group of people with personal and professional experience of cancer. Trained staff provide telephone and written information about cancer, including practical and emotional help. A freephone Asian cancer information helpline for Asians in the United Kingdom is also available. A variety of booklets and leaflets in minority ethnic languages as well as in English has been prepared by CancerLink and they are freely available to cancer patients. A Directory of Useful Organizations produced by CancerLink includes addresses of the head offices of national organizations for information about specific types of cancer, counselling, hospice care, and bereavement services.

Other organizations

In the United States, the government-sponsored National Cancer Institute (NCI) runs a free service called the Cancer Information

Service (http://cis.nci.nih.gov), from 19 regional offices. The service, which can provide information in English and Spanish, is available to patients, their relatives, health-care professionals, and the general public. Callers are put in touch with operators in the office closest to his or her geographical area. Operators may consult the Physician Data Query database (PDQ) which is the NCI's comprehensive computerized cancer information database. PDQ contains the most up-to-date information available about detection, treatment (including availability of clinical trials and second opinions), and prevention of cancer. Access to PDQ is also available to the general public upon obtaining a member identification number and payment of a fee. The NCI's CancerNET Cancer Information Web page (http://wwwicic.nci.nih.gov) has useful information for patients on all aspects of cancer. The NCI Information Services also produces publications which are free to callers.

The American Cancer Society (ACS) is a non-profit organization which sponsors research into cancer and provides information to the public. The ACS produces many publications on all aspects of cancer. Local chapters of the ACS also provide services to patients such as transportation to medical appointments, support groups, and financial assistance. These services can be accessed by telephone or via the ACS web page.

Organizations in other countries also offer cancer information services, for example the Anti-Cancer Council of Victoria, in Australia, although their scope may not be as extensive as others mentioned here. A list of those organizations is provided at the end of this chapter.

Other information services deal with specific types of cancer. Breast Cancer Care in the United Kingdom, for example, offers women specific information about breast cancer and its treatment, breast prostheses, breast reconstruction, concealing blemishes after radiotherapy, etc. The association has a useful list of the many shops around Britain which stock prostheses and related items as well as several mail order firms. Breast Cancer Care operates a telephone helpline 5 days a week. It also produces its own selection of books and leaflets on topics such as breast surgery, lymphoedema, and breast self-examination which are freely available to individuals.

The Hodgkin's Disease and Lymphoma Association provides information and support to sufferers and relatives of those with Hodgkin's disease or non-Hodgkin's lymphoma. Support groups are run by local branches of the association and patient-to-patient and relative-to-relative contact schemes can be arranged. Relevant literature, including a quarterly newsletter and videos and tapes, are available for loan.

The British Colostomy Association aids the rehabilitation of those who have had a colostomy. It provides a telephone and postal advice service and also welcomes personal callers. It can arrange home and hospital visits by patients already experienced in living with colostomies. Services are free of charge. There are 22 area organizers throughout Britain. The British Colostomy Association publishes a series of leaflets on living with a colostomy, how to cope with constipation and diarrhoea, travelling, etc. Advice is given on the suitability and availability of various appliances.

The National Association of Laryngectomee Clubs has 95 British clubs which aid rehabilitation of those who have had a laryngectomy. As well as providing useful literature for patients, such as a handbook for laryngectomy patients, laryngectomy stoma care, emergency resuscitation, speaking tips for laryngectomees, the association can also arrange preoperative and postoperative visiting of patients and provide ongoing social support.

In the United States, the ACS sponsors a number of organizations such as Candlelighters which provides emotional support and information for parents of children with cancer, the International Association of Laryngectomees, and the United Ostomy Association.

Only some of the large British and United States cancer information and support services are mentioned here. Many smaller, regional and local cancer organizations also exist in these countries and in many others. A comprehensive list of all the information and support services in the United Kingdom is available through CancerBACUP and CancerLink.

Befriending

Many of the charitable organizations operate a system of visiting patients in hospital or in their own homes. Visitors are usually volunteers who have had personal experience of cancer themselves. Patients often find it difficult to confide in relatives who may be overly involved or very distressed and may find it easier to talk to someone who shares a common experience and who can provide support in a caring but more objective manner. Breast Cancer Care in the United Kingdom has a list of volunteer helpers who can be called upon to visit women undergoing breast surgery or later at home. Reach to Recovery is a similar volunteer visitation scheme in the United States. The visitor is carefully chosen and trained for her volunteer role. In as much as is possible she is matched to the patient on surgery, treatment, age, marital status, etc.

The British Colostomy Association (BCA) also operates a personal visiting system. The volunteers are often selected by stoma care nurses located in general hospitals and are then registered with the BCA after a period of training. Members of the National Laryngectomee Association Clubs in Britain, which promote the rehabilitation of laryngectomy patients, are frequently invited by surgeons and nursing staff to lecture and demonstrate speech aids and to talk to patients before and after their operation to show what can be achieved. The Leukaemia Care Society is an organization in Britain set up by parents and children who have had leukaemia. It provides a range of services such as visiting at home and in hospital, financial assistance, holidays, and support in times of stress.

Financial support

In the United Kingdom, cancer treatments are freely available to patients on the National Health Service (NHS) whatever their income or financial status, but in other countries, for example the United States and many countries in Europe, patients may be liable for the costs of their medical care. Many patients will have privately-funded or work-related medical insurance schemes. In the United States, Medicaid, funded by the federal and state governments, pays the medical expenses of those patients who are on low income or on welfare and those who are disabled. Patients must apply at a local social services office. Medicare is a federal health insurance scheme for those who are over 65, those in receipt of social security disability benefits for at least 2 years, and those with permanent kidney failure. Eligible veterans and their families may receive cancer treatment at a Veterans Administration Medical Center. Most developed countries will have similar types of government-assisted schemes for the needy. In underdeveloped countries, such schemes are at best patchy and many patients and their families will often have to make huge sacrifices for medical treatment or go without. Local communities may raise the costs of medical treatment through fund-raising activities.

In spite of private medical and government insurance schemes, many patients and their families, particularly if the patient is the main provider in the family, experience considerable financial difficulty as a result of loss of income and the many unplanned expenses that a chronic illness can incur. Sometimes it is the additional stresses, such as inadequate housing or financial worry, that lead to emotional decompensation. Many oncology units and hospitals have medical social workers or welfare rights workers who are able to advise sick patients about benefits to which they may be entitled.

In the United Kingdom, patients may contact their local Citizens Advice Bureau or the Benefits Agency Benefit Enquiry Line. The opportunities for backdating benefits are very limited so patients should be encouraged to seek advice promptly. In the United Kingdom, patients may qualify for income support and Housing Benefits if they satisfy certain criteria. Those on Income Support automatically qualify for free NHS prescriptions, free NHS wigs and fabric supports, free NHS sight tests and dental treatment and the refund of necessary travel costs to and from hospital for NHS treatment. If patients need help with personal care because of their illness or disability then they may be eligible for Attendance Allowance (for the over 65s) or Disability Living Allowance (for those aged 0–65). There are 'Special Rules' for people who are terminally ill; by this the Benefits Agency means those who are not expected to live more than 6 months. A form completed by the patient's doctor must accompany an application under the 'Special Rules'. In these situations the Benefits Agency is usually able to deal with claims within 10 days. These allowances are not means tested or contributions based and are not taxable. More information is available from the Benefits Agency website at http://www.dss.gov.uk/ba.

Some of the national cancer charities provide financial assistance to cancer patients in need. The American Cancer Society, for example, may offer reimbursements for transportation, medicine, and medical supplies. British organizations such as Sargent Cancer Care for young people up to the age of 21, and Macmillan Cancer Relief for adults, make grants available to patients to meet a wide variety of needs including travelling expenses, clothing, fuel bills, telephone installation, furniture, short-term care, and convalescence. Both bodies take the patient's means into account and require applications to be made via the patient's medical or social carers.

Various charitable, religious, and philanthropic agencies such as The Lions Club may also be able to help.

Some of the cancer information services provide valuable information about mortgages, personal insurance, and holiday insurance. The Association of British Insurers can also provide cancer patients with advice and guidance on insurance matters.

Specialized oncology units

The organization and provision of psychosocial support services has been greatly facilitated by the recent development of specialized oncology units which concentrate medical and paramedical expertise. Many of these units have their own counsellors, social workers, and psychiatrists or psychologists who are skilled in the use of the psychotherapeutic and social interventions outlined earlier in this chapter. They are also familiar with the wide range of services in the community such as the cancer information and counselling services, to which they can direct patients.

Specialized oncology units constitute minisupport systems in their own right because patients quickly build up relationships with the other patients as well as with members of staff. Thus, they help to alleviate the alienation experienced by so many cancer patients on general wards. They also function as the nucleus for supportive activities, often run by the patients themselves (for example support groups, relaxation groups, fund-raising concerns, etc.).

Specialized oncology units generally have strong links with local community medical and nursing services, community support teams, and local hospices, thus ensuring continuity of care from shortly after diagnosis through to the final stages of the illness.

Conclusion

Malignant disease is the second commonest cause of death in adults in the developed countries. Modern technology has produced significant advances in the treatment of some types of cancer, but has done little so far to alter the prognosis of the commonly occurring ones. It is vitally important that cancer research continues. Society demands a cure for cancer and it is hoped that current advances in our understanding of this disease will result in a steady improvement in outcome. It is equally important that we deal with the needs of those patients today who may not be fortunate enough to benefit from curative technologies. It is essential that the resources are made available to provide adequately for them. Supplying accurate, consistent information, tailored to the patient's needs, and providing emotional support in the form of psychotherapy and counselling, support groups, and social services has beneficial psychological effects and helps patients and their families to cope with what is undoubtedly a most traumatic experience.

Useful addresses—United Kingdom

Association of British Insurers
51 Gresham Street, London EC2V 7HQ

020–7600 3333
http://www.abi.org.uk/

Breast Cancer Care
Kiln House, 210 New King's Road, London SW6 4 NZ
13a Castle Terrace, Edinburgh, EH1 2DP
Suite 2/8, 65 Bath Street, Glasgow, G2 2BX

020–7384 2984
0131–221 0407
0141–353 1050
Free national helpline 0500 245 345

British Association for Counselling
1 Regent Place, Rugby, Warwickshire, CV21 2PJ

0788 550899

British Colostomy Association
15 Station Road, Reading, Berkshire RG1 1LG

01734 391537

CancerBACUP
3 Bath Place, Rivington Street, London EC2A 3JR
30 Bell Street, Glasgow G1 1LG
CancerBACUP Information Service

020–7696 9003
0141–553 1553
020–7613 2121
Freephone 0800 181199
http://www.cancerbacup.org.uk

CancerLink
11–21 Northdown Street, London N1 9BN
9 Castle Terrace, Edinburgh, EH1 2DP

020–7833 2818
0131–228 5557

Hodgkin's Disease and Lymphoma Association
PO Box 275, Haddenham, Aylesbury, Bucks HP17 8JJ

01844 291500

Leukaemia Research Fund
43 Great Ormond Street, London WC1N 3JJ
37 Whittinghame Drive, Glasgow G12 0YH

020–7405 0101
0141 339 1101
http://www.leukaemia.demon.co.uk/

Macmillan Cancer Relief
Anchor House, 15–19 Britten Street, London SW3 3TZ
National information line

020–7351 7811
0845 601 6161
http://www.macmillan.org.uk/

Marie Curie Cancer Care
28 Belgrave Square, London SW1X 8QG

020–7235 3325
http://www.mariecurie.org.uk/

National Association of Laryngectomee Clubs
Ground floor, 6 Rickett Street, Fulham, London SW6 1RU

020–7381 9993
http://members.aol.com/nalcuk/index.htm

Sargent Cancer Care for Children
14 Abingdon Road, London W8 6AF

020–7565 5100
http://www.ncl.ac.uk/~nchwww/sargent/

Tak Tent Cancer Support–Scotland
Block C20, Western Court, 100 University Place, Glasgow G12 6 SQ

0141 211 1930/1/2

Tenovus Cancer Information Centre
College Buildings, Courtenay Road, Splott, Cardiff CF1 1SA

029 2049 7700
Freephone helpline 0800 526527

Ulster Cancer Foundation
40–42 Eglantine Avenue, Belfast BT9 6 DX

Helpline 028 9066 3439
Admin 028 9066 3281

Useful addresses—International

AMERICA	American Cancer Society 1599 Clifton Road NE Atlanta Georgia 30329–4251 1–800-ACS-2345	http://www.cancer.org
	National Cancer Institute 31 Center Drive MSC 2580 Bethesda, MD 20892 2580 1–800–4CANCER	http://wwwicic.nci.nih.gov
AUSTRALIA	Anti-Cancer Council of Victoria Cancer Information and Support Service I Rathdown Street Carlton South 3053 Victoria	Helpline 61 3 92792 1129 http://www.accv.org.au/
CANADA	Canadian Cancer Society Cancer Information Service Suite 200 10 Alcorn Avenue Toronto Ontario M4V 3B1	Freeline 1 888 939 3333 http://www.cancer.ca
DENMARK	Kraeftens Bekaempelse The Danish Cancer Society Strandboulevarden 49 DK-2100 Copenhagen 0	Helpline 45 80 30 10 30 http://www.cancer.dk
FRANCE	Ecoute Cancer La Ligue Nationale Contre le Cancer 13 Avenue de la Grande Armee 75116 Paris	Helpline 33 1 45 00 15 15
GERMANY	Krebsinformationsdienst: KID Deutsches Krebsforschungszentrum Im Neuenheimer Feld 280 69120 Heidelberg 1	Helpline 49 6221 41 01 21 http://www.krebsinformation.de
IRELAND	CancerHelp Line Irish Cancer Society 5 Northumberland Road Dublin 4	Helpline 353 1 668 18 55 Freeline 353 1 800 200 700
ITALY	Instituto Europeo di Oncologia Via Ripamonti 435 20141 Milan	Helpline 39 2 57 48 93 10 http://www.ieo.it
INDIA	Cancer Information Service Sitaram Bhartia Institute of Science Research B-16, Mehrauli Institutional Area New Delhi 110 016	Helpline 011 686 7435
ISRAEL	Cancer Information Service Israel Cancer Association Beit Mati PO Box 437 Givatayim 53104	Helpline 972 3 572 16 16 http://www.cancer.org.il

THE NETHERLANDS Nederlandse Kankerbestrijding Helpline 31 0800 022 66 22
Koningin Wilhemina http://www.kankerbestrijding.nl
Fonds International:
Dutch Cancer Society
8 Sophialaan
1075 BR Amsterdam

SWEDEN Cancer Information Service Helpline 46 8 729 43 16
Oncologic Centre
Radiumhemmet
Karolinska Hospital
S-171 76 Stockholm

References

1. Maguire P. Psychological and social consequences of cancer. *Recent Advances in Clinical Oncology*, 1982; **1**: 376.

2. Fallowfield L. Editorial: Psychosocial interventions in cancer. *British Medical Journal*, 1995; **311**: 1316–17.

3. Bloom JR. Social support systems and cancer: a conceptual view. In: Cohen J, Cullen JW, Martin LR, eds. *Psychosocial aspects of cancer*. New York: Raven Press, 1982: 129–49.

4. Wortman CB. Social support and the cancer patient. *Cancer*, 1984; **53** (Suppl.):2339–60.

5. Rainey LC. Cancer counseling by telephone helpline: the UCLA psychosocial cancer counselling line. *Public Health Reports*, 1985; **100**: 308–15.

6. Liang LP, Dunn SM, Gorman A, Stuart-Harris R. Identifying priorities of psychosocial need in cancer patients. *British Journal of Cancer*, 1990; **62**: 1000–3.

7. Slevin ML, Nichols SE, Downer SM, *et al.* Emotional support for cancer patients: what do patients really want? *British Journal of Cancer*, 1996; **74**: 1275–9.

8. Morton J. Personal view. *British Medical Journal*, 1987; **295**: 1482.

9. Slevin ML. Talking about cancer: how much is too much? *British Journal of Hospital Medicine*, 1987; **38**: 56, 58–9.

10. Hughes KK. Decision-making by patients with breast cancer: the role of information in treatment selection. *Oncology Nursing Forum*, 1993; **20**: 623–8.

11. McHugh P, Lewis S, Ford S, Newlands E, Rustin G, Coombes C, Smith D, O'Reilly S, Fallowfield L. The efficacy of audiotapes in promoting psychological well-being in cancer patients: a randomised, controlled trial. *British Journal of Cancer*, 1995; **71**: 388–92.

12. Meredith C, Symonds P, Webster L, *et al.* Informational needs of cancer patients in West Scotland: cross sectional survey of patients' views. *British Medical Journal*, 1996; **313**: 724–6.

13. Slevin ML, *et al.* BACUP-the first two years: evaluation of a national cancer information service. *British Medical Journal*, 1988; **297**: 669–72.

14. Fallowfield L, Ford S, Lewis S. No news is not good news: Information preferences of patients with cancer. *Psycho-Oncology*, 1995; **4**: 197–202.

15. Dunkel-Schetter C. Social support and cancer: findings based on patient interviews and their implications. *Journal of Social Issues*, 1984; **40**: 77–98.

16. Buckman R. Breaking bad news: why is it still so difficult? *British Medical Journal*, 1984; **288**: 1597–9.

17. Maguire P, Faulkner A. How to do it: communicate with cancer patients: 1. Handling bad news and difficult questions. *British Medical Journal*, 1988; **297**: 907–9.

18. Maguire P, Faulkner A. How to do it: communicate with cancer patients: 2. Handling uncertainty, collusion and denial. *British Medical Journal*, 1988; **297**: 972–4.

19. Maguire P, Booth K, Elliott C, Jones B. Helping health professionals involved in cancer care acquire key interviewing skills—the impact of workshops. *European Journal of Cancer*, 1996; **32A**: 1486–9.

20. Gordon WA, Freidenbergs I, Diller L, *et al.* Efficacy of psychosocial intervention with cancer patients. *Journal of Consulting and Clinical Psychology*, 1980; **48**: 743–59.

21. Fawzy NW. A psychoeducational nursing intervention to enhance coping and affective state in newly diagnosed malignant melanoma patients. *Cancer Nursing*, 1996; **18**: 427–38.

22. Fawzy FI, Fawzy NW, Canada AL. Psychoeducational intervention programs for patients with cancer. In: Perry M, ed. American Society of Clinical Oncology Educational Book. Alexandria, Virginia: American Society of Clinical Oncology, 1998: 396–411.

23. Maguire P, Tait A, Brooke M, Thomas C, Sellwood R. Effects of counselling on the psychiatric morbidity associated with mastectomy. *British Medical Journal*, 1980; **281**: 1454–6.

24. Worden JW, Weisman AD. Do cancer patients really want counselling? *General Hospital Psychiatry*, 1980; **2**: 100–3.

25. Ramirez AJ. Liaison psychiatry in a breast cancer unit. *Journal of the Royal Society of Medicine*, 1989; **82**: 15–17.

26. Goldberg D. Cognitive therapy for depression. *British Medical Journal*, 1982; **284**: 143–4.

27. Moorey S, Greer S. *Psychological therapy for patients with cancer: a new approach.* London: Heinemann, 1989.

28. Greer S, Moorey S, Baruch JD, *et al.* Adjuvant psychological therapy for patients with cancer: a prospective randomised trial. *British Medical Journal*, 1992; **304**: 675–80.

29. Moorey S, Greer S, Bliss J, Law M. A comparison of adjuvant psychological therapy and supportive counselling in patients with cancer. *Psycho-Oncology*, 1998; **7**: 218–28.

30. Plant H, *et al.* Evaluation of a support group for cancer patients and their families and friends. *British Journal of Hospital Medicine*, 1987; **38**: 317–22.

31. Fawzy FI, Fawzy NW, Arndt LA, Pasnau RO. Critical review of psychosocial interventions in cancer care. *Archives of General Psychiatry*, 1995; **52**: 100–13.

32. Yalom ID, Greaves C. Group therapy with the terminally ill. *American Journal of Psychiatry*, 1977; **134**: 396–400.

33. Spiegel D, Bloom JR, Yalom I. Group support for patients with metastatic cancer. A randomized outcome study. *Archives of General Psychiatry*, 1981; **38**: 527–33.

34. Bottomly A, Hunton S, Roberts G, *et al.* A pilot study of cognitive behavioural therapy and social support group interventions for newly diagnosed cancer patients. *Journal of Psychosocial Oncology*, 1996; **14**: 65–83.

35. Meyer TJ, Mark MM. Effects of psychosocial interventions with adult cancer patients: a meta-analysis of randomized experiments. *Health Psychology*, 1995; **14**: 101–8.

36. Fletcher C. Listening and talking to patients. *British Medical. Journal*, 1980; **281**: 994–6.

37. **Venn MJ, et al.** The experience and impact of contacting a cancer information service. *European Journal of Cancer Care*, 1996; 5: 38–42.

38. **Lechner L, De Vries H.** The Dutch cancer information helpline: experience and impact. *Patient Education and Counseling*, 1996; 28; 149–57.

39. **Butow P, et al.** Information booklets about cancer: factors influencing patient satisfaction and utilization. *Patient Education and Counseling*, 1998; 33: 129–41.

40. **Clement-Jones V.** Cancer and beyond: the formation of BACUP. *British Medical Journal*, 1985; 291: 1021–3.

Complementary medicine: challenges, lessons, and patients' expectations

Robert Buckman

Introduction

Complementary or alternative remedies have stimulated a dramatic increase in both public interest and patients' demands over the last two decades.[1],[2] There are many reasons for this increase, some due to the philosophical attractions of complementary medicine, and others due to the claims or promises of benefit: both of these will be addressed in this chapter.

The issue of complementary medicine is particularly important in oncology, because the cancer patient is in a more vulnerable position than most other patients. The word 'cancer' triggers a deep-seated fear in most people, and cancer patients and their families often feel a sense of hopelessness and desperation about their situation (sometimes inappropriately). As a result of the desperation, they may be prey to false hopes or promises of any kind, and may be particularly tempted if a complementary remedy offers apparent cure or remission without side-effects. Claims of this nature have been made frequently by complementary practitioners, and even though regulations in many countries are controlling such false claims, news stories about such remedies are widely reported in the press and on television. Hence, complementary medicine is a topic that every oncologist is going to be asked about frequently.

The claims of complementary medicine put the oncologist (and any other health-care professional involved) in a difficult position. The health-care professional has a continuing, clinical relationship with the patient, and so has to maintain a practical and supportive approach to these issues while still being truthful and honest in dealing with facts and data, or lack of them.

It may seem at first that these two objectives—of maintaining a supportive relationship with the patient, while still respecting facts and truth—are mutually exclusive and must lead to confrontation.[3] Fortunately, this is not inevitable and there is an approach that can achieve both goals: this strategy will be presented at the end of this chapter.

Definitions and terminology

There is considerable controversy as to what to call 'non-conventional medicine'. This is made even more difficult since there are few common features shared by every type of non-conventional remedies —other than the fact that they are not conventional medicine. For the purposes of this chapter, the term 'complementary medicine' will be used simply as a global phrase to include all complementary, alternative, unproven, unconventional, or folk remedies.

As regards the distinction between conventional medicine and complementary medicine, we may define that in practical terms. Pragmatically, we can define conventional physicians as 'doctors who have been trained in medical schools licensed by the governments of their countries, and who practice medicine in a manner approved by the regulatory boards supervising medical practice'. We may then define conventional treatments as 'treatments given by those conventional doctors or physicians (and their associated health-care professionals including nurses, physiotherapists, psychotherapists, and so on) which would be regarded as acceptable by the majority of their peers'.

Complementary medicine may then be defined as 'all actions or interventions which are not conventional medicine and which are carried out to try and help or heal a patient'.

These definitions carry a significant implication: namely that not every intervention performed by a conventional health-care professional is *de facto* conventional medicine. If a conventionally qualified physician decides to prescribe a naturopathic remedy, for example, instead of an antibiotic for a patient with bacterial lobar pneumonia, this would not mean that the naturopathic remedy is by definition a conventional treatment for pneumonia. In fact, in some countries a physician who did that would be censured and might lose his or her license to practise.

At any point in time, what comprises conventional medicine is a consensus opinion. It is what most conventional practitioners would do in those circumstances (as regulated by the authorities or bodies set up to regulate medical practice). This, therefore, is how current practice is defined, and it is altered by new data incorporating new treatments and research findings, and discarding disproven ones. The boundaries of conventional medicine are not, and have never been, rigid. As shall be discussed, the hallmark or touchstone of current, conventional medicine is the use of testing—and attempting to disprove—a theory or a new treatment.

Objective assessment of effectiveness

It is important to recognize that there are objective differences in approach between most areas of contemporary conventional medicine and the practice of complementary medicine. That conventional medicine, and particularly oncology, is an evolving and changing practice does not mean that it is based solely on current fashion, whim, or arbitrary choice. Nor does it mean that the only difference between conventional medicine and complementary medicine is merely a personal choice of what to believe. Many (although not all) treatments in conventional medicine are based on scientific practice, an objective basis congruent with what is termed the hypothetico-deductive model of science.

The central principle of all scientific endeavours, as delineated in Karl Popper's hypotheticodeductive model is the attempt to disprove the proposed hypothesis.[4] (A brief and digestible description is Kuhn's excellent overview).[5] Deductions are derived from the original hypothesis (by closely defined rules or criteria) and then tested in experiments. If the experiments fail to disprove the deductions, then the original hypothesis continues to be valid.

Hence in all areas of investigation, it is the act of attempting to disprove a theory that makes the outcome scientific. In medicine, there are several ways of testing a hypothesis in a 'disprovable' way. The randomized, clinical trial is one such example. Selective collection of anecdotal data, without prospectively defined criteria, is not.

It is often stated by many complementary medicine practitioners that their particular remedy or treatment approach simply cannot be tested in a clinical trial. This is not true. Any remedy or intervention, conventional or complementary, can be tested in any disease or symptom in an appropriately designed clinical trial (see Chapter 7.1). The appropriate design and performance of a trial—including the definition of entry criteria, the measurements or assessments to be performed, and defining the outcome criteria and so on—is simply a matter of thought and work. (One study cited below, a randomized trial of a traditional Chinese medicine mixture compared to a specifically manufactured placebo in the treatment of childhood eczema, is an excellent example of trial design and execution).

The attractions of complementary medicine

Complementary medicine continues to attract large numbers of people and there is no sign that the rise in consultations and use of these remedies is decelerating. In several surveys of the general public, it has been estimated that one-quarter to one-third of the general public have consulted with a complementary practitioner or have used a complementary remedy within the previous year.[1] In oncology clinics, the figure may be higher.[6]

The reasons for this are complex and multifactorial. A recent survey showed that many of the reasons concern lifestyle choices of the patients and philosophical attractions as well as perceived benefits of the treatment. Dissatisfaction with the care given by conventional physicians does not seem to be as prominent a factor as was thought previously.[7],[8]

Perhaps the central element underlying the lifestyle and philosophical attractions of complementary medicine is the perception of control. Contemporary social norms strongly suggest to the public that they deserve, and should strive for, control over all aspects of their lives. While this personal control may be achievable in many areas of career, home life, recreation, information gathering, and so on, it often does not apply to illness. One of the most unpleasant aspects of illness, particularly a cancer, is that it is beyond the control of the patient. This is often perceived by the patient as an intellectual rebuff or insult. Furthermore the diagnosis and treatment are also perceived as being beyond the control of the individual (who cannot decide for himself or herself precisely what should be done, but can only consent or refuse the suggestions made by the clinical team).

This is not the case with complementary medicines. The single feature that unites many aspects of the attractions of complementary medicine is that the patient has a genuine feeling of control. He or she makes the decision to go to this particular clinic, or to try this remedy, or to go on to this diet.

Granted that a feeling of control underlies many of the attractions, they may be grouped under 11 main headings (Table 1). Patients differ in their affinities to the different features of complementary remedies—some like the idea that the remedy has been used since ancient times and get comfort from a perception of ancient mystical wisdom. Others like the idea of a solo genius who has discovered the cure for cancer when the billion-dollar ranks of conventional cancer research could not—the David-and-Goliath perception. (Current examples include the treatments promoted by Di Bella in Italy, Gaston Naessens in Canada, Burzynski in the United States, Alivizatos in Greece, and many others. An excellent historical review of some typical practitioners is available).[9] Other attractions include the perception that a treatment is natural (ignoring the fact that most cancers are quite natural too) and may in some way enhance the body's own natural healing forces which have been paralysed by some aspect of the illness or by conventional treatment.

A more detailed analysis of these factors has been made previously.[10] However, one major factor is that most patients believe that the remedy they are using (or are about to use) works and is effective against cancer. Since this element is so important in most patients' decisions, the next sections will deal with the factual data concerning complementary remedies in cancer, and an analysis of why the public have come to perceive these remedies as effective.

Are any complementary remedies effective in the treatment of cancer?

To date, no complementary medicines have been shown to be effective in the treatment of cancer in randomized or even case–control studies. Most of them have not been tested in a systematic fashion, and in many cases there has not even been an attempt at collection of data.[11] However, the ones that have been tested systematically in the treatment of cancer have not been shown to have any effect on the disease or on the survival of patients.

It should be noted, since many patients are aware of this, that in diseases other than cancer, a few non-conventional treatments have been methodically tested and have been found to have some effect. (They are: (a) a specific traditional Chinese medicine found to be effective in childhood eczema;[12] (b) chiropractic manipulation for low back pain;[13],[14] (although some studies have been negative); (c) acupuncture as an analgaesic;[15] and (d) St John's wort as an antidepressant.[16]) It could be legitimately said that any therapy such as these which has been tested in a reliable and reproducible fashion and has been found to be effective is, from that point on, scientifically valid treatment, whether its origins were once regarded as complementary medicine or not.

However, in the treatment of patients with any of the cancers, no complementary medicine so far has been shown to be effective despite initial publicity and many (often hundreds) of anecdotal claims. Table 2 shows the studies that have not shown any effect for the

Table 1 Some of the attractions of complementary medicine

Aspect of remedy	Rationale
Control	Complementary remedies are (usually) under the control of the patient, instead of the health-care professional; this underlies many of the other factors
Concept of health	Remedy or treatment not only conquers disease but establishes positive health
Concept of force or energy	Basis is often a universal hypothesis of natural forces
Unifying hypothesis of disease	All diseases are caused by an imbalance or negative force(s)
Self-healing	Forces are accessible within the patient which can reverse course of disease
Natural	Inherent advantage of the remedy is derived from natural products over synthetic
Traditional	Based on centuries of folk wisdom: knowledge that ancestors had which was lost
Exotic	Imported from different culture—previously unavailable to people of this culture
David and Goliath	Answer to major question (e.g. cancer) has been found by 'little man' where the powers of national or industrial bodies have failed
Justice	Cure is available to those whose attitudes and beliefs show them to be worthy of it
Success stories	Every complementary practitioner has many anecdotes (sometimes thousands) of patients who were told the prognosis was grim but who then experienced apparently miraculous or unexpected remissions or cures

following medicines (in treatment of established disease or prevention): laetrile,[17] hydrazine,[18],[19] vitamin C,[20] beta-carotene supplements,[21]–[23] the Di Bella multitherapy,[24] and shark cartilage.[25]

Other studies have not shown any effect in prolonging survival at the following complementary medicine centres: the Livingston–Wheeler Clinic (California),[26] the E-Caps approach of Dr Bernie Siegel (Connecticut, United States),[27],[28] and the Bristol Cancer Help Centre (United Kingdom).[29] These latter studies, together with the results of Dr David Spiegel's studies in Stanford, California, will be discussed below.

So why do so many people believe that complementary medicines work? Part of the answer lies in the philosophical attractions listed above, but much of the enthusiasm is fuelled by stories and anecdotes of apparent remissions, responses, or cures.[6],[8] Since they are such an important component in the decision-making it is worth detailing how some of these stories have conventional and straightforward explanations.

Conventional explanations of apparently miraculous responses

Over a period of 2 years, the author investigated many examples of miraculous or unexpected responses to complementary medicine. Most of these case histories were submitted in response to advertisements (in Britain and in Canada) for examples of significant encounters with complementary medicine.[10] In all cases, there was a conventional (often straightforward or even simple) explanation for the apparently miraculous outcome. They can be classified under eight main headings (summarized in Table 3), and a typical history is included within each category as an example.

No tissue diagnosis

In many cases there had not been a tissue diagnosis. This apparently simple part of a case story was frequently missing—but its absence

was often obscured by a large amount of compelling personal detail, sometimes repeated over a long period of time. The following is an example:

A woman in her mid-50s telephoned a television company's researcher (in response to an advertisement) to say that she had been cured of bowel cancer by herbal treatments. She stated that her treatment had been recommended to her by an iridologist 7 years earlier, after she had previously been seen at a local hospital by a (conventional) gastroenterologist who had done a biopsy and told her that she had bowel cancer and required surgery. The iridologist had confirmed this diagnosis instantly from appearance of the patient's iris, and started her on herbal therapy. Seven years later she was disease free and completely well.

Contact with that hospital's pathology department and a detailed and protracted search did not locate any biopsy specimen taken at the time stated by the patient. When the author discussed this with the patient (not having spoken to her previously) she demurred, saying that she had not had a biopsy 'as such' but that the gastroenterologist had told her that he 'did not like the look of her colon'.

Perhaps this woman was not deliberately misleading the researcher, but she certainly indulged in wishful thinking. Appreciating the attention and support of her iridologist she was probably trying to amplify the benefit of what she thought the iridologist had achieved. Yet the television researcher and two other senior members of the television company's staff who heard the first version of this patient's story were convinced that it represented unarguable proof that cancer could be cured by herbal remedies.

Premature statements

Anecdotes may also be misleading, particularly to non-medical audiences, because of statements that are made prematurely. Patients frequently state that they have been cured, or that an unexpected or

Table 2 Complementary remedies or approaches that have been tested in the treatment of cancer patients

Treatment or approach		N	Trial design	Survival difference and P value	Reference
Laetrile		178	Phase II: response analysis and cohort survival	Median survival 4.8 months; 1-year survival = 0% (1 partial response)	17
Hydrazine sulphate:	1.	127	RCT (hydrazine vs placebo)	4.3 months hydrazine 4.7 months placebo No regressions. NSD	1. 18
	2.	243	RCT (Cisplatin, etoposide placebo, vs Cisplatin, etoposide, hydrazine)	5.8 months hydrazine 8.0 months placebo NSD	2. 19
Vitamin C		130	RCT (vitamin C vs placebo)	Vit. C 2 months Placebo 2 months NSD	20
Beta carotene	1. 2.	22 701 physicians 18 314 smokers	1. RCT beta-carotene, placebo 2. RCT beta-carotene, placebo	1. NSD 2. NSD in incidence of lung cancer, cardiovascular disease	1. 21 2. 22
Shark cartilage		60	Phase II single-arm: response analysis	Median time to progression 28 weeks No complete or partial remissions	25
Di Bella cocktail		386	Phase II Single-arm: response analysis (4 individual trials)	At 6-month follow-up: N = 3 partial remissions 12% had stable disease 52% progressive disease 25% deaths	24
Livingston–Wheeler		78 case–control pairs	Case–control study: Livingston-Wheeler clinic vs University of Pennsylvania Cancer Center	Median survival 15 months both groups NSD	26
E-Caps (Dr Bernie Siegel)	1.	?N = 40			1. 27
	2.	34 cases 102 controls	Case–control study: 24 E-Caps, 102 patients in same area of Connecticut	NSD in survival	2. 28
Bristol Cancer Help Centre		334 cases, 461 controls	Case–control study: 334 patients with breast cancer at Bristol, 461 controls at 3 conventional cancer centres	Relapse-free survival (126 matched pairs) Bristol 21; control 6 (P = 0.0004) Overall survival with metastases at entry (92 matched pairs) Bristol 55; control 73; NSD Overall survival (initially disease free) 9126 matched pairs) Bristol 8; control 2; (P=0.01)	29
Dr David Spiegel		86	RCT; patients with metastatic breast cancer: 1-year psychotherapeutic group intervention vs control	Median survival (study entry to death) Psychotherapy: 36.6 months Control 18.9 months (P= <0.00001)	47

RCT = randomized, controlled trial; NSD = no significant difference

miraculous remission has occurred, while the data may be well within the natural history of that particular tumour. Although this type of statement may not cause intrinsic harm to the patient himself or herself, and may even be of benefit in terms of coping strategies and attitudes, the story may mislead other people into believing that treatment has a genuine effect when it does not. Perhaps the most widely known is the story of the much-loved film star Steve McQueen.[30]

Table 3 Alternative explanations of unexpected or miraculous responses to complementary medicine

Possible explanation	Examples (see text)
No facts	Patient stated that biopsy was done when it was not
Premature statements	Patient reports cure after complementary medicine or immediately following conventional adjuvant therapy for breast cancer, or early in low-grade lymphoma
Wrong diagnosis error in conventional medicine error in complementary medicine	No evidence of cancer, or of recurrence; e.g. 'there are no cancer cells in the ascites'
Natural history of condition	Biological variability not widely understood
Concurrent conventional therapy	Patient taking, e.g. tamoxifen, without realizing this is conventional cancer therapy
Misinterpretation of information	(a) Prognosis was not stated as '3 months'. (b) CT scan showed pleural nodules
Spontaneous remission	Rare but well documented in most malignancies
Feeling better versus getting better	Almost every patient taking complementary medicines feels better

Steve McQueen had an abdominal mesothelioma, which did not respond to any conventional therapy. He went to a complementary clinic in Mexico and was given several different treatments including herbal remedies, colonic irrigation, diet supplements, and meditation. McQueen was so impressed by the experience that he broadcast his gratitude on Mexican public radio to the President and the people of Mexico for allowing the clinic to exist and allowing him to be cured of his disease. On the recording, he was clearly very ill, and in fact died a few weeks later after an ill-advised laparotomy and 'debulking' at the clinic.

Stories such as this (premature statements) are common. In a Mexican complementary medicine clinic, several women were interviewed who had had recent surgery for breast cancer followed by adjuvant chemotherapy. They stated that that the breast cancer had been cured by the laetrile and other complementary medicines given after the conventional treatment. Although their statements would be compelling to a lay audience, they are premature from a medical viewpoint.

Wrong diagnosis

Errors in diagnosis are not common, but the impact of even a few anecdotes is important, because such stories become widely disseminated.

Error in conventional assessment

In some cases, the diagnosis by conventional practitioners is wrong. For example four patients were identified among the long-term survivors in a palliative care unit. All of them had been admitted with a diagnosis of terminal illness, but review of the histopathology showed that the initial diagnosis was erroneous.[31] This is probably uncommon, but it does occur from time to time, particularly with those malignancies in which distinguishing a true cancer from a similar non-malignant condition, or a less aggressive malignancy, may be difficult. For example small-cell lung cancer may be difficult to distinguish from a condition with a far better prognosis, small-cell neuroendocrine carcinoma.[32]

Occasionally, a set of unusual circumstances contribute to a misdiagnosis in the course of follow-up, even after the initial diagnosis was correct.

A woman in her late 50s had breast cancer 14 years previously. Five years after diagnosis she developed lymphadenopathy in the left supraclavicular fossa: biopsy showed recurrent breast cancer. (This biopsy has since been reviewed several times and is undoubtedly recurrent adenocarcinoma of breast in a lymph node.) At that time, the standard treatment for metastatic breast cancer was oophorectomy, which was then performed. Shortly after the oophorectomy, however, she developed another mass in the neck (this time in the left posterior triangle). This was monitored for several years and did not change in size. It was believed by the medical team that was further recurrence of the breast cancer that, for some unknown reason, remained stable. When she moved house, she changed to another oncology centre where a new baseline assessment was done. This showed that the mass in the left neck was not lymphadenopathy but a cervical rib.

Had this patient been taking any complementary medicine remedies, her case might have been widely publicized as a case of metastatic breast cancer, held in check for many years by that remedy. As it was, she had probably been cured of metastatic breast cancer, although such cases are very rare, (by the excision of the supra-clavicular recurrence and/or oophorectomy) and had a non-malignant cause of her second cervical mass.

Error in complementary assessment

Complementary practitioners may sometimes assess a clinical condition in a way that is over-optimistic, fanciful, or simply wrong. Often patients are not under simultaneous follow-up with a conventional practitioner, so there is rarely a chance to review or investigate the complementary practitioner's claims. However, there are many documented cases in which, for example, a chest-wall recurrence enlarged while the patient was receiving a complementary remedy and was being told by the complementary practitioner that the lesion was shrinking, a bone scan which showed progressive disease was reported as showing improvement, increasing size of an axillary node mass and increasing arm girth were reported by a complementary practitioner as improvement and so on.[33]

A woman with ovarian carcinoma went to Athens for a complementary remedy after completing conventional chemotherapy. After the complementary treatment, she was told by the Athens doctor that she was now cured. A few months later, however, (having now returned to Toronto) she developed ascites. By coincidence her complementary practitioner happened to be visiting Toronto at the time: he told her and her husband that the ascites was not a sign of recurrence and that, if tested, there would be no malignant cells in the fluid. A diagnostic paracentesis was done (by the author) the following day and malignant cells were clearly present. The patient died a few weeks later of the disease and was extremely disappointed in having been deceived by her complementary medicine practitioner.

There are often additional social or psychological reasons why a patient may feel better, and this may assist a complementary practitioner to make an erroneous and over-optimistic assessment.

At a recent faith-healing demonstration in Britain (filmed as part of an investigative documentary into claims of faith healing), a faith healer brought a 9-year-old girl onto the stage who, it later turned out, had widespread metastatic neuroblastoma. She was on high-doses of morphine and could walk only with difficulty. In the presence of an audience of 10 000 people, the healer encouraged her to get out of her wheelchair, which she did. She walked across the stage and the healer announced that the next time she saw her doctor, she would be told she had 'no cancer in the bones'. This was not the case, and the patient died a few weeks later.

According to medical staff at the hospital where she was an inpatient, the patient had usually been able to take a few steps out of the wheelchair, although of course the audience at the healing demonstration did not know this. Despite the claims made by this healer, the patient's ability to walk a few steps was not a miracle nor even outside her usual range of mobility. Because of the healer's clams, most people in the audience might well have believed, and probably still believe, that they had been present at a miraculous cure.

Variation in the natural history of the condition

Another possible and straightforward explanation of unexpected outcomes is the variability in the natural history of many tumours. The average survival from any disease is precisely that—an average. All bell curves have a tail, and in some tumours the variability is considerable. There have always been occasional patients, for example, with biopsy-proven hepatic metastases from melanoma who survive for several years despite steadily increasing hepatomegaly. Although such patients are rare, their stories are striking and memorable, and a complementary practitioner may need only one or two such cases to develop a considerable reputation as a healer. Variability of natural history is not a concept easily understood by the general public, and a patient who is doing well will be regarded as a compelling witness to the efficacy of whatever remedy he or she is taking.

Concurrent conventional therapy

Another, and probably quite common, explanation for an apparently unexpected or miraculous remission is that the patient was receiving conventional treatment at the same time as the complementary medicine remedy. This can happen even without the patient consciously realizing it.

The cofounder of a complementary cancer help centre in Britain developed breast cancer and wrote a book detailing the various complementary medicine remedies that she had used. A few years after initial surgery she developed chest wall recurrence. The recurrence was oestrogen-receptor-positive and tamoxifen was recommended. In her book she detailed the various herbs and other treatments that she used and said that her conventional doctor was later very surprised to find the chest wall recurrence was regressing. She wrote that her conventional doctor was at a loss to explain what was causing the remission or stabilization, but encouraged the patient to continue doing whatever it was she was doing. It turned out that she had in fact been taking tamoxifen for several years during this whole period.[34]

This patient did not apparently realize that tamoxifen was an anticancer drug, nor that it causes regression of disease in approximately 60 per cent of cases of oestrogen-receptor-positive recurrence. Although her book gave the contrary impression, the course of her disease was exactly as one would have expected in those circumstances.

A man with Kaposi's sarcoma recently wrote a magazine article about his treatment.[35] He had multiple Kaposi's sarcoma lesions in both lungs and had been taking an extract of shark cartilage. The tumours progressed and his radiation oncologist gave radiotherapy to one lung. The tumours in the irradiated lung regressed, whereas those in the non-irradiated lung did not. The patient's interpretation was that the shark cartilage must have caused the regression (despite the fact the shark cartilage was taken by mouth and therefore reached the lesions in both lungs). He wrote that the radiotherapy clearly could not have been the cause of the improvement (despite the fact that only the irradiated lung showed improvement), because he thought that small doses of radiotherapy could not be of value. He did not know of the radiosensitivity of Kaposi's sarcoma.

In another case, a patient with a soft-tissue sarcoma was treated with radiotherapy. Two non-oncologist physicians reported that at the end of the radiotherapy course there was 'no immediate benefit'. The following day, the patient started taking a homoeopathic remedy. A few weeks later the physicians noted a regression of the sarcoma (a time course that is normal after radiotherapy) but attributed the regression to the homoeopathic remedy.

Many complementary medicine clinics (in Mexico, for example) routinely and openly use conventional treatment: their patients regularly receive chemotherapy and radiotherapy in addition to their complementary remedies. Hence any statements about the efficacy of complementary remedies (as opposed to a conventional treatments) need to be evaluated carefully, since so many patients receive (knowingly or unknowingly) conventional treatment at the same time.

Misinterpretation of information

There are several ways in which it is possible to misinterpret what a health-care professional says, and this may lead to an apparently unexpected outcome.

Selective recall

Discussion of the prognosis is an extremely emotionally charged conversation. As a result, what is recalled and recounted may not be necessarily what was said. Since many patients ask directly 'How long have I got?' many physicians feel an (appropriate) obligation to give an honest answer and not simply avoid the discussion. While accurate prediction is not possible, it is usually possible to give a range of likely possibilities. For example if the median survival is, say, 12 months, with 15 per cent of patients alive at 2 years and 5 per cent at 5 years, it would be fair to say to the patient something such as 'The prognosis is probably measured in a small number of years for most people, but a few people will do better than that'. The patient may then ask whether that means the prognosis could be less than a year or 2 years. Since a small percentage of patients in this situation will die of the disease in a short time, say less than 6 months, the physician might say 'Yes, this could happen but it is not very likely'. The patient might then ask 'Do you mean I might not be around in 3 months?' and the doctor may reply 'Well, that is not very likely, but it could happen'. The patient might then say to a friend or relative who asks 'That doctor gave me 3 months'.

If the patient then uses a complementary medicine remedy and is alive at 1 year (as half of all such patients would be anyway) the credit for that apparent extension of survival is given to the complementary remedy.

Most people do not realize that a statement such as 'only 5 per cent of patients are alive 5 years after diagnosis' means that 1 in 20 patients will survive longer than 5 years.

Misinterpretation

Sometimes, the patient may misinterpret or forget what the medical team actually said:

> A patient wrote to say that, 4 years previously, he had had a rhabdomyosarcoma of the left thigh. CT scan of his lungs, according to his letter, had shown metastases. His doctors had treated the primary on his thigh (with surgery and radiotherapy) but had given him no treatment for the secondaries. He then embarked on a major lifestyle change—and took up intensive prayer, meditation, psychotherapy, dietary change, and exercise. Four years later, he was completely well. In fact, the first CT scan had shown two small (3 mm) subpleural nodules that the radiologist and the oncologist had both interpreted as consistent with metastases but which could be non-malignant in origin. The radiation oncologist and the medical oncologist had each explained this to the patient, and had said they would repeat the scans every 3 months. In all the follow-up scans the lesions remained the same size. It turned out that the man had had exposure to asbestos when he was younger, a likely cause of the pleural lesions. In subsequent interviews the patient stated that he now did remember being told that the lesions had remained the same size and therefore were not secondaries.

It would have been easy to accept at face value (without reviewing the CT scans and interviewing the oncologists) this patient's first written version of events, and therefore to believe that there was evidence that metastatic sarcoma was controllable by lifestyle changes.

Spontaneous remissions

Spontaneous remission (or spontaneous regression) is defined as complete disappearance of all disease (and without new tumours developing) without any therapy. Boyd collected a large series[36] and further cases were documented by Everson and Cole.[37] From these series it is estimated that approximately one in every 100 000 cases of cancer will show spontaneous regression. In these publications more than half of the proven cases of spontaneous regression came from four cell types: renal cell carcinoma, melanoma, neuroblastoma, and choriocarcinoma. In the other half of the cases, there were one or two examples of almost every type of cancer.

These data show that almost any type of cancer can regress without apparent cause, and secondly, that spontaneous regression is much more common among four relatively rare types of cancer than it is among all the others.

Feeling better versus getting better

The above explanations may account for the unexpected outcome in many cases, but do not account for the widespread, almost universal, feelings of satisfaction and benefit that most patients experience when they use complementary remedies. That so many users feel well while taking complementary medicines is taken as further evidence of efficacy. Most people do not clearly distinguish between objective regression of disease ('getting better') and improvement in subjective symptoms ('feeling better'), and therefore believe that if a patient is feeling better he or she must be getting better. Feelings of improvement are, of course, an end-point or outcome in themselves ('feeling good is good in itself') yet are often regarded as synonymous with tumour regression.

These explanations of apparently unexpected remissions—and, in particular, the clear distinction between disease regression and the subjective feeling of improved well being—provide a practical and acceptable foundation on which conventional physicians may base their responses to complementary medicine. Some guidelines will follow in the final section of this chapter. However, it is also important to review in this chapter another area that is often regarded as part of complementary medicine—namely the mind and psychological factors, and whether or not they have any interactions with cancer and its behaviour.

Cancer and the mind

There are two distinct issues here: firstly, whether or not patients' attitudes, the psychological events in their lives, or their personality may contribute to causing a cancer (or protecting against it). Secondly, whether the mind can affect the outcome of cancer: in other words, if a person has cancer, whether or not a change in attitude or personality will, of itself, alter the progress of the disease.

Can the mind cause cancer?

There is a widespread idea that cancer is in some way the consequence of an unhealthy mental attitude or of major, psychologically stressful incidents in the person's life. Healers, doctors, writers, patients, and people from every different discipline and part of our society suggest, or even state as a proven fact, that by some means cancer is the outward expression of unresolved emotional processes, involving either mood or life events (or both). There are many variations on this theme but, in general, they all suggest that the person who later develops cancer has partly contributed to causing it (other than by smoking or other risk-enhancing activity) by bottling up emotions, by not expressing anger, by allowing external stresses to build up internally, or by some other psychological process.

Clearly, if this were proven to be true, then the world might be regarded by some people as a more understandable place, and possibly more fair and just. It would, in some people's view, be a symbol of justice or order if the people who held 'unhealthy' attitudes (unrelated to any high-risk physical actions) had a high risk of developing cancer, and if the people who had the 'correct' attitudes or beliefs could thereby reduce the chances of getting the disease.

By and large, support for that concept comes from individual stories or case histories, but some research on larger groups of people is available and does not support the role of psychological factors in carcinogenesis.

Individual stories and case histories

Almost every member of the public knows someone, or knows of someone, who developed a cancer shortly after a time of great stress. A man's wife dies and 3 months later he is found to have cancer of the bowel; a woman nurses her dying mother through the last year of her life, and a shortly afterwards finds a breast lump that turns out to be malignant; a lawyer is suddenly 'let go' after 15 years, and following depression, he is found to have lung cancer.

Stories such as these make intuitive sense to the general public. It seems logical that a catastrophic stress—a divorce, bereavement, dismissal—should be followed by a catastrophic illness such as cancer. Several factors contribute to the intuitive believability of individual stories, of which the most common is 'set thinking'.

The phrase 'set thinking' describes the pattern that we all have of putting things we see into groups, in other words filing our experiences in sets of data. Almost everybody falls into set thinking from time to time. (If you have just bought a blue sports car, for example, then every time you see another blue sports car, you notice it. It now has particular significance and it may seem to you that there is a sudden surge in popularity of blue sports cars. It is much more likely that the number of blue sports cars on the road has not altered, it is just that you are now noticing the ones that are there.)

This is true of individual case histories, and the apparent connection between life events and cancer. Everyone notices any link that makes intuitive sense—the divorce, bereavement, unemployment, and so on. However, the reverse cases remain unnoticed—nobody systematically or routinely recalls the number of people who have recently experienced divorce (or bereavement or dismissal) and who have not developed cancer, nor those people who have developed cancer who have not had a recent psychological stress. Hence the importance of epidemiological studies to establish whether or not there is any relationship between psychological factors and carcinogenesis.

In addition to set thinking, there are often other important factors missing from individual case histories (for example the person dismissed after 20 years of work might have been a heavy smoker for 30 years). For these reasons, then, epidemiological studies are required in order to demonstrate any link (or lack of it) between life events and carcinogenesis.

Epidemiological studies

Several epidemiological studies have examined the hypothesis that either the affect of the person or life events contribute to the cause of cancer. So far, these studies have not shown that there is a causal relationship. A few examples will be detailed here, but there are excellent reviews available:[38]

Depression

One major study evaluated communities in five cities and compared the incidence of cancer after a period of 10 years.[39] If depression was even a minor contributory cause to cancer, the study had a very high chance of showing that connection. In fact, there was no link, and the people with diagnosed clinical depression had the same chance of developing cancer as the general population.

Bereavement

In terms of psychological stress, it has long been known that bereavement is one of the most stressful. A study in Israel looked for an increase in cancer among parents who had lost a child. No increase in cancer was found.[40] A study among widows in Britain came to the same conclusion.[41]

Can the mind change the outcome?

The idea that the mind can change the outcome of cancer is as important, and as popular, as the idea that the mind can cause cancer in the first place. The hypothesis is also intellectually appealing—the attitude or personality of the person with cancer may alter the progress of the cancer. This is also congruent with the perception of the individual (by choosing how to think and feel) having some control over the disease. Because of the importance of this issue, some of the most important studies in this area will be discussed.

Attitudes and breast cancer (United Kingdom, 1979)

A prospective study, in 1979, showed some remarkable findings during follow-up of a small group of patients after primary surgery for breast cancer.[42] Using semistructured interviews, the investigators assessed the attitudes that the patients had to their illness before surgery and then correlated those attitudes to their survival after surgery (using those with a benign diagnosis at surgery as a control group). They found that patients who were extremely angry and those patients who went into denial had significantly longer survival than those who simply coped with the disease and carried on as best they could, or those who went into a helpless/hopeless state. This paper was widely publicized, and the methodology (of classifying patients' reaction in this particular way) has been used in several studies since. However, the results have never been repeated in another study. This is unusual since the original study was on a small group of patients and would not be difficult to repeat. Therefore, to date, this study remains a single interesting observation.

Bristol Cancer Help Centre

The Bristol Cancer Help Centre is Britain's best known complementary medicine centre for cancer patients. The treatment there includes a wide range of excellent psychological support services as well as spiritual techniques and (until recently) a stringent diet. In their early publications the centre had claimed that their treatments 'can and do prolong life'.[43] After several years, they collaborated with conventional physicians in a study of people with advanced breast cancer. Patients at the Bristol centre were matched with approximately twice the number of patients at conventional centres. To prevent potential bias as a result of patients who felt extremely ill being more likely to go to Bristol than less ill patients, the study censored from analysis any patients who had died within 3 months of arrival at the Bristol centre.

The data showed that the chance of dying was higher at the Bristol centre than in the conventional centres.[29] The publication of this paper caused immense political furore. Undoubtedly, some of the contractual agreements between the participants about how and when the results were to be published had not been honoured. Also, there was no attention paid in the publication to the quality of life of the patients. Furthermore, the patients in the study were only informed of the results of the study after publication. Eventually, after major political activity, the sponsoring charity apologized for these omissions.

Nevertheless, the data (after some minor adjustments) clearly showed that patients did not live longer when they attended the Bristol centre. The conclusions in this paper are strikingly similar to those of a similar study which compared the survival and quality of life of patients at a complementary medicine clinic in the United States with patients in a conventional centre.[26] Furthermore, the same conclusion is supported by the two Siegel studies discussed below.

Dr Bernie Siegel

Dr Bernie Siegel (he prefers the use of his first name) is a surgical oncologist who has written several popular books on the psychological aspects of serious illness, particularly cancer. He states that in his experience certain psychological characteristics and behaviour patterns seemed to be associated with a longer survival, and characterized such patients as 'exceptional cancer patients' or E-CaPs. He founded therapy groups and meetings of E-CaPs and of those who wanted to be E-CaPs, and has written several popular books on the subject. The books contain much good and sound advice about coping with illness, and organizing one's life. However, through the stories and examples in the book, he implies that psychological attitudes are a determinant of survival.

He was an investigator in a study that led to two publications[27],[28] neither of which showed that attending E-Cap groups had any effect on survival. (In fairness it has to be said that although those studies do not show any effect, his participation in this research is admirable and creditable. The fact that there was no demonstrable benefit in terms of survival does not diminish the support value that the groups have for the people who attend.)

However, at the time many patients accepted, and many still do, as a proven fact that positive attitudes will prolong survival. There are several myths and apocryphal stories which have been propagated uncritically and which send patients the message that the effect of attitude on survival is an established fact. It is worth quoting one of these, since it demonstrates how an apparently proven fact can be generated from a misunderstanding.

At one of Siegel's lectures (attended by the author) he talked appropriately and helpfully about caring and coping, giving clear, sensible, and useful guidelines and anecdotes. However, he mentioned only two pieces of medical data, the first being the Spiegel study from California (see below). Immediately following that, Bernie mentioned another piece of surprising data (the following is a transcript from the tape of that lecture):[44]

> When I just think of the word 'hope' there were two oncologists who wrote something about the work they were doing, because each one started a new protocol with four drugs, and the first letter of the drugs were E-P-H-O. And what one noticed was that approximately three-quarters of the patients who he was treating had their cancer respond. And the other noticed that only one-fourth of the patients he was treating responded. All doing the same thing with the same drugs. When they met and started talking they discovered one significant difference in what they were doing. One took the E,P,H, and O and called his protocol HOPE —and the other called it EPHO. And HOPE was significant and symbolic.

The audience was impressed with the effect of an attitude—hope—on the response of cancer to chemotherapy. However, it seemed highly unlikely that these data were true. There are no recent studies involving the use of a chemotherapy combination with the acronym EPHO (or HOPE for that matter). Secondly, the drugs

mentioned suggested that the tumour was non-small cell lung cancer: any therapy in that disease with a response rate of 75 per cent would be far beyond current response rates. Thirdly, there are no recent studies of any chemotherapy in any epithelial tumour that show as large as a three-fold difference between two drug regimens.

On further investigation, the quotation was traced to an article in which the author reported a conversation that he said he had overheard at an oncology conference.[45] The author of that article, a medical oncologist in California, said in response to specific inquiries, that he had written the story as an example or illustration, not as fact. The article was actually a parable (and a rather witty and tongue-in-cheek one) which had the objective of telling physicians that there is more to treating cancer patients than giving drugs. Specifically, the author of the article said that: (a) there never was a drug combination called EPHO (or HOPE); (b) he had not overheard two oncologists describing their papers to be presented at a major conference; (c) a response rate of 75 per cent in non-small cell lung cancer would indeed be extraordinary; and (d) he had invented the whole anecdote in its entirety to illustrate the point he wanted to make.

The point of this example is to illustrate the power of an anecdote if it reflects what we all want to believe, and how easily it may be propagated and later emerge as a scientifically proven fact.

Dr David Spiegel

Dr David Spiegel (first names are being used to avoid confusion with Dr Bernie Siegel), a psychiatrist at Stanford, published a paper in 1989 which is of considerable importance.[46] In the late 1970s and early 1980s, Spiegel set up structured psychotherapy support groups for patients with metastatic breast cancer. These group sessions were carefully designed, and did not encourage the participants to take a 'positive attitude' or even to hope that the prognosis would improve if they did.

First, the participants in the groups were actively encouraged to face the clinical facts of their situation, and to confront, and cope with, the possibility, for example, of dying of their disease. Secondly, the groups were encouraged to develop networking and social contacts between the participants outside the group sessions. Although the groups met formally only once a week, the individual participants met more frequently and often became close friends. They visited each other's homes, and supported each other when things went badly (for example visited each other in hospital). Thirdly, there were additional aspects to the support system, such as support for the husbands and new techniques for pain control. The patients were never told, nor encouraged to believe, that any of these techniques could improve their survival.

The original study was designed to see if sessions such as these could improve the quality of life, and it showed that these techniques did improve coping strategies and the quality of life.[47] Several years later, when Bernie Siegel's concept of hope as a therapeutic agent became popular, David Spiegel reanalysed and updated his own data to determine the survival of the original patients, and whether the group sessions had had any effect. He found that the women who had attended these groups survived longer than the controls (medians 36.6 months in the therapy group versus 18.9 months in the control group). This was the first, and so far the only, piece of evidence derived from a randomized, prospective study which shows that survival might be affected by psychological and social factors. However, the study was small ($n = 86$; $n = 50$ intervention; $n = 36$ controls, no intervention) and the result might have been obtained by chance (see also Chapter 6.1).

Spiegel immediately set up replication studies at other centres. When those studies are published, there will be a definitive answer. If the replication studies do confirm Spiegel's original data, then there will be strong evidence that group support can prolong life in advanced breast cancer. If they do not show the same results as the 1989 findings, then it will mean that either the 1989 results were a chance finding, or there is some factor that was at work in Stanford in 1989 which cannot be reproduced or translated to other centres.

Life events and recurrence of breast cancer

In addition to studies on the patients' reactions to illness and to the use of complementary approaches, there have been several studies of the impact of life events on the survival of patients after the diagnosis of breast cancer. Two studies at one hospital in the United Kingdom showed a possible influence.[48],[49] However, these were based on the recall of past life events by patients after the time of relapse. Clearly, the process of recalling past stresses at the time of an event as serious as relapse has the potential for introducing bias. One's ability to recall past events might well increase if one thought that those events may have played a role in one's current medical situation. By contrast, a larger prospective study in the United Kingdom (designed to exclude this recall bias) showed that there was no connection between life events and survival. Those researchers re-examined their data after 10-years follow-up and again found no connection between life events and survival.[50]

Psychoneuroimmunology

If it were established that the mind can influence either the cause or the course of cancer, then there would be no difficulty in thinking of possible mechanisms by which this could occur. Many investigators are looking at mechanisms by which psychological factors influence various physiological parameters, particularly the immune system. A label has already been attached to the field: psychoneuroimmunology.

Much of the work that is labelled as psychoneuroimmunology concerns the effects of mood, stress, or personality on some measurable aspect of a body system (T lymphocytes, stress hormones, and other parameters). Many of these studies have shown a relationship between psychological states and the parameter under investigation. This may be important, but it is not known whether or not this has any role in serious or chronic diseases, and particularly in cancer. It is quite possible that changes in lymphocyte levels or other immune function tests may affect some aspects of some disease. For example there is some evidence (although there are contradictory studies) that major stress may marginally increase the chance of getting a cold after intranasal application of rhinovirus.[51] However, there is a major difference between getting a cold and developing (or altering the course of) malignant disease.

At present, the label 'psychoneuroimmunology' is valid description of an active area of research. However, it is not a proven phenomenon in oncology, although many well-informed patients assume (partly because of the sound of the label) that it is.

Blaming the patient

It is possible that contemporary attitudes about the mind and cancer are part of a long tradition in humankind's attitude to apparently mysterious illness, namely to blame the patient.

Blaming the patient helps healthy family members and friends to feel safe. If we, the healthy, can identify something the patient has done, and has chosen to do, that has caused the cancer, then we will not get that cancer if we avoid doing the same thing. Hence the widespread urge to find things in patients' lives that set them apart from the healthy ones. Many examples from the past illustrate this basic trait of human behaviour. It was believed until several decades ago that tuberculosis would selectively strike artists and sensitive people (the personality type was actually labelled 'the phthisical personality'). It was also believed, until more recently, that people with obsessional personalities were more prone to ulcerative colitis ('the colitic personality'). In Victorian times, Down's syndrome was thought to be due to the parents being intoxicated at the moment of conception! It was believed, until a few years ago, that gastric ulcers were caused by stress coupled with a Type A personality. When the association with *Helicobacter pylorii* was discovered, it was found that if the bacterium is absent, the chance of developing an ulcer is minimal.

Many people's attitudes to possible psychological causes of cancer demonstrate the same social phenomenon. There are of course some cancers where a patient's actions are a known contributing factor (smoking in causing cancers of the lung, mouth, larynx, oesophagus, bladder, pancreas, kidney, etc., sunlight in skin cancers, and so on) but most cancers arrive mysteriously and, in the light of current knowledge, apparently randomly. Human beings find randomness difficult to cope with, and often impose a (spurious) order on the events to explain them. This underlies the phenomenon of blaming the patient: it is humankind's time-honoured way of dealing with its own discomfort in the face of the unknown.

Practical guidelines for responding to issues concerning complementary medicine

For all the above reasons, it may be possible that any remedy, whether it is a medication and/or a course in attitude-changing, may be hailed as effective against cancer, but may in fact be of no value against the disease process. If that is the case, how should the clinician advise the patient?

The important principle in discussing complementary medicine with the patient is to maintain consistently (but gently) the distinction between subjective and objective factors, while at the same time acknowledging and responding to the patient's emotions. In general, patients respond negatively to interviews when their emotions have been ignored, (which is why a brusque statement 'Of course garlic pills don't work—your disease is incurable.' may be true but is unhelpful and unkind). Fortunately, there are established techniques that can be used to acknowledge the patient's feelings, without compelling the physician to agree with (or even pronounce on) any statements or expectations that are not true (see also Chapters 6.1 and 6.2).

This is not an easy interview to have with a patient who may be ready to go anywhere to try a complementary remedy, and it is made worse if the patient refuses to have conventional therapy in those situations in which the chance of benefit is great. Nevertheless, there

Table 4 Some practical hints in conducting an interview about complementary medicine

1.	Maintain a clear distinction (in your own mind at least) between subjective 'feeling better' and objective 'getting better'.
2.	Elicit the patient's expectations of the complementary remedy.
3.	Acknowledge (using the empathic response) the patients feelings about the complementary remedy.
4.	Do not 'own' or accept responsibility for statements about the complementary remedy or its possible side-effects; these are the domain of the complementary medicine practitioner to whom the patient should be addressing those questions (serious consequences or interactions are theoretically possible but are rare in practice—particularly in comparison with the sequelae of conventional therapy).
5.	Stay as realistic and as cool as possible when explaining the potential benefits and potential side-effects of the proposed conventional treatment.
6.	Explore the 'how'—rather than the 'whether'—of trying the complementary remedy.
7.	Explore a possible negotiated compromise (for example delaying conventional treatment for 2 or 3 weeks to see if the complementary remedy produces any effect).
8.	Stay close to the concept that the patient is making his or her own choice: your job is to provide information about what can realistically be expected from conventional treatment (this is sometimes called 'disinvesting in the outcome'); ultimately the patient will come to decide what information is credible.

are techniques that can be used in these interviews, and the central components are as follows (see also Table 4):

1. Maintain a clear distinction (in your own mind at least) between subjective 'feeling better' and objective 'getting better'.

2. Elicit the patient's expectations of the complementary remedy.

3. Acknowledge (using the empathic response) the patients feelings about the complementary remedy.

4. Do not 'own' or accept responsibility for statements about the complementary remedy or its possible side-effects. These are the domain of the complementary medicine practitioner to whom the patient should be addressing those questions. (Serious consequences or interactions are theoretically possible but are rare in practice—particularly in comparison with the sequelae of conventional therapy.)[23],[52],[53]

5. Stay as realistic and as cool as possible when explaining the potential benefits and potential side-effects of the proposed conventional treatment.

6. Explore the 'how'—rather than the 'whether'—of trying the complementary remedy.

7. Explore a possible negotiated compromise (for example delaying conventional treatment for 2 or 3 weeks to see if the complementary remedy produces any effect).

8. Stay close to the concept that the patient is making his or her own choice: your job is to provide information about what may be realistically expected from conventional treatment. (This is sometimes called 'disinvesting in the outcome'.) Ultimately, the patient will come to decide what information is credible.

Details of how this may be achieved in practice are illustrated in scenarios with simulated patients on a CD-ROM set (and videotapes derived from it) which set out an overall approach to all clinical interviews, and particularly illustrate the use of the empathic response as a communication skill.[54] The details of using empathic response in responding to the emotional content of a clinical interview are also set out in a textbook,[55] and there are several case reports which include details of different aspects of these discussions.[56] For the patient and family there is also some written material available on

this subject which discusses patient's attitudes to complementary medicine and how unrealistic hopes may eventually be damaging.

In a few cases, the clinician may choose to compromise and delay treatment for a few weeks in order to give the patient a chance to try out the complementary medicine, before proceeding with conventional treatment if there is no success. From the point of view of oncology practice, this may not be ideal, but in some cases it may be the only alternative to a confrontation ending with the patient refusing all conventional treatment. Furthermore, the passage of time often allows the patient to accept gradually that the complementary medicine is not working, an attitude that may not be achievable in the first interview.

Finally, it is worth saying a little more about exploring the 'how' rather than the 'whether'. One possible way of expressing this difficult point (taken from a book written for the patient and family) is something like this:

> If you go to try a complementary medicine remedy with the attitude that it would be nice if it worked, and would not be a disaster if it didn't, and if you can afford it (in terms of money and time), then you will lose nothing by going—and may feel a fair bit better in yourself for doing it. If, on the other hand, you feel desperate and want more than anything else to be cured, and are prepared to sell anything and go anywhere to get a cure, then you are lining yourself up for serious disappointment and you may find that you have lost time and money when both are scarce. In some respects, the most important question to ask yourself is not 'shall I go?' but 'what are my feelings about going and what am I expecting?'

Conclusion

The central view of this chapter has been found to be useful in practice. Recently, a committee of the College of Physicians and Surgeons of Ontario was mandated to define the role and responsibility of the College regarding complementary medicine. The committee's report was based on the stance set out above.[57] It was unanimously accepted by the College and drew widespread approval from the general public when it was released. Furthermore, it did not precipitate any major conflict (or litigation) from practitioners of complementary medicine. The same stance has also been presented to the Council on Scientific Affairs (M. Karlan, personal communication, November 1996).

The central principle is a simple one. The 'patient' consists of the sum of 'the disease' and 'the person'. Complementary medicine practitioners have always been good at supporting the person: conventional physicians have, until recently, been good only at looking after the disease. If we in conventional medicine insist (correctly) that complementary medicine practitioners must stop making untrue and unsubstantiated claims, then by the same token we should learn to be better at 'person doctoring'.

'Getting better' is quite distinct from 'feeling better', but in the care of the cancer patient both are important.

References

1. Eisenberg DM, Kessler RC, Foster C, Norlock FE, Calkins DR, Delbanco TL. Unconventional medicine in the United States. *New England Journal of Medicine*, 1993; **328**: 246–52.

2. Eisenberg DM, Davis RB, Ettner SL, Appel S. Trends in alternative medicine use in the United States, 1990–1997. *Journal of the American Medical Association*, 1998; **280**: 1569–75.

3. Angell M, Kassirer JP. Alternative medicine—the risks of untested and unregulated remedies. *New England Journal of Medicine*, 1998; **339**: 839–41.

4. Popper KR. *The logic of scientific discovery*. New York: Basic Books, 1959.

5. Kuhn TE. *The structure of scientific revolutions*. Chicago: Phoenix Books, 1962.

6. Fernandez CV, Stutzer CA, MacWilliam L, Fryer C. Alternative and complementary therapy use in pediatric oncology patients in British Columbia: prevalence and reasons for use and nonuse. *Journal of Clinical Oncology*, 1998; **16**: 1279–86.

7. Cassileth BR. Historical trends and patient characteristics. In: Barrett S, Cassileth B, eds. *Dubious cancer treatments*. Tampa, Florida: American Cancer Society, Florida Division, 1991.

8. Astin JA. Why patients use alternative medicine. *Journal of the American Medical Association*, 1998; **279**: 1548–53.

9. Wilson BR. Dubious science and spurious degrees. In: Barrett S, Cassileth B, eds. *Dubious cancer treatments*. Tampa, Florida: American Cancer Society, Florida Division, 1991.

10. Buckman R, Sabbagh K. *Magic or medicine? An investigation of healing*. London: Macmillan, 1993.

11. Tannock IF, Warr DG. Unconventional therapies for cancer: A refuge from the rules of evidence? *Canadian Medical Association Journal*, 1998; **159**: 801–2.

12. Sheehan MP, Atherton DJ. A controlled trial of traditional Chinese medicinal plants in widespread non-exudative atopic eczema. *British Journal of Dermatology*, 1992; **126**: 179–84.

13. Meade TW, Dyer S, Browne W, Townsend J, Frank AO. Low back pain of mechanical origin: randomised comparison of chiropractic and hospital outpatient treatment. *British Medical Journal*, 1990; **300**: 1431–7.

14. Koes BW, Bouter LM, van Mameren H, *et al.* Randomised clinical trial of manipulative therapy and physiotherapy for persistent back and neck complaints: results of one year follow up. *British Medical Journal*, 1992; **304**: 601–5.

15. ter Riet G, Kleijnen J, Knipschild P. Acupuncture and chronic pain: A criteria-based meta-analysis. *Journal of Clinical Epidemiology*, 1990; **43**: 1191–9.

16. Linde K, Ramirez G, Mulrow CD, Pauls A, Weidenhammer W, Melchart D. St John's wort for depression—an overview and meta-analysis of randomised clinical trials. *British Medical Journal*, 1996; **313**: 253–8.

17. Moertel CG, Fleming TR, Rubin J, *et al.* A clinical trial of amygdalin (laetrile) in the treatment of human cancer. *New England Journal of Medicine*, 1982; **306**: 201–6.

18. Loprinzi CL, Kuross SA, O'Fallon JR, *et al.* Randomized placebo-controlled evaluation of hydrazine sulfate in patients with advanced colorectal cancer. *Journal of Clinical Oncology*, 1994; **12**: 1121–5.

19. Loprinzi CL, Goldberg RM, Su JQ, *et al.* Placebo-controlled trial of hydrazine sulfate in patients with newly diagnosed non-small-cell lung cancer. *Journal of Clinical Oncology*, 1994; **12**: 1126–9.

20. Moertel CG, Fleming TR, Creagan ET, Rubin J, O'Connell MJ, Ames MM. High-dose vitamin C versus placebo in the treatment of patients with advanced cancer who have had no prior chemotherapy. *New England Journal of Medicine*, 1985; **312**: 137–41.

21. Hennekens CH, Buring JE, Manson JE, *et al.* Lack of effect of long-term supplementation with beta carotene on the incidence of malignant neoplasms and cardiovascular disease. *New England Journal of Medicine*, 1996; **334**: 1145–9.

22. Omenn GS, Goodman GE, Thornquist MD, *et al.* Effects of a combination of beat carotene and vitamin A on lung cancer and cardiovascular disease. *New England Journal of Medicine*, 1996; **334**: 1150–5.

23. Markman M. Medical complications of 'alternative' cancer therapy. *New England Journal of Medicine*, 1985; **312**: 1640.

24. Raschetti R. Evaluation of an unconventional cancer treatment (the Di Bella multitherapy): results of phase II trials in Italy. *British Medical Journal*, 1999; **318**: 224–8.

25. Miller DR, Anderson GT, Stark JJ, Granick JL, Richardson D. Phase I/II trial of the safety and efficacy of shark cartilage in the treatment of advanced cancer. *Journal of Clinical Oncology*, 1998; **16**: 3649–55.

26. Cassileth BR, Lusk EJ, Guerry D, *et al.* Survival and quality of life among patients receiving unproven as compared with conventional cancer therapy. *New England Journal of Medicine*, 1991; **324**: 1180–5.

27. Morganstern H, Gellert GA, Walter SD, Ostfield AM, Siegel BS, The impact of a psychosocial support program on survival with breast cancer. *Journal of Chronic Diseases*, 1984; **37**: 273.

28. Gellert GA, Maxwell RM, Siegel BS. Survival of breast cancer patients receiving adjunctive psychosocial support therapy: A 10-year follow-up study. *Journal of Clinical Oncology*, 1993; **11**: 66–9.

29. Bagenal FS, Easton DF, Harris E, Chilvers CED, McElwain TJ. Survival of patients with breast cancer attending the Bristol Cancer Help Centre. *Lancet*, 1990; **336**: 606–10.

30. Chowka PB. Steve McQueen—legacy of a medical outlaw. *New Age Magazine*, 1981; **1981**: 28–36.

31. Rees WD, Dover SB, Low-Beer TS. 'Patients with terminal cancer' who have neither terminal illness nor cancer. *British Medical Journal*, 1987; **295**: 318–9.

32. Warren WH, Memoli VA, Jordan AG, Gould VE. Reevaluation of pulmonary neoplasms resected as small cell carcinomas. Significance of distinguishing between well-differentiated and small cell neuroendocrine carcinomas. *Cancer*, 1990; **65**: 1003–10.

33. Zavertnik JJ. Immuno-augmentative therapy. In: Barrett S, Cassileth B, eds. *Dubious cancer treatments*. Tampa, Florida: American Cancer Society, Florida Division, 1991.

34. Buckman R, Sabbagh K. *Magic or medicine?* (TV series). London, Channel Four, 1993.

35. Callen M. A miracle cure? *QW Magazine*, 1992: 35–8.

36. Boyd W. *The spontaneous regression of cancer*. Springfield, Ill: Charles C Thomas, 1966.

37. Everson TC, Cole WH. *Spontaneous regression of cancer.* Philadelphia: WB Saunders, 1966.

38. Fox BH. Psychogenic factors in cancer, especially its incidence. In: Maes S, Spielberg CD, Defares PB, Sarason IG, eds. *Topics in health psychology.* Chichester: John Wiley and Sons, 1988: 37–55.

39. Zonderman AB, Costa PT, McRae RR. Depression as a risk for cancer morbidity and mortality in a nationally representative sample. *Journal of the American Medical Association,* 1989; **262**: 1191–5.

40. Levar I, Friedlander Y, Kark J, Peritz E. An epidemiological study of mortality among bereaved parents. *New England Journal of Medicine,* 1988; **319**: 457–61.

41. Jones DR, Goldblatt PO, Leon DA. Bereavement and cancer: some data on the deaths of spouses from the longitudinal study of office of population censuses and surveys *British Medical Journal,* 1984; **289**: 461–4.

42. Greer S, Morris T, Pettingale KW. Psychological response to breast cancer: effect on outcome *Lancet,* 1979; **ii**: 785–7.

43. Bristol Cancer Help Centre. *Cancer and its non-toxic treatment.* Bristol: Bristol Cancer Help Centre, 1985.

44. Siegel B. *Lecture June 25th 1990 Toronto.* (Audiocassette). Toronto: Speaker's Cassette Library, 1990.

45. Buchholtz WM. The medical uses of hope. *Western Journal of Medicine,* 1988; **1**: 148.

46. Spiegel D, Bloom JR, Kraemer HC, Gottheil E. Effect of psychosocial treatment on survival of patients with metastatic breast cancer. *Lancet,* 1989; **ii**: 888–91.

47. Spiegel D, Bloom JR, Yalom I. Group support for patients with metastatic cancer. *Archives of General Psychiatry,* 1981; **36**: 527–33.

48. Ramirez AJ, Craig TJK, Watson JP, Fentimen IA. Stress and relapse of breast cancer. *British Medical Journal,* 1989; **298**: 292–3.

49. Ramirez AJ, Richards MA, Gregory WM. Life events and breast cancer prognosis. *British Medical Journal,* 1992; **304**: 1632.

50. Barraclough J, Osmond C, Taylor I. Life events and breast cancer prognosis. *British Medical Journal,* 1993; **307**: 325.

51. Cohen S, Tyrrell DAJ, Smith AP. Psychological stress and susceptibility to the common cold. *New England Journal of Medicine,* 1991; **325**: 606–12.

52. Eisele JW, Reay DT. Deaths related to coffee enemas. *Journal of the American Medical Association,* 1980; **244**: 1608–9.

53. Epidemiologic reports. Isolation of HTLV-III/LAV from serum proteins for cancer therapy in the Bahamas. *Canadian Medical Association Journal,* 1986; **134**: 148.

54. Buckman R, Baile W, Korsch B. *A Practical Guide to communication skills in clinical practice* (CD-ROM set). Toronto: Canada Medical Audio-Visual Communication, 1998.

55. Buckman R, Kason Y. *How to break bad news.* Baltimore: Johns Hopkins University Press, 1992.

56. Jenkins CA, Scarfe A, Bruera E. Integration of palliative care with alternative medicine in patients who have refused curative cancer therapy: A report of two cases. *Journal of Palliative Care,* 1998; **14**: 55–9.

57. College of Physicians and Surgeons of Ontario Ad Hoc Committee on Complementary Medicine. *Report to Council. Members' Dialogue* (Nov/Dec 1997), 1997: 8–14.

6.6 Care of patients who are dying, and their families

Irene J. Higginson and Eduardo Bruera

Introduction

While many treatments aim to cure or to extend the life of cancer patients, and some cancers (notably testicular cancers and lymphomas) are now curable, the majority of people with cancer will die from it. This is particularly true for patients with lung cancer—representing one-third of all cancers. But it also includes many patients with gastrointestinal, genitourinary, ear, nose, and throat, and breast cancers. Cancers discovered at an advanced stage or where early treatment is not effective are most commonly in this category.

Much can be done for patients whose cancer is not curable to control symptoms, to improve the quality of remaining life, the quality of dying, and to support patients and their family. Ideally, these approaches begin early in care: with symptom control and 'total' care for the patient's physical, emotional, social, spiritual, and service needs and for their family. Controlling symptoms and improving the quality of life for patients, even at the end of life, can enhance their existence, and, in some instances, may extend it.[1] Thus, the phrase 'nothing more can be done' should be outlawed. There is always something more that can be done to aim to support patients and their families and to improve the control of symptoms.

Concepts in care for patients who are dying and their families

Dying in society

Despite the fact that we all will die, dying remains a taboo in many societies. How death is handled and where it takes place reflect societal values and priorities. Increasingly in advanced industrial societies, death is concentrated among older age groups. Three-quarters of the 1.34 million cancer deaths in England between 1985 and 94 were aged over 65 years: the mean age at death increased over the period from 69.9 in 1985 to 71.3 in 1994.[2] The decline in mortality among younger age groups means that less and less people meet death. At younger ages death may be seen as a rarity, unfair, a tragedy, a problem, something society should strive to prevent; even at older ages it can be seen as something unexpected and unwelcome and much effort and resources are devoted to trying to postpone it.[3] These attitudes affect patients, their families, carers, friends, and children and many of the staff in health, social, and other services that encounter them.

Dying and cancer

Globally, death from cancer continues to increase. Much of this is due to the ageing population, and to increases in cigarette smoking in many countries. Global predictions of mortality, which adjust for likely changes in lifestyle and demography and advances in treatments, suggest that cancers of the lung, trachea, and bronchus will rise from being the 10th common cause of death in 1990, to being the fifth most common in 2020. World-wide, stomach cancer is predicted to rise from the 14th most common cause of death to the eighth.[4] In the 10 years between 1985 and 1994 more than 1.3 million people died from cancer in England. Epidemiologically-based assessments of need suggest that within a population of 1 million, with a similar age and sex distribution to that of industrialized countries, there would be approximately 2800 cancer deaths per year.[5] Of these, in the last year of life, 2400 people will experience pain that requires treatment, 1300 will have trouble with breathing, and 1400 will have symptoms of vomiting or feeling sick: many other symptoms are also present, and many symptoms can occur at the same time. These problems and many others need to be managed effectively.

The patient and family as the unit of care

Concern for the patient and family as the unit of care is an essential element in the care of people who are dying. The term 'family' is meant in its broad sense and encompasses close relatives (often a spouse, children, or siblings), a partner, and close friend(s) who are significant for the patient. They should have every available option to meet their choices, and expert recognition of their cultural and individual needs. Not everyone will have the time to embark on long family discussions, but everyone can recognize the family or carers by name and accept them as an integral part of the team caring for the patient. This includes acknowledging the concerns of the family or friends, and finding mechanisms for these to be heard and discussed, whether care is at home, in hospital, or in a hospice. The evidence supporting this approach is two-fold. Firstly, there is evidence from descriptive studies of dissatisfaction and problems when such an approach does not occur,[6,7] and secondly there is evidence from comparative and descriptive studies in Europe and the United States of higher satisfaction among carers when services do provide this.[8,9] A systematic review of both comparative studies[10,11] and randomized trials[12,13] affirmed this but many of the studies were small, retrospective, and used matched rather than randomly-allocated groups (level of evidence ranged from 2 to 5).[14] A second, systematic review

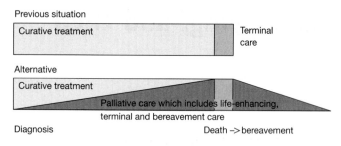

Fig. 1 Models of palliative and terminal care.

did not find improved quality of life among patients, although it questioned the appropriateness of the scales used.[15]

When do palliative and terminal care begin, and are these different from earlier care?

Palliative care is the total care for patients with progressive, advanced disease, and for their families and or carers. It is concerned with physical, psychosocial, and spiritual care, focusing on both the quality of the remaining life of the patient and on the support of the family and those close to the patient. Terminal care occurs when the patient's condition suggests that it is extremely likely that death will occur within a matter of days. Common signs of impending death include: profound weakness, being confined to bed, drowsiness for extended periods, lack of interest in food and fluids, disorientation with respect to time, limited attention span, and difficulty in swallowing medication.

Palliative care services focused initially on the care of dying cancer patients, that is terminal care. Modern concepts of palliative care include terminal care and bereavement care as well as care throughout the trajectory of advanced illness. Three levels of care are proposed: the palliative care approach employed ideally by every doctor and nurse; palliative care procedures and techniques (important adjuncts to care that are undertaken by relevant specialists); and specialist palliative care—where doctors, nurses, and other clinicians are specially trained. As Fig. 1 indicates, terminal care continues from, and is part of, good palliative care. The trajectory towards dying can vary: a patient may appear reasonably stable and then deteriorate, but then become stable again, although weaker.

Changing gear towards the end of life

Evidence based guidelines have reviewed the need to 'change gear' when managing the care of patients towards the end of life. Although many of the studies are descriptive, they represent the best information on which to base practice (level of evidence 3 to 5).[16] During the terminal phase the goals of care are redefined towards the alleviation of symptoms and distress and support for the patient and family at the time of death. Existing symptoms may change or new symptoms arise, which require management. A review of medication is needed. Some medications, such as those for pre-existing heart or respiratory disorders, or any other non-essential mediation may become inappropriate, particularly if these are difficult for the patient to take. Patients may choose to die in different ways. Some will aim for a peaceful death with the family around, many patients will die as they

have lived. A patient who has fought all through their illness may prefer to die fighting, as this is their right. Close to death, a small observational study suggested that patients may focus their hopes on being, including relationships with others, rather than doing.[17]

Patients and their family will often ask about the prognosis and may be concerned about the process of death itself. The family many need to be warned about a deterioration, and may be resentful if they miss an opportunity for farewells, which can lead to considerable grief. Based on a sociological study, Weisman defined 'appropriate death' as 'an absence of suffering, preservation of important relationships, an interval for anticipatory grief, relief of remaining conflicts, belief in timeliness, exercise of feasible option in activities, and consistency with physical limitations, all within the scope of one's ego ideal'.[18] Kellehear described the features of a modern 'good death' as 'awareness of dying, social adjustments and personal preparations, public preparations (legal, financial, religious, funeral, medical), work or activities reduced, and farewells'.[19] While these definitions are based on descriptive studies (level of evidence, 5) they suggest that death is an individual experience which includes not only symptom and emotional concerns, but spiritual and social concerns including future planning and farewells. Thus, attention needs to be focused on the needs and wishes of the individual person and those close to him or her. Pain and symptom management are essential. Alongside these, care needs to be orientated towards enabling the patient to 'live' with dignity until death. This can involve a wide and very individual range of aspects, such as new achievable activities, the creative activities of hospice day care, attention to appearance (hair, teeth), the environment and surroundings, family gatherings or attending important functions, a reconciliation of existential and spiritual meanings. 'You are important because you are you', as coined by Cicely Saunders, is the underpinning philosophical principle of modern palliative care.

Place of care at the end of life?

Trends

Much of the care in the last year of life occurs at home but there has been an increasing trend towards the hospitalization of death in many countries, although this has now reached a plateau (level of evidence ranges 3 to 5). In England, studies based on random samples of deaths (excluding those with no prior warning or illness) showed that the proportions of patients who died in institutions increased between 1969 and 1987, from 46 per cent to 50 per cent in hospitals and from 5 per cent to 18 per cent in hospices and other institutions, including residential care homes.[20] There was also an increase in the proportions living in institutions and being admitted to hospitals during the last year of life. Meanwhile, the proportion that died at home fell from 42 per cent to 24 per cent. Analysis of more recent trends indicates that death in hospital is now decreasing. In England, between 1985 and 1994, the percentage of cancer deaths in an National Health Service hospital or nursing home (including National Health Service hospices) fell gradually from 58 per cent (1985) to 47 per cent (1994) while the percentage who died in non-National Health Service hospitals, nursing homes, voluntary hospices, and communal establishments increased (Fig. 2). Approximately 17 per cent of cancer deaths were in voluntary or National Health Service hospices, and this number is steadily increasing.[21] Voluntary hospices represent 82 per cent of all hospice beds in the United Kingdom.[22] The

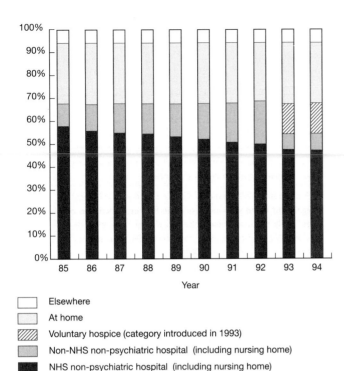

Elsewhere

At home

Voluntary hospice (category introduced in 1993)

Non-NHS non-psychiatric hospital (including nursing home)

NHS non-psychiatric hospital (including nursing home)

Fig. 2 Trends in place of death in England.

percentage that died at home remained largely unchanged at around 26 per cent.

In the United States, Mann *et al.* found that, between 1980 and 1990, 22 per cent of 468 patients with gynaecological cancer died at home. Examination of the variable year of death demonstrated that the likelihood of death in the hospital generally increased from 1980 to 1990, despite aggressive efforts by caregivers to facilitate and encourage death at home.[23]

Preferences of patients, families, and professionals

Bowling has argued against the 'institutionalization' of death because home death is more natural and a person has more chance to influence their quality of life.[24] Miller and Fins proposed restructuring hospital care, to provide a more hospice or home like atmosphere.[25] Studies of preferences support this. A literature review identified 14 studies of preferences, in different developed countries. Although response rates and study designs varied (levels of evidence 3 to 5), between 50 and 70 per cent of cancer patients preferred to be cared for at home for as long as possible and to die at home (Table 1, level of evidence 3 to 5).[26]–[30] In a longitudinal study, under existing circumstances Townsend *et al.*[31] found that 34 out of 59 (58 per cent) patients wished to die at home. Had there been a limited increase in community care, 41 out of 59 (67 per cent) patients would have wished to die at home. Only 17 of those patients who wished to die at home achieved this. In a study of patients in the care of a hospice home care team, Hinton found that as death approached some patients appeared to change their preferences and opt for hospice care rather than home care.[29] However, home care was still the preference of over half of the patients in the last week of life. 'Realistic' (Hinton's word) preferences for home care fell steadily from 100 per cent to 54 per cent of patients and to 45 per cent of relatives. Reasons for these changes in preference were not explored. Family members often have slightly lower preferences for home care than do patients, and in a few recent studies there has been an increasing preference for hospice care among both patients and families. Health professionals also usually favour home care, although views vary (Table 1).

Assessment of patients and their families

Appropriate assessment

Assessment of the patient is the critical aspect of care in palliative care, just as at other times of care. However, measurement of pulse, blood pressure, temperature, and functional status are often inappropriate because they do not help to plan care. Appropriate assessment should emphasize pain and symptom control,[43] the quality of life for the patient,[44]–[46] fears and anxiety, psychological, social, and spiritual concerns,[47] any future wishes, and the family members or carers.[48],[49] This breadth of assessment requires a multiprofessional approach to care (see below).

Clinical records should include a body chart (see Chapter 5.8) on which pain and other symptoms are recorded at each visit. However, these are often charted only when patients are first seen, and reassessment is missed. This can be improved by continued monitoring. Several suitable assessment systems are available. Examples of assessment systems in common use are: the Support Team Assessment Schedule (STAS),[50] Edmonton Symptom Assessment System (ESAS), and the Palliative Care Assessment (PACA).[51] In addition, quality of life measures may be useful (see Chapter 6.3). The challenge is to find measures that are sufficiently short and practical for routine use, are useful when patients are towards the end of life, encompass the family, and are validated in this setting. Note that many traditional quality of life measures show consistently low values in palliative patients, because of the emphasis on physical function in these measures. Assessment and quality of life measures specific to palliative care (Table 2) have been developed, as well as cancer-specific or symptom measures (see Chapter 5.8).

The Support Team Assessment Schedule (STAS)[53],[54] includes 17 items covering: 2, pain and symptoms; 3, patient anxiety, insight, and spiritual; 2, family anxiety and insight; 2, planning affairs; 3, communication; 3, home services; 2, support of other professionals. Development was by means of collaboration with five support teams, and revised in light of presentations at professional meetings, observation of palliative care, and interviews with patients and families. The STAS is used by more than 100 registered users including home, hospital, and hospice settings in at least nine countries. Time to complete ratings for one patient averages 2 min. Its reliance on professionals' assessments may be a weakness, but the STAS was validated to ensure that professional ratings reasonably reflected patient views.[55],[56] Recently, a new shortened version, the Palliative Outcome Scale (POS),[57] which includes patient completed assessments and open questions, has become available. Extra items, such as individual symptoms, can be added.[58]–[60] An example of one patient's monitoring during care is shown in Fig. 3.

The Edmonton Symptom Assessment System[61] includes nine visual analogue scales: pain, activity, nausea, depression, anxiety,

Table 1 Some studies that aimed to describe preferences for place of care and death

Author, year, country	Patient population and study design	Results	Grade of evidence
Addington-Hall and MacDonald, 1991[32] UK	Setting: Inner London health district All patients admitted to hospital with cancer and a prognosis of less than 1 year were eligible; 80 carers participated	Most carers (72%) of home death patients felt home was correct place of death because patient expressed preference for home Most carers (95%) of hospital death patients felt hospital was correct place of death when patient needed treatment not available at home (weak evidence)	III
Ashby M et al., 1993[28] Australia	Setting: metropolitan 462 adults chosen at random	Most people (60%) want to die at home (weak evidence) Significant trend with increasing age for respondents to be less likely to want to die at home (χ^2 (trend) $= 19.8$, df $= 1$, $p<0.001$) and more likely to want to die in hospital (χ^2 (trend) $= 11.4$, df $= 1$, $p<0.001$)	III
Beckingham, 1996[33] UK	Setting: urban health district Preference for place of death of 78 patients of district nurses matched against actual place of death; cross-sectional study	Study 1—67.9% want to die at home; 10.3% want to die in hospice (weak evidence) Fewer patients died at home (43.3%) than preferred home death (67.9%) More patients died in hospital (33.3%) than preferred (1.3%) More patients died in hospice (23.1%) than preferred (10.3%)	IV
Brent and Harrow Health Agency, 1994[34] UK	Setting: Outer London health district 4 surveys, no details of study design Studies 1–3 preferences for place of death (94, 84, and 191 patients) Study 4 actual place of death versus preference (82 deaths)	Studies 2 and 3—Preferences for place of death: home 25–29%; hospital 19–31%; hospice 38–52%; other 2–4% 25% of continuing care patients want to die at home, 40% in hospice, 25% in hospital (weak evidence) Study 4—80% died in preferred location	IV
Charlton, 1991[35] UK	Setting: 10 GP waiting rooms 4117 completed questionnaires; control group (n = 100) chosen at random	Majority would prefer to die at home—sample: home 63%, hospice 16%; control: home 53%, hospice 13% (moderate evidence) People with personal experience of dying more likely to prefer hospice (33% home, 23% hospice)	III
Gilbar, Steiner, 1996[36] Israel	Setting: patients with cancer in home care unit 171 patients and their families Retrospective study, independent variables correlated with preference for home death	Patient preference for home care associated with women, patients > 60 years, families who talk about illness and death (weak evidence)	IV
Hinton, 1994[29] UK	Setting: hospice Prospective, study of randomized sample of 232 patients Patients' and relatives' preference for place of care recorded at intervals	Patients' preference for home decreases as death approaches (90→50%), replaced by preference for hospice (10→40%) (moderate evidence) Relatives' preference for home decreases as death approaches (92→40%), replaced by preference for hospice (8→40%) (moderate evidence)	III
McWhinney et al., 1995[37] Canada	Setting: palliative care inpatient unit with home support team in large chronic care hospital 75 patients who died at home, 75 patients who died in hospital Retrospective case–control chart review, preferences from medical records, no information on medical status when preference stated	Patients who died at home expressed a preference for dying at home (62.7%) (moderate evidence) 37.7% expressed a strong preference for dying at home; 16.0% expressed a conditional preference for dying at home; patients who died at home expressed a much higher preference for dying at home ($p<0.001$)	III
Neubauer, Hamilton, 1990[38] US	Setting: Atlanta Telephone survey of 253 adults selected at random Description of hospice care given before attitudes to hospice care sought	Majority would rather die at home than in hospital (weak evidence); white people more likely to want to die at home than black people (81.5 vs. 62.2%); 70–75% would want hospice care if terminally ill	IV
Spiller and Alexander, 1993[39] UK	Setting: palliative care unit 18 consecutive patients and their caregivers Prospective survey, structured interview	Patients' preferences for place of terminal care do not differ from carers' preferences (moderate evidence)	III

Table 1 *continued*

Author, year, country	Patient population and study design	Results	Grade of evidence
Toscani and Cantoni, 1991[40] Italy	Setting: Italian population sample 964 people interviewed by telephone using questionnaire	64% would prefer to die at home; 12.3% in hospital; 10.7% rather not think about it; 7.3% makes no difference; 5.7% don't know/can't answer (weak evidence)	IV
Townsend et al., 1990[31] UK	Setting: hospital and community care 84 patients with cancer expected to live less than 1 year randomly selected Patients interview at intervals and carer interviewed after death to compare actual with preferred place of death	As the disease progressed, preference for home death decreased (58→49%), with increases in preference for hospital (20→24%) and hospice (20→24%) (moderate evidence) Given ideal rather than existing circumstances, home death preference increased (67→70%) and hospice (15→18%), with decrease in preference for hospital (16→10%) (moderate evidence)	III
Ward, 1974[41] UK	Setting: terminal care unit 279 patients who died of cancer Death certificates examined, medical staff interviewed, carer approached for interview	75% of carers were positive about place of death (either home or hospital) (weak evidence) 17% of hospital carers would have preferred death to be at home; 23% of home carers preferred hospital; 88% of GPs preferred home	III
Zusman, Tschetler, 1984[42] US	Representative sample of 500 interviews from census of general population in North Carolina	Financial reasons most likely to be given for preferring to die at home, followed by individual, family, and health considerations Those who preferred home were more likely to be young, white, educated, dissatisfied with medical services, considered their health excellent, afraid of hospitals	IV

drowsiness, appetite, well being, shortness of breath. Assessments are completed by the patient, and if this is not possible a family member or nursing staff complete the ratings. See Fig. 4 for an example of assessments during care.

Assessment and management of some common symptom complexes

Epidemiology and interactions of symptoms and problems

Determining the prevalence of symptoms at the end of life is made difficult because most of the studies rely on data collected in selected populations, who are referred to a particular service such as a pain clinic or palliative care team. The referral suggests that this group of patients had more problems than average. Thus, estimates of prevalence from prospective studies may overestimate that among all patients at the end of life. Also, because of difficulties in prognostication, it is difficult to collect data in the period before death.

An alternative approach is to use the reports of bereaved carers after the death. This has the advantage that the population can be identified and randomly selected from death registrations, but has the problem that reports may be influenced by their own grief, by

recall, and by how much contact they had with the patient (especially if the patient was in hospital). Relatives tend to report problems as more severe than do patients,[62] and during bereavement there is some evidence that their views alter again.[63],[64]

Some findings are consistent across all studies. Firstly, pain, weakness (or asthenia, and associated cachexia), breathless, and constipation are all common symptoms, that require management. Secondly, symptoms are usually multiple and interact with each other. For example depression may lead to anorexia or exacerbate pain. Symptoms also interact with emotional, social, and spiritual problems, so that pain can be exacerbated by worry, lack of information, fears, anxiety, or any unresolved matters. The systems of comprehensive assessment, described above, allow analysis of the range of problems and the potential interactions. Table 3 gives estimates of symptom prevalence, based on the views of bereaved carers.

Cancer pain

Pain affects approximately 80 per cent of cancer patients before death.[65] While it is the result of tumour involvement in three out of four patients, it can also be related to anticancer treatments, or unrelated to cancer and its treatment. The patient may also have several different types of cancer pain. Despite the many guidelines for appropriate pain management, many cancer patients experience considerable pain and approximately half of them receive inadequate

Table 2 Most useful measures for assessing the outcome of palliative care for people with advanced cancer

Measure (author and year)	Number of items and domains	Validity	Reliability	Responsiveness to change	Appropriateness of format:		
					Setting	Time	Administration
Edmonton Symptom Assessment Schedule, ESAS (Bruera, 1993)[43],[61]	9 (patient); pain activity, nausea, depression, anxiety, drowsiness, appetite, well being, shortness of breath	Correlates with STAS (except for activity)	Inter-rater (0.5–0.9)	Improvement demonstrated in palliative care	Inpatient	Few min	Patient completion or with nurse assistance
McGill Quality of Life Questionnaire, MQOL (Cohen et al., 1997)[52]	17 (patient); physical symptoms, psychological symptoms, outlook on life and meaningful existence	Correlates with Spitzer Quality of Life and SIS	Internal consistency (0.89)	Distinguishes between patients	Inpatient, outpatient	Not known	Patient completion
Palliative Care Assessment, PACA (Ellershaw et al., 1995)[51]	12 (patient and relatives); symptom control, insight and future placement	Symptom scores correlate with the McCorkle Symptom Distress Scale	Inter-rater (0.44–1)	Improvement demonstrated in palliative care	Inpatient	Few min	Professional completion
Palliative Outcome Scale, POS	10 (patient and family); pain, symptom, anxiety, information, well being, practical, plus two self-determined problems	Correlates with Support Team Assessment Schedule and EORTC-QLQ C30 for similar domains; patient free-report assessment of important concerns	Inter-rater (0.5–0.8); internal consistency (0.7)	Improvement and deterioration demonstrated in individual and groups of patients	Hospital inpatient, outpatient community hospital, primary care, hospice, inpatient, home care, day care	5 min	Separate patient and professional completion possible
Support Team Assessment Schedule, STAS (Higginson, 1993)[54]–[56]	17 (patient and carer); pain and symptom control, insight, psychosocial, family needs, planning affairs, home services, communication, support of other professionals	Correlates with patients' and families' ratings and with HRCA-QL	Inter-rater (0.65–0.94); internal consistency (0.68–0.89); test–retest (0.36–0.76)	Improvement and deterioration demonstrated in different groups of patients in palliative care	Community hospice	2 min	Professional completion

EORTC-QLQ = European Organization for Research into Treatment of Cancer—Quality of Life Questionnaire.

HRCA—QL = Hebrew Rehabilitation Centre for Ageing—Quality of Life Index.

SIS = Single Item Scale of Quality of Life.

analgesia (see Chapter 5.8). A review of pain management in nursing homes in the United States identified poor management of pain, even when the symptom was detected.[66]

Pharmacological treatment based on the regular use of oral opioids results in excellent pain control in the majority of patients (see Chapter 5.8). The World Health Organization analgesic ladder proposes non-opioid analgesics as the first step, followed by a mild opioid (step 2) or strong opioids (step 3) in patients with persistent pain (level of evidence 2–4) (Fig. 5).[67]–[70] Non-opioid drugs (including NSAIDs) are effective analgesics for patients with mild cancer pain and can be

DATE:										
WEEK:	0	1	2	3	4	5	6	7	8	9
Pain control	3	2	2	2	1	1	1	1	0	1
Other symptom control	2	1	1	1	3	1	1	2	0	0
Patient anxiety	3	2	2	1	1	1	0	0	0	0
Family anxiety	3	3	3	1	1	1	1	3	0	0
Patient insight	1	1	1	1	1	1	1	1	1	1
Family insight	1	1	1	1	1	1	1	1	0	0
Comm. between family and patient	0	0	0	0	0	0	0	0	0	0
Comm. between professionals	4	1	1	2	0	0	0	1	0	0
Comm. profs to patient and family	2	1	1	1	0	0	0	0	0	0
TOTAL – CORE 9 ITEMS	19	12	12	10	8	6	5	9	1	2
*Planning	0	0	0	0	0	0	1	2	0	0
*Practical	0	0	2	0	2	0	0	0	0	0
*Financial	0	0	0	0	0	0	0	0	0	0
*Wasted time	4	0	0	0	0	0	0	0	0	0
*Spiritual	0	0	0	0	0	0	0	0	0	0
*Professional anxiety	1	1	1	1	0	0	0	1	0	0
*Advising profs	1	4	2	1	2	1	0	1	0	1
TOTAL – ALL ITEMS	25	17	17	12	12	7	6	13	1	3
OTHER MAIN SYMPTOM:	DVT Leg ulcer	"	"	→mobility	Urine obstruction	"	Double vision	Vomit	/	/
KARNOFSKY	060	060	060	040	040	040	040	030	020	020
DAYS IN: home	1	1	1	1	0	0	0	1	0	0
hospital	0	0	0	0	0	0	0	7	7	7
hospice	0	0	0	0	0	0	0	0	0	0
CONTACT WITH TEAMS: Face to face with: patient/family	2	2	1	1	2	2	1	2	2	3
professionals	1	1	2	0	2	0	1	1	1	0
Calls: patient/family	0	1	1	1	0	1	1	0	1	0
professionals	0	0	0	1	1	0	0	1	0	1
KEY TEAM WORKER:	02	02	02	03	02	02	05	05	02	03
COMMENTS:				→Catheter needed	Catheterised			Syringe driver started		

Fig. 3 Example of STAS assessments for Mr T—the weekly STAS scores of a 76-year-old man with metastatic cancer of the prostate. His wife was partially sighted and suffered from diabetes. They lived in a ground floor home. His main problems were pain due to a deep vein thrombosis, a leg ulcer, and bone metastasis, and frustration because he felt he was wasting a great deal of time with radiotherapy. In STAS each item is rated 0–4, with high scores indicating severe and low or 0 scores no problems. The chart shows scores over 9 weeks, from referral until he died. During care, pain due to his deep vein thrombosis and bone metastasis were resolved, but pain continued to be rated as 1 (mild), due to his ulcer. Practical needs occurred on two occasions during his care when he deteriorated. This can be seen when the scores for practical needs increase to 2 in week 2 and again in week 4. Initially, there was a need to improve communication between the hospital and community staff (indicated by a score of 4), because the general practitioner had not been aware of the treatment given in the hospital, and several different hospital consultants were involved. The decrease in scores in STAS shows how the team was able to improve many of Mr T's problems, and help his wife; most of his problems were alleviated in the last few weeks before he died. However, his symptoms and the concerns of his wife were only fully resolved after he was admitted to hospital in week 7.

combined with opioids in patients with moderate to severe pain.[71],[72] Regular opioid analgesics are the main stay of therapy for chronic cancer pain, and oral morphine remains the drug of choice, but other opioid agonists, such as hydromorphone and oxycodone, exhibit similar pharmokinetic and pharmacodynamic properties in cancer pain.[73] Slow-release oral morphine preparations are available in many countries. These preparations are used for the maintenance of analgesia in patients who have been appropriately titrated, usually

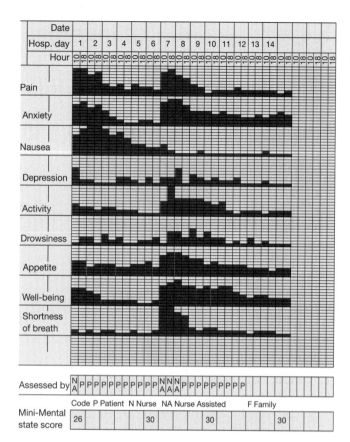

Fig. 4 Edmonton Symptom Assessment System assessments for one patient—a 64-year-old woman with advanced carcinoma of the breast with multiple bone metastases who was admitted because of poor control of pain and nausea. Note pulmonary embolism on day 7. After an increase in the dose of morphine and the institution of both metoclopramide and dexamethasone, good pain control was achieved. Unfortunately, during day 7, she presented with sudden onset of severe dyspnoea and chest pain. The diagnosis of pulmonary embolism was made and oxygen, subcutaneous heparin, and an increase in the dose of morphine were administered. Her dyspnoea progressively improved over the next few days. Her appetite, sensation of well being, and activity deteriorated significantly as a result of the pulmonary embolism and progressively improved after successful treatment with anticoagulation.

using rapid-release opioid analgesics[74],[75] and all patients should be allowed intermittent extra doses (5–20 per cent of regular 24-h oral dose) of rapid-release opioids for breakthrough pain.[76]

Adjuvant drugs

Opioid analgesics may not completely control pain syndromes in some patients, particularly in instances of neuropathic pain (see Chapter 5.8). Coanalgesics such as tricyclics[77],[78] and neuroleptics[79] can be used for neuropathic pain, although there are no randomized, controlled trials in advanced cancer (level of evidence 2–4). If patients are unable to take oral medication, it is often difficult to find alternative routes for these adjuvant drugs, and they may have to be discontinued when patients are at the very end of life.

Table 3 Cancer patients: prevalence of problems (per 1 000 000 population)

Symptom	Percentage with symptom in last year of life*	Estimated number in each year per million population
Pain	84	2357
Trouble with breathing	47	1318
Vomiting or feeling sick	51	1431
Sleeplessness	51	1431
Mental confusion	33	926
Depression	38	1065
Loss of appetite	71	1992
Constipation	47	1318
Bedsores	28	785
Loss of bladder control	37	1038
Loss of bowel control	25	701
Unpleasant smell	19	533
Total deaths from cancer		2805

*As per studies of Cartwright and Seale based on a random sample of deaths and using the reports of bereaved carers[20]

Note: Patients usually have several symptoms.

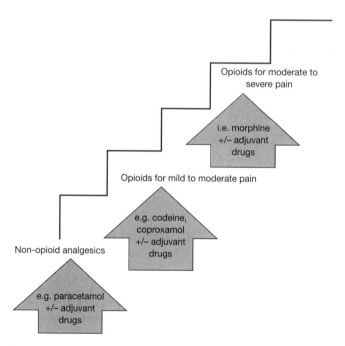

Fig. 5 WHO analgesic ladder.

Pain control when patients are dying

While patients are dying, and even when they become unconscious, pain control using regular analgesics is still required if it was needed

Table 4 Issues in pain control in dying cancer patients

Need for alternate opioid routes (e.g. subcutaneous, rectal)

Borderline cognition (for tolerance of adjuvant psychotropics)

Dehydration, decreased renal function (accumulation of opioid metabolites)

Fluctuating consciousness, sedation, delirium (difficult pain assessment)

Need to support family assessment of pain and its treatment

Mechanical factors
- **Disease within the lung**, e.g. primary or secondary tumour, mesothelioma, lymphangitis carcinomatosis, lung collapse or consolidation, infection, emphysema, chronic obstructive airways disease, asthma, bronchospasm, fibrosis post-radiotherapy;
- **Disease outside the lung**, e.g. pleural effusion, ascites, hepatomegaly, mediastinal or paratracheal lymphadenopathy, superior vena cava obstruction, pericardial effusion.

Impaired diffusion of respiratory gases—e.g. pulmonary embolism, pulmonary oedema, ischaemic heart disease.

Biochemical factors—anaemia, uraemia.

Psychogenic factors—anxiety, fear, depression, hyperventilation syndrome (characteristics are dyspnoea plus tingling or muscle tremors, faintness, dizziness, and sometimes sweating, palpitations and angina).

Fig. 6 Mechanisms of breathlessness.

at an earlier stage of illness. Table 4 shows some of the special problems in pain management in dying cancer patients. A common difficulty is that patients become too weak to swallow oral medication. The 24-h morphine dose can then be recalculated to provide a subcutaneous dose, and other medication can also be provided by this route. The most useful sites to insert the butterfly needle for subcutaneous infusions are the upper chest, outer aspect of the arm, abdomen, and thighs. Ambulatory infusion devices, syringe drivers, and other continuous delivery systems allow either a continuous or regular infusion of opioid, thus avoiding repeated injection. Patient controlled and spring operated delivery systems are also available and are particularly useful in countries where batteries to operate the delivery system cannot be obtained. The 24-h dose for subcutaneous delivery should be calculated based on prior treatment. Because of the unique difficulties outlined in Table 4, patients should undergo frequent assessment of pain, cognition, and other symptoms. The dose of opioids and other adjuvants should be frequently titrated in order to prevent metabolite accumulation or drug interactions contributing to agitated delirium.

Opioid side-effects

The most common side-effects of opioid analgesics are sedation, nausea, and constipation. Stool softeners and laxatives should be prescribed routinely. Sedation and nausea are frequent complications of initial doses, but usually subside spontaneously upon continuation of the opioid and are rarely a cause for halting analgesic treatment. There is no consistent evidence that one particular opioid agonist has significantly lower prevalence or intensity of sedation, nausea, or constipation compared to other opioid agonists, but individual patients may sometimes benefit from a change in the type of opioid. Occasionally, patients who have received high doses of opioids may develop cognitive impairment, severe sedation, hallucinations, or even myoclonis/grand mal seizures, and hyperalgesia. These side-effects are probably due to a combination of non-opioid effects due to the accumulation of excitory-active opioid metabolites and opioid effects of the parent compounds.[80] Some authors recommend a change in the opioid if the side-effects occur, such as from morphine to hydromorphone or methadone. This should only be undertaken by experienced clinicians.[81],[82] Other measures that can assist in the treatment of acute episodes of opioid toxicity include dose reduction, hydration in order to increase the elimination of hydrosoluble active metabolites, and drugs for the management of agitation (see below).

Breathlessness

Breathlessness (or dyspnoea) is an uncomfortable awareness of breathing. Like pain, it is a subjective sensation that is universally experienced at some time or other. The mechanisms of breathlessness are shown in Fig. 6. Cancer patients present with breathlessness as a consequence of either abnormality of the blood gases or stimulation of their mechanoreceptors. Breathlessness is expressed differently among patients with similar levels of function. Therefore, the goal of treatment should be to improve the subjective sensation as experienced by the patient, rather than to improve abnormalities in blood gas or pulmonary function.

Breathlessness has many causes and occurs in 20 to 70 per cent of patients with advanced cancer before death.[83] The prevalence of breathlessness may increase in the last weeks of life, and is often difficult to control. Indeed, two studies suggest that since pain control has improved, breathlessness is the most prevalent severe symptom at the end of life.[84],[85] It can be due to lung cancer or metastases, pleural effusion, pulmonary embolism, muscle weakness, anaemia, pneumonia, chronic heart failure, chronic obstructive pulmonary disease, and/or psychological distress.[86]

Treatment of breathlessness

Specific causes of breathlessness, such as pulmonary embolism or pneumonia, should be treated if they are causing symptoms. General measures include ensuring that the patient is comfortable, providing information and discussion, and ensuring that the room is well ventilated. In some instances a fan is helpful.[87] Other supportive measures include modification in the activity level and the use of bathroom aids, walking aids, and portable oxygen. Physiotherapy assessment is often helpful and the patient can learn breathing and relaxation exercises, and family massage. This will improve performance and increase the autonomy of patients and their families, as well as relieve the symptoms. It also gives the family a positive role during acute attacks. Although generally advocated, these types of supportive measures have been tested only in descriptive and case studies.

Drug therapy

Several randomized, controlled trials have indicated beneficial effects of systemic opioids for breathlessness in cancer patients[88]–[90] (level of evidence 2). However, the optimal type, dose, and modality of administration has not yet been determined. In most practice, a therapeutic trial of a small dose of opioid is given. Nebulized opioids have attracted interest, because of the possibility that they will act locally, avoiding systemic side-effects. However, as yet the evidence is controversial. A retrospective chart review by Farncombe *et al.* of 40 patients suggested symptomatic benefit of nebulized opioids,[91] but a recent, randomized trial by Davis did not shown any benefit as opposed to placebo.[92]

Bronchodilators and methylxanthines (for example aminophylline) are indicated in patients with airways obstruction. A recent study demonstrated that almost half of 57 consecutive patients with lung cancer had evidence of airways obstruction and only four of these were receiving bronchodilators.[93] Thus, airways obstruction is commonly present among patients with bronchial cancer and is strongly associated with breathlessness, and is undertreated.

Corticosteroids may be effective in the management of breathlessness including that due to carcinomatosis lymphangitis and superior vena cava obstruction.[94] Benzodiazepines and other anxiolytics are commonly used in the management of cancer-related breathlessness, but two of the three randomized, controlled trials of these agents in chronic obstructive pulmonary disease found no significant benefit.[95]–[97] There are no trials in advanced cancer, although the drugs might be useful when anxiety is present.

Oxygen

Several randomized, controlled trials have suggested that oxygen has symptomatic benefits in patients with chronic obstructive pulmonary disease. The number of studies in cancer patients is small, but two randomized, controlled trials, which selected patients with cancer who had hypoxia and compared inspiration of oxygen and air, found that oxygen had a significant symptomatic benefit.[98],[99] If it is felt that oxygen may be of benefit, a therapeutic trial is worth considering.

Nursing interventions, relaxation, physiotherapy

A recent study suggested that a multifactoral intervention, which included information and explanation, support, lifestyle and home modification, development of strategies (such as relaxation) to deal with breathlessness, as well as a review of medications, has demonstrated benefits over a control group of oncology patients who did not receive this intervention.[100] In the trial the intervention was led by nurses, but it could be led by other professionals, such as physiotherapists.

Cachexia–anorexia

This syndrome consists of progressive weight loss, lipolysis, loss of visceral and skeletal protein mass, and profound anorexia. A majority of patients experience this devastating complication before dying of cancer and AIDS. It is most prevalent among patients with cancers of lung and pancreas, and least prevalent among patients with cancer of the breast.[101] Weight loss is an independent risk of poor survival, and cachectic patients have a higher incidence of complications after surgery, radiation therapy, and chemotherapy. In addition, cachexia aggravates weakness, associated with anorexia and chronic nausea, and is a source of psychological distress for patients and families because of the associated symptoms and the change in body image.

This syndrome was interpreted previously as the result of increased energy demands from the growing tumour mass. Recent research has demonstrated that cachexia occurs mostly as a result of major metabolic abnormalities including profound lipolysis and loss of skeletal and visceral proteins due to immune mediators such as tumour necrosis factor and interleukin-6, as well as tumour by-products including lipolytic hormone. Anorexia is an almost universal component of cachexia and should be interpreted as a result of the metabolic abnormalities rather than the main cause of cachexia.

Treatment

Unfortunately, studies of aggressive nutritional support, including enteral and parenteral nutrition, generally found no significant improvement in patient survival or tumour shrinkage, and limited effects on the complications associated with surgery, radiotherapy, or chemotherapy. Since most studies failed to assess patients' symptoms, it is not clear if intensive nutrition has any symptomatic benefits (level of evidence 2 to 5).[102] Intensive nutrition may be appropriate in certain clinical situations such as patients recovering from surgery and awaiting chemotherapy, or patients with slow-growing tumours and bowel obstruction in whom starvation due to lack of intake rather than metabolic abnormalities appear to be the main cause of cachexia.[103]

A number of drugs have been found to have beneficial effects on the symptoms of cachexia, and some have effects on patients' nutritional status.

Corticosteroids

A number of randomized, placebo-controlled trials have demonstrated the symptomatic effects of different types of corticosteroids.[104] All researchers have shown a limited effect of up to 4 weeks on appetite, food intake, sensation of well being, and performance status. None of the studies has demonstrated gain in body weight. Corticosteroids have also been found to improve nausea, asthenia,[105],[106] and pain control[107] and are useful in a wide variety of patients, especially those with short expected survival (level of evidence 3 to 5). The most effective type, dose, and route of administration has not been established and should be addressed in randomized, controlled trials.

Progestational drugs

These drugs have demonstrated dose-related effects on appetite, caloric intake, weight gain (mainly fat), and sensation of well being, with an optimal dose of megestrol acetate ranging from 480 to 800 mg/day administered orally. Recent studies involving terminally ill patients have found that the symptomatic improvement (appetite, fatigue, sensation of well being) occurs even in the absence of significant weight gain (level of evidence 2 to 4).[108],[109] Both megestrol and medroxyprogesterone can induce thromboembolic phenomena, breakthrough vaginal bleeding, peripheral oedema, hyperglycaemia, hypertension and Cushing's syndrome, alopecia, adrenal suppression, and adrenal insufficiency if the drug is abruptly discontinued. However, in most clinical trials, patients rarely needed to stop these drugs because of adverse effects. In patients requiring high-dose progestational drugs, financial cost may be very high.

Recent research suggests that, in the future, it may be possible to treat cancer cachexia with combined drug therapy focusing simultaneously on the release of immune by-products, the rate of protein breakdown in muscles, and the central causes of loss of appetite. Table 5 summarizes emerging drugs for the management of cancer cachexia.

The main outcome of the treatment of cancer cachexia should focus on the symptoms and quality of life rather than on nutritional

Table 5 Emerging drugs for cancer cachexia

Drug	Mechanism of action
Pentoxyfilline	↓Tumour necrosis factor-α
β₂-Adrenoreceptor agents (clenbuterol)	↓muscle protein breakdown
Anabolic androgenic steroids	protein synthesis through androgen receptor
Melatonin	↓Tumour necrosis factor-α; cytokine modulation
Thalidomide	↓Tumour necrosis factor-α; cytokine modulation
Cannabinoids	Central nervous system
ω-3 Fatty acids (fish oil)	↓Interleukin-6; tumour prolytic factors
Non-steroid anti-inflammatory drugs	↓Interleukin-6

Table 6 Drugs for the treatment of chronic nausea in cancer patients

Prokinetic agents	Metoclopramide Domperidone Cisapride
Corticosteroids	Dexamethasone Methylprednisolone
5HT₃ Antagonist	Ondansetron Granisetron
Decreased gastrointestinal secretion and mobility	Octreotide Hyoscine butylbromide
Other drugs	Haloperidol Dimenhydrinate Prochlorperazine

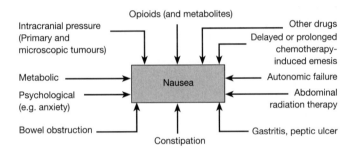

Fig. 7 Mechanisms of chronic nausea.

endpoints, since the survival of cachectic cancer patients is usually limited to weeks or months due to the incurable nature of the underlying malignancy.

Chronic nausea

Nausea lasting for longer than 4 weeks is very frequent in terminal cancer patients. It is a complex syndrome whose causes include autonomic dysfunction, which is frequent in advanced cancer patients, gastroparesis, and opioid analgesics, which can cause nausea by direct central effects, as well as by aggravated delayed gastric emptying, vestibular stimulation, and constipation (Fig. 7).

Treatment

When an underlying cause is identified, attempts should be made to correct it, including the management of metabolic abnormalities, aggressive bowel care, and treatment of metastases.

Symptomatic treatment includes antiemetics, summarized in Table 6 (see also Chapter 4.11). In patients with no bowel obstruction, metoclopramide is an effective agent due to its combination of central

and gastric emptying effects.[110] One study has suggested that slow-release metoclopramide is more effective than rapid-release metoclopramide in the control of chronic nausea (level of evidence grade 2).[111] Dexamethasone and other corticosteroids can potentiate the antiemetic effects of metoclopramide. In patients with contraindications to these two agents or who have bowel obstruction, a number of centrally-active agents can be administered including haloperidol or dimenhydrate. In patients with bowel obstruction, drugs capable of decreasing the amount of gastrointestinal secretions and motility, such as octreotide, can have a role in the control of nausea and vomiting.[112]

Unfortunately, while there has been much research into the pharmacological management of chemotherapy-induced emesis, chronic nausea has received minimal attention and, therefore, our understanding of the mechanisms and treatment of this syndrome continues to be limited.

Asthenia and weakness

This syndrome consists of profound tiredness upon usual or minimal efforts, accompanied by an unpleasant anticipatory sensation of generalized weakness. Asthenia and weakness are the most frequent symptoms associated with advanced cancer. The three main mechanisms are direct tumour effects, tumour-induced products, and accompanying conditions including anaemia, paraneoplastic syndromes, and chronic infections. Figure 8 summarizes the most common mechanisms of asthenia.

The relationship between asthenia and cachexia is complex. Many patients with advanced cancer have both symptoms, but some patients, such as those with breast cancer or lymphoma, may present with severe asthenia in the absence of malnutrition.

Management

Figure 9 summarizes a clinical approach to the management of asthenia. Whenever specific causes are identified, their correction will lead to improvement in asthenia. General non-pharmacological measures, such as adapting activities of daily living and occupational therapy, will help match clinical function and symptom status with the expectation of patients and families. Counselling may be of help to those patients in whom asthenia is an expression of affective

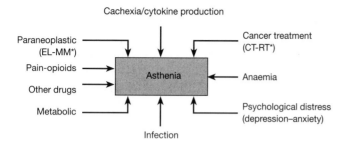

Fig. 8 Mechanisms of asthenia. *CT: chemotherapy; RT: radiotherapy; EL: Eaton–Lambert; MM: myasthenia, myocytes.

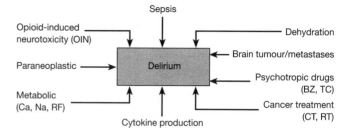

*CT: chemotherapy; RT: radiation therapy; RF: renal failure; TC: tricyclic antidepressant; BZ: benzodiazepines

Fig. 10 Mechanism of delirium. *CT: chemotherapy; RT: radiotherapy; RF: renal failure; TC: tricyclic antidepressants; BZ: benzodiazepines.

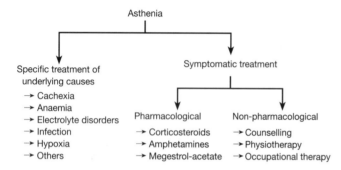

Fig. 9 Clinical approach to the management of asthenia.

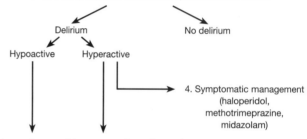

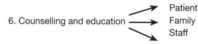

Fig. 11 Clinical approach to delirium in cancer patients.

disorders such as anxiety or depression. Consistent with the management of asthenia in chronic fatigue syndrome, in some instances gentle activity rather than rest can be helpful. Physiotherapy can help patients to make the most of their available strength. Most hospices now have physiotherapists who work with inpatients, and those attending day care and in the community. This helps to break the cycle of increased rest leading to increased muscle wasting leading to increased asthenia and fatigue.

General pharmacological measures include corticosteroids and amphetamines. Corticosteroids can decrease asthenia, either by inhibiting the release of tumour-induced substances or by a central euphoriant effect. Amphetamines have been found to antagonize opioid-induced sedation and fatigue. These drugs have also been proposed for the management of hypoactive–hypoalert delirium and fatigue, but their use tends to be confined to North America.

Delirium

Delirium, sometimes known as acute confusional state or acute brain syndrome, is characterized by acute onset cognitive impairment. It is distinguished from dementia by its acute rather than chronic onset, and its remitting rather than progressive nature. Patients experiencing delirium are often aware and they and their family are very anxious because of the delirium. Thresholds of detecting delirium vary, but some cognitive impairment, changing sleep–wake cycle, and fluctuating consciousness are common in terminal stages. Delirium is frequently undiagnosed[113] and it is important to check the more distressing manifestations of delirium, such as misinterpretations, psychomotor agitation, hallucinations, delusions, and other

abnormalities of perception. Frequent causes include: infection, dehydration, metabolic abnormalities, toxicity of opioids, benzodiazepines and other drugs, and cytokine production (Fig. 10). Figure 11 summarizes the clinical approach for the treatment of delirium of patients with advanced cancer.

Approximately 30 per cent of patients treated for cancer-related delirium experience complete improvement in cognition (level of evidence 4).[114] The remaining patients will usually continue in hypoactive delirium or will progressively become hypoactive if they were in hyperactive or mixed delirium. A small minority of patients may remain in a state of chronic hyperactive or mixed delirium and require chronic psychotropic medication.

Haloperidol is indicated in the symptomatic management of patients presenting with hyperactive forms of delirium, including psychomotor agitation, delusions, or hallucinations (level of evidence 4–5).[115] Haloperidol should be considered a temporary measure while other strategies such as change in the type of opioid, hydration, or the management of metabolic or infectious complications are introduced. In most patients, the hyperactive symptoms improve within 3 to 5 days.

Patients who failed to improve with at least two courses of neuroleptics may require aggressive sedation including the use of subcutaneous infusions of midazolam (level of evidence 4–5).[116] This highly liposoluble benzodiazepine is very potent and has a short half-life, allowing for rapid titration. As for other neuroleptics, the use of midazolam should normally be considered a short-term measure, while causes of reversible delirium are investigated and treated.

Constipation

Constipation is a frequent concomitant of terminal illness. Impacted faeces may simulate abdominal malignancy. Once this impaction is relieved and bowel mobility restored, the patient's condition frequently improves dramatically.

Causes of constipation include inactivity, weakness, dehydration, diminished food intake, low fibre diet, and direct or indirect effects from cancer such as narrowing of the gut, hypercalcaemia, or nerve damage. Constipation may also result as a side-effect of medication, such as opioids, iron, anticonvulsants, diuretics, vincristine, or anti-muscarinics, such as hyoscine.

A history with abdominal examination (including rectal examination if indicated) is needed to clarify the changes in bowel habit and characteristics of the stools.

If intestinal obstruction is a possibility, only laxatives with a predominantly softening action, such as lactulose or docusate sodium, should be used in order not to cause intestinal cramps. Otherwise in terminal illness a large dose of laxatives is usually needed. The bulk stimulants are less frequently used because patients are often reluctant to take copious fluid and these also can aggravate the situation if intestinal motility is impaired. However, patients can be improved if they can drink extra fluid, particularly fruit drinks. Supportive measures are often very important. These include ensuring privacy in hospital units, taking the patient to the toilet area, even if using a commode, rather than expecting the patient to use a bedpan in the area where she or he is eating and sleeping, and raising the toilet seat or, if possible, installing hand rails in the home. Rectal measures, such as suppositories and enemas, may be needed despite oral laxatives. Constipation needs to be anticipated, enquired about, and treated throughout the course of illness.

Communication and information

Poor communication is one of the most common reasons for litigation and complaint, and poor communication results in dissatisfaction and increased comorbidity of both the cancer patient and their family or carers (see Chapter 6.2).

Towards the end of life, patients and their families or carers may have specific concerns that they wish to discuss, or at least express. These may related to the diagnosis, or prognosis, or to particular things that they wish to do or sort out before she or he dies. The skills needed for effective communication in palliative care include: listening, assessment, facilitation, techniques for handling difficult questions, and self-awareness (see Chapter 6.2 for further details). When they become very frail, patients may need more time to express their concerns. Concerns can range widely, but some of the difficult issues may relate to fears about the process of death, how dying will happen, and what will happen afterwards. Some people may wish to plan their funerals in advance, but others may not wish to discuss death at all.

Psychological and emotional concerns

Psychological and emotional problems are common in terminal illness but are often ignored or dismissed by the patient's family and by professionals. In depth discussion is often needed to identify the causes of the problems and these may be quite different from what one might expect. There are many interwoven factors that may include the family, finances, spiritual needs, guilt, anger, fear of dying, or unrelieved physical symptoms. All staff are relevant but the appropriate chaplain, pastor, and/or social worker can have important roles in supporting the anxious and frightened patient. A psychiatrist or psychologist will be needed for more complicated problems or to assess psychiatric morbidity such as depression or severe anxiety states (see Chapter 6.1).

The patient may employ different defence mechanisms and coping strategies including:

- regression—becoming more child-like;
- denial—to blot out or ignore some realities;
- rationalization—providing an alternative everyday explanation for symptoms or feelings rather than the true one;
- intellectualization—becoming theoretical (often used by doctors and nurses in painful situations);
- projection—pushing the problem on to others;
- displacement—displacing emotional energy into other thoughts and activities;
- introjection—looking within oneself to find solutions;
- repression—unconscious suppression of painful memories;
- withdrawal and avoidance—withdrawing from and avoiding painful situations.

Understanding these mechanisms can help staff to explain and empathize with a patient's behaviour. It is only when the mechanisms are in excess that problems occur—for example excessive introjection can result in self-blame, isolation and depression; excessive projection can result in alienation of friends and family members or paranoid states; excessive displacement can lead to complete exhaustion followed by severe depression or anxiety.

The stress of prolonged illness or the shock of a recent diagnosis of terminal cancer can predispose a person to psychiatric and psychological problems, particularly if they have few external supports (for example if they live alone, have few friends, or are very poor), have limited communication skills (such as in learning difficulties or impaired vision or hearing), or if they have a history of mental health problems.

Fear and anxiety

Fear and anxiety in a patient can be recognized. The face generally expresses their emotions. Some patients attempt to disguise their feelings by a fixed smile and there is often a tightening of the facial muscles, particularly the forehead.

In depth discussion is often needed over a period of time and any causes for anxiety (such as poor pain control) should be dealt with. Some patients find comfort from living each day for what pleasures, joys, and comforts can be achieved in that day, or by keeping a diary and recording their enjoyments, looking always for the positive uplifting events.

Benzodiazepines (such as diazepam, 2–5 mg, two or three times daily, or the shorter-acting lorazepam) can be helpful, particularly if the patient has a chronic anxiety state and was already taking a small dose of these medications. Benzodiazepines with a long half-life, such as diazepam, are sedating and tend to accumulate in frail or elderly people, but, short-acting benzodiazepines, although less sedating, have more withdrawal phenomena. Extreme agitation may require a neuroleptic such as haloperidol, and in small doses this may also help milder anxiety. Sedating antidepressants, such an amitriptyline and dothiepin, are increasingly used in anxiety states and imipramine is helpful if there are panic attacks.

Non-pharmacological techniques such as relaxation therapy, aromatherapy, exercises in breathing control (especially if hyperventilation is a problem), and massage may sometimes allow drug treatment to be withdrawn.

Depression

Recent research suggests that, although adjustment disorders are common (25–35 per cent of patients), a minority (5–15 per cent) of patients become seriously depressed.[117] Depression often goes undetected, partly because patients do not readily volunteer the symptoms and partly because it is often difficult to decide where natural sadness ends and depression begins (see Chapter 6.1). Too often it is assumed that depression in terminal illness is to be expected or is untreatable. Depression causes considerable suffering for the patient and their family and therefore should be rigorously treated. Depression is usually characterized by a gradual onset of the following symptoms and signs:

- depressed mood or irritability;
- loss of interest and enjoyment;
- agitation or retardation;
- self-neglect or self-mutilation;
- cognitive triad—self is worthless, outside world meaningless, and future hopeless;
- diurnal mood swings (low mood in the morning);
- early morning wakening;
- change in behaviour—becoming indecisive, withdrawn, arguing.

Often the physical symptoms of depression such as weight loss, anorexia, fatigue, and constipation cannot be used for diagnosis because these may be present due to the terminal illness. Depression should also be distinguished from an adjustment disorder—a maladaptive reaction to a stress that occurs within 3 months and persists for no more than 3 months. The symptoms of an adjustment disorder are less specific than those of depression and often fluctuate from day to day; in general it will respond to psychological support.

Management should include (see also Chapter 6.1):

- consideration of possible organic causes of depression including drugs such as diuretics and antihypertensives, cimetidine, metoclopramide, methotrexate, orvinblastine, if possible, these should be stopped;
- emotional and psychological support;
- antidepressant drugs.

Serotonin uptake inhibitors (such as fluoxetine, 20 mg daily) are effective antidepressants and are less sedating and have fewer antimuscarinic and cardiovascular side effects than tricyclics. Tricyclic antidepressant drugs are sometimes used, especially if these are also being considered for their effect in neuropathic pain. These start at a low dose and gradually increase to the therapeutic range; amitriptyline is useful if sedation is required: the newer drugs such as trazodone (sedating) and lofepramine (less sedating) are reported to have fewer antimuscarinic and cardiovascular adverse effects and so are often recommended in very elderly or debilitated patients. All antidepressants have some adverse effects, most commonly dry mouth, blurred vision, hesitancy of micturition, and constipation, and it is wise to warn patients in advance of these symptoms. All of the antidepressants take 2 to 3 weeks to elevate mood, although patients may benefit from the anxiolytic or sedative effects much earlier.

Family or carer concerns

Little is known about the psychosocial impact of caring for a dying relative on carers: most research has focused on carers in the bereavement stage. However, in the advanced phase of illness the family and those close to the patient can experience heightened symptoms of depression, anxiety, psychosomatic symptoms, restriction of roles and activities, strain in relationships, and poor physical health. Some studies have reported spouses as experiencing the same level of distress and anxiety as patients. A longitudinal study suggested that a substantial group of caregivers experience distress one year after diagnosis and that mental health status declined for 30 per cent of carers.[118] In a recent study, 32 per cent of carers were rated as having severe anxiety at the time of referral of the patient to six specialist palliative home care teams, and anxiety remained severe for 26 per cent of carers in the patient's last week of life.[119] Therefore, it is not only during bereavement that carers need support. Interventions designed specifically for carers have rarely been evaluated and a range of models of support exist, from replacement services, such as respite care and day care, to individualized discussions and group support. Respite care for patients often aims to relieve the carers of the burden of care in the home but the extent to which these services achieve this goal has not yet been evaluated in comparative studies. In a United States randomized, controlled trial, Toseland et al. evaluated a 6-week carer support intervention of 1.5 h per week for 80 spouses of cancer patients.[120] Fear of the spouse dying was the most common pressing problem reported. The study found improvements in physical aspects, role, and social functioning of the carers with the most distress in the intervention group compared to the control group. Coping strategies in the form of support, information, and coping skills were the most effective. This study needs to be replicated,

Table 7 How effective are specialist palliative care services?

Specialist palliative care service	Studies	Findings: compared with conventional care
Inpatient	1 RCT, >5 comparative quasi-experimental studies versus conventional care	Equal or improved symptoms, improved satisfaction
Multidisciplinary home-care team	3 RCTs, >5 comparative quasi-experimental studies versus conventional care	Longer time at home, equal or improved symptoms, improved satisfaction
Multidisciplinary hospital team	Descriptive studies	Symptoms and problems improve during care (as for home care and inpatient)

Source: Higginson, Radcliffe Medical Press, 1997;[123] Hearn and Higginson, 1998.[14]

especially where reactions to group therapies and psychosocial needs may differ from the United States. Stress and appraisal of events is individual and carers will differ in the extent to which they find coping methods useful. Therefore, interventions that take an eclectic approach may prove the most beneficial.

Specialist palliative care services

Hospices and specialist palliative care services have increased rapidly in number world-wide. In 1998, there were over 1400 hospice or palliative care services in 35 countries in Europe, almost 600 in Canada, approximately 3000 in the United States, and over 240 in Australasia.[121] In the United Kingdom, there were over 210 inpatient hospices, over 400 home-care teams, and over 260 palliative care teams working in hospitals. Palliative services and hospices usually offer a shared model of care. In the United Kingdom, just over 50 per cent of cancer patients who die receive care from some kind of palliative care team or nurse.[122]

Multiprofessional team

The specialists who may be included in a multiprofessional palliative care team are doctors, clinical nurse specialists, social workers, chaplains, therapists, and psychologists or psychiatrists. The team aims to:

- achieve accurate and speedy assessment and diagnosis of the problems;
- plan and implement effective integrated treatment and care;
- communicate effectively with the patient, family, and with all other professionals and agencies involved in the care of the patient, and within itself;
- audit its activities and outcomes.

A systematic review of the effectiveness of specialist palliative care multiprofessional teams identified 18 relevant studies. These included randomized, controlled trials and comparative or observational studies. When specialist multidisciplinary care is compared to conventional care, four of the five randomized, controlled trials and the majority of the comparative studies indicate that the specialist, co-ordinated approach resulted in similar or improved outcomes in terms of patient satisfaction, the patient being cared for where they wished, family satisfaction, and better control of family anxiety and the patient's pain and other symptoms (see Table 7). Those studies that

examined costs showed a tendency for a reduction in hospital inpatient days, more time spent at home, and equal or lower costs. There were no worse outcomes associated with specialist multidisciplinary care, although the early studies carried out by Parkes[7],[10] showed more pain in patients cared for at home compared to hospital or hospice; in these studies specialist multidisciplinary teams were operating in both home and hospice.

Only one study attempted to examine the 'team' effect separately from the general effect of a palliative care service.[124],[125] In this observational study (level 4) of 207 patients who had died at home, no combination of health-care professionals was consistently effective but a general practitioner provided the poorest overall care. In this study no general practitioner working alone provided financial advice to patients or families, and the combination of a specialist nurse and general practitioner failed to provide advice about other local sources of support. This study reported that for those carers needing training with simple nursing tasks, teams which contained a district nurse provided such training more often than those which did not, and for symptom control the specialist nurse, general practitioner, and district nurse combined appeared to provide the highest relief.

Summary

Care for people who are dying from cancer is an important part of cancer care. The patient and the family should be regarded as the unit of care: the term 'family' is taken in its broad sense and encompasses close relatives, a partner, and close friends. Care is concerned with physical, emotional, social, and spiritual problems for patients and families. It focuses on the quality of remaining life of the patient and on the support of the family and those close to the patient. Care at the end of life continues from good earlier care. Control of pain, using WHO guidelines and based usually on regular opioid medication, and the management of other symptoms are important component of care. Needs of the family are commonly overlooked and often require specific attention. The multiprofessional palliative care team, usually through specialist palliative care services, has been proven an effective means of meeting more closely the needs of patients and families.

References

1. **Hanratty J.** *Palliative care of the terminally ill.* Oxford: Radcliffe Medical Press, 1989.

2. **Higginson IJ, Astin P, Dolan S.** Where do cancer patients die? Ten-year trends in the place of death of cancer patients in England. *Palliative Medicine*, 1998; **12**: 353–63.

3. **Cartwright A.** Dying. In: Ebrahim S, Kalache A, eds. *Epidemiology in old age.* London: BMJ Publications, 1996: 408–14.

4. **Murray CJ, Lopez AD.** Alternative projections of mortality and disability by cause 1990–2020: Global Burden of Disease Study. *Lancet*, 1997; **349**: 1498–504.

5. **Higginson IJ.** Health care needs assessment: palliative and terminal care. In: Stevens A, Raftery J, eds. *Health care needs assessment.* 2nd Series. Oxford: Radcliffe Medical Press, 1997.

6. **Cartwright A, Hockey L, Anderson JL.** *Life before death.* London: Routledge and Kegan Paul, 1973.

7. **Parkes CM.** Home or hospital? Terminal care as seen by surviving spouses. *Journal of the Royal College General Practitioners*, 1978; **28**: 19–30.

8. **Morris JN, Sherwood S, Wright SM, Gutkin CE.** The last weeks of life: does hospice make a difference? In: Mor V, Greer DS, Kastenbaum R, eds. *The hospice experiment.* Baltimore: John Hopkins University Press, 1988:109–32.

9. **Higginson I, Wade A, McCarthy M.** Palliative care: views of patients and their families. *British Medical Journal*, 1990; **301**: 277–81.

10. **Parkes CM.** Terminal care: evaluation of in-patient service at St Christopher's Hospice. Part II. Self-assessments of effects of the service on surviving spouses. *Postgraduate Medical Journal*, 1979; **55**: 523–7.

11. **Greer DS, Mor V.** An overview of national hospice study findings. *Journal of Chronic Disease*, 1986; **39**: 5–7.

12. **Kane RL, Klein SJ, Bernstein L, Rothenberg R, Wales J.** Hospice role in alleviating the emotional stress of terminal patients and their families. *Medical Care*, 1985; **23**: 189–97.

13. **Zimmer JG, Groth-Juncker A, McCusker J.** Effects of a physician-led home care team on terminal care. *Journal of the American Geriatric Society*, 1984; **32**: 288–92.

14. **Hearn J, Higginson IJ.** Do specialist palliative care teams improve outcomes for cancer patients? A systematic literature review of the evidence. *Palliative Medicine*, 1998; **12**: 317–32.

15. **Salisbury C, Bosanquet N, Wilkinson EK, Franks PJ, Kite S, Lorentzon M, Naysmith A.** The impact of different models of specialist palliative care on patients' quality of life: a systematic literature review. *Palliative Medicine*, 1999; **13**: 3–17.

16. **Working party on Clinical Guidelines in Palliative Care.** *Changing Gear. Guidelines for managing patients at the end of life.* London: National Council for Hospice and Specialist Palliative Care Services, 1997.

17. **Heath K.** Fostering hope in terminally ill people. *Journal of Advanced Nursing* 1990; **15**: 1250–9.

18. **Weisman AD.** The psychiatrist and the inexorable. In: Feifel JC, ed. *New meanings of death.* New York: McGraw-Hill, 1977.

19. **Kellehear A.** *Dying of cancer. The final year of life.* London: Harwood, 1990.

20. **Cartwright A.** Changes in life and care in the year before death 1969–1987. *Journal of Public Health Medicine*, 1991; **13**: 81–7.

21. **Higginson IJ, Astin P, Dolan S.** Where do cancer patients die? Ten year trends in the place of death of cancer patients in England. *Palliative Medicine*, 1998; **12**: 353–63.

22. **Hospice Information Service.** *Directory of hospice and palliative care services for the United Kingdom and Ireland.* London: Hospice Information Service, St Christopher's Hospice, 1999.

23. **Mann WJ, Loesch M, Shurpin KM, Chalas E.** Determinants of home versus hospital terminal care for patients with gynaecological cancer. *Cancer*, 1993; **71**: 2876–9.

24. **Bowling A.** The hospitalisation of death: should more people die at home? *Journal of Medical Ethics*, 1983; **9**: 158–61.

25. **Miller FG, Fins JJ.** A proposal to restructure hospital care for dying patients. *New England Journal of Medicine*, 1996; **334**: 1740–2.

26. **Sen-Gupta GJA, Higginson IJ.** Home care in advanced cancer: a systematic literature review of preferences for and associated factors. *Psycho-Oncology*, 1998; **7**: 57–67.

27. **Dunlop R, Davies RJ, Hockley JM.** Preferred versus actual place of death: a hospital palliative care support team study. *Palliative Medicine*, 1989; **3**: 197–201.

28. **Ashby M, Wakefield M.** Attitudes to come aspects of death and dying, living wills and substituted health care decision-making in South Australia: public opinion survey for a parliamentary select committee. *Palliative Medicine*, 1993; **7**: 273–82.

29. **Hinton J.** Can home care maintain an acceptable quality of life for patients with terminal cancer and their relatives? *Palliative Medicine*, 1994; **8**: 183–96.

30. **Costantini M, Camoirano E, Madeddu L, Bruzzi P, Verganelli E, Henrique F.** Palliative home care and place of death among cancer patients: a population based study. *Palliative Medicine*, 1993; **7**: 323–31.

31. **Townsend J, Frank AO, Fermont D, Dyer S, Karran O, Walgrove A, Piper M.** Terminal cancer care and patients' preference for place of death: a prospective study. *British Medical Journal*, 1990; **301**: 415–17.

32. **Addington-Hall J, MacDonald LD.** Dying from cancer: the views of bereaved family and friends about the experiences of terminally ill patients. *Palliative Medicine*, 1991; **5**: 207–14.

33. **Beckingham A.** *Palliative care in Bexley and Greenwich for people with cancer.* Part 1. A study of effectiveness, quality and coverage, Vol. 1. London: Department of Public Health, Bexley and Greenwich, 1996: 1–55.

34. **Brent and Harrow Health Authority.** *Review of palliative care services.* London: Brent and Harrow Health Authority, 1994:1–67.

35. **Charlton RC.** Attitudes towards the care of the dying: A questionnaire survey of general practice attenders. *Family Practice*, 1991; **8**: 356–9.

36. **Gilbar O, Steiner M.** When death comes: where should patients die? *Hospital Journal* 1996; **11**: 31–48.

37. **McWhinney IR, Bass MJ, Orr V.** Factors associated with location of death (home or hospital) of patients referred to a palliative care team. *Canadian Medical Association Journal*, 1995; **152**: 362–7.

38. **Neubauer BJ, Hamilton CL.** Racial differences in attitudes towards hospice care. *Hospice Journal*, 1990; **6**:.37–48.

39. **Spiller JA, Alexander DA.** Domiciliary care: a comparison of the views of terminally ill patients and their family caregivers. *Palliative Medicine*, 1993; **7**: 109–15.

40. **Toscani F, Cantoni L.** Death and dying: perceptions and attitudes in Italy. *Palliative Medicine*, 1991; **5**: 334–43.

41. **Ward AWM.** Terminal care in malignant disease. *Social Science and Medicine*, 1974; **8**: 413–20.

42. **Zusman ME, Tschetler P.** Selecting whether to die at home or in a hospital setting. *Death Education*, 1984; **8**: 365–81.

43. **Bruera E, MacDonald S.** Audit methods: The Edmonton symptom assessment system. In: Higginson I, ed. *Clinical audit in palliative care.* Oxford: Radcliffe Medical Press, 1993.

44. **Cella DF.** Measuring the quality of life in palliative care. *Seminars in Oncology*, 1986; **79**: 165–9.

45. **Bullinger M.** Quality of life assessment in palliative care. *Journal of Palliative Care*, 1992; **8**: 34–9.

46. **Finlay IG, Dunlop R.** Quality of life assessment in palliative care. *Annals of Oncology*, 1994; **5**: 13–18.

47. **Miller RD, Walsh TD.** Psychosocial aspects of palliative care in advanced cancer. *Journal of Pain and Symptom Management*, 1991; **6**: 24–9.

48. **McCarthy M, Higginson IJ.** Clinical audit by a palliative care team. *Palliative Medicine*, 1991; **5**: 215–21.

49. **Higginson I.** *Quality, standards, clinical and organisational audit for*

palliative care. London: National Council for Hospice and Specialist Palliative Care Services, 1992.

50. Higginson I, McCarthy M. Validity of a measure of palliative care—comparison with a quality of life index. *Palliative Medicine*, 1994; **8**: 282–90.

51. Ellershaw JE, Peat SJ, Boys LC. Assessing the effectiveness of a hospital palliative care team. *Palliative Medicine*, 1995; **9**: 145–52.

52. Cohen SR, Mount BM, Bruera E, Provost M, Rowe J, Tong K. Validity of the McGill Quality of Life Questionnaire in the palliative setting: a multicentre Canadian study demonstrating the importance of the existential domain. *Palliative Medicine*, 1997; **11**: 3–20.

53. Higginson I, Wade A, McCarthy M. Effectiveness of two palliative support teams. *Journal of Public Health Medicine*, 1992; **1**: 50–6.

54. Higginson I. Audit methods: a community schedule. In: Higginson I, ed. *Clinical audit in palliative care*. Oxford: Radcliffe Medical Press, 1993.

55. Higginson I, McCarthy M. Validity of the support team assessment schedule: do staffs' ratings reflect those made by patients or their families? *Palliative Medicine*, 1993; **7**: 219–28.

56. Higginson I. Audit methods: validation and in-patient use. In: Higginson I, ed. *Clinical audit in palliative care*. Oxford: Radcliffe Medical Press, 1993.

57. Hearn J, Higginson IJ. The process of conducting a multi-centre study to validate a core outcome measure in palliative care settings. *Journal of Pain and Symptom Management* 1998; **15**: S10.

58. McKee E. Audit experience: a nurse manager in home care. In: Higginson I, ed. *Clinical audit in palliative care*. Oxford: Radcliffe Medical Press, 1993.

59. Edmonds PM, Stuttaford JM, Penny J, Lynch AM, Chamberlain J. Do hospital palliative care teams improve symptom control? Use of modified STAS as an evaluation tool. *Palliative Medicine*, 1998; **12**: 345–51.

60. Higginson I. Clinical teams, general practice, audit and outcomes. In: *Outcomes into clinical practice*. London: British Medical Association, 1994.

61. Bruera E, Kuehn N, Miller M, Selmser P, MacMillan K. The Edmonton symptom assessment system (ESAS): A simple method for the assessment of palliative care patients. *Journal of Palliative Care*, 1991; **7**: 6–9.

62. Field D, Douglas C, Jagger C, Jagger D, Jagger P. Terminal illness: views of patients and their lay carers. *Palliative Medicine*, 1995; **9**: 45–54.

63. Higginson I, Priest P, McCarthy M. Are bereaved family members a valid proxy for a patient's assessment of dying? *Society of Scientific Medicine*, 1994; **38**: 553–7.

64. Hinton J. How reliable are relative's retrospective reports of terminal illness? Patients and relatives accounts compared. *Society of Scientific Medicine*, 1996; **43**: 1229–36.

65. Hearn J, Higginson IJ. *Epidemiology of pain in cancer*. London: Department of Palliative Care and Policy.

66. Bernabei R, *et al.* Management of pain in elderly patients with cancer. *Journal of the American Medical Association*, 1998; **279**: 1877–82.

67. Ventafridda V, Tamburini M, Caraceni C, DeConno F, Naldi F. A validation study of the WHO method for cancer pain relief. *Cancer*, 1987; **59**: 850–6.

68. Walker VA, Hoskin PJ, Hanks GW, White ID. Evaluation of WHO analgesic guidelines for cancer pain in a hospital-based palliative care unit. *Journal of Pain and Symptom Management*, 1988; **3**: 145–9.

69. Twycross RG. Cancer pain a global perspective. In: Twycross RG, ed. *The Edinburgh symposium on pain and medical education*. Royal Society of Medicine International Symposium Series (149), London, 1989:3–16.

70. Takeda F. Results of field-testing in Japan of the WHO draft interim guidelines of relief of cancer pain. *Pain Clinic*, 1986; **1**: 83–9.

71. Pace V. The use of non-steroidal anti-inflammatory drugs in cancer. *Palliative Medicine*, 1995; **9**: 273–86.

72. Portenoy RK. Adjuvant analgesics in pain management. In: Doyle D, Hanks GWC, MacDonald N, eds. Oxford: *Oxford textbook of palliative medicine*. Oxford University Press, 1993:229–44.

73. Schug SA, Zech D, Dorr U. Cancer pain management according to WHO analgesic guidelines. *Journal of Pain and Symptom Management*, 1990; **5**: 27–32.

74. Walsh TD, McDonald N, Bruera E, Shepherd KV, Michaud M, Zanes R. A controlled study of sustained-release morphine sulphate tablets in chronic pain from advanced cancer. *American Journal of Clinical Oncology (CCT)*, 1992; **15**: 268–72.

75. Bruera E, Sloan P, Mount B, Scott J, Suarez-Almazor M. A randomised double blind double dummy crossover trial comparing the safety and efficacy of oral sustained-release hydromorphone with immediate release hydromorphone in patients with cancer pain. Canadian Palliative Care Clinical Trials Group. *Journal of Clinical Oncology*, 1996; **14**: 1713–7.

76. Coluzzi P. A titration study of oral transmucosal phentonyl citrate for breakthrough pain in cancer patients. *Proceedings of the American Society of Clinical Oncology*, 1997; (Abstract 134) **16**: 325..

77. McQuay HJ, Tramer M, Nye BA, Carroll D, Wiffen PJ, Moore RA. A systematic review of antidepressants in neuropathic pain. *Pain*, 1996; **68**: 217–27.

78. McQuay HJ, Moore RA. Antidepressants and chronic pain. *British Medical Journal*, 1997; **314**: 763–4.

79. McQuay H, Carroll D, Jadad AR, Wiffen P, Moore A. Anticonvulsant drugs for management of pain: a systematic review. *British Medical Journal*, 1995; **311**: 1047–52.

80. Ripamonti C, Bruera E. CNS adverse effects of opioids in cancer patients. Guidelines for treatment. *Central Nervous System Drugs*, 1997; **8**: 21–37.

81. Lawler PG, Turner KS, Hanson J, Bruera ED. Dose ratio between morphine and methadone in patients with cancer pain. *Cancer*, 1998; **82**: 1167–73.

82. Bruera E, Pereira J, Watanabe S, Belzile M, Cuehn N, Hanson J. Opioid rotation in patients with cancer pain. A retrospective comparison of dose, ratios between methadone, hydromorphone and morphine. *Cancer*, 1996; **78**: 852–7.

83. Heyse-Moore L, Ross V, Mulles M. How much of a problem is dyspnoea in advanced cancer? *Palliative Medicine*, 1991; **5**: 20–6.

84. Higginson IJ, McCarthy M. Measuring symptoms in terminal cancer: are pain and dyspnoea controlled? *Journal of the Royal Society of Medicine*, 1989; **82**: 264–7.

85. Reuben DB, Mor V. Dyspnea in terminally ill cancer patients. *Chest*, 1986; **89**: 234–6.

86. Simon PM, *et al.* Distinguishable types of dyspnea in patients with shortness of breath. *American Review of Respiratory Disease*, 1990; **142**: 1009–14.

87. Schwartzstein RM, *et al.* Cold facial stimulation reduces breathlessness induced in normal subjects. *American Review Respiratory Disease*, 1987; **136**: 58.

88. Bruera E, *et al.* Subcutaneous morphine for dyspnoea in cancer patients. *Archives of Internal Medicine*, 1993; **119**: 906–7.

89. Cohen MH, *et al.* Continuous intravenous infusion of morphine for severe dyspnea. *Southern Medical Journal*, 1991; **84**: 229–34.

90. Bruera E, *et al.* The effects of morphine on the dyspnoea of terminal cancer patients. *Journal of Pain and Symptom Management*, 1990; **5**: 341–4.

91. Farncombe M, Chater S, Gillin A. The use of nebulised opioids for breathlessness: a chart review. *Palliative Medicine*, 1994; **8**: 306–12.

92. Davis C. The role of nebulised drugs in palliating respiratory symptoms. *European Journal of Palliative Care*, 1995; **2**: 9–15.

93. Congleton J, Mures MF. The incidence of airflow obstruction in bronchial carcinoma, its relation to breathlessness and response to bronchodilator therapy. *Respiratory Medicine*, 1995; 89: 291–6.

94. Weir DC, *et al.* Corticosteriods trials in non-asthmatic chronic airflow obstruction: a comparison of oral prednisolone and inhaled beclomethasone diproprionate. *Thorax*, 1991; 45: 112–7.

95. Man GCW, Sproule BJ. Effect of alprazolam on exercise and dyspnea in patients with chronic obstructive pulmonary disease. *Chest*, 1986; 90: 832–6.

96. Woodcock AA, Gross ER, Geddes DM. Drug treatment of breathlessness: contrasting effects of diazepam and promethazine in pink puffers. *British Medical Journal*, 1981; 283: 343–6.

97. Mitchell-Heggs P, *et al.* Diazepam in the treatment of dyspnoea in the pink puffer syndrome. *Quarterly Journal of Medicine*, 1980; 69: 9–20.

98. Bruera E, *et al.* The effects of oxygen on the intensity on dyspnoea in hypoxemic terminal cancer patients. *Lancet*, 1993; 343: 13–14.

99. Bruera E, Schoeller T, MacEachern T. Symptomatic benefit of supplemental oxygen in hypoxemic patients with terminal cancer: the use of the N1 randomised controlled trial. *Journal of Pain and Symptom Management*, 1992; 7: 365–8.

100. Bredin M, Corner J, Krishnasamy M, Plant H, Bailey C, A'Hern R. Multicentre randomised controlled trial of nursing intervention for breathlessness in patients with lung cancer. *British Medical Journal*, 1999; 318: 901–4.

101. Bruera E. ABC of palliative care: anorexia, cachexia and nutrition. *British Medical* Journal, 1997; 315: 1219–22.

102. Vigano A, Bruera E. Enteral and parenteral nutrition in cancer patients. In: Bruera E, Higginson I, eds. *Cachexia-anorexia in cancer patients*. Oxford: Oxford Medical Publications, Oxford University Press, 1996:110–27.

103. Twomey PL. Cost-effectiveness of total parenteral nutrition. In: JL Rombeau, MD Caldwell, eds. *Clinical nutrition, parenteral nutrition*. 2nd edn. Philadelphia: Saunders, 1993: 401–8.

104. Fainsinger RL. Pharmacological approach to cancer anorexia and cachexia. In: Bruera E, Higginson I, eds. *Cachexia-anorexia in cancer patients*. Oxford: Oxford Medical Publications, Oxford University Press, 1996:128–40.

105. Neuenschwander H, Bruera E. Asthenia. In: Doyle D, Hanks GWC, MacDonald N, eds. *Oxford textbook of palliative medicine*, 2nd edn. Oxford: Oxford University Press, 1998:573–81.

106. Farr W. The use of corticosteroids for symptom management in terminally ill patients. *American Journal of Hospice Care*, 1990; 1: 41–6.

107. Watanabe S, Bruera E. Corticosteroids as adjuvant analgesics. *Journal of Pain and Symptom Management*, 1994; 9: 442–5.

108. Beller E, *et al.* Improved quality of life with megestrol acetate in patients with endocrine-insensitive advanced cancer: a randomised placebo-controlled trial. *Annals of Oncology*, 1997; 8: 277–83.

109. Bruera E, Ernst S, Hagen N, Spachynski K, Belzile M, Hanson J. Symptomatic effects of megestrol acetate (MA): a double-blind, crossover study. *Proceedings of the American Society for Clinical Oncology*, 1996; 1716:531.

110. Bruera E, Seifert L, Watanabe S, Babul N, Darke A, Harsanyi Z, Suarez-Almazor M. Chronic nausea in advanced cancer patients: a retrospective assessment of a metoclopramide-based antiemetic regimen. *Journal of Pain and Symptom Management*, 1996; 11: 147–53.

111. Bruera E, *et al.* Comparison of the efficacy, safety and pharmacokinetics of controlled release and immediate release metoclopramide for the management of chronic nausea in patients with advanced cancer. *Cancer*, 1994; 74: 3204–11.

112. Mercadante S. The role of octreotide in palliative care. *Journal of Pain and Symptom Management*, 1993; 9: 406–11.

113. Bruera E, Miller L, McCallion J, Macmillan K, Krefting L, Hanson J. Cognitive failure in patients with terminal cancer: a prospective study. *Journal of Pain and Symptom Management*, 1992; 7: 192–5.

114. Pereira J, Hanson J, Bruera E. The frequency and clinical course of cognitive impairment in patients with terminal cancer. *Cancer*, 1997; 79: 835–42.

115. Breitbart W, *et al.* A double-blind trial of haloperidol, chlorpromazine, and lorazepam in the treatment of delirium in hospitalized AIDS patients. *American Journal of Psychiatry*, 1996; 153: 231–7.

116. Bruera E, Pereira J. Neuropsychiatric toxicity of opioids. In: Jensen TS, Turner JA, Wiesenfeld-Hallen Z, eds. *Proceedings of the 8th world congress on pain. Progress in pain research and management*, Vol 8. Seattle: IASP Press, 1997:717–38.

117. Cody M. Depression and the use of antidepressants in patients with cancer. *Palliative Medicine*, 1990; 4: 271–8.

118. Ell K, Nishimot R, Mantell J, Hamovitch M. Longitudinal analysis of psychological adaptation among amily members of patients with cancer. *Journal of Psychomatic Research*, 1999; 32: 429.

119. Hodgson CS, Higginson IJ, McDonnell M, Butters E. Family anxiety in advanced cancer. *British Journal of Cancer*, 1997; 76: 1211–14.

120. Toseland RW, Blanchard CG, McCallion P. A problem solving intervention for caregivers of cancer patients. *Society of Scientific Medicine*, 1995; 40: 517–28.

121. Hospice Information Service. *Palliative Care Services Worldwide*. January 1998. London: Hospice Information Service, 1998.

122. Eve A, Smith AM, Tebbitt P. Hospice and palliative care in the UK 1994–5, including a summary of trends 1990–5. *Palliative Medicine*, 1997; 11: 31–43.

123. Higginson IJ. Health care needs assessment: palliative and terminal care. In: Stevens A, Raftery J, eds. *Health care needs assessment*. 2nd Series. Oxford: Radcliffe Medical Press, 1997.

124. Jones RVH. Teams and terminal cancer care at home: do patients and carers benefit? *Journal of Interprofessional Care*, 1993; 7: 239–45.

125. Jones RVH, Hansford J, Fiske J. Death from cancer at home: the carers' perspective. *British Medical Journal*, 1993; 306: 249–51.

7

Assessment of the results of cancer treatment

7.1 Clinical trials and data management

Valter Torri

Clinical trials

Introduction

A clinical trial can be defined as a prospective study conducted on patients with the aim of acquiring knowledge on the therapeutic usefulness of a particular treatment. Clinical trials are used for all kinds of clinical intervention. Given the importance of pharmacological intervention, this chapter will focus in particular on clinical trials of drugs. The general aspects discussed also apply to other treatments.

Assessment of the potential therapeutic value of a treatment requires the planning of a series of steps. Before being tested on patients, treatments have to pass a preclinical screening phase that helps to select the more promising treatment and provide some information on dosage. However, the exact magnitude of risks and benefits can only be estimated after clinical assessment.

The first step of evaluation in humans is aimed at obtaining information on pharmacokinetics of the drug, its toxicity, and dose-finding (phase I). The second step focuses on studying the clinical activity of the drug (phase II). The third step aims at comparing the new treatment versus a control arm to obtain information on its relative efficacy (phase III).

Each of these steps follows precise methodological and practical rules to properly answer the particular question posed at each phase. The aim of this chapter is to highlight the importance of the methodology of the clinical research, and to discuss critical aspects of the design, conduct, and analysis of clinical trials.

General aspects

Although clinical trials are important tools for gaining scientific knowledge, they are inherently inefficient compared with laboratory experimentation. Human evaluation trials have to tackle the problems of human heterogeneity, complex organization (many studies are multidisciplinary and can be run in different settings), and ethical issues (informed participation of patients). Moreover, for comparative trials, patients in the control arm should receive the 'best optimal standard care', although the anticipated effect of the treatment may not be large. Designs that maximize differences among treatment characteristics are, in general, not feasible. Finally, clinical trials may require complex data management for collecting and analysing large amounts of data and for co-ordinating all aspects related to a clinical study.

Choice of the clinical question and study design

The value of a clinical study is determined largely by the clinical importance of the question to be answered. The question to be tested in a clinical trial should satisfy various criteria of relevance, such as better comprehension of the mechanism of action, biological activity, safety and benefit for the patient, in terms of better survival or quality of life, symptom relief, and feasibility. The details of the type of design, the criteria for patient selection, the number of patients needed, the number and type of data to be collected, largely depends on the nature of the question being posed. The objective, design, and practical issues can identify each phase of the clinical study.

Phase I trials

Phase I clinical trials represent the first step in evaluating a new anticancer agent for use in humans. They are not comparative and are not randomized. They are conducted on a small number of patients and, due to the lack of information concerning the risk/benefit profile of the agent, it is preferable to select patients for which conventional therapies have ceased to be successful, in order to give the patients a further possibility of care. Besides this aim, three other purposes of such studies can be identified:

- determination of qualitative (which organ is involved) and quantitative (predictability, extent, duration, and reversibility) toxicity of the new drug;
- investigation of basic clinical pharmacology, including measurement of pharmacokinetics and pharmacodynamic effects;
- identification of the maximum tolerated doses (**MTD**) that will be used to establish the appropriate dose in early phase II studies. The MTD can be defined as the dose associated with serious but reversible side-effects, offering the best estimate of a favourable therapeutic ratio on a given schedule via a given route of administration.

The selection criteria of patients for phase I trials include that the patient has a tumour at a stage which is not eligible for standard therapy. It is appropriate to include patients with a non-measurable disease, which is an otherwise usual requirement for later phases' testing of the drug's anti-tumour activity. Other eligibility criteria may be a good performance status, as well as the absence of clinically relevant cardiac, hepatic, renal, or haematological impairment due to the high risk of side-effects. For the same reason, patients who have suffered from toxicity caused by previous therapies are not generally included in such studies.

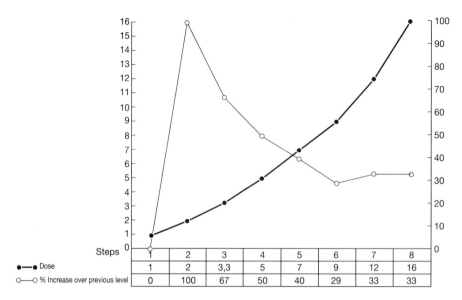

Steps	1	2	3	4	5	6	7	8
●—● Dose	1	2	3,3	5	7	9	12	16
○—○ % Increase over previous level	0	100	67	50	40	29	33	33

Fig. 1 Modified Fibonacci dose-escalation scheme.

A phase I study might follow an adaptive, sequentially increasing dose design: the decision to use a next higher dose depends upon the result observed at the current dose. In a typical phase I design, three patients, who previously have never been treated with the agent under investigation, receive the drug at a given dose-level. If none of them suffers toxicity, generally measured by means of toxicity scales,[1] the next three subjects will receive the next higher dose. However, if even one patient suffers toxicity the same dose will be administered to three more patients. Escalation of dose will continue if only one of these six patients has had side-effects. If more than one patient has experienced toxicity, the dose will be identified as the MTD. The starting dose, as well as the following ones, is usually chosen on the basis of previous preclinical experiments.[2] One of the most common procedures is to start with a dose equal to one-tenth of the LD10,[3] which is the lethal dose for 10 per cent of rodents. This is followed by the administration of higher doses according to the 'modified' Fibonacci scheme, considered as the standard method. In a typical assessment the percentage increment from the starting dose will be the following: 100, 67, 50, 40, 29, 33, 33. The initial escalation is rapid, with smaller increments the closer the toxic range is approached (Fig. 1). Modifications are made according to the results of preclinical studies[4],[5] and the properties of the studied drug.[6]

Alternative designs have recently been developed, in order to reduce both the number of patients receiving a dose below the biologically active level and to increase the speed at which trials are completed. They also increase the amount of information obtained, providing an estimate of the distribution of the MTD population and of the degree of cumulative toxicity.[7],[8] These targets are achieved by doubling the doses until the MTD is reached and by escalating the intrapatient dose.

The approaches described are particularly useful for classic cytotoxic therapies. However, one of the most active areas of research in recent years has been the identification of new compounds, such as biological-response modifiers (interferon, interleukins, and angiogenesis inhibitors). From a general point of view, such agents are designed to improve the therapeutic benefit by modifying the host response to the tumour and/or cytotoxic drugs. The phase I trials described above are often inappropriate for these treatments, because the maximum tolerated dose may not be the optimum dose. Phase I trials of these agents should attempt to determine the maximum effective dose, that is the maximum modification in the host biological response, rather than, for example, myelotoxicity, as a requirement for therapeutic activity. Appropriate designs for development phases are still under study to address these questions.

Phase II trials

Once a safe dose and schedule has been established, it must be used in a phase II trial to determine whether the new agent has sufficient antitumour activity to be worthy of large-scale studies. Agents shown to be active and with acceptable toxicity may then be incorporated in combination chemotherapy regimens. Phase II trials of combined chemotherapy regimens are not primarily concerned with the assessment of activity, since each single agent has already been shown to be active and tolerated, but the goal is to achieve a certain better level of activity. Therefore, once the tolerability has been demonstrated by small pilot studies, under the assumption that the combination is better than the single agents (i.e. there is a higher probability of tumour regression) randomized, controlled trials can be conducted. The aim is to obtain reasonably precise estimates of the activity of the treatment under study, with appropriate early stopping rules in case the experimental arm is not effective.[9]

Usually, patients relapsing in a phase III trial are offered treatment in a phase II trial. However, for some tumours (such as advanced, non-small-cell, lung cancer, for which there is no effective standard chemotherapy regimen), untreated patients are preferable for inclusion in phase II trials, since there is a better chance that a new regimen's potential activity will be better detected in such patients. Patients who have been previously treated, and in whom the disease is progressing, have a smaller chance of response because of the development of drug resistance. Since these resistance mechanisms are often common to different classes of drugs, the possibility exists of underestimating the antitumour activity of the agent studied. The most commonly used outcome of activity for phase II trials is tumour-mass reduction (response). Consequently, patients must have measurable lesions to allow this assessment of drug activity. From a methodological point of view, it is necessary, before the start of the study, to describe in detail the criteria for the assessment of the outcome (see Chapter 7.2). Generally, it is preferable to use standard, internationally accepted, classification methods (WHO criteria, see Chapter 7.2; or those recently revised, e.g. RECIST[10]), to allow comparison of the results from different studies. The use of tumour markers has recently been suggested, which allows the response to treatment to be evaluated in a different and complementary way (see Chapter 3.4).[11]

Design and sample size for phase II trials

The determination of the appropriate sample size for a phase II trial, usually between 40 and 60 patients, is aimed at treating as few patients as possible, while at the same time determining whether the new agent is effective or shows insufficient antitumour activity. If effective, a phase III study will be performed; if not, the development of the drug will usually be interrupted.

The classic approach, proposed by Gehan,[12] is a two-stage trial in which the first stage is conducted on a cohort of evaluable patients. If none of them show an objective response to treatment the study is stopped; if activity is seen, more subjects are treated in order to obtain a more precise estimate of the antitumour effect. Once the minimum acceptable level of activity is stated at a response rate of, for example, 20 per cent, then the stopping rule is based on the idea that if no response was obtained in the first 14 patients, then the probability of getting at least a 20 per cent response is very low, calculated as $(1-0.20)^{14} = 0.044$. If at least one response is observed, then the probability of getting more then 20 per cent is 5 per cent or more, and the second cohort of patients is enrolled, of which the number depends on the desired precision of the estimate and the results of the first stage. For example, with a total number of 45 patients the interval confidence limits will be plus or minus 15 per cent.

Since 1961, the year of its presentation, Gehan's design has been subject to various modifications in order to increase its internal validity and efficiency. In fact it is important to note that in a screening phase, such as a phase II trial, it is essential to ensure that errors are not made when interpreting the results. At this stage of the investigation of a drug it is very important to avoid the risk of false-negative results. A false-positive study will probably be corrected in subsequent trials, while a false-negative trial is rarely repeated. Moreover, the issue of heterogeneity in phase II studies needs important consideration. In fact, there is often great variability in the response rates reported from different phase II studies of the same agent. Patient selection, response criteria, interobserver variability in response assessment, dosage modification, and protocol compliance, may contribute to this variability. For this reason, multiple-step procedures and randomized, comparative designs (which provide multiple comparisons) have been proposed not only to allow the trial to be interrupted early, but also to select the most promising among several experimental treatments.[14] Randomized, phase II studies allocate patients into two or more treatment arms, each arm testing a new agent. The sample size is established to ensure that if a treatment is superior to all the others by a given amount, then it will be selected with a defined probability. This approach provides unbiased comparisons among groups and, using a selection-theory approach as an alternative to testing the null hypothesis of equivalence, the agent producing the highest response rate can be chosen for phase III testing.[15]

Phase III trials

Phase III trials represent the most important test for assessing the efficacy of new treatments. In these studies formal comparison is made between new treatment and standard therapies. Phase III studies potentially apply to all patients in every stage of disease. Efficacy can be assessed by choosing outcome measures related directly to patient benefits (survival, time to progression, improvement in symptoms, or in health status indicators related to treatment effect). If intermediate endpoints correlated to long-term patient benefit are available (in some cancers, this might be the response to treatment) these might be used as surrogate endpoints. However, given the great importance for defining treatments for the population as a whole, it is important emphasize the methodological aspects of phase III trials.

Defining the question

The value of a clinical trial is largely determined by the importance of the question. Operatively, it means that solid rational criteria have to be followed to determine the type of control group and the purposes of the comparison.

Choice of control group

The choice of control group is a critical decision in designing a clinical trial, since it affects the inferences that can be drawn from the trial, the degree to which bias in conducting and analysing the study can be minimized, and the types of subjects that can be recruited.

Control groups allow the outcome caused by the experimental treatment to be discriminated from outcomes caused by other factors, such as other treatments, or the natural progression of the disease. If the course of a disease were predictable from patient characteristics such that outcome could be predicted reliably for any group of subjects, the results of treatment could be compared with a similar group of patients previously studied ('historical control'). In most situations, however, a concurrent control group is needed because it is impossible to predict outcome with adequate accuracy.

A concurrent control group is one chosen from the same population as the experimental group and treated in a defined way as part of the same trial that studies the experimental treatment.

Control groups can be classified on the basis of the type of treatment received: no active treatment (no treatment, placebo); or active treatment (different dose or regimen of the study treatment, different active treatment).

Purposes of the comparison

Phase III trials are comparative: the goal is the assessment of the relative efficacy, safety, benefit/risk relationship, or utility between experimental and control treatments.

A study may demonstrate efficacy of the experimental treatment by showing that it is superior to the control (placebo, low dose, and active drug) or by showing the new drug to be similar in efficacy to a known effective therapy. Clinical studies designed to show that a new drug is similar in efficacy to a standard agent are defined 'equivalence' trials.[16] Because in this case the finding of interest is one-sided, these are actually non-inferiority trials, attempting to show that the new drug is not less effective than the control by more than a defined amount. As the fundamental assumption of such studies is that showing non-inferiority is evidence of efficacy, caution in conducting and interpreting non-inferiority trials is needed.

A particularly important issue in this context is the choice of the non-inferiority margin (that is to say, the degree of inferiority of the experimental treatment compared to the control), that the trial will attempt to exclude statistically. This margin can only be derived on past experience. Therefore, a different patient population and a different selection and timing of the endpoint may affect the interpretation of the results.

The choice of the control group, the purpose of the trial, the selection of dosage, the patient population, and the clinical relevant difference to be detected are therefore key issues that should be taken into account when setting up a comparative study, particularly for equivalence trials.

Assuring comparability among treatment groups

Validity is based essentially on the capability to determine whether the tested treatment is different in terms of efficacy compared to the standard treatment and to obtain a reliable estimate of the magnitude of this difference. The study design should ensure that other factors (patient selection, difference in ancillary therapies, difference in patient evaluation) do not influence the evaluation. For this reason the only studies considered valid are those using a concurrent, randomized control arm. Comparison with historical or non-randomized groups are unreliable and should be abandoned. The key point of randomization is in ensuring that the researcher cannot know the treatment to be assigned to any future patient. In this way, patients will receive the treatment independently of their prognostic factors or of clinician preferences. *The ethical basis for this approach is that, in the context of a therapeutic clinical trial, the clinician does not know which treatment is the most appropriate for the patient and, with the patient's consent, can justifiably randomize the allocation (uncertainty principle).*[13] *If on the other hand he knows, or thinks to know, which option is best for the patient, then the patient should receive that option and not participate in the trial.* From this point of view, ethical problems may arise in equivalence trials. In this case, patients are randomized to a treatment which, by definition, is assumed to be somewhat worse than the comparator, to show at last that this is not the case. If no advantage for patients is foreseen, the practice of randomization is not ethical, as it exposes patients to unknown—however unlikely—risks, while hopefully offering the same effect that other available treatment would provide anyway. Even if the trial succeeds in verifying equivalence or non-inferiority, this means no advantage for the patients. Therefore, randomization in equivalence/non-inferiority trials is acceptable only if some benefit for patients can be hypothesized, carefully considered, and reliably tested. In consequence, the testing of drugs supposed to be as effective as those available is acceptable only if related trials can address other potential advantages over current therapies. Equivalence trials must prove the new drug to be safer, more tolerable, easier to use, or cheaper.

There are several techniques for randomization (simple randomization, stratified randomization, minimization), these differ substantially in their capability to control the balance between the comparison groups with respect to baseline characteristics that can affect the outcome measures.[17]

The aim of avoiding biases has to continue not only during the treatment allocation phase, but also during the treatment period and follow-up; adopting, when possible and appropriate, blinding techniques. Blindness can be achieved using a placebo for the control arm and/or ensuring that the responsibility for assessing the intervention lies with someone other than the investigator(s). This is particularly important if the evaluation of outcome can be affected by subjective judgement ('soft endpoint'). In cancer clinical trials, blinding may play a role in the evaluation of ancillary therapies where subjective factors may play a part, such as analgesic or antiemetic treatments. A similar way of monitoring patients should be adopted in the treatment being compared, in order to avoid bias in the assessment of the endpoint. Finally, analysis should be conducted considering all the patients according to the treatment group assigned by randomization (intention-to-treat analysis). This avoids the bias introduced by a differential dropout from the study. The intention-to-treat approach should be always used for the evaluation of primary endpoints. For example, when assessing overall survival it is best that all patients are included in the analysis, irrespective of the treatment received after randomization. However, for other secondary endpoints, such as a comparison of toxicity, it may be important to compare only those patients receiving at least some clearly predefined number of cycles of therapy.

Assuring precision of results

Once scientific validity is achieved, the next step is to define, with as much precision as possible, the magnitude of the effect. This could be achieved with an adequate sample of patients and a sufficient follow-up for the determination of the events of interest. Sample size is one of the crucial considerations affecting the feasibility of the studies and their design and organization. To understand the importance of calculating sample size, it is necessary to introduce the concepts of 'significance test' and 'power'.

A statistical test is performed to compare the treatments under investigation. In general, the hypothesis, which is being tested, called the 'null hypothesis', is that all treatments are equivalent. The statistical test calculates the probability, under the null hypothesis, of results being equal to or more extreme than those observed. This probability is called the statistical significance of the tests, or p value. If p is less than the significance level-α, which was specified before the trial, the test is said to be statistically significant and the null hypothesis of treatment-equivalence is rejected. If the null hypothesis of treatments is not true, then the alternative hypothesis must be true. The alternative hypothesis specifies the difference between the treatments.

The statistical power of a comparative trial is the probability of detecting a postulated treatment-difference if, in truth, it exists. The power is a function of the magnitude of postulated benefit: the same trial may have a high probability to detect a large difference, but little power to detect small differences. Therefore, it is important to specify the magnitude of clinical benefits that are considered to be important to be detected, and to define a realistic difference that must be detected if it exists. In this respect, the role of systematic overviews is valuable for indicating the size of expected differences for new trials testing similar strategies. In general, the anticipated benefit is modest. The systematic reviews on the role of chemotherapy in non-small-cell lung cancer provide a good example. At the outset of this review there was considerable pessimism about the role of chemotherapy in non-small-cell lung cancer. In particular, no trials had detected a significant result in favour of adjuvant chemotherapy. The review instead showed that the results for regimens containing cisplatin favoured chemotherapy. Trials comparing surgery versus surgery plus chemotherapy gave a 13 per cent reduction in the risk of death, equivalent to an absolute benefit of 5 per cent at 5 years.[18] None of the trials involved was planned with a sufficient power for detecting a difference of this magnitude. These results provided the basis for planning multicentre international trials of adequate size.

From a general point of view, the sample size for a particular comparative group can be evaluated through the following equation:

$$n \simeq \left[\frac{(z_\alpha + z_\beta) \cdot \sigma}{\mu} \right]^2$$

where z_α and z_β are the normal deviates related to the α and β levels, μ is the measure of the relevant clinical difference to be detected and s is the standard deviation of the observations.[17] In the case of survival analysis, the parameter more frequently used in cancer trials, σ/μ depends on the model assumptions, the accrual time, and the overall study duration.

In general, for survival analysis, the summary measure of interest is the hazard ratio (HR),[20] the ratio of the risk of event in the two groups, estimated by:

$$HR = \frac{\log \lambda_t}{\log \lambda_c}$$

where λ_t and λ_c are the instantaneous event rates for the treatment and control groups, respectively. Assuming proportional hazards, the relationship between HR and the absolute difference in survival at a defined time can be defined as:

$$\pi_e = e^{(\log \pi_c \cdot HR)}$$

where π_e and π_c are the survival at a given year in the experimental and control groups, respectively. Therefore, if an anticipated value of π_e and HR are provided, an anticipated value of π_e can be calculated. Figure 2 shows the relationship between HR and the absolute difference $\pi_e - \pi_c$ for different π_c.

The formula providing the number of events required using the HR, for a test comparing two survival experiences (logrank test[21],[22]) is:

$$E = \frac{(HR + 1)^2 \cdot (z_\alpha + z_\beta)^2}{(HR - 1)^2}$$

and the total number of patients is:

$$N = \frac{2E}{(2 - \pi_c - \pi_e)}$$

The formula can be also generalized for the proportion of allocated patients different than 1 and for taking withdrawals into account.[23] Figure 3 reports the number of patients needed for a range of difference and different power according to the previous formula. Table 1 provides the number of patients required for different study durations, and the difference to be detected at a power = 0.80 with

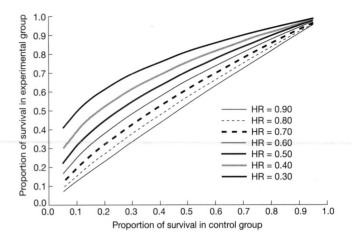

Fig. 2 Relationship between survival in the experimental arm and the hazard ratio (HR), for a different survival in the control arm.

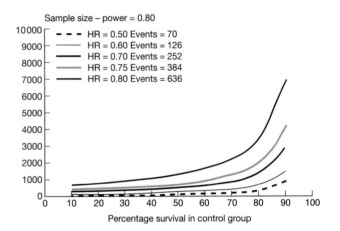

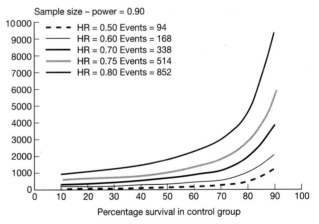

Fig. 3 Sample size needed for different hazard ratios (HR) and power.

$\alpha = 0.05$ (two sides), using an approach that allows for considering follow-up time.[24]

Sample size for equivalence trials may imply a greater precision in the estimate of the effect, hence statistical considerations must be adapted accordingly.[25]

Table 1 Number of subjects for comparison of survival rates

5-year survival (%)			Patients required if accrual lasts 4 years			
Control arm	Expected in experimental arm if:		Minimum follow-up = 1 year	Minimum follow-up = 3 years	Minimum follow-up = 1 year	Minimum follow-up = 3 years
	HR = 0.75	HR = 0.50	HR = 0.75		HR = 0.50	
20	30	45	706	522	146	106
40	50	63	1038	710	218	148
60	68	77	1696	1100	350	226
80	85	89	3494	2170	754	468

Event required:

- Hazard ratio = 0.75: 384
- Hazard ratio = 0.50: 70

Assuring efficiency—design

Trials in cancer are often expensive and require a long duration for the accrual and evaluation of results. Efficiency may be improved by statistical design and by trial management. From the statistical point of view, one of the most useful approaches is the factorial design. With a factorial design it is possible to answer different questions in the same study. The simplest factorial design is a 2 × 2 balanced study, in which patients have the same chance of receiving treatment A, or treatment B, or both A and B, or no treatment. Within one study it is therefore possible to answer the question regarding the efficacy of treatment A and the efficacy of treatment B and whether they add together. Factorial designs should be employed when it is reasonable to exclude any important interactions of treatment, in terms of toxicity and in terms of efficacy.[26] If the study is aimed instead at detecting a clinical interaction then the factorial designs are the most appropriate, but in this case the number of patients needed to detect a statistically significant interaction increases considerably.

Assuring efficiency—conduct of study

The feasibility and quality of a study depends crucially on the quality of information gathered. In this sense, it is important to select the essential information and consider only variables that are crucial for the question of interest. The choice of the type of information will depend on the type of question: trials of early phases of new drugs will focus mostly on safety and tolerability data, while public-health oriented trials, comparing therapeutic strategies already used, will focus mostly on a survival endpoint. It is possible to maintain the efficiency of trials by adopting approaches that allow timely changes in the protocol. Monitoring the results from a continuing trial, especially when it is expected to last for a long time, is appropriate for reasons connected with both toxicity and efficacy. First of all, a high incidence of unexpected and serious adverse events might lead to stopping the study early, this is also case with evidence strongly supporting the advantage or disadvantage of the studied treatment. Furthermore, poor quality of data, a low rate of patient compliance, or a low accrual rate can convince the researchers to interrupt it earlier. On the other hand, the possibility of obtaining a more precise estimate of the study objective, of performing subgroup analyses, of testing the effect of eventual prognostic factors, as well as of increasing

the power of assessing secondary endpoints, are reasons to continue the study for as long as possible.

Monitoring implies multiple looks at the data. Generally, a study protocol should define types, modalities, and time for the analysis. It is important to note that the more statistical tests are performed, the higher the probability of false-positive results. If five statistical tests are performed, the probability of a significant result, due to repetition, is more than 20 per cent instead of 5 per cent. However, approaches for controlling the inflation of false-positive results can be adopted. The most widely used approaches to study monitoring are the frequentist methods[27] that, controlling for a type I error, allow for repeated testing. Besides these approaches, likelihood-based methods, Bayesian approaches, and decision theory can be used. In contrast to the classical monitoring of trials, which requires adjustment of the inference for the stopping rule used, the Bayesian method provides a flexible framework for monitoring of clinical trials. Basically, the state of knowledge before the study (prior probability) about the treatment effect, is updated by the results of an interim analysis to yield the state of knowledge after the analysis (posterior probability), and inference in this case requires no adjustment. Flexibility allows that information from clinical trial and other sources can be combined and used explicitly to calculate a predictive probability for future observation and in drawing conclusions. Applications of these methods have been more frequent in the recent years.[28]–[31]

Beside the statistical tools for controlling multiple comparisons, it is necessary to build up a committee to evaluate the safety and efficacy of trials. This is the reason for a wider adoption of independent 'Data Monitoring Committees' composed of experts in clinical and methodological fields, these experts do not participate in the study but they do have the commitment of giving suggestions relevant to the conduct of the trial.

Conducting the statistical analysis

Statistical analysis involves all the aspects of a clinical trial. Besides statistical aspects related to the study design, the choice of procedures for allocating a patient to a particular treatment group, the planning of sample size, and interim analyses (discussed above), an appropriate analysis should consider all the information regarding the balancing of study groups, the definition of the possible different statistical

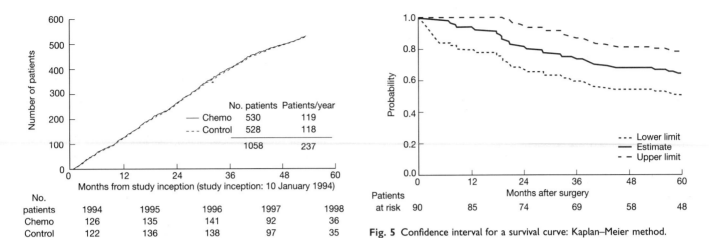

Fig. 4 Patient accrual over time—the ALPI trial.

Fig. 5 Confidence interval for a survival curve: Kaplan–Meier method.

approaches for a selected patient population, the thorough description of toxicity and compliance, and the use of appropriate methods for the analysis of efficacy endpoint.

Analysis of balancement of the study groups

The assessment of the balancement of the treatment groups is useful either in the phase of patient's accrual and in the phase of final analysis. Possible unbalancement happening during recruitment may help in discovering problems during the randomization procedure. Figure 4 shows the plot of accrual by treatment arm in the Adjuvant Lung Project Italy (**ALPI**) trial:[32] in this case, the accrual was similar in the two groups overall and at each particular time. Tables presenting the distribution by group of baseline factors that may affect outcome are also useful, since they give an idea of the quality of balance provided by the randomization procedure and indicate different approaches for the analysis.

Definition of the patient population and approach to the analysis

Another important point is the definition of the subset that is eligible ·and evaluable for the particular kind of analysis being conducted. As an example, for efficacy analysis, all eligible patients may be analysed according to the intention-to-treat approach, that is to say in the group assigned by randomization. However, for safety analysis, only patients treated for a minimum defined number of cycles may be considered, since in this case the intention-to-treat approach may fail to identify potential toxicity problems.

Analysis of compliance with the treatment protocol and safety

Analysis of treatment compliance provides insights into the feasibility of the protocol treatment and on the interpretation of efficacy results. Usually a complete description of those patients who modified or interrupted the treatment plan, together with the reason for non-compliance, should be presented. A description of the distribution of the number of cycles given, the total dosage, and the dose intensity is generally useful.

Analysis of efficacy endpoint

Usually, the type of data most frequently used for an efficacy analysis in oncology is survival data. Here, the outcome variable is the time from the study beginning (usually the time from randomization) to

a specifically critical event, such as death or progression of the disease. It should be taken into account that the distribution of survival time is unlikely to be normal and that the observation may be censored. Censored observation arises in patients for whom, at the end of the study, the critical event has not yet occurred. It may happen:

- because the patients is still alive (if the endpoint is the death) when the trial analysis is performed;
- because the patients was lost to follow-up before the end of the trial; or
- because the patient died of some cause unrelated to the disease in question.

Techniques allowing for censoring patients should be preferred to other (continuous or categorical) data analysis. Commonly, the survival data are displayed using a Kaplan–Meier survival plot, and group comparisons can be made using the log-rank test or semi-parametric regression models.[33] Figure 5 shows a Kaplan–Meier plot with the confidence interval for the survival distribution. It can be noted that the Kaplan–Meier curves are a step function, and that the tail of the survival curve became unstable (larger confidence interval) when there are few patients at risk. This is the reason why it is recommended that the number of subjects at risk at key time points are displayed.[34]

Interpreting and presenting the results

Summary statistics and graphical methods are important tools for interpreting the results. Regarding summary statistics, it is important to provide the appropriate measures with their degree of precision. For example, for continuous data, the mean and standard deviation should be presented; if the data have an asymmetrical distribution then the median and interquartile ranges may be appropriate. For categorical and ordered categorical data, the proportion in each category should be reported. The presentation of results should include the value of the appropriate test statistics and the p value. Confidence intervals for the main summary measures should be given. Confidence intervals are to be preferred to the presentation of the p value—because it is from these statistics that it is possible to form an opinion on the precision of effect, since clinical relevance is a complex judgement than can not be measured only by statistical significance. Confidence intervals allow the extrapolation of the single

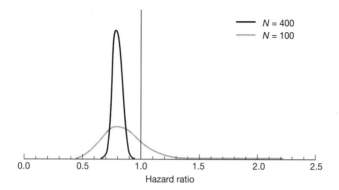

Fig. 6 Normal distribution for the results of two hypothetical studies. Hazard ratio = 0.80 in both studies. Number of events = 100 and 400, respectively.

result (such as an hazard ratio) to a range of values that are considered to be plausible for the population. The width of the confidence interval associated with a sample statistic depends on its standard error and on the degree of confidence related to the resulting interval. Figure 6 represents the relationship between the normal distribution, the confidence intervals, and the *p* values. The criteria of presentation of the results are also important. Results may be expressed by measuring the absolute or relative reduction of unfavourable events or the number of patients needed to be treated to avoid such events. Depending on the type of measurements, the interpretation of research data may differ.[35]

Assuring generalizability

The generalizability in clinical trial results depends on how restricted is the population under study and the nature of the restrictions. If only a small proportion of available patients are permitted to participate, any extrapolation of results to the remaining patients should be viewed with caution. Reasons for patient exclusion can vary: not only patients' characteristics (eligibility criteria) but also institutional factors (characteristics of participating centres) and physician or patient preferences may play an important role in selecting a biased sample of the general patient population, thus reducing the applicability of the findings.[36]

Eligibility criteria are patient-specific characteristics that define and limit the class of patient that can be treated in the trial.[34] Restriction of eligibility is justified for scientific and safety reasons. It seems reasonable and appropriate to impose eligibility requirements that reflect the scientific objectives of the trial, such as diagnostic restrictions.[37] In addition, there may be reason to believe that the therapies under study cannot possibly benefit certain types of patients or, alternatively, are likely to benefit only a defined type of patient.[37] However, increasing diagnostic restriction may increase the precision of the study, but it reduces the number of patients available. There are also other limitations (poor anticipated compliance, reduced access to a medical facility, legal requirements) that may contribute to reduce the pool of eligible patients. In addition, limitations on generalizability means that the trial does not mimic clinical practice, and that it increases complexity and cost and reduces accrual.

There are important problems in selection related to the institution or to patient/physician preferences. Studies performed only in specialized centres may produce results that are non-immediately applicable to community centres. In studies focused on accrual patterns it has been consistently shown that, among patients eligible for inclusion in the protocol, the primary motivation for non-participation was a physician preference for a particular therapy or alternative treatment.[38],[39]

The limitation of generalizability therefore becomes a major issue in clinical trials. This is particularly true if one considers that, although a well-conducted randomized trial provides the highest quality information in clinical debates, it still represents aggregates of information from many patients who are diverse, even in narrowly restricted study, in terms of prognosis and side-effects.

Possible measures for reducing the problem may be the promotion of large collaborative trials, with limited restriction criteria (which also include community hospitals) and the incorporation of the uncertainty principle as major criteria for patient selection. Efforts for comparing the prognosis of patients from clinical trials with a general population, using registries, might be helpful in evaluating the discrepancies and the dimension of the bias. Moreover, extrapolation from a clinical trial to clinical practice should be based on all the best evidence available, more than on the results of a single trial. In this sense, evidence-based medicine[40],[41] should be encouraged.

Evaluating the results in the context of available evidence

Once the trial results are available the next step is evaluating the findings in the context of all the evidence available on the same or similar strategies. This process of evaluation, called systematic review, has developed in the recent years and is now recognized as a methodological discipline for the synthesis of evidence. The statistical approach for synthesizing evidence of a systematic review is called meta-analysis.[42]

The systematic review analyses all the available evidence, avoiding consideration of data derived from selected studies that may not correctly represent all the available evidence (publication bias). Single, randomized clinical trials are usually inconclusive and, due to the insufficient sample, they may be imprecise in the estimate of any size difference. Properly collecting and analysing all the available evidence may therefore improve precision and allow a greater extrapolation of results, since the patients included in all the studies may better represent the general population of patients eligible for the therapy under investigation than the patients included in a single, selected, small trial.

Because the aim is exhaustivity and objectivity, a systematic review can be considered as a real research project, having need of a formal design for the conduct and analysis of the study. Study objectives, a research strategy for collecting evidence, eligibility criteria for including relevant trials, criteria for evaluating the quality of the study, and statistical methods for combining the results should be planned in advance. Regarding the statistical method, a general approach may be as follows: once the data are extracted and appropriate summary statistical measures retrieved (for example, the relative odds of death in each relevant study), the first analysis is to evaluate the degree of homogeneity of the results. If the results among studies are inconsistent, then it could be important to 'explain' heterogeneity, stratifying trials in planned subgroups (for example, by treatment schemes defined according to the presence or absence of relevant drugs), and then to produce summary estimates of the effect in these subgroups. If, on the other hand, homogeneity is met, then the overall summary result can be considered as the best estimate for all trials. These summary estimates of treatment effect are usually weighted means of the results gathered from each single trial, with the weights being related to the sample size of each trial.

However, since the systematic review is, by definition, mostly a retrospective exercise, its quality depends on the quality of included trials. Nevertheless, with the cautions related to retrospective studies, the results of systematic reviews, particularly those based on the analysis of individual patient data, have influenced practice and research in recent years.[43],[44]

Data management

Introduction

Over the last 20 years the 'technology' of clinical trials has become increasingly complex. This has been largely due to the diffusion of large-scale studies, which is investigation conducted at the national or even international level involving the participation of several centres.

The advent of large-scale clinical trials represents a major achievement in clinical research, making it possible to identify relatively small (but still relevant in terms of public-health implications) benefits of therapeutic interventions. Large-scale trials also have an educational impact, fostering networking among centres, standardization of procedures and patient management, and the interdisciplinary exchange of skills and experiences.

Another factor increasing the complexity of clinical trials has been legislation. This has been driven by several concerns related to the need to avoid scientific misconduct as well as of ensuring respect of patients' rights.

These changes have many implications, one of these is the increasing professionalism required for the design and conduct of a clinical trial. The successful conduct of a study therefore results from the interaction of different skills and expertise, ranging from the clinician statisticians to the data managers. To be fruitful, the interaction of these different professional components has to be embedded in a proper organizational environment, combining the ability to co-ordinate the work of the many people involved (a task requiring a certain degree of flexibility) to the maintenance of the necessary scientific rigour.

A great deal of this central co-ordinating task is devoted to handling and managing the information collected at the peripheral level by the participating institutions. The co-ordinating centre is the place from where the research question stems, and from where it is translated into an operational working protocol. It is at the co-ordinating centre that clinical investigators share their preliminary ideas, discuss the clinical issues of interest, and face the possible options. In this early phase of the birth of a trial the role of the co-ordinating centre is not just to host the debate, but to shape it in such a way as to make the different options translatable into answerable research questions. At the trial centre statisticians and data managers can work with clinicians and help to foresee the implications and feasibility of the proposals put forward by the clinical investigators.

They will help to decide what is the required sample size, what type of information is to be collected and how, and the length of the study.

The data management system

Data management is the process of systematically collecting data, in a standardized way, and ensuring and maintaining their quality. The process of data management involves sending the information back to the clinical personnel involved in the study to give a sense of the importance of the data they collect, to reinforce their own involvement, and to indicate and respond to problems encountered in the clinic.

Each item of information to be collected has different implications, including its relevance to the study goals, its translation on to a form, and its possible legal implications (such as conflict with the right of confidentiality). The process of data management therefore involves a multidisciplinary team, as these aspect can be addressed only if clinical, data managing, and the statistical expertise are involved.

Data collection

Data collection is the core activity of the whole data management process, and can be divided into four stages:

(1) identification of data worth collecting;
(2) collecting and recording the data on a paper collection form;
(3) coding and classifying the information collected;
(4) converting the information into electronic records suitable for the analysis.

Identification of data worth collecting

Generic data are not related to the goals of the study, but have to be collected to ensure the identification of individual patients and of the institution where they were cared for. These data include: the institution code number; the patient's initials, date of birth, and code number; the name of the principal investigator; and the date of written informed consent.

Specific data are those directly related to the goal of the study, the nature of the clinical issues of interest, and the specific disease addressed. All the data concerning the clinical characteristics of the patients are included within this category, as well as the type of diagnostic and therapeutic management they received, the type of follow-up, and the clinical outcome.

In particular, the temptation to collect information on every aspect of care perceived as 'potentially relevant' by clinicians must be resisted, and every effort should be made to focus on items of information really important to the conduct of the study.[45] Each item of information has an 'opportunity cost', in the sense that each piece of information collected not only takes up space on the form, but also other people's time and effort. The greater the amount of information to be collected, the greater the complexity of the form on which it must be gathered. The data collection form has to be kept simple, user friendly, and not time consuming, if the clinicians are to be persuaded to collaborate.

Collecting and recording the data through a form

Others have already pointed out some key aspects of the design of a form, providing some guidelines on this issue.[46] It is useful to think of a data collection form as a series of items, each aimed at obtaining a single response, and composed of text and a response field. The basic function of the data collection form is to ask for specific items of information, which can be done using different approaches. The text should be kept as simple as possible and clearly phrased using words familiar to the user. Each patient needs to be identified by a single set of information (i.e. institution number, code number, patient initials, and their date of birth), and these should be reported on every single page of the form. The form should be designed in such a way as to foresee the possibility that a specific item of information may not be available. This can be done through inclusion of 'unknown' or 'not applicable' options, and it will allow the possibility of distinguishing whether information is missing, if this represents non-applicability/availability, rather than being simply overlooked by the user. The form should look as appealing as possible, without being distracting. The forms are generally divided into different sections, that is groups of items related to the same aspects (i.e. patient sociodemographic data, etc.). Time is important in the data collection process. The timing and frequency of data collection should be driven by the research protocol, and is usually based upon key moments in the patient-care process: time of randomization, conclusion of the planned treatment, follow-up visits, occurrence of events of interest.

Coding and classifying the information collected

Free-text should be coded centrally using an *ad-hoc* dictionary, either one that is standard or internal. Before coding, a clinical supervisor should verify the appropriateness of the free-text in the context and choose the most appropriate definition.

Designing a computer system for data management

For data management, the selection of appropriate hardware and software should be taken into account when defining/implementing a clinical protocol study. Different selections may be made, depending on the type of study and the amount of data management undertaken by each group,[45] especially in the choice of the operating system and the software used to collect study information. Moreover, supplementary technology, such as a network and different methods of data transmission, could also be considered.[48]

The software for managing the database should be selected with the primary goal of ensuring that all required functionality is available. The choice of the database management system (**DBMS**), the software for managing data, should satisfy at least the following criteria: support for data entry, development of customized data entry screens, support for *ad-hoc* queries, and representation of missing values. Moreover, aspects such as data backup, recovery, security, table look-up for the implementation of a data dictionary, multiuser access, etc., are becoming essential.

Many types of commercial software satisfy these basic features and they are becoming much more easier to use than in the past, even if they are built for general purpose. More recently, more specific software for the management of clinical trials has been developed. These software help the user to design a complete system for data management, without knowing any 'theoretical' model of the data; it is also becoming much easier to implement standards and ensure GCP rules. These software, due to their high costs, are equally suitable for an environment where many trials are conducted or for a specific large project.[49]–[53]

Assuring data quality and data validation

It is commonly accepted that the need for detailed plans and a system for ensuring protocol adherence and the collection of uniform data will certainly influence the quality of the final statistical analysis.[54]–[56]

Implementation of quality assurance procedures, however, is costly. Therefore, when considering the methods to be adopted, a reasonable decision should be made on how to keep the effectiveness of the whole system.

Many studies reported in the scientific literature have focused on the problem of the quality of data and the commonly accepted methods that have been investigated. Training the personnel involved in the practice of the data management (both clerks and data managers), is an essential point.[57] Duplicate data-entry can result in a reduction in the data-entry errors, but it will double the time for completing data-entry activities (double input and correction); a more thorough check of the main important field, such as main outcomes, is therefore suggested.[58] In spite of all the sophisticated techniques used to control data quality some information could be anomalous; therefore quality assurance needs to be part of the data-management system to ensure the detection and solution of anomalous data.

The quality assurance and monitoring programme should include periodic reports to the participating centres on consistency, reliability, completeness, and timeliness of data. Possible sources of errors in data are misinterpretation/deviation from the study protocol and incomplete, inaccurate, or illegible data recording.

A complete 'validation' plan for the quality control should be designed and revised by all the personnel involved in the trial at the co-ordinating centre (clinical researcher, data-manager, statistician, and computer programmer) before the inception of data-collection. Site visits are useful for evaluating protocol compliance, accuracy, and reliability of data. Accrual, adherence to eligibility criteria, and the completeness and accuracy of the study forms should be monitored to detect possible 'outlier' institutions. Many studies have investigated differences in the quality of data between 'major' and 'minor' participants, but the results have been difficult to interpret.[59]–[61]

Standardization is an essential feature of a 'multiple' study site, where many studies, (concomitant or not, in the same field or not) are conducted. Standard operating procedures (**SOPs**) are formal documents where every process related to the conduct of a study is described (then applied). These have become essential in the pharmaceutical industry, research institutes, or in contract research organizations (**CROs**) (see Table 2). Standardization can involve many different activities, for example the use of standard forms and coding systems across different studies, or the definition of a standard 'dictionary' and system to define medical terms by code numbers. Recently, the use of a standard, official dictionary system created by professional societies has become a common approach.[62],[63] Classification of diseases—the ICD-10 developed by the World Health Organization (**WHO**) is the most used standard dictionary for classifying morbidity and mortality; other systems developed by other professional societies provide glossaries and/or classifications to assist in the diagnosis of disease and treatment of patients.

Dictionaries of adverse reactions—standardization for this topic has been less applicable due to the wide range of existing dictionaries developed by individual companies, professional societies, and health and regulatory agencies. The World Health Organization (WHO)

Table 2 List of SOPs

Planning the randomization system
Designing, reviewing, printing, and shipping the case report forms
Standard CRFs
Management of security access to information
Creating, validating, and adapting a data-management system
Management of CRFs at the co-ordinating centre
Standard Data Entry Convention
Double data-entry and source comparison
Quality control of data-entry activities
Management and correction of errors
Site visit
Validating source data
Freezing a database
General rules for archiving data
Data management report writing
Security management of computer data
Updating software and hardware

Standardization of a group's activities is a way of documenting how the data, and all related activities, are conducted: the definition of the 'Standard Operating Procedures' (SOPs), is a formal document where every process related to the conduct of a study is described (then applied).

Adverse Reaction Terminology,[64] COSTART,[65] and FDA[66] systems are the most used worldwide.

References

1. **Miller AB, et al.** Reporting results of cancer treatment. *Cancer*, 1981; **47**: 207–14.

2. **Grieshaber CK, Marsoni S.** Relation of preclinical toxicology to findings in early clinical trials. *Cancer Treatment Report*, 1986; **70**: 65–72.

3. **Rozencweig M, et al.** Animal toxicology for early clinical trials with anticancer agents. *Cancer Clinical Trials*, 1981; **4**: 21–8.

4. **Williams CJ, Carter SK.** Management of trials in the development of cancer chemotherapy. *British Journal of Cancer*, 1978; **37**: 434–47..

5. **Ratain MJ, Mick R, Schilsky RL, Siegler M.** Statistical and ethical issues in the design and conduct of phase 1 and 2 clinical trials of new anticancer agents. *Journal of National Cancer Institute*, 1993; **85**: 1637–43.

6. **Mitchell MS.** Combining chemotherapy with biological response modifier in treatment of cancer. *Journal of the National Cancer Institute*, 1988; **80**: 1445–50.

7. **Mani S, Ratain M.** New phase I trial methodology. *Seminars in Oncology*, 1997; **24**: 253–61.

8. **Simon R, Freidlin B, Rubinstein L, Arbuck SG, Collins J, Christian MC.** Accelerated titration designs for phase I clinical trials in oncology. *Journal of the National Cancer Institute*, 1997; **89**: 1138–47.

9. **Simon R, Wittes RE, Ellemberg SS.** Randomised phase II clinical trials. *Cancer treatment report*, 1985; **69**: 1375–81.

10. **Therasse P, Arbuck SG, Eisenhauer EA, et al.** New guidelines to evaluate the response to treatment in solid tumors. European Organization for Research and Treatment of Cancer, National Cancer Institute of the United States, National Cancer Institute of Canada. *Journal of the National Cancer Institute* 2000; **92**: 205–16.

11. **Rustin GJS, van der Burg MEL, Berek JS.** Tumor markers. *Annals of Oncology*, 1993; **4**: 71–7.

12. **Gehan EA.** The determination of the number of patients required in a preliminary and follow-up trial of a new chemotherapic agent. *Journal of Chronic Diseases*, 1961; **13**: 346–53.

13. **Peto R.** Trials: the next 50 years. *British Medical Journal*, 1998; **317**: 1170–1.

14. **Simon R, Wittes RE, Ellemberg SS, Shrager R.** Optimal two stage designs for clinical trials with binary response. *Statistics in Medicine*, 1988; **7**: 571–9.

15. **Anonymous.** Phase II trials in the EORTC. The Protocol Review Committee, the Data Center, the Research and Treatment Division, and the New Drug Development Office, European Organization for Research and Treatment of Cancer. *European Journal of Cancer*, 1997; **33**: 1361–3.

16. **Jones B, Jarvis I, Lewis JB, Ebbur, AJ.** Trials to assess equivalence: the importance of rigorous methods. *British Medical Journal*, 1996; **313**: 36–9.

17. **Friedman L, Furberg K, DeMets D.** *Fundamentals of clinical trials* (3rd edn). St Louis: Mosby, 1996: 61–81.

18. **Non-small Cell Lung Cancer Collaborative Group.** Chemotherapy in non-small cell lung cancer: a meta-analysis using updated data on individual patients from 52 randomised clinical trials. *British Medical Journal*, 1989; **311**: 899–909.

19. **Lachin JM.** An introduction to sample size determination and power analysis for clinical trials. *Controlled Clinical Trials*, 1981; **2**: 93–113.

20. **Parmar MKB, Torri V, Stewart L.** Extracting summary statistics to perform meta-analyses of the published literature for survival endpoints. *Statistics in Medicine*, 1998; **17**: 2815–34.

21. **Peto R, et al.** Design and analysis of randomised clinical trials requiring prolonged observation of each patient. I Introduction and design. *British Journal of Cancer*, 1976; **34**: 585–12.

22. **Peto R, et al.** Design and analysis of randomised clinical trials requiring prolonged observation of each patient. II Analysis and examples. *British Journal of Cancer*, 1977; **35**: 1–39.

23. **Freedman LS.** Table of the number of patients required in clinical trials using the logrank test. *Statistics in Medicine*, 1982; **1**: 121–9.

24. **Lachin JM. Foulkes MA.** Evaluation of sample size and power for analyses of survival with allowance for nonuniform patient entry, losses to follow-up, noncompliance, and stratification. *Biometrics*, 1986; **42**: 507–19.

25. **Blackwelder WC.** 'Proving the null hypothesis' in clinical trials. *Controlled Clinical Trials*, 1982; **3**: 345–53.

26. **Freedman LS, Green SB.** Statistical design for investigating several interventions in the same study: methods for cancer prevention trials. *Journal of the National Cancer Institute*, 1990; **82**: 910–14.

27. **Demets DL.** Practical aspects in data monitoring: a brief review. *Statistics in Medicine*, 1987; **6**: 753–60.

28. **Berry D.** A case for Bayesianism in clinical trials. *Statistics in Medicine*, 1993; **12**: 1377–93.

29. **Etzioni R, Kadane J.** Bayesian statistical methods in public health and medicine. *Annual Review of Public Health*, 1995; **16**: 23–41.

30. **Parmar MKB, Spiegehalter DJ, Freedman LS.** The chart trials: Bayesian design and monitoring in practice *Statistics in Medicine*, 1994; **12**: 1297–1312.

31. **Fayers PM, Ashby D, Parmar MKB.** Tutorial in biostatistics: bayesian data monitoring in clinical trials. *Statistics in Medicine*, 1997; **16**: 1413–30.

32. Clerici M, on behalf of the Adjuvant Lung Project Italy (ALPI) trial. Randomised study of adjuvant chemotherapy for stage I–II–IIIa non-small cell lung cancer (NSCLC): report on the ALPI trial. *Proceedings of the American Society for Clinical Oncology*, 1995; **1141**, 370.

33. Altman DG. *Practical statistics for medical research*. London: Chapman and Hall, 1991.

34. Brown J, Machin D. Statistics and clinical oncology. *Clinical Oncology*, 1996; **8**: 71–4.

35. Bobbio M, Demichelis B, Giustetto G. Completeness of reporting trial results: effect on physicians' willingness to prescribe. *Lancet*, 1994; **343**: 1209–11.

36. Begg CB. Selection of patients for clinical trials. *Seminars in Oncology*, 1988; **15**: 434.

37. George SL. Reducing patient eligibility criteria in cancer clinical trials. *Journal of Clinical Oncology*, 1996; **14**: 136.

38. Hunter CP, *et al.* Selection factors in clinical trials: results from the community clinical oncology program physician's patient log. *Cancer Treatment Report*, 1987; **71**: 559.

39. Begg CB, *et al.* Cooperative groups and community hospitals: measurement of impact in the community hospital. *Cancer*, 1983; **52**: 1760.

40. Lomas J, *et al.* The role of evidence in the consensus process. Results from a Canadian consensus exercise. *Journal of the American Medical Association*, 1988; **259**: 3001.

41. Grimmshaw J, Russel I. Achieving health gain through clinical guidelines. 1 Developing scientifically valid guidelines. *Quality Health Care*, 1993; **2**: 243.

42. D'Agostino R, Weintraub M. Meta-analysis: a method for synthesizing research. *Clinical Pharmacology and Therapeutics*, 1995; **58**: 605–16.

43. Early breast cancer trialists collaborative group. Effect of adjuvant tamoxifen and cytotoxic therapy on mortality in early breast cancer. *New England Journal of Medicine*, 1988; **319**: 1681–92.

44. Non-small cell lung cancer collaborative group. Chemotherapy in non-small cell lung cancer: a meta-analysis using updated data on individual patients from 52 randomised clinical trials. *British Medical Journal*, 1995; **311**: 899–909.

45. Verter J. How much data should we collect in a randomized clinical trial? *Statistics in Medicine*, 1990; **9**: 103–13.

46. Spilker B, Schoenfelder J. *Data collection forms in clinical trials*. New York: Raven Press, 1991.

47. McFadden ET, LoPresti F, Bailey LR, Clarke E, Wilkins PC. Approaches to data management. *Controlled Clinical Trials*, 1995; **16**: 30S–65S.

48. Christiansen DH, Hosking JD, Dannenberg AN, Williams OD. Computer-assisted data collection in epidemiology research. *Controlled Clinical Trials*, 1990; **11**: 101–15.

49. MACRO. ©Integral Solution Limited. http://www.infermed.com/

50. Clintrial®. Domain pharma Corporation. http://www.Domain.pharma.com/

51. SAS/PH-Clinical® Software. SAS Institute Inc., Cary, NC. http://www.sas.com/.

52. IMPACT. Fraser Williams. www.fraser-williams.com/impact/

53. Oracle Pharmaceuticals®. Oracle Corporation. http://www.oracle.com/.

54. Pocock SJ. *Clinical trials: a practical approach*. New York: Wiley, 1983.

55. Martinez YN, McMahon A, Barnell GM, Wigodsky HS. Ensuring data quality in medical research through an integrated data management system. *Statistics in Medicine*, 1984; **3**: 101–11.

56. Renard J, Van Glabbeke M. Quality control and data handling. In *Data management and clinical trials* (ed. N Rotmensz, K Vantogelen, J Renard). New York: Elsevier, 1989: 147–62.

57. Neaton JD, Duchene AG, Svendsen KH, Wentworth D. An examination of the efficiency of some quality assurance methods commonly employed in clinical trials. *Statistics in Medicine*, 1990; **9**: 115–24.

58. Day S, Fayers P, Harvey D. Double data entry: what value, what price? *Controlled Clinical Trials*, 1998; **19**: 15–24.

59. Flann M, Tinazzi A, Torri V. Weeding out bad apples: monitoring data quality in RCTs. *Controlled Clinical Trials*, 1996; **17**(2S): 116. [Abstract]

60. Sylvester RJ, *et al.* Quality of institutional participation in multicenter clinical trials. *New England Journal of Medicine*, 1981; **305**: 852–5.

61. Eastern Co-operative Oncology Group. Participation of community hospital in clinical trials: analysis of five years of experience in the Eastern Co-operative Oncology Group. *New England Journal of Medicine*, 1982; **306**: 1076–80.

62. Cote RA, Robboy S. Progress in medical information management: Systematised nomenclature of medicine (SNOMED). *Journal of the American Medical Association*, 1980; **243**: 756–62.

63. DUMC Duke University Medical Centre. Health Informatics Standards. http://www.mcis.duke.edu/standards/termcode/codehome.htm.

64. Sills J. World Health Organisation Adverse Reaction Terminology Dictionary. *Drug Information Journal*, 1989; **23**: 211–16.

65. Joseph M, Schoeffler K, Doi Pa, Yefko H, Engle C, Nissman E. An automated COSTART coding scheme. *Drug Information Journal*, 1991; **25**: 97–108.

66. Forbes MB, Perez AE, Gelberg A. FDA's adverse drug reaction drug dictionary and its role in post-marketing surveillance. *Drug Information Journal*, 1986; **20**: 135–45.

7.2 Endpoints

Andrew Kramar

The choice of criteria for assessing the results of cancer treatment is an important part in the evaluation of treatments or therapeutic strategies. Many different criteria can be defined or constructed, but they will always fall into two main categories: (1) efficacy, which symbolizes the potential capability of the treatment to cure the patient's disease or to improve his/her well being; and (2) toxicity, the potential capability of the treatment to avoid adverse harmful effects to the patient. However, just what is meant by a success or a failure will depend on the particular clinical experimental situation. In some situations, a primary and secondary endpoint may be used simultaneously in expressing treatment efficacy. A balance between all these measures will often be used as an overall evaluation of the treatment strategy. In all cases, the criterion used should be clinically meaningful and easily reproducible from one study type to another.

In phase I trials, the objective is to study the clinical pharmacology and the relationship between toxicity and the treatment dose schedule in search of a maximum tolerated dose (**MTD**), which will in turn determine a lower recommended dose for phase II studies. Cancer patients with advanced stages of the disease, who have either failed to respond to other treatments or for whom no other therapies exist, are usually included in such trials. From the experimenter's point of view, a success can be defined as having reached the MTD; although from the patient's point of view, experiencing toxicity will not in general be considered a success. In such trials, the probability for the patient experiencing toxicity is much more likely than experiencing efficacy. A review of 7960 patients treated in 228 phase I trials over a 14-year period estimated a 6 per cent response rate. The authors concluded that, although the response rate is indeed low, it was unlikely that the drug would be used in the clinic if no responses were noted in these phase I studies.[1]

Phase II studies are initiated in order to identify promising treatments for specific tumour sites. In these studies, a success is usually defined as a complete or significant decrease in tumour size or in the size of metastatic lesions after a specified evaluation time. In these types of studies, there is more chance of observing increased therapeutic response rates than in phase I studies. This is because the patient population is more homogeneous and a potential clinical benefit is expected for the patients who are now treated at the dose recommended from the results of the phase I trial. These studies are performed on a relatively small number of patients in order to decide whether the treatment ought to be studied in large-scale comparative trials. Precise definitions of response need to be used, since response is the main criterion in phase II studies. The experimental design of most phase II trials now evaluate response in at least two stages, with

the possibility of rejecting a drug early if it is unlikely to show sufficient activity.[2],[3]

In trials containing a small number of patients, it may be difficult to make decisions on whether or not to continue the trial based on the number of responses observed after the first stage, especially if the definition of response is imprecise. The decision rules for choosing the number of responses and the number of patients is determined in such a way as to satisfy the error associated with: (1) rejecting a promising treatment (alpha risk, usually as 10 per cent); and (2) not rejecting an invaluable treatment (beta risk, usually taken as 5 per cent). Declaring a treatment as promising after a phase II trial will consequently lead to further study in phase III. If in fact, this treatment is no better than the standard, then this phase III trial will have been undertaken unnecessarily. On the other hand, declaring a treatment as insufficiently active after a phase II trial will consequently mean the abandonment of further development. If in fact, this treatment is a worthwhile option, then patients will not be given the chance to benefit from this treatment. In most planning stages of phase II trials the beta error rate is considered much more important than the alpha error rate. Phase II studies also provide supplementary data on toxicity.

In phase III studies, success may be defined in many ways. The usual main endpoint for such studies is the duration of survival. It is an objective measure, being clinically meaningful and easy to update. However, success in this case concerns the vital status of the patient, which will obviously change over time with more follow-up. From a particular patient's point of view, the treatment can only be considered a success as long as the patient is alive. From the investigator's point of view, the treatment can be considered a viable option if the probability of living longer is increased in comparison to another standard or reference treatment. So from a technical point of view, it is time to failure, rather than time to success, which is considered the main endpoint in this situation. However, even though time to death is a final ultimate measure, time to treatment failure may be more readily used in such studies.

Other measures such as tumour progression, local recurrence, distance metastases, second malignancies, treatment-related complications, or quality of life in general are also widely used. From these definitions, other endpoints—such as progression-free survival, relapse-free survival, disease-free survival, event-free survival, failure-free survival, complication-free survival, or quality-adjusted survival—have appeared in the literature and are used regularly in evaluating treatments. However, it is not always clear as to what are the differences or similarities between these measures, and why one particular endpoint is chosen as the main judgement criterion for a particular study.

In studies designed to investigate treatment efficacy, many endpoints will generally be reported simultaneously. However, before launching a trial the primary endpoint must be chosen in order to calculate sample size. Since the interpretation of the data relies heavily upon the vocabulary used, the terminology needs to be clearly defined so that the same names refer to the same criteria and different names refer to different criteria. The following sections present definitions commonly used for response, non-response, and toxicity and describe how these measures are then summarized to form indices useful in evaluating therapeutic strategies.

Response

Clinical response

Percentage changes in tumour size before and after treatment are used in defining clinical response in many cancer-treatment trials. The definition of response according to the World Health Organization (WHO) falls into four main categories:[4]

- complete disappearance of tumour (complete response, CR);
- a more than 50 per cent decrease in tumour size (partial response, PR);
- no change in tumour size (stable disease, SD); and
- a more than 25 per cent increase in tumour size (progressive disease, PD).

The designation of minor response should be avoided. So, according to the WHO definitions of stable disease, tumours which decrease by less than 50 per cent are considered as having stabilized in the same way as tumours which increase by no more than 25 per cent.

For patients with metastatic disease, change in the size of lesions, measurable in two perpendicular diameters, follow the same pattern of definitions. The per cent change can be calculated from the product of the bidimensional measurements of each lesion taken individually, but in most cases it is calculated from the sum of the products of all bidimensional measurements among all target lesions within the same organ site. For malignant disease measurable only in one dimension, such as abdominal, mediastinal, or hilar mass, the evaluation of tumour size is less reliable.

An example for calculating response evaluation is presented in Table 1. Consider a patient with two thoracic node lesions and three pulmonary lesions measurable in two dimensions. The first lesion in the thoracic-node organ site measured 952 mm² at baseline. After chemotherapy, this lesion measured 418 mm², resulting in a 56 per cent decrease. Per cent change in the sum of the products of the perpendicular dimensions within each organ site result in a 51 per cent and 59 per cent decrease in the thoracic nodes and lung lesions, respectively. This patient is thus classified as a partial responder. Had the per cent **decrease** in thoracic nodes been less than 50 per cent, this patient would have been classified with stable disease. Had the per cent **increase** in thoracic nodes been more than 25 per cent, this patient would have been classified with progressive disease.

However, no matter what response is observed for the selected target lesions, patients are none the less classified as having progressive disease if new lesions appear. Proposed modifications by the Southwest Oncology Group (**SWOG**) classify patients as having progressive disease when a more than 50 per cent increase in tumour size or

metastatic lesions is observed. These modifications were motivated by concerns regarding the ease with which a patient may be considered mistakenly to have disease progression by the current criteria, primarily because of measurement error. For this and other reasons, such as the arbitrary definition of a partial response, Response Evaluation Criteria in Solid Tumors (RECIST) guidelines have been proposed.[5] These guidelines will probably supersede the WHO criteria. In summary, these guidelines propose to use unidimensional instead of bidimensional measurements and to compare the change in the sum of the longest diameter for all target lesions from baseline instead of the sum of the products of the longest diameter with its perpendicular diameter for all target lesions from baseline. Definition of response then falls into the four following main categories: complete response—the disappearance of all target lesions; partial response—at least a 30 per cent decrease in the sum of the longest diameter of target lesions as compared to baseline; progressive disease—at least a 20 per cent increase in the sum of the longest diameter as compared to the smallest sum longest diameter recorded since treatment started or the appearance of one or more new lesions; and stable disease: (SD) as neither sufficient shrinkage to qualify for partial response nor sufficient increase to qualify for progressive disease, taking as reference the smallest sum longest diameter since the treatment started.[5]

For patients with non-measurable organ sites, such as bone metastases, change from baseline is not very easy to measure and treatment response can be highly biased. Examples of non-measurable evaluable lesions include the following: ill-defined pelvic or abdominal masses; lymphangitic lung metastases; malignant ascites or pleural effusion uninfluenced by diuretics; ill-defined skin metastases; and bone metastases. Due to the slow evolution of these latter lesions, response needs to be defined according to other terminology, such as those adopted by the European Organization for Research and Treatment of Cancer (**EORTC**) or the SWOG.[6] In such cases, stabilizing the spread of bone metastases may be considered a success. The notion of response (non-response) thus depends on which definition is used for assessing success (or failure). Similar difficulties occur for patients who present a multitude of metastatic lesions, where the appreciation of the appropriate clinical response category may be more difficult and subjective. For instance, the SWOG classifies patients with uncontrolled hypercalcaemia or increasing skeletal involvement, as manifested by an increasing number of lytic lesions on bone scan, as patients with progressive disease.

Assessing response can be made more difficult with the continual improvement of imaging techniques. To obtain an unbiased assessment of tumour response, a second-party review by a panel of experts, exterior to the study, is recommended and has become standard practice in many clinical trials.[7]

For practical reasons, certain oncology groups restrict the type of lesions, which are considered eligible for response evaluation, by imposing a minimum size for the bidimensional lesions. For example, skin metastases of at least 2.5 cm, lung metastases of at least 2 cm not adjacent to any other structure, and liver metastases or soft tissue lesions of at least 2.5 cm measured by ultrasound or computed tomography (**CT**) scan. The RECIST criteria categorize tumour lesions as either measurable in at least one dimension if the longest diameter is 20 mm or more with conventional techniques or is 10 mm or more with spiral CT scan.[6] All other tumour lesions are categorized as non-measurable if the longest diameter is less than 20 mm with conventional techniques or is less than 10 mm with spiral CT scan,

Table 1 Example of response calculation for a patient presenting several bidimensional measurable lesions in two different organ sites

Organ sites	Pretreatment			Post-treatment			% Change
	mm^1	mm^2	Product	mm^1	mm^2	Product	
Thoracic nodes							
Lesion 1	34	28	952	22	19	418	−56
Lesion 2	43	40	1720	37	24	888	−48
Sub-total			2672			1306	−51
Lung							
Lesion 1	24	17	408	14	10	140	−66
Lesion 2	30	19	570	23	12	276	−52
Lesion 3	21	19	399	15	10	150	−62
Sub-total			1377			566	−59

or as truly non-measurable. They do not recommend to use the term 'evaluable' in reference to measurability since it does not provide additional meaning or accuracy. Truly non-measurable lesions include bone lesions, leptomeningeal disease, ascites, pleural/pericardial effusion, inflammatory breast disease, lymphangitis cutis/pulmonis, abdominal masses that are not confirmed and followed by imaging techniques, and cystic lesions.

These restrictions are usually applied to phase II studies, since the per cent change in these measurements is the main criterion for assessing treatment effect. In phase III studies, no limit is usually imposed as to the minimum measurements used in defining response when this measurement criterion is not the main endpoint.

Some authors may be stricter in their definition of response and include only the absence of either a complete or partial response as a failure—commonly referred to as an objective response. This definition is preferred by many due to the subjective nature of the definition of a partial response, the frequency of assessment, as well as the duration of response.[8] To reduce misclassification errors, it has been suggested that the criteria be assessed at least 1 month apart.[9] If this second evaluation is incorporated in the definition of response, it can be used in many ways. First of all, it is usually performed on patients who are in complete or partial response in order to confirm the response. For instance, patients are only considered to have a complete response if it lasts at least 1 month. The SWOG is even stricter in their definition of partial response. They classify patients into this category if a decrease of at least 50 per cent in measurable lesions has been observed for at least 3 months. If this is the case, then the date of complete response corresponds to the date of the first evaluation and the second evaluation only serves as confirmation. Non-confirmed complete responses will either need to be reviewed or ignored. If differences are observed between the two evaluations, then patients will usually be classified in the worst category at the reported date of the corresponding response. Patients with a partial response at the first evaluation and a complete response at the second evaluation will usually be classified as showing a complete response at the date of the second evaluation. Knowledge of these dates are important for calculating the response duration.

Since tumour recurrence can be observed to occur in patients who showed a complete response, it is important to study the duration of response as a complete response of short duration may not be

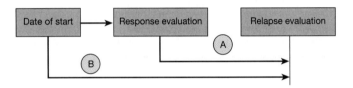

Fig. 1 Assessing the duration of response to therapy.

considered a long-lasting success. On the other hand, patients with long-lasting stable disease may progress after a much longer period. It is important to evaluate not only the percentage of patients who respond to treatment but also the duration of response. When speaking of response duration, it seems logical to define response duration only among patients who respond, whether completely or partially, and to calculate the duration between the onset of response and the date when progressive disease is first noted. However, these two response categories may be treated differently depending on whether complete, partial, or overall response durations are to be reported. Difficulties in defining response duration are linked to the fact that a responding patient may undergo a period of continuing improvement and eventually reach a complete response. The duration of complete response will then be calculated from the date of the complete response until relapse (corresponding to A in Fig. 1), but the duration of partial response is be calculated from the start of treatment (corresponding to B in Fig. 1).[10] However, this method is not employed by all, since it may imply a shorter response duration for complete than for partial responders. These difficulties have been encountered in the reporting of outcomes in Hodgkin's disease and lymphoma.[11] For instance, the EORTC has adopted the same response-duration definition for complete and partial responders, and start the clock running from either the date of randomization or from the start of treatment in non-randomized studies (corresponding to B in Fig. 1). This method eliminates part of the bias linked to the imprecision in date of a complete response, as well as the fact that is inappropriate to subset patients using a time-dependent outcome measure and then measure 'time-to-event' from the onset of therapy.[11] The RECIST recommend to measure the duration of objective response from either complete or partial response, whichever status is recorded first, until the first date that recurrent or progressive disease is objectively documented, taking as reference for progressive disease the smallest measurements recorded since the treatment started.[6] In any case, the definition used should be clearly stated in the protocol and/or in the resulting publications.

Response definitions, which take into account a second measurement, are stricter, in the sense that they may avoid misclassifying patients who are at the frontier of the cut-off point used in defining response. Nevertheless, some difficulties will occur and will have to be handled appropriately. What to do with patients who do not have a second evaluation? What to do with patients who have a second evaluation less than 1 month after the first evaluation or much later than 1 month? It is important for the reader to be aware of these difficulties when evaluating response rates for a particular study.

Marker response

In some cases it may be necessary to rely on the evaluation of validated biochemical tumour markers in defining response, either to reduce the need for regular scanning or simply because clinical response may be difficult to measure. However, these recommendations will usually only be applied to phase III studies. For instance, a decrease in prostate-specific antigen (PSA) may be used as a parameter of response evaluation for patients with prostate cancer. The serum tumour markers α-fetoprotein (AFP) and human chorionic gonadotropin (hCG) are critical to the choice of therapy and monitoring of patients with germ-cell tumours of the testis.[13] These proteins are concordant with the growth of the tumour and disappear from the serum following effective surgery and chemotherapy.[14] As a result, these tumour markers are actually used in conjunction with clinical evaluation in defining response to treatment, especially in patients with advanced disease.[15] The false-negative rate is very low, and normal levels of hCG in choriocarcinoma reliably indicate the presence of fewer than 10^5 tumour cells.[16] The estimation of the marker half-life for patients undergoing chemotherapy may be used as a way of detecting drug resistance. If the marker does not decline sufficiently during the first cycles of therapy this may indicate the need to change to a more intensive treatment protocol.[17],[18]

Several authors have attempted to formally define marker response in tumour sites where no such 'magic' markers have yet been found. These definitions are based on the correlation between the per cent change in marker levels from baseline with clinical tumour-response criteria. A more precise correlation may be obtained through the use of more precise tumour measurements of specific metastatic sites for patients with advanced disease. These definitions, however, need to be easy enough to be used in practice, but precise enough for evaluating treatments in clinical trials. For example, definitions based on serial CA-125 levels used to measure the response of ovarian carcinoma in patients receiving first-line chemotherapy have been proposed.[19] Other examples include the comparison of the per cent change in the carcinoembryonic antigen (CEA), the clinical response to chemotherapy for patients with gastrointestinal cancers,[20] and for patients with advanced colorectal cancer.[21] Most definitions of marker response and marker progression are based on criteria similar to the WHO, Eastern Cooperative Oncology Group (ECOG)[22] and EORTC definitions of clinical response, in that they involve defining a cut-off point for the per cent change in marker values from baseline.

It is also possible to apply stricter definitions for marker response by defining a complete marker response for those patients who maintain normal marker levels for at least 4 weeks. Recommendations by the EORTC incorporate biochemical markers in the overall response evaluation, in so far as a clinical complete response is only considered complete if marker levels have also been normalized. Clinical partial response is only considered a partial response if marker levels have decreased by at least 90 per cent, and a 25 per cent rise in marker level means progression. Of course, the use of markers in defining response should only refer to validated markers in specific tumour sites.

Similar methodological problems arise for the definition of marker response as for the definitions used for clinical response. One difficulty has to do with defining whether the per cent change should be calculated on an arithmetic or logarithmic scale, the latter being more appropriate when the measurements follow a log-normal distribution. However, this question is never brought up for clinical response, although it could be. It is also important to determine how often the measurements should be made, and how measurements that exhibit a 'yo-yo' effect should be handled. Apart from measurement error associated with biological measurements, this effect may be associated with the timing of the initial value, which should not be taken too long before the start of initial treatment. In some cases, if the marker values are correlated with the extent of disease and if the initial measurement was taken too early before the start of treatment, the markers may be seen to increase under therapy when in fact they are decreasing. When two or more markers are used in defining response, as with hCG and AFP in germ-cell tumours, then strict definitions for complete marker response will require both markers to be normalized. Progressive marker response will require that at least one marker increases by, say, at least 25 per cent.

Some patients will present difficulties to the assessment of clinical response and/or marker response. Considerable variation is observed in response rates across many studies of the same treatment, which could be explained not only by the differences in patient characteristics but also by the different methods used in assessing response, as well as by measurement errors.[23] Methods for calculating the duration of response, and whether or not an external review panel is used to confirm the response, may influence many of the overall results. Data representations on different selected patient populations may also contribute to some of the discrepancies observed. Guidelines for the use of tumour markers in breast and colorectal cancer in clinical practice have recently been adopted by the American Society for Clinical Oncology Tumour Marker Expert Panel.[24]

Recommendations by the RECIST working group provide recent guidelines concerning the evaluation of overall response which take into account target, non-target, and new lesions, the frequency of re-evaluation especially for phase II trials, as well as the need for confirmation of objective response in order to avoid the over-estimation of the response rate observed. An editorial concerning these recent recommendations insist on the fact that these new criteria should be continuously evaluated since even small differences in response rates could affect the conduct of phase I and phase II trials.[25]

Representation of data for response

Data for response evaluation will usually be descriptive in nature, beginning with an assessment of how many patients responded to

Table 2 Examples of various response-rate calculations depending on the patient population

	Whole population (n = 48)		Eligible only (n = 45)		Eligible and evaluable (n = 39)	
Objective response	13	27%	13	29%	13	33%
95% CI	[15%–41%]		[16%–44%]		[19%–50%]	
Stable disease	18		15		15	
Progressive disease	11		11		11	
Non-evaluable	6		6		—	

treatment (complete and partial), how many had stable disease, and how many progressed at the time of evaluation. Sometimes the best response is also reported. The number of ineligible and non-evaluable patients should also accompany the tables for response, along with reasons for their ineligibility and non-evaluability. The per cent objective response in phase II trials is usually provided along with 95 per cent confidence intervals (CI) obtained from the binomial distribution. Tables for such calculations are readily available. The true response rate should lie within this interval 95 per cent of the time. The denominator used in the calculation should be described, since response rates are calculated as the ratio of the number of patients who respond relative to the total patient population at risk of responding, which is usually taken as the whole population. This implies treating non-evaluable patients as non-responders. The per cent response obtained for the whole patient population is generally referred to as an 'intent-to-treat analysis'. However, the use of different patient populations in the denominator will give different response rates, the least favourable rate usually being the one calculated for the entire patient population. If no responses are observed among ineligible and non-evaluable patients, then it is easy to verify that $R/N < R/(N–K)$ where R corresponds to the number of responses, N is the number of patients, and K is the number of ineligible and non-evaluable patients. Response rates, calculated only on the population who received the full treatment, should be avoided, since these rates will not provide a true picture of the feasibility of the protocol when eventually applied in clinical practice.

For example, suppose the following results were observed in a phase II trial. Of the 48 patients entered, 3 were considered ineligible due to an error in diagnosis. These three patients were evaluated for response and had stable disease. Some six patients were considered non-evaluable for response since they dropped out of the study before response could be evaluated (two for toxicity, three for refusal to continue, and one lost to follow-up). Table 2 presents the results for the whole population, eligible patients only, and eligible and evaluable patients only.

The response rate increases from 27 per cent to 29 per cent to 33 per cent depending on the patient population (Table 2) The least favourable are observed in the intent-to-treat analysis. Among the eligible patients only, the results obtained consider non-evaluable patients as non-responders. Among the eligible and evaluable patients only, the results obtained consider non-evaluable patients as re-sponders in the same proportion as evaluable patients.

Toxicity and adverse events

The evaluation of toxicity and adverse events is the main criterion in the search for the maximum tolerated dose in phase I studies. The information gathered in these studies is thus very detailed. Acute toxicity is usually evaluated in phase II and phase III trials to complement information about the treatment. Late adverse events are essentially evaluated in phase III trials where patients are followed for many years.

Acute effects

No matter which part of the drug development process is being studied, it is important to choose the most appropriate toxicity grading system: WHO, EORTC, National Cancer Institute of Canada—Common Toxicity Criteria (**NCIC-CTC**), SWOG, Radio-therapy Oncology Group (**RTOG**), etc. The choice of the most appropriate scale will depend on the known effects of the drug. For instance, a new drug which presents known gastrointestinal effects may supplement the usual toxicity grading systems with a much more complete daily account of adverse events.

Once the choice of the appropriate scale of measurement is made, the frequency of assessment needs to be defined. Haematological toxicity, if evaluated only at the beginning of each chemotherapy cycle, will not be sufficient in calculating the nadir nor the duration of aplasia. Studies specifically designed to evaluate the effects of growth factors on haematological toxicity or studies with new cytotoxic agents will need to be stringent in defining the frequency of assessment. Studies where the frequency of assessment differs between treatment arms may produce biased comparisons.

Late effects

Late effects are one of the major endpoints in studies that evaluate treatment with some form of radiation therapy. It is well known from radiobiology that increased dose rates influence late effects to a greater extent than early effects. So in trials which compare different dose rates, it is imperative to use late-effects scoring systems and to follow patients regularly in order to be able to capture these effects. Late effects associated with radiotherapy have been coded into a system with 'subjective, objective, management, and analytical' (**SOMA**) components for the evaluation of 'late effects on normal tissue (**LENT**).[26] Scoring systems have also been developed for specific cancer sites such as gynaecological cancers.[27] Chemotherapy pro-tocols, which include anthracyclines, have been associated with an increased risk of cardiac events. Therapy for Hodgkin's disease may result in severe infections, thyroid, cardiovascular, pulmonary, di-gestive, or gonadal dysfunction. It may also result in secondary malignancy, which is considered to be the most serious com-plication.[28]

Representation of data for toxicity

Data for toxicity evaluation will usually be descriptive in nature, beginning with an assessment of how many and what percentage of patients presented a specific toxic event. These toxic events are usually separated into haematological and non-haematological toxicity by grade. Data can also be presented by cycle for patients undergoing chemotherapy. In some instances, percentages are presented with the total number of grade 3 or more toxic events observed divided by the total number of cycles. This measure may be meaningful as an economic measure, but it does not take into account the fact that the same patient may be continually presenting the same toxic event for each cycle. Confounding data from all cycles will consider a patient who experiences four grade 3 toxicities in the same way as four patients experiencing one grade 3 toxicity.

Time-to-event data

As already mentioned in the Introduction, in cancer studies it is unfortunately much easier to rely on a definition of failure than it is to rely on the definition of a success, especially in the long term. Even for complete responses which present no images of disease on the CT scan, a few tumour cells may still be present just waiting to recur in the near or distant future. For studies where overall survival is the major endpoint, it is obvious that treatment will be evaluated by comparing survival curves and not just the number of deaths, since if the investigator waits long enough and receives regular follow-up information on all patients, all the patients will eventually die. The percentage of successes will thus be zero, ignoring those lost to follow-up of course. This will not necessarily be the case for intermediate endpoints—such as local failure, distant failure, second malignancies, or death from cancer—since these events will not be observed to occur in all patients no matter how long the investigator waits. Just how these events will be accounted for in the analysis of each one of these individual events will, of course, influence the results if many competing events of different types are likely to occur.

Overall survival

Time to death is an easy quantity to measure as long as patients are followed and information is regularly communicated to the statistical centre. Overall survival thus constitutes an ultimate indicator of treatment success or failure. Some studies use **cancer-specific** survival analysis by considering deaths from other causes as part of the independent censoring mechanism. If the probability of deaths from other causes are highly likely, then it will be important to consider methods relating to competing risks in order to obtain an overall picture of the treatment effect.[29]

One rational for focusing attention on death from cancer is that differences in treatment efficacy may be masked by deaths from other causes, especially if they are numerous and/or unequally distributed between treatment groups. However, it is not always easy to classify patients into causes of death related or not related to cancer. Death from myocardial infarction, for example, can be related to chemotherapy.

Even though time to death is a final ultimate measure, it may not necessarily be well adapted to all situations. For studies of adjuvant therapy, the obvious main endpoint is tumour recurrence, since the aim of the therapy is to improve the probability that the patient has been cured of his neoplastic disease.[30] Overall survival in these situations should nevertheless be investigated as a secondary endpoint, since potential adverse consequences to these therapies may include second malignancies such as leukaemia and other myelodysplastic disorders.[31]

External comparisons using overall mortality data can also be used to correct for non-cancer deaths and thus to obtain net survival estimates. Relative survival can be defined as the ratio of the observed survival of a given cohort of patients to the survival that the group would have experienced based on the life table of the population from which they were diagnosed.[32] Interpretation in this setting can allow an estimation of the time to cure, thus correcting for overall mortality adjusted for age and gender. However, this method has some disadvantages since it is heavily influenced by the initial age distribution of the cohort and by its evolution with time. It is also influenced by the heterogeneity of life expectancy within the cohort. Thus it cannot be reliably used for comparisons between populations. This method can produce increasing survival rates, which may be even greater than 100 per cent in some cases, thus suggesting that cancer patients receive better medical care than the general population. A more logical explanation has to do with the fact that there will be an increasing dominance of individuals with the longest life expectancy. For some cancers, net survival is better for those diagnosed at a younger age. A maximum likelihood approach using modelling techniques for computing net survival rather than relative survival has been suggested,[32] which avoids some of these problems.

Progression-, relapse-, and disease-free survival

Treatment failure can be defined by a multitude of events such as disease progression, local recurrences, distant metastases, or second malignancies. There are no international definitions for disease-free survival, relapse-free survival, or progression-free survival. Most authors, however, do seem to know what they are referring to when they refer to these endpoints. Disease progression is used as a category for failure when no response has been observed. A patient who fails 'locally' is said to have a local recurrence, whereas a patient who develops metastases is said to have a distant recurrence. These definitions are quite standard. The main difficulty, however, lies in the fact that it is not always clear which patient population is used in the calculation of survival rates for these endpoints. Similar difficulties are encountered when describing the number of patients who have 'no evidence of disease' (**NED**). It is not always clear whether a 1-year 50 per cent NED rate refers to the patient population, which has not yet failed at all, or whether it also encompasses patients who have initially failed but who are in a state of NED at 1 year after a second intervention. Minimum follow-up of patients is of importance when reporting results in this way.

For the calculation of disease-free survival, some authors may censor patients who develop second malignancies, considering these patients as no longer at risk of a relapse once a second malignancy has been observed. In estimating disease-free survival rates, however, it is much better to include all events (including local and distant relapses, second cancers, or death, whichever comes first) and to describe the pattern of events. Disease-free survival, by its name, refers to a period during which the patient no longer has any clinical manifestation of the disease. This implies that the starting point for estimating disease-free survival rates is the date of a complete response. To represent the disease-free survival rate over time, some authors have suggested that survival estimates are applied in the usual way, and that non-complete responses are counted as failures at time 0. This has the effect of representing the complete response rate on the same graph as the disease-free survival curve.[33]

For relapse-free survival, the same care needs to be taken in defining which events should be used and how they are taken into account. Relapse-free survival, by its name, refers to a period during which the patient has not yet relapsed but is at risk of failing treatment. This implies that the starting point for estimating relapse-free survival rates is the first date of treatment, or the date of randomization in randomized trials. The end date is the date of relapse, death, or the last follow-up, whichever comes first. Events such as second cancers or death from causes other than cancer are usually treated as censored observations in this context. Due to the lack of a consensus in the definition of these types of endpoints, it has become necessary to describe the definitions in sufficient detail in the Methods sections of all protocols and publications.

Local control

Many studies, which evaluate the effects of 'locally applied' treatment, such as surgery or radiotherapy, use local control as the main endpoint for evaluating treatment. In this context, it is easier to define local failure rather than local control since failure can easily be considered a failure, whereas local control may eventually become a failure with sufficient follow-up. Nevertheless, there are pitfalls associated with the identification of local failure endpoints, especially for cancer sites such as localized prostate cancer, which base a risk in the PSA markers as a surrogate for local failure.[34]

There are two types of local failure. The first of which concerns those patients who never respond. The second type of local failure refers to patients who fail locally after a first response was observed. It can also refer to patients who fail locally a second time after a successful treatment intervention rendered the patient disease-free after the first local failure. Local failure can thus be thought of as a process containing several components. At any point in time, the local control rate can represent the percentage of patients who have not yet failed locally. This percentage is usually small, since it is calculated as a simple ratio of the number of patients who failed locally (at least once) to the total number of patients. However, this percentage does not reflect the percentage of patients who are in a state of local control at any point in time, since patients who previously failed locally can be in a state of local control after a successful second intervention. Similar arguments hold for the NED status mentioned previously. This percentage also does not reflect the estimate of the local control rate, had other patients not experienced distant failure, nor died from their disease. These events will interfere with an estimate of the net local control rate. Comparisons between studies with different local control rates will depend heavily on the distribution and the timing of the occurrence of other events. Usual Kaplan–Meier survival methods of analysis of time to local failure are thus not always pertinent. Two populations with exactly the same number of local failures occurring at exactly the same event times will show different local control rates if patients in one group experience metastases at an earlier rate.[35]

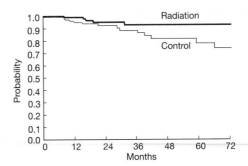

Fig. 2 Naive Kaplan–Meier curves (assuming independent censoring) for time to local failure for patients with breast cancer randomized to radiation or observation (control) after mastectomy plus adjuvant chemotherapy; distant failure counted as censored observations. (From Gelber *et al.* 1990[33] with permission.)

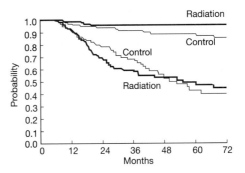

Fig. 3 Bounds for time to local failure curves (when independent censoring is not assumed) for breast cancer patients in Fig. 2; any curve falling inside these bounds is as good an estimate as the naive Kaplan–Meier curve. (From Gelman *et al.* 1990[33] with permission.)

Gelman *et al.*[35] present an example showing the 'naive' Kaplan–Meier curves for the time to local failure of patients with breast cancer randomized to radiation or observation after mastectomy plus adjuvant chemotherapy. These curves assume independent censoring. Patients who fail first in distant sites or die without local failure are counted as censored observations. Figure 2 tends to favour radiation therapy over observation.

Figure 3 shows the bounds for the Kaplan–Meier curves for the time to local failure with two assumptions: (1) the lower bounds of the curves assume that all patients who first fail distantly are destined to fail locally shortly after their distant failure—if this were the case, then adjuvant radiotherapy would be considered an ineffective means of improving local control. (2) The upper bounds assume that all patients who first fail distantly are destined to never fail locally. This example illustrates that the effects of therapy on local control depend on the extent to which a correlation exists between local and distant failure.

There is thus a methodological problem in analysing time to local failure with the use of readily available survival analysis software, since the censoring mechanism incorporates deaths without local failure and possibly distant metastases. The same problem occurs when analysing cancer-specific death by censoring deaths from other

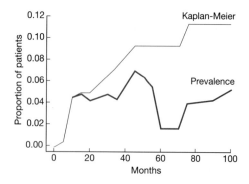

Fig. 4 Plot of the proportion of patients estimated to have complications (prevalence) as a function of time after treatment. Also shown is the Kaplan–Meier plot of the cumulative probability of experiencing a complication. (From Peters *et al.* 1995[36] with permission.)

causes. Considering these endpoints as independent of one another, when in fact dependency exists, may lead to contradictory and counterintuitive results. This phenomenon should be considered when interpreting data analyses involving competing risks.[36] In overall survival analyses, a censored observation will eventually become a death with more follow-up, but early deaths will 'prevent' the observation of local recurrences. It is recommended that time to local failure should be analysed using methods adapted from competing-risk methodology, especially if the probability of observing other events is relatively high. The occurrence of events such as distant failures or early deaths can mask the potential benefits or harms of chemoradiotherapy associations. The cumulative incidence estimates so obtained provide straightforward probability estimates, but these should be interpreted simultaneously with other events.[37]

Complications

If acute and chronic toxicities or complications constitute another mode of failure, this event can be incorporated as another failure type. An analysis of the time to the first complication using cumulative incidence observations provides information as to the time distribution of the first complication, but it is insufficient in describing the reversible nature of these events. Not all treatment complications are permanent: some resolve spontaneously and others are amenable to correction. This may also occur in succession and be of varying severity. None of the commonly used methods for reporting results makes the distinction between **experiencing** a complication at some point and **having** a complication at a subsequent timepoint.[38] One possibility for representing long-term reversible complications over time is to evaluate the prevalence of complications, by considering multiple entries into a complication state over time among patients still alive.

Figure 4 shows an example of how the Kaplan–Meier estimate of cumulative probability overestimates the likelihood that at any given time a surviving patient will have a complication.[38] The use of nonparametric methods for taking a cure state into account provides a much better picture of the reversible nature of these events, since these curves can decrease either because of recovery from complication or because those patients with complications die more rapidly than those without. The prevalence estimate provides an indication of the

percentage of patients in a state of complication at each specific point in time. In situations where complications states are regularly collected according to a validated scoring system, these prevalence estimates can be weighed according to degrees of severity.[39]

Representation of time-to-event data

When analysing time-to-event data, descriptive statistics provide an indication as to the total number of events that have occurred, but this crude method does not take time into account. To take time into account, it is necessary to define the event of interest, a starting date, and an end date. There are many statistical methods for estimating survival rates for time-to-event data, the most common one in clinical trial and prognostic factor studies is the Kaplan–Meier method.[40] This method is non-parametric in the statistical sense, in that no specific parametric assumptions need to be made about the distribution of the time-to-event data. The term 'actuarial survival' is also employed, but it should only be used on large data sets or when data is only available in grouped form. In general, the univariate comparison of survival rates between two or more groups are performed using the log-rank test.[41] Other linear-rank test procedures are available which give more weight to early events. When many covariables may influence survival time, such as tumour stage or lymph-node involvement, multivariate comparison of survival rates between two or more treatment groups are performed using the Cox proportional hazard's regression model.[42] This method allows an adjusted comparison between treatment groups when any imbalances in prognostic factors are observed. However, the use of this multivariate model is not without difficulties, which are associated with the selection of variables, selection of the appropriate coding of the variables, and verification of the model assumptions.

Many computer programs are commercially available for estimating and comparing survival curves. However, the graphical representations are not always presented in an informative fashion. It is our recommendation that overall survival and time-to-treatment failure curves are plotted in such a way that the censoring distributions between groups can be readily compared. This has the advantage of providing the reviewer with the results, as well as the potential reader of the published article with an indication as to whether or not a survival analysis was not performed too early. Also, confidence intervals around selected timepoints are a helpful indicator of the magnitude and precision of the treatment effect. Studies should indicate how time-to-treatment failure was calculated and which events were included in its definition. Time origins should also be specified. The time from randomization to time of occurrence of the first event should be the recommended definition of time-to-treatment failure.[43]

Quality of life

The evaluation of cancer therapies have historically been focused on endpoints such as tumour response, disease-free and overall survival, and treatment-related toxicities or complications.[44] In situations where the use of new therapies is not expected to increase the duration of overall survival, focus on the evaluation of treatment will need other measurement instruments. It may be reasonable to ask the question whether a few weeks' or months' survival time can be sacrificed for a relatively better 'quality of life' (QoL). Studies that collect data on quality of life invariably do so to examine trade-offs between the quantity and quality of life. Combined therapy in many disease sites is usually associated with more toxic effects, raising the question of whether the treatment benefits justify its quality-of-life costs for the individual patient. This situation applies to patients with a relatively short expected survival time. It can also apply to situations where patients in two different treatment groups have a relatively long expected survival time.

Quality of life rather than duration of life will be an important question and its evaluation is becoming more and more important in medical research.[45] However, it is not easy to define just what is meant by the term 'quality of life'. In clinical trials, the patient's general performance status was and still is evaluated using the Karnofsky[46] or ECOG scales.[47] However, these measures are usually used before and during therapy, with the evaluation being performed by the clinician. In phase II and III trials, the measurement of toxicity follows well-defined scales of measurement. However, they do not encompass notions related to the burden that these toxicities impose on the patient. Due to the subjective nature of QoL, another approach was necessary.

Scales of measurement

Even though there is no consensus in the literature on how the concept of QoL is to be defined, it is well accepted that QoL is multidimensional. The WHO has defined quality of life as an individual's perception of their position in life in the context of the culture and value systems in which they live and in relation to their goals, expectations, standards, and concerns.[48] The assumptions in developing such an instrument implies that the term 'quality of life' encompasses a broad entity, and that the various components could serve to measure the effect of specific health interventions on quality of life. The general purpose of a QoL assessment in medicine is to provide a more accurate estimation of the well being of individuals. The WHOQoL instrument encompasses five domains: physical health (bodily states and functions); psychological health; level of independence; social relationships; and environment. This instrument, however, is not necessarily well adapted to patients with cancer. More specific instruments have been developed: Cancer Rehabilitation Evaluation System (CARES);[49] Functional Living Index—Cancer (FLIC);[50] Linear Analog Self Assessment (LASA);[51] Nottingham Health Profile (NHP);[52] Psychological Adjustment to Illness Scale (PAIS);[53] Quality of Life Index (QLI);[54] Quality of Life Index (QL-Index);[55] Rand Health Insurance Study (HIS)[56] Scales; and the Sickness Impact Profile (SIP).[57]

The EORTC Quality of Life Study Group has developed and validated many quality-of-life modules for patients with cancer—the most common being the QLQ-C36[58] and QLQ-C30,[59] which is a cancer-specific core questionnaire. Details concerning the methods used for validation have been published.[60] This instrument is multidimensional, cancer-specific, patient-based, and is designed for self-administration. It is intended for application across a range of cancer diagnoses: lung cancer (QLQ-LC13); head and neck cancer (QLQ-H&N35); breast cancer (QLQ-BR23); colorectal cancer (QLQ-CR38); oesophageal cancer (QLQ-OE24); and prostate cancer (QLQ-PR25). It is also a short questionnaire and has been translated into more than 20 languages. The dimensions include five functioning scales

(physical, role, emotional, cognitive, and social); three symptom scales (fatigue, pain, nausea and vomiting); an overall health and an overall quality-of-life scale; six single items (dyspnoea, sleep disturbance, loss of appetite, constipation, diarrhoea, financial difficulties). For studies where quality of life is considered an important criterion in assessing treatment outcome, the first step is to choose a validated system of measurement.

For a particular study, not only will the instrument have to be chosen, but also the frequency of use will need to be defined. It is preferable to collect quality-of-life data alongside the collection of clinical data from both practical and analytical perspectives. It is recommended that quality of life is assessed three or four times during a clinical trial. The first assessment should be performed before treatment, the second assessment during treatment when treatment-related side-effects are expected to be at their height, and the third assessment at the time when the treatment benefit is expected to be at its maximum. In some cases, it may be important to capture long-term effects, in which case additional assessments may be made. It is important to space these evaluations (similarly for the different treatment arms) during intervals which correspond to changes in the disease process and treatment adaptation. These QoL questionnaires should not be spaced too closely together in order to minimize the workload and increase compliance of both the patients and institutions.

Representation of quality-of-life data

The quantity of information gathered on quality-of-life data will need to be appropriately summarized using a procedure for obtaining scores, since some items are correlated. Missing values will also need to be accounted for. The EORTC scoring manual contains the necessary code for summarizing the data and provides ways of imputing missing values. Interpretation of these scores in the clinical setting has recently been undertaken.[61] One procedure uses unweighted summated scales, but current methodological research is investigating other methods of analysis, namely Rasch models.[62]

One such method combines both quality and quantity of life into a single measure such as quality-adjusted life years (QALY). One approach, known as 'quality-adjusted time without symptoms or toxicity' (Q-TWiST), defines a series of health states, and uses a partitioned survival analysis to calculate the average amount of time spent in each state.[63] Each state is then weighted according to a utility score to account for a possible decrement in quality of life. A weighted sum of the health-state durations is then used as a measure of quality-adjusted time.[64] This one measure is then compared between treatment groups for evaluating short- and long-term treatment effects.

A recent study, comparing postoperative combined radiotherapy and chemotherapy to adjuvant radiotherapy alone in poor-prognosis patients with rectal cancer, reported a reduced risk of relapse and overall death but an increased amount of time spent in toxicity and a shorter survival after relapse in the combined therapy group.[65] This trade-off, measured by the Q-TWiST method, concluded in favour of the combined modality treatment. Outcome was improved in terms of delayed recurrence and increased survival despite more time spent with early and late toxic effects. An example of a partitioned survival plot for data from this randomized trial is presented in Fig. 5.[65]

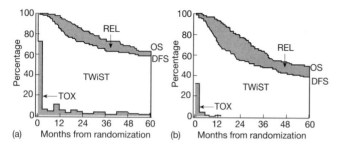

Fig. 5 Partitioned survival plots for patients with poor-prognosis resectable rectal cancer treated with (a) adjuvant chemotherapy and radiation therapy or (b) adjuvant radiation therapy alone. Overall survival (OS) up to 5 years from random assignment to treatment is partitioned by curves for the time with toxicity (TOX, either early or late) and disease-free survival (DFSD). These curves divide the 5 years since random assignment to treatment into three periods: time with toxicity (TOX), time without symptoms or toxicity (TWiST), and time after relapse (REL). (From Gelber et al. 1996[65] with permission.)

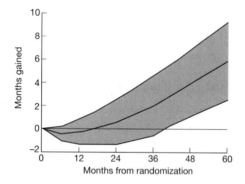

Fig. 6 Q-TWiST (quality-adjusted time without symptoms or toxicity) gain function for patients with poor-prognosis resectable rectal cancer treated with adjuvant chemotherapy and radiotherapy or adjuvant radiation therapy alone. The vertical axis indicates the average months of Q-TWiST gained with the combined therapy compared with radiation therapy alone. The horizontal axis shows the time since random assignment to treatment. The bold line indicates the months gained for Q-TWiST evaluated with arbitrary utility coefficients of $U_{tox} = U_{rel} = 0.5$, and the shaded region shows the regions for any selection of utility coefficients between 0 and 1. By 5 years, depending on the selection of utility coefficient values, between 2 and 9 months of quality-adjusted survival was gained for the combined-treatment group compared with the radiotherapy-alone group. (From Gelber et al. 1996[65] with permission).

Another representation can be obtained by plotting the number of months gained for one treatment group against the other.[65] Figure 6 shows a clear benefit for the combined treatment modality seen 5 years from randomization, ranging from 2 to 9 months depending on the choice of the utility coefficients.

A meta-analysis of 3920 patients aged 50 years or older with node-positive breast cancer treated with combination chemotherapy plus tamoxifen compared to patients treated with adjuvant tamoxifen did not give a better Q-TWIST, despite a modest benefit of increased relapse-free and overall survival rates for patients who received chemotherapy.[66]

Intermediate endpoints

The use of intermediate endpoints in making decisions about treatment outcome is very appealing, as conclusions based on these parameters can save time, money, and patients. However, the validity of a potential alternative endpoint for cancer is determined primarily by the extent to which the intermediate endpoint is a necessary event on the causal pathway to cancer.[67] If the positive results are indeed true, then new patients may benefit earlier from the results of this research. If the negative results are true, then new patients are spared from participating in a negative study and other clinical trials can be initiated earlier. If the data are inconclusive, more data will need to be collected. When disease progression or relapse are used as intermediate endpoints to describe early treatment failure, many questions can arise as to the appropriateness of these endpoints as alternative parameters for estimating overall survival. For example, survival time is usually quite short after disease progression in patients with non-small-cell lung cancer, and this intermediate endpoint may be quite suitable for treatment evaluation. In other cases, such as young patients with germ-cell tumours, disease progression after first-line therapy does not necessarily correlate with survival, since patients with this highly curable disease can go on to second-, third-, or fourth-line therapy. The use of these alternative endpoints for estimating survival rates assumes that they are good predictors of overall survival. Thus more information on the effect of treatment will be obtained after a shorter observation time, and results may be arrived at with a smaller number of patients. Conclusions can be drawn without the disadvantage of having to explain the possible dilution effect obtained by using a criterion obtained from an amalgam of several different event types used to define treatment failure.

Time to the occurrence of the first of these events can then be used as the main endpoint or as an intermediate endpoint in defining treatment outcome. As long as the events used are clearly defined, this amalgam of failure types may provide an overall answer to the global question of treatment effect. However, specific questions, linked to a particular type of treatment failure, may be necessary in cases where unexplainable or contradictory results are observed between the overall survival curves and the failure-free survival curves. Other incentives for breaking down the failure-free survival curves into separate components lie in the fact that certain treatment modalities may only influence specific event types such as local failure. For instance, it may well be that 'locally applied treatment', such as surgery or radiotherapy, may influence local control or local failure to a greater extent than chemotherapy, which in turn may inhibit to a greater extent the occurrence of distant failure. Hypotheses about the biology of the disease may be generated when the separate components, including different treatment strategies, are correctly analysed. If treatments are interrupting disease via different mechanisms of action, there is no guarantee that an earlier measure of outcome will equally reflect the overall effects of these treatments.

One intermediate endpoint often used is response to treatment. This measure of early treatment success may or not be a good indicator of long-term success. Many journals still publish survival curves for responding and non-responding patients, implying that a significant result in favour of a prolonged survival for responders justifies the use of 'response' as an alternative parameter for survival. Many authors have criticized this approach and have shown that it is biased.[68] The principal bias involved in comparing the survival of responders to that of non-responders lies in the fact that a patient has to have lived long enough in order to be classified a responder. So, responders already have a guaranteed survival time that non-responders do not have—it is obvious that the responders' survival will be longer. The other bias involves the fact that patients who respond may have a better prognostic profile and consequently their survival may also be increased. More appropriate methods include the use of the landmark method or survival methods using techniques with time-dependent covariates.[69]

The landmark method ignores all data before a preselected time-point, say 4 months, corresponding to the minimum survival time to qualify as a responder. An example for patients with advanced colorectal cancer showed that a response to chemotherapy is associated with a longer survival, after correction for the guarantee time effect and the distribution of prognostic variables.[70] It is important to note in cases where all patients who are destined to respond actually do respond before any failures are observed in the group of non-responding patients, that conventional methods and methods which correctly account for guarantee time will give exactly the same test results.

In certain cancer sites, such as lung cancer or colorectal cancer, failure-free survival and overall survival are indeed correlated, since death invariably occurs for patients who either locally or distantly relapse. In many curable disease sites in oncology, such as germ-cell tumours, early breast cancer, or certain paediatric tumours, it is necessary to wait many years before enough events are observed to estimate survival curves. In these cases, even when relapses do occur, patients may still be submitted to curable second-, third-, or even fourth-line therapy. So when overall survival is used in the evaluation of first-line treatment strategies in these patients, it is important to keep in mind that a comparison of overall survival involves the comparison not only of the results of first-line treatment but also of the subsequent therapy applied to patients who fail.

Multiple endpoints

In most clinical studies a lot of data is usually gathered. Not only are patient demographic data, clinical, biological, and treatment data collected, but outcome in terms of response, relapse, survival, as well as acute and chronic toxicity are also reported. Covariables, measured in a continuous scale, are usually grouped into categories and any analysis of all this data creates a problem of multiplicity. The main difficulty lies in the value of the statistical tests and concerns essentially inflated p-values, which measure the strength of an association.[71] Even in the absence of a difference, spurious statistical differences will occur just by chance. This phenomenon is not only associated with subgroup analysis but also with multiple endpoints. One possible remedy is to adjust the p-value to the number of tests performed and not to consider anything significant unless the observed p-value is corrected. However, this method is very difficult to apply, because tests are not really independent, and it is not usually known ahead of time how many tests will be performed. Another possibility for hypothesis testing for multiple endpoints is to construct some linear combination of important endpoints and to use this newly defined endpoint within the framework of a composite hypothesis.[72]

The best way to avoid many of the problems associated with multiple comparisons and multiple endpoints is to perform a well-designed study with a protocol that defines the main objectives, the population under study, the main endpoints, and the sample size needed to detect a clinically worthwhile difference with sufficient power. The use of multiple endpoints in a study will influence the required sample size. These problems can be addressed by designing sound protocols with defined endpoints that take into account population selection, prespecified cut-off points for continuous variables, and eventually the number of prognostic factors to be tested.[73]

Whether it be for survival, treatment failure, local control, complications, or quality of life it is important clearly to define the criteria being used, how there were assessed, what were the starting and end timepoints used, and how censored observations are defined and accounted for. Statistical methods for estimating and comparing effects should be indicated, as well as the computer software used for data analysis.

References

1. **Von Hoff DD, Turner J.** Response rates, duration of response, and dose response effects in phase I studies of antineoplastics. *Investigational New Drugs*, 1991; **9**: 115–22.

2. **Gehan EA.** The determination of the number of patients required in preliminary and follow-up trials of a new chemotherapy agent. *Journal of Chronic Diseases*, 1961; **13**: 346–53.

3. **Simon R.** Optimal two-stage designs for phase II clinical trials. *Controlled Clinical Trials*, 1989; **10**: 1–10.

4. **Miller AB, Hoogstraten B, Staquet M, Winkler A.** Reporting results of cancer treatments. *Cancer*, 1981; **47**: 207–14.

5. **Therasse P, Arbuck SG, Eisenhauer EA,** *et al.* New guidelines to evaluate the response to treatment in solid tumors. *Journal of the National Cancer Institute*, 2000; **92**: 205–16.

6. **Green S, Weiss GR.** Southwest Oncology Group standard response criteria, endpoint definitions and toxicity criteria. *Investigational New Drugs*, 1992; **10**: 239–53.

7. **Simon R, Wittes RE.** Methodologic guidelines for reports of clinical trials. *Cancer Treatment Reports*, 1985; **69**: 1–3.

8. **Warr D, McKinney S, Tannock I.** Influence of measurement error on assessment of response to anticancer chemotherapy: proposal for new criteria of tumor response. *Journal of Clinical Oncology*, 1984; **2**: 1040–6.

9. **Baar J, Tannock I.** Analyzing the same data in two ways: a demonstration model to illustrate the reporting and misreporting of clinical trials. *Journal of Clinical Oncology*, 1989; **7**: 969–78.

10. **Hayward JL, Carbone PP, Heuson JC, Kumaoka S, Segaloff A, Rubens RD.** Assessment of response to therapy in advanced breast cancer. *Cancer*, 1977; **39**: 1289–94.

11. **Dixon DO,** *et al.* Reporting outcomes in Hodgkin's disease and lymphoma. *Journal of Clinical Oncology*, 1987; **5**: 1670–2.

12. **Anderson JR, Propert KJ, Harrington DP.** Guidelines for reporting outcomes of lymphoma trials. *Journal of Clinical Oncology*, 1988; **6**: 559.

13. **Bosl GJ, Chaganti RS.** The use of tumor markers in germ cell malignancies. *Hematology Oncology Clinics of North America*, 1994; **8**: 573–87.

14. **Vogelzang NJ, Lange PH, Goldman A, Vesseta RH, Fralet EE, Kennedy BJ.** Acute changes of α-fetoprotein and human chorionic gonadotropin during induction chemotherapy of germ cell tumor. *Cancer Research*, 1982; **42**: 4855–61.

15. **Bates S.** Clinical applications of serum tumor markers. *Annals of Internal Medicine*, 1991; **115**: 623–38.

16. **Searle F,** *et al.* A human choriocarcinoma xenograft in nude mice: a

model for the study of antibody localization. *British Journal of Cancer*, 1981; **44**: 137–44.

17. **Toner GC, Geler NL, Tan C, Nisselbaum, J, Bosl GJ**. Serum tumor marker half-life during chemotherapy allows early prediction of complete response and survival in nonseminomatous germ cell tumors. *Cancer Research*, 1990; **50**: 5904–10.

18. **Murphy BA, *et al.*** Serum tumor marker decline is an early predictor of treatment outcome in germ cell tumor patients treated with cisplatin and ifosfamide salvage chemotherapy. *Cancer*, 1994; **73**: 2520–6.

19. **Rustin GJS, *et al.*** Defining response of ovarian carcinoma to initial chemotherapy according to serum CA 125. *Journal of Clinical Oncology*, 1996; **14**: 1545-51.

20. **Ychou M, Duffour J, Kramar A, Grenier J**. Value of serial carcinoembryonic antigen levels in evaluating the response to chemotherapy in patients with advanced digestive cancers. *Oncology Reports*, 1998; **5**: 1245–50.

21. **Ward U, *et al.*** The use of tumour markers CEA, CA-195 and CA-242 in evaluating the response to chemotherapy in patients with advanced colorectal cancer. *British Journal of Cancer*, 1993; **67**: 1132-5.

22. **Oken MM, *et al.*** Toxicity and response criteria of the Eastern Cooperative Oncology Group. *American Journal of Clinical Oncology*, 1982; **5**: 649–55.

23. **Moertel GG, Hanley JA**. The effect of measurement error on the results of therapeutic trials in advanced cancer. *Cancer*, 1976; **38**: 388–94.

24. **American Society for Clinical Oncology Tumor Marker Expert Panel**. Clinical practice guidelines for the use of tumor markers in breast and colorectal cancer. *Journal of Clinical Oncology*, 1996; **14**: 2843-77.

25. **Gehan EA, Tefft MC**. Will there be resistance to the RECIST (Response Evaluation Criteria in Solid Tumors)? *Journal of the National Cancer Institute*, 2000; **92**: 179–81.

26. **Pavy JJ, *et al.*** EORTC Late Effects Working Group. Late effects toxicity scoring: the SOMA scale. *Radiotherapy and Oncology*, 1995; **35**: 11–15.

27. **Chassagne D, *et al.*** A glossary for reporting complications of treatment in gynecological cancers. *Radiotherapy and Oncology*, 1993; **26**: 195–202.

28. **Henry-Amar M, Joly F**. Late complications after Hodgkin's disease. *Annals of Oncology*, 1996; 7(Suppl. 4): 115–26.

29. **Pepe MS, Mori M**. Kaplan-Meier, marginal or conditional probability curves in summarizing competing risks failure time data?. *Statistics in Medicine*, 1993; **12**: 737–51.

30. **Ellenberg SS, Hamilton JM**. Surrogate endpoints in clinical trials: cancer. *Statistics in Medicine*, 1989; **8**: 405-13.

31. **Boice JD**. Leukemia and preleukemia after adjuvant treatment of gastrointestinal cancer with semustine (Methyl-CCNU). *New England Journal of Medicine*, 1983; **309**: 1079–84.

32. **Estève J, Benhamou E, Croasdale M, Raymond L**. Relative survival and the estimation of net survival: elements for further discussion. *Statistics in Medicine*, 1990; **9**: 529–38.

33. **Pignon JP, Arriagada R**. Treatment evaluation. In *Comprehensive textbook of thoracic oncology* (ed. J Aisner, R Arriagada, MR Green, N Martini, MC Perry). Baltimore: Williams and Wilkins, 1996: 188–214.

34. **Schellhammer P, *et al.*** Assessment of endpoints for clinical trials for localized prostate cancer. *Urology*, 1997; **49**: 27–38.

35. **Gelman R, Gelber R, Craig Henderson I, Norman Coleman C, Harris JR**. Improved methodology for analyzing local and distant recurrences. *Journal of Clinical Oncology*, 1990; **8**: 548–55.

36. **Slud E, Byar D**. How dependent causes of death can make risk factors appear protective. *Biometrics*, 1988; **44**: 265–9.

37. **Kramar A, Arriagada R**. Analyzing local and distant recurrences. *Journal of Clinical Oncology*, 1990; **8**: 2086–7. [Correspondence]

38. **Peters LJ, Withers HR, Brown BW**. Complicating issues in complication reporting. *International Journal of Radiation Oncology, Biology, Physics*, 1995; **31**: 1349–51.

39. **Lancar R, Kramar A, Haie-Meder C**. Nonparametric methods for analysing recurrent complications of varying severity. *Statistics in Medicine*, 1995; **14**: 2701–12.

40. **Kaplan EL, Meier P**. Nonparametric estimation from incomplete observations. *Journal of the American Statistical Association*, 1958; **53**: 457–81.

41. **Peto R, Peto J**. Asymptotically efficient rank invariant test procedures (with discussion). *Journal of the Royal Statistical Society A*, 1972; **135**: 185–206.

42. **Cox DR**. Regression models and life tables (with discussion). *Journal of the Royal Statistical Society B*, 1972; **34**: 187–220.

43. **Anderson JR, Propert KJ, Harrington DP**. Guidelines for reporting outcomes of lymphoma trials. *Journal of Clinical Oncology*, 1988; **6**: 559–60. [Correspondence]

44. **Aaronson NK, Cull A, Kaasa Stein, Sprangers MAG, for the EORTC Study Group on Quality of Life**. The European Organisation for Research and Treatment of Cancer (EORTC) modular approach to quality of life assessment in oncology: an update. In *Quality of life and pharmacoeconomics in clinical trials* (2nd edn) (ed. B Spiker). New York: Raven Press, 1996: 179–89.

45. **Schumacher M, Olschewski M, Schulgen G**. Assessment of quality of life in clinical trials. *Statistics In Medicine*, 1991; **10**: 1915–30.

46. **Karnofsky DA, Burchenall JH**. The clinical evaluation of chemotherapeutic agents in cancer. In *Evaluation of chemotherapeutic agents* (ed. MC Macleod). New York: Columbia University Press, 1949: 199–205.

47. **Zubrod CG, *et al.*** Appraisal of methods for study of chemotherapy of cancer in man: comparative therapeutic trial of nitrogen mustard and triethylene thiophosphamide. *Journal of Chronic Diseases*, 1960; **11**: 7–33.

48. **WHOQoL Group**. Study protocol for the World Health Organisation project to develop a quality of life assessment instrument (WHOQoL). *Quality of Life Research*, 1993; **2**: 153–9.

49. **Schag CC, Heinrich RL**. Development of a comprehensive quality of life measurement tool: CARES. *Oncology*, 1990; **4**: 135–8.

50. **Schipper H, Clinch J, McMurray A, Levitt M**. Measuring the quality of life of cancer patients. *Journal of Clinical Oncology*, 1984; **2**: 472–83.

51. **Priestman TJ, Baum M**. Evaluation of quality of life in patients receiving treatment for advanced breast cancer. *Lancet*, 1976; **24**: 899–901.

52. **Hunt SM, McKenna SP, McEwen J, Williams J, Papp E**. The Nottingham health profile: subjective health status and medical consultations. *Social Science Medicine*, 1981; **15**: 221–9.

53. **Morrow GR, Chiarello RJ, Derogatis LR**. A new scale for assessing patient's psychological adjustment to medical illness. *Psychology Medicine*, 1978; **8**: 605–10.

54. **Padilla GV, Presant C, Grant MM, Metter G, Lipsett J, Heide F**. Quality of life index for patients with cancer. *Research Nursing Health*, 1983; **6**: 117–26.

55. **Spitzer WO, *et al.*** Measuring the quality of life of cancer patients: a concise QL-index for use by physicians. *Journal of Chronic Diseases*, 1981; **34**: 585–97.

56. **Brook RH, *et al.*** Overview of adult health status measures in Rand's health insurance study. *Medical Care*, 1979; **17**: 1–13.

57. **Bergner M, Bobbitt RA, Carter WB, Gilson BS**. The sickness impact profile: development and final revision of a health status measure. *Medical Care*, 1981; **10**: 787–805.

58. **Aaronson NK, Bullinger M, Ahmedzai S**. A modular approach to quality-of-life assessment in cancer clinical trials. *Recent Results of Cancer Research*, 1988; **3**: 231–49.

59. **Tchekmedyian NS, Cella DF**. Quality of life in current oncology practice and research. Appendix A. *Oncology*, 1990; **4**: 215.

60. **Ringdal GI, Ringdal K.** Testing the EORTC quality of life questionnaire on cancer patients with heterogeneous diagnoses. *Quality of Life Research*, 1993; **2**: 129–40.

61. **King MT.** The interpretation of scores from the EORTC quality of life questionnaire QLQ-C30. *Quality of Life Research*, 1996; **5**: 555–67.

62. **Wang WC, Wilson M, Adams RJ.** Measuring individual differences in change with multidimensional Rasch models. *Journal of Outcome Measures*, 1998; **2**: 240–65.

63. **Gelber RD, Gelman RS, Goldhirsch A.** A quality-of-life oriented endpoint for comparing therapies. *Biometrics*, 1989; **45**: 781–95.

64. **Glasziou PP, Simes RJ, Gelber RD.** Quality adjusted survival analysis. *Statistics in Medicine*, 1990; **9**: 1259–76.

65. **Gelber RD, Goldhirsch A, Cole BF, Wieand HS, Schroeder G, Krook JE.** A quality-adjusted time without symptoms or toxicity (Q-TWiST) analysis of adjuvant radiation therapy and chemotherapy for resectable rectal cancer. *Journal of the National Cancer Institute*, 1996; **88**: 1039–45.

66. **Gelber RD, *et al.*** Adjuvant chemotherapy plus tamoxifen compared with tamoxifen alone for postmenopausal breast cancer: meta-analysis of quality-adjusted survival. *Lancet*, 1996; **347**: 1066–71.

67. **Schatzkin A, Freedman LS, Dorgan J, McShane L, Schiffman MH, Dawsey SM.** Using and interpreting surrogate end-points in cancer research. *International Agency for Research on Cancer Scientific Publication*, 1997; **142**: 265–71.

68. **Anderson JR, Cain KC, Gelber RD.** Analysis of survival by tumor response. *Journal of Clinical Oncology*, 1983; **1**: 710–19.

69. **Mantel N, Byar D.** Evaluation of response-time data involving transient states: an illustration using heart-transplant data. *Journal of the American Statistical Association*, 1974; **69**: 81–6.

70. **Graf W, Påhlman L, Bergström R, Glimelius B.** The relationship between an objective response to chemotherapy and survival in advanced colorectal cancer. *British Journal of Cancer*, 1994; **70**: 559–63.

71. **Pocock SJ, Geller N, Tsiatis AA.** The analysis of multiple endpoints in clinical trials. *Biometrics*, 1987; **43**: 487–98.

72. **Tang DI, Geller NL, Pocock SJ.** On the design and analysis of randomized clinical trials with multiple endpoints. *Biometrics*, 1993; **49**: 23–30.

73. **Pocock SJ.** Clinical trials with multiple outcomes: a statistical perspective on their design, analysis, and interpretation. *Controlled Clinical Trials*, 1997; **18**: 530–45 (discussion 546–9).

7.3 The nature of evidence that can be used to make decisions in cancer care

Christopher J. Williams

Introduction

Western medicine has for the last several centuries striven to base its treatments on a rational scientific foundation. It is this that, in some people's minds, has separated it from other systems of medical care used in the past or those currently in use in different parts of the world. The success of such an approach is evident, though some mourn the loss of some of the perceived 'strengths' of other non-science-based systems. This chapter will examine how we use evidence to take scientifically based treatments developed in the laboratory and apply them in the cancer community.

In the last few years the term 'evidence-based medicine' (EBM) has been coined and attempts made to exploit the aims of this movement. Sackett and Haynes have defined these as: 'the practice [of EBM] is a process of life-long, problem-based learning in which care for our own patients creates the need for evidence about diagnosis, prognosis, therapy and other clinical and health care issues'.[1]

The term 'evidence-based medicine' has attracted criticism. This is partly because it can be taken to imply that we did not use evidence in the past—perhaps a more accurate, though more cumbersome, expression should be 'medicine based on better evidence', for the strength of EBM is its transparent use of the best currently available data. A second fear of EBM is that it will be used to describe a prescription which doctors should use to treat all patients. This is clearly not the intention of this approach.

It is the use of the best available evidence that has to be married, at least, with information on the patients overall condition, the clinical experience of the clinician, the availability of treatments, and the wishes of the patient, before we can arrive at a wise decision for that individual.

Currently, the available information on treatment efficacy and short- and long-term side-effects of therapy is often inconclusive or frankly contradictory. In this situation we can continue to allow doctors to decide for themselves what the data mean, or we can try to organize all the data in such a way that it gives the most reliable evidence which we can use in planning treatment and new trials. Continuing to rely on doctors' personal appraisal of the literature is likely to fail—current evidence has shown, for instance, that the decision to start antihypertensive therapy is more closely linked to the number of years since the doctor graduated from medical school than the severity of the patient's target organ damage.[2]

The following sections of this chapter will look at the steps needed to gather and systematically appraise data, and, in particular, will critically review how we handle evidence at present and how we could improve. In view of this remit we shall concentrate on showing the potential flaws in current methodology in order to identify the areas that need attention.

Clinical trials

It is not the main aim of this chapter to discuss clinical trials in detail since parts of this topic are included in other chapters. However, if we are to consider how we synthesize evidence from the clinical literature we need to look at the building blocks that we are going to use. Since the main theme will be how we take treatments into the clinic, we shall concentrate on trials testing the efficacy of treatments where we already have some evidence that the treatment has activity. Such phase III trials are frequently randomized controlled trials (RCTs). More recently, there has also been a trend towards carrying some phase II trials in a randomized fashion.

Questions that we shall address include:
What is the **evidence** that we need to use data from RCTs, whenever possible? In addition, how reliable are the RCTs that we have done to date? We shall also tackle the issue of what to do if there are a number of trials asking the same question—how do we synthesize this information?

Evidence that RCTs are more reliable

Although it has been commonly accepted for several decades that RCTs are the preferred method for carrying out clinical research, there is remarkably little systematic evidence as to whether this conclusion is valid. However, the available historical data[3] for a variety of conditions strongly supports the contention that un-randomized trials or those using an historical control are more likely to be biased. In his landmark paper Sacks and his colleagues[3] examined the outcomes in a series of trials, randomized and historically controlled, asking six different therapeutic questions. When the outcomes are examined according to whether the treatment was allocated randomly or not (that is to say, the control was historical), it is very apparent that historically controlled trials (HCTs) grossly overestimate the treatment effect (Table 1).

Misinformation from uncontrolled trials does not just hinder progress, it can cause real harm. One of the questions addressed by Sacks *et al.*[3] in their paper was the use of diethylstilboestrol (DES) to prevent habitual abortion. In the 1960s, several historically controlled trials purported to show that diethylstilboestrol given in pregnancy could increase the chances of a woman, who had had several

Table 1 A study of the comparative results of RCTs and HCTs asking the same questions (reproduced with permission from ref. 6)

6 therapies, 50 RCTs and 56 HCTs
44 of 56 HCTs (79%) found the 'new' therapy to be significantly better than the control
10 of 50 RCTs (20%) found the 'new' therapy to be significantly better than the control
The outcomes for new treatments were similar regardless of whether they were from RCTs or HCTs
Outcomes were clearly worse for control patients in HCTs when compared with control patients in RCTs

RCTs, randomized controlled trials; HCTs, historically controlled trials.

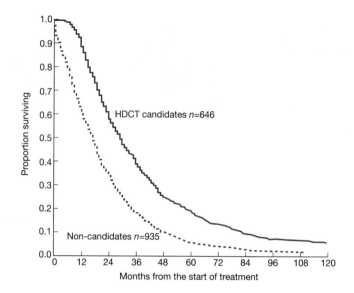

Fig. 1 Survival of patients with breast cancer eligible for inclusion in trials of high-dose chemotherapy compared with non-eligible patients.

abortions, subsequently having a healthy baby. This information led to the wide-scale international use of diethylstilboestrol for this indication. Three subsequent RCTs clearly show that this treatment does not work—interestingly, the only difference in the results of these RCTs and non-RCTs is that the outcome in the control group of the non-RCTs is considerably worse than control arm of the RTCs (Table 2). When the issue of bias was addressed by 'matching' patients in one trial the overall conclusion was unchanged, though all the results of this small trial are very much more than the other trials.

Latter surveillance and follow-up of these RCTs established that there are major side-effects associated with the use of diethylstilboestrol in pregnancy. The finding of clear-cell cancers of the vagina in the daughters of women treated with DES in pregnancy was a devastating unexpected consequence of this unproved treatment.[4]–[6] Further long-term experience from RCTs addressing this question have also shown that male and female offspring of treated women have a much higher incidence of depression, and that male offspring are much less likely to form stable long-term relationships.[4]–[6]

A more recent example of how the failure to use RCTs could be misleading is the series of historically controlled trials of adjuvant high-dose therapy, supported with autologous-marrow or peripheral blood stem-cell transfusion, in the treatment of women with breast cancer at very high risk of recurrence.[7],[8] The original reports were of meticulous trials with carefully matched control groups. They showed a very large benefit resulting in a major delay in time to disease progression and improved overall survival. However, such treatments are complex, toxic, and expensive and, fortunately, there was a demand that RCTs be carried out. Whilst these were awaited, analyses of two retrospective cohorts of consecutive patients,[9],[10]

comparing those who would have been eligible for inclusion in high-dose therapy trials with those who were ineligible, led to further doubt about the safety of the results of the original historically controlled trials (Fig. 1). The use of inclusion criteria (computed tomography (**CT**) scan, bone marrow biopsy, ability to comply with the protocol, and living within a specified distance of the centre, for instance) that would not have been applied in the control groups of the original trials could have led to a biased comparison.

Despite the lack of RCT evidence and the doubt engendered by the two retrospective studies, use of adjuvant high-dose chemotherapy with stem-cell support for patients with high-risk breast cancer became commonplace, particularly in North America where there was severe pressure for medical insurance companies to pay for such treatment. In March 1999, the National Cancer Institute (**NCI**) made a clinical announcement [http://rex.nci.nih.govmassmedia/pressreleases/inter-imqa.html] that preliminary evidence from RCTs,[11]–[13] presented at the 35th Annual Meeting of the American Society of Clinical Oncology (**ASCO**), showed no clear benefit from high-dose therapy in the treatment of breast cancer (Table 3). Only one of these RCTs provided evidence of benefit from high-dose chemotherapy and an audit of this trial subsequently showed it to be fraudulent.[13] Further long-term follow-up and data from other RCTs is needed before a definitive

Table 2 Comparison of the results of RCTs and HCTs testing the ability of diethylstilboestrol to prevent recurrent abortion (reproduced with permission from ref. 3)

Type of trial	No. of trials	No. of patients	% Live infants DES- treated	Control
RCT	3	2175	87.3	87.6
HCT	4	2358	85.3	56
HCT [matched]	1	216	45	8

Table 3 Interim analysis of RCTs of adjuvant high-dose chemotherapy for high-risk breast cancer

Organization	Median follow-up (months) at time of EFS and S analysis	EFS or RFS (high versus lower-dose)	Survival or death (high versus lower-dose)	Recurrences of breast cancer at last analysis (high versus low-dose)
CALDGB (US Intergroup)	37	EFS: 68% vs. 64%	S: 78% vs. 80%	78/394 pts vs. 107/389 pts
Scandinavian	20.2		D: 40 pts vs. 40 pts	78 pts vs. 50 pts
South Africa	70	RFS*: 400 vs. 190 weeks	*S: 400 vs. 320 weeks *D: 8/75 vs. 28/79 pts	* 19/75 pts vs. 52/79 pts

*The asterisk indicates that the differences shown are considered significantly different by a statistical test. an audit has subsequently shown this trial to be fraudulent.

EFS, event-free survival; RFS, recurrence-free survival; S, survival; D, death; pts, patients.

The two largest studies, United States and Scandinavian, do not demonstrate a difference in survival between the high- and lower-dose groups. In contrast, the South African study, subsequently shown to be fraudulent, does show a significant decrease in the number of breast cancer recurrences and a significant improvement in survival in favour of the high-dose treatment. It is also noteworthy that the high-dose group in the United States trial has fewer recurrences of breast cancer. The Scandinavian and US trial results should be viewed as preliminary because the median follow-up on these studies is not long.

In weighing these results, it is important to keep in mind the side-effects of these treatments. Details of the toxicity in the two treatment groups are not yet available. However, the US trial reports that the high-dose therapy was associated with 29 therapy-related deaths versus none on the lower-dose therapy. The Scandinavian trial had two therapy-related deaths in the high-dose group, but in the lower-dose group (a group that received 5-FU, epirubicin, and cyclophosphamide with G-CSF tailored to the individual's blood counts), eight cases of secondary acute leukaemia/myelodysplasia developed.

statement can be made, but in the meantime this treatment should be regarded as experimental.

These old and new data show that there is nearly always a need for RCTs if we are to be sure that new treatments really are advances. Failure to carry out RCTs (radical mastectomy, for instance) and lack of formal appraisal of all the evidence is likely to result in misleading conclusions, which may mean that we fail to adopt a useful therapy or that we use a potentially harmful approach (Fig. 2). Despite this, there are still many unrandomized trials carried out in cancer care. Although randomized trials comparing different chemotherapy and radiotherapy approaches are relatively common, such trials in surgery, palliative care, nursing and supportive care are often uncontrolled. Although it has been claimed that it is often impossible to perform RCTs in these areas, there are good examples of such trials having been carried out successfully.

Where synthesis of the literature is to be carried out (see below) it is paramount that the conclusions are based on the strength of the evidence. Systematic reviews of unrandomized trials will always suffer from the unreliability of the primary data, and the accumulation of data from large numbers of patients in uncontrolled trials should not be allowed to lend potentially biased data undeserved credibility. This is not to say that uncontrolled trials have no utility, but that any conclusions drawn must be tentative and are best used to develop hypotheses to be tested, whenever possible, in RCTs.

How well have we carried out RCTs?

The main rationale for carrying out formal RCTs is twofold—one, to use random allocation of the treatments to avoid bias, and secondly to accrue sufficient patients to reduce chance findings. Secure randomization and large numbers of patients reaching the endpoint in the trial are the cornerstone of reliable clinical research.

Studies that have looked at the safety of randomization have shown that where there is uncertainty over safety of randomization there is a strong tendency for those trials to be much more positive than reports of trials with safe randomization. Schulz et al.,[14] in a study of 250 trials from 33 systematic reviews, found that the odds ratio for treatment effect was inflated by 30 per cent when concealment of treatment allocation prior to randomization was unclear (poorly described), and 41 per cent when concealment was clearly inadequate (randomization by month of birth, for instance). In this study, randomization by the sealed-envelope method was accepted as adequate, though unpublished data from meta-analyses of individual patient data (see below) suggest that this is not the case. Only telephone randomization by an independent third party appears safe.

Examination of the cancer literature shows that there have been far too many small trials that were grossly underpowered and were never likely to answer the question that they were addressing. The individual patient data meta-analysis of 52 RCTs of chemotherapy for non-small-cell lung cancer[15] found that only 9387 patients had been treated with chemotherapy in such trials over the past three decades. During this period some 15 to 20 million patients will have died from this cancer. None of the trials was large enough to give reliable answers, and the mean size of the treatment arms was less than 100. This finding, for the commonest tumour in industrialized countries, is not unique. Trial size has been grossly inadequate for nearly all tumour types to date. The proportion of patients with adult solid tumours who enter clinical trials is less than 3 per cent in Western countries.

In addition to a failure to include adequate numbers, RCTs have also often failed to include appropriate comparative groups and endpoints. In the meta-analysis of chemotherapy for non-small-cell lung cancer the intent of chemotherapy in nearly all the trials was palliative in nature. Despite this, the meta-analysis failed to find

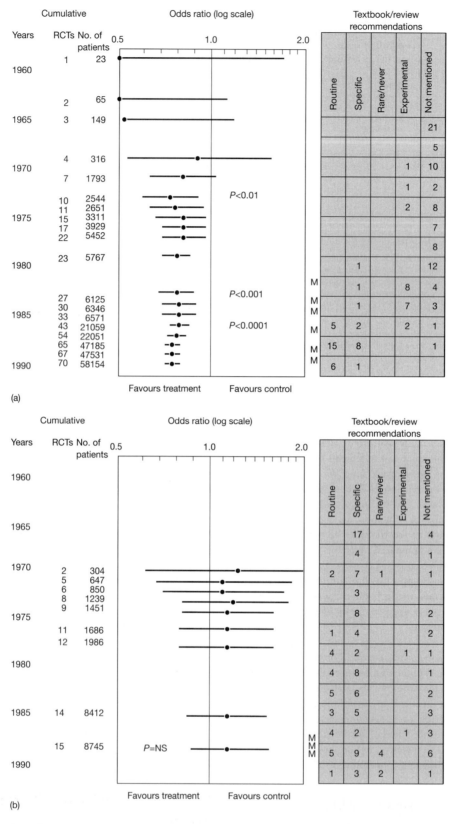

Fig. 2 Cumulative meta-analysis of two treatments for acute myocardial infarction compared with treatment recommendations from reviews and textbooks. (a) This summarizes the situation for thrombolytic therapy and (b) the use of lidocaine (lignocaine). The meta-analysis for thrombolytic therapy shows that there was good evidence for the use of this treatment from the early 1970s, but it was only in the late 1980s and early 1990s that it was recommended at all or used routinely. In contrast, there has never been any evidence to support the use of lidocaine (if anything, the evidence suggests that it may be harmful), but it was routinely recommended throughout this period.

useful data on quality of life (**QoL**) or symptom control in any of the RCTs. Although recent RCTs have moved to include QoL, there is still a paucity of data on the degree of patient benefit when therapy is palliative in nature. Where QoL has been measured in RCTs it is very common to only do this for the period of therapy—whereas such comparative trials should be recording QoL throughout the course of the disease. This is because the application of a single therapy at one point in time cannot be isolated from consequences of that treatment on the latter course of the patient's disease and its subsequent treatments (see also Chapter 6.3).

Thus, for example, the use of effective chemotherapy may be toxic in the short term but result in disease control and very good palliation for many months, the patient subsequently relapsing and dying with no further response to treatment. Such patients may have a relatively poor QoL during treatment and in the period when they fail to respond to further treatment and are dying, whereas they have a good QoL whilst they are off treatment when their disease is controlled. In an alternative scenario, ineffective chemotherapy may be less toxic and not substantially worsen QoL. However, the patient never gains disease control or a very good QoL. They receive subsequent chemotherapies with minor responses and no gain in QoL, eventually dying after a duration similar to the first patient. If QoL were only measured during the treatment period, an RCT comparing these treatments would conclude that the first treatment worsens QoL and has no survival advantage and should be avoided,[16] see also **Q-TWiST** (quality-adjusted time without symptoms of disease and toxicity of treatment) analysis in Chapter 7.4. If the RCT were to have measured QoL throughout the course of the disease, the result would look very different. Survival would be similar; but patients receiving the first treatment would have a substantial period of good QoL off treatment compared with a generally poor QoL throughout the course of the disease with the second, less-toxic therapy. The need for long-term measurement of QoL, however, makes the use of such methods more time-consuming and expensive.

In addition to the failure to collect data on QoL in non-small-cell lung cancer, there has been a relative paucity of trials comparing chemotherapy with no chemotherapy in an era when there was no evidence of benefit from chemotherapy. Instead, many randomized trials compared different chemotherapy regimens—nearly always showing that the regimes produced similar survival patterns.

A further problem for those reviewing reports of clinical trials is the poor quality of some reports. Many do not report important information or they fail to define the terms used. Moher and Schulz[17] have reported on appraisals of the quality of reports of clinical trials in cancer and general medicine. Thus adequate definitions of randomization only appear in 30 to 50 per cent of trial reports, and data on sample size, confidence intervals, and adequate statistical analysis are only available in a minority of papers. Systematic review (see below) of reports of clinical trials may help to improve the quality of reporting by underlining the deficiencies in current practice. Insistence by journals that reports of clinical trials conform to the Consolidated Standards of Reporting Trials (**CONSORT**) statement[18] would vastly improve the current situation. Table 4 shows the main factors included in the CONSORT checklist for those preparing, publishing, and reading reports of RCTs.

We have come a long way in the 50 years since the first true RCT, but there is much that we can do to improve the reliability, applicability, and usefulness of current RCTs and their reports. As we become more successful with our treatments the complexity of running RCTs will increase. Crude endpoints, such as tumour response and survival, will no longer suffice and there will also be a need for long-term surveillance for adverse treatment effects. In addition, there will be a continuing need to carry out large pragmatic trials that give clear answers to important questions. Given the very low proportion of patients entering clinical trials, there is a need to integrate RCTs into routine care—the current situation of often treating patients without sound evidence is unacceptable. A significant proportion of patients would be willing to be entered into RCTs, knowing that the data from studies shows that treatment in a trial or using a set treatment protocol is likely to be more effective than *ad hoc* treatments.[19]

Given the current situation of multiple small trials that cannot give reliable results, what can the clinician do with the mass of data that they have generated? The next section describes one approach to making the best of a bad job.

Systematically reviewing the literature

The emphasis during medical training is to stress the importance of peer-reviewed publications of RCTs. Oncologists are encouraged to read these and to base their practise on their reading and understanding of the literature. These aims are laudable, but are they attainable? There are many obstacles in the way of those carrying out a personal review of the literature, or indeed in preparing such a review for publication. It is only in the last few years that we have woken up to some of these problems.

Why do we need reviews?

The simple answer is that there is a need to give information to the non-specialist and that there is just too much data out there for even the specialist to keep up with (23 000 biomedical journals publishing 2 000 000 papers a year). A study of the information needs of general physicians has estimated that the average practitioner needs to identify and read 19 peer-reviewed papers every day for 365 days a year—a total of 6935 papers a year.[20] A United Kingdom study found, in contrast, that medical practitioners spent about 30 minutes a week reading such papers, and an informal survey in Oxford of those attending medical grand rounds showed that more than half had not read a peer-reviewed paper in the previous week (Sackett, personal communication). Even enthusiastic clinical teachers only self-reported that they read peer-reviewed papers for 2 hours a week.

Such data underlines the pressures that doctors work under and the gap between their information needs and what can currently be achieved. At the same time, there is data suggesting that clinicians need a new, clinically important piece of evidence as often as twice for every three patients.[21]

What are the problems with current narrative reviews?

The concept of writing reviews advising on current clinical practice is hardly new, so it is only sensible to change the methods used if they can be shown to be failing. There have been a number of studies of the methodology used in narrative reviews in general medicine

Table 4 Items that should be included in reports of randomized trials

Heading	Subheading	Descriptor
Title		Identify the study as a randomized trial
Abstract		Use a structured format
Introduction		State prospectively defined hypothesis, clinical objectives, and planned subgroup or covariate analyses
Methods	Protocol	*Describe the:*
		Planned study population, together with inclusion or exclusion criteria
		Planned interventions and their timing
		Primary and secondary outcome measure(s) and the minimum important difference(s), and indicate how the target sample size was projected
		Rationale and methods for statistical analyses, detailing the main comparative analyses and whether they were completed on an intention-to-treat basis
		Prospectively defined stopping rules (if warranted)
	Assignment	*Describe the:*
		Unit of randomization (e.g. individual, cluster, geographic)
		Method used to generate the allocation schedule
		Method of allocation concealment and timing of assignment
		Method to separate the generator from the executor of assignment
	Masking (blinding)	*Describe the:*
		Mechanism (e.g. capsules, tablets)
		Similarity of treatment characteristics (e.g. appearance, taste)
		Allocation schedule control (location of code during trial and when broken)
		Evidence for successful blinding among participants, person doing intervention, outcome assessors, and data analysts
Results	Participant flow and follow-up	Provide a trial profile (see Fig. 1) summarizing participant flow, numbers and timing of randomization assignment, interventions, and measurements for each randomized group
	Analysis	State estimated effect of intervention on primary and secondary outcome measures, including a point estimate and measure of precision (confidence interval)
		State results in absolute numbers when feasible (e.g. 10/20, not 50%)
		Present summary data and appropriate descriptive and interferential statistics in sufficient detail to permit alternative analyses and replication
		Describe prognostic variables by treatment group and any attempt to adjust for them
		Describe protocol deviations from the study as planned, together with the reasons
Discussion		State specific interpretation of study findings, including sources of bias and imprecision (internal validity) and discussion of external validity, including appropriate quantitative measures when possible
		State general interpretation of the data in light of the totality of the available evidence

and cancer. Bramwell and Williams[22] used methods developed by Cynthia Mulrow[23] to assess the quality of narrative reviews published in the *Journal of Clinical Oncology* from its inception in 1983 through to the end of 1995. These types of studies have consistently shown that many narrative reviews are potentially flawed. Examination of the potential flaws is instructive in that it shows the potential strengths and weaknesses of the currently popular approach to appraising medical information. The paper from Bramwell and Williams identified a number of weaknesses that we shall examine in some detail. The main areas we will discuss are: (1) data identification, (2) selection of data to be included, (3) assessment of the validity of that data, and (4) quantitative synthesis of the data, where appropriate. Each of these, and the ramifications of not attending to them, will be discussed separately.

Searching for reports of trials

In their review, Bramwell and Williams found that only 12 out of 106 reviews stated how the authors identified the papers that they had analysed. Even where they recorded that reviewers had stated a search strategy, they allowed a bare assertion that an electronic search of a database (usually MEDLINE) had been done as sufficient. Lack of any, or provision of little, information on how trial reports were found means that readers of such reviews have no way of assessing the adequacy of the methods used. This is a key question since publication bias is a very real problem. It pervades the literature from beginning to end and some of it is subtle, though many of the main problems have come from our failure to pay any attention to obvious biases.

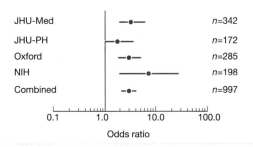

Fig. 3 Meta-analysis of four studies examining the association between significant results and publication (unadjusted odds ratio and 95 per cent confidence intervals). The overall OR for the four studies including 997 trials is 2.88 (from ref. 24 with permission).

The first and most unacceptable bias is the failure to publish the results of clinical research. It is difficult to find out how often this happens, but is appears to be relatively common. Were such failure to report results randomly distributed, its impact would be less worrying. However, there is good evidence that unreported trials are very much more likely to show that a new treatment is no better (or is worse) than a control.

Dickersin and Min,[24] in a paper about the publication record of 293 National Institutes of Health (NIH) trials that had been funded in 1979, found that an encouraging 93 per cent of those complete 5 years before their paper was written had been published. However, even with the NIH's very good publication record, trials with a 'significant' result were more likely to have been published than those showing 'non-significant' results (adjusted odds ratio 12.30—95 per cent confidence interval (CI) 2.54 to 60.00). The reason for non-publication appeared to rest with the investigators most of the time (63 per cent). The commonest explanation being that the results were considered uninteresting or that there was insufficient time to analyse and write up the trial. These findings are similar to other studies (Fig. 3), except that the proportion of unpublished trials was unusually low in the NIH series (most studies show that trials funded by outside bodies and multi-institution RCTs are more likely to be published). Non-publication rates in the four studies[24] shown in Fig. 3 range from 7 to 34 per cent. Since these trials were all from prestigious institutions, the rate of non-publication may be even higher in the medical community in general. There are few data on non-publication rates for papers on cancer, but the Early Breast Cancer Trialists' Collaborative Group found that 22 per cent of trials relevant to their early reviews were unpublished.[25] Failure to publish 'negative' results of RCTs is the most pernicious form of bias and has been described as medical fraud by Iain Chalmers and others.[26]

Even where RCTs have been reported in abstract form at international meetings, many of these are not subsequently published in a peer-reviewed journal. Scherer and her colleagues[27] found that only 51 per cent of 2391 abstracts of RCTs in 11 studies were fully published (Table 5). Full publication appeared to be associated with 'significant' results. The publication record in the only oncology study showed results that were similar to other areas of medicine—only 58 per cent of 197 abstracts appeared as full papers. Time to publication in eight of the studies shows that nearly all the abstracts had been converted into full publication by 36 months, few new publications appearing after that time (Fig. 4).

Where reports of RCTs are published there still is a bias, in that 'significant' trials are generally reported on average 2 years earlier that 'non-significant' trials. The bias towards later publication of 'non-significant' trials is apparent at every stage in the process towards publication (Table 6). Thus early publication of a cohort of 'significant' results may be misleading, since a further cohort of 'non-significant' studies may follow 2 or 3 years later—possibly too late to appropriately influence opinion.

Calls for an international register of RCTs in cancer[28] are at last being acted upon so that the identification and tracking of the publication record of clinical research will be easier. There are also plans to introduce a unique identification number for all randomized clinical trials (International Standard Randomised Clinical Trial Number—ISRCTN) that will allow the publication history of a trial to be tracked over time (http://controlled-trials.com).

However, more subtle biases exist and care will still need to be taken to avoid publication bias. For instance, most narrative medical reviews only include English language reports. Research has, however, shown that non-English researchers who publish reports of trials in English and their own language tend to report their 'statistically significant' trials in English and their 'non-significant' trials in their own language. In a study of bilingual (German/English) researchers by Egger et al.[29] only 35 per cent of German-language papers, compared to 62 per cent of English-language papers, reported 'significant' results. The odds ratio for the publication of significant results in English was 3.75 (95 per cent CI, 1.25 to 11.3).

Another, sometimes subtle, bias is the reporting of an RCT on more than one occasion. Thus in Egger's study, 31 per cent of the eligible reports were excluded since they were duplicate reports written in German and English. Where duplication is covert (masked by a change of authors, of language, and adding extra data) it may seriously bias the literature. For instance, when Tramer[30] and colleagues carried out a meta-analysis of data from RCTs of ondansetron as a postoperative antiemetic they found that 17 per cent of reports were covert duplications, and that this resulted in 28 per cent of the patient data being duplicated. Duplication led to an overestimation of ondansetron's efficacy of 23 per cent (Table 7), since reports of trials showing a greater treatment effect appeared more likely to have been duplicated.

Thus, great care needs to be taken if we are to avoid the pitfalls of publication bias. Whilst the use of a single electronic database search is an improvement on no search, there is good evidence that this will not give a full and balanced view of the literature. The Cochrane Cancer Network is helping in the process of hand-searching the world's literature to identify as many reports of controlled and randomized trials as possible. This includes searching for trials in journals already included in current electronic databases. In a study comparing the number of RCTs found by hand-searching specific journals with those found by searching MEDLINE using the tag 'RCT' in 'Publication Type' the findings were:

- *International Journal of Radiation Oncology, Biology, and Physics* (1976–1997)—589 reports of RCTs were found by hand-searching and only 273 tagged as such on MEDLINE;
- *British Journal of Cancer* (1977–1997)—388 reports of RCTs by hand-searching compared with 197 tagged as RCT on MEDLINE;
- *European Journal of Surgical Oncology* (1984–1997) and its precursor *Clinical Oncology* (1975–1984)—131 reports of RCTs found by hand-searching and only 46 tagged as RCT on MEDLINE.

Table 5 Reports assessing full publication of results initially presented as abstracts*

Reference	Specialty	Type of sample	Follow-up (months)	Abstracts (No.)	Published in full (No. (%))
Dudley 1978[1]	Surgery	All	36	51	29 (57)
Goldman and Loscatzo 1980[2]	Cardiology	Random sample	37	276	137 (50)
Meranze et al. 1982[3]	Anaesthesiology	All	27	379	122 (32)
McCormick and Holmes 1985[4]	Paediatrics	Selected sessions	36	355	172 (48)
Chalmers et al. 1990[5]	Perinatology	All	48	176	64 (36)
Juzych et al. 1991[6]	Vision research	Random sample	54	175	105 (60)
De Beliefeuille et al. 1992[7]	Oncology	Random sample	66	197	115 (58)
Juzych et al. 1993[8]	Vision research	Random sample	78	327	206 (63)
Yentis et al. 1993[9]	Anaesthesiology	Random sample	60	215	108 (50)
Dirk 1993[10]	Anaesthesiology	All from 1 department	45	147	79 (54)
Present study	Vision research	All verified RCTs	36	93	61 (66)
Total				2391	1198
Weighted mean (95% CI)					51 (45–57)
Range					32–66%

*RCT, randomized controlled trial; CI, confidence interval.

Complete details for the references quoted in Table 5 can be obtained from Scherer et al.[27]

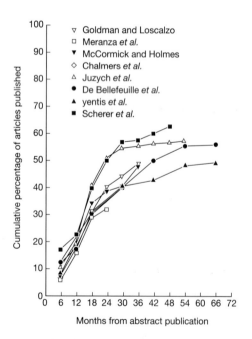

Fig. 4 Proportion of total abstracts published over time, calculated from individual studies (from ref. 27 with permission).

Legend:
▽ Goldman and Loscalzo
□ Meranza et al.
▼ McCormick and Holmes
◇ Chalmers et al.
△ Juzych et al.
● De Bellefeuille et al.
▲ yentis et al.
■ Scherer et al.

Y-axis: Cumulative percentage of articles published
X-axis: Months from abstract publication

Table 6 Publication record of trials submitted to the Royal Prince Alfred Hospital Ethics Committee between 1979 and 1988,[41] correlation with significant outcome

- 748 eligible studies
- 520 (70%) replied to the survey
- 218 trials included tests of significance
- Those with positive outcomes were significantly more likely to have been published than negative results (HR, 2.32; 95% CI, 1.47–3.66; $p = 0.0003$)
- This result was even stronger for the 130 clinical trials (HR, 3.13; 95% CI, 1.76–5.58; $p +0.0001$)
- Time to publication of the 218 trials was shorter for those with positive outcomes than those with negative results (median 4.8 vs. 8.0 years)
- The results for time to publication for the 130 clinical trials was similar (median 4.7 vs. 8.0 years)

Because of the late introduction of tagging for clinical trials and other technical problems, together with the fact that MEDLINE only includes about 4000 of the 23 000 biomedical journals published each year, there is a need to examine a number of databases to find the greatest number of RCTs. Searches should generally be carried out by an information specialist, since there is plenty of data to suggest that a skilled searcher using an optimal strategy will find at least twice as many pertinent reports as a clinical researcher without specific searching skills. In addition, the unskilled searcher is likely to find many more reports that are of no interest, but which have to be read. Searches should also attempt to find as many unpublished RCTs as possible. This is done by searching meeting abstracts, registers of

Table 7 Treatment efficacy (number needed to treat (NNT) to prevent emesis) in RCTs of ondansetron for the prevention of postoperative emesis. Results of all RCTs and those published more than once. Adding duplicates to the originals produced an overestimation of treatment efficacy of 23% [(6.4 − 4.9)/6.4] (data reproduced with permission from ref. 30)

16 RCTs not duplicated	NNT 9.5 (95% CI 6.9–15)
Original report of 3 duplicated RCTs	NNT 3.9 (95% CI 3.3–4.8)
6 duplicates of 3 original trials	NNT 3.3 (95% CI 2.8–3.8)
All 9 reports of duplicated RCTs	NNT 3.5 (95% CI 3.2–4.0)
All 19 original trials combined	NNT 6.4 (95% CI 5.3–7.9)
All 25 original and duplicated reports of RCTs	NNT 4.9 (95% CI 4.4–5.6)

theses, contacting known researchers, pharmaceutical companies, and other funders of trials.

Failure to use a formal search strategy will inevitably result in a biased set of data—in addition to the structural problems described, the tendency of reviewers to use their own carefully gathered reference material is likely to be flawed. Clinicians more often read prestigious journals (which more often publish 'significant' reports) and the decision to retain a copy of a paper may be influenced by it showing a significant result. Clinicians are also more likely to retain a paper that is of interest to them—possibly reflecting their bias or supporting their own research. A paper by Hunt and colleagues discusses the problems of searching in more detail.[31]

The inclusion of data from unpublished sources, abstracts, and less prestigious journals does not mean that reviewers need to accept original research of poorer quality. However, blinded studies of trial quality using explicit criteria have not shown that trials from such sources are technically poorer. The job of the reviewer is to identify poor-quality research, whatever its source, and they should not exclude trials from sources stereotyped as of poorer quality because of the lack of a peer review.

Selection of data to be included

It is a paradox that we insist that clinical trials be randomized and based on a written protocol, whilst at the same time we are very happy to read and write reviews, based on these trials, that make no attempt to avoid bias and which do not use explicit methods. Having identified the trials that have been carried out, the next step in a review is deciding which trials to include and what data to use from each trial. There is clearly a potential for bias at both of these stages.

Bramwell and Williams found that predetermined criteria for inclusion and exclusion of trials was rarely used. Only 10 per cent of 106 reviews appeared to use such criteria, though there was evidence that selection of certain publications and omission of others was taking place. In an analysis of 56 reviews of chemotherapy for advanced ovarian cancer, Williams and Lodge[32] found that the mean number of reports of RCTs discussed in each review was five. Examination of the literature suggests that there are in excess of 70 RCTs that would potentially be of interest to many

of these reviews. None of the papers examined stated how they selected the reports to be discussed or tabulated the reports that were excluded. None appeared to use prespecified criteria when making these decisions.

Assessment of validity

Mulrow described this as 'a standardized methodological assessment of the data'. She makes the point that if authors are to describe the quality of the report or the trial itself, these assessments should be based on validated instruments rather than *post hoc* criticism. Bramwell and Williams found that only 8 per cent of reviews in the *Journal of Clinical Oncology* used such explicit methods. However, the majority of reviews criticized some studies and compared and contrasted results and trial methodology in their discussion. Since in nearly all cases little or no data were presented, readers were left to accept these judgements or to go back and read all the papers in order to form their own opinion—defeating the object of the review for many readers.

Another aspect of data validity is the accuracy with which data is extracted from papers. Because of the nature of the work and the inadequacy of the reporting of trials, two or more individuals extracting data will often come to different conclusions. This may be on key points of trial design, such as whether the trial is randomized or not, or the quantitative data recorded in the report. Surprising though it may seem, some trial reports are so poorly presented that it is very difficult and occasionally impossible to tell if the trial, for instance, is randomized or not. Similarly, some data is obscure and difficult to find, or is contradictory in different parts of a paper. Added to this is the fatigue and subsequent inaccuracies that affect reviewers reading multiple papers at one sitting. None of the reviews in the study of the quality of reviews in advanced ovarian cancer[32] reported that the data had been extracted by two or more individuals and any disagreements sorted out by discussion.

Quantitative assessment of the literature

Where appropriate, meta-analytic techniques can be used to combine the results of individual trials to give a summary statistic for that intervention. Bramwell and Williams[22] found that only one of 106 reviews in the *Journal of Oncology* used meta-analytic techniques. In contrast, all the reviews used qualitative methods of integrating the data from a variety of sources, although without using any explicit criteria. None of the reviews of chemotherapy for ovarian cancer used quantitative analytical techniques.

Summary and conclusions

Despite failing to use methods designed to avoid bias, 101 of the 106 reviews in the study of Bramwell and Williams reported conclusions and/or a summary. In addition, 76 per cent of the reviews addressed the issue of future directions for research and clinical practice. In the review of chemotherapy for advanced ovarian cancer,[32] all but 3 of the 56 reviews included explicit or implied conclusions. These varied widely over time and in the platinum era were always in favour of platinum combinations. Looking at the situation prior to the recent introduction of paclitaxel, it is interesting that by far the largest trial testing these approaches (ICON 2—2075 patients) failed to show that a platinum combination was more effective than single-agent platinum.[33] A meta-analysis of this trial and of others asking the same question is likely to come to the same conclusion. Data from a meta–analysis of all the other trials combined (1095 patients) only suggested that platinum combinations may improve survival (hazard ratio (HR) 0.91, $p = 0.206$) by a small amount.[34] Thus, it may be that the conclusions of all the narrative reviews identified may not be supported by a systematic review of the data from 3165 patients in trials asking this specific question.

Individual patient data (IPD) meta-analysis

Most systematic reviews have been based on published data, often supported with additional data collected from the authors of trials by the reviewer. However, there is good evidence that an even more rigorous approach to collecting the data should be regarded as the safest method of meta-analysis.[35]

In an individual patient data meta-analysis the reviewer identifies those researchers who have carried out the RCTs in the question of interest. Having done this, the reviewers will need to contact all the researchers to ask for their co-operation in undertaking the review based on the draft protocol that has been developed. He or she will collect a copy of the protocol for each RCT and the raw data from each trial. Ideally this data should have been updated. This will be analysed in the meta-analysis using an agreed protocol. The reviewer will, in addition, need to make every attempt to contact researchers who have carried out research which has not yet been published.

Use of this process is time-consuming but has great advantages. Any errors in the data provided can be identified and corrected (mistype resulting in death before the patient was randomized, for instance). The analysis can be carried out by intention to treat, possession of the raw data allows the reviewer to restore in-appropriately excluded patients. The updating of data means that IPD meta-analyses often have long-term follow-up which was never reported for each trial. Although fraud is rare, this can be checked for by an independent appraisal of each trial. Are there major imbalances of prognostic information across groups in a trial, for example? Is the pattern of randomization consistent with the society where the trial was carried out (for example, randomization is uncommon on Sundays in Christian countries whilst it is common in Jewish and Moslem cultures).

Many in the field of evidence-based medicine feel that IPD meta-analysis is the 'gold standard' to which to aspire, but that it is not possible to do such rigorous reviews for all questions. Comparisons of systematic reviews of published data and individual patient data suggest that there may be differences in the results.[36],[37] In some instances the findings of a systematic review of published data may stimulate the setting up of an IPD meta-analysis.

Quality of evidence

It is implicit in Western medicine that we use the very best evidence when making decisions. However, this brief chapter seeks to show that there is much that we could do to improve the quality of the evidence that we use. While this is generally accepted, there is a lack of will to change and improve the way we gather and use information. This may partly stem from a need to acknowledge the poor quality of what we do at present and the uncertainty about the quality of the care we deliver that follows on from this.

A number of studies about the way clinical decisions are made have found that specialists feel that there are only a few times during a week when they need further evidence to help them to make a decision. However, when they are taken through each case asking them to justify each decision, it is clear that in many individual consultations there are one or more questions where the data supporting decisions are unclear and when further evidence is really required.[21] It may be that the discomfort of this realization causes clinicians to compensate by being overconfident of the data that they act upon.

One way that this may manifest itself is in differences in the interpretation of the same data-set by members of different medical specialist groups. A good example of this is the way that data from RCTs of postoperative radiotherapy versus no radiotherapy for women who had undergone a radical mastectomy for breast cancer were interpreted. A study of narrative reviews found that two out of three radiotherapists concluded that such radiotherapy improved survival, whereas one out of three non-radiotherapists concluded that radio-therapy had no effect on survival. A contemporary systematic review of the data from these trials in fact suggested that neither conclusion was right—a meta-analysis showed that patients who had received radiotherapy had a worse survival.[38] A subsequent meta-analysis[39] has shown that the situation is even more complex—there was a reduction in the number of deaths from cancer, but this was at least offset by an excess number of deaths from cardiac disease (presumably related to irradiation of the left ventricle).

Where does this leave us in the real world?

The aims described here are idealistic, setting goals for what we could achieve by a careful balanced use of the literature. However, not every decision can be made in the light of such an exhaustive process. As well as the lack of time, the human factor needs to be taken into account. What is the role of the clinician as an individual and how do they interact with the patient and their family?

Effective healthcare requires that all aspects of patient care be attended to. This means that in any one patient's care decisions are constantly being made. Some of these are obvious, whether or not to use adjuvant chemotherapy for instance, whilst others are 'routine' and become invisible. Some of the invisible decisions are clinical, whether to do a follow-up test for example, while others are about the process of how we deliver care. This chapter has concentrated mainly of the big 'obvious' decisions, but even here we need to consider what we do in the absence of reliable information to help us make decisions.

When patients and clinicians come to make 'big' decisions there are a number of factors that need to be taken into account, regardless of what the evidence shows:

- What is the clinical experience and attitude of the clinician?
- What can the healthcare system provide?
- What can the individual hospital provide?
- What are the wishes of the patient and his or her carers?

Each of these factors will still come into play when there is good evidence for an intervention, but they may be even more important when there is little reliable evidence. How do we make a decision in practical terms? Say an operation is clearly indicated, but there is little evidence to tell us whether this should be a simple or radical operation, what do we do? Currently the decision is influenced by some of the following factors—personal experience with the techniques or problem, peer pressure, pressure from hospital 'management' and other staff, habit, and the patient's wishes. Often these are all conflated into a 'personal' decision, where the individual components are largely subconscious.

Sometimes this will result in a 'good' decision, but in other cases the decision might not be optimal. Regardless of the quality of the decision, it will often not be questioned. However, it is increasingly likely that the veracity of decisions will be questioned by audit, management, and, most importantly, by patients. Although I put the wishes of patients and carers at the bottom of the bulleted list above, I believe that they should have the most important say in what is appropriate for them. However, they need to be informed if they are to do this most usefully. The advent of information technology means that far more patients are in a position to be knowledgeable about their care. Some will have the motivation and far more time than any doctor to find out the answer to the question that they are asking. However, sometimes they may be unable to put this into an appropriate context, since they may not have a sufficient level of general background expertise. On other occasions they will find highly pertinent information that can be used to 'improve' a decision. One of the challenges for the future is to find the best ways to share decision-making between the patient and doctor/nurse, both in terms of knowledge provision as well as what is appropriate to them as an individual.

In the case of the surgical question posed above, the bulleted list of pressures above may result in a variety of decisions:

- The doctor is not experienced in performing the radical operation and recommends the simple procedure.
- The doctor is very experienced in undertaking the radical operation and likes the challenge and kudos that it gives, and recommends the radical option.
- The healthcare system may have guidelines supporting, or not, the radical operation.
- The hospital may have issues regarding operating time that may persuade the surgeon that simple surgery is appropriate, given that extra benefit from radical surgery has yet to be shown.
- The patient may have specific wishes about 'leaving no stone unturned' or wishing to avoid unnecessary side-effects at all costs, which lead them to request radical or simple surgery.
- The patient may occasionally find information (Internet/journals/guidelines, etc.) that may put the question in a different light, changing their own or the clinician's decision.

The bottom line is that in nearly all decisions in medicine there is no 'right' answer. Very often the evidence will be equivocal and open to interpretation. Even when the evidence points one way, the patient's or clinician's experience may lead justifiably to another choice. The main purpose of this chapter, however, is to stress that oncologists should be striving to ensure that the best evidence is made available and used as often as possible.

Conclusions

The chapter brings to the attention of oncologists some of the flaws in the way that we carry out research and then assemble and use evidence. The quality of RCTs has improved enormously over the past two decades, but there has been a lack of understanding of the potential flaws inherent in combining and comparing data from different RCTs. This has sometimes resulted in a failure to identify effective treatments, the adoption or continuation of ineffective or dangerous treatment, and a general lack of continuity in planning rational clinical research and therapy for individual patients. The development of information technology now gives us the opportunity of closing some of the loopholes, but clinicians will need to increase their appraisal and review skills to make the best of these opportunities.

In the meantime, patients and their carers now have more access to good-quality review information, guidelines, and primary research. Many have the motivation and time to work to understand this data and have the ability to become very knowledgeable. They are only concerned with their own problem and because of this will always be able to devote more time than their physician to finding and appraising information. The increased emphasis on best evidence will inevitably mean that the dialogue between patient and physician will change from one of directive decision-making to both making shared decisions.

References

1. **Sackett DL, Haynes RB.** On the need for evidence-based medicine. *Evidence-Based Medicine*, 1995; **1**: 5–6.
2. **Evans CE,** *et al.* Educational package on hypertension for primary care physicians. *Canadian Medical Association Journal*, 1984; **130**: 719–22.
3. **Sacks HS, Chalmers TC, Smith H.** Randomised versus historical controls for clinical trials. *American Journal of Medicine*, 1982; **72**: 233–40.
4. **Beral V, Colwell L.** Randomised trial of high doses of stilboestrol and ethisterone therapy in pregnancy: long-term follow up of the children. *Journal of Epidemiology and Community Health*, 1981; **35**: 155–60.
5. **Baird DD, Wilcox AJ, Herbst AL.** Self-reported allergy, infection and autoimmune diseases in women exposed *in utero* to diethylstilboestrol. *Journal of Clinical Epidemiology*, 1996; **49**: 263–6.
6. **Meara J, Vessey M, Fairweather DV.** A randomised double-blind controlled trial of diethylstilboestrol in pregnancy: 35 year follow-up in mothers and their offspring. *British Journal of Obstetrics and Gynaecology*, 1989; **96**: 620–2.
7. **Antman K,** *et al.* High dose combination alkylating agent preparative regime with autologous bone marrow support: the Dana-Farber/Beth Israel hospital experience. *Cancer Treatment Reports*, 1987; **71**: 119–25.
8. **Peters WD,** *et al.* High dose combination alkylating agents with bone marrow support as initial management for breast cancer. *Journal of Clinical Oncology*, 1988; **6**: 1368–76.
9. **Rahman ZU, Frye DK, Buzdar AU.** Impact of selection process on response rate and long-term survival of potential high-dose chemotherapy candidates treated with standard-dose doxorubicin containing chemotherapy in patients with metastatic breast cancer. *Journal of Clinical Oncology*, 1997; **15**: 3171–7.
10. **Garcia-Carbanero R,** *et al.* Patient selection in high-dose chemotherapy trials: relevance in high-risk breast cancer. *Journal of Clinical Oncology*, 1997; **18**: 3178–84.
11. **Peters W,** *et al.* A prospective, randomized comparison of two doses of combination alkylating agents as consolidation after CAF in high-risk

breast cancer involving ten or more axillary lymph nodes: preliminary results of CALGB 9082/SWOG 9114/NCIC MA-13. *Proceedings of the American Society of Clinical Oncology*, 1999; **18**: 2. [Abstract.]

12. **The Scandinavian Breast Cancer Study Group 9401.** Results from a randomized adjuvant breast cancer study with high dose chemotherapy with CTCb supported by autologous bone marrow stem cells versus dose escalated and tailored FEC therapy. *Proceedings of the American Society of Clinical Oncology*, 1999; **18**: 3. [Abstract.]

13. **Bezwoda WR.** Randomised, controlled trial of high dose chemotherapy (HD-CNVp) versus standard dose (CAF) chemotherapy in high-risk surgically treated breast cancer. *Proceedings of the American Society of Clinical Oncology*, 1999; **18**: 4. [Abstract.]

14. **Schulz KF, Chalmers I, Haynes RB, Altman DG.** Empirical evidence of bias: dimensions of methodological quality associated with estimates of treatment effects in controlled trials. *Journal of the American Medical Association*, 1995; **273**: 408–12.

15. **Non-Small Cell Lung Cancer Collaborative Group.** Chemotherapy in non-small cell lung cancer: a meta-analysis using updated data on individual patients from 52 randomised trials. *British Medical Journal*, 1995; **311**: 899–909.

16. **Coates A, et al.** Improving the quality of life during chemotherapy for advanced breast cancer. A comparison of intermittent and continuous treatment strategies. *New England Journal of Medicine*, 1987; **317**: 1490–5.

17. **Moher D, Schulz KF.** Randomized clinical trials in cancer: improving the quality of their reports will also facilitate better conduct. *Annals of Oncology*, 1998; **9**: 483–8.

18. **Begg C, et al.** Improving the quality of reporting randomised controlled trials. The CONSORT statement. *Journal of the American Medical Association*, 1996; **276**: 637–9.

19. **Stiller C.** Survival of patients in clinical trials and at specialist centres. In *Introducing new treatments for cancer: practical, ethical and legal problems* (ed. CJ Williams). Chichester: John Wiley, 1992: 119–36.

20. **Davidoff F, Haynes RB, Sackett D, Smith R.** Evidence-based medicine. A new journal to help doctors identify the information that they need. *British Medical Journal*, 1995; **310**: 1085–6.

21. **Covell DG, Uman GC, Manning PR.** Information needs in office practice: are they being met? *Annals of Internal Medicine*, 1985; **103**: 596–9.

22. **Bramwell VCH, Williams CJ.** Do authors of review articles use systematic methods to identify, assess and synthesize information? *Annals of Oncology*, 1997; **8**: 1185–96.

23. **Mulrow CD.** The medical review article: state of the science. *Annals of Internal Medicine*, 1987; **106**: 485–8.

24. **Dickersin K, Min YI.** NIH clinical trials and publication bias. *Online Journal of Current Clinical Trials*, 1993.

25. **Early Breast Cancer Trialists' Collaborative Group.** *Treatment of early breast cancer. Volume 1. Worldwide evidence 1985–1990.* Oxford: Oxford University Press, 1990.

26. **Chalmers I, Gray M, Sheldon T.** Handling scientific fraud. Prospective registration of health care research would help. *British Medical Journal*, 1995; **311**: 262.

27. **Scherer RW, Dickersin K, Langenberg P.** Full publication of results initially reported in abstracts. A meta-analysis. *Journal of the American Medical Association*, 1994; **272**: 151–62.

28. **Horton R, Smith R.** Time to register randomised trials. *British Medical Journal*, 1999; **319**: 864–5.

29. **Egger M, et al.** Language bias in randomised controlled trials in English and German. *Lancet*, 1997; **350**: 326–9.

30. **Tramer MR, Reynolds DJ, Moore RA, McQuay HJ.** Impact of covert duplicate publication on meta-analysis: a case study. *British Medical Journal*, 1997; **315**: 635–40.

31. **Hunt DL, Haynes RB, Browman GP.** Searching the medical literature for the best evidence to solve clinical questions. *Annals of Oncology*, 1998; **9**: 377–83.

32. **Williams CJ, Lodge M.** Poor quality of reviews of randomised clinical trials of chemotherapy for advanced ovarian cancer: need for action. *Proceedings of the American Society of Clinical Oncology*, 1997; **16**: 1534. [Abstract.]

33. **ICON Collaborators.** ICON 2: randomised trial of single agent carboplatin against three-drug combination of CAP in women with ovarian cancer. *Lancet*, 1998; **352**: 1571–6.

34. **Advanced Ovarian Cancer Trialists' Group.** Chemotherapy for ovarian cancer (Cochrane Review). In *The Cochrane Library*. Oxford: Update Software, 1999: Issue 4.

35. **Clarke M, Stewart L, Pignon JP, Bijnens L.** Individual patient data meta-analysis in cancer. *British Journal of Cancer*, 1998; **77**: 2036–44.

36. **Stewart LA, Parmar MKB.** Meta-analysis of the literature or individual patient data: is there a difference? *Lancet*, 1993; **341**: 418–22.

37. **Parmar MKB, Stewart LA, Altman DG.** Meta-analysis of randomised trials: when the whole is more than just the sum of the parts. *British Journal of Cancer*, 1996; **74**: 496–501.

38. **Cuzick J, et al.** Overview of randomized trials of postoperative adjuvant radiotherapy in breast cancer. *Cancer Treatment Reports*, 1987; **71**: 15–29.

39. **Early Breast Cancer Trialists' Collaborative Group.** Effects of radiotherapy and surgery in early breast cancer: an overview of randomised trials. *New England Journal of Medicine*, 1995; **333**: 1444–55.

40. **Embracing patient partnership.** *British Medical Journal*, 1999; **319**: 719–94.

41. **Stern JM, Simes RJ.** Publication bias: evidence of delayed publication in a cohort study of clinical research projects. *British Medical Journal*, 1997; **315**: 640–5.

Economic considerations for cancer clinicians

Jane Hall and M. H. N. Tattersall

Introduction

Cancer is one of the leading causes of death in developed countries and is growing in importance in the developing countries. Advances in treatment and early diagnosis and new possibilities for prevention are enabling more to be done in cancer control and care. But even in the richest countries, more money could be spent on cancer control and research. So clinicians find themselves confronting questions of how much should be spent on cancer control, how cancer services should be organized, what treatments should be used, and being increasingly responsible for clinical budgets.

Health economics has much to offer in understanding and addressing these problems. The scope of health economics includes the measurement of the burden of illness, the measurement of health outcomes including quality of life, understanding decision-making, considering health service structures and organization, assessing the effects of different methods of payment, and investigating access to services and equity. In addition, health economics can work alongside clinical epidemiology so that evidence of efficiency can be considered with evidence of effectiveness.

This chapter provides a brief introduction to health economics for cancer clinicians. First, it discusses the broader considerations of the economics of healthcare; second, it reviews the principles of economic evaluation; and third, it considers economic evaluations relating to some common cancers and supportive care treatments. The chapter ends by discussing the relationship of economic analysis and evidence based medicine.

Cancer treatment and health economics

Healthcare expenditure accounts for between 6 per cent and 10 per cent of **GDP** (Gross Domestic Product, a measure of the total value of goods and services produced in a country) in most developed countries. The United States spends more on healthcare than any other nation and there healthcare spending amounts to almost 14 per cent of GDP.[1] So healthcare is big business. Yet in even in countries with market-based systems of healthcare, governments play a major role in regulating, financing, and, in some cases, directly providing healthcare. So healthcare is as much part of the political agenda as it is a matter of economics (for further discussion see ref. 2).

Healthcare is often discussed in terms of rights and entitlements. Good health is a precondition for the exercise of many other functions.

But government cannot guarantee 'good health for all'; what it can provide is access to healthcare. So healthcare itself can be seen as a human right, and not something to be left to individuals' ability to pay for it. Further, individuals as purchasers of healthcare frequently face a vulnerability not faced by consumers in other markets. Emergency care can be a matter of 'life and death'. Delays in getting the appropriate care can affect the chance of survival and recovery. For these, and possibly other reasons, there is a stronger sense of altruism in healthcare than other aspects of life.

There are other reasons, too, why healthcare is quite different to other commodities that can be bought and sold in markets. Healthcare is not valued in itself; who would choose a stay in hospital or endure chemotherapy treatment if they thought they did not 'need' it? People cannot predict and therefore plan their purchases of healthcare. And they rarely have the knowledge required to be informed consumers. (Further discussion can be found in ref. 2). Those who plan, pay for, and provide healthcare face a perplexing situation.

First, there is not a simple relationship between healthcare 'need' and healthcare spending. Countries with similar populations and similar disease patterns spend quite different amounts on healthcare; and within countries, apparently similar communities use quite different levels of health services. So something other than health 'need' determines the level of spending.

Second, the potential demand for healthcare seems, if not unlimited, then at least very large. Changing epidemiology has seen the emergence of diseases with a long natural history, and chronic disease and disability. These require more and ongoing healthcare compared to acute episodes of illness. Developments in medical technology have increased the range of interventions. Many new technologies are described as 'half-way' technology; that is, they improve survival and quality of life but they do not cure the disease or eliminate all its problems. So more people are living longer with treatable conditions while the range and expense of possible treatments is increasing rapidly.

Third, more healthcare spending does not yield better health outcomes; or even more satisfied customers. Therefore, those who pay for healthcare are questioning the value they get for the money. And taxpayers are questioning what and how governments spend their funds. Worldwide, there is a reluctance to increase the size of government budgets.

What does this mean for clinicians? They work in health systems where the budgets cannot support everything that could be done. Changing and restructuring health systems is a continuing phenomenon. And they are asked to justify how they want to provide

Table 1 Potential effects on health benefits and costs

Costs	Benefits		
	More	Same	Less
Less	a	b	c
Same	d	e	f
More	g	h	i

Programmes which cost less for more of the same health benefits are clearly better, as programmes which cost more for the same or fewer health benefits are clearly worse. Thus new programmes which fall in (a), (b), or (d) are better than the alternative, while those which fall in (f), (h), or (i) are worse.

services, and clinical treatment itself, on the basis of its effectiveness and efficiency. To tackle that we turn to the principles and practice of economic evaluation.

Principles of economic evaluation

Economic evaluation is the systematic comparison of the costs and benefits of an intervention with the alternative use of those resources so as to maximize efficiency. Efficiency is often used synonymously and erroneously with cost-cutting. It means getting the most from scarce resources.[3] Cutting costs is not more efficient unless (1) the same output at the same quality is produced at less cost, or (2) the resources saved can be used with greater benefit somewhere else. In healthcare, the limit on resources is evident through controls on healthcare budgets. However, resource scarcity is not just monetary. Trained healthcare professionals and high technology facilities are also scarce. It takes time to train new doctors or to construct new hospitals, so providing more money may not make resources less scarce.

The comparison of costs and benefits of alternatives can be illustrated diagrammatically (see Table 1). A programme may cost more, less, or the same as the alternative use of funds and it may provide greater, fewer, or the same health benefits. Clearly, if a new programme can reduce costs but yield the same health outcomes it is more efficient. It is not difficult to decide that the new programme is preferable to the old way of doing things and is therefore better. The programmes that give unequivocally more health gains per pound are preferable to their alternatives (cells a, b, and d). Programmes that give clearly less health gains per pound than their alternatives are not to be preferred (cells f, h, and i). When a new treatment or programme offers improved health outcomes but at a higher cost it is more difficult to judge. Here it is important to focus on the margin, or an incremental analysis. In other words, to ask whether the additional cost is worth the additional benefits.

These methods have been applied across many areas of public sector decision-making;[4] what is particular to its use in evaluating health programmes is the conceptualization and measurement of benefits.

Types of economic appraisal

Economic evaluation is generally regarded as comprising three techniques: cost-effectiveness analysis, cost-utility analysis, and cost-benefit analysis (Table 2). Sometimes, a fourth technique is included,

cost-minimization analysis. Cost-minimization analysis is the comparison of the costs of alternatives. It is often described as a partial economic evaluation as it considers only costs and ignores benefits. However, it is an appropriate form of analysis if the outcomes of the alternatives have already been shown to be equivalent.

What distinguishes the different types is the approach to measuring benefits. Both cost-effectiveness analysis and cost-utility analysis investigate efficiency (that is, health outcomes related to costs) and can answer the question as to which of the alternatives is the best buy. Therefore, it follows that no programme considered alone can be 'cost-effective'; it can only be more, or less cost-effective than an alternative. Cost-benefit analysis, by valuing benefits in units of money, shows whether the benefits are worth more than the costs and, hence, can answer the question 'Is this programme worthwhile'? There are a number of guides to the application of economic evaluation in healthcare, including those by Drummond et al.,[5] Gold et al.,[6] and Sloan.[7]

Cost-effectiveness analysis

With cost-effectiveness analysis (CEA), benefits are measured in their naturally occurring clinical units, most usually life years saved, although it could be heart attacks prevented, cases of cancer diagnosed, and so on. CEA was developed primarily by the United States military which also met the problem of valuing human life, although with a rather different objective than the health services! The phrase 'more bang for the buck' is a reminder of the military contribution. The clinical units used to measure benefits have to be common to the programmes being compared. How do you choose between £5000 for a heart attack prevented and £150 for a cancer detected? This can be overcome if the outcomes can be transformed into the same measure of health benefit, such as life years saved. It allows a wide range of interventions to be compared on the basis of cost per life years saved. CEA has been much more widely used in healthcare evaluation than the other techniques.

Cost-utility analysis

Measuring benefits as life years saved does not take into account potentially important differences in quality of life. Improving quality of life is the primary aim of many cancer treatments. Research has shown that there are health states, such as being unconscious or confined to bed on life-support systems in severe pain, which are widely regarded as worse than death. Concern with quality has prompted the development of another technique of economic evaluation: cost-utility analysis or CUA.[8] In this form of analysis, life years saved are counted but they are weighted according to their quality. This provides an outcome measure which, in a single score, combines both survival and health-related quality. The resultant outcome measure is known generally as quality-adjusted life years (QALYs) or healthy-year equivalents (HYEs), and the results of the analysis are presented as a cost per QALY or HYE.[9]

Cost-benefit analysis

QALYs are a major advance over life years saved in that they allow for a broader concept of benefits. Even so, the question arises as to whether QALYS or similar health outcomes capture all the relevant benefits. In many encounters, aspects such as reassurance, being treated with dignity, being involved in treatment decisions, may be

Table 2 Types of economic appraisal

Type	Benefits	Analysis	Advantages	Disadvantages
Cost-benefit	All benefits measured in money	Is this programme workable?	Programmes with different aims can be compared. One programme can be considered versus doing nothing	Difficult to measure health in monetary terms. Intangible benefits often omitted
Cost-effectiveness	Benefits measured in clinical units; for example, life years saved, deaths averted, cases detected	Comparison of programmes with same health aims	Life and health do not have to be valued. Wide range of alternative health programmes can be considered	Ignores quality of life. Cannot compare health programmes with other programmes
Cost-minimization	Benefits not measured	Comparison of programmes with same aims and level of benefits	Estimates of cost only required	Ignores benefits
Cost-utility	Benefits measured in QALYs	Comparison of health programmes	Incorporates quality and quantity of life. All health programmes can be	Cannot compare health programmes with other programmes. Problems in measuring quality of life

valued as benefits. Screening programmes are a particular case where the concept of benefits should be defined more broadly than health outcomes. The immediate 'product' of screening is information. For the true positives, the information can be used to modify risk factors or institute early treatment, and this intervention may improve health outcomes. For the true negatives, the information will not lead to improved health outcomes; none the less, the reassurance provided by a negative test result may be valued by the recipient. Those with a false-positive test result may be made concerned and anxious by the information, as well as having to go through further tests. In this case the value of the information may be negative.

The need to measure a wider range of benefits has led to renewed interest in cost-benefit analysis (**CBA**) which requires that all benefits are measured and valued in money. Valuing both benefits and costs in monetary terms provides a straight answer to the question of whether the additional benefits are worth their costs. Current approaches emphasize estimating individuals' willingness to pay. However, many people find it difficult to place a price on better health outcomes, or are unfamiliar with the true cost of health services. New empirical approaches to eliciting valid estimates are being tested.

Cost-minimization analysis

Cost-minimization analysis compares the costs of one or more alternative programmes. The level of benefits achieved by each programme are not explicitly considered, so this is sometimes termed a partial economic evaluation. A full economic evaluation considers both costs and benefits. Some texts do not include cost-minimization as a form of economic evaluation because of this exclusion of benefits. It is only a useful and valid type of economic analysis if the benefits of the alternatives have been demonstrated to be quantitatively equivalent. There are many examples of such studies in the literature in which equivalence is assumed rather than demonstrated. Also, it is not unusual to find cost-minimization analyses (incorrectly) labelled as cost-benefit or cost-effectiveness analyses.[10]

Counting the costs

In all types of economic appraisal, resource use is measured in costs. Money is a convenient means of counting costs, but it is important to remember that it is resource use and the opportunity-costs of those resources that is of interest. The key issue in measuring the costs of a cancer treatment or any other healthcare service is to compare the resource use in a world with that service with those in a world without it. The difference is the relevant figure. In calculating this, it is more important to have an imprecise estimate of the 'right' cost than a precise, but quite wrong, figure.

Costs often match expenditure, but not always. The prices charged for healthcare services, such as the charge per day in hospital or the charge for a chest radiograph, are often set with more consideration of health insurance arrangements than the opportunity-cost of resources. In costing hospital services, the mean *per diem* rate is frequently but inappropriately used. The problem with the *per diem* rate is that it is generally calculated by including all the hospital expenditure and dividing by all hospital days. This would be satisfactory if all hospital days were equally expensive. However, as *per diem* rates cannot distinguish obstetric patients from cardiac surgical patients or days in the intensive-care ward from days in the medical ward, they rarely measure opportunity-costs for any particular ward, patient group, or type of treatment. The development of case-mix measures (such as Diagnostic Related Groups, **DRGs**) and of case-mix adjusted standardized costs have made the estimation of costs and the comparison of estimates across studies much easier. However, even DRG costs may not represent the true opportunity-cost and must be used with caution.

The resource use that is most readily identified is that directly associated with the programme or treatment. These are not the total costs. It is important to include all the 'downstream' costs, that is costs that would not have been incurred if the programme did not exist.

Screening is a helpful example here. The costs of the screening programme are the costs of recruiting people, taking the test, and communicating the result. But these are not the total costs as there are several 'downstream' costs. Those people with positive screening tests will require further tests to confirm or rule out a diagnosis. Those diagnosed will require treatment and ongoing follow-up. Screening may identify some conditions, which, while not malignant, may require some intervention. All these costs are consequences of the initial screening and so should be considered as part of the total costs. However, there may also be some cost-savings. Screening may detect disease at an earlier stage. As that disease would commonly have become symptomatic in time, then treatment costs would have been incurred eventually. So future treatment costs avoided are a cost-saving. Total costs should be net costs.

Other aspects of costs

It is erroneous, but not uncommon, to categorize all the positive effects as benefits and all the negative ones as costs. It is important to remember that costs are the opportunity-costs of resources. Costs are what is limited or constrained; that is, resources. Benefits are what is being maximized. So both costs and benefits can be positive and negative. This is not just an issue of logic. The results of economic evaluation are often presented as ratios, a cost per unit of benefit, and changing whether a particular item is classified as a 'cost' or a 'benefit' can alter the results. Consequently, classifying costs and benefits correctly is crucial.

This discussion of healthcare costs has focused on costs from the point of view of the health sector, as do most cost-analyses. This is appropriate as these are the major costs of detecting and treating cancer and caring for those who have it. However, the costs of treating cancer can also comprise non-health service costs, such as the cost for the patient travelling to the treatment centre, or time spent by the patient in treatment, or time spent by family members looking after the patient. Where these have an opportunity-cost (that is, the resources could be used in some other beneficial way), then they should be taken into account.

It is particularly important to consider costs outside the health sector when the extent of these varies significantly from one programme to another. A good example is community care for the elderly, which is often proposed as a cheaper alternative to institutional care.

However, these analyses rarely take into account the costs borne by those providing the care at home, often the wives and daughters.

If one of two alternative treatments returns patients to work sooner, should the earning generated by the earlier return to work be counted as cost-savings? This is not just an issue of how comprehensive a range of costs is included. Its resolution rests on defining the objective of healthcare programmes, that is what healthcare is seeking to maximize. If the maximand is population health, then productivity gains as such are not relevant in the measure of benefits. If the maximand is social welfare, then the question is how well does GDP (or any other measure of economic activity) measure that. However, it should be noted that these productivity gains, sometimes called indirect benefits, are frequently as large or larger than the value of resource use, so that their inclusion will significantly affect the results.

Return to work is sometimes suggested as a measure of recovery, an indicator of return to normal activities. Whilst this may be so, actual return to work will depend on social and economic circumstances such as the availability of jobs and the provision of pensions, as well as physical and mental function. In our view, the capacity to resume normal activities is better measured through estimating health gains and treated as a benefit in QALY terms.

It is sometimes suggested that the cost of providing pensions or social-security benefits should also be counted as cost-savings. Although these payments are costs to the government, it is generally agreed that they are not opportunity-costs. From the viewpoint of society as a whole, they represent not a loss of production but a transfer of purchasing power from one group to another. These are known as transfer payments.

The term 'economic costs of illness' is sometimes used to refer to the sum of the direct costs and the earning losses due to premature mortality and morbidity. Illness *per se* does not cost society anything; it is what society chooses to do about it that uses resources. Therefore, the term 'cost of illness' is misleading. In addition, this notional sum is not relevant to the approach of evaluating health interventions described here—that is, making explicit the incremental health gains and costs of new or alternative healthcare programmes.

The Global Burden of Disease Study is a major research effort sponsored by the World Health Organization and the World Bank.[11] It is attempting to monitor health status across the world by developing a sophisticated measure of the burden of illness. In particular, this project has developed a new health measure, the 'disability-adjusted life year' or **DALY**. This can be considered as a variant of the QALY;[12] however, DALYs are a measure of the healthy life lost disaggregated by disease. DALYs are calculated by estimating the years of life lost due to a disease, estimating the loss of quality of life due to that disease, weighting those losses to reflect the social value of people at different ages, and applying a discount rate to reflect social preference for benefits delivered sooner rather than later. However, DALY estimates do not attempt to assess the current costs of treating disease and do not purport to be a measure of the costs of illness. That said, DALYs focus on notional losses attributed to disease rather than the outcomes of intervention, and so are not a measure of incremental benefits. Therefore, many of the same criticisms of cost-of-illness studies can be applied to DALYs.

Benefits (and risks)—health outcomes

The benefits of healthcare programmes are primarily health outcomes. Cancer is often a life-threatening disease. Consequently, the first and often the most important health benefit is survival. Earlier cancer treatment might also improve quality of life if improved function or less radical surgery is required. However, in some instances more intensive treatment that detracts from quality of life carries a better probability of long-term survival. Here, there may be a trade-off between quantity and quality of life. Very few medical interventions come with no risks or side-effects. Consequently, both positive and negative effects on health outcomes should be considered.

The measurement of quality of life, or more accurately health-related quality of life, is increasingly accepted as an important component of the evaluation of cancer treatment. It is so important that a number of specific instruments have been developed to measure quality of life in cancer patients. One measure which has been used is 'time without symptoms or toxicity' (TWiST).[13] This recognizes that there is a difference between the gain in survival in good health and that while experiencing symptoms or the side-effects of treatment. TwiST can be regarded as a very simple measure of quality of life. In general, quality-of-life measures are subjective and multi-dimensional, often encompassing physical, emotional, and social aspects of health status. Frequently, these are expressed as an arbitrary numeric score on a scale of 1 to 100; and, in general, these are not combined to give a single score. The quality-of-life measures needed for outcome measures in economic evaluation differ from clinically familiar measures in several important ways. The multiple dimensions must be reduced to a single score; the numerical scale must have particular properties; and the scale must be anchored at 0 and 1. The anchor points of the scale must be equivalent to death (no life years) and full health (one year of good health). The scale itself must have interval properties, that is the difference between 0.3 and 0.5 must have the same meaning as the difference between 0.6 and 0.8, so that the arithmetical manipulation of life years and weights is valid. This approach can also be used with TwiST data; TwiST time can be assigned a maximum utility of 1 and different utilities can be applied to the different health states during treatment (Fig. 1).

Estimating the weights required to calculate QALYs can be approached in two ways. One can start with a generalized health-status measure. The specific health outcomes of the programme being evaluated have to be described in terms of the selected health-status measure. Generalized measures often have existing weighting scales derived from some form of community survey. One measure that is gaining widespread acceptance is the SF36,[14] although this does not, as yet, provide summary scores which have the scaling characteristics required to estimate QALYs. The EuroQol was developed for the specific purpose of economic evaluation and has now been tested in a range of European countries.[15]

Alternatively, one can estimate the weights directly from empirical work. The specific health outcomes of the programme being evaluated have to be described in ways that can be used in survey. The values for these different health states are determined by a survey; those surveyed might be a community sample or potential patients and/or patients. The main estimation approaches are the standard gamble and the time trade-off. These techniques are fully described by Drummond et al.[8]

Cost-benefit analysis, which allows for a wider range of benefits, requires that those benefits be valued in money terms. The human capital approach estimates the value of life as an individual's contribution to national productivity, as measured by his or her lifetime earnings. It does not account for differences in the quality of life beyond an individual's capacity to work. It values those with a working lifespan ahead of them more highly than the old. The human capital value of life years saved is not accepted as a valid estimate of the value of saving life. Further, estimating the benefits of health programmes only in terms of life years saved, even when a dollar value can be placed on those years, ignores differences in quality of life.

Beyond health outcomes

As yet, cost-effectiveness analysis remains the most widely applied form of economic evaluation. The development of cost-utility analysis, which depends on outcome measures that incorporate both survival

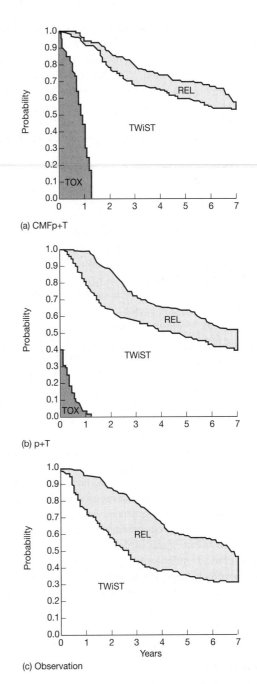

(a) CMFp+T

(b) p+T

(c) Observation

Fig. 1 Partitioned survival plots. Survival plots are shown for three endpoints, from left to right: TOX, SDFS, and survival. This divides the 7 years since randomization into the three stages, TOX, TWiST and REL, indicated. TOX, any reversible subjective toxic effect of any grade reported during a cycle or month of treatment; REL, any relapse or second primary breast cancer; SDFS, systemic disease-free survival (excluding local recurrence or contralateral breast cancer).

and quality of life, has been a major methodological advance in economic evaluation, and has extended the potential usefulness of economics in evaluating cancer programmes. However, QALYs, although a broader measure of benefit, still restrict the benefits of health programmes to health outcomes. But is there more to healthcare than health outcomes?

There are a number of other effects which may be considered as benefits (or as disbenefits) of receiving healthcare. These include being treated with dignity, a feeling of being cared for, and the ability and opportunity to be involved in treatment decisions. Such factors are generally what seems to be meant by the goal of 'patient-centred healthcare', or 'customer-focused services'. The need to move beyond health outcomes is particularly relevant where the evaluation of screening programmes is being considered. Screening in itself does not produce improved health outcomes; rather it produces information. The same is true for diagnostic tests, but an important difference is that screening targets well people. The information produced is useful if it leads to some change, earlier treatment, or perhaps modification of risk factors, that will in turn lead to better health outcomes. The information itself may have a positive or a negative value. For those individuals with true-positive results, the information may produce anxiety and, unless there is a true survival advantage, give them a longer period of living with disease. For those with a false-negative result, there is needless anxiety. Similarly, a negative test result may give people a significant sense of reassurance and the confidence to get on with their lives.

The desire to include a much broader range of benefits, such as information, reassurance, and being treated with dignity, has also led to interest in new ways to estimate the value of benefits. From this, there follows interest in exploring the relative importance of different types of benefit and, for this, researchers are turning to choice-modelling. Choice-modelling uses the following approach. The product to be evaluated is broken down into several attributes; for example, a trip from home to work can be a combination of travel time, waiting time, comfort, and cost. Respondents are asked to consider different combinations of these attributes. Preferences are elicited by asking them to rank or rate alternatives or to make discrete choices among alternatives. The data generated from carefully designed experiments can be used to evaluate the value of different attributes. If cost is included as one of the attributes, then willingness to pay for changes in product attributes can be estimated. This provides an alternative approach to valuing benefits for cost-benefit analysis.

These empirical techniques are well established in marketing, transport, and environmental economics but have yet to be used extensively in healthcare applications.

Estimating costs

Clinicians and health administrators often want to know the cost of healthcare services. So how can clinicians estimate costs? The steps to follow are summarized in Table 3 and described below.

Step 1—Specify the question

The first answer to the question 'How do I calculate the cost of my new improved course of chemotherapy?' is another question: 'Why do I want to know?' Is it to compare the cost of one chemotherapeutic regimen with that of another? Or to compare chemotherapy with radiotherapy? Or will the new regimen provide treatment for patients who were not previously treated with curative intent? The key issue, as stated, is defining the difference in resource use/benefits forgone in a world with this activity and a world without it. Therefore the alternative must be specified.

Table 3 Estimated health service costs

Step 1	Specify the question
Step 2	Identify the point of view
Step 3	Identify the relevant inputs
Step 4	Count the quantities of each input
Step 5	Estimate an opportunity-cost for each input
Step 6	Calculate cost estimates: total costs = (opportunity-cost × quantity)

Step 2—Identify the point of view

Whose costs are to be considered? The costs of healthcare fall on four main groups: patients, insurers, providers, and governments. From the providers' viewpoint the cost of a hospital stay is a measure of the resources that could otherwise be available to other patients. From the patients' viewpoint the cost of a hospital stay is the charge raised for that stay, and the patient is interested in how much of that will be paid by the insurance fund and how much remains to be met by himself or herself.

Step 3—Identify the relevant inputs

What resources are used in the services being considered and how will they change? For example, from the providers' viewpoint the surgical treatment of oesophageal cancer involves operating theatre time, days occupying a hospital bed, and antibiotic and chemotherapeutic agents (see ref. 16 for an example of estimating costs following these steps). It includes the treatment of complications in a proportion of patients. If patients with oesophageal cancer were not treated at all, these resources would be available for other patients.

Some resources 'used' by these patients may not be released for other applications, at least not immediately. These are fixed costs; that is to say, costs which do not vary with changes in workload. If the workload in a hospital ward drops suddenly because of a surgeons' strike, there will be few cost-savings. Nursing and other staff will still be in the wards; cleaning, lighting, and power will still be provided. However, the longer the surgeons are on strike, the fewer the costs that are fixed. In a week, almost all costs are fixed; over 20 years almost everything, even hospital buildings, can be varied.

Step 4—Count the quantities of the inputs

The amount of each input used should be measured in its naturally occurring unit. For example, hours of operating theatre time, hours of doctor time, number of doses of drugs, and number of fields of radiation therapy should be counted. Wherever possible, these quantities should be derived from actual amounts used rather than from subject estimates, which are usually unreliable. The information can be collected from review of patients' records or direct observation, or from both.

Step 5—Estimate the opportunity-cost for each input

A unit value for each input must be determined. This can usually be based on the prices of inputs, such as the hourly wage rate of nurses, cost of drugs, or cost of meals, where the inputs can be identified for the particular group of patients being considered. Prices are appropriate when they reflect the opportunity-cost of the resources being used. However, there are some inputs whose use is shared commonly by several groups of patients. These are known as joint costs. In a hospital, for example, the services of the personnel department, the power and lighting, and the information and reception desks are used by all and cannot be identified for particular patient groups. They are, by definition, shared. They can be apportioned to different patient groups and there are several accepted conventions for doing this.[8] In estimating incremental costs, shared costs are often fixed and therefore irrelevant (to economists anyway; economists and accountants will almost always differ on this point).

A piece of equipment, such as a linear accelerator, will be used over a long period and for many patients. Its acquisition price is paid only once. Opportunity-cost is important in determining how much of the capital value of a piece of equipment, or land, or building is used in any given timespan. Could the building or piece of equipment have been used for anything else? If not, the opportunity-cost is zero. If it could, the opportunity-cost is its value in that alternative use. When the opportunity-cost is zero, the amount already paid for it is irrelevant, it is a sunk cost. If there is an opportunity-cost—in other words, if there are benefits forgone because more patients wait to use the machine beyond the group now using it—how should the value of the use of the linear accelerator be calculated? Although the payment is once only, the value of the capital is regarded as decreasing over time and with use. The opportunity-cost of capital needs to be expressed in terms of the building or equipment use. For example, the capital depreciation of a linear accelerator may be converted to the cost per treatment field given. (A detailed discussion of calculating depreciation is given by Drummond *et al.* in ref. 8.)

Step 6—Calculate cost-estimates

Calculating cost-estimates is now a matter of simple arithmetic (opportunity-cost multiplied by quantity).

Economic studies of cancer control and supportive care

The following section overviews some published economic studies of cancer-control strategies for common cancer types, and economic evaluations of supportive-care measures.

Cancer control

Economic studies in breast cancer

The economic studies in breast cancer have covered a wide range, from screening mammography, local treatment options in early breast cancer, adjuvant systemic endocrine and cytotoxic treatment, the frequency of follow-up visits for patients with breast cancer to the care of women with advanced disease. Studies of mammographic screening and the assessment of abnormalities have examined the cost per QALY of mammography-screening services and the cost:benefit ratio of different screening frequencies and different ages of screenees, the number of radiographic views, and the status of double-film reading.

The financial costs of treating women with node-negative breast cancer with or without adjuvant systemic therapy has been determined by Hillner.[17] Using data from the Early Breast Cancer Trialists' Collaboration, the estimated annual risk of recurrence was 4 per cent, which was reduced by 39 per cent with combination chemotherapy. The paper presents baseline data for 45 to 60-year-old women, and shows an average gain in overall survival from systemic adjuvant therapy of 0.92 years. When adjusted for quality of life (TWiST), the gain from treatment is 0.43 quality-adjusted life years, resulting in a cost per QALY of $US15 400 for a 45-year-old woman and $US18 800 for a 60-year-old woman.

Smith and Hillner studied the cost-efficacy of adjuvant chemotherapy in premenopausal women with node-positive or -negative, oestrogen receptor-positive or -negative early breast cancer.[18] Treatment options considered were (1) no adjuvant treatment, (2) endocrine treatment (tamoxifen), (3) cyclophosphamide, methotrexate, and fluorouracil (CMF), and (4) CMF + tamoxifen. The incremental benefit of each treatment strategy was calculated. The incremental cost-benefit for chemotherapy or tamoxifen compared with no adjuvant therapy was equivalent, a survival gain of about 5.5 months for node-positive patients and 3.5 months for node-negative patients. The clinical and incremental cost:effectiveness ratio for combined chemotherapy and tamoxifen was limited whatever the nodal status and hormone-receptor status (from 0.2 to 2.1 months) and the resulting cost:effectiveness ratio varied between $US14 700 and $US80 700.

Advanced breast cancer

The costs of managing advanced breast cancer have been reported by Richards *et al.*[19] and Hurley *et al.*[20] The mean duration of survival from the diagnosis of metastatic disease was 27 months in the Richards study, and patients spent a mean duration of 32 inpatient days. The distribution of costs were as follows: inpatient care, 57 per cent; outpatient visits, 12 per cent; surgical treatment, 2 per cent; tamoxifen, 2 per cent; chemotherapy drugs, 8 per cent; radiotherapy, 7 per cent; imaging tests, 9 per cent; and laboratory investigations, 3 per cent. The most common imaging tests were bone and chest radiographs (eight and six per patient, respectively), but the most costly imaging was radionuclide scans (2.9 per patient) accounting for 41 per cent of the imaging costs.

Launois *et al.* have reported a cost-utility analysis of three different, second-line, single-agent chemotherapy regimens in metastatic breast cancer.[21] Vinorelbine was compared with paclitaxel and docetaxel, though no randomized trials comparing these three treatments have been reported. The clinical data were taken from pooled phase II trials. A median survival of 12 months was assumed with the three treatments. The total treatment costs, calculated from the viewpoint of the third-party payer and including the patient's transportation costs, etc. were very similar, though the treatment and follow-up costs for docetaxel were more than double the amount for vinorelbine. However, the costs of treatment-related complications were similar, while the costs of disease-related complications were 20 per cent lower with docetaxel. There is no evidence at this stage that the newer agents such as taxanes are more cost-effective than standard drugs such as anthracyclines.

Lung cancer

Lung cancer is the leading cause of cancer deaths in the developed world and is estimated to account for 20 per cent of all the

Table 4 Total direct healthcare costs for small-cell lung cancer (SCLC) and non-small-cell lung cancer (NSCLC) in the Canadian healthcare system

SCLC Stage	Average cost per case (1988 Canadian $)	NSCLC stage	Average cost per case (1988 Canadian $)
Limited	29 864	1	21 400
Extensive	23 789	11	23 881
		111a	22 131
		111b	19 366
		1V	16 501
Overall	25 988		19 781

Note: Costs include direct medical care costs, costs from diagnosis to death, exclude non-medical direct and indirect costs.

cancer-care costs in the United States. Lung cancer costs the United States Health System about $US8 billion annually. The treatment of lung cancer is of limited efficacy, and the majority of patients with inoperable disease do not survive 2 years. There has been much attention in the past few years to calculating the economics of tobacco smoking and the costs of treating tobacco-related ill health. Tobacco is estimated to cause one-third of deaths in middle age in the developed world, and will become the leading cause of death in the developing world during the first third of the twenty-first century. By 2030, it is estimated that tobacco will be responsible for 10 million deaths annually worldwide. This vast economic burden is a major public health concern, which has prompted not only the tobacco litigation, particularly in the United States, but also the examination of governments' attitudes to raising tobacco taxation and withdrawing support from tobacco growers.

The important role of family physicians in promoting smoking cessation cannot be overestimated. It can be argued that all medical practitioners have a role in not only publicizing the health costs of tobacco consumption, but also in supporting the Public Health lobby in support of tobacco taxation and against tobacco advertising to children.

Economic evaluations of lung cancer treatment have ranged from documenting the costs of treating small-cell- and non-small-cell lung cancer to measuring the costs of staging, and palliative cancer chemotherapy. Rosenthal et al.[22] conducted an institution-based evaluation of the direct healthcare costs of diagnosing and treating small-cell lung cancer. They reported a cost per case of 18 234 Australian dollars ($A) for limited-stage and $A13 177 for extensive-stage cancer. Hospitalization accounted for 42 per cent of costs, chemotherapy for 18 per cent, and radiotherapy for 11 per cent. Terminal-care costs were not included. Evans et al. used a population-based health model to estimate overall direct healthcare costs with the management of both small-cell and non-small-cell lung cancer (see Table 4).[23],[24] Together, these reported costs per case are large, and because of the high incidence of lung cancer they translate into high overall costs.

Several groups have reported cost-effectiveness analyses of the different approaches to staging lung cancer. These studies support

the use of computed tomography (CT) scanning to examine the mediastinum of patients with potentially operable non-small-cell lung cancer, and suggest that positron-emission tomography (PET) scanning may also have a role. Richardson et al. developed an algorithm for staging small-cell lung cancer patients and reported an optimal sequence of performing these procedures.[25] Although the ordering sequence is important, it is less so than ceasing the work-up when a metastasis had been detected.

The increasing use of chemotherapy in palliation of patients with non-small-cell lung cancer has led to a series of economic evaluation that compare the costs and benefits of different treatments. Hillner and Smith[26] conducted a cost-effectiveness analysis of vinorelbine chemotherapy versus vinorelbine plus cisplatin and vindesine plus cisplatin. Compared with vinorelbine, the addition of cisplatin cost $US17 700 per life year gained (an incremental cost per patient of $US2700; mean survival gain 8 weeks), whereas the cost of vindesine plus cisplatin was $US22 100 per life year gained (incremental cost $US1150; mean survival gain 2.7 weeks). These regimens are cost-effective compared with many other widely used medical treatments (Table 5). Recently, Earle and Evans examined the cost-effectiveness of combination chemotherapy with cisplatin and either etoposide or paclitaxel in patients with advanced non-small-cell lung cancer.[28] The primary survival and resource utilization outcomes were obtained from a large randomized trial in which patients given paclitaxel-containing treatment had a median survival of 9.7 months compared to 7.4 months for the etoposide-containing regimen. As administered in the trial, paclitaxel-containing regimens cost 76 370 Canadian dollars ($C) per life year gained (**LYG**) relative to etoposide and cisplatin. When modelled as an outpatient regimen, paclitaxel cost $C30 619 per LYG.

Goodwin and Shepherd concluded in their review of economic issues in lung cancer that effective treatments in lung cancer also tend to be cost-effective when compared with other commonly used medical interventions.[29] However, they caution that a focus on costs alone, rather than a comparison of costs to benefit, may have led to a different conclusion. The costs of chemotherapy in the treatment of lung cancer is not the major cost in the management of advanced lung cancer; hospitalization is still the major cost in care.

Cancer of the large bowel

The economic evaluations of the control of large bowel cancer cover a range of topics from analyses of screening programmes to the management of different stages of cancer of the rectum and large bowel. The costs of initial care (first 6 months after diagnosis) of patients with large bowel cancer increase with the tumour stage, but costs of care during the last 6 months of life did not vary by stage, comorbidity, age, or sex.[30],[31] The initial diagnostic costs in cases detected by screening programmes was higher than for symptomatic cases in the report of Whynes et al. Although the costs of managing Dukes stage C cases were greater than in earlier stages, there is no support for the belief that treatment costs will be reduced if screening programmes are introduced.

Brown et al. investigated some of the consequences of an increased use of adjuvant chemotherapy in patients with Dukes stage C, large bowel cancer. The gain in expected survival of 1.9 years per treated patient was adjusted by assuming utility weights of 0.8 for time with toxicity and 0.5 for survival time after relapse. The final cost per

Table 5 Comparison of incremental cost-effectiveness

Intervention	Incremental cost-effectiveness $/additional year of life (1994 $US)
Liver transplantation versus medical management	251000
Mammography at 50 years of age or younger	245000
ABMT versus standard chemotherapy for metastastic breast cancer	123000
Dialysis versus supportive care for end-stage renal disease	53000
Mammography aged 50–70 years	37000
Vindesine/cisplatin versus vinorelbine alone for NSCLC	23000
Vinorelbine/cisplatin versus vindesine/cisplatin for NSCLC	16000
Chemotherapy versus best supportive care for NSCLC	4900
CAV + EP versus CAV alone for metastatic SCLC	4900
Smoking cessation counselling	1400

After ref. 27, with permission.

Abbreviations: ABMT, autologous bone-marrow transplantation; CAV, cyclophosphamide, daunorubicin, vincristine; EP, etoposide, cisplatin; NSCLC, non-small-cell lung cancer; SCLC, small-cell lung cancer.

QALY after discounting the cost per life year saved by 6 per cent was $US2260. Recently, some new drugs with activity in colorectal cancer have been marketed, and there are claims of similar activity and comparable or reduced toxicity to fluorouracil, though drug costs are greater.

Supportive care

Antiemetics

Developments in supportive care in the past decade have had a major impact not only on the operating budgets of cancer-treatment units but also on patients' quality of life. From the perspective of the patient, nausea and vomiting have been major side-effects to consider when contemplating palliative cancer chemotherapy.[32] With the introduction of serotonin antagonists, acute vomiting has been better controlled, permitting more outpatient treatment and enhanced treatment compliance and patient well being. The overall effect of serotonin antagonists has been to displace vomiting from its status of the most feared side-effect of cancer chemotherapy.[33] There have been several reports of economic explorations of the costs and benefits of improved emetic control using serotonin antagonists. Jones et al. analysed the impact on the pharmacy budget of different policies for using serotonin antagonists for controlling vomiting after chemotherapy.[34] Increases in the total costs of chemotherapy varied from 3 to 10 per cent if only used for acute emesis (first 24 h after chemotherapy) to 12 to 34 per cent if used for acute and delayed vomiting. The authors argue that with a less than 4 per cent increase in the pharmacy budget, about one-third of all patients on chemotherapy can receive serotonin antagonists, which in their view is well justified by the improvement in vomiting control.

Zbrozek et al. reported an economic evaluation of ondansetron versus metoclopramide in patients treated with high-dose cisplatin.[35] The antiemetic efficacy was taken from a meta-analysis which included randomized trials and case series. Based on reasonable definitions of success and failure, the expected number of emetic episodes was 3 for ondansetron and 2.7 for metoclopramide. For cost-utility calculations it was assumed that the reduction in emesis was worth 5 units on a quality-of-life scale running from 1 to 100 (sustained for 24 h). This gain was translated into 0.00014 QALYs and the incremental cost per QALY was estimated to be $US40 000 per average-sized adult. The appropriateness of QALY to measure antiemetic benefit must be questioned, though additional data on patients' quality of life when receiving antiemetic treatment is clearly required.

Growth factors

The development of bone-marrow and, more recently, other growth factors that ameliorate the duration and severity of cancer chemotherapy effects on the marrow and mucosa has led to the rapid adoption of these agents in cancer treatment. Bone-marrow growth factors have been shown to reduce the duration and severity of neutropenia after cytotoxic treatment and to permit the safe administration of higher treatment doses. There have been several economic assessments of the use of granulocyte colony-stimulating factors (G-CSFs) in the treatment of small-cell lung cancer in patients with fever and neutropenia, three of them using efficacy data from a clinical trial reported by Crawford et al.[36] In this trial, prophylactic administration of G-CSF or placebo was started on day 4 of each chemotherapy cycle, and continued until the neutrophil count rose to more than 1000 cells/μl. Patients whose temperature rose above 38.2 °C when their neutrophil count was less than 1000 cells/μl were admitted to hospital and treated with empirical antibiotics. From the perspective of the payer, the use of G-CSF resulted in a net saving of $US1250 per cycle,[37] while in the cost model, in which true costs were estimated by multiplying each hospital's charges with individual cost-to-charge ratio, the use of G-CSF resulted in an additional cost of $US140 per cycle.

The American Society of Clinical Oncology has published guideline recommendations for the use of G-CSFs.[38] These guidelines refer to a cost-effectiveness study reporting a cost-saving if the anticipated incidence of febrile neutropenia after cancer chemotherapy is more than 40 per cent. Neymark[39] has observed that this unreferenced statement appears to draw on the study of Lyman *et al.*,[40] and he remarks that either of two other studies on the same question for the same group of patients would have led to quite different threshold values in the recommendations.

The use of G-CSFs had added considerably to the pharmacy costs of cancer chemotherapy, and there are differing policies in different countries, and different hospitals. The report of Frampton and Faulds indicates that in different academic health centres in the United States, there were appropriate indications for about 70 per cent of G-CSF use, though the 'correct' dosages as recommended by the manufacturer were used in only 50 per cent of cases.[41]

Economic analysis and evidence-based medicine

Medical practice according to the best evidence based on comprehensive and systematic review of all available data is increasingly being advocated, both to improve quality of care and to reduce costs. Evidence-based treatment guidelines for many cancer situations have been developed and disseminated. As yet, evidence-based guidelines rarely consider costs or efficiency in terms of health outcomes.[42]

However, incorporating an economic evaluation within a clinical trial is becoming more frequent. This allows the relevant data on costs and outcomes to be collected prospectively, at a usually modest cost. Data can be collected in more detail at a patient level, which therefore allows analysis of how costs and outcomes vary together. However, there are also disadvantages. Clinical trials are designed to maximize internal validity, while economic analysis requires external validity or generalizability. The patients who are accepted into the trial are unlikely to be representative of the patients for whom the treatment will eventually be prescribed. Nor are the doctors who participate in trials representative. For the economic analysis, costs and outcomes for a much longer period than that of the trial may be required. The multinational nature of many modern trials can present a problem. Simply converting one currency into another using foreign exchange rates is not adequate. While the use of purchasing price parities allows for the purchasing power of one currency against another, this does not take into account differences in practice. The relevant unit prices will differ from one healthcare setting to another even in the same country, and the costs may vary greatly even if resource use is similar.

The alternative to building an economic analysis into a prospective trial is to use a simulated decision analysis, drawing probabilities from a review of the literature. It is also possible to use a decision analytic approach to extend the results of a particular trial and to model the future course of costs and outcomes.

Systematic reviews of the economic evaluation literature are beset by the problems of pooling data, as discussed above. Neymark concluded that the main advantage of conducting systematic reviews of economic evaluations of particular healthcare interventions is to enhance the likelihood that all the factors of relevance for the transferability of the results are taken into account. A further problem

Table 6 Features of a good economic evaluation

- Terminology should be correct
- Alternatives being compared should be clearly described
- Perspective of the study should be clearly stated, societal perspective is preferred
- All costs and consequences should be included
- Future costs should be discounted
- Impact of uncertainty should be analysed

with comparing results from different economic evaluations is to ensure that the methods used are comparable. Reviews of the literature have shown substantial variation in methods and approach used.[43] This has led some commentators to call for the use of a standardized methodology. There are two reasons why methods should not be completely standardized. Some differences in approach are legitimate differences of analytical viewpoint. Where there are differences in the viewpoint or context of a study, differences in approach may be appropriate. In addition, the methods of data collection and analysis are still developing; and imposing methodological constraints my limit debate and further development. However, there are many examples in the literature of poorly designed and executed studies. As a result, there have been several attempts to develop critical checklists to guide authors and reviewers, such as that produced by the *British Medical Journal*,[44] and the United States Panel on Cost-effectiveness in Health and Medicine.[45] From these and other commentaries, it can be seen that there are several issues on which health economists are agreed and which should be taken as hallmarks of a good-quality study (these are summarized in Table 6).

Conclusions

The number of published economic evaluations has been increasing, reflecting the growing interest of decision-makers throughout health systems. The conceptual and methodological basis of economic evaluation has been in existence for decades. Health-service planners, managers, and clinicians were at first slow to adopt economic evaluation in their decision-making 'tool-kit'. Surveys, such as that by Ross,[46] pointed out that most decision-makers remained unfamiliar with the methods of economic evaluation and felt that economic analysts were too distant from the decision-making context. There are many factors which influence health-policy decisions including political factors, feasibility, existing programmes, and considerations of equity, as well as efficiency. And clinicians have been reluctant to acknowledge that cost and resource implications might play a role in determining treatment.

One of the developments in health-system reform has been the separation of the role of purchasing healthcare on behalf of a population group from that of providing that care. Purchasers have been faced with a fixed and constrained budget; and the need to maximize the benefits obtained from that. They have turned to economic evaluation as a means of helping to determine the 'best buys' for their population. More generally, health bureaucrats have also turned to economic evaluation when faced with the need to determine whether to fund new technologies or new programmes. Some governments have attempted to incorporate such evaluation into their ongoing decision-making.

The role of the clinician is changing. Clinicians now often find themselves as budget holders, responsible for managing resources for a group of patients and charged with determining the best health outcomes. Clinicians are also involved in developing population-based strategies for cancer prevention and control, again working with fixed budgets and having to assess the competing demands for limited resources. Whenever clinicians face real opportunity-costs, then a working knowledge of economics will be useful.

References

1. **Anderson GF, Poullier JP.** Health spending, access, and outcomes: trends in industrialized countries. *Health Affairs*, 1999; **18**(3): 178–92.

2. **Hall J, Viney R.** The political economy of health sector reform. In *Health reform in Australia and New Zealand* (ed. A Bloom). Melbourne: Oxford University Press, 2000.

3. **Mankiw NG.** *Principles of economics.* Orlando, FL: Dryden Press, 1998.

4. **Williams A, Giadina E.** *Efficiency in the public sector: the theory and practice of cost-benefit analysis.* Aldershot, UK: Edward Elgar, 1993.

5. **Drummond MF, O'Brien B, Stoddart GL, Torrance GW.** *Methods for the economic evaluation of health care programmes* (2nd edn). Oxford: Oxford University Press, 1997.

6. **Gold MR Siegal JE, Russell LB, Weinstein MC.** (ed.). *Cost-effectiveness in health and medicine.* New York: Oxford University Press, 1996.

7. **Sloan F.** (ed.). *Valuing health care.* New York: Cambridge University Press, 1995.

8. **Drummond MF, O'Brien B, Stoddart GL, Torrance GW.** *Methods for the economic evaluation of health care programmes* (2nd edn). Oxford: Oxford University Press, 1997.

9. **Mehrez A, Gafni A.** Quality-adjusted life-years, utility theory and healthy years equivalents. *Medical Decision Making*, 1989; **9**: 142–9.

10. **Udvarhelyi S, Cloditz GA, Rai A, Epstein AM.** Cost-effectiveness and cost-benefit analyses in the medical literature. Are methods being used correctly? *Annals of Internal Medicine*, 1992; **116**: 238–44.

11. **Murray CJ, Lopez AD.** *The global burden of disease: a comprehensive assessment of mortality and disability from diseases, injuries, and risk factors in 1990 and predicted to 2020.* Harvard, MA: Harvard University Press, 1996. [Published by the Harvard School of Public Health on behalf of the World Health Organisation and the World Bank.]

12. **Williams A.** Calculating the global burden of disease: time for a strategic reappraisal? *Health Economics*, 1999; **8**(1): 1–8.

13. **Goldhirsch A, Gelber RD, Simes RJ, Glasziou P, Coates AS.** Costs and benefits of adjuvant therapy in breast cancer: a quality-adjusted survival analysis. *Journal of Clinical Oncology*, 1989; **7**: 36–44.

14. **Ware JE, Sherbourne CD.** The MOS 36 item short form health survey SF-36. Conceptual framework and item selection. *Medical Care*, 1992; **30**(6): 473–83.

15. **EuroQol Group.** EuroQol—a new facility for the measurement of health-related quality of life. *Health Policy*, 1990; **16**(3): 199–208.

16. **Walker QJ, et al.** The management of oesophageal carcinoma: radiotherapy or surgery? Cost considerations. *European Journal of Cancer and Clinical Oncology*, 1989; **25**(11): 1657–62.

17. **Hillner B.** Financial costs, benefits and patient preferences in node negative breast cancer: insights from a decision analysis model. In *Recent results in cancer research*, Vol. 127 (ed. Senn H-J, Gelber RD, Goldhirsch A, Thurlimann B.) Berlin: Springer Verlag, 1993; **127**: 277–84.

18. **Smith T, Hillner B.** The efficacy and cost-effectiveness of adjuvant therapy of early breast cancer in premenopausal women. *Journal of Clinical Oncology*, 1993; **11**: 771–6.

19. **Richards M, et al.** Advanced breast cancer: use of resources and cost implications. *British Journal of Cancer*, 1993; **67**: 856–60.

20. **Hurley S, et al.** The costs of breast cancer recurrence. *British Journal of Cancer*, 1992; **65**: 449–55.

21. **Launois R, et al.** A cost utility analysis of second line chemotherapy in metastatic breast cancer. Docetaxel versus paclitaxel versus vinorelbine. *Pharmacoeconomics*, 1996; **10**: 504–21.

22. **Rosenthal M, et al.** The cost of treating small cell lung cancer. *Medical Journal of Australia*, 1992; **156**: 605–10.

23. **Evans WK, et al.** Estimating the cost of lung cancer diagnosis and treatment in Canada. *Canadian Journal of Oncology*, 1995; **5**: 408–19.

24. **Evans WK, et al.** The economics of lung cancer management in Canada. *Lung Cancer*, 1996; **14**: 19–29.

25. **Richardson GE, et al.** Application of an algorithm for staging small cell lung cancer can save one third of the initial evaluation costs. *Archives of Internal Medicine*, 1993; **153**: 329–37.

26. **Hillner BE, Smith TJ.** Cost effectiveness analysis of three regimens using vinorelbine for nonsmall cell lung cancer. *Seminars in Oncology*, 1996; **23**: 25–30.

27. **Smith TJ, Hillner BE, Desch CE.** Efficacy and cost effectiveness in oncology: Rational allocation of cancer care resources. *Journal of the National Cancer Institute*, 1993; **85**: 1460–74.

28. **Earle CC, Evans WK.** Cost-effectiveness of paclitaxel plus cisplatin in advanced non-small-cell lung cancer. *British Journal of Cancer*, 1999; **80**: 815–20.

29. **Goodwin PJ, Shepherd FA.** Economic issues in lung cancer: a review. *Journal of Clinical Oncology*, 1998; **16**: 3900–12.

30. **Taplin S, et al.** Stage, age, comorbidity and direct costs of colon, prostate and breast cancer care. *Journal of the National Cancer Institute*, 1995; **87**: 417–26.

31. **Whynes D, et al.** Screening and the costs of colorectal cancer. *British Journal of Cancer*, 1993; **68**: 965–8.

32. **Coates AS, et al.** On the receiving end—patient perception of the side effects of cancer chemotherapy. *European Journal of Cancer and Clinical Oncology*, 1983; **19**: 203–8.

33. **Griffin A-M, et al.** On the receiving end. V: Patient perceptions of the side effects of cancer chemotherapy in 1993. *Annals of Oncology*, 1996; **7**: 189–95.

34. **Jones A, Lee G, Bosanquet N.** The budgetary impact of 5-HT3 receptors in the management of chemotherapy-induced emesis. *European Journal of Cancer*, 1992; **29A**: 51–6.

35. **Zbrozek A, et al.** Pharmacoeconomic analysis of ondansetron versus metaclopramide for cisplatin induced nausea and vomiting. *American Journal of Hospital Pharmacy*, 1994; **51**: 1555–63.

36. **Crawford J, et al.** Reduction by granulocyte colony stimulating factor of fever and neutropenia induced by chemotherapy in patients with small-cell lung cancer. *New England Journal of Medicine*, 1991; **325**: 164–70.

37. **Glaspy J, et al.** The impact of therapy with filgastrim on the health care cost associated with chemotherapy. *European Journal of Cancer*, 1993; **29A**(Suppl. 7): S23–S30.

38. **American Society of Clinical Oncology.** Update of recommendations for the use of hematopoietic colony stimulating factors: evidence-based clinical practice guidelines. *Journal of Clinical Oncology*, 1996; **14**: 1957-60.

39. **Neymark N.** *Assessing the economic value of anticancer therapies. Recent results in cancer research.* Berlin: Springer Verlag, 1998; **148**: 1–285.

40. **Lyman G, et al.** Decision analysis of hematopoietic growth factors in patients receiving cancer chemotherapy. *Journal of the National Cancer Institute*, 1993; **85**: 488–93.

41. **Frampton J, Faulds D.** Filgastrim—a reappraisal of pharmacoeconomic

considerations in the prophylaxis and treatment of chemotherapy induced neutropenia. *Pharmacoeconomics*, 1996; **9**: 76–96.

42. **Maynard A.** Evidence based medicine: an incomplete method for informing treatment choices. *Lancet*, 1997; **349**: 126–8.

43. **Drummond M, Brandt A, Luce B, Rovira J.** Standardizing methodologies for economic evaluation in health care: practice, problems and potential. *International Journal of Technology Assessment in Health Care*, 1993; **9**(1): 26–36.

44. **Drummond MF, Jefferson TO, on behalf of the BMJ Economic Evaluation Working Party.** Guidelines for authors and peer reviewers of economic submissions to the BMJ. *British Medical Journal*, 1996; **313**: 275–83.

45. **Weinstein MC, Siegel JE, Gold MR, Kamlet MS, Russell LB.** Recommendations of the panel on cost-effectiveness in health and medicine. *Journal of the American Medical Association*, 1996; **276**(15): 1253–8.

46. **Ross J.** The use of economics evaluation in health care: Australian decision makers' perceptions. *Health Policy*, 1995; **31**(2): 103–10.

8

Melanoma and skin cancer

8.1 Cutaneous malignant melanoma

Alexander M. M. Eggermont, Philippe Autier, and Ulrich Keilholz

Introduction

The invasive cutaneous malignant melanoma (referred to as 'melanoma' in this chapter) arises from the epidermal melanocyte. During embryogenesis, melanocytes migrate from the neural crest to the skin. After birth, melanocytes produce the melanin. Knowledge about the genetic and biochemical defects that transform the melanocyte into an often aggressive and fatal tumour has considerably increased over the last 10 years.

With incidence rates doubling every 10 to 15 years over the past 40 to 50 years, melanoma is an important health problem for countries with populations of European (Caucasian) origin. Except for lung cancer in women, no other tumour incidence rate has been on a steeper rise. One worrying aspect about this trend is the relative youth of the adult population involved. The median age of patients treated for this condition is in the region of 50 years. In the United States, the lifetime risk of developing melanoma has more than doubled in the past 20 years and reached 1 in 75 in 2000. In some regions of Australia and New Zealand, it is already as high as 1 in 30. As the sharp increase in 'suntanning behaviour' over the last three decades is most probably the main cause for the current 'melanoma epidemic', primary and secondary prevention programmes need to be put in place to curb the present trends.

The prognosis for the majority of patients with melanoma is directly related to the depth of invasion of the primary lesion at the time of diagnosis and treatment. A simple excision is curative in its early stage. However, no currently available treatment reliably affects the course of disease once a melanoma metastasizes. Awareness needs to be promoted of the classic clinical signs associated with melanoma (change in colour, recent enlargement, nodularity, pruritus, ulceration or bleeding), and also of the more subtle clinical characteristics (such as irregular or angular borders or variations in colour) as these latter characteristics often signal minimally invasive, early, and curable melanomas.

Epidemiology and aetiology

Incidence and mortality

Incidence

Before 1950, melanoma was a rare tumour. In the second half of the twentieth century, it became one of the fastest growing cancers in incidence, with a doubling in the number of melanoma cases every 15 to 20 years in fair-skinned populations of Australia, North America, and Western Europe. At the end of the twentieth century, melanoma represented between 3 and 5 per cent of all cancers occurring in White populations of Western Europe and North America, and 8 to 13 per cent of cancers occurring in Australian White populations.

If melanoma is rare in the under 20-year age group, it does occur earlier in life than other common solid tumours. The median age at diagnosis is 50 to 55 years, which makes it one of the most frequent malignancies diagnosed in White subjects between the ages of 20 and 50 years. In some areas, melanoma seems more frequent in men than women (Queensland State in Australia, United States), while the reverse is observed in other areas (Victoria State of Australia, Canada, Norway, France). More refined examination of the data show that, globally, before 60 years of age, melanoma is somewhat more frequent among women, being equivalent in older people.

At the end of the twentieth century, the melanoma incidence rates were still rising in all countries (Fig. 1). The highest incidence and mortality rates are reported in Queensland, Australia, a tropical area where subjects of European Celtic ancestry migrated. Incidence rates are lower in Victoria, a more Southern State of Australia with a population of similar origin, indicating that the incidence of melanoma parallels the year-round intensity of solar irradiation. In contrast, the reverse situation is observed in Europe, with higher incidence rates observed in Scandinavian countries (like Norway) than in France. In Mediterranean countries, incidence rates are lower than in France, but the rising trend in incidence is also present in those populations.

A closer look at incidence data suggests that, the yearly increase in melanoma incidence is less manifest in some countries than it was during the 1970s or 1098s (for example, in Canada and Norway, and women in the United States). A Scottish report described a stabilization in melanoma incidence among women under than 65-years old.[5] However, the shape of the incidence curves indicates that the epidemic is unlikely to stabilize soon in most fair-skinned populations, since many melanomas occur in older people who were not well informed about the harmful effects of excessive sun-exposure when they were young.

The increase in melanoma incidence is not confined to fair-skinned populations. In Japan, although mortality from melanoma is lower in absolute terms than in most fair-skinned populations, increasing trends in mortality are present.[6]

Melanoma is rare among black people (less than 0.5 cases of melanoma per 100 000 per year in the United States), occurring almost exclusively as acral melanoma of the hands and feet. There is no evidence of a changing melanoma incidence in black populations.

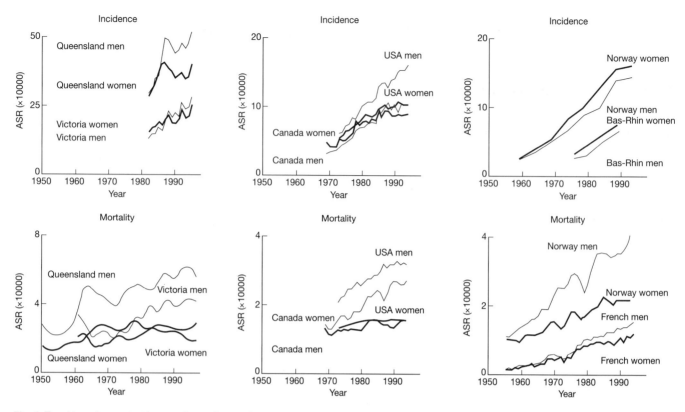

Fig. 1 Trend in melanoma incidence and mortality in selected countries (data sources: World Health Organization Cancer Mortality Data Bank; Refs 1–4). Mortality data were available for a longer period than incidence data. ASR is the age-standardized rate per 100 000 persons per year. Note the differences in ASR scales between countries.

Mortality

After 1950, sharp increases in the number of deaths due to melanoma were observed in most fair-skinned populations (Fig. 1).[6],[7] However, increases in melanoma mortality have never been as great as for its incidence; a slowing down of melanoma mortality was observed in several countries after 1985. More specifically, in Australia, the United States, Canada, Scandinavian countries, and Scotland, melanoma mortality rates seem to have stabilized or started to fall in women of all ages,[5],[8]–[10] while deaths due to melanoma are still increasing in men. A feature common to these countries is the stabilization (and sometimes the reduction) of mortality rates in more recent generations (mainly in women born after 1940), indicating that most deaths from melanoma observed after 1990 tends to be of older subjects, mainly in men 60-years old or more.

In Southern and Central Europe, melanoma mortality rates resemble the situation prevailing in France (Fig. 1), where steep, almost linear, increases are still present for both men and women.[7],[11] Trends in mortality rates in the United Kingdom and The Netherlands present features in between those of Scandinavian countries and France. The different patterns in melanoma mortality trends could result from the time differences in the instigation of sun-protection promotion and the surveillance of pigmented skin lesions between countries.

The lower increase in the mortality rate relative to that of incidence is principally due to the improved survival of patients with melanoma.

Increased survival does not seem to be attributable to better disease management, but more to other factors. First, the proportion of melanomas diagnosed when they are thin (Breslow thickness < 1.5 mm) has steadily increased, principally in young females.[12] It should not be overlooked, however, that, generally speaking, the absolute numbers of thick melanomas (Breslow thickness ≥ 3 mm) has remained unchanged over the last two decades. Because thick melanomas are usually more frequent in people 60-years old or more (mainly men), mortality from that disease is still on the rise in this segment of White populations.

Second, the increase in incidence has been more manifest for superficial spreading melanoma (SSM) than for nodular melanoma (NM)—SSM has a better prognosis than NM. Third, changes have probably occurred in the disease itself with the appearance of less aggressive forms of melanoma,[13]–[15] but this hypothesis needs further research.

The more pronounced decrease in mortality in women could be due to two factors. First, irrespective of the stage at detection, melanoma has a worse prognosis in men than in women.[16] In men, the increase in melanoma incidence has been more marked for the trunk and for the head and neck; moreover, SSM or NM melanomas detected in these sites have a poorer prognosis than melanomas detected elsewhere. In women, the increase in melanoma incidence has been greater for the legs, where melanomas have a better prognosis and are easier to detect by self-examination. Second, women seem more receptive to prevention messages than men, and thus women consult earlier when they observe a suspicious pigmented skin lesion.[17]

Patient characteristics associated with melanoma

Occupational and socioeconomic status

There is a strong positive relationship between melanoma incidence and increasing socioeconomic status. Melanoma is less frequent among occupational groups whose work is mainly outdoors.

Individual history of melanoma

Between 3 and 7 per cent of patients with a primary melanoma will develop a second primary melanoma that will usually appear within 5 years from the first. Multiple melanomas in the same patient are not uncommon in hereditary forms of the disease.[18] Second or third primary melanomas are always much thinner than the first primary melanoma, probably because of the continuing surveillance of these patients.

Common and atypical naevi

Naevi (moles) result from a clonal expansion of melanocytes. The number of naevi is the strongest predictor that an individual (without prior melanoma) may develop a melanoma. Adults with more than 100 naevi, with one dimension equal to or greater than 2 mm, have an increased melanoma risk of 15 or more.

Naevi are rare at birth, but their number increases steeply during childhood and adolescence, reaching a peak in early adulthood. After 25 years of age, the number of naevi steadily decreases, and after 50 years old that number is less than half it was 30 years before.

Atypical naevi (also known as dysplastic naevi) are large naevi with irregular borders and varied pigmentation. There is a strong positive correlation between the presence of atypical naevi (AN) and a large number of common naevi. The presence of multiple AN in with or without other signs (such as more than 100 naevi > 2 mm, naevi in the anterior scalp, pigmented lesion in the iris), has been termed the dysplastic naevus syndrome (DNS) phenotype, or the atypical mole syndrome (AMS) phenotype.[19],[20] The AMS phenotype is often present in subjects belonging to families with multiple cases of melanoma (see below), but it is also encountered outside the context of familial melanoma.

In the past, histological examination of clinically suspicious naevi was regarded as providing the best evidence for the presence of atypia. But histology requires biopsies, and interobserver agreement for the recognition of atypical naevi remains unsatisfactory. Therefore, recognition of the AN and AMS phenotype is now based on clinical criteria. However, controversies persist with regard to the characterization of the AN and AMS phenotype. Despite disparities in the definitions used, studies consistently show that subjects presenting with a single AN already have a two- to threefold increased risk of developing melanoma. Subjects with several AN, or with an overt AMS phenotype, have their melanoma risk increased by a factor 10 or more.[21]–[23] The risk of melanoma associated with the number of AN or with the AMS phenotype seems to be independent of the total number of common naevi.

Histological and longitudinal studies with pictures of patients, indicate that 40 to 80 per cent of melanomas do not develop from pre-existing naevi. Furthermore, there is only a weak correlation between the number of common naevi, or of AN, on a given body site and the diagnosis of a melanoma on that site. These observations suggest that naevi and AN would be rather markers of both genetic background and exposure to UV-light, than precursor lesions of melanoma.

Natural sensitivity to sunlight (skin phototype)

Pigmentary traits such as red-blond hair, blue eyes, and a light skin complexion are all associated with a greater susceptibility to sunlight and higher melanoma risk. Subjects who tan poorly and sunburn at mid-day on a sunny Spring day are at a higher risk for melanoma. Natural reaction to sunlight can be classified according to skin type,[24] from: 'always burn, never tan' (skin type I) to 'always tan, never burn' (skin type IV). Skin type V comprises Asian people and those with brown skins, and skin type VI comprises people with black skins.

A propensity to develop freckles when in the sun is another marker of natural sun sensitivity, which is associated with melanoma independently from the naevi–melanoma association.

The Celtic type

The 'Celtic type' is a term often used to describe fair-skinned subjects who have a high sensitivity to sunlight. Celtic type subjects have red-blond hair and a pale skin. These subjects have a high propensity to sunburn, tan poorly, and frequently develop freckles. Many Europeans who migrated to Australia were of Celtic type, partly elucidating why melanoma became such a frequent disease among White Australians.

Hereditary factors

About 10 per cent of patients with melanoma have a family history of the disease. Melanoma occurring in two or more family members suggests an aggregation of melanoma possibly related to genetic factors. In some families with multiple cases of melanoma, patients with melanoma as well as their relatives were found to harbour atypical naevi. The family aggregation of melanoma and of subjects with AN has been described as the familial atypical multiple mole and melanoma (FAMMM), or the dysplastic naevus syndrome (DNS), and, more recently, the atypical mole syndrome (AMS). The AMS phenotype is found with a higher frequency in these families than in the general population.

In melanoma-prone families, onset of the first melanoma occurs about 10 years earlier than in sporadic patients with melanoma. Melanoma-prone family members with AN have a nearly 50 per cent chance of developing a melanoma by the time they are 50 years of age.[25] However, these subjects do not seem to have a higher risk of developing other types of cancer. In contrast, those without AN but who belong to melanoma-prone families seem to have a melanoma risk equivalent to subjects without a family history of melanoma.[26]

CDKN2

In those melanoma-prone families with a high frequency of AN, investigations have identified the CDKN2 gene (also known as the MTS1 or p16INK-4A gene) as possibly being involved in the hereditary forms of melanoma.[27] CDKN2A is a tumour-suppressor gene located on chromosome 9p21, which encodes for the p16 protein. The p16 protein inhibits the cyclin-dependent kinases CDK4 and CDK6 involved in cell-cycle regulation. Since 1993, a search for *CDKN2A* alterations in patients with melanoma has been performed in many communities worldwide. Germline mutations of *CDKN2A* have been found in 10 to 30 per cent of families with a predisposition to melanoma, and in 15 per cent of patients with multiple primary melanomas.[18] Specific *CDKN2A* mutations are associated with a higher probability of developing a pancreatic cancer, while other mutations are not.[28] Inactivation (by deletion or mutation) of the *CDKN2A* gene is described in 10 to 30 per cent cases of sporadic melanoma. Germline mutation of the *CDK4* gene (rendering it resistant to control by p16) has also been described in two American and one French families.[29],[30]

However, the relationships between *CDKN2A* alterations, the AMS phenotype, and melanoma occurrence remain far from understood. Transcription of the *CDKN2A* gene is complex as it encodes for two different proteins (p16 and p19ARF). Germline *CDKN2A* mutations have been found in only 8 per cent of Swedish melanoma-prone families,[31] and in only 0.2 per cent of all melanoma cases diagnosed in Queensland, Australia, the world area with the highest melanoma incidence.[32]

Subjects with multiple AN or with the AMS phenotype seem to be deficient in their ability to repair DNA damage induced by UV-light or X-rays, particularly if they belong to melanoma-prone families.[33],[34] However, if AMS subjects are found more frequently in families with germline *CDKN2A* mutations, no particular link seems to exist between the AMS phenotype and alteration of the *CDKN2A* gene.[35] This absence of a link suggests that acquisition of the AMS phenotype could reflect the biological steps in melanoma genesis occurring earlier than the inactivation of the p16 protein. It could also reflect the presence of other alterations in the vicinity of the coding sequences of the *CDKN2A* gene, which could be associated with both the AMS phenotype and the lower ability to repair radiation-induced DNA damage. Hence, new investigations are exploring the possibility that another gene located on the 9p21 chromosome could be involved in familial and sporadic melanoma.[36]

A test for detecting mutations in the *CDKN2A* gene is commercially available. The utility of the test is, however, questionable, as it does not screen out all possible alterations implicated in inherited melanoma. For instance, a number of melanoma-prone families have a clear-cut linkage with the 9p21 locus, but do not carry detectable *CDKN2A* mutations. Thus, a negative test may be falsely reassuring. If a test turns out to be positive, it does not predict whether the subject carrying the mutation will actually develop a melanoma (unknown gene penetrance). Furthermore, knowledge of proneness to melanoma on the basis of a documented family history is itself sufficient to warrant genetic counselling; therefore, with our present state of knowledge, testing for some *CDKN2A* gene mutations is unlikely to affect the management of such family members.

Melanoma and other diseases

Xeroderma pigmentosum (XP) is a rare, recessive hereditary disease characterized by defects in the ability to repair UV-induced DNA damage. The risk of skin cancer (including non-melanoma skin cancers and melanoma) is increased by about 1000 in patients with XP. The higher incidence of melanoma in these patients supports an important role for DNA damage in the pathogenesis of melanoma. An alteration or suboptimal functioning of genes encoding for DNA repair could increase the occurrence of melanoma. However, some syndromes associated with defective DNA repair do not lead to an increased melanoma risk.

Immune processes are thought to play a key role in melanoma development. Evidence that immunosuppressed patients have more naevi[37] suggests that melanoma could be more frequent in immunocompromised subjects. However, to date, no report has documented an increased melanoma incidence in immunocompromised patients.

Subjects with a previous non-melanoma skin cancer (squamous-cell or basal-cell skin cancer) and those presenting with numerous solar keratoses have a higher incidence of melanoma. Since non-melanoma skin cancer and keratoses generally occur among older subjects, surveillance for head and neck melanoma is particularly relevant in these subjects.

Environmental causes of melanoma

Exposure to sunlight

The epidemic of melanoma observed in most fair-skinned populations over the last 50 years cannot be explained by genetic changes. The worldwide increase in the incidence and mortality of melanoma among fair-skinned populations is regarded as being the consequence of increasing sun-exposure in people sensitive to the harmful effects of sunlight.[38] However, it has not yet been possible to reproduce human melanoma in animal models using only UV irradiation. It is thus essential to note that all the available evidence supporting a sun–melanoma association is based on epidemiological data. If epidemiological studies over the last 10 years have provided a more consistent picture of the sun–melanoma association, they also show the complexity of this association. Moreover, some observations seem to contradict the hypothesis of increased sun-exposure as a cause for the melanoma epidemic. First, melanoma is very rare on the hands, a usually sun-exposed site. Second, melanoma is found more frequently among indoor than among outdoor workers—the former typically spend only a few weeks per year in sunny areas (usually during holidays), while the latter may accumulate large amounts of sun-exposure over their lifetime. Furthermore, subjects with high occupational sun-exposure (for instance, farmers, construction workers) were sometimes found to be at lower risk for melanoma. Third, in Europe, melanoma incidence is highest in Scandinavian countries, and lowest in Mediterranean countries. Fourth, in the early epidemiological investigations, no clear relationship emerged between total lifetime sun-exposure and melanoma occurrence.

The first evidence that sunlight could be implicated in the development of melanoma came from studies of migrants into highly sunny areas.[39] These studies described a lower melanoma risk in subjects born in less sunny areas. In the early 1980s, following the finding that sunburn were associated with melanoma occurrence,[40],[41] the concept of 'intermittent sun-exposure was forged.[42] Intermittent sun-exposure refers to those sun-exposures typical of indoor workers taking holidays in sunny areas, eager to acquire a tanned skin through sunbathing, or to have their children playing almost naked on the beach. In these circumstances, skin areas usually covered by clothes are brutally sun exposed—

particularly when such exposure takes place around midday when solar UV irradiation reaches its peak value.

More than 30 epidemiological studies support the hypothesis that it is the repetition of intermittent sun-exposure, and not lifetime chronic sun-exposure, which is the main environmental factor implicated in melanoma occurrence.[43] Intermittent sun-exposure would be more efficient in triggering melanoma because such individuals are naturally sun-sensitive and attracted by holidays in more southern sunny areas. This would explain why, in Europe, the incidence of melanoma is highest in Nordic populations.[44] Also, wealthier people are more likely to be able to afford longer holidays in southern sunny areas, which would explain the positive correlation between melanoma and higher socioeconomic status.

The intermittent sun-exposure hypothesis is mainly relevant for melanoma occurring on those body sites usually covered by clothes, such as the trunk and shoulders, and, to some extent, the legs in women. The sharpest increase in melanoma incidence is observed on these body sites in all fair-skinned populations, and it parallels the dramatic expansion of recreational sun-exposure that took place after the second World War. However, a number of observations (listed below), suggest that intermittent sun-exposure would be less important for melanoma arising on body sites usually sun-exposed, and that the susceptibility of melanocytes (or of factors in their immediate vicinity—for example, surrounding keratinocytes, the local immune response) to sunlight would differ according to body site:

1. The incidence of melanoma of the trunk reaches its maximum around 40 to 50 years of age, and tends to stabilize and decrease after 70 years, while the incidence of head and neck melanoma steadily increases with age, being highest after 60 years of age.[45] As a matter of fact, recreational sun-exposure is highly prevalent among the younger age groups, while ageing is a surrogate for lifetime chronic sun-exposure of the head and neck.

2. A stronger association exists between the number of solar keratoses on the forearm (an indicator of chronic lifetime sun-exposure) and head and neck melanoma than with melanoma of the trunk.[46]

3. Trunk melanoma more frequently originates from pre-existing naevi than does head and neck melanoma.[47]

Anatomical differences in susceptibility to UV-light could also explain why melanoma is rare on usually sun-exposed sites such as the hands.

The few available data on risk factors for acral melanoma of the soles and palms indicate that these melanomas have similar risk factors as other melanoma. But in addition, they are associated with a history of a penetrating injury, exposure to agrochemicals, and the presence of naevi on the toes and soles of the feet.[48]

Childhood is a critical time for the onset of melanoma, as shown by studies in migrants[39] and in White subjects who spent part of their life in sunny climates.[49] A closer look at the respective impact of sun-exposure both during childhood and adulthood (Fig. 2) indicates that, regardless of levels of sun-exposure in adults, melanoma development seems difficult in the absence of significant sun-exposure during childhood. Hence, it is probable that childhood is a period of greater vulnerability to some sun-induced biological alterations essential for the occurrence of melanoma in adult life. Thus, restricting a child's exposure to the sun could represent the most efficient way of reducing the incidence of melanoma. It is likely that the stabilization

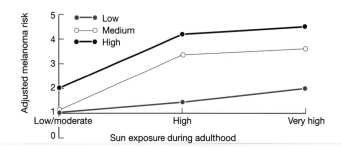

Fig. 2 Joint effect on melanoma risk of amounts of sun-exposure during childhood and during adulthood. Melanoma risk is adjusted for age, sex, skin type, and hair colour. (Figure was drawn from data in ref. 13, with permission of the publisher; for clarity, 95 per cent confidence limits are not displayed in the figure.)

in melanoma incidence observed in younger people in some countries (for example, in Australia and Scotland) could partly be due to the adoption of more prudent sun habits in recent generations. Finally, it can be speculated that the importance of sun-exposure has been underestimated because of the difficulty in accurately exploring the sun-exposure habits of adults before they were 20 years of age.

The data in Fig. 2 can also shed light on the common observation that the melanoma risk is reduced in subjects who have a long history of occupational sun-exposure.[43] Outdoor workers are generally of lower socioeconomic status, and those with a long history of occupational sun-exposure are likely to be old. It is therefore not improbable that when they were a child or adolescent (that is to say, pre-1940 in most studies examining this question), outdoor workers with high chronic sun-exposure had fewer opportunities to enjoy holidays in sunnier climates. As a consequence, relative to patients with melanoma known to be of higher socioeconomic status, people with high occupational sun-exposure could appear as being at a lower risk for developing melanoma, but this impression would be largely artefactual.

Laboratory studies suggest that it is the UV component of the solar spectrum that is capable of triggering melanoma in humans. UV radiation reaching the Earth's surface comprises UVB (280–315 nm) and UVA (315–340 nm). The UV wavelength(s) involved in melanoma occurrence, and the way in which these wavelengths would have the greatest efficiency for triggering melanoma, are still unknown.

Ultraviolet radiation exposures other than the sun

Fluorescent lamps

Fluorescent lighting contains a small proportion of UV radiation. These small amounts could represent a theoretical hazard as fluorescent lighting is in widespread use. However, epidemiological studies have not produced data consistent with such an effect.[38]

Sunlamps or sunbed use

Indoor tanning has become a significant source of exposure to UV radiation since the 1980s; between 10 and 50 per cent of adolescents in North America and Europe report having used these devices, sometimes for a considerable number of hours. The term 'UVA-tanning' is improper as most tanning devices emit 2 to 5 per cent of their UV spectrum in the UVB wavelength: this UVB fraction is known to cause the majority of the DNA damage associated with sunbed use.[50]

Epidemiological studies up to 1993, which specifically examined the association between melanoma and indoor tanning, failed to demonstrate an increased risk of melanoma due to indoor tanning, but new data are awaited to resolve this issue.[51] However, the association between sunbed use and melanoma displays several key features: the existence of a dose–effect relationship; stronger associations with sunbed exposures that took place years before a diagnosis of melanoma; and the highest risk of melanoma in people who experienced skin burns caused by the UV lamps. These results are consistent with the hypothesis of a delayed impact of sunbed use on melanoma incidence—due to the latency period of several decades between exposure to a carcinogen and the occurrence of cancer. With available data, it is impossible to establish a limit below which indoor tanning would not lead to an increased risk of melanoma.

An increased melanoma risk has been observed in patients suffering from severe psoriasis treated with a combination of UVA and psoralens (namely, PUVA therapy).[52] It is, however, impossible to ascertain which treatment component was implicated in the higher melanoma risk, since psoralens are potent photocarcinogens and these patients received a variety of other potentially carcinogenic treatments (for example, coal tar).

In any case, data about the potential harmful effects of indoor tanning continue to accumulate, and sunbed use should be discouraged.

Gene–gene and gene–environment interactions

Pigmentary traits, skin phototype, propensity to develop freckles when in the sun, naevi number, and the presence of atypical naevi seem to have independent, and synergistic, effects on melanoma risk. These observations support the hypothesis that pigmentary traits, skin type, naevi number, and the presence of AN could be phenotypic makers of yet largely unknown genetic lesion(s) or polymorphisms governing an individual's predisposition to melanoma. Interactions between these phenotypic traits would reflect gene–gene interactions. UV-light is capable of causing a large variety of cell damage, and of disturbing local and systemic immune responses. Consequently, an individual's propensity for developing melanoma would be critically linked to an inherited ability to resist and/or repair the diverse alterations caused by UV-light. The ability to resist and/or to repair would probably diminish with accumulation of host characteristics associated with an increased melanoma risk.

Interactions also seem to exist between phenotypic traits and sun-exposure, as similar sun-exposure may have a dramatic impact on the melanoma risk of a Celtic-type individual, but almost none in an individual with a dark complexion who tans easily. Naevi, AN, AMS phenotype, and melanoma have common epidemiological characteristics, such as increased frequency with increasing sun-exposure or with increasing natural susceptibility to sunlight.[53],[54] Hence, if naevi number or acquisition of the AMS phenotype are known to have a strong genetic determinism,[19],[55] levels of sun-exposure will influence the expression of these genetic factors.[56]–[58] Hence, associations between naevi number, presence of AN, and melanoma may exist outside the context of a familial aggregation of melanoma. Conversely, a familial aggregation of melanoma may exist without evidence of high numbers of naevi or of AN in family members.

Some studies have looked at relationships between naevi numbers, melanoma occurrence, and some genetic characteristics, finding, for instance, that sun-exposure could increase the melanoma incidence among families carrying CDKN2 mutations,[59] or that the inter-individual variability in naevi number is better explained by genetic factors than by variable levels of sun-exposure.[55] These studies, however, tell little, if anything, about the kind and magnitude of interactions possibly existing between genes and sun-exposure. However, investigations on gene–gene and gene–environment interactions in melanoma are still in their preliminary stages.

Primary prevention of melanoma

There is some evidence from epidemiological studies that sun protection, particularly wearing clothes when in the sun, decreases the risk of melanoma.[53],[60] This is particularly true for sun protection during childhood.

The role of sunscreens in melanoma prevention is controversial. Data from retrospective and prospective studies on naevi development and melanoma in both children and adults not only showed no protective effect associated with sunscreen use, but suggested an increased melanoma risk associated with increasing sunscreen use, not explainable by a higher sun sensitivity of sunscreen users.[53],[61],[62] Since modern sunscreens are known to be safe products tested for a wide range of potential phototoxic effects,[63] a direct carcinogenic effect of sunscreens was unlikely to explain the sunscreen–naevi or sunscreen–melanoma associations.

A double-blind, randomized trial of young healthy volunteers demonstrated that use of a potent sunscreen induced recreational sun-exposures of longer duration, and encouraged sun-exposure during hours of peak UV irradiation.[64] With the increased usage of sunscreens, people sunbathe for longer, without burning, and ultimately are at higher risk of developing a melanoma. The longer sun-exposure allowed by sunscreen use is an unconscious phenomenon. Although these findings do not suggest that people should not use sunscreens, consumers should be warned that sunscreen use may unconsciously increase their exposure to the sun, and thus, probably, their melanoma risk.

Melanoma prevention advice should put the emphasis on reducing the time spent in the sun and on wearing sun-protective clothing.

Early detection of melanoma

Melanoma is a visible skin lesion so that a skin examination does not require invasive procedures. Moreover, removal of melanoma at an early stage (namely, a Brewslow thickness of about 0.75 mm) cures the disease. Therefore, melanoma is a potentially eradicable disease. Despite this apparent simplicity, the best strategy for detecting melanomas when they are at an early curable stage is still debated.

One population-based, case-control study in the United States showed some evidence that skin self-examination may reduce the incidence of advanced stages of melanoma, and thus probably also, of melanoma mortality.[65] These results are in agreement with the observation of decreasing melanoma thickness over time in many communities, which, to a large extent, seems attributable to increasing melanoma awareness and spontaneous skin surveillance (by individuals and/or by their doctor).

A consequence of increasing thinner lesions is that although melanoma incidence is still rising in most fair-skinned populations,

Table 1 Regular skin examinations are recommended to subjects who have the following characteristics associated with an increased risk for the development of melanoma

- AMS phenotype (with or without evidence for hereditary disease)

- High naevi number, i.e. 100 naevi having one dimension greater or equal to 2 mm

- Presence of one atypical naevus

- Belonging to a family with an aggregation of melanoma cases

- History of non-melanoma skin cancer

- Extensive skin damage due to exposure to ultraviolet light (e.g. solar keratoses)

- Immunocompromised patients, regardless of the underlying cause of immune depression

- Psoriasitic patients treated with PUVA therapy (oral psoralen combined with ultraviolet A irradiation)

- Subjects who used sunscreens or suntan lotions prepared with the 5-methoxypsoralen, a tanning activator, but also a known photocarcinogen[66]

- History of disease known to be, or deemed to be, associated with higher risk of melanoma (e.g. xeroderma pigmentosum, chronic lymphocytic leukaemia)

the clinical appearance of the disease has changed towards lesions more resembling benign skin lesions. This shift in clinical presentation has increased the possibility of confusion between benign and malignant skin-pigmented lesions, and increased the number of unnecessary removals of clinically suspect naevi.

Because of more widespread skin self-surveillance, and because of the difficult clinical recognition of a benign versus a malignant lesion (even by expert eyes), large-scale population screening for melanoma is not regarded as a relevant option. For, most probably, little gain in extra years of life, a screening programme would be costly (body examination, excision of suspect lesions, and eventual plastic surgery) and would generate considerable overtreatment with cosmetic damage (scars). Screening would also transform many healthy subjects into 'cancer patients' because of the discovery of a melanoma *in situ* that would almost certainly never evolve into invasive disease.

However, further efforts are needed for the early detection of melanoma. First, the absolute number of thick melanomas (those with poorer prognosis) remains unchanged, mainly in older men. Also, a large proportion of melanomas in men arises on body sites where they are difficult to see, for instance on the back. Hence, promotion of skin surveillance should now give priority to educating adult men and older people. Second, efforts should be directed towards known high-risk subjects. Regular skin examination should be recommended to adult having with the characteristics summarized in Table 1.

Pathology

Melanocytic precursor lesions and tumour progression

Melanocytes arise from the neural crest and migrate to their final destinations in the skin, uveal tract, meninges, and ectodermal mucosa. The vast majority of melanomas arise from cutaneous sites where normally most melanocytes are situated at the epidermal–dermal junction of the skin. Benign melanocytic tumours such as common acquired naevi, dysplastic naevi, and congenital naevi may evolve into malignant melanomas in a stepwise fashion, a process called tumour progression.

Dysplatic naevi are the major potential precursor lesions (in about one-third of all melanomas), and markers of individuals at increased risk for melanoma. The development of a melanoma, whether *de novo* (70 per cent) or within pre-existing naevi (30 per cent), is associated with acquisition of the property of clinically more-or-less inexorable growth, with vertical growth-phase lesions as the hallmark of malignancy and metastatic potential.

Precursor lesions

As discussed above, it is clear that the risk of melanoma is related to a number of readily observable host characteristics such as fair skin, fair/red hair, blue eyes, sunburning rather than suntanning capacity of the skin, the tendency to freckle, and the presence and number of benign melanocytic naevi (especially the presence of atypical or dysplastic naevi). Characteristics of various types of naevi, their role as precursor lesions, and the process of tumour progression are discussed below.

Common acquired naevi

The number of acquired naevi and the tendency to freckle correlate with the risk of developing a melanoma.[67] The risk is modest in comparison to the formal precursor lesions discussed below. Acquired naevi are classified as junctional, compound, or dermal, depending on the type of naevus cells and the site of melanocyte concentration in the skin. Almost all melanomas associated with naevi arise from the intraepidermal or junctional component.

Atypical moles or dysplastic naevi

An atypical mole or dysplastic naevus is characterized by architectural disorder and cytological atypia. It is a recognized precursor lesion of melanoma. Especially in the setting of the dysplastic naevus syndrome (DNS) or atypical mole syndrome (AMS), the risk of developing a malignant melanoma is greatly increased.[67] Surprisingly, this increased risk is independent of known risk factors such as hair and eye colour, freckling, and family history.[68] The familial AMS or DNS syndrome is characterized by the occurrence of multiple, large (6 mm or greater diameter) macular moles with irregular borders and often variable shades of brown, black, and red. Dysplastic naevi have both macular and papular components and may appear anywhere on the body, but especially on the trunk. Substantial asymmetry, excessive pigmentary variegation, focal black areas, or grey areas suggestive of partial regression should prompt a biopsy to rule out melanoma. Characteristic histological features of dysplastic naevi are the presence of an immature or disordered pattern of growth, of focal ('random') cytological atypia in melanocytes, and of a lymphocytic host response. Melanoma may arise from the dysplastic naevi or from apparently normal skin remote from any naevi. Melanomas found in association with dysplastic naevi are of the superficial spreading type and are often relatively thin.

Congenital naevi

Congenital melanocytic naevi, present at birth, are usually classified as small or giant congenital naevi. Congenital naevi are collections of naevus cells in pigmented skin lesions, with an irregular surface, increased pigmentation in varying shades of brown, and hypertrichosis. They are considered markers for an inherent predisposition to malignant melanoma.[69] The lifetime risk of melanoma in patients presenting with congenital naevi approaches 20 per cent.

Tumour progression in histopathological terms

Clark classified the steps of primary neoplasia as Classes I through III.[70] Class I or 'precursor' lesions are characterized by stability, indolence, or regression, except for those rare lesions that progress to the next step. The Class I melanocytic lesions include common acquired melanocytic naevi (Class IA); melanocytic naevi with an abnormal pattern of intraepidermal melanocytic growth ('aberrant differentiation', Class IB); and melanocytic naevi with dysplasia (Class IC).

Class I lesions

In the Clark model these lesions are limited in their ability to invade tissue and their capacity for cell proliferation is self-limited. Class I lesions rarely progress to Class II lesions, which are limited in their ability to invade tissue, but their lesional cells tend to proliferate inexorably in the epidermal compartment of their origin.

Class II lesions

These include radial growth phase (**RGP**) melanoma *in situ* (Class IIA), and invasive radial growth phase or 'microinvasive' melanoma (Class IIB). During the period of radial growth, malignant cells grow in a radial fashion, either above or just below the basal lamina. The RGP is not associated with the ability to metastasize.[71],[72] The RGP may last many years for superficial spreading melanoma, lentigo maligna melanoma, and acral lentiginous melanoma.

Class III lesions

Such lesions tend to proliferate inexorably, may invade and form tumour masses in stromal tissue compartments, and may have competence for metastasis. Class III melanocytic tumours include primary malignant melanomas with growth in the mesenchyme as well as in the epithelium of the primary site, lesions termed 'vertical growth

phase' (**VGP**) or 'tumorigenic' melanoma in this model. Because it is the first step in tumour progression that is associated with the potential for metastasis, VGP is the pivotal lesion in melanocytic tumour biology. Interobserver agreement for the diagnoses of VGP has been studied by a pathology panel established by the British Cancer Research Campaign.[73] It was concluded that the findings 'emphasized the possibility of recognizing more threatening melanomas not only by thickness, but also by the VGP'. This panel also supported the use of the term 'microinvasion', as discussed above.

Tumour progression in terms of molecular progression

Tumour progression represents mutational events that affect attributes of the neoplastic phenotype, such as cell proliferation, invasion, migration, and metastasis. A number of phases can be distinguished in this process, which are described below.[74]

First phase: genetic instability

The disruption of genetic integrity, which induces sustained genetic instability within the genome of the melanocyte, is the first critical step in the development of melanoma. The usual situation for normal melanocytes is one of non-proliferation and genetic stability. Genetic damage of melanocytes (by, for instance, UV-light exposure), is normally repaired by DNA-repair mechanisms, but self-limiting proliferation may occur and lead to the induction of naevi with or without atypia. Repeated damage may then lead to the induction of genetic instability and to the onset of deregulated proliferation.

Second phase: deregulated proliferation

Critical to the expansion of the cells with deleterious mutations or other genetic defects is the development of deregulated proliferation. In contrast to the self-limiting proliferation in the various types of naevi, the genetic instability results in the induction of deregulated proliferation and leads to *in situ* or superficial spreading primary melanomas. This stage of tumour progression is still in the non-invasive, non-metastatic phase.

Third phase: development of invasive potential

The melanoma cells, which in the radial growth phase are restricted to growth in the epidermis, now undergo a spontaneous acquisition of an invasive phenotype, enabling them to penetrate the underlying dermal layer and demonstrate the vertical growth phase. This change requires melanoma-directed dysregulation of the surrounding normal tissue interactions and architecture allowing physical invasion, the ability of melanoma cells to abrogate or attenuate inhibitory growth from the normal tissue, and the production by melanoma cells of paracrine and autocrine growth factors and cytokines (and their receptors) thereby allowing altered growth and differentiation.[75] For invasion to occur, the melanoma cell must disrupt the extracellular matrix (**ECM**) of the dermis, which is also a crucial step towards metastatic spread.[76]

Fourth phase: development of metastatic potential

Numerous biological pathways are involved in the ability of melanoma cells to invade tissue, survive and migrate through that tissue, escape from the inflammatory response, develop blood vessels and enter and survive in the lymph and bloodstream, and finally invade and survive in other organs. One of the most important steps in the metastatic process is the tumour-directed growth of new blood vessels required for the expansion of the tumour mass, as well as serving as a conduit for tumour cells into the systemic circulation.[75]–[79] The development of melanoma-mediated angiogenesis is associated with the development of metastases and poor clinical prognosis in melanoma. During progression, melanoma cells acquire the capacity to produce angiogenic factors directly. Several of these angiogenic factors are vascular endothelial growth factor (**VEGF**), tumour growth factor-β1 (**TGF-β1**), tumour necrosis factor (**TNF**), and the basic group, fibroblast growth factor (**bFGF**).

Diagnosis, classification, and staging

Introduction

The American Joint Committee on Cancer (**AJCC**) identifies four different forms of cutaneous melanoma occurring in humans: superficial spreading melanoma, nodular melanoma, lentigo maligna melanoma, and acral lentiginous melanoma. The two other forms of melanoma are mucosal melanoma and ocular melanoma. In the National Cancer Data Base (**NCDB**) report on almost 85 000 cases diagnosed between 1985 through 1994, the percentages of melanomas that were cutaneous, ocular, mucosal, and unknown primaries were 91.2 per cent, 5.2 per cent, 1.3 per cent, and 2.2 per cent, respectively.[80] For cutaneous melanomas, the proportion of patients presenting with AJCC Stages 0, I, II, III, and IV were 14.9 per cent, 47.7 per cent, 23.1 per cent, 8.9 per cent, and 5.3 per cent, respectively.

Diagnosis

It can be very hard to distinguish a melanoma from various forms of naevi, especially a dysplastic naevus, as discussed above. The **ABCD** signs that raise suspicion are: Asymmetry, Border irregularities, Colour variation, and a Diameter of more than 6 mm. The ABCD can be extended to **ABCDEF** by adding Evolution (clinical change) and risk Factors (fair hair/skin, the atypical moles syndrome, high naevi count, etc.)

Closer dermatoscopic examination of the lesion can provide much useful information for the diagnostician, enabling an accurate judgement to be made about disease status. Skin-surface microscopy and epiluminescence microscopy (**ELM**) magnify lesions up to 50-fold and can be used by experienced operators to successfully identify over 90 per cent of malignant lesions. In the hands of untrained individuals, however, these techniques have led to an overabundance of false-negative results. Computer technology is also starting to play a part in the analysis of skin lesions. Digital forms of ELM, which enhance images and allow comparison of surface features with those from a stored database, are now being used experimentally at various sites across Europe and North America. A group of German researchers has also reported a success rate of over 90 per cent for an automated process of classifying stored images. Other imaging techniques being assessed as diagnostic tools include ultrasound and spectrophotometry. All these systems are, however, still in the early stages of development and their benefits need to be properly proven in the clinic.

As yet, none of these techniques can provide sufficient information on precursor lesions to identify them before they progress to malignancy. The majority of malignant lesions develop *de novo* on the skin, with the transformation of dysplastic naevi being responsible in less than 40 per cent of cases. Targeted preventive measures will remain a dream until the identification of such lesions becomes possible.

Classification

The forms of cutaneous melanoma in order of frequency are superficial spreading melanoma, nodular melanoma, and lentigo maligna melanoma. These different forms of melanoma represent distinct pathological entities that have different clinical and biological characteristics.

Superficial spreading melanoma (SSM)

SSM is the most common form of cutaneous melanoma, accounting for approximately 70 per cent of all melanomas. The alarming rise in incidence in cutaneous melanoma is mostly of the SSM type. SSM generally arises in a pre-existing naevus and is often associated with the pigmented atypical mole syndrome or dysplastic naevi syndrome. SSM may typically have the long natural history of a naevus, exhibiting minor change over several years. Early in their evolution, SSMs usually are flat, muticoloured lesions, with irregular borders. Amelanotic areas often represent areas of regression. As the lesion grows, it may develop an irregular surface. SSMs occur throughout adulthood, with a peak incidence in the fifth decade of life. Most commonly they occur on the head, neck, and trunk in males and on the extremities in females (Fig. 3 and Plate 1).

Nodular malignant melanoma (NM)

NM is the second most common growth pattern, comprising about 15 per cent of all cutaneous melanomas. NM arises mostly *de novo* and not in a previously present naevus. NM is diagnosed most commonly on the trunk of men, but may develop on any body

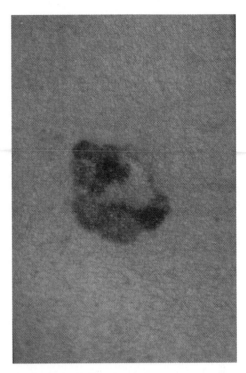

Fig. 3 Superficial spreading melanomas. Note irregular border, variations in colour, and area of partial regression (see also Plate 1).

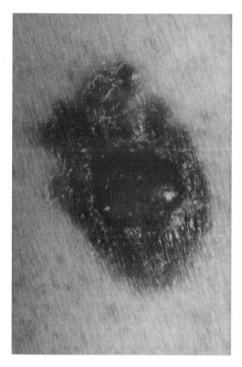

Fig. 4 Nodular melanomas tend to be thicker, more high-risk lesions (see also Plate 2).

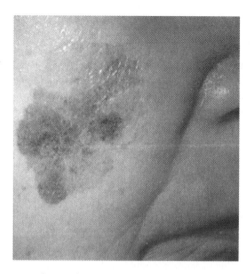

Fig. 5 Lentigo maligna melanoma with a nodular area of accelerated growth (see also Plate 3).

surface area. NM is biologically more aggressive than SSM. Clinically, the lesion is often dark and most often uniform in colour. Histologically, NM is notable for the complete absence of melanocytic abnormalities in the adjacent epidermis. Approximately 5 per cent of NM are amelanotic. NM does not have a radial growth phase and is associated with rapid evolution to vertical growth and invasion of the dermis. For this reason, nodular melanomas tend to be thicker, more high-risk lesions (Fig. 4 and Plate 2).

Lentigo maligna melanoma (LMM)

LMM (about 10 per cent of all melanomas) arises from lentigo maligna (precancerous melanosis of Dubreuilh). It occurs in elderly people (median age 70 years). LMM lesions are usually flat large lesions (more than 3 cm in diameter) with irregular borders and a variety of shades of tan to dark-brown on sun-exposed skin (see Fig. 5 and Plate 3). A nodular melanoma can arise in an LMM. Hypopigmented areas in the lesion represent areas of regression. The precursor lesion, lentigo maligna, has usually been present for long periods (5 to 15 years) prior to the development of invasive (nodular) melanoma.

Acral lentiginous melanoma (ALM)

ALM is found on the palms, soles, and subungual regions. It represents approximately 3 to 5 per cent of all cutaneous melanomas. This melanoma occurs in older individuals (median 60 years) and in a higher relative frequency in dark-skinned individuals and has a relatively poor prognosis. Subungual melanoma most commonly occurs on the great toe or thumb. ALM often appears as a tan to dark brown macule with an irregular border, but in advanced lesions it may be ulcerating or may present as a fungating mass. Although

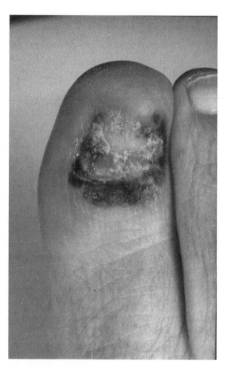

Fig. 6 Acral lentiginous melanoma (see also Plate 4).

similar in clinical appearance to LMM, ALM is a biologically much more aggressive lesion, with a relatively short evolution to the vertical growth phase (Fig. 6 and Plate 4).

Non-cutaneous melanoma

Ocular melanoma

Of the ocular melanomas, which comprise about 5 per cent of all melanomas, 85 per cent are uveal, 4.8 per cent are conjunctival, and 10.2 per cent occur at other sites.[80]

Table 2(a) American Joint Committee on Cancer Tumour (T), Node (N), Metastasis (M) classification system for melanoma*

	Current 1992	Proposed 2000	
T stage			
T0	Tis	Tis	
T1	<0.76	<1.0	A. No ulceration; B: ulceration or level IV or V
T2	0.76–1.5	1–2	
T3	2.6–4.0	2–4	
T4	>4	>4	
N stage			
N1	1	One lymph node	A: micrometastasis; B: macrometastasis
N2	2–4	2–3 lymph nodes	A: micrometastasis; B: macrometastasis; C: in-transit disease without positive nodes
N3	5 or more	4 or more metastatic lymph nodes, matted nodes, ulcerated melanoma, and metastatic lymph node(s), or nodal diseaseand in-transit or satellite lesions	
M stage			
M1	Any systemic metastasis	Any systemic metastasis	A: Distant skin, soft tissue, or nodal metastasis; B: pulmonary metastasis; C: all other visceral involvement or any patient with elevated blood levels of lactic dehydrogenase

Tis, tumour *in situ*.

*Proposed year 2000 version and current version. Micrometastases are diagnosed after elective or sentinel lymphadenectomy. Macrometastases are defined as clinically detectable lymph node metastases confirmed by therapeutic lymphadenectomy or when any lymph node metastasis exhibits extracapsular extension.

Mucosal melanoma (**MM**)

MM can occur in a variety of mucosal sites, including the oral cavity, oesophagus, anus, vagina, and conjunctiva. For mucosal melanomas, the distribution of head and neck, female genital tract, anal/rectal, and urinary tract sites was 55.4 per cent, 18 per cent, 23.8 per cent, and 2.8 per cent, respectively.[80] Mucosal melanomas are associated with a particularly poor prognosis.

Clinical staging

Meaningful comparisons between treatment centres and databases can only be drawn if a uniform classification system exists and is widely adopted. The most commonly used classification and staging system for melanoma is that of the American Joint Committee on Cancer (**AJCC**), pTNM (primary tumour, node, and metastases), which is used throughout this chapter. In this system localized disease without nodal involvement is classified as stage I or II (depending on the thickness of the primary tumour). Regional lymph node involvement and/or in-transit metastases is classified as stage III. Systemic metastases are classified as stage IV. Prognosis rapidly declines with increasing stage. The 10-year survival rates for the thin (< 1.5 mm) stage I melanomas is about 90 per cent; for stage II melanomas (> 1.5 mm) about 70 per cent; for stage III melanomas with regional metastases (lymph nodes; in-transit metastases) about 30 per cent; and for stage IV distant melanoma metastases less than 5 per cent.

The 1992 American Joint Committee on cancer staging system for cutaneous melanomas is presented in detail in Table 2(a) and (b), together with the new staging proposal, as presented at the end of the year 2000. This proposal simplifies the T staging by tumour thickness, and most importantly recognizes ulceration of the primary

as a very important independent prognostic factor throughout the staging system. In the N category, it recognizes that microscopic versus macroscopic node involvement and the number of involved nodes are of major importance. Moreover, it puts in-transit metastases into the N category.[288]

Molecular staging

The aim of identifying very small numbers of tumour cells in lymph nodes and peripheral blood for a more sensitive staging of patients with melanoma has led numerous investigators to develop and explore **RT-PCR** (reverse transcriptase-polymerase chain reaction)-based assays. PCR techniques allow the identification of very small copy numbers of specific DNA or RNA species. Since no consistent genetic abnormality has been identified for melanoma, the molecular assays rely on tissue-specific gene expression. This means that lymph node and blood samples are investigated for the expression of genes which are usually expressed in melanocytes and melanoma cells, but not in the lymph nodes or peripheral blood of healthy individuals or non-melanoma patients.

The technical issues have been summarized in a recent review.[81] Table 3 summarizes the genes that are expressed in melanoma cells but usually not in unaffected peripheral blood or lymph nodes. An ideal marker gene should be continuously expressed in all tumour cells, and the level of expression should not decrease during tumour progression. By far the most widely used gene is that coding for tyrosinase, which has several features of an ideal marker gene. Tyrosinase is expressed in approximately 80 per cent of all melanomas throughout all clinical stages, and the percentage of tyrosinase-expressing melanoma cells increases with tumour progression. Another gene coding for a melanosomal protein, Melan-AIMART1, has

Table 2(b) American Joint Committee on Cancer Tumour (T), Node (N), Metastasis (M) stage grouping for cutaneous melanoma*

Pathological stage	T	N	M	Clinical stage	T	N	M
0	Tis	N0	M0	0	Tis	N0	M0
IA	T1a	N0	M0	IA	T1a	N0	M0
IB	T1b	N0	M0	IB	T1b	N0	M0
	T2a	N0			T2a	N0	M0
IIA	T2b	N0	M0	IIA	T2b	N0	M0
	T3a	N0			T3a	N0	M0
IIB	T3b	N0	M0	IIB	T3b	N0	M0
	T4a	N0			T4a	N0	M0
IIC	T4b	N0	M0	IIC	T4b	N0	M0
IIIA	T1–4a	N1a	M0	IIIA	Any T1–4a	N1b	M0
IIIB	T1–4a	N1b	M0	IIIB	Any T1–4a	N2b	M0
	T1–4a	N2a					
IIIC	Any T	N2b, N2c	M0	IIIC	Any T	N2c	M0
	Any T	N3			Any T	N3	M0
IV	Any T	Any N	M1	IV	Any T	Any N	M1

*Clinical staging includes microstaging of the primary melanoma and clinical and radiological evaluation. It should be used after complete excision of the primary melanoma with clinical assessment for regional and distant metastasis. Pathological staging includes microstaging of the primary melanoma and pathological information about the regional nodes after partial or complete lymphadenectomy, except for pathological stage 0 or stage 1A patients, who do not need pathological evaluation of their lymph nodes.

Table 3 Marker genes used for diagnostic PCR

Marker gene	Expression during tumour progression	Illegitimate expression in blood	Expression in tissue by other cells
Tyrosinase	↑	–	–
MelanA/MART1	↑	–	–
gp100	↓	–	–
MAGE3	?	(+)	(+)
MUC1	?	(+)	+

similar features, whereas the third gene of this group, encoding gp100, is frequently lost during tumour progression and illegitimately expressed in peripheral blood and tissues. Theoretically, a multimarker PCR would be more sensitive than a PCR assay testing for the expression of a single marker gene. However, since the expression of tyrosinase and MART1 is rather concordant, the increase in sensitivity should be only modest and, in principle, the risk of false-positive results increases with the number of marker genes analysed.

All the clinical results of RT-PCR assays described below have been obtained in single laboratories with in-house assays. There is currently no standardization of assay systems and assay controls to ensure reliability of results obtained on a per sample basis. This may explain many of the discrepancies, especially with regard to the investigation of peripheral blood samples. A first quality-assurance initiative was performed by the EORTC Melanoma Cooperative Group.[82] This study revealed concordant results and high sensitivity in five out of nine laboratories, whereas the remaining four laboratories suffered from low sensitivity and/or false-positive results in several or all of the samples analysed. Furthermore, it is evident from this initiative that the disparities originated from pre-PCR processing of samples (RNA extraction, cDNA synthesis) rather than from the PCR amplification itself.

Each of the studies described below employed qualitative PCR assays. The advent of more widely available quantitative PCR instruments may increase the informative value of these assays in the future and, at the same time, solve some of the quality-assurance problems. None the less, it has to be taken into account that without internal standards suitable for assessing the reliability of all steps of the RT-PCR assay, the variability of pre-PCR sample processing will still have a major impact on quantitative assessment of gene expression.

Suitable internal standards that can be added to the clinical sample prior to processing[83] are under development to circumvent this important limitation.

RT-PCR on lymph nodes

The rationale for applying RT-PCR analysis on lymph nodes is to increase the sensitivity of tumour-cell detection. If robust and reliable RT-PCR assays can be developed, these could also eliminate the need to investigate multiple sections of a given lymph node by immunohistology. Compared to such an immunohistological assessment, the RT-PCR assays are less laborious and less costly.

The molecular investigation of lymph nodes is of greatest interest for the evaluation of sentinel lymph nodes. Several studies have shown that the sensitivity of an RT-PCR assay is higher compared to the sensitivity of immunohistology. One study revealed that the detection of tyrosinase transcripts in sentinel lymph nodes is of prognostic importance,[84] and several confirmatory studies are underway. However, since no therapeutic implications can be based on the molecular analysis of sentinel lymph nodes (the same is generally true for histological and immunohistological examinations), molecular staging of sentinel lymph nodes is currently only useful in the context of clinical trials, although the results may be informative for assessing a patient's risk of developing regional and/or systemic recurrences.

RT-PCR assays on peripheral blood

There is currently no evidence that melanocytes circulate in peripheral blood, and, therefore, the detection of RNA species usually expressed in melanocytes and melanoma cells, especially tyrosinase, has been accepted as indicating the presence of melanoma cells in the blood. There are numerous studies evaluating RT-PCR-based melanoma-cell detection in peripheral blood. Smith and colleagues initially described a nested RT-PCR assay with two sets of primers that detected tyrosinase transcripts.[85] Subsequent investigations by other groups using the same primers and nested PCR reported that the frequency of tyrosinase RNA detection is correlated with the stage of disease,[86],[87] that the presence of tyrosinase mRNA is a prognostic marker for systemic recurrences,[87] and that the prognostic value is independent of known prognostic factors.[88] Subsequent investigations did, in part, duplicate these results, whereas other reports failed to confirm these findings. The conflicting literature emphasizes the need for rigid quality-control measures to be implemented in all laboratories performing diagnostic PCR assays. Quantitative assays may, in the future, increase the consistency of results obtained by different laboratories and, at the same time, may add to the informative value of RT-PCR assays for the detection of melanoma cells in peripheral blood.

This type of molecular staging investigating peripheral blood theoretically facilitates the detection of haematogenous spread prior to the development of visible distant metastases. Ideally, systemic treatment should be implemented during this early period. Presently, however, there are no treatment modalities for melanoma with proven survival benefit. Therefore, molecular detection of circulating melanoma cells is currently only applicable within clinical trials. However, the recent development of antigen-specific tumour vaccines, which may be most efficient in the adjuvant setting, has led to continued interest in the early detection of tumour spread.

Currently, the detection of circulating melanoma cells in patients with metastatic disease has pure scientific value. In patients with distant melanoma metastases, the investigation of circulating melanoma cells may increase our knowledge of tumour biology, and quantitative assessment may help predict recurrences in the fraction of patients enjoying remission of distant metastases.

Prognostic factors

Of about 85 000 cases registered between 1985 and 1994 in the National Cancer Data Base (**NCDB**), the proportion of patients presenting with AJCC stages 0, I, II, III, and IV were 14.9 per cent, 47.7 per cent, 23.1 per cent, 8.9 per cent, and 5.3 per cent, respectively. Factors associated with decreased survival included more advanced stage at diagnosis, nodular or acral lentiginous histology, increased age, male gender, non-White race, and lower income. Multivariate analysis identified stage, histology, gender, age, and income as independent prognostic factors.

Prognostic factors in stage I–II

Microstaging methods, such as the measurement of thickness of the primary tumour as established by Breslow, and determination of the level of (epi)dermal invasion according to Clark are the most powerful prognostic factors in stage I–II melanomas. Breslow's microstaging method uses an ocular micrometer to measure the vertical thickness of the primary tumour from the granular layer of the epidermis, or the base of an ulcer, to the deepest identifiable contiguous melanoma cell.[89] Easier and more reproducible than Clark's level of invasion, it has become the generally accepted and preferred method of microstaging the primary tumour. The thicker the melanoma, the greater the risk for developing metastatic disease. Clark's method of microstaging is based upon five increasing levels of penetration through the dermis to the subcutaneous fat:[90] level I, intraepidermal; level II, penetration into papillary dermis; level III involves the papillary dermis and may extend to the papillary–reticular dermis interface; level IV, extension into the reticular dermis; level V, extension into the subcutaneous fat. It has been well established that the deeper the level of penetration, the poorer the prognosis. In patients with stage I–II disease, those factors with prognostic impact are: ulceration of the primary and signs of regression of the primary, possibly as both events may lead to an underestimation of the true thickness of the primary. Other factors also play a role—sex (females do better than males); tumour site (extremity melanomas have a better prognosis than head and neck and truncal melanomas; and age (younger patients have a better prognosis than older patients).[91]–[93] It has long been believed that pregnancy was associated with a particular poor outcome, but when results were corrected for thickness this belief was proven incorrect.[94]

Overriding prognostic significance of sentinel node status in patients with stage II tumours

The diagnostic power and accuracy of the sentinel node (**SN**) procedure in patients with stage I–II disease is such that up to 50 per cent of patients with thick, stage II primaries can now be classified as 'high-risk (but early) stage III patients' and no longer as intermediate-risk stage II patients. This is discussed in greater detail in the paragraphs on the surgical management of melanoma. Sentinel node staging is completely changing the landscape in melanoma management. Stage I–II patients who are sentinel node-negative have an excellent prognosis with expected survival rates above 90 per cent, whereas sentinel node-positive (formerly stage I–II patients) have expected survival rates below 50 per cent. The sentinel node status overrides all other prognostic factors.[95] The prognosis for a stage II SN-negative patient is excellent, whereas the prognosis of a stage II SN-not staged patient is unclear and dubious. This means that patients should be now staged and classified as either SN-positive or -negative.

Prognostic factors in stage III

Once patients have regional metastatic disease their prognosis sharply deteriorates. The number of positive lymph nodes (or in-transit metastases) is the strongest prognostic factor in patients with stage III disease,[95],[96] overriding the prognostic factors that are important in stage I–II. Sex remains of importance, as females do better at all stages than males.

Prognostic factors in stage IV

The following factors are of independent prognostic relevance for patients with distant metastases: serum lactate dehydrogenase (**LDH**) levels reflecting tumour volume, performance status, site of metastatic lesions, and/or the number of metastatic sites. This is discussed at greater length below in the section on stage IV disease.

Screening for distant spread

Radiological screening/staging procedures in patients with stage I–II melanoma have been shown to be of very little value. Kersey and co-workers[97] showed that the use of various diagnostic investigations (blood tests, chest radiographs, CT-scans, bone scans) in 393 patients with resected stage I–II melanoma is associated with substantial false-positive findings and of little to no value.

Buzaid and colleagues came to the same conclusion regarding the routine use of CT-scans in stage III melanoma.[98] The use of a **FDG-PET** (fluorodeoxyglucose-positron emission tomography) scan is also not recommended for detecting occult regional or distant metastases in patients with stage I–II melanoma.[99] In many countries, the routine use of CT, MRI, or PET scan for patients with stage III disease is advised against because of the lack of treatment options when distant metastases are discovered. The search for asymptomatic distant metastases without a clear therapeutic option results in an 'early verdict of death' and is generally not in the interest of most patients.[100] In patients with stage IV tumour, a CT scan of thorax and abdomen is usually performed to assess prognosis. Moreover, an MRI scan of the brain is useful in determining the patient's short-term prognosis and treatment options, especially in case of solitary brain metastasis. In stage I–II patients the sentinel node procedure is much more sensitive and specific than any other method. Additional tests in sentinel node-negative, stage I–II patients are very unlikely to yield any valuable information.

Surgical management of malignant melanoma

Surgical management of primary melanoma

Diagnostic biopsy

An excisional biopsy is the appropriate diagnostic procedure for a skin lesion suspected of being a melanoma, provided it is anatomically, functionally, and cosmetically feasible. Punch biopsy, incisional or shave biopsy, and excochleation are discouraged for a variety of reasons. A punch or incisional biopsy may well be justified in the case of a melanoma arising in a very large naevus, M. du Breuihl, or any other situation where an excisional biopsy causes functional or cosmetic problems.

The advantages of an excisional biopsy are that it provides the pathologist with the optimal chance of making the correct diagnosis and proper microstaging. It avoids the possibility that 'the wrong' part of a naevus has been removed, thereby leading to an incorrect diagnosis in those cases where a melanoma arises in a pre-existing naevus; it avoids an incorrect assessment of the Breslow thickness as well as the Clark level of invasion due to a tangential, prior incisional biopsy; and it avoids problems with an assessment of ulceration of the primary.

Margins of excision

In parallel with developments in the management of breast cancer, the extent of the surgical procedures to manage the primary tumour has been reduced. The dogma of using a wide excision of 5 cm or more, as introduced by Handley,[101] lost its rationale once Breslow had clearly shown that the thickness of the melanoma was closely related to prognosis.[102] Thus the concept of the necessity of a 5-cm margin was challenged[103],[104] and evaluated in a number of phase III trials. Several randomized trials were conducted of patients with thin melanomas less than 2 mm. In the French Trial[105] (319 patients) and the Scandinavian Trial[106] (769 patients), patients were randomized to undergo an excision with margins of 2 versus 5 cm, while in the WHO-Melanoma Program Trial-10[107],[108] (623 patients) margins of 1 versus 3 cm were employed. The Intergroup Trial in the United States[109],[110] (486 patients) compared different margins (2 versus 4 cm) in the management of thicker melanomas (between 1 and 4 mm) (Table 4). All trials had very similar results: local recurrence rates, disease-free survival (**DFS**) and overall survival (**OS**) were virtually identical in the narrow excision and the wide excision arm in all four trials. The conclusion from these trials is that a 1-cm margin is sufficient for melanomas under 2 mm, and that a margin of 2 cm is adequate for melanomas between 1 and 4 mm in size. A non-randomized study, based on 278 cases treated at the M.D. Anderson and the Lee Moffit Cancer Center,[111] demonstrated a lack of impact of wider than 2-cm excision margins on the local recurrence rate in patients with melanomas thicker than 2 mm and showed identical DFS and OS rates in both treatment groups. Taken together, it can be stated that a 2-cm margin can be considered adequate for all melanomas thicker than 2 mm. This means that virtually all melanomas at any site can be treated by excision and primary closure. Whether in the end it will be proven that a 1-cm margin is adequate for all melanomas, irrespective of their thickness, will depend on the outcome of the continuing UK-MCG trial,[112] which compares 1-cm versus 3-cm excision margins in patients with melanomas thicker than 2 mm. Given the outcome in all the randomized trials so far conducted, which have shown that the narrower margin was as good as the wider margin, we should not be surprised should the UK trial eventually bring an end to the myth that primary melanomas need wide excision margins. At the present time, a conservative approach should be recommended on the basis of the data above. A 0.5-cm margin should be considered adequate for *in situ* melanomas; for melanomas under 2 mm, a 1-cm margin is adequate; for melanomas

Table 4 Margins and primary melanoma

Trial (ref.)	Margin	Pts	NE LR	WE LR	NE DFS	WE DFS	NE OS	We OS	At
	(%)	(%)	(%)	(%)	(%)	(%)	(yrs)		
Melanoma < 2 mm									
WHO-10[107],[108]	1 vs 3	623	2.5	1.0	81	81	87	87	10
French Trial[105]	2 vs 5	319	–	–	91	87	93	90	4
Scandinavian[106]	2 vs 5	769	0.8	1.0	76	80	90	93	5
Melanoma 1–4 mm									
Intergroup Trial[109]	2 vs 4	486	0.8	1.7	n.s.	n.s.	80	82	6
Update[110]	2 vs 4	470	2.1	2.6	n.s.	n.s.	n.s.	n.s.	8
Melanoma > 2 mm									
Non-randomized study[111]	< 2 vs 3–5	278	8	16	30	28	58	50	5
UK-MCG Trial[112]	1 vs 3 >	800	–	–	–	–	–	–	

Ref, reference; Pts, patients; NE, narrow excision; WE, wide excision; LR, local recurrence; DFS, disease-free survival; OS, overall survival; yrs, years.

Table 5 Recommended margins

In-situ melanoma	0.5 cm
Melanoma < 2 mm	1.0 cm
Melanoma > 2 mm	2.0 cm*

*Narrower margins should be considered at sites with anatomical, functional, or cosmetic constraints.

thicker than 2 mm, a 2-cm margin is adequate. Narrower margins should be considered as very reasonable in all those areas where a 2-cm margin would meet with anatomical, functional, or cosmetic constraints (Table 5). It should stand to reason that histopathologically free margins should be adequate, that primary closure is the rule, and that split skin grafts will be something of the past.

Elective lymph node dissection

Immediate or elective lymph node dissection (**ELND**) has been practised widely, based on the hypothesis that micrometastases from the primary melanoma disseminate sequentially from the primary tumour to regional lymph nodes and then to distant sites. Thus survival should be increased if nodal metastases are removed before they spread further. As in breast cancer, it is now acknowledged that, in the vast majority of the patients, lymphatic spread occurs in parallel with haematogenous spread. Thus lymph node metastases are 'indicators rather than governors of survival'.[113] Of note is the report by Cascinelli and co-workers that only half of the patients demonstrate regional lymph node metastases prior to metastases at other sites.[114] It is therefore very unlikely that removal of lymph nodes containing micrometastases changes the prognosis, as widespread micrometastatic disease is most often present.[115]

Retrospective studies usually demonstrated a survival benefit in patients treated by excision of the primary followed by immediate regional lymph node dissection.[116]–[119] The use of historical controls and databases often suffers from selection bias and differences in staging procedures in use at different times. Hence, they can only be used for hypothesis building, but they rarely, if ever, have the power to provide proof of a concept. This problem can partly be overcome when controls from the same time period are used instead of historical controls, which usually eliminates major differences in the accuracy of staging procedures. Three large studies comprising some 10 000 patients, which did not compare results between different periods—one by Drepper and co-workers in Germany,[120] the careful analysis of the very large Duke University database by Slingluff *et al.*,[121] and the methodologically correct reanalysis of the Australian database by Coates and co-workers[122]—failed to show an overall benefit of ELND, not even in those patients with a primary of intermediate thickness. Only in some subgroups, with no logical pattern or biologically plausible explanation, was a small benefit of ELND sometimes observed. Only properly conducted, prospective, phase III trials can provide an answer. Thus far four trials have been conducted, but have failed to demonstrate a significant effect of ELND on overall survival. In the first two trials, the large WHO-10 trial[123],[124] and the much smaller Mayo Clinic Trial,[125],[126] no benefit was observed for the ELND arm of the studies. Patients with microscopically involved lymph nodes in the ELND arm fared no better than the patients who underwent a delayed lymph node dissection for clinically positive nodes. The overall outcome of the United States Intergroup trial of patients with intermediate primaries between 1 and 4 mm in thickness was also negative, in spite of the title of the report of this trial.[127] No benefit of ELND was seen in the 2- to 3-mm or 3- to 4-mm thick melanomas, but a benefit was observed in those patients with relatively thin melanomas of between 1 and 2 mm in thickness. This was in contrast to predictions and the reason is not well understood. The observation that a benefit for ELND was observed in patients younger than 60 years of age, whereas almost the reverse was seen in patients over 60 years old, is not understood; quite likely it results from the many subgroup analyses performed, with or without proper stratification in the design of the trial. Unfortunately, the crucial analysis comparing the outcome in patients with micrometastases who underwent an ELND to the outcome in patients who did not undergo ELND but underwent a delayed lymph node dissection (**DLND**) once nodal involvement had become clinically evident has not been done. The recently reported WHO-14 trial in patients with primary truncal melanomas thicker than 1.5 mm also showed no significant benefit of ELND in the overall population.[128] However, in this trial, patients with micrometastases in the lymph nodes discovered after ELND fared better than those who underwent a delayed lymph node dissection for clinically positive nodes. This observation differs from the results of the much larger WHO-10 trial on ELND in patients with melanomas of the extremities.[123],[124] In the extremity trial, standard axillary and groin dissections were performed and no lymphoscintigraphies were needed to identify the correct lymph node basin, which of course is much more problematic in a truncal melanoma trial. In the WHO-10 trial, the survival curve of patients who underwent an ELND and were microscopically positive, overlapped fully with the survival curve of patients who did not undergo an ELND but who later underwent a DLND when regional nodal metastasis had become clinically evident. In patients with thick primaries (> 1.5 mm), only an estimated 20 to 25 per cent will harbour micrometastatic disease in regional lymph nodes; even in these patients, immediate lymph node dissection has only been shown to have some impact in one out of the four trials. Anyway, routine ELND is a gross overtreatment of the patient population and should be abandoned.

Sentinel node procedure

Intraoperative lymphatic mapping and selective lymphadenectomy is also called 'the sentinel node procedure'. The sentinel node (SN) procedure presents an attractive option for circumventing the problem of overtreatment and for inflicting morbidity on the whole patient population. The SN procedure relies on the concept that regions of the skin have specific patterns of lymphatic drainage, not only to the regional lymphatic basin but also to a specific lymph node (the sentinel lymph node) in the basin. If lymphatic spread to the regional lymph nodes has occurred, then the sentinel node is the first node to be involved; thus to have the best chance of detecting microscopic spread to the regional lymph node(s), this is the node on which to concentrate all staging efforts.

The method, using a blue dye only, was promulgated for the management of melanoma by Morton.[129] The methodology has gained much in accuracy from the use of a radiolabelled colloid and a hand-held probe for intraoperative SN identification, as well as preoperative use of lymphoscintigraphy, resulting in an almost 100 per cent identification rate of the SN.[130]–[134]

The chance of identifying microscopic foci using these procedures is also considerably higher than by evaluating a large number of involved nodes from full ELND material. It is now clear that missing microscopic disease by routine histopathological evaluation of an ELND explains the observation in the WHO-1 trial, that patients who underwent ELND and remained free of overt metastases to the regional lymph nodes had a significantly better survival curve than the patients who underwent an ELND and were found to have no such microscopic nodal involvement. SN-mapping with meticulous histopathological work-up (haematoxylin and eosin (H&E) in combination with immunohistochemical staining) of that one or those few sentinel nodes will be associated with a much lower rate of false-negative diagnoses. In the near future, RT-PCR on negative nodes may complete the diagnostic work-up as a last step in determining whether tumour cells are present in the sentinel node. From the initial reports it could be shown that the SN-PCR positive rate corresponded most closely to the relapse and death rates in patients, as

they do with Breslow thickness.[135] By H&E and immunohistochemical evaluation of the SN, a false-negative rate was only observed in 4.1 per cent of 243 patients. Re-evaluation of those SNs revealed that in 75 per cent of cases the diagnosis would have been made had more sections of the sentinel node been examined.[136]

It is unlikely that selective lymph node dissection (SLND) will improve survival by itself. But it has been demonstrated to be the best prognostic factor, outperforming all other prognostic factors to the point that even Breslow thickness is no longer an independent prognostic factor in SN-positive patients![137] The use of SN-mapping dissects the heterogeneous groups of patients (stage IIA–IIB) into truly node-positive and truly node-negative populations, both with very different prognoses: SN-negative patients have a 5-year survival better than 90 per cent, while for SN-positive patients it is less than 50 per cent. SN-mapping may well be beneficial in selecting patients for adjuvant treatment once a confirmed active adjuvant treatment has been identified.

Treatment of symptomatic regional lymph nodes

Surgery is the treatment of choice for metastatic disease in the regional lymph nodes. Full regional lymph node dissections for metastases in the head and neck region, the axilla, and the groin offer the only chance for cure and locoregional control. The 5-year survival rates after therapeutic lymph node dissections vary from 25 to 40 per cent, with the higher the number of involved lymph nodes the poorer the survival.[138]–[140] For clinically involved inguinal lymph nodes, it is has been demonstrated that a deep or ilioinguinal groin dissection achieves the best local control. However, it is not superior in terms of survival rates after surgery when compared to superficial or inguinal lymph node dissection only.[141] Yet, even patients with clear involvement of iliac and obturator nodes without signs of systemic disease can occasionally be cured by a deep groin dissection.[141],[142]

A brief description of the standard lymphadenectomies follows.

Axillary lymphadenectomy

A complete axillary lymph node dissection should be performed, including those nodes at levels I, II, and III. The boundaries of the dissection should include the axillary vein superiorly, beginning at the thoracic outlet and coursing to the latissimus dorsi tendon. The lateral border of the dissection is the anterior edge of the latisimus dorsi muscle. The posterior boundary is the subscapular muscle. The anterior border of the resection is the pectoralis major group. The inferior boundary of the dissection should be the juncture of the latissimus dorsi and the serratus anterior muscles. The contents within these boundaries should be completely removed, with the exception of the long thoracic nerve and the thoracodorsal nerve which should be identified during the dissection and preserved throughout. The pectoralis minor muscle may be divided or sacrificed with the specimen at the discretion of the surgeon. Care should be exercised that the anterior pectoral nerve is not injured in the superior part of the dissection. The preferred approach to the axilla is through a horizontal incision in the line of the skin crease, 3 or 4 cm below the apex of the skin fold of the axilla.

Inguinal lymphadenectomy

A superficial femoral node dissection should be performed by excising all the nodes inferior to the inguinal ligament and bounded by the medical border of the sartorius muscle in the lateral border of the adductor magnus muscle. The fatty and lymphatic tissues should be dissected carefully off the femoral vessels and nerves all the way up to the inguinal canal and for 3 cm superior to the inguinal ligament. This area can be entered through a curvilinear incision starting laterally over the inguinal ligament and curving medially and inferiorly ending over the midpoint of the adductor magnus muscle. Transposition of the sartorius muscle can be used to protect the vessels in case of missing soft tissue and skin coverage.

Deep inguinal and external iliac node dissection

This area can be most easily approached by incising the abdominal wall musculature 3 or 4 superior to the inguinal ligament. This incision is taken down through the external oblique, internal oblique, and transversus muscles, and the surgeon at that point stays extraperitoneally as in the approach to the iliac vessels for renal transplantation. With this approach, the external, internal, and common iliac arteries are exposed and the lymphatics crossing along the iliac vessels are excised. Patients undergoing an ilioinguinal lymph node dissection, which is the preferred management of patients with palpable positive nodes in the inguinal area or when Cloquet's node is positive, may preferably have two separate incisions made following the skin lines. One incision 3 cm above Poupart's ligament for the ilio-obturator nodes part of the dissections, and one 4 cm distal to Poupart's ligament for the inguinal/femoral triangle part of the lymph node dissection. This approach is associated with much less wound and seroma problems than a vertical S-shaped incision approach spanning the whole ilioinguinal area.

(Modified) radical neck dissection

A classic, but preferably modified, radical neck dissection may be performed for patients with melanoma of the head and neck. Patients with melanoma located on the ear and anterior scalp and face will require superficial parotidectomy along with a radical neck procedure. The boundaries of the radical neck dissection are inferiorly the clavicle; the mandible, the mastoid, and the tail of the parotid gland superiorly; the anterior border of the trapezius muscle posteriorly; and the strap muscle of the larynx anteriorly. The sternocleidomastoid muscle is preferably preserved. For posterior lesions, the radical neck incision must be extended posteriorly, or a second incision must be made so that the suboccipital nodal group can be sampled.

Complications of lymphadenectomy

The most common complications associated with lymph node dissection are those related to the wound itself, which may lead to prolongation of hospital stay. However, the severity and type of the complication vary with the site of node dissection. Most complications occur after (ilio)inguinal lymph node dissections. Significant oedema may occur in up to 10 per cent of the patients, particularly if the iliac and obturator nodes are removed with the superficial inguinal nodes and those of the femoral triangle. Wound infections occur as well as lymphatic fistulas in up to 25 per cent of cases. Elevating the leg while recumbent and wearing elastic compression stockings for 6 to 8 weeks after surgery may minimize morbidity. Morbidity associated with axillary and neck dissections is generally less, but sometimes lesions to a nerve (ramus marginalis of the facial nerve!) can be a serious complication. Wound seroma and infection are relatively infrequent in axillary node dissection, while significant arm oedema occurs in approximately 1 per cent of patients.

Prophylactic isolated limb perfusion

The technique of regional isolated limb perfusion (ILP) utilizing an extracorporeal circuit was pioneered by Creech and co-workers.[143] The advantage of this treatment modality is that a high dose of a cytostatic drug can be delivered to the tumour-bearing extremity without producing systemic side-effects. ILP permits regional cytostatic concentrations 15 to 20 times higher than those reached after systemic administration.[144] The standard drug in this setting is melphalan (l-phenylalaninemustard).[145]

Isolated limb perfusion was believed to have an impact on survival in the treatment of high-risk primary melanoma through the mechanism of ridding the extremity of in-transit micrometastases (in-transit on their way to form regional lymph node metastases) and established in-transit metastases in the (sub)cutaneous compartment. Macroscopic in-transit metastases are known to develop in 5 to 8 per cent of patients with a high-risk primary melanoma.

Retrospective studies suggested that a prophylactic ILP (just like ELND) improved outcome in patients with high-risk primary melanoma.[146],[147] However a well-conducted, retrospective study in a large matched-controlled population, which evaluated the effect of adjuvant ILP after excision of a primary melanoma more than 1.5 mm thick, showed no significant benefit.[148] The results of a randomized, prematurely closed, trial, claiming a survival benefit after ILP, are very questionable because of sample size and the unusually unfavourable outcome in the control arm.[149],[150] Another randomized trial, aborted after 51 patients had been recruited. The only valid study on high-risk primary melanoma of the extremity is the Intergroup trial of the EORTC-WHO and NAPG (North American Perfusion Group). A total of 852 patients were randomized to the trial over a period of 10 years, 832 of whom were evaluable at a median follow-up of 6.4 years.[151] ILP had only a regional effect, but a significant reduction in the appearance of in-transit metastases was noted (from 6 per cent to 3 per cent). A reduction in regional lymph node metastases (or a delay in their appearance) was noted (from 16.7 per cent to 12.6 per cent), with no effect on the appearance of distant metastases. Thus prophylactic ILP had no significant effect ($RR = 1.03$; $p = 0.822$) on overall survival and should no longer be performed.

Treatment of in-transit metastases of the extremities

Melanoma recurs locally in the extremities, mostly in the form of in-transit metastases (in 5 to 8 per cent of patients with melanoma), and can present an appalling problem to the patient. Various locoregional treatment options exist, but effective management remains a challenge. The choice depends primarily on the number and size of the lesions and on the general condition of the patient. Treatments vary from (multiple) excision(s), laser-evaporation, intralesional injection of interferons, regional chemotherapy, namely isolated limb infusions and isolated limb perfusions.[152]

A single or only a few in-transit metastases are initially generally treated by surgical excision. Carbon-dioxide laser management of recurrences only seems successful in the management of small nodules (less than 1.5 cm in thickness).[153] Intralesional injections with interferons yield modest response rates of short duration. Intra-arterial or systemic chemotherapy is mostly ineffective.

Isolated limb perfusion is the treatment of choice for bothersome multiple in-transit metastases and is the most effective option, providing excellent local control but no clear survival benefit.[154] However, about 25 per cent of the patients with stage II–IIIa are alive at 5 to 10 years.[155] Thus ILP can be curative. A single ILP with melphalan yields an overall response rate of about 80 per cent (40 per cent complete response (CR); 40 per cent partial response (PR)).[156] Hyperthermia may improve response rates, but at the cost of increased regional toxicity.[157] The addition of tumour-necrosis factor-alpha (TNF-α) to melphalan has proven most effective in term of response rate: yielding a 70 to 80 per cent complete response rate, and an overall response rate of up to 100 per cent.[158]–[160]

Whether TNF also significantly improves the time to local recurrence or progression is not yet clear. TNF is most effective and beneficial in case of bulky (sarcoma-like) disease.[161] This is in line with the spectacular effects on irresectable, soft-tissue extremity sarcomas.[162] Another important development is the hypoxic ILI procedure. This short, simple, easily repeatable, and cheap procedure seems to be as effective as a standard ILP with melphalan, and results may be further improved by adding TNF.[163] A serious shortcoming of many reports in the literature is that often the duration of local tumour control is not reported, in spite of the fact that this is the most important measure of success.

Surgery of (isolated) distant metastases

Despite the well-recognized tendency of melanoma to disseminate widely, surgical excision of metastases can provide excellent palliation, and sometimes long-term survival in selected patients. Excision of multiple metastases from multiple organ sites does not improve outcome. But some patients with multiple metastases in the same organ, such as the lung, may enjoy long-term survival. Soft-tissue sites are usually associated with a more favourable prognosis that visceral sites (see Table 12).

Subcutaneous and lymph node metastases

Metastatic deposits in subcutaneous sites and lymph nodes are frequent in patients with disseminated melanoma and may represent the only manifestation of disease. Surgical excision of these clinically involved sites can be of palliative value in order to prevent local problems, and may be associated with prolonged disease-free periods and a median survival as long as 29 months.[164]

Lung metastases

Occasionally, patients present with a solitary pulmonary nodule as the only manifestation of recurrent melanoma. The value of thoracotomy or sternotomy in this setting remains controversial and depends on the biological behaviour of the tumour, such as a slow doubling time.[163] However, 5-year survival rates of up to 35 per cent have been reported in patients with apparently solitary pulmonary metastases.[165]–[168]

Gastrointestinal metastases

Gastrointestinal metastases from a metastatic melanoma may produce blood loss or symptoms of acute obstruction due to an intussusception

segment of small bowel. Indications for surgery are most frequently associated with acute bowel obstruction from an intussuscepting small bowel or from chronic gastrointestinal bleeding.[169] Surgery is of palliative value and may sometimes be followed by a long asymptomatic period, but prolonged survival is unusual.

Brain metastases

Solitary brain metastases are preferentially treated by stereotactic radiation therapy. Surgical removal of solitary brain metastases may relieve associated symptoms and occasionally results in long-term survival.[170],[171] Postoperative cranial radiotherapy is generally considered of value since other occult lesions may exist.

Follow-up after surgery

There is a general agreement that follow-up of patients with stage I–II cutaneous melanoma after treatment of the primary melanoma is advisable because: about 75 to 80 per cent of all first melanoma recurrences are local or locoregional in nature[172]–[174] and can generally be treated by surgery with curative intent; between 3 and 6 per cent of the patients develop a second primary melanoma, and up to 30 per cent of individuals from melanoma-prone families.[175] These second primary melanomas may be diagnosed at an early stage by regular follow-up.[176] Furthermore, between 4 and 5 per cent of the patients develop basal-cell carcinomas of the skin, for which there is simple treatment when diagnosed timely.

Ideally, the optimal follow-up schedule should be tailored to the risk of recurrence or the risk of development of a second primary lesion.

The majority of recurrences (up to 70 per cent) in patients with stage I–II melanoma is discovered by the patient in between follow-up visits to his physician.[174],[177],[178] In a landmark publication on the value of follow-up investigations in patients with stage I melanoma, Kersey and colleagues[177] reported that, out of 394 patients with at least a median follow-up of 3 years, 64 patients developed metastatic melanoma. Of these 64 patients, 36 (56.3 per cent) identified their own recurrence to the physician. Thus history alone identified more than half of the recurrences. The physician only discovered recurrent melanoma in a further 22 patients (34.3 per cent) on physical examination. Thus a history together with a physical examination was responsible for 90.6 per cent of the detection of recurrent disease. Furthermore, five patients developed second primary melanomas, which were all detected by the patient and/or the physician. This publication demonstrates the lack of efficacy of using various diagnostic procedures routinely during follow-up.[177] Moreover, now that the sentinel node staging procedure will classify most stage III patients as 'truly node-negative', the chance for a regional recurrence is only about 4 per cent.[135] This also means that follow-up schedules can be simplified to 6-monthly intervals in patients with SN-negative stage I–II disease; confirming the National Cancer Institute's (NCI) consensus advice on the follow-up frequency for patients with thin melanomas (< 1.0 mm)—6-monthly check-ups during years 1 and 2, and thereafter follow-up at 12-monthly intervals for up to 5 or 10 years depending on concomitant risk factors.

In patients with stage III disease, the most frequently adopted follow-up schedule is every 3 months during years 1 and 2, every 6 months during years 3 and 5, and every 6 or 12 months during years

6 to 10. Lifelong follow-up may be reserved for patients with an atypical mole syndrome or other high-risk factors.

Adjuvant therapy of malignant melanoma

Locoregional adjuvant procedures

Adjuvant therapies in the management of primary malignant melanoma can be locoregional or systemic in nature. Locoregional adjuvant therapies are surgical procedures performed in addition to the simple excision of the primary melanoma, in the absence of clinical evidence of the presence of locoregional disease. These procedures are: (1) re-excision of the excisional biopsy area to obtain wide excision margins; (2) elective lymph node dissection (ELND) of the regional lymph nodes; (3) adjuvant ILP with cytostatic drug(s). These procedures have been discussed above. It has become obvious that adjuvant surgical procedures are of little value and that a simple excision of the primary, with an adequate margin, suffices as the primary management of melanoma.

The most useful staging procedure to assess the risk of the patient having (often widespread) micrometastatic disease has proven to be sentinel node mapping. It clearly divides the melanoma population between SN-negative patients with very little risk for relapse and SN-positive patients with a very high risk for relapse.

Systemic adjuvant therapy

Systemic adjuvant therapies have the goal of eradicating micrometastatic deposits throughout the body after surgical management of primary melanomas that have a high risk of systemic dissemination, but without clinical evidence of the presence of metastatic disease. In this chapter we will only discuss the situation on the basis of data from randomized phase III trials.

Results of various non-IFN-α adjuvant therapy trials in stage II–III melanoma

Numerous phase III trials evaluating adjuvant therapy of stage II/III malignant melanoma with various agents have been performed over the last three decades. In terms of impact on disease-free survival (DFS) and on overall survival (OS), all trials—with the exception of only one trial with *Corynebacterium parvum*, one trial with interferon-α (IFN-α), and a few small inconclusive trials—virtually all trials have failed to show any impact of the adjuvant therapeutic strategy on survival.

Adjuvant chemotherapy, aspecific immunotherapy, and combined chemoimmunotherapy

In the absence of virtually any significant action of cytostatic agents in stage IV melanoma, efforts in the development of adjuvant therapies for melanoma have generally focused on the modulation and activation of the immune system. In the early years the focus was on aspecific immunostimulation by agents such as bacille Calmette–Guérin (BCG) or *C. parvum*. Studies were performed in patients with stage II and III melanoma, in which regimens of chemotherapy alone, immunotherapy alone, or immunochemotherapy combinations were compared to observation of the patients. To date, 11 trial reports have been published on the efficacy of adjuvant therapy with chemotherapy alone (DTIC (dacarbazine) or CCNU (lomustine) or BCNU (carmustine)), or with BCG alone, or with the combination of chemoimmunotherapy and BCG;[179]–[189] three negative trials on the use of *C. parvum* alone or in combination with DTIC;[190]–[192] and one positive trial report[193] on the use of *C. parvum* alone compared with BCG. On the use of another aspecific immunostimulant, levamisole, three negative and one partially positive trial reports have been published.[194]–[197]

Vitamin A

A Southwest Oncology Group (SWOG) phase III trial, comprising 252 patients, failed to demonstrate any impact on survival with the use of adjuvant vitamin A treatment.[198]

Hormonal

One very small randomized trial has been conducted in patients with stage II–III disease using megestrol acetate 800 mg, four times daily. There were only 33 patients in the treatment arm and 34 patients in the control arm. A surprising outcome showed a median survival of 7.6 years in the treatment arm and 2.6 years in the control arm ($p = 0.03$). The inadequate size of the trial does not allow for any conclusions. The NCCTG has undertaken efforts to run a confirmatory trial, but no data have so far been reported.

Cytokines other than interferon-α (IFN-α) (Table 6)

Interferon-gamma (IFN-γ)

Results of another SWOG trial on adjuvant therapy with interferon-gamma (IFN-γ)[200] as well as the EORTC 18771 trials have been reported.[201] In the SWOG trial, the patients in the IFN-γ arm did significantly worse than in the observation arm. In the EORTC 18771/DKG-80 trial, disease-free and overall survival rates in the IFN-γ arm were no different from the observation arm. Quite importantly, this trial also showed that the mistletoe extract 'Iscador', which is a popular 'alternative medicine' preparation in central Europe prescribed to many cancer patients, had absolutely no positive impact on DFS or OS when administered in the adjuvant setting to high-risk patients with melanoma.

Interleukin-2 (IL-2)

IL-2 has modest activity in stage IV melanoma, but so far has not been widely evaluated in the adjuvant setting for the treatment of melanoma. A Swiss–German phase III trial reported no impact on DFS or OS with the use of low doses of IL-2 and IFN-α to treat patients with stage II melanoma.[202]

Adjuvant specific (tumour-cell vaccines) immunotherapy

Experience with vaccines that are supposed to induce a specific antimelanoma immune response has so far been very limited. No significant impact on DFS or OS was reported from three sizeable 'active specific immunotherapy' trials of whole tumour-cell vaccines.[203]–[205] One trial in the United States comprising 251 patients treated with a viral oncolysate of melanoma cells[206] and one very large trial in Australia with a viral oncolysate[207],[208] were also negative.

Ganglioside GM2 vaccine Gangliosides such as GM2 that characterize melanomas, have been well described as differing from those of normal melanocytes and as having limited expression on most normal

Table 6 Various phase III, non-IFN-α adjuvant therapy trials in stage II/III melanoma

Randomized phase III trials	DFS/OS
Aspecific immunotherapy and/or chemotherapy	
BCG/C. parvum/levamisole ± chemotherapy: 18 trials:	
Adjuvant chemotherapy (DTIC, CCNU, BCNU), or	–/–
Aspecific immunotherapy (BCG, C. parvum, levamisole), or	–/–
Combined chemoimmunotherapy	–/–
(Various authors: 1981–1991[179]–[197])	
Vitamin A	
SWOG trial (Meyskens 1994[198])	–/–
Hormonal	
Megestrol acetate[199]	+/+
(* only 33 vs 34 patients)	
Cytokines other than IFN	
IFN-γ	
SWOG trial (Meyskens 1995[200])	–/–
EORTC 18771/ DKG-80 (Kleeberg 1999[201])	–/–
Interleukin-2:	
IL-2 (SC) + IFN (SC) (Hauschild 1997[202])	–/–
Tumour-specific vaccines	
Adjuvant-specific (tumour-cell vaccines) immunotherapy	
BCG + allogeneic tumour cells (Morton 1982,[203] Terry 1982[204])	–/–
BCG + allogeneic tumour cells (Morton 1986[205])	–/–
Viral oncolysate vaccines	
Wallack et al. 1995[206]	–/–
Hersey et al. 1993,[207] 1997[208]	–/–
Ganglioside GM2 vaccine	
GM2/BCG vs BCG MSK-Trial (Livingston 1994[210])	+/+

DFS, disease-free survival; OS, overall survival.

tissues.[284] Serological studies of melanoma have suggested a favourable prognosis for patients with pre-existing or vaccine-induced antibody titres against GM2.[285] Autologous antibodies against GM2 are, however, infrequently detected in unimmunized patients.

Livingston and co-workers evaluated a series of autologous and allogeneic tumour vaccine regimens, and more recently purified ganglioside combined with immunological adjuvants. The combination of BCG with ganglioside GM2 has been shown to induce the formation of IgM antibodies in the majority of treated melanoma patients.[209]

A randomized trial of GM2/BCG adjuvant therapy following surgery for AJCC stage III melanoma was conducted in 122 patients at Memorial Sloan-Kettering Cancer Center (**MSKCC**) between 1987 and 1988.[210] This trial demonstrated the induction of anti-GM2 IgM antibodies in the majority of treated patients, and the presence of natural antibodies against GM2 in a small subset of the control unvaccinated group of patients. Serological responses against GM2 were again demonstrated to be a favourable prognostic factor. In addition, the vaccinated group of patients showed a borderline prolongation of relapse-free survival, confounded by the unanticipated presence of anti-GM2 antibodies among six patients in the control group. With the removal of these confounding results from patients who had a prestudy serological reactivity to GM2, the impact of GM2/BCG vaccination upon relapse-free survival was significant ($p = 0.02$). It was recently reported from

a study of the polyvalent melanoma-cell vaccine that survival was significantly prolonged in patients who developed significant GM2 IgM antibody titres.[211]

Results of phase III trials regarding adjuvant therapy with IFN-α

IFN-α is a cytokine with direct and indirect antitumour effects. The direct antitumour effects are mediated by the antiproliferative, protein synthesis–inhibiting, and prodifferentiative effects of IFN. The indirect antitumour effects are mediated by immunomodulatory effects, on the one hand, such as the activation of host immune cells and augmentation of the expression of tumour cell-surface antigens on tumour cells, and by antiangiogenic effects on the other hand. The potential impact of this cytokine has been investigated in many phase I–II studies in stage IV melanoma and in multiple randomized phase III trials in AJCC stage II and stage III melanomas.

High-risk melanoma (stage IIB–III)

Over the last decade, many trials of IFN have been performed in patients with stage II–III melanoma. However, many have been underpowered, have suffered from the fact that mixed populations were studied (node-negative and node-positive patients in one and the same trial), and have investigated a variety of doses and durations of treatment. The various trials are summarized in Table 7.

Table 7 IFN-α adjuvant therapy phase III trials in stage IIA–IIB or IIB–III melanoma

Study	IFN-α regimen	Outcome
ECOG EST 1684[212] n = 280 IIB–IIIB	20 MU/m² IV 5 days per week for 4 weeks (induction) 10 MU/m² SC, tiw for 48 weeks (maintenance) *versus* observation	Significant DFS benefit (5-yr RFS: IFN, 37%; obs, 26%) Significant OS benefit (5-yr OS rate: IFN, 46%; obs, 37%) At 10 years: no OS benefit
NCCTG 83-7052[213] n = 262 T > 1.7 mm N0M0 TxN1-2M0	20 MU/m² IM, tiw for 3 months *versus* observation	No significant difference in DFS or OS
WHO-16[214] n = 427 TxN1-2M0	3 MU SC, tiw for 3 years *versus* observation	No significant difference in DFS or OS
EORTC 18871 n = 830 T > 3 mm N0M0 TxN1-2M0[201]	1 MU IFNα-2b SC on alternate days *or* IFN-gamma SC on alternate days *or* Iscador *or* observation	No significant difference in DFS or OS
ECOG 1694 n = 642 IIB–IIIB[216]	20 MU/m² IV 5 days per week for 4 weeks (induction) 10 MU/m² SC tiw for 48 weeks (maintenance) *versus* vaccination with GM2-KLH/QS-21 (2 years)	No observation arm Early unblinding at 1.3 years follow-up HDI significant impact on DFS and OS at early analysis
EORTC-MCG Trial 18952 n = 1418 IIB–III	Arm A and Arm B: induction therapy with IFN-2b, 10 MU, SC, 5 d/week, for 4 weeks *followed by*: maintenance therapy Arm A: 10 MU, SC, tiw, 1 year Arm B: 5 MU, SC, tiw, 2 years Arm C: Observation	First analysis at end of 1999 at 1.5 years follow-up Significant impact on distant metastasis free interval (DMFI) for 2-year treatment arm B p = 0.145 at early analysis
French MCG[218] n = 499 IIA–IIB	3 MU SC tiw for 18 months *versus* Observation	Significant DFS benefit: Trend for OS IFN, 100 pts; Obs., 119 pts: IFNα-2a, 43%; Obs., 51 %
Austrian MCG[217] n = 311 IIA–IIB	3 MU SC daily for first 3 weeks and 3 tiw for 11 months *versus* observation	Significant DFS benefit: IFN 37 pts (24%); observation 57 pts (57%) No OS benefit (too early for analysis)

OS, overall survival; DES, disease-free survival; RFS, relapse-free survival; Obs, observation; tiw, three times per week; SC, subcutaneously; IM, intramuscularly; IV, intravenously.

In only one rather small trial comprising 280 patients (ECOG 1684), was a significant benefit on DFS and OS observed after high-dose IFN treatment (HDI) with IFN-2α for 1 year; treatment consisted of 4 weeks of a daily intravenous administration of 20 MU/m², followed by 48 weeks of 10 MU/m², subcutaneously, three times a week.[212] In the NCCTG trial (262 patients) it was demonstrated that the same high dose when administered intramuscularly, three times a week for only 12 weeks, gave no significant impact on survival in this mixed population of stage II patients with primaries thicker than 1.7 mm and patients with stage III melanoma.[213] Both HDI regimens were associated with significant grade III–IV toxicity in about 75 per cent of the patients, requiring dose reductions and interruptions of the treatment schedules.

Low-dose IFN-α treatment (LDI) was evaluated in the WHO-16 trial. In this trial 427 patients with stage III melanoma were evaluated after randomization into either the observation arm or the LDI-treatment arm (3 MU, subcutaneously, three times per week, for 3 years). Although a temporary effect on DFS was observed in the treatment arm, in the final analysis no DFS or OS benefit was observed

in this WHO-16 trial.[214] Another low-dose IFN regimen (1 MU, subcutaneously, on alternative days for 1 year) was evaluated in the EORTC-18871 trial, which showed no trend for a benefit.[201] Unfortunately the impact on overall survival by high-dose IFN therapy was not confirmed by the ECOG 1690 study, in spite of a significant benefit on DFS.[215] Low-dose IFN treatment at 3 MU for 2 years in the ECOG 1690 trial did not demonstrate a benefit for either DFS or OS, just as in the WHO-16 trial. Overall, it can be stated that observations have been inconsistent on the efficacy of IFN-α in the adjuvant treatment setting for high-risk melanoma. Dose intensity as well as duration of treatment are not clearly defined, and the efficacy of any regimen has yet to be demonstrated or confirmed by more than one trial. The largest trial by far in high-risk patients with melanoma (stage IIB–III) is the EORTC 18952 trial in 1418 patients. This trial evaluates the impact of intermediate doses of IFN where an induction period (of 4 weeks, 5 days per week, 10 MU subcutaneously) is followed by a maintenance period of 10 MU subcutaneously, three times per week, for 1 year versus 5 MU, subcutaneously, three times per week, for 2 years, versus observation.

This trial will be analysed in the autumn of the year 2000. Table 7 summarizes the experience with IFN in adjuvant phase III trials up to 2000.

Immature data from the Intergroup trial 1694 in the United States and from the EORTC 18952 trial have recently been reported. These data should be interpreted with caution as the median follow-up for the reports of these trials were 1.3 years for the 1694 and 1.5 years for the 18952 trial.

The Intergroup 1694 trial was unblinded early and reported early[286] because of a significant difference for DFS as well as OS between the HDI arm and the GM2-vaccine arm in 880 randomized stage IIB-III patients. Whether these differences in survival will continue to be significant must be awaited, especially in the light of the the ECOG 1690 experience. The EORTC 18952 first analysis will be reported at the 37th Annual Meeting of ASCO. A significant impact on the primary endpoint of distant metastasis-free interval (DFMI) will be reported with respect to the 2-years treatment arm ($p = 0.145$).[287] Again these data should be interpreted with greatest caution as many 'early positive reports' have seen the light in the history of phase III trials.

Phase III trials in intermediate-risk melanoma stage IIA–IIB

In patients with stage II primary melanomas more than 1.5 mm, clinically node-negative, three trials in Europe have completed accrual. The trials are similar in design, all using IFN-2a at low doses of 3 MU for 6 months (Scottish Trial),[216] 12 months (Austrian Trial),[217] or 18 months (French Trial).[218] A preliminary report on the Scottish trial has not demonstrated a benefit in disease-free survival or overall survival,[216] whereas, in the Austrian study, 12 months' treatment has been reported to result in a significant benefit on relapse rate.[217] The Austrian study has not reached maturity and so far no significant impact on overall survival has been observed. The French trial has reached maturity and a significantly prolonged DFS was observed in the IFN-arm. The impact on overall survival failed to reach significance but demonstrated a favourable trend.[218] The NCCTG trial, which evaluated the impact of high-dose IFN, intramuscularly, three times per week for 3 months, was negative both for DFS and OS in the stage II population of this mixed stage II–III trial.[213] Moreover, both ECOG 1684 and ECOG 1690 did not show a significant impact of HDI on DFS or OS in the stage IIB population of these trials.[212],[215] In the ECOG 1690 trial, no effect on DFS or OS was observed in the LDI arm for the stage IIB patients. Also in the EORTC/DKG-80 trial, the very low dose of 1 MU, subcutaneously, three times per week for 1 year, yielded no impact on DFS or OS in the stage II patients in this trial. So, in review, we can state that, in patients with stage II melanoma, in only two trials was an impact of IFN on DFS observed, whereas in three other low-dose trials as well as in three high-dose trials this has not been the case. In not a single trial has a significant benefit on OS been reported.

Overall the data on the impact of treatment with IFN are still unclear, especially whether the treatment will have any sizeable effect on overall survival. The EORTC-Melanoma Cooperative Group has preferred to investigate a treatment option with considerable less side-effects in this stage II patient population, which, as a consequence of the increasing use of SN staging, will be transformed into a population with a much better prognosis and lower risk for relapse. The prognosis in SN-negative patients is so excellent that it will no longer justify (even the evaluation of) toxic adjuvant therapy.[180],[216]

Hence, in the EORTC-18961 trial, comprising 1300 patients, the efficacy of vaccination with the ganglioside vaccine GM2-KLH/QS-21 will be compared to the outcome in patients receiving standard care (observation).[216]

Ongoing and future trials (Table 8)

On the basis of the results with IFN in stage II patients, and on the basis of the observation of a rebound in relapse rates in the IFN-treated patients in a number of trials (WHO-16 trial in stage III, French trial in stage II), the hypothesis has been raised that IFN needs to be administered for very long periods to be effective. This hypothesis is also based on the antiangiogenic mode of action of IFN, as demonstrated by Fidler and others.[219],[220]

The EORTC-Melanoma Cooperative Group will evaluate the effects of long-term interferon therapy compared with standard care (observation) in patients with stage III melanoma. Long-term therapy has two prerequisites: low toxicity and easy administration. Therefore a pegylated form[221] of interferon-α (Peg-Intron) will be evaluated, as this agent needs only to be administered subcutaneously once a week, for a total treatment period of 5 years. Roughly 50 per cent of the total population of about 900 patients are expected to enter the trial as patients with microscopic metastatic involvement of regional lymph node(s), as a consequence of the steady increase in SN-mapping. The other 50 per cent will be patients with clinically overt (palpable) regional node involvement after node dissection.

At present, the ECOG (1694 trial) is evaluating the GM2-KLH/QS-2 1 vaccine in patients with stage IIB–III disease. In this trial 851 patients are randomized into either HDI (ECOG 1684 schedule) or the vaccine arm. The ECOG in trial 1697 is evaluating the impact of 4 weeks of IFN, 20 MU/m^2, intravenously, for 4 weeks versus observation in 1420 patients. These huge numbers of patients are necessary because of the tremendous impact of SN-mapping and the excellent prognosis of SN-negative patients. In the United States, two more very large adjuvant trials are ongoing. The Sunbelt trial is evaluating the impact of SN-staging and the use of RT-PCR methods on SN evaluation, and HDI (ECOG 1684 schedule) in a multiarm trial in 3000 patients.[222] Morton's Polyvalent Melanoma-cell Vaccine (PMV), a melanoma cell line-based vaccine that so far has only been studied in uncontrolled trials,[223],[224] is now being evaluated in a large multicentre trial comprising 750 patients with stage III disease—BCG + PMV treatment will be compared to treatment with BCG alone.

Stage IV melanoma (distant metastases)

Site and pattern of metastases

In principle, metastatic lesions can be found in every tissue. Predominant sites (Table 9) are: skin, subcutaneous tissue, lymph nodes; lungs; liver; brain; and bone.[225] The frequency of mucosal involvement, especially in the gastrointestinal tract, is difficult to assess, but is higher than clinically evident. Most of the distant tumour deposits can be identified by careful clinical examination, chest radiographs, and abdominal ultrasound; although CT or MRI imaging of the brain, thorax, and abdomen and radionuclide bone scintigraphy

Table 8 Large ongoing and future phase III trials in stage IIA–IIB or IIB–III melanoma

Study	IFN-α regimen	Remarks
Stage III		
EORTC 18991	PEG-IFN-α$_{2b}$ for 5 years SC, once a week	Observation arm
Stage III	(first 8 weeks at 6.0 µg/kg, remaining period at 3.0 µg/kg	in Stage III
n = 900	*versus* observation	
JWCI	BCG + polyvalent melanoma vaccine	Observation arm
Stage III	*versus*	(BCG + placebo to be regarded as 'no
n = 750	BCG + placebo	treatment arm')
Stage II		
ECOG 1697	IFN-α$_{2b}$, IV, 5 days a week for 4 weeks	Large numbers in Stage II
Stage IIA	*versus*	
n = 1420	Observation	
EORTC 18961	GM2-KLH/QS-21 vaccination for 3 years	Large numbers in Stage II
n = 1300	*versus*	
IIA-IIB	Observation	
Stage I-II-III		
Sunbelt Trial	In clinically node negative patients with primary melanoma>1.0 mm	Multiple arms
n = 3000	If SN negative (H&E, IHC, and PCR negative): observation	Will answer impact,
Stage I-II-III	If SN positive (H&E, IHC, and PCR positive): CLND + high dose IFN	of SN-mapping, SN-PCR, CLND, and of
	If SN-only 1 node positive: CLND alone *versus* CLND + high dose IFN	HDI if only very limited SN involvement
	If SN-only PCR positive: observation *versus* CLND *versus* CLND + high dose IFN	

SC, subcutaneously; IV, intravenously; H&E, haematoxylin and eosin staining; IHC, immunohistochemistry; PCR, polymerase chain reaction.

Table 9 Common distant sites of metastatic melanoma*

Site	Clinical series* (%)	Autopsy series* (%)
Skin, subcutaneous, lymph nodes	42–59	50–75
Lungs	18–36	70–87
Liver	14–20	54–77
Brain	12–20	36–54
Bone	11–17	23–49
Gastrointestinal tract	1–7	26–58

Adapted with permission from Balch CM, Milton GW. Diagnosis of metastatic melanoma at distant sites. In *Cutaneous melanoma: clinical management and treatment results world-wide* (ed. CM Balch, GW Milton). Philadelphia: JB Lippincott, 1985: 221.

may reveal many more sites of asymptomatic disease manifestations. Therefore, the latter investigations are required for inclusion in most systemic treatment trials.

Prognostic factors

Several reports are available describing multifactorial analyses of possible prognostic factors for the survival of patients with a stage IV melanoma. Of the larger analyses, three investigated patients with melanoma regardless of their treatment,[226]–[228] whereas one investigation included only patients treated with interferons[229] and another, only patients with high-dose IL-2-based regimens.[230] The

results of the three largest analyses are summarized in Table 10. The most consistent independent prognostic factors for survival are the site of metastatic lesions and/or number of metastatic sites, serum LDH, and performance status. One investigation revealed that serum LDH and the number of metastatic lesions are related, and that the additive informative value of serum LDH is highest in patients with the lowest number of metastatic sites and vice versa.

Although it is possible to predict the probability with which a given patient should respond to chemotherapy or cytokine treatment, there is no consensus on how to base treatment decisions on prognostic factors in patients with distant melanoma metastases. Currently, the prognostic factors can safely be used in counselling patients with metastatic disease, and as stratification factors for randomized trials.

The survival data of the larger reports on the multifactorial evaluation of prognostic factors are summarized in Table 11. One analysis suggested treatment modality as a prognostic factor for survival, describing improved survival if IFN-α was added to high-dose IL-2 and a further trend for improvement by adding chemotherapy. These hypotheses need to be tested in randomized trials. The other reports did not indicate a relationship between the type of treatment (chemotherapy or interferon alone) and survival. The survival rates in reports on chemotherapies and interferons are below 10 per cent 2 years after the detection of distant metastases and below 2 per cent after 5 years. The report by Barth and colleagues[228] describe somewhat higher survival rates. However, it has to be taken into account that this patient series contains a high percentage of patients who were referred to a large clinical centre for surgical resection of single distant metastases, which may have led to a positively selected patient population. The survival rates in the study investigating patients on high-dose IL-2-based treatment programmes

Table 10 Independent prognostic factors for patients with stage IV melanoma; results of three multifactorial analyses

Ref. n Treatment	Balch et al.[226] 198 Various	Barth et al.[228] 1521 Various	Keilholz et al.[230] 631 IL-2 based
Performance status	n.r.	n.r.	+
Site of metastases	+	+	+
Number of sites	+	n.r.	+
Serum LDH	n.r.	n.r.	+
Interval from diagnosis to distant metastases	+	+	n.r.
Age	−	−	−
Gender	−	−	−
Treatment modality	−	−	+

n.r., not reported.

Table 11 Survival analysis for patients with advanced melanoma

First author	No. of assessable patients	Treatment	Median survival (months)	Survival rate (%) at:		
				1 year	2 year	5 year
Balch[226]	198	Various	6	−	8	2
Ahmann[227]	503	Chemotherapy	−	−	9	2
Creagan[229]	191	Interferons	6	24	9	2
Barth[228]*	1521	Various	7.5	32	14	6
Keilholz[230]	631	IL-2-based	10.5	41.2	19.9	10.4

*Patient collection not based on intent to treat.

are higher in comparison to all other reports. This may be a consequence of treatment and/or a consequence of patient selection for IL-2-based treatment regimens. Current randomized trials are addressing this question.

Surgery of distant metastases

Numerous patients present with a limited number of distant metastases in skin, subcutaneous tissue, and clinically assessable lymph nodes. In this patient population, simple surgical excision of tumour lesions may offer quick and sometimes long-lasting palliation (Table 12). Whether this type of surgery has an impact on the time until further recurrences or on the length of survival has not been proven in comparative trials (see above).

The presentation with single visceral metastases amenable for surgical excision is rare in patients with melanoma. Several clinical series report prolonged recurrence-free survival rates for patients in whom single visceral metastases were resected. Comparative studies proving an effect of the surgical removal of visceral metastases on

time to progression and on survival are not available and are difficult to perform.

Due to the very limited data available, surgical excision of distant melanoma metastases should be reserved for carefully selected patients. Easily accessible lesions can be simply excised if they are disturbing for the patient or for palliative reasons. If visceral metastases are accessible only by major surgery, a thorough evaluation of the patient has to be completed to exclude other asymptomatic tumour manifestations. Observation for several weeks, or even months, is a useful strategy for further patient selection. If during this observation period additional tumour lesions emerge, local treatment options are of limited value, and major surgery is not indicated; whereas patients who do not develop further visible tumour lesions during this observation period may be better candidates for visceral surgery. Of course this 'wait-and-watch' strategy can only be applied for patients with asymptomatic tumour lesions.

Another, perhaps more promising, strategy in patients with a limited number of distant metastases is to await the results of systemic

Table 12 Median survival of melanoma patients after complete surgical resection of distant metastases

Site	Survival in months (no. patients)			
	M.D. Anderson Cancer Center	Memorial Hospital	University of Alabama Hospitals	Roswell Park Institute
Skin, subcutaneous	23 (64)	25 (12)	17 (13)	31 (25)
Lung	16 (26)	19 (17)	9 (17)	9 (13)
Brain	15 (16)	7.5 (5)	8 (17)	5 (4)
Gastrointestinal (excluding liver)	18 (9)	15 (12)	8 (5)	8 (3)
Overall 2-year survival rate	15%	21%	16%	31%

*Table taken with permission from DeVita VT Jr, Hellman S, Rosenberg SA (ed.). *Cancer: principles and practice of oncology* (5th edn). Philadelphia: Lippincott-Raven, 1997.[231]

treatment and reconsider the patient for surgery if at least a minor response has been achieved. This empirical approach will limit major surgery to patients with melanomas that are principally responsive to systemic treatment, which is associated with a better long-term prognosis.

Radiation treatment

Melanoma is rather radiation-resistant. Reasonable response rates have only been obtained with the use of larger radiation doses per fraction than the normal 2 Gy given five times per week in conventional radiation therapy.[232] Consequently, irradiation of melanoma metastases is useful only if they are located in rather radiation-resistant tissue. Organ sites most amenable for palliative radiation treatment are therefore the brain and bones.

However, there are no larger prospective studies available on the results of the irradiation of bone lesions. Because of the limited toxicity and discomfort for the patient, the irradiation of bone lesions, which puts a patient at risk for fracture, should be performed if the patient's prognosis is not limited by disease evolution in other sites.

Basically, the prognosis of patients with melanoma brain metastases is poor. Until the late-1980s the strategy has been to administer whole-brain irradiation when handling multiple metastatic sites and to offer surgical excision for single accessible metastases. The availability of stereotactic irradiation has changed this approach. There are several reports describing excellent palliative results in patients with stereotactic irradiation of single or few brain metastases.[233] Because of its high response rate, stereotactic irradiation of brain metastases is sometimes termed radiosurgery. Another advantage of stereotactic irradiation for the patient is that the total dose can be delivered in a single treatment. It is currently unclear whether stereotactic irradiation of a limited number of cerebral metastases should be followed by adjuvant whole-brain irradiation to prevent outgrowth of micrometastases.[234]

Chemotherapy

Melanoma is characterized by its poor responsiveness to cytotoxic agents. Active agents are summarized in Table 13. None of these compounds have reproducibly produced response rates exceeding 20 per cent in patients with advanced melanoma. Since there is no study indicating a survival benefit from the use of any of these drugs, the chemotherapy of advanced melanoma should be regarded as palliative.

Single-agent chemotherapy

DTIC Dacarbazine (DTIC) is the best-studied single agent used for the treatment of melanoma. This non-classical alkylating agent must be administered intravenously and is metabolically transformed in the liver to mitozolomide, the active metabolite. The response rate of up to 20 per cent has led to the licensing of this compound for the treatment of advanced melanoma in many countries. Patients with skin, subcutaneous tissue, and lymph node metastases respond more frequently than patients with visceral metastases.[245],[246] The median duration of response is approximately 6 months in patients continuing treatment. Complete responses are rare and usually confined to subcutaneous and lymph node metastases. The 5-year survival rate in patients with advanced melanoma treated with dacarbazine is approximately 2 per cent.[226],[227]

The mostly used treatment schedule is the administration of 850 to 1000 mg/m^2 on a single day every 3 to 4 weeks, **or** 250 mg/m^2 per day for 5 consecutive days every 3 weeks. The predominant acute side-effect of this drug is severe nausea. The introduction of 5-HT3 antagonists for the treatment of nausea has considerably eased the use of DTIC. Haematological toxicity is mild, and neutropenic fever rarely develops. Because of the high tolerability, DTIC is today still the preferred cytotoxic agent for patients with melanoma treated outside of clinical trials.

Temozolomide Temozolomide is 100 per cent absorbed after oral administration and can also be administered intravenously. This compound is spontaneously converted *in vivo* to mitozolomide, also the active metabolite of DTIC. In contrast to DTIC, temozolomide crosses the blood–brain barrier, thereby having efficacy in brain metastases.[247] A recent randomized trial comparing DTIC and temozolomide in patients with advanced melanoma did not show a significant survival difference between these two agents, but suggested a trend towards a lower frequency of cerebral metastatic development during or following temozolomide treatment.[240] The ease of application and the potential efficacy of temozolomide in the brain may lead to the preferred use of this agent instead of DTIC in the future.

Table 13 Randomized trials of chemotherapy in advanced melanoma: various cytotoxic agents, tamoxifen

Reference	Regimen	n	RR (%)	CR (%)	Median time to progression (months)	Median survival (months)
Various cytotoxic agents						
Wittes 1978[235]	D/cyclophosphamide	29	24	7	n.r.	5.5
	D/V	34	18	6	n.r.	5.0
	D/procarbazine	32	13	0	n.r.	3.0
Costanzi 1982[236]	(a) BCNU/hydroxyurea/D	95	31	9	n.r.	5.0
	(b) BCNU/hydroxyurea/D/	161	27	12	n.r.	6.9
	BCG	130	18	7	n.r.	7.1
	(c) D/BCG		$p(a{:}c) = 0.04$			n.s.
			$p(b{:}c) = 0.05$			
Luikart 1984[237]	D	28	14	7	2.0	4.2
	V/C/bleomycin	41	10	0	2.0	3.6
Buzaid 1993[238]	D	45	11	0	n.r.	n.r.
	C/V/D	46	24	0	n.r.	n.r.
Jungnelius 1998[239]	D/V	165	21	10	2.2	5.9
	D/V/C	161	31	16	4.2	7.2
			n.s.	n.s.	$p = 0.0068$	$p = 0.22$
Middleton, ASCO 1999[240]	D	149	12.1	n.r.	1.5	5.7
	Temozolomide	156	13.5	n.r.	1.9	7.9
					$p = 0.012$	$p = 0.06$
Tamoxifen						
Cocconi 1992[241]	D	52	12	6	n.r.	6
	D/T	60	28	7	n.r.	11
			$p = 0.03$	n.s.		$p = 0.02$
Rusthoven 1996[242]	Carmustine/D/C	100	21	6	3	6
	Carmustine/D/C/T	104	30	3	3	6
			$p = 0.187$	$p = 0.33$	$p = 0.86$	$p = 0.52$
Agarwala 1999[243]	C/D	28	11	4	n.r.	7.0
	C/D/T	28	14	4	n.r.	4.6
						n.s.
Saxman 1999[244]	D	120	9.9	n.r.	n.r.	6.3
	D/C/T/BCNU	120	16.8	n.r.	n.r.	7.7

Abbreviations: CR, complete response; RR response rate; D, dacarbazine; C, cisplatin; V, vinblastine; T, tamoxifen; n.r., not reported; n.s., not significant.

Cisplatin Cisplatin[248]–[250] and the sister compound carboplatin[251] are further active drugs used for the treatment of advanced melanoma. Most investigators feel that cisplatin is more active than carboplatin, although there are no comparative investigations. The association of cisplatin with severe nausea and renal toxicity has limited its use as a palliative agent. In most treatment protocols, 100 mg/m² of cisplatin is administered every 3 to 4 weeks, either as a single dose or divided over 3 days.

The concomitant administration of amifostine to cisplatin has been shown to decrease renal toxicity, haemotoxicity, and neurotoxicity (which may become permanent with the prolonged use of cisplatin). Two studies have shown that higher doses of cisplatin can be administered to patients with melanoma if coadministered with amifostine. One study used up to 150 mg/m² cisplatin,[252] while another study investigated 100 mg/m² cisplatin administered on day

1 and day 8 of a 4-week cycle.[253] Both studies used 740 mg/m² of amifostine. It may be possible to increase the response rate obtained by cisplatin with this modification; however, the subjective toxicity remains high and the response duration is usually brief. An alternative cisplatin schedule includes weekly 50 to 80 mg/m² administration.[254] This dose can be administered without vigorous hyperhydration and is associated with less subjective toxicity; however, clinical experience of this regimen in the treatment of melanoma is limited.

Nitrosureas Nitrosureas are another group of active cytotoxic agents in melanoma. Response rates vary between 10 per cent and 20 per cent. The most interesting nitrosurea is fotemustine because it penetrates the blood–brain barrier. Fotemustine does not yield an advantage over DTIC or cisplatin in terms of response rate, but it has been found to be additionally active in brain metastases.[247],[255] The major problematic side-effect of fotemustine (and the other nitrosureas) is prolonged and cumulative haemotoxicity. The subjective toxicity of this group of compounds is low.

Fotemustine and the other nitrosureas have to be administered intravenously. A typical administration schedule of fotemustine is an introduction period of 100 mg/m² weekly for 4 consecutive weeks, followed by a pause of 5 weeks, followed by the subsequent administration of 100 mg/m² every 4 weeks, if not prohibited by haemotoxicity.

Treosulfan Treosulfan, a non-classical alkylating agent used for decades for the treatment of ovarian carcinoma, has recently been found to be active as a single agent *in vitro* and *in vivo* in melanoma.[256] Treosulfan can be administered orally and intravenously; it is associated with few subjective side-effects, mild haemotoxicity, and basically no other toxicity. This toxicity profile makes treosulfan an interesting agent for further studies.

Taxanes Among the new generation of cytotoxic compounds, only taxanes have been shown to have activity against melanoma in small phase II trials. However, the response rates obtained for both compounds, docetaxel and paclitaxel, as single agents have been below 20 per cent.

Combination chemotherapies (Table 14)

There are numerous phase II studies suggesting that the response rate that can be achieved with combination chemotherapies exceeds the response rate of single-agent chemotherapy. This is probably true, although only supported by relatively few, and mostly small-sized, randomized investigations. However, in all these investigations, the rate of complete responses was low, and the objective response rate (partial and complete responses) usually ranged between 10 per cent and 30 per cent. It has to be further taken into account that the early studies used the old WHO criteria for response assessment, which did not require confirmation of an objective remission by two independent investigations at least 4 weeks apart. Therefore, the old studies contain a fraction of responses that would not qualify for an objective remission in the newer studies. Using the new response criteria, the improvement in objective response rates by combination chemotherapies in comparison to single-agent treatment (usually dacarbazine) is modest at best.

In most of the studies dacarbazine was administered to all patients, and various agents were additionally administered. Among the other agents, cisplatin most consistently increased the response rate. Conversely, there is no study evaluating whether the inclusion of DTIC in combination chemotherapies impacts on the response rate.

The ability of tamoxifen to improve the outcome of patients receiving chemotherapies for advanced melanoma has been extensively studied. This attention arose out of evidence from phase I and phase II trials that the addition of tamoxifen, especially to cisplatin-based treatment regimens, may increase the efficacy of chemotherapy. In one small Italian randomized trial, the addition of tamoxifen to dacarbazine actually did significantly increase the response rate; however, this effect could not be duplicated in any other comparative study.[241]

In most trials there is, considering the lack of efficacious combination chemotherapies, no rigid evaluation of the time to progression. However, in one trial a significant increase in time to progression was shown with the combination of dacarbazine, vinblastine, and cisplatin in comparison to the combination of dacarbazine and vinblastine alone.[239]

The major dampening of all enthusiasm for using combination chemotherapies in patients with advanced melanoma is the drawback that none of these studies have suggested any impact on survival. Thus, combination chemotherapy cannot be used as an accepted standard treatment for advanced melanoma. In most trials, dacarbazine is used as the standard treatment arm. However, the use of dacarbazine is only justified by its history and modest toxicity, and not by any study suggesting an impact of dacarbazine on time to progression or survival.

In conclusion, chemotherapy of advanced melanoma should be regarded as purely palliative, with a low rate of objective responses and without proof of survival benefit. As evident from several large analyses, most responses to chemotherapy are not durable, the expected 2-year survival rate is below 10 per cent, and only very few patients will survive more than 5 years.

Cytokines

The frequent observation of regression zones in primary melanoma, histologically characterized by heavy lymphocytic infiltrate, and the rare observation of spontaneous regression in metastatic disease have fuelled studies on immunological treatment approaches to melanoma for decades. For metastatic melanoma, the cytokines IFN-α and IL-2 are most extensively investigated (Table 15). Because of insufficient clinical data, other cytokines will not be discussed in this chapter.

IFN-α

IFN-α has been extensively studied for the adjuvant treatment of primary melanoma (see above), whereas only few small studies have reported on its use as a single agent the treatment of advanced metastatic disease. In these studies, various treatment regimens of IFN-α have produced some objective responses, serving as a basis for inclusion of IFN-α in combination therapies.

IL-2

IL-2 is a potent immunostimulatory agent with direct effects on T lymphocytes, B lymphocytes, monocytes/macrophages, and natural killer (**NK**) cells. Further indirect effects are mediated via secreted secondary cytokines on a variety of other cell types. Recombinant IL-2 has been extensively tested for its effect in the treatment of advanced melanoma. Administered as a single agent, IL-2 can produce objective responses in up to 25 per cent of patients with stage IV melanoma. This response rate is in the same order as the response rates observed with the most active cytotoxic agents; however, a considerable fraction of IL-2-mediated responses will be long-lasting, unlike most responses achieved with cytotoxic drugs. As a consequence of its ability to induce durable results, IL-2 has been licensed for use in advanced melanoma in some countries.

A variety of treatment regimens have been used. The four most widely tested regimens are:

(I) administration of repeated bolus injections every 8 h for a maximum of 5 days;

(II) continuous intravenous infusion for 5 days;

Table 14 Randomized trials of chemotherapy in advanced melanoma: IFN-α, IFN-α/IL-2, chemotherapy

Reference	Regimen	n	RR (%)	CR (%)	Median time to progression (months)	Median survival (months)
IFN-α						
Falkson 1991[257]	D	32	20	6	2.53	9.6
	D/IFN-α	32	53	35	8.96	17.6
			p = 0.007		p < 0.01	p < 0.01
Thomsom 1993[258]	D	83	17	2	n.r.	8.8
	D/IFN-α	87	21	7	n.r.	7.5
Bajetta 1994[259]	(a) D	82	20	5	3	11
	(b) D/IFN-α: 9 MIU, 3 × /wk	76	28	8	7.6	13
	(c) D/IFN-α: 3 MIU, 3 × /wk	84	23	7	5.5	11
					p(a:b) = 0.02	
					p(a:c) = 0.09	
Falkson 1998[260]	D	66	15	2	2.3	10.0
	D/IFN-α	60	21	6	3.0	9.3
	D/T	62	18	2	1.9	8.0
	D/IFN-α/T	62	19	3	2.6	9.5
Sparano 1993[261]	IL-2	44	5	0	n.r.	10.2
	IL-2/IFN-α	41	10	0	n.r.	9.7
Dorval 1999[262]	C/IL-2	57	16	6	n.r.	10.4
	C/IL-2/IFN-α	60	25	3	n.r.	10.6
			n.s.			n.s.
IFN-α/IL-2						
Johnston 1998[263]	BCNU/D/C/T	30	27	0	3	5.5
	BCNU/D/C/T/ IFN-α/IL-2	35	22	2	2	5.0
Rosenberg 1999[264]	C/D/T	52	27	8	n.r.	15.8
	C/D/T/IFN-α/IL-2	50	44	6	n.r.	10.7
			p = 0.071			p = 0.052
Chemotherapy						
Keilholz 1997[265]	IFN-α/IL-2	66	18		1.7	9.2
	IFN-α/IL-2/C	60	33		3.0	9.2
			p = 0.04		0.02	n.s.

Abbreviations: CR, complete response; RR response rate; D, dacarbazine; C, cisplatin; V, vinblastine; T, tamoxifen; n.r., not reported; n.s., not significant.

(III) a 'decrescendo' schedule of continuous intravenous infusion starting with a high initial dose, which is tapered in a stepwise fashion to a low maintenance dose; and

(IV) intermittent or prolonged subcutaneous applications of a variety of doses (Box 1).

All these regimens have now been included into combination therapies, but there is no comparative study available of two or more of the different regimens.

Combination immunotherapy

The rationale of combining IL-2 and IFN-α is based on *in vitro* observations, where IFN-α upregulates the expression of HLA class I molecules in tumour cells and synergizes with IL-2 in activating immunological effector cells. In larger phase II studies, the objective response rates of the combination treatment was between 11 per cent and 41 per cent.[276]–[278] However, the role of IFN-α in addition to IL-2 was never proven. The only randomized trial investigating IL-2

alone versus IL-2 plus IFN-α was terminated because of low response rates in both treatment arms; in this study, a rather low dose of IL-2 had been administered.[261] With respect to single-agent IL-2, a proportion of patients was observed with durable remissions in most other trials.

To investigate the role of treatment duration, two sequential studies have been carried out with either a 5-day regimen of bolus IL-2 and IFN-α or a 3-day regimen.[270] In this study, the 5-day regimen resulted in prohibitive cardiotoxicity and central nervous system toxicity. The 3-day regimen was associated with manageable toxicity. However, the response rate of the 5-day regimen was substantially higher (41 per cent) than the 3-day regimen (20 per cent).

The addition of IFN-α to a continuous intravenous infusion of IL-2, however, does not significantly increase toxicity, and the response rates range from 10 per cent to 20 per cent. A higher response rate of 41 per cent was observed with the combination of a 'decrescendo' IL-2 regimen and IFN-α.[269]

Table 15

Reference	IL-2 administration and concomitant treatment	No. of patients	Response rate (%)
IL-2 only[266],[267],[268] (7 trials 1989–1996)	ivb or civ	265	range 3–24
IL-2 + IFN-α Keilholz 1993[269]	(a) civ + IFN-α	27	18
	(b) descrescendo + IFN-α	27	41
Sparano 1993*[261]	ivb (reduced dose) + IFN-α	41	10
Kruit 1996[270]	(a) ivb + IFN-α (5 days)	17	41
	(b) ivb + IFN-α (3 days)	25	20
Keilholz 1997*[265]	descrescendo + IFN-α	66	18
IL-2 + chemotherapy Flaherty 1990[271]	civ + D 1 g/m²	32	22
Dummer 1995[272]	civ + D 850 mg/m²	57	25
Demchak 1991[273]	ivb, + C 150 mg/m²	27	37
Flaherty 1993[274]	sc + C + D	27	41
Atkins 1994[275]	ivb + T, C + D	38	42
IL-2 + IFN-α + chemotherapy Richards 1992[276]	ivb + IFN-α + C + D + BCNU + T	74	57
Khayat 1993[277]	civ + IFN-α + C + T	39	54
Buzaid 1994[278]	ivb + IFN-α + C + D	151	54
Keilholz 1997*[265]	descrescendo + IFN-α + C	60	33

Abbreviations: ivb, intravenous bolus; civ, continuous intravenous infusion; sc, subcutaneous; D, dacarbazine; C, cisplatin; T, tamoxifen. *Randomized study.

Box 1 High-dose IL-2 regimens with confirmed activity in advanced melanoma

I *High-dose bolus application*
720 000 IU/kg IV over 15 min repeated every 8 h for a maximum of 5 days

II *Continuous infusion*
18×10^6 IU/m² per 24 h for 5 days

III *'Decrescendo' schedule*
18×106 IU/m² over 6 h   immediately followed by:
18×106 IU/m² over 12 h   immediately followed by:
18×106 IU/m² over 24 h   immediately followed by:
13.5×106 IU/m² over 72 h .

IV *Intermittent or prolonged SC administration*
of a variety of doses

Chemotherapy, cytokine combinations: chemoimmunotherapy

Response rates exceeding 50 per cent were achieved in several phase II trials combining cytotoxic agents and IL-2 with or without IFN-α. Combinations of cytokines with single-agent chemotherapy as well as polychemotherapy have been tested. Comparing all published phase II data, it is apparent that with regimens containing the three drugs—cisplatin, IFNα and IL-2—with or without further agents, the response rates were consistently above 50 per cent. These observations prompted several phase III trials investigating the effects of various chemoimmunotherapy components.

EORTC-database

To develop solid hypotheses for designing phase III trials, the EORTC collected a database on higher dose IL-2-based treatments with the emphasis on the long-term results of patients with melanoma who had received IL-2 alone, in combination with IFN-α, or with cytotoxic drugs. Response and survival data are summarized in Table 16. The basic results of this database are that the addition of cytotoxic agents to cytokines doubled the response rate, and the addition of IFN-α to IL-2 was associated with a prolonged overall survival; there was a trend towards an additional effect of chemotherapy on overall survival, this was, however, not significant. The survival rate of 23 per cent at 2 years and 13 per cent at 5 years contrast with earlier similar analyses of patients receiving chemotherapy or interferons without IL-2.

Table 16 EORTC database: response rates of different treatment modalities

Treatment	CR + PR (%)	95% CI	p
IL-2 only	14.9	8.9–22.8	
IL-2 + ct	20.8	10.5–35.0	n.s.
IL-2 + IFN-α	23.0	16.6–30.5	n.s.
IL-2 + ct + IFN-α	44.9	39.3–50.6	< 0.001

Abbreviations: CR, complete response; PR, partial response; CI, confidence interval; ct, chemotherapy; n.s., not significant.

However, these survival data need to be prospectively evaluated in randomized trials.

Data from randomized trials

To date, only one larger randomized study has addressed the question of whether the addition of chemotherapy would improve the results of cytokine treatment. This trial was performed by the EORTC and evaluated a treatment regimen with IFN-α and 'decrescendo' IL-2 with or without a single dose of cisplatin.[265] Some 86 per cent of patients accrued into this trial had visceral metastatic disease, indicating an advanced disease stage in the majority of patients. In this trial, a response rate above 50 per cent, as reported in phase II studies, could not be confirmed. Nevertheless, the response rate doubled with the addition of cisplatin to the cytokine combination. In accordance, the median time to progression was also almost doubled by the addition of cisplatin. However, this palliative benefit did not translate into a survival benefit. The conclusion of this study is that the addition of cisplatin offers valuable palliation, but only short-term.

The results of two phase II studies are available that investigated the role of the combination of IFN-α and IL-2 in addition to chemotherapy. The first trial performed at the Royal Marsden Hospital, London, investigated a regimen of rather low doses of IL-2 and IFN-α in addition to polychemotherapy. In this study, the addition of cytokines did not affect the response rate and survival. The second trial performed at the National Cancer Institute, Bethesda, investigated the addition of IFN-α and high-dose bolus IL-2 to cisplatin, DTIC, and tamoxifen. Although the response rate increased from 27 per cent with chemotherapy alone to 44 per cent with the chemotherapy/cytokine combination, the median survival showed a trend in favour of the arm without cytokines. Taken together, these studies potentially indicate that only intensive cytokine regimens may be able to increase the response rate achieved by chemotherapy alone. This notion is confirmed by a recent, randomized, phase II study investigating different doses of IL-2 in this context, where a significant increase in response rate was observed with high-dose IL-2 as compared to a low-dose regimen.

Two larger phase III trial are currently being performed to investigate the effect of IL-2 regimens, with confirmed activity in several phase II studies, on the survival of patients with advanced melanoma. The EORTC protocol randomizes patients to receive DTIC, cisplatin, IFN-α with or without the 'decrescendo' regimen of IL-2. The ECOG is evaluating the combination of cisplatin, vinblastine, DTIC with or without IFN-α and continuous intravenous infusion of IL-2. These trials will clarify whether the addition of cytokines to chemotherapy has an impact on the survival of patients with advanced melanoma.

Before the results of the randomized co-operative group trials are known, the treatment of advanced melanoma with cytokines with or without chemotherapy should only be performed within controlled trials.

Vaccines

The development of specific melanoma vaccines is an exciting and rapidly expanding field of applied tumour immunology. The identification of melanoma antigens recognized by T lymphocytes has opened several strategies for the construction of vaccines to specifically elicit cellular immune responses. Strategies include: the use of whole melanoma cells or melanoma cell lysates as a source for a variety of possible tumour antigens; recombinant proteins or synthetic peptides to induce immune responses against specific targets; anti-idiotype monoclonal antibodies as a means of mimicking specific antigens; and so-called 'gene therapy' transducing the expression of defined melanoma antigens into antigen-presenting cells in vitro or in vivo.

Numerous phase I and small phase II trials have been performed using all these approaches; however, these studies are not reviewed in this chapter because each approach is still experimental. With the current information, it can only be concluded that all the vaccine approaches produce only minimal toxicity, and that, with most of the approaches, occasional anti-tumour responses have been observed in patients with metastatic melanoma.

The recent development of reliable assays to monitor the induction of a T cell-mediated immune response will hopefully improve our understanding of vaccination approaches.[289],[281] It is of crucial importance to clarify whether the efficacy of tumour vaccines to induce an immune response is related to the tumour load of a given patient. From our current understanding, and as indicated by animal experimental data, melanoma vaccines may be more useful in the adjuvant setting than in metastatic disease.

References

1. **Institute for Epidemiological Cancer Research.** *The cancer registry of Norway. Cancer in Norway 1996.* Oslo, 1996.

2. **Parkin DM, Whelan SL, Ferlay J, Raymond L, Young I.** *Cancer incidence in five continents,* Vol. VII. Lyon: IARC Scientific Publications, 1997: No. 143.

3. **Ries LAG, Kosary CL, Hankey BF, Miller BA, Harras A, Edwards BK (ed.).** *SEER Cancer Statistics Review, 1973–1994.* Bethesda, MD: National Cancer Institute, 1997: NIH Publ. No. 97-2789.

4. **National Cancer Institute of Canada.** *Canadian cancer statistics 1998.* Toronto, Canada: NCIC, 1998.

5. **MacKie RM et al.** Cutaneous malignant melanoma in Scotland: incidence, survival, and mortality, 1979–1994. *British Medical Journal,* 1997; **315:** 1117–21.

6. **Armstrong BK, Kricker A.** Cutaneous melanoma. *Cancer Surveys,* 1994; **19:** 219–40.

7. **Swerdlow AJ.** International trends in cutaneous melanoma. *Annals of the New York Academy of Sciences,* 1990; **609:** 235–51.

8. **Giles GG, Armstrong BK, Burton RC, Staples MP, Thursfield V.** Has mortality from melanoma stopped rising in Australia? Analysis of trends between 1931 and 1994. *British Medical Journal,* 1996; **312:** 1121–5.

9. **Roush GC, McKay L, Holford TR.** A reversal in long-term increase in deaths attributable to malignant melanoma. *Cancer,* 1992; **69:** 1714–20.

10. Scotto J, Pitcher H, Lee JAH. Indications of future decreasing trends in skin melanoma mortality among Whites in the United States. *International Journal of Cancer*, 1991; **49**: 490–7.

11. Balzi O, Carli P, Geddes M. Malignant melanoma in Europe: changes in mortality rates (1970–90) in European Community countries. *Cancer Causes and Control*, 1997; **8**: 85–92.

12. Smith JAE, Whatley PM, Redburn IC. Improving survival of melanoma patients in Europe since 1978. *European Journal of Cancer*, 1998; **34**: 2197–203.

13. Autier P, Doré IF for the EPIMEL, EORTC Melanoma Co-operative group. Influence of sun exposures during childhood and during adulthood on melanoma risk. *International Journal of Cancer*, 1998; **77**: 533–7.

14. Masbach A, Westerdahl I, Ingvar C, Olsson H, Jonsson N. Cutaneous malignant melanoma in South Sweden 1965, 1975, and 1985. *Cancer*, 1994; **73**: 1625–30.

15. Burton R, Armstrong BK. Recent incidence trends imply a non-metastasising form of invasive melanoma. *Melanoma Research*, 1994; **4**: 107–13.

16. Thörn M, Ponten F, Bergström R, Sparen P, Adami HO. Clinical and histopathological predictors of survival in patients with malignant melanoma: a population-based study in Sweden. *Journal of the National Cancer Institute*, 1994; **86**: 761–9.

17. MacKie RM, Hole H. Audit of public education campaign to encourage earlier detection of malignant melanoma. *British Medical Journal*, 1992; **304**: 1012–15.

18. Monzon I et al. CDKN2A mutations in multiple primary melanoma. *New England Journal of Medicine*, 1998; **338**: 879–87.

19. Slade J, Marghoob AA, Salopek TG, Rigel DS, Kopf AW, Bart RS. Atypical mole syndrome: risk factor for cutaneous melanoma and implications for management. *Journal of the American Academy of Dermatology*, 1995; **32**: 479–94.

20. Newton JA et al. How common is the atypical mole syndrome in apparently sporadic melanoma? *Journal of the American Academy of Dermatology*, 1993; **29**: 989–96.

21. Grob JJ et al. Count of benign melanocytic naevi as a major indicator for non- familial nodular and superficial spreading melanoma. *Cancer*, 1990; **66**: 387–95.

22. Bataille V et al. Risk of cutaneous melanoma in relation to the numbers, types and sites of naevi: a case-control study. *British Journal of Cancer*, 1996; **73**: 1605-ll.

23. Tucker MA et al. Clinically recognized dysplastic naevi. A central risk factor for cutaneous melanoma. *Journal of the American Medical Association*, 1997; **277**: 1439–44.

24. Fitzpatrick TB. The validity and practicability of sun-reactive skin types I through VI. *Archives of Dermatology*, 1988; **124**: 869–71.

25. Tucker MA, Fraser MC, Goldstein AM, Elder DE, Guerry D, Organic SM. Risk of melanoma and other cancers in melanoma-prone families. *Journal of Investigative Dermatology*, 1993; **100**: 3505–55.

26. Carey WP et al. Dysplastic naevi as a melanoma risk factor in patients with familial melanoma. *Cancer*, 1994; **74**: 3118–25.

27. Haluska FG, Hodi FS. Molecular genetics of familial cutaneous melanoma. *Journal of Clinical Oncology*, 1998; **16**: 670–82.

28. Goldstein A et al. Increased risk of pancreatic cancer in melanoma-prone kindreds with p16INK4 mutations. *New England Journal of Medicine*, 1995; **333**: 970–4.

29. Zuo L et al. Germline mutations in the p16INK4a binding domain of CDK4 in familial melanoma. *Nature Genetics*, 1996; **12**: 97–9.

30. Soufir N et al. Prevalence of p16 and CDK4 germline mutations in 48 melanoma-prone families in France. The French familial Melanoma Study Group. *Human Molecular Genetics*, 1998; **7**: 209–16.

31. Platz A et al. Screening for germline mutations in the CDKN2A and CDKN2B genes in Swedish families with hereditary cutaneous melanoma. *Journal of the National Cancer Institute*, 1997; **89**: 697–702.

32. Aitken J et al. CDKN2A variants in a population-based sample of Queensland families with melanoma. *Journal of the National Cancer Institute*, 1999; **91**: 446–52.

33. Moriwaski SI, Tarone RE, Tucker MA, Goldstein AM, Kraemer KH. Hypermutability of UV-treated plasmids in dysplastic nevus/familial melanoma cell lines. *Cancer Research*, 1997; **57**: 4637–41.

34. Sanford KK, Parshard R, Price FM, Tarone RE, Thompson I, Guerry D. Radiation-induced chromatid breaks and DNA repair in blood lymphocytes of patients with dysplastic naevi and/or cutaneous melanoma. *Journal of Investigative Dermatology*, 1997; **109**: 546–9.

35. Puig S et al. Inherited susceptibility to several cancers but absence of linkage between dysplastic nevus syndrome and CDKN2A in a melanoma family with a mutation in the CDKN2A (P16INK4A) gene. *Human Genetics*, 1997; **101**: 359–64.

36. Van der Velden PA, Sandhuijk LA, Bergman W, Hille ET, Frants RR, Gruis NA. A locus linked to p16 modifies melanoma risk in Dutch familial atypical multiple mole melanoma (FAMMM) syndrome families. *Genome Research*, 1999; **9**: 575–80.

37. Grobb JJ et al. Excess of naevi related to immunodeficiency: a study in HIV-infected patients and renal transplants recipients. *Journal of Investigative Dermatology*, 1996; **107**: 694–7.

38. International Agency for Research on Cancer. *Solar and ultraviolet radiation. Monographs on the evaluation of the carcinogenic risk of chemicals to humans.* Lyon: IARC, 1992: Vol. 55.

39. Holman CDA, Armstrong Bk. Cutaneous malignant melanoma and indicators of total accumulated exposure to the sun: an analysis separating histogenic types. *Journal of the National Cancer Institute*, 1984; **73**: 75–82.

40. Sober AL, Lew RA, Fitzpatrick TB, Marvell R. Solar exposure patterns in patients with cutaneous melanoma—a case control series. *Clinical Research*, 1979; **27**: 536A.

41. MacKie RM, Aitchison T. Severe sunburns and subsequent risk of primary cutaneous malignant melanoma in Scotland. *British Journal of Cancer*, 1982; **46**: 955–60.

42. Elwood JM, Gallagher RP, Hill GB, Pearson JCG. Cutaneous melanoma in relation to intermittent and constant sun exposure—The Western Canada Melanoma Study. *International Journal of Cancer*, 1985; **35**: 427–33.

43. Elwood M, Jopson J. Melanoma and sun exposure: an overview of published studies. *International Journal of Cancer*, 1997; **73**: 198–203.

44. Bentham G, Aase A. Incidence of malignant melanoma of the skin in Norway, 1955–89: associations with solar ultraviolet radiation, income and holidays abroad. *International Journal of Epidemiology*, 1996; **25**: 1132–8.

45. Osterlind A, Hou-Jensen K, Moller Jensen O. Incidence of cutaneous malignant melanoma in Denmark 1978–82. Anatomic site distribution, histologic types, and comparison with non-melanoma skin cancer. *British Journal of Cancer*, 1998; **58**: 385–91.

46. Bataille V et al. Solar keratoses: a risk factor for melanoma but negative association with melanocytic naevi. *International Journal of Cancer*, 1998; **78**: 8–12.

47. Green A. A theory of site distribution of melanomas: Queensland, Australia. *Cancer Causes and Control*, 1992; **3**: 513–16.

48. Green A, McCredie M, MacKie R, Giles G, Young P, Morton C. A case-control study of melanomas of the soles and palms. *Cancer Causes and Control*, 1999; **10**: 21–5.

49. Autier P et al. Melanoma and residence in sunny areas. *British Journal of Cancer*, 1997; **76**: 1521–4.

50. Woollons A et al. The 0.8 per cent ultraviolet B content of an ultraviolet A sunlamp induces 75 per cent of cyclobutane pyrimidine dimers in human keratinocytes *in vitro. British Journal of Dermatology*, 1999; **140**: 1023–30.

51. Swerdlow AJ, Weinstock MA. Do tanning lamps cause melanoma? An

epidemiologic assessment. *Journal of the American Academy of Dermatology*, 1998; **38**: 89–98.

52. Stern RS, Nichols KT, Vakeva LH. Malignant melanoma in patients treated for psoriasis with methoxsalen (psoralen) and ultraviolet A radiation (PUVA). The PUVA Follow-up Study. *New England Journal of Medicine*, 1997; **336**: 1041–5.

53. Autier P *et al.* for the EORTC Melanoma Group. Sunscreen use, wearing clothes and naevi number in 6- to 7-year-old European children. *Journal of the National Cancer Institute*, 1998; **90**: 1873–81.

54. Abadir MC, Marghoob AA, Slade I, Salopeck TG, Yadav S, Kopf AW. Case-control study of melanocytic naevi on the buttocks in atypical mole syndrome: role of solar radiation in the pathogenesis of atypical moles. *Journal of the American Academy of Dermatology*, 1995; **33**: 31–6.

55. Zhu G *et al.* A major quantitative-trait locus for mole density is linked to the familial melanoma gene CDKN2A: a maximum-likelihood combined linkage and association analysis in twins and their sibs. *American Journal of Human Genetics*, 1999; **65**: 483–92.

56. Bataille V *et al.* The association between naevi and melanoma in populations with different levels of sun exposure: a joint case-control study of melanoma in the United Kingdom and Australia. *British Journal of Cancer*, 1998; **77**: 505–10.

57. Kelly JW, Rivers JK, MacLennan R, Harrisson S, Lewis AE, Tate BI. Sunlight: a major factor associated with the development of melanocytic naevi in Australian schoolchildren. *Journal of the American Academy of Dermatology*, 1994; **30**: 40–8.

58. Fritschi L, McHenry P, Green A, MacKie R, Green L, Siskind V. Naevi in schoolchildren in Scotland and Australia. *British Journal of Dermatology*, 1994; **130**: 599–603.

59. Goldstein A *et al.* Sun-related risk factors in melanoma-prone families with CDKN2A mutations. *Journal of the National Cancer Institute*, 1998; **90**: 709–11.

60. Autier P, Doré JF, Lejeune F. Sun protection in childhood or early adolescence and reduction of melanoma risk in adults: an EORTC case-control study in Germany, Belgium and France. *International Epidemiology and Biostatistics*, 1996; **1**: 51–7.

61. Autier P *et al.* Melanoma and use of sunscreens: an EORTC case-control study in Germany, Belgium and France. *International Journal of Cancer*, 1995; **61**: 749–55.

62. Autier P *et al.* Melanoma and sunscreen use: need for studies representative of actual behaviours. *Melanoma Research*, 1997; **7**(Suppl. 2): S115–20.

63. Gasparro FP, Mitchnick M, Nash IF. A review of sunscreen safety and efficacy. *Photochemistry and Photobiology*, 1998; **68**: 243–56.

64. Autier P *et al.* Sunscreen use and duration of sun exposure: a double blind randomized trial. *Journal of the National Cancer Institute*, 1999; **15**: 1304–9.

65. Berwick M, Begg CB, Fine JA, Roush GC, Barnhill RL. Screening for cutaneous melanoma by skin self-examination. *Journal of the National Cancer Institute*, 1996; **88**: 17–23.

66. Autier P, Doré JF, Césarini JP, Boyle P. Should subjects who used psoralen suntan activators be screened for melanoma? *Annals of Oncology*, 1997; **8**: 435–7.

67. Swerdlow AJ, Green A. Melanocytic naevi and melanoma:an epidemiological perspective. *British Journal of Dermatology* 1987; **117**: 137–46

68. Bliss JM *et al.* Risk of cutaneous melanoma associated with pigmentation characteristics and freckling: systematic overview of ten case-control studies. *International Journal of Cancer*. 1995; **67**: 367–76.

69. Rhodes AR, Melski JW. Small congenital nevocellular naevi and risk of cutaneous melanoma. *Journal of Pediatrics*, 1982; **100**: 219–24.

70. Clark WH. Tumour progression and the nature of cancer. *British Journal of Cancer*, 1991; **64**: 631–44

71. Elder DE *et al.* Invasive malignant melanomas lacking competence for

metastasis. *American Journal of Dermatopathology*, 1984; **6**(Suppl.): 55–61.

72. Guerry D, IV *et al.* Lessons from tumor progression: the invasive radial growth phase of melanoma is common, incapable of metastasis, and indolent. *Journal of Investigative Dermatology*, 1993; **100**: 342S–5S.

73. Cook MG *et al.* The evaluation of diagnostic and prognostic criteria and the terminology of thin cutaneous melanoma by the CRC Melanoma Pathology Panel. *Histopathology*, 1996; **28**: 497–512.

74. Hart IR, Goode NT, Wilson RE. Molecular aspects of the metastatic cascade. *Biochimica Biophysica Acta*, 1989; **989**: 65–71.

75. Stetler Stevenson WG, Aznavoorian S, Liotta LA. Tumor cell interactions with the extracellular matrix during invasion and metastasis. *Annual Review of Cell Biology*, 1993; **9**: 541–79.

76. Liotta LA, Steeg PS, Stetler Stevenson WG. Cancer metastasis and angiogenesis: an imbalance of positive and negative regulation. *Cell*, 1991; **64**: 327–35.

77. Seftor REB, Seftor EA, Stetler-Stevenson WG, Hendrix MJC. The 72 kDa type IV collagenase is modulated via differential expression of αvβ3 and α5β1 integrins during human melanoma cell invasion. *Cancer Research*, 1993; **53**: 3411–16.

78. de Vries TJ *et al.* Plasminogen activators, their inhibitors, and urokinase receptor emerge in late stages of melanocytic tumor progression. *American Journal of Pathology*, 1994; **144**: 70–6.

79. Edward M. Integrins and other adhesion molecules involved in melanocytic tumor progression. *Current Opinion in Oncology*, 1995; **7**: 185–205.

80. Chang AE, Karnell LH, Menck HR. The National Cancer Data Base report on cutaneous and non-cutaneous melanoma: a summary of 84,836 cases from the past decade. The American College of Surgeons Commission on Cancer and the American Cancer Society. *Cancer*, 1998; **83**: 1664–78.

81. Keilholz U *et al.* PCR detection of circulating tumour cells. *Melanoma Research*, 1997; **7**: 5133–41.

82. Keilholz U *et al.* Reliability of reverse transcription-polymerase chain reaction (RT-PCR)- based assays for the detection of circulating tumour cells: a quality-assurance initiative of the EORTC Melanoma Cooperative Group. *European Journal of Cancer*, 1998; **34**: 750–3.

83. Willhauck M. Vogel S, Keilholz U. Internal control for quality assurance of diagnostic RT-PCR. *Biotechniques*, 1998; **25**: 656–9.

84. Reintgen D. Conrad A. Detection of occult melanoma cells in sentinel lymph nodes and blood. *Seminars in Oncology*, 1997; **24**(Suppl. 4): 1 1–15.

85. Smith B *et al.* Detection of melanoma cells in peripheral blood by means of reverse transcriptase and polymerase chain reaction. *Lancet*, 1991; **338**: 1227–9.

86. Brossart P *et al.* Hematogenous spread of malignant melanoma cells in different stages of disease. *Journal of Investigative Dermatology*, 1993; **101**: 887–90.

87. Battyani Z *et al.* PCR detection of circulating melanocytes as a prognostic marker in patients with melanoma. *Archives of Dermatology*, 1995; **131**: 443–7.

88. Mellado B *et al.* Detection of circulating neoplastic cells by reverse-transcriptase polymerase chain reaction in malignant melanoma: association with stage and prognosis. *Journal of Clinical Oncology*, 1996; **14**: 2091–7.

89. Breslow A. Prognostic factors in the treatment of cutaneous melanoma. *Journal of Cutaneous Pathology*, 1979; **6**: 208–16.

90. Clark WH Jr, From L, Bernardino EA, Mihm MC Jr. The histogenesis and biologic behavior of primary human malignant melanoma of the skin. *Cancer Research*, 1969; **29**: 705–10.

91. Balch CM, Wilkerson JA, Murad TA, Soong S-J, Ingalls AL, Maddox WA. The prognostic significance of ulceration of cutaneous melanoma. *Cancer*, 1980; **45**: 3012–17.

92. Balch CM, Soong S-J, Shaw HM, Urist MM, McCarthy WH. An analysis of prognostic factors in 8500 patients with cutaneous melanoma. In *Cutaneous melanoma: clinical management and treatment results worldwide* (ed. CM Balch, AN Houghton, GW Milton, Al Sober, S-I Soong). Philadelphia: Lippincott, 1985: 321–30.

93. Gershenwald JE *et al.* Multi-institutional melanoma lymphatic mapping experience: value of sentinel lymph node status in 612 stage I or stage II melanoma patients. *Journal of Clinical Oncology*, 1999; **17**: 976–83.

94. MacKie RM, Bufalino R, Morabito A, Sutherland C, Cascinelli N. Lack of effect of pregnancy on outcome of melanoma. *Lancet*, 1991; **337**: 653–7.

95. Balch CM, Soong S-J, Murad TM, Ingalls AL, Maddox WA. A multifactorial analysis of melanoma: III. Prognostic factors in melanoma patients with lymph node metastases (stage II). *Annals of Surgery*, 1981; **193**: 77.

96. Morton DL, Wanek LA, Nizze JA, Elashoff RM, Wong JH. Improved long-term survival after lymphadenectomy of melanoma metastatic to regional nodes. *Annals of Surgery*, 1991; **214**: 491–7.

97. Kersey PA *et al.* The value of staging and serial follow-up investigations in patients with completely resected, primary, cutaneous malignant melanoma. *British Journal of Surgery*, 1985; **72**: 614–17

98. Buzaid AC *et al.* Role of computed tomography in the staging of primary melanoma. *Journal of Clinical Oncology*, 1995; **8**: 2104–8.

99. Wagner JD *et al.* Prospective study of FOG-PET imaging of lymph node basins in melanoma patients undergoing sentinel node biopsy. *Journal of Clinical Oncology*, 1999; **17**: 1508–15.

100. Rümke P, van Everdingen JJE. Consensus on the management of melanoma of the skin in the Netherlands. *European Journal of Cancer*, 1992; **28**: 600–4.

101. Handley WS. The pathology of melanotic growths in relation to their operative treatment. Lancet, 1907; **i**: 927–33.

102. Breslow A. Thickness, cross-sectional areas and depth of invasion in the prognosis of cutaneous melanoma. *Annals of Surgery*, 1970; **172**: 902–8.

103. Day CL. Narrower margins for clinical stage I melanoma. *New England Journal of Medicine*, 1982; **306**: 479–81.

104. Ackerman AB. How wide and deep is wide and deep enough? *Human Pathology*, 1983; **14**: 743–4.

105. Banzet P *et al.* Wide versus narrow surgical excision in thin (<2 mm) stage I primary cutaneous malignant melanoma: long term results of a French multicentric prospective randomized trial on 319 patients. *Proceedings of the American Association of Clinical Oncology*, 1993; **12**: 387.

106. Ringborg U *et al.*: Resection margins of 2 versus 5 cm for cutaneous malignant melanoma with a tumor thickness of 0.8 to 2.0 mm: randomized study by the Swedish Melanoma Study Group. *Cancer*, 1996; **77**: 1809–14.

107. Veronesi U *et al.* Thin stage I primary cutaneous malignant melanoma. Comparison of excision with margins of 1 or 3 cm. *New England Journal of Medicine*, 1988; **318**: 1159–62. [Published erratum appears in *New England Journal of Medicine*, 1991; **325**: 292.]

108. Cascinelli N. Update WHO-10 trial. *WHO-program meeting*, May 1995, Albany, NY: pp. 317–21.

109. Balch CM *et al.* Efficacy of 2-cm surgical margins for intermediate-thickness melanomas (1 to 4 mm). Results of a multi-institutional randomized surgical trial. *Annals of Surgery*, 1993; **218**: 262–7; discussion 267–9. [See comments.]

110. Karakousis CP *et al.* Local recurrence in malignant melanoma: long-term results of the multiinstitutionat randomized surgical trial. *Annals of Surgical Oncology*, 1996; **3**: 446–52.

111. Heaton KM *et al.* Surgical margins and prognostic factors in patients with thick (>4 mm) primary melanoma. *Annals of Surgical Oncology*, 1998; **5**: 322–8.

112. Ball AS, Thomas J. Surgical management of malignant melanoma. *British Medical Bulletin*, 1995; **51**: 584–608.

113. Cady B. Lymph node metastases. Indicators, but not governors of survival. *Archives of Surgery*, 1984; **119**: 1067–72.

114. Cascinelli N. Metastatic spread of stage I melanoma of the skin. *Tumori*, 1983; **69**: 449–54.

115. Cady B. 'Prophylactic' lymph node dissection in melanoma: does it help? *Journal of Clinical Oncology*, 1988; **6**: 24. [Editorial]

116. Balch CM *et al.* Tumor thickness as a guide to surgical management of clinical stage I melanoma patients. *Cancer*, 1979; **43**: 883–8.

117. Balch CM *et al.* A comparison of prognostic factors and surgical results in 1,786 patients with localized (stage I) melanoma treated in Alabama, USA, and New South Wales, Australia. *Annals of Surgery*, 1982; **196**: 677–84.

118. Milton GW *et al.* Prophylactic lymph node dissection in clinical stage I cutaneous malignant melanoma: results of surgical treatment in 1319 patients. *British Journal of Surgery*, 1982; **69**: 108–11.

119. Reintgen DS *et al.* Efficacy of elective lymph node dissection in patients with intermediate thickness primary melanoma. *Annals of Surgery*, 1983; **198**: 379–85.

120. Drepper H *et al.* Benefit of elective lymph node dissection in subgroups of melanoma patients. Results of a multicenter study of 3616 patients. *Cancer*, 1993; **72**: 741–9.

121. Slingluff CL Jr *et al.* Surgical management of regional lymph nodes in patients with melanoma. *Annals of Surgery*, 1994; **219**: 120–30.

122. Coates AS *et al.* Elective lymph node dissection in patients with primary melanoma of the trunk and limbs treated at the Sydney Melanoma unit from 1960 to 1991. *Journal of the American College of Surgeons*, 1995; **180**: 402–9. [See comments]

123. Veronesi U *et al.* Inefficacy of immediate node dissection in stage 1 melanoma of the limbs. *New England Journal of Medicine*, 1977; **297**: 627–30.

124. Veronesi U. Delayed regional lymph node dissection in stage I melanoma of the skin of the lower extremities. *Cancer*, 1982; **49**: 2420–30.

125. Sim FH. A prospective randomized study of the efficacy of routine elective lymphadenopathy in management of malignant melanoma; preliminary results. *Cancer*, 1985; **41**: 948–51.

126. Sim FH. Lymphadenectomy in the management of stage I malignant melanoma: a prospective randomized study. *Mayo Clinic Proceedings*, 1986; **61**: 697–705.

127. Balch CM *et al.* Efficacy of an elective regional lymph node dissection of 1 to 4 mm thick melanomas for patients 60 years of age and younger. *Annals of Surgery*, 1996; **224**: 255–63; discussion 263–6.

128. Cascinelli N, Morabito A, Santinami M, MacKie RM, Beth F. Immediate or delayed dissection of regional nodes in patients with melanoma of the trunk: a randomised trial. *Lancet*, 1998; **351**: 793–6.

129. Morton DL *et al.* Technical details of intraoperative lymphatic mapping for early stage melanoma. *Archives of* Surgery, 1992; **127**: 392–9.

130. Albertini JJ *et al.* Intraoperative radiolymphoscintigraphy improves sentinel lymph node identification for patients with melanoma. *Annals of Surgery*, 1996; **223**: 217–24.

131. Thompson JF *et al.* Sentinel lymph node status as an indicator of the presence of metastatic melanoma in regional lymph nodes. *Melanoma Research*, 1995; **5**: 255–60.

132. Gershenwald JE *et al.* Improved sentinel lymph node localization in primary melanoma patients with the use of radiolabeled colloid. *Surgery*, 1998; **124**: 203–10.

133. Krag DN *et al.* Minimal-access surgery for staging of melanoma. *Archives of Surgery* 1995; **130**: 654–8.

134. Uren RF *et al.* Lymphoscintigraphy to identify sentinel lymph nodes in patients with melanoma. *Melanoma Research*, 1994; **4**: 395–9.

135. Gershenwald JE *et al.* Patterns of recurrence following a negative sentinel lymph node biopsy in 243 patients with stage I or II melanoma. *Journal of Clinical Oncology*, 1998; 16: 2253–60.

136. Gershenwald JE *et al.* Multi-institutional melanoma lymphatic mapping experience: value of sentinel lymph node status in 612 stage I or stage II melanoma patients. *Journal of Clinical Oncology*, 1999; 17: 976–83.

137. Shivers SC *et al.*. Molecular staging of malignant melanoma: correlation with clinical outcome. *Journal of the American Medical Association*, 1998; 28(16): 1410–15.

138. Balch CM *et al.* A multifactorial analysis of melanoma: III. Prognostic factors in melanoma patients with lymph node metastases (stage II). *Annals of Surgery*, 1981; 193: 377–88.

139. Callery C *et al.* Factors prognostic for survival in patients with malignant melanoma spread to the regional lymph nodes. *Annals of Surgery*, 1982; 196: 69–75.

140. Morton DL *et al.* Improved long-term survival after lymphadenectomy of melanoma metastatic to regional nodes. Analysis of prognostic factors in 1134 patients from the John Wayne Cancer Clinic. *Annals of Surgery*, 1991; 214: 491–9; discussion 499–501.

141. Mann GB, Coit DG. Does the extent of operation influence the prognosis in patients with melanoma metastatic to inguinal nodes? *Annals of Surgical Oncology*, 1999; 6: 263–71.

142. Strobbe LJA *et al.* Positive iliac and obturator nodes in melanoma: survival and prognostic factors. *Annals of Surgical Oncology*, 1999; 6: 255–62.

143. Creech DG. Chemotherapy of cancer: regional perfusion utilizing an extracorporeal circuit. *Melanoma Research*, 1958; 4: 616–32.

144. Benckhuijsen C *et al.* Regional perfusion treatment with melphalan for melanoma in a limb: an evaluation of drug kinetics. *European Journal of Surgical Oncology*, 1988; 14: 157–63.

145. Thompson JF, Gianoutsos MP. Isolated limb perfusion for melanoma: effectiveness and toxicity of cisplatin compared with that of melphalan and other drugs. *World Journal of Surgery*, 1992; 16: 227–33.

146. McBride CM, Sugarbaker EV, Hickey RC. Prophylactic isolation–perfusion as the primary therapy for invasive malignant melanoma of the limbs. *Annals of Surgery*, 1975; 182: 316–24.

147. Martijn H *et al.* Comparison of two methods of treating primary malignant melanomas Clark IV and V, thickness 1.5 mm and greater, localized on the extremities. Wide surgical excision with and without adjuvant regional perfusion. *Cancer*, 1986; 57: 1923–30.

148. Franklin HR *et al.* To perfuse or not to perfuse? A retrospective comparative study to evaluate the effect of adjuvant isolated regional perfusion in patients with stage I extremity melanoma with a thickness of 1.5 mm or greater. *Journal of Clinical Oncology*, 1988; 6: 701–8.

149. Ghussen F *et al.* A prospective randomized study of regional extremity perfusion in patients with malignant melanoma. *Annals of Surgery*, 1984; 200: 764–8.

150. Ghussen F. Hyperthermic perfusion with chemotherapy in melanoma of the extremities. *World Journal of Surgery*, 1989; 13: 598–604.

151. Koops HS *et al.* Prophylactic isolated limb perfusion for localized, high-risk limb melanoma: results of a multicenter randomized phase III trial. *Journal of Clinical Oncology*, 1998; 16: 2906–12.

152. Eggermont AM. Treatment of melanoma in-transit metastases confined to the limb. *Cancer Surveys*, 1996; 26: 335–49.

153. Hill S, Thomas JM. Use of the carbon dioxide laser to manage cutaneous metastases from malignant melanoma. *British Journal of Surgery*, 1996; 83: 509–12.

154. Hafstrom L *et al.* Regional hyperthermic perfusion with melphalan after surgery for recurrent malignant melanoma of the extremities. Swedish Melanoma Study Group *Journal of Clinical Oncology*, 1991; 9: 209–14.

155. Klaase JM *et al.* Limb recurrence-free interval and survival in patients with recurrent melanoma of the extremities treated with normothermic isolated perfusion. *Journal of the American College of Surgeons*, 1994; 178: 564–72.

156. Vrouenraets BC, Nieweg OE, Kroon BB. Thirty-five years of isolated limb perfusion for melanoma: indications and results. *British Journal of Surgery*, 1996; 83: 1319–28.

157. Vrouenraets BC *et al.* Toxicity and morbidity of isolated limb perfusion. *Seminars in Surgical Oncology*, 1998; 14: 224–31.

158. Lienard D *et al.* High-dose recombinant tumor necrosis factor alpha in combination with interferon gamma and melphalan in isolation perfusion of the limbs for melanoma and sarcoma. *Journal of Clinical Oncology*, 1992; 10: 52–60.

159. Lienard D *et al.* Isolated perfusion of the limb with high-dose tumour necrosis factor- alpha (TNF-alpha), interferon-gamma (IFN-gamma) and melphalan for melanoma stage III. Results of a multi-centre pilot study. *Melanoma Research*, 1994; 4(Suppl. 1): 21–6.

160. Kettelhack C, Hohenberger P, Schlag PM. Die Isolierte Extremitatenperfusion mit Tumornekrosefaktor alpha und Melphalan beim malignen Melanom. *Deutsche Medizinische Wochenschrift*, 1997; 122: 177–81.

161. Fraker DL *et al.* Palliation of regional symptoms of advanced extremity melanoma by isolated limb perfusion with melphalan and high-dose tumor necrosis factor. *Cancer Journal from Scientific American*, 1995; 1: 122.

162. Lienard D *et al.* Isolated limb perfusion in primary and recurrent melanoma: indications and results. *Seminars in Surgical Oncology*, 1998; 14: 202–9.

163. Thompson JF *et al.* Isolated limb infusion with cytotoxic agents: a simple alternative to isolated limb perfusion. *Seminars in Surgical Oncology*, 1998; 14: 238–47.

164. Karakousis CP *et al.* Metastasectomy in malignant melanoma. *Surgery*, 1995; 115: 295–300.

165. Tafra L *et al.* Resection and adjuvant immunotherapy for melanoma metastatic to the lung and thorax. *Journal of Thoracic and Cardiovascular Surgery*, 1995; 110: 119–25,

166. Cahan WG. Excision of melanoma metastases to the lung. Problems in diagnosis and management. *Annals of Surgery*, 1973; 178: 703–9.

167. Mathisen DJ, FIye MN, Peabody J. The role of thoracotomy in the management of pulmonary metastases from malignant melanoma. *Annals of Thoracic Surgery*, 1975; 27: 295–301.

168. Marincola FM, Mark JBD. Selective factors resulting in improved survival after surgical resection of tumors metastatic to the lung. *Archives of Surgery*, 1990; 135: 1387–92.

169. Worman ILd *et al.* Surgery as palliative treatment for distant metastases of melanoma. *Annals of Surgery*, 1986, 204: 181–5.

170. Fell DA, Leavens ME, McBride CM. Surgical versus non-surgical management of metastatic melanoma to the brain. *Neurosurgery*, 1980; 7: 230–5.

171. Patchell RA *et al.* A randomized trial of surgery in the treatment of single metastases to the brain. *New England Journal of Medicine*, 1990; 322: 494–9.

172. Fusi S, Ariyan S, Sternlicht A. Data on first recurrence after treatment for malignant melanoma in a large patient population. *Plastic and Reconstructive Surgery*, 1993; 91: 94–8.

173. Martini L, Brandani P, Chiarugi C, Reali UM. First recurrence analysis of 8403 cutaneous melanomas: a proposal for a follow-up schedule. *Tumori*, 1994; 80: 188–97.

174. Baughan CA, Hall VL, Leppard BJ, Perkins PJ. Follow-up in stage I cutaneous malignant melanoma: an audit. *Clinical Oncology*, 1993; 5: 174–80.

175. Frank W, Rogers GS. Melanoma update. Second primary melanoma. *Journal of Dermatologic Surgery and Oncology*, 1993; 19: 427–33.

176. Brandt SE, Welvaart K, Hermans J. Is long-term follow-up justified after excision of a thin melanoma (≤ 1.5 mm)? A retrospective analysis of 206 patients. *Journal of Surgical Oncology*, 1990; 43: 157–60.

177. Kersey PA *et al.* The value of staging and serial follow-up investigations in patients with completely resected, primary, cutaneous malignant melanoma. *British Journal of Surgery*, 1985; **72**: 614–17.

178. Regan MW, Reid CD, Griffiths RW, Briggs JC. Malignant melanoma, evaluation of clinical follow up by questionnaire survey. *British Journal of Plastic Surgery*, 1985; **38**: 11–14.

179. Hill GJ II *et al.* DTIC and combination therapy for melanoma. *Cancer*, 1981; **47**: 2556–62.

180. Pinsky CM, Oettgen HF. Surgical adjuvant for malignant melanoma. *Surgical Clinics of North America*, 1981; **61**: 1259–66.

181. Fisher RI *et al.* Adjuvant immunotherapy or chemotherapy for malignant melanoma: preliminary report of the National Cancer Institute randomized clinical trial. *Surgical Clinics of North America*, 1981; **61**: 1267–77.

182. Veronesi U *et al.* A randomized trial of adjuvant chemotherapy and immunotherapy in cutaneous melanoma. *New England Journal of Medicine*, 1982; **307**: 913–16.

183. Jacquillat C, Banzet P. Maral J Clinical trials of chemotherapy and chemoimmunotherapy in primary malignant melanoma. *Recent results in Cancer Research*, 1982; **80**: 254–8.

184. Quirt IC *et al.* Randomized controlled trial of adjuvant chemoimmunotherapy with DTIC and BCG after complete excision of primary melanoma with a poor prognosis or melanoma metastases. *Canadian Medical Association Journal*, 1983; **128**: 929–36.

185. Paterson AH, Willans DJ, Jerry LM, Hanson J, McPherson T. Adjuvant BCG immunotherapy for malignant melanoma. *Canadian Medical Association Journal*, 1984; **131**: 744–8.

186. Wells, HB *et al.* A randomized trial of adjuvant chemotherapy and immunotherapy in Stage I and Stage II cutaneous melanoma. An interim report. *Cancer*, 1985; **55**: 707-l2.

187. Loutfi A *et al.* Double blind randomized prospective trial of levamisole/placebo in stage I cutaneous malignant melanoma. *Clinical and Investigative Medicine*, 1987; **10**: 325–8.

188. Tranum BL *et al.* Lack of benefit of adjunctive chemotherapy in stage I malignant melanoma: A Southwest Oncology Group study. *Cancer Treatment Reports*, 1987; **71**: 643–4.

189. Czarnetzki BM, Macher E, Suciu S, Thomas D, Steerenberg PA, Rumke Ph. Long-term adjuvant immunotherapy in stage I high risk malignant melanoma, comparing two BCG preparations versus non-treatment in a randomised multicentre study (EORTC PROTOCOL 18781). *European Journal of Cancer* 1993; **29A**: 1237–42.

190. Karakousis CP *et al.* Chemoimmunotherapy (DTIC and *Corynebacterium parvum*) as adjuvant treatment in malignant melanoma. *Cancer Treatment Reports*, 1979; **63**: 1739–43.

191. Balch CM *et al.* A randomized prospective trial of adjuvant *C. parvum* immunotherapy in 260 patients with clinically localized melanoma (stage I): prognostic factors analysis and preliminary results of immunotherapy. *Cancer*, 1982; **49**: 1079–84.

192. Thatcher N *et al.* Randomized study of *Corynebacterium parvum* adjuvant therapy following surgery for (stage II) malignant melanoma. *British Journal of Surgery*, 1986; **73**: 111–15.

193. Lipton A *et al. Corynebacterium parvum* versus BCG adjuvant immunotherapy of stage II malignant melanoma. *Journal of Clinical Oncology*, 1991; **9**: 1151–6.

194. Loufti A *et al.* Double blind randomised prospective trial of levamisole/placebo in stage I cutaneous malignant melanoma. *Clinical and Investigative Medicine*, 1987; **10**: 325–8.

195. Lejeune FJ *et al.* An assessment of DTIC versus levamisole and placebo in the treatment of high risk stage I patients after removal of a primary melanoma of the skin: a phase III adjuvant study. EORTC PROTOCOL 18761. *European Journal of Cancer and Clinical Oncology*, 1988; **24**: 881–90.

196. Quirt IC *et al.* Improved survival in patients with poor prognosis malignant melanoma treated with adjuvant tevamisole: a phase III study by the National Cancer Institute of Canada Clinical Trials Group. *Journal of Clinical Oncology*, 1991; **9**: 729–35.

197. Spitler LE. A randomized trial of levamisole versus placebo as adjuvant therapy in malignant melanoma. *Journal of Clinical Oncology*, 1991; **9**: 736–40.

198. Meyskens FL *et al.* Randomized trial of vitamin A versus observation as adjuvant therapy in high-risk primary malignant melanoma: a Southwest Oncology Group Study I. *Clinical Oncology*, 1994; **12**: 2060–5.

199. Creagan ET *et al.* A prospective randomized controlled trial of megesterol acetate among high risk patients with resected malignant melanoma. *American Journal of Clinical Oncology*, 1989; **12**: 152–5.

200. Meyskens FL *et al.* Randomized trial of adjuvant human interferon-gamma versus observation in high risk cutaneous melanoma: a Southwest Oncology Group Study. *Journal of the National Cancer Institute*, 1995; **87**: 1710–13.

201. Kleeberg U *et al.* EORTC 18871 adjuvant trial in high risk melanoma patients IFNa vs IFNgamma vs Iscador vs observation. *European Journal of Cancer*, 1999; **35**(S4): 264. [Abstract]

202. Hauschild A, Burg G, Dummer R. Prospective randomized multicenter trial on the outpatient use of subcutaneous interleukin 2 and interferon 2b in high risk melanoma patients. *Melanoma Research*, 1997; **7**(Suppl, 1): abstract.

203. Morton DL *et al.* Adjuvant immunotherapy: results of a randomized trial in patients with lymph node metastases. In *Immunotherapy of human cancer* (ed. WD Terry, SA Rosenberg). New York: Elsevier North Holland, 1982: 245–9.

204. Terry WD *et al.* Treatment of stage I and II malignant melanoma with adjuvant immunotherapy or chemotherapy: preliminary analysis of a prospective randomized trial, In *Immunotherapy of human cancer* (ed. WD Terry, SA Rosenberg). New York: Elsevier North Holland, 1982: 252–7.

205. Morton DL. Adjuvant immunotherapy of malignant melanoma: status of clinical trials at UCLA. *International Journal of Immunotherapy*, 1986; **2**: 31–6.

206. Wallack MK *et al.* A phase III randomized, double-blind, multiinstitutional trial of vaccinia melanoma oncolysate–active specific immunotherapy for patients with stage II melanoma. *Cancer*, 1995; **75**: 34–42.

207. Hersey P, Coates P, McCarthy WH. Active immunotherapy following surgical removal of high risk melanoma. Present status and future prospects. *Proceedings of the Society for Biologic Therapy*, 1993; **24**: abstract.

208. Hersey P. Coates P. Tyndall L. Is adjuvant therapy worthwhile? *Melanoma Research*, 1997; **7**(Suppl.): 14.

209. Livingston PO *et al.* Vaccines containing purified GM2 ganglioside elicit GM2 antibodies in melanoma patients. *Proceedings of the National Academy of Sciences, USA*, 1987; **84**: 2911–15.

210. Livingston PO *et al.* Improved survival in stage III melanoma patients with GM2 antibodies: a randomised trial of adjuvant vaccination with GM2 ganglioside. *Journal of Clinical Oncology*, 1994; **12**: 1036–44.

211. Takahashi T, Johnson TD, Nishinaka Y, Morton DL, Irie RF. IgM anti-ganglioside antibodies induced by melanoma cell vaccine correlate with survival of melanoma patients. *Journal of Investigative Dermatology*, 1999; **112**: 205–9.

212. Kirkwood JM, Strawderman MH, Ernstoff MS, Smith TJ, Borden EC, Blum RH. Interferon-2b adjuvant therapy of high-risk resected cutaneous melanoma: the Eastern Cooperative Oncology Group Trial EST 1684. *Journal of Clinical Oncology*, 1996; **14**: 7–17.

213. Creagan ET *et al.* Randomized surgical adjuvant clinical trial or recombinant interferon-alfa-2a in selected patients with malignant melanoma. *Journal of Clinical Oncology*, 1995; **13**: 2776–83.

214. Cascinelli N. Evaluation of efficacy of adjuvant rIFN 2A in regional node metastases. *Proceedings of the American Society of Clinical Oncology*, 1995; **14**: 410. [Abstract]

215. **Kirkwood JM** *et al.* Preliminary analysis of the E1690/S9111/C9190 Intergroup Postoperative Adjuvant Trial of High- and Low-Dose IFNalpha2b (HDI and LDI) in high-risk primary or lymph node metastatic melanoma. *Proceedings of the American Society of Clinical Oncology*, 1999; **18**: 2072. [Abstract]

216. **Eggermont AMM.** The Current Melanoma Cooperative Group adjuvant trial programme on malignant melanoma: prognosis versus efficacy, toxicity and costs. *Melanoma Research*, 1997; 7(Suppl. 2): 127–31.

217. **Pehamberger H** *et al.* Adjuvant interferon a-2a treatment in resected primary stage II cutaneous melanoma. *Journal of Clinical Oncology*, 1998; **16**: 1425–9.

218. **Grob JJ** *et al.* Randomised trial of interferon a-2a as adjuvant therapy in resected primary melanoma thicker than 1.5 mm without clinically detectable node metastases. *Lancet*, 1998; **351**: 1905–10.

219. **Singh RK, Gutman M, Bucana CD, Sanchez R, Llansa N, Fidler IJ.** Interferons alpha and beta down-regulate the expression of basic fibroblast growth factor in human carcinomas. *Proceedings of the National Academy of Sciences, USA*, 1995; **92**: 4562–6.

220. **Dinney CP, Bielenberg DR, Perrotte P, Reich R, Bucana CD, Fidler IJ.** Inhibition of basic fibroblast growth factor expression, angiogenesis and growth of human bladder carcinoma in mice by systemic interferon-alpha administration. *Cancer Research*, 1998; **58**: 808–14.

221. **Nucci M** *et al.* The therapeutic value of poly(ethylene glycol)-modified proteins. *Advances in Drug Delivery Reviews*, 1991; **6**: 133–51.

222. **Ross MR.** Prospective randomized trials in melanoma: defining contemporary surgical roles. *Cancer Treatment and Research*, 1997; **90**: 1–27.

223. **Morton DL** *et al.* Prolongation of survival in metastatic melanoma after active specific immunotherapy with a new polyvalent melanoma vaccine. *Annals of Surgery*, 1992; **216**: 463–70.

224. **Morton DL** *et al.* Polyvalent melanoma vaccine improves survival of patients with metastatic melanoma. *Annals of the New York Academy of Sciences*, 1993; **690**: 120–4.

225. **Balch C, Milton G (ed.)** *Diagnosis of metastatic melanoma at distant sites.* Philadelphia, PA: JB Lippincott, 1985.

226. **Balch C, Soong S, Murad T, Smith J, Maddox W, Durant I.** A multifactorial analysis of melanoma. IV. Prognostic factors in 200 melanoma patients with distant metastases (stage III). *Journal of Clinical Oncology*, 1983; **1**: 126–34.

227. **Ahrnann D, Creagan E, Hahn R, Edmonson J, Bisel H, Schaid D.** Complete responses and long-term survivals after systemic chemotherapy for patients with advanced malignant melanoma. *Cancer*, 1989; **3**: 224–7.

228. **Barth A, Wanek L, Morton D.** Prognostic factors in 1,521 melanoma patients with distant metastases. *Journal of the American College of Surgeons*, 1995; **181**: 193–201.

229. **Creagan E, Schaid D, Ahmann D, Frytak S.** Disseminated malignant melanoma and recombinant interferon: analysis of seven consecutive phase II investigations. *Journal of Investigative Dermatology*, 1990; **95**: 188S–192S.

230. **Keilholz U** *et al.* Results of IL-2-based treatment in advanced melanoma: a case-record based analysis of 631 patients. *Journal of Clinical Oncology*, 1998; **16**: 2921–9.

231. **DeVita VT Jr, Hellman S, Rosenberg SA.** Cancer: *Principles and practice of oncology* (5th edn). Pennsylvania, PA: Lippincott-Raven, 1997.

232. **Overgaard J, Overgaard M, Hansen PV, von der Maase H.** Some factors of importance in the radiation treatment of malignant melanoma. *Radiotherapy and Oncology*, 1986; **5**: 183–92.

233. **Engenhart R** *et al.* Long-term follow-up for brain metastases treated by percutaneous stereotactic single high dose irradiation. *Cancer*, 1992; **71**: 1353.

234. **Fuller BG, Kaplan ID, Adler J, Cox RS, Bagshaw MA.** Stereotaxic radiosurgery for brain metastases: the importance of adjuvant whole brain irradiation. *International Journal of Radiation Oncology, Biology, Physics*, 1992; **23**: 413–18.

235. **Wittes RE, Wittes JT, Golbey RB.** Comination chemotherapy in metastatic malignant melanoma: a randomized study of three DTIC-containing combinations. *Cancer*, 1978; **42**: 415–21.

236. **Costanzi JJ** *et al.* Combined chemotherapy plus BCG in the treatment of disseminated malignant lymphoma: a Southwest Oncology Group study. *Medical Pediatric Oncology*, 1982; **10**: 251–8.

237. **Luikart SD, Kennealey GT, Kirkwood JM.** Randomized phase III trial of vinblastine, bleomycin, and *cis*-dichlorodiammine-platinum versus dacarbazine in malignant melanoma. *Journal of Clinical Oncology*, 1984; **2**: 164–8.

238. **Buzaid A** *et al.* Cisplatin, vinblastine, and dacarbazine versus dacarbazine alone in metastatic melanoma. *Proceedings of the American Society of Clinical Oncology*, 1993; **1993**: 1389.

239. **Jungnelius U** *et al.* Dacarbazine–vindesine versus dacarbazine–vindesine–cisplatin in disseminated malignant melanoma. a randomised phase III trial. *European Journal of Cancer*, 1998; **34**: 1368–74.

240. **Middleton M** *et al.* A randomized phase III study of temozolamide (TMZ) versus dacarbazine (DTIC) in the treatment of patients with advanced metastatic melanoma. In *Proceedings of ASCO: Melanoma and sarcoma; 1999*: 536a. [Abstract]

241. **Cocconi G** *et al.* Treatment of metastatic malignant melanoma with dacarbazine plus tamoxifen. *New England Journal of Medicine*, 1992; **327**: 516–23.

242. **Rusthoven** *et al.* Randomized, double-blind, placebo controlled trial comparing the response rates of carmustine, dacarbazine, and cisplatin with and without tamoxifen in patients with metastatic melanoma. *Journal of Clinical Oncology*, 1996; **14**: 2083–90.

243. **Agarwala SS, Ferri W, Gooding W, Kirkwood JM.** A phase III randomized trial of dacarbazine and carboplatin with and without tamoxifen in the treatment of patients with metastatic melanoma. *Cancer*, 1999; **85**: 1979–84.

244. **Saxman S** *et al.* A phase III multicenter randomized trial of DTIC, cisplatin, BCNU and tamoxifen versus DTIC alone in patients with metastatic melanoma. In *Proceedings of the American Society of Clinical Oncology (ASCO): Melanoma and sarcoma*, 1999: 536a. [Abstract]

245. **Ryan L, Kramar A.** Borden E. Prognostic factors in metastatic melanoma. *Cancer*, 1993; 71(1O): 2995.

246. **Comis R.** DTIC (NSC-453 88) in malignant melanoma: a perspective. *Cancer Treatment Reports*, 1976; **64**: 1123.

247. **Jacquillat C** *et al.* Final report of the French multicenter phase II study of the nitrosourea fotemustine in 153 evaluable patients with disseminated malignant melanoma including patients with cerebral metastases. *Cancer*, 1990; **66**: 1873–8.

248. **Al-Sarraf M** *et al.* Cisplatin hydration with and without mannitol diuresis in refractory disseminated malignant melanoma: a Southwest Oncology Group study. *Cancer Treatment Reports*, 1982; **66**: 31–5.

249. **Mechl Z, Krejci P.** Cis-diamminedichloroplatinum in the treatment of disseminated malignant melanoma. *Neoplasma*, 1983; **30**: 371–7.

250. **Rosenthal MA** *et al.* Synchronous cisplatin infusion during radiotherapy for the treatment of metastatic melanoma. *European Journal of Cancer*, 1991; **27**: 1564–6.

251. **Casper ES, Bajorin D.** Phase II trial of carboplatin in patients with advanced melanoma. *Investigative New Drugs*, 1990; **8**: 187–90.

252. **Glover D, Glick JH, Weiler C, Fox K, Guerry D.** WR-2721 and high-dose cisplatin: an active combination in the treatment of metastatic melanoma. *Journal of Clinical Oncology*, 1987; **5**: 574–8.

253. **Buzaid AC, Murren J, Durivage HJ.** High-dose cisplatin plus WR-2721 in a split course in metastatic malignant melanoma. A phase II study. *American Journal of Clinical Oncology*, 1991; **14**: 203–7.

254. **Planting AS, van der Burg ME, de Boer-Dennert M, Stoter G, Verweij**

J. Phase I/II study of a short course of weekly cisplatin in patients with advanced solid tumours. *British Journal of Cancer*, 1993; **68**: 789–92.

255. **Kleeberg UR et al.** Palliative therapy of melanoma patients with fotemustine. Inverse relationship between tumour load and treatment effectiveness. A multicentre phase II trial of the EORTC-Melanoma Cooperative Group (MCG). *Melanoma* Research, 1995; **5**: 195–200.

256. **Neuber K, tom Dieck A, Blodorn-Schlicht N, Itschert G, Karnbach C.** Treosulfan is an effective alkylating cytostatic for malignant melanoma *in vitro* and *in vivo*. *Melanoma Research*, 1999; 125–32.

257. **Falkson C, Falkson G, Falkson H.** Improved results with the addition of interferonalfa-2b to dacarbazine in the treatment of patients with metastatic malignant melanoma. *Journal of Clinical Oncology*, 1991; **9**: 1403–8.

258. **Thompson D et al.** Interferon-alfa 2a does not improve response or survival when combined with dacarbazine in metastatic malignant melanoma: results of a multi-institutional Australian trial. *Melanoma Research*, 1993; **3**: 133–8.

259. **Bajetta E et al.** Multicenter randomized trial of dacarbazine alone or in combination of two different doses and schedules of interferon alfa-2a in the treatment of advanced melanoma. *Journal of Clinical Oncology*, 1994; **12**: 806–11.

260. **Falkson CI, Ibrahim J, Kirkwood JM, Atkins MB, Blum RH.** Phase III trial of dacarbazine versus dacarbazine with interferon alpha-2b versus dacarbazine with tamoxifen versus dacarbazine with interferon alpha-2b and tamoxifen in patients with metastatic malignant melanoma: an Eastern Cooperative Oncology Group study. *Journal of Clinical Oncology*, 1998; **16**: 1743–51.

261. **Sparano J et al.** Randomized phase III trial of treatment with high-dose interleukin-2 either alone or in combination with interferon-alfa2a in patients with advanced melanoma. *Journal of Clinical Oncology*, 1993; **11**: 1969–77.

262. **Dorval T et al.** Randomized trial of treatment with cisplatin and interleukin-2 either alone or in combination with interferon-alpha-2a in patients with metastatic melanoma: a Federation Nationale des Centres de Lutte Contre le Cancer Multicenter, parallel study. *Cancer*, 1999; **85**: 1060–6.

263. **Johnston S et al.** Randomized phase II trial of BCDT with or without interferon alpha and interleukin-2 in patients with metastatic melanoma. *British Journal of Cancer*, 1998; **77**: 1280–6.

264. **Rosenberg SA et al.** Prospective randomized trial of the treatment of patients with metastatic melanoma using chemotherapy with cisplatin, dacarbazine, and tamoxifen alone or in combination with interleukin-2 and interferon alfa-2b. *Journal of Clinical Oncology*, 1999; **17**: 968–75.

265. **Keilholz U et al.** IFNα/IL-2 with or without cisplatin in metastatic melanoma: a randomized trial of the EORTC Melanoma Cooperative Froup. *Journal of Clinical Oncology*, 1997; **15**: 2579–88.

266. **Thatcher N, Dazzi H, Gosh A, Johnson R.** Recombinant IL-2 given intrasplenically and intravenously in advanced malignant melanoma: a phase I/II study. *Cancer Treatment Reports*, 1989; **16** (Suppl. A): 49–52.

267. **Parkinson D et al.** Interleukin-2 therapy in patients with metastatic malignant melanoma: a phase II study. *Journal of Clinical Oncology*, 1990; **8**: 1650–6.

268. **Legha S, Gianan M, Plager C, Eton O, Papadopoulous N.** Evaluation of interleukin-2 administered by continuous infusion in patients with metastatic melanoma. *Cancer*, 1996; **77**: 89–96.

269. **Keilholz U et al.** Interferon-α and interleukin-2 in the treatment of malignant melanoma: a comparison of two phase II trials. *Cancer*, 1993; **72**: 607–14.

270. **Kruit W et al.** Dose-efficacy study of two schedules of high-dose bolus administration of interleukin-2 and alpha-interferon in patients with metastatic melanoma. *British Journal of Cancer*, 1996; **74**: 951–5.

271. **Flaherty L et al.** A phaseI-II study of dacarbazine in combination with outpatient interleukin-2 in metastatic malignant melanoma. *Cancer*, 1990; **65**: 2471–7.

272. **Dummer R et al.** A multicenter phase II clinical trial using dacarbazine and continuous infusion of interleukin-2 in metastatic melanoma: clinical data and immunomonitoring. *Cancer*, 1995; **75**: 945–8.

273. **Demchak P, et al.** Interleukin-2 and high-dose cisplatin in patients with metastatic melanoma: a pilot study. *Journal of Clinical Oncology*, 1991; 9:1821–30.

274. **Flaherty L et al.** A phase II study of dacarbazine and cisplatin in combination with outpatient administered interleukin-2 in metastatic malignant melanoma. *Cancer*, 1993; **71**: 3250–5.

275. **Atkins M et al.** Multiinstitutional phase II trial of intensive combination chemotherapy for metastatic melanoma. *Journal of Clinical Oncology*, 1994; **12**: 1553–60.

276. **Richards J, Mehta N, Ramming K, Skosey P.** Sequential chemoimmunotherapy in the treatment of metastatic melanoma. *Journal of Clinical Oncology*, 1992; **10**: 1338–43.

277. **Khayat D et al.** Sequential chemoimmunotherapy with cisplatin, interleukin-2 and interferon alfa-2 for metastatic melanoma. *Journal of Clinical Oncology*, 1993; **11**: 2173–80.

278. **Buzaid, Legha S.** Combination of chemotherapy with interleukin-2 and interferon-alpha for the treatment of advanced melanoma. *Seminars in Oncology*, 1994; **6**(Suppl. 14): 23–8.

279. **Rosenberg S et al.** Combination therapy with interleukin-2 and alpha-interferon for the treatment of patients with advanced cancer. *Journal of Clinical Oncology*, 1989; **7**: 1863–74.

280. **Kruit W et al.** Clinical experience with the combined use of recombinant interleukin-2 (IL-2) and interferon-alpha-2a (IFN alpha) in metastatic melanoma. *British Journal of Haematology*, 1991; **79** (Suppl.): 84–6.

281. **Dillman R et al.** Inpatient continuous-infusion interleukin-2 in 788 patients with cancer. The National Biotherapy Study Group experience. *Cancer*, 1993; **71**: 2358–70.

282. **Scheibenbogen C, Lee K, Moebius U, Herr W, Rammensee H, Keilholz U.** A sensitive ELISPOT assay for detection of HLA class I restricted CD8+ T lymphocytes specific for influenza peptides in the blood of healthy donors and melanoma patients. *Clinical Cancer Research*, 1997; **3**: 221–6.

283. **Herr W, Schneider J, Lohse AW, Meyer zum Buschenfelde KH, Wolfel T.** Detection and quantification of blood-derived CD8+ T lymphocytes secreting tumor necrosis factor alpha in response to HLA-A2.1-binding melanoma and viral peptide antigens. *Journal of Immunological Methods*, 1996; **191**: 131–42.

284. **Hamilton WB, Helling F, Lloyd KO, Livingston PO.** Ganglioside expression on human malignant melanoma assessed by quantitiative immune thin layer chromatography. *International Journal of Cancer*, 1993; **53**: 566-73.

285. **Jones PC, Sze LL, Liu PY.** Prolonged survival for melanoma patients with elevated IgM antibody to oncofetal antigen. *Journal of the National Cancer Institute*, 1981; **66**: 249–54.

286. **Kirkwood JM, Ibrahim J, Sondak VK, Sosman JA, Ernstoff MS.** Relapse-free and overall survival are significantly prolonged by high-dose IFN alpha 2b (HDI) compared to vaccine GM2-KLH with QS21 (GMK, Progenics) for high-risk resected stage IIB-III melanoma: results of the Intergroup Phase III study E1694/S9512/C503801. *Annals of Oncology*, 2000; **11** (Suppl. 4): 4.

287. **Eggermont AMM, Kleeberg UR, Ruiter DJ, Suciu S.** The European Organization for Research and Treatment of Cancer Melanoma Group trial experience with more than 2000 patients, evaluating adjuvant therapy treatment with low or intermediate doses of interferon alpha-2b.. Educational Book of 37th Annual Meeting, 2001. *American Society of Clinical Oncology*, 2001: in press.

288. **Balch CM et al.** A new American Joint Committe on cancer staging system for cutaneous melanoma. *Cancer*, 2000; **88**: 1484–91.

8.2   Melanoma of the eye and orbit

John Hungerford

The overwhelming majority of malignant melanomas in the orbital region are primary tumours and most arise within the eye in the pigmented structures of the uveal tract. Less commonly, malignant melanoma may develop outside the eye in the conjunctiva, occasionally in the skin of the eyelids, and, rarely, in the orbit itself. Metastatic spread of cutaneous melanoma to the eye and to the ocular adnexa does occur, though it is rare.[1] Direct spread of conjunctival melanomas to the orbit and to the skin of the eyelids is not uncommon and direct extraocular extension of uveal melanoma to the orbit is all too frequent. There are many similarities and some differences between melanomas in all ocular sites and their cutaneous counterparts. Just as they are in the skin, ocular and adnexal melanomas may be of variable pigmentation and may exhibit a superficial spreading or nodular growth pattern. Like skin melanomas, ocular and adnexal melanocytic tumours are easily visible either on direct inspection for lesions of the eyelids, conjunctiva, and iris or with the ophthalmoscope for those of the ciliary body and choroid. The diagnosis is usually based on clinical appearance and confirmed by biopsy of accessible lesions and non-invasive imaging of inaccessible tumours. The pattern of metastatic spread of melanomas of the conjunctiva and eyelid skin is similar to that of cutaneous melanomas, mainly because they have access to the lymphatics. A TNM staging system would be possible for ocular adnexal melanomas but, because of the rarity of the disease and the multiplicity and complexity of the prognostic factors, an evaluation of this approach did not recommend its use.[2] There is therefore very little TNM-based outcome data relating to eyelid and conjunctival melanoma. There are, however, no lymphatics in the eye and orbit, and primary uveal and orbital melanomas do not spread to regional glands. Rather, they exhibit haematogenous spread and the target organs affected are significantly different from those involved by cutaneous, eyelid, and conjunctival melanomas, with the liver being almost universally involved. It is partly for this reason that the TNM staging for uveal melanoma, proposed by the UICC, has not gained wide acceptance. It is rarely used by specialists in ocular oncology and there is, therefore, barely any outcome data published in this format for melanoma of the uveal tract.

Malignant melanoma of the eyelids

Primary melanoma of the skin of the eyelids is very uncommon and accounts for no more than 1 per cent of all lid tumours.[3],[4] Most eyelid melanomas arise as direct extensions from conjunctival tumours or in association with primary acquired conjunctival melanosis

(PAM).[5] Occasionally, an eyelid melanoma may be the first sign of unsuspected PAM.[6] It is important to search the whole conjunctiva for PAM when an eyelid melanoma is discovered. A metastatic deposit from a distant primary cutaneous malignant melanoma may occasionally be seen in the eyelid. Metastatic melanomas in the eyelid tend to be subcutaneous, and this clinical feature and the presence or history of a distant primary skin tumour serves to distinguish them from the rare primary neoplasms. Primary melanoma of the eyelid usually presents as a pigmented lesion with an irregular outline, and is sometimes associated at or soon after diagnosis with pre-auricular or submandibular lymph node metastases depending, respectively, on whether the upper or lower eyelid is involved. The degree of pigmentation may vary from area to area within an individual tumour and between lesions. Many eyelid melanomas are amelanotic. Clinically, an eyelid melanoma may be raised or fairly flat and, histologically, the incidence of these tumours is approximately equally divided between nodular and superficial spreading lesions.[4] The neoplasm may arise de novo or it may develop in a pre-existing naevus or in an area of lentigo maligna and must be distinguished from these lesions. Corresponding naevi may be present at the lid margin on both upper and lower eyelids. These divided or 'kissing' naevi arise from a single lesion when the eyelids divide in embryonic life, and rarely undergo malignant change.

Another condition that must be differentiated from malignant melanoma of the eyelid is oculodermal melanocytosis (naevus of Ota). This congenital disorder occurs predominantly in individuals of Asian and Mediterranean extraction and may be distinguished from malignant melanoma by the associated involvement of the episclera and the uveal tract of the ipsilateral eye. Being sub-conjunctival, the episcleral element has a characteristic slate-grey rather than a brown colour. Uveal tract involvement is most noticeable in individuals with light-coloured eyes in whom the iris of the affected eye is much darker than that of its fellow. Involvement of the choroid is apparent as a much darker red reflex on the affected side than on the other. The eyelid skin involvement diagnostic of naevus of Ota may be absent, in which case the disorder is defined as ocular melanocytosis. This variant is commoner in the United Kingdom than full-blown naevus of Ota and seems to affect lighter skinned individuals. As with the oculodermal variant, the whole eye is usually involved but in a forme fruste of the condition that seems to be commoner when the eye alone is affected, segmental involvement of the episclera, iris, and choroid may be seen occasionally. Malignant melanomas may arise in any of the tissues affected by oculodermal or ocular melanosis. By far the majority of examples of such malignant change take place in the uveal tract element, and it is fascinating to note that, in the segmental form, the tumour will always arise in the area of affected choroid. Pigmented seborrhoeic keratosis is common and may be mistaken for melanoma. It has a much more regular outline and is more uniformly pigmented than a malignant melanoma.

The diagnosis of eyelid melanoma should be established by a wide excision, which may also serve as the definitive treatment. It may be followed by a plastic repair of the eyelid if necessary. Local recurrence is infrequent when this approach is adopted for small melanomas, but very large or recurrent lesions are best managed by exenteration of the orbit. Nodular malignant melanomas of the eyelid skin have a worse prognosis than superficial spreading variants, although the outlook is better than for cutaneous melanomas in general.[4] It is probable that, as with cutaneous melanomas elsewhere, Breslow thickness is the single most significant predictor of prognosis for survival from an eyelid melanoma.

Malignant melanoma of the conjunctiva

Primary malignant melanoma occurs between 20 and 40 times less frequently in the conjunctiva than in the uveal tract and comprises approximately 2 per cent of all ocular malignancies.[7]–[9] The tumour occurs almost exclusively in adults and mainly in fair-skinned Whites. A primary malignant melanoma may arise in the bulbar conjunctiva, which covers the anterior sclera of the eye, in the palpebral conjunctiva covering the inner, tarsal, surface of the eyelids, or in the upper or lower fornix where the bulbar conjunctiva is reflected on to that covering the tarsus. The tumour may also arise in the plica semi-lunaris, which represents the vestigial nictitating membrane and, rarely, in the caruncle at the inner canthus. The caruncle is composed of epidermal tissue with hair follicles and has more affinity with skin than does the conjunctiva. The outlook is much better for tumours involving the bulbar conjunctiva than for those elsewhere in the conjunctiva or caruncle, presumably because they have less easy access to lymphatics. The growth pattern may be of superficial spreading or nodular type and the degree of pigmentation varies between intensely pigmented and amelanotic.

Unlike in the skin, there is no known association with solar exposure but host factors are prominent in the aetiology of conjunctival malignant melanoma. Most tumours develop in an area of pre-existing conjunctival pigmentation.[10] Some 18 per cent arise in a conjunctival naevus and these tumours, like occasional melanomas that arise de novo, tend to be solitary and circumscribed. Formerly it was held that a larger proportion of conjunctival melanomas arose in naevi, but this is no longer considered to be so: some apparent naevi which are thought subsequently to have undergone malignant change may originally have been undiagnosed melanomas in a radial growth phase.[11] Approximately 57 per cent of melanomas arise in PAM and these tumours are usually multifocal and often diffuse (Fig. 1). Some melanomas that appear at first to be arising de novo or in a naevus eventually show signs of PAM, possibly indicating that naevus formation may be a step in the development of malignancy in some individuals with melanosis. Clinically, conjunctival melanoma must be distinguished from extrascleral extension of an anterior uveal-tract melanoma, from a conjunctival naevus, from racial conjunctival pigmentation and acquired melanosis, from ocular melanocytosis,

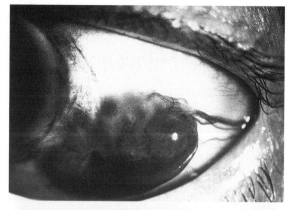

(a)

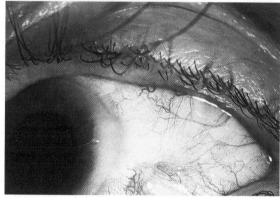

(b)

Fig. 1 (a) Small malignant melanoma of the bulbar conjunctiva arising at the limbus in primary acquired melanosis. (b) The appearance of the same eye 1 year later, after block excision with a superficial keratectomy and sclerectomy.

and from a staphyloma, subconjunctival haemorrhage, or foreign body.

In most reports, the survival rate is better in melanomas arising in a pre-existing naevus than in those that arise de novo or in PAM,[12] though this feature has not been observed in all series.[13] The worse outcome for melanomas arising in PAM can be explained by the tendency for individuals with this condition to develop multifocal malignancies, one or more of which is likely ultimately to involve a high risk area of conjunctiva.

Conjunctival naevus

Conjunctival naevi are rarely if ever visible at birth but appear during the first few years of life. They may darken and enlarge around the time of puberty and give cause for concern. This is rarely an indication of malignant change in an adolescent, and usually results from increased pigmentation of the naevus cells and from epithelial down-growth into the tumour with cyst formation. Cystic change is a characteristic feature of conjunctival naevi and helps to distinguish them clinically from conjunctival melanomas. In the rare instances when cysts are seen with a histologically proven malignant conjunctival melanoma, they provide convincing evidence of the origin of that particular tumour from a pre-existing naevus. Naevi without cysts may be misdiagnosed histologically as malignant because of the presence of bizarre cells and inflammation. It was the correction of such errors that led Jay[14] to reclassify as naevi 43 tumours initially diagnosed histologically as melanomas. Very occasionally, a Spitz naevus may be encountered in the conjunctiva. This variant usually arises in the caruncle, perhaps because of this structure's similarity to skin.

Primary acquired melanosis

Pigmentation of the conjunctiva may be congenital and a racial characteristic, or it may be acquired. Congenital limbal conjunctival pigmentation first becomes noticeable in early life. It is almost universal in Blacks, occurs in some 50 per cent of Oriental and Hispanic individuals, and is seen in only 10 per cent of Whites. The brown pigmentation is present within the epithelium and must be distinguished from the grey colour of ocular or oculodermal melanocytosis, conditions that are also first evident in youth. The malignant potential of melanocytosis is confined to the tissue in which it arises: because the conjunctival epithelium is not involved, there is no propensity to conjunctival malignant melanoma.

By contrast, PAM usually presents in middle life as a flat, granular, intraepithelial, reddish-brown pigmentary change which is clinically similar to racial pigmentation. Typically, the pigment is first observed in the bulbar conjunctiva. A tendency for PAM to progress through a premalignant to a frankly malignant phase has long been recognized. The histological correlate of this progression begins with the appearance of atypical melanocytes in the basal layer. A benign variant of acquired melanosis without atypia has been categorized histopathologically and is said not to progress to the precancerous form, but, in clinical practice, acquired melanosis with atypia is much commoner than without. 'PAM with atypia' is the current term for the premalignant variant first described by Reese[15] and to which he gave the name precancerous conjunctival melanosis. PAM is strictly a pathological rather than a clinical description. Confusingly, by common usage, the term has come to mean the atypical variety, leaving no current term for the entity without abnormal cells, except, perhaps, 'PAM without atypia'.

Clinically, the course of PAM is variable. In PAM with atypia, the abnormal melanocytes spread contiguously or non-contiguously, and, over a period of years, extend to involve the palpebral conjunctiva, that of the fornices and plica, and the corneal epithelium.[16] Pigmentation may extend around the eyelid margin and into the lid skin. Discrete skin pigmentation may be seen that is non-contiguous with the conjunctival changes, and may have histological appearances ranging from benign through lentigo maligna to frank malignant melanoma.[5] The incidence and time scale of malignant change in PAM is difficult to estimate because most patients with acquired melanosis do not present until they have developed their first melanoma. As the number of individuals with as yet undiagnosed PAM is unknown, the denominator of the fraction who develop malignancy is uncertain. Moreover, many patients with melanoma describe the presence of a reddish discoloration of the conjunctiva suggestive of PAM for decades. This is often mistaken for inflammation and treated as such for long periods, making it difficult to be certain how long melanosis has been present. Reese[17] estimated that approximately 17 per cent of patients with precancerous melanosis followed for more than 5 years developed malignant change, whilst Folberg et al.[12] showed that approximately 50 per cent of examples of PAM with atypia will develop one or more invasive melanomas. Ultimately,

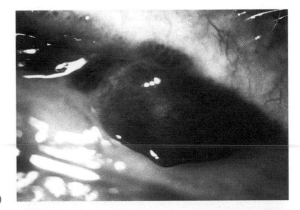

(a)

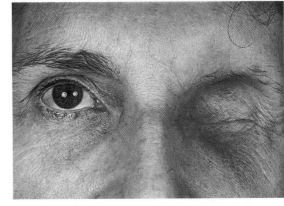

(b)

Fig. 2 (a) Large malignant melanoma of the conjunctiva arising in the upper fornix in primary acquired melanosis, and (b) the appearance 6 months after lid-splitting orbital exenteration.

multifocal melanoma will probably arise in most individuals with PAM who avoid death from another cause and survive long enough for the conjunctival disease to run its full course. Malignant tumours arise sequentially over a long period and may be nodular or superficial spreading in character, and pigmented or amelanotic. Both pigmented and non-pigmented melanomas may develop at random in the same individual with PAM. Initially, the interval between tumours may be measured in years and each lesion is commonly solitary. With time, however, the interval between new melanomas tends to shorten and more than one new tumour may develop simultaneously. Sooner or later, the disease enters an aggressive phase with very rapid development of new tumours, sometimes at intervals of only a few weeks (Fig. 2).

The degree of pigmentation observed in PAM may vary with time, and the waxing and waning characteristic of the disorder may be so extreme that it seems to disappear. Apparent spontaneous resolution is rarely sustained. This feature of PAM, and the fact that multifocal melanomas have been reported to arise in amelanotic PAM,[18] suggests that the disappearance of pigmentation is due to altered melanin production rather than to a loss of the atypical pigment cells. Pigmentation may also vary in the same individual during pregnancy and, in this respect, it may be relevant that some 40 per cent of conjunctival melanomas have been found to contain oestrogen receptors.[19] There is recent evidence to suggest that PAM may be a manifestation of the atypical mole syndrome.[20]

Attempts have been made to eliminate acquired melanosis, because at least 20 per cent of patients with the condition and 50 per cent of those who have atypia will ultimately develop a life-threatening malignant tumour. Excision of early and circumscribed areas of PAM is always frustrated by the reappearance of the condition sooner or later at another site in what was apparently healthy conjunctiva. It is not yet clear whether this happens because of spread from the initial focus of the melanocytes destined to proliferate, or whether there is a field-change involving all the melanocytes in the conjunctiva of the affected eye. It is not technically possible to carry out a block excision of the whole conjunctiva and corneal epithelium with preservation of the integrity of the eye and, to date, no completely successful panconjunctival treatment for PAM has been reported. Since melanocytes are susceptible to freezing, attempts have been made to destroy the atypical cells by cryotherapy.[21] Cryotherapy is certainly followed by depigmentation of the treated area and is claimed to be able to destroy naevus and melanoma cells,[22],[23] but there is insufficient experience of this approach at present to determine how effective it will be. Present evidence suggests that it cannot prevent all new melanomas and that the best we can hope for is that it may be able to postpone malignant change and reduce the number of new tumours. Moreover, there are no clinical means of detecting areas of amelanotic PAM and this entity defies any form of prophylactic treatment at present. Extensive cryotherapy to the limbus destroys the stem cells responsible for populating the corneal epithelium. For this reason, panconjunctival cryotherapy is not a practical proposition. Treating only visible melanosis misses areas of amelanotic PAM, which probably accounts for at least some of the new melanomas that still arise after prophylactic cryotherapy.

The particular risk factors associated with PAM contribute significantly to the high mortality rate of conjunctival melanoma. Lifelong follow up is therefore necessary for PAM, with an interval of no longer than 6 months for the individual who has not yet developed a melanoma and 4 months for the patient who has already had an invasive tumour, looking for evidence of malignant change. At each visit the upper eyelid should be double-everted so that the whole conjunctiva may be thoroughly searched. Patients should be encouraged to report any changes between visits. Although PAM with atypia is commoner than that without, it is difficult to differentiate clinically between the two and the diagnosis should be confirmed histologically to justify time-consuming follow-up. Impression cytology may be helpful if it gives a positive result,[24] but a possibility of false-negatives exists and cytological absence of melanocytic atypia requires confirmation by incisional biopsy.

It is at least as important to be alert to the possibility of malignant change in any area of pigmented conjunctiva as it is in melanocytic lesions of the skin. Clinical features of malignant change are increased thickness, a change in pigmentation, the appearance of prominent blood vessels feeding a tumour, and tethering of the conjunctiva to the underlying sclera in areas where it is usually mobile. In adolescence, a short period of benign enlargement due to epithelial downgrowth and cyst formation can be ignored, but increase in size later in life and particularly sustained growth should be regarded with suspicion. Melanomas arising de novo tend to present in the bulbar conjunctiva exposed in the interpalpebral fissure where they may soon be noticed by the patient. By contrast, melanomas arising in PAM may develop anywhere within the conjunctiva and particularly in areas hidden from view. Such tumours may become very large before they are noticed, either because of a lump in the eyelid or because of bleeding or a mass protruding under the eyelid. When a conjunctival melanoma presents at a site other than the interpalpebral fissure, it almost always does so in PAM so that a particularly careful search should be made for melanosis in any patient with a melanoma in an area of conjunctiva normally hidden by the eyelids.

Malignant melanoma

The treatment of an invasive conjunctival malignant melanoma is essentially surgical. Any new, raised, pigmented patch appearing in the conjunctiva of an adult and any area of increased thickness or vascularity within a pre-existing naevus or area of PAM should be excised, if possible with a 3-mm margin. Usually, excision biopsy of this type will also serve as the definitive treatment. Bulbar conjunctival melanomas not involving the corneoscleral limbus are amenable to simple excision with a low chance of recurrence. Most apparent recurrences are, in reality, new foci of melanoma arising in PAM. The development of multiple local recurrences in a patient not yet diagnosed as having PAM should always raise suspicion of this disorder. The interpalpebral limbus is a frequent site for conjunctival melanoma. At the limbus, the conjunctiva is adherent to the underlying sclera and melanomas arising in this location tend to recur if they are not adequately excised. Melanomas show little tendency to invade the corneal and scleral lamellae, and the incidence of this type of recurrence may be greatly reduced by performing a block excision of the tumour with the underlying superficial one-third of the adjacent cornea and sclera (Fig. 1). Separation of the corneal epithelium at the tumour margin is facilitated by the application of absolute alcohol. In the unlikely event that corneal invasion occurs significantly beyond the limbus, transparency may be maintained by replacing lost corneal tissue with a lamellar graft.[16] After incomplete excision, the recurrence rate may be reduced by adjunctive treatment either by radiotherapy[25] or cryotherapy.[26] Beta-radiotherapy using a strontium-90 surface applicator is preferred and the total surface dose should be at least 50 Gray (Gy), given as 10 Gy per day for 5 days. As with PAM, strenuous efforts should be made to avoid irradiating or freezing the whole limbus to minimize the risk of stem-cell failure.

Robertson et al.[5] reported a mortality rate of 26 per cent in patients with conjunctival melanoma but without eyelid involvement who were followed for between 5 and 25 years. An identical figure was reported by Folberg et al.[12] in patients followed for more than 8 years, and others have observed similar outcomes.[14] Involvement of the eyelid skin has a very adverse influence on survival, with a mortality rate which at 70 per cent is more akin to that of cutaneous melanoma.[5] Survival rates are much better for solitary, circumscribed, thin melanomas arising in the bulbar conjunctiva and not arising in PAM than for multifocal and thick tumours that develop in unfavourable locations, including the palpebral conjunctiva, the fornices, the plica, and the caruncle, and which are associated with acquired melanosis.[10] Melanomas arising in high-risk locations have twice the mortality rate of epibulbar tumours, mixed-cell lesions containing epithelioid cells have three times the mortality rate of spindle-cell tumours.[10] The overall 5-, 10-, and 20-year survival probabilities have been estimated at 83, 70, and 68 per cent, respectively.[10] Differences in access to the lymphatics may be the underlying reason why some locations are less favourable than others—histological evidence of lymphatic invasion increases the mortality rate fourfold compared with tumours that show no such involvement of lymph channels.[10] The development of new tumours in PAM may contribute to the greater mortality rates seen the longer patients are followed.[5],[12],[14] These risk factors conspire to make melanoma associated with PAM a much more serious disease than that which arises *de novo* or develops in a naevus. Because of these differences, solitary melanomas of the bulbar conjunctiva have been managed by conservative local excision, but multifocal melanomas developing elsewhere in the conjunctiva have tended to be treated by orbital exenteration.

Melanomas arising in the palpebral conjunctiva, the fornices, the plica, and the caruncle are more difficult to eradicate, partly because adjunctive treatments are more difficult to apply in these locations. It is for this reason that standard treatment has tended towards orbital exenteration for such lesions and particularly for neglected, large, extensive, or multiple tumours. A recent study in London, however, suggests that an attempt at conservative excision is legitimate before resorting to exenteration if this approach fails.[27] Two groups of exenterated patients have been compared retrospectively. The indications for orbital exenteration were similar in both, namely conjunctival melanoma in an unfavourable location for conservative excision. One group of patients underwent orbital exenteration as the primary treatment of their conjunctival melanomas, whilst the other group were exenterated only when conservative excision failed. Survival rates were similar in both groups: the key to survival appeared to be the thickness of the largest tumour rather than the treatment method. The melanoma-related mortality rate in this series of patients with a poor prognosis ranged between zero in tumours with a maximum thickness of 1 mm and 50 per cent in those in excess of 2 mm thick. A particularly poor outcome was recorded for melanoma of the caruncle, with six out of seven patients dying despite primary exenteration. Orbital exenteration, frequently advocated for caruncular melanoma, is an illogical operation for tumours in this location because it can achieve a clearance margin of only a millimetre or two, does not give a good survival prospect, and has a severe cosmetic deficit. In London, caruncular melanomas have been managed recently by excision followed by local radiotherapy to the tumour bed with protons and to the nasal passages with photons. This approach has achieved a local control rate as good as exenteration and the survival rate so far is better.

Most conservatively treated patients with PAM will survive simple excision of their initial tumours and, initially at least, will keep an eye which is cosmetically satisfactory, comfortable, and enjoys near-normal visual function. Many will remain in this happy situation for years but the proportion of patients who will survive ultimately to enter the aggressive phase is high. Orbital exenteration continues to play an important part in the management of patients in whom conservative therapy has failed. Indeed, 95 of the reported London series of 256 patients (37 per cent) eventually required exenteration.[10],[27] Exenteration may be required as the primary treatment of others who present with massive neglected melanomas. There is no need to exenterate the posterior orbit, as the procedure can almost always be achieved through a lid-splitting approach with primary closure of skin and orbicularis muscle salvaged from the eyelid. If one eyelid is extensively involved, it is usually possible to close the defect resulting from exenteration with skin and orbicularis muscle from the other lid, especially in the elderly patient with lax eyelid skin (Fig. 2). Following exenteration the patient may be fitted with a spectacle-mounted prosthesis. Younger patients may benefit from an osseous-integrated prosthesis, but this is always best carried out as a secondary procedure. Osseous integration is not advised for patients who have received adjuvant radiotherapy because there is a risk of postoperative bone necrosis.

Advanced melanomas ultimately invade the lymphatics and spread to preauricular, submandibular, and cervical nodes before disseminating locally to the parotid gland or widely, usually to the liver, subcutaneous tissues, or brain. Although patients about to undergo exenteration should have a metastatic evaluation including chest radiographs, liver function tests, and abdominal ultrasound as well as a routine computed tomography (CT) scan of the head and orbits prior to surgery, many will require the operation for palliation even in the presence of asymptomatic metastases. Patients who develop spread to regional glands or the parotid are best managed by excision of all visible local disease followed by radiotherapy to the neck. In this way unpleasant local recurrence may be avoided. Although this treatment is unlikely to prevent eventual dissemination, there have been some very long-term survivors.

Following exenteration, recurrence in the orbit, nasal passages, and paranasal sinuses has been noted in some patients.[5],[28] Orbital recurrence tends to occur following treatment of large, neglected lesions and nasal recurrence after that of inner canthal tumours, presumably because of implantation of tumour cells shed down the nasolacrimal duct. In London, patients exenterated for large melanomas are now offered postoperative adjunctive orbital radiotherapy, and those who have undergone exenteration for inner canthal melanomas are prescribed radiotherapy to the ipsilateral nasal passages in the hope of eliminating local recurrence. It may be that prevention of nasal recurrences explains the better outlook currently achieved for caruncular melanoma treated by local excision and radiotherapy rather than by exenteration without radiation.

Conjunctival melanomas may respond to radiotherapy as the primary treatment,[29] but high doses in the region of 100 Gy are required to achieve tumour regression. However, this amount of radiation cannot be given to the whole conjunctiva using an external-beam approach without intolerable side-effects. Beta-irradiation of small, circumscribed melanomas of the bulbar conjunctiva using strontium-90 surface applicators has been found to be effective,[30] but shrinkage may take several years and, since these tumours are very visible, most ocular oncologists prefer to excise them and to employ radiotherapy, where appropriate, in an adjuvant setting. Practical physical considerations make it difficult to apply brachytherapy using beta-applicators to diffuse and superficially spreading melanomas associated with PAM and to melanomas of the palpebral conjunctiva, the fornix, the plica, and the caruncle. Proton-beam radiotherapy alone may be effective for treating inner canthal melanomas, but combinations of charged-particle therapy and brachytherapy using gamma emissions from cobalt-60 plaques have been tried for the treatment of extensive melanomas elsewhere in the bulbar and palpebral conjunctiva. Cobalt plaques have the advantage of almost equal gamma emissions from both their inner and outer surfaces—a useful property when treating juxtaposed areas of involved bulbar and palpebral conjunctiva. The plaque is positioned in the conjunctival fornix between the adjacent layers of affected conjunctiva and secured with sutures through the conjunctival tissue and into the underlying sclera. Unfortunately, the dose distribution of protons is not favourable in such locations because there is no superficial sparing effect for lesions close to the surface. This, together with the high penetrance of gamma emissions from cobalt-60 and the large doses required, means that these treatments result in considerable damage to the eye, to normal eyelid structures, and to the lacrimal apparatus, though the full effect of such changes may not be apparent for several years. Radiation may induce uveitis and painful neovascular glaucoma which demands enucleation. Such eyes as are retained are dry and uncomfortable. Radiation-induced telangiectasia make these eyes chronically red and unsightly. Permanent loss of eyelashes occurs and depigmentation is noticeable in dark-skinned patients. When the upper eyelid is irradiated, keratinization leads to abrasion of the cornea and subsequently to corneal vascularization and opacification which is not amenable to treatment. In general, therefore, radiotherapy is not a satisfactory substitute for orbital exenteration in advanced conjunctival melanoma because it rarely results in a seeing eye, the cosmetic appearance is often worse than that achieved with a prosthesis, and, perhaps most important of all, the irradiated eye is chronically painful.

From the foregoing it will be apparent that the life prognosis of a patient with conjunctival melanoma will depend significantly on the thickness and location of their presenting tumour and that, except for individuals who present early with PAM alone, these factors are beyond the control of the surgeon. It should also be clear that, having achieved complete clearance of the first tumour, it is vital that the clinician maintains an adequate level of surveillance of the patient so that any new tumours are detected before they reach a thickness of more than 1 mm. The surgeon should treat any new lesions aggressively and, if conservative options fail to control new melanomas, should not hesitate to offer radical treatment by orbital exenteration. This is particularly important for patients who have presented initially with good-prognosis lesions. For others, the surgeon may be able to offer only palliative therapy.

Malignant melanoma of the uveal tract

The uveal tract comprises the iris, the ciliary body, and the choroid and is by far the most common site for the development of a malignant melanoma in the orbital region. The annual incidence of all uveal melanomas has been estimated to be between five and seven cases per million per year in the United States and Europe.[8],[9],[31] Uveal melanomas can arise at any age and congenital lesions have been reported. The peak incidence is in late middle age: in one study there were only three cases per million per year in those under 50 years of age, whereas there were 21 per million per year in those aged 50 years or more.[32] Uveal melanoma is predominantly a tumour of fair-skinned Whites. It is uncommon in Orientals and extremely rare in Blacks. There is no convincing evidence that exposure to sun predisposes to uveal melanoma; in one study from Denmark there had been no increase in the frequency of the ocular tumour during a period when cutaneous melanoma had increased five to six times.[33] Just as they do in conjunctival melanoma, host factors also play an important part in the aetiology of this tumour within the eye. Most examples probably arise in pre-existing choroidal naevi, which have been reported in up to 2 per cent of eyes in clinical examination and 6.5 per cent at autopsy, though the chance of malignant change has been estimated to be less than 1 in 500 during a 10-year period.[34]

Naevi are frequently seen in the iris but rarely in the ciliary body, perhaps because they are very difficult to detect in this location. Malignant transformation may also take place in a melanocytoma.[35] This tumour usually arises in the substance of the optic nerve head but may occasionally be seen in the choroid, ciliary body, or iris. Optic nerve-head melanocytomas were formerly regarded as juxtapapillary melanomas that were invading the nerve but it is now recognized that they represent a particular type of benign magnocellular naevus.[36] Melanocytomas are seen predominantly in people of Black or Oriental extraction and in darker skinned Whites. They are probably congenital but may grow slowly. Malignant change in a melanocytoma may account for a significant proportion of the relatively few melanomas that occur in these racial groups, in which the tumour is otherwise rare. The uveal tract is the site of election for melanoma arising in ocular or oculodermal melanocytosis. Intraocular melanomas arising in these conditions tend to develop in the choroid or ciliary body and only rarely in the iris.

There have been reports of a familial incidence[37] and of bilateral uveal melanomas. Some of these cases have been linked to the atypical mole syndrome (AMS),[38] which is dominantly inherited and in which there is an increased incidence of uveal naevi[39] as well as of dysplastic cutaneous moles and malignant melanomas. Opinions vary as to whether people with AMS have a higher incidence of ocular melanoma than those without the disorder. Greene et al.[40] found no association, but Bataille et al.[41] reported that the relative risk for ocular melanoma increased with the number of atypical naevi. Ocular melanoma patients with a family history of ocular or cutaneous melanoma should be screened for (AMS).

An association has been observed between breast and ovarian cancer and ocular melanoma. Observations of families with BRCA2-linked breast cancer suggest an approximately 20-fold increase in the risk of ocular melanoma. It is hoped that identification of genes conferring an increased risk of ocular melanoma will provide insights into the pathogenesis of the tumour, as well as identifying individuals at high risk who might benefit from targeted surveillance. However, at present, the identification of such people is restricted to the small number belonging to families possessing the BRCA2 gene and those with the atypical mole syndrome.[42]

Clinically, the single most important indicator of a poor prognosis for survival in uveal melanoma is large tumour size.[43] Histologically, tumours containing a high proportion of epithelioid cells have a worse outlook than those consisting predominantly of spindle cells.[44],[45] The clinical and histopathological features may not be independent predictors of outcome because it has been shown that a large tumour volume is closely associated with an epithelioid-cell content.[46] Furthermore, although there is an increased risk of death from metastatic melanoma in the presence of extrascleral extension, it has been demonstrated that this too is a feature of epithelioid-cell tumours,[47] and multivariate analysis fails to confirm the presence of an independent adverse effect of extrascleral extension on survival rate.[48]

The survival rate is significantly better for melanomas of the iris than for those arising in the ciliary body and choroid. Iris melanomas are easily detected by the patient and their better prognosis is due, at least in part, to early recognition and treatment. However, a higher proportion of malignant melanocytic iris tumours have a relatively benign, spindle-cell histology when compared with their counterparts in the ciliary body and choroid.[49] Choroidal melanomas may be detected when they are quite small because they produce an early disturbance of vision, particularly if they arise close to the optic nerve or macula. Asymptomatic posterior choroidal melanomas are relatively easy to see ophthalmoscopically and are often detected at an early stage during a routine eye examination. By contrast, melanomas of the ciliary body are difficult to see with the ophthalmoscope and may not disturb vision until quite late in their evolution because of their greater distance from the optic nerve and macula. These two clinical features conspire to delay detection of most ciliary body melanomas until they are larger, on average, than choroidal melanomas. The large size reached by many anterior melanomas before detection undoubtedly contributes to the relatively poor prognosis of tumours located anterior to the equator of the eye. However, anterior location has been observed to have an adverse effect on survival rate independent of tumour size.[45] This effect may be related to their relatively easy access to the large vortex veins draining the choroid: the presence of melanoma within a vortex vein is strongly associated with the subsequent development of metastases.

The ophthalmic surgeon trying to define the appropriate management of an inaccessible, posterior intraocular tumour that may be a malignant melanoma is frequently faced with a difficulty similar to that of the neurosurgeon faced with a deep-seated brain tumour. In attempting to obtain material for a tissue diagnosis he runs the risk of defeating the object of subsequent conservative therapy, producing irreparable damage to the function of the organ that he hopes to preserve. Under these circumstances, the surgeon must rely on clinical diagnostic criteria aided by non-invasive tests. Fortunately, using such techniques, clinicians specializing in ocular oncology can distinguish melanomas from simulating lesions with an accuracy approaching 98 per cent.[50],[51] Anterior and some posterior tumours are nowadays more amenable to modern biopsy techniques with little risk of damage.

Malignant melanoma of the choroid

Some 80 per cent of uveal melanomas arise in the choroid. Most large tumours have a very characteristic appearance and present no difficulty in diagnosis to the experienced clinician. The typical choroidal melanoma is of a brownish-grey colour rather than black because it is normally viewed through the overlying retina. It has a fairly steeply rising contour as it emerges from the surrounding healthy choroid. As the tumour grows, it eventually ruptures Bruch's inner limiting membrane of the choroid, and commonly bursts through the retinal pigment epithelium to mushroom beneath the neurosensory retina in the subretinal space. This growth pattern leads to the characteristic collar-stud appearance of many choroidal melanomas (Fig. 3). At the time that Bruch's membrane is breached the tumour may bleed through the retina into the vitreous, but such haemorrhages usually resolve spontaneously and rarely recur. The retinal pigment epithelium is hypertrophied over some melanomas, and amelanotic tumours may appear as dark as the pigmented variants. However, the element of an amelanotic melanoma that protrudes through Bruch's membrane and through the retinal pigment epithelium shows the true pale colour of the neoplasm. The clinical significance of this feature of some choroidal melanomas is that the darker tumour at the base of the 'collar-stud' may be overlooked by the inexperienced observer so that the true size and extent of the lesion may be

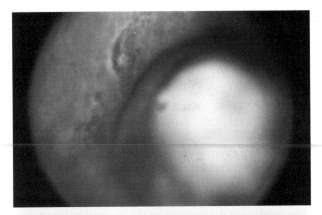

(a)

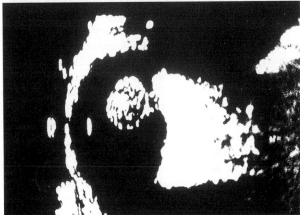

(b)

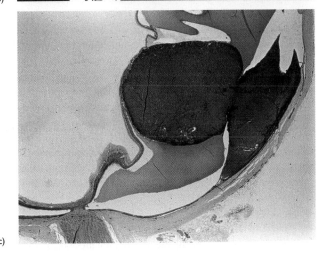

(c)

Fig. 3 (a) Fundus photograph of a typical, large malignant melanoma of the choroid; (b) B-scan ultrasound; and (c) histological section of the same tumour showing a 'collar-stud' contour.

underestimated. After rupture of Bruch's membrane, and with continued tumour growth, the overlying retina may be infiltrated. A pigmented melanoma that has grown through the retina has a brown, velvety appearance similar to that of this tumour in the ciliary body where it is not covered by overlying retinal tissue. The typical collar-stud choroidal melanoma is the equivalent of nodular melanoma in the skin or conjunctiva. Occasionally, however, the growth pattern of a choroidal tumour will parallel that of a superficial spreading melanoma. Such tumours are termed diffuse or *en plaque* melanomas. By convention, a diffuse melanoma must be less than 5 mm thick and involve at least 25 per cent of the uveal tract.[52] Diffuse melanomas have a more pronounced tendency to local extrascleral extension than the nodular variant. Larger, actively growing melanomas tend to leak fluid under the retina and thereby to produce a serous retinal detachment. Growth of a melanoma or extension of its retinal detachment towards the macular area produces symptoms of distortion of vision of 'metamorphopsia' that lead to detection of the tumour. Alternatively, the lesion may impair vision by producing a visual defect or by bleeding into the vitreous. Smaller melanomas are often asymptomatic and discovered on routine eye examination.

The clinical appearance of a large pigmented melanoma is so characteristic that it is most unlikely to be mistaken for anything else when the optic media are clear enough to obtain a good ophthalmoscopic view. When there is haemorrhage or other opacity in the media or when there is extensive retinal detachment over the tumour, it may be difficult to see the outline of the lesion. CT scanning and magnetic resonance imaging (**MRI**) are relatively unhelpful in the biometry and diagnosis of uveal melanoma because the target is small and these tests rely on taking a series of 'cuts'. Because of this they do not give an accurate estimate of tumour size and, furthermore, the internal characteristics of the tumour are less specific with these tests than with ultrasound. Because it is a dynamic test, B-scan ultrasonography has a superior ability to define the precise contour and extent of a tumour. Consequently, it is the most useful ancillary investigation for a large melanoma (Fig. 3). It has the added advantage of being able to distinguish one type of tumour from another on the basis of its internal reflectivity characteristics, to measure the height of a lesion very precisely, and to detect unexpected extrascleral extension or optic nerve invasion. The most important and difficult distinction to make is that between a small melanoma and a benign choroidal naevus. Ultrasonography is less helpful in this respect because small melanomas rarely have a collar-stud contour. Ultrasound may help diagnostically by categorizing the internal reflectivity or by showing choroidal excavation, a characteristic feature of many melanomas. Melanocytic tumours tend to have low internal reflectivity. Additionally, it may be helpful by simply measuring its height. A significant proportion of melanocytic choroidal tumours under 3 mm thick are benign, whereas tumours in excess of this limit are almost always malignant.[53] Because of this, and because of the relative difficulty in obtaining tissue for histological analysis, it used to be standard practice to document the growth of lesions less than 3 mm thick before categorizing them as definite melanomas requiring active treatment. Many small melanomas are indistinguishable from choroidal naevi but certain features have been identified that are predictive of subsequent growth and categorization as a malignant tumour. These include a thickness greater than 1.5 mm and the presence of retinal detachment or clumps of orange lipofuscin pigment on the surface of the tumour.[54] The finding on fluorescein angiography of intrinsic vasculature or of pinpoint or late vascular leakage is suggestive of malignancy, but this test has a diagnostic accuracy rate of less than 50 per cent.[51] When a small tumour exhibits all the features indicative of malignancy, it may be treated promptly as a melanoma without incurring delay by waiting to document enlargement. Hypertrophy or hyperplasia of the retinal pigment epithelium are common conditions that may be mistaken for a small pigmented melanoma, and a benign melanocytoma may

be seen, usually next to the optic disc in darker skinned individuals.

A solitary metastatic deposit from an as yet undetected primary carcinoma may be mistaken for an amelanotic melanoma, and up to half of the patients presenting with such a lesion do so as the first sign of their malignancy.[55] The most common primary sites for choroidal metastases are breast, lung, and kidney. Often, choroidal metastases are multifocal and so are easily distinguished from a primary melanoma. They tend to have a shelving rather than a steeply rising contour, best seen on ultrasound, and medium internal reflectivity. In cases of doubt that cannot be resolved by ultrasound, choroidal biopsy, or systemic evaluation, a brief period of observation will commonly settle the issue. It is most unusual for a small melanoma to grow in under 3 months but many metastatic carcinomas will. Other pale lesions that must be distinguished from amelanotic melanoma are choroidal haemangioma and choroidal osteoma, both of which show high internal reflectivity on ultrasound.

Radioactive tracers and particularly ^{32}P were used for many years to localize ocular melanomas, but the limitations of this test restricted its popularity and it has fallen out of fashion.[56] Radio-immunoscintigraphy using ^{99}Tc^{m}-labelled F(ab')$_2$ fragments of monoclonal antibody raised against cutaneous melanoma can distinguish between a metastatic carcinoma or choroidal haemangioma and a melanocytic tumour. However, the antibodies currently available recognize common antigens on the surfaces of naevi as well as on melanomas and cannot therefore categorize a pigmented tumour as benign or malignant.[57]

It has been estimated that between 20 and 50 per cent of patients with a posterior uveal melanoma will ultimately die a metastatic death,[58] with a mean interval between treatment of the primary tumour and clinical evidence of metastases ranging from 34 to 43 months.[59],[60] The survival rate of individuals with choroidal melanoma in relation to the size of their tumour has been difficult to establish precisely because of problems in estimating tumour volume accurately. Using a mathematical model, it has been shown that 82 per cent of patients having an eye enucleated for a choroidal melanoma with a volume of less than 600 mm^3 will survive 5 years and that over 90 per cent of tumours in this category are spindle-cell lesions. The 5-year survival rate for tumours of 900 mm^3 and over falls to 50 per cent. In a multivariate analysis, tumour volume was found to be more important in predicting outcome than cell type.[48] It has been suggested that the higher proportion of epithelioid cells seen in larger melanomas results from the transformation of spindle-cell tumours to lesions with a more aggressive cell type and growth pattern.[43] It is more probable that epithelioid-cell tumours are often found to be large because they grow rapidly and remain small for a shorter time.[48] Although extrascleral extension of a choroidal melanoma reduces the 5-year survival rate from 67 per cent without this finding to 34 per cent with, tumours which spread locally outside the eye tend to contain epithelioid cells more often than those that do not. It is by no means certain, therefore, that increased mortality is due to the event of extrascleral spread rather than to the histologically more aggressive type of melanoma that exhibits this sort of behaviour.

Once the diagnosis of choroidal melanoma has been established clinically beyond reasonable doubt or histopathologically by biopsy, systemic metastatic evaluation should be undertaken. Far the most common site for metastases from a choroidal primary is the liver, followed by the lungs.[31] When carrying out these investigations, it should be borne in mind that very few patients will be found to have detectable metastatic melanoma at the time of diagnosis of their intraocular primary. This is especially so for small melanomas, and only 1 in 40 patients with a lesion large enough to warrant surgical intervention will be found to have metastases at the initial staging.[61] By contrast, some 50 per cent of patients with a large melanoma will have metastases 5 years after treatment. At the time of the initial diagnosis, there is no sensitive screening test for metastatic uveal melanoma. Although some advocate whole-body scans, it pays to concentrate on high-risk areas. In a recent study of a series of 245 patients with uveal melanoma 22 per cent of whom had died, all screening investigations performed at diagnosis were found to have a low yield but the most sensitive were those for gamma-glutamyl transpeptidase (γ-GT; sensitivity 21 per cent), and alkaline phosphatase (sensitivity 25 per cent), with γ-GT being more specific (specificity 92 per cent). No blood test had a positive predictive power greater than 50 per cent. The chest radiograph and liver ultrasound were both 100 per cent specific but had sensitivities of only 2 and 14 per cent, respectively.[62]

Because of the limitations of treating metastatic melanoma, the main aim of staging patients with an ocular tumour is to avoid unnecessarily intensive treatment of an ocular primary should a patient have metastatic disease. With the possible exception of individuals whose lifespan is limited by intercurrent disease and the very elderly patient with a melanoma that is growing slowly (if at all), everyone with a definite melanoma and no detectable metastases should be offered active treatment. For the otherwise healthy patient, the only indication for serial observation of a melanocytic tumour is to establish, by documenting growth, that it is a malignant tumour if this is in doubt at presentation. Once such a lesion has grown, observation should be discontinued and treatment commenced.

Formerly, enucleation of the eye was the standard treatment for all patients with choroidal melanoma. However, in most specialist centres this mutilating procedure has been largely replaced for all except the largest melanomas and recurrent tumours, by techniques that aim to conserve the globe, often with good visual function. The popularity of the newer approach stems mainly from the poor record of enucleation in preventing metastatic spread. Whether or not a conservative treatment has been successful in achieving sustained local tumour control may not be known for months or years and some patients find this disturbing. These individuals are best enucleated.

Treatment options

The choice of treatment depends on a number of factors, including the size and location of the tumour, the presence or absence of an associated retinal detachment or extrascleral extension, the visual status of the contralateral eye, and, very occasionally, the presence of metastases at diagnosis. It is important to realize that the interface between treatment options is by no means absolute. A surprising proportion of patients with uveal melanoma have lost the contralateral eye or have defective vision in it. In such patients with posterior melanomas, radiation may destroy central vision in the better eye. With the aim of preserving vision, and only on an informed basis, such patients may be offered non-radiational therapy even though the local tumour control rate may not be quite so good. In rare cases where liver metastases are detected at diagnosis, the eye is not enucleated unless it is painful. Lung and cutaneous metastases are compatible with longer survival times and conservative treatment

may be considered in such patients who have no apparent liver involvement.

Photocoagulation

Very small melanomas may be destroyed by coagulation, using either a xenon arc[63] or laser. After first sealing off the choroidal blood supply of the tumour by photocoagulation of healthy tissue outside its margin, the lesion itself is treated heavily until it is replaced by a flat scar (Fig. 4). Several treatment sessions are usually required. This approach is contraindicated for melanomas that are more than 3 mm thick, amelanotic, located within the papillomacular bundle of nerve fibres or immediately adjacent to the fovea or optic disc, crossed by large retinal blood vessels, or over which there is an extensive retinal detachment. In the long term, the method has an inferior local tumour control rate compared with radiotherapy for larger tumours. In London, after 5 years of follow-up, only 67 per cent of melanomas up to 3 mm thick were controlled by photocoagulation compared with 97 per cent of tumours up to 8 mm thick treated by radiotherapy using plaque or proton beam. Most melanomas small enough for this treatment are asymptomatic tumours detected on routine examination and close to the optic disc or macula. What is more, as will be apparent from the treatment size criteria, at least some suitable lesions may really be naevi! Probably the only remaining indication for this treatment method is to destroy a very small melanoma that fulfils all the criteria for the diagnosis of a malignant tumour and that is located on the nasal side of the optic disc, not touching the margin of the disc, but too close to avoid sight loss from ischaemic optic neuropathy if radiotherapy is employed. When photocoagulation is applied close to the macula, retinal shrinkage occurs with visual loss due mainly to macular hole formation.

The undoubted limitations of photocoagulation have recently led to the exploration of other non-radiational treatment methods for small and sometimes for larger melanomas. Microwave-induced hyperthermia was first used as an adjunct to radiotherapy. Later, employing infrared radiation at 810 nm generated by a diode laser, Oosterhuis increased the temperatures used to levels higher than normally employed for hyperthermia and coined the term 'transpupillary thermotherapy' (TTT). As with photocoagulation, heat is generated from diode laser emissions mainly by absorption into melanin pigment. It is claimed that diode laser-generated infrared radiation produces less side-effects on normal structures than conventional photocoagulation. Oosterhuis[64] still intended the method mainly as an adjunct to radiation, with the aim of reducing the dose of radiotherapy needed to regress a tumour. He observed that the penetration of laser emissions, and therefore of heat, into thicker melanomas was strictly limited, but the method has been widely adopted by others as a single-agent treatment on the basis of relatively short follow-up data.[65] Originally, heat was applied within the confines of small pigmented tumours but the technique has been extended to treat larger lesions and, using chromatophores, non-pigmented melanomas. Because of edge relapses, treatments have been extended beyond the margins of tumours into healthy tissue and treatment energies have been increased to levels that produce visible coagulation. These treatments are not really thermotherapy but in fact photocoagulation by another method. It remains to be seen whether tumour control rates will approach those provided by radiation. The issue is of considerable importance, because if a long-term systemic cure can be achieved for any choroidal melanoma it will be for smaller

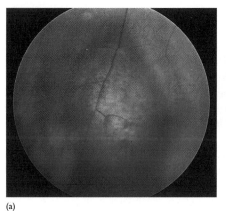
(a)

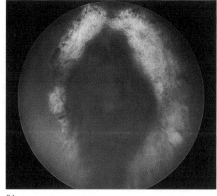
(b)

Fig. 4 Small choroidal malignant melanoma (a) before and (b) after treatment by xenon-arc photocoagulation.

lesions. Treatments that fail to achieve adequate local control of small melanomas are potentially particularly dangerous.

Scleral plaque radiotherapy

It used to be held that melanomas could not be destroyed by radiation. This is not so, but they are very radioresistant neoplasms that require what is effectively a tumour-necrosis dose to bring about regression. The dose necessary is well in excess of that which would produce irreversible and blinding radiation damage to the retina, choroid, and optic nerve if the whole eye were to be irradiated. It was for this reason that the first successful radiation treatments of choroidal melanoma employed brachytherapy techniques that concentrated the high dose in that part of the eye containing the neoplasm. This allowed the radiation to be rapidly attenuated away from the tumour margin because of the effects of the inverse square law.[66] Provided that it is distant from the optic disc and macula, a melanoma may be destroyed by this method with preservation of vision.

The radiation sources used initially were radon seeds[67] and, later, ^{60}Co incorporated into an applicator or 'plaque' shaped to the contour of the external surface of the sclera and provided with suture holes for attachment to the globe.[66] These high-energy, gamma-ray sources cannot be shielded on their external surfaces and produce side-effects on the ocular adnexa, particularly on the lacrimal apparatus.[68],[69] They have been largely replaced by shielded low-energy sources employing the same principles. Low-energy gamma emissions from ^{125}I seeds are shielded externally by gold and used to treat melanomas up to 8 mm in thickness (Fig. 5).[70]–[72] Beta-emissions from [106]Ru/[106]Rh are shielded externally by silver and used to treat lesions up to 5 mm thick (Fig. 6).[73] The tumour is localized during a surgical operation, usually by casting its shadow on the scleral surface by fibre-optic transillumination and marking the outline. The sutures are placed using a Plexiglas dummy applicator so that the position can be checked by repeat transillumination (Fig. 7). The dummy applicator is then replaced by the active plaque (Fig. 8), which is left in place long enough to deliver a dose of between 80 and 120 Gy to the apex of the tumour, as measured by ultrasound and allowing an extra millimetre for the scleral thickness. Treatment takes from 2 to 10 days. The source is renewed when the dose rate threatens to fall below 45 cGy/h at the tumour apex.

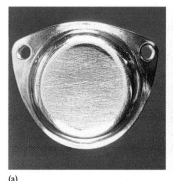
(a)

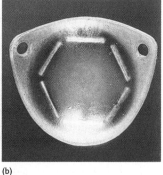
(b)

Fig. 5 (a) External and (b) internal view of a ^{125}I scleral applicator of the pattern in use at St Bartholomew's Hospital. Six ^{125}I seeds are embedded in epoxy resin in a recess in the internal surface of a gold carrier.

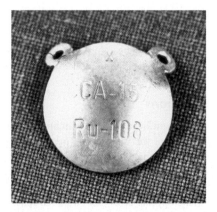

Fig. 6 [106]Ru/[106]Rh scleral applicator.

The goal of radiotherapy for uveal melanoma is to prevent further cell division in the treated tumour. Following treatment, a tumour-associated serous retinal detachment will usually disappear between 1 and 3 months. The pattern of tumour regression is variable but shrinkage is rarely apparent before 3 months have elapsed after

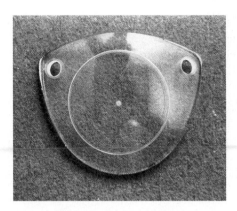

Fig. 7 Perspex dummy applicator for use with the ^{125}I applicator.

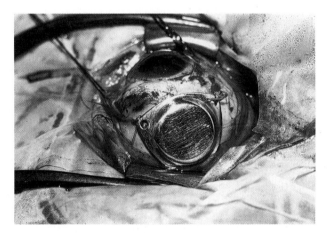

Fig. 8 ^{125}I applicator in place, sutured to sclera over a medium-sized ciliochoroidal malignant melanoma within the eye.

treatment. The tumour is monitored by serial ultrasound measurements of its height and photographs of its outline. Tumours under 5 mm thick may regress to a flat scar (Fig. 9), but there is usually some permanent residual thickness detectable after treatment of thicker melanomas. Regression may continue, sometimes episodically,

for 2 or more years. Structures adjacent to the plaque may suffer radiation damage. Lens opacity may follow treatment of anterior tumours. Damage to blood vessels produces late ischaemic changes that will affect vision, particularly if they involve the optic disc and macula. Because of the dose distribution of radiation from plaques, these vascular effects are felt most when the technique is used to treat thicker and more posteriorly located melanomas. Conversely, the best visual results are obtained when plaques are used to treat tumours at, or anterior to, the equator of the globe, especially on the nasal side away from the macula. Severe ischaemia, particularly that associated with persistent retinal detachment, may lead to neovascular glaucoma. Cataract, ischaemic maculopathy, and neovascular glaucoma are all less common after [106]Ru/[106]Rh- than after ^{125}I-plaque therapy, partly because of the less-penetrating radiation from ruthenium applicators and partly because they are generally used to treat thinner tumours.

Plaque radiotherapy has a good record for long-term preservation of the eye, though enucleation is still indicated for continued tumour growth or painful neovascular glaucoma. In a group of 330 patients treated, in London, by modern, low-energy plaques and followed for a median period of 4 years, 7 per cent required enucleation.[74] Of 1019 patients with posterior uveal melanoma treated, in Philadelphia, by plaque, 6 per cent required enucleation, though the median follow-up interval was not reported.[75] The mean interval from treatment to removal of the eye was 29 months. Most eyes (51 per cent) were removed for tumour growth. In an older series, conducted in London, of 123 patients treated by cobalt plaque and followed for a median period of 16 years, 78 per cent of patients retained the treated eye. Vision in retained eyes was 6/12 or better in 25 per cent, 6/18 to 6/60 in 35 per cent, and less than 6/60 in 40 per cent, depending mainly on the location of the tumour within the eye. In a modern series of 64 patients treated by iodine-125 plaque, but with a mean follow-up period of only 65 months, 45 per cent retained 20/100 vision or better and 28 per cent kept a visual acuity within two Snellen lines of the value before treatment.[72]

To date, no study has shown a worse survival rate after plaque therapy than after enucleation when patients have been properly matched for other risk factors such as tumour size and location. However, such studies as have been done have all been retrospective.[76]–[78]

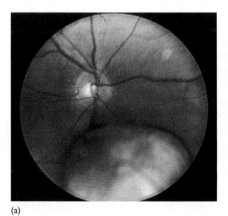

(a)

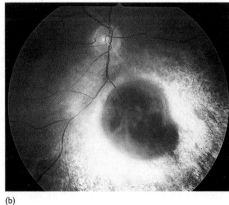

(b)

Fig. 9 (a) Choroidal melanoma before treatment by ^{125}I scleral applicator and (b) 1 year after plaque radiotherapy. The tumour has regressed to a flat, pigmented scar and is surrounded by a zone of radiation-induced atrophy of the choroid and retina.

Charged-particle radiotherapy

It is now possible to deliver a pencil beam of radiation to a melanoma within the eye using positively charged particles, either protons[79] or helium ions,[80] accelerated by a cyclotron. The dose distribution of the beam is theoretically ideal for the treatment of uveal-tract melanomas. It has a very well-defined edge, with the isodoses falling rapidly to below the 50 per cent level within 2 mm. Furthermore, the radiation dose first rises as the beam passes through the tissues and as the particles decelerate and release their energy. It then falls rapidly to zero as the particles come to a halt. This sudden release of energy is termed the Bragg peak. The effects of the Bragg peak are to minimize the entry dose and virtually to eliminate any exit dose.

In order to direct the beam precisely to a tumour within the eye, a surgical operation is first performed to attach inert tantalum marker clips to the sclera around its base (Fig. 10). The technique of localization used is the same as for insertion of a radioactive plaque. The clips do not need to be removed after radiotherapy. The distances are recorded from each clip to the tumour margin, from one clip to another, and from the clips to the corneoscleral limbus. The dimensions of the eye to be treated are established from measurements of the corneal diameter and by ultrasonic biometry of the axial length of the globe. These measurements are then collated with information from a B-scan ultrasound about the tumour contour and dimensions and from retinal photographs and drawings defining its location within the eye, using a three-dimensional computer planning program (Fig. 10). A treatment plan is thereby generated which records the gaze co-ordinates that must be viewed by the patient during therapy for correct targeting with minimum ocular side-effects, details of the collimator required, and the information necessary to spread a series of Bragg peaks throughout the tumour and to maximize the superficial sparing effect. The plan also predicts the orthogonal and lateral radiographic projections of the metal clips when the eye is correctly positioned for treatment. Simulation is then undertaken with the patient viewing a fixation target at the given co-ordinates and with head movement eliminated by a face mask and bite block (Fig. 11). The patient is ready for treatment when the disposition of the clips on the radiographs matches the computer prediction. A total of 60 Gy is given in four equal fractions over 4 consecutive days.

In principle, charged-particle therapy is suitable for the treatment of ocular melanomas of any size because, in contrast to plaque therapy, the radiation dose is distributed evenly throughout the tumour. In practice, however, the volume of normal ocular tissue that receives a high dose when treating a small posterior melanoma is unnecessarily large, and side-effects are less when such melanomas are treated with plaques. In London, therefore, charged-particle therapy has been reserved for tumours more than 8 mm thick and for those arising in locations where the dose distribution from a plaque may be suboptimal, such as adjacent to the optic disc.

The success rates for preservation of the eyes with large, medium-sized, and small melanomas are reported from Boston, United States, to be 90, 96, and 98 per cent, respectively.[81] Overall, in the Boston series, only 6.4 per cent of a series of 994 eyes required enucleation during a median follow-up period of 2.7 years.[82] Time from treatment to enucleation averaged 13 months. Some 89 per cent of enucleations after proton therapy are performed within 3 years of treatment[81] and none more than $5\frac{1}{2}$ years after treatment.[82] Continued tumour growth occurs in very few eyes. In Boston, only 1.9 per cent of 1077 eyes exhibited continued tumour growth during a mean follow-up

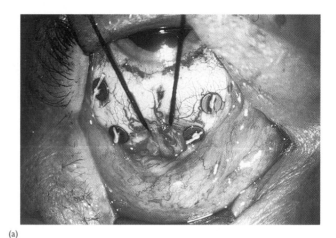

(a)

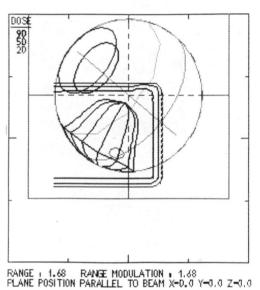

87265   LEFT EYE   5-JUL-88
PLANE WITHIN THE EYE
FIXATION LIGHT: POLAR 51 AZIMUTHAL 44 TWIST 0
EYE CENTRE IS AT   0.00   0.70   0.00
APERTURE IS : APER
LID SURF. AT 0.00 cm IN FRONT OF EYE SURFACE

RANGE : 1.68   RANGE MODULATION : 1.68
(b)   PLANE POSITION PARALLEL TO BEAM X=0.0 Y=0.0 Z=0.0

Fig. 10 (a)(b) (a) Tantalum clips sutured to the sclera around a large ciliary-body melanoma to mark its position before proton-beam radiotherapy. (b) Black and white image of the three-dimensional, colour computergraphic proton-treatment plan generated from the tantalum clip data, from B-scan, ultrasound biometry, and from fundus photographs.

period of 4 years.[83] In contrast to plaque therapy, most melanoma eyes requiring enucleation after charged-particle therapy are removed because of neovascular glaucoma—with only 25 per cent due to tumour growth.[82] A study of London patients showed that the main risk factors for this development are large tumour size and retinal detachment.[84] Eyes containing small melanomas without retinal detachment have only a 10 per cent chance of glaucoma. When a melanoma is either too large for plaque therapy or associated with a retinal detachment the risk is 36 per cent, but when both risk factors are present 90 per cent of eyes will develop glaucoma. Approximately one-third of eyes with rubeotic glaucoma require enucleation for pain and the remainder are chronically red and uncomfortable.

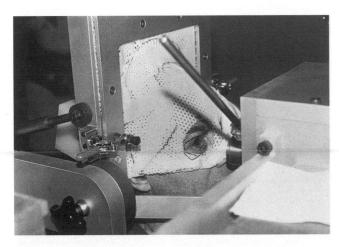

Fig. 11 Proton-beam radiotherapy set-up: the patient is seated in an electrically powered chair and views a target whilst his head is held rigid by a tailor-made mask and bite block.

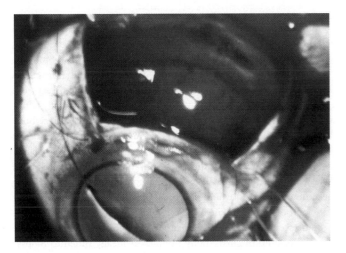

Fig. 12 Intraoperative view of surgical resection of choroidal melanoma.

Consequently, charged-particle therapy is inadvisable when the risk of glaucoma is high. The visual results have been reported after helium-ion radiotherapy: with a median follow-up of 27 months, 49 per cent of patients had 20/200 vision or better in the treated eye.[85]

Choroidal resection

In selected patients, a choroidal melanoma may be resected surgically. Two alternative surgical techniques have been described. The tumour may be excised under an autogenous lamellar or full-thickness scleral flap (Fig. 12),[86],[87] or the whole eye wall including the melanoma may be resected and the defect closed by a homograft of sclera.[88] The former technique has gained greater acceptance. The choroid is the most vascular tissue in the body and profound vascular hypotension is required during anaesthesia to achieve a successful resection, particularly when the scleral flap method is used. This limits the procedure to young individuals who have no history of cardiovascular disease. Nevertheless, cerebrovascular accidents have occurred. Constant electroencephalography (EEG) monitoring during the operation is recommended and occasionally the procedure has to be abandoned intraoperatively. Choroidal resection is one of the only eye operations to pose a serious threat to the health of the patient and should not be undertaken lightly, especially in older patients and when the other eye is healthy.

By combining the operation with vitrectomy, it is possible to excise very posterior tumours. A margin of at least 1 millimetre of normal tissue should be allowed. The method has a much higher intraoperative and acute postoperative complication rate than plaque or charged-particle procedures, the main risks being intraocular haemorrhage and retinal detachment. Approximately one-third of patients require a second operation to reattach a detached retina. The visual results are better for tumours situated more posteriorly and nasally than for those in anterior and temporal locations. The main factor limiting success in terms of local tumour control is the base diameter of the melanoma, and not its thickness as in plaque therapy or its volume as in charged-particle therapy. Local tumour control rates after choroidal resection alone have been substantially lower than those following radiotherapy[89] and, consequently, adjuvant plaque therapy to the excision site is now recommended. A ruthenium plaque of diameter greater than the surgical resection is applied at the end of the operation and the dose should be prescribed to the post-resection thickness of the sclera, choroid, and retina rather than to the pre-resection height of the whole tumour. This approach may reduce the high, edge relapse rate that has bedevilled choroidal resection, though such recurrences can often be managed by photocoagulation or laser hyperthermia.

As the requirement for profound, hypotensive anaesthesia has undoubtedly limited the popularity of trans-scleral resection of posterior uveal melanomas, there is increasing interest in internal or 'endoresection', using techniques developed in general ophthalmology for internal reattachment of ordinary retinal detachments.[90],[91] This technique is in its infancy.

Enucleation

Enucleation is advised for continued tumour growth that cannot be controlled by conservative methods and for painful complications after conservative therapy. It is also indicated as the primary treatment of eyes with very large or diffuse melanomas, particularly if the eye is blind or painful or if it has raised intraocular pressure. There is no contraindication during enucleation to the primary insertion of an orbital implant. The implant may be integrated with the extraocular muscles to impart realistic movement to the artificial eye that is fitted as a secondary procedure.

The presence of a massive extrascleral extension is an indication for enucleation, but small extrascleral nodules can be excised to allow for insertion of a plaque or can be incorporated into the treatment plan for charged-particle therapy. Extrascleral extension has a highly significant adverse effect on local tumour control and 50 per cent of melanomas will recur in the orbit when the extension is non-encapsulated or surgically transected.[47] It has been shown that adjuvant orbital radiotherapy to a dose averaging 50 Gy is effective in reducing the local recurrence rate.[92] The need for postenucleation radiotherapy is not a contraindication to the insertion of an integrated orbital implant.

Orbital exenteration

This radical operation is now rarely indicated for uveal melanoma. Nevertheless, it still provides the most effective means of establishing local tumour control in massive extrascleral extension of a neglected melanoma. It was once the standard treatment for extrascleral extension of any degree but is no longer held to improve the survival rate in this situation.[93] Exenteration may be the best choice for an extensive orbital recurrence, though a small amount of recurrent or residual melanoma in the orbit may best be excised locally, preserving the socket, and before giving adjuvant orbital radiotherapy and fitting a conventional artificial eye.

When planning exenteration, it is important to obtain CT or MRI scans to ensure that the tumour does not extend out of the orbit posteriorly and is resectable. A systemic metastatic evaluation should be undertaken, but even if it is negative the operation is unlikely to achieve a cure. In the presence of metastatic disease, exenteration may still be indicated for palliative reasons. If the eyelids are not involved by tumour, they may be split surgically to provide skin and orbicularis muscle for primary closure. This approach assures rapid rehabilitation by allowing early fitting of a spectacle-mounted or adhesive prosthesis.

Malignant melanoma of the ciliary body

Some 12 per cent of uveal melanomas arise in the ciliary body in front of the ora serrata, which marks the anterior limit of the retina and underlying choroid. Melanomas of the ciliary body have a more definite brown tinge than their choroidal counterparts because their surface colour is not obscured by overlying retina. Bruch's inner limiting membrane of the choroid also ceases at the ora serrata, with the result that melanomas confined to the ciliary body never have a collar-stud contour. As they grow, some melanomas extend posteriorly from the ciliary body under the retina into the choroid and vice versa. The ora serrata can be seen crossing the surface of such 'ciliochoroidal' melanomas and they exhibit clinical features dependent on their combined sites of origin. Less frequently, a lesion of the ciliary body may grow forwards, displacing the root of the iris and presenting in the anterior chamber where it may be confused with a primary melanoma of the iris (Fig. 13). The ciliary body counterpart of the diffuse variant of choroidal melanoma is one that is relatively flat and extends ultimately to involve the entire circumference of the anterior uveal tract. This variant is termed a 'ring melanoma'. It often involves the iris root and trabecular meshwork and, consequently, it usually presents with raised intraocular pressure. Ring melanomas are very difficult to detect but should be suspected in any patient with intractable unilateral glaucoma and abnormal iris pigmentation.[94]

Melanomas of the ciliary body tend to present late because their peripheral location means that they do not involve the macular area either directly, or indirectly by means of a retinal detachment, until very large. They are also extremely difficult to visualize ophthalmoscopically during a routine eye examination unless a need is seen to dilate the pupil. A ciliary-body melanoma may be detected because it disturbs vision by inducing astigmatism or a cataract, by producing a retinal detachment, by impinging on the visual axis, or by elevating the intraocular pressure. Additionally, or alternatively, it may become externally visible through invasion of the iris root or by extending extrasclerally, where it may easily be seen as an episcleral

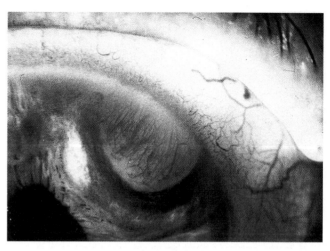

Fig. 13 Malignant melanoma of the ciliary body eroding the iris root and presenting in the anterior chamber of the eye.

nodule because if its anterior location. Finally, it may be found because large feeder or 'sentinel' vessels are seen in the episclera, where they may initially be mistaken for ocular inflammation.

The lesions that can be confused with a ciliary-body melanoma are, for the most part, rare and cannot usually be distinguished from a melanocytic tumour by any non-invasive clinical test. Ultrasonography is less helpful in confirming the diagnosis of ciliary-body than of choroidal melanoma because of the absence of both a collar-stud contour and choroidal excavation in the anterior variant. Ultrasound may reveal that the lesion is cystic but, although epithelial cysts are not uncommon, the finding cannot be regarded as excluding melanoma: ciliary-body and choroidal melanomas may both appear cystic on occasion. The site of ciliary-body melanomas is inaccessible for fluorescein angiography but isotope scans my be informative. The anterior location of ciliary-body tumours is ideally suited to biopsy.

There are many pitfalls in the clinical diagnosis, but most of the lesions that must be differentiated from an anterior melanoma are benign. Consequently, incisional and, where possible, excisional biopsy should always be considered for doubtful lesions. Metastatic lesions are uncommon in the ciliary body and tend to favour the posterior uveal tract. A pale mass in the ciliary body in a child or young person may be a medulloepithelioma, though this tumour has been reported in older people.[95] In an adult it may be a leiomyoma.[96] A very dark lesion may prove to be a melanocytoma, particularly in a dark-skinned individual and when there is raised intraocular pressure due to pigment dispersion[97] or an adenoma of the pigmented ciliary epithelium if the pressure is normal. Adenomas can also occur in the retinal pigment epithelium and masquerade as choroidal melanomas, but they are more often located anteriorly.[98]

In general, the indications for the treatment of a ciliary-body melanoma are the same as those for a choroidal melanoma. The therapeutic techniques are similar but the outcomes are significantly different. All treatment methods other than photocoagulation may be employed. The physical limitations placed on plaque therapy by tumour size are the same as for choroidal melanoma. It is difficult to define the tumour edges during surgery of melanomas in the ciliary body because of the dense shadow normally cast by that structure during transillumination. Furthermore, edge recurrences are difficult to detect and treat. It is particularly important, therefore, to use a large plaque that more than covers the tumour edge when carrying out plaque radiotherapy for anterior melanomas. It is also important to use a modern, shielded plaque when treating a ciliary-body lesion if radiation damage to the eyelids and lacrimal apparatus are to be avoided. If they cannot be retracted during treatment, the eyelids are more likely to suffer damage during charged-particle therapy for an anterior melanoma than for a posterior one because of loss of the superficial sparing effect of the Bragg peak. Keratinization of the eyelid margin is a particular problem following charged-particle therapy for anterior melanomas and is at its most troublesome when the central portion of the upper eyelid receives a high dose. Keratinization in this location leads to severe corneal-surface disease and an irritable eye that is not easily relieved by lubricants. As a result, proton therapy is no longer used in London to treat superior, anterior melanomas. Cataract is a common, direct effect of irradiating a tumour in the anterior segment of the eye. Ruthenium plaques are much less likely to produce cataract than iodine applicators when used to treat anterior lesions. Cataract may follow surgical resection suggesting that, like neovascular glaucoma, another a complication of treatment of anterior tumours, it may also follow disturbance of the physiology of the anterior segment.

Ciliary-body tumours may be excised surgically. Invasion of the iris root is difficult to assess and the tumour is usually removed with a corresponding sector of iris in the procedure known as 'iridocyclectomy'. Although more accessible and therefore technically easier to remove than more posterior lesions, the results are not as good. Again, the tumour edges are hard to define so that late relapse is common. Also, if removal of the tumour and a margin of healthy tissue involves more than one-third of the ciliary body hypotony usually follows, leading in turn to visual loss from macular oedema. Unlike tumours in the choroid, ciliary-body melanomas are not separated from the vitreous gel by the intervening retina. This means that iridocyclectomy may be complicated by vitreous loss or incarceration, haemorrhage, and late progressive-tractional retinal detachment. Defective vision in the other eye may justify treating a melanoma extending for more than one-third of the ciliary circumference with charged particles. However, since attempts to treat lesions involving more than half of the anterior portion of the eye in this way almost always leads to painful glaucoma, scleritis, or keratitis, such globes are therefore best enucleated, whatever the state of the fellow eye. Enucleation is the only treatment for a ring melanoma and any area of extrascleral extension should be given a wide surgical margin in order to avoid adjuvant radiotherapy. Though it is generally accepted that anterior melanomas have a worse life prognosis than posterior lesions, even when correcting for the fact that they tend to present later and are therefore larger than their choroidal counterparts, there are no data on survival rates for pure ciliary-body melanomas.

Malignant melanoma of the iris

Approximately 8 per cent of uveal melanomas arise in the iris, which is the least frequent site of origin for this tumour within the eye. Iris melanomas are more common in light-coloured than in dark irides[97] and show a distinct predilection for the inferior portion of the structure. They are externally visible, which probably accounts for

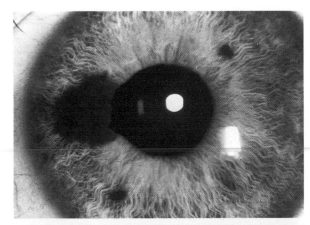

(a)

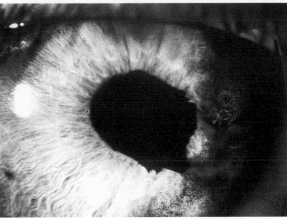

(b)

Fig. 14 (a) Circumscribed malignant melanoma of the iris with satellite lesions and (b) diffuse malignant melanoma of the iris. Local resection was contraindicated for both tumours and the eyes were enucleated after malignant epithelioid cells were demonstrated by biopsy.

their tendency to present in younger people[99] and when they are smaller than melanomas elsewhere in the eye.[100] Like other uveal melanomas, those affecting the iris may be circumscribed or diffuse (Fig. 14). Circumscribed tumours may have satellite lesions. Both circumscribed and diffuse tumours at the iris root must be distinguished from neoplasms of the ciliary body invading the anterior chamber of the eye. The degree of pigmentation of an iris melanoma may range from intensely black to white. Some pale, iris melanomas have an appearance similar to tapioca, though this feature has no apparent prognostic significance. A circumscribed, pigmented iris melanoma in an adult must be distinguished from a naevus, a melanocytoma, or a solitary cyst of the iris pigment epithelium. A circumscribed pale melanoma of the iris must be differentiated from a deposit of metastatic carcinoma or lymphoma, a neurofibroma, or a leiomyoma, although the existence of the latter tumour in the iris has recently been called into question.[101] In a child, the pale lesion must be distinguished from a medulloepithelioma or juvenile xanthogranuloma, both of which, though rare, are commoner than melanoma in this age group.

The most frequent and important, but at the same time the most difficult, distinction to draw clinically is that between an iris naevus and a malignant melanoma.[49] An iris naevus, in turn, must be distinguished from the iris freckles that are seen on almost all pale-coloured irides. Freckles tend to be small, flat, and multiple and they do not distort the underlying stroma of the iris. An iris naevus, on the other hand, is usually more than 1 mm in diameter and can be up to 1 mm thick. Like melanomas they may show all variations of pigmentation and may invade the underlying stroma. Formerly, a melanocytic tumour of the iris was regarded as clinically malignant when it was large or documented to grow or when it distorted the pupil, invaded intraocular structures, or produced secondary glaucoma, but these clinical criteria are now considered much less clear-cut. Histologically, iris melanomas are notable for having few epithelioid cells and a preponderance of naevoid or spindle A cells of doubtful malignant potential. The histopathological division between benign and malignant is much less distinct than it is elsewhere in the uveal tract, such that one pair of investigators reclassified 87 per cent of a group of iris melanocytic tumours, previously categorized as malignant on histological criteria, as being naevi.[102] It is now known from the histological evaluation of many such lesions excised on clinical grounds that benign naevi may grow and exhibit invasive features.[100] Conversely, many iris lesions of alarming clinical and histological appearance have been present, unchanged, for a long time. In one series, fewer than 5 per cent of melanocytic iris tumours with a clinical appearance suggestive of melanoma were documented to grow over a mean follow-up period approaching 5 years.[103]

The overall mortality rate of iris melanomas has been reported to be between 3 and 5 per cent but this figure rises towards 10 per cent when only tumours with epithelioid cells are considered, albeit a finding based on a very small series.[100] It follows that there is a need to distinguish clinically between naevoid tumours which require no treatment and the rare, truly malignant iris melanomas which pose a threat to life. This is especially important because of the tendency of iris melanomas to present very early in their evolution. Unfortunately, there are no reliable clinical hallmarks of malignancy. We have seen that even growth and invasion may be observed in benign lesions, whilst malignant ones may not change over a long observation period. Malignant iris melanomas do tend to have prominent vascularity and this is seen most easily in the amelanotic tumours. Using this feature, attempts have been made to correlate the fluorescein-iris angiographic features of iris melanocytic tumours with malignancy. The ability of the test to predict whether a tumour is frankly malignant or not is uncertain and in one study it was considered helpful in only 50 per cent of cases.[104] Fluorescein iris angiography is now rarely used as a diagnostic tool because the abnormal vessels suggestive of malignancy can be seen perfectly well on slit-lamp examination without angiography in pale tumours—and with neither technique in heavily pigmented ones!

Because of the benign histological appearances of many excised iris melanomas, there has been a trend away from immediate surgical excision and towards a policy of serial photographic observations of suspicious lesions to document their growth before intervening. Qualitative diagnostic ultrasound has no place in the appraisal of iris lesions and is less precise than photographs in detecting change. This approach requires a definition of the term 'suspicious'. Any iris lesion that has significant thickness on slit-lamp biomicroscopy or which measures 3 mm or more in diameter should be followed in this way. Clearly, there is a spectrum of disease and some early melanomas will not be subjected to reappraisal. Furthermore, by adhering to this scheme, some benign lesions that grow may be excised, whilst others

that have epithelioid cells but do not grow will be ignored. Nevertheless, this approach represents the best compromise that can be achieved at present for smaller iris lesions in the absence of a better clinical indicator of malignancy.

It will be wise to qualify this scheme by defining a category of probable melanomas that do require urgent treatment. This group should include all extensive or highly vascular lesions, those in excess of 1 mm in thickness, especially when they touch the corneal endothelium, and those with satellite lesions, extensive invasion of the trabecular meshwork producing glaucoma, or extrascleral extension via the iris root. Where possible, such lesions may be excised but, where not, an incisional biopsy may be justifiable before resorting to enucleation if any cells are found which are not unequivocally naevoid.[105]

Circumscribed melanomas that do not extend to the iris root and have no satellite lesions are very amenable to excision by sector iridectomy. It is technically possible to include a small portion of the adjacent iris root, trabecular meshwork, and ciliary body in such an excision, but there may be local recurrence and tumours invading the ciliary body may have a worse prognosis.[106] Because most iris melanomas arise in the inferior portion of the iris, the resultant defect is rarely covered by the upper eyelid. This means that it is cosmetically noticeable, especially in a light-coloured iris, and, more seriously, that the operation may be followed by troublesome photophobia. Some have advocated excision for tumours involving up to half the surface of the iris. Though technically feasible, eyes that have been subjected to very large resections usually develop intractable glaucoma from disturbance of the trabecular meshwork, rarely retain useful vision for long, and have usually been managed by enucleation, often after confirmatory biopsy. The various disadvantages of surgical resection of iris melanomas have led to the increasing use of radiotherapy, either by plaque or charged particles, in the treatment of iris melanomas of all sizes, though it remains to be seen whether the side-effects of radiation in such an anterior location will be outweighed by those of surgical resection.

Malignant melanoma of the orbit

Most melanomas of the orbit are extensions of tumours arising in the conjunctiva or uveal tract and are managed according to their origin and extent. Primary malignant melanoma of the orbit is rare.[107] In younger patients this tumour tends to arise in a cellular blue naevus,[108],[109] whilst in older individuals there is a tendency for it to develop in association with ocular or oculodermal melanocytosis,[110]–[112] where it may arise in a Black patient.[113] The presence of melanocytosis may help in the diagnosis of primary orbital melanoma in a patient presenting with proptosis, which may be of rapid or slow onset. The dark tumour may be visible beneath the conjunctiva and may be confused with haemorrhage from an orbital varix.

Clinically, primary orbital melanoma is well circumscribed on CT and a posterior lesion may be confused with a meningioma. When it arises in a cellular blue naevus, the orbital primary may be relatively benign and, if circumscribed, may be excised locally by orbitotomy with preservation of the eye. Melanomas arising in melanocytosis are more malignant: these and poorly circumscribed or recurrent melanomas should be excised by orbital exenteration if CT shows them to be resectable. There are few data on survival rates following treatment of this rare tumour.

Summary

Many aspects of the management of melanomas of the eye and orbit remain controversial. The relative rarity of conjunctival melanoma and the difficulty of eradicating primary acquired melanosis completely without risking loss of the eye have hampered progress in this particular tumour. Uveal melanomas, however, are common and there is a compelling need to confirm objectively the clinical impression that survival rates are no worse after treatments that aim to conserve the eye than they are after enucleation. It is to be hoped that prospective, randomized treatment trials in progress will answer this vexed question. Finally, effective adjuvant treatments and therapy for metastatic disease still seem as far off now as ever they have been.

References

1. Stephens RF, Shields JA. Diagnosis and management of cancer metastatic to the uvea: a study of 70 cases. *Ophthalmology*, 1979; **86**: 1336–49.

2. de Wolff-Rouendaal D. Conjunctival melanoma in the Netherlands: a clinicopathological and follow-up study. Den Haag: CIP-gegevens Koninklijke Bibliotheek, 1990: 127–36. [Thesis]

3. Aurora A, Blodi F. Lesions of the eyelids: a clinicopathologic study. *Survey of Ophthalmology*, 1970; **15**: 94–104.

4. Garner A, Koorneef L, Levene A, Collin JRO. Malignant melanoma of the eyelid skin: histopathology and behaviour. *British Journal of Ophthalmology*, 1985; **69**: 180–6.

5. Robertson DM, Hungerford JL, McCartney A. Pigmentation of the eyelid margin accompanying conjunctival melanoma. *American Journal of Ophthalmology*, 1989; **108**: 435–9.

6. Hicks C, Liu C, Hiranandani M, Garner A, Hungerford J. Conjunctival melanoma after excision of a lentigo malignant melanoma in the ipsilateral eyelid skin. *British Journal of Ophthalmology*, 1994; **78**: 317–18.

7. Verhoeff FH, Loring RG. A case of primary epibulbar sarcoma, with secondary growths in limbus and sclera, and invasion of choroid, ciliary body, and iris. *Archives of Ophthalmology*, 1903; **32**: 97–122.

8. Keller AZ. Histology, survivorship and related factors in the epidemiology of eye cancers. *American Journal of Epidemiology*, 1973; **97**: 386–93.

9. Scotto J, Fraumeni JF Jr, Lee JA. Melanomas of the eye and other non-cutaneous sites: epidemiological aspects. *Journal of the National Cancer Institute*, 1976; **56**: 489–91.

10. Paridaens ADA, Minassian DC, McCartney ACE, Hungerford JL. Prognostic factors in primary malignant melanoma of the conjunctiva: a clinicopathological study of 256 cases. *British Journal of Ophthalmology*, 1994; **78**: 252–9.

11. Jakobiec FA. Conjunctival melanoma. *Archives of Ophthalmology*, 1980; **98**: 1378–84.

12. Folberg R, McLean IW, Zimmerman LE. Malignant melanoma of the conjunctiva. *Human Pathology*, 1985; **16**: 136–43.

13. Liesegang TJ, Campbell RJ. Mayo Clinic experience with conjunctival melanomas. *Archives of Ophthalmology*, 1980; **98**: 1385–9.

14. Jay B. Naevi and melanomata of the conjunctiva. *British Journal of Ophthalmology*, 1965; **49**: 169–204.

15. Reese AB. Precancerous and cancerous melanosis of the conjunctiva. *American Journal of Ophthalmology*, 1955; **39**: 96–100.

16. Paridaens ADA, McCartney ACE, Hungerford JL. Recurrent malignant melanoma of the corneal stroma: a case of 'black cornea'. *British Journal of Ophthalmology*, 1992; **76**: 444–6.

17. Reese AB. Precancerous and cancerous melanosis. *American Journal of Ophthalmology*, 1966; **61**: 1272–7.

18. Paridaens ADA, McCartney ACE, Hungerford JL. Multifocal amelanotic conjunctival melanoma and acquired melanosis *sine pigmento*. *British Journal of Ophthalmology*, 1992; **76**: 163–5.

19. Paridaens ADA, Alexander RA, Hungerford JL, McCartney ACE. Oestrogen receptors in conjunctival malignant melanoma: immunocytochemical study using formalin fixed paraffin wax sections. *Journal of Clinical Pathology*, 1991; **44**: 840–3.

20. Bataille V, Boyle J, Hungerford JL, Newton JA. Three cases of primary acquired melanosis of the conjunctiva as a manifestation of the atypical mole syndrome. *British Journal of Dermatology*, 1993; **128**: 86–90.

21. Brownstein S, Jakobiec FA, Wilkinson RD, Lombardo J, Jackson B. Cryotherapy for precancerous melanosis atypical melanocytic hyperplasia of the conjunctiva. *Archives of Ophthalmology*, 1981; **99**: 1224–31.

22. Jakobiec FA, Brownstein S, Albert W, Schwarz F, Anderson R. The role of cryotherapy in the management of conjunctival melanoma. *Ophthalmology*, 1982; **89**: 502–15.

23. Jakobiec FA, Rini FJ, Fraunfelder FT, Brownstein S. Cryotherapy for conjunctival primary acquired melanosis and malignant melanoma. Experience with 62 cases. *Ophthalmology*, 1988; **96**: 1058–69.

24. Paridaens ADA, McCartney ACE, Curling OM, Lyons CL, Hungerford JL. Impression cytology of conjunctival melanosis and melanoma. *British Journal of Ophthalmology*, 1992; **76**: 198–201.

25. Lederman M, Wybar K, Busby E. Malignant epibulbar melanoma: natural history and treatment by radiotherapy. *British Journal of Ophthalmology*, 1984; **68**: 605–17.

26. Collin JRO, Allen LH, Garner A, Hungerford JL. Malignant melanoma of the eyelid and conjunctiva. *Australian and New Zealand Journal of Ophthalmology*, 1986; **14**: 29–34.

27. Paridaens ADA, McCartney ACE, Minassian DC, Hungerford JL. Orbital exenteration in 95 cases of primary conjunctival malignant melanoma. *British Journal of Ophthalmology*, 1994; **78**: 520–8.

28. Paridaens ADA, McCartney ACE, Lavelle RJ, Hungerford JL. Nasal and orbital recurrence of conjunctival melanoma 21 years after exenteration. *British Journal of Ophthalmology*, 1992; **76**: 369–71.

29. Lederman M. Radiotherapy of epibulbar malignant melanomata. *Transactions of the Ophthalmological Society of the United Kingdom*, 1953; **73**: 399–413.

30. Lommatzsch PK. Beta-ray treatment of malignant epibulbar melanoma. *Albrecht von Graefes Archive für Klinische und Experimentelle Ophthalmologie*, 1978; **209**: 111–24.

31. Jensen OA. Malignant melanomas of the uvea in Denmark, 1943–1952. *Acta Ophthalmologica*, 1963; **75**(Suppl.): 57–220.

32. Wilkes SR, Robertson DM, Kurland LT, Campbell JR. Incidence of uveal malignant melanoma in the resident population of Rochester and Olmsted County, Minnesota. *American Journal of Ophthalmology*, 1979; **87**: 639–41.

33. Østerlind A. Trends in incidence of ocular malignant melanoma in Denmark 1943–1982. *International Journal of Cancer*, 1987; **40**: 161–4.

34. Ganley JP, Constock GW. Benign nevi and malignant melanomas of the choroid. *American Journal of Ophthalmology*, 1973; **76**: 19–25.

35. Apple DJ, *et al.*. Malignant transformation of an optic nerve melanocytoma. *Canadian Journal of Ophthalmology*, 1984; **9**: 20–5.

36. Zimmerman LE, Garron LK. Melanocytoma of the optic disc. *International Ophthalmology Clinics*, 1962; **2**: 431–40.

37. Canning CR, Hungerford J. Familial uveal melanoma. *British Journal of Ophthalmology*, 1988; **72**: 241–3.

38. Oosterhuis JA, Went LN, Lynch HT. Primary choroidal and cutaneous melanomas, bilateral choroidal melanomas, and familial occurrence of melanomas. *British Journal of Ophthalmology*, 1982; **66**: 230–3.

39. Rodriguez-Sains RS. Ocular findings in patients with dysplastic nevus syndrome. *Ophthalmology*, 1986; **93**: 661–5.

40. Greene MH, Sanders RJ, Chu FC. The familial occurrence of cutaneous melanoma, intraocular melanoma and the dysplastic nevus syndrome. *American Journal of Ophthalmology*, 1983; **96**: 238–45.

41. Bataille V, Sasieni P, Cuzick, Hungerford JL, Swerdlow A. Risk of ocular melanoma in relation to cutaneous and iris naevi. *International Journal of Cancer*, 1995; **60**: 622–6.

42. Houlston RS, Damato BE. Genetic predisposition to ocular melanoma. *Eye*, 1999; **13**: 43–6.

43. Flocks M, Gerende JH, Zimmerman LE. The size and shape of malignant melanomas of the choroid and ciliary body in relation to prognosis and histological characteristics. A statistical study of 210 tumors. *Ophthalmology*, 1955; **59**: 740–58.

44. McLean IW, Foster WD, Zimmerman LE. Prognostic factors in small malignant melanomas of the choroid and ciliary body. *Archives of Ophthalmology*, 1977; **95**: 48–58.

45. Shammas HF, Blodi FC. Prognostic factors in choroidal and ciliary body melanomas. *Archives of Ophthalmology*, 1977; **95**: 63–9.

46. Davidorf FH, Lang JR. The natural history of melanoma of the choroid: small versus large tumours. *Ophthalmology*, 1975; **79**: 310–20.

47. Starr HJ, Zimmerman LE. Extrascleral extension and orbital recurrence of malignant melanoma of the choroid and ciliary body. *International Ophthalmology Clinics*, 1962; **2**: 369–84.

48. Kidd MN, Lyness RW, Patterson CC, Johnston PB, Archer DB. Prognostic factors in malignant melanoma of the choroid: a retrospective survey of cases occurring in Northern Ireland between 1965 and 1980. *Transactions of the Ophthalmological Society of the United Kingdom*, 1986; **105**: 114–21.

49. Hungerford J. Prognosis in ocular melanoma. *British Journal of Ophthalmology*, 1989; **73**: 689–90. [Editorial]

50. Robertson DM, Campbell RJ. Errors in the diagnosis of malignant melanoma of the choroid. *American Journal of Ophthalmology*, 1979; **87**: 269–75.

51. Char DH, *et al.* Diagnostic modalities in choroidal melanoma. *American Journal of Ophthalmology*, 1980; **89**: 223–30.

52. Font RL, Spaulding AG, Zimmerman LE. Diffuse malignant melanoma of the uveal tract: a clinicopathologic report of 54 cases. *Transactions of the American Academy of Ophthalmology and Otorhinolaryngology*, 1968; **72**: 877–95.

53. Naumann GOH, Yanoff M, Zimmerman LE. Histogenesis of malignant melanoma of the uvea. I. Histopathologic characteristics of nevi of the choroid and ciliary body. *Archives of Ophthalmology*, 1966; **76**: 784–96.

54. Augsburger JJ, Schroeder RP, Territo C, Gamel JW, Shields JA. Clinical parameters predictive of enlargement of melanocytic choroidal lesions. *British Journal of Ophthalmology*, 1989; **73**: 911–17.

55. Ferry AP, Font RL. Carcinoma metastatic to the eye and orbit. *Archives of Ophthalmology*, 1974; **92**: 276–86.

56. Hagler WS, Jarrett WH, Killian JH. The use of ^{32}P test in the management of malignant melanoma of the choroid: a five year follow-up study. *Transactions of the American Academy of Ophthalmology*, 1977; **83**: 49–60.

57. Bomanji J, Hungerford JL, Granowska M, Britton KE. Radioimmunoscintigraphy of ocular melanoma with ^{99m}Tc labelled cutaneous melanoma antibody fragments. *British Journal of Ophthalmology*, 1987; **71**: 651–8.

58. Shields JA. Current approaches to the diagnosis and management of choroidal melanomas. *Survey of Ophthalmology*, 1977; **21**: 443–63.

59. Jensen OA. Malignant melanomas of the posterior uvea: a recent follow-up of cases in Denmark, 1943–1952. *Acta Ophthalmologica*, 1970; **48**: 1113–28.

60. Einhorn LH, Burgess MA, Gottlieb JA. Metastatic patterns of choroidal melanoma. *Cancer*, 1974; **34**: 1001–4.

61. Wagoner MD, Albert DM. The incidence of metastases from untreated ciliary body and choroidal melanoma. *Archives of Ophthalmology*, 1982; **100**: 939–40.

62. Hicks C, Foss AJE, Hungerford JL. Predictive power of screening tests in uveal melanoma. *Eye*, 1998; **12**: 945–8.

63. Vogel MH. Treatment of malignant melanomas with photocoagulation: evaluation of 10-year follow-up data. *American Journal of Ophthalmology*, 1972; **74**: 1–11.

64. Oosterhuis JA, Journée-de-Korver JG, Keunen JEE. Transpupillary thermotherapy: results in 50 patients with choroidal melanoma. *Archives of Ophthalmology*, 1998; **116**: 157–62.

65. Shields CL, Shields JA, Cater J, Lois N, Edelstein C, Gündüz K, Mercado G. Transpupillary thermotherapy for choroidal melanoma: tumour control and visual results in 100 consecutive cases. *Ophthalmology*, 1998; **105**: 581–90.

66. Stallard HB. Radiotherapy for malignant melanoma of the choroid. *British Journal of Ophthalmology*, 1966; **50**: 147–55.

67. Moore RF. Choroidal sarcoma treated by the intraocular insertion of radon seeds. *British Journal of Ophthalmology*, 1930; **14**: 145–52.

68. Bedford MA. The use and abuse of cobalt plaques in the treatment of choroidal malignant melanomata. *Transactions of the Ophthalmological Society of the United Kingdom*, 1973; **93**: 139–43.

69. MacFaul PA. Local radiotherapy in the treatment of malignant melanoma of the choroid. *Transactions of the Ophthalmological Society of the United Kingdom*, 1977; **97**: 421–7.

70. Sealy R, LeRoux PLM, Rapley F, Hering E, Shackleton D, Sevel D. The treatment of ophthalmic tumours with low energy sources. *British Journal of Radiology*, 1976; **49**: 551–4.

71. Harnett AN, Thomson ES. An iodine-125 plaque for radiotherapy of the eye: manufacture and dosimetric considerations. *British Journal of Radiology*, 1988; **61**: 835–8.

72. Packer S, Stoller S, Lesser ML, Mandel FS, Finger PT. Long-term results of iodine 125 irradiation of uveal melanoma. *Ophthalmology*, 1992; **99**: 767–74.

73. Lommatzsch P. β-Irradiation of choroidal melanoma with ^{106}Ru/^{106}Rh applicators: 16 years' experience. *Archives of Ophthalmology*, 1983; **101**: 713–17.

74. Wilson MW, Hungerford JL. Comparison of episcleral plaque and proton beam radiotherapy for the treatment of choroidal melanoma. *Ophthalmology*, 1999; **106**: 1579–87.

75. Shields CL, Shields JA, Karlsson U, Markoe AM, Brady LW. Reasons for enucleation after plaque radiotherapy for posterior uveal melanoma. Clinical findings. *Ophthalmology*, 1989; **96**: 919–24.

76. Gass DM. Comparison of prognosis after enucleation vs cobalt-60 irradiation of melanomas. *Archives of Ophthalmology*, 1985; **103**: 916–23.

77. Augsburger JJ, Gamel JW, Sardi VF, Greenberg RA, Shields JA, Brady LW. Enucleation vs cobalt plaque radiotherapy for malignant melanomas of the choroid and ciliary body. *Archives of Ophthalmology*, 1986; **104**: 655–61.

78. Adams KS, *et al.*. Cobalt plaque versus enucleation for uveal melanoma: comparison of survival rates. *British Journal of Ophthalmology*, 1988; **72**: 494–7.

79. Gragoudas ES, *et al.* Proton irradiation of small choroidal malignant melanomas. *American Journal of Ophthalmology*, 1977; **83**: 665–73.

80. Char DH, *et al.* Helium ion charged particle therapy for choroidal melanoma. *Ophthalmology*, 1980; **87**: 565–70.

81. Munzenrider JE, *et al.* Conservative treatment of uveal melanoma: probability of eye retention after proton treatment. *International Journal of Radiation Oncology and Biological Physics*, 1988; **15**: 553–8.

82. Egan KM, *et al.* The risk of enucleation after proton beam irradiation of uveal melanoma. *Ophthalmology*, 1989; **96**: 1377–83.

83. Gragoudas ES, Egan KM, Seddon JM, Walsh SM, Munzenrider JE. Intraocular recurrence of uveal melanoma after proton beam irradiation. *Ophthalmology*, 1992; **99**: 760–6.

84. Foss AJE, *et al.* Predictive factors for the development of rubeosis following proton beam radiotherapy for uveal melanoma. *British Journal of Ophthalmology*, 1997; **81**: 748–54.

85. Linstadt D, *et al.*. Vision following helium ion radiotherapy of uveal melanoma: a Northern California Oncology Group Study. *International Journal of Radiation Oncology and Biological Physics*, 1988; **15**: 347–52.

86. Stallard HB. Partial choroidectomy. *British Journal of Ophthalmology*, 1966; **50**: 660–2.

87. Foulds WS. Local excision of choroidal melanomas. *Transactions of the Ophthalmological Society of the United Kingdom*, 1974; **93**: 343–6.

88. Peyman GA, Apple DJ. Local excision of a choroidal melanoma, full thickness eye wall resection. *Archives of Ophthalmology*, 1974; **92**: 216–18.

89. Damato BE, Paul J, Foulds WS. Risk factors for residual and recurrent uveal melanoma after trans-scleral local resection. *British Journal of Ophthalmology*, 1996; **80**: 102–8.

90. Kertes PJ, Jonson JC, Peyman GA. Internal resection of posterior uveal melanoma. *British Journal of Ophthalmology*, 1998; **82**: 1147–53.

91. Damato B, Groenwald C, McGalliard J, Wong D. Endoresection of choroidal melanoma. *British Journal of Ophthalmology*, 1998; **82**: 213–18.

92. Hykin PG, McCartney ACE, Plowman PN, Hungerford JL. Postenucleation orbital radiotherapy for the treatment of malignant melanoma of the choroid with extrascleral extension. *British Journal of Ophthalmology*, 1990; **74**: 36–9.

93. Kersten RC, Tse DT, Anderson RL, Blodi FC. The role of orbital exenteration in choroidal melanoma with extrascleral extension. *Ophthalmology*, 1985; **92**: 436–43.

94. Lee V, Cree IA, Hungerford JL. Ring melanoma—a rare cause of refractory glaucoma. *British Journal of Ophthalmology*, 1999; **83**: 194–8.

95. Canning CR, McCartney ACE, Hungerford J. Medulloepithelioma diktyoma. *British Journal of Ophthalmology*, 1988; **72**: 764–7.

96. White V, Stevenson K, Garner A, Hungerford J. Mesectodermal leiomyoma of the ciliary body: a case report. *British Journal of Ophthalmology*, 1989; **73**: 12–18.

97. Shields JA, Annesly WH, Spaeth GL. Necrotic melanocytoma of iris with secondary glaucoma. *American Journal of Ophthalmology*, 1977; **84**: 826–9.

98. Chang M, Shields JA, Wachtel DL. Adenoma of the pigment epithelium of the ciliary body simulating a malignant melanoma. *American Journal of Ophthalmology*, 1979; **88**: 40–4.

99. Ashton N. Primary tumours of the iris. *British Journal of Ophthalmology*, 1964; **48**: 650–68.

100. Geisse LJ, Robertson DM. The prognosis of primary tumors of the iris treated by iridectomy. *Archives of Ophthalmology*, 1985; **99**: 638–48.

101. Foss AJ, Pecorella I, Alexander RA, Hungerford JL, Garner A. Are most intraocular 'leiomyomas' really melanocytic lesions? *Ophthalmology*, 1994; **101**: 919–24.

102. Jakobiec FA, Silbert G. Are most iris 'melanomas' really nevi? *Archives of Ophthalmology*, 1981; **99**: 2117–32.

103. Territo C, Shields CJ, Shields JA, Augsburger JJ, Schroeder RP. Natural course of melanocytic tumors of the iris. *Ophthalmology*, 1988; **95**: 1251–5.

104. Dart JK, Marsh RJ, Garner A, Cooling RJ. Fluorescein angiography of anterior uveal and melanocytic tumours. *British Journal of Ophthalmology*, 1988; **72**: 326–37.

105. Kersten RC, Tse DT, Anderson R. Iris melanomas: nevus or malignancy? *Survey of Ophthalmology*, 1985; **29**: 423–33.

106. McGalliard JN, Johnston PB. A study of iris melanoma in Northern Ireland. *British Journal of Ophthalmology*, 1989; **73**: 591–5.

107. Shields JA, Bakewell B, Augsburger JJ, Flanagan JC. Classification and incidence of space-occupying lesions of the orbit. A survey of 645 biopsies. *Archives of Ophthalmology*, 1984 **102**: 1606–11.

108. Rottino A, Kelly AS. Primary orbital melanoma. Case report with review of the literature. *Archives of Ophthalmology*, 1942; **27**: 934–49.

109. Wolter JR, Bryson JM, Blackhurst RT. Primary orbital melanoma. *Ear Nose and Throat Journal*, 1966; **45**: 64–7.

110. Jay B. Malignant melanoma of the orbit in a case of oculodermal melanosis naevus of Ota. *British Journal of Ophthalmology*, 1965; **49**: 359–63.

111. Hagler WS, Brown CC. Malignant melanoma of the orbit arising in a nevus of Ota. *Transactions of the American Academy of Ophthalmology and Otorhinolaryngology*, 1966; **78**: 817–22.

112. Haim T, Meyer E, Kerner H, Zonis S. Oculodermal melanocytosis nevus of Ota and orbital malignant melanoma. *Annals of Ophthalmology*, 1982; **14**: 1132–6.

113. Wilkes SR, Uthman EO, Thornton CN, Randall EC. Malignant melanoma of the orbit in a black patient with ocular melanocytosis. *Archives of Ophthalmology*, 1984; **102**: 904–6.

Skin cancer other than melanoma

David S. Soutar and A. G. Robertson

Introduction

The skin is the largest organ in the body and the site most often affected by tumours. By far the most common skin malignancy encountered in clinical practice is basal cell carcinoma. This, however, is not recorded routinely in cancer registries and therefore the true incidence of skin cancer remains unknown. In many areas of the world primary carcinoma of the skin is increasing.[1],[2] Traditionally, non-melanoma skin cancer has included tumours arising from the surface epithelium and adnexal structures and comprises basal cell carcinoma, squamous cell carcinoma, and adnexal tumours including Merkel cell carcinoma and sebaceous gland tumours. It should, however, be remembered that other malignancies such as Kaposi's sarcoma, cutaneous lymphoma, a variety of malignant vascular tumours and neural tumours, and secondary metastases from distant primary sites, for example renal carcinoma, can affect the skin.

Aetiology

Ultraviolet radiation from exposure to sunlight is the most common aetiological factor for both melanoma and non-melanoma skin cancer. The carcinogen in sunlight is UV-D (280 to 320 nm), shorter wavelengths being filtered by the atmosphere. Non-melanoma skin cancer is more common in outdoor workers and the incidence, particularly of basal cell carcinoma, increases with proximity to the equator.[3],[4] This supports the concept of chronic sun exposure and total dose being related to the development of these tumours in adult life. However, as for melanoma, the question of childhood sensitivity and the amount of exposure in childhood may also contribute to the risk in later life.[5],[6]

The majority of tumours occur on sun-exposed sites, which further supports the idea that ultraviolet radiation is the major aetiological factor. Ionizing radiation, either from radiotherapy or atomic fall-out, has also been associated with an increase in non-melanoma skin cancer.[7],[8] Exposure to a variety of chemical agents, such as nitrates, arsenicals, soot, and oils, has been associated with non-melanoma skin cancer, but many of these agents are now of historical interest only. Immunosuppression is now a most important factor in the development of skin cancer, with increased incidence largely related to improved survival of transplant patients, particularly those with renal transplants, and to the emergence of AIDS.[9]

The susceptibility of certain skin types associated with non-melanoma skin cancer and the geographical variation in incidence suggest that certain individuals have a genetic predisposition. Evidence is provided by a group of genetic diseases which are associated with the development of multiple primary tumours. Naevoid basal cell carcinoma syndrome (Gorlin's syndrome) is an autosomal familial cancer syndrome in which multiple basal cell carcinomas appear at an early age. The gene responsible is on chromosome 9q22–31.[10],[11] Recently attention has focused on the human homologue of the drosophila polarity gene—the *patched* gene.[12],[13] This gene is considered to act as a tumour suppressor gene. Bazex's syndrome is a rare crosslinked syndrome which predisposes individuals to multiple basal cell carcinomas. This disease has been mapped to chromosome Xq24–27.[14] Non-melanoma skin cancer in childhood occurs in individuals with xeroderma pigmentosum, a rare autosomal recessive genetic disease. Squamous cell carcinoma has been linked to a particular family in the form of the self-healing squamous cell carcinoma known as Ferguson-Smith disease and sebaceous or adnexal tumours are seen in Muir–Torre syndrome, usually in association with colonic tumours.[15],[16]

Although skin cancers share many common aetiological factors (Table 1), their behaviour and natural history is greatly variable and it is worth considering more closely the three most common non-melanoma skin cancers, namely basal cell carcinoma, squamous cell carcinoma, and skin appendage tumours (adnexal tumours).

Basal cell carcinoma

Basal cell carcinoma is the commonest malignant tumour affecting the skin. Clinically, it is a slow-growing locally invasive and locally destructive tumour in which distant metastases rarely occur. Several types are described based on their physical appearance, and there are a variety of clinical classifications. The essential component determined by clinical investigation is the extent of the tumour and in this regard the classification described by Emmett (Table 2) is useful.[17] Localized tumours generally have a clear cut-off point from tumour to normal tissue and the margins can be well defined. The papulonodular variety fits the classical description of the rodent ulcer with a rolled, pearly edge which often develops central ulceration (Fig. 1). The solid type almost appears to grow out of the skin in an exophytic way and frequently has telangiatatic vessels coursing across its surface. The cystic variety can appear as a thin cyst, particularly around the eyelids, and sometimes also has telangiatatic vessels.

In the diffuse type, the pattern of spread is insidious, and defining the tumour margins can be difficult. The infiltrating type is clearly not purely an exophytic growth and infiltration of adjacent tissues can be demonstrated by palpation. The multifocal variety appears to

Table 1 Skin cancer aetiology

Aetiology	Premalignant condition	Malignancy
UV radiation/PUVA	Actinic keratosis	BCC, SCC
	Bowen's disease	SCC
Radiotherapy	Radiation keratosis	SCC
		Angiosarcoma/Lymphangiosarcoma
Immunosuppresion	Keratosis	All types of NMSC
Chemicals	Chemical keratosis, e.g. arsenic	SCC, BCC
Chronic inflammation	Erythroplasia of Queyrat	SCC glans penis
Genetic disorders	Variable	BCC, SCC
Chronic skin damage/scar	Variable	Marjolin's ulcer, SCC, BCC

BCC = basal cell carcinoma. SCC = squamous cell carcinoma, NMSC = non-melanoma skin cancer. PUVA = photochemotherapy with ultraviolet A light.

Table 2 Clinical classification of basal cell carcinoma based on Emmetts classification[17]

Type	Subtype
Localized	Papulonodular
	Solid
	Cystic
Diffuse	Infiltrating
	Multifocal
	Cilatrizing
	Morphoeic
	Metatypical

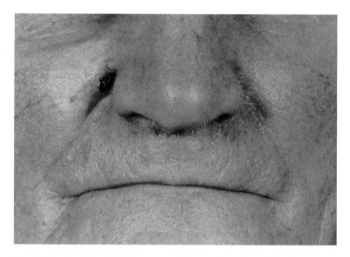

Fig. 2 Morphoeic basal cell carcinoma. Notice the pallor of the skin and the small area of ulceration.

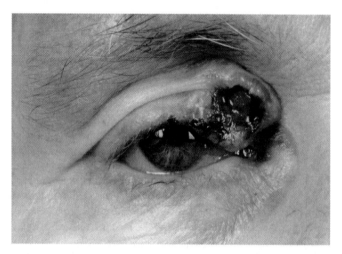

Fig. 1 Basal cell carcinoma of the upper right eyelid, showing pearly edge and ulceration.

have areas of almost normal looking skin which may represent healing of a previously ulcerated area. These multifocal lesions may be superficial or can infiltrate in depth. The morphoeic type of basal cell carcinoma infiltrates the dermis and produces a dense stromal reaction with stromal fibrosis. This gives the skin a characteristic white plaque-like appearance which is stiff, hence the term morphoea. The difficulty lies in determining the lateral extent of these tumours because of the dense stromal reaction (Fig. 2). Metatypical basal cell carcinomas commonly appear as large, ulcerating, often exophytic, lesions. Characteristically they look very similar to squamous cell carcinomas but have a long history (Fig. 3). It is the length of history that usually differentiates these tumours. Patients may present with more than one primary basal cell carcinoma which may be associated with a syndrome as discussed previously. Patients who have a basal cell carcinoma show a high incidence of a second lesion compared with the normal population. Second basal cell carcinomas frequently develop in the first year (16 per cent) and the incidence then falls to approximately 10 per cent over the next 4 years.[18]

In addition to the physical appearance of primary basal cell carcinoma, there are three other clinical pictures which are encountered, namely recurrent basal cell carcinoma, aggressive or horrifying basal cell carcinoma, and metastatic basal cell carcinoma.

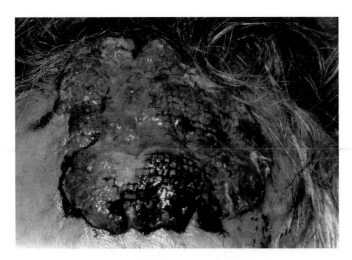

Fig. 3 Metatypical basal cell carcinoma of the forehead.

Recurrent basal cell carcinoma

The clinical appearance of recurrent basal cell carcinoma is very variable and is often dependent on previous treatment. The margins are difficult to determine but recurrence should always be regarded as having a diffuse pattern. Patients at risk of developing recurrence include those who have already presented with recurrent basal cell carcinoma, those with basal cell carcinomas showing an aggressive histological pattern, and lesions arising at cosmetically sensitive sites where tissue is scarce.[19]

Horrifying basal cell carcinoma

This is the most dangerous basal cell carcinoma, characterized clinically by deep invasion and widespread destruction of adjacent tissues. The terminology is somewhat confusing, since it is also termed aggressive basal cell carcinoma, but this latter term applies to the histological appearance rather than the clinical appearance and behaviour. These tumours tend to occur in young individuals; they are large (> 3 cm) and often appear in the region of the head and neck, particularly the scalp.[20],[21] Inadequate primary treatment is cited as an important factor in the development of horrifying basal cell carcinoma, particularly deep tumour extension following radiotherapy. The diffuse infiltrative type of basal cell carcinoma has been implicated in the development of these horrifying lesions, with a high incidence in morphoeic or metatypical basal cell carcinomas and those with adenoid differentiation.[22],[23] Unusual aetiologies such as arsenic, immunosuppression, and X-ray-induced tumours have also been implicated.[24]

The clinical danger of these tumours, particularly those arising in the head and neck, is their capacity to infiltrate through bone and into the central nervous system causing widespread local destruction.

Metastatic basal cell carcinoma

The development of a distant metastasis from a basal cell carcinoma is exceptionally rare, so much so that it remains worthy of a single case report. The incidence is reported as varying from 0.0028 per cent to 0.55 per cent.[25] Characteristically, patients have a large basal cell carcinoma, usually of long standing, which has proved resistant to treatment at the local site. Metatypical basal cell carcinoma with squamous differentiation has been associated with metastases.[26] Facial basal cell carcinomas tend to metastasize to regional nodes, but a wide variety of organs have also been reported as showing metastasis including lung, liver, brain, heart, and pericardium.[27] The histological variations that occur in basal cell carcinoma continue to fuel the debate as to whether basal cell carcinomas do indeed metastasize or whether these tumours are variants of adnexal tumours.

Pathological features

One of the major problems with basal cell carcinoma is that the cell of origin and the histogenesis have not been accurately determined. The keratin phenotype of basal cell carcinoma would suggest an origin in the hair follicles.[28] If this is indeed the case, then basal cell carcinoma is a type of adnexal tumour; however, because of its frequent occurrence it has been classified separately. Unlike many other tumours there does not appear to be a premalignant phase for basal cell carcinoma arising de novo. Possible exceptions are tumours in sebaceous naevi (Borst–Jadassohn epithelioma) and the fibro-epithelioma of Pinkus.

Basal cell carcinomas are composed of islands or nests of basophilic cells which resemble miniature basal cells of the epidermis lying in a connective tissue stroma. Typically the cells pack together in a regular manner to produce peripheral palisading. The cellular islands and nests within the stroma give them different patterns, and this has led to a variety of classifications. In an attempt to marry the pathological features with the clinical variants, Sexton et al. proposed the classification shown in Table 3.[29] From the clinical perspective, it is the pattern and degree of infiltration and the arrangement of cells within the stroma that is most important rather than the degree of differentiation or number of mitoses present.

Squamous cell carcinoma

As with other skin cancers, the incidence of squamous cell carcinoma is increasing.[1] Actinic (solar) skin damage is a major aetiological factor. The epidermal keratinocytes appear to be more sensitive to solar radiation than adnexal keratinocytes. Immunosuppression or the presence of chronically damaged skin as the result of trauma, burns, or previous radiotherapy are also important factors. Unlike basal cell carcinoma, there does appear to be a progression through dysplasia, carcinoma in situ, to frankly invasive squamous cell carcinoma. This is particularly true where there is solar damage which can result in a focal lesion, termed actinic keratosis. These lesions appear as red scaly patches indicative of abnormal keratinization, which can persist for many years without apparently progressing. Removal of the scale can produce a superficial ulcer, the depth of which is dependent on the depth at which the scale separates. A true actinic keratosis is superficial and any depth or induration and infiltration should raise clinical suspicion of progression to carcinoma in situ or invasive carcinoma. Sometimes, the focal lesion appears to extend superficially, appearing as a red scaly area that can be confused with basal cell carcinoma. Histological examination of such lesions, particularly those arising on the legs, can show intraepidermal squamous cell carcinoma, sometimes known as Bowen's disease. Alternatively

Table 3 Classification of basal cell carcinomas based on Sexton Jones et al.[29]

Type	Histology
Superficial	Tumour abuts or penetrates the papilliary dermis
Nodular	Rounded mass of tumour cells with well defined peripheral papillary dermis
Micronodular	Tumour islands with retained uniform contour
Infiltrative	Tumour islands with irregular contour and spike formation. Poorly developed peripheral pallisading
Morphoeic	Narrow strands or cords of cells Sclerotic stroma

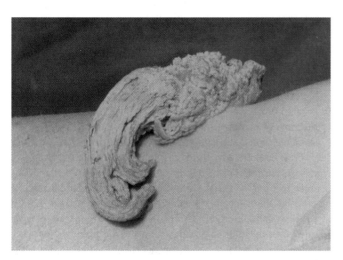

Fig. 4 Keratin horn.

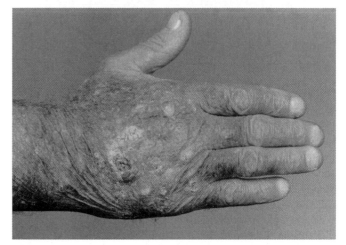

Fig. 5 Typical appearance of an immunosuppressed patient showing widespread skin damage with 1.5 cm indurated squamous cell carcinoma.

a focal lesion can present with a similar appearance to a wart except that it is composed of keratin and dried serous discharge. If there is abundant keratin, the lesion may appear as a keratin horn (Fig. 4). Removal of the horn will reveal an ulcerating base more typical of a squamous cell carcinoma.

The second clinical picture is that of a much more rapidly growing lesion which quickly ulcerates. Growth may be exophytic, resulting in a cauliflower-like ulcerating mass with little infiltration in the base. Alternatively, infiltration will proceed through the layers of the skin resulting in an ulcer with a rolled edge and an indurated margin. Unlike basal cell carcinoma, the history is measured in months rather than years and the degree of ulceration is indicative of tumour necrosis as its growth outstrips its blood supply. Tumours arising in apparently normal skin have this faster ulcerative growth pattern and should raise clinical suspicion (Fig. 5).

Metastases usually arise in the regional lymph nodes. They are associated with rapidly growing infiltrative lesions with a short history. Metastases from squamous cell carcinomas arising in sun-damaged skin are relatively infrequent.[30] The lip, columella, and ear show a higher incidence of metastases than other sites. Other dangerous areas are tumours arising at mucocutaneous junctions, in normal undamaged skin, or in areas of chronic damage such as sepsis, scarring, burns, or irradiation.[31] There is yet a further complication to the clinical presentation of squamous cell carcinoma, namely the

so-called self-healing squamous cell carcinoma which presents as keratoacanthoma or as the familial disease termed Ferguson-Smith disease.[15],[16]

Keratoacanthoma is histologically identical to squamous cell carcinoma but its clinical picture is of a lesion that grows rapidly over a period of approximately 6 weeks and subsequently undergoes regression to leave a small pitted scar on the skin surface. Such lesions are usually single, but multiple keratoacanthomas have been reported. In the familial disease, multiple lesions are present, often in differing stages. The familial disease has been linked to a particular family in the west of Scotland but has a different histological picture to keratoacanthoma. Again, lesions may regress to leave pitted scars on the skin. The management of keratoacanthoma and Ferguson-Smith disease remains a significant clinical problem because of the difficulty in differentiating these conditions from frankly invasive squamous cell carcinoma.

Pathological features

Solar damage to the epidermal keratinocytes produces epithelial dysplasia, first in the basal layers and then throughout the epidermis as a whole. This disordered growth with abnormal maturation and keratinization is associated with cellular atypia with subsequent progression to frank neoplasia. The severity of dysplasia can increase to a level where the appearance is that of squamous cell carcinoma *in situ* delineated by an intact basement membrane. Subsequent invasion of the dermis is indicative of frankly infiltrative squamous cell carcinoma. The degree of differentiation is regarded by some as a prognostic factor, and perineural spread, although relatively uncommon, is associated with a poorer prognosis.[32],[33] Keratoacanthoma is primarily a clinical diagnosis where there is great expansion of the dermis but infiltration does not penetrate deeper than the sweat glands. In Ferguson-Smith disease, the histological pattern is almost identical to invasive squamous cell carcinoma with penetration into the dermis and even into the subcutaneous fat. To date, there has been little evidence that the morphological characteristics of squamous cell carcinoma are indicative of prognosis, and clinicians have to rely on a high index of suspicion related to the site of the lesion, clinical history, and clinical examination.

Adnexal tumours

This group of tumours arise from skin appendages, although the cell of origin is often difficult to determine. Such tumours may arise from eccrine sweat glands, hair follicles, sebaceous and apocrine glands, and the apud system. They are clinically indistinguishable from many other cutaneous lesions and are often only diagnosed once histology is available. The majority of tumours from adnexal structures are benign, but there are malignant counterparts. In the eccrine glands, for example, there is a malignant porocarcinoma and eccrine carcinoma. Eccrine carcinoma infiltrates locally and metastasizes. Eccrine carcinoma can show tubular histological formation, and the histological diagnosis is frequently that of anaplastic squamous cell carcinoma. The behaviour of eccrine carcinoma in fact mirrors that of squamous cell carcinoma. Some tumours arising from eccrine glands are similar to salivary gland tumours and show features of adenoid cystic carcinoma. Malignant tumours of the sebaceous glands are frequently found in the eyelids. A feature of local spread is that of padgetoid migration of tumour cells through the epithelium. Anaplastic sebaceous carcinoma often resembles squamous cell carcinoma in its histological appearance and also in its clinical behaviour.

Merkel cell carcinoma has a very distinctive histological appearance. It is thought to arise from cells which have granules similar to those found in cells derived from the apud system.[34] Such tumours are thought to be of neuroendocrine origin and behave in a similar fashion to malignant melanoma, developing satellite lesions and lymph node metastasis. The commonest clinical presentation is of a painless indurated non-ulcerative skin nodule which is often red in colour. It may also appear as a cystic or ulcerated lesion, most commonly in the head and neck, and is predominantly a disease of the elderly. It shows local recurrence rates of around 40 per cent, with lymph node metastasis in around 40 to 65 per cent of cases.[35]–[37] Surgical treatment is wide local excision but there has been considerable debate concerning the management of lymph nodes in view of the high risk of lymph node metastasis. As in management of this problem in melanoma, the detection of lymph node metastasis can be improved by sentinel node biopsy (for details see Chapter 8.1).[38] Merkel cell carcinoma is also a radioresponsive tumour, with good response in patients treated by this modality alone.[39],[40] This has led several authors to adopt a policy of wide local excision with or without neck dissection followed by postoperative radiotherapy as

combined modality treatment, with reported improvements in locoregional control.[40]–[42] The role of chemotherapy remains under debate, but with Merkel cell carcinoma having a significant incidence of distant metastasis approaching 30 per cent, and probably much greater in those cases in which there is loss of locoregional control, work is continuing on improved treatment modalities including combined chemotherapy and chemoradiotherapy.[43],[44]

It is difficult to diagnose adnexal tumours clinically and treatment is dependent on accurate histological diagnosis. Adnexal skin tumours are relatively rare in clinical practice and there are few identifiable clinical features which differentiate them from the more common forms of skin cancer.

Miscellaneous lesions

The main types and variants of non-melanoma skin cancers have been described above. It should be remembered that other conditions affect the skin which can present clinically as skin tumours. These include cutaneous lymphoma, a variety of sarcomas including Kaposi's sarcoma, dermal tumours such as dermatofibrosarcoma protruberans, malignant fibrous histiocytoma, vascular tumours such as angiosarcoma, neural tumours, and secondary metastases. Furthermore, malignancy of the skin has to be differentiated from benign lesions and from tumour-like lesions such as nodular fasciitis and atypical fibroxanthoma. Malignant fibrous histiocytoma is the commonest soft tissue sarcoma in adult life. It presents as a nodule with a wide variety of histological appearances but in essence is a pleomorphic high-grade sarcoma. Prognosis is related to the size of the primary tumour and in the skin it requires wide local excision.

Dermatofibrosarcoma protruberans (see Chapter 16.1) presents as a slow-growing multinodular lesion which is fixed to the skin. It commonly appears in the trunk in young adults and is more common in males and in Blacks. The major problem with this tumour is local recurrence; metastases are very rare. The treatment of choice is wide local surgical excision.

Angiosarcomas are malignant tumours of endothelium which may show haemangiomatous or lymphatic differentiation. The term, therefore, is often widely used to include both angiosarcomas of vascular endothelium and lymphangiosarcomas developing from lymphatic endothelium but containing typically haemorrhagic and blood-filled spaces lined by vascular endothelium. The exact classification is dependent on the pathological appearance but two types of angiosarcoma can be distinguished clinically. Angiosarcomas without lymphoedema occur almost exclusively on the face and scalp in adults over the age of 50. The skin is typically discoloured with a blue/red hue within which there are nodules or areas of ulceration. Local recurrence is common as is disseminated metastasis, particularly to the lungs. Despite aggressive treatment with surgery and radiotherapy, the mortality approaches 80 per cent in five years.

The other clinical picture is angiosarcoma with lymphoedema—lymphangiosarcoma. A recent review has shown that patients with a history of breast cancer have a 59-fold increased risk of developing upper extremity angiosarcoma.[45] The angiosarcoma may arise in the chest and breast following treatment with radiotherapy or in the upper extremity following a history of chronic lymphoedema. The incidence of lymphangiosarcoma in postmastectomy lymphoedema

Table 4 TNM classification of skin carcinoma

T	Primary tumours
Tx	Primary tumour cannot be assessed
T0	No evidence of primary tumour
Tis	Carcinoma *in situ*
T1	Tumour 2 cm or less in greatest dimension
T2	Tumour more than 2 cm but not more than 5 cm in greatest dimension
T3	Tumour more than 5 cm in greatest dimension
T4	Tumour invades deep extradermal structures, i.e. cartilage, skeletal muscle, or bone In the case of multiple simultaneous tumours, the tumour with the highest category will be classified and the number of separate tumours will be indicated in parethesis, e.g. T2(5)
N	Regional lymph nodes
Nx	Regional lymph nodes cannot be assessed
N0	No regional lymph node metastasis
N1	Regional lymph node metastasis
M	Distant metastasis
Mx	Presence of distant metastasis cannot be assessed
M0	No distant metastasis
M1	Distant metastasis

TNM classification of malignant tumours, 4th edn, 2nd revision.

has been well recognized and is known as the Stewart–Treves syndrome. Lymphangiosarcomas also carry a poor prognosis, with a tendency to both lymphatic and haematogenous metastases. Radical surgery often involving amputation is the treatment of choice, with postoperative irradiation showing some promising results. In limbs, isolated limb perfusion can also be considered.[46]

The wide variety of conditions that can affect the skin demand clearly defined protocols for the investigation and management of suspected skin tumours. This involves clinical diagnosis, histological diagnosis, and treatment protocols.

Clinical diagnosis

Some of the clinical features of particular non-melanoma skin cancers have been previously discussed. The length of history is often an indication of the type and nature of the disease. The site and size of the skin lesion are clearly important, and in many centres the TNM classification is used to define treatment protocols (Table 4). Close clinical inspection with palpation and stretching of the skin can help to identify the extent of local infiltration. This can be greatly assisted by the use of magnification. Attention should be paid to skin type, presence or absence of actinic damage, or evidence of other previously induced skin damage. Inquiry should also be made to identify any

association with familial genetic syndromes or early genetic susceptibility. Problems still persist, particularly in the identification of the rarer adnexal tumours, but experienced clinicians can have a high degree of clinical diagnostic accuracy. A review of basal cell carcinoma in the West of Scotland Regional Plastic Surgery Unit showed that the clinical diagnosis of basal cell carcinoma was confirmed histologically in 98.2 per cent of cases.[47] Overall the diagnosis of basal cell carcinoma was made clinically in 96 per cent and prior biopsy was only required in 9.4 per cent. There may, however, be problems in differentiating between Bowen's disease and basal cell carcinoma, and further difficulties arise when lesions are pigmented. In malignant skin disease, examination of the regional lymph nodes is mandatory and completes the TNM staging process. Special investigations such as computed tomography, magnetic resonance imaging, and lymphoscintigraphy are only used in specific cases of either an unusual malignancy or advanced disease. Cutaneous ultrasound, or high-resolution ultrasound, can help in determining the thickness of cutaneous tumours. It is, however, virtually never used in surgical practice and only very occasionally in the planning of radiotherapy.

Histological diagnosis

Fine-needle aspiration cytology is not used in the diagnosis of skin lesions. Punch biopsy is a common and simple technique which can be performed under local anaesthetic and provides sufficient tissue to allow for histological diagnosis. Tissue diagnosis is essential if field ablative or destructive treatments are proposed where there is no excision with a subsequent specimen for full pathological examination.

Biopsy is not essential if treatment is going to be surgical and where there is sufficient clinical expertise; many lesions can be cured by simple excisional biopsy, providing both a diagnosis and cure in one operation.

Treatment modalities

Surgical excision remains the mainstay for treatment of skin cancer, the aim being to excise the tumour completely and ensure that the margins of tumour clearance are satisfactory. The alternative method is to ablate the tumour and the surrounding tissue and not attempt to define tumour clearance by examining the ablation edge. Such techniques include radiotherapy, photodynamic therapy, laser surgery, cryotherapy, and topical chemotherapy with 5-fluorouracil for example.

Surgical management

Complete excision of the tumour is the aim of surgical procedures. The wide variety of tumour types necessitate differing tumour margins of excision. Several methods are currently in use to determine the completeness of excision.

Frozen section

Tissue can be sampled at the margins, whether laterally or in depth, and examined at the time of operation using frozen section techniques. Problems include sampling error and prolongation of operating time as each specimen is examined to identify the presence or absence of tumour, but in difficult situations frozen section can be useful. An alternative is to use techniques based on Mohs' micrographic chemosurgery. In the 1930s, Dr Frederick Mohs developed a technique for fixing skin cancer tissue *in situ*, excising this fixed tissue in layers and examining each layer or slice as a horizontal section. This technique can now be incorporated into frozen section analysis and allows for a horizontal section of the whole excision area to be examined in one sitting.[48] This can therefore allow for identification of the tumour, both in depth and laterally. Such techniques are most useful in difficult situations of repeatedly recurrent tumours or in the aggressive or horrifying types of basal cell carcinoma. An alternative is to excise the skin tumour with what is regarded clinically as an adequate margin and to simply pack off the defect with no attempt at reconstruction. Full histological examination can usually be completed within 48 h. If clear, then the case can return to theatre for formal reconstruction. If there is inadequate clearance, the original procedure can be repeated, or frozen sections used as described above. Clearly, this technique can only be used where vital structures such as nerves, vessels, bone etc. are not exposed.

Incomplete excision, when reported, is a difficult clinical problem, particularly in basal cell carcinoma. Not all incompletely excised basal cell carcinomas recur and this may reflect orientation of histological specimens.[49] The clinician may be influenced to re-excise in certain situations:

(i) Where the site of the lesion is potentially dangerous should it recur.

(ii) Where there is an aggressive infiltrative morphological pattern.

(iii) Where incomplete excision is reported in depth.

(iv) Where there is a history of previous treatment, particularly radiotherapy.

(v) Where the method of reconstruction could potentially mask the clinical recurrent disease.

In our own experience, surgery is a very effective method of management.[19] In primary tumour excision recurrence rates vary from 5 to 10 per cent, with recurrence rates being higher for recurrent disease (15 to 25 per cent).[49],[50] Our experience has shown a recurrence rate of 1.9 per cent for completely excised basal cell carcinomas compared with a recurrence rate of 24.1 per cent following incomplete excision.[19],[47] Accepting the problems of histological accuracy with regard to orientation and tissue sampling, there is evidence to support further surgery when there is a report of incomplete excision, particularly in danger areas as mentioned above.

It is the responsibility of the surgeon to assist the pathologist in orientating the specimen. This is most readily done by placing a suture at a particular point. In difficult situations, a long and a short suture can be used. A further method is to tattoo areas of concern with methylene blue. It is important to impregnate the dermis rather than just mark the skin surface, since the latter marking is readily destroyed when the sample is placed in formalin.

As an aid to help avoid distortion in formalin, difficult specimens can be pinned on to a cork board. An alternative is to place the tissue sample on a piece of filter paper prior to insertion in formalin. This helps fix the tissue specimen with minimal distortion.

Radiotherapy

Advances in dermatological and surgical techniques, especially plastic surgical reconstruction, over the past few decades (Fig. 6) have led to a reduction in the use of radiotherapy in the management of skin cancers. Radiotherapy, however, still has an important role in the management of appropriately selected skin tumours. It should be used in situations where it can produce superior cosmetic or functional results and equivalent or better local tumour control rates.

Radiotherapy has advantages in the management of selected tumours arising on the eyelids, external ear, and nose, especially if the normal tissue framework is not disturbed prior to the initiation of treatment. The resulting immediate cosmetic effect, after the eradication of the tumour, is usually superior to that of surgery even with the recent advances in reconstructive techniques. Furthermore treatment margins can be as wide as thought necessary when treating with radiotherapy in contrast to surgery where wide margins will lead to greater disfigurement.

There is only one prospective randomized trial comparing radiotherapy and surgery in the management of basal cell carcinoma.[51] In this trial 347 patients underwent surgery and the remaining 173 patients had radiotherapy. The 4-year actuarial failure rate was 0.7 per cent for surgery compared with 7.5 per cent for radiotherapy. The study concluded that recurrence rates and cosmesis were both superior at 4 years for surgery. In another study, the cosmetic outcomes in patients following either surgery or radiotherapy have been compared over a 15-year period following radiotherapy.[52] Between the first and fifteenth years the percentage of patients having either an excellent or good cosmetic result following radiotherapy declined by 20 per cent. This was due to the late development of varying degrees of atrophy, hyperpigmentation, and telangectasia. In contrast there was no cosmetic deterioration in those who underwent surgery or curettage. There is no specific cut-off age for these changes. Patients older than 55 years are more appropriate candidates for radiotherapy than those younger as the late cosmetic changes are less likely to be unacceptable. Elderly debilitated patients or those who are considered inoperable can be treated with radiotherapy without the need for anaesthesia. The treatment course can be limited to a few fractions, but it must be remembered that using higher doses per fraction and fewer treatment sessions will cause worse permanent normal tissue damage than using lower doses per fraction and more sessions.

The radiotherapy modality chosen will depend on the thickness of the lesion. If lesions are treated with megavoltage photons the dose to the underlying structures is high. The dose to these structures can be reduced by using superficial X-rays or electrons. Orthovoltage therapy uses 75 to 125 kV photons which have favourable beam characteristics for skin tumours less than 5 mm thick. An electron beam is more complex to use than orthovoltage photons.

When planning treatment a margin should be allowed around the tumour to encompass subclinical extension into the surrounding tissues. The size of the margin depends upon the size and site of the tumour and its histology. If the lesion is small (less than 0.5 cm in diameter) with a well defined edge, a margin of 0.5 cm is satisfactory. Where the lesion is larger and ulcerated, the minimum margin is 1 cm. Slightly larger margins have to be allowed if electron therapy is adopted to allow for the divergence of the beam edge to ensure that the edge of the tumour receives 100 per cent of the dose. To allow for the reduced dose at the edge of the electron beam the field can be collimated on the surface of the skin. The final choice of electron energy depends on the depth of tumour infiltration. Field sizes should not be less than 4 cm as the beam flatness is lost. Superficial lesions overlying cartilage sites such as the nose, ear,

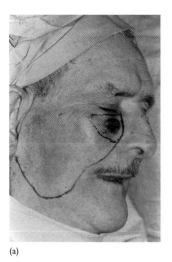 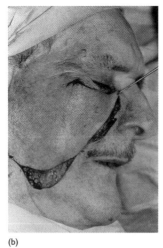 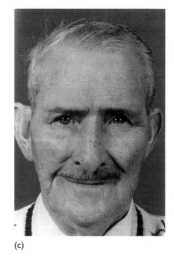 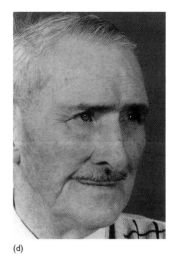

(a)   (b)   (c)   (d)

Fig. 6 (a) Basal cell carcinoma of the right cheek with the excision marked and an extensive cervical facial flap. (b) The flap is transposed to fill the defect. (c, d) Result at 2 months following surgery.

dorsum of the hand, and the scalp should be treated with electrons rather than superficial photons. The latter release more energy to bone and cartilage due to the photoelectric effect.

The incidence of necrosis can be greatly limited or even prevented by choosing the appropriate modality and an appropriate treatment schedule—total dose, fraction (fraction size), overall treatment time—to cater for the area of tissue being treated.[53],[54]

The radiotherapy treatment schedule that should be adopted depends upon the size of the lesion. It has to be appreciated that radiotherapy has cosmetic side-effects. If doses such as 18 to 20 Gy are given as a single fraction then a white atrophic area will result. For larger lesions fractionated therapy is adopted and a treatment schedule of 35 Gy in five fractions over 7 days or 50 Gy in 16 fractions over 22 days can be used. If the lesion is greater than 49 cm^2 in area a treatment schedule of 60 Gy in 30 fractions over 42 days may be prescribed. The object of therapy is to cure the lesion with the minimum of morbidity.

Radiotherapy is an effective treatment for skin carcinomas overlying the nose and ear. The cartilage in those areas tolerates therapeutic doses of radiation. Hayter et al. reviewed 130 cases of skin carcinoma (68 basal cell carcinoma, 62 squamous cell carcinoma) overlying the pinna.[54] Patients were treated using 100, 150 and 250 kVp, and received 17.5 to 64 Gy in 1 to 48 days. The commonest schedule used was 35 Gy in five fractions. They found that the use of high doses per fraction and short treatment times led to an unacceptable incidence of necrosis in 16 to 18 per cent of patients. When the dose per fraction was reduced below 6 Gy the incidence of necrosis fell to 2 per cent. This is in keeping with general observation that the incidence of necrosis depends upon the primary tumour size, the field area, and the total dose.[54],[55]

Petrovitch et al. reviewed a series of 896 patients with skin lesions arising in the lip and head and neck area treated over a period of 20 years.[56] In this group of patients 362 had squamous cell carcinomas, of which 250 arose on the nose. Early in the study, patients were treated with 250 to 300 kV photons; later 6 and 9 MV electrons were used. Initially patients received 30 Gy in three fractions, this was changed to 48 Gy in 12 fractions and eventually modified to 51 Gy

in 17 fractions over 21 days. The surrounding normal tissue was protected either by lead masks or appropriate shields, especially when treating lesions around the mouth, eyelids, and periorbital tissues. Of those responding, 53 per cent had stage 4 disease at the time of presentation. The control rate was related to the size of the lesion. Ten-year survival was 98 per cent for those with lesions less than 2 cm and 79 per cent for those with lesions of 2 to 5 cm (5-year survival 92 per cent). Where the lesion was larger than 5 cm the 8-year survival was 53 per cent and the 5-year survival was 60 per cent.

It is estimated that radiotherapy is only used as the primary treatment for basal cell carcinoma in approximately 8 per cent of patients in the United Kingdom.[57] Radiotherapy, however, does have an important role to play in the more unusual and aggressive tumours, particularly of the adnexal variety, and where there is escape either in the form of satellite lesions or nodal metastases. Lymph node metastasis, particularly with extracapsular spread, is a particularly difficult problem which benefits from postoperative radiotherapy.

Cryosurgery

The use of liquid nitrogen has been reported to have a high success in the treatment of basal cell carcinoma.[58] Fraunfelder et al. have shown a 7.5 per cent recurrence rate in basal cell carcinomas and noted that recurrence was high in larger tumours of the infiltrative variety.[59]

There is no doubt that cryotherapy is an effective method of treatment, particularly when surgery is not an option. It is a primary treatment for actinic keratosis and superficial well localized lesions. Single-cycle treatment is sufficient for most superficial tumours and double-cycle treatment for deeper tumours, particularly those 3 mm or more in depth. Cure rates of 97 to 99 per cent for skin cancers have been reported, with good cosmetic results.[60]

Curettage and electrodesiccation

This technique obtains a sample for histological diagnosis, debulking the tumour by using a curette. The remaining tumour cells are then electrodesiccated to produce a char which again can be curetted. This can be repeated two or three times. The disadvantage is that the depth of the wound where electrodesiccation is performed does not have accurate histology. Curettage can also be combined with cryotherapy, the latter technique replacing the previous electrodesiccation. In a study where basal cell carcinomas were treated by the triple electrodesiccation technique and the defect subsequently excised, residual tumour was found in 8.3 per cent of cases in the trunk and extremities and 46 per cent of lesions on the face.[61] The overall recurrence rate using this technique is not as high (3 to 10 per cent), presumably due to further destruction with progressive necrosis and inflammation. The technique should be limited to superficial, well-defined lesions and not used in cases of recurrent tumour or in difficult situations.

Laser surgery

The laser can be used as a cutting tool, replacing the knife, or as an ablative instrument for vaporizing tumour. It can also be used to supply the light to activate photosynthesizing agents in the treatment known as photodynamic therapy (see Chapter 4.29). Carbon dioxide laser ablation has been advocated for superficial basal cell carcinoma and a low incidence of recurrence in the short term has been reported.[62],[63] A balance has to be struck between vaporization, thermal damage, depth of damage, and subsequent healing by contraction and fibrosis.

Photodynamic therapy

Few studies have been carried out to investigate the value of photodynamic therapy in the management of skin cancer using systemic or topical porphyrins. The introduction of photoactivated agents which can be applied topically—for example δ-aminolaevulinic acid applied under occlusive foil to enhance tissue penetration—reduces photobleaching and other systemic side-effects and this is a more appealing approach.[64],[65] However, laser exposure causes erythema, severe burning, and pain especially if the area being treated is on the face. Healing occurs within 10 to 14 days, with cosmetic results equal or superior to those of the other treatment modalities. Absorption of δ-aminolaevulinic acid right to the base of deep lesions is poor. In superficial squamous cell carcinomas one to three sessions of photodynamic therapy may be necessary to clear the tumour. Further studies are necessary before the true value of this modality can be identified. It is more likely that it will be of more value in treating superficial lesions than thickened ones.

Chemotherapy

5-fluorouracil has been used for many years in topical form in the treatment of superficial skin malignancies. It is available in 2 per cent or 5 per cent strengths and is usually applied twice daily to the lesion and its margins. 5-fluorouracil primarily affects atypical cells and dysplastic cells, including those in actinic keratosis, and the surrounding skin tends to be spared. Systemic chemotherapy is restricted to metastatic disease in which combination chemotherapy provides some useful palliation.

The effect of oral retinoids has been evaluated in a number of prospective, double-blind, placebo-controlled studies to prevent the development of skin carcinomas in patients with xeroderma pigmentosum and those undergoing a renal transplant.[66] They have been reported as being of benefit, though agents such as isotretinoin are recognized to have marked side-effects especially when used over a prolonged time period. In patients with previously treated skin carcinomas retinoids may not be so beneficial. A review of the role of retinoids as an agent ot prevent cancer has been published.[67] This study involved 525 subjects with a 4-year history of four or more basal cell carcinomas and/or squamous cell carcinomas who were treated for 3 years with either vitamin A, isotretinoin, or placebo. No benefits were derived from any form of intervention. It was concluded that the chemopreventative effects of retinoids were more pronounced in patients with the early stages of cancer, e.g. actinic keratosis, and that further research into the value of newer retinoids was required both from the point of view of efficacy and side-effects.

Non-melanoma skin cancer comes in various clinical guises with markedly differing patterns of invasion and clinical course. Surgical excision remains the most common form of treatment, although a wide variety of other methods are currently under investigation. By far the majority of skin cancers are simply treated but the clinician must be alert to the danger signs of recurrence, aggressive behaviour and dissemination, which in a small number of cases can prove fatal.

References

1. **Glass AE, Hoover RN.** The emerging epidemic of melanoma and squamous cell carcinoma. *Journal of the American Medical Association*, 1989; **262**: 2097.

2. **Emmett AJJ, O'Rourke O.** *Malignant skin tumours* (2nd edn). Edinburgh, Churchill Livingstone, 1991.

3. **Marks R, Jolley D, Dorevitch AP, Selwood TS.** The incidence of non-melanocytic skin cancers in an Australian population: results of a five-year prospective study. *Medical Journal of Australia*, 1989; **150**: 475–8.

4. **Stone JL, Elpern DJ, Reizner G, Farmer ER, Scotto J, Pabo R.** Incidence of non-melanoma skin cancer in Kauai during 1983. *Hawaii Medical Journal*, 1986; **45**: 281–2, 285–6. (Erratum in *Hawaii Medical Journal*, 1986; **45**: 378.)

5. **Marks R.** The epidemiology on non-melanoma skin cancer: who, why and what can we do about it. *Journal of Dermatology*, 1995; **22**: 853–7.

6. **Marks R.** An overview of skin cancers. Incidence and causation. *Cancer*, 1995; **75**: 607–12.

7. **Albert DM, McGhee CN, Seddon JM, Weichelbaum RR.** Development of additional primary tumours after 62 years in the first patient with retinoblastoma cured by radiation therapy. *American Journal of Ophthalmology*, 1984; **97**: 189–96.

8. **Ron E, Modan B, Preston D, Alfandary E, Stovall M, Boice JD.** Radiation-induced skin carcinomas of the head and neck. *Radiation Research*, 1991; **125**: 318–25.

9. **Hardie IR, *et al.*** Skin cancer in Caucasian renal allograft recipients living in a subtropical climate. *Surgery*, 1980; **87**: 177.

10. **Gorlin RJ, Goltz RW.** Multiple nevoid bassal cell epithelioma, jaw cysts, and bifid ribs. *New England Journal of Medicine*, 1960; **262**; 908–12.

11. **Farndon PA, Del Mastro RG, Evans DG, Kilpatrick MW.** Location of gene for Gorlin syndrome. *The Lancet*, 1992; **339**: 581–2.

12. **Gailani MR, Leffell DJ, Ziegler EG, Bale AE.** Relationship between sunlight exposure and a key genetic alteration in basal cell carcinoma. *Journal of the National Cancer Institute*, 1996; **88**: 349–54.

13. **Bale AE, Gailani MR, Leffell DJ.** The Gorlin sydrome gene: a tumour suppressor active in basal cell carcinogensis and embryonic

development. *Proceedings of the Association of American Physicians*, 1997; **107**: 253–7.

14. Vabres P, *et al.* The gene for Bazex-Dupre-Christol syndrome maps to chromosome Xq. *Journal of Investigative Dermatology*, 1995; **105**: 87–91.

15. Sommerville J, Milne JA. Familial primary self-healing squamous epithelioma of the skin. *British Journal of Dermatology*, 1950; **62**: 485.

16. Ferguson-Smith MA, Wallace DC, James ZH, Renwick JH. *Birth Defects*, 1971; **7**: 157.

17. Emmett AJ. Surgical analysis and biological behaviour of 2277 basal cell carcinomas. *Australia and New Zealand Journal of Surgery*, 1990; **60**: 855–63.

18. Marghoob M, *et al.* Risk of another basal cell carcinoma developing after treatment of a basal cell carcinoma. *Journal of the American Academy of Dermatology*, 1993; **28**: 22–8.

19. Soutar DS, Tiwari R. The skin. In: Soutar DS, Tiwari R (ed.) *Excision and reconstruction in head and neck cancer.* London: Churchill Livingstone, 1994: 369–87.

20. Jackson R, Adams RH. Horrifying basal cell carcinoma: a study of 33 cases and a comparison with 435 non-horror cases and a report on four metastatic cases. *Journal of Surgical Oncology*, 1973; **5**: 431–63.

21. Leffell DJ, Headington JT, Wong DS, Swanson NA. Aggressive-growth basal cell carcinoma in young adults. *Archives of Dermatology*, 1991; **127**: 1663–7.

22. Randle HW, Roenigk RK, Brodland DG. Giant basal cell carcinoma (T3). Who is at risk? *Cancer*, 1993; **72**: 1624–30.

23. Vico P, Fourez T, Nemec E, Andry G, Deraemaecker R. Aggressive basal cell carcinoma of head and neck areas. *European Journal of Surgical Oncology*, 1995; **21**: 490–7.

24. Oram Y, Orengo I, Griego RD, Rosen T, Thornby J. Histologic patterns of basal cell carcinoma based upon patient immunostatus. *Dermatological Surgery*, 1995; **21**: 611–14.

25. Snow SN, *et al.* Metastatic basal cell carcinoma. Report of five cases. *Cancer*, 1994; **73**: 328–35.

26. Von Domarus H, Stevens PJ. Metastatic basal cell carcinoma. Report of five cases and review of 170 cases in the literature. *Journal of the American Academy of Dermatology*, 1984; **10**: 1043–60.

27. Weedon D, Wall D. Metastatic basal cell carcinoma. *Medical Journal of Australia*, 1975; **2**: 177.

28. Asada O, *et al.* Solid basal cell epithelioma (BCE) possibly originates from the outer root sheath of the hair follicle. *Acta Dermatologica Venereologica*, 1993; **73**: 286–92.

29. Sexton M, Jones DB, Maloney ME. Histologic pattern analysis of basal cell carcinoma. Study of a series of 1039 consecutive neoplasms. *Journal of the American Academy of Dermatology*, 1990; **23**: 1118–26.

30. Lund HZ. How often does squamous cell carcinoma of the skin metastasise? *Archives of Dermatology*, 1965; **92**: 635.

31. Moller R, Reymann F, Hou-jensen K. Metastasis in dermatological patients with squamous cell carcinoma. *Archives of Dermatology*, 1979; **115**: 703.

32. Goepfert H, *et al.* Perineural invasion in squamous cell skin carcinoma of the head and neck. *American Journal of Surgery*, 1984; **148**: 542.

33. Mendenhall WM, *et al.* Carcinoma of the skin of the head and neck with perineural invasion. *Head and Neck*, 1989; **11**: 301.

34. Tang CK, Toker C. Trabecular carcinoma of the skin: An ultrastructural study. *Cancer*, 1978; **42**: 2311–21.

35. Silva EG, Mackay B, Goepfept H, Burgess MA, Fields RS. Endocrine carcinoma of the skin (Merkel cell carcinoma). *Pathology Annals*, 1984; **19**: 1–30.

36. Shaw JHF, Rumball E. Merkel cell tumour: Clinical behaviour and treatment. *British Journal of Surgery*, 1991; **78**: 138–42.

37. O'Brien PC, Denham JW, Leong AS. Merkel cell carcinoma: A review

of behaviour patterns and management strategies. *Australian and New Zealand Journal of Surgery*, 1987; **57**: 847–50.

38. Hill ADK, Brady MS, Coit DG. Intraoperative lymphatic mapping and sentinel node biopsy for merkel cell carcinoma. *British Journal of Surgery*, 1999; **86**: 518–21.

39. Hasel H. Merkel cell carcinoma: the role of primary treatment with radiotherapy. *Clinical Oncology*, 1991; **3**: 114–16.

40. Pacella J, *et al.* The role of radiotherapy in the management of primary cutaneous neuro-endocrine tumours. Experience at the Peter Maccallum Cancer Institute. *International Journal of Radiation Oncology and Biological Physics*, 1988; **14**: 1077–84.

41. Wilder RB, *et al.* Merkel cell carcinoma. Improved local regional control with postoperative radiation therapy. *Cancer*, 1991; **68**: 1004–8.

42. Bourne RG and O'Rourke MG. Management of merkel cell tumour. *Australia and New Zealand Journal of Surgery*, 1988; **58**: 971–4.

43. Fenig E, *et al.* The treatment of advanced merkel cell carcinoma. A multi-modality chemotherapy and irradiation therapy treatment approach. *Journal of Dermatological Surgery and Oncology*, 1993; **19**: 860–4.

44. Yiengpruksawan A, Coit DG, Thaler HT, Urmacher C, Knapper WK. Merkel cell carcinoma. Prognosis and management. *Archives of Surgery*, 1991; **126**: 11514–19.

45. Cozen W, Bernstein L, Wang F, Press MF, Mack TM. The risk of angiosarcoma following primary breast cancer. *British Journal of Cancer*, 1999; **81**: 532–6.

46. Stewart NJ, *et al.* Lymphangiosarcoma following mastectomy. *Clinical Orthopaedics and Related Research*, 1995; **320**: 135–41.

47. El-Sheemy MA. The surgical management of basal cell carcinoma: an analysis of 563 lesions. MSc. thesis, Glasgow University, 1991.

48. Mohs FE. Chemosurgery for skin cancer: fixed tissue and fresh tissue techniques. *Archives of Dermatology*, 1976; **112**: 211–15.

49. Richmond JD, Davie RM. The significance of incomplete excision in patients with basal cell carcinoma. *British Journal of Plastic Surgery*, 1987; **40**: 63–7.

50. Hayes H. Basal cell carcinoma. The East Grinstead experience. *Plastic and Reconstructive Surgery*, 1962; **30**: 273.

51. Avril M-F, Auperin A, Margulis A, Gerbaulet A, Al E. Basal cell carcinoma of the face: Surgery or radiotherapy? Results of a randomised study. *British Journal of Cancer*, 1997; **76**: 100–6.

52. Lovett RD. External irradiation of epithelial skin cancer. *International Journal of Radiation Oncology and Biological Physics*, 1990; **19**: 235–42.

53. Hunter RD, Pereira DTM, Pointon RCS. Megavoltage electron beam therapy in the treatment of basal and squamous cell carcinoma of the pinna. *Clinical Radiology*, 1982; **33**: 341–5.

54. Hayter CRR, Lee KHY, Groome PA, Brundage MD. Necrosis following radiotherapy for carcinoma of the pinna. *International Journal of Radiation Oncology and Biological Physics*, 1996; **36**: 1033–7.

55. Abbatucci JS, Boulier N, Laforge T, Lozier JC. Radiation therapy of skin carcinomas: Results of a hypofraction schedule in 675 cases followed more than 2 years. *Radiotherapy and Oncology*, 1989; **14**: 113–19.

56. Petrovich Z, Parker RG, Luxston G, Kuist H, Jepson J. Carcinoma of the lip and selected sites of head and neck skin. The clinical study of 896 patients. *Radiotherapy and Oncology*, 1987; **8**: 11–17.

57. Motley RJ, Gould DJ, Douglas WS, Simpson NB. Treatment of basal cell carcinoma by dermatologists in the United Kingdom. British Association of Dermatologists Audit Subcommittee and the British Society for Dermatological Surgery. *British Journal of Dermatology*, 1995; **132**: 437–40.

58. Kuflick EG. Cryosurgery for cutaneous malignancy: an update. *Dermatological Surgery*, 1997; **23**: 1081–7.

59. Fraunfelder FT, Zacarian SA, Wingfield DL and Limmen BL. Results

of cryotherapy for eyelid malignancies. *Transactions of the American Academy of Ophthalmology and Otolarnygology*, 1984; **97**: 184–8.

60. **Graham GF.** Cryosurgery. In: McGrath MH, Turner ML (ed.) *Clinics in plastic surgery*. Philadelphia: Saunders, 1993: 131–47.

61. **Suhge D'Aubermont PC, Bennett RG.** Failure of curettage and electrodesiccation for removal of basal cell carcinoma. *Archives of Dermatology*, 1984; **120**: 1456–60.

62. **Adams EL, Price NM.** Treatment of basal cell carcinomas with a carbon-dioxide laser. *Journal of Dermatology, Surgery and Oncology*, 1979; **5**: 803–6.

63. **Wheeland RG, Bailin PL, Ratz JL, Roenigk RK.** Carbon dioxide laser vaporisation and curettage in the treatment of large or multiple superficial basal cell carcinomas. *Journal of Dermatology, Surgery and Oncology*, 1987; **13**: 119–25.

64. **Wolf P, Rieger E, Kerl H.** Topical photodynamic therapy with endogenous porphyrins after application of 5-aminolevulinic acid; an alternative treatment modality for solar keratosis, superficial squamous cell carcinomas and basal cell carcinomas? *Journal of the American Academy of Dermtology*, 1993; **28**: 17–21.

65. **Calzavara-Pinton PG.** Repetitive photodynamic therapy with topical δ-aminolaevulinic acid as an appropriate approach to the routine treatment of superficial non-melanoma skin tumours. *Journal of Photochemistry and Photobiology B*, 1985; **29**: 53–7.

66. **Bavick JN, *et al*.** Prevention of skin cancer and reduction of keratotic skin lesions during acitretin therapy in renal transplant patients: a double blind, placebo–controlled study. *Journal of Clinical Oncology*, 1995; **13**: 1933–8.

67. **Moon TE, *et al*.** Effect of retinol to prevent squamous cell skin cancer in moderate-risk subjects: a randomised, double-blind controlled trail. *Cancer Epidemiology Biomark Preview*, 1997; **6**: 949–56.

9

Head and neck cancer

9.1.1 Epidemiology of premalignant and malignant lesions

N. W. Johnson

Descriptive epidemiology

Definitions of head and neck cancer

This chapter covers malignancies of the upper aerodigestive tract, most of which share common risk factors. Most are squamous-cell carcinomas (**SCC**) arising in the mucous membranes of the mouth, pharynx, and larynx. Indeed, of all oropharyngeal malignancies reported to the Surveillance, Epidemiology and End Results (**SEER**) registries in the United States between 1973 and 1987, apart from lesions of salivary glands, gingivae, nasopharynx, nasal cavity, and sinuses, more than 95 per cent were SCC.[1] Upper aerodigestive tract alcohol- and tobacco-related SCC are thus the major head and neck cancers. They constitute a major public health problem and the major workload of head and neck oncologists. Because these cancers sometimes arise out of longstanding, potentially malignant lesions and conditions, so-called premalignant lesions of mucous membranes are also considered here.

Less coverage is given to other lesions. Neoplasms arise from all the constituent tissues of the head and neck: bone, blood vessels, nerves, fibrous tissue, fat, muscle, and mucous glands. Furthermore, we have the odontogenic tumours. Because these are uncommon, no strong epidemiological data exist. Leukaemias and lymphomas, which so often involve the head and neck, are dealt with elsewhere.

Most international databases employ the World Health Organization's (**WHO**) International Classification of Diseases coding system, and most data currently available are expressed in the 9th revision (ICD-9): there is, however, a steady trend towards the 10th revision (ICD-10). It is important to define these codes and to be clear how many of these precise anatomical sites are included in any particular dataset (Table 1). Neoplasms of the major salivary glands have quite distinct natural histories, ill-understood aetiologies, and distinct management protocols compared to mucosal cancers. Similarly, nasopharyngeal malignancies are usually Epstein–Barr virus-related carcinomas (**NPC**, nasopharyngeal carcinoma) distinctly

different from the more widespread alcohol- and tobacco-related SCCs of the upper aerodigestive tract. Care is needed when examining datasets, as to whether or not malignancies of the major salivary glands and nasopharynx are included as 'oral' cancers. Many datasets make a distinction between lip and intraoral cancer, and we have to be clear whether 'oral cancer' is taken to include the oropharynx and hypopharynx. Fortunately, data for the larynx are usually recorded separately.

Incidence rates and trends worldwide

Much of the world produces no data and, in other regions, often amongst the most populous, data may come from localized, atypical areas. Hospital-based cancer registries gather only cases which present to hospital, so those in many developing countries may not come to attention, either because of fear or the inability of poor people to access hospital services. Death rates may be even more unreliable because the follow-up of treated cases and death certification are incomplete—compounded by the limited international standardization of cause of death, let alone calibration of those signing death certificates.

Figure 1 plots the estimated numbers of new cases of the most common cancers by anatomical site in males and females, comparing so-called developed countries with developing countries. There are striking differences. For both sexes combined cancer of the mouth and pharynx ICD-9 (140–149) ranks sixth overall in the world, behind lung, stomach, breast, colon and rectum, and cervix plus corpus uteri. The mouth and pharynx are the third most common site amongst males in developing countries and the fourth amongst females. The same ranking applies within the European Union.[3] If one adds the larynx (ICD-9, 161), these head and neck cancers become the fifth most common anatomical site in the world—hardly a rare and unimportant public health issue! There were half a million incident cases of oral and pharyngeal plus laryngeal cancer worldwide in 1990 (Table 2). This is a substantial disease burden, with high mortality rates—54 per cent overall: death to registration (**D/R**) ratios range from 0.47 to 0.65 according to site.

Effectively, the highest rates in the world for oral cancer are found in France, the Indian subcontinent, Brazil, and central and eastern Europe. The ostensibly extremely high rates for oral and pharyngeal cancer in the relatively small Pacific Island populations have not been researched in detail and may relate to chewing and smoking habits. Hong Kong and the adjoining Guandung Province of China, together with other South East Asian countries with high immigrant populations from Southern China, have the highest incidence rates of

Much of this information has been published in *Oral cancer* by Shah J, Johnson NW, Batsakis J. Oxford: Isis Medical, 2001.

Table 1 ICD-9 and -10 equivalents for the sites considered in this chapter

ICD-9 equivalent	Description	ICD-10 code
140–49	Malignant neoplasms of the lip, oral cavity, and pharynx	C00–14
140.0–140.9	Lip	C00
141.0	Base of tongue	C01
141.1–141.9	Other and unspecified parts of the tongue	C02
143.0–143.9	Gum	C03
144.0–144.9	Floor of the mouth	C04
145.2–145.5	Palate	C05
145.0–145.1, 145.6–145.9	Other and unspecified parts of the mouth	C06
142.0	Parotid gland	C07
142.1–142.9	Other and unspecified major salivary glands	C08
146.0–146.2	Tonsil	C09
146.3–146.9	Oropharynx	C10
147.0–147.9	Nasopharynx	C11
148.1	Pyriform sinus	C12
148.0, 148.2–148.9	Hypopharynx	C13
149.0–149.9	Other and ill-defined sites in the lip, oral cavity, and pharynx	C14
160.0–160.1	Nasal cavity and middle ear	C30
160.2–160.9	Accessory sinuses	C31
161.0–161.9	Larynx	C32

NPC. For laryngeal cancer, the top 15 countries are widely scattered, including many in Europe, related to the high smoking prevalences in these populations in recent decades. In India, Bangladesh, Pakistan, and Sri Lanka oral cancer is the most common site and accounts for about a third of all cancers.

There is a dramatic increase in mouth cancer incidence (ICD-9 143–149) for both sexes in Japan, which more than doubled between 1973 and 1985 and is still rising at 30 per cent or more every 5 years, at least within the Miyagi and Osaka registries.[5] The national data for Japan show this trend to be strongest for males, to be continuing through 1993, and to be strongest for floor of the mouth and oropharyngeal cancers. A cohort effect in males born from about 1920 onwards is apparent.[6] Figure 2 shows the leading sites of the new cancer cases and of deaths for the United States in 1997. 'Oral cavity' cancer here includes all 140–149 sites: in males there were 20 900 new cases and 5600 estimated deaths; for females 9850 new cases and 2840 deaths. This represents a death-registration ratio of 0.274. In other words, even in an advanced society like the United States, nearly one in three people with oral cancer in time die with or as a result of their disease. Elsewhere in North America, notably in the Maritime Provinces of Canada, there is a steep increase in cumulative risk of males developing mouth cancer, increasing in successive birth cohorts, which is reflected in mortality trends.[5] There is also an upward trend for both males and females in Australia and amongst the non-Maori population in New Zealand.

The pattern in Europe, more so than in North America, gives cause for concern. Data from Denmark[8] and from Scotland[9] first drew our attention to dramatically rising trends in the incidence of oral and pharyngeal cancer, particularly of the tongue amongst young adult males. This has now been well documented in many countries, and is reflected in growing mortality rates. It is most striking in central and eastern Europe: in Slovakia, for example, oropharyngeal cancer increased from a rate of 6.8 per 100 000 per annum between 1968 and 1970 to a staggering 47.9 per 100 000 between 1987 and 1989 in 35- to 64-year-old males.[10]

For all these cancer sites, demographic trends, both overall population increases in developing countries and an increasing proportion of older citizens worldwide, will increase the number of cases substantially.

Age distribution

Incidence increases with age in all countries. In the West, 98 per cent of oral and pharyngeal cases are found in patients over 40 years of age (Fig. 3). In high-prevalence areas, cases occur prior to the age of 35 due to heavy abuse of various forms of tobacco. Furthermore, a number of cases of oral mucosal SCC occur in both young and old

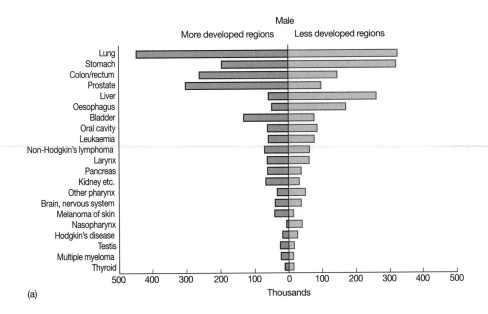

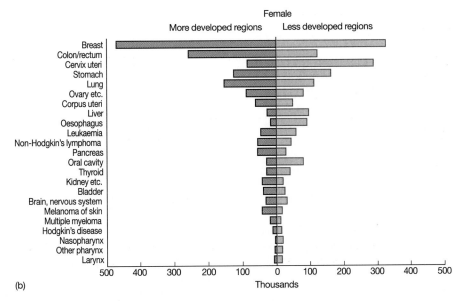

Fig. 1 Estimated numbers of new cases (thousands) of 21 cancers in men (A), and 23 cancers in women (B), in developed and developing parts of the world. The estimates are for 1990. (Redrawn from ref. 2 with permission.)

patients, often in the absence of traditional alcohol- and tobacco-risk factors, and these may pursue a particularly aggressive course.

Sex distribution

In industrialized countries, men are affected two to three times as often as women, largely due to their higher indulgence in the risk factors—such as heavy alcohol and tobacco consumption for intraoral and laryngeal cancer and sunlight for lip cancer in those who work outdoors. However, the incidence of tongue and other intraoral cancers for women can be greater than or equal to that for men in high-incidence areas such as India, where tobacco chewing and sometimes smoking are also common amongst women. In the United States, from 1991 to 1993 the death rate per 100 000 of the population

for oral and pharyngeal cancer was 4.4 for males and 1.6 for females, down from 5.9 and 1.9, respectively, in 1971 to 1973. Note, however, that because the population of the United States has become larger (a 22 per cent increase from 1973 to 1993 alone) and older, the actual number of deaths has risen over the past 25 years, more so in women (Table 3).

Ethnic variations

Ethnicity strongly influences prevalence rates due to social and cultural practices, as well as death rates due to socioeconomic differences. Where these represent risk factors, their continuation by emigrants from high-incidence regions to other parts of the world results in comparatively high rates in immigrant communities. Among Indians

Table 2 Estimated number of cases and deaths worldwide in 1990 (from refs 2 and 4 with permission)

(ICD-9)	Female		Male		Total		D/R
	All ages Incidence	Mortality	All ages Incidence	Mortality	All ages Incidence	Mortality	
Oral cavity (140–5)	70 135	34 096	140 860	65 939	210 995	100 035	0.47
Nasopharynx (147)	17 659	10 778	39 701	24 292	57 360	35 070	0.61
Other pharynx (146, 8–9)	17 335	11 565	76 645	49 992	93 980	61 557	0.65
Larynx (161)	17 282	8939	118 380	64 598	135 662	73 537	0.54
Total	122 411	65 378	375 586	204 821	497 997	270 119	0.54

D/R, Death to registration ratio.

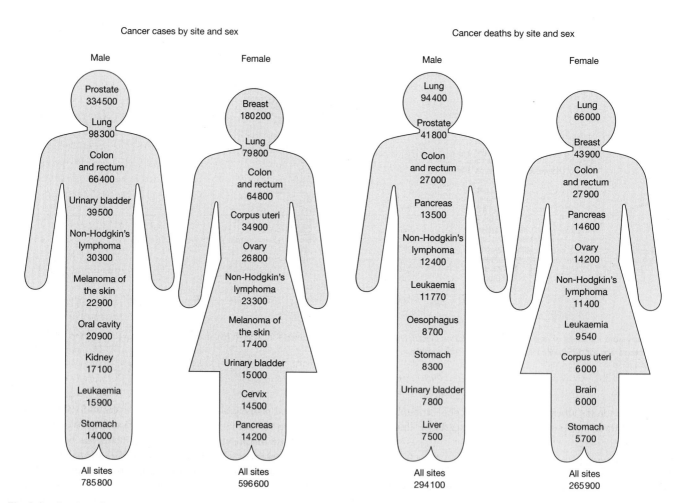

Fig. 2 Leading sites of new cancer cases and deaths in the United States. Estimates are for 1997, and exclude basal- and squamous-cell skin cancer and *in situ* carcinomas except for bladder. (Data derived from ref. 7.)

in the Malay Peninsular, for example, oral cancer has long been considerably more common than amongst Malays or Chinese.[12] Similar trends are noted among Indian migrants from India to Natal.[13] There is a significant correlation between the percentage of the population described as Asian and the incidence rate for oral and pharyngeal cancer in the North Thames[14] and Midlands regions of

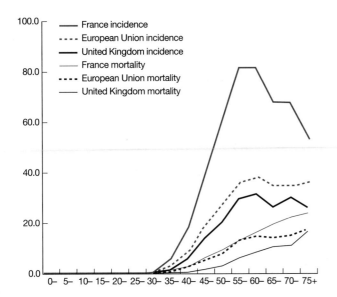

Fig. 3 Age-specific incidence rates (per 100 000 population per year) for oral cancer in the UK, in France (where rates are much higher), and for the European Union overall, as an example of the pattern in the Western world. Data refer to the situation in 1990, and for all ICD-9 sites 140–149. (From ref. 11 with permission.)

Table 3 Actual numbers of deaths from oral and pharyngeal cancer in the US, by sex, 1973–1997 (Source: Various tables from American Cancer Society Inc.)

	1973	1993	1997
Males	5553	5515	5600
Females	2269	2726	2840
Total	7822	8341	8440

England.[15] Swerdlow *et al.*[16] have recently shown that mortality rates for 1979 to 1985 from oral cancer in Indian migrants to England and Wales are increased above the rates for those born in England (odds ratio (**OR**) 2.2; 95 per cent confidence interval (**CI**), 1.5–3.1). We have recently confirmed this using data from 7222 patients with head and neck cancers registered in SE England from 1986 to 1991. Immigrants from India, Pakistan, Bangladesh, Nepal, and Sri Lanka (95/232 cases) had significantly higher rates of intraoral cancer, and residents of Chinese origin (45/67 cases) had significantly higher rates of nasopharyngeal cancer, than the remainder of the local population; furthermore, cancer at these sites presented, on average, 10 to 15 years earlier in these groups.[17]

In the United States, both the incidence and mortality rates for alcohol- and tobacco-related cancers in Black Americans are substantially higher than for Whites. Blacks are not enjoying the same downward trends in mortality rates. The incidence for Black males in the United States is so high, 20.4 per 100 000 per annum, that

oral/pharyngeal cancer becomes the fourth most common site for malignant disease (Table 4).

Mortality rates and trends

Mortality rates show major changes over time. In the United States there have been substantial declines in deaths from stomach cancer in both sexes over the past half century, with dramatic rises in deaths from lung cancer due to the smoking epidemic! The female epidemic is some 20 years behind; however, death rates continue to rise in females, although they are now beginning to fall in males. There has been a fall in deaths from oral cancer, from 6.0 per 100 000 per annum in 1962 to 4.5 in 1990–1992, in males and a steady rate of 1.6 in females. Recently the SEER programme reported a 22.6 per cent overall fall in the mortality rate from oral cancer between 1973 and 1993 (Table 5). However, there has been a considerable rise in mortality amongst Black males (10.3 per cent), more so in those aged 65 and over (16.4 per cent), an even larger rise in older Black females (19.1 per cent), and a smaller but significant rise amongst older White females (3.4 per cent). Furthermore, the 5-year survival rate for males of all races has declined from 53.5 per cent in 1974 to 47.5 per cent in 1988: rates range from a high of 72.1 per cent for White females in Utah to a low of 24.8 per cent for Black males in metropolitan Atlanta. These are striking differences, which are probably explained by socioeconomic condition, age, stage at diagnosis, continued presence or absence of environmental risk factors, and access to hospital and community care.

Within continental United States there is a more than fivefold regional interstate variation in mortality rates (Fig. 4) due to ethnic mix, socioeconomic mix, and variations in risk factors, including the use of oral smokeless tobacco in the south. Striking variations are also seen across the European Union (Fig. 5).[19] There is likely to be a doubling in deaths from oral cancer in the EU between 1970 and 2000 fuelled by younger age groups, and which therefore will probably continue well into the next century. The highest mortality rates in the world for laryngeal cancer in men are found in Hungary, Poland, Slovakia, and Romania.[20]

Rising trends in incidence and mortality are seen for oral cancer in many other parts of the world[21] and for laryngeal, lung, and other tobacco-related cancers in most of the world, especially in developing countries.[5] The data show a strong cohort effect in individuals born from the 1920s onwards,[22] as clearly seen for Eastern European countries outside the European Union (**EU**) (Fig. 6). The increases are particularly striking in young and middle-aged men. Table 6 lists the increase in risk for 19 countries, in which this risk is consistently demonstrable from the WHO's mortality database.

A more detailed analysis for intraoral cancer in males in England and Wales between 1901 and 1990 is shown in Fig. 7. For laryngeal cancer there are similar but less marked trends: again countries of central and eastern Europe show the most disturbing rises.

In population terms, survival rates around the world show little improvement. Cure and survival rates are better in highly specialized, high-volume treatment institutions. But such expert management is not uniformly available. Examples of survival curves from one well-documented, western-industrialized area, the Yorkshire Cancer Registry in the United Kingdom, are shown in Fig. 8. There is

Table 4 Incidence rates for the five most commonly diagnosed cancers in males in the United States, 1988–92, for Whites and African-Americans (from ref. 7 with permission)

African-Americans		Whites	
Prostate	180.6	Prostate	134.7
Lung	117.0	Lung	76.0
Colon and rectum	60.7	Colon and rectum	56.3
Oral/pharyngeal	20.4	Urinary bladder	31.7
Stomach	17.9	Non-Hodgkin's lymphoma	18.7

Rates per 100 000 per annum, age-adjusted to the 1970 US standard population.

Table 5 Mortality trends for oral and pharyngeal cancer in the United States between 1973 and 1993, by race and sex (from ref. 18 with permission)

	All races			Whites			Blacks		
	Total	Males	Females	Total	Males	Females	Total	Males	Females
All ages									
% change	−22.6	−26.2	−16.3	−26.7	−31.6	−17.5	2.9	10.3	−8.8
Est. ann %	−1.4*	−1.7*	−1.0*	−1.7*	−2.1*	−1.1*	−0.1	0.2	−0.3
Under 65									
% change	−26.7	−24.5	−34.0	−33.2	−32.3	−37.5	−1.6	7.3	−21.5
Est ann %	−1.8*	−1.6*	−2.3*	−2.2*	−2.1*	−2.6*	−0.4	0.0	−1.2*
65 and over									
% change	−18.2	−26.8	3.7	−20.4	−31.1	3.4	12.6	16.4	19.1
Est ann %	−1.1*	−1.8*	0.2	−1.3*	−2.1*	0.1	0.6*	0.7*	1.4*

*Indicates that the estimated annual percentage change in rate is statistically significantly different from zero.

no significant overall difference by age or sex; lip cancer is, biologically, a much less aggressive neoplasm than intraoral cancer and is more readily eradicated. The apparently large differences by treatment modality reflect the fact that smaller and more readily curable lesions will form a proportion of those for whom surgery is the main approach, whereas large, perhaps inoperable, lesions will form a proportion of those treated primarily by radiotherapy. Furthermore, these curves do not distinguish the effects of combined-modality therapy. The major determinants of survival are discussed elsewhere.[26] They include:

- patient factors at diagnosis: age, sex, socioeconomic status, nutritional status and intercurrent disease, and continuing presence of risk factors (see ref. 27);
- tumour factors: site, size, differentiation, and biological behaviour of the neoplasm, including host immune response, and the extent of regional and distant metastases;
- management factors: treatment modality and thoroughness, with smaller components derived from the quality and extent of supportive care and aftercare, the treating institution (facilities—including team work, experience—including case load and case mix).

Epidemiology of potentially malignant lesions and conditions

Definitions

Although in common use, the term(s) 'precancerous/premalignant lesion(s)' of upper aerodigestive tract mucosa' are unsatisfactory because they imply that irreversible steps in the multistage process of genetic alterations leading to invasive carcinoma have taken place. However, the risk of a lesion becoming malignant within the lifespan of the patient is highly unpredictable and low. Furthermore, such lesions may regress. Additionally, in much of the West, most carcinomas arise without the patient or clinician being aware of a pre-existing lesion. In high-incidence areas of the world, notably South Asia, the reverse is the case—tobacco or areca nut chewing habits result in chronic lesions and the majority of oral cancers arise from these; the carcinomas have a distinctive natural history that is less aggressive than those arising *de novo* in the West. A preferable term is 'potentially malignant lesions and conditions', amongst which there is a greater risk of malignant change. This broad group is generally classified under 'lesions' and 'conditions'; the latter being more generalized and widespread, and accompanied by significant systemic

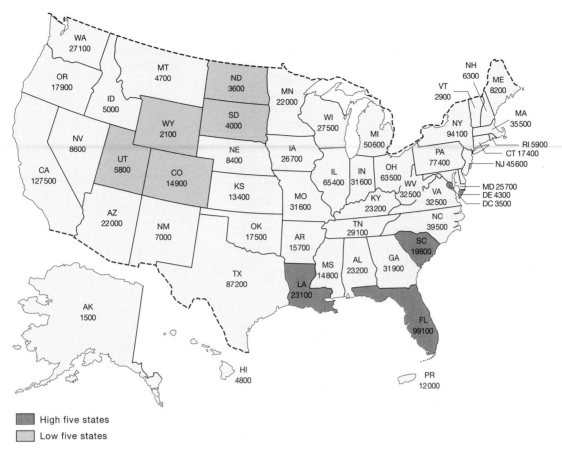

Fig. 4 Average age-adjusted mortality rates per 100 000 population pa for oral and pharyngeal cancer in each state of the United States, 1989–93, both sexes combined. The highest five states and the lowest five states are shaded as indicated. (Data from the United States National Centre for Health Statistics, as published in ref. 18; reproduced with permission (see legend to Fig. 6).)

involvement. These 'conditions' are associated with mucosal atrophy and altered mucosal homeostasis without a discrete lesion being visible clinically. We generally consider the potentially malignant 'lesions' to include leucoplakia and erythroplakia of various clinical presentations (such as homogenous, verrucous, nodular, or speckled (mixed lesions)). Potentially malignant 'conditions' are usually taken to include sideropenic dysphagia (mucosal atrophy associated with chronic iron-deficiency anaemia), erosive lichen planus, oral sub-mucous fibrosis, discoid lupus erythematosus, tertiary syphilis, and actinic kerotosis.

The term 'leucoplakia' has long been loosely used by clinicians specializing in oral diseases, in otorhinolaryngology, and in gynaecology. Dentists have tended to follow an old WHO definition as 'a white patch which cannot be rubbed off and cannot be characterized clinically or histologically as any other lesion'. The term should only be used as a clinical descriptor of a white patch or plaque and never used once histological information is available (see refs 28, 29). Biopsy of such lesions is essential to establish diagnosis and to estimate the degree of epithelial dysplasia, which has value for predicting malignant potential. Biopsy will indicate whether a cancer is already present or not—provided the biopsy site or sites are carefully chosen. Histology may lead to diagnosis of a specific lesion such as lichen planus, chronic candidiasis, or lupus erythematosus. Histology helps to characterize

tobacco-induced lesions and assists in differentiating these from idiopathic plaques in which no causal factor is evident.

As many as possible of the descriptors given in Table 7 should be recorded for every lesion and condition. Diagnostic labels should not be applied until all information is available. 'White patch not otherwise specified (**NOS**)' is a better term for undiagnosable lesions, which probably represent a large, ill-understood spectrum. 'Keratosis without', or 'keratosis with mild/moderate/severe dysplasia' are acceptable diagnostic labels for these lesions.

Prevalence and incidence

Because of these unsatisfactory definitions, and the way in which they have changed over time, a very wide range of figures are reported in the literature. That pertaining to the mouth is summarized in the paper by Johnson, Ranasinghe, and Warnakulasuriya.[30]

Malignant transformation rates

Data are limited and difficult to interpret because of variable follow-up, disease definitions, diagnostic criteria, and treatment interventions. The literature gives rates from 0.3 to 17.5 per cent for oral leucoplakia; consensus range from 3 to 6 per cent. Schepman *et al.*[31] describe 20/166 (12 per cent) transforming after 6 to 201

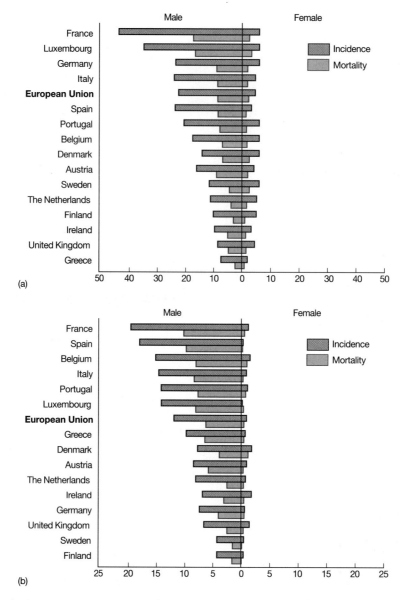

Fig. 5 The marked variability in incidence and mortality rates (per 100 000 pa) for oral plus pharyngeal (a) and for laryngeal cancer (b) across the European Union. Crude rates, all ages. (Data reproduced from ref. 11 with permission.)

months (median 32 months) in a hospital-based population in the Netherlands—representing a rate of 2.9 per cent per annum. Women without smoking habits were at significantly higher risk. Importantly, patients who had received any form of active treatment did not have a statistically significantly decreased risk of malignant transformation. This latter observation is repeatedly alluded to in the literature and demands extensive multicentre prospective trials of the efficacy of various treatment modalities.[32]

Interestingly, the rates tend to be on the low side for tobacco-associated lesions such as those common in South Asia where the oral cancer incidence is high. Idiopathic leucoplakias in Europe and America carry a higher risk. Van der Waal *et al.*[28] give, in arbitrary order, the following features as being associated with malignant transformation in oral leucoplakia:

- sex; females appear to be at higher risk;
- duration of the lesion;
- lack of obvious risk factors, so-called idiopathic leucoplakia;
- location: e.g. floor of the mouth or the tongue seem to be high-risk sites (but this is influenced by risk habits)—in the Amsterdam study[31] the site was not a risk factor;
- non-homogenous types;
- colonization by fungi, usually *Candida albicans*;
- presence of epithelial dysplasia.

For laryngeal leucoplakia, the largest and longest study in the United States (mean follow-up of 7.2 years) gives a transformation rate for dysplastic lesions of 36 per cent.[33] Controversy continues over the presence of concomitant leucoplakia in patients with oral

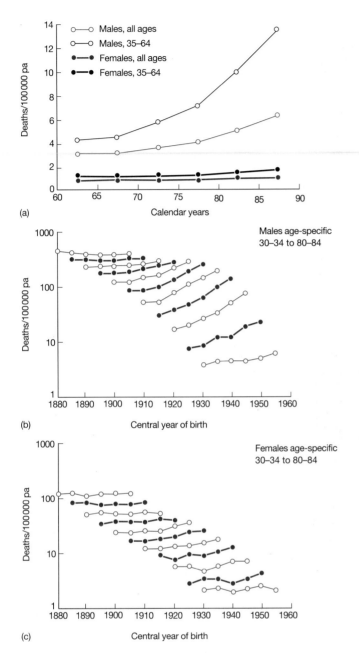

Fig. 6 Age-standardized death rates of oral and pharyngeal cancer in Eastern Europe (countries outside the EEC), 1963–87. There are substantial rises in males, with a strong cohort effect. (From ref. **23** with permission.)

not always adequate information on the patients' smoking and drinking habits. There have always been arguments that the two diseases appeared coincidentally (see, for example, refs 38–40). A study from Greece demonstrated the development of SCC in a mean time of 6.5 years in 4 of 326 patients followed up from 6 months to 10 years: three had the erosive form, one papular/atrophic, and none had a family history of cancer, alcohol or tobacco habits, or nutritional disturbances.[37] Muzio et al.[41] describe 14/263 (5.32 per cent) of their cases transforming between 3 and 10 years of the diagnosis of OLP. The two recent single case reports of SCC[42] and of verrucous carcinoma[43] developing in hepatitis C-related OLP, in the absence of traditional risk factors, add to both knowledge and confusion. Perhaps a significant factor in the controversy over the malignant potential in OLP is too loose a histological definition of lichen planus.

Oral submucous fibrosis clearly has a significant malignant potential, rates as high as 7 per cent over 15 years being reported from the extensive studies in India.[44]

Epidemiology of other mucosal neoplasms

The minor salivary glands give rise to neoplasms, in most series from the West these represent about 10 per cent of all salivary tumours (5 per cent in the large British series of 1403 patients treated between 1947 and 1992[45]). Most information on site prevalence, however, comes from hospital series and these inevitably demonstrate bias. For example, an early study from Bombay showed 110 of 355 salivary neoplasms seen between 1941 and 1965 to be in the minor glands,[46] and in Nigeria, 94 of 295 were also intraoral:[47] it is not known whether this reflects real racial or ethnic differences. Importantly, up to 50 per cent of minor gland neoplasms are malignant.[48] Most occur around the junction of the hard and soft palate, followed by the upper lip or cheek, less commonly the lower lip or tongue (as, for example, in the Brazilian series of 164 cases[49]). Tumours of the sublingual gland are relatively rare and nearly all are malignant in most of the populations described (for example, in Israel[50]).

Pleomorphic adenomas are most common, followed by mucoepidermoid and adenoid cystic carcinomas.[51] There may be ethnic and/or geographical differences, for instance in Black South Africans. Whilst benign mixed tumours comprised 48 per cent of a case series of 70 patients, polymorphous low-grade adenocarcinoma was the most frequent malignant tumour.[52] With the more overtly malignant tumour types, survival is significantly influenced by clinical stage and histological grade: 5-, 10-, and 15-year survival rates of 75 per cent, 62 per cent, and 56 per cent, respectively, were reported from a large series of malignant cases treated at the Memorial Hospital, New York, between 1966 and 1991.[53]

Insufficient evidence exists to give precise age or sex distributions, but cases are seen between the third and the seventh decades of life, and they tend to present later than do comparable lesions in the major glands, particularly if they are benign and slow growing (as, for example, in the African series reported by Arotiba[54]).

Evidence for risk factors is limited. For tumours of the major glands exposure to ionizing radiation, even decades earlier, has been implicated.[55] Long-term follow-up of the survivors of the Nagasaki and Hiroshima bombs show a dose–response effect for both benign and, especially, malignant tumours, most of the effect of which is accounted for by mucoepidermoid carcinoma.[56],[57] One study has

carcinoma. Schepman et al.[34] report its presence in 47 per cent of cases in Amsterdam (n = 100), whereas in Berlin a recent report[35] gives only 19 per cent (n = 102). The latter figure is closer to the published retrospective studies, which emphasize that the majority of oral carcinomas develop in apparently normal-looking mucosa—at least in the Western world.

Controversy continues over oral lichen planus (**OLP**).[36] Many reports describe transformation, ranging from zero to 5.6 per cent of patients, particularly in those with erosive and ulcerative forms (see the bibliography in ref. 37). But insufficient evidence is presented in many of these cases to confirm the original diagnosis, and there is

Table 6 Age–period–cohort modelling of oral cancer mortality rates in 19 countries with increasing risk (from ref. 21 with permission)

Country	Birth cohort with lowest risk	Relative risk for 1940 cohort
Federal Republic of Germany	1900	10.12
Hungary	1905	9.32
Czechoslovakia	1905	6.14
Austria	1910	4.80
Spain	1905	3.56
Poland	1910	3.41
Scotland	1915	2.82
Denmark	1910	2.61
Ireland	1915	2.11
Italy	1910	2.09
Switzerland	1910	1.97
England and Wales	1910	1.90
Northern Ireland	1910	1.88
The Netherlands	1905	1.82
Norway	1915	1.62
Canada	1900	1.61
New Zealand	1905	1.47
Portugal	1915	1.46
Australia	1905	1.44

shown smokers to have eight times the risk of developing Warthin's tumour of the parotid, compared to cases of pleomorphic adenoma,[58] but the former are not minor salivary gland tumours. Given the strong effect of local risk factors for carcinoma arising from the surface epithelium, and because of the permeability of duct epithelium and the closeness of minor salivary glands to the surface, one might suspect tobacco and alcohol to be important factors in the genesis of minor salivary gland neoplasms. Against this, however, is the low rate of malignant transformation of stomatitis nicotina of the hard palate, a condition with marked reactive changes in minor glands.

The majority of malignant melanomas are found on the skin[59] where exposure to ultraviolet light is the main aetiological agent. Fair-skinned races are more susceptible and episodes of acute sunburn, perhaps decades earlier, are especially dangerous. The incidence of *de novo* melanomas, or malignant transformation of naevi, shows a clear association with outdoor occupations and with latitude for fair-skinned races, for instance on the coast of Queensland, Australia. Melanomas do, nevertheless, develop in mucosal membranes, particularly in the eye, the vulva and vagina, the anus and rectum, the upper respiratory tract, and occasionally in the oral cavity and lip. The aetiology of oral melanoma remains obscure. It is presumably not related to exposure to ultraviolet light: indeed Barrett and colleagues have recently argued, on the basis of clinical, histological, and immunohistochemical features, that oral melanoma should be

regarded as a separate entity and not as a subtype of cutaneous melanoma.[60] A recent review indicates that the mouth may be the primary site for between 0.2 and 8.0 per cent of melanomas.[61] They are always sinister, so that any pigmented patch on mucosa of the head and neck demands full investigation, including biopsy.[62] Most present on the hard palate or maxillary gingivae during the fifth to the seventh decades,[63] with a male predominance.[64] They appear to be more common in dark-skinned races[65] and in Japanese people,[66] which raises further questions about predisposing and aetiological factors. Population incidence data are available for oral and nasal melanoma combined from nine Cancer Registries in the United States, which show an average low rate of 0.041 per 100 000 per annum, increasing over the 1973 to 1991 period.[67] Both sites were equally fatal, with a 5-year survival of only 25 per cent.

Analytical epidemiology: aetiology and risk factors

Introduction and terminology

Aetiology (from the Greek and late Latin) deals with the causes of disease. All diseases have predisposing and direct causes. Predisposition is always partly inherited; it can also result from a complex societal, cultural, and environmental amalgam. *Pathogenesis* (Greek:

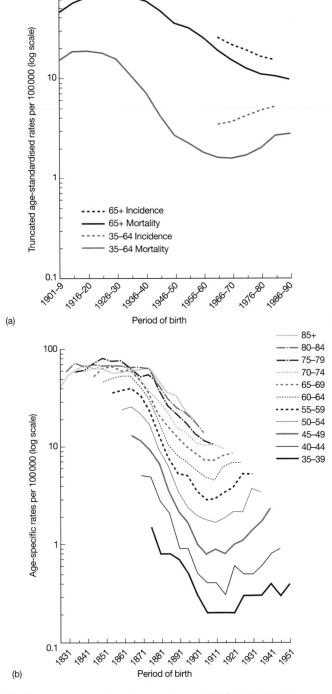

(a)

(b)

Fig. 7 Trends in age-adjusted intraoral cancer (ICD-9: 141, 143–6) incidence and mortality rates for males in England and Wales, 1901–1900. Note the downward trends this century for older individuals, but the rising trends since the mid-60s for those aged 35–64 years. A, truncated ages; B, by birth cohorts. (From ref. 24 with permission.)

pathways complex, with several routes to a critical outcome such as malignant transformation of a clone of cells, care needs to be taken to ascribe proper weight to all the factors involved.

Here we define a 'risk factor' as an agent, attribute, or behaviour that is part of the causal chain of the disease. A 'risk marker' or 'risk indicator' is associated with the disease, and may or may not be causal: it will have power to predict the presence or likely future occurrence of disease, but may not explain the mechanisms. Socioeconomic status is an example of the latter: it is associated with many diseases, certainly with head and neck cancer, but is not of itself causal—the higher prevalence of smoking, alcohol abuse, and poorer nutrition are the relevant factors. Social class is therefore described as a 'confounder' in epidemiological studies of aetiopathogenesis. In order of importance, risk is dominated by tobacco use, alcohol abuse, and nutritional insufficiencies, all which have heavy confounds with socioeconomic, cultural, religious, occupational, racial, and geographical variables. For the larynx, a recent review also includes radiation risk.[68] We begin this section with a look at genetic factors followed by a discussion of environmental factors; principally considering SCC and its precursor lesions and conditions, where the risk factors are relatively well understood. We know little about the aetiology of neoplasms of salivary glands, other soft tissues, bone, and the odontogenic apparatus.

Familial and genetic predisposition

The effect is not strong. Lip cancer is amongst the sites which show the strongest cancer clustering within families in the genealogical records of the Utah (Mormon church) database, the others being leukaemia, lobular breast cancer, early melanoma, and adenocarcinomas of the lung in females.[69] Holloway and Sofaer[70] studied surname distributions from the Scottish Cancer Registry. For cancer of the lip there was a slightly increased isonomy in patients both within and between regions. This suggests some genetic predisposition; but it also reflects the fact that families tend to have the same occupation, in this case outdoor work (such as farming, fishing, and forestry) with its attendant exposure to ultraviolet light. For tongue cancer there was some increased isonomy within but not between regions. Whilst this could result from inherited susceptibility, a more likely explanation is that environmental risk factors such as tobacco and alcohol will be common to families. For cancer of the salivary glands there was increased isonomy both within and between regions, again suggesting—but not proving—that genetic factors are involved: this is consistent with reports of the familial occurrence of malignant salivary gland tumours.[71]

Studies from Kerala, South India, revealed a familial association in 0.94 per cent of the total oral cancers accrued between January and July 1995, consistent with an autosomal inheritance pattern.[72] No constitutional chromosomal abnormalities were detected. However, there was a significant difference between the patients with oral cancer and their unaffected relatives in the sensitivity of their chromosomes to bleomycin damage: one unaffected member who showed enhanced bleomycin sensitivity later went on to develop an oral cancer.[73] Of course, a common environmental source of DNA damage is not excluded.

In The Netherlands, Copper et al.[74] took 617 first-degree relatives of 105 patients with head and neck cancer and found 31 cases amongst them of cancer of the respiratory and upper digestive tract, versus

production or development of disease) is used for the mechanisms involved. Causes and mechanisms may be described together as *aetiopathogenesis*. As all diseases are multifactorial and all mechanistic

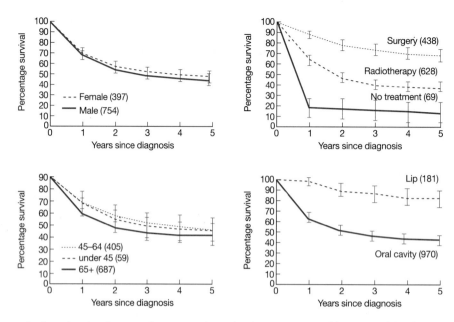

Fig. 8 Overall survival curves for lip and oral cavity cancer by age, sex, site, and major treatment modality, averaged for the years 1979–88, as reported to the Yorkshire Cancer Registry in the United Kingdom. (From ref. 25 with permission.)

Table 7 Descriptors of white, red, and related oral mucosal lesions (from ref. 29 with permission)

Clinical markers	Aetiological factors or associations	Histological features
White; Red;	Friction; Tobacco; Restorations	Epithelial atrophy; Hyperplasia;
Grey/brown; Mixed	Iron and other deficiencies	Keratinization; Dysplasia
Ulcerative	Fungi; viruses	Connective tissue:
Verruciform	Idiopathic	Fibrosis/elastosis;
Nodular		Nature and intensity of immune
Papilloma; Inverted		inflammatory infiltrate;
papilloma		Vascularity/angiogenesis

10 cases in the control group composed of first-degree relatives of the index patients' spouses ($n = 617$). This produced a relative risk (RR) of 3.5 ($p = 0.0002$) for first-degree relatives, and of 14.6 ($p = 0.0001$) for siblings. This group also found the mutagen sensitivity of lymphocytes to be increased in patients with multiple head and neck cancers. There was no relationship to smoking and drinking histories, implying a constitutional factor affecting the way genotoxic compounds are dealt with.

It is important to control for environmental factors in such studies. This was carefully done in a large case-control study of oral and pharyngeal cancer in the United States.[75] A similar proportion of cases (46 per cent, $n = 487$) and controls (41 per cent, $n = 485$) reported cancer in a parent or sibling and, although trends were apparent, most were not statistically significant. The strongest elevated risk was of oral or pharynx cancer among those whose sisters developed other cancers, but here the odds ratios were only 1.6 (95 per cent CI, 1.1–2.2). We have to conclude therefore that a genetic predisposition to these cancers is small.

Occupational and risk factors

Solar radiation

Outdoor workers, for instance farmers, fishermen, foresters, and postal delivery workers, are at risk of developing lip cancer as a result of exposure to ultraviolet light (UV) in countries at high latitudes with clean air through which UV penetrates easily, albeit for only part of the year, such as Finland[76] and from countries closer to the equator with regular long hours of sunshine, such as rural Greece where the lip can account for 60 per cent of oral cancers.[77] A study from California shows that the risk of lip cancer for women is strongly related to their lifetime solar-radiation exposure, but that lipstick and other sunscreens are protective:[78] well-differentiated SCCs arise out of longstanding solar keratoses.

The effects of early life exposure are longstanding, for instance New Zealanders have a fourfold, or more, RR of developing cutaneous melanoma and lip cancer than residents of England and Wales—migrants in both directions retain intermediate risks.[79]

Table 8 Risk of upper aerodigestive cancer from domestic fuels (from ref. 81 with permission)

	Odds ratio	p Value	95% CI
Larynx (164 cases: 656 controls)			
Heating with fossil fuel > 40 years	2.0	0.02	1.10–3.46
Cooking with fossil fuel > 40 years	1.4	0.3	0.76–2.41
Pharynx (105 cases: 420 controls)			
Heating with fossil fuel > 40 years	3.3	0.0005	1.43–7.55
Cooking with fossil fuel > 40 years	2.5	0.05	1.03–6.30
Oral cavity (100 cases: 400 controls)			
Heating with fossil fuel > 40 years	2.4	0.008	1.26–4.40
Cooking with fossil fuel > 40 years	1.6	0.1	0.90–2.97

Atmospheric pollution

Part of the urban and rural difference in the incidence of head and neck cancer relates to atmospheric pollution. In parts of England, mean sulphur dioxide and smoke concentrations in the atmosphere are positively correlated with SCC of the larynx and, to a lesser extent, the pharynx.[80] There is growing concern about air pollution in cities and the impact on public health, especially of oxides of sulphur and nitrogen, carbon monoxide and dioxide, and hydrocarbon particulates (e.g. **PM 10s**; particulate material of less than 10 μm in diameter, mostly from diesel exhausts). The dramatic rise in incidence and severity of asthma around the world is related to poor air quality. Malignancies of the lower respiratory tract may also increase.

In German studies, the increased risks for air pollution in the workplace, traffic jams on the way to work, high traffic emissions in residential areas, and outdoor air pollution in residential areas were present for all head and neck cancer sites, but they were not statistically significant. However, household heating and cooking with fossil fuels produced statistically significant increased risks (Table 8). After adjusting for tobacco and alcohol consumption, RRs of between 1.4 and 3.3 were obtained. Socioeconomic differences were excluded as confounders. Polycyclic aromatic hydrocarbons, cadmium, and tetrachlorethylenes bound to respirable particles were found to be important factors. Hard coal products are most dangerous. In a suburb of Rome with a large waste-disposal site, a waste incinerator plant, and an oil refinery, mortality from laryngeal cancer declines with distance from the sources of pollution, after correcting for socioeconomic conditions.[82] Chronic exposure to paint, varnish, and lacquer is a definite risk factor for cancers of the larynx ($RR = 2.3$) and oral cavity ($RR = 3.6$): these are significant values after correction for alcohol and tobacco use.[83]

The importance of fossil-fuel combustion at work is confirmed in a large study in four areas in the United States (1114 cases, 1268 controls), with ORs of approximately 2.0 for pharyngeal sites. Male carpet installers emerged as being at risk, with an OR of 7.7 (95 per cent CI, 2.4–24.9; 23 cases, 4 controls).[84] Asbestos, pesticide exposures, and mists from strong inorganic acids (OR 1.8 95 per cent CI 1.1–2.9 for the latter) were shown for laryngeal cancer in Uruguay.[85] The risk of laryngeal cancer from acid mists in the steel industry is confirmed in a United States study of 1031 exposed men.[86]

Immunosuppression

Individuals with HIV/AIDS are at increased risk for a limited number of neoplasms, especially Kaposi's sarcoma, which commonly presents in the mouth,[87] and lymphoma, which occasionally presents as an oral mucosal or intraboney lesion in the jaws.[88] SCCs of the upper aerodigestive tract are not, however, more common in these patients, and the characteristic oral hairy leucoplakia of HIV disease does not undergo malignant transformation. Nevertheless, HIV-positive patients with one of these cancers have a poorer prognosis, after adjusting for the effects of age, stage, and tumour site.[89]

Immunosuppressed, organ-transplanted patients are at an increased risk of developing lip cancer. However, this is principally due to the effects of ultraviolet light, although the effects of smoking, if present, continue to play their role.[90]

Tobacco use

Globally, tobacco is the major cause of cancer. Alcohol synergizes with tobacco as a risk factor for upper aerodigestive tract SCC: this is supermultiplicative for the mouth, additive for the larynx, and between additive and multiplicative for the oesophagus.[91] Sorting the independent effects is difficult because habits overlap. Many believe that the rising incidence of oral cancer in Europe is largely due to rising alcohol consumption (see below). In many developing countries, particularly in Moslem communities, accurate data on alcohol consumption are impossible to obtain because of religious and cultural inhibitions. Taken together, the effects of tobacco use, heavy alcohol consumption, and poor diet probably explain over 90 per cent of the cases of head and neck cancer. The preventive approach is therefore clear.

According to Doll et al.,[92] using data from the long-term study of male British doctors, about half of all regular smokers will be killed by their habit (Table 9). Among men in industrialized countries, smoking is estimated to be the cause of 40 to 45 per cent of all cancer deaths, 90 to 95 per cent of lung cancer deaths, over 85 per cent of oral cancer deaths, 75 per cent of chronic obstructive lung-disease deaths, and 35 per cent of cardiovascular-disease deaths in those aged between 35 and 69 years. Thus, whilst upper aerodigestive tract cancers figure prominently, lung cancer and other pulmonary and

Table 9 The major causes of smoking-related deaths

Cancers: of the lung, bladder, pancreas, mouth, oesophagus, pharynx, and larynx
Chronic obstructive pulmonary and other respiratory diseases
Vascular diseases, including coronary artery and peripheral arterial diseases
Peptic ulceration

cardiovascular diseases should be the starting point for anti-tobacco counselling.

Types of tobacco use: a global perspective

Smoking of tobacco as factory-made cigarettes, cigars, and cheroots, and loose tobacco in pipes or hand-made cigarettes is familiar to all. There is great variation in tar, nicotine, and nitrosamine content depending on species, curing additives, and method of combustion. Such smoking habits are the predominant form of tobacco use in the West, and in growing millions of people in developing countries. With government regulation of tobacco advertising, restrictions on smoking in public transport and public places, and the awarding of damages to individuals and health authorities, manufacturers are increasingly targeting developing countries for tobacco sales, especially of their higher tar varieties.

Smokeless tobacco

Much of the tobacco in the world is consumed without combustion, by placing it in contact with mucous membranes through which nicotine is absorbed to provide the pharmacological lift. Use of nasal stuff, popular in the last century, is returning. Other forms of snuff, loose or packeted, placed in the oral vestibule, are common in Scandinavia and the United States. Tobacco is also prepared in blocks or flakes for chewing. In developing countries, tobacco is mostly consumed mixed with other ingredients (Table 10). The very extensive

evidence for the carcinogenicity of these mixtures is covered exhaustively by Daftary et al.[93] and Gupta et al.[94]

Toombak, the form used in Sudan, contains very high levels of tobacco-specific nitrosamines (**TSNs**). A study of 375 patients with SCC of the lip, buccal cavity, and floor of the mouth and 271 patients with similar cancers of the tongue, palate, and maxillary sinus, compared with 204 non-squamous oral and non-oral malignant neoplasms, and with 2820 disease-free individuals showed overall adjusted ORs associated with toombak dipping of 7.3 and 3.9, respectively, for the first oral cancer group, compared to hospital and population controls. These effects rise to 11.0 and 4.3, respectively, in long-term users. No significant ORs were found for the second cancer group where the agent is not in direct contact with the cancer site.[95] Distinctive forms of leucoplakia are common in habitués but, interestingly, these show a low prevalence of epithelial dysplasia, hence longitudinal studies are necessary to establish the rate of malignant transformation.[96]

Betel quids

The recommended terminology is that of Zain et al.[97] Quids are prepared form areca nuts, which are cured or sun-dried, and then chopped. These are usually placed on a leaf of the *Piper betel* vine, although the inflorescence is used by some, for example in Papua New Guinea. Slaked lime is an essential ingredient. It lowers the pH and accelerates the release of alkaloids from both tobacco and the nut, and gives an enhanced pharmacological 'lift'. The lime is prepared by baking limestone where available: near coasts from seashells or snail shells (such as Kerala and Sri Lanka) or from coral (as in the Pacific Islands). Customs vary widely. In Papua New Guinea, the areca nut is chewed directly, the lime being smeared on the oral mucosa itself: tobacco is rarely added, though cigars of rough local tobacco are commonly smoked[98] and cigarette consumption is growing. The spread of oral cancer from the coasts to the highlands in Papua New Guinea has followed the trade in coast-grown areca nuts.

Chewing of areca is deeply embedded in the social and cultural history of India, Sri Lanka, Pakistan, Bangladesh, Myanmar, Thailand, Cambodia, Malaysia, Singapore, Indonesia, The Philippines, New

Table 10 Some common forms of oral smokeless tobacco

Habit	Ingredients	Population
Pan/paan/betel quid	Areca nut, betel leaf/inflorescence, slaked lime, catechu, condiments, with or without tobacco	Indian subcontinent, Southeast Asia, Papua New Guinea, part of South America
Khaini	Tobacco and lime	Bihar (India)
Mishri	Burned tobacco	Maharashtra (India)
Zarda	Boiled tobacco	India and Arab countries
Gadakhu	Tobacco and molasses	Central India
Mawa	Tobacco, lime, and areca	Bhavnagar (India)
Nass	Tobacco, ash, cotton or sesame oil	Central Asia, Iran, Afghanistan, Pakistan
Naswar/niswar	Tobacco, lime, indigo, cardamom, oil, menthol, etc.	Central Asia, Iran, Afghanistan, Pakistan
Shammah	Tobacco, ash, and lime	Saudi Arabia
Toombak	Tobacco and sodium bicarbonate	Sudan

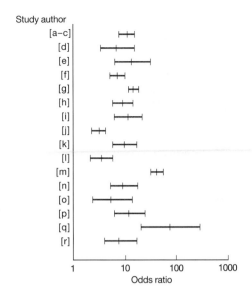

Fig. 9 Summary of crude odds ratios and 95% CIs for the development of oral cancer in populations chewing betel quid in any form, irrespective of smoking habits. (From ref. 102 with permission; a–r, refs 103–120, respectively.)

Guinea, Taiwan, and China, and in emigrant communities therefore. Its use appears in ancient Sanskrit literature. Areca nuts contain potent cholinergic muscurinic alkaloids, notably arecoline and guavacoline, with parasympatheticomimetic effects. They promote salivation and the passage of wind through the gut, they raise the blood pressure and pulse rate, and elicit euphoria due to γ-aminobutyric acid (**GABA**) receptor inhibitory activity—properties which contribute to habituation and dependence. There are also bronchoconstrictor effects, and evidence for the exacerbation of asthma and diabetes.[99] The historical, social, and general health aspects of betel quid use are well discussed by Bedi and Jones.[100] Daftary et al.[101] set out the evidence for the carcinogenicity of betel quid in considerable detail, and an excellent meta-analysis is summarized in Fig. 9. Table 11 shows the importance of adding tobacco, and Table 12 the efficacy of habit intervention.

Areca nut alone as an oral carcinogen

Although the IARC[122] concluded that: 'there was insufficient evidence that the chewing of betel quid without tobacco was carcinogenic to man', this is a probability. Areca nut is certainly the main aetiological agent in oral submucous fibrosis,[123] but in this case-control study 12 of the 14 concurrent patients with oral cancer and submucous fibrosis also used tobacco.

In Guam, where areca nut is chewed alone or with leaf only, there is apparently no increase in oral cancer.[124] Conversely in Taiwan, most heavy chewers of betel quids do not include tobacco, yet oral cancer is clearly associated.[125] Importantly, the synergistic role of alcohol has not been evaluated in these studies.[126] Increased micronucleated epithelial cells, as an intermediate marker of oral cancer risk, has been reported in users of areca nut without tobacco in The Philippines,[127] and in India.[128] Strong evidence that the chewing of areca alone produces oral cancer comes from South Africa: amongst the Indian immigrant community of the Eastern Cape, 39/57 with

cheek cancer and 21/25 with tongue cancer were nut chewers who did not use tobacco.[13] Finally, a small but well-designed case (n = 40): control (n = 160) study in Taiwan clearly showed a strong carcinogenic effect of the local quids, with an OR of 58.4 after adjusting for cigarette and alcohol use.[129] Importantly, this study also showed a strong dose–response relationship: adjusted ORs rose to 276 when more than 20 quids were consumed per day, and to 398 with more than 40 years of chewing. Nevertheless, 18/40 people drank alcohol and the majority, 32/40, also smoked, so that multiple risk factors are clearly operating in this community.[129]

In evaluating the dangers of these complex mixtures it is important to remember that betel leaf is protective:[130] at least two compounds have been identified—β-carotene and hyroxychavicol, an astringent antiseptic.

Oral snuff in Scandinavia and North America

Brown et al.[131] described 'snuff dippers' cancer' in the SE United States due to the habit of placing snuff in the labial sulcus. This was the basis for the classical description of verrucous carcinoma by Ackermann[132] and that was later confirmed by McCoy and Waldron.[133] Females in the textile industry here have a high prevalence of snuff dipping and elevated death rates from oral cancer.[134]

There is concern about the use of factory-produced, portion-packed snuff and the oral cancers it might cause, particularly amongst adolescents in the United States.[135] Chewing tobacco and packaged snuff habits are practised by some prominent sportsmen, many of whom are role models for the young.[136] The United States Department of Health and Human Services[137] concluded that such use constituted a significant risk to health from oral cancer and other oral lesions, and that it could lead to nicotine addiction and dependence. The United States Congress banned the advertising of smokeless tobacco on radio and television in 1986 and required health warnings on packages and printed advertisements. The European Union banned the sale of portion and loose snuff in all its member states in 1992: when Sweden joined the EU in 1995 it was exempted from the ban on sales, but exports were banned.[138] The IARC[122] stated that: 'there was sufficient evidence that snuff causes cancer' and the Swedish Government requires warning labels on such products.

This habit is addictive and can produce hyperkeratotic lesions in the area of habitual contact.[139] In the United States, 2.9 per cent of males and 0.1 per cent of females from a survey of 17 027 schoolchildren aged between 12 and 17 years had lesions associated, in a dose-dependent fashion, with snuff (particularly) and chewing tobacco.[140] However, there is limited evidence that malignancies follow, though there may be a long latent period. Current evidence that this is a high-risk activity is equivocal. An ecological study, based on combined data from the 1986 United States National Mortality Followback Survey[141] (n = 16 598) and the coincident National Health Interview Survey of 1987,[142] concluded that the use of smokeless tobacco, either as snuff or chewing tobacco, does not increase the risk of oral or other digestive cancers, but the number of reliable observations was small. Most importantly, alcohol emerged as a major risk factor for oral cancer with a strong dose–response relationship, as it did to a lesser extent with other digestive cancers. Smoking was associated with a risk of oral but not other digestive cancers (Table 13). This view of the lower cancer risk of smokeless tobacco in the United States has led to a movement to advocate the

Table 11 Relative risks (RR) of oral cancer from betel quid with or without tobacco

Reference	Cases/controls	Betel quid with tobacco	Betel quid without tobacco	No chewing habit
116	Oral cancer	219	33	25
	Controls	35	144	99
	RR	24.8*	0.9	1
112	Oral cancer	138	46	135
	Controls	61	70	256
	RR	4.34*	1.24	1
110	Oral cancer	190	35	9
	Controls	215	16	102
	RR	9.1*	1.2	1
109	Oral cancer	339	40	88
	Controls	474	216	1690
	RR	13.7*	3.6*	1

*$p < 0.01$

Table 12 Effect of cessation of tobacco use on the incidence of oral mucosal lesions in a 10-year, follow-up study of 12 212 users (from ref. 121 with permission)

Stopped	Incident cases	Incidence/ 100 000*	Incident cases	All others Incidence/ 100 000*	Incidence ratio
Leukoplakia					
Men	7	92	183	219	0.42
Women	5	63	54	201	0.31
Lichen planus					
Men	7	107	111	143	0.75
Women	19	396	93	294	1.35

*Age-adjusted

practice as a less-dangerous alternative to smoking, and an aid to nicotine withdrawal in those addicted to smoking.[144]

Chewing tobaccos are distinctly different from snuff. Snuff as manufactured and used in Europe and North America is very different from the snuff-like products used in the Middle East, which are made locally in a variety of small-scale industries by individual vendors or directly by the users. Products such as Toombak, in the Sudan and the Shammah of Arabia have exceptionally high TSN contents. There is, however, a paradox in that the characteristic hyperkeratotic lesions of Toombak users show a low prevalence of epithelial dysplasia,[96] as do those described in the United States and Scandinavia: in the case of the Sudan this might be because those users most susceptible to cancer have already succumbed.

In Scandinavia it is clear that local snuff is not a major risk factor: two recent case-control studies of oral cancer cases in Sweden have failed to show an association[145] (Table 14).

Might snuff be used to help smokers quit? This approach has been condemned on the grounds that it can lead to nicotine addiction, that it ignores the potential role of snuff in other cancers and in cardiovascular diseases, and that other ethically accepted forms of

nicotine-replacement therapy (such as chewing gums, skin patches, inhalators, and nasal sprays) are widely available. Note, therefore, two recent Swedish studies: 585 cases of myocardial infarction with 10 per cent snuff users and 589 controls with 15 per cent snuff users showed a relative risk of myocardial infarction of 0.89 (95 per cent CI, 0.62–1.29) in snuff users, compared to 1.87 (95 per cent CI, 1.40–2.48) in smokers.[147] Another study from health screenings of 135 036 construction workers identified 6297 snuff users. The relative risk for death due to cardiovascular disease was 1.4 (1.2–1.6) for this group, compared to 1.9 (1.7–2.2) for smokers.[148] No increased risk amongst snuff users who had never smoked was found among men with Crohn's disease and ulcerative colitis, in a case-control study.[149] The possibility of an increased risk of cancer at other sites has not yet been fully addressed. Nevertheless, on present evidence, snuff habits as they exist in Scandinavia and, probably in the United States, carry low risks of serious health hazards, including oral cancer. As Axell points out,[150],[151] however, this does not mean that oral snuff should be encouraged: it almost always produces mucosal lesions, often affects salivary flow, causes gingival recessions, and creates nicotine dependence and addiction.

Table 13 Relative risks and confidence intervals for oral cancer (ICD-9: 140–149) (multiplicative model; from ref. 143 with permission)

Sex		
Male	1.00	
Female	0.52	0.27–1.00
Race		
White	1.00	
Non-white	2.63	1.31–5.27
Age (years)		
25–44	1.00	
45–64	47.22	6.07–367.19
65–84	84.88	10.7–666.38
85+	206.03	20.0–2122.83
Lifetime smoking (packs)		
0–19	1.00	
20–11 999	1.07	0.48–2.38
12 000+	2.85	1.14–5.77
Annual drinking		
0.52 (less than 1/week)	1.00	
53–365 (less than 1/day)	2.75	1.26–5.99
366+	7.20	3.74–13.88
Occupation		
Professional/managerial/clerical	1.00	
Blue collar/service/technical	1.06	0.62–1.83
Smokeless tobacco		
0–99 (non-user)	1.00	
100–9999 times	0.92	0.25–3.42
10 000+	1.21	0.32–4.63

Table 14 Oral cancer in Swedish snuff users

Ref. and user	No. of pairs	RR	95% CI
Schildt *et al.*, 1998[145]			
Current users	410	0.6	0.3–1.1
Previous users		1.4	0.7–2.8
Lewin *et al.*, 1998[146]			
Current users	128	1.0	0.7–1.6
Previous users		1.2	0.6–1.9

RR, relative risk; CI, confidence interval.

Smoking and head and neck cancer

The most comprehensive source of evidence for the carcinogenicity of tobacco smoke remains the IARC publication of 1986. This is summarized by the United States Surgeon General's Report of 1989 (Table 15), which stated that: 'upper aerodigestive sites have the highest ARs [attributable risks] in males, of all the many sites influenced by smoking'.[153]

Pipe smoking has long been associated with lip cancer, where the nature of the stem and its permeability and, maybe, heat are cofactors. Some literature suggests that pipe and cigars are less risky for the development of oral cancer than cigarettes,[154] but the study from North Italy[91] shows higher risks associated with these practices for cancer of the mouth and oesophagus than cigarettes.

A major difficulty in accurately quantifying smoking risks for aerodigestive tract cancer is its strong synergism with alcohol (Table 16). A large case-control study from the United States provides good evidence of a dose–response relationship for both tobacco and alcohol (Table 17; Fig. 10).

The relationship between the anatomical site of oral cancer and smoking is less clear-cut than with smokeless tobacco. Pooling of carcinogens in saliva gives cancers in the 'gutter' area—the floor of the mouth and the ventral and lateral aspects of the tongue. Mashberg and Meyers[158] reported, in a United States population, that 201/207 asymptomatic, primarily erythroplastic carcinomas were found in three locations: floor of mouth (101), ventral or lateral tongue (36), and soft palate (64). In the Amsterdam series,[155] the floor of mouth and retromolar area were significantly more related to tobacco use than cancers of the tongue and cheek. However, in another series (comprising 359 United States male veterans), smoking was more strongly associated with soft palate cancers than anterior sites, and alcohol was associated with floor-of-mouth lesions.[159] This is interesting because the long-recognized lesions of stomatitis nicotina (synonym: Smokers' palate) have a low malignant potential (except in reverse smokers). These lesions predominantly affect the hard palate, producing hyperkeratosis without significant epithelial dysplasia, with plugging of the orifices of minor salivary glands and associated inflammation. Stomatitis nicotina, in the West, is most commonly associated with pipe smoking and both the hard and soft palate are relatively uncommon sites of squamous cell carcinoma.

A high frequency of dysplastic, potentially malignant, lesions and of SCC is found among reverse (ie with the lighted end inside the mouth) chutta smokers in India along the coasts of Visakhapatnam and Srikakulam[160] and in rural Andrha Pradesh.[161] In the state of Goa, The Caribbean, South America, and The Philippines, however, palatal cancer is not commonly reported in reverse smokers.[162]

The mechanisms of tobacco carcinogenesis

Over 300 carcinogens have been identified in tobacco smoke or in its water-soluble components which will leach into saliva.[152] The major, and most studied of these (Table 18) are the aromatic hydrocarbon benzpyrene (benzo[*a*]pyrene) and the tobacco-specific nitrosamines (**TSNs**): *N*′-nitrosonornicotine (**NNN**), *N*′-nitrosopyrrolidine (**NPYR**), *N*′-nitrosodimethylamine (**NDMA**), and 4-(methylnitrosamino)-1-(3-pyridyl)-1-butanone (**NNK**).

We have known since the 1920s that polycyclic aromatic hydrocarbons were the carcinogens present in tars, thus the interest in 'low tar' smoking materials. Benzpyrene is a powerful carcinogen, there being 20 to 40 nanograms per cigarette.[164] The role of *N*-nitrosamines is reviewed by Hoffman and Hecht.[165] Mainstream cigarette smoke can contain 310 ng of NNN and 150 ng of NNK. These are generated primarily during pyrolysis, but also endogenously from some smokeless tobacco. They act locally, on keratinocyte stem cells, and are absorbed and act in many other tissues in the body. They produce DNA adducts, principally O^6-methylguanine, which interfere with DNA replication. There is damage to all replicating cells, including those of the immune system.

Metabolism of these carcinogens usually involves oxygenation by p450 enzymes in cytochromes, and then conjugation, which involves the enzyme glutathione-*S*-transferase (**GST**). Polymorphisms of the

Table 15 Cancer deaths due to smoking in the United States, 1985

Site	Attributable deaths (%)		Numbers of deaths per annum
	Men	**Women**	
Lung	90	79	106 000
Lip, oral cavity, pharynx	92	61	7000
Oesophagus	78	75	7000
Bladder	47	37	4000
Kidney	48	12	3000
Larynx	81	87	3000

Table 16 Alcohol and tobacco habits of 690 consecutive cases of oral cancer in Amsterdam, 1971–1991 (from ref. 155 with permission)

Tobacco and alcohol	56%
Tobacco only	14%
Alcohol only	5%
Neither	25%

p450 and GST genes are currently under active study in the search for genetic markers of a susceptibility to head and neck cancer, and indeed to tobacco-related cancers at many other body sites;[166] not all results are consistent, however.

Marijuana use and head and neck cancer

Recreational use of extracts of the plant *Cannabis satava*, is widespread. It may be smoked in three ways: (1) as marijuana, derived from macerated flowers mixed with tobacco (under which circumstances the concentration of the active intoxicant, Δ^9-tetrahydrocannabinol (**THC**), is of the order of 1–6 per cent, mass/volume (**m/v**)); (2) as hashish (that is, dried resin), placed in a pipe (THC 6–10 per cent m/v); or (3) as hash oil (THC 30–60 per cent), from flowers of the female plant. When burned, the cannabinoids are absorbed and many potential carcinogens are released, including polycyclic aromatic hydrocarbons, benzopyrene, phenols, phytosterols, acids, and terpenes, including nitrosamines at similar levels to those found in tobacco smoke.[167] There are, of course, the products of the tobacco itself.

Reports of aerodigestive tract cancer in marijuana users have been reviewed.[168] Recreational users of marijuana often also enjoy alcohol

Table 17 Odds ratios for oral and pharyngeal cancer in US males, adjusted for race, age, study location, and respondent status (95% CI) (from ref. 156 with permission)

Smoking rate	Number of alcoholic drinks per week					
	< 1	**1–4**	**5–14**	**15–29**	**30+**	**Total**
Non-smoker	1.0	1.3	1.6	1.4	5.8	1.0
Short duration/former smoker	0.7	2.2	1.4	3.2	6.4	1.1 (0.7–1.7)
1–19/day for 20+ years	1.7	1.5	2.7	5.4	7.9	1.6 (0.9–2.7)
20–39/day for 20+ years	1.9	2.4	4.4	7.2	23.8	2.8 (1.8–4.3)
40+/day for 20+ years	7.4	0.7	4.4	20.2	37.7	4.4 (2.7–7.2)
Pipe and cigar only	0.6	1.0	3.7	4.7	23.0	1.9 (1.1–3.4)
Total	1.0 (0.7–2.0)	1.2 (1.0–2.7)	1.7 (2.0–5.4)	3.3 (5.4–14.1)	8.8	

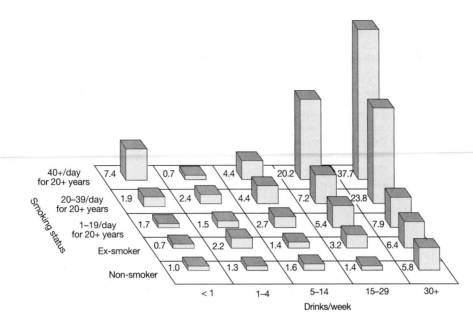

Fig. 10 Relative risks of oral and pharyngeal cancer in the United States in relation to alcohol and tobacco consumption. (Redrawn from ref. 157 with permission.)

and tobacco, and tobacco usually forms part of the marijuana smoking mix. It is thus impossible at present to discern an independent risk for the smoking of cannabis products themselves though, because of their composition, a theoretical risk certainly exists.

Little evidence exists on the risk of marijuana smoking for the development of potentially malignant oral lesions though, as with more conventional tobacco smokers, leucoedema, nicotinic stomatitis, denture-related stomatitis, angular cheilitis, and median rhomboid glossitis are more common.[169]

Alcohol and head and neck cancer

Pure ethanol has never been shown to be carcinogenic *in vitro* or in animal studies.[170] It is presumed to act in concert with other, more direct, carcinogens in the beverage—so-called congeners—and with other environmental carcinogens, especially from tobacco. Nevertheless, an increased risk of upper aerodigestive tract cancer associated with alcohol drinking in non-smokers has been demonstrated.[171]

The interaction of alcohol with smokeless tobacco is not easily quantified because where betal quid, with or without tobacco, and other traditional forms of smokeless tobacco are commonly used, there are often religious or social inhibitions: indeed drinking alcohol is banned by law in some of these societies. Where it is used, it is likely to be produced illicitly and may contain impurities that add to the risk.

The increase in oral cancer in the western world has been related to rising alcohol use. In England and Wales alcohol consumption per capita fell from the turn of the century to the 1930s but has more than doubled since. Using mortality from liver cirrhosis as a surrogate measure of damage to health from alcohol, Hindle[172] has plotted trends over this century and shown how they closely match the trends in oral cancer mortality (Fig. 11(a)). Taking deaths from lung cancer as a measure of tobacco damage, it is striking how the trends for oral cancer move, both down and up this century, in opposite directions

(Fig. 11(b)): strong circumstantial evidence that alcohol rather than tobacco is the major factor in the observed trends in oral cancer mortality and, by inference, incidence.

All forms of alcoholic drinks are dangerous if heavily consumed, the most dangerous reflecting the predominant habit in the population under study. Thus there is evidence for the role of beer,[156],[173] wine,[91],[174] and spirits,[175] which some[176] have taken to implicate ethanol itself. A recent report from Uruguay comparing 471 cases of oral and pharyngeal cancer with 471 controls, showed slightly higher odds ratios for 'pure hard liquor' drinking (3.6; 95 per cent CI, 2.1–6.2) than for 'pure wine' drinking (2.1; 1.3–3.3).[177]

Good evidence for the very significant role of alcohol again comes from Northern Italy (Table 19). It is notable that the 95 per cent CIs for ORs for all beverages cross unity until the total consumption is really quite high—above 55 drinks per week. This is consistent with data from Paris (Table 20). When the tobacco effect is adjusted for, heavy alcohol consumption itself produces considerable risks, with ORs or RRs of 17, 23, 33, and 70 appearing for oral cancer in the different studies. For these high rates of alcohol use/abuse, the risks are greater than for tobacco, adjusted for alcohol. Self-reported alcohol consumption tends to be underestimated, implying that alcohol may be even more important. Table 21 shows the tobacco/alcohol synergism to be supermultiplicative for the oral cavity and pharynx, between additive and multiplicative for the oesophagus, and close to additive for the larynx. Simplistically, this relates to both agents being present in the mouth, alcohol being present in the oesophagus with smaller amounts of tobacco products, and tobacco products contacting the larynx with few constituents of the beverage.

Alcohol contributes to head and neck cancer in several ways:

- Ethanol increases the permeability of oral mucosa to water[180] and to many water-soluble molecules including important carcinogens: increased passage of NNN has been demonstrated *in vitro*.[181] The effect is greater at 15 per cent of ethanol than at 5 per cent, but is

Table 18 A list of confirmed carcinogens in tobacco smoke (see ref. 163)

Class	Compound
Aromatic hydrocarbons Monocyclic	Benzene Benz[a]anthracene
Dicyclic and polycyclic	Benzo[b]fluoranthene Benzo[j]fluoranthene Benzo[k]fluoranthene Benzo[a]pyrene Dibenz[a,h]anthracene Dibenzo[a,e]pyrene Dibenzo[a,h]pyrene Dibenzo[a,i]pyrene Dibenzo[a,l]pyrene Ideno[1,2,3-c,d]pyrene 5-Methylchrysene
Aldehydes	Acetaldehyde Formaldehyde
Nitrogen compounds N-nitroso compounds	(4-Methylnitrosamino)-1-(3-pyridyl)-1-butanone (NNK) N'-Nitrosodimethylamine (NDMA) N-Nitrodiethylamine N-Nitroso-N-methylethylamine (NEMA) N-Nitrosonornicotine (NNN) N-Nitrosopyrrolidine (NPYR) N-Nitrosopiperidine N-Nitroso-n-butylamine N-Nitrosodi-n-propylamine
Polycyclic aza-arenes	Dibenz[a,h]acridine Dibenz[a,j]acridine
Miscellaneous nitrogen compounds	4-Aminobiphenyl ortho-anisidine 1, 1-Dimethylhydrazine 2-Naphthylamine 2-Nitropropane Urethane

not further enhanced at 40 per cent, suggesting the mechanism is related to rearrangement of the epithelial permeability barrier rather than to lipid extraction.[182] It implies a solvent action on keratinocyte membranes, with enhanced penetration of carcinogens into proliferating cells where they may exert a direct mutagenic action.[183] Rats fed ethanol by stomach tube showed a decreased synthesis of lipids contributing to the intercellular permeability barrier, perhaps because of liver damage.[184]

- The immediate metabolite of ethanol, acetaldehyde, may be formed locally and damage cells.[185] Indeed, considerable amounts can be found in saliva after moderate alcohol consumption, due to the action of bacterial alcohol dehydrogenases. Production is significantly reduced after 3-days' use of an antiseptic mouthwash, which is consistent with poor oral hygiene being an independent risk factor for oral cancer in some studies.[186]

- Alcoholic liver disease is common in heavy drinkers and this reduces the detoxification of active carcinogens.[171]

- Alcohol is high in calories, which suppresses appetite. Those with a serious drinking problem become socially fractured, and many choose to spend their available cash on drink rather than on food.

All this contributes to an inadequate diet. Metabolism is further damaged by liver disease. As a result nutritional deficiencies are common.[187]

Mouthwash use and risk of oral cancer

Drawing 866 cases from Californian, Atlanta, and New Jersey registries, and matching with 1249 controls, Winn et al.[188] found increased risks associated with regular use of a mouthwash, of 40 per cent for men and 60 per cent for women, after adjusting for alcohol drinking and tobacco use. Risks generally increased in proportion to frequency and duration of mouthwash use, and were only apparent when the alcohol content of the mouthwash exceeded 25 per cent: the effects were stronger in women revealing a maximum OR of 2.4 (1.5–3.9) in females who began regular use before the age of 20. In most published studies, rarely do ORs exceed 2 with, in most cases 95 per cent CIs spanning unity. Several published reviews (see, for example, refs 189 and 190) have helped the British, Canadian, and American Dental Associations to endorse products of this type for controlling dental plaque and gingivitis. It seems prudent, however, to keep the

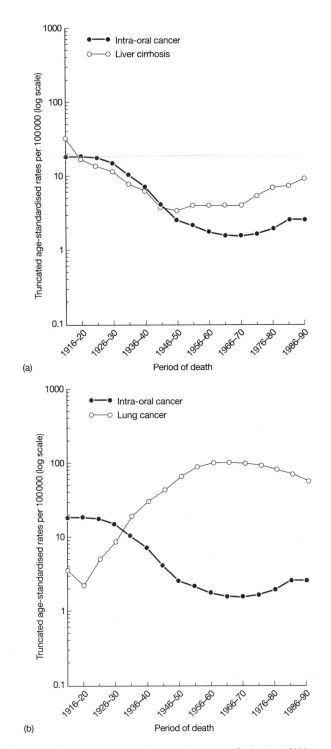

Fig. 11 (a) Trends in mortality of intraoral cancer in England and Wales, compared to trends in mortality from liver cirrhosis, 1911–1990 for males aged 35–64. (b) Trends in mortality of intraoral cancer in England and Wales, compared to lung cancer mortality, 1911–1990 for males aged 35–64. (Figures from ref. 172 with permission.)

alcohol content as low as possible (alcohol is necessary to dissolve some of the antimicrobial agents) and to state the full composition on the label.

The levels of alcohol in proprietary mouthwashes are unlikely to influence legal proceedings based on exhaled air analyses.[191]

Head and neck cancer in non-users of tobacco and/or alcohol

A minority of patients develop a cancer in the apparent absence of one or both of these risk factors. Clearly other factors are operating in people who have cancer without the decades of exposure associated with high-risk individuals. Lifelong abstainers from both alcohol and tobacco are uncommon and little is known about their wider lifestyle. Do they have unusual dietary practices? We may suspect hereditary and other environment factors, such as infection. Rich and Radden[192] found that Australian patients with oral cancer who had never used tobacco or alcohol developed their carcinomas particularly on the buccal mucosa and upper alveolar ridge, and the Amsterdam data[155] are consistent with this. Hodge *et al.*,[193] in a Kentucky population, described 33 of 945 cases (3.4 per cent) of head and neck cancers in non-users of tobacco. A definite majority of women, especially older women, were non-users of both tobacco and alcohol and had comparatively few cancers of the floor of the mouth. Other findings with oral cancer in non-user American cohorts are:[194]

- a low incidence of second primaries;
- a higher level of differentiation of the primary lesions;
- a lower frequency of associated oral candidiasis;
- importantly; **no better overall survival.**

A retrospective study of 59 tobacco non-users with SCCs of the head and neck also contained significantly more women,[195] had significantly more tongue cancers, and a relatively high rate of second primaries in the head and neck. Most importantly, this group had a high exposure to ETS (passive smoking). In a Spanish study, patients without a history of tobacco and alcohol use who developed laryngeal cancer were on average 10 years older, showed no male predominance, and had lesions mainly on the glottis, which permitted earlier diagnosis and a better survival rate.[196]

None of these studies on the rare cases which occur in non-users of tobacco and/or alcohol dilute the evidence that these are far and away the major risk factors. Viral infections and nutritional inadequacies, which are addressed next, are the main hypothetical factors in this group of patients.

Viruses and head and neck cancer

Viral oncogenesis

About 15 per cent of all human cancers may have an aetiological relationship to viruses (Table 22). This is, however, difficult to establish because there may be a latent period of one or more decades between the time of initial infection and the appearance of the malignancy:[197] the fingerprint of the virus may have left the affected cells (the so-called 'hit and run' mechanism) or be difficult to detect because distinctive parts of the viral genome rarely become integrated into human tissues. Table 23 lists those proliferative mucosal lesions of the head and neck putatively caused by viruses.

Table 19 Odds ratios for oral and pharyngeal cancer in males, according to alcohol habits: Northern Italy, 1984–1989 *(95% CI) (from ref. 178 with permission)

	Oral cavity (n = 157)		**Pharynx (n = 134)**	
Wine (drinks/week)				
≤ 20	1		1	
21–34	1.1	(0.5–2.3)	0.7	(0.3–1.6)
35–55	1.9	(0.9–3.7)	1.9	(0.9–3.7)
56–83	4.9	(2.6–9.5)	3.1	(1.6–6.1)
84 +	8.5	(3.6–20.2)	10.9	(4.7–25.3)
Beer (drinks/week)				
0	1		1	
1–13	1.0	(0.6–1.8)	0.5	(0.3–1.0)
14 +	0.8	(0.5–1.4)	0.9	(0.5–1.5)
Spirits (drinks/week)				
0	1		1	
1–6	0.7	(0.4–1.3)	0.4	(0.2–0.9)
7 +	0.9	(0.6–1.3)	1.2	(0.8–1.8)
Total (drinks/week)				
≤19	1		1	
20–34	1.1	(0.5–2.5)	0.9	(0.4–2.0)
35–59	3.2	(1.6–6.2)	1.5	(0.8–3.1)
60 +	3.4	(1.7–7.1)	3.6	(1.8–7.2)

Adjusted for age, area of residence, education, occupation, and smoking.

The human papillomaviruses (HPV)

Papillomaviruses are species- and tissue-specific. The HPVs, of which over 75 types have so far been described with some 26 potential new types awaiting classification, are all epitheliotropic, specifically for squamous epithelia. Over half are related to skin, the remainder with mucosal lesions: mucocutaneous junctions of the anogenital and oral regions are commonly involved. They are DNA viruses with about 7900 base pairs arranged in a double-stranded circular genome encapsulated within an icosahedral protein shell (the capsid), 55 nm in diameter.

Papillomaviruses and disorders of epithelial proliferation

Many are highly infectious and responsible for hyperproliferative lesions like the common wart (verruca vulgaris) and anogenital warts

Table 20 Relative risk of developing upper aerodigestive tract cancer by alcohol and tobacco habits: Paris registry 1975–1982 (from ref. 179 with permission)

	Tobacco g/day (adjusted for alcohol)			**Alcohol** g/day* (adjusted for tobacco)		
	10–19	**20–29**	**> 30**	**40–99**	**100–159**	**> 160**
Oropharynx	4.0	7.6	15.2	2.6	15.2	70.3
Hypopharynx	7.1	12.6	35.1	3.3	28.6	143.1
Supraglottis	6.1	19.6	48.8	2.6	11.0	42.1
Glottis	3.0	9.5	28.4	0.8†	1.5†	6.1
Epilarynx	1.7†	6.7	14.8	1.9†	18.7	101.4
Lips	4.5	9.7	21.5	1.8†	4.9	10.5
Mouth	3.9	8.6	15.4	2.7	13.1	70.3

*15 g alcohol is approximately one unit.

< 9 g tobacco/day and < 40 g alcohol/day taken as RR of 1, respectively.

Confidence limits excluded for clarity, but all except † do not cross unity and are thus significant at the 5% level.

Table 21 Odds ratios for upper aerodigestive cancer in males according to smoking and drinking habits: Northern Italy, 1986–89 (from ref. 91 with permission)

Smoking practice	Alcohol intake—drinks/week			
	< 35	35–69	60 +	Total
Oral cavity/pharynx				
non-smokers	1	1.6	2.3	1
light	3.1	5.4	10.9	3.7
intermediate	10.9	26.6	36.4	14.1
heavy	17.6	40.2	79.6	25.0
Total	1	2.3	3.4	
Larynx				
non-smokers	1	1.6	–	1
light	0.9	5.0	5.4	1.0
intermediate	4.5	7.1	9.5	5.4
heavy	6.1	10.4	11.7	6.7
Total	1	1.4	2.8	
Oesophagus				
non-smokers	1	0.8	7.9	1
light	1.1	7.9	9.4	2.5
intermediate	2.7	8.8	16.7	4.0
heavy	6.4	11.0	17.5	6.6
Total	1	3.1	5.7	

Table 22 Viruses clearly related to human cancers

Virus	Associated neoplasm
DNA viruses	
Epstein–Barr	Burkitt's lymphoma
	Nasopharyngeal carcinoma
	Lymphomas in the immunosuppressed
Human herpesvirus-8 (KSHV)	Kaposi's sarcoma
Hepatitis B	Hepatocellular carcinoma
Papillomaviruses	Benign papillomas and warts
	Anogenital (incl. cervical) cancer
	?? Head and neck cancers
RNA viruses	
Human T-cell leukaemia virus (HTLV-1)	Adult T-cell leukaemia
HTLV-2	Hairy-cell leukaemia
HTLV-3	Cutaneous T-cell leukaemia

or condylomata. Most are benign, the HPVs associated with them being termed 'low-risk' types.[198]

Conversely, 'high-risk' HPV types are those associated with premalignant lesions and SCC.[198],[199] Their viral genomes can become integrated and transcriptionally active in tumour cells, such that the IARC has classified HPV-16 and -18 as carcinogenic (Group 1), HPV-31 and -33 as probably carcinogenic (Group 2a), and some others as possibly carcinogenic in man (Group 2b): the latest evaluations can be found at the IARC homepage: *http://www.iarc/fr/*). Detection of

HPV infection may be a useful risk marker for subsequent malignancy: indeed detection and typing of HPV in routine uterine cervical smears is becoming common.

The E6 and E7 open reading frames of the high-risk HPVs are important because they encode transforming proteins, and can be regarded as viral oncogenes. They bind to, and inactivate, the important cell-cycle regulatory tumour suppressor gene proteins p53 and pRb, respectively.[200] They thus act by 'taking the brakes off' the control of cell proliferation, and by inhibiting apoptosis (Fig. 12).[201] As a result, spontaneous or induced mutations are not eliminated and a transformed state can become established.[202]

Papillomaviruses and head and cancer

HPV-16 is the most common type associated with cervical and oral cancers.[203] *In vitro* studies show that primary human oral epithelial cells can be immortalized by high-risk HPV types;[204],[205] however, exposure to tobacco-related chemicals was required for these cells to progress to a fully malignant phenotype.[206]

That infection with high-risk HPV, and even demonstrable integration of known viral oncogenes, is neither necessary nor sufficient for the development of head and neck cancer is supported by our observations that p53 mutations (but not overexpression) correlate with the **absence** of HPV-16 E6.[207] This is consistent with data from Riethdorf *et al.*[208] who showed that only about 40 per cent of head and neck squamous carcinomas carrying p53 mutations also carried high-risk HPV, and only about 40 per cent of HPV-positive tumours showed p53 mutations.

The question of the predictive value of HPV infection in at-risk individuals with or without a detectable potentially malignant lesion is important. High-risk HPVs have frequently been detected in benign oral lesions and in clinically and histologically normal mucosa.[201],[209] Whether or not detecting them adds to the utility of oral screening is unknown and requires substantial further work.

Studies of HPV in patients with oral cancer report prevalences from 0 per cent[210] to 100 per cent.[211] The literature to 1997 is summarized in Table 24. The higher prevalences, unsurprisingly, are reported by studies using the more sensitive techniques and fresh tissue.

Our own work using a highly sensitive, nested-PCR method, with two sets of HPV consensus primers to the L1 region, detected HPV DNA in 14/28 (50 per cent) oral SCCs and 4/12 (33 per cent) cases of dysplastic mucosa peripheral to the tumours. HPV-16 was found in 13/28 cancers; five of these also harboured HPV-7 and one HPV 6 alone; thus 14 of the 28 cancers (50 per cent) had no detectable HPV. HPV-16 was the type detected in all 4 of the 11 potentially malignant tissues (two of which also harboured HPV-6). No other types were found.[212] These results confirm the trend apparent in Table 24, namely that HPV-16, a high-risk HPV, is that most commonly associated with oral cancer and, possibly, with its immediate precursor stages.

Several important findings emerge from reviewing this considerable, rapidly growing, and often inconsistent literature:

- There appears to be a real trend in the prevalence of HPV infection from normal oral mucosa in healthy patients, through mucosa distant to an oral lesion, through dysplastic or otherwise potentially malignant mucosa, to oral cancer itself.

- The detection rate in oral cancer (perhaps 30–50 per cent) is

Table 23 Proliferative mucosal lesions of the head and neck associated with viruses (as far as possible the order in which the types are listed implies frequency of isolation)

Normal mucosa	HPV-33, 18, 6, 2; EBV; HSV; CMV, and many others
Papilloma	HPV-6, 11, 16
Verruca vulgaris	HPV-2, 4, 6, 11
Condyloma acuminatum	HPV-6, 11, 13, 32
Focal epithelial hyperplasia (Heck's disease)	HPV-13 (1, 32, 6, 11)
Keratoacanthoma	?HPV-37
Leucoplakia	HPV-11, 16
Proliferative verrucous carcinoma	HPV-16
Koilocytic dysplasia	HPV-31, 33, 35; 16, 18; 6, 11
Squamous-cell carcinoma	HPV-16, 18, 6, 2, 57; ?EBV, ?HSV, ?HHV-6
Carcinoma of the uterine cervix	*HPV-31, 33, 35*

NB: that for HPVs, currently the most studied family, types 6, 11, 13, and 32 are regarded as 'low risk' and types 16, 18, 31, 33, 35, and 39 as 'high risk'.

HPV, human papillomavirus; EBV, Epstein–Barr virus; HSV, herpes simplex virus; CMV, cytomegalovirus; HHV, human herpesvirus.

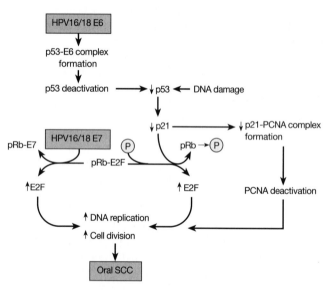

Fig. 12 An outline of how high-risk HPVs may promote oral carcinogenesis. The E6 protein of these viruses binds to and deactivates p53. When DNA damage occurs p53 and p21 cannot then be upregulated and hence there is no inhibition of proliferative-cell nuclear antigen (**PCNA**) activity or of pRb phosphorylation: Phosphorylated pRb releases activated E2F transcription factors, thus encouraging DNA replication. The E7 protein of HPVs binds directly to pRb with the same effect. (Adapted with permission from ref. 201.)

considerably lower than that reported in cervical carcinoma (85–90 per cent) and virus seems less likely to become integrated.

- HPV types 31, 33, and 35, commonly associated with cervical cancer, are not found in oral carcinomas, in which HPV-16 and -18 are the most common.

- There may be a correlation of HPV-16 and -18 with the aggressiveness of oral mucosal neoplasms, as these seem to be present at lower prevalences in verrucous carcinomas and in keratoses (see above and ref. 213) For example, in the now well-recognized entity proliferative verrucous leucoplakia (**PVL**), a condition whose appearance and natural history suggest HPV involvement, Palefsky et al.[214] found that eight out of nine lesions from seven patients contained HPV-16: in patients in the United Kingdom we found only 2/36 samples from seven patients to be positive.[215]

- There may be important geographical differences in HPV infection rates. For example, we have found, using *in situ* hybridization (**ISH**),[216] a surprisingly low prevalence in Sudanese Toombak-induced oral mucosal lesions.

- The finding of these types of normal oral mucosa may suggest that HPV can be latent for long periods. When involved in the carcinogenic process, HPV infection may be an early event.

- There is no apparent relationship between clinical stage and HPV status in SCC of the head and neck. This adds credence to the postulate that HPV involvement is not a late event in the evolution of these cancers.[199],[217],[218]

- There may be a predilection of HPV infection for patients with tonsillar carcinoma and elsewhere in Waldeyer's ring.[219]

- There may be a significant association with smoking. This has not, however, been found in all studies.[220]

- There may be a significant inverse correlation between HPV presence and age: patients older than 60 years have a lower prevalence of HPV in their tumours.[221] This relates to the aetiology of oral cancer in younger patients without a typical history of long exposure to tobacco and alcohol.

- No clear or consistent associations between HPV presence and survival or other behavioural outcomes have been demonstrated.

Table 24 Summary of HPV types described in oral SCC and normal mucosa with all methodologies combined (from ref. 201 with permission)

HPV type	Oral SCC		Normal oral mucosa	
	No.	%	No.	%
1	0/6	0		
2	4/45	9	33/479	7
3	1/28	4	0/33	0
4	1/39	3		
5	0/6	0		
6	62/642	10	90/973	9
7			1/262	<1
11	68/644	10	30/593	5
13	1/103	1	0/300	0
16	252/1156	22	84/852	10
17	0/6	0		
18	124/881	14	58/535	11
20	0/6	0		
30	0/52	0		
31	0/198	0	8/109	7
32	0/23	0	0/5	0
33	0/231	0	10/67	15
35, 42–44	0/73	0		
45	0/99	0		
51, 52, 56	0/73	0		
57	1/28	4	0/33	0

• The marked differences described for HPV prevalence rates for SCC of the oesophagus from high- and low-risk geographical areas[222] may apply to oral cancer—hence the importance of the ongoing multinational, descriptive, molecular epidemiological studies.

HPV and laryngeal papillomas and leucoplakia

E6-specific PCR was used to determine the prevalence of HPV in these lesions. HPV-6 and -11 were found in **all** (17/17) juvenile laryngeal papillomas and in 7/11 (63 per cent) of laryngeal leucoplakias. The high oncogenic-potential types, HPV-16, -18, -33 were present in none of the juvenile lesions, 6/27 (22 per cent) of the adult papillomas, and 4/11 (36 per cent) of the laryngeal leucoplakias.[223] These latter may be at risk of malignant transformation, but longitudinal studies are lacking. In contrast Poljak *et al.* found only 2/88 laryngeal epithelial lesions to be positive.[224]

The herpesviruses and head and neck cancer

Herpes simplex viruses

The epidemiology of cancer of the uterine cervix suggests an infective component, for example this disease is rare in celibates (such as nuns), and shows a relationship to the number of sexual partners (not to frequency of intercourse). For some time this focused attention on a possible role for HSV type-2, a common genital tract infection in women, and transfection of epithelial cultures with HSV can immortalize such cells. By implication, a role for HSV-1 (and -2 which can be carried in the mouth) was sought in oral carcinogenesis. Animal studies show that HSV can act as a co-carcinogen with tobacco or other chemical carcinogens[225] and that immunization against HSV can inhibit the co-carcinogenic effect induced by dimethyl-benzanthracene.[226]

Serum IgA antibodies to HSV-1 are higher in smokers, and higher again in smokers with head and neck cancers, suggesting that prolonged exposure to HSV may sensitize the mucosa to tobacco carcinogens. A more likely explanation, however, is that the generalized immunosuppression, particularly of natural killer-cell (**NK**) activity, which is induced by smoking, favours the acquisition or chronicity of HSV infections and/or carriage, with consequent raised antibody titres.[227]

Stronger, but still circumstantial, evidence comes from a case-control study of 410 pairs from northern Sweden. Univariate analysis showed ORs of 1.9 (0.7–4.5, and therefore not significant) for groups with a clearly stated ('certain') history of HSV-1 infection and 3.3 (1.6–6.5, therefore significant) for groups with a highly suspected ('certain plus probable') HSV-1 infection. Because most reports were of recurrent herpes labialis, lip cancer was analysed separately—revealing ORs of 4.6 (1.7–13) for the highly suspected group. These associations remained in multivariate analysis, which showed HSV infection (OR 3.8; 2.0–7.0), liquor use (OR 1.5; 1.0–2.3), and current smoking (OR 1.5; 0.9–2.5) to be major influences.[145]

Epstein–Barr virus (**EBV**)

Because of the very clear relationship of EBV to nasopharyngeal cancer in man,[228] to Burkitt's lymphoma which characteristically affects the jaws,[229] and to lymphomas in immunosuppressed patients, many have sought evidence for a role in SCC at other head and neck sites. Natural infection with EBV occurs worldwide and affects more than 90 per cent of many populations, either subclinically or as infectious mononucleosis during teenage years. Spread is mainly by oral contact. The major salivary glands harbour EBV and the virus can be recovered from the saliva of otherwise healthy seropositive individuals. EBV exhibits dual tropism, infecting both lymphocytes and epithelial cells, particularly those of the nasopharynx. Entry of the virus is facilitated by an envelope glycoprotein binding to the C3d receptor on the cell membrane of B cells and to either this or a closely related epitope of the surface of epithelial cells. In oral mucosa this is expressed on cells of the prickle-cell layer.

EBV has transforming properties *in vitro* and many lymphoblastoid cell lines (for example, Raji) are driven in this way. EBV DNA has been detected in some tonsillar carcinomas, supraglottic laryngeal carcinomas, and some salivary gland carcinomas.[230] However, although we could detect EBV receptors on malignant as well as normal oral keratinocytes,[231] we could not detect viral DNA in oral cancer by ISH. Given the high proportion of individuals who will be secreting EBV in saliva, methods involving the wholesale processing of tissue (such as DNA extraction from biopsies) cannot avoid salivary contamination. Nevertheless, an extensive study from India on DNA samples has recently been reported, using PCR to amplify a 239-bp fragment of the BamH1L region of the EBV genome, followed by

Southern blot hybridization with an EBV oligonucleotide probe.[232] EBV was detected in 25/103 oral cancer samples (25 per cent), 13/100 (13 per cent) of non-malignant oral lesions (predominantly leucoplakia), only 3/76 (4 per cent) of normal mucosal specimens from the contralateral side of patients with oral lesions, and from 10/141 (7 per cent) samples of peripheral blood cells (50 oral cancer patients and 50 with other oral lesions). This is a substantial sample and shows a clear prevalence trend. In a smaller study of Dutch patients using primers for the BamH1W repeat, EBV was found in 100 per cent of the SCCs ($n = 36$), 78 per cent of premalignant lesions ($n = 9$), and 8 per cent of clinically normal mucosa ($n = 12$). Using primers for the single-copy BNLF-1 gene, a region of the EBV genome with oncogenic potential, EBV was detected in only 50 per cent of the SCCs and none of the other tissues. These latter authors accept that saliva or infiltrating leucocytes could be the source of the EBV detected, possibly due to tumour-associated immunosuppression in these patients resulting in increased shedding of EBV. They, and others, have been unable to demonstrate the clonal presence of EBV in the neoplastic cells of oral SCC. Thus, all the above is circumstantial evidence, but it leaves alive the possibility that EBV may contribute as one of the multiple factors in oral carcinogenesis, at least in a proportion of patients. The evidence continues to grow of a key role for EBV in the pathogenesis of nasopharyngeal carcinoma. EBV is detected in all cells in the majority of NPC cases, regardless of geographic origin, though there may be strain variation between endemic (such as South China) and non-endemic regions.[233] A limited number of EBV genes are expressed, and LMP-1 is probably the major oncogene. B cells are probably the major reservoir, the mechanism of transfer to other cells remaining poorly understood.[234] There may be coexistence of HPV and EBV.[235]

HHV-6

This member of the Herpesviridae family also has primary tropism for CD4 lymphocytes but has a productive phase in salivary-duct epithelial cells. Primary infection is usually asymptomatic, but it can cause severe febrile illnesses in children. Reactivation in later life may be associated with a variety of conditions that show immunological dysfunction. Following description of the frequent detection of HHV-6 in a small series of oral cancers from India, and elevated levels of anti-HHV-6 antibodies in these patients' sera, one group has now reported a study on Malaysian patients. Up to 80 per cent of oral SCCs contained HHV-6 DNA (by both PCR: 19/24 cases, and ISH: 33/42 cases) or antigen (by immunocytochemistry: 41/51 cases), with a lower proportion in potentially malignant lesions (leucoplakia and lichen planus): none out of seven normal oral tissues were positive by any method.[236] These associations do not establish a role for this virus in oral carcinogenesis, but do justify further research.

HHV-8 and Kaposi's sarcoma

Kaposi's sarcoma (**KS**) and non-Hodgkin's lymphoma (**NHL**) are common in AIDS patients. EBV is implicated in the cause of up to half of the systemic NHLs and perhaps all central nervous system lymphomas in these patients. There is growing evidence that another herpesvirus, HHV-8 (or **KSHV**—KS-associated herpesvirus) is implicated in KS. One group has found it at prevalences approaching 100 per cent in KS from all body sites and in all epidemiological groups with KS, including non-HIV positive 'classical' cases.[237] It has been detected in about half of oral KS lesions and oral ulcers in HIV-positive patients by others.[238] Porter et al.[239] discuss possible pathogenic mechanisms involving the virus producing homologues of human gene products that dysregulate cell-cycle arrest and inhibit apoptosis and cell-mediated immune responses.

Fungal infections

Several species of *Candida*, especially *C. albicans* are common commensals of the oral cavity. They become opportunistic pathogens when there is local (for example, associated with the use of steroid inhalers) or systemic (for example, use of drugs in transplant patients, or HIV disease) immunosuppression, reduction of competing oral flora (such as seen with the long-term use of antibiotics), or local changes favouring their proliferation and adherence to oral mucosa: these latter include poor denture hygiene, and surface roughening and/or hyperkeratosis. A proportion of leucoplakias are superficially invaded by fungal hyphae,[240] particularly nodular leucoplakias, and these have a higher risk of malignant transformation. Of 4724 oral mucosal biopsies accessed by one service in London between 1991 and 1995, PAS-positive fungal hyphae were found in 223 (4.7 per cent) with a significant positive association with moderate or severe dysplasia.[241] There is also a clear association between smoking and the risk of candidal infection in the mouth:[242] this also applies to HIV-positive individuals, thus compounding the risk.[243] Patients with iron deficiency, clearly at increased risk for oral cancer (see below), are also more prone to oral candidiasis, indicating an interactive, multifactorial process in oral carcinogenesis.

It remains uncertain as to whether *Candida* spp. invade oral potentially malignant lesions as a secondary event, or whether they are causal in the lesion and/or subsequent cancer. However, a mechanism clearly exists, as these organisms have the necessary enzymes to promote the nitrosation of dietary substrates.[244]

Diet and nutrition in the aetiology of head and neck cancer

Interest here relates to the roles of iron, of the antioxidant or free-radical scavenging vitamins A, C, and E, and to trace elements such as zinc and selenium, for which there is evidence of a protective effect.

There is a high incidence of upper gastrointestinal tract cancer in middle-aged women with chronic anaemia, with dysphagia, glossitis, and atrophy of associated mucosae—the Plummer–Vinson or Patterson–Brown–Kelly syndrome. In animals rendered experimentally iron deficient by venesection and a low-iron diet there is contradictory evidence of the effect on epithelial-cell kinetics, with some studies showing increased turnover, theoretically increasing the risk of mutational error,[245] and others a decrease.[246] This results in epithelial atrophy[247] and increased cancer risk, clearly shown when such animals are challenged with chemical carcinogens.[248] On the other hand, there is surprisingly little information on the risks of oral cancer associated with anaemia and sideropenia in human studies. Anaemias of chronic blood loss following hookworm infections and other chronic diseases are common in those parts of south Asia where oral

Table 25 Odds ratios (OR) for oral and pharyngeal cancer according to certain food groups, Pordone, Italy, 1984–89. Includes corrections for age, sex, occupation, smoking, and drinking (from ref. 178 with permission)

OR for frequency of consumption by tercile: (Low consumption is reference category with OR set at 1)		
	Intermediate	High
Pasta or rice	1.1	1.4
Polenta	1.2	1.8
Cheese	1.0	1.7
Eggs	1.4	1.6
Pulses	1.4	1.9
Carrots	0.8	0.7
Fresh tomatoes	0.7	0.5
Green peppers	0.6	0.5

cancer prevails, as is mucosal atrophy, which presumably makes tissues more susceptible to tobacco carcinogens.[249]

Food groups

Of 13 case-control studies which have examined the association between fruit and vegetable consumption and oral/pharyngeal cancer, 11 report a meaningful inverse association.[250]–[252] The reduction in risk with fruits, from the highest to the lowest intake, varies from 80 per cent to 20 per cent[253] and is evident for tongue, mouth, and pharynx cancers.[254] There is similar protection from vegetables rich in carotenes.[255]–[257] Table 25 summarizes the data from the high-risk area in Northern Italy, based on 302 cases and 699 controls. A high intake of maize revealed a two- or threefold risk compared with a low maize intake, possibly because it is less nutritious than other grains and may cause deficiencies of B group vitamins. In Milan, an area of intermediate risk, high intakes of milk, meat, and cheese were associated with a reduced risk. This is somewhat surprising in view of the well-established increased risk associated with these foods for bowel, breast, and other cancers; however, they probably indicate the better nourished individuals. Again in Milan, carrots (OR 0.4 for the highest versus the lowest tercile), green vegetables (OR 0.6), and fresh fruit (OR 0.2) were strongly protective, and the effect is clear when expressed in terms of β-carotene intake. A strong protective effect is evident for carotenoids and vitamin C from vegetables and fruit, and of fibre intake in oral cancer risk in an important study from Beijing, China.[258]

La Vecchia *et al.*[178] estimate that approximately 15 per cent of oral and pharyngeal cancers in Europe can be attributed to dietary deficiencies or imbalances, perhaps accounting for 5000 avoidable deaths per year. Similar conclusions can be drawn from studies of laryngeal cancer.[259] In the presence of tobacco and/or alcohol, a low intake of fruit and vegetables has been estimated to account for between 25 and 50 per cent of cases amongst men.[260] Artificial supplementation with micronutrients is discussed later: however, obtaining these nutrients from natural foods is more effective than taking dietary supplements.

Dental factors in the aetiology of head and neck cancer

Clinicians have long noticed an association between poor oral hygiene and poor dental status and oral cancer. 'Dentition' (recorded as the number of natural teeth, appliances, sharp or fractured teeth) appears as a correlate in several studies (see, for example, ref. 261). As these are certain to be confounded by socioeconomic, tobacco, alcohol abuse, nutritional, and other correlates of cancer risk, it requires carefully designed, and large, case series and case-control studies to evaluate the importance of dental factors. Furthermore, it is well known in chemical carcinogenesis experiments in animals that repeated traumatizing of mucosa localizes the site at which the tumour appears, increases the yield, and reduces the latent period. Many human cases have been described of an oral cancer at the site of chronic trauma arising from a broken tooth, a denture clasp or an ill-fitting denture flange, or excrescence.

There have been three recent studies indicating that denture wearing *per se* is not a risk factor, but that chronic ulceration from an unsatisfactory appliance may promote a neoplasm in the presence of other risk factors. A large study in Brazil, based on 717 cases of mouth, pharynx, and larynx cancer, and 1434 controls, reports an OR of 2.3 (1.2–4.6) for cancer of the mouth and, interestingly, of 2.7 (1.1–6.2) for cancer of the pharynx with a history of oral sores caused by ill-fitting dentures.[262] This study also showed that less than daily toothbrushing was associated with an increased risk of tongue neoplasms of 2.1 (1.0–4.3), or of other parts of the mouth of 2.4 (1.0–5.4)—in all cases the logistic regression analyses being carefully controlled for factors such as age, sex, tobacco and alcohol, ethnicity, income, and education. Micro-organisms from dental plaque may contribute to chemical carcinogenesis, for example nitrosating enzymes: it is also likely that infrequent or inadequate oral hygiene fails to dilute tobacco-derived and other carcinogens that are present. Data from the northern Sweden study[145] and from a smaller study in the United States[263] also show no increased risk associated with fillings, dentures or fixed prostheses, nor, importantly, in the Swedish study, with dental X-ray exposure.

Aetiological factors in potentially malignant lesions and conditions

In summary (setting aside simple frictional keratoses), several types of leucoplakias are strongly associated with tobacco use in all its forms. Paradoxically, although tobacco is undeniably one of the two major aetiological agents, it is not the tobacco-associated lesions that have the highest risk of malignant transformation, but those which appear idiopathic. Papillomavirus infection is likely to be very important, possibly especially so in the larynx. Oral submucous fibrosis is clearly caused by areca nut chewing in genetically predisposed individuals: malignant transformation is enhanced by tobacco use and nutritional insufficiencies, but can occur without a history of tobacco. The precipitating antigen in the cell-mediated (auto)immune response of lichen planus remains an enigma: transformation is enhanced by traditional risk factors for oral cancer, but can occur in their absence.

Prevention of head and neck cancer

Primary prevention

Taken together tobacco, heavy alcohol consumption, and poor diet probably explain over 90 per cent of cases. The preventive approach is clear, and all healthcare professionals have an obligation and many opportunities to contribute to prevention. Major international and national agencies are active in this field (WHO,[264] CDC,[265] United States DHHS,[137] DH,[266] and see their websites).

Health promotion can be directed at whole communities, targeted at: sectors such as youth; prepared specifically for defined populations such as employees of a business; or delivered to individual 'clients' such as dental patients, those attending a health centre, antenatal clinic, physician's office, etc. Dentists and doctors can obtain literature suitable for use in their offices or hospitals from many sources, including national medical and dental associations, national health promotion groups, and cancer prevention agencies. Much excellent material can be found on the Internet, by inserting simple terms like 'oral cancer', 'larynx cancer', 'tobacco' or 'alcoholism' into one of the common search engines (see Appendix).

Deaths through tobacco use

A critical, concise analysis of the role of tobacco in health and disease, and of the approaches to prevention, is presented by the Department of Health for England.[267] Worldwide, somebody dies every 10 seconds due to tobacco usage. In developed countries tobacco is responsible for 24 per cent of all male deaths and 7 per cent of female deaths, rising to over 40 per cent for men in some of the former socialist countries and 17 per cent for women in the United States. This represents an average loss of life for all cigarette smokers of 8 years and, for those whose deaths are directly attributed to tobacco, of 16 years.[268]

> . . . for every 1000 20-year-old smokers it is estimated that one will be murdered, six will die in road accidents and 250 will die in middle age from smoking.

Deaths attributed to smoking in developing countries are lower, about 21 per cent for men and only 4 per cent for women. However, these proportions are rising as the fall in tobacco consumption in the West is matched by growth in developing countries. Indeed, of the vast majority of the 1100 million smokers in the world, 800 million live in developing countries, 300 million in China alone! Globally, some 3 million deaths a year are attributable to smoking, rising to 10 million a year in 30 to 40 years time when some 7 million will be in developing countries.[269],[270] When the use of oral smokeless tobacco is added to these figures, and the deaths it contributes through oral and pharyngeal and oesophageal cancer, the seriousness of the global epidemic of tobacco-related diseases is even more staggering.

About half of all regular smokers will be killed by their habit[92] (see Table 9). Among men in industrialized countries, smoking is estimated to be the cause of 40 to 45 per cent of all cancer deaths, 90 to 95 per cent of lung cancer deaths, over 85 per cent of oral cancer deaths, 75 per cent of chronic obstructive lung-disease deaths, and 35 per cent of cardiovascular-disease deaths in those aged between 35 and 69 years. Thus, whilst oral and pharyngeal cancer figure prominently, prevention of lung cancer, other pulmonary diseases,

Table 26 Estimated smoking prevalence among men and women, 15 years of age and over, in selected countries with very high rates (from ref. 270 with permission)

	Men	Women
Republic of Korea	68.2	6.7
Latvia	67.0	12.0
Russian Federation	67.0	30.0
Dominican Republic	66.3	13.6
Tonga	65.0	14.0
Turkey	63.0	24.0
China	61.0	7.0
Bangladesh	60.0	15.0
Fiji	59.3	30.6
Japan	59.0	18.4
Sri Lanka	54.8	0.8
Algeria	53.0	10.0
Indonesia	53.0	4.0
Samoa	53.0	18.6
Saudi Arabia	52.7	n/a
Estonia	52.0	24.0
Kuwait	52.0	12.0
Lithuania	52.0	10.0
South Africa	52.0	17.0
Poland	51.0	29.0

and cardiovascular diseases should be the starting points for anti-tobacco counselling.

Data are available from the WHO which rank smoking prevalence around the globe. The top 20 nations are listed in Table 26. Sweden is the only country in the world to have reached the goal of having just 20 per cent of its adult population smoking. In the United Kingdom and many other countries the decline in smoking prevalence has plateaued. Even in those countries which have been relatively successful there are increases in the proportion of teenagers taking up smoking, particularly females. Many of these will go on to smoke all their lives. Females are at greater risk than male smokers of developing the most lethal form of bronchogenic carcinoma—small-cell lung cancer.

The cost-effectiveness of approaches to tobacco (principally smoking) prevention/intervention are ranked. Individual action by doctors and dentists is clearly important, as can be seen in Table 27. The effectiveness of brief individual action by doctors and dentists is strikingly shown in Table 28.

Adolescent smoking is a particular concern. A comprehensive review of the world literature concludes that there is no single cause, and that personal, sociocultural, and environmental factors all encourage smoking uptake. All three types of influence need to be addressed, yet there is evidence for modest success for interventions

Table 27 An hierarchy of the cost-effectiveness of approaches to smoking cessation (from ref. 271 with permission)

- Imposition/raising of taxes
- Legislation against advertising and sponsorship
- Legislation for smoke-free areas in public places, transport, etc.
- Medical action: advice/intervention by healthcare professionals
- Education/health promotion at: national; state; school; workplace; etc.
- Dedicated quitting group activities
- Dedicated individual quitting activities

via schools, mass media, community-based programmes, and environmental measures covering controls on advertising, packaging, pricing, retailing, and smoking policies.[273]

Clinicians and tobacco control

Members of the health professions can be active in influencing politicians and community leaders to adopt appropriate legislative approaches. All professional associations are urged to adopt a policy on tobacco and health (Table 29).

Healthcare professionals can work within their clinical environment to great effect. General medical practitioner advice to quit tobacco use is respected by the majority of patients, and dentists can be equally effective (Table 30). This is achieved by following the simple scheme of the 4As (expanded here to 5As), widely used around the world (Table 31). Clinicians involved in oral healthcare have a natural entry to discussions of tobacco-related diseases because of the oral signs of tobacco use and its influence on many oral diseases and conditions (Table 32).[281] The malignant and potentially malignant lesions and conditions are important, but are not common and give rise to limited opportunities for primary prevention. The socially

important changes—bad breath and tooth staining—are often sufficient to focus on the desirability of quitting. Because periodontal diseases are so common, increased severity and extent of disease, and limitations in response to treatment, can be an important 'hook' for involving an affected patient in tobacco-usage control.[282] The scientific evidence on the harm to general and oral health of tobacco use, with special emphasis on oral cancer and precancer, oral candidiasis, other mucosal diseases, periodontal diseases, salivary flow rate and composition, susceptibility to dental caries, impact on wound healing, and the success or failure of dental implants is summarized in a report of the EU Working Group on Tobacco and Oral Health, 1998.[283]

Clinicians of many specialities are willing to receive training in tobacco-control methods. This may involve advice to clients on the use of nicotine replacement to help over the period of withdrawal. Nicotine, is 10 times more addictive than heroin.[284] An important study in the United Kingdom has shown that the use of nicotine skin patches can double the rate of smoking cessation when handled through a medical practitioner, from 5 per cent to 10 per cent of recruits.[277] This played a role in the comparable 11 per cent quit rate we have recently demonstrated as possible in dental practice.[280] The California tobacco survey shows that such patches are significantly important aids to smokers who want to quit when used as an adjuvant to other forms of assistance.[285] Nicotine replacement is available as tablets for dissolving under the tongue, as skin patches, chewing gums, nasal sprays, or as inhalators fashioned like a cigarette (which then helps with the oral and tactile stimulation that is part of smoking addiction). All have a role to play in appropriate circumstances.[286] These devices deliver nicotine with different pharmacokinetic consequences. Advice on their appropriate use, including dosages and contraindications, are included in the training literature referred to above, and from the manufacturers. In some countries these products are available over the counter, with detailed instructions: pharmacists/drug stores can also be consulted by doctors, dentists, or patients for advice.

Table 28 Life-years gained over 45 for a western population of approx. 500 000 smoking at a 27 per cent prevalence, and estimated costs per life year gained

Intervention	Effectiveness (%)	Population reached (%)	Life-years gained	Cost per life-year (£)
(undiscounted)				
Primary health care intervention				
Brief advice	2	80	3034	94
Additional gains and costs on top of brief advice from:				
Brief counselling	2	70	2665	545
Nicotine gum	8	50	7601	463
Community interventions				
Local 'No smoking' days	0.15	90	284	21
Broader community-wide	0.50	100	948	54
programmes	0.10	100	190	271
	0.05	100	95	541

Data from ref. 272 with permission.

Table 29 Position statement on tobacco

Tobacco in daily use

- The use of tobacco is harmful to general health, as it is a common cause of addition, preventable illness, disability, and death. The use of tobacco also causes an increased risk for oral cancer, periodontal disease,and other deleterious oral conditions and it adversely affects the outcome of oral healthcare.
- The FDI urges its member associations and all oral health professionals to take decisive actions to reduce tobacco use and nicotine addiction among the general public.
- The FDI also urges all oral health professionals to integrate tobacco-use prevention and cessation services into their routine and daily practice.

Tobacco in education

- Brief interactions, for example by identifying users, giving direct advice, supportive material, and follow-up, all have significant impact on the patients' use of tobacco products.
- The FDI urges all oral health institutions and all continuing education providers to integrate tobacco-related subjects into their programmes.

Protecting the children

- The adverse consequences of environmental tobacco smoke are particularly severe for children—and lifelong.
- The FDI strongly endorses and promotes public and professional education and policies, which prevent and/or reduce the exposure to tobacco smoke for infants, children, and young people.

Prevent the initiation

- More than 80% of adults who use tobacco started their use of tobacco before the age of 18. Use of tobacco among children and youths easily produces nicotine dependency, the risk of which is vastly underestimated by the young people themselves.
- The FDI vigorously supports all measures that endeavour to prevent the initiation of tobacco use.

Table 30 A selection of smoking cessation trials in primary care

References	Country	Year	Setting	No.	Method	Period	Quit rate (%)
275	USA	1989	Private dentist	374	Dentist training + brief advice	1 year	7.7
					+ nicotine gum	1 year	16.3
					+ reminders on notes +	1 year	8.6
					gum and reminders	1 year	16.9
276	Italy	1991	GMP	923	Minimal intervention	1 year	4.8
					Repeated Counselling	1 year	5.5
					Counselling and gum	1 year	7.5
					Counselling and spirometry	1 year	6.5
277	UK	1993	GMP	400	Brief advice + nicotine patches	1 year	9.3
				200	Brief advice + placebo patches	1 year	5.0
278	UK	1995	GMP	800	Nicotine patches	1 year	9.6
				400	Placebo patches	1 year	4.8
279	UK	1996	Hospital periodontal clinic	98	Dental Health Education + advice against smoking	3–6 months	13.3
					Dental Health Education only	3–6 months	5.3
280	UK	1998	GDP	154	Brief advice + optional nicotine patches	9 months	11.0

GMP, general medical practitioner; GDP, general dental practitioner.

There is no doubt that primary prevention by habit intervention is the most cost-effective approach to the management of oral cancer. This is strikingly demonstrated in a model of the situation in Sri Lanka (Fig. 13).

Passive smoking

Several critical meta-analyses of the world literature, by Hackshaw *et al.*,[287] the California Environmental Protection Agency,[288] and the United States Environmental Protection Agency,[289] show conclusively that exposure to environmental tobacco smoke (ETS) is a major cause of serious illness. In the United States it is responsible for 3000 deaths from lung cancer each year, 35 000 to 62 000 deaths from ischaemic heart disease (tobacco smoke has a marked effect on platelet biology even at low doses), 150 000 to 300 000 cases of bronchitis or pneumonia in infants and children up to 18 months of age (of whom a proportion die), 8000 to 26 000 new cases of asthma and exacerbation

Table 31 Five As

- **A**sk patients about their tobacco habits
- **A**dvise them on the importance of quitting
- **A**gree with them a quit date
- **A**ssist them in achieving this
- **A**rrange follow-up

Table 32 Easily visible tobacco-induced and associated conditions of the upper aerodigestive tract

Oral cancer

Leukoplakia
Homogeneous leukoplakia
Non-homogeneous leukoplakia
Verrucous leukoplakia
Nodular leukoplakia
Erythroleukoplakia

Other tobacco-induced oral mucosal conditions
Snuff dipper's lesion
Smoker's palate (nicotinic stomatitis)
Smoker's melanosis

Tobacco-associated effects on the teeth and supporting tissues
Tooth loss (premature mortality)
Staining
Abrasion
Periodontal diseases:
Destructive periodontitis
Focal recession
Acute necrotizing ulcerative gingivitis

Other tobacco-associated oral conditions
Gingival bleeding
Calculus
Halitosis
Leucoedema
Chronic hyperplastic candidiasis (candidal leucoplakia)
Median rhomboid glossitis
Hairy tongue

Possible association with tobacco
Oral clefts
Dental caries
Dental plaque
Lichen planus
Salivary changes
Taste and smell

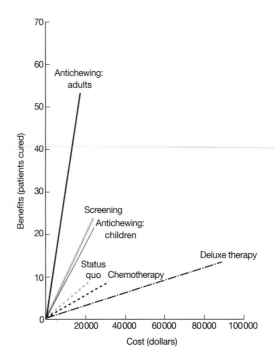

Fig. 13 Cost–benefit analysis of oral cancer in Sri Lanka.

of asthma in up to a million children, 9700 to 18 600 cases of low birth weight, and 1900–2700 sudden infant deaths. The *International consultation on environmental tobacco smoke (ETS) and child health*, published by the WHO in 1999,[290] points out that almost half the world's children are regularly exposed to ETS. Preventing this will lead to improved child, adolescent, and ultimately adult health. All health professionals, should set an example by not smoking (seeking help if we are current smokers), and by ensuring that the work environment is smoke-free.

Clinicians and the management of heavy alcohol consumption

Excessive alcohol consumption is a major cause of individual morbidity, mortality, and damage to society. In the United States, alcohol-related diseases contribute 100 000 excess deaths each year.[291] Tobacco and alcohol abuse are more significant than hard drugs, when measured by outcomes such as person-years of life lost or bed days occupied in hospital (Fig. 14). All healthcare clinicians have a responsibility to help patients, colleagues, and students use alcohol sensibly: students and staff in medical institutions are amongst the highest risk groups for dangerous drinking.[292]

Many primary-care clinicians are inhibited from taking alcohol histories, but such questioning is directed at genuine concerns for their patients' general and oral health. Oral and other upper aerodigestive tract cancers, and potentially malignant lesions, are the major concerns of head and neck clinicians. The rise in incidence and mortality of these cancers in many countries, particularly in Europe, is related to rising alcohol consumption. Differences in alcohol consumption (particularly amongst those who also smoke) explain most of the increasingly higher rates of oral cancer amongst Blacks, as compared to Whites in the United States.[293] Projections of disease levels based on trends in alcohol consumption lead to disturbing predictions of future cancers at these sites (Fig. 15).[294] In addition, alcohol contributes to dental and maxillofacial injuries; secondary events following liver damage and, often, undernutrition, comprise adverse effects on periodontal health, wound healing, and resistance to infection.[187]

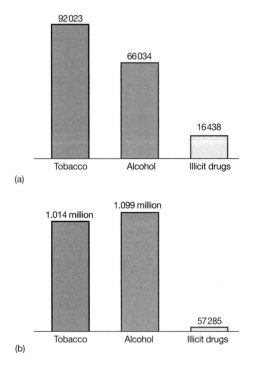

(a)

(b)

Fig. 14 Person-years of life lost (ages 0–69) due to tobacco, alcohol, and illicit drug use, Australia 1986. (b) Hospital bed-days occupied due to tobacco, alcohol, and illicit drug use (ages 0–69). (Figure by courtesy of Dr Nigel Gray, UICC and Anticancer Council of Victoria, Australia.)

All clinicians can see these facial and intraoral signs in their patients, and suspicion may be aroused by patient behaviour. There are well-established tools for the estimation of problem drinking in

patients. These include the so-called CAGE (*c*ut down, *a*nnoyed by criticism, *g*uilty about drinking, *e*ye-opener drinks) and AUDIT (Alcohol Use Disorders Identification Test) questionnaires, of which a recent study showed the AUDIT to be marginally superior.[295] We have validated the AUDIT questionnaire, as developed by the WHO.[296] In a study of 107 south London misusers, over half of whom consumed more than 200 units of alcohol per week and 80 per cent of whom also smoked, eight subjects had oral mucosal lesions, including two previously treated carcinomas in one individual. Dental caries experience did not differ from an age-matched national sample, but periodontal disease was more severe and was related to both smoking and undernutrition, as recorded by Body Mass Index and mid-arm muscle circumference measurements. Clearly such individuals are a priority group for preventive counselling.[187] A policy of **Ask, Advise** ought to be followed, accepting that **Referral** is wise for patients with a suspected alcohol problem, given the complexity of the addictive process and the therapeutic challenges in this demanding, specialized field. Dedicated groups, agencies, and clinics exist in most countries, and practitioners should be aware of local networks. Serious alcohol dependence often requires inpatient and/or day-stay treatment, which is both demanding and expensive.[297] Again much professional advice, and access to self-help and support groups for individuals with alcohol problems and their families, can be found on the Internet.

Specific training can enhance the effectiveness of primary-care physicians in detecting and managing hazardous drinking habits in their patients, and direct contact with trainers is more effective than using mailed training kits.[298] In a study in Sydney, Australia, 36 trained general medical practitioners recruited 179 patients with an alcohol problem over 3 months, 32 per cent of whom reported reduced drinking to the researchers.[299] As with tobacco control, education and health promotion interventions need to be taken at

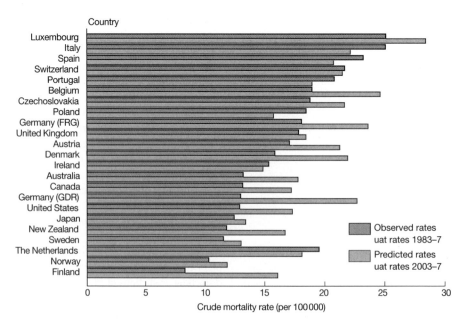

Fig. 15 The projected rise in mortality from aerodigestive tract cancer over the current year timeframe, modelled from risk factor trends in a number of industrialized countries. (From ref. 294 with permission.)

Table 33 The major causes of death from alcohol abuse

Stroke

Cardiomyopathy

Cancer (several sites)

Liver cirrhosis

Pancreatitis

Accidents

Suicide

Homicide

all levels of society, and many governments around the world are working to improve their utility.[300]

Moderate alcohol consumption may be beneficial, for example in reducing the risk of cardiovascular disease. The so-called J-shaped curve relationship between alcohol consumption and total mortality has been established for some years.[301] The lowest mortality occurs in those who consume one or two drinks per day. In teetotallers or very occasional drinkers the mortality rate is higher than those who take one or two drinks per day: In those who take three or more drinks per day, mortality rises rapidly in a dose-dependent manner. The major causes of death are listed in Table 33. The protection against coronary heart disease provided by one or two drinks per day is in the order of 30 to 59 per cent,[302] and there is less atherosclerosis in moderate drinkers, visible at catheterization or at autopsy. This effect seems to be independent of confounders such as smoking and poor diet. It is generally considered[303] that about half of the protective effect is mediated through increased levels of HDL-C (high-density lipoprotein-cholesterol), which carries cholesterol from arterial walls back to the liver.[304] Other beneficial effects are mediated through a reduction in clotting factors and platelet activity, and/or clot lysis.[305]

Other protective substances have been identified, such as anti-oxidants in wine derived from grape skins[306] and in dark beer.

However, the epidemiological evidence does not show any particular beverage to be consistently more effective in reducing coronary heart disease, perhaps because of the considerable variability in confounding factors such as smoking, diet, and age.[307] The frequency of consumption is also important. Studies in eastern Europe, where patterns of alcohol use and heart disease are different from western areas, show binge-drinking to be dangerous: such individuals do not have raised HDLs—indeed raised levels of low-density lipoprotein (LDLs)—and they show a tendency to increased thrombosis after cessation of drinking.[308]

What therefore constitutes potentially unhealthy levels of alcohol consumption? Many governments and agencies suggest a healthy limit of 21 units of alcohol a week for men and 14 for women, with at least two alcohol-free days per week. A unit of alcohol is taken to be a single glass (approximately 284 ml) of average strength beer or lager, a single measure (approximately 25 ml) of spirits, or a single standard (approximately 113 ml) glass of wine or aperitif (50 ml).[309]

Healthy eating in the prevention of head and neck cancer

Clinicians usually enquire about the dietary habits of patients because they are interested in their likely adverse effects on cardiovascular health, or—for dentists—in their possible cariogenicity. Adequate (neither under nor over) nutrition is essential to host resistance against all diseases and this is strongly true of cancer. Table 34 summarizes dietary measures suggested for the prevention of cancer, based on a critical review by Sir Richard Doll—the epidemiologist who has made perhaps the greatest single contribution to our knowledge of the causes and prevention of cancer this century.[310] He believes that the overall risk of cancer can be reduced by a third or more by modifying the diet. The protective role of diets adequate in trace elements, minerals, and vitamins (particularly the antioxidant or free-radical scavenging vitamins A, C, and E) has been emphasized.[178],[311],[312] Many studies have shown that an intake of protective nutrients is more effective when these are derived from natural foodstuffs rather than from synthetic food supplements. Thus, the advice we should give to our patients, which is part of every nation's health promotion guidelines, is summarized in Table 35.

Table 34 Dietary measures suggested for the prevention of cancer (modified from Doll, 1989)

Measure	Type of cancer affected
Reduce:	
Calories (avoid obesity)	Gall bladder, body of uterus, possibly breast
Fat	Breast, colon and rectum, prostate, and endometrium
Smoked and grilled food	Stomach, perhaps others
Salt-cured food	Stomach
Nitrates	Stomach, possibly others
Saccharin	Possibly bladder
Increase:	
Fibre	Colon and rectum
Vegetables	Colon and rectum: many sites, including head and neck
Fruit	Colon and rectum: many sites including head and neck
Vitamins A, C, E	Many sites, including head and neck
Beta-carotene	Many sites, including head and neck
Selenium	Many sites, including head and neck

Table 35 American Cancer Society (1996) guidelines on diet, nutrition, and cancer, adapted for head and neck cancer

1.	Choose most of the foods you eat from plant sources
	• Eat five or more servings of fruit and vegetables each day
	• Eat other foods from plant sources, such as breads, cereals, grain products, rice, pasta, or beans several times a day
2.	Limit your intake of high-fat foods, particularly from animal sources
	• Choose foods low in fat
	• Limit consumption of meats, particularly high-fat meats
3.	Be physically active: achieve and maintain a healthy weight
	• Be moderately active for 30 min or more on most days of the week
	• Stay within your healthy weight range
4.	Limit consumption of alcoholic beverages, if you drink at all
AND	
	• Avoid sexually transmitted infections
	• Do not use tobacco

Table 36 The basic principles of screening for disease

• The condition should be an important health problem

• Its natural history should be understood

• There should be an accepted and proven intervention

• There should be a suitable and accepted diagnostic test

• The cost of screening should be balanced in relation to other healthcare expenditure

Adapted from ref. 315 with permission.

Table 37 Potential advantages of screening for head and neck cancer and precancer

• Reduced mortality

• Reduced incidence of invasive cancers

• Improved prognosis for individual patients

• Reduced morbidity from earlier treatment

• Identification of high risk-individuals/groups allowing targeted prevention

• Reassurance for those screened as negative

• Cost savings from expensive treatments

Secondary prevention: screening for head and neck cancer and potentially malignant lesions

Rationale and utility

Screening for disease is a very precise science[314] and must follow established principles (Table 36).[315] Head and neck cancer meets some, but not all, these criteria. Moreover, although there are clear potential advantages for screening (Table 37), there are also potential disadvantages (Table 38).

The rationale for screening is based on the fact that these cancers may be asymptomatic and localized for a period of their natural history, and are preceded by potentially malignant lesions and conditions such as leucoplakia, erythroplakia, and submucous fibrosis, when they might be detected by simple systematic clinical examinations. This is important because habit intervention,[121] dietary intervention,[316] and surgical treatment[28],[317] may result in their resolution or elimination.

However, population screening cannot be recommended[318],[319] because there is inadequate understanding of natural history[320] and

Table 38 Potential disadvantages of screening for head and neck cancer and precancer

• Detection of cases already incurable may increase morbidity for some

• Unnecessary treatment for premalignant lesions which might not progress

• Psychological trauma to those with a false-positive result

• Reinforcing bad habits amongst some individuals screened as negative

• Costs

there is insufficient evidence of utility[321] or cost-effectiveness. Oral-cancer screening programmes have been carried out on several hundreds of thousands of individuals in developing countries (mostly Sri Lanka, India, and Cuba) and several thousands in developed countries (mostly the United States, United Kingdom, and Italy)—the evidence

Table 39 Results of oral cancer/precancer screening programmes

Investigators (ref.)	Year	Country	Sample	Cancer		Precancer	
				No		**No**	**%**
Ross and Gross[323]	1971	USA	12 868	1	8	339	2.6
Folsom et al.[324]	1972	USA	158 996	120	75	803	0.5
Axell et al.[325]	1976	Sweden	20 333	1	5	732	3.6
Mehta et al.[326]	1969	India	50 915	26	51	881	1.7
Warnakulasuriya et al.[322]	1983	Sri Lanka	28 295	4	14	1220	4.2
Bouquot and Gorlin[327]	1986	USA	23 616	22	93	682	2.9
Ikeda et al.[328]	1991	Japan	3 131	None	—	77	2.5
Banoczy and Rigo[329]	1991	Hungary	7 820	1	13	104	1.3

from these is reviewed by Warnakulasuriya and Johnson[322] (Table 39) and by Franceschi et al.[320] In the high-incidence parts of the world, a substantial proportion of suspicious lesions has been found (ranging from 2 to 16 per cent in south Asia) but the compliance of patients to attend follow-up was poor. The yield is substantially lower in the West. For example, the largest study group comprised over 23 000 adults in Minnesota over 30 years of age whose mouths were examined by dentists between 1957 and 1972. Although more than 10 per cent of those screened had an oral lesion, these were mostly benign: 'precancer' was encountered in 2.9 per cent and cancer in less than 0.1 per cent.

A stronger case may be made for targeting screening to at-risk populations—for head and neck cancer perhaps to smokers and heavy drinkers over the age of, say, 40 years. Such individuals can be identified from the records of family medical practitioners, or occupational health records. Even so, studies of this kind conducted in the United Kingdom[330] and in Japan[331] have shown high non-attendance rates for the initial oral examination. This, together with the low prevalence of lesions, makes even this type of screening of dubious utility. In studies conducted by ear, nose, and throat specialists in Northern Italy between 1994 and 1998, the yield was substantially increased by adding inspections of the pharynx and larynx (with appropriate instrumentation) and by aiming the programme at smokers and/or heavy drinkers, relying on general practitioners for the identification of these high-risk individuals. Even so, only 1564 out of 4419 (35 per cent) individuals complied with the examination: this yielded 152 (9.7 per cent) 'precancerous' lesions (mostly low-risk flat leucoplakias), and 20 (1.3 per cent) cancers at any of these upper aerodigestive sites.

The Oral Cancer Screening Group at the Eastman Dental Institute, London, has carried out an outstanding series of investigations in recent years. They have shown that the sensitivity and specificity of lesion detection is comparable to that of oral examination by the use of artificial intelligence systems to compute all known risk factors for oral cancer (Table 40). This is an exciting way forward for the future, but bringing these individuals to early treatment will remain a problem.

In a simulation model, estimates of quality-adjusted life years (**QALYs**) and of lives gained from screening were obtained, compared with the *status quo* of no screening. Participants were a notional population of 100 000 adults of average age 55 years and 20 years' life expectancy. The basic assumptions were a 50 per cent attendance of the eligible population, a prevalence of oral cancer of 0.998 per cent and of precancer 2.57 per cent, a positive predictive value of the screening test of 0.67, and a negative predictive value of 0.99. The cancers were assumed to be 40 per cent at Stage 1, 60 per cent at Stage 2 + without screening, and 60 per cent Stage 1 and 40 per cent Stage 2 + with screening. Patients with oral precancer were assumed to have a survival of 19.2 years, with Stage 1 cancer 14.6 years, and Stage 2 + cancer 10.8 years. The public's perceived utilities were 0.92 for precancer and 0.88 and 0.68 for Stage 1 and Stage 2 + cancer, respectively, compared to a utility of 1.0 for health. One cycle of the programme was modelled over 1 year in a dental practice setting. The cost benefits obtained under these circumstances are shown in Table 41.

This estimate of a cost per life saved by screening a high-risk population for oral cancer, £8333, compares favourably with costs estimated for other, more common, cancers,[332] for which population screening programmes already exist in many countries (Table 42). Indeed, the longest established cancer screening programmes in the world, those for cancer of the uterine cervix, are extremely expensive and controversial. They have never been evaluated by means of a randomized controlled trial and, although changes in incidence make it difficult to estimate the effect of a screening programme quantitatively, the impact on this disease is less than hoped for.

Opportunistic screening—in other words, offering a screening test for an unsuspected disorder at a time when a person presents to a doctor, or a dentist, or any other suitably trained primary healthcare professional for another reason—is rational and cost-effective.[333] The clinical identification of suspect lesions by direct vision and palpation is a skill which can be taught, at least for the mouth, to any primary healthcare worker—even those with quite basic training.[334] An encouraging outcome of such studies comes from the Oral Cancer Case Finding Programme in Cuba. Between 1983 and 1990, 10 167 999 subjects were examined nationwide when they attended stomatological clinics: only 8259 out of 30 480 patients (27 per cent) with suspect lesions complied with referral, and of these there were 3220 potentially malignant lesions, 581 SCCs, and 127 other malignancies. However,

Table 40 Screening for oral cancer and potentially malignant lesions

Location	Lesion	Prevalence (%)	Sensitivity	Specificity
Dental Hospital	1042	3.00	0.81	0.99
Medical practice	985	2.22	0.64	0.99
Company HQ	309	5.5	0.71	0.99
Neural network	365	2.74	0.80	0.77

Based on clinical and digital examination of the oral mucosa by dentists, with confirmation by an oral medicine specialist. The first three studies provided the data for training the neural network.

Table 41 Hypothetical cost-benefits of oral cancer screening programmes (assuming the cost of a screening examination to be £5.00)

Screening of whole population
- Cost of screening 100 000 = £500 000
- Lives saved = 5.6
- Cost per life saved = £89 286

Screening a high-risk population
- Cost of screening 25 000 = £125 000
- Lives saved = 15
- Cost per life saved = £8 333

Table 42 Costs per life saved for cancer screening programmes

• Breast cancer	£80 000*
• Cervical cancer	£300 000*
• Colon cancer	£6 500*
• Oral cancer (high risk)	£8 883

Data from ref. 332 with permission.

although at considerable cost, the programme was shown to be effective because there was 'downstaging' of the cancers seen: Stage I lesions rising from 22.8 per cent to 48.2 and Stages II, III, and IV lesions falling from 77.2 per cent to 51.8 per cent.[335] This study used specially trained stomatologists. In spite of their lower cost and comparable accuracy to dentists, use of auxiliaries for population screening still cannot be recommended because there is no evidence yet available of the efficacy of such an approach in reducing the incidence and mortality of head and neck cancer.

Toluidine Blue (tolonium chloride)

The use of Toluidine Blue dye as a mouthwash or topical application is receiving attention as an aid to the diagnosis of oral cancer and potentially malignant lesions. It has a place, with appropriate training, in screening high-risk subjects and in helping to define the site for biopsy. The method has good sensitivity, with a very low false-negative rate. However, most studies have taken both overtly invasive carcinomas and severe (or even moderate) dysplasia as true-positive lesions under the umbrella 'oral cancer'. Although 100 per cent of invasive lesions will stain, most studies show that only 50 per cent or less of dysplasias are detected. The false-positive rate is likely to be very low in patients presenting with perfectly healthy mucosae, but areas of inflammation, ulceration, or erosion stain positively whatever their cause. False-positives may be as high as 48 per cent following a single application, but repeating the stain 10 to 14 days later to allow acute ulcerative or traumatic lesions to heal can reduce this to 11 per cent. The dorsum of the tongue always stains positively, due to retention of dye in crevices between the papillae, making it of limited value for studying lesions at this site, unless the lesion arises out of an atrophic area. Likewise, crevices and cracks within thick keratotic plaques retain dye and produce a false-positive result.

Good clinical judgement, training, and experience in the use of Toluidine Blue staining, ensure the rational use of this diagnostic aid. Biopsy remains the 'gold standard' for diagnosing oral cancer and potentially malignant lesions. False-positives are of less concern that false-negatives. All positive stain reactions require biopsy, as do any suspicious lesions which do not stain.

The use of Toluidine Blue,[274] in expert and experienced hands, is recommended for:

- monitoring suspicious lesions over time;
- screening for oral mucosal malignancy and premalignancy in high-risk individuals and population groups;
- follow-up of patients already treated for upper aerodigestive tract cancer;
- helping to determine an optimal site for biopsy when a suspicious lesion or condition is present; and
- intraoperative use during surgery for upper aerodigestive tract malignancy as an application to help judge the borders of the neoplasm.

Molecular screening

It is possible to analyse tissue, and any body fluid, including saliva, for aberrations in oncogenes or tumour suppressor genes or their protein products. It is also possible to screen chromosomes from exfoliated epithelial cells in health, from potentially malignant lesions, and from overt cancers and to record abnormalities such as loss, amplification, or transposition of parts of the genome important in carcinogenesis.

It is not known precisely how many 'hits' or aberrations are necessary to render a clone of cells malignant, though a figure of around six is often quoted. This has led to models for the development of head and neck cancer.[336] Such models should not be taken to imply that precisely this series of abnormalities, in precisely that order, are necessary or sufficient for a cancer to develop: the number, type, and order may differ from patient to patient. Nevertheless, the accumulation of such changes indicates an increasing risk of malignant transformation and this information will, in the future, be put to use in:

- screening clinically normal patients who are heavy smokers and drinkers to determine their risk of a future cancer;
- screening potentially malignant lesions and conditions in order to assess how far the path to malignancy has been travelled, and thus to focus intervention for the individual patient;
- determining completeness of excision/killing by radiotherapy/ chemotherapy, by sampling tissue *in situ* after treatment for an overt cancer, in order to assess the risk of recurrence or second primary—this encompasses the concepts of 'field change' and of 'residual disease';
- screening peripheral blood or bone marrow for malignant cells disseminated from the primary lesion;
- screening blood or saliva for the presence of a marker indicative of the presence of neoplasm—residual or recurrent primary, new primary, or metastatic disease.

Tertiary prevention: preventing recurrence of further primary cancers and minimizing morbidity

When a patient treated for a head and neck cancer develops further cancer in the region, months or years after apparently successful treatment, it is often unclear whether the new lesion is a recurrence— arising from incomplete removal of the primary lesion—or a second primary lesion, arising in a field of altered mucosa. The concept of 'field cancerization' is that the patient's genetic predisposition—plus the lifelong accumulation of potentially carcinogenic insults from risk factors—renders the patient, and the anatomical area, at increased risk of cancer. This applies whether the second cancer is synchronous with the first, or arises later (metachronous). An alternative view is that a clone of genetically damaged, and therefore 'premalignant' cells migrates in the anatomical area and may give rise to second tumours.[337] Either way, the whole of the upper aerodigestive tract can be regarded as the susceptible field.[338] Unsurprisingly, therefore, the risk of a further cancer is high once a patient has been treated, amounting to some 20 per cent of patients over a 5-year period. This is especially so if the tobacco, alcohol, and dietary risk factors continue to be present. Therefore all the above primary prevention approaches are especially important at this stage, including supplementation with antioxidants such as vitamin A[339] or retinoids.[340]

Chemoprevention of malignant transformation of oral pre-cancerous lesions (leucoplakia has been most extensively investigated as it is the commonest, even if variably and loosely defined) and conditions by dietary supplementation is another exciting field under active investigation.

The current position has been thoroughly evaluated by San-karanarayanan et al.,[341] from which the following summary is partly derived. Both the experimental animal evidence and the then published clinical trials were thoroughly analysed by Tanaka in 1995.[342] Many

field studies have been conducted in India on pan or other smokeless tobacco-associated lesions, with or without beedi (a small amount of dried leaf and tied with a cotton thread) smoking and alcohol as cofactors. Those from the West relate to smoking- and alcohol-related cancers. The essential conclusions are:

- In the primary prevention of upper aerodigestive tract cancers, a substantial reduction in risk can be obtained by increasing fruit and vegetable consumption.[250],[343] This is quite distinct from the use of nutritional supplements in secondary and tertiary prevention.
- Retinoids and β-carotene have been shown to result in the regression of oral leucoplakia, but the lesions soon recur after stopping the chemopreventive agents.[344]
- Lower frequencies of malignant transformation have been observed in a small number of subjects with leucoplakia receiving retinoids compared to subjects receiving β-carotene.[345]
- Supplementation has not been shown to reduce the risk of loco-regional recurrence in patients treated for head and neck cancer.
- A reduction in the frequency of second primaries has been observed with 13-*cis*-retinoic acid[346] but not with etretinate.[347]
- Although retinoids seem to be effective in inhibiting head and neck carcinogenesis, compared with β-carotene, the synthetic retinoids are quite toxic, which limits their usefulness.[345]
- Retinoids have the potential to enhance carcinogenesis under certain conditions, perhaps due to an angiogenic effect, so their use cannot yet be justified outside clinical trials.[348]
- There is insufficient evidence to evaluate the chemopreventive effects of vitamin E or of selenium in head and neck cancer. Some early results on combinations of vitamin E and β-carotene are encouraging.[349]
- None of the potential intermediate biomarkers studied for the effect of chemopreventive regimes have yet been fully validated. Amongst these micronucleated epithelial cells have received the most attention: Prasad et al.[350] and Sankaranarayanan et al.[341] conclude that this method has value in monitoring compliance amongst patients.
- Many other potential biomarkers are under investigation. These include DNA adducts,[350] cell-proliferation markers such as Ki67 and PCNA, EGFR (epidermal growth-factor receptor), and erbB expression, aberrations of the *p53* gene or its protein, HPV gene expression or integration. In respect of studies on retinoid chemo-prevention it may be possible to use nuclear retinoic acid receptors for this purpose.[351]
- Attempts at chemoprevention of head and neck cancer should only be made in the context of well-planned, preferably multicentre, clinical trials. Many of these are ongoing.

Further secondary prevention (by screening) is also especially important. Treated patients should be monitored regularly to ensure that their mastication, swallowing, speaking, smiling, and other functions as well as their physical appearance and their social integration are as good as the cancer-care team can manage, and to screen for new lesions. Toluidine Blue application may have utility here. The cost-effectiveness of regular upper aerodigestive tract endoscopy has yet to be established. Nowhere is teamwork in cancer care more important than with treated patients, in order to maximize the quality of life for those afflicted and to ensure the best possible quality of death.

Appendix Sources of information on tobacco cessation programmes

Useful addresses	Useful websites
• US Department of Health and Human Services, Public Health Services, Agency for Health Care Policy and Research, 2101 East Jefferson St, Suite 501, Rockville, MD 20852, USA	• Lifesaver *http://www.lifesaver.co.uk* An interactive HEA website designed to offer the support and motivation smokers may need to quit for life
• The European Union Working Group on Tobacco and Oral Health, c/o Danish Dental Association, Amaliegarde 17, PO Box 143, DK-1004, Copenhagen K, Denmark; Tel: +45 33 15 77 11; Fax: +45 33 15 31 37	• The Quit Guide to Stopping Smoking *http://healthnet.org.uk/quit/guide.htm* Advice and tips on quitting
• The Health Education Authority, Trevelyan House, 30 Great Peter St., London SW1P 2HW, UK; Tel: +44 171 222 5300; Fax: +44 171 413 2632	• Quit Now *http://quitnow.info.au* One-stop shop advice on quitting and information on the overall Australian National Tobacco Campaign
• The British Dental Association, 64 Wimpole St, London W1M 8AL, UK; Tel: +44 171 305 0875; Fax: +44 171 487 5232	• How to Quit Smoking *http://www.cdc.gov/nccdphp/osh/tobacco.htm* The US Centre for Disease Control's Tobacco Information and Prevention Source
• The International Agency for Research on Cancer (UICC), 3 rue du Conseil-General, 1205 Geneva, Switzerland; Tel: +41 22 809 1830; Fax +41 22 809 1810; e-mail: *education@uicc.ch*	• Health Education Authority *http://www.hea.org.uk*
	• World Health Organization *http:www.who.ch*
	• International Union Against Cancer *http://www.uicc.ch*
	• British Dental Association *http://www.bda-dentistry.org.uk*
	• FDI World Dental Federation *http://www.fdi.org.uk/worldental*
	• Cancer Research Campaign *http://www.crc.org.uk*
	• Oral Cancer Information Centre *http://www.oralcancer.org*

References

1. **Muir C, Welland L.** Upper aerodigestive tract cancers. *Cancer*, 1995; 75; 1(Suppl.): 147–53.

2. **Parkin DM, Pisani P, Ferlay J.** Estimates of the worldwide incidence of twenty-five major cancers in 1990. *International Journal of Cancer*, 1999; 80: 827–41.

3. **Black RJ, Bray F, Ferlay J, Parkin DM.** Cancer incidence and mortality in the European Union. *European Journal of Cancer*, 1997; 33: 1075–107.

4. **Ferlay J, Parkin DM, Pisani P.** *Globocan 1: cancer incidence and mortality worldwide.* Lyon: IARC Press, 1998. [CD-rom]

5. **Coleman MP, Esteve J, Damiecki P, Arslan A, Renard H.** *Trends in cancer incidence and mortality.* Lyon: IARC, 1993: Scientific Publication No 121.

6. **Zheng Y, Kirita T, Kurumatani N, Sugimura M, Yonemasu Y.** Trends in oral cancer mortality in Japan: 1950–1993. *Oral Diseases*, 1999; 5: 3–9.

7. **American Cancer Society.** *Cancer facts and figures.* 1997

8. **Moller H.** Changing incidence of cancer of the tongue, oral cavity and pharynx in Denmark. *Journal of Oral Pathology and Medicine*, 1989; 18: 224–9.

9. **Macfarlane GJ, Boyle P, Scully C.** Oral cancer in Scotland: changing incidence and mortality. *British Medical Journal*, 1992; 305: 1121–3.

10. **Plesko I, Macfarlane GJ, Evstifeeva TV, Obsitnikova A, Kramarova E.** Oral and pharyngeal cancer incidence in Slovakia 1968–1989. *International Journal of Cancer*, 1994; 56: 481–6.

11. **Ferlay J, Black RJ, Pisani P, Valdivieso MT, Parkin DM.** *Eucan 90: Cancer in the European Union IARC Cancerbase No 1. Electronic Database.* Lyon: IARC, 1996.

12. **Ramanathan K, Lakshmi S.** Oral cancer in Chinese males. *Asian Journal of Medicine*, 1974; 10: 3–7.

13. **van Wyck CW, Stander I, Padayachee A, Grobler-Rabie AF.** The areca nut habit and oral squamous cell carcinoma in South African Indians. *South African Dental Journal*, 1992; 83: 425–9.

14. **Thames Cancer Registry.** Cancer in South-eastern England, 1995.

15. **Edwards D.** PhD Thesis: University of London, 1998.

16. **Swerdlow AJ, Cooke KR, Skegg DC, Wilkinson J.** Cancer incidence in England and Wales and New Zealand and in migrants between the two countries. *British Journal of Cancer*, 1995; 75: 236–43.

17. **Warnakulasuriya KAAS, Johnson NW, Linklater KM, Bell J.** Cancer of mouth, pharynx and nasopharynx in Asian and Chinese immigrants resident in Thames regions. *Oral Oncology*, 1999; 35: 471–5.

18. **Surveillance, Epidemiology and End Results.** Cancer statistics and review. Bethesda, MD: National Cancer Institute, 1997.

19. **Smans M, Muir CS, Boyle P.** *Atlas of cancer mortality in the European Economic Community.* Lyon: IARC, 1992: Scientific Publication No. 107.

20. **Zatonski W, Smans M, Tyczynski J, Boyle P.** *Atlas of cancer mortality in Central Europe.* Lyon: IARC, 199?: Scientific Publication No. 134.

21. Macfarlane GJ, Boyle P, Evstifeeva V, Robertson C, Scully C. Rising trends in oral cancer mortality among males worldwide: the return of an old public health problem. *Cancer Causes and Control*, 1994; 5: 259–63.

22. Negri E, La Vecchia C, Levi F, Franceschi S, Serra-Majem L, Boyle P. Comparative descriptive epidemiology of oral and oesophageal cancers in Europe. *European Journal of Cancer Prevention*, 1996; 5: 267–80.

23. Franceschi S, Levi F, La Vecchia C, Lucchini F, Negri E. Comparison of cancer mortality trends in major European areas, 1960–89. *European Journal of Cancer Prevention*, 1994; 3: 145–206.

24. Hindle I, Downer MC, Speight PM. The epidemiology of oral cancer. *British Journal of Oral and Maxillofacial Surgery*, 1996; 34: 471–6.

25. Joslin C, Rider L, Crellin A. *Cancer in Yorkshire: Cancer registry Special Report Series 2. Head and Neck Cancer.* Leeds: Yorkshire Cancer Organisation, 1995.

26. Edwards D, Johnson NW. Treatment of upper aerodigestive tract cancers in the United Kingdom and its effect on survival. *British Journal of Cancer*, 1999; 81: 323–9.

27. Macfarlane GJ, Macfarlane TV, Lowenfels AB. The influence of alcohol consumption on worldwide trends in mortality from upper aerodigestive tract cancers in males. *Journal of Epidemiology and Community Health*, 1996; 50: 636–9.

28. van der Waal I, *et al.* Oral leukoplakia: a clinicopathological review. *Oral Oncology*, 1997; 33: 291–301.

29. Johnson NW, van der Waal, Axell T. Oral leukoplakia. *Oral Diseases*, 1997; 3: 47–8.

30. Johnson NW, Ranasinghe AW, Warnakulasuriya KAAS. Potentially malignant lesions and conditions of the mouth and oropharynx: a natural history—cellular and molecular markers of risk. *European Journal of Cancer Prevention*, 1993; 2(Suppl. 2): 31–51.

31. Schepman KP, van der Meij EH, Smeele LE, van der Waal I. Malignant transformation of oral leukoplakia: a follow-up study of a hospital-based population of 166 patients with oral leukoplakia from the Netherlands. *Oral Oncology*, 1998; 34: 270–5.

32. Marley JJ, *et al.* A comparison of the management of potentially malignant oral mucosal lesions by oral medicine practitioners and oral and maxillofacial surgeons in the UK. *Journal of Oral Pathology and Medicine*, 1998; 27: 489–93.

33. Issing WJ, Struck R, Naumann A, Kasternbauer E. High concentrate A-mulsin, a new therapy concept in laryngeal leukoplakia. *Laryngorlinootologie*, 1996; 75: 29–33.

34. Schepman KP, van der Meij EH, Smeele LE, van der Waal I. Concomitant leukoplakia in patients with oral squamous cell carcinoma. *Oral Diseases*, 1999; 6.

35. Scheifele C, Reichart PA. Oral leukoplakia in 102 patients with oral squamous cell carcinoma. *Oral Diseases*, 2000; 6: [In press.]

36. Barnard NA, *et al.* Oral cancer development in patients with oral lichen planus. *Journal of Oral Pathology and Medicine*, 1993; 22: 421–4.

37. Markopoulos AK, Antoniades D, Papanayotou P, Trogonidis G. Malignant potential of oral lichen planus: a follow-up study of 326 patients. *Oral Oncology*, 1997; 33: 263–9.

38. Kovesi G, Banoczy J. Follow up studies in oral lichen planus. *International Journal of Oral Surgery*, 1973; 2: 13–19.

39. Fulling HJ. Cancer development in oral lichen plaus: a follow up study of 327 patients. *Archives of Dermatology*, 1973; 108: 667–9.

40. Krutchoff DJ, Cutlert L, Laskowski S. Oral lichen planus: the evidence regarding malignant transformation. *Journal of Oral Pathology*, 1978; 7: 1–7.

41. Lo Muzio L, Mignnogna MD, Favia G, Procaccini M, Testa NF, Bucci E. The possible association between oral lichen planus and oral squamous cell carcinoma: a clinical evaluation on 14 cases and a review of the literature. *Oral Oncology*, 1998; 34: 2349.

42. Porter SR, Di Alberti L, Kumar N. Human herpes virus 8 (Kaposi's sarcoma herpesvirus). *Oral Oncology*, 1998; 34: 5–14.

43. Carrozzo M, Carbone M, Gandolfo S, Valente G, Colombatto P, Ghisetti V. An atypical verrucous carcinoma of the tongue arising in a patient with oral lichen planus associated with hepatitis C virus infection. *Oral Oncology*, 1997; 33: 220–5.

44. Murti PR, Bhonsle RB, Pindborg JJ, Daftary DK, Gupta PC, Mehta FS. Malignant transformation rate in oral submucous fibrosis over a 17-year period. *Community Dentistry and Oral Epidemiology*, 1985; 13: 340–1.

45. Renehan A, Gleave EN, Hancock BD, Smith P, Mcgurk M. Long-term follow up of over 1000 patients with salivary gland tumours treated in a single centre. *British Journal of Surgery*, 1996; 83: 1750–4.

46. Potdar GG, Paymaster JC. Tumours of minor salivary glands. *Oral Surgery, Oral Medicine, Oral Pathology*, 1969; 28: 310–19.

47. Abiose BO, Oyejide O, Ogunniyi J. Salivary gland tumours in Ibadan, Nigeria: a study of 295 cases. *African Journal of Medical Sciences*, 1990; 19: 195–9.

48. van der Waal I. Salivary gland neoplasms. In *Oral diseases in the Tropics* (ed. R Prabhu *et al.*). Oxford: Oxford University Press, 1991: Chapter 41.

49. Loyola AM, de-Araujo VC, de-Sousa SO, de-Araujo NS. Minor salivary gland tumours: a retrospective study of 164 cases. *European Journal of Cancer, B Oral Oncology*, 1995; 31B: 197–201.

50. Nagler RM, Laufer D. Tumours of the major and minor salivary glands: a review of 25 years experience. *Anticancer Research*, 1997; 17: 701–7.

51. Rivera-Bastidas H, Ocanto RA, Acevedo AM. Intra-oral salivary gland tumours: a retrospective study of 62 cases in a Venezualan population. *Journal of Oral Pathology and Medicine*, 1996; 25: 1–4.

52. van Heerden WF, Raubenheimer EJ. Intraoral salivary gland neoplasms: a retrospective study of seventy cases in an African population. *Oral Surgery, Oral Medicine, Oral Pathology*, 1991; 71: 579–82.

53. Spiro RH, Thaler HT, Hicks WF, Kher UA, Huvos AH, Strong EW. The importance of clinical staging of minor salivary gland carcinoma. 1991; 162: 330–6.

54. Arotiba GT. Salivary gland neoplasms in Lagos, Nigeria. *West African Journal of Medicine*, 1996; 15: 11–17.

55. Shore-Freedman E, Abrahams C, Recant W, Schneider AB. Neurilemmomas and salivary gland tumours of the head and neck following childhood irradiation. *Cancer*, 1983; 51 2159–63.

56. Land CE, Saku T, Hayashi Y, Takahara O, Matsuura H, Tokuoka S. Incidence of salivary gland tumours among atomic bomb survivors. *Radiation Research*, 1996; 146: 28–3.

57. Saku T, *et al.* Salivary gland tumours among atomic bomb survivors, 1950–1987. *Cancer*, 1997; 79: 1465–75.

58. Kotwall CA. Smoking as an aetiologic factor in the development of Warthin's tumour of the parotid gland. *American Journal of Surgery*, 1992; 164: 646–7.

59. Eneroth CM. Malignant melanoma of the oral cavity. *International Journal of Oral Surgery*, 1975; 4: 191–7.

60. Barrett AW, Bennett JH, Speight PM. A clinicopathological and immunohistochemical analysis of primary oral mucosal melanoma. *European Journal of Cancer: B Oral Oncology*, 1995; 31B: 100–5.

61. Bovo R, Farruggio A, Agnoletto M, Galceran M, Polidoro F. Primitive malignant melanoma of the base of the tongue. *Acta Otorhinolaryngologica Italica*, 1996; 16: 371–4.

62. Manganaro AM, Hammond HL, Dalton MJ, Williams TP. Oral melanoma: case reports and review of the literature. *Oral Surgery, Oral Medicine, Oral Pathology, Oral Radiology, and Endodontics*, 1995; 80: 670–6.

63. Soman CS, Sirsat MV. Primary malignant melanoma of the oral cavity in Indians. *Oral Surgery, Oral Medicine, Oral Pathology*, 1974; 38: 426–34.

64. Chaudry AP, Hampel A, Gorlin RJ. Primary malignant melanoma of the oral cavity; a review of 105 cases. *Cancer*, 1958; **11**: 923–8.

65. Goubran GF, Adekeye EO, Edwards MB. Melanoma of the face and mouth in Nigeria: a review and comment of three cases. *International Journal of Oral Surgery*, 1978; 7: 453–62.

66. Umeda M, Shimada K. Primary malignant melanoma of the oral cavity: its histological classification and treatment. *British Journal of Oral and Maxillofacial Surgery*, 1994; **32**: 39–47.

67. Chiu NT, Weinstock MA. Melanoma of oronasal mucosa. Population based analysis of occurrence and mortality. *Archives of Otolaryngology—Head and Neck Surgery*, 1996; **122**: 985–8.

68. Koufusan JA, Burk AJ. The aetiology and pathogenesis of laryngeal carcinoma. *Otolaryngology Clinics of North America*, 1997; **30**: 1–19.

69. Canon-Albright LA, *et al.* Familiarity of cancer in Utah. *Cancer Research*, 1994; **54**: 2378–85.

70. Holloway SM, Sofaer JA. Coefficients of relationship by isonomy among oral cancer registrations in Scottish males. *Community Dentistry and Oral Epidemiology*, 1992; **20**: 284–7.

71. Merrick Y, Albeck H, Nielsen NH, Hansen HS. Familial clustering of salivary gland carcinoma in Greenland. *Cancer*, 1986; **57**: 2097–112.

72. Ankathil R, *et al.* Mutagen sensitivity as a predisposing factor in familial oral cancer. *International Journal of Cancer*, 1996; **69**: 265–7.

73. Ankathil R, Mathew A, Joseph F, Nair MK. Is oral cancer susceptibility inherited? Report of five oral cancer families. *European Journal of Cancer: B Oral Oncology*, 1996; **32B**: 63–7.

74. Copper MP, *et al.* Role of genetic factors in the aetiology of squamous cell carcinoma of the head and neck. *Archives of Otolaryngology—Head and Neck Surgery*, 1995; **121**: 157–60.

75. Goldstein AM, *et al.* Familial risk in oral and pharyngeal cancer. *European Journal of Cancer, B Oral Oncology*, 1994; **30B**: 319–22.

76. Pukkala E, Notkola V. Cancer incidence among Finnish farmers, 1979–93. *Cancer Causes Control*, 1997; **8**: 25–33.

77. Antoniades DZ, Styanidis K, Papanayatou P, Trigonidis G. Squamous cell carcinoma of the lips in a northern Greek population: evaluation of prognostic factors on five year survival rate. *European Journal of Cancer: B Oral Oncology*, 1995; **31B**: 333–9.

78. Pogoda JM, Preston-Martin S. Solar radiation, lip protection and lip cancer risk in Los Angeles county women. *Cancer Causes and Control*, 1996; 7: 458–63.

79. Swerdlow AJ, Marmot MG, Grunlicj AE. Cancer mortality in Indian and British ethnic immigrants from the Indian subcontinent to England and Wales. *British Journal of Cancer*, 1995; **72**: 1312–19.

80. Wake M. The urban/rural divide in head and neck, cancer—the effect of atmospheric pollution. *Clinical Otolaryngology*, 1993; **18**: 298–302.

81. Dietz A, Senneweld E, Maier H. Indoor air pollution by emissions of fossil fuel single stoves: possibly a hitherto underrated risk factor in the development of carcinomas in the head and neck. *Otolaryngology—Head and Neck Surgery*, 1995; **112**: 308–15.

82. Michelozzi   P, Fusco D, Forastiere F, Ancona C, Dell'Orco V, Perucci CA. Small area study of mortality among people living near multiple sources of air pollution. *Occupational and Environmental Medicine Journal*, 1998; **55**: 611–15.

83. Maier H, Tisch M, Enderle G, Dietz A, Weidauer H. Berufliche Exposition gegenuber Farben, Lacken und Losungsmittein und Krebsrisiko intramuscular Bereich des oberen Aerodigestivtraktes. *HNO*, 1997; **45**: 905–8.

84. Huebner WW, *et al.* Oral and pharyngeal cancer and occupation: a case-control study. *Epidemiology*, 1992; 3: 300–9.

85. De Stefani E, Boffeta P, Oreggia F, Ronco F, Kogevinas M, Mendilaharsu M. Occupation and the risk of laryngeal cancer in Uruguay. *American Journal of Industrial Medicine*, 1998; **33**: 537–42.

86. Streenland K. Laryngeal cancer among workers exposed to acid mists. *Cancer Causes and Control*, 1997; **8**: 34–8.

87. Epstein JB. Management of oral Kaposi's sarcoma and a proposal for clinical staging. *Oral Diseases*, 1997; 3(Suppl. 1): S124–S128.

88. Jordan RCK, Chong L, DiPierdomenico S, Satita F, Main JHP. Oral lymphoma in HIV infection. *Oral Diseases*, 1997; 3(Suppl. 1): S135–137.

89. Singh B, Balwally AN, Shaha AR, Rosenfeld RM, Har-El G, Lucente FE. Upper aerodigestive tract squamous cell carcinoma. The human immunodeficiency virus connection. *Archives of Otolaryngeal and Head and Neck Surgery*, 1996; **122**: 639–43.

90. King GN, *et al.* Increased prevalence of dysplastic and malignant lip lesions in renal transplant recipients. *New England Journal of Medicine*, 1995; **332**: 1052–8.

91. Franceschi S, *et al.* Smoking and drinking in relation to cancers of the oral cavity, pharynx, larynx and oesophagus in Northern Italy. *Cancer Research*, 1990; **50**: 6502–7.

92. Doll R, *et al.* Mortality in relation to smoking: 40 years observations on male British doctors. *British Medical Journal*, 1994; **309**: 901–11.

93. Daftary DK, Murti PR, Bhonsle RB, Gupta PC, Mehta FS, Pindborg JJ. Risk factors and risk markers for oral cancer in high incidence areas of the world. In *Risk markers for oral diseases*, Vol. 1: *Oral cancer* (ed. NW Johnson). Cambridge: Cambridge University Press, 1991: 29–63.

94. Gupta PC, Hamner JE, Murti PR. *Control of tobacco-related cancers and other diseases*. Delhi: Oxford University Press, 1992.

95. Idris AM, Ahmed HM, Malik MAO. Toombak dipping and cancer of the oral cavity in the Sudan: a case control study. *International Journal of Cancer*, 1995; **63**: 477–80.

96. Idris AM, Warnakulasuriya KAAS, Ibrahim YE, Nilsen R, Cooper D, Johnson NW. Toombak associated oral mucosal lesions in Sudanese show a low prevalence of epithelial dysplasia. *Journal of Oral Pathology and Medicine*, 1996; **25**: 239–44.

97. Zain RB, Gupta PC, Warnakulasuriya S, Shrestha P, Ikeda N, Axell T. Oral lesions associated with betel quid and tobacco chewing habits. *Oral Diseases*, 1997; 3: 204–5.

98. MacLennan R, Paissat D, Ring A, Thomas S. Possible aetiology of oral cancer in Papua New Guinea. *Papua New Guinea Medical Journal*, 1985; **28**: 3–8.

99. Boucher BJ. Betel quid, smokeless tobacco and general health. In *Betel quid and tobacco chewing among the Bangladeshi community in the United Kingdom; usage and health issues* (ed. R Bedi, P Jones). London: Centre for Transcultural Oral Health, 1995.

100. Bedi R, Jones P. (ed.) *Betel-quid and tobacco chewing amongst the Bangladeshi community in the United Kingdom—usage and health issues*. London: Centre for Transcultural Oral Health, 1995.

101. Daftary DK, Murti PR, Bhonsle RB, Gupta PC, Mehta FS, Pindborg JJ. In *Oral diseases in the Tropics* (ed. SR Prabhu, DF Wilson, DK Daftary, NW Johnson). Oxford: Oxford Medical, 1992: 402–48.

102. Thomas S, Wilson, A. A quantitative evaluation of the role of betel quid in oral carcinogenesis. *Oral Oncology*, 1993; **29B**: 265–71.

103. Sankaranarayanan R, Duffy SW, Day NE, Nair MK, Padmakumary G. A case control investigation of cancer of the oral tongue and the floor of the mouth in Southern India. *International Journal of Cancer*, 1989, **44**: 617–21.

104. Sankaranarayanan R, Duffy SW, Padmakumary G, Day NE, Nair MK. Risk factors for cancer of the buccal and labial mucosa in Kerala, Southern India. *Journal of Epidemiology and Community Health*, 1990; **44**: 286–92.

105. Sankaranarayanan R, Duffy SW, Padmakumary G, Day NE, Padmanabhan TK. Tobacco chewing, alcohol and nasal snuff in cancer of the gingiva in Kerala, India. *British Journal of Cancer*, 1989; **60**: 638–43.

106. Notani PN. Role of alcohol in cancers of the upper alimentary tract, use of models in risk assessment. *Journal of Epidemiology and Community Health*, 1988; **42**: 187–92. [For hospital based controls.]

107. Idem—for community controls.

108. Jussawalla DJ, Deshpande VA. Evaluation of the risk in tobacco chewers and smokers, an epidemiologic assessment. *Cancer*, 1971; **28**: 244–52.

109. Jafarey NH Zaidi SH. Carcinoma of the oral cavity and oropharynx in Karachi, Pakistan—An appraisal. *Tropical Doctor*, 1976; **6**: 63–7.

110. Hirayama T. An epidemiological study of oral and pharyngeal cancer in central and southeast Asia. *Bulletin of the World Health Organisation*, 1966; **34**: 41–69.

111. Shanta V Krisnamurti S. Further studies on the aetiology of carcinomas of the upper alimentary tract. *British Journal of Cancer*, 1963; **17**: 8–23.

112. Chandra A. Different habits and their relation with cancer of the cheek. Chittaranjan Cancer Hospital, Calcutta National Cancer Research Centre. *Bulletin*, 1962; 33–36.

113. Sanghvi LD Rao KCM, Khanolkar VR. Smoking and chewing of tobacco in relation to cancer of the upper alimentary tract. *British Medical Journal*, 1955; **1**: 1111–14.

114. Simarak S, *et al.* Cancer of the oral cavity, pharynx/larynx and lung in North Thailand, case-control study and analysis of cigar smoke. *British Journal of Cancer*, 1977; **36**: 130–40.

115. Wahi PN, Kehar U, Lahiri B. Factors influencing and oropharyngeal cancers in India. *British Journal of Cancer*, 1965; **19**: 642–60.

116. Shanta V, Krishnamurti S. A study of aetiological factors in oral squamous cell carcinomas. *British Journal of Cancer*, 1959; **13**: 381–8.

117. Khanolkar VR. Oral cancer in India. *Unio Int Contra Cancrum. Acta*, 1959; **15**: 67–77.

118. Khanna NN, Pant GC, Tripathi FM, Sanyal B, Gupta S. Some observations on the aetiology of oral cancer. *Indian Journal of Cancer*, 1975; **12**: 77–83.

119. Orr IM. Oral cancer in betel nut chewers in Travancore, its aetiology, pathology and treatment. *Lancet*, 1933; **2**: 575–80.

120. Sarma SN. A study into the incidence and aetiology of cancer of the larynx and adjacent parts in Assam. *Indian Journal of Medical Research*, 1958; **46**: 525–33.

121. Gupta PC, Murti PR, Bhonsle RB, Mehta FS, Pindborg JJ. Effect of cessation of tobacco use on the incidence of oral mucosal lesions in a ten year follow up of 12212 users. *Oral Diseases*, 1995; **1**: 54–8.

122. International Agency for Research on Cancer. Tobacco habits other than smoking; Betel quid and areca nut chewing, and some related nitrosamines. *IARC Monographs for the Evaluation of Carcinogenic Risks to Humans*, Vol 37. Lyon: IARC, 1985.

123. Maher R, Lee AJ, Warnakulasuriya KAAS, Lewis JA, Johnson NW. Role of areca nut in the causation of oral submucous fibrosis: a case-control study in Pakistan. *Journal of Oral Pathology and Medicine*, 1994; **23**: 65–9.

124. Stich HF, Rosin MP, Brunnermann KD. Oral lesions, genotoxicity and nitrosamines in betel quid chewers with no obvious increase in oral cancer risk. *Cancer Letters*, 1986; **31**: 15–25.

125. Ko YC, Chiang TA, Chang SJ, Hsieh SF. Prevalence of betel quid chewing habit in Taiwan and related socio-demographic factors. *Journal of Oral Pathology and Medicine*, 1992; **21**: 261–4.

126. Thomas S, Kearsley J. Betel quid and oral cancer: a review. *Oral Oncology*, 1993; **29B**: 251–5.

127. Stich HF, Stich W, Parida BB. Elevated frequency of micronucleated cells in the buccal mucosa of individuals at high risk for oral cancer: betel quid chewers. *Cancer Letters*, 1982; **17**: 125–34.

128. Dave BJ, Trivedi AH, Adhvaryu SD. Role of areca nut in the cause of oral cancers. *Cancer*, 1992; **70**: 1017–23.

129. Lu CT. A case-control study of oral cancer in Changhua County, Taiwan. *Journal of Oral Pathology and Medicine*, 1996; **25**: 245–8.

130. Nagabhushan M, Amonkar AAJ, DeSouza AV. Nonmutagenicity of betel leaf and its anti-mutagenic action against environmental mutagens. *Neoplasma*, 1987; **34**: 159–68.

131. Brown RL, Shu JM, Scarborough JE, Wilkins SA, Smith RR. Snuff dippers intraoral cancer: clinical characteristics and response to therapy. *Cancer*, 1965; **18**: 2–13.

132. Ackerman LV. Verrucous carcinoma of the oral cavity. *Surgery*, 1948; **23**: 670–8.

133. McCoy JM, Waldron CA. Verrucous carcinoma of the oral cavity. *Oral Surgery, Oral Medicine, Oral Pathology*, 1981; **52**: 623–9.

134. Winn DM, Blot W, Shy CM, Pickle LW, Toledo A, Fraumeni JF. Snuff dipping and oral cancer amongst women in the southern United States. *New England Journal of Medicine,*. 1981; **304**: 749–95.

135. Winn DM. Smokeless tobacco: the epidemiological evidence. *CA: A Cancer Journal for Clinicians*, 1988; **38**: 236–43.

136. Connolly GN, Orleans CT, Kogan M. Use of smokeless tobacco in major league baseball. *New England Journal of Medicine*, 1998; **318**: 1281–5.

137. US Department of Health and Human Services. *The health consequences of using smokeless tobacco: a report of the advisory committee to the Surgeon General*. Bethesda, MD: National Institutes of Health, Public Health Service, 1986: NIH Publication No. 86–2874.

138. McCarten B. Smokeless tobacco: the Irish and EU experience. *Oral Diseases*, 1998; **4**: 56–7.

139. Grady D, *et al.* Oral mucosal lesions found in smokeless tobacco users. *Journal of the American Dental Association*, 1990; **121**: 117–23.

140. Tomar SL, Winn DM, Swango PA, Giovino GA, Kleinman DV. Oral smokeless tobacco lesions among adolescents in the United States. *Journal of Dental Research*, 1997; **76**: 1277–86.

141. *US National Mortality Followback Survey*. National Centre for Health Statistics, USA, 1986.

142. *National Health Interview Survey*. National Centre for Health Statistics, USA, 1987.

143. Sterling TD, Rosenbaum WL, Weinkam JJ. Analysis of the relationship between smokeless tobacco and cancer based on data from the national mortality followback survey. *Journal of Clinical Epidemiology*, 1992; **42**: 223–31.

144. Rodu B. *For smokers only: how smokeless tobacco can save your life*. New York: Sulzberger and Graham, 1995.

145. Schildt E-B, Eriksson M, Hardell L, Magnuson A. Oral infections and dental factors in relation to oral cancer: a Swedish case-control study. *European Journal of Cancer Prevention*, 1998; **6**: 201–6.

146. Lewin F, *et al.* Smoking tobacco, oral snuff and alcohol in the aetiology of squamous cell carcinoma of the head and neck: a population based case–referent study in Sweden. *Cancer*, 1998; **82**: 1367–75.

147. Huhtasaari F, Asplund K, Lundberg V, Stegmyr B, Wester PO. Tobacco and myocardial infarction: is snuff less dangerous than cigarettes? *British Medical Journal*, 1992; **305**: 1252–6.

148. Bolinder G, Alfresson L, Englund A, de Faire U. Smokeless tobacco use and increased cardiovascular mortality. *American Journal of Public Health*, 1994; **84**: 399–404.

149. Persson G, Hellers G, Ahlbom A. Use of moist snuff and inflammatory bowel disease. *International Journal of Epidemiology*, 1993; **22**: 1101–3.

150. Axell TE. Oral mucosal changes related to smokeless tobacco usage: research findings in Scandinavia. *European Journal of Cancer: Oral Oncology*, 1993; **29B**: 299–302.

151. Axell TE. Smokeless tobacco and oral health: the Swedish experience. *Oral Diseases*, 1998; **4**: 55–6.

152. International Agency for Research on Cancer. Tobacco smoking. *IARC Monographs on the evaluation of Carcinogenic Risks to Humans*, Vol 38. Lyon: IARC, 1986.

153. US Surgeon General's Report 1989

154. Wynder EL, Mushinski MH, Spivah JC. Tobacco and alcohol

consumption in relation to the development of multiple primary cancers. *Cancer*, 1977; **40**: 1872–8.

155. Javonovich A, Schulten EAJM, Kostense PJ, Snow GB, van der Waal I. Tobacco and alcohol related to the anatomic site of oral squamous cell carcinoma. *Journal of Oral Pathology and Medicine*, 1993; **22**: 459–62.

156. Blot WJ, *et al.* Smoking and drinking in relation to oral and pharyngeal cancer. *Cancer Research*, 1988; **48**: 3282–7.

157. Blot WJ. Alcohol and cancer. *Cancer Research*, 1992; **52**(Suppl.): 2119–23.

158. Mashberg A, Meyers H. Anatomical site and size of 222 early asymptomatic oral squamous cell carcinomas: a continuing prospective study of oral cancer II. *Cancer*, 37: 2149–57.

159. Bofetta P, *et al.* Carcinogenic effect of tobacco smoking and alcohol drinking on anatomic sites of the oral cavity and oropharynx. *International Journal of Cancer*, 1992; **52**: 530–3.

160. Gupta PC, *et al.* Incidence rates of oral cancer and natural history of oral precancerous lesions in a 10-year follow up study of Indian villagers. *Community Dentistry and Oral Epidemiology*, 1980; **8**: 287–333.

161. van der Eb MM, Leyten EM, Gavarasana S, Vandenbroucke JP, Kahn PM, Cleton FJ. Reverse smoking as a risk factor for palatal cancer: a cross-sectional study in rural Andhra Pradesh, India. *International Journal of Cancer*, 1993; **54**: 754–8.

162. Ortiz GM, Pierce AM, Wilson DF. Palatal changes associated with reverse smoking in Filipino women. *Oral Diseases*, 1996; **2**: 232–7.

163. Davidson BJ, Hsu TC, Schantz SP. The genetics of tobacco-induced malignancy. *Archives of Otolaryngology—Head and Neck Surgery*, 1995; **121**: 157–60.

164. Hecht SS, Carmella SG, Murphy SE, Foiles PG, Chung FL. Carcinogen biomarkers relating to smoking and upper aerodigestive tract cancer. *Journal of Cellular Biochemistry*, 1993; **7F**(Suppl.1): 27.

165. Hoffman D, Hecht SS. Nicotine derived *N*-nitrosamines and tobacco-related cancer: current status and future directions. *Cancer Research*, 1985; **45**: 935–44.

166. Lafuente A, *et al.* Glutathione and glutathione *S*-transferases in human squamous cell carcinomas of the larynx and GSTM1-dependent risk. *Anticancer Research*, 1998; **18**: 107–11.

167. Nahas G, Latour C. The human toxicity of marijuana. *Medical Journal of Australia*, 1993; **156**: 495–7.

168. Firth NA. Marijuana use and oral cancer: a review. *Oral Oncology*, 1997; **6**: 398–401.

169. Darling MR, Arendorf TM. Effects of cannabis smoking on oral soft tissues. *Community Dentistry and Oral Epidemiology*, 1993; **21**: 78–81.

170. International Agency for Research on Cancer. Alcohol drinking. In *IARC monographs on the evaluation of carcinogenic risks to humans*. Lyon: IARC, 1988.

171. Kato I, Nomura AM. Alcohol in the aetiology of upper aero-digestive tract cancer. *European Journal of Cancer: Part B Oral Oncology*, 1994; **30B**: 75–81.

172. Hindle I. PhD thesis: University of London, 1997.

173. Bundgaard T, Wildt J, Frydenberg M, Elbrond O, Nielson JE. Case-control study of squamous cell cancer of the oral cavity in Denmark. *Cancer Causes and Control*, 1995; **6**: 57–67.

174. Andre K, Schraub S, Mercier M, Bontemps P. Role of alcohol and tobacco in the aetiology of head and neck cancer: a case-control study in the Doubs region of France. *European Journal of Cancer: Part B Oral Oncology*, 1995; **31**: 301–9.

175. Zheng T, *et al.* Tobacco smoking, alcohol and risk of oral cancer: a case-control study in Beijing, People's Republic of China. *Cancer Causes and Control*, 1990; **1**: 173–9.

176. Boyle P, *et al.* European School of Oncology Advisory Report to the European Commision for the Europe Against Cancer Programme: oral carcinogenesis in Europe. *European Journal of Cancer: Part B Oral Oncology*, 1995; **31**: 75–85.

177. De Stefani E, Boffeta P, Oreggia F, Fierro L, Mendilaharsu M. Hard liquor drinking is associated with higher risk of cancer of the oral cavity and pharynx than wine drinking. A case-control study in Uruguay. *Oral Oncology*, 1998; **34**: 99–144.

178. La Vecchia C, Tavani A, Franceschi S, Levi F, Corragao G, Negri E. Epidemiology and prevention of oral cancer. *Oral Oncology*, 1997; **33**: 302–12.

179. Brugere J, Guenel P, Leclerc A, Rodrigues J. Differential effects of tobacco and alcohol in cancer of the larynx, pharynx and mouth. *Cancer*, 1986; **57**: 391–5.

180. Hsu TC, Furlong C, Spitz MR. Ethyl alcohol as a co-carcinogen with special reference to the aerodigestive tract: a cytogenetic study. *Anticancer Research*, 1991; **11**: 1097–102.

181. Squier CA, Cox P, Hall BK. Enhanced penetration of nitrosonornicotine across oral mucosa in the presence of ethanol. *Journal of Oral Pathology*, 1986; **15**: 276–9.

182. Trigkas TK, Cruchley AT, Williams DM, Wertz P, Squier CA. Human oral mucosal permeability is increased by short term exposure to ethanol. *Journal of Dental Research*, 1993; **72**: 694.

183. McCoy GD, Wynder EL. Etiological and preventive implications in alcohol carcinogenesis. *Cancer Research*, 1979; **39**: 2844–50.

184. Squier CA, Kremer M, Wertz PW. Ingestion of ethanol increases epithelial permeability in the rat. *Journal of Dental Research*, 1995; **74**: 476.

185. Enwonwu CO, Meeks VI. Bionutrition and oral cancer in humans. *Critical Reviews in Oral Biology and Medicine*, 1995; **6**: 5–17.

186. Homann N, Jousimies-Somer H, Jokelainen K, Heine R, Salaspuro M. High acetaldehyde levels in saliva after ethanol consumption: methodological aspects and pathogenetic implications. *Carcinogenesis*, 1997; **18**: 1739–43.

187. Harris C, Warnakulasuriya KAAS, Gelbier S, Johnson NW, Peters TJ. Oral and dental health in alcohol misusing patients. *Alcoholism: Clinical and Experimental Research*, 1997; **21**: 1707–9.

188. Winn DM, *et al.* Mouthwash use and oral conditions in the risk of oral and pharyngeal cancer. *Cancer Research*, 1991; **51**: 3044–7.

189. Elmore JG, Horwitz RI. Oral cancer and mouthwash use: evaluation of the epidemiologic evidence. *Otolaryngology—Head and Neck Surgery*, 1995; **113**: 153–261.

190. Shapiro S, Castellana JV, Sprafka JM. Alcohol-containing mouthwashes and oropharyngeal cancer: a spurious association due to underascertainment of confounders? *American Journal of Epidemiology*, 1996; **144**: 1091–5.

191. Bhatti SA, Walsh TF, Douglas CWI. Ethanol and pH levels of proprietary mouthwashes. *Community Dental Health*, 1994; **11**: 71–4.

192. Rich AM, Radden BG. Squamous cell carcinoma of the oral mucosa: a review of 244 cases in Australia. *Journal of Oral Pathology*, 1984; **13**: 459–71.

193. Hodge KM, Flynn MB, Drury T. Squamous cell carcinoma of the upper aerodigestive tract in nonusers of tobacco. *Cancer*, 1985; **55**: 1232–5.

194. Ng SKC, Kabat GC, Wynder EL. Oral cavity cancer in non-users of tobacco. *Journal of the National Cancer Institute*, 1993; **85**: 743–5.

195. Tan E-H, Adelstein DJ, Droughton MLT, van Kirk MA, Lavertu P. Squamous cell head and neck cancer in non-smokers. *American Journal of Clinical Oncology*, 1997; **20**: 146–50.

196. Agudelo D, Quer M, Leon X, Diez S, Burgues J. Laryngeal carcinoma in patients without a history of tobacco and alcohol use. *Head and Neck*, 1997; **19**: 200–4.

197. Vineis P, Brandt-Rauf PW. Mechanisms of carcinogenesis: chemical exposure and molecular changes. *European Journal of Cancer*, 1993; **29A**: 1344–7.

198. **zur Hausen H.** Human papillomaviruses in the pathogenesis of anogenital cancer. *Virology*, 1991; **184**: 9–13.

199. **Snijders PJF,** *et al.* Prevalence of mucosatropic human papillomaviruses in squamous cell carcinomas of the head and neck. *International Journal of Cancer*, 1996; **66**: 464–9.

200. **Bernard H-U, Apt D.** Transcriptional control and cell type specificity of HPV gene expression. *Archives of Dermatology*, 1994; **130**: 210–15.

201. **Sugerman PB, Shilitoe EJ.** The high risk human papilloma viruses and oral cancer: evidence for and against a causal relationship. *Oral Disease*, 1997; **3**: 130–47.

202. **Bauer G.** Interference of papilloma viruses with p53-dependent and –independent apoptotic pathways. Clues to viral oncogenesis (Review-hypothesis). *Oncology Reports*, 1997; **4**: 273–5.

203. **Woods KV, Shillitoe EJ, Spitz MR, Storthz K.** Analysis of human papillomavirus DNA in oral squamous cell carcinomas. *Journal of Oral Pathology and Medicine*, 1993; **22**: 101–8.

204. **Park NH, Min BM, Li SL, Haung MZ, Cherrick HM, Doniger J.** Immortilisation of normal human oral keratinocytes with type 16 human papillomavirus. *Carcinogenesis*, 1991; **12**: 1627–31.

205. **Sexton CJ,** *et al.* Characterisation of the factors involved in human papilloma virus type 16-mediated immortalisation of oral keratinocytes. *Journal of General Virology*, 1993; **74**: 755–61.

206. **Shin K-H, Tannyhill RJ Liu X, Park NH.** Oncogenic transformation of HPV-immortalised human oral keratinocytes is associated with genetic instability of cells. *Oncogene*, 1996; **12**: 1089–96.

207. **Penhallow J,** *et al.* p53 alterations and HPV infections are common in oral SCC: p53 gene mutations correlate with the absence of HPV-16-E6 DNA. *International Journal of Oncology*, 1998; **12**: 59–68.

208. **Riethdorf S,** *et al.* p53 mutations and HPV infection in primary head and neck, squamous cell carcinoma do not correlate with overall survival: a long term follow up study. *Journal of Oral Pathology and Medicine*, 1997; **26**: 315–21.

209. **Miller CS, White DK.** Human papillomavirus expression in oral mucosa, premalignant conditions, and squamous cell carcinoma. A retrospective review of the literature. *Oral Surgery, Oral Medicine, Oral Pathology, Oral Radiology and Endodontics*, 1996; **82**: 57–68.

210. **Ogura H, Watanbe S, Fukushima K, Masuda Y, Fujiwara T, Yebe Y.** Human papillomavirus DNA in squamous cell carcinomas of the respiratory and upper digestive tracts. *Japanese Journal of Clinical Oncology*, 1993; **23**: 221–5.

211. **Yeudall WA, Paterson IC, Patel V, Prime SS.** Presence of human papillomavirus sequence in tumour derived human oral keratinocytes expressing mutant p53. *European Journal of Cancer: Part B Oral Oncology*, 1995; **2**: 136–43.

212. **Elamin F, Steingrimsdottir H, Warnakulasuriya S, Johnson NW, Tavassoli M.** Prevalence of human papillomavirus infection in premalignant and malignant lesions of the oral cavity in UK subjects: a novel method of detection. *Oral Oncology*, 1998; **34**: 191–7.

213. **Nielsen H, Norrild B, Vedtofte P, Praetorius F, Reibel J, Homstrup P.** Human papillomavirus in oral premalignant lesions. *European Journal of Cancer: Part B Oral Oncology*, 1996; **32B**: 264–70.

214. **Palefsky JM, Silverman SS, Abdel-Salaam M, Daniels TE, Greenspan JS.** Association between proliferative verrucous leukoplakia and infection with human papillomavirus type 16. *Journal of Oral Pathology and Medicine*, 1995; **24**: 193–7.

215. **Warnakulasuriya KAAS, Speight PM, Tavassoli M, Elamin F, Penhallow J, Johnson NW.** Association between proliferative verrucous leukoplakia, p53 protein and HPV infection. *Oral Diseases*, 1997; **3**(Suppl. 1): S28.

216. **Ibrahim SO, Warnakulasuriya KAAS, Idris AM, Hirsch JM, Johnson NW, Jahannessen AC.** Expression of keratin 13, 14 and 19 in oral hyperplastic and dysplastic lesions from Sudanese and Swedish snuff-dippers: association with human papilloma virus infection. *Anticancer Research*, 1998; **18**: 635–45.

217. **Mao EJ, Schwartz SM, Daling JR, Oda D, Tickman L, Beckmann AAM.** Human papilloma virus and p53 mutations in normal, premalignant and malignant oral epithelia. *International Journal of Cancer (Prev. Oncol.)*, 1996; **69**: 152–8.

218. **Haraf DJ,** *et al.* Human papilloma virus and p53 in head and neck, cancer: clinical correlates and survival. *Cancer Research*, 1996; **2**: 755–62.

219. **Paz IB, Cook N,** 1997. Human papillomavirus (HPV) in head and neck, cancer. An association of HPV-16 with squamous cell carcinoma of Waldeyer's tonsilar ring. *Cancer*, 79: 595–604.

220. **McKaig RG, Baric RS, Olshan AF.** Human papilloma virus and head and neck, cancer: epidemiology and molecular biology. *Head and Neck*, 1998; **20**: 260–5.

221. **Cruz IBF,** *et al.* Age-dependence of human papillomavirus DNA presence in oral squamous cell carcinoma. *European Journal of Cancer, Part B Oral Oncology*, 1996; **32B**: 55–62.

222. **Turner JR, Sheen LH, Crum CP, Dean PJ, Odze RD.** Low prevalence of human papillomavirus infection in esophageal squamous cell carcinomas from North America. *Human Pathology*, 1997; **28**: 174–8.

223. **Arndt O, Johannes A, Zeise K, Brock J.** *Laryno Otologie*, 1997; **76**: 142–9.

224. **Poljak M, Gale N, Kambia V.** Human papillomaviruses: a study of their prevalence in the epithelial lympoplastic lesions of the larynx. *Acta Oto-Laryngologica Suppl. (Stockholm)*, 1997; **527**: 66–9.

225. **Larsson PA, Johansson SL, Vahlne A, Hirsch JM.** Snuff tumorigenesis: effects of long term snuff administration after initiation with 4-nitroquinoline *N*-oxide and herpes simplex virus type 1. *Journal of Oral Pathology and Medicine*, 1989; **18**: 187–92.

226. **Park K, Cherrick H, Min B-M, Park NH.** Active HSV-1 immunisation prevents the co-carcinogenic activity of HSV-1 in the oral cavity of hamsters. *Oral Surgery, Oral Pathology, Oral Medicine*, 1990; **70**: 186–91.

227. **Larsson PA, Edstrom S, Westin T, Nordkrist A, Hirsch JM, Vahlne A.** Reactivity against herpes simplex virus in patients with head and neck cancer. *International Journal of Cancer*, 1991; **49**: 14–18.

228. **De-The G.** The Epstein–Barr virus in neoplasms of the head and neck. In *Oral cancer: detection of patients and lesions at risk* (ed. NW Johnson). Cambridge: Cambridge University Press, 1991: 88–95.

229. **Shapira J, Peylan-Ramu N.** Burkitt's lymphoma. *Oral Oncology*, 1998; **34**: 15–23.

230. **Boulter A, Johnson NW, Birnbaum W, Teo CG.** Epstein–Barr virus (EBV) associated lesions of the head and neck. *Oral Diseases*, 1996; **2**: 117–24.

231. **Talacko AA, Teo CG, Griffin BE, Johnson NW.** Epstein–Barr virus receptors but not viral DNA are present in normal and malignant oral epithelium. *Journal of Oral Pathology and Medicine*, 1991; **20**: 20–5.

232. **D'Costa J, Saranath D, Sanghvi V, Mehta AR.** Epstein–Barr virus in tobacco-induced oral cancers and oral lesions from India. *Journal of Oral Pathology and Medicine*, 1998; **27**: 78–82.

233. **Sung NS, Edwards RH, Seiller-Moiseiwcitsch F, Perkins AG, Zeng F, Raab-Traub N.** Epstein–Barr virus strain variation in nasopharyngeal carcinoma from the endemic and non-endemic regions of China, 1998.

234. **Griffin BE, Xue SA.** Epstein–Barr virus infections and their association with human malignancies: some key questions. *Annals of Medicine*, 1998; **30**: 249–59.

235. **Rassekh CH,** *et al.* Combined Epstein–Barr virus and human papilloma virus infection in nasopharyngeal carcinoma. *Laryngoscope*, 1998; **108**: 362–7.

236. **Yadav M, Arivanathan M, Chandrashekran A, Tan BS, Hashim BY.** Human herpesvirus-6 (HHV-6) DNA and virus-encoded antigen in oral lesions. *Journal of Oral Pathology and Medicine*, 1997; **26**: 391–401.

237. **Boshoff C, Whitby D, Talbot S, Weiss RA.** Etiology of AIDS-related Kaposi's sarcoma and lymphoma. *Oral Diseases*, 1997; **3**(Suppl. 1): S129–S132.

238. Di Alberti L, *et al.* Detection of human herpesvirus-8 DNA in oral ulcer tissues of HIV infected individuals. *Oral Diseases,* 1997; **3**(Suppl. 1): S133–S144.

239. Porter SR, Lodi G, Chandler K, Kumar N. Development of squamous cell carcinoma in hepatitis C virus-associated lichen planus. *Oral Oncology,* 1997; **33**: 58–9.

240. Rindum JL, Stenderup A, Holmstrup P. Identification of candida albicans types related to healthy and pathological oral mucosa. *Journal of Oral Pathology and Medicine,* 1994; **23**: 406–12.

241. Barrett AW, Kingsmill VJ, Speight PM. The frequency of fungal infection in biopsies of oral mucosal lesions. *Oral Diseases,* 1998; **4**: 26–31.

242. Arendorf TM, Walker DM. Tobacco smoking and denture wearing as local aetiological factors in median rhomboid glossitis. *International Journal of Oral Surgery,* 1994; **13**: 511–15.

243. Galai N, Park LP, Wesch J, Visscher B, Riddler S, Margolick JB. Effect of smoking on the clinical progression of HIV-1 infection. *Journal of the Acquired Immune Deficiency Syndrome and Human Retrovirology,* 1997; **14**: 451–8.

244. Keogh P, Hald B, Holmstrup P. Possible mycological aetiology of oral mucosal carcinoma: catalytic potential of infecting *Candida albicans* and other yeasts in the production of *N*-nitrosobenzylmethylamine. *Carcinogenesis,* 1987; **8**: 1543–8.

245. Rennie JS, MacDonald DG. Cell kinetics of hamster ventral tongue epithelium in iron deficiency. *Archives of Oral Biology,* 1984; **29**: 195–9.

246. Ranasinghe AW, Johnson NW, Scragg MA. Iron deficiency depresses cell proliferation in hamster cheek pouch epithelium. *Cell and Tissue Kinetics,* 1987; **20**: 403–12.

247. Ranasinghe AW, Johnson NW, Scragg MA, Williams RA. Iron deficiency reduces cytochrome concentrations of mitochondria isolated from hamster cheek epithelium. *Journal of Oral Pathology and Medicine,* 1989; **18**: 582–5.

248. Prime SS, MacDonald DG, Rennie JS. The effect of iron deficiency on experimental carcinogenesis in the rat. *British Journal of Cancer,* 1983; **47**: 413–18.

249. Ranasinghe AW, Warnakulasuriya KAAS, Tennekoon GE, Seneviratne B. Oral mucosal changes in iron deficiency anaemia in Sri Lankan female population. *Oral Medicine, Oral Pathology* 1983; **55**: 29–32.

250. La Vecchia C, Tavani A. Fruit and vegetables and human cancer. *European Journal of Cancer Prevention,* 1998; **7**: 3–8.

251. Block G, Patterson B, Subar A. Fruit, vegetables and cancer prevention: a review of the epidemiological evidence. *Nutrition and Cancer,* 1992; **18**: 1–29.

252. Potter JD, Steinmetz K. Vegetables, fruit and phytoestrogens as preventive agents. In *Principles of chemoprevention* (ed. BW Stewart, D McGregor, O Kleihues). Lyon: IARC, 1996: Scientific Publication No. 139, 61–90.

253. Winn DM. Diet and nutrition in the aetiology of oral cancer. *American Journal of Clinical Nutrition,* 1995; **61**: 437S–445S.

254. McLaughlin JK, Gridley G, Block G, Winn DM, Preston-Martin S, Schoenberg JB. Dietary factors in oral and pharyngeal cancer. *Journal of the National Cancer Institute,* 1988; **80**: 1237–43.

255. Franceschi S, Bidoli E, Baron AE, *et al.* Nutrition and cancer of the oral cavity and pharynx in north-east Italy. *International Journal of Cancer,* 1991; **47**: 20–5.

256. Franceschi S, Barra S, LaVecchia C, Bidoli E, Negri E, Talimini R. Risk factors for cancer of the tongue and the mouth. A case-control study from northern Italy. *Cancer,* 1992; **70**: 2227–33.

257. Franco EL, Kowalski LP, Oliveira BV, *et al.* Risk factors for oral cancer in Brazil: a case-control study. *International Journal of Cancer,* 1989; **43**: 992–1000.

258. Zheng T, *et al.* A case-control study of oral cancer in Beijing, People's Republic of China. Associations with nutrient intakes, foods and food groups. *European Journal of Cancer Oral Oncology,* 1993; **29B**: 45–55.

259. Nomura AM, Ziegler RG, Stemmerman GN, Chyou PH, Craft NE. Serum micronutrients and upper aerodigestive tract cancer. *Cancer Epidemiological Biomarkers and Prevention,* 1997; **6**: 407–12.

260. Riboli E, Kaaks R, Esteve J. Nutrition and laryngeal cancer. *Cancer Causes and Control* 1990; **1**: 147–56.

261. Zheng T, Boyle P, Hu HF. Dentition, oral hygiene and risk of oral cancer: a case-control study in Beijing, People's Republic of China. *Cancer Causes and Control,* 1990; **1**: 235–41.

262. Velly AM, *et al.* Relationship between dental factors and risk of upper aerodigestive tract cancer. *Oral Oncology,* 1998; **34**: 284–91.

263. Lockhart PB, Norris CM, Pulliam C. Dental factors in the genesis of squamous carcinoma of the oral cavity. *Oral Oncology,* 1998; **34**: 133–9.

264. World Health Organisation. *Tobacco Control Initiative: rationale, update and progress.* Geneva: WHO, 1998.

265. Centres for Disease Control and Prevention. Preventing and controlling oral and pharyngeal cancer: recommendations from a National Strategic Planning Conference (*http: //www.cdc.gov/epo/mmwr/preview/mmwrhtml/00054567.htm*). *Morbidity and Mortality Weekly Reports,* 1998; **47**: RR-14.

266. Department of Health. *Smoking kills: a White paper on tobacco.* London: HMSO, 1998.

267. Department of Health. *Report of the Scientific Committee on Tobacco and Health.* London: HMSO. 1998.

268. Peto R, *et al.* Mortality from smoking worldwide. *British Medical Bulletin,* 1996; **52**: 12–21; and *Tobacco or health: a global status report.* Geneva: WHO, 1997.

269. Peto R, Lopez AD, Boreham J. *Mortality from smoking in developing countries 1950–2000—Imperial Cancer Research Fund and World Health Organisation.* Oxford University Press. 1994

270. World Health Organisation. *Tobacco or health: a global status report.* Geneva: WHO, 1997.

271. *British Journal of Addiction,* 1992; **87**: 527–8.

272. Health Education Authority and University of York. *Cost effectiveness of smoking cessation interventions.* London: Centre for Health Economics, 1998.

273. Stead M, Hastings G, Tudor-Smith C. Preventing adolescent smoking: a review of options. *Health Education Journal,* 1996; **55**: 31–54.

274. FDI World Dental Federation. *Statements on oral cancer, Toluidine Blue and on tobacco.* (*http//www.worldserver.pipex.com/worldental*). 1999.

275. Cohen SJ, *et al.* Helping smokers quit: a randomised controlled trial with private practice dentists. *Journal of the American Dental Association,* 1989; **118**: 41–5.

276. Segnan N, Ponti A, Battista RN, *et al.* A randomised trial of smoking cessation interventions in general practice in Italy. *Cancer Causes and Control,* 1991; **2**: 239–46.

277. Russell MA, *et al.* Targeting heavy smokers in general practice: randomised controlled trial of transdermal nicotine patches. *British Medical Journal,* 1993; **306**: 1308–12.

278. Stapleton JA, *et al.* Dose effects and predictors of outcome in a randomised trial of transdermal nicotine patches in general practice. *Addiction,* 1995; **90**: 31–42.

279. Macgregor IDM. Efficacy of dental health advice as an aid to reducing cigarette smoking. *British Dental Journal,* 1996; **180**: 292–6.

280. Smith SE, Warnkaulasuriya KAAS, Feyrabend C, Belcher M, Cooper DJ, Johnson NW. A smoking cessation programme conducted through dental practices in the UK. *British Dental Journal,* 1998; **185**: 299–303.

281. Mecklenburg RE, Greenspan D, Kleinman DV. Tobacco effects in the mouth. Washington DC: US Dept of Health and Human Services, 1996: NIH Publication No. 96–3330.

282. American Academy of Periodontology Position Paper: Tobacco use and the periodontal patient. *J Periodontal* 1996; **67**: 51–6.

283. EU Working Group on Tobacco and Oral Health. *Oral Diseases,* 1998; **4**: 48–67.

284. **Sachs DPL.** Advances in smoking cessation treatment. In *Current pulmonology*, Vol. 12 (ed. ?? Simmons). Chicago: Year Book Publishers, 1991: 139–98.

285. **Pierce JP, Gilpin E, Farkas AJ.** Nicotine patch use in the general population: results from the 1993 California tobacco survey. *Journal of the National Cancer Institute*, 1995; **87**: 87–93.

286. **Silagy C, Mant D, Fowler G, Lodge M.** Meta-analysis on efficacy of nicotine replacement therapies in smoking cessation. *Lancet*, 1994; **343**: 139–42.

287. **Hackshaw AK, Law MR, Wald NJ.** The accumulated evidence on lung cancer and environmental tobacco smoke. *British Medical Journal*, 1997; **315**: 980–8.

288. **California Environmental Protection Agency, Office of Environmental Health Hazard Assessment.** *Health effects of environmental exposure to tobacco smoke* (http://www.calepa.cahwnet.gov/oehha/docs/finalets.htm). Sacramento, CA: California Environmental Protection Agency, 1997.

289. **US Environmental Protection Agency.** *Respiratory health effects of passive smoking: lung cancer and other disorders.* Washington DC: EPA, 1992: Publication EPA/600/6–90/006F.

290. **World Health Organisation.** *International consultation on environmental tobacco smoke (ETS) and child health.* Geneva: WHO, 1999.

291. **McGinnis JM, Foege WH.** Actual causes of death in the United States. *Journal of the American Medical Association*, 1993; **270**: 2207–12.

292. **Gray JD, Bhopal RS, White M.** Developing a medical school policy. *Medical Education*, 1998; **32**: 138–42.

293. **Day GL, et al.** Racial differences in risk of oral and pharyngeal cancer: alcohol, tobacco and other determinants. *Journal of the National Cancer Institute*, 1993; **85**: 465–73.

294. **Macfarlane GJ, Sharp L, Porter S, Franceschi S.** Trends in survival from cancers of the oral cavity and pharynx in Scotland: a clue as to why the disease is becoming more common. *British Journal of Cancer*, 1996; **73**: 805–8.

295. **Bradley KA, Bush KR, McDonell MB, Malone T, Fihn SD.** Screening for problem drinking: comparison of CAGE and AUDIT. Ambulatory Care Quality Improvement Project (ACQUIP). Alcohol Use Disorders Identification Test. *Journal of General Internal Medicine*, 1998; **13**: 379–88.

296. **Saunders JB, Aasland OG, Babor TF, De La Fuente JR, Grant M.** Development of alcohol use disorders identification test (AUDIT): WHO collaborative project on early detection of persons with harmful alcohol consumption—11. *Addiction*, 1993; **88**: 791–804.

297. **Long CG, Williams M, Hollin CR.** Treating alcohol problems: a study of programme effectiveness and cost effectiveness according to length and delivery of treatment. *Addiction*, 1998; **93**: 561–71.

298. **Gomel MK, Wutzke SE, Hardcastle DM, Lapsley H, Reznik RB.** Cost-effectiveness of strategies to market and train primary health care physicians in brief intervention techniques for hazardous alcohol use. *Social Science and Medicine*, 1998; **47**: 203–11.

299. **Richmond RL, G-Novak K, Kehoe L, Calfas G, Mendelsohn CP, Wodak A.** Effect of training on general practitioners' use of brief intervention for excessive drinkers. *Australian and New Zealand Journal of Public Health*, 1998; **22**: 206–9.

300. **Subcommittee on Health Services Research, National Advisory Council on Alcohol Abuse and Alcoholism.** *Improving the delivery of alcohol treatment and prevention services: executive summary.* Bethesda MD: National Institute on Alcohol Abuse and Alcoholism, National Institutes of Health, Department of Health and Human Services, 1997: NIH Publication No. 4224.

301. **Klatsky AL, Armstrong MA, Friedman GD.** Alcohol and mortality. *Annals of Internal Medicine*, 1992; **117**: 646–54.

302. **Gazioano JM, et al.** Moderate alcohol intake, increased levels of high density lipoprotein and its sub-fractions, and decreased risk of myocardial infarction. *New England Journal of Medicine*, 1993; **329**: 1829–34.

303. **Pearson TA.** Alcohol and heart Disease. *Circulation*, 1995; **94**: 3023–25.

304. **Suh I, Shaten BJ, Cutler JA, Kuller LH.** Alcohol use and mortality from coronary heart disease: the role of high-density lipoprotein cholesterol—for the Multiple Risk Factor Intervention Trial Research Group. *Annals of Internal Medicine*, 1992; **116**: 881–7.

305. **Ridker PM, Vaughan DE, Stampfer MJ, Glynn RJ, Hennekens CH.** Association of moderate alcohol consumption and plasma concentration of endogenous tissue-type plasminogen activator. *Journal of the American Journal Of Medicine*, 1994; **272**: 929–33.

306. **Jang M, et al.** Cancer chemopreventive effect of resveratrol, a natural product derived from grapes. *Science*, 1997; **275**: 218–20.

307. **Rimm EB, Klatsky A, Grobbee D, Stampfer MJ.** Review of moderate alcohol consumption and reduced risk of coronary heart disease: is the effect due to beer, wine or spirits. *British Medical Journal*, 1996; **312**: 731–6.

308. **McKee M, Britton A.** The positive relationship between alcohol and heart disease in Eastern Europe: potential physiological mechanisms. *Journal of the Royal Society of Medicine*, 1998; **91**: 402–7.

309. **Health Education Authority.** *That's the limit—a guide to sensible drinking.* London: HEA, 1992.

310. **Doll R.** The prevention of cancer: opportunities and challenges. In *Reducing the risk of cancers* (ed. T Heller, B Davey, L Bailey). London: Hodder and Stoughton, 1989.

311. **Hakama M, Beral V, Buiatti E, Faivre J, Parkin DM (ed.).** *Chemoprevention in cancer control.* Lyon: IARC, 1996: Scientific Publication No. 136.

312. **Stewart BW, McGregor D, Kleihues P (ed.).** *Principles of chemoprevention.* Lyon: IARC, 1996: Scientific Publication No. 139.

313. **American Cancer Society Advisory Committee on Diet, Nutrition and Cancer Prevention.** Guidelines in diet, nutrition and cancer prevention: reducing the risk of cancer with healthy food choices and physical activity. *CA: A Cancer Journal for Clinicians*, 1996; **46**: 325–41.

314. **Chamberlain J, Moss S.** *Focus on cancer: evaluation of cancer screening.* London: Springer, 1996.

315. **Wilson JMG, Jungner G.** *Principles and practice of screening for disease.* WHO: Geneva, 1968: Public Health Paper No. 34.

316. **Sankaranarayanan R, et al.** Chemoprevention of oral leukoplakia with vitamin A and beta carotene: an assessment. *Oral Oncology*, 1977; **33**: 231–6.

317. **Tradati N, et al.** Oral leukoplakias: to treat or not? *Oral Oncology*, 1997; **33**: 317–21.

318. **Speight PM, Downer MC, Zakrzewska JM (ed.)** Screening for oral cancer and precancer: report of a UK working group. *Community Dental Health*, 1993; **10**(Suppl. 1): 1–89.

319. **Rodrigues VC, Moss SM, Tuomainen H.** Oral cancer in the UK: to screen or not screen. *Oral Oncology*, 1998; **34**: 454–65.

320. **Franceschi S, Barzan L, Talamini R.** Screening for cancer of the head and neck: if not now, when? *Oral Oncology*, 1997; **33**: 313–16.

321. **Downer MC, Jullien JA, Speight PM.** An interim determination of health gain from oral cancer and prescreening: 1. Obtaining health state utilities. *Community Dental Health*, 1997; **14**: 139–42.

322. **Warnakulasuriya KAAS, Johnson NW.** Strengths and weaknesses of screening programmes for oral malignancies and potentially malignant lesions. *European Journal of Cancer Prevention*, 1996; **5**: 93–8.

323. **Ross NM, Gross E.** Oral findings based on an automated multiphasic health screening programme. *Journal of Oral Medicine*, 1971; **26**: 21–6.

324. **Folsom PC, White CP, Bromer L.** Oral exfoliative cytology. Review of literature and a report of a three year study. *Oral Surgery*, 1972; **33**: 61–74.

325. **Axell TE.** A prevalence study of oral mucosal lesions in an adult Swedish population. Thesis. *Odontologisk Revy*, 1976; **27**: Suppl. 36.

326. **Mehta FS, Pindborg JJ, Gupta PC, et al.** Epidemiologic and histologic

study of oral cancer among 50 915 villagers in India. *Cancer*, 1969; **24**: 832–49.

327. Bouquot JE, Gorlin RJ. Leukoplakia, lichen planus and other oral keratoses in 23,616 White Americans over the age of 35 years. *Oral Surgery*, 1986; **61**: 378–81.

328. Ikeda N, Ishi T, Iida S, Kawai T. Epidemiological study of oral leukoplakia based on mass screening for oral mucosal diseases in a selected Japanese population. *Community Dentistry and Oral Epidemiology*, 1991; **19**: 160–3.

329. Banoczy J, Rigo O. Prevalence study of oral precancerous lesions within a complex screening system in Hungary. *Community Dentistry and Oral Epidemiology*, 1991; **19**: 265–7.

330. Jullien JA, *et al.*. Attendance and compliance at an oral cancer screening programme in a general medical practice. *Oral Oncology, European Journal of Cancer* 1995**31B**: 202–206.

331. Ikeda N, *et al.* Characteristics of participants and non-participants in annual mass screening for oral cancer in 60 year old residents of Tokoname city, Japan. *Community Dental Health*, 1995; **12**: 83–8.

332. Roberts CJ, Farrow SC, Charny MC. How much can the NHS afford to spend to save a life or avoid a severe disability? *Lancet*, 1985; **1**: 89–91.

333. Sankaranarayanan R. Health care auxiliaries in the detection and prevention of oral cancer. *Oral Oncology*, 1997; **33**: 149–54.

334. Warnakulasuriya KAAS, Pindborg JJ. Reliability of oral precancer screening by primary health care workers in Sri Lanka. *Community Dental Health*, 1990; **7**: 73–9.

335. Santana JC, *et al.* Oral cancer case finding programme (OCCFP). *Oral Oncology*, 1977; **33**: 10–12.

336. Califano J, *et al.* Genetic progression model for head and neck cancer; implications for field cancerisation. *Cancer Research*, 1996; **56**: 2488–92.

337. Partridge M, Emilion G, Pateromichelakis S. Field cancerisation of the oral cavity: comparison of the spectrum of molecular alterations in cases presenting with both dysplastic and malignant lesions. *Oral Oncology*, 1997; **33**: 332–7.

338. Ogden GR. Field cancerisation in the head and neck. *Oral Diseases*, 1998; **4**: 1–3.

339. Jyothirmayi R, *et al.* Efficacy of vitamin A in the prevention of loco-regional recurrence and second primaries in head and neck cancer. *European Journal of Cancer: Part B Oral Oncology*, 1996; **32B**: 373–6.

340. Lippman SM, *et al.* Strategies for chemoprevention study of premalignancy and second primary tumours in the head and neck. *Current Opinion in Oncology*, 1995; **7**: 234–41.

341. Sankaranarayanan R, *et al.* Chemoprevention of cancers of the oral cavity and the head and neck. In *Principles of chemoprevention* (ed. BW Stewart, D McGregor, P Kleihues). Lyon: IARC, 1996: IARC Scientific Publication No. 139.

342. Tanaka T. Chemoprevention of oral carcinogenesis. *Oral Oncology*, 1995; **31B**: 3–15.

343. De Stefani E, Deneo-Pelligrini H, Mendilaharsu M, Ronco A. Diet and risk of cancer of the upper aerodigestive tract—1. Foods; II. *Oral Oncology*, 1999; **35**: 17–21.

344. Stich HF, Mathew B, Sankaranarayanan R, Krishnan Nair M. Remission of oral precancerous lesions of tobacco/areca nut chewers following administration of β-carotene or vitamin A, and maintenance of the protective effect. *Cancer Detection and Prevention*, 1991; **15**: 93–8.

345. Lippman SM, *et al.* Comparison of low dose isotretinoin with beta carotene to prevent oral carcinogenesis. *New England Journal of Medicine*, 1993; **328**: 15–20.

346. Benner SE, Pajak TF, Lippman SSM, Earley C, Hong WK. Prevention of second primary tumours with isotretinoin in patients with squamous cell carcinoma of the head and neck: long term follow up. *Journal of the National Cancer Institute*, 1994; **86**: 140–1.

347. Bolla M, *et al.* Prevention of second primary tumours with etretinate in squamous cell carcinoma of the oral cavity and oropharynx. Results of a multicentric double blind randomised study. *European Journal of Cancer*, 1994; **30A**: 767–72.

348. Schwartz JL, Shklar G. Retinoid and carotenoid angiogenesis: a possible explanation for enhanced oral carcinogenesis. *Nutrition and Cancer*, 1997; **27**: 192–9.

349. Garewell H. Antioxidants in oral cancer prevention. *American Journal of Clinical Nutrition*, 1995; **62**(Suppl.): S1410–S1416.

350. Prasad MPR, Mukundan MA, Krishnaswamy K. Micronuclei and carcinogen DNA adducts as intermediate end points in nutrient intervention trail of precancerous lesions in the oral cavity. *Oral Oncology*, 1995; **31B**: 155–9.

351. Khuri FR, Leppman SSM, Spitz MR, Lotan R, Hong WK. Molecular epidemiology and chemoprevention of head and neck cancer. *Journal of the National Cancer Institute*, 1997; **39**: 199–211.

9.1.2 Pathology of head and neck cancers

Andrew Gallimore

General considerations

The head and neck region is host to a multitude of both benign and malignant tumours, including an enormous variety of types of carcinoma, lymphomas, and tumours of the bone and soft tissues. It is fair to say that almost all tumours occurring elsewhere in the body may be seen in the head and neck. Such a cornucopia of pathology and differential diagnosis requires pathologists to open their minds to all possibilities when dealing with neoplasms in this region.

For most cases experience and awareness are all that are required in reaching a diagnosis, but in other instances the use of ancillary diagnostic techniques, such as immunohistochemistry, is invaluable. A prime example of this is in the diagnosis of small round cell tumours in the nasal cavity, where, in some cases, the differential diagnosis of malignant melanoma, undifferentiated sinonasal carcinoma, olfactory neuroblastoma, lymphoma, and embryonal rhabdomyosarcoma requires such special techniques.

Tissue for pathological examination may be obtained by a number of means, including biopsy under direct vision or endoscopically, by excision needle biopsy, or by fine needle aspiration. The latter is used for obtaining samples for cytological examination. Cytology has a particularly prominent role in the preoperative diagnosis of salivary gland lesions and for lumps in the neck. Other methods of obtaining tissue are avoided in the latter situation, for fear of implanting malignant tumour locally.

Although the head and neck is a source of an enormous diversity of pathology, by far the commonest tumour of mucosal surface origin in the region is squamous carcinoma. As in the bronchus and uterine cervix, preinvasive dysplastic lesions may be recognized.

Epithelial hyperplasia, dysplasia, and carcinoma *in situ*

Epithelial hyperplasia occurs as a reaction to injury. It is a common finding in smokers and, in the larynx, in those who abuse their voice. When arising in the respiratory epithelium of the supraglottis and subglottis the epithelium is thickened by a proliferation of reserve cells which, in the early stages, is covered by columnar epithelium, but later on this progresses to complete squamous metaplasia. That arising in the stratified squamous epithelium of the glottis is characterized by surface hyperkeratosis or parakeratosis. The latter lesion is known as keratosis, and appears clinically as a thickened white vocal cord. Lesions with a warty appearance are referred to as verrucous keratosis.

Leukoplakia is a clinical term which describes a white patch on the mucosal surface. In the oral mucosa, this is subclassified into homogeneous, nodular, erosive, and papillary verrucous forms. The histology underlying the mucosal change common to all types of leukoplakia is acanthosis, associated with hyperkeratosis and parakeratosis. The critical feature is the presence and degree of epithelial dysplasia since this may progress to invasive squamous carcinoma. There is some correlation with the clinical appearance of such mucosal abnormalities. Dyplasia is rarely present in homogeneous leukoplakia and is most often seen in the papillary verrucous form. Erythroplakia denotes a reddened mucosal lesion. Histologically this is defined by epithelial atrophy and vascular dilatation within the mucosa and either dysplasia or invasive carcinoma is present in most cases of erythroplakia.

Dysplasia commonly occurs on a background of epithelial hyperplasia, and includes nuclear atypia and a loss of epithelial maturation and stratification. Epithelial dysplasia implies a genetic event conferring a risk of frank malignant change, proportional to the severity of the dysplasia. The classification of laryngeal dysplasia as proposed by the World Health Organization (**WHO**) Collaborating Centre is broadly similar to that established for intraepithelial neoplasia of the uterine cervix, and grades the severity of dysplasia on the proportion of the epithelial thickness involved.[1] Unlike that for the cervix, the grading of laryngeal dysplasia separates severe dysplasia and carcinoma *in situ*, but the distinction is somewhat arbitrary.

Dysplasia in oral mucosa is graded in a similar fashion to that occurring in the larynx. The diagnostic problems are overdiagnosis of mild degrees of dysplasia, which may be difficult to distinguish from inflammatory changes, and underestimation of the more severe degrees of dysplasia. The latter arises because in the epithelium of the upper aerodigestive tract severe dysplastic changes may be associated with differentiation in the superficial epithelial layers. The classic full-thickness change, as seen in carcinoma *in situ* in the cervix, is rarely encountered in the mucosa of the upper aerodigestive tract. In the oral cavity, the majority of dysplastic lesions arise in a high-risk area of mucosa which includes the floor of the mouth, the lateral–ventral tongue, the soft palate, the retromolar trigone, and the anterior tonsillar pillar.[2] This mucosa is continuously bathed in saliva, and so suffers the greatest exposure to carcinogens.

Invasive carcinoma

Histological features with prognostic significance

The great majority of invasive carcinomas are moderately differentiated, and so histological grade has little bearing on prognosis. The growth pattern is of greater importance: carcinomas growing in poorly cohesive strands or cords, with jagged edges or as single cells, have a greater propensity to metastatic spread than those with a cohesive, rounded, pushing margin.[3] The tumour thickness or depth of invasion is an independent variable influencing prognosis. Tumours less than 4 mm thick metastasize in about 8 per cent of cases. Thirty-five per cent of tumours between 4 and 8 mm thick metastasize, and those thicker than 8 mm metastasize in 83 per cent of cases.[4] The finding of vascular or perineural invasion is also correlated with risk of metastasis.[4],[5]

Adequate surgical clearance is of prime importance in avoiding local recurrence. Recurrence is likely when the tumour is present within 5 mm of the margin or severe dysplasia is present. Intraoperative frozen section assessment of resection margins is an essential component to surgical management, since the prognosis for patients with positive surgical margins is very poor.

Histological variants of squamous carcinoma

Verrucous carcinoma accounts for 5 per cent of oral carcinomas. The common sites are the buccal mucosa, gingiva, tongue, palate, and tonsillar pillar. It presents as a warty mass which may be painful or tender. Alcohol is not implicated in aetiology, but most sufferers either smoke heavily or chew tobacco. Papillary squamous carcinoma differs from verrucous carcinoma in that it shows a greater degree of cytological atypia amounting to carcinoma *in situ* or invasive carcinoma.

Spindle cell carcinoma arises on the vermilion border of the lip, the tongue, the alveolar ridge, and the gingiva. Predisposing factors include smoking, alcohol, poor oral hygiene, and previous irradiation. Basaloid squamous carcinoma occurs at the tongue base and the tonsil. These aggressive neoplasms occur typically in male smokers and drinkers. Cervical lymph node metastases are present at diagnosis in the majority of cases.

Adenosquamous carcinoma is also an aggressive, and rare, carcinoma. In this region it occurs in the tongue and the floor of mouth. It may also arise in the nasal cavity and the larynx. It has a strong predilection for males, usually presenting in the elderly, although younger adults may be affected. The tumour, which may appear as an ulcer or a submucosal nodule, arises from seromucous gland ducts. Histologically, there are foci of squamous carcinoma, adenocarcinoma, and a mixed pattern. Also, there is severe dysplasia of surface and duct epithelium.

Pathology per head and neck site

Oral cavity and oropharynx

Approximately 90 per cent of malignant tumours of the oral cavity and oropharynx are typical squamous carcinoma or a variant on the theme. The majority of the remaining 10 per cent represent salivary-type adenocarcinomas, discussed elsewhere.

Larynx

Squamous carcinoma and variants

Squamous carcinoma comprises more than 90 per cent of laryngeal malignancy, which itself represents approximately 2 per cent of cancer in men and 0.5 per cent in women.

The structural framework of the larynx includes tough fibroelastic membranes which act as a barrier impeding the spread of carcinoma. These barriers enable a division of the larynx into topographical areas, each with different clinicopathological behaviour in relation to squamous carcinoma. These anatomical compartments are incorporated into the two most commonly used staging systems for laryngeal carcinoma, those of the International Union Against Cancer and the American Joint Committee on Cancer Staging and End Results Reporting.[6],[7]

Supraglottic

Supraglottic tumours, representing 30 to 35 per cent of the total, include those arising from the epiglottis, the false cord, the aryepiglottic fold, and the arytenoid body. Carcinomas of the saccule are also included in this category. Because the laryngeal airway is wide at this point, supraglottic tumours tend to present at a relatively late stage, usually with local pain or otalgia. Early tumours respect the elastic barriers at the level of the ventricle and the anterior commissure, and only 1 per cent of tumours involve the glottis. The thyroid cartilage is protected from invasion so long as the inferior edge of the tumour remains above the ventricle and anterior commissure. Anterior extension does occur, and epiglottic tumours arising below the hyoid bone penetrate into the pre-epiglottic space. Those above this level may involve the free edge of the epiglottis. The hyoid bone is protected by the thyrohyoid membrane. The laryngeal mucosa of the supraglottis is rich in lymphatics and the incidence of cervical lymph node metastases is high, about 40 per cent overall. Approximately one-third of patients with no clinically detectable disease in the neck are found to have nodal disease pathologically.

Glottic

Squamous carcinoma of the vocal fold is the commonest clinicopathological type, accounting for 60 to 65 per cent of laryngeal carcinoma. Tumours induce hoarseness, and usually present early. Extension beyond the superficial tissues is impeded by the conus elasticus and the thyroglottic ligament. Metastatic disease is restricted by the paucity of lymphatics at this site.

Subglottic

Subglottic carcinoma is defined as that in which there is tumour involving the vocal cord with greater than 1 cm subglottic extension or tumour located below the cord only. This is an uncommon site of origin, representing less than 5 per cent of the total. Entirely subglottic disease, with no cord involvement, is distinctly rare. Involvement of the thyroid and cricoid cartilages and anterior spread through the thyrocricoid membrane into prelaryngeal tissues is common. Metastatic disease to cervical lymph nodes occurs in up to 20 per cent of cases.

Transglottic

Transglottic carcinomas are not included in the two main staging systems. These are large tumours, probably originating in the glottis, which span the ventricle. There is invasion of the laryngeal cartilages and a high incidence of cervical lymph node metastases.

Hypopharyngeal carcinoma

Squamous carcinoma of the hypopharynx, although not of laryngeal origin, is in close proximity and has a profound effect on the larynx. The majority of these lesions arise within the pyriform sinus, and a smaller number develop in the postcricoid region and lateral wall of the hypopharynx. Pyriform sinus tumours spread medially, beneath intact mucosa, to infiltrate the supraglottic larynx. Involvement of the arytenoid cartilage, the posterior edge of the thyroid cartilage, or the upper part of the cricoid cartilage is common. The degree of lateral spread and laryngeal involvement is best determined by examination of horizontal slices of the larynx.

Pathological appearances of laryngeal and hypopharyngeal cancers

Laryngeal squamous carcinoma is an ulcerated, fungating lesion. At presentation, tumours are usually in the region of 3 to 5 cm in diameter. Vocal fold carcinomas are quite often keratotic, and will appear white. Some tumours have a distinctly papillary appearance, and a proportion of these will be found to be verrucous squamous carcinomas. Rarely, carcinomas are polypoid, a typical macroscopic appearance of spindle cell carcinoma. Squamous carcinomas of the larynx, as at other sites, may be graded on the basis of nuclear features, degree of keratinization, and the presence of intercellular bridges into well, moderately, and poorly differentiated neoplasms. Although important, the histological grade of the tumour is of secondary significance in comparison to stage in determining prognosis.

Verrucous carcinoma is a well-differentiated variant of squamous carcinoma. The lesion has an exophytic, papillary architecture and is composed of a proliferation of squamous epithelium which shows cytological atypia only in basal and parabasal cells. Cells in the prickle layer are typically large with glassy, eosinophilic cytoplasm and indistinct cell borders. The surface shows spires of parakeratosis and hyperkeratosis. This lesion shows superficial infiltration of the underlying stroma along a broad front, and metastases are rare. This lesion, which represents fewer than 5 per cent of laryngeal squamous carcinomas, must be distinguished from benign verrucous hyperplasia or squamous papilloma on the one hand and from a well differentiated papillary carcinoma on the other, a difficult task when presented with a small, superficial biopsy. The latter distinction has therapeutic implications, since irradiation of verrucous carcinoma has been shown to be, at best, relatively ineffective and, in some cases, may promote the development of dedifferentiation to anaplastic carcinoma.[8]

Spindle cell carcinoma is an uncommon entity which shows a predilection for the upper aerodigestive tract. The most common laryngeal location is the subglottis, where, it appears as a polypoid mass. The histological appearance is biphasic, comprising a relatively minor component of squamous carcinoma, which may be invasive or *in situ*, associated with a dominant spindle cell component. The latter may be cytologically bland or malignant. In the latter case this may resemble malignant fibrous histiocytoma, osteosarcoma, or some other specific sarcoma. The surface is often ulcerated and it is not uncommon for the epithelioid component to be inconspicuous or even absent. In most cases there is at least focal evidence of epithelial differentiation in the spindle cells, which may be derived from immunohistochemical or ultrastructural studies, and it is accepted that these neoplasms are sarcomatoid carcinoma.[9] An earlier demonstration of positivity for α_1-chymotrypsin and α_1-antitrypsin, and the conclusion that this infers fibrohistiocytic differentiation, is discounted on the basis of the lack of specificity of these markers.[10] Prognosis for spindle cell carcinoma is better for polypoid tumours than for deeply invasive lesions.[11] Metastatic disease may take the form of monophasic carcinoma, or of a biphasic deposit. Purely sarcomatoid metastases are rarely encountered.

Another variant of squamous carcinoma is basaloid squamous carcinoma. This shows *in situ* or invasive squamous carcinoma together with invasion by groups of small, hyperchromatic basaloid cells which show peripheral palisading and central, comedo-like necrosis. Typically, the stroma is hyalinized. These highly malignant tumours are also found in the pharynx, hypopharynx, oesophagus, and tongue.

Neoplasms with neuroendocrine differentiation

Small cell carcinoma of the larynx is rare, comprising less than 0.5 per cent of laryngeal malignancy. Presenting in elderly male smokers, it is identical in appearance to the homologous lung tumour and is equally aggressive.[12] Both regional nodal metastases and distant dissemination are common.

Large cell neuroendocrine carcinoma is also a highly malignant neoplasm which presents in elderly male smokers. The majority of tumours are polypoid and arise in the submucosa of the supraglottis, close to the arytenoid cartilage. They are composed of large, argyrophilic polyhedral cells, arranged in trabeculae and tubules which show immunoreactivity for chromogranin, calcitonin, and other neuroendocrine markers and possess dense-core granules.[13] Morphological features of malignancy include nuclear pleomorphism, hyperchromasia, mitotic activity, and necrosis.

Typical carcinoid tumour may also arise in the supraglottic larynx, but this is less common. As with the bronchial homologue, prognosis is favourable.

Another unusual laryngeal neoplasm with neuroendocrine differentiation is paraganglioma. As elsewhere, these have a complement of chief cells, which show immunopositivity for neuroendocrine markers and a peripheral population of S100-positive sustentacular cells. Located in the supraglottis they often involve the aryepiglottic fold. Metastatic disease develops in approximately 20 per cent of cases.

Salivary-type neoplasms

These lesions arise from the seromucous glands of the supraglottis and, occasionally, the subglottis. The most common type is adenoid cystic carcinoma, which, like its counterpart in the salivary glands, has a long natural history with poor long-term survival.[14] Spread along nerves and haematogenous spread are typical. Other salivary-type malignancies, such as mucoepidermoid and acinic carcinoma, are rare.

Sarcomas

Sarcomas of the larynx are unusual. The commonest are cartilaginous neoplasms, which have a predilection for the cricoid lamina. As determined by cellularity, nuclear features, and mitotic activity, the great majority are low-grade chondosarcomas.[15] Behaviour is generally indolent, local recurrence is the rule, and metastases are distinctly uncommon. Dedifferentiation to high-grade sarcoma has been documented but this is exceptional.[16]

The full range of soft tissue sarcomas may be represented in the larynx, but all are rare. These include malignant fibrous histiocytomas and fibrosarcomas, some of which, at least, probably represent spindle cell carcinoma in which the epithelial component has not been recognized.

Prognosis

Histological grade, using a variation on Broders' criteria, although subordinate to stage, has independent prognostic significance.[17] Flow cytometry studies have concluded that aneuploidy is correlated with the risk of recurrence.[18] Other morphological features have been investigated for their impact on survival. The presence of stromal Langerhans cells, which are antigen-presenting cells, at the tumour interface has been proposed to be of benefit to survival.[19] Characterization of the type of keratins elaborated by squamous carcinoma, however, has not yielded any significant findings.[20]

Nasal cavity and paranasal sinuses

Squamous carcinoma

Squamous carcinoma is twice as common in males as in females and accounts for 3 per cent of all head and neck cancer and for 1 per cent of all cancer deaths. Approximately 90 per cent of cases arise in the maxillary antrum or nasal cavity, with the remainder distributed in the ethmoid, sphenoid, and frontal sinuses. There is a well-established association of squamous carcinoma of the nasal cavity with cigarette smoking and exposure to nickel ore, chromium, radium, and isopropyl alcohol. Exposure to the radiological contrast medium thorotrast, on the other hand, is a risk factor in the development of squamous carcinoma of the maxillary antrum. Sinonasal squamous carcinoma may develop within an inverted papilloma, occurring in 6 to 14 per cent of cases.[21],[22] The role of human papilloma virus is controversial, but genomic material of human papilloma virus 16/18 has been identified in tumour cells, by *in situ* hybridization techniques and polymerase chain reaction in up to 14 per cent of cases.[23]

The majority of sinonasal squamous carcinomas are keratinizing and easily recognized. Cylindric cell, or transitional cell, carcinoma is a non-keratinizaing variant which has a papillomatous architecture, and is often low grade, creating the opportunity for confusion with inverted or exophytic papilloma. This lesion behaves no differently from typical squamous carcinoma. Verrucous carcinoma and spindle cell squamous carcinoma may both arise in the sinonasal region.

Adenocarcinoma

Adenocarcinoma accounts for 10 to 20 per cent of sinonasal malignancy and occurs in non-salivary and salivary types. The former may be further subclassified into low-grade and intestinal-type adeno-carcinoma.

Low-grade adenocarcinoma may occur over a wide age range, from childhood to old age, with a median incidence in the sixth decade. Both sexes are equally affected. The majority of cases arise in the nasal cavity or ethmoid sinus, and only a minority develop in the maxillary antrum, the commonest site of squamous carcinoma. There is no known association with exogenous carcinogens. Local recurrence is common, occurring in a third of cases, but long-term survival is good. Deaths are due to local extension and metastases are unusual. The histological appearance is bland, with closely packed glandular structures lined by a single layer of uniform columnar or cuboidal cells. Mitotic figures are sparse in the majority of cases. Both cytoplasmic and extracellular mucin is often demonstrable.

Approximately 20 per cent of cases of intestinal-type adeno-carcinoma occur in individuals who have had long-term industrial exposure to hard-wood dust, an experience which confers a high relative risk of developing adenocarcinoma.[24] These patients are almost invariably male and the lesion has a high predilection for the ethmoid sinus. Intestinal adenocarcinoma in non-exposed patients is more common in females and occurs preferentially in the maxillary antrum.

Morphologically, intestinal-type adenocarcinoma mimics virtually normal or neoplastic small or large bowel mucosa. The most common type is colonic adenocarcinoma, in which tubular structures featuring epithelium with varying grades of nuclear atypia, replete with goblet cells, invade the sinonasal mucosa. Enteric-type adenocarcinoma includes cellular components found in the small bowel, including goblet, absorptive, Paneth, and argentaffin endocrine cells. Mucinous adenocarcinomas feature a variable proportion of signet ring cells and pools of extracellular mucin. Attempts at relating morphology to prognosis have shown that a tubulopapillary architecture confers a more favourable outcome. Exclusion of the possibility that intestinal sinonasal adenocarcinoma represents metastasis from a gut primary is advisable, since this differentiation is not possible on histological grounds.

Adenoid cystic carcinoma is the commonest salivary-type adeno-carcinoma. This has an affinity for the maxillary antrum, although it may occur elsewhere in the nasal cavity or paranasal sinuses. Mucoepidermoid carcinoma ranks second in frequency followed by acinic carcinoma. These tumours behave in a similar fashion to their counterparts in minor salivary gland tissue elsewhere.

Small cell carcinoma may arise within the paranasal sinuses or the nasal cavity. These locally aggressive tumours show a relative reluctance to disseminate.

Sinonasal undifferentiated carcinoma

An aggressive neoplasm, undifferentiated sinonasal carcinoma may present at any time in adulthood. It is a disease which has a marginal predilection for females and is most often found in the nasal cavity, maxillary antrum, or ethmoid sinus. Extension into the sphenoid and frontal sinuses, orbit, or cranial cavity is common. These are rapidly fatal neoplasms for which surgical resection is rarely possible and radiotherapy and chemotherapy offer little benefit. Survival is meas-ured in weeks or months.[25]

The histological appearance is of nests, cords, ribbons, or trabeculae or moderately large epithelial cells which possess a moderately pleo-morphic, hyperchromatic nucleus with a conspicuous nucleolus.

Mitotic activity is plentiful, as is apoptosis and confluent necrosis, and vascular invasion is typical. There is no suggestion of either squamous or glandular differentiation, but there is usually some evidence of neuroendocrine features with immunohistochemistry or electron microscopic evaluation.[30] Foci of severe dysplasia or carcinoma *in situ* may be evident in surface epithelium.

Olfactory neuroblastoma

The reserve cell of the olfactory epithelium in the roof of the nasal cavity is thought to be the progenitor cell of olfactory neuro-blastoma.[26] This tumour, which shows a variable combination of epithelial and neuronal differentiation, may present at any age. Incidence peaks in adolescence and again in middle age and both sexes are affected equally. Tumours present as a vascular polypoid mass in the roof of the nasal cavity or ethmoid sinus, causing nasal obstruction and epistaxis.

Two main growth patterns are seen, either rounded nests of cells separated by stroma rich in thin-walled blood vessels, or as diffuse sheets of cells. The tumour cells possess a small round nucleus with fine chromatin and sparse cytoplasm. There is only a mild to moderate degree of pleomorphism, but mitotic figures may be scanty or abund-ant. A characteristic feature is the presence of eosinophilic, fibrillary matrix which contains neurofilaments. Other useful diagnostic fea-tures include the presence of Homer-Wright or Flexner-type rosettes. Immunohistochemistry shows positivity for neurone specific enolase (NSE), synaptophysin, and neurofilaments in a high proportion of cases.[27] S100-positive sustentacular cells are also common, located at the periphery of the cell nests. Some cases show a greater degree of epithelial differentiation, with more abundant cytoplasm, intercellular cohesion, and a lack of fibrillary matrix. Overall, about 30 per cent of cases show immunopositivity for low-molecular-weight cyto-keratins.[20] Electron microscopy confirms neuronal differentiation with dense-core granules and cell processes containing neurofilaments or tubules.

Malignant melanoma

Melanoma of the nasal cavity and paranasal sinuses represents 1 per cent of all melanomas. Most occur in the nasal cavity, and those arising in the sinuses do so in the maxillary antrum or, less often, in the ethmoid sinus. There is no sex predilection and, as for cutaneous melanoma, tumours may present at any age, although the great majority occur in the sixth decade and beyond. Presentation is usually with nasal obstruction or epistaxis.

The gross appearance is of a fleshy mass, which may be sessile or pedunculated and which is often darkly pigmented. The histological appearance is of a cellular neoplasm which, in many cases, is ulcerated. The tumour cells may be small and round, spindle shaped, epithelioid, or pleomorphic. Melanin pigmentation is demonstrated in ap-proximately 70 per cent of cases. Nests of melanocytes at the epithelial–stromal junction are an infrequent finding, possible a consequence of ulceration, but Pagetoid spread, particularly within respiratory-type epithelium, is not uncommon.

Immunostains are positive for S100 and HMB45; the former is less specific but more sensitive than the latter.[28] Positivity, at least focally, is also found for epithelial membrane antigen, and the plasma cell marker VS38c, a potential source of confusion with poorly differentiated carcinoma and plasmacytoma respectively.

The prognosis for sinonasal melanoma is dismal. Surgical resection is the mainstay of therapy, but repeated recurrence is characteristic, the overall 5-year survival being no more than 10 per cent; most patients succumb within 2 years.[29]

Sarcomas

The full range of malignant neoplasms of bone and soft tissue may present in the nasal cavity or paranasal sinuses. All are uncommon and most are rarities. The head and neck region is a common site for rhabdomyosarcoma, but they are more often located in the orbit or nasopharynx. Spindle cell sarcomas, usually of low grade, are occasionally seen, and these may represent fibrosarcomas, malignant fibrohistiocytic tumours, or peripheral nerve sheath neoplasms.

Nasopharynx

Nasopharyngeal carcinoma

The WHO recognizes three categories of nasopharyngeal carcinoma: keratinizing squamous carcinoma, differentiated non-keratinizing carcinoma, and undifferentiated carcinoma. The last two categories are closely related in aetiology, epidemiology, and response to treatment. In endemic areas the great majority of cases are represented by undifferentiated carcinoma. This has a characteristic appearance of groups and islands of cells with a large, vesicular nucleus and prominent nucleolus and a pale basophilic cytoplasm with indistinct cell borders. There is a prominent lymphoid stroma, composed of T cells, which is either admixed with the epithelial cells (Schmincke pattern), or surrounds the tumour cell islands (Regaud pattern). The differentiated non-keratinizing type shows some features of maturation, with more distinct cell borders and a pavementing architecture. Both these types share a strong association with Epstein–Barr virus infection and sensitivity to radiotherapy. Keratinizing squamous carcinoma, of similar appearance to squamous carcinoma at other sites, does not have the same association with Epstein–Barr virus and responds poorly to therapy.

The association of Epstein–Barr virus, a ubiquitous virus for which evidence of infection may be found in most adults worldwide, with undifferentiated nasopharyngeal carcinoma has been well known for some years. Early studies relied on serological evidence of elevated titres of antibodies to Epstein–Barr virus-associated proteins.[30] This has evolved to using serological investigation as a surveillance and screening tool in high-risk populations and to monitor disease progression in affected individuals. More recently, advances in molecular biological techniques, particularly in situ hybridization, have enabled the demonstration of genomic material of the Epstein–Barr virus within tumour cells.[31] Further, the finding that this DNA is clonal strongly implicates Epstein–Barr virus in oncogenesis.[32] There is also evidence of a genetic predisposition, in that inheritance of HLA A2 and Bsin2 antigens on the same chromosome confers an increased risk of developing carcinoma, whereas the possession of HLA A11 affords a degree of protection.[33] Cytogenetic studies have shown an array of chromosomal abnormalities in undifferentiated nasopharyngeal carcinoma, most consistently in chromosome 3. It is suggested that a deletion of a recessive oncogene on the short arm of this chromosome is involved in the pathogenesis of undifferentiated nasopharyngeal carcinoma.[34] Environmental factors are undoubtedly also important; in endemic areas the consumption of salted fish is positively correlated with risk of developing nasopharyngeal carcinoma.[35]

Miscellaneous malignant tumours

Adenocarcinomas of salivary and non-salivary type may arise in the nasopharynx, but are uncommon. Of the former, adenoid cystic carcinoma and mucoepidermoid carcinoma head the list. Rhabdomyosarcoma and lymphoma are important nasopharyngeal malignancies, described elsewhere.

Salivary glands

The pathology of the salivary glands is a large and complex topic, reflecting the rich diversity of salivary gland tumours. A discussion of the general features of malignant salivary gland tumours will be given in this chapter.

Tumour classification

Tumours are classified on the basis of the type of cells which comprise the tumour and the architectural pattern. The purpose of such histological classification is to enable prediction of biological behaviour in order to choose the most appropriate mode of therapy for a given case. A number of classification schemes have been proposed for salivary gland tumours. A recent and widely adopted scheme was proposed in 1991 by WHO, itself a revision of an earlier version. In this, there are 18 categories of primary epithelial malignancy, some of which may be further divided into subtypes.[36] By and large, malignant salivary tumours are not assigned a histological grade, a notable exception being mucoepidermoid carcinoma, which can usefully be described as being of high, low, or intermediate grade.

For many tumours, such as acinic cell carcinoma, variations in morphology have no bearing on behaviour, and other aspects such as the size and extent of the tumour are more important parameters influencing prognosis.[37] For others, designation as a particular histological type implies a certain stereotypic behaviour. Polymorphous low-grade adenocarcinoma of minor salivary glands, for example, is invariably an indolent tumour, whereas salivary duct carcinoma is, by definition, highly malignant.

In adults, the ratio of benign to malignant salivary tumours varies from between 54 to 80 per cent benign to 21 to 46 per cent malignant. In children there is an almost equal proportion of benign and malignant tumours. Series with a greater number of minor salivary gland tumours show a higher incidence of malignancy. This reflects the fact that minor gland tumours are more likely to be malignant than tumours of the major glands.

Approximately 33 per cent of neoplasms of the major salivary glands are malignant, compared with 50 per cent of minor gland neoplasms. Further, minor salivary gland tumours from different sites show a varying propensity for malignancy. About 70 per cent of tumours of the sublingual gland are malignant, rising to 90 per cent in the retromolar area.

The commonest histological type overall is mucoepidermoid carcinoma, representing 33 per cent of carcinomas, followed by acinic cell carcinoma, adenocarcinoma NOS (not otherwise specified), and adenoid cystic carcinoma. In children, mucoepidermoid carcinoma and acinic cell carcinoma are the most frequent histological types. The frequency of a particular histological type of neoplasm varies with site in the minor salivary glands. Acinic cell carcinoma, for example, represents 1.4 per cent of palatal salivary tumours, but 10.3 per cent of salivary neoplasms of the buccal mucosa. Similarly, adenoid cystic carcinoma accounts for 8.3 per cent of palatal tumours and 17.1 per cent of lingual neoplasms.

Aetiology

Little is known of the aetiology of malignant salivary gland neoplasms. Undifferentiated carcinoma has a similar morphology and epidemiological association with Epstein–Barr virus infection as undifferentiated nasopharyngeal carcinoma. Although it is reasonable to assume that the Epstein–Barr virus has an aetiological role in tumorigenesis, this entity has not been as extensively studied as its nasopharyngeal counterpart.

Irradiation, both environmental, as in those exposed to the fallout of the atomic bombs at Hiroshima and Nagasaki, and therapeutic, has been implicated in the development of salivary carcinomas. The relative risk of developing a malignant salivary tumour in those exposed to the atomic bombs has been estimated at 11 times that of unexposed individuals, with the greatest risk to those closer to the centre of the blast.[38] The peak incidence of carcinomas occurred 12 to 16 years after exposure. In the past, therapeutic irradiation to the head and neck was employed for a number of benign conditions, such as acne, hyperplastic tonsils and adenoids, or for treating keloid scars. This resulted in a relative risk of up to 40 for the development of salivary gland carcinoma.[39] In addition to salivary neoplasms, these patients are at risk of developing a second primary tumour, usually within the field of irradiation. Such tumours include thyroid, parathyroid, and lung neoplasms.

Only a few malignant salivary tumours have been studied for chromosomal abnormalities. The findings suggest that some cases of adenoid cystic carcinoma, mucoepidermoid carcinoma, squamous carcinoma, undifferentiated carcinoma, and adenocarcinoma NOS have deletions of the long arm of chromosome 6, where the c-*myb* proto-oncogene is found, loss of the Y chromosome, or trisomy 8.[40] None of these changes are specific, since they are observed in some cases of acute lymphoblastic leukaemia, non-Hodgkin's lymphoma, melanoma, and ovarian carcinoma.

Frozen sections and fine needle aspiration cytology

Overall, the accuracy of diagnosis of salivary gland tumours at frozen section is in the region of 96 per cent.[41] This figure is lower for malignant tumours, around 86 per cent, than for benign tumours. The commonest lesion responsible for a false positive diagnosis of carcinoma is a pleomorphic adenoma. Less often, lymphoepithelial cysts are diagnosed as lymphoma or as mucoepidermoid carcinoma. False negative diagnoses are most often seen with low-grade mucoepidermoid carcinomas, acinic cell carcinomas, adenoid cystic carcinomas, and carcinoma ex pleomorphic adenoma. False negative diagnoses are often a result of inadequate tissue sampling. Accuracy is improved if the pathologist receives the resection specimen intact, enabling sampling of macroscopically suspicious areas.

Fine needle aspiration cytology is attractive in the diagnosis of salivary gland tumours because of its low cost, low morbidity, speed of diagnosis, and the high level of accuracy. The latter, in the determination of whether a tumour is benign or malignant, is high—98 per cent for benign tumours and 93 per cent for malignant tumours. In a recent study, the false positive rate was found to be 1.2 per cent and false negatives were diagnosed in 4.5 per cent of cases.[42]

Cytological analysis has the disadvantage, compared with evaluation of histological biopsy specimens, that the tumour architecture cannot be assessed, nor can the appearance of the tumour–stroma interface, a feature important in the determination of invasion. These limitations reduce the reliability of fine needle aspiration cytology in reaching a definitive classification of a neoplasm. Particular difficulties arise with the similar cytological appearances of pleomorphic adenoma, adenoid cystic carcinoma, and polymorphous low-grade adenocarcinoma. Similarly, it is not possible to distinguish between basal cell adenoma and basal cell adenocarcinoma on cytological grounds, since the distinction relies on the identification of stromal invasion. In many cases these limitations are of little importance since the type and extent of the surgical procedure is more dependent on the size and extent of tumour spread than on its precise histological classification.

External auditory canal and middle ear

Squamous carcinoma may arise in the external auditory canal or the middle ear cleft. Tumours of the canal often cause destruction of the wall and penetrate the tympanic membrane and extend into the middle ear. Tumours are difficult to treat, and in one series the mortality was 50 per cent. Squamous carcinoma arising in the middle ear itself is a disease of late middle age, presenting with deafness, otalgia, and a bloody discharge. Synchronous carcinoma of the canal is common. Tumour spreads into the carotid canal, mastoid air spaces, and internal auditory meatus. Intracranial involvement is a late manifestation and a common cause of death.

Glandular neoplasms of the external canal arise from the ceruminous glands. Adenocarcinoma is often well differentiated and may be difficult to distinguish from anadenoma. Such tumours often recur locally and may lead to regional or distant metastases. Adenoid cystic carcinoma may arise in the canal, and has the typical morphology and behaviour of its counterpart in the salivary glands. Perineural infiltration is a common finding and dissemination to distant sites, particularly the lungs, is a common mode of spread. A 50 per cent mortality is associated with this neoplasm.

So-called adenoma of the middle ear is a controversial entity. This tumour presents over a wide age range and has no sex predilection. Its commonest presentation is with conductive deafness. Grossly it appears as a circumscribed lesion behind an intact tympanic membrane. It is firm, grey, and not vascular. Histologically it is composed of uniform, bland cuboidal cells arranged in small sheets, trabeculae, cords, or glands.

Cytoplasm is eosinophilic and demonstrates argyrophilia. Mucin may be demonstrated within glandular lumina. There is no mitotic activity or necrosis. Ultrastructural studies and immunohistochemistry demonstrate neuroendocrine differentiation in a high proportion of cases. Such cases with dense-core granules and positivity for neuroendocrine markers, such as chromogranin, NSE, and some peptide hormones have been categorized by some as carcinoid tumours.[43] The prevailing view, however, is that they are all part of the spectrum of middle ear adenoma, and are benign neoplasms.

Certainly, simple surgical excision leads to cure in the majority of cases.

Adenocarcinoma of the middle ear cleft is very rare. This is composed of bland glandular cells, arranged on a vascular, papillary stroma. Some cases have the appearance of thyroid follicles and others show clear cell change and resemble metastatic renal cell carcinoma. The entity, also vanishingly rare, described as low-grade adenocarcinoma of the endolymphatic sac may be related. Adenocarcinoma typically infiltrates the temporal bone and is very difficult to treat.

Paragangliomas arise from either the jugular bulb or the promontory of the middle ear cleft. They are commoner in females and usually present in middle age, with conductive deafness. Some patients experience pain, tinnitus, and a bloody discharge, or develop a facial nerve palsy. The gross appearance is of a vascular, sprouting mass. The histological findings are characteristic. Nests of chief cells are surrounded by flat, spindle-shaped sustentacular cells. The latter may be identified by their positive immunohistochemical staining with S100 protein. Local recurrence is common, occurring in up to 50 per cent of cases, but metastatic disease is rare.

Rhabdomyosarcoma of the middle ear is rare and confined to the paediatric population. Tumours are of embryonal or botryoid type. Extension into the external canal, mastoid cavity, and the cranial cavity are common developments.

Orbit

Malignant tumours within the orbit arise from the soft tissues, the optic nerve, or the lachrymal gland.

Rhabdomyosarcoma is the commonest primary neoplasm of childhood. The favoured site is the upper, medial part of the orbit, often presenting as a swelling of the upper eyelid. Set within an oedematous matrix the tumour cells are small and spindle shaped, with a densely staining nucleus. Occasional strap cells with visible cytoplasmic striations are commonly present. It is common for there to be a condensation of tumour cells beneath the surface, forming the cambium layer, characteristic of the botryoid subtype of embryonal rhabdomyosarcoma. Diagnosis may be confirmed with the immunohistochemical demonstration of desmin or myoglobin, or the ultrastructural finding of thick myosin filaments. The prognosis for all types of rhabdomyosarcoma is poor, but the alveolar type, less common than the embryonal form, is especially aggressive.

Haemangiopericytoma is a sarcoma which may present at any age from early adulthood to old age. It is a vascular, spindle cell neoplasm which may appear as a pulsatile orbital swelling. These are usually circumscribed tumours in which there is a characteristic staghorn pattern of blood vessels. They may behave in a benign or malignant fashion, which is difficult to predict from the histological appearance, although nuclear pleomorphism, abundant mitotic activity, necrosis, and haemorrhage all point to potential malignancy. Overall about 30 per cent of haemangiopericytomas recur locally and 15 per cent of patients die from the effects of metastatic disease. Recurrence or metastasis may occur many years after the initial presentation.

Other sarcomas such as alveolar soft part sarcoma, osteosarcoma, leiomyosarcoma, fibrosarcoma, and angiosarcoma may arise in the orbit, but they are rarities.

Gliomas of the optic nerve represent about 3 per cent of orbital neoplasms, and the majority occur in childhood. These lesions expand the nerve within the dural covering and extend into the cranial cavity. The optic chiasm is often involved. About 25 per cent are associated with neurofibromatosis. The histological appearance is of a low-grade juvenile pilocytic astrocytoma, composed of thin astrocytes arranged in a parallel or random array. An eosinophlic swelling of the cell processes, forming Rosenthal fibres is typical, and calcification and microcystic change may also be seen. Although they cause blindness, biologically, these tumours behave in a benign fashion, but the adult counterpart is usually an aggressive, high-grade malignant tumour, most often glioblastoma multiforme.

Approximately 40 to 50 per cent of primary epithelial neoplasms of the lachrymal gland are malignant. In descending order of frequency of carcinoma are adenoid cystic carcinoma, carcinoma ex pleomorphic adenoma, adenocarcinoma NOS, and mucoepidermoid carcinoma. Adenoid cystic carcinoma spreads along nerves and invades the bone of the orbital wall. The cribriform pattern is the commonest histological pattern; such tumours have a better outlook than those with a solid, basaloid appearance. As elsewhere, adenoid cystic carcinoma may run a protracted course, but the outlook for long-term survival is poor. Other types of carcinoma have a very poor prognosis.

Conclusion

It is clear that the head and neck region is host to a great variety of pathological tumour types, both benign and malignant. It is also true, however, that numerically the most prevalent malignancy in the region as a whole is squamous cell carcinoma. Pathological diagnosis is not usually problematic, except for the case of well-differentiated papillary squamous lesions. Numerous laboratory techniques have been employed, from time to time, in an attempt to provide objective assessments of likely behaviour and prognosis in individual cases. Nonetheless, the most valuable assessment for this purpose is the accurate documentation of tumour stage, and nothing else can replace this.

There is little application for screening for premalignant disease, except perhaps for serological tests in areas endemic for nasopharyngeal carcinoma. In the future, it may be that it will be possible to identify individuals who are carriers of particular genes which confer an excess risk of developing carcinoma. Risk may be reduced by surveillance or adopting lifestyles which avoid compounding risk factors, such as smoking or alcohol. At present, the most important role of the diagnostic histopathologist is in the accurate diagnosis and meticulous and standardized documentation of disease grade and stage, in order that individual patients receive proper treatment and pathological databases to study disease trends and effectiveness of therapies can be created.

References

1. **Shanmugaratnam K, et al.** Histological typing of tumours of the upper respiratory tract and ear. *World Health Organisation international histological classification of tumours* (2nd edn). Berlin: Springer, 1991.

2. **Shafer WG.** Oral carcinoma *in situ*. *Oral Surgery*, 1975; **39**: 227–38.

3. **Crissman JD, Liu WY, Gluckman JL, Cummings G.** Prognostic value of histopathologic parameters in squamous cell carcinoma of the oropharynx. *Cancer*, 1984; **54**: 2995–3001.

4. **Shingaki S, Suzuki I, Nakajima T, Kawasaki T.** Evaluation of histopathologic parameters in predicting cervical lymph node

metastasis of oral and oropharyngeal carcinoma. *Oral Surgery*, 1988; **66**: 683–8.

5. Carter RL, Tanner NS, Clifford P, Shaw HJ. Perineural spread in squamous cell carcinomas of the head and neck: A clinicopathologic study. *Clinical Otolaryngology*, 1979; **4**: 271–81.

6. Union Internationale Contre Cancer. *TNM classification of malignant tumours* (2nd edn). Geneva: Union Internationale Contre Cancer, 1974.

7. American Joint Committee on Cancer. *Staging of cancer of head and neck sites and of melanoma.* Chicago: American Joint Committee on Cancer, 1980.

8. Ferlito A, Recher G. Ackerman's tumor (verrucous carcinoma) of the larynx: a clinicopathologic study of 77 cases. *Cancer*, 1980; **46**: 1617–30.

9. Zarbo RJ, Crissman JD, Venkat H, Weiss MA. Spindle-cell carcinoma of the uper aerodigestive tract mucosa. An immunohistologic and ultrastructural study of 18 biphasic tumors and comparison with 7 monophasic spindle-cell tumors. *American Journal of Surgical Pathology*, 1986; **10**: 741–53.

10. Ellis GL, Langloss JM, Heffner DK, Hyams VJ. Spindle–cell carcinoma of the aerodigestive tract. An immunonohistochemical analysis of 21 cases. *American Journal of Surgical Pathology*, 1987; **11**: 335–42.

11. Weidner N. Sarcomatoid carcinoma of the upper aerodigestive tract. *Seminars in Diagnostic Pathology*, 1987; **4**: 157–68.

12. Gnepp GR, Hyams V. Primary anaplastic small cell (oat cell) carcinoma of the larynx. *Cancer*, 1983; **51**: 1731–45.

13. Woodruff JM, Senie RT. Atypical carcinoid tumor of the larynx. A critical review of the literature. *ORL Journal of Otorhinolaryngology and Related Specialties*, 1991; **53**: 194–209.

14. Olofsson J, Van Norstrand AWP. Adenoid cystic carcinoma of the larynx. A report of four cases and a review of the literature. *Cancer*, 1977; **40**: 1307–13.

15. Goethals PL, Dahlin DC, Devine KD. Cartilaginous tumors of the larynx. *Surgery Gynaecology Obstetrics*, 1963; **117**: 77–82.

16. Branwein N, Moore S, Som P, Biller H. Laryngeal chondrosarcomas: A clinicopathologic study of 11 cases, including two 'dedifferentiated chondrosarcomas'. *Laryngoscope*, 1992; **102**: 858–67.

17. Wiernik G, Millard PR, Haybittle JL. The predictive value of histopathological classification into degrees of differentiation of sqaumous carcinoma of the larynx and hypopharynx compared with the survival of patients. *Histopathology*, 1991; **14**: 411–17.

18. Westerbeek HA, Mooi WJ, Hilgers FJ, Baris G, Begg AC, Balm AJ. Ploidy status and the response of T1 glottic carcinoma to radiotherapy. *Clinical Otolaryngology*, 1993; **18**: 98–101.

19. Gallo O, *et al.* Langerhans cells related to prognosis in patients with laryngeal carcinoma. *Archives of Otolaryngology Head and Neck Surgery*, 1991; **117**: 1007–10.

20. Mallofre C, *et al.* Expression of cytokeratins in squamous cell carcinoma of the larynx. Immunohistochemical analysis and correlation with prognostic factors. *Pathology Research and Practice*, 1993; **189**: 275–82.

21. Laser A, Rothfield PR, Shapiro RS. Epithelial papilloma and squamous carcinoma of the nasal cavity and paranasal sinuses. *Cancer*, 1976; **38**: 2503–10.

22. Smith O, Gullane PJ. Inverting papilloma of the nose: Analysis of 48 cases. *Journal of Otolaryngology*, 1987; **16**: 154–6.

23. Furata Y, *et al.* Detection of human papillomavirus DNA in carcinomas of the nasal cavities and paranasal sinuses by the polymerase chain reaction. *Cancer*, 1992; **69**: 353–7.

24. Demers PA, *et al.* Wood dust and sino-nasal cancer: Pooled reanalysis of twelve case-controlled studies. *American Journal of Industrial Medicine*, 1995; **28**: 151–66.

25. Frierson HF Jr, Mills SE, Fechner RE, Taxy JB, Levine PA. Sinonasal undifferentiated carcinoma. An aggressive neoplasm derived from schneiderian epithelium and distinct from olfactory neuroblastoma. *American Journal of Surgical Pathology*, 1986; **10**: 771–9.

26. Mills SE, Frierson HF Jr. Olfactory neuroblastoma. A clinicopathologic study of 21 cases. *American Journal of Surgical Pathology*, 1985; **9**: 317–27.

27. Frierson HF Jr, Ross GW, Mills SE, Frankfurter A. Olfactory neuroblastoma. Additional immunohistochemical characterisation. *American Journal of Clinical Pathology*, 1990; **94**: 547–53.

28. Franquemont DW, Mills SE. Sinonasal malignant melanoma. A clinocopathologic and immunohistochemical study of 14 cases. *American Journal of Clinical Pathology*, 1991; **96**: 689–97.

29. Gallagher JC. Upper respiratory melanoma: pathology and growth rate. *Annals of Otology Rhinology and Laryngology*, 1970; **79**: 551–6.

30. Pearson GR, *et al.* Application of Epstein–Barr virus (EBV) serology to the diagnosis of North American nasopharyngeal carcinoma. *Cancer*, 1983; **51**: 260–8.

31. Brousset P Butet V, Chittal S, Selves J, Delsol G. Comparison of *in situ* hybridisation using different nonisotopic probes for detection of Epstein–Barr virus in nasopharyngeal carcinoma and immunohistochemical correlation with anti-latent membrane protein antibody. *Laboratory Investigation*, 1992; **67**: 457–64.

32. Sun Y, *et al.* An infrequent point mutation of the p53 gene in human nasopharyngeal carcinoma. *Proceedings of National Academy of Sciences of the USA*, 1992; **89**: 6516–20.

33. Simons MJ, *et al.* Immunogenetic aspects of nasopharyngeal carcinoma:IV. Increased risk in Chinese of naspharyngeal carcinoma associated with a Chinese-related HLA profile (A2, Singapore 2). *Journal of the National Cancer Institute*, 1976; **57**: 977–80.

34. Huang DP, *et al.* Loss of heterozygosity on the short arm of chromosome 3 in nasopharyngeal carcinoma. *Cancer Genetics and Cytogenetics*, 1991; **54**: 91–9.

35. Yu MC, *et al.* Preserved foods and nasopharyngeal carcinoma: A case-control study in Guangxi, China. *Cancer Research*, 1988; **48**: 1954–61.

36. Seifert G, Sobin LH: The World Health Organisation's Histological Classification of Salivary Gland Tumours. A commentary on the second edition. *Cancer*, 1992; **70**: 379–85.

37. Lewis JE, Olsen KD, Weiland LH: Acinic cell carcinoma. Clinicopathologic review. *Cancer*, 1991; **67**: 172–9.

38. Merrick Y, Albeck H, Neilsen NH, Hansen HS. Familial clustering of salivary gland carcinoma in Greenland. *Cancer*, 1986; **57**: 2097–102.

39. Shore-Freedman E, Abrahams C, Recant W, Schneider AB. Neurilemomas and salivary gland tumors of the head and neck following childhood irradiation. *Cancer*, 1983; **51**: 2159–63.

40. Sandros J, Mark J, Happonen RP, Stenman G. Specificity of 6q-markers and other recurrent deviations in human malignant salivary gland tumors. *Anticancer Research*, 1988; **8**: 637–44.

41. Gnepp DR, Rader WR, Cramer SF, Cook LL, Sciubba J. Accuracy of frozen section diagnosis of the salivary gland. *Otolaryngology Head and Neck Surgery*, 1987; **96**: 325–30.

42. Layfield LJ, Tan P, Glasgow BJ. Fine-needle aspiration of salivary gland lesions: Comparison with frozen sections and histologic findings. *Archives of Pathological Medicine*, 1987; **111**: 346–53.

43. Krouse JH, Nadol JB, Goodman ML. Carcinoid tumors of the middle ear. *Annals of Otology, Rhinology and Laryngology*, 1990; **99**: 547–52.

9.1.3 Imaging of head and neck tumours

R. Sigal

Since the advent of modern cross sectional imaging, computed tomography (CT) and magnetic resonance (MR) imaging, there is no doubt, both to clinicians and radiologists, that imaging plays an essential role in the management of head and neck cancers. At present, questions focus on the advantages and drawbacks of these techniques and their complementary role at the various stages of the disease, on the exact role of ultrasound (US) and on the potential for new imaging techniques such as positron emission tomography (PET). Technical progress is permanent, as exemplified by MR imaging which allows more images to be obtained, faster, with better spatial resolution, and new types of contrast, or even information (MR angiography, MR spectroscopy, MR therapy).

However, this continuous improvement is causing two problems: in the literature, clinical series dealing with application of new technicalities often comprise limited numbers of patients; in addition, they may be partially obsolete at the time of publication. Therefore, as with treatment protocols, imaging preferences and protocols vary from one institution to another. Moreover, in a cost constraint environment, the high investment and running costs of these techniques has created the incentive to define cost-effective imaging strategies. Although still in the early stages in most countries, there is little doubt that this trend will deeply affect the practice of medical imaging in the future. As before, the radiologist must perform the best possible examination and provide adequate image interpretation. However, more and more his or her role is to act as a consultant by helping to select the optimal imaging technique and to define cost-effective imaging strategies. In this context, one can never sufficiently emphasize the value of daily co-operation between clinicians and head and neck radiologists:[1] common reading of imaging files, participation in clinical rounds, and multidisciplinary meetings ensure pertinent formulation of clinical questions and appropriate radiological answers. With the advent of new therapeutic techniques, such as conformal radiotherapy, this co-operation is enforced by the common use of dedicated workstations. Finally, it should be mentioned that specific training and experience are particularly important in head and neck radiology. This area, more than any other, is regarded by most radiologists as very challenging, both anatomically and technically, and often represents only a marginal proportion of their activity. One of the tasks of experienced head and neck radiologists is to promote this subspecialty among their colleagues.

Diagnostic imaging techniques

Conventional techniques

Standard dental views, which include dental occlusal films and plain film panoramic view, present three main advantages: they yield the best information on the patient's dentition, they are not degraded by dental amalgam artefacts, and they are familiar to clinicians. However, conventional radiographs cannot show small erosion of the inner cortex and give no information on the medullary bone; therefore they can hardly be considered as more than a screening examination. In oral cancer, CT and MR are more effective in deciding the need and the type of mandibulectomy.[2]

Barium swallow studies may be useful for evaluating the extension of a hypopharyngeal tumour (particularly located into the postcricoid area) to the cervical oesophagus.[3] Studies with water soluble contrast medium are also useful to identify post-treatment pharyngocutaneous fistula and aspiration into the trachea. Cineradiography and video-pharyngography may reveal pharyngeal and oesophageal dysfunction due to post-treatment fibrosis.[4]

Sialography should no longer be used when a parotid or sub-mandibulary gland tumour is suspected or certain.

Computed tomography

Careful, symmetrical installation of the patient is important in order to avoid generating images that simulate or obfuscate disease. The chin and/or forefront should be immobilized, or at least maintained by using dedicated strips. In the axial plane, images must cover the area extending from the skull base down to the thoracic inlet in order to assess the primary tumour, to perform lymph node survey, and to identify a possible synchronous tumour. With modern CT units, working in spiral mode rather than in conventional mode, acquisition of this set of images requires less than 5 min. Avoiding dental material often requires acquisition of two series with different gantry obliquity. The scout view must be printed in order to help the clinician to identify the level and inclination of each image. Slice thickness should not exceed 3 mm, and must be reduced to 1 to 2 mm for high-detail work. Contiguous sections are needed not only to avoid missing a small lesion but because they allow reformatted views to be obtained. The choice of the field of view (10 to 18 cm) and of the matrix size (512 × 512) must ensure that the pixel size (smallest picture element) is below 1 mm. Acquisitions are performed either breath hold or with quiet breathing. A modified Valsalva manoeuvre is particularly useful to open the pyrifom sinuses (Fig. 1). Intravenous injection of contrast material is mandatory, and there is no need for a non-contrast study. If a patient presents a history of severe contrast medium allergy, MR imaging should be consider rather than CT. Iodine injection helps delineate the tumour extent and differentiate between lymph nodes and adjacent vessels. It s therefore essential that all vessels (arteries and veins) are completely and constantly opacified from the first to the last image of the examination. This can be obtained when rapid scanning of the head and neck is performed synchronously with bolus injection performed via a power injector. Double windowing (soft tissue and bone algorithms) is always needed for analysis of bones and cartilages (Fig. 2). Undermagnification, at the neck level, and overmagnification, when the thoracic inlet is reached, should be avoided by properly adjusting the magnification factor.

Dental CT programmes, which include CT reformatting programmes,[5] allows evaluation of dental aspects of the oral cavity, including implants, periodontal disease, odontogenic tumours, and osteoradionecrosis.

CT-guided biopsy is currently used, including in lesions of the suprahyoid deep spaces and skull base.[6],[7] Fine-needle aspiration has gained general acceptance because of its safety, high accuracy rate, and cost effectiveness. More recently, the diagnostic accuracy has been increased by the use of core needle biopsies, which provide more tissue for pathological examination.[8],[9]

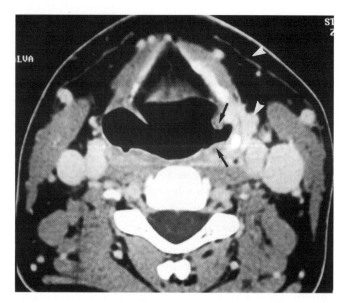

Fig. 1 CT manoeuvres. Pyriform sinus squamous cell carcinoma. Contrast-enhanced axial CT scan. The scan was acquired with the patient performing a modified Valsalva manoeuvre. The left pyriform sinus opens incompletely; tumour invasion of the internal and external walls (arrows) is demonstrated. Extrapharyngeal spread is also visible (arrowhead).

CT scan is also currently used for radiation therapy treatment planning, with a specific positioning and immobilizing device. It will play an essential role, along with MR, in the development of conformal radiation therapy.[10]

On-going developments in hardware and software have resulted in the production of more images in less time, with data manipulation such as three-dimensional reconstruction (Fig. 3) and reformation into multiple planes. These are particularly useful for sinonasal cavities, skull base, and nasopharynx imaging when direct coronal scanning cannot be performed (because the patient does not stand hyperextension positioning). In the neck it allows reconstruction of the spirally acquired sections with good anatomical information, provided that breathing and swallowing motion remain limited (Fig. 4). These manipulations are performed on dedicated workstations. At present, radiologists are devoting more and more energy to these time-consuming tasks and to the selection of appropriate images for the referring clinicians since a typical CT currently totals more than 100 images.

Magnetic resonance imaging

MR presents two main differences from CT. Firstly, it is a multi-dimensional acquisition technique which allows images to be acquired directly in any plane (whereas CT is restricted to one acquisition plane, usually axial). Secondly, MR is a multiparameter technique: each point of the image or voxel (volume element) depends on at least four parameters: proton density, T1 relaxation time, T2 relaxation time, and flow,[11] whereas CT is only dependent on one parameter: the attenuation of the X-ray beam. For a given level, several kinds of contrast can be generated, depending on the contributing parameter(s). This explains why MR is more difficult to perform and interpret, but also more sensitive than CT.

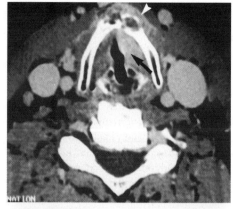

(a)

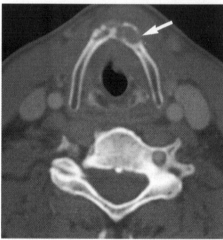

(b)

Fig. 2 CT soft tissue and bone window setting. Left vocal cord squamous cell carcinoma. (a) Contrast-enhanced axial CT scan. The tumour enhances with contrast (arrow). Tumour enhancement is also seen in the anterior strap muscle (arrowhead). (b) Same level, bone window setting, shows blowing of the thyroid cartilage (arrow), with disruption of the outer cortex, indicating tumour invasion.

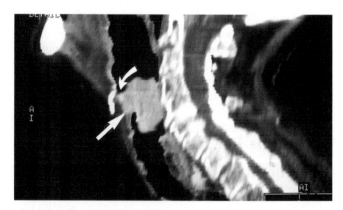

Fig. 3 CT reformatted view. Epiglottic squamous cell carcinoma. Contrast-enhanced CT scan, sagittal reformatted view. The exophytic component of the tumour obstructs the airway. The tumour invades the pre-epiglottic space (arrow) and the vallecula (curved arrow), but spares the base of the tongue.

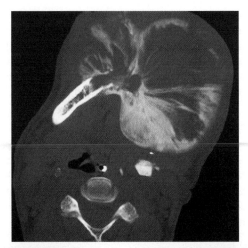

(a)

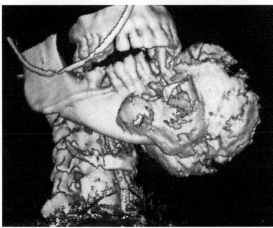

(b)

Fig. 4 (a)(b) CT three-dimensional display. Mandibular osteosarcoma. (a) Axial CT scan, bone window setting, displays a large mass invading the mandible with osteogenic components indicating a probable osteosarcoma. Diagnosis was confirmed at histology. (b) Three-dimensional reconstruction does not offer additional diagnostic information, but can be used by surgeons for surgical planning.

These advantages, superior tissue contrast and multiplanar views, are to be balanced with potential technical limitations. In head and neck imaging, motion artefacts due to swallowing, respiration, and blood circulation are especially troublesome. The ability to overcome these inconvenience by using appropriate 'counter measures' (flow compensation, in-plane and out-of-plane saturation, gating, etc.) are the hallmark of high quality MR units and experienced radiographers and radiologists. In cancer of the oral cavity, dental fillings (amalgams and moreover bridges) may degrade the image, creating so-called 'susceptibility artefacts'. However, what matters is the distance between the fillings and the area to be examined. If the fillings are located in an incisor, a tumour of the tongue base will be assessable, at least with sequences that minimize this type of artefacts (spin echo T1-weighted sequence). Claustrophobia and the impossibility to remain supine in obstructed airway patients account for a few percentages of technical failure. Education of the patient is essential. The patient should be reminded to maintain quiet breathing and to minimize swallowing during sequence acquisition.

MR study of the suprahyoid regions can be done with the head coil, which is standard on all MR units. This coil, however, does not cover the neck. A dedicated head and neck coil capable of covering the area from the skull base to the thoracic inlet is preferable. This type of coil is not available on all MR sites. Specialized coils developed for MR angiography of the supra aortic vessels are an excellent alternative since they allow the area between the aortic arch and the circle of Willis to be visualized.

The study comprises a combination of sagittal, coronal, and axial views. Image protocols include at least one T1-weighted sequence and one T2-weighted sequence, (acquired with spin-echo, fast-spin-echo or gradient echo techniques). Although not mandatory, intravenous injection of a contrast medium (compound) is highly recommended in cancer evaluation because it helps increase the conspicuity of the primary tumour and because it is the only reliable technique to detect perineural extension. After gadolinium injection, T1-weighted acquisition is performed in two or three orthogonal planes, one of them at least with a fat suppression technique. This technique allows the signal of fatty tissues (which normally appears bright on T1-weighted images) to be nullified, making recognition of abnormal contrast take up easier. Unenhanced, T1-weighted sequences are always needed to assess the medullary bone of the mandible and skull base correctly. As a general rule, no single sequence can give all the necessary information by itself and it always necessary to use more than one technique.[12]

The choice of the field of view, matrix size, slice thickness, and number of excitations is a compromise between signal-to-noise ratio, spatial resolution, and scanning time.[13] The basic field strength of the machine is an important determinant of the image quality. Most MR machines are either middle field units (between 0.5 and 1 tesla) or high field units (up to 2 teslas). Low field units (down to approximately 0.1 tesla) are cheaper but image quality is generally considered problematic in the head and neck area. T1-weighted images lead to optimal anatomical information provided that sufficient spatial resolution is programmed. This is routinely achieved by the use of a 15-cm field of view, 4-mm slice thickness, and 512 × 256 matrix. T2-weighted sequences are aimed at identifying abnormal tissue contrast (usually an increase in water content that will appear as an increased signal intensity area). This can be obtained by the use of a 20 to 25-cm field of view, 4-mm slice thickness, and 256 × 256 matrix.

For cancer evaluation, MR angiography has not obtained the status it has reached in the evaluation of carotid stenoses. It has been used to demonstrate flow within lesions and represents a familiar imaging display for surgical planning.[14] MR angiography is probably not useful in predicting carotid artery invasion by head and neck masses, since standard MR can directly image both the mass and the lumen.[15]

Ultrasound

Sonography is performed with a high frequency probe (7.5 to 13 MHz). Colour Doppler and power Doppler sonography help to differentiate a true vascular mass from a mass adjacent to, or displacing, surrounding structures. Not all radiological teams use sonography (other than for evaluation of thyroid and orbital pathology). This technique has several drawbacks: it does not explore the deep structures, it is operator dependent, and it does not provide standardized reference images for the clinicians. Its main advantages are low cost and easily accessible technique, which can easily guide a fine-needle aspiration.

Several studies, particularly from The Netherlands, have shown the benefit of ultrasound-guided fine-needle aspiration in the diagnosis of lymph node metastasis,[16],[17] with a specificity superior to 95 per cent.

Radionuclide studies

There is no routine indication for radionuclide studies in the head and neck area (besides thyroid and parathyroid). In the evaluation of the mandible, bone scan suffers from a lack of specificity, which is particularly prejudicial in a population with poor dental status, as dental abscesses and infection can simulate neoplastic infiltration.

Angiography

Because of the availability of CT, MRI, and MR angiography, indications for diagnostic angiography have almost completely ceased in the recent years. Diagnostic angiography is still the first step when endovascular therapy is needed (i.e. chemodectoma).

Special techniques—work in progress

Positron emission tomography

Positron emission tomography (PET) is a cross-sectional technique that maps the location and concentration of various radiopharmaceuticals. In cancer evaluation, 2-deoxy-2-[^{18}F]fluoro–D-glucose (FDG) has been mainly used. FDG-PET assesses tissue glucose metabolism, which increases with tumour growth.[18] Tumour uptake is unrelated to the histological grade. This technique has shown interesting results in the detection of head and neck cancers[19] and lymph node metastasis.[20] Another advantage is the capability to differentiate post-treatment changes from recurrence,[21],[22] a problem largely unsolved with other techniques. PET presents several drawbacks. The radiopharmaceuticals have a short half-life (110 min for FDG) and must be produced by a cyclotron located close to the imaging site, or even on site for new tracers under investigation such as thymidine, methionine, or tyrosine labelled with C^{11} (half-life: 20 min). Investment and running cost are high, and the number of machines is restricted. Spatial resolution is limited to 3 mm, which prevents microdeposits being seen and leads to anatomically poorly defined images. This last inconvenience may be obviated by the use of precise coregistration between MR or CT anatomical and PET functional images.[23] At present, FDG-PET has been proposed as a pretherapy exam when results from other modalities are ambiguous.[24] Further studies are needed to define the role of PET in the post-treatment period.[25]

Single photon emission CT (SPECT)[26] is a cheaper alternative to PET, but with worse spatial resolution. This problem has been partially overcome by the introduction of a dual-head coincidence gamma camera.[27] Other classical pharmaceuticals have been tested for the detection of occult primary and recurrences, such as thallium-201 SPECT[28] and for monitoring of nasopharyngeal carcinoma, such as Tc-99m-Sestamibi SPECT.[29]

Dynamic MRI

Sequential registration of MR images after bolus administration of gadolinium compound has been advocated as a means to differentiate between tumour recurrence, which enhances rapidly, and post-therapeutic changes, which present a delayed contrast take up.[30],[31] This method is not sufficiently reliable, even with the help of specialized image analysis software.[32] Dynamic MR has also been proposed to differentiate paragangliomas with an early vascular peak, from vascular nerve sheath tumours with a slightly delayed peak.[33]

MR therapy

Since the mid 90s, intraoperative MRI scanners have appeared on the market. These machines present an 'open configuration' with a space between the scanner's coils which gives access to the patient while imaging. These units have been used both for biopsy[34] and laser-induced thermotherapy,[35] with dedicated non-ferromagnetic instrumentation.

MR spectroscopy

The data available are limited. A study from Mukherji[36] shows that proton MR spectroscopy can help differentiate primary squamous cell carcinoma and nodal metastases from normal tissue both *in vitro* and *in vivo*. In the latter case, this technique necessitates a large sample (voxel size: $2 \times 2 \times 2$ cm) and is very sensitive to the so-called 'susceptibility' artefacts, which are frequent in the head and neck.

New MR contrast agents

The commonly used MR contrast agent, gadolinium, is non-specific: tumour, infection, and inflammation take contrast. Dextran-coated, ultrasmall, superparamagnetic iron oxide is a new contrast agent with the aim of performing lymphography.[37] The contrast medium is injected intravenously. The iron particles are taken up by macrophages in the reticuloendothelial system, and this translates into a signal reduction on T2-weighted images. If the normal lymph node is replaced by metastatic tissue, the lymph node shows a high signal intensity. The preliminary results of Anzai seem promising in the differentiation between metastatic disease and benign hyperplasia with a specificity of 84 per cent and a sensitivity of 95 per cent.[38] Further studies are needed to confirm the value of this product.

Teleradiology

Head and neck radiology, a highly specialized field of radiology, is a typical field for the development of teleradiology.[39] Head and neck teleradiology will probably deal less with primary diagnosis (i.e. the examination is performed by a radiographer and interpreted by a radiologist) than second opinion (i.e. difficult cases are submitted to subspecialty experts). The speed of development of teleradiology will depend on several factors: technical (image format and image exchange protocol standardization, image speed transmission, security, and confidentiality), legal (liability), and economical (software and hardware costs, transmission costs, reimbursement), with the additional difficulty that some of them vary from one country (or state) to another.[40] In fact, teleradiology will tend to be one of the many activities which will be made possible by the development of imaging networks, (inter- or intra-institutional), hospital information systems, and picture archive and communication systems. The electronic patient record should enhance the capability to mix, share, and store data of various sources (clinical data, biology, radiology, pathology).

Table 1 Clinical information needed by the radiologist

1. Patient status
   initial workup
   treatment monitoring (i.e. evaluation after several regimen of chemotherapy)
   follow-up
   suspicion of relapse
   complication of treatment

2. Area(s) involved

3. Histological diagnosis (suspected or confirmed)

4. Previous head and neck treatment(s), with the date of completion of the last treatment

5. Results of physical examination

6. Results of endoscopic examination (if available)

7. Results of previous imaging examinations (in particular for follow-up)

8. UICC or AJCC staging (if available)

UICC = Union Internationale Contre le Cancer; AJCC = American Joint Committee on Cancer.

Internet will play an increasing role, at least in the education domain (reference image databases; teaching files).

Initial stage imaging and post-treatment imaging

It is critically important to the head and neck radiologist to get accurate clinical information about the patient referred for imaging workup whatever the stage of disease (Table 1). Imaging of the lung, liver, and bones is required to detect metastasis: a presentation of these techniques, results, and indications is beyond the scope of this chapter. The information will help the radiologist to select the appropriate imaging modality, to focus technically the examination onto the suspected area, and to interpret the images.

Initial stage

The majority of cancers of the head and neck are squamous cell carcinoma arising from the epithelium of the mucosa. Most often the lesion is identified by the clinician, and therefore the radiologist plays a minor role in the detection of the disease. In this situation, performing tissue characterization with the help of imaging data is not necessary: pathology, which is mandatory, is easy when the lesion is accessible to biopsy. The role of the radiologist is to define the exact spread of the mucosal lesion in deeper tissues. This task, called tumour mapping, is a key stage in the therapeutic planning. Imaging plays a complementary role with physical and endoscopic examination. CT and/or MR may show disease spreading beyond what is seen or palpated by the clinician: extension to the orbits, skull base, brain (Fig. 5), or identification of retropharyngeal nodes. But imaging may also help to identify the site of origin when patients are difficult to examine (trismus) or when the mucosa is hidden beyond lymphoid tissue (squamous cell carcinoma lying deep in the crypts

of the faucial or lingual tonsils). Superficial spread along the mucosa, such as in carcinoma *in situ*, is not visible at imaging. Discrepancies between imaging and physical data can therefore occur in both sides: imaging ignores superficial extension, and physical examination often underestimates deep spread. For instance, the subglottic mucosal extension of a glottic squamous cell carcinoma may be unseen radiologically; but the same tumour may involved the pre-epiglottic space and cartilages and be only disclosed at imaging (Fig. 2).

Imaging is an indispensable tool in patients with clinical suspicion of submucosal mass. CT and MR imaging can establish the positive diagnosis by showing a true mass versus a pseudomass (such as a tortuous internal carotid artery or a vertebral body osteophyte displacing the pharyngeal posterior wall). Imaging can guide a biopsy, or conversely prevent a procedure that can be hazardous in case of hypervascularized mass. By evidencing the exact space of origin of the lesion (see below) and its characteristics (CT density, MR signal, homo- or heterogeneity, contour, contrast enhancement), imaging can anticipate the correct diagnosis.[41] It should, however, be clearly stated that probably the main limitation of CT and MR is their lack of specificity (Fig. 6). Contrast enhancement (either iodine or gadolinium) is common to benign and malignant neoplasms but also to inflammation and infection. This is particularly troublesome in the head and neck area where these conditions frequently coexist. Although work in progress have been done to overcome this inconvenience (see above), this is still the routine situation and this underscores the absolute need for histological proof when a treatment is considered.[42] In the head and neck, biopsy is almost always feasible, albeit sometimes aggressive. Often, the correct diagnosis is ensured by comparing imaging results with clinical, pathological, and biological data.

Spaces

Tumour mapping supposes a precise anatomical knowledge. Modern cross sectional imaging has deeply modified the perception of the anatomy of the head and neck because it permits direct identification of the main deep structures. A reappraisal of the anatomy has been proposed by H.R. Harnsberger[43] and has become common ground among head and neck radiologists (although other descriptions exist).[44] The concept of space is superimposed on the traditional presentation of areas (oropharynx, nasopharynx, oral cavity, etc.). French anatomists originally described these spaces in the nineteenth century;[45] they are defined by the course of the three layers of the deep cervical fascia (not directly visualized), superficial layer (investing fascia), middle layer (buccopharyngeal fascia), and deep layer (prevertebral fascia). The different spaces and their critical content are presented in Tables 2, 3, and 4 and Fig. 7. The mucosal space is located on the airway side of the pharynx and therefore is not completely fascia-enclosed. The advantage of using this terminology is that it allows tumour spread in the deep tissues to be described using precise anatomical landmarks (Figs 8 and 9), as well as specific differential diagnoses for each space.

It is noteworthy that, in the literature, the term 'parapharyngeal space' (or even infratemporal fossa) has been used to describe a large area that includes the carotid space, the masticator space, and the small area described by Harnsberger as the parapharyngeal space. This parapharyngeal space is an important landmark with three distinct features: it is central (with respect to the masticator, carotid, and parotid spaces), it is symmetrical, and it is essentially composed

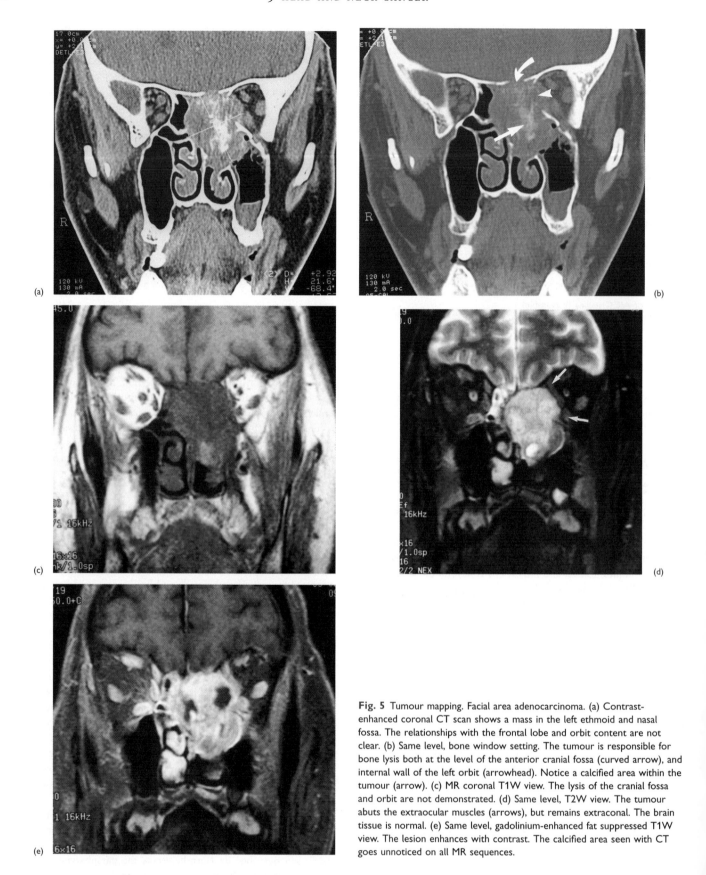

Fig. 5 Tumour mapping. Facial area adenocarcinoma. (a) Contrast-enhanced coronal CT scan shows a mass in the left ethmoid and nasal fossa. The relationships with the frontal lobe and orbit content are not clear. (b) Same level, bone window setting. The tumour is responsible for bone lysis both at the level of the anterior cranial fossa (curved arrow), and internal wall of the left orbit (arrowhead). Notice a calcified area within the tumour (arrow). (c) MR coronal T1W view. The lysis of the cranial fossa and orbit are not demonstrated. (d) Same level, T2W view. The tumour abuts the extraocular muscles (arrows), but remains extraconal. The brain tissue is normal. (e) Same level, gadolinium-enhanced fat suppressed T1W view. The lesion enhances with contrast. The calcified area seen with CT goes unnoticed on all MR sequences.

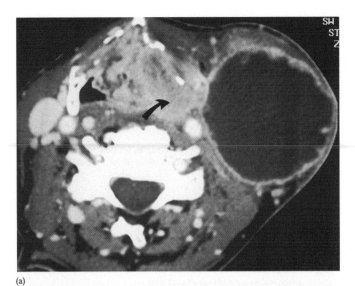

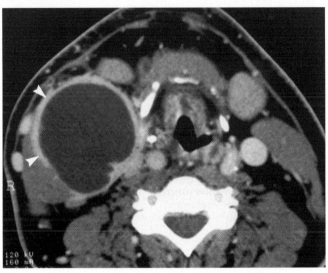

Fig. 6 Lack of specificity. Low attenuation neck masses. (a) Contrast-enhanced axial CT scan shows a large necrotic lymph node adjacent to a left pyriform sinus cancer (curved arrow). (b) In another patient contrast-enhanced axial CT scan shows a low attenuation mass, which was a second branchial cyst. Notice that the cyst wall slightly enhances with contrast (arrowheads), but is more regular than in the previous case.

of fat, which characteristically exhibits high signal intensity on T1-weighted images and low attenuation on CT. The main characteristic of most of these spaces is their verticality: the carotid, retropharyngeal, and perivertebral spaces extend both across the infra- and the suprahyoid neck (down to T3 for the retropharyngeal space). The parapharyngeal and masticator spaces are related to the oropharynx and nasopharynx. This substantiates the need to explore any cancer from the skull base to the thoracic inlet. These spaces have been compared to vertical elevator shafts, which represent natural routes for tumour or infectious spread.[43] The fascia can be transpierced by malignant tumours; however, these spaces tend, at least initially, to channel tumour growth and to confine even high-grade tumours.[46]

Primary tumour: basic CT and MR patterns

CT

On plain CT, the density of most tumours is very closed to that of surrounding muscles. For this reason non-contrast-enhanced CT is useless. After intravenous injection of iodine, most tumours take contrast. Hypervascularized lesions usually correspond to chemodectoma (located in the carotid space) or vascular schwannoma. It is noteworthy that many cancers only enhance mildly, resulting in a poor differential contrast with surrounding muscles. In this situation, careful analysis of the various spaces is essential to identify the disease and to analyse its extension. The larger the tumour, the more likely it is to be non-homogeneous, with a mixture of 'active' hyperintense areas and necrotic hypointense sectors. Careful attention to the fatty, hypodense tissues is important for detecting asymmetry of the parapharyngeal space, extracapsular spread of lymph node metastasis, or pre-epiglottic space invasion. Metastatic lymph nodes do not enhance with contrast. In fact, the best indicator of tumour invasion is the presence of central, low-density necrosis, whatever the size of the node. The presence of hypodense central tissue has been regarded as a predictor of poor response to chemotherapy.[47]

Bone window setting images allow visualization not only of calcification, but also thin bones, such as the cribrifom plate or the lamina papyracea, two key elements in the diagnostic workup of facial area tumours which are not seen with MR.

MR

As a rule, T1-weighted images do not provide a good tumour-to-tissue contrast because both the tumour and the surrounding muscles exhibit the same signal intensity. T1-weighted images offer the best contrast between tumour and fat (i.e. tumour extension into the orbital fat). This type of image is also essential to depict the medullary portion of the mandible and skull base. Medullary bone in adults is essentially made of fat and exhibits a characteristic high signal on T1-weighted images. Tumour invasion causes replacement of normal marrow and translates into an area of low signal intensity; this aspect, however, is non-specific and is seen in cases of infection or inflammation. Areas of low signal intensity are particularly frequent in the horizontal branch of the mandible since many cancer patient have a poor dental status with dental infection.[2] Lipoma can be identified thanks to their signal hyperintensity.

T2-weighted images usually provide excellent tumour-to-muscle contrast. Muscles are displayed with relatively low signal intensity. The signal intensity of the tumour depends on its internal architecture, and particularly on the degree of cellularity and water content. Tumours with a low nucleocytoplasmic ratio or cystic components or areas of necrosis exhibit a high signal intensity. This is the case with most of the squamous cell carcinoma arising from the oral mucosa. Salivary gland tumours (such as pleomorphic adenomas and Whartin's tumours), cystic haemangioma and lymphangioma, and chordoma exhibit a marked, high signal intensity. Adenoid cystic carcinoma presentation varies from low to high signal intensity, and this is partly related to the histological subtype: solid, cribriform, or tubular.[48] Fibro-osseous tumours and most facial area tumours (squamous cell carcinoma and adenocarcinoma) exhibit a low signal intensity because they have few water protons. In the sinonasal area, T2-weighted sequences are especially interesting because they allow differentiation between tumour extension, which appears with low signal intensity, and oedematous mucosa and trapped secretions, which are displayed

Table 2 Spaces and content of the suprahyoid neck (adapted from Ref. 43)

Space	Extent	Contents	Differential diagnosis
Mucosal	Skull base to lower hypoharynx	Lymphoid tissue (adenoids, faucial, and lingual tonsils) Superior, middle constrictor muscles Salpingopharyngeal muscle Levator palatini muscle[a] Torus tubarius[a]	*Pseudotumour* Asymmetric fossa of Rosenmuller, postinfectious or postirradiation mucosal inflammation *Congenital* Tornwaldt's cyst *Inflammatory* Adenoid or faucial tonsil hypertrophy, tonsilitis or abscess Postinflammatory dystrophic calcification or retention cyst *Benign tumour* Benign mixed tumour of minor salivary gland *Malignant tumour* Squamous cell carcinoma (SCC), non-Hodgkin lymphoma, minor salivary gland malignancy
Parapharyngeal	Skull base to hyoid bone	Fat Branches of cranial nerve V3 Internal maxillary artery Ascending pharyngeal artery	*Pseudomass* Asymmetric pterygoid venous plexus *Congenital* Atypical second branchial cleft cyst *Infectious* Pleomorphic adenoma, lipoma *Malignancies* Tumour spread from mucosal, parotid, or masticator spaces
Masticator	External temporal fossa to angle of the mandible	Lateral pterygoid muscle Medial pterygoid muscle Masseter muscle Inferior alveolar nerve (branch of cranial nerve V3) Ramus and body of mandible	*Pseudomass* Accessory parotid gland, benign masseteric hypertrophy *Congenital* Haemangioma, lymphangioma *Infectious* Odontogenic abscess *Benign tumour* Osteoblastoma, leiomyoma, neural sheath tumour *Malignancies* Soft tissue sarcoma, chondrosarcoma, osteosarcoma Rhabdomyosarcoma (children) Non-Hodgkin lymphoma SCC from oropharynx (retromolar trigone).
Parotid	External auditory canal to angle of the mandible	Parotid gland Facial nerve (VII) Retromandibular vein External carotid and internal maxillary arteries Intraparotid lymph nodes	*Congenital* First branchial cleft cyst Haemangioma, lymphangioma (children) *Infectious or inflammatory* Abscess, reactive lymphadenopathy, benign lymphoepithelial lesions (AIDS), sarcoid *Benign tumour* Pleomorphic adenoma, Whartin's tumour, oncocytoma, lipoma, facial nerve schwannoma or neurofibroma *Malignant tumour* Mucoepidermoid carcinoma, adenoic cystic carcinoma, non-Hodgkin lymphoma Metastatic lymph nodes from skin SCC and melanoma
Submandibular	Between mylohyoid muscle and hyoid bone; communicates with the sublingual and parapharyngeal spaces	Fat Anterior belly of digatric muscle Superficial portion of submandibular gland Submandibular and submental lymph nodes Facial artery and vein Inferior loop of cranial nerve XII	*Pseudomass* V3 nerve motor atrophy *Congenital* Second branchial cleft cyst, cystic hygroma, lymphangioma, haemangioma, suprahyoid thyroidal duct cyst *Infectious* Ludwig's angina, cellulitis, abscess, submandibular gland inflammation, diving ranula *Benign tumour* Lipoma, epidermoid, dermoid, benign mixed tumour of submandibular gland *Malignant tumour* Tumour spread from tongue or floor of the mouth SCC, submandibular gland carcinoma Nodal metastasis of oral cavity and face SCC, nodal lymphoma

Table 2 continued

Space	Extent	Contents	Differential diagnosis
Sublingual	Between mylohyoid muscle and geniohyoid/genioglossus muscles	Lingual nerve (branch of cranial nerve V3) Cranial nerves IX and XII Lingual artery and vein Sublingual gland and ducts Deep portion of submandibular gland Wharton's duct	*Pseudotumour* Hypoglossal nerve motor atrophy *Congenital* Haemangioma, lymphangioma, epidermoid, dermoid, lingual thyroid *Infectious* Ludwig's angina, cellulitis, abscess, dilated Wharton's duct due to calculus or stenosis *Benign tumour* Benign mixed tumour of sublingual gland *Malignant tumour* Tumour spread from tongue or floor of the mouth SCC Sublingual gland carcinoma
Retropharyngeal	Skull base to aortic arch	See Table 4	See Table 4
Perivertebral	Skull base to mediastinum	See Table 4	See Table 4
Carotid	Skull base to mediastinum	See Table 4	See Table 4

ª originates outside space.

with high signal intensity (because they contain a high number of water protons). In facial area tumours, intracerebral extension is identified because they are responsible for a high signal intensity oedema on T2-weighted images.

After gadolinium injection, enhancement patterns parallel what is observed on contrast-enhanced CT—enhancement grossly reflects the degree of vascularity of a tumour. Contrast take-up occurs not only in tumours but also in inflammation and infection. Physiological mucosal enhancement is clearly seen at the three levels of the pharynx. On gadolinium MR, it may be difficult to recognize abnormal high signal intensity enhancement in a lesion located close or into a fatty tissue, since fat also exhibits physiologically high signal intensity on T1-weighted images. The solution comes from the so-called 'fat saturation' technique: during image acquisition, a specific radio-frequency pulse is emitted which nullifies the signal of fat; as a result, fatty tissues display a low signal intensity, allowing better delineation of the limits of contrast take-up. Fat saturation techniques are especially interesting in the neck, where fat is always present, and if extension into the orbits is suspected[12],[49] (Fig. 5).

One the main interests of injecting gadolinium is the recognition of perineural spread, a characteristic feature of adenoid cystic carcinoma, and a frequent finding in squamous cell carcinoma (Fig. 10). MR has been shown to have a sensitivity of 95 per cent, although it may fail to depict microscopic foci of perineural tumour infiltration.[50] Cranial nerve V and VII are particularly at risk in cases of facial area and parotid tumours respectively. gadolinium-MR enables the diagnosis by showing enlargement and abnormal contrast enhancement.[51]–[53] MR can show both anterograde and retrograde extension. In case of trigeminal invasion, MR clearly analyses the foramen ovale (mandibulary nerve V3), the foramen rotundum and pterygopalatine fossa (maxillary nerve V2), and the Gasserian ganglion (and cavernous sinus). In nasopharyngeal carcinoma, for instance,

MR was able to demonstrate trigeminal perineural invasion in more than 50 per cent of patients with no facial pain or paresthesia.[53]

In facial area tumours with intracranial extension, meninges appear thickened and enhancing when they are invaded (Fig. 11). Linear enhancement is a poor predictor of dural invasion (40 per cent accuracy). Focal nodules and dural enhancement wider than 5 mm or pial enhancement are good predictors of tumour spread with an accuracy superior to 80 per cent.[54]

Exophytic, infiltrative, and necrotic tumours

The growth of malignancies arising from the mucosa can follow several patterns. These four patterns can coexist (Fig. 12):

- Superficial spread is characterized by the respect of the basal membrane. This pattern is seen in *in situ* carcinoma. This type of lesion cannot be evidenced at imaging because the depth of penetration is not sufficient.

- By definition, squamous cell carcinoma are infiltrative lesions extending beyond the basal membrane. If the chorion is minimally invaded, the lesion is histologically characterized as a microinvasive carcinoma and is usually not seen at imaging. When the carcinoma invade the various underlying soft tissues, it is clearly identified at imaging.

- Exophytic tumours grow in the lumen of the sinonasal cavities, nasopharynx, oropharynx, oral cavity, hypopharynx, and larynx.

- Ulceration is frequent; necrosis is usually associated with large lesions.

The upper aerodigestive tract presents several sulci in which tumours may grow or originate (i.e. glossotonsillar sulcus, gingivo-buccal sulcus, sulcus lying between the undersurface of the tongue and the floor of the mouth). Since imaging examinations are performed on patients with closed mouth, sulci become virtual and it may be

Table 3 Spaces and content of the infrahyoid neck (adapted from Ref. 43)

Space	Extent	Contents	Differential diagnosis
Visceral	Hyoid bone to mediastinum	Thyroid gland Parathyroid glands Larynx Trachea Hypopharynx Oesophagus Recurrent laryngeal nerves Lymph nodes (paratracheal)	*Pseudomass* Thyroid pyramidal lobe or prominent isthmus *Congenital* Thyroid gland: thyroglossal duct cysts *Infectious* Thyroid gland: thyroiditis *Benign neoplasms* Thyroid gland: goiter, colloid cyst, adenoma Parathyroid glands: adenoma, cyst Larynx: laryngocele Oesophagus: Zenker's diverticulum *Malignancies* Thyroid: carcinoma (papillary, follicular, anaplastic), non-Hodgkin lymphoma, metastasis Larynx and hypopharynx: squamous cell carcinoma Oesophagus: carcinoma Lymph nodes: metastases from thyroid and subglottic laryngeal carcinoma, lymphoma
Posterior cervical	Skull base to clavicles	Fat Spinal accessory nerve (cranial nerve XI) Spinal accessory lymph nodes Preaxillary brachial plexus	*Congenital* Lymphangioma, haemangioma, third branchial cleft cysts *Infectious* Abscess, spinal accessory cervical chain adenopathy *Benign neoplasms* Lipoma, neural sheath tumour *Malignancies* Spinal accessory cervical chain adenopathy, liposarcoma
Retropharyngeal	Skull base to aortic arch	See Table 4	See Table 4
Perivertebral	Skull base to mediastinum	See Table 4	See Table 4
Carotid	Skull base to mediastinum	See Table 4	See Table 4

difficult to assess precisely the site of origin and the structures invaded by a tumour. A typical example is given by tumours of the glossotonsillar sucus: it is sometimes difficult to evaluate whether or not a tumour has invaded the base of the tongue and/or the tonsillar fossa (Fig. 13). In addition, this assessment greatly depends on the exophytic or infiltrative characteristics of the lesion. A purely exophytic lesion will displace the base of the tongue and tonsillar fossa, whereas an infiltrative tumour may invade one or two sides. Clinical information becomes essential in such situation. Similar difficulties are encountered in lesions arising from a recess or reaching it (i.e. fossa of Rosenmuller, pyriform sinus, valleculae). The Valsalva maneuver is routinely used to open the pyriform sinuses (Fig. 1) but is not always successful.

Benign versus malignant appearance

The problem of establishing whether a lesion has a benign or a malignant appearance only arise in a submucosal mass. Ultimately, the diagnosis is confirmed by biopsy. Imaging, however, can anticipate the diagnosis by displaying the exact space of origin of the lesion and its CT/MR characteristics. A good example is given by salivary gland tumours (Figs 14 and 15). If a lesion presents as a homogeneous,

well-circumscribed, high signal intensity on T2-weighted images, the diagnosis of pleomorphic adenoma is likely. However, intraparotid lymph nodes, other benign tumours, low-grade malignancies, and even some adenoid cystic carcinoma (cribriform subtype) may share the same features. Conversely, a lesion presenting as a ill-defined mass, poorly marginated, extending outside the gland, with low signal intensity on T2-weighted images is highly suspicious of being a high-grade, aggressive lesion. If lymph nodes and/or perineural spread along cranial nerve VII is seen, malignancy becomes certain (although exact diagnosis needs to be established histologically). In summary, one can say that, at imaging, a diagnosis of benignancy is never certain, but a diagnosis of malignancy is often accurate.

Bone and/or cartilage destruction certainly constitutes one of the best indicators of cancer. Lysis of the bone cortex and cartilage are best seen with CT, whereas T1-weighted MR images are optimal to show abnormal signal within the medullary part of the bones, either in the skull base or mandible (Figs 16 and 17). Bone remodelling or cartilage sclerosis is not specific and can be seen in benign tumours. In fact, a combination of diagnostic criteria should be used to predict tumour invasion. For instance in laryngeal tumours, Becker

Table 4 Spaces common to the suprahyoid and infrahyoid neck (adapted from Ref. 43)

Space	Extent	Contents	Differential diagnosis
Carotid	Skull base (jugular foramen) to aortic arch	Common carotid artery Internal jugular vein Vagus nerve (cranial nerve X) Sympathetic chain Deep cervical lymph nodes	*Pseudomass* Carotid bulb and internal jugular vein asymmetry. Carotid artery ectasia *Congenital* Second branchial cleft cyst *Infectious* Deep cervical chain adenopathy, abscess *Benign neoplasms* Carotid body tumour, neural sheath tumour *Malignancies* Deep cervical chain adenopathy *Vascular* Internal jugular vein thrombosis, asymmetric internal jugular vein; carotid artery dissection and pseudoaneurysm
Retropharyngeal	Skull base to mediastinum (T3)	Fat Medial and lateral lymph nodes at the suprahyoid level	*Pseudomass* Tortuous carotid artery *Congenital* Lymphangioma, haemangioma *Infectious* Adenopathy, cellulitis, abscess *Benign neoplasms* Lipoma *Malignancies* Direct invasion from primary pharyngeal squamous cell carcinoma
Perivertebral	Skull base to mediastinum	*Prevertebral portion* Prevertebral and scalene muscles Brachial plexus roots Phrenic nerve Vertebral artery and nerve Vertebral body and pedicle *Paraspinal portion* Paraspinal muscles Posterior elements	*Pseudomass* Vertebral body osteophyte, cervical rib, levator scapulae hypertrophy, anterior disk herniation *Infectious* Vertebral spondylodiscitis *Benign neoplasms* Neural sheath tumour (brachial plexus), chordoma and other vertebral body benign tumour *Malignancies* Vertebral body and epidural metastasis, non-Hodgkin lymphoma, vertebral body malignant tumour, sarcoma (including brachial plexus neurosarcoma)

recommends the use of the following criteria: extralaryngeal tumour and erosion or lysis in the thyroid, cricoid, and arytenoid cartilages and sclerosis in the cricoid and arytenoid (but not thyroid) cartilages. This combination yields a sensitivity of 82 per cent and a specificity of 79 per cent.[55]

Growth patterns may help to establish differential diagnosis.[1] Benign lesions tend to grow slower than malignant ones. It is therefore legitimate, if there is a doubt on a deeply sited submucosal mass, to follow the patient at imaging. However, as stated by Mancuso, one should resist the temptation to universally link gross morphology and growth patterns to histology. Benign inflammatory lesions may have an aggressive growth pattern, and malignant tumour may have an indolent appearance.[1] One should also bear in mind that low-grade malignancies may mimic benign lesions both in terms of presentation and growth pattern, and that benign lesions may become malignant.

Lymph nodes

Imaging plays an important role in lymph node survey, especially in adipose or short-neck patients. In patients presenting with clinical evidence of lymph node disease, imaging often modifies the clinical staging by showing additional nodes, ipsi- or contralateral, or by showing multiple, matted ganglions instead of one unique node.

Imaging can detect clinically occult, metastastic lymph nodes, either located at the cervical or retropharyngeal level (Fig. 18). This is particularly important in the 25 per cent or more of patients presenting with no palpable neck disease (N0 stage). The performance

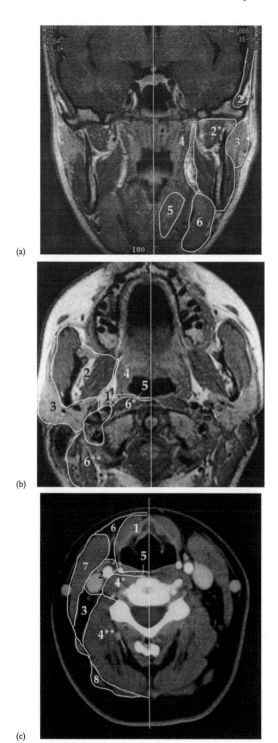

Fig. 7 Anatomy of the deep spaces. White line represents the different layers of the deep cervical fascia. (a) Supra-hyoid level, proton density weighted coronal MR view.1: parapharyngeal space; 2*: masticator space, infrazygomatic portion; 2**: masticator space, suprazygomatic portion; 3: parotid space; 4: mucosal space; 5: sublingual space; 6: submandibulary space. (b) Supra-hyoid level, axial T1-weighted MR view. 1: parapharyngeal space; 2: masticator space; 3: parotid space; 4: mucosal space; 5: retropharyngeal space; 6*: paravertebral space, anterior compartment; 6**: paravertebral space, posterior compartment. (c) Infrahyoid neck, contrast-injected axial CT scan. 1: visceral space; 2: carotid space; 3: posterior cervical space; 4*: perivertebral space, anterior portion; 4**: perivertebral space, posterior portion; 5: retropharyngeal space; 6: anterior cervical space; 7: sternocleidomastoid muscle; 8: trapezius muscle.

of CT and MR remains, however, unsatisfactory since micrometastases are found in up to 25 to 40 per cent of radiographically normal nodes.[56] Identification of metastatic lymph nodes remains a difficult challenge, both with CT and MR. At present, CT is considered the most reliable technique to detect lymph nodes,[57] although one can expect that technical improvement will rapidly put MR on an equal footing. The best criteria for tumour invasion is the identification of intranodal necrosis and microdeposits, whatever the size of the lymph node, which appear as low attenuated areas in CT,[58] and high signal intensity areas on T2-weighted images.[59] Hypodensity has been used as a predictor of response to cisplatin-based chemotherapy.[47] Extracapsular spread can be identified by subtle modification of the perinodal fat, including small-sized nodes.[58] Indirect evidence of nodal metastases includes nodal enlargement, a grouping of three or more borderline-sized nodes in the primary drainage pathway, and a spherical rather than an elliptical shape. The size criteria has a poor predictive value. Traditionally, radiologists take 1-cm diameter as the limit between normal and abnormal lymph nodes (other than the upper jugulodigatric node with a 1.5-cm diameter). A recent study suggests that a minimal axial diameter of 7 mm in level II nodes and 6 mm for the rest of the neck represent the optimal compromise between specificity and sensitivity in necks without palpable metastases.[60]

MR or CT? [1],[3]

Although the aim should be to perform only one modality, in some situation both MR and CT should be done. In fact, what matters is the choice of the first step examination in each clinical situation. In practice, this choice is often made by clinicians. Ideally it should be the results of a common strategy defined by clinicians and radiologists. With the results of the first step examination, the radiologist should then decide whether or not complementary radiological information is needed. One can see the importance of co-operation between radiologists and clinicians in this process.[61] Although the establishment of imaging guidelines should be favoured, it should be clear that one universal guideline cannot exist: the choice between CT and MR is still unsettled in many clinical situations. In addition, it depends on several local factors such as CT and MR availability and familiarity of non-radiologists with MR. Another factor is the effective use of the information provided by each technique for treatment planning. One example is given by the ability of MR imaging to show subtle invasion of the muscles of the tonsillar region (anterior and posterior pillars, and pharyngeal constrictor muscle), information not provided by CT. This data is only relevant in centres where treatment planning will be modified by this kind of information (i.e. the choice between surgery and irradiation).

The general advantages and inconvenience of CT and MR are presented in Table 5. With time, the trend for MR has been to establish its superiority from top to bottom. It is now the practice of most radiologists to favour MR as the primary modality in cancer of the nasopharynx, facial area, skull base, and anytime that there is potential perineural spread or extension to the brain and meninges. MR is tending to become the modality of choice in the evaluation of parotids, oral cavity, and oropharynx. The next step will be to determine whether state-of-the-art MR (performed with a dedicated coil and appropriate artefacts reduction techniques) will confirm the promising results in neck disease, including larynx[62],[63] and hypopharynx. In lymph node disease, it will have to be demonstrated

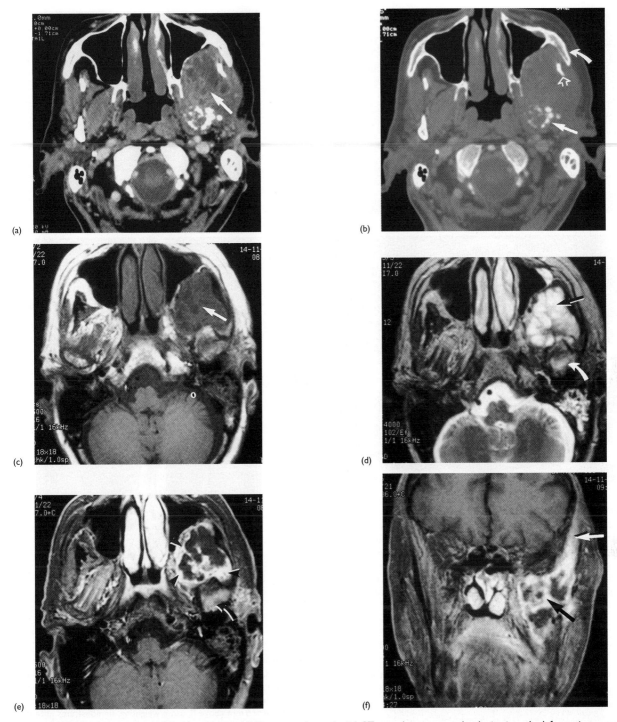

Fig. 8 Tumour of the masticator space. Chondrosarcoma. (a) Contrast-enhanced axial CT scan shows a mass developing into the left masticator space (arrow), with mass effect on the posterior wall of the maxillary sinus. The tumour only mildly enhances with contrast, making identification of its medial and lateral limits difficult. (b) Same level, bone window setting. Pop corn calcifications in the area of the ramus (arrow) indicate a possible cartilaginous component. The tumour abuts the zygomatic arch, which remains intact (curved arrow), and slightly displaces the coronoid process (open arrow). (c) MR T1W view. Muscle-to-tumour contrast is poor. The lesion is slightly heterogeneous. The zygomatic arch and the coronoid process are not identified. (d) Same level, T2W view. Muscle-to-tumour contrast is excellent: the anterior portion of the lesion displays a heterogeneous, increased signal intensity. The posterior portion is displayed with lower signal intensity (curved arrow). (e) Same level, axial gadolinium-enhanced, fat-suppressed, T1W view. The active portion of the lesion markedly enhances with contrast (arrowheads), whereas central portions do not. The calcificied areas seen at CT are not identified, but MR allows 'active' enhancing tissue in this area to be identified (curved arrow). (f) Coronal view, same weighting as (e), demonstrates that the lesion invades both the infrazygomatic (black arrow) and suprazygomatic parts of the masticator space, since abnormal contrast take up is seen in the upper part of the temporal muscle (white arrow).

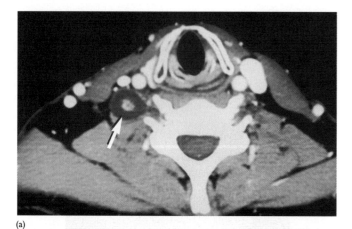

(a)

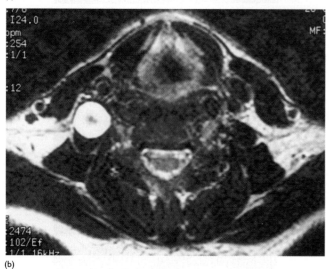

(b)

Fig. 9 Tumour of perivertebral space. Cystic schwannoma. (a) Contrast-enhanced axial CT scan shows a well-circumscribed lesion (arrow) located in the perivertebral space, and extending to the adjacent cervical posterior space. (b) MR T2W view. The lesion presents a high signal intensity peripheral area indicating a cystic component, and a central low intensity portion. The space of origin and the CT/MR characteristics make the diagnosis of cystic schwannoma likely. The diagnosis was confirmed at histology.

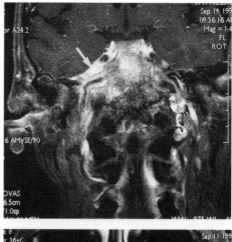

(a)

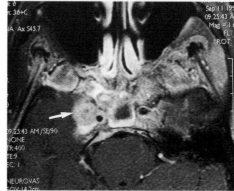

(b)

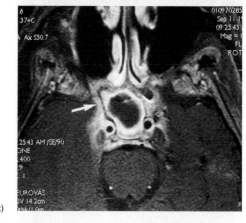

(c)

Fig. 10 Perineural spread. (a) Coronal gadolinium-enhanced, fat-suppressed, T1W view shows perineural retrograde invasion of the mandibulary nerve (V^3), above the foramen ovale (arrow). (b) Axial view, same weighting, demonstrates invasion of the Gasserian ganglion (arrow). (c) Axial view 5 mm above B, same weighting, demonstrates anterograde extension along maxillary nerve (V^2) (arrow).

that the excellent results achieved with MR in the detection of retropharyngeal adenopathy[64] can be obtained at the cervical level, which is still not the case.[57]

Post-treatment

Imaging plays an important role in the management of patients after treatment, who are often difficult to examine clinically.

Expected changes

Surgery

The presentation of site-specific changes is beyond the scope of this chapter. It is important for the radiologist to be familiar with the results of the main surgical procedures, particularly partial surgery of the larynx,[65] neck dissection,[66] and reconstructive surgery with

myocutaneous flaps.[67],[68] As stated by Mancuso, the word 'scar' should refer to the end product of the inflammatory response.[1] This collagenous, poorly hydrated tissue is displayed, when compared to muscles, with low signal intensity on T2-weighted images, and shows no contrast enhancement (either gadolinium or iodine). In contrast, granulation tissue corresponds to the ongoing inflammatory response: it appears with moderately to markedly increased signal intensity on

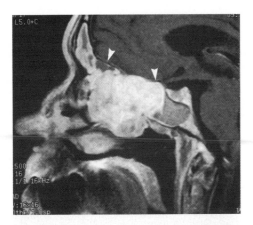

Fig. 11 Meningeal enhancement. Sagittal, gadolinium-enhanced, T1W view. A large facial area adenocarcinoma abuts the anterior cranial fossa. Enhancement of the duramater (arrowheads) constitutes an indirect evidence of bony disruption.

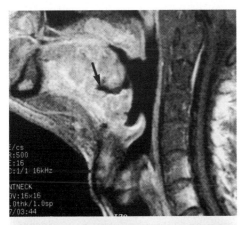

(a)

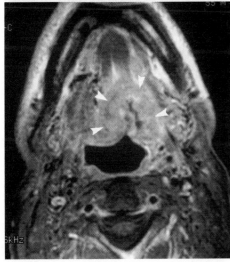

(b)

Fig. 12 Infiltrative pattern. Squamous cell carcinoma of the base of the tongue. (a) Sagittal, T1W view. The ulcerative portion of the tumour is seen as a markedly decreased signal intensity area (arrow). (b) Axial, gadolinium-enhanced, T1W view. The infiltrative portion invades both geniohyoid/genioglossus complex and neurovascular bundles of the tongue, indicating the need for a total glossectomy (if surgery is considered).

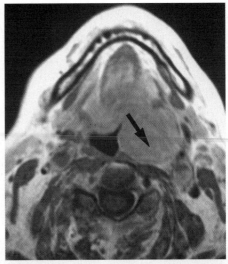

(a)

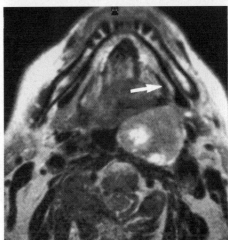

(b)

Fig. 13 Exophytic pattern. Glossotonsillar synovial sarcoma. (a) Axial, T1W view. The tumour (arrow), displayed with a signal intensity comparable to that of surrounding muscle, protrudes into the oropharyngeal lumen. (b) Axial, T2W view. The tumour displaces rather than infiltrates the hyoglossus muscle (arrow). The well-circumscribed, smoothly marginated, non-infiltrative characteristics do not reflect the clinical and histological aggressiveness of this neoplasm.

T2-weighted images and enhances with contrast. Contrast take up is maximum in the weeks following surgery and lasts more with MR than with CT, because MR is a more sensitive technique. Enhancement diminishes and disappears in the first 3 months following surgery. It is therefore useless and confusing to make a baseline scan during this period since areas showing increased signal intensity on T2-weighted images and contrast enhancement may correspond either to tumour or inflammation. Postoperative infection typically presents as an ill-defined, poorly marginated, heterogeneous, contrast-enhanced lesion. Imaging helps to differentiate abscess, which presents with at least one fluid cavity, and even gas bubbles. In practice however, infection and tumour may coexist along with acute inflammation and are almost indistinguishable at imaging. Follow-up imaging under high-dose antibiotics can help solve the problem.

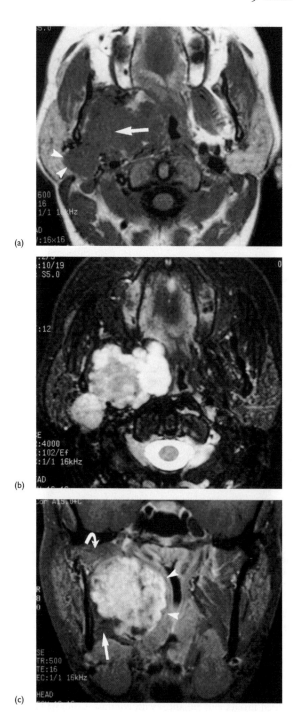

(a)

(b)

(c)

Fig. 14 Benign pattern. Parapharyngeal pleomorphic adenoma. (a) Axial, T1W view. The tumour (arrow) displays a non-specific, intermediate signal intensity, which makes it indistinguishable from the pterygoid muscles. The relationship with the deep portion of the parotid gland (arrowheads) indicates that the tumour did not originate from this gland. (b) Same level, T2W view. The tumour has relatively smooth margins. Although heterogeneous, it predominantly contains increased signal intensity areas, indicating a probable salivary gland origin. (c) Coronal, gadolinium-enhanced, fat-suppressed, T1W view. Despite substantial mass effect, the lateral pterygoid muscle (curved arrow), medial pterygoid muscle (arrow), and mucosal space (arrowheads) do not enhance with contrast indicating probable preservation of these structures.

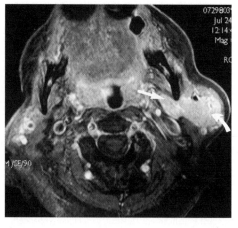

Fig. 15 Benign pattern. Left parotid pleomorphic adenoma. Axial, gadolinium-enhanced, fat-suppressed, T1W view. The tumour (curved arrow) is smoothly marginated and extends across the stylomandibular foramen in the deep portion of the gland (arrow).

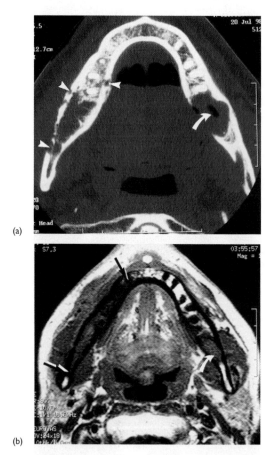

(a)

(b)

Fig. 16 Bone lysis. Active osteoradionecrosis. (a) Axial CT, bone window setting. Multiple areas of bone lysis are visible on the cortex of the right horizontal branch of the mandible (arrowheads). Contralateral bone lysis is due to an old dental abscess (curved arrow). (b) Axial, T1W view. Medullary bone abnormally low signal intensity extends almost from the symphisis menti to the angle of the mandible (arrows). On the left side, the dental abscess is also depicted as a low signal intensity area (curved arrow).

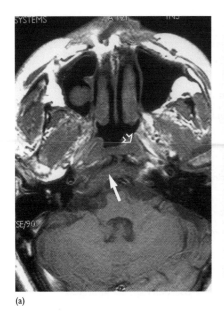
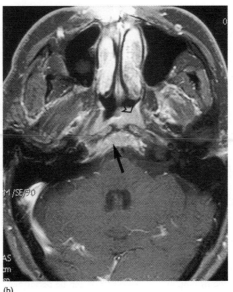

(a)　　　　　　　　　　　　(b)

Fig. 17 Tumour spread to medullary bone. Nasopharyngeal carcinoma with extension to the skull base. (a) Axial, T1W view. The body of the sphenoid shows a decreased signal intensity, indicating tumour invasion (arrow). The left fossa of Rosenmuller is obliterated (open arrow), but the tumour is not visible. (b) Same level, gadolinium-enhanced, fat-suppressed, T1W view. The medullary bone within the body of the sphenoid strongly enhances with contrast (arrow). The tumour (open arrow) enhances in a similar fashion to the mucosa, demonstrating the absence of extension in the deep extracranial tissues (parapharyngeal and masticator spaces).

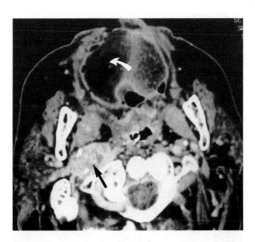

Fig. 18 Retropharyngeal lymph node. Contrast-enhanced, axial CT scan showing a right retropharyngeal node (arrow). Invasion of the XII hypoglossal nerve is attested by the fatty degeneration of the ipsilateral side of the tongue (curved arrow).

Radiotherapy

Changes induced by radiation therapy depend on technical factors such as total dose to, and volume of, irradiated tissue, size of daily fractions, and the time interval between fractions.[69],[70] These changes are also time dependent. It is critically important to have this information to correctly schedule and interpret an examination.

At the end of therapy, changes are maximum: the tumour is necrotic and oedematous and cannot be differentiated from peritumoural oedema, thus forming a heterogeneous mass with predominant areas of increased signal intensity on T2-weighted images and increased contrast enhancement. When therapy is successful, the tumour area shrinks and gives place to fibrosis. Endstage fibrosis does not retain contrast: it presents with a CT density and a MR signal close to muscle. It is best identified by comparison with fatty tissues.

Normally, fibrosis occurs in the first 3 months following therapy and will keep developing for years. Contrast enhancement may persist beyond this period if internal microvasculature is developed, or when the healing process is slow or delayed. In fact, such a situation is more frequently seen with MR because this technique is more sensitive than CT to contrast take up.

Alterations in soft tissues are dose dependent. Under 50 Gy, changes are transient and not visible at CT or MR 2 to 3 months after the end of therapy. Over 65 Gy, permanent damages are visible. The skin and the platysma are thickened. The subcutaneous and deeper fat is infiltrated, probably by perilymphatic fibrosis and thickening of pre-existing fibrous septa.[1] The mucosa is thickened and enhances with contrast, particularly in the pharynx and larynx.[71] In this latter site, mucosal thickening associated with deep-sited lymphoedema is responsible for the narrowing of the airway. Salivary glands moderately enhance with contrast. The maxillary sinus and mastoid cells often contain inflammatory secretions typically displayed as high signal intensity areas on T2-weighted images. Skull base lysis does not heal. In the cervical vertebral bodies, the irradiated medullary bone is replaced by fat (this can help to delineate the limits of the irradiated volume on T1-weighted images).

Chemotherapy

At present, changes induced by most current chemotherapy regimen are milder than those seen with radiation therapy. However, one can speculate that this situation will change with the increase in use of chemotherapy and the introduction of new, more aggressive, chemotherapy regimen.

Follow-up policies; detection of relapse

There is no need to perform an imaging study during radiation therapy or chemotherapy, unless imaging can modify the therapeutic planning (change of chemotherapy regimen, change of irradiated volume, or boost).

Table 5 CT and MR: advantages and drawbacks

CT	MR
Simple to perform	Technically challenging
No specific hardware needed	Dedicated coil needed for the examination of infrahyoid neck
Short examination time (typical study length: 15 min)	Long examination time (typical study length: 30–45 min)
Widely available	Restricted number of machines
Low cost	High cost (typically twice as CT)
Adapted to the study of critically ill patients, or those requiring anaesthesia	Specialized non-magnetic monitoring and anaesthesic material needed for the study of severely ill patients
Study failure almost nil	Study failure limited, but one or more sequences can be hampered by artefacts
Familiar to clinicians	Unfamiliar to clinicians (new type of image contrast coming with new sequences)
Typical irradiation is 2–5 mGy per examination	Non-ionizing technique
Information acquired in one plane (axial or coronal)	Information acquired in any plane
Reformation along any plane possible, but can be degraded by motion of pharyngolarynx	Reformation can be performed if direct acquisition has not been done
Single parameter information (X-ray beam attenuation)	Multiparameter information (proton-density, T1, T2, Gadolinium enhanced, fat-suppressed T1 Gadolinium enhanced sequences)
Excellent detection of calcification and air (necrosis)	Excellent detection of haemorrhage, perineural spread
Excellent analysis of cortical bone and cartimages	Excellent analysis of medullary bone
Dental artefacts only	Numerous kinds of artefacts
Specific contraindication: severe allergia to iodine contrast agent	Specific contraindication: claustrophobia, pacemakers, schrapnels, ferromagnetic clips

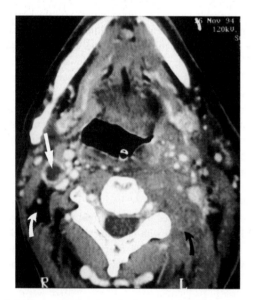

Fig. 19 Relapse: cervical lymph node. Contrast-enhanced, axial CT scan shows a right jugulodigastric node, with central hypodensity (arrow). The patient initially presented with a left tonsillar squamous cell carcinoma and ispsilateral nodes. These areas are now filled with a non-specific, non-enhancing tissue presenting the same attenuation (black curved arrow) as surrounding muscles. The exact extent can be evaluated by comparison with the right fatty posterior cervical space (white curved arrow).

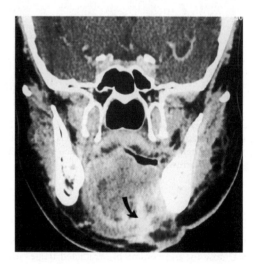

Fig. 20 Early complication—post-treatment infection. The patient was operated 6 months earlier for a squamous cell carcinoma of the posterior floor of the mouth, and had a 65 Gy irradiation. Contrast-enhanced coronal CT scan shows an ill-defined area in the left sublingual/submandibular spaces (arrow), with extension to the subcutaneous tissue. This aspect is non-specific and could correspond to inflammation or early relapse.

In the post-treatment period, reference baseline scans are recommended in patients at risk of tumour relapse, particularly when the primary was located in a clinically non-accessible area (skull base,

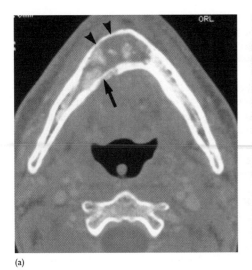

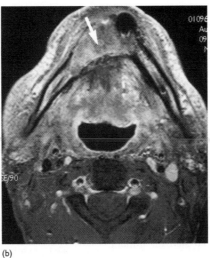

Fig. 21 Long-term complication—mandibular osteoradionecrosis. (a) Axial CT scan, bone window setting, shows thinning of the outer cortex (arrowheads), and focal disruption of the inner cortex (arrow). (b) Same level, gadolinium-enhanced, fat-suppressed, T1W view shows that the medullary bone is replaced by a non-specific enhancing tissue (arrow).

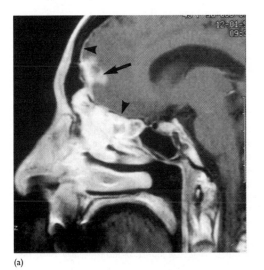

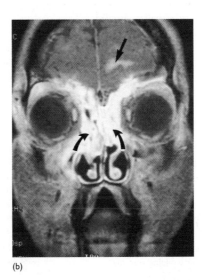

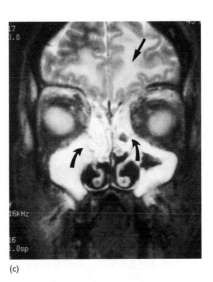

Fig. 22 Long-term complication—post-irradiation brain toxicity. (a) Sagittal, gadolinium-enhanced, T1W view shows an area of contrast take-up in the frontal lobe (arrow), close to the meninges, which are also enhancing (arrowheads). (b) Coronal, gadolinium-enhanced, fat-suppressed, T1W view shows the inflammatory area (arrow). A non-specific enhancing tissue is filling the upper part of the sinonasal area (curved arrows). (c) Coronal, T2W view demonstrates increased signal intensity brain oedema (arrow). Increased signal intensity areas are seen in the sinonasal area (curved arrows), which is in favour of post-irradiation inflammatory changes.

nasopharynx, sinonasal cavities) or when post-treatment oedema or pain prevent a good physical examination. Performing a baseline scan for every patient at risk is important because the patterns of post-treatment temporal changes are highly variable from one subject to another. The baseline study should be performed no sooner than 3 months after completion of all treatments, at a time when acute and subacute inflammatory changes should have disappeared.[1] In practice, the comparison between successive examinations often constitutes the clue to diagnosis by showing abnormal reappearance of contrast enhancement with or without associated mass effect. As at the initial stage, imaging may miss superficial or small-sized tumour. Therefore, the diagnostic of tumour relapse can only be made by biopsy. Biopsy sometimes involves the risk of necrosis and should be

only decided with reference to a body of clinical, biological, and imaging information.

Relapses may occur in lymph nodes, with or without relapse at the primary site (Fig. 19). The metastatic nodes may show the same pattern as seen at the pretherapeutic stage. In the neck however, because of neck dissection and irradiation, lymph nodes tend to present as poorly marginated, heterogeneous masses. Recurrences also occur in the retropharyngeal space, even when the primary was initially located at the infrahyoid level, and this justifies scanning from the skull base to the clavicles, as in the initial workup.

The choice between MR and CT varies from one institution to another, and depends on the site of origin and type of tumour,[72] machine availability, examination cost, and sometimes health-care policies. The frequency of imaging follow-up is also controversial. In summary, follow-up imaging tends to be routine in cancer patients. However, further studies are needed to demonstrate the benefits of the various imaging strategies and the exact role of FDG-PET and other metabolic imaging techniques in overall survival and disease-free survival.[22]

Complications

Imaging can display early complications, such as infection, abscess (Fig. 20), haematoma, or necrosis. Long-term complications due to radiation therapy[4] may occur in the head and neck area. Pharyngo-cutaneous fistula and swallowing disorders due to cervical and pharyngeal muscles are evidenced on swallow studies. Laryngeal osteochondronecrosis and bone necrosis of the mandible are best seen with CT. Contrast-enhanced MR shows intramedullary abnormal signal intensity, which is non-specific and should alert for tumour recurrence (Fig. 21). CT, MR imaging, and colour Doppler are excellent modalities for the detection of carotid stenoses induced by radiation arteriopathy. Cranial nerve paralysis usually involves the hypoglossal nerve and translates into lingual atrophy, equally visible on CT and MR. Finally MR is the best choice to visualize delayed neurotoxicity either to the spinal cord or to the brain (Fig. 22).

References

1. Mancuso A. Imaging in patients with head and neck cancer. In: Million R, Cassisi N, eds. *Management of head and neck cancer. A multidisciplinary approach.* 2nd edn. Philadelphia: JB Lippincott, 1994: 43–59.

2. Sigal R, Zagdanski A, Schwaab G, *et al.* CT and MR imaging of squamous cell carcinoma of the tongue and floor of the mouth. *Radiographics*, 1996; **16**: 787–810.

3. Tamler B, Kligerman M. Diagnostic imaging aides to head and neck radiation oncology. *Radiology Clinics of North America*, 1996; **6**: 515–30.

4. Becker M, Schroth G, Zbären P, *et al.* Long-term changes induced by high-dose irradiation of the head and neck region: imaging findings. *Radiographics*, 1997; **17**: 5–26.

5. Abrahams J. Dental implants and multiplanar imaging of the jaw. In: Som PM, Curtin HD, eds. *Head and neck imaging*. 3rd edn. Baltimore: Mosby, 1996:350–74.

6. Robbins K, vanSonnenberg E, Casola G, Varney R. Image-guided needle aspiration of inacessible head and neck lesions. *Archives of Otolaryngology Head and Neck Surgery*, 1990; **116**: 957–61.

7. Yousem D, Sack M, Scanlan K. Biopsy of parapharyngeal space lesions. *Radiology*, 1994; **193**: 619–22.

8. Mukherji S, Turestsky D, Tart R, Mancuso A. A technique for core biopsies of head and neck masses. *American Journal of Neuroradiology*, 1994; **15**: 518–20.

9. Tu A, Geyer C, Mancall A, Baker R. The buccal space: a doorway for percutaneous CT-guided biopsy of the parapharyngeal region. *American Journal of Neuroradiology*, 1998; **19**: 728–31.

10. Eisbruch A, Marsh L, Martel M, *et al.* Comprehensive irradiation of head and neck cancer using conformal multisegmental fields: assessment of target coverage and noninvolved tissue sparing. *International Journal of Radiation Oncology Biology Physics*, 1998; **41**: 559–68.

11. Wehrli F. Principles of magnetic resonance imaging. In: Starck D, Bradley W, eds. *Magnetic resonance imaging*. 3rd edn. St Louis: Mosby, 1999:1–14.

12. Ross R, Schomer D, Chappel P, Enzmann D. MR imaging of head and neck tumors: comparison of T1 weighted contrast-enhanced fat-suppressed images with conventional T2-weighted and fast spin-echo T2-weighted images. *American Journal of Roentgenology*, 1994; **163**: 173–8.

13. Hendrick R. Image contrast and noise. In: Starck D, Bradley W, eds. *Magnetic resonance imaging*. 3rd edn. St Louis: Mosby, 1999:49–67.

14. Colletti PM, Terk MR, Zee CS. Magnetic resonance angiography in neck masses. *Computerized Medical Imaging and Graphics*, 1996; **20**: 379–88.

15. Yousem DM, Hatabu H, Hurst RW, *et al.* Carotid artery invasion by head and neck masses: prediction with MR Imaging. *Radiology*, 1995; **195**: 715–20.

16. Takes R, Knegt P, Manni J, *et al.* Regional metastases in head and neck squamous cell carcinoma: revised value of US with US-guided FNAB. *Radiology*, 1996; **198**: 819–23.

17. van den Brekel M. US-guided fine-needle aspiration cytology of neck nodes in patients with N0 disease. *Radiology*, 1996; **201**: 580–1.

18. McGuirt WF, Greven K, Williams D, *et al.* PET scanning in head and neck oncology: a review. *Head and Neck*, 1998; **20**: 208–15.

19. Jabour B, Choi H, Hoh C, *et al.* Extracranial head and neck: PET imaging with 2-[f18] fluoro-2-deoxy-D-glucose and MR imaging correlation. *Radiology*, 1993; **186**: 27–35.

20. Braams J, Pruim J, Freling N, *et al.* Detection of lymph node metastases of squamous-cell cancer of the head and neck with FDG-PET and MRI. *Journal of Nuclear Medicine*, 1995; **36**: 211–6.

21. Anzai Y, Carroll W, Quint D, *et al.* Recurrence of head and neck cancer after surgery or irradiation : prospective comparison of 2-deoxy-2- (F-18) fluoro-D-glucose PET and MR imaging diagnoses. *Radiology*, 1996; **200**: 135–41.

22. Fischbein N, Aassa O, Caputo G, *et al.* Clinical utility of positron emission tomography with18F-fluorodeoxyglucose in detecting residual/recurrent squamous cell carcinoma of the head and neck. *American Journal of Neuroradiology*, 1998; **19**: 1189–96.

23. Wahl R, Quint L, Cieslak R, Aisen A, Koeppe R, Meyer C. 'Anatomometabolic' tumor imaging: fusion of FDG PET with CT or MRI to localize foci of increased activity. *Journal of Nuclear Medicine*, 1993; **34**: 1190–7.

24. Keyes JJ, Watson NJ, Williams Dr, Greven K, McGuirt W. FDG PET in head and neck cancer. *American Journal of Roentgenology*, 1997; **169**: 1663–79.

25. Goodwin W. PET and recurrent squamous cell carcinoma of the head and neck: a surgeon's view. *American Journal of Neuroradiology*, 1998; **19**: 1197.

26. Mukherji S, Drane W, Mancuso A, Parsons J, Mendenhall W, Stringer S. Occult primary tumors of the head and neck: detection with 2-(F-18) fluoro-2-deoxy-d- glucose SPECT. *Radiology*, 1996; **199**: 761–6.

27. Shreve P, Steventon R, Deters E, Kison P, Gross M, Wahl R. Oncologic diagnosis with 2-[fluorine-18]fluoro-2-deoxy-D-glucose imaging: dual-head coincidence gamma camera versus positron emission tomographic scanner. *Radiology*, 1998; **207**: 431–7.

28. Valdès Olmos RA, Balm AJM, Hilgers FJM, *et al.* Thallium-201 SPECT in the diagnosis of head and neck cancer. *Journal of Nuclear Medicine*, 1997; **38**: 873–9.

29. Kostakoglu L, Uysal U, Ozyar E, *et al.* Monitoring response to therapy with Thallium-201 and Technetium-99m-Sestamibi SPECT in nasopharyngeal carcinoma. *Journal of Nuclear Medicine*, 1997; **38**: 1009–14.

30. Takashima S, Noguchi Y, Okumura T, Aruga H, Kobayashi T. Dynamic MR imaging in the head and neck. *Radiology*, 1993; **189**: 813–21.

31. Baba Y, Furusawa M, Murakami R, *et al.* Role of dynamic MRI in the evaluation of head and neck cancers treated with radiation therapy.

International Journal of Radiation Oncology Biology Physics, 1997; **37**: 783–7.

32. Zagdanski A, Sigal R, Bosq J, Bazin J, Vanel D, Di Paola R. Factor analysis of medical image sequences in MR of head and neck tumors. *American Journal of Neuroradiology*, 1994; **15**: 1359–68.

33. Vogl T, Mack M, Juergens M. Skull base tumors: Gadodiamide injection-enhanced MR imaging- drop-out effect in the early enhancement pattern of paragangliomas versus different tumors. *Radiology*, 1993; **188**: 339.

34. Fried MP, Hsu L, Jolesz FA. Interactive magnetic resonance imaging-guided biopsy in the head and neck: initial patient experience. *Laryngoscope*, 1998; **108**: 488–93.

35. Vogl T, Mack M, Müller P, *et al.* Recurrent nasopharyngeal tumors: preliminary clinical results with interventional MR imaging-controlled laser-induced thermotherapy. *Radiology*, 1995; **196**: 725–33.

36. Mukherji K, Schiro S, Castillo M, Kwock L, Muller E, Blackstock W. Proton MR spectroscopy of squamous cell carcinoma of the extracranial head and neck: *in vitro* and *in vivo* studies. *American Journal of Neuroradiology*, 1997; **18**: 1057–72.

37. Anzai Y, Prince M. Iron oxide-enhanced MR lymphography: the evaluation of cervical lymph node metastases in head and neck cancer. *Journal of Magnetic Resonance Imaging*, 1997; **7**: 75–81.

38. Anzai Y, Blackwell K, Hirschowitz S, *et al.* Initial clinical experience with dextran-coated superparamagnetic iron oxide for detection of lymph node metastases in patients with head and neck cancer. *Radiology*, 1994; **192**: 709–15.

39. Baum S, Caplan A. Teleradiology: friend or foe? *Radiology*, 1996; **201**: 16–7.

40. Berlin L. Malpractice issues in radiology. Teleradiology. *American Journal of Roentgenology*, 1998; **170**: 1417–22.

41. Yousem D, Montone K. Head and neck lesions. Radiologic-pathologic correlations. *Radiology Clinics of North America*, 1998; **36**: 983–1014.

42. Yousem D. Dashed hopes for MR imaging of the head and neck: the power of the needle. *Radiology*, 1992; **184**: 25–6.

43. Harnsberger HR. *Handbook of head and neck imaging.* 2nd edn. St Louis: Mosby, 1995.

44. Som P, Curtin H. Fasciae and spaces. In: Som P, Curtin H, eds. *Head and neck imaging.* 3rd edn. Baltimore: Mosby, 1996:738–46.

45. Charpy A. Aponévroses du cou. In: Poirier P, ed. *Traité d'anatomie humaine.* Paris: L. Bataille et Cie, 1906:410–31.

46. Som P, Curtin H, Silvers A. A re-evaluation of imaging criteria to assess aggressive masticator space tumors. *Head and Neck*, 1997; **19**: 335–41.

47. Janot F, Cvitkovic E, Piekarski JD, *et al.* Correlation between nodal density in contrasted scans and response to cisplatin-based chemotherapy in head and neck squamous cell cancer: a prospective validation. *Head and Neck*, 1993; **15**: 222–9.

48. Sigal R, Monnet O, de Baere T, *et al.* Adenoid cystic carcinoma of the head and neck: evaluation with MR imaging and clinical-pathologic correlation in 27 patients. *Radiology*, 1992; **184**: 95–101.

49. Dubin M, Teresi L, Bradley WJ, *et al.* Conspicuity of tumors of the head and neck on fat-suppressed MR images: T2-weighted fast-spin-echo versus contrast-enhanced T1-weighted conventional spin-echo sequences. *American Journal of Roentgenology*, 1995; **164**: 1213–21.

50. Nemzek W, Hecht S, Gandour-Edwards R, Donald P, McKennan K. Perineural spread of head and neck tumors: how accurate is MR imaging. *American Journal of Neuroradiology*, 1998; **19**: 701–6.

51. Laine FJ, Braun IF, Jensen ME. Perineural tumor extension through the foramen ovale : evaluation with MR imaging. *Radiology*, 1990; **174**: 65–71.

52. Chong V, Fan Y. Pterygopalatine fossa and maxillary nerve infiltration in nasopharyngeal carcinoma. *Head and Neck*, 1996; **19**: 121–5.

53. Su CY, Lui CC. Perineural invasion of the trigeminal nerve in patients with nasopharyngeal carcinoma. *Cancer*, 1996; **78**: 2063–9.

54. Eisen M, Yousem D, Montone K, *et al.* Use of preoperative MR to predict dural, perineural, and venous sinus invasion of skull base tumors. *American Journal of Neuroradiology*, 1996; **17**: 1937–45.

55. Becker M, Zbären P, Delavelle J, *et al.* Neoplastic invasion of the laryngeal cartilage : reassessment of criteria for diagnosis at CT. *Radiology*, 1997; **203**: 521–32.

56. van den Brekel M, van der Waal I, Meijer C, Freeman J, Castelijns J, Snow G. The incidence of micrometastases in neck dissection obtained from elective neck dissections. *Laryngoscope*, 1996; **106**: 987–91.

57. Curtin HD, Ishwaran H, Mancuso AA, Dalley RW, Caudry DJ, McNeil BJ. Comparison of CT and MR in staging of neck metastases. *Radiology*, 1998; **207**: 123–30.

58. Yousem D, Som P, Hackney D, Schwaibold F, Hendrix R. Central nodal necrosis and extracapsular neoplastic spread in cervical lymph nodes : MR imaging versus CT. *Radiology*, 1992; **182**: 753–9.

59. Chong V, Fan Y, Khoo J. MRI features of cervical nodal necrosis in metastatic disease. *Clinical Radiology*, 1996; **51**: 103–9.

60. van den Brekel M, Castelijns J, Snow G. The size of lymph nodes in the neck on sonograms as a radiologic criterion for metastasis: how reliable is it? *American Journal of Neuroradiology*, 1998; **19**: 695–700.

61. Mukherji S, Pillsbury H, Castillo M. Imaging squamous cell carcinomas of the upper aerodigestive tract : what clinicians need to know. *Radiology*, 1997; **205**: 629–46.

62. Becker M, Zbaren P, Laeng H, Stoupis C, Porcellini B, Vock P. Neoplastic invasion of the laryngeal cartilage: comparison of MR imaging and CT with histopathologic correlation. *Radiology*, 1995; **194**: 661–9.

63. Williams DWI. Imaging of laryngeal cancer. *Otolaryngology Clinics of North America*, 1997; **30**: 35–58.

64. Lam W, Chan Y, Leung S, Metreweli C. Retropharyngeal lymphadenopathy in nasopharyngeal carcinoma. *Head and Neck*, 1997; **19**: 176–81.

65. Maroldi R, Battalia G, Nicolai P, *et al.* CT appearance of the larynx after conservative and radical surgery for carcinomas. *European Radiology*, 1997; **7**: 418–31.

66. Som P. Postoperative neck. In: Som P, Curtin H, eds. *Head and neck imaging.* Baltimore: Mosby, 1996:992–1005.

67. Hudgins P, Burson J, Gussack G, Grist W. CT and MR appearance of recurrent malignant head and neck neoplasms after resection and flap reconstruction. *American Journal of Neuroradiology*, 1994; **15**: 1689–94.

68. Wester DJ, Hansman Whiteman ML, Singer S, Bowen BC, Goodwin WJ. Imaging of the postoperative neck with emphasis on surgical flaps and their complications. *American Journal of Roentgenology*, 1995; **164**: 989–93.

69. Mukherji S, Mancuso A, Kotzur I, *et al.* Radiologic appearance of the irradiated larynx. Part I. Expected changes. *Radiology*, 1994; **193**: 141–8.

70. Parsons J. The effect of radiation on normal tissues of the head and neck. In: Million R, Cassisi N, eds. *Management of head and neck cancer. A multidisciplinary approach.* Philadelphia: JB Lippincott, 1994: 245–89.

71. Mukherji S, Mancuso A, Kotzur I, *et al.* Radiologic appearance of the irradiated larynx. Part II. Primary site response. *Radiology*, 1994; **193**: 149–54.

72. Chong VFH, Fan YF. Detection of recurrent nasopharyngeal carcinoma: MR imaging versus CT. *Radiology*, 1997; **202**: 463–70.

9.1.4 Therapeutic principles in the management of head and neck tumours

William M. Mendenhall, Nicholas J. Cassisi, Scott P. Stringer, and Scott P. Tannehill

Introduction

In this overview of therapeutic principles in the treatment of head and neck cancer, general principles in the management of the primary tumour are discussed. A more comprehensive review is found in site-specific chapters. Because management of the neck and of cases with an unknown primary site is not discussed in detail elsewhere, these topics are reviewed in this chapter.

Anatomy

The incidence of lymph node metastases at the time of diagnosis is related to the relative density of the capillary lymphatic network at the primary site. The nasopharynx and pyriform sinus have the most profuse capillary lymphatic networks, whereas the paranasal sinuses, middle ear, and true vocal cords have either sparse or no capillary lymphatics.

The location of the various lymph node groups in the head and neck is depicted in Fig. 1.[1] Under normal conditions, the right and left lymphatic networks do not shunt lymph from one side to the other.

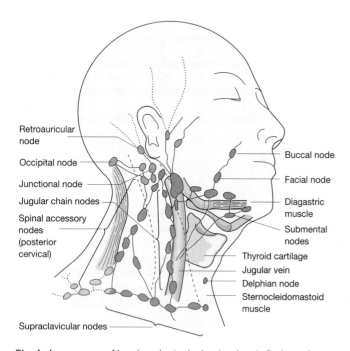

Fig. 1 Arrangement of lymph nodes in the head and neck. Redrawn from Rouvière H. *Anatomy of the human lymphatic system*, p. 27. Tobias MJ, translator. Ann Arbor, Edwards Brothers, 1938.[1]

The internal jugular chain lymph nodes are adjacent to the internal jugular vein and extend from the skull base to the clavicles. The most superior group of lymph nodes in this chain lies near the base of the skull in the posterior aspect of the lateral pharyngeal space and is referred to as the parapharyngeal or junctional lymph nodes. These lymph nodes lie deep to the sternocleidomastoid muscle, the posterior belly of the digastric muscle, and the tail of the parotid gland. The remainder of the internal jugular chain lymph nodes are artificially divided into three groups: subdigastric (level II—from the junctional nodes to the level of the hyoid bone), middle jugular (level III—from the level of the hyoid bone to the omohyoid muscle), and lower jugular (level IV—from the level of the omohyoid muscle to the clavicle).

The spinal accessory chain lymph nodes (level V) are distributed along the course of cranial nerve XI in the posterior triangle of the neck. The superior nodes of this group blend with the upper internal jugular chain nodes

The supraclavicular lymph nodes merge laterally with the spinal accessory chain lymph nodes and medially with the lower internal jugular chain lymph nodes.

There are three to six submandibular lymph nodes that may be either preglandular or postglandular; there are no lymph nodes in the substance of the submandibular gland. The submental lymph nodes lie in the midline between the anterior bellies of the digastric muscles, anterior to the hyoid bone and external to the mylohyoid muscle. The submandibular and submental lymph nodes are referred to as level I nodes.

The lateral retropharyngeal lymph nodes lie within the retropharyngeal space, which is bounded anteriorly by the pharyngeal constrictor muscles, superiorly by the skull base, and posteriorly by the prevertebral fascia. They are usually at the level of the C1 and C2 vertebral bodies, but may be found as inferiorly as C3. The medial retropharyngeal nodes are small, inconstant intercalated nodes that are located near midline and empty into the lateral retropharyngeal lymph nodes.

Level VI lymph nodes are defined as those that are bounded by the hyoid bone, the sternum, and the common carotid arteries and include the paratracheal, pretracheal, precricoid (Delphian), and tracheoesophageal groove nodes.

Natural history

The risk of lymph node metastases is influenced by the primary site, the degree of histological differentiation, the size of the lesion (T stage), depth of invasion, and the density of capillary lymphatics. The estimated risk of subclinical disease in the clinically negative neck as a function of primary site and T stage is shown in Table 1.[2] Locally recurrent lesions have a higher risk of lymphatic involvement than untreated lesions.

The N stage distribution at diagnosis by primary site and T stage is shown in Table 2.[3] The most commonly involved lymph nodes in the head and neck are the subdigastric (level II) lymph nodes, followed by the midjugular (level III) lymph nodes. Lesions that are well lateralized usually spread first to the ipsilateral neck nodes; those that are on or near the midline, as well as lateralized base of tongue and nasopharyngeal lesions, may spread to both sides of the neck.

Table 1 Definition of risk group

Group	Estimated risk of subclinical neck disease (%)	Stage	Site
I Low risk	<20	T1	Floor of mouth, retromolar trigone, gingiva, hard palate, buccal mucosa
II Intermediate risk	20–30	T1	Oral tongue, soft palate, pharyngeal wall, supraglottic larynx, tonsil
		T2	Floor of mouth, oral tongue, retromolar trigone, gingiva, hard palate, buccal mucosa
III High risk	>30	T1–4	Nasopharynx, pyriform sinus, base of tongue
		T2–4	Soft palate, pharyngeal wall, supraglottic larynx, tonsil
		T3–4	Floor of mouth, oral tongue, retromolar trigone, gingiva, hard palate, buccal mucosa

Modified from Mendenhall and Million. *International Journal of Radiation Oncology Biology Physics*, 1986; **12**: 741–6.[2]

Patients who have clinically positive lymph nodes in the ipsilateral side of the neck may be at risk for contralateral lymph node spread if the metastatic nodes significantly obstruct the lymphatic trunks. Additionally, in patients who have undergone previous surgery on one side of the neck, lymph is shunted across the submental region to the opposite side of the neck. When contralateral lymph node metastases occur, the level II lymph nodes are most frequently involved, followed by the level III and level IV nodes.

As tumour grows within a lymph node, the node becomes indurated, rounded, and enlarged. Tumour eventually extends through the capsule of the lymph node and invades surrounding structures. Extension to the neurovascular bundle is common and may produce a mass that is fixed to palpation. The incidence of tumour involvement and the probability of capsular penetration versus lymph node size are shown in Table 3.[4]

The risk of lateral retropharyngeal lymph node involvement is related to primary site and neck stage; the medial retropharyngeal nodes are almost never the site of metastatic disease. The incidence of positive retropharyngeal nodes based on pretreatment computed tomography (CT) and, in selected cases, magnetic resonance imaging (MRI) is shown in Table 4.[5]

The incidence of distant metastases at presentation is relatively low. The probability of distant metastases developing after treatment is related to neck stage and location of positive nodes in the neck (Table 5).[6],[7]

Initial evaluation

History and physical examination

The history and physical examination focuses on the location and extent of the tumour, the patient's medical condition, and factors that may influence treatment decisions, such as prior operations, radiation therapy, and significant medical problems such as emphysema and heart disease.

The preferred position for neck examination is with one hand on the side of the neck and the other tilting the head toward the side that is to be examined in order to relax the sternocleidomastoid muscle. The index finger is placed in the sternal notch; normally, nothing should be palpable except the anterior wall of the trachea. Clinically positive nodes, often metastatic from thoracic or abdominal tumours, are sometimes found in this area. Often only the top or side of the node can be appreciated. Next, the thumb and index finger encircle the sternocleidomastoid muscle to palpate the internal jugular nodes, which are adjacent to the jugular vein and deep to the muscle (Fig. 2).[8] As one proceeds up the neck from the sternal notch, the thumb and index finger are in constant motion in a 'wiggle-waggle' manoeuvre.

Positive internal jugular nodes are often small and deep and may feel like a firm pea or bean sliding between the thumb and index finger. The carotid bulb and artery are identified because they are pulsatile. It may be difficult to distinguish a calcified carotid bulb from a positive node; aggressive palpation may cause syncope and collapse secondary to a vasovagal response. The jugulodigastric node is located at the angle of the mandible; a metastatic lymph node in this area may be deep, with only its external surface palpable. The junctional lymph nodes are high in the neck and are often difficult to palpate, particularly in men, because the sternocleidomastoid muscle and posterior belly of the digastric muscles intervene, and the attachment of these muscles to the mastoid tip restricts the examining fingers. The spinal accessory (level V) and supraclavicular lymph nodes may be appreciated by moving the finger over the skin in a circular movement; the lymph nodes are relatively superficial, and positive nodes are identified as they slide under the examining fingers. The submental and submandibular lymph nodes (level I) are palpated bimanually with one finger placed in the floor of mouth and the other palpating the external aspect of the submandibular and submental areas. It may be difficult to distinguish an obstructed submandibular gland from an enlarged node; in the former case, the gland is often tender to palpation, and saliva cannot be expressed from Wharton's duct. CT of the neck is the most accurate method of making this distinction.

Preauricular lymph node examination may reveal enlarged metastatic nodes due to skin cancer or, rarely, nasopharyngeal cancer. These are often small and just anterior to the tragus. Facial lymph nodes may be involved secondary to cancer of the upper lip or nasal vestibule and are adjacent to the facial neurovascular bundle in the cheek. They are best appreciated by bimanual palpation.

The larynx is moved laterally; the 'thyroid click' is caused by movement of the thyroid cartilage against the prevertebral musculature. Loss of the thyroid click is due to anterior displacement of the larynx, often by a hypopharyngeal tumour. The group VI nodes are usually not palpable and may be involved by carcinomas of the thyroid and advanced laryngeal cancers.

Table 2 Clinically detected nodal metastases on admission, by T stage

Primary site	T stage	N0 (%)	N1 (%)	N2–N3 (%)
Oral tongue[a]	T1	86	10	4
	T2	70	19	11
	T3	52	16	31
	T4	24	10	66
Floor of mouth[a]	T1	89	9	2
	T2	71	18	10
	T3	56	20	24
	T4	46	10	43
Retromolar trigone/ anterior tonsillar pillar[b]	T1	88	2	9
	T2	62	18	20
	T3	46	21	33
	T4	32	18	50
Soft palate[b]	T1	92	0	8
	T2	64	12	24
	T3	35	26	39
	T4	33	11	56
Tonsillar fossa[b]	T1	30	41	30
	T2	32	14	54
	T3	30	18	52
	T4	10	13	76
Base of tongue[b]	T1	30	15	55
	T2	29	14	56
	T3	26	23	52
	T4	16	8	76
Oropharyngeal walls[b]	T1	75	0	25
	T2	70	10	20
	T3	33	22	44
	T4	24	24	52
Supraglottic larynx[c]	T1	61	10	29
	T2	58	16	26
	T3	36	25	40
	T4	41	18	41
Hypopharynx[d]	T1	37	21	42
	T2	30	20	49
	T3	21	26	54
	T4	26	15	58
Nasopharynx[e]	T1	8	11	82
	T2	16	12	72
	T3	12	9	80
	T4	17	6	78

2044 patients, MD Anderson Hospital, Houston, 1948–1965. Modified from Lindberg, *Cancer*, 1972; **29** : 1446–9.[3]

[a] T stage defined by Lindberg, *Cancer*, 1972; **29** : 1446–9.[3]

[b] T stage defined by Fletcher et al. in: *Cancer of the head and neck*, Williams and Wilkins, 1967: 185.[71]

[c] T stage defined by Fletcher et al., *American Journal of Roentgenology, Radium Therapy, and Nuclear Medicine*, 1970; **108** : 19–26.[72]

[d] T stage defined by MacComb et al., in: *Cancer of the head and neck*, Williams and Wilkins, 1967: 232.[73]

[e] T stage defined by Chen and Fletcher, *Radiology*, 1971; **99** : 165–71.[74]

After the neck examination, the mucosal surfaces of the oral cavity and oropharynx are inspected with a headlight and two tongue blades. The tongue, floor of mouth, and tonsils are palpated; early tumours of the base of tongue and tonsil may be palpable before being visible and are often missed on physical examination. Submucosal asymmetry of the hard palate, particularly the posterolateral aspect of the palate, may indicate the presence of a minor salivary gland tumour. Retropharyngeal lymph nodes are usually located anterolateral to the C1–C2 vertebral bodies and are often involved secondary to nasopharyngeal cancers and, less frequently, pharyngeal wall malignancies.[5] A positive

Table 3 Relationship between node size, the presence of tumour in the node, and capsular penetration in 519 nodes[a]

	Size of node (cm)				
	1	**2**	**3**	**4**	**5**
Number of nodes	177	183	84	17	58
Percentage positive	33	62	81	88	100
Percentage positive with capsular penetration	14	26	49	71	76

[a] Institut Gustave-Roussy (Villejuif, France). Modified from Richard et al. Laryngoscope, 1987; **97**: 97–101.[4]

Table 4 Incidence of positive retropharyngeal nodes for various primary sites and clinical neck stages (794 tumours)[a]

Primary site	Clinical neck stage		
	N0 neck (%)	**N+ neck (%)**	**Overall (%)**
Nasopharynx	2/5 (40)	12/14 (86)	74
Pharyngeal wall	6/37 (16)	12/56 (21)	19
Soft palate	1/21 (5)	6/32 (19)	13
Tonsillar region	2/56 (4)	14/120 (12)	9
Pyriform sinus or postcricoid area	0/55 (0)	7/81 (9)	5
Base of tongue	0/31 (0)	5/90 (6)	4
Supraglottic larynx	0/87 (0)	4/109 (4)	2

[a] Detected on pretreatment computed tomography (CT) and/or magnetic resonance imaging (MRI). From McLaughlin et al., Head and Neck, 1995; **17**: 190–8, with permission.[5]

N+ = neck nodes clinically involved (stages N1–N3B).

Table 5 Five-year risk of distance metastases as a function of neck stage and node location (455 patients)[a]

N stage	Upper neck only (%)	Lower neck ± upper neck (%)	Significance level
N1	12	34	p = 0.129
N2A	19	55	p = 0.230
N2B	21	22	p = 0.127
N3A	45	71	p = 0.024
N3B	19	35	p = 0.022

[a] Calculated by the life-table method.

From Ellis et al. International Journal of Radiation Oncology Biology Physics, 1989; **17**: 293–7, with permission.[6]

retropharyngeal node is sometimes seen as a submucosal mass behind the anterior tonsillar pillar. Glomus vagale tumours may also present as submucosal parapharyngeal space masses. The location and

condition of the teeth and their relationship to potential radiation therapy portals are documented.

Next, the hypopharynx and larynx are examined with a mirror. The mobility of the vocal cords is appreciated. Fixation of a vocal cord may indicate tumour invasion of the cricoarytenoid joint, recurrent laryngeal nerve, and/or vocalis muscle. If mirror examination is suboptimal, the examination is repeated using a flexible fiberoptic endoscope.

The nasal vestibules and nasal cavity are examined with a nasal speculum. The nasopharynx is examined with a flexible fiberoptic endoscope passed along the floor of the nasal cavity lateral to the septum and below the inferior turbinate. The fossa of Rosenmüller is the most common location of a primary nasopharyngeal carcinoma and is carefully visualized. The external ear canals are examined with an otoscope and the tympanic membranes are inspected to determine whether there is evidence of fluid or a mass in the middle ear.

The cranial nerves are examined; cranial nerve deficits may be the presenting sign or symptom of patients with nasopharyngeal cancer invading the cavernous sinus and patients with advanced skin cancers. The most common cranial nerves involved by skin cancers with perineural invasion are the second division of the fifth nerve and the seventh nerve.[9] These patients usually have a history of a squamous

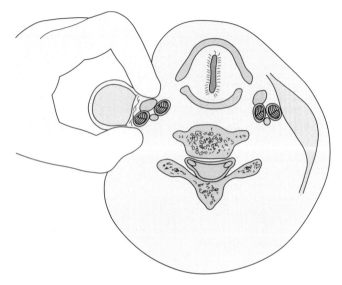

Fig. 2 Diagram of neck examination. The thumb and index finger form a C to palpate beneath the sternocleidomastoid muscle. From Million RR, Cassisi NJ, Mancuso AA, Stringer SP, Mendenhall WM, Parsons JT. Management of the neck for squamous cell carcinoma. In: Million RR, Cassisi NJ. *Management of head and neck cancer: a multidisciplinary approach.* 2nd edn. Philadelphia: JB Lippincott, 1994: 75–142, with permission.[8]

Table 6 Biopsy-proven primary site versus physical and radiographic findings

Patient	Number of patients with biopsy-proven primary site/ number of patients evaluated[a]
PE?/RAD?	7/42 (17%)
PE?/RAD⊕	29[b]/56 (52%)
PE⊕/RAD?	5/9 (56%)
PE⊕/RAD⊕	15[c]/23 (65%)
Total	56/130 (43%)

[a] Significance levels: 7/42 versus 34/65, $p = 0.00023$; 7/42 versus 15/23, $p = 0.00012$; 34/65 versus 15/23, $p = 0.20413$.

[b] One of 29 patients had a positive 2-[flourine-18]-2-deoxy-D-glucose (FDG) single photon emission computed tomography (SPECT) scan and a negative computed tomography (CT) of the head and neck; the remaining 28 patients had a positive CT and/or magnetic resonance imaging (MRI) scan.

[c] Two of the 15 remaining patients had a positive FDG-SPECT scan and a negative CT of the head and neck; the remaining 13 patients had a positive CT and/or MRI scan.

PE? = no suggestive findings on physical examination; PE⊕ = suggestive of a primary site, but not definitely positive; RAD? = no suggestive findings on radiographic studies; RAD⊕ = radiographic studies suggestive of primary site.

Adapted from Mendenhall *et al. Head and Neck*, 1998; **20**: 739–44.[10]

cell carcinoma of the midface and the insidious onset of numbness or weakness and are sometimes misdiagnosed as having a Bell's palsy.

Radiographic evaluation

The radiographic workup is obtained after the history and physical examination so that the studies may be selected based on the initial evaluation (see Chapter 9.1.3). In the United States, CT is preferred by many clinicians to complement staging of the neck; ultrasonography has proven to be an accurate alternative. MRI is preferred to CT for evaluating retropharyngeal lymph nodes.

The radiographic evaluation of the unknown head and neck primary site includes a chest radiograph and CT scan from the skull base to the clavicles. The results of the radiographic workup followed by panendoscopy and directed mucosal biopsies for a series of 130 patients evaluated at the University of Florida are depicted in Table 6.[10] More than 80 per cent of the primary sites detected were in the tonsillar fossa or base of tongue.

Nuclear medicine studies have also been used in a limited number of patients to detect unknown head and neck primary sites. The rationale for these tests is that tumour, with a higher metabolic rate than surrounding normal tissues, preferentially takes up a radioactive tracer, such as fluorodeoxy-glucose (FDG), and the lesion appears as an area of increased uptake on the scan. Because only limited data are available pertaining to these studies, it is difficult to evaluate their usefulness. Our limited experience with FDG single photon emission computed tomography indicates that few patients will benefit from the test.[10]

Dental evaluation

A dental evaluation is obtained before initiating treatment in dentulous patients. This consists of an examination and dental radiographs, usually including pantomography. If the patient is to receive irradiation, teeth deemed to be in marginal condition that will receive 45 Gy or more in 25 fractions over 5 weeks, or its biological equivalent, are extracted and radiation therapy may commence 10 to 14 days thereafter. Impacted third molars are not removed if they are covered by bone; otherwise, they are extracted if that portion of the jaw is anticipated to receive a high irradiation dose. Teeth that are retained are at a higher risk for developing dental caries if the patient has xerostomia because of the decreased saliva and altered pH of the saliva that remains. Fluoride trays are fashioned and the patient is instructed to use a fluoride gel nightly before going to bed. Patients have follow-up every 3 months by a dentist for evaluation and cleaning. If the patient wants dentures after radiation therapy to the oral cavity and/or oropharynx, it is desirable to wait at least 6 to 12 months after treatment. The dentures should fit well and not abrade the alveolar ridge because of the risk of inducing a bone exposure and subsequent osteonecrosis.

Nutritional evaluation

Patients who have lost more than 10 per cent of their body weight and those who are very lean and are anticipated to have difficulty maintaining their weight during radiation therapy have a percutaneous gastrostomy tube placed before initiating irradiation. If a surgical procedure is planned to follow radiation therapy, placement of the feeding tube may be influenced by the planned reconstruction. Nasogastric feeding tubes are infrequently used because they are difficult to maintain for long periods of time. A dietitian evaluates the patients undergoing radiation at least once weekly; most patients will be placed on a dietary supplement during and after therapy to maintain a daily caloric intake of 2000 or more calories. Intravenous fluids are a 'quick

Table 7 UICC and AJCC neck staging[11],[12]

Stage		Definition
NX		Regional lymph nodes cannot be assessed
N0		No regional lymph node metastasis
N1		Metastasis in a single ipsilateral lymph node, 3 cm or less in greatest dimension
N2		Metastasis in a single ipsilateral lymph node, more than 3 cm but not more than 6 cm in greatest dimension; or in multiple ipsilateral lymph nodes, none more than 6 cm in greatest dimension; or in bilateral or contralateral lymph nodes, none more than 6 cm in greatest dimension
	N2a	Metastasis in single ipsilateral lymph node, more than 3 cm but not more than 6 cm in greatest dimension
	N2b	Metastasis in multiple ipsilateral lymph nodes, none more than 6 cm in greatest dimension
	N2c	Metastasis in bilateral or contralateral lymph nodes, none more than 6 cm in greatest dimension
N3		Metastasis in a lymph node more than 6 cm in greatest dimension

fix' for the dehydrated patient who cannot swallow secondary to the acute effects of radiation therapy, but they are not a long-term solution. Patients who have not had a gastrostomy placed before irradiation and who lose more than 4.5 kg and/or become dehydrated undergo a percutaneous gastrostomy before their nutritional status further deteriorates.

Staging

The purpose of a staging system is to facilitate reporting and comparison of the end results. It is imperative not to compare the end results of clinically staged patients with results of those who are pathologically staged after an operation. The latter group will almost always contain a significant subset of patients who are 'upstaged' and thus bias any comparison against those who are clinically staged.

Staging is based on the physical findings and the radiographic evaluation. The two major staging systems are the Union Internationale Contre le Cancer (UICC)[11] and the American Joint Committee on Cancer (AJCC).[12] The two systems are similar and are based on the TNM definition of tumour extent. The stage of the primary lesion (T stage) is based on the size of the tumour, extension to adjacent sites, and/or invasion of structures such as bone and cranial nerves. Although tumour volume is highly predictive of outcome for some tumour sites, it is not included in the staging system.[13]–[15] The neck stage (N stage) is based on the number and size of positive lymph nodes. Node mobility is an important parameter but is not included because of significant interobserver variability. The UICC and the AJCC N-staging systems are the same (Table 7). The M stage is based on the presence of distant metastases. The overall stage is based on the T and N stage and is depicted in Table 8 for both the UICC and the AJCC. Stage IV is particularly heterogeneous and can be stratified into favourable and unfavourable subsets;[16] both of the current UICC and AJCC staging systems include a stratification of stage IV (Table 8).

Multidisciplinary consultations

The patient is evaluated by all of the physicians who may participate in his or her care, and a plan is formulated before proceeding with treatment. A paradigm for this process is the multidisciplinary head

Table 8 UICC and AJCC stage grouping[11],[12]

Stage 0	Tis	N0	M0
Stage I	T1	N0	M0
Stage II	T2	N0	M0
Stage III	T3	N0	M0
	T1	N1	M0
	T2	N1	M0
	T3	N1	M0
Stage IVA	T4	N0	M0
	T4	N1	M0
	Any T	N2	M0
Stage IVB	Any T	N3	M0
Stage IVC	Any T	Any N	M1

and neck conference, which occurs weekly at our institution. Patients are presented, their pathology and radiographic studies are reviewed, and head and neck examinations are performed by multiple physicians. Conference participants weigh treatment options and arrive at a recommendation that is discussed with the patient who makes the decision.

Treatment selection

General considerations

The parameters that influence treatment selection include the location and extent of the primary tumour, the presence and extent of regional adenopathy, the presence of distant metastases, synchronous second primary cancers, and the medical condition and wishes of the patient. Physician availability in various subspecialties also influences choice of treatment.

Patients who have advanced disease at the primary site and in the neck and those who are in very poor medical condition are often treated with palliative intent. A short course of palliative irradiation is often the most expedient and inexpensive option to afford relief of symptoms. Patients with advanced disease with a remote chance of cure may also be treated with chemotherapy. However, the side-effects of treatment may occasionally be severe enough to adversely affect the quality of life more than the cancer, and the response to chemotherapy is frequently less than 3 to 4 months. Surgical procedures, such as placement of a tracheostomy or gastrostomy, may be necessary if the airway is compromised or the patient is unable to swallow.

Synchronous primary tumours of the upper aerodigestive tract occur in a small subset of patients at presentation and influence the choice of treatment. Patients with two or three early-stage primary cancers in sites that could be treated either with irradiation or surgery, such as the oropharynx or supraglottis, may be more likely to be treated with radiation therapy because of ease of treating a large volume of mucosal tissue and both sides of the neck.

Selection of treatment for the primary tumour

The major treatment modalities for local and regional disease are surgery and radiation therapy. Chemotherapy has an adjuvant role in some situations. Early-stage tumours (T1–T2) are best treated by one modality, whereas combined irradiation and surgery often produce better cure rates for T3 and T4 cancers. Advanced lesions (T3–T4) in some sites (e.g. oropharynx)[17] have local control rates after radiotherapy alone that are similar to those observed after surgery and irradiation but with fewer complications. On the other hand, treatment of tumours in some sites (e.g. nasal cavity)[18] by combined modality therapy may yield cure rates similar to those obtained with irradiation alone but produce fewer complications.

Combination surgery and radiation therapy

Preoperative irradiation

The most common reason for giving radiation therapy before resection of the primary site is that a tumour is thought to be incompletely resectable, usually because of fixed metastatic adenopathy. Less often, a marginally resectable primary tumour may be treated in the hope that it may be rendered resectable by preoperative irradiation.[19] Radiation therapy is also given before surgery when it is desirable to avoid irradiating a graft used for reconstruction, such as the transposed stomach after a total laryngopharyngectomy and gastric transposition.[20] An additional reason to give preoperative irradiation is to reduce the extent of a resection that would otherwise be excessively morbid. Examples of this latter approach include high-dose radiation therapy of an advanced oral tongue cancer, followed by 'nidusectomy' of residual disease, and high-dose radiation therapy of an advanced nasal vestibule cancer with limited invasion of the premaxilla, followed by a partial maxillectomy.[21]

Preoperative irradiation usually consists of 45 to 50 Gy at 1.8 to 2.0 Gy per fraction (or its radiobiological equivalent) followed by a boost (if necessary) to areas of disease that were initially unresectable. The final dose is often in the range of 65 to 75 Gy, depending on the response to radiation therapy. The major disadvantage of preoperative irradiation is an increased risk of complications, such as wound breakdown and fistulae. The risk of postoperative complications can be minimized by limiting the areas boosted above 45 to 50 Gy to only those sites where the tumour is thought to be unresectable.

Postoperative irradiation

The strongest predictors for local–regional recurrence after surgery alone are positive margins and extracapsular extension.[22]–[24] The probability of salvage after local–regional failure is often low, depending on the site and extent of the tumour. Additionally, salvage treatment is often more extensive and morbid than initial treatment so that if there is a significant risk of local–regional recurrence after surgery, postoperative irradiation is indicated. Additional indications for postoperative irradiation includes close margins (≤5 mm), multiple positive neck nodes, 1-cm or greater subglottic extension, invasion of the primary tumour into the soft tissues of the neck, perineural invasion, endothelial-lined-space invasion, bone invasion, and cartilage invasion.[25]

Although 45 to 50 Gy at 1.8 to 2.0 Gy per fraction is highly effective in eradicating subclinical disease in the patient who has not had surgery, higher doses are necessary in the postoperative setting.[23] After surgery, it is likely that tumour is trapped in hypoxic compartments and relatively more resistant to irradiation. Although it may be tempting to irradiate only those sites thought to be at high risk, tumour may be seeded throughout the entire operative bed. Both the primary site and neck should be irradiated with the dose to areas at highest risk boosted to the final tumour dose.[25] The doses employed at our institution are based on the suspected amount of residual disease: negative margins, 60 Gy in 30 fractions; microscopically positive margins, 66 Gy in 33 fractions; and gross residual disease, 70 Gy in 35 fractions. Treatment is administered once daily in a continuous course.[26] If a dose per fraction of 1.8 Gy is used, the total doses are increased by 5 Gy. Patients with oral cavity primary tumours who have positive margins have poor local control rates with once-daily irradiation and may benefit from altered fractionation schedules.[27] The dose is lowered in some situations because the risk of postoperative complications may be unacceptably high with the dose-fractionation schedule outlined above. Patients who have undergone a supraglottic laryngectomy who require postoperative irradiation are given 55 Gy at 1.8 Gy per fraction.[28] Because the usual indication for irradiation in this setting is extensive neck disease, the dose to the involved side(s) of the neck may be boosted to a higher dose. Treatment is often administered with ^{60}Co or 4-MV X-rays because tumour may be located under the skin flaps and underdosed with higher energy beams. If it is necessary to use high-energy beams (≥6 MV photons) and tumour is suspected to be in a relatively superficial location, a 'beam spoiler' or bolus may be necessary to ensure adequate coverage.

The most convincing data supporting the use of postoperative irradiation is from the Medical College of Virginia.[22] Patients were operated on by two distinct groups of surgeons, and whether they received postoperative irradiation depended on the treatment policy of the surgical team: patients operated on by otolaryngologists who had positive margins and/or extracapsular extension received postoperative irradiation, whereas those operated on by general surgical oncologists had only follow-up. One hundred and twenty-five patients were treated, 54 with surgery and irradiation and the remainder with surgery alone. The 3-year rates of local–regional control and survival

Table 9 Three-year results of surgery alone compared with surgery and postoperative irradiation: Medical College of Virginia (125 patients)

Parameter	Surgery (%) 71 patients	Surgery and irradiation (%) 54 patients	p value
Local control–ECE	31	66	0.03
positive margins	41	49	0.04
ECE and positive margins	0	68	0.001
Disease-free survival	25	45	0.0001
Cause-specific survival	41	72	0.0003

ECE = extracapsular extension.

Data from Huang et al. International Journal of Radiation Oncology Biology Physics, 1992; **23**: 737–42.[22]

were significantly higher in the group of patients who received postoperative irradiation (Table 9).[22]

Treatment selection for specific tumour sites

Treatment selection for various tumour sites will be addressed in site-specific chapters. The treatment philosophy and results at the University of Florida may be found elsewhere.[17],[18],[29]–[38]

Management of the neck

Neck surgery

Standard radical neck dissection involves removal of the superficial and deep cervical fascia with its lymph nodes in levels I to V in continuity with the sternocleidomastoid muscle, omohyoid muscle, internal and external jugular veins, spinal accessory nerve, and submandibular gland. Sacrifice of cranial nerve XI usually results in atrophy of the trapezius muscle, with shoulder drop and discomfort.

Modified radical neck dissection (functional neck dissection) removes the superficial and deep cervical fascia with its enclosed lymph nodes and leaves one or more of the non-lymphatic structures such as the sternocleidomastoid and digastric muscles, internal jugular vein, and spinal accessory nerve. This procedure is performed when the likelihood of control of neck disease is thought to be equivalent to that obtained by a radical neck dissection. Currently, the vast majority of patients undergoing a neck dissection at the University of Florida undergo this operation with at least preservation of cranial nerve XI. The advantages of the functional neck dissection are less cosmetic deformity and better function (primarily the latter).

For a selective neck dissection, one or more of lymph node groups I to V are not removed. The advantage of the selective neck dissection is that it provides equivalent efficacy and less morbidity in appropriately selected cases. Supraomohyoid neck dissection removes the lymph nodes in levels I to III and is most commonly used for patients with small oral cavity cancers and a clinically negative neck. The lateral neck dissection entails removal of levels II to IV nodes and is most often used in the treatment of laryngeal, oropharyngeal, and hypopharyngeal cancers. If significant metastatic adenopathy is encountered during a selective neck dissection, it should be converted to a radical or modified radical dissection.

Bilateral neck dissections may be done simultaneously or separately in patients with bilateral neck disease as long as one internal jugular vein is preserved. At one time, simultaneous neck dissection appeared to be associated with a higher incidence of complications when compared with staged neck dissections. Our more recent experience suggests that this is no longer the case.

Complications of neck dissection

Complications of neck dissection include haematoma, seroma, lymphoedema, wound infection, wound dehiscence, chyle fistula, damage to cranial nerves VII, X, XI, and XII, carotid exposure, and carotid rupture. The incidence of complications is higher when neck dissection is combined with resection of the primary lesion or when it follows a course of radiation therapy. The postoperative mortality rate for unilateral neck dissection after radiation therapy was 3 per cent for patients treated between 1964 and 1982.[39]

The incidence of postoperative complications in a series of 143 patients treated with radiation therapy to the primary lesion and neck followed by unilateral neck dissection was 23 per cent; 17 patients (12 per cent) required a second operation.[39] The incidence of complications was higher for maximum subcutaneous doses over 60 Gy. Taylor et al.[40] updated the University of Florida experience with an analysis of the incidence of moderate (2+) and severe (3+) wound complications in a series of 205 patients who underwent a planned unilateral neck dissection after radiation therapy. Radiation therapy was given once daily in 123 patients, twice daily in 80 patients, and with both techniques in the remaining two patients. The incidence of wound complications had a trend to increase with total dose and dose per fraction (Fig. 3).[40] The incidence of postoperative complications for patients undergoing a bilateral neck dissection after irradiation to the primary lesion and neck is increased compared with those who undergo a unilateral neck dissection.[39]

Radiation therapy of the neck

Radiation therapy may be used in the treatment of cervical lymph node metastases as elective treatment when there are no palpable lymph nodes, as the only treatment for clinically positive lymph nodes, or as preoperative or postoperative treatment in combination with neck dissection for clinically positive lymph nodes.

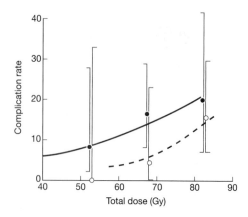

Fig. 3 Complication rate (2+ or 3+) versus total dose, with a separate analysis for once-a-day (solid curve) and twice-a-day (dashed curve) radiotherapy. Data are plotted at the midpoints of the ranges 45 to 60 Gy, 60 to 70 Gy, and 75 to 90 Gy. Error bars denote 95 per cent confidence intervals. The curves are the results of separate logistic regression analyses. From Taylor JMG, Mendenhall WM, Parsons JT, Lavey RS. The influence of dose and time on wound complications following post-radiation neck dissection. *International Journal of Radiation Oncology Biology Physics*, 1992; **23**: 41–6, with permission.[40]

Elective radiation therapy of cervical lymph nodes when the primary tumour is treated by radiation therapy

The factors that influence the decision to irradiate the neck electively are site and size of the primary lesion, histological grade, difficulty in neck examination, relative morbidity for adding lymph node coverage, likelihood of the patient's returning for follow-up examinations, and suitability of the patient for a radical neck dissection if the tumour appears in the neck at a later date. Patients in whom the primary lesion is to be treated by radiation therapy, who have clinically negative nodes, and in whom the risk of subclinical disease is 20 per cent or greater receive elective neck irradiation to a minimum dose equivalent to 45 to 50 Gy over 4.5 to 5 weeks. Patients with T1–T2 vocal cord cancers[41] and those with lesions arising in the lip, nasal vestibule, nasal cavity, or paranasal sinuses have a low risk of subclinical neck disease, and the neck is not treated electively unless the lesion is recurrent, advanced, or poorly differentiated.[21]

The lateral treatment portals used to encompass cancers in the oropharynx, supraglottic larynx, and hypopharynx incidentally include the upper internal jugular and often the midjugular chain lymph nodes. Radiation portals used for primary lesions of the oral cavity, nasopharynx, glottis, nasal cavity, and paranasal sinuses must be enlarged if one intends to irradiate the lymph nodes. The treatment portals for irradiation of the cervical lymph nodes must be designed in such a way as to minimize additional mucosal radiation therapy. A common error in irradiating oropharyngeal and nasopharyngeal cancers is to enlarge the lateral (primary) portals inferiorly to unnecessarily include all of the larynx in the lateral portals (Fig. 4 and Plate 1).[42] Because the midneck is smaller in circumference than the upper neck, the total dose and dose per fraction are higher in the larynx than along the central axis of the beam, leading to 'double trouble'. Treating an unnecessarily large field increases the acute and late effects of radiation therapy and, by increasing the risk of an unplanned split, reduces the probability of disease control.

Elective neck irradiation for early oral cavity lesions includes the submaxillary and subdigastric lymph nodes. The midjugular and low jugular lymph nodes are treated as well, by using a narrow anterior field. For primary lesions located in the oropharynx, nasopharynx, supraglottic larynx, and hypopharynx, the lower neck nodes are also routinely irradiated. The low neck is treated with a single anterior field (Figs 5[42] and 6 and Plates 2, 3). A tapered midline larynx/ trachea shield is added to protect the spinal cord, the larynx, and the pharynx. For primary lesions lying below the thyroid notch, a small midline tracheal block is placed in the low-neck field, primarily to avoid field overlap at the spinal cord. A 5-mm wide midline block made of Lipowitz's metal may be used to shield the trachea, oesophagus, and spinal cord below the level of the cricoid; this results in a 16 to 17-mm midline gap between the 90 per cent isodose lines for 6-MV X-ray when the block is placed 15 to 18 cm above the patient (source-to-skin distance 100 cm). Great care must be used to ensure that this block does not shield the midjugular and low jugular lymph nodes. The schema for treatment of the clinically negative neck at the University of Florida is summarized in Fig. 7.[43]

Treatment of clinically positive cervical lymph nodes when the primary tumour is treated by radiation therapy

The dose required to control a clinically positive lymph node that is included within the radiation portals depends on the size of the lymph node and, to some degree, on its histology. For squamous cell carcinoma, the recommended minimum doses (at 2 Gy per fraction, five fractions per week) for lymph nodes of various sizes are: 1.0 cm, 60 Gy; 1.5 to 2.0 cm, 66 Gy; 2.5 to 3.0 cm, 70 Gy; and 3.5 to 6.0 cm, 74 Gy. If the treatment is delivered at 1.8 Gy per fraction, five fractions per week, the total dose is increased approximately 5 Gy. The dose is not reduced when early, complete regression occurs during fractionated therapy.

The decision to add a neck dissection after radiation therapy for multiple, unilateral positive nodes or bilateral lymph node disease is individualized and is based on the diameter of the largest node, node fixation, number of clinically positive nodes in the neck, and the dose received by the nodes. If clinically positive lymph nodes receive full-dose irradiation and disappear completely during radiation therapy, the likelihood of control by radiation therapy alone is improved, and a neck dissection may be withheld.[23],[44],[45] However, if multiple nodes at multiple levels are involved, it is usually safer to perform the neck dissection immediately after radiation therapy because detection of lymph node recurrence may be made difficult by fibrosis of subcutaneous tissues of the neck and because the likelihood of successful salvage after recurrence in the neck is 5 per cent or less. Data have been published from the Medical College of Virginia that show that the risk of isolated failure in the neck is approximately 5 per cent if there has been a complete response in the neck after an aggressive altered-fractionation schedule for oropharyngeal cancer.[45] Results from M. D. Anderson Cancer Center,[44] which also suggest that neck dissection may be safely withheld, are based on patients who received very aggressive radiation therapy (72 Gy over 6 weeks) to the neck, and the conclusion may not be generalizable to patients who receive less aggressive fractionation schedules. Limited data also suggest that neck dissection may be safely withheld in patients who experience a complete response to induction chemotherapy followed by high-dose radiation therapy.[46],[47] The schema for treatment of the clinically

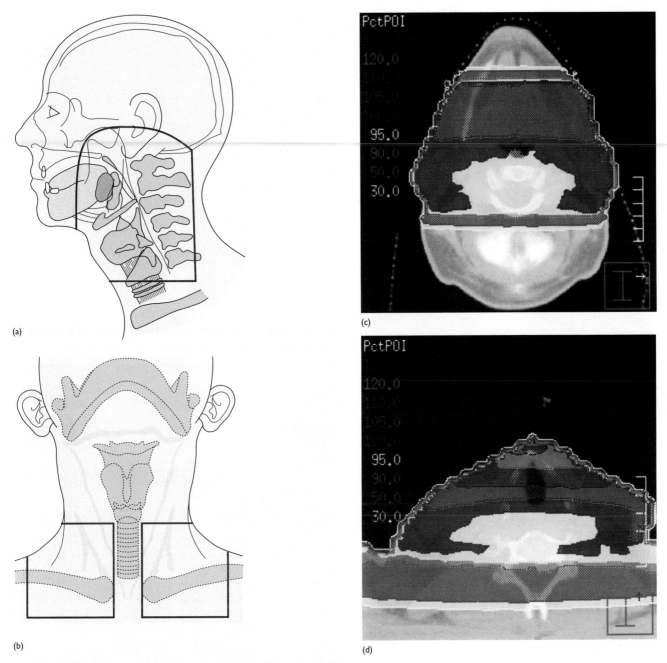

Fig. 4 Carcinoma of the base of tongue: large radiation portals. (a) Parallel-opposed lateral portals include the primary lesion, larynx, hypopharynx, most of the cervical spinal cord, and the upper portion of the trachea and cervical oesophagus. Treatment through this portal tangentially irradiates the skin of the anterior neck unnecessarily. If an anterior field is not used to irradiate the low neck, the inferior border of the lateral field may be placed near the clavicle (dashed line). (b) Anterior low-neck portal. The wide midline tracheal block partially shields the low internal jugular lymph nodes, which are located adjacent to the trachea. The supraclavicular lymph nodes, which are less likely to be involved with tumour than the low jugular nodes, are adequately covered. (c) Central axis dosimetry at the level of the base-of-tongue primary lesion. The dose distribution was obtained using parallel-opposed 6-MV X-ray fields weighted equally. (d) Off-axis contour through larynx. The minimum dose to most of the larynx is 5 per cent higher than the minimum tumour dose specified at the central axis, and a small amount of the anterior larynx receives approximately 25 per cent more irradiation. If the base-of-tongue tumour dose is specified as 50 Gy at 2 Gy per fraction, the maximum larynx dose will be in excess of 62.5 Gy at 2.5 Gy per fraction. (a) and (b) from Mendenhall WM, Parsons JT, Million RR. Unnecessary irradiation of the normal larynx (Editorial). *International Journal of Radiation Oncology Biology Physics*, 1990; **18**: 1531–3, with permission.[42] (See also Plate 1).

positive neck at the University of Florida is shown in Fig. 8.[43] Some patients who undergo surgery as the initial treatment and who have one or no positive nodes and no extracapsular extension may require postoperative irradiation because of indications relating to the primary tumour site (that is, close or positive margins, perineural invasion, etc.).

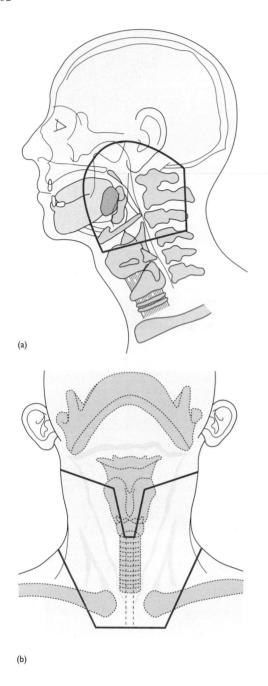

(a)

(b)

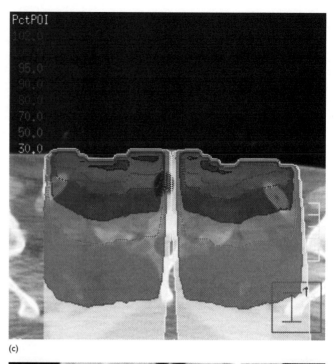

(c)

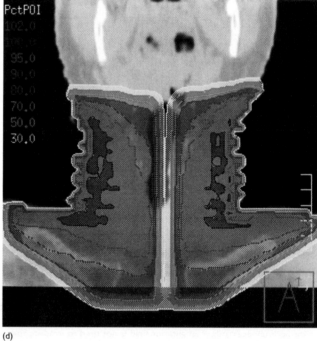

(d)

Fig. 5 Carcinoma of the base of tongue: radiation portals sparing the larynx. (a) Parallel-opposed fields include the primary lesion with a 2 to 3 cm inferior margin. The lower border of the field is placed at the thyroid notch and slants superiorly as the junction line proceeds posteriorly. This substantially reduces the amount of mucosa, larynx, and spinal cord included in the primary treatment portals. (b) *En face* low portal with tapered midline larynx block. It is not necessary to treat the supraclavicular fossa unless clinically positive nodes are found in that particular hemineck. A 5-mm midline tracheal block may be placed in the low-neck portal (dashed line). (c) Axial and (d) sagittal. Dose distribution under a 5-mm midline tracheal block with an anterior 6-MV X-ray field. (a) and (b) from Mendenhall WM, Parsons JT, Million RR. Unnecessary irradiation of the normal larynx (Editorial). *International Journal of Radiation Oncology Biology Physics*, 1990; **18**: 1531–3, with permission.[42] (See also Plate 2.)

If a neck dissection is to follow radiation therapy in patients with clinically positive lymph nodes, the preoperative dose varies with the size and location of the lymph nodes, fixation, and response to radiation therapy. Preoperative doses of 50 Gy are sufficient for mobile lymph nodes 3 to 4 cm in size, but a dose of 60 Gy or more is recommended for nodes of 5 to 6 cm and for fixed nodes. Lymph

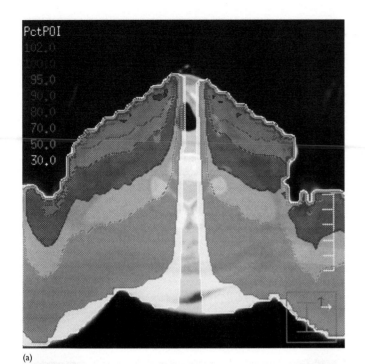

(a)

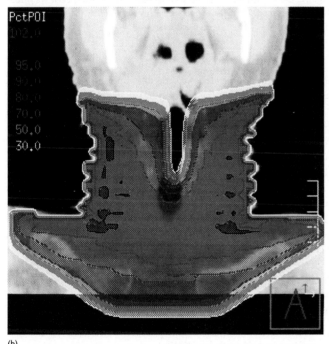

(b)

Fig. 6 Dose distribution for an anterior 6-MV X-ray field to the lower neck. (a) Axial contour through the level of the thyroid notch. (b) Sagittal contour. The source-to-skin distance (SSD) marker is placed on the anterior surface of the sternocleidomastoid opposite the cricoid cartilage. The internal jugular chain lymph nodes receive a minimum dose that is 80 to 85 per cent of the maximum dose. When 50 Gy is administered to the depth of maximum dose (Dmax), these nodes receive more than 40 Gy. The larynx and spinal cord are shielded by an anterior lead block. (See also Plate 3.)

nodes measuring 7 to 8 cm are almost always fixed to adjacent structures and often require doses of 70 to 75 Gy for the surgeon to

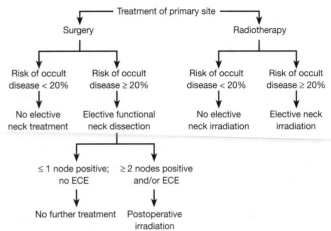

Fig. 7 Schema for treatment of the clinically negative neck. ECE = extracapsular extension. From Mendenhall WM, Parsons JT. Squamous cell carcinoma of the head and neck: Management of the neck and the unknown primary site. In Gunderson LL, Tepper JE, eds. *Clinical radiation oncology.* New York: Churchill Livingstone, 1998, with permission.[43]

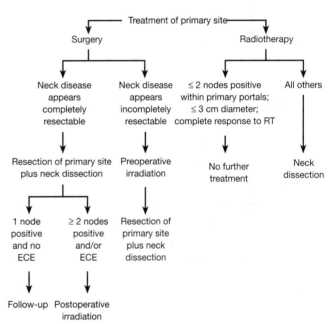

Fig. 8 Schema for treatment of the clinically positive neck. ECE = extracapsular extension. From Mendenhall WM, Parsons JT. Squamous cell carcinoma of the head and neck: Management of the neck and the unknown primary site. In: Gunderson LL, Tepper JE, eds. *Clinical radiation oncology.* New York: Churchill Livingstone, 1998, with permission.[43]

achieve a complete resection. If the lymph node lies behind the plane of the spinal cord, electrons may be used to boost the dose after the primary fields have been reduced off the spinal cord after 45 to 50 Gy.

Another technique commonly used for boosting the dose to the neck mass, after spinal cord tolerance has been reached and the treatment to the primary lesion has been completed, is opposed

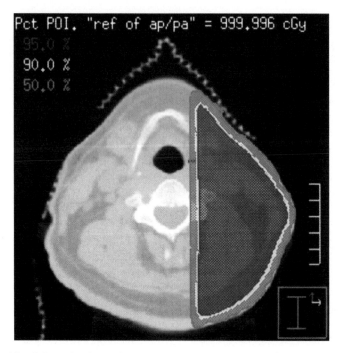

Pct POI. "ref of ap/pa" = 999.996 cGy

95.0 %

90.0 %

50.0 %

Fig. 9 Dose distribution for anterior and posterior wedge 6-MV X-ray portals, both fields weighted 1.0. This technique can be used to boost the dose to one or both sides of the neck. (See also Plate 4.)

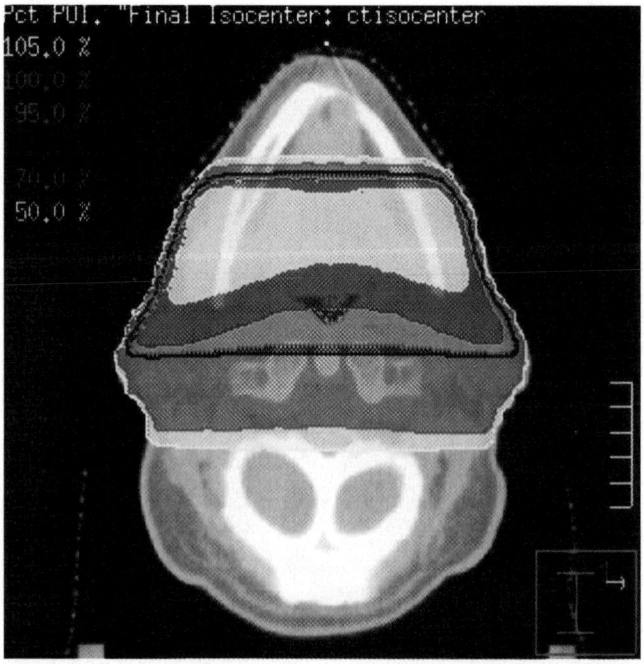

Pct POI. "Final Isocenter: ctisocenter

105.0 %

100.0 %

95.0 %

70.0 %

50.0 %

Fig. 10 Dose distribution for parallel-opposed ⁶⁰Co portals, each weighted 1.0, with reduced 6-MV X-ray portals, each weighted 0.4. (See also Plate 5.)

anterior and posterior fields with wedges. The final dose to the neck node (not to the entire neck) may be 70 to 80 Gy without exceeding the spinal cord tolerance (Fig. 9 and Plate 4). The anterior and posterior wedge-pair technique is preferable to an appositional electron boost field because high-energy electron beams increase the dose to the skin and underlying structures such as the mucosa and spinal cord. The technique is well suited for the patient with a small or unknown primary tumour where the mucosal dose may be in the range of 55 to 60 Gy, after which the dose to the node may be boosted as necessary.

When the cervical lymph nodes are located superficially, sometimes within 1 cm of the skin or fixed to it, treatment with high-energy photon beams (≥ 6 MV) may underdose these nodes. Treatment should be initiated with ⁶⁰Co or 4-MV X-rays for the initial 45 to 50 Gy, after which a higher energy photon beam can be used to continue radiation therapy to the primary tumour if the neck nodes are clinically negative or if a neck dissection is planned to follow radiation therapy (Fig. 10 and Plate 5). Parallel-opposed 6-MV X-ray beams may adequately treat the upper neck nodes included in the primary treatment fields; however, the supraclavicular nodes in the *en face* low-neck field may be underdosed with a 6-MV beam in very thin patients. Although electrons alone may be used to treat cervical nodes, it is preferable to combine them with photons because of the high surface dose and resultant fibrosis that may occur if electrons are the sole modality. In Fig. 11 (and see Plate 6), use of both 20-MeV electrons and 6-MV X-rays is compared with treatment by 20-MeV electrons alone in a patient with a lateralized lesion of the oropharynx. The addition of the 6-MV X-rays to the 20-MeV electrons decreases the surface dose while still adequately irradiating the cervical nodes that are within the primary field. The addition of

the X-ray beam also produces a dose distribution that is less affected by bone than that from the electron beam alone.

Large lymph nodes may not show much regression during the course of radiation therapy, but they often show a major regression from completion of treatment to the time that the patient returns for neck dissection, usually after 4 to 6 weeks. The mass often has a thick capsule that facilitates its removal at the time of neck dissection.

Patients with bilateral neck disease require individualized treatment planning jointly by the radiation oncologist and the surgeon. If disease is minimal on one side, radiation therapy alone may be used to control the disease on that side of the neck, and a neck dissection may be used on the side with more disease. If major bilateral disease is present, bilateral neck dissections should follow radiation therapy. It has been our experience that a tracheostomy should be electively performed when the larynx has been included in the irradiation portals. This can eventually be removed a few weeks postoperatively.

Complications of neck irradiation

The complications of neck irradiation include subcutaneous fibrosis and lymphoedema of the larynx and submentum. The latter complication may be minimized by sparing an anterior strip of skin when designing the parallel-opposed lateral portals used to encompass the primary lesion. Clothespins may be used to retract additional skin and subcutaneous tissues out of the radiation field and thereby further decrease the risk of laryngeal oedema (Fig. 12)[48] by allowing a route by which the fluids may escape, a situation analogous to 'sparing a strip' in patients with soft tissue sarcoma. The probability of complications is directly related to radiation dose and volume with little, if any, morbidity observed with the doses used for elective radiation therapy of the neck.

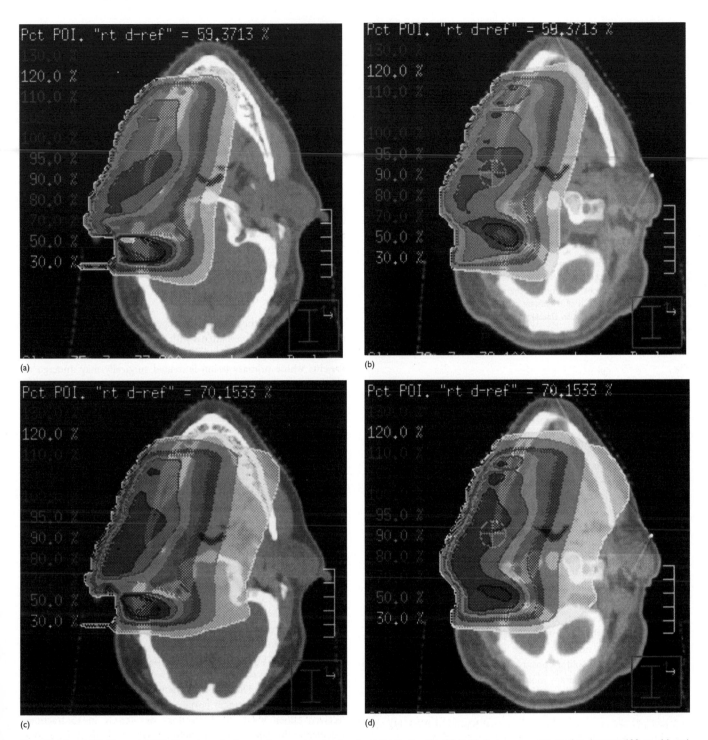

(a) (b) (c) (d)

Fig. 11 (a) and (b). Two axial CT slices through the oropharynx showing the dose distribution for 20-MeV electrons, source-to-skin distance 100 cm. (c) and (d) The same two axial CT slices showing the dose distribution for 20-MeV electrons and 6-MV X-rays, source-to-skin distance 100 cm for both. The given doses are weighted 3:2. The addition of the 6-MV X-ray beam reduces the surface dose and gives a dose distribution that is affected less by bone with a minimally increased exit dose to the contralateral side. (See also Plate 6.)

In patients who receive radiation therapy in conjunction with resection of the primary lesion and a neck dissection, complications of neck treatment are essentially the same as those occurring after neck dissection. However, they occur with an increased incidence depending on the radiation dose and extent of surgery.

Treatment of the neck after incisional or excisional biopsy

Open biopsy of a clinically positive neck node before definitive treatment potentially spills tumour cells along tissue planes that may

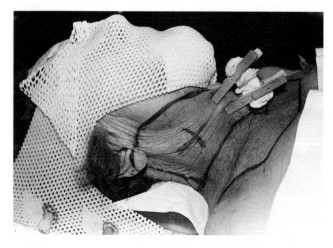

Fig. 12 Parallel-opposed portals with clothes-pegs used to increase the amount of tissue spared anteriorly. From Mendenhall WM, Million RR, Cassisi NJ. Squamous cell carcinoma of the supraglottic larynx treated with radical irradiation: Analysis of treatment parameters and results. *International Journal of Radiation Oncology Biology Physics*, 1984; **10**: 2223–30, with permission.[48]

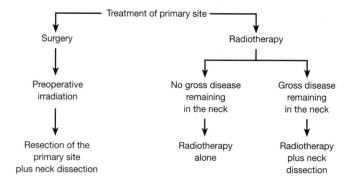

Fig. 13 Schema for treatment of the neck after incisional/excisional biopsy. From Mendenhall, Parsons. Squamous cell carcinoma of the head and neck: Management of the neck and the unknown primary site. In: Gunderson LL, Tepper JE, eds. *Clinical radiation oncology.* New York: Churchill Livingstone, 1998, and reproduced with permission.[43]

not be removed with a radical neck dissection. McGuirt and McCabe[49] reported that incisional or excisional biopsy of positive neck nodes before definitive surgery increased the risk of neck failure and worsened the prognosis for patients with squamous cell carcinoma of the head and neck. Investigators from the University of Florida reported their experience with incisional or excisional biopsy of positive neck nodes followed by radiation therapy as the initial step in the treatment of the patient.[7],[50],[51] After excisional biopsy of a single lymph node, radiation therapy alone to the primary lesion and to the neck resulted in a 95 per cent rate of control of neck disease.[51] If residual disease remained in the neck after biopsy, radiation therapy followed by neck dissection was more successful than radiation therapy alone for controlling neck disease.

If the primary lesion is to be treated surgically, the patient is treated with preoperative radiation therapy to the primary lesion and neck, followed by resection. If the primary lesion is to be treated with radiation therapy, the patient's neck also is treated with radiation therapy. If there is no gross disease remaining in the neck after excisional biopsy of a solitary positive node (N_{EXC}), the neck may be treated with radiation therapy alone. Virtually all such patients have palpable induration secondary to haematoma. CT is very useful in determining whether the residual induration is due to haemorrhage and oedema versus tumour. If an incisional biopsy of the node has been performed or if other positive nodes remain after an excisional neck node biopsy, radiation therapy is followed by a neck dissection (Fig. 13).[43]

Results of neck treatment

Clinically negative nodes

Elective neck dissection and elective neck irradiation are equally effective in controlling subclinical disease. The decision regarding whether to use surgery or radiation therapy for the purpose of electively treating the neck nodes depends on the method used to treat the primary lesion. Patients with a relatively early primary lesion and clinically negative nodes should be treated with one modality. Patients whose primary lesion is treated surgically may undergo an elective neck dissection, and those whose primary lesion is to be treated with radiation therapy should be considered for elective neck irradiation.

The results of elective neck irradiation at the University of Florida for patients with squamous cell carcinoma of the head and neck in whom the primary lesion was controlled are shown in Table 10.[2] Patients were stratified into three risk categories based on the estimated risk of subclinical disease in the neck, as follows: group I—low risk (<20 per cent likelihood of occult disease); group II—moderate risk (20–30 per cent risk of occult disease); and group III—high risk (>30 per cent likelihood of occult disease). There were six neck failures in 28 patients (21 per cent) who did not receive elective neck irradiation and eight neck failures (5 per cent) in 162 patients who received elective neck irradiation. Of the eight failures in patients receiving elective neck irradiation, two occurred within the irradiation fields, one at the field margin, and five outside the irradiation fields. No correlation was found between the control rate in the first-echelon lymph nodes and the radiation dose for doses ranging from 40 to 55 Gy or greater. Only one failure occurred in the first-echelon lymph nodes, and this was after 48 Gy in 25 fractions using continuous-course irradiation. The low neck, defined as that part of the neck located below the treatment portals used to treat the primary lesion, received either 50 Gy in 25 fractions or 40.5 Gy in 15 fractions, specified at the depth of maximum dose (Dmax). Both of these dose-fractionation protocols were equally effective in sterilizing subclinical disease in the low neck.[52] Elective neck irradiation is equally efficacious for squamous cell carcinoma arising from various head and neck primary sites.

If the primary lesion recurs, there is a renewed risk of lymphatic spread to the neck, even after elective neck irradiation has been administered, because of the possibility of reseeding the neck lymphatics. In patients in whom primary failure occurs in addition to failure in the clinically negative nodes, the chances of surgical salvage are poor. In patients in whom the primary lesion is controlled and in whom failure develops in the initially negative neck, the chances of

Table 10 Control of disease in the clinically negative neck with elective neck irradiation (number controlled/ number treated)

Risk group	No ENI	Partial ENI	Total ENI
I (<20%)	13/15 (87%)	16/17 (94%)	1/1
II (20–30%)	6/9 (67%)	34/38 (89%)	10/11 (91%)
III (>30%)	3/4 (75%)	32/33 (97%)	61/62 (98%)

ENI = elective neck irradiation.

From Mendenhall et al. International Journal of Radiation Oncology Biology Physics, 1986; **12**: 741–6, with permission.[2]

Table 11 Failure of initial ipsilateral neck treatment versus stage:[75] 596 patients with carcinoma of the tonsillar fossa, base of tongue, supraglottic larynx, or hypopharynx

Treatment	N0			N1	N2A	N2B	N3A	N3B
	No treatment	Partial treatment	Complete treatment					
Irradiation		15%	2%	15%	27%	27%	38%	34%
Surgery	55% (16/29)	35%	7%	11%	8%	23%	42%	41%
Combined		1/5	0/6	0	0	0	23%	25%

MD Anderson Hospital data; patients treated 1948–1967.

Modified from Barkley et al. American Journal of Surgery, 1972; **124**:462–7.[58]

Table 12 Five-year rate of neck control according to the 1983 AJCC[75] stage and treatment (459 patients; 593 heminecks[a])

Stage	Radiotherapy alone		Radiotherapy + neck dissection		Significance
	Number of heminecks	Control (%)	Number of heminecks	Control (%)	
N1	215	86	38	93	$p = 0.28$
N2A	29	79	24	68	$p = 0.6$
N2B	138	70	80	91	$p < 0.01$
N3A	29	33	40	69	$p < 0.01$

[a] Excludes 67 heminecks on which incisional or excisional biopsy was done before treatment.

University of Florida data; patients treated 10/64–10/85; analysis 12/88 by Eric R. Ellis.

From Mendenhall et al. In: Perez CA, Brady LW, eds. Principles and practice of radiation oncology, 2nd edn., 1992: 790–805, with permission.[59]

Table 13 Cervical metastasis appearing in the contralateral N0 neck: 596 patients with carcinoma of the tonsillar fossa, base of tongue, supraglottic larynx, or hypopharynx

Treatment	Cervical metastasis (%)				
	N0	N1	N2A	N2B	N3A
Irradiation	4	2	9	7	0
Surgery	25	17	23	43	33
Combined	0	0	0	11	0

M. D. Anderson Hospital data; patients treated 1948–1967.

Adapted from Barkley et al. American Journal of Surgery, 1972; **124**: 462–7.[58]

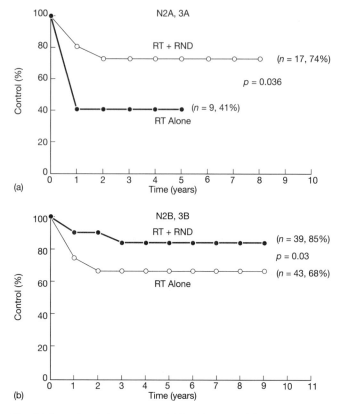

(a)

(b)

Fig. 14 Rate of neck disease control (life table method) for patients treated with twice-daily irradiation alone (RT) or combined with neck dissection (RT + RND) for clinically positive neck nodes. (A) N2A, N3A. (B) N2B, N3B. From Parsons JT, Mendenhall WM, Cassisi NJ, Stringer SP, Million RR. Neck dissection after twice-a-day radiotherapy: Morbidity and recurrence rates. *Head and Neck*, 1989; **11**: 400–4, with permission.[60]

salvage with neck dissection are approximately 50 to 60 per cent.[53]

Although elective neck irradiation significantly reduces the risk of neck recurrence, there is no definite evidence that it improves survival rates. It would be necessary to conduct a large, randomized trial to detect a survival difference, if one exists. Another problem is that the first-echelon lymph nodes are often included in the treatment portals used to treat the primary lesion, so that it is often impossible to avoid at least partial elective neck irradiation. Therefore, such a trial would have to be restricted to primary sites where the portals would have to be enlarged to electively irradiate the neck or to patients treated with elective neck dissection rather than elective neck irradiation. Vandenbrouck *et al.*[54] and Fakih *et al.*[55] have conducted randomized trials comparing elective neck dissection with no elective neck treatment for patients with oral cavity carcinoma and oral tongue cancer. No survival advantage was noted for patients undergoing elective neck dissection in either study. However, because of the small number of patients in both trials, it is likely that even if a survival difference existed, it would have been missed.

Dearnaley *et al.*[56] reported a series of 148 patients treated at the Royal Marsden Hospital (London) with an interstitial implant, alone or combined with external-beam irradiation, for cancer of the tongue or floor of mouth. Of 131 patients with negative neck nodes at diagnosis, 59 patients (45 per cent) received elective neck irradiation to a dose of 40 Gy. A multivariate analysis revealed that elective neck irradiation significantly improved survival and reduced the risk of dying from cancer. Piedbois *et al.*[57] reported a series of 233 patients with T1–T2N0 carcinoma of the oral cavity treated with interstitial iridium brachytherapy. One hundred and twenty-three patients received no elective neck treatment, and 110 patients underwent an elective neck dissection. Patients who received an elective neck dissection tended to have more advanced primary lesions. Although the ultimate rates of neck control were similar, a multivariate analysis revealed that elective neck dissection was significantly associated with improved survival.

Clinically positive nodes

The incidence of treatment failure in the neck by N stage and treatment category has been reported by the M. D. Anderson Cancer Center in Houston (Table 11)[58] and the University of Florida (Table 12).[59] In patients in whom the neck is treated with combined modalities, radiation therapy precedes surgery when the primary site is to be treated with irradiation or when the node is fixed. Surgery precedes radiation therapy when the primary site is to be treated operatively and the nodes are resectable.

When the initial treatment is surgery, a neck dissection is sufficient treatment for patients with a single positive lymph node unless there

Table 14 Effect of neck-node biopsy on 5-year rate of neck control (660 heminecks)

Hemineck stage	No neck biopsy		Neck biopsy		Significance of difference between curves
	Number of heminecks	Probability of hemineck control (%)	Number of heminecks	Probability of hemineck control (%)	
N1	253	87 ± 3	12	100	$p = 0.22$
N2A	53	73 ± 8	15	93 ± 6	$p = 0.18$
N2B	218	78 ± 3	23	72 ± 11	$p = 0.86$
N3A	69	54 ± 7	17	81 ± 10	$p = 0.30$

From Ellis *et al. Head and Neck*, 1991; **13**: 177–83, with permission.[7]

Table 15 Prognostic factors, in order of their importance, for predicting the time to occurrence of various events

Event	Rank order	Factor	Level of significance
Recurrence in neck (n = 660 heminecks)	1	Increasing N stage	$p = 0.0001$
	2	Treatment of neck with RT alone	$p = 0.0001$
	3	Fixed nodes	$p = 0.0001$
	4	T stage[a]	$p = 0.0350$
Death with disease present (n = 508 patients)	1	Recurrence above clavicles	$p = 0.0001$
	2	Increasing N stage	$p = 0.0003$
	3	Fixed nodes	$p = 0.0053$
	4	Treatment of neck with RT alone	$p = 0.0121$
Distant metastasis (n = 508 patients)	1	Recurrence above clavicles	$p = 0.0001$
	2	Increasing N stage	$p = 0.0003$
	3	Fixed nodes	$p = 0.0704$
	4	Nodes below thyroid notch	$p = 0.1023$

RT = radiation therapy.

[a] This factor is thought to be correlated with the censoring pattern.

From Ellis *et al. Head and Neck*, 1991; **13**: 177–83, with permission.[7]

Table 16 Diagnostic workup for cervical lymph node metastases: unknown primary tumour

General
History
Physical examination
Careful examination of the neck and supraclavicular regions
Examination of oral cavity, pharynx, and larynx (indirect laryngoscopy)

Radiographic studies
Chest radiograph
Computed tomography and/or magnetic resonance imaging scans of head and neck (special attention to nasopharynx, pharynx, and larynx)
Upper gastrointestinal series and barium enema (in patients with adenocarcinoma involving supraclavicular lymph nodes)

Laboratory studies
Complete blood cell count
Blood chemistry profile

Direct endoscopy and directed biopsies
Nasopharynx, both tonsils, base of tongue, both pyriform sinuses, and any suspicious or abnormal mucosal areas
Fine needle aspirate or core needle biopsy of the cervical node

From Mendenhall *et al.* In: Perez CA, Brady LW, eds. *Principles and practice of radiation oncology*, 2nd edn. Philadelphia: J.B. Lippincott, 1992: 790–805, with permission.[59]

is extracapsular spread of disease. Radiation therapy may be added for control of subclinical disease in the contralateral side of the neck (Table 13).[58] The presence of multiple positive nodes in the surgical specimen is an indication for postoperative radiation therapy of the neck, especially when positive nodes are found at more that one level.

Olsen *et al.*[24] reported a series of 284 patients who underwent neck dissection at the Mayo Clinic (Rochester, MN) for pathological stage N1 and N2 squamous cell carcinoma of the head and neck; no patient received adjuvant therapy. Neck-recurrence-free survival rates at 5 years were as follows: N1, 76 per cent; N2, 60 per cent; and overall, 69 per cent. A multivariate analysis revealed that four or more positive nodes ($p = 0.005$), invasion of lymphatic and/or vascular spaces ($p = 0.003$), invasion of soft tissue ($p = 0.0008$),

and a desmoplastic stromal pattern ($p = 0.0001$) were significantly associated with an increased risk of recurrence in the neck.

The postoperative dose prescribed is usually 60 Gy in 30 fractions to 65 Gy in 35 fractions over 6 to 7 weeks for patients with negative margins; higher doses may be prescribed when residual disease is present in the neck. If radiation therapy is to be added after surgery, it is usually initiated within 4 to 6 weeks after the operation, although it has been reported that a delay to 10 weeks is not associated with an increased risk of neck failure.

Radiation therapy alone is sufficient for patients with N1 and early N2B disease as long as the fraction size (2 Gy) and the total dose are sufficient. Radiation therapy followed by neck dissection has provided better rates of disease control than radiation therapy alone for patients with more advanced neck disease. The rate of neck disease control

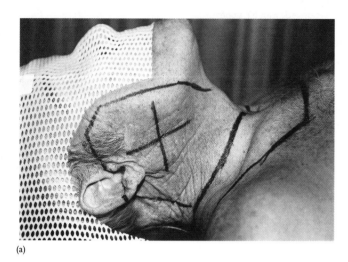
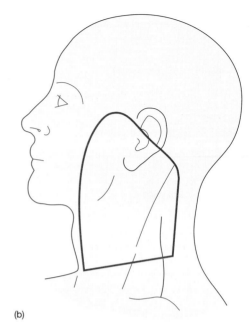

(a)

(b)

Fig. 15 Parallel-opposed lateral fields are used to treat an unknown head and neck primary lesion. (a) Patient set up for treatment showing that a strip of skin is spared anteriorly over the larynx, and clothespins are used to increase the amount of unirradiated tissue in this area. (b) Diagram of treatment field. From Mendenhall WM, Parsons JT, Mancuso AA, Stringer SP, Cassisi NJ, Million RR. Head and neck: Management of the neck. In Perez CA, Brady LW, eds. *Principles and practice of radiation oncology*, 2nd edn. Philadelphia: J.B. Lippincott, 1992: 790–805, with permission.[59]

Table 17 Metastatic cervical lymph nodes, unknown primary site: 3-year disease-free absolute survival rates

Stage	Type of treatment		
	Surgery	Radiation therapy	Combination therapy
NX	31/39 (79%)	8/9 (89%)	3/3
N1	4/6 (67%)	1/3	1/3
N2	10/22 (45%)	3/4	5/9
N3	14/37 (38%)	13/36 (36%)	4/13 (31%)
Total	59/104[a] (57%)	25/52[b] (48%)	13/28[b] (46%)

MD Anderson Hospital; 184 patients, July 1948–June 1968.

[a] Salvage in 8 patients by radiation therapy and in 6 patients by surgery.

[b] Salvage in 1 patient by surgery

From Jesse et al. Cancer, 1973; **31**: 854–9, with permission.[68]

for patients treated with twice-daily irradiation, alone or followed by neck dissection, is depicted in Fig. 14,[60] which shows a significant improvement in the control rates when neck dissection was added in selected cases. As shown in a multivariate analysis by Ellis *et al.*,[7] the addition of neck dissection after radiation therapy is independently related to a significantly decreased risk of dying of cancer. At least 50 Gy should be given preoperatively to the lymph nodes, although doses vary according to the size and degree of fixation of the lymph node. The likelihood of disease control in the neck after irradiation

and neck dissection is decreased when the node is fixed before treatment or when residual tumour is found in the pathological specimen.[39] No difference is seen in the rate of control as a function of the interval between radiation therapy and neck dissection when comparing patients who have surgery within 6 weeks with those who have neck dissection more than 6 weeks after radiation therapy. In the event of a subsequent local recurrence, prior combined treatment of the neck does not diminish the chance of successful surgical salvage of the patient. Some authors have reported that the likelihood of

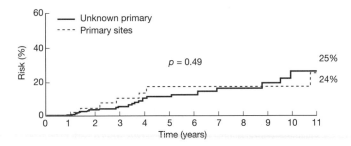

Fig. 16 Incidence of mucosal site failure or second head and neck primary lesions after mucosal radiation therapy for unknown head and neck primary site (dashed lines) compared with incidence of metachronous second primary head and neck cancer after radiation therapy for squamous cell carcinoma of the tonsillar area, supraglottic larynx, pyriform sinus, and pharyngeal wall (solid line). From Harper CS, Mendenhall WM, Parsons JT, Stringer SP, Cassisi NJ, Million RR. Cancer in neck nodes with unknown primary site: Role of mucosal radiotherapy. *Head and Neck*, 1990; **12**: 463–9, with permission.[69]

local control after radiotherapy is inversely related to neck stage; others have not observed this finding.[61]–[63] If such a relationship exists, it is likely to be a weak one.[64]

Clinically positive nodes with incisional or excisional biopsy

Patients who have undergone an incisional or excisional biopsy of a metastatic lymph node before referral do not have an increased risk of neck failure or a decreased cure rate if radiation therapy is the next step in their treatment (see Fig. 13).[43] The likelihood of control and the cure rate are probably diminished if an operation without prior radiation therapy follows incisional or excisional biopsy of a metastatic neck node because of the risk that the biopsy procedure disseminated tumour cells into tissues not removed by neck dissection.

Ellis *et al.*[7] reported 508 patients with 660 positive heminecks treated at the University of Florida with radiation therapy alone or followed by a planned neck dissection. Pretreatment node biopsy did not influence outcome when irradiation was the next step in treatment (Table 14). The results of the forward stepwise log-rank tests of prognostic factors for predicting time to recurrence are shown in Table 15.

Cervical lymph node metastasis with unknown primary tumour

In a small percentage of patients with enlarged cervical lymph nodes, the primary lesion cannot be found, even after extensive evaluation. Patients with enlarged lymph nodes in the upper neck have a good prognosis when treated aggressively, compared with those with enlarged lymph nodes in the low internal jugular chain or supraclavicular fossa. The latter group is more likely to have a primary lesion located below the clavicles, which carries with it a dismal prognosis. The majority of patients have either squamous cell carcinoma or poorly differentiated carcinoma. Those with adenocarcinoma almost always have a primary lesion below the clavicles, although if the nodes are located in the upper neck, one must exclude a salivary gland, thyroid, or parathyroid primary tumour. This section deals with patients who

have squamous cell or poorly differentiated carcinoma in the upper or middle neck.

Patients should be evaluated with a thorough physical examination including careful evaluation of the head and neck. A needle biopsy of the lymph node should be performed. A fine-needle aspirate is preferred to a biopsy because it is less traumatic and there is a lower likelihood of seeding tumour cells along the needle track. Limited data suggest that evaluation of the neck node biopsy for Epstein–Barr virus (EBV) DNA, via polymerase chain reaction, may be useful in detecting a nasopharyngeal primary tumour.[65] Tumours testing positive for EBV DNA are likely to be nasopharyngeal in origin. After chest roentgenography, CT or MRI of the head and neck is obtained to detect an unknown primary lesion arising from the mucosa of the head and neck. Direct endoscopy and examination under anaesthesia are performed with directed biopsies of the nasopharynx, tonsils (including an ipsilateral or bilateral tonsillectomy), base of tongue, and pyriform sinuses, and of any abnormalities noted on CT or MRI or suspicious mucosal lesions noted during endoscopy. If the primary lesion is not found on repeated physical examination by multiple examiners or on the CT or MRI of the head and neck, a small subset of patients will have their primary sites detected by directed biopsies. The diagnostic evaluation for the patient with cervical metastasis from an unknown head and neck primary lesion is summarized in Table 16.[59]

Some patients may be cured with treatment directed only to the involved area of the neck;[66],[67] however, we usually irradiate the nasopharynx, oropharynx, hypopharynx, and larynx as well as both sides of the neck. It is not necessary to irradiate the oral cavity unless the patient has submandibular adenopathy, in which case we either do a neck dissection and observe the patient or irradiate the oral cavity and oropharynx and not the nasopharynx, larynx, or hypopharynx. Patients are treated with parallel-opposed fields at 1.8 Gy per fraction to a midline dose of 55.8 Gy with reduction off the spinal cord at 45 Gy tumour dose (Fig. 15).[59] The lower neck is treated through a separate *en face* anterior field. Dosimetry is obtained at the level of the central axis (which usually corresponds to the oropharynx), the nasopharynx, and the larynx. Within the past year, we have limited the mucosal sites included in the lateral portals to the oropharynx and nasopharynx because the most common primary sites are the tonsillar fossa and tongue base. Although the nasopharynx is a relatively low-risk site, it is necessary to treat the skull base to include the retropharyngeal nodes, which means that some of the nasopharynx is already within the irradiation fields. The hypopharynx is included if the patient has a group III or IV node. Because the dose to the nasopharynx is usually 3 to 5 Gy lower than the central axis dose, a nasopharynx boost must be added to bring the dose up to 55 Gy. If there is a suspected primary site, an additional 5 Gy may be delivered to that site as well. Treatment of the neck depends on the extent and location of the adenopathy.

One hundred eighty-four patients with squamous cell carcinoma from an unknown head and neck primary site were treated at the M. D. Anderson Cancer Center.[68] The relationship of primary site appearance versus treatment revealed: surgery alone, 21/104 (20 per cent); radiation therapy, 3/52 (6 per cent); and irradiation plus surgery, 4/28 (14 per cent).[68] When the primary lesion appeared, the survival rate was 50 per cent lower than when the primary lesion did not appear after treatment of the neck. The absolute survival rate at

3 years as a function of treatment group and disease stage is shown in Table 17.[68]

The incidence of subsequent mucosal primary lesions was compared by Harper et al.[69] for patients with a known primary site and a series of 69 patients treated for an unknown primary site at the University of Florida. The incidence for both groups was approximately 25 per cent at 10 years, suggesting either that mucosal irradiation significantly reduced the risk of primary site failure, or that patients with unknown primary sites have a much lower risk of a second primary head and neck cancer developing subsequently (Fig. 16).[69]

Reddy and Marks[70] reported 52 patients treated to the neck alone (16 patients) or the neck and potential head and neck primary sites (36 patients). Failure in the head and neck mucosa occurred in 44 per cent of those who underwent treatment to the neck alone, compared with 8 per cent in those who underwent irradiation of the head and neck mucosa ($p = 0.0005$). The 5-year survival rates were similar for the two treatment groups.

The main complication of radiation therapy for patients treated for an unknown head and neck primary tumour is xerostomia. The complications of treatment of the neck, which have been discussed previously, depend on whether a neck dissection is added.

References

1. Rouvière H. Anatomy of the human lymphatic system. (Tobias M, translator). Ann Arbor, MI: Edwards Brothers, 1938: 1–28, 77–8.
2. Mendenhall WM, Million RR. Elective neck irradiation for squamous cell carcinoma of the head and neck: Analysis of time-dose factors and causes of failure. International Journal of Radiation Oncology Biology Physics, 1986; 12: 741–6.
3. Lindberg R. Distribution of cervical lymph node metastases from squamous cell carcinoma of the upper respiratory and digestive tracts. Cancer, 1972; 29: 1446–9.
4. Richard JM, Sancho-Garnier H, Micheau C, Saravane D, Cachin Y. Prognostic factors in cervical lymph node metastasis in upper respiratory and digestive tract carcinomas: Study of 1,713 cases during a 15-year period. Laryngoscope, 1987; 97: 97–101.
5. McLaughlin MP, Mendenhall WM, Mancuso AA, et al. Retropharyngeal adenopathy as a predictor of outcome in squamous cell carcinoma of the head and neck. Head and Neck, 1995; 17: 190–8.
6. Ellis ER, Mendenhall WM, Rao PV, Parsons JT, Spangler AE, Million RR. Does node location affect the incidence of distant metastases in head and neck squamous cell carcinoma? International Journal of Radiation Oncology Biology Physics, 1989; 17: 293–7.
7. Ellis ER, Mendenhall WM, Rao PV, et al. Incisional or excisional neck-node biopsy before definitive radiotherapy, alone or followed by neck dissection. Head and Neck, 1991; 13: 177–83.
8. Million RR, Cassisi NJ, Mancuso AA, Stringer SP, Mendenhall WM, Parsons JT. Management of the neck for squamous cell carcinoma. In: Million RR, Cassisi NJ, eds. Management of head and neck cancer: a multidisciplinary approach. Philadelphia: J.B. Lippincott, 1994: 75–142.
9. Mendenhall WM, Parsons JT, Mendenhall NP, Brant TA, Stringer SP, Cassisi NJ, et al. Carcinoma of the skin of the head and neck with perineural invasion. Head and Neck, 1989; 11: 301–8.
10. Mendenhall WM, Mancuso AA, Parsons JT, Stringer SP, Cassisi NJ. Diagnostic evaluation of squamous cell carcinoma metastatic to cervical lymph nodes from an unknown head and neck primary site. Head and Neck, 1998; 20: 739–44.
11. International Union Against Cancer. Sobin LH, Wittekind Ch., eds. TNM classification of malignant tumours. New York: Wiley-Liss, 1998: 17–47.
12. American Joint Committee on Cancer. AJCC cancer staging handbook. Philadelphia: Lippincott-Raven Publishers, 1998: 25–61.
13. Mendenhall WM, Parsons JT, Mancuso AA, Pameijer FA, Stringer SP, Cassisi NJ. Definitive radiotherapy for T3 squamous cell carcinoma of the glottic larynx. Journal of Clinical Oncology, 1997; 15: 2394–402.
14. Pameijer FA, Mancuso AA, Mendenhall WM, Parsons JT, Kubilis PS. Can pretreatment computed tomography predict local control in T3 squamous cell carcinoma of the glottic larynx treated with definitive radiotherapy? International Journal of Radiation Oncology Biology Physics, 1997; 37: 1011–21.
15. Pameijer FA, Mancuso AA, Mendenhall WM, et al. Evaluation of pretreatment computed tomography as a predictor of local control in T1/T2 pyriform sinus carcinoma treated with definitive radiotherapy. Head and Neck, 1998; 20: 159–68.
16. Mendenhall WM, Parsons JT, Million RR, Cassisi NJ, Devine JW, Greene BD. A favorable subset of AJCC stage IV squamous cell carcinoma of the head and neck. International Journal of Radiation Oncology Biology Physics, 1984; 10: 1841–3.
17. Parsons JT, Mendenhall WM, Million RR, Stringer SP, Cassisi NJ. The management of primary cancers of the oropharynx: Combined treatment or irradiation alone? Seminars in Radiation Oncology, 1992; 2: 142–8.
18. Parsons JT, Bova FJ, Fitzgerald CR, Mendenhall WM, Million RR. Radiation optic neuropathy after megavoltage external-beam irradiation: Analysis of time-dose factors. International Journal of Radiation Oncology Biology Physics, 1994; 30: 755–63.
19. Wang ZH, Million RR, Mendenhall WM, Parsons JT, Cassisi NJ. Treatment with preoperative irradiation and surgery of squamous cell carcinoma of the head and neck. Cancer, 1989; 64: 32–8.
20. Mendenhall WM, Sombeck MD, Parsons JT, Kasper ME, Stringer SP, Vogel SB. Management of cervical esophageal carcinoma. Seminars in Radiation Oncology, 1994; 4: 179–91.
21. Mendenhall WM, Stringer SP, Cassisi NJ, Mendenhall NP. Squamous cell carcinoma of the nasal vestibule. Head and Neck, 1999; 21: 385–93.
22. Huang DT, Johnson CR, Schmidt-Ullrich R, Grimes M. Postoperative radiotherapy in head and neck carcinoma with extracapsular lymph node extension and/or positive resection margins: a comparative study. International Journal of Radiation Oncology Biology Physics, 1992; 23: 737–42.
23. Peters LJ, Goepfert H, Ang KK, Byers RM, Maor MH, Guillamondegui O, et al. Evaluation of the dose for postoperative radiation therapy of head and neck cancer: First report of a prospective randomized trial. International Journal of Radiation Oncology Biology Physics, 1993; 26: 3–11.
24. Olsen KD, Caruso M, Foote RL, et al. Primary head and neck cancer. Histopathologic predictors of recurrence after neck dissection in patients with lymph node involvement. Archives of Otolaryngology – Head and Neck Surgery, 1994; 120: 1370–4.
25. Amdur RJ, Parsons JT, Mendenhall WM, Million RR, Stringer SP, Cassisi NJ. Postoperative irradiation for squamous cell carcinoma of the head and neck: An analysis of treatment results and complications. International Journal of Radiation Oncology Biology Physics, 1989; 16: 25–36.
26. Amdur RJ, Parsons JT, Mendenhall WM, Million RR, Cassisi NJ. Split-course versus continuous-course irradiation in the postoperative setting for squamous cell carcinoma of the head and neck. International Journal of Radiation Oncology Biology Physics, 1989; 17: 279–85.
27. Parsons JT, Mendenhall WM, Stringer SP, Cassisi NJ, Million RR. An analysis of factors influencing the outcome of postoperative irradiation for squamous cell carcinoma of the oral cavity. International Journal of Radiation Oncology Biology Physics, 1997; 39: 137–48.

28. Lee NK, Goepfert H, Wendt CD. Supraglottic laryngectomy for intermediate-stage cancer: U.T. M.D. Anderson Cancer Center experience with combined therapy. *Laryngoscope*, 1990; **100**: 831–6.

29. Fein DA, Mendenhall WM, Parsons JT, *et al.* Carcinoma of the oral tongue: a comparison of results and complications of treatment with radiotherapy and/or surgery. *Head and Neck*, 1994; **16**: 358–65.

30. Rodgers LW, Stringer SP, Mendenhall WM, Parsons JT, Cassisi NJ, Million RR. Management of squamous cell carcinoma of the floor of the mouth. *Head and Neck*, 1993; **15**: 16–9.

31. Mendenhall WM, Van Cise WS, Bova FJ, Million RR. Analysis of time-dose factors in squamous cell carcinoma of the oral tongue and floor of mouth treated with radiation therapy alone. *International Journal of Radiation Oncology Biology Physics*, 1981; **7**: 1005–11.

32. Mendenhall WM, Parsons JT, Mancuso AA, Stringer SP, Cassisi NJ. Radiotherapy for squamous cell carcinoma of the supraglottic larynx: An alternative to surgery. *Head and Neck*, 1996; **18**: 24–35.

33. Parsons JT, Mendenhall WM, Stringer SP, Cassisi NJ, Million RR. Salvage surgery following radiation failure in squamous cell carcinoma of the supraglottic larynx. *International Journal of Radiation Oncology Biology Physics*, 1995; **32**: 605–9.

34. Parsons JT, Mendenhall WM, Stringer SP, Cassisi NJ. T4 laryngeal carcinoma: Radiotherapy alone with surgery reserved for salvage. *International Journal of Radiation Oncology Biology Physics*, 1998; **40**: 549–52.

35. Mendenhall WM, Parsons JT, Stringer SP, Cassisi NJ, Million RR. Radiotherapy alone or combined with neck dissection for T1-T2 carcinoma of the pyriform sinus: An alternative to conservation surgery. *International Journal of Radiation Oncology Biology Physics*, 1993; **27**: 1017–27.

36. Fein DA, Mendenhall WM, Parsons JT, Million RR. T1-T2 squamous cell carcinoma of the glottic larynx treated with radiotherapy: A multivariate analysis of variables potentially influencing local control. *International Journal of Radiation Oncology Biology Physics*, 1993; **25**: 605–11.

37. Parsons JT, Kimsey FC, Mendenhall WM, Million RR, Cassisi NJ, Stringer SP. Radiation therapy for sinus malignancies. *Otolaryngologic Clinics of North America*, 1995; **28**: 1259–68.

38. Million RR, Cassisi NJ, eds. *Management of head and neck cancer: a multidisciplinary approach.* Philadelphia: J.B. Lippincott, 1994.

39. Mendenhall WM, Million RR, Cassisi NJ. Squamous cell carcinoma of the head and neck treated with radiation therapy: The role of neck dissection for clinically positive neck nodes. *International Journal of Radiation Oncology Biology Physics*, 1986; **12**: 733–40.

40. Taylor JMG, Mendenhall WM, Parsons JT, Lavey RS. The influence of dose and time on wound complications following post-radiation neck dissection. *International Journal of Radiation Oncology Biology Physics*, 1992; **23**: 41–6.

41. Mendenhall WM, Parsons JT, Million RR, Fletcher GH. T1-T2 squamous cell carcinoma of the glottic larynx treated with radiation therapy: Relationship of dose-fractionation factors to local control and complications. *International Journal of Radiation Oncology Biology Physics*, 1988; **15**: 1267–73.

42. Mendenhall WM, Parsons JT, Million RR. Unnecessary irradiation of the normal larynx [Editorial]. *International Journal of Radiation Oncology Biology Physics*, 1990; **18**: 1531–3.

43. Mendenhall WM, Parsons JT. Squamous cell carcinoma of the head and neck: Management of the neck and the unknown primary site. In: Gunderson LL, Tepper JE, eds. *Clinical radiation oncology.* New York: Churchill Livingstone, 2000; 549–63.

44. Peters LJ, Weber RS, Morrison WH, Byers RM, Garden AS, Goepfert H. Neck surgery in patients with primary oropharyngeal cancer treated by radiotherapy. *Head and Neck*, 1996; **18**: 552–9.

45. Johnson CR, Silverman LN, Clay LB, Schmidt-Ullrich R. Radiotherapeutic management of bulky cervical lymphadenopathy in

squamous cell carcinoma of the head and neck: Is postradiotherapy neck dissection necessary? *Radiation Oncology Investigations*, 1998; **6**: 52–7.

46. Armstrong J, Pfister D, Strong E, *et al.* The management of the clinically positive neck as part of a larynx preservation approach. *International Journal of Radiation Oncology Biology Physics*, 1993; **26**: 759–65.

47. Wolf GT, Fisher SG. Effectiveness of salvage neck dissection for advanced regional metastases when induction chemotherapy and radiation are used for organ preservation. *Laryngoscope*, 1992; **102**: 934–9.

48. Mendenhall WM, Million RR, Cassisi NJ. Squamous cell carcinoma of the supraglottic larynx treated with radical irradiation: Analysis of treatment parameters and results. *International Journal of Radiation Oncology Biology Physics*, 1984; **10**: 2223–30.

49. McGuirt WF, McCabe BF. Significance of node biopsy before definitive treatment of cervical metastatic carcinoma. *Laryngoscope*, 1978; **88**: 594–7.

50. Parsons JT, Million RR, Cassisi NJ. The influence of excisional or incisional biopsy of metastatic neck nodes on the management of head and neck cancer. *International Journal of Radiation Oncology Biology Physics*, 1985; **11**: 1447–54.

51. Mack Y, Parsons JT, Mendenhall WM, Stringer SP, Cassisi NJ, Million RR. Squamous cell carcinoma of the head and neck: Management after excisional biopsy of a solitary metastatic neck node. *International Journal of Radiation Oncology Biology Physics*, 1993; **25**: 619–22.

52. Mendenhall WM, Parsons JT, Million RR. Elective lower neck irradiation: 5000 cGy/25 fractions versus 4050 cGy/15 fractions. *International Journal of Radiation Oncology Biology Physics*, 1988; **15**: 439–40.

53. Mendenhall WM, Million RR, Cassisi NJ. Elective neck irradiation in squamous-cell carcinoma of the head and neck. *Head and Neck Surgery*, 1980; **3**: 15–20.

54. Vandenbrouck C, Sancho-Garnier H, Chassagne D, Saravane D, Cachin Y, Micheau C. Elective versus therapeutic radical neck dissection in epidermoid carcinoma of the oral cavity. Results of a randomized clinical trial. *Cancer*, 1980; **46**: 386–90.

55. Fakih AR, Rao RS, Borges AM, Patel AR. Elective versus therapeutic neck dissection in early carcinoma of the oral tongue. *American Journal of Surgery*, 1989; **158**: 309–13.

56. Dearnaley DP, Dardoufas C, A'Hearn RP, Henk JM. Interstitial irradiation for carcinoma of the tongue and floor of mouth: Royal Marsden Hospital experience 1970–1986. *Radiotherapy and Oncology*, 1991; **21**: 183–92.

57. Piedbois P, Mazeron JJ, Haddad E, *et al.* Stage I-II squamous cell carcinoma of the oral cavity treated by iridium-192: Is elective neck dissection indicated? *Radiotherapy and Oncology*, 1991; **21**: 100–6.

58. Barkley HT, Jr, Fletcher GH, Jesse RH, Lindberg RD. Management of cervical lymph node metastases in squamous cell carcinoma of the tonsillar fossa, base of tongue, supraglottic larynx, and hypopharynx. *American Journal of Surgery*, 1972; **124**: 462–7.

59. Mendenhall WM, Parsons JT, Mancuso AA, Stringer SP, Cassisi NJ, Million RR. Head and neck: Management of the neck. In: Perez CA, Brady LW, eds. *Principles and practice of radiation oncology.* Philadelphia: J.B. Lippincott, 1992: 790–805.

60. Parsons JT, Mendenhall WM, Cassisi NJ, Stringer SP, Million RR. Neck dissection after twice-a-day radiotherapy: Morbidity and recurrence rates. *Head and Neck*, 1989; **11**: 400–4.

61. Wall TJ, Peters LJ, Brown BW, Oswald MJ, Milas L. Relationship between lymph nodal status and primary tumor control probability in tumors of the supraglottic larynx. *International Journal of Radiation Oncology Biology Physics*, 1985; **11**: 1895–902.

62. Withers HR, Peters LJ, Taylor JM, *et al.* Local control of carcinoma of the tonsil by radiation therapy: An analysis of patterns of fractionation

in nine institutions. *International Journal of Radiation Oncology Biology Physics*, 1995; **33**: 549–62.

63. Freeman DE, Mendenhall WM, Parsons JT, Million RR. Does neck stage influence local control in squamous cell carcinomas of the head and neck? *International Journal of Radiation Oncology Biology Physics*, 1992; **23**: 733–6.

64. Mendenhall WM, Parsons JT, Siemann DW. Does neck stage predict local control after irradiation for head and neck cancer? *Oncology (Huntington)*, 1996; **10**: 381–4.

65. Macdonald MR, Freeman JL, Hui MF, *et al.* Role of Epstein-Barr virus in fine-needle aspirates of metastatic neck nodes in the diagnosis of nasopharyngeal carcinoma. *Head and Neck*, 1995; **17**: 487–93.

66. Coster JR, Foote RL, Olsen KD, Jack SM, Schaid DJ, DeSanto LW. Cervical nodal metastasis of squamous cell carcinoma of unknown origin: Indications for withholding radiation therapy. *International Journal of Radiation Oncology Biology Physics*, 1992; **23**: 743–9.

67. Weir L, Keane T, Cummings B, *et al.* Radiation treatment of cervical lymph node metastases from an unknown primary: An analysis of outcome by treatment volume and other prognostic factors. *Radiotherapy and Oncology*, 1995; **35**: 206–11.

68. Jesse RH, Perez CA, Fletcher GH. Cervical lymph node metastasis: Unknown primary cancer. *Cancer*, 1973; **31**: 854–9.

69. Harper CS, Mendenhall WM, Parsons JT, Stringer SP, Cassisi NJ, Million RR. Cancer in neck nodes with unknown primary site: Role of mucosal radiotherapy. *Head and Neck*, 1990; **12**: 463–9.

70. Reddy SP, Marks JE. Metastatic carcinoma in the cervical lymph nodes from an unknown primary site: Results of bilateral neck plus mucosal irradiation vs. ipsilateral neck irradiation. *International Journal of Radiation Oncology Biology Physics*, 1997; **37**: 797–802.

71. Fletcher GH, Jesse RH, Healey JE Jr, Thoma GW Jr. Oropharynx. In: MacComb WS, Fletcher GH, eds. *Cancer of the head and neck.* Baltimore: Williams and Wilkins, 1967: 179–212.

72. Fletcher GH, Jesse RH, Lindberg RD, Koons CR. The place of radiotherapy in the management of the squamous cell carcinoma of the supraglottic larynx. *American Journal of Roentgenology, Radium Therapy, and Nuclear Medicine*, 1970; **108**: 19–26.

73. MacComb WS, Healey JE, Jr, McGraw JP, Fletcher GH, Gallager HS, Paulus DD. Hypopharynx and cervical esophagus. In: MacComb WS, Fletcher GH, eds. *Cancer of the head and neck.* Baltimore: Williams and Wilkins, 1967: 213–40.

74. Chen KY, Fletcher GH. Malignant tumors of the nasopharynx. *Radiology*, 1971; **99**: 165–71.

75. American Joint Committee on Cancer. *Manual for staging of cancer.* Philadelphia: J.B. Lippincott, 1983: 37–42.

9.2 Chemotherapy for head and neck cancer

Alastair J. Munro

Introduction

It is a fact, as remarkable as it is melancholy, that cancers of the head and neck respond dramatically to chemotherapy and yet chemotherapy contributes but little to the cure of these tumours. Chemotherapy can, even for advanced tumours, produce dramatic regressions—even within a week or so of treatment. This is no mean feat. A $3 \times 2 \times 3$ cm tumour contains approximately 20 billion cells, a tumour that is barely detectable contains about 0.1 billion cells. This means, that to produce a dramatic clinical response 19.9 billion cells have to disappear fairly rapidly. The intriguing biological question is: if cell killing is this impressive, why does it not translate into improved cure? The answer may lie in the biology of cancers of the head and neck.

These tumours arise from squamous epithelium. Cell loss is a feature of epithelial surfaces: the majority of skin cells produced by the basal cell layer being lost by desquamation. The London Underground employs people to clear skin squames shed by customers and electrostatically attracted to the live rails. If they did not, the live rails would attract their own insulating layer of shed squames and the trains wouldn't run. Tumours of squamous surfaces are no different. Cell loss is part of their repertoire. When the potential doubling time of a squamous carcinoma, estimated from the cell-cycle time and proliferative fraction, is compared with the observed doubling time then the proportion of cells lost can be calculated. Between 95 per cent and 99 per cent of the cells produced by a squamous carcinoma may be lost. This means that even small carcinomas of the head and neck may be, comparatively speaking, genetically ancient. In the absence of cell loss it would take only about 35 generations to progress from a single cell to a palpable tumour. If cell loss is incorporated into the calculations, then it could take 1500 generations. With each successive generation there is an exponential increase in the number of cell divisions and each cell division provides an opportunity for mutation to take place. Thus, even by the time they are diagnosed, and before any treatment has been given, head and neck cancers may contain clones of cells that have spontaneously acquired resistance to treatment. These resistant clones might, ultimately, limit cure of the tumour.

There is another implication of high cell loss: rapid regression following treatment. If the majority of the cells that are produced are lost, then any temporary disruption of production will cause rapid shrinkage of the tumour. The dramatic loss of cells is a function of the biological behaviour of the tumour rather than a reflection of the effectiveness of the treatment at killing cells.

The basic biology of head and neck cancer, particularly cell loss, might explain both the rapid initial response to chemotherapy and the ultimate failure of such treatment to eradicate the disease. Mainly because of this tantalizing, but undelivered, promise, the role of chemotherapy in the management of head and neck cancer is controversial (Box 1).

A recent survey of practice amongst non-academic (community-based) cancer specialists in the United States shows a wide variation in the use of chemotherapy for head and neck cancer. The reasons for choosing to give treatment are intriguing: over 30 per cent of specialists use chemotherapy simply to 'maintain spirit of multidisciplinary care' (Box 2).[3]

When a subject is dominated by dogma the only sane approach is to go back to the data and attempt to draw conclusions based on evidence and facts rather than received wisdom or unsubstantiated opinion. A structured, systematic approach is essential. However, there are major problems in adopting an evidence-based approach for the use of chemotherapy in head and neck cancer. Only a small proportion of patients with head and neck cancer are entered into clinical trials. These patients tend to be fitter, younger, and less socially disadvantaged than the majority of patients with head and neck cancer. The evidence we have available, which we would like to apply to the formulation of policies for treating all patients, has been obtained from an untypical minority. A treatment which is effective for a fit patient with excellent social support may be ineffective or even dangerous for an unfit, socially isolated, patient. In a current study in the United Kingdom of head and neck cancer there have been several unexpected toxic deaths in patients treated with synchronous methotrexate and radiotherapy. Alcoholics seem to be particularly

Box 1

- '... phase III studies have established a role for induction chemotherapy and chemo-radiotherapy in the multidisciplinary treatment of patients with locally advanced but potentially curable (M0) squamous cell carcinoma of the head and neck region.'[1]
- 'Why has so much chemotherapy done so little in head and neck cancer?'[2]

Box 2 Use of chemotherapy[3]

- 4 per cent used synchronous radiotherapy and chemotherapy
- 61 per cent used neoadjuvant chemotherapy then radiotherapy
- 36 per cent used surgery then radiotherapy

Reasons for the use of chemotherapy[3]
- 67 per cent—to improve locoregional control
- 56 per cent—to improve survival
- 34 per cent—to be co-operative
- 29 per cent—to improve quality of life
- 26 per cent—to decrease distant metastases

Box 3

- '… the total number of newly diagnosed SCCHN patients during the study period was 1,215. However, due to religious barriers, low education level, and poor socio-economic status less that half of the patients accepted treatment … only 54 patients remained for inclusion in this study.'[4]
- '… 58 black patients suffering from advanced head and neck cancer … mostly middle-aged males who were heavy smokers and drinkers. Positive Wasserman reactions were common.'[5]

Box 4 Problems specific to the chemotherapy of head and neck cancer

Patients are often in poor general condition:
- heavy smokers
- alcohol abuse
- poor nutrition

Patients may not comply with complex treatment programmes:
- may have poor social support (indigent, living rough, socially isolated, alcohol abuse)
- may have concurrent medical problems (heart disease, chronic obstructive airways disease, alcoholic liver disease)

Treatment-related toxicity may go undetected and unreported

susceptible—the supposition being that there is an interaction between alcoholic liver disease and methotrexate, probably affecting drug metabolism, that potentiates the toxicity of the drug and produces excessive myelosuppression.

There are major problems with simply translating the evidence-base into clinical practice. The management of head and neck cancer is no different from any other branch of oncology: decision-making should involve a consideration of the patient as an individual, clinical judgement and respect for the autonomy of the individual are every bit as important as any 'scientific' application of the available evidence. It is worth reminding ourselves of the problems with 'evidence', namely: the evidence we have is not what we need; the evidence we need we are unable to obtain; and the evidence we want is not always the evidence we need.

The main reason for using chemotherapy to treat patients with head and neck cancer is to improve survival. A further potential benefit is that, by improving local control and without compromising survival, chemotherapy may permit surgery to be less radical or to be avoided altogether—the so-called organ-conservation approach. There is nothing novel in this concept. Radiotherapy has, for many years, and for precisely this reason, been used in the primary management of selected patients with head and neck cancer. Chemotherapy, in this context, is not necessarily a replacement for radiotherapy but it might be a useful adjunct.

The social milieu within which treatment for head and neck cancer is given is very different from that for other cancers such as breast cancer or ovarian cancer. Patients with head and neck cancer are typically heavy smokers and heavy drinkers and may have poor social support. The very factors which contributed to the cause of their cancer in the first place may compromise their ability to withstand aggressive treatment. This has obvious consequences for individual patients, but it also calls into question the general applicability of results obtained from clinical trials in this type of cancer. Patients entered into studies may be highly selected or untypical (Box 3).

There is no reason to suppose, for example, that treatment effects demonstrated in relatively fit patients with excellent social support will be achievable in socially isolated patients in poor physical condition.

There are also important international differences in the causes of head and neck cancer which may have implications for treatment response. Oral cancers in India are largely due to the habit of chewing betel nut, and the biology of nasopharyngeal cancer is very different in patients from North Africa when compared with patients from the Far East. It is against this complex background that the evidence-base for the utility of chemotherapy of head and neck cancer must be interpreted (Box 4).

Chemotherapy for head and neck cancer can be classified according to a simple system which takes account of both the timing of the drug treatment, in relation to any definitive treatment, and its purpose (Box 5).

The definition of the potential advantages and disadvantages of chemotherapy for head and neck cancer provides a framework which can be used systematically to assess the evidence concerning the role of chemotherapy in this cancer (Boxes 6 and 7).

Specific questions arise from the issues so far raised:

Box 5 Classification of chemotherapy for head and neck cancer

Palliative:
- given with the prime intention of relieving symptoms, any improvement in survival is a secondary benefit

Curative:
- given with the intention of improving the rate of cure and/or survival, may permit less aggressive locoregional treatment to be used without compromising cure

Neoadjuvant:
- chemotherapy given before definitive locoregional therapy (surgery and/or radiotherapy)

Synchronous:
- chemotherapy given at the same time as definitive locoregional treatment with radiotherapy

Adjuvant:
- chemotherapy given after definitive locoregional therapy (surgery and/or radiotherapy)

Box 6 Summary of the potential advantages of chemotherapy in head and neck cancer

Improved survival:
- improving local control
- decreasing the incidence of distant metastases

Decreased need for radical surgery:
- improving local control

Relieving symptoms:
- decreasing tumour size

- Does chemotherapy improve survival for patients with head and neck cancer?
- Is there an optimal sequence for timing chemotherapy in relation to other interventions (surgery, radiotherapy)?
- Does chemotherapy given before radiotherapy or surgery have any adverse effect on local control and/or survival?
- Does chemotherapy given before surgery decrease the number of radical resections required (without jeopardizing survival)?
- Does chemotherapy improve local control?

Box 7 Potential disadvantages of chemotherapy for head and neck cancer

- may increase the rate of treatment-related deaths
- may increase toxicity and the overall burden of treatment
- may, falsely, convince clinicians that appropriate surgery can safely be omitted
- may, through clonal selection of resistant cells, impair the effectiveness of subsequent treatment

- Does chemotherapy increase the rate of treatment-related deaths?
- Does chemotherapy decrease the rate of distant metastases?
- Does chemotherapy increase treatment-related toxicity?
- What are the response rates to chemotherapy, and is any one chemotherapy regimen clearly superior when assessed in terms of tumour response?
- Is nasopharyngeal carcinoma a special case?
- Does palliative chemotherapy significantly relieve symptoms and improve overall quality of life in patients with advanced disease?

In an attempt to find evidence to answer at least some of these questions, a previous overview[6] of randomized controlled trials of adjuvant chemotherapy in head and neck cancer has been revised and updated—the results of which are summarized in Tables 1, 2, 3, and 4. This is a literature-based analysis and, as such, will tend to overestimate the benefits of chemotherapy. The advantages of meta-analyses based on individual patient data over those based on published data have been well described.[7] One important, but often neglected, advantage of the literature-based approach is that results can be obtained earlier than with the more painstaking approach—this has advantages when it comes to planning further randomized trials. A meta-analysis of the effect of chemotherapy in head and neck cancer has been performed by the MACH-NC investigators and some of the results have recently been published[8] (Table 1(b)). The results of the two meta-analyses are in broad agreement: there is a significant improvement in survival when chemotherapy is added to standard locoregional treatment. The improvement is related to the timing of the chemotherapy, being greater for synchronous treatment and less for neoadjuvant treatment. Adjuvant chemotherapy, given after primary treatment with surgery and/or radiotherapy has been little used in the management of head and neck cancer. Only three randomized trials have followed this approach: the results show no improvement in survival compared to locoregional therapy alone.

The individual patient meta-analysis[8] also suggests that the benefit from chemotherapy is relatively less in older patients. Presumably the balance of competing risks, improved tumour control versus treatment-related mortality, shifts with increasing age.

Table 1(a) Survival data from a literature-based overview of randomized trials of adjuvant chemotherapy in head and neck cancer

Survival	No. of trials	No. of patients	Rate difference (%)	Low (%)	High (%)	Control (%)	Chemotherapy (%)
All trials	73	11 355	8	5	11	39	46
Neoadjuvant	43	6205	4	2	6	37	41
Synchronous	28	3910	16	11	21	31	47
Postadjuvant	3	326	−9	−22	4	65	56

Survival is defined at a minimum of 2 years. The rate difference is calculated according to the method of DerSimonian and Laird[9] and full details of the methodology can be found in the paper by Munro.[6] The rates for control and chemotherapy are crude calculations and, because of the weighting used, the subtraction of the one from the other will not always agree with the DerSimonian and Laird calculation of the rate difference.

Table 1(b) Survival data from the individual patient meta-analysis performed by the MACH-NC group[8]

Survival	No. of trials	No. of patients	Relative risk of death	95% CI low	95% CI high
All trials	65	10 850	0.90	0.85	0.94
Neoadjuvant	31	5269	0.95	0.88	1.01
Synchronous	26	3727	0.81	0.76	0.88
'Adjuvant'	8	1854	0.98	0.85	1.19

CI, confidence interval.

Table 2 Data on locoregional control from a literature-based overview of randomized trials of adjuvant chemotherapy in head and neck cancer

	No. of trials	No. of patients	Rate difference (%)	Low (%)	High (%)	Control (%)	Chemotherapy (%)
Locoregional control (synchronous)	14	2484	19	9	29	49	62
Locoregional control (neoadjuvant)	26	4726	−2	−7	2	61	60
Radical surgery required (neoadjuvant)	19	2652	−15	−27	−3	65	45

[a] Locoregional control is defined as the long-term control of both primary tumour and regional nodes according to clinical assessment.

Table 3 Data on treatment-related toxicity and mortality from a literature-based overview of randomized trials of adjuvant chemotherapy in head and neck cancer[a]

	No. of trials	No. of patients	Rate difference (%)	Low (%)	High (%)	Control (%)	Chemotherapy (%)
Mucositis (synchronous)	24	3453	16	10	21	15	28
Treatment-related death (synchronous chemoradiotherapy)	22	2966	0.6	−4	+5	0.1	0.7
Treatment-related death (neoadjuvant)	27	4709	2.0	1.0	3.0	2.0	4.0

[a] Mucositis is defined as a mucosal reaction ≥3 by WHO criteria. Treatment-related deaths includes deaths related to chemotherapy (sepsis, etc.) as well as deaths occurring in the perioperative period in those patients undergoing surgery.

Table 4 Data on metastases from a literature-based overview of randomized trials of adjuvant chemotherapy in head and neck cancer[a]

Distant metastases	No. of trials	No. of patients	Rate difference (%)	Low (%)	High (%)	Control (%)	Chemotherapy (%)
All trials	35	6153	−6	−8	−3	19	13
Neoadjuvant trials	25	4420	−7	−11	−4	22	14
Synchronous chemoradiotherapy	13	1890	1	−4	+7	20	21

[a] The rate of metastasis is calculated as an absolute rate and includes all patients with metastases, whether or not locoregional failure was also present.

Does chemotherapy improve survival for patients with head and neck cancer?

Adjuvant chemotherapy

A systematic review of randomized trials involving the use of adjuvant chemotherapy for the treatment of patients with head and neck cancer suggest that there may be a modest survival benefit from adding adjuvant chemotherapy to definitive treatment for such patients. The improvement is about 8 per cent (95 per cent CI, 5 to 11 per cent). The baseline survival is around 39 per cent, adding chemotherapy improves this to 47 per cent. The implication being that, in order to prevent one death, it is necessary to treat 13 patients with chemotherapy. The confidence interval on this figure, the number needed to treat (NNT) is from 9 to 20 patients. These figures are based on data from 73 randomized comparisons involving a total of 11 355 patients.

Chemotherapy alone

Very few patients have been treated with chemotherapy as the sole treatment for localized, operable disease. In one series from Paris, 121 patients were treated with chemotherapy alone (cis-platinum and 5-fluorouracil) for localized squamous-cell carcinoma (SCC) of the head and neck.[10],[11] Although 20 patients eventually required surgery, 101 patients did not. The overall survival for the whole group was 71 per cent, disease-free survival 60 per cent, at 5 years. The results of such a limited study must be interpreted with caution, and certainly cannot be used as the basis for changing the current emphasis on surgery and/or radiotherapy for the primary treatment of localized cancers of the head and neck.

Although many thousands of patients with metastatic cancer of the head and neck have been treated with chemotherapy, there are no long-term, disease-free survivors. Any improvements in survival have been relatively modest, typically an increase of 12 weeks or so. There are very few randomized trials comparing chemotherapy with no active treatment in patients with far advanced (inoperable or metastatic) disease. Survival in such patients is poor: 90 per cent of patients are dead within 2 years. Early randomized studies by Morton and Stell[12] suggested that chemotherapy did little to improve survival. Patients randomized to chemotherapy did, however, spend more time at home than patients randomized to supportive care (RP Morton, personal communication). Survival is, in any event, an inappropriate endpoint for this group of patients. With currently available therapies there is no prospect of cure. Treatment is therefore, by definition, palliative and the quality of survival will be more important than its duration. The intriguing biological question remains: if these tumours can show response rates to chemotherapy similar to those observed in lymphomas, why are they not, like lymphomas, curable by chemotherapy?

Using survival as the outcome measure, is there an optimal sequence for timing chemotherapy in relation to other treatments (surgery, radiotherapy)?

The majority of randomized studies have assessed the contribution of neoadjuvant chemotherapy: 43 studies, 6205 patients. The survival benefit is 4 per cent (CI, 2 to 6 per cent) in favour of chemotherapy. The control-arm survival rate is 37 per cent, rising to 41 per cent with neoadjuvant chemotherapy. The NNT is 25 (95 per cent CI, 16 to 50). Studies on synchronous chemotherapy have, until recently, been less popular: 28 studies involving 3910 patients. This is surprising since the results are very much more impressive. The absolute difference in survival rate is 16 per cent in favour of chemotherapy; the survival rate with radiotherapy alone is 31 per cent compared to 47 per cent for radiotherapy and synchronous chemotherapy. The confidence interval on the rate difference is from 11 per cent to 21 per cent. The NNT is 6 (95 per cent CI, 5 to 10). Chemotherapy given after initial definitive treatment has not been extensively studied, with data only being available from three studies. The results suggest that, if anything, survival is worse with chemotherapy given after initial therapy: the survival rate is 9 per cent lower, but the confidence interval is wide, from −22 per cent to +4 per cent.

A wide variety of regimens have been used in phase III trials of synchronous chemotherapy versus radiotherapy alone. Although no clearly superior regimen emerges, 5-fluorouracil (5-FU) as a single agent appears to be surprisingly effective (Table 5). However, this conclusion is influenced by one trial,[13] and when this trial is excluded the rate difference falls to 18.5 per cent (95 per cent CI, 7 to 30 per cent).

The results of randomized trials of chemotherapy for the treatment of head and neck cancer suggest that, in terms of survival, the following conclusions can be drawn:

Table 5 Survival according to chemotherapy regimen in trials comparing synchronous chemotherapy and radiotherapy with radiotherapy alone

Regimen	Rate difference (%)	95% CI	Studies	No. of patients
Bleo alone	17	2 to 32	5	670
Plat + 5FU	19	11 to 27	5	983
5FU alone	24	17 to 32	4	846

Bleo, bleomycin; Plat, cisplatinum; 5Fu, 5-fluorouracil; CI, confidence interval.

1. Adjuvant chemotherapy can improve survival.
2. Chemotherapy is more effective when given synchronously with radiotherapy than when given as neoadjuvant therapy.
3. Chemotherapy has a limited effect on the survival of patients with advanced disease.

Does chemotherapy given before radiotherapy or surgery have any effect on locoregional control and/or survival?

Locoregional control, in this context, can be defined as the long-term control, when assessed clinically, of the primary tumour and regional nodes. Of the 43 studies of neoadjuvant treatment, only 27 report data relevant to this question (see Table 2). The difference in locoregional control is 1 per cent in favour of the control group: crude rates are 60 per cent with neoadjuvant chemotherapy versus 61 per cent with locoregional treatment alone. This difference is neither statistically nor clinically significant: the confidence limits on the rate difference are from −7 per cent to +2 per cent.

The fact that a treatment which can produce dramatic tumour shrinkage fails to improve local control is intriguing. Are surgeons so impressed by tumour regression that they perform a less radical procedure and thereby compromise locoregional control? They should not be fooled into altering their surgical approach: the operation and its margins should be dictated by the size of the tumour before, rather than after, any chemotherapy. If regression is anticipated, then the tumour margins should be tattooed before chemotherapy to ensure that the scope and extent of the subsequent operation is appropriate. Indirect evidence, used to answer the next question, suggests that surgeons may be inappropriately limiting the extent of surgical resection in patients treated initially with chemotherapy.

Another possible explanation for the failure of neoadjuvant chemotherapy to improve local control is that, through mutation and clonal selection, the tumour cells left after chemotherapy are biologically more aggressive than the cells initially present. This is the 'leaner and meaner' argument of Rosenthal et al.[14] These two explanations are not, of course, mutually exclusive. A partially resected, biologically aggressive tumour is more likely to recur than a similarly resected, less aggressive tumour. Hence, it is likely that surgical margins will

be more secure for less aggressive tumours than they will be for more aggressive tumours.

Does chemotherapy given before surgery decrease the number of radical resections required (without jeopardizing survival)?

A radical resection can be defined as an operation performed with the intention of removing all viable tumour. The data from randomized comparisons suggests that the need for radical surgical procedures is significantly reduced by neoadjuvant chemotherapy. Table 2 shows the relevant data obtained from 15 trials (2652 patients). The rate of radical surgery was 65 per cent in the control patients but only 45 per cent in the patients given neoadjuvant chemotherapy. The absolute rate difference was 15 per cent, with confidence limits from 3 per cent to 27 per cent. As many of these studies did not formally require that radical resection be avoided in patients with an excellent response to chemotherapy, these figures will therefore underestimate the effectiveness of chemotherapy in preventing the need for potentially mutilating surgery. The survival data show a minor benefit, as opposed to detriment, from the use of neoadjuvant chemotherapy. The suggestion from these data is that aggressive surgery may be avoided if chemotherapy is used and that, overall, there is no survival disadvantage to this approach.

A contradictory picture emerges when only those trials directly comparing radical surgery with an 'organ conserving' approach are considered. The meta-analysis of chemotherapy in head and neck cancer (**MACH-NC**),[15] on pooled data from individual patients, shows an inferior 5-year survival for the conservatively treated patients: 39 per cent versus 45 per cent in the patients randomized to radical surgery. This difference is not statistically significant ($p = 0.1$), and therefore the 'difference' in survival may be spurious. However, even with pooling, the sample size is small—only a total of 602 patients randomized in three separate studies—so that this may simply be an example of a type II statistical error. If there is a genuine difference in survival then this needs to be reconciled with the conclusion from the literature-based analysis suggesting that chemotherapy can reduce the requirement for radical surgery and can do so without compromising survival. One explanation could simply be that, in patients with advanced disease, chemotherapy produces sufficient tumour regression to provide adequate palliation without the need to resort to surgery. Radical surgery is avoided, most of these patients die, regardless of the treatment given, and there is therefore no demonstrable survival disadvantage from chemotherapy. The organ-conserving studies deal with less advanced tumours and so a detectable survival disadvantage might occur, perhaps based on the 'leaner and meaner' argument mentioned previously.[14]

Does chemotherapy given synchronously with radiotherapy improve local control?

The addition of chemotherapy to radical radiotherapy produces a significant improvement in local control. There are 14 studies, involving 2484 patients, which report relevant data (Table 2). The locoregional control rate with radiotherapy alone is 49 per cent, but this rises to 62 per cent with synchronous chemotherapy and radiotherapy. The rate difference is 19 per cent, 95 per cent CI from 9 per cent to 29 per cent, in favour of combined treatment.

Does chemotherapy increase the rate of treatment-related deaths?

There is some evidence that neoadjuvant chemotherapy increases the risks of treatment-related death (Table 3). When deaths in the perioperative period, as well as deaths directly attributable to chemotherapy, are included then the treatment-related mortality increases from 1.2 per cent to 4 per cent. This corresponds to an absolute difference of 2 per cent (95 per cent CI, 1 per cent to 3 per cent), a difference that is significant both clinically and statistically. Thus some of the improvement in survival that might be expected to be achieved from the use of neoadjuvant chemotherapy may be offset by the increased mortality associated with treatment. This problem may be avoided, in part at least, by the careful selection of patients for treatment and more vigorous supportive care at and around the time of chemotherapy and surgery.

Based on an analysis of 2966 patients in 22 trials, there is no evidence that chemotherapy when given synchronously with radiotherapy increases the treatment-related mortality. The absolute rate difference is 0.6 per cent (CI, from −4 per cent to +5 per cent).

Does chemotherapy decrease the rate of distant metastases?

There is no evidence that adding synchronous chemotherapy to radiotherapy decreases the rate of distant metastasis. Regardless of treatment, the rate is around 20 per cent when the results of 13 randomized studies (1890 patients) are pooled (see Table 4). An estimate based on data from 25 studies involving 4420 patients (see Table 4) indicates that neoadjuvant chemotherapy does, however, appear to have a significant effect in lowering the rate of distant metastases—14 per cent when neoadjuvant chemotherapy is used, compared with 22 per cent when locoregional treatment alone is used. This absolute rate difference of around 7 per cent has a confidence interval from 4 per cent to 11 per cent. Distant metastases, as the sole cause of failure, are a relatively unimportant cause of treatment failure in the management of head and neck cancer. Synchronous chemoradiotherapy produces a greater survival advantage than neoadjuvant chemotherapy, even though the latter decreases the rate of distant metastases. The main mechanism whereby synchronous chemotherapy and radiotherapy improves survival appears to be through its ability to improve locoregional control.

Does chemotherapy increase treatment-related toxicity?

This question is really only relevant when the potential benefits of synchronous chemotherapy and radiotherapy are being considered.

The main acute toxicity from radiotherapy to the head and neck is mucositis. If the radiation dose is increased then, given the steep relationship between dose and response, we can expect an increase in both tumour response and mucositis. If the addition of chemotherapy increases both local control and mucositis then it is entirely possible that a similar effect could have been achieved simply by increasing the dose of radiation.

Data on severe (grade 3 or 4) mucositis is available for 24 of the randomized studies comparing radiotherapy alone with radiotherapy plus synchronous chemotherapy. The rate of severe mucositis is almost doubled, from 15 per cent to 28 per cent, when combined treatment is given. The absolute rate difference is 16 per cent, confidence interval 10 per cent to 21 per cent (see Table 3). This magnitude of difference is almost exactly the same as the survival benefit. This suggests that, when the therapeutic ratio is assessed using survival and mucositis as the two endpoints, there is little to be gained from adding synchronous chemotherapy to radiotherapy.

Data on quality-of-life (**QoL**) measurements obtained from a randomized comparison of radiotherapy alone versus radiotherapy plus synchronous chemotherapy, suggests that overall quality of life may be better with chemoradiotherapy.[16] However there are problems with the interpretation of these data—mainly because of a higher laryngectomy rate, with its consequent effects on QoL, in the group treated with radiation alone.

What are the response rates to chemotherapy, and is any one chemotherapy regimen clearly superior when assessed in terms of tumour response?

There are insufficient data available from randomized studies to address questions concerning the nuances of chemotherapeutic response. In order to improve the sample size, and hence the precision of any estimates, a systematic review of published phase II studies of chemotherapy in head and neck cancer has been performed. Trials have been reviewed applying the Cochrane principle: that in order to avoid bias, even the most obscure publications should be included and that particular attention should be given to obtaining data previously only published in meeting abstracts. Data are available from 616 trials published between 1966 and 1998. Since there is a widespread belief that nasopharyngeal cancer responds differently to chemotherapy, it has been considered separately.

Complete response has been defined clinically as all demonstrable disease disappearing completely for at least 8 weeks. The complete response rates are summarized in Table 6. It is impossible to extract useful data on the response of metastatic disease, since many trials define as 'advanced disease' tumours that are either locally advanced or metastatic. Trials that include patients with metastatic disease usually also include a proportion of patients who have advanced, but non-metastatic, disease. Nevertheless, the complete response rate is much lower (9 per cent) in trials that include patients with metastatic disease than in trials where only those patients with localized disease are included: complete response rate 29 per cent. Many studies have combined chemotherapy and radiation, either sequentially or

Table 6 Pooled response data from phase 2 and phase 3 trials of chemotherapy for squamous carcinoma of the head and neck (excluding nasopharyngeal carcinoma)

Group	Rate (%)	95% CI	No. of patients
CR chemotherapy alone	29	28–30	9482
CR chemotherapy + radiotherapy	61	60–62	5330
CR any chemotherapy	40	39–40	15 353
CR chemotherapy only, no platinum	17	15–19	1961
CR chemotherapy only, with platinum	32	31–33	7461
CR chemotherapy, 5-FU-based	34	33–35	5302
CR chemotherapy, platinum and 5-FU	37	35–38	4439
CR chemotherapy, 5-FU no platinum	21	18–24	863
CR chemotherapy, neither 5-FU nor platinum	22	21–23	4180
CR chemotherapy only, local phase 2	36	34–37	5188
CR chemotherapy only, local phase 3	20	19–22	4294
CR chemotherapy local	29	28–30	9482
CR local to taxanes, naïve	49	45–54	421

CR, complete response; 5-FU, 5-fluorouracil.

Table 7 Pooled data (from both phase 2 and phase 3 studies) on the complete response rates at the primary site and in lymph nodes

Group	CR rate (%)	95% CI	No. of studies	No. of patients
Primary tumour	33	30–36	14	1086
Nodes	28	25–32	8	702

CR, complete response; assessed clinically.

Table 8 Pooled data from phase 2 and 3 trials of chemotherapy for head and neck cancer: squamous-cell carcinomas excluding nasopharyngeal carcinoma

Group	Response rate (%)	95% CI	No. of patients
RR local	63	63–63	12 691
RR local naïve	64	63–65	11 603
RR local non-naïve	51	44–58	204
RR local to taxanes	70	64–74	392
RR metastatic disease	33	32–33	5159

RR, response rate; patients showing complete or partial response to treatment.

synchronously. The addition of radiation to chemotherapy appears to double the response rate from 29 per cent to 61 per cent. The complete response rates defined in phase II studies overestimate the treatment effect demonstrated in phase III studies. For local disease, the pooled complete response rate in phase II studies was 36 per cent (CI, 34 per cent to 37 per cent) compared with 20 per cent (CI, 19 per cent to 22 per cent) for phase III studies.

There appears to be no major difference between the response of the primary tumour and the response of nodal disease to chemotherapy. There are surprisingly few data to address this question as interpretation is complicated by other treatment, such as surgery or radiotherapy. The most useful data come from studies using chemotherapy as the sole treatment and in which the complete response rate is reported (Table 7). There is no major difference in response rate, the trend suggests that the primary responds rather better than the nodes but the difference, perhaps because of small numbers, is not significant.

The evolution of effective chemotherapy can be studied in two ways—by looking at changes over time or by assessing the impact of individual drugs upon results. The clear message that emerges is the importance of *cis*-platinum. Early studies (before 1985) produced a

complete response rate of 16 per cent; subsequently the complete response rate has risen to 36 per cent (CI, 35 per cent to 38 per cent; see Table 6). The CR rate to regimens without platinum is 17 per cent (CI, 15 per cent to 19 per cent) compared to 32 per cent (CI, 31 per cent to 33 per cent) for platinum-based regimens. The taxanes have recently been introduced into the treatment of head and neck cancer and the early results suggest that they may have an important role (Tables 6 and 8). The CR with taxane-based regimens is 49 per cent (CI, 45 per cent to 54 per cent), suggesting an incremental improvement equivalent to that produced by *cis*-platinum. However, these data are based on only 421 patients treated, all in phase II studies, and the longer term results are unlikely to be as impressive as the preliminary data.

There is no evidence that carboplatin is inferior to *cis*-platinum in the treatment of head and neck cancer—the CR rate for carboplatin-based regimens is 28 per cent (26 to 31 per cent), whereas the CR

Table 9 Pooled data on complete response obtained in trials of chemotherapy for head and neck cancer: squamous-cell carcinomas excluding nasopharyngeal carcinoma

Group	Studies	Rate (%)	95% CI	No. of patients
Carboplatin	47	28	26–31	1839
Platinum (all)	334	32	31–33	15 895
Platinum (phase 2)	228	40	39–41	9349
Platinum (phase 3)	106	21	20–22	6545

Carboplatin includes all carboplatin-based regimens, platinum includes all cisplatinum-based regimens. Note that the response rate for platinum-based regimens is twice as high in phase 2 studies as it is in phase 3 studies.

Table 10 Pooled data on complete response rates from phase 2 and phase 3 studies of chemotherapy for carcinoma of the nasopharynx

Group	No. of patients	Rate (%)	95% CI
Chemotherapy alone	2045	27	25–29
Chemotherapy (local)	1354	33	31–36
Radiotherapy + chemotherapy (local)	359	81	77–85
Chemotherapy (metastatic)	664	13	11–16

Complete response assessed clinically.

rate for platinum-based regimens is 32 per cent (31 to 33 per cent) (Table 9).

Overall response rates, complete and partial responses, of head and neck cancer to chemotherapy are high, namely 63 per cent for locoregional disease and 33 per cent for metastatic disease Table 8. The frustration is, as outlined above, that these impressive results have not produced unequivocal clinical benefit.

Is nasopharyngeal carcinoma a special case?

There is a widespread belief that nasopharyngeal carcinoma is more responsive to chemotherapy than squamous cancers of the head and neck arising at other sites. Nasopharyngeal carcinomas are certainly both epidemiologically and histologically distinct from other cancers of the head and neck. Indeed, even within nasopharyngeal cancer, there is a variety of histological patterns and clinical presentations. The disease as it presents in the Far East appears very different from nasopharyngeal carcinoma affecting people of North African origin. This latter group appear to have a form of the disease that is particularly likely to spread systemically, with involvement of bone, bone marrow, liver, and lungs. These important clinical differences have clear implications for the effectiveness of locoregional, as opposed to systemic, therapies.

The results of chemotherapy for carcinoma of the nasopharynx are summarized in Tables 10 and 11. The response data are very similar to those for other head and neck cancers and there is no evidence that nasopharyngeal cancer is particularly susceptible to treatment with cytotoxic drugs.

There are only four published studies on randomized comparisons of radiotherapy alone versus chemotherapy plus radiotherapy for nasopharyngeal carcinoma (Table 12). There are two neoadjuvant studies, one study of synchronous therapy and one early study of chemotherapy given as adjuvant treatment after radiotherapy.

Pooling the results from these studies shows that, overall, there is no evidence of survival benefit from chemotherapy (Table 12). The rate difference is 7 per cent in favour of chemotherapy, but the 95 per cent confidence interval extends from –9 per cent to +23 per cent, indicating no statistically significant difference. The one published synchronous study is, however, strongly positive: there is a 32 per cent improvement in survival with the addition of chemotherapy to radiotherapy (95 per cent CI 17 per cent to 47 per cent).[17] The rate of mucositis was not significantly increased by the combined treatment (rate difference 9 per cent; 95 per cent CI, –6 per cent to +24 per cent). The poor survival in the control arm of this study is noteworthy; however, the survival rate in the chemotherapy arm is similar to that observed in other studies.

A series of publications from the Institute Gustave Roussy report their extensive experience with the investigation and treatment of patients, predominantly of North African origin, with carcinoma of the nasopharynx.[21] These patients have histologically undifferentiated carcinoma of nasopharyngeal type (**UCNT**) and which is almost always associated with evidence of Epstein–Barr virus (**EBV**) infection. The incidence of occult metastatic disease is high: 23 per cent have bone marrow invasion; 30 per cent have liver metastases; 63 per cent have bone metastases; and 20 per cent have lung metastases. Over

Table 11 Pooled data on response rates from phase 2 and phase 3 studies of chemotherapy for carcinoma of the nasopharynx

Group	No. of patients	Rate (%)	95% CI
Chemotherapy alone	2213	72	70–74
Chemotherapy (local)	1414	82	80–84
Radiotherapy + chemotherapy (local)	237	95	91–97
Chemotherapy (metastatic)	799	54	51–58

Table 12 Survival data from randomized trials comparing radiotherapy alone with radiotherapy plus chemotherapy in nasopharyngeal cancer

Trial	No. of patients	Rate difference (%)	95% CI	Radiotherapy alone	Radiotherapy plus chemotherapy
Intergroup synchronous[17]	147	32	17 to 47	46	78
VUMCA neoadjuvant [18]	339	7	−3 to 18	52	59
Chan neoadjuvant[19]	77	−2	−20 to 17	80	78
Rossi postadjuvant [20]	229	−8	−21 to 3	67	58
Pooled[a]	792	7	−9 to 23	58	64

[a] The pooled result shows no statistically significant benefit from chemotherapy.

90 per cent of patients who present with clinical N3 disease die from systemic metastases. Given these findings, it is important to distinguish these patients from patients with the more straightforward squamous carcinomas of the nasopharynx, where systemic spread is unusual and locoregional treatment may be curative.

Patients with UCNT may benefit from aggressive chemotherapy, although the question of scheduling has not been adequately addressed. The available evidence suggests that, for this particular type of nasopharyngeal carcinoma, the most active regimen is a combination of bleomycin, epirubicin and *cis*-platinum. This regimen is prohibitively toxic when combined with synchronous radiotherapy and its use has been mainly confined to neoadjuvant studies.

Does palliative chemotherapy significantly relieve symptoms and improve overall quality of life in patients with advanced disease?

It is a sorry indictment of clinical research that there are virtually no objective data available to address the question of whether palliative chemotherapy is of any benefit in relieving the symptoms of patients with cancer of the head and neck. Over 15 000 patients have been treated in phase II studies of chemotherapy for advanced head and neck cancer, but fewer than 3000 had a complete response to chemotherapy alone. In the remaining 12 000 patients treatment,

when assessed in terms of tumour response, was only of partial benefit or less. In not one of these studies was the issue of benefit, as perceived by the patients, addressed. We simply cannot tell whether or not any of these patients obtained useful relief of symptoms.

Common sense dictates that if a locally advanced head and neck tumour shrinks, even slightly, as a result of treatment then the patient's symptoms should be relieved. However, important questions remain: is any benefit sufficient to justify the side-effects and inconvenience of treatment? Is any benefit of sufficient duration? Is the treatment, from the patient's point of view, worthwhile? Chemotherapy produces high overall response rates in head and neck cancer, these responses can be rapid and the effective, and the regimens have toxicity that is both manageable and acceptable. Effective palliation should therefore be possible: the challenge is to prove that this is the case. Research in this area needs to move from the obsessional measurement of tumour size to an approach that is centred more upon the hopes, expectations, and experiences of the patients.

Data obtained from patients about to start radical therapy for head and neck cancer suggest, as might be expected, that such patients rank cure and longevity as the highest priority.[22] However, other factors of more relevance to palliative treatment are also considered important,[22] namely:

- having no pain;
- being able to swallow all foods/liquids;
- having normal amounts of energy;
- returning to activities quickly;
- keeping natural voice;

- having speech understood easily;
- keeping normal sense of taste or smell;

Chemotherapy for carcinomas of the salivary glands

Tumours of the salivary glands are histologically distinct from other cancers of the head and neck. In terms of their response to chemotherapy, most behave as well-differentiated adenocarcinomas and hence the regimens used to treat these tumours are not those used to treat the squamous carcinomas of the head and neck. Malignant salivary tumours, particularly the adenoid cystic and mucoepidermoid types, are associated with a prolonged natural history: 5-year survival data may mislead, and so 10-year and 15-year survival rates are required to assess survival benefit. Unfortunately, these are rarely available.

There are only 18 published trials of chemotherapy for salivary carcinomas, 16 of which involve patients with metastatic disease. The complete response rate, from pooled data, is 6 per cent (CI, 4 per cent to 10 per cent) with an overall response rate of 30 per cent (CI, 25 per cent to 36 per cent). The most widely used regimens combine platinum with an anthracycline and cyclophosphamide, which give a complete response rate of 13 per cent (CI, 7 per cent to 21 per cent) and an overall response rate of 45 per cent (CI, 35 per cent to 55 per cent).

Summary and conclusions

It is quite remarkable that in spite of over 30 years of clinical trials we know as little as we do about the role of chemotherapy in head and neck cancer. This is partly due to the fact that head and neck cancers involve a variety of different sites and subsites and thus there is considerable heterogeneity. This lack of uniformity is further compounded by differences in treatment philosophy. In the United States and many European centres the primary emphasis is on surgical removal of the tumour, with radiotherapy relegated to a supportive role. In the United Kingdom, Scandinavia, and Canada there has been more emphasis on the use of radiotherapy as the primary treatment, with surgical removal being held in reserve for those tumours which are not controlled by radiotherapy. Chemotherapy has had to seek its niche amidst considerable confusion. These problems have been compounded by the lack of a systematic approach to the introduction of chemotherapy. As new drugs appear they have been added to existing regimens in an *ad hoc* fashion, reflecting the fact that the optimal regimen has not yet been defined—the widespread use of platinum and 5-fluorouracil (**5-FU**) is based as much on habit as upon any methodical acquisition of evidence.

There is a bewildering combinatorial expansion of drugs, doses, routes, and schedules. Even though the first trials of 5-FU were published in the early 1960s we still don't know whether it is essential to infuse 5-FU for the treatment of head and neck tumours or whether bolus administration is adequate. One point clearly emerges from the confusion: the most effective single agent for the non-surgical treatment of localized head and neck cancer is radiotherapy.

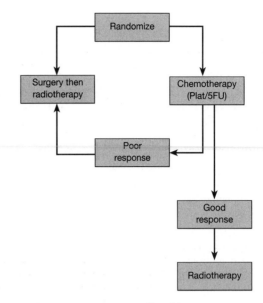

Fig. 1 VA study: Laryngeal cancer stage III or IV.

The currently fashionable approach of organ conservation can be regarded, in one sense, as reflecting the belated discovery by certain head and neck surgeons that some tumours, T3 tumours of the larynx for example, can be cured without surgery.

The potentially curative role of radiotherapy alone has long been recognized and primary radiotherapy has, in many countries, long been the initial treatment of choice for these tumours. It is difficult to identify the contribution, if any, of chemotherapy in this context. The VA study[23] has been much quoted and has been highly influential (Fig. 1), but it did not really address an important question: does chemotherapy add anything to a primarily radiotherapeutic approach to the treatment of laryngeal cancer? Could equivalent results have been achieved, in this group of patients, by simply treating with radical radiotherapy and reserving surgery for those patients whose tumours failed to respond or recurred after treatment? Was the chemotherapy simply a pragmatic way of defining, in advance of radiotherapy, those tumours destined to respond well to irradiation?

The VA study demonstrates that laryngeal conservation may be a safe option at least for some carefully selected patients, although it does not help with defining either the most effective conservative treatment or which patients might safely be treated with a conservative approach. Laryngeal tumours, staged as T3, are a very mixed group of tumours. An infiltrating supraglottic tumour will behave differently from an exophytic tumour at the same site. Cord fixation in T3 glottic tumours can arise by different mechanisms: a large tumour fixing the cord by sheer bulk; a smaller tumour causing cord fixation through damage to the intrinsic laryngeal musculature. A further study, with detailed prospective recording of pretreatment host-related and tumour-related factors, followed by randomization between radiotherapy alone and radiotherapy plus chemotherapy will be required. The available evidence suggests that the most effective way to combine radiotherapy and chemotherapy would be to give them synchronously. However, the use of synchronous treatment has the potential disadvantage of eliminating the ability to use a chemotherapeutic response as a predictor of a radiotherapeutic response. There is certainly evidence to suggest that those cancers of the head and neck which fail to respond to chemotherapy have a decreased likelihood of responding well to radiotherapy. The chemotherapy can, in this context, be regarded as an *in vivo* predictive assay for a radiation response. The concern here is that initial treatment with chemotherapy may, through clonal selection, modify the biological behaviour of a tumour so that it is more aggressive and less likely to respond well to subsequent treatment (the leaner-and-meaner argument[14]). A predictive test that carries the risk of making a tumour more aggressive is, fundamentally, unsafe. In order to improve therapeutic decision-making we need assays that can produce results in real time, either before radiotherapy or in the first few days of treatment, and that are capable of predicting, with reasonable accuracy, the likelihood of a response to radiotherapy. It is impossible, on the available evidence, to recommend neoadjuvant chemotherapy outwith a randomized controlled trial.

The most effective regimens are platinum-based, and the combination of *cis*-platinum and 5-FU is a reasonable choice. The addition of a taxane to this combination may improve the response rate but at considerable extra cost, both financial and in terms of toxicity.

The question of whether chemotherapy should be routinely added to radical radiotherapy for treating patients with head and neck cancer is an extremely difficult one. There is clear evidence that survival is improved, but at the price of increased toxicity. A further generation of trials is required. We need to do more than assess survival and local control, we need high-quality data on regimen-related toxicity. This new generation of studies could take two different approaches: one would be to use the same dose of radiation in both the chemotherapy + radiotherapy arm and the radiotherapy arm, another approach would be to compare a conventional dose of radiotherapy plus synchronous chemotherapy to a slightly higher dose of radiotherapy alone.

Chemotherapy undoubtedly has an important role to play in the palliation of symptoms in patients with advanced tumours of the head and neck. Again a new generation of studies is required, looking explicitly at the trade-offs between symptoms produced by the treatment and the relief of tumour-related symptoms. In the meantime the combination of *cis*-platinum, or analogue, and 5-FU offers a reasonable compromise between effectiveness and toxicity. As orally active long-term inhibitors of thymidylate synthetase become available then outpatient treatment, with its obvious benefits, will become more feasible.

With a clearer appreciation of the advantages and limitations of chemotherapy for head and neck cancer, we are finally in a position to put its investigation on to a more rational basis. In the meantime, however, our clinical decision-making has to be based on evidence that is, at best, imperfect and, more usually, irrelevant.

References

1. **Clark JR, et al.** Induction chemotherapy with cisplatin, fluorouracil, and high-dose leucovorin for squamous cell carcinoma of the head and neck: long-term results. *Journal of Clinical Oncology*, 1997; 15: 3100–10.

2. **Taylor SG.** Why has so much chemotherapy done so little in head and neck cancer. *Journal of Clinical Oncology*, 1987; 5: 1–3.

3. **Harari PM.** Why has induction chemotherapy for advanced head and neck cancer become a United States community standard of practice? *Journal of Clinical Oncology*, 1997; 15: 2050.

4. **Maipang T, Maipang M, Geater A, Panjapiyakul C, Watanaarepornchai S, Punperk S.** Combination chemotherapy as induction therapy for advanced resectable head and neck cancer. *Journal of Surgical Oncology*, 1995; 59: 80–5.

5. **Bezwoda WR, deMoor NG, Derman DP.** Treatment of advanced head and neck cancer by means of radiation therapy plus chemotherapy—a randomised trial. *Medical and Pediatric Oncology*, 1979; 6: 353–8.

6. **Munro AJ.** An overview of randomised controlled trials of adjuvant chemotherapy in head and neck cancer. *British Journal of Cancer*, 1995; 71: 83–91.

7. **Clarke M, Stewart L, Pignon JP, Bijnens L.** Individual patient data meta-analysis in cancer. *British Journal of Cancer*, 1998; 77: 2036–44.

8. **Pignon JP, Bourhis J, Domenge C, Designè L, on behalf of the MACH-NC collaborative group.** Chemotherapy added to locoregional treatment for head and neck squamous-cell carcinoma: three meta-analyses of updated individual data. *Lancet*, 2000; 355: 949–55.

9. **DerSimonian R, Laird N.** Meta-analysis in clinical trials. *Controlled Clinical Trials*, 1986; 7: 177–88.

10. **Belpomme D, Troutoux J, Bassot V, Aidan D, Elbez M.** Chemocurability of a subset of patients with head and neck squamous carcinoma (HNC), exclusively treated by short-term cisplatin–fluorouracil continuous infusion (PFU-CI). *ASCO Abstracts*, 1998; 17: 1517. [Abstract]

11. **Laccourreye H.** Limited cancers of the glottic stage of the larynx and exclusive chemotherapy—15 years of experience. *Bulletin of the Academy of National Medicine*, 1997; 181: 641–9.

12. **Morton RP, Stell PM.** Cytotoxic chemotherapy for patients with terminal squamous carcinoma—does it influence survival? *Clinical Otolaryngology*, 1984; 9: 175–80.

13. **Sanchiz F, et al.** Single fraction per day versus two fractions per day versus radiochemotherapy in the treatment of head and neck cancer. *International Journal of Radiation Oncology, Biology and Physics*, 1990; 19: 1347–50.

14. **Rosenthal DI, Pistenmaa DA, Glatstein E.** A review of neoadjuvant chemotherapy for head and neck cancer: partially shrunken tumors may be both leaner and meaner. *International Journal of Radiation Oncology, Biology and Physics*, 1993; 28: 315–20.

15. **Lefebvre JL, et al.** Meta-analysis of chemotherapy in head and neck cancer (MACH-NC): (2) larynx preservation using neoadjuvant chemotherapy (CT) in laryngeal and hypopharyngeal carcinoma. *ASCO Abstracts*, 1998; 17: 1473. [Abstract]

16. **Larto MA, et al.** A randomized trial comparing radiation therapy alone with chemoradiotherapy for squamous cell cancer of the head and neck (SCHNC): Quality of Life (QOL) assessment. *ASCO Abstracts*, 1998; 17: 1471. [Abstract]

17. **Al-Sarraf M, et al.** Chemoradiotherapy versus radiotherapy in patients with advanced nasopharyngeal cancer: phase III randomized intergroup study 0099. *Journal of Clinical Oncology*, 1998; 16: 1310–17.

18. **International Nasopharynx Cancer Study Group: VUMCA I Trial.** Preliminary results of a randomized trial comparing neoadjuvant chemotherapy (cisplatin, epirubicin, bleomycin) plus radiotherapy vs. radiotherapy alone in Stage IV (> = N2, M0) undifferentiated nasopharyngeal carcinoma: a positive result on progression-free survival. *International Journal of Radiation Oncology, Biology and Physics*, 1996; 35: 463–9.

19. **Chan AT, et al.** A prospective randomized study of chemotherapy adjunctive to definitive radiotherapy in advanced nasopharyngeal carcinoma. *International Journal of Radiation Oncology, Biology and Physics*, 1995; 33: 569.

20. **Rossi A, et al.** Adjuvant chemotherapy with vincristine, cyclophosphamide and doxorubicin after radiotherapy in loco-regional

nasopharyngeal cancer: results of a 4-year multicenter randomized study. *Journal of Clinical Oncology*, 1988; **6**: 1401–10.

21. **Altun M, Fandi A, Dupuis O, Cvitkovic E, Krajina Z, Eschwege F.** Undifferentiated nasopharyngeal cancer (UCNT): current diagnostic and therapeutic aspects. *International Journal of Radiation Oncology, Biology and Physics*, 1995; **32**: 859–77.

22. **List MA, *et al.*** Head and neck cancer (HNC) patients: how do patients prioritize potential treatment outcomes? *ASCO Abstracts*, 1998; **17**: 1472.

23. **Dept VA.** Laryngeal Cancer Study Group. Induction chemotherapy plus radiation compared with surgery plus radiation in patients with advanced laryngeal cancer. *New England Journal of Medicine*, 1991; **324**: 1685–90.

Tumours of the nasal cavity and paranasal sinuses

David J. Howard and Anna M. Cassoni

Introduction

Neoplasms of the nasal cavity and paranasal sinuses are rare, comprising some 3 per cent of head and neck cancers and, except where there is a strong occupational component in the aetiology, the male: female incidence is 2:1. There is an association between adenocarcinoma and woodworkers with hard woods, such as mahogany, where particles produced are greater than 5 micrometres in diameter.[1],[2] They provide a considerable therapeutic challenge and, like all head and neck cancers, are best managed by a multidisciplinary group providing surgery, radiotherapy, chemotherapy, prosthetics, speech and swallowing rehabilitation, and psychological support.

Tumours often present late and so it is difficult to be precise about the site of origin. Several staging systems have been proposed,[3] but are of limited usefulness as they do not fully take into account the impact of modern imaging techniques in staging, nor the effect on prognosis of modern surgical techniques. Most are T4 at presentation, but the effect of such a staged tumour close to the cranial cavity, for example, differs from one in the floor of the antrum.

The concept of benign and malignant is not always helpful. Nodal and distant metastases are uncommon, even in histologically malignant tumours. Local involvement is of overwhelming importance and benign tumours may run an aggressive course and require invasive treatment because of their proximity to vital structures.

Finally, tumours at these sites and their treatment can have a major impact on the patient's quality of life through both cosmesis and function.[4]

Pathology

The sinonasal area produces a great diversity of histological subtypes, including tumours of idiosyncratic behaviour. The majority of malignant tumours are squamous-cell carcinomas. Malignant tumours of salivary glands comprise some 10 to 15 per cent of all sinonasal tumours. Adenocarcinoma is uncommon, but workers in the woodworking and shoe industries are at increased risk. Aesthesioneuroblastoma arises from olfactory neuroepithelium, and at all ages. It tends to arise close to the cribriform plate, with a high risk of microscopic spread at this site involving the anterior cranial cavity. Mucosal malignant melanoma occurs, but accounts for less than 1 per cent of tumours in the nasal cavity and paranasal sinuses combined (Tables 1 and 2).

A wide range of sarcomas may present here, including rhabdomyosarcoma, osteosarcoma, chondrosarcoma, Ewing's/PNET (peripheral neuroepithelioma) and soft-tissue sarcoma; however, these are uncommon. Lymphoma may also, rarely, involve this area.

Table 1 Range of histology in resected malignant sinonasal tumours

	No.		No.
Adenocarcinoma	42	Malignant fibrous histiocytoma	2
Olfactory neuroblastoma	26	Spindle-cell sarcoma	1
Squamous-cell carcinoma	25	Carcinosarcoma	1
Chondrosarcoma	19	Osteogenic sarcoma	1
Adenoid cystic	15	Angiosarcoma	1
Anaplastic	10	Haemangiopericytoma	1
Malignant melanoma	8	Alveolar soft-part sarcoma	1
Cylindric-cell carcinoma	5	Malignant schwannoma	1
Rhabdomyosarcoma	3	Mucoepidermoid carcinoma	1
Metastasis	3	Ewing's sarcoma	1

Histological diagnosis in 167 patients undergoing craniofacial resection for sinonasal neoplasia at the Royal National Throat, Nose and Ear Hospital, London. There is a preponderance of nasal cavity and ethmoid lesions, but it demonstrates the considerable histological diversity.

Table 2 Range of benign histology

	No.		No.
Meningioma	7	Neurofibroma	2
Fibro-osseous disease	6	Angioma	2
Osteoma	5	Angiofibroma	2
Phycomycete granuloma	3	Cholesterol granuloma	1
Reparative granuloma	2	Pseudotumour	1
Osteoblastoma	2	Dermoid	1
Leiomyoblastoma	2	Pleomorphic adenoma	1
Meningoencephalocoele	2	Haemangioma	1
Osteomyelitis	2		

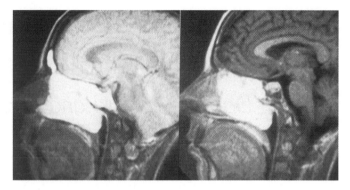

Fig. 1 T1-weighted MRI sagittal sections with and without gadolinium (right and left, respectively) showing olfactory neuroblastoma, clearly defined in contrast to fluid in the frontal and sphenoid sinuses and inflamed mucosa in the anterior nasal cavity.

Diagnosis

The maxilla is the commonest site, but as lesions often arise in the middle meatus, the ethmoids, nasal cavity, and antrum are often involved. Nasal obstruction is a common symptom, as is rhinorrhoea, which may be bloodstained. These symptoms may be attributed to infection.

Tumours of the maxillary antrum may present in a variety of ways:

(1) nasal symptoms—due to medial spread;

(2) oral symptoms—with pain in the upper jaw, swelling, loosening of teeth, or problems with dentures: these symptoms occur at presentation in about 15 per cent of cases;

(3) ocular—swelling, pain, epiphora, or diplopia: these symptoms are due to extension through the roof, occurring in some 5 per cent of cases;

(4) facial—with spread anteriorly into the cheek or involvement of the infraorbital nerve causing pain and paraesthesia;

(5) posterolateral spread—if into the pterygoid area it may produce trismus.

Tumours of the ethmoid may present with nasal obstruction, a blood-stained discharge, or broadening of the bridge of the nose.

In addition to the ENT and ophthalmic examinations, both flexible and rigid nasendoscopy now aid earlier the detection of neoplasia and accurate biopsy.

The combination of computed tomography (**CT**) and magnetic resonance imagery (**MRI**) is most effective in determining the extent of a tumour. Contrast-enhanced CT best defines bone destruction and early involvement of the cribriform plate and the ethmoid roof. Gadolinium **DTPA** (diethylenetriaminepenta-acetic acid)-enhanced MRI is most accurate in defining soft-tissue tumour extent[5] (Figs 1 and 2 and see also Plate 1).

A histological diagnosis is necessary in all patients, and endoscopy allows effective biopsy in most patients. A Caldwell Luc is best avoided. Biopsy is contraindicated if an angiofibroma is suspected because of the high risk of severe bleeding.

Cervical lymphadenopathy occurs in 10 to 20 per cent of cases and is associated with a poor prognosis, as are distant metastases at presentation.

There is relatively little resistance to spread into the orbit around the infraorbital canal. The posterior wall is thin and involvement

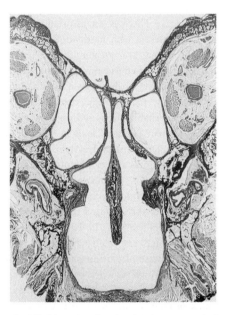

Fig. 2 Coronal midfacial section showing the close anatomical relationship, and therefore pathway of spread from the nose and paranasal sinuses to the orbit, cribriform plate, and anterior cranial fossa (see also Plate 1).

through this to the pterygoid and infratemporal region is associated with a poor prognosis (Fig. 3 and see Plate 2).

The ethmoids often contain secretions due to osteal obstruction, which need to be distinguished from a tumour. Once the sphenoid is involved, there is a risk of cavernous sinus and middle cranial fossa involvement (Fig. 4 and see Plate 3).

Although the lamina papyracea may have natural areas of dehiscence, and they provide an easy route of spread, the orbital periosteum provides a significant barrier. The roof of the ethmoid is variable, and above the cribriform plate, but tumour may enter the anterior cranial fossa relatively easily via either structure. The dura is relatively resistant, and though its involvement is not a contraindication to operation, frank involvement of the frontal lobes carries a very poor prognosis[6] (Fig. 5 and see Plate 4).

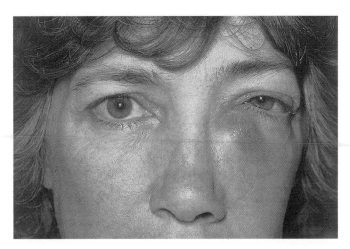

Fig. 3 Clinical photograph showing squamous cell carcinoma of left maxilla involving anterior soft tissues of cheek and medial canthus with extension into the inferomedial orbit (see also Plate 2).

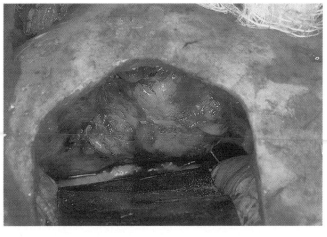

Fig. 5 Intraoperative photograph of an anterior craniotomy showing a chondrosarcoma extending through the cribriform plate and ethmoid sinus to involve the dura (see also Plate 4).

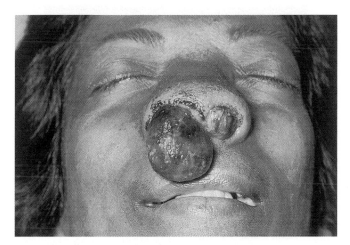

Fig. 4 Clinical photograph showing a poorly differentiated squamous-cell carcinoma occupying both nasal cavities (see also Plate 3).

Staging

Staging of nasal cavity and paranasal sinus carcinomas is not as well established as for other head and neck tumours. Only the maxillary sinus and ethmoid sinus have a staging system agreed on by the American Joint Committee on Cancer (**AJCC**). For cancer of the maxillary sinus and the ethmoid sinus, the AJCC has designated staging by the TNM classification.[7]–[9]

TNM definitions

Maxillary sinus
Primary tumour (T):

TX: Primary tumour cannot be assessed

T0:   No evidence of primary tumour

Tis: Carcinoma *in situ*

T1:   Tumour limited to the antral mucosa with no erosion or destruction of bone

T2:   Tumour causing bone erosion or destruction, except for the posterior antral wall, including extension into the hard palate and/or the middle of the nasal meatus

T3:   Tumour invades any of the following: bone of the posterior wall of the maxillary sinus, subcutaneous tissues, skin of the cheek, floor or medial wall of the orbit, infratemporal fossa, pterygoid plates, ethmoid sinuses

T4:   Tumour invades the orbital contents beyond the floor or medial wall, including any of the following: the orbital apex, cribriform plate, base of the skull, nasopharynx, sphenoid, frontal sinuses

Ethmoid sinus
Primary tumour (T):

T1:   Tumour confined to the ethmoid with or without bone erosion

T2:   Tumour extends into the nasal cavity

T3:   Tumour extends to the anterior orbit, and/or maxillary sinus

T4:   Tumour with intracranial extension, orbital extension including apex, involving the sphenoid, and/or frontal sinus and/or skin of external nose

Regional lymph nodes and distant metastasis (M): see Chapter 9.1.4.

AJCC stage groupings

Stage 0
Tis, N0, M0

Stage I
T1, N0, M0

Stage II
T2, N0, M0

Stage III
T3, N0, M0
T1, N1, M0

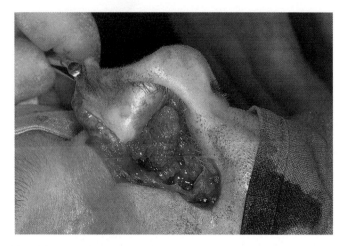

Fig. 6 Intraoperative photograph showing the exposure obtained by lateral rhinotomy to reveal a primary mucosal malignant melanoma (see also Plate 5).

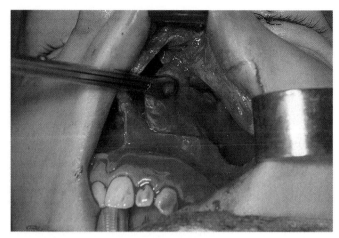

Fig. 7 Intraoperative photograph showing mobilization of an angiofibroma from the left nasal cavity, nasopharynx, and left pterygomaxillary region via a midfacial degloving approach (see also Plate 6).

T2, N1, M0

T3, N1, M0

Stage IVA

T4, N0, M0

T4, N1, M0

Stage IVB

Any T, N2, M0

Any T, N3, M0

Stage IVC

Any T, Any N, M1

Management

Surgical techniques

The comments in this section are based upon a distillation of the literature and the personal experience of over 500 cases of sinonasal neoplasia by the surgical co-author (DJH).

The majority of patients undergo some form of surgery: lateral rhinotomy and medial maxillectomy, midfacial degloving, partial or total maxillectomy, total rhinectomy, or craniofacial resection with or without orbital clearance.

Lateral rhinotomy gives good access to the nasal cavity, the frontal–ethmoid–sphenoidal complex and the medial maxilla, and, by limiting the superior extent of the incision, the cosmesis is good. However, except perhaps for melanoma and other nasal cavity tumours in the elderly, it has been largely superseded by midfacial degloving[10] (Fig. 6 and see Plate 5).

Midfacial degloving combines bilateral sublabial incisions with elevation of the soft tissues of the mid-third of the face with cartilaginous nasal incisions, and offers greater exposure without external scars[11] (Figs 7 and 8 and see Plates 6 and 7).

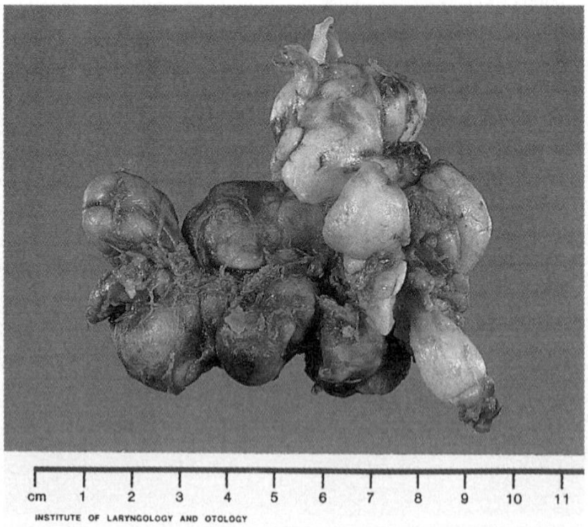

Fig. 8 Operative specimen showing an extensive angiofibroma with components that occupied the posterior nasal cavity, nasopharynx, sphenoid, pterygomaxillary, and infratemporal fossa regions (see also Plate 7).

Craniofacial resection is used for all malignant tumours involving the anterior skull base. This method provides a superior approach to that of total maxillectomy and orbital clearance, and gives better clearance and improved cosmesis. It also allows evaluation at operation of the orbital periosteum by frozen section, allowing preservation, in a proportion of patients, of the eye. If the periosteum is breached, an orbital clearance is usual with conservation of skin and orbicularis oculi, to produce a skin-lined socket suitable for a prosthesis. An extended lateral rhinotomy or midfacial degloving with a bicoronal incision is used to provide access to the anterior cranial fossa. The frontal lobes are retracted and a wide dissection of the dura is performed with *en bloc* removal of the ethmoid complex, cribriform plate, and additional structures as appropriate. Where the medial bony wall of the orbit is breached, but the orbital periosteum is

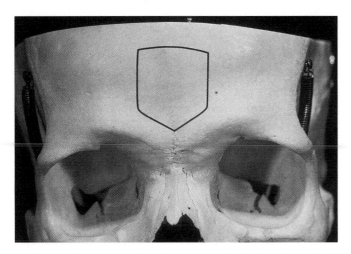

Fig. 9 Anterior craniotomy undertaken at craniofacial resection.

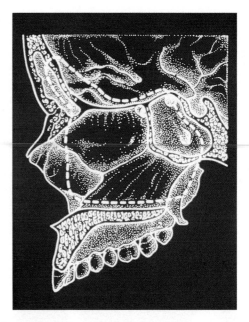

Fig. 11 Diagram to illustrate the extent of resection in a midline sagittal view at anterior craniofacial resection.

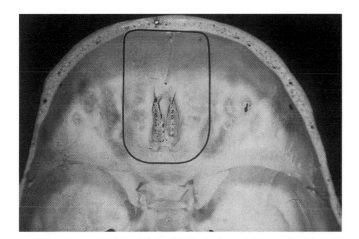

Fig. 10 Outline of osteotomies allowing removal of the floor of the anterior cranial fossa.

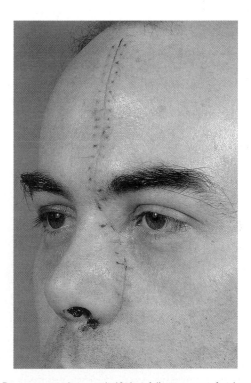

Fig. 12 Postoperative photograph 10 days following craniofacial resection (and see also Plate 8).

intact, the area may be excised and the defect repaired with a split skin graft, thereby preserving a fully functional eye. Dura is repaired with fascia lata and a split skin graft or a vascularized periosteal flap[10] (Figs 9, 10, 11, 12, and 13 and see Plates 8 and 9).

Reconstruction and rehabilitation

Sinonasal surgery has cosmetic and functional effects that are obvious and difficult to hide. Orbital exenteration and radical maxillectomy are perceived as the most severe facial disfigurement after surgery, with mandibulectomy and rhinectomy also scoring highly.[12] Fatigue levels, headaches, and visual, taste, and smell abnormalities are common complications.[4] Expert maxillofacial prosthodontics are necessary. Preoperative assessment and manufacture of a temporary prosthesis, which can be placed into a maxillectomy cavity at the completion of surgery, allows early resumption of relatively normal speech and nutrition. This prosthesis should be provided for all those undergoing radical maxillectomy, and should subsequently be replaced

by a permanent denture-bearing prosthesis. A permanent obturator is provided later (Figs 14 and 15 and see Plates 10 and 11).

Osseointegration techniques using titanium screws,[13] which become integrated into the skeleton, allow firm attachment of a prosthesis. However, radiotherapy may slow this integration, which may

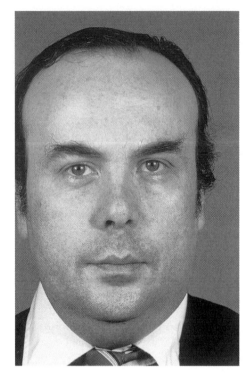

Fig. 13 Photograph of the same patient 22 months later (and see also Plate 9).

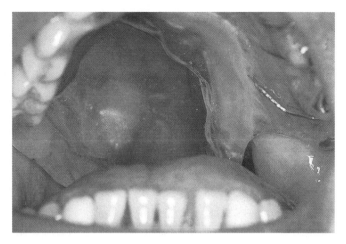

Fig. 15 Clinical photograph of a maxillary obturator fitted orally (and see also Plate 11).

then take up to a year in the orbit. The availability of these specialized techniques have dramatically improved the postoperative rehabilitation of these patients[14] (Figs 16 and 17).

Rhinectomy is occasionally required for extensive nasal tumours. The defect is repaired with a prosthesis suspended on spectacles or osseointegrated implants, or by skin and soft tissue flaps (Figs 18 and 19).

Complications of surgery

Complications of sinonasal surgery include cerebrospinal fluid leak, meningitis, frontal lobe abscess, cerebrovascular accident, diabetes insipidus, convulsions, nasolacrimal duct blockage with epiphora, diplopia, and serous otitis media. About 40 per cent of patients experience morbidity. In modern practice, serious complications are

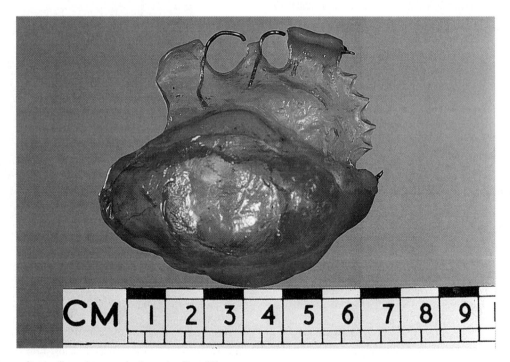

Fig. 14 Lightweight acrylic maxillary obturator (and see also Plate 10).

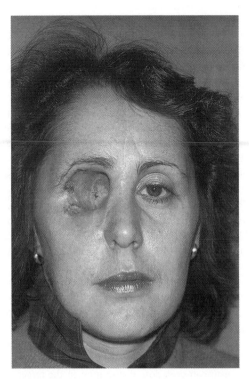

Fig. 16 Postoperative photograph showing a patient after craniofacial resection and right orbital clearance for an adenoid cystic carcinoma.

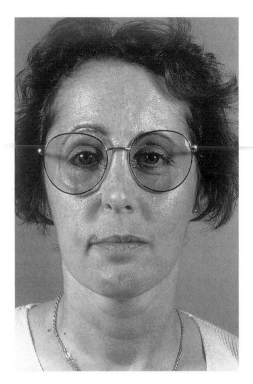

Fig. 17 Photograph of the same patient with an osseointegrated orbital prosthesis.

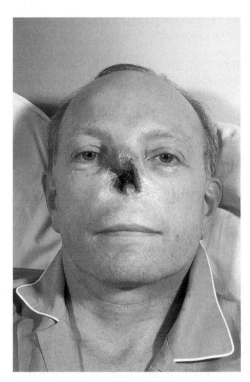

Fig. 18 Photograph showing early postoperative appearances after total rhinectomy.

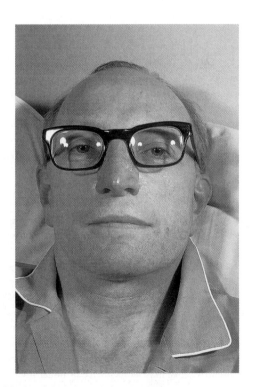

Fig. 19 Nasal prosthesis mounted on spectacles.

few and hospital stays vary from 4 to 18 days. Perioperative mortality is of the order of 2 per cent for major craniofacial surgery.[6]

Radiotherapy

Before radiotherapy, a dental evaluation should be performed and appropriate conservation work carried out. Any teeth clearly needing extraction in the near future should be extracted and a regular preventive programme of hygiene and daily fluoride topical gel application commenced.

As for irradiating all tumours of the head and neck, the patient must be immobilized in an appropriate, individually made cast. In the majority of tumours the lower border of the tumour volume will be at the level of the commissure. It is usual to insert a gag to depress the tongue and lower oral cavity out of the radiation field. The proximity of target volumes to sensitive structures (such as the eye, optic chiasm, and brainstem) requires accuracy and reproducibility of the set-up. The development of conformal techniques requires errors no greater than 2 to 3 mm and 2 degrees of rotation. Where possible, the fields in the various phases of therapy should be decided at the outset to allow the cast in the incident beam to be cut out, as far as is compatible with stability and accuracy, to maximize skin sparing.

Conventional techniques include quite wide margins, especially along mucosal planes. Conformal techniques encourage the definition of the GTV (gross target volume), that is the visible tumour defined by clinical, radiological, and pathological means. The clinical target volume (CTV) adds to this any sites considered at significant risk of microscopic spread. This includes draining lymph glands and a margin around the GTV. There is little information on how wide this should be, especially in relation to the complex anatomy of this region, but 0.5 to 1 cm seems usual. Having defined the CTV, a further 0.5 to 1 cm is added to account for uncertainties in localization and variability in the set-up.[15]

CT planning should be used for the majority of tumour plans in this area. Conventional planning using the simulator and based on bony landmarks may lead to a geographical miss. The presence of air-filled cavities perturbs the dose distribution and CT planning will give a more accurate representation.

Three-dimensional planning techniques may allow better preservation of unaffected structures, especially parts of the globe on both sides, but the optic nerve on the affected side remains at risk.[15],[16]

Irradiation techniques

Supervoltage irradiation with electron or photon beams is used. A variety of techniques are available, depending on the precise site and extent.

Antrum—in the unusual case of a lesion confined to the infrastructure being treated, the ethmoid may be excluded. However, the target volume is usually the whole maxillary antrum and ipsilateral ethmoid as mucosal spread throughout is common. The nasopharyngeal vault, the sphenoid sinus, and the pterygoid fossa are also included. The medial and inferior walls of the orbit are included, but the extent to which the orbital contents must be irradiated will depend on the degree of tumour extension. The incidence of nodal involvement is up to 20 per cent, but elective treatment of the clinically negative neck is not employed.

The volume is covered by an anterior and usually two lateral fields, the contralateral field being narrower and serving to prevent the dose 'falling off' in the posteromedial corner of the volume. The anterior field is weighted 1.5 to 3 with respect to the lateral fields, and the ipsilateral field is angled a few degrees posteriorly to avoid an exit beam through the opposite lens.

Orbit—shielding should be used where possible for sensitive orbital contents. The lacrimal gland should always be shielded where the globe may be preserved at surgery—the risk of loss of the eye later from ulceration with infection is high, carrying with it a risk of sympathetic ophthalmopathy of the other eye. Where possible, this shielding should be extended to cover the cornea and part of the retina. Whenever the ethmoid is treated, the medial quarter to third of the orbit is irradiated. Following enucleation, the dose to the temporal lobe is increased. This could be reduced by placing a tissue-equivalent bolus in the cavity during therapy, but it will produce a very marked acute reaction.

Nasal septum—most lesions are relatively superficial and can be treated with a single electron beam. For lesions of the anterior vestibule, nasolabial fold, or columella, a single, direct anterior electron field of appropriate energy may be used. A margin of 1 to 1.5 cm deep to the skin is necessary. In this case, a tissue-equivalent bolus should be applied anteriorly, and wax placed in the nostrils during therapy to ensure an even dose distribution in the target volume. In view of the constriction of the electron isodoses at depth, a wide portal must be used. However, this technique will produce a marked skin reaction. This technique is also appropriate where there is spread on to the cheek (Fig. 20).

More extensive or posteriorly placed lesions—these may be treated satisfactorily by two anterior, wedged fields, allowing the target volume to extend posteriorly into the premaxilla. The superior borders are placed below the eyes. In both these approaches, the buccal mucosa and gum will be irradiated. Doses of 60 to 70 Gy in 2-Gy fractions, or equivalent, are required.

Brachytherapy

This may be suitable for early lesions or occasionally as a boost technique for bulky lesions. Iridium wires are inserted into the septum, floor of the nasal cavity, and the nasal alae, depending on the precise target volume. As sole treatment, a dose of 60 Gy over 6 days is given. When used as a boost, 30 Gy may be given by external beam, followed by 30 to 35 Gy brachytherapy.

Late effects of radiation therapy

Optic

If in or close to the radiation volume, the lens, cornea, lacrimal gland, retina, optic nerve, and chiasm may be at risk. Opacities of the ipsilateral lens may occur even if the cornea is shielded. If the lacrimal gland and cornea can be shielded, the risk to vision is small. This also spares a significant proportion of the retina. Where the cornea is spared by requiring the patient to look laterally, more of the posterior retina receives the high dose with a significant incidence of retinopathy. There is a risk of optic nerve damage of the order of 8 per cent at doses of 60 Gy and over. Retinopathy, where the entire retina has been treated to more than 60 Gy, has a latency of 2 to 3 years, longer with lower doses; optic nerve damage is manifested later.

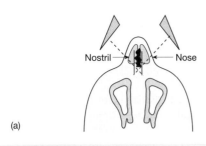

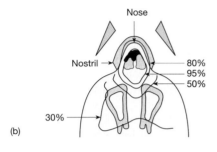

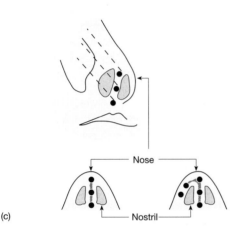

Fig. 20 Radiotherapy techniques for nasal cavity. (a) Tumour of the septum: anterior oblique wedge pair; hinge angle 90 degrees. (b) Advanced tumour; anterior oblique wedge pair; hinge angle 90 degrees with tissue equivalent bolus. (c) Interstitial implant to the septum.

Neurological

The volume for the ethmoid/antrum includes part of the frontal lobes. About 10 per cent of patients will develop a temporary syndrome including vertigo, lethargy, and somnolence at about 2 to 3 months' postirradiation, which lasts for 1 to 2 months. If cerebral symptoms develop, the possibility of meningitis, secondary to chronic infection, should be borne in mind.

Aural

Temporary serous otitis media may occur after, during, or soon after therapy, although most cases resolve spontaneously.

Nasal

Synechiae may develop following the successful treatment of tumours of the nasal cavity. These may cause nasal block, irritation, and crusting. The symptoms may be relieved by salt-water douches. Tumours of the septum may resolve leaving septal perforations, for which no therapy is required.

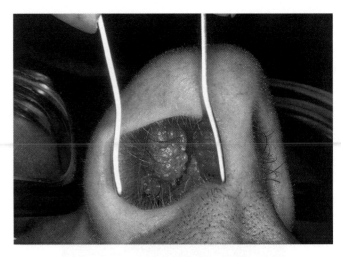

Fig. 21 Photograph of an everted papilloma in the nasal vestibule.

Dental

The risk of osteoradionecrosis is less in the maxilla than the mandible due to its better blood supply. Nevertheless, the usual precautions should be taken before irradiating teeth that will be retained, in other words removing those which would need extraction in the near future and instituting a regular preventive programme of hygiene and daily lifetime fluoride-gel topical applications.

Palliation

Any untreated malignancy of this area is painful, disfiguring, and difficult to palliate. Especially in tumours with a long natural history, such as adenoid cystic tumours or chondrosarcoma, judiciously planned and timed surgery may keep the patient relatively symptom-free for prolonged periods, even if the chances of cure are small.[18]

Management and results per specific sites

A good example of a concise management proposal can be found in the PDQ statements for paranasal sinuses and nasal cavity cancer on the NCI website (http://cancernet.nci.nih.gov) The latest AJCC stage grouping is also available on the same webpage.

Nasal vestibule

The majority of tumours here are squamous-cell carcinomas, but basal-cell carcinomas, adnexal tumours, and melanomas also occur. The approach to therapy is similar, but with surgery being especially favoured for adnexal tumours and melanomas.

While, overall, surgery and radiotherapy both produce high cure rates, radiotherapy is often chosen for a better cosmetic result in all but the smallest lesions which are treated by primary excision, with surgery otherwise reserved for salvage. Excision usually involves removal of underlying cartilage (Figs 21 and 22).

Tumours of the vestibule may invade the alar and septal cartilages and, occasionally, the skin of the nose or upper lip. Tumours at this

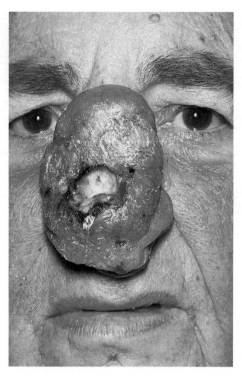

Fig. 22 Clinical photograph showing an extensive squamous-cell carcinoma of the nasal vestibule.

site are often more extensive than they appear. Posterior spread occurs late. The clinical target volume is the visible lesion plus a margin for microscopic spread. In view of the anatomy the directions of spread may be quite complex so that the fields and technique will need to be individualized. Of special concern is deep spread into underlying tissues posterior to the columella and in the nasolabial fold where the lesion is close to these areas.

Results

For T1/T2 N0 tumours, local control by radiotherapy alone is achieved in 80 to 90 per cent of cases.[19] In selected patients treated with brachytherapy, control rates were 97 per cent (T1, N0) and 79 per cent (T2, N0).[20] Disease-free survival for T3 is reported as being 40 per cent.[17] The tumour grade has an impact on survival, with 83 per cent of patients with grade 1 tumours surviving disease-free, while only 20 per cent of patients with higher grades did so.[21],[22] About 20 per cent of patients develop nodal metastases, generally these are bilateral, and this may be associated with local relapse.

Nasal cavity

A variety of benign tumours occur in this area including inflammatory polyps, giant-cell reparative granuloma, and benign salivary and odontogenic tumours. Malignant tumours high in the septum and posterior nasal cavity tend to be of a higher grade than those in the inferior and anterior areas. In the former areas, the mucosa is closely adherent to periosteum and perichondrium and tumours here tend to invade these structures early.

Here also, the results of surgery and radiotherapy are similar in terms of tumour control when used for similar stages. In practice,

surgery is used for smaller lesions, especially those of the septum. More advanced lesions are treated with combined modality therapy or radiotherapy alone. Most lesions are less than 5 cm in diameter.[19]

Surgery

Lateral rhinotomy and midfacial degloving techniques provide good access to this area and allow the resection of suitable tumours with good cosmetic results.

Radiotherapy

The clinical target volume will depend on the precise site and extent of tumour involvement, the histological type and grade, and whether radiation is delivered postoperatively or is the sole treatment modality. Target volume will include the medial wall of the maxillary antrum, the ethmoids, medial orbital wall, nasopharynx, sphenoid, and base of the skull.

The routes of spread are similar for most types of tumours, but adenoid cystic carcinomas may have a greater tendency to perineural spread. A technique of anterior field irradiation with one or two lateral portals, with shielding to the eyes, is usually suitable.

A dose of 60 to 65 Gy in 2-Gy fractions is given, with a reduction in the target volume to that of the gross disease with a smaller margin at 50 Gy. Postoperative radiotherapy is given to 60 Gy. Prophylactic treatment to the cervical lymph glands is not usual in view of the low risk of spread.

Results of therapy are often reported combined with those of paranasal sinuses. Local failure rates are high at 40 to 60 per cent, and cure rates are in the order of 45 per cent.[17],[23]

Paranasal sinuses

Most tumours of the paranasal sinuses only present when they are relatively advanced, early symptoms often being mistaken for inflammatory disease. About 80 per cent of such tumours arise in the maxillary antrum and 10 to 15 per cent in the ethmoids; however, tumours involving the sphenoid or frontal sinuses alone are uncommon. Over 50 per cent of tumours affecting the paranasal sinuses are squamous-cell carcinomas.

Whilst surgery alone may be sufficient for treating T1 and T2 tumours of the inferior maxilla, for most tumours a planned combined approach with surgery and radiotherapy is usual. Where surgery has been performed, the following are clear indications for postoperative radiotherapy: positive or close margins; perineural invasion; tumour spillage; or the inability to perform an *en bloc* resection. There are theoretical advantages to preoperative radiotherapy: increased resectability; sterilization of the tumour bed with a reduced risk of seeding; and less hypoxia at the viable periphery, as the microvasculature has not been surgically disrupted. Postoperative radiotherapy allows the pathology findings to be taken into account, although the whole tumour bed requires radiotherapy. The degree and significance of radiotherapy on postoperative healing is debated. There is, however, no clearly demonstrated advantage to pre- as opposed to postoperative radiotherapy.[6] Tumours involving the nasopharynx, sphenoid, base of the skull, and the infratemporal fossa may or may not be considered resectable, depending on the surgeon's level of expertise, but patient's with such tumours are likely to be given radiotherapy first. The possibility of conservation of the eye at surgery is a particular issue for the radiotherapist offering preoperative radiotherapy; this should be discussed before treatment planning so that sensitive structures, that may be preserved, can be shielded as much as possible.

Squamous-cell carcinomas often breach more than the medial wall and therefore require radical maxillectomy by a conventional Weber–Ferguson incision, or preferably a midfacial degloving procedure. Orbital clearance may also be required, in which case the socket is lined by the skin of the eyelids.

Lesions involving the superior ethmoids and cribriform are treated with craniofacial resection, which allows accurate assessment of the orbit and, with frozen section, permits conservation of the eye.

Radiotherapy

Tumours of the ethmoids alone are rare and treatment generally involves the whole ipsilateral maxilloethmoid complex.

The clinical target volume includes the maxilla or the residual cavity, the orbit, and the ipsilateral nasal cavity and ethmoid. If the posterior wall is breached, the whole pterygoid fossa is included.

Field placement is usually with an anterior and ipsilateral field, often with a small contralateral field to top up the dose to the posteromedial portion of the volume. The ipsilateral field is positioned with its anterior border at the lateral orbital margin, in order to spare the ipsilateral anterior chamber, and angled a few degrees posteriorly to spare the contralateral lens from the exit beam. The optic chiasm and pituitary gland may be shielded throughout, unless the posterior ethmoids, cribriform plate, or sphenoid are involved. The dose to the optic chiasm should be kept as low as possible using modern 3D-treatment planning. The aim is to prevent hot spots arising when a dose of 70 Gy is delivered in 35 fractions over 7 weeks, or when a biologically equivalent dose with a shorter overall treatment time or a larger dose per fraction is planned. Where possible, the lacrimal gland and anterior chamber are shielded; this will also shield part of the retina. Care needs to be taken in placing this shielding as the roof of the maxilla extends superiorly within the orbit. The anterior field is weighted with respect to the lateral 2.5 B 3:1. Following enucleation, there will be an increased dose to the temporal lobe. This could be reduced by placing tissue-equivalent bolus in the cavity, but this would lead to a very marked acute reaction. A dose of 60 to 65 Gy in 2-Gy fractions is usual.

Results

Tumours of the infrastructure and superolateral antrum have the best prognosis of this group. For the whole group, survival is in the order of 35 to 60 per cent.[6],[15],[24]–[26] Radiotherapy alone is generally associated with survival in the order or 33 per cent or less. Patients treated in such a way usually have more advanced tumours. However, selected series report higher response rates: Waldron et al.,[23] from Toronto, report a 39 per cent 5-year survival for patients with ethmoid tumours treated with radiotherapy alone, and an associated 52 per cent local failure rate, which they consider acceptable.

In one study of 39 patients using conformal techniques, those treated with postoperative radiotherapy had no recurrence if treated for close margins, 21 per cent if the margins were microscopically positive, and 80 per cent if there was a gross residual tumour. Radiotherapy alone for inoperable disease produces local control rates of 32 per cent at 3 years. This group was given doses of 68.4 Gy.[15]

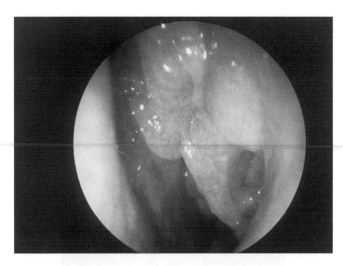

Fig. 23 Endoscopic photograph of an inverted papilloma in the middle meatus (and see Plate 12).

Follow-up

Careful follow-up is important as recurrence may be salvaged by second-line therapy, or symptoms prevented or delayed. Follow-up is usually by routine physical examination, including endoscopy and examination under anaesthesia with biopsy. Where visual access is limited, a postoperative CT scan and enhanced MR imaging with subtraction techniques provide excellent post-treatment imaging.[27]

Special tumour types

Inverted papilloma

This is an uncommon lesion which arises from the mucosa of the sinonasal tract. Although classified as benign, it may have a very aggressive course (with multiple recurrences, bone destruction, and extensive local invasion) and may transform to carcinoma in approximately 2 per cent of cases.[28] It occurs more frequently in males over 40 years of age. As its name suggests, its microscopic appearance is of a papilloma growing into stroma, rather outwards from the epithelium (Fig. 23 and see Plate 12).

Local resection is associated with recurrence rates of 40 to 80 per cent. Radical resection results in local control rates of 90 per cent.

Radiotherapy may be added in unresectable lesions and those associated with frank histological malignancy.

Aesthesioneuroepithelioma (olfactory neuroblastoma)

This rare tumour arises from the olfactory epithelium. It most commonly presents with nasal obstruction, epistaxis, and an impaired sense of smell. It may spread into the orbit, antrum, or ethmoid. Its proximity to the cribriform plate confers a risk of intracranial spread. It may affect all ages, but is most commonly reported in the second and third decades of life (Fig. 24).

Its behaviour is unpredictable and may recur locally and with metastatic disease. Cervical node involvement has been reported in up to 20 per cent of cases at some time during the course of the disease.

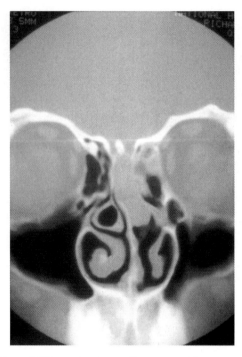

Fig. 24 Coronal CT scan showing an olfactory neuroblastoma involving the superior nasal cavity, septum, and cribriform plate.

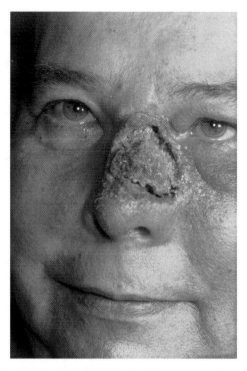

Fig. 25 Clinical photograph showing a T-cell lymphoma of the nose (and see also Plate 13).

There are few data on the most appropriate management. Where possible, radical craniofacial resection should be performed.[6] Post-operative radiotherapy is recommended with techniques such as those described, dependent on the sites involved. Despite its resemblance to neuroblastoma, it is not particularly radiosensitive and a dose of between 55 and 60 Gy is advised.

T-cell lymphoma of the nose and sinuses (midline destructive granuloma)

This causes extensive ulceration and necrosis of the nasal cavity and ethmoids and is due to a T-cell lymphoma. Treatment is with combination chemotherapy and local radiotherapy (Fig. 25 and see Plate 13).

Other treatments

The role of chemotherapy as neoadjuvant, adjuvant, or concurrent therapy has not been widely studied in the group, although some patients have been included in studies of several tumour sites. Where reported separately, response rates in the order of 40 per cent are suggested.[26] The role of chemotherapy in the treatment of head and neck malignancies is addressed elsewhere. It may be that in squamous-cell lesions the chemotherapeutic effect is similar to that for other sites, that is there is a small advantage.

Chemotherapy, especially platinum-based, may have a good palliative effect, with up to 60 per cent of patients experiencing a response, which is usually associated with an improvement in symptoms. Unfortunately, patients experiencing a complete response may then decline to undergo the surgery that offers them a chance of a complete cure.[29] In combination with radiotherapy, chemotherapy may act as

a radiosensitizer and decrease the need for surgery, but it has not been shown to increase survival rates.[30],[31]

Knegt *et al.*[32] have described the use of topical 5-fluorouracil for treating adenocarcinoma of the nose and sinuses, packing the limited surgical cavity on repeated occasions following local debridement. This approach is not generally accepted.

Except in some vestibule tumours, brachytherapy has a limited role, but it is occasionally useful in the form of gold or yttrium implants into recurrent tumours in the skull base, or for high dose-rate afterloading. In squamous tumours in some sites, altered fractionation schedules, acceleration by a variety of schemes, and dose escalation by hyperfractionation have been used; in some studies they shown an advantage, but not specifically in these sites.

At the time of writing, none of the management strategies outlined above are based on level I evidence from controlled trials. Although some are reports of relatively large series, they still mainly rely on individual institution experience. It is to be hoped that a large national or multinational, prospective randomized study incorporating the best elements of surgery, radiotherapy, and chemotherapy may provide us with more definite answers. Until such time, these rare cases should be treated by experienced teams in major centres with maximum support facilities for the patients.

References

1. **Wilhelmsson B, Drettner B.** Nasal problems in wood furniture makers. A study of symptoms and physiological variables. *Acta Otolaryngologica*, 1984; **98**: 548–55.
2. **Drettner B, Wilhelmsson B, Lund LB.** Experimental studies on

carcinogens in the nasal mucosa. *Acta Otolaryngologica*, 1985; **99**: 205–7.

3. **Lund VJ, Howard DJ.** Tumours of the paranasal sinuses. In *Diseases of the sinuses* (ed. ME Gershwin, GA Incaudo). New Jersey: Humana Press, 1996: 291–310.

4. **Jones E, Lund VJ, Howard DJ, Greenberg MR, McCarthy M.** Quality of life of patients treated surgically for head and neck cancer. *Journal of Laryngology and Otolology*, 1992; **106**: 238–42.

5. **Lund VJ, Howard DJ, Lloyd GAS, Cheesman AD.** Magnetic resonance imaging of paranasal sinus tumours for craniofacial resection. *Head and Neck Surgery*, 1989; **11**: 279–83.

6. **Lund VJ, Howard DJ, Wei WI, Cheesman AD.** Craniofacial resection for tumours of the nasal cavity and paranasal sinuses—a 17-year experience. *Head and Neck Surgery*, 1998; March: 97–105.

7. **Schantz SP, Harrison LB, Forastiere AA.** Tumors of the nasal cavity and paranasal sinuses, nasalpharynx, oral cavity, and oropharynx. In *Cancer: principles and practice of oncology* (5th edn) (ed. VT DeVita Jr, S Hellman, SA Rosenberg). Philadelphia, PA: Lippincott–Raven, 1997: 741–801.

8. **Laramore GE (ed.).** *Radiation therapy of head and neck cancer.* Berlin: Springer-Verlag, 1989.

9. **Maxillary sinus.** In *American Joint Committee on Cancer: AJCC cancer staging manual* (5th edn). Philadelphia, PA: Lippincott–Raven, 1997: 47–52.

10. **Howard DJ, Lund VJ.** Surgical options in the management of nose and sinus neoplasia. In *Tumours of the upper jaw* (ed. DFN Harrison, VJ Lund). Edinburgh: Churchill Livingstone, 1993: 329–36.

11. **Howard DJ, Lund VJ.** The mid-facial degloving approach to sino-nasal disease. *Journal of Laryngology and Otology*, 1992; **106**: 1059–62.

12. **Dropkin MJ, Malgady RG, Scott DW, Oberst MT, Strong EW.** Scaling of disfigurement and dysfunction in post-operative head and neck patients. *Head and Neck Surgery*, 1983; **6**: 559–70.

13. **Manderson RD.** Prosthetics in head and neck surgery. In *Head and neck surgery Part 2* (4th edn) (ed. IA McGregor, DJ Howard). London: Butterworth–Heinemann, 1992: 576–92.

14. **Tjellstrom A.** Osseo-integrated systems and their application in the head and neck. *Archives of Otolaryngology, Head and Neck Surgery*, 1989; **3**: 39–70.

15. **Roa WHY, *et al.*** Results of primary and adjuvant CT-based 3-dimensional radiotherapy for malignant tumours of the paranasal sinuses. *International Journal of Radiation Oncology, Biology and Physics*, 1994; **28**: 857–65.

16. **Martel MK, *et al.*** Dose-volume complication analysis for visual pathway structures of patients with advanced paranasal sinus tumours. *International Journal of Radiation Oncology, Biology and Physics*, 1997; **38**: 273–84.

17. **Wang CC.** *Radiation therapy for head and neck neoplasms.* New York: John Wiley, 1997.

18. **Howard DJ, Lund VJ.** Reflections on the management of adenoid cystic carcinoma of the nose and paranasal sinuses. *Otolaryngology—Head and Neck Surgery*, 1985; **93**: 338–40.

19. **Wong CS, Cummings BS, Elhakim T.** External irradiation of squamous carcinoma of the nasal vestibule. *International Journal of Radiation Oncology, Biology and Physics*, 1986; **12**: 1943–6.

20. **Levendag PC, Pomp J.** Radiation therapy of squamous cell carcinoma of the nasal vestibule. *International Journal of Radiation Oncology, Biology and Physics*, 1990; **19**: 1363–7.

21. **Mak ACA, van Andel JG, van Woerkan.** Radiation therapy for carcinoma of the nasal vestibule. *European Journal of Cancer*, 1980; **16**: 81–5.

22. **Haynes WD, Tapley N.** Radiation treatment of cancer of the nasal vestibule. *American Journal of Roentgenology, Radiation and Therapeutic Medicine*, 1974; **120**: 595–612.

23. **Waldron JN, *et al.*** Ethmoid sinus cancer: twenty-nine cases managed with primary radiation therapy. *International Journal of Radiation Oncology, Biology and Physics*, 1998; **41**: 361–9.

24. **Harbo G, *et al.*** Cancer of the nasal cavity and paranasal sinuses. A clinico-pathological study of 277 patients. *Acta Oncologica*, 1997; **36**: 45–50.

25. **Jakobsen MH, Larsen SK, Kirkegaard J, Hansen HS.** Cancer of the nasal cavity and paranasal sinuses. Prognosis and outcome of treatment. *Acta Oncologica*, 1997; **36**: 27–31.

26. **Roux, *et al.*** Ethmoid sinus carcinomas: results and prognosis after neoadjuvant chemotherapy and combined surgery—a 10-year experience. *Surgical Neurology*, 1994; **42**: 98–104.

27. **Lund VJ, Lloyd GAS, Howard DJ, Cheesman AD, Phelps PD.** Enhanced magnetic resonance imaging and subtraction techniques in the post-operative evaluation of craniofacial resection of sino-nasal malignancy. *Laryngoscope*, 1996; **106**: 553–8.

28. **Lund VJ.** Papillomas of the nasal cavity and paranasal sinuses. In *Tumours of the upper jaw* (ed. DFN Harrison, VJ Lund). Edinburgh: Churchill Livingstone, 1993: 73–80.

29. **Jacobs J, *et al.*** Induction chemotherapy in advanced head and neck cancer. A Radiation Therapy Oncology Group Study. *Archives of Otolaryngology—Head and Neck Surgery*, 1987; **113**: 193–7.

30. **Choi K, *et al.*** Locally advanced paranasal sinus and nasopharynx tumours using hyperfractional radiation and concomitant infusion cisplatin. *Cancer*, 1991; **67**: 2748–52.

31. **Schuller D, *et al.*** Preoperative chemotherapy in advanced resectable head and neck cancer. Final report of The South West Oncology Group. *Laryngoscope*, 1988; **98**: 1205–11.

32. **Knegt P, *et al.*** Carcinoma of the paranasal sinuses. *Cancer*, 1985; **62**: 1–5.

9.4 Tumours of the nasopharynx

Roberto Molinari, Cesare Grandi, Laura Lozza, Silvana Pilotti, and Gabriella Della Torre

The nasopharynx is the site of origin of various benign and malignant tumours. There are many histological types, but usually one or two predominate in a series. Among the benign tumours, only juvenile angiofibroma is prevalent, whereas undifferentiated carcinoma, squamous-cell carcinoma, and lymphomas account for almost 95 per cent of malignancies.

From the clinical point of view, nasopharyngeal carcinoma has a peculiar natural history and a good response to radiation treatment, thus giving it distinctive features among head and neck cancers.

Anatomy and anatomical relationships

The nasopharynx is part of the upper respiratory passage, intercalated between the nasal and oropharyngeal cavities (Fig. 1). The lateral walls are in close relationship with the upper parapharyngeal space and the skull base, where the internal carotid artery enters the carotid canal from the anterior foramen lacerum to the interior of the skull. In addition to the internal carotid artery and jugular vein, the region also contains several nervous formations: motor branches to the peristaphylin and pterygoid muscles, the IXth, Xth, XIth, and XIIth cranial nerves, the sympathetic trunk, and the otic ganglion.

Other anatomical structures surround the nasopharynx: anteriorly the ethmoid and, through this, the medial wall of the orbit and the antrum; and superiorly, the sphenoid sinus, whose lateral walls are in strict relation to the cavernous sinuses and their contents (VIth, IVth, IIIrd ophthalmic nerves) (Fig. 2).

Histopathology

Carcinomas are the predominant nasopharyngeal malignancy. Except for a small number of adenocarcinomas, adenoid cystic carcinomas, and other rare types, malignant epithelial tumours are represented essentially by nasopharyngeal carcinoma. In spite of its relative frequency, this carcinoma has provoked a longstanding controversy about its subdivision into distinct histological subtypes and their clinical significance.[1]–[4] The World Health Organization (WHO) classification subdivides nasopharyngeal carcinoma into three variants

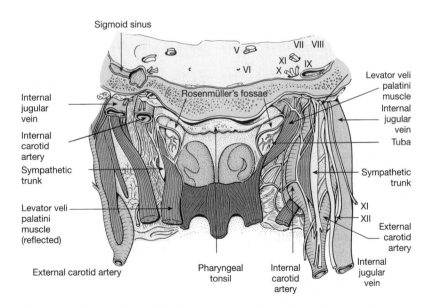

Fig. 1 Frontal section of the cranium through the nasopharynx showing the anatomical relationships with surrounding structures, with particular emphasis on the pharyngeal recess and upper parapharyngeal spaces and their content. V, sensitive branches of the trigeminal nerve; VI, abducent nerve; VII, facial nerve; VIII, vestibular and cochlear nerves; IX, glossopharyngeal nerve; X, vagus nerve; XI, accessory spinal nerve; XII, hypoglossal nerve.

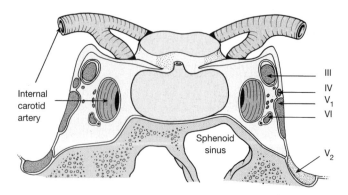

Fig. 2 Frontal section through the cavernous sinus, with the course of the first cranial nerves in its lateral walls. III, oculomotor nerve; IV, trochlear nerve; V$_{1-2}$, first and second branches of the trigeminal nerve; VI, abducent nerve.

according to the predominant histological pattern: keratinizing, non-keratinizing, and undifferentiated types. On the basis of electron-microscopic findings, all types may be regarded as variants of squamous-cell carcinoma.[5]

The three histological variants of nasopharyngeal carcinoma may be reduced to two—squamous-cell carcinoma (*i*) and undifferentiated carcinoma (*i* and *iii*)—for clinical and prognostic purposes. In contrast to squamous-cell carcinoma, undifferentiated carcinoma of naso-phyaryngeal type (**UCNT**) is characterized by occurrence at a younger age, the smaller size of the primary tumour, more extensive cervical lymph-node involvement, higher radiosensitivity, better survival when analysed by stage, and late recurrences. Recurrences are more common in cervical lymph nodes for UCNT than in the primary site as for squamous-cell carcinoma.[6]

From the aetiological point of view, all three varieties of naso-pharyngeal carcinoma appear to be Epstein–Barr virus (EBV)-related.[7] The availability of recombinant EBV DNA fragments as probes for Southern blot analysis showed that all types of naso-pharyngeal carcinoma (*i*, *ii*, and *iii*), and not only UCNT,[8]–[10] contain EBV DNA, even though the number of genome equivalents is high in UCNT and low in squamous-cell carcinoma.[7]

Epidemiology

Nasopharyngeal carcinoma and especially UCNT show striking pe-culiarities as regards several features: geographical distribution, racial and hereditary factors, aetiological agents, including EBV, and en-vironmental factors such as dietary habits, exposure to household carcinogens, plant extracts, and chronic nasal infections.

Geographical distribution of nasopharyngeal carcinoma

The incidence of nasopharyngeal carcinoma in different countries throughout the world shows striking variability.[11] Chinese pop-ulations show the highest incidence in the world, with rates that are 15 to 30 times higher than those found in most other populations. Nasopharyngeal carcinoma is also very frequent in other regions of South-east Asia, among Chinese emigrants in other countries, and in a few scattered regions of the world.

Emigrant Chinese populations in several countries continue to show a remarkably higher incidence of nasopharyngeal carcinoma (approximately 20-fold in the United States) than the respective indigenous populations. In Chinese born abroad, these rates are lower than for those born in China and tend to further decrease in subsequent generations. In contrast, racial groups at low risk for the carcinoma and residing in high-risk countries do not show any increase in incidence.

All these remarks indicate, besides racial factors, an interference by environmental agents.

Race and heredity

Racial factors cannot be considered as directly chromosome linked. Like most cancers, nasopharyngeal carcinoma can be assumed to arise as a consequence of genetically determined responses to environmental stimuli. A strong association has been found between specific *HLA-A* gene types and nasopharyngeal carcinoma.[12]

Environmental factors

For many years, dietary habits have been put forward as an explanation of the high incidence rates in some populations. Cantonese salted fish consumed in Hong Kong by the Chinese population since childhood was found to increase the risk for nasopharyngeal car-cinoma by a factor as high as 17 times compared with non-con-sumers.[13],[14]

Household exposure to fumes in poorly ventilated homes has also been suspected to be a risk factor, as has exposure to fumes, smoke, and chemicals in the environment.

Special mention should be made about a series of studies on herbs and plants that are widespread in China and some African regions and used for medical purposes. In particular, phorbol and related diterpene esters, which are present in Euphorbiaceae and Thymelaceae, have been extensively investigated. Their role in nasopharyngeal carcinoma could be linked to their ability to activate latent EBV genomes in previously infected cells.[15]

EBV and nasopharyngeal carcinoma

In comparison to all other head and neck cancers, nasopharyngeal carcinoma stands out for the unique feature of a 100 per cent association with a latent EBV infection. Many studies have been performed to elucidate the mechanisms of viral carcinogenesis (see Chapters 2.2 and 2.9). There is cumulative evidence that tumorigenesis of nasopharyngeal carcinoma follows a multigene/multistage process and is of clonal evolution.[16] Specific genetic changes on multiple chromosomes have been found, involving the locus of various tumour-suppressor genes, also including overexpression of *ras*, c-*myc*, and *bcl*-2, enhancing cell proliferation and cell survival.[17] Whether specific genetic changes follow the development of latent EBV infection or precede it is debated, as is how EBV enters nasopharyngeal carcinoma cells or other epithelial cells. EBV DNA in invasive nasopharyngeal carcinoma was found be present in a clonal population of cells, and, more interestingly, even in preinvasive lesions.[18] Such findings are consistent with the hypothesis that EBV infection is a very early, and possibly initiating, event in the development of nasopharyngeal carcinoma.

Immunological reactions

The EBV genome inside infected cells codes for several molecular antigenic complexes,[19] including enzymes useful for viral DNA replication. In the latent state, only small parts of the genome are transcribed, expressing nuclear antigens (EBNA, Epstein–Barr nuclear antigens) and lymphocyte-determined membrane antigens. After reactivation of the viral genome and during a productive cycle, additional parts of the genome (approximately 40 per cent) are actively transcribed. During the early replicative stage, early antigens (EA) and DNA enzymes (DNA polymerase and deoxyribonuclease), both necessary for viral DNA synthesis, are synthesized. EA consist of restricted and diffuse (d) components, based on their different location in the infected cells and sensitivity to methanol fixation. In the late replicative stage, two major late antigens, viral capsid antigen (VCA) and membrane antigens (MA), are identified. The antigens are indispensable for the formation of virions.[20]

Almost all patients with diagnosed nasopharyngeal carcinoma, particularly UCNT, carry EBV genomes in tumour epithelial cells[7],[8],[21] and exhibit a broad spectrum of serum antibodies to EBV antigens. Such antibodies are characteristic of the disease and differ from those seen in healthy individuals previously infected with EBV. The main serological features of nasopharyngeal carcinoma are the antibody response to the d component of the EA antigenic complex[20] and the almost uniform presence of IgA antibodies[22] to VCA and often also to the diffuse component of early antigens (EAd). Antibodies to EA are detectable during acute EBV infection and then disappear as the virus enters a phase of latency. In contrast, antibodies to other antigens (VCA and EBNA) remain elevated during viral latency.[23] The reappearance of anti-EA antibodies signals viral reactivation, and their presence in patients with nasopharyngeal carcinoma suggests that an active viral replication is associated with or closely precedes the tumour. Like the anti-EAd antibody response, EBV-related IgA antibodies are very rarely observed in healthy controls.

A vast literature describes the serological screening for IgG and IgA antibodies to VCA and EAd in patients with nasopharyngeal carcinoma, and proves the value of their determination as a means of early detection and monitoring of the tumour.[24] Serological examinations, mainly done by immunofluorescence, have indicated that positivity for anti-VCA IgG antibodies is very high in patients with nasopharyngeal carcinoma and in healthy individuals. This response is not diagnostically useful owing to its low specificity. In contrast, for the anti-VCA IgA antibodies, a high percentage (more than 90 per cent) of patients are positive compared to almost none of the normal individuals. Similarly, anti-EAd IgG antibodies are present in 80 to 85 per cent of patients, but they are less specific than anti-VCA IgA. For the anti-EAd IgA antibodies, only approximately 50 to 70 per cent of patients are positive, whereas normal individuals lack IgA to the antigen. Thus, no single antibody differentiates clearly between patients and healthy controls, and all three antibodies should be determined to obtain an optimal diagnostic evaluation. The anti-VCA IgA response provides the best combination between sensitivity and specificity, and the anti-EAd IgA response is the most specific but the least sensitive. It has been observed that, in high-risk populations, anti-EAd IgA antibodies can only be detected in anti-VCA IgA-positive individuals. However, only a small percentage of anti-VCA IgA-positive individuals eventually become anti-EAd IgA-positive. Moreover, the specificity of the test is high with newer immunoenzymatic and immunoautoradiographic methods,[25] which have revealed anti-EAd IgA antibodies in 80 and 96 per cent of patients with nasopharyngeal carcinoma, respectively. The anti-EAd IgA test can therefore be used to complement the anti-VCA IgA test and both antibodies may serve as specific screening markers for the carcinoma. The usefulness of their determination has been demonstrated in mass surveys in endemic areas of China,[26],[27] with detection of nasopharyngeal carcinoma at a very early stage.

The titres of the various antibodies in nasopharyngeal carcinoma are dependent on the entity of tumour burden, as reflected by the stage of the disease and the treatment given.[28] When the tumour in the primary or metastatic sites is successfully treated, anti-VCA IgG titres decline, whereas the corresponding IgA as well as anti-EAd IgG and IgA may become gradually undetectable. When the tumour responds only transiently or partially to treatment, the patients maintain or develop high antibody titres and the increases are noted well in advance of the detection of recurrent tumours or metastases.

Natural history of nasopharyngeal carcinoma

Local growth and spread

All malignant tumours of the nasopharynx initially grow asymptomatically, with different tendencies to early infiltration depending on their histological type. Squamous keratinizing carcinoma shows the maximum propensity for local aggressiveness, with rapid infiltration of the bone, although its growth may be slower than that of UCNT. UCNT can also rapidly invade the bone, but the most frequent route of spread is through the lateral wall of the nasopharynx, with early invasion of the upper parapharyngeal space.

During their growth and local spread, all nasopharyngeal tumours progressively invade several surrounding structures, causing a complex and variable series of signs and symptoms. If treatment is unsuccessful, death by local progression may be due to several causes: massive haemorrhage from rupture of the internal carotid artery; thrombosis of the same artery or of the cavernous sinus with thromboembolism; invasion of the brain with endocranial hypertension; pathological fracture of the base of the skull; and involvement of the upper spinal cord.

Lymphatic spread

Lymph-node metastases are very frequent in malignant tumours of the nasopharynx and are commonly the first sign of the illness. It is difficult to assess the frequency of involvement of the upper retropharyngeal lymph nodes in the absence of high-definition, computed tomography (CT) or magnetic resonance imaging (MRI). The first palpable node metastases are usually located in the subdigastric and upper spinal lymph nodes, between the mastoid and the posterior edge of the mandible. From these nodes, metastatic spread can follow, separately or frequently contemporaneously, the route of the jugular chain or the lymphatic chain along the accessory spinal nerve (posterior triangle).

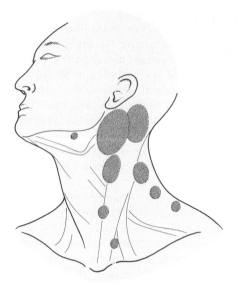

Fig. 3 Distribution of neck node metastases in nasopharyngeal carcinoma. The size of the nodes is proportional to the frequency of involvement of the different lymph-node groups.

The distribution and frequency of neck node metastases in naso-pharyngeal carcinoma are peculiar (Fig. 3). A common feature of the metastases is a progressive downward involvement of multiple echelons, as far as the supraclavicular lymph nodes. From these, axillary and mediastinal neck nodes may also be reached. Inguinal lymph-node metastases can also occur. Table 1 lists the frequency of neck node metastases from nasopharyngeal carcinoma at the time of diagnosis as reported in several published series.

The lymphatic spread of nasopharyngeal carcinoma is frequently bilateral, not only when the primary tumour spans the midline, but also when it seems to be strictly unilateral. Within the single lymph node, metastatic growth can reach considerable size, more frequently than in other head and neck cancers. The growth of metastatic lymph nodes may be very slow and a patient may have borne an asymptomatic mass in the neck for several years by the time a diagnosis of nasopharyngeal carcinoma is made.

Distant metastases

At autopsy,[37] metastases from nasopharyngeal carcinoma have been found with the same frequency (nearly 50 per cent of cases) in liver and bones, in 38 per cent in the lung, and in 10 per cent in the spleen. During the course of the disease, the first clinical manifestation of distant metastases is usually in the bones. This is probably because in this location metastases are symptomatic earlier and easier to detect than in the liver.

Unusual locations of metastases have been described. Apart from direct involvement by the primary tumour, no case of brain metastasis has been recorded.[38]

Distant metastases have been reported with variable frequency in the literature. They are rare at the time of diagnosis in almost all published series (3 to 9 per cent). In contrast, distant metastases occur with increasing frequency during the course of the disease, even after successful treatment of the primary tumour and neck nodes, but mainly in the case of locoregional recurrence. Table 2 summarizes the rates of appearance of distant metastases, alone or combined with locoregional recurrences, in the most substantial published series.

In spite of a certain variability from series to series, the frequency of distant spread is significantly higher than in other head and neck cancers. A correlation with nodal metastases has been demonstrated:

Table 2 Appearance of distant metastases, alone or combined with locoregional relapses

Reference	Total no. of cases	Percentage with metastases
Bedwinek and Perez[39]	111	34.0
Brugère et al.[30]	122	20.0
Chen and Fletcher[40]	181	27.6
Ellouz et al.[31]	733	62.0
Hoppe et al.[41]	113	11.5
Hsu and Tu[42]	966	22.2
Huang et al.[43]	1206	13.0
Petrovich et al.[44]	256	36.0
Qin et al.[45]	1379	48.2

Table 1 Frequency and main features of clinical neck node metastases at diagnosis in several series

Reference	No. of cases	Neck nodes (%)	Bilateral (%)	Fixed (%)
Ahmad and Stefani[29]	256	80.5	28.5	51.0
Brugère et al.[30]	296	74.0	NR	50.0
Ellouz et al.[31]	939	79.0	51.0	63.0
Huang[32]	1605	78.6	48.0	NR
Mesic et al.[33]	131	88.0	45.0	NR
Molinari et al.[34]	410	71.2	40.5	33.3
Pontvert et al.[35]	139	68.0	NR	44.0
Vikram et al.[36]	107	73.1	30.0	NR

NR, not reported.

particularly the lower the level of involved neck nodes, the higher the rate of distant metastases.[6],[31],[38],[46],[47]

The probability of haematogenous spread is also related to the histological type. UCNT has the highest metastatic rate, followed by adenoid cystic carcinoma and adenocarcinoma, then squamous-cell carcinoma.

Duration of the disease

Nasopharyngeal carcinoma, and especially UCNT, have clinical courses that can be very different. In some cases the disease evolves very rapidly, with early involvement of multiple lymph nodes in all levels of the neck, the appearance of distant metastases, and death within a year. More frequently, UCNT has a more indolent course, with local recurrence 3 to 5 years after radiation treatment of the primary. Relapses occurring after 7 or 8 years are not unusual.[32],[38]

Characteristics of the patients

Age

UCNT can occur at all ages, although it shows a specific peak in the fifth decade. In some countries (for example, Tunisia),[31],[48] two peaks of incidence have been found, in infancy and in middle age, but the finding has not been reported for other countries. Squamous-cell carcinoma is prevalent in patients late in life, especially in women.

Sex

The male:female ratio is 2:1 or 3:1 in almost all series, especially in those countries where nasopharyngeal carcinoma is frequent. Like all head and neck cancers, the ratio can be 1:1 or even 1:2 in northern Europe.

Clinical history and symptoms

Early symptoms and signs

Owing to the anatomical structure and site of the nasopharynx, any tumour there can grow initially with no symptom or sign, except for the relatively uncommon onset on the tubal ostium or in its vicinity. Unilateral hearing loss is the most frequent first local symptom reported by the patient when an accurate case history is obtained.

Bleeding is also a common initial sign, although real epistaxis is rare. The finding of postnasal bleeding during examination or traces of blood in a nasal mucous discharge should be considered very significant for an early diagnosis.

Nasal obstruction is very common but not really an early symptom.

In countries where nasopharyngeal carcinoma is uncommon, it is not rare to see patients treated for a long time with anti-inflammatory therapies or even operated on (polypectomy, nasal septum surgery, transtympanic drainage) before a correct diagnosis is made.

Cervical adenopathy is perhaps the most frequent first sign of nasopharyngeal carcinoma reported in the literature. It is typically in the upper part of the neck, deep under the sternomastoid muscle, but subdigastric nodes are also frequently involved first.

Diagnostic work-up

Local clinical examination

An exhaustive examination of the nasopharynx is mandatory, especially in the presence of symptoms or signs even remotely suggestive of a nasopharyngeal tumour.

When the only sign in asymptomatic patients is an enlarged neck node, the eventual primary lesion is presumably small and examination of the nasopharynx should be extremely thorough. Even under local anaesthesia, anatomical reasons or a patient's poor cooperation can hamper a correct view. In the past, several devices have been set up to overcome such difficulties. At present, they have been substituted by cold-light fibre-optic endoscopes, which may be rigid or flexible. Two models of rigid endoscopes exist: one large, the other thin (Fig. 4). The advantage of the large type is its magnification power (3 ×), which allows a complete view of the entire cavity from only one viewpoint. It should be used exactly as a laryngoscope, rotated for 180 degrees upward, introduced through the mouth, in contact with the posterior pharyngeal wall. Surface anaesthesia is useful but unnecessary in many cases. The thin, rigid model is introduced through the nasal cavities after surface local anaesthesia.

The flexible, thin nasopharyngolaryngoscope is introduced through the nasal cavities and positioned in the nasopharynx, where its tip may be orientated to explore the entire cavity. An important advantage of some models is the possibility of directly taking aimed biopsies by means of a small forceps inserted into the instrument.

Biopsy is mandatory in any case. It can be done under local anaesthesia with forceps introduced through the mouth (upward angled forceps) or the nasal cavity (right forceps). Mounting a small cotton or gauze swab on the same forceps allows the collection of adequate material for cytological examination. Biopsy is not always a simple procedure, especially in the presence of small lesions where the aim is difficult and swabbing the entire cavity can be advantageous. At present, flexible endoscopes with forceps ensure a correct histological diagnosis in practically all cases.

Visualization of the nasopharynx is sometimes very difficult or even impossible for anatomical reasons or psychological distress. In such cases, the patient should be examined under general anaesthesia. Although in this way visualization of nasopharyngeal lesions is more imprecise, palpation and multiple biopsies are greatly facilitated.

Radiodiagnostic work-up

An accurate radiological examination of head and neck structures is extremely important for a reliable assessment of tumour extension and nodal involvement. The accuracy of the investigation is an essential premise for a correct staging and adequate irradiation.

All conventional radiological examinations used in the past should be considered obsolete since they can only detect large tumours filling the nasopharynx or evident bone involvement. Once the diagnosis of nasopharyngeal tumour is made or even suspected, CT scan is today considered the minimum level of radiological study mandatory for staging and treatment planning.[49],[50] However, its prime role mainly depends on problems of cost and availability of other imaging techniques, such as MRI (Fig. 5(a), (b)). In fact, CT has some limitations due to a relative lack of sensitivity in detecting skull-base involvement, perineural infiltration, and early intracranial spread. These weak points of CT are the strengths of MRI, so that the two

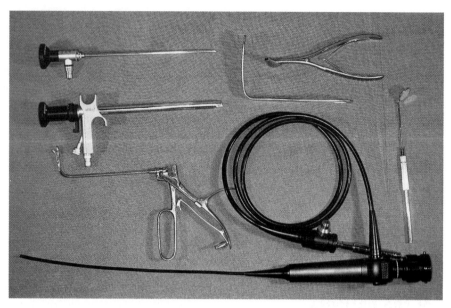

Fig. 4 Updated equipment for nasopharyngeal examination and biopsy.

methods should be considered complementary. MRI is more sensitive than CT in detecting bone marrow changes in the skull base, although it has some limitation in discriminating between neoplastic infiltration, inflammatory reactions, or a combination of both. In addition, MRI is far more sensitive than CT in the detection of perineural tumour spread, especially along the branches of the trigeminal nerve (V2 and V3) (foramen ovale).[49] CT can easily detect early cortical erosion of the skull base, which is best seen with high-resolution bone windows. Dural involvement can be detected earlier with MRI than with CT.[51]

Newer, functional imaging techniques such as positron emission tomography (PET), single photon emission computed tomography (SPECT) and magnetic resonance spectroscopy imaging (MRSI) can provide additional biological information regarding tumour metabolic activity and physiological state.[52]

Additional examinations

Other examinations should be planned when a nasopharyngeal carcinoma has been diagnosed. These are indicated in Table 3. A thorough examination of the entire neck is always necessary. All palpable nodes should be recorded on a map, noting their side, size, location by levels, and characteristics (mobility or fixation). In the presence of nodes in the lower level, palpation of the axillae is also opportune.

A lymph-node biopsy frequently precedes the diagnosis of naso-pharyngeal carcinoma. Its histological features are often so typical that the primary tumour is sought in the nasopharynx.

Besides the clinical examination, ultrasonography and, mainly, CT scan can be very helpful in staging the disease. Fine-needle aspiration biopsy is sometimes useful for such a purpose, especially in the case of unusual locations of some nodes or for a more precise staging (doubtful nodes in supraclavicular or axillary fossae).

Serological investigation can reveal the existence of high titres of anti-EBV antibodies in patients with nasopharyngeal carcinoma. It can therefore be used in difficult cases to exclude or confirm the existence of a tumour, for example in the case of neck node metastases from poorly differentiated or undifferentiated carcinoma with an unknown primary origin.

An exhaustive staging of nasopharyngeal carcinoma requires the search for possible distant metastases, which have some frequency of occurrence even at the onset, especially in UCNT. Systematic diagnostic work-up should include chest radiographs, a liver ultrasound scan, and a bone scintiscan.

Prognostic factors

The knowledge and weight of the prognostic factors are essential to define a valid clinical classification. Nasopharyngeal carcinoma has many peculiar characteristics that distinguish it from all other head and neck malignancies. Such differences are so important that most of the features used for other neoplasms are inadequate for this tumour.

Host-related factors

Age

There is almost general agreement in the literature about an inverse correlation between age and survival.[34],[45],[53] The significance of the factor varies from series to series but is uniformly very high in univariate and multivariate analyses. The only debated point is the evaluation of disease in childhood (under 15 years of age). This category of patients is usually treated by paediatric oncologists, who report the disease as particularly aggressive so that a multimodal treatment is usually recommended.[54],[55]

Tumour-related factors

Histology

The 5-year specific and overall survival is significantly better in groups 2 and 3 of the WHO classification than in group 1 (squamous-cell carcinoma), in univariate and in multivariate analyses.

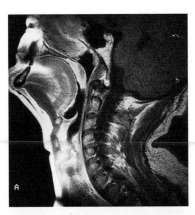

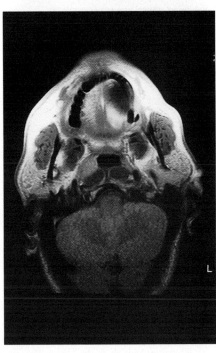

Fig. 5 Midplane sagittal (a) and axial (b) MRI scans showing a nasopharyngeal carcinoma.

Table 3 Diagnostic work-up for nasopharyngeal carcinoma

History
  Duration
  Symptoms

Physical examination (head and neck)
  Indirect (or direct) nasopharyngoscopy
  Neck palpation
  Biopsy (on T, N, T + N), cytology
  Cranial nerve evaluation
  External ear inspection

Radiological imaging
  Locoregional
    Lateral tomography (basic approach)
    CT scan of nasopharynx, base of skull, neck (after diagnosis of nasopharyngeal
      carcinoma), or skull-base tomograms
    MRI (for special cases)
  General
    Chest radiograph
    Liver scintiscan (in more advanced cases)
    Bone scintiscan (in more advanced cases)
    Bone radiography (in symptomatic patients or with a positive
      scintiscan)

Laboratory studies
  Haematological analyses (WBC, RBC, alkaline phosphatase, liver function
    studies, etc.)
  EBV serology (VCA-IgA, EAd-IgG, etc.)
  Bone marrow biopsy (in more advanced cases)

Primary tumour extent

The advent of imaging techniques has prompted reliable means to directly evaluate the extent of the primary tumour outside the nasopharyngeal cavity, which is present in two-thirds of the cases. A significant difference at multivariate analysis was found only between intrinsic nasopharyngeal cancers (previous T1 and T2 lesions, now grouped in the T1 category) and tumours extending outside the nasopharynx.[53] Bone erosion (paranasal sinuses and base of the skull) shows a moderately negative impact on local control. Involvement of cranial nerves, intracranial extension, and invasion of the orbit, oropharynx and/or infratemporal fossa are associated with a significantly worse prognosis in all outcome aspects.

Regional extent

Level: extension to the lower neck is a highly significant prognostic factor, with 30 to 50 per cent of patients developing distant metastases.

Laterality: there is no difference between ipsilateral or contralateral neck node involvement, whereas bilateral metastasis implies worse nodal control and survival.

Multiplicity: there is no difference in regional control rates, but distant failures and survival are worse in the case of multiple node metastases.

Fixation: patients with fixed nodes have a significantly worse prognosis than those whose nodes are not fixed, but such a factor may be correlated with size.

Size: differences in survival are found to depend on size, but they are very significant only for neck metastases greater than 6 cm in diameter.[56]

Distant metastases

The significance of the factor is overwhelming. However, some recent reports[57] have shown that survival can be relatively prolonged by chemotherapy.

Titres of anti-EBV cytotoxic antibodies

The initial titre of commonly tested EBV antibodies (VCA, EAd, EBNA-IgA, IgG) did not show a strong prognostic influence after adequate locoregional treatment. However, an increase in EA-IgA and IgG in complete responders during follow-up is highly predictive of relapses.[58] Neel *et al.*[59] reported a significant relationship between titres of antibody-dependent cellular cytotoxicity and survival. This

Table 4 UICC classification of nasopharyngeal cancer

T:	*primary tumour*	
	Tis:	*In situ* carcinoma
	T1:	Tumour confined to nasopharynx
	T2:	Tumour extending outside the cavity to soft tissues of oropharynx and/or nasal fossae
		T2a: Without parapharyngeal extension
		T2b: With parapharyngeal extension
	T3:	Tumour invading bony structures and/or paranasal sinuses
	T4:	Tumour with intracranial extension and/or involvement of cranial nerves, extension to infratemporal fossa, hypopharynx or orbit
N:	*regional lymph nodes*	
	Nx:	Regional lymph nodes cannot be assessed
	N0:	No regional lymph-node metastasis
	N1:	Unilateral metastasis in lymph node(s), less than 6 cm in the greatest dimension, above supraclavicular fossa
	N2:	Bilateral metastases in lymph node(s), less than 6 cm in the greatest dimension, above supraclavicular fossa
	N3:	Metastases in lymph node(s)
		(a) more than 6 cm in greatest dimension
		(b) in the supraclavicular fossa

Stage grouping

Stage	0:	Tis N0 M0
	I:	T1 N0 M0
	IIA:	T2a N0 M0
	IIB:	T1 N1 M0
		T2a N1 M0
		T2b N0, N1 M0
	III:	T1 N2 M0
		T2a–b N2 M0
		T3 N0,N1,N2 M0
	IVA:	T4 N0,N1,N2 M0
	IVB:	any T, N3 M0
	IVC:	any T, any N, M1

From Sobin and Wittekind.[11]

is related to the presence of high titres of anti-EBV antibodies (VCA) of the IgG class and seems to show a favourable prognostic influence.[60]

Clinical classification

More clinical classifications have been created for nasopharyngeal carcinoma than for any other cancer of the head and neck. During the past 20 years, a progressive succession of technological improvements has involved endoscopic instrumentation (various fibre-optic devices) and imaging systems (CT, MRI), thereby allowing an earlier diagnosis and more accurate evaluation of the local extent of the primary tumour into soft tissues and bone and the involvement of neck nodes, including retropharyngeal nodes. Meanwhile, a more thorough knowledge of clinical and histological prognostic factors and a more objective retrospective comparison of the long-term results achieved in very large series treated around the world have settled some divergencies existing between the previous clinical classifications, mainly regarding the criteria used in staging lymphatic spread.

The UICC[11] has recently elaborated a new classification which represents a reasonable assembling of most relevant prognostic factors related to the extent of the disease (Table 4). The main variations deal, first of all, with the procedures to be applied for the definition of T and N categories. Besides clinical examination, imaging is mandatory as the only tool fit for the evaluation of extra-nasopharyngeal extensions, which is the key to the classification of the primary tumour.

The efficiency of the new UICC TNM classification system is still to be demonstrated in large series of patients, with special regard to the stage-grouping categories.

About this point, two recent studies have presented a scoring method to identify categories of patients with different risks of dying from the disease. Both studies have many conclusions in common.[59],[61] Table 5 presents the classification of the Milan group which attempts to join an anatomical description of the tumour (classical TN stage) with a prognostic score.

Treatment

Treatment of benign nasopharyngeal tumours or those of low-grade malignancy is almost always surgical, with various approaches and technical procedures. In contrast, primary surgery is not indicated in nasopharyngeal carcinoma for various reasons. First, it has very few chances of resulting in radical removal of the primary tumour and neck metastases, owing to the hardly accessible location of the former and the frequency of clinical and subclinical involvement

Table 5 Classification with a prognostic score as proposed by the Istituto Nazionale Tumori of Milan

	Score
A: Age	
A_0 = Patient 50 years or younger	0
A_1 = Patient older than 50 years	1
H: Histology	
H_0 = Undifferentiated carcinoma	0
H_1 = Differentiated carcinoma	1
Stage of primary	
T_0 = Tumour confined to the nasopharynx	0
T_1 = Tumour extended beyond the nasopharynx	1
N: nodal involvement	
N_0 = No clinically positive node	0
N_1 = Clinically positive nodes at the first or second level of the neck	1
N_2 = Clinically positive nodes at more levels or at the third level of the neck	2
Prognostic groups	
Stage	
0 = Sum of the scores 0	
1 = Sum of the scores 1	
2 = Sum of the scores 2	
3 = Sum of the scores 3	
4 = Sum of the scores 4 or 5	

From Grandi et al.,[61] with permission.

of retropharyngeal nodes on both sides. Second, nasopharyngeal carcinoma shows a high radioresponsivity and a good radiocurability, although high doses are required for a satisfactory locoregional control. Surgery can reasonably succeed in radically removing only small primary lesions, which are easily controlled by radiotherapy.

As regards neck metastases, they show the same radioresponsivity as the primary, whereas their surgical removal with standard neck dissection gives rise to several problems: retropharyngeal nodes are not removed, the dissection is frequently done bilaterally, with few reasonable indications for functional procedures, a correct planning of the following radiotherapy can be hampered and, finally, the patient will face the sum of all possible late complications of both approaches. As a consequence, radiotherapy represents the major modality of primary treatment.

Chemotherapy had been used in the past for palliative treatment of recurrent or metastatic nasopharyngeal carcinomas. Many drugs had been tested alone and methotrexate (MTX), doxorubicin (ADM), bleomycin (BLM), 5-fluorouracil (5-FU), mytoxantrone, epirubicin (EpiADM) showed a certain activity. Higher response rates were achieved using combination schemes, and cisplatin (CDDP) + 5-FU, CDDP + ADM, CDDP + EpiADM + BLM showed the strongest activity, with up to 80 per cent complete (CR) and partial response (PR) rates.[62],[63] A number of these chemotherapy courses were subsequently used as the primary treatment in locoregionally advanced cases and were followed by standard radiotherapy. At the end of a full combined treatment, the final response rates seemed to be higher than those achieved with radiotherapy alone in historical series. Based on such remarks, and in accordance with the results achieved in other head and neck cancers, chemotherapy was introduced in a

multimodality approach for the treatment of more advanced cases, especially aiming at preventing distant metastases. Since the second half of the 1980s, several phase II studies have been conducted[64],[65] using sequential neoadjuvant chemotherapy and, more recently, concurrent radiochemotherapy.

First-line radiotherapy

During the last 15 years, there have been several technical improvements, which have had a true impact on allowing concentration of the dose to the primary and its regional spread area, without increasing the rate of complications. Precision in the pretreatment staging of patients affected with nasopharyngeal carcinoma represents the basic step to successful treatment.[66] The fast evolution of accurate tumour imaging has certainly helped the adjustment of more refined treatment planning with optimization of the ratio of tumour-to-normal tissue volume in the radiation field.[49],[67],[68] Thanks to the possibility of beam shielding with fashioned blocks and of checking the treatment volume by means of control port films, geographic misses are avoided and the dose to the neighbouring structures (temporal lobes, brainstem and spinal cord, pituitary gland, eyes, and oral cavity) is reduced.

Perhaps in the future, integration of the data obtained from different sophisticated imaging modalities (such as PET, SPECT, and MRSI) into the treatment planning system will improve the accuracy in determining a tumour's target volume.[69] Recent developments in CT and MRI, as well as software and hardware technology for three-dimensional (3D) radiotherapy treatment planning and treatment delivery, have allowed the realization of 3D conformal radiotherapy.[70]

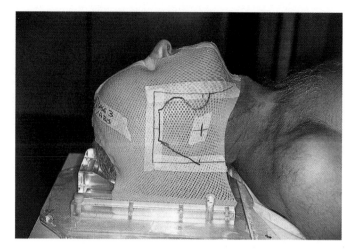

Fig. 6 The patient is immobilized in an individual moulded thermoplastic shell, which allows a quick, accurate, and reproducible set-up. Treatment marking can also be drawn on the shell, sparing skin tattoos.

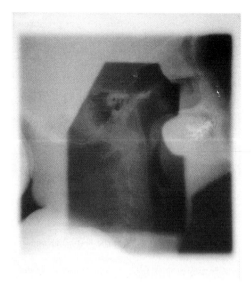

Fig. 7 Localization film of upper lateral portal showing shieldings for the oral cavity and brainstem.

It is a very complex technique used to deliver a high radiation dose to a volume conforming to the 3D shape of the tumour target volume, allowing the possibility for tumour dose escalation with respect to the surrounding normal tissues. Such technical characteristics make 3D conformal radiotherapy a very interesting tool when planning the treatment of an area with a very complex anatomy, such as the nasopharynx and surrounding normal tissues.[71] Whether the improvements in treatment planning will result in increased local control and survival should be evaluated in phase III studies.

Multiple arch stereotactic irradiation with 4- to 6-MV linear accelerators[72],[73] and brachytherapy, realized by means of radioactive seed implants (gold-198, cobalt-60) or self-designed endocavitary applicators (iridium-198, caesium-137), also make it possible to customize the dose distribution around complex lesions and to spare critical tissues close to the tumour.[74],[75] Both the techniques can be used when a boost is required after the initial radiotherapy.

Even if each centre has its own methods of treatment according to their experience, planning facilities, devices for patient positioning and field shaping (Fig. 6), and ultimately the ability of the staff to realize a highly accurate treatment, some mandatory rules for correct radiation planning have been clearly defined and can be applied to practically all cases of nasopharyngeal carcinoma.[33],[41],[45],[76]–[78] Only very early and definitely limited lesions may be candidates for less extensive radiological treatment. The primary tumour is generally treated to a total dose of 64 to 72 Gy with two opposed lateral fields. The margins of the fields must be wide and encompass every direct extension of the tumour, as evaluated with CT or MRI, to reduce the risk of marginal recurrences. A third anterior field is used when the tumour has a marked anterior or nasal extension. The upper lymphatic stations, retropharyngeal and subdigastric, are treated within the lateral fields. After 40 to 45 Gy, the spinal cord is shielded and the posterior nodes are treated with electron beams. The lower neck and supraclavicular area are irradiated with a single anterior field matched with the lateral fields: a median shield protects the larynx and the spinal cord. When a dose of 50 Gy is reached, the initially involved lymph nodes are boosted to 65 to 70 Gy. Fields are adequately shaped at the beginning of treatment and carefully modified during its course

(Figs 7 and 8(a,b)). To reduce the incidence of toxicity, single daily doses do not exceed 1.8 to 2 Gy.

Evaluation of the response to radiotherapy is very important during the treatment and after its completion. A reliable indication of the definitive response can be made 3 to 4 weeks after the end of treatment, when mucosal reactions begin to reduce and minor residual disease in the nasopharynx or cervical nodes have progressively disappeared.

An additional dose of between 10 and 25 Gy, if required, is usually given through endocavitary brachytherapy (Fig. 9(a,b)) or by means of external multiple fields.[74],[77],[79]–[81] In the case of residual cervical adenopathy at the end of treatment, an additional dose can be given to a small volume with photons or electrons, but the surgical approach should be evaluated as an alternative chance.

The importance of overall radiotherapy time in determining local control, particularly in patients with advanced disease, has been strongly emphasized in retrospective studies, and the negative impact of an increase in total treatment time has been pointed out.[82]–[84] A continuous course of irradiation over 7 to 8 weeks, five fractions a week, is considered more effective than a split-course treatment.[85] An interruption of 10 to 15 days may be necessary only in cases of severe and painful mucositis, which is usually complicated by a mycotic infection, and an adjustment of the total dose is consequently suggested for these patients. Because lengthening the course of radiotherapy has been shown to reduce the therapeutic results, accelerated fractionation (two or three fractions per day, smaller fraction dose, and shorter overall treatment time, maintaining the total dose the same as in conventional fractionation) has been tested in selected patients, aiming to overcome the tumour proliferation that persists during radiotherapy and to improve local control and survival.[86]–[88]

A dose–control relationship has also been demonstrated,[89] and it is now a rule to consider the extension of the disease before planning the total dose: T1 N0–1 patients are generally treated to 64 to 66 Gy (54 Gy to the initial target volume plus a boost of 14 to 16 Gy), whereas higher doses to 70 to 72 Gy (a boost of 16 to 18 Gy after

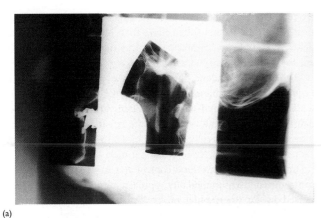

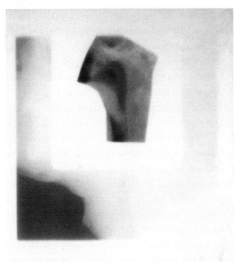

Fig. 8 (a) Simulation radiograph showing reduced lateral portals to deliver additional dose to residual tumour in the nasopharynx. (b) Localization film of the same portal.

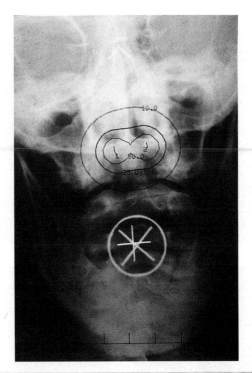

(a)

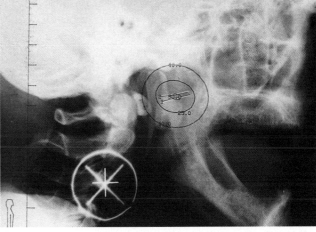

(b)

Fig. 9 (a) and (b) Radiographs illustrate an intracavitary application in the nasopharynx with two iridium sources. Superimposed is the isodose curve showing the dose rate (cGy/h).

54 Gy) are recommended in more advanced disease. An unacceptable rate of complications was reported when more than 90 Gy were given.[90] A 5 per cent reduction dose may be applied to undifferentiated carcinoma because of its greater radiosensitivity.

Acute and late toxicity

Despite efforts to limit toxicity, some radiation-induced side-effects cannot be avoided. Patients need careful and frequent examination during the treatment. Poor appetite, modified salivary gland function, alterations of taste, and mucosal injury are the main causes of weight loss: adequate diet and hydration should be maintained. Pain, bacterial and fungal infection that may occur need to be promptly treated. All patients should be submitted to dental evaluation prior to radiotherapy and informed on prophylactic measures to reduce subsequent dental problems.[91]–[93]

In adequately treated patients, radiotherapy for nasopharyngeal carcinoma is not without late complications due to the large volume of irradiation generally applied. When coping with symptoms suggesting radiation damage, every effort must be made to exclude other possible causes, tumour recurrence in particular. Mucous membranes, muscles, bones, subcutaneous tissues, and the central nervous system may be involved. Almost all patients suffer for xerostomia. Trismus, caused by fibrosis of masseter muscles and the temporomandibular joint, is particularly frequent and affects between 10 and 15 per cent of patients. Otological complications are also common, and persistent sensorineural hearing loss develops in about 24 per cent of irradiated patients.[94]

Less frequent late effects, related to the type of fractionation, the dose of radiation, and the size of the fields or to re-irradiation, may be necrosis of the temporal bones and of the mandibular angle, fibrosis of cervical soft tissues, encephalopathy, myelitis, palsy of posterior cranial nerves, and ocular lesions.[95]–[97] Disorders of the hypothalamic–pituitary axis are often detectable only by biological

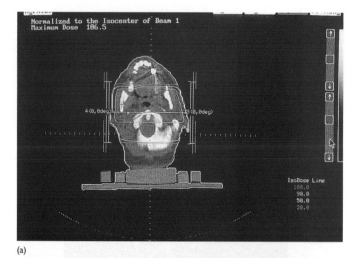

Normalized to the Isocenter of Beam 1
Maximum Dose 106.5

IsoDose Line
100.0
90.0
50.0
20.0

(a)

IsoDose Line
6000.0
5700.0
5400.0
4500.0

(b)

Fig. 10 (a) and (b) Examples of dose distribution for lateral portals with 6 MV photons to deliver definitive irradiation to a nasopharyngeal carcinoma. A total dose to 70 Gy can be given to the target with reducing fields. (See also Plate 1.)

tests.[(33),(98)] Radiation-induced malignancies, mostly osteosarcomas, have been reported.[(99)]

Owing to the evolution and refinement of treatment techniques and dose calculation, and above all the development of CT-based dosimetry planning, severe treatment-related complications are increasingly more uncommon (Fig. 10(a, b) and Plate 1).

Results of therapy

Because of the progress in imaging and irradiation techniques in recent years,[(66),(83)] locoregional control and overall survival rates have improved.

Considering all stages, the 5- and 10-year survival rates are about 50 per cent and 40 per cent, respectively (Table 6). For undifferentiated carcinomas results are even better, with a survival rate between 20 and 30 per cent higher than that for squamous-cell carcinomas.[(33),(56),(103)]

An impressive discrepancy in data is seen in the literature, and evaluations are difficult, especially when old series are compared with

more recent ones. Moreover, when the impact on survival of well-known prognostic factors (often more than one are present in each patient) is considered, complex statistical models are required to assess the actual influence of a single factor.

With radiotherapy alone, the prognosis at 10 years for T1 to T2 N0 squamous-cell carcinoma is good, with 85 per cent local control and less than 10 per cent distant failure. Different probability of local and distant failure depends on the tumour extent, the local recurrence rate being greatly increased in the case of T3 to T4 tumours and the distant spread in that of N2 to N3 nodal metastases.

In an effort to improve local control and survival, chemotherapy was introduced in a multimodality approach for the treatment of more advanced disease, where a high probability of micrometastases at presentation is known. Recently, a controlled study of 339 patients,[(104)] comparing induction chemotherapy with cisplatin, epirubicin, and bleomycin followed by radiotherapy to radiotherapy alone, showed an advantage for the use of neoadjuvant chemotherapy, with a significant difference in disease-free survival (47 per cent in the chemoradiotherapy arm versus 30 per cent in the radiotherapy arm) but not in overall survival. However, there is a need for staging information regarding the patient selection in this study.

The value of chemotherapy after definitive radiotherapy has also been tested,[(63),(105)] but it still needs to be clarified. The only randomized study on adjuvant chemotherapy reported no benefit in terms of relapse-free and overall survival when six courses of chemotherapy were added to radiation.[(106)] It was noted that the chemotherapy regimen employed did not include cisplatin, and the drug doses administered may be considered insufficient by current standards.

Concurrent chemotherapy and radiotherapy is another approach to consider in treating locally advanced nasopharyngeal carcinoma: its rationale is based on the sensitivity of the neoplasm to chemotherapy and radiation as well as to the radiosensitizing actions of some agents, such as cisplatinum and 5-fluorouracil. An advantage when cisplatinum was used concomitantly with radiotherapy has been shown in a few studies.[(63),(107),(108)]

Recently, a randomized RTOG study[(109)] compared radiotherapy alone to a combination of cisplatin and fluorouracil given during and after radiotherapy: a statistical superiority of the chemoradiotherapy arm in progression-free and overall survival was found: 46 per cent 3-year survival rate in the radiotherapy arm versus 76 per cent in the chemoradiotherapy arm.

Even though it is still unclear whether this advantage is due to concomitant or adjuvant chemotherapy, as a result of this study a combined approach in locoregional advanced nasopharyngeal cancer (T4 and/or N2–N3) should be considered the standard treatment at a level 2 of evidence. Owing to the high toxicity of the concurrent regimen, a careful patient selection and available supportive measures are prerequisites before starting such a treatment.

The optimal combination of chemotherapy and radiotherapy must be confirmed in well-designed trials, which requires the collaboration of medical and radiation oncologists.

At a level 4 of evidence, the standard treatment in the case of more limited lesions (T1–T2–T3, N0–N1) still remains radiotherapy alone.

Management of recurrences

Despite the good radioresponsivity of nasopharyngeal carcinoma, large fields of irradiation, and high total doses to the primary tumour

Table 6 Survival rates reported in the literature

Reference	No. of cases	Stage	5-year survival (%)
Chen and Fletcher[40]	229	All	35
Hsu and Tu[42]	966	All	43
Huang et al.[43]	1032	All	56
		I, II, III	79, 63, 44
Mesic et al.[33]	251	All	52
Grandi et al.[61]	410	All	53
Qin et al.[45]	1379	I, II, III, IV	86, 59, 45, 29
Lee et al.[100]	4128	All	43 (10-year)
Olmi et al.[101]	165 (1978–1991)	All	53
	143 (1960–1978)	All	41
Perez et al.[102]	143	All	40 (10-year)

area and to nodal sites of the whole neck, a substantial number of cases (between 15 and 30 per cent) present local and/or regional recurrences, most of them diagnosed within 2 years of treatment. Regular follow-up needs accurate clinical examination and imaging assessment and may detect early relapses that are still salvageable. The optimal re-treatment modality remains to be established.

Recurrence of the primary tumour can be treated with surgery or a second radiation treatment. Surgery is rarely feasible, with limitations depending on the site and size of the recurrence and on the initial extent of the tumour (bone or intracranial involvement, extrapharyngeal spread). Different surgical approaches have been attempted: transpalatal,[110] transpalatal and cervical,[111] infra-temporal,[112] transtemporal,[113] anterolateral with maxillary swing,[114] and cervicomandibular.[115] All these experiences dealt with relatively few cases and reported 2- or 3-year survival rates higher than those achieved with radiotherapy re-treatment. However, the selection of patients as candidates for surgical salvage was very restrictive and hardly comparable to the series of cases receiving a second radiation treatment, which included more heterogeneous clinical situations. The surgical treatment is affected by different degrees of complications and late consequences depending on the technique used.

When patients are unsuitable for surgery, a second course of radiotherapy should be considered because of the exceptional radiosensitivity of the disease, despite the risk of additional side-effects.[116],[117] The target should be very carefully defined through CT and MRI, and treatment planning should consider multiple, small portals, adequately tailored according to the characteristics of the previous treatment and the present situation, the patient's general condition, and the availability of equipment and expertise. Published results are encouraging, showing 25 to 35 per cent of patients to be alive and disease-free at 5 years after the second course of radiotherapy.[118],[119]

A dose of at least 50 Gy should be given with conventional fractionation, external radiotherapy. Higher doses are limited by the surrounding normal tissues that have already been compromised by the previous irradiation. However, by means of brachytherapy it is possible to deliver a booster dose to mainly mucosal disease with a markedly reduced dose to the critical tissue. Due to the fact that brachytherapy cannot give a sufficient dose to tumours distant from the radioactive source, patients with deep-seated lesions, such as the skull base or the cavernous sinus, can today be treated with stereotactic radiotherapy, which allows selective irradiation of deep and irregular structures.[73] Because of the multiple arching around the isocentre in a 3D setting, normal tissues are spared to an extent that has never been achieved before in classical irradiation practice.[120]

Neck node recurrences are usually accessible to radical surgery (radical neck dissection), which provides good results.[34],[110] Even if a re-irradiation of the neck is not usually recommended because of the high incidence of complications, for patients who are unsuitable for surgery or when disease cannot be completely resected, small volumes of the neck can be given a second irradiation by means of external radiotherapy or brachytherapy.

Recently, the role of particle beam radiotherapy has been tested in a small series of patients with recurrent disease: the modality seems to be effective, but it is expensive, limited in availability, and not feasible for most patients.[121] The actual trend in recurrent disease is to add chemotherapy, including cisplatinum, to radiotherapy in order to achieve the best tumour control.[122] In summary, there is no standard indication for recurrent disease, and each treatment must be individualized according to the particular clinical situation and previous therapies.

Radiotherapy of metastases

The distant metastasis rate is between 20 and 35 per cent at 5 years, and it is correlated with the T and N stage. Most of the failures occur during the first 3 years after treatment and commonly affect the bone (20 per cent), lung (13 per cent), and liver (9 per cent).[29],[123] A high response rate (70 to 80 per cent) has been demonstrated with cisplatinum-based combination chemotherapy,[124],[125] offering a good palliative treatment choice, with a small but constant (10 per cent) proportion of long-term, disease-free survivors. Radiotherapy can play an important role again, mainly for painful bone lesions, bulky adenopathies, spinal cord compression, and obstructive jaundice. A palliative dose of between 36 and 40 Gy, according to the clinical situation, can improve the quality of life of the patients.

Conclusions

Advances in technology have allowed accurate determination of disease extent and high-quality radiation dosimetry and treatments, but some effort is still needed to reduce the incidence of failures for nasopharyngeal carcinoma. Several approaches to enhance the efficacy of radiation have been tested: altered fractionated radiotherapy and the use of combined chemoradiotherapy after the introduction of cisplatinum have shown promising results and are being extensively investigated.

Grouping patients according to their risk of local or distant spread is essential when conducting future clinical trials: different types of local therapy intensification (altered fractionation, radiation dose escalation by conformal radiotherapy, intracavitary or stereotactic boost) and concurrent chemoradiotherapy should be addressed to patients with the highest risk of local relapse, whereas patients at high risk for distant spread are more suitable for testing the efficacy of new chemotherapy regimens.

As regards therapy of locally or regionally recurrent disease, many possibilities are available: for residual or recurrent cervical nodes, neck dissection is the current treatment and the results reported are quite good.

Re-irradiation of local recurrence is still the standard therapy, even though surgical salvage of local failure (which was considered only exceptionally in the past) has been re-evaluated in selected cases.

The complexity of management of the disease is well known: only the cooperation of a multidisciplinary team, where specific competencies of surgeons and medical and radiation oncologists are continuously shared, can give the patients the best results.

References

1. Liang PC, Chen CC, Chu CC, Hu YF, Chu KM, Tsung YS. The histopathologic classification, biologic characteristics and histogenesis of nasopharyngeal carcinoma. *Chinese Medical Journal*, 1962; **81**: 629–58.

2. Yeh S. A histological classification of carcinomas of the nasopharynx with a critical review as to the existence of lymphoepitheliomas. *Cancer*, 1962; **15**: 895–920.

3. Shanmugaratnam K. The pathology of nasopharyngeal carcinoma: a review. In *Oncogenesis and herpes viruses II* (ed. PM Biggs, G de-Thé, LN Payne). Lyon: IARC, 1972: 239–48.

4. Micheau C, Rilke F, Pilotti S. Proposal for a new histopathological classification of the carcinomas of the nasopharynx. *Tumori*, 1978; **64**: 513–18.

5. Gazzolo L, de-Thé G, Vuillaume M, Ho HC. Nasopharyngeal carcinoma. Ultrastructure of normal mucosa, tumor biopsies, and subsequent epithelial growth *in vitro*. *Journal of the National Cancer Institute*, 1972; **48**: 73–86.

6. Zucali R, Milani F. Storia naturale dei carcinomi della rinofaringe. In *I. Tumori della testa e del collo* (ed. U Veronesi, E Bocca, R Molinari, H Emanuelli). Milan: Casa Editrice Ambrosiana, 1979: 243–54.

7. Raab-Traub N, *et al.* The differentiated form of nasopharyngeal carcinoma contains Epstein–Barr virus DNA. *International Journal of Cancer*, 1987; **39**: 25–9.

8. Wolf H, zur Hausen H, Becker V. EB viral genomes in epithelial nasopharyngeal carcinoma cells. *Nature (New Biology)*, 1973; **244**: 245–7.

9. Pagano JS, Huang CH, Klein G, de-Thé G, Shanmugaratnam K, Yang CS. Homology of Epstein–Barr virus DNA in nasopharyngeal carcinomas from Kenya, Taiwan, Singapore, and Tunisia. In *Oncogenesis and herpes viruses II* (ed. G de-Thé, MA Epstein, H zur Hausen). Lyon: IARC, 1975: 179–90.

10. Andersson-Anvret M, Forsby N, Klein G. Relationship between the Epstein–Barr virus genome and nasopharyngeal carcinoma in Caucasian patients. *International Journal of Cancer*, 1979; **23**: 762–7.

11. Sobin L, Wittekind C. *UICC-TNM classification of malignant tumours* (5th edn). New York: Wiley–Liss, 1997.

12. Chan SH, Day NE, Kunara T, Nam N, Chia KB, Simons MJ. HLA and nasopharyngeal carcinoma in Chinese. A further study. *International Journal of Cancer*, 1983; **32**: 171–6.

13. Ho JHC. An epidemiologic and clinical study of nasopharyngeal carcinoma. *International Journal of Radiation Oncology, Biology, Physics*, 1978; **4**: 183–98.

14. Huang DP, Ho JHC. Salted fish and nasopharyngeal carcinoma. In *Carcinogens and mutagens in the environment*, Vol. II: *Natural occuring compounds* (ed. HF Stich). Boca Raton, FL: CRC Press, 1982.

15. Ito Y. Vegetable activators of the viral genome of EBV and the causation of Burkitt's lymphoma and nasopharyngeal carcinoma. In *The Epstein–Barr virus: recent advances* (ed. MA Epstein, BG Achong). London: Heineman Medical, 1986: 207–36.

16. Jiang X, Sao KT. The clonal progression in the neoplastic process of nasopharyngeal carcinoma. *Biochemical and Biophysical Research Communications*, 1996; **221**: 122–8.

17. Lu QL, Elia G, Lucas S, Thomas JA. Bcl-2 protooncogene expression in Epstein–Barr virus-associated nasopharyngeal carcinoma. *International Journal of Cancer*, 1993; **53**: 29–35.

18. Pathmanathan R, Prasad U, Sadler R, Flynn K, Raab-Traub N. Clonal proliferation of cells infected with Epstein–Barr virus in pre-invasive lesions related to nasopharyngeal carcinoma. *New England Journal of Medicine*, 1995; **333**: 693–8.

19. Ooka T. The molecular biology of Epstein–Barr virus. *Biomedicine and Pharmacotherapy*, 1985; **39**: 59–66.

20. Henle G, Henle W, Klein G. Demonstration of two distinct components in the early antigen complex of Epstein–Barr virus-infected cells. *International Journal of Cancer*, 1971; **8**: 272–83.

21. Desgranges C, *et al.* Nasopharyngeal carcinoma. X. Presence of Epstein–Barr genomes in separated epithelial cells of tumours in patients from Singapore, Tunisia and Kenya. *International Journal of Cancer*, 1975; **16**: 7–15.

22. Henle G, Henle W. Epstein–Barr virus-specific IgA serum antibodies as an outstanding feature of nasopharyngeal carcinoma. *International Journal of Cancer*, 1976; **17**: 1–7.

23. Henle G, Henle W, Horowitz CA. Antibodies to Epstein–Barr virus-associated nuclear antigen in infectious mononucleosis. *Journal of Infectious Diseases*, 1974; **130**: 231–9.

24. Glaser R, Zhang HY. The importance of viral markers in the study of Epstein–Barr virus-associated illness. *Bulletin de l'Institut Pasteur*, 1989; **85**: 189–200.

25. Zeng Y, Gong CH, Jan MG, Fun Z, Zhang LG, Li HY. Detection of Epstein–Barr virus IgA/EA antibody for diagnosis of nasopharyngeal carcinoma by immunoautoradiography. *International Journal of Cancer*, 1983; **31**: 599–601.

26. Zeng Y, *et al.* Serological mass survey for early detection of nasopharyngeal carcinoma in Wuzhou City, China. *International Journal of Cancer*, 1982; **29**: 139–41.

27. de-Thé GB, Zeng Y. Population screening for EBV markers: toward improvement of nasopharyngeal carcinoma control. In *The Epstein–Barr virus: recent advances* (ed. MA Epstein, BG Achong). London: Heinemann Medical, 1986: 247–9.

28. Henle W, Ho JHC, Henle G, Chau JCW, Kwan HC. Nasopharyngeal carcinoma: significance of changes in Epstein–Barr virus-related antibody patterns following therapy. *International Journal of Cancer*, 1977; **20**: 663–72.

29. Ahmad A, Stefani S. Distant metastases of nasopharyngeal carcinoma. A study of 256 male patients. *Journal of Surgical Oncology*, 1986; **33**: 194–7.

30. Brugère J, Eschwège F, Schwaab G, Micheau C, Cachin Y. Les

carcinomes du nasopharynx (cavus): aspects cliniques et évolutifs. *Bulletin du Cancer*, 1975; **62**: 319–30.

31. Ellouz R, *et al.* Le cancer du cavum en Tunisie. Paper presented at the XV Congrès Medical Maghrèbien. Institut Salah Azaiz, Tunis, 1986.

32. Huang SC. Nasopharyngeal cancer: a review of 1605 patients treated radically with cobalt 60. *International Journal of Radiation Oncology, Biology, Physics*, 1980; **6**: 401–7.

33. Mesic JB, Fletcher GH, Goepfert H. Megavoltage irradiation of epithelial tumors of the nasopharynx. *International Journal of Radiation Oncology, Biology, Physics*, 1981; **7**: 447–53.

34. Molinari R, Grandi C, Boracchi P, Mezzanotte G, Marubini E. Prognostic factors in nasopharyngeal carcinoma. Uni- and multivariate analysis of 410 cases from a multicentric study. In *Head and neck oncology research* (ed. GT Wolf, TE Carey). Kugler, Amsterdam; Berkeley/Ghedini Editor, Milan. 1988: 495–504.

35. Pontvert D, Bataini P, Brugère J, Jaulerry C, Brunin F. Carcinomes du rhinopharynx de l'adulte. *Bulletin du Cancer*, 1987; **74**: 415–25.

36. Vikram B, Strong EW, Manolatos S, Mishra UB. Improved survival in carcinoma of the nasopharynx. *Head and Neck Surgery*, 1984; **7**: 123–8.

37. Teoh TB. The pathologist and surgical pathology of head and neck tumours. *Journal of the Royal College of Surgeons of Edinburgh*, 1971; **16**: 117–34.

38. Choa G. Cancer of the nasopharynx. In *Cancer of the head and neck* (ed. JY Suen EN Myers). New York: Churchill Livingstone, 1981: 372–414.

39. Bedwinek JM, Perez CA. Carcinoma of nasopharynx. In *Principles and practice of radiation oncology* (ed. CA Perez, LW Brady). Philadelphia, PA: Lippincott, 1987: 479–98.

40. Chen KY, Fletcher GH. Malignant tumors of the nasopharynx. *Radiology*, 1971; **99**: 165–71.

41. Hoppe RT, Williams J, Warnke R, Goffinet DR, Bagshaw MA. Carcinoma of the nasopharynx—the significance of histology. *International Journal of Radiation Oncology, Biology, Physics*, 1978; **4**: 199–205.

42. Hsu MM, Tu SM. Nasopharyngeal carcinoma in Taiwan: clinical manifestation and results of therapy. *Cancer*, 1983; **52**: 362–8.

43. Huang SC, Lui LT, Lynn TC. Nasopharyngeal cancer: study III. A review of 1206 patients treated with combined modalities. *International Journal of Radiation Oncology, Biology, Physics*, 1985; **11**: 1789–93.

44. Petrovich Z, Cox JD, Middleton R, Ohanian M, Paige C, Jepson J. Advanced carcinoma of the nasopharynx. 2. Pattern of failure in 256 patients. *Radiotherapy and Oncology*, 1985; **4**: 15–20.

45. Qin D, *et al.* Analysis of 1379 patients with nasopharyngeal carcinoma treated by radiation. *Cancer*, 1988; **61**: 1117–24.

46. Ho JHC. *Stage classification of nasopharyngeal carcinoma: a review.* Lyon: IARC Scientific Publications, 1978: No. 20, 99–113.

47. Baker SR, Wolfe RA. Prognostic factors of nasopharyngeal malignancy. *Cancer*, 1982; **49**: 163–9.

48. Cammoun M, Hoerner GV, Mourali N. Tumors of the nasopharynx in Tunisia. *Cancer*, 1974; **33**: 184–92.

49. Chong VFH, Fan YF. Skull base erosion in nasopharyngeal carcinoma: detection by CT and MRI. *Clinical Radiology*, 1996; **51**: 625–31.

50. Chong VFH, Fan YF. Pterygopalatine fossa and maxillary nerve infiltration in nasopharyngeal carcinoma. *Head and Neck*, 1997; **19**: 121–5.

51. Eisen MD, Yousem DM, Montone T. Use of preoperative MR to predict dural, perineural and venous sinus invasion of skull base tumors. *American Journal of Neuroradiology*, 1996; **17**: 1937–45.

52. Kuszyk BS, Ney DR, Fishman EK. The current state of the art in three dimensional oncologic imaging: an overview. *International Journal of Radiation Oncology, Biology, Physics*, 1995; **33**: 1029–39.

53. Teo P, *et al.* Significant prognosticators after primary radiotherapy in 903 nondisseminated nasopharyngeal carcinomas evaluated by computed tomography. *International Journal of Radiation Oncology, Biology, Physics*, 1996; **36**: 291–304.

54. Lobo-Sanahuja F, Garcia I, Carranza A, Camacho A. Treatment and outcome of undifferentiated carcinoma of the nasopharynx in childhood: a 13-year experience. *Medical and Pediatric Oncology*, 1986; **14**: 6–11.

55. Gasparini M, Lombardi F, Rottoli L, Ballerini E, Morandi F. Combined radiotherapy and chemotherapy in stage T$_3$ and T$_4$ nasopharyngeal carcinoma in children. *Journal of Clinical Oncology*, 1988; **6**: 491–4.

56. Sanguineti G, *et al.* Carcinoma of the nasopharynx treated by radiotherapy alone: determinants of local and regional control. *International Journal of Radiation Oncology, Biology, Physics*, 1997; **37**: 985–96.

57. Cvitkovitch E. UCNT: chemocurable sometimes, but not very often. *Annals of Oncology*, 1997; **8**: 723–5.

58. de Vathaire F, *et al.* Prognostic value of EBV markers in the clinical management of nasopharyngeal carcinoma (NPC): a multicenter follow-up study. *International Journal of Cancer*, 1988; **42**: 176–81.

59. Neel HB III, Taylor WF, Pearson GR. Prognostic determinants and a new view of staging for patients with nasopharyngeal carcinoma. *Annals of Otology, Rhinology, and Laryngology*, 1985; **94**: 529–37.

60. Neel HB III, Pearson GR, Taylor WF. Antibody-dependent cellular cytotoxicity: relation to stage and disease course in North American patients with nasopharyngeal carcinoma. *Archives of Otolaryngology*, 1984; **110**: 742–7.

61. Grandi C, *et al.* Analysis of prognostic factors and proposal of a new classification for nasopharyngeal cancer. *Head and Neck Surgery*, 1990; **12**: 31–40.

62. Bachouchi M, *et al.* High complete response in advanced nasopharyngeal carcinoma with bleomycin, epirubicin and cisplatin before radiotherapy. *Journal of the National Cancer Institute*, 1990; **82**: 616–20.

63. Tsuji H, *et al.* Improved results in the treatment of nasopharyngeal carcinoma using combined radiotherapy and chemotherapy. *Cancer*, 1989; **63**: 1668–72.

64. Geara FB, *et al.* Induction chemotherapy followed by radiotherapy versus radiotherapy in patients with advanced nasopharyngeal carcinoma. *Cancer*, 1997; **79**: 1279–86.

65. Chan AT, Teo PM, Leung Tw, Johnson PJ. The role of chemotherapy in the management of nasopharyngeal carcinoma. *Cancer*, 1998; **82**: 1003–12.

66. Olmi P, *et al.* Computed tomography in nasopharyngeal carcinoma. Part I: T stage conversion with CT staging. Part II: Impact on survival. *International Journal of Radiation Oncology, Biology, Physics*, 1990; **19**: 1171–82.

67. Sham JST, *et al.* Nasopharyngeal carcinoma: CT evaluation of patterns of tumor spread. *American Journal of Neuroradiology*, 1991; **12**: 265–70.

68. Olmi P, Fallai C, Colagrande S, Giannardi G. Staging and follow-up of nasopharyngeal carcinoma: magnetic resonance imaging vs computerized tomography. *International Journal of Radiation Oncology, Biology, Physics*, 1995; **32**: 795–800.

69. Sailer SL, *et al.* Improving treatment planning accuracy through multimodality imaging. *International Journal of Radiation Oncology, Biology, Physics*, 1996; **35**: 117–24.

70. Emarni B, *et al.* 3D conformal radiotherapy in head and neck cancer. The Washington University experience. *Frontiers of Radiation Therapy and Oncology*, 1996; **29**: 207–20.

71. Kutcher GJ, *et al.* Three-dimensional photon treatment planning for carcinoma of the nasopharynx. *International Journal of Radiation Oncology, Biology, Physics*, 1991; **21**: 169–82.

72. Kondziolka D, Lundsford LD. Stereotactic radiosurgery for squamous cell carcinoma of the nasopharynx. *Laryngoscope*, 1991; **101**: 519–22.

73. Cmelak AJ, *et al.* Radiosurgery for skull base malignancies and

nasopharyngeal carcinoma. *International Journal of Radiation Oncology, Biology, Physics,* 1997; **10:** 2241–9.

74. Wang CC. Improved local control of nasopharyngeal carcinoma after intracavitary brachytherapy boost. *American Journal of Clinical Oncology. Cancer Clinical Trials,* 1991; **14:** 5–8.

75. Rong JM. Preliminary study on HDR brachytherapy for nasopharyngeal carcinoma. *Chinese Journal of Clinical Oncology,* 1994; **21:** 736–9.

76. Cellai E, Chiavacci A, Olmi P. Carcinoma of the nasopharynx. *Acta Radiologica: Oncology,* 1982; **21:**   fasc. 2.

77. Hwang HN. Nasopharyngeal carcinoma in the People's Republic of China: incidence, treatment, and survival rates. *Radiology,* 1983; **149:** 305–9.

78. Perez CA. Nasopharynx. In *Principles and practice of radiation oncology,* 2nd edn. (ed. CA Perez, LW Brady). Philadelphia, PA: Lippincott, 1992: 617–43.

79. Amornmarn R, Prempree T, Selwchand W, Jaiwatana J. Radiation management of advanced nasopharyngeal cancer. *Cancer,* 1983; **52:** 802–7.

80. Vikram B, Hilaris H. Transnasal permanent interstitial implantation in carcinoma of the nasopharynx. *International Journal of Radiation Oncology, Biology, Physics,* 1984; **10:** 153–5.

81. Chang JT, *et al.* The role of brachytherapy in early stage nasopharyngeal carcinoma. *International Journal of Radiation Oncology, Biology, Physics,* 1996; **36:** 1019–24.

82. Fowler JF, Lindstrom MJ. Loss of local control with prolongation in radiotherapy. *International Journal of Radiation Oncology, Biology, Physics,* 1992; **23:** 457–67.

83. Lee AW, *et al.* Effect of time, dose, and fractionation on local control of nasopharyngeal carcinoma. *Radiotherapy and Oncology,* 1995; **36:** 24–31.

84. Kwong DL, *et al.* The effect of interruptions and prolonged treatment time in radiotherapy for nasopharyngeal carcinoma. *International Journal of Radiation Oncology, Biology, Physics,* 1997; **39:** 703–10.

85. Marcial VA, Hanley JA, Chang C, Davis LW, Moscol JA. Split-course radiation therapy of carcinoma of the nasopharynx: results of a national collaborative clinical trial of the Radiation Therapy Oncology Group. *International Journal of Radiation Oncology, Biology, Physics,* 1980; **6:** 409–14.

86. Wang CC. Accelerated hyperfractionated radiation therapy for carcinoma of the nasopharynx. Techniques and results. *Cancer,* 1989; **63:** 2461–7.

87. Ang KK, *et al.* Concomitant boost radiotherapy schedules in the treatment of carcinoma of oropharynx and nasopharynx. *International Journal of Radiation Oncology, Biology, Physics,* 1990; **19:** 1339–45.

88. Overgaard J, *et al.* Conventional radiotherapy as the primary treatment of squamous cell carcinoma of the head and neck. A randomized multicenter study of 5 versus 6 fractions per week. Preliminary report from DAHANCA 7 trial. *International Journal of Radiation Oncology, Biology, Physics,* 1997; **39:** S188.

89. Marks JE, Bedwinek JM, Lee F, Purdy JA, Perez CA. Dose-response analysis for nasopharyngeal carcinoma. An historical perspective. *Cancer,* 1982; **50:** 1042–50.

90. Yan JH, *et al.* Management of local residual primary lesion of nasopharyngeal carcinoma: are higher doses beneficial? *International Journal of Radiation Oncology, Biology, Physics,* 1989; **16:** 1465–9.

91. Horiot JC, *et al.* Dental preservation in patients irradiated for head and neck tumors: a ten-year experience with topical fluoride and a randomized trial between two fluoridation methods. *Radiotherapy and Oncology,* 1983; **1:** 77–82.

92. Copeland EM, Ellis LM. Nutritional management in patients with head and neck malignancies. In *Management of head and neck cancer: a multidisciplinary approach,* 2nd edn (ed. RR Million, NJ Cassisi). Philadelphia, PA: Lippincott, 1994: 193–202.

93. Singh N, Scully C, Joyston-Bechal S. Oral complications of cancer therapies: prevention and management. *Clinical Oncology,* 1996; **8:** 15–24.

94. Grau C, Overgaard J. Postirradiation sensorineural hearing loss: a common but ignored late radiation complication. *International Journal of Radiation Oncology, Biology, Physics,* 1996; **36:** 515–17.

95. Bedwinek JM, Shukovsky LJ, Fletcher GH, Daley TE. Osteonecrosis in patients treated with definitive radiotherapy for squamous cell carcinoma of the oral cavity and naso- and oropharynx. *Radiology,* 1976; **119:** 665–7.

96. Marks JE, Davis CC, Gottsma VL, Purdy JE, Lee F. The effects of irradiation on parotid salivary function. *International Journal of Radiation Oncology, Biology, Physics,* 1981; **7:** 1013–19.

97. Parsons JT. The effects of radiation on normal tissues of the head and neck. In *Management of head and neck cancer: a multidisciplinary approach,* Vol. 14 (ed. RR Million, NJ Cassisi). Philadelphia, PA: Lippincott, 1984: 173–207.

98. Lam KSL, *et al.* Symptomatic hypothalamic–pituitary dysfunction in nasopharyngeal carcinoma patients following radiation therapy: a retrospective study. *International Journal of Radiation Oncology, Biology, Physics,* 1987; **13:** 1343–50.

99. Dickens P, Wei WI, Sham JST. Osteosarcoma of the maxilla in Hong Kong Chinese postirradiation for nasopharyngeal carcinoma: a report of four cases. *Cancer,* 1990; **66:** 1924–6.

100. Lee AW, *et al.* Retrospective analysis of 5037 patients with nasopharyngeal carcinoma treated during 1976–1985. Overall survival and patterns of failure. *International Journal of Radiation Oncology, Biology, Physics,* 1992; **23:** 261–70.

101. Olmi P, Cellai E, Fallai C. Nasopharyngeal carcinoma: an analysis of 308 patients treated with curative radiotherapy. *IVth International IST Symposium: Interaction of chemotherapy and radiotherapy in solid tumors.* Genova, 1992: 27. [Abstract]

102. Perez CA, *et al.* Carcinoma of the nasopharynx: factors affecting prognosis. *International Journal of Radiation Oncology, Biology, Physics,* 1992; **23:** 271–80.

103. Fletcher GH, Million R. Nasopharynx. In *Textbook of radiotherapy,* 3rd edn (ed. GH Fletcher). Philadelphia, PA: Lee and Febiger, 1980: 364–83.

104. VUMCA (International Nasopharyngeal Cancer Study Group). Preliminary results of a randomized trial comparing neoadjuvant chemotherapy (cisplatin, epirubicin, bleomycin) plus radiotherapy vs radiotherapy alone in stage IV (> or = N2, M0) undifferentiated nasopharyngeal carcinoma: a positive effect on progression-free survival. *International Journal of Radiation Oncology, Biology, Physics,* 1996; **35:** 463–9.

105. Rahima M, Rakowsky E, Barzilay J, Sidi J. Carcinoma of the nasopharynx: an analysis of 91 cases and a comparison of differing treatment approaches. *Cancer,* 1986; **58:** 843–9.

106. Rossi A, *et al.* Adjuvant chemotherapy with vincristine, cyclophosphamide and doxorubin after radiotherapy in local-regional nasopharyngeal cancer: results of a 4-years multicenter randomized study. *Journal of Clinical Oncology,* 1988; **58:** 1401–10.

107. Marcial VA, *et al.* Concomitant cisplatin chemotherapy and radiotherapy in advanced mucosal squamous cell carcinoma of the head and neck. *Cancer,* 1990; **66:** 1861–8.

108. Souhami L, Babinowits M. Combined treatment in carcinoma of the nasopharynx. *Laryngoscope,* 1998; **98:** 881–3.

109. Al Sarraf M, *et al.* Chemoradiotherapy versus radiotherapy in patients with advanced nasopharyngeal cancer: phase III randomized Intergroup Study 0099. *Journal of Clinical Oncology,* 1998; **16:** 1310–17.

110. Tu G, Hu Y, Ye N. Salvage surgery for nasopharyngeal carcinoma. *Archives of Otolaryngology, Head and Neck Surgery,* 1988; **114:** 328–9.

111. Fee W, Robertson JB, Goffinet DR. Long-term survival after surgical resection for recurrent nasopharyngeal cancer after radiotherapy

failure. *Archives of Otolaryngology, Head and Neck Surgery*, 1991; **117**: 1233–6.

112. Fish U. The infratemporal approach for nasopharyngeal tumors. *Laryngoscope*, 1983; **93**: 36–44.

113. Panje WR, Gross CE. Treatment of tumors of the nasopharynx: surgical therapy. In *Comprehensive management of head and neck tumors*, Vol. 1 (ed. SE Thawley, WR Panje). Philadelphia, PA: WB Saunders. 1987: 662–3.

114. Wey WI, *et al.* Maxillary swing approach for resection of tumors in and around the nasopharynx. *Archives of Otolaryngology, Head and Neck Surgery*, 1995; **121**: 638–42.

115. Morton RP, Liavaag PG, McLean M, Freeman JL. Transcervico-mandibulo-palatal approach for surgical salvage of recurrent nasopharyngeal cancer. *Head and Neck*, 1996; **18**: 352–8.

116. Pryzant RM, Wendt CD, Delclos L, Peters LJ. Retreatment of nasopharyngeal carcinoma in 53 patients. *International Journal of Radiation Oncology, Biology, Physics*, 1992; **22**: 941–7.

117. Lee AW, *et al.* Reirradiation for recurrent nasopharyngeal carcinoma: factors affecting therapeutic ratio and ways for improvement. *International Journal of Radiation Oncology, Biology, Physics*, 1997; **38**: 43–52.

118. Yan JH, Hu YH, Gu XZ. Radiation therapy of recurrent nasopharyngeal carcinoma: report on 219 patients. *Acta Radiologica: Oncology*, 1983; **22**: 23–8.

119. Wang CC. Re-irradiation of recurrent nasopharyngeal carcinoma treatment techniques and results. *International Journal of Radiation Oncology, Biology, Physics*, 1987; **13**: 953–6.

120. Buatti JM, Friedman WA, Bova FJ, Mendenhall WM. Linac radiosurgery for locally recurrent nasopharyngeal carcinoma: rationale and technique. *Head and Neck*, 1995; **17**: 14–19.

121. Feehan PE, *et al.* Recurrent locally advanced nasopharyngeal carcinoma treated with heavy charged particle irradiation. *International Journal of Radiation Oncology, Biology, Physics*, 1992; **23**: 881–4.

122. Altun M, *et al.* Undifferentiated nasopharyngeal cancer (UCNT). Current diagnosis and therapeutic aspects. *International Journal of Radiation Oncology, Biology, Physics*, 1995; **32**: 859–77.

123. Sham JST, Cheung YK, Chan FL, Choy D. Nasopharyngeal carcinoma: pattern of skeletal metastases. *British Journal of Radiology*, 1990; **63**: 202–5.

124. Choo R, Tannock I. Chemotherapy for recurrent or metastatic carcinoma of the nasopharynx: a review of the Princess Margaret Hospital experience. *Cancer*, 1991; **68**: 2120–4.

125. Chi KH, Chan WK, Cooper DL. A phase II study of outpatient chemotherapy with cisplatinum, 5-fluorouracil, and leucovorin in nasopharyngeal carcinoma. *Cancer*, 1994; **73**: 247–52.

9.5 Oral cavity

Jean-Jacques Mazeron, Cesare Grandi, and Alain Gerbaulet

Anatomy

Externally, the oral cavity includes the upper and lower lips; internally it comprises the floor of mouth, the anterior two-thirds of the tongue, the buccal mucosa, upper and lower gingiva, and the hard palate.

The alveolar ridge of the maxilla, which is covered by the mucosa and the teeth and continues with the hard palate, forms the upper gingiva. The lower gingiva covers the mandible from the gingivobuccal sulcus to the mucosa of the floor of mouth. It continues posteriorly with the retromolar trigone and above with the maxillary tuberosity. The buccal mucosa covers the internal surface of the lips and checks.

The floor of mouth is U-shaped and extends from the anterior inner aspect of the lower gingiva to the insertion of the anterior tonsillar pillar into the tongue. It continues internally with the mobile tongue, which is separated posteriorly of the base of tongue by the circumvallate papillae with a V configuration.

The lymphatics of the upper lip mostly drain to the submaxillary lymph nodes, and occasionally to the periauricular and parotid lymph nodes. The lymphatic drainage of the lower lip is to submaxillary and subdigastric lymph nodes. Lesions located near the midline drain to the submental nodes or to either side of the submaxillary lymph nodes. The lymphatic drainage of the buccal mucosa goes primarily to the submaxillary and subdigastric lymph nodes.

Lymph node drainage of the lower gingiva and floor of mouth goes to submaxillary and subdigastric lymph nodes. Submental nodes are seldom involved. Nodal extension is bilateral in lesions located near or crossing the midline. Primary lymphatic drainage of the oral tongue goes to the subdigastric and submaxillary lymph nodes, and is often bilateral.

Epidemiology and aetiological factors

Thirty-thousand new cases of oral cavity cancers occurred in United States in 1991.[1] In France, 6100 new cases of oral cavity cancers were observed in males and 900 in females between 1983 and 1987. The incidence rates were 25.3/100 000 and 2.7/100 000, and the mortality rates 7.5/100 000 and 1/100 000, respectively. The primary tumours were located in the oral tongue for 37 per cent of patients, floor of mouth for 22 per cent, lip for 11 per cent, salivary glands for 11 per cent, alveolar ridge for 3 per cent, in others sites of the oral cavity in 18 per cent, and site remained unknown for 18 per cent. These rates were slightly higher than in the other European countries in females and markedly higher in males. Between 1981 to 1985 and 1986 to 1990, there were a 3.7 per cent per year decrease

in incidence of tongue cancer in males and a 2.9 per cent per year increase in females, due to a decreased alcohol consumption in male and an increased alcohol consumption in female.

The relation between tobacco exposure and disease development and a dose–response relationship have been demonstrated (see Chapter 9.1.1). The mucosal areas that are exposed to prolonged contact with alcohol are also at increased risk of cancer development

Others factors must be considered. Genetic susceptibility may be the most significant variable. Genetic factors associated with increased risk include mutagen sensitivity, which potentially reflects an underlying DNA repair deficiency. Xeroderma pigmentosum, Fanconi anaemia, and ataxia telangiectasia, all diseases characterized by mutagen sensitivity, have been associated with increased risk of oral cancer.

Additional factors include diet. Vitamin A deficiency is associated with an increased risk for oral cancer, while high consumption of fruit and vegetable is considered to provide a protective effect. Intensive use of mouth wash, poor dental hygiene, syphilis, and marijuana smoking are also considered as risk factors. Herpes simplex type 1 (HSV-1) has been considered as an aetiological factor, but its role in still under discussion. Human papilla virus has also been incriminated.

Pathology

Squamous cell carcinoma represents at least 90 per cent of all oral cavity cancers. Its variants include well differentiated (more than 75 per cent keratinization) to moderately differentiated carcinoma (25–75 per cent keratinization), and poorly differentiated carcinoma (less than 75 per cent keratinization). Additionally, cancers can arise from minor salivary glands, including adenoid cystic, mucoepidermoid, and adenocarcinoma. Rare, soft tissue neoplasm include mucosal melanoma, plasmocytoma, and soft tissue sarcoma. There also exist some cancers arising from bone, including osteosarcoma, and neoplastic lesions that are not truly malignant disorders of bone growth, such as amenoblastoma.

Clinical features

Premalignant lesions

Most frequent locations include the cheek mucosa and the commissures. The borders of the tongue, floor of the mouth, and the alveolar ridge are less commonly involved, while the hard palate and gingiva are seldom involved. Leucoplakia is either localized and well circumscribed or diffuse and multiple. Carcinoma *in situ* or invasive carcinoma may be present, in particular when a burning sensation is reported by the patient.

Oral leucoplakia can be classified as homogenous (flat and non-indurated) or a non-homogenous. The latter, which more often leads to malignant transformation, can be further subdivided into erythroleucoplakia, erosive leucoplakia, nodular leucoplakia, and verrucous leucoplakia.

Malignant lesions

The mean duration of symptoms is approximately 4 to 5 months, ranging from a few weeks to 1 year. Early carcinomas, less than 1 cm, may be asymptomatic and discovered during routine dental examination. They often show erythroplastic changes, without induration. However, most tumours measure more than 1 to 2 cm, are symptomatic, and present as an indurated area of ulceration. They also can be exophytic, papillary, or verrucous. Uncommonly, they can grow submucosally, causing an ulceration at a late stage of the disease.

Lip

Patients often present with an exophytic or ulcerative, slow growing lesion of the vermilion border of the lower lip, which is occasionally associated with bleeding and pain. At a late stage, tumour may involve the skin of the chin, progress along the dental nerve, and extend to the foramen of the mandible, leading to bone destruction. Five to 10 per cent of patients develop nodal involvement.

Alveolar ridge and retromolar trigone

Pain, exacerbated by chewing, is usually the first symptom. Bleeding and loose teeth are less frequent. In edentulous patients, the principal symptom is ill-fitting dentures. These lesions are associated with lymph nodes in approximately 30 per cent of cases, and in 70 per cent for T4.

Floor of the mouth

Cancer of the floor of the mouth typically presents as an exophytic and often painful lesion. These lesions may extend interiorly to bone, deeply infiltrating the muscles, and posteriorly to invade the tongue. Lymph node spread occurs in approximately 10 per cent of T1 lesions, 30 per cent of T2, and 50 per cent of T3–4.

Mobile tongue

Tongue cancer may be exophytic or infiltrative, and is often painful, with occasional difficulties in speech and deglutition. Reduced mobility of the tongue is less common. Evolution is often more rapid than with other oral cancers. An history of lasting leucoplakia may precede the symptoms. Lymph node metastasis is observed in 15 to 75 per cent of cases, and is bilateral in 25 per cent.

Investigations

All patients undergoing resections for oral cancer require a detailed examination of the head and neck region as well as a thorough general physical examination. In addition, routine blood examination is made and a chest radiograph and an electrocardiogram taken. With the exception of patients with very advanced lesions, no routine bone scan or ultrasonographic examination of the liver is indicated, as the risk of liver and bone metastases is very low.

In most patients, especially for tumours of the posterior part of the oral cavity, an examination under general anaesthesia, preferably in combination with panendoscopy in order to rule out synchronous second primary tumours, is made.[2],[3] Panencodoscopy includes bronchial and oesophageal examination with brushing cytological tests and biopsies of any lesion, and a vital staining with toluidine blue. It yields some 2 per cent synchronous tumours, which would not otherwise have been detected at that time. As no major complications are associated with this procedure, it is generally accepted to include it as a part of the initial work-up even in the absence of a demonstrated cost/benefit or cost/efficacy advantage.

Computed tomography (CT) and magnetic resonance imaging (MRI) are both useful. The CT scan shows both soft tissue and bone, and is better than MRI for evaluating nodes. MRI is better in detecting muscle infiltration, because of a better tumour–muscle contrast. MRI is also more sensitive than CT scan at showing invasion of the medullary space of the mandible and tumour spread along the inferior alveolar nerve. Three dimensional visualization of the tumour volume is also easier with MRI.

Both CT and MRI are particularly useful in tumours of the retromolar trigone, which spread along the pterygomandibular raphe. MRI is particularly indicated in infiltrating and/or ulcerating tumours of the mobile tongue for visualizing deep extension to the muscle of the tongue, which may be clinically undetectable.

CT has a high sensitivity for diagnosis of metastatic cervical nodes, These nodes typically have a specific image, with a central hypodensity and an enhancing peripheral rim. However, the density of the node may be homogeneous, and only the size is of significance. The maximal normal limit of size for submandibular and subdigastric nodes is approximately 1.5 cm. The systematic use of CT imaging often results in nodal upstaging by showing metastatic nodes in N0 patients or by detecting additional nodes in patients whose clinical examination has shown metastatic spread to the neck.

Cervical ultrasonography is a non-invasive technique, which has a high sensitivity for diagnosis and measurement of subclinical adenopathies. It also is the more appropriate technique to detect invasion or thrombosis of neck blood vessels.

An evaluation of oral hygiene and dental status should always be made. Mandibular panoramic radiographs, to provide information about the height and the structure of the mandible as well as radiographic evidence of bone destruction, are indicated (see below). When radiotherapy is planned, a complete evaluation of the dental and periodontal status will be made by the oral surgeon:

- Teeth with caries should be restored. Teeth with deep caries or poor periodontal support must be removed and complete healing obtained before starting radiotherapy.[4]

- Customized dental carriers should be made for daily topical fluoride gel applications (5 to 10 min/day) for the rest of the patient's life to prevent the occurrence of dental caries.[5]

- A prosthesis including a lead shielding should be made when brachytherapy is planned close to the mandible to reduce the dose to the mandible and prevent osteoradionecrosis.[6]

Staging

The Tumour, Node, and Metastasis (TNM) classification is given in Table 1.

Management

Management of premalignant lesions

Oral cancer is, in a large proportion of cases, preceded by premalignant lesions such as leucoplakia and erythroplakia. Leucoplakia is by far the most common one. Malignant transformation of oral leucoplakia, if untreated, takes place in 5 to 10 per cent of all cases. Malignant transformation almost exclusively occurs in cases where epithelial dysplasia is present in the biopsy. Spontaneous regression is exceptional.

Several treatments are available. In cases in which there is no clinical suspicion of cancer, the primary treatment of leucoplakia is aimed at the elimination of the possible cause. When no causative factors seem to be present or when no regression is obtained within 2 to 3 months after the elimination of such factor(s), further diagnostic work up and treatment are indicated.

For a solitary leucoplakia of less than 2 to 3 cm in diameter, an excisional biopsy can be done. In leucoplakia of the vermilion border of the lower lip, a vermillectomy or lip shave may be done (see Fig. 4). The taking of an incisional biopsy followed by cold-knife surgery, laser surgery,[8] or cryosurgery is another common approach. Active treatment is always required in the presence of epithelial dysplasia, especially if there is moderate or severe dysplasia.

For multiple or extensive (larger than 2–3 cm) leucoplakia, in which one or more biopsies have not shown epithelial dysplasia, a wait-and-see policy may be followed. Of course this carries the potential risk of malignant transformation within an indefinite period.

This is even more true for multiple or extensive leucoplakias in which moderate or severe epithelial dysplasia has been demonstrated and in which removal by cold-knife surgery or laser cannot be accomplished. In extensive leucoplakia when biopsies show dysplasia, some prefer excision of large areas of involved mucosa, with 'resurfacing' by split skin or flaps.

Chemoprevention of oral leucoplakia may be of value in patients with multiple and/or extensive lesions, irrespective of the presence of epithelial dysplasia. Several chemoprevention trials have demonstrated the efficacy of retinoids, retinal, and/or β-carotene in reversing oral leucoplakia;[9]–[12] 13-cis-retinoic acid produced remissions in 65 to 80 per cent of patients;[9],[10] leucoplakia is reported to respond to β-carotene, 30 mg/day, (partial and complete remissions) in 71 per cent of cases.[12] Similar results have been reported with vitamin A in a study conducted in India.[11] However, in all studies the lesions recurred when treatment was discontinued.

Management of malignant lesions: treatment techniques

The currently used treatments for oral cancer consist of various kinds of surgical excision, electrocoagulation, laser, radiotherapy, and immunotherapy. For treatment with curative intent, surgery and radiation therapy are the two most important modalities. The role for chemotherapy in therapy of cancer of the oral cavity is not established so far. Chemoradiotherapeutic approaches with organ preservation finalities, which are very promising for other sites (larynx, hypopharynx, and oropharynx) yielded less encouraging results for the oral cavity.[13] For this reason, chemotherapy should not be planned as a standard therapy for operable tumours or be delivered in controlled clinical research trials.

Surgical approaches

Five approaches are possible: (i) transoral, (ii) lower cheek flap, (iii) mandibulotomy, (iv) upper cheek flap, and (v) visor flap (Fig. 1).

Small lesions located anteriorly in the oral cavity, without deep infiltration in the muscles of the floor of the mouth, can be excised transorally. Larger lesions and tumours of the tongue or floor of mouth located more posteriorly, and tumours of the retromolar trigone and buccal mucosa, often require a splitting of the lower lip (Fig. 2) and the raising of a cheek flap, sacrificing the ipsilateral mental nerve.

In midline cancers of the anterior part of the floor of mouth and ventral part of the anterior tongue with deep infiltration, a visor flap can be used. Thus a visible scar on the chin and lower lip is avoided. Depending on the site of the tumour and the height of the mandible, it is sometimes possible to preserve both mental nerves when the visor flap is not raised above their level.

In (larger) tumours of the posterior part of the oral cavity, zigzag splitting of the lower lip or encircling the chin prominence and mandibulotomy are used.[14] Its advantage is good exposure for posteriorly localized lesions while preserving both mental nerves.

In tumours of the palate and superior alveolar process, an upper cheek flap (modified Weber–Fergusson incision) is indicated.

Extent of the resection

A 2-cm circumferential surgical margin should be taken in tongue and floor-of-mouth cancer, as experience has taught that submucosal and perineural spread and spread along muscular planes occur frequently.[15],[16] Whenever surgical margins are doubtful, frozen sections should be obtained, as histologically-positive margins in patients treated with surgery alone result in a high rate of local recurrence. Looser et al.[17] found considerable differences in local recurrence rates between patients with inadequate margins and those with tumour-free margins (71 versus 32 per cent), as also was found by Byers et al. (12–18 versus 80 per cent).[18]

Reconstruction

During the last decades, considerable progress in reconstruction of the oral cavity has been made. Reconstruction aims at restoration of function and cosmesis. A wide variety of methods is available today. In general, immediate reconstruction is preferred. Depending on the specific area and extent of the defect, direct suturing, free skin grafts, skin flaps, myocutaneous flaps, and free flaps are used.

Direct suturing is used in small defects. Split skin grafts are used to cover mucosal defects in which no bulk is required, on surfaces that are sufficiently vascular to accept such grafts. Occasionally, skin flaps, such as the forehead flap, the nasolabial flap, and the deltopectoral flap, can be indicated. Myocutaneous ('composite') flaps are island flaps with a skin paddle overlying a muscular component. The pectoralis major muscle flap provides both skin and volume. It is used so often that it is regarded as the 'workhorse' of reconstruction

Table 1 TNM classification

Histopathological grading

After surgery, the analysis of the specimen will allow a pathological staging, pT, pN, and pM using the same definition.

pN0—histological examination of a selective neck dissection specimen will ordinarily include 6 or more lymph nodes and of a radical or modified radical neck dissection specimen 10 or more lymph nodes.

GX—grade of differentiation cannot be assessed

G1—well differentiate

G2—moderately differentiated

G3—poorly differentiated

G4—undifferentiated

Additional descriptors

For identification of special cases the y, r, a, and m symbols are used. Although they do not affect the stage grouping, they indicate cases needing separate analysis.

y—In those cases in which classification is performed during or following initial multimodality therapy, the TNM or pTNM categories are identified by a y prefix

prefix r—recurrent tumours, when staged after a disease-free interval

a—The prefix indicatesthat classification is first determined at autopsy

suffix m in parentheses—multiple primary tumours at a single site

Optional descriptors

L—lymphatic invasion: LX, lymphatic invasion cannot be assessed; L0, no lymphatic invasion; L1, lymphatic invasion

V—venous invasion: VX venous invasion cannot be assessed; V0, no venous invasion; V1, microscopic venous invasion; V2, macroscopic involvement of the wall of veins, with no tumour within the veins; V2n, macroscopic venous invasion

C-factor or certainty factor—validity of classification according to the diagnosis methods employed, definitions are:

C2—evidence obtained by special diagnosis means (e.g. radiographic imaging in special projection, tomography, computerized tomography, ultrasonography, lymphography, angiography; scintigraphy, magnetic resonance imaging; endoscopy, biopsy, and cytology)

C3—evidence from surgical exploration, including biology and cytology

C4—evidence of an extent of disease following definitive surgery and pathological examination of the resected specimen

C5—evidence from autopsy

TNM clinical classification is equivalent to C1, C2, and C3 in varying degrees of certainty, while the pT pathological classification generally is equivalent to C4

Lip and oral cavity

Tx—primary tumour cannot be assessed

T0—no evidence of primary tumour

Tis—carcinoma *in situ*

T1—tumour 2 cm or less in greatest dimension

T2—tumour more than 2 cm but not more than 4 cm in greatest dimension

T3—tumour more than 4 cm in greatest dimension

T4 lip—tumour invades adjacent structures, e.g. through cortical bone, inferior alveolar nerve, floor of mouth, skin of face

T4 oral cavity—tumour invades adjacent structures, e.g. though cortical bone, into deep (intrinsic) muscle of tongue, maxillary sinus, skin (superficial erosion alone of bone/tooth socket by gingival primary is not sufficient to classify as T4)

Nx—regional lymph nodes cannot be assessed

N0—no regional lymph node metastasis

N1—metastasis in a single ipsilateral lymph node, 3 cm or less in greatest dimension

N2—metastasis in a single ipsilateral lymph node, more than 3 cm but not more than 6 cm in greatest dimension; or in multiple ipsilateral lymph nodes, none more than 6 cm in greatest dimension; or in bilateral or contralateral lymph nodes, none more than 6 cm in greatest dimension

N2a—metastasis in a single ipsilateral lymph node, more than 3 cm but not more than 6 cm in greatest dimension

N2b—metastasis in multiple ipsilateral lymph nodes, more than m cm in greatest dimension

N2c—metastasis in bilateral or contralateral lymph nodes, none more than 6 cm in greatest dimension

N3—metastasis in a lymph node more than 6 cm in greatest dimension (midline nodes are considered ipsilateral nodes)

MX—distant metastasis cannot be assessed

M0—no distant metastasis

M1—distant metastasis

Stage grouping

Stage 0—TisN0M0

Stage I—T1N0M0

Stage II—T2N0M0

Stage III—T3N0M0, T1N1M0, T2N1M0, T3N1M0

Stage IVA—T4N0M0, T4N1M0, any T N2M0

Stage IVB—any T N3M0

Stage IVC—any T any N M1

The classification applies only to carcinoma. The fifth International Against Cancer (UICC) TNM classification of malignant tumours of oral cavity is identical to that published by the American Joint Committee on Cancer (AJCC).[7]

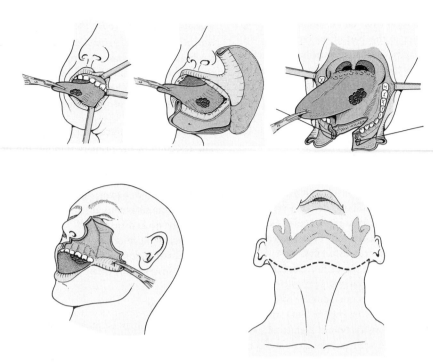

Fig. 1 Surgical approaches to the mouth: (1) transoral, (2) lower cheek flap, (3) mandibulotomy, (4) upper cheek flap, and (5) visor flap.

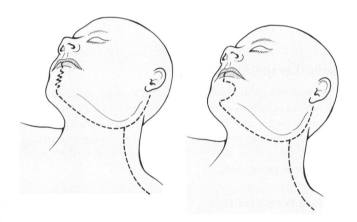

Fig. 2 Lip-splitting incisions. The lip and the chin are divided by a midline incision. Division of the lower lip in zigzag fashion or encircling the chin prominence gives a better cosmetic result than the classic vertical incision. The incision can be continued with the neck dissection incision.

in head and neck surgery. This flap can only be used when a radical neck dissection is made, because the flap cannot be tunnelled under the skin in the neck otherwise. Free flaps are increasingly used in intraoral reconstruction. The radial forearm flap is more often used than any other free flap. Based on the radial artery and either the cephalic vein or the venae commitantes, this flap may be transferred as a composite flap containing vascularized bone, vascularized tendon, or sensory nerves. Its thin, pliable skin with rich vascularity permits a high flexibility in design and a high degree of reliability. Unquestionably, its best indication is in the restoration of oral mucosal defects following ablative surgery. It has been used in virtually every portion of the oral cavity,[19],[20] and particularly helps to preserve the mobility of the residual tongue following ablative surgery. It is probably the reconstruction of choice when the mandibular arch is preserved.

Management of the mandible

In addition to examination under general anaesthesia, panoramic and dental radiographs are helpful in determining bone invasion, although apparently normal radiographic findings do not exclude bone involvement. As many as 30 per cent of patients with cancer of the oral cavity encroaching on the mandible and normal radiographic findings have microscopic bone invasion.[21] The high incidence of microscopic invasion of the periosteum and cortical layer of the mandible, even with normal radiological findings, is part of the rationale for the surgical management of the mandible. Tumours that encroach on the mandible and do not provide an adequate margin of normal intervening tissue usually require that at least a portion of the mandible would be sacrificed. A marginal resection of the upper part of the mandible or of the outer or inner cortical plate may provide an adequate margin around the tumour while still preserving mandibular continuity.[22]–[25] When bone invasion is present on radiographic examination, bone preservation is usually not possible and segmental mandibulectomy is indicated. Whether marginal mandibulectomy is feasible and oncologically safe depends to a large extent on whether the patient is dentate or edentulous. In case of bone invasion, one should be aware that the inferior alveolar canal can be involved as well, thus requiring large segmental resection. In an edentulous mandible, the remaining part of the mandible is usually so thin that preservation of bone is impossible. In addition, bone invasion usually occurs above the mylohyoid line. In the edentulous mandible the proximity of the mylohyoid line to the occlusal ridge implies a rapid spread of tumour to this part of the bone.

After segmental mandibulectomy, when it is felt that reconstruction is needed, the decision must be taken regarding the timing of the reconstruction (immediate versus planned secondary procedure) and the surgical technique: the available options are alloplastic devices, non-vascularized bone graft, and vascularized bone graft. In spite of improved devices, reconstruction plates remain a second-choice solution and are mainly used in severely debilitated patients or when surgery has a purely palliative intent,[26],[27] as the failure rate over a 4-year period are reported near to 25 per cent and the fate of the plate in the long run is uncertain. For many years, arguments against primary reconstruction of segmental mandibular defects were raised. Success rates of primary reconstruction with non-vascularized bone graft, mesh trays, or pedicled osteomyocutaneous flaps ranged from 40 per cent to 70 per cent. Secondary reconstruction with similar techniques was 80 per cent to 90 per cent successful. The functional quality of secondary reconstruction was, however, limited by fibrosis of remaining masticatory muscles and of perimandibular soft tissues. Few patients were able to wear dentures or resume a normal diet. Substantial advantages of primary reconstruction of segmental mandibular defect have now been reported with vascularized bone composite free flaps with a success rate greater than 95 per cent.[28] To date, the superiority of primary reconstruction with vascularized bone graft in terms of appearance and functional results is unquestionable. Satisfactory results are reported both with fibula and iliac crest free flaps, the choice depending on the type of resection (amount of bone and soft tissues removed), and the surgeon's preference and skill.[28],[29]

Neck dissection

Treatment of the primary tumour and the neck are intimately associated in oral cancer. The surgical management of the neck is discussed elsewhere (see Chapter 9.1.4). Only some general comments on the particular situation of oral cancer will be given here.

Treatment of N0 neck in T1/T2 tumours

Primary cancer is usually treated with brachytherapy or transoral resection. Twenty to 40 per cent of these patients present occult regional disease.[30]–[32] To date, there is no reliable criteria to identify these patients, even if some biological predictors of neck metastases have been reported: (depth of muscle invasion, double DNA aneuploidy, and histological differentiation of the tumour.[33] The decision should be made between an elective neck dissection or to limit to a 'watchful waiting' policy. There is no randomized study demonstrating an advantage in survival with either of these policies, but the salvage rate of a subsequent therapeutic dissection is shown to be about 50 per cent only.[34]–[37] For this reason, although a strict follow-up (monthly) may be still considered acceptable, the patient should be counselled of the potential increased risk and an elective neck dissection proposed since expected compliance to follow-up is doubtful.

Selective versus complete neck dissection

Nodal metastases in level V are rare in oral cavity cancer, and negligible in N0 patients, but frequent 'skip diffusion' in level IV has been reported.[38] As a consequence, a dissection of levels I to IV should be always performed, adding a level V dissection in case of clinically evident neck disease.

Indication of postoperative radiotherapy after a neck dissection

An increased local–regional control with postoperative radiotherapy has been shown in cases of multiple metastatic nodes or presence of capsular rupture, but not for intranodal metastases.[39],[40] Therefore postoperative radiotherapy should be considered the standard option in the former clinical situation.

In continuity versus discontinuous neck dissection

The resection of the primary tumour and of the neck nodes should preferably be done in continuity. In oral cancer in particular, however, this may be considered too mutilating, as it would resect too much normal tissue. A higher rates of recurrence in the neck has been shown in simultaneous discontinuous neck dissections than in in-continuity neck dissections.[41] When a discontinuous dissection is preferred, a staging procedure is recommended (for example, 2–3 weeks after resection of the primary tumour) when the stage of the neck justifies this delay, before doing the neck dissection.

Tracheotomy

A tracheotomy may be indicated for various reasons. Postoperative swelling of the posterior part of the oral cavity may result in a compromised airway. Loss of support for the tongue after segmental mandibulectomy or large bulky myocutaneous flaps may also necessitate a tracheotomy. Patients with a poor pulmonary condition or in danger of aspiration as in near-total glossectomy need a tracheotomy as well. In all these circumstances the tracheotomy is a temporary safety measure and will be closed in the postoperative period.

Radiotherapeutic approach

The target volume is irradiated by external beam megavoltage radiation. The radiation source is outside the patient. Localized radiation treatment can be carried out with brachytherapy by temporarily or permanently placing radioactive material in the tumour (interstitial therapy). The sources used for head-and-neck tumours are mostly ^{192}Ir wires or iodine seeds.

External beam irradiation

The target volume for external beam irradiation encompasses the tumour plus safety margins and the regional lymph nodes, which are in the submaxillary regions for the upper lip (sometimes including the preauricular and parotid nodes) (ICRU 50 report). The submandibular and subdigastric nodes drain the lower lip, gingiva, floor of the mouth, oral tongue, and buccal mucosa.[42]

Tumours of the oral cavity are irradiated by two opposed lateral fields, equally weighted; in lateralized tumours, the dose delivered to the ipsilateral side should be increased, for example giving two-thirds of the dose to that field and one-third to the opposite field. Another possibility is the use of two wedged fields, either perpendicular or at an angle chosen according to dosimetry and site. A cobalt source or an accelerator are used. Electrons with energies varying from 4 to 32 MeV are chosen to treat superficial lesions (lip) or to treat (electively) the posterior neck in order to reduce the dose to the spinal cord. Tumours of the floor of the mouth or mobile tongue can, in a few cases, be an indication for the intraoral cone technique, which delivers orthovoltage X-rays or electrons.[43]

The patient is treated in the supine position. The head must be positioned each day as during the simulation session. Even in a complete, customized head-and-neck mask there is room for 3 to 5 mm of movement. Generally, two lateral opposed fields are used for the primary and the upper neck and the lower neck is treated with an anterior field. The following critical organs must be considered:

1. Spinal cord—this should be excluded after a maximum dose of 40–45 Gy to prevent radiation myelitis or spared if treatment of the posterior neck is necessary.

2. Parotid gland—a dry mouth after external beam therapy is almost unavoidable; however, the use of a tongue depressor can considerably reduce the upper margin of the field, thereby saving some of the parotid gland.

3. The larynx should be shielded when an anterior field is used, to prevent unwarranted oedema, chondritis, or necrosis.

4. Exclusion of the temporomandibular joint should be planned at about 50 Gy, whenever relevant, to prevent the late relevance of trismus.

5. Mandible—increasing dose exposes the patient to an increasing risk of osteoradionecrosis.

The field margins are chosen as follows:

1. The anterior margin must stay behind the lower lip except in the case of an anterior, localized tumour.

2. The superior margin depends on the tumour extent for carcinoma of the buccal mucosa. A tongue depressor (if not too painful) can be used to lower the upper margin, thereby saving a part of the parotid gland. The upper margin passes through the tip of the mastoid. The external ear is shielded.

3. The inferior margin, including the submandibular region, lies at the level of the hyoid. Posteriorly, the margin is at the level of the mastoid point, to include the posterior neck nodes whenever justified.

4. When an anterior field is added, in order to treat the middle and lower neck, the larynx is shielded with a midline block.

Total dose will vary upon the treatment aim and strategy:

1. External beam as the sole treatment with curative intent: 70–75 Gy to the tumour and clinically-positive nodes; elective neck-node irradiation 45–50 Gy.

2. External beam combined with brachytherapy: external beam therapy to the tumour and primary nodes is started at a dose of up to 45–50 Gy, followed by an interstitial implant (1–2 weeks later) with iridium wires delivering a boost dose of 25–30 Gy.

3. External beam followed by surgery: 45–50 Gy is given to the tumour and neck nodes with a double aim—to reduce the tumour bulk and to kill tumour cells that are spilled during the operation, thereby reducing the risk of locoregional failure. When surgical margins are insufficient, a 20–25 Gy boost is given postoperatively.

4. Postoperative radiotherapy: depending on the pathological findings, the external beam therapy should preferably be started within 3–4 weeks after surgery. Decreased survival is observed when radiotherapy starts later than 6 weeks postsurgically.[44],[45]

    (a) When the local resection is sufficient (clear margins) no postoperative radiation is given, with one exception—after surgery of T3–4 tumours (tumour diameter > 5 cm and/or involvement of bone and/or soft tissue) a dose of 60 Gy reduces the risk of local recurrence.

    (b) When there are positive neck nodes, 50–55 Gy is sufficient to control the neck but the dose must be increased to 60–65 Gy when there is capsular rupture or perineural spread, and when the surgeon suspects that tumour spillage occurred during the operation.

    (c) In incomplete resections (microscopically or macroscopically), radiotherapy is given up to 70 Gy, depending on the tumour bulk and pathological findings. The rate of relapse after postoperative radiotherapy in local and regional sites is dose dependent.[17],[46]–[49]

    (d) If a high rate of relapse is expected in the N0 neck nodes (depending on the size and site of the tumour), 45–50 Gy to the neck will prevent neck relapse.[50],[51]

    (e) When a tumour is considered surgically or radiotherapeutically 'incurable', a few high-dose fractions may be given in order to decrease (temporarily) symptoms such as pain or bleeding (palliative radiotherapy, e.g. 20 Gy in five fractions or 30 Gy in 10 fractions).

The 'classical' fractionation schedules prescribe a fraction dose of 1.8 to 2 Gy per session, 5 days a week, so that a total dose of 70 Gy is reached in 7 weeks overall treatment time. Split-course regimens should be avoided. It is known from experimental and clinical data that the tumour starts repopulation during the second or third week of treatment, and regeneration would take place during the rest period in the split schedule. From clinical data, an average dose of 0.6 Gy per day should compensate the accelerated repopulation. After a split of 10 days, a dose of 6 Gy is lost due to tumour regrowth by accelerated repopulation.[52]–[54] To shorten the overall time, attempts have been made to increase the dose per day. Hyperfractionation is necessary to prevent late complications. The interval between twice-daily (or even thrice-daily) fractions must be at least 6 h to allow complete repair of sublethal damage in normal tissues.

Brachytherapy

The dose delivered by interstitial iridium wires can be high and well localized due to rapid fall off around the sources, thus delivering a maximal dose to the tumour and sparing as much as possible surrounding normal structures. The dose is classically delivered at low dose rate in the Paris and Manchester systems. This implies that with dose-rate ranges from 40 to 60 cGy/h, the overall time to deliver 65 to 70 Gy varies between 4 and 8 days. Iodine-125 seeds are used as permanent implants, especially in failures occurring in previously irradiated areas. The total dose is delivered over 1 year. Recently, attempts have been made to replace low-dose-rate brachytherapy by high-dose-rate brachytherapy (> 12 Gy/h) or pulsed-dose-rate brachytherapy. Results obtained with high-dose-rate brachytherapy are controversial and only preliminary results are available with pulsed-dose-rate brachytherapy.

Radiobiology of brachytherapy[55],[56]

1. Repair of sublethal damage—depending on the dose rate used, repair may occur, thereby protecting normal tissues prone to develop late radiation damage. The tissues that profit most from continuous, low-dose-rate irradiation are those that are also

sensitive to changes in fraction dose. These are the late-reacting tissues with a low α/β ratio.

2. Due to reoxygenation during treatment, hypoxic cells may become more 'radiosensitive'. This effect is, however, much more clearly demonstrated in daily fractionated external irradiation.

3. Repopulation does not occur, as the overall treatment time is too short.

4. Redistribution is a phenomenon that is discussed extensively[57] but although it is known that due to the irradiation cells are blocked in the G2-phase when a dose sufficient to stop cell division is delivered, this does not mean that, over the period of the treatment, the tumour is forced into a more sensitive phase.

5. Low-dose-rate implants generally involve a range of dose rates varying from 0.3 to 1.5 Gy/h. It has been a matter of debate as to whether such a variation in dose rate has any impact on clinical results. Experimental radiobiological data imply a significant change in biological effectiveness in this range of dose rates with a greater variation for normal tissue late effect than for tumour control. Recent clinical studies also suggested that in the dose-rate range from 0.3 to 1 Gy/h, the overall treatment duration affects treatment outcome. In order to maximize local control and minimize late effects, and consequently increase therapeutic ratio, it has been recommended that the total dose should be kept high and the dose rate low, that is in the range 0.3 to 0.6 Gy/h.[6],[58],[59]

Guide-gutter (Pierquin's technique) (Figs. 3(a and b), 4(a and b))

Single or double guide-gutters, with lengths varying from 30 to 50 mm, are available.[60] The guides are usually implanted under local anaesthesia, sometimes under sedative analgesia, or exceptionally under general anaesthesia. Fluoroscopy serves to check the equidistance and parallelism of the gutters. Sutures are placed under the horizontal bar. When the gutters are satisfactorily in place, an iridium pin is inserted into the guide. While holding the transverse portion of the pin against the tissue, the gutter is removed and the sutures are tied over the hairpin. Indications for this technique are lesions of the floor of the mouth and lateral portion of the mobile tongue.

Plastic tube (Henschke's technique) (Fig. 5(a and b))

Stainless steel needles are implanted under general or sedative anaesthesia through the skin, subdermal tissues, and muscles covering the tumour and its safety margins. The rules of equidistance and parallelism must be followed. A heavy nylon monofilament (0.8 mm) is then inserted in the needles. Loops must be made, with careful avoidance of kinks. The needles are removed and the plastic outer tubes are threaded over the monofilaments; the plastic tubes are clamped to the monofilament and together they are pulled through the tissue; the monofilaments are taken out, leaving in place the hollow plastic tubes. The plastic tubes are rinsed with dilute heparin solution to clear blood clots. The procedure is completed by placing spacers and immobilization buttons over the ends of the plastic tubes. After radiographic control the desired lengths of the sources can be determined and the sources placed in the plastic tubes, manually or

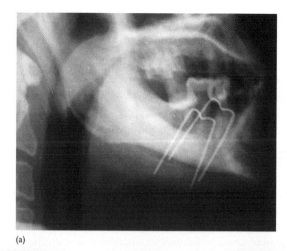

(a)

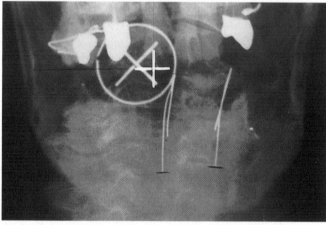

(b)

Fig. 3 (a)(b) Guide-gutter implant in carcinoma of the floor of the mouth.

by remote afterloading. Indications for this technique are tumours of the mobile tongue, floor of mouth, lip, and buccal mucosa.

Hypodermic needle (Pierquin's technique)

Short hypodermic needles with variable lengths from 3 to 10 cm, 0.8 mm outer diameter, 0.5 mm inner diameter, serve to contain the iridium wires (0.3 mm diameter). The hypodermic needles remain in place and are kept parallel and equally spaced by retaining plates or plastic-tube spacers. The needles must be sufficiently long to cover the tumour plus its safety margin. Carcinoma of the lower lip is especially suitable for this technique.

Dosimetry of interstitial implantation

Paris system This system is based on the following principles:[60]

- radioactive lines must be rectilinear, parallel, and with their centres in the same plane perpendicular to the direction lines—this is known as the central plane;
- same linear reference air Kerma rate;
- adjacent sources must be equidistant.

The basal dose rates are calculated as the minimum dose rate in the central plane between each group of adjacent sources, either by computer or by using graphs. The different basal dose rates should

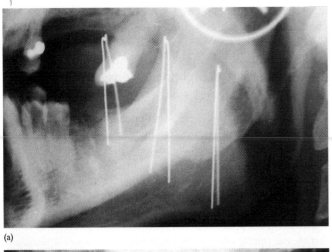

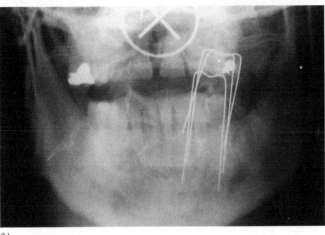

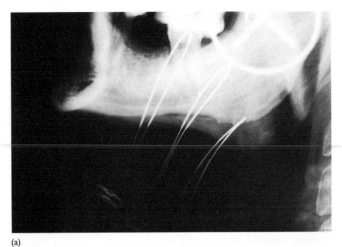

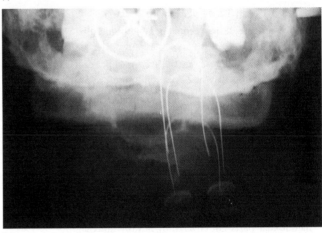

Fig. 4 (a)(b) Guide-gutter implant in carcinoma of the mobile tongue.

Fig. 5 (a)(b) Plastic tube implant in carcinoma of the mobile tongue.

not differ by more than 10 per cent from the mean. The reference isodose is calculated at 85 per cent of the basal dose rate. The reference isodose must encompass the target volume (i.e. the tumour plus the safety margin) and defines the 'treatment volume'.

Manchester system For this method of calculation, the effective minimum dose is taken as 10 per cent above the absolute minimum dose in a plane or volume. In contrast to the Paris system, where the chosen length of the sources is sufficient to have the isodose covering the whole length of the target volume, the Manchester system uses 'crossing needles' perpendicular to, and at the active ends of, the plane of sources, so that the active length actually determines the target length.

Acute reactions

Mucositis

The so-called 'tumoritis' occurs around 20 Gy. Symptoms are treated with saline mouthwashes and a modified diet. Stopping alcohol intake and smoking during (and hopefully after) treatment are strongly recommended.

Dry mouth and taste loss

After a few Gy a reduction of salivary flow occurs. Dry mouth develops during treatment and can be permanent. Total dose and volume of salivary glands localized in the treatment volume[61],[62] are responsible for the severity of xerostomia. A lifetime direct consequence of dry mouth is dental decay (caries). To prevent this, daily topical fluoride applications are necessary.[5] There is no effective treatment for dry mouth or taste loss. The effects of sialogogues are under investigation.[63] Pilocarpine stimulates the remaining salivary glands and increases comfort in about 50 per cent of irradiated patients.[64] Daily pretreatment (200 mg/m^2 intravenously) with amifostine reduces the incidence of both acute and chronic xerostomia during head and neck radiotherapy.[65] Antitumour efficacy is preserved. Candidiasis can develop on the mucosa, which must be treated by topical application of a fungicide.

Dysphagia and dyspnoea

Dysphagia may sometimes occur, necessitating the insertion of a naso-oesophageal tubing.

Skin

Erythema starts developing after 20 to 30 Gy and dry and wet epidermolysis can occur at doses of 50 Gy or more. More severe and earlier reactions are often seen after induction or concomitant chemotherapy, especially with bleomycin-containing regimens, sometimes necessitating interruption of treatment. Treatment consists of topical corticosteroids, eucerine, or eosin solution.

Late complications

Soft tissue necrosis

This may sometimes occur, with fistulation. It can be seen after delivering a high dose, especially when a large fraction size is used. Poorly vascularized tissue is more susceptible to the development of necrosis. Soft tissue necrosis is more frequent after interstitial irradiation than with external beam techniques. Predisposing factors include increased total dose, increased dose rate,[6],[58],[59] increased treated volume,[6] and increased intersource spacing.[66] In a population of 134 T1 and 145 squamous cell carcinoma of mobile tongue and floor of mouth definitively treated with ^{192}Ir at the Henri Mondor Hospital, actuarial necrosis rates at 5 years were:

- T1: 33 per cent; T2: 44 per cent ($p = 0.07$);
- mobile tongue: 28 per cent; floor of the mouth: 58 per cent ($p < 0.001$);
- dose >62.5 Gy and dose rate >0.5 Gy/h: 44 per cent; dose >62.5 Gy and dose rate <0.5 Gy/h: 24 per cent; dose <62.5 Gy and dose rate >0.5 Gy/h: 37 per cent; dose <62.5 Gy and dose rate < 0.5 Gy/h: 5 per cent ($p < 0.001$);
- intersource spacing 9–14 mm: 33 per cent; intersource spacing 15–20 mm: 46 per cent ($p = 0.04$).

Osteoradionecrosis of the mandible

Predisposing factors are:

- the dose delivered to the mandible;
- mandibular parts not covered by healthy mucosa;
- dental extractions done within 10 days of the brachytherapy;
- interstitial implants during which three or more iridium lines are in close contact with the bone.

Osteoradionecrosis can be prevented by a lead-shielded dental mould, worn by patient during brachytherapy or during direct external beam irradiation for lip cancer.[6] Conservative treatment of osteoradionecrosis consists of high doses of antibiotics. Good results were reported with treatment with hyperbaric oxygen.[67] If the necrosis persists, necrotic bone should be removed surgically. In more advanced cases, segmental hemimandibulectomy should be justified.

Hypothyroidism

This may be due to irradiation of the thyroid gland, and is either clinically manifest or occult. Therefore, before irradiation of the neck and during postradiation follow-up, thyroid function must be tested.[68]

Chemotherapy

Chemotherapy as the sole treatment for head-and-neck cancer is not curative. The Meta-Analysis of Chemotherapy on Head and Neck Cancer (MACH-NC) group[69] performed a meta-analysis using updated individual data from 63 randomized trials (1965–1993) including 10 717 patients, comparing locoregional treatment to the same treatment plus chemotherapy in locally advanced head and neck squamous cell carcinoma. No effect of adjuvant or neoadjuvant chemotherapy was demonstrated on survival, but a significant effect of concomitant chemotherapy was shown on locoregional control and survival. These results are not site specific since the trials included all head and neck sites.

Management of malignant lesions: treatment indications

The chosen treatment will depend on tumour's site, pathological type and extent, the patient's general condition, age and social status, the physician experience and skill, and the patient's and physician's personal preference. The therapy should be tailored to the individual case by a treatment team (head and neck surgeons, radiation therapists, medical oncologists, oral surgeons, stomatologists, etc.), so that not only is the cancer optimally treated, but important aspects of function and cosmesis are preserved.[70] In small tumours, surgery and radiotherapy are equally effective; in larger tumours, surgery if feasible is superior, whereas in many instances, a combination of the two will be indicated, not only for the primary tumour, but also for the regional lymph nodes.

There is no evidence in the literature that histological tumour differentiation may be a valid guideline for choosing treatment: moreover anaplastic tumours and poorly differentiated squamous cell cancers, usually considered more suitable for radiotherapy, are relatively rare in the oral cavity.

The results of radiotherapy, namely brachytherapy, and surgery for T1 and T2 oral cancers in eradicating the disease are comparable. Therefore, the choice of treatment is to a large extent dependent on the morbidity of surgery and radiotherapy in each clinical situation. Cancers of the anterior two-thirds of the tongue, floor of mouth, and cheek all have different biological behaviours, while the sequelae of treatment are also different for these various sites. General rules are therefore difficult to give. In general, however, every effort should be made to conserve function and to limit cosmetic damage to a minimum.

Postoperative complications depend on the site of the tumour within the oral cavity. When taking surgical margins,[16] the result defect, even in small oral cancers, can be considerable. A 5-cm removal of tongue to remove a 1-cm tumour produces significant problems in speech, chewing, and swallowing.[71] When speech is likely to be severely impaired by surgery, radiotherapy should be favoured. In other instances, there are few long-term complications after surgery.

When radiotherapy is successful, there is no cosmetic alteration in the patient's appearance. The presumed advantage of radiotherapy is preservation of tissue and function. Other disadvantages exist, however. Acute reactions consist of mucositis, ulceration, dry mouth, loss of taste, dysphagia, xerostomia, and erythema of the skin. Soft tissue necrosis can cause serious problems. The functional long-term sequelae of radiotherapy are unavoidable and may alter quality of life. A permanent dry mouth and loss of taste cause lifelong morbidity. Second primaries are a serious threat in young patients; however very few are radiation induced. Osteoradionecrosis of the mandible is a serious hazard of radiotherapy in oral cancer.[72] When the bone has been invaded by cancer, it is generally accepted that radiotherapy should not be used.[73]

The results of primary surgery are far superior to radiotherapy in advanced oral cancers (T3–T4), as the recurrence rate after radiotherapy is much higher than in others head and neck sites.[74]

Surgery is mandatory in infiltrative cancers, especially when they are attached or adjacent to the mandible. The majority of oral cancers are already larger than 2 cm at the time of detection. In such cases, treatment of the neck will also be needed (see below). A combined surgical and radiotherapeutic treatment is currently employed in these cases. Indication for postoperative radiotherapy depend on local and/or regional tumour extension. There is no randomized study demonstrating a survival advantage with this policy, but postoperative radiotherapy increases local regional control in patients with surgical margins involved by tumour and/ or with spread in nodes and capsular rupture. In case of inadequate surgical margins both external radiotherapy and brachytherapy are effective.[40],[75]–[77] Postoperative radiation therapy should be based on the pathological findings: inadequate margins, extranodal and perineural spread, and two or more pathologically positive nodes are indications for postoperative irradiation. Whenever the above conditions are not present, surgery alone may be considered as the treatment of choice.[78]

In general, well-defined and accessible T1–T2 tumours are an excellent indication for brachytherapy. The results of local control are at least as good as those from surgery. In larger tumours (T3) or ill-defined lesions, treatment can be started by external beam up to a dose of 45 to 50 Gy in order to make the tumour accessible for brachytherapy, which gives a boost of 25 to 35 Gy in 2 to 4 days. In recurrent disease in a previously irradiated area, an attempt can be made to control the disease with brachytherapy at low or very low dose rate (20 cGy/h or less), when primary salvage surgery is not feasible. The advantages of brachytherapy in recurrent disease are the preservation of organs and treatment of a well-defined volume. Patients with recurrent disease often develop a second primary in the head-and-neck area. Treating the first tumour by brachytherapy alone may facilitate curative surgical or even radiation treatment of a second primary tumour emerging near the site of the first tumour.

As recurrence of oral cavity cancer is frequently local or regional, salvage surgery is often the only chance of cure. After a radiotherapy failure the salvage rate of a subsequent surgery is reported to be 40 per cent.[37],[79] A second surgery after a first failure, even when feasible, has less than 10 per cent cure rate.[37],[80]

For relapsing tumours, when salvage surgery is not feasible and when the patient has not been previously irradiated, salvage radiation therapy can be tried, although often with poor outcome due to tumour bulk, poor vascularization, and the patient's general condition. When radiation has already be given it is, in selected cases, possible to again irradiate recurring tumours or nodes using interstitial and/ or external techniques.[81]

Treatment indications and results by site

Lip

Lip cancer behaves more like a skin cancer than an oral cavity cancer. For tumours of 4 cm or less, equally effective local control is obtained by surgery or radiotherapy,[60],[84] and neck treatment is indicated only in case of clinical suspicions. Localized external radiotherapy by electrons provides more than 90 per cent local control in small lesions.

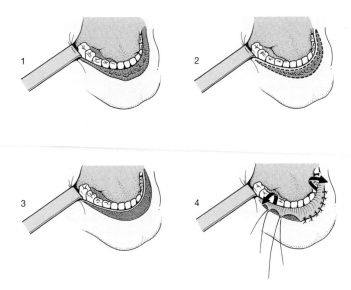

Fig. 6 'Lip shave' or vermillionectomy is done in dysplastic lesions or carcinoma *in situ* of the lower lip.

When there is invasion of neighbouring structures such as gum or bone, surgery must be performed, with postoperative radiotherapy. The goal of surgery is eradication of the disease, with establishment of a competent oral sphincter with an adequate buccal sulcus, minimization of deformity, and restoration of a cosmetically acceptable appearance.[83]

Dysplastic lesions and carcinoma *in situ* can be managed by a lip shave (Fig. 6). T1 lesions can be excised with 1-cm margins in a 'V' wedge with primary closure. Cryosurgery or laser excision is also possible. Surgical excision of T2 lesions is usually more extensive and may require a shield- or square-shaped excision, with reconstruction by lip-switch procedures such as the Abbe or Estlander flaps (Fig. 7). T3 and T4 lesions are of surgical pertinence and may require resection of 50 to 100 per cent of the lip, with reconstruction by a Karapandzic flap or full-thickness cheek advancement flaps. Comprehensive overviews are provided by Tiwari and Holt.[82],[83]

Brachytherapy provides excellent cosmetic outcome.[85],[86] Careful attention must be paid to tumours of the labial commissure with a slightly elevated risk of necrosis after radiotherapy; in particular, the total dose should not exceed 65 Gy. When brachytherapy is used in tumours of 5 cm or more, a dose of 75 to 85 Gy must be delivered using two applications, 2 to 3 weeks apart. Brachytherapy can be applied after external beam radiotherapy, after tumour shrinkage and elective node radiotherapy.

If strict follow-up is guaranteed no further treatment of regional nodes is necessary in small tumours. In other cases, a neck node dissection must be made. Operable positive neck nodes should be managed by surgery followed by external beam radiotherapy; the dose given is 50 or 65 Gy (depending on histological type). Inoperable nodes are treated by external beam radiation to deliver 70 Gy. Local control rated obtained with definitive brachytherapy (^{192}Ir) are high:[60] T1 (<2 cm) 98.4 per cent; T2 (>2–<4 cm) 96.6 per cent; T3 (>4 cm) 89.9 per cent. The overall 5-year survival rate is 85 per cent. When nodes are positive, the survival rate drops to 50 to 70 per cent.[87]

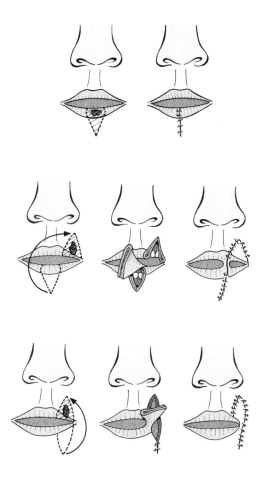

Fig. 7 T1 lesions are excised with a 'V' wedge with primary closure. T2 lesions may require a shield- or square-shaped excision, with reconstruction by lip-switch procedures such as the Abbe or Estlander flaps.

Floor of mouth

Results are similar for surgery and radiotherapy (usually brachytherapy alone), in T1–T2 tumours. The therapeutic choice should be based on functional considerations. In the best series the 5-year survival rates approach 80 per cent.[88] Surgery, sometimes with postoperative radiotherapy, remains the best treatment for more advanced lesions with reported 5-year survivals of about 50 per cent.[89]–[91] The survival drops markedly when nodes are positive.

Small tumours of the anterior floor of the mouth can be resected per orally with primary closure or with a split skin graft. Shah *et al.* prefer to leave the wound open.[92] Marginal or segmental mandibulectomy may be necessary.[22]–[25] For small tumours (that is 2 cm if close to the mandible or 3 cm if remote from the mandible) brachytherapy is the alternative treatment. With brachytherapy, up to 95 per cent local control is obtained for T1 tumours and 70 to 75 per cent for T2 tumours.[88],[93] The local control rate is strongly dose dependent. Salvage surgery is kept for recurrent local disease.

In advanced, deeply infiltrating or posteriorly localized lesions, a composite resection must be done. The reconstructive possibilities after 'en bloc surgery' have improved considerably during the last decades. In most instances, in particular vascularized flaps, the cosmetic and functional results are acceptable. The surgery comprises local excision with en bloc resection of the lymph nodes. Depending on the histological findings, postoperative radiotherapy is delivered. This is definitely indicated in case of positive resection margins, multiple positive nodes, and/or extranodal spread.

Where surgery is contraindicated or the tumour is inoperable a full course of external beam radiotherapy may be proposed. In small lesions treated by brachytherapy or transoral surgery and with negative neck, a strict monthly follow-up of the regional nodes may be sufficient, although 20 to 40 per cent of patients have subclinical neck disease. Alternatively, a delayed neck dissection (3 or 4 weeks after primary treatment) may be proposed even if it must be bilateral when the tumour is median or paramedian. When the tumour is treated by a combination of external beam and brachytherapy, the regional lymph nodes receive 50 Gy, which is enough to control subclinical disease. In cases of operable, positive nodes a neck dissection is mandatory, followed by external beam radiotherapy depending on the pathology findings.

When the treatment plan for the tumour consists of external beam and brachytherapy, lymph node dissection is done after 50 Gy. After exclusive external beam radiotherapy, surgical removal of residual nodes can be done at 8 weeks in patients with the primary under control. Inoperable lymph node metastases should be treated by external beam radiotherapy, which must be given up to 70 Gy using shrinking field techniques and electron beam boosts.

Mobile tongue

Cancer of the tongue is a highly aggressive disease, both in its local behaviour and the occurrence of cervical lymph node metastases. Small tumours can be treated equally effectively with radiation or surgery, whereas the results of surgery are superior in more advanced lesions.[94]–[96]

For T1 and T2 exophytic lesions, the results of surgery for local control, by means of transoral partial glossectomy, are 90 and 70 per cent, respectively.[72],[97]–[100] After a wedge resection or hemiglossectomy, the wound can usually be closed in an anteroposterior fashion. The effect on speech and swallowing is usually minimal and, in our opinion, less serious than the potential complications of radiation in these particular patients.

Small lesions represent excellent indication for interstitial treatment, except for ill-defined lesions or those surrounded by dysplasia; in this case, a partial glossectomy must be proposed. Wang[101] reported excellent results with the intraoral cone external radiotherapy technique. The 5-year overall survival rate is 69 per cent for T1 patients and 41 per cent for T2 patients.[59] Five-year local control rates were 80 to 95 per cent with ^{192}Ir implantation alone of T1–2N0 cancers. Results obtained with brachytherapy alone of T1–T2 tumours were higher than those following combined external beam and brachytherapy boost.[59],[102]–[104] Minor or moderate soft tissue necrosis occurred in 25 per cent and minor or moderate bone necrosis in 10 per cent of cases. Recent retrospective analyses have shown that optimization of modalities of low-dose-rate brachytherapy for these indications should result in an increase in therapeutic ratio, namely a higher local control rate and/or a lower necrosis rate. It is recommended that the tumour should be exclusively treated by ^{192}Ir, with a total dose of 65 to 70 Gy, a dose rate of 0.3 to 0.6 Gy/h, and intersource spacing of 1 to 1.4 cm, and using a customized lead gutter prosthesis to shield the mandible during irradiation.[6],[58],[66]

The overall results in advanced lesions are not as good, which to a large extent is related to the frequency of positive lymph nodes in the neck. Five-year survival rates in stage III–IV patients range from 18 to 55 per cent according to different authors.[91],[105] T3 and T4 lesions usually require a cheek flap or mandibulotomy and, depending on the extent of the tumour, marginal or segmental mandibulectomy. A reconstruction procedure is generally necessary to obtain an adequate function and appearance, the choice among a pectoralis-major flap, forearm free flap, or fibula or iliac crest osteocutaneous flaps depending on whether the mandible is removed or not and on the patient's age, general condition, and expectancies. External beam radiotherapy must be given to all cases.

Forty per cent of patients with carcinoma of the mobile tongue have clinical or occult neck node metastases.[50] The policy for the neck nodes is similar to that for floor-of-mouth tumours.

Buccal mucosa

Even in the case of small tumours (T1–T2), the choice between surgery and radiotherapy should be done according to functional outcome and treatment morbidity. When the amount of removed tissue allows for direct mucosa suture without significant gum retraction, surgery is considered to be the optimal treatment. Brachytherapy will be preferred in larger tumours.

Small, superficial T1 and T2 tumours of the buccal mucosa can be resected and primarily closed by means of a split skin graft or may be left open. Small lesions (< 5 cm) are also good indication for interstitial therapy. Good local control can be obtained without mutilating surgery.

For T3–T4 tumours, surgery eventually followed by radiotherapy will be the treatment of choice. Brachytherapy is no longer indicated when there is involvement of the gum or the intermaxillary commissure. In this case, surgery is the primary choice, followed by external beam radiotherapy; this is given systematically where there is bony involvement and/or incomplete resection. Advanced lesions will be approached by a lower or upper cheek flap; considerable defects of soft tissue and bone can result. These defects must be closed to avoid retracting scars and gum fibrosis and consequent trismus (using local cutaneous, myocutaneous, or revascularized free flaps). When the tumour proves to be inoperable or when the patient's condition does not allow surgical intervention, external beam treatment is given up to a dose of 70 Gy. The approach to regional lymph nodes is similar to that for the mobile tongue and floor of mouth.

The mean overall 5-year survival rate is around 40 per cent, varying from 77 to 18 per cent[86] from stage I to stage IV.[106],[107] The 5-year disease-free survival rate was 61 to 46 per cent for T1–T2, 33 per cent for T3, and 10 per cent for T4 tumour patients. Krishna Nair et al.[108] concluded that elective neck node irradiation probably did not improve the treatment results. For positive nodes the survival dropped to 43 per cent, compared to 75 per cent for negative nodes.

Mandibular alveolar mucosa/gingiva

Radiotherapy is not the first treatment of choice for these tumours for the following reasons: interstitial therapy is not possible; external beam has only an elevated risk of osteoradionecrosis and proves to be less effective in bony involvement. Surgery is the best initial treatment for these tumours. It ranges from local, limited excision with conservation of the continuity of the mandible[109] to (when there is invasion of the mandibular bone) partial resection, with simultaneous monobloc dissection of the neck nodes. Clinically-positive nodes are always resected in one block with the primary tumour. N0 patients can undergo a ispilateral or bilateral supra-omohyoidal neck dissection at the same time as the local excision of the tumour.

Cancer of the hard palate and upper alveolar ridge

These represent the least common tumours of the oral cavity. No large series of tumours exclusively located to the hard palate has been published. Five-year survival rates vary according to the stage, and this subsite presents better outcome than tongue and floor of the mouth.[110],[111]

Superficial lesions can be treated with excision of mucosa alone. Only early lesions without involvement of the bone can be treated by radiotherapy (external beam or with surface moulds[112] for superficial lesions, or the guide-gutter technique); by two opposed lateral fields a dose of 60 Gy can be delivered, eventually boosted by intraoral cone up to 70 Gy. For more extensive disease, for epithelial as well as glandular tumours, surgery is the treatment of first choice. The specific problem at this site is involvement of the maxilla, necessitating partial or total maxillectomy with subsequent placement of a palatal obturator. As this tumour does not tend to give early metastatic nodes, a clinically negative neck may be left for strict follow-up.

Retromolar trigone

Due to strict bone contiguity, radiotherapy may only be indicated for this subsite in small superficial tumours. Surgery will be the best treatment in most cases.[113] In the majority of tumours of the retromolar trigone, a portion of the mandible must be resected. In tumours of moderate dimension (T2 and small T3 lesions), a marginal resection may suffice, with reconstruction by a masseter flap;[82] in larger or deeper infiltrating lesions a segmental mandibulectomy may have to be done, with reconstruction by a pectoralis major island flap or by a composite free flap.

Five-year survival of patients treated with surgery and postoperative radiotherapy is 80 per cent for T1 lesions; for T4 tumours it exceeded 50 per cent, as reported by Kowalski et al.,[114] and it ranged from 27 to 40 per cent as reported by Berktold.[115] As 50 per cent of patients have ipsilateral neck disease, treatment of the neck is also indicated. More extensive disease should be treated by primary surgery.

Minor salivary gland tumours (see Chapter 9.8 for more details)

Treatment of carcinoma of the minor salivary glands is surgical. If radiation treatment is given, the field is adapted to the site.[116]

Conclusion

Most oral cavity cancers are induced by excessive alcohol and/or tobacco habits. Current treatment strategies include surgery and/

Table 2 Proposed standards, options (alternative treatments), and recommendations

	Standard	Options	Recommendations
T1–T2	Surgery Brachytherapy	External radiation therapy	No brachytherapy if tumour close to the bone Postoperative radiotherapy if positive or close margins
T3–T4	Surgery	Radiation therapy +/− brachytherapy Chemoradiotherapy Chemotherapy + surgery	Postoperative radiotherapy if positive or close margins Chemoradiotherapy under investigation Chemotherapy + surgery under investigation in controlled clinical trials
N0 neck	Elective neck dissection Close follow-up	Radiotherapy	'Wait and see' to be discussed with the patient for possible increased risk Postoperative radiotherapy for multiple positive nodes or extranodal spread
N1–N3 operable neck	Surgery	Radiotherapy Chemoradiotherapy	Postoperative radiotherapy for multiple positive nodes or extranodal spread Chemoradiotherapy under investigation
N1–N3 inoperable neck	Radiotherapy +/− surgery	Chemoradiotherapy +/− surgery	Chemoradiotherapy under investigation in controlled clinical trials
Follow-up	No standard		Clinical examination: every 3 months, years 1–2 every 6 months, years 3–5 yearly after 5 years Chest radiograph yearly

or radiation and, more recently, concomitant chemoradiation in moderately advanced and advanced cases. Very few randomized studies have been published.[34],[69] As a result, there is no consensus on standard treatment and there are a number of controversies on optimal management. Table 2 summarized the consensus and alternative management in most oral cavity tumours. We consequently recommend that each patient should be seen in a multidisciplinary clinic before any treatment, and that the management should be tailored to the clinical presentation. Treatment failures remain frequent despite improvements in clinical and radiological investigation, and in surgical and radiotherapeutic techniques. New primaries in the head and neck region, bronchus, and oesophagus are also frequent.

References

1. **Menk HR, *et al.***Preliminary report of the national data base CA 41. 1991: 7–39.

2. **Tepperman BS, Fitzpatrick PJ.** Second respiratory and upper digestive tract cancers after oral cancer. *Lancet*, 1981; ii: 547–9.

3. **de Vries N, *et al.*** Multiple primary tumours in oral cancer. *International Journal of Oral and Maxillofacial Surgery*, 1986; **15**: 85–7.

4. **Daly TE.** Dental care in the irradiated patients. In: Fletcher GH, ed. *Text book of radiotherapy.* 2nd edn. Philadelphia: Lea and Feabiger, 1973: 157–65.

5. **Horiot JC, Schraub S, Bone MC, *et al.*** Dental preservation in patients irradiated for head and neck tumors: a ten-year experience with topical fluoride and a randomized trial between two fluoridation methods. *Radiotherapy and Oncology*, 1983; **1**: 77–82.

6. **Pernot M, *et al.*** Complications following definitive irradiation for cancers of the oral cavity and the oropharynx (in a series of 1134 patients). *International Journal of Radiation Oncology Biology Physics*, 1997; **37**: 577–85.

7. **Flemming ID, *et al.***AJCC cancer manual. Philadephia: Lippincott, 1997.

8. **Roodenburg JL, *et al.*** CO_2-laser surgery of oral leukoplakia. *Oral Surgery, Oral Medicine, Oral Pathology*, 1991; **71**: 670–4.

9. **Shah JP, *et al.*** Effect of retinoids on oral leukoplakia. *American Journal of Surgery*, 1983; **146**: 466–70.

10. **Hong WK, *et al.***13-Cis retinoic acid in the treatment of oral leukoplakia. *New England Journal of Medicine*, 1986; **315**: 1501–5.

11. **Stitch HF, *et al.*** Response of oral leukoplakias to the administration of vitamin A. *Cancer Letters*, 1988; **40**: 93–101.

12. **Garewal HS, *et al.*** Response of oral leukoplakia to beta-carotene. *Journal of Clinical Oncology*, 1990; **8**: 1715–20.

13. **Taylor SG, *et al.*** Concomitant cisplatin/5FU infusion and radiotherapy in advanced head and neck cancer: 8-year analysis of results. *Head and Neck*, 1997; **19**: 684–91.

14. **Spiro RH, *et al.*** Mandibular swing approach for oral and oropharyngeal tumors. *Head and Neck Surgery*, 1981; **3**: 371–8.

15. **Ballantyne AJ.** Current controversies in the management of cancer of the tongue and floor of mouth. In: Kagan AR, Miles JW, ed. *Head and neck oncology, controversies in cancer treatment.* Boston: Hall, 1981: 86–97.

16. **Westbury G.** Carcinoma of the tongue. In: Rob C, Smith R, ed. *Operative surgery: head and neck.* London: Butterworth, 1981: 664–71.

17. **Looser KG, *et al.*** The significance of 'positive' margins in surgically resected epidermoid carcinomas. *Head and Neck Surgery*, 1978; **1**: 107–11.

18. **Byers M, *et al.*** The prognostic and therapeutic value of frozen section determinations in the surgical treatment of squamous carcinoma of the head and neck. *American Journal of Surgery*, 1989; **136**: 525–8.

19. Martin IC, *et al*. Free vascularized fascial flap in oral cavity reconstruction. *Head and Neck*, 1994; **16**: 45–50.

20. Soutar DS, *et al*. The radial forearm flap in intraoral reconstruction: the experience of 60 consecutive cases. *Plastic and Reconstructive Surgery*, 1989; **78**: 1–8.

21. Baker SR. Malignant neoplasms of the oral cavity. In: Cummings CW, *et al*. ed. *Otolaryngology-head and neck surgery*. St Louis: Mosby, 1990: 1281–343.

22. Novack AJ. The surgical management of malignant lesions of the floor of the mouth. *Otolaryngologic Clinics of North America*, 1979; **12**: 97–113.

23. Applebaum EL, *et al*. Carcinoma of the floor of mouth. *Archives of Otolaryngology*, 1980; **106**: 419–22.

24. Schramm VL, *et al*. Surgical management of early epidermoid carcinoma of the anterior floor of mouth. *Laryngoscope*, 1980; **90**: 207–10.

25. Beecroft WA, *et al*. Mandible preservation in the treatment of cancer of the floor of the mouth. *Journal of Surgical Oncology*, 1982; **19**: 171–5.

26. Koch WM, *et al*. Advantages of mandibular reconstruction with the titanium hollow screw osseointegrating reconstruction plate (THORP). *Laryngoscope*, 1994; **104**: 545–52.

27. Irish JC, *et al*. Primary mandibular reconstruction with the titanium hollow screw reconstruction plate: evaluation of 51 cases. *Plastic and Reconstruction Surgery*, 1995; **96**: 93–9.

28. Urken ML. Composite free flaps in oromandiular reconstruction. Review of the literature. *Archives of Otolaryngology Head and Neck Surgery*, 1991; **117**: 724–32

29. Hidalgo DA, *et al*. A review of 60 consecutive fibula free flap mandible reconstructions. *Plastic and Reconstructive Surgery*, 1995; **96**: 597–602.

30. Marchetta FC, *et al*. Management of localised oral cancer. *American Journal of Surgery*, 1977; **134**: 448–9.

31. Whitehurst JO, Drouilas A. Surgical treatment of squamous cell carcinoma of the oral tongue. *Archives of Otolaryngology*, 1987; **103**: 212–15.

32. Shah JP, *et al*. The patterns of cervical lymph node metastases from squamous carcinoma of the oral cavity. *Cancer*, 1990; **66**: 109–13.

33. Byers M, *et al*. Results of treatment for squamous carcinoma of the lower gum. *Cancer*, 1989; **47**: 2236–8.

34. Van den Brouck C, *et al*. Elective versus therapeutic radical neck dissection in epidermoid carcinome of the oral cavity. *Cancer*, 1980; **46**: 386–90.

35. Lydiatt DD, *et al*. Treatment of stage I and II oral tongue cancer. *Head and Neck*, 1993; **15**: 308–12.

36. Piedbois P, *et al*. Stage I–II squamous cell carcinoma of the oral cavity treated by iridium-192: is elective dissection indicated ? *Radiotherapy and Oncology*, 1991; **21**: 100–6.

37. Yuen AP, *et al*. Results of surgical salvage of locoregional recurrence of carcinoma of the tongue after radiotherapy failure. *Annals of Otology, Rinology and Laryngology*, 1997; **106**: 779–82.

38. Byers RM, *et al*. Can we detect the presence of occult nodal metastases in patients with squamous carcinoma of the oral tongue? *Head and Neck*, 1997; **20**: 138–44.

39. Cachin Y, Eschwège F. Combination of radiotherapy and surgery in head and neck cancers. *Cancer Treatment Review*, 1975; **2**: 177.

40. Bartelink H, *et al*. The value of postoperative radiotherapy as an adjuvant to radical neck dissection. *Cancer*, 1983; **52**: 1008–13.

41. Leemans C, *et al*. Discontinuous neck dissection in carcinoma of the oral cavity. *Archives of Otolaryngology, Head and Neck Surgery* 1991; **117**: 1003–6.

42. Million RR, Cassisi MM, Wittes RE. Cancer of the head and neck. In: De Vita VT, Hellman S, Rosenberg SA, ed. *Cancer principles and practice of oncology*. 2nd edn. Philadelphia: Lippincott, 1985.

43. Wang CC, *et al*. Intra-oral cone radiation therapy for selected carcinomas of the oral cavity. *International Journal of Radiation Oncology Biology Physics*, 1988; **9**: 1185–9.

44. Vikram B. Importance of the time interval between surgery and postoperative radiation therapy in the combined management of head and neck cancer. *International Journal of Radiation Oncology Biology Physics*, 1979; **5**: 1837–40.

45. Robertson AS, *et al*. Post-operative radiotherapy in the management of advanced intra-oral cancers. *Clinical Radiology*, 1986; **37**: 173–8.

46. Mirimanoff RO, Wang CC, Doppke KP. Combined surgery and postoperative radiation therapy for advanced laryngeal and hypopharyngeal carcinomas. *International Journal of Radiation Oncology Biology Physics*, 1985; **11**: 499–504.

47. Admur RJ, *et al*. Split-course versus continuous-course irradiation in the postoperative setting for squamous cell carcinoma of the head and neck. *International Journal of Radiation Oncology Biology Physics*, 1989; **17**: 179–85.

48. Admur RJ, *et al*. Postoperative irradiation for squamous cell carcinoma of the head and neck: and analysis of treatment results and complications. *International Journal of Radiation Oncology Biology Physics*, 1989; **16**: 25–36.

49. Peters LJ, *et al*. Evaluation of the dose for postoperative radiation therapy of head and neck cancer: first report of a prospective randomized trial. *International Journal of Radiation Oncology Biology Physics*, 1993; **26**: 3–11.

50. Decroix Y, Ghossein NA. Experience of the Curie Institute in treatment of cancer of the mobile tongue. I. Treatment policies and result. *Cancer*, 1981; **47**: 496–502.

51. Richaud P, *et al*. Cancers de la cavité buccale sans adénopathie palpable: valeur de l'irradiation externe exclusive. *Annals of Oto-laryngology*, 1985; **102**: 593–5.

52. Maciejewski B, *et al*. The influence of the number of fractions and of overall treatment time on local control and late complication rate in squamous cell carcinoma of the larynx. *International Journal Of Radiation Oncology Biology Physics*, 1983; **9**: 321–9.

53. Withers HR, Mason KA. The kinetics of recovery in irradiated colonic mucosa of the mouse. *Cancer*, 1974; **34**: 896–903.

54. Withers HR, *et al*. The hazard of accelerated tumor clonogen repopulation during radiotherapy. *Acta Oncologia*, 1988; **27**: 131–45.

55. Hall EJ. Radiation dose-rate: a factor of importance in radiobiology and radiotherapy. *British Journal of Radiology*, 1972; **45**: 81–97.

56. Hall EJ, Brenner DJ. The dose-rate in interstitial brachytherapy; a controversy resolved. *British Journal of Radiology*, 1992; **65**: 242–7.

57. Mitchell JB, *et al*. Dose-rate effects on the cell cycle and survival of S3 HeLa and V79 cells. *Radiation Research*, 1979; **79**: 520–36.

58. Mazeron JJ, *et al*. Effect of dose rate on local control and complications in definitive irradiation of T1–2 squamous cell carcinoma of the mobile tongue and floor of mouth with interstitial Iridium 192. *Radiotherapy Oncology*, 1991; **21**: 39–47.

59. Pernot, *et al*. The study of tumoral, radiobiological and general health factors that influence results and complications in a series of 448 oral tongue carcinomas treated exclusively by irradiation. *International Journal of Radiation Oncology Biology Physics*, 1994; **29**: 673–9.

60. Pierquin B, Wilson JF, Chassagne D (ed). *Modern brachytherapy*. New York: Masson, 1987.

61. Cheng VSJ, *et al*. The function of the parotid gland following radiation therapy for head and neck cancer. *International Journal of Radiation Oncology Biology Physics*, 1981; **7**: 253–8.

62. Mira JG, *et al*. Some factors influencing salivary function when treating with radiotherapy. *International Journal of Radiation Oncology Biology Physics*, 1981; **7**: 535–41.

63. Norberg LE, Lundquist PG. Aspects of salivary gland radiosensitivity: effects of sialogogues and irradiation. *Archives of Otorhinolaryngology*, 1989; **246**: 200–4.

64. **Horiot JC, et al.** Radiotherapy for head and neck cancers including chemotherapy. *Current Opinion Oncology*, 1994; **6**: 272–6.

65. **Brizel DM, et al.** Final report of a randomized trial of amifostine as a radioprotectant in head and neck cancer. *International Journal of Radiation Oncology Biology Physics*, 1999; **45** (Suppl. 1):147–8.

66. **Simon JM, et al.** Effect of intersource spacing on local control and complications in brachytherapy of mobile tongue and floor of mouth. *Radiotherapy Oncology*, 1992; **26**: 19–25.

67. **Hart CGB, Mainous EG.** The treatment of radiation necrosis with hyperbaric oxygen (OHP). *Cancer*, 1976; **37**: 2580–5.

68. **Wilhelm KR, Schulz-Wendtland R.** Auswirkung der Bestrahlung von Mund-, Rachen- und Larynxtumoren auf die Schildrüsenfunktion. *Strahlentherapie and Onkologie*, 1988; **164**: 270–7.

69. **Bourhis J, et al.** Meta-analysis of chemotherapy in head and neck cancer (MACH-NC): (1) loco-regional treatement vs same treatment + chemotherapy. *Proceedings of the American Society of Clinical Oncology*, 1998; **17**: 386a.

70. **Byers RM.** Factors afecting choice of initial therapy in oral cancer. *Seminar in Surgical Oncology*, 1995; **11**: 183–9.

71. **Fuller D, et al.** Speech and swallowing rehabilitation for head and neck tumour patients. In: Thawley SE, Panje WR, ed. *Comprehensive management of head and neck tumours*. Philadelphia: Saunders, 1987: 100–31.

72. **Marks JE, et al.** Floor of mouth cancer: patient selection and treatment results. *Laryngoscope*, 1983; **93**: 475–80.

73. **Henk JM.** Management of the primary tumour. In: JM Henk JM, Langdon JD, ed. *Malignant tumours of the oral cavity*. London: Arnold, 1985.

74. **Levendag PC, et al.** Local tumor control in radiation therapy of cancer in the head and neck. *American Journal of Clinical Oncology*, 1996; **19**: 469–77.

75. **Parsons JT, et al.** An analysis of factors influencing the outcome of postoperative irradiation for squamous cell carcinoma of the oral cavity. *International Journal of Radiation Oncology Biology Physics*, 1997; **39**: 137–48.

76. **Pernot, et al.** Epidermoid carcinomas of the floor of mouth treated by exclusive irradiation: statistical study of a series of 207 cases. *Radiotherapy Oncology*, 1995; **35**: 177–85.

77. **Chao KS, et al.** The impact of surgical margins status and use of an interstitial implant on T1, T2 oral tongue after surgery. *International Journal of Radiation Oncology Biology Physics*, 1996; **36**: 1039–43.

78. **Hicks WL Jr, et al.** Surgery as a single modality therapy for squamous cell carcinoma of the oral tongue. *American Journal of Otolaryngology*, 1998; **19**: 24–8.

79. **Llewelyn J, et al.** Survival of patients who needed salvage surgery for recurrence after radiotherapy for oral carcinoma. *British Journal of Maxillofacial Surgary*, 1997; **35**: 424–8.

80. **Fang FM, et al.** Combined modality therapy for squamous carcinoma of the buccal mucosa: treatment results and prognostic factors. *Head and Neck*, 1997; **19**: 506–12.

81. **Langlois D, et al.** Salvage irradiation of oropharynx and mobile tongue about iridium 192 brachytherapy in Centre Alexis Vautrin. *International Journal of Radiation Oncology Biology Physics*, 1988; **14**: 849–54.

82. **Tiwari RM.** Masseter cross over flap in primary closure of oro or oropharyngeal defects. *Journal of Laryngology and Otology*, 1987; **101**: 72–8.

83. **Holt GR.** Surgical therapy of oral cavity tumors: lip tumors. In: Thawley SE, Panje WR, ed. *Comprehensive management of head and neck tumors*. Philadelphia: Saunders, 1987: 536–51.

84. **Antoniades DZ, et al.** Squamous cell carcinoma of the lips in a northern Greek population. Evaluation of prognostic factors on 5-year survival rate. *European Journal of Cancer*, 1995; **31B**: 333–9.

85. **Mazeron JJ, Richaud P.** Compte rendu de la XVIIIème Réunion du Groupe Européen de Curiethérapie. Session consacrée aux cancers de la lèvre. *Journal Européen de Radiothérapie*, 1984; **5**: 50–6.

86. **Gerbaulet A, Pernot M.** Le carcinomé pidermoide de la face interne de joue. A propos de 748 malades. *Journal Européen de Radiothérapie*, 1985; **6**: 1–4.

87. **Zitsch RP, et al.** Outcome analysis for lip carcinoma. *Otolaryngology Head and Neck Surgery*, 1995; **113**: 589–96.

88. **Pernot M, et al.** Indications, techniques and results of postoperative bracytherapy in cancer of the oral cavity. *Radiotherapy and Oncology*, 1995; **35**: 186–92.

89. **Grandi C, et al.** Surgery versus combined therapies for cancer of the anterior floor of mouth. *Head and Neck Surgery*, 1983; **6**: 653–9.

90. **Guillamondegui OM, et al.** Surgical treatment of advanced carcinoma of the floor of mouth. *American Journal of Roentgenology*, 1980; **126**: 1256–9.

91. **Zelefsky MJ, et al.** Postoperative radiotherapy for oral cavity cancer: impact of anatomic subsite on treatment outcome. *Head and Neck*, 1990; **12**: 470–5.

92. **Shah JP, et al.** Surgical therapy of oral cavity tumours: buccal mucosa, alveolus, retromolar trigone, floor of mouth, hard palate, and tongue tumours. In: Thawley SE, Panje WR, ed. *Comprehensive management of head and neck tumours*. Philadelphia: Saunders, 1987: 551–63.

93. **Grimard L, et al.** Iridium-192 curietherapy for T1 and T2 epidermoid carcinomas of the floor of mouth. *International Journal of Radiation Oncology Biology Physics*, 1990; **18**: 1299–306.

94. **Frazell EL.** A review of the treatment of cancer of the mobile portion of the tongue. *Cancer*, 1971; **28**: 1178–81.

95. **White D, Byers RM.** What is the preferred initial method of treatment for squamous carcinoma of the tongue? *American Journal of Surgery*, 1980; **149**: 553–5.

96. **Fein DA, et al.** Carcinoma of the oral tongue: a comparison of results and complications of treatment with radiotherapy and/or surgery. *Head and Neck*, 1994; **16**: 358–65.

97. **Spiro RH, Strong EW.** Epidermoid carcinoma of the tongue: treatment by partial glossectomy alone. *American Journal of Surgery*, 1971; **122**: 707–10.

98. **Spiro RH, Strong EW.** Discontinuous partial glossectomy and radical neck dissection in selected patients with epidermoid carcinoma of the mobile tongue. *American Journal of Surgery*, 1973; **126**: 544–6.

99. **Lam KH, et al.** Carcinoma of the tongue: factors affecting the results of surgical treatment. *British Journal of Surgery*, 1980; **67**: 101–5.

100. **Marks JE, et al.** Carcinoma of the tongue: a study of patient selection and treatment results. *Laryngoscope*, 1981; **91**: 1548–59.

101. **Wang CC.** Radiotherapeutic management and results of T1N0, T2N0 carcinoma of the oral tongue: evaluation of boost techniques. *International Journal of Radiation Oncology Biology Physics*, 1989; **17**: 287–91.

102. **Menderhall WM, et al.** T2 oral tongue carcinoma treated with radiotherapy: analysis of local control and complications. *Radiotherapy and Oncology*, 1989; **16**: 245–52.

103. **Benk V, et al.** Iridium 192 implantation for T1 and T2 squamous cell carcinomas of the mobile tongue. *Radiotherapy and Oncology*, 1990; **18**: 339–47.

104. **Wendt CD, et al.** Primary radiotherapy in the treatment stage I and II oral tongue cancers: importance of the proportion of therapy delivered with interstitial therapy. *International Journal of Radiation Oncology Biology Physics*, 1990; **18**: 1287–92.

105. **Callery CD, et al.** Changing trends in the management of squamous carcinoma of the tongue. *American Journal of Surgery*, 1984; **148**: 449–52.

106. **Vegers JWM, et al.** Squamous cell carcinoma of the buccal mucosa. A review of 85 cases. *Archives of Otolaryngology*, 1979; **105**: 192–5.

107. **Bloom ND, Spiro RH.** Carcinoma of the cheek mucosa, a retrospective analysis. *American Journal of Surgery*, 1980; **149**: 556–9.

108. **Nair MK,** *et al.* Evaluation of the role of radiotherapy in the management of carcinoma of the buccal mucosa. *Cancer*, 1988; **61**: 1326–31.

109. **Byers M,** *et al.* Results of treatment for squamous carcinoma of the lower gum. *Cancer*, 1981; **47**: 2236–8.

110. **Evans JF, Shah JP.** Epidermoid carcinoma of the palate. *American Journal of Surgery*, 1981; **142**: 451–5.

111. **Kovalic JJ, Simpson JR.** Carcinoma of the hard palate. *Journal of Otolaryngology*, 1993; **22**: 118–20.

112. **Pernot M.** Hard and soft palate. In: Pierquin B, Wilson JF, Chassagne D, ed. *Modern brachytherapy*. New York: Masson, 1987.

113. **Genn MG,** *et al.* Cost benefit management decisions for carcinoma of the retromolar trigone. *Head and Neck*, 1995; **17**: 419–24.

114. **Kowalski LP,** *et al.* End results of 114 extended 'commando' operations for retromolar trigone. *American Journal of Surgery*, 1993; **166**: 374–9.

115. **Berktold RE.** Carcinoma of the oral cavity. Selective management according to site and stage. *Olaryngologic Clinics of North America*, 1985; **18**: 445–50.

116. **Simpson JR.** Cancer of the salivary glands. In: Perez CA, Brady LW, ed. *Principles and practice of radiation oncology*. Philadelphia: Lippincott, 1987.

Tumours of the oropharynx

J. C. Horiot, R. Sigal, and J. L. Lefebvre

Anatomy (see Fig. 1)

The oropharynx has five walls: two lateral, one anterior, one posterior, and one superior. The lateral walls include the tonsils and tonsillar fossa and the anterior and posterior faucial pillars. The base of the tongue inferior to the vallate papillae, the vallecula, and the anterior part of the suprahyoid epiglottis make up the anterior wall. The soft palate and uvula form the superior wall. The posterior pharyngeal wall runs parallel to those structures, forming the anterior wall. The posterior wall and adjacent lateral pharyngeal walls constitute the mesopharynx.

The oropharynx is not a region defined by specific embryological or anatomical criteria. It consists of the structures located between the oral cavity, nasopharynx, and hypopharynx. Anteriorly, the retromolar trigone is often included in the faucial arch, although located in the oral cavity. The lower boundary is delineated by the free margin of the suprahyoid epiglottis and pharyngoepiglottic folds. Superiorly and anteriorly, the limits with the nasopharynx are at the free margin of the soft palate and uvula. The posterior wall and the lateral walls behind the posterior faucial pillar are in direct continuity, upwards to the nasopharynx and downwards to the hypopharynx. The anterior and posterior pillars are folds of mucous membranes over the glosso-palatine and pharyngopalatine muscles, whereas the tonsillar fossa is covered laterally by the superior constrictor, stylopharyngeus, and pharyngopalatine muscles.

The parapharyngeal (or lateral pharyngeal) space lies between the pharynx and the masticator space, the latter containing the muscles of mastication. The poststyloid (retrostyloid) parapharyngeal space contains the internal carotid artery, internal jugular vein, hypoglossal, vagus, accessory, glossopharyngeal nerves, and the sympathetic plexus. The retropharyngeal space lies between the pharynx and prevertebral musculature. The lateral retropharyngeal nodes (of Rouvière) lie at the boundary between the parapharyngeal and retropharyngeal spaces just medial to the carotid artery.

The rich lymphatic network of the tonsillar fossa, faucial arch, and base of the tongue drains primarily into the subdigastric (upper internal jugular) nodes. There are also lymphatic connections with para- and retropharyngeal nodes. In addition, the anterior pillar and retromolar trigone drain to the submandibular nodes. The lymphatics of the posterior pillar and posterior wall drain primarily to the para- and retropharyngeal nodes as well as the upper internal jugular and spinal accessory nodes.

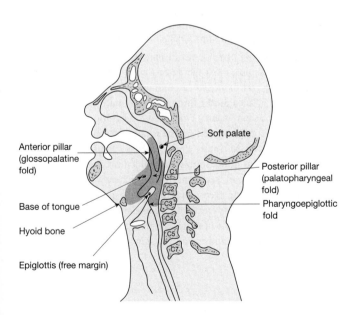

Anterior pillar
(glossopalatine
fold)

Soft palate

Posterior pillar
(palatopharyngeal
fold)

Pharyngoepiglottic
fold

Base of tongue

Hyoid bone

Epiglottis (free margin)

C1
C2
C3
C5
C7

Fig. 1 Sagittal section through the oropharynx. The coloured area represents the limits of this part of the pharynx (see description in the text and imaging section for frontal and axial representation). (Redrawn with permission from MacComb and Fletcher *Cancer of the head and neck* (Baltimore: Williams and Wilkins).)

Epidemiology

Some difficulties arise from the lack of uniformity in definitions of the oropharynx: some tumour registries include the oropharynx in the pharynx section, thus making the distinction from hypopharyngeal tumours impossible, whereas others add together the figures for the oral cavity and oropharynx. In addition, it is not always stated whether the figures contain all types of cancers or just epithelial tumours. Referring to epithelial tumours of the oropharynx only, the age-adjusted incidence rate (standardized incidence, world age-standardized incidence rate) per 100 000 population varies from 0.2 (females from Connecticut, United States) to 13.9 (males from Calvados, France), to a maximum of 23 in the tumour registry of the French 'Departements du Nord et du Pas de Calais'.[1],[2] Surprising differences are observed in Western Europe, with low figures of 0.6 and 0.7 in Denmark and the United Kingdom (Birmingham) and high figures of 11.6 in France. Including the base of the tongue in the oropharynx, the incidence rises to 15.8 (for males, Doubs, France). Table 1 shows

Table 1 Tumour registry of Doubs (France); crude incidence 1978–87 (per 100 000 residents) (by courtesy of S. Schraub (Besançon) (personal communication, 1990) and Muir and Waterhouse[1])

	Males	Females
Oropharynx	11.64	0.74
Base of tongue	4.19	0.28
Retromolar tongue	0.67	0.20
Total	16.5	1.22

In this tumour registry the oropharynx includes cancers of all pathologies from the following subsites: tonsillar fossa, anterior pillar, vallecula, soft palate (as well as oropharynx without known subsite of origin).

the incidence by sex and subsites for the tumour registry of the Doubs.[1]

Oropharyngeal carcinomas represent 0.5 per cent of all cancers in the United States versus 1 to 1.5 per cent in France. As with all squamous carcinomas of the head and neck, oropharyngeal cancers occur more often in males, the sex ratio (male:female) varying from 4:1 in the United States to 9:1 in France. Most oropharyngeal cancers appear after 40 years of age, with a peak incidence between the sixth and seventh decades of life.

Aetiological factors (see also Chapter 9.1.1)

Carcinogenesis in the head and neck is multifactorial, being affected by several environmental factors, and exhibits considerable inter-individual variation. Aetiological factors for oropharyngeal carcinomas are common to all epithelial tumours of the head and neck: excessive alcohol consumption, a long history of smoking, and, to a lesser extent, poor oral hygiene and its related conditions. The risk is strongly enhanced by the synergistic action of smoking and drinking. Considering the risk of an abstinent individual to be 1, the relative risks are about 5, 18, and 40 for light drinkers or heavy smokers, light smokers and heavy drinkers, and heavy smokers and heavy drinkers, respectively.[3] Although such figures are approximate, they reflect the fact that more than 90 per cent of patients with oropharyngeal carcinoma have a long history of tobacco smoking and alcohol intake.

Ethnic factors have been suggested but are not supported by reliable data. The role of premalignant mucosal changes is more difficult to assess. Leucoplakia is often observed in combination with invasive carcinoma of the anterior pillar and soft palate. However, there are no data on the incidence of oropharyngeal cancers developing from pre-existing leucoplakia. Conversely, premalignant changes are likely to play an important part in the development of multiple primary cancers, either simultaneous or sequential, that are reported in 10 to 15 per cent of patients with oropharyngeal cancers.

Several types of human papilloma virus have been identified in the aetiology of epithelial cancers such as cervical, anal, perianal, vulvar, and penile carcinoma (see also Chapter 2.2). There is emerging evidence that more than 20 per cent of oropharyngeal cancers also contain DNA from human papilloma viruses, mainly the tumorigenic human papilloma virus HPV16.[4],[5] Molecular mechanisms of human papilloma virus-mediated carcinogenesis are not yet fully understood. They probably include modifications in host cell genes engaged in the control of human papilloma virus gene expression in proliferating cells. The mode of transmission of human papilloma virus to the upper airway is unclear and has not yet been related to oral sex. The presence of human papilloma virus in preinvasive and invasive disease suggests that the viral presence precedes the mucosal changes. To confirm this hypothesis, a prospective seroepidemiological study of exposure to human papilloma virus with sufficient follow-up is needed to detect and register early disorders of epithelial proliferation, premalignant, and malignant disease. Human papilloma virus-positive tumours seem to have a better prognosis than human papilloma virus-negative tumours. Evidence of this observation needs to be confirmed by multifactorial analysis of population-based registries. Confirmation of the role of human papilloma virus in the carcinogenesis of head and neck cancers could lead to the development of antipapilloma therapies and preventive methods with vaccines and gene therapy.

Pathology (see Chapter 9.1.2)

Squamous cell carcinoma represents 90 to 95 per cent of malignant oropharyngeal lesions. Its variants include well-differentiated to moderately well-differentiated carcinoma (40 to 50 per cent), and poorly differentiated carcinoma (30 to 40 per cent), arising mostly from the tonsillar fossa. A subvariant of the latter, sometimes reported as lymphoepithelioma, is a poorly differentiated carcinoma with diffuse lymphoid infiltration. Verrucous carcinoma and adenocarcinoma are rare (1 to 3 per cent). Malignant lymphoma represents 5 to 10 per cent of oropharyngeal malignancies and is excluded from this review.

Pathological diagnosis of the primary tumour is obtained by biopsy, usually taken during examination under sedative analgesia or general anaesthesia. It should be taken at the border of the primary and normal tissues in order to avoid sampling a necrotic part of the tumour. This will also allow the detection of subclinical extensions of microinvasive and/or *in situ* carcinoma at the edges of the visible tumour, which is a common finding in carcinoma of the anterior faucial pillar and soft palate. Fine needle aspiration is a safe and efficient way to confirm nodal spread in clinically suspicious nodes, but it will only be of value when positive. Incisional and even excisional biopsies of nodes should be avoided because they interfere with further sequences of treatment by comprehensive neck dissection and/or radiotherapy, or even jeopardize the patient's prognosis; an incisional biopsy of a node creates the equivalent of a capsular rupture and may sometimes result in an accelerated growth of cancer in the nodes, dermal invasion, and metastatic skin nodules.

Biology

Head and neck cancers, like most cancers, are genetic diseases. A sequence of genetic aberrations is involved in carcinogenesis, locoregional growth, and metastatic spread. Susceptibility genes, cell cycle control genes, DNA repair mechanisms, and induction of apoptosis are involved in the initiation of carcinogenesis and disease progression.

The most frequent chromosome abnormalities are deletions affecting 3p, 5q, 8p, 9p, and 18q. Less common consistent changes are amplifications in 3q, 5p, 7p, 8q, and 11q. Loss of heterozygosity on chromosome 18q in metastatic and locally recurrent tumours, but not in primary tumours from the same patients, suggests that a tumour suppressor gene in this region may be important in the progression of head and neck cancers.

Mutated or inactivated p53 may also be involved in head and neck carcinogenesis. Benzopyrene in cigarette smoke can induce such changes in this tumour suppressor gene, thus enhancing proliferation of cancer cells. Abnormal p53 is also associated with increased resistance to radiotherapy.

Correlations between the overexpression or underexpression of certain biomarkers (Bcl-X_L, p53, and Bcl-X_S) and clinical response justify more translational research on new biomarkers as prognostic indicators. In addition to tissues, serum samples also provide a source of prognostic indicators. Antibodies to p53 are proving to be of value in predicting the clinical course of disease.[6],[7] Epidermal growth factor receptor is overexpressed in head and neck cancers (see also Chapter 1.4). The level of expression of epidermal growth factor receptor increases with the severity of dysplasia. The immunohistochemical detection of increased tumour levels of transforming growth factor-α or epidermal growth factor receptor allows a statistically significant prediction of decreased disease-free survival, independent of nodal stage. Upregulation of both the receptor and the ligand (transforming growth factor-α) are primarily a consequence of enhanced gene transcription and can be modulated by retinoic acid. Cell signalling through epidermal growth factor receptor involves selective activation of Stat (signal transducers and activators of transcription) proteins. New drug development is now producing chimeric antibodies to antiepidermal growth factor receptor which have been evaluated in phase I and II trials in patients with recurrent disease.

Genetic instability probably plays a key-role in explaining the interindividual variation in response to environmental factors. Future research is likely to involve the determination of genetic instability mechanisms using in vivo model systems, head and neck cancers developing in young patients with low exposure to carcinogens, and those in non-smokers. Candidate genes include cyclin D1 and other cyclins, cell cycle genes, p16, CDK4 and CDK6, aurora-like kinases, apoptosis-related genes such as Bcl-X_L and Bcl-X_S, and the human papilloma virus related genes E6 and E7. Combinations of genes are probably involved. The development of strategies for reducing or reversing genetic instability mechanisms by targeting treatment of unstable cells and tissues with relevant genes is an exciting challenge for prevention of cancer in this high-risk population.

Angiogenesis also plays an important role in the growth and spread of head and neck cancers. Various angiogenesis inhibitors are being evaluated in clinical trials. Inhibitors of matrix metalloproteinases may markedly affect invasion, metastasis, and angiogenesis. These inhibitors act by preventing the degradation of the extracellular matrix, thus reducing the growth and metastasis of cancer cells. They might also influence angiogenesis by inhibiting the ability of the matrix metalloproteinases to facilitate proliferation of capillaries at tumour margins.

These biological considerations highlight the tremendous progress achieved in the last decade in our understanding of carcinogenesis as well as its consequences for translational research and emerging novel therapies.

Clinical experience

The natural history and responsiveness to treatment of carcinoma of the oropharynx differs somewhat from that of other head and neck cancers. Conflicting statements have been made about whether tumour differentiation has a favourable influence or a detrimental effect on local control. Bataini et al. showed that undifferentiated tumours had better local control ($p = 0.01$) than well-differentiated tumours:[8] this is not an independent prognostic factor and is correlated with the higher proportion of undifferentiated tumours in the most favourable oropharyngeal subsite, the tonsillar fossa. Similar observations can be drawn for nodal involvement: In a series of more than 1000 cases from the Institut Curie, the nodal failure rate is similar in well-differentiated and poorly differentiated tumours (respectively 9 and 11 per cent).[9]

Cell kinetics

Although the volume of tumour is an overwhelming risk factor, it is obvious that a subset of small tumours may present with a recurrence after 'tumouricidal' radiation, while some large primaries can be unexpectedly controlled. Variations in intrinsic radiation sensitivity, in the proportion of hypoxic cells, and of the reoxygenation process during fractionated radiotherapy, relating to growth fraction and cell kinetics, are invoked to explain the different responses observed (see Chapter 4.2). Individual data on the kinetics of tumour cells (labelling index, duration of the S phase, and potential doubling time) can be obtained from biopsy specimens.[10],[11] The potential doubling time (T_{pot}) has been proposed as the most relevant variable for assessing tumour repopulation during treatment (see Chapter 1.7). T_{pot} was estimated in the European Organisation for Research on Treatment of Cancer (EORTC) protocol 22851 comparing accelerated fractionation with conventional fractionation.[10]–[12] The median T_{pot} of these tumours was 4.2 days (range 1.5 to 15.5 days), 24 per cent of patients having tumours with a T_{pot} of less than 2 days. Initial data had suggested better 2-year local control differences in favour of longer T_{pot} and in patients with short T_{pot} treated with accelerated fractionation, but were not confirmed with larger accrual and longer follow-up.

A large multicentre analysis was undertaken of the value of pretreatment cell kinetics parameters as predictors of the outcome of radiotherapy in head and neck cancers treated by conventional dose/fractionation regimens (60 Gy in at least 6 weeks using a single fraction per day).[13] A higher labelling index LI and not T_{pot} was the single parameter most significantly associated with poorer local control ($p = 0.02$) in univariate analysis, but neither LI nor T_{pot} were predictive for survival and LI lost significance in a multivariate analysis of local control. Tumour cell proliferation was also assessed in 115 head and neck cancer patients entered in the CHART regimen of accelerated radiotherapy (see also Chapter 4.2);[14] no parameter related to cell kinetics predicted the outcome of patients treated with the accelerated regimen, in keeping with the view that tumour repopulation during treatment was minimized by that regimen. Univariate analysis of the effects of individual parameters on cause-specific outcome was not significant. Variations of tumour response are multifactorial, and tumour repopulation during treatment is one of many factors. Present research projects involve the evaluation of a combination of improved individual cell kinetics parameters, as well as assays of inherent radiosensitivity and hypoxia.

Clinical features

Symptoms and signs common to all oropharyngeal subsites

The first symptoms are often ignored by heavy smokers and heavy drinkers who are used to accepting the inconveniences of chronic mucosal inflammatory changes of the upper aerodigestive tract. They include mild discomfort and the sensation of a foreign body, sometimes associated, even at an early stage, with odynophagia and otalgia, via the anastomotic tympanic nerve of Jacobson. At more advanced stages, spread to the masticator space causes trismus and temporal headache, and sometimes posterolateral spread to the poststyloid parapharyngeal space causes involvement of the cranial nerve. Enlarged lymph nodes in the neck may be the first symptom noticed by the patient and are present in 50 to 60 per cent of cases at first presentation.

Subsites of origin of oropharyngeal carcinoma

The initially or predominantly involved subsite is important:

(1) for understanding the routes of extension
(2) for evaluating the areas at risk for microscopic spread
(3) for selection of the optimum therapy
(4) for defining the areas to be included in radiotherapeutic target volumes
(5) for analysing results and prognostic factors.

In the report by Bataini, of 1313 cases of oropharyngeal carcinoma, 67 per cent arose from the lateral pharyngeal walls (including the tonsillar fossae) and soft palate, 32.5 per cent from the glossoepiglottic area (or anterior wall), and only 1.5 per cent from the posterior wall.[15] A similar distribution was observed by Rider, who also reported that, in the tonsillar area, 45 per cent of carcinomas seemed to arise from the fossa and 55 per cent from the pillars, mostly from the anterior.[16]

Tonsillar fossa

Early symptoms usually consist of a unilateral sore throat persisting despite symptomatic care. There may be associated ear pain, even at an early stage. Then the lesions involve neighbouring structures, mainly the soft palate, the anterior faucial pillar, and the glossotonsillar sulcus.

Soft palate

The site of any sore throat is ill defined, and it is worsened by food and drink. Destruction of the uvula may be responsible for vocal change. Advanced lesions cause problems in swallowing.

Anterior faucial pillar

Leucoplakia and/or carcinoma *in situ*, often asymptomatic, are occasionally diagnosed during routine examinations by dentists and physicians. Lesions extending to the retromolar trigone are discovered because of pain or chronic irritation caused by ill-fitting dentures. At a later stage, pain is the major symptom, resulting from spread along the buccinator and pterygoid muscle, or from infiltration and/or ulceration of the glossotonsillar sulcus. Various degrees of trismus are observed, depending upon extension into the masticator space. Infiltrating lesions can easily adhere to the ascending ramus of the mandible. At a later stage, they invade the outer table of the bone and the pterygomandibular space. They can then spread upwards along the lingual and inferior alveolar nerve, and sometimes progress to the base of the skull by a perineural route.

Base of the tongue

Small tumours are rare because of the scarcity of early symptoms. Most tumours will be diagnosed because of difficulties in swallowing, ear pain, and often swelling of the neck due to adenopathies. In advanced stages, the lesions infiltrate the deep muscles, producing fixation of the tongue, painful ulceration, and haemorrhage.

Vallecula (glossoepiglottic sulcus)

Lesions of the vallecula or lesions of the suprahyoid epiglottis are usually diagnosed at an earlier stage because they give early symptoms of difficulty or pain on swallowing. Most tumours of the vallecula are moderately infiltrating and have a tendency to lateral spread towards pharyngoepiglottic folds or to the pre-epiglottic space when deeply ulcerated. In contrast, most suprahyoid epiglottic tumours are exophytic and can sometimes become bulky without much impairment of deglutition or compromise of the airway as they do not tend to infiltrate the base of tongue or the epilarynx.

Nodal spread

The incidence and topography of nodal spread are correlated with the volume and subsite of the primary tumour. In the series from the Institut Curie, the overall incidence of positive neck nodes was 63 per cent.[9] Fletcher and Lindberg showed a progressive increase in incidence of positive nodes for the following subsites: retromolar trigone, anterior faucial pillar, soft palate (45 per cent), oropharyngeal walls (59 per cent), tonsillar fossa and base of tongue (77 per cent).[17],[18] In all series, the subdigastric area is the first and most commonly involved nodal location. The overall occurrence of contralateral nodal spread is about 20 per cent but varies with the origin of the primary: 6 per cent for the retromolar trigone and anterior faucial pillar, 20 per cent for the soft palate and tonsillar fossa, 25 per cent for the oropharyngeal walls, and 34 per cent for the base of the tongue. Bilateral nodal involvement occurs mainly with midline primary subsites (up to 40 per cent in tumours of the soft palate and base of the tongue) and its incidence increases with the size of the primary tumour. The lower and midjugular nodes are also often involved. Surgery, when undertaken, will usually be limited to a supraomohyoid modified neck dissection, sometimes with a sampling of contralateral nodes. Knowing the pattern and incidence of nodal spread, radiotherapy is the only treatment able to cover all the potential areas, and initial neck surgery will rarely prevent the need for postoperative radiotherapy.

Investigations

Imaging techniques (see also Chapter 9.1.3)

In patients with a superficial biopsy-proven lesion, the role of imaging is to visualize the extent of the tumour as accurately as possible, and in particular to assess involvement of the deeper tissues.

In patients presenting with a submucosal mass the aims of imaging are:

(1) To confirm the clinical diagnosis by showing a true mass versus a pseudomass.

(2) To guide a biopsy, or conversely to prevent a potentially hazardous procedure.

(3) To demonstrate the subsite and/or space of origin of the lesion and its characteristics (computed tomography (CT) density, magnetic resonance (MR) signal, homogeneity versus heterogeneity, contour, contrast enhancement).

Both CT and MR scans suffer from a lack of specificity. Tumour, infection, and inflammation may share the same CT and MR characteristics. This emphasizes the need for pathological confirmation of the diagnosis before planning of treatment. The correct diagnosis is often ensured by pooling imaging results with clinical, pathological, and biological data. Hence, close co-operation between radiologists and clinicians is a key factor in success.

Computed tomography

Computed tomography should be performed in the axial plane, parallel to the mandible. The study should extend from the skull base to the thoracic inlet in order to map tumour spread, to identify or rule out the presence of a second primary head and neck site, and to establish the lymph node status. Contrast injection is mandatory. With CT, most lesions enhance with contrast, usually moderately. It can be useful to compare a suspicious area with the contralateral site to demonstrate subtle invasion. Coronal views can help to define extension to the deep spaces, and should be performed in tumours of the soft palate. However, they are technically feasible in only about two-thirds of patients because of discomfort in positioning patients or because of dental amalgam artefacts. Spiral CT is useful when coronal views are not feasible. Double windows (soft tissue and bone algorithms) of the mandible and skull base are always necessary.

Magnetic resonance imaging

Magnetic resonance imaging is performed with a head coil or, if available, a specialized head and neck coil capable of covering both the suprahyoid regions and the neck. The patient should be reminded to maintain quiet breathing and to minimize swallowing during sequence acquisition. The study comprises a combination of sagittal, coronal, and axial views. The imaging protocol should include at least one T_1-weighted spin echo sequence and one T_2-weighted sequence. Gadolinium is routinely injected to detect perineural extension. Using T_1-weighted MR sequences, tumours show an intermediate signal intensity, comparable with that of the muscles, making identification of small tumours difficult. Using T_2-weighted sequences, the signal intensity of a tumour may range from hypo- to hyperintensity depending on the degree of cellularity and water content. For the same reason, contrast enhancement after gadolinium injection may be more or less heterogeneous. In general, larger tumours are more likely to be necrotic and heterogeneous. Sagittal views are particularly important for tumours of the base of the tongue and soft palate. The axial plane is optimal for assessment of the tonsillar fossa, glossotonsillar sulcus, retromolar trigone, and deep spaces. Coronal views are useful to evaluate the deep spaces. Magnetic resonance angiography can be used any time there is a suspicion of vascular lesion (glomus tumour). The usefulness of MR angiography to exclude invasiveness of the carotid arteries has not been established.

The choice between CT and MR is controversial and depends on several factors (see Chapter 9.1.3). Many head and neck radiologists advocate the use of MR as the examination of first choice because it best displays extension to the deep spaces. CT is not necessary if MR is technically satisfactory, unless mandibular invasion is suspected. In such a case, CT with a bone window setting is needed. Many teams continue to perform CT as the examination of first choice, either because MR is not available or because CT images are more familiar to clinicians.

Other techniques

Ultrasound imaging cannot evaluate the oropharynx itself, but it can be used to assess lymph node status, particularly when combined with fine needle aspiration.

Posteroanterior and lateral chest radiographs are used to detect lung metastasis or lung cancer. Computed tomography is more sensitive, but there is no cost–benefit analysis showing the advantage of using this technique rather than conventional radiographs.

Fluorodeoxyglucose positron emission tomography has shown promising results in discriminating between metastatic and hyperplastic lymph nodes.[19] Moreover, after treatment it can differentiate between tumour residue or relapse and posttherapeutic changes.[20]

Imaging findings per oropharyngeal subsite

Computed tomography and MR may be negative in squamous cell carcinomas with limited superficial spread. Conversely, imaging can demonstrate tumours spreading in patients without clinical symptoms or specific physical findings.

The oropharynx is located between the oral cavity, nasopharynx, hypopharynx, and larynx. Although interconnected and covered by the same mucosa, each subsite has its own specific clinical and radiological characteristics.

The tonsillar fossa (Figs 2, 3, and 4)

Tonsillar cancer usually causes tonsillar enlargement, but this finding is not specific since normal tonsils may be asymmetric. Imaging may help to identify a squamous cell carcinoma lying deep in the crypts of the faucial tonsils. Magnetic resonance is able to directly visualize the tonsils and to detect invasion of the posterior faucial pillar. Normally, the pillar appears as a thin, rounded structure with low signal intensity on T_2-weighted axial images. When invaded by tumour it is either thickened or not visible. Treatment planning may depend on this information. Invasion of the pharyngeal constrictor muscles can also be evidenced by MR. Extension to the deep spaces can be depicted in the axial and coronal planes: tumour first invades the

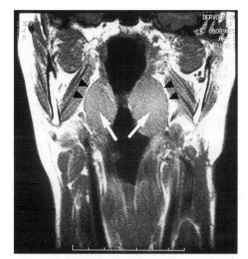

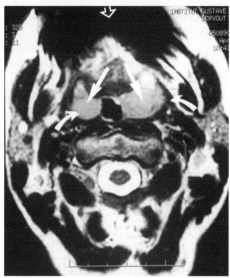

Fig. 2 Bilateral tonsillar lymphoma. (a) Coronal T_1-weighted view. Both tonsils are markedly enlarged, smoothly marginated, and homogeneous (arrows). The parapharyngeal spaces are spared (arrowheads). (b) Axial T_2-weighted view. The tonsils are displayed with increased signal intensity (straight arrows). The pharyngeal constrictor muscle (straight arrows) and posterior pillar are not invaded by the tumour. A large 'susceptibility' artefact due to dental amalgam precludes analysis of the oral cavity (open arrow).

parapharyngeal space, which is easily identified because of its fatty content, and then spreads to the carotid space and/or the masticator space. In the masticator space, special attention should be paid to the angle and the ramus of the mandible. Both CT and MR are useful in this regard. Computed tomography can detect cortical lysis whereas MR is able to recognize medullary bone invasion, which appears as an area of low signal intensity. Once a tumour invades the deep spaces, clinically occult extension can occur superiorly towards the skull base (beneath the nasopharyngeal mucosa) or anteriorly towards the retromolar trigone. Tumours invading the faucial pillars may reach the soft palate and the nasopharynx via the levi palatini muscles. Extension to the tongue is specific to the anterior pillar (since the muscular portion of this pillar is the palatoglossus muscle). Extension

to the hypopharynx is specific to the posterior pillar (since the muscular portion of this pillar is the palatopharyngeal muscle).

The retromolar trigone (Fig. 5)

This region is difficult to identify radiologically. The landmark is the pterygomandibular raphé that extends vertically from the posterior aspect of the horizontal branch of the mandible to the hamulus of the pterygoid plate. However, this raphé cannot be visualized directly, even by MR. It is located with respect to the posterior border of the mylohyoid muscle, the anterior aspect of the ramus, and the pterygoid plate. Physical examination of the lower part of the retromolar trigone is easy when a patient correctly opens his mouth. In contradistinction, tumours located in the superior part can be overlooked clinically. Axial CT and MR show this type of deep spreading, and possible extension into the buccal space (buccinator muscle) and masticator space (medial pterygoid and masseter muscles).

The glossotonsillar sulcus

It may be difficult to identify radiologically the site of origin of a lesion located in the glossotonsillar sulcus. A tumour arising from the glossotonsillar sulcus may mimic a lesion of the lateral border of the posterior third of the tongue, or an exophytic tumour of the tonsillar fossa. Such a lesion extends medially to the base of tongue, posteriorly to the vallecula, anteriorly to the posterior part of the floor of the mouth, and inferiorly to the submandibular space and even the upper neck. This latter extension may be clinically occult.

The base of the tongue (Fig. 6)

Physiologically, the lingual tonsil enhances strongly after contrast injection (iodine or gadolinium). In addition, the lymphoid tissue presents marked variation in shape and size and may protrude into the valleculae. Therefore, it may be difficult to depict the exact boundaries of a tumour since a neoplasm may be indistinguishable from the lingual tonsil after contrast enhancement. $T2$-weighted images are useful because most squamous cell carcinomas exhibit a lower signal intensity than the lymphoid tissue. Sagittal MR is superior to CT in showing anterior extension into the lingual muscles (geniohyoid and genioglossus). Imaging can depict the lingual artery and can therefore show the course of the neurovascular bundle of the tongue, and this is critical information for deciding the type of glossectomy. With CT, the lingual artery is directly visualized, provided that an adequate technique of contrast infusion is used. With MR, the artery is located because it courses medial to the hyoglossus muscle (and lateral to the genioglossus muscle more anteriorly). Direct identification with serpigineous flow of low signal intensity is not warranted. The sagittal plane is also useful when inferior extension to the pre-epiglottic space is suspected (this is rare, however, because the hyoepiglottic ligament which separates the valleculae from the pre-epiglottic space is relatively resistant to tumour extension, although direct extension via the thyrohyoid ligament is possible).

The soft palate

Imaging of this region is difficult. The soft palate is approximately concave in all directions, and therefore there is no ideal imaging plane,

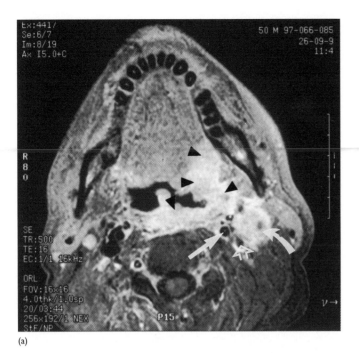
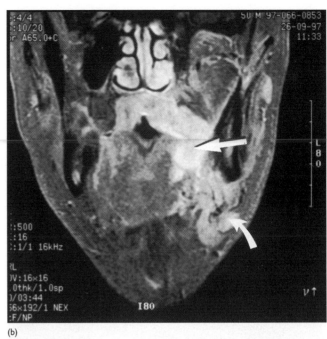

Fig. 3 Squamous cell carcinoma of the left tonsil. (a) Axial gadolinium-enhanced fat-suppressed *T*1-weighted view. The tumour (arrowheads) extends beyond the tonsillar fossa. Anteriorly, it extends into the posterior floor of the mouth, abutting the mandible. However, there is no abnormal enhancement within the medullary bone. Laterally, the middle pterygoid muscle shows subtle enhancement (compared with the contralateral side) indicating probable invasion. Posteriorly, the lesion extends into the posterior pharyngeal wall, crossing the midline. The tumour also abuts the internal carotid artery that still demonstrates the typical flow void pattern (arrows) indicating patency. The internal jugular vein is partially thrombosed (open arrow) because of an adjacent jugulodigastric metastatic lymph node (curved arrow). (b) Coronal view, same weighting, demonstrating superior extension along the tonsillar pillars (straight arrow). The soft palate is invaded, but it is not possible to clearly differentiate between the normal portion, which physiologically enhances with contrast, and the tumour. A submandibular metastatic lymph node is seen (curved arrow).

either on CT or MR. Pseudothickening may be due to asymmetric positioning of the patient in the axial and coronal plane. Moreover, the soft palate physiologically enhances with contrast (iodine and gadolinium) and this may explain difficulties in delineating enhancing tumours. Imaging can demonstrate lateral extension when the fatty parapharyngeal space is invaded by tumour. More laterally, it can show invasion of the middle and superior parts of the retromolar trigone. Retropharyngeal lymph nodes, which are often associated with this localization, are more easily detected. Extension to the skull base can occur via the veli palatini muscles.

The posterior wall (Fig. 7)

If a tumour invades the retropharyngeal space it may extend as in a liftshaft, from the base of the skull downwards to the mediastinum. Spread of the tumour into the anterior compartment of the para-vertebral space is rare (longus colli and longus capiti muscles). Laterally, both carotid spaces may be invaded.

Submucosal masses

Imaging plays an essential role in demonstrating the space in which the lesion develops (with specific differential diagnoses for each space), and in guiding the biopsy. The majority of these lesions bulge into the tonsillar region. Computed tomography and MR at best demonstrate the exact space of origin (masticator, parapharyngeal,

carotid, and even parotid spaces), guide the biopsy, or help in selecting the appropriate surgical approach.

Lymph nodes

As for other sites of head and neck cancer, identification of metastatic lymph nodes is essential. More than 60 per cent of patients have positive lymph nodes at initial presentation. In practice, CT is often first used to explore the oropharynx and neck. Magnetic resonance will not be necessary in most cases. Availability of equipment and experience still make CT the most reliable technique for detecting lymph nodes, although technical improvements should soon put MR on an equal footing. In fact, MR could be used as a single imaging procedure for the primary tumour and neck provided that a specific neck MR coil is available. The best criteria to predict tumour invasion include central low CT attenuation (or increased signal intensity on T_2-weighted images using MR), which represents nodal necrosis, focal tumour deposits, and peripheral rim enhancement. Indirect evidence of nodal metastases includes nodal enlargement, a grouping of three or more borderline-sized nodes in the primary drainage pathway, and a spherical rather than an elliptical shape. Size criteria are particularly poor in terms of specificity and sensitivity. The size criteria currently in use are 10 mm (and even 15 mm for level II). A recent study conducted by van den Brekel *et al.* has shown that a minimal axial diameter of 7 mm in level II nodes and 6 mm for the rest of the neck constitutes the best compromise between specificity and sensitivity.[21]

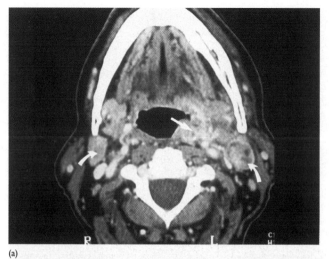

(a)

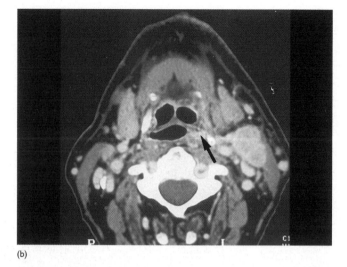

(b)

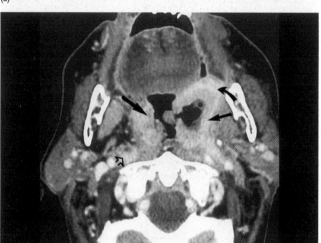

(c)

Fig. 4 Squamous cell carcinoma of the left tonsil. (a) Contrast-enhanced axial CT scan. The tumour (arrow) enhances with contrast, making a distinction from the surrounding muscles. It extends into the posterior pharyngeal wall. Invasion in the posterior faucial pillar is not directly seen. Notice bilateral subdigastric lymph nodes (curved arrows). (b) Same patient, 20 mm below. The tumour (arrow) has reached the upper left pyriform sinus, by invading the palatopharyngeal muscle. (c) Same patient, 50 mm above. The tumour (arrows) has reached the soft palate by invading faucial pillars. The palate has undergone partial necrosis. It extends anteriorly and laterally towards the retromolar trigone (curved arrow). Notice a right retropharyngeal lymph node (open arrow).

As shown by several studies conducted in The Netherlands, ultrasound-guided fine needle aspiration can make a diagnosis of lymph node metastasis with a specificity of greater than 95 per cent. This technique is operator-dependent.

Other investigations

These are part of the routine work-up of head and neck cancer at any site. They include a careful general examination of the patient, chest radiographs, electrocardiogram, and blood tests. In addition, the following procedures can be grouped together to save time and reduce the number of anaesthetics given:

- Complete examination of the head and neck in order to confirm the findings of the standard examination, especially when pain is present (for example when the glossopharyngeal area and base of tongue are involved), and to eliminate the presence of a second primary head and neck site.
- Bronchial and oesophageal endoscopic examinations with brushings for cytology and/or biopsies of any mucosal abnormalities. The systematic practice of panendoscopy combined with vital staining

with toluidine blue can detect up to 19 per cent of concomitant primaries of the upper aerodigestive tract at the time of initial work-up.[22]

Extraction of teeth not amenable to restoration by the usual conservative means, for example for deep caries or for advanced periodontal disease. Teeth in good condition are preserved, provided the patient is given a fluoride gel for systematic daily topical application or uses a toothpaste with a high fluoride content. These methods have led to a 96 per cent successful preservation of teeth in good condition in irradiated patients.[23]

Staging

General rules (see Chapters 3.5 and 9.1.4)

With regard to head and neck cancers in general and oropharyngeal cancers in particular there is no significant change between the 1987 and the 1997 editions of the UICC TNM staging system.[24] The 1987 UICC TNM staging (Table 2) was a definite improvement over

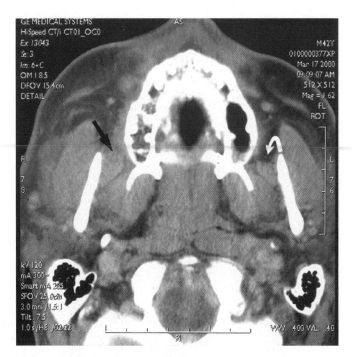

Fig. 5 Squamous cell carcinoma of the retromolar trigone. Contrast-enhanced axial CT scan. The tumour (arrow) does not enhance with contrast. Distinction from surrounding muscles is difficult. Comparison with the contralateral side shows evidence of abnormal obliteration of the buccal fat pad (curved arrow). The fat is easily recognized because of its low attenuation.

the previous edition, mostly because the size of lymph nodes was taken into account as well as the multiplicity of nodes involved. However, some problems arise when attempting to compare previous data based upon the new classification with published reports using the 1983 or earlier TNM editions, which were based on laterality and fixation rather than size.

Management

Radiotherapy and surgery, used alone or combined, are the reference strategies for stages I and II oropharyngeal cancer. Altered fractionation radiotherapy schemes and synchronous chemoradiotherapy, are emerging as the two most promising new strategies for carefully selected patients with stages III to IV disease. Hence, the main clinical decisions to be made by multidisciplinary teams are in selecting:

(1) radiotherapy or surgery as a single treatment;

(2) which should come first in the case of combination treatment;

(3) which patients should be proposed for new strategies;

(4) which new strategy;

(5) what to do in advanced disease not amenable to these new strategies.

These questions are not easy to answer since level I evidence is seldom available.

Radiotherapy will simultaneously treat the primary tumour and all nodal areas. It will also allow, from the first day, treatment of both macroscopic and microscopic disease. Surgery, even in the most

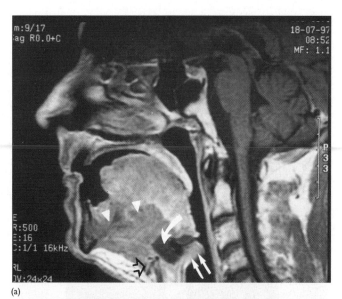

(a)

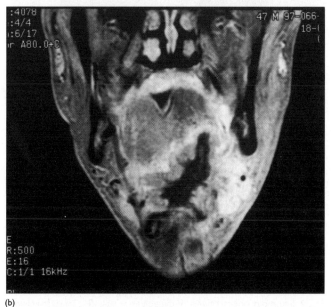

(b)

Fig. 6 Squamous cell carcinoma of the base of the tongue. (a) Sagittal gadolinium-enhanced T_1-weighted image. The tumour contains a limited necrotic area (curved arrow) which almost reaches the hyoid bone (open arrow), and a vast portion which extends to the anterior floor of the mouth by infiltrating the geniohyoid and genioglossus muscles (arrowheads). The free epiglottis is thickened (double arrows), but the pre-epiglottic space is spared, as shown by the normal high-signal-intensity aspect of the fatty component. (b) Coronal gadolinium-enhanced fat-suppressed T_1-weighted image. The tumour extends bilaterally, indicating invasion of both neurovascular bundles of the tongue.

radical excisions, will expose the patient to potential microscopic residues both in the neighbourhood of the primary tumour and in the nodal areas, and in situations where adjuvant radiotherapy will be necessary. It is therefore very important to set up a multidisciplinary discussion at the end of the work-up, not only to select the most appropriate treatment or sequence but also in order to avoid an unnecessary burden for the patient, and to save time, cost, and effort

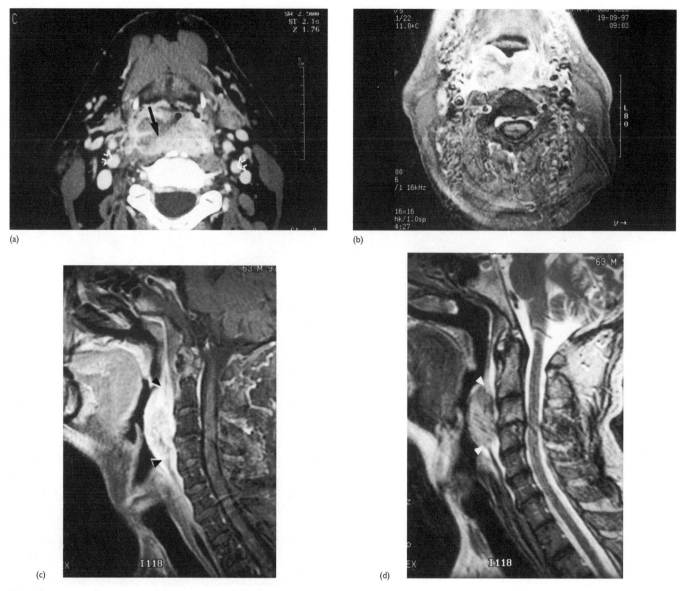

Fig. 7 Squamous cell carcinoma of the posterior wall. (a) Contrast-enhanced axial CT scan. The tumour protrudes anteriorly; laterally it remains separated from both internal carotid arteries (arrows). Posteriorly, the tumour abuts the anterior compartment of the paravertebral space (longus capiti muscles, arrows). (b) Axial gadolinium-enhanced fat-suppressed T_1-weighted image provides the same information. (c) Sagittal gadolinium-enhanced fat-suppressed T_1-weighted image and (d) sagittal T_2-weighted view allows precise delineation of the superior and inferior extent of the tumour (arrowheads). The vertebral bodies display a normal appearance on all MR sections, confirming the absence of tumour spread into the paravertebral space.

for the physicians, whenever similar results can be expected from different approaches.

Radiotherapy technique[25]-[27]

Target volumes (see Chapter 4.3)

Primary tumour

As a general rule the entire oropharynx should be included, regardless of the size and site of the primary. Tumours located in border areas (for example the anterior pillar or the vallecula) will require an extension of the target volume to other regions (for example the

posterior third of the oral cavity and the epilarynx). A safety margin of 3 cm should be allowed around the macroscopic limits of the primary tumour in order to encompass the subclinical epithelial and/or submucosal extensions around the primary. When the posterior wall is involved, adequate coverage of the prevertebral muscles requires inclusion of the spinal cord in the irradiated volume to a maximum cord dose of about 40 Gy in 20 fractions. The exclusion of parts of the oropharynx may be possible when small tumours (T_1) are lateralized (for example tumours of the anterior pillars) using special techniques (oblique wedged photons, three-dimensional treatment planning). The rationale is to spare the opposite salivary glands and

Table 2 TNM clinical classification

Primary tumour

T_x	Primary tumour cannot be assessed
T_0	No evidence of primary tumour
T_{is}	Carcinoma *in situ*
T_1	Tumour 2 cm or less in greatest dimension
T_2	Tumour > 2 cm but < 4 cm in greatest dimension
T_3	Tumour > 4 cm in greatest dimension
T_4	Tumour invades adjacent structures, for example through cortical bone, soft tissue of neck, deep (extrinsic) muscle of tongue

Regional lymph nodes

N_x	Regional lymph nodes cannot be assessed
N_0	No regional lymph node metastasis
N_1	Metastasis in a single ipsilateral lymph node, 3 cm or less in greatest dimension
N_2	Metastasis in a single ipsilateral lymph node, > 3 cm but < 6 cm in greatest dimension, or in multiple ipsilateral lymph nodes, none > 6 cm in greatest dimension, or in bilateral or contralateral
N_{2a}	Metastasis in single ipsilateral lymph nodes, > 3 cm but < 6 cm in greatest dimension
N_{2b}	Metastasis in multiple ipsilateral lymph nodes, none > 6 cm in greatest dimension
N_{2c}	Metastasis in bilateral or contralateral lymph nodes, none > 6 cm in greatest dimension
N_3	Metastasis in lymph nodes > 6 cm in greatest dimension

avoid subsequent xerostomia. This functional advantage should be carefully balanced against the risk of a geographical miss, for example because of insufficient coverage of the soft palate, of ignoring multiple microscopic primaries arising on the opposite side, and/or of a lack of treatment of the contralateral risk of nodal spread.

Nodal areas

The best control of nodal spread will be obtained by the inclusion of all neck nodes in the nodal target volume. Partial neck irradiation, excluding for instance some initially clinically negative areas of the neck, would expose the patient to a sixfold greater risk of recurrence in these areas as compared with the risk of recurrence in these N_0 areas when irradiation of the whole neck is systematically performed.[28]

There are some exceptions to this general recommendation; it is not necessary to irradiate the contralateral posterior neck in an N_0 lesion arising from the anterior pillars, or to include the submental areas when subdigastric and submaxillary areas are clinically negative. The presence of clinically involved nodes, regardless of their site, is a strong argument for including the whole neck in the nodal target volume. The entire pharynx, and the para- and retropharyngeal spaces to the base of the skull, will be part of the target volume when clinically positive nodes are present in the upper neck or when nodes are seen in CT slices in areas that are not accessible to palpation (for example the retropharyngeal space). It is also advisable to extend the target volume to the base of the skull when the primary tumour arises from the lateral or posterior pharyngeal wall, even when there is no palpable node.

Dose prescription

Different dose levels should be prescribed: potential areas of microscopic spread should receive doses of about 50 Gy in 25 fractions over 5 weeks; this dose will ensure a 90 per cent probability of local control in these areas.[29],[30] Both primary and nodal target volumes should then be reduced to the areas of the clinically demonstrable tumour, again with a 2 to 3 cm margin of safety to encompass

subclinical disease present in the immediate vicinity of these sites. The cumulative dose will then vary from 60 to 75 Gy depending upon the initial volume of disease (for example 60 to 65 Gy when the tumour is lees than 2 cm in diameter; 65 to 70 Gy when it is 2 to 4 cm; and 70 Gy and above when it is larger than 4 cm). A second reduction in target volume is sometimes advisable in cases of good regression and when total doses of 70 Gy or above are planned. Total doses above 75 Gy are not advised unless special techniques are used (two fractions per day or a boost with interstitial brachytherapy). In curative radiotherapy, the dose per fraction should not exceed 2 Gy per fraction in order to minimize the risk of late damage to slowly proliferating normal tissues (see Chapter 4.3). Doses per fraction of 1.7 to 1.8 Gy are prescribed when target volumes include a significant area of the oral mucosa (for example more than one-third) and/or when the target volume needs to include the supraglottic larynx. A review of results of radical radiation therapy for head and neck cancer indicates a significant loss of local control when the administration of radiation therapy is prolonged; hence lengthening of standard treatment schedules should be avoided whenever possible.[31] Weekly doses of 10 Gy using 2 Gy per fraction are still a widely used and recommendable standard. The use of multiple fractions per day either in pure hyperfractionated regimes or in hyperfractionated and accelerated regimes is discussed later in the section on the results of treatment.

Treatment planning

The 'conventional' approach is no longer recommended for accurate curative treatment planning. The patient set-up was done directly in the simulator room. Standardized anatomical landmarks adapted to clinically defined target volumes were used to delineate the portal sizes, later checked and corrected, when needed, from the portal films. Then contours were recorded and dose distributions were calculated in the central plane of the beams and off-axis in other planes of interest when reliable computer programs were available.

These procedures were repeated each time the irradiated volume was modified. This 'conventional' approach is often associated with variations between the prescribed dose and the actual dose distribution obtained in each patient.

The 'modern' approach involves the use of digital imaging data transferred to computerized treatment planning systems. This gives access to individualized three-dimensional treatment planning and conformal radiotherapy approaches whenever indicated. They involve the following steps:

(1) Computed tomography slices are obtained in a sufficient number of planes, representative of the various target volumes in the treatment position, on a flat treatment couch similar to that used for radiotherapy.

(2) Immobilization and the reproducibility of the patient's position are best realized by customized casts directly shaped on the patient's head and neck, using thermoplastic materials. Frontal and lateral 'scout films' visualize the projection of the planes of the selected CT slices. These anatomical data are then analysed directly in the treatment planning system used for dose calculations.

(3) The radiation oncologist delineates the various target volumes and critical organs in each plane and confirms the prescribed dose to each.

(4) The radiation oncologist and the radiation physicist then agree upon the technical choices (beam qualities, angles, and weights for the dose distribution to be as close as possible to the prescribed dose at different parts of the irradiated volumes and at different times of the treatment).

(5) From these choices, the dimensions and location of the portals will be projected on to the patient's outer contours, materialized, and finally checked on the simulator.

Usual beam arrangements and beam qualities (see Chapter 9.1.4)

In the radiotherapeutic techniques most commonly used for oropharyngeal carcinoma, the primary tumour and upper neck nodes are encompassed with parallel, opposed portals. Upper posterior cervical nodes may either be included in the volume irradiated with these two portals up to the safe tolerance dose of the spinal cord (for example 40 Gy in 20 fractions over 4 weeks) or be treated from the beginning with electron-beam 'strips' using an electron beam energy (for example 7 to 13 MeV) adapted to the depth of the target volume. Once the spinal cord dose of 40 Gy is reached, the target volume is reduced posteriorly to the midvertebral body. Electron beam fields are then designed to deliver the missing dose to reach the prescribed dose to the upper posterior neck. Additional care is needed to spare the spinal cord, brain, and peripheral nerves (brachial plexus) when accelerated radiotherapy is planned. In that case, the spinal cord dose should be kept as low as possible and in no instance should it be above 36 Gy over 5 weeks.[32]

Patients who smoke during radiation therapy appear to have lower response rates and shorter survival duration than those who do not; this may relate to induction or worsening of tumour hypoxia.[33] Patients should be strongly advised to stop smoking before beginning radiation therapy, and of course to maintain that resolution after treatment.

Brachytherapy (see Chapter 4.3.3)

The technique of interstitial brachytherapy using ^{192}Ir in plastic tubes is an elegant method for delivering a high dose to a limited target volume with a very steep dose gradient outside the implanted area. Brachytherapy is of particular interest for delivering a boost in patients with clinically negative nodes after 50 to 55 Gy given by external radiotherapy. Tumours of the soft palate offer an excellent indication for brachytherapy, allowing a high local dose (70 to 80 Gy when needed) to be reached without increasing the contribution to the temporomandibular joint and the muscles of mastication. Brachytherapy techniques have been described to cover adequately the tonsillar fossa, tonsillar pillars, and glossopalatine sulcus using loops of polyethylene tubing inserted through the submental area.

Interstitial brachytherapy of the base of the tongue is probably the easiest brachytherapy technique of any oropharyngeal location. Unfortunately, this site is often associated with large ulcerating tumours and bilateral nodes, so that the usefulness of the technique is limited because it boosts only part of the target volume. Conversely, the use of interstitial brachytherapy as a boost technique is highly recommended in T_1 to T_2 disease, where it provides the best way of reaching a high dose to the target volume without including the mandibular bone. The boost dose in brachytherapy depends upon the dose previously delivered with external irradiation and upon the initial and residual volume of disease. It usually ranges from a minimum of 20 Gy (for example after 45 Gy of external irradiation in favourable T_1 to T_2 disease) to 30 to 35 Gy (in larger tumours), thus participating in a total cumulative dose (with external irradiation) of 80 to 85 Gy. Computer dosimetry is mandatory because most of these implants are made with curved radioactive lines.

Surgery

Primary site

Treatment of the primary site can be divided into three main technical procedures, all requiring general anaesthesia:

(1) Transoral procedures should only be considered for wide local excision of very small malignant tumours and/or of lesions with borderline histological appearance (for example severe dysplasia). They do not usually require a temporary tracheostomy or a nasogastric tube. The resection is done with an electric surgical knife and rarely with a CO_2 laser. The anterior pillar, soft palate, and tonsillar fossa are the only oropharyngeal sites amenable to transoral procedures.

(2) Transmaxillary resections need at least a temporary tracheostomy. A simple mandibular section (mandibular swing) may sometimes allow good access to the lesions. At the opposite end of the spectrum, a hemimandibulectomy (the so-called commando procedure) may be necessary when there is direct spread to bone or when the tumour infiltrates the lateral pharyngeal spaces. Simple lateral resections of the mandible are feasible when tumour extension remains distant from the bone (for example when there is no spread to the outer part of the glossopharyngeal sulcus). This type of mandibular resection is also used to reach the posterior oropharyngeal wall after sagittal section of the tongue to the valleculae.

(3) Anterior cervicotomies require either a temporary or a permanent tracheostomy and, in all cases, a nasogastric feeding tube. They

give access to the base of the tongue and the valleculae, and depending upon tumour extension may be extended to the laryngeal vestibule and pre-epiglottic space by either a subglossal–supraglottic laryngectomy or a total subglottic laryngectomy. Histopathological examination of the margins of resection is mandatory: in fact, there are major difficulties in appreciating clinically the safety margins in the thickness of lingual muscles, as well as the superficial mucosal spread. Multiple biopsies with proper identification must be examined carefully during the operative procedure by an experienced pathologist.

Surgical management of neck nodes

Except for early lesions amenable to transoral surgical procedures, neck surgery, when done, is always combined with resection of the primary tumour. When surgery is planned first, neck procedures should be bilateral when the primary tumour reaches or extends beyond the midline structures.

Surgical reconstruction

Mandibular swing repairs are done with simple osteosyntheses. The repair of a hemimandibulectomy requires a difficult procedure. Free bony transplants (from the iliac crest, scapula, or fibula) combined with microvascular anastomoses or titanium plus bone-substitute (mixed with spongy bone) prostheses do not give the same quality of result as when used as part of reconstructive surgery after facial trauma. The long delay in healing is often inconsistent with the need for early postoperative radiotherapy, whereas this type of surgery may be impossible or hazardous in heavily irradiated tissues. The use of myocutaneous flaps (from pectoralis major, latissimus dorsalis, or trapezius) is of great value in repairing large mucosal defects and/or to compensate for large resections of the oral tongue and/or base of the tongue. The presence of a muscular pedicle allows efficient protection of the carotid axis and is of particular relevance when performing salvage surgery for radiotherapeutic failures.

Chemotherapy (see also Chapter 9.2)

Chemotherapy *per se* has relatively limited effects against squamous cell carcinomas of the head and neck. Some drugs, however, are able to produce regression of tumours, although complete responses are rare and of short duration. Cisplatin used alone or in combination with 5-fluorouracil is the most commonly used drug in head and neck cancer. The sequencing of chemotherapy with other treatments is described below.

Indications for various treatment techniques

Surgery alone

Except for the rare indication for purely intraoral surgery, the surgical techniques used for oropharyngeal carcinoma require the removal of part of the ascending ramus of the mandible and/or of a portion of the lateral pharyngeal wall, tongue, and soft palate. As a consequence, various degrees of swallowing, speech, and chewing problems will occur. The majority (up to 75 per cent) of patients who have had surgery are unable to return to a normal solid diet.[34] It is therefore essential to restrict surgery as the initial treatment of oropharyngeal carcinoma to clinical situations in which the probability of local

control with radiotherapy is low and/or to those cases where radiotherapy would be associated with a high risk of severe complications. Infiltrating carcinoma arising in the functional area within the oral cavity and/or involving the mandibular bone and/or producing trismus may be considered as the optimal indications for surgical resection (as primary treatment or after preoperative radiotherapy).

Combinations of surgery and radiotherapy[35]

Except for very small lesions, most indications for surgery will also be indications for adjuvant radiotherapy. The risk of subclinical extension beyond the surgical margins and of subclinical disease in the neck (regardless of the extent of nodal surgery) is high, and surgery alone in large oropharyngeal carcinomas will be associated with a high rate of locoregional failure. In addition, the site of failure after surgical reconstruction with myocutaneous flaps is often hidden, thus delaying the time of diagnosis until the recurrence is large.

Should radiotherapy be pre- or postoperative?

Radiobiological rationale favours preoperative radiotherapy. A preoperative radiation dose is likely to be more effective than the same dose given postoperatively. Earlier killing of cancer cells and reduction of the overall treatment time decreases the risk of tumour repopulation during treatment. In addition, fibrosis of the tumour bed, often associated with hypoxia, increases radiation resistance when radiotherapy is planned postoperatively. Early disease progression in the tumour bed and local recurrences seem less frequent when locally advanced disease is managed with preoperative radiotherapy. Some surgeons, however, claim that preoperative radiotherapy makes surgery more difficult. It may also increase healing time and perioperative complications. Other surgeons prefer to operate after radiotherapy. Preoperative doses (40 to 45 Gy in 20 to 25 fractions over 4 to 5 weeks) are usually lower than postoperative radiotherapy doses (60 to 70 Gy to areas of high risk). Unfortunately, no randomized trial has addressed this question in operable, moderately advanced oropharyngeal cancers. Thus, the level of evidence is based upon convergent experiences and historical comparisons. Except for a single report showing no difference between pre- and postoperative radiotherapy in oropharyngeal and oral carcinomas, there are no convincing data available and the sequence of treatment remains a matter of preference within multidisciplinary teams.[36] This question may soon become obsolete with the increasing use of initial concurrent radiochemotherapy schemes.

Indications by subsite

Base of the tongue

In the rare cases of early lesions of the base of the tongue, surgery and radiotherapy are able to provide equally good results. However, the functional results with radiotherapy alone are better. Hence, radiotherapy alone is the recommended as the first treatment, with salvage surgery being considered for treatment of recurrences.

Vallecula

Small lesions are amenable to satisfactory control either by radiotherapy alone or by surgery. Most surgical techniques will require a supraglottic laryngectomy, provided there is no extension to the pharyngoepiglottic fold and that the removal will not exceed 80 per cent of the base of tongue. A bilateral neck dissection is needed. However, most of these tumours also extend to the base of the tongue and radiotherapy is often preferred to avoid the risk of insufficient surgical margins. Adjuvant radiotherapy is necessary when positive microscopic margins are found on the pharyngeal section and/or when positive nodes are present in the neck dissection. Radiotherapy alone will treat this microscopic risk on both sides and is associated with fewer complications in swallowing than surgery. Larger tumours of the vallecula and/or base of tongue are rarely indications for surgery because they are often associated with bilateral neck nodes. A primary surgical procedure may be discussed in the case of a well-lateralized N_0 or N_1 lesion, or in large infiltrating and ulcerating lesions of the base of the tongue with destruction of the epiglottic cartilage and/or infiltration of the pre-epiglottic space. Needless to say, these procedures should be done only in patients with a reasonably good general condition and without large bilateral nodes.

Tonsillar fossa

Transoral surgical techniques are recommended when the differential diagnosis between inflammation, leukoplakia, and malignant tumour remains questionable. A tonsillectomy, sometimes extended to part of the anterior or posterior pillar, may provide a better specimen for pathology and be safer than a simple biopsy in the case of non-malignant lesions and/or severe dysplasia with or without intra-epithelial or microinvasive components. However, radiotherapy alone will be the most suitable treatment in most cases with invasive carcinoma to widely encompass the primary tumour and adjacent areas of potential local and regional spread. The indications for surgery in larger tumours are only justified when there is a deep extension to the mandible with trismus and/or destruction of the bony table. It then requires a wide excision of the adjacent mandible and of a portion of the tongue and soft palate. Myocutaneous flaps are necessary to close the defect.

Soft palate

Transoral surgical procedures are feasible in small (less than 10 mm) lesions of the soft palate and uvula. Larger resections would result in problems of speech and swallowing, and should be reserved for salvage surgery after radiotherapeutic failures.

Results of treatment

A review of the literature precludes any valid comparison between the various reports for miscellaneous reasons: variations in endpoints for reporting (local control alone, regional control alone without mentioning locoregional control figures), variations in statistical methods used for analysis, and, finally, variations in the proportion of oropharyngeal subsites and/or missing data on results per subsite. We shall often refer to the findings of the Institut Curie which provide a large series of patients treated according to a homogeneous strategy and reviewed with multivariate methods of analysis.[37],[38]

Results of radiotherapy

Primary tumour

About 90 per cent of the failures observed in the primary tumour and/or in the neck occur within the first 3 years of follow-up. The tumour stage is the most significant prognostic factor for local control ($p < 0.0001$): local control figures are about 89 per cent for T_1, about 84 per cent for T_2, about 63 per cent for T_3, and about 43 per cent for T_4 tumours. Numerous reports indicate the overwhelming importance of tumour volume in tumour control. The initial tumour subsite ($p < 0.001$) is the second most significant prognostic factor for local control:[15] an increasing risk of primary tumour failure is observed with the following sequence—tonsillar fossa, posterior pillar (about 23 per cent), anterior pillar (about 34 per cent), glosso-pharyngeal sulcus (about 50 per cent), lateral and posterior pharyngeal walls, base of tongue (over 50 per cent). Barker and Fletcher, reporting 190 cases of T_1, T_2, and T_3 tumours of the retromolar trigone and/or anterior faucial pillar, showed that there was not much difference in local control per stage (respectively 15, 19, and 15 per cent).[39] They explained this finding by the pattern of superficial spread often observed in these subsites in which tumour stage does not correlate with marked changes in tumour volume. They stress the importance of a generous anterior margin for the target volume, as failures due to geographical misses mostly occurred on the gum and/or buccal mucosa.

Altered fractionation schemes (see also Chapters 4.2 and 4.3)

Hyperfractionation

Conventional fractionation schemes of radiotherapy alone already offer a high chance of local control for most patients with T_1, T_2, T_3, N_0, N_1 oropharyngeal carcinomas, so these patients were often selected for testing possible improvements in radiotherapy by taking advantage of an increased therapeutic gradient using two fractions per day instead of one. This scheme allows an increase in total dose of about 15 per cent without enhancing late radiation damage to normal tissues. Pure hyperfractionation involves a similar overall treatment time to conventional fractionation.

Horiot et al., in an EORTC randomized trial (EORTC 22791) of 366 patients with T_2, T_3, N_0, N_1 oropharyngeal cancers, demonstrated an improvement in 5-year local control ($p < 0.01$) and overall survival ($p = 0.05$) by delivering 80.5 Gy in 70 fractions over 7 weeks compared with 70 Gy in 35 fractions over 7 weeks, without an increase in the rate of complications (Fig. 8).[40],[41]

Accelerated radiotherapy

The time factor plays a determinant role in the probability of local control (see also Chapter 4.2). The decrease in local control with prolongation of the overall treatment time beyond 5 weeks was shown to be as large as 20 to 25 per cent for every 10 days' prolongation in 465 cases of tonsillar carcinoma reported by Bataini et al. and Fowler et al.[8],[37] These observations are consistent with a very short doubling times (2 to 4 days) for repopulation of surviving cells during radiotherapy. It also constitutes the biological basis for accelerated radiotherapy whereby a significant shortening of the overall treatment time is aimed at reducing the effect of tumour repopulation during treatment.

The EORTC trial 22851 compared a standard radiotherapy regimen (70 Gy in 35 fractions over 7 weeks) with an accelerated split-course regimen of 72 Gy in 45 fractions over 5 weeks.[32] Sixty four per cent of the 511 patients had stage II, III, or IV oropharyngeal carcinoma. Patients in the accelerated fractionation arm did significantly better with regard to locoregional control ($p = 0.02$) resulting at 5 years

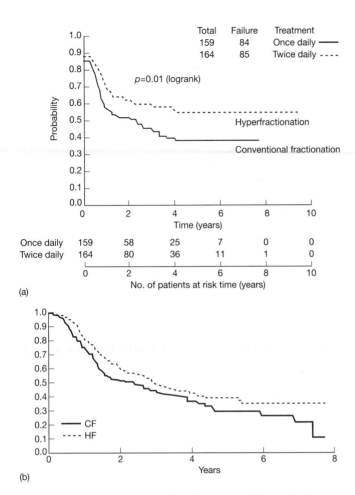

Fig. 8 (a) Probability of remaining free of locoregional disease. (b) Overall survival: patients receiving hyperfractionation show a significant improvement ($p = 0.05$).

A four-arm prospective randomized RTOG phase III trial (RTOG 90–03) was designed to investigate, in the same study, standard fractionation, one hyperfractionated, and two accelerated radiation therapy regimens.[42] Conventional radiotherapy (70 Gy in 35 fractions over 7 weeks, **SFX**) was compared with hyperfraction (**HFX**) of 81.6 Gy in 68 fractions over 7 weeks, accelerated fractionation with split course treatment (**AFX-S**) of 67.2 Gy in 42 fractions over 6 weeks, and accelerated fractionation with concomitant boost (**AFX-C**) of 72 Gy in 42 fractions over 6 weeks. A 1.2 Gy dose per fraction was administered twice daily with a minimum interval of 4 h, 5 days per week. Patients with stage III and IV carcinomas of the oral cavity, oropharynx, nasopharynx, hypopharynx, and supraglottic larynx were stratified by site, presence or absence of nodal metastases, and performance status. This trial confirmed the results of the EORTC 22791 hyperfractionation trial with an improved locoregional control of the HFX arm compared with the SFX arm ($p = 0.045$). The AFX-C regimen was also superior to the SFX arm ($p = 0.05$) with regard to locoregional control. Both altered regimes showed a trend towards a better disease-free survival compared with SFX (respectively $p = 0.067$ and $p = 0.054$). The AFX-C regimen was comparable to the standard SFX regimen.

Results and indications for delivering the radiotherapy boost with interstitial brachytherapy

Very high control rates (80 to 95 per cent in T_1, T_2; 74 per cent in T_3) have been reported when an additional dose of 20 to 30 Gy is delivered with interstitial brachytherapy after 45 to 50 Gy of external irradiation.[43]–[45] All reports consistently point out that the best selection of patients for interstitial brachytherapy is represented by those with tumours of the tonsillar area and/or soft palate with limited residual volume and no palpable nodes after external irradiation. There are no randomized controlled trials, but comparisons with historical controls do not suggest improved local control with this technique in tumours which deeply infiltrate the retromolar trigone, the glosso-tonsillar sulcus, and the base of the tongue. Complications include superficial mucosal necrosis in about 20 per cent of cases, most of which heal spontaneously, and bone necrosis in 5 per cent; only 1 of 269 patients reported by Pernot et al. died from complications.[45] In summary, interstitial brachytherapy is likely to improve the chance of local control in a selected group of patients with a favourable tumour and subsite presentation. If planned in continuity with or with a short time gap between the course of external irradiation, it allows a significant reduction in the overall treatment time and combines the rationales of accelerated and conformal radiotherapy.

Nodal control

As for the primary tumour, comparison of results is difficult due to variation in the criteria used for analysis: isolated nodal failures versus failures occurring both at the primary site and in nodes, ultimate control after salvage of failures, methods of analysis, etc. However, some general conclusions can be drawn: when treated with radiotherapy alone, the 5-year actuarial control rate of N_0, N_1 disease is high (80 to 90 per cent) and does not differ significantly for N_0 or N_1 (unilateral, < 3 cm); 85 per cent 5-year regional control in 323 patients with N_0, N_1 disease was reported by Horiot et al., including all nodal failures.[40] The figures reported by Bataini (98 per cent in N_0 and 90 per cent in N_1 disease) are given only at 3 years in patients with their primary tumour under control.[37] When this criterion for

in a 13 per cent gain (95 per cent confidence interval: 3 to 23 per cent gain) in locoregional control over the conventional fractionation arm. This improvement is of a larger magnitude in patients with a poorer prognosis (N_2 to N_3 any T, T_4 any N) than in patients with more favourable stage. Multivariate analysis confirmed accelerated fractionation as an independent prognostic factor for locoregional control ($p = 0.03$). Disease-specific survival shows a trend ($p = 0.06$) in favour of the accelerated fractionation arm. A higher late toxicity was observed in the accelerated fractionation arm compared with the conventional fractionation arm, respectively 15 per cent versus 2 per cent for severe fibrosis, 13 per cent versus 5 per cent for severe mucosal damage, seven cases of peripheral neuropathies and two cases of transverse myelitis observed in the accelerated fractionation arm only. This late normal tissue damage seems to correlate with the large daily dose used in a split-course regimen with a small number of treatment days (4.8 Gy per day in three fractions of 1.6 Gy delivered with a 4 h interval between fractions and over 15 treatment days). Several schemes of continuous accelerated fractionation delivering 60 to 70 Gy over 5 to $5\frac{1}{2}$ weeks, using two fractions per day or concomitant boost in the last 2 weeks, do not seem associated with increased late toxicity.

analysis is used, high 3-year control rates are also observed for N_2 (88 per cent) and N_3 (71 per cent) disease. Such data support the rationale for radiotherapy alone for oropharyngeal tumours of moderate volume regardless of nodal stage, using modified neck dissection only for salvage of nodal failures. There is a sharp dose–control relationship for nodes larger than 3 cm.[17],[37] Doses of 70 Gy in 35 fractions over 7 weeks are adequate for nodes of size less than 3 cm. However, doses of 75 to 80 Gy are necessary to obtain high control rates in nodes larger than 3 cm, 80 per cent for nodes of 3 to 6 cm, and 70 per cent for nodes larger than 6 cm, provided that an adequate radiotherapeutic technique is used, delivering high doses within the shortest possible time. In large and/or rapidly growing nodes, the boost dose should be delivered during the treatment, using the principle of the concomitant boost technique, preferably with accelerated fractionation.[46] Boosting residual nodes after an overall treatment time of 8 weeks does not provide the same benefit, and a 2-month, delayed, modified neck dissection or 'lumpectomy' should be preferred when large, non-fixed residual nodes are still present after 50 Gy. Factors other than size influence nodal control:

(1) Node mobility results in a 6 per cent failure of treatment versus 13 per cent in fixed nodes in 1035 patients with their primary controlled.[9]

(2) Control of the primary tumour.

It is of interest, however, that the rate of isolated nodal failures is independent of the oropharyngeal subsite of origin (about 5 per cent in anterior faucial pillar, tonsillar fossa, and base of the tongue), although being significantly lower in the oropharynx than in the hypopharynx and larynx (10 per cent; $p < 0.01$).[9]

Results of surgery

There are fewer reports of surgery alone than of radiotherapy alone for T_1 or T_2 oropharyngeal carcinoma. In addition, the number of patients in surgical series is usually very small and does not allow a reliable comparison with series from radiotherapy alone comprising several hundreds of patients. Good results can be achieved in small selected groups; Maltz et al., in 36 patients, reported 80 per cent 5-year survival for T_1 and 69 per cent for T_2 disease.[47]

Most surgical series combine radiotherapy (either pre- or postoperative) and surgery, or keep surgery for salvage of radiotherapeutic failures. This general trend is illustrated in the series of 809 cases reported by Lefebvre et al., in which 20 cases (2.5 per cent) had surgery alone, 589 (73 per cent) had radiotherapy alone, and 119 (15 per cent) underwent a combination of surgery and radiotherapy.[48]

Lefebvre et al. also report a series of 403 cases of carcinoma of the tonsillar area treated surgically by buccopharyngectomy and hemimandibulectomy.[34] There were 52 T_2, 188 T_3, and 163 T_4 tumours representing 40 stage II, 164 stage III, and 199 stage IV patients; 274 had indications for initial surgery and postoperative radiotherapy, 29 had preoperative radiotherapy, and in 100 cases surgery was done as a salvage treatment for recurrent tumour. A more extensive procedure than originally planned was performed in about one-third of cases, and ultimately the resection was considered inadequate in only 6 per cent of cases. Locoregional failures occurred in 31 per cent of the postoperative radiotherapy group (5-year survival 42 per cent), 59 per cent of the preoperative radiotherapy group (5-year survival 16 per cent), and in 61 per cent of the salvage treatment group (5-year survival 17 per cent). Perez et al. reported 120 cases

treated by preoperative radiotherapy (30 to 40 Gy) and surgery.[49] The local failure rate was: 22 per cent in T_1, N_0; 15 per cent in T_1, T_2, N_1, N_2; about 30 per cent in T_3 or T_1, T_2, T_3, N_3; and 78 per cent in T_4 disease.

Geoffray et al. reported 90 cases of tonsillar carcinoma (one T_1, 34 T_2, 49 T_3, and six T_4) treated with radical surgery and postoperative radiotherapy to 50 Gy.[50] Local failures occurred in 25 per cent of cases (17 per cent in T_2, 27 per cent in T_3, and four patients out of six in T_4); the local failure rate rose to 39 per cent (9/23) after discovery of inadequate margins. The radiotherapy dose was also an important indicator, with 37 per cent of failures when doses were less than 40 Gy and 16 per cent when doses of 50 Gy and above were used. Inadequate margins are not necessarily associated with a poorer prognosis when postoperative radiotherapy is given at sufficient doses (17 per cent failure rate above 65 Gy versus 58 per cent for doses below 65 Gy).

As the base of the tongue carries the highest risk of local failure with radiotherapy of all oropharyngeal subsites, it is of interest to compare the results of surgery and of a combination of surgery and radiotherapy for this subsite. Harrold and Whicker et al., in a large series of patients treated with surgery alone, reported 56 and 37 per cent local failure rates, whereas Thawley et al. and Riley et al., using surgery and radiotherapy, report lower figures (40 and 22 per cent respectively).[51]–[54] Surgery (with or without radiotherapy) does not improve the outcome as compared with radiotherapy alone, which can also be applied to a less selected group of patients with regard to age and general condition. The posttherapy performance status of patients with primary tumours of the base of the tongue appears to be better following radiation therapy than following surgery.[55] Local control and survival being similar, the better preservation of function (swallowing and speech) provided by radiotherapy is consistent with a better quality of life and social reintegration after treatment.

Results of chemotherapy (see also Chapter 9.2)

A recently published patient-based meta-analysis of 63 controlled clinical trials for head and neck cancers has shown no improvement with adjuvant or induction chemotherapy regimens compared with standard therapies without chemotherapy in the curative management of head and neck cancers.[56] However, this analysis demonstrates a significant benefit in locoregional control and survival with concomitant radiochemotherapy regimens, and trials undertaken more recently that were not included in the meta-analysis have tended to confirm this.

Concomitant chemoradiotherapy at present appears to be the only approach, together with accelerated radiotherapy, which offers a chance of circumventing the risk of tumour repopulation during treatment and which avoids the selection of resistant cells that occurs when induction chemotherapy is used.

Results of randomized trials of concomitant radiochemotherapy

There are a very few trials of concomitant radiochemotherapy for oropharyngeal cancers only. In the French ARCORO trial, 226 patients with stages III and IV oropharyngeal carcinoma were randomized to radiotherapy alone (70 Gy in 35 fractions) or to the same radiotherapy

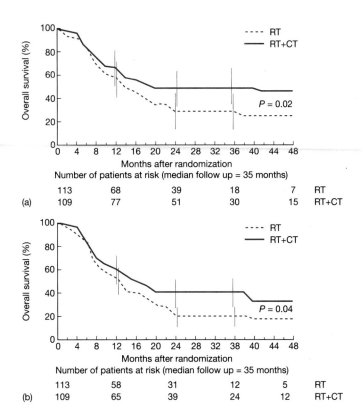

(a)

(b)

Fig. 9 Significant overall survival and disease-free improvement in patients receiving concomitant chemoradiotherapy compared with standard radiotherapy alone. (From Calais et al.[57])

Table 3 Absolute 5-year survival of carcinoma of the tonsillar area (including anterior and posterior pillar). (Adapted from Bataini et al.[15])

Stage	Number of cases	Survival (%)
$T_1 N_0 N_1$	18/27	67
$T_2 N_0 N_1$	36/79	46
$T_3 N_0 N_1$	36/128	28
$T_4 N_0 N_1$	28/124	23
$T_1 T_2 N_2 N_3$	9/48	19
$T_3 T_4 N_2 N_3$	23/151	15
Total	150/557	27

An increased risk of late damage to normal tissues seems likely to occur in trials of concurrent radiochemotherapy and may outweigh the expected benefit. Finally, most trials of chemotherapy include all head and neck subsites together (often without stratification), thus making them difficult to analyse when looking for a reliable comparison in a specific site (or subsite) and stage.

with concomitant chemotherapy consisting of three cycles of a 4-day continuous infusion regimen containing carboplatin (70 mg/m² per day) and 5-fluorouracil by (600 mg/m² per day).[57] Grade 3 to 4 mucositis and haematological toxicity were significantly higher in the combination regimen. Three-year overall actuarial survival and disease-free survival rates (Fig. 9) were improved in the radiochemotherapy arm compared with radiotherapy alone—51 per cent versus 31 per cent and 42 per cent versus 20 per cent ($p = 0.02$ and 0.04 respectively). The locoregional control rate was also improved (66 per cent versus 42 per cent).

A similar approach was evaluated by Jeremic et al., although with less specific entry criteria (unresectable head and neck cancers).[58] One hundred and fifty nine patients with stage III/IV (M_0) squamous cell carcinoma of the head and neck were randomized to receive standard fraction radiotherapy (70 Gy, group 1) or the same radiotherapy plus either 6 mg/m² of cisplatin (group 2) or 25 mg/m² of carboplatin (group 3), both given daily during radiotherapy. Groups 2 and 3 had significantly longer median survival times and higher 5-year survival rates than group 1 (31 months versus 16 months, $p = 0.002$). Median time to local recurrence and 5-year local recurrence-free survival were significantly higher for the radiochemotherapy regimens when compared with radiotherapy alone. There was no difference between the three treatment groups regarding control of regional lymph nodes and distant metastasis. Acute high-grade (greater than or equal to 3) haematological toxicity was significantly higher in the two radiochemotherapy groups.

Survival

As for all other head and neck cancers, causes of death other than the primary cancer greatly deteriorate the 5-year survival rate, even in patients with a high rate of locoregional control. In the series of 809 cases described by Lefebvre et al., with 29 per cent T_1, T_2, and 71 per cent T_3, T_4 disease, 497 (61 per cent) died from the initial cancer (or from its metastases), 57 (7 per cent) from a second primary, and 97 (12 per cent) from intercurrent disease or an unknown cause.[48] The incidence of second primaries was as high as 28 per cent (8 per cent before, 10 per cent simultaneously, and 10 per cent after the oropharyngeal cancer). Of course, the combination of tumour and nodal stages strongly influences the 5-year survival rate, as shown by Bataini et al.[15] in 557 cases of carcinoma of the tonsillar area (Table 3), falling from 67 per cent in the best group (T_1, N_0, N_1) to 15 per cent in the worst group (T_3, T_4, N_2, N_3). The cause of death in 157 of 356 patients (44 per cent) of T_2, T_3, N_0, N_1 entered in the EORTC trial 22791 was as follows: primary cancer 33 per cent, intercurrent disease 13 per cent, other cancer 6 per cent, unknown 4 per cent, complications of treatment 1 per cent.[40] In spite of that burden, overall survival was improved as a consequence of the large benefit in locoregional control brought about by the higher total dose hyperfractionation regimen. The only other phase III trial strategy resulting in an improved survival is synchronous radiochemotherapy. Thus there are two conclusions: some hyperfractionated regimens and some radiochemotherapy regimens can improve locoregional control and survival in stage III/IV oropharyngeal cancers. However, in both instances, theses trials were for patients in good to excellent general condition: this indicates a selection process that should be kept in mind when extrapolating these results to standard practice.

Complications

Radiotherapy

The main detrimental effect of major acute intolerance is to preclude the delivery of the planned radiotherapeutic dose. However, this should remain a rarity when adequate supportive care (including admission to hospital, nasogastric or G-tube feeding, intravenous fluids) is offered to patients suffering such acute mucositis that an oral diet is precluded. In EORTC trial 22791, only 6 per cent of patients could not receive the prescribed dose, despite the aggressiveness of the scheme (80.5 Gy in 7 weeks and 70 fractions). In the same trial, using an actuarial method, at 3 years, 70 per cent of patients were free of late grade 2, 3 complications consisting of bone and mucosal necrosis (6 per cent), fibrosis (15 per cent), and oedema (15 per cent); several complications often occurred in a single patient.

Surgery

Resection of the mobile portion of the tongue is mostly responsible for speech troubles, while that of the base of the tongue produces problems in swallowing. Hemimandibulectomies without reconstructive procedures are followed by an off-centring of the remaining hemimandible, thus rendering inefficient most efforts to restore chewing and swallowing functions. There is a high incidence (about 30 to 40 per cent) of hypothyroidism in patients who have received external beam irradiation to the entire thyroid gland or to the pituitary gland. Although the inclusion of these glands in the target volume of oropharyngeal cancers is seldom justified, thyroid function testing of patients in whom high-dose irradiation of these glands cannot be avoided must be considered as part of post-treatment follow-up.

Functional complications constitute the major burden of late postsurgical damage; 77 per cent of the 403 patients in the series of Lefebvre et al. could not return to normal feeding habits, while 39 per cent presented with significant sequelae or complete loss of laryngeal function.[34] According to Lefebvre et al., this risk should restrict the role of surgery to T_3, T_4 disease extended to the intermaxillary commissure, anterior pillar, and retromolar trigone, all other cases being offered radiotherapy with surgical salvage of failures.

Treatment of failures

Simultaneous failures at the primary and nodal sites are rarely amenable to a second treatment with curative intent and most cases will be submitted to experimental approaches with various chemotherapeutic regimens or other palliative treatments. Conversely, isolated failures, either at the tumour or node, can often be proposed for a salvage surgical procedure. Treatment failures in the tonsillar fossa and anterior pillar are best suited to transmaxillary buccopharyngectomies and can yield 5-year survival rates of up to 30 per cent.[59] Small recurrences on the soft palate can sometimes be salvaged with interstitial brachytherapy.[45]

The optimal choice of treatment strategies

There is no clear-cut evidence for superior survival obtained by any therapeutic strategy proposed in this chapter.

A few basic concepts must be kept in mind regarding the choice of therapeutic strategy. The oropharynx is a complex anatomical region of utmost functional importance for breathing, swallowing, and speaking. Each subsite of oropharyngeal cancer has a specific natural history and each treatment has specific functional consequences depending upon the orpharyngeal subsite. Hence the accurate identification of the subsite of origin and tumour extension is mandatory. Knowledge of the tumour and nodal extension is markedly improved by the systematic use of modern imaging techniques.

Choice of the treatment strategy must be made within the framework of a multidisciplinary panel and adequate information about functional and cosmetic consequences must be given to the patient when several treatment choices are followed by a similar oncological outcome.

Radiotherapy and surgery can be used with similar chances of cure for T_1 and T_2 tumours. Functional results are usually better with radiotherapy, especially for tumours of the faucial arch. Except for superficial lesions, elective treatment (either surgery or radiotherapy) should be given to the N_0 upper neck, sometimes bilaterally (uvula, base of the tongue). Patients with N_1 disease should receive either radiotherapy or surgery according to the choice made to treat the primary tumour. In practice most of these clinical presentations are amenable to radiotherapy alone. Patients with N_2 or N_3 disease will most often need combinations of radiotherapy and surgery.

Radiotherapy is at present the most widely used initial approach for patients with T_2,T_3, or T_4 oropharyngeal carcinoma, except when tumours are infiltrating muscles of mastication and/or the ascending ramus of the mandible and/or the retromolar trigone, when wide surgical resection is indicated, using various flaps for closure. Pre- or postoperative radiotherapy remains necessary. The same type of surgery is indicated to treat local failures after radiotherapy.

A few recent comparative studies of therapeutic options seem to suggest that concomitant radiochemotherapy regimens (cisplatinum based) provide better local control and disease-free survival than radiotherapy alone in patients with stage III/IV oropharyngeal cancers who are in good general condition. Unfortunately, there are few well-conducted studies, and none of them is of large scale. These results, added to a similar conclusion from a large meta-analysis, at least provide the background for future research trials:

(1) To compare improved radiotherapy regimens (hyperfractionation, accelerated radiotherapy, alone or combined with chemotherapy) with the standard radiochemotherapy regimens (conventional radiotherapy and chemotherapy).

(2) To evaluate new drugs (taxanes) or new drug combinations during radiotherapy.

(3) To test new radiosensitizers and to improve tumour oxygenation during treatment (erythropoietin).

(4) To evaluate the newly developed predictive factors of tumour resistance, cell kinetics, and inherent radioresistance.

It is probable that in the near future the therapeutic choice will depend on a careful review of each case consisting not only of a more accurate staging of the neoplasm, but also based upon the pretherapeutic individual assessment of which strategy will be more likely to give the best chance of cure to a particular patient. Progress in understanding head and neck carcinogenesis should also result in the emergence of new predictive biomarkers of tumour response for current standard therapies. Novel therapies (vaccines, gene therapy) should also be proposed in the coming decade in patients with newly identified aetiological factors.

References

1. **Muir C, Waterhouse J (ed.)** *Cancer incidence in five continents*, vol. V, no. 8. Lyon: IARC, 1987.

2. **Adenis L, et al.** Registre des cancers des voies aérodigestives supérieures des départements du Nord et du Pas de Calais 1984–1986. *Bulletin du Cancer*, 1988; **75**: 745–50.

3. **Rothman K, Keller A.** The effect of joint exposure to alcohol and tobacco on risks of cancer of the mouth and pharynx. *Journal of Chronic Diseases*, 1972; **25**: 711–16.

4. **Gillison ML, et al.** Evidence for a causal assocoation between human Papillomavirus and a subset of head and heck cancers. *Journal of the National Cancer Institute*, 2000; **92**: 709–20.

5. **Zur Hausen H.** Papillomaviruses causing cancer: Evasion from host-cell control in early events in carcinogenesis. *Journal of the National Cancer Institute*, 2000; **92**: 690–8.

6. **Bosch FX, Homann N, Conradt C, Dietz A, Erber R.** p53 mutations/p53 protein overexpression. Differential significance for the progression of head-neck carcinomas. *HNO*, 1999; **47**: 833–48.

7. **Sittel C, Eckel HE, Damm M, von Pritzbuer E, Kvasnicka HM.** Ki-67 (MIB1), p53, and Lewis-X (LeuM1) as prognostic factors of recurrence in T1 and T2 laryngeal carcinoma. *Laryngoscope*, 2000; **110**: 1012–17.

8. **Bataini JP, et al.** A multivariate primary tumor control analysis in 465 patients treated by radical radiotherapy for cancer of the tonsillar region: clinical and treatment parameters as prognostic factors. *Radiotherapy and Oncology*, 1989; **14**: 265–77.

9. **Bernier J, Bataini JP.** Regional outcome in oropharyngeal and pharyngo-laryngeal cancer treated with high dose per fraction radiotherapy. Analysis of neck disease response in 1646 cases. *Radiotherapy and Oncology*, 1986; **6**: 87–103.

10. **Moonen L, et al.** Cell kinetic study in human tumors using IrdR labelling and flow cytometry. *International Journal of Radiation Oncology, Biology, Physics*, 1989; **17** (suppl. 1): abstract 33.

11. **Begg AC, et al.** The predictive value of cell kinetic measurements in a European trial of accelerated fractionation in advanced head and neck tumors: An interim report. *International Journal of Radiation Oncology, Biology, Physics*, 1990; **19**: 1449–53.

12. **Horiot JC, et al.** Hyperfractionated compared with conventional radiotherapy in oropharyngeal carcinoma: An EORTC randomized trial. *European Journal of Cancer*, 1990; **26**: 779–80.

13. **Begg AC, et al.** The value of pretreatment cell kinetic parameters as predictors for radiotherapy outcome in head and neck cancers: A multicenter analysis. *Radiotherapy and Oncology*, 1999; **50**: 13–23.

14. **Wilson GD, Dische S, Saunders MI.** Studies with bromodeoxyuridine in head and neck cancer and accelerated radiotherapy. *Radiotherapy and Oncology*, 1995; **36**: 189–97.

15. **Bataini JP, et al.** Cancer épidermoide de la région amygdalienne. Résultats de la radiothérapie et analyse multifactorielle du pronostic. *Journal Européen de Radiothérapie*, 1986; **7**: 139–40.

16. **Rider WD.** Epithelial cancer of the tonsillar area. *Radiology*, 1962; **78**: 760–4.

17. **Fletcher GH.** Oral cavity and oropharynx. In: *Textbook of radiotherapy* (3rd edn). Philadelphia, PA: Lea and Febiger, 1980: 286–329.

18. **Lindberg RD.** Distribution of cervical lymph node metastasis from squamous cell carcinoma of the upper respiratory and digestive tracts. *Cancer*, 1972; **29**: 1446–9.

19. **Keyes JJ, Watson NJ, Williams DR, Greven K, McGuirt W.** FDG PET in head and neck cancer. *American Journal of Roentgenology*, 1997; **169**: 1663–79.

20. **Anzai Y, Carroll W, Quint D, et al.** Recurrence of head and neck cancer after surgery or irradiation: prospective comparison of 2-deoxy-2- (F-18) fluoro-D-glucose PET and MR imaging diagnoses. *Radiology*, 1996; **200**: 135–41.

21. **van den Brekel M, Castelijns J, Snow G.** The size of lymph nodes in the neck on sonograms as a radiologic criterion for metastasis: how reliable is it? *American Journal of Neuroradiology*, 1998; **19**: 695–700.

22. **Pradoura JP.** Bilan préthérapeutique d'un malade porteur d'un cancer des VADS ou d'une adénopathie cervicale sans port d'entrée. In: Brugère J (ed.) *Cancers des voies aéro-digestives supérieures-progrès en cancérologie*. Paris: Doin Editeurs, 1986: 15–30.

23. **Horiot JC, et al.** Dental preservation in patients irradiated for head and neck tumors: a 10-year experience with topical fluoride and a randomized trial between two fluoridation methods. *Radiotherapy and Oncology*, 1983; **1**: 77–82.

24. **UICC (International Union Against Cancer).** Sobin LH, Wittekind Ch (ed.) *TNM classification of malignant tumors* (5th edn). New York: Wiley-Liss, 1997.

25. **ICRU (International Commission on Radiation Units and Measurements).** Prescribing, recording, and reporting photon beam therapy. *ICRU report 50*. Washington, DC: International Commission on Radiation Units and Measurements, 1993.

26. **ICRU (International Commission on Radiation Units and Measurements).** Dose and volume specification for reporting interstitial therapy. *ICRU report 58*. Washington, DC: International Commission on Radiations Units and Measurements, 1997.

27. **ICRU (International Commission on Radiation Units and Measurements).** Prescribing, recording, and reporting photon beam therapy (supplement to ICRU report 50). *ICRU report 62*. Washington, DC: International Commission on Radiation Units and Measurements, 1999.

28. **Berger DS, et al.** Elective irradiation of the neck lymphatics for squamous cell carcinoma of the nasopharynx and oropharynx. *American Journal of Roentgenology*, 1971; **111**: 66.

29. **Fletcher GH.** Squamous cell carcinoma of the oropharynx. *International Journal of Radiation Oncology, Biology, Physics*, 1979; **5**: 2076.

30. **Fletcher GH.** Clinical dose response curves of human malignant epithelial tumors. *British Journal of Radiology*, 1973; **46**: 1–12.

31. **Fowler JF, et al.** Further analysis of the time factor in squamous cell carcinoma of the tonsillar region. *Radiotherapy and Oncology*, 1990; **19**: 237–44.

32. **Horiot JC, et al.** Accelerated fractionation (AF) compared to conventional fractionation (CF) improves locoregional control in the radiotherapy of advanced head and neck cancers : results of the EORTC 22851 randomized trial. *Radiotherapy and Oncology*, 1997; **24**: 111–21.

33. **Browman GP, Wong G, Hodson I, et al.** Influence of cigarette smoking on the efficacy of radiation therapy in head and neck cancer. *New England Journal of Medicine*, 1993; **328**: 159–63.

34. **Lefebvre JL, et al.** Composite resection with mandibulectomy in the treatment of posterolateral oral cavity and lateral oropharynx squamous cell carcinoma. *American Journal of Surgery*, 1993; **166**: 435–9.

35. **Lefebvre JL, et al.** L'association chirurgie suivie d'irradiation dans le traitement des cancers de la région amygdalienne. *Journal Européen de Radiothérapie*, 1988; **7**: 138–9.

36. **Snow GB, et al.** Comparison of pre- and post-operative radiotherapy for patients with carcinoma of the head and neck (interim report). *Acta Otolaryngologica*, 1981; **91**: 611.

37. **Bataini JP, et al.** Primary radiotherapy of squamous cell carcinoma of the oropharynx and pharyngolarynx: Tentative multivariate modelling system to predict the radiocurability of neck nodes. *International Journal of Radiation Oncology, Biology, Physics*, 1988; **14**: 635–42.

38. Bataini JP, *et al.* Impact of cervical disease and its definitive radiotherapeutic management on survival: experience in 2013 patients with squamous cell carcinoma of the oropharynx and pharyngolarynx. *Laryngoscope*, 1990; **100**: 716–23.

39. Barker JL, Fletcher GH. Time, dose and tumour volume relationships in megavoltage irradiation of squamous cell carcinoma of the retromolar trigone and anterior tonsillar pillar. *International Journal of Radiation Oncology, Biology, Physics*, 1977; **2**: 407.

40. Horiot JC, *et al.* Hyperfractionation versus conventional fractionation in oropharyngeal carcinoma: final analysis of a randomized trial of the EORTC cooperative group of radiotherapy. *Radiotherapy and Oncology*, 1993; **4**: 231–41.

41. Horiot JC, *et al.* New radiotherapy fractionation schemes in head and neck cancers: The EORTC trials: A benchmark. In: Kogelnik HD, Sedlmayer F (ed.) *Progress in radio-oncology VI*. Bologna: Monduzzi Editore, 1998: 735–41.

42. Fu KK, *et al.* A Radiation Therapy Oncology group (RTOG) phase III randomized study to compare hyperfractionation and two variants of accelerated fractionation to standard fractionation radiotherapy for head and neck squamous cell carcinomas: first report of RTOG 9003. *International Journal of Radiation Oncology, Biology, Physics*, 2000; **48**: 7–16.

43. Mazeron JJ, *et al.* Interstitial radiation therapy for squamous cell carcinoma of the tonsillar region: the Creteil experience (1971–1981). *International Journal of Radiation Oncology, Biology, Physics*, 1986; **12**: 895–900.

44. Mazeron JJ, *et al.* Definitive radiation treatment for early stage carcinoma of the soft palate and uvula: the indications for iridium 192 implantation. *International Journal of Radiation Oncology, Biology, Physics*, 1987; **13**: 1829–37.

45. Pernot M, *et al.* Palato-tonsillar lesions: treatment of 269 cases with associated external irradiation and brachytherapy [abstract]. *Journal of Cancer Research and Clinical Oncology*, 1990; suppl. 116 (II): 796.

46. Peters LJ, *et al.* Accelerated fractionation in the radiation treatment of head and neck cancer. *Acta Oncologica*, 1988; **27**: 185–94.

47. Maltz R, *et al.* Carcinoma of the tonsil: results of combined therapy. *Laryngoscope*, 1974; **81**: 2172.

48. Lefebvre JL, *et al.* Les cancers des voies aéro-digestives supérieures. Etude globale de 2418 dossiers. *Bulletin du Cancer*, 1989; **76**: 763–70.

49. Perez CA, *et al.* Carcinoma of the tonsillar fossa. A non-randomized comparison of preoperative radiation and surgery or irradiation alone: long term results. *Cancer*, 1982; **50**: 2314–22.

50. Geoffray B, *et al.* Combined treatment of cancer of the posterior oral cavity and oropharynx. *Clinical Otolaryngology*, 1987; **12**: 429–39.

51. Harrold C. Surgical treatment of cancer of the base of the tongue. *American Journal of Surgery*, 1967; **114**: 247.

52. Whicker JH, *et al.* Surgical treatment of squamous cell carcinoma of the base of the tongue. *Laryngoscope*, 1972; **82**: 1853.

53. Thawley SE, *et al.* Preoperative irradiation and surgery for carcinoma of the base of the tongue. *Annals of Otology, Rhinology and Laryngology*, 1983; **92**: 485.

54. Riley RW, *et al.* Squamous cell carcinoma of the base of the tongue. *Otolaryngology, Head and Neck Surgery*, 1983; **91**: 143.

55. Harrison LB, Zelefsky MJ, Armstrong JG. Performance status after treatment for squamous cell cancer of the base of tongue—a comparison of primary radiation therapy versus primary surgery. *International Journal of Radiation Oncology, Biology, Physics*, 1994; **30**: 953–7.

56. Pignon JP, Bourhis J, Domenge C, Designé L. Chemotherapy added to locoregional treatment for head and neck squamous-cell carcinoma: three meta-analyses of updated individual data. *The Lancet*, 2000; **355**: 949–55.

57. Calais G, Alfonsi M, Bardet E, *et al.* Randomized trial of radiation therapy versus concomitant chemotherapy and radiation therapy for advanced-stage oropharynx carcinoma. *Journal of the National Cancer Institute*, 1999; **91**: 2081–6.

58. Jeremic B, Shibamoto Y, Stanisavljevic B, Milojevic L, Milicic B, Nikolic N. Radiation therapy alone or with concurrent low-dose daily either cisplatin or carboplatin in locally advanced unresectable squamous cell carcinoma of the head and neck: a prospective randomized trial. *Radiotherapy and Oncology*, 1997; **43**: 29–37.

59. Vandenbrouck C, *et al.* Chirurgie de rattrapage après radiothérapie. In: Veronesi U *et al.* (ed.) *I tumori della testa e del collo*. Milan: Ambrosiana, 1979.

Pharyngeal walls, hypopharynx, and larynx

J. L. Lefebvre, D. Chevalier, and F. Eschwege

Malignancies of the larynx, hypopharynx, and pharyngeal walls represent about half the cases of cancers arising along the upper aerodigestive tract. The vast majority of these tumours are squamous-cell carcinomas.

Squamous carcinomas of the hypopharynx and pharyngeal walls carry one of the most dismal prognoses of all tumours of the upper aerodigestive tract. Occurring in an anatomical region where clinical access is difficult, these carcinomas are frequently advanced at the time of diagnosis. They have a particularly high propensity for lymphatic and metastatic spread and tend to occur in debilitated patients with a long and important history of alcohol and tobacco abuse. The survival rate is poor despite aggressive surgery and radiotherapeutic treatments. Published data show a wide variation in 5-year survival rates—from 10 to 60 per cent. Extension of disease at first presentation is the most important prognostic factor. Thanks to the constant progress made both in diagnosis and treatment, an increasing numbers of patients are now cured. Therapeutic approaches are less mutilating and consistent with a better quality of life. Long-term overall results, however, remain disappointing.

Conversely, laryngeal cancers occur in less-debilitated patients, with earlier symptoms. Several surgical and radiotherapeutic strategies allow individual adjustments. In general, results are good in terms of locoregional control (above 90 per cent in vocal-cord carcinoma). Distant metastases are less frequent than in pharyngeal tumours but the risk is rather high (bronchial carcinomas in particular).

Epidemiology (for more information, see Chapter 9.1.1)

The descriptive epidemiology of larynx cancers is well documented, because they are reported separately. Larynx cancers occur with the highest incidence in Latin Europe.[1] In France,[2] the incidence is twice as high in males than the mean incidence in the rest of the European Community.

Conversely, hypopharynx cancers are often found mixed in the larger group of pharyngeal cancers. However, the incidence is high in some French areas (Northern France, Alsace, Normandy, and Brittany) as well as in some areas of India.[1]

Cancers of the larynx and hypopharynx occur mainly in males (at least 80 per cent of the cases, up to 95 per cent in hypopharynx cancers). Age at diagnosis ranges between 40 and 70 years, with a peak around 55 years for males and 60 years for females. They occur mostly in poorly educated populations with a low sociocultural level, particularly the case for hypopharyngeal cancers.

Aetiology and pathogenesis (for more information, see Chapter 9.1.1)

Extensive tobacco smoking is a common feature in these patients. As in other head and neck sites, a frequent association with alcohol abuse is found. Alcoholic profiles vary according to the primary site: the daily consumption and the total consumption of ethanol before diagnosis are higher for cancers of the hypopharynx than for the supraglottic larynx and higher for cancers of the supraglottis than for the glottis.[3]

More frequent occurrences in blue-collar workers employed in particular areas, such as metallurgy, have been reported,[4],[5] but the almost constant association with alcohol and tobacco abuse compromises the evaluation of possible environmental and professional factors.

The frequency of precancerous changes prior to invasive cancer is also subject to discussion since not all precancerous lesions are diagnosed. However, at least some patients with glottic lesions report a long history of dysphonia before a diagnosis of cancer is made—leading to the assumption of a progressive evolution, with a first stage of chronic laryngitis. Knowledge of such a natural history could be of use in the decision to treat by surgery or irradiation, but this is still unclear. In the same way, there are increasing data about a probable viral role in some cases (in particular, the herpes simplex virus and the human papilloma virus).

Anatomy

Normal anatomy

Hypopharynx and pharyngeal walls (Figs 1, 2, and 3)

The inferior segment of the aerodigestive tract, the hypopharynx or low pharynx, is the portion of the pharynx between the oropharynx and the cervical oesophagus. Its superior margin is at the level of the hyoid bone, its inferior margin is at the level of the lower border of the cricoid cartilage. Anteriorly, the hypopharynx projects on to the posterior aspect of the larynx; posteriorly, it is related to the prevertebral fascia. The hypopharynx is separated from the laryngeal orifice by the epilarynx: the free border of the epiglottis and the

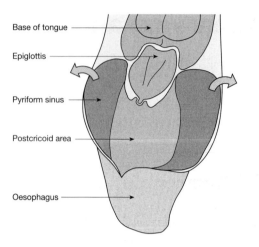

Fig. 1 Anatomy of the hypopharynx, posterior view of the pharyngolarynx.

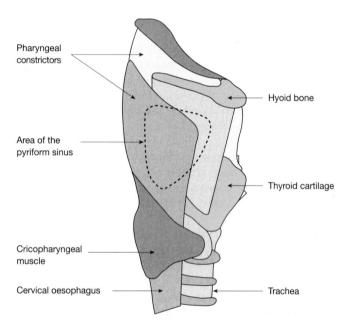

Fig. 2 Anatomy of the hypopharynx, lateral view.

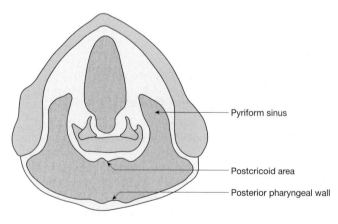

Fig. 3 Anatomy of the hypopharynx, transverse section.

suprahyoid epiglottis, aryepiglottic fold, arytenoids, and interarytenoid fold.

The hypopharynx can be subdivided into three anatomical sites: the pyriform sinus, the postcricoid area, and the posterior pharyngeal wall.

The pyriform sinuses extend laterally, on either side of the larynx, from the pharyngoepiglottic fold superiorly to the apex at the level of the cricoid cartilage inferiorly. The pyriform sinuses can be subdivided into the membranous pyriform sinus (the superior portion related to the thyrohyoid membrane and the pre-epiglottic space) and the cartilaginous pyriform sinus (the lower portion between the thyroid ala laterally and the cricoid and arytenoid cartilages medially).

The postcricoid pharynx corresponds to the posterior aspect of the arytenoid and cricoid cartilages. Laterally, it is intimately related to the apex of each pyriform sinus; inferiorly, it is related to the superior border of the cervical oesophagus.

The posterior pharyngeal wall is related to the anterior surface of the cervical vertebrae. Between the constrictor muscle and the prevertebral fascia there is a thin layer of loose areolar tissue, the retropharyngeal space. The posterior hypopharyngeal wall is continuous with the posterior oropharynx wall above and with the cervical oesophagus below. Laterally, it joins the pyriform fossae.

Larynx

The larynx is the portion of the respiratory tract between the oropharynx and the nasal cavities and the trachea. Its superior margin is at the level of the hyoid bone, its inferior margin at the level of the sixth. cervical vertebra. Anteriorly, the larynx is protected by the thyroid cartilage. The upper part of the epiglottis partially covers its superior orifice, while the cricoid calibrates the larynx.

The larynx can be subdivided into three anatomical sites (Figs 4 and 5): the supraglottis, the glottis, and the subglottis. These regions differ in their origin.

The supraglottic larynx is made of the superior margin of the larynx, the epilarynx (suprahyoid epiglottis, aryepiglottic folds, and arytenoids), and the laryngeal vestibule (false vocal cords, infrahyoid epiglottis, and ventricles). It responds, anteriorly, to the fatty space called the pre-epiglottic space.

The glottic larynx is made of the two true vocal cords. Their anterior union forms the anterior commissure. Laterally, they respond to the paraglottic spaces.

The subglottic larynx is limited superiorly by the inferior face of the true vocal cord and, inferiorly, by the superior limit of the trachea.

Pathology (for more information, see Chapter 9.1.2)

The vast majority of laryngeal and hypopharyngeal cancers are squamous-cell carcinomas. Premalignant lesions (leucoplakia, erythroplakia) precede some of them, particularly in the larynx.

Histological types

Squamous-cell carcinoma

Macroscopic examination distinguishes four types of tumours with different patterns of spread.

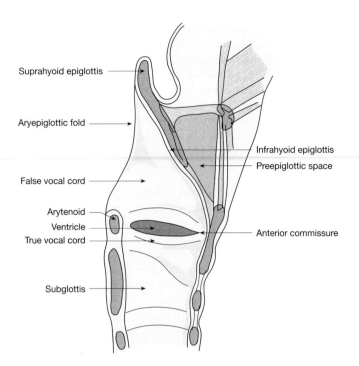

Fig. 4 Anatomy of the larynx, sagittal section. Suprahyoid epiglottis, aryepiglottic fold, false vocal cord, infrahyoid epiglottis, pre-epiglottic space, arytenoid, ventricle, true vocal cord, anterior commissure, subglottis.

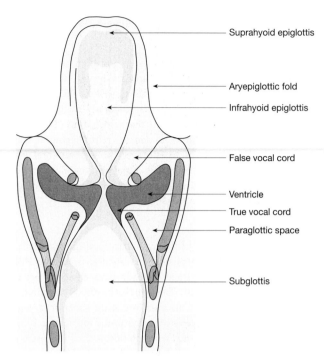

Fig. 5 Anatomy of the larynx, frontal section. Suprahyoid epiglottis, aryepiglottic fold, infrahyoid epiglottis, false vocal cord, ventricle, true vocal cord, paraglottic space, subglottis.

1. Infiltrating or ulcerating-infiltrating lesions, the most frequent type, are well circumscribed and tend to spread in depth to underlying structures (muscles, membranes, and cartilage). The pattern of spread depends on the site of the primary tumour and the resistance of neighbouring anatomical elements to invasion.

2. Bulky tumours are less frequent. They occur mainly on the aryepiglottic folds and the false vocal cords.

3. Superficially spreading lesions ('carpet carcinoma'), confined to the mucosa, can involve all or part of the hypopharyngeal epithelial lining. The possibility of a concurrent oropharyngeal or oesophageal tumour explains cases of recurrent disease at a distance from the primary tumour. This type of tumour is mainly found on the hypopharyngeal mucosa

4. Association of invasive and preneoplastic lesions, in particular at the glottic level.

Microscopically, these epidermoid carcinoma may be well, moderately, or poorly differentiated. As with the nasopharynx they are rarely undifferentiated. Adenosquamous carcinoma or carcinosarcoma are also rare.

Other types of malignancies

Occasionally, tumours of the seromucinous glands (mucoepidermoid tumour, adenoid cystic carcinoma, adenocarcinoma), neuroendocrine tumours (carcinoid tumours, small-cell undifferentiated carcinoma, so-called 'oat-cell carcinoma'), melanomas, lymphomas, or sarcomas may be diagnosed in the larynx or the hypopharynx.

Routes of spread

Hypopharynx and pharyngeal walls

The pattern of spread of hypopharyngeal squamous-cell carcinoma depends on the site of the primary tumour.[6],[7]

Local growth

Pyriform sinus Tumours of the medial wall may spread superficially towards the marginal area of the larynx, the aryepiglottic fold, and the arytenoids; they may infiltrate deeply to the pharyngolaryngeal wall, including the thyroarytenoid and cricoarytenoid muscles and the cricoarytenoid joint. Involvement of the paraglottic and preepiglottic spaces explains the frequency of early vocal-cord fixation. Tumours may also involve the recurrent laryngeal nerve beneath the mucosa of the pyriform sinus to immobilize the hemilarynx.

Tumours of the lateral wall spread rapidly to the ala of the thyroid cartilage and having penetrated this structure they invade the homolateral thyroid lobe. Tumours of the lateral pyriform sinus may extend to the apex of the pyriform sinus and to the posterior pharyngeal wall; spread often takes place by a submucosal route.

Advanced tumours of the pyriform sinus are very frequent; they invade both the thyroid cartilage and the larynx.

Postcricoid area Because of their anatomical site, these tumours are rarely diagnosed at an early stage. They frequently invade posterior cricoarytenoid muscles and cricoid and arytenoid cartilages. The apex of the pyriform sinus terminates in the postcricoid area and is often invaded early. Furthermore, advanced tumours could encircle the hypopharyngeal lumen.

Posterior pharyngeal wall These tumours are often ulcerating-infiltrating lesions that spread both superficially and submucosally to the entire posterior pharyngeal wall as well as the hypo- and oropharyngeal walls. Superiorly, they spread early to the posterior tonsillar pillars and can extend into the nasopharynx. Posteriorly, they spread to prevertebral muscles and the retropharyngeal space, but prevertebral fascia seems to effectively protect vertebral bone against tumour extension. Carcinomas of the pharyngeal wall spread laterally to the pyriform sinuses, but they seldom affect the laryngeal structures and then only at a late stage.

Lymphatic metastasis

The rich lymphatic network of the hypopharyngeal mucosa explains the high propensity of hypopharyngeal carcinomas for metastatic spread (three-quarters of patients already have clinically positive nodes at initial presentation). The lymphatic vessels draining the pyriform sinuses follow the same trajectory as the superior laryngeal nerves and vessels as they penetrate the thyrohyoid membrane. Lymph vessels also course through the thin anterior wall of the pyriform sinus with the nerve. Drainage of the lymphatics in this area occurs primarily into the subdigastric lymph node and the middle jugular node; the spinal accessory lymph nodes may also be involved. Drainage from the posterior wall of the hypopharynx is to the jugular chain and the retropharyngeal lymph nodes. A tumour may extend superiorly to involve the high-lying nodes at the base of the skull. The lower hypopharynx drains to the paraoesophageal nodes, the paratracheal nodes, and nodes of the supraclavicular fossa.

Distant metastases

Distant metastases are a common feature during the evolution of a hypopharyngeal carcinoma—figures as high as 50 per cent have been reported in the literature. As for most of the upper aerodigestive tract tumours, patients with locally advanced diseases and/or lymph-node metastases have the highest risk for distant metastases (mainly in the lung, thereafter in the liver, on bones, or in the brain).

Larynx

The growth and spread of laryngeal carcinoma is, to a great extent, determined by the site of origin of the tumours and has been well described.[6]–[9]

Local growth

Glottic carcinomas Most glottic carcinomas arise from the free border of the vocal cords, which is normally covered with a squamous epithelium. They may extend along the vocal cord to involve or to cross the anterior commissure. They may be located in and around the anterior commissure only. Posteriorly, the tumour may extend to the arytenoid cartilage or deeper, when it may then lie very close to the mucosa of the piriform sinus. Subglottic extension to the subsurface of the vocal cords or supraglottic extension towards the ventricle are common findings.

Tumours arising or invading the anterior commissure are characterized by their tendency to extend subglottically. There is a high risk for early invasion of the thyroid cartilage and for spreading through the cricothyroid membrane to outside the larynx. Less

frequent is the superior extension towards the very inferior part of the pre-epiglottic space through the thyroepiglottic ligament.

When the thyroid cartilage is invaded, tumour invasion occurs primarily in the ossified parts of the cartilage.

Vocal cord fixation means the invasion of the vocal cord muscles and, in a high percentage of cases, destruction of the laryngeal framework and/or spread outside the larynx. Initially, the term 'transglottic' meant that the tumour surrounded the ventricle,[7],[10] but nowadays the term often refers to tumours involving all regions of the larynx and often with a fixed hemilarynx ('3-story cancer').

Supraglottic carcinomas Tumours arising in the supraglottic region are often located on the posterior surface of the epiglottis and anterior parts of the false vocal cords or on the aryepiglottic folds. Pre-epiglottic space invasion is frequent.

Supraglottic carcinomas often remain within the supraglottic region and may extend either upwards to the base of the tongue or laterally to the piriform sinus; they do not always respect the glottic region. They may either be exophytic or more ulcerofungating, or often grow with pushing margins. If ulcerated, they may extend down below the anterior commissure and when doing so they may invade the thyroid cartilage.[11]

Subglottic carcinomas Primary subglottic carcinomas are rare and often grow circumferentially within the subglottis. They may extend superiorly towards the vocal cord, anteriorly through the cricothyroid membrane, anteriorly or posteriorly through the cricotracheal space, and caudally to involve the trachea.

Lymph-node involvement The free margins of the vocal cords have little lymphatic drainage, which explains the low incidence of cervical metastases for tumours confined to the vocal cords (less than 10 per cent of cases). However, the supraglottis is rich in lymphatics, this being one explanation of the high incidence of lymph-node metastases for carcinomas arising in this area (in around one-third of cases).

The incidence of nodal metastases increases with the size and extent of the primary tumour, being about 50 per cent for transglottic tumours.

Distant metastases

Few patients present with distant metastases at the time of diagnosis of their laryngeal carcinoma. Distant metastases are more common in the lung particularly. Patients with poorly differentiated, necrotic tumours, with lymph-node metastases have the highest risk for pulmonary metastases.

Second primary tumours

As with other tumours of the upper aerodigestive tract, there is a special risk for multiple primaries. Indeed, the complete mucosal field, which has been exposed to the carcinogenic effects of tobacco and alcohol, may develop multiple primaries either concomitantly or successively. These multiple tumours are mainly located on the upper aerodigestive tract itself, or on the oesophagus, or in the lung. Lung metachronous cancers are particularly frequent in patients with cancer of the larynx, while pharyngeal or oesophageal cancers are more often associated with hypopharyngeal cancers. The earlier the stage of the first primary (that is to say the better the prognosis), the higher is the risk of metachronous cancer.

Clinical presentation

Hypopharynx and pharyngeal walls

Either a sore throat or a neck mass reveals the majority of hypopharyngeal tumours.

Dysphagia

Dysphagia is the most common symptom. Initially, the patient complains of intermittent difficulties when swallowing saliva. Symptoms persist and gradually become chronic. Questioning the patient will often reveal that it feels as though there is a foreign body in the throat. Dysphagia progressively increases in severity, initially for solid foods and later for liquids. Severe dysphagia is a hallmark symptom for a tumour invading the lower hypopharynx and cervical oesophagus. A persistent sore throat, particularly in patients with known risk factors for cancer in this region (alcohol and/or tobacco abuse), requires a careful physical examination of the upper aerodigestive tract by an ENT specialist. Dysphagia is frequently associated with odynophagia.

Concurrent clinical symptoms

Hoarseness may be due to either direct laryngeal invasion or to recurrent laryngeal nerve infiltration in the postcricoid or cervical oesophagus areas. Dyspnoea, hypersialorrhoea, significant weight loss are observed with more advanced tumour.

Cervical adenopathy

Nearly one-third of patients with a hypopharyngeal tumour consult because of a neck mass. These painless, often mobile, cervical adenopathies, have a predilection for the subdigastric and mid-jugular nodal levels.

Larynx

Hoarseness

Hoarseness is the most frequent and earliest symptom for primary glottic lesions, but a late one for supraglottic and subglottic tumours, where it often indicates glottic involvement. A persistent hoarseness (particularly in patients with known risk factors) requires a careful physical examination of the upper aerodigestive tract by an ENT specialist.

Concurrent clinical symptoms

Dysphagia, odynophagia, irritation, and coughing are characteristic symptoms of supraglottic lesions. Dyspnoea may be the first sign of subglottic cancer or an advanced tumour.

Cervical adenopathy

Nodal metastasis is uncommon in glottic carcinoma, although the incidence increases with advancing stage. In supraglottic carcinoma, it is observed in up to 30 per cent of cases, often bilaterally.

Screening, diagnosis, and staging

Physical examination

Pharyngolaryngoscopy

Dynamic visual examination is required of the entire pharyngolaryngeal region by pharyngolaryngoscopy, which remains the basic diagnostic procedure. The patient must be examined during respiration, phonation, and in Valsalva's' manoeuvre. Depending on the examiner's preferences and individual patient factors, examination may be made with a laryngeal mirror, a Bercy–Ward type of rigid endoscope, or a fibrescope. Stroboscopy is a pertinent examination in the diagnosis of early glottic tumours. Pharyngolaryngoscopy assesses the site of origin, the extension, the size of the tumour, and the mobility of the vocal cords.

Examination of the cervical region

Careful, cervical palpation is necessary to detect adenopathies. The jugulocarotid, spinal, and supraclavicular node chains must be explored bilaterally. The size and site of all enlarged nodes must be mapped. Cervical examination must also search for signs of extralaryngeal spread to the homolateral thyroid lobe or to the thyroid cartilage. Involvement of the thyroid cartilage may cause pain when pressure is applied to its external border, after rotation of the larynx towards the opposite site.

Direct pharyngolaryngoscopy

Direct endoscopic examination under general anaesthesia is the main diagnostic technique and allows:

(1) multiple biopsies at the level of the tumour for histological examination;

(2) an accurate determination of superficial tumour spread, essential for selection of therapy;

(3) detection of synchronous cancers or premalignant conditions, which requires a systematic endoscopic examination of the entire ENT sphere (oral cavity, oropharynx, nasopharynx, larynx), oesophagus;

(4) more detailed information about findings obtained from cervical palpation, in particular on a possible continuity between a neck mass and the primary tumour.

Microlaryngoscopy may be useful for small lesions of the true vocal cord, and the use of optical instruments is recommended to assess the anterior commissure, the epiglottis, or the subglottic extension of glottic cancer.

Imaging (for more detailed information, see Chapter 9.1.3)

Computed tomography (CT) of the pharynx and the larynx

CT is the single best, radiological technique for assessing the depth of invasion of pharyngeal or laryngeal tumours. Thin slices must be obtained in phonation, slow respiration, and during Valsalva's manoeuvre, with injection of contrast medium. Helicoidal CT is at least as good as conventional CT and allows multiplanar reconstruction.[12] The systematic use of CT to evaluate laryngeal or pharyngeal tumours also provides information about the neck. CT has a high sensitivity for the diagnosis of metastatic cervical nodes, when a rather specific image (central hypodensity with an enhancing peripheral rim) is present.

Magnetic resonance imaging (MRI)

MRI is more sensitive than CT in detecting neoplastic invasion of cartilage. Its inability to differentiate between non-neoplastic inflammatory changes from a tumour may lead to an overestimation of neoplastic invasion.

Cervical ultrasonography

This technique is simple, non-invasive, rapid and has a high sensitivity for the diagnosis of an accurate measurement of subclinical adenopathies. It is useful for follow-up.

Clinical staging

The T definition varies according to the primary site while N and M definitions are similar for all sites.

Primary site

Whatever the primary site

TX   primary tumour cannot be assessed
T0   no evidence of primary tumour
Tis   carcinoma *in situ*

Hypopharynx and pharyngeal walls

T1   tumour limited to one subsite of the hypopharynx
T2   tumour invades more than one subsite or an adjacent site, without fixation of the hemilarynx
T3   tumour invades more than one subsite of the hypopharynx or an adjacent site, without fixation of the hemilarynx
T4   tumour invades adjacent structures, e.g. cartilage or soft tissues of the neck

Supraglottis

T1   tumour limited to one subsite of the supraglottis, with normal vocal cord mobility
T2   tumour invades more than one subsite of the supraglottis or glottis, with normal vocal cord mobility
T3   tumour limited to the larynx with vocal cord fixation and/or invades the postcricoid area, medial wall of piriform sinus, or pre-epiglottic tissues
T4   tumour invades through the thyroid cartilage and/or extends to other tissues beyond the larynx, e.g. to the oropharynx and soft tissues of the neck

Glottis

T1   tumour limited to the vocal cord(s) (may involve anterior or posterior commissures) with normal mobility
T1a   tumour limited to one vocal cord
T1b   tumour involves both vocal cords
T2   tumour extends to the supraglottis and/or glottis, and/or with impaired vocal cord mobility
T3   tumour limited to the larynx with vocal cord fixation
T4   tumour invades through the thyroid cartilage and/or extends to other tissues beyond the larynx, e.g. to the oropharynx and soft tissues of the neck

Subglottis

T1   tumour limited to the subglottis
T2   tumour extends to the vocal cord(s) with normal or impaired mobility
T3   tumour limited to the larynx with vocal cord fixation
T4   tumour invades through the thyroid cartilage and/or extends to other tissues beyond the larynx, e.g. to the oropharynx and soft tissues of the neck

Nodal extension

NX   regional lymph nodes cannot be assessed
N0   no regional lymph-node metastasis
N1   metastasis in a single ipsilateral lymph node, 3 cm or less in greatest dimension
N2   metastasis in a single ipsilateral lymph node, more than 3 cm but not more than 6 cm in greatest dimension, or in multiple ipsilateral lymph nodes, none more than 6 cm in greatest dimension, or in bilateral or contralateral lymph nodes, none more than 6 cm in greatest dimension
N2a   metastasis in a single ipsilateral lymph node, more than 3 cm but not more than 6 cm in greatest dimension
N2b   metastasis in multiple ipsilateral lymph nodes, none more than 6 cm in greatest dimension,
N2c   metastasis in bilateral or contralateral lymph nodes, none more than 6 cm in greatest dimension,
N3   metastasis in a lymph node more than 6 cm in greatest dimension

Distant metastasis

MX   presence of distant metastasis cannot be assessed
M0   no distant metastasis
M1   distant metastasis

Stage grouping

Stage 0	Tis	N0	M0
Stage I	T1	N0	M0
Stage II	T2	N0	M0
Stage III	T3	N0	M0
	T1	N1	M0
	T2	N1	M0
Stage IV	T4	N0, 1	M0
	any T	N2, 3	M0
	any T	any N	M1

Treatment techniques

Surgery

Hypopharynx and pharyngeal walls

Partial surgical procedures (Fig. 6)

Several partial procedures may be performed using a temporary tracheostomy.

Partial lateral pharyngectomy (Fig. 6(a)) Using a lateral pharyngotomy, the cornu major of the hyoid bone and the posterior two-thirds of the thyroid ala are resected as well as the lateral wall of the pyriform sinus and the underlying deep fascia, including the thyrohyoid muscle. Primary closure of the pharyngostome is usually possible, but may require a local flap. This procedure is indicated for limited tumours of the lateral wall of the pyriform sinus. Local control is excellent but 5-year survival does not exceed 50 per cent[13] due to intercurrent diseases, distant metastases, and metachronous cancers.

Posterior partial pharyngectomy (Fig. 6(b)) The pharynx is approached anteriorly, through the hyoid bone, which may be either transected or resected. Retractors pushing the base of the tongue

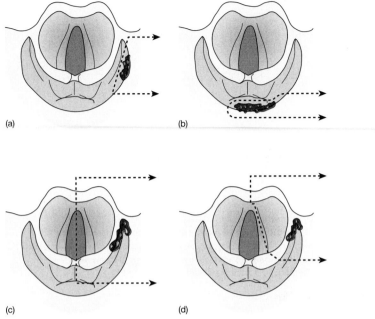

(a)

(b)

(c)

(d)

Fig. 6 Partial surgery of the hypopharynx. (a) Partial lateral pharyngectomy; (b) posterior partial pharyngectomy; (c) hemilaryngopharyngectomy (partial pharyngolaryngectomy; (d) supraglottic hemilaryngopharyngectomy.

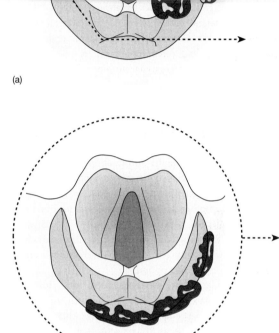

(a)

(b)

Fig. 7 Surgery of the hypopharynx including total laryngectomy. (a) Total laryngopharyngectomy, (b) circumferential total laryngopharyngectomy.

upwards and the larynx laterally expose the hypopharyngeal wall. The tumour is resected down to the prevertebral fascia. A skin graft or a flap is required for repairing the defect. This narrow approach may be replaced by a median labiomandibular glossotomy; the mandible is split along the midline, bisecting the tongue in the median raphe. Exposure of the pharynx is better and primary closure is usually achieved, with good functional and cosmetic results. This procedure is indicated for limited tumours of the two superior thirds of the posterior hypopharyngeal wall.

Partial pharyngolaryngectomy (Fig. 6(c)) A lateral cervicotomy is performed to allow resection of the hemithyroid cartilage and hemi-hyoid bone. The entire pyriform sinus and corresponding hemilarynx above the cricoid cartilage are sacrificed; this removes the vocal cord and its arytenoid, the ventricle and the ventricular strip, half of the epiglottis and of the pre-epiglottic spaces, the marginal area of the larynx, and the adjacent pyriform sinus. After mucosal covering of the remaining arytenoid and the margin of resection of the suprahyoid epiglottis, the defect is repaired by apposition of the edges, after mobilization of the prevertebral insertions and myoplasty. This procedure is indicated for limited tumours of the medial wall of the pyriform sinus without impaired mobility of the larynx and those located above the superior border of the cricoid. Local control is excellent, but the 5-year survival is between 45 and 50 per cent.[14]

Supraglottic hemipharyngolaryngectomy This variant, inspired by the technique of Alonzo, differs from the previous procedure only in that the glottic stage is conserved (Fig. 6(d)). Cartilage resection is limited to the upper half of the homolateral thyroid ala; apposition of the mucosal edges or use of a subhyoid muscle flap achieves closure. This technique has about the same indications and results.[15],[16]

Procedures including total laryngectomy (Fig. 7)

Total laryngopharyngectomy (Fig. 7(a)) This procedure combines total laryngectomy and partial hypopharyngectomy; the extent of pharyngeal resection varies, but allows pharyngo-oesophageal restoration by simple tubulization. Lateral cervicotomy is performed for *en bloc* resection of the larynx and the first tracheal rings, the apex and both walls of the pyriform sinus, and sometimes even part of the postcricoid mucosa. The remaining hypopharyngeal mucosa is sutured around a nasogastric tube. A definitive tracheostomy is created. All published series report over 80 per cent local control and a 35 per cent 5-year survival. Most patients die from distant metastases.

Circumferential total laryngopharyngectomy (Fig. 7(b)) This procedure is used for more widespread tumours massively invading the postcricoid area or the posterior pharyngeal wall, thus requiring complete resection of the hypopharyngeal mucosa over a variable distance. Repair techniques used for pharyngo-oesophageal restoration include free or pedicle flaps, skin or myocutaneous flaps, and visceral transposition with vascular microanastomoses. The most commonly used free flaps for reconstruction of the pharynx and cervical oesophagus are the third jejunum and the pedicle antebrachial flap.

Total oesophagopharyngolaryngectomy This procedure is indicated for lesions involving and infiltrating the cervical oesophagus. It associates circumferential pharyngolaryngectomy and total oesophagectomy; transposition of a colon segment or gastric transposition into the oesophageal space obtains pharyngo-oesophageal restoration.

For cases requiring a partial or a total ablation of the oesophagus, the 5-year survival rate barely exceeds 10 to 15 per cent.

Cervical region

As a rule, partial surgical techniques are always combined with radical or modified homolateral neck dissection. Contralateral dissection is necessary if the lesion involves the midline. Bilateral cervical dissection, including the mediastinal recurrent chains, is also performed in circumferential total pharyngolaryngectomies.

Larynx

Partial laryngeal procedures

Laser surgery Endoscopic techniques to treat laryngeal carcinoma have gained importance since the introduction of the CO_2 laser. This technique is now a well-accepted therapeutic modality for early glottic carcinoma. It produces cure rates equivalent to those of external cordectomy and radiotherapy for the treatment of T1a tumour of the mid-true vocal cord with normal mobility.[17]–[19] However, the resulting voice is not usually as good as it is after radiotherapy.[20] Microlaryngoscopic surgery for T1 glottic carcinoma can also be considered as a cost-effective option.[21]

Transoral CO_2 laser has also been used with curative intent in larger laryngeal carcinomas.[19],[22],[23] This surgery is becoming increasingly popular, particularly in Germany. Although published local control can be as high as 80 per cent, it must be emphasized that this surgery requires a particular expertise, and that it does not allow a real assessment of surgical margins or an *en bloc* resection of the primary tumour with cervical lymph nodes. These concerns are of importance for advanced glottic, transglottic, or hypopharyngeal cancers.

Endoscopic surgery Another option for very early disease is to resect the tumour during a direct laryngoscopy under general anaesthesia. The purpose of such endoscopic resections is either to remove suspicious lesions and to obtain a fair pathological diagnosis (for example, for superficial lesions of the vocal cords resembling precancerous changes) or to perform the treatment itself provided that these lesions are both small and perfectly accessible (small lesions of the mid-third of a vocal cord or of the suprahyoid epiglottis, for example).

External partial surgery External partial procedures (Fig. 8) are performed using a temporary tracheotomy.

Cordectomy via the laryngofissure (Fig. 8(a)): In this technique the larynx is opened by a vertical section of the thyroid cartilage on the midline. One vocal cord is then resected, with the adjacent paraglottic space, from the anterior commissure to the vocal process of the arytenoid. A simple suture of both thyroid cartilage ala thereafter ensures the closure of the larynx. This technique is indicated for lesion of the vocal cord remaining at a distance both from the anterior commissure and the arytenoid. When properly indicated (T1a of the mid-true vocal cord) this surgery is able to control 94 per cent of cases; but each time this surgery is extended either to the anterior

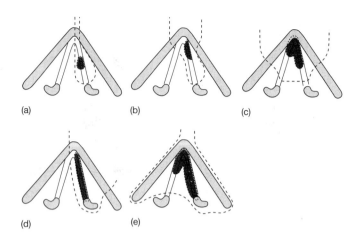

Fig. 8 Partial surgery of the glottic larynx. (a) Cordectomy, (b) frontolateral laryngectomy, (c) anterior frontal partial laryngectomy, (d) hemilaryngectomy, (e) supracricoid partial laryngectomy with cricohyoidoepiglottopexy (CHEP).

commissure or the arytenoid, local control may decrease to 72.5 per cent.[24]

Frontolateral laryngectomy (Fig. 8(b)): In this technique the anterior commissure is included with the resection, by making the mucosal incision through the anterior part of the contralateral vocal cord. This technique is indicated for T1a lesions that approach the anterior commissure. Published data mention a 5-year local control of 82 per cent and a survival of 87 per cent.[25]

Anterior frontal partial laryngectomy with epiglottoplasty (Fig. 8(c)): The larynx is approached anteriorly, and an anterior frontal partial laryngectomy performed. If necessary, one arytenoid cartilage should be resected. The anterior part of the larynx is reconstructed with the epiglottis, which is pulled inferiorly and mobilized by separating the anterior soft tissue and ligament attachments. Hence the epiglottis reaches the cricoid cartilage and is sutured laterally to the thyroid ala and inferiorly to the cricothyroid membrane. This technique is indicated for the treatment of T1b and T2 glottic cancer without patterns of deep invasion in the paraglottic space. Published local control rates range from 93 per cent for T1 to 79 per cent for T2.[26]

Hemilaryngectomy (Fig. 8(d)): In this procedure the thyroid ala, the arytenoid, and mucosa from the aryepiglottic fold to the cricothyroid membrane are resected. Various techniques of hemilaryngectomy alone or with reconstruction have been described (cartilage, skin, muscle). Initially, hemilaryngectomy was indicated to treat glottic cancer involving the posterior part of the larynx and/or with invasion of the floor of the ventricle. A compilation of published data shows that the overall cure rate ranges from 72 to 87 per cent.[7],[27]

Supracricoid partial laryngectomy with cricohyoidoepiglottopexy (CHEP)(Fig. 8(e)): This procedure removes the entire thyroid cartilage both true and false vocal cord, and, if necessary, one arytenoid cartilage. The larynx is reconstructed, performing a cricohyoidoepiglottopexy, thus moving the cricoid cartilage up to the hyoid bone and base of the tongue. Functional results are obtained with the remaining arytenoid cartilage and its mobility against the epiglottis and the base of the tongue. The goal of this technique is to remove the entire paraglottic space on the tumour side and is indicated for T2 and selected T3 but with a mobile arytenoid cartilage. Reports

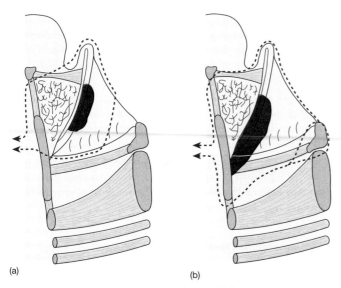

Fig. 9 Partial surgery of the supraglottic larynx. (a) Supraglottic partial laryngectomy, (b) supracricoid partial laryngectomy with cricohyoidopexy (CHP).

give a 95 per cent 5-year local control and a 77 per cent 5-year survival.[28],[29]

Supraglottic partial laryngectomy (Fig. 9(a)): The larynx is exposed after a bilateral dissection. The larynx is entered superiorly through the valeculla. An incision is made to remove both false vocal cords, the entire epiglottis, and the superior part of the thyroid cartilage. Both true vocal cords and arytenoids are spared. Closure is achieved by suturing the thyroid cartilage and the base of tongue. In the case of upper spread, the procedure can be extended superiorly and a part of the base of tongue resected. The larynx, however, must be entered inferiorly through the ventricle to prevent injury to the true vocal cords. Local control is excellent (90 per cent), but 5-year survival is quite disappointing (69 per cent) due to distant metastases and second primaries.[30]

Supracricoid partial laryngectomy with cricohyoidopexy (CHP)(Fig. 9(b)). This procedure removes the entire thyroid cartilage, both true and false vocal cords, the epiglottis with the pre-epiglottic space, and, if necessary, one arytenoid cartilage. Closure is achieved as in the CHEP technique by impacting the cricoid cartilage against the hyoid bone and the base of the tongue. Again despite impressive reported local control (97 per cent), 5-year survival does not exceed 79 per cent due to second primaries and distant metastases.[29],[31]

Total laryngectomy

This procedure is indicated for the surgical treatment of T3 and T4 carcinomas of the larynx with patterns of deep and massive invasion (fixation of the true vocal cord and the arytenoid cartilage, massive invasion of the pre-epiglottic space, invasion through the thyroid cartilage with external extension). In the case of upper spread, the procedure can be extended superiorly and a part of the base of tongue resected. If a tumour invades the subglottic area, several tracheal rings are resected with the larynx.

Cervical region Glottic cancer. A modified or radical neck dissection is performed for the T3 or T4 tumours. Usually T1 or T2 carcinomas

are also N0 and are treated with a partial laryngeal procedure without neck dissection.

Supraglottic cancer. Bilateral neck dissection is necessary due to the high risk of contralateral neck metastasis.

Subglottic extension. A bilateral dissection is also necessary, including along the mediastinal recurrent nerve.

Radiotherapy

Definitive irradiation

The irradiation techniques used to treat hypopharyngeal and laryngeal cancers are intimately related to the anatomy of this region and the pathways of tumour and nodal extension. The frequency of submucosal spread in hypopharyngeal cancers, often overlooked by endoscopy, justifies treatment of the entire hypopharynx. Depending on the tumour site, irradiation of the oropharynx and cervical oesophagus may also be indicated. Furthermore, the high propensity of hypopharyngeal tumours for nodal invasion makes treatment of the bilateral cervical node-bearing regions mandatory, whether radiotherapy is used as the sole procedure or is given postoperatively. In laryngeal tumours the radiotherapy technique varies according to a subsite. Supraglottic tumours require larger target volumes than glottic cancers encompassing primary and lymph-node areas. Target volumes of subglottic tumours or subglottic spread may be extended down to the upper mediastinum because of the risk of nodal extension along the recurrent chains. Conversely, tumours limited to the glottic area may by treated by only irradiating the primary site. Treatment planning will follow the ICRU 62 report recommendations.[32]

Hypopharynx and pharyngeal walls

Patients are treated in a supine position. Proper treatment planning includes patient immobilization in customized masks used on simulator CT scans and treatment tables.

The standard technique usually consists of two opposed parallel fields covering the primary site and both the superior and middle nodal-level target volumes.

Megavoltage equipment will be used, either cobalt-60 or photon-X of 4- to 6-MV linear accelerators. The spinal cord may be included in the first part of the treatment and excluded after 40 to 42 Gy of the nodal volume. The posterior neck is then treated by an electron beam of 8 to 10 MeV, or higher when justified The anterior part of the primary target volume continues to be treated by X-photon or gamma beams.

An anteroposterior/posteroanterior (AP/PA) beam treats the lower cervical nodes. When an extension to the cervical oesophagus is suspected, midline protection is not used before a dose of 45 Gy has been delivered.

For each patient, dosimetry is calculated and validated, not only at the centre of the target volume, but at each reference level. The usual dose is 70 Gy in 35 fractions, 2 Gy per fraction for the tumour and nodes. For non-metastatic, cervical node areas, the usual dose is 50 Gy in 5 weeks. Higher doses with conventional fractionation have not improved results. Modification of fractionation allows an increase of the total dose with a diminution of the dose by fraction (hyperfractionation) or a reduction of the overall treatment time (accelerated radiotherapy). No randomized studies have included enough hypopharyngeal cancers to draw conclusions on these fractionated regimes for this specific site. Most of the studies incorporate the larynx and hypopharynx, and few studies are able to demonstrate results for the hypopharyngeal cancers.

After definitive radiotherapy, disease control as well as survival vary considerably according to the tumour stage. For T1/T2 lesions, published data report about 50 per cent local control to be around 50 per cent, while the 5-year survival rate is between 11 and 49 per cent.[(33)–(35)] For T3 and T4 lesions, local control is around 33 per cent with a 5-year survival below 20 per cent[(33),(34)] and 6 to 7 per cent in patients considered as inoperable due to locoregional extension and/or performance status.[(35),(36)]

Larynx

Cancer of the larynx was one of the first tumours to be treated and cured by radiotherapy. Reliable positioning and immobilization of the patient is needed to ensure good reproducibility. Patients are treated in a supine position in relative neck hyperextension. Treatment immobilization, use of simulators, dosimetry, and dose calculation are identical to those used for hypopharyngeal cancers.

Cancer of the glottis For a T1 lesion, the target volume is limited to the glottic larynx since lymph-node involvement is very rare. Most often the treatment is delivered through two small lateral opposed fields (5×5 cm to 6×6 cm). The fields' limits are the upper border of the thyroid cartilage, the inferior border of the cricoid cartilage, and the anterior border of the vertebral bodies. A posterior reduction is possible for anterior tumours. Use of wedges, daily clinical examination, weekly portal films, or electronic portal imaging are needed. The 5-year local control ranges from 75 per cent to 94 per cent, and 5-year survival from 65 per cent to 94 per cent.[(37)–(46)]

In T2 tumours, the subclinical nodal involvement is also very rare and the fields are often basically the same as for T1, margins being adapted to the supraglottic or subglottic extension of the tumour. For T2 tumours the impaired laryngeal mobility, subdigastric and mid-jugular lymph nodes are treated in most institutions, with doses of 70 Gy over 7 weeks (five fractions of 2 Gy per week). Conservation of the overall treatment time without gaps during the treatment is a prognostic factor as is the cessation of smoking. The 5-year local control is between 60 per cent and 83 per cent and 5-year survival between 41 per cent and 93 per cent.[(42),(47)–(54)]

Cancer of the supraglottis The target volume includes the primary tumour and bilateral jugular chains and supraclavicular areas. As for hypopharynx cancers, opposed lateral fields are used with spinal reduction and, whenever possible, further primary field reduction after 50 to 55 Gy. Supraclavicular areas are treated with an anterior field. For T1 and T2 lesions, published data mention control rates between 88 per cent for T1 and 65 per cent for T2,[(55),(56)] or 57 to 68 per cent for T1 and T2 together,[(57),(58)] while survival has been reported to be around 75 per cent for stages 1 and 2.[(59)]

Cancer of the subglottis The treated volume is adapted to the tumour extension. Due to the possible lymphatic involvement along the recurrent chains, anterior and posterior fields are frequently used to treat the primary tumour and the lower cervical and upper mediastinal lymph nodes when necessary. After 40 to 45 Gy, field reductions are needed. There are very few reports focusing on radiation therapy of this subsite and published series only include a small number of patients.[(60)–(62)] Local control is about 80 per cent and this decreases to less than 30 per cent for T4.

Advanced larynx cancer It is quite impossible to find data about transglottic carcinomas. Papers often refer to 'advanced laryngeal cancers' (namely, T3–T4 or stages III–IV). Reports of local control vary widely between 23 and 67 per cent;[(63)–(70)] this wide range is due to the fact that this description comprises totally different scenarios. Some cases are resectable. Surgery is, in most cases, 'mutilating' (removes the entire larynx) but it is efficient. Generally, radiation therapy is slightly less efficient but, in many instances, it does allow preservation of the larynx (see the discussion on larynx preservation below). Other cases are unresectable. Radiation therapy is most often given with palliative intent but the results are rather poor. Both situations indicate the need for ongoing research to provide better treatment regimens.

Status on ongoing research

The past two decades have seen an impressive wealth of clinical research aimed at improving the results of radiotherapy. Globally, two approaches were followed: either modification of the fractionation and the total treatment duration or the addition of chemotherapy. Unfortunately, there are few data comparing these new approaches with conventional irradiation and few studies focusing on larynx and hypopharynx cancer. A three-arm randomized study from Spain[(71)] compared conventional irradiation with one fraction per day versus two fractions per day versus concurrent chemoradiotherapy. Response rates were higher in the two experimental arms for the subset of larynx cancers (310 cases) and, moreover, for the subset of hypopharynx cancers (119 cases). A randomized trial[(72)] comparing conventional irradiation versus continuous, hyperfractionated accelerated irradiation (three fractions a day for 12 successive days) was carried out in the United Kingdom (CHART trial). The experimental arm achieved much better results only for larynx cancers and only for T3 and, moreover, T4 diseases. A large meta-analysis[(73)] showed that concomitant chemoradiotherapy led, in published randomized trials, to a better survival. These new developments are indisputably of interest but to date remain in the field of clinical research. On the one hand, large trials are more and more difficult to complete or are stopped before completion, and, on the other hand, there is an infatuation with chemotherapy-based protocols which compromise the assessment of irradiation-alone (with different fractionation protocols).

Postoperative irradiation

After partial laryngectomy, the target volume is usually limited to the lymphatics (using anteroposterior fields with shielding of the larynx). The role of postoperative radiotherapy when surgical margins are positive remains the subject of discussion. Few studies have been published with few patients treated, no randomized studies have been published. Some of the studies have reached contradictory conclusions: if postoperative irradiation is not mandatory for some authors, it is recommended by others for patients with insufficient margins, without solid arguments. After total laryngectomy, the target volumes include the tumour bed and bilateral cervical lymph nodes. When surgical margins are clean, the total dose is limited to 50 Gy. A boost of 10 to 15 Gy is delivered on limited volumes to the sites of extracapsular spread.

Supportive care in radiotherapy

Although indispensable, the same preirradiation dental care is not required for patients with hypopharyngeal tumours as for those with oral and oropharyngeal lesions. Any carious tooth that cannot be treated must be extracted. Prior to treatment, topical fluoride should be applied daily to avoid caries caused by the modification of salivary flow.[74] Swallowing may become difficult during radiotherapy. A nasogastric feeding tube may be required to maintain normal calorie intake.

Chemotherapy (for more information, see Chapter 9.2)

Chemotherapy in protocols with curative intent

A new era in the management of head and neck tumours was initiated in the early 1980s with the appearance of platinum-based chemotherapeutic regimens. Impressive response rates in previously untreated patients led to the evaluation of chemotherapy in phase III trials. In the early 1990s, it appeared obvious that this approach had not translated into any improvement in outcome for most patients. This was clearly demonstrated by the meta-analysis carried out at the Institut Gustave Roussy (MACH-NC analysis),[73] which included more than 10 000 patients enrolled in randomized trials comparing conventional treatment to the same treatment with chemotherapy. The conclusion of this meta-analysis was that adjuvant chemotherapy produced a non-significant increase in survival (1 per cent) and induction chemotherapy a 4 per cent increase, while concomitant chemoradiotherapy resulted in a significant increase in survival of 8 per cent.

Nevertheless, chemotherapy had an indisputable impact on the management of advanced, but resectable, larynx and hypopharynx squamous carcinoma. Often, chemosensitive tumours are also radiosensitive. This led some teams to assess the possibility of avoiding the total ablation of the larynx (total laryngectomy with or without partial pharyngectomy, so-called 'mutilating surgery') by using induction chemotherapy followed in good responders by irradiation or, in poor responders, by the initially planned surgery. Unfortunately, most attempts at larynx preservation were carried out in non-controlled trials with historical comparisons from surgical series. Only four randomized trials have been published: three of which had the same design (but not the same eligibility criteria). The Veterans' trial on larynx cancers was the first to be published.[75],[76] In this trial, 332 patients were randomly assigned to receive either 'mutilating surgery' or two cycles of cisplatinum and 5-fluorouracil, followed in responders (partial or complete responders) by a third cycle and irradiation, or by surgery in non-responders. There was no significant difference in survival between both arms and, at 4 years, two-thirds of the survivors in the chemotherapy arm had retained their larynx, representing one-third of the patients who had been randomized in this experimental arm. Another trial was recently published by a French group (GET-TEC).[77] Here, the selection was different from the American study since all tumours were classified T3 and more cases were glottic or transglottic tumours. Patients were randomized to receive either the standard treatment (total laryngectomy) or three cycles of induction chemotherapy followed by irradiation when a greater than 80 per cent clinical response was observed, or by total laryngectomy in the other cases. Locoregional control and survival were significantly higher

in the surgery arm. Unfortunately, only 68 patients were enrolled and CT scans were not routinely performed to assess the tumour extension nor the tumour response to chemotherapy or radiotherapy, thus limiting the power of this trial. The third trial was conducted by the EORTC[78] in patients with hypopharynx tumours who were only eligible for total laryngectomy with partial pharyngectomy. A total of 202 patients were enrolled in this study, which was designed to compare the standard treatment (surgery and postoperative irradiation) versus two or three cycles of chemotherapy followed in clinically complete responders at the primary site by irradiation or, for other patients, by conventional treatment. There was no significant difference in survival, despite a notable difference in median survival favouring the experimental arm (44 months) when compared with the surgery arm (25 months). This difference in median survival was only explained by the fact that distant metastases appeared much later after chemotherapy, leading to a better survival at 3 years which was not shown at 5 years. Finally, at 3 and 5 years half the survivors in the chemotherapy arm had retained a functional larynx. These three trials had a similar design and used the same chemotherapy regimen (the classical cisplatinum and 5-fluorouracil combination). Hence, they were compiled in a specific analysis[79] of the meta-analysis mentioned above. A non-significant trend for a 6 per cent poorer survival was observed in the chemotherapy arms, but the results varied according to the anatomical subsite.

The fourth trial,[80] in resectable hypopharynx tumours only amenable to mutilating surgery, compared the outcome of patients randomly assigned to receive either: (1) induction chemotherapy followed by surgery and postoperative irradiation; or (2) induction chemotherapy followed by irradiation, with surgery held in reserve for salvage. In both arms, the design was applied irrespective of the tumour response to chemotherapy. With a median follow-up of 92 months in the 92 randomized patients, it appeared that a better 5-year survival (37 per cent) and a better local control (63 per cent) was achieved in the surgery arm when compared with the radiotherapy arm (respectively, 19 per cent and 39 per cent). The comparison of this trial with the EORTC trial suggests that tumour chemosensitivity must be taken into account before deciding on subsequent radiation therapy instead of surgery.

Apart from these four randomized trials, which were tailored to assess the larynx, the possibility of larynx preservation is nowadays unquestionable. However, this approach must be considered as still under investigation. Induction chemotherapy with such a goal cannot be considered as the new standard approach for the treatment of advanced larynx and/or hypopharynx squamous-cell carcinoma[81],[82] and must be compared with other irradiation approaches with or without modification of the fractionation, with or without concurrent chemotherapy. In addition, it is clear that whenever a partial surgical procedure is still possible, this option must be preferred as the first approach, without chemotherapy.

Palliation chemotherapy

When previously untreated patients with unresectable disease are not good candidates for irradiation (massive laryngeal structure destruction, large necrotic nodes, etc.), chemotherapy is sometimes proposed with the aim that tumour reduction may improve the response to subsequent irradiation. The most common induction chemotherapy consists of the cisplatinum and 5-fluorouracil regimen. In general, three courses are delivered before evaluation of the response and a possible change in therapeutic decision. Another, and probably more efficient, approach is concurrent chemoirradiation. However, tolerance is worse, requiring a thorough selection of patients and intensive medical support. These approaches should be considered in the clinical research stage.

In the case of unresectable recurrent or metastatic diseases for which re-irradiation cannot be delivered, chemotherapy remains the sole treatment that can be proposed (supportive care only being the alternative approach). Median survival is about 6 months regardless of the approach. Chemotherapy should be discussed according to the patient's wishes and performance status. New drugs or new administration modalities are often assessed in these clinical situations, again in the framework of phase I and phase II clinical research trials.

Management and prognosis

General considerations

Therapeutic approaches to larynx and hypopharynx cancers may vary according to numerous parameters.

For early disease, the choice is between partial surgery or definitive irradiation, while chemotherapy has no role to play. This choice is based on:

- the patient's characteristics (age, occupation, performance status, pulmonary function) and preferences;
- tumour characteristics (anatomical site, size, presence of surrounding premalignant changes, infiltration of natural spaces, extension to cartilage, larynx mobility);
- nodal extension and/or distant metastases;
- the surgeon's and radiotherapist's expertise; and
- institutional policies.

For advanced disease, the choice is between 'mutilating' surgery, with or without postoperative irradiation, or definitive irradiation with surgery held in reserve for salvage. This choice is based on rather similar parameters but is strongly influenced by the discussion on larynx-preserving approaches (some of them including chemotherapy) which still are under evaluation. For more advanced and unresectable disease, the choice is between irradiation alone with different fractionations and chemoirradiation regimens in the framework of clinical research.

After partial surgery of properly selected larynx or hypopharynx cancers, a 90 per cent local control is achieved, regardless of the surgical procedure. The 5-year survival rate ranges from 50 per cent for hypopharynx cancer to 80 per cent for larynx cancer. The quality of pharyngolaryngeal function (phonation, breathing, and swallowing) is rarely assessed. After radical surgery, local control is around 85 per cent with a 5-year survival rate of between 40 per cent for hypopharynx cancers and 60 per cent for larynx cancer.[81] It is obvious that there is always a favourable patient selection in surgical series, while radiotherapy series contain a mixture of favourable and unfavourable cases.

Treatment selection

Regardless of the clinical context, the decision process requires a multidisciplinary approach. Except for advanced stages, the absence of randomized trials comparing different strategies leaves an open

debate on the most appropriate approach. We miss a fair comparison of both surgical and non-surgical approaches as regards carcinologic and functional results. Retrospective studies carried out on selected subsets of patients do not provide the basis for decision-making founded on the available evidence; this explains the many management options offered for tumours of similar stage and location.

Primary tumour management recommendations

Hypopharynx and pharyngeal walls cancer

T1T2
- membranous portion of the piriform sinus: definitive irradiation or partial surgery with postoperative irradiation;
- cartilaginous portion of the piriform sinus: partial surgery with postoperative irradiation;
- lateral pharyngeal walls: definitive irradiation;
- posterior pharyngeal wall: definitive irradiation or partial surgery with postoperative irradiation.

T3T4
- resectable: radical surgery with postoperative irradiation or larynx-preserving approach (clinical research).
- resectable tumour involving the oesophageal sphincter: wide surgery with free-flap reconstruction or gastric pull-up and postoperative irradiation (patients with good performance status and limited nodal involvement), or hyperfractionated irradiation, or concurrent chemoirradiation (in the other cases);
- unresectable: hyperfractionated irradiation or concurrent chemoirradiation.

Larynx

Supraglottic cancer

T1
- endoscopic (laser) surgery, or conventional partial surgery, or, preferably, definitive irradiation.

T2
- false vocal cord: definitive irradiation;
- laryngeal aspect of the epiglottis without extension to the anterior commissure nor impaired mobility: definitive irradiation;
- extension to the anterior commissure or impaired mobility: definitive irradiation or, preferably, partial surgery.

T3
- due to larynx rigidity: radical surgery or larynx-preserving approach (clinical research);
- due to limited pre-epiglottic space invasion: definitive irradiation or partial surgery;
- due to massive pre-epiglottic space invasion: radical surgery or larynx-preserving approach (clinical research).

T4
- radical surgery with postoperative irradiation or larynx-preserving approach (clinical research).

Glottic cancer

T1
- endoscopic (laser) surgery, or partial surgery, or definitive irradiation.

T2
- due to extension to the anterior commissure: superficially: definitive irradiation or partial surgery, deeply: partial surgery;
- due to arytenoid extension: partial surgery or definitive irradiation.

T3T4
- resectable: radical surgery or larynx-preserving approach (clinical research);
- unresectable: definitive irradiation with or without chemotherapy.

Transglottic cancer (all are either T3 or T4)

T3T4
- resectable: radical surgery or larynx-preserving approach (clinical research);
- unresectable: definitive irradiation with or without chemotherapy.

Subglottic cancer

T1T2
- superficial: definitive irradiation;
- infiltrating: if resectable: radical surgery or cautious larynx-preserving approach (clinical research); if unresectable: definitive irradiation with or without chemotherapy.

T3T4
- resectable: radical surgery or larynx-preserving approach (clinical research);
- unresectable: definitive irradiation with or without chemotherapy.

Neck management recommendations

Hypopharynx, pharyngeal walls, and supraglottic cancer

Whatever the primary site and the T classification, the neck is systematically treated whether there are palpable lymph nodes or not. Management of the neck is similar to the primary management (surgery or irradiation). In the particular case of a limited primary tumour with a massive nodal involvement (T1N3, for example), a radical neck dissection may be performed prior to irradiation if the primary is to be treated by irradiation.

Neck management, whether surgical or radiotherapeutic, is bilateral each time the primary is located on the supraglottic larynx, the posterior pharyngeal wall, or arises in the midline.

When a neck dissection is performed, postoperative irradiation is delivered in the case of multiple nodal involvement or in the case of capsular rupture. There are ongoing studies assessing whether concurrent postoperative chemoirradiation, in the case of massive nodal involvement, could improve the outcome.

Glottic cancer

The neck is treated only when there are palpable lymph nodes or when the primary is classified more than T2. The treatment is similar, in this case, to that for the hypopharynx, pharyngeal walls, and supraglottic cancer (see above).

Subglottic or transglottic cancer

A neck dissection is systematically performed, including the recurrent chains.

Distant metastases

When these metastases are isolated and if the short-term prognosis is not unfavourable, metastasectomy may be performed. In other cases, chemotherapy or supportive care may be the treatment of choice.

Local or nodal recurrence

Surgery, irradiation, or re-irradiation should be proposed whenever the patients' performance status is compatible with such treatments. If not, the patients may be treated by either chemotherapy or supportive care according to each individual case.

Follow-up

The reliability of an appropriate follow-up remains an open debate. Early detection of locoregional failure gives a better chance for ultimate cure with salvage treatment. Conversely, the cost-effectiveness of screening for distant metastases and second primaries is not proven. The problem is really complex since these patients are exposed to various events such as locoregional recurrences, second primaries, and treatment side-effects, which may present with similar symptoms. The frequency of associated morbidity related to lifestyle brings additional complexity to this follow-up.

A regular clinical examination remains the best solution. There is no biological marker, and imaging is sometimes unable to differentiate local failures and post-therapeutic modifications. If a CT scan or MRI may be of use, then new tools (such as positron-emission tomography (PET) scanning) could, in the future, be more reliable at detecting persistent diseases; however, to date, they remain investigational tools. As a result, a physical examination complemented by a careful history is still recommended. Follow-up examinations are recommended monthly or every 2 months for the first 3 years after treatment, then every 3 months for 3 more years, and finally every 6 months in subsequent years.

The follow-up schedule must not only keep convalescence in mind, but also, ultimately, rehabilitation resulting in a return to as near-normal condition as possible. Rehabilitation of patients following treatment for hypopharyngeal cancer is especially difficult, due to their poor general condition and the radical therapies used. Nutritional support, speech therapy, or intensive physical therapy after radical surgery and neck dissection must often be continued for long periods, despite acute psychosocial problems. Successful physical and psychological readaptation (with true familial and social reintegration, including a return to professional activities) is seldom achieved, even though many patients consider resumption of their former occupation the unquestionable proof of their cure. Account must always be taken of the various long-term effects of irradiation or cervical surgery (sclerosis, hyposialia, etc.) in physical therapy programmes aimed at improving functional status. In addition, attention must be paid to educating patients in order to modify their lifestyles and behaviours.

Conclusions

Larynx and hypopharynx cancers are frequent in developed countries and, in particular, in Latin Europe. These cancers are mainly due to tobacco consumption, often associated with alcohol abuse. They are potentially preventable diseases. Modern imaging has considerably improved the quality of pretherapeutic work-up, allowing a more appropriate treatment selection. Both functional surgery and irradiation refinements have improved the outcome thanks to better local control, functional results, and quality of life. To date, the place of chemotherapy remains controversial. If adjuvant chemotherapy has failed to improve any aspect of the outcome, then induction chemotherapy, even though it has been unable to improve survival, has reopened the discussion on the preservation of larynx function. Nevertheless, induction chemotherapy cannot be considered as standard for larynx and hypopharynx treatment with curative intent. Finally, ongoing studies should, in the future, establish the role and place of concurrent chemoradiotherapy.

References

1. **International Agency for Research on Cancer.** *Cancer incidence in five continents*, Vol. VI. Lyon: IARC Scientific Publications, 1992: No. 120.

2. **Jensen OM, Esteve J, Moller H, Renard H.** Cancer in the European Community and its member states. *European Journal of Cancer*, 1990; **26**: 1167–256.

3. **Lefebvre, et al.** Epilarynx: pharynx or larynx? *Head and Neck*, 1995; **17**: 377–81.

4. **Brugere J, Guenel P, Leclerc A, Rodriguez J.** Differential effects of tobacco and alcohol in cancer of the larynx, pharynx and mouth. *Cancer*, 1986; **57**: 391–5.

5. **Brugere J, Guenel P, Rodriguez J, Leclerc A, Point D.** Facteurs exogenes et socio-professionnels dans les cancers de l'hypopharynx. In *Cancers de l'hypopharynx* (ed. JP Bataini, J Leroux-Robert). Paris: Masson, 1989: 10–17.

6. **Olofsson J, van Nostrand AWP.** Growth and spread of laryngeal and hypopharyngeal carcinoma with reflections on the effect of preoperative irradiation. *Acta Oto-Laryngologica*, 1973; Suppl. 308.

7. **Kleinsasser O.** *Tumors of the Larynx and the Hypopharynx.* Stuttgart: Georg Thieme Verlag, 1988.

8. **Ogura JH.** Surgical pathology of cancer of the larynx. *The Laryngoscope*, 1955; **65**: 867–926.

9. **Kirchner JA.** One hundred laryngeal cancers studied by serial section. *Annals of Otology Rhinology and Laryngology*, 1969; **78**: 689–709.

10. **McGavran MH, Bauer WC, Ogura JH.** The incidence of cervical lymph node metastases from epidermoid carcinoma of the larynx and their relationship to certain characteristics of the primary tumour. A study based on clinical and pathological findings for 96 patients treated by primary *en bloc* laryngectomy and radical neck dissection. *Cancer*, 1961; **14**: 55–66.

11. **Kirchner JA, Som ML.** Clinical and histological observations on supraglottic cancer. *Annals of Otology Rhinology and Laryngology*, 1971; **80**: 638–45.

12. **Robert Y, Rocourt N, Chevalier D, Duhamel A, Carcasset S, Lemaitre L.** Helical CT of the larynx: a comparative study with conventional CT scan. *Clinical Radiology*, 1996; **51**: 882–5.

13. **Castelain B, Vankemmel B, Coche-Dequeant B, Lefebvre JL, Prevost B.** Les cancers de l'hypopharynx T1T2. Places respectives de la chirurgie et de la radiothérapie au Centre Oscar Lambret. In *Cancers de l'hypopharynx* (ed. JP Bataini, J Leroux-Robert). Paris: Masson, 1989: 112–16.

14. **Laccourreye H, et al.** Les hemilaryngopharyngectomies. Resultats fonctionnels et carcinologiques. *Annales d'Otolaryngologie et de Chirurgie Cervico-faciale*, 1988; **105**: 443–7.

15. **Gehanno P, Barry B, Guedon C, Depondt J.** Lateral supraglottic pharyngolaryngectomy with arytenoidectomy. *Head and Neck*, 1996; **18**: 494–500.

16. **Chevalier D, Watelet JB, Darras JA, Piquet JJ.** Supraglottic hemilaryngopharyngectomy plus radiation for the treatment of early lateral margin and pyriform sinus carcinoma. *Head and Neck*, 1997; **19**: 1–5.

17. **Remacle M, Lawson G, Jamart J, Minet M, Watelet JB, Delos M.** CO_2 laser in the diagnosis and treatment of early cancer of the vocal cord. *European Archives of Otorhinolaryngology*, 1994; **254**: 169–76.

18. **Shapsay SM, Hybels RL, Bohigian RK.** Laser excision of early vocal cord carcinoma: indications, limitations, and precautions. *Annals of Otology, Rhinology and Laryngology*, 1990; **99**: 46–50.

19. **Rudert HH, Werner JA.** Endoscopic resections of glottic and supraglottic carcinomas with the CO_2 laser. *European Archives of Otorhinolaryngology*, 1995; **252**: 146–8.

20. **Rydell R, Schallen L, Fex S, Elner A.** Voice evaluation after excision vs radiotherapy of T1 a glottic carcinoma. *Acta Otolaryngologica (Stockholm)*, 1995; **115**: 560–5.

21. **Myers EN, Wagner RL, Johnson JT.** Microlaryngoscopic surgery for T1 glottic lesions: a cost-effective option. *Annals of Otology, Rhinology and Laryngology*, 1994; **103**: 28–30.

22. **Eckel HE.** Endoscopic laser resection of supraglottic carcinoma. *Archives of Otolaryngology – Head and Neck Surgery*, 1997; **117**: 682–7.

23. **Iro H, Waldfahrer F, Altendorf-Hofmann A, Weidenbecher M, Sauer R, Steiner W.** Transoral laser surgery of supraglottic cancer. *Archives of Otolaryngology – Head and Neck Surgery*, 1998; **124**: 1245–50.

24. **Lefebvre JL, Vankemmel B, Buisset E, Desaulty-Cousin A, Adenis L.** La cordectomie dans le traitement des cancers de la corde vocale. A propos de 200 cas. *Journal Français d'Oto-Rhino-Laryngologie*, 1987; **36**: 415–21.

25. **Leroux-Robert J.** A statistical study of 620 laryngeal carcinomas of the glottic region personally operated upon more than five years ago. *The Laryngoscope*, 1950; **105**: 1440–52.

26. **Zanaret M, Giovanni A, Gras R, Cannoni M.** Near total laryngectomy with epiglottic reconstruction: long-term results in 57 patients. *American Journal of Otolaryngology*, 1993; **14**: 419–25.

27. **Silver CE, Moisa II, Stern WBR.** Surgical therapy. In *Neoplasms of the larynx* (ed. A Ferlito). Edinburgh: Churchill Livingstone, 1993: 451–92.

28. **Piquet JJ, Chevalier D.** Subtotal laryngectomy with cricohyoidoepiglottopexy for the treatment of extended glottic carcinomas. *American Journal of Surgery*, 1991; **162**: 357–61.

29. **Lefebvre JL, Chevalier D.** Supracricoid partial laryngectomy. In *Advances in Otolaryngology-Head and Neck Surgery*, Vol. 12 (ed. EN Myers). St Louis, MO: Mosby, 1998: 1–15.

30. **Chevalier JJ, Thill C, Darras JA, Piquet JJ.** Les résultats du traitement des cancers de l'étage sus-glottique. *Annales d'Otolaryngologie et de Chirurgie Cervico-faciale*, 1993; **110**: 7–51.

31. **Chevalier D, Piquet JJ.** Subtotal laryngectomy with cricohyoidopexy for supraglottic carcinoma: a review of 61 cases. *American Journal of Surgery*, 1994; **168**: 472–3.

32. **ICRU report 62.** *Prescribing, recording and reporting photon beam therapy* (Supplement to ICRU Report 50). Library of Congress ISBN 0–913394–61–0.

33. **Bataini P, et al.** Results of radical radiotherapeutic treatment of carcinoma of the pyriform sinus: experience of the Institut Curie. *International Journal of Radiation Oncology, Biology, Physics*, 1982; **8**: 1277.

34. **Dubois JB, Guerrier B, Di Ruggiero JM, Pourquier H.** Cancer of the piriform sinus: treatment by radiation therapy alone and with surgery. *Radiology*, 1993; **160**: 377.

35. **Vandenbrouck C, et al.** Squamous cell carcinoma of the pririform sinus. A retrospective study of the management and results of 351 cases treated at the Institut Gustave Roussy. *Head and Neck*, 1987; **1**: 4–13.

36. Castelain B, Prevost B, Coche-Dequéant B, Lefebvre JL, Vankemmel B. Résultats de la radiothérapie exclusive dans le traitement des cancers inopérables de l'hypopharynx. In *Cancers de l'hypopharynx* (ed. JP Bataini, J Leroux-Robert). Paris: Masson, 1989: 117–22.

37. Lusinchi A, Dube P, Wibault P, Kunkler I, Luboinski B, Eschwège F. Radiation therapy in the treatment of early glottic carcinoma: the experience of Villejuif. *Radiotherapy Oncology*, 1989; 15: 313–19.

38. Terhaard CHJ, Snippe K, Ravasz LA, van der Tweel I, Hordjik GJ. Radiotherapy in T1 laryngeal cancer: prognostic factors for locoregional control and survival, uni- and multivariate analysis. *International Journal of Radiation Oncology, Biology, Physics*, 1991; 21: 1179–86.

39. Mendenhall WM, Parsons JT, Million RR, Fletcher GH. T1–T2 squamous cell carcinoma of the glottic larynx treated with radiation therapy: relationship of dose-fractionation factors to local control and complications. *International Journal of Radiation Oncology, Biology, Physics*, 1988; 15: 1267–73.

40. Cellai E, Chiavacci A, Olmi P. Causes of failure of curative radiation therapy in 205 early glottic cancers. *International Journal of Radiation Oncology, Biology, Physics*, 1990; 19: 1139–42.

41. Akine Y, *et al.* Radiotherapy of T1 glottic cancer with 6 MeV X-rays. *International Journal of Radiation Oncology, Biology, Physics*, 1991; 20: 1215–18.

42. Olszewski SJ, Vaeth JM, Green JP, Schroeder AF, Chauser B. The influence of field size, treatment modality, commisure involvement and histology in the treatment of early vocal cord cancer with irradiation. *International Journal of Radiation Oncology, Biology, Physics*, 1985; 11: 1333–7.

43. Pelliteri PK, Kennedy TL, Vrabec DP, Beiler D, Hellstrom M. Radiotherapy. The mainstay in the treatment of early glottic carcinoma. *Archives of Otolaryngology – Head Neck Surgery*, 1991; 117: 297–301.

44. Robson NLK, Oswal VH, Flood LM. Radiation therapy of laryngeal cancer: a twenty year experience. *Journal of Laryngology and Otology*, 1990; 104: 699–703.

45. Fein DA and al. Pretreatment hemoglobin level influences local control and survival of T1-T2 squamous cell carcinomas of the glottic larynx. *Journal of Clinical Oncology*. 1995; 13: 2077–83.

46. Rudoltz MS, Benammar A, Mohiuddin M. Prognostic factors for local control and survival in T1 squamous cell carcinoma of the glottis. *International Journal of Radiation Oncology, Biology, Physics*, 1993; 26: 767–72.

47. Harwood AR, Beale FA, Cummings BJ, Keane TJ, Rider WD. T2 glottic cancer: an analysis of dose–time–volume factors. *International Journal of Radiation Oncology, Biology, Physics*, 1981; 7: 1501–5.

48. Slevin NJ, Vasanthan S, Dougal M. Relative influence of tumour dose versus dose per fraction on the occurrence of late normal tissue morbidity following larynx radiotherapy. *International Journal of Radiation Oncology, Biology, Physics*, 1992; 25: 23–8.

49. Wang CC. Factors influencing the success of radiation therapy for T2 and T3 glottic carcinomas. *Journal of Clinical Oncology*, 1986; 9: 517–20.

50. Turesson I, Sandberg N, Mercke C, Johansson KA, Sandin I, Wallgren A. Primary radiotherapy for glottic laryngeal carcinoma stage I and II. *Acta Oncologica*, 1991; 30: 357–62.

51. Fein DA, Mendenhall WM, Parsons JT, Stringer SP, Cassisi NJ, Million RR. Carcinoma *in situ* of the glottic larynx: the role of radiotherapy. *International Journal of Radiation Oncology, Biology, Physics*, 1993; 27: 379–84.

52. Howell-Burke D, Peters LJ, Goepfert H, Oswald MJ. T2 glottic cancer. *Archives of Otolaryngology Head Neck Surgery*, 1990; 116: 830–5.

53. Schwaab G, Mamelle G, Lartigau E, Parise Jr O, Wibault P, Luboinski B. Surgical salvage treatment of T1/T2 glottic carcinoma after failure of radiotherapy. *American Journal of Surgery*. 1994; 168: 474–5.

54. van den Bogaert W, Ostyn F, Van der Shueren E. The significance of extension and impaired mobility in cancer of the vocal cord. *International Journal of Radiation Oncology, Biology, Physics*, 1983; 9: 181–4.

55. Spaulding CA, Krochak RJ, Shin Hahn S, Constable WC. Radiotherapeutic management of cancer of the supraglottis. *Cancer*, 1986; 57: 1292–8.

56. Mendenhall WM, Parsons JT, Mancuso AA, Stringer SP, Cassisi NJ. Radiotherapy for squamous cell carcinoma of the supra glottic larynx: an alternative to surgery. *Head and Neck*, 1996; 18: 24–35.

57. Levendag PC, Hoekstra CJM, Eukenboom WMH, Reichgelt BA, Van Putten WLJ. Supraglottic larynx cancer, T1–4 N0, treated by radical radiation therapy. *Acta Oncologica*, 1988; 27: 253–60.

58. Inoue Ta., Matayoshi Y, Inoue To, Ikeda H, Teshima T, Murayama S. Prognostic factors in telecobalt therapy for early supraglottic carcinoma. *Cancer*, 1993; 72: 57–61.

59. Glinsky B, Reinfuss M, Walasek T, Skolyszewski J. Radiothérapie exclusive de 250 cancers du larynx sus-glottique stade I–II. *Bulletin du Cancer/Radiotherapie*. 1996; 83: 177–9.

60. Haylock BJ, Deutsch GP. Primary radiotherapy for subglottic carcinoma. *Journal of Clinical Oncology*, 1993; 5: 143–6.

61. Warde P, Harwood AR, Keane T. Carcinoma of the subglottis. Results of initial radical radiation. *Archives of Otolaryngology Head and Neck Surgery*, 1987; 113: 1228–9.

62. Guedea F, Parsons JT, Mendenhall WM, Million RR, Stringer SP, Cassisi NJ. Primary subglottic cancer: results of radical radiation therapy. *International Journal of Radiation Oncology, Biology, Physics*, 1991; 21: 1607–11.

63. Lindelov B, Hansen HS. Advanced squamous cell carcinoma of the larynx. *Acta Oncologica*, 1990; 29: 505–8.

64. Meredith AP, Randall CJ, Shaw HJ. Advanced laryngeal cancer: a management perspective. *Journal of Laryngology and Otology*, 1987; 101: 1046–54.

65. Karim ABMF, Kralendonk JH, Njo KH, Tierie AH, Hasman A. Radiation therapy for advanced (T3T4N0-N3M0) laryngeal carcinoma: the need for a change of strategy: a radiotherapeutic viewpoint. *International Journal of Radiation Oncology, Biology, Physics*, 1987; 13: 1625–33.

66. Davidson J, Briant D, Gullane P, Keane T, Rawlinson E. The role of surgery following radiotherapy failure for advanced laryngopharyngeal cancer. *Archives of Otolaryngology Head and Neck Surgery*, 1994; 120: 269–76.

67. Terhaard CHJ, *et al.* Local control in T3 laryngeal cancer treated with radical radiotherapy, time dose relationship: the concept of nominal standard dose and linear quadratic model. *International Journal of Radiation Oncology, Biology, Physics*, 1991; 20: 1207–14.

68. Harwood AR, Rawlinson E. The quality of life of patients following treatment for laryngeal cancer. *International Journal of Radiation Oncology, Biology, Physics*, 1983; 9: 335–8.

69. Eschwège F, Ghilezan M, Mamelle G, Wibault P, Lusinchi A, Luboinski B. Results of T3, T4 laryngeal cancers treated by exclusive external radiotherapy. Experience of the Institute Gustave Roussy (IGR). In *Laryngeal cancer* (ed. R Smee, GP Bridger). Amsterdam: Elsevier, 1994: 536–8.

70. van den Bogaert W, Ostyn F, van der Schueren E. The primary treatment of advanced vocal cord cancer: laryngectomy or radiotherapy? *International Journal of Radiation Oncology, Biology, Physics*, 1983; 9: 329–4.

71. Sanchiz F, *et al.* Single fraction per day versus two fractions per day versus radiochemotherapy in the treatment of head and neck cancer. *International Journal of Radiation Oncology, Biology, Physics*, 1990; 19: 1347–50.

72. Dische S, Sauders M, Barrett A, Harvey A, Gibson D, Parmar M. A randomised multicentre trial CHART versus conventional radiotherapy in head and neck cancer. *Radiotherapy and Oncology*, 1997; 44: 123–36.

73. Bourhis J, Pignon JP, Designe L, Luboinski M, Guerin S, Domenge C. Meta-analysis of chemotherapy in head and neck cancer (MACH-NC): 1 loco-regional treatment vs same treatment + chemotherapy (CT). *Proceedings of the American Society of Clinical Oncology*, 1998; Abstract 1468.

74. Horiot JC, *et al.* Dental preservation in patients irradiated for head and neck tumors: a ten-year experience with topical fluoride and a randomized trial between two fluoridation methods. *Radiotherapy and Oncology*, 1983; **1**: 77–82.

75. The Department of Veterans Affairs Laryngeal Cancer Study Group. Induction chemotherapy plus irradiation compared with surgery plus irradiation in patients with advanced laryngeal cancer. *New England Journal of Medicine*, 1991; **324**: 1685–90.

76. Wolf GT, Hong WK, Department of Veterans Affairs Laryngeal Cancer Study Group. Induction chemotherapy as part of a new treatment strategy to preserve the larynx in advanced laryngeal cancer. In *Head and neck cancer*, Vol. 3 (ed. JT Johnson, MS Didolkar). Amsterdam: Excerpta Medica, 1993: 27–35.

77. Richard JM, *et al.* Randomized trial of induction chemotherapy in larynx carcinoma. *Oral Oncology*, 1998; **34**: 224–8.

78. Lefebvre JL, Chevalier D, Luboinski B, Kirkpatrick A, Collette L, Sahmoud T. Larynx preservation in pyriform sinus cancer: preliminary results of a European Organization for Research and Treatment of Cancer phase III study. *Journal of the National Cancer Institute*, 1996; **13**: 890–9.

79. Lefebvre JL, *et al.* Meta-analysis of chemotherapy in head and neck cancer (MACH-NC): 2 larynx preservation using neoadjuvant chemotherapy (CT) in laryngeal and hypopharyngeal carcinoma. *Proceedings of the American Society of Clinical Oncology*, 1998; Abstract 1473.

80. Beauvillain C, *et al.* Final results of a randomized trial comparing chemotherapy plus radiotherapy with chemotherapy plus surgery plus radiotherapy in locally advanced resectable carcinomas. *The Laryngoscope*, 1997; **107**: 648–53.

81. Lefebvre JL. Larynx preservation: the discussion is not closed. *Otolaryngology-Head and Neck Surgery*, 1998; **118**: 389–93.

82. Eschwege F, Bourhis J, Luboinski B, Lefebvre JL. La conservation d'organes en cancerologie ORL: mythe ou realite. A propos de la conservation laryngée. *Cancer Radiotherapy*, 1998; **2**: 437–45.

Salivary glands

C. B. Croft and R. W. R. Farrell

Introduction

Epidemiology

Tumours of the salivary glands are relatively rare, comprising slightly less than 3 per cent of all head and neck neoplasms.[1] Their relative infrequency and tendency to histological variability continue to contribute to a grave lack of hard data on which to pursue an 'evidence-based approach' to the subject. There are no published prospective controlled studies of differing methods and modalities of management other than in advanced malignant disease.

Although a majority of salivary gland tumours arise in the major or parotid salivary glands, approximately 10 to 20 per cent of all salivary gland tumours arise outside the major salivary glands, occurring in the mucous glands of the palate, lips, tongue, nasopharynx, paranasal sinuses, and pharynx. Salivary gland tumours also occur in minor salivary glands associated with the lacrimal glands and may rarely occur in the tracheobronchial tree, oesophagus, breast, and skin.[2],[3]

The propensity for tumours originating in the minor salivary glands to be malignant is a consistent feature in large retrospectively reviewed series from major tertiary centres.[4] Jones *et al.* report an 'incidence of malignant tumours of 68 per cent' in their series of 145 minor salivary gland tumours, the majority of these tumours (70 per cent) being adenoid cystic carcinoma.[5]

The occurrence of malignant salivary gland tumours has been associated with radiation exposure, genetic factors, and carcinoma of the breast.[6]–[8]

However, a majority of salivary gland tumours occur in the parotid gland, with 75 to 85 per cent of all tumours being of parotid origin and 80 per cent of such tumours being benign pleomorphic adenomas.[9] Data from the British salivary Gland Tumour Panel confirm that the incidence of malignancy rises to 35 per cent in tumours of the submandibular salivary glands and to 86 per cent in the very small number of sublingual gland tumours.[10]

Presentation

Salivary gland tumours, whether benign or malignant, will present as a solitary mass developing within the substance of the affected gland. Global or recurrent enlargement of the affected gland suggests calculus or inflammatory disease and a rare global major salivary gland enlargement is seen in systemic disorders such as diabetes mellitus, myxoedema, Cushing's syndrome, and alcoholism. General enlargement of the parotid glands is also seen in anorexia nervosa.[11]

Patients with benign or low-grade malignant tumours may present with a slowly growing mass present for many years (Fig. 1).

Rapid growth of the mass and pain related to the lesion suggests malignant transformation, but is not diagnostic. Involvement of the facial nerve (VII) is generally an indicator of malignancy, although this feature is present at initial presentation in only 3 per cent of all parotid tumours, and generally indicates a poor prognosis. The authors have seen partial interference of the facial nerve function in large benign parotid tumours intimately related to the nerve, although such a finding is extremely rare, but direct involvement of some part of the facial nerve may be demonstrated in as many as 40 to 67 per cent of high-grade parotid malignancies.[12] Malignant tumours of the parotid gland tend to extend to the retromandibular area of the parotid and invade the so-called deep lobe, passing into the parapharyngeal space. Here, involvement of the lower cranial nerves may occur with the development of dysphagia, pain, and ear symptoms. Further involvement of the surrounding structures may involve the petrous bone, external auditory canal, and temporomandibular joint.

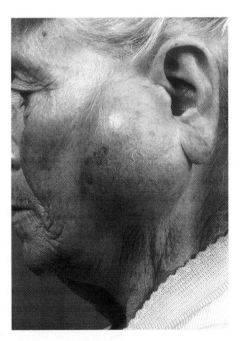

Fig. 1 A large parotid pleomorphic adenoma. The mass has been present for more than 5 years.

Malignant tumours metastasize to lymph nodes within the parapharyngeal space and to the deep jugular chain and the pre- and postfacial nodes.

However, the incidence of lymph node enlargement at presentation is low, but highly significant in terms of survival. Data from Armstrong *et al.* demonstrate that 16 per cent of patients with parotid tumour and 8 per cent of patients with submandibular or sublingual tumour had clinically involved lymph nodes at presentation.[13] Nodal involvement increases with the T-stage and with tumour grade. Armstrong *et al.* showed that 49 per cent of patients with high-grade tumours (44/91) had subclinical disease on elective neck dissection compared with 7 per cent in patients with low- or intermediate-grade tumours.

Investigations

Examination

Several and various pathologies can mimic a salivary gland tumour. It is important to palpate the gland bimanually, particularly the submandibular gland, to try and differentiate a salivary gland from a lymph node or other extrinsic lesion. Evaluation of skin fixation, facial nerve function, and intraoral examination for parotid deep lobe extension are routine. Systemic palpation of the neck for lymphadenopathy and the rare bilateral Warthin's tumour should be undertaken. A list of alternative pathologies is given below:

- metastatic lymph node disease
- reactive lymph nodes
- HIV infection
- sarcoidosis
- masseteric hypertrophy
- prominent transverse cervical process of C1
- chronic parotitis
- lymphangioma (paediatric)
- haemangioma.

Imaging

Although plain films and sialography are useful in calculous and non-neoplastic salivary gland disease, plain films and sialography have virtually no role to play in the evaluation of salivary gland tumours. Sialography provides no useful information regarding the position and relations of a salivary tumour. There are no typical sialographic features peculiar to any particular tumour type. The authors feel that routine sialography in salivary gland tumours can be discarded.

Advanced imaging techniques are unnecessary if the salivary gland tumour is mobile, discrete, and/or superficial. If there is concern that the mass is extrinsic to the salivary gland in question, then computed tomography (**CT**) scanning and magnetic resonance imaging (**MRI**) are the preferred imaging procedures (Fig. 2), providing information on:

- location of the mass
- true extension within the gland and possible relationship to the facial nerve
- demonstration of features suggestive of malignancy and malignant infiltration of surrounding structures and the facial nerve.

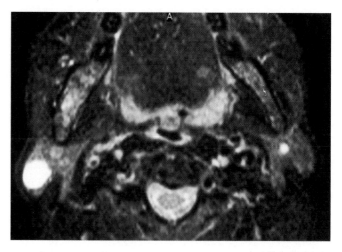

Fig. 2 T_2-weighted MRI image showing well-defined margins, high signal, and superficial lobe location of a parotid mass, characteristic of a benign lesion. The diagnosis is of a lymphoepithelial cyst.

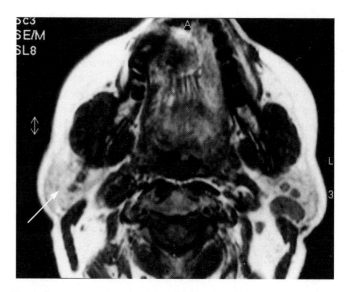

Fig. 3 T_1-weighted MRI image showing low signal mass with well-defined margins within both superficial and deep lobes of the parotid. The facial nerve cannot be distinguished, but its course is inferred (L) by the line between the retromandibular vein and stylomastoid foramen.

Detailed imaging is also helpful in order to stage the disease and in the evaluation of recurrent and deep lobe parotid tumours and where a facial nerve palsy is present. Recent studies have compared MRI with CT in the evaluation of salivary gland neoplasia. MRI has been shown to be superior, although it cannot always differentiate tumour boundaries from surrounding tissues, and the position of the facial nerve cannot be reliably predicted, although its position in relation to a particular tumour can be inferred (Fig. 3).[14]

Extension of the tumour to the base of the skull with erosion of the bone or osteolysis is most usefully evaluated by CT scanning.

Detailed information on imaging techniques can be obtained elsewhere in this textbook.

Ultrasound and fine needle aspiration cytology

The prime role for ultrasound in the investigation of salivary gland tumours is in association with fine needle aspiration cytology. Fine needle aspiration cytology has become an ever-increasingly popular diagnostic investigation.[15]–[18] Initial concerns regarding tumour seeding within the needle track have been unfounded.[19]

Recent data suggest that in experienced hands fine needle aspiration cytology has an overall sensitivity in salivary neoplasms of 93 per cent. The specificity for the absence of neoplasm is 99 per cent and the predictive value of a positive aspiration for neoplasm is 98.3 per cent.[20] Certain individual tumours are difficult to diagnose using this technique, particularly low-grade or well-differentiated mucoepidermoid carcinoma, because of the absence of true malignant features in well-differentiated or mucoid areas of the tumour. However, from both the surgeon's and the patient's point of view, a preoperative diagnosis is helpful in formulating a surgical strategy and clarifying the degree of urgency which might be required. It also provides a useful guide to the need for further investigation, i.e. detailed imaging, and may give important information in relation to tumour type and the facial nerve. The presence of an aggressive high-grade tumour greatly increases the chance of partial or complete facial nerve sacrifice and a positive fine needle aspirate gives the surgeon and the patient an opportunity to discuss the full implications of facial nerve resection. It would be inappropriate to suggest that the facial nerve should be surgically sacrificed on the basis of a cytopathological diagnosis, but with frozen section support and the gross relationship of tumour and nerve displayed at surgery, the correct and best decision in the patient's interest can be reached.

However, as John Conley has said, 'if the pathology is uncertain or if there is disagreement between the surgeon and the pathologist or if the clinical condition does not correlate with the analysis of either surgeon or pathologist, prudence should be exercised in planning a mutilating procedure'. The authors strongly adhere to the policy that the facial nerve should be preserved in its entirety as far is technically possible.

Biopsy

Any form of incisional biopsy is absolutely contraindicated in tumours of the major salivary glands, although biopsy may be considered in fungating tumours and tumours of the minor salivary glands as commonly seen in palatal biopsy.

Surgical pathology of salivary gland tumours

Primary tumours of the salivary gland display a heterogeneity that is almost unique. They also have a great diversity of morphological features. Classification of salivary gland tumours is, therefore, difficult, and this is reflected by its continual refinement. The latest WHO classification is the one most commonly used and is shown in Table 1. The most frequently occurring tumours of the salivary glands will be discussed. We will not make any reference to the rare and esoteric.

Staging

This section describes the TNM classification system for malignant salivary tumours in the major glands.[22]

Table 1 Tumour type: the morphology code is that of the International Classification of Diseases for oncology (ICD-O) and the Systematized Nomenclature of Medicine (SNOMED). (From Seifert and Sobin.[21])

1	**Adenomas**
1.1	Pleomorphic adenoma
1.2	Myoepithelioma (myoepithelial adenoma)
1.3	Basal cell adenoma
1.4	Warthin's tumour (adenolymphoma)
1.5	Oncocytoma (oncocytic adenoma)
1.6	Canalicular adenoma
1.7	Sebaceous adenoma
1.8	Ductal papilloma
1.8.1	Inverted ductal papilloma
1.8.2	Intraductal papilloma
1.8.3	Sialadenoma pililliferum
1.9	Cystadenoma
1.9.1	Papillary dystadenoma
1.9.2	Mucinous cystadenoma
2	**Carcinomas**
2.1	Acinic cell carcinoma
2.2	Mucoepidermoid carcinoma
2.3	Adenoid cystic carcinoma
2.4	Polymorphous low-grade adenocarcinoma (terminal duct adenocarcinoma)
2.5	Epithelial–myoepithelial carcinoma
2.6	Basal cell adenocarcinoma
2.7	Sebaceous carcinoma
2.8	Papillary cystadenocarcinoma
2.9	Mucinous adenocarcinoma
2.10	Oncocytic carcinoma
2.11	Salivary duct carcinoma
2.12	Adenocarcinoma
2.13	Malignant myoepithelioma (myoepithelial carcinoma)
2.14	Carcinoma in pleomorphic adenoma (malignant mixed tumour)
2.15	Squamous cell carcinoma
2.16	Small cell carcinoma
2.17	Undifferentiated carcinoma
2.18	Other carcinomas
3	**Non-epithelial tumours**
4	**Malignant lymphomas**
5	**Secondary tumours**
6	**Unclassified tumours**
7	**Tumour-like lesions**
7.1	Sialadenosis
7.2	Oncocytosis
7.3	Necrotizing sialometaplasia (salivary gland infarction)
7.4	Benign lymphoepithelial lesion
7.5	Salivary gland cysts
7.6	Chronic sclerosing sialadenitis of submandibular gland (Kuttner's tumour)
7.7	Cystic lymphoid hyperplasia in acquired immunodeficiency syndrome (AIDS)

Primary tumour (T)

- Tx: primary tumour cannot be assessed.
- T0: no evidence of primary tumour.
- T1: tumour 2 cm or less in greatest dimension.
- T2: tumour more than 2 cm but not more that 4.0 cm in greatest dimension.
- T3: tumour more than 2 cm but not more that 6.0 cm in greatest dimension.
- T4: tumour less than 6 cm in greatest dimension.

   All categories can be subdivided into:

   (a) no local extension
   (b) evidence of local extension.

Local extension is defined as clinical evidence of invasion of either skin, soft tissue, bone, or nerve.

Regional lymph nodes (N)

- Nx: regional lymph nodes cannot be assessed.
- N0: no regional lymph node metastases.
- N1: metastases in a single ipsilateral lymph node, 3 cm or less in greatest dimension.
- N2: metatstases in a single ipsilatreal lymph node less than 3 cm but not more than 6 cm in greatest dimension, or in multiple ipsilateral lymph nodes none more than 6 cm in greatest dimension, or bilateral or contralateral lymh nodes none more than 6 cm in greatest dimension.

   (a) MN2a: metastasis in single ipsilateral lymph node less than 3 cm but not more than 6 cm in greatest dimension.
   (b) N2b: metastasis in multiple ipsilateral lymph nodes, none more that 6 cm in greatest dimension.
   (c) N2c: metastasis in bilateral or contralateral lymph nodes, none more than 6 cm in greatest dimension.

- N3: metastasis in a lymph node more than 6 cm in greatest dimension.

Distant metastases (M)

- Mx: presence of distant metastases cannot be assessed.
- M0: no distant metastases.
- M1: distant metastases.

Stage grouping

Stage I	T1a	N0	M0
	T2a	N0	M0
Stage II	T1b	N0	M0
	T2b	N0	M0
	T3a	N0	M0
Stage III	T3b	N0	M0
	T4a	N0	M0
	T less than 4b	N1	M0
Stage IV	T4b	Any N	M0
	Any T	N2, N3	M0
	Any T	Any N	M1

All categories are subdivided, 'a' being no local extension and 'b' with local extension.

Management

Discussion and debate with regard to the management of salivary gland tumours is complicated by the dearth of properly conducted controlled trials into any of the aspects of treatment of salivary gland tumours. At a recent review of the management of parotid pleomorphic adenoma where over 300 references were surveyed, 70 of which were analysed fully, there were no randomized controlled trials dealing with the management of parotid pleomorphic adenoma, and all but two papers were retrospective or descriptive in nature. The important issue of whether a pleomorphic adenoma can best be managed by total superficial parotidectomy or by partial superficial parotidectomy cannot be answered with our present state of knowledge. Many of the tumours of the salivary glands are rare and their behaviour is not yet known for certain. Although surgery in good hands offers the best chance for cure, and even in high-grade tumours a good chance of tumour control at the primary site, we are faced with the difficulties posed by management of the facial nerve and by the fact that the alternative therapeutic modalities of radiotherapy and chemotherapy do not offer a radical treatment alternative. Currently there is no firm evidence that radiotherapy is satisfactory as the primary treatment of any salivary gland tumour other than lymphoma. However, individual high-grade tumours, as already indicated, are partially radiosensitive and radiotherapy should constitute part of a combined regimen of treatment.[23] Improved success rates have been claimed for neutron beam therapy,[24] though the small numbers of salivary gland tumours thus far treated and the period of follow-up being so short, there are no current results that reach statistical significance (see below).

Patients presenting with salivary gland tumours may present *de novo* with an undiagnosed and untreated salivary gland mass. As already discussed, such patients may present with clinically apparently benign tumours or alternatively clinically suspicious tumours with a history of rapid growth or local pain or, lastly, clinically malignant tumours where there is loss of facial nerve function and fixation to skin or other surrounding tissues. There are also patients who present for management, following previous surgical intervention, who require further management of a previously unsuspected malignancy. This group of complicated patients includes those cases referred after incomplete resection of the tumour, and, lastly, the unfortunate patient who presents with recurrence after surgical excision of either a benign or malignant salivary gland tumour.

The investigation of patients presenting with an undiagnosed salivary gland mass has already been discussed. We have found fine needle aspiration cytology biopsy to be the gold-standard investigation in patients presenting with a salivary gland lesion. Accurate diagnosis using fine needle aspiration cytology requires the support of a cytopathologist skilled and interested in the diagnosis of head and neck neoplasms in general, and salivary gland tumours in particular. However, over the past decade fine needle aspiration biopsies have become standard procedures with high degrees of sensitivity, as already stated.[25] We have already mentioned that the we do not routinely use CT or MRI scanning in straightforward clinically benign salivary gland tumours, although imaging of tumours of the submandibular and sublingual glands would be desirable if there is any hint of fixation. Imaging is reserved for those patients with a complicated presentation of either previous or incomplete surgery, damage to the facial nerve, or recurrent disease. Lastly, prior to considering the various treatment options in detail, it is worth considering the patient's age. Many patients presenting with salivary gland tumours are extremely elderly, and there is naturally a reluctance to offer surgical intervention to patients nearing the end of their natural span, i.e. greater than 75 years. Our practice is, in an elderly or frail patient, to routinely perform fine needle aspiration cytological examination; and if the lesion is benign, consider placing the patient on a regular follow-up basis. Naturally the patient must be fully informed about the potential for malignant change, typically in a pleomorphic adenoma. Our view is that this decision can best be made with full participation and with full information given to the patient.

There are at present no indications for the enucleation of any tumour of any salivary gland.[26] However, the indications for a limited excision are primarily for the treatment of small benign tumours typically found in the lower pole of the parotid gland or tumours of the minor salivary glands. As already mentioned. the pendulum has swung away from facial nerve resection in the vast majority of tumours of the parotid gland, and the commonly held view is that the facial nerve should be spared as far as possible.

The prime indications for postoperative radiotherapy for salivary gland tumours are in cases of known residual disease, recurrent malignant tumours, and as adjuvant therapy for high-grade and advanced stage malignancies.[27],[28] Radiotherapy is also indicated in tumours that are either inoperable or where resection is technically impossible, and the dosage in these situations is 70 Gy.[29]

Benign neoplasms of the salivary glands

Pleomorphic adenoma

This common tumour constitutes 90 per cent of benign tumours of the parotid gland and 50 per cent of benign tumours of the submandibular gland. It is an epithelial tumour composed of both epithelial and myoepithelial elements, and displays a wide variety of histopathological patterns. However, its most clinically important feature is the fact that it grows and develops by expansion and does not have a true capsule developing both macroscopic and microscopic bosselations. Salivary gland tissue surrounding the tumour becomes compressed as a result of pressure exerted by the enlarging tumour and together with the surface layer of fibrous tissue surrounding the tumour it forms a capsule. The presence of this apparent capsule has led surgeons in the past to attempt removal of the tumour by enucleation. The work of Patey and Thackray has demonstrated that at the junctional zone between the pleomorphic adenoma and its capsule, the tumour grows not only by uniform expansion but by repeated localized infiltration through the pseudocapsule.[26] During enucleation procedures these extra-capsular extensions may be broken off from the main bulk of the tumour accounting for recurrence and the tendency for recurrent pleomorphic adenoma to be multiple.[26] Pleomorphic adenomas grow by expansion rather than by invasion, and this accounts for their lack of fixation to the surrounding tissues. They do, however, distort and displace the facial nerve considerably at times and the we have dealt with deep lobe tumours that by expanding laterally have so compressed overlying parotid tissue that the facial nerve is separated from the skin by only a few millimetres of compressed salivary tissue. This variability of the position of the facial nerve in large pleomorphic adenoma greatly increases the importance of formal dissection and recognition of the facial nerve as the main starting point of any form of parotidectomy. Where the tumour can be found to splay or distort the facial nerve, as has been described, it is invariably possible to dissect the involved branches of the facial nerve cleanly and safely from a pleomorphic adenoma. However, any attempt to enucleate the tumour without a cuff of normal parotid tissue results in unacceptable recurrence rates of up to 40 per cent.[30] Tumours arising in the deep lobe of the parotid gland pass between the stylohyoid membrane and the posterior edge of the mandibular ramus into the parapharyngeal space. By displacing the medial pterygoid they push into the lateral wall of the oropharynx. Recurrence may be less common with these tumours due to the acquisition of a more substantial capsule and this does allow true enucleation of benign tumours involving the deep lobe and parapharyngeal space. Management of pleomorphic adenoma necessitates superficial parotidectomy in the majority of cases, and in those rare cases involving the deep lobe a total parotidectomy with facial nerve preservation is necessary.

Radiotherapy for pleomorphic adenoma

The prime modality for these tumours is surgery in view of the patient's age, benign pathological behaviour, the remote possibility of developing a radiation-induced malignancy, and the other complications of radiotherapy. Definite indications for postoperative irradiation include:[31]

1. Deep lobe tumours which compromise the resection margin sharing the facial nerve.
2. Two or more benign recurrences.
3. Lesions greater than 5 cm in size.
4. Microscopically positive margins.
5. Malignant transformation of a benign tumour.
6. Significant tumour spillage.

Radiotherapy should include the entire parotid bed and it is usually necessary to include the subdigastric or retroparotid lymphatic bed. A dosage of 50 to 60 Gy is usually adequate to gain tumour control. The cumulative risk of recurrence following surgery and radiotherapy for tumours of the parotid gland is 8 per cent at 20 years.[32]

Monomorphic adenoma

The majority of these tumours are adenolymphomas or oxyphilic adenomas. They occur much less frequently than pleomorphic adenomas and characteristically arise in the superficial and peripheral aspects of the parotid gland. The lesions are frequently cystic and fluctuent.

Adenolymphoma—Warthin's tumour

Warthin's tumour represents 6 to 10 per cent of all parotid gland tumours, second in frequency only to pleomorphic adenoma. It occurs most frequently in the lower pole of the gland, proximate to the angle of the mandible. Because of its superficial position within the parotid gland, it infrequently comes into contact with the facial nerve, and if this conjunction does occur it is usually with the lower branches of the cervicofacial trunk. The tumours arise from ductal epithelial elements incorporated in lymphoid tissue outside of and

Table 2 Relative frequencies and sites of occurrence of salivary gland tumours. (Data from Eveson and Cawson.[33])

Tumour type	Parotid	Submandibular	Sublingual	Minor
Benign				
Pleomorphic adenoma	63.3	59.5	0.0	42.9
Adenolymphoma	14.0	0.8	0.0	0.0
Oxyphil adenoma	0.9	0.4	0.0	0.0
Other monomorphics	7.1	1.9	14.2	11.0
Malignant				
Mucoepidermoid carcinoma	1.5	1.6	0.0	8.9
Acinic cell tumour	2.5	0.4	0.0	1.8
Adenoid cystic carcinoma	2.0	16.8	28.6	13.1
Adenocarcinoma	2.6	5.0	14.2	12.2
Epidermoid carcinoma	1.1	1.9	0.0	1.2
Undifferentiated carcinoma		1.8	3.9	14.2
Carcinoma ex pleomorphic adenoma	3.2	7.8	28.6	7.1
Total number of cases	1756	257	7	336

within the parotid capsule. The lesions are well defined, soft, or fluctuent and are frequently cystic with a compressible texture. The combination of lymphoid tissue in a cystic space increases the tumour's susceptibility to inflammation which can result clinically in rapid growth or fluctuation in size and local pain and discomfort. However, it is rare for the cystic component of the tumour to form an abscess. Warthin's tumours are also frequently associated with a second tumour and the most frequent combination appears to be a Warthin's tumour associated with a pleomorphic adenoma. Such occurrences may involve the ipsilateral or contralateral gland and may be synchronous. These tumours are satisfactorily managed surgically with a partial lateral lobectomy after appropriate dissection and display of the relevant branches of the facial nerve. Recurrence of the tumour is extremely rare and malignant transformation has been reported only in patients subjected to previous irradiation to the neck.

Oxyphilic adenoma

Oxyphilic adenomas are rare benign tumours composed of large epithelial cells. They account for 1 per cent of all salivary gland lesions, and occur late in life with an almost equal sex distribution. They usually arise in the parotid gland and tend to be multifocal. The presence of bilateral tumours has been reported. Surgical excision via a superficial parotidectomy is the treatment of choice, bearing in mind the multifocal origin of these tumours.

Malignant tumours of the salivary glands

Table 2 gives a breakdown for comparison purposes of the relative frequencies and sites of occurrence.

Mucoepidermoid carcinoma

Mucoepidermoid carcinomas constitute 9 per cent of all salivary gland tumours.[12] Ninety per cent of the tumours are found in the parotid gland, with 8 per cent occurring the submandibular gland, and 1 per cent in the sublingual gland. Mucoepidermoid carcinoma constitutes the most common salivary gland tumour in children. The sex incidence is equal and the tumour usually presents in the fifth decade. A distinctive microscopic feature of this tumour, as the name implies, is the presence of both mucus and epidermoid cells and commonly multiple microcysts. The tumour may be divided into low-grade and high-grade categories on the basis of histological appearance and clinical behaviour. The majority (80 per cent) of the tumours are low grade. These tumours tend to have abundant mucus cells and mucin production, and although they can occasionally show invasive and metastatic potential, their predominant behaviour pattern is of gradual local growth within the affected gland; their behaviour and prognosis is similar to that of pleomorphic adenoma. In the series of Seifert et al. none of the well-differentiated mucoepidermoid carcinomas metastasized, whereas 50 per cent of the poorly differentiated tumours metastasized to regional lymph nodes.[12] Further attempts at histopathological classification have been undertaken by Batsakis and Luna who suggested grading mucoepidermoid carcinoma into three grades;[34] and although low grade or grade 1 and high grade or grade 3 behave in the manner already discussed, the behaviour of intermediate grade 2 tumours cannot be correlated with outcome. Tumours that may be expected to have a poor prognosis are those which are predominantly solid and have a preponderance of epidermoid cells. The data of Seifert et al. suggest that 5-year survival for high-grade mucoepidermoid carcinoma is only 40 per cent, whereas 5-year survival for low-grade tumours is approximately 85 per cent.[12]

Management of low-grade mucoepidermoid carcinoma is via a complete superficial parotidectomy where the tumour is localized lateral to the facial nerve. A more extensive low-grade tumour would require a total conservative parotidectomy with facial nerve preservation where possible. In high-grade tumours, radical parotidectomy with sacrifice of the facial nerve plus supraomohyoid or full functional neck dissection is required. Mucoepidermoid carcinomas do manifest a degree of radio-sensitivity and radiotherapy should form part of the management of malignant high-grade tumours with radical postoperative radiotherapy being administered to the parotid field and ipsilateral neck. It is also important to note that high-grade tumours may metastasize to the lungs, skeletal system, and brain. Patients may survive for long periods with pulmonary metastasis and the presence of metastases should not inhibit attempts at local control of the tumour.

The overall recurrence rate for all grades and all treatment modalities is 35 per cent, but within the high-grade group the recurrence rate approaches 75 per cent.[35] The majority of tumours recur locally within the first year following treatment.[35]

Metastases commonly arise from tumours within the submandibular gland. Distant metastases are uncommon but do include lung, skeleton, and brain. Interestingly, better survival is seen in young female patients.[35] Five-year survival rates have little relevance in this tumour and consideration must be given to the 15-year survival of both intermediate and high-grade tumours, which is in the region of 33 per cent.

Acinic cell carcinoma

This tumour accounts for around 2 per cent of all salivary gland lesions and most commonly affects the parotid gland. It is rarely bilateral and is more often found in females. The mean age of occurrence is 45 years. These tumours are divided into high- and low-grade lesions, with the low grade having a variety of solid, papillary, and microcystic forms. The high-grade tumours are usually well differentiated and little indication is given as to how they will behave clinically. The only histological factors that appear to give an indication of occurrence of the potential to metastasize were given by Ellis and Corio when they described multinodularity, stromal hyalinization, and widespread mitotic activity as frequently seen in clinically aggressive lesions.[36]

Optimal management of this tumour is via total conservative parotidectomy with preservation of the uninvolved facial nerve. If the final histological report indicates a poorly differentiated and potentially aggressive lesion then surgery should be followed by postoperative radiotherapy treatment to the surgical field and ipsilateral neck.

Adenoid cystic carcinoma

This tumour arises very frequently in the minor salivary glands in addition to fair representation in the major glands. Twenty-five per cent occur in the parotid gland, 15 per cent in the submandibular gland, and the remainder (60 per cent) occur in the minor salivary glands. Many of these minor salivary gland tumours arise in the mouth; the area of the hard and soft palate constituting a particularly likely site for this interesting and perplexing tumour. The major feature of adenoid cystic carcinoma is its marked tendency to perineural spread, accounting for the association of local and referred pain in the area of the primary tumour. Adenoid cystic carcinomas also invade bone by direct extension, although there may be little radiological evidence of osteolysis in such cases. Lymph node involvement is often by direct extension and only 15 per cent of adenoid cystic carcinomas metastasize to lymph nodes. However, the tumour is distinguished by its tendency to distant metastasis, often after several local recurrences at the primary site. Metastases involve lungs, brain, and the skeletal system. Single-site distant metastases are compatible with prolonged survival, and it may be worth treating the metastasis aggressively if there is evidence of control at the primary site. Microscopically the tumour may be distinguished by cribriform-hyaline, tubular, and solid (basaloid) types. Attempts to correlate the histology with prognosis have indicated that the solid or basaloid tumours correlate with increased incidence of lymph node metastasis, i.e. 33 per cent of cases with solid tumour types versus 4 per cent of cases with cribriform tumours,[12] and that ultimately median survival was shorter in those patients with solid type histology and increasing T stage.[37]

Management of adenoid cystic carcinomas presents a particular challenge for surgeons and oncologists. The propensity of the tumour to invade bone and to spread perineurally means that the tumour has often extended well beyond its macroscopic boundaries. It is generally agreed that radiotherapy improves local control, and although response of adenoid cystic carcinoma to radiotherapy can be idiosyncratic, every patient with this tumour should be considered for combination therapy. Where appropriate, initial surgical treatment would include radical resection of the affected gland with sacrifice of the facial nerve with immediate cable grafting. Resection of surrounding tissues may be required, according to the results of the frozen section, including resection of the mandible, mastoid process, and lateral temporal bone with the contents of the infratemporal fossa. This procedure should be accompanied by a supraomohyoid neck dissection extended to a full functional neck dissection if lymph nodes are found to be involved on frozen section. Surgery should be followed at an appropriate interval by radical radiotherapy to the primary site and neck. Patients with more extensive disease pose a particular dilemma. It is far from certain that any excision, however wide, would actually produce a tumour-free margin and scarcely justify the extensive functional and cosmetic defects that would result. Such cases may be best managed by limitation of their treatment to a radical parotidectomy with facial nerve resection and cable grafting followed by postoperative radiotherapy. Finally, it is important to realize that patients with adenoid cystic carcinoma must be followed up for life. Survival is progressively reduced by recurrence of the disease and ultimately by metastasis. The 5-year survival rate is quoted at 68 per cent, with 10-year survival of 43 per cent, reducing at 15 years to 26 per cent.[23] Follow-up is for life.

Squamous cell carcinoma

Primary squamous carcinoma of the parotid gland is rare and usually occurs in elderly men.[38] There is a range of differentiation from well to poorly differentiated tumours. Aggressive, infiltrative invasion of surrounding tissues is typical. These tumours have a poor prognosis as they tend to spread rapidly by local infiltration.

The 5-year survival rate is 40 per cent. Careful preoperative assessment is mandatory, with MRI scanning to include the neck, as lymph node metastases are frequent. The possibility of the lesion being a secondary deposit from a primary site in the head and neck must always be considered, and we would recommend a positron emission tomography scan when there is any doubt. Treatment is by radical parotidectomy, appropriate neck dissection, and postoperative radiotherapy to the primary site and ipsilateral neck.

Carcinoma arising in a pleomorphic adenoma (carcinoma ex pleomorphic adenoma)

There is convincing evidence that carcinoma can arise from a long-standing pleomorphic adenoma, and this is one of the most common types of carcinoma of the salivary glands (20 per cent).[12],[39] Clinically, suspicion is raised when a long-standing lesion becomes symptomatic, typically undergoing a sudden increase in size accompanied by local pain. The relative risk of this tumour undergoing malignant change rises from 1.5 per cent at 5 years to 10 per cent at 15 years.[39] The biological behaviour of these tumours is more aggressive than for carcinoma arising *de novo*, with infiltration at the periphery of the tumour, a relatively high incidence of lymph node metastasis (25 per cent), and an incidence of distant metastasis of 30 per cent. Although the prognosis in carcinoma ex pleomorphic adenoma is poor, with a quoted 5-year survival rate of only 25 per cent,[12] treatment should include radical parotidectomy with supraomohyoid neck dissection extended to full neck dissection in the presence of involved lymph nodes.

Salivary gland lymphoma

The parotid gland contains 20 to 30 follicles and lymph nodes with a rich network of interconnecting lymph vessels. Periparotid lymph nodes are found on the external surface of the gland and are numerous in the pretragal and supratragal areas. The intraglandular and periglandular nodes are in free communication with and drain into the upper cervical deep lymph node chain. The submandibular chain has a broadly similar structure with six to eight periglandular lymph nodes in the submandibular triangle. Any of these focal areas of lymphatic tissue may be involved in primary lymphoma. They may also be the site of metastatic tumour spread from surrounding structures and malignant melanomas and squamous cell carcinomas dominate the tumour types.

An interesting association in the development of lymphoma in relation to salivary gland disease is the association of Sjögren's syndrome, particularly those cases with xerostomia and kerato-conjunctivitis sicca, known as the 'sicca syndrome', occurring in the absence of any associated collagen disease. These appear to have lymphoid and immunological hyperactivity predisposing to the development of lymphoma. These patients either develop localized lymphoma in the affected salivary glands or in the cervical lymph nodes or may present with a generalized lymphadenopathy.[40]

Lymphomas of the salivary glands are classified as either low or high grade. The low-grade tumours include MALT lymphoma (mucosa-associated lymphoid tissue), and prognosis is usually good.[41] Treatment of stage I and II disease is by surgery or radiotherapy. Rarely, a localized low-grade lymphoma of the parotid gland may be treated by surgery alone. Regular follow-up is mandatory in these cases. Advanced stage III and IV disease with low-grade lymphomas (70 per cent of cases) will require a chemotherapeutic approach with radiotherapy for locally symptomatic disease. Doses of 30 to 40 Gy over 4 to 5 weeks are required to treat the primary tumour site.

High-grade tumours of whatever stage always require chemotherapy. Adjuvant radiotherapy, i.e. 40 to 50 Gy, would be added to control localized bulky disease.

Surgery of the parotid gland

There has been considerable confusion in the literature as to what constitutes a parotidectomy, and much confusion over the terminology used for operations on the parotid gland. In principle there are five named operations:

1. Enucleation: implies the removal of the parotid tumour by capsular dissection without exposure of the facial nerve. This is an unacceptable option due to the fact that few tumours have a true capsule and microscopic deposits of tumour may be left behind. (See the section on pleomorphic adenoma.)

2. Partial lateral lobectomy: following identification of the facial nerve trunk and its relevant branches, the tumour is excised with a cuff of normal parotid tissue. A portion of uninvolved and apparently normal parotid is left behind.

3. Superficial parotidectomy: this is removal of all parotid tissue lying lateral to the facial nerve encompassing the tumour.

4. Total conservative parotidectomy: removal of all parotid tissue both superficial and deep to the facial nerve with conservation of the nerve.

5. Radical parotidectomy: complete excision of the parotid gland with facial nerve and any surrounding, involved structures, i.e. mandible, petrous bone.

The terminology is confusing and in part deficient. A partial lateral parotidectomy which is usually performed for benign tumours may often include part of the deep lobe. Furthermore, the tumour may 'bow string' a branch of the facial nerve, which implies that the surgeon has to perform an extra-capsular dissection in order to preserve the nerve. However, it is vitally important to be clear about the various procedures and to record as precisely as possible the procedure undertaken.

Management of tumours of the salivary glands

General issues

The management of low- and intermediate-grade tumours

A summary of tumours in this group was given earlier in Table 2. The management of all low- and intermediate-grade tumours should be surgically conservative. The choice of operation depends on the location of the tumour, and a definitive preoperative diagnosis is useful in planning surgery and in counselling patients.

In the majority of cases these tumours are best treated by either a partial lateral lobectomy or a superficial parotidectomy. Partial lateral lobectomy is reserved for small tumours where it is possible to remove the lesion with a cuff of normal tissue, and leave a significant portion of the gland and related facial nerve undisturbed, i.e. Warthin's tumour.

Superficial parotidectomy is performed when the disease is completely, or almost completely, lateral to the facial nerve. This operation may also be performed in order to clearly identify the facial nerve when there are tumours arising either in the overlying skin or the external auditory meatus, and which require wide excision or where the facial nerve is deemed to be at risk.

Total conservative parotidectomy is only indicated if the tumour involves both lobes or arises within the deep lobe of the parotid gland and expands into the parapharyngeal space. In treating deep lobe tumours, the superficial lobe must be resected in order to provide adequate visualization of the facial nerve and exposure of the deep lobe. If the tumour is large and access difficult, then anterior dislocation of the mandible at the temporomandibular joint improves surgical access, and permits excision of the tumour.

Tumour spillage, which may occur whilst removing a pleomorphic adenoma from the region of a branch of the facial nerve, is best treated at the time of surgery by irrigation with normal saline of the tissues directly involved and the surrounding region. If, in the surgeon's opinion, tumour spillage has been significant, then radiotherapy in the early postoperative period must be considered. Factors that influence this decision are the patient's age, sex, and the extent of wound contamination.

The facial nerve should be preserved as far as possible in tumours in these categories even if the tumour has to be dissected directly off the facial nerve.[23]

Recurrent tumours of low and intermediate grades

The management of recurrent low-grade tumours of the parotid gland is by surgical excision as far as is technically possible. However, recurrent tumour, as in pleomorphic adenoma, most commonly presents with multiple areas of recurrence due to seeding of the tumour in the surgical field and skin. It is then necessary to perform a total conservative parotidectomy, and in this situation a repeat dissection of the facial nerve can be extremely difficult and testing and the surgery may well be followed by a facial nerve deficit. It is, however, necessary to resect the area of recurrence *in toto* together with the affected overlying skin. Closure of the surgical defect can often be effected primarily but may on occasion require a cervical rotation flap.

Wherever possible, it is essential to maintain the integrity of the facial nerve when operating for recurrent benign disease. However, when the nerve has previously been properly dissected it is more liable to be involved with scar formation or encapsulation by tumour, and damage to part or all of the nerve is possible. The significant risk of damage to the facial nerve can be reduced somewhat with the use of facial nerve monitoring in these difficult recurrent cases. Our practice is routinely to approach the trunk of the facial nerve in the classical manner, but all too often this area is heavily involved with scar tissue and recurrent tumour. In these instances identification of the peripheral branches of the facial nerve with retrograde dissection provides the optimal technique and reduces the potential for inadvertent facial nerve trunk damage. The incidence of facial nerve deficit in surgery for recurrent disease is 28 per cent.[42] Therefore, both surgeon and patient should be prepared for this outcome, and the real possibility of the patient requiring a cable graft or other reanimation procedure.

In general, recurrence of these tumour types is best treated by a total conservative parotidectomy as far as is technically possible. Postoperative radiotherapy should be considered in all patients if it has not been employed in primary treatment.

The management of high-grade tumours

High-grade tumours with their propensity for local recurrence and metastasis over a period of years are optimally treated by a combination of radical surgery with postoperative radiotherapy. High-grade tumours may be divided into two groups. Firstly, the unsuspected high-grade malignancy in which conventional partial parotidectomy has been undertaken, but paraffin sections reveal a high-grade malignancy. Although such cases will require reoperation with completion to total parotidectomy, there is an increasing tendency to be as conservative as possible with the facial nerve. Firstly, the deficit that results from facial nerve sacrifice is considerable with significant functional and cosmetic deformity. If there is an adequate description of the intraoperative findings in relation to the facial nerve and tumour, at the previously performed surgery, then it is reasonable to perform a total parotidectomy preserving any uninvolved portion of the facial nerve, relying on postoperative radiotherapy to supplement tumour control at the primary site. In more advanced presentations where there is preoperative evidence of facial nerve involvement, in the presence of a high-grade tumour, radical parotidectomy with facial nerve resection should be undertaken. Radical resection with frozen section control in these cases may necessitate extending the procedure with removal of the posterior third of the mandible and related musculature, and possibly including partial resection of the petrous temporal bone. A supraomohyoid neck dissection should be undertaken, and if there is frozen section evidence of positive nodes then completion to a radical neck dissection should be performed. Reconstruction in these advanced cases necessitates an immediate reanimation procedure, with facial nerve grafting, ideally using a donor Sural nerve graft. Reconstruction of the defect at the primary site may require a myocutaneous flap. Reconstruction of the deficit in patients severely compromised by the radical surgery described requires a team approach with involvement of plastic and reconstructive surgeons who will support the efforts of the oncological surgical team whose primary role is to secure as wide a tumour clearance as possible. The total facial palsy resulting from radical excisional surgery results in ectropion with the potential for corneal ulceration. A lateral tarsorrhaphy or gold weight implant into the upper eyelid at the time of surgery should be undertaken to protect the cornea.

After a suitable interval to allow wound healing, radical external beam radiotherapy should be undertaken, as discussed later in the section on radiotherapy of salivary tumours.

Submandibular gland tumours

The presence of a mass in the submandibular gland or increasing enlargement of the gland necessitates surgical removal of the gland for therapeutic and diagnostic reasons. Preoperative investigations should include fine needle aspiration cytology and, in the submandibular gland in particular, imaging with CT and MRI scanning may be useful in defining tumour involvement of extraglandular tissues. Management of malignant submandibular gland tumours should include combination surgery and radiotherapy with appropriate ipsilateral neck dissection. The lymph nodes of the submandibular gland drain into the submental triangle, and the accompanying neck dissection should be extended anteriorly to include the submental triangle nodes. Radical surgery will involve clearance of the submandibular triangle, possibly including the mandibular branch of the facial nerve, but the underlying lingual and hypoglossal nerves may require sacrifice with the underlying hyoglossus muscle. Wound closure can usually be obtained primarily, but may require a cervical rotation flap or myocutaneous flap.

Chemotherapy

The efficacy of chemotherapy in the treatment of lymphomas arising in salivary glands is proven and has already been discussed. However, considerable uncertainty remains with respect to the known effectiveness of chemotherapeutic agents in primary epithelial salivary gland tumours. There is very little evidence to suggest that combination chemotherapy can be effective in high-grade tumours such as mucepidermoid, adenoid cystic, and undifferentiated carcinoma. The most widely favoured drugs used in combinations have included cisplatinum, 5-fluorouracil, and doxorubicin. However, there are few prospective trials of chemotherapy in salivary gland tumours and most studies have involved patients who have already undergone primary treatment with surgery, radiotherapy, or combinations of these modalities. Jones *et al.* recently published results of a randomized phase II trial of epirubicin and 5-fluorouracil versus cisplatinum in recurrent, malignant salivary gland tumours.[43] The authors reported a single partial response in the cisplatinum group, and concluded that chemotherapy using these favoured agents had no place in the treatment of advanced malignant salivary gland tumours.

Spiro *et al.* have suggested that the only role for chemotherapy in salivary gland tumours is in the palliation of patients with unresectable tumours.[44]

Radiotherapy

Radiation therapy techniques

The most frequently employed radiotherapy approach utilizes unilateral homolateral fields over about 7 weeks and Gy per fraction; 25–12–18 MeV with 12 to 16 MeV electrons, either alone or in combination with photons.[32] The generally accepted ratio consists of about two-thirds electrons and one-third photons. This ratio may vary depending on the individual patient, patient anatomy, and depth of the target volume. The rationale for this combination is to partially spare the upper orodigestive tract (thus reducing a huge mucositis) and opposite salivary glands (to reduce the incidence of postirradiation sarcoma). An alternative technique uses just photons (cobalt-60; 4 to 6 MV), with oblique AP-PA wedged beams. This technique may be preferred when the target volume includes the inframaxillary and upper posterior cervical nodes.

Patients with minimal disease following surgery should be treated with 50 to 60 Gy over 5 to 6 weeks utilizing 2 Gy per fraction. The entire surgical bed must be included in the irradiated volume. The volume is also determined by the pathological findings such as perineural invasion of a major nerve, and its pathway should be included in the target volume. In irradiating parotid tumours it is important to include ipsilateral subdigastric nodal areas, as the inferior pole of the parotid lies within this region. The ipsilateral neck should be treated following a neck dissection, and should be electively treated in patients with recurrent or high-grade tumours over 5 weeks. The standard dose for such treatments is 50 Gy over 5 weeks. The underlying spinal cord must be spared by using tangential fields which also avoid high-dose radiation to the contralateral parotid gland. Low-grade lesions do not require elective neck radiation. Treatment of the submandibular gland is similar, except that when the tumour extends towards the midline, lateral fields may be required. Treatment dosage ranges from 50 Gy for microscopic residual disease up to 65 Gy for high-grade malignancy or advanced disease.

A CT scan following surgery is essential to customize the target volume. Three-dimensional reconstruction-based treatment planning is useful in controlling dose distribution and ensuring homogeneity within the planned target volume, and to control steep fall-off of the dose distribution in critical organs.

Acute side effects and late complications of radiotherapy

Partial xerostomia is not infrequently seen following treatment of salivary gland tumours with radiotherapy, and may be permanent. A laterized acute mucositis usually occurs from the third week of radiotherapy and intensifies up until the week following the end of treatment. A normal appearance is recovered within 3 to 5 weeks of treatment. Trismus is unusual, and occurs due to fibrosis of the temporomandibular joint or of the masseteric muscles. Whenever possible, the target volume should exclude the temperomandibular joint after 50 Gy. Necrosis of the oropharyngeal mucosa should no longer be seen with appropriate data management and dose distribution.

Ear complications are rare, the most common being otitis media with effusion. Osteoradionecrosis of the temporal bone is unusual and may occur after a delay of many years.

References

1. **Leegard T, Lindeman H.** Salivary gland tumours. Clinical picture and treatment. *Acta Otolaryngologica*, 1970; **263**: 155–9.
2. **Eneroth CM.** Salivary gland tumours in the parotid gland, submandibular gland and the palate region. *Cancer*, 1971; **27**: 1415–27.
3. **Spiro RH, Spiro JD.** Cancer of the salivary glands. In: *Cancer of the head and neck.* 645.
4. **Spiro RH.** Salivary neoplasms: Overview of a 35 year experience with 2,807 patients. *Head and Neck Surgery*, 1986; **8**: 177–85.
5. **Jones AS, Beasley NJ, Houghton DJ, Helliwell TR, Husband DJ.** Tumours of the minor salivary glands. *Clinical Otolaryngology*, 1998; **23**: 27–33.
6. **Belsy JL, Tachikawa K, Chihak RW, Yamamato T.** Salivary gland tumours in atomic bomb survivors. Hiroshima–Nagasaki. 1957–1970. *Journal of the American Medical Association*, 1972; **2/9**: 804–68.
7. **Deguch H, Hamano H, Hayashi, Y.** C-Myc, ras p 21 and p53 expression in pleomorphic adenoma, and is malignant form, of the human salivary glands. *Acta Pathologica*, 1993; **43**: 413–22.
8. **Berg JW, Hutter RVP, Foote FWJ.** The unique association between salivary gland cancer and breast cancer. *Journal of the American Medical Association*, 1968; **204**: 771–7.
9. **Batsakis JG.** *Tumours of the head and neck* (2nd edn). Baltimore: Williams and Wilkins, 1982: 64–194.
10. **Cawson RA, Gleeson MJ, Eveson JW.** British Salivary Gland Tumour Panel data apnoea quoted in 'Pathology and surgery of the salivary glands'. *Isis Medical*, 1997, 117–18.
11. **Walsh BT, Croft CB.** Salivary gland enlargement in anorexia nervosa. *International Journal of Psychiatric Medicine*, 1981; **11**: 255–7.
12. **Seifert G, Miehlke A, Haubrich J, Chilla R.** *Diseases of the salivary glands.* Stuttgart: Georg Thieme, 1986.
13. **Armstrong JG, Harrison LB, Thaler HT,** *et al.* The indications for the elective treatment of the neck in cancer of the major salivary glands. *Cancer*, 1992; **69**: 615–19.
14. **Chaudhuri R, Bingham JB, Grossman JE, Gleeson MJ.** Magnetic resonance imaging of the parotid gland using the STIR sequence. *Clinical Otolaryngology*, 1992; **17**: 211–17.
15. **McGurck M, Hussain K.** Role of fine needle aspiration cytology in the

management of the discrete parotid lump (review). *Annals of the Royal College of Surgeons of England*, 1997; **79**: 198–202.

16. Kocjan G, Nayagam M, Harris M. Fine needle aspiration cytology of salivary gland lesions: advantages and pitfalls. *Cytopathology*, 1990, **1**: 269–75.

17. Young JA, Smallman LA, Thompson H, Proops DW, Johnson AP. Fine needle aspiration cytology of salivary gland lesions. *Cytopathology*, 1990, **1**: 25–33.

18. Shaha AR, Webber C, DiMaio T, Jaffe BM. Needle aspiration biopsy in salivary gland lesions. *American Journal of Surgery*, 1990; **160**: 373–6.

19. Batsakis JG, Sneige N, El-Naggar AK. Fine needle aspiration biopsy of salivary glands. *Laryngoscope*, 1991; **101**: 245–9.

20. Orell SR. Diagnostic difficulties in the interpretation of fine needle aspirates of salivary gland lesions: the problem revisited. *Cytopathology*, 1995; **6**: 285–300.

21. Seifert G, Sobin LH. The World Health Organization's histological classification of salivary gland tumours. *Cancer*, 1992; **70**: 379–85.

22. Beahrs OH, Henson DE, Hutter RVP, Kennedy BJ (ed.). *American Joint Committee of Cancer: manual for staging of cancer* (4th edn). Philadephia: Lippincott, 1992: 49.

23. Wyatt MG, Coleman N, Eveson JW, Webb AJ. Management of high grade parotid carcinomas. *British Journal of Surgery*, 1989; **76**: 1275–7.

24. Duncan W, Orr JA, Arnott SJ, Jack WJ. Neutron therapy for malignant tumours of the salivary glands. A report of the Edinburgh experience. *Radiotherapy Oncology*, 1987; **8**: 99–104.

25. Frable MAS, Frable WJ. Fine needle aspiration biopsy of salivary glands. *Laryngoscope*, 1991; **101**: 245–9.

26. Patey DH, Thackray AC. The treatment of parotid tumours in the light of pathological study of parotidectomy material. *British Journal of Surgery*, 1958; **45**: 477–87.

27. Matsuba HM, Thawley SE, Devineni VR, *et al.* High grade malignancies of parotid gland: Effective use of planned combined surgery and irradiation. *Laryngoscope*, 1985; **95**: 1059.

28. Sykes AJ, Logue JP, Slevin NJ, Gupta NK. An analysis of radiotherapy management of 104 patients with parotid carcinoma. *Clinical Oncology*, 1995; **7**: 16–20.

29. Borthne A, Kjellevold K, Kaalhus O, *et al.* Salivary gland malignant neoplasms: Treatment and prognosis. *International Journal of Radiation Oncology, Biology and Physics*, 1986; **12**: 747–54.

30. Donovan DT, Conley JJ. Capsular significance in parotid tumour

surgery: reality and myths of lateral lobectomy. *Laryngoscope*, 1984; **94**: 324–9.

31. Liu F-F, Rotstein L, Davison AJ, *et al.* Benign parotid adenomas: A review of the Princess Margaret Hospital experience. *Head and Neck Journal*, 1995; **17**: 177–83.

32. Soni SC, Kahn FR, Paul JM, *et al.* Electron beam treatment of malignant tumours of salivary glands. *Journal of Radiology*, 1997; **48**: 677.

33. Eveson JW, Cawson RA. British Salivary Gland Tumour Panel data, 1985

34. Batsakis JG, Luna MA. Histological grading of salivary gland neoplasms: Mucoepidermoid carcinoma. *Annals of Otolaryngology*, 1990, **99**: 835–8.

35. Kane MJ, McCaffrey TV, Olsen KD, Lewis JE. Primary parotid malignancies—a clinical and pathologic review. *Archives of Otolaryngology and Head and Neck Surgery*, 1991; **117**: 307–15.

36. Ellis GL, Corio RL. Acinic cell adenocarcinoma: A clinicopathologic analysis of 294 cases. *Cancer*, 1983; **52**: 542–9.

37. Hamper K, Lazal F, Diteal M, *et al.* Prognostic factors for adenoid cystic carcinomas of the head and neck, a retrospective evaluation of 96 cases. *Journal of Oral Pathology and Medicine*, 1990; **19**: 101–7.

38. Ellis GL, Auclair PL, Gnepp DR. *Surgical pathology of the salivary glands*. Philadelphia: Saunders, 1991: ch. 19.

39. Eneroth CM, Blanck C, Jakobsson PA. Carcinoma in pleomorphic adenoma of the parotid gland. *Acta Otolaryngologica*, 1968; **66**: 477–92.

40. Sinn SS, Sheiban IK, Fishleder A, *et al.* Monocytoid B cell lymphoma in patients with Sjögrens syndrome: A clinicopatholgic study of 13 patients. *Human Pathology*, 1991; **22**: 422–30.

41. Chan JKC, Banks PM, Cleary ML, *et al.* A proposal for clarification of lymphoid neoplasms (by the International Lymphoma Study Group). 1994; **25**: 517–36.

42. Woods JE. The facial nerve in parotid malignancy. *American Journal of Surgery*, 1983; **146**: 493–6.

43. Jones AS, Phillips DE, Cook JA, Helliwell TR. A randomised phase II trial of Epirubicin and 5-Fluorouracil versus cis platinum in the palliation of advanced and recurrent malignant tumours of the salivary glands. *British Journal of Cancer*, 1994; **69**(1): 1182–3.

44. Spiro IJ, Wang CC, Montgomery MW. Carcinoma of the parotid gland. Analysis of treatment results and patterns of failure after combined surgery and radiation therapy. *Cancer*, 1993; **71**: 2699–705.

9.9 Temporal bone malignancies

Andrew S. Jones and Tristram H. J. Lesser

There is a diffuse group of malignant neoplasms that originate in or involve the temporal bone. They consist of primary tumours, together with local involvement of tumours from adjacent organs and tumours metastasizing to the area. The most common primary tumour is the squamous-cell carcinoma, accounting for some 80 to 90 per cent of cases (Fig. 1). Adenoid cystic carcinomas, adenocarcinomas, and sarcomas make up the majority of the rest. Local malignancies, such as parotid neoplasms (Fig. 2),[1] nasopharyngeal neoplasms, and intracranial malignancies may invade directly into the temporal bone. Distant metastases originate from sites such as the lung, breast (Fig. 3), kidney, prostate, and almost anywhere else in the body,[2] including the vagina.[3]

As well as the highly malignant tumours there is a group of locally invasive tumours which involve the temporal bone; for example, glomus jugulare chemodectomas, hydradinomas (ceruminomas), parotid tumours, and chondrosarcomas to name but a few. Benign neoplasms, including teratomas, choristomas, and cholesteatomas, also involve the temporal bone. These two groups of tumours, along with metastases and diseases such as tuberculosis and Wegener's disease, are part of the differential diagnosis of malignant tumours of the temporal bones. They are referred to below, but are not comprehensively covered. Malignancies such as rhabdomyosarcomas (the most common childhood sarcoma) are rare, but, although 7 per cent involve the temporal bone, they are similarly beyond the scope of this chapter.

Primary squamous-cell carcinoma of the temporal bone has an incidence of between 0.9 and 2.0 per million of the population per year, and a female to male ratio of 1.2:1.[4] However, this generally quoted incidence is based on very small numbers. The incidence of all tumours affecting the external auditory canal, middle ear, mastoid, and temporal bone is much higher at six per million.

Squamous-cell carcinoma is a disease of adulthood, with a peak age of presentation between 65 and 75 years.[4],[5] The aetiology is unknown in most cases, but the most frequently cited factor is chronic inflammation.[4] As many as 85 per cent of all patients with middle-ear cancers have currently discharging ears, and many authorities consider that the carcinoma has much in common with Marjolin's

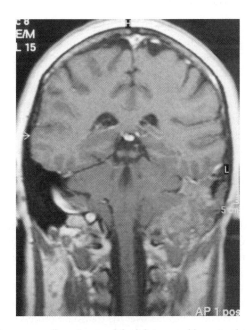

Fig. 1 Squamous-cell carcinoma of the left temporal bone involving dura.

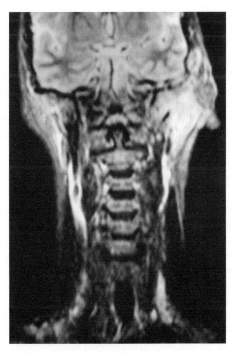

Fig. 2 Parotid carcinoma involving the temporal bone.

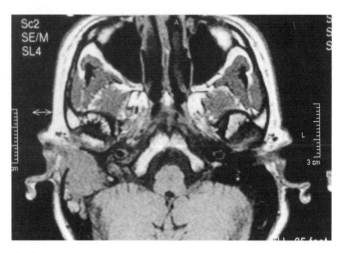

Fig. 3 Metastatic breast adenocarcinoma involving the right temporal bone.

ulcer.[6] The history may include previous mastoidectomy or radiation injury, either in the form of repeated treatment of otitis externa or the treatment of adjacent malignancies, such as parotid or nasopharyngeal tumours.[7]

In a series of 300 patients with radium poisoning, 8 developed carcinoma of the mastoid. The patients were either radium-dial painters or people who had received radium water or radium-like salts for therapeutic purposes.[7]

It has been suggested that indigenous microbial flora may produce carcinogens. For example, aflatoxin B is a highly potent carcinogen produced by *Aspergillus flavus*, which is a common contaminant of the ear canal and mastoid cavities. Cerumen itself may also contain carcinogens. In addition, the local use of chlorinated disinfectants may also be associated with the development of squamous-cell carcinoma in a mastoid cavity.

About one-third of middle-ear cancers occur simultaneously with cholesteatomas. Interestingly, squamous-cell carcinoma develops spontaneously in the ear canal and middle ear of ageing gerbils, and one dose of azoxymethane administered to a rat induces squamous carcinoma of the external auditory canal glands in 15 per cent of animals. In humans, human papillomavirus types 16 and 18 have been found in 80 per cent of a group of middle-ear carcinomas associated with chronic otitis media. To date, all reports suggest that chronic middle ear-disease is the most common aetiological factor.

Pathology

The distinction between tumours arising in the ear canal and middle ear is difficult but important. The prognosis for cancers of the two areas is different: some 50 per cent of patients with external auditory meatus tumours survive to 5 years, but this figure drops to only 25 per cent for those with middle-ear tumours.[5]

Small tumours (T1) of the ear canal or middle ear can easily be differentiated on examination. However, once the tumour has spread beyond the site of origin, especially if chronic infection or previous surgery has altered the anatomy, the differentiation between tumours of the middle ear and those of the external auditory canal is somewhat arbitrary and could just as well be considered a continuum.

The staging of these tumours was originally suggested by Lewis, altered by Stell[4] and then by Clark *et al.*,[8] and has since been updated by the Pittsburgh team[9] and validated in 1994.[10] There is, however, no internationally accepted staging. The most frequently used staging system[10] consists of a T stage for tumours, where T1 tumours are limited to the site of origin with no bone destruction and no evidence of soft tissue extension. T2 tumours have limited bony erosion, not full thickness, and radiographic evidence of soft tissue involvement of less than 0.5 cm. T3 tumours either erode the osseous external auditory canal throughout its full thickness, involving the middle ear and/or mastoid, or present with a facial paralysis. T4 tumours erode the cochlear, extend into the surrounding tissues by more than 0.5 cm, or involve the dura, base of the skull, parotid gland, temporomandibular joint, jugular foramen, or carotid canal. Nodal involvement automatically places the patient in an advanced stage of the disease.

When a tumour has spread beyond the temporal bone to involve the areas mentioned above, it appears that the 3-year survival rate is reduced from 80 per cent to 26 per cent and that a facial palsy converts a 50 per cent survival rate down to 25 per cent. The presence of neck nodes will convert a 65 per cent survival to 40 per cent at 3 years.[5]

In contrast, a previous mastoidectomy appears to confer some benefit; perhaps because, in many cases, the patient is kept under review and hence a tumour may be found earlier.[5]

Presentation of tumours

A chronic discharge, sometimes bloody, occurs in 70 per cent of patients. Pain occurs in 70 per cent and facial nerve palsy in approximately 50 per cent. Swelling around the ear, deafness, cranial nerve palsies, and nodal metastasis also cause patients to present.

Spread of tumours

Tumours originating in the ear canal, particularly in the cartilaginous portion, spread easily because the cartilaginous walls present little resistance to tumour spread. Spread tends to be either posteriorly into the postauricular sulcus or anteriorly into the parotid gland. As the cartilage of the external auditory canal may be regarded as an inward migration of the cartilage of the pinna, tumours spread readily into the concha. The bony portion of the canal is surrounded by dense bone, which provides an effective initial barrier to tumour spread; however, tumours tend to spread along the canal into the middle ear.

Once a tumour is in the middle ear there are several pathways readily available for its medial spread into the petrous apex. The oval and round windows are a theoretical, but uncommon, pathway; more importantly are tracks of cells leading above, below, and behind the labyrinth into the petrous apex. The tumour can therefore gain access to the petrous pyramid lying medially to the mastoid genu of the internal carotid artery.

The lower cranial nerves are not infrequently involved in cancer of the middle ear—in some cases because the tumour has metastasized to Rouvière's node, which lies over the transverse process of the atlas in the lateral compartment of the parapharyngeal space, or possibly by direct extension into the jugular bulb causing the jugular foramen syndrome. The Eustachian tube may act as a conduit and thereby compromise the carotid artery canal, and the tumour may also spread via the mastoid air cells into the internal auditory meatus. It is surprising how tumours may grow around the labyrinth leaving the otic capsule spared. Spread into the Eustachian tube bone will also lead to involvement of the trigeminal or ocular motor nerves in the lateral wall of the cavernous sinus. Lymphatic spread can occur in three directions: anteriorly to the parotid gland lymph nodes, and especially to the gland in front of the tragus; inferiorly to the lymph glands that lie along the external jugular vein and those under the sternocleidomastoid; and posteriorly to the mastoid lymph nodes.

Tumour types other than squamous-cell carcinomas

Tumours of the external auditory canal

Glandular tumours, basal-cell carcinoma, and rare entities such as sebaceous gland carcinoma, melanoma, syringocystadenomata papilliferum, myxomas (as part of Carney's syndrome), B-cell lymphoma, histiocytosis X, and amyloidosis are amongst the lesions occurring in the external ear canal.

The glandular tumours invading the ear canal may be benign, cause obstruction, but no pain, and require local excision. Those arising in the ceruminous glands are now called hydradinomas (see below). The ceruminous glands of the external auditory canal are typical apocrine sweat glands. These glands do not secrete wax, which is produced by the sebaceous glands, but a watery fluid devoid of lipids. The hydradinomas comprise four distinct types.

1. The ceruminous adenoma, which is a well-differentiated, but benign, localized glandular tumour with cystic and papillary variants.

2. Ceruminous adenocarcinoma is similar, but invasive, and has a wide histological spectrum of glandular adenoid tubular and adenoid cystic patterns; the basic pattern being one of an adenocarcinoma with two layered eosinophilic glands.

3. Adenoid cystic carcinoma is histologically the same as the tumour found in the salivary glands.

4. Pleomorphic adenoma appears as a nest of epithelial cells in a mixoid pseudocartilaginous stroma containing mucin, exactly as a salivary gland tumour.

The terms 'hydradinoma' and 'ceruminoma' are synonymous. However, hydradinoma is a better term because ceruminoma is a misnomer, the so-called ceruminous glands being modified sweat glands (see above).

Basal-cell carcinomas arise primarily in the external auditory meatus and are rare. More commonly, they are extensions of the tumours involving the pinna.

The incidence of sebaceous-cell carcinoma is extremely uncommon, with less than a 100 cases anywhere in the body having been described. Although the tumours can occur anywhere, they most frequently occur in the head and neck, mainly on the concha and the nose. There are said to be three types: sebaceous adenoma; basal-cell carcinoma; and true sebaceous carcinoma.

Middle-ear tumours

A long list of benign and non-squamous malignant tumours can affect this site. The malignant ones include: adenoid cystic carcinoma, adenocarcinoma, aggressive papillary middle-ear tumour (adenocarcinoma), sarcomas, osteogenic and chondrosarcomas, undifferentiated carcinomas, secondary carcinomas, and some rarer tumours such as verrucous carcinoma, plasmacytoma, leiomyosarcoma, and histiocytosis X.

The benign tumours include dermoid or congenital cholesteatomas, glomus tumours, choristomas, hamartomas, teratomas, middle-ear adenomas, carcinoid tumours, haemangiomas, pleomorphic adenomas, fibrous dysplasias, eosinophilic granulomas, schwannomas of the cranial nerves, and meningiomas to name but a few!

Choristoma

A choristoma is formed of normal tissue in an inappropriate site. They rarely occur in the middle ear and when they do they are usually salivary gland choristomas. The patients present with deafness and there are often other associated abnormalities of the middle ear. These abnormalities include absence of the stapes and an abnormal course of the facial nerve. The tumour itself can be left *in situ*, as attempts to remove it frequently put the facial nerve and other middle-ear structures at risk.

Adenoma

Benign adenomas of the middle ear occur equally between the sexes, with a maximum age incidence between 40 and 50 years. The usual symptom is unilateral progressive deafness, which is conductive. The external canal is usually normal, with many patients having an intact tympanic membrane. Radiologically, a mass is observed in the middle ear or mastoid with no bony destruction. The tumour can be excised by simple surgical removal. This must not be mistaken for the aggressive papillary middle-ear tumours which also affect adults of both sexes. These similarly look histologically benign tumours, but they have a very aggressive destructive behaviour and require radical surgery. Often, they will have a long history and if not treated aggressively will erode the petrous bone and extend intracranially, damaging the cranial nerves.

Adenocarcinomas of the middle ear are even rarer than adenocarcinomas of the external auditory meatus, which is surprising since the middle ear is lined with glandular epithelium. They have a poor prognosis.

Assessment of tumours

Local assessment is designed to identify the extent of the tumour, particularly those factors which render the tumour incurable.

Clinical examination can assess the external soft tissue spread, the local lymph-node metastases, and a search can be made for distant metastases. The cranial nerves are examined and assessment made of facial paralysis, trismus, fullness of the parotid gland, fullness of the infratemporal fossa, and perichondritis of the auricle.

Further assessment and staging is achieved radiologically. CT scans will show bony involvement well, but MRI scanning is required to demonstrate soft tissue involvement, in particular involvement of the dura. Care must be taken to look for temporomandibular joint articular fossa erosion and it is useful to assess whether the thin bone between the Eustachian tube and the carotid artery is involved. Lymph nodes in the neck and retropharyngeal space can be demonstrated both on CT and MRI scans, although these cannot be definitive as nodes may be present because of chronic inflammation.

Carotid angiography with a venous phase is required if the sigmoid sinus or jugular bulb are to be sacrificed at surgery, as venous crossflow needs to be demonstrated to avoid the possibility of life-threatening cerebral oedema. The differential diagnosis of metastatic disease as well as tuberculis otitis, necrotizing otitis externa, and glomus jugular tumours and Wegener's disease must also be borne in mind.

Treatment

Published reports generally refer to those patients who are treated, but inevitably there must be untreatable patients. Clearly, a poor general condition may preclude major surgery and distant metastases contraindicate treatment. The extent of disease may also be a contra-indication and this will be discussed below.

In terms of the level of evidence for treatment, no large randomized trial or meta-analysis has been conducted, not even a small randomized trial of treatment. No studies have been reported using non-randomized contemporary controls and none with historical controls. Thus, we are left with only level-5 evidence—in other words, that from case series.

There have been two recent papers bringing together the published case series: one by Prasad and Janecka,[5] who reviewed 144 patients, and the other by Donald,[11] who found 262 analysable cases from nine centres in the United States of what were termed middle fossa skull-base cancer resections. This, however, was a mixed bunch of tumours, including nasopharyngeal cancers extending into the middle fossa. Therefore most of the evidence is from a review of the case series.

Radiotherapy

Radiotherapy alone has seldom been recommended, except by the Christie Hospital in Manchester,[6] and no papers have reported sufficient numbers of patients treated solely with radiotherapy for this to be a treatment of choice. In a recent case series, adjuvant radiotherapy was used to treat patients with T1 and T2 tumours (as defined above) of the external auditory meatus. Patients who underwent an unspecified surgical resection alone had a cure rate of 57 per cent. In those who received adjuvant radiotherapy the cure rate was 100 per cent.[12] The dose of radiotherapy and the technique of radiotherapy have altered survival figures. Megavoltage equipment (linear accelerators) using wedge pair arrangements, delivering a dose of between 45 and 55 Gy over a period of 3 to 4 weeks, has been used in the United Kingdom.[6] With more protracted radiotherapy, the radiation dosage can be increased to 65 Gy, often with a 4:1 ratio in favour of electrons for a more selective irradiated volume and wider fields. When used as an adjunct to surgery, this modality improved the 5-year cure rate of tumours with extension beyond the temporal bone from 9 per cent to 65 per cent.[13] The type of radiotherapy has a significant part to play in the cure rate for these tumours.

Moreover, modern radiotherapy treatment-planning techniques, based upon 3D reconstruction from CT slices, allow a much better delineation of the planned target volume and a steep dose gradient for sparing neighbouring critical structures.

Before leaving the subject of radiotherapy and considering surgery specifically, it is worth mentioning the effects of radiation on the ear. Normally, radiotherapy alters the wax in the external ear canal, and makes it thicker and drier. The tympanic membrane becomes red and congested, particularly in the region of the handle of the malleus, and oedema occurs, particularly anterior inferiorly. A moisture producing radiation membrane is seen to form along the floor of the ear canal, but discharge from the mastoid cavity tends to diminish with radiotherapy. At the end of treatment the cavity becomes lined with radiation membrane. The vestibular apparatus tends to be relatively immune to radiation damage and vestibular symptoms are unusual.

Complications of radiotherapy

The external ear canal may become stenosed or may develop osteoradionecrosis. Neural complications result in damage to the temporal lobe, brainstem, or eyes. Osteoradionecrosis is difficult to differentiate from residual disease. It is impossible to irradiate the petrous temporal bone and much of the middle cranial fossa without irradiating cerebral tissue. Fortunately, the brain seems to be relatively resistant to radiation damage; but damage is more likely to occur in the elderly, possibly because of a compromised microvasculature. It is extremely unusual for the facial and auditory nerves in their extracranial course to be damaged by therapeutic irradiation. Post-irrradiation conductive deafness may occur in patients who have been successfully treated for carcinoma of the external auditory canal; this is possibly due to thickening of the mucus in the nasopharynx which then blocks the Eustachian opening, and atresia of the Eustachian orifices due to necrosis of the Eustachian cartilage. This tends to be characterized by severe earache and trismus, and, in addition, fibrosis of the fascia spaces surrounding the levator palatine muscle may occur.

Surgery

Surgery has been performed as a radical mastoidectomy before radiotherapy, as a primary form of treatment, as part of combined treatment, or occasionally as salvage after failed radiotherapy.

Most recent case reports involve a combination of radiotherapy and surgery. They state that if surgery can be performed to remove the tumour *in toto* and is followed by radical radiotherapy, this carries the best prognosis. However, there is no definitive evidence to back this up.

Prasad and Janecka's review of the literature was merely able to conclude that when a carcinoma is confined to the external canal, it appears that mastoidectomy or lateral, or subtotal, temporal bone resection yield similar survival rates when used in combination with radiotherapy.[5] However, following lateral temporal bone resection there appeared to be no advantage in giving radiotherapy. Once a tumour involves the middle ear, subtotal temporal bone resection has led to a better survival than lateral temporal bone resection or mastoidectomy. There is too little information available to be able to comment on post-treatment survival figures in patients with carcinomas involving the petrous apex.

Resection of involved dura does not appear to improve survival; however, the influence of negative margins on resection requires further study. Experience regarding resections of an involved internal carotid artery or the brain is too limited for any conclusions to be drawn. There have been two separate reports of tumours invading the brain in the middle cranial fossa where the patients have survived for 5 years,[14] but, as yet, there are no case reports of a 5-year survival in patients following resection of the carotid artery.

Primary surgery dates back to 1945 with the first petrousectomy reported by Parsons and Lewis. Lewis was mainly responsible for the development of surgery in this area, and described the block resection of the involved portion of the auditory canal, middle ear, mastoid process, petrous bone, temporomandibular joint, parotid gland, base of the zygoma, the auricle, and surrounding skin.[15]

The type of incision is dictated by the need to excise previous incisions made for biopsy or mastoidectomy.[16] Preferably, a pre-auricular S-shaped incision is used, similar to a parotidectomy incision, but with a superior extension for the middle fossa exposure and inferior extension to the neck. The neck extension is for node sampling and great vessel control, and for microvascular anastamosis for the free flap. This incision heals more rapidly and avoids delay to postoperative radiotherapy. The flaps are raised and the part of the pinna involved connected to the specimen, the canal is closed over to avoid tumour spillage. It is surprising how much pinna can be kept; even if only a small bridge of skin connects it to its blood supply, it will usually be of some cosmetic value. A temporal craniotomy is undertaken early in the procedure to assess invasion of the dura and the apex of the petrous pyramid. Invasion of a small part of the dura is not an indication of non-resectability, but deep invasion of the petrous apex may well be. The dura and brain are separated from the underlying bone, and the procedure continues if resectability is confirmed. Parotidectomy with tagging of the peripheral branch of the facial nerve is undertaken followed by division of the temporomandibular joint and zygomatic arch. This is then followed by division of the styloid process to define the position of the carotid artery and division of the posterior border of the mastoid process lateral or medial to the lateral sinus. Next, the floor of the middle ear and the bulb of the jugular vein are divided. The deep cuts are made by transection of the petrous pyramid lateral and posterior to the internal carotid artery using a Giggly saw or curved chisels. Thus a block of tissue containing the tumour is removed. Any further resection of the petrous apex or Eustachian tube is achieved by removing separate blocks of tissue.

Once surgical tumour removal has been confirmed on frozen section, the facial nerve is reconstructed using a primary nerve graft from the facial nerve stump to the peripheral nerve branches using the greater auricular nerve or sural nerve. If for some reason this is not available, a facial hypoglossal anastomosis can be carried out, providing the hypoglossal nerve does not form part of the resection. There is a large hole to fill, so, as a minimum, a free abdominal fat graft and vascularized temporalis muscle are used to obliterate the cavity. Usually, if some of the auricle or any skin or dura has been resected or breached, a free flap is necessary to repair the defect. The rectus abdominus free flap is the most commonly used, followed by the latissimus dorsi. In closing the defect, care must be taken to separate the nasopharynx/Eustachian tube from the cranial defect.

Lymph-node metastases are unusual. However, nodes are sampled in the procedure and a neck dissection may need to be carried out to remove the lymph nodes.

Complications of surgery

The incidence of bleeding has been reduced dramatically by using drills for dissection under direct revision. Preoperatively, the area is often infected with Gram-negative organisms in patients with longstanding chronic otitis media and therefore appropriate anti-microbial therapy is required. Deafness and vertigo occur following surgery. Vertigo can be a problem, taking a number of weeks before compensation occurs. Carotid artery thrombosis may occur due to trauma of the carotid vessels and this has occasionally led to hemiplegia; damage to the lower cranial nerves requires speech and swallowing rehabilitation. Cerebrospinal fluid leakage, pneumocephalus, and meningitis are much less of a problem with free-flap repair, but there may still be a need for lumbar drains if no vascularized tissue is used. As stated above, it is important for the cut end of the Eustachian tube to be carefully closed, particularly if the patient is likely to be bagged or ventilated postoperatively.

Choice of treatment

As stated above, the place of radiotherapy is well defined. If used as a primary treatment the cure rate is poor, if combined with mastoidectomy this improves, but best results are obtained from some kind of radical removal followed by radiotherapy. En-bloc resection is often impractical. Normal practice appears to entail removing the block lateral and posterior to the internal carotid artery and then removing the petrous apex as a further block.

When do patients become incurable?

Patients with brain or carotid artery involvement are considered to be incurable. This may be obvious at presentation, but sometimes the scans over- and underestimate the extent of the tumour.

The literature records two patients, each with a tumour involving the brain, who survived for more than 5 years following partial excision of the temporal lobe. Another report has described a patient who survived for 2 years after removal of the internal carotid artery and petrous apex.

The prognosis for a squamous-cell carcinoma of the external meatus is better than that for the middle ear, but when the prognostic significance of histological appearance of squamous carcinoma has been assessed, none of the factors studied, including the degree of differentiation, was found to have any effect on survival, although the patient's general condition and the presence of lymph nodes were all significant predictors of survival.

Thus, once faced with a carcinoma of the temporal bone it appears that all but the smallest and most superficial cancers of the external auditory canal require some sort of temporal bone resection followed by radical irradiation.

References

1. Horowitz SW, Leonetti JP, Azar-Kai B, Fine M, Izquierdo R. CT and MR of temporal bone malignancies primary and secondary to parotid carcinoma. *American Journal of Neuroradiology*, 1994; **15**: 142–3.

2. **Streitmann MJ, Sismanis A.** Metastatic carcinoma of the temporal bone. *American Journal of Otology*, 1996; **17**: 780–3.

3. **Corey JP, Nelson E, Craford M, Riester JW, Geiss R.** Metastatic vaginal carcinoma to the temporal bone. *American Journal of Otology*, 1991; **12**: 128–31.

4. **Stell PM.** Carcinoma of the external auditory meatus and middle ear. *Clinical Otolaryngology*, 1984; **9**: 281–99.

5. **Prasad S, Janecka IP.** Efficacy of surgical treatments for squamous cell carcinoma of the temporal bone: a literature review. *Otolaryngology Head and Neck Surgery*, 1994; **110**: 270–80.

6. **Birzgalis AR, Keith AO, Farrington WT.** Radiotherapy in the treatment of middle ear and mastoid carcinoma. *Clinical Otolaryngology*, 1992; **17**: 113–16.

7. **Ruben RJ, Thaler SB, Holzer N.** Radiation induced carcinoma of the temporal bone. *Laryngoscope*, 1997; **87**: 1613–21.

8. **Clark LJ, Narula AA, Morgan DA, Bradley PJ.** Squamous carcinoma of the temporal bone: a revised staging. *Journal of Laryngology and Otology*, 1991; **105**: 346–8.

9. **Arriaga M, Cartin H, Hirsch, BE, Takahashi H, Kamaren D.** Staging proposal for external auditory meatus carcinoma based on preoperative clinical examination and CT findings. *Annals of Otolaryngology, Rhinology, and Laryngology*, 1990; **99**: 714–21.

10. **Austin JR, Stewart KL, Fawzi N.** Squamous cell carcinoma of the external auditory canal. *Archives of Otolaryngology, Head and Neck Surgery*, 1994; **120**: 1228–32.

11. **Donald PJ.** Skull base surgery; combined results of treatment of malignant disease. *Skull Base Surgery*, 1992; **2**(2): 76–9.

12. **Pfreundneer L, et al.** Carcinoma of the external auditory canal and middle ear. *International Journal of Radiation Oncology, Biology, Physics*, 1999; **44**: 777–88.

13. **Spector JG.** Management of temporal bone carcinomas: a therapeutic analysis of two groups of patients and long-term followup. *Otolaryngology Head and Neck Surgery*, 1991; **104**: 58–66.

14. **Moffat DA, Grey P, Ballagh RH, Hardy DG.** Extended temporal bone resection for squamous cell carcinoma. *Otolaryngology Head and Neck Surgery*, 1997; **116**: 617–23.

15. **Lewis JS.** Temporal bone resection: a review of 100 cases. *Archives of Otolaryngology*, 1975; **79**: 23–5.

16. **Lesser THS.** Petrosectomy. In Bleach N, Mifford, C, van Hasselt A, eds. *Operative Otolaryngology*, 1997. Oxford: Blackwell Science.

Rare head and neck tumours

J. M. Henk

Aesthesioneuroblastoma

Aesthesioneuroblastoma is a rare tumour arising from the olfactory neuroepithelium that is situated in the roof of the nasal cavity, on the upper third of the nasal septum, and on the superior turbinate. It was originally described in 1924 and termed 'aesthesio-neuroepitheloma';[1] since then its histological variability has led to a number of different names. Aesthesioneuroblastoma is now the generally accepted term, as the tumour arises from basal neural cells of the olfactory mucosa that retain mitotic activity throughout life.[2] It has been classified in the past as a primitive neuroectodermal tumour, but is best regarded as a separate entity as it is a tumour of adults, is usually slow-growing, and has a relatively low propensity to metastasize. It should not be confused with neuroblastoma of childhood.

Aetiology

Aesthesioneuroblastoma comprises approximately 3 per cent of nasal neoplasms, excluding benign polyps. In North America and western Europe its incidence is about 0.15 cases per million population per year. The sex incidence is approximately equal. The tumour occurs at all ages from infancy to 90, but is very rare under the age of 10 or over the age of 70, with a peak incidence between the ages of 50 and 60. There are no known causative factors.

Pathology

Typically, the tumour consists of small or medium-sized round cells with uniform nuclei, scant cytoplasm, and few mitoses. The cells tend to form rosettes or pseudorosettes. The stroma consists of intercellular fibrils (Fig. 1). Pathognomonic histological features may be difficult to find. Consequently, the tumour may be confused with other round cell tumours that occur in the nose, including undifferentiated carcinoma, lymphoma, and melanoma. It is probably underdiagnosed.

Immunohistochemistry is helpful but is not absolutely specific.[3] Nearly all the tumours are positive for neurone-specific enolase. The S-100 stain is also frequently positive. The absence of cytokeratin and desmin confirms the non-epithelial origin. Electron microscopy shows neurosecretory granules, cytoplasmic filaments, and dendritic cell processes, features that clinch the diagnosis.

Behaviour

The tumour grows slowly in most cases and initially is confined to the upper part of the nasal cavity, and as it grows it begins to invade adjacent structures. The ethmoid sinus, the orbit, the maxillary sinus, the infratemporal fossa, and the anterior cranial fossa may all eventually be involved. Lymph nodes are involved in about 20 per cent of cases. The incidence of blood-borne metastases is also about 20 per cent; the lungs and bones are the commonest sites.

Clinical features

Most cases present with nasal symptoms, especially unilateral obstruction and epistaxis. There is often a long history of nasal symptoms before the diagnosis is made. Invasion of the orbit may lead to complaints of pain, epiphora, diplopia, or blurred vision. Intracranial extension may cause headache and cerebrospinal fluid leak.

Treatment

Aesthesioneuroblastoma is a radioresponsive tumour, although less radiosensitive than most neuro-ectodermal tumours. Local control rates of approximately 50 per cent can be achieved from radical radiotherapy given to maximum tissue tolerance dosage.[4]

The optimum treatment is total surgical removal followed by radiotherapy. Craniofacial resection is necessary to remove a tumour of the cribriform plate; smaller lesions confined to the nasal cavity can be removed via a lateral rhinotomy. Even quite small tumours often recur after surgery alone, so postoperative radiotherapy is now

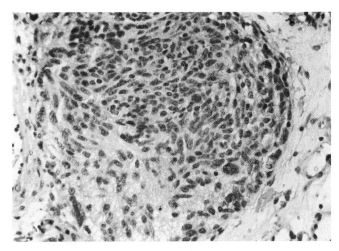

Fig. 1 Aesthesioneuroblastoma. An island of cells with peripheral differentiation into glial elements (× 350).

recommended for all cases.[5] Unresectable tumours are treated by radical radiotherapy alone. Lymph node metastases should be managed by neck dissection and postoperative radiotherapy. Elective treatment of the clinically negative neck is not warranted in view of the low incidence of nodal metastases.

The value of chemotherapy in advanced or inoperable disease has not yet been established. Responses to a variety of agents, including cyclophosphamide, vincristine, doxorubicin, and dacarbazine have been reported but the response rates are not high enough to suggest that chemotherapy should be a routine part of the management of locally advanced disease.[6] Chemotherapy is worth trying in patients with distant metastases or inoperable local recurrence.

Prognosis

As with all rare tumours, reported series are small and results differ widely. A literature review of 945 cases (reported up to 1994) revealed a steady improvement in prognosis in recent years with increasing use of combined treatment.[7] The overall 5-year survival rate is now about 65 per cent, ranging from over 80 per cent in patients with localized operable tumours to 40 per cent for inoperable tumours. However, this is a slowly-growing tumour, and at least a third of deaths from disease occur more than 5 years after presentation,[8] so the long-term prognosis is uncertain.

Juvenile angiofibroma

Juvenile angiofibroma is a rare, benign, but troublesome lesion occurring in adolescent or young adult males. It arises at the posterior end of the nasal cavity whence it spreads to neighbouring structures. Some authorities regard it as essentially hamartomatous rather than truly neoplastic. Nevertheless it can produce serious problems, especially profuse haemorrhage, so treatment is nearly always indicated. The optimum treatment, especially for advanced lesions with intracranial extension, remains controversial.

Aetiology

Most series report an exclusively male incidence with an age range of 7 to 30 with a peak at 14 years. A few cases have been reported in females and older adults, but these reports were nearly all over 20 years ago. It is possible that these cases were misdiagnosed, and were in fact low-grade vascular tumours of a different type.

Pathology

Juvenile angiofibroma consists of vascular channels of varying diameter lined by epithelial cells. Between the vessels is a fibrous stroma consisting of fibroblasts and collagen fibres. Farag et al.[9] drew attention to the histological resemblance of juvenile angiofibroma to the erectile tissue of the penis, and postulated that it is a developmental defect consisting of ectopic erectile tissue that is stimulated into growth by androgens at puberty. They found specific androgen receptors in all the lesions that they examined, but oestrogen receptors have not been found.[10]

Behaviour

The tumour arises in the lateral part of the roof of the posterior choanal margin at the superior margin of the sphenopalatine foramen. It grows forward to fill the nasal cavity on the same side, displacing the septum to the opposite side and flattening the turbinates. Posteriorly it grows into the lumen of the nasopharynx, eventually filling it and displacing the soft palate downwards. Laterally it can extend to the pterygoid fossa, which it probably enters through the sphenopalatine foramen. From there it can invade the infratemporal fossa and the posterior part of the orbit via the inferior orbital fissure. Adjacent bone can be destroyed by pressure erosion, allowing intracranial extension. The major blood supply is from the maxillary artery, but as the tumour grows and invades it may pick up supplies from other arteries.

The natural history of juvenile angiofibroma is not clear, It was formerly believed that spontaneous regression took place a few years after puberty, but this is no longer widely accepted. All cases are now treated, so confirmation of spontaneous regression cannot be obtained. However, some instances of regression after incomplete removal have been documented.[11]

Three cases have been reported that claim to be instances of sarcomatous transformation,[12] attributed to the effect of radiation. Two of the patients were unusual in that they were both adults aged 48 at the time of initial diagnosis. These cases may have been radiation-induced sarcomas arising in the stroma or adjacent soft tissues, rather than malignant change in the angiofibroma.

Clinical features

The most frequent symptoms are nasal obstruction and epistaxis that occur in most cases. Other symptoms are less frequent as they result from extensive disease. These include headache, facial deformity, deafness, and swelling of the palate. Epistaxis tends to be frequent, heavy, and sometimes life-threatening. On examination a vascular haemorrhagic mass is visible in the nasal cavity on one side, and in the nasopharynx. Swelling of the cheek indicates extension into the maxilla or infratemporal fossa. Proptosis indicates spread to the orbit.

Diagnosis

The diagnosis can nearly always be made with reasonable certainty by clinical examination and computed tomography (CT) scanning (Fig. 2). When a firm clinical diagnosis of juvenile angiofibroma has been made the next step should be angiography, which gives a characteristic picture and also serves to identify the arterial supply as an aid to subsequent surgery (Fig. 3). Biopsy is hazardous; it often causes severe haemorrhage which is difficult to control, so it should be reserved for cases where clinical examination and radiology leave doubt about the diagnosis.

Treatment

The tumour should be removed surgically whenever possible. The major problem with surgery is intra-operative bleeding, especially if resection is incomplete.

Embolization is an effective way of reducing vascularity pre-operatively and is now used almost routinely,[13] although in one series there was a suggestion that the risk of recurrence was increased

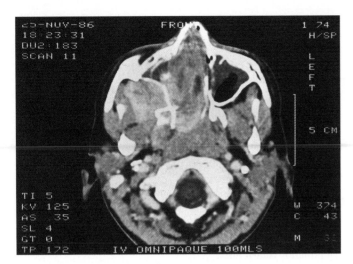

Fig. 2 CT scan of a 10-year-old boy with juvenile angiofibroma invading the nasal cavity and infratemporal fossa.

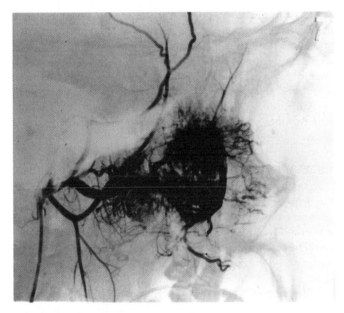

Fig. 3 Subtraction angiogram of the same patient as in Fig. 2.

by embolization.[14] Most angiofibromas derive their blood supply principally from the maxillary artery, which can be embolized safely. Tumours with a substantial supply from the internal carotid system are unsuitable for embolization.

The management of larger lesions, especially with intracranial or orbital extension, is more controversial. At the Mayo Clinic (Rochester, Minnesota) partial excision via a lateral rhinotomy approach is recommended.[11] In 40 patients so managed there were no deaths; residual disease mostly remained asymptomatic or actually regressed.

The alternative to surgery in advanced cases is radiotherapy. Cummings et al.[15] reported 55 patients treated with radiotherapy to doses of 35 Gy in 3 weeks. Follow-up was between 3 and 26 years. Cure was achieved in 80 per cent. Recurrences in the remaining 20 per cent were successfully treated by either surgery or re-irradiation. Morbidity was low; two patients in whom the orbit was involved by tumour developed unilateral cataract. One patient developed hypopituitarism after re-irradiation, otherwise there were no endocrine effects. There were two subsequent malignancies, a basal cell carcinoma of the face 13 years after irradiation, and a carcinoma of the thyroid arising outside the radiotherapy field 14 years after treatment. There were no deaths from the disease or from complications of treatment.

The management of the large tumour should be the subject of discussion between surgeon, radiologist, and radiotherapist. The relative risks of surgery and radiotherapy must be considered in each patient. In skilled hands the risks of embolization and surgery are slight. Up to 1970 there were reports of an operative mortality of 2 to 3 per cent, but in recent years operative deaths have become exceedingly rare. Postoperative complications depend on the extent of surgery. Cerebrospinal fluid leak, nasal sequestrum, or cranial nerve palsies are all rare complications.

If radiotherapy is carefully planned and no more than 35 Gy given it should not cause any side-effects; the only risk is radiation-induced neoplasia, the magnitude of which is still unknown but is probably no more than 5 per cent in the patient's lifetime; however, in general it is prudent not to use radiotherapy as the primary treatment except for very extensive intracranial tumours, or for progressive symptomatic recurrence after partial removal.

Paraganglioma

Paragangliomas are rare tumours. In the head and neck region they are of the non-chromaffin type and are believed to arise principally from chemoreceptor cells, hence the alternative term 'chemodectoma'. They arise at four sites in the head and neck:

1. the carotid body
2. the middle ear (glomus tympanicum)
3. the jugular bulb (glomus jugulare)
4. the nodose ganglion of the vagus nerve (glomus vagale)

These tumours are nearly always benign, and have a low mortality. They are sometimes confused histologically with metastases in the base of skull from renal carcinoma; therefore, some reports of fatal cases in the past may have been incorrect. The anatomical sites make surgical removal difficult. Recent developments in surgical technique have improved the operability rate, but the management of the larger lesions remains controversial.

Aetiology

Paragangliomas occur in adults over a wide age range, from 20 to 90 years, with a peak incidence in the fourth and fifth decades. They are commoner in females than males, especially glomus jugulare tumours of which over 80 per cent occur in females. Some cases, especially carotid body tumours, are familial. Grufferman et al.[16] in a literature review of 900 patients with carotid body tumours reported that 4 per cent of unilateral tumours and 32 per cent of bilateral tumours were familial. They considered that data collected from a few families suggested autosomal dominant transmission. However, in some families these tumours are inherited only from fathers,

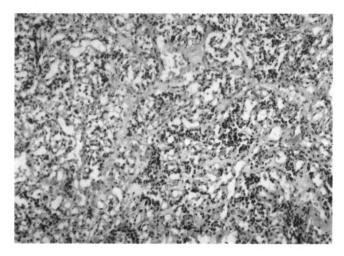

Fig. 4 Paraganglioma. Aggregates of uniform cells in a vascular stroma (× 150).

suggesting genomic imprinting.[17] The gene responsible maps to chromosome 11q23-qter.

Pathology

The histological pattern of paraganglioma is uniform and similar in the tumours at all sites (Fig. 4). The tumours consist of nests of cuboidal cells separated by a highly vascular fibrous stroma. The cells contain neurosecretory granules. Mitoses are scanty. The cells are usually non-chromaffin, although occasionally chromaffin-positive secretory granules can be seen, especially in carotid body tumours. Some tumours behave in the same manner as phaeochromocytoma of the adrenal gland, producing catecholamines causing hypertension. Nearly all these tumours are benign, although very occasionally a malignant variant with an invasive pattern and more mitoses is seen.

Behaviour

Carotid body tumours

These arise in the carotid body, a collection of chemoreceptor tissue approximately 5 mm in diameter situated within the adventitia of the posteromedial surface of the common carotid bifurcation. The tumour forms a rubbery, well-circumscribed mass that enlarges slowly. The external and internal carotid arteries become displaced around it, and the carotid bifurcation becomes splayed. If the tumour is not removed it can eventually become quite large, indenting the lateral pharyngeal wall and reaching the skull base. Distant metastases occur in about 5 per cent of cases.

Glomus vagale

This is the rarest type of head and neck paraganglioma. It arises from chemoreceptor cells within the sheath of the vagus nerve, most frequently at the level of the angle of the mandible, but occasionally in the supraclavicular region. It expands the vagus nerve; nerve fibres become splayed around the mass. The tumour may eventually reach the base of the skull at the jugular foramen, and if not removed it may extend intracranially It is the most likely of the head and neck

paragangliomas to become malignant; the incidence of malignancy is approximately 20 per cent.[18] Metastases may be found in lymph nodes, bone, and lungs.

Glomus tympanicum

This tumour arises from chemoreceptor cells in the tympanic branches of the glossopharyngeal or vagus nerve. Initially it forms a mass within the middle ear cavity. As it grows, first it invades the mastoid bone, then the petrous bone. Malignancy is very rare.

Glomus jugulare

This tumour arises from chemoreceptor cells in the adventitia of the jugular bulb. It grows initially within the jugular foramen, and therefore involves cranial nerves at an early stage. It invades the petrous bone, and often grows through the jugular foramen to enter the posterior cranial fossa.

Clinical features

Carotid body and glomus vagale tumours

These present as a painless slow-growing lump in the neck. The carotid body tumour is palpable in the mid-neck at the carotid bifurcation. It is of rubbery consistency, attached to the carotid but not pulsatile. It usually has limited mobility in a vertical direction, but is more freely mobile in the anteroposterior plane. Glomus vagale tumour has similar features but is usually palpable at a higher level in the neck or presents as a parapharyngeal swelling; vagus nerve function is usually preserved until the tumour involves the jugular foramen, when it produces a clinical picture similar to that of a glomus jugulare tumour (see below).

Glomus tympanicum and glomus jugulare

These tumours most commonly present as deafness. Pulsatile tinnitus is a characteristic symptom, but is not present in all cases. Other common symptoms include vertigo, throbbing headache, and pain in the ear. Facial palsy is quite common. Lesions of the lower four cranial nerves occur because of tumour at the jugular foramen, and are therefore common with glomus jugulare tumours. On examination no mass can be felt. Tumour in the middle ear is visible as a bluish-red discoloration of the tympanic membrane, or as a pulsating mass visible through the tympanum; these features occur in glomus tympanicum tumours, and in more advanced glomus jugulare tumours that have extended into the petrous bone. When the disease is advanced it may not be possible to distinguish between a glomus tympanicum and a glomus jugulare tumour.

Diagnosis and investigation

The diagnosis should be made on the basis of the clinical and radiological findings. Incisional biopsy should be avoided because of the vascularity of these tumours. Contrast-enhanced high-resolution CT scanning is the best way to diagnose and delineate glomus tympanicum and glomus jugulare tumours. These tumours show marked contrast enhancement because of their vascularity, and bone erosion can be demonstrated. They also show enhancement on magnetic resonance imaging following gadolinium administration. Carotid body tumours cause splaying of the internal and external carotid arteries at the bifurcation of the common carotid artery; this feature, together with high vascularity, can be demonstrated on angiography or CT scanning. In the case of the glomus vagale tumour, CT shows a densely enhancing mass high in the parapharyngeal space.

Treatment and prognosis

Complete extirpation of a paraganglioma can only be achieved by total surgical removal. However, the site and extent of many of these tumours make surgical removal difficult or hazardous. It is not always justified to risk postsurgical neurological deficit to remove a benign lesion, so that in some cases either radiotherapy or no treatment is preferable.

Carotid body tumours are usually amenable to surgery. They are removed by subadventitial dissection of the tumour from arterial walls. It is usually possible to preserve the carotid system intact, but occasionally the external carotid must be sacrificed. Intraluminal shunting may be advisable to maintain cerebral blood flow during the operation. Meyer et al.[19] recommend studies of cerebral blood flow pre-operatively to assess the need for intraluminal shunting, together with electroencephalogram monitoring during the operation. Relative contra-indications to surgery are the presence of multiple tumours, invasion of the base of skull, and cerebrovascular disease especially in older patients. It is reasonable to withhold treatment in an older patient with a slow-growing tumour and no symptoms other than the lump in the neck.

Radiotherapy has not been widely used, so there is lack of adequate evidence of its efficacy. It has long been regarded as ineffective, but there are some recent reports of good tumour control; e.g. Lybeert et al.[20] achieved regression in all nine tumours irradiated, with no regrowth observed in a follow-up period of 4 to 16 years. Shrinkage of the mass was slow and continued for several months. In some patients a residual asymptomatic lump persisted. Radiotherapy is worth trying in a patient with symptomatic or progressive disease who is considered unsuitable for surgery.

Glomus tympanicum and jugulare tumours confined to the middle ear and mastoid with no sign of invasion of the petrous bone or intracranial extension should be excised. The management of more extensive tumours, especially of the glomus jugulare, is controversial. Radiotherapy has been the most commonly used treatment for many years. Regression of tumour after radiotherapy occurs in nearly all cases, but is slow and continues for many months or even years. Regression results from mitotic death in the slowly-dividing tumour cells with their long cell-cycle times. It may also be due in part to a similar effect on endothelial cells in the stromal blood vessels, but this is probably not the major factor as some have claimed. Some clinical and radiological signs of tumour often persist indefinitely. Symptoms are relieved in over 90 per cent of patients. Long-term follow-up studies suggest that tumour regrowth occurs during the lifetime of only about 10 per cent of patients. Wang et al.[21] reviewed the results of radiotherapy in 244 patients in 13 publications; the overall local control rate was 91 per cent.

The persistence of signs of disease for a long period have led some surgeons to regard radiotherapy as an unsatisfactory method of treatment, and the small risk of a radiation-induced tumour must be considered in a young patient.[22] In the past the recurrence rate after surgery was higher than that after radiotherapy, 40 per cent in eight publications reviewed by Wang et al.[21] The development of techniques for operating on the base of the skull, and the reduction in vascularity that can be obtained by prior arterial embolization, have led to increased enthusiasm for surgery. It is now possible to excise tumours invading the petrous bone or extending intracranially that were formerly considered inoperable. Nevertheless the morbidity remains rather high even in the best hands, with recent surgical series reporting up to a 50 per cent incidence of new or exacerbated cranial nerve lesions and hearing loss in patients treated for advanced tumours.[23],[24]

At the present state of our knowledge radiotherapy still seems the better option for advanced glomus jugulare tumours, except in younger patients. Surgery should not be attempted unless there is an excellent chance of complete removal. There is no logic to combined treatment; if radiotherapy is going to be necessary the patient will do just as well without surgery.

Glomus vagale tumours should always be treated surgically whenever possible because of the risk of malignancy. Inoperable tumours are treated by radiotherapy.

The radiotherapy dose for paraganglioma need not be to the maximum tissue tolerance level. In most reported series 40 to 50 Gy in 2 Gy daily fractions was used. Cummings et al.[25] achieved a 93 per cent local control rate from 35 Gy in 15 fractions. The morbidity of radiotherapy at this dose is negligible, consisting of dryness and crusting in the external auditory meatus and a small area of temporary epilation. Major morbidity, i.e. temporal bone necrosis and brain stem injury, has been reported from 60 Gy or more, but it now known that there is no need to use such a high dose.

Metastases from malignant paraganglioma occasionally take up meta-iodobenzylguanidine, which when labelled with radioactive iodine is useful for detection of metastases, and if the uptake is high, for treatment.

Soft tissue sarcoma of head and neck

Between 10 and 15 per cent of soft tissue sarcomas occur in the head and neck but they comprise less than 1 per cent of head and neck cancer.[26] They occur mainly in adults, with the exception of embryonal rhabdomyosarcoma, a disease of children with a very different behaviour from the other histological types, and will therefore not be considered under this heading.

Aetiology

In most reported series the mean age is between 40 and 50, i.e. lower than that of carcinoma. The reported male/female ratio varies between 1 : 1 and 2 : 1. Some cases are associated with various genetic disorders, e.g. retinoblastoma, neurofibromatosis, and Gardener's syndrome, and a few are radiation induced. In the majority of cases no causative factor can be identified.

Pathology

All histological types may be found in the head and neck. The commonest is malignant fibrous histiocytoma, which now includes many tumours previously classified as fibrosarcoma. Sarcomas vary in their histological grade; about 50 per cent in the head and neck are of low grade. Aggressive fibromatosis is probably a type of low-grade sarcoma.

Behaviour

Sarcomas can arise anywhere in the extracranial soft tissues; for example, the neck, parapharyngeal space, scalp, orbit, or paranasal sinuses. The rate of growth of the primary tumour depends on the histological grade; volume doubling times can be as short as 2 weeks or as long as 2 years. The tumour invades locally and may produce a pseudocapsule from compression of the surrounding tissues; this capsule, however, will always contain tumour cells, so that an attempt to 'shell-out' the tumour will always be followed by recurrence.

Lymph node metastases are rare; they may occasionally occur in synovial, epithelioid, or angiosarcoma. Blood-borne metastases are seen rather less commonly than from sarcomas elsewhere in the body. Only about one-third of patients develop metastases, mainly to the lungs.

Treatment

If there is no evidence of distant metastases the primary tumour should be excised with as wide a margin of normal tissue as possible. Postoperative radiotherapy to a dose of 60 Gy in 6 weeks is probably advisable in most cases; even when the excision appears to be complete. In a series of 130 patients treated at the Royal Marsden Hospital (London, UK) the local control rate at 10 years was 50 per cent in those patients who received postoperative radiotherapy compared with 24 per cent in those who did not ($p = 0.004$), despite the fact that radiotherapy was more often used when surgery was considered incomplete.[27] Cure of inoperable tumours by radiotherapy alone is rare.

Chemotherapy has not been shown to have any value as adjuvant therapy in patients with operable tumours. It may bring about temporary regression of inoperable tumours or metastases.

The major prognostic factors are stage and histological grade. Localized and well-differentiated tumours are associated with 5-year survival rates over 80 per cent. All histopathological types have a similar prognosis, with the exception of angiosarcoma, for which 5-year survival is only about 10 per cent.[28]

Granular cell tumour

Granular cell tumours are rare lesions that can occur in all parts of the body, but have a predilection for head and neck sites. The tongue is the commonest site; this tumour has also been reported in the larynx, trachea, cheek, pharyngeal muscles, and orbit.[29] Multiple tumours of this type are occasionally seen. The tumour is commoner in females than males and the peak incidence is in young adults. The cell of origin is not known for certain. It was formerly believed to be skeletal muscle, hence the old term 'myoblastoma', which is almost certainly a misnomer. Histochemical studies now suggest a probable neuroendocrine origin.[30]

Pathology

Granular cell tumours consist of nests of round or oval cells with small central nuclei. The cytoplasm contains periodic acid-Schiff-positive granules (Fig. 5). They may be associated with pseudo-epitheliomatous hyperplasia and consequently may be misdiagnosed as squamous cell carcinoma. Some of these tumours may infiltrate

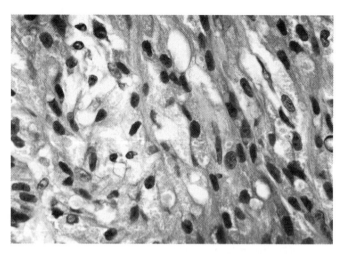

Fig. 5 Granular cell tumour of the tongue, showing intracellular granules ($\times$ 400).

surrounding tissues, but the true incidence of malignancy is difficult to assess. Metastases to regional lymph nodes have been reported but are exceedingly rare.

Clinical features

The commonest presentation is as a smooth firm non-ulcerated swelling, immediately below the mucosa of the tongue, most often on the dorsum near the mid-line. There are no features to distinguish granular cell tumours from other benign tumours.

Treatment

The treatment is wide local excision. The recurrence rate is about 5 per cent, so follow-up is advisable.

Meibomian gland carcinoma

Carcinoma of the Meibomian gland is the rarest type of malignant tumour of the eyelid, accounting for about 1 per cent of the total. It has a histological structure identical to sebaceous carcinoma of the skin, but behaves in a more aggressive manner. It presents as a yellowish swelling at the lid margin, and must be distinguished from a basal cell carcinoma or a Meibomian cyst. It occurs with equal frequency on the upper and lower lid.

Spread is by local invasion of the orbit, and metastases to regional lymph nodes. In a series of 88 patients reported by Boniuk and Zimmerman,[31] 17 per cent had orbital involvement, and lymph node metastases occurred in 28 per cent. The mortality from the tumour was 30 per cent at 5 years.

The treatment of the primary tumour is surgical. A small lesion can be excised locally and the eyelid reconstructed. Larger tumours require orbital exenteration. Involved lymph nodes are managed by radical neck dissection. This tumour is not very radio-responsive; local control is rarely achieved by radiotherapy. Postoperative radiotherapy to the neck is indicated if there is extensive lymph node involvement.

References

1. **Berger L, Luc R.** L'Esthésioneuroépithéliome olfactif. *Bulletin de l'Association Français pour l'Etude de Cancer*, 1924; **13**: 410–21.

2. **Michaeu C.** A new histochemical and biochemical approach to olfactory esthesioneuroma: a nasal tumor of neural crest origin. *Cancer*, 1976; **40**: 314–18.

3. **Taxy JB, *et al.*** The spectrum of olfactory neural tumors. *American Journal of Surgical Pathology*, 1986; **10**: 687–95.

4. **Parsons JT, *et al.*** Malignant tumors of the nasal cavity and ethmoid and sphenoid sinuses. *International Journal of Radiation Oncology, Biology, Physics*, 1988; **14**: 11–22.

5. **Foote RL, *et al.*** Esthesioneuroblastoma: the role of adjuvant radiation therapy. *International Journal of Radiation Oncology, Biology, Physics*, 1993; **27**: 835–42.

6. **Wade PM, Smith RE, Johns ME.** Response of esthesioneuroblastoma to chemotherapy. *Cancer*, 1984; **53**: 1036–41.

7. **Broich G, Pagliari A, Ottaviani F.** Esthesioneuroblastoma: a general review of the cases published since the discovery of the tumour in 1924, *Anticancer Research*, 1997; **17**: 2683–706.

8. **Bailey BJ, Barton S.** Olfactory neuroblastoma: management and prognosis. *Archives of Otolaryngology*, 1975; **101**: 1–5.

9. **Farag MM, Ghanimah SE, Regaie A, Saleem TH.** Hormonal receptors in juvenile nasopharyngeal angiofibroma. *Laryngoscope*, 1987; **97**: 208–11.

10. **Johns ME, MacLeod RM, Cantrell RW.** Estrogen receptors in nasopharyngeal angiofibromas. *Laryngoscope*, 1980; **90**: 628–34.

11. **Jones GC, De Santo LW, Bremer JW, Neel HB.** Juvenile angiofibroma: behaviour and treatment of extensive and residual tumors. *Archives of Otolaryngology Head and Neck Surgery*, 1986; **112**: 1191–3.

12. **Chen KTK, Bauer FW.** Sarcomatous transformation of nasopharyngeal angiofibroma. *Cancer*, 1982; **49**: 369–71.

13. **Davis KR.** Embolization of epistaxis and juvenile nasopharyngeal angiofibromas. *American Journal of Roentgenology*, 1987; **148**: 209–18.

14. **McCombe A, Lund VJ, Howard DJ.** Recurrence in juvenile angiofibroma. *Rhinology*, 1990; **28**: 97–102.

15. **Cummings BJ, *et al.*** Primary radiation therapy for juvenile nasopharyngeal angiofibroma. *Laryngoscope*, 1984; **94**: 1599–611.

16. **Grufferman S, *et al.*** Familial carotid body tumours. *Cancer*, 1980; **46**: 2116–22.

17. **van der Mey AGL, *et al.*** Genomic imprinting in hereditary glomus tumours: evidence for new genetic theory. *Lancet*, 1989; **ii**: 1291–4.

18. **Persson AV, *et al.*** Vagal body tumour: paraganglioma of the head and neck. *CA: A Cancer Journal for Clinicians*, 1985; **35**: 232–7.

19. **Meyer FB, Sundi TM, Pearson BW.** Carotid body tumors: a subject review and suggested surgical approach. *Journal of Neurosurgery*, 1986; **64**: 377–85.

20. **Lybeert MLM, *et al.*** Radiotherapy of paragangliomas. *Clinical Otolaryngology* 1984; **9**: 105–9.

21. **Wang ML, *et al.*** Chemodectoma of the temporal bone: a comparison of surgical and radiotherapeutic results. *International Journal of Radiation Oncology, Biology, Physics* 1988; **14**: 643–8.

22. **Lalwani AK, Jackler RK, Gutin PH.** Lethal fibrosarcoma complicating radiation therapy for benign glomus jugulare tumor. *American Journal of Otology*, 1993; **14**: 398–402.

23. **Lawson W, *et al.*** Complications in the management of large glomus jugulare tumors. *Laryngoscope*, 1987; **97**: 152–7.

24. **Gjuric M, Rudiger Wolf S, Wigand ME, Weidenbecher M.** Cranial nerve and hearing function after combined-approach surgery for glomus jugulare tumors. *Annals of Otology, Rhinology and Laryngology*, 1996; **105**: 949–54.

25. **Cummings BJ, *et al.*** The treatment of glomus tumors in the temporal bone by megavoltage radiation. *Cancer*, 1984; **53**: 2635–40.

26. **Weber RS, *et al.*** Soft tissue sarcomas of the head and neck in adolescents and adults. *American Journal of Surgery*, 1986; **152**: 386–92.

27. **Eeles RA, *et al.*** Head and neck sarcomas: prognostic factors and implications for treatment. *British Journal of Cancer*, 1993; **68**: 201–7.

28. **Willers H, *et al.*** Adult soft tissue sarcomas of the head and neck treated by radiation and surgery or radiation alone: patterns of failure and prognostic factors. *International Journal of Radiation Oncology, Biology, Physics*, 1995; **33**: 585–93.

29. **Alessi DM, Zimmerman MC.** Granular cell tumors of the head and neck. *Laryngoscope*, 1988; **98**: 810–14.

30. **Williams HK, Williams DM.** Oral granular cell tumours: a histological and immunocytochemical study. *Journal of Oral Pathology and Medicine*, 1997; **26**: 164–9.

31. **Boniuk M, Zimmerman LE.** Sebaceous carcinoma of the eyelid, eyebrow, caruncle and orbit. *Transactions of the American Academy of Ophthalmology and Otolaryngology*, 1968; **72**: 619–42.

9.11 Tumours of the orbit

J. M. Henk

This chapter concerns neoplasms of the orbit and eye, excluding intraocular melanoma and retinoblastoma which are covered in Chapters 8.2 and 17.3.

The orbit is a pyramidal space enclosed within bony walls. It contains the eyeball and its associated extrinsic muscles, nerves, and glands. For practical surgical and oncological purposes it can be divided into two anatomical spaces—the intraconal space, which lies within the cone formed by the extrinsic eye muscles and fascia, and the peripheral space lying between the cone and the orbital periosteum. The cone acts as a barrier to spread of tumours, so that it is unusual for a tumour to involve both spaces in the early stages.

The orbit contains muscle, fat, neural, lymphoid, and glandular tissues. Hence a wide variety of primary tumour types can occur Each tumour type is exceedingly rare. Incidence figures for primary orbital tumours as a group are not available, as they are not classified separately by cancer registries. Secondary tumours are seen more frequently than primaries: metastases from virtually every type of tumour have been reported in the orbit. However, most orbital swellings are non-neoplastic and have many causes so that the diagnosis of an orbital tumour can be difficult.

The more frequently occurring orbital neoplasms are listed in Table 1. The common non-neoplastic causes of orbital swellings and masses which may produce clinical features similar to those of a tumour are listed in Table 2.

Clinical diagnosis

The presenting symptom of an orbital tumour is usually swelling of an eyelid, protrusion of the eye, or visual disturbance. When taking the history attention must be paid to features such as duration of symptoms, occurrence of thyroid disease, sinus disease, head injury, systemic illnesses, or tumour elsewhere in the body.

Examination

Both orbits should be inspected noting any localized or general swelling of the eyelids. It is important to look for bilateral oedema of the lids with retraction or lid lag, which will suggest a diagnosis of dysthyroid eye disease. Proptosis is looked for and measured. Both orbits should be palpated simultaneously comparing the resistance of corresponding quadrants. If there is proptosis present, the normal lacrimal gland may be easily palpated above and lateral to the globe and mistaken for a tumour. Eye movements must be checked; a tumour will often affect the function of the eye muscle it is adjacent to or involves, so that there is limitation of movement of the eye towards the tumour. Full examination of the eye is necessary. Regional lymph nodes must be palpated and a general examination of the patient performed, looking for evidence of a systemic disease which may affect the orbit, for example thyrotoxicosis, sarcoidosis, or a malignancy elsewhere.

Investigation

Magnetic resonance is the best method of imaging the orbit if a tumour is suspected. The intraocular structures and visual pathways

Table 1 Orbital neoplasms

Benign	Malignant
Dermoid	Lymphoma
Neurilemmoma	Melanoma
Neurofibroma	Connective tissue
Meningioma	rhabdomyosarcoma
Lymphangioma	fibrous histiocytoma
Optic nerve glioma	fibrosarcoma etc.
Lacrimal gland	Lacrimal gland
pleomorphic adenoma	adenoid cystic carcinoma
	adenocarcinoma
	malignant mixed tumour
	Haemangiopericytoma
	Metastases

Table 2 Non-neoplastic causes of proptosis and orbital masses

Dysthyroid eye disease
Vascular malformations
  capillary haemangioma
  varices
Inflammatory
  mucocoele of ethmoid sinus
  Wegener's granuloma
  lymphoid hyperplasia
  pseudotumour
  cellulitis
Sarcoidosis
Langerhans histiocytosis

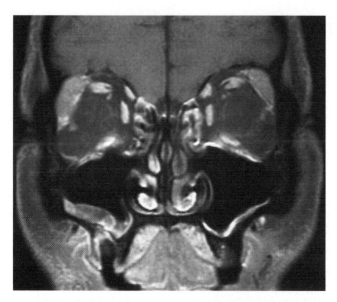

Fig. 1 Coronal MRI scan showing lymphoma involving both lacrimal glands.

can be demonstrated with high resolution, and it has the advantage of multiplanar evaluation (Fig. 1). It has now largely supplanted other methods of imaging; however CT remains superior for demonstrating abnormalities in the bone, and for radiotherapy planning.

Histology is essential for diagnosis. A tumour in the anterior part of the orbit is easily accessible to biopsy through an incision in the eyelid or conjunctival fornix. Access to lesions in the posterior part of the orbit is obtained via a lateral orbitotomy approach. Biopsy of a mass in the intraconal space behind the globe is hazardous and carries some risk of optic nerve damage and visual loss. Often only a small amount of tissue can be obtained for biopsy so that histological diagnosis may be difficult.

Needle aspiration cytology under CT guidance is a useful technique for detecting malignancy but may not yield a precise histological diagnosis, It is especially useful for diagnosing orbital metastases in a patient known to have malignant disease.[1]

Treatment principles

Surgery

Surgery is indicated for benign tumours, and for malignant tumours not amenable to cure by radiotherapy. Whenever possible the aim of surgery should be to remove the tumour and preserve useful vision. The type of operation is determined by the position of the tumour within the orbit. In general, a lateral orbitotomy approach provides the best access, especially for lacrimal gland tumours.

Radiotherapy

Radiotherapy is preferable to surgery for radical treatment of radio-sensitive tumours such as lymphoma and rhabdomyosarcoma. It also has a role in the management of lacrimal gland and neural tumours, and in palliation of incurable tumours and metastases to the orbit. The objective of radiotherapy to the orbit is to deliver to the tumour

a dose of radiation high enough to offer a chance of cure while at the same time keeping the dose to the vulnerable, normal tissues in the eye and orbit within tolerance levels. This ideal may not be attainable in the case of large lesions, but can be achieved in the treatment of many tumours, perhaps more often than generally realized.

Radiation tolerance of normal tissues

The lens of the eye is the most radiosensitive structure in the orbit. The effect of radiation is to cause cell death in the germinative zone, the ring of mitotically-active cells at the periphery of the lens. Degenerate fibres and debris from the killed cells migrate to the posterior pole of the lens and cause opacities. If only a few cells are affected, the opacity may remain static and does not impair vision. If a larger number of cells are killed, the opacities increase leading to cataract formation and consequent visual impairment.

Information on radiation tolerance of the lens is derived mainly from estimates of lens dose in patients who received radiotherapy to the orbit, based on measurements in tissue-equivalent phantoms. Merriam and Focht[2] studied patients treated by a variety of radio-therapy techniques; they observed lens opacities after doses as low as 400 roentgens (approximately 3.6 Gy). Patients whose lenses had received more than 1150 roentgens (approximately 10.5 Gy) invariably developed progressive cataract. Bessell et al.[3] studied patients treated with megavoltage irradiation for orbital lymphoma using corneal shielding. No opacities were seen when the germinative zone received doses of 10 Gy or less in 15 fractions. Subsequent follow up of the same group of patients has shown that 15 Gy in 15 fractions gave an approximately 50 per cent incidence of lens opacity at 8 years after treatment. At doses higher than 15 Gy all patients eventually developed a cataract.[4]

The cornea is the second most radiovulnerable structure in the eye. Data on radiation tolerance are scanty. The cornea has a radio-sensitivity similar to that of other surface epithelia. Clinical experience suggests that surface doses of 30 Gy or more in 2-Gy daily fractions may lead to acute keratitis, but at doses below 50 Gy late sequelae are unlikely. A dose of 50 Gy or more usually causes scarring or perforation, often with an associated iridocyclitis, and secondary glaucoma may supervene. Corneal damage is probably the chief mechanism producing the shrunken atrophic or 'phthisic' globe seen after very high doses of radiation.

Radiation injury to the retina results from endothelial cell death in small vessels leading to ischaemic changes, producing the characteristic clinical picture of radiation retinopathy.[5] Changes seen on oph-thalmoscopy include microaneurysms, new vessel formation, haem-orrhages, cotton wool exudates, and pallor. As with most vascular radiation effects, there is a latent period of from 18 to 36 months after radiotherapy before retinopathy becomes symptomatic. The severity of retinopathy is strongly dose related. At doses below 35 Gy the incidence of retinal effects is low and the changes are slight or absent.[3],[6] Visual impairment is rare at doses below 50 Gy in 25 fractions. Above 50 Gy the risk of visual impairment from retinopathy rises steeply.[5] Thompson et al.[7] reported that seven out of 10 patients whose retinas received between 60 and 70 Gy lost vision, although Shukovsky and Fletcher[8] found no case of visual loss from retinopathy at doses up to 68 Gy.

The optic nerve is an extension of the white matter of the central nervous system and therefore has a radiation tolerance similar to that

Table 3 Radiation tolerance of structures in the orbit for fraction sizes of ≤2 Gy

Germinal epithelium of lens	10 Gy
Lacrimal and conjunctival glands	30 Gy
Cornea	50 Gy
Retina	50 Gy
Optic nerve	55 Gy

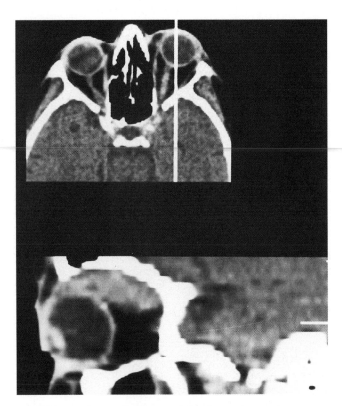

Fig. 2 CT scan of orbit of a patient with lymphoma, showing the tumour limited to the superior part of the orbit. This patient was treated with anterior and lateral fields, with the anterior field angled 10° caudally so that the shadow of the corneal shield passed below the posterior extent of the tumour.

of the brainstem. The risk of optic nerve injury is low below 56 Gy in 2-Gy fractions;[5] with higher doses the incidence of damage is dependent on fraction size. Parsons and colleagues[5] found that with fraction sizes of 1.9 Gy or less the incidence of optic nerve damage was only 8 per cent at total doses between 60 and 75 Gy.

The lacrimal, meibomian, and other glands in the conjunctiva responsible for forming the tear film have a radiation sensitivity similar to that of other mucus and sebaceous glands in the body. A dose of up to 40 Gy to the whole orbit is unlikely to cause a severe dry eye syndrome.[3],[5] Higher doses lead to failure of formation of the tear film with a risk of severe corneal damage as a consequence. Most of the glands producing the tear film are in the upper eyelid, so shielding of a portion of the upper lid when the orbit is irradiated can prevent a dry eye syndrome.

Radiation tolerance levels for structures in the orbit are summarized in Table 3.

Radiotherapy techniques

It is important to delineate the exact position and extent of tumour in the orbit before planning radiotherapy. CT scanning with reconstruction of images in the coronal and sagittal planes or MRI are helpful (Fig. 2).

Fortunately, the majority of tumours suitable for radiotherapy rarely penetrate the intraconal space behind the globe. Accordingly, the plan shown in Fig. 3 is suitable for most patients. Three-dimensional conformal CT planning is valuable in more difficult cases to improve the dose distribution while preserving vision. For example if the tumour is on the roof of the orbit the anterior field is inclined inferiorly so that the shadow of the corneal shield passes below the orbital apex, hence avoiding an underdosed area in the tumour.

If the tumour surrounds the globe, the entire orbital contents must be irradiated uniformly, so cataract is inevitable. A suitable technique in such a situation is to use superior and inferior oblique fields (Fig. 4). This method avoids any risk of irradiation of the opposite eye. The patient is treated with the eye open looking into the beam so that the surface-sparing can keep the corneal dose within tolerance. An alternative technique, suitable for a more sensitive tumour such as a lymphoma, where homogeneity of dose within the orbit is less important, is to use a 20 MeV electron beam with a corneal shield; side scatter of electrons causes a build up of dose behind the lens so that the dose in the intraconal space is no less than 60 per cent of the applied dose.[9]

Tumours of the intraconal space and posterior half of the globe are treated using lateral fields. For low dose or palliative treatment,

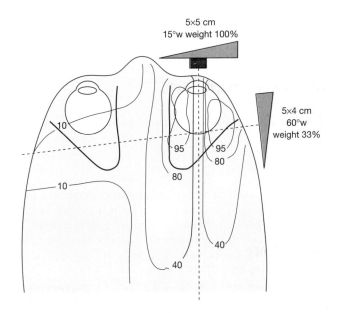

5×5 cm
15°w weight 100%

5×4 cm
60°w
weight 33%

Fig. 3 Two-field plan suitable for treatment of most orbital tumours using either a cobalt unit or a 5 MV linear accelerator.

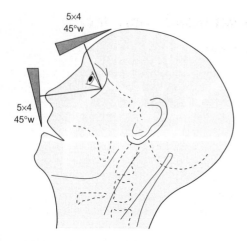

Fig. 4 Technique for treating orbital tumours in the sagittal plane, avoiding the contralateral orbit.

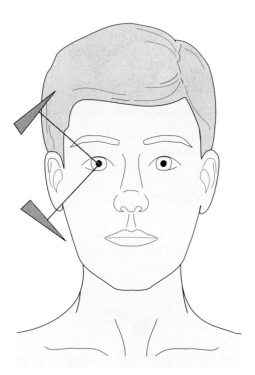

Fig. 5 Technique of irradiation of tumours in the posterior half of the orbit.

for example a lymphoma or choroidal metastases treatment, a single lateral field is used, in the same position as the lateral field in Fig. 3 so that both lenses are avoided. If a higher dose is required, for example intraconal rhabdomyosarcoma treatment, superolateral and inferolateral fields can be used, so avoiding any exit dose to the opposite eye (Fig. 5).

The technique shown in Fig. 4 is suitable for postoperative irradiation after orbital exenteration, for example for malignant fibrous histiocytoma or adenocarcinoma of the lacrimal gland. The technique is also applicable to a tumour confined to the medial wall of the orbit, for example an infiltrating basal-cell carcinoma. The fields are narrow with the their lateral edges just medial to the cornea.

Lymphoma

The orbit may be the site of origin of a lymphoma, or orbital involvement may be the presenting symptom of a generalized lymphoma. The orbit may become involved at a later stage of the disease in a patient with systemic lymphoma. This section will deal with lymphoma presenting as an orbital tumour and therefore deemed 'primary'.

Lymphoma may present with a variety of symptoms; usually swelling of an eyelid, proptosis, conjunctival redness, discomfort in the eye, or diplopia. Visual acuity is rarely affected. Commonly, there is a rubbery mass arising anteriorly in the orbit, more often superiorly than inferiorly. This enlarges slowly producing the appearance of expansion of the eyelid and eventually displacement of the globe and proptosis. There is often subconjunctival infiltration which may reach the limbus and partly or completely surround the cornea. In some cases, especially in children and young adults, the tumour grows more rapidly and either takes on an inflammatory appearance or becomes fixed to the skin and periosteum. It is unusual for lymphoma to arise posteriorly in the orbit; when it does so it produces a painless proptosis.

Pathology

All histological types and grades of lymphoma have been reported in the orbit. Only about 20 per cent fall into the intermediate or high-grade categories.[10] The higher grades of lymphoma occur at all ages. Lymphoblastic lymphoma is occasionally seen in children but is very rare and must be distinguished from granulocytic sarcoma, that is an orbital presentation of acute myeloid leukaemia. Centroblastic and mixed types are found in young and middle-aged adults, whereas in the elderly the immunoblastic type predominates.

At least 80 per cent of orbital lymphomata are of low grade and present over the age of 40 years. The commonest histological picture is diffuse lymphocytic. Nodular lymphoma is rarely diagnosed on an orbital biopsy because of the small amount of tissue obtained, but it is not unusual to find a nodular pattern in subsequently involved lymph nodes. Some tumours, especially of the conjunctiva, are of the MALT (mucosa-associated lymphoid tissue) type.[11]

Orbital lymphoma must be distinguished from lymphoid hyperplasia. Often a biopsy contains sheets of small lymphocytes with a mixture of other cells of the lymphoid series but with no clear histological features of malignancy, in which case it is not possible to say for certain on histological grounds whether the lesion is benign lymphoid hyperplasia or a lymphoma. The term 'indeterminate lymphocytic lesion'[12] has been applied to this kind of lesion. Other terms sometimes used are 'pseudolymphoma', which should be discarded as it implies a non-neoplastic condition, and 'pseudotumour', which is inappropriate as it is a term usually applied to inflammatory masses of uncertain origin that mimic tumours.

The majority of lymphoid masses in the orbit consist of a monotypic B cell proliferation, indicating low-grade lymphoma. However, some polytypic lesions formerly assumed to be hyperplasia progress to disseminated lymphoma.[13] Immunoglobulin gene rearrangements can be found in nearly all indeterminate lymphocytic lesions, whether monotypic or polytypic, indicating their essentially neoplastic nature.[14] It now seems likely that the vast majority of lymphoid masses presenting in the orbit which show an indeterminate or pseudolymphomatous histological pattern are actually low-grade lymphomata.

Staging

Orbital lymphoma is staged in the same way as other lymphomata. It is often associated with lymphoma at other extranodal sites, so clinical examination must include inspection of the skin and examination of the pharynx. Full staging investigations are essential in a patient with high or intermediate grade lymphoma. However, the value of investigations such as abdominal CT and bone marrow biopsy in older patients with low grade orbital lymphoma is questionable, as treatment is not normally given for occult disseminated disease in the absence of symptoms.

Natural history

Of patients presenting with orbital lymphoma who are subjected to full staging investigations, about 50 per cent of high and intermediate grade and 80 per cent of low grade prove to be stage 1. If only local treatment is given, high and intermediate grade tumours will show evidence of disseminated lymphoma within 5 years in about 70 per cent of cases.[10] The corresponding 5-year dissemination rate of low grade lymphoma and indeterminate lymphocytic lesions is of the order of 20 per cent, but systematic lymphoma can sometimes appear much later after the initial orbital presentation.

Treatment

High and intermediate-grade lymphoma in children and young adults should be treated by chemotherapy regardless of stage. In older patients it is reasonable to treat initially by radiotherapy keeping chemotherapy in reserve until dissemination appears. A dose of 40 Gy in 20 fractions in 4 weeks seems sufficient, as in the Royal Marsden Hospital series there have been no local recurrences.[10]

In low-grade lymphoma there is little or no evidence that early institution of treatment influences survival . Treatment is therefore largely symptomatic. The majority of patients are concerned by their ocular symptoms and require treatment. For stage 1 a dose of 30 Gy in 15 fractions in 3 weeks results in 100 per cent local control. In a patient with disseminated, low-grade lymphoma a smaller dose, 15 to 20 Gy, is adequate to obtain palliation of ocular symptoms.

The morbidity of radiotherapy is low.[3] The most frequent complication is dryness of the eye which may require regular use of artificial tears. The risk of cataract formation depends on the radiotherapy technique used; provided there is adequate shielding that reduces the dose to the germinative zone at the periphery of the lens to less than 10 Gy, cataract is unlikely to occur.[4]

Prognosis

The prognosis is the same as that of extranodal lymphoma at other sites. Stage 1 low-grade orbital lymphoma patients have the same life expectancy as the normal population of the same age regardless of whether or not dissemination occurs.

Lacrimal gland tumours

Presentation

Lacrimal gland tumours are extremely rare. They occur predominantly in young and middle-aged adults with a 2:1 male preponderance. They present as a swelling of the upper eyelid often with visual symptoms resulting from displacement or reduced mobility of the eye. On examination a mass is palpable in the superolateral quadrant of the orbit.

There are many other causes of swelling in the lacrimal fossa, which occur more commonly than tumours. The commonest cause of enlargement of the gland itself is chronic inflammation. Lymphoma, pseudotumour, dacrocele, dermoid, and granuloma all occur at this site and must be distinguished from lacrimal gland tumours. Shields et al.[15] in a review of 142 lacrimal gland biopsies found that 16 per cent of lacrimal gland swellings were primary epithelial neoplasms.

Pathology

The same histological types of tumour occur in the lacrimal gland as in the salivary glands. The commonest is the benign pleomorphic adenoma. This is a tumour mainly of young and middle-aged adults. The most frequently occurring malignant tumours are the adenoid cystic carcinoma, which has a peak incidence in young adults, and the adenocarcinoma, which is mainly a tumour of the elderly. Hence malignant lacrimal gland tumours tend to have a bimodal age distribution. Other malignant types, such as mucoepidermoid carcinoma, malignant mixed tumour, acinic cell carcinoma, and anaplastic carcinoma, occur rarely.

Diagnosis and investigation

In a patient presenting with a lacrimal gland mass it is important to try to make a clinical diagnosis, because it is essential that pleomorphic adenoma is totally removed with its capsule intact and without a preliminary biopsy.[16]

A pleomorphic adenoma characteristically grows slowly, producing a painless swelling of the upper eyelid. The patient often does not seek medical advice immediately and a history of at least a year before presentation is usual. On clinical examination a hard, smooth, nontender mass is palpable in the lacrimal fossa. Radiological investigation shows a clearly demarcated mass of uniform density without calcification. There may be pressure erosion or sclerosis of underlying bone, but there is no destruction or invasion of the bone.

Malignant lacrimal gland tumours grow more rapidly and often produce pain. The length of history at presentation is usually less than 1 year. A hard mass is palpable often with diffuse induration and sometimes inflammatory signs. Radiological investigation may show a diffuse mass, sometimes with calcification. There may be destruction of bone and invasion of structures outside the orbit. The clinical presentation is similar to that of inflammatory lesions such as chronic dacroadenitis and pseudotumour, and of other malignant tumours, so an incisional biopsy is mandatory.

Natural history

Adenoid cystic carcinoma of the lacrimal gland progresses in a similar manner to adenoid cystic carcinoma of major and minor salivary glands. It usually grows fairly slowly but spreads widely. The lacrimal gland is adjacent to the bony wall of the orbit, so invasion of bone may occur. The major route of spread, however, is along perineural spaces. Growth occurs along the roof of the orbit to the orbital apex and through the superior orbital fissure. Eventually, there is widespread intracranial extension. The supraorbital nerve may be invaded so that tumour deposits appear on the scalp. Nearly all these tumours eventually recur after attempted removal,[17] mostly within 10 years, but sometimes as long as 25 years later. Lung metastases occur in about 25 per cent of cases;[18] they grow slowly and usually remain asymptomatic for several years.

Adenocarcinoma and other types of malignant lacrimal gland tumours usually grow more rapidly than adenoid cystic carcinoma. They spread mostly by local invasion of adjacent orbital structures and then through the orbital walls to the anterior cranial fossa and paranasal sinuses. Metastases to regional lymph nodes and to distant sites occur occasionally. Recurrences after treatment mostly appear within 3 years.

Treatment

In a patient with a lacrimal gland swelling in whom the clinical features suggest the possibility of pleomorphic adenoma, the mass must be excised with its capsule intact. This necessitates removal of the lacrimal gland and the overlying periosteum. If the capsule is breached, tumour cells seed into the surrounding tissues so that there is a high risk of recurrence.

Recurrence appears as multiple nodules throughout the orbit and leads eventually to loss of the eye; the only treatment is orbital exenteration. Postoperative radiotherapy is therefore advisable in any patient in whom the capsule is breached at operation or who has had an incisional biopsy before excision. A high dose is advisable; at least 50 Gy in 25 fractions is necessary to give the best chance of preventing recurrence. If the cornea and lens are shielded, this dose can be administered without ocular complications.

Malignant lacrimal gland tumours should be treated by surgical excision whenever possible. Radical surgery involves orbital exenteration and usually removal of at least the rim and part of the lateral bony wall of the orbit. This is justified for adenocarcinoma and malignant mixed tumour where it may be curative. Postoperative radiotherapy to a dose of 60 Gy in 30 fractions should be given whenever there is any doubt about the completeness of the surgical excision.

Adenoid cystic carcinoma is rarely if ever cured by radical surgery; the results of more conservative surgery followed by radiotherapy to a dose of 60 Gy in 30 fractions or equivalent seem as good in terms of local tumour control and survival. A useful eye can often be preserved by such a policy.[19]

Soft tissue tumours

Rhabdomyosarcoma

Approximately 10 per cent of all childhood rhabdomysarcomata arise in the orbit. The peak age incidence is between 6 and 8 years. They are nearly all of the embryonal type. Rhabdomyosarcoma is covered elsewhere. However, when this tumour occurs in the orbit it presents special problems in management because of its very good prognosis at this site, and the necessity to preserve vision and avoid facial deformity as much as possible.

Clinical features

The tumour arises in the soft tissue of the orbit, usually anteroinferiorly or anterosuperiorly and therefore presents as a swelling in the conjunctival fornix or in the eyelid. Rapid growth occurs so that the mass takes on an inflammatory appearance and spreads deeper into the orbit, producing proptosis and chemosis. About 10 per cent arise within the muscle cone posterior to the globe, in which case proptosis is the presenting symptom. In untreated cases there is local spread to the soft tissues surrounding the orbit, the paranasal sinuses, and the middle cranial fossa. Meningeal involvement may occur if there is extension to the ethmoid sinus or through the sphenoid fissure. Lymph node metastases in the neck occur only occasionally; blood-borne metastases eventually appear, but tend to occur at a later stage in this disease than is the case with rhabdomyosarcoma arising in other parts of the body.

Diagnosis and staging

The tumour must be distinguished from other causes of acute orbital swelling, for example cellulitis, leukaemic deposit, or metastatic neuroblastoma. A biopsy is essential, and can usually be obtained quite simply through an anterior incision. However, in the case of the posterior intraconal tumours, a lateral orbitotomy approach is necessary.

The local extent of the disease must be ascertained by clinical examination and CT or MRI scan. Investigations to detect distant metastases should include clinical examination, chest radiograph, bone marrow, and isotope bone scan.

Treatment

Prior to 1960, the standard treatment was orbital exenteration. Success was obtained only in the case of small tumours, and the local control rate was less than 50 per cent.[20] Treatment by biopsy and radiotherapy gave slightly better results, with local control rates between 50[21] and 100 per cent.[22] In patients in whom the local disease was controlled, distant metastases were relatively uncommon. Those who succumbed from the disease mostly had local recurrence, regional spread, and distant metastases. The addition of induction and adjuvant chemotherapy to radiotherapy improved long-term survival rates to over 90 per cent.[23] The United States Inter-Group Rhabdomyosarcoma (IRS) study III showed that the combination of vincristine and actinomycin D is as effective as any other and avoids the toxicity and long-term risks of anthracyclines or alkylating agents.[24]

Data on optimum radiotherapy dosage are scanty. Without chemotherapy a dose of 60 Gy appeared to give the best control.[21] For the treatment of microscopic residual disease after chemotherapy there is no evidence of a dose effect above 35 Gy, although 45 Gy in 25 fractions is most commonly given. The IRS IV study suggested a better local control rate with 50.4 Gy compared to 45 Gy given in IRS III, but in the former there was better compliance with the radiotherapy protocol, and also more aggressive chemotherapy was given to some of the patients.[25]

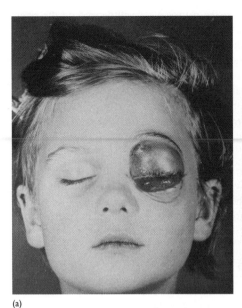 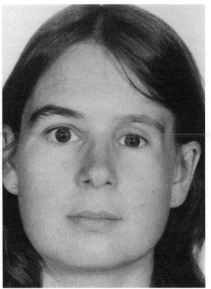

(a) (b)

Fig. 6 (a) Six-year old girl with orbital rhabdomyosarcoma in 1961. She was treated solely by radiotherapy. (b) The same patient aged 32. She has had no surgery, and vision remains 6/6 in both eyes.

The major drawback of radiotherapy to the orbit in childhood is disturbance of growth of the bony walls of the orbit and adjacent parts of the maxilla and mandible, leading to facial deformity as the child grows; the younger the child when treated the greater is the eventual deformity. Irradiation at the age of 8 or older causes only mild facial asymmetry (Fig. 6), but if treatment is given below the age of 5 frequent reconstructive operations become necessary during the period of growth in order to maintain an acceptable facial appearance.

Another risk of radiotherapy is ocular damage. In the early IRS studies, 90 per cent of patients suffered some ocular complication.[26] However, if normal orbital anatomy is restored by prior chemotherapy, these complications can be avoided by careful radiotherapy technique as described above.

Of 12 patients over the age of 4 years treated in this manner at the Royal Marsden Hospital between 1979 and 1988 and followed for a minimum of 10 years, 11 had completely normal vision and facial deformities were slight.

The radiation sequelae in the early studies led the International Society of Paediatric Oncology to investigate the use of more intensive chemotherapy, reserving radiotherapy for residual disease. Survival was slightly less than in the IRS studies, 86 per cent at 4 years. There was a 30 per cent local recurrence rate, and one chemotherapy-related death.[27] In view of these results the optimum treatment outside the context of a clinical trial remains the combination of vincristine and actinomycin-D with radiotherapy.

Other sarcomata

Most types of soft tissue sarcoma have been reported to occur in the orbit. They include fibrous histiocytoma, liposarcoma, angiosarcoma, haemangiopericytoma, and alveolar soft part sarcoma. The behaviour and management is similar to that of these tumour types elsewhere in the head and neck region (see Chapter 9.10).

Neural tumours

Intraorbital optic nerve glioma

Pathology

Optic nerve glioma is a rare tumour of childhood, involving the optic nerve or chiasm. Some arise in the intraorbital part of the nerve and therefore present as orbital tumours. The nature of the tumour is controversial. It often shows no signs of progression over many years, so that it has been suggested that it is a hamartoma rather than a true neoplasm.[28] However, it usually enlarges slowly and causes increasing morbidity. The histological picture is that of a grade I or grade II pilocytic astrocytoma, often with extracellular mucoid material and surrounding meningeal reaction.

Most cases occur in childhood from infancy to 18 years, with a median age of between 4 and 5 years. The occasional case presents in adult life. About 50 per cent are associated with neurofibromatosis-1.[29]

Diagnosis

The usual presenting symptom is deterioration of vision. Proptosis may be noticed, especially in a young child who does not complain of visual loss. On examination there is reduced visual acuity, a relative afferent pupillary defect, and either a pale or a swollen optic disc. Radiographs show enlargement of the optic canal and CT shows expansion of the optic nerve.

Treatment

Initially the patient should be observed to determine if there is evidence of progression. Monitoring is by visual acuity, visual fields, and degree of proptosis. Progression is more likely if the patient does not have neurofibromatosis-1.[29] Biopsy is not advisable; it is likely to cause further visual deterioration and small amounts of tissue from the nerve are difficult to interpret histologically.

Treatment is indicated if there are signs of progressive enlargement of the tumour. The optic nerve and chiasm are inspected through a frontal craniotomy approach. If the chiasm appears normal the whole length of the optic nerve from globe to chiasm is excised. If the chiasm is involved no attempt should be made to excise the tumour.

The value of radiotherapy in progressive, inoperable tumours is difficult to assess because of the very slow rate of growth of the tumours, and there have been no controlled trials. Jenkin et al. in a multivariate analysis of prognostic factors in 87 patients, found that radiotherapy was a significantly favourable factor for survival ($p =$ 0.03), although the effect was in more posteriorly situated tumours which are those most likely to be inoperable.[30] In children below the age of 5 years, chemotherapy using carboplatin or etoposide has been used in an attempt to arrest progression of the tumour, thereby enabling radiotherapy to be delayed in order to minimize the ill-effects of radiotherapy in very young children.[31]

Optic nerve sheath meningioma

Pathology

Meningioma may arise within the orbit from the arachnoid cells around the intraorbital portion of the optic nerve. The same histological types of meningioma can occur at this site as in other parts of the central nervous system.

Optic nerve sheath meningioma is a rare tumour. It occurs predominantly in middle-aged women. The relative incidence in females compared to males is at least 4:1. The age range is from 11 to 86, with a median of about 55 years. The mean age in males is lower than in females. However, the tumour occasionally presents during pregnancy, as is the case for meningioma at other sites.

Clinical features

The tumour grows initially within the dura covering the optic nerve, causing pressure on the nerve and consequent visual disturbance. The enlarged nerve becomes more rigid than normal, interfering with ocular movement and so causing diplopia. As the tumour enlarges it causes proptosis. Eventually it may grow through the dura into the space within the muscle cone. Intracranial extension is rare, as is malignant change.

The first symptom is visual deterioration, consisting of diminished acuity, field defects, and loss of colour vision. Proptosis and diplopia occur later.

Diagnosis

The optic disc is always abnormal, showing either atrophy or swelling. Visual loss in the absence of proptosis suggests a lesion of the optic nerve rather than a tumour outside the dural sheath, which usually causes proptosis before affecting vision.

CT scanning shows a contrast enhancing mass within the optic nerve, often with calcification. If the diagnosis can be made from the clinical and radiological features, biopsy is best avoided.

Treatment

When a clinical and radiological diagnosis of optic nerve meningioma has been made there is usually no need for urgent treatment, unless there is large mass with a relatively short history of increasing proptosis which suggests an aggressive tumour needing immediate resection.

In the majority of cases the management will depend on the extent of visual loss at presentation.

In a patient with useful vision remaining in the affected eye, surgical decompression of the optic nerve is rarely successful.[32] Radiotherapy should be considered as an alternative. Kennerdell et al.[33] reported six patients who received 55 Gy; vision improved in all six. If the eye is blind it is probably wise to excise the tumour with the affected portion of the nerve, in order to prevent extension of the tumour outside the orbit at a later date.

Prognosis

Without treatment vision in the affected eye is inevitably lost, usually within 2 years. Mortality is low, most patients having a normal life span. Death from intracranial extension or malignant change occurs rarely, mostly many years after the initial symptoms.

Neurilemmoma

Pathology

Neurilemmoma, also known as Schwannoma, arises from nerve sheaths. It can therefore arise anywhere in the orbit, but is found most frequently along the course of the supraorbital nerve. It consists of spindle cells with intercellular fibrils. There are solid areas with a palisades or whorls of cells (Antoni A type) and areas of looser texture with no pattern (Antoni B type). Malignancy is very rare.

Diagnosis

CT shows a well-demarcated mass, with only slight contrast enhancement, unlike more vascular tumours such as meningioma.

Treatment

The tumour is usually amenable to local excision with preservation of the eye.[34] The type of operation is dictated by the site of the tumour and its attachments to adjacent structures. There are too few reported cases for meaningful survival figures to be quoted, but in general the behaviour and prognosis of neurilemmoma in the orbit is the same as in other parts of the body. Malignant tumours tend to spread through the supraorbital fissure and therefore have a poor prognosis.

Metastases to the orbit

Direct spread

Basal-cell carcinoma of the eyelid is usually superficial and easily treated by local excision or superficial radiotherapy. A minority are of a more infiltrative type and may invade the orbit. Those arising at the medial canthus are especially likely to behave in this way. When a patient presents with a basal-cell carcinoma at the medial canthus which feels indurated or attached to deep tissues a CT scan is advisable, as there may be spread along the medial wall of the orbit. If a basal-cell carcinoma involves the medial wall or floor of the orbit but the eye is unaffected, treatment should be by radiotherapy, with shielding of the cornea and lens. This gives a high probability of tumour control with a good prospect of preserving vision. If there is involvement of extraocular muscles or fixation of the eyelids it is not possible to control the tumour by radiotherapy without destroying the eye, so orbital exenteration may be preferable.

Squamous carcinoma of the eyelids may also invade the orbit if neglected, and also spread to regional lymph nodes. Upper lid tumours tend to spread initially to preauricular nodes, lower lid tumours to the facial node. Management of the primary tumour is similar to that of basal-cell carcinoma. Radical neck dissection is necessary if there is lymph node involvement.

Tumours of the adjacent paranasal sinuses and nasal cavity may invade the orbit. Carcinoma of the ethmoid sinus spreads through the medial wall of the orbit at an early stage, and often presents with proptosis, as may carcinoma of the lacrimal sac. Carcinoma of the maxillary antrum sometimes spreads through the floor of the orbit. Nasal and nasopharyngeal tumours may reach the orbit via the pterygoid fossa and inferior orbital fissure: these include naso-pharyngeal carcinoma, plasmacytoma, and juvenile angiofibroma.

Invasion of the posterior orbit by intracranial tumours is rare. Sometimes sphenoidal-ridge meningioma may do this.

Blood-borne metastases

Nearly all malignant tumours have been known to metastasize to the orbit. Metastases are commonest in the bony wall of the orbit, but may also be found in the soft tissues. They cause pain, proptosis, and displacement of the globe. Sometimes an orbital metastasis is the presenting sign of malignancy.

The commonest primary tumours to metastasize to the orbit are carcinoma of the bronchus and carcinoma of the breast. The latter usually metastasizes to bone, but can affect the soft tissues which become diffusely infiltrated by scirrhous tumour producing a characteristic clinical picture of enophthalmos and fixation of the eye. Another rare but characteristic sign is the bilateral periocular ecchymosis produced by metastases from adrenal neuroblastoma.

Leukaemic deposits in the orbit are fairly common. Acute myeloid leukaemia sometimes presents as an orbital swelling, the so-called granulocytic sarcoma. This tumour must not be confused with lymphoma or rhabdomyosarcoma, from which it can be distinguished histologically by the use of the non-specific esterase stain.

Intraocular tumours

Metastases

Blood-borne metastases are occasionally found in the eye. The majority occur in the choroid at the posterior pole. Metastases in other parts of the uveal tract, in the retina, and in the conjunctiva have been described but are very rare. The presenting symptoms are blurred vision or a field defect which often progresses rapidly to total visual loss. There may be pain from secondary glaucoma.

Ophthalmoscopy shows yellowish or greyish patches with localized areas of retinal detachment. At least 50 per cent of all choroidal metastases arise from carcinoma of the breast.[35] They are frequently bilateral and usually associated with metastases in other organs, especially the lung. The prognosis is poor; median survival times from presentation of choroidal metastases between 7 and 17 months have been reported. The lung is the second commonest primary site. Choroidal metastases from most sites and types of malignant tumour have been reported but are all rare.

Palliative radiotherapy is indicated in all patients except those in the terminal stage. Using a linear accelerator, unilateral metastases are treated with a single lateral 4 × 4 cm field; the anterior margin is at the lateral bony margin of the orbit and the beam is directed 5° posteriorly to avoid the lens. For bilateral metastases lateral opposed fields are used; care must be taken to avoid an exit dose to the lenses from the contralateral fields, so the beams should either be angled 5 to 10° posteriorly or, if asymmetric collimators are available, the beams can be lateral opposed with the anterior field edges at the central axis of the beam. Tumour doses in the range of 30 Gy in 10 fractions to 40 Gy in 15 fractions have been reported to be effective. The higher doses should be given to patients in good general condition with a prospect of 1 or 2 years survival.

Symptomatic improvement is seen in the majority of patients treated by radiotherapy. Vision returns to its presymptomatic state in about a third of cases.[36] Provided the condition is diagnosed and treated before there is gross retinal detachment some useful vision in the affected eye can usually be preserved.

Juvenile xanthogranuloma

Xanthogranuloma may involve the iris of infants. Unlike those in the skin, the lesions in the iris do not resolve spontaneously without leaving serious sequelae. They frequently cause secondary glaucoma and loss of the eye unless treated.

Most cases occur in the first year of life. The infant is noticed to have a clouding of the cornea or yellowish discoloration of part of the iris. On ophthalmalogical examination the iris appears thickened; there may be blood in the anterior chamber and raised intraocular pressure.

Low-dose radiotherapy is highly effective in bringing about resolution of the lesion and lowering intraocular pressure to normal. It is more effective and has less risk or morbidity than surgery or steroid therapy. The eye is irradiated by a single anterior field using superficial X-rays of half value layer 2 to 3 mm Al. Most reports are of fractionated radiotherapy to a dose of 3 to 4 Gy in three to six fractions.[37] However, general anaesthesia is usually needed for radiotherapy because of the age of the patient, in which case a single exposure of 2 Gy is adequate. Long-term sequelae of this treatment have not been published but cataract from this low dose is unlikely.

References

1. **Czerniak B**, *et al.* Diagnosis of orbital tumours by aspiration biopsy guided by computerized tomography. *Cancer*, 1984; **54**: 2385–9.
2. **Merriam GR, Focht EF.** A clinical study of radiation cataracts and relationship to dose. *American Journal of Roentgenology*, 1957; **77**: 759–85.
3. **Bessell EM, Henk JM, Whitelocke RAF, Wright JE.** Ocular morbidity after radiotherapy of orbital and conjunctival lymphoma. *Eye*, 1987; **1**: 90–6.
4. **Henk JM, Warrington AP, Whitelocke RAF.** Radiation dose to the lens and cataract formation. *International Journal of Radiation Oncology Biology Physics*, 1993; **25**: 815–20.
5. **Parsons JT, Fitzgerald CR, Hood CI,** *et al.* The effects of irradiation on the eye and optic nerve. *International Journal of Radiation Oncology Biology Physics*, 1983; **9**: 609–22.
6. **de Schryver A, Wachtmeister L, Baryd I.** Ophthalmologic observations

on long-term survivors after radiotherapy for nasopharyngeal tumours. *Acta Radiologica (Ther)*, 1971; **10**: 193–209.

7. **Thompson GM, Migdal CS, Whittle RJM.** Radiation retinopathy following treatment of posterior nasal space carcinoma. *British Journal of Ophthalmology*, 1983; **67**: 609–14.

8. **Shukovsky LJ, Fletcher GH.** Retinal and optic nerve complications in a high dose irradiation technique of ethmoid sinus and nasal cavity. *Radiology*, 1972; **104**: 629–34.

9. **Vikayakumar S, McCarthy W, Thomas F, *et al.*** Radiotherapy of orbital neoplasms: advantages of using photons plus electrons with 'anterior chamber' block. *International Journal of Radiation Oncology Biology Physics*, 1986; **12** (Suppl. 1):101–2.

10. **Bessell EM, Henk JM, Wright JE, Whitelocke RAF.** Orbital and conjunctival lymphoma; treatment and prognosis. *Radiotherapy and Oncology*, 1988; **13**: 237–44.

11. **Wotherspoon AC, *et al.*** Primary low-grade B-cell lymphoma of the conjunctiva: a mucosa-associated lymphoid tissue type lymphoma. *Histopathology*, 1993; **23**: 417–24.

12. **Morgan G, Harry J.** Lymphocytic tumours of indeterminate nature; a 5-year follow-up of 98 conjunctival and orbital lesions. *British Journal of Ophthalmology*, 1978; **62**: 381–3.

13. **Alper MG, Bray M.** Evolution of a primary lymphoma of the orbit. *British Journal of Ophthalmology*, 1984; **68**: 225–60.

14. **Medeiros LJ, Andrade RE, Harris NL, *et al.*** Lymphoid infiltrates of the orbit and conjunctiva: comparison of immunologic and gene rearrangement data. *Laboratory Investigation*, 1989; **60**: 61A.

15. **Shields CL, Shields JA, Eagle RC, Rathwell JP.** Clinicopathological review of 142 cases of lacrimal gland lesions. *Ophthalmology*, 1989; **96**: 431–5.

16. **Wright JE.** Factors affecting survival of patients with lacrimal gland tumours. *Canadian Journal of Ophthalmology*, 1982; **17**: 3–9.

17. **Font RL, Smith SL, Bryan RG.** Malignant epithelial tumors of the lacrimal gland: a clinicopathologic study of 21 cases. *Archives of Ophthalmology*, 1998; **116**: 613–6.

18. **Janecka I, *et al.*** Surgical management of tumours of the lacrimal gland. *American Journal of Surgery*, 1984; **148**: 539–41.

19. **Brada M, Henk JM.** Radiotherapy for lacrimal gland tumours. *Radiotherapy and Oncology*, 1987; **9**: 175–83.

20. **Jones IS, Reese AB, Krout J.** Orbital rhabdomyosarcoma: an analysis of sixty-two cases. *Transactions of the Ophthalmological Society*, 1965; **63**: 223–65.

21. **Lederman M, Wybar K.** Embryonal sarcoma. *Proceedings of the Royal Society of Medicine*, 1976; **69**: 895–903.

22. **Sagerman RH, Tretter P, Ellsworth RM.** The treatment of orbital rhabdomyosarcoma of children with primary radiation therapy. *American Journal of Roentgenology*, 1972; **114**: 31–4.

23. **Abramson DH, Ellsworth RM, Tretter P, *et al.*** The treatment of orbital rhabdomyosarcoma with irradiation and chemotherapy. *Ophthalmology*, 1979; **86**: 1330–5.

24. **Crist W, *et al.*** The third inter-group rhabdomyosarcoma study. *Journal of Clinical Oncology*, 1995; **13**: 610–30.

25. **Wharam MD, Anderson JR, Laurie F, Glicksman AS, Maurer HM.** Failure-free survival for orbit rhabdomyosarcoma patients on intergroup rhabdomyosarcoma study IV (IRS-IV) is improved compared to IRS-III. *Proceedings of the American Society of Clinical Oncology*, 1997; **16**: 518a.

26. **Heyn R, *et al.*** Late effects of therapy in orbital rhabdomyosarcoma in children. *Cancer*, 1986; **57**: 1738–43.

27. **Rousseau P, Flamant F, Quintona E, Voute PA, Gentet JC.** Primary chemotherapy in rhabdomyosarcomas and other malignant mesenchymal tumors of the orbit: results of the International Society of Pediatric Oncology MMT 84 study. *Journal of Clinical Oncology*, 1994; **12**: 516–21.

28. **Hoyt WF, Baghdassarian SA.** Optic nerve glioma in childhood: natural history and rationale for conservative management. *British Journal of Ophthalmology*, 1969; **53**: 793–8.

29. **Wright J E, McDonald WI, Call NB.** Management of optic nerve gliomas. *British Journal of Ophthalmology*, 1980; **64**: 545–52.

30. **Jenkin D, Angyalfi S, Becker L, *et al.*** Optic glioma in children: surveillance, resection or irradiation? *International Journal of Radiation Oncology Biology Physics*, 1993; **25**: 215–25.

31. **Janss AJ, Grundy R, Cnaan A, *et al.*** Optic pathway and hypothalamic/ chiasmatic gliomas in children younger than age 5 years with a 6-year follow-up. *Cancer*, 1995; **75**: 1051–9.

32. **Wright JE, Call NB, Liaricos S.** Primary optic nerve meningioma. *British Journal of Ophthalmology*, 1980; **64**: 553–8.

33. **Kennerdell JS, Maroon JC, Malton M, Warren FA.** The management of optic nerve sheath meningiomas. *American Journal of Ophthalmology*, 1988; **106**: 450–7.

34. **Carroll GS, Halk BG, Fleming JC, *et al.*** Peripheral nerve tumours of the orbit. *Radiology Clinics of North America*, 1999; **37**: 195–202.

35. **Freedman MI, Folk JC.** Metastatic tumours to the eye and orbit. *Archives of Ophthalmology*, 1987; **105**: 1215–9.

36. **Thatcher N, Thomas P.** Choroidal metastases from breast carcinoma; a survey of 42 patients and the use of radiation therapy. *Clinical Radiology*, 1975; **26**: 549–53.

37. **Müller RP, Busse H.** Strahlentherapie bei juvenilem Xanthogranulom der Iris. *Klinische Monatsblätter für Augenheilkunde*, 1986; **189**:15–8.

Index

Note: Alphabetical order is letter-by-letter. Page numbers in *italic* refer to figures and/or tables.

anaemia *(continued)*
  of chronic disease (ACD) 945, 959–60
  in the elderly 865
  Fanconi
    association with acute leukaemia 2217
    association with oral cavity cancer 1391
    genetics *142*, 145
  and gastric cancer 1521
  haemolytic 945, 2267
  in hairy cell leukaemia 2269
  and head and neck cancer 1272–3
  in Hodgkin's disease 2315
  iron deficiency 961, 1554
  leucoerythroblastic 960, 2250–1
  in lung cancer 2080
  megaloblastic 960, 2221
  microangiopathic haemolytic 948, 962, 967
  in multiple myeloma 2428, 2437
  pernicious 1520
anal canal 1591
anal cancer
  adenocarcinoma 1592
  aetiology and pathogenesis 1591
  brachytherapy 438–9
  chemoradiotherapy 350, 388, 500, 1594–7
  clinical presentation 1592
  colloid 1591
  definition 1591
  diagnosis 1592
  effect of disease/therapy on male sexual function 2061
  epidemiology 1591
  follow-up 1599
  inguinal area management 1598–9
  lymphatic extension 1593
  lymphoma 1592
  management 1594–1594*10*
  melanoma 1592
  pathology 1591–2
  radiotherapy 1594, *1595*, 1597–8
  sarcoma 1592
  small-cell carcinoma 1591
  squamous cell carcinoma 1591
  staging 1592–3, *1594*
  surgery 1599
analgesic ladder 1021, 1108, *1110*
analgesics 1019, 1021–5
  adjuvant 1019, 1021, 1025–7
  as carcinogens *132*
  in spinal metastatic disease 983
anal margin/verge 1591
anaplastic lymphoma kinase (ALK) 2342, 2386, 2597–8
anastrozole 825, *1770*, *1771*, 1773
androblastoma 1818–20
androgen receptors in prostate cancer 829–30, 1941
androgens
  blockade
    complete 828
      in prostate cancer 828–9, 1959, 1964–5
      in metastatic breast cancer *1770*
  production by sex-cord–stromal tumours 1817, 1819
  in prostate cancer 828–9
aneuploidy 79, *80*, 84, 1727
  in oesophageal cancer 1486–7
angiocardiography during anthracycline therapy 719
angiofibroma 1464–5, 2676
angiogenesis 53, 89
  animal models 89
  control 94–6
  cytokine inhibitors 750
  in head and neck cancer 1411
  mechanism 90
  melanoma-mediated 1182–3
  and metastasis 103–4
  in multiple myeloma 2427
  natural inhibitors 93–4, 749
  as prognostic factor in breast cancer 1728
  role of extracellular matrix 92–3
  stimulators 90–2

as therapeutic target 96–9, 571, 749–50
angiogenin *90*
angiography
  carotid 1460
  cerebral 2713
  CT 256
  head and neck cancer 1304
  pancreatic cancer 324
  spinal arteries 2739
  see also magnetic resonance angiography
angioimmunoblastic lymphadenopathy with
    dysproteinaemia (AILD) 970–1
angioma, spinal 2738
angiomyxoma, vulval 1918
angiopoietin *50*, 54, 91, *93*
angiosarcoma 2499
  bone 2579–80
  cutaneous 1237–8
  female genital system 1918–19
  liver 199, 1638
  pleural 2171
  pulmonary 2168
angiostatin 93–4, 98, 110, 749
animal models
  angiogenesis 89
  carcinogenesis 131–4
  colorectal cancer 210
  medullary thyroid carcinoma 2776
  use in cytotoxic drug screening 782
anion gap 917
ANNA-1 *see* anti-Hu antibodies
ANNA-2 *see* anti-Ri antibodies
annexin V 71
anorexia
  in cancer 935–6, 1007
  dietary management 1011
  in hypercalcaemia 902
  palliation 1112–13
anovulation 1856, 1927
anterior cervical space *1312*
anterior faucial pillar 1409
  tumours 1412
anthophyllite 2125
anthracenediones 721–2
anthracyclines 715–21
  in acute myeloid/myeloblastic leukaemia 2201–2,
      2226–7
  adverse effects 1758, 2633
    congestive heart failure 629
    leukaemia 2192
  in breast cancer 1748–9
  drug interactions 732
  in ovarian cancer 1798
  synthetic compounds related to 721–3
anthrapyrazoles *721*, 722–3
anthropometric variables in breast cancer 1685
antiamphiphysin antibodies *939*, 941, 942, 972
antiandrogens
  non-steroidal 1964
  in prostate cancer 828–9, 1028, 1963–4, 1966
    withdrawal 1966
antiangiogenic therapy 96–8, 630
  advantages 96
  in combination 99
antibiotics
  in acute leukaemia 2223
  antitumour *567*, 715–27
  in chemotherapy-induced neutropenia 579, 583–4
  prophylactic
    in acute leukaemia 2200
    before surgery for colorectal cancer 1562
    in chemotherapy-induced neutropenia 579
    in lymphoma 2408
    postsplenectomy 963
antibodies 853
  bispecific 859–60
  conjugation 855, 858
  engineered *855*

genetic fusion 855
glycosylation 855
non-immunogenic 856, *857*
radiolabelling 855
see also specific antibodies
antibody-dependent cell-mediated cytotoxicity (ADCC)
    842
antibody-directed enzyme prodrug therapy (ADEPT)
    653, 859
anti-CD20 antibodies
  in lymphoma
    B-cell 856–7
    childhood 2408
    follicular 2358–9
    mantle cell 2359
anti-CD34 antibodies 802
anti-CD40 antibodies 843
anti-CEA antibodies 2781
anti-c-erbB2 *see* Herceptin
antichymotrypsin 311, 1914
anticonvulsants
  interactions with chemotherapy 630
  in pain relief 1025, 1027
anti-CV2 antibodies 972
antidepressants 1041
  as analgesics 1025, 1027, 1110
  in anxiety states 1116
  in palliative care 1116
antidiuretic hormone *see* arginine vasopressin
anti-EBV antibodies 1375, 1379–80
antiemetics 593–5, 596
  economic studies 1169
  rescue therapy 595
antifolates 664–73
  see also methotrexate
antifungal agents
  in chemotherapy-induced neutropenia 579–80, 584–5
  prophylactic
    in acute leukaemia 2200
    in chemotherapy-induced neutropenia 579–80
antigen-loss tumour variants 840
antigen-presenting cells 840, 2327–8, 2457
antigens
  differentiation 122, *123*, 233
  from genes overexpressed in tumours 121–2
  immunization against 124
  lymph node response to 2327–8
  processing and presentation 115, 116–17, 840, *841*
  recognition by autologous antibodies 124–5
  recognition by T cells 115–24
  resulting from mutations 122–4
  tumour-specific
    classification 120
    genetic mechanisms 118
    identification 120, *121*
    shared 120–1, *122*
    transplantation 117–18
  viral 124
antigen supplementation 841
anti-GM1 antibodies 970
anti-hCG antibodies 1876, *1878*
anti-Hu antibodies 934, 971
  in cerebellar degeneration 938–9
  in encephalomyelitis 937, 938
  in lung cancer 2080
  in opsoclonus–myoclonus 941
  in subacute sensory neuronopathy 942
anti-idiotype antibodies 857
anti-idiotype responses *843*
anti-IL-6 antibodies 2424
anti-MAG antibodies *939*, 970
antimetabolites 663
  combinations 690–5
  discovery and development 781
  mechanisms of action *567*
  targets 663–4
  see also specific agents
antineuronal antibodies 934, *939*, 971

determinants of disease 185, 188
DEXA (dual-energy X-ray absorptiometry) 2435
dexamethasone
  as adjuvant analgesic 1026
  in brain tumour 2716–17
  in chemotherapy-induced emesis 593, 59372594
  in Cushing's syndrome *921*, 922
  effects on hypothalamic–pituitary–adrenal axis *921*
  in spinal metastatic disease 979, 980–1, 983
dexamethasone suppression test 2802, 2805
dexrazoxane (ICRF 187) 717, 719
dextromoramide 1024
dextropropoxyphene 1022
dFdC *see* gemcitabine
DHFR *see* dihydrofolate reductase
diabetes insipidus (DI)
  in brain tumour 2712
    childhood 2696
  central
    aetiology *911*
    pathophysiology 911–12
  cranial 2795
  in craniopharyngioma 2789
  diagnosis 912, 2795
  differential diagnosis *913*
  investigation 2794–5
  in Langerhans cell histiocytosis 2461, 2465
  nephrogenic
    diagnosis 2795
    pathophysiology 912
  in pituitary tumours 2789, 2792–3
  postoperative 2793
  treatment 2796
diabetes mellitus
  in acromegaly 2799
  and endometrial cancer 1856
  and pancreatic cancer 1604
diacylglycerol 60
Diagnostic Related Groups 1163
3,4-diaminopyridine 944
diamorphine 1023
diaphragmatic paralysis in lung cancer 2078
diarrhoea
  chemotherapy-induced 629, 1579
  in colorectal cancer 1554
  following surgery for neuroblastoma 2609
  management 1012
  primary tumours 2171
  radiotherapy-induced 389, 1568
  secretory 2822
diazepam
  as adjuvant analgesic 1027
  in anxiety states 1116
  in muscle spasms 1027
diaziquone (AZQ)
  adverse effects *650*
  chemistry 640
  clinical pharmacology 649–50
  dosage and administration *650*
  indications *650*
  structure *650*
Di Bella multitherapy 1091, *1092*
dibromoiducitol 2697
DIC (disseminated intravascular coagulation) 947–8, 967,
    968, 2220, 2223
diclofenac 1026
dideoxy-chain termination 9–10
dideoxynucleotide triphosphates 9–10
diencephalic syndrome 2696
diet
  alternative/complementary 1014
  and breast cancer 1686–8
  and colorectal cancer 1546–7
  and head and neck cancer 1272–3, 1279, *1280*
  iodine content 2757
  and oesophageal cancer 1483, 1484
  and pancreatic cancer 1604
  relationship with cancer incidence 130, 198, *199*

  therapeutic 1013–14
dietary fibre intake
  and risk of breast cancer 1688
  and risk of colorectal cancer 1546
diethylstilboestrol
  as carcinogen *132*
  clinical trials 1149–50
  and endometrial cancer 1856
  in metastatic breast cancer *1770*
  in prostate cancer 828, 1963, 1964
  and testicular cancer 2008
  and vaginal cancer 1889, 1891, 2683
2'2'-difluoro-2'-deoxycytidine *see* gemcitabine
digital rectal examination in prostate cancer 276, 1948–9
dihydrocodeine 1022
dihydrofolate reductase (DHFR)
  inhibition by methotrexate 668
  and methotrexate resistance 757–8, 766
dihydrolenperone 782
dihydropyrimidine dehydrogenase 677
5α-dihydrotestosterone 828
dihydrotestosterone receptors 1941
1,25-dihydroxyvitamin D *see* calcitriol
dimerization partner proteins 68
dimethyl xanthenone acetic acid 468, 856
dioxins and soft tissue sarcoma 2495
dipipanone 1024
diploidy 84, 1727
disability-adjusted life year 1164
discoidin 1 54
disialoganglioside 2607
disseminated intravascular coagulation 947–8, 967, 968,
    2220, 2223
distamycin A 740
distancing 1038–9
distress 1043
distribution of disease 187–8
diuretics
  adverse effects 912
  in ascites 892
  in hypercalcaemia 904
  in prevention of tumour lysis syndrome 2397
  in SIADH 910
diverticular disease and colorectal cancer 1548
DLI, in chronic myeloid leukaemia 2245–6
DMDC (2-deoxy-2-methylidenecytidine) 684
DMXAA (dimethyl xanthenone acetic acid) 468, 856
DNA
  alkylation 641–2, *643*
    cellular consequences 642–3
  amplification 4
  analysis of abnormalities 230–1
  characterization 3, *4*
  complementary (cDNA)17.5 *232*
  damage
    background 129
    by anthracyclines 716–17
    by ionizing radiation 167, *168*, 169, 365–6
    by ultraviolet radiation 177–9
    consequences 138–41
    detection and quantitation methods 136, *137*
    endogenous 136
    exogenous agent-induced 136–7, *138*, *139*, *140*
    human 137–8, *140*
    processing 366
    replication following 135–6
    reversal 141, *142*
    sensors 139, 140–1
    sites 136, *138*, *140*
    strand scission 723
  interstrand crosslinks 641–2, *643*
    agents 653
    repair 642–3
  intracellular injection in gene therapy 844–5
  minor-groove binders 740
  ploidy analysis in cytological samples 248
  probes 6
  promoter regions 845

  protein crosslinks 641–2
  rejoining 366
  repair 141–5, 366
    adduct removal 141
    base excision repair 141–2, *143*
    following alkylation 642–3
    global genome repair 142–3, *144*
    human syndrome gene involvement *142*
    inhibition 366, 489–90
    long-patch 142
    nucleotide excision repair 142, *144*, 177, 657
    postreplication mismatch repair 145
    recombination repair 145
    short-patch 142, *143*
    transcription-coupled repair 143, 145
  replication 68–9
  sequencing 9–10
  as target for carcinogen action 135–7, *138*, *139*, *140*
  as target of new drug development 740–1
DNA-activated protein kinase 26
DNA ligase I 142, *143*
DNA ligase III 142
DNA mismatch repair genes 18
DNA-PK 26
DNA polymerase 81
DNA polymerase β 142
DNA polymerase β 142
DNA repair genes *16*, 227, 614
DNA viruses, oncogenic 152, *153*
dNTPs (deoxynucleotides) 5
docetaxel
  clinical pharmacology 732
  clinical use *733*
  drug interactions 732–3
  mechanism of action 731–2
  in metastatic melanoma 1201
  in non-small-cell lung cancer 2098–9
  in ovarian cancer 1802
  resistance to 732
  structure *731*
Doege–Potter syndrome 2171
dolasetron 593
dolastatin 742
donor-lymphocyte infusion, in chronic myeloid
    leukaemia 2245–6
l-dopadecarboxylase 2111
dopamine receptors in chemotherapy-induced emesis 591
Doppler imaging 258, 1874–5
dose-response curves
  carcinogens 133
  chemoradiotherapy 489–90, 490–1
  chemotherapy 565, 773, 797–8
  hyperthermia with radiotherapy 516–17
  radiotherapy 367–8, 379
dothiepin 1041, 1116
double labelling techniques 81
down-staging 319
Down syndrome and leukaemia 2192, 2217
doxazosin 2815
doxifluridine 679
doxil 720
doxorubicin 715
  adverse effects 717, 718–19
    nausea and vomiting 592–4
  clinical efficacy 718–19
  clinical pharmacology 718, *719*
  in combination 718, 733
  in combination with radiotherapy 491, 492
  coupled with integrins 98
  dose-modifying effects *492*
  effects on nutritional status *1011*
  effects on testicular function 609
  in hepatocellular carcinoma 1636
  inhibition of radiation-induced damage 490
  intra-arterial 792
  liposomal formulations 720, 854, 1803, 2483
  mechanism of action 716–17
  mechanisms of resistance 717–18